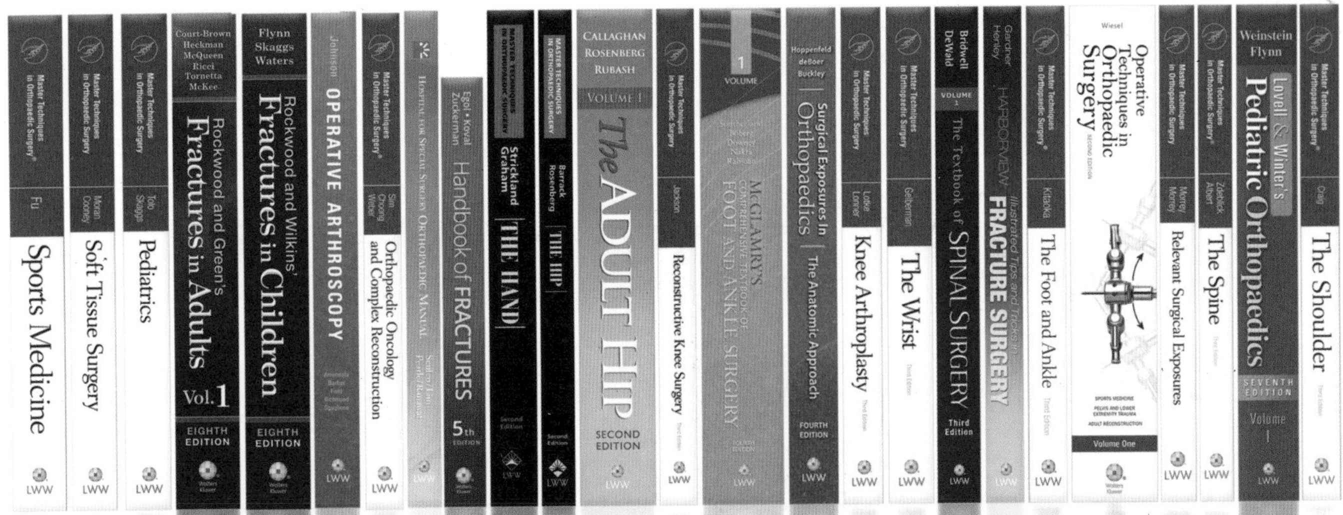

Want **Trial Access** to Lippincott's LWW Health Library: Orthopaedic Surgery Collection?

Try the brand New ***LWW Health Library: Orthopaedic Surgery Collection***, **free for 30 days**. **Search** across the **newest editions** of over **25 gold-standard titles** in an **easy-to-use portal** on your **computer**, **tablet**, or **smartphone**.

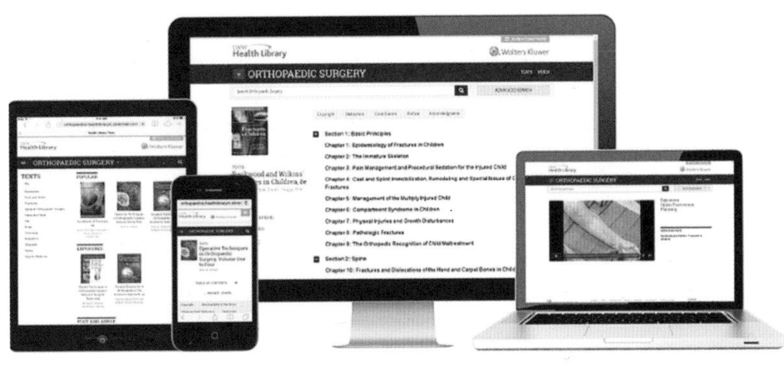

Go to

http://lwwhealthlibrary.com/orthopaedicsurgery

and enter the access code on the adjoining page to start your free 30-day trial!

Note: The same code will activate both the enhanced ebook and the 30 day trial of the LWW Health Library

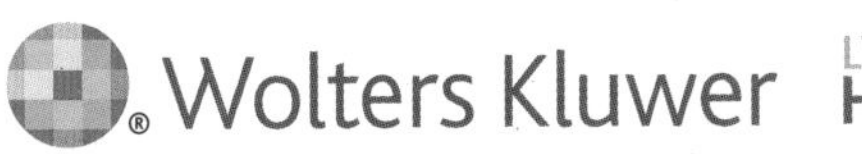

Subscriptions to the LWW Health Library are available for institutional purchase only. Details available at lwwhealthlibrary.com/orthopaedicsurgery.

Questions, Concerns? We are happy to help. Please contact us at 1-800-468-1128 or techsupp@lww.com

Operative Techniques in Hand, Wrist, and Elbow Surgery

SECOND EDITION

Also Available In This Series

OPERATIVE TECHNIQUES IN FOOT AND ANKLE SURGERY, Second Edition
Editor: **Mark E. Easley**
Editor-in-Chief: **Sam W. Wiesel**

OPERATIVE TECHNIQUES IN PEDIATRIC ORTHOPAEDIC SURGERY, Second Edition
Editors: **John M. Flynn & Wudbhav N. Sankar**
Editor-in-Chief: **Sam W. Wiesel**

OPERATIVE TECHNIQUES IN ORTHOPAEDIC TRAUMA SURGERY, Second Edition
Editor: **Paul Tornetta III**
Editor-in-Chief: **Sam W. Wiesel**

OPERATIVE TECHNIQUES IN SHOULDER AND ELBOW SURGERY, Second Edition
Editors: **Gerald R. Williams, Jr., Matthew L. Ramsey, & Brent B. Wiesel**
Editor-in-Chief: **Sam W. Wiesel**

OPERATIVE TECHNIQUES IN SPORTS MEDICINE SURGERY, Second Edition
Editor: **Mark D. Miller**
Editor-in-Chief: **Sam W. Wiesel**

OPERATIVE TECHNIQUES IN JOINT RECONSTRUCTION SURGERY, Second Edition
Editors: **Javad Parvizi & Richard H. Rothman**
Editor-in-Chief: **Sam W. Wiesel**

OPERATIVE TECHNIQUES IN SPINE SURGERY, Second Edition
Editors: **John M. Rhee & Scott D. Boden**
Editor-in-Chief: **Sam W. Wiesel**

OPERATIVE TECHNIQUES IN ORTHOPAEDIC SURGICAL ONCOLOGY, Second Edition
Editors: **Martin M. Malawer, James C. Wittig, & Jacob Bickels**
Editor-in-Chief: **Sam W. Wiesel**

Operative Techniques in Hand, Wrist, and Elbow Surgery

SECOND EDITION

Thomas R. Hunt III, MD, DSc
EDITOR
Professor and Chairman
Wilhelmina Arnold Barnhart Endowed Chair
Joseph Barnhart Department of Orthopedic Surgery
Baylor College of Medicine
Houston, Texas

Brian D. Adams, MD
ASSOCIATE EDITOR
Professor
Joseph Barnhart Department of Orthopedic Surgery
Baylor College of Medicine
Houston, Texas

Sam W. Wiesel, MD
EDITOR-IN-CHIEF
Chairman and Professor
Department of Orthopaedic Surgery
Georgetown University Medical School
Washington, DC

With select chapters from:

Sports Medicine edited by
Mark D. Miller, MD

Shoulder and Elbow edited by
Gerald R. Williams, Jr., MD
Matthew L. Ramsey, MD
Brent B. Wiesel, MD

Pediatrics edited by
John M. Flynn, MD
Wudbhav N. Sankar, MD

Oncology edited by
Martin M. Malawer, MD, FACS
James C. Wittig, MD
Jacob Bickels, MD

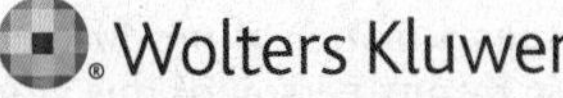

Philadelphia • Baltimore • New York • London
Buenos Aires • Hong Kong • Sydney • Tokyo

Acquisitions Editor: Brian Brown
Product Development Editor: Dave Murphy
Marketing Manager: Daniel Dressler
Production Project Manager: Bridgett Dougherty
Design Coordinator: Holly McLaughlin
Manufacturing Coordinator: Beth Welsh
Prepress Vendor: Absolute Service, Inc.

2nd edition

9 8 7 6 5 4 3 2 1

Printed in China

Library of Congress Cataloging-in-Publication Data

Names: Hunt, Thomas R., editor. | Adams, Brian D., editor. | Wiesel, Sam W., editor.
Title: Operative techniques in hand, wrist, and elbow surgery / [edited by] Thomas R. Hunt III, Brian D. Adams ; editor-in-chief, Sam W.Wiesel.
Other titles: Operative techniques in hand, wrist, and forearm surgery
Description: Second edition. | Philadelphia : Wolters Kluwer, [2016] | Preceded by Operative techniques in hand, wrist, and forearm surgery / Thomas R. Hunt III, editor ; Sam W. Wiesel, editor-in-chief. c2011. | Includes bibliographical references and index.
Identifiers: LCCN 2015040291 | ISBN 9781451193053 (alk. paper)
Subjects: | MESH: Hand—surgery. | Arm Injuries—surgery. | Hand Injuries—surgery. | Upper Extremity—surgery.
Classification: LCC RD731 | NLM WE 830 | DDC 617.4/7—dc23 LC record available at http://lccn.loc.gov/2015040291

This work is provided "as is," and the publisher disclaims any and all warranties, express or implied, including any warranties as to accuracy, comprehensiveness, or currency of the content of this work.

This work is no substitute for individual patient assessment based on healthcare professionals' examination of each patient and consideration of, among other things, age, weight, gender, current or prior medical conditions, medication history, laboratory data, and other factors unique to the patient. The publisher does not provide medical advice or guidance, and this work is merely a reference tool. Healthcare professionals, and not the publisher, are solely responsible for the use of this work including all medical judgments and for any resulting diagnosis and treatments.

Given continuous, rapid advances in medical science and health information, independent professional verification of medical diagnoses, indications, appropriate pharmaceutical selections and dosages, and treatment options should be made and healthcare professionals should consult a variety of sources. When prescribing medication, healthcare professionals are advised to consult the product information sheet (the manufacturer's package insert) accompanying each drug to verify, among other things, conditions of use, warnings, and side effects and identify any changes in dosage schedule or contraindications, particularly if the medication to be administered is new, infrequently used, or has a narrow therapeutic range. To the maximum extent permitted under applicable law, no responsibility is assumed by the publisher for any injury and/or damage to persons or property, as a matter of products liability, negligence law or otherwise, or from any reference to or use by any person of this work.

LWW.com

CCS0116

Dedication

To my cherished wife Teri and our four extraordinary children, Thomas, William, Caitlin, and Christopher, for their love and understanding, and especially for their endless supply of smiles, laughter, and fun!

—TRH

Contents

SECTION X ARTHRITIS

SECTION XI COMPARTMENT SYNDROME, VASCULAR DISORDERS, AND INFECTION

Contributors

Joseph A. Abboud, MD
Associate Professor
Thomas Jefferson University Hospital
Rothman Institute
Philadelphia, Pennsylvania

Joshua M. Abzug, MD
Assistant Professor
Department of Orthopaedics
University of Maryland School of Medicine
Baltimore, Maryland

Brian D. Adams, MD
Professor
Joseph Barnhart Department of Orthopedic Surgery
Baylor College of Medicine
Houston, Texas

Laith M. Al-Shihabi, MD
Resident
Department of Orthopedic Surgery
Rush University Medical Center
Chicago, Illinois

Owen L. Ala, MD
Orthopedic Surgeon
Orthopedic Physicians Anchorage
Anchorage, Alaska

Christopher H. Allan, MD
Associate Professor
Hand and Microsurgery
Department of Orthopaedics
Harborview Medical Center
University of Washington School of Medicine
Seattle, Washington

Aymeric André, MD
Resident
Department of Plastic Surgery
University Hospital Rangueil
Paul-Sabatier University
Toulouse, France

Harikrishna Ankem, MBBS, MS (Ortho), DNB(Orth), MRCS(Edin, UK)
Consultant Shoulder and Elbow Surgeon
Apollo Health City
Hyderabad, India

Edward A. Athanasian, MD
Associate Attending Orthopaedic Surgeon
Chief of the Hand and Upper Extremity Service
Hospital for Special Surgery
Associate Professor of Clinical Orthopaedic Surgery
Weill Cornell Medical College
New York, New York

Cameron T. Atkinson, MD
Orthopedic Hand Surgeon
Arlington Orthopedic Associates, P.A.
Arlington, Texas

Luke S. Austin, MD
Assistant Professor of Orthopaedic Surgery
Thomas Jefferson University Hospital
Rothman Institute
Philadelphia, Pennsylvania

Mark N. Awantang, MD
Hand Surgeon
Upper Extremity and General Orthopedic Surgery
Southern Orthopedic Specialists, P.A.
Panama City, Florida

Alejandro Badia, MD, FACS
Hand and Upper Extremity Surgeon
Badia Hand to Shoulder Center
Doral, Florida
Chief of Hand Surgery
Baptist Hospital
Miami, Florida

Donald S. Bae, MD
Associate Professor
Department of Orthopaedic Surgery
Harvard Medical School
Attending Physician
Department of Orthopedic Surgery
Boston Children's Hospital
Boston, Massachusetts

Carla Baldrighi, MD
Department of Reconstructive Microsurgery
Ospedale CTO
Azienda Ospedaliero-Universitaria Careggi
Florence, Italy

Keith D. Baldwin, MD, MSPT, MPH
Assistant Professor
Neuromuscular Orthopedic and Orthopedic Trauma
Division of Orthopedics
The Children's Hospital of Philadelphia
Philadelphia, Pennsylvania

Mark E. Baratz, MD
Orthopaedic Surgeon
Department of Orthopaedic Surgery
University of Pittsburgh Medical Center
Pittsburgh, Pennsylvania

Asheesh Bedi, MD
Harold and Helen W. Gehring Early Career Professor of Orthopaedic Surgery
Assistant Professor of Sports Medicine and Shoulder Surgery
Department of Orthopaedic Surgery
University of Michigan
Ann Arbor, Michigan

Michael S. Bednar, MD
Professor
Chief, Division of Hand Surgery
Department of Orthopaedic Surgery & Rehabilitation
Loyola University, Stritch School of Medicine
Maywood, Illinois

Pedro K. Beredjiklian, MD
Associate Professor of Orthopaedic Surgery
Thomas Jefferson University Hospital
Chief of Hand Surgery
Rothman Institute
Philadelphia, Pennsylvania

Jacob Bickels, MD
The National Unit of Orthopedic Oncology
Tel-Aviv Sourasky Medical Center
Professor of Orthopedic Surgery
Sackler Faculty of Medicine
Tel-Aviv University
Tel-Aviv, Israel

Randy R. Bindra, FRCS
Professor of Orthopaedic Surgery
Griffith University and Gold Coast University Hospital
Southport, Australia

Philip E. Blazar, MD
Associate Professor of Orthopedic Surgery
Brigham and Women's Hospital
Harvard Medical School
Boston, Massachusetts

Nicolas Bonnevialle, MD
Clinical Assistant in Orthopedic Surgery
Department of Orthopedics and Traumatology
University Hospital Purpan
Paul-Sabatier University
Toulouse, France

Martin I. Boyer, MD FRCS(c)
Carol B. and Jerome T. Loeb Professor
Department of Orthopaedic Surgery
Washington University School of Medicine
St. Louis, Missouri

David J. Bozentka, MD
Chief of Hand Surgery
Associate Professor
Department of Orthopaedic Surgery
Perelman School of Medicine at the University of Pennsylvania
Philadelphia, Pennsylvania

Jay T. Bridgeman, MD, DDS
Adjunct Clinical Professor
University of Missouri Health System School of Medicine
Columbia, Missouri

John S. Bucchieri, MD
Lake Orthopaedic Associates
Willoughby, Ohio

Jeffrey E. Budoff, MD
Director, Orthopaedic Hand and Upper Extremity Service
Houston Veterans Administration Medical Center
Southwest Orthopaedic Group
Houston, Texas

Reuben A. Bueno, Jr., MD
Associate Professor of Plastic Surgery
Department of Plastic Surgery
Vanderbilt University Medical Center
Nashville, Tennessee

Ryan Calfee, MD, MSc
Associate Professor
Department of Orthopaedic Surgery
Washington University School of Medicine
St. Louis, Missouri

John T. Capo, MD
Professor
Department of Orthopaedics
Director of Research
Division of Hand Surgery
NYU Langone Medical Center Hospital for Joint Diseases
New York, New York
Chief of Hand Surgery
Jersey City Medical Center
Jersey City, New Jersey

Robert Carrigan, MD
Assistant Professor of Clinical Orthopaedic Surgery
Perelman School of Medicine at the University of Pennsylvania
Attending Orthopaedic Surgeon
Division of Orthopedics
The Children's Hospital of Philadelphia
Philadelphia, Pennsylvania

Charles Cassidy, MD
Orthopaedist in Chief
Associate Professor
Chairman
Tufts University School of Medicine
Boston, Massachusetts

Andrea Celli, MD
Department of Orthopaedic Surgery
Shoulder and Elbow Unit
Hesperia Hospital
Modena, Italy

Nilesh M. Chaudhari, MD
Assistant Professor
Codirector of Hand and Upper Extremity Fellowship Program
University of Alabama at Birmingham
Birmingham, Alabama

Emilie Cheung, MD
Associate Professor of Orthopaedic Surgery
Stanford University Medical Center
Stanford, California

Andrew Chin, MD, FRCS
Consultant Hand Surgeon
Hand Surgery Unit
Singapore General Hospital
Singapore

Paul D. Choi, MD
Assistant Professor
Department of Orthopaedic Surgery
University of Southern California
Faculty
Children's Orthopaedic Center
Children's Hospital Los Angeles
Los Angeles, California

Joshua Choo, MD
Resident
Plastic and Reconstructive Surgery
Department of Surgery
University of Louisville School of Medicine
Louisville, Kentucky

Kevin C. Chung, MD, MS
Assistant Dean for Instructional Faculty
Professor
Department of Surgery
University of Michigan Medical School
Ann Arbor, Michigan

Michael Ciccotti, MD
The Everett J. and Marian Gordon Professor of Orthopaedic Surgery
Chief, Division of Sports Medicine
Director, Sports Medicine Fellowship and Research
Department of Orthopaedic Surgery
Rothman Institute
Sidney Kimmel Medical College at Thomas Jefferson University
Head Team Physician, Philadelphia Phillies and Saint Joseph's University
Senior Medical Consultant, Philadelphia 76ers
Philadelphia, Pennsylvania

Jason M. Clark
University of Southern Florida

Mark S. Cohen, MD
Professor
Director, Hand and Elbow Section
Director, Orthopaedic Education
Department of Orthopaedic Surgery
Rush University Medical Center
Chicago, IL

Patrick Cole, MD
Orthopedic Hand Fellow
Department of Orthopedic Surgery
Baylor College of Medicine
Houston, Texas

Evan D. Collins, MD
Orthopedic Surgeon
Houston Methodist Hospital
Vice Chairman
Houston Methodist Center for Performing Arts Medicine
Houston, Texas

Garet Comer, MD
Department of Orthopaedic Surgery
Stanford University Medical Center
Palo Alto, California

Patrick M. Connor, MD
OrthoCarolina
Sports Medicine Center - Charlotte
Charlotte, North Carolina

John E. Conway, MD
Private Practice
Fort Worth, Texas

Roger Cornwall, MD
Associate Professor
Department of Orthopaedic Surgery
University of Cincinnati College of Medicine
Clinical Director of Pediatric Orthopaedics
Department of Orthopaedic Surgery
Cincinnati Children's Hospital Medical Center
Cincinnati, Ohio

Alex Cowey, MRCS, FRCS(T&O), HandDipSurg
Consultant Orthopaedic and Hand Surgeon
Department of Orthopaedics
The Royal United Hospital
Bath, United Kingdom

Andrew W. Cross, MD, DVM
The Hand Center
Greenville Health System
Greenville, South Carolina

Randall W. Culp, MD
Professor of Orthopaedics, Hand & Microsurgery
The Philadelphia Hand Center
Thomas Jefferson University Hospital
Philadelphia, Pennsylvania

Catherine M. Curtin, MD
Associate Professor
Department of Plastic Surgery
Palo Alto Veterans Hospital
Palo Alto, CA

John R. Dawson, MD
Assistant Professor
Chief of Orthopedics, Ben Taub General Hospital
Joseph Barnhart Department of Orthopedic Surgery
Baylor College of Medicine
Houston, Texas

Jorge I. de la Torre, MD, FACS
Professor and Chief
Division of Plastic Surgery
University of Alabama at Birmingham
Birmingham, Alabama

Niloofar Dehghan, MD
Department of Orthopaedic Surgery
St. Michael's Hospital
University of Toronto
Toronto, Ontario, Canada

Rafael J. Diaz-Garcia, MD
Attending Surgeon
Department of Surgery
Allegheny Health Network
Clinical Assistant Professor
Department of Plastic Surgery
University of Pittsburgh School of Medicine
Pittsburgh, Pennsylvania

Brandon P. Donnelly, MD
Hand Surgery Fellow
The Philadelphia Hand Center
Thomas Jefferson University Hospital
Philadelphia, Pennsylvania

Christopher Doumas, MD
Orthopaedic Surgeon
Hand & Upper Extremity Surgery
University Orthopaedic Associates
Somerset, New Jersey

Christopher J. Dy, MD
Resident Physician
Department of Orthopaedic Surgery
Hospital for Special Surgery
New York, New York

Thomas Ebinger, MD
Hand, Wrist, and Elbow Specialist
Steindler Orthopedic Clinic
Iowa City, Iowa

J. Ollie Edmunds, Jr., MD
Professor of Orthopaedics
Director of Hand and Upper Extremity Service
Chief of Orthopaedic Surgery at Charity Hospital
New Orleans, Louisiana

John C. Elfar, MD
Assistant Professor
Department of Orthopaedic Surgery
University of Rochester Medical Center
Rochester, New York

Jennifer Etcheson, BS, MS
Medical Student
Dartmouth Medical School
Hanover, New Hampshire

Peter J. Evans, MD
Director
Upper Extremity Center
Department of Orthopaedic Surgery
Cleveland Clinic
Cleveland, Ohio

Marybeth Ezaki, MD
Professor of Orthopaedic Surgery
Department of Orthopaedic Surgery
UT Southwestern Medical Center
Director of Hand Surgery
Texas Scottish Rite Hospital for Children
Dallas, Texas

Paul Feldon, MD
Associate Clinical Professor of Orthopaedic Surgery
Tufts University School of Medicine
Boston, MA

John J. Fernandez, MD
Assistant Professor
Rush University Medical Center
Chicago, Illinois

Diego Fernandez, MD
Specialist in Orthopaedic Surgery and Surgery of the Hand (FMH)
Department of Orthopaedic Surgery
Lindenhof Hospital
Bern, Switzerland

Angel Ferreres, MD
Codirector of the Fellowship in Hand Surgery of the University of Barcelona
Full-time Consultant
Hand and Upper Extremity Surgery
Institut Kaplan
Barcelona, Spain

Rimma Finkel, MD
Private Practice
Chandler, Arizona

John M. Flynn, MD
Chief of Orthopedic Surgery
The Children's Hospital of Philadelphia
Professor of Orthopaedic Surgery
Perelman School of Medicine at the University of Pennsylvania
Philadelphia, Pennsylvania

Christopher L. Forthman, MD
Consultant
Curtis National Hand Center
Staff
Johns Hopkins Medical Institutions
Baltimore, Maryland

Jeffrey B. Friedrich, MD, FACS
Associate Professor of Surgery and Orthopedics
University of Washington
Seattle, Washington

Sam Fuller, MD
Resident
Department of Surgery
Section of Plastic and Reconstructive Surgery
University of Chicago Medical Center
Chicago, Illinois

Marc García-Elías, MD, PhD
Consultant in Hand Surgery
Institut Kaplan
Barcelona, Spain

William B. Geissler, MD
Alan E. Freeland Chair of Hand Surgery
Professor and Chief
Division of Hand and Upper Extremity Surgery
Chief, Section of Arthroscopic Surgery and Sports Medicine
Director, Hand and Upper Extremity Fellowship
Department of Orthopaedic Surgery and Rehabilitation
The University of Mississippi Medical Center
Jackson, Mississippi

Harris Gellman, MD
Voluntary Clinical Professor
Departments of Plastic and Orthopaedic Surgery
University of Miami
Coral Springs, Florida

Filippos S. Giannoulis, MD, PhD
Hand Surgery-Upper Limb and Microsurgery Department
Kat Hospital
Athens, Greece

Grey Giddins, FRCS (Orth)
Consultant
Orthopaedic and Hand Surgeon
Visiting Professor
University of Bath
Bath, United Kingdom

Steven Z. Glickel, MD
Director of Hand Surgery
St. Luke's-Roosevelt Hospital Center
Director
The CV Starr Hand Surgery Center
Clinical Professor of Orthopaedic Surgery
Icahn School of Medicine at Mount Sinai
New York, New York

Charles A. Goldfarb, MD
Professor of Orthopaedic Surgery
Department of Orthopaedic Surgery
Washington University School of Medicine
St. Louis, Missouri

Mark Goleski, MD
Fellow
Division of Cardiovascular Medicine
Keck School of Medicine of the University of Southern California
Los Angeles, California

Peter Goljan, MD
Clinical Research Fellow
The Philadelphia Hand Center
Philadelphia, Pennsylvania

Christopher R. Goll, MD
Chief
Hand Surgery Division
Southeast Orthopedic Specialists
Jacksonville, Florida

Christine M. Goodbody, MD
The Children's Hospital of Philadelphia
Perelman School of Medicine at the University of Pennsylvania
Philadelphia, Pennsylvania

Adam M. Goodyear, MD
Orthopedic Surgeon
Department of Orthopedic Surgery
The University of Kansas Medical Center
Kansas City, Kansas

Yair Gortzak, MD
Head of the Orthopedic Oncology Clinic
Tel Aviv Sourasky Medical Center
Tel Aviv, Israel

Thomas J. Graham, MD
Chief Innovation Officer
Justice Family Chair in Medical Innovations
Vice Chair, Department of Orthopaedic Surgery
Cleveland Clinic
Cleveland, Ohio

Jennifer Green, MD
Orthopaedic Surgeon
Department of Orthopaedics
Hand and Upper Extremity Surgery
Mount Auburn Hospital
Cambridge, Massachusetts

Jeffrey A. Greenberg, MD, MS
Physician
Indiana Hand to Shoulder Center
Indianapolis, Indiana

Eyal Gur, MD
Director, Unit of Microsurgery
Head, Department of Reconstructive and Aesthetic Surgery
Department of Plastic Surgery
Tel Aviv Sourasky Medical Center
Senior Lecturer
Sackler School of Medicine, Tel Aviv University
Tel Aviv, Israel

Yung Han, MD
Orthopaedic Surgeon
Kerlan-Jobe Orthopaedic Clinic
Los Angeles, California

Douglas P. Hanel, MD
Professor of Orthopaedics and Sports Medicine
University of Washington
Head, Pediatric Hand Surgery Program
Children's Hospital Medical Center
Seattle, Washington

Scott L. Hansen, MD
Associate Professor of Surgery
Departments of Surgery and Orthopaedic Surgery
Chief, Hand and Microvascular Surgery
University of California, San Francisco
Chief, Plastic and Reconstructive Surgery
San Francisco General Hospital
San Francisco, California

Colin Harris, MD
Orthopedic Spine Surgeon
Syracuse Orthopedic Specialists Spine Center
Syracuse, New York

Robert U. Hartzler, MD, MS
Orthopaedic Surgeon
Shoulder and Elbow Surgery
The San Antonio Orthopaedic Group
San Antonio, Texas

George Frederick Hatch III, MD
Assistant Professor of Orthopaedic Surgery
Department of Orthopaedic Surgery
Keck School of Medicine of the University of Southern California
Los Angeles, California

Kathryn A. Heim, MD
Orthopedic Hand and Upper Extremity Surgeon
Holy Cross Medical Group
Fort Lauderdale, Florida

Carlos Heras-Palou, MD, FRCS(Trau&Orth)
Pulvertaft Hand Centre
Royal Derby Hospital
Derby, England

Levi Hinkelman, MD
Orthopedic Surgery Resident
Grand Rapids Medical Education Partners
Michigan State University College of Human Medicine
Grand Rapids, Michigan

K. J. Hippensteel, MD, LT, MC, USNR
Orthopaedic Surgery Resident
Department of Orthopaedic Surgery
Washington University in St. Louis
St. Louis, Missouri

Matthew E. Hiro, MD
Assistant Professor of Plastic Surgery
Department of Surgery
Emory University School of Medicine
Atlanta, Georgia

Eric P. Hofmeister, MD, CAPT, MC, USN
Associate Professor
Uniformed Services University of the Health Sciences
Naval Medical Center San Diego
San Diego, California

Harry A. Hoyen, MD
Associate Professor
Department of Orthopaedic Surgery
MetroHealth Medical Center
Case Western Reserve University
Cleveland, Ohio

Thomas B. Hughes, MD
Clinical Associate Professor of Orthopaedic Surgery
Department of Orthopaedic Surgery
University of Pittsburgh Medical Center
Pittsburgh, Pennsylvania

Thomas R. Hunt III, MD, DSc
Professor and Chairman
Wilhelmina Arnold Barnhart Endowed Chair
Joseph Barnhart Department of Orthopedic Surgery
Baylor College of Medicine
Houston, Texas

Asif M. Ilyas, MD, FACS
Program Director of Hand and Upper Extremity Surgery Fellowship
Rothman Institute
Associate Professor of Orthopaedic Surgery
Thomas Jefferson University
Philadelphia, Pennsylvania

Joseph E. Imbriglia, MD
Chairman, Hand & UpperEx Center
Clinical Professor of Orthopaedic Surgery
Department of Orthopaedic Surgery
Director of the Hand and Upper Extremity Fellowship Program
University of Pittsburgh School of Medicine
Pittsburgh, Pennsylvania

Matthew Iorio, MD
Hand Surgeon
Division of Plastic and Reconstructive Surgery
Department of Orthopaedics
Harvard Medical School
Beth Israel Deaconess Medical Center
Boston, Massachusetts

John M. Itamura, MD
Associate Professor
Clinical Professor of Orthopaedic Surgery
Keck School of Medicine of the University of Southern California
Orthopaedic Surgeon
Kerlan-Jobe Orthopaedic Clinic
Los Angeles California

Peter J.L. Jebson, MD
Associate Professor
Michigan State College of Human Medicine
Clinical Instructor
Grand Rapids Medical Education Partners
Department of Orthopaedic Surgery
Spectrum Health Medical Group
Grand Rapids, Michigan

Nelson L. Jenkins, MD
Plastic Surgeon
Cleveland Plastic and Hand Surgery
Shelby, North Carolina

Christopher M. Jones, MD
Assistant Professor of Orthopaedics
Jefferson Medical College,
Thomas Jefferson University
Rothman Institute
Philadelphia, Pennsylvania

Marci D. Jones, MD
Associate Professor
Department of Orthopedics
University of Massachusetts Medical School
Worcester, Massachusetts

Neil F. Jones, MD
Professor of Orthopedic Surgery
Director, UC Irvine Hand Center
Irvine, California

Abhishek Julka, MD
Faculty
University of Wisconsin School of Medicine and Public Health
Madison, Wisconsin

Jesse B. Jupiter, MD
Hansjorg Wyss/AO Professor of Orthopaedic Surgery
Harvard Medical School
Massachusetts General Hospital
Boston, Massachusetts

Michael Kalisvaart, MD
Fellow
Orthopaedic Sports Medicine
Stanford University
Redwood City, California

Check C. Kam, MD
Hand Surgeon
South Florida Orthopaedics & Sports Medicine
Stuart, Florida

Srinath Kamineni, MBBCH, BSc, FRCS, FRCS-Orth1Tr
Elbow and Shoulder Specialist
Department of Orthopaedic Surgery and Sports Medicine
University of Kentucky
Elbow Shoulder Research Centre
Lexington, Kentucky

Morton Kasdan, MD
Clinical Professor
Division of Plastic and Reconstructive Surgery
Department of Surgery
University of Louisville School of Medicine
Louisville, Kentucky

Leonid I. Katolik, MD
Orthopaedic Surgeon
The Philadelphia Hand Center
Jefferson Medical College,
Thomas Jefferson University
Philadelphia, Pennsylvania

Yoav Kaufman, MD
Medical Resident
Plastic Surgery Division
Baylor College of Medicine
Houston, Texas

Mohamed Khalid, MD
Fellow, UAB Hand and Upper Extremity Fellowship
Department of Orthopaedic Surgery
University of Alabama at Birmingham
Birmingham, Alabama

Prakash Khanchandani, MD
Additional Senior Consultant
Department of Orthopaedics
Sri Sathya Sai Institute of Higher Medical Sciences
Prasanthigram, Puttaparthi, India

Thomas R. Kiefhaber, MD
Hand Surgery Specialists
Cincinnati, Ohio

Nayoung Kim, BS
Research Fellow
The Rothman Institute Hand and Wrist Research
Philadelphia, Pennsylvania

Richard Y. Kim, MD
Director of Hand Surgery
Departments of Plastic & Reconstructive Surgery and Orthopaedic Surgery
Hackensack University Medical Center
Hackensack, New Jersey

Hervey L. Kimball III, MD, MS
Assistant Clinical Professor Orthopaedic Surgery
Tufts University School of Medicine
New England Baptist Hospital
Boston, Massachusetts

Elizabeth King, MD
Resident Surgeon
Department of Orthopaedic Surgery
University of Michigan
Ann Arbor, Michigan

Graham J. W. King, MD, MSc, FRCSC
Director, Roth | McFarlane Hand and Upper Limb Centre
Chief of Surgery, St. Joseph's Health Centre
Professor of Orthopaedic Surgery and Biomedical Engineering
Western University
London, Ontario, Canada

Melissa A. Klausmeyer, MD
Assistant Professor
Surgery-Plastic & Recon Surgery, Orthopedics
University of Colorado School of Medicine
Aurora, Colorado

Kyle P. Kokko, MD, PhD
Assistant Professor
Department of Orthopaedics
Medical University of South Carolina
Charleston, South Carolina

Yehuda Kollender, MD
Department Director
Attending Surgeon, National Unit of Orthopedic Oncology
Tel Aviv Sourasky Medical Center
Senior Lecturer
Sackler School of Medicine,
Tel Aviv University
Tel Aviv, Israel

Thomas J. Kovack, DO
Orthopedic Surgeon
OhioHealth Orthopedic Surgeons
Hilliard, Ohio

Scott H. Kozin, MD
Chief of Staff
Shriners Hospitals for Children—Philadelphia
Clinical Professor
Department of Orthopaedic Surgery
Temple University School of Medicine
Philadelphia, Pennsylvania

Mark A. Krahe, DO
Professor of Orthopaedic Surgery
Hamot Hospital
Erie, Pennsylvania

Leo T. Kroonen, MD
Orthopaedic Surgeon
Department of Orthopaedic Surgery
Kaiser Permanente
San Diego, California

Kate Kuhlman-Wood, MD
Hand Fellow
Division of Plastic Surgery
Department of Orthopedic Surgery
Baylor College of Medicine
Houston, Texas

Amy L. Ladd, MD
Professor (MCL) of Orthopedic Surgery
Stanford University School of Medicine
Stanford, California

Jeffrey Lawton, MD
Associate Professor
Chief, Division of Elbow, Hand and Microsurgery
Department of Orthopaedic Surgery
University of Michigan
Ann Arbor, Michigan

Byung J. Lee, MD
Orthopedic Surgeon
Irving Orthopedics and Sports Medicine
Irving, Texas

L. Scott Levin, MD FACS
Paul B. Magnuson Professor and Chairman of the Department of Orthopaedic Surgery
Professor of Surgery (Plastic Surgery)
Perelman School of Medicine at the University of Pennsylvania
Philadelphia, Pennsylvania

Fred Liss, MD
Hand and Wrist Surgeon
Rothman Institute
Thomas Jefferson University
Philadelphia, Pennsylvania

Bryan J. Loeffler, MD
OrthoCarolina
Hand Center - Charlotte
Charlotte, North Carolina

Joseph M. Lombardi, MD
Department of Orthopedic Surgery
New York Presbyterian Hospital
Columbia University Medical Center
New York, New York

James N. Long, MD
Plastic Surgeon
Department of Plastic Surgery
The Kirklin Clinic of UAB Hospital
Birmingham, Alabama

Dean Louis, MD
Professor Emeritus (Surgery)
University of Michigan
Consultant
Ann Arbor Veterans Hospital
Ann Arbor, Michigan

John D. Lubahn, MD
Orthopaedic Surgeon
Department of Orthopaedic Surgery
Hand Microsurgery & Reconstructive Orthopaedics, LLP
Erie, Pennsylvania

David M. Lutton, MD
Orthopaedic Surgeon
Washington Circle Orthopaedic Associates, P.C.
Washington, DC

David H. MacDonald, DO, FAOAO
Hand and Upper Extremity Specialist
Hughston Clinic, P.C.
Columbus, GA
Program Director
Jack Hughston Memorial Hospital
Orthopaedic Residency
Phenix City, Alabama

Anna-Lena Makowski, Histotechnologist, HTL
Miami International Hand Surgical Services
North Miami Beach, Florida

Martin M. Malawer, MD, FACS
Director of Orthopedic Oncology
Professor, Orthopedic Surgery
George Washington University School of Medicine
Professor (Clinical Scholar) of Orthopedics and Professor of Pediatrics (Hematology and Oncology)
Georgetown University School of Medicine
Washington, District of Columbia
Consultant, Pediatric and Surgery Branch
National Cancer Institute
National Institutes of Health
Bethesda, Maryland

Kevin J. Malone, MD
Assistant Professor
Department of Orthopaedic Surgery
MetroHealth Medical Center
Case Western Reserve University School of Medicine
Cleveland, Ohio

Pierre Mansat, MD, PhD
Professor of Orthopedics
Toulouse Medical School
University Hospital of Toulouse
Department of Orthopedics and Traumatology
Pierre Paul Riquet Hospital
Toulouse, France

Alexander M. Marcus, MD
Orthopedic Associates of Central Jersey, PA
Edison, New Jersey

Andrew D. Markiewitz, MD, MBA
Hand Surgery Specialist
Trihealth Orthopedic and Spine Institute
Cincinnati, Ohio

Paul A. Martineau, MD, FRCSC
Assistant Professor
Section of Sport Medicine
Section of Upper Extremity Surgery
Department of Orthopaedic Surgery
McGill University Health Center
Montreal, Quebec, Canada

Jun Y. Matsui, MD
Hand and Upper Extremity Surgery
Department of Orthopaedic Surgery
Kaiser Permanente
San Leandro, California

Evan McGlinn, BS
Section of Plastic Surgery
University of Michigan Health System
Ann Arbor, Michigan

Michael D. McKee, MD, FRCS(c)
Professor
Upper Extremity Reconstructive Service
Department of Surgery
Division of Orthopaedics
St. Michael's Hospital and the
University of Toronto
Toronto, Ontario, Canada

Kenneth R. Means, Jr., MD
Director, Clinical Research
Curtis National Hand Center
MedStar Union Memorial Hospital
Baltimore, Maryland

Robert J. Medoff, MD
Associate Clinical Professor
John A. Burns School of Medicine
University of Hawai'i at Mānoa
Honolulu, Hawaii

Charles T. Mehlman, DO, MPH
Professor, Pediatric Orthopaedics
University of Cincinnati College of Medicine
Director
Pediatric Musculoskeletal Outcomes Research
Pediatric Orthopaedic Resident Education
Cincinnati Children's Hospital Medical
Center
Cincinnati, Ohio

Chris Mellano, MD
Clinical Fellow
Department of Sports Medicine
Rush University Medical Center
Chicago, Illinois

Greg Merrell, MD,
Physician
Indiana Hand to Shoulder Center
Clinical Assistant Professor
Department Orthopaedic Surgery
Indiana University
Indianapolis, Indiana

Raymond J. Metz, Jr., MD
Orthopedic Hand Surgeon
CORE Orthopedics and Sports Medicine
Elk Grove Village, Illinois

Frederick N. Meyer, MD
Professor and Chairman
Department of Orthopaedic Surgery
University of South Alabama College
of Medicine
Mobile, Alabama

Alex M. Meyers, MD
Orthopaedic Surgeon
Reconstructive Hand to Shoulder
of Indiana
Carmel, Indiana

Mark A. Mighell, MD
Instructor of Surgery
Uniformed School of Health Sciences
Bethesda, Maryland
Associate Professor
Department of Orthopaedic Surgery
University of South Florida
Florida Orthopaedic Institute
Tampa, Florida

Alexander D. Mih, MD
Associate Professor of Orthopaedic Surgery
Indiana University School of Medicine
Staff Surgeon
Indiana Hand to Shoulder Center
Indianapolis, Indiana

Joshua T. Mitgang, MD
Orthopedic Surgeon
Orlin & Cohen Orthopedic Group
Lynbrook, New York

Nathan A. Monaco, MD
Resident
Department of Orthopaedic Surgery
UPMC Hamot
Erie, Pennsylvania

Bruce A. Monaghan, MD
Chief, Section of Orthopaedics
Vice Chairman, Department of Surgery
Inspira Health Network
Woodbury, New Jersey

Bernard F. Morrey, MD
Professor and Emeritus Chair
Department of Orthopedic Surgery
Mayo Clinic
Rochester, Minnesota
Professor of Orthopedics
The University of Texas Health Science
Center at San Antonio
San Antonio, Texas

Chaitanya S. Mudgal, MD
Program Director
Hand Surgery Fellowship Program
Hand & Upper Extremity Orthopaedic
Surgeon
Assistant Professor of Orthopaedic Surgery
Harvard Medical School
Boston, Massachusetts

Michael T. Mulligan, MD
Assistant Professor
Associate Residency Program Director
Division of Orthopaedic Surgery
Albany Medical College
Albany, New York

Peter M. Murray, MD
Professor of Orthopaedic Surgery
Mayo Clinic
Jacksonville, Florida

Anand M. Murthi, MD
Chief, Shoulder and Elbow Surgery
Attending Orthopaedic Surgeon
Department of Orthopaedics & Sports Medicine
MedStar Union Memorial Hospital
Baltimore, Maryland

Sameer Nagda, MD
Assistant Professor of Clinical Orthopaedic
Surgery
Georgetown University School of Medicine
Washington, DC
Sports Medicine and Shoulder Specialist
The Anderson Orthopaedic Clinic
Arlington, VA

Mitchell E. Nahra, MD
Lake Orthopaedic Associates, Inc.
Lake Health Medical Center
Willoughby, Ohio

Sanjiv Naidu, MD, PhD
Pinnacle Hand Center
Mechanicsburg, Pennsylvania

Brian Najarian, MD
Associate Clinical Professor
Department of Orthopaedic Surgery
St. John Providence Hospital & Medical
Center
Southfield, Michigan

Michael N. Nakashian, MD
Orthopedic Surgeon
Brielle Orthopedics
Brick, New Jersey

David Netscher, MD
Clinical Professor
Department of Orthopedic Surgery
Division of Plastic Surgery
Baylor College of Medicine
Houston, Texas
Adjunct Professor of Clinical Surgery
Weill Cornell Medical College
New York, New York

José M. Nolla, MD
Orthopaedic Surgeon
Kelsey-Seybold Clinic
Houston, Texas

Matt Noyes, MD, PT
Shoulder/Elbow Service
Department of Orthopaedic Surgery
Western Reserve Hospital
Cuyahoga Falls, Ohio

Michael J. O'Brien, MD
Assistant Professor
Department of Orthopaedics
Tulane University School of Medicine
New Orleans, Louisiana

Nikhil Oak, MD
Resident Surgeon
Department of Orthopaedic Surgery
University of Michigan Health and Hospital Systems
Ann Arbor, Michigan

Scott N. Oishi, MD
Associate Professor
Department of Plastic Surgery
Department of Orthopaedic Surgery
UT Southwestern Medical Center
Head Surgeon
Hand Surgery Department
Texas Scottish Rite Hospital for Children
Dallas, Texas

A. Lee Osterman, MD
Professor of Hand and Orthopaedic Surgery
Thomas Jefferson University
Orthopaedic Surgeon
The Philadelphia Hand Center
Philadelphia, Pennsylvania

Meredith N. Osterman, MD
Orthopaedic Surgeon
The Philadelphia Hand Center
Philadelphia, Pennsylvania

E. Anne Ouellette, MD
Hand Surgeon
Ouellette Group Physicians
Mount Sinai Medical Center
Miami Beach, Florida

Patrick Owens, MD
Assistant Professor of Clinical Orthopaedics
Hand and Upper Extremity Surgery
University of Miami Leonard M. School of Medicine
Miami, Florida

Loukia K. Papatheodorou, MD, PhD
Orthopaedic Surgeon
University of Pittsburgh Medical Center
Orthopaedic Specialists - UPMC
Pittsburgh, Pennsylvania

Bradford O. Parsons, MD
Associate Professor
Department of Orthopaedics
Mount Sinai Hospital
New York, New York

Alexander H. Payatakes, MD
Assistant Professor
Penn State Hershey Bone and Joint Institute
Hershey, Pennsylvania

Sebastian C. Peers, MD
Orthopedic Fellow
Cleveland Clinic
Cleveland, Ohio

Jason Petrungaro, MD
Plastic Surgeon
Petrungaro Plastic Surgery
Munster, Indiana

Craig S. Phillips, MD
Hand and Upper Extremity Surgery
Microvascular Surgery
Illinois Bone & Joint Institute
Fellowship Director
Hand and Upper Extremity Surgery
NorthShore University Health System
Associate Editor

The Journal of Hand Surgery
Clinical Assistant Professor of Surgery
Department of Surgery
Section of Orthopaedic Surgery
The University of Chicago Pritzker School of Medicine
Chicago, Illinois

Kristan A. Pierz, MD
Assistant Professor
Department of Pediatric Orthopaedics
Medical Director, Center for Motion Analysis
Connecticut Children's Medical Center
Hartford, Connecticut

Samantha L. Piper, MD
Assistant Professor
Hand, Elbow and Upper Extremity
Department of Orthopaedic Surgery
University of California, San Francisco
San Francisco, California

Vimala Ramachandran, MD
Northern Arizona Orthopaedics
Flagstaff, Arizona

Rey N. Ramirez, MD
Orthopaedic Surgeon
Hand Microsurgery & Reconstructive Orthopaedics, LLP
Erie Shriners Ambulatory Surgery Center and Outpatient Specialty Care Center
Erie, Pennsylvania

Matthew L. Ramsey, MD
Professor and Vice Chairman of Orthopaedic Surgery
Sidney Kimmel College of Medicine at Thomas Jefferson University
Chief, Shoulder and Elbow Service
Rothman Institute
Philadelphia, Pennsylvania

Ghazi Rayan, MD
Clinical Professor of Orthopedic Surgery
Adjunct Professor of Anatomy/Cell Biology
University of Oklahoma
Director of Oklahoma Hand Surgery Fellowship Program
Chair, Department of Hand Surgery
INTEGRIS Baptist Medical Center
Oklahoma City, Oklahoma

Lee M. Reichel, MD
Assistant Professor
Joseph Barnhart Department of Orthopedic Surgery
Baylor College of Medicine
Houston, Texas

Ross J. Richer, MD
Orthopaedic Specialty Group
Fairfield, Connecticut

David Ring, MD, PhD
Chief of Hand Surgery
Massachusetts General Hospital
Professor of Orthopaedic Surgery
Harvard Medical School
Boston, Massachusetts

Kyle P. Ritter, MD
Orthopedic Surgeon
Hendricks Orthopedics and Sports Medicine
Danville, Indiana

Michael Rivlin, MD
Orthopaedic Surgeon
Department of Orthopaedic Surgery
Thomas Jefferson University Hospital
Rothman Institute
Philadelphia, Pennsylvania

Marco Rizzo, MD
Professor of Orthopedics
Department of Orthopedic Surgery
Mayo Clinic
Rochester, Minnesota

Susanne Roberts, MD
Orthopaedic Surgery Resident
Harvard Combined Orthopaedic Residency Program
Massachusetts General Hospital
Boston, Massachusetts

Matthew J. Robon, MD
Orthopaedic Surgeon
Proliance Orthopaedics and Sports Medicine
Bellevue, Washington

Anthony A. Romeo, MD
Professor
Departments of Orthopedic Surgery
Program Director
Shoulder and Elbow Fellowship
Section Head, Shoulder and Elbow Surgery
Division of Sports Medicine
Rush University Medical Center
Team Physician, Chicago White Sox and Bulls
Chief Medical Editor, *Orthopedics Today*
Chicago, Illinois

Yishai Rosenblatt, MD
Head of the Elbow Service
The Unit of Hand Surgery, Division of Orthopaedic Surgery
Tel-Aviv Sourasky Medical Center
Tel Aviv, Israel

Melvin P. Rosenwasser, MD
Carroll Professor of Orthopedic Surgery
Columbia University Medical Center
Director Hand and Microsurgery
Director of Orthopedic Trauma
New York Presbyterian Hospital
New York, New York

Marc Safran, MD
Professor
Department of Orthopaedic Surgery
Stanford University
Redwood City, California

Jason C. Saillant, MD
Orthopaedic Surgeon
The Philadelphia Hand Center
Philadelphia, Pennsylvania

Rodrigo Santamarina, MD
Assistant Professor
Department of Surgery
University of Massachusetts Medical School
Pittsfield, Massachusetts

Keith A. Segalman, MD
CNHC Faculty
Curtis National Hand Center
Baltimore, Maryland

Apurva S. Shah, MD
Assistant Professor
Department of Orthopaedics and Rehabilitation
University of Iowa
University of Iowa Hospitals & Clinics
Iowa City, Iowa

David B. Shapiro, MD
Department of Orthopaedic Surgery
Cleveland Clinic
Cleveland, Ohio

Joseph M. Sherrill, MD
Orthopaedic Surgeon
Sherrill Orthopedics Sports and Hand Center
Birmingham, Alabama

Eon K. Shin, MD
Assistant Professor
Department of Orthopaedic Surgery
Thomas Jefferson University Hospital
Philadelphia, Pennsylvania

Alexander Y. Shin, MD
Professor and Consultant
Department of Orthopedic Surgery
Division of Hand Surgery
Mayo Clinic
Rochester, MN

David L. Skaggs, MD
Professor
Department of Orthopaedic Surgery
Keck School of Medicine of the University of Southern California
Chief of Orthopaedic Surgery
Department of Orthopaedic Surgery
Children's Hospital Los Angeles
Los Angeles, California

Emily Slate, MD
Hand Surgery Fellow
The Philadelphia Hand Center
Philadelphia, Pennsylvania

Robert R. Slater, Jr., MD, FACS
Clinical Professor
Department of Orthopaedic Surgery
University of California, Davis
Folsom, California

David J. Slutsky, MD
Hand Surgeon
The Hand and Wrist Institute
Associate Professor
Department of Orthopedics
Harbor-UCLA Medical Center
Torrance, California

Brian G. Smith, MD
Professor
Department of Orthopedics
Yale University
Director
Pediatric Orthopedics
Yale-New Haven Children's Hospital
New Haven, Connecticut

Joaquin Sanchez-Sotelo, MD, PhD
Consultant and Professor of Orthopedic Surgery
Director, Shoulder and Elbow Fellowship
Vice Chair, Adult Reconstruction
Mayo Clinic
Rochester, Minnesota

Dean G. Sotereanos, MD
Clinical Professor of Orthopaedic Surgery
University of Pittsburgh School of Medicine
Orthopaedic Specialists - UPMC
Pittsburgh, Pennsylvania

Vikram Sathyendra, MD
Orthopaedic Surgeon
Steel Valley Orthopaedics and Sports Medicine
Jefferson Hills, Pennsylvania

Felix H. Savoie III, MD
Professor of Clinical Orthopaedics
Chief of Sports Medicine
Tulane University School of Medicine
New Orleans, Louisiana

Edwin E. Spencer, Jr., MD
Attending Surgeon
Shoulder and Elbow Center
Knoxville Orthopaedic Clinic
Knoxville, Tennessee

Robert J. Strauch, MD
Professor of Clinical Orthopaedic Surgery
Columbia University Medical Center
New York, New York

Philipp N. Streubel, MD
Assistant Professor
Hand and Upper Extremity Surgery
Shoulder and Elbow Surgery
Department of Orthopaedic Surgery and Rehabilitation
University of Nebraska College of Medicine
Omaha, Nebraska

Robert M. Szabo, MD, MPH
Professor of Orthopaedics and Plastic Surgery
Chief, Hand and Upper Extremity Service
Department of Orthopaedic Surgery
University of California Davis School of Medicine
Sacramento, California

Jane S. Tan, MD
Orthopaedic Surgeon
Resurgens Orthopaedics
Covington, Georgia

John S. Taras, MD
Associate Professor
Department of Orthopaedic Surgery
Thomas Jefferson University
Chief of the Division of Hand Surgery
Drexel University College of Medicine/Hahnemann Hospital
Philadelphia, Pennsylvania

Andrew L. Terrono, MD
Chief of Hand Surgery
New England Baptist Hospital
Clinical Professor of Orthopedic Surgery
Tufts University School of Medicine
Boston, Massachusetts

Joseph J. Thoder, MD
Orthopaedic Surgery and Sports Medicine
John W. Lachman Professor
Program Director, Hand Surgery
Temple University School of Medicine
Philadelphia, Pennsylvania

Beverlie L. Ting, MD
Department of Orthopedic Surgery
Brigham and Women's Hospital
Boston, Massachusetts

E. Bruce Toby, MD
Professor
Peltier/Reckling Chair of Orthopedic Surgery
Department of Orthopedic Surgery
University of Kansas Medical Center
Kansas City, Kansas

Matthew M. Tomaino, MD, MBA
Tomaino Orthopaedic Care for Shoulder, Hand, and Elbow
Rochester, New York

Rick Tosti, MD
Resident
Temple University School of Medicine
Philadelphia, Pennsylvania

Richard L. Uhl, MD
Professor of Surgery
Division of Orthopaedic Surgery
Albany Medical Center
Albany, New York

Thomas F. Varecka, MD
Assistant Professor of Orthopaedic Surgery
University of Minnesota
Director, Hand and Microsurgery
Hennepin County Medical Center
Minneapolis, Minnesota

Luis O. Vásconez, MD, FACS
Program Director
Fellowship Program
University of Alabama at Birmingham
Birmingham, Alabama

Carley Vuillermin, MBSS, FRACS
Orthopedic Surgery Department
Boston Children's Hospital
Boston, Massachusetts

Eric R. Wagner, MD
Department of Orthopedic Surgery
Mayo Clinic
Rochester, Minnesota

Thanapong Waitayawinyu, MD
Associate Professor
Nonthavej Hospital
Nonthaburi, Thailand

Jennifer Waljee, MD, MS
Assistant Professor of Surgery
Section of Plastic Surgery
Department of Surgery
University of Michigan
Ann Arbor, Michigan

John J. Walsh IV, MD
Professor and Chairman
Department of Orthopaedics
University of South Carolina School of Medicine
Columbia, South Carolina

Lance G. Warhold, MD
Division Director
Hand and Upper Extremity Surgery
Department of Orthopaedic Surgery
Dartmouth-Hitchcock Medical Center
Associate Professor of Orthopaedic Surgery
Geisel School of Medicine at Dartmouth
Hanover, New Hampshire

Peter M. Waters, MD
John E. Hall Professor
Department of Orthopaedic Surgery
Harvard Medical School
Surgeon-in-Chief
Department of Orthopedic Surgery
Boston Children's Hospital
Boston, Massachusetts

Barrett Weiss, AB
Brown University
Providence, Rhode Island

Arnold-Peter Weiss, MD
R. Scot Sellers Scholar of Hand Surgery
Vice Chairman and Professor
Department of Orthopaedics
Warren Alpert Medical School of Brown University
Providence, Rhode Island

James A. Wilkerson, MD
Orthopaedic Surgeon
OA Centers for Orthopaedics
Portland, Maine

Gerald R. Williams, Jr., MD
John M. Fenlin, Jr., MD, Professor of Shoulder and Elbow Surgery
Department of Orthopaedic Surgery
Rothman Institute
Sidney Kimmel Medical College at Thomas Jefferson University
Philadelphia, Pennsylvania

Rafael M. M. Williams, MD
Wilson, Wyoming

Chris J. Williamson, MD
Orthopaedic Surgeon
Department of Orthopaedic Surgery
Einstein Medical Center
Philadelphia, Pennsylvania

Andrew Wong, MD
Assistant Clinical Professor
Loma Linda University Medical Center
Loma Linda, California
Orthopaedic Surgeon
Arrowhead Orthopaedics
Riverside, California

Robert W. Wysocki, MD
Assistant Professor
Department of Orthopedic Surgery
Rush University Medical Center
Chicago, Illinois

Jeffrey Yao, MD
Associate Professor of Orthopaedic Surgery and Surgery
Robert A. Chase Hand and Upper Limb Center
Stanford University Medical Center
Redwood City, California

Ravit Yanko-Arzi, MD
Attending Surgeon
Department of Plastic Surgery
Tel Aviv Sourasky Medical Center
Tel Aviv, Israel

Arik Zaretski, MD
Head of the Micro-Surgery Division of the Plastic Surgery Department
Tel Aviv Ichilov Hospital
Tel Aviv Sourasky Medical Center
Tel Aviv, Israel

Benjamin S. Zellner, MD, BA
Medical Resident
Orthopedic Surgery
Baylor College of Medicine
Houston, Texas

David S. Zelouf, MD
Assistant Professor
Thomas Jefferson University Hospital
Orthopaedic Surgeon
The Philadelphia Hand Center
Philadelphia, Pennsylvania

Elvin G. Zook, MD
Professor Emeritus
Division of Plastic Surgery
Department of Surgery
Southern Illinois University School of Medicine
Springfield, Illinois

Foreword

Since the pioneering exploration of hand surgery 60 years ago by Erik Moberg in Sweden and Guy Pulvertaft in the United Kingdom, the evolution of diagnostic and treatment techniques for hand, wrist, and elbow-related problems has been truly amazing. As a result of the many well-designed anatomic, biomechanical, traumatologic, and clinical studies conducted over the years, the knowledge base in our field is enormous. The challenge for upper limb surgeons is to safely and uniformly incorporate this acquired knowledge into everyday practice in the emergency department, in the clinic, and in the theaters.

Operative Techniques in Hand, Wrist, and Elbow Surgery provides us a framework to meet this challenge! Thoughtful, yet practical, chapters submitted by acclaimed experts from around the globe and edited by Professor Thomas R. Hunt III has resulted in a superb volume; one which will facilitate mastery of the newer, most effective surgical approaches and procedures for the hand, wrist, and elbow. It provides precise guidance for surgeons seeking instruction in specific surgical procedures within this anatomic area. The combination of illustrative clinical images and color drawings along with step-by-step descriptions of a myriad of operative procedures ranging from open to arthroscopic to microsurgical presented in a user-friendly, bullet-pointed format will make this volume the key reference allowing busy surgeons to quickly review management options and prepare for cases. An extremely valuable feature within each chapter is a table highlighting "pearls and pitfalls." By raising awareness of critical components and potential obstacles, these tables will help the surgeon be effective and "do no harm!"

It is a privilege and a great pleasure to introduce this book to upper limb surgeons around the world! It is an enjoyable, informative, and particularly thorough textbook, which will be a highly valued reference for countless surgeons and departments! It will make the learning curve less steep for those in training, and it will be a source for reference and inspiration for all. Professor Hunt has undertaken a monumental task, and he is to be commended for his contribution to this complex field! I am convinced that *Operative Techniques in Hand, Wrist, and Elbow Surgery* will become a "must-have" textbook for all those interested in the treatment of hand, wrist, and elbow conditions.

Tommy Lindau, MD, PhD

Foreword

from the First Edition

Next to the Brain, the Hand is the greatest asset to man and to it is due the development of man's handiwork."

—Sterling Bunnell

I am honored to write the foreword for Operative Techniques in Hand, Wrist, and Forearm Surgery, edited by Thomas R. Hunt.

First, I am proud as a father acknowledging his son's accomplishment. Tom was a hand fellow with Bill Bora and me at The University of Pennsylvania. His enthusiasm in learning the field of upper extremity surgery translated naturally to a dedication to teaching the discipline. His skill at this is reflected by his rise to become the Chair of Orthopaedic Surgery and the Director of the Hand Surgery Service at the University of Alabama, Birmingham. His skill in editing this text required the coordination of over 175 authors from around the world. The orchestration of this many surgical egos is no easy task and corralling from them a coherent and worthwhile text demanded attention to thousands of details by a dedicated mentor. Congratulations, Tom, you have more than earned it.

Secondly, I am proud to be have been included among the talented collection of authors whose chapters cover the gamut of operative techniques from the hand to the elbow. The book is a practical guide and an invaluable reference to a hand surgeon, whether novice hand trainee or wizened practitioner. It offers insights into old standards and solutions to new and evolving hand conditions. In clear detail, each chapter defines a strategy and technique to expand the reader's confidence.

I particularly like the fact that most chapters emphasize anatomy because the highly technical procedures described here require an intimate knowledge of upper extremity anatomy. In the 14th century, Guy de Chauliac complained, "A surgeon ignorant of anatomy carves the body as a blind man carves wood." Seven centuries later, this work puts that complaint to rest. Each procedure in the book is presented with a detailed description of the surgical anatomy and a clear delineation of the indications and critical steps to ensure successful surgery. This book allows the hand surgeon who uses it to provide knowledgeable care to their patient. One can demand no more of a book than that.

A. Lee Osterman, MD

Preface

On the pages that follow you will find a detailed description of effective surgical procedures for the treatment of most hand, wrist, and elbow disorders in both the pediatric and adult populations, written by a diverse cadre of experts in the field. This volume's 155 chapters are grouped into fourteen sections based primarily on the type of pathology, age of the patient and, when appropriate, the anatomic location. Each chapter provides a brief description of the essential anatomy, pathogenesis, natural history, physical and radiographic examination, and non-operative management. However, the majority of the content is dedicated to providing the reader a detailed step-by-step operative guide supplemented with carefully chosen clinical images and color drawings. The chapters conclude with a concise listing of critical operative pearls and pitfalls as well as a discussion of the post-operative rehabilitation and the expected patient outcomes. The references are limited to those few articles and chapters that directly relate to the disorders and treatments discussed.

Though the practical advice and expert opinion provided in this volume should serve as a valuable resource for a wide array of readers, it is specifically designed for orthopaedic, plastic, and general surgeons in training as well as those in practice. The brevity and focus of the chapters together with the precise procedural format makes *Operative Techniques in Hand, Wrist, and Elbow Surgery* an excellent text to review when preparing for a specific case. The operative procedures described are not included for historical interest, rather they are chosen by the experts based on their extensive experience and assessment of their patient's outcomes.

The final product seen herein represents the end result of heroic efforts by numerous individuals. First and foremost, the authors generously donated their time and expertise in the production of these template-based chapters. Dr. Brian Adams, a consummate educator, devoted hours as the Associate Editor of this volume. The talented editorial staff and artists worked tirelessly and patiently assisting the many authors and somehow managed to keep all documents, figures and tables related to the numerous chapters organized and moving toward completion. Finally, the Editor-in-Chief Dr. Sam Wiesel, and the Executive Editor Mr. Brian Brown, provided the vision, direction and support necessary to make this book, and others in this series, a reality.

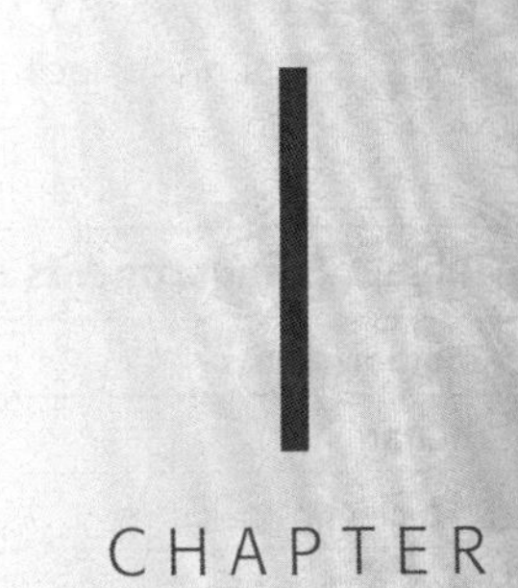

Anatomy and Surgical Approaches of the Forearm, Wrist, and Hand

Melissa A. Klausmeyer, Asif M. Ilyas, and Chaitanya S. Mudgal

DEFINITION

- Safe surgical dissection and exposure require an in-depth knowledge of anatomy. In no place is this more relevant than in the surgical approaches to the hand, wrist, and forearm.
- The critical aspect of successful surgical approaches in the forearm and wrist is the use of internervous planes.
  - These planes lie between muscles that are innervated by different nerves.
  - Dissection through internervous planes allows extensive mobilization and exposure without risk of muscle denervation.
- Unique to the hand, wrist, and forearm is the complex relationship of not only the muscles overlying bone but also the close proximity and delicate balance of accessory anatomic structures, including tendons, vessels, and nerves. Consideration of postoperative function of the extremity should start with preoperative surgical planning.
  - Elective incisions should not cross flexion creases (antecubital fossa, wrist, or digit creases) to avoid scar contracture.
  - If necessary, a transverse limb or zigzag incision should be incorporated to avoid crossing flexion creases perpendicularly.

ANATOMY

- The anatomy of the hand, wrist, and forearm is intricate and can be discussed in many ways and in extensive detail. For the discussion in this chapter, anatomy will focus on the compartments of the hand and forearm and their relevance to surgical approaches (Table 1).

SURGICAL MANAGEMENT

- All surgical approaches to the hand, wrist, and forearm warrant sound understanding of surface and deep anatomy, internervous planes, and surgical technique.
- Planning the surgical approach begins by identifying reliable surface anatomy.

Preoperative Planning

- Arrangements for instruments, sutures, microscope, imaging support, implants, and assistants should be made before the day of surgery.
- Anatomy, radiographic templating, surgical approach, procedure, and alternatives should be reviewed.

Positioning

- Most approaches to the hand, wrist, and forearm can be performed with the patient supine and the operative extremity extended on a hand table and the surgeon and assistants seated.
- The hand table should be stable and well secured. It should allow adequate space for both the operative limb and the surgeon's elbow and forearm to minimize fatigue and enhance stability and is usually placed so that the patient's shoulder is level with the cephalad third of the table, allowing the hand to be placed on the table without undue abduction of the shoulder.
- The stool should be stable and comfortable, with the height set such that the knees are level with the hips and the feet are resting flat on the ground.
- The lights should be angled directly over the hand table and not from behind the surgeon or assistant's shoulder to prevent shadows on the operative field.
- Loupe or microscope magnification is often essential for good visualization in upper extremity surgery.
- The use of a pneumatic tourniquet (either sterile or unsterile) is advised to maintain a bloodless field and clear visualization of all anatomic structures.

Approach

- Multiple approaches to the hand, wrist, and forearm exist and are best divided into the anatomic site and direction of exposure.
- The approach should be chosen based on the indication for surgery.

Table 1 Compartments of the Hand and Forearm

Compartments	Origin	Insertion	Innervation
Thenar			
Abductor pollicis brevis	Trapezium/scaphoid	Radial base of thumb P1	Median (recurrent motor branch)
Flexor pollicis brevis	Trapezium	Base of thumb P1	Median (recurrent motor branch)
Opponens pollicis	Trapezium	Radial base of thumb P1	Median (recurrent motor branch)
Adductor			
Adductor pollicis	Capitate/third metacarpal	Ulnar base of thumb P1	Ulnar
Hypothenar			
Abductor digiti minimi	Pisiform	Ulnar base of small P1	Ulnar
Flexor digiti minimi brevis	Hook of hamate	Base of small P1	Ulnar
Opponens digiti minimi	Hook of hamate	Ulnar base of small P1	Ulnar
Interosseous			
Dorsal interossei (4)	#2, 3, 4, 5 metacarpals	Radial or ulnar base of P1	Ulnar
Volar interossei (3)	#2, 4, 5 metacarpals	Radial or ulnar base of P1	Ulnar
Carpal Tunnel			
Flexor digitorum profundus and superficialis tendons, lumbricals, flexor pollicus longus tendon, median nerve	Hook of hamate	Scaphoid tubercle	
Superficial Volar Forearm			
Pronator teres	Medial epicondyle	Mid-third of radius	Median
Flexor carpi radialis	Medial epicondyle	Base of #2 MC	Median
Palmaris longus	Medial epicondyle	Palmar fascia of hand	Median
Flexor carpi ulnaris	Medial epicondyle	Pisiform/base of #5 MC	Median
Flexor digitorum superficialis	Medial epicondyle	Base of #2, 3, 4, 5 P2	Median
Deep Volar Forearm			
Flexor digitorum profundus	Ulna/interosseous membrane	Base of #2, 3, 4, 5 P3	#2, 3 – Median (ant. interosseous branch) #4, 5 – Ulnar nerve
Flexor pollicis longus	Distal third of radius	Base of thumb P2	Median (ant. interosseous branch)
Pronator quadratus	Distal third of ulna	Distal third of radius	Median (ant. interosseous branch)
Dorsal Forearm			
Abductor pollicis longus	Mid-third dorsal radius	Radial base of thumb MC	Radial (post. interosseous branch)
Extensor pollicis brevis	Mid-third dorsal radius	Dorsal base of thumb P1	Radial (post. interosseous branch)
Extensor pollicis longus	Dorsal ulna	Dorsal base of thumb P2	Radial (post. interosseous branch)
Extensor digitorum communis	Lateral epicondyle	Dorsal base of #2, 3, 4, 5 P3	Radial (post. interosseous branch)
Extensor indicis proprius	Dorsal ulna	Dorsal base of #2 P3	Radial (post. interosseous branch)
Extensor digiti quinti	Lateral epicondyle	Dorsal base of #5 P3	Radial (post. interosseous branch)
Extensor carpi ulnaris	Lateral epicondyle	Dorsal base of #5 MC	Radial (post. interosseous branch)
Supinator	Lateral epicondyle	Proximal third of radius	Radial (post. interosseous branch)
Mobile Wad			
Brachioradialis	Lat. condyle humerus	Distal radius styloid	Radial
Extensor carpi radialis longus	Lat. condyle humerus	Dorsal base of #2 MC	Radial
Extensor carpi radialis brevis	Lat. condyle humerus	Dorsal base of #3 MC	Radial (post. interosseous branch)

P1, proximal phalanx; P2, middle phalanx; P3, distal phalanx; ant., anterior; MC, metacarpal; post., posterior; lat., lateral.

Skin Incisions of the Hand

- Incisions should be outlined by sterile surgical markers before making the actual incision to confirm appropriate position, to confirm the adequacy of skin bridges should multiple incisions be used, and to help guide closure.
- Incisions can be made in skin creases on the volar aspect of the hand, but incisions in deep creases should be avoided due to the thin subcutaneous tissue, tendency for maceration due to moisture, and tendency toward poor apposition of skin edges on closure.
- Incisions perpendicular to a volar flexion crease should be avoided to prevent scar formation and secondary skin contractures that can lead to loss of motion and functional impairment (**TECH FIG 1A,B**).
- Incisions on the dorsal surface of the hand can be smaller due to the more mobile and loose nature of the dorsal skin (**TECH FIG 1C**).
  - Vertical, horizontal, and curved incisions can all be used with good facility as long as adequate skin bridges are maintained.
- Fingers can be exposed dorsally, volarly, or midaxially.
  - Dorsal incisions can be longitudinal or curvilinear.
  - Volar incisions are best facilitated by a zigzag pattern (Bruner incision) that cross creases laterally and at angles.
  - Midaxial incisions are best placed at the junction of glabrous and nonglabrous skin, with attention being paid to the neurovascular bundle that sits in the plane of the flexor sheath. The neurovascular bundle can be taken volarly with the volar flap or can be left in place by carrying the dissection superficial to it.

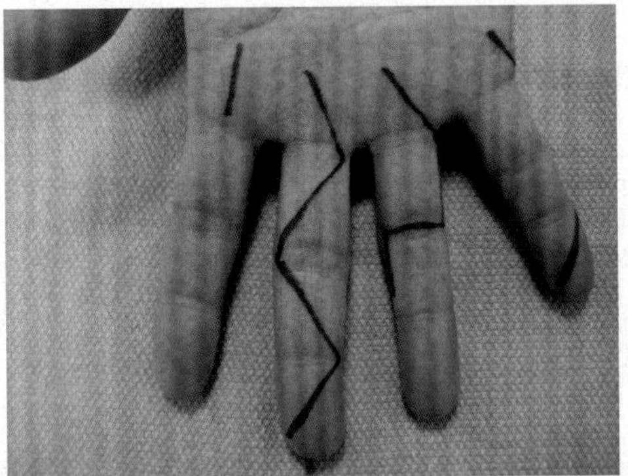
A

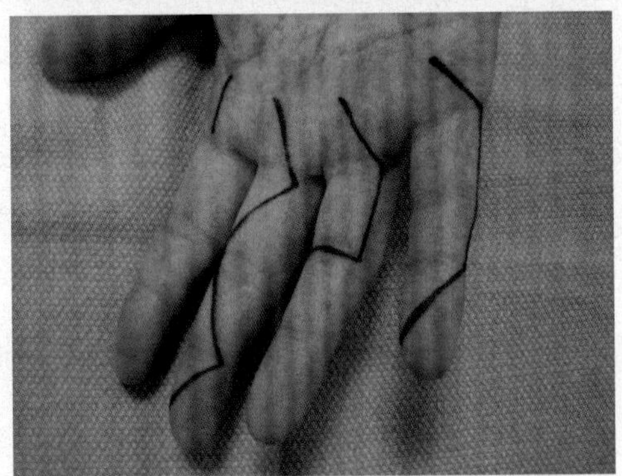
B

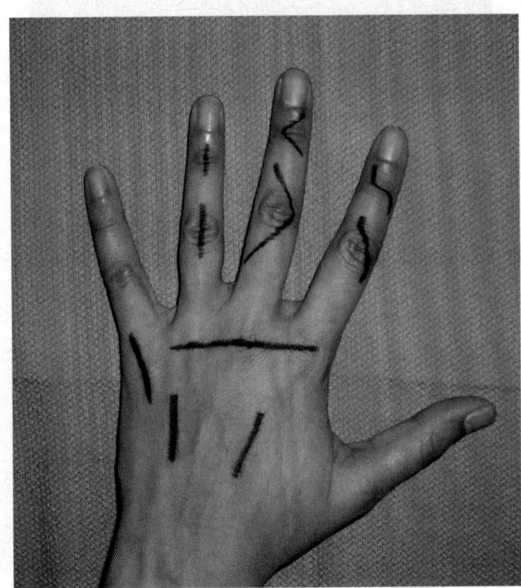
C

TECH FIG 1 • Examples of volar (**A,B**) and dorsal (**C**) incisions for the hand and digits.

Approach to the Nail Bed

- The nail plate is removed bluntly from the underlying sterile matrix and overlying eponychium.
- Longitudinal incisions are made at the radial and ulnar edges of the eponychium to expose the proximal nail bed and germinal matrix.

Approach to the Interphalangeal Joints

- Straight dorsal longitudinal incisions can be made or a variety of curved incisions can be used, including an S-type and a chevron style (**TECH FIG 2A**).
- In the distal interphalangeal joint, an H-type incision may also be used for exposure. It is critical to be aware of the location of the germinal matrix, which is about 1 mm distal to the attachment of the extensor tendon.
- At the proximal interphalangeal joint, the extensor mechanism should be immediately evident (**TECH FIG 2B**).

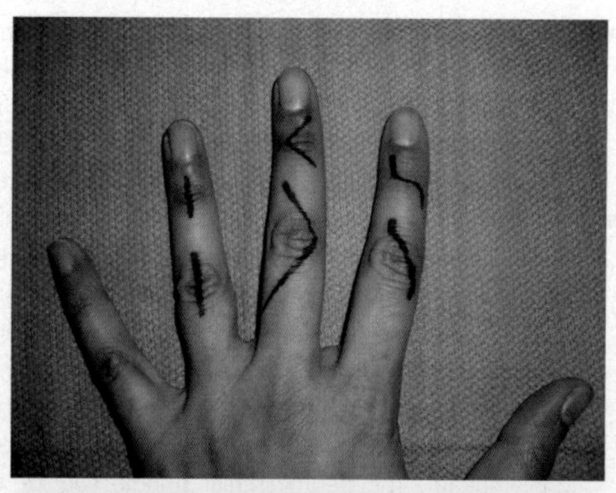

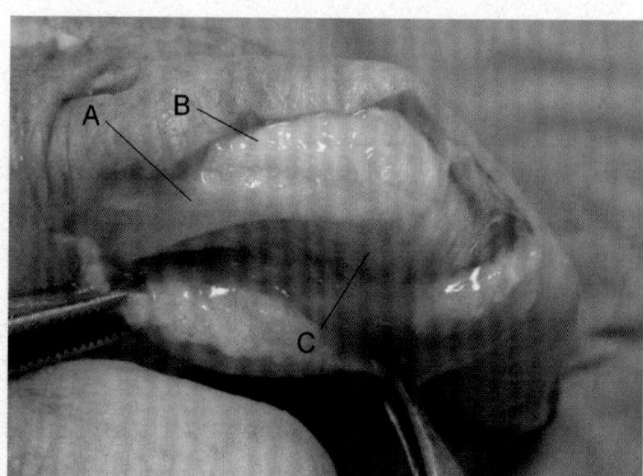

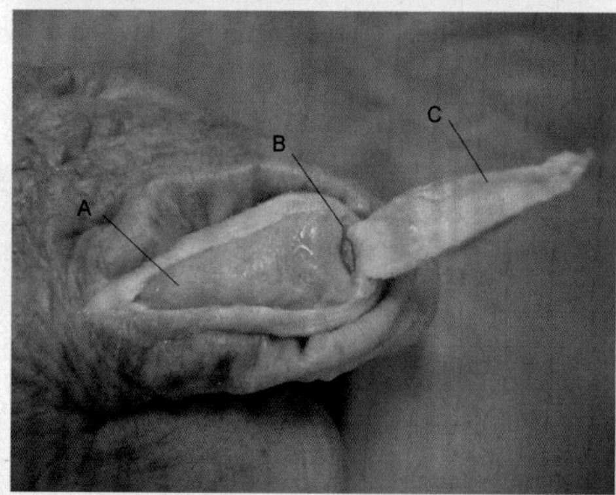

TECH FIG 2 • **A.** Examples of dorsal proximal and distal interphalangeal joint skin incisions. **B.** Extensor mechanism at the proximal interphalangeal joint. *A*, lateral band; *B*, extensor mechanism; *C*, proximal interphalangeal joint. **C.** Exposure of the proximal interphalangeal joint by a distally based V-flap elevation of the extensor mechanism. *A*, proximal phalanx; *B*, proximal interphalangeal joint; *C*, reflected extensor tendon.

- The integrity of the central slip inserting onto the middle phalanx guides exposure of the proximal interphalangeal joint. It is critical not to detach the central slip distally and to maintain continuity of the extensor mechanism through the lateral bands on each side (**TECH FIG 2C**).
- Three techniques can be employed to approach the joint dorsally:
  - The lateral bands can be freed and gently retracted dorsally, allowing a lateral approach into the joint.
  - When more exposure is required, the lateral bands can be incised in line with the extensor mechanism and repaired later.
  - Lastly, to maximize exposure of the joint, the extensor mechanism is cut dorsally in a long distally based V-shaped flap, raised, and later repaired (the Chamay approach).
- The "shotgun" technique can be employed to approach the joint volarly.
  - A zigzag incision is used to expose the tendon sheath overlying the joint.
  - The sheath and pulleys (C1, A3, and C2) are divided longitudinally; do not divide the A2 or A4 pulley.
  - The flexor tendons are retracted radially or ulnarly.
  - Propagation of the split in the flexor digitorum superficialis aids in retraction of the profundus tendon making the shotgun of the joint much easier.
  - The collateral ligaments are divided longitudinally from the volar plate.
  - The joint is hyperextended to expose the joint surfaces.[3]

Approach to the Metacarpophalangeal Joint

- With the metacarpophalangeal joint flexed, identify the extensor tendon and the apex of the joint, which is the metacarpal head.
- Make a straight dorsal longitudinal incision centered over the metacarpophalangeal joint.
  - If multiple joints are being approached, a transverse incision centered dorsally connecting each of the joints may be used (**TECH FIG 3A**).
- The extensor mechanism should be immediately evident. Sensory branches of either the radial or ulnar nerve, depending on which joint is being approached, should be identified and protected (**TECH FIG 3B**).
- Three techniques can be employed to approach the metacarpophalangeal joint:
  - The sagittal band that runs like a sling around the joint can be freed and retracted distally, exposing the dorsal capsule of the metacarpophalangeal joint.
    - This technique is best used for a dorsal capsulotomy or capsulectomy.
  - When further exposure is required, the extensor mechanism is incised centrally and longitudinally through the substance of the tendon. Extensile exposure of the joint will be obtained immediately deep to the tendon.
    - This technique maintains balance of the extensor mechanism and avoids postoperative subluxation and deviation.

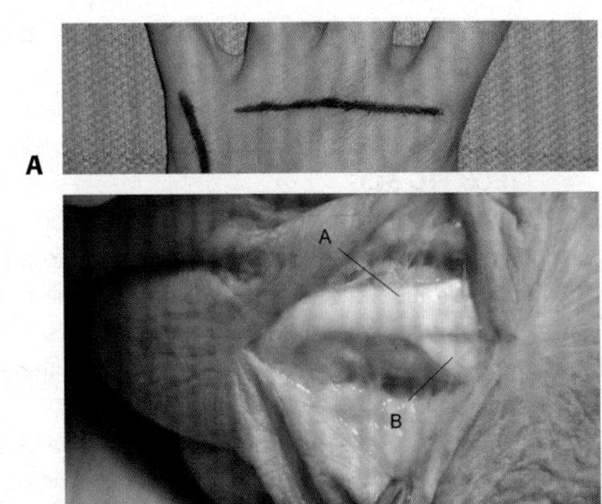

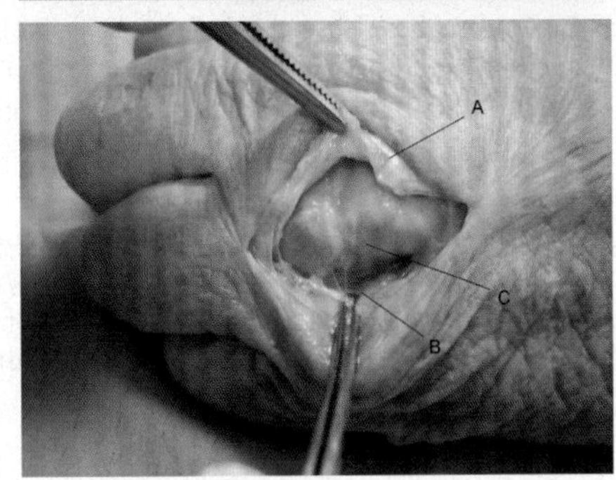

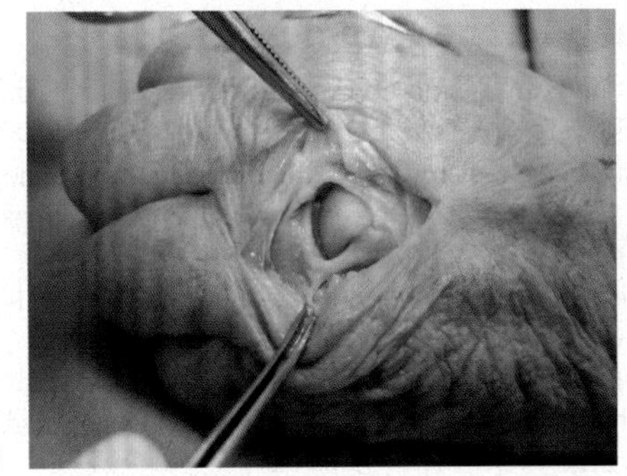

TECH FIG 3 • A. Examples of metacarpophalangeal skin incisions. A straight longitudinal incision can be placed over each joint. If multiple joints are being approached, a single straight transverse incision can be used. **B.** Extensor mechanism overlying the metacarpophalangeal joint. *A*, extensor tendon; *B*, ulnar sagittal band. **C.** The ulnar sagittal band is incised in line with the extensor mechanism revealing the metacarpophalangeal joint. *A*, extensor tendon; *B*, reflected ulnar sagittal band; *C*, metacarpophalangeal joint. **D.** The metacarpophalangeal joint is arthrotomized dorsally to the collaterals.

  - The tendon split should stop before the level of the proximal interphalangeal joint to avoid compromise of the central slip.
- The extensor mechanism can be incised along the ulnar sagittal band in line with the tendon.
  - Release of the radial sagittal band should be avoided to prevent postoperative ulnar subluxation of the tendon.
  - This technique also provides extensile exposure of the metacarpophalangeal joint as well as the collateral ligaments but risks postoperative tendon subluxation or finger deviation (**TECH FIG 3C,D**).

Approach to the Metacarpals

- Palpate the metacarpal subcutaneously. Identify overlying extensor tendons.
- Make a straight dorsal longitudinal incision over the metacarpal. If more than one metacarpal is being approached, then place the incision between adjacent metacarpals (**TECH FIG 4**). An incision between the metacarpals rather than directly over them may minimize postoperative scar adhesion between the skin incision and the underlying extensor tendon.
- Overlying extensor tendons must be identified and protected.
- Juncturae tendinae may cross over the field while connecting two tendons. They should be maintained if possible; if not, they should be released and tagged for repair before closure.
- Dorsal interossei are attached to either side of the metacarpal.
- Incise the periosteum of the metacarpal longitudinally along its exposed dorsal ridge and raise the interossei medially and laterally in a subperiosteal fashion.

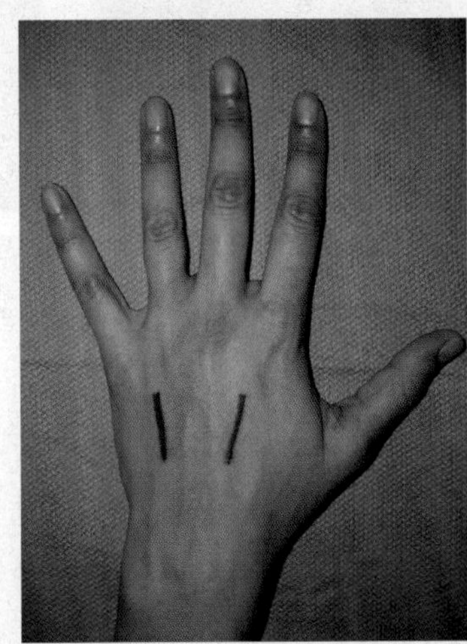

TECH FIG 4 • Incision for approaching multiple metacarpals.

Approach to the Carpal Tunnel

- The carpal tunnel is an enclosed fibro-osseous tunnel that contains nine flexor tendons and the median nerve. Its borders include the transverse carpal ligament (the roof), the carpal bones (the floor), the hook of hamate (ulnar wall), and the scaphoid (radial wall).
  - The proximal extent of the tunnel lies at the level of the distal wrist crease.
- Identify the interthenar depression, which lies between the thenar eminence radially and the hypothenar eminence ulnarly (**TECH FIG 5A**).
- Palpate the hook of hamate and pisiform bone along the ulnar base of the hand.
- Determine the cardinal line of Kaplan, the estimated distal extent of the transverse carpal ligament.[5] The cardinal line of Kaplan runs from the base of the first web space (with the thumb abducted in the plane of the palm) parallel to the proximal palmar crease toward the hook of hamate.
- The extent of the incision can vary depending on the surgeon's preference, ranging from a limited approach (**TECH FIG 5B**) to an extensile one.
- The incision should be centered within the interthenar depression and in line with the third web space to avoid injury to the palmar cutaneous branches of the median and ulnar nerves.[9]
- The internervous plane occurs between the palmar cutaneous branches of the ulnar and median nerves.
- Incise the subcutaneous fat in line with the skin incision. Deep to the fat lies the longitudinally oriented superficial palmar fascia (**TECH FIG 5C**).
  - Incise this fascia in line with the incision.
  - Avoid raising flaps radially or ulnarly to prevent skin devitalization and injury to branches of the palmar cutaneous branch of the median and ulnar nerves.
- Deep to the superficial palmar fascia lies the thick transverse carpal ligament.
  - Release this ligament in line with the skin incision, paying attention to the median nerve lying deep to it as well as being cautious of the recurrent motor branch of the median nerve, which could cross through or across the transverse carpal ligament (**TECH FIG 5D**).
- Confirm the release of the transverse carpal ligament both proximally and distally.
  - Distal release is confirmed on visualization of the "sentinel" pad of fat, which has a distinct yellow color different from that of the subcutaneous fat.
  - Proximal release is confirmed both visually and by feel and usually corresponds to the confluence of the transverse carpal ligament with the deep forearm fascia (antebrachial fascia), generally located at the level of the distal wrist crease.

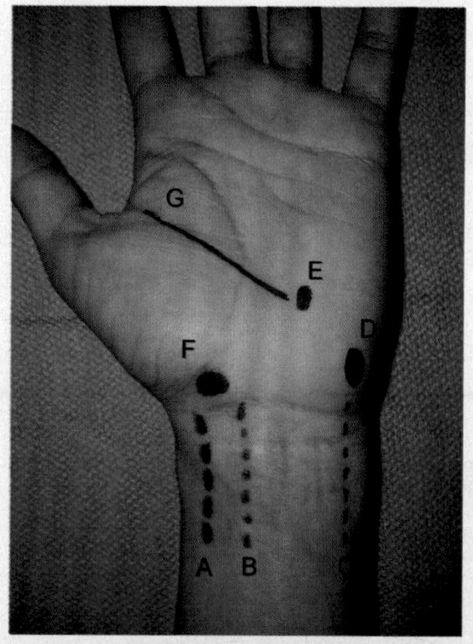

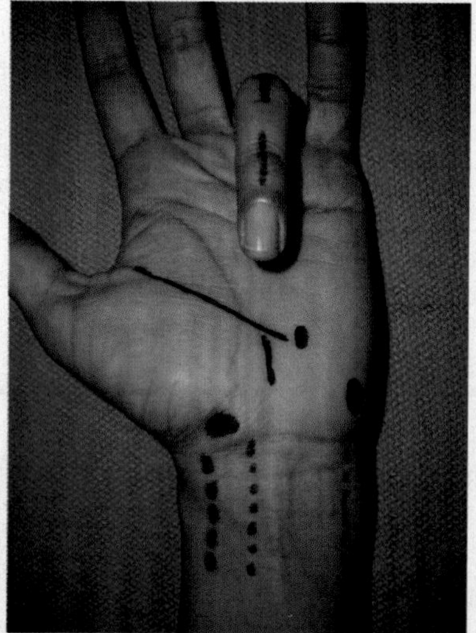

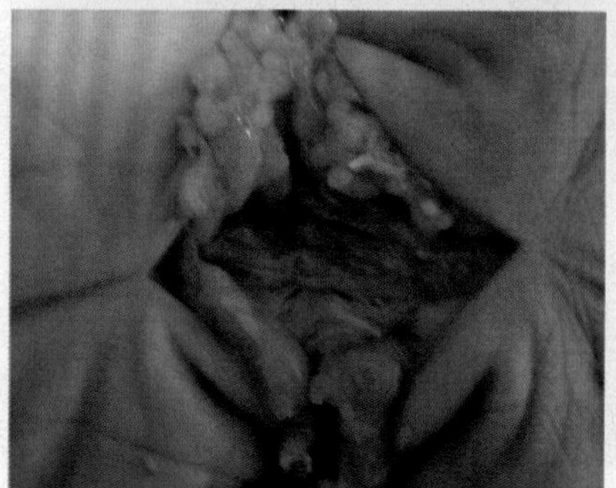

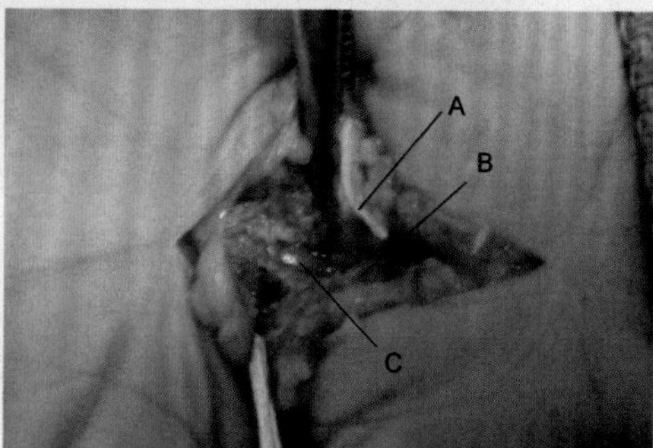

TECH FIG 5 • A. Surface anatomy of the volar hand. *A*, radial artery; *B*, flexor carpi radialis tendon; *C*, flexor carpi ulnaris tendon; *D*, pisiform; *E*, hook of hamate; *F*, distal pole of scaphoid; *G*, cardinal line of Kaplan. **B.** Incision for the limited incision carpal tunnel approach. **C.** Superficial palmar fascia of the hand. **D.** Partial release of the transverse carpal ligament with the median nerve lying deep to it. *A*, retracted superficial palmar fascia; *B*, partially released transverse carpal ligament; *C*, median nerve.

Approach to Canal of Guyon

- The canal of Guyon is an enclosed fibro-osseous space at the ulnar base of the hand through which the ulnar neurovascular structures travel.
  - Its borders include the volar carpal ligament (the roof), the transverse carpal ligament (the floor), the pisiform (ulnar wall), and the hook of hamate (radial wall).
- Palpate the pisiform bone, which lies subcutaneously at the ulnar base of the hand immediately distal to the wrist flexion crease in line with the flexor carpi ulnaris (see **TECH FIG 5A**).
- Palpate the hook of hamate, which lies about 2 cm distal and 2 cm radial to the pisiform bone.
  - This may be difficult to palpate in patients with large hands or those with well-developed hypothenar musculature.
- Palpate the flexor carpi ulnaris tendon, which runs along the ulnar aspect of the forearm and inserts into the pisiform upon crossing the wrist flexion crease.
- Make a zigzag or curved incision between the pisiform and hook of hamate and extend it proximally (**TECH FIG 6A**).
  - Avoid crossing the wrist flexion crease perpendicularly. Extend it proximally along the radial border of the flexor carpi ulnaris tendon (**TECH FIG 6B**).
- Identify the flexor carpi ulnaris proximal to the wrist flexion crease and mobilize it ulnarly by releasing the fascia along its radial border. The ulnar artery and nerve will lie just deep and radial to the tendon, with the nerve more superficial and ulnar to the artery.
- Follow the ulnar artery and nerve distally into the hand.
  - In the hand, the flexor carpi ulnaris tendon will insert into the pisiform and the ulnar artery and nerve will dive deep to the volar carpal ligament.
- Releasing the volar carpal ligament radial to the pisiform opens the roof of the canal of Guyon and decompresses the ulnar artery and nerve. In the canal of Guyon, the nerve splits into its motor and sensory branches. The motor branch of the ulnar nerve dives below a fibrous arch formed by the hypothenar musculature originating from the hook of hamate (**TECH FIG 6C**).
- There is a high frequency of anatomic variations of the ulnar neurovascular structures within the canal of Guyon, and a release of the canal must include not only the roof but also the distal extent of it as it enters below the fibrous arch below the hypothenar muscles.[6]

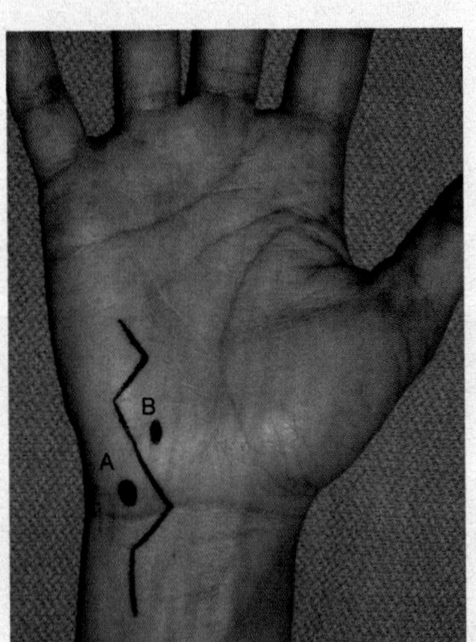

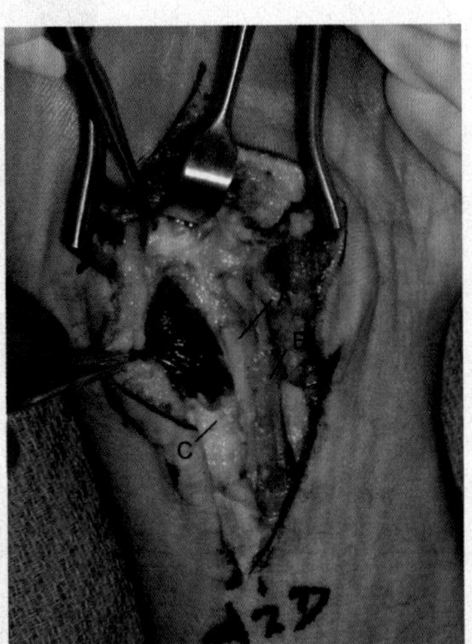

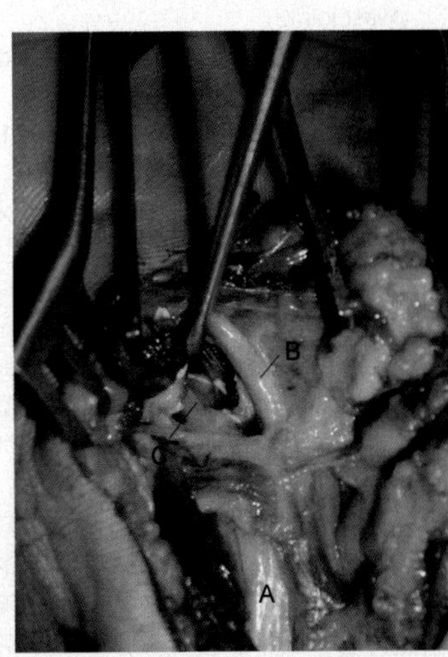

TECH FIG 6 • A. Surface anatomy and incision for the approach to the canal of Guyon. *A*, pisiform; *B*, hook of hamate. **B.** The ulnar neurovascular structures in the base of the hand after release of the volar carpal ligament. *A*, ulnar nerve; *B*, ulnar artery and vein; *C*, pisiform with origin of the hypothenar muscles. **C.** Fibrous arch formed by the hypothenar muscles over the motor branch of the ulnar nerve. *A*, ulnar nerve; *B*, sensory branch of ulnar nerve; *C*, motor branch of ulnar nerve.

Volar Approach to the Radius

- Identify the flexor carpi radialis at the wrist flexion crease distally and follow it proximally (**TECH FIG 7A**). Its tendinous nature will give way to the muscle at roughly the middle of the forearm or approximately 8 to 10 cm proximal to the distal wrist crease.
- Identify the brachioradialis, which originates along the lateral epicondylar ridge of the distal humerus and is the most superficial muscle mass along the lateral forearm. Distally and laterally, it has a broad insertion along the flare of the radial border of the radius.
- Identify the biceps tendon, which is the broad and taut extension of the biceps tendon that crosses anterior to the elbow joint and dives toward its insertion into the radius medial to the brachioradialis.
- Identify the radial artery at the wrist. It is found between the flexor carpi radialis and brachioradialis tendons.
- With the forearm supinated, begin the incision proximal to the wrist flexion crease and immediately radial to the flexor carpi

radialis tendon and extend the incision proximally parallel to the tendon.
   - The incision can end lateral to the biceps tendon and distal to the elbow flexion crease.
   - The incision can be extended as shown by the dotted extensions in **TECH FIG 7A**.
   - The length of the incision depends on the extent of bone that needs to be exposed.
- As described by Henry,[4] the internervous plane distally occurs between the flexor carpi radialis (median nerve) and the brachioradialis (radial nerve). Proximally, it occurs between the pronator teres (median nerve) and the brachioradialis (radial nerve).
   - Distally, the interval between the flexor carpi radialis and the brachioradialis is developed (**TECH FIG 7B**).
   - The radial artery lies just ulnar to the brachioradialis tendon and lies underneath the brachioradialis in the middle of the forearm.
   - Dissection should not drift ulnar to the flexor carpi radialis for the median nerve lies just deep and ulnar to this tendon.
   - The superficial radial sensory nerve exits from under the brachioradialis at the middle of the forearm, about 8 to 10 cm proximal to the radial styloid, and travels adjacent to the tendon distally.[1] The nerve arborizes proximal to the wrist joint.
   - Proximally, the interval between the pronator teres and brachioradialis is developed.
- An alternative to the volar approach of Henry is the transflexor carpi radialis approach.
   - In this approach, the incision is placed directly over the flexor carpi radialis tendon.
   - The flexor carpi radialis sheath is opened sharply in line with the tendon. The incision in the sheath is best placed in the radial half of the sheath, so as to avoid any injury to the palmar cutaneous branch of the median nerve, which runs alongside the flexor carpi radialis tendon starting approximately 5 cm proximal to the distal wrist crease.
   - The tendon is retracted ulnarly, and the floor of the tendon sheath is opened sharply, leading directly into the deep layer between the finger flexors and the pronator quadratus, also known as the *space of Parona*.[7]
- Several muscles lie over the radius in the deep layer. Distally, the pronator quadratus and flexor pollicis longus cover the radius (**TECH FIG 7C**). On the middle third of the radius lie the flexor carpi radialis and pronator teres.
- To expose the radius, these muscles are released along the volar radial aspect of the radius and are raised in a subperiosteal fashion ulnarly.
- Proximally, the supinator muscle covers the radius. Through its substance travels the posterior interosseous nerve as it travels to the dorsal compartment of the forearm.
- To expose the radius proximally, the forearm must be fully supinated, and the supinator is released along the ulnar border of the radius and raised radially. The forearm must be kept fully supinated to protect the posterior interosseous nerve.

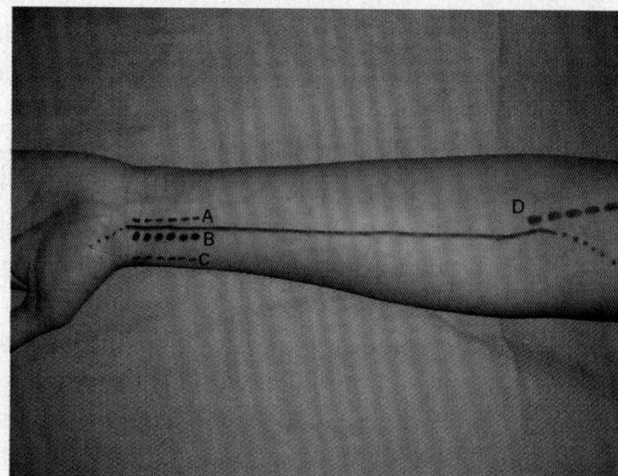

A

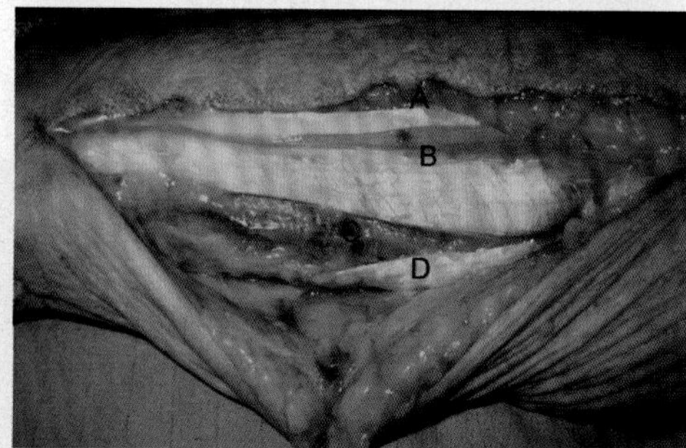

B

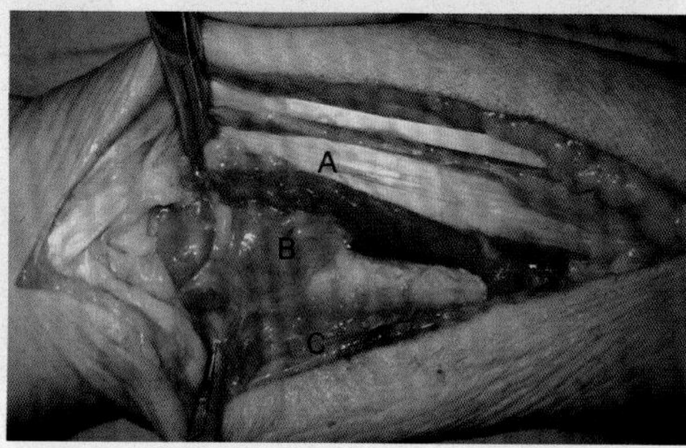

C

TECH FIG 7 • A. Surface anatomy and incision of the volar forearm. *A*, flexor carpi radialis; *B*, radial artery; *C*, brachioradialis; *D*, biceps tendon. **B.** Superficial exposure of the volar radius showing the palmaris longus (*A*) and the internervous plane between the flexor carpi radialis (*B*) and the brachioradialis (*D*). *C*, radial artery. **C.** Deep exposure of the volar distal radius showing the pronator quadratus (*B*) covering the distal radius. *A*, flexor carpi radialis; *C*, radial artery.

Dorsal Approach to the Radius

- Identify the tubercle of Lister at the distal and radial aspect of the radius. It is the most prominent bony protuberance on the dorsal distal radius, and the extensor pollicis longus tendon curves around it ulnarly (**TECH FIG 8A**).
- Identify the "mobile wad of three," which is the common muscle mass composed of the brachioradialis and the extensor carpi radialis longus and brevis.[4]
- Identify the lateral epicondyle of the distal humerus, which is the bony prominence most easily palpable proximal to the radial head along the lateral aspect of the elbow.

- With the forearm pronated, make the incision from the tubercle of Lister and extend it proximally along the ulnar border of the "mobile wad" toward the lateral epicondyle.
  - The length of the incision depends on the extent of bone that needs to be exposed (**TECH FIG 8A**).
  - The wrist can be partially denervated by performing a neurectomy of the posterior interosseous nerve, which lies on the radial floor of the fourth dorsal compartment.
- As described by Thompson,[8] the internervous plane distally occurs between the extensor carpi radialis brevis (radial nerve, posterior interosseous nerve, or both) and the extensor pollicis longus (posterior interosseous nerve).
  - Proximally, it occurs between the extensor carpi radialis brevis (radial nerve; inconsistent innervation) and the extensor digitorum communis (posterior interosseous nerve).
- Distally, develop the interval between the extensor carpi radialis brevis and the extensor pollicis longus with the tubercle of Lister positioned between them (**TECH FIG 8B**).
- Exposing proximally, the interval between the extensor carpi radialis brevis and the extensor digitorum communis is identified by the emergence of the outcropping abductor pollicis longus and the extensor pollicis brevis (**TECH FIG 8C**).
- Distally, the radius sits immediately below the superficial extensor tendons.
  - To expose the distal radius, the extensor retinaculum and the sheath of the extensor pollicis longus tendon is opened, and the tendon is retracted radially.
  - The floor of the tendon sheath is incised longitudinally, and the extensor tendons are raised subperiosteally, with the extensor carpi radialis longus and brevis taken radially and the finger extensors taken ulnarly.
- Proximally, the abductor pollicis longus and extensor pollicis brevis cover the middle third of the radius.
  - To expose the radius, these muscles are released along their radial border, to avoid denervation, and raised ulnarly.
  - The proximal third of the radius is covered by the supinator. Within its substance and between its two heads runs the posterior interosseous nerve.
- Exposure of the dorsal radius proximally requires exposure and protection of this nerve before elevating the supinator off the radius.
  - First, identify the nerve as it exits between the two heads of the supinator.
  - Follow the nerve proximally through the substance of the supinator's superficial head while taking care to preserve all its branches.
  - Once the nerve is identified along its entire course, the supinator can be released along its radial border and raised ulnarly.

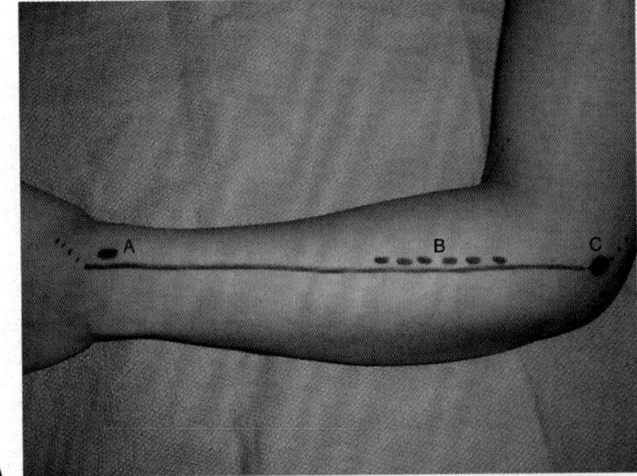

A

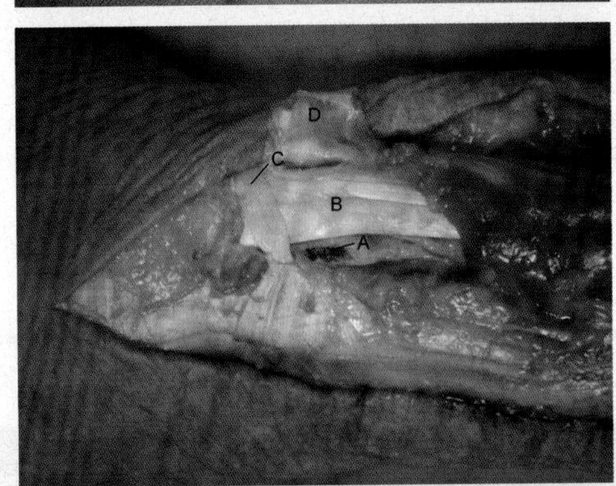

B

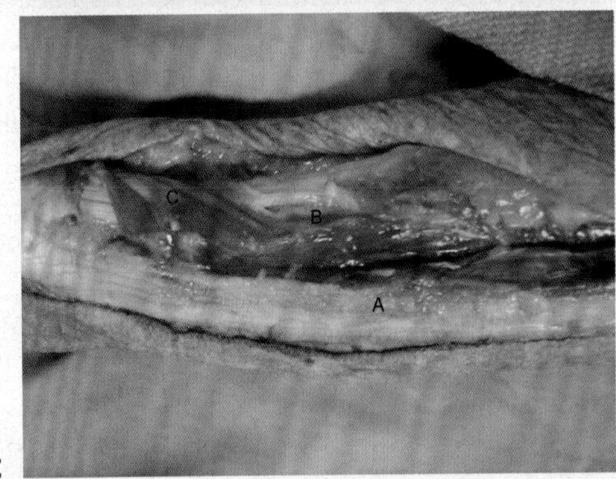

C

TECH FIG 8 • A. Surface anatomy and incision of the dorsal forearm. *A*, tubercle of Lister; *B*, ulnar border of the mobile wad of three; *C*, lateral epicondyle. **B.** Superficial exposure of the dorsal distal radius. *A*, tubercle of Lister; *B*, extensor carpi radialis longus and brevis; *C*, extensor pollicis longus; *D*, reflected extensor retinaculum. **C.** Musculature of the dorsal forearm. *A*, extensor digitorum communis; *B*, extensor carpi radialis brevis; *C*, abductor pollicis longus and extensor pollicis brevis.

Approach to the Ulna

- Identify the ulnar head and styloid distally with the forearm in neutral rotation (**TECH FIG 9**).
- Identify the subcutaneous border of the ulna.
- Identify the tip of the olecranon proximally.
- With the forearm in neutral rotation, begin the incision at the level of the head of the ulna but proximal to the styloid. Extend the incision across the subcutaneous border of the ulna proximally toward the olecranon. The length of incision depends on the extent of the bone that needs to be exposed.
- Distally, the internervous plane occurs between the flexor carpi ulnaris (ulnar nerve) and the extensor carpi ulnaris (posterior interosseous nerve).
  - Proximally, at the level of the olecranon, the internervous plane occurs for a short length between the flexor carpi ulnaris (ulnar nerve) and the anconeus (radial nerve).

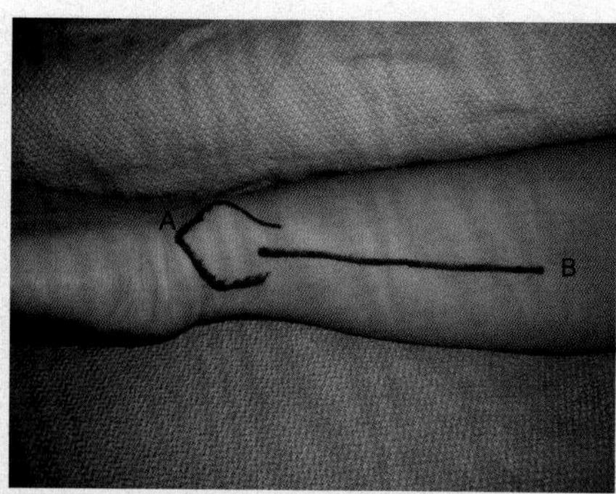

TECH FIG 9 • Surface anatomy and incision for the ulnar shaft. *A*, ulnar head and styloid; *B*, subcutaneous border of ulna.

- Distally, the interval between the flexor carpi ulnaris and the extensor carpi ulnaris occurs along the subcutaneous border of the ulna.
  - Both muscles can be raised volarly and dorsally off the ulna, respectively, in a subperiosteal fashion.
- The ulnar artery and nerve travel deep and radial to the flexor carpi ulnaris. The nerve is protected by careful subperiosteal elevation of the flexor carpi ulnaris.
- The dorsal branch of the ulnar nerve branches about 8 cm proximal to the pisiform and crosses the subcutaneous border of the ulna as it travels dorsally about 5 cm proximal to the pisiform.[2]
- Proximally, the interval remains along the subcutaneous border of the ulna.
- The triceps tendon inserts on the proximal aspect of the ulna.
- When exposing the ulna proximally during deep dissection, the integrity of the triceps tendon is maintained by incising the tendon in line with its fibers across the border of the ulna and raising it medially and laterally in a subperiosteal fashion.
- The ulnar nerve travels around the medial epicondyle and dives between the two heads of the flexor carpi ulnaris.
- Before exposing the ulna's most proximal and medial portion, the ulnar nerve should be identified and protected, followed by subperiosteal elevation of the flexor carpi ulnaris.

PEARLS AND PITFALLS

Approach to the interphalangeal joints (proximal and distal)	▪ Protect the germinal matrix and terminal tendon at the base of the distal phalanx. ▪ Protect the central slip at the base of the middle phalanx.
Approach to the metacarpophalangeal joints	▪ If necessary, release the ulnar sagittal band at the joint. Avoid releasing the radial sagittal band.
Approach to the carpal tunnel	▪ Protect branches of the palmar cutaneous branch of the median and ulnar nerves in the subcutaneous tissue by centering the incision in the interthenar eminence. ▪ Remain vigilant for a transligamentous recurrent motor branch of the median nerve.
Volar approach to the radius	▪ Dissection should not drift ulnar to the flexor carpi radialis tendon to protect the median nerve and its cutaneous branches.
Dorsal approach to the radius	▪ The posterior interosseous nerve ends at the level of the wrist dorsally in line with the fourth metacarpal and is easily approached for denervation for postoperative pain relief.

REFERENCES

1. Abrams RA, Brown RA, Botte MJ. The superficial branch of the radial nerve: an anatomic study with surgical implications. J Hand Surg Am1992;17(6):1037–1041.
2. Botte MJ, Cohen MS, Lavernia CJ, et al. The dorsal branch of the ulnar nerve: an anatomic study. J Hand Surg Am 1990;15(4):603–607.
3. Eaton RG, Malerich MM. Volar plate arthroplasty of the proximal interphalangeal joint: a review of ten years' experience. J Hand Surg Am 1980;5(3):260–268.
4. Henry AK. Extensile Exposure, ed 2. Edinburgh: E&S Livingstone, 1966.
5. Kaplan EB. Functional and Surgical Anatomy of the Hand, ed 2. Philadelphia: JB Lippincott, 1965.
6. Konig PS, Hage JJ, Bloem JJ, et al. Variations of the ulnar nerve and ulnar artery in Guyon's canal: a cadaveric study. J Hand Surg Am 1994;19(4):617–622.
7. Parona F. Dell'oncotomia negli accessi profundi diffuse dell'avambracchio. Annali Universali di Medicina e Chirurgia Milano, 1876.
8. Thompson JE. Anatomical methods of approach in operations on the long bones of the extremities. Ann Surg 1918;68(3):309–329.
9. Watchmaker GP, Weber D, Mackinnon SE. Avoidance of transection of the palmar cutaneous branch of the median nerve in carpal tunnel release. J Hand Surg Am 1996;21(4):644–650.

Surgical Approaches to the Elbow

Luke S. Austin, Joseph A. Abboud, Matthew L. Ramsey, and Gerald R. Williams, Jr.

2

CHAPTER

ELBOW APPROACHES

- The surgical exposures described for the elbow are divided into posterior, medial, and lateral approaches. These descriptions denote the deep surgical interval employed (Table 1).
- Often, these deep approaches can be performed through a direct medial or lateral skin incision. Alternately, a midline posterior incision can be used and then subcutaneous flaps can be created to access the deeper medial or lateral intervals.

POSTERIOR APPROACH TO THE ELBOW

- Releasing the triceps attachment to the olecranon is not advisable, owing to the difficulty of adequate repair and possible disruption during rehabilitation. Today, there are four choices of posterior exposure:
  - Triceps splitting
  - Triceps reflecting
  - Triceps preserving
  - Olecranon osteotomy

Triceps-Splitting Approaches

Posterior Triceps-Splitting Approach (Campbell)

- Care must be exercised to maintain the medial portion of the triceps expansion over the forearm fascia in continuity with the flexor carpi ulnaris.
- Laterally, the anconeus and triceps are more stable, with less chance of disruption.

Indications

- Total elbow arthroplasty
- ORIF of distal humerus fracture
- Removal of loose bodies
- Capsulectomies
- Posterior exposure of the joint for ankylosis, sepsis, synovectomy, and ulnohumeral arthroplasty

Approach

- Skin incision begins in the midline over the triceps, about 10 cm above the joint line, and is generally placed laterally or medially across the tip of the olecranon. It continues distally over the lateral aspect of the subcutaneous border of the proximal ulna for about 5 to 6 cm (**FIG 1A**).
- Triceps is exposed, along with the proximal 4 cm of the ulna.
- A midline incision is made through the triceps fascia and tendon as it is continued distally across the insertion of the triceps tendon at the tip of the olecranon and down the subcutaneous crest of the ulna (**FIG 1B**).
- Triceps tendon and muscle are split longitudinally, exposing the distal humerus.
- The anconeus is then reflected subperiosteally laterally, whereas the flexor carpi ulnaris is similarly retracted medially.
- Insertion of the triceps is carefully released from the olecranon, leaving the extensor mechanism in continuity with the forearm fascia and muscles medially and laterally (**FIG 1C**).
- Ulnar nerve is visualized and protected in the cubital tunnel.
- Closure of the triceps fascia is required only proximal to the olecranon, but the insertion should be repaired to the olecranon with a suture passed through the ulna.
- The incision is then closed in layers.

Triceps-Splitting, Tendon-Reflecting Approach (Van Gorder)

- A variation of the technique described earlier
- Allows lengthening of the triceps if necessary
- Has been largely abandoned in favor of the triceps-reflecting techniques

Table 1 Indications and Recommended and Alternative Surgical Approaches

Indication	Recommended Approach	Alternative Approach
Total elbow arthroplasty	Bryan-Morrey, extended Kocher	Gschwend et al, Campbell, and Wadsworth
Soft tissue reconstruction	Global	Kocher, Bryan-Morrey, and Hotchkiss
T intercondylar fracture	MacAusland with chevron olecranon osteotomy	Alonso-Llames
Radial head fracture	Kocher	Kaplan
Capitellum fracture	Kaplan extended lateral approach	Kocher with or without Kaplan
Coronoid fracture	Taylor and Scham	Hotchkiss
Extra-articular distal humerus fracture	Alonso-Llames	Bryan-Morrey, Campbell
Monteggia fracture-dislocation	Gordon	Boyd
Radioulnar synostosis excision	Kocher or Gordon	Boyd or Henry

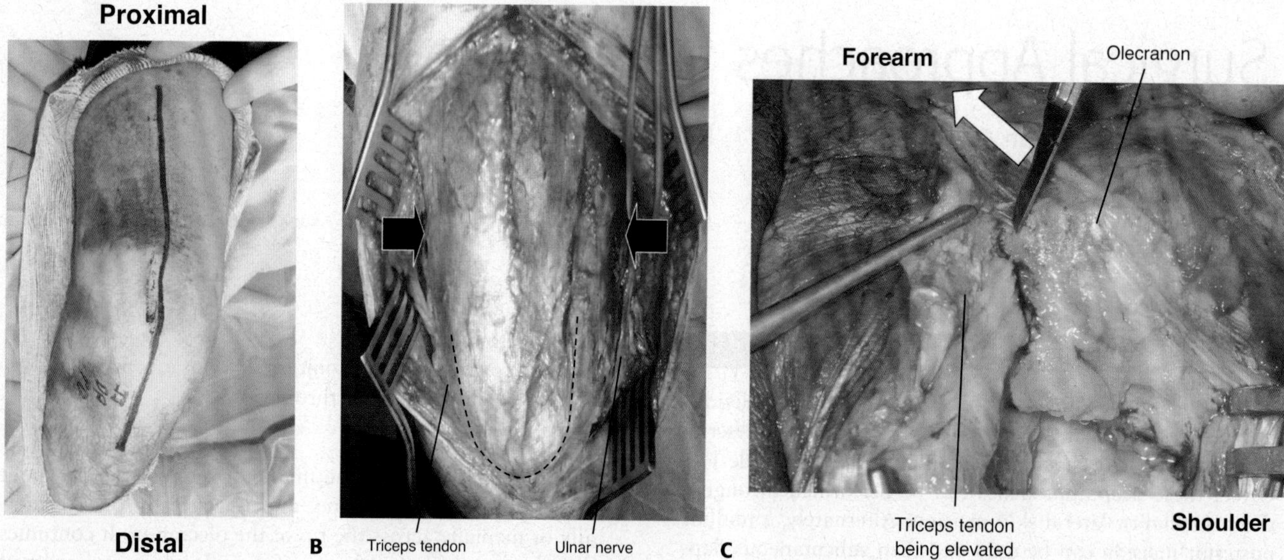

FIG 1 • **A.** Skin incision for the posterior triceps-splitting approach. **B.** Medial and lateral flaps are elevated, allowing full access to the triceps tendon. The ulnar nerve is isolated along the medial border with a vessel loop. **C.** The insertion of the triceps being elevated off the olecranon from medial to lateral. (**A:** Courtesy of Asif M. Ilyas, MD, and Jesse B. Jupiter, MD; **B,C:** Courtesy of Srinath Kamineni, MD.)

Indications

- Same as those for midline-splitting approach described earlier

Approach

- A posterior midline incision begins 10 cm proximal to the olecranon and extends distally onto the subcutaneous border of the ulna between the anconeus and the flexor carpi ulnaris.
- Triceps fascia and aponeurosis are exposed along the tendinous insertion into the ulna.
- Tendon is reflected from the muscle in a proximal to distal direction, freeing the underlying muscle fibers while preserving the tendinous attachment to the olecranon (**FIG 2**).
- Triceps muscle is then split in midline, and the distal humerus is exposed subperiosteally.
- Periosteum and triceps are elevated for a distance of about 5 cm proximal to the olecranon fossa, exposing the posterior aspect of the joint.
- If more extensive exposure is desired, the subperiosteal dissection is extended to the level of the joint, exposing the condyles both medially and laterally.
- Ulnar nerve should be identified and protected.
- After the procedure, if an elbow contracture has been corrected, the joint should be maximally flexed.
- The tendon slides distally from its initial position, and the proximal muscle and tendon are reapproximated in the lengthened relationship.
- The distal part of the triceps is then securely sutured to the fascia of the triceps expansion, and the remainder of the wound is closed in layers.

Triceps-Reflecting Approaches

- The triceps mechanism may be preserved in continuity with the anconeus and simply reflected to one side or the other.
- Three surgical approaches have been described that preserve the triceps muscle and tendon in continuity with the distal musculature of the forearm fascia and expose the entire joint.

Bryan-Morrey Posteromedial Triceps-Reflecting Approach

- Developed to preserve the continuity of the triceps with the anconeus

Indications

- Total elbow arthroplasty
- Interposition arthroplasty

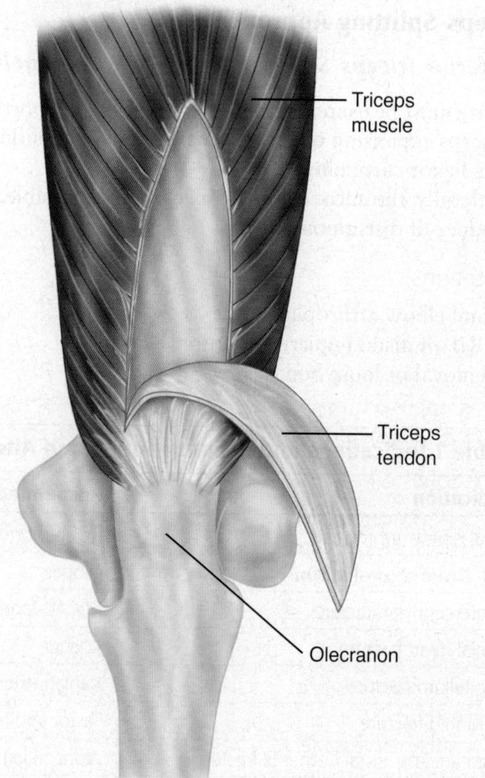

FIG 2 • Triceps-splitting, tendon-reflecting approach. The tendon is reflected from the muscle in a proximal to distal direction.

- Surgical treatment of elbow dislocations
- ORIF of distal humerus fracture
- Synovial disease
- Infection

Approach

- A straight posterior incision is made medial to the midline, about 9 cm proximal and 8 cm distal to the tip of the olecranon (**FIG 3A**).
- The ulnar nerve is identified proximally at the margin of the medial head of the triceps and, depending on the procedure, is either protected or carefully dissected to its first motor branch and transposed anteriorly.
- The medial aspect of the triceps is elevated from the posterior capsule.
- The fascia of the forearm between the anconeus and the flexor carpi ulnaris is incised distally for about 6 cm.
- The triceps and the anconeus are elevated as one flap from medial to lateral, skeletonizing the olecranon and subcutaneous border of the ulna (**FIG 3B**). This should be performed at 20 to 30 degrees of flexion to relieve tension on the insertion, thereby facilitating dissection.
- The collateral ligaments may be released from the humerus for exposure as needed (**FIG 3C**).
  - If stability is important, these ligaments should be preserved or anatomically repaired at the conclusion of the surgery.
  - When performing a linked total elbow replacement, it is not necessary to preserve or repair the collateral ligaments.
- The triceps attachment can be thin at the attachment to the ulna, and it is not uncommon for a buttonhole to be created when reflecting the triceps.
  - To prevent this, the flap can be raised as an osteoperiosteal flap (see osteoanconeus flap approach).
  - A small osteotome is used to elevate the fascia with the petals of bone.
  - The flap is mobilized laterally, elevating the anconeus origin from the distal humerus until it can be folded over the lateral humeral condyle.
  - At this point, the radial head can be visualized.
- The tip of the olecranon can be excised to help expose the trochlea.

Osteoanconeus Flap Approach

- This provides excellent extension and reliable healing of the osseous attachment to the olecranon.
- This approach exposes only the ulnar nerve, whereas the Mayo approach translocates the nerve.

Indications

- This is a triceps-reflecting approach similar in concept to the Bryan-Morrey triceps-reflecting approach.
- Most often used for joint replacement or distal humeral fractures

Approach

- A straight posterior incision is made medial to the midline, about 9 cm proximal and 8 cm distal to the tip of the olecranon.
- The ulnar nerve is identified and protected but not translocated.
- The triceps attachment is released from the ulna by osteotomizing the attachment with a thin wafer of bone.
  - This is the essential difference from the Bryan-Morrey approach.

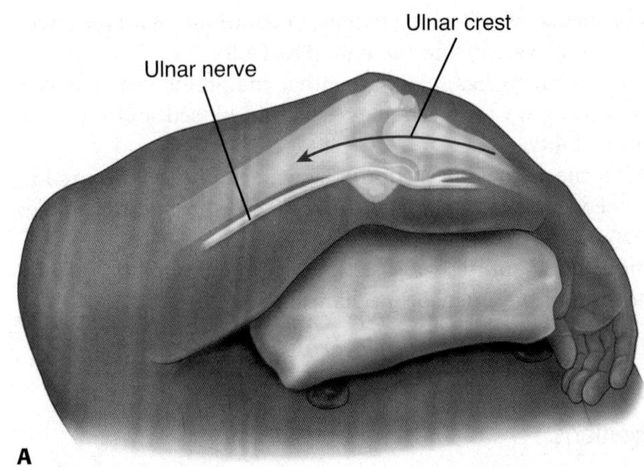

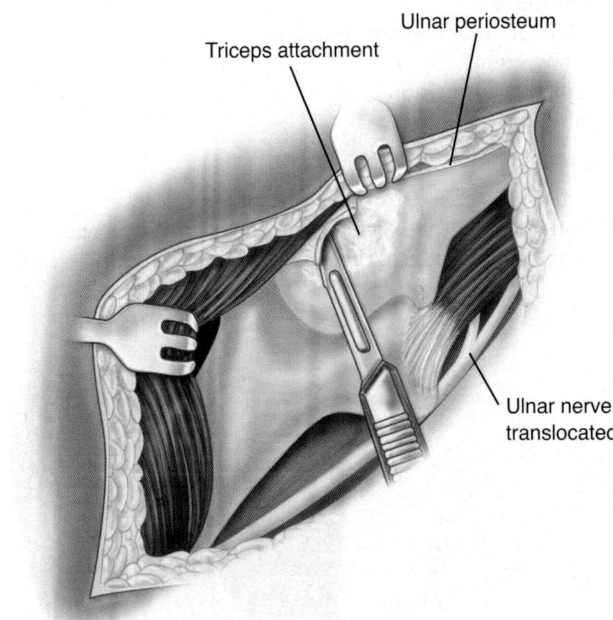

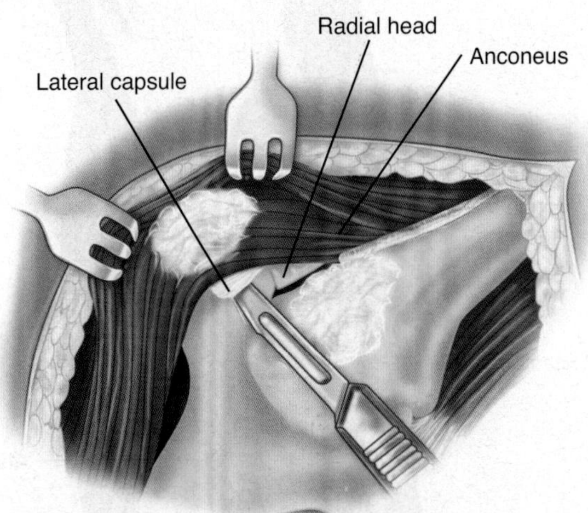

FIG 3 • The Bryan-Morrey posterior approach. **A.** Straight posterior skin incision. **B.** The ulnar nerve has been translocated anteriorly. The medial border of the triceps is identified and released, and the superficial forearm fascia is sharply incised to allow reflection of the fascia and periosteum from the proximal ulna. **C.** The extensor mechanism has been reflected laterally, and the collateral ligaments have been released.

- The medial aspect of the triceps, in continuity with the anconeus, is elevated from the ulna (**FIG 4A,B**).
- The collateral ligaments are either maintained or released, depending on the pathology being addressed and the need for stability.
- After the surgical procedure, the wafer of bone is secured to its bed by nonabsorbable sutures placed through bone holes (**FIG 4C**).
- Interrupted sutures are used to repair the remaining distal portion of the extensor mechanism.

Extensile Kocher Posterolateral Triceps-Reflecting Approach

Indications

- Joint arthroplasty
- Ankylosis
- ORIF of distal humerus fractures
- Synovectomy
- Radial head excision
- Infection

Approach

- Extensile exposure from the Kocher approach
- Skin incision begins 8 cm proximal to the joint just posterior to the supracondylar ridge and continues distally over the Kocher interval between the anconeus and extensor carpi ulnaris about 6 cm distal to the tip of the olecranon.
- Proximally, the triceps is identified and freed from the brachioradialis and extensor carpi radialis longus along the intramuscular septum to the level of the joint capsule.
- The interval between the extensor carpi ulnaris and the anconeus is identified distally.
- The triceps in continuity with the anconeus is subperiosteally reflected. Sharp dissection frees the bony attachment of the triceps expansion to the anconeus from the lateral epicondyle.
- The triceps remains attached to the tip of the olecranon.
- The lateral collateral ligament complex is released from the humerus.
- The joint may be dislocated with varus stress. If additional exposure is necessary, the anterior and posterior capsule can be released.
- Routine closure of layers is performed, but the radial collateral ligament should be reattached to the bone through holes placed in the lateral epicondyle.

Mayo Modified Extensile Kocher Approach

- The extensile Kocher approach and the Mayo modification of the extensile Kocher approach provide sequentially greater exposure from the initial Kocher approach.

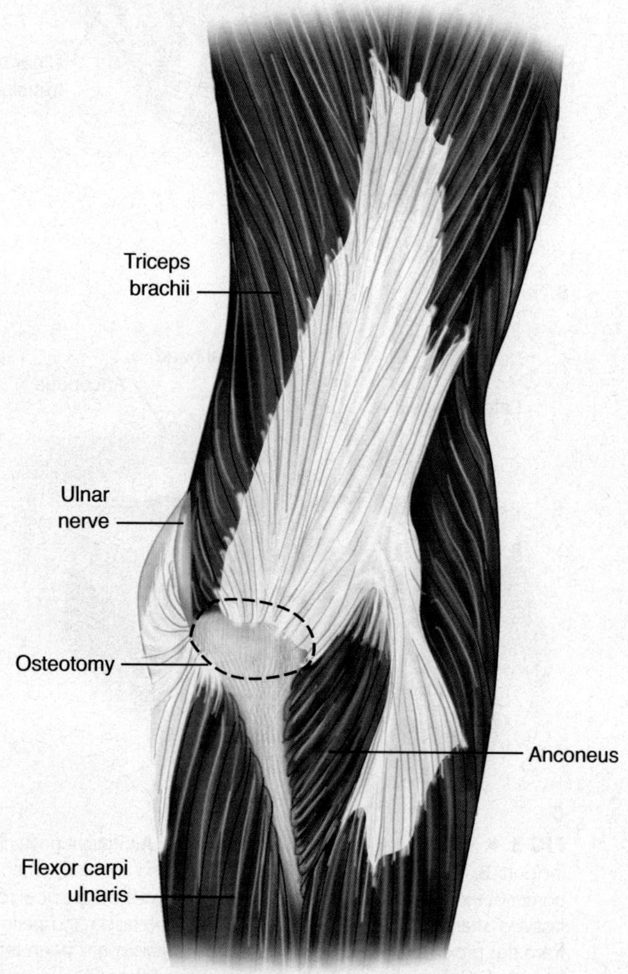

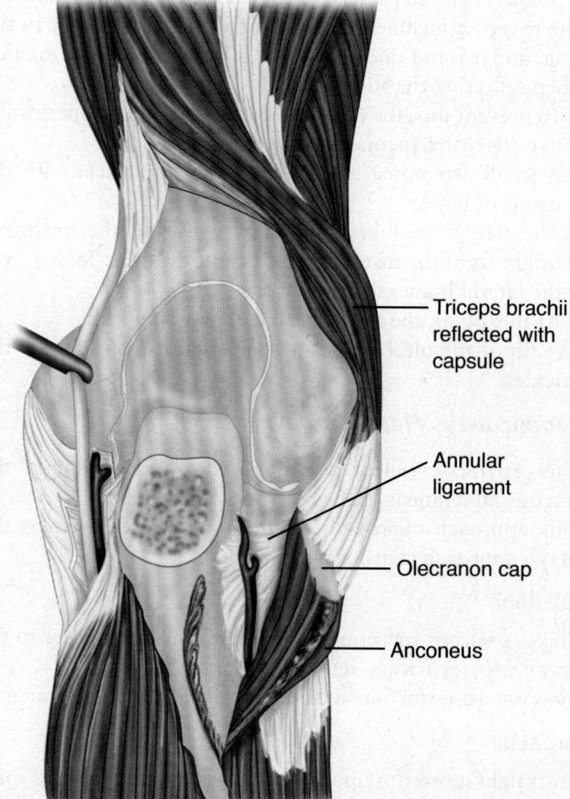

FIG 4 • Posterior view of the right elbow demonstrates a straight fascial incision to the lateral aspect of the tip of the olecranon. **A.** The line of release after the ulnar nerve has been identified and protected. **B.** The olecranon has been osteotomized and the triceps swept from medial to lateral in continuity with the anconeus and forearm fascia. *(continued)*

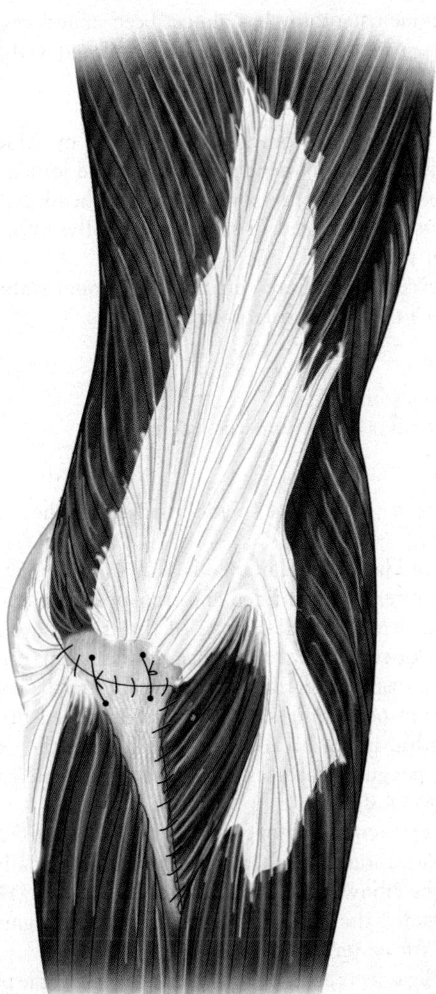

FIG 4 • *(continued)* **C.** Closure with sutures placed through bone and the distal extensor mechanism is done with interrupted sutures.

Indications

- Release of ankylosed joint
- Interposition arthroplasty
- Replacement arthroplasty

Approach

- A modification of the extensile Kocher approach consists of reflecting the anconeus and triceps expansion from the tip of the olecranon by sharp dissection.
- The extensor mechanism (triceps in continuity with the anconeus) may be reflected from lateral to medial.
- The ulnar nerve should be decompressed or transposed if an extensile lateral approach is used.
- The triceps is reattached in a fashion identical to that described for the Mayo approach.

Triceps-Preserving Approaches

Posterior Triceps-Sparing Approach

- Because the triceps is not elevated from the tip of the olecranon, rapid rehabilitation is possible.

Indications

- Tumor resection
- Joint reconstruction for resection of humeral nonunion
- Joint replacement

Approach

- A posterior incision is made medial to the tip of the olecranon.
- Medial and lateral subcutaneous skin flaps are elevated.
- The ulnar nerve is identified and transposed anteriorly.
- The medial and lateral aspects of the triceps are identified and developed distally to the triceps attachment on the ulna (**FIG 5**).
- For distal humerus fractures fixation
  - The common flexors and common extensors are partially released from the distal humerus to expose the supracondylar column for plate fixation.
- For total elbow arthroplasty or tumor resection
  - The common flexors and extensors are fully released from the medial and lateral epicondyle. The collateral ligaments and capsule are released and the distal humerus is excised.
  - The distal humerus is exposed by bringing it through the defect along the lateral margin of the triceps (**FIG 6**).
  - The ulna is exposed by supinating the forearm.
  - After the implant has been inserted, the joint is articulated.
- There is no need to close or repair the extensor mechanism with this approach.

Olecranon Osteotomy

- Worldwide, the transosseous approach is probably the exposure most often used, especially for distal humeral fractures.

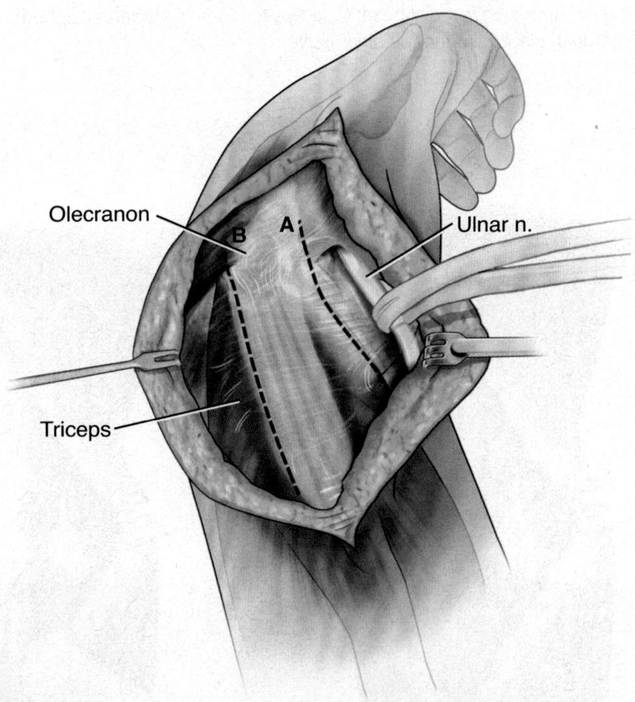

FIG 5 • Posterior triceps-sparing approach. (*A*) Medial window begins distally between the olecranon and flexor carpi ulnaris and proceeds proximally between the triceps and the intramuscular septum. The ulnar nerve should be transposed anteriorly. (*B*) Lateral window begins distally between the olecranon and the anconeus and proceeds proximally, splitting the lateral head of the triceps.

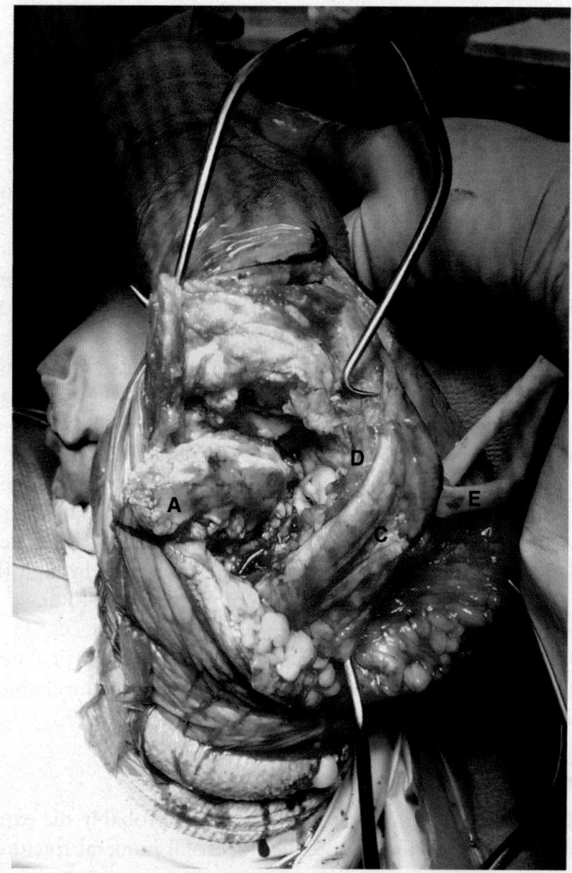

FIG 6 • Exposure of the distal humerus through the lateral window. *A*, distal humerus; *B*, radial head; *C*, triceps tendon; *D*, olecranon; *E*, penrose drain placed around the ulnar nerve.

The oblique osteotomy has almost been abandoned, and the transverse osteotomy has largely been replaced by the chevron.

Chevron Transolecranon Osteotomy

- Intra-articular osteotomy, first described by MacAusland, was originally recommended for ankylosed joints.
- It has been adapted by some for radial head excision and synovectomy and used or modified by others for T and Y condylar fractures.
- The chevron osteotomy enhances rotational stability compared to a transverse osteotomy.

Indications

- Ankylosed joints
- Intra-articular distal humerus fractures

Approach

- A posterior incision is made medial to the tip of the olecranon.
- Medial and lateral subcutaneous skin flaps are elevated.
- The ulnar nerve is identified and transposed anteriorly.
- The medial and lateral aspects of the triceps are identified and developed distally to the triceps attachment on the ulna.
- An apex-distal chevron or V osteotomy is performed with a thin oscillating saw but not completed through the subchondral bone. An osteotome completes the osteotomy, creating irregular surfaces that interdigitate increasing stability (**FIG 7A,B**).
- The triceps tendon, along with the osteotomized portion of the olecranon, may then be retracted proximally, and by flexing the elbow joint, the joint can be exposed (**FIG 7C**).
- Occasionally, the medial or lateral collateral ligaments are released for better exposure.
  - These ligaments are then repaired at the end of the procedure.
- At the completion of the procedure, the tip of the olecranon is secured via tension band, screw, or plate fixation.

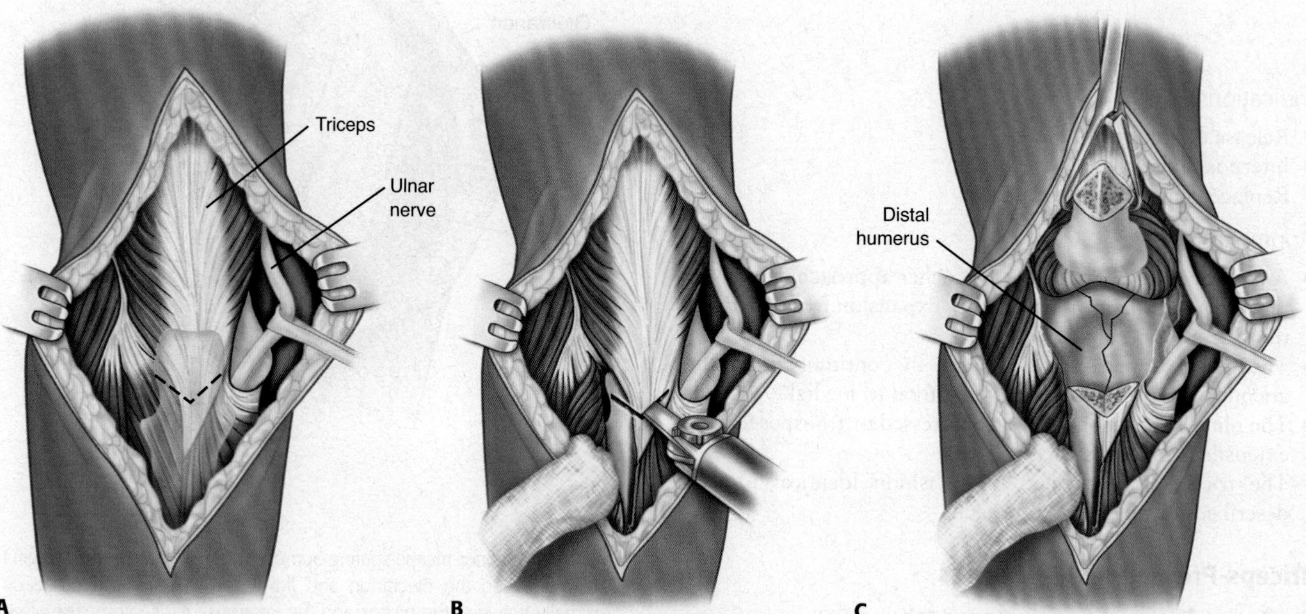

FIG 7 • Olecranon osteotomy. **A.** The triceps is released medially and laterally, whereas the ulnar nerve is protected. **B.** A chevron osteotomy with a distal apex is initiated with an oscillating saw. **C.** The proximal portion containing the olecranon osteotomy and triceps tendon is retracted proximally, exposing the elbow joint.

PEARLS AND PITFALLS

Ulnar nerve	■ The ulnar nerve must be identified and protected whenever performing a posterior approach to the elbow.
Radial nerve	■ The radial nerve is in danger when proximal exposure exceeds 10 cm from the lateral epicondyle.
Triceps insufficiency	■ Triceps insufficiency typically occurs due to fixation failure (tendon or osteotomy). Performing a triceps-sparing approach is the best method of preventing this complication.

LATERAL APPROACH TO THE ELBOW

- Lateral exposures to the elbow are widely used to treat a variety of elbow pathologies. The exposures differ according to the deep interval used.
- With any of the lateral exposures to the joint or to the proximal radius, the surgeon must be constantly aware of the possibility of injury to the posterior interosseous or recurrent branch of the radial nerve.

Anterolateral Approach to the Elbow (Kaplan)

Indications

- Anterior capsular release
- Posterior interosseous nerve exposure
- Capitellar/lateral column fractures

Approach

- Deep interval for the anterolateral approach lies between the extensor digitorum communis and the extensor carpi radialis longus muscles. (Intermuscular interval is best found by observing where vessels penetrate the fascia along the anterior margin of the extensor digitorum communis aponeurosis.)
- Fascia is split longitudinally between the extensor digitorum communis and the extensor carpi radialis longus. (As the dissection is carried deep through the extensor carpi radialis longus, the extensor carpi radialis brevis is encountered.)
- Deep to the extensor carpi radialis brevis, the transversely oriented fibers of the supinator are encountered, along with the posterior interosseous nerve. The posterior interosseous nerve defines the distal extent of the exposure. Pronation moves the radial nerve away from the surgical field.
  - If required, proximal dissection with elevation of the extensor carpi radialis longus, extensor carpi radialis brevis, and brachioradialis anteriorly from the lateral supracondylar ridge of the humerus provides exposure of the anterior joint capsule.

Modified Distal Kocher Approach

Indications

- Reconstruction of the lateral ulnar collateral ligament

Approach

- The skin incision begins just proximal to the lateral epicondyle of the humerus and extends obliquely for about 6 cm in line with the fascia of the anconeus and extensor carpi ulnaris muscles (**FIG 8A**).
- The Kocher interval between the anconeus and extensor carpi ulnaris is incised (**FIG 8B**).
- Development of the Kocher interval reveals the lateral joint capsule.
- The anconeus is then reflected posteriorly off the joint capsule distally to expose the crista supinatoris.
- The extensor carpi ulnaris and the common extensor tendon are released from the lateral epicondyle and reflected anteriorly, exposing the lateral capsule. The radial nerve is at a safe distance from the dissection, and it is protected by the extensor carpi ulnaris and extensor digitorum communis muscle mass (**FIG 8C**).
- A longitudinal incision is made through the capsules to expose the radiocapitellar joint.

Boyd (Posterolateral) Approach

- Radioulnar synostosis may occur as the proximal radius and ulna are exposed subperiosteally.

Indications

- Monteggia fracture-dislocations
- Radial head fractures
- Resection of radioulnar synostosis

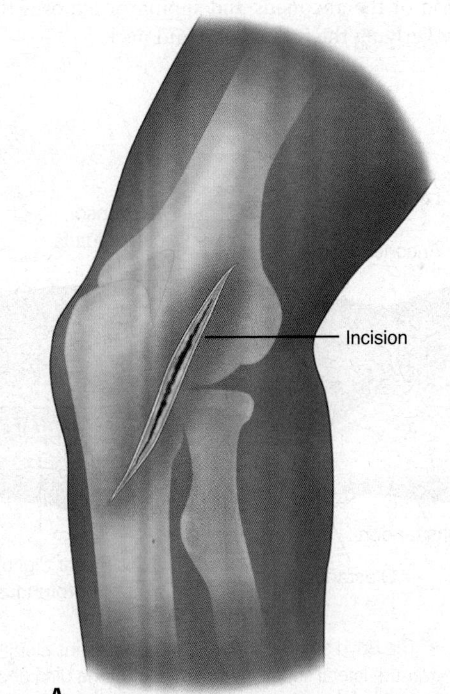

FIG 8 ● Distal Kocher approach. **A.** The incision begins about 2 to 3 cm above the lateral epicondyle over the supracondylar ridge and extends distally and posteriorly for about 4 cm. *(continued)*

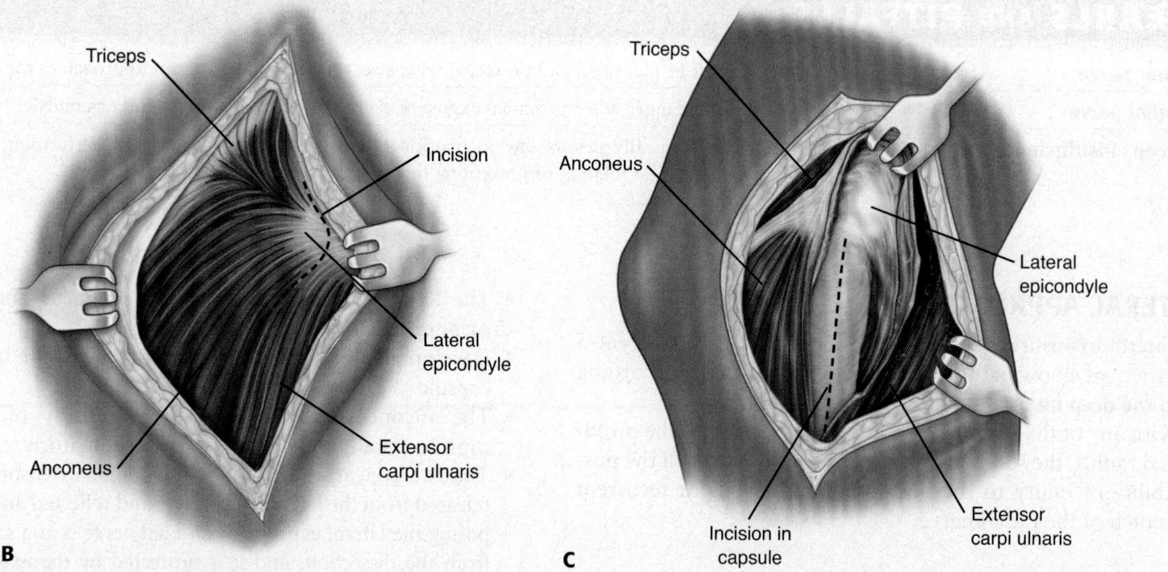

FIG 8 • *(continued)* **B.** The interval between the anconeus and the extensor carpi ulnaris is identified. **C.** Development of this interval reveals the capsule.

Approach

- The incision begins just posterior to the lateral epicondyle lateral to the triceps tendon and continues distally to the lateral tip of the olecranon and then down to the subcutaneous border of the ulna.
- The anconeus and supinator are subperiosteally elevated from the subcutaneous border of the ulna (anconeus and supinator) (**FIG 9A,B**).
- Retraction of the anconeus and supinator exposes the joint capsule overlying the radial head and neck.
- The supinator muscle protects the posterior interosseous nerve.
- This lateral capsule contains the lateral ulnar collateral ligament, and its division can lead to posterolateral rotatory instability.
- To expose the radial shaft, the incision may be continued along the subcutaneous ulnar border, elevating the muscles off the lateral aspect of the ulna (extensor carpi ulnaris, abductor pollicis longus, and extensor pollicis longus).
- The posterior interosseous and recurrent interosseous arteries may need ligation.

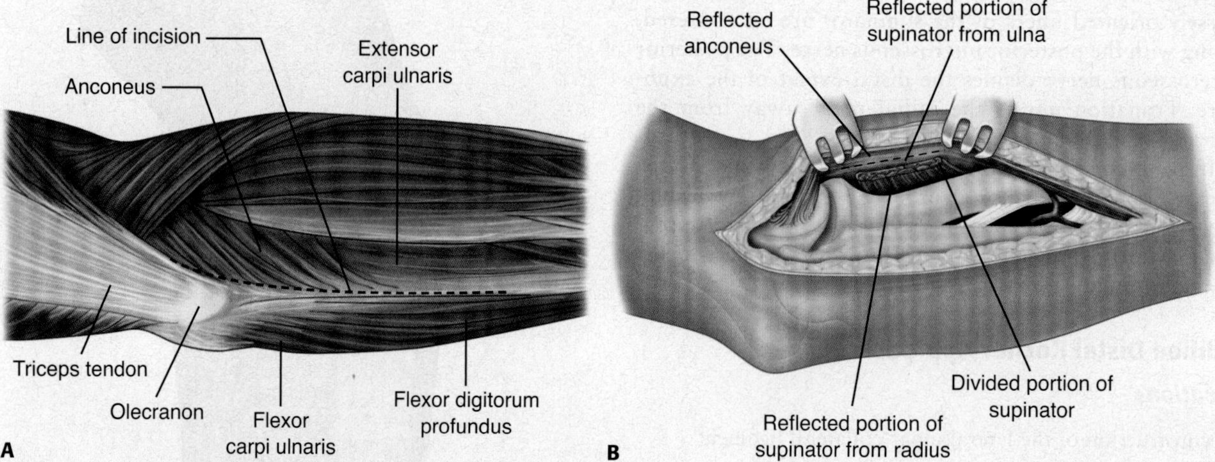

FIG 9 • The Boyd approach. **A.** The incision begins along the lateral border of the triceps about 2 to 3 cm above the epicondyle and extends distally over the lateral subcutaneous border of the ulna about 6 to 8 cm past the tip of the olecranon. The ulnar insertion of the anconeus and the origin of the supinator muscle are elevated subperiosteally. More distally, the subperiosteal reflection includes the abductor pollicis longus, the extensor carpi ulnaris, and the extensor pollicis longus muscles. The origin of the supinator at the crista supinatoris of the ulna is released, and the entire muscle flap is retracted radially, exposing the radiohumeral joint. **B.** The posterior interosseous nerve is protected in the substance of the supinator.

PEARLS AND PITFALLS

Posterior interosseous nerve	▪ The posterior interosseous nerve prevents distal extension of the lateral exposure. Pronation of the forearm can help protect the nerve. It is at most risk with the Kaplan approach.
Lateral ulnar collateral ligament	▪ Incision through the lateral capsule can disrupt the lateral ulnar collateral ligament and lead to posterior lateral rotatory instability.

MEDIAL APPROACH TO THE ELBOW

- There are relatively few indications for medial exposure of the elbow joint. This has been superseded by arthroscopic approaches.
- The most valuable contribution to medial joint exposure is that described by Hotchkiss. This extensile exposure provides greater flexibility, particularly for exposure of the coronoid and for contracture release.

Extensile Medial Over-the-Top Approach

- Excellent visualization of the anteromedial and posteromedial elbow
- Not a sufficient approach for excision of heterotopic bone on the lateral side of the joint
- Does not provide adequate access to the radial head

Indications

- Coronoid fractures
- Contracture release (when ulnar nerve exploration required)
- Anterior and posterior access to the joint
- May be converted to a triceps-reflecting exposure of Bryan-Morrey

Approach

- Superficial dissection
  - Skin incision can vary between the boundaries of a pure posterior skin incision and midline medial incision (**FIG 10A**).
  - Subcutaneous skin is elevated.
  - The medial supracondylar ridge of the humerus, the medial intramuscular septum, the origin of the flexor pronator mass, and the ulnar nerve are identified.

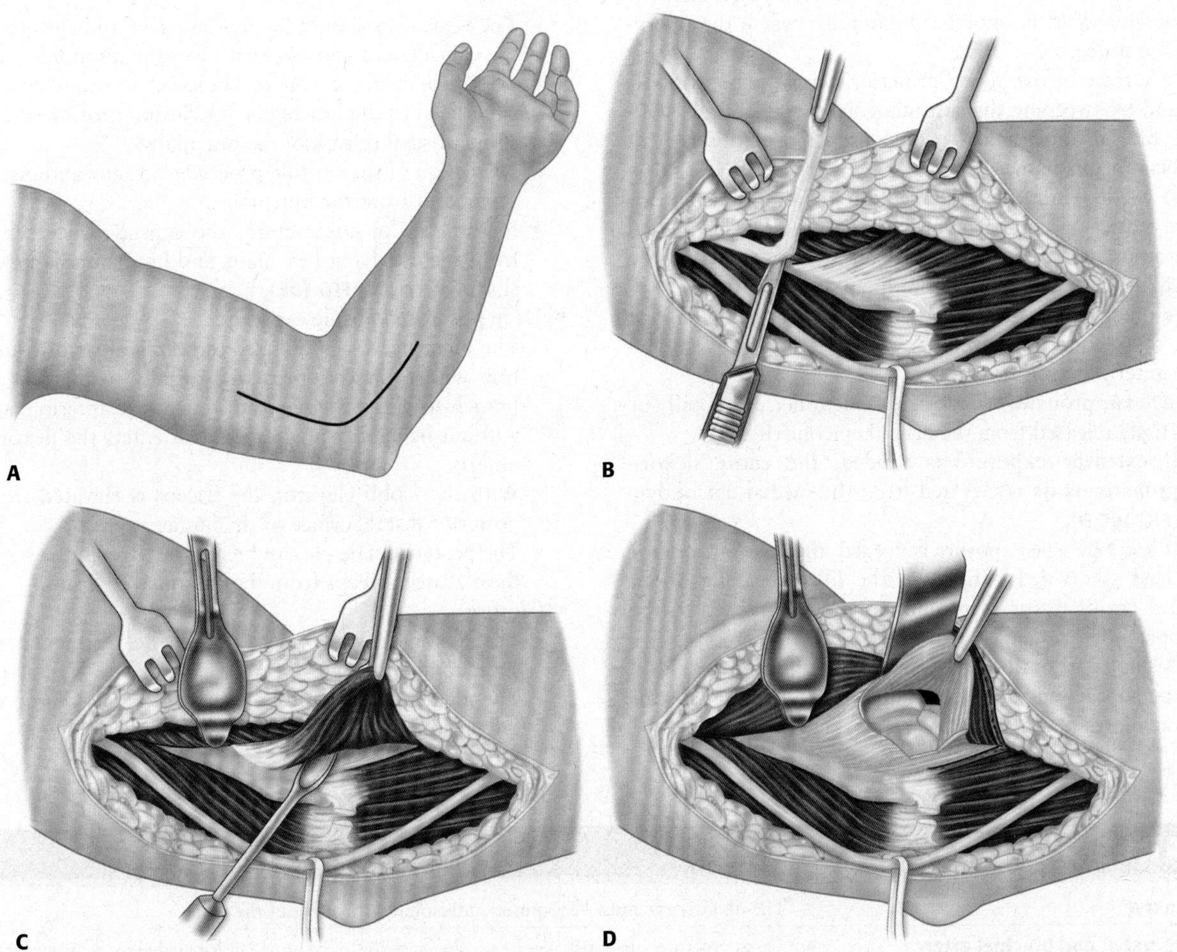

FIG 10 ● **A.** Medial skin incision along the midline. **B.** The medial intermuscular septum (*light blue*) is excised from the medial epicondyle to 5 cm proximal to it. The ulnar nerve is shown tagged with a suture loop. **C,D.** If the extensile exposure is needed, the entire flexor pronator muscle mass is elevated from the medial epicondyle. *(continued)*

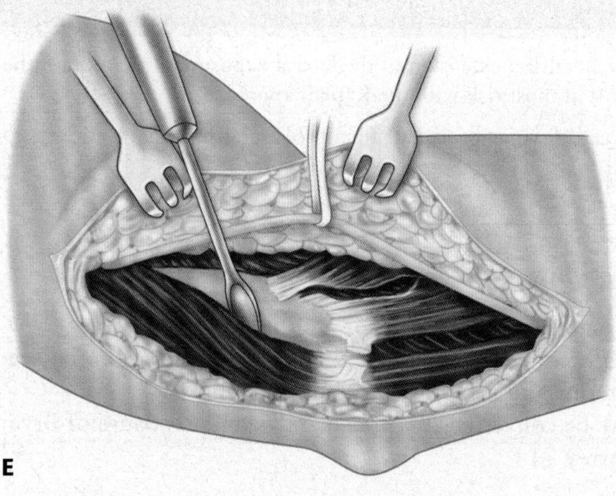

E

FIG 10 • *(continued)* **E.** The capsule can be sharply excised in cases of capsular contracture.

- Anterior to the septum, running just on top of the fascia (not in the subdermal tissue), the medial antebrachial cutaneous nerve is identified and protected.
- The ulnar nerve is identified. If the patient previously had surgery, the ulnar nerve should be identified proximally before the surgeon proceeds distally.
  - If anterior transposition was performed previously, the nerve should be mobilized carefully before the operation proceeds.
- The surface of the flexor–pronator muscle mass origin is found by sweeping the subcutaneous tissue laterally with the medial antebrachial cutaneous nerve in this flap of subcutaneous tissue.
- The medial intramuscular septum divides the anterior and posterior compartments of the elbow. The medial intramuscular septum is ultimately excised from the medial epicondyle to 5 cm proximal to it (**FIG 10B**).
- The ulnar nerve is protected, and the veins at the base of the septum are cauterized.

- Deep anterior exposure
  - The flexor pronator mass origin is identified and totally or partially released from the medial epicondyle.
    - If extensile exposure is needed, the entire flexor–pronator mass is elevated from the medial epicondyle (**FIG 10C,D**).
    - If less extensile exposure is needed, the flexor–pronator mass is divided parallel to the fibers, leaving about 1.5 cm of flexor carpi ulnaris tendon attached to the epicondyle.
    - A small cuff of fibrous tissue of the origin can be left on the supracondylar ridge as the muscle is elevated; this facilitates reattachment when closing.
  - The flexor–pronator origin should be dissected down to the level of bone but superficial to the joint capsule. As this plane is developed, the brachialis muscle is encountered from the underside.
  - The brachialis muscle is identified along the supracondylar ridge and released in continuity with the flexor–pronator mass.
  - These muscles should be kept anterior and elevated from the capsule and anterior surface of the distal humerus.
  - The median nerve and the brachial vein and artery are superficial to the brachialis muscle and protected with the subperiosteal release of the brachialis.
  - Dissection of the capsule proceeds laterally and distally to separate it from the brachialis.
  - In the case of contracture, the capsule, once separated from the overlying brachialis and brachioradialis, can be sharply excised (**FIG 10E**).
- Deep posterior capsule exposure
  - The ulnar nerve is mobilized to permit anterior transposition with a dissection carried distally to the first motor branch to allow the nerve to rest in the anterior position without being sharply angled as it enters the flexor carpi ulnaris.
  - With the Cobb elevator, the triceps is elevated from the posterior distal surface of the humerus.
  - The posterior capsule can be separated from the triceps as the elevator sweeps from the proximal to distal.
- Closure
  - The flexor–pronator mass should be reattached to the supracondylar ridge.
  - The ulnar nerve should be transposed and secured with a fascial sling to prevent posterior subluxation.

PEARLS AND PITFALLS

Ulnar nerve	■ The ulnar nerve must be exposed and isolated throughout the case.
Median nerve and brachial artery	■ These structures are at risk when exposing anterior to the brachialis or medial to the pronator teres.
Medial antebrachial cutaneous nerve	■ This nerve should be identified just superficial to the fascia and protected to prevent injury and possible neuroma formation.

ANTERIOR APPROACH TO THE ELBOW

- Because of the vulnerability of the brachial artery and median nerve, the anteromedial approach to the elbow is not recommended.
- The extensile exposure described by Henry, and modified by Fiolle and Delmas, is best known and is the most useful for anterior exposure of the joint. Minor modifications of the Henry approach have been described, and a limited anterolateral exposure has been described by Darrach.

Modified Anterior Henry Approach

Indications

- Anteriorly displaced fracture fragments
- Excision of tumors in this region
- Reattachment of the biceps tendon to the radial tuberosity
- Exploration of nerve entrapment syndromes
- Anterior capsular release for contracture

Approach

- The skin incision begins about 5 cm proximal to the flexor crease of the elbow joint and extends distally along the anterior margin of the brachioradialis muscle to the flexion crease.
- At the elbow flexion crease, the incision turns medially to avoid crossing the flexor crease at a right angle. The incision continues transversely to the biceps tendon and then turns distally over the medial volar aspect of the forearm (**FIG 11A**).
- The fascia is released distally between the brachioradialis and pronator teres.
- The interval between the brachioradialis laterally and the biceps and brachialis medially is identified. This interval is entered proximally, and gentle, blunt dissection demonstrates the radial nerve coursing on the inner surface of the brachioradialis muscle (**FIG 11B**).
- Care is taken to avoid injury to the superficial sensory branch of the radial nerve.
  - Because the radial nerve gives off its branches laterally, it can safely be retracted with the brachioradialis muscle.
  - At the level of the elbow joint, as the brachioradialis is retracted laterally and the pronator teres is gently retracted medially, the radial artery can be observed where it emerges from the medial aspect of the biceps tendon, giving off its muscular and recurrent branches in a mediolateral direction.
- The muscle branch is ligated, but the recurrent radial artery should be sacrificed only if the lesion warrants an extensive exposure.
- The posterior interosseous nerve enters the supinator and continues along the dorsum of the forearm distally.
- Dissection continues distally, exposing the supinator muscle, which covers the proximal aspect of the radius and the anterolateral aspect of the capsule (**FIG 11C**).

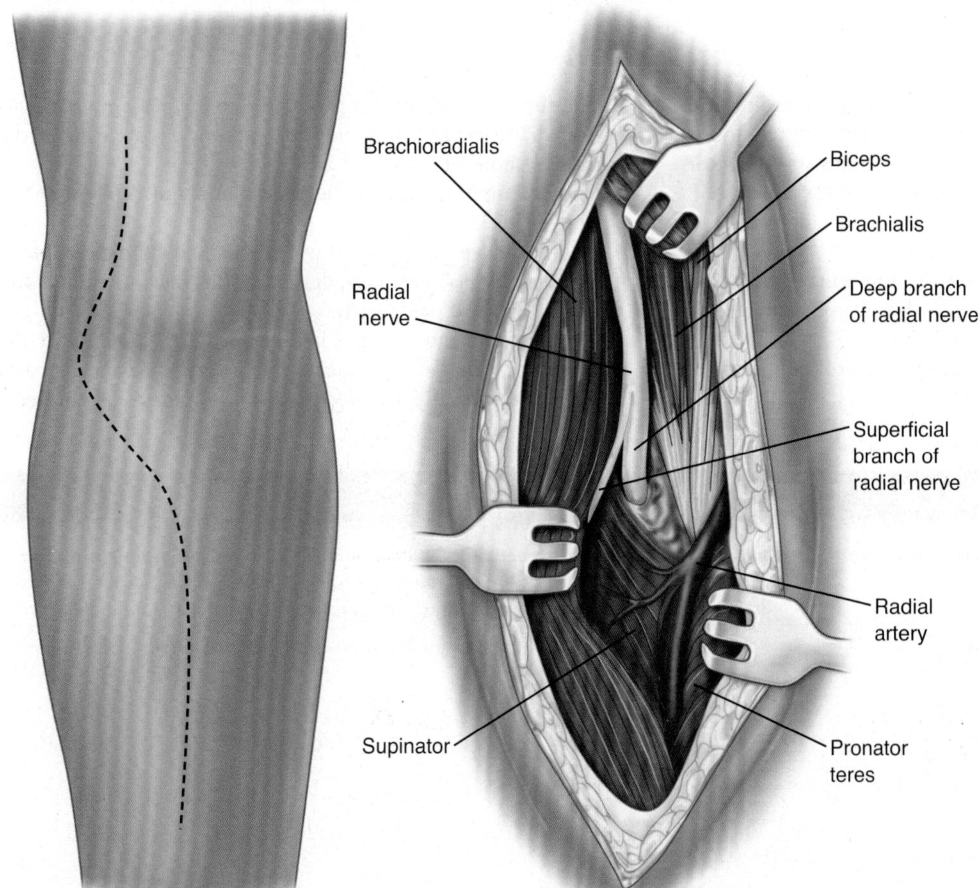

FIG 11 • The anterior Henry approach. **A.** An incision is made about 5 cm proximal to the elbow crease on the lateral margin of the biceps tendon. It extends transversely across the joint line and curves distally over the medial aspect of the forearm. The interval between the brachioradialis and brachialis proximally and the biceps tendon and pronator teres in the distal portion of the wound is identified. The radial nerve is protected and retracted along with the brachialis. **B.** The supinator muscle is released from the anterior aspect of the radius, which is fully supinated. *(continued)*

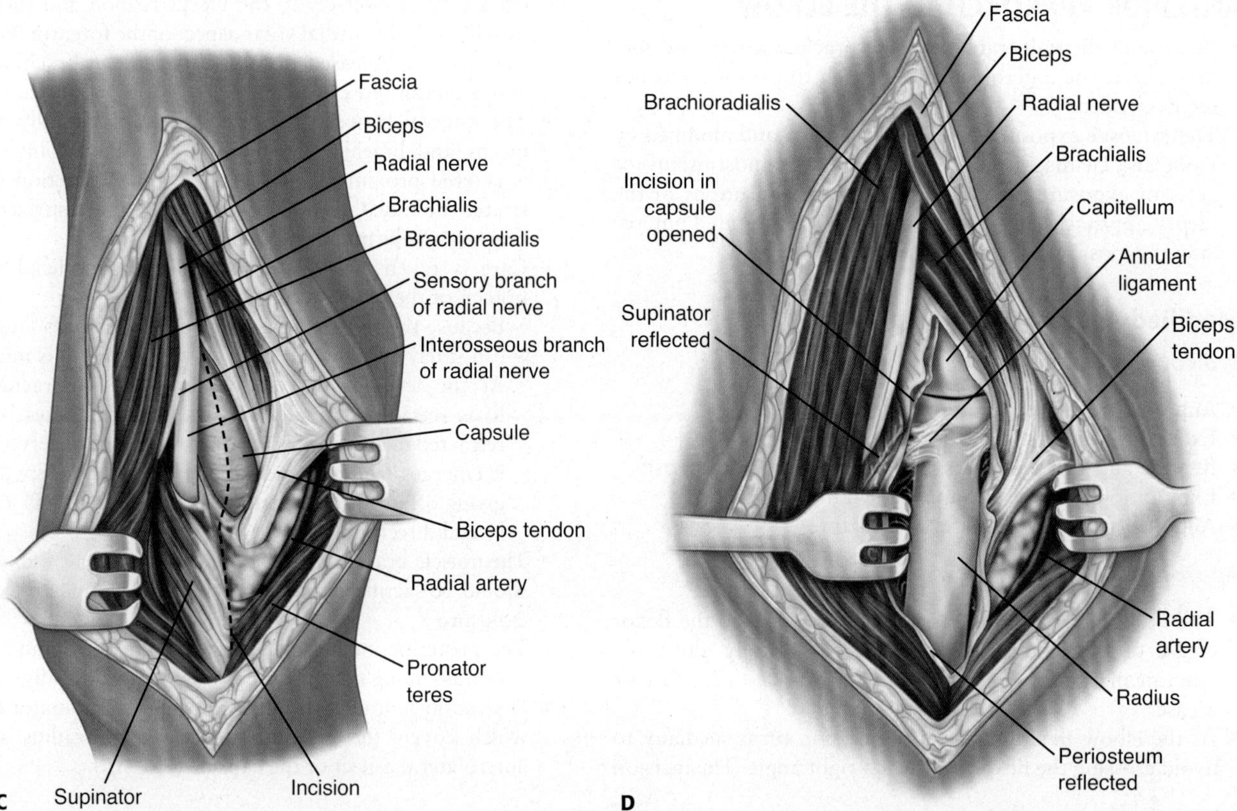

FIG 11 • *(continued)* **C.** The radial recurrent branches of the radial artery and its muscular branches are identified and sacrificed if more extensive exposure is required. The biceps tendon is retracted medially along with the brachialis muscle. **D.** This interval may now be developed to expose the anterior aspect of the elbow joint.

- Muscle attachments to the anterior aspect of the radius and those distal to the supinator include the discrete tendinous insertion of the pronator teres and the origins of the flexor digitorum sublimis and the flexor pollicis longus.
- The brachialis muscle is identified, elevated, and retracted medially to expose the proximal capsule.
- If more distal exposure is needed, the forearm is fully supinated, demonstrating the insertion of the supinator muscle along the proximal radius.
  - This insertion is incised, and the supinator is subperiosteally retracted laterally (**FIG 11D**).
- The supinator serves as a protection to the deep interosseous branch of the radial nerve, but excessive retraction of the muscle should be avoided.
- The proximal aspect of the radius and the capitellum are thus exposed.
- Additional visualization may be obtained both proximally and distally because the radial nerve has been identified and can be avoided proximally.
- The posterior interosseous nerve is protected distally by the supinator muscle, and the radial artery is visualized and protected medially if a more extensile exposure is required.

PEARLS AND PITFALLS

Radial nerve and posterior interosseous nerve	■ The radial nerve runs beneath the brachioradialis, and the posterior interosseous nerve branches off just distal to the radial head and courses laterally around the radial neck. Excessive retraction or improper retractor placement may injure the nerve.
Radial recurrent artery	■ Radial recurrent artery should be ligated if distal exposure is required.

Arthroscopy of the Wrist: Preparation and Techniques

3

CHAPTER

David J. Slutsky

BACKGROUND

- Since its inception, wrist arthroscopy has continued to evolve. The initial emphasis on viewing the wrist from the dorsal aspect arose from the relative lack of neurovascular structures as well as the familiarity of most surgeons with dorsal approaches to the radiocarpal joint.
- Anatomic studies provided a better understanding of both the interosseous ligaments as well as carpal kinematics, which led to the development of midcarpal arthroscopy.
- Innovative surgeons continue to push the envelope through the development of techniques for treating intracarpal pathology, which in turn has culminated in a plethora of new accessory portals.

ANATOMY

- The standard portals for wrist arthroscopy are dorsal (**FIG 1A–C**). This is in part due to the relative lack of neurovascular structures on the dorsum of the wrist as well as the initial emphasis on assessing the volar wrist ligaments. The dorsal portals that allow access to the radiocarpal joint are so named in relation to the tendons of the dorsal extensor compartments.
  - The 1-2 portal lies between the first extensor compartment tendons, which include the extensor pollicis brevis and the abductor pollicis longus, and the second extensor compartment, which contains the extensor carpi radialis brevis (ECRB) and extensor carpi radialis longus (ECRL) (**FIG 1D**).
  - The 3-4 portal is named for the interval between the third dorsal extensor compartment, which contains the extensor pollicis longus tendon, and the fourth extensor compartment, which contains the extensor digitorum communis (EDC) tendons.
  - The 4-5 portal is located between the EDC and the extensor digiti minimi (EDM).
  - The 6R portal is located on the radial side of the extensor carpi ulnaris (ECU) tendon; the 6U portal is located on the ulnar side.
- The midcarpal joint is assessed through two portals, which allows triangulation of the arthroscope and the instrumentation.
  - The midcarpal radial portal is located 1 cm distal to the 3-4 portal and is bounded radially by the ECRB and ulnarly by the EDC.
  - The midcarpal ulnar portal is similarly located 1 to 2 cm distal to the 4-5 portal and is bounded by the EDC and the EDM.
- The triquetrohamate portal enters the midcarpal joint at the level of the triquetrohamate joint ulnar to the ECU tendon. The entry site is both ulnar and distal to the midcarpal ulnar

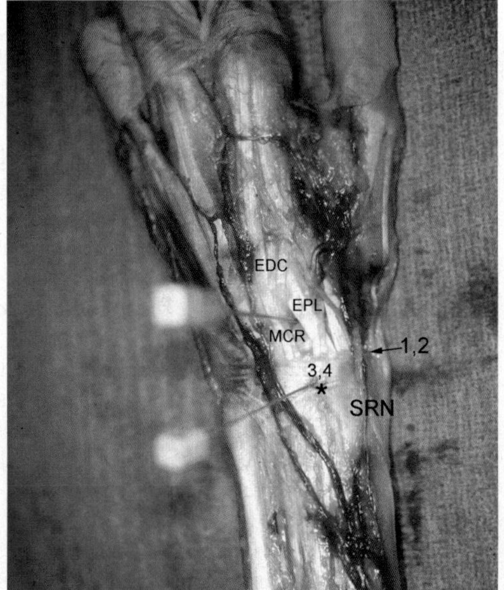

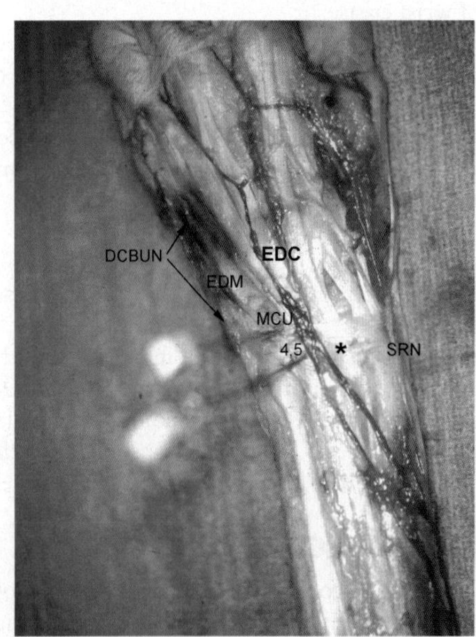

FIG 1 • Dorsal portal anatomy. **A.** Cadaver dissection of the dorsal aspect of a left wrist demonstrating the relative positions of the dorsoradial portals. *EDC*, extensor digitorum communis; *EPL*, extensor pollicis longus; *MCR*, midcarpal radial; *SRN*, superficial radial nerve; *asterisk*, tubercle of Lister. **B.** Relative positions of the dorsoulnar portals. *EDM*, extensor digiti minimi; *DCBUN*, dorsal cutaneous branch of the ulnar nerve. *(continued)*

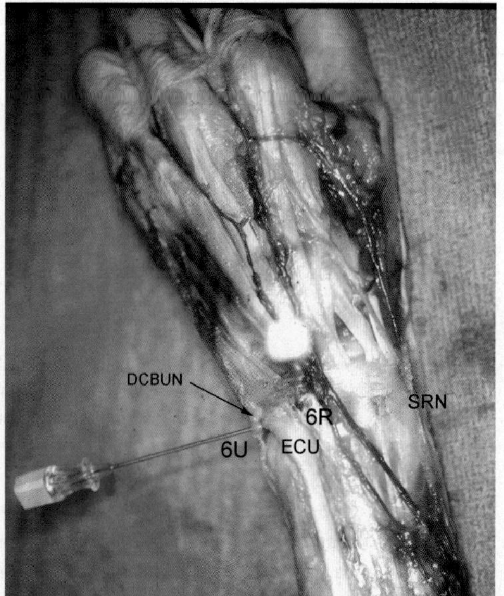

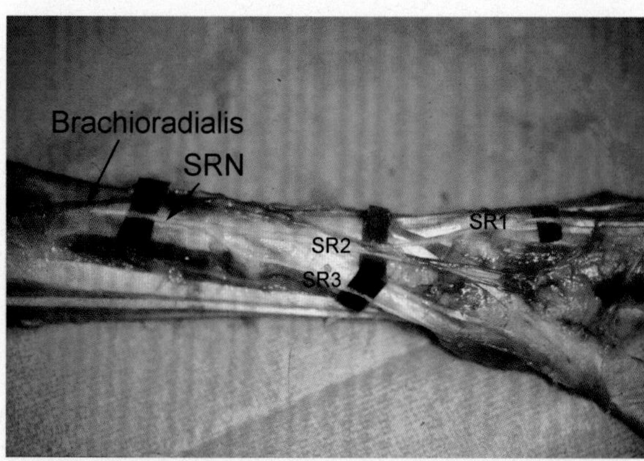

FIG 1 • *(continued)* **C.** Positions of the 6R and 6U portals. *ECU*, extensor carpi ulnaris. **D.** Branches of the superficial radial nerve (SRN). *SR1*, minor dorsal branch; *SR2*, major dorsal branch; *SR3*, major palmar branch. (From Slutsky DJ. Wrist arthroscopy portals. In: Slutsky DJ, Nagle DJ, eds. Techniques in Hand and Wrist Arthroscopy. Philadelphia: Elsevier, 2007.)

portal. Branches of the dorsal cutaneous branch of the ulnar nerve are most at risk (**FIG 2A**).

- The dorsal radioulnar joint portal lies between the ECU and the EDM tendons. Transverse branches of the dorsal cutaneous branch of the ulnar nerve are the only sensory nerves in proximity to the dorsal radioulnar portal at a mean of 17.5 mm distally (range 10 to 20 mm) (**FIG 2B,C**).
- There are two volar portals that can be used to access the radiocarpal joint.
  - The volar radial portal is accessed through the floor of the flexor carpi radialis (FCR) tendon sheath at the level of the proximal wrist crease.[4,7,9]
    - Anatomic studies revealed that there is a safe zone free of any neurovascular structures equal to the width of the FCR tendon plus at least 3 mm in all directions.
    - The volar aspect of the midcarpal joint can be accessed through the volar radial midcarpal portal. The same skin incision is used but the capsular entry point is about 1 cm distal.
  - The volar ulnar portal is located underneath the ulnar border of the flexor tendons at the level of the proximal wrist crease.[6]
- The volar aspect of the distal radioulnar joint (DRUJ) can be accessed through the volar distal radioulnar portal using the same skin incision, but the capsular entry point for the volar distal radioulnar portal lies 5 mm to 1 cm proximal to the ulnocarpal entry point (**FIG 2D,E**).

NONOPERATIVE MANAGEMENT

- In general, wrist arthroscopy is indicated as a diagnostic technique in any patient with persistent wrist pain that has not responded to an appropriate trial of conservative measures:
  - Nonsteroidal anti-inflammatories and activity modification
  - Cortisone injection
- Wrist arthroscopy is used as an adjuvant procedure for the treatment of acute fractures of the distal radius or scaphoid or for staging degenerative disorders involving the carpus.

Indications

- The indications for the use of the standard dorsal portals are intertwined with the indications for wrist arthroscopy and depend largely on the condition that is being treated.
  - A typical arthroscopic examination of the wrist will include variable combinations of the 3-4 portal, the 4-5 portal, and the 6R and 6U portals.
  - The 3-4 and 4-5 portals are the main viewing portals for the radial aspect of the radiocarpal joint and for instrumentation.
  - The 4-5 and 6R portals are used to access the ulnocarpal joint.
  - The 6U portal is typically used for outflow.
- The volar radial portal is indicated for the evaluation of the dorsal radiocarpal ligament (DRCL) and the palmar portion of the scapholunate interosseous ligament (SLIL). The volar radial portal also facilitates arthroscopic reduction of intra-articular fractures of the distal radius fractures by providing a clear view of the dorsal rim fragments.
- The volar ulnar portal is indicated for visualizing and débriding palmar tears of the lunotriquetral ligament. It also aids in the repair or débridement of dorsally located triangular fibrocartilage (TFC) tears because the proximity of the 4-5 and 6R portals makes triangulation of the instruments difficult.
- Midcarpal arthroscopy through the dorsal midcarpal portals is essential in making the diagnoses of scapholunate and lunotriquetral instability.
  - The grading scale reported by Geissler and colleagues[2] provides a means for staging the degree of instability and provides an algorithm for treatment.

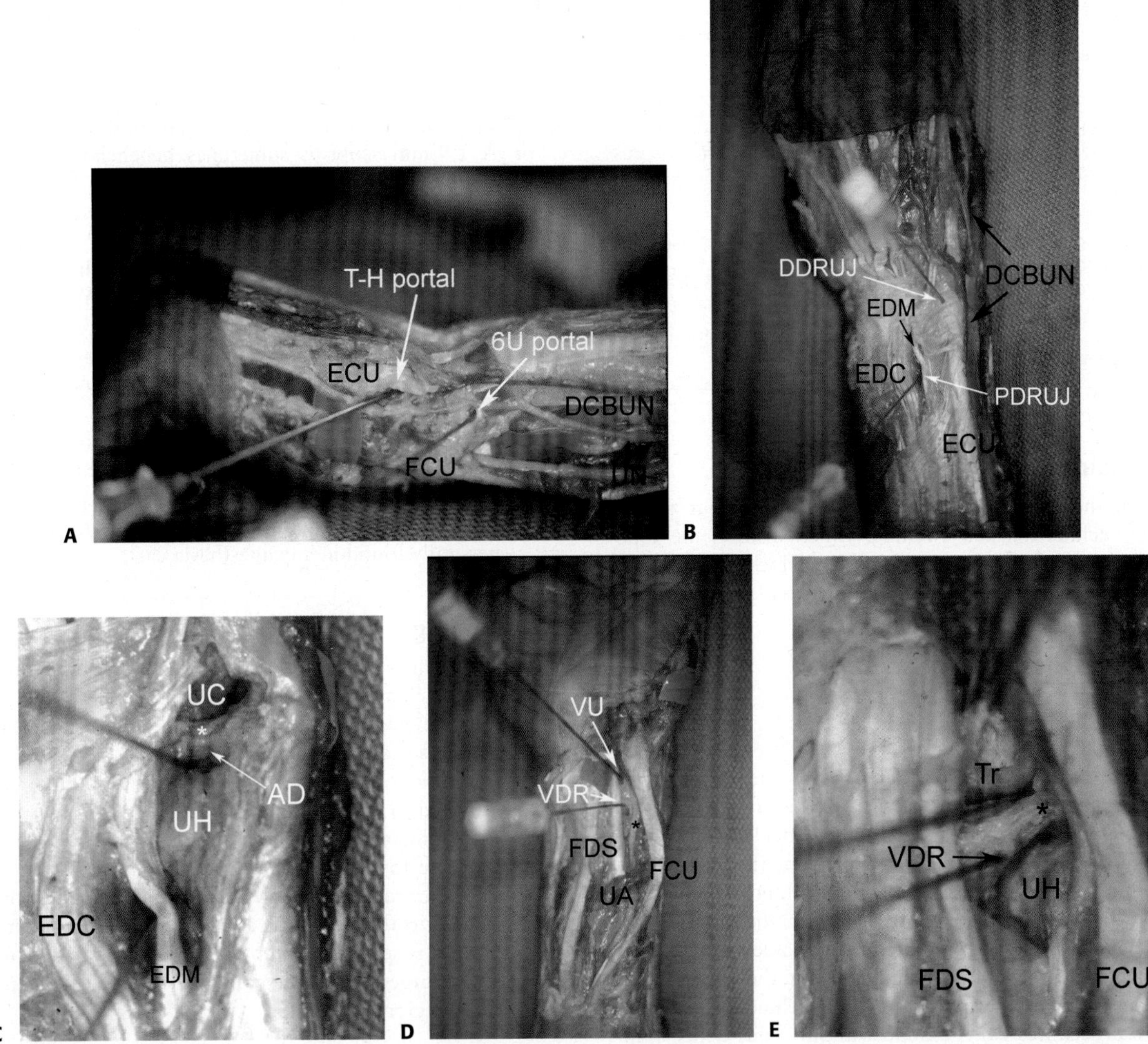

FIG 2 • **A.** Ulnar aspect of a left wrist demonstrating the relative positions of the triquetrohamate (T-H) portal and the 6U portal. *ECU*, extensor carpi ulnaris; *FCU*, flexor carpi ulnaris; *DCBUN*, dorsal cutaneous branch of the ulnar nerve; *UN*, ulnar nerve. **B,C.** Dorsal DRUJ portal anatomy. **B.** Relative position of the proximal DRUJ (PDRUJ) and distal DRUJ (DDRUJ) portals. **C.** Close-up with the dorsal capsule removed demonstrating the position of the needles in relation to the dorsal radioulnar ligament (*asterisk*). *UC*, ulnocarpal joint; *AD*, articular disc; *UH*, ulnar head; *EDC*, extensor digitorum communis; *EDM*, extensor digiti minimi. **D,E.** Volar DRUJ portals. **D.** Volar aspect of a left wrist demonstrating the relative positions of the volar ulnar (*VU*) and volar DRUJ (*VDR*) portals in relation to the ulnar nerve (*asterisk*) and ulnar artery (*UA*). *FDS*, flexor digitorum sublimis; *FCU*, flexor carpi ulnaris. **E.** Close-up view after the volar capsule is removed showing position of needles in relation to the volar radioulnar ligament (*asterisk*). *Tr*, triquetrum. (From Slutsky DJ. Wrist arthroscopy portals. In: Slutsky DJ, Nagle DJ, eds. Techniques in Hand and Wrist Arthroscopy. Philadelphia: Elsevier, 2007.)

  - Midcarpal arthroscopy is likewise employed for the assessment and treatment of chondral lesions of the proximal hamate.
  - The triquetrohamate joint can also be accessed through another special-use midcarpal portal.[1]
- The volar radial midcarpal portal is occasionally used as an accessory portal for visualizing the palmar aspects of the capitate and hamate in cases of avascular necrosis or osteochondral injury.
  - This portal facilitates visualization of the palmar aspect of the capitohamate interosseous ligament, which is important in minimizing translational motion and has an essential role in providing stability to the transverse carpal arch.
- The volar DRUJ portal is useful for assessing the deep foveal attachment of the triangular fibrocartilage complex (TFCC), which would normally require an open capsulotomy.
  - It may be employed if the suspicion of a peripheral TFCC detachment remains despite the absence of any visible TFCC tears through the standard ulnocarpal portals.
- The dorsal DRUJ portal may be used in concert with the volar DRUJ portal to more completely assess the status of the articular cartilage of the ulnar head and sigmoid notch as well as for instrumentation.
- The number of conditions amenable to arthroscopic treatment continues to grow. Many arthroscopic procedures are now common, whereas others await clinical validation. Table 1 provides a list of the more standard procedures.

Table 1 Arthroscopic Wrist Procedures

Ganglion resection: volar and dorsal
Release of wrist contracture
Arthroscopic synovectomy
Staging of degenerative arthritis (scapholunate advanced collapse or scaphoid nonunion advanced collapse, Kienbock disease)
Radial styloidectomy
Proximal pole of hamate resection
Dorsal radiocarpal ligament repair
Evaluation and treatment of carpal instability: scapholunate, lunotriquetral, midcarpal
Triangular fibrocartilage tears: repair versus débridement
Arthroscopic wafer resection
Arthroscopic reduction and internal fixation of distal radius fractures
Arthroscopic-guided fixation of scaphoid fractures

Contraindications

- Contraindications to the use of dorsal or volar portals would include marked swelling, which distorts the topographic anatomy; large capsular tears, which might lead to extravasation of irrigation fluid; neurovascular compromise; bleeding disorders; or infection.
- Unfamiliarity with the regional anatomy is a relative contraindication.

SURGICAL MANAGEMENT

- It is useful to have a systematic approach to viewing the wrist.
- The structures that should be visualized as a part of a standard examination include the radius articular surface; the proximal scaphoid, lunate, and triquetrum; the SLIL and lunotriquetral interosseous ligament (LTIL), both palmar and dorsal; the radioscaphocapitate ligament; the long radiolunate ligament; the radioscapholunate ligament; the ulnolunate ligament; the ulnotriquetral ligament; the articular disc; and the radial and peripheral TFCC attachments.
- Many procedures can be done without fluid, which minimizes the amount of swelling and fluid extravasation. Intermittent irrigation with a 10-mL syringe attached to the inflow portal of the arthroscope followed by suction with the full radius resector can help clear the field.
- The volar radial portal is used in patients with radial-sided and dorsal wrist pain to visualize the palmar SLIL and the DRCL.
- In patients with ulnar-sided wrist pain, the volar ulnar portal is used to assess the palmar LTIL and dorsal radioulnar ligament, the region of the ECU subsheath, and the radial TFCC attachment.
  - The scope is then inserted in the 3-4 portal followed by various combinations of the 4-5 portal and 6R portal. The 6U portal is mostly used for outflow, but it may be used for instrumentation when débriding palmar LTIL tears.
- Midcarpal arthroscopy is then performed to probe the SLIL and LTIL joint spaces for instability, the capitohamate interosseous ligament, and to look for chondral lesions on the proximal capitate and hamate and loose bodies.
  - The special-use portals such as the dorsal and volar DRUJ portals and the 1-2 portal are used as needed.

Preoperative Planning

- A 2.7-mm, 30-degree angled scope along with a camera attachment is used.
  - Table 2 describes the typical field of view as seen through a 2.7-mm arthroscope under ideal conditions.[1,3]
  - A 1.9-mm scope is sometimes beneficial, especially for evaluation of the DRUJ.
- A 3-mm hook probe is needed for palpation of intracarpal structures.
- A motorized shaver or diathermy unit such as the Oratec probe (Smith & Nephew, New York, NY) is useful for débridement.
- Ancillary equipment is largely procedure dependent.
  - A motorized 2.9-mm and 3.5-mm burr is needed for bony resection.
  - There are a variety of commercially available suture repair kits, including the TFCC repair kit by Linvatec (ConMed Linvatec, Corp., Largo, FL). Ligament repairs can also be facilitated by use of a Tuohy needle, which is generally found in any anesthesia cart.

Positioning

- The patient is positioned supine on the operating table with the involved arm abducted on an arm table.
- A tourniquet is placed as far proximal on the arm as feasible.
- Traction is useful:
  - A shoulder holder along with 5- to 10-pound sandbags attached to an arm sling
  - A commercially available traction tower such as the Linvatec tower (ConMed Linvatec Corp., Utica, NY) or the ARC traction tower (Arc Surgical LLC, Hillsboro, OR)
- For the dorsal portals, the surgeon faces the dorsum of the wrist and is seated by the patient's head. For the volar portals, the surgeon faces the palm and is seated in the patient's axillary region.

Approach

- Portals are established by palpating and identifying anatomic landmarks and then inserting a 22-gauge needle into the joint space. The joint can be injected with 5 mL of saline. The ability to draw the saline back into the syringe serves as evidence that the needle is in the joint. This is not necessary for dry arthroscopy.
- Shallow incisions avoid injury to sensory nerve branches and tendons. Soft tissues are dissected using a blunt mosquito clamp or a pair of small tenotomy scissors. The dorsal capsule is pierced with these same instruments, providing access to the joint.
- A blunt trocar is used to introduce the scope cannula, which will house the scope and the inflow.
- An 18-gauge needle is placed in the 6U portal for outflow, but this is not needed with dry arthroscopy.
- Synovitis, fractures, ligament tears, and a tight wrist joint may limit the field of view and necessitate the use of more portals to adequately assess the entire wrist.

Table 2 Field of View

Portal	Radial	Central	Volar	Dorsal /Distal	Ulnar
1-2	Scaphoid and lunate fossa, dorsal rim of radius	Proximal and radial scaphoid, proximal lunate	Oblique views of RSC, LRL, SRL	Oblique views of DRCL	TFCC poorly visualized
3-4	Scaphoid and lunate fossa, volar rim of radius	Proximal scaphoid and lunate, dorsal and membranous SLIL	RSC, RSL, LRL, ULL	Oblique views of the DRCL insertion onto the dorsal SLIL	TFCC radial insertion, central disc, ulnar attachment, PRUL, DRUL, PTO, PSR
4-5	Lunate fossa, volar rim of radius	Proximal lunate, triquetrum, dorsal and membranous LTIL	RSL, LRL, ULL	Poorly seen	TFCC radial insertion, central disc, ulnar attachment, PRUL, DRUL, PTO, PSR
6R	Poorly seen	Proximal lunate, triquetrum, dorsal and membranous LTIL	ULL, ULT	Poorly seen	TFCC radial insertion, central disc, ulnar attachment, PRUL, DRUL, PTO, PSR
6U	Sigmoid notch	Proximal triquetrum, membranous LTIL	Oblique views of ULL, ULT	Oblique views of DRCL	TFCC oblique views of the radial insertion, central disc, ulnar attachment, PRUL, DRUL
Volar radial	Scaphoid and lunate fossa, dorsal rim of radius	Scaphoid and lunate fossa, dorsal rim of radius	Palmar scaphoid and lunate, palmar SLIL	Oblique views of RSL, LRL, ULL	Oblique views of the radial insertion, central disc, ulnar attachment, PRUL, DRUL
Midcarpal radial	Scaphotrapeziotrapezoidal joint, distal scaphoid pole	SLIL joint, distal scaphoid, distal lunate	Radial limb of arcuate ligament (ie, continuation of the RSC ligament)	Proximal capitate, CHIL, oblique views of proximal hamate	LTIL joint, partial triquetrum
Midcarpal ulnar	Distal articular surface of the lunate and triquetrum and partial scaphoid	SLIL joint	Volar limb of arcuate ligament (ie, continuation of the triquetrocapitolunate)	Oblique views of proximal capitate, CHIL, proximal hamate	LTIL joint, triquetrum
Dorsal distal radioulnar joint	Sigmoid notch, radial attachment of TFCC	Ulnar head	Palmar radioulnar ligament	Proximal surface of articular disc	Limited view of deep DRUL
Volar distal radioulnar joint	Sigmoid notch, radial attachment of TFCC	Ulnar head	Dorsal radioulnar ligament	Proximal surface of articular disc	Foveal attachment of deep fibers of TFCC (ie, DRUL,PRUL)

RSC, radioscaphocapitate ligament; LRL, long radiolunate ligament; SRL, short radiolunate ligament; DRCL, dorsal radiocarpal ligament; TFCC, triangular fibrocartilage complex; SLIL, scapholunate interosseous ligament; RSL, radioscapholunate ligament; ULL, ulnolunate ligament; PRUL, palmar radioulnar ligament; DRUL, dorsal radioulnar ligament; PTO, pisotriquetral orifice; PSR, prestyloid recess; LTIL, lunotriquetral interosseous ligament; ULT, ulnotriquetral ligament; CHIL, capitohamate ligament.
Adapted from Slutsky DJ. Wrist arthroscopy portals. In: Slutsky DJ, Nagle DJ, eds. Techniques in Hand and Wrist Arthroscopy. Philadelphia: Elsevier, 2007.

3-4 Portal

- The concavity overlying the lunate between the extensor pollicis longus and the EDC is located just distal to the tubercle of Lister in line with the second web space.
- The radiocarpal joint is identified with a 22-gauge needle that is inserted 10 degrees palmar to account for the volar inclination of the radius.
- The vascular tuft of the radioscapholunate ligament (**TECH FIG 1A**) is directly in line with this portal. Superior to the radioscapholunate ligament is the membranous portion of the SLIL.
- By rotating the scope dorsally while looking in an ulnar direction, the insertion of the dorsal capsule onto the dorsal aspect of the SLIL can often be visualized. This is a common origin for the stalk of a dorsal ganglion.
- The radioscaphocapitate ligament and the long radiolunate ligament are radial to the portal and can be probed with a hook in the 4-5 portal (**TECH FIG 1B**).
- The LTIL, TFCC, and ulnolunate ligament are ulnar to the portal.

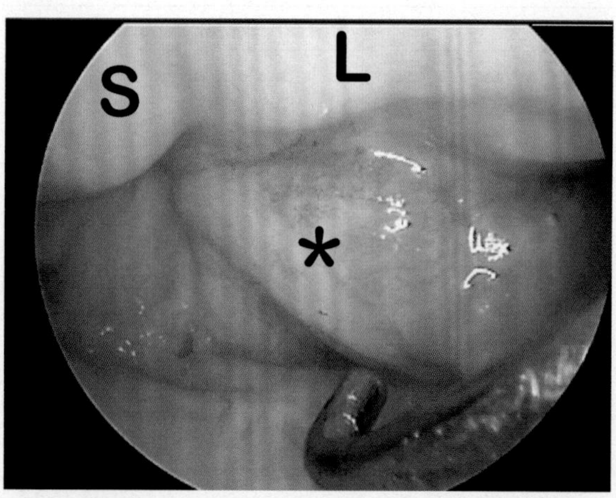

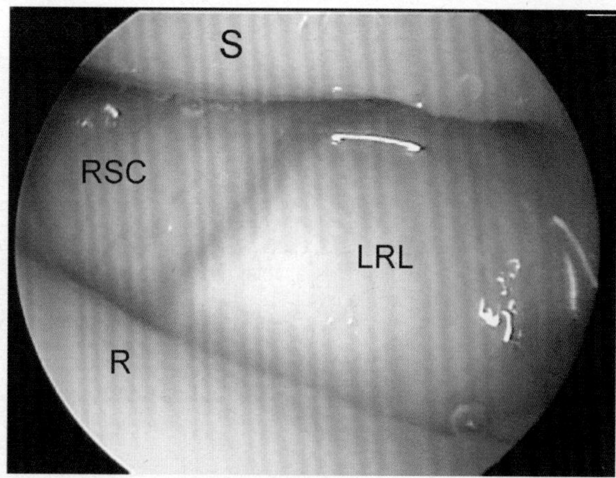

TECH FIG 1 • **A.** View of the radioscapholunate ligament (*asterisk*) from the 3-4 portal. *S*, scaphoid; *L*, lunate. **B.** View of the radioscaphocapitate (*RSC*) and long radiolunate ligament (*LRL*) from the 3-4 portal. *S*, scaphoid; *R*, radius.

4-5 Portal

- The interval for the 4-5 portal is identified with the 22-gauge needle between the EDC and EDM in line with the ring metacarpal.
- Because of the normal radial inclination of the distal radius, this portal lies slightly proximal and about 1 cm ulnar to the 3-4 portal.
- Care must be taken when inserting the scope because the LTIL lies directly ahead of this portal.
- One encounters the ulnar half of the lunate when moving the scope radially, and the oblique surface of the triquetrum in a superior and ulnar direction.
- The LTIL is seen obliquely from this portal and is often difficult to differentiate from the carpal bones without probing, unless a tear is present (**TECH FIG 2A**).
- The ulnolunate ligament and the ulnotriquetral ligament can be seen on the far end of the joint.
- Proximally, the radial insertion of the TFCC blends imperceptibly with the sigmoid notch of the radius, but it can be palpated with a hook probe in either the 3-4 or 6R portal.
- The peripheral insertion of the TFCC slopes upward into the ulnar capsule. Peripheral TFCC tears are often located ulnarly and dorsally.
- The palmar radioulnar ligament can be probed and visualized (especially if torn), but the dorsal radioulnar ligament is poorly seen.
- The pisotriquetral recess can sometimes be identified by a small tuft of protruding synovium and when probed may yield views of the articular facet of the pisiform (**TECH FIG 2B**).

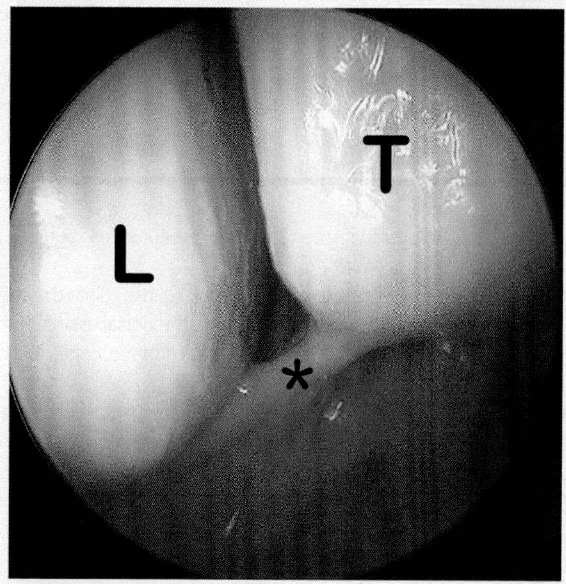

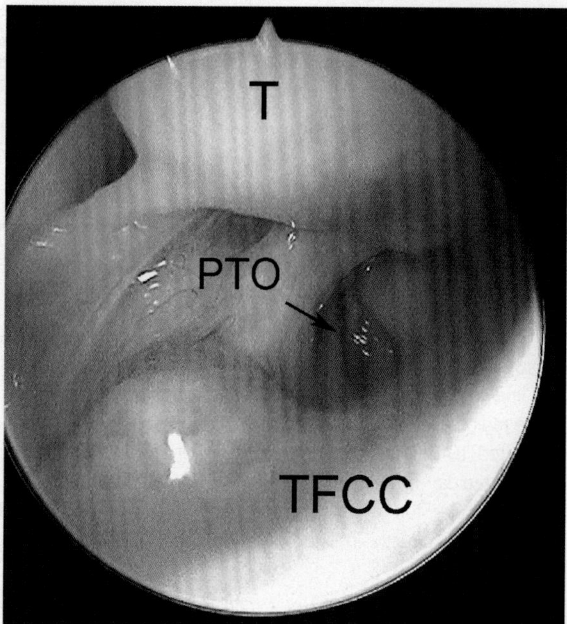

TECH FIG 2 • **A.** View of a lunotriquetral ligament tear (*asterisk*) from the 6R portal. *L*, lunate; *T*, triquetrum. **B.** View of the pisotriquetral orifice (*PTO*) from the 6R portal. *T*, triquetrum; *TFCC*, triangular fibrocartilage.

6R and 6U Portals

- The 6R portal is identified on the radial side of the ECU tendon, just distal to the ulnar head.
  - The scope should be angled 10 degrees proximally to avoid hitting the triquetrum. The TFCC is immediately below the entry site.
  - The LTIL is located radially and superiorly, whereas the ulnar capsule is immediately adjacent to the scope.
- The 6U portal is found on the ulnar side of the ECU tendon. Angling the needle distally and ulnar deviation of the wrist helps avoid running into the triquetrum.
  - This portal can be used to view the dorsal rim of the TFCC or for instrumentation when débriding the palmar LTIL.

1-2 Portal

- The relevant landmarks in the snuff box are palpated and outlined, including the distal edge of the radial styloid, the abductor pollicis longus, extensor pollicis brevis, extensor pollicis longus tendons, and the radial artery in the snuff box.
- To minimize the risk of injury to branches of the superficial radial nerve and the radial artery, the 1-2 portal should be no more than 4.5 mm dorsal to the first extensor compartment and within 4.5 mm of the radial styloid (**TECH FIG 3**).[10]
- A blunt trocar and cannula are inserted with the wrist in ulnar deviation to minimize damage to the proximal scaphoid.

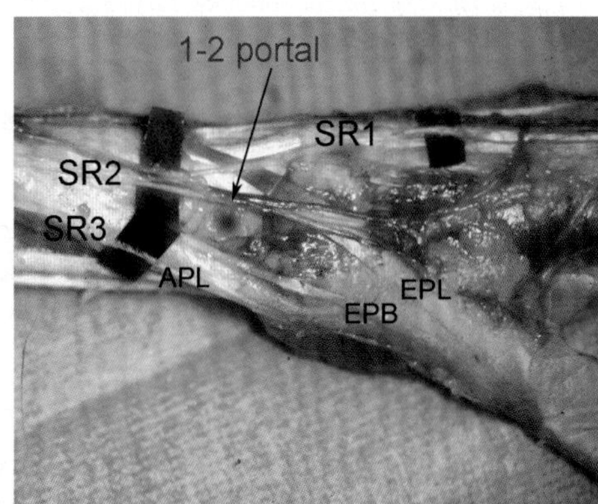

A

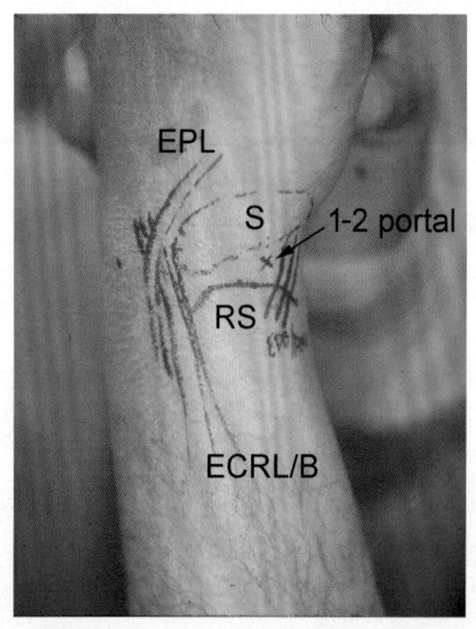

B

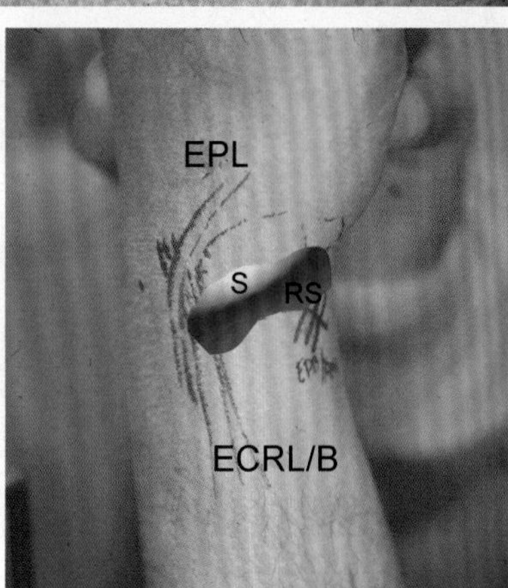

C

TECH FIG 3 ● Landmarks for the 1-2 portal. **A.** Cadaver dissection demonstrating the placement of the 1-2 portal. *SR*, superficial radial nerve branches; *EPL*, extensor pollicis longus; *EPB*, extensor pollicis brevis; *APL*, abductor pollicis longus. **B.** Surface landmarks for 1-2 portal. *S*, scaphoid; *ECRL/B*, extensor carpi radialis longus and brevis. **C.** Superimposed intra-articular field of view. (From Slutsky DJ. Wrist arthroscopy portals. In: Slutsky DJ, Nagle DJ, eds. Techniques in Hand and Wrist Arthroscopy. Philadelphia: Elsevier, 2007.)

Midcarpal Radial Portal

- The midcarpal radial portal is found 1 cm distal to the 3-4 portal.
- Flexing the wrist and firm thumb pressure helps identify the soft spot between the distal pole of the scaphoid and the proximal capitate.
- The scaphotrapezial trapezoidal joint lies radially and can be seen by rotating the scope dorsally.
- The scapholunate articulation can be seen proximally and ulnarly; it can be probed for instability or step-off. Further ulnarly, the lunotriquetral articulation is visualized.
- Moving the scope superiorly yields oblique views of the proximal surface capitate and hamate as well as the capitohamate interosseous ligament.
- The continuation of the radioscaphocapitate ligament, which forms the radial arm of the arcuate ligament (ie, the scaphocapitate ligament) can occasionally be seen across the midcarpal space.

Midcarpal Ulnar Portal

- The midcarpal ulnar port is found 1 cm distal to the 4-5 portal and 1.5 cm ulnar and slightly proximal to the midcarpal radial portal in line with the ring metacarpal axis.
- This entry site is at the intersection of the lunate, triquetrum, hamate, and capitate with a type I lunate facet and directly over the lunotriquetral joint with a type II lunate facet.[11]
  - This portal provides preferential views of the lunotriquetral articulation.
- Directly anteriorly, the ulnar limb of the arcuate ligament (**TECH FIG 4**) (ie, the triquetro-hamate-capitate ligament) can be seen as it crosses obliquely from the triquetrum, across the proximal corner of the hamate to the palmar neck of the capitate.
  - This is especially important in midcarpal instability.
  - Normally, there is very little step-off between the distal articular surfaces of the scaphoid and lunate.
  - Direct pressure from the scope combined with traction may force the carpal joints out of alignment.

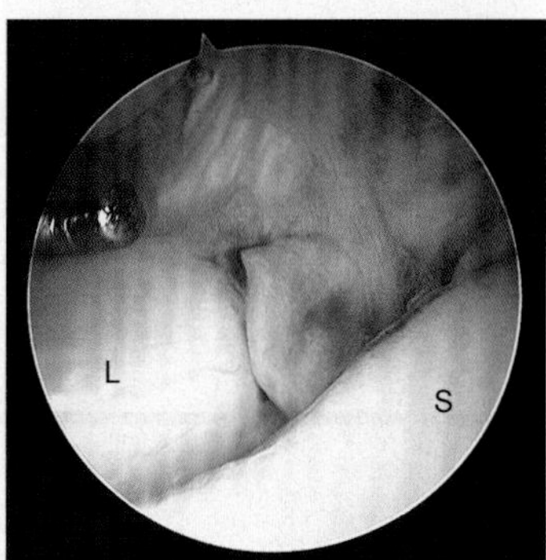

TECH FIG 4 • View of the arcuate ligament from the midcarpal radial portal. *S*, scaphoid; *L*, lunate

- The traction should be released, and the scapholunate joint should be viewed with the scope in the midcarpal ulnar portal, whereas the lunotriquetral joint should be viewed with the scope in the midcarpal radial portal.

Volar Radial Portal

- A 2-cm transverse or longitudinal incision is made in the proximal wrist crease overlying the FCR tendon. The portal is established in the usual manner (**TECH FIG 5**).
- It is not necessary to specifically identify the adjacent neurovascular structures, provided that the anatomic landmarks are adhered to.
- A hook probe is inserted through the 3-4 portal and used to assess the palmar aspect of the SLIL and the DRCL.
- A useful landmark when viewing from the volar radial portal is the intersulcal ridge between the scaphoid and lunate fossae.
  - The radial origin of the DRCL is seen immediately ulnar to this, just proximal to the lunate.

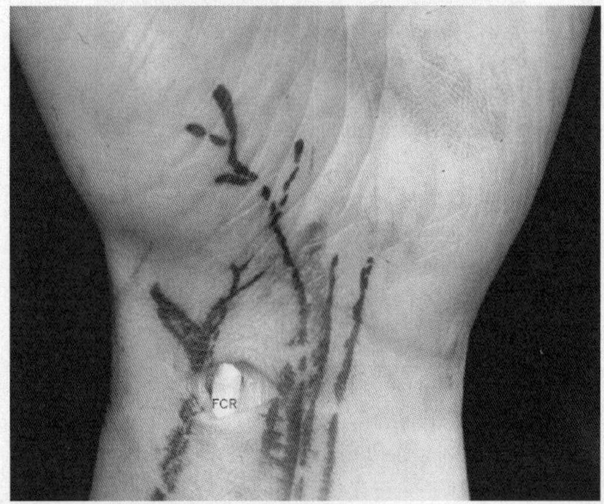

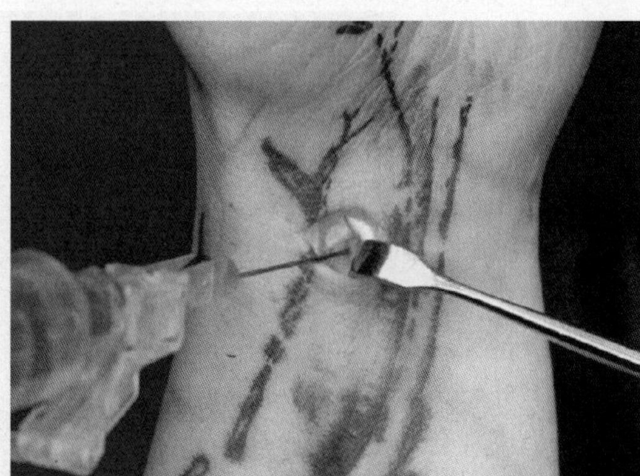

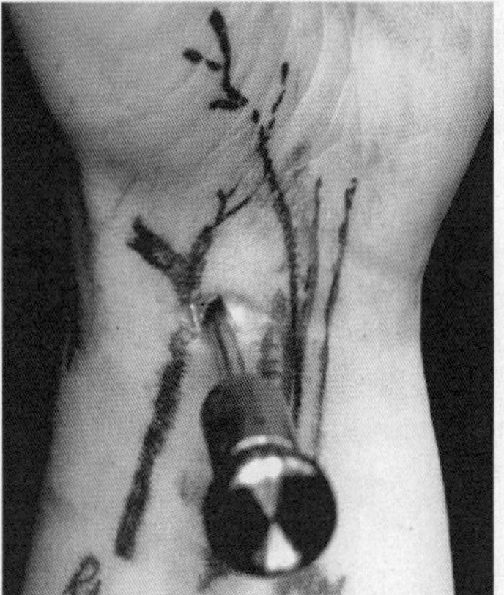

TECH FIG 5 • Technique for volar radial portal. **A.** Skin incision for volar radial portal. *FCR*, flexor carpi radialis tendon. **B.** Saline injection of radiocarpal joint. **C.** Insertion of cannula through floor of the FCR sheath. (From Slutsky DJ. Volar portals in wrist arthroscopy. J Am Soc Surg Hand 2002;2:225–232.)

Volar Radial Midcarpal Portal

- The volar aspect of the midcarpal joint can be accessed through the same skin incision as the volar radial portal.
- The capsular entry site through the volar radial midcarpal portal is entered by angling the trocar 1 cm distally and about 5 degrees ulnarward to the radiocarpal site.
- A hook probe can be inserted dorsally in the midcarpal radial portal for palpation.
- With tears of the palmar SLIL, one can see the intact dorsal fibers and the volar surface of the capitate.

Volar Ulnar Portal

- The volar ulnar portal is established via a 2-cm longitudinal incision centered over the proximal wrist crease along the ulnar edge of the finger flexor tendons (**TECH FIG 6**).
- The tendons are retracted to the radial side and the radiocarpal joint space is identified with a 22-gauge needle.
- Care is taken to situate the portal underneath the ulnar edge of the flexor tendons and to apply retraction in a radial direction alone to avoid injury to the ulnar nerve and artery.
- The median nerve is protected by the interposed flexor tendons.
- The palmar region of the LTIL can usually be seen slightly distal and radial to the portal.
- A hook probe is inserted through the 6R or 6U portal.

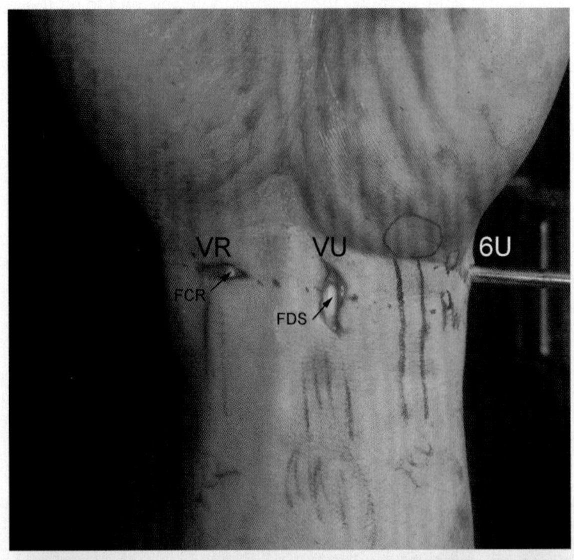

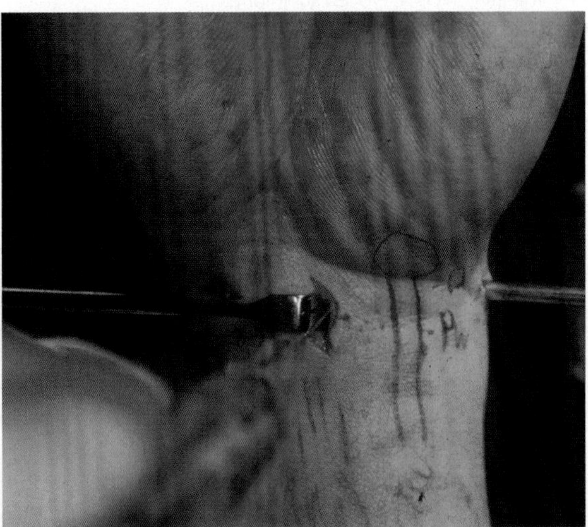

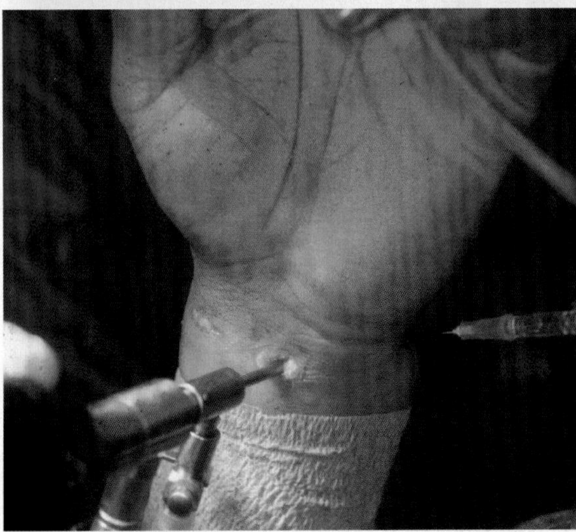

TECH FIG 6 • Technique for volar ulnar portal. **A.** Skin incision for volar ulnar portal. *VR*, volar radial portal; *VU*, volar ulnar portal; *FCR*, flexor carpi radialis tendon; *FDS*, flexor digitorum sublimis. **B.** FDS retracted, saline injection of radiocarpal joint. **C.** Insertion of cannula through capsule deep to FDS tendons. (From Slutsky DJ. The use of a volar ulnar portal in wrist arthroscopy. Arthroscopy 2004;20:158–163.)

Distal Radioulnar Joint Portals

Volar Distal Radioulnar Joint Portal

- The volar DRUJ portal is accessed through the volar ulnar skin incision (**TECH FIG 7A–E**).
  - The joint is entered by angling the 22-gauge needle 45 degrees proximally.
    - It is useful to leave a needle or cannula in the ulnocarpal joint for reference.
  - Alternatively, a probe can be placed in the distal DRUJ portal and advanced through the palmar incision to act as a switching stick over which the cannula can be threaded.[5]
- Initially, the space appears quite limited, but over the course of 3 to 5 minutes, the fluid irrigation expands the joint space, which improves visibility.
- A 3-mm hook probe is inserted through the dorsal distal DRUJ portal for palpation.
  - A burr or thermal probe can be substituted as necessary.
- Direct visualization of the foveal attachment prevents accidental injury to this structure.
- The articular disc is seen superiorly.
- Proximal surface tears of the TFCC, which are usually caused by severe axial load, may be detected through this portal.
- The dome of the ulnar head lies inferiorly.
- The TFCC attachment to the sigmoid notch can be palpated with a hook probe in the distal dorsal DRUJ portal as it penetrates the dorsal DRUJ capsule.
- The deep attachments of the dorsal radioulnar ligament can be seen as it inserts into the fovea.
- In ideal cases, the conjoined tendon of the dorsal radioulnar ligament, ulnar collateral ligament, and palmar radioulnar ligament can be visualized.

Dorsal Distal Radioulnar Joint Portal

- The dorsal aspect of the DRUJ can be accessed through proximal and distal portals.
- The proximal DRUJ portal is located in the axilla of the joint, just proximal to the sigmoid notch and the flare of the ulnar metaphysis.
  - This portal is easier to penetrate and should be used initially to prevent chondral injury from insertion of the trocar.
  - The forearm is held in supination to relax the dorsal capsule, to move the ulnar head volarly, and to lift the central disc distally from the head of the ulna.
  - Reducing the traction to 1 to 2 pounds permits better views between the ulna and the sigmoid notch by reducing the compressive force caused by axial traction.

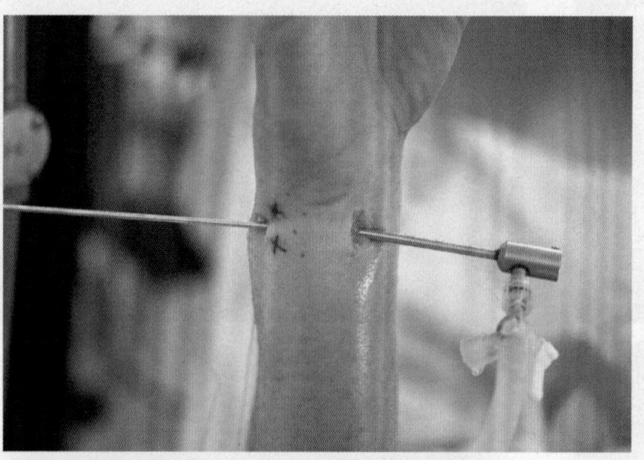
A

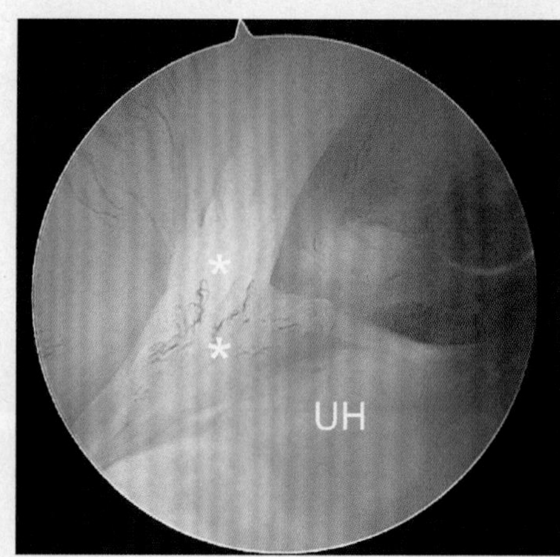

B

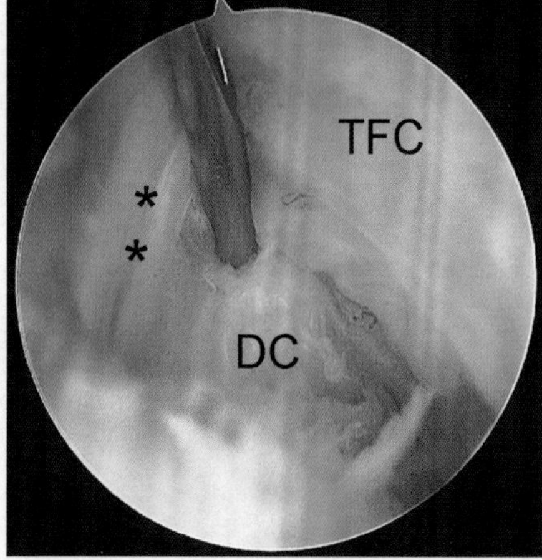

C

TECH FIG 7 • **A.** Arthroscopic cannula is inserted in the volar DRUJ portal with a hook probe in the 6R portal. **B.** View of the foveal ligament attachment (*asterisks*) from the VDRU portal. *UH*, ulnar head. **C.** View of the undersurface of the triangular fibrocartilage (*TFC*). A 22-gauge needle is used to tension the foveal ligaments (*asterisks*). *DC*, dorsal capsule.*(continued)*

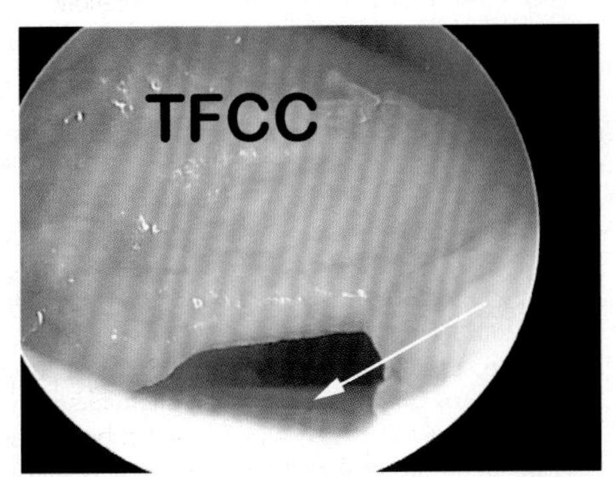

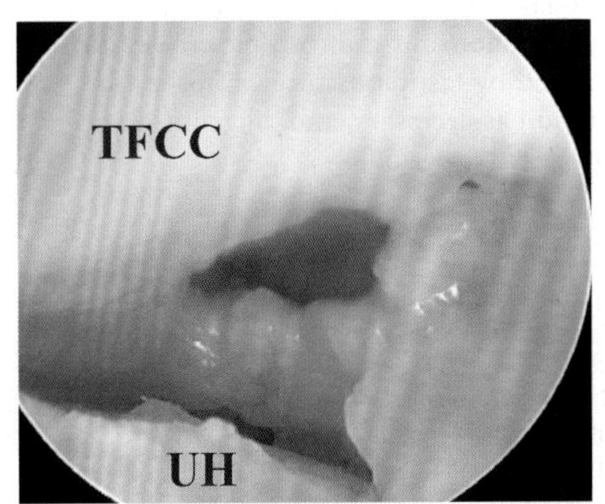

TECH FIG 7 • *(continued)* **D.** View of a radial TFC tear from the 4-5 portal under dry arthroscopy. Note the exposure of the ulnar head (*arrow*). *TFCC*, triangular fibrocartilage complex. **E.** View of the same TFC tear from the VDRU. *UH*, ulnar head.

- The joint space is entered by inserting a 22-gauge needle horizontally at the neck of the distal ulna.
  - Fluoroscopy facilitates needle placement.
- The distal dorsal DRUJ portal is identified 6 to 8 mm distally with the 22-gauge needle and just proximal to the 6R portal.
  - This portal can be used for outflow drainage or for instrumentation.
  - It lies on top of the ulnar head but underneath the TFCC and so is difficult to use in the presence of positive ulnar variance.
  - The TFCC has the least tension in neutral rotation of the forearm, which is the optimal position for visualizing the articular dome of the ulnar head, the undersurface of the TFCC, and the proximal radioulnar ligament from its attachment to the sigmoid notch to its insertion into the fovea of the ulna.
  - Because of the dorsal entry of the arthroscope, the course of the dorsal radioulnar ligament is not visible until its attachment into the fovea is encountered.
  - Entry into this portal provides views of the proximal sigmoid notch cartilage and the articular surface of the neck of the ulna.

PEARLS AND PITFALLS

- Use shallow skin incisions.
- Use the wound spread technique to protect surrounding sensory nerves.
- If the trocar does not insert easily, reposition to avoid chondral injury.
- Wrist traction often diminishes during the procedure and should be readjusted as needed to avoid scraping the articular surface.
- Use of a standard methodologic approach ensures a complete and thorough examination.

POSTOPERATIVE CARE

- The postoperative rehabilitation depends on the specific procedure that is performed.
- After diagnostic arthroscopy, with or without débridement, the patient is splinted for comfort for a brief period of 4 to 7 days.
- Active wrist motion is encouraged after this period and patients are allowed activities of daily living, followed by gradual strengthening.
- If a ligament repair or TFCC repair has been performed or if there is interosseous pinning, the protocol is adjusted as necessary and typically involves an initial period of immobilization before instituting wrist motion.

COMPLICATIONS

- Most of the complications related to use of the dorsal portals are related to injury to the sensory branches of the superficial radial nerve and the dorsal cutaneous branch of the ulnar nerve.
  - The palmar cutaneous branch of the ulnar nerve is at risk with the volar radial portal, although the interposed FCR tendon mitigates this risk.
  - There is no true internervous plane when using the volar ulnar portal; hence, sensory branches of the palmar cutaneous branches of the ulnar nerve or nerve of Henle are always at risk. Thus, proper wound spread technique is paramount.
  - The ulnar neurovascular bundle is also potentially at risk with overzealous retraction or poor portal placement.

- Venous bleeding, loss of wrist motion (especially forearm supination), complications related to fluid extravasation, and infection are general risks attendant to any arthroscopic procedure.
  - These can be minimized by fastidious surgical technique, aggressive rehabilitation as necessary, and diligent follow-up in the early postoperative period.

REFERENCES

1. Berger RA. Arthroscopic anatomy of the wrist and distal radioulnar joint. Hand Clin 1999;15(3):393–413.
2. Geissler WB, Freeland AE, Savoie FH, et al. Intracarpal soft-tissue lesions associated with an intra-articular fracture of the distal end of the radius. J Bone Joint Surg Am 1996;78(3):357–365.
3. Slutsky DJ. Arthroscopy portals: volar and dorsal. In: Budoff J, Slade JF, Trumble TE, eds. Master's Techniques in Wrist and Elbow Arthroscopy. Chicago: American Society for Surgery of the Hand, 2006.
4. Slutsky DJ. Clinical applications of volar portals in wrist arthroscopy. Tech Hand Up Extrem Surg 2004;8(4):229–238.
5. Slutsky DJ. Distal radioulnar joint arthroscopy and the volar ulnar portal. Tech Hand Up Extrem Surg 2007;11:38–44.
6. Slutsky DJ. Management of dorsoradiocarpal ligament repairs. J Am Soc Surg Hand 2005;5:167–174.
7. Slutsky DJ. Volar portals in wrist arthroscopy. J Am Soc Surg Hand 2002;2:225–232.
8. Slutsky DJ. Wrist arthroscopy portals. In: Slutsky DJ, Nagel DJ, eds. Techniques in Hand and Wrist Arthroscopy. Philadelphia: Elsevier, 2007.
9. Slutsky DJ. Wrist arthroscopy through a volar radial portal. Arthroscopy 2002;18:624–630.
10. Steinberg BD, Plancher KD, Idler RS. Percutaneous Kirschner wire fixation through the snuff box: an anatomic study. J Hand Surg Am 1995;20:57–62.
11. Viegas SF. Midcarpal arthroscopy: anatomy and portals. Hand Clin 1994;10(4):577–587.

Elbow Arthroscopy: The Basics

John E. Conway

CHAPTER 4

DEFINITION

- Elbow arthroscopy involves the use of an arthroscope to examine the interior of the elbow joint and provides the opportunity to perform minimally invasive diagnostic and therapeutic procedures.
- Elbow arthroscopy has evolved to allow the definitive care of more than a dozen complex elbow conditions.
- Despite an expanded understanding of the surrounding neurovascular anatomy, essential portal placement for access to the elbow joint continues to present a level of risk for injury that exceeds that seen in other joints.[4,6,7,14]
- The safe application of this treatment modality requires that the surgeon have a solid grasp of the relative anatomy, fellowship or laboratory training in treatment techniques, experience as an arthroscopist, and an objective assessment of his or her own level of skill.

ANATOMY

- Neurovascular injury risk is relatively high and a three-dimensional grasp of elbow anatomy is essential for safe and successful elbow arthroscopy (**FIG 1**).[1,3,5–8,10–12,15]
- Miller et al[8] showed that the bone-to-nerve distances in the 90-degree-flexed elbow increased with joint insufflation an average of 12 mm for the median nerve, 6 mm for the radial nerve, and 1 mm for the ulnar nerve.
  - The capsule-to-nerve distance changes very little with insufflation, however, and the protective effect of insufflation is lost when the elbow is in extension.
- Miller et al[8] also showed that in the insufflated, 90-degree-flexed elbow, both the radial and median nerves passed within 6 mm of the joint capsule and that the radial nerve was on average 3 mm closer to the capsule than the median nerve. The ulnar nerve was essentially on the capsule.
  - Others have also shown the close proximity of the radial nerve to the joint capsule and stressed the greater risk to this nerve during both portal placement and capsular resection.[2,3,6,8,12]
- Stothers et al[11] emphasized the importance of elbow flexion during portal placement and showed that the portal-to-nerve distances decreased an average of 3.5 to 5.1 mm laterally and 1.4 to 5.6 mm medially when the elbow was in extension.
  - For the distal anterolateral portal, the distance from the sheath to the radial nerve averaged 1.4 mm (range 0 to 4 mm) in extension and 4.9 mm (2 to 10 mm) in flexion.
- Field et al[3] compared three anterolateral portals and reported a statistically significant difference in portal-to-radial nerve distance, with greater safety shown with the more proximal locations.

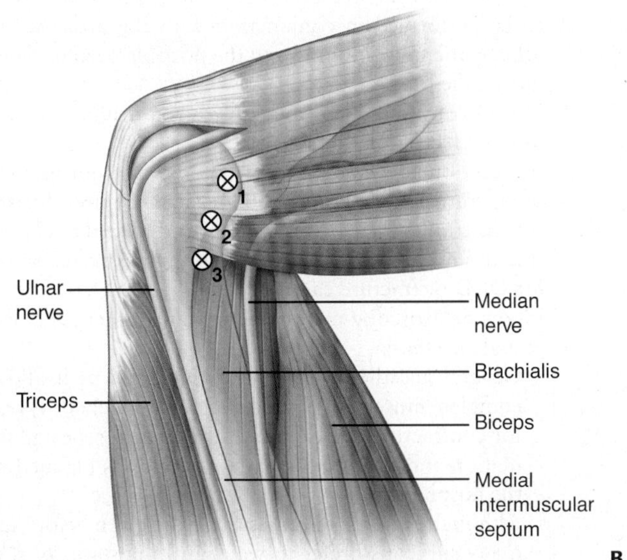

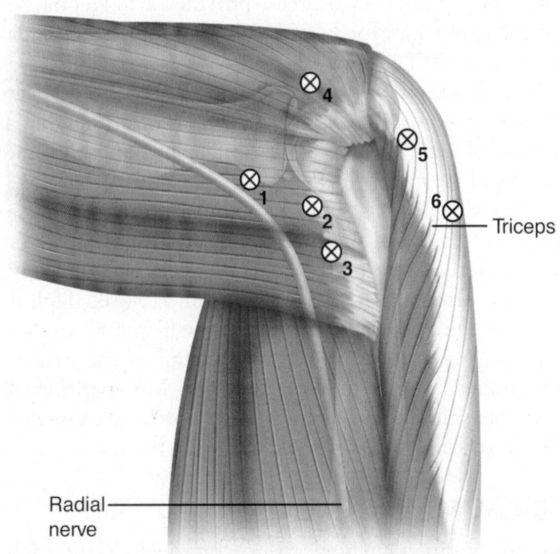

FIG 1 • **A.** Relative anatomy of the medial elbow and the arthroscopic portal sites: *1*, standard anteromedial; *2*, midanteromedial; and *3*, proximal anteromedial. **B.** Relative anatomy of the lateral and posterior elbow and the arthroscopic portal sites: *1*, distal anterolateral; *2*, midanterolateral; *3*, proximal anterolateral; *4*, direct posterolateral; *5*, posterolateral; and *6*, posterior central.

- Anatomic studies suggest three guidelines for neurovascular safety:
  - Portal placement is safer when the elbow is flexed 90 degrees than when it is in extension.[11]
  - Maximal joint distention before portal placement increases the safety during placement by increasing the nerve-to-portal distance.[3,5,6,11]
  - The nerve-to-portal distance is greater for the more proximal anterior portals than for the more distal anterior portals.

PATIENT HISTORY AND PHYSICAL FINDINGS

- This chapter does not address a specific condition but instead offers a broad view of the basic considerations and setup issues for a surgical treatment that may be applied to many different elbow problems.
- A complete review of the numerous clinical tests described for the diagnostic evaluation of the elbow would exceed the scope of this chapter.

IMAGING AND OTHER DIAGNOSTIC STUDIES

- Routine preoperative elbow radiographs should include a true lateral view, a standard anteroposterior (AP) view, and an AP view of both the distal humerus and proximal forearm when joint motion loss prevents full joint extension.
- Additional radiographic views include the cubital tunnel view, the posterior impingement view, the capitellum view, and the radial head view.
  - The cubital tunnel view, an AP projection of the humerus with the elbow maximally flexed, provides a clear view of the medial epicondyle and cubital tunnel groove.
  - The posterior impingement view is also an AP projection of the humerus with the elbow maximally flexed, but the humerus is rotated into 45 degrees of external rotation. This image offers better assessment of the posteromedial edge of the olecranon tip and the medial epicondyle apophysis.
  - The capitellum view, an AP projection of the ulna with the elbow flexed 45 degrees, provides a tangential view of the capitellum for better evaluation of osteochondritis dissecans (OCD) lesions.
  - The radial head view is an oblique view of the 90-degree-flexed elbow with the beam passing between the ulna and the radial head. It allows for clear imaging of both the radial head and the radial–ulna interval.
- Although this point is sometimes argued, computed tomography is often useful when resection of intra-articular bone is considered as a part of contracture release arthroscopy.
- Magnetic resonance (MR) imaging in a closed high-field magnet with thin-section, optimized, high-spatial-resolution sequences may provide exceptional detail of the structures surrounding the elbow joint; however, MR arthrography, with either saline or gadolinium, will improve the assessment of intra-articular structures such as loose bodies.

SURGICAL MANAGEMENT

- The indications for elbow arthroscopy include the evaluation and treatment of septic arthritis, lateral synovial plica syndrome, systemic inflammatory arthritis, loose bodies, synovitis, OCD, degenerative arthritis, posterior impingement, traumatic arthritis, trochlea chondromalacia, arthrofibrosis, lateral epicondylitis, joint contracture, posterolateral rotatory instability, and olecranon bursitis.
- Treatment options for these conditions include diagnostic evaluation, loose body removal, synovial biopsy, partial or complete synovectomy, plica excision, extensor carpi radialis brevis tendon débridement, capsule release, capsulotomy, capsulectomy, exostosis excision, ulnohumeral arthroplasty, contracture release, chondroplasty, microfracture chondroplasty, percutaneous drilling or fixation of OCD lesions, capitellum osteochondral transplantation, radial head excision, internal fixation of fractures, lateral ulnar collateral ligament plication, ulnar nerve decompression, and finally, olecranon bursoscopy and bursectomy.
- The relative contraindications for elbow arthroscopy include recent joint or soft tissue infection; developmental changes; previous trauma or surgery that significantly alters the normal neurovascular, bony, or soft tissue anatomy of the elbow; extensive extracapsular heterotopic ossification; complex regional pain syndrome; and conditions that prevent distention of the elbow capsule.
- Previous ulnar nerve transposition usually requires exposure of the ulnar nerve before the creation of an anteromedial portal.

Preoperative Planning

- As with all medical conditions, the importance of the information gained from a careful and complete history and examination for establishing an accurate diagnosis cannot be overemphasized.
- Plain radiographs are also essential, but some authors suggest that computed tomography and MR imaging offer little in the preoperative assessment.
  - In contrast, the exact location of intra-articular, capsular, and extra-articular bone; the thickness of the joint capsule; the integrity of the cartilage covering an OCD lesion; and the presence of stress fractures or loose bodies unseen on radiographs are a few examples of how additional imaging may direct or modify care.
- The surgeon should consider how associated procedures to be performed in conjunction with the arthroscopy will affect patient positioning and the possible need to reposition during the case.
- Fluoroscopy should be available when drilling, pinning, or internal fixation is considered.
- In addition to standard arthroscopic instrumentation, the preoperative plan should also consider the need for specialized instruments such as retractors and special biters for contracture release surgery and small fragment fixation devices for OCD or fracture care.
- Elbow arthroscopy may be done using either general or regional anesthesia.
  - General anesthesia is typically preferred as it allows for complete muscle relaxation. Regional blockade is reserved for contracture release procedures where repeated manipulation and continuous passive motion is planned during the hospitalization.
  - Although regional anesthesia may be given before surgery, many surgeons prefer to wait until the status of the neurovascular structures is established in the recovery setting.
  - Indwelling catheter regional anesthesia is described and sometimes recommended for contracture release procedures, but not all centers are comfortable or experienced

with these techniques, and repeated regional anesthesia during the hospitalization appears to be equally effective.
- The use of ultrasound during injection may decrease the morbidity associated with regional anesthesia.

Positioning

- The four patient positions for elbow arthroscopy are the supine cross-body position, the supine suspended position, the lateral decubitus position, and the prone position.
  - Although the latter two positions are most popular today, experience with one of the supine positions still offers advantages. For example, a surgeon who prefers the prone position may elect to use the supine cross-body position when arthroscopic and open procedures are combined, preventing the need for repositioning.
- Supine cross-body position
  - Arthroscopy in this position may be done with one of several commercially available arm-holding devices but is performed equally well with an assistant acting as the arm holder (**FIG 2A**).
  - Because the elbow is not rigidly stabilized in this position, complex procedures may be more challenging and present a greater level of risk for injury.
  - The supine cross-body position is a safe and effective position for elbow arthroscopy regardless of the complexity of the procedure and provides the opportunity to convert to either an open cross-body approach or an open abducted-on-arm board approach.
- Supine suspended position
  - This position requires the use of a traction device from which the arm is hung. Capture of the hand or wrist is necessary, and finger traps on the index and long fingers work well in this regard (**FIG 2B**).
  - The elbow is not stabilized against either a post or pad, which allows considerable movement of the elbow beneath the hand.
  - Two potential disadvantages of this position are the unexpected withdrawal of the arthroscope from the freely swinging joint and the almost vertical position of the arthroscope during arthroscopy of the posterior compartment.
- Lateral decubitus position
  - This position for elbow arthroscopy is typically set up the same as for shoulder surgery except that the arm is draped across a padded horizontal post attached to the table (**FIG 2C**).
  - The advantage of this position over the supine positions is that a stable platform is created on which the upper arm rests. There is equal access to the anterior and posterior compartments.
  - The advantage of this position over the prone position becomes apparent when management of the airway is at issue. If prone positioning is a concern, such as in patients with a high body mass index or compromised lung

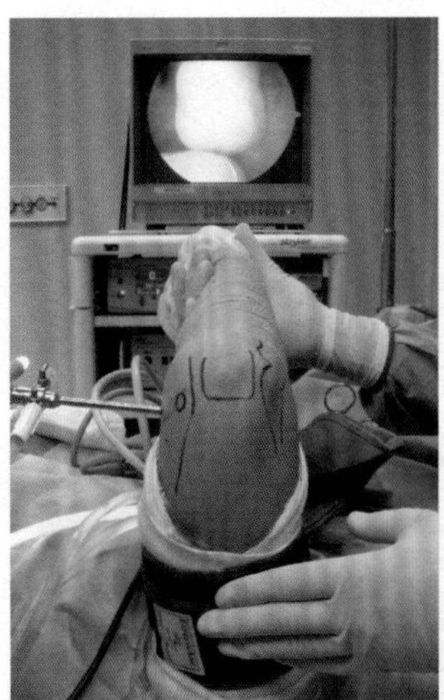
A

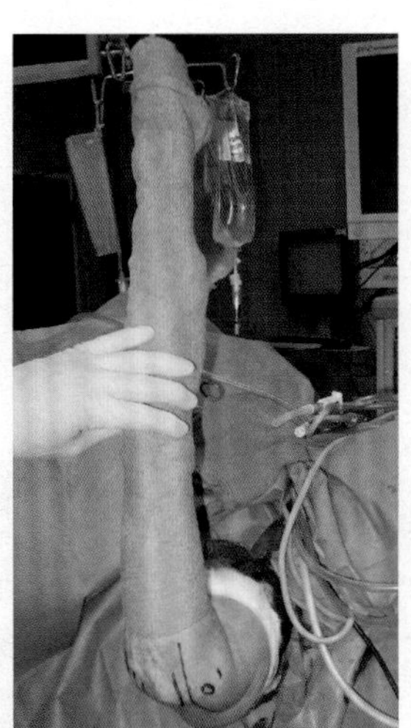
B

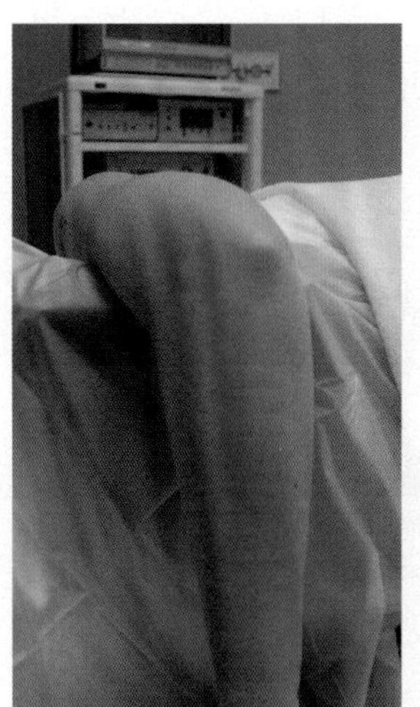
C

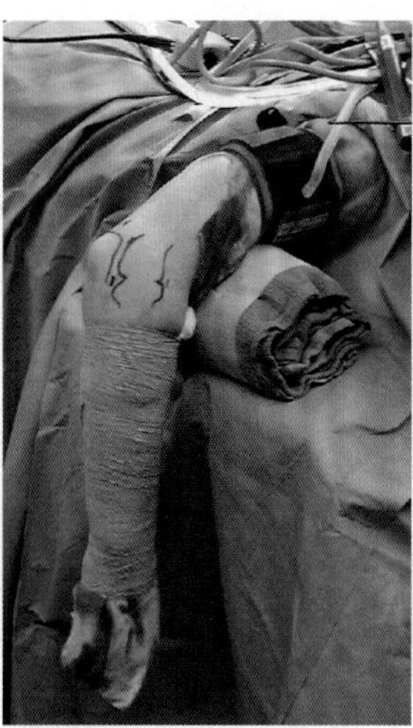
D

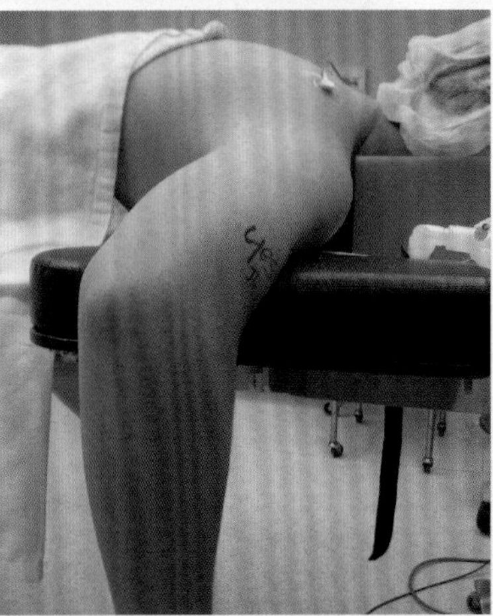
E

FIG 2 • Positioning. **A.** Left elbow draped in the supine cross-body position. An arthroscope is in the proximal anteromedial portal and a loose body is shown on the monitor. **B.** Left elbow draped in the supine suspended position. Sterile towels and elastic wrap are used to cover finger traps attached to the index and long fingers. **C.** Left elbow in the lateral decubitus position. **D.** Right elbow draped in the prone position. A roll of towels is placed between the upper arm and a shortened arm board aligned with the table. **E.** Right elbow draped over a shortened padded arm board.

volume, the case is probably best done in the lateral decubitus position.
- One disadvantage of this position is that small patients, such as gymnasts with OCD lesions, are difficult to position laterally and still maintain full access to the arm.
- Prone position
  - Many surgeons, because of the stability and access provided, prefer the prone position. However, careful attention to positioning is essential to avoiding complications (**FIG 2D**).
  - The airway must be secure and the face should be well padded.
  - Chest rolls are used to lift the chest and abdomen from the table, decreasing the airway pressure required for ventilation.
  - The knees are padded and the feet are elevated.
  - The nonoperative arm is placed on a well-padded arm board, with attention to the ulnar nerve, and the operative arm is allowed to hang over a shortened, padded arm board positioned along the side of the table (**FIG 2E**).
  - Pulses in all four extremities are confirmed.
  - After draping, a small roll of towels is placed beneath the upper arm to align the humerus in the coronal plane of the body and to allow the elbow to flex to 90 degrees.

Approach

- The first arthroscopic portal is anterior except when the entire procedure is accomplished through posterior portals. Occult conditions may exist in the anterior compartment, and a complete diagnostic assessment of the joint requires anterior portals.
- Whether the initial anterior portal should be medial or lateral is debatable but usually determined by surgeon preference and patient diagnosis. Good arguments may be made for either approach.[1,9,14]
- The second anterior portal may then be created with either outside-in or inside-out methods. We prefer to make the medial portal first and then create the lateral portal with an outside-in method.
- Instruments
  - A standard 4.0-mm, 30-degree offset arthroscope may be used for virtually all elbow arthroscopic procedures. On rare occasion, both a 4.0-mm, 70-degree offset arthroscope and a 2.7-mm arthroscope may be helpful. Because it is often necessary to maintain the tip of the arthroscope just a few millimeters through the capsule, an arthroscope sheath without side flow ports is preferred and minimizes fluid extravasation into soft tissues.
  - Essential instruments include an 18-gauge spinal needle, a hemostat, a Wissinger rod, switching rods, and both standard and small mechanical shavers (**FIG 3A,B**).
  - Specialized instruments have recently become available from several sources and include a series of curved and straight arthroscopic retractors, curettes, and osteotomes. Hand biters, designed to resect the anterior capsule more safely, are very useful during contracture release surgery (**FIG 3C**).

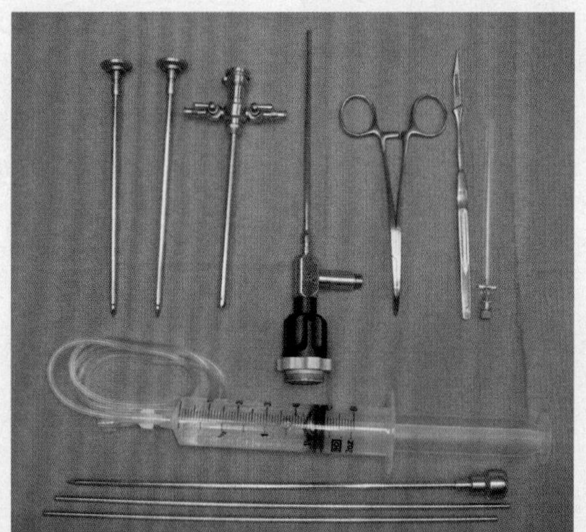
A

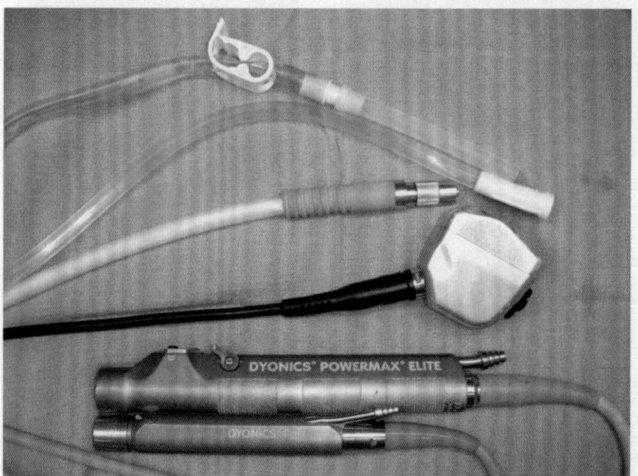

B

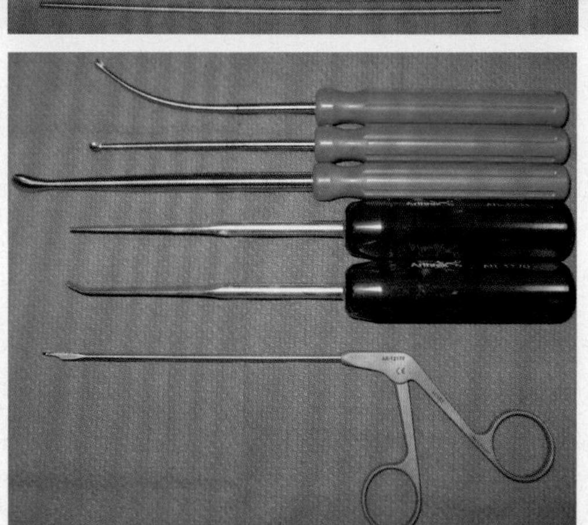
C

FIG 3 • **A,B.** Basic instruments used in elbow arthroscopy. **A.** A standard 4.0-mm, 30-degree offset arthroscope, an arthroscope sheath with sharp and dull trocars, an 18-gauge spinal needle, a 60-mL saline in large syringe with connector tubing, a hemostat, a Wissinger rod, and switching rods. **B.** A standard mechanical shaver, a mini mechanical shaver, an arthroscope camera, a light cord, inflow tubing, and suction tubing. **C.** Specialized instruments for elbow arthroscopy: a hand biter and curved and straight arthroscopic retractors, curettes, awls, and osteotomes.

Limb Preparation

- Setup and portal positions are shown in the supine cross-body position.
- After the administration of general anesthesia, the operative-arm shoulder is relocated to extend just over the edge of the surgical table, affording access to the whole extremity and limiting the reach required for the surgeon.
  - Both the shoulder and the entire arm are prepared and draped and a sterile tourniquet is applied as proximally as possible.
- After limb exsanguination, the tourniquet is elevated and an elastic compression wrap is applied tightly to the forearm, extending from distal to proximal and ending just distal to the radial head.
  - The elastic wrap will limit fluid extravasation into the subcutaneous tissues and the muscle compartments of the forearm and potentially decrease the risk of compartment syndrome.
- Landmarks about the elbow and the proposed arthroscopic portal sites are marked.
- Before portal placement, the joint is distended with saline using an 18-gauge spinal needle passed through the posterolateral "soft spot" (**TECH FIG 1**).
  - The soft spot is located at the center of the triangle formed by the olecranon prominence, the lateral epicondyle prominence, and the lateral margin of the radial head.
- Connector tubing attached to a 60-mL syringe allows an assistant to maintain joint distention during the creation of the initial portal without obstructing the surgeon's access.

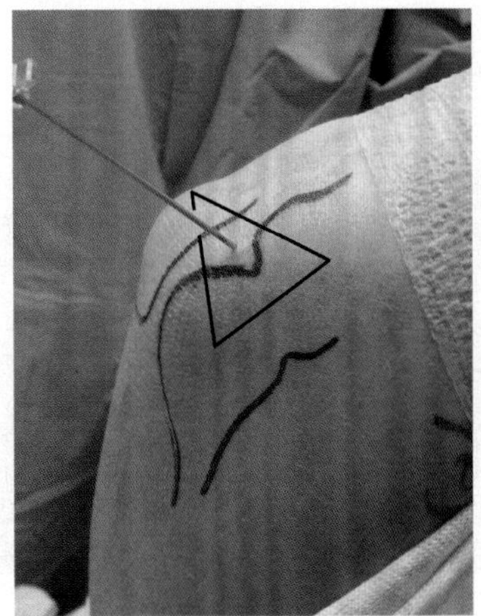

TECH FIG 1 • Left elbow joint in the supine cross-body position being inflated with saline through the posterolateral soft spot with an 18-gauge spinal needle. The soft spot is found at the center of a triangle formed by the olecranon tip, the lateral epicondyle prominence, and the lateral margin of the radial head.

Order of Portal Placement

- Anterior or posterior
  - Neurovascular risk is the most important factor to be considered when determining the order of portal placement.
  - Soft tissue swelling and loss of the capacity to distend the joint would be expected after the creation of the posterior portals and would place both the median and radial nerves closer to the path of the anterior portals.
  - Most surgeons choose to begin the arthroscopy with the anterior portals.
- Medial or lateral
  - The order is usually determined by surgeon preference and the nature of the conditions requiring treatment.
  - The sheath-to-nerve distance for the midanteromedial portal averages 23 mm,[5] that for the distal anterolateral portal averages 3 mm,[5] and that for the proximal anterolateral portal averages 14.2 mm.[3]
  - Because the nerve-to-sheath distance is greater for the anteromedial portals than for the anterolateral portals, it has been argued that the initial approach to the joint is safer when medial.
- Once the medial portal is established, the lateral portal can be made with an outside-in technique and an 18-gauge spinal needle[11,12] or with an inside-out technique and a Wissinger rod.[5]
  - Both methods are relatively safe techniques, but the outside-in method affords greater control of the angle into the joint and potentially greater access to the anterior humerus.

Anteromedial Portals

- There are three commonly described anteromedial portals: standard, mid, and proximal (**TECH FIG 2A**).
- The nerve at greatest risk for injury is the medial antebrachial cutaneous nerve. This risk diminishes when the depth of the portal incision avoids cutting the subcutaneous tissues.[6]
- Dissection to the flexor fascia with a blunt-tipped hemostat allows mobilization of the cutaneous nerves away from the portal for additional protection.
  - Up to six branches are described crossing the medial elbow, and on average, at least one branch is within 1 mm (range 0 to 5 mm) of the portal (**TECH FIG 2B**).
- Both the median nerve and the brachial artery are also at risk during medial portal placement.
  - Continuing the hemostat dissection to the medial joint capsule (**TECH FIG 2C**), introducing the arthroscope sheath with a blunt trocar, and finally penetrating the capsule with a sharp trocar will allow safe medial capsule penetration and avoid extracapsular arthroscope placement.
  - Some authors argue that sharp trocars have no role in elbow arthroscopy; however, blunt trocars are more inclined to penetrate the capsule laterally or, even less desirably, to remain extracapsular. Modifying a sharp trocar by blunting the tip provides a safe and effective compromise.

Standard Anteromedial Portal

- Andrews and Carson[2] described the standard anteromedial portal as located 2 cm anterior and 2 cm distal to the prominence of the medial epicondyle. They reported that the median nerve-to-sheath distance was 6 mm.
  - The path of the portal penetrates the common flexor origin as well as the flexor carpi radialis and the pronator muscles.
  - In some patients, the portal also penetrates the medial border of the brachialis muscle.

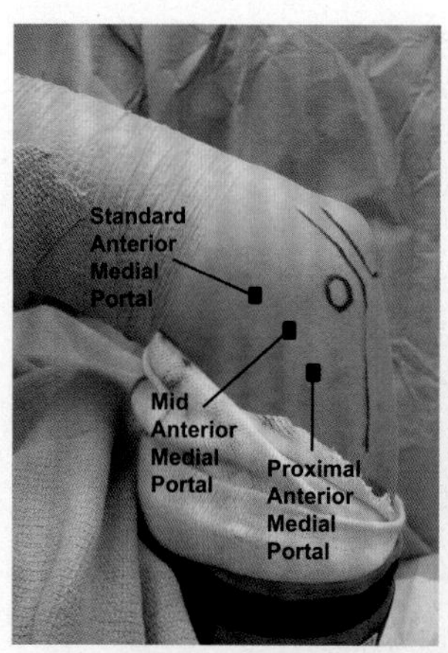

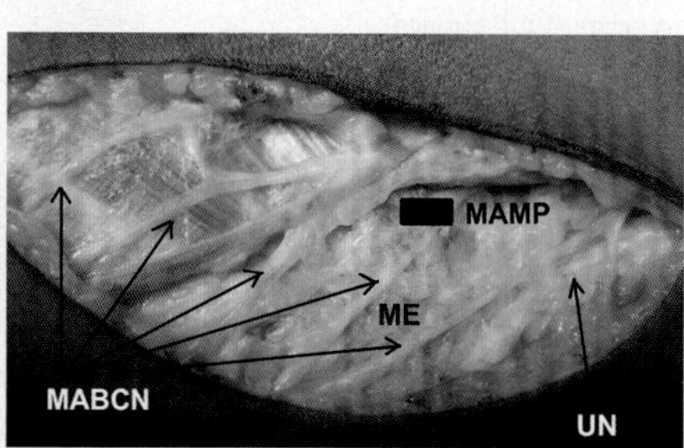

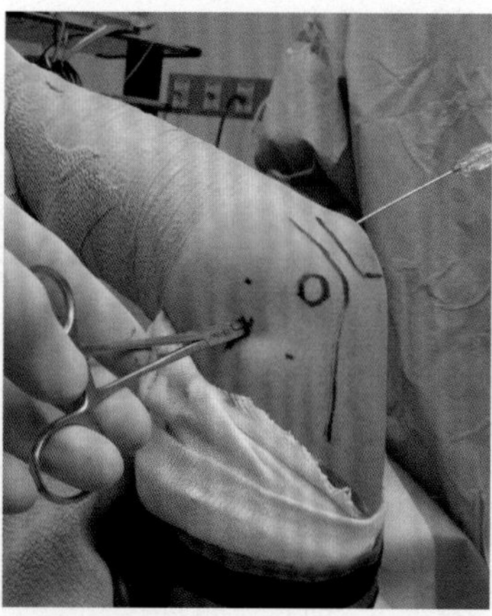

TECH FIG 2 • **A.** Medial surface of the left elbow in the supine cross-body position. Locations of the standard and proximal anteromedial portals are shown. **B.** Medial elbow showing multiple branches of the medial antebrachial cutaneous nerve (*MABCN*). **C.** Anteromedial portal being created with hemostat dissection through the skin, subcutaneous tissues, fascia, and muscle to the medial capsule. *ME*, medial epicondyle; *MAMP*, midanteromedial portal; *UN*, ulnar nerve.

- Lynch et al[6] showed that with joint distention and 90-degree elbow flexion, this portal averaged 14 mm from the median nerve. However, Stothers et al[11,12] showed that the median nerve-to-sheath distance averaged only 7 mm (range 5 to 13 mm) and that the brachial artery-to-sheath distance was just 15 mm (range 8 to 20 mm).
- The standard anteromedial portal may be created with either medial (outside in) or lateral (inside out) methods. Some authors suggest that it is more safely created using the latter method with a rod exchange technique.
- Although this portal offers excellent visualization of the anterolateral contents of the elbow joint, it is now most commonly recommended as an accessory portal for capsular retractors.

Proximal Anteromedial Portal

- The proximal anteromedial portal, popularized by Poehling et al,[10] is described as 2 cm proximal to the prominence of the medial epicondyle and just anterior to the medial intermuscular septum.
  - Others have subsequently described this portal as up to 2 cm anterior to the septum.[9]
- The locations of both the septum and the ulnar nerve must be established before portal placement and the path of the portal must remain anterior to the septum.
- Arthroscope sheath contact with the anterior humerus is advised to further protect the median nerve.[10]
- In this location, at 90 degrees of flexion and with joint distention, the portal averages 12.4 mm (range 7 to 20 mm) from the median nerve, 18 mm from the brachial artery, 12 mm (range 7 to 18 mm) from the ulnar nerve, and 2.3 mm (range 0 to 9 mm) from the medial antebrachial cutaneous nerves.
- This portal also provides visual access to the lateral elbow joint structures, but viewing the superior capsular structures, the lateral capitellum, and the radiocapitellar joint space is limited compared to the standard anteromedial portal.[11,12]

Midanteromedial Portal

- A modification of the proximal anteromedial portal was described by Lindenfeld[5] as located 1 cm proximal and 1 cm anterior to the prominence to the medial epicondyle.
- The portal is directed distally into the center of the joint to preserve the protection afforded by the proximal location and was shown to average 22 mm from the median nerve.

Anterolateral Portals

- Although at less risk for injury than the medial antebrachial cutaneous nerve, the anterior branch of the posterior antebrachial nerve crosses the lateral elbow and may be injured during portal placement. Limiting the depth of the skin incision and using the arthroscope to cast a silhouette of the nerve may provide reasonable protection.
- There are three anterolateral portal locations: distal, mid, and proximal (**TECH FIG 3A**).

Distal Anterolateral Portal

- Andrews and Carson[2] were first to describe an anterolateral portal and recommended placement 3 cm distal and 1 cm anterior to the prominence of the lateral epicondyle. Their work documented that the radial nerve averaged 7 mm from the arthroscope sheath when the elbow was flexed 90 degrees.
- Others have reported that the nerve-to-sheath distance was less, averaging only 3 to 4.9 mm,[5,11,12] and that in extension, this distance was just 1.4 mm.
  - Field et al[3] showed that Andrew and Carson's recommendation located the portal near or directly over the radial head in all specimens studied, and that for smaller patients, these measurements would potentially place the portal distal to the radial head.
- To lessen the risk of radial nerve injury, landmarks, rather than measurements, are used to determine that the portal is proximal to the radial head.[3]

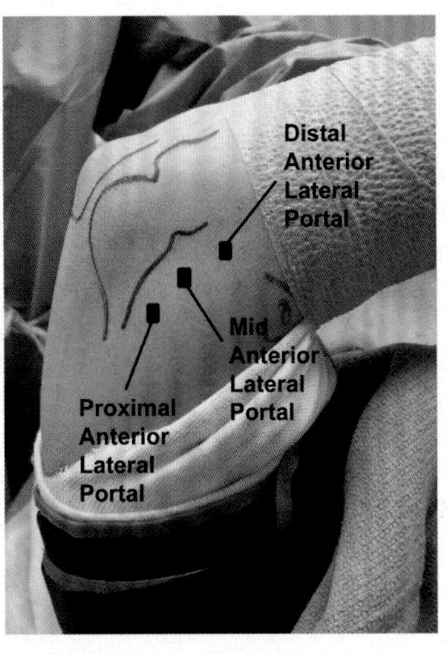

A

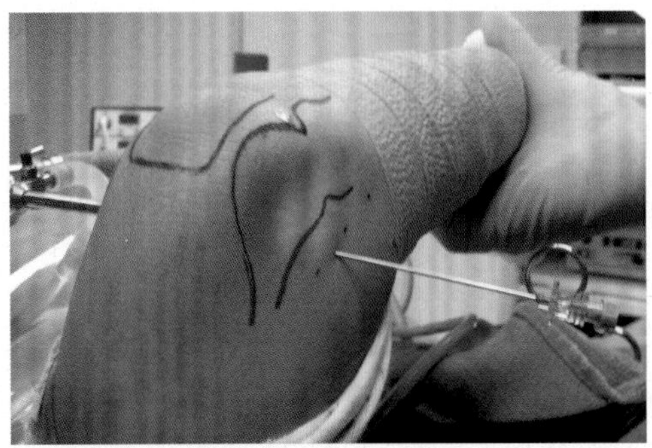

B

TECH FIG 3 • **A.** Lateral surface of the left elbow in the supine cross-body position. Locations of the distal, mid, and proximal anterolateral portals are shown. **B.** Lateral surface of the left elbow with a midanterolateral portal being created using an outside-in method. The spinal needle defines the path of the portal.

- Because of safety concerns, this portal is much less commonly used than the more proximal portals and is typically reserved for a blunt retractor.
- An outside-in method is effective and probably safest.
  - With the elbow at 90 degrees, the forearm in slight pronation, and the joint maximally distended, an 18-gauge spinal needle is placed just anterior to the radial head and directed proximally toward the center of the radiocapitellar joint (**TECH FIG 3B**).
  - A hemostat is then used to dissect through the capsule and a blunt-tipped retractor is introduced to mobilize the anterior capsule.
  - The arthroscope and working instruments are placed in more proximal portals.
- Superficially, the anterior branch of the posterior antebrachial cutaneous nerve was shown to lie on average 7.6 mm (range 0 to 20 mm) from the portal entry and was in contact with the sheath in 43% of elbows studied.[11]

Midanterolateral Portal

- The midanterolateral portal is safer and used more commonly than the distal anterolateral portal.
- Field et al[3] compared distal, mid, and proximal anterolateral portals and found that the more proximal portals were statistically farther from the sheath than the distal portal. They described the location of the midanterolateral portal as 1 cm anterior to the prominence of the lateral epicondyle and just proximal to the anterior margin of the radiocapitellar joint space.
- At 90 degrees of flexion, the radial nerve-to-sheath distance was reported to average 9.8 mm without joint distention and 10.9 mm with distention. This was more than twice the distance reported for the distal portal.
- Both inside-out and outside-in methods are effective and safe means to establish this portal. This portal is most useful for visualization of the medial elbow and débridement of the anterior radiocapitellar joint surfaces.

Proximal Anterolateral Portal

- Stothers et al[11,12] described the location of the proximal anterolateral portal as 1 to 2 cm proximal to the prominence of the lateral epicondyle, with the path of the portal along the surface of the anterior humerus. The sheath is directed toward the center of the elbow joint, penetrating the brachioradialis, brachialis, and extensor carpi radialis muscles before passing through the joint capsule.
- Several studies have shown that the radial nerve-to-sheath distance averaged 9.9 to 14.2 mm in the 90-degree-flexed and distended elbow.[3,11] This represents a statistically significant increase in the distance from the nerve to the sheath compared to either the mid or the distal portal.
- The anterior branch of the posterior antebrachial cutaneous nerve averaged 6.1 mm from the portal, with the trocar in contact with the nerve 29% of the time.[11]
- The proximal anterolateral portal may be made before or after the anteromedial portal, and an outside-in method is most commonly recommended.
- Although the view of the anteromedial structures was similar for all three anterolateral portals, the proximal anterolateral portal was consistently described as providing a more extensive evaluation of the joint, particularly when viewing the radiocapitellar joint.[11,12,15]

Dual Anterolateral Portals

- When the ulnar nerve has been previously transposed into either a submuscular or subcutaneous position, the creation of an anterior medial portal may be done by palpating or dissecting the nerve prior to portal placement; however, at times, it will be safer and as effective to use two anterior lateral portals.
- The first portal is created in the midanterior lateral portal position as described earlier.
- A proximal anterolateral portal is then created after the midanterolateral portal is established and a 70-degree scope may be used to ensure portal entry position.

Single Portal Dual Cannula Anterolateral Portal

- Single portal dual cannula instrumentation will soon be available, allowing the creation of a single 7-mm portal with dual cannulas for the camera lens and the necessary instruments and shaver blades.
- A single portal dual cannula portal will avoid the need for dual anterolateral portals.

Posterior Portals

- Compared with the anterior portals, all posterior portals are relatively safe[11] (**TECH FIG 4A**).
- Laterally, the posterior antebrachial cutaneous nerve is at risk, and there are anecdotal reports of injury to the radial nerve branch to the anconeus muscle.
- The ulnar nerve is the closest major nerve to any posterior portal and has been described as no closer than 15 to 25 mm from the posterior central portal.[11]
  - This nerve is typically at risk only during posteromedial capsule resection for joint contracture release; however, even with safely performed perineural capsulectomy, recovery of flexion for patients with less than 110 degrees of preoperative elbow flexion still exposes the ulnar nerve to traction injury.
  - In this setting, nerve transposition is advised.
- The posterior portals may be established with the elbow between 45 and 90 degrees of flexion.[11,12]
  - Less flexion is recommended and is thought to decrease the tension in the posterior tissues, expand the olecranon fossa, and provide greater access to the medial and lateral recesses.

Posterior Central Portal

- The posterior central portal, also called the *straight posterior portal*, has been described by many authors and is usually located 2 to 4 cm proximal to the olecranon prominence and halfway between the medial and lateral condyles.
- This is commonly the initial posterior portal and provides good visualization of the olecranon fossa, the olecranon tip, the posterior trochlea, and the medial recess. The lateral recess, the central trochlea, and the radiocapitellar joint are less well seen.
- Although the ulnar nerve-to-sheath distance is consistently described as 15 mm or more,[11] the nerve should always be palpated and outlined before portal placement.
- Sharp dissection and sharp trocars are often discouraged when establishing anterior portals; however, a no. 11 blade may be used safely to create the posterior central portal and probably limits triceps tendon trauma.
  - An 18-gauge needle is first used to confirm the location of the fossa, and the blade is then directed toward the center of the fossa and in line with the tendon fibers.
  - For patients with arthrofibrosis, the portal may be more easily created with a sharp trocar.
- An intercondylar foramen is found in some patients, so caution is advised when establishing this portal.
  - Transhumeral access to the anterior compartment is possible through the foramen.
  - In patients without a foramen, a fenestration technique using a small-headed reamer is described for anterior access.
  - Use of the posterior central portal for anterior compartment visualization is recommended only for those well experienced in elbow arthroscopy, however.

Single Portal Dual Cannula Posterior Central Portal

- A single portal dual cannula portal will allow the management of posterior compartment pathology, such as posterior impingement, trochlea chondromalacia, and loose bodies, without the need to create a posterolateral portal.
- As the posterolateral portal is the most likely portal to drain and often slowest to close and become nontender,[4] avoiding the need for an posterolateral portal may allow the patient a more rapid return to unrestricted activities.

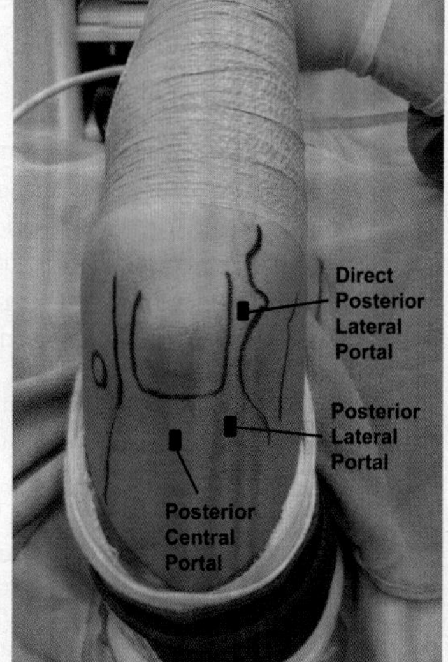

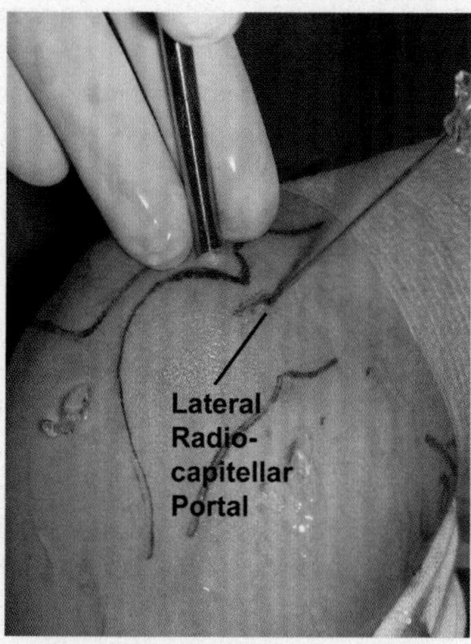

TECH FIG 4 • A. Posterior surface of the left elbow in the supine cross-body position. Locations of the posterior central, posterolateral, and direct posterolateral portals are shown. **B.** Posterolateral surface of the left elbow with the arthroscope in the direct posterolateral portal and an 18-gauge spinal needle being used to determine the appropriate location for the accessory direct radiocapitellar portal.

Posterolateral Portal

- Andrews and Carson[2] described the posterolateral portal as 3 cm proximal to the olecranon and through the lateral border of the triceps tendon.
- More distally, accessory portals may be safely placed anywhere between the proximal posterolateral portal and the soft spot.[1,12] The location of the portal is determined by the intended purpose.
  - For procedures performed in the posteromedial region of the elbow, a more proximal portal will provide greater access and visualization.
  - In contrast, a more distal portal will facilitate procedures confined to the posterolateral recess.
- An 18-gauge needle is used to confirm proper access to the olecranon fossa and the lateral gutter.
  - The scope is established in the olecranon fossa while remaining directly on the lateral column of the humerus to avoid capture of the posterior fat pad.
- When properly placed, this portal provides a clear view of the olecranon fossa, the olecranon tip, the posterior and central trochlea, the medial recess, the lateral recess, and the posterior radiocapitellar joint.
- A second, more proximal posterolateral portal may be used for a curved retractor when needed.

Direct Posterolateral Portal

- The direct posterolateral portal is typically the site used for joint inflation before anterior portal placement. The location is defined as the center of a triangle formed by the prominence of the lateral epicondyle, the prominence of the olecranon, and the radial head (see **TECH FIG 1**).
- Also known as the *midlateral portal*, the *dorsal lateral portal*, and more commonly, the *soft spot portal*, this portal penetrates the anconeus muscle and consistently provides the best view of the radiocapitellar joint.

Single Portal Dual Cannula Direct Posterolateral Portal

- A single portal dual cannula direct posterolateral portal can be used in place of any of the other described posterolateral portals and in some cases allow for elbow arthroscopy with just one portal.

Lateral Radiocapitellar Portal

- O'Driscoll and Morrey[9] described the standard midlateral portal, also called the *lateral radiocapitellar portal*, and noted that this portal is difficult to create because of limited space.
- This portal is best used when a very small mechanical shaver blade may be employed in the management of OCD capitellum lesions and radiocapitellar chondral injury.
- An 18-gauge needle is used to determine appropriate portal location (**TECH FIG 4B**).

Distal Posterolateral Portal

- van den Ende K et al[13] described a distal posterolateral portal called the *distal ulnar portal*.
- This portal provides a more direct perpendicular approach to either the capitellum surface or a capitellum osteochondral defect and is useful for microfracture chondroplasty, osteochondral fragment fixation, and osteochondral graft implantation.

PEARLS AND PITFALLS

Preparation	■ The surgeon should know the structural and neurovascular anatomy of the elbow well. ■ The surgeon should work within his or her experience and acknowledge his or her limitations. ■ A thoroughly considered surgical plan is mandatory.
Neurovascular risk	■ All bony landmarks and portal sites are outlined before starting. ■ Depth of all skin incisions is limited. ■ The elbow joint is maximally distended with fluid before creating the anterior portals. ■ The elbow is maintained at 90 degrees during anterior portal placement and capsular resection. ■ More proximal portal sites should be used for the anterior portals. ■ The location of the medial intermuscular septum must be confirmed, and the surgeon must remain anterior to it while creating the proximal anteromedial portal. ■ Retractors are used for visualization and protection during synovectomy and capsulectomy. ■ Suction is avoided during mechanical resection of the capsule. ■ Previous trauma or surgery may alter the location of neurovascular structures. ■ Ulnar nerve subluxation may reposition the nerve directly beneath the proximal medial portal. ■ Postoperative vascular compromise from either direct vascular injury or compartment syndrome is difficult to assess after regional anesthesia.
Fluid management and tissue swelling	■ The amount of fluid extravasation into the soft tissues is limited with an end-flow arthroscope sheath, low-pressure gravity inflow, and a forearm compression wrap.

POSTOPERATIVE CARE

- Wounds are routinely closed with simple sutures.
- Synovial–subcutaneous and synovial–cutaneous fistulas have been described and most commonly occur in the posterolateral portals along the lateral margin of the triceps tendon.[4]
  - Deep absorbable sutures placed in the fascia of the lateral triceps along with locking mattress sutures in the skin will minimize the risk for this complication.
- Unless contraindicated by the procedure performed, the elbow is splinted near full extension to minimize swelling.
- The arm is elevated overnight and the splint is removed the following day.
- Passive and active range-of-motion exercises are started as soon as the procedure performed will allow.
- For patients undergoing contracture release surgery, an axillary regional block is performed early the next day.
  - The elbow is gently taken through a full arc of motion and then placed into continuous passive motion.
- Based on the extent of the release, the amount of swelling, and the level of pain, the patient is hospitalized for 1 to 3 days.
- Postoperative static progressive range-of-motion braces and physical therapy are also used to recover motion.

COMPLICATIONS

- The incidence of neurologic complications after elbow arthroscopy has been reported to be 0% to 14%.[4]
  - Transient as well as incomplete and complete permanent nerve palsies, including iatrogenic nerve resection injuries, have also been described for the radial, ulnar, and median nerves.
- Kelly et al[4] retrospectively reviewed 473 consecutive arthroscopy procedures and found an overall complication rate of 7%.
  - Transient neurapraxia was the most common immediate minor complication and included radial nerve, ulnar nerve, posterior interosseous nerve, anterior interosseous nerve, and medial antebrachial cutaneous nerve palsies.
    - Risk factors include autoimmune disorder, contracture, capsulectomy, and possibly prolonged tourniquet time.
  - Prolonged clear or serous drainage from anterolateral and midlateral portal sites was the most common minor complication and was reported to occur in 5% of patients.
  - Deep infection occurred in 0.8% of patients; all the cases occurred in patients who had received intra-articular corticosteroids at the end of the procedure.
  - Mild postsurgical contracture occurred in 1.6% of patients.[1,4]

REFERENCES

1. Abboud JA, Ricchetti ET, Tjoumakaris F, et al. Elbow arthroscopy: basic setup and portal placement. J Am Acad Orthop Surg 2006;14:312–318.
2. Andrews JR, Carson WG. Arthroscopy of the elbow. Arthroscopy 1985;1:97–107.
3. Field LD, Altchek DW, Warren RF, et al. Arthroscopic anatomy of the lateral elbow: a comparison of three portals. Arthroscopy 1994;10:602–607.
4. Kelly EW, Morrey BF, O'Driscoll SW. Complications of elbow arthroscopy. J Bone Joint Surg Am 2001;83A:25–34.
5. Lindenfeld TN. Medial approach in elbow arthroscopy. Am J Sports Med 1990;18:413–417.
6. Lynch GJ, Myers JF, Whipple TL, et al. Neurovascular anatomy and elbow arthroscopy: inherent risks. Arthroscopy 1986;2:191–197.
7. Marshall PD, Fairclough JA, Johnson SR, et al. Avoiding nerve damage during elbow arthroscopy. J Bone Joint Surg Br 1993;75B:129–131.
8. Miller CD, Jobe CM, Wright MH. Neuroanatomy in elbow arthroscopy. J Shoulder Elbow Surg 1995;4:168–174.
9. O'Driscoll SW, Morrey BF. Arthroscopy of the elbow: diagnostic and therapeutic benefits and hazards. J Bone Joint Surg Am 1992;74A:84–94.
10. Poehling GG, Whipple TL, Sisco L, et al. Elbow arthroscopy, a new technique. Arthroscopy 1989;5:222–281.
11. Stothers K, Day B, Regan W. Arthroscopy of the elbow: anatomy, portal sites, and a description of the proximal lateral portal. Arthroscopy 1995;11:449–457.
12. Stothers K, Day B, Regan W. Arthroscopic anatomy of the elbow: an anatomical study and description of a new portal. Arthroscopy 1993;9:362–363.
13. van den Ende KI, McIntosh AL, Adams JE, et al. Osteochondritis dissecans of the capitellum: a review of the literature and a distal ulnar porta. Arthroscopy 2011;27(1):122–128.
14. Verhaar J, van Mameren H, Brandsma A. Risks of neurovascular injury in elbow arthroscopy: starting anteriomedially or anteriolaterally? Arthroscopy 1991;7:287–290.
15. Woods GW. Elbow arthroscopy. Clin Sports Med 1987;6:557–564.

Pediatric Elbow and Forearm Fractures and Dislocations

Closed Reduction and Percutaneous Pinning of Supracondylar Fractures of the Humerus

5 CHAPTER

Paul D. Choi and David L. Skaggs

DEFINITION

- Supracondylar fractures of the humerus are common injuries in children. As many as 67% of children hospitalized with elbow injuries have supracondylar fractures; supracondylar fractures of the humerus represent 3% to 17% of all childhood fractures.[7,10,11] The annual incidence of supracondylar fractures has been estimated at 177.3 per 100,000.[9]
- The peak age at fracture is 5 to 7 years.
- The cause of injury is most commonly trauma to the elbow, most often resulting from a fall from height (70%) or related to sports activities.
- Nearly all (98%) supracondylar fractures of the humerus are of the extension type.[1] Flexion-type injuries also occur.
- Open injuries occur in 1% of cases. Concurrent fractures, most commonly involving the distal radius, scaphoid, and proximal humerus, occur in 1% of cases. Associated neurovascular injuries can occur, with nerve injury existing in 11% of cases and vascular insufficiency present in up to 20% of cases.[1,2,10] Anterior interosseous nerve injury is the most common nerve injury associated with extension-type supracondylar fractures of the humerus.

ANATOMY

- The periosteum most commonly fails anteriorly with extension-type supracondylar fractures of the humerus.
  - With posteromedial displacement, the periosteum also fails laterally.
    - Therefore, with posteromedially displaced fractures, forearm pronation can aid in the reduction (**FIG 1**).
  - With posterolateral displacement, the periosteum also fails medially.
    - Forearm supination usually aids in the reduction of these posterolaterally displaced fractures.
- The direction of displacement has implications for which neurovascular structures are at risk from the penetrating injury of the proximal metaphyseal fragment (**FIG 2**).
  - Medial displacement of the distal fragment places the radial nerve at risk.
  - Lateral displacement of the distal fragment places the median nerve and brachial artery at risk.
- The ulnar nerve courses through the cubital tunnel posterior to the medial epicondyle. It is at particular risk with flexion-type fractures or when a medial pin is placed for fracture fixation.
  - The ulnar nerve subluxates anteriorly as the elbow is flexed. Therefore, the elbow should be relatively extended if a medial pin is placed for fracture fixation.

PATHOGENESIS

- Supracondylar fractures of the humerus generally occur as a result of a fall onto an outstretched hand with the elbow in full extension.
- The distal humerus is very thin at the supracondylar region, a critical factor in producing a consistent injury pattern and failure in the supracondylar humeral region.
  - During a fall with the elbow in full extension, the olecranon in its fossa acts as a fulcrum.
  - The capsule, as it inserts distal to the olecranon fossa and proximal to the physis, transmits an extension force to this region, resulting in failure and fracture.

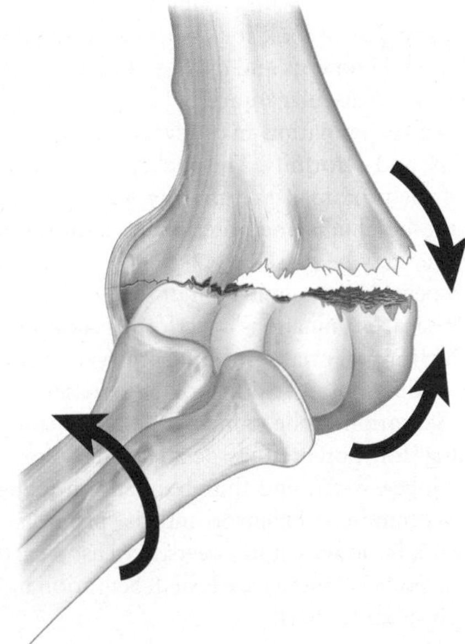

FIG 1 • Reduction of a posteromedially displaced supracondylar fracture of the humerus. Pronation of the forearm closes the hinge and aids in reduction.

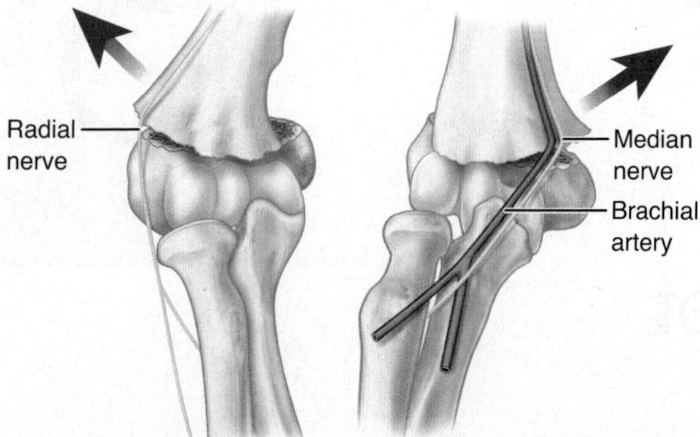

FIG 2 • Relationship to neurovascular structures. The proximal metaphyseal spike penetrates laterally with posteromedially displaced fractures and places the radial nerve at risk. With posterolaterally displaced fractures, the spike penetrates medially and places the median nerve and brachial artery at risk.

- With the elbow in full extension and the elbow becoming tightly interlocked, bending forces are concentrated in the distal humeral region.
- Increased ligamentous laxity, leading to hyperextension of the elbow, may be a contributing factor to this injury pattern.

NATURAL HISTORY

- The physis of the distal humerus contributes little to the overall growth of the humerus (20% of the humerus); therefore, the remodeling capacity of supracondylar fractures of the humerus is limited. Near-anatomic reduction of these fractures is important.
- The majority of supracondylar fractures of the humerus (other than extension type I fractures) are unstable; therefore, stabilization in the form of cast immobilization or, preferably, operative fixation is usually necessary.

PATIENT HISTORY AND PHYSICAL FINDINGS

- Evaluation of the child with an elbow injury must include an overall assessment to look for associated trauma (especially in the proximal humerus and distal radius regions) as well as associated neurovascular injury.
- The physical examination may reveal swelling, tenderness, ecchymosis, and deformity. The pucker sign, which occurs as a result of the proximal fracture fragment spike penetrating through the brachialis and anterior fascia into the subcutaneous tissue, may be present.
- Thorough neurologic examination of the involved extremity is critical. Physical examinations to perform include the following:
  - Assessing for potential associated injury to the ulnar nerve. Finger abduction and adduction (interossei) strength are tested. Sensation in the palmar little finger is tested.
  - Assessing for potential associated injury to the radial nerve. Finger, wrist, and thumb extension (extensor digitorum communis, extensor indicis proprius, extensor carpi radialis longus and brevis, extensor carpi ulnaris, extensor pollicis longus) are tested. Sensation in the dorsal first web space is tested.
  - Assessing for potential associated injury to the median nerve. Thenar strength (abductor pollicis brevis, flexor pollicis brevis, opponens pollicis) is tested. Sensation in the palmar index finger is tested.
  - Assessing for potential associated injury to the anterior interosseous nerve. Index distal interphalangeal flexion (flexor digitorum profundus index) and thumb interphalangeal flexion (flexor pollicis longus) are tested.
- Accurate vascular assessment of the involved extremity is also critical. Examinations to perform include the following:
  - Palpation of distal radial pulse
  - General evaluation of perfusion: capillary refill, skin temperature and color
  - The role of modalities like Doppler ultrasonography and pulse oximetry is still unclear.
  - Preoperative angiography is not usually warranted.

IMAGING AND OTHER DIAGNOSTIC STUDIES

- Initial imaging studies should include plain radiographs of the elbow—anteroposterior (AP), lateral, and sometimes oblique views.
- Comparison views of the contralateral elbow are sometimes helpful.
  - The fat pad sign, particularly posterior, represents an intra-articular effusion and can be associated with a supracondylar fracture of the humerus (53% of the time) (**FIG 3A**).[10]
  - On the AP view, the Baumann angle correlates with the carrying angle and should be 70 to 78 degrees or symmetric with the contralateral elbow (**FIG 3B**).
  - On the lateral view, the anterior humeral line (line drawn along the anterior aspect of the humerus) should intersect the capitellum (**FIG 3C**).
    - This line crosses the middle third of the capitellum in most healthy children older than 4 years.
    - In children younger than 4 years, this line may cross the anterior one-third of the capitellum.[1]
- The most commonly used classification system, the Gartland classification, is based on plain radiographic appearance:
  - Extension type I: nondisplaced
  - Extension type II: capitellum displaced posterior to anterior humeral line with variable amount of extension and angulation; posterior cortex of the humerus is intact
  - Extension type III: completely displaced with no cortex intact
  - A multidirectionally unstable type IV fracture has more recently been described. These fractures are unstable in both flexion and extension because of complete circumferential loss of a periosteal hinge.[1,10]
  - Flexion type

DIFFERENTIAL DIAGNOSIS

- Fracture of elbow (other than involving the supracondylar humeral region)
  - Salter-Harris fractures involving the elbow
- Nursemaid's elbow
- Infection

NONOPERATIVE MANAGEMENT

- Recent clinical practice guidelines by the American Academy of Orthopaedic Surgeons (AAOS) recommend nonsurgical immobilization of the injured limb for nondisplaced fractures (type I) meeting the following criteria[4,9]:
  - The anterior humeral line transects the capitellum on the lateral radiograph.

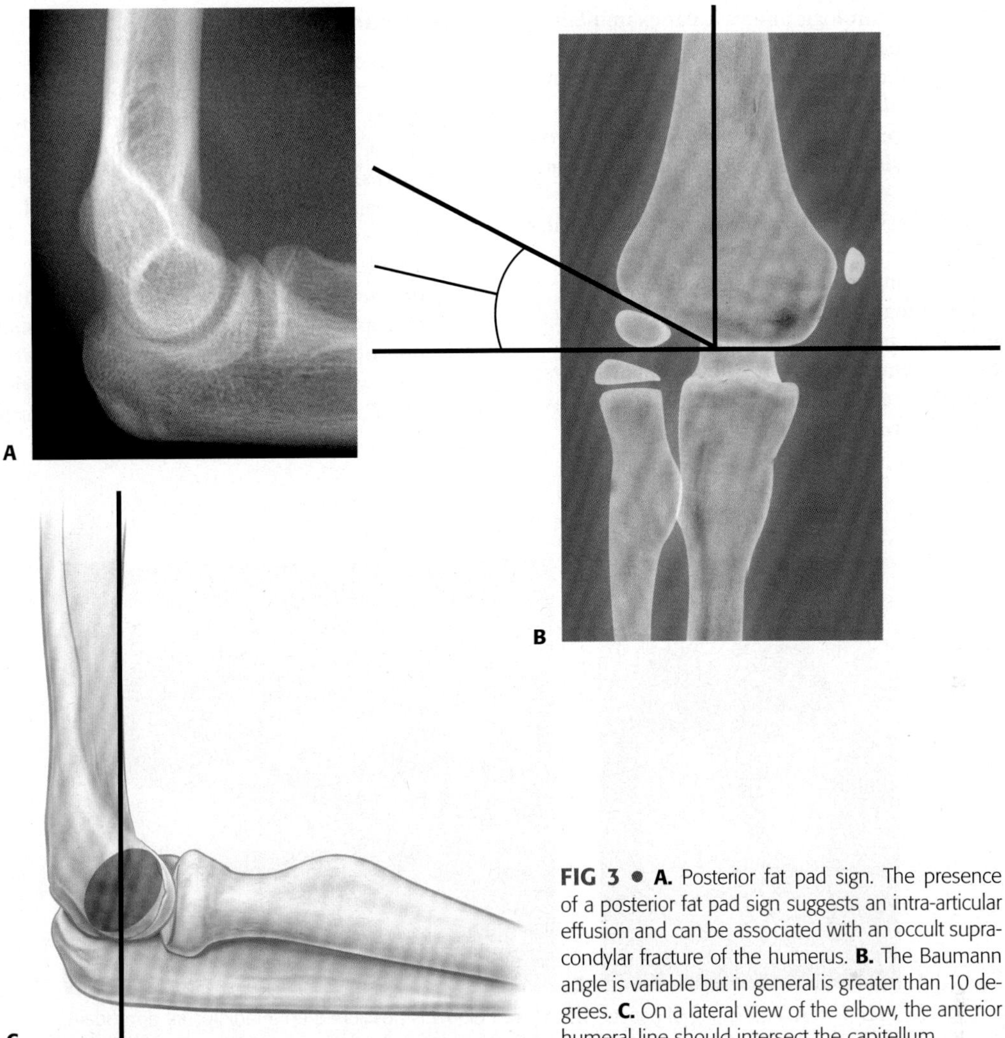

FIG 3 • **A.** Posterior fat pad sign. The presence of a posterior fat pad sign suggests an intra-articular effusion and can be associated with an occult supracondylar fracture of the humerus. **B.** The Baumann angle is variable but in general is greater than 10 degrees. **C.** On a lateral view of the elbow, the anterior humeral line should intersect the capitellum.

- The Baumann angle is greater than 10 degrees or equal to the other side.
- The olecranon fossa and medial and lateral cortices are intact.
- Nonoperative management consists of immobilization of the elbow in no more than 90 degrees of flexion in a splint or cast.
  - As the brachial artery becomes compressed with increasing flexion of the elbow, the clinician must ensure that the distal radial pulse is intact and that there is adequate perfusion distally.

SURGICAL MANAGEMENT

- Clinical practice guidelines by the AAOS advocate closed reduction and percutaneous pin fixation for most displaced supracondylar fractures of the humerus.[9]
- The two main options for percutaneous pin fixation are the lateral entry pin and crossed-pin techniques.
- Most fractures can be stabilized successfully by the lateral entry pin technique.[5,9,12]
  - Two pins are usually adequate for type II fractures; three pins are recommended for type III fractures.
- Biomechanical studies have revealed comparable stability in the lateral entry and crossed-pin techniques.
- An advantage of the lateral entry pin technique is the significantly lower risk of iatrogenic nerve injury. The ulnar nerve is at risk when pins are inserted medially (5% to 6% risk).
- The crossed-pin technique may be indicated if persistent instability is noted intraoperatively after placement of three lateral entry pins.

Preoperative Planning

- Displaced supracondylar fractures of the humerus (including Gartland type II and III) require reduction. Usually, reduction can be achieved by closed means. The preferred method for fixation is percutaneous pinning.
- Indications for open reduction of supracondylar fractures of the humerus are limited but include open injuries, fractures irreducible by closed means, and fractures associated with persistent vascular compromise even after adequate closed reduction.
  - One may consider open reduction and early antecubital fossa exploration in the setting of displaced supracondylar fractures of the humerus with vascular compromise and median nerve injury—as higher risk of nerve and/or vascular entrapment at the fracture site has been reported.[6]
- All imaging studies are reviewed. A high index of suspicion for associated fractures, especially of the forearm, is important; if present, there is an increased risk of compartment syndrome.

- Complete preoperative neurologic and vascular examination is performed and documented.
- The contralateral arm should be examined, and the carrying angle of the contralateral arm should be noted.
- The timing of surgery remains controversial. Recent retrospective evidence suggests that a delay in treatment of some supracondylar fractures may be acceptable.[1,3,8]
- Fractures with "red flags" usually require urgent treatment.
  - Significant swelling
  - Antecubital skin tenting, puckering, or ecchymosis
  - Neurologic or vascular compromise (except an isolated anterior interosseous nerve injury)
  - Concern for compartment syndrome (firm compartments, increasing analgesic requirements, increased anxiety, associated forearm fracture ["floating elbow"])

Positioning

- The patient is positioned supine on the operating room table.
- The fractured elbow is placed on a radiolucent arm board (**FIG 4A**). The arm should be far enough onto the arm board to allow for complete visualization of the elbow and distal humerus. In smaller children, the child's shoulder and head may need to rest on the arm board as well.
  - The wide end of a fluoroscopy unit is sometimes used as a table.
  - In cases of severe instability of the fracture, use of the fluoroscopy unit as an arm board is suboptimal because reduction of the fracture is frequently lost with rotation of the arm, which is needed for AP and lateral views of the elbow.
  - The fluoroscopy monitor is placed opposite to the surgeon for ease of viewing (**FIG 4B**).

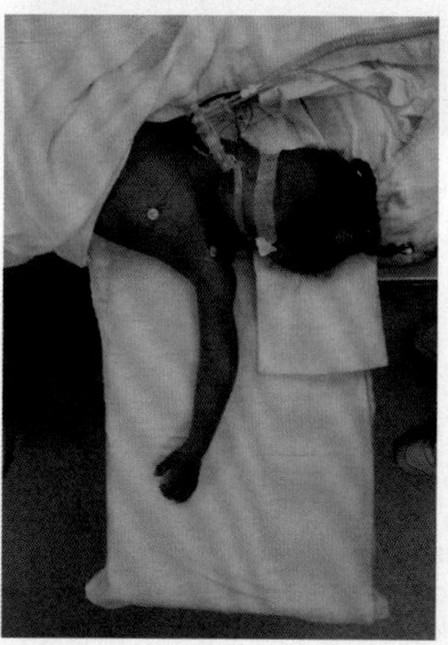

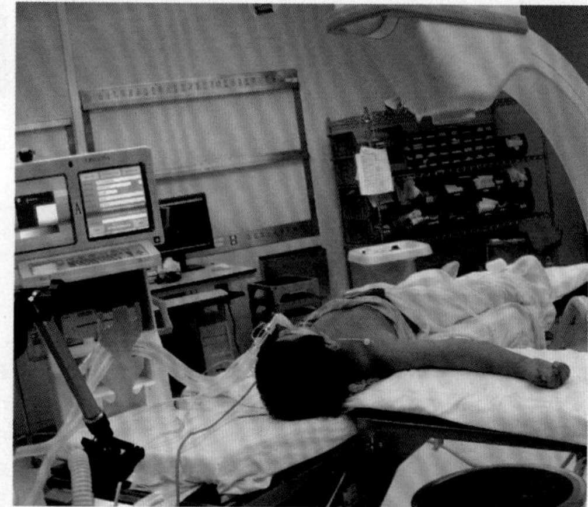

FIG 4 • A. Positioning of patient. The injured elbow is positioned on a radiolucent arm board. In smaller children, the child's shoulder and head may also need to rest on the arm board to allow full views of the elbow and distal humerus. **B.** Positioning the fluoroscopy monitor on the opposite side of the bed allows the surgeon to see the images easily while operating.

TECHNIQUES

Closed Reduction

- Traction is applied with the elbow in 20 to 30 degrees of flexion (**TECH FIG 1A**) to prevent tethering of the neurovascular structures over the anteriorly displaced proximal fragment.
- For severely displaced fractures, where the proximal fragment is entrapped in the brachialis muscle, the "milking maneuver" is performed (**TECH FIG 1B**).
  - The soft tissue overlying the fracture is manipulated in a proximal to distal direction.
- Once length is restored, the medial and lateral columns are realigned on the AP image.
  - Varus and valgus angular alignment is restored.
  - Medial and lateral translation is also corrected.
- For the majority of fractures (ie, extension type), the flexion reduction maneuver is performed next (**TECH FIG 1C**).
  - The elbow is gradually flexed while applying anteriorly directed pressure on the olecranon (and distal condyles of the humerus) with the thumbs.
- The elbow is held in hyperflexion as the reduction is assessed by fluoroscopy.
- Reduction is adequate if the following criteria are fulfilled:
  - The anterior humeral line crosses the capitellum.
  - The Baumann angle is greater than 10 degrees or comparable to the contralateral side.
  - Oblique views show intact medial and lateral columns.
- The forearm is held in pronation for posteromedial fractures.
- The forearm is held in supination for posterolateral fractures.
- For unstable fractures, the fluoroscopy machine instead of the arm is rotated to obtain lateral views of the elbow (**TECH FIG 1D**).

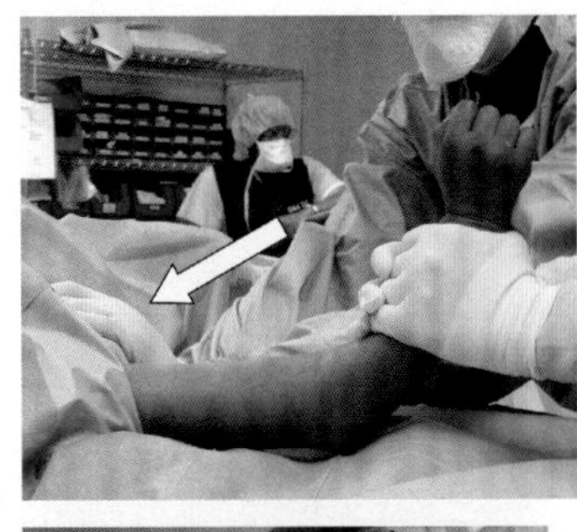

A

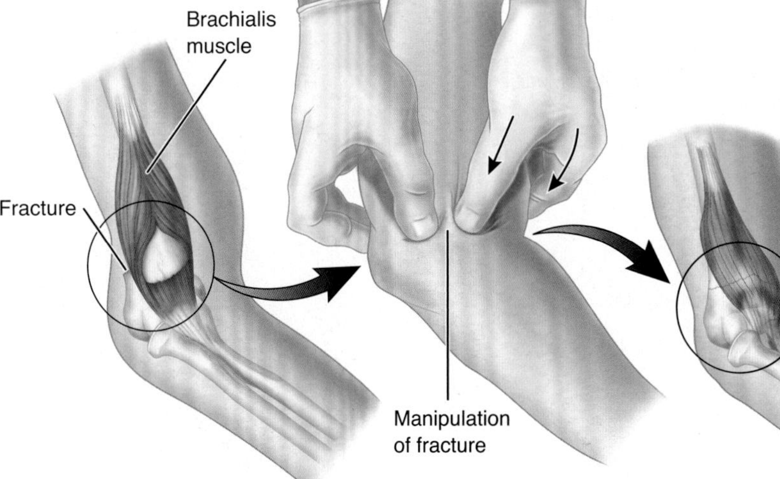

B

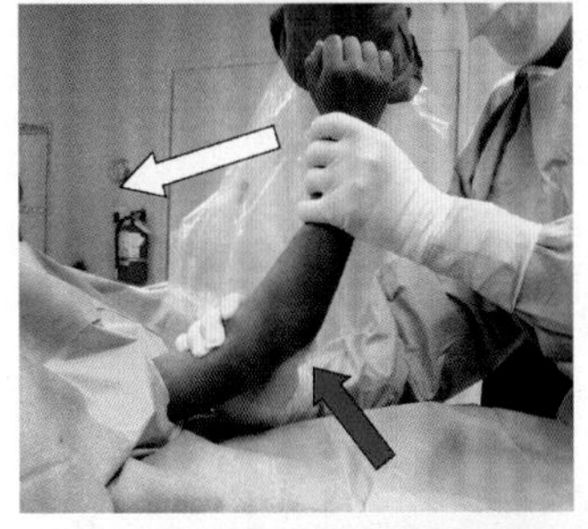

C

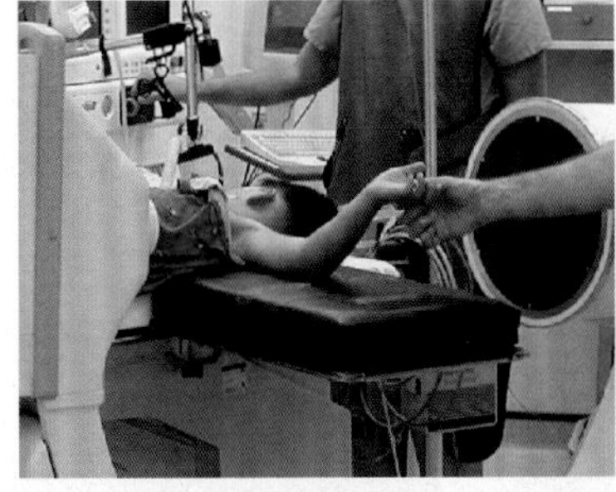

D

TECH FIG 1 • **A.** Reduction. Traction is applied with the elbow flexed 20 to 30 degrees. Countertraction should be provided by the assistant with pressure applied to the axilla. **B.** If the fracture is difficult to reduce, the proximal fracture fragment may be interposed in the brachialis muscle. The milking maneuver is performed to free the fracture from the overlying soft tissue. **C.** The elbow is flexed while pushing anteriorly on the olecranon with the thumbs. **D.** For unstable fractures, the fluoroscopy unit instead of the arm is rotated to obtain lateral views of the elbow.

Lateral Entry Pin Technique

- Once satisfactory reduction is obtained, K-wires can be inserted percutaneously for fracture stabilization.
  - A 0.062-inch smooth K-wires are commonly used.
  - Smaller or larger sizes may be used depending on the size of the child.
- The goals of the lateral entry pin technique are to maximally separate the pins at the fracture site and to engage both the medial and lateral columns (**TECH FIG 2A–C**).
  - The pins can be divergent or parallel.
  - Sufficient bone must be engaged in the proximal and distal fragments.
  - Pins may cross the olecranon fossa.
- As a general rule, two pins are adequate for type II fractures; three pins are recommended for type III fractures.
- The K-wire is positioned against the lateral condyle without piercing the skin (**TECH FIG 2D**).
  - The starting point is assessed under AP fluoroscopic guidance.
  - The K-wire is held freehand to allow maximum control.
- Once a satisfactory starting point and trajectory are confirmed, the K-wire is pushed through the skin and into the cartilage.
  - The cartilage of the distal lateral condyle functions as a pincushion.
- The starting point and trajectory are assessed by AP and lateral fluoroscopic guidance.
- When satisfactory starting point and trajectory are confirmed, the pin is advanced with a drill until at least two cortices are engaged.
- At this point, the reduction is again assessed.
  - The reduction must appear satisfactory on AP, lateral, and two oblique views.
  - The elbow is rotated to allow for oblique views of the medial and lateral columns.
- Additional pins are inserted (**TECH FIG 2E–H**).
- The elbow is stressed under live fluoroscopy in both the AP and lateral planes.
- Once satisfactory reduction and stability are confirmed, the vascular status is again assessed.
- Upon completion, the pins can be bent and cut approximately 1 to 2 cm off the skin.

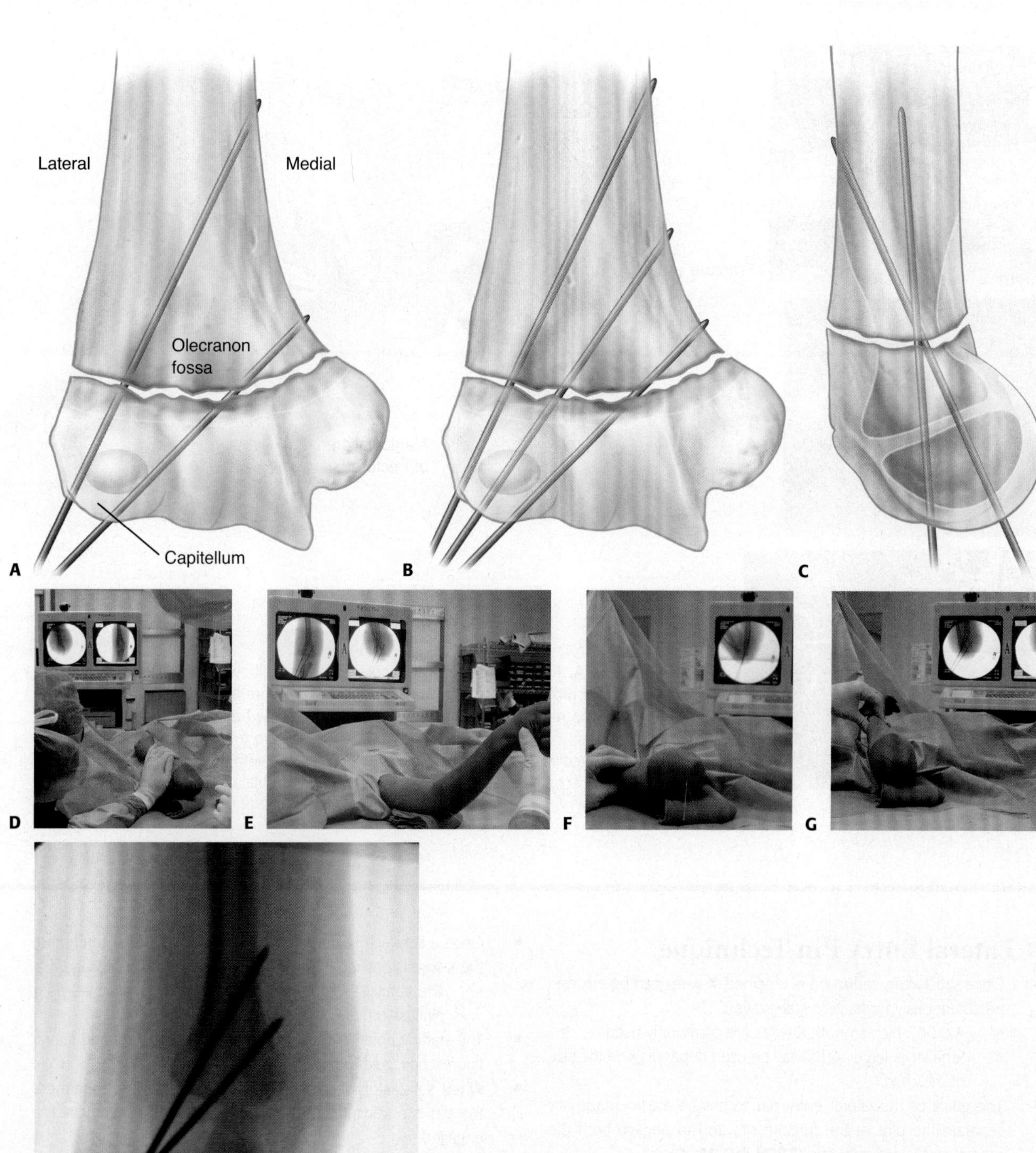

TECH FIG 2 • A–C. Lateral entry pin technique: optimal pin configuration. The pins are separated at the fracture site to engage the medial and lateral columns. **A.** Optimal pin configuration for two pins (AP view). **B.** Optimal pin configuration for three pins (AP view). **C.** Optimal pin configuration (lateral view). **D.** The pin is held freehand. Once starting point and trajectory are confirmed under fluoroscopic guidance, the pin is pushed through the skin and into the cartilage. **E,F.** Assessment of coronal alignment on AP and lateral views. **G.** Externally and internally rotated oblique views are used to assess the medial and lateral columns. **H.** Stress fracture. The elbow should be stressed under live fluoroscopy to confirm adequate stability.

Crossed-Pin Technique

- If satisfactory stability cannot be achieved by lateral entry pins or if the surgeon is more comfortable with lateral and medial entry pins, the crossed-pin technique can be performed.
- The lateral entry pins are inserted first: This will allow the elbow to be extended when placing the medial entry pins.
  - The ulnar nerve subluxates anteriorly with increasing flexion of the elbow; therefore, the ulnar nerve may be at risk when medial entry pins are placed with the elbow in 90 degrees or more of flexion.
- After insertion of the lateral entry pins, the elbow is extended to 20 to 30 degrees of flexion (**TECH FIG 3A**).
- A small incision is made over the medial epicondyle.
- Blunt dissection is performed down to the level of the medial epicondyle.
- A pin is positioned on the medial epicondyle (**TECH FIG 3B**).
- The starting position and trajectory are assessed under fluoroscopic guidance.
- When a satisfactory starting point and trajectory are confirmed, the pin is advanced with a drill until at least two cortices are engaged (**TECH FIG 3C,D**). The medial column should be engaged.
  - Ideally, the pin should be separated from the other pins maximally at the fracture site.
- The reduction and stability of the fracture are assessed just as with the lateral entry pin technique. The vascular status is similarly evaluated.

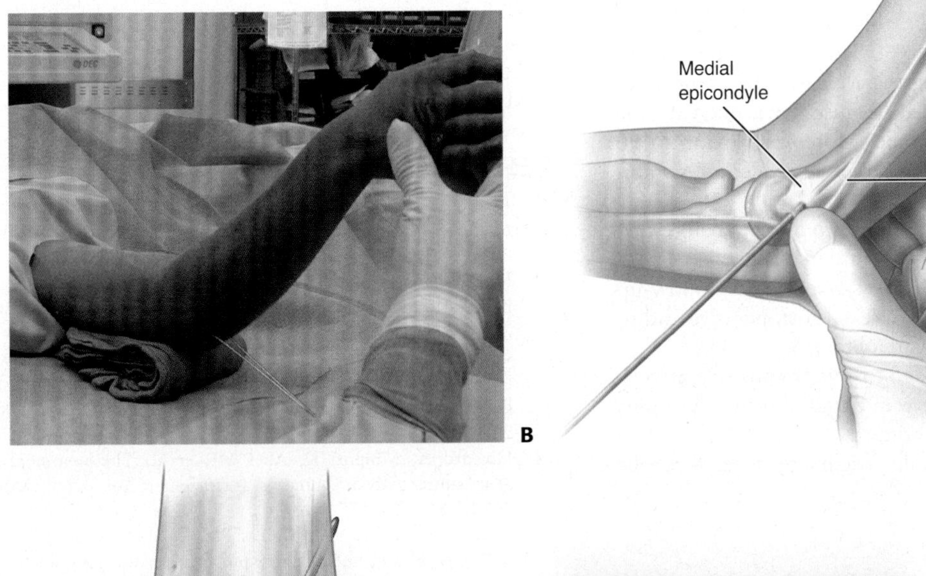

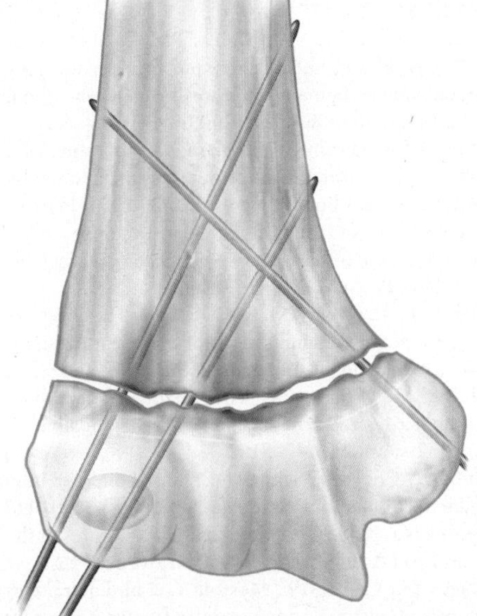

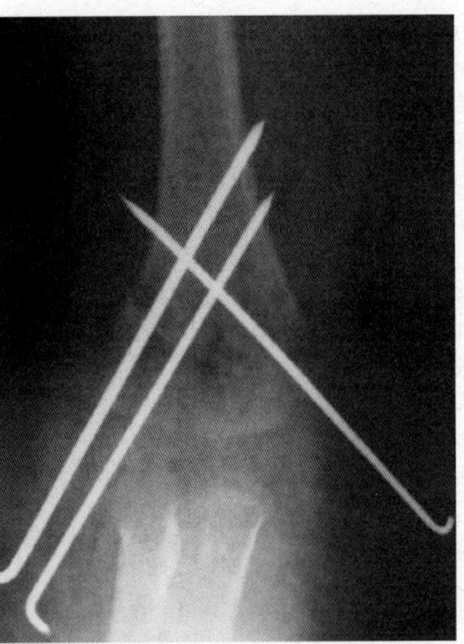

TECH FIG 3 • Crossed-pin technique. **A.** To minimize risk of iatrogenic injury to the ulnar nerve, the elbow is extended to 20 to 30 degrees of flexion before the pins are inserted medially. **B.** The starting point is on the medial epicondyle. **C,D.** The medial pin should engage the medial column and at least two cortices.

PEARLS AND PITFALLS

Clinical examination	▪ A thorough preoperative neurologic and vascular examination should be performed and documented. ▪ The surgeon should look for red flags such as ecchymosis, excessive swelling, puckering of skin, and associated fractures, which may be indications for an urgent reduction.
Indications	▪ Nondisplaced (type I) fractures can be treated nonoperatively with splint or cast immobilization. ▪ Fractures with medial comminution or impaction should be treated operatively to avoid cubitus varus. ▪ Displaced fractures require reduction (usually closed) and operative fixation (usually percutaneous pinning).
Reduction	▪ Traction is applied with the elbow in 20–30 degrees of flexion.
Lateral entry pin placement	▪ Maximal pin separation at the fracture site to engage the medial and lateral columns is the goal. ▪ For type II fractures, two pins are usually adequate; for type III fractures, additional fixation with a third pin is usually indicated.
Medial entry pin placement	▪ Lateral entry pins are inserted first so that the elbow can be extended to 20–30 degrees of flexion, allowing for safer insertion of medial entry pins.

POSTOPERATIVE CARE

- The arm is immobilized, preferably in a cast (sometimes a splint), with the elbow in 45 to 60 degrees of flexion.
  - Flexing the elbow to 90 degrees, as is used for most other casting, is not recommended because it will increase the risk of compartment syndrome. Moreover, flexion to 90 degrees is not needed since the fracture reduction is stabilized by the pins, not the cast.
  - Sterile foam may be directly applied to the skin before cast application to allow for postoperative swelling.
- The arm is immobilized for 3 to 4 weeks, with follow-up evaluations at 1 and 3 (or 4) weeks. Postoperative radiographs (AP and lateral views) are obtained.
- Pins are usually discontinued at 3 to 4 weeks postoperatively.
- Range-of-motion exercises are initiated shortly after pins and immobilization are discontinued.
- Return to full activity typically occurs by 6 to 8 weeks postoperatively.

OUTCOMES

- The AAOS has reported improved outcomes (radiographic, clinical, and functional) following closed reduction and percutaneous pin fixation of most displaced supracondylar fractures of the humerus (type 2, type 3, flexion).[4,9]
- Multiple studies have reported on the efficacy and high safety profile of the lateral entry pin technique.[4,5,9,12,13]
  - No significant difference in loss of reduction between lateral entry and crossed-pin techniques
  - No significant difference in radiographic outcome (Baumann angle, Baumann angle change)
  - Significantly lower risk of iatrogenic nerve injury (ulnar) with lateral entry technique
- Studies have suggested that treatment of some supracondylar fractures may be delayed without significant added risk in appropriately selected patients.[1,3,8]

COMPLICATIONS

- Elbow stiffness
- Infection
- Vascular injury
- Neurologic injury
- Malunion
- Nonunion
- Avascular necrosis
- Myositis ossificans

REFERENCES

1. Abzug JM, Herman MJ. Management of supracondylar humerus fractures in children: current concepts. J Am Acad Orthop Surg 2012;20(2):69–77.
2. Franklin CC, Skaggs DL. Approach to the pediatric supracondylar humeral fracture with neurovascular compromise. Instr Course Lect 2013;62:429–433.
3. Gupta N, Kay RM, Leitch K, et al. Effect of surgical delay on perioperative complications and need for open reduction in supracondylar humerus fractures in children. J Pediatr Orthop 2004;24(3):245–248.
4. Howard A, Mulpuri K, Abel MF, et al. The treatment of pediatric supracondylar humerus fractures. J Am Acad Orthop Surg 2012;20(5):320–327.
5. Kocher MS, Kasser JR, Waters PM, et al. Lateral entry compared with medial and lateral entry pin fixation for completely displaced supracondylar humeral fractures in children. A randomized clinical trial. J Bone Joint Surg Am 2007;89(4):706–712.
6. Mangat KS, Martin AG, Bache CE. The "pulseless pink" hand after supracondylar fracture of the humerus in children: the predictive value of nerve palsy. J Bone Joint Surg Br 2009;91(11):1521–1525.
7. Mangwani J, Nadarajah R, Paterson JM. Supracondylar humeral fractures in children: ten years' experience in a teaching hospital. J Bone Joint Surg Br 2006;88(3):362–365.
8. Mehlman CT, Strub WM, Roy DR, et al. The effect of surgical timing on the perioperative complications of treatment of supracondylar humeral fractures in children. J Bone Joint Surg Am 2001;83-A(3):323–327.
9. Mulpuri K, Wilkins K. The treatment of displaced supracondylar humerus fractures: evidence-based guideline. J Pediatr Orthop 2012;32(suppl 2):S143–S152.
10. Omid R, Choi PD, Skaggs DL. Supracondylar humeral fractures in children. J Bone Joint Surg Am 2008;90(5):1121–1132.
11. Otsuka NY, Kasser JR. Supracondylar fractures of the humerus in children. J Am Acad Orthop Surg 1997;5(1):19–26.
12. Skaggs DL, Cluck MW, Mostofi A, et al. Lateral-entry pin fixation in the management of supracondylar fractures in children. J Bone Joint Surg Am 2004;86-A(4):702–707.
13. Woratanarat P, Angsanuntsukh C, Rattanasiri S, et al. Meta-analysis of pinning in supracondylar fracture of the humerus in children. J Orthop Trauma 2012;26(1):48–53.

Open Reduction of Supracondylar Fractures of the Humerus

6 CHAPTER

Christine M. Goodbody and John M. Flynn

DEFINITION

- A supracondylar fracture that requires open reduction is one that cannot be treated with closed reduction and percutaneous pinning.

ANATOMY

- The neurovascular anatomy to consider for an open reduction includes the following:
  - The ulnar nerve passes behind the medial epicondyle.
  - The radial nerve courses from posterior to anterior just above the olecranon fossa.
  - The brachial artery and median nerve pass through the antecubital fossa and are often immediately subcutaneous anteriorly because of fracture displacement, putting them at risk during the skin incision.

PATIENT HISTORY AND PHYSICAL FINDINGS

- The patient history is the same for supracondylar fractures being treated by closed methods.
- A careful neurovascular examination must also be performed.

SURGICAL MANAGEMENT

- Indications for open treatment of a supracondylar fracture include an open fracture, a fracture that proves irreducible by closed techniques, and a compromised vascular supply to the hand that does not reconstitute with closed reduction.
- The timing for surgical intervention has been a matter of debate. Many surgeons believe that prompt reduction is optimal. Other studies show no significant increase in complication rates with delayed treatment.[2,3]

Preoperative Planning

- For children with a severe, potentially irreducible fracture, it is helpful to make a provisional attempt at fracture reduction immediately after the induction of anesthesia.
- After milking the fracture from its entrapment in the brachialis muscle, standard reduction maneuvers are performed to reduce the distal fragment into generally good alignment.
- Although time should not be spent perfecting the reduction (which will likely be lost during prepping and draping), this provisional reduction of severe fractures after induction can alert the surgical team that open reduction may be necessary, allowing time to gather equipment (such as a sterile tourniquet) and to obtain and place a radiolucent table to facilitate open reduction.

Positioning

- The patient is placed supine on the operating table. A hand table attachment is valuable when open reduction is needed.
- A sterile tourniquet is placed on the child's arm after preparation and draping.
- The surgeon should make sure that the portable image intensifier can be moved easily into and out of the operative field to assist with pinning of the fracture.

Approach

- In general, a transverse anterior incision through the antecubital fossa is the most useful and cosmetic.
- If more visualization is needed, this incision can be extended medially or laterally based on displacement, but this is rarely necessary.
- Extension of the incision on the opposite side of the displacement of the distal fragment allows for removal of soft tissue obstacles to reduction.
- If there is a suspicion of neurovascular compromise, the anterior approach provides the best extensile exposure to explore these structures.
- An inability to reduce the fracture may indicate that the proximal fragment has buttonholed through the brachialis muscle. Again, an anterior approach provides the most useful exposure to reduce this deformity.

■ Open Reduction through an Anterior Approach

Incision and Dissection

- Once the patient has been prepared and draped, the tourniquet is inflated.
- A transverse incision is made across the antecubital fossa (**TECH FIG 1A**). Care must be taken in dissecting, as the neurovascular bundle may be in a nonanatomic location–typically immediately subcutaneous and at risk for damage during the initial dissection (**TECH FIG 1B**).
- Dissection proceeds until the metaphyseal spike is encountered. It is often covered by a small amount of tissue and parts of the brachialis muscle that may be torn (**TECH FIG 1C**).
- It is at this point that the neurovascular bundle should be located, if it has not yet been identified. This usually involves dissecting across the anterior aspect of the metaphyseal spike. This step should not be omitted even if there is no vascular compromise. Once the vessels are identified, they should be retracted out of the field.

Fracture Reduction

- Defining the outline of the distal fragment can be the most challenging aspect of the procedure. It is usually posterior and lateral, and the periosteum is folded over its surface (**TECH FIG 2**).
- Reduction is obtained by reaching into the fracture site with a hemostat and getting hold of the cut edge of the periosteum. This cut edge is extended with scissors to increase the size of the buttonhole and to help free up the distal fragment. The distal fragment is then brought anteriorly and reduced to the shaft fragment, which is maneuvered back through the buttonhole into its resting position posterior to the brachialis muscle.
- Alternatively, the surgeon can hold his or her thumb on the proximal fragment and push downward while an assistant applies traction to the forearm with the elbow flexed at 90 degrees.[1] A periosteal elevator can be used as a lever to assist the reduction.

Pinning

- Once a reduction has been obtained, the fracture is fixed with smooth Kirschner wires. This is accomplished in the same manner as closed reduction with percutaneous pinning.
- Three divergent, lateral entry pins are placed as described in Chapter 5.

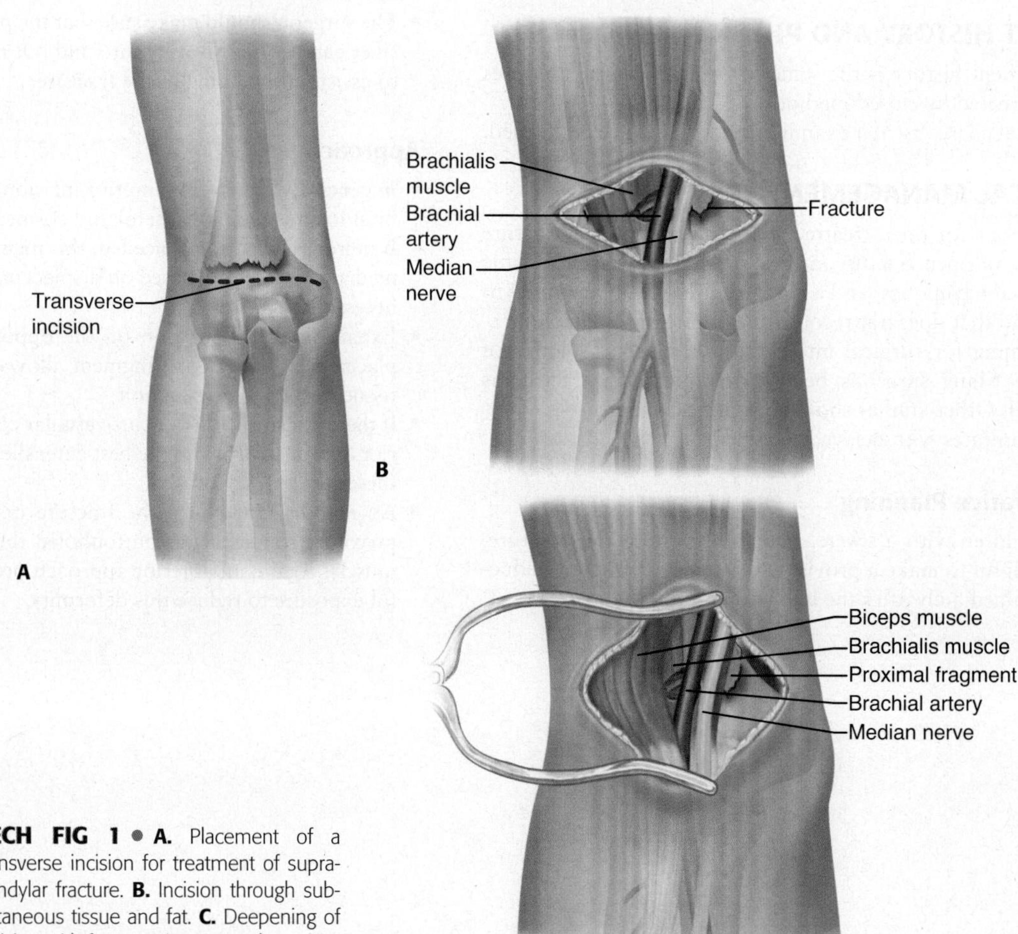

TECH FIG 1 • **A.** Placement of a transverse incision for treatment of supracondylar fracture. **B.** Incision through subcutaneous tissue and fat. **C.** Deepening of incision with fracture site exposed.

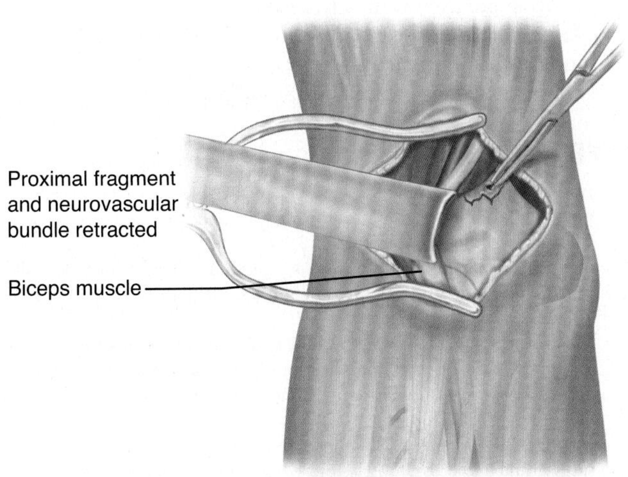

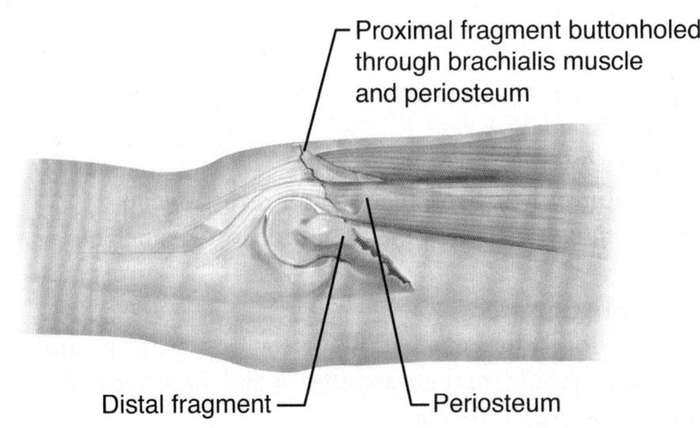

TECH FIG 2 • **A.** Proximal fragment is retracted to expose distal fragment. **B.** Sagittal view of fracture with proximal fragment shown buttonholing muscle and periosteum.

- Alternatively, a cross-pinning strategy can be used with medial and lateral entry pins. Ideally, both the medial and lateral pins should cross proximal to the fracture site. The surgeon must be sure to engage both the medial and lateral columns of the distal fragment.
- The surgeon checks pin placement and reduction with fluoroscopy. If acceptable, the pins are bent, cut, and left out of the skin. Once healed, they can easily be removed in the office.
- The incision is closed with absorbable sutures.

PEARLS AND PITFALLS

Indications	▪ The primary indications for an open reduction are interposed tissue in the fracture site preventing closed reduction and vascular compromise that does not improve with closed reduction and percutaneous pinning.
Neurovascular structures	▪ The neurovascular bundle can be located anywhere within the operative field and must be identified even if there is no suspicion of compromise.
Reduction of the fracture	▪ The distal fragment often can be palpated but not seen, as it is hidden by the overlying periosteum. The surgeon should expand the buttonhole through the periosteum for better visualization.
Fracture pinning	▪ Pins should be maximally separated at the fracture site if three lateral pins are used. Convergent pins are not stable. If medial and lateral pins are used, the surgeon should engage the medial and lateral columns of the distal fragment.

POSTOPERATIVE CARE

- Sterile dressings are applied over the incision.
- A strip of Xeroform dressing is wrapped around the pins, followed by soft dressings.
- The elbow is splinted in 60 to 90 degrees of flexion with a neutral forearm.
- The patient is admitted overnight for observation. Often, a long-arm cast can be placed safely the next day, with the arm flexed about 80 degrees. This cast can be maintained until the pins are removed 3 or 4 weeks after surgery.
  - Supracondylar fractures in children reliably heal in 3 weeks, but when open reduction is used, healing may be delayed by an additional week. It is wise to get an x-ray with the cast off but the pins still in at 3 weeks after injury. If the fracture is not completely healed, cast protection for an additional week is recommended.
- The patient can then be placed back into a sling and started on gentle range-of-motion exercises out of the sling for another 2 weeks.
- The child can then start to use the arm normally.
- Formal physical therapy is usually not necessary.

OUTCOMES

- It is generally agreed that prompt attention to reduction and stabilization of supracondylar fractures results in better outcomes and fewer complications.[4,5]
- Postoperative loss of reduction is uncommon.[7] However, children with supracondylar fractures that have been treated with open reduction generally take longer to regain their elbow motion than children treated with closed pinning. Families should be advised about this longer period of elbow stiffness in the immediate postoperative period.
- A 2001 study of 862 supracondylar fractures, 65 of which were treated with open reduction, found 55% excellent results, 24% good results, 9% fair results, and 12% poor results 5.8 months after injury in those treated with open reduction.[6]

COMPLICATIONS

- Complications can result from the injury itself or from surgery.
- The risk of infection is decreased with the use of perioperative antibiotics.
- Iatrogenic neurovascular injury
  - Identification of neurovascular structures is crucial.
  - The ulnar nerve is susceptible to injury if a medial pin is used.
- Compartment syndrome
  - The child should be kept overnight for observation, and the surgeon should make sure that serial neurovascular examinations are performed.
  - The first sign of compartment syndrome in a child is usually increased pain or increased pain medication requirements.
  - The children most at risk are those who had compromised blood flow to the hand immediately after injury.
  - Children who have compartment syndrome in the setting of a median nerve injury often do not complain of pain because of the sensory deficit.
- Loss of motion
  - Although rare, some loss of full extension has been reported.
  - If there is excessive posterior angulation at the time of healing, some loss of full flexion can occur.
- Cubitus valgus and cubitus varus
  - Varus angulation is mostly cosmetic.
  - Valgus deformity can cause loss of full elbow extension and can result in tardy ulnar nerve palsy.
- Myositis ossificans is rare and should resolve in 1 to 2 years.

REFERENCES

1. Ay S, Akinci M, Kamiloglu S, et al. Open reduction of displaced supracondylar humeral fractures through the anterior cubital approach. J Pediatr Orthop 2005;25:149–153.
2. Leet AI, Frisancho J, Ebramzadeh E. Delayed treatment of type 3 supracondylar humerus fractures in children. J Pediatr Orthop 2002;22: 203–207.
3. Mehlman CT, Strub WM, Roy DR, et al. The effect of surgical timing on the perioperative complications of treatment of supracondylar humeral fractures in children. J Bone Joint Surg Am 2001;83-A(3): 323–327.
4. Morrisy RT, Weinstein SL. Open reduction of supracondylar fractures of the humerus. In: Atlas of Pediatric Orthopaedic Surgery, ed 3. Philadelphia: Lippincott Williams & Wilkins, 2001:63–67.
5. Otsuka NY, Kasser JR. Supracondylar fractures of the humerus in children. J Am Acad Orthop Surg 1997;5:19–26.
6. Reitman RD, Waters P, Millis M. Open reduction and internal fixation for supracondylar humerus fractures in children. J Pediatr Orthop 2001;21:157–161.
7. Sankar WN, Hebela NM, Skaggs DL, et al. Loss of pin fixation in displaced supracondylar humeral fractures in children: causes and prevention. J Bone Joint Surg Am 2007;89(4):713–717.

Open Reduction and Internal Fixation of Fractures of the Medial Epicondyle

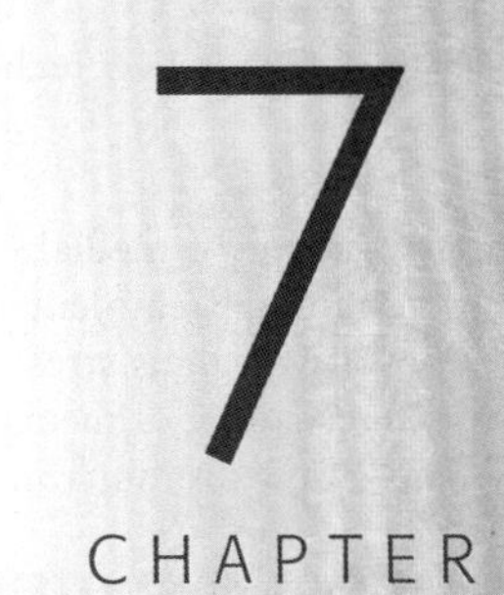

Brian G. Smith and Kristan A. Pierz

DEFINITION

- Trauma to the medial aspect of the elbow may cause a medial epicondyle fracture, which is an injury to the apophysis of the medial epicondyle.

ANATOMY

- Medial epicondylar fractures involve the medial epicondylar apophysis on the posteromedial aspect of the elbow.
- The flexor–pronator muscle mass arises from this apophysis, including the palmaris longus, the flexor carpi ulnaris and radialis, the flexor digitorum superficialis, and one part of the pronator teres and the ulnar collateral ligament (**FIG 1**).[3]

PATHOGENESIS

- A direct blow to the medial aspect of the elbow may cause a fracture to the medial epicondyle, but this is rare.
- More commonly, a fall on an outstretched arm causes an avulsion of the medical epicondyle via tension generated by stretch of the muscles attaching to it. Elbow dislocation is frequently associated with a medial epicondyle fracture and may occur with spontaneous reduction at the time of the injury (**FIG 2**).
- Considerable force applied to the arm may cause elbow dislocation and associated disruption of the ulnar collateral ligament. This ligament, the principal stabilizing ligament of the elbow, can avulse the medial epicondyle, and the apophyseal fragment may sometimes become lodged in the elbow joint.[3]
- Overuse may cause a chronic stress-type injury or an apophysitis, an example of which would be Little League elbow.

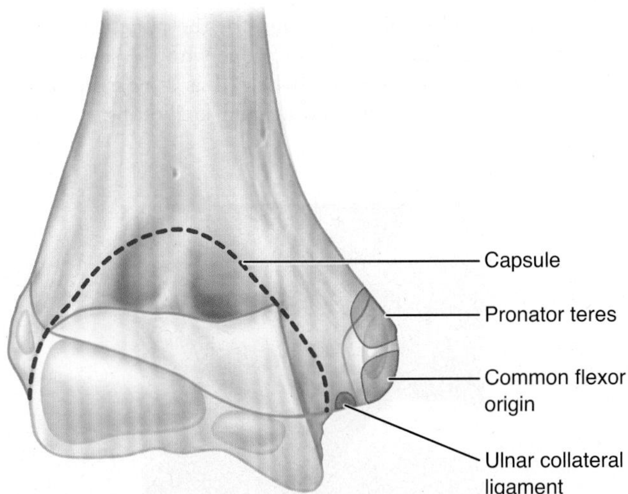

FIG 1 • Anatomic landmarks and site of muscle and ligament attachments on medial epicondyle.

NATURAL HISTORY

- The outcome of medial epicondyle fractures is related to the amount of fracture displacement and also the demands placed on the elbow by the patient.
- Minimally displaced fractures treated nonoperatively generally do well, especially if the patient is not an athlete or if the fracture involves the patient's nondominant arm.
- Untreated displaced fractures may lead to chronic medial elbow instability and even recurrent elbow dislocations.
  - Throwing athletes may have significant impairment in their sports activities.[9]

PATIENT HISTORY AND PHYSICAL FINDINGS

- For any elbow injury, the mechanism of injury should be sought, with particular attention to the details of a fall. In children, this may be difficult to elicit, but often, a witness may be available. Medial epicondyle fractures frequently arise from a fall.
- The two most important issues in the physical examination are to document neurovascular status and to assess for elbow stability. Determination of stability includes determination of whether the elbow is dislocated, which can be assessed clinically and confirmed radiographically.

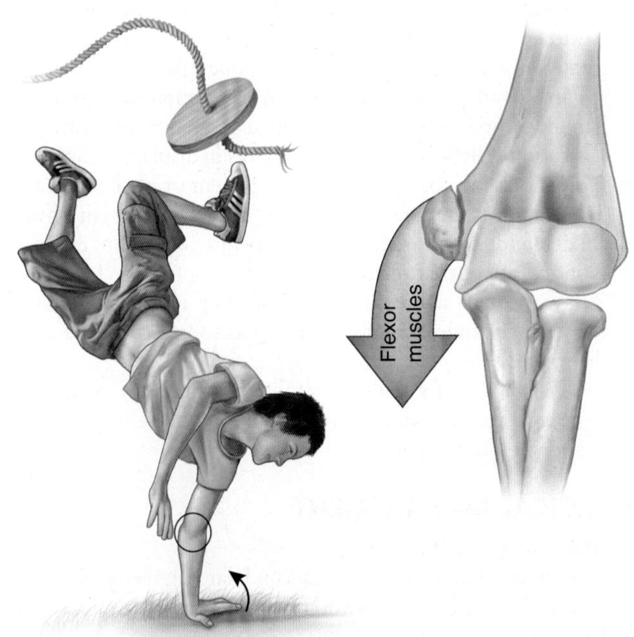

FIG 2 • A common mechanism of injury: a fall on an outstretched arm causing either a "pull-off" or a "push-off" avulsion of the medial epicondyle.

- Assessment of medial elbow stability is often important in determining treatment.
- A positive valgus stress test confirms medial elbow instability. Persistence of medial elbow instability may cause significant elbow disability in athletes or those doing heavy labor.

IMAGING AND OTHER DIAGNOSTIC STUDIES

- Standard anteroposterior (AP) and lateral radiographs of the elbow are required, but oblique views are often helpful to visualize the medial epicondyle, which is on the posteromedial aspect of the distal humerus.
- Widening of the apophysis may be the only sign of injury, so comparison views of the unaffected elbow are often helpful to assess and determine subtle degrees of displacement.
- If there is radiographic absence of the medial epicondyle and suspected joint incarceration, an arthrogram, computed tomography (CT) scan, or magnetic resonance imaging (MRI) may occasionally be needed.

DIFFERENTIAL DIAGNOSIS

- Medial condylar fractures
- Supracondylar fractures
- Elbow dislocation

NONOPERATIVE MANAGEMENT

- Smith in 1950 became a strong advocate of nonoperative management of this injury, pointing out that the fracture involved an apophysis rather than a physis and thus future growth was not compromised. He also documented that imperfect reduction or even nonunion was not automatically associated with a poor outcome in terms of elbow function and strength.[3]
- A more recent study from Sweden where all patients were treated nonoperatively showed 96% good to excellent results. Over 60% of the patients had a fibrous union or nonunion.[3]
- Two studies have compared nonoperative and operative treatment. Bede and associates[1] found that nonoperative treatment had better outcomes than operative treatment.
  - Farsetti and coworkers[5] demonstrated similar results of nonoperative treatment and open reduction and internal fixation (ORIF) with Kirschner wires in displaced fractures.
- Indications for nonoperative management of medial epicondyle fractures include patients who do not place high physical demands on their elbows and most nondominant elbows.
- Nonoperative treatment encompasses splinting for 5 to 7 days or until acute soft tissue swelling resolves and then early active range of motion starting as soon as possible after the injury.
  - Physical therapy may be required if range of motion is slow to return, but passive stretch may cause more injury and should be avoided.

SURGICAL MANAGEMENT

- Absolute indications
  - Incarceration of the medical epicondylar fragment in the joint
  - Associated elbow dislocation with ulnar nerve dysfunction
- Relative indications
  - Elbow dislocation in a high-demand patient
  - A displaced fracture with medial elbow instability in a high-demand patient

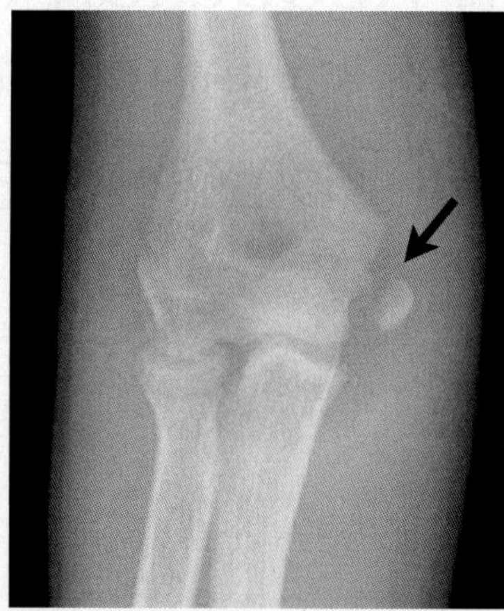

FIG 3 • Injury film. The medial epicondylar fragment is displaced and located in the joint.

PREOPERATIVE PLANNING

- Careful review of radiographs is done to assess the elbow joint for reduction and to assess the amount of displacement of the medical epicondylar fracture (**FIG 3**). Recent research indicates plain radiography may underestimate the actual displacement of medical epicondyle fractures based on imaging by CT scans.[4]
- A complete assessment of neurovascular status of the upper extremity is performed, with particular attention to the ulnar nerve examination.
- A valgus stress test is performed to assess for medial elbow instability, typically under sedation or anesthesia.

Positioning

- The patient is placed supine on the operating table with the arm abducted 90 degrees at the shoulder and placed on a radiolucent hand table. The arm is externally rotated such that the medial aspect of the elbow is accessible (**FIG 4**).
- Alternatively, a C-arm image intensifier base may serve as the operating table for a smaller child or based on the surgeon's preference.
- The surgeon should be positioned in the patient's axilla for surgery.
  - Another option for positioning for the patient has been proposed: Placing the patient prone with the shoulder internally rotated has been advocated as a means of relaxing the flexor–pronator group and facilitating reduction of the fracture.[6]

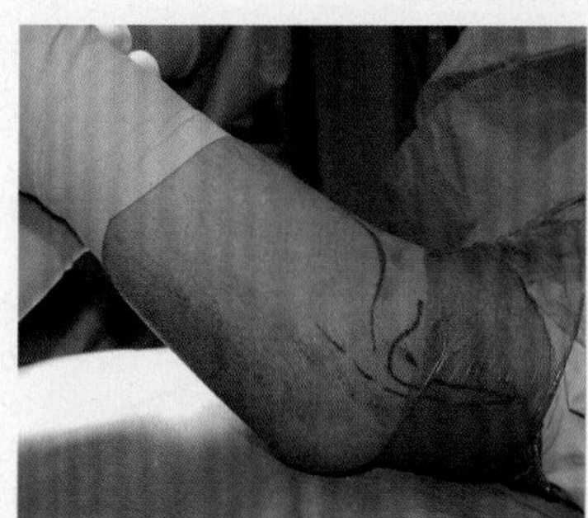

FIG 4 • Arm positioning and approach to the medial epicondyle, with the ulnar nerve course marked out.

Open Reduction and Internal Fixation with Cannulated Screw

- A skin incision about 4 cm long is made centered over the medial epicondyle after exsanguination of the limb and inflation of a tourniquet on the upper arm (**TECH FIG 1A**). Often with displaced injuries, the fractured fragment is just subcutaneous and little dissection is required.
- The ulnar nerve should be identified and carefully protected. Most experts do not recommend routine mobilization or transposition of the nerve.
- The fracture is identified, and any organized hematoma is removed (**TECH FIG 1B**).
- The fracture is reduced with a towel clip. Elbow flexion, forearm pronation, and wrist flexion aid in reducing the fracture.
- Some surgeons suggest curettage of the apophyseal cartilage to expedite healing of the fracture, which may persist as a healed apophysis if this is not done. This tip may be especially advantageous in the throwing athlete who is eager to return to sports as soon as possible.
- The fracture is stabilized with one or two guide pins from the 4.0-mm cannulated screw set. An 18-gauge needle may even be used as the second pin.[7]
- An alternative method of placing the pin is to drill from the inside of the medial epicondyle fracture fragment out, cut the pin to achieve a beveled edge at the fracture margin, and use it as a joystick to help reduce the fragment back to the humeral metaphysis and drill it into place.[7] Some surgeons will even predrill the metaphyseal side of the humerus to make fracture reduction easier.
- Radiographs are checked to assess reduction and pin placement.
- The pin selected for overdrilling should not be in the olecranon fossa. The second pin provides rotational stability of the fragment during drilling and screw placement.
- An appropriate-length screw is selected and inserted over the guide pin, stabilizing the fracture.
  - A washer may be used to provide a wide surface area of fixation and prevent screw head migration.
- AP and lateral intraoperative radiographs should confirm reduction and screw placement position (**TECH FIG 1C–G**).
- Elbow stability should be checked and full range of motion confirmed before closure.
- Standard skin closure is carried out, and the arm is splinted or casted at 90 degrees of elbow flexion.

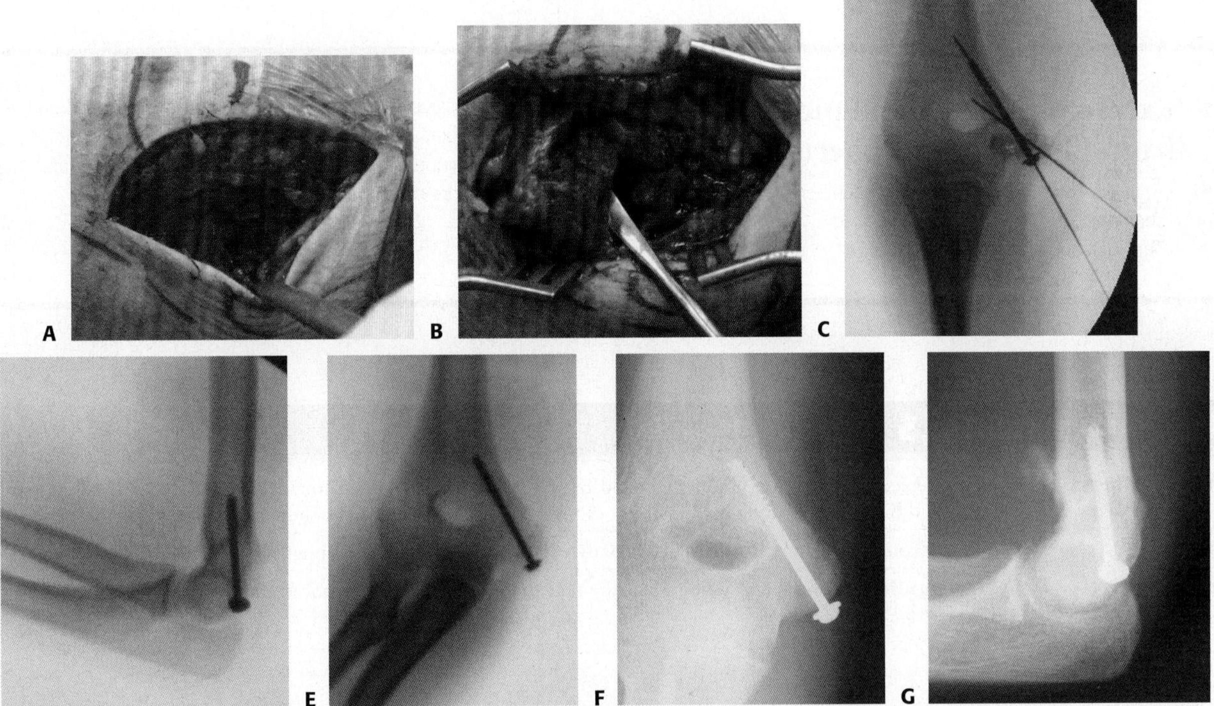

TECH FIG 1 • **A.** Incision with ulnar nerve identified. **B.** The fracture fragment is mobilized. **C.** Fluoroscopic image showing two pins spanning the fracture fragment for rotational stability. **D,E.** Cannulated screw fixation shown fluoroscopically. **F,G.** Radiographs showing healed fracture. Heterotopic bone formation anteriorly can be seen on the lateral radiograph.

Suture or K-Wire Fixation

- Should the fracture cause comminution of the medial epicondyle, repair with sutures may be warranted in a high-demand patient or one with medial instability.
- This would involve sutures placed directly in the tendinous tissue and secured to the periosteum adjacent to the bed from which the epicondyle was avulsed.
- K-wires may be used as a means of fixation in the presence of comminution or if the epicondyle fragment is too small for a screw (**TECH FIG 2**).

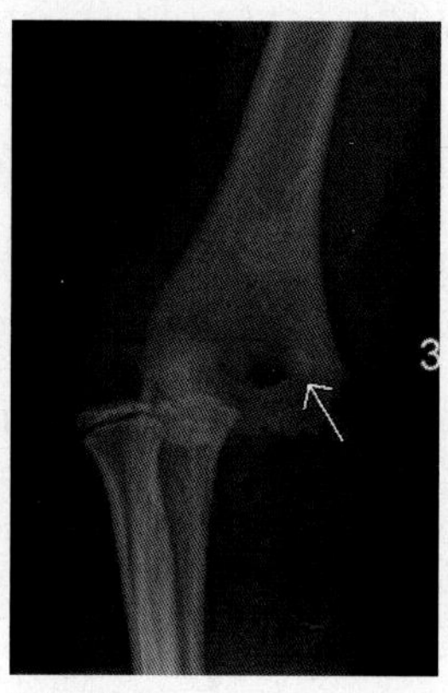
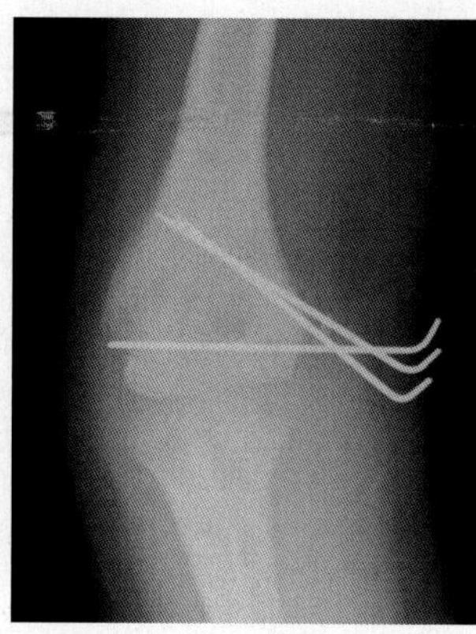
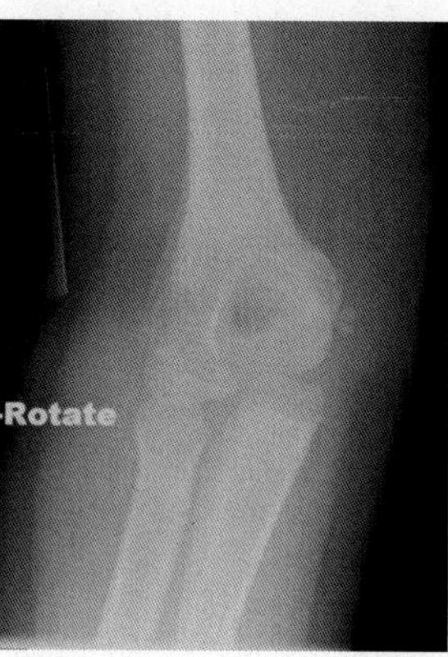

TECH FIG 2 • A. AP radiograph of an almost 8-year-old boy with an elbow fracture-dislocation and a displaced medial epicondyle fracture; *arrow* identifies the fracture fragment. **B.** Because of the small size of the fragment, K-wire fixation was selected to stabilize the fracture fragment. **C.** Follow-up radiograph at 7 weeks postoperatively. (Courtesy of Felicity Fishman, MD.)

Extraction of Medial Epicondyle from Elbow Joint: Roberts Technique

- A valgus stress is applied to the elbow with the forearm supinated.
- The wrist and fingers are dorsiflexed.
- As the position is reached, the fragment should be dislodged from the joint.
- This technique is most effective in the first 24 hours after the injury, before much muscle spasm occurs.[3]

PEARLS AND PITFALLS

Postoperative stiffness	■ Medial epicondyle fracture fragment should be fixed with a cannulated screw if possible rather than pins to have rigid fixation permitting early motion. Elbow motion is encouraged as soon as possible.
Recognition	■ The surgeon must beware of a medial epicondyle that is absent on radiography: It may be trapped in the joint.
Loss of extension	■ The surgeon must document radiographically that the internal fixation is not in the olecranon fossa, where it may block elbow extension.

POSTOPERATIVE CARE

- Postoperative management after open reduction of medial epicondyle fractures depends on the type and stability of the fixation of the epicondylar fragment.
- For ORIF with screws, initial splinting for 3 to 5 days in about 50 to 60 degrees of flexion is recommended, followed by early active range of motion.
- Some authors recommend a removable brace preventing valgus stress but permitting full flexion and extension for 4 weeks.[2]
- In one recent series on young athletes with this injury repaired with screw fixation, active range of motion out of the brace continued from weeks 5 to 8 postoperatively. At 8 weeks, noncontact sports were allowed, and return to full activity was possible at 12 weeks after surgery.[2]

OUTCOMES

- Eight adolescent athletes undergoing ORIF with screw fixation for this fracture had excellent results with no residual valgus instability and full return to all sports. One patient had a loss of 5 degrees of hyperextension, but all other patients had recovery of full range of motion.[2]
- In another series, 21 of 23 patients treated operatively had recovery of full movement, whereas only 14 of 20 patients treated nonoperatively had full range of motion.[10]
- A recent series of operative treatment and early motion in 25 patients with displaced fractures showed good to excellent results in all patients.[9]
- Similarly, another study of competitive athletes found excellent results in 20 patients, 6 treated nonoperatively and 14 operatively. All overhead athletes were able to return to their sport.[7,8]

COMPLICATIONS

- Failure to diagnose joint entrapment of the medial epicondyle fracture
- Ulnar nerve dysfunction
- Loss of range of motion
- Nonunion
- Myositis ossificans

REFERENCES

1. Bede WB, Lefebvre AR, Rosman MA. Fractures of the medial humeral epicondyle in children. Can J Surg 1975;18:137–142.
2. Case SL, Hennrikus WL. Surgical treatment of displaced medial epicondyle fractures in adolescent athletes. Am J Sports Med 1997;25: 682–686.
3. Chambers HG, Wilkins KE. Medial apophyseal fractures. In: Rockwood CA, Wilkins KE, Beaty JH, eds. Fractures in Children, ed 6. Philadelphia: Lippincott-Raven, 1996:800–819.
4. Edmonds EW. How displaced are "nondisplaced" fractures of the medial humeral epicondyle in children? Results of a three-dimensional computed tomography analysis. J Bone Joint Surg Am 2010;92(17):2785–2791.
5. Farsetti P, Potenza V, Caterini R, et al. Long-term results of treatment of fractures of the medial humeral epicondyle in children. J Bone Joint Surg Am 2001;83-A(9):1299–1305.
6. Glotzbecker MP, Shore B, Matheney T, et al. Alternative technique for open reduction and fixation of displaced pediatric medial epicondyle fractures. J Child Orthop 2012;6:105–109.
7. Gottschalk HP, Eisner E, Hosalkar, HS. Medial epicondyle fractures in the pediatric population. J Am Acad Orthop Surg 2012;20:223–232.
8. Lawrence JT, Patel NM, Macknin MD, et al. Return to competitive sports after medial epicondyle fractures in adolescent athletes. Am J Sports Med 2013;41:1152–1157.
9. Lee HH, Shen HC, Chang JH, et al. Operative treatment of displaced medial epicondyle fractures in children and adolescents. J Shoulder Elbow Surg 2005;14:178–185.
10. Wilson NI, Ingram R, Rymaszewski L, et al. Treatment of fractures of the medial epicondyle of the humerus. Injury 1988;19:342–344.

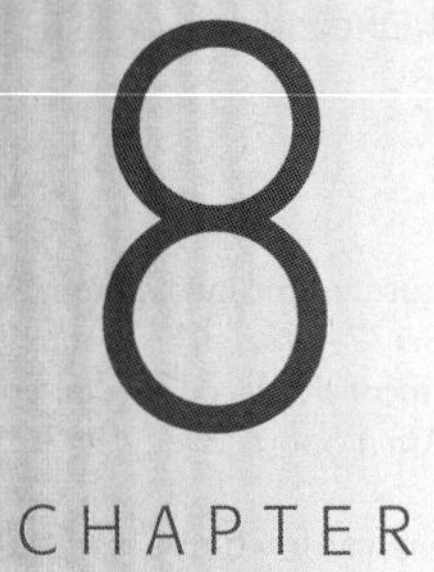

CHAPTER

Open Reduction and Internal Fixation of Displaced Lateral Condyle Fractures of the Humerus

Kristan A. Pierz and Brian G. Smith

DEFINITION

- Lateral condyle fractures refer to fractures of the outer (lateral) aspect of the distal humerus and may involve any or all of the following: metaphysis, physis, epiphysis, and articular surface.
- Fractures of the lateral condyle of the distal humerus account for 10% to 15% of all pediatric elbow fractures, second in frequency only to supracondylar distal humerus fractures.[6]
- Nondisplaced fractures may hinge on the articular cartilage, making them more stable than their unstable, displaced counterparts.

ANATOMY

- Proximally, lateral condyle fractures almost always include some portion of the posterolateral metaphysis and then propagate along the physis before exiting through or around the ossification center of the capitellum.
- The articular cartilage may or may not be violated.
- The extensor carpi radialis longus and brevis muscles and lateral collateral ligament typically remain attached to the distal fragment.
- Anterior and posterior portions of the elbow joint capsule may be torn if there is significant displacement.
- Milch[11] classified lateral condyle fractures based on the distal portion of the fracture line (**FIG 1**).
  - Milch type I fractures (the less common) traverse the metaphysis and physis as well as extend across the ossification center of the lateral condyle.
  - Milch type II fractures (the more common) extend from the metaphysis, through the physis, and exit in the unossified trochlea, medial to the capitellum ossification center. Displacement of the trochlear crista allows lateral translation of the forearm and increases the instability of this pattern.
- It is difficult to apply the Salter-Harris classification system to lateral condyle fractures because portions of the distal humeral epiphysis may not yet be ossified.
  - A fracture propagating from the metaphysis through the physis and then through the capitellum ossification center (Milch I) is analogous to a Salter-Harris type IV fracture.
  - A fracture that extends from the metaphysis through the physis and exits through the unossified trochlea medial to the capitellar ossification center (Milch II) may appear radiographically analogous to a Salter-Harris type II fracture, but its involvement of the articular cartilage is analogous to Salter-Harris types III and IV.
- A numeric classification system identifies fractures based on displacement.[8,13]
  - Stage I fractures involve the metaphysis and physis but often do not violate the articular cartilage, thus limiting their ability to displace. Displacement is less than 2 mm.
  - Stage II fractures cross the articular surface but are minimally displaced. Displacement is 2 to 4 mm.
  - Stage III fractures are displaced fractures that cross the metaphysis, physis, and articular surface, frequently resulting in rotation of the distal fragment (**FIG 2**).

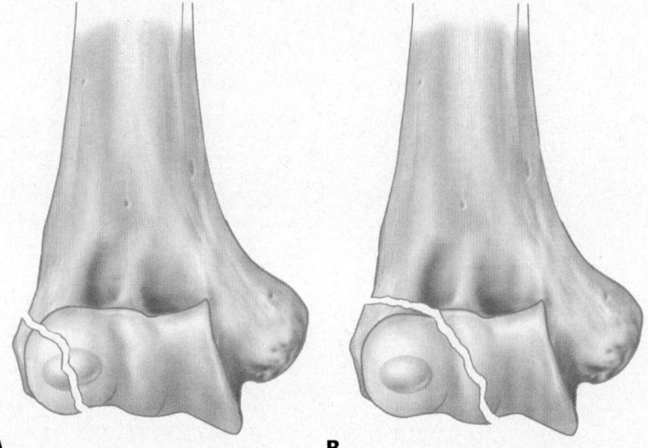

FIG 1 • Milch classification of lateral condyle fractures is based on location. **A.** Type I fracture line passes through the ossific nucleus of the capitellum. **B.** Type II fracture line passes medial to the capitellar ossific nucleus into the trochlear groove.

PATHOGENESIS

- The typical mechanism for a lateral condyle fracture is a fall on an outstretched hand.
- Adduction of a supinated forearm with the elbow extended can result in avulsion of the lateral condyle.
- Axial load of the forearm combined with valgus force can also propagate a fracture through the lateral condyle.
- Lateral condyle fractures usually occur as isolated injuries, although elbow joint subluxation and radial head or olecranon fractures may be associated.

NATURAL HISTORY

- The natural history of lateral condyle fractures depends on the fracture displacement as well as the long-term viability of the growing physis.[5]
- Completely nondisplaced lateral condyle fractures may heal regardless of treatment.
- Nondisplaced fractures can displace over time if the articular cartilage is violated or if there is significant associated soft tissue injury.
- Delayed union can occur even in nondisplaced fractures and may be due to poor metaphyseal circulation, bathing of the

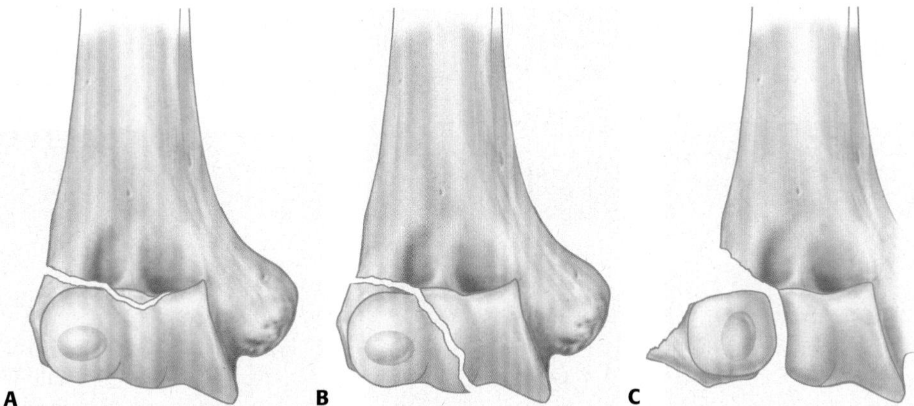

FIG 2 • Numeric classification of lateral condyle fractures is based on displacement. **A.** Stage I fractures are nondisplaced and do not violate the articular surface. **B.** Stage II fractures violate the articular surface but are minimally displaced (0 to 2 mm). **C.** Stage III fractures are displaced more than 2 mm and may be rotated.

fracture in synovial fluid, or tension on the condylar fragment by attached muscles.

- Fractures that heal in near-anatomic alignment can yield excellent functional and cosmetic outcomes.
- Lateral condyle fractures associated with lateral physeal arrest can result in valgus deformity and tardy ulnar nerve palsy.
- Lateral condyle fractures associated with central physeal arrest can result in a "fishtail" deformity due to continued growth medially and laterally but limited growth in between.

PATIENT HISTORY AND PHYSICAL FINDINGS

- Most patients report a fall, either on an outstretched hand or from some height, resulting in pain and inability to fully move the elbow.
- It may be difficult to obtain a history from a young child; therefore, parents or caregivers may need to be questioned.
- The clinician should be patient during the physical examination. Young children may be very fearful. The clinician should ask the child to point to what hurts most, and this part should be examined last. This allows the clinician to establish the patient's trust and rule out other associated injuries.
- The clinician should look for obvious deformity, swelling, ecchymosis, and open wounds about the elbow.
- The clinician should assess for pulses and capillary refill.
- Sensation is assessed by comparison with the uninvolved side. Rather than stroking a finger and asking a young child, "Do you feel this?", the clinician can rub the same site on both hands and ask, "Does it feel the same or different?"
- Motor function is assessed by observing for spontaneous movement during the entire encounter. A scared child may refuse to move when asked by a physician but may demonstrate voluntary movement when asked by a parent or sibling. Being playful during the examination can help. For example, when testing for ulnar nerve function, asking a 5-year-old to show you how old he or she is may be more rewarding than asking the child to spread his or her fingers.
- The wrist and shoulder are palpated before touching the elbow.
- A single finger is used to gently palpate the olecranon, medial epicondyle, posterior humerus, lateral condyle, and radial head to try to localize the specific site of injury. Crepitus suggests displacement and instability of the fracture fragment.
- Increased motion during varus stress testing suggests instability of the fracture. Due to pain, however, this test can rarely be done on an awake child. It is often reserved for intraoperative assessment rather than preoperative diagnosis.

IMAGING AND OTHER DIAGNOSTIC STUDIES

- Radiographs of a suspected lateral condyle fracture should include anteroposterior (AP), lateral, and internal oblique views (**FIG 3A–C**).
- Valgus and varus stress radiographs can provide information about the stability of the fracture. Because such films are poorly tolerated in an awake child, they are rarely obtained outside of the operating room.
- For nondisplaced or minimally displaced fractures, magnetic resonance imaging (MRI) can be used to determine whether the articular surface is violated[7] (**FIG 3D**).
  - Such studies, however, are expensive, are rarely needed for surgical decision making, and frequently require sedation in young children, so they are not obtained routinely.
- Arthrograms can provide detail about the articular congruity of lateral condyle fractures but are typically reserved for intraoperative assessment[10] (**FIG 3E**).

DIFFERENTIAL DIAGNOSIS

- Contusion
- Lateral collateral ligament strain or sprain
- Radial head or neck fracture
- Supracondylar distal humerus fracture
- Transphyseal fractures
- Medial condyle fractures
- Proximal ulnar or Monteggia fractures
- Elbow dislocation
- Child abuse

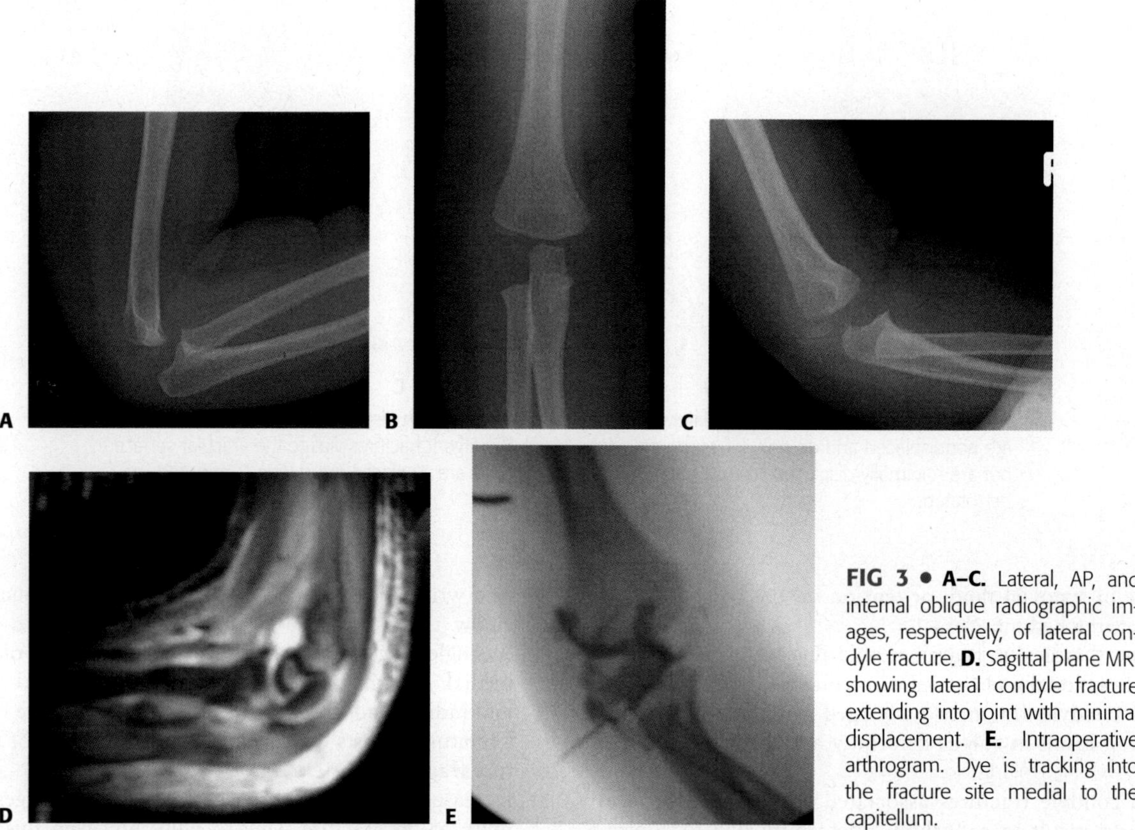

FIG 3 • A–C. Lateral, AP, and internal oblique radiographic images, respectively, of lateral condyle fracture. **D.** Sagittal plane MRI showing lateral condyle fracture extending into joint with minimal displacement. **E.** Intraoperative arthrogram. Dye is tracking into the fracture site medial to the capitellum.

NONOPERATIVE MANAGEMENT

- Nonoperative management of lateral condyle fractures is typically reserved for nondisplaced or minimally displaced (<2 mm) fractures.
- The upper extremity is immobilized in a long-arm splint or cast with the elbow flexed 90 degrees and the forearm in neutral.
  - Casts that are excessively heavy or short on the upper arm tend to slide down, thus increasing the risk of later displacement.
- Follow-up radiographs should be obtained in 3 to 5 days to assess for further displacement.
- If displacement occurs, operative treatment is indicated.
- If the fracture remains nondisplaced, long-arm casting is continued for another week, and then repeat radiographs are obtained.
  - If still nondisplaced, the fracture is maintained in a long-arm cast until there is radiographic evidence of fracture union, typically at 4 to 6 weeks.
- Delayed union may occur, requiring up to 12 weeks of immobilization. Poor vascularization of the fracture fragment and bathing of the fragment in articular fluid may contribute to this phenomenon.

SURGICAL MANAGEMENT

- Surgery is recommended for lateral condyle fractures with more than 2 mm of displacement or rotational deformity that occurs acutely or during the early follow-up period of nonoperative treatment.[1]
- Closed techniques with percutaneous pinning are reserved for minimally displaced fractures, with a congruous articular surface confirmed by arthrography.
- Open surgery is required for displaced fractures.

Preoperative Planning

- Preoperatively, a careful neurovascular examination should be performed and documented. Fortunately, unlike supracondylar fractures, isolated lateral condyle fractures rarely have any associated neurovascular injury.
- Plain radiographs, including AP, lateral, and internal oblique views, should be adequate to make the decision to operate.
  - Displacement of more than 2 mm indicates the need for surgical intervention.
- Displacement of more than 2 mm on two or more views suggests instability and often requires open treatment.
- Displacement of more than 2 mm on only one view suggests that the fracture may be hinging on intact articular cartilage and may be treatable by percutaneous techniques.
- Fractures with borderline displacement (2 to 3 mm) may be better assessed under anesthesia, where stress radiographs or an arthrogram can guide treatment.

Positioning

- The patient is placed in the supine position on the operating table, and general anesthesia is induced.
- The child should be brought to the edge of the operating table to facilitate fluoroscopic imaging of the operative limb (**FIG 4**).

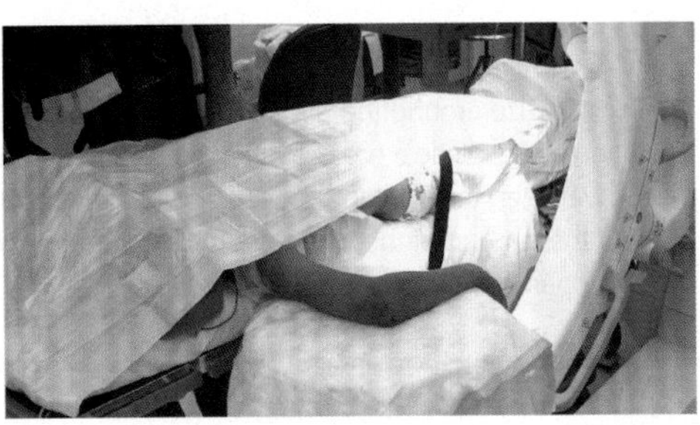

FIG 4 • Positioning the patient on the edge of the table allows easy access for fluoroscopy. The base of the unit may be used as an arm table.

- Care must be taken to prevent the patient's head from rolling off the table's edge. Placing a foam doughnut under the head can provide stability. Additionally, a small arm board may be attached to the proximal side of the operating table to help support the head.
- The receiving end of a standard fluoroscopy unit can be used as the operative table for the involved limb. Bringing the fluoroscopy unit up from the foot of the bed allows room for the surgeon and assistant to access the lateral side of the elbow.
  - Alternatively, a hand table may be used, and the fluoroscopy unit can be brought in after draping.
- For open cases, a sterile tourniquet is recommended to allow full access to the elbow after draping.

TECHNIQUES

Closed Reduction and Percutaneous Pinning

- This technique is reserved for minimally displaced (2 to 4 mm) fractures.
- Fracture stability should be assessed under anesthesia with varus stress radiographs and/or arthrography.
- Two divergent smooth pins are recommended. Although 0.062-inch Kirschner wires are usually adequate, 5/64-inch Steinmann pins may be used in larger children.
- The first wire is placed through the skin into the lateral condyle to engage the metaphyseal fragment distally (bicortical purchase).
  - The wire should be directed from distal lateral to proximal medial, penetrating the cortex medially.
- A second wire is then placed in a similar manner, diverging at the fracture site.
  - Increasing the distance between the wires at the fracture site increases stability[2] (**TECH FIG 1A**).
- Wires may cross the ossification center of the capitellum to improve divergence (**TECH FIG 1B,C**).

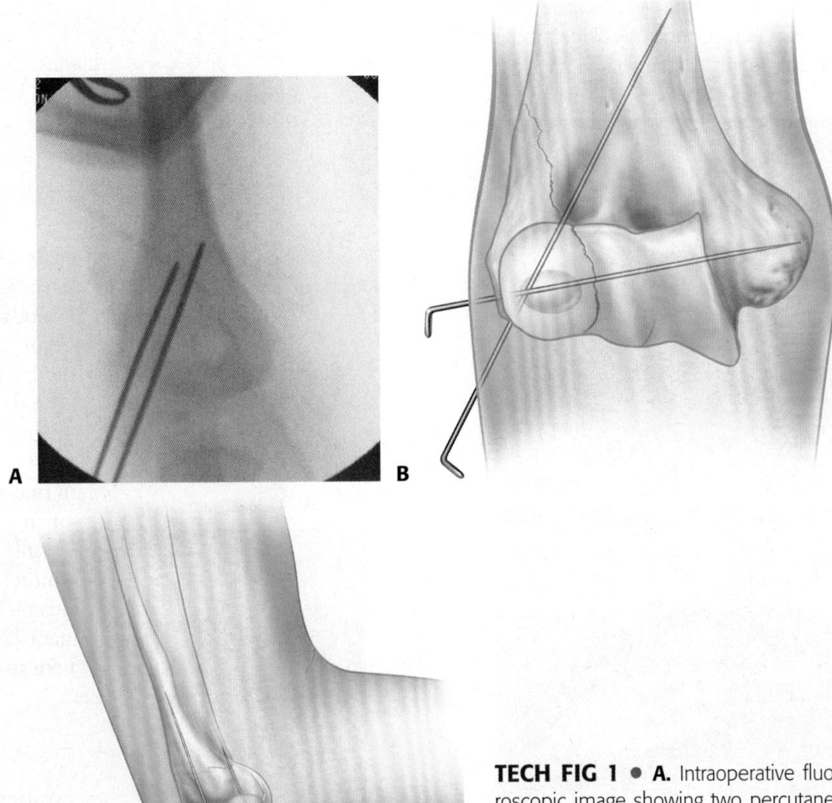

TECH FIG 1 • **A.** Intraoperative fluoroscopic image showing two percutaneously placed Kirschner wires stabilizing a lateral condyle fracture. **B,C.** AP and lateral views of fracture treated with two divergent Kirschner wires.

- Occasionally, a third wire is needed. This wire is added if, after placing the first two wires, there is still motion at the fracture site when the elbow is varus stressed under fluoroscopy.
- The wires can be cut and bent 90 degrees outside of the skin.
- Wrapping gauze around the pin as it exits the skin may limit pin migration and provide a protective barrier. Sterile felt can also be placed between the skin and the cut end of the wire. This helps prevent the cut end of the wire from digging into the skin during the postoperative swelling phase.

Open Reduction and Internal Fixation

- Unstable fractures usually require open treatment. This includes acutely displaced fractures as well as originally nondisplaced fractures that displace during early follow-up.[9] Although one can attempt a closed reduction of an unstable fracture, open reduction should be performed if any displacement persists.[14]

Exposure

- The lateral Kocher approach is used, although the dissection is typically facilitated by the rent in the brachioradialis that leads directly to the lateral condyle.
- A 5- to 6-cm curvilinear incision is used, with two-thirds of the incision proximal and one-third distal to the elbow joint (**TECH FIG 2A**).
- The interval is between the brachioradialis and the triceps down to the lateral humeral condyle. The anterior articular surface of the elbow joint is exposed by working from proximal to distal and retracting the soft tissues of the antecubital fossa anteriorly.[15]
  - Although the fracture hematoma can obscure distinct muscular planes, a tear in the aponeurosis of the brachioradialis may lead directly to the fracture site.
- Dissection is kept anteriorly. Care should be taken to avoid stripping any of the soft tissues from the posterior aspect of the fracture fragment while the soft tissues are elevated off the anterior distal humerus because this contains the blood supply to the lateral condyle epiphysis[18] (**TECH FIG 2B**).
- Exposure is complete when the trochlear or medial extent of the fracture can be assessed anteriorly.

Fracture Reduction

- The goal of reduction is to achieve a congruent articular surface without any step-off.
- Lifting the anterior soft tissues with a Zenker retractor or similar instrument can allow direct visualization and inspection of the articular surface.
  - A Zenker retractor is narrow and angled, which makes it useful for lifting and retracting the anterior soft tissues without unnecessary stretch (**TECH FIG 3A**).

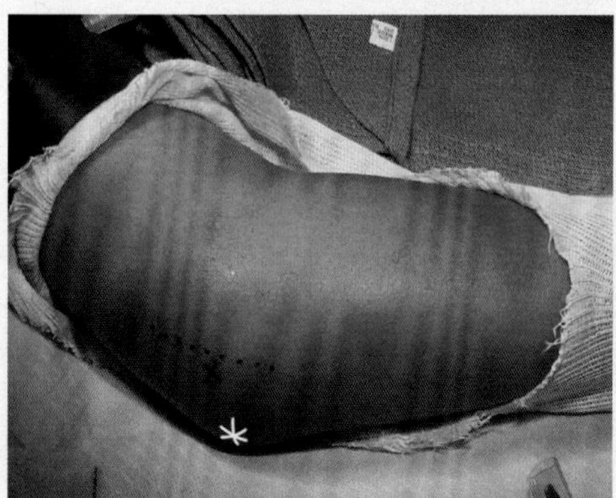

A

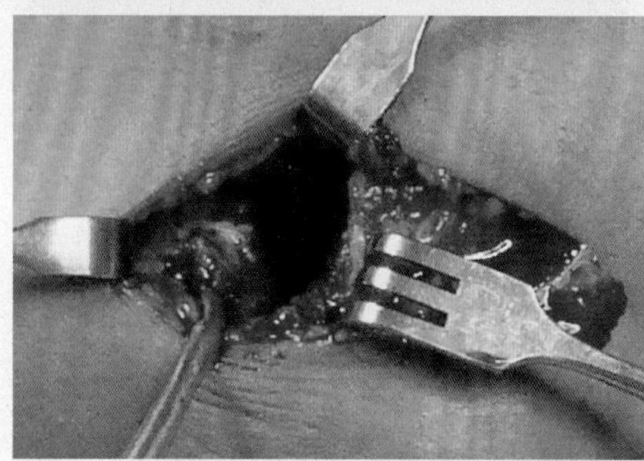

B

TECH FIG 2 • A. Kocher-type lateral incision is marked by *dotted line*. *X* marks lateral condyle. The *asterisk* marks olecranon. **B.** Dissection is carried out anteriorly to expose the articular surface.

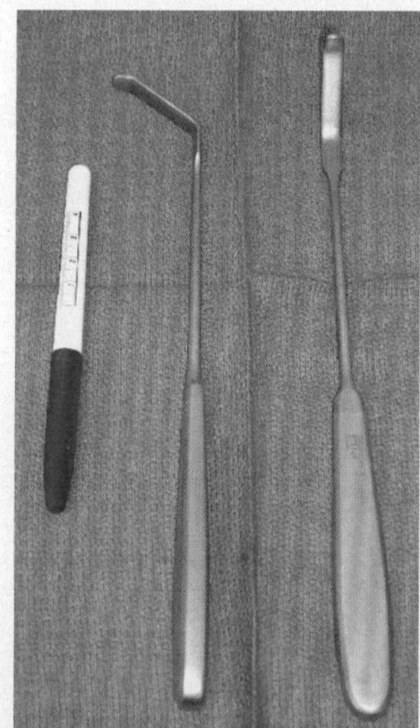

A

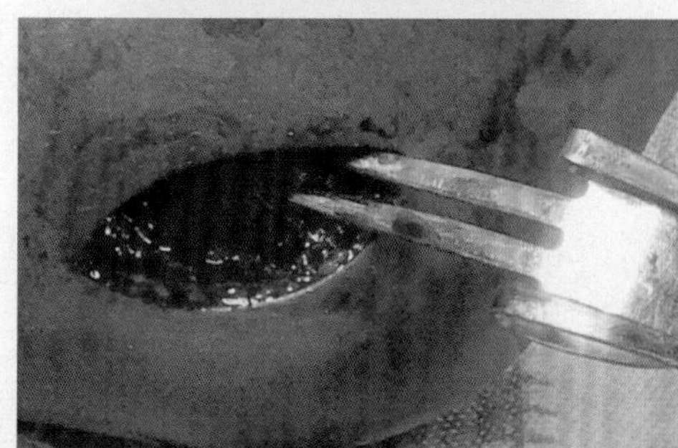

B

TECH FIG 3 • A. The Zenker retractor is narrow and angled, making it ideal to elevate the anterior soft tissues. A pen is shown for reference. **B.** A sterilized standard kitchen fork can be a useful reduction tool.

- A small finger or elevator can be placed into the anterior elbow joint to palpate the trochlear–capitellar junction.
- A sterilized common kitchen fork can be a useful instrument in this case.
  - Bending the outer tines back decreases the width of the fork and allows the central tines to fit into a small wound.
  - The central tines can be used to engage the distal fragment, which is then rotated and pushed into position.
- Gaps between the tines allow room for placement of Kirschner wires (**TECH FIG 3B**).
- Alternatively, a Kirschner wire can be placed into the distal fragment and used as a joystick to help control the reduction.

Fixation

- Once the fragment is reduced, a smooth Kirschner wire is advanced from the metaphyseal portion of the distal fragment, across the fracture site, and into the medial cortex proximal to the fracture.
- A second Kirschner wire (or the original joystick wire) can now be advanced across the fracture site into the medial cortex.
- The wires can be cut and bent 90 degrees outside the skin to facilitate easy removal in the office in about 4 weeks (3 to 6 weeks depending on appearance of healing on radiographs).[3,17]
  - Alternatively, they can be cut very short and bent under the skin. This technique has not been proven to decrease the risk of deep infections, and it requires a return to the operating room for removal; hence, it may not be as cost effective as leaving the pins exposed[4] (**TECH FIG 4**).
- If the wires are to be cut and bent outside the skin, the wires enter the skin through a separate stab site posterior to the incision.
  - If a wire needs to be placed through the incision, it can be cut and the posterior skin can be pulled up and over the sharp cut end before closure.
- Increasing the space between the wires at the fracture site increases rotational control.
  - Recently, bioresorbable implants have been tried, but long-term results are limited.[16]
- In older children with a larger metaphyseal fragment, a compression screw can be used rather than wires.
  - The screw head may be prominent under the skin and symptomatic after healing, however, thus requiring a return to the operating room for removal.
  - Compressive threads across immature cartilage can potentially impede growth in younger children.
  - This technique, therefore, is usually reserved for older patients or delayed unions or nonunions.
- In many cases, closure of the lateral periosteum may be possible with sutures. Such closure may lessen the chance of lateral spur formation, add stability, and speed healing.

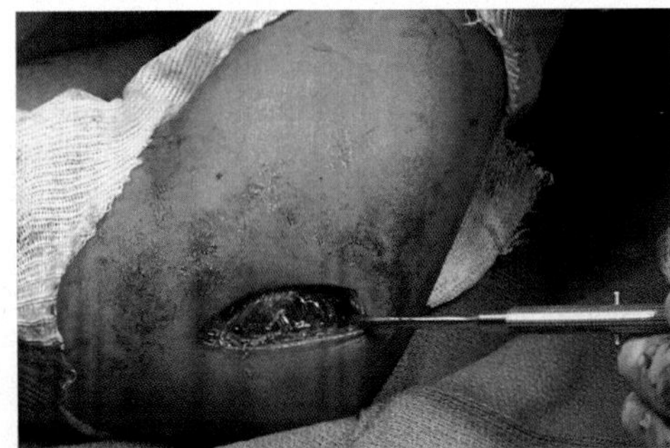

TECH FIG 4 ● After reduction and pinning, Kirschner wires may be cut and bent. Here, they are to be buried under the skin.

PEARLS AND PITFALLS

Nonoperative management	■ Follow-up radiographs should be obtained within 3 to 5 days. ■ Any loss of reduction suggests instability and prompts the need for operative intervention.
Postoperative bone spur	■ A posterior or posterolateral metaphyseal bone spur frequently forms postoperatively. This is best seen on lateral radiographs. The bony prominence may give the clinical appearance of cubitus varus. Fortunately, this tends to improve over time and rarely requires intervention. Warning the parents initially of the probability of the occurrence can reduce anxiety later.
Postoperative swelling	■ Placing felt over the cut, bend ends of the wires onto the skin decreases the risk of skin swelling over or pressing into their sharp tips while in the cast. ■ Bivalving the cast decreases the risk of postoperative compartment syndrome.
Delayed union and nonunion	■ This occurs more commonly in fractures treated nonoperatively. ■ Prolonged casting of up to 12 weeks may be needed. ■ If the fracture does not heal, open reduction with bone grafting may be necessary.
Cubitus valgus and tardy ulnar nerve palsy	■ Premature closure of the lateral physis may lead to gradual deformity as the medial side continues to grow. ■ Anatomic reduction decreases the risk. ■ Follow-up radiographs can reveal the deformity. ■ Nerve symptoms can take years to develop; therefore, patients should be counseled about signs and symptoms of ulnar nerve stretch.
Cubitus varus	■ Unstable fractures treated nonoperatively can displace proximally and laterally, allowing the elbow to drift into a varus position. ■ Doing careful early follow-up and fixing unstable fractures should prevent this.

POSTOPERATIVE CARE

- The arm is placed in a long-arm cast with the elbow flexed 90 degrees and the forearm in neutral to slight pronation.
- If there is significant swelling, the cast can be bivalved in the operating room and overwrapped the following week.
- Radiographs are obtained in 1 week to look for any loss of reduction.
- Wires can usually be pulled in 4 weeks.
  - Authors have debated the exact timing. Although some have shown adequate healing by 3 weeks, a period of 4 to 6 weeks is generally required; the decision should be based on radiographic evidence of early callus.
- Gentle early active range of motion is encouraged after wire removal.
- A removable posterior splint can be made for children who will not comply with activity modifications.
- Physical or occupational therapy is rarely needed in children but may be recommended for those who fail to show improved range of motion.

OUTCOMES

- Patients who are treated quickly and whose fractures heal in an anatomic position with no subsequent growth arrest can expect excellent (90%) function and range of motion. Approximately, 10% have minor loss of extension (10 to 15 degrees) at 1 to 2 years.[17]
  - Complications are three times as likely to occur in fractures with displaced articular cartilage than in those with an intact articular surface.[19]
- Outcome studies following patients into adulthood are lacking.
- Patients who are treated with open reduction at 3 or more weeks after fracture are at greater risk for loss of range of motion (about 34 degrees), premature physeal closure, valgus deformity, tardy ulnar nerve palsy, and avascular necrosis, thus emphasizing the need for early treatment.[8]

COMPLICATIONS

- Pin tract infections can occur but usually resolve after wire removal and oral antibiotics.
- Posterior or posterolateral metaphyseal bone spurs frequently form postoperatively and are best seen on lateral radiographs (**FIG 5**). The size of the spur has been associated with the initial fracture displacement.[12] Fortunately, these tend to smooth over time and are rarely symptomatic; thus, they usually require no treatment.
- Delayed union and nonunion are more common with nonoperative treatment than with surgical treatment.
- Malunion may occur in unstable fractures treated nonoperatively or in those with premature growth arrest.
- Avascular necrosis is more common after operative treatment than nonoperative management and is likely due to excessive posterior stripping that disrupts the epiphyseal blood supply.
- Tardy ulnar nerve palsy can develop slowly with progressive valgus deformity following premature growth arrest or nonunion.

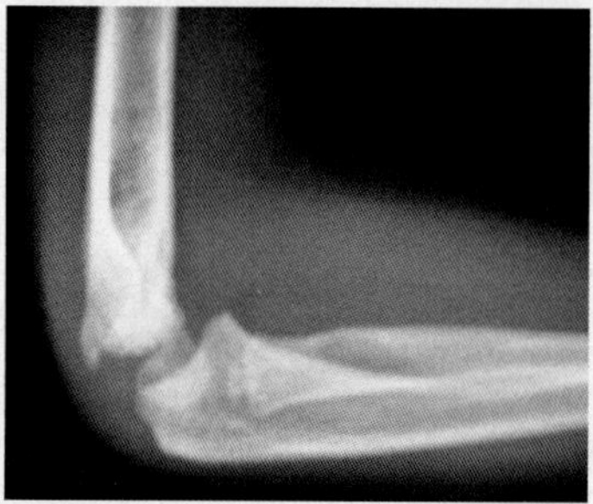

FIG 5 • Lateral radiograph showing postoperative bone spur projecting from posterior metaphysis.

REFERENCES

1. Bhandari M, Tornetta P, Swiontkowski MF. Displaced lateral condyle fractures of the distal humerus. J Orthop Trauma 2003;17:306–308.
2. Bloom T, Chen LY, Sabharwal S. Biomechanical analysis of lateral humeral condyle fracture pinning. J Pediatr Orthop 2011;31:130–137.
3. Cardona JI, Riddle E, Kumar SJ. Displaced fractures of the lateral humeral condyle: criteria for implant removal. J Pediatr Orthop 2002;22:194–197.
4. Das De S, Bae DS, Waters PM. Displaced humeral lateral condyle fractures in children: should we bury the pins? J Pediatr Orthop 2012;32:573–578.
5. Flynn JC, Richards JF Jr, Saltzman RI. Prevention and treatment of nonunion of slightly displaced fractures of the lateral humeral condyle in children. An end-result study. J Bone Joint Surg Am 1975;57(8):1087–1092.
6. Gorgola GR. Pediatric humeral condyle fractures. Hand Clin 2006;22:77–85.
7. Horn BD, Herman MJ, Crisci K, et al. Fractures of the lateral humeral condyle: role of the articular hinge in fracture stability. J Pediatr Orthop 2002;22:8–11.
8. Jakob R, Fowles JV, Rang M, et al. Observations concerning fractures of the lateral humeral condyle in children. J Bone Joint Surg Br 1975;57:430–436.
9. Launay F, Leet AI, Jacopin S, et al. Lateral humeral condyle fractures in children: a comparison of two approaches to treatment. J Pediatr Orthop 2004;24:385–391.
10. Marzo JM, D'Amato C, Strong M, et al. Usefulness and accuracy of arthrography in management of lateral humeral condyle fractures in children. J Pediatr Orthop 1990;10:317–321.
11. Milch H. Fractures and fracture-dislocations of the humeral condyles. J Trauma 1964;4:592–607.
12. Pribaz JR, Bernthal NM, Wong TC, et al. Lateral spurring (overgrowth) after pediatric lateral condyle fractres. J Pediatr Orthop 2012;32:456–460.
13. Rutherford A. Fractures of the lateral humeral condyle in children. J Bone Joint Surg Am 1985;67:851–856.
14. Song KS, Kang CH, Min BW, et al. Closed reduction and internal fixation of displaced unstable lateral condylar fractures of the humerus in children. J Bone Joint Surg Am 2008;90:2673–2681.
15. Sullivan JA. Fractures of the lateral condyle of the humerus. J Am Acad Orthop Surg 2006;14:58–62.
16. Takada N, Otsuka T, Suzuki H, et al. Pediatric displaced fractures of the lateral condyle of the humerus treated using high strength, bioactive, bioresorbable F-u-HA/PLLA pins: a case report of 8 patients with at least 3 years of follow-up. J Orthop Trauma 2013;27(5):281–284.
17. Thomas DP, Howard AW, Cole WG, et al. Three weeks of Kirschner wire fixation for displaced lateral condylar fractures of the humerus in children. J Pediatr Orthop 2001;21:565–569.
18. Wattenbarger JM, Gerardi J, Johnston CE. Late open reduction internal fixation of lateral condyle fractures. J Pediatr Orthop 2002;22:394–398.
19. Weiss JM, Graves S, Yang S, et al. A new classification system predictive of complications in surgically treated pediatric humeral lateral condyle fractures. J Pediatr Orthop 2009;29:602–605.

Open Reduction and Internal Fixation of Pediatric T-Condylar Fractures

CHAPTER 9

Keith D. Baldwin and John M. Flynn

DEFINITION

- T-condylar fractures of the distal humerus in children and adolescents are relatively rare occurrences. They are thought to represent 2% of all pediatric elbow fractures.[5]
- The proposed mechanism is similar to that of pediatric supracondylar fractures but with a higher energy mechanism of injury.[6]
- The olecranon acts as a wedge during hyperextension and creates a Y- or T-shaped fracture with the center in the olecranon fossa.
- These fractures are less likely to be comminuted than in adults.
- In younger children, an acceptable result can often be obtained with closed reduction and pinning, although this is generally not as straightforward as in a standard supracondylar humerus fracture (**FIG 1**).

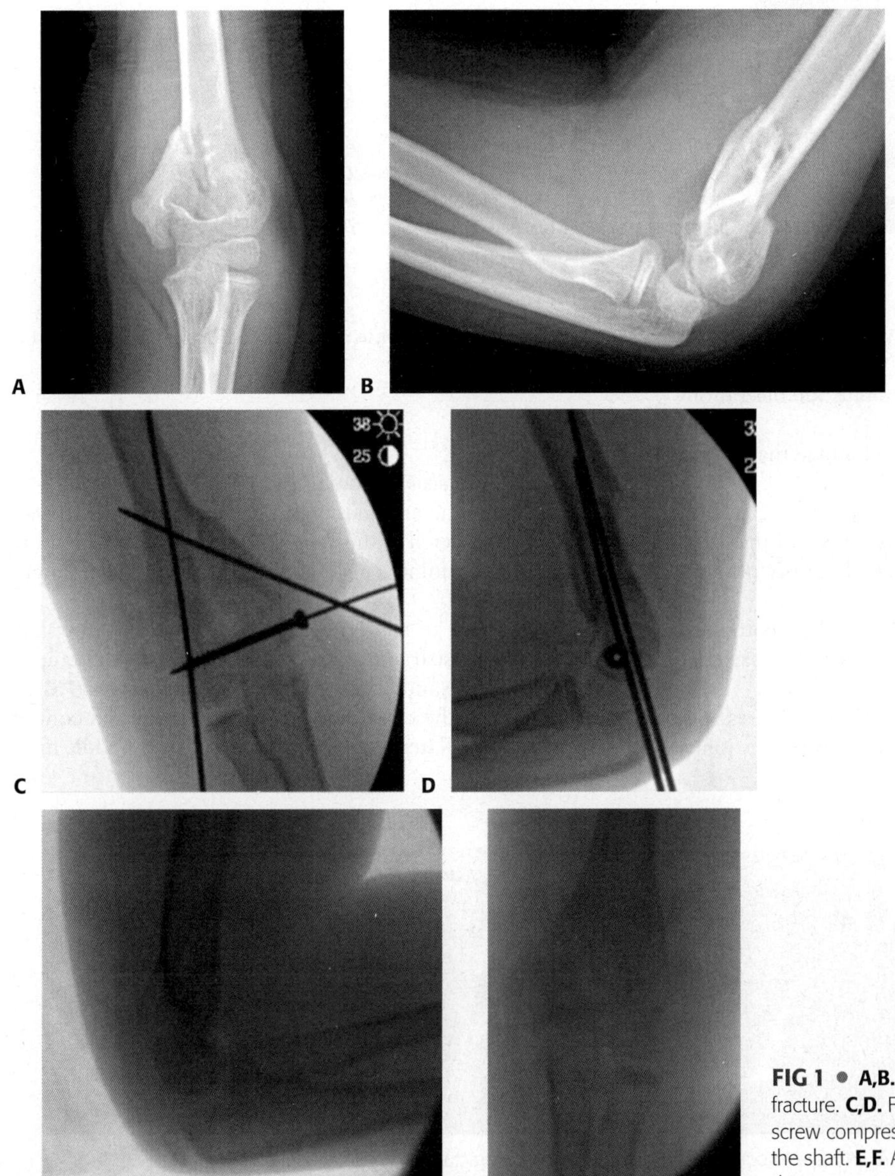

FIG 1 • **A,B.** An 8-year-old boy with T-condylar distal humerus fracture. **C,D.** Fixed with mini-open reduction with intercondylar screw compression and K-wire fixation of the distal humerus to the shaft. **E,F.** After hardware removal, the patient had 0 to 140 degrees range of motion with no pain.

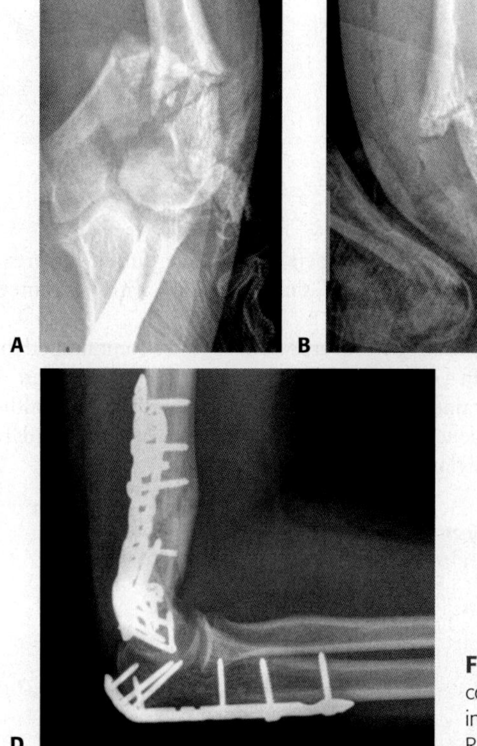

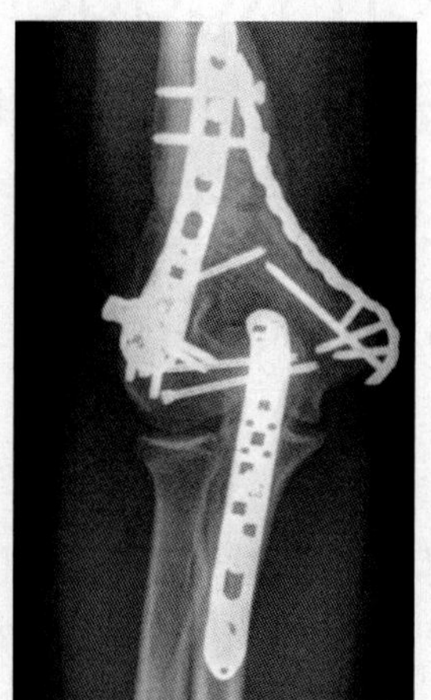

FIG 2 • A,B. A 15-year-old boy with type IIIA open distal humerus comminuted T-condylar humerus fracture. **C,D.** Three months following open reduction and internal fixation with olecranon osteotomy. Range of motion 0 to 140 degrees with no pain.

- Older children and young adolescents will often require an open approach.
- Comminution in the fossa may necessitate an olecranon osteotomy (**FIG 2**).
- Generally, pediatric fractures are less comminuted than adult fractures and may not require a full osteotomy.
  - A Morrey slide approach is used in such a case where the triceps and ulnar periosteum are elevated off the ulna medially to expose the distal humerus without performing an osteotomy.[3]
  - It was originally described to avoid olecranon osteotomies in cases where total elbow replacement would be a salvage operation.
  - It can be useful in adolescents because the fractures are not as comminuted, but excellent visualization of the joint is desirable to provide anatomic reduction and restoration of elbow function.

ANATOMY

- The distal humerus is a complex articulation.
- The ulnohumeral articulation is the articulation which needs to be reconstructed in this type of fracture. Occasionally, the radiocapitellar joint is also damaged with capitellar comminution (**FIG 3A**).
- The remainder of the limb should be carefully examined. Coexisting wrist fractures can increase the risk of compartment syndrome and other soft tissue complications (**FIG 3B**).
- Conceptually, the distal humerus is a hinge which contains a medial and a lateral column connected by a middle hinge.

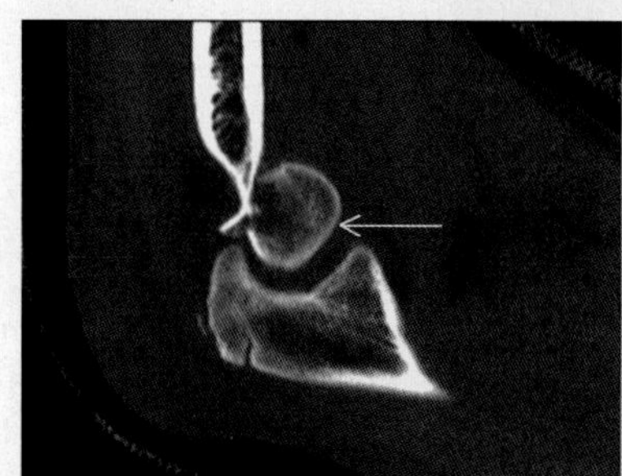

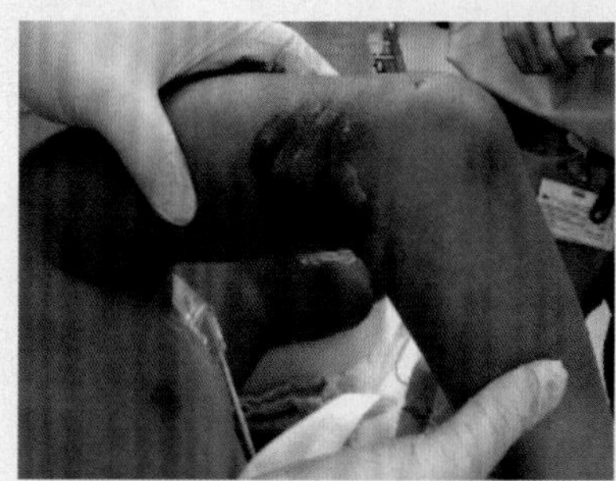

FIG 3 • A. A 13-year-old boy with a T-condylar humerus fracture with coronal split of the capitellum. **B.** Fracture blisters result from severe soft tissue injury.

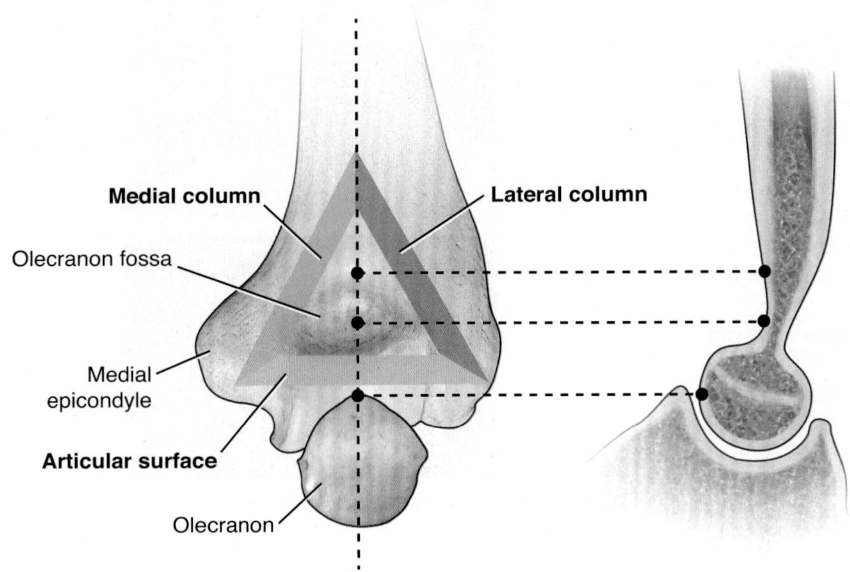

FIG 4 • Triangle of stability concept. The mechanical properties of the distal humerus are based on a triangle of stability, comprising the medial and lateral columns and the articular surface. (Adapted from Bonczar MR, Rikli D, Ring D. Distal humerus 13-C1 open reduction; perpendicular [biplanar] plating. AO Foundation Web site. Available at: http://bit.ly/1wEegQS. Published June 21, 2007. Accessed November 1, 2013.)

This creates a "triangle of stability," which must be recreated in order for fixation to be successful in T-condylar humerus fractures.[2] Regardless of the fixation strategy, this concept must be followed (**FIG 4**).

- Posteromedially, the ulnar nerve travels through a groove in the distal humerus called the *cubital tunnel*. The nerve must be exposed along the medial border of the triceps down to the first motor branch, which pierces the flexor carpi ulnaris.
- The triceps covers the distal humerus and attaches to the proximal ulna at the olecranon process.
- The olecranon obscures the view of the distal humerus articular surface, with the elbow in extension.
- To visualize the fracture line with the Morrey slide, the elbow must be flexed past 90 degrees.
- Also important, the distal fracture fragments typically rotate with the apex anteriorly, which is important to remember when reducing the joint surface.

PATHOGENESIS

- The mechanism of injury is a direct impact of the semilunar notch or coronoid process of the olecranon. Either of these structures can wedge into the trochlea, causing a split in the condyles.
- This most frequently occurs with a fall of the flexed elbow.

NATURAL HISTORY

- The natural history of this fracture without anatomic restoration is characterized by stiffness, varus malunion, and chronic elbow dysfunction.

PATIENT HISTORY AND PHYSICAL FINDINGS

- Mechanism of injury is important to obtain, higher energy injuries suggest an increased risk for compartment syndrome
- A careful neurovascular examination should be performed, with particular attention to the median, ulnar, and radial nerves.
- The limb should be inspected for open wounds. High-energy T-condylar fractures are often open injuries.

IMAGING AND OTHER DIAGNOSTIC STUDIES

- Quality anteroposterior (AP) internal and external oblique views can be useful if the diagnosis is in question.
- Traction views can often be useful in fractures where shortening is present, although children and adolescents will often tolerate these poorly.
- Computed tomography (CT) can be useful, but the coronal and sagittal reconstructions must be rendered in the plane of the joint or perpendicular to it (normal AP and lateral planes); otherwise, the information obtained will be difficult to interpret.
- Coronal fragments may be missed if high-quality imaging is not obtained (see **FIG 3A**).

DIFFERENTIAL DIAGNOSIS

- T-condylar fractures must be differentiated from other fractures of the distal humerus in children and adolescents because the treatment will differ.
- High-quality radiographs are generally sufficient to make this diagnosis.
- A CT or traction views can be helpful if the diagnosis is in question or if a coronal shear fragment is suspected on plain radiographs.

NONOPERATIVE MANAGEMENT

- Initial management includes a well-padded splint following adequate physical examination.
- If the injury is open, an intravenous (IV) first-generation cephalosporin should be administered as soon as the injury is identified. If there is excessive contamination, comminution, or soft tissue injury, IV gentamicin is also recommended.
- There is limited value in nonsurgical management with the exception of patients with nonfunctional upper limbs at baseline.

SURGICAL MANAGEMENT

- Open injuries should be addressed surgically within 24 hours; closed injuries may be addressed semielectively.
- Attention is given to the distal radius; "floating elbows," in which both the distal humerus and distal radius and/or ulna are affected, are not uncommon. These injuries should be identified early, as they are at increased risk for compartment syndrome.
- The soft tissue envelope is an important consideration. Fracture blisters (see **FIG 3B**) can be present, which can compromise the sterility and the closure of the procedure.
- The vast majority of T-condylar humerus fractures require operative treatment.
- In younger children, a percutaneous or mini-open approach may be possible.
- In older children and adolescents, an open posterior approach offers direct visualization and anatomic reduction and fixation of fracture fragments.

Preoperative Planning

- High-quality AP and lateral radiographs are mandatory prior to surgery.
- Internal and external oblique views may be useful in identifying columnar comminution.
- CT scan can be useful in identifying coronal shear fragments.
- Method of fixation should be chosen by patient age, degree of displacement, and amount of comminution.
  - Specialized distal humeral plating systems are available from several different manufacturers to allow either bicolumn or "90:90" plating.

Positioning

- We prefer positioning in a lateral position.
- The patient is intubated supine and then flipped to a lateral position over a beanbag.
- The bony prominences of the lateral malleolus and fibular head are carefully padded. A pillow is placed between the legs.
- The beanbag is inflated holding the patient in lateral decubitus, and an axillary roll is placed.

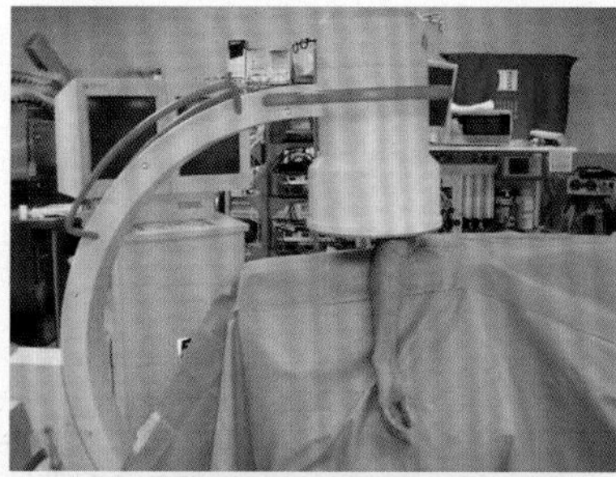

A

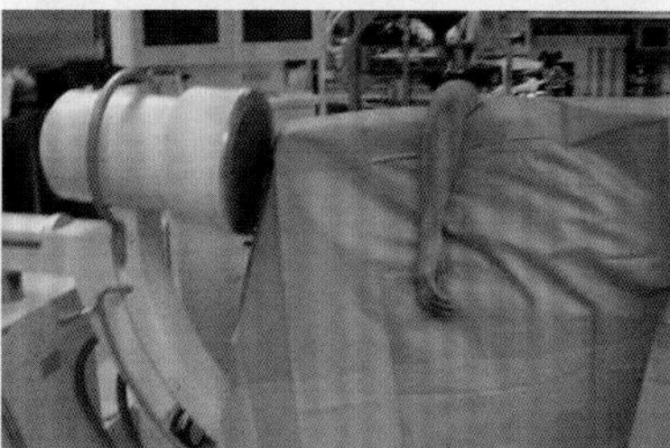

B

FIG 5 • **A,B.** Patient positioning for distal humerus fractures. (Courtesy of Samir Mehta, MD.)

- The contralateral arm is flexed at the shoulder and elbow to 90 degrees and placed on an arm board that is rotated so it is flush with the bed. This arm is then secured to the arm board.
- The operative arm is laid over a radiolucent arm board or paint roller so that the elbow is flexed 90 degrees (**FIG 5**).
- C-arm is brought in to assure that AP and lateral x-rays are adequate.
- The arm is then prepped and draped sterilely.
- A sterile tourniquet is used if one is desired.
- A "brain bag" is placed under the arm to be used to catch any blood or irrigant that comes from the field.
- The Bovie and suction are also placed in this bag for use.

Approach

- As described in the following text. A posterior incision is used.

TECHNIQUES

Exposure

- In highly comminuted fractures, an olecranon osteotomy is recommended for full joint visualization and reduction of comminuted pieces.
- A long posterior midline incision is used, the skin incision curves medially around the olecranon and then proceeds along the posterior border of the ulna. The incision is around 7 cm distal to the olecranon and 9 cm proximal as originally described.
- Then the dissection is carried deeply until the fascia is identified.

Morrey Slide

- The fascia is then divided and the ulnar nerve identified proximally in the perineural fat adjacent to the medial head of the triceps. The ulnar nerve is then dissected free of the cubital tunnel and traced back distally to its first motor branch.
- After identification of the ulnar nerve, the superficial fascia of the forearm is incised to the distal extent of the incision. The periosteum of the medial ulna is incised 6 cm below the tip of the olecranon (**TECH FIG 1A**).
- The periosteum and fascia are preserved together as a unit and reflected in a subperiosteal fashion off the bone (**TECH FIG 1B**).
- At the insertion of the triceps, Sharpey fibers connect the triceps to the olecranon (**TECH FIG 1C**). A modification of the Morrey technique exists in which a small wafer of bone is detached with

the periosteal sleeve at this point in order to have bone-to-bone healing and not to risk disconnecting the tendon altogether (**TECH FIG 1D**).

- If the bone wafer technique is not employed, the arm should be extended to 20 to 30 degrees to relieve tension and allow safe release of the entire triceps mechanism with the periosteal sleeve.
- Following release of the triceps, the remainder of the periosteum/fascial sleeve is slid laterally.
- This allows for visualization of the elbow joint. If access to the radial head is desired for capitellar comminution, the anconeus can be elevated off of the lateral ulna. The tip of the olecranon can also be excised if joint exposure is insufficient (**TECH FIG 1E**).

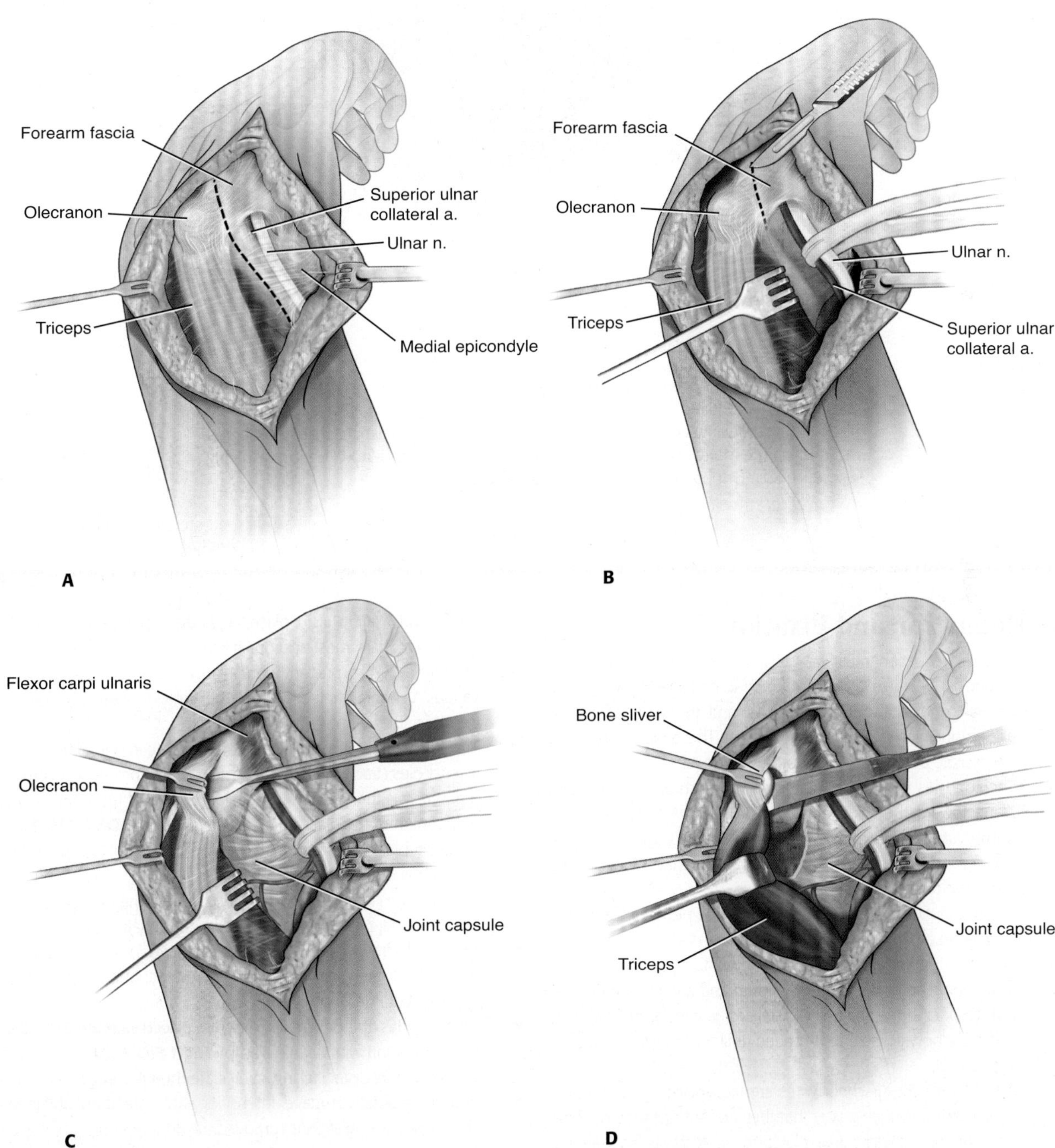

TECH FIG 1 • **A.** Superficial exposure. **B.** Elevation of the triceps off of the ulna. **C.** Medial periosteal flap being created. **D.** Morrey slide technique with bone wafer modification. *(continued)*

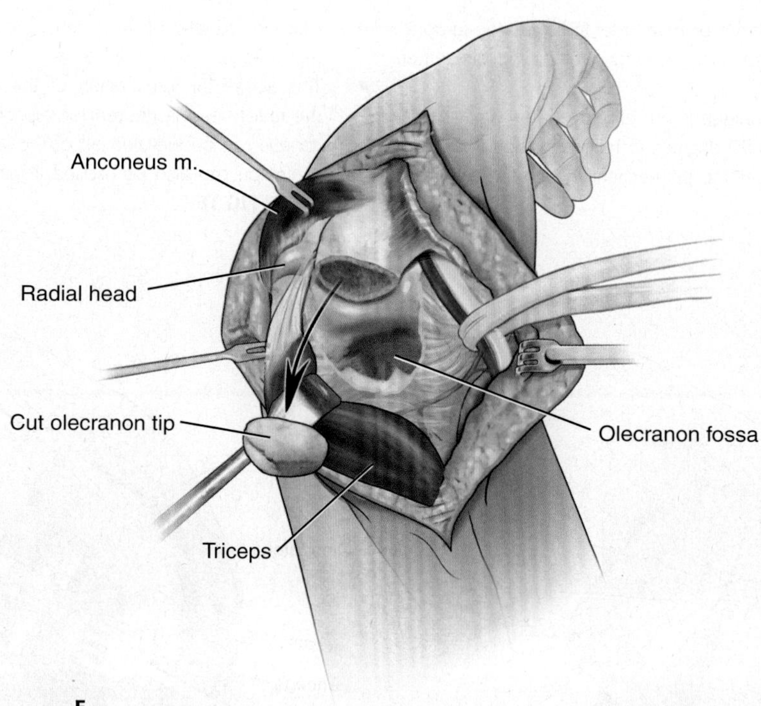

TECH FIG 1 • *(continued)* **E.** The tip of the olecranon can be resected if more joint visualization is required. Additionally, the anconeus can be subperiosteally reflected if access to the radial head is necessary in the case of a coronal capitellar split. (Adapted from Bryan RS, Morrey BF. Extensive posterior exposure of the elbow: a triceps-sparing approach. Clin Orthop Relat Res 1982;[166]:188–192.)

Reduction and Fixation

- Articular reduction must be accomplished first. In adolescent T-condylar fractures, there tend to be three large fragments, the medial condyle, the lateral condyle, and the shaft. Occasionally, coronal splits or comminution exist. These will occasionally necessitate an olecranon osteotomy approach.
- The condyles tend to be rotated toward each other in the axial plane toward the midline (**TECH FIG 2A**). A large reduction clamp can be placed on each epicondyle and used to reduce and compress the condyles. The condyles are then provisionally fixed with Kirschner wires.
- If comminution exists, generally the joint is provisionally reconstructed in an anterior to posterior direction.[4]
- The shaft is then reduced to the now intact and provisionally fixed joint. The joint is generally flexed and anteriorly translated with respect to the shaft. The distal arm is translated posteriorly and the elbow flexed and extended until an anatomic reduction is obtained.
- A 5/64 or 7/32 Kirschner wires are then placed in a cross-pin configuration in such a way that they are out of the way of the final fixation (usually dual plates in adolescents). When the provisional fixation is in place, a medial and lateral plate are selected that are most appropriate for the patient's bone.
- Of note, 2.7-mm precontoured plates are now available from various vendors that allow for the smaller sizes needed in pediatric-sized elbows.
- The plates are provisionally fixed on the bone in one of the distal screw holes (traditionally hole 2 from distal to proximal). A proximal screw is then placed in the slotted hole of the more proximal portion of the plate but not fully tightened (**TECH FIG 2B**).
- Fluoroscopic shots are obtained at this point to assure that the provisional reduction is adequate.
- A large bone clamp is then used to compress the bone between the plates (ie, placed from the medial to the lateral plate).
- Two distal screws (one medial and one lateral) are then placed using the locking towers. These screws should engage the opposite column of bone.[4]
- Following this, the proximal screws are placed with the condyles in compression with a large clamp (**TECH FIG 2C,D**).
- The remaining distal locking screws are then placed.
- Final intraoperative image intensifier shots are then obtained after provisional fixation is removed.

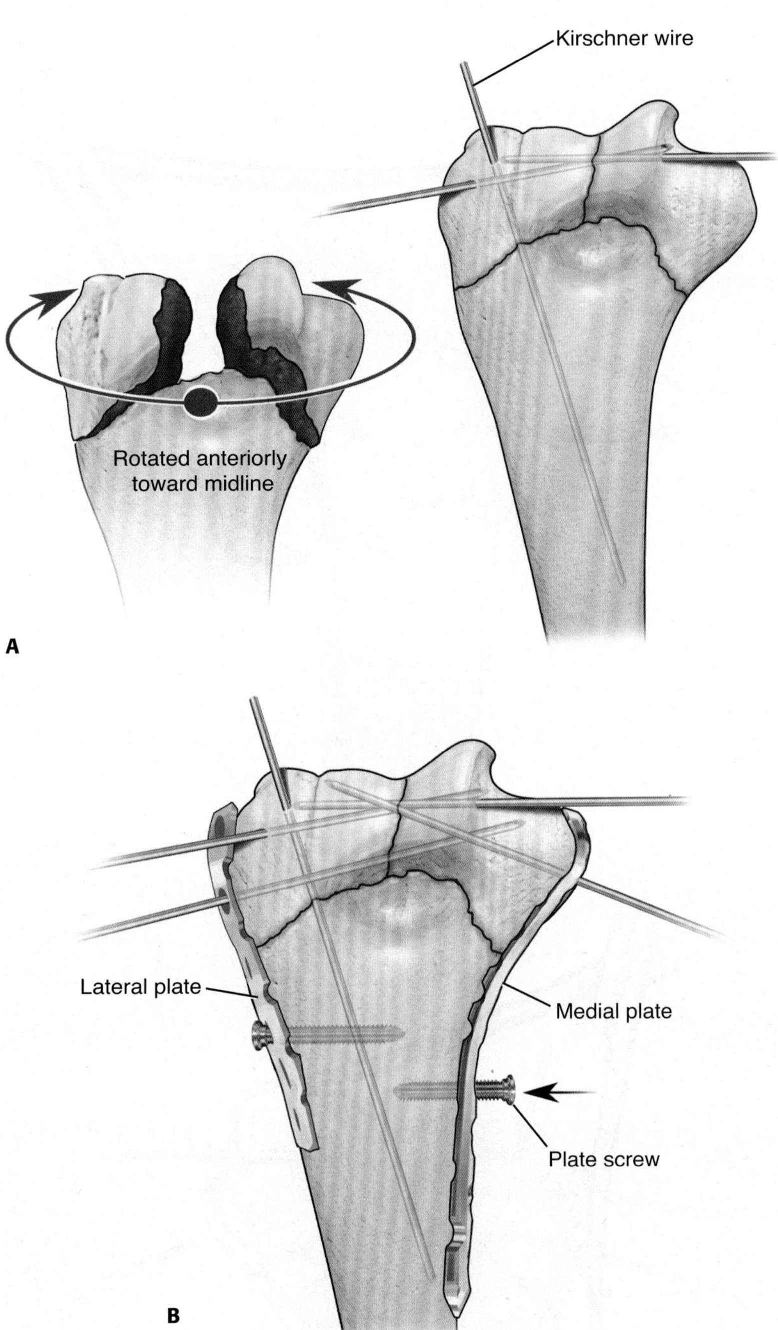

TECH FIG 2 • **A.** Fragments tend to be rotated anteriorly toward the midline. **B.** Plates are provisionally held on with Kirschner wires and shaft screws. *(continued)*

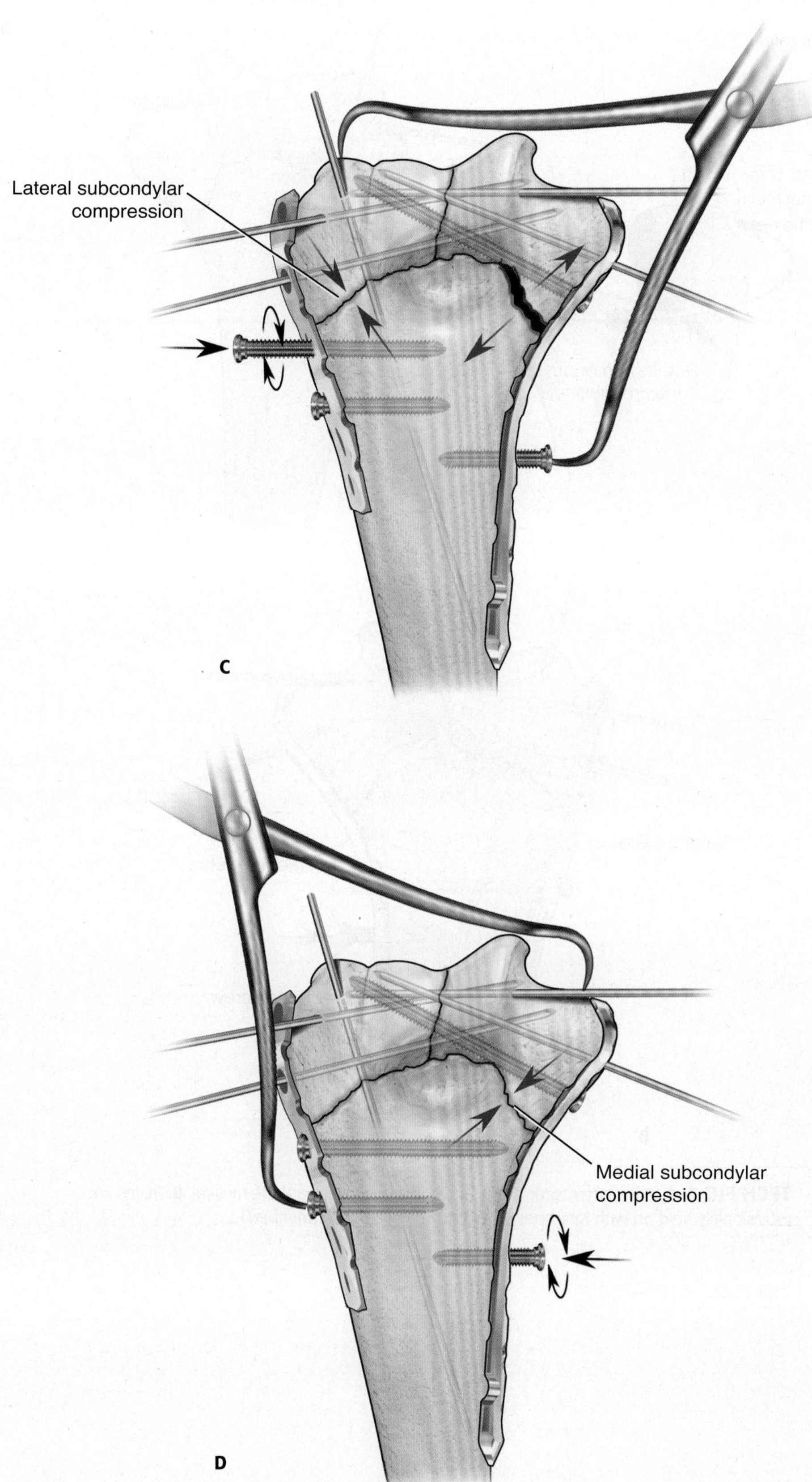

TECH FIG 2 • *(continued)* Supracondylar compression is accomplished first laterally (**C**) then medially (**D**). (Adapted from O'Driscoll SW. Green's Operative Hand Surgery, ed 4. New York: Churchill Livingstone, 1999:339.)

Closure

- The surgical field is carefully irrigated with 3 L of normal saline solution.
- If the bone wafer technique is used, the wafer is replaced anatomically using heavy, transosseous nonabsorbable suture. If the elevation is used, the triceps is repaired to the bone through transosseous sutures (**TECH FIG 3**).
- The ulnar nerve is not routinely transposed unless there appears to be pressure on the nerve from the plate.
- The fascia/periosteum layer is carefully repaired to itself using heavy Vicryl suture.
- A 10F Jackson-Pratt drain is routinely placed.
- A subcutaneous loose closure of 2-0 Vicryl is then used.
- Last, the skin is closed with simple nylon stitches if the closure appears to be complex or if it is simple and loose, absorbable monofilament simple stitches may be placed, although the patient should be advised that they take several months to reabsorb and fall off.

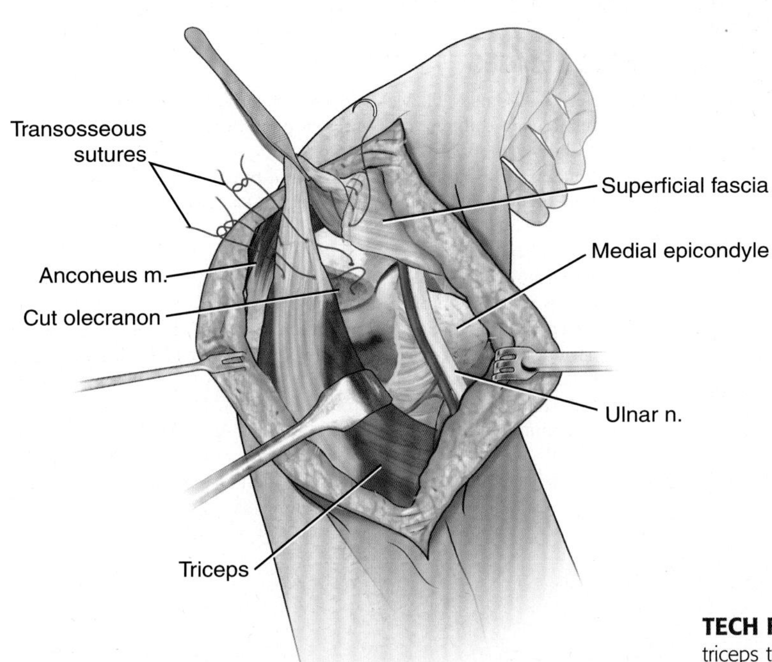

TECH FIG 3 • Transosseous sutures are used to repair the triceps to the olecranon. The defect in the fascia/periosteum unit is then repaired. (Adapted from Bryan RS, Morrey BF. Extensive posterior exposure of the elbow: a triceps-sparing approach. Clin Orthop Relat Res 1982;[166]:188–192.)

PEARLS AND PITFALLS

Visualizing the fracture	■ The C-arm should be brought in prior to draping to assure that adequate imaging can be obtained intraoperatively. A radiolucent arm board is quite helpful in this regard.
Preoperative planning	■ A CT scan or traction x-rays can be helpful preoperatively to assess the degree of comminution or presence of coronal split fracture lines which could impede reduction at the time of surgery.
Obtaining the reduction	■ The articular block should be reconstructed first; in adolescents, there is generally less comminution than in adults, so this block can generally be reconstructed into one large fragment. After this fragment is reduced, the articular block can be reduced to the shaft segment.
Preventing stiffness	■ The goal of surgery is to provide a stable enough construct that immediate motion or, at the very least, motion within 3 weeks is possible. Often, adolescents are nonadherent to self-therapy regimens, and frequent follow-up is necessary to prevent elbow stiffness or need for arthrolysis. Consider a continuous passive motion (CPM) postoperatively. Patients should be advised that usually 10 degrees of extension loss can be expected.
Closure	■ Closure with staples or nylon stitches is advised; remove every other day at 10–14 days. These will allow for wound care with early motion.
Follow-up	■ Follow-up once a week for 4–6 weeks for motion checks. Multiple x-rays are unnecessary, but monitoring the early motion is essential.

POSTOPERATIVE CARE

- A well-padded posterior splint in about 70 degrees of flexion is placed, and a sling applied.
- The patient is kept in house for 24 to 48 hours; the drain is pulled when less than 20 mL of drainage per shift is recorded.
- In open fractures, antibiotics are given for 48 hours. In closed fractures, antibiotics are stopped after 24 hours.
- Patients are sent home in a posterior splint which is removed five times a day for active and active-assisted range of motion (30 repetitions each session). They may also shower at this point.
- The patient is seen back in 2 weeks for a wound check.
- At 6 weeks, all immobilization is removed, and the patient is started on home low load prolonged stretching exercises and formal physical therapy.
- No gym or sports are allowed for 3 months or until the maximum range of motion (or full range of motion) has occurred and physical therapy has cleared the patient for activity.

OUTCOMES

- Re et al[6] reported a series of T-condylar humerus fractures in children and adolescents and reported that the Bernard Morrey approach resulted in significantly better motion than the more traditional triceps-splitting approach. This group also reported that early motion resulted in better final flexion and earlier functional range of motion than when range of motion was delayed.
- Beck et al[1] reported on 26 children and adolescents who had T-condylar fractures who were operatively treated. Approximately, one-third had elbow stiffness at final follow-up. Early range of motion resulted in earlier return to motion.

COMPLICATIONS

- Stiffness is quite common in T-condylar humerus fractures; preventing stiffness can be achieved by adequate stabilization to allow early motion.
- Symptomatic hardware is common; in adolescents, we do not routinely remove hardware unless the patient complains of it.
- Infection is more common in open injuries but still quite rare.
- Nerve injuries are generally neurapraxias and resolve spontaneously in 3 to 6 months.

REFERENCES

1. Beck NA, Ganley TJ, McKay S, et al. T-condylar fractures of the distal humerus in children: does early motion affect final range of motion? J Child Orthop 2014;8:161–165.
2. Bonczar MR, Rikli D, Ring D. Distal humerus 13-C1 Open reduction; perpendicular (biplanar) plating. AO Foundation Web site. Available at: http://bit.ly/1wEegQS. Published June 21, 2007. Accessed November 11, 2013.
3. Bryan RS, Morrey BF. Extensive posterior exposure of the elbow. A triceps-sparing approach. Clin Orthop Relat Res 1982;(166):188–192.
4. Green DP, Hotchkiss RN, Pederson WC; Dr. D. Sergeant Pepper Memorial Fund. Green's Operative Hand Surgery, ed 4. New York: Churchill Livingstone, 1999.
5. Maylahn DJ, Fahey JJ. Fractures of the elbow in children: review of three hundred consecutive cases. J Am Med Assoc 1958;166:220–228.
6. Re PR, Waters PM, Hresko T. T-condylar fractures of the distal humerus in children and adolescents. J Pediatr Orthop 1999;19:313–318.

Closed, Percutaneous, Intramedullary, and Open Reduction of Radial Head and Neck Fractures

Roger Cornwall

DEFINITION

- Radial neck fractures are extra-articular fractures of the radius proximal to the bicipital tuberosity.
- Radial neck fractures are most common in children 9 to 12 years old and represent 14% of elbow fractures in children.[17] The physis is typically involved as a Salter-Harris I or II pattern (**FIG 1**), yet Salter-Harris III and IV patterns also occur. Alternatively, the fracture can be extraphyseal through the metaphysis.[1,33]
- Intra-articular radial head fractures are less common elbow injuries in patients with open physes than in skeletally mature patients (7% vs. 52%).[18]
- The Wilkins classification of radial head and neck fractures is based on the mechanism of injury and the pattern of the fracture, specifically whether there is physeal or articular involvement[34]:
  - Type I: valgus injury
    - A: physeal injury—Salter-Harris I or II
    - B: intra-articular—Salter-Harris III or IV
    - C: metaphyseal fracture
  - Type II: elbow dislocation
    - D: fracture occurred during reduction
    - E: fracture occurred during dislocation
- The O'Brien and Judet classifications of radial neck fractures are based on degree of angulation.
  - O'Brien classification[22]
    - Type I: less than 30 degrees
    - Type II: 30 to 60 degrees
    - Type III: more than 60 degrees
  - Judet classification[14] (**FIG 2**)
    - Type I: undisplaced
    - Type II: less than 30 degrees
    - Type III: 30 to 60 degrees
    - Type IVa: 60 to 80 degrees
    - Type IVb: more than 80 degrees

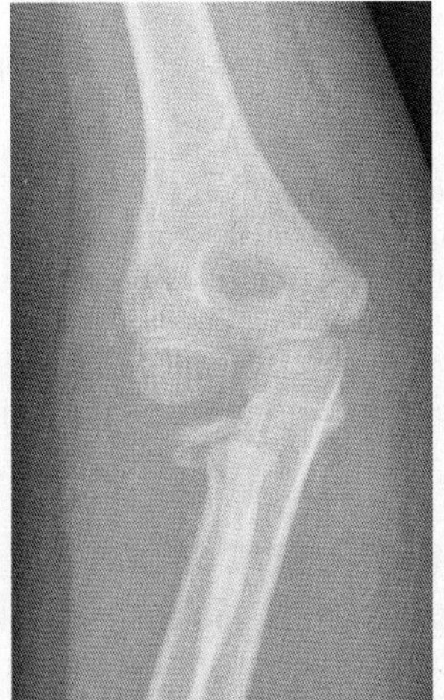
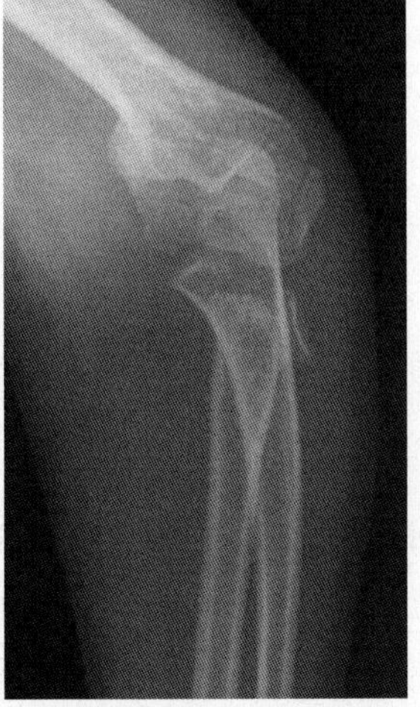

FIG 1 • Displaced radial neck fractures. **A.** Salter-Harris type II. **B.** Salter-Harris type I.

ANATOMY

- The radial head articulates with the capitellum and the radial notch of the ulna. The radial neck is extra-articular and has a normal 15 degrees of angulation on anteroposterior (AP) and 5 degrees on lateral radiographic views. The radial head ossific nucleus appears at about 4 years of age.
- Ossification of the proximal radial epiphysis (radial head) occurs by 4 years of age, at which time the radial head and neck have assumed their adult shape. The proximal radial physis closes at 14 years in girls and 17 years in boys.
- The proximal radioulnar joint is stabilized by the annular ligament and the accessory collateral ligament.
- There are no muscular attachments to the radial neck. The blood supply is derived from the adjacent periosteum.
- The radial nerve gives rise to the superficial radial nerve and the posterior interosseous nerve at the level of the lateral condyle. The posterior interosseous nerve travels distally anterior to the radial head and neck, enters the arcade of Frohse 2.6 cm distal to the radial head (**FIG 3**), and submerges between the superficial and deep fibers of the supinator 6.7 cm distal to the radial head.[5] The radial recurrent artery originates from the radial artery and travels toward the lateral epicondyle in the opposite direction along the path of the radial nerve on the anteromedial surface of the supinator.

PATHOGENESIS

- The most common mechanism of radial neck fractures is a valgus and axial force to the elbow caused by a fall on an outstretched hand. This mechanism results in a lateral compression and a medial traction injury. The actual plane of maximal radial head angulation depends on the forearm position of supination or pronation at the time of impact.[12]
- The other mechanism of injury is an elbow dislocation where the fracture occurs either during the dislocation (radial head anterior) or during the elbow reduction (radial head posterior).[12]
- Associated injuries, such as medial collateral ligament rupture or occult elbow dislocation, occur in 30% to 50% of radial neck fractures.[28]

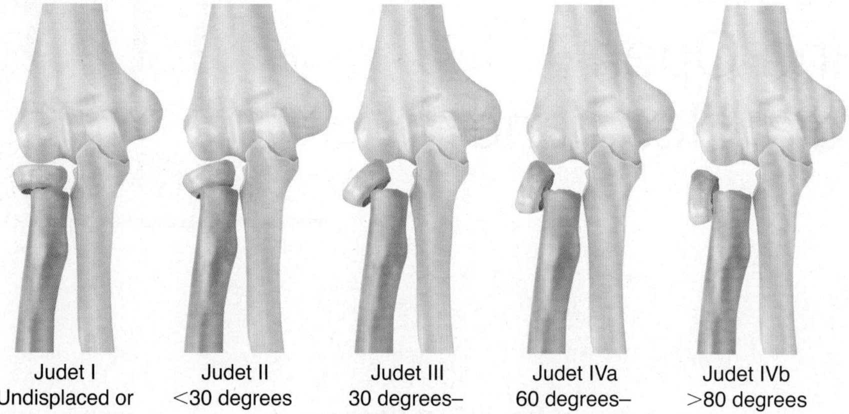

FIG 2 • Judet classification of radial neck fractures in children.

- A posteriorly displaced radial neck fracture can occur during the spontaneous reduction of a posterior elbow dislocation.[11]
- Alternatively, an unrecognized (undisplaced) radial neck fracture can be displaced posteriorly during the manipulative reduction of a posterior elbow dislocation. During the reduction maneuver, if the elbow is flexed, the distal humerus (lateral condyle) strikes the radial head, knocking it posteriorly off the metaphysis (**FIG 4**).
- Chronic stress fractures of the radial head and neck can occur with repetitive valgus loading, such as overhead throwing.

NATURAL HISTORY

- The prognosis for radial neck fractures depends on the energy of injury, the amount of displacement, and the presence of any associated injuries.
- Most radial neck fractures are minimally displaced or undisplaced. These heal uneventfully.
- The greater the degree of angulation or translation, the greater the disruption in the relationship of the radiocapitellar joint, which may be associated with a decrease in the range of pronation and supination.[3]
- The upper limit of acceptable angulation (0 to 60 degrees) is unclear and may be age-dependent.[24] Most believe that angulation less than 30 degrees is unlikely to cause a clinically (functionally) significant loss of motion.
- Other reported consequences include avascular necrosis of the radial head, heterotopic ossification, radioulnar synostosis, and premature physeal closure, which may result in pain, crepitus, and valgus deformity and stiffness.[3,13,24,26,27]
  - These outcomes may be associated with age, severity of displacement, presence of associated injuries, or delay in treatment.
- Some of these might be a complication of the treatment (poor reduction, open treatment, or internal fixation) rather than the natural history.
- Overall, poor results have been reported in up to 15% to 33% of all radial neck fractures in children.[7,10,13,27,30]

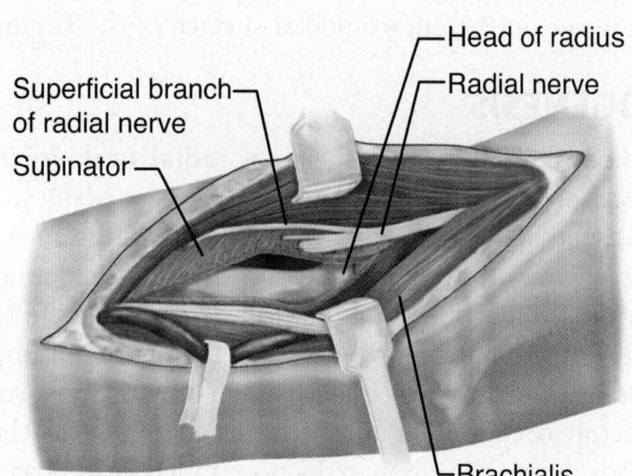

FIG 3 • The posterior interosseous nerve courses volarly to the radial head and neck and enters the arcade of Frohse about 2.6 cm distal to the articular surface of the radial head.

PATIENT HISTORY AND PHYSICAL FINDINGS

- Elucidating the mechanism of injury is important to truly understand the personality of the fracture, which can help in directing treatment. Higher energy mechanisms are more likely to be associated with concomitant injuries. Elbow dislocations that have reduced before presentation are not uncommon, so it is helpful to ask the patient and family whether a marked deformity was noted at the time of injury.
- Carefully palpating each anatomic area in the elbow to find the points of maximal tenderness helps diagnose the fracture as well as additional injuries. Associated injuries include medial collateral ligament tears, medial epicondyle fractures, ulnar fractures, and supracondylar humerus fractures. A neurologic evaluation assesses distal radial, medial, and ulnar nerve motor and sensory function.
- Assessing elbow stability and range of motion can help determine the need for treatment.
  - Valgus instability indicates a medial elbow injury in addition to an unstable radial neck fracture.
  - Blocks in forearm rotation, in particular pronation, are typically due to loss of congruity of the radioulnar joint and indicate a need for reduction.
  - Stability and range-of-motion assessment may necessitate either an intra-articular anesthetic injection or an examination under anesthesia.

IMAGING AND OTHER DIAGNOSTIC STUDIES

- AP, lateral, and oblique radiographs often show radial neck fractures well (**FIG 5A,B**). However, the true extent of fracture angulation can be underestimated on plain radiographs, as orthogonal views may fail to capture the true plane of angulation.

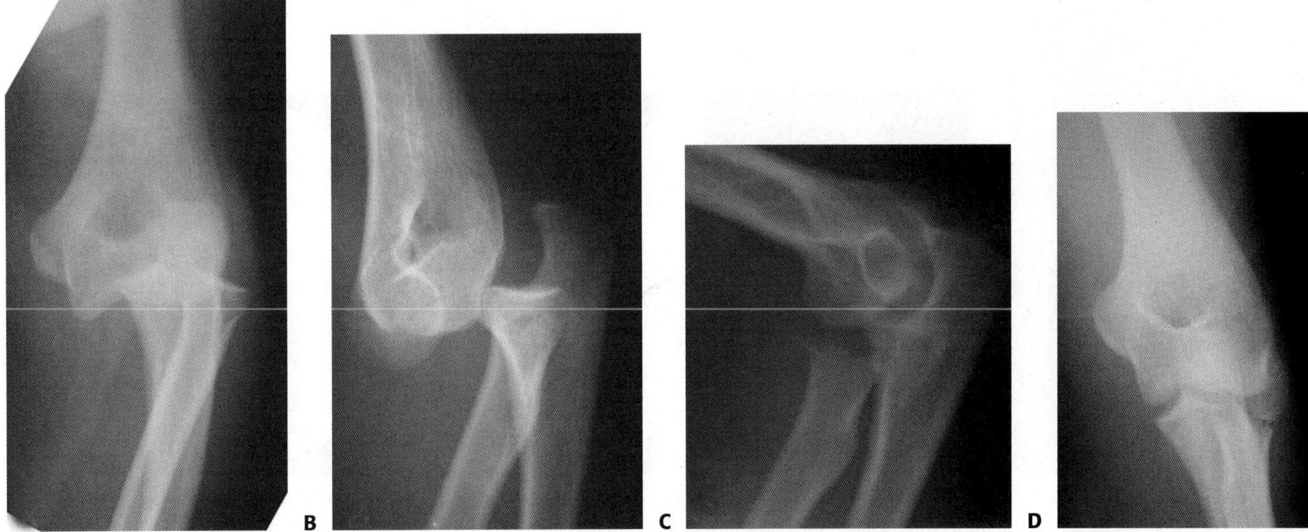

FIG 4 • Posteriorly displaced radial neck fracture produced during the reduction of a posterior elbow dislocation. **A,B.** AP and lateral views of the elbow dislocation. **C.** The radial head is no longer visible on the lateral view after elbow reduction. **D.** Displaced radial head apparent on AP view.

- The clinician should carefully rule out associated injuries such as fractures of the olecranon (intra-articular) (**FIG 5C,D**), proximal ulna, medial epicondyle, or lateral condyle or elbow dislocation.
- In posterior elbow dislocations, the clinician should carefully examine the radial neck for an occult fracture that is at risk for displacement during the reduction maneuver.
- Radial neck fractures can occur before the ossification of the radial head, without clear evidence of fracture on plain radiographs.
  - Ultrasound, magnetic resonance imaging (MRI) (**FIG 5E**), and arthrography (**FIG 5F,G**) are useful for diagnosing and evaluating radial neck fractures in young patients with nonossified radial heads.
  - In the operating room, arthrography is useful in outlining the nonossified radial head when monitoring and verifying reduction.

DIFFERENTIAL DIAGNOSIS

- The diagnosis of a radial neck fracture is usually easily made with appropriate imaging. However, the presence or absence of the following associated injuries should be ascertained:
  - Medial collateral ligament rupture
  - Medial epicondyle fracture
  - Olecranon fracture
  - Monteggia equivalent type IV fracture

NONOPERATIVE MANAGEMENT

- Ultimately, the objective is to obtain and maintain a congruent joint with restored elbow range of motion in all planes. Most consider up to 30 degrees of angulation and 3 mm of translation as limits of an acceptable reduction.

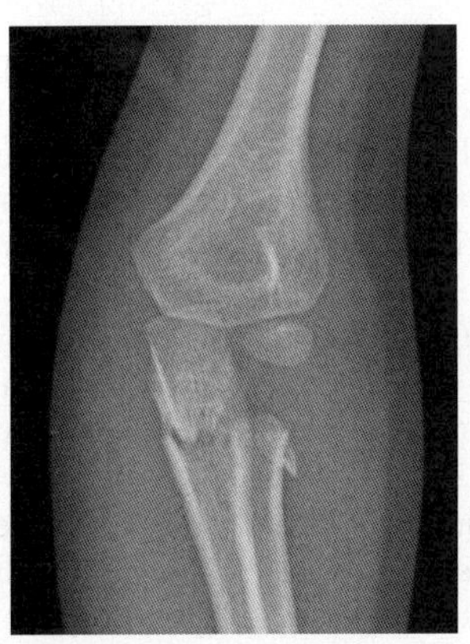

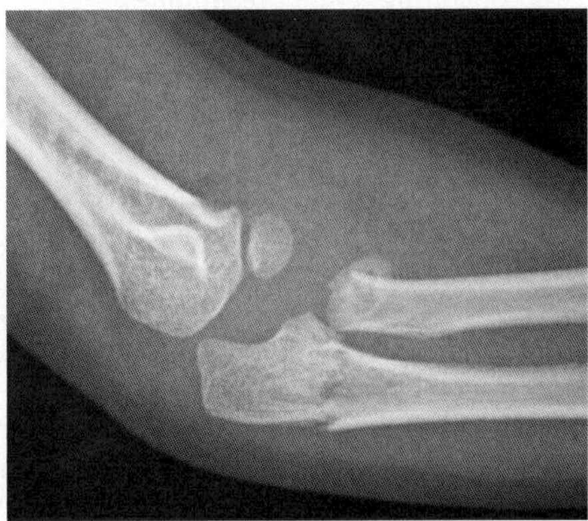

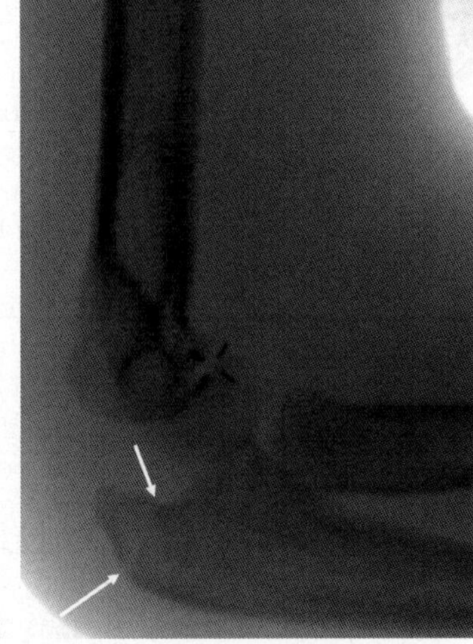

FIG 5 • **A,B.** AP and lateral radiographs demonstrate an ulnar fracture and radial neck fracture in a 3-year-old child with a nonossified radial head. However, it is difficult to discern the degree of angulation on plain radiographs. MRI is useful when evaluating radial neck fractures in children with nonossified radial heads. **C.** Radial neck fracture with associated intra-articular fracture of the olecranon. Olecranon fracture (*arrows*) appears minimally displaced on lateral view. *(continued)*

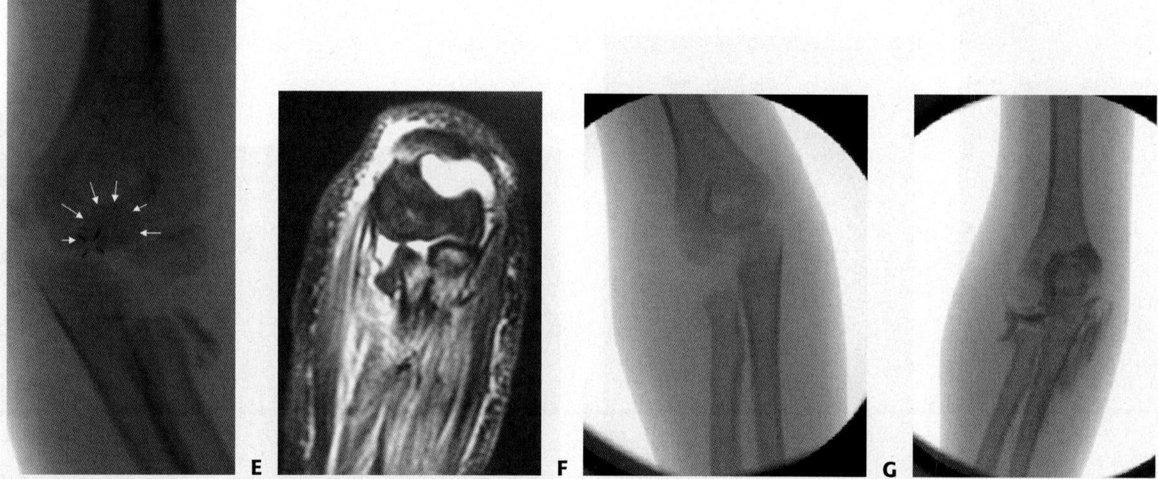

FIG 5 • *(continued)* **D.** Significant displacement of the proximal olecron fragment (*arrows*) is seen on AP view. **E.** MRI from patient in **A** and **B** clearly shows the 60-degree radial neck angulation not defined on plain films. **F,G.** Arthrography demonstrates a 90-degree displaced radial neck fracture not seen on plain films. It is also useful to monitor and verify reduction intraoperatively.

Controversy exists regarding the exact numbers, however, with reported acceptable angulation ranging from 20 to 60 degrees.[1,3,15,21,26,30–34]

- Two things partially account for the controversy:
  - The accuracy of the radiographic measurement is variable and depends on whether the radiographic beam is perpendicular to the true plane of the fracture.
  - Twenty-five degrees of fracture angulation can have variable effects on the congruity of the radioulnar joint, depending on the direction of angulation.
- It is therefore important to base the decision of treatment on the functional effects of the angulation rather than a specific number. Any block of pronation or supination warrants a reduction of the fracture, no matter what the radiographic angulation is.

- As remodeling potential decreases with advancing skeletal maturity, less residual angulation is acceptable (15 to 20 degrees).[9,32]
- Closed reduction is recommended if there is more than 30 degrees of angulation or 3 mm of translation or if there is any block to range of motion. Reduction can be done either with sedation in the emergency room or in the operating room. The advantage of the latter is the immediate ability to proceed to a percutaneous reduction technique should the closed techniques fail, which is more likely in cases with severe displacement.
- The nature and duration of immobilization depend on the fracture pattern, the presumed stability, and the maturity of the patient. For example, a 17-year-old reliable patient with a nondisplaced stable radial neck fracture can be treated with a sling and early range of motion. Physeal fractures, fractures needing reduction, and fractures in young patients usually need immobilization in a cast for 3 weeks, however.
  - When clinical and radiographic signs of healing are lacking, the cast may remain for an additional 2 weeks, followed by a reevaluation of the healing progress.

SURGICAL MANAGEMENT

- If closed reduction fails, the next step is to proceed to a percutaneous reduction technique. Techniques using a Steinmann pin to push or lever are described in detail in the Techniques section.
- Every attempt to achieve a closed or percutaneous reduction is made, as the rates of complications, including avascular necrosis, heterotopic ossification, and nonunion, are higher with an open approach.[3,21,36]
- The markedly displaced floating fragments associated with elbow dislocations often require an open approach, whereas most angulated radial head fractures can be reduced by a combination of closed and percutaneous techniques.

Preoperative Planning

- It is essential to obtain proper elbow and forearm radiographs and diagnose all injuries before proceeding to the operating room.
- Familiarity with all of the closed and percutaneous reduction techniques described in the Techniques section is useful, as each fracture behaves and responds differently to different techniques.
- It is prudent to advise both the parents and the operating room staff that a range of techniques from closed to open may be employed to obtain reduction. Doing so eliminates any element of surprise. The surgeon should ensure the availability of elastic titanium nails, Kirschner wires, and Steinmann pins if needed.
- Elbow range of motion and stability are assessed under anesthesia. The elbow is then pronated and supinated under fluoroscopy to find the maximum plane of angulation before reduction (**FIG 6**).
- Several different techniques of closed and percutaneous reduction make up the "reduction ladder" covered in the Techniques section, much like the plastic surgeon's reconstructive ladder. These tools may be used in stepwise progression or in conjunction as needed.

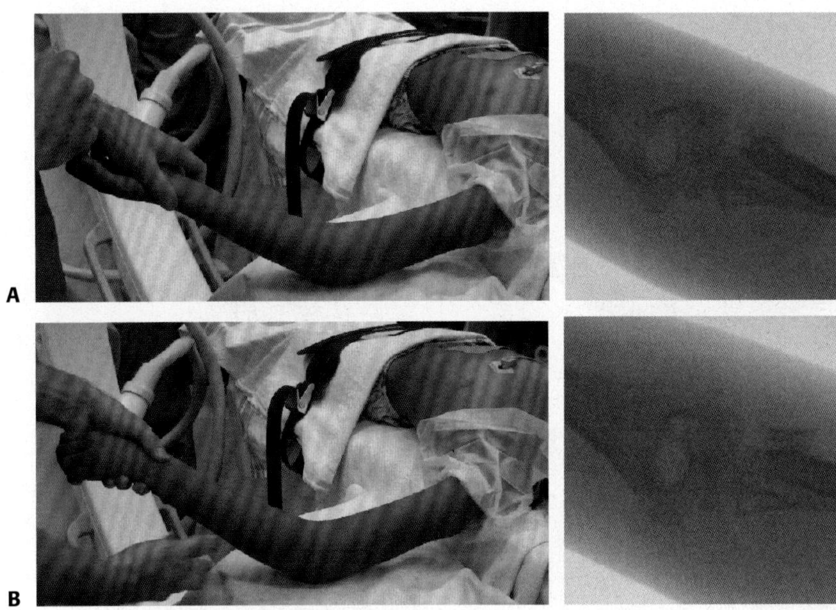

FIG 6 • The maximal angle of displacement is found with fluoroscopy imaging through the ranges of full supination (**A**) to pronation (**B**). In this case, maximal angulation is noted with 50 degrees of pronation.

Positioning

- The patient is positioned supine on the operating room table, with the elbow on the fluoroscopy C-arm and the arm positioned on the collimator of the C-arm (**FIG 7**).
- The imaging monitor is placed at the opposite side of the bed for easy visualization.
- Alternatively, the patient may be positioned supine with the injured arm positioned over a radiolucent arm board and the image intensifier positioned parallel to the operating table to allow the C-arm to be moved freely from the AP to lateral position.

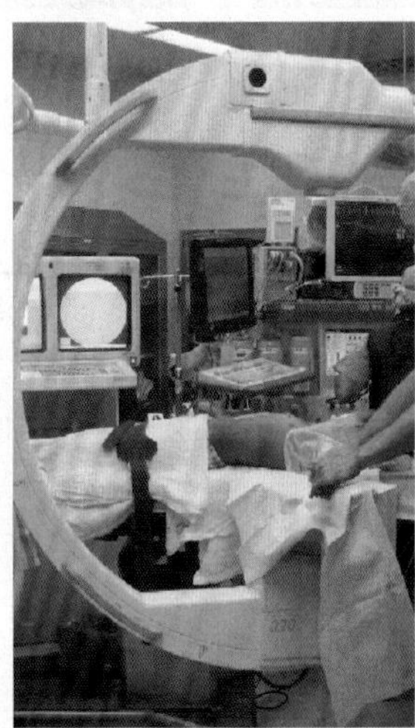

FIG 7 • After sterile preparation, the arm is draped out using the C-arm as an operating table. The imaging monitor is placed for easy visualization on the other side of the bed.

Approach

- The posterolateral Kocher approach is used for open reduction of severely displaced floating fragments. The approach is further described in the Techniques section.

TECHNIQUES

Closed Reduction

Israeli or Kaufman Technique

- Kaufman et al[15] described a closed reduction technique with the elbow flexed 90 degrees.
- Fluoroscopy is used to establish the forearm position demonstrating maximal angulation (see **FIG 6**).
- One hand is used to control forearm rotation, and the other hand is used to provide lateral pressure to the displaced radial head with the thumb (**TECH FIG 1A–C**).
- After reduction, fracture stability and range of motion are assessed (**TECH FIG 1D–G**).

Patterson Technique

- With the elbow extended and forearm supinated, varus stress is applied to the elbow by an assistant. The surgeon reduces the fragment with lateral digital pressure (**TECH FIG 2**).
- Drawbacks of this technique include the need for a knowledgeable assistant providing countertraction and varus stress and the potential difficulty in palpating the radial head in this position.

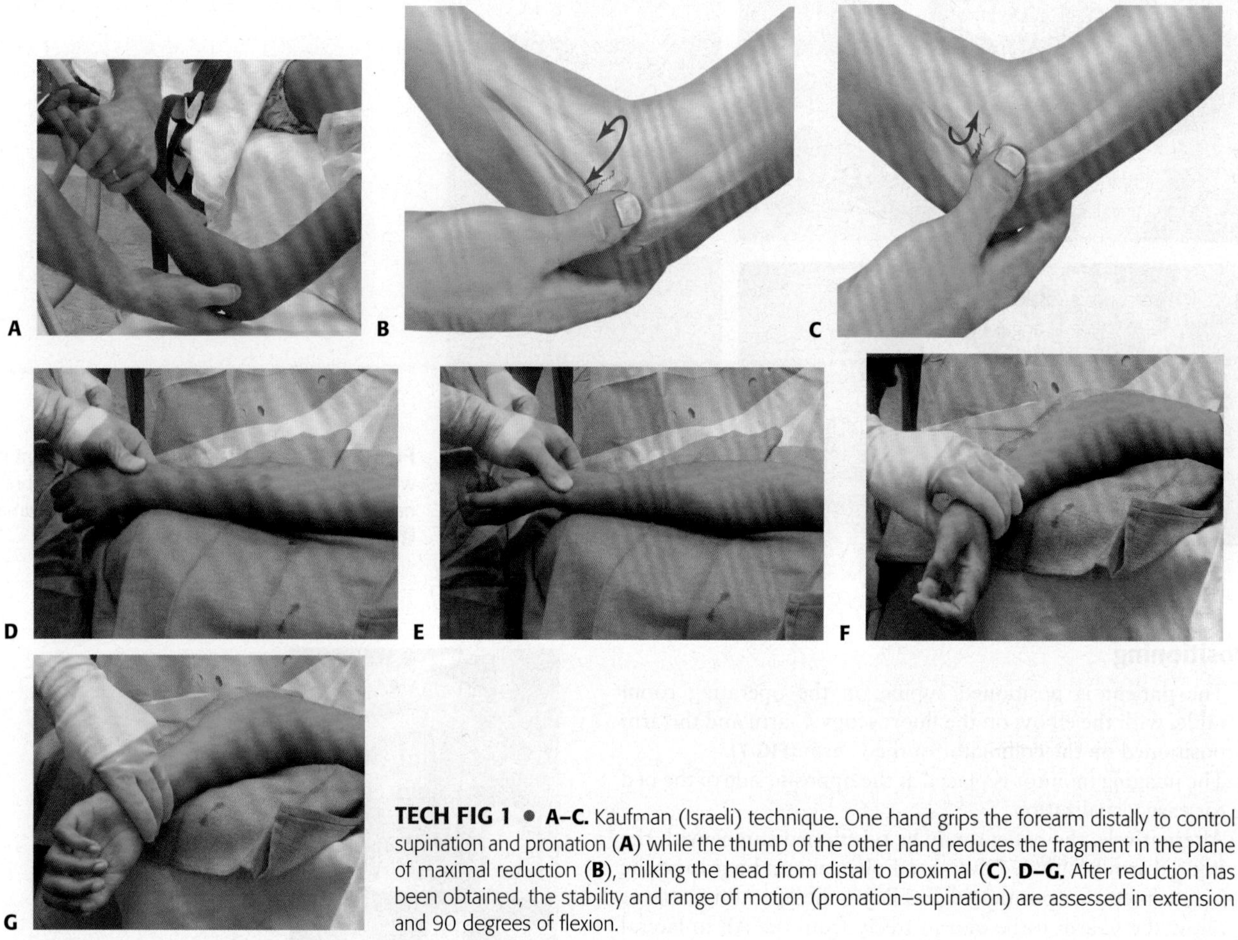

TECH FIG 1 • **A–C.** Kaufman (Israeli) technique. One hand grips the forearm distally to control supination and pronation (**A**) while the thumb of the other hand reduces the fragment in the plane of maximal reduction (**B**), milking the head from distal to proximal (**C**). **D–G.** After reduction has been obtained, the stability and range of motion (pronation–supination) are assessed in extension and 90 degrees of flexion.

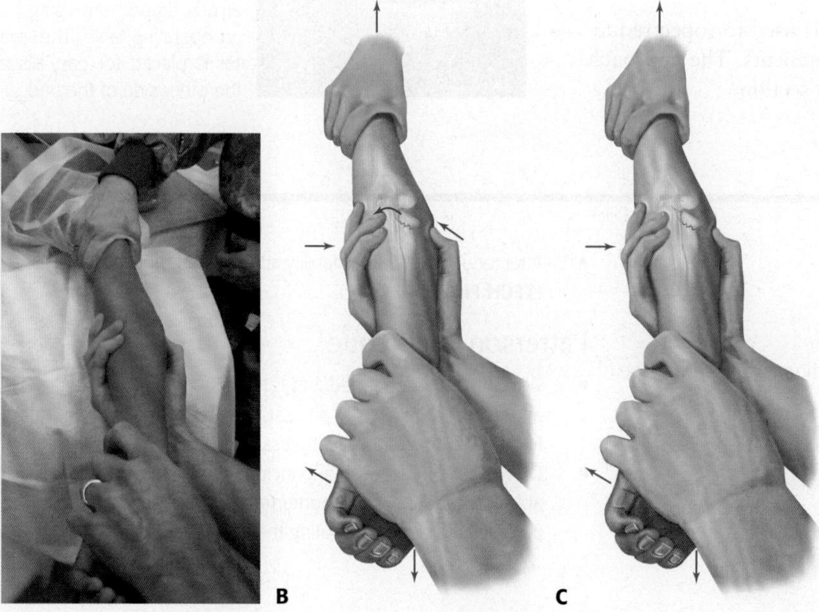

TECH FIG 2 • Patterson technique. **A.** The assistant helps with positioning the elbow in extension, applying a varus force while holding the forearm in supination. **B,C.** Digital pressure from the thumb is applied to the radial head to achieve reduction.

Percutaneous Reduction with a Kirschner Wire or Steinmann Pin

- If closed reduction fails, a Kirschner wire or a Steinmann pin can be used to directly push or lever the radial head into anatomic position.
- The surgeon must beware of the posterior interosseous nerve coursing volarly and distally over the radial head. The radial head can be protected by pronating the forearm and by using a posterolateral pin approach (**TECH FIG 3**).
- The forearm is rotated using fluoroscopic guidance so that the plane of maximal angulation is visualized.

Push Technique

- The blunt end of a larger Kirschner wire, 0.062 inch or larger, is percutaneously inserted through the skin distal to the fracture and just off the lateral border of the ulna (**TECH FIG 4A,B**) through a 2-mm incision.
- With fluoroscopic guidance, the pin is placed against the posterolateral aspect of the proximal fragment, and the radial head is pushed into place (**TECH FIG 4C,D**).
- Axial traction and rotation of the forearm can dislodge an impacted fracture and assist in the reduction.

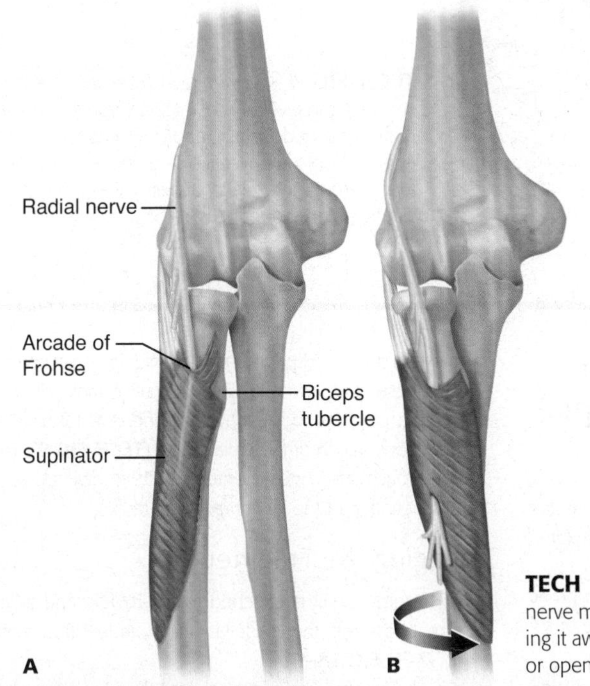

TECH FIG 3 • A,B. The posterior interosseous nerve moves volarly and medially with pronation, moving it away from the working area during percutaneous or open treatment of radial head and neck fractures.

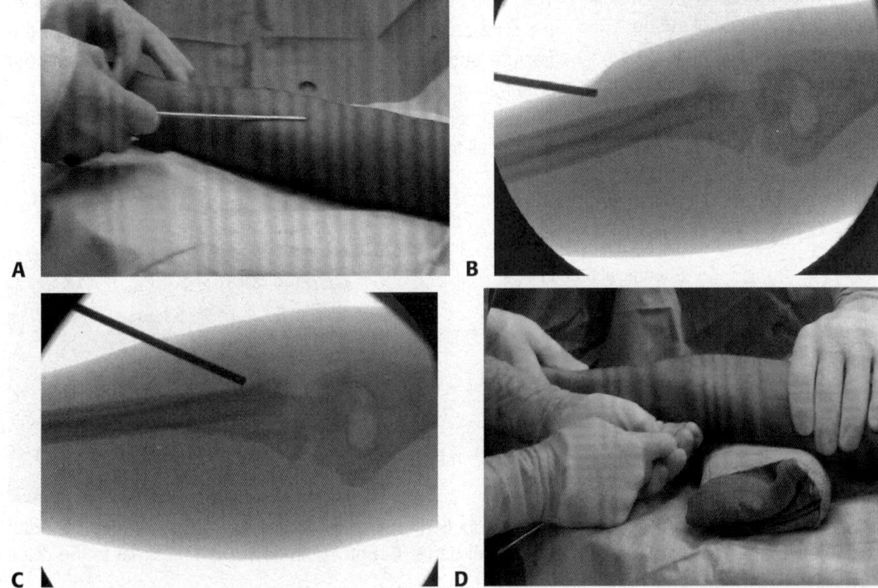

TECH FIG 4 • Push technique for percutaneous reduction of radial neck fracture. A,B. Imaging is used to plan the trajectory of the push pin. The pin is inserted posterolaterally, avoiding the volar posterior interosseous nerve. **C,D.** Using imaging as guidance, the radial head fragment is pushed into reduction.

Lever Technique

- Alternatively, the pin (or a Freer elevator) can be used as a lever. When doing so, the skin entry site of the pin must be placed more proximally, however, at the level of the fracture site (**TECH FIG 5A**).
- With the pin just through the skin, the pin is pulled distally (applying tension to the skin) to allow a retrograde approach to the fracture.
- The deeper soft tissues are then pierced, the fracture site is entered (**TECH FIG 5B**), and the proximal fragment is levered proximally to correct the angulation while translation is corrected with simultaneous lateral digital pressure. During the levering maneuver, the tensioned skin relaxes, thus making the reduction easier (**TECH FIG 5C**).
  - If the skin instead were entered distally for the lever maneuver, however, the skin tension during the reduction maneuver would make the reduction substantially more difficult.
- After percutaneous reduction, fracture stability in all planes is assessed. If unstable, pin fixation of the fragment is recommended.

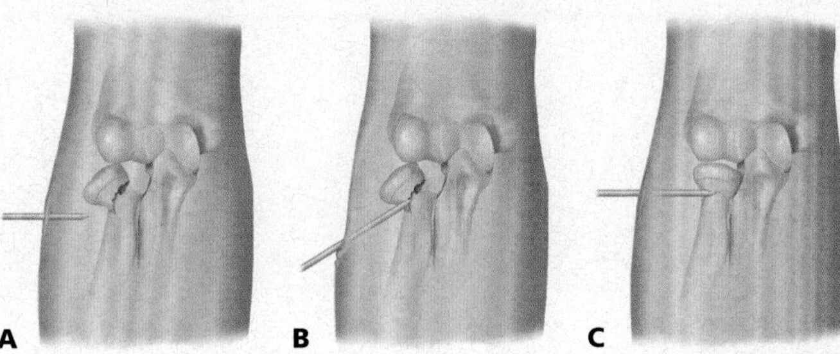

TECH FIG 5 • Lever technique. **A.** The lever pin is inserted at the level of the fracture through the skin. **B.** The pin is then pushed distally, applying tension to the skin before approaching the physeal side of the fracture and (**C**) levering the fragment into place, allowing the built-up tension of the skin to aid in the reduction.

Closed Intramedullary Reduction and Fixation (Metaizeau Technique)

Description

- Metaizeau described an intramedullary reduction and fixation technique for the treatment of displaced radial neck fractures[9] that has been widely adopted.[4,6,8,16,20,23,25,29]
- The intramedullary manipulation of the radial head can be accomplished by an elastic titanium nail or a Kirschner wire of sufficient length, the tip of which is bent about 30 degrees.
- The diameter of the elastic nail or Kirschner wire is usually 2 mm. A 2.5-mm nail may be suitable in some children older than 10 years. The curved nail tip can be bent additionally.
- The entry point for the nail can either be a radial or dorsal site on the radius as described for radial shaft fracture flexible intramedullary nailing. On the dorsal side, the entry site is immediately proximal to Lister tubercle between the second and third extensor compartments. The bare cortical area can be reliably identified between these compartments by avoiding retraction of the tendons in these compartments. The alternative radial entry site is 1.5 to 2 cm proximal to the physis, taking care to avoid injury to the sensory branch of the radial nerve (**TECH FIG 6**). Through either approach, the cortex is entered with an awl, taking care to avoid penetration of the far cortex of the radius.

Engaging the Fragment

- The elastic nail is attached to a T-handle and advanced proximally through the medullary canal under fluoroscopic guidance (**TECH FIG 7A–C**).
  - The forearm is rotated until the plane of maximum deformity is visualized.
- The curved tip of the nail or the Kirschner wire is directed toward the displaced proximal fragment and gently advanced across the fracture until the tip engages the epiphyseal fragment without penetrating the articular surface (**TECH FIG 7D–F**).
- AP and lateral radiographs are obtained to confirm the position of the nail tip in the epiphyseal fragment.

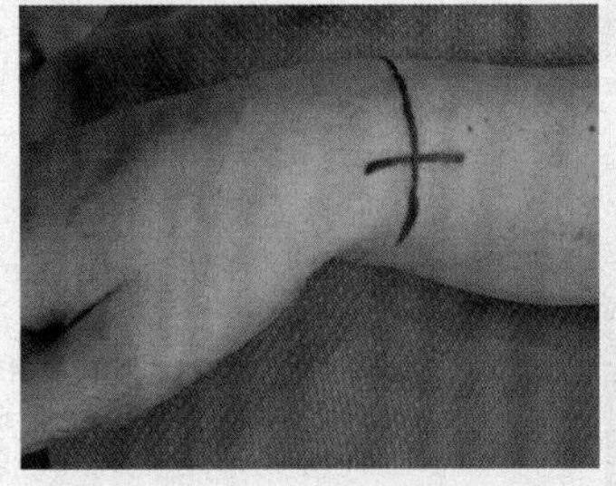

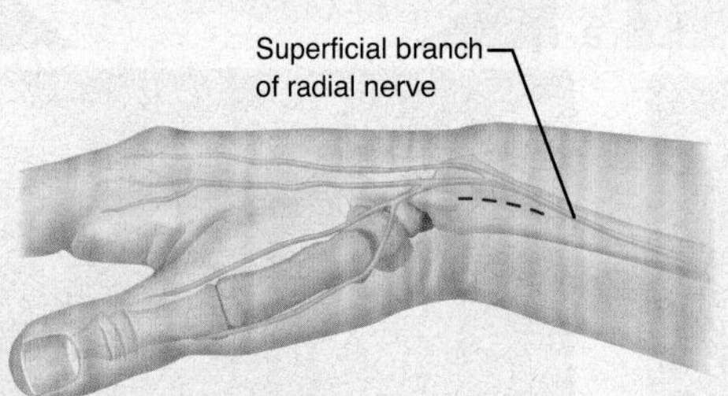

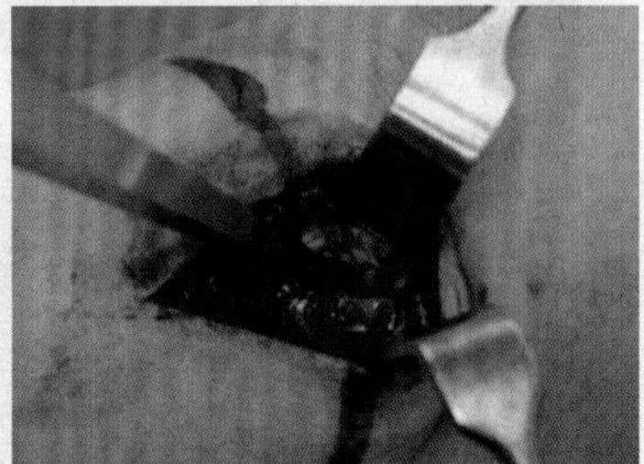

TECH FIG 6 • **A–F.** Radial-side entry point for elastic nail for centromedullary reduction technique. **A.** Incision centered over the distal radial physis. **B.** The surgeon should avoid injury to the superficial branch of the radial nerve. **C.** Entry point is 1.5 cm proximal to the distal radial physis. *(continued)*

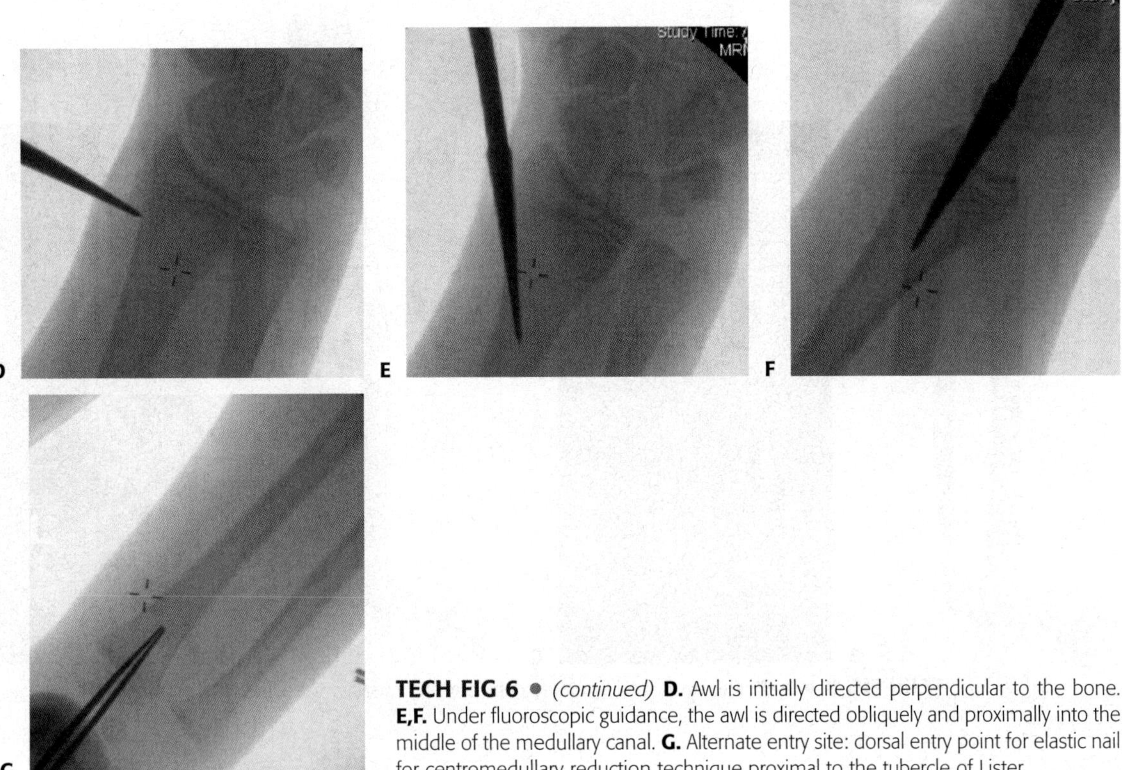

TECH FIG 6 • *(continued)* **D.** Awl is initially directed perpendicular to the bone. **E,F.** Under fluoroscopic guidance, the awl is directed obliquely and proximally into the middle of the medullary canal. **G.** Alternate entry site: dorsal entry point for elastic nail for centromedullary reduction technique proximal to the tubercle of Lister.

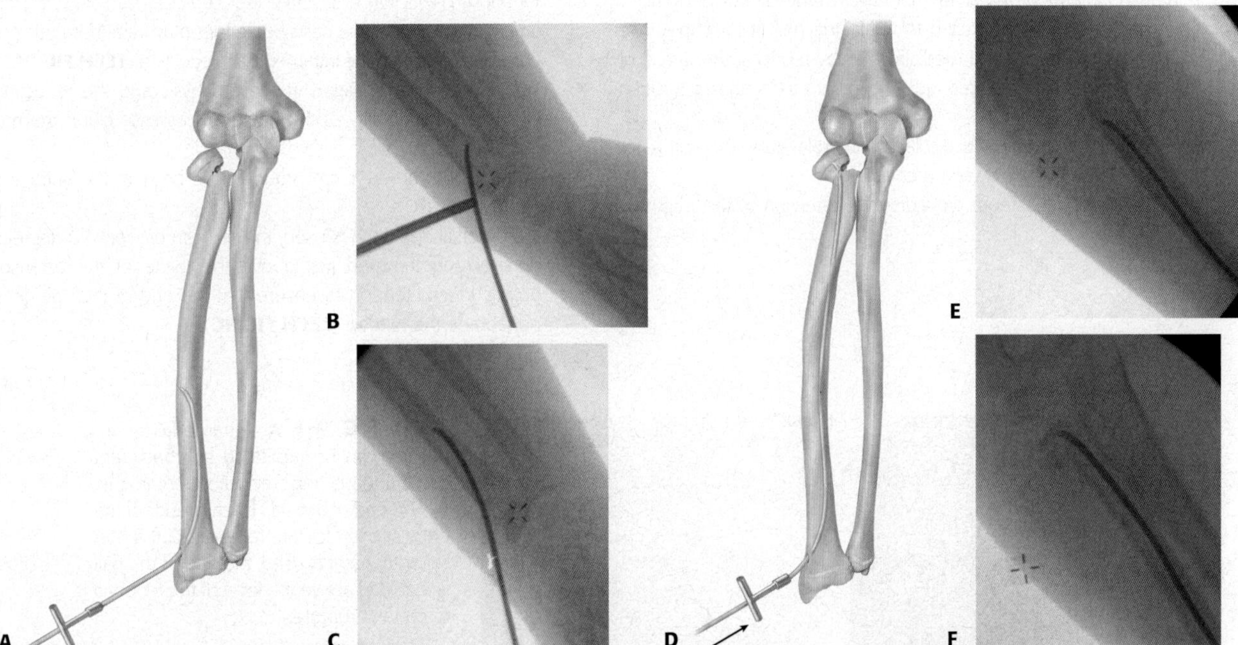

TECH FIG 7 • Closed intramedullary reduction and fixation technique of Metaizeau with an elastic nail. **A–C.** Proximal advancement of elastic nail through the medullary canal. **D–F.** The curved tip is directed toward and advanced into the displaced epiphyseal fragment.

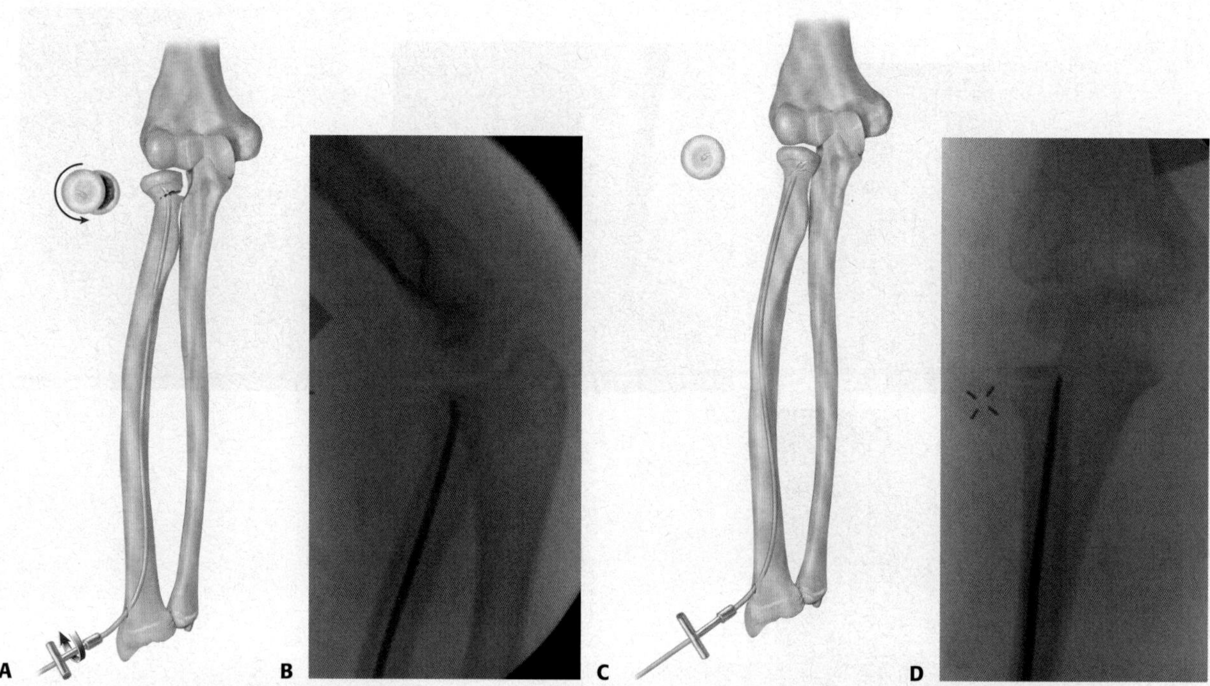

TECH FIG 8 • A–D. The elastic nail is rotated anteriorly and medially to reduce the radial head.

Rotating the Fragment into Place

- The nail tip is used to elevate the fragment to reduce the tilt anchoring the proximal fragment against the lateral condyle.
- The T-handle is then used to rotate the nail or Kirschner wire typically anteriorly and medially, thereby reducing the lateral or posterolaterally displaced radial head back to its normal location (**TECH FIG 8**).
  - If the epiphysis is displaced anterolaterally, the nail is rotated posteriorly and medially.
- The intact periosteum prevents overcorrection of the fragment medially.

Completing the Procedure

- The reduction maneuver may be facilitated with a prior or concurrent closed reduction. In severely displaced radial neck fractures, the percutaneous technique described earlier may be performed concurrently to facilitate the intramedullary reduction (**TECH FIG 9A**).
- With the nail tip engaged in the epiphysis and the reduction complete, the stability of the fracture is assessed, and the nail is left in situ.
- The nail is trimmed 1 cm proud of the bone at the entry site (**TECH FIG 9B**).
- If the dorsal approach is used, the nail can be bent 90 degrees dorsally and trimmed just above the plane of the extensor pollicis longus tendon to ensure that the end of the nail does not abrade the tendon (**TECH FIG 9C**).

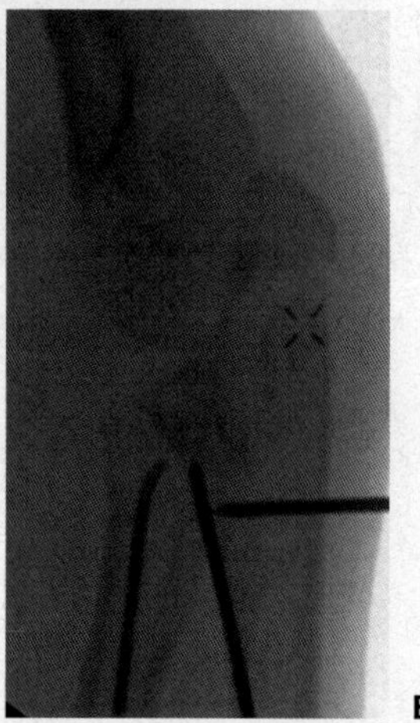

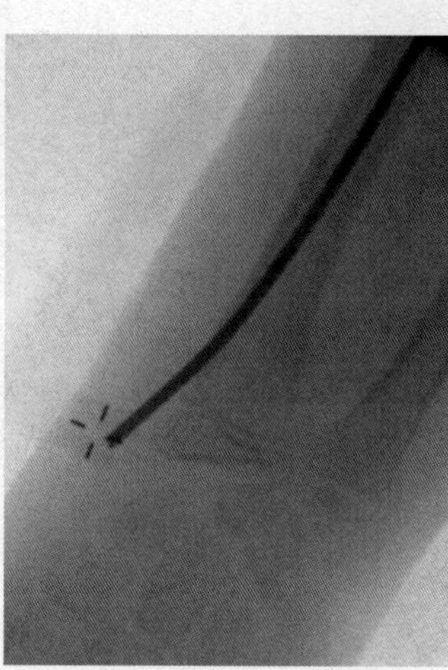

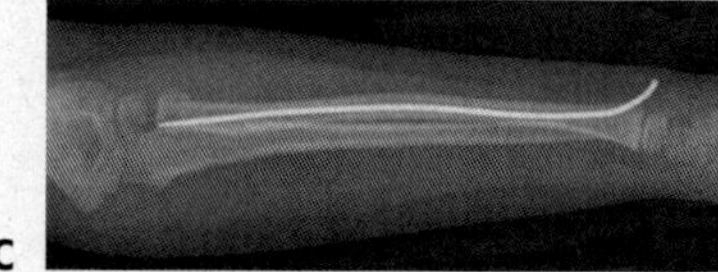

TECH FIG 9 • A. Intramedullary reduction can be facilitated by concurrent percutaneous pin reduction technique. **B.** The end of the nail is left proud off the entry site to facilitate removal. **C.** If a dorsal entry point is used, the end of the nail is trimmed above the level of the tendons to prevent rupture.

Open Reduction

- Kocher posterolateral approach to the radial head is used. Pronating the forearm brings the posterior interosseous nerve further anteromedially, away from the surgical field.
- A skin incision about 5 cm long is made, centered over the posterolateral aspect of the radial head (**TECH FIG 10A**). The interval between the anconeus (radial nerve) and the extensor carpi ulnaris (posterior interosseous nerve) is developed (**TECH FIG 10B**).
- A longitudinal incision is made along the capsule, unless the capsule has not already been torn open by the injury causing trauma (**TECH FIG 10C**).
- The proximal fragment is identified and reduced under direct visualization and fluoroscopic guidance. If the annular ligament has been injured, it should be repaired.
- Occasionally, the fracture is widely displaced anteromedially, necessitating further exposure before identification. In such a case, a more extensile approach is recommended as well as a formal proximal identification of the radial nerve and posterior interosseous nerve.
- If the fracture requires open reduction, internal fixation is recommended.
  - A retrospective review of radial neck nonunions noted that they were commonly associated with an early loss of fixation, related to either displacement or premature removal of pins.[33]
  - Options for internal fixation include pins placed obliquely through the radial head in an ice cream cone pattern throughout the safe zone. Absorbable pins can also be used. Radial head fixation can be achieved with epiphyseal–metaphyseal interrupted, circumferentially placed absorbable sutures.[2] For skeletally mature children, headless screws or a T-plate in the safe zone can be used.
  - Although seldom indicated, Leung and Tse[19] described a lateral mini-plate buttress technique for the open physis. The plate is anchored distally in the radial neck with 2-mm screws and left unattached proximally, providing a buttress preventing lateral dislocation of the radial head.
  - Transcapitellar pin fixation has been described, but it provides poor distal fixation and is associated with pin breakage at the radiocapitellar joint.[3]

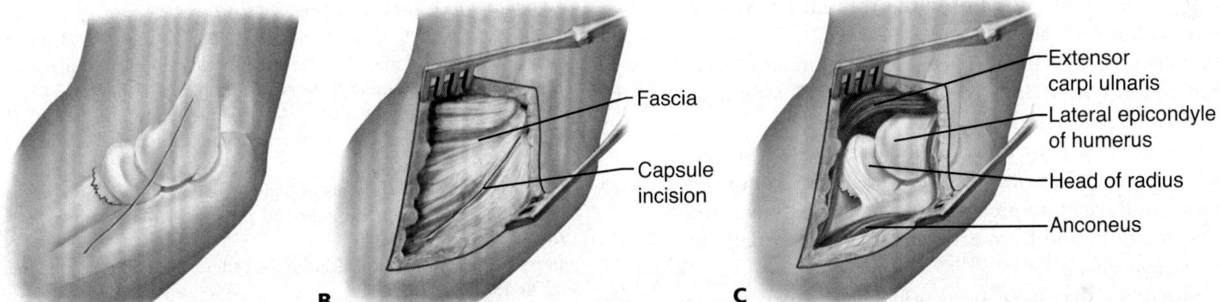

TECH FIG 10 • **A.** The Kocher posterolateral approach to the elbow uses the interval between the anconeus and the extensor carpi ulnaris. **B.** The capsule is incised longitudinally. **C.** The radial head fragment may be readily visualized after exposure, unless medially or posteriorly displaced.

PEARLS AND PITFALLS

Indications	▪ The surgeon should have a discussion with the family and alert the operating room staff regarding the "reduction ladder" and the various techniques that may be employed.
Operative technique	▪ Although percutaneous reduction can be a tedious and time-consuming procedure, open reduction should be avoided if at all possible. ▪ A mini-open approach using a Freer elevator as a shoehorn can sometimes reduce the fragment when percutaneous Steinmann pin reduction is unsuccessful. ▪ For intramedullary reduction and fixation, in the radial approach, the surgeon should avoid injury to the sensory branch of the radial nerve. If the dorsal approach is used, the nail is bent away from Lister tubercle and trimmed above the dorsal aspect of the extensor tendons so as not to abrade it. ▪ If an open reduction is necessary, fixation is necessary. ▪ Transarticular pins should be avoided, as they may break at the joint. ▪ Radial head excision is contraindicated in children because of valgus elbow deformity, longitudinal forearm instability, and high incidence of overgrowth.
Imaging	▪ After achieving reduction, the surgeon should verify improved range of motion and make sure that the reduction is a true change in alignment and not simply a radiograph taken out of the plane with maximal angulation. ▪ The surgeon should beware of reversal of radial head position during radial head reductions and should make sure on plain radiographs that the radial head is properly reduced and not flipped 180 degrees.[35]
Follow-up	▪ Clinical or radiographic signs of fracture healing should be present before removing pin fixation. The period of pin fixation or immobilization should be longer for unstable, high-energy injuries.

POSTOPERATIVE CARE

- After reduction, the elbow is immobilized in 90 degrees of flexion in the position of supination–pronation that is most stable for 3 weeks.
- If a splint is used postoperatively because of swelling, it is changed to a cast at 1 week.
- At follow-up, the cast is removed for radiographic and clinical examination. If healing is inadequate (which is more likely in higher energy injuries in older children), the cast (and the pins if used) is continued for 2 more weeks, after which patient is reevaluated for healing.
- If pin fixation is used, no elbow motion is allowed until pins are removed.
- Graduated range-of-motion exercises begin when the cast is removed.

OUTCOMES

- Many series have shown a good to excellent outcome in 76% to 94% of children with radial neck fractures.[1,3,26,28,30]
  - Indicators for a favorable prognosis include younger age (younger than 10 years), isolated low-energy injury, closed reduction, early treatment, less than 30 degrees of initial angulation, less than 3 mm of initial translation, and reduction within parameters discussed earlier.[3,21,28]
- Poor outcomes, such as limitations in range of motion, have been reported in 6% to 33% of patients, usually after a severely displaced radial neck fracture.
  - Risk factors for a poor outcome include severe displacement, associated injuries, delayed treatment, poor reductions, old age, fractures needing open treatment and internal fixation, and intra-articular fractures in patients with an open physis.[18,21,26,28,33,36]
  - Poor outcomes that have been noted with open procedures are partially due to a selection bias, where patients needing open procedures are more likely to have had high-energy injuries with additional vascular and soft tissue trauma.

COMPLICATIONS

- Loss of joint congruity, fibrous adhesions, and radial head overgrowth result in a loss of elbow motion. In order of decreasing frequency, pronation, supination, extension, and flexion are affected.[28]
- Radial head overgrowth is observed in 20% to 40% of cases due to presumed increased vascularity stimulating the physis. Premature physeal closure can occur and is seldom symptomatic, but it can accentuate a valgus deformity. Delayed appearance of the ossific nucleus is possible after a fracture occurring before ossification.
- Avascular necrosis of the radial head occurs in 10% to 20% of patients.[3,21] Seventy percent of cases occur in cases of open reduction.[3]
- Radial neck nonunions are rare but have been reported and are often associated with premature loss of fixation.[33]
- Posttraumatic radioulnar synostosis occurs in 0% to 10% of cases,[3,21,26] typically in association with open reductions, extensive dissection, residual displacement, and concurrent ulnar fracture. Exostectomy of synostosis is a technically demanding procedure with a variable success rate.
- Heterotopic ossification (6% to 25% of cases)[3,21] can occur as myositis ossificans in the supinator or as ossification within the capsule. Surgical treatment is rarely indicated.

REFERENCES

1. Bernstein SM, McKeever P, Bernstein L. Percutaneous reduction of displaced radial neck fractures in children. J Pediatr Orthop 1993;13:85–88.
2. Chotel F, Vallese P, Parot R, et al. Complete dislocation of the radial head following fracture of the radial neck in children: the Jeffery type II lesion. J Pediatr Orthop B 2004;13:268–274.
3. D'Souza S, Vaishya R, Klenerman L. Management of radial neck fractures in children: a retrospective analysis of one hundred patients. J Pediatr Orthop 1993;13:232–238.
4. Eberl R, Singer G, Fruhmann J, et al. Intramedullary nailing for the treatment of dislocated pediatric radial neck fractures. Eur J Pediatr Surg 2010;20:250–252.
5. Ebraheim NA, Jin F, Pulisetti D, et al. Quantitative anatomical study of the posterior interosseous nerve. Am J Orthop 2000;29:702–704.
6. Endele SM, Wirth T, Eberhardt O, et al. The treatment of radial neck fractures in children according to Metaizeau. J Pediatr Orthop B 2010;19:246–255.
7. Fowles JV, Kassab MT. Observations concerning radial neck fractures in children. J Pediatr Orthop 1986;6:51–57.
8. González-Herranz P, Alvarez-Romera A, Burgos J, et al. Displaced radial neck fractures in children treated by closed intramedullary pinning (Metaizeau technique). J Pediatr Orthop 1997;17:325–331.
9. Green NE. Fractures and dislocations of the elbow. In: Green NE, Swiontkowski MF, eds. Skeletal Trauma in Children. Philadelphia: Saunders, 2003.
10. Henrikson B. Isolated fractures of the proximal end of the radius in children epidemiology, treatment and prognosis. Acta Orthop Scand 1969;40:246–260.
11. Jeffery CC. Fractures of the head of the radius in children. J Bone Joint Surg Br 1950;32-B:314–324.
12. Jeffery CC. Fractures of the neck of the radius in children. Mechanism of causation. J Bone Joint Surg Br 1972;54:717–719.
13. Jones ER, Esah M. Displaced fractures of the neck of the radius in children. J Bone Joint Surg Br 1971;53:429–439.
14. Judet H, Judet J. Fractures et Orthopedique de L'enfant. Paris: Maloine, 1974.
15. Kaufman B, Rinott MG, Tanzman M. Closed reduction of fractures of the proximal radius in children. J Bone Joint Surg Br 1989;71:66–67.
16. Klitscher D, Richter S, Bodenschatz K, et al. Evaluation of severely displaced radial neck fractures in children treated with elastic stable intramedullary nailing. J Pediatr Orthop 2009;29:698–703.
17. Landin LA, Danielsson LG. Elbow fractures in children. An epidemiological analysis of 589 cases. Acta Orthop Scand 1986;57:309–312.
18. Leung AG, Peterson HA. Fractures of the proximal radial head and neck in children with emphasis on those that involve the articular cartilage. J Pediatr Orthop 2000;20:7–14.
19. Leung KS, Tse PY. A new method of fixing radial neck fractures: brief report. J Bone Joint Surg Br 1989;71:326–327.
20. Metaizeau JP, Lascombes P, Lemelle JL, et al. Reduction and fixation of displaced radial neck fractures by closed intramedullary pinning. J Pediatr Orthop 1993;13:355–360.
21. Newman JH. Displaced radial neck fractures in children. Injury 1977;9:114–121.
22. O'Brien PI. Injuries involving the proximal radial epiphysis. Clin Orthop Relat Res 1965;41:51–58.
23. Prathapkumar KR, Garg NK, Bruce CE. Elastic stable intramedullary nail fixation for severely displaced fractures of the neck of the radius in children. J Bone Joint Surg Br 2006;88:358–361.
24. Radomisli TE, Rosen AL. Controversies regarding radial neck fractures in children. Clin Orthop Relat Res 1998;(353):30–39.

25. Schmittenbecher PP, Haevernick B, Herold A, et al. Treatment decision, method of osteosynthesis, and outcome in radial neck fractures in children: a multicenter study. J Pediatr Orthop 2005;25:45–50.
26. Steele JA, Graham HK. Angulated radial neck fractures in children. A prospective study of percutaneous reduction. J Bone Joint Surg Br 1992;74:760–764.
27. Steinberg EL, Golomb D, Salama R, et al. Radial head and neck fractures in children. J Pediatr Orthop 1988;8:35–40.
28. Tibone JE, Stoltz M. Fractures of the radial head and neck in children. J Bone Joint Surg Am 1981;63:100–106.
29. Ugutmen E, Ozkan K, Ozkan FU, et al. Reduction and fixation of radius neck fractures in children with intramedullary pin. J Pediatr Orthop B 2010;19:289–293.
30. Vahvanen V, Gripenberg L. Fracture of the radial neck in children. A long-term follow-up study of 43 cases. Acta Orthop Scand 1978;49:32–38.
31. Vocke AK, Von Laer L. Displaced fractures of the radial neck in children: long-term results and prognosis of conservative treatment. J Pediatr Orthop B 1998;7:217–222.
32. Waters PM. Injuries of the shoulder, elbow and forearm. In: Abel MF, ed. Orthopaedic Knowledge Update: Pediatrics 3. Rosemont, IL: American Academy of Orthopaedic Surgeons, 2006.
33. Waters PM, Stewart SL. Radial neck fracture nonunion in children. J Pediatr Orthop 2001;21:570–576.
34. Wilkins KE. Fractures of the neck and head of the radius. In: Rockwood CA, Wilkins KE, King RE, eds. Fractures in Children. Philadelphia: Lippincott, 1984.
35. Wood SK. Reversal of the radial head during reduction of fracture of the neck of the radius in children. J Bone Joint Surg Br 1969;51:707–710.
36. Zimmerman RM, Kalish LA, Hresko MT, et al. Surgical management of pediatric radial neck fractures. J Bone Joint Surg Am 2013;95: 1825–1832.

CHAPTER

Reconstruction for Missed Monteggia Lesion

Apurva S. Shah and Peter M. Waters

DEFINITION

- Monteggia fracture-dislocations are rare complex traumatic upper limb injuries defined by fracture of the ulna associated with proximal radioulnar joint dissociation and radiocapitellar joint dislocation. These injuries typically affect patients between 4 and 10 years of age.[19]
- The diagnosis of an acute Monteggia fracture-dislocation is often missed by skilled radiologists, emergency room physicians, pediatricians, and orthopaedic surgeons.[4,21]
- Late presentation of a previously undetected traumatic dislocation of the radial head occurs.
  - In children with a seemingly isolated dislocation of the radial head, scrutiny of forearm radiographs often demonstrates plastic deformation or fracture malunion of the ulna (**FIG 1**). The combination of these radiographic findings establishes the diagnosis of a chronic Monteggia fracture-dislocation or chronic Monteggia lesion, as opposed to a congenital dislocation of the radial head.[4]
- Patients with chronic Monteggia lesions can present for evaluation at a variety of time points.[21]
  - In some children, radial head dislocation is first noted several weeks after initiating treatment for a misdiagnosed, isolated ulnar fracture.
  - In other patients, the diagnosis may not be established for months to years following injury due to the development of pain, loss of motion, and/or valgus malalignment.
- Even a few weeks after injury, treatment of a Monteggia lesion is much more complicated than acute recognition and treatment.[21]
  - Nonetheless, due to pain, restriction of motion, and functional disability, most patients with chronic Monteggia lesions are offered surgical correction.

ANATOMY

- Understanding the anatomy of the radiocapitellar joint and proximal radioulnar joint is crucial for understanding safe and appropriate treatment of chronic Monteggia lesions.
- The bony architecture, joint contour, and periarticular ligaments all contribute to stability of radial head and congruity of the radiocapitellar and proximal radioulnar joints.
- The radial head exhibits an asymmetric cylindrical shape with a concavity in the midportion to accommodate its articulation with the convex capitellum.
  - The radial head also articulates with the lesser sigmoid or radial notch of the proximal ulna. This complex pair of articulations permits forearm rotation in addition to elbow flexion and extension.
- The annular ligament is the principal stabilizer of the radial head during forearm rotation. The annular ligament originates on the anterior margin of the lesser sigmoid notch of the proximal ulna and encircles the radial neck before inserting on or adjacent to the posterior margin of the lesser sigmoid notch (**FIG 2**).[16]
  - The annular ligament occupies 80% of the fibro-osseous ring.[16]
  - The annular ligament is one component of the Y-shaped lateral ligamentous complex and maintains the radial head in contact with the ulna at the proximal radioulnar joint (**FIG 3**).

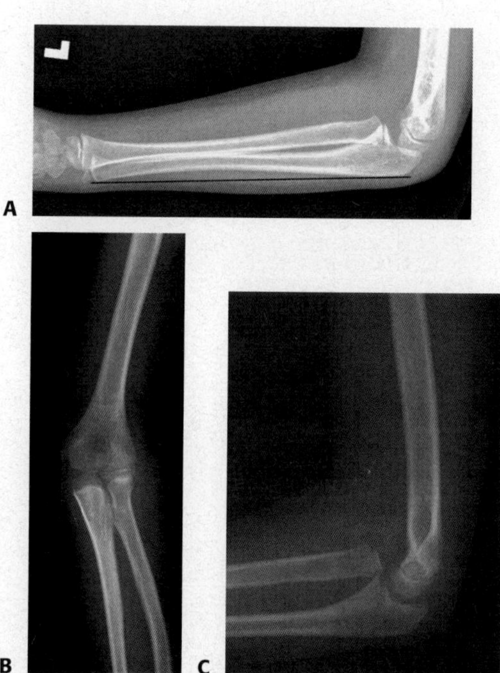

FIG 1 • Chronic Monteggia lesion in a 7-year-old girl with a 5-week history of elbow pain and loss of motion following trauma. **A.** Initial lateral forearm radiograph demonstrates an abnormal ulnar bow line, or deviation of the ulna from its normally straight dorsal border, and is suggestive of plastic deformation. Anterior dislocation of the radial head is also noted. These findings were not detected in the emergency department where dedicated elbow films were not obtained, and the child was diagnosed with an elbow sprain. **B.** AP elbow radiograph 5 weeks after injury demonstrates a normal radiocapitellar line with a poorly characterized calcification overlying the lateral aspect of the capitellum. On the AP view, the radiocapitellar line is often normal in acute or chronic Bado type I Monteggia lesions. **C.** Lateral elbow radiograph 5 weeks after injury demonstrates disruption of the radiocapitellar line and anterior translation of the radial head. There is calcification of the displaced annular ligament and anterior elbow capsule, which can be mistaken for heterotopic ossification.

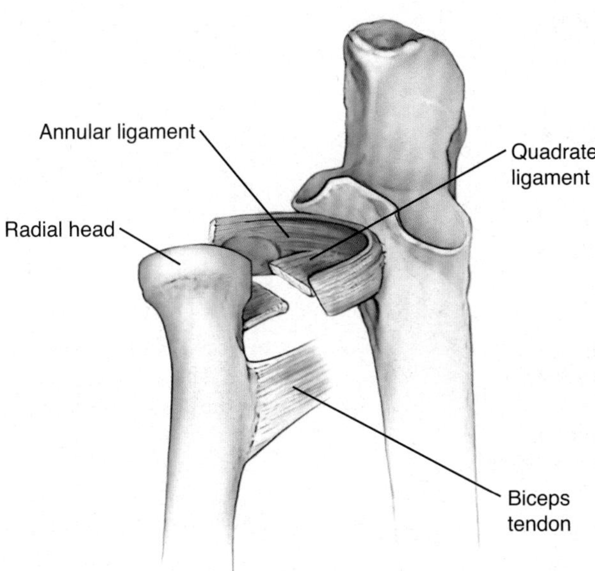

FIG 2 • Ligamentous anatomy of the proximal radioulnar joint. The annular ligament is the principal stabilizer of the radial head during forearm rotation. In supination, the annular and quadrate ligaments are taught and increase stability of the proximal radioulnar joint.

- Because the radial head is not perfectly cylindrical, the annular ligament has been found to tighten anteriorly in forearm supination and posteriorly in forearm pronation.[16]
- The quadrate ligament lies just distal to the annular ligament and connects the proximal ulna and the radial neck (see **FIG 2**).
  - The anterior portion of the quadrate ligament is stronger and denser than the posterior portion, whereas the central portion is relatively thin.
  - The anterior portion stabilizes the proximal radioulnar joint in maximum supination and the weaker posterior portion stabilizes the joint in maximum pronation.[24]
- The oblique cord is a small, inconsistent fibrous bundle that originates from the lateral side of the ulna just distal to the lesser sigmoid notch and inserts just distal to the bicipital tuberosity of the radius.[27] The oblique cord progressively tightens in supination and also stabilizes the proximal radioulnar joint. This structure is not thought to be clinically relevant.[27]
- The radial head is most stable with the forearm in a position of supination.[24] Although the bony architecture provides little inherent stability to the proximal radioulnar joint, the elliptical shape of the radial head contributes to ligament function. In forearm supination, the long axis of the radial head is perpendicular to the lesser sigmoid notch, causing the annular ligament and the anterior segment of the quadrate ligament to tighten (**FIG 4**).
- The posterior interosseous nerve passes under the arcade of Frohse and through the supinator (**FIG 5**). The proximity of

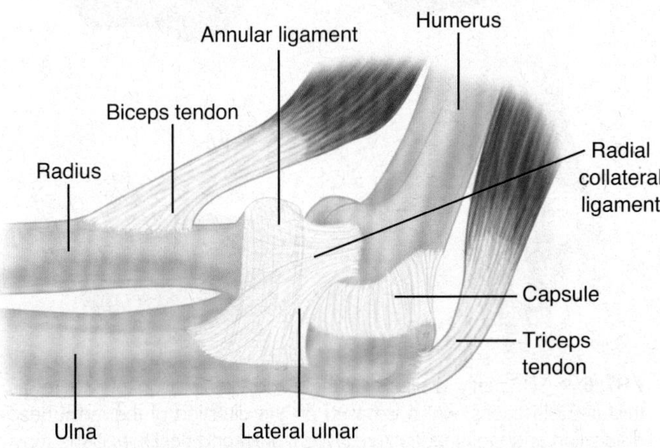

FIG 3 • The Y-shaped lateral ligamentous complex of the elbow consists of the radial collateral ligament, the lateral ulnar collateral ligament, and the annular ligament.

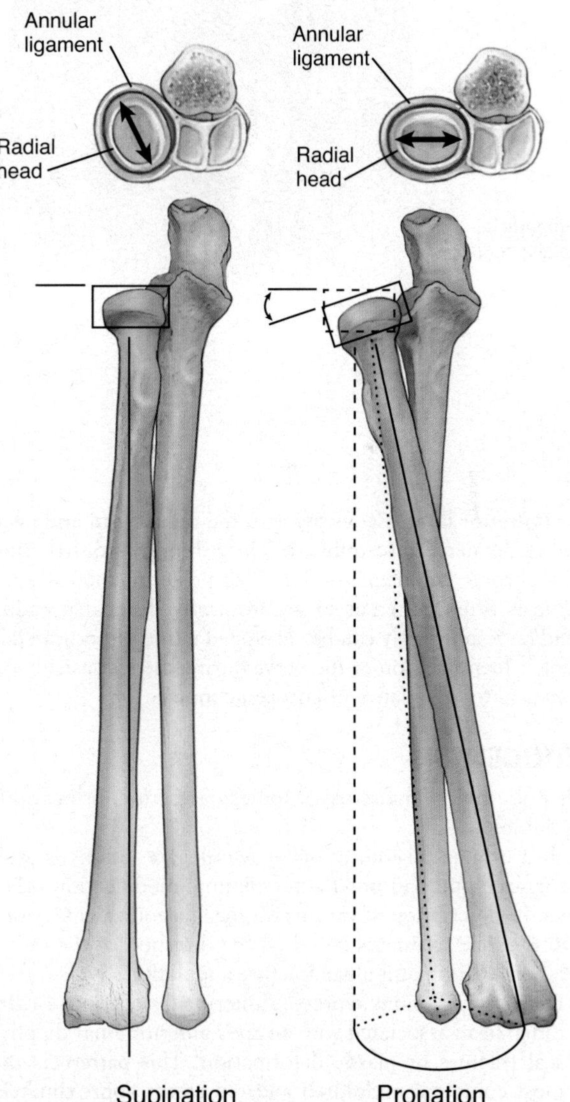

FIG 4 • The radial head is most stable with the forearm in a position of supination. The radial head is elliptical and is stabilized at the proximal radioulnar joint by the annular ligament. In forearm supination, the long axis of the radial head is perpendicular to the lesser sigmoid notch, causing the annular ligament and the anterior segment of the quadrate ligament to tighten and maximize stability.

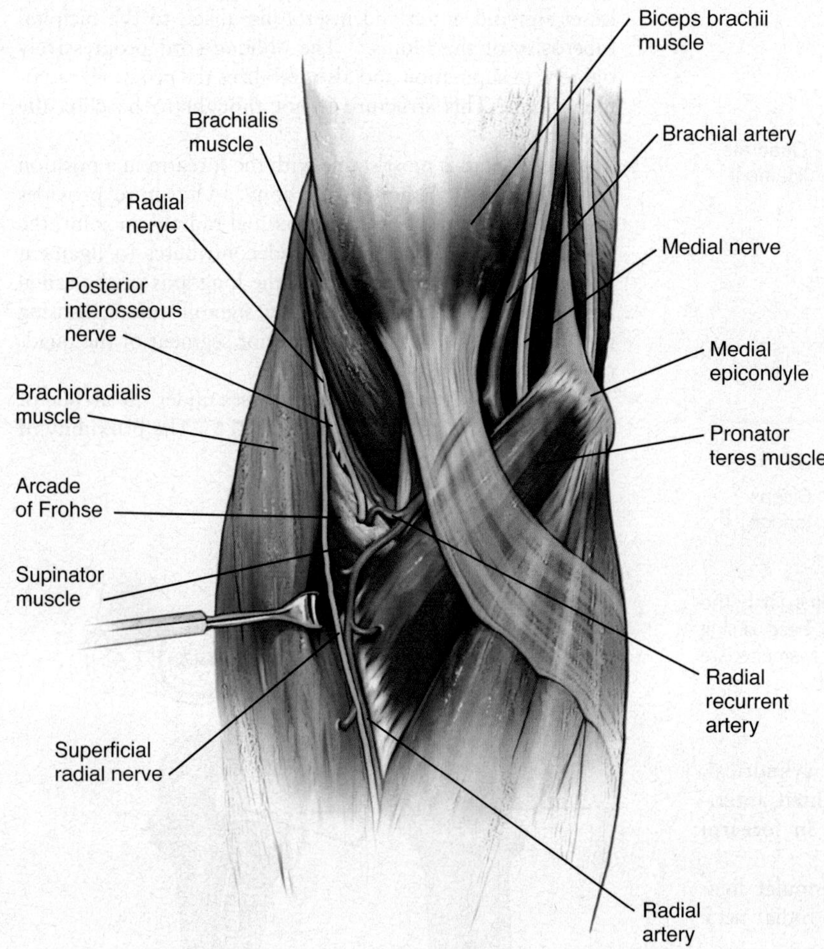

FIG 5 • Diagram of the anterior elbow. The radial nerve emerges above the elbow in the interval between the brachioradialis and the brachialis. The radial nerve divides into the superficial sensory branch and the posterior interosseous branch. The posterior interosseous nerve passes under the arcade of Frohse and through the supinator. The proximity of the posterior interosseous nerve to the radial head and neck makes the nerve susceptible to injury during reconstruction of a chronic Monteggia lesion.

the posterior interosseous nerve to the radial head and neck makes the nerve susceptible to injury during reconstruction of a chronic Monteggia lesion. The posterior interosseous nerve is often adherent to a chronically dislocated radial head/neck and rarely can be entrapped in the radiocapitellar joint.[21] Identification of the nerve during the reconstruction is critical for avoidance of iatrogenic injury.

PATHOGENESIS

- There are multiple patterns of Monteggia fracture-dislocations in children.
- Bado's original classification of Monteggia lesions is well recognized and had undergone minimal modification other than the description of various Monteggia equivalent lesions (**FIG 6**).[1] The scheme is based on the direction of the radial head dislocation and ulnar fracture angulation.
  - Bado type I lesions represent anterior dislocations of the radial head associated with an apex anterior ulnar diaphyseal fracture or plastic deformation. This pattern is the most common in children and represents approximately 70% to 75% of all injuries.[19]
    - Type I lesions can occur secondary to direct blow, hyperpronation, or hyperextension.
    - The most common mechanism is fall on an outstretched hand that forces the elbow into maximal extension with the forearm in relative pronation.[26] Due to the laxity of

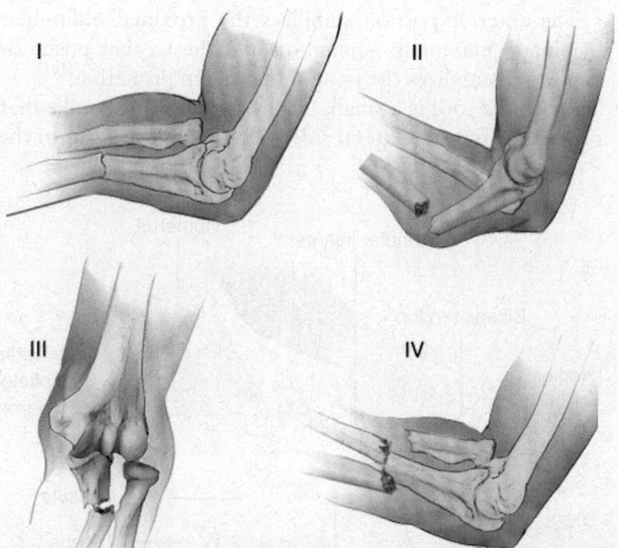

FIG 6 • Schematic diagram of the Bado classification of Monteggia fracture-dislocations, which is based on the direction of the radial head dislocation and the ulnar fracture. Type I, anterior dislocation, is the most common pattern in children. Type II is posterior dislocation. Type III, lateral dislocation, is the second most common Monteggia lesion in children. Type IV is anterior dislocation with radial shaft fracture distal to the associated ulnar fracture.

the annular and quadrate ligaments in pronation, the stability of the radial head is tenuous and the anterior bending force combined with reflexive contraction of the biceps brachii results in anterior dislocation of the radial head. Due to the continued bending moment, the ulna undergoes plastic deformation or tension failure of the anterior cortex.

- Bado type II lesions are characterized by posterior or posterolateral dislocation of the radial ahead associated with a posterior ulnar diaphyseal or metaphyseal fracture. This is the most common pattern in adults but represents approximately 5% of Monteggia lesions in children.[19]
- Bado type III lesions demonstrate lateral dislocation of the radial head and are associated with an apex lateral (varus) fracture of the proximal ulna. This is the second most common Monteggia lesion in children and represents nearly 30% of all pediatric injuries.[19]
- Bado type IV lesions are characterized by anterior dislocation of the radial head and fractures of both the radius and ulna. Type IV lesions are rare in children.

- The initial diagnosis of a Monteggia fracture-dislocation is often missed by qualified physicians.[4,21] Because the ulna heals rapidly in children, a chronic Monteggia lesion can develop over a period of 3 to 4 weeks. Due to the frequency of Bado type I lesions, most chronic Monteggia lesions in children are characterized by anterior dislocation of the radial head and apex anterior ulnar fracture malunion or plastic deformation.[13,21]
- Suboptimal treatment of the ulnar fracture in an acute Monteggia lesion can also result in unrecognized or late subluxation or dislocation of the radial head, resulting in a chronic Monteggia lesion.[19]
  - In general, only plastic and greenstick ulnar fractures should be treated with closed reduction and casting. All complete fractures should be treated surgically to avoid late instability.[20]
  - Transverse or short oblique ulnar fractures should be treated with intramedullary pin fixation and long oblique or comminuted fractures should be treated with open reduction and plate fixation.[20]
  - Always obtain dedicated elbow radiographs to evaluate congruency of the radiocapitellar reduction following reduction of the ulnar fracture.
- Chronic Monteggia lesions can result in substantial loss of function and are far more complex than acute injuries in terms of surgical decision making and management.[21]

NATURAL HISTORY

- Initial reports on chronic Monteggia fracture-dislocations suggested that the natural history of the untreated lesion was not problematic. In these reports, results from late surgical reconstruction were complicated by scarring, arthrosis, and loss of motion. For these reasons, the classic treatment was neglect and radial head excision at skeletal maturity if necessary.
- More recent data suggests that most chronic Monteggia lesions are not tolerated well over time.[6,21] Patients can develop pain, arthrosis and loss of motion, functional impairment, progressive cubitus valgus, and late neuropathy even if initial symptoms are mild.[2,6,21] Loss of elbow flexion and forearm pronation can occur.[21] The best treatment for this problem remains preventative.
- Tardy ulnar, median, and posterior interosseous nerve palsy have been reported secondary to cubitus valgus and radial head dislocation in the setting of chronic Monteggia lesions.[3,11]

PATIENT HISTORY AND PHYSICAL FINDINGS

- Most patients presenting with a chronic Monteggia lesion note a distinct history of trauma. The traumatic episode often involves significant force and is frequently characterized by a fall on to an outstretched hand with the elbow in extension and the forearm in pronation.
  - A history of trauma aids in distinguishing a traumatic radial head dislocation form a congenital radial head dislocation.
  - A history of acute elbow pain and temporary loss of motion in a child younger than 4 years of age secondary to minor trauma should prompt consideration of radial head subluxation or nursemaid's elbow. Radiographs will reveal an aligned radial head and no ulnar fracture or deformity. Children with a nursemaid's elbow usually have prompt resolution of discomfort and restoration of movement following closed reduction maneuvers.
- The timing of the injury and nature of prior medical treatment should be clarified. Patients presenting within 2 weeks of injury may still be candidates for standard treatment strategies for acute Monteggia fracture-dislocations.
- Physical examination may reveal cubitus valgus as well as loss of forearm rotation and elbow flexion. Nerve functional testing should be performed.
  - On inspection, anterior fullness in the cubital fossa may be detected. This corresponds to a palpable anterior dislocation of the radial head. The dislocated radiocapitellar joint should be palpated during forearm rotation to detect crepitation or other signs of elbow arthrosis.
  - The elbow carrying angle should be evaluated. The carrying angle in normal children increases with age and averages 9.3 degrees in males and 11.5 degrees in females.[7] Patients with chronic Monteggia lesions frequently demonstrate cubitus valgus and can present with carrying angles that exceed 30 degrees.[21] For some patients and families, this represents a significant aesthetic concern.
  - Elbow motion and forearm rotation should be precisely assessed. Normal elbow motion varies by child and averages 4 degrees of hyperextension to 145 degrees of flexion.[7] Loss of elbow motion is common, particularly in chronic Bado type I Monteggia lesions where anterior dislocation of radial head results in abutment against the humerus.[21] Elbow flexion is limited in the majority of patients with chronic Bado type I lesions and averages 110 degrees.[13] Terminal elbow flexion may be associated with visible discomfort. Loss of forearm rotation, particularly pronation, is also common.[21] Many children with chronic Monteggia lesions demonstrate compensatory radiocarpal and midcarpal rotation which can obscure assessment of true forearm rotation. In order to careful track true forearm rotation, the examiner must assess rotation of the radial styloid relative to the axis of the ulna.

- A detailed neurologic examination should be performed to assess peripheral nerve function, including the ulnar nerve, median nerve, and posterior interosseous nerve (see Exam Table at the end of the volume). Sensibility can be assessed subjectively with light touch or objectively with two-point discrimination in a cooperative child older than 5 years of age. Hand and wrist strength is tested.
  - In tardy ulnar nerve palsy, patients may demonstrate diminished sensibility at the volar pad of the small finger (autonomous zone). Patients may also present with intrinsic muscle atrophy, clawing of the small finger and ring finger, diminished digital abduction strength, a positive Froment sign, or a positive Wartenberg sign.[3]
  - Patients with a tardy posterior interosseous nerve palsy will demonstrate weakness with finger metacarpophalangeal joint extension and thumb retropulsion.[11] Because the extensor carpi radialis longus is innervated by the radial nerve, patients may demonstrate preserved wrist extension with a tendency toward radial deviation. Sensation at the first dorsal web space is typically normal.

IMAGING AND OTHER DIAGNOSTIC STUDIES

- The standard evaluation of a suspected chronic Monteggia lesion includes anteroposterior (AP) and lateral radiographs of the forearm and elbow.
  - Any disruption of the ulna, including subtle ulnar bowing, should alert the clinician to scrutinize the radiocapitellar joint (see **FIG 1A**). As noted, radial head subluxation or dislocation is often missed in the acute setting, particularly when the ulnar plastic deformation or greenstick fracture.[4]
  - Forearm radiographs are not a substitute for dedicated elbow radiographs when attempting to precisely characterize radiocapitellar alignment.
- Radiocapitellar alignment should be carefully scrutinized on the AP and lateral elbow radiographs.
  - In a chronic Bado type I Monteggia lesion, the radiocapitellar alignment may appear normal on an AP radiograph (see **FIG 1B**) despite demonstrating obvious anterior translation of the radial head on the lateral radiograph (see **FIG 1C**).
  - In a chronic Bado type III Monteggia lesion, the radiocapitellar alignment may appear normal on a lateral radiograph despite demonstrating obvious lateral or anterolateral translation of the radial head on the AP radiograph.
  - Radiocapitellar alignment can be assessed through marking of the radiocapitellar line on both the lateral (**FIG 7**) and AP radiograph. A line drawn through the center of the radial neck and head passes through the capitellum in 95% of normal elbows.[15] However, in contrast to early reports, the radiocapitellar line does not reliably interest the middle third of the capitellum and measurement can be affected by clinician bias, patient age, and forearm rotation.[15] For this reason, disruption of the radiocapitellar line suggests, but is not pathognomonic, for subluxation or dislocation of the radial head. Contralateral radiographs are often useful for comparison. Despite limitations, the radiocapitellar line should be used as a tool for evaluating radiocapitellar alignment. If subtle radiocapitellar subluxation is suspected, magnetic resonance imaging (MRI) should be obtained to visualize cartilaginous articular congruity.

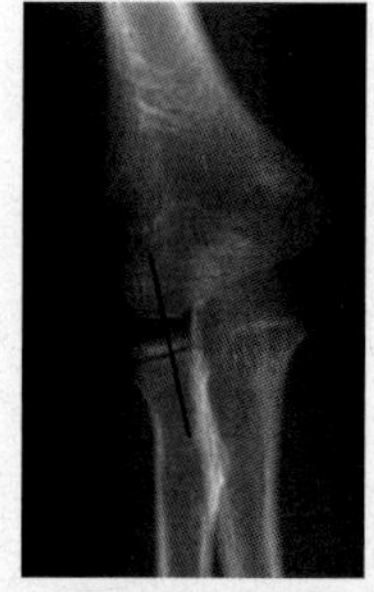

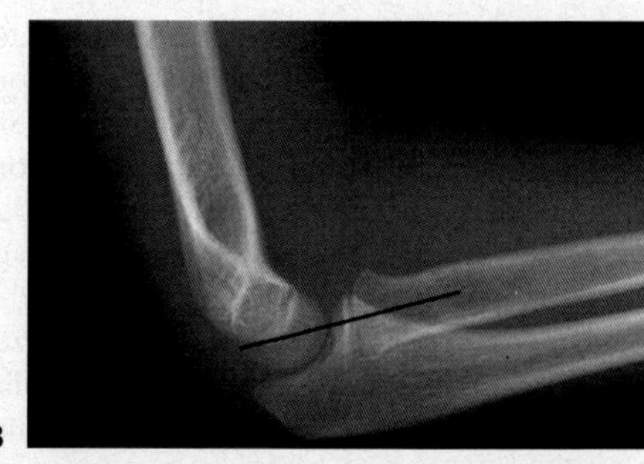

FIG 7 • In a normal elbow, the radiocapitellar line generally bisects the capitellum. A disruption of the radiocapitellar line is concerning for radial head subluxation or dislocation but due to variation in the normal pediatric population is not pathognomonic for a Monteggia lesion. **A.** AP elbow radiograph in a 7-year-old girl demonstrating a normal radiocapitellar line. **B.** Lateral elbow radiograph in a 7-year-old girl demonstrating a normal radiocapitellar line.

- With late presentation of a chronic Monteggia lesion, congruency of the radial head and capitellum should be evaluated on plain radiographs and, if necessary, MRI. If the radial head is no longer centrally concave or the capitellum appears irregularly convex, joint congruity may not be achievable with surgical reduction.
- Elbow radiographs may demonstrate calcification of the displaced annular ligament or anterior elbow capsule and can be misinterpreted as heterotopic ossification (see **FIG 1**). This calcification may appear within weeks of the initial trauma and its presence is not a contraindication to surgical reconstruction.
- Distinguishing traumatic and congenital radial head dislocations can be difficult (**FIG 8**). When there is clear disruption of

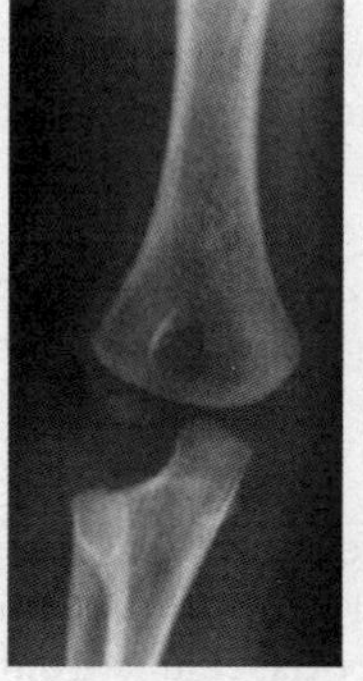

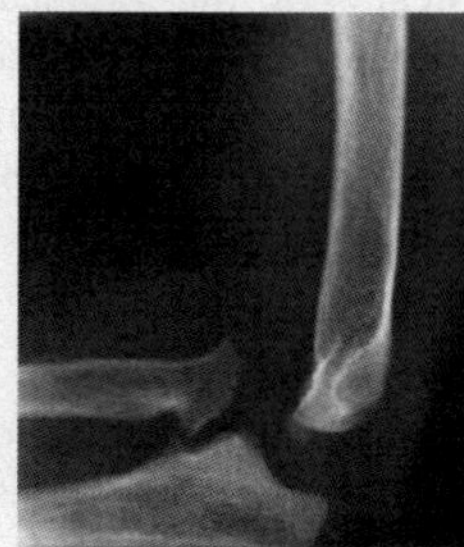

FIG 8 • Congenital dislocation of the radial head in a 7-year-old boy with limited forearm rotation. **A.** AP radiograph demonstrates an abnormal radiocapitellar line. **B.** Lateral elbow radiograph also demonstrates an abnormal radiocapitellar line with anterior dislocation of the radial head. The dysplasia of the radial head and hypoplastic appearance of the capitellum are consistent with a congenital etiology despite the anterior radial head dislocation which is more frequently seen following trauma. (From Shah AS, Waters PM. Monteggia fracture-dislocation in children. In: Rockwood and Wilkins' Fractures in Children, ed 8. Philadelphia: Lippincott Williams & Wilkins. In press.)

radiocapitellar alignment on plain radiographs, it is important to inspect the shape of the radial head and capitellum. Hypoplasia of the capitellum and convex deformity of the radial head are usually indicative of a congenital radial head dislocation. Congenital radial head dislocation can be associated with ulnar dysplasia, radioulnar synostosis, and a variety of syndromes including nail patella syndrome. Congenital radial head dislocations are frequently posterior and may be bilateral. If there is no history of trauma or the force of described trauma seems minimal, a congenital etiology should be considered. Chronic anterior dislocations of the radial head are most frequently associated with a traumatic etiology.

DIFFERENTIAL DIAGNOSIS

- Congenital radial head dislocation (see **FIG 8**)
- Nursemaid's elbow (pulled elbow, radial head subluxation)
- Isolated traumatic radial head dislocation
- Traumatic elbow dislocation

NONOPERATIVE MANAGEMENT

- The indications for reconstruction of a chronic Monteggia lesion are not well defined in the literature.
- Nonoperative management can be considered in an asymptomatic child, but yearly clinical and radiographic follow-up is recommended.
- There are important contraindications for chronic Monteggia reconstruction. Some surgeons have advocated patient age (before age 12 years) or time from injury (<3 years) as discriminating factors for surgical consideration,[10,17] but it is more important to consider the morphology of the radial head and the capitellum.[18,22,25] In older patients or more chronic lesions, MRI can be obtained to further delineate cartilage quality and potential joint congruity. Patients with radial head enlargement or deformity, flattening of the capitellum, or joint arthrosis are not candidates for reconstruction.[10,22,25] In these patients, radial head excision can be considered if pain does not resolve with nonoperative means but does place the patient at risk of developing wrist pain or progressive cubitus valgus.

SURGICAL MANAGEMENT

- At present, there is limited evidence and conflicting retrospective literature on the management of chronic Monteggia lesions. Evidence regarding management of chronic Monteggia lesions is limited to small, single-center retrospective case series.
- Unless there is concern regarding the morphology of the radial head or capitellum, we believe that symptomatic patients with chronic Monteggia lesions are candidates for surgical reconstruction.
- Descriptions of surgical reconstructions for patients with chronic Monteggia lesions include annular ligament repair or reconstruction alone,[2,8,12,13,21,22] ulnar osteotomy alone,[5,9,10,12,14,21,23] combined ulnar osteotomy and annular ligament repair/reconstruction,[8,12–14,17,21,22,25,28] and radial osteotomy.[12,13,25] The relative merit of each surgical technique has not been well elucidated and is likely to vary by patient and lesion. However, almost every series advocates for an ulnar realignment osteotomy when reconstructing a chronic Monteggia lesion. The principal controversy revolves around whether an annular ligament reconstruction should be performed in addition to the ulnar osteotomy.
- The technique for open reduction of the radial head and annular ligament reconstruction in the setting of a chronic Monteggia fracture-dislocation is attributed to Bell Tawse.[2] This technique for radiocapitellar reduction in chronic Monteggia lesions employed the Boyd approach and reconstructed the annular ligament by turning down a strip of triceps fascia.
- Our overall approach for surgical treatment of chronic Monteggia lesions includes an open osteotomy of the ulna with plate fixation, open reduction of radiocapitellar joint, and repair or reconstruction of the annular ligament.
  - To avoid potential complications of posterior interosseous nerve injury and compartment syndrome, the reconstruction is performed via an extensile posterior approach that permits identification and protection of the posterior interosseous nerve and prophylactic forearm fasciotomies.
- There are surgeons who advocate extra-articular osteotomy of the ulna alone, including use of external or intramedullary fixation of the ulna.

Preoperative Planning

- The morphology of the radial head and capitellum should be evaluated on plain radiographs and, if necessary, on MRI to define the concavity of the radial head and the reducibility of the proximal radioulnar joint and radiocapitellar joints. A normal concave radial head articular surface and normal convex capitellar articular surface are requirements for reconstruction. Three-dimensional imaging in children with radial head dislocation more than 3 years from injury can reveal flattening of the radial head and even development of a dome-shaped deformity.[18] Corresponding flattening of the lesser sigmoid notch can also be observed.[18]
- Preoperative elbow flexion–extension and forearm supination–pronation should be measured and recorded.

Positioning

- General anesthesia is preferred over a regional block to allow postoperative assessment of peripheral nerve function and compartment syndrome.
- The patient is placed in a supine position on the operating table with the elbow, forearm, and hand outstretched onto a hand table. The entire upper limb including the axilla should be included in the surgical field.
- A sterile pneumatic tourniquet is employed to maximize access to the upper arm, which is required for the extensile surgical approach.

Approach

- One of two surgical intervals, the Boyd (extensile posterior) or the Kocher (posterolateral), can be employed for open reduction of the radiocapitellar joint and repair or reconstruction of the annular ligament (**FIG 9**).
  - Either approach can be extended distally along the subcutaneous border of the ulna which can be exposed in the interval between the extensor carpi ulnaris and the flexor carpi ulnaris.

- Either approach can also be extended proximally to help identify the radial nerve and expose the triceps fascia if required for reconstruction of the annular ligament.
- The Boyd or extensile posterior approach to the elbow requires development of an interval between the anconeus and the ulna and permits excellent visualization of the radiocapitellar joint.
- The Kocher or posterior approach to the elbow is developed between the anconeus and the extensor carpi ulnaris.

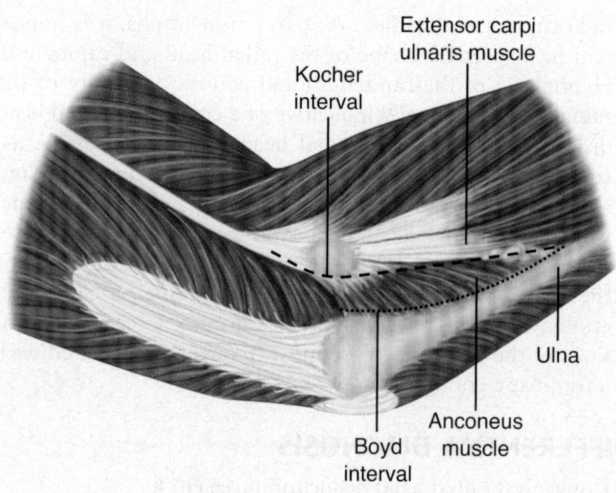

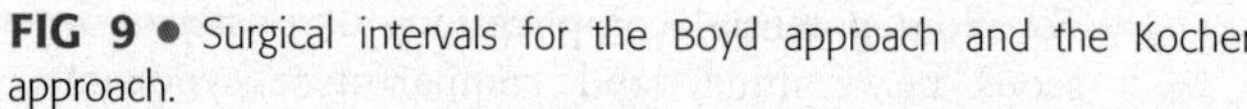

FIG 9 • Surgical intervals for the Boyd approach and the Kocher approach.

Extensile Posterolateral Approach

- An extensile curvilinear posterolateral incision is planned (**TECH FIG 1A**).
- The midportion of the incision permits access to the radiocapitellar joint through the Kocher interval, defined as the interval between the anconeus and the extensor carpi ulnaris.
- The incision can be extended proximally which allows identification and decompression of the radial nerve and harvesting of the triceps fascia if required for annular ligament reconstruction.
- The incision can be extended distally toward the subcutaneous border of the ulna for the ulnar opening wedge osteotomy. The ulna is exposed between the extensor carpi ulnaris and the flexor carpi ulnaris.
- Initially, only the proximal and midportion of the incision is opened.
  - The radial nerve should be identified between the brachioradialis and the brachialis and can be traced distally as it bifurcates into its sensory and motor (posterior interosseous) branches (**TECH FIG 1B**).
  - As noted earlier, the posterior intraosseous nerve can be adherent to the anterior elbow joint capsule which itself is distorted by the dislocated radial head.
  - Identification of the posterior interosseous nerve allows for its protection during joint reduction and annular ligament repair/reconstruction.
- In the midportion of the incision, the interval between the anconeus and the extensor carpi ulnaris is then developed (**TECH FIG 1C**).
  - If necessary for visualization, the extensor–supinator mass can be elevated off of the anterior lateral epicondyle and lateral supracondylar ridge as a single soft tissue sleeve.
  - Placement of marking sutures will facilitate anatomic repair of the extensor–supinator origin during closure.
  - The elbow capsule is incised anterior to the lateral ulnar collateral ligament to preserve the integrity of lateral ligamentous complex and ulnohumeral stability.

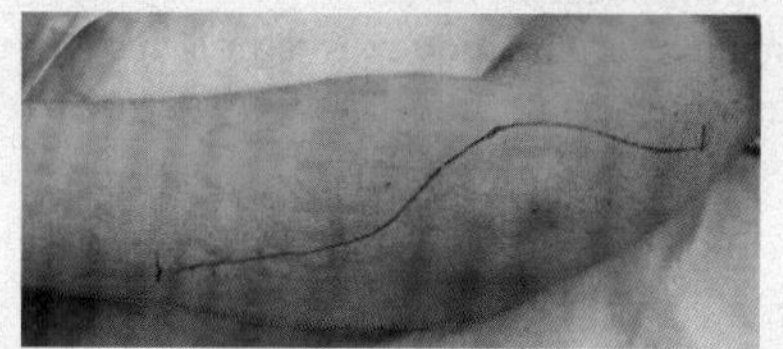
A

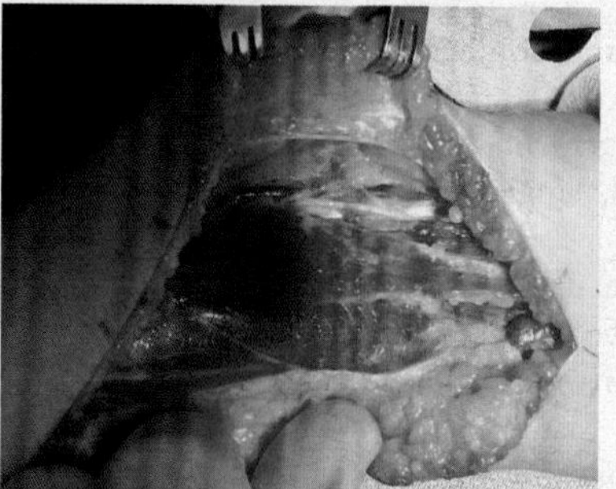
B

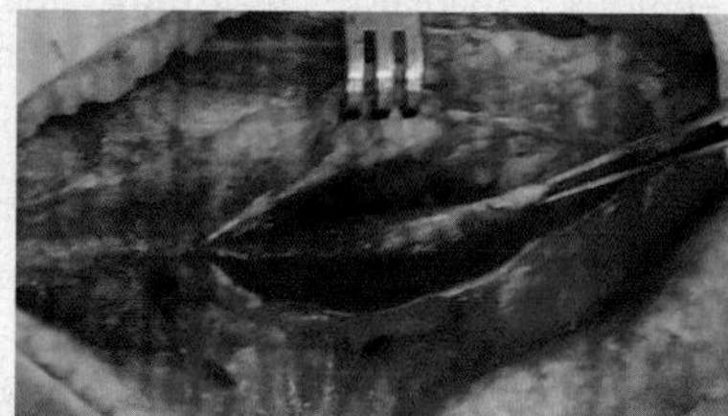
C

TECH FIG 1 • Surgical exposure for reconstruction of a chronic Monteggia lesion. **A.** A curvilinear posterolateral approach to the elbow is planned. The proximal and distal extent of the incision is used as necessary. **B.** The posterior interosseous nerve should be identified at its bifurcation from the radial nerve and traced distally. The posterior interosseous nerve should be carefully dissected off of the anterior elbow capsule to avoid iatrogenic injury during radiocapitellar reduction. **C.** The interval between the anconeus and the extensor carpi ulnaris is used to access the radiocapitellar joint. (© COSF, Boston. From Flynn J, ed. Pediatric Hand and Upper Limb Surgery. Philadelphia: Lippincott Williams & Wilkins, 2012.)

Open Reduction of the Radiocapitellar Joint

- Inspection of the radiocapitellar joint is initially obscured by fibrosis and synovitis. The radial head is typically dislocated anteriorly with a wall of anterior capsule and annular ligament blocking reduction.
- Pulvinar and synovitis are carefully débrided from the radiocapitellar joint to permit visualization of the radial head, annular ligament, and capitellum (**TECH FIG 2**). The lesser sigmoid notch should also be thoroughly débrided to permit reduction of the proximal radioulnar joint. Thorough débridement of this region is critical to anatomic joint reduction and stabilization.
- Protection of the posterior interosseous nerve is necessary during joint débridement.
- Although tedious, the annular ligament can generally be identified. The central aperture of the annular ligament may not be readily appreciated, but careful dissection and dilation of its aperture allows reconstitution of its typical ring shape.
  - Dilation is performed by making small radial incisions extending from the center toward the periphery.
  - At this stage, a decision must be made about whether the native annular ligament can be salvaged. The native ligament is generally usable.
- If the annular ligament cannot be reduced over the radial head, the ligament may be incised along its posterior insertion (at or adjacent to the posterior rim of the lesser sigmoid notch) and repaired following reduction of the radial head.
  - If necessary, repair of the annular ligament is completed through ulnar periosteal tunnels with braided 2-0 polyester suture (Ethibond, Ethicon, Inc., Somerville, NJ).
- If the annular ligament can be salvaged, the reduction of the radial head is evaluated with fluoroscopy.
- If there is anatomic restoration of radiocapitellar alignment, annular ligament repair (or reconstruction) alone may be sufficient.
  - This is very unusual, and typically, ulnar osteotomy is required.
- If the annular ligament cannot be salvaged, its remnant is sharply excised in preparation for subsequent annular ligament reconstruction, usually with a strip of triceps or extensor–supinator fascia.

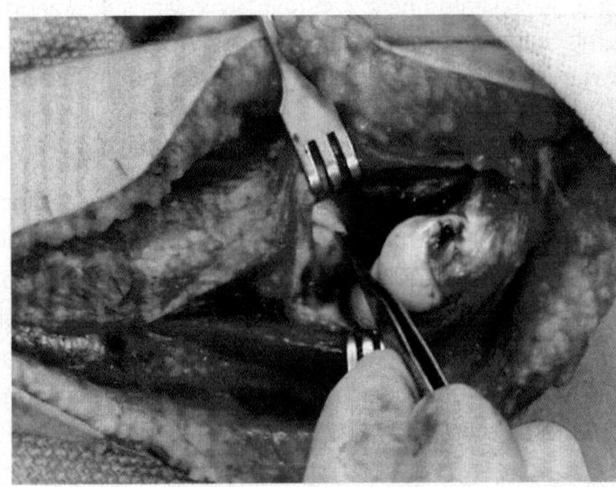

TECH FIG 2 • The dislocated radial head and the collapsed annular ligament are identified. (© COSF, Boston. From Flynn J, ed. Pediatric Hand and Upper Limb Surgery. Philadelphia: Lippincott Williams & Wilkins, 2012.)

Ulnar Osteotomy

- In general, annular ligament repair or reconstruction alone does not result in a congruent, stable radiocapitellar reduction due to the deforming force created by concomitant ulnar malunion.
- An opening wedge osteotomy of the ulna is normally required. Some surgeons only perform an extra-articular reconstruction with ulnar osteotomy and do not routinely obtain an open reduction of the radiocapitellar joint or perform an annular ligament reconstruction.
- The ulna is exposed in the extensor carpi ulnaris–flexor carpi ulnaris interval. Osteotomy of the ulna is planned at the apex of the malunion (**TECH FIG 3A**).
  - When the ulnar injury is characterized by plastic deformation, the osteotomy can be made proximal to the apex and closer to the elbow to more effectively correct of radiocapitellar malalignment.
  - Fluoroscopy is used to localize the site of the intended osteotomy, and a subperiosteal exposure is obtained.
- An oscillating saw is used to create an osteotomy with preservation of the far cortex. Copious irrigation with saline is used to minimize thermal necrosis. A laminar spreader is used to create an opening wedge. Partial overcorrection of the ulna is suggested to avoid late radial head dislocation.[14]
- Temporary pinning of the radiocapitellar joint can help determine the size of the opening wedge osteotomy. In this technique, the radiocapitellar and proximal radioulnar joints are anatomically reduced. A smooth 0.045- to 0.062-inch Kirschner wire is temporarily inserted across the radiocapitellar joint to stabilize the reduction.
  - Anatomic reduction of the radial head allows the ulnar osteotomy to open the necessary amount to maintain the reduction.
- When the radial head is anatomically reduced, the ulnar osteotomy is provisionally stabilized with appropriately contoured plate and screw fixation (**TECH FIG 3B**). We typically use double-stacked one-third tubular plates in younger patients and a 3.5-mm dynamic compression plate in larger patients (Synthes, West Chester, PA).
  - Other options include external fixation or intramedullary fixation.

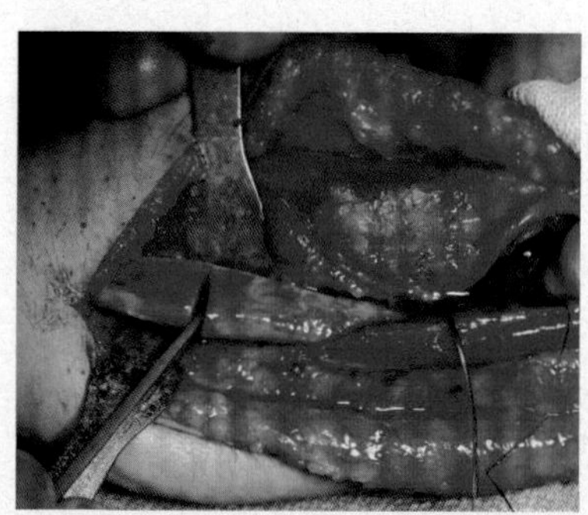
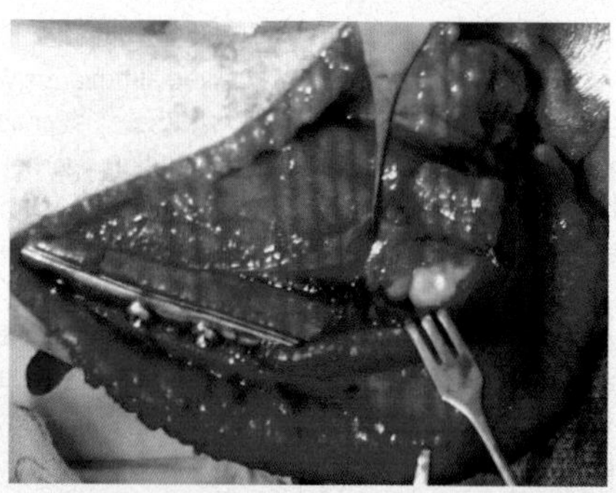
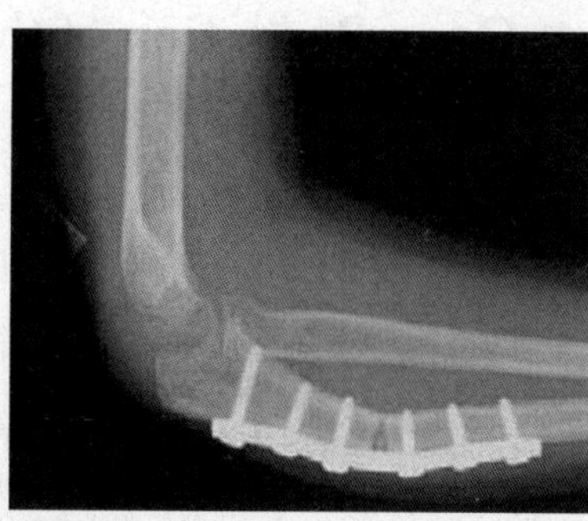

TECH FIG 3 • Ulnar osteotomy. **A.** An osteotomy of the ulna is performed at the apex of the malunion using an oscillating saw. **B.** The ulnar osteotomy is stabilized with appropriately contoured plate and screw fixation. In younger children, double-stacked one-third tubular plates are employed as illustrated in this case. **C.** Four to six cortices of fixation should be obtained on either side of the ulnar osteotomy. Overcorrection of the ulna, as illustrated here, can help avoid late subluxation of the radial head. (© COSF, Boston. **A,B:** From Flynn J, ed. Pediatric Hand and Upper Limb Surgery. Philadelphia: Lippincott Williams & Wilkins, 2012; **C:** From Shah AS, Waters PM. Monteggia fracture-dislocation in children. In: Rockwood and Wilkins' Fractures in Children, ed 8. Philadelphia: Lippincott Williams & Wilkins. In press.)

- The temporary Kirschner wire is removed. Further testing under direct visualization and fluoroscopy is performed to confirm that the correct angle and degree of osteotomy was selected for maintenance of radiocapitellar and proximal radioulnar joint alignment.
  - If correct, the fixation is completed. Four to six cortices of fixation should be achieved proximal and distal to the osteotomy site (**TECH FIG 3C**).
- If available at the malunion site, fracture callous and periosteal bone can be used for local graft after completion of the osteotomy. Periosteal repair is performed to expedite bone healing.
- As mentioned, an alternative to plate and screw fixation is external fixation.[5,9] External fixation can be used with an acute opening wedge osteotomy[9] or by gradual lengthening and angulation.[5]

Annular Ligament Reconstruction

- In our opinion, annular ligament repair or reconstruction is indicated. This involves either suture repair of the reduced annular ligament to the proximal ulna or, if an annular ligament repair is not feasible, use of local fascia for reconstruction.
  - Although this is supported by many surgeons, several investigators report success with isolated ulnar osteotomy. Sufficient evidence does not exist to demonstrate a clear advantage to either approach.
- A strip of triceps fascia may be used to perform an annular ligament reconstruction. While preserving its attachment to the olecranon, an 8-cm strip of the central triceps fascia is elevated off the muscle in a proximal to distal fashion, all the way to the level of the radial neck. The extensor–supinator fascia may be used as an alternative.
- Careful dissection is required to avoid inadvertent amputation of the triceps fascia from olecranon apophysis.
- The fascial strip is then passed around the radial neck in order to recreate the annular ligament.
- The reconstructed ligament can be passed through drill holes created in the ulna or reapproximated to the ulnar periosteum using braided 2-0 polyester suture.
  - Often, periosteal repair is sufficient in the young child.
- Seel and Peterson[22] advocate use of two crossing drill holes in the proximal ulna placed at the anterior and posterior margins of the lesser sigmoid notch. Although this procedure increases the technical difficulty, the resulting reconstruction may prevent the more posteriorly directed force that can occur with the Bell Tawse technique (**TECH FIG 4**).[2,22]
  - To facilitate annular ligament reconstruction using the Seel and Peterson technique, we recommend provisionally suturing the triceps fascia and using a wire loop for suture passage.
- Overtensioning of the reconstruction should be avoided in order to prevent notching of the radial neck in the long term.

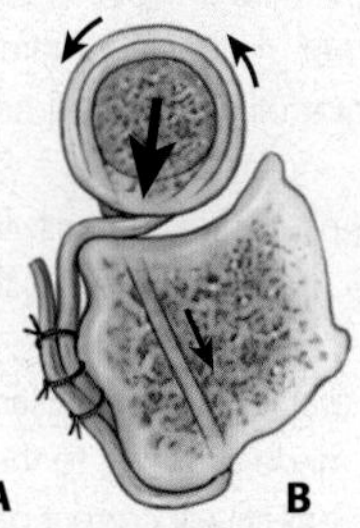
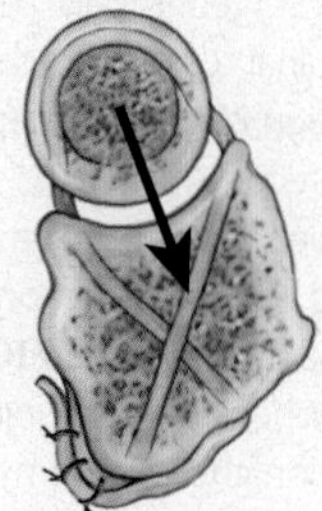

TECH FIG 4 • Schematic representation of annular ligament reconstruction techniques. **A.** The Bell Tawse reconstruction which results in a posteriorly directed force.[2] **B.** The technique suggested by Seel and Peterson. In this technique, crossing drill holes are created at the anterior and posterior rim of the lesser sigmoid notch. The resulting reconstruction may improve stability of the radial head.[22] (Adapted from Seel MJ, Peterson HA. Management of chronic posttraumatic radial head dislocation in children. J Pediatr Orthop 1999;19:306–312.)

Prophylactic Forearm Fasciotomies

- Under direct visualization, limited prophylactic fasciotomies of the volar and dorsal compartments are performed to minimize risk of postoperative compartment syndrome.
- Prophylactic fasciotomies have the secondary advantage of facilitating periosteal closure.

Final Evaluation of Reduction and Wound Closure

- Final orthogonal fluoroscopy images should be obtained to verify stable reduction of the radiocapitellar and proximal radio-ulnar joints.
- Continued wire fixation of the radiocapitellar joint is rarely needed if the ulnar osteotomy and annular ligament repair/reconstruction are performed correctly.
  - In our experience, this has been occasionally necessary in revision reconstruction of a chronic Monteggia lesion where reconstructive options are more limited.
  - In this case, a wire of sufficient size is mandatory to avoid fatigue and breakage. As always, a smooth wire should be used to avoid physeal injury. The wire is typically removed 3 to 4 weeks postoperatively.
- Following radiocapitellar reduction, annular ligament repair or reconstruction, and ulnar osteotomy, a layered wound closure is performed. The periosteum overlying the ulna is repaired to expedite bone healing.
- The capsule is repaired and the extensor–supinator origin is reattached to the lateral epicondyle and lateral supracondylar ridge of the humerus. Intermuscular intervals are reapproximated, and the wound is closed over a Jackson-Pratt drain.

PEARLS AND PITFALLS

Distinguish congenital and traumatic dislocation of the radial head	■ Hypoplasia of the capitellum and convex deformity of the radial head is indicative of a congenital radial head dislocation.
Avoidance of compartment syndrome	■ Avoid preoperative regional block to monitor the child following reconstruction. ■ Prophylactic volar and dorsal forearm fasciotomies can be performed to minimize risk of postoperative compartment syndrome. ■ Wounds should be closed over a drain if there is a concern for hemostasis.
Protection of the posterior interosseous nerve	■ When planning an intra-articular reconstruction of a long-standing lesion or in the presence of a preoperative radial neuropathy, the radial nerve should be identified in the brachioradialis–brachialis interval and then followed distally as it branches into the superficial radial nerve and the posterior interosseous nerve. ■ The posterior interosseous nerve can be adherent to the joint capsule and displaced radial head or incarcerated at the radiocapitellar joint. Careful identification and protection of the posterior interosseous nerve during surgical exposure can help avoid iatrogenic injury during the reconstruction.
Late subluxation of the radial head	■ Combined annular ligament reconstruction and ulnar osteotomy is advocated. ■ After completion of the ulnar osteotomy, setting the radiocapitellar alignment first is helpful as this determines the amount of ulnar correction needed to maintain a stable reduction. ■ Overcorrection of the ulna is often required for stable reduction of the radial head. ■ Carefully scrutinize the reduction with intraoperative fluoroscopy, and do not accept subtle malalignment. ■ Serial radiographs should be obtained 2–6 weeks after surgical intervention in order to detect unexpected loss of reduction early.
Ulnar nonunion	■ If an oscillating saw is used for the osteotomy, copious irrigation should be employed to minimize thermal necrosis. ■ Plate fixation is mandatory to avoid loss of fixation. ■ Fracture callous and periosteal bone at the site of the malunion can be used as local bone graft after completion of the osteotomy. ■ If needed, allograft bone is added to the osteotomy site.

POSTOPERATIVE CARE

- Following wound closure, a bivalved long-arm cast is applied, typically with the elbow in 80 to 90 degrees of flexion and the forearm in 60 to 90 degrees of supination to maximize stability of the radiocapitellar and proximal radioulnar joints.
- All children should be admitted overnight for pain control and neurovascular monitoring.
- Casting is discontinued 4 to 6 weeks after surgical reconstruction and children are transitioned to a protective long-arm splint for an additional 3 to 4 weeks. Splint removal for active motion, particularly forearm rotation, is important. Formal rehabilitation is initiated and maximal recovery is anticipated at 6 months. Elbow flexion and extension return more rapidly than forearm rotation.

OUTCOMES

- Data on outcomes following reconstruction of chronic Monteggia lesions is limited to small, retrospective case series. Most reports lack long-term follow-up and fail to report validated functional outcome measures.
- Nakamura et al[17] reported long-term clinical and radiographic outcomes in 22 children that underwent combined ulnar osteotomy and annular ligament reconstruction, at an average follow-up of 84 months.
  - The radial head remained stable in nearly 80% of patients and was subluxated (but not frankly dislocated) in approximately 20% of patients, which is representative of other results reported in the literature.[8,12,21,23]
  - Postoperative functional outcomes (Mayo Elbow Performance Index) reliably improved, with the vast majority of patients experiencing excellent (19 of 22) or good (2 of 22) results.
  - Average elbow flexion improved from 124 to 138 degrees. Average postoperative forearm pronation exceeded 65 degrees. Improvement in elbow motion is reliable and similar results have been described by other investigators. Loss of some forearm rotation, particularly pronation, can be expected.[8,12,13,21,23]
- The complication rate for chronic Monteggia reconstruction is high and includes late radial head subluxation, notching of the radial neck, osteoarthritis, delayed ulnar union, ulnar nonunion, compartment syndrome, peripheral nerve injury, and stiffness, amongst others.[17,21]
- Good results can more reliably be obtained in children younger than 12 years of age or within 3 years of injury.[17]

COMPLICATIONS

- Restricted elbow or forearm motion, particularly pronation
- Postoperative compartment syndrome can occur. Routine perioperative neurovascular monitoring is recommended for early detection. Pain out of proportion to examination or increasing narcotic requirements represent early signs of compartment syndrome and should prompt immediate evaluation. Prophylactic intraoperative forearm fasciotomies are advocated to lessen the risk.
- Posterior interosseous nerve palsy can occur following reconstruction. If the nerve was identified and protected during surgery, expectant management is recommended. Serial clinical examination will demonstrate an advancing Tinel sign and progressive return of motor function. Failure of recognizable clinical recovery by 6 months is a relative indication for surgical exploration.
- Ulnar nerve palsy can occur with extensive lengthening of the ulna and may be an indication for decompression.
- Recurrent subluxation or dislocation of the radial head does occur and negates the original purpose for surgical reconstruction. This is not an operation for the uninitiated.
- Notching of the radial neck if the annular ligament reconstruction is too taut.[17]
- Ulnar nonunion can occur. An incomplete hinged osteotomy, supplemental bone grafting, stable fixation, and periosteal repair lessen the risk.

REFERENCES

1. Bado JL. The Monteggia lesion. Clin Orthop Relat Res 1967;50:71–86.
2. Bell Tawse AJ. The treatment of malunited anterior Monteggia fractures in children. J Bone Joint Surg Br 1965;47:718–723.
3. Chen WS. Late neuropathy in chronic dislocation of the radial head. Report of two cases. Acta Orthop Scand 1992;63:343–344.
4. Dormans JP, Rang M. The problem of Monteggia fracture-dislocations in children. Orthop Clin North Am 1990;21:251–256.
5. Exner GU. Missed chronic anterior Monteggia lesion. Closed reduction by gradual lengthening and angulation of the ulna. J Bone Joint Surg Br 2001;83:547–550.
6. Fahey JJ. Fractures of the elbow in children. Instr Course Lect 1960;17:13–46.
7. Golden DW, Jhee JT, Gilpin SP, et al. Elbow range of motion and clinical carrying angle in a healthy pediatric population. J Pediatr Orthop B 2007;16:144–149.
8. Gyr BM, Stevens PM, Smith JT. Chronic Monteggia fractures in children: outcome after treatment with the Bell-Tawse procedure. J Pediatr Orthop B 2004;13:402–406.
9. Hasler CC, Von Laer L, Hell AK. Open reduction, ulnar osteotomy and external fixation for chronic anterior dislocation of the head of the radius. J Bone Joint Surg Br 2005;87:88–94.
10. Hirayama T, Takemitsu Y, Yagihara K, et al. Operation for chronic dislocation of the radial head in children. Reduction by osteotomy of the ulna. J Bone Joint Surg Br 1987;69:639–642.
11. Holst-Nielsen F, Jensen V. Tardy posterior interosseous nerve palsy as a result of an unreduced radial head dislocation in Monteggia fractures: a report of two cases. J Hand Surg Am 1984;9:572–575.
12. Horii E, Nakamura R, Koh S, et al. Surgical treatment for chronic radial head dislocation. J Bone Joint Surg Am 2002;84-A(7):1183–1188.
13. Hui JH, Sulaiman AR, Lee HC, et al. Open reduction and annular ligament reconstruction with fascia of the forearm in chronic monteggia lesions in children. J Pediatr Orthop 2005;25:501–506.
14. Inoue G, Shionoya K. Corrective ulnar osteotomy for malunited anterior Monteggia lesions in children. 12 patients followed for 1-12 years. Acta Orthop Scand 1998;69:73–76.
15. Kunkel S, Cornwall R, Little K, et al. Limitations of the radiocapitellar line for assessment of pediatric elbow radiographs. J Pediatr Orthop 2011;31:628–632.
16. Martin BF. The annular ligament of the superior radio-ulnar joint. J Anat 1958;92:473–482.
17. Nakamura K, Hirachi K, Uchiyama S, et al. Long-term clinical and radiographic outcomes after open reduction for missed Monteggia fracture-dislocations in children. J Bone Joint Surg Am 2009;91:1394–1404.
18. Oka K, Murase T, Moritomo H, et al. Morphologic evaluation of chronic radial head dislocation: three-dimensional and quantitative analyses. Clin Orthop Relat Res 2010;468:2410–2418.
19. Ramski DE, Hennrikus WP, Bae DS, et al. Pediatric Monteggia fractures: a multicenter examination of treatment strategy and early clinical and radiographic results. J Pediatr Orthop 2015;35(2):115–120.
20. Ring D, Waters PM. Operative fixation of Monteggia fractures in children. J Bone Joint Surg Br 1996;78:734–739.

21. Rodgers WB, Waters PM, Hall JE. Chronic Monteggia lesions in children. Complications and results of reconstruction. J Bone Joint Surg Am 1996;78:1322–1329.
22. Seel MJ, Peterson HA. Management of chronic posttraumatic radial head dislocation in children. J Pediatr Orthop 1999;19:306–312.
23. Song KS, Ramnani K, Bae KC, et al. Indirect reduction of the radial head in children with chronic Monteggia lesions. J Orthop Trauma 2012;26:597–601.
24. Spinner M, Kaplan EB. The quadrate ligament of the elbow—its relationship to the stability of the proximal radio-ulnar joint. Acta Orthop Scand 1970;41:632–647.
25. Stoll TM, Willis RB, Paterson DC. Treatment of the missed Monteggia fracture in the child. J Bone Joint Surg Br 1992;74:436–440.
26. Tompkins DG. The anterior Monteggia fracture: observations on etiology and treatment. J Bone Joint Surg Am 1971;53:1109–1114.
27. Tubbs RS, O'Neil JT Jr, Key CD, et al. The oblique cord of the forearm in man. Clin Anat 2007;20:411–415.
28. Wang MN, Chang WN. Chronic posttraumatic anterior dislocation of the radial head in children: thirteen cases treated by open reduction, ulnar osteotomy, and annular ligament reconstruction through a Boyd incision. J Orthop Trauma 2006;20:1–5.

12

CHAPTER

Intramedullary Fixation of Forearm Shaft Fractures

Charles T. Mehlman

DEFINITION

- Forearm shaft fractures represent the third most common fracture encountered in the pediatric population.[5]
- Closed fracture care is successful in the large majority of children who sustain forearm shaft fractures (especially the common greenstick fracture pattern).[4]
- For children who are 8 to 10 years of age and older with complete fracture patterns, the limits of acceptable displacement (angulation, rotation, and translation) become more strict and the likelihood of surgical intervention increases.[1,13]

ANATOMY

- The forearm represents a largely nonsynovial, two bone joint with a high-amplitude range of motion (roughly 180 degrees). In the fully supinated anteroposterior (AP) plane, the radius bows naturally out and away from the relatively straight ulna, whereas both bones are predominantly straight in the lateral plane.
- Anatomically, the shaft of the radius extends from the most proximal aspect of the tubercle of Lister (which approximates the distal metaphyseal–diaphyseal junction) to the proximal base of the bicipital tuberosity. The shaft of the ulna corresponds to these same points on the radius (**FIG 1**).[11,13]
- In unfractured bones, the normal orientation of the radial styloid and bicipital tuberosity is slightly less than 180 degrees from one another, whereas the ulnar styloid and coronoid process come closer to a true 180-degree relationship.
- Classically, forearm shaft fractures are divided into distal third (pronator quadratus region), central third (pronator teres region), and proximal third (biceps and supinator region). These anatomic relationships offer insight into the deforming forces acting on the fractured forearm (**FIG 2**).

PATHOGENESIS

- Forearm shaft fractures most commonly occur secondary to a fall on an outstretched arm and usually involve both bones. Forward falls tend to involve a pronated forearm, and backward falls involve a supinated forearm.
- Single-bone forearm shaft fractures should raise significant suspicion regarding the presence of a Galeazzi or Monteggia-type injury (see Chap. 11).
- Mechanisms of injury that involve little rotational force result in forearm fractures at nearly the same levels, whereas greater rotational force results in fractures at rather different levels.

NATURAL HISTORY

- The remodeling potential of the pediatric forearm shaft has been well documented and is considered to be most predictable in children younger than about 8 to 10 years of age.
- Spontaneous correction and improvement of malaligned shaft fractures are considered to occur in young children via three mechanisms:
  - Adjacent physes produce "straight bone" via normal growth.
  - Physeal orientation tends to "right its horizon" via the Hueter-Volkmann law.[12]
  - True shaft remodeling occurs via Wolff law.[15]

PATIENT HISTORY AND PHYSICAL FINDINGS

- The clinician should gather as much pertinent information as possible regarding the mechanism of injury (eg, a fall from the bottom step of the playground sliding board may be much different from a fall from the top step of the same sliding board).
- The clinician should determine whether the patient has any other complaints of pain beyond the forearm shaft region (eg, wrist or elbow tenderness). Any perceived deformity or pain to palpation should trigger dedicated radiographs of the problematic region.
- The clinician should elicit any past history of fracture or bone disease in the patient or the patient's family.
- Physical examination of the skin of the child's forearm should be performed to rule out the presence of an open fracture. Any wound, no matter how small or seemingly superficial, should be carefully evaluated. Persistent bleeding or oozing from a small suspicious wound should be considered an open fracture until proven otherwise.
- The environment of the injury has special significance for open fracture management. For instance, farm-related injuries may alter the treatment regimen for the patient.
- Multiple trauma or high-energy trauma scenarios dictate that a screening orthopaedic examination be performed to help rule out injuries to the other extremities as well as the spine.
- Brachial, radial, and ulnar pulses should be palpated, and distal capillary refill should be assessed.
- Sensory examination should include, at minimum, light touch sensation testing (or pinprick testing if necessary)

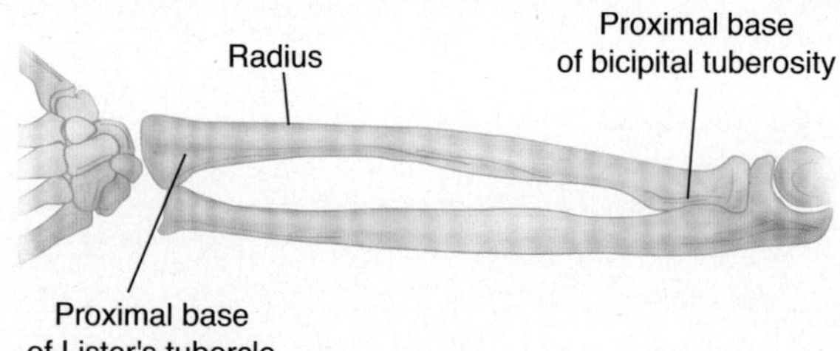

FIG 1 • The radial diaphysis extends from the most proximal aspect of the tubercle of Lister to the proximal base of the bicipital tuberosity. The ulnar diaphysis corresponds to these same points on the radius.

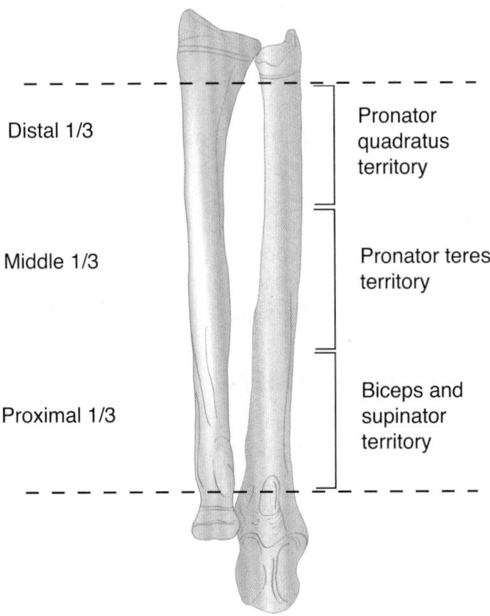

FIG 2 ● Forearm shaft fractures are divided into distal third (pronator quadratus region), central third (pronator teres region), and proximal third (biceps and supinator region).

of the autonomous zones of the radial, ulnar, and median nerves. Older children may be able to comply with formal two-point discrimination testing.

- It has been said that you need only a thumb to test the motor function of all three major nerves: radial nerve = extensor pollicis longus, ulnar nerve = adductor pollicis, median nerve = opponens pollicis.
- Peripheral nerves in the fractured extremity are assessed with the "rock–paper–scissors" method.
  - The radial nerve (really the posterior interosseous nerve in the forearm) is tested with "paper"—extension of the fingers and wrist well above a zero-degree wrist position. The autonomous zone is the dorsal web space between the thumb and index finger. There is a risk of iatrogenic injury during surgical exposure of the proximal radial shaft.
  - The ulnar nerve is tested with "scissors"—adducted thumb, abducted fingers, and flexor digitorum profundus function to ring and pinky. The autonomous zone is palmar tip pinky finger. This is the most common iatrogenic nerve injury after internal fixation of forearm shaft fractures.
  - The median nerve is tested with "rock." The autonomous zone is palmar tip index finger. The median is the most commonly injured nerve after closed or open forearm shaft fractures.
- The anterior interosseous nerve is tested with the "okay" sign. Flexion of the distal interphalangeal of the index finger and the interphalangeal of the thumb herald flexor digitorum profundus and flexor pollicis longus function of these digits. This is a motor branch only (it has no cutaneous innervation, only articular). Isolated palsy has been reported secondary to constrictive dressings and after proximal ulnar fracture.

IMAGING AND OTHER DIAGNOSTIC STUDIES

- AP and lateral radiographs (two orthogonal views) that include the entire radius and ulna are essential for proper diagnosis of forearm shaft fractures in children (**FIG 3**). If suspicion exists for compromise of the distal or proximal radioulnar joints (Galeazzi or Monteggia injuries), dedicated wrist and elbow radiographs are also indicated.

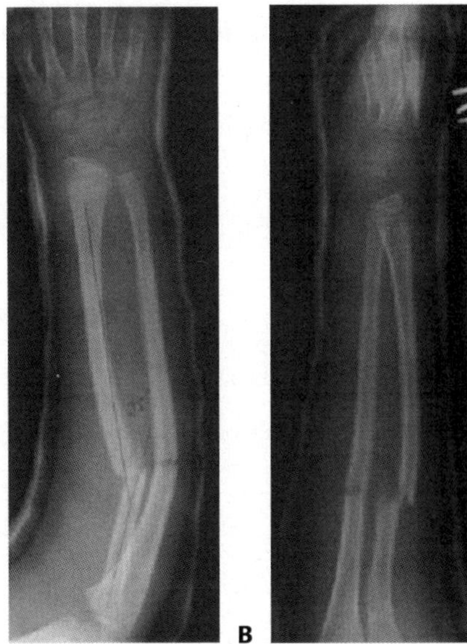

FIG 3 ● AP (**A**) and lateral (**B**) radiographs of a boy age 9 years and 11 months with a forearm shaft fracture.

- If fracture angulation is noted on both orthogonal forearm views, the true fracture angulation exceeds that measured on either individual view (**FIG 4**).
- The radiographs should be used to classify the forearm fracture in a practical fashion with respect to two bones, three

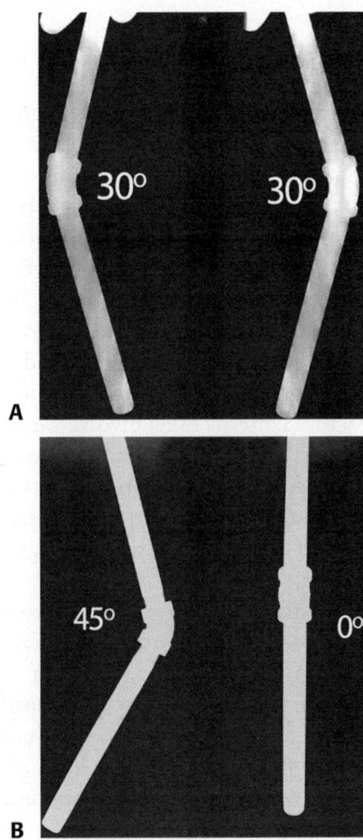

FIG 4 ● **A.** Out-of-plane AP and lateral views of a 45-degree angulated iron pipe. **B.** True AP and lateral views of the same pipe.

Table 1 Practical Classification of Forearm Shaft Fractures

Bones: Single-bone fractures occur but both-bone injuries predominate.
- Radius
- Ulna

Level: Fracture level has bearing on nonoperative versus operative decision making.
- Distal third
- Middle third
- Proximal third

Pattern: Fracture pattern has bearing on nonoperative versus operative decision making.
- Bow (also known as *plastic deformation*)
- Greenstick
- Complete
- Comminuted

levels, four fracture patterns (Table 1). This is akin to describing bone tumors in terms of matrix, margins, and so forth.

DIFFERENTIAL DIAGNOSIS

- Galeazzi injury (concomitant distal radioulnar joint disruption)
- Monteggia injury (concomitant proximal radioulnar joint disruption)
- Coexisting distal humeral fracture (eg, supracondylar humeral fracture, also known as *floating elbow*)
- Open fracture (the clinician must be beware of small, innocuous-appearing wounds)
- Compartment syndrome (more common in setting of floating elbow and extended efforts at indirect reduction of difficult to reduce fractures)[3]

NONOPERATIVE MANAGEMENT

- Nonoperative (closed) fracture management is used in the vast majority of pediatric forearm shaft fractures.[4]
- Successful nonoperative treatment requires an eclectic mix of anatomic knowledge, skillful application of reduction techniques, appreciation for remodeling potential, and respect for the character of the soft tissue envelope.
- Greenstick fracture patterns retain a degree of inherent stability; intentional completion of these fractures is *not* recommended. Davis and Green[7] reported a 10% loss of reduction rate with greenstick fractures and a 25% rate with complete fractures.
- Greenstick fracture patterns often involve variable amounts of rotational deformity such that when the forearm is appropriately derotated, reduction of angulation occurs simultaneously.
- Apex volar greenstick fractures are considered to represent supination injuries that require a relative degree of pronation to effect reduction.
- Apex dorsal greenstick fractures are considered to be pronation injuries that require supination to aid reduction.
- Classic finger-trap and traction reduction techniques are probably best reserved for complete both-bone fracture patterns. When dealing with complete both-bone shaft fractures, respect should be paid to the level of the fractures when choosing a relatively neutral, pronated, or supinated forearm position.
- Price et al[14] has suggested that estimated rotational malalignment should not exceed 45 degrees. The related concepts of maintenance of an appropriate amount of radial bow and interosseous space on the AP radiograph must also not be forgotten, but precise criteria do not exist at this time.
- Initial above-elbow cast immobilization is the rule for all forearm shaft fractures, as this appropriately controls pronation–supination as well as obeying the orthopaedic maxim of immobilizing the joints above and below the fracture. An extra benefit of above-elbow immobilization relates to the activity limitation it imposes; in some instances, this may increase the chances of maintaining a satisfactory reduction in an otherwise very active customer.

SURGICAL MANAGEMENT

- Flexible intramedullary nail treatment of pediatric forearm shaft fractures focuses predominantly on displaced complete fractures, many of which may have minor comminution (butterfly fragments usually <25% of a shaft diameter).
- When efforts at closed fracture management do not achieve and maintain fracture reduction within accepted guidelines, surgical treatment is indicated.
- When complete fractures occur in children younger than about 8 to 10 years of age with angulation of at least 20 degrees in the distal third, 15 degrees in the central third, or 10 degrees in the proximal third, risk–benefit discussions are appropriate regarding further efforts at fracture reduction and possible internal fixation.[8,17]
- Lesser measured angulation associated with significant forearm deformity (as defined in a discussion between the orthopaedic surgeon and the parents) may also prompt intervention in selected children.
- Complete forearm shaft fractures in children older than 8 to 10 years of age should be evaluated very critically with the intention to accept no more than 10 degrees of angulation at any level.[8,17] Compromise (loss) of interosseous space should also be considered as well as rotational malalignment (difficult to assess precisely) when debating the merits of continued cast treatment versus flexible intramedullary nail fixation.
- Single bone fixation of pediatric forearm shaft fractures has been described by some authors but is *not* advocated due to increased risk of redisplacement.[6]

Preoperative Planning

- Rotational alignment of the radius and ulna should be assessed and estimated using the guidelines mentioned in the Anatomy section. Concern is increased if greater than 45 degrees of rotational malalignment is judged to be present.
- Measurement of the narrowest canal diameter of the radius (usually midshaft) and ulna (usually distal third) will aid in the selection of appropriately sized intramedullary nails. Implants 2 mm in diameter or smaller are commonly used, and the same-sized nail is used in each bone. It is far worse to select implants that are too big rather than too small.
- Assessment of existing or impending comminution is prudent. Significant comminution may lead the surgeon to choose plate fixation over intramedullary fixation for one or both bones.
- Assessment of the soft tissue envelope of the forearm is important. Tense swelling of the forearm certainly increases suspicion for compartment syndrome, and the surgeon should be prepared to measure compartment pressures accordingly.

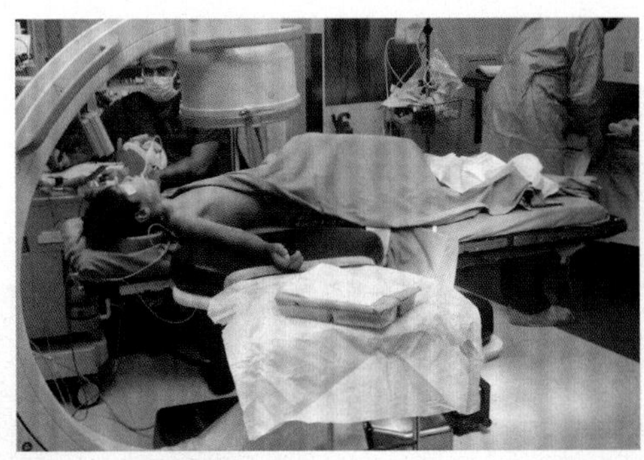

FIG 5 ● My preferred operating room setup, with the injured arm on the radiolucent hand table and the C-arm properly positioned.

Positioning

- The patient is placed in a supine position on the operating room table with the involved extremity positioned on a sturdy hand table to allow easy, unobstructed radiographic visualization of the entire forearm (**FIG 5**).
- In general, the monitor for the portable fluoroscopy unit should be positioned near the end of the operating table, opposite the imaging unit (C-arm).
- A nonsterile tourniquet may be applied about the upper arm (near the axilla) before preparation and draping, but it is *not* routinely inflated.
- The limb is appropriately prepared and draped, with care being taken to ensure that the first layer is a sterile impervious one (eg, blue plastic U-drape). The C-arm is also appropriately protected with a C-arm sterile plastic drape and an additional sterile skirt (usually a sterile paper half-sheet). Without this sterile skirt, certain limb positions and certain surgical maneuvers occur far too close to nonsterile territory.

Approach

- Physeal-sparing distal radial entry is routinely obtained via the floor of the first dorsal compartment (alternately, the interval between the second and third dorsal compartments near the proximal base of the tubercle of Lister may be used).
- Physeal-sparing proximal ulnar entry is typically achieved via an anconeus starting point just off the posterolateral ridge of the olecranon. The true tip of the olecranon is avoided as an entry point because it needlessly violates an apophyseal growth plate, and a subcutaneous nail in this region often leads to painful olecranon bursitis.
- In complete both-bone fractures, the radius is routinely approached first, as it is considered to be the more difficult bone to reduce.
- No power instruments are required for completion of the procedure. Key instruments are a stout sharp-tipped awl and T-handled chucks that achieve a firm grip on the flexible nail such that it can be rotated as needed (**FIG 6**).

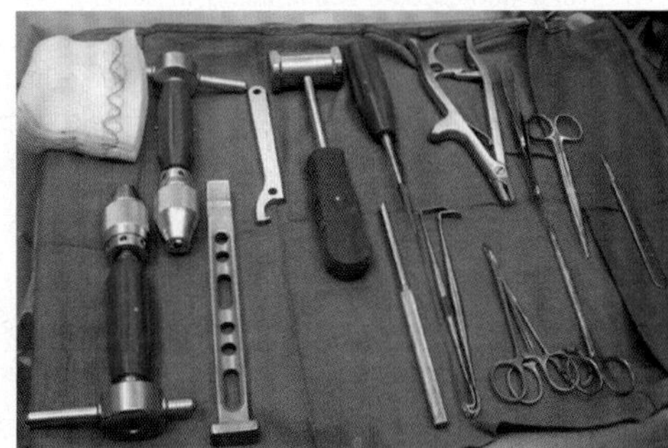

FIG 6 ● Valuable tools for intramedullary nailing of pediatric forearm fractures.

TECHNIQUES

Distal Radial Entry Point (Physeal Sparing)

- Using fluoroscopy (C-arm), a physeal-sparing distal radial incision is fashioned overlying the first dorsal compartment (**TECH FIG 1A**).
- Care is taken to protect branches of the superficial radial nerve. A short portion of the first dorsal compartment is opened.
- The tendons within the first dorsal compartment are retracted and protected before the awl engages the distal radius (**TECH FIG 1B**).

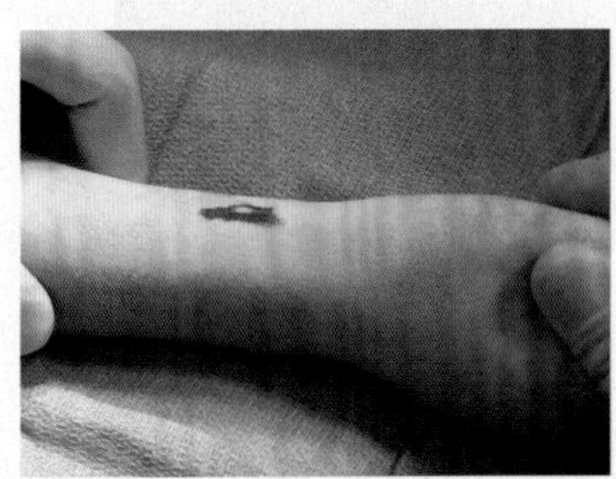

A

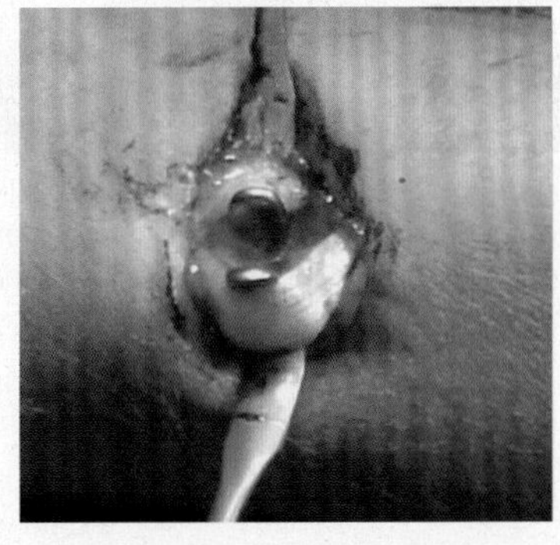

B

TECH FIG 1 ● Repair of forearm fracture of the patient in **FIG 3**. **A.** Physeal-sparing incision fashioned with fluoroscopic assistance. **B.** The surgeon must identify and protect the abductor pollicis longus and extensor pollicis brevis. *(continued)*

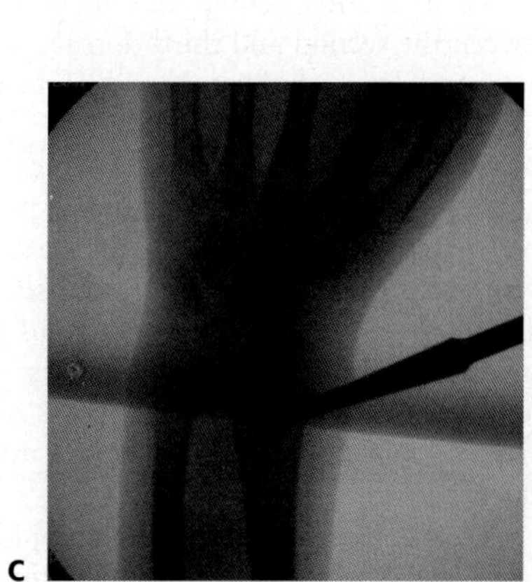

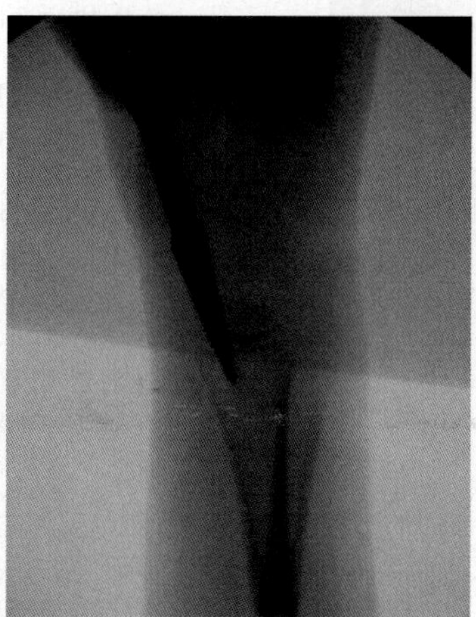

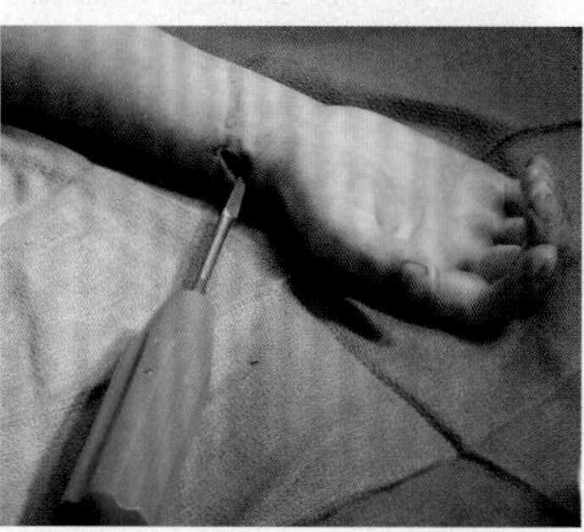

TECH FIG 1 • *(continued)* **C,D.** AP and lateral fluoroscopic confirmation of entry point. **E.** Well-seated and slightly angulated awl.

- After fluoroscopic confirmation of starting awl position, partial right and left rotations (not full turns) are used to gain satisfactory distal radial entry. A two-handed awl technique is used.
- Satisfactory intramedullary awl position is confirmed by a gentle "bounce" against the far cortex as well as fluoroscopic AP and lateral projections (**TECH FIG 1C–E**).
- The awl is temporarily left in its intraosseous position before insertion of the radial flexible intramedullary nail. Thus, the surgeon's ability to judge both the portal location and the angle of nail entry will be facilitated by immediate sequential awl removal and nail tip insertion.

Reduction and Nail Passage within the Radius

- The flexible nail for the radius is contoured such that it will reestablish appropriate radial bow. Nail contouring is gradual, smooth, and substantial. Acute bends in the nail should *not* be apparent (**TECH FIG 2A–C**).
- Entry into the distal radius entry site should be directly visualized, and the feel of the nail within the intramedullary canal offers distinct tactile feedback called scrape. Entry is further confirmed fluoroscopically (**TECH FIG 2D**).
- The radial nail is gently advanced up to the level of the fracture. Reduction is achieved via a combination of longitudinal traction and judicious use of AP compression with a radiolucent tool such as a vinyl Meyerding mallet (**TECH FIG 2E**).
- The nail is rotated to optimize nail passage across the fracture site (**TECH FIG 2F–H**), and then it is advanced to an appropriate depth within the proximal fragment (**TECH FIG 2I**).

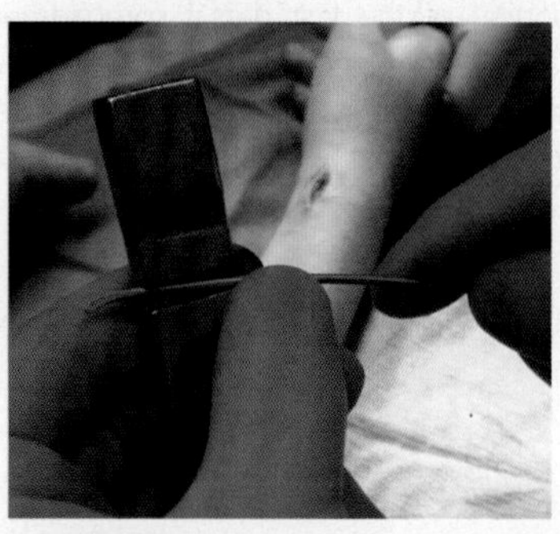

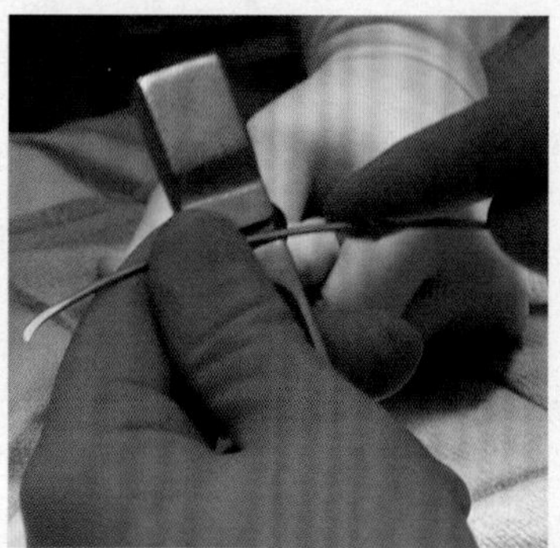

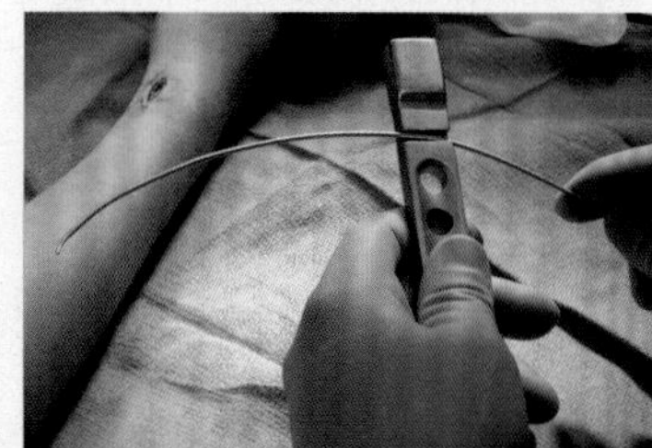

TECH FIG 2 • Insertion and passing of the radial nail. **A.** Gentle contouring of the distal aspect of the radial nail is important, as overbending effectively increases the diameter of the implant and may lead to nail incarceration. **B.** The "channel bender" is an effective tool for creating a properly contoured radial nail. **C.** The apex of the contoured nail should be placed so as to recreate appropriate radial bow (slightly distal of midshaft radius). *(continued)*

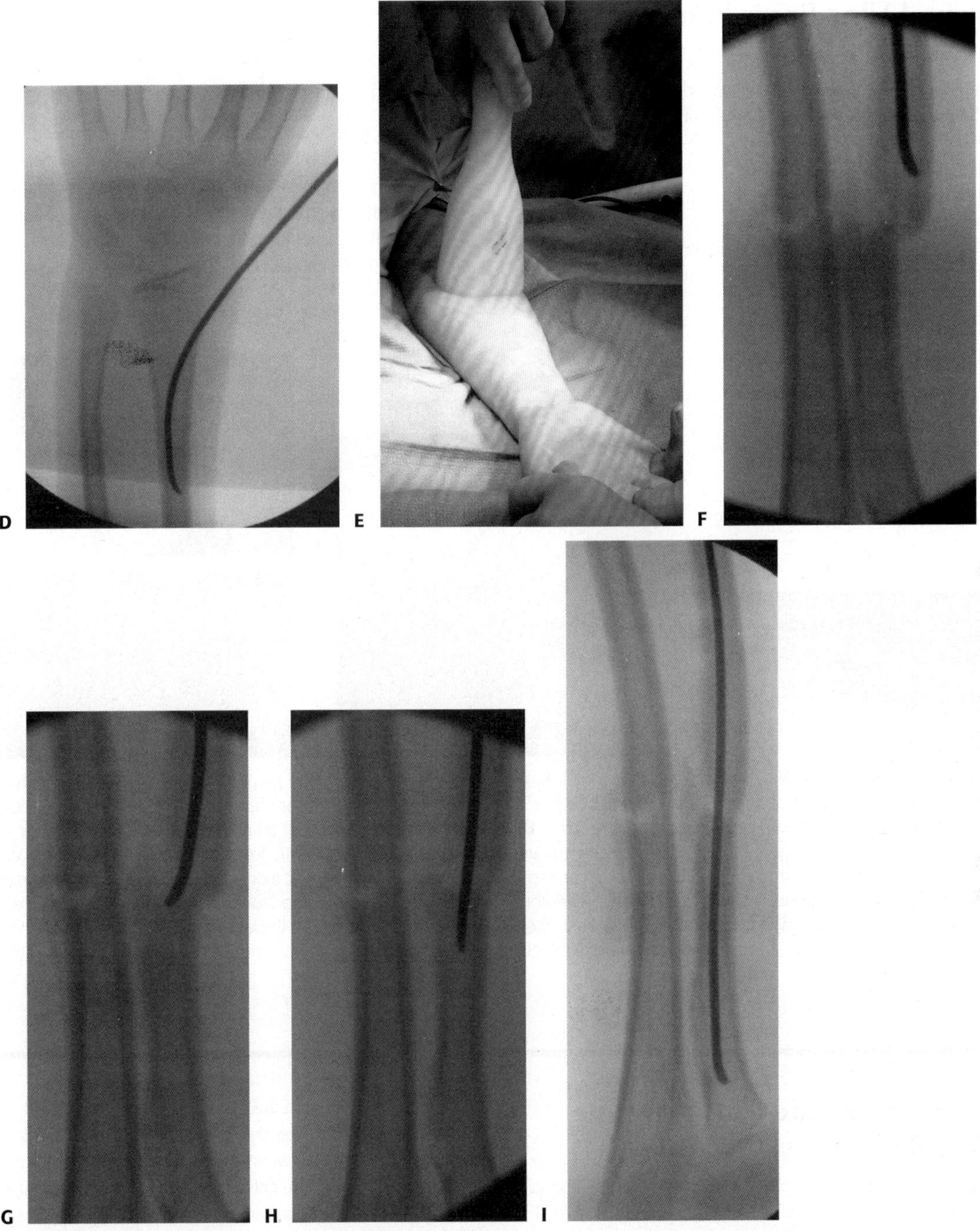

TECH FIG 2 • *(continued)* **D.** Under direct visualization, the contoured radial nail is manually inserted into the previously prepared entry point. Distinctive intramedullary tactile feedback (scrape) should be detected, and the implant advanced as far as possible using only the surgeon's hands. Note the trajectory of the nail (tip points radially), as this nail orientation should be maintained during most of the procedure. **E.** Appropriate longitudinal traction needs to be applied by an assistant as well as supplemental reduction forces such as that provided by the broad flat surface of a vinyl Meyerding mallet. **F.** The bent tip of the nail (the "fang") approaches the fracture site after being advanced as far as possible without using a hammer. "Manual forces only" should be used as much as possible to advance the nail within the canal using a properly tightened T handle or similar chuck. **G.** As the fang crosses the fracture site, proximal fragment intramedullary canal entry is often facilitated by nail rotation. At this point, finesse is much, much more important than brute strength. **H.** Once the nail properly enters the proximal fragment, the position is radiographically confirmed, and the nail is rotated back toward its "entry trajectory." **I.** The nail is advanced to an appropriate level in the region of the radial neck and rotated so as to properly recreate radial bow. Restoration of radial bow can be quite striking when visualized under live C-arm imaging. When radial nail contouring is preserved during the insertion process, the nail should be rotated 180 degrees such that the fang points in an ulnar direction. If this position does *not* optimize radial bow, then live C-arm imaging will allow the surgeon to choose the nail rotation that does.

Proximal Ulna Entry Point (Physeal-Sparing)

- An entry point is selected on the lateral edge of the subcutaneous border of the proximal ulna. The skin is touched but not pierced by the awl (**TECH FIG 3A**).
- Once correct position is confirmed fluoroscopically, the awl is used to gain percutaneous entry to the intramedullary canal of the proximal ulna (**TECH FIG 3B**).
- A mildly contoured (ie, nearly straight) flexible nail is inserted into the proximal ulna intramedullary canal (**TECH FIG 3C**).
- Proper position within the proximal ulna is confirmed fluoroscopically (**TECH FIG 3D**).

Reduction and Nail Passage within the Ulna

- The ulna is reduced, and the nail is passed across the fracture site in a manner similar to the radius. If open reduction becomes necessary, a simple Müller (AO-type) approach to the ulna is used (exploiting the interval between the extensor carpi ulnaris and the flexor carpi ulnaris).
- The ulnar nail is cut such that it is subcutaneous yet easily palpable.

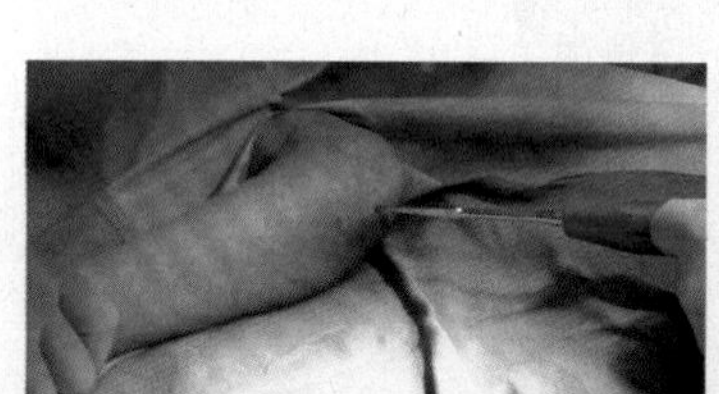
A

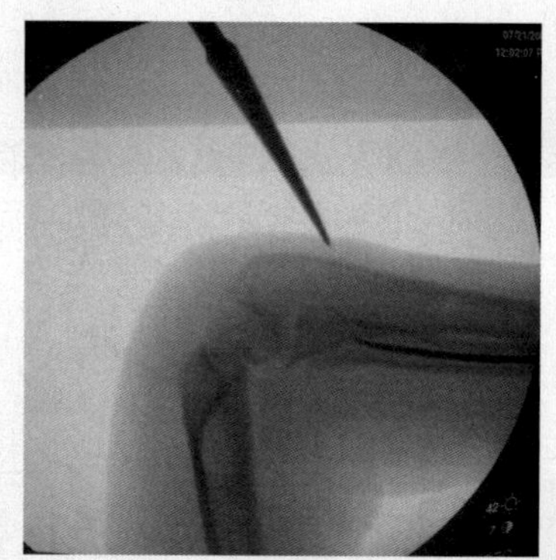
B

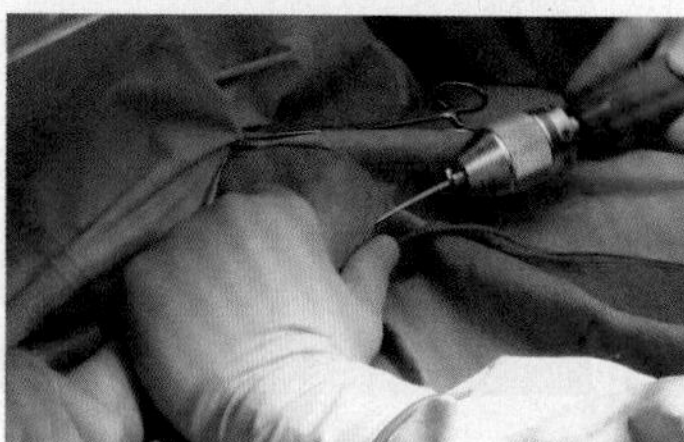
C

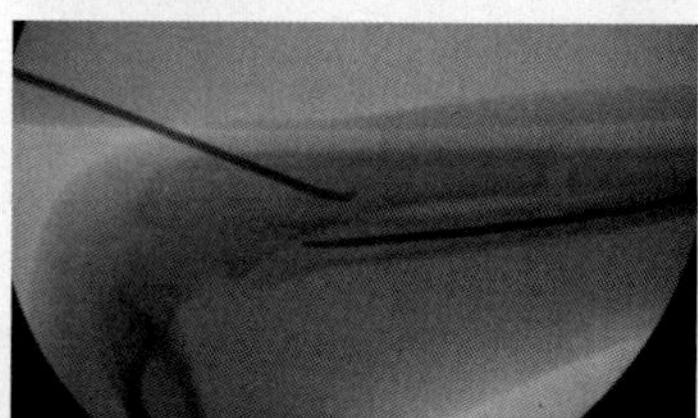
D

TECH FIG 3 • Insertion and passing of the ulnar nail. **A.** As opposed to the radial entry point where a true incision is very important to allow protection of nerves and tendons, true percutaneous entry is an option for the anconeus starting point (distal to olecranon physis and just lateral off the ridge of the ulna). **B.** Radiographic confirmation of an acceptable awl entry point as well as awl trajectory is necessary. Anconeus entry is preferred over true tip-of-the-olecranon entry for two reasons: the anconeus entry point avoids unnecessary physeal injury and also decreases the likelihood of large painful olecranon bursae. **C.** The ulnar nail is contoured in a far more gentle fashion, as the ulna is a predominantly straight bone compared to the radius. After manual nail entry, the ulnar nail is advanced with the use of a chuck. Note the 90-degree flexed position of the elbow and the 90-degree external rotation of the shoulder. **D.** Similar nail advancement technique is used for the ulna, with the exception of any dramatic nail rotation maneuver at the end of nail insertion.

Final Rotation and Cutting of the Radial Nail

- The precontoured radial nail is rotated so as to optimize and normalize the anatomic bow of the radial shaft. This step is most dramatic when performed under several seconds of live fluoroscopic imaging.
- Appropriate full-length forearm imaging must be performed at the end of the case to ensure an acceptable rotational relationship between the radial styloid and the bicipital tuberosity as well as the ulnar styloid and the coronoid process.
- Care must be taken when cutting the radial nail. If the nail is too short, removal will be difficult, and dorsal compartment tendons adjacent to a sharp nail edge will be at risk. Thus, the nail should be cut to protrude beyond the tendons while still remaining subcutaneous.

Closure, Dressing, Splinting, and Aftercare

- Closure of the radial entry site is performed with absorbable subcutaneous and subcuticular suture and Steri-Strips. Care is taken to protect branches of the superficial branch of the radial nerve (**TECH FIG 4A,B**).
- Light Xeroform, sterile gauze, and Tegaderm dressings are applied to the surgical sites (**TECH FIG 4C–E**).
- A removable forearm fracture brace may also be applied to increase patient comfort (**TECH FIG 4F**).

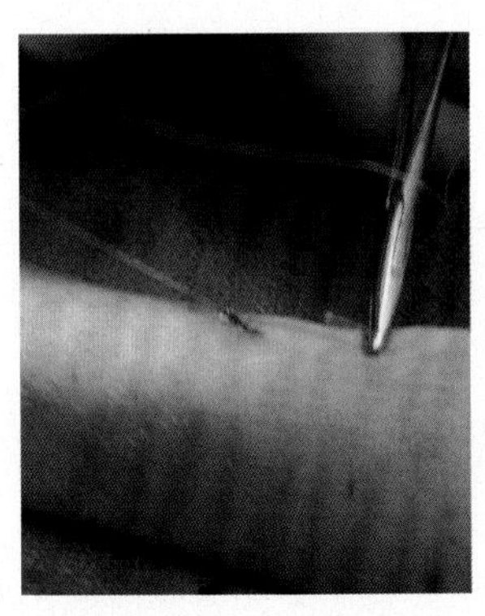
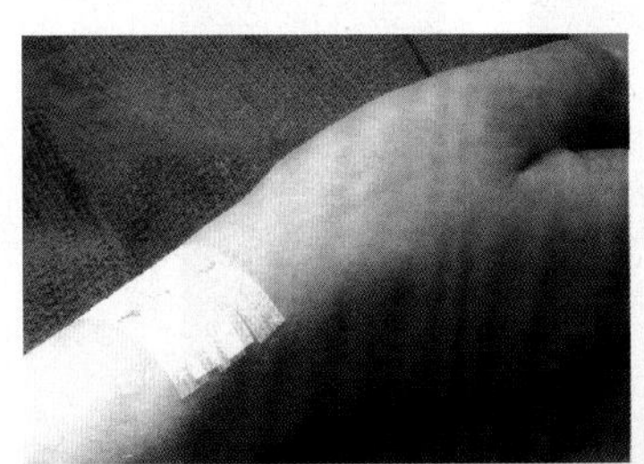
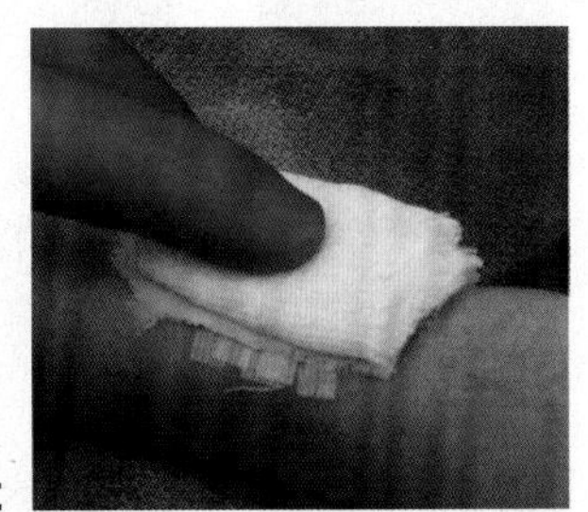
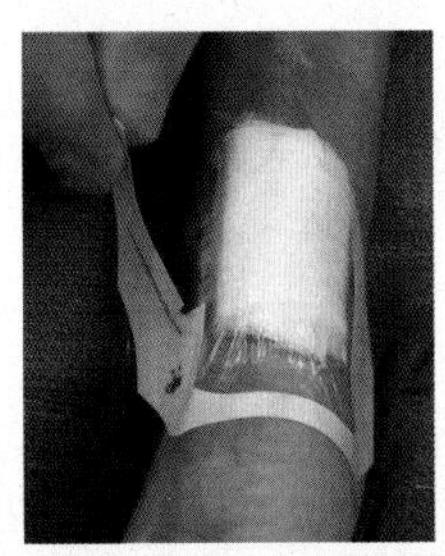
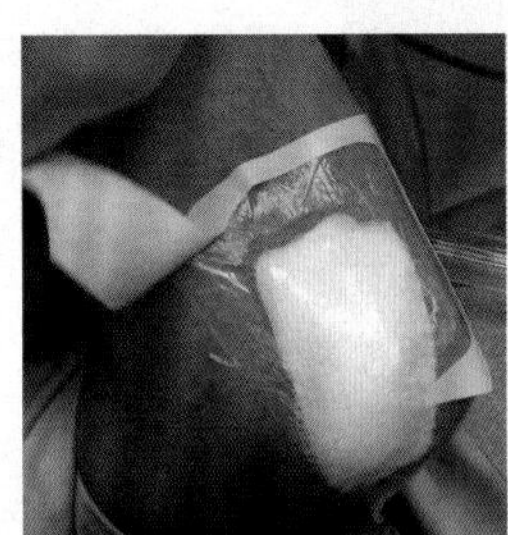
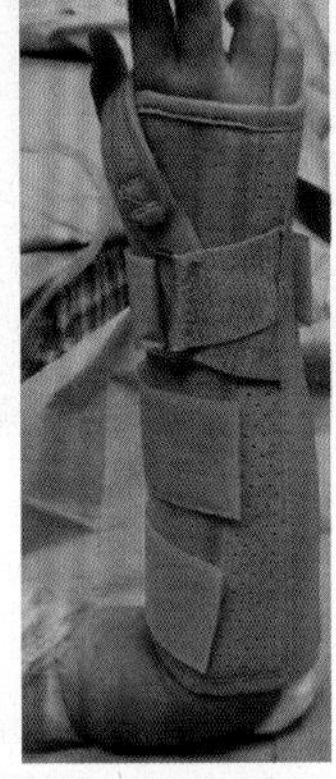

TECH FIG 4 • My preferred closure, dressing, and splinting technique. **A.** Several interrupted absorbable sutures (typically 3-0 Vicryl) are used for closure of the subcutaneous and subcuticular portion of the radial wound. Steri-Strips are added for final wound closure (**B**), followed by Xeroform and sterile gauze (**C**), and a Tegaderm dressing (**D**). **E.** A similar dressing consisting of Xeroform, sterile gauze, and Tegaderm is applied to the proximal ulnar wound. **F.** A removable Velcro forearm fracture brace is applied at the end of the procedure.

PEARLS AND PITFALLS

Which bone to reduce and fix first?	■ Once one bone is successfully reduced and stabilized via indirect techniques, achieving the same for the second bone will be more difficult. Thus, the radius should be stabilized first, as it is "deeper." Then, if required, exposure of the nearly subcutaneous ulna is relatively easy.
How much flexible nail should be left extruding from the bone?	■ If it is too long, soft tissue adjacent to sharp nail edges is at risk. If it is too short, nail removal will be needlessly difficult.
At what point should efforts at closed reduction be abandoned in favor of a limited open reduction?	■ The author use the "three strikes and you're out" rule (three low-amplitude shots at crossing the fracture site) or the "11-minute rule." Once either or both are violated, the author convert the case to an open reduction. Remember, cases of forearm compartment syndrome have been attributed to extended efforts at indirect reduction.
What if an intramedullary nail seems to become incarcerated after crossing the fracture site?	■ The surgeon should remove the nail and convert to one of a smaller diameter before creating new comminution or distracting the fracture site. Distracted fracture fragments may lead to nonunion.
What if sterile intraoperative radiographs suggest malrotation of one or both of the forearm bones?	■ The surgeon should back the offending nail up a bit and see if improved rotational alignment of the fracture fragments can be obtained via forearm rotation and T-handle chuck manipulation. The surgeon then readvances the nail to hold position. If this does not work, the surgeon should consider switching to a smaller diameter nail, as intramedullary interference fit may be excessive.
When should the flexible nails be removed?	■ The originators of this technique suggest nail removal by about the sixth postoperative month. Forearm shaft fractures have the highest refracture rate (about 12%) of all pediatric fractures.

POSTOPERATIVE CARE

- Other than patients with open fracture, flexible nailing of the forearm can be performed as an outpatient procedure so long as there are absolutely no concerns about swelling or compartment syndrome.
- Oral prophylactic antibiotics may be continued for several doses postoperatively if desired, but usually, an appropriately administered preoperative intravenous antibiotic (within 2 hours of the surgical incision) is all that is required.
- The patient is allowed immediate active elbow and hand motion. Concerns about rotational stability after flexible nail stabilization seem to have been vastly overstated, and above-elbow immobilization is not required.
- As there are no sutures to remove, outpatient follow-up may occur in 4 to 6 weeks (**FIG 7A,B**).
- The originators of this procedure have suggested that the nails be removed by about the sixth postoperative month (**FIG 7C,D**).

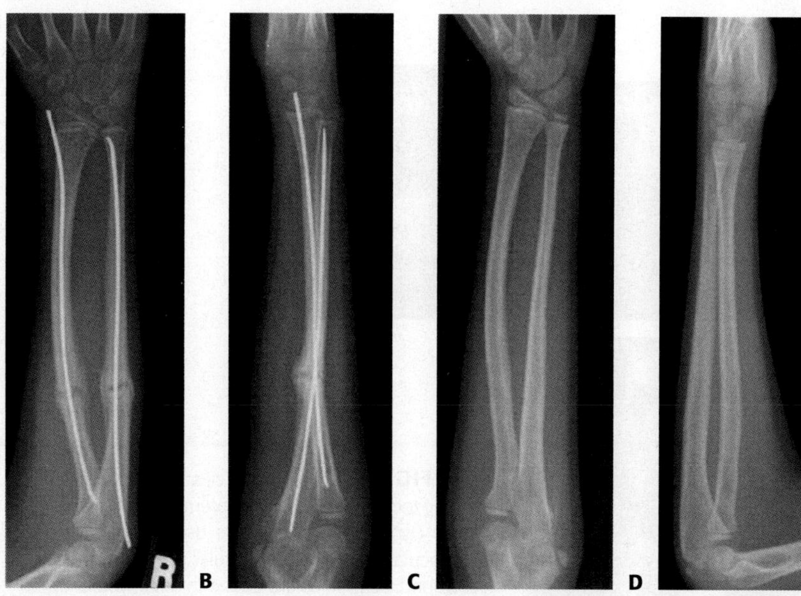

FIG 7 • Postoperative AP and lateral radiographs at 4 weeks (**A,B**) and 1 year (**C,D**) of the patient in **FIG 3** and all techniques figures.

OUTCOMES

- At this time, no randomized trials comparing flexible intramedullary nailing of forearm shaft fractures versus cast treatment have been conducted.
- A systematic review of English-language reports comparing flexible nailing to cast treatment found a significantly lower risk of forearm stiffness with nailing (25% stiffness with casting vs. 5% with flexible nailing). This comes at the price of a higher rate of minor complications (21%) with surgery versus casting (6%).[13]
- One of the largest published series[4] of pediatric forearm shaft fractures treated using flexible intramedullary nailing showed 92% excellent results with full range of motion at an average of 3.5 years of follow-up.[10]

COMPLICATIONS

- Sensory neurapraxia (usually the superficial branch of the radial nerve) occurs at a rate of at least 2% after flexible intramedullary nailing. These deficits are almost always temporary, resolving over weeks to months. The branching pattern of this nerve is such that it presents itself throughout the region of the first, second, and third extensor compartments (**FIG 8**).[2]
- The deep infection rate (osteomyelitis) after flexible intramedullary nailing of pediatric forearm shaft fractures is less than 0.5%; this can be compared to the reported 5% rate of osteomyelitis after plate fixation of similar fractures.[13]
- Extensor tendon injury (especially the extensor pollicis longus) has been reported by multiple authors and may occur during nail insertion or nail removal as well as when tendons repetitively glide past a sharp nail tip (slowly sawing the tendon in two). Radial entry through the floor of the first compartment may minimize this complication (vs. entry between the second and third compartments).[9,16]
- In the clinical setting of forearm shaft fractures coexisting with ipsilateral humeral fracture (floating elbow), the incidence of compartment syndrome may be as high as 33%. When longer operative times are required (about 2 hours), a 7.5% rate of compartment syndrome has also been reported.[18]

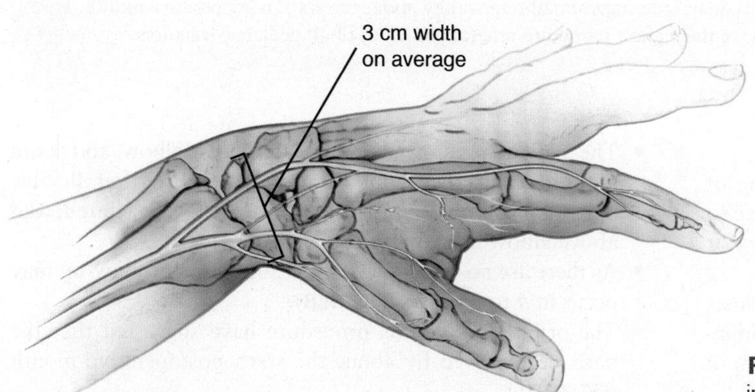

FIG 8 • Relevant anatomy of superficial branch of the radial nerve in the region of the first, second, and third extensor compartments.

- Delayed union and nonunion are decidedly rare after flexible intramedullary nailing of pediatric forearm fractures. If either delayed union or nonunion occurs, there is usually some explanation, such as a technical error (eg, too large an intramedullary implant distracting the ulnar fracture site), infection, or neurofibromatosis.
- There should be a 5% or less chance of long-term forearm stiffness (defined as exceeding a 20 degree loss of pronation or supination) after flexible intramedullary forearm shaft fixation.[1]

REFERENCES

1. Antabak A, Luetic T, Ivo S, et al. Treatment outcomes of both-bone diaphyseal paediatric forearm fractures. Injury 2013;44(suppl 3):S11–S15.
2. Auerbach DM, Collins ED, Kunkle KL, et al. The radial sensory nerve. An anatomic study. Clin Orthop Rel Res 1994;(308):241–249.
3. Blackman AJ, Wall LB, Keeler KA, et al. Acute compartment syndrome after intramedullary nailing of isolated radius and ulna fractures in children. J Pediatr Orthop 2014;34(1):50–54.
4. Bowman EN, Mehlman CT, Lindsell CJ, et al. Nonoperative treatment of both-bone forearm shaft fractures in children: predictors of early radiographic failure. J Pediatr Orthop 2011;31:23–32.
5. Cheng JC, Ng BK, Ying SY, et al. A 10-year study of the changes in the pattern and treatment of 6,493 fractures. J Pediatr Orthop 1999;19:344–350.
6. Colaris J, Reijman M, Allerma JH, et al. Single-bone intramedullary fixation of unstable both-bone diaphyseal forearm fractures in children leads to increased re-displacement: a multicenter randomized controlled trial. Arch Orthop Trauma Surg 2013;133:1079–1087.
7. Davis DR, Green DP. Forearm fractures in children: pitfalls and complications. Clin Orthop Relat Res 1976;(120):172–183.
8. Johari AN, Sinha M. Remodeling of forearm fractures in children. J Pediatr Orthop B 1999;8:84–87.
9. Kravel T, Sher-Lurie N, Ganel A. Extensor pollicis longus rupture after fixation of radius and ulna fracture with titanium elastic nail (TEN) in a child: a case report. J Trauma 2007;63:1169–1170.
10. Lascombes P, Prevot J, Ligier JN, et al. Elastic stable intramedullary nailing in forearm shaft fractures in children: 85 cases. J Pediatr Orthop 1990;10:167–171.
11. Mehlman CT. Fractures of the forearm, wrist, and hand. Orthopaedic Knowledge Update 9. Rosemont, IL: AAOS, 2008.
12. Mehlman CT, Araghi A, Roy DR. Hyphenated history: the Hueter-Volkmann law. Am J Orthop 1997;26:798–800.
13. Mehlman CT, Wall EJ. Injuries to the shafts of the radius and ulna. In: Beaty JH, Kasser JR, eds. Rockwood and Wilkins' Fractures in Children, ed 6. Philadelphia: Lippincott Williams & Wilkins, 2006:399–441.
14. Price CT, Scott DS, Kurzner ME, et al. Malunited forearm fractures in children. J Pediatr Orthop 1990;10:705–712.
15. Schock CC. The crooked straight: distal radial remodeling. J Ark Med Soc 1987;84:97–100.
16. Sproule JA, Roche SJ, Murthy EG. Attritional rupture of extensor pollicis longus tendon: a rare complication following elastic stable intramedullary nailing of a paediatric radial fracture. Hand Surg 2011;16:69–72.
17. Younger AS, Tredwell SJ, Mackenzie WG, et al. Accurate prediction of outcome after pediatric forearm fracture. J Pediatr Orthop 1994;14:200–206.
18. Yuan PS, Pring ME, Gaynor TP, et al. Compartment syndrome following fixation of pediatric forearm fractures. J Pediatr Orthop 2004;24:370–375.

13 CHAPTER

Elbow Fractures and Dislocations

Management of Simple Elbow Dislocation

Bradford O. Parsons and David M. Lutton

DEFINITION

- Simple elbow dislocation is a dislocation of the ulnohumeral joint without concomitant fracture.
- Complex instability denotes the presence of a fracture associated with dislocation.
- The elbow is the second most commonly dislocated large joint.

PATHOANATOMY

- Elbow stability is conferred by highly constrained osseous anatomy and the ligamentous anatomy.
- Essentially, there are three primary stabilizers of the elbow.[9,12]
  - The osseous architecture of the ulnohumeral joint, including the coronoid process and greater sigmoid notch of the ulna, and the trochlea of the humerus
  - The anterior band of the medial collateral ligament (aMCL) resists valgus stress. The aMCL originates on the anterior inferior face of the medial epicondyle and inserts on the sublime tubercle of the ulna.
  - The lateral ulnar collateral ligament (LUCL) resists varus stress. The LUCL originates from an isometric point on the lateral supracondylar column and traverses across the inferior aspect of the radial head, inserting on the supinator crest of the ulna.[8] Unlike the aMCL, the LUCL originates in the precise center of rotation of the elbow; this is important when reconstructing the ligament.
- Secondary stabilizers include the radial head and dynamic constraints such as the flexor and extensor muscles of the forearm.
  - When the elbow is extended, the anterior joint capsule contributes about 15% of varus–valgus stability.[9]
  - The radial head does not resist physiologic valgus stress in the presence of an intact aMCL; however, it plays a major role in the presence of aMCL insufficiency.
- O'Driscoll has described the term *ring of disability* to describe series of pathologic events that result in ulnohumeral dislocation.
  - A simple elbow dislocation begins with an extension varus stress that disrupts the LUCL and progresses medially with tearing of the anterior and posterior capsules. This allows the ulna to "perch" on the distal humerus. Further soft tissue or osseous injury results in dislocation[13] (**FIG 1A**).
    - Most traumatic injuries to the LUCL result in avulsion of the ligament from the lateral humerus (**FIG 1B**).
  - As forces continue from lateral to medial across the joint, the anterior and posterior capsular tissues and eventually the medial collateral ligament (MCL) may be disrupted; however, it is theoretically possible to dislocate the ulnohumeral joint with disruption of the LUCL and preservation of the aMCL.[12]
- O'Driscoll et al[12] has proposed the term *posterolateral rotatory instability* (PLRI) to describe the condition of chronic LUCL insufficiency resulting in rotatory recurrent ulnohumeral instability.
- Fractures may occur with elbow dislocations, and the risk of recurrent instability increases significantly with complex dislocations. These fractures commonly include radial head or neck and coronoid fractures, although any fracture about the elbow may be observed.
  - Radial head fractures are usually readily apparent on plain radiographs.
  - Coronoid fractures may be subtle, and even a "fleck" of coronoid is often a hallmark of a more significant injury (eg, "terrible triad" injury), and its importance should not be underestimated.
  - Recently, a variant of elbow instability termed *posteromedial rotatory instability* (PMRI) has been described. PMRI is the sequela of a LUCL injury and a medial coronoid facet fracture. This injury pattern is most commonly observed without radial head fracture, making it potentially very subtle on plain radiographs. A computed tomography (CT) scan can delineate this injury in detail and should be obtained if any suspicion exists (**FIG 1C–E**).[2,11]

ETIOLOGY AND CLASSIFICATION

- Most elbow dislocations occur with a fall on an outstretched arm.
- Forces of valgus, extension, supination, and axial compression across the joint can result in the ulna rotating away from the humerus, disrupting lateral anterior soft tissues initially, and dislocating the elbow.
- Simple elbow dislocations are classified by the direction of displacement of the ulna in reference to the humerus, with posterolateral dislocation the most common.
  - Less common variants include anterior, medial, or lateral dislocations.

PATIENT HISTORY AND PHYSICAL FINDINGS

- History is aimed at determining the timeline and mechanism of injury, frequency of dislocations, and previous treatment.
- Unlike the shoulder, recurrent instability of the elbow is rare after an initial simple dislocation that was treated expediently.
  - Recurrent instability is more common in association with fractures (eg, the terrible triad injury).
  - Chronic instability, although rare in the United States, does occasionally occur, and management often requires reconstructive surgery or elbow replacement. Closed treatment is rarely successful in these patients.

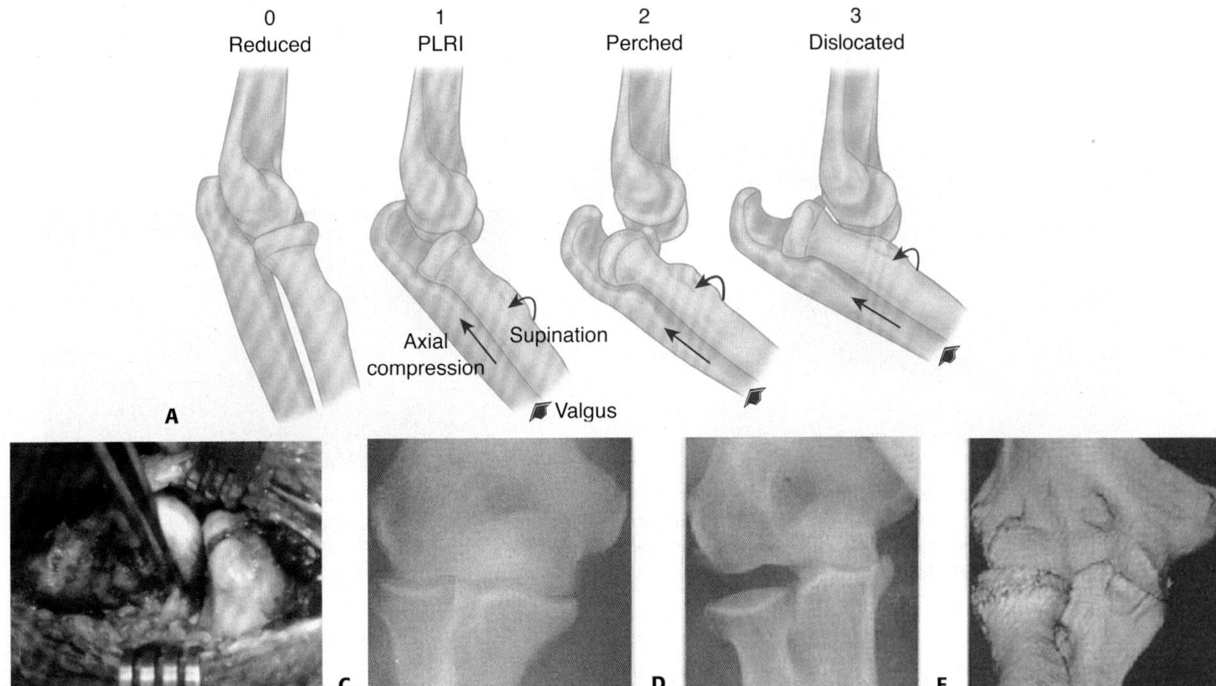

FIG 1 • A. PLRI follows a typical progression of disruption, allowing the joint to become perched and then dislocate as soft tissue injury progresses. **B.** Intraoperative photograph demonstrating avulsion of the origin of the LUCL after traumatic dislocation of the elbow. The origin of the LUCL and the extensor muscles are avulsed as one layer, held by the forceps. **C–E.** PMRI is a variant of elbow instability in which the elbow dislocates, rupturing the LUCL, and the medial coronoid sustains an impaction fracture. **C,D.** In this injury pattern, the radial head remains intact, making appropriate diagnosis of the severity of the injury difficult on standard radiographs. CT scans help better delineate the injury pattern. **E.** Impaction fracture can be seen on the 3-D CT reconstruction. (**A:** Adapted from O'Driscoll SW, Morrey BF, Korinek S, et al. Elbow subluxation and dislocation: a spectrum of instability. Clin Orthop Relat Res 1982;280:194; **C–E:** Copyright the Mayo Foundation, Rochester, MN.)

- Iatrogenic injury of the LUCL (during procedures such as open tennis elbow release or radial head fracture management) is a known cause of recurrent PLRI. However, these patients often complain of subtle lateral elbow pain due to subluxation of the joint with activities, such as rising from a chair, but rarely have recurrent dislocation.
- Examination at the time of injury requires attention to the neurovascular anatomy.
  - Nerve injury can occur after elbow dislocation, and a thorough neurologic examination of the extremity is mandatory before any treatment of the dislocation.
    - Most nerve injuries are neurapraxia that often resolve.
    - The ulnar nerve is most frequently involved, although median or radial nerve injury may also occur.[14]
- The dislocated elbow has obvious deformity, with the elbow typically held in a varus position and the forearm supinated.
- After initial reduction, the neurovascular status of the limb is reevaluated. Loss of neurologic function after closed reduction is rare but can be an indication for surgical exploration to rule out an entrapped nerve.
- Stability of the joint is assessed based on the amount of extension obtainable and association of pronation or supination with instability.
  - It is helpful to evaluate the stability throughout the elbow range of motion while the patient is still anesthetized, as this may guide treatment (examination under anesthesia).
  - Stressing of the lateral soft tissues is performed with the lateral pivot shift maneuver, which can be performed under anesthesia and with fluoroscopic imaging[12] (**FIG 2**).
    - This test can be used to assess the degree of PLRI and may aid in determining treatment.
- Medial ecchymosis may be a sign of an aMCL injury and often is apparent 3 to 5 days after dislocation when the MCL has been injured.

IMAGING AND OTHER DIAGNOSTIC STUDIES

- Standard orthogonal radiographs of the elbow are obtained before and after reduction to assess for fracture and confirm relocation of the joint.
  - Congruency of the trochlea–ulna and radial head–capitellum is assessed.
  - Slight widing of the ulnohumeral joint (drop sign) or posterior displacement of the radial head relative to the capitellum should be noted.
- Valgus stress views, once the joint is reduced, may help demonstrate an aMCL injury.
  - With the elbow flexed 30 degrees and the forearm in pronation, a valgus stress is placed under fluoroscopic evaluation to see if the medial ulnohumeral joint opens compared to the resting state.
- Varus stress views are often not helpful.
- CT scans with three-dimensional (3-D) reconstructions are obtained in any situation where a fracture may be

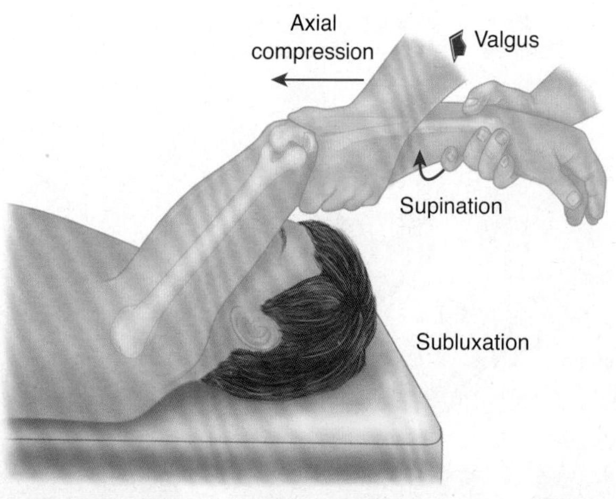

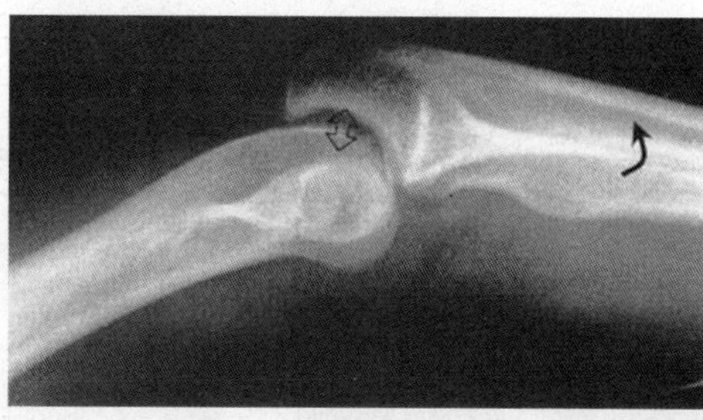

A B

FIG 2 • **A.** The lateral pivot shift maneuver is performed with the patient's arm positioned overhead, and a supination valgus stress is applied. As the elbow is brought into flexion, the joint reduces, often with a clunk. **B.** When performed under fluoroscopy, subluxation of the radial head posterior to the capitellum can be observed, consistent with PLRI. (**B:** From O'Driscoll SW, Bell DF, Morrey BF. Posterolateral rotatory instability of the elbow. J Bone Joint Surg Am 1991;73[3]:440–446.)

suspected, as it is critical to identify PMRI variants or subtle coronoid fractures, which may be an indication for surgical management.

- Magnetic resonance imaging (MRI) is usually not necessary in the management of acute simple dislocation; however, it can be useful in the case of recurrent PLRI.

NONOPERATIVE MANAGEMENT

- Most simple dislocations may be managed nonoperatively with splinting or bracing, guided by the degree of instability determined during the examination under anesthesia after reduction.[12]
- Once reduced, elbow stability is assessed during flexion–extension in neutral forearm rotation.
  - If the elbow is stable throughout an arc of motion, it is immobilized in a sling or splint for 3 to 5 days for comfort and then range-of-motion exercises are initiated.
  - If instability is present in less than 30 degrees of flexion, the forearm is pronated and stability is reassessed.
    - If pronation confers stability, then a hinged orthosis that maintains forearm pronation is used, after 3 to 5 days of splinting, to allow protected range of motion.
- Elbows that sublux (confirmed by fluoroscopic imaging) in less than 30 degrees of flexion and pronation of the forearm are managed with a brief period of splinting, followed by a hinged orthosis that controls rotation of the forearm and has an extension block.
- Elbow instability above 30 degrees of flexion can be an indication for surgical stabilization.
- Hinged bracing is maintained for 6 weeks, with progressive advancement of extension and rotation, as allowed by stability of the joint.
  - Weekly radiographs are needed to ensure maintenance of a congruent joint during the first 4 to 6 weeks.
- After 6 weeks, bracing is discontinued, and terminal stretching to regain motion is used if flexion contractures exist.

SURGICAL MANAGEMENT

Indications

- Surgical management is indicated in elbows that are unstable, even when placed in flexion (more than 30 degrees) and pronation, elbows that recurrently subluxate or dislocate during the treatment protocol, or those with associated fractures ("complex" instability).
- Management of simple dislocation requires repair or reconstruction of the ligamentous structures leading to the instability. By definition, simple dislocation occurs without fracture.
- An algorithmic approach to ligament repair is used to stabilize the elbow. LUCL insufficiency is felt to be the primary lesion with simple dislocations and is therefore addressed first.
- The LUCL usually avulses from the humerus and can be repaired in the acute setting.
  - Repair may be performed via bone tunnels in the humerus or with suture anchors, depending on the surgeon's preference.
  - Reconstruction of the LUCL is rarely needed in acute management but is often needed in chronic instability. Reconstruction is performed with autograft (either palmaris or gracilis) or allograft.
    - Repair or reconstruction of the LUCL typically confers stability, even in the face of MCL injury, as the intact radial head is a secondary stabilizer to valgus instability.
- Persistent instability after LUCL repair is rare and is more commonly observed with fracture-dislocations or chronic instability.
  - If persistent instability exists, the MCL is repaired or reconstructed. A hinged external fixator may be placed to protect the repair.

Preoperative Planning

- Planning should include preparing for the possibility of reconstruction of the LUCL which requires either autograft or allograft tendon.
  - If autograft is to be harvested, a tendon stripper is needed.
  - For allograft, we routinely use semitendinosus tendon.

- A hinged external fixator should be available in the rare case that the elbow remains unstable after ligamentous repair or reconstruction.
- A 2.0- and 3.2-mm drill bits or burrs are used to make bone tunnels for LUCL repair or reconstruction.
  - Some surgeons prefer suture anchor repair of ligament avulsions; if desired, these should be available.
- Fluoroscopy is useful for confirming reduction and is required for placement of a hinged external fixator.
- A sterile tourniquet is used to provide a bloodless surgical field.

Patient Positioning

- Patients are positioned supine with the arm on a radiolucent hand table.
- A small bump is placed under the scapula to aid in arm positioning.
- The forequarter is draped free to ensure the entire brachium is kept in the surgical field.
- If hamstring autograft is to be used for LUCL, the leg should be draped free, and a bump is placed under the hemipelvis to aid in exposure.

Lateral Ulnar Collateral Ligament Repair

Surgical Approach and Arthrotomy

- Tourniquet control is used during this procedure.
- A fluoroscopic examination under anesthesia is performed to allow for an accurate assessment of the instability pattern
- Two different surgical approaches may be used to manage elbow instability.
- A posterior midline skin incision is versatile and can be used to gain access to both the medial and lateral aspects of the joint.
  - Alternatively, a "column" incision, centered over the lateral epicondyle, may be used (**TECH FIG 1A**). If medial-sided exposure is needed, a similar column incision may be made over the medial epicondyle to gain access.
  - There are benefits to both approaches, and currently, no data exist delineating which approach is better.
    - For simple dislocation, we routinely use a lateral column approach.
- After skin incision, skin flaps are raised anteroposterior at the level of the deep fascia.
- In the acute setting, the lateral soft tissues are usually avulsed off the epicondyle, exposing the joint. Occasionally, however, the extensor origin is intact with an underlying ligament injury.
  - If the extensor muscles are intact, the interval between the extensor carpi ulnaris (ECU) and anconeus (the Kocher approach), which directly overlies the LUCL, is used. This interval is often readily identified by the presence of a "fat stripe" in the deep fascia (**TECH FIG 1B**). The anconeus is reflected posteriorly, and the ECU is reflected anteriorly to expose the capsuloligamentous complex.
- The elbow joint is then exposed by incising the proximal capsule along the lateral column of the humerus, continuing distally along the radial neck (through the supinator muscle and underling capsule) in line with the ECU–anconeus interval.
  - The posterior interosseous nerve (PIN) is at risk with this exposure, and therefore, the forearm is kept in pronation to protect the PIN.
- The radiocapitellar joint and coronoid are inspected to confirm no fractures are present and that no soft tissue is interposed in the joint, preventing reduction.
- Once the joint is clear of debris, the ability to obtain a concentric reduction is confirmed with fluoroscopy.

Ligament Repair

- The origin of the LUCL is identified.
  - Often, the LUCL is avulsed from the isometric point on the lateral capitellum, and the origin can be identified by a "fold" of tissue on the deep surface of the capsule (**TECH FIG 2A**).
- Starting at the origin, a running no. 2 nonabsorbable Krackow locking suture is placed along the anterior and posterior aspect of the ligament. Once placed, the suture–ligament construct is tensioned to confirm the integrity of the insertion onto the ulna.
  - A common mistake is to start the repair at the level of the proximal origin of the superficial tissue, which is not the origin of the LUCL but part of the extensor origin.

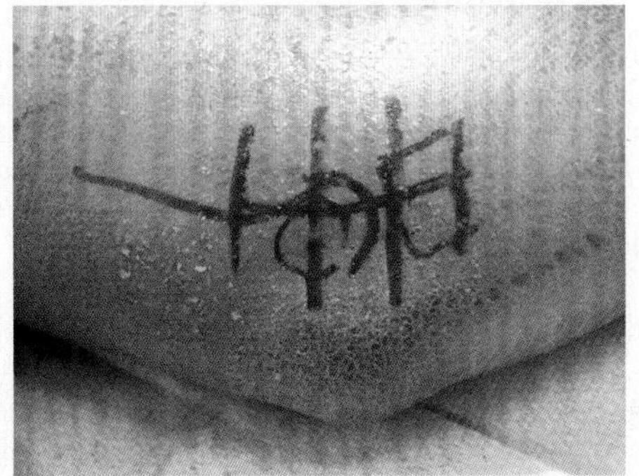

A

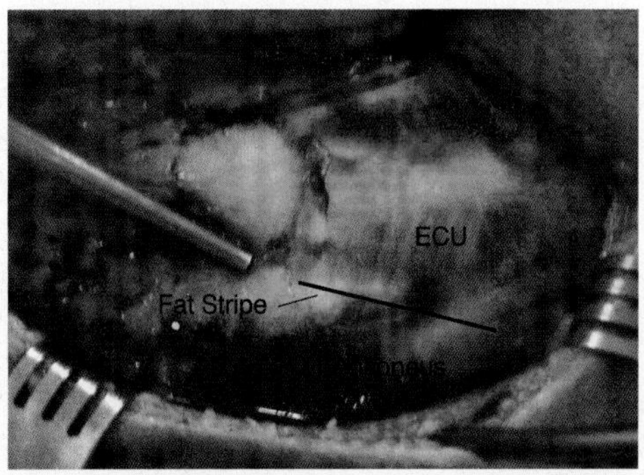

B

TECH FIG 1 • **A.** Lateral column skin incision. The lateral incision is centered over the epicondyle and radiocapitellar joint and is often the primary incision, as the LUCL rupture is thought to be the primary injury in simple dislocations. **B.** The deep interval between the ECU and anconeus is used to gain exposure to the joint. This is often identified by a fat stripe in the fascia. Care should be taken not to violate the LUCL, which traverses in line with this interval deep to the fascia and supinator muscle.

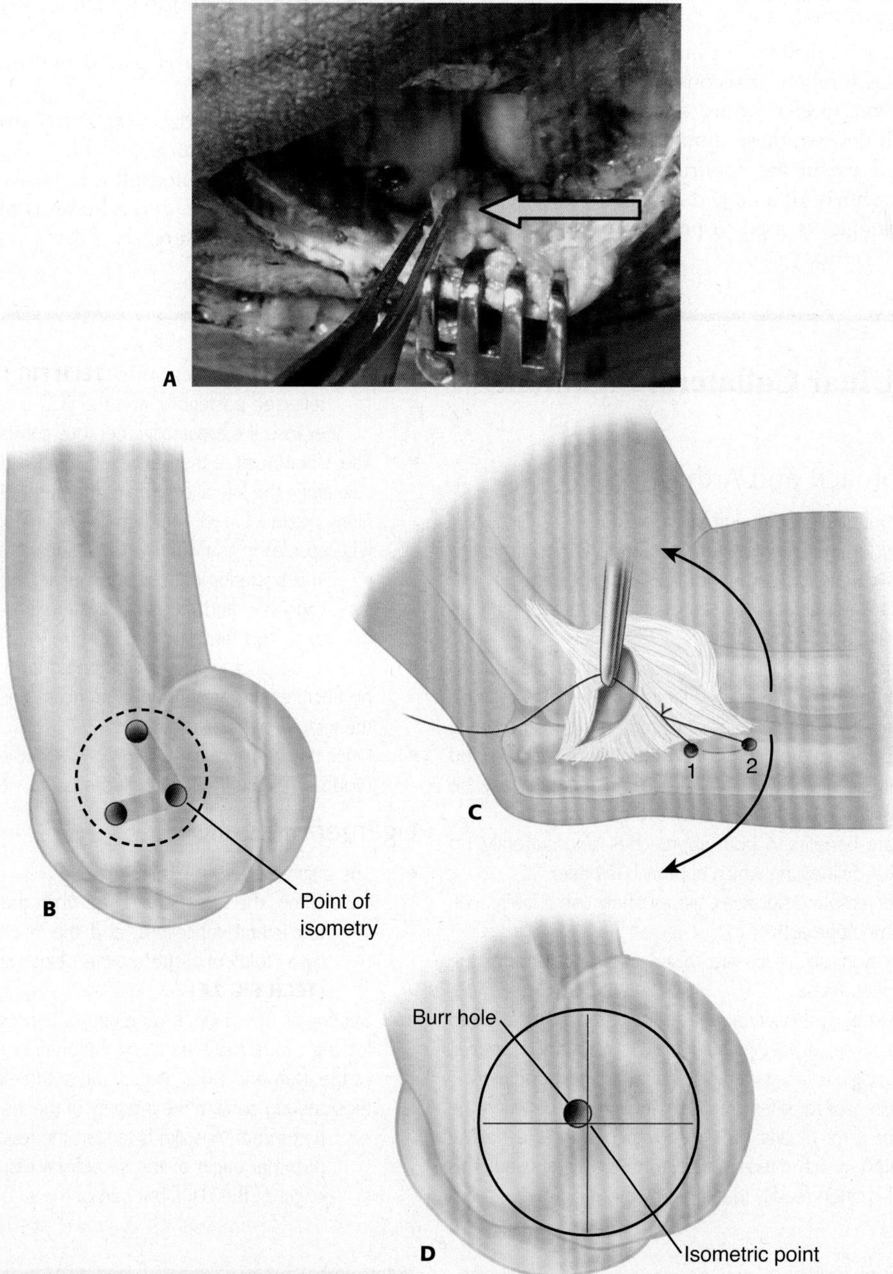

TECH FIG 2 • A. The origin of the LUCL, which often avulses during elbow dislocation, is identified by a fold of tissue on the deep surface of the capsule. The isometric point of the joint is in the center of rotation of the capitellum (**B**), and confirmation is made using the previously placed sutures in the ligament remnant to ensure that an isometric repair will be obtained (**C**). **D.** It is important to make the humeral tunnel so that the most anterior aspect of the tunnel is placed at the isometric point. Exit holes for the humeral tunnel are made anterior and posterior to the lateral supracondylar ridge (**B**).

- The isometric origin on the humerus is then identified in the center of the capitellum, not the lateral epicondyle (**TECH FIG 2B,C**).
  - Confirmation of the isometric point is made by clamping the limbs of the running suture at the point of isometry and then flexing and extending the elbow to confirm proper placement.
- A 2.0-mm burr is used to make a humeral bone tunnel.
  - It is critical to make the most anterior aspect of the bone tunnel at the isometric point, not the center of the tunnel, as this small translation can result in a lax LUCL repair (**TECH FIG 2D**).
- Two “exit” tunnels (in a Y configuration), one anterior and one posterior to the lateral column, are then made with a 2.0-mm

drill bit or burr, connected to the distal humeral tunnel at the isometric point.

- Once the humeral tunnels are completed, the limbs of the running suture are passed through the humeral tunnels.
- The joint is concentrically reduced with fluoroscopic confirmation, and the LUCL repair sutures are then tied with the joint reduced and the elbow in 30 degrees of flexion and neutral rotation.
- The elbow is ranged through an arc of motion to assess stability, with careful attention placed on the radial head's articulation with the capitellum, looking for posterior sag in extension, indicating either a lax LUCL or a nonisometric repair.
- If the elbow is stable through an arc of motion, the extensor origin is repaired with interrupted, heavy (no. 0) nonabsorbable suture, and the skin is closed in layers.

Lateral Ulnar Collateral Ligament Reconstruction

- Occasionally, the native LUCL is damaged beyond repair (more often with iatrogenic PLRI than with primary instability) or attenuated after recurrent or chronic elbow instability, and reconstruction is necessary.
- Autograft palmaris, autograft gracilis, or allograft may be used.
- Autograft and allograft options should be discussed with the patient and decisions made preoperatively. We routinely use semitendinosus allograft unless the patient desires autograft.

Bone Tunnel Preparation

- We use a "docking" technique, similar to those described for MCL reconstruction,[1] for LUCL reconstruction.
- The insertion of the LUCL is at the supinator crest of the ulna, and reconstruction begins with creation of the ulnar tunnels at the supinator crest.
- Reflecting the supinator origin from the ulna posterior to the radial head exposes the supinator crest.
  - The forearm is held in pronation to protect the PIN.
- Once the crest is exposed, the ulnar tunnel is made at the level of the radial head using two 3.4-mm burr holes placed 1 cm apart. Care is taken to connect the holes using small curettes or awls without fracturing the roof of the tunnel (**TECH FIG 3**).
- Once the ulnar tunnel is made, a suture is placed in the tunnel to aid in graft passage and to help identify the isometric point on the humerus, similar to the technique described with ligament repair.
- Once the isometric origin on the humerus is confirmed, humeral bone tunnels are made as mentioned in the LUCL Repair section.
  - With LUCL reconstruction, the isometric tunnel is deepened to about 1 cm to allow graft docking.
  - Furthermore, the docking tunnel is widened using a 3.4-mm burr to be able to accept both limbs of the graft.
  - It is important to widen the docking hole anterior and proximal to the isometric point, as the most posterior aspect of the tunnel needs to be at the isometric point.

Graft Preparation

- One end of the graft is freshened and tubularized using a no. 2 nonabsorbable suture in a running Krackow fashion.
- The graft is then passed through the ulnar bone tunnels using the passage suture previously placed.
- The limb of the graft with locking suture is then fully docked into the humeral origin, and the joint is reduced.
- The final length of the graft is determined by tensioning the graft and identifying the point at which the free limb of the graft meets the isometric origin. This point is marked on the graft.
  - Care should be taken to ensure appropriate graft tension and length by fully docking the first limb and then marking the free limb at the point of initial contact with the humerus, thereby allowing some overlap of graft limbs in the humeral tunnel but minimizing the likelihood of slack in the final construct.
- The marked graft end is then freshened and tubularized in an identical fashion as the other limb.

Final Reconstruction

- Once the graft is placed and ready for final tensioning and fixation, the capsule and remnant of the LUCL is repaired back to the humerus in an effort to make the ligament reconstruction extra-articular, if possible.
- Each limb of the graft is then placed into the isometric docking tunnel on the humerus with corresponding limbs from each locking suture exiting the proximal humeral tunnels.
  - Both limbs of locking suture from one end of the graft are passed through one proximal tunnel in the humerus, followed by the limbs from the other end of the graft through the second proximal tunnel.

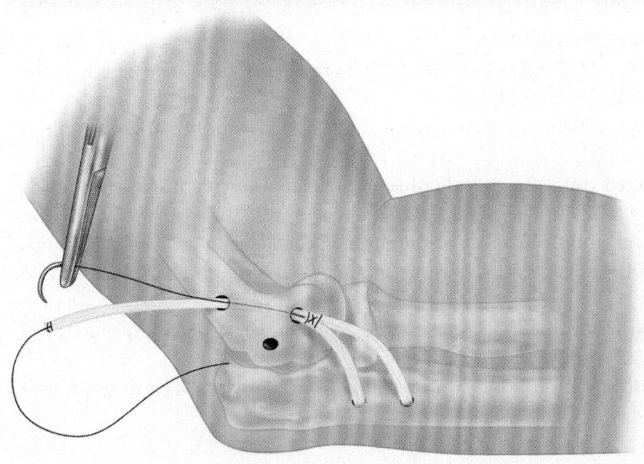

TECH FIG 3 • The insertion of the LUCL is the supinator crest of the ulna. Reconstruction uses an ulnar tunnel in the supinator crest made at the level of the radial head. Holes are made about 1 cm apart and connected to form a tunnel.

- The joint is then reduced, and the graft is finally tensioned to ensure there is no slack and neither graft end has "bottomed out" in the humeral docking tunnel.
- The locking sutures are then tied together over the lateral column of the distal humerus with the joint concentrically reduced in 30 degrees of flexion and neutral rotation.
- The joint is then ranged and stability assessed. If the joint is stable, no further reconstruction is necessary, and the extensor muscles are repaired using a nonabsorbable interrupted stitch, followed by skin closure.

Hinged External Fixation

- A hinged fixator may be necessary in chronic dislocations, some fracture-dislocations, or rarely in patients with persistent instability after LUCL repair or reconstruction for simple dislocation.[4,16]
- Once any soft tissue blocking reduction is removed and a concentric reduction can be obtained, the fixator is placed.
- All hinged elbow fixators are constructed around the axis or rotation of the elbow to allow range of motion to occur while maintaining a concentric reduction.
  - Most implants are built around an axis pin, placed in this center of rotation.
  - The center of rotation is identified as the center of the capitellum on a lateral aspect of the elbow, and on the medial side, it is just anteroinferior to the medial epicondyle, in the center of curvature of the trochlea (**TECH FIG 4**).
  - The axis pin is placed through both of these points, parallel to the joint surface, and the position is confirmed by fluoroscopy.
- After placement of the axis pin, the humeral and ulnar pins are placed after confirmation of concentric reduction of the elbow is made.
- Once the external fixator is fully constructed, the elbow is taken through an arc of motion, and maintenance of reduction is confirmed.
- Fixators are kept on for 6 to 8 weeks.
- Meticulous pin care is necessary to minimize pin tract infections or loosening.

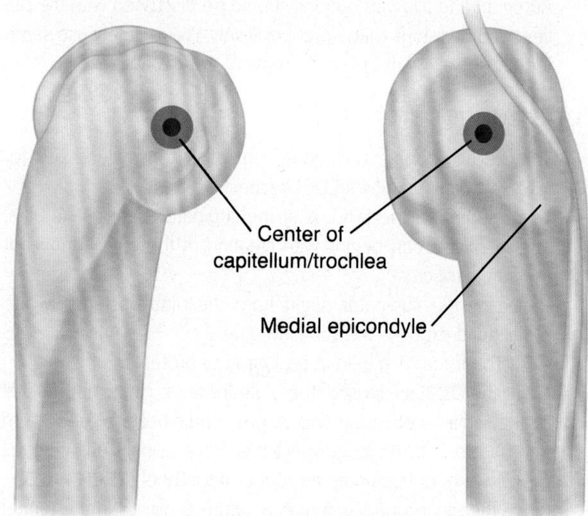

TECH FIG 4 • The center of rotation of the elbow, along which an axis pin for hinged fixators is placed, is identified by the center of the capitellum and just anteroinferior to the medial epicondyle.

PEARLS AND PITFALLS

- LUCL avulsion is the primary ligamentous injury in most simple dislocations of the elbow.
- If the radial head and coronoid are intact (as is the case in a simple dislocation), the MCL rarely needs to be repaired or reconstructed, as the radial head acts as a secondary stabilizer in the elbow with a repaired lateral ligament complex.
- The LUCL origin can be identified by a capsular fold of tissue. This is the point at which repair sutures should be placed, not at the origin of the more superficial extensor tendons.
- The isometric origin of the LUCL is in the center of the capitellum, as projected onto the lateral column, and repair or reconstruction needs to be brought to this point to have an isometric ligament.
- Bone tunnels in the humerus for repair or reconstruction are made so the anteroinferior aspect of the tunnel is at the isometric origin.
- A hinged external fixator may be necessary in management of elbow dislocation, especially chronic or recurrent situations, and should be available.
- All hinged fixators are constructed around the axis of rotation of the elbow, identified by a line between the isometric point on the lateral capitellum, and the center of rotation of the trochlea on the medial aspect of the joint.
- Stiffness is the most common adverse sequela of elbow dislocation, and therefore, range of motion should be started as soon as soft tissue and skin healing allows, with care taken to avoid varus or valgus stress.

POSTOPERATIVE CARE

- After operative stabilization without external fixation, the elbow is splinted in 90 degrees of flexion for 3 to 5 days to allow wound healing.
- Range-of-motion exercises are then begun in flexion, extension, and rotation, with care taken to avoid varus or valgus stress.
  - A hinged orthosis can be helpful in protecting the ligament repair or reconstruction.
- Active and passive motion is continued for 6 weeks, when strengthening is added.
- Residual contractures, often loss of extension, can be managed with static splinting and terminal stretching.
- Most patients return to full activity by 4 to 6 months.

OUTCOMES

- Most series have reported the results of closed management of simple dislocation.
  - Mehlhoff and colleagues[7] reported the results of 52 simple dislocations managed, with most patients having normal elbows. Length of immobilization, especially greater than 3 weeks, was found to be more likely to result in persistent loss of extension.
  - Similarly, Eygendaal and colleagues[3] reported the long-term results of 50 patients after closed management of simple dislocations. Sixty-two percent of patients described their elbow function as good or excellent, and 24 of 50 (48%) patients had loss of extension of 5 to 10 degrees.
- Some series have examined the surgical management of PLRI, often as a result of recurrent instability after traumatic dislocation.
  - Nestor and colleagues[10] reported the results of 11 patients with recurrent PLRI managed with either repair or reconstruction of the LUCL. Ten of 11 (91%) remained stable and 7 of 11 (64%) had an excellent result.
  - More recently, Sanchez-Sotelo and colleagues[15] reported the results of 44 patients treated for recurrent PLRI (9 occurred after simple dislocation). Thirty-two (75%) of the patients had an excellent result by Mayo score.
  - Lee and Teo[5] found that in patients with chronic PLRI, reconstruction offered more predictable outcomes than repair.

COMPLICATIONS

- Stiffness[3,7]
- Heterotopic ossification[6]
- Neurovascular injury[14]
- Recurrent instability[3,7]
- Compartment syndrome
- Hematoma or infection

REFERENCES

1. Dodson CC, Thomas A, Dines JS, et al. Medial ulnar collateral ligament reconstruction of the elbow in throwing athletes. Am J Sports Med 2006;34:1926–1932.
2. Doornberg JN, Ring DC. Fracture of the anteromedial facet of the coronoid process. J Bone Joint Surg Am 2006;88(10): 2216–2224.
3. Eygendaal D, Verdegaal SH, Obermann WR, et al. Posterolateral dislocation of the elbow joint. Relationship to medial instability. J Bone Joint Surg Am 2000;82(4):555–560.
4. Jupiter JB, Ring D. Treatment of unreduced elbow dislocations with hinged external fixation. J Bone Joint Surg Am 2002;84-A(9): 1630–1635.
5. Lee BP, Teo LH. Surgical reconstruction for posterolateral rotatory instability of the elbow. J Shoulder Elbow Surg 2003;12: 476–479.
6. Linscheid RL, Wheeler DK. Elbow dislocations. JAMA 1965;194: 1171–1176.
7. Mehlhoff TL, Noble PC, Bennett JB, et al. Simple dislocation of the elbow in the adult. Results after closed treatment. J Bone Joint Surg Am 1988;70(2):244–249.
8. Morrey BF, An KN. Functional anatomy of the ligaments of the elbow. Clin Orthop Relat Res 1985;(201):84–90.
9. Morrey BF, Tanaka S, An KN. Valgus stability of the elbow. A definition of primary and secondary constraints. Clin Orthop Relat Res 1991;(265):187–195.
10. Nestor BJ, O'Driscoll SW, Morrey BF. Ligamentous reconstruction for posterolateral rotatory instability of the elbow. J Bone Joint Surg Am 1992;74(8):1235–1241.
11. O'Driscoll SW. Acute, recurrent, and chronic elbow instabilities. In: Norris TR, ed. Orthopaedic Knowledge Update: Shoulder and Elbow 2. Rosemont: American Academy of Orthopaedic Surgeons, 2002:313–323.
12. O'Driscoll SW, Bell DF, Morrey BF. Posterolateral rotatory instability of the elbow. J Bone Joint Surg Am 1991;73(3):440–446.
13. O'Driscoll SW, Morrey BF, Korinek S, et al. Elbow subluxation and dislocation. A spectrum of instability. Clin Orthop Relat Res 1992;(280):186–197.
14. Rana NA, Kenwright J, Taylor RG, et al. Complete lesion of the median nerve associated with dislocation of the elbow joint. Acta Orthop Scand 1974;45:365–369.
15. Sanchez-Sotelo J, Morrey BF, O'Driscoll SW. Ligamentous repair and reconstruction for posterolateral rotatory instability of the elbow. J Bone Joint Surg Br 2005;87(1):54–61.
16. Tan V, Daluiski A, Capo J, et al. Hinged elbow external fixators: indications and uses. J Am Acad Orthop Surg 2005;13:503–514.

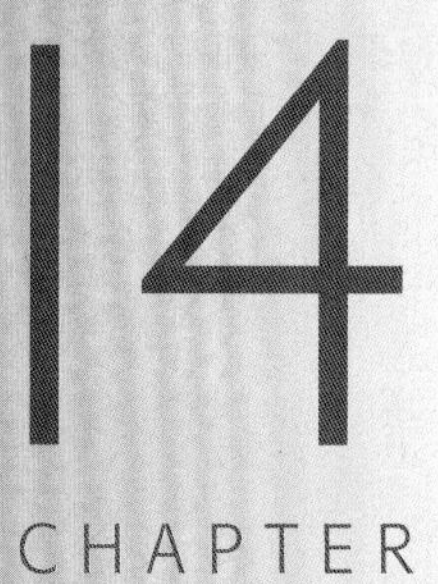

Arthroscopic Treatment of Chondral Injuries and Osteochondritis Dissecans

Marc Safran and Michael Kalisvaart

DEFINITION

- Osteochondritis dissecans (OCD) is a progressive form of osteochondrosis involving focal injury to the subchondral bone or its blood supply. It may occur in many different areas of the adolescent skeleton.
- The knee is the most common location for OCD, but it may occur in several locations of the elbow, including the radial head, the trochlea, and the capitellum (the most common location within the elbow).
- The injury to the subchondral bone results in loss of structural support for the overlying articular cartilage. As a result, degeneration and fragmentation of the articular cartilage and underlying bone occur, often with the formation of loose bodies.
- The histopathology of the subchondral bone in OCD is consistent with osteonecrosis.
- Articular cartilage injury may also occur anywhere in the elbow, especially after trauma. More common locations of nonarthritic chondral injury include the radial head and capitellum.

ANATOMY

Bony Anatomy

- The bony anatomy of the elbow allows for two complex motions: flexion–extension and pronation–supination.
- The ulnohumeral articulation of the elbow is almost a true hinge joint with its constant axis of rotation through the lateral epicondyle and just anterior and inferior to the medial epicondyle. This well-fitted hinge joint allows for little excessive motion or toggle.
- The radius articulates with the proximal ulna and rounded capitellum of the distal humerus. The radiocapitellar joint and the proximal radioulnar joint allow for pronation–supination (**FIG 1A**). The ulnohumeral joint allows for flexion–extension of the elbow.
- The ulnohumeral joint has 11 to 16 degrees of valgus. This results in increased compressive force in the lateral elbow (radiocapitellar joint) with axial loading.

Ligamentous Anatomy

- The ligaments of the elbow are divided into the radial and ulnar collateral ligament complexes.
  - The lateral or radial collateral ligamentous complex provides varus stability. These ligaments are rarely stressed in the athlete.
  - The ulnar or medial collateral ligament complex consists of three ligaments: the anterior oblique, the posterior oblique, and the transverse.
- The ulnar collateral ligament complex, particularly the anterior oblique ligament, resists valgus force, such as occurs with throwing, whereas the radiocapitellar joint is a secondary restraint to valgus force (**FIG 1B**).

Intraosseous Vascular Anatomy

- There are two nutrient vessels in the lateral condyle of the developing elbow.

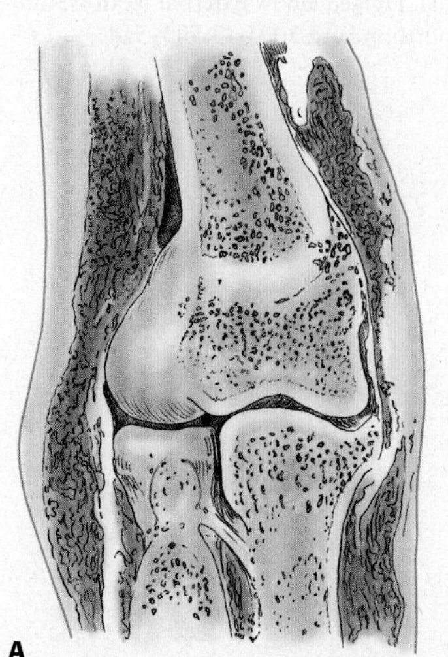

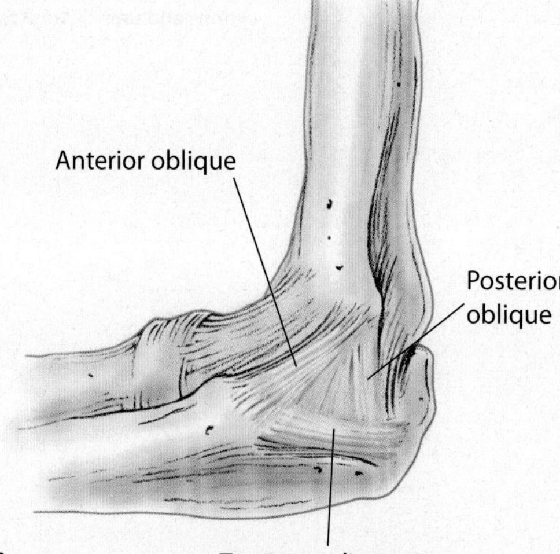

FIG 1 • **A.** Cross-section of the elbow showing the round, convex capitellum and the matching concave radial head. **B.** Anatomy of the medial elbow ligamentous complex. The ulnar collateral ligament complex comprises three ligaments: the anterior oblique, posterior oblique, and transverse ligaments.

- Each vessel extends into the lateral aspect of the trochlea, with one entering proximal to the articular cartilage and the other entering posterolaterally at the origin of the capsule.
- Although these two vessels communicate with each other, they do not do so with the metaphyseal vasculature. The rapidly expanding capitellar epiphysis in the developing elbow thus receives its blood supply from one or two isolated transchondroepiphyseal vessels that enter the epiphysis posteriorly.
- These vessels function as end arteries passing through the cartilaginous epiphysis to the capitellum.
- Metaphyseal vascular anastomoses do not make significant contributions to the capitellum until approximately 19 years of age, placing this region at risk for vascular injury.

PATHOGENESIS

- The cause of OCD is unclear and controversial.
- OCD typically affects the dominant extremity of adolescents and young adults, with onset of symptoms between 11 and 16 years of age.
- Most cases are seen in high-level athletes who experience repetitive valgus stress and lateral compression across the elbow (eg, overhead-throwing athletes, gymnasts, weightlifters).
- The lesion usually affects only a portion of the capitellum.
- Genetic factors, trauma, and ischemia have been proposed as causes.
- Most authors believe that the primary mechanism of injury is repetitive microtrauma in a genetically predisposed individual's developing elbow that results in vascular injury due to the tenuous blood supply.
- The capitellum is softer than the radial head.
- Repeated microtrauma, such as axial loading in the extended elbow or repeated throwing that produces valgus forces on the elbow, results in increased force in the radiocapitellar joint.
  - The repetitive microtrauma caused by these forces has been proposed to weaken the capitellar subchondral bone and result in fatigue fracture.
  - Should failure of bony repair occur, an avascular portion of bone may then undergo resorption with further weakening of the subchondral architecture. This is consistent with the characteristic rarefaction often seen at the periphery of the lesion.
  - The altered subchondral architecture can no longer support the overlying articular cartilage, rendering it vulnerable to shear stresses, which may lead to fragmentation.
- The tenuous blood supply of the end arterioles in the capitellum may become injured with the repetitive microtrauma, resulting in OCD.
- Although a genetic predisposition to OCD has been proposed in the literature, convincing scientific evidence of OCD as a heritable condition does not currently exist. Some individuals are more susceptible than others, and this may be genetically based.

NATURAL HISTORY

- The natural history of capitellar OCD is unpredictable. No reliable criteria exist for predicting which lesions will collapse with subsequent joint incongruity and which will go on to heal without further sequelae.
- If healing is going to take place, it usually occurs by the time of physeal closure.
- If healing is not going to take place, repetitive microtrauma and shear stresses to the articular surface of a lesion that has lost its subchondral support may result in further subchondral collapse and deformation with joint incongruity as well as articular cartilage injury, fragmentation, and loose body formation.
- In advanced cases, degenerative changes accompanied by a decreased range of motion are likely to develop.

PATIENT HISTORY AND PHYSICAL FINDINGS

- The classic patient with OCD is an adolescent athlete who experiences repetitive valgus stress and lateral compression across the elbow (eg, overhead-throwing athletes, gymnasts, weightlifters).
  - The patient usually complains of the insidious onset of poorly localized, progressive lateral elbow pain in the dominant arm.
  - He or she may also note a flexion contracture.
- The throwing athlete may note a reduction in throwing distance or velocity or both.
- Prodromal pain is not always present.
- Typically, pain is exacerbated with activity and relieved by rest.
- In advanced cases in which a fragment has become unstable or loose body formation has occurred, mechanical symptoms of elbow locking, clicking, or catching may be present.
- Physical examination methods
  - On examination, there may be tenderness to palpation and crepitus over the radiocapitellar joint.
  - Effusion indicates intra-articular irritation and may be consistent with a loose or unstable OCD lesion or loose body.
  - Swelling, palpated in the posterolateral gutter (soft spot), may be appreciated.
  - Crepitus may be present on range-of-motion testing.
  - Loss of 10 to 20 degrees of extension is common, and mild loss of flexion and forearm rotation may also be seen. Loss of pronation is less common.
  - Provocative testing includes the "active radiocapitellar compression test," which consists of forearm pronation and supination with the elbow in full extension in an attempt to reproduce symptoms.
- The examiner should rule out radiocapitellar overload as the result of ulnar collateral ligament insufficiency using the milking maneuver, modified milking maneuver, valgus stress test, or moving valgus stress test.

IMAGING AND OTHER DIAGNOSTIC STUDIES

- Diagnostic evaluation of the elbow for OCD begins with plain radiographs—an anteroposterior (AP) view, lateral view, oblique views, and a 45-degree flexion AP view, which is particularly good at revealing the lesion.
- Radiographs typically show the classic radiolucency (**FIG 2A**) or rarefaction of the capitellum (**FIG 2B**) in addition to irregularity or flattening of the articular surface.
- The lesion frequently appears as a focal rim of sclerotic bone surrounding a radiolucent crater with rarefaction located in the anterolateral aspect of the capitellum.

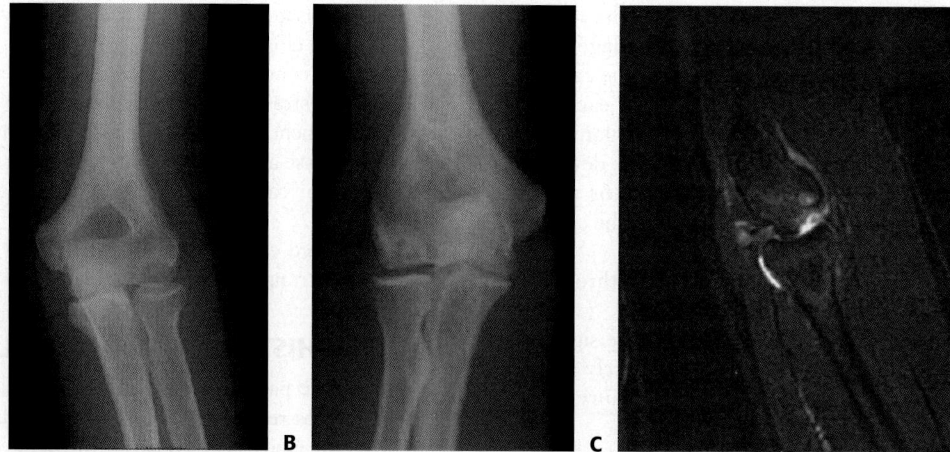

FIG 2 • **A.** Radiograph of a 15-year-old baseball pitcher with OCD of the capitellum of the dominant elbow. Clear lesion and sclerosis of the bony bed are shown. **B.** OCD in a 15-year-old gymnast with rarefaction of the capitellar lesion on oblique radiograph of the elbow. **C.** MRI of the elbow of a baseball pitcher, revealing OCD with loss of overlying articular cartilage and loose body.

- Radiographs, however, may not reveal the osteochondral lesions in the earlier stages. They are not of much benefit for truly chondral lesions.
- In advanced cases, articular surface collapse, loose bodies, subchondral cysts, radial head enlargement, and osteophyte formation may be seen.
- Further diagnostic imaging of OCD lesions primarily consists of magnetic resonance imaging (MRI), although ultrasonography and bone scintigraphy have been used.
- MRI is especially valuable in assessing the integrity of the articular cartilage overlying the OCD lesion as well as in diagnosing OCD in its early stages and identifying loose bodies (**FIG 2C**).
- Controversy exists over the use of contrast-enhanced magnetic resonance arthrography. This technique, however, can potentially provide additional information regarding the status of the articular cartilage and identification of loose bodies.
- Bone scintigraphy is very sensitive for identifying osteoblastic activity or increased vascularity at the site of an OCD lesion. However, it is nonspecific and has limited usefulness in diagnosis.
- Computed tomography can help define bony anatomy and identify loose bodies.
- Ultrasonography can also help in the assessment of capitellar lesions, including early stages, but ultrasound is technician dependent.

DIFFERENTIAL DIAGNOSIS

- Panner disease
- Infection
- Lateral epicondylosis
- Lateral epicondylar apophysitis
- Radial head osteochondrosis
- Radial head or neck injury
- Radiocapitellar overload and chondromalacia due to ulnar collateral ligament injury
- Posterolateral rotatory instability

NONOPERATIVE MANAGEMENT

- The choice of conservative or surgical management depends on the patient's age, symptoms, size of the lesion, and stage of the lesion, specifically the integrity of the cartilage surface.
- The goal of treatment for OCD of the elbow is to prevent the progression of the disorder, detachment of the osteochondral lesion, and degenerative changes of the articular cartilage.
- Small, nondisplaced lesions with intact overlying articular cartilage in younger (skeletally immature) athletes are best managed conservatively with relative rest and activity modification, ice, and nonsteroidal anti-inflammatories, particularly if the bone scan shows increased bony activity.
- Activity modification consists of avoiding throwing activities and weight bearing on the involved arm.
- Short-term immobilization (less than 2 to 3 weeks, depending on symptoms) may be considered.
- Serial radiographs, at 10- to 12-week intervals, are obtained to monitor healing.
- Activity modification is continued until the radiographic appearance of revascularization and healing.
- Radiographic findings of OCD may persist for several years. As a result, after conservative management, the most important issue in terms of an athlete's ability to return to sports is symptom resolution.
- Most patients can return to full activity after 6 months.

SURGICAL MANAGEMENT

- The indications for surgical treatment include persistent symptoms despite conservative management, symptomatic loose bodies, articular cartilage fracture, displacement of the osteochondral lesion, and cold bone scan.
- The surgeon must assess the size, stability, and viability of the fragment and decide whether to remove the fragment or attempt to surgically reattach it.
- Most fragments cannot be reattached and therefore are excised, followed by local débridement.

- Arthroscopic abrasion chondroplasty or subchondral drilling may be performed to encourage healing.
- Although symptoms usually improve, about half of all patients will continue to have chronic pain or limited range of motion.
- In general, many athletes cannot return to their prior levels of competition.
- Surgical indications for operative management of stable lesions with intact articular cartilage include radiographic evidence of lesion progression and failure of symptom resolution despite a 6-month trial of a conservative, nonoperative regimen.
  - Arthroscopic examination, débridement as needed, and drilling or microfracture of the OCD lesion (with or without in situ pinning) are usually the surgical treatments of choice.
- Unstable lesions, characterized by overlying articular cartilage injury and instability as well as collapse or disruption of the subchondral bone architecture, and those with loose bodies are usually managed surgically.
  - These lesions are frequently flap lesions. They characteristically present with more advanced radiographic changes (including a well-demarcated fragment surrounded by a sclerotic margin).
  - There is controversy whether simple fragment excision or reduction (open or arthroscopic) and internal fixation is the preferred treatment. Many authors advocate excision of displaced fragments, often augmented by drilling or microfracture.
- Critical considerations in operative planning include the size and integrity (viability) of the fragment, the subchondral architecture on the fragment and the opposing bony bed, the potential for anatomic restoration of the articular surface, and the method of fixation if attempted.
- Internal fixation of the fragment may be performed using metallic screws, bioabsorbable screws or pins, Kirschner wire, bone pegs, and dynamic staple fixation.
- There have been a few reports of osteoarticular autograft or allograft plugs in the treatment of more advanced lesions, but experience with this method is limited. The current recommendations are for lesions that involve the lateral column.

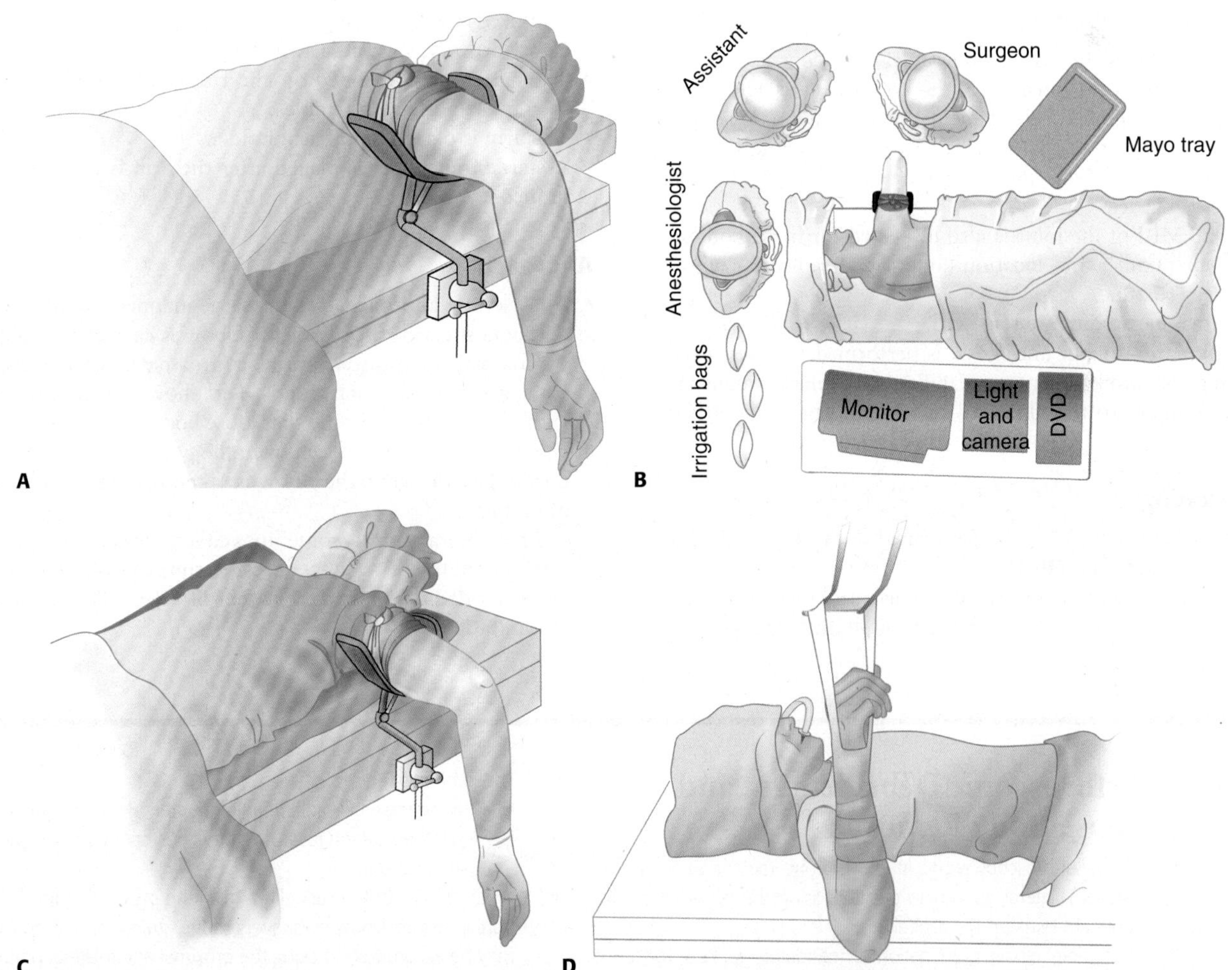

FIG 3 • **A.** Lateral positioning for elbow arthroscopy, including tourniquet placement. **B.** Setup in the operating room for the lateral position. **C.** Prone position of the patient. This is the preferred position, particularly due to the ease of posterior elbow access. The setup of the room is the same and the relative position of the elbow for the surgeon is similar between the prone and lateral positions. **D.** Supine position of the patient. Some surgeons prefer this position because it is easier to convert to open surgery and easier anesthesia management; however, posterior arthroscopic access is more difficult in this position.

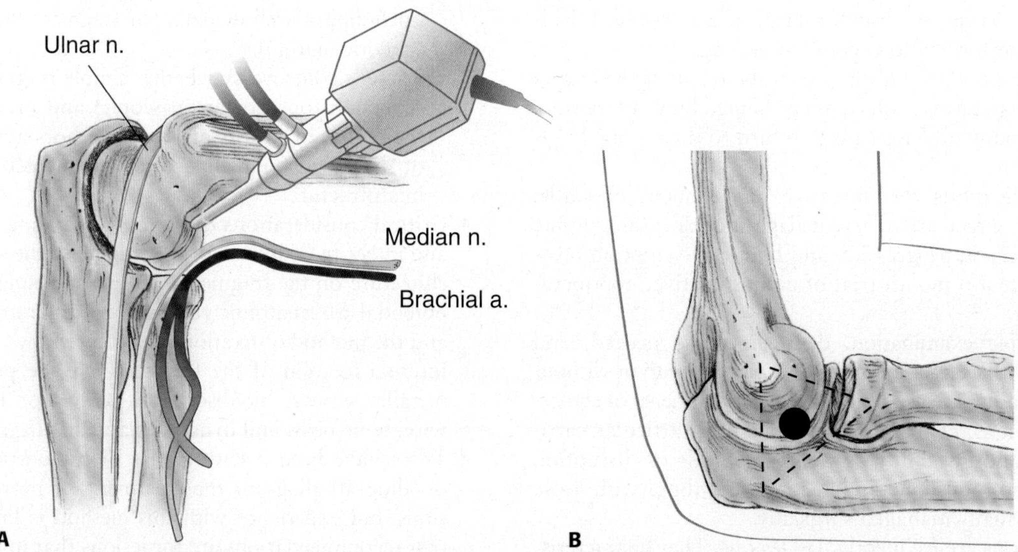

FIG 4 • **A.** The elbow arthroscope is brought in from the proximal anteromedial portal that provides a direct view of the anterior capitellum and radial head. **B.** Position of the direct lateral soft spot portal.

Preoperative Planning

- Before surgery, an MRI, preferably with contrast, can be used to assess the integrity of the articular cartilage to help determine whether débridement, loose body removal, and drilling may be needed or more advanced techniques, such as reduction and internal fixation or osteochondral transfer, may be needed.
  - The MRI of the joint is also inspected for loose bodies—their number and location (anterior vs. posterior elbow) (see **FIG 2C**).
- All imaging studies are reviewed.
- Examination under anesthesia is performed to assess range of motion and ligamentous stability, particularly valgus laxity, as injury to the ulnar collateral ligament in the athlete may increase the load on the radiocapitellar joint.

Positioning

- Elbow arthroscopy can be performed in the supine, lateral, or prone position (**FIG 3**).
- Prone positioning is preferred because it allows easy access to the elbow and reduces the risk of sterility breaks if the arm needs to be in a finger-trap device, as needed for supine elbow arthroscopy and arthroscopy.
- The patient is positioned on chest rolls and padding under the knees and feet and ankles.
- The arm is placed on an arm holder.
- A sterile tourniquet is placed after the arm is prepared and draped.

Approach

- All cases are approached in the same manner initially.
  - Diagnostic arthroscopy of the elbow is carried out using a proximal anteromedial portal, a proximal anterolateral portal, and two posterior portals. This allows for assessment of the entire joint to ensure that loose bodies are not missed.
- The capitellum may be seen from the proximal anteromedial portal (**FIG 4A**) while the elbow is taken through a full range of motion.
- A direct lateral portal (sometimes called the *soft spot portal*) is then used to allow direct access to the radiocapitellar joint and is needed to confirm the extent of the OCD or chondral lesion (**FIG 4B**).

TECHNIQUES

Arthroscopic Débridement and Loose Body Removal

- Elbow arthroscopy is begun in the prone (senior author's preference), lateral, or supine position using the proximal medial portal to visualize the capitellum.
- Complete elbow examination is mandatory to look for loose bodies:
  - Proximal anteromedial portal
  - Proximal anterolateral portal
  - Posterior central portal
  - Posterolateral portal
  - Direct lateral portal
- Loose bodies tend to hide:
  - In the proximal radioulnar joint anteriorly or the gutters
  - In the olecranon fossa or gutters posteriorly, particularly the lateral gutter
- When looking at the capitellum from the proximal anteromedial portal, instrumentation (shavers, burrs, graspers, and curettes) may be accomplished using the proximal anterolateral portal.
- Flexion and extension of the elbow allow for enhanced visualization of the capitellum.
- Loose bodies and chondral fragments may be removed via the anterior portals (**TECH FIG 1A,B**).
- Then the arthroscope is brought in from the posterior portals to look for loose bodies.

- The direct lateral ("soft spot") portal is used for complete evaluation of the capitellum.
  - This portal is mandatory to fully evaluate the extent of the lesion and to allow for adequate débridement of loose cartilage.
  - Often, loose bodies will be found using this portal.
- Débridement is performed using shavers, curettes, graspers, and rongeurs to remove loose bodies and any loose, scaly, or fragmented cartilage (**TECH FIG 1C**).

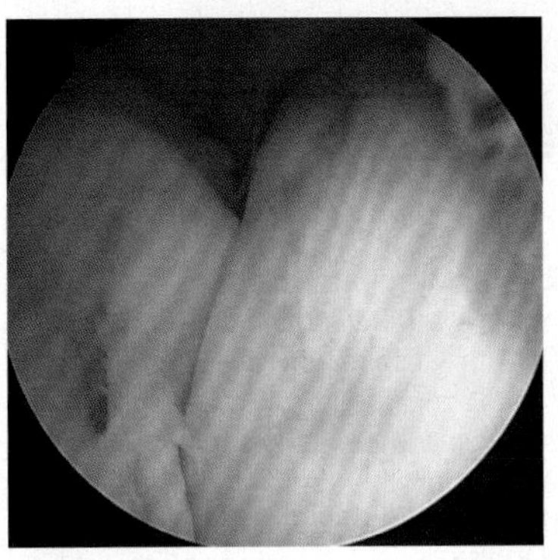

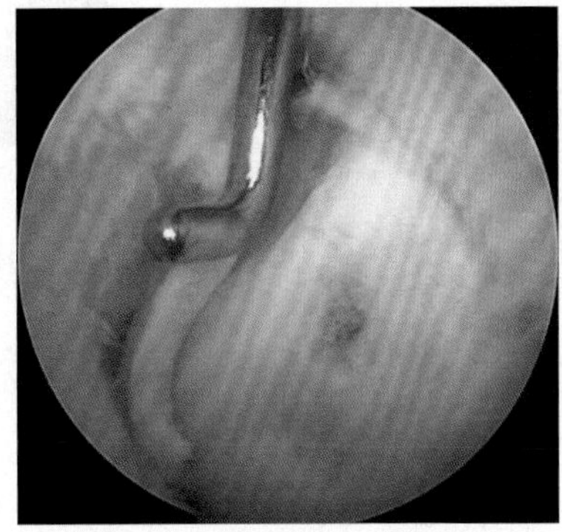

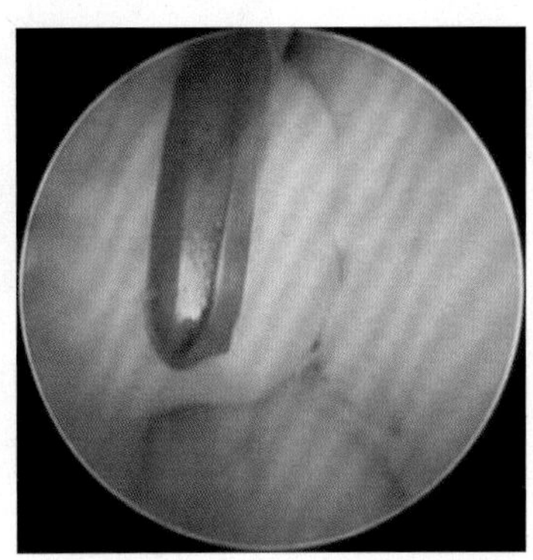

TECH FIG 1 • OCD of the capitellum. **A.** View from the proximal anteromedial portal reveals a flap of cartilage from the capitellum (*left*) and a slightly deformed radial head (*to the right*). **B.** Probe on the flap of chondral tissue from the capitellum of this same patient. **C.** Grasper removing a loose body as viewed from the direct lateral portal.

Microfracture and Abrasion Arthroplasty

- When the OCD fragment is loose and it is not possible to fix the lesion back to the bony bed, then microfracture or abrasion arthroplasty may be indicated to stimulate a fibrocartilaginous growth in the bony defect.
- The principle is to stimulate cartilage-like regeneration based on the formation of a superclot that is progressively invaded by multipotent cells from the marrow.
- This is achieved by complete débridement of all unstable and damaged cartilage in the lesion and the preservation of the subchondral layer for chondral lesions based on experience of the treatment of knee chondral injuries.
- Elbow arthroscopy is begun in the prone (senior author's preference), lateral, or supine position using the proximal medial portal to visualize the capitellum.
- Complete elbow examination using all four standard and the additional direct lateral arthroscopic portals is mandatory to look for loose bodies.
- When looking at the capitellum from the proximal anteromedial portal, instrumentation (shavers, burrs, graspers, and curettes) may be done using the proximal anterolateral portal.
- Flexion and extension of the elbow allow for enhanced visualization of the capitellum.
- All underlying bone is débrided with an arthroscopic shaver or burr or manually with curettes or pituitary rongeurs.
- Next, the arthroscope is brought in from the posterior portals to look for loose bodies.
- The direct lateral (soft spot) portal is used for complete evaluation of the capitellum.
  - This portal is mandatory to fully evaluate the extent of the lesion and to allow for adequate débridement of loose cartilage and may allow for a good direction for microfracturing the bed.
- Abrasion is carried out from either anterolateral or direct lateral portals to the complete lesion. This may be done with a shaver on high speed or burr.
- For chondral lesions, abrasion arthroplasty involves removal of the zone of calcified cartilage then use of a burr to lightly remove only a partial thickness of the subchondral bone to expose subchondral arterioles to bring blood into the lesion. The key is not to go too deep into the cancellous bone.
- For OCD with a cartilage cap that is not intact, abrasion is done lightly to remove only a little bone to allow bleeding into the bony bed.
- Microfracture or drilling can also be used to bring blood into the defect when the OCD or chondral lesion results in an exposed bony bed, with the theoretical benefit of microfracture being that less bone is lost and there is no heat production, which may be seen with drilling.
- The bone is pierced every 3 to 4 mm for a 4-mm depth with an awl for microfracture or 0.062 Kirschner wire for drilling (**TECH FIG 2**).
- If the anterolateral or direct lateral portals do not allow for adequate directionality of the drilling or microfracture, an additional outside-in portal may be made based on the known anatomy and using a spinal needle.

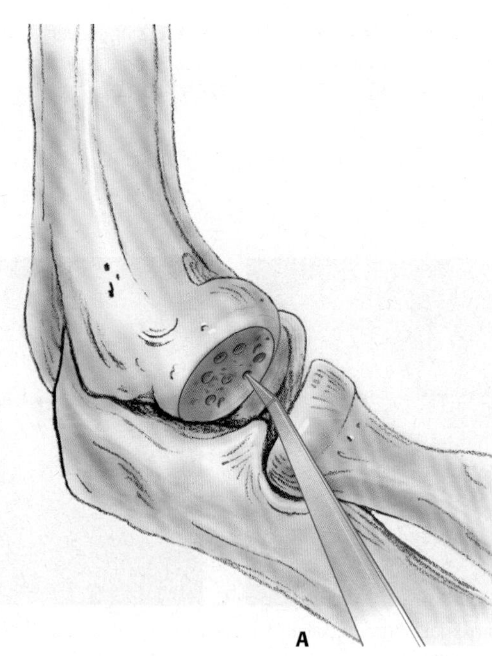

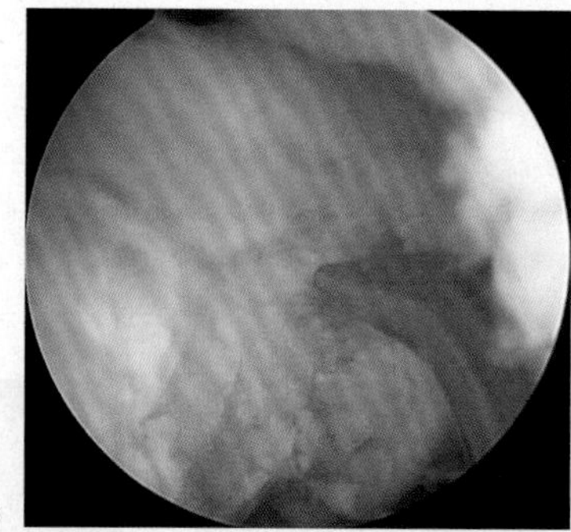

TECH FIG 2 • **A.** Microfracture of the capitellum, making several small perforations within the capitellum about 4 mm apart and 4 mm deep. **B.** Intraoperative arthroscopic photograph from the direct lateral portal with a microfracture awl at the edge of the OCD lesion after removing the zone of calcified cartilage.

Drilling for Intact Osteochondritis Dissecans Lesions

- When the OCD lesion has an intact overlying chondral surface, then drilling may enhance or stimulate a healing response of the lesion, although this is not frequently needed.
- The key is to try to prevent violation of the OCD cartilage cap, although some surgeons drill from outside-in, trying to avoid injury to the articular cartilage and some drill from the joint, which will perforate the articular cartilage.
- Elbow arthroscopy is begun in the prone (senior author's preference), lateral, or supine position using the proximal medial portal to visualize the capitellum.
  - Complete elbow examination using all four standard portals and the additional direct lateral arthroscopic portals is mandatory to look for loose bodies.
- When looking at the capitellum from the proximal anteromedial portal, instrumentation (shavers, burrs, graspers, and curettes) may be done using the proximal anterolateral portal.
- Flexion and extension of the elbow allow for enhanced visualization of the capitellum.
- Next, the arthroscope is brought in from the posterior portals to look for loose bodies.
- The direct lateral (soft spot) portal is then used for complete evaluation of the capitellum.
- OCD lesions with intact articular cartilage, subchondral softening, fibrillated cartilage, or cartilage character change may be identified visually or palpably using a probe (**TECH FIG 3**) or alternatively using fluoroscopic imaging.
- Drilling through the cartilage and through the sclerotic subchondral bone is done in an effort to promote healing.
- Attempts are made to limit the number of perforations through the intact cartilage, but the subchondral plate should be penetrated multiple times.
  - This may be accomplished by redirecting the drill in different directions from the same single (or a few) perforations through the articular cartilage.
- The lesion is pierced with an 0.062 Kirschner wire for drilling.
- If the anterolateral or direct lateral portals do not allow for adequate directionality of the drilling, an additional outside-in portal may be made based on the known anatomy and using a spinal needle.

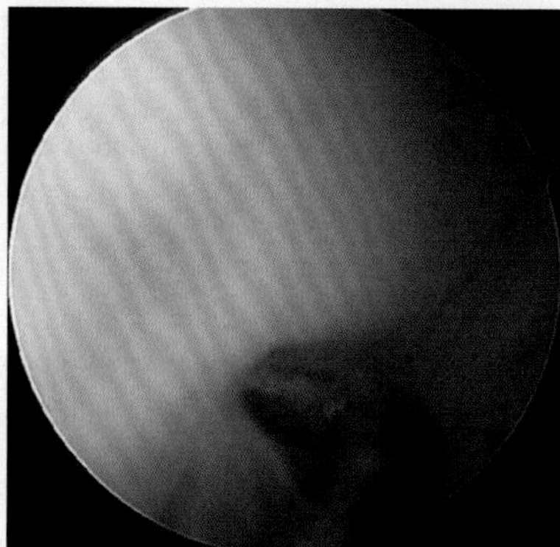

TECH FIG 3 • View from the direct lateral portal of an OCD lesion with intact articular cartilage. The probe is deforming the intact cartilage owing to the lack of subchondral support.

TECHNIQUES

Drilling for Intact Osteochondritis Dissecans Lesion: Outside-In Technique

- When the OCD lesion has an intact overlying chondral surface, then drilling may enhance or stimulate a healing response of the lesion.
- The key is to try to prevent violation of the OCD cartilage cap, although some surgeons drill from outside-in, trying to avoid injury to the articular cartilage and some drill from the joint, which will perforate the articular cartilage.
- Elbow arthroscopy is begun in the prone (senior author's preference), lateral, or supine position using the proximal medial portal to visualize the capitellum.
  - Complete elbow examination using all four standard and the additional direct lateral arthroscopic portals is mandatory to look for loose bodies.
- When looking at the capitellum from the proximal anteromedial portal, instrumentation (shavers, burrs, graspers, and curettes) may be done using the proximal anterolateral portal.
- Flexion and extension of the elbow allow for enhanced visualization of the capitellum.
- Next, the arthroscope is brought in from the posterior portals to look for loose bodies.
- The direct lateral (soft spot) portal is then used for complete evaluation of the capitellum.
- OCD lesions with intact articular cartilage, subchondral softening, fibrillation of the cartilage, or cartilage character change may be identified visually or palpably (see **TECH FIG 3**) or alternatively using fluoroscopy.
- Fluoroscopy is then brought in to identify the lesion.
- Using an anterior cruciate ligament tibial guide or posterior cruciate ligament femoral guide can be useful to help aim the drill bit from outside the elbow toward the lesion.
- Depending on the location of the lesion, the drill is brought from proximal and slightly anterior to the lateral epicondyle or posteriorly on the distal humerus.
- A small incision is made at the proposed drilling entry site and blunt dissection is done to bone.
- The lesion is drilled with a 0.062 Kirschner wire for drilling while watching with fluoroscopy or arthroscopy to ensure the articular cartilage is not violated.
- Multiple passes with the Kirschner wire should be performed to enhance healing throughout the lesion.

Internal Fixation

- When the OCD fragment is partially detached or completely detached but not malformed and there is significant bone on the cartilage fragment, consideration for reattachment is recommended.
- The principle is to stimulate healing and to stabilize the fragment within the bony bed.
- Elbow arthroscopy is begun in the prone, lateral, or supine position, using the proximal medial portal to visualize the capitellum.
- If it is likely the patient will need internal fixation of a partially detached OCD fragment, and there is a possibility that an arthrotomy is needed, the senior author has found that performing the surgery in the lateral position is a bit easier.
- Complete elbow examination using all four standard and the additional direct lateral arthroscopic portals is mandatory to look for loose bodies.
- When looking at the capitellum from the proximal anteromedial portal, instrumentation (shavers, burrs, graspers, and curettes) may be done using the proximal anterolateral portal.
- Flexion and extension of the elbow allow for enhanced visualization of the capitellum.
- All underlying bone is débrided with an arthroscopic shaver or burr or manually with curettes or pituitary rongeurs.
- Next, the arthroscope is brought in from the posterior portals to look for loose bodies.
- The direct lateral (soft spot) portal is used for complete evaluation of the capitellum.
  - This portal is mandatory to fully evaluate the extent of the lesion and to allow for adequate débridement and preparation of the bed.
- The osteochondral flap or undersurface of the fragment is elevated and the underlying sclerotic bone is curetted and débrided of fibrous tissue (**TECH FIG 4A**). Drilling of the base is also performed to stimulate healing.
- The abrasion and drilling are carried out from either anterolateral or direct lateral portals to the complete lesion. This may be done with a curette, a shaver on high speed, or a burr and a drill or Kirschner wire to gently débride the bed without removing much bone.
- The flap is then replaced within the bed.
- Retrograde pinning of the lesion with threaded or unthreaded wires can be performed with the wires exiting the lateral epicondyle for later removal (**TECH FIG 4B,C**).
  - The ends of the pins should be positioned below the articular surface so that the wires do not penetrate the joint space.
- Bioabsorbable pins and bioabsorbable screws have been used as an alternative (**TECH FIG 4D**).
- Further, some surgeons will place metallic screws for fixation. These can either be headless variable-pitched screws that are buried beneath the articular surface or regular-headed screws, which some prefer for better compression but must be removed.
- If the anterolateral or direct lateral portals do not allow for adequate directionality of the drilling or microfracture, an additional outside-in portal may be made based on the known anatomy and using a spinal needle.
- An arthrotomy may be necessary to perform the débridement or internal fixation.

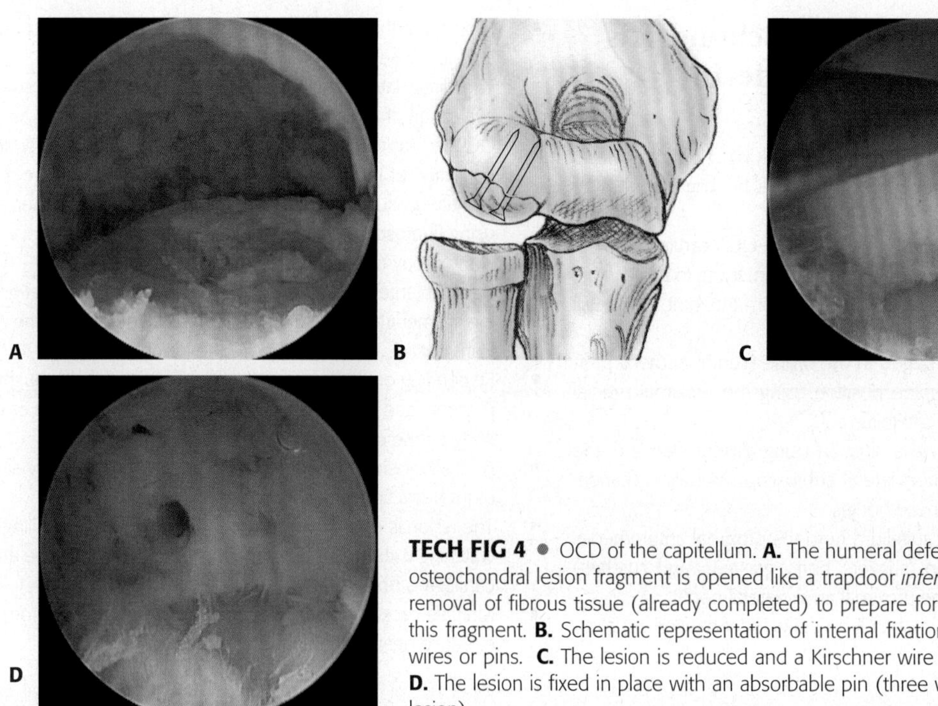

TECH FIG 4 ● OCD of the capitellum. **A.** The humeral defect is *above*, and the osteochondral lesion fragment is opened like a trapdoor *inferiorly*. This allows for removal of fibrous tissue (already completed) to prepare for repair or fixation of this fragment. **B.** Schematic representation of internal fixation of the lesion with wires or pins. **C.** The lesion is reduced and a Kirschner wire holds the fragment. **D.** The lesion is fixed in place with an absorbable pin (three were used to fix this lesion).

Osteochondral Autograft Implantation

- When the OCD fragment is loose and it is not possible to fix the lesion back to the bony bed, and there is a large crater, particularly if it involves the lateral column, then consideration is given to inserting osteochondral autograft plugs into the defect to eliminate or reduce edge loading and loss of lateral support for the joint.
- This is achieved by taking osteochondral plugs from the knee and implanting them into the capitellum.
- Elbow arthroscopy is begun in the prone, lateral, or supine position, using the proximal medial portal to visualize the capitellum. Because insertion of the plugs often requires an arthrotomy and the grafts must come from the knee, the supine position is preferred.
- Complete elbow examination using all four standard and the additional direct lateral arthroscopic portals is mandatory to look for loose bodies.
- When looking at the capitellum from the proximal anteromedial portal, instrumentation (shavers, burrs, graspers, and curettes) may be done using the proximal anterolateral portal.
- Flexion and extension of the elbow allow for enhanced visualization of the capitellum.
- A posterior or posterolateral approach may be used.
- The radiocapitellar joint is approached anteriorly by splitting the intermuscular plane between the extensor digitorum communis and the extensor carpi radialis longus and brevis, exposing the anterior capsule, which is then incised.
- The posterior approach uses a posterior longitudinal skin incision with the elbow in full flexion. Then the anconeus and posterior capsule are divided, providing direct access to the OCD lesion.
  - The posterolateral Kocher approach uses the interval between the anconeus and extensor carpi ulnaris. The lateral collateral ligament complex is protected and preserved, allowing exposure of the posterior radiocapitellar joint.
- A commercially available osteochondral graft harvesting system is used.
- The size of the lesion is assessed to decide how many grafts and of which size are necessary, although usually, less than 100% fill is achieved.
- Recipient sockets are created in the lesion with the recipient graft harvesting tool.
- Occasionally, the sclerotic bed makes it difficult to use the recipient harvesting tool and a cannulated drill is needed to make the recipient bed.
- Drilling is carried out at the base of the socket before inserting the graft to allow for marrow stimulation and enhance healing potential.
- Osteochondral grafts about 10 mm long are then harvested arthroscopically or with miniarthrotomy from the knee intercondylar notch or periphery of the non–weight-bearing portion of the lateral femoral condyle.
- There are only a few case reports of this technique. Some use multiple 3.5-mm plugs and some use single larger osteochondral plugs.
- Depth of the recipient socket is measured with a calibrated depth gauge or alignment stick.
- The length of the osteochondral autograft plug is matched to the depth of the recipient socket.
- The graft is seated flush with the surrounding intact cartilage.
- Complete coverage of the lesion usually is not possible, although coverage of 80% to 90% of the lesion size should be achieved.

PEARLS AND PITFALLS

Nerve injury	■ The greatest risk of elbow arthroscopy, for OCD or any other diagnosis, is nerve injury. Knowledge of elbow neuroanatomy, particularly as it relates to the arthroscopic portals, is of paramount importance. It is safest to use the proximal medial portal and the proximal lateral portals anteriorly. Distending the joint, using the outside-in technique, and using blunt instruments after skin incision only all help to reduce iatrogenic nerve injury.
Direct lateral portal	■ Familiarity with the direct lateral portal is critical for the evaluation and treatment of chondral and osteochondral lesions of the capitellum. The posterior radial head and capitellum are best seen with this portal, and loose bodies from OCD occasionally may only be seen from this portal. Full appreciation of the lesion cannot be made without the use of this portal.
Converting to an open procedure	■ Occasionally, synovitis or lack of working space makes visualization of the lesion difficult. Further, fixation of the lesion may be difficult arthroscopically. If visualization or fixation is difficult arthroscopically, there should be a low threshold to converting the procedure to open. The threshold of conversion to open should be based on experience and comfort with arthroscopy.

POSTOPERATIVE CARE

- After elbow arthroscopy for débridement or loose body removal:
  - Early range-of-motion exercises are encouraged to prevent loss of elbow motion. Other early goals include reducing swelling, pain, and muscular atrophy.
  - As motion becomes full and the soft tissues are healing with minimal swelling, rehabilitation concentrates on strengthening and endurance of the joint as well as normalization of arthrokinematics of the elbow. This usually begins after 2 weeks.
  - After 4 weeks, the athlete is prepared to return to functional activities with more strengthening, endurance, and flexibility. However, some believe that individuals with OCD lesions who have a defect should not return to sports activities because of the risk of arthritic change in the elbow.
- After in situ drilling, return to sports is usually delayed until 3 to 6 months postoperatively, when there is good radiographic evidence of bony incorporation and healing.
- After microfracture or internal fixation:
  - Range of motion is encouraged, but some clinicians put their patients in a range-of-motion brace positioned in varus to reduce stress over the radiocapitellar joint.
  - Some also consider adding the use of continuous passive motion to help in cartilage nourishment to encourage the microfracture clot or the healing surface of a fixed lesion to reduce adhesions. In these scenarios, strengthening is usually not initiated for at least 6 weeks.
  - Return to gymnastics or throwing sports is delayed until 6 months postoperatively.
- Following the autograft transfer procedure:
  - The joint is immobilized until 2 weeks postoperatively, when the cast or splint is discontinued.
  - Beginning week 3, range-of-motion exercises are started.
  - Strengthening of the elbow and forearm is begun at 3 months postoperatively, and a throwing program is initiated at 6 months, with full return to participation at 10 to 12 months postoperatively.

OUTCOMES

- Reports in the literature on follow-up of the conservative and surgical management of OCD are difficult to compare and interpret because there is a lack of a universally accepted classification system, the numbers of patients in most series is limited, and there are disparities in age at presentation, symptoms, lesion size, location, stability, and viability. Further, there are differences in the method of diagnostic imaging used, surgical technique, and length of follow-up.
- A consensus exists in the literature on the need to limit continual high-stress loading of the radiocapitellar joint in patients treated (even successfully) with OCD to prevent the deterioration of the frequently obtained short-term favorable results. As a result, most pitchers are counseled to move to other positions and gymnasts are advised of the difficulty in returning to continued high-level competitive gymnastics.
- Conservative treatment of OCD does not provide uniformly successful results.
- Takahara et al[6,7] presented the results of nonoperative management of early OCD lesions with an average follow-up of 5.2 years and reported that more than half of these patients had pain with activities and fewer than half of the lesions showed radiographic improvement.
- Surgery also does not result in uniformly good outcomes.
- In one of the longest follow-up studies available in the elbow OCD literature, Bauer et al[1] presented the results of 31 patients (23 of whom were treated surgically with lesion or loose body excision) with capitellar OCD followed for an average of 23 years. At follow-up, the most common complaints were decreased range of motion (average 9 degrees of flexion loss, 2 degrees of extension loss, and 6 degrees of pronation–supination loss) and pain with activity. Radiographic evidence of degenerative changes involving the elbow joint was present in 61% and radial head enlargement in 58%.
- McManama et al[4] presented data on 14 adolescents with radiocapitellar OCD lesions treated with excision via a lateral arthrotomy with average follow-up of 2 years. Lesions were not sized, but 93% had good or excellent results.
- Jackson et al[3] reported on the roughly 3-year follow-up of OCD lesions in 10 female gymnasts treated primarily with curettage of loose cartilage, drilling, and loose body excision. All of the patients reported symptomatic relief, but only 1 patient returned to competition, and she did so with discomfort. Average loss of extension at follow-up in this series was 9 degrees, which is consistent with other reports.
- Ruch et al[5] presented the follow-up at an average of 3.2 years after arthroscopic débridement alone for management of

elbow OCD in 12 adolescents. The average flexion contracture improved 13 degrees (23 degrees preoperatively to 10 degrees postoperatively). All patients had capitellar remodeling on follow-up radiographs, and approximately 42% had associated radial head enlargement. Ninety-two percent of the patients in this series were highly satisfied, with minimal symptoms. Of note, 5 patients (42%) had a triangular lateral capsular avulsion fragment (seen radiographically but not at arthroscopy), which had a statistically significant association with a worse subjective outcome.

- Baumgarten et al[2] presented an average 4-year follow-up (range 24 to 75 months) on 17 elbows with OCD treated in 16 patients. Their results showed that the average flexion contracture improved 14 degrees, approximately 24% had pain, 7 of 9 (78%) throwers and 4 of 5 (80%) gymnasts were able to return to sport, and no patient had demonstrable degenerative joint disease.

COMPLICATIONS

- The complications seen with OCD treated surgically or not include flexion contracture, elbow pain, arthritis, and inability to return to sports.
- Loose bodies may develop in elbows treated nonoperatively.
- Surgical intervention, particularly arthroscopy, has the added risk of nerve injury because the neural structures are so close to the usual elbow arthroscopy portals.

REFERENCES

1. Bauer M, Jonsson K, Josefsson PO, et al. Osteochondritis dissecans of the elbow: a long-term follow-up study. Clin Orthop Relat Res 1992;284:156–160.
2. Baumgarten TE, Andrews JR, Satterwhite YE. The arthroscopic classification and treatment of osteochondritis dissecans of the capitellum. Am J Sports Med 1998;26:520–523.
3. Jackson D, Silvino N, Reimen P. Osteochondritis in the female gymnast's elbow. Arthroscopy 1989;5:129–136.
4. McManama GB Jr, Micheli LJ, Berry MV, et al. The surgical treatment of osteochondritis of the capitellum. Am J Sports Med 1985;13:11–21.
5. Ruch DS, Cory JW, Poehling GG. The arthroscopic management of osteochondritis dissecans of the adolescent elbow. Arthroscopy 1998;14:797–803.
6. Takahara M, Ogino T, Fukushima S, et al. Nonoperative treatment of osteochondritis dissecans of the humeral capitellum. Am J Sports Med 1999;27:728–732.
7. Takahara M, Ogino T, Sasaki I, et al. Long-term outcome of osteochondritis dissecans of the humeral capitellum. Clin Orthop Relat Res 1999;363:108–115.

Open Reduction and Internal Fixation of Supracondylar and Intercondylar Fractures

15 CHAPTER

Joaquin Sanchez-Sotelo

PATIENT HISTORY AND PHYSICAL FINDINGS

- Distal humerus fractures occur in two age groups:
  - Younger patients who sustain high-energy trauma
  - Older patients with underlying osteopenia
- Comminution is the dominant feature of supracondylar and intercondylar fractures and complicates internal fixation. The complicated skeletal geometry of the distal humerus also contributes.
- The goals of the initial evaluation are to
  - Understand the fracture pattern
  - Determine the existence of previous symptomatic elbow pathology
  - Determine the extent of associated soft tissue (open fractures)
  - Identify associated musculoskeletal or neurovascular injuries

IMAGING AND OTHER DIAGNOSTIC STUDIES

- Elbow radiographs in the anteroposterior and lateral planes are the first imaging studies obtained and should be carefully scrutinized to identify the fracture lines and fragments as well as the extent of comminution. It is also important to look for associated injuries in the proximal radius and ulna.
  - A complete understanding of the fracture pattern is difficult to obtain based only on simple radiographs because of the complex geometry of the distal humerus and fragment overlapping (**FIG 1A,B**).
- Computed tomography (CT) with three-dimensional reconstruction is extremely helpful, especially in the more complex cases. It allows the surgeon to look for specific fractured fragments at the time of fixation, facilitating accurate fracture reduction (**FIG 1C,D**).
- Traction radiographs obtained in the operating room with the patient under anesthesia just before surgery also can be helpful, especially if a CT scan is not available.

SURGICAL MANAGEMENT

- Internal fixation is the treatment of choice for most fractures of the distal humerus.
- Modern fixation techniques seem to benefit from the following:
  - Fixation strategies designed to improve the mechanical stability of the construct
  - Use of precontoured periarticular plates
  - Use of screws locked to the plates
- Elbow arthroplasty should be considered in elderly patients with previous elbow pathology or in very low comminuted fractures in patients with osteopenia.[12,14] However, internal fixation can be successful even in low transcondylar fractures.[18]
- The goal of the internal fixation technique is to achieve a construct stable enough to allow immediate unprotected motion without fear of redisplacement.[15,16] This can be attained in most distal humerus fractures—even the most complex—provided the following principles are adhered to the following (**FIG 2**):
  - Plates used for internal fixation are applied so that fixation in the distal fragments is maximized.

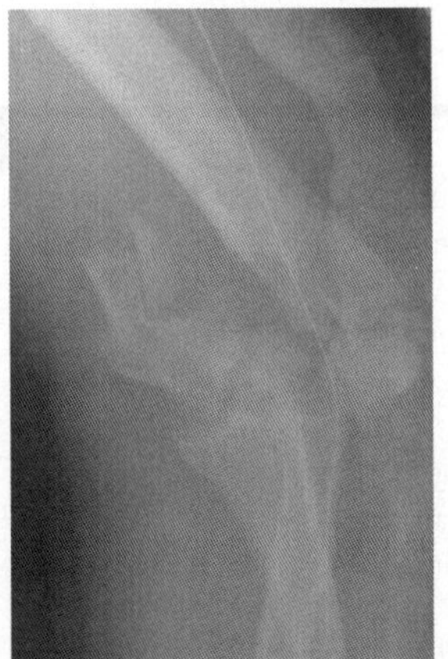
A

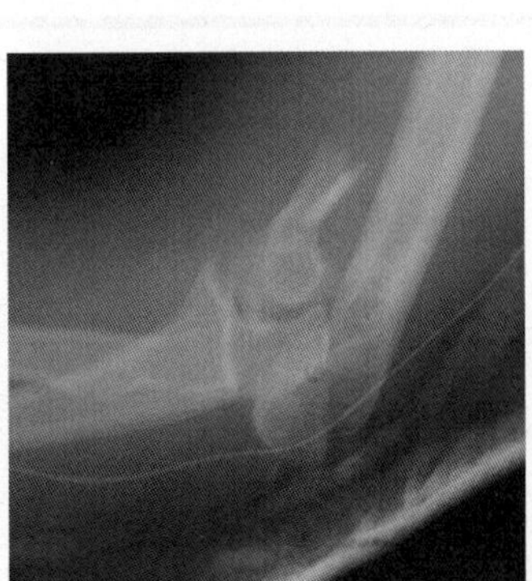
B

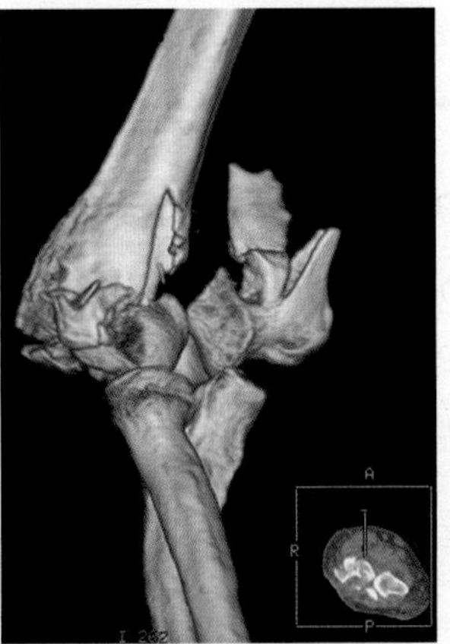
C

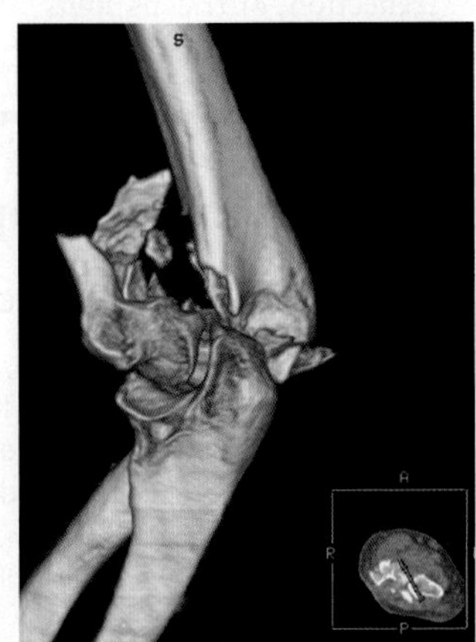
D

FIG 1 • **A,B.** Anteroposterior (AP) and lateral radiographs showing a comminuted intra-articular supraintercondylar fracture of the distal humerus. The complexity of the fracture is difficult to appreciate fully because of the geometry of the distal humerus, fracture comminution, and fragment overlapping. **C,D.** The use of CT with three-dimensional reconstruction and surface rendering helps understand the fracture configuration and anticipate the surgical findings.

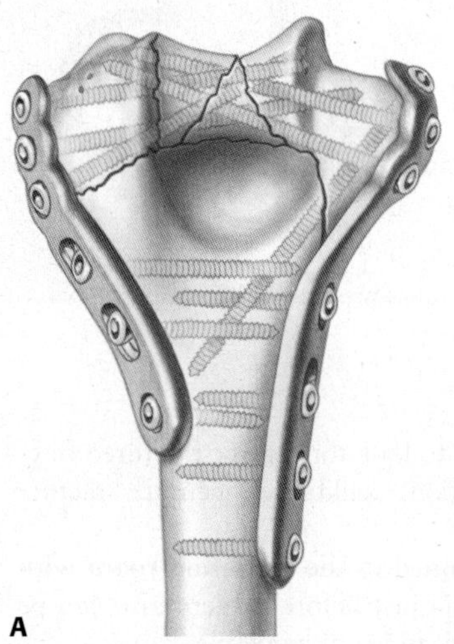

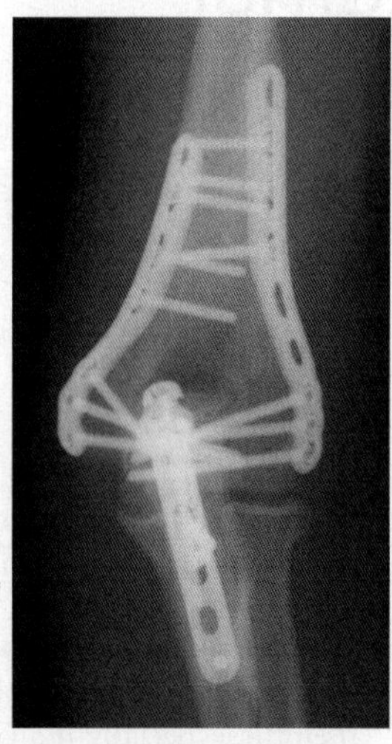

FIG 2 • A. Internal fixation using two parallel medial and lateral plates allows maximal fixation of the plates in the distal fragments and increased stability at the supracondylar level. **B.** This postoperative AP radiograph shows anatomic reduction of a complex distal humerus fracture and stable fixation using the principles and technique described in this chapter. The olecranon osteotomy was fixed with a plate. (**A:** Copyright Mayo Clinic.)

- Distal screw fixation contributes to stability at the supracondylar level, where true interfragmentary compression is achieved.

Approaches

- Adequate exposure is necessary to achieve satisfactory reduction and fixation.
- The management of the ulnar nerve is controversial; some surgeons favor routine subcutaneous transposition, whereas others prefer to leave the nerve in its anatomic location at the end of the procedure. A number of patients will develop a transitory or permanent ulnar neuropathy, mostly sensitive, regardless of nerve management; preoperative counseling is important in this regard.
- Most fractures require mobilization of the extensor mechanism of the elbow through an olecranon osteotomy, triceps reflection, or triceps split.
- Simple fractures occasionally may be addressed working on both sides of the triceps without mobilization of the extensor mechanism.
- Olecranon osteotomy is the preferred surgical approach for internal fixation for most distal humerus fractures.[13]
  - Advantages
    - Provides excellent exposure
    - Offers the potential of bone-to-bone healing, thereby limiting the risk of triceps dysfunction
  - Disadvantages
    - Complications: nonunion, intra-articular adhesions
    - Hardware removal may be needed.
    - Limits the ability for intraoperative conversion to elbow arthroplasty
    - May devitalize the anconeus muscle
    - The proximal ulna cannot be used as a template to judge reduction and motion.
- Triceps reflection and triceps split[9] allow preservation of the intact ulna.
  - Avoid complications related to olecranon osteotomy.
  - Facilitate intraoperative conversion to total elbow arthroplasty.
  - Allow use of the proximal ulna as a template for reduction of the distal humerus articular surface.
  - Allow assessment of extension deficit after fracture fixation, which is especially useful in fractures requiring metaphyseal shortening.
- Bilaterotricipital approach[1]
  - Goals and indications
    - The goal is to provide adequate exposure for fracture fixation without violating the extensor mechanism.
    - This approach is used only for the more simple fracture patterns (eg, extra-articular or simple intra-articular distal humerus fractures [AO/OTA A, C1, C2]) or when elbow arthroplasty is being considered.
  - Advantages
    - This approach avoids complications related to the extensor mechanism.
    - No postoperative protection is needed.
    - Surgical time is decreased.
  - Disadvantage
    - The procedure provides limited exposure of the articular surface.

TECHNIQUES

Surgical Approach

Olecranon Osteotomy

- Chevron osteotomy provides increased stability (**TECH FIG 1A**).
- The distal apex of the chevron osteotomy is centered with the bare area of the olecranon articular surface.
- The anconeus is divided with electrocautery in line with the lateral limb of the osteotomy.
  - Alternatively, the anconeus may be preserved by dissecting it free on its distal aspect and reflecting it proximally attached to the proximal ulnar fragment.[2]
- Start the osteotomy with a thin oscillating saw; use of a thick saw blade removes bone excessively, which may make it more difficult to obtain interfragmentary compression at the time of olecranon osteotomy fixation and thus increase the risk of olecranon osteotomy nonunion.
- Complete the osteotomy with an osteotome.
  - Decreases risk of damage to the articular cartilage on ulna and humerus
  - Creates irregularities at the opposing cut surfaces, which may increase interdigitation
- Mobilize the fragment to facilitate exposure (**TECH FIG 1B**).
- Fixation (**TECH FIG 1C**)
  - Some biomechanical studies support the combination of a 7.3-mm cancellous screw and tension band over either a screw alone or K-wires plus tension band; others have found no differences.

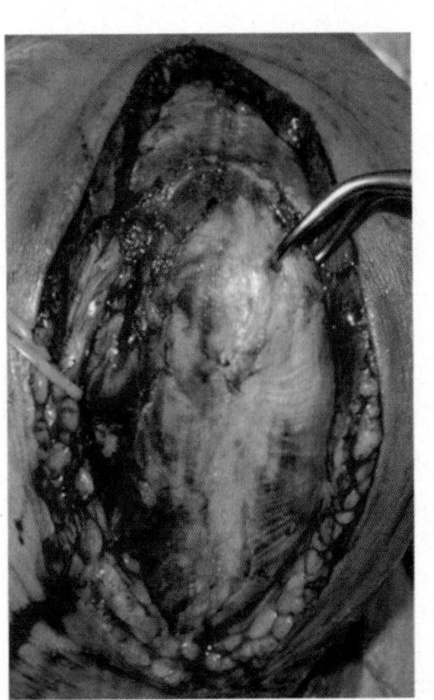
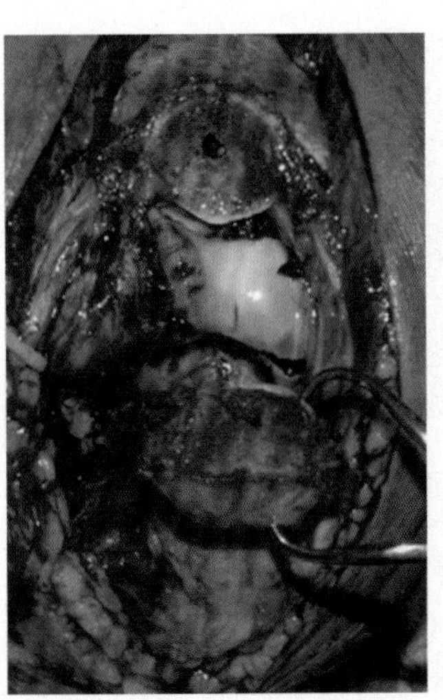
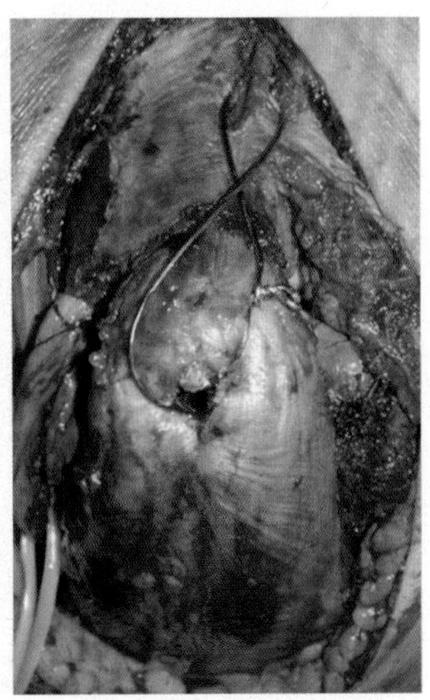

TECH FIG 1 • Olecranon osteotomy provides an excellent exposure for distal humerus fracture fixation. **A.** A chevron osteotomy is initiated with a microsagittal saw and completed with an osteotome. Drilling and tapping before performing the osteotomy facilitates fixation of the osteotomy if screw fixation is selected. **B.** Proximal mobilization of the osteotomized fragment and triceps allows ample exposure of the articular surface and columns. **C.** Fixation may be performed with a cancellous screw and tension band, wires and a tension band, or a plate.

- The author's preferred method uses K-wires plus a tension band in patients with good bone quality and plate fixation in patients with osteopenia.
- If screw fixation is planned, drill and tap the ulna before performing the osteotomy.
- Plate fixation provides improved fixation, but the risk of wound complications is increased.
- There is substantial interest in the development of intramedullary fixation devices locked proximally and distally; they would combine the benefits of stability and intramedullary location, which could lead to a decreased rate of wound complications and painful hardware requiring removal.

Triceps Reflection and Triceps Split

- Bryan-Morrey triceps-sparing approach (**TECH FIG 2**)
  - The triceps is elevated from the medial intermuscular septum and the posterior aspect of the humeral shaft.
  - The forearm fascia and periosteum are incised just lateral to the flexor carpi ulnaris.
  - The triceps, forearm fascia, and anconeus are elevated in continuity from medial to lateral.
  - When this approach is used for fracture fixation, the anterior bundle of the medial collateral ligament and the lateral ulnar collateral ligament must be preserved to avoid postoperative instability.
- Mayo-modified extensile Kocher approach
  - The triceps is elevated from the lateral intermuscular septum and the posterior aspect of the humeral shaft.
  - The triceps and anconeus are elevated in continuity from lateral to medial.
  - As noted earlier, the anterior bundle of the medial collateral ligament and the lateral ulnar collateral ligament must be preserved to avoid postoperative instability.

Bilaterotricipital Approach

- The triceps is elevated from the medial and lateral intermuscular septae.
- Lateral dissection can be extended anterior to the anconeus muscle (**TECH FIG 3**).
- The arthrotomy is performed posterior to the medial collateral ligament and lateral collateral ligament complex.

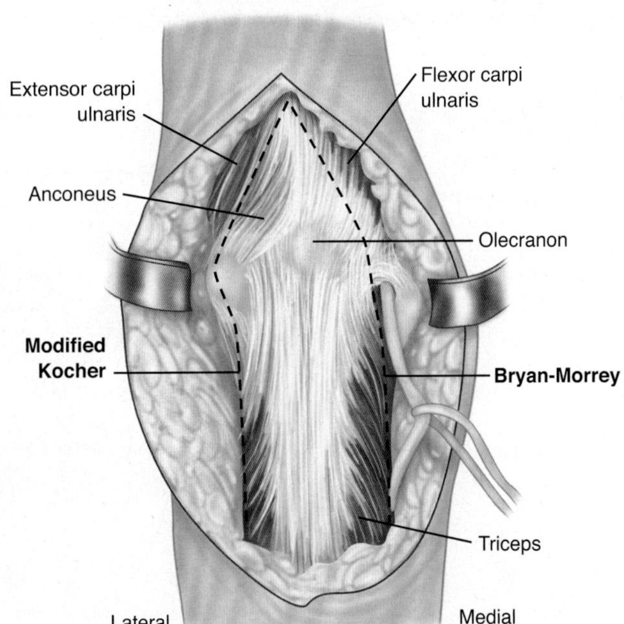

TECH FIG 2 • The extensor mechanism (ie, triceps, anconeus, and forearm fascia) may be elevated off the ulna subperiosteally in continuity from medial to lateral (Bryan-Morrey approach) or from lateral to medial (Mayo-modified extensile Kocher approach).

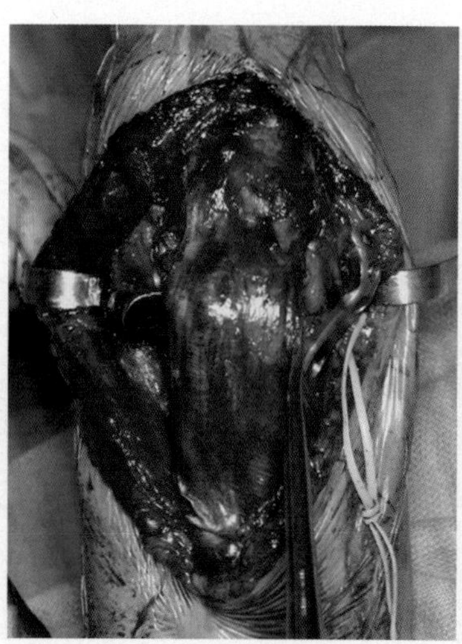

TECH FIG 3 • Fractures with no or limited articular involvement may be fixed working on both sides of the triceps. As shown in this image, the extensor mechanism is left mostly undisturbed.

Internal Fixation

Technical Objectives

- Screws in the distal fragments (articular segment) should be placed according to the following principles:
  - Every screw should pass through a plate.
  - Each screw should engage a fragment on the opposite side that also is fixed to a plate.
  - As many screws as possible should be placed in the distal fragments.
  - Each screw should be as long as possible.
  - Each screw should engage as many articular fragments as possible.
  - The screws should lock together by interdigitation within the distal segment, thereby rigidly linking the medial and lateral columns together, creating an architectural structure similar to that of an arch or dome.
- Plates are used for fixation.
  - Plates should be applied such that compression is achieved at the supracondylar level for both columns.
  - Plates must be strong enough and stiff enough to resist breaking or bending before union occurs at the supracondylar level.

Provisional Assembly of the Articular Surface and Plate Placement

- Reduce the articular surface fragments anatomically.
  - The proximal ulna and radial head may be used as templates.
- Rotational alignment should be carefully assessed.
- Use smooth K-wires to maintain the reduction provisionally (**TECH FIG 4A**).

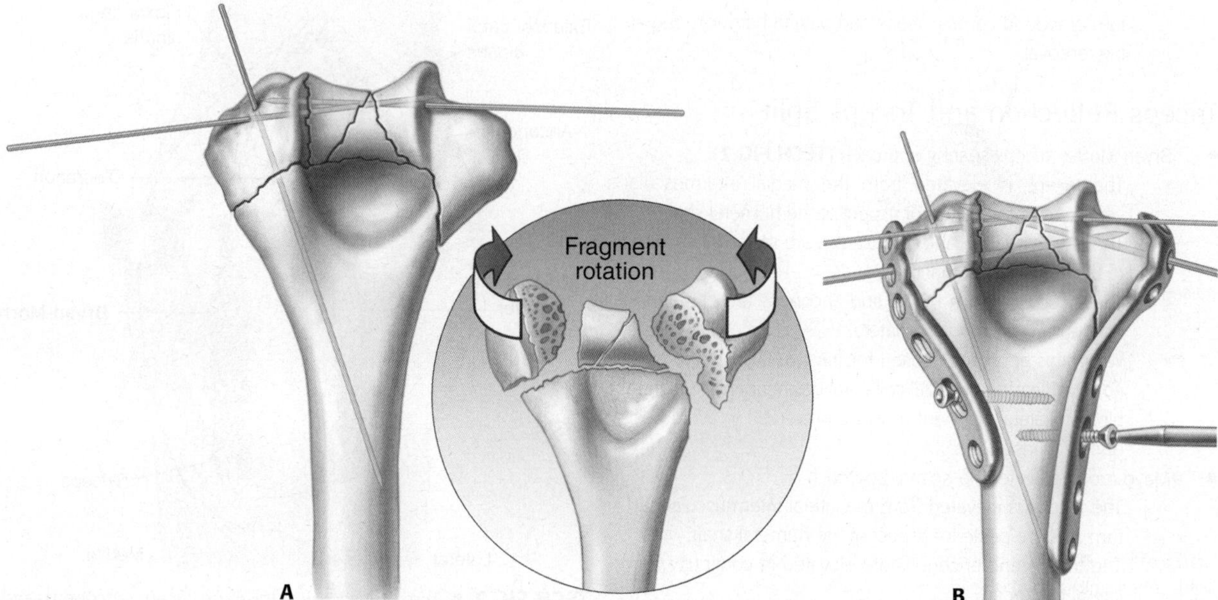

TECH FIG 4 • **A.** Anatomic reduction of the articular surface is maintained provisionally with fine wires placed so that they will not interfere with plate and screw application. **B.** The medial and lateral plates are held in place provisionally with two distal 2.0-mm pins (which later will be replaced by screws) and two proximal screws through an oval hole to allow small adjustments in plate positioning. (Copyright Mayo Clinic.)

- Two 2.0-mm smooth wires introduced at the medial and lateral epicondyles facilitate provisional placement of the plates and can be replaced by screws later.
- Fine-threaded wires, absorbable pins or very small screws may be used for definitive fixation of small fracture fragments.
- Medial and lateral plates are placed so that one of the distal holes of each plate slides over the medial and lateral 2.0-mm smooth wires introduced at the medial and lateral epicondyles (**TECH FIG 4B**).
- One cortical screw is loosely introduced into a slotted hole of each plate to hold the plates in place; use of slotted holes for these screws facilitates later adjustments in plate positioning.

Articular and Distal Fixation

- Two or more distal screws are inserted through the plates medially and laterally. As noted, the screws should be as long as possible and engage fragments on the opposite column.
  - Before screw application, a large bone clamp is used to compress the articular fracture lines, unless there is comminution of the articular surface.
- The two 2.0-mm smooth pins may be replaced with distal screws without previous drilling to avoid accidental breakage of the drill when contacting the other screws. Usually, these last screws will interdigitate with the previously applied distal screws, thereby increasing the stability of the construct (**TECH FIG 5**).

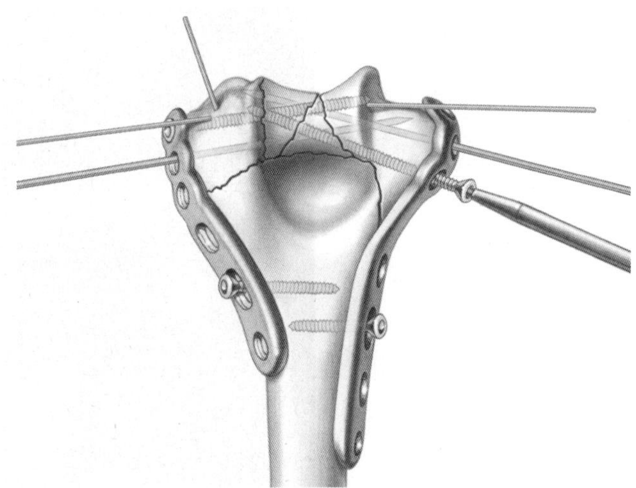

TECH FIG 5 • Maximal distal plate anchorage is then achieved by insertion of multiple long screws through the plates and into the distal fragments. Usually, the screws from the medial and lateral directions will engage, creating an interlocked structure that increases fracture stability. (Copyright Mayo Clinic.)

Supracondylar Compression and Proximal Plate Fixation

- The proximal screw on one side is backed out, and a large bone clamp is applied distally on that side and proximally on the opposite side to apply maximum compression at the supracondylar level. Compression is maintained by application of one proximal screw in the compression mode (**TECH FIG 6A,B**).
- The same steps are followed on the opposite side.
- The remaining diaphyseal screws are then introduced, providing additional compression as they push the undercontoured plates to gain intimate contact with the underlying bone (**TECH FIG 6C**).
- Small posterior fragments can be fixed with threaded wires or absorbable pins.
- Provisional wires are removed.
- The elbow is put through range of motion. Motion should be smooth. If extension is limited, part of the tip of the olecranon may be removed.

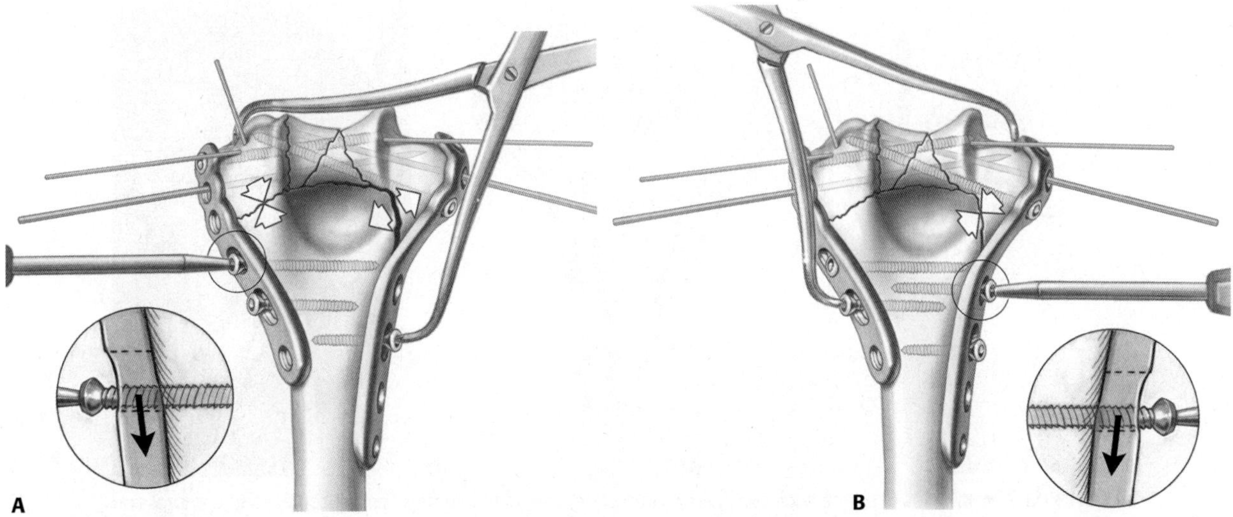

TECH FIG 6 • **A,B.** Supracondylar compression is achieved with the use of a large clamp, insertion of screws in the compression mode, and slight undercontouring of the plates. The same technique is applied laterally and medially. *(continued)*

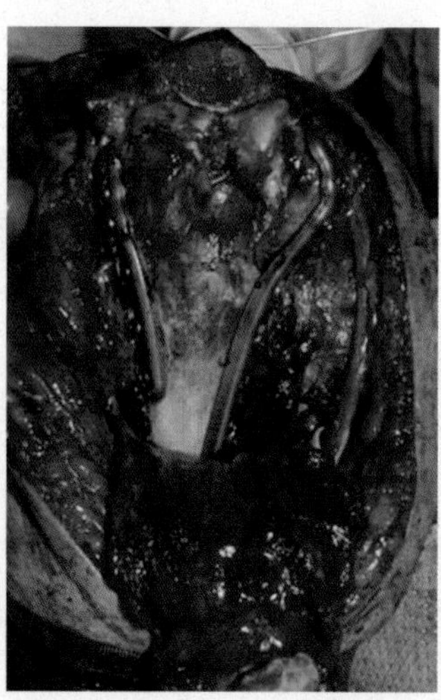

TECH FIG 6 • *(continued)* **C.** Internal fixation of a complex distal humerus fracture. (**A,B:** Copyright Mayo Clinic.)

Supracondylar Shortening

- In cases with supracondylar comminution (ie, bone loss), compression at the supracondylar level cannot be achieved unless the humerus is shortened into a nonanatomic reduction that will provide adequate bone contact (**TECH FIG 7A,B**).
  - The humerus may be shortened between a few millimeters and 2 cm with only minor losses in extension strength.[10]
- Bone is trimmed from the diaphysis to ensure adequate bone contact with the distal fragments. The distal fragments are typically already small, and further removal from these distal fragments should be avoided.
- The distal fragments are translated proximally and anteriorly. Anterior translation is necessary to create room for the radial head and the coronoid in flexion.
- The fracture is fixed in the desired position using the technique described previously.
- A new deep and wide olecranon fossa is created by removing bone from the distal and posterior aspect of the diaphysis (**TECH FIG 7C**). Otherwise, extension will be restricted.

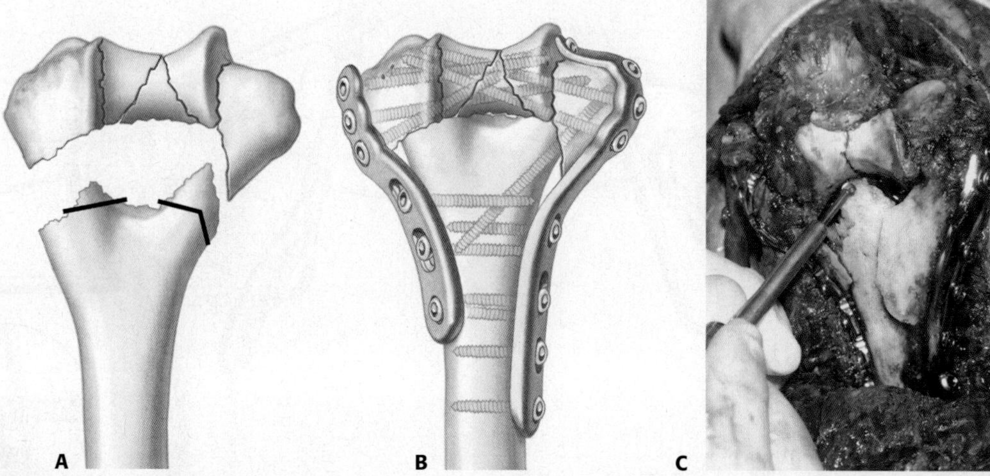

TECH FIG 7 • In cases of severe supracondylar comminution, adequate interfragmentary contact and compression takes priority over anatomic reduction. The humerus may be shortened anywhere from a few millimeters to 2 cm by trimming the bony spikes of the diaphysis (**A**), advancing the distal segment proximally and anteriorly, and fixing it in a nonanatomic fashion (**B**). **C.** The olecranon fossa is recreated in this case by removing bone from the posterior aspect of the diaphysis with a burr. (**A,B:** Copyright Mayo Clinic.)

PEARLS AND PITFALLS

Olecranon osteotomy	▪ Position the apex of the osteotomy distally. ▪ Use a thin oscillating saw to minimize bone loss. ▪ If plate fixation is preferred, consider drilling the holes for the plate before beginning the osteotomy. This facilitates plate fixation of the osteotomy at the conclusion of the surgery. ▪ Similarly, if tension band fixation with an intramedullary screw is preferred, predrill and tap the screw hole.
Triceps reflection and triceps split	▪ Subperiosteal detachment of the extensor mechanism is critical to preserve its thickness and facilitate a strong reattachment. ▪ Reproduce anatomic reattachment of the extensor mechanism. ▪ Use heavy, nonabsorbable suture (no. 5 Ethibond [Ethicon, Inc., Somerville, NJ] or no. 2 FiberWire [Arthrex, Inc., Naples, FL]) through bone. ▪ Protect extension against resistance for 6 weeks.
Bilaterotricipital approach	▪ Separate the triceps from the underlying medial and lateral joint capsules. ▪ Resect the posterior capsule and fat pad to improve visualization.

POSTOPERATIVE MANAGEMENT

- After closure, the elbow is placed in a bulky, noncompressive dressing with an anterior plaster splint to maintain the elbow in extension, and the upper extremity is kept elevated.
  - In patients with severe swelling, open fractures or compromised soft tissues consideration should be given to an incisional or standard vacuum-assisted closure device.
- Motion is initiated according to the extent of soft tissue damage. Motion usually can be initiated on the first or second postoperative day, but it may be necessary to wait for several days in the case of open fractures or severe soft tissue damage.
- Most patients benefit from a program of continuous passive motion for the first week or two after fixation; some may benefit from a longer period of passive motion.
- When postoperative motion fails to progress as expected, a program of patient-adjusted static flexion and extension splints is implemented.
- Treatment with indomethacin or single-dose radiation to the soft tissues shielding the fracture site may be considered for patients with high risk of heterotopic ossification, such as those with associated head or spinal trauma as well as those who require several surgeries in a short period of time. However, failure to shield the fracture site or the olecranon osteotomy seems to lead to a higher rate of nonunion.

OUTCOMES

- The results of internal fixation for fractures of the distal humerus using modern techniques are summarized in Table 1.
  - The results of the different studies are difficult to interpret because the severity of the injuries included cannot be compared, and there may be variations in the accuracy of range-of-motion measurements.
- Improvements in fixation techniques have resulted in a decreased rate of hardware failure and nonunion, but range of motion is not reliably restored in every patient. In addition, other complications remain relatively common[8] as detailed below.

COMPLICATIONS

- Infection
- Nonunion
- Stiffness, with or without heterotopic ossification
- Need for removal of the hardware used for fixation of the olecranon osteotomy
- Ulnar neuropathy
- Posttraumatic osteoarthritis or avascular necrosis requiring interposition arthroplasty or elbow replacement

Table 1 Results of Internal Fixation for Distal Humerus Fractures Affecting the Humeral Columns

Study	No.	Mean Age (Range) (y)	Follow-up (mo)	Fracture Type (no.) (AO Classification)	Open	Mean Degrees ROM (range)	Overall results	Complications (no.)	Reoperations (no.)
Jupiter et al[5]	34	57 (17–79)	70 (25–139)	C1 (13) C2 (2) C3 (19)	14 (41%)	76% achieved at least 30–120	79% satisfactory*	Nonunion (2) Refracture (1) Olecranon osteotomy nonunion (2) Class II HO (1) Ulnar neuropathy (4) Median neuropathy (1)	Hardware removal (24) Capsulectomy (3) HO removal (1) Nerve decompression (4)
Henley et al[4]	33	32 (15–61)	18.3	C1 (23) C2 (8) C3 (2)	14 (42%)	Mean extension, 19; mean flexion, 126	92% satisfactory* (only 25 patients evaluated)	Hardware failure (5) Infection (2) Olecranon osteotomy nonunion (2) Class II HO (2)	Repeat ORIF (2) TBW removal (6) Olecranon osteotomy repeat ORIF (2)
Sanders et al[17]	17	51 (12–85)	>24	C1 (4) C2 (3) C3 (10)	7 (41%)	108 (55–140)	76% satisfactory*	Delayed union (2) Infection (2) Pulmonary embolism (1) Ulnar neuropathy (1)	Hardware removal (3) Ulnar nerve decompression (1)
McKee et al (closed fractures)[7]	25	47 (19–85)	37 (18–75)	C (25)	None	108 (55–140)	Mean DASH: 20 (0–55)	Ulnar neuritis (3) Transient radial nerve palsy (1) Nonunion (1) Malunion (1)	TBW removal (3) Repeat ORIF (1) Elbow release (2)
McKee et al (open fractures)[6]	26	44 (17–78)	51 (10–141)	C1 (5) C2 (13) C3 (8)	100%	97 (55–140)	Mean DASH: 23.7 (0–57.5) 60% satisfactory MEPS	Septic nonunion (1) Delayed union (4) Transient radial nerve palsy (1)	Repeat ORIF (3)
Pajarinen et al[11]	21	44 (16–81)	24 (10–41)	C1 (6) C2 (12) C3 (3)	5 (24%)	107 (98–116)	56% satisfactory OTA	Deep infection (1) Nonunion (2) Traumatic nerve injuries (3) Olecranon osteotomy nonunion (1)	Repeat ORIF (2)
Gofton et al[3]	23	53 (16–80)	45 (14–89)	C1 (3) C2 (11) C3 (9)	7 (30%)	122 (extension loss, 19 ± 12; flexion,142 ± 6)	Mean DASH: 12 (0–38) Subjective satisfaction: 93% 87% satisfactory MEPS	Deep infection (1) Olecranon osteotomy nonunion (2) Class II HO (3) Avascular necrosis (1) Reflex sympathetic dystrophy (1) Capitellar nonunion (1)	Olecranon osteotomy repeat ORIF (2) Elbow release (3) Capitellar ORIF (1)
Soon et al[19]	15	43 (21–80)	12 (2–27)	B (3) C1 (4) C2 (4) C3 (4)	None	109 (45–145)	86% satisfactory MEPS	Transient ulnar neuritis (2) Hardware failure (3) Nonunion (1)	Total elbow arthroplasty (1) Repeat ORIF (3) Elbow manipulation or release (4)
Sanchez-Sotelo et al[15]	32	58 (16–99)	24 (12–60)	A3 (3) C2 (4) C3 (25)	13 (44%)	Mean extension: 26 (0–55) Mean flexion: 124 (80–150)	83% satisfactory MEPS	Delayed union (1) Ulnar neuropathy (6) Class II HO (5) Infection (1)	Wound débridement or coverage (4) Bone grafting (1) HO removal (4) HO removal and distraction arthroplasty (1) Triceps reconstruction (1)

ROM, range of motion; Class II HO, heterotopic ossification restricting motion; ORIF, open reduction and internal fixation; TBW, tension band wiring; DASH, Disabilities of the Arm, Shoulder and Hand questionnaire; MEPS, Mayo Elbow Performance Score; OTA, Orthopaedic Trauma Association.
*According to the Jupiter rating system.

REFERENCES

1. Alonso-Llames M. Bilaterotricipital approach to the elbow. Its application in the osteosynthesis of supracondylar fractures of the humerus in children. Acta Orthop Scand 1972;43:479–490.
2. Athwal GS, Rispoli DM, Steinmann SP. The anconeus flap transolecranon approach to the distal humerus. J Orthop Trauma 2006;20: 282–285.
3. Gofton WT, Macdermid JC, Patterson SD, et al. Functional outcome of AO type C distal humeral fractures. J Hand Surg Am 2003;28:294–308.
4. Henley MB, Bone LB, Parker B. Operative management of intra-articular fractures of the distal humerus. J Orthop Trauma 1987;1:24–35.
5. Jupiter JB, Neff U, Holzach P, et al. Intercondylar fractures of the humerus. An operative approach. J Bone Joint Surg Am 1985;67:226–239.
6. McKee MD, Kim J, Kebaish K, et al. Functional outcome after open supracondylar fractures of the humerus. The effect of the surgical approach. J Bone Joint Surg Br 2000;82(5):646–651.
7. McKee MD, Wilson TL, Winston L, et al. Functional outcome following surgical treatment of intra-articular distal humeral fractures through a posterior approach. J Bone Joint Surg Am 2000;82-A(12): 1701–1707.
8. Lawrence TM, Ahmadi S, Morrey BF, et al. Wound complications after distal humerus fracture fixation: incidence, risk factors and outcome. J Shoulder Elbow Surg 2014;23(2):258–264.
9. Morrey BF. Anatomy and surgical approaches. In: Morrey BF, ed. Joint Replacement Arthroplasty. Philadelphia: Churchill-Livingstone, 2003:269–285.
10. O'Driscoll SW, Sanchez-Sotelo J, Torchia ME. Management of the smashed distal humerus. Orthop Clin North Am 2002;33:19–33.
11. Pajarinen J, Björkenheim JM. Operative treatment of type C intercondylar fractures of the distal humerus: results after a mean follow-up of 2 years in a series of 18 patients. J Shoulder Elbow Surg 2002;11:48–52.
12. Popovic D, King GJ. Fragility fractures of the distal humerus: what is the optimal treatment? J Bone Joint Surg Br 2012 94(1):16–22.
13. Ring D, Gulotta L, Chin K, et al. Olecranon osteotomy for exposure of fractures and nonunions of the distal humerus. J Orthop Trauma 2004;18:446–449.
14. Sanchez-Sotelo J. Distal humeral fractures: role of internal fixation and elbow arthroplasty. J Bone Joint Surg Am 2012;94(6):555–568.
15. Sanchez-Sotelo J, Torchia ME, O'Driscoll SW. Complex distal humeral fractures: internal fixation with a principle-based parallel-plate technique. J Bone Joint Surg Am 2007;89(5):961–969.
16. Sanchez-Sotelo J, Torchia ME, O'Driscoll SW. Principle-based internal fixation of distal humerus fractures. Tech Hand Upper Extremity Surg 2001;5:179–187.
17. Sanders RA, Raney EM, Pipkin S. Operative treatment of bicondylar intraarticular fractures of the distal humerus. Orthopedics 1992;15: 159–163.
18. Simone JP, Streubel PN, Sanchez-Sotelo J, et al. Low transcondylar fractures of the distal humerus: results of open reduction and internal fixation. J Shoulder Elbow Surg 2014;23(4):573–578.
19. Soon JL, Chan BK, Low CO. Surgical fixation of intra-articular fractures of the distal humerus in adults. Injury 2004;35:44–54.

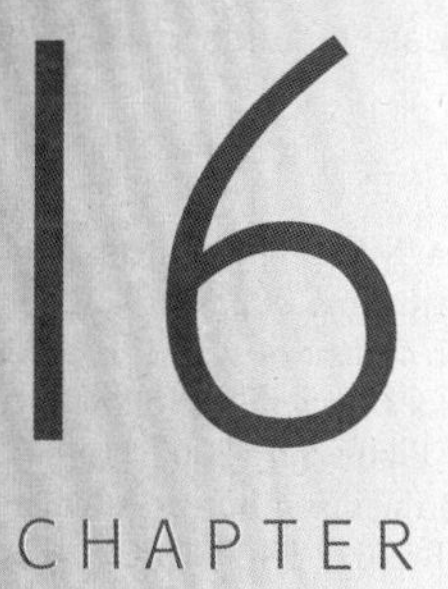

Open Reduction and Internal Fixation of Capitellum and Capitellar–Trochlear Shear Fractures

Asif M. Ilyas, Michael Rivlin, and Jesse B. Jupiter

DEFINITION

- Capitellar fractures are uncommon, accounting for less than 1% of all elbow fractures and 6% of all distal humerus fractures.[4]
- They often are associated with radial head fractures and posterior elbow dislocations.
- A classification system for capitellar fractures has been proposed by Bryan and Morrey[4] and modified by McKee:
  - Type 1: complete fractures of the capitellum[14]
  - Type 2: superficial subchondral fractures of the capitellar articular surface[29]
  - Type 3: comminuted fractures[2]
  - Type 4: coronal shear fractures that include a portion of the trochlea as well as the capitellum as one piece[21] (**FIG 1**)
- Ring et al[25] have proposed a new classification, expanding on the growing understanding that isolated capitellum fractures are rare and often are involved as part of articular shear fractures of the distal humerus. The classification includes five anatomic components, with type 1 articular injuries encompassing the capitellum and capitellar–trochlear shear patterns (**FIG 2**):
  - Type 1: capitellum and lateral aspect of the trochlea
  - Type 2: lateral epicondyle
  - Type 3: posterior aspect of the lateral column
  - Type 4: posterior aspect of the trochlea
  - Type 5: medial epicondyle
- More recently, Dubberley and colleagues[8] introduced a classification system based on radiographic pattern of injury taking posterior comminution into account.
  - Type 1: fracture of the capitellum (with or without trochlear ridge involvement)
  - Type 2: capitellum and trochlea fracture that remain as one fragment
  - Type 3: capitellum and trochlea as separate fragments
  - Type A: no posterior condyle comminution
  - Type B: posterior condyle comminution present

ANATOMY

- The two condyles of the distal humerus diverge from the humeral shaft to form the lateral and medial columns, which support the trochlea between them. The anterior aspect of the lateral column is covered with articular cartilage, forming the capitellum. Distally, these two condyles can be visualized as forming a triangle at the end of the humerus.
- The capitellum is the first epiphyseal center of the elbow to ossify.

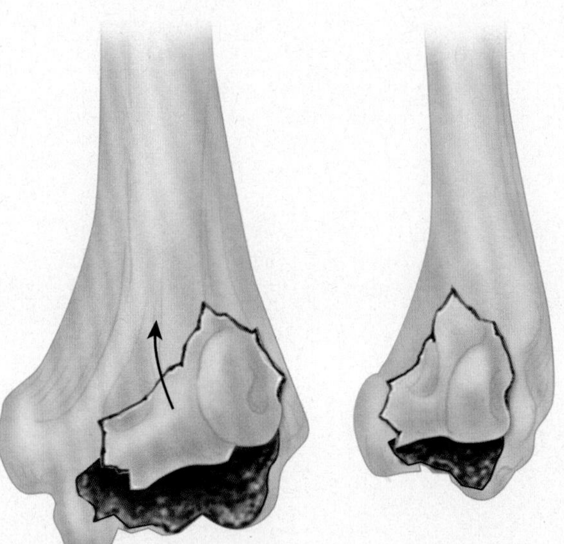

FIG 1 • Type 4 coronal shear fractures of the distal humerus. (Adapted from McKee MD, Jupiter JB, Bamberger HB, et al. Coronal shear fractures of the distal end of the humerus. J Bone Joint Surg Am 1996;78[1]:49–54.)

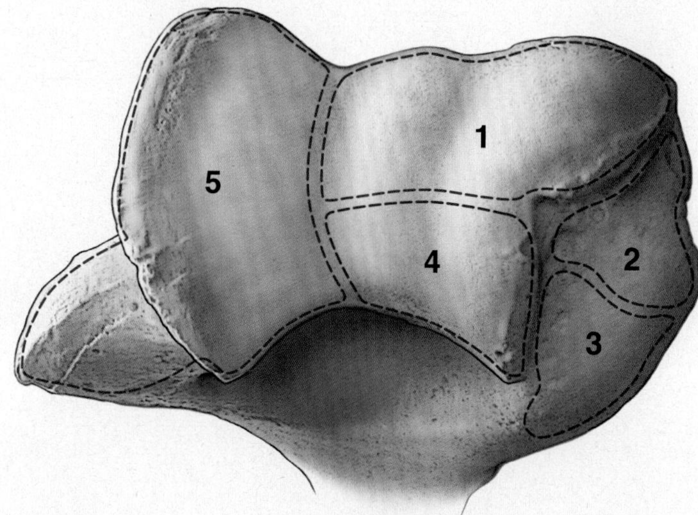

FIG 2 • Articular fractures of the distal part of the humerus, including type 1 fractures that encompass capitellum and capitellar–trochlear shear fractures. (Adapted from Ring D, Jupiter JB, Gulotta L. Articular fractures of the distal part of the humerus. J Bone Joint Surg Am 2003;85-A[2]:232–238.)

- It is covered by articular surface anteriorly but devoid of it posteriorly.
- The capitellum is directed distally and anteriorly at an angle of 30 degrees to the long axis of the humerus.
- The radial head rotates on the anterior surface of the capitellum in elbow flexion and articulates with its inferior surface in elbow extension.
- The lateral collateral ligament inserts next to the lateral margin of the capitellum.
- The blood supply of the capitellum is derived posteriorly. It arises from the lateral arcade, which is the anastomosis of the radial collateral arteries of the profunda brachii and the radial recurrent artery.[30]

PATHOGENESIS

- Capitellum and capitellar–trochlear shear fractures involve impaction of the radial head against the lateral column of the distal humerus in a partially extended position, resulting in shearing of the articular cartilage of the distal humerus.
- Fracture fragments vary in size and displace superiorly and anteriorly into the radial fossa, resulting in impingement with elbow flexion.
- Associated injuries include proximal and distal radial as well as carpal fractures; ligamentous injuries include collateral ligament (lateral more common than medial) and triceps ruptures.[8]

NATURAL HISTORY

- Capitellar fractures occur almost exclusively in adults. These fractures do not occur in children because in that age group, the capitellum is largely cartilaginous, and a similar mechanism of injury would instead cause a supracondylar or lateral condyle fracture.
- Capitellar fractures are more common in females, a finding that can be attributed to the increased carrying angle of the female elbow.
- Displaced fractures that go untreated can be expected to have a poor outcome owing to the progressive loss of motion from the mechanical block to flexion, potential longitudinal instability of the forearm, and the likely development of subsequent posttraumatic arthrosis from the residual articular incongruity.
- Capitellar and trochlear fractures are prone to nonunion if multiple articular fragments are present or the posterior column is involved.[3]

PATIENT HISTORY AND PHYSICAL FINDINGS

- Symptoms of capitellar fractures are similar to those of radial head fractures, including pain and swelling along the lateral elbow and pain with elbow motion.
- Although there may be variable loss of forearm rotation, loss of flexion and extension is most common, often accompanied by crepitus and pain.
- The association of concomitant radial head fractures and ligamentous injuries with capitellar fractures is high.[22]
- The shoulder and wrist should also be examined for concomitant injury.

IMAGING AND OTHER DIAGNOSTIC STUDIES

- Standard radiographs are often inadequate for accurate assessment of capitellar fractures.
- Lateral radiographs are best for obtaining an initial evaluation of capitellar fractures.
- Anteroposterior views do not reliably show the fracture because the outline of the distal humerus is not consistently affected.
- The radial head–capitellum view can help identify fractures of the capitellum. This view is a lateral oblique projection taken with the x-ray beam pointing 45 degrees dorsoventrally, thereby eliminating the ulno- and radiohumeral articulation shadows.[13]
  - A type 1 fracture appears as a semilunar fragment sitting superiorly with its articular surface pointing up and away from the radial head in most cases.
  - Type 2 fractures are more difficult to diagnose, depending on the amount of subchondral bone accompanying the articular fragment. They may appear as a loose body lying in the superior part of the joint.
  - Type 3 fractures display variable amounts of comminution.
  - Coronal shear fractures show a characteristic "double arc" sign on lateral radiographic views (**FIG 3A**).
- Computed tomography (CT) scans can provide excellent characterization of the fracture, and we subsequently recommend routine use of it for preoperative planning.
  - CT scanning of the elbow should be done at 1- to 2-mm intervals using axial or transverse cuts.

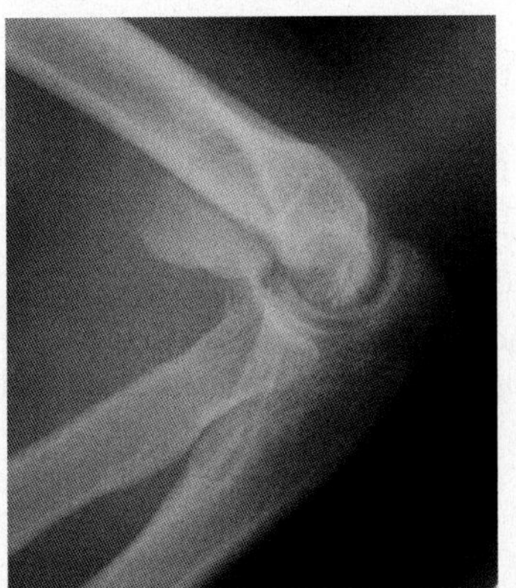
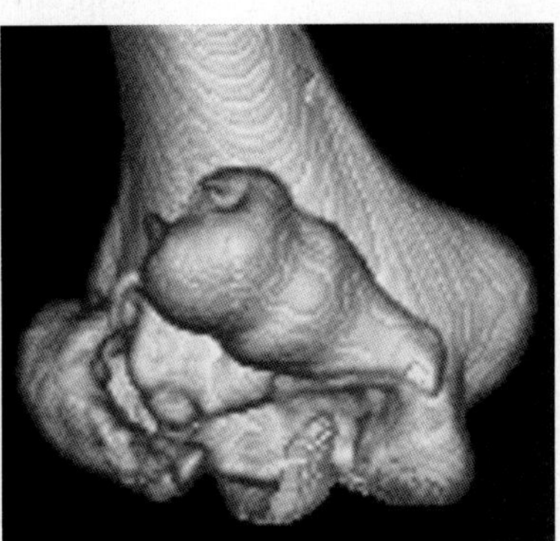
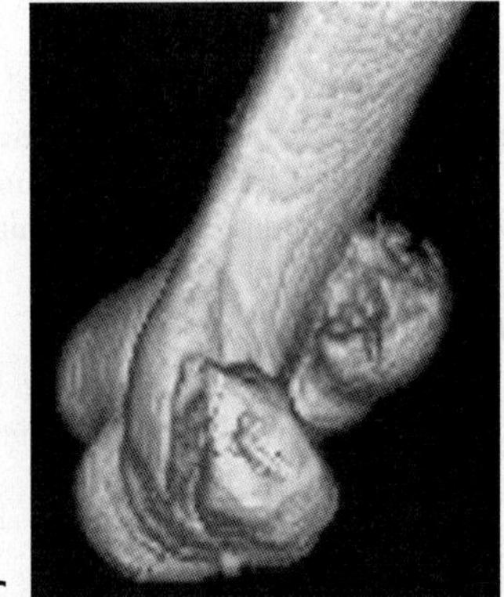

FIG 3 • **A.** Characteristic double arc sign on lateral radiographs of coronal shear fractures. **B,C.** 3-D CT reconstructions of a coronal shear fracture of the distal humerus.

- Three-dimensional (3-D) CT reconstructions provide the best detail and ability to appreciate the anatomic orientation of the fracture patterns and should be considered if 3-D imaging is available (**FIG 3B,C**).

DIFFERENTIAL DIAGNOSIS

- Radial head fracture
- Distal humeral lateral condyle fracture
- Elbow dislocation

NONOPERATIVE MANAGEMENT

- We recommend operative management for capitellum and capitellar–trochlear shear fractures.
- Truly nondisplaced and isolated capitellum fractures can be splinted for 3 weeks, followed by protected motion. However, close supervision is required, as this fracture is inherently unstable and prone to displacement.
- Closed reduction techniques, which have been described in the literature, should be performed with caution, and only complete anatomic reduction should be accepted for nonoperative management.[5,23]
- Capitellar–trochlear shear fractures should not be treated nonoperatively because of their inherent instability and the expectant loss of motion and posttraumatic arthrosis from residual articular incongruity.

SURGICAL MANAGEMENT

- The short-term goal of surgery is anatomic reduction and stable fixation of the fracture to allow for early motion without mechanical block.
- The long-term goals of surgery are a pain-free elbow with maximal motion, minimal stiffness, and avoidance of posttraumatic arthrosis.
- Capitellar fractures are uncommon, and the wide array of treatment options presented in the literature is based on relatively small series.
  - Treatment options include closed reduction,[5,23] open excision,[1,10,20] open reduction and internal fixation (ORIF), and arthroplasty.[6,11]
- With the improvement in techniques for fixation of small fragments and management of articular surfaces, ORIF has become the mainstay of treatment.
  - Advantages of ORIF include restoration of the native anatomy and function.
  - Disadvantages include stiffness and possible failure of fixation.
- In elderly patients, we do consider total elbow arthroplasty for complex intra-articular distal humerus fractures.[15,17]
  - Advantages include early return to function and motion.
  - Disadvantages include functional limitations.

Preoperative Planning

- Before proceeding with surgery, a thorough understanding of the fracture and its orientation should be obtained with the help of a CT scan, and if possible, 3-D reconstructions.
- The timing of surgery is important. Fractures preferably should be approached within 2 weeks, before osseous healing sets in, but after swelling has diminished.
- Ensure that the necessary implants and hardware are available.
- Reduction and fixation of the fracture will require minimum K-wires, articular or headless screws, and small fragment AO screws.
- Additional implants to consider include lateral column periarticular locking plates.
- An image intensifier should be used during surgery to confirm reduction of the fracture and proper positioning of implanted hardware.

Positioning

- General anesthesia is recommended for maximum soft tissue relaxation.
- The patient usually is positioned supine on the operating table, with the arm extended onto a radiolucent hand table, facilitating the lateral approach.
- Alternatively, a lateral or prone position can be considered, with the anterior surface of the elbow supported by a padded bolster if a posterior approach is planned.

Approach

- Either a lateral or posterior midline incision should be used.
- A lateral incision allows for direct visualization to a lateral approach to the elbow.
- A posterior incision also allows for access to the lateral approach to the elbow but also facilitates access to the posterior and medial approaches to the elbow, if necessary.
- Multiple intervals can be used in the lateral approach to the elbow, including the Kocher, Hotchkiss, and Wagner approaches.
  - We advocate the Wagner approach, which uses the interval between the extensor carpi radialis longus (ECRL) and the extensor digitorum communis (EDC), as it provides ready access to the anterolateral aspect of the radiocapitellar joint while protecting the insertion of the lateral collateral ligament complex.
  - To increase exposure, the lateral collateral ligament complex can be raised posteriorly sharply with a scalpel or osteotomized with a wedge of lateral epicondyle for subsequent suture anchor repair or internal fixation, respectively.
- Alternatively, the Kocher approach, which uses the interval between the extensor carpi ulnaris (ECU) and the anconeus can provide access to the capitellum while affording greater protection of the posterior interosseous nerve.
- In many cases, a capsular violation has occurred. This can be exploited and used as the interval to expose the fracture, thereby avoiding the need to cause an additional soft tissue defect.

Capitellar Fractures

Exposure

- The incision should begin 2 cm proximal to the lateral epicondyle and extend 3 to 4 cm distally toward the radial neck.
- If no large soft tissue or capsular defect is present, a direct lateral Wagner approach between the ECRL and EDC interval is recommended.
- The remaining common extensor origin is sharply raised off the lateral epicondyle and reflected anteriorly to expose the anterolateral elbow joint.
  - The capitellar fracture will most likely be found displaced anteriorly and proximally.
  - Care must be taken to avoid excessive proximal dissection and injury to the radial nerve traveling between the brachialis and brachioradialis.
  - Care must also be taken to avoid excessive distal dissection and injury to the posterior interosseous nerve by limiting dissection to only the radial neck. In addition, the forearm should be kept pronated, and no retractors should be placed anteriorly around the radial neck.
- Often, the lateral ligamentous complex will be avulsed from the distal aspect of the humerus, with or without some aspect of the lateral epicondyle.
  - This ligamentous violation can be exploited to improve exposure by hinging open the joint on the medial collateral ligament with a varus stress.
- The capitellar fracture fragment will typically be displaced anteriorly and proximally (**TECH FIG 1**).
- The fracture fragment will also typically be devoid of any soft tissue attachments and therefore prone to displacing out of the joint with excessive manipulation. Hence, care must be taken to avoid losing the fragment off the surgical field.

Reduction and Fixation

- The fragment is reduced under direct visualization, held with reduction tenaculums, and provisionally fixed with 0.045-inch K-wires. Alternatively, the guidewires that will be used for cannulated screw fixation can be used for provisional fixation as well.
- Internal fixation options include fixation with (1) headless compression screws from either an anterior or posterior direction, (2) cancellous screws from a posterior direction, (3) posterolateral column locking plate fixation, or (4) a hybrid construct using any or all of these techniques.
- Headless compression screws allow for guidewire-directed placement, direct fracture reduction, and maximal compression of the fracture fragment. Similarly, headless compression screws may be particularly useful in cases with fragments with less subchondral bone, such as type 2 and small type 1 fracture fragments (**TECH FIG 2A**). However, anterior screw placement can be challenging due to the thick anterior soft tissue envelope that will be present with an intact lateral collateral ligament complex. Alternatively, headless compression screws can be placed retrograde from a posterior direction to ease hardware placement (**TECH FIG 2B**). However, this direction does not achieve maximum fracture compression and can risk fracture distraction.
- Cancellous screws are best for fracture fragments with a large subchondral component as with type 1 fracture fragments. However, extending the dissection posteriorly around the lateral column

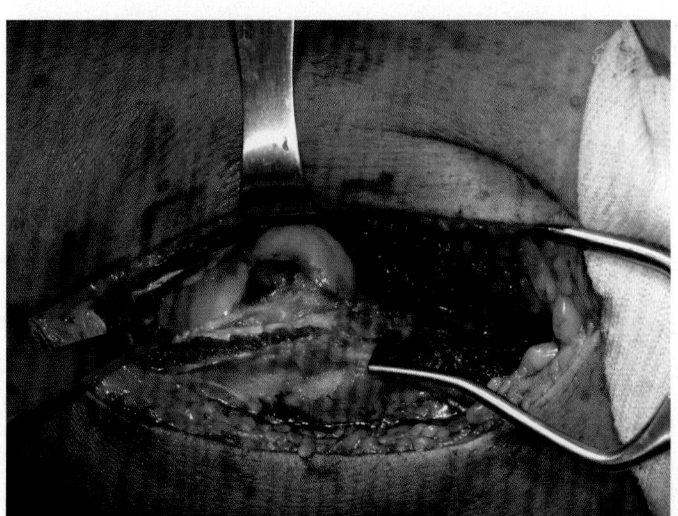

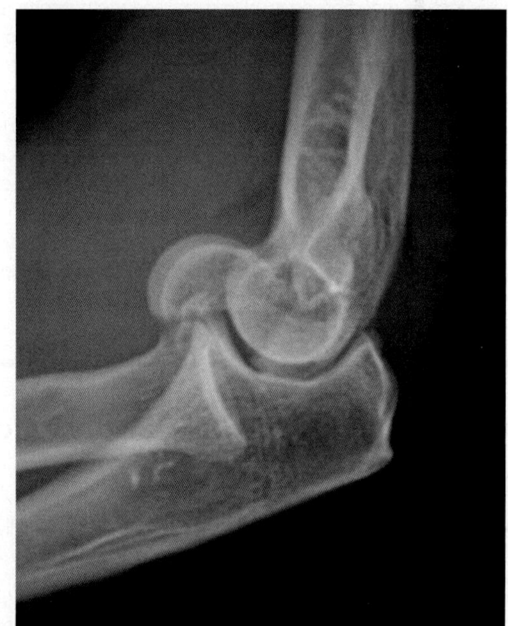

TECH FIG 1 • **A,B.** The displaced capitellar fracture fragment will typically be displaced anteriorly and proximally and will be devoid of any soft tissue attachments.

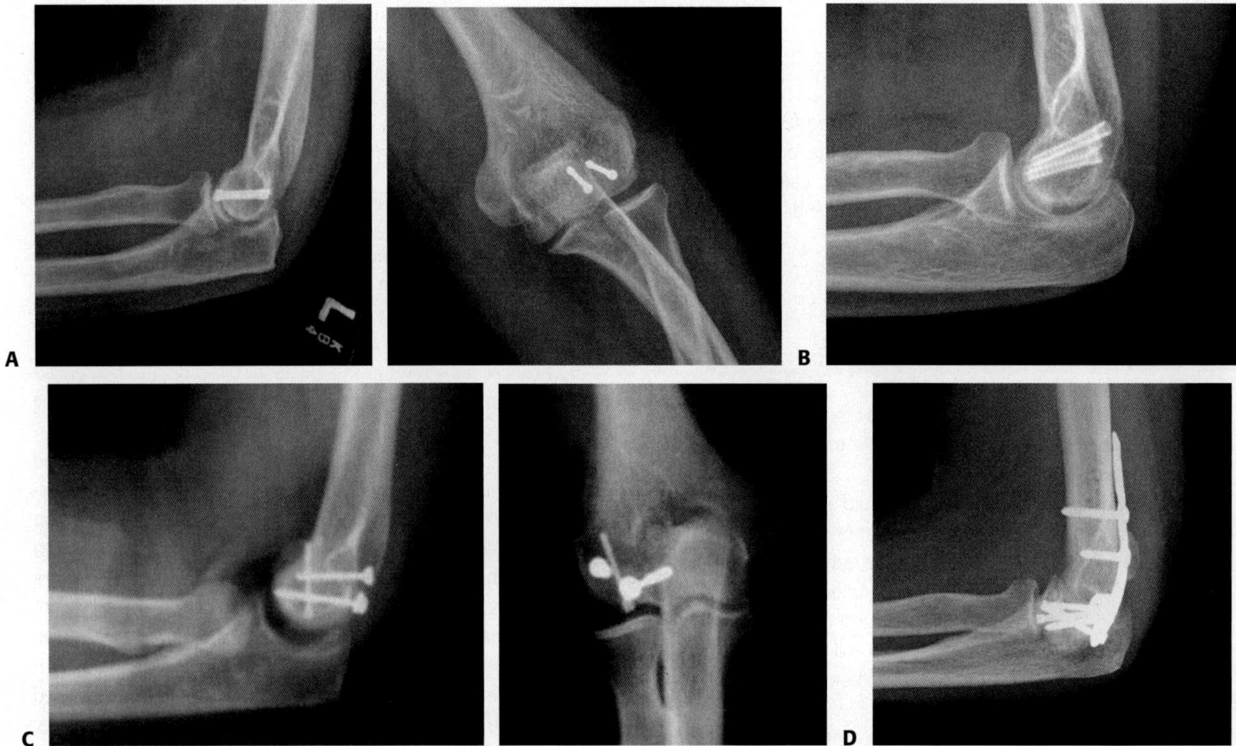

TECH FIG 2 • Fixation of capitellar fractures with (**A**) anteriorly placed headless compression screws, (**B**) posteriorly placed headless compression screws, (**C**) combination of a headless screw anteriorly and cancellous screws posteriorly, and (**D**) hybrid fixation using anteriorly placed headless compression screws followed by neutralization of the fracture with a locked periarticular plate applied posteriorly.

theoretically increases the risk of osteonecrosis (**TECH FIG 2C**). We recommend using partially threaded cannulated screw to optimize fracture reduction, screw placement, and fracture compression.

- Use of a periarticular locking plate alone or in a hybrid construct with headless compression screws can be of value to improve the stability of the construct (**TECH FIG 2D**). This technique will require greater posterior dissection, therefore increasing the theoretical risk of osteonecrosis. However, application of a posterolateral plate can provide posterior stability in cases with posterior cortical extension or comminution.
- Excision of fracture fragments can be considered in type 2 fractures with small, thin articular pieces and type 3 comminuted fractures where the fragments are not amenable to internal fixation.
- Fragment reduction and hardware position should be confirmed by image intensifier.
- Unrestricted forearm rotation and elbow flexion–extension without mechanical block or catching should be confirmed intraoperatively.
- If the lateral collateral ligament complex is found to be avulsed, it should be repaired back to the lateral epicondyle with drill holes and heavy nonabsorbable sutures or suture anchors.
- The capsule should be closed.
- The retracted extensor origin should be relaxed and closed to the surrounding soft tissue.

Capitellar–Trochlear Shear Fractures

Exposure

- A posterior midline incision should be used, but initially, a lateral approach to the joint will be performed.
  - A posterior incision provides extensile exposure, access to both sides of the elbow, and ease of osteotomy, if necessary (**TECH FIG 3A**).
- A direct lateral Wagner approach between the ECRL and EDC interval is recommended.
- The remaining common extensor origin is sharply raised off the lateral epicondyle and reflected anteriorly to expose the anterolateral elbow joint. Alternatively, a capsular violation may be present that can be exploited (**TECH FIG 3B**).
- The capitellar–trochlear shear fracture will most likely be found displaced anteriorly and proximally.
  - Care must be taken to avoid excessive proximal dissection and injury to the radial nerve traveling between the brachialis and brachioradialis.
  - Care must also be taken to avoid excessive distal dissection and injury to the posterior interosseous nerve by limiting dissection to only the radial neck. In addition, the forearm should be kept pronated, and no retractors should be placed anteriorly around the radial neck.

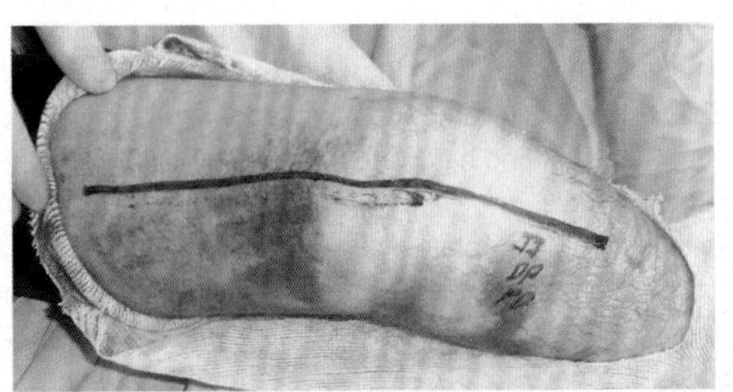
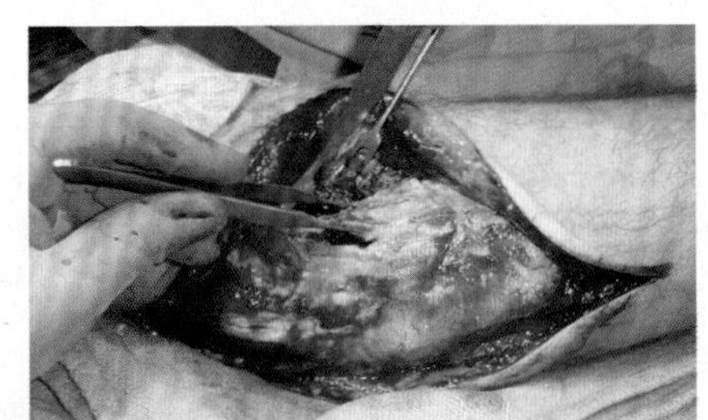
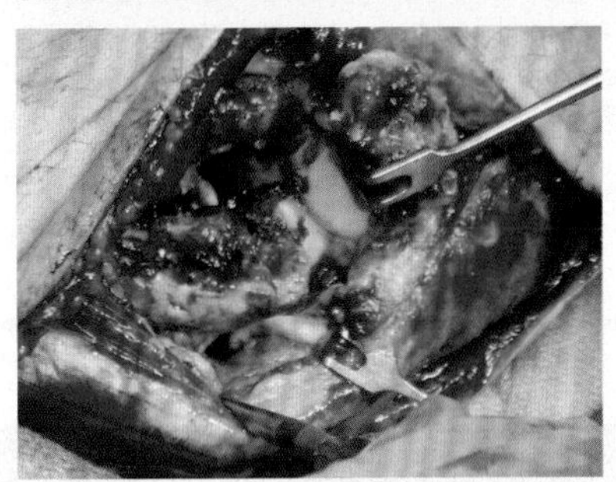
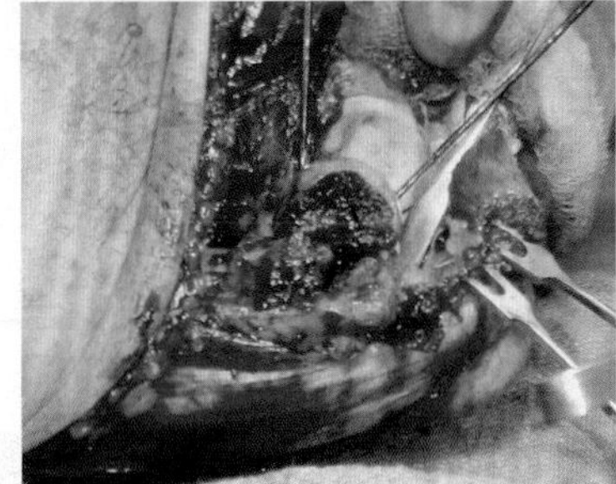

TECH FIG 3 • A. Posterior midline incision used for capitellar–trochlear shear fractures. **B.** Deep lateral approach to the elbow using the capsular violation to enter the radiocapitellar joint. **C.** The fracture fragments tend to displace proximally and internally rotate. Note, avulsion of the lateral epicondyle with subsequent retraction allowing for excellent visualization. **D.** The fracture is reduced and provisionally pinned with 0.045-inch K-wires.

- Often, the lateral ligamentous complex will be avulsed from the distal aspect of the humerus, with or without some aspect of the lateral epicondyle.
  - This ligamentous violation can be exploited to improve exposure by hinging open the joint on the medial collateral ligament with a varus stress.
  - Alternatively, a formal lateral epicondyle osteotomy can be performed to enhance visualization while maintaining the integrity of the lateral ligamentous complex.
  - Additionally, a formal olecranon osteotomy may be performed to improve visualization and fixation of fractures extending medially and posteriorly.
- The fracture fragments should now be visualized and accounted for. They are most commonly displaced proximally and internally rotated (**TECH FIG 3C**).

Reduction and Fixation

- The fragment is reduced under direct visualization, held with reduction tenaculums, and provisionally fixed with 0.045-inch K-wires (**TECH FIG 3D**).
- Inability to reduce the fracture anatomically may represent fracture impaction, requiring either disimpaction or bone grafting, or both.
- Internal fixation options include fixation with (1) headless compression screws from either an anterior or posterior direction, (2) cancellous screws from a posterior direction, (3) posterolateral column locking plate fixation, or (4) a hybrid construct using any or all of these techniques.
- Headless compression screws allow for guidewire-directed placement, direct fracture reduction, and maximal compression of the fracture fragment (**TECH FIG 4A**). Similarly, headless

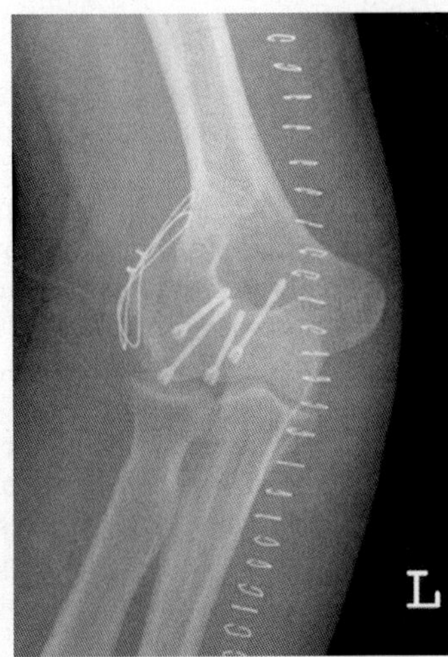

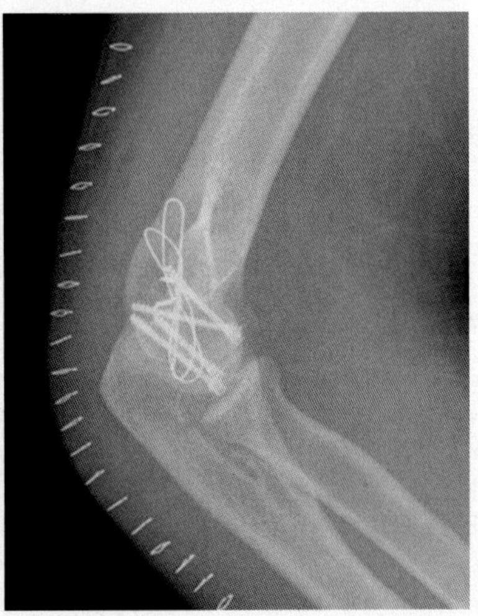
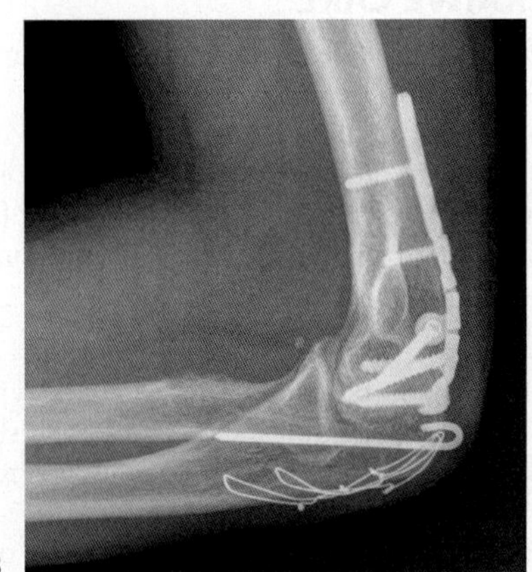

TECH FIG 4 • Postoperative radiographs illustrating (**A**) repair of the lateral epicondyle and anterior fixation of a capitellar–trochlear shear fracture with multiple headless compression screws. Alternatively, (**B**) note repair of a different capitellar–trochlear shear fracture using a periarticular locking plate applied to the posterolateral aspect of the distal humerus, facilitated with an olecranon osteotomy.

compression screws may be particularly useful in cases with fragments with less subchondral bone, such as type 2 and small type 1 fracture fragments.

- Cancellous screws are best for fracture fragments with a large subchondral component as with type 1 fracture fragments. However, extending the dissection posteriorly around the lateral column theoretically increases the risk of osteonecrosis. We recommend using partially threaded cannulated screw to optimize fracture reduction, screw placement, and fracture compression.
- Use of a periarticular locking plate alone or in a hybrid construct with headless compression screws can be of value to improve the stability of the construct (**TECH FIG 4B**). This technique will require greater posterior dissection, therefore increasing the theoretical risk of osteonecrosis. However, application of a posterolateral plate can provide posterior stability in cases with posterior cortical extension or comminution.
- Fragment reduction and hardware position should be confirmed by image intensifier.
- Unrestricted forearm rotation and elbow flexion–extension without mechanical block or catching should be confirmed intraoperatively.
- The lateral epicondyle, if avulsed or osteotomized, should be repaired with a tension band technique or plate and screws.
- The capsule should be closed.
- The interval and released extensor origin should be relaxed and closed to the surrounding soft tissue.

PEARLS AND PITFALLS

Diagnosis	■ Diligence should be paid to identifying concomitant injuries such as elbow dislocations, radial head fractures, and ligamentous instability.
Imaging	■ Plain radiographs are insufficient, and a CT scan should be considered routinely. ■ Order 3-D reconstructions if possible.
Nonoperative management	■ Nonoperative management should be chosen cautiously. Anatomic and stable reduction of the fracture is necessary. Otherwise, a painful elbow with restricted motion may result. ■ We do not recommend nonoperative management of any capitellar–trochlear shear fractures.
Surgical management	■ Lateral epicondyle osteotomy can enhance exposure. ■ A posterior skin incision will afford access to both sides of the joint and an olecranon osteotomy, if necessary. ■ Inability to reduce the fracture anatomically may represent impaction of the lateral column and require disimpaction or bone grafting. ■ Excision of small comminuted fragments that cannot be fixed internally is preferred over nonanatomic reduction and malunion. ■ Concomitant fractures and ligamentous injuries should be treated simultaneously to optimize outcomes.
Postoperative management	■ Stable fixation should be sought to facilitate early motion. ■ Heterotopic ossification is common after elbow fractures, and prophylaxis with nonsteroidal anti-inflammatory drugs should be considered.

POSTOPERATIVE CARE

- If secure fixation has been obtained, immediate mobilization can be initiated postoperatively.
- If fixation is tenuous, splint or cast the elbow for 3 to 4 weeks, followed by active and assisted range-of-motion exercises. Some advocate the use of hinged external fixator for complex articular fractures or with severe ligamentous injuries.[12]

OUTCOMES

- Focusing initially on outcomes after ORIF of types 1 and 2 capitellar fractures, multiple small series have shown good results using Herbert screws in an anterior to posterior direction.[7,16,18,24]
- More recently, Mahirogullari et al[19] reported on 11 cases of type 1 capitellum fractures treated with Herbert screws, which yielded 8 excellent and 3 good results. They recommended fixation in a posterior to anterior direction with at least two Herbert screws.
- Reported outcomes on type 4 capitellar–trochlear shear fractures are limited. McKee et al[21] originally described this pattern and reported on 6 cases.
  - Each case involved an extended lateral Kocher approach and fixation with Herbert screws from an anterior to posterior direction. Good or excellent results were achieved in all cases, with average elbow motion of 15 to 141 degrees, and forearm rotation of 83 degrees pronation, and 84 degrees supination.
- Ring and Jupiter examined 21 cases of articular fractures of the distal humerus treated with Herbert screw fixation and found 4 excellent results, 12 good results, and 5 fair results.
  - All of the fractures healed and had an average range of motion of 96 degrees. No ulnohumeral instability, arthrosis, or osteonecrosis was reported.
- The authors stressed the importance of proper evaluation of these fractures and awareness that apparent capitellum fractures often are complex articular fractures of the distal humerus.[25]

- Dubberley et al[8] further subclassified type 4 fractures in their series of 28 cases. They achieved an average range of motion of flexion–extension of 25 degrees less than the contralateral elbow and 4 degrees of supination–pronation less than the contralateral elbow.
  - Two comminuted cases required conversion to a total elbow arthroplasty.
  - Varied fixation methods were used, including Herbert screws, cancellous screws, absorbable pins, and supplementation with K-wires.
- Ruchelsman and colleagues[26,27] reported a case series of 16 patients that were treated with ORIF.
- All patients achieved full forearm rotation and all but two had functional arc of elbow range of motion.
- They reported 15 good to excellent results and one fair result.
- The authors did not find association between concomitant radial head fracture and worse outcomes.
- Sen and colleagues[28] reported internal fixation of isolated trochlear fractures with promising results in a small case series.
- Comminuted fractures (Dubberley type B) have been shown to be more prone to inferior outcomes complicated by avascular necrosis, degenerative arthritis, and heterotopic ossification.[9]

COMPLICATIONS

- The most common complication of capitellar fractures is loss of elbow motion and residual pain. The compromised motion most commonly is manifested in loss of flexion and extension.
- Ulnar neuropathy has been noted after ORIF, and some recommend routine ulnar nerve decompression.[25] This is especially important in capitellar–trochlear shear fractures, as hinging of the elbow on the medial side increases the risk of ulnar nerve compression.
- Osteonecrosis may occur from the initial fracture displacement or surgical exposure. Blood is supplied to the capitellum from a posterior to anterior direction and may be compromised by surgical dissection.
  - In symptomatic cases in which revascularization after fixation has not occurred, delayed excision is indicated.
- Malunions may occur when the patient has delayed seeking treatment, when inadequate reduction or loss of closed reduction occurs, or after ORIF. Malunions result in loss of motion and may require excision of the fragment and soft tissue releases.
- Nonunions may occur, although this is uncommon. They most likely result secondary to inadequate reduction or lack of revascularization of the fragment.

REFERENCES

1. Alvarez E, Patel M, Nimberg P, et al. Fractures of the capitulum humeri. J Bone Joint Surg Am 1975;57(8):1093–1096.
2. Broberg MA, Morrey BF. Results of delayed excision of the radial head after fracture. J Bone Joint Surg Am 1986;68(5):669–674.
3. Brouwer KM, Jupiter JB, Ring D. Nonunion of operatively treated capitellum and trochlear fractures. J Hand Surg Am 2011;36(5): 804–807.
4. Bryan RS, Morrey BF. Fractures of the distal humerus. In: Morrey BF, ed. The Elbow and Its Disorders. Philadelphia: WB Saunders, 1985:302–399.
5. Christopher F, Bushnell L. Conservative treatment of fractures of the capitellum. J Bone Joint Surg 1935;17:489–492.
6. Cobb TK, Morrey BF. Total elbow arthroplasty as primary treatment for distal humerus fractures in elderly patients. J Bone Joint Surg Am 1997;79(6):826–832.
7. Collert S. Surgical management of fracture of the capitulum humeri. Acta Orthop Scand 1977;48:603–606.
8. Dubberley JH, Faber KJ, Macdermid JC, et al. Outcome after open reduction and internal fixation of capitellar and trochlear fractures. J Bone Joint Surg Am 2006;88(1):46–54.
9. Durakbasa MO, Gumussuyu G, Gungor M, et al. Distal humeral coronal plane fractures: management, complications and outcome. J Shoulder Elbow Surg 2013;22(4):560–566.
10. Fowles JV, Kassab MT. Fracture of the capitulum humeri. Treatment by excision. J Bone Joint Surg Am 1975;56(4):794–798.
11. Garcia JA, Mykula R, Stanley D. Complex fractures of the distal humerus in the elderly. The role of total elbow replacement as primary treatment. J Bone Joint Surg Br 2002;84(6):812–816.
12. Giannicola G, Sacchetti FM, Greco A, et al. Open reduction and internal fixation combined with hinged elbow fixator in capitellum and trochlea fractures. Acta Orthop 2010;81(2):228–233.
13. Greenspan A, Norman A. The radial head, capitellum view: useful technique in elbow trauma. AJR Am J Roentgenol 1982;138:1186–1188.
14. Hahn NF. Fall von einer besonderes Varietat der Frakturen des Ellenbogens. Z Wund Geburt 1853;6:185.
15. Kamineni S, Morrey BF. Distal humeral fractures treated with noncustom total elbow replacement. Surgical technique. J Bone Joint Surg Am 2005;87(suppl 1)(pt 1):41–50.
16. Lansinger O, Mare K. Fracture of the capitulum humeri. Acta Orthop Scand 1981;52:39–44.
17. Lee JJ, Lawton JN. Coronal shear fractures of the distal humerus. J Hand Surg Am 2012;37(11):2412–2417.
18. Liberman N, Katz T, Howard CV, et al. Fixation of capitellar fractures with Herbert screws. Arch Orthop Trauma Surg 1991;110:155–157.
19. Mahirogullari M, Kiral A, Solakoglu C, et al. Treatment of fractures of the humeral capitellum using Herbert screws. J Hand Surg Br 2006;31:320–325.
20. Mazel MS. Fracture of the capitellum. J Bone Joint Surg 1935;17: 483–488.
21. McKee MD, Jupiter JB, Bamberger HB. Coronal shear fractures of the distal end of the humerus. J Bone Joint Surg Am 1996;78(1):49–54.
22. Milch H. Fractures and fracture-dislocations of the humeral condyles. J Trauma 1964;13:882–886.
23. Ochner RS, Bloom H, Palumbo RC, et al. Closed reduction of coronal fractures of the capitellum. J Trauma 1996;40:199–203.
24. Richards RR, Khoury GW, Burke FD, et al. Internal fixation of capitellar fractures using Herbert screw: a report of four cases. Can J Surg 1987;30:188–191.
25. Ring D, Jupiter JB, Gulotta L. Articular fractures of the distal part of the humerus. J Bone Joint Surg Am 2003;85-A(2):232–238.
26. Ruchelsman DE, Tejwani NC, Kwon YW, et al. Open reduction and internal fixation of capitellar fractures with headless screws. J Bone Joint Surg Am 2008;90(6):1321–1329.
27. Ruchelsman DE, Tejwani NC, Kwon YW, et al. Open reduction and internal fixation of capitellar fractures with headless screws. Surgical technique. J Bone Joint Surg Am 2009;91(suppl 2, pt 1):38–49.
28. Sen RK, Tripahty SK, Goyal T, et al. Coronal shear fracture of the humeral trochlea. J Orthop Surg 2013;21(1):82–86.
29. Steinthal D. Die isolirte Fraktur der eminentia Capetala in Ellengogelenk. Zentralk Chir 1898;15:17.
30. Yamaguchi K, Sweet FA, Bindra R, et al. The extraosseous and intraosseous arterial anatomy of the adult elbow. J Bone Joint Surg Am 1997;79(11):1653–1662.

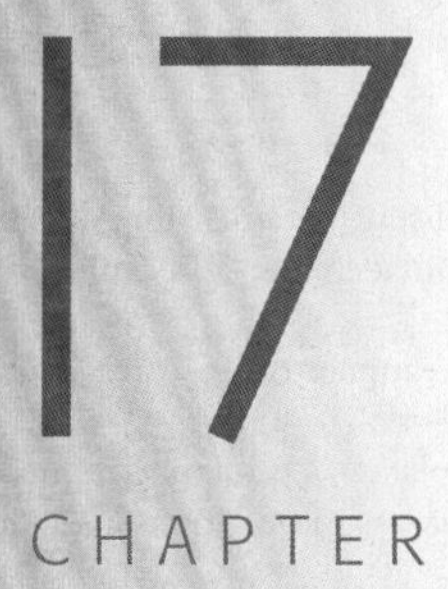

CHAPTER 17

Elbow Replacement for Acute Trauma

Srinath Kamineni and Harikrishna Ankem

DEFINITION

- Most comminuted elbow fractures have associated soft tissue injuries, which are often of equal or greater importance to the bony injury.
- The goal when treating acute elbow fractures is that of anatomic open reduction and internal fixation (ORIF) with management of any soft tissue injuries.
- An acute elbow arthroplasty should be considered only if ORIF is unlikely to achieve a predictably good functional outcome in the older age groups.
- In the majority of cases, elbow replacements for the treatment of acute fractures should be limited to the physiologically elderly patient with low functional demands.

ANATOMY

- The bony anatomy of the elbow consists of the distal humerus, proximal ulna, and proximal radius.
- Important soft tissue stabilizers include the medial and lateral ligamentous complexes and surrounding musculature, especially the brachialis, common flexor and common extensor masses, and triceps.
- The ulnar nerve is tethered to the medial condylar–epicondylar fragment by the cubital tunnel retinaculum distally and the arcade of Struthers proximally.

PATHOGENESIS

- Elbow injuries are often the result of direct impact—for example, a direct blow on the elbow during a fall.
- Knowing the energy of the fracture is important to gauge the likelihood of associated injuries.
- Less energy is required to create a comminuted fracture in elderly and osteoporotic individuals, but muscular injuries of the triceps and brachialis are common, with a subsequent influence on the functional outcome.
- The ulnar nerve displaces with the medial fragment. As a consequence, the nerve may kink, leading to a local nerve injury. Nerve lacerations are an uncommon consequence of comminuted distal humeral fractures.

NATURAL HISTORY

- Most distal humeral fractures are treatable with either nonoperative management or ORIF. Challenging fracture subgroups include fractures that involve articular surfaces and are highly comminuted, although younger patients (younger than 65 years old) are generally not considered candidates for total joint replacements, partial joint replacements are an emerging solution.[22]
- Many direct and indirect soft tissue complications may ensue, including neurovascular entrapment,[8,12] muscle tears leading to myositis ossificans,[12,18,23] and soft tissue contracture with joint stiffness.
- There is some evidence to suggest that congruently reducing and fixing a comminuted intra-articular distal humeral fracture does not eliminate the risk of posttraumatic arthritis,[13] although, where possible, ORIF with anatomic congruity should remain the primary goal.

PATIENT HISTORY AND PHYSICAL FINDINGS

- The physical examination (**FIG 1**) should be performed gently in the presence of fractures, especially when comminution suggests the possibility of neurovascular injury.
- A complete examination of the elbow should also include evaluation of associated injuries. It should begin away from the elbow, progressing toward it, for example, shoulder/wrist with progression toward the elbow.
- The following associated injuries should be ruled out:
  - Distal radial and scaphoid fractures: Because the most common mechanism of injury is a fall onto an outstretched hand, the energy transfer of the fall begins in the extended wrist, through the distal radius and scaphoid. Direct palpation of the distal radius should be done, and anatomic snuffbox tenderness should be elicited. Palpation of the

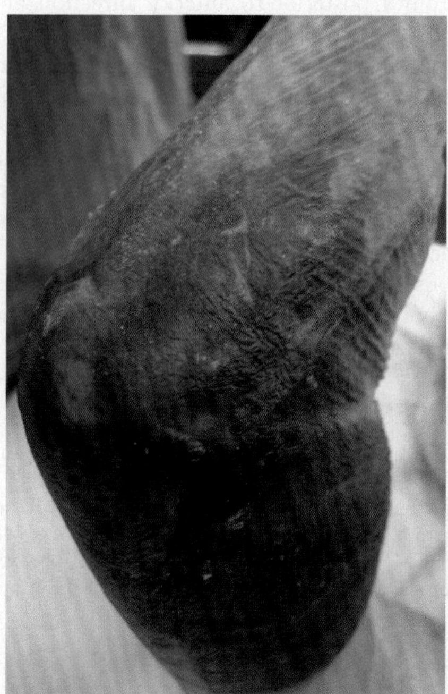

FIG 1 • Typical appearance of an elbow with an underlying fracture with extensive swelling and bruising.

scaphoid tubercle and ulnar and radial deviation of the wrist may also identify a scaphoid injury.

- Distal radioulnar joint disruption: Ballottement of the ulnar head should be done in the volar and dorsal directions, in pronation and supination. A disrupted joint is often painful with such ballottement, and the ulnar head may be prominent with the forearm in pronation.
- Fracture extension beyond the elbow: The examiner should palpate the ulnar shaft, along its subcutaneous border, from the wrist to the olecranon.
- Interosseous membrane injury: Palpating the interval between the bones of the forearm is not a sensitive examination but can raise suspicion for an Essex-Lopresti injury, leading to further imaging. If an interosseous membrane disruption is present, this will influence the type of implant used for elbow replacement (one with a radial head replacement), but the pathology is not commonly described.

IMAGING AND DIAGNOSTIC STUDIES

- Plain radiographs, including anteroposterior (AP) and lateral views (**FIG 2**) of the elbow and both wrists, should be obtained. The elbow view may have to be taken in a protective splint or plaster backslab for patient comfort.
- Elbow radiographs will allow initial assessment of the degree of comminution and may indicate the presence of decreased bone mineral density.
- Bilateral wrist views will indicate the presence of an axial (interosseous membrane) injury if the ulnar head is in positive variance compared to the contralateral uninjured wrist.
- Plain tomograms are of use in improving the understanding of the fracture configuration, but an alternative would be a computed tomography (CT) scan. With the latter, the surgeon can view a three-dimensional reconstruction, which is a useful surgical planning tool for ORIF.
- If there is evidence on physical examination of a neurologic injury, it is prudent to document its extent with a carefully performed neurologic examination.

DIFFERENTIAL DIAGNOSIS

- Nonunion
- Ligamentous disruption
- Fracture-dislocation

NONOPERATIVE MANAGEMENT

- The "bag-of-bones" technique is a nonoperative method of treatment described by Eastwood[7] that encourages the compressive molding of the comminuted distal humeral fracture fragments.
- Subsequent rehabilitation with collar and cuff support achieves substandard but acceptable results only in the elderly and debilitated group of patients who have almost no demand on elbow function.
- This type of treatment does not achieve acceptable results with respect to stability and strength in younger patients.

SURGICAL MANAGEMENT

Open Reduction and Internal Fixation

- ORIF has been widely documented for comminuted fractures of the distal humerus.
- Some reported series demonstrate good results with fixation of such challenging fractures, with better results predominantly in the younger age groups.[19,24] Rarely are good results achieved in the elderly, osteoporotic group.[13]
- Many series report less than satisfactory outcomes in the elderly treated by operative fixation.[19]
- A direct comparison of internal fixation to primary total elbow replacement in the elderly osteoporotic group revealed that replacement produced no poor results and no need for revision surgery at 2 years of follow-up. The internal fixation group produced three poor results requiring revision to a total elbow replacement.[10]

Elbow Arthroplasty

- When a distal humerus fracture is not reliably reconstructable, arthroplasty becomes a valid treatment option.
- Elbow replacement following a failed attempt at fixation has proven to have a significantly worse outcome than if the arthroplasty was performed initially.[9]
- There are a number of studies that support the concept of an acute total elbow arthroplasty in select patients with comminuted fractures of the distal humerus.[6,9,16]
- The more traditional form of replacement for the elderly and low-demand population with an unreconstructable distal humerus fracture is the total elbow arthroplasty.

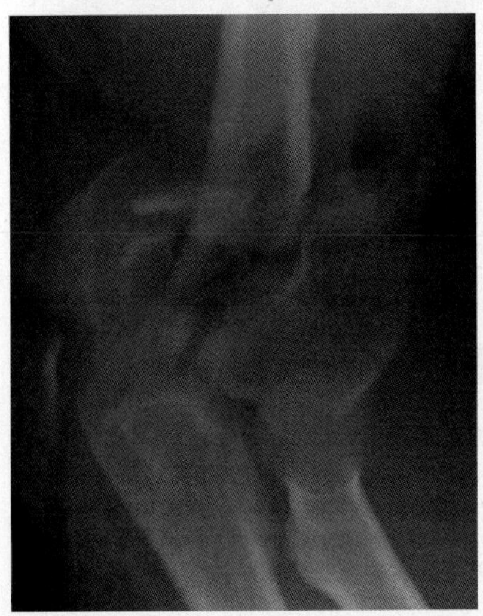

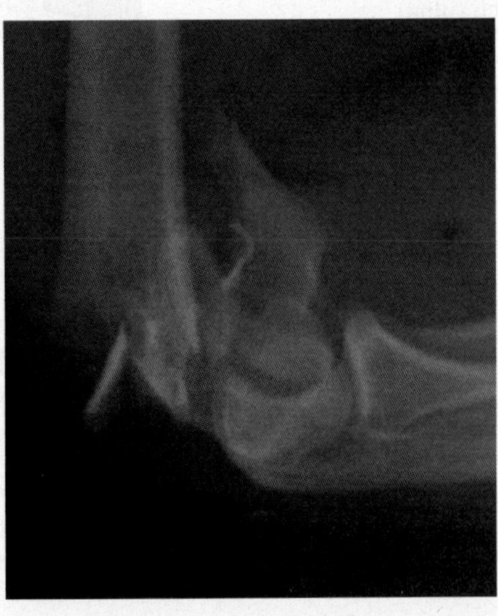

FIG 2 • Standard AP (**A**) and lateral (**B**) plain radiographs.

- A more recent innovation has been the replacement of the distal humerus (hemiarthroplasty) to preserve an intact ulna and radial head.[20] This procedure is not U.S. Food and Drug Administration (FDA) approved and so should be considered experimental and not for general consideration, especially because the elbow joint is variable and highly congruent in its topography, which differs from many of the standard implants used for acute fractures. However, there is a definite place within the algorithm of acute fracture management for such a surgical technique and implant and is still available outside the United States for this indication.

Indications and Contraindications (Total Elbow Arthroplasty)

- Indications for acute total elbow arthroplasty
  - Comminuted, unreconstructable distal humerus fracture
  - Physiologically elderly patient
  - Low-demand patient
  - Poor quality/injured cartilage of ulna
- Absolute contraindications for acute joint replacement (total or hemi)
  - Infection (overt)
  - Lack of soft tissue coverage (skin, muscle)
- Relative contraindications for acute joint replacement
  - Infection in distant body part
  - Contaminated wound
  - Neurologic injury involving the elbow flexors

Indications and Contraindications (Distal Humeral Hemiarthroplasty)

- Indications for acute elbow hemiarthroplasty
  - Unreconstructable distal humeral fracture (C3)
  - Unreconstructable combined fractures of capitellum and trochlea
  - Well-preserved cartilage of ulna
  - Very low bicondylar T fracture of distal humerus
    - Young patient
    - Active patient
  - Repairable or intact collateral ligaments (may require reconstruction of the medial and lateral supracondylar columns)
  - Repairable or intact radial head
- Contraindications for acute elbow hemiarthroplasty
  - Unreconstructable medial/lateral columns
  - Articular damage to greater sigmoid notch (ulna)
  - Osteoporotic/osteopenic ulna (relative)

Preoperative Planning

- Standard radiographs should be obtained (AP and lateral).
- If doubt exists regarding the ability to anatomically repair the fracture, then a CT scan should be requested to assess the degree of comminution and the fracture line orientation.
- An assessment of humeral shaft bone loss is important in planning the implant design that might be considered. If the degree of loss is greater than the articular condylar fragments, an implant that has the ability to restore humeral length will be more appropriate. If an unreconstructable fracture of the humeral articular surfaces without humeral shaft bone loss is encountered, an implant with the ability to resurface the articular surfaces as a hemiarthroplasty or a resurfacing ulnotrochlear replacement can be considered, but the former implantation technique should be regarded as an off-label and experimental procedure.
- Humeral shaft length loss of 2 cm can be tolerated and standard implants used.
- Humeral shaft length loss of greater than 2 cm can be restored with implant designs with anterior flanges, especially those with extended flanges that allow restoration of humeral length.
- The surgeon should assess the intramedullary canal dimensions of the humerus and ulna. This will help to plan the requirement of extra small diameter.
- Neurovascular status of the limb should be fully assessed and documented in the clinical notes.

Patient Positioning

- Two methods of patient positioning can be used, depending on surgeon comfort and the access required.
  - Supine: The arm is draped for maximum maneuverability. During the procedure, the arm is supported on a large rolled towel placed on the patient's upper thorax, carefully avoiding the endotracheal tube, stabilized by an assistant. In this position the surgeon stands on the side of the patient's injured limb (**FIG 3A**).
  - Lateral decubitus: The arm is positioned on an arm support, thereby minimizing the need for an assistant, but this setup is less maneuverable. In this position, the surgeon stands on the opposite side of the patient's injured limb (**FIG 3B**).

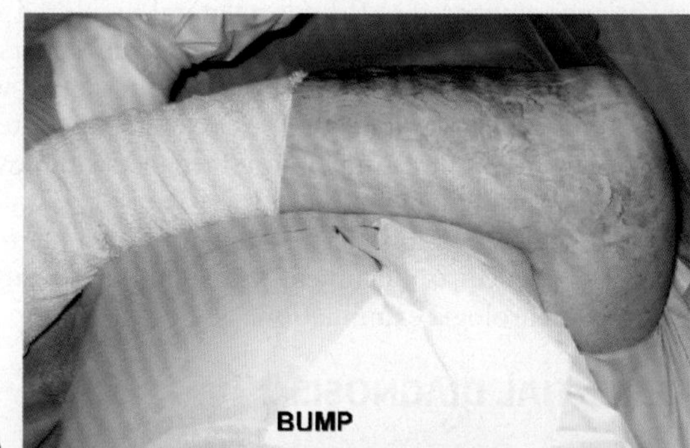

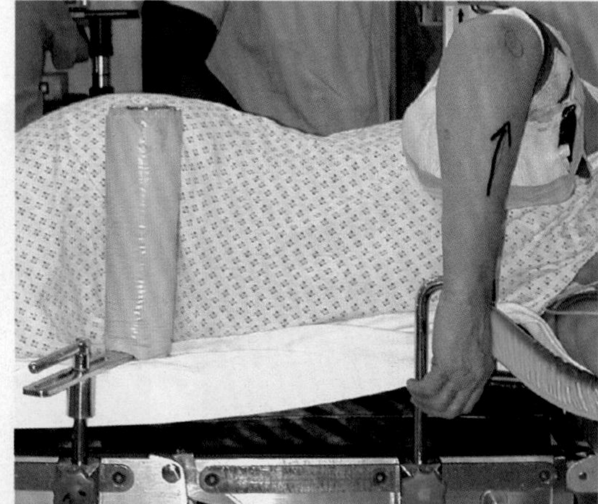

FIG 3 • **A.** Patient positioned in a supine position. The elbow is isolated and placed on a roll of towel placed on the patient's chest and stabilized by an assistant. The surgeon must take care to avoid the neck and anesthetic equipment. **B.** Patient positioned in a lateral decubitus position with the elbow draped over an arm support.

Surgical Approach

- Two main surgical approaches are useful for acute total elbow arthroplasty:
  - "Triceps on" (eg, Alonso-Llames, paratricipetal)
  - "Triceps off" (eg, Bryan-Morrey)
- The triceps should be carefully managed in either approach, and it often has a thin tendon, especially in older patients and those with rheumatoid arthritis. The triceps tendon should be dissected from the olecranon with a small curved scalpel blade, maintained perpendicular to the interface between the tendon and bone.

Incision and Dissection

- Make a midline longitudinal skin incision (**TECH FIG 1A**), with a gentle curve to avoid the olecranon weight-bearing prominence. Extend the incision 5 cm distal to and proximal to the prominence of the olecranon tip.
- Develop the full-thickness medial and lateral skin flaps (**TECH FIG 1B**) and define the medial and lateral borders of the triceps (**TECH FIG 1C,D**).
- At the medial border, define and partially neurolyse the ulnar nerve, and mark and handle it with a tied vessel loop (without an attached hemostat because its constant weight may cause inadvertent nerve injury) (**TECH FIG 1E**).
- Remain in the medial gutter to extend the dissection distally to define the medial fracture fragment. Release the flexor–pronator mass and medial collateral ligament from the medial epicondyle and resect this bony fragment (**TECH FIG 1F**).

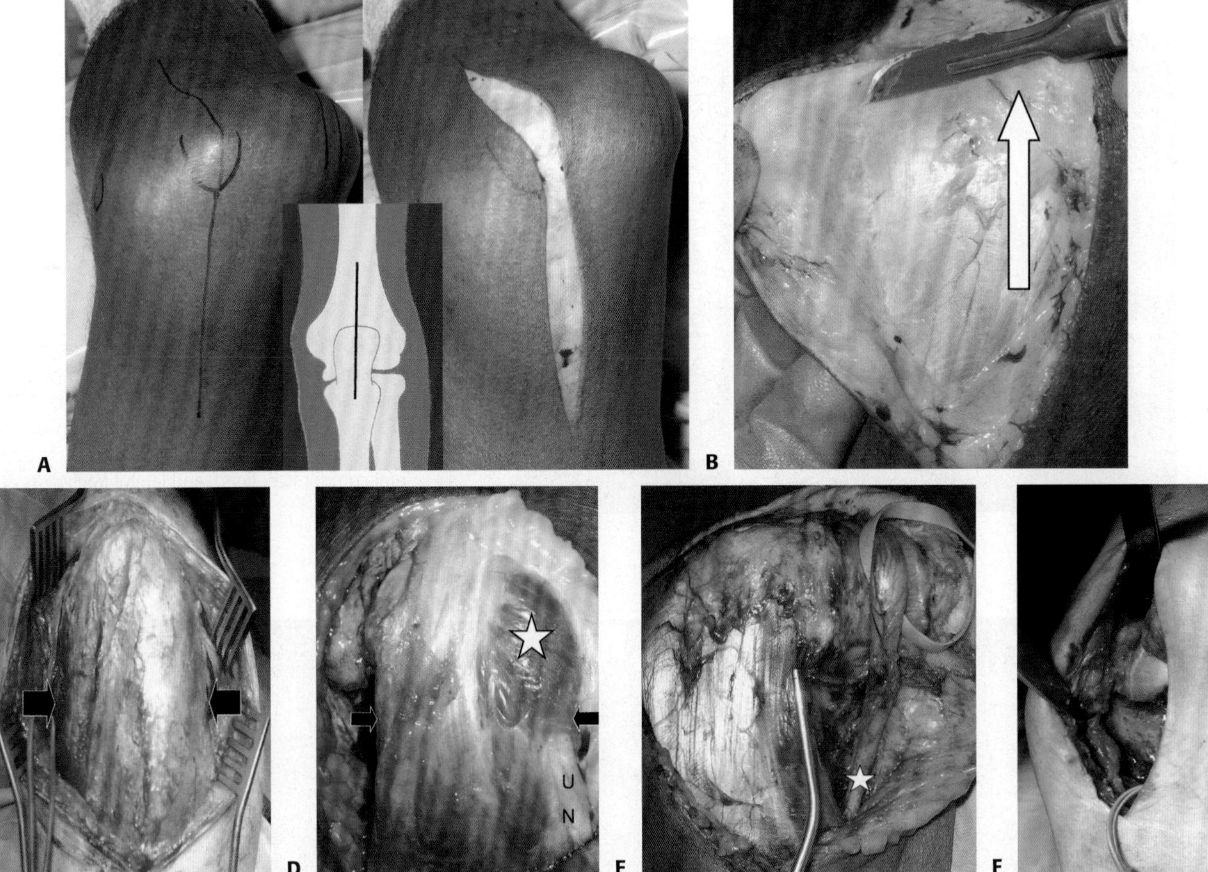

TECH FIG 1 • **A.** Skin incision is posteriorly longitudinal, with or without a small diversion to avoid the "point" of the olecranon. **B.** Raising the skin should aim to maintain the full thickness of the flaps by using the "flat knife" technique. **C.** The medial and lateral borders of the triceps are defined (*arrows*). **D.** This patient had an anconeus epitrochlearis (*star*) in relation to the ulnar nerve (*UN*). **E.** A vessel loop is used to maneuver the nerve without an attached clip. **F.** The medial fragment of the fracture is removed once all the soft tissues are released from it, and the nerve is gently retracted to ensure tension-free removal.

Triceps Management

Triceps On (Triceps Preserving)

- With the ulnar nerve gently medially retracted, use a periosteal elevator to define the plane between the medial triceps and the posterior humerus, proximally to the triceps attachment at the olecranon. Carry the dissection across the posterior humerus to the lateral aspect of the triceps, exiting posteriorly to the lateral intermuscular septum. Use the elevator to lift the triceps, with blunt dissection, by sliding the shaft of the elevator proximal and distal in the interface (**TECH FIG 2A**).
- Develop the lateral triceps–lateral intermuscular septum margin to the lateral attachment of the triceps on the olecranon. Release the common extensors and lateral collateral ligament complex from the lateral fracture fragment. Resect the lateral fracture fragments, having firstly cleared them of soft tissue attachments (**TECH FIG 2B**).
  - While in the lateral corridor, visualize the radial head and resect sufficient head to prevent abutment on the prosthesis.
- From the lateral margin of the humeral shaft, raise the brachialis from 2 to 3 cm of the anterior surface.
- An alternative approach when considering a hemiarthroplasty is ulnar osteotomy and triceps reflection. This is relatively a simple exposure, but the osteotomy will need to be fixed with a plate and screw construct.

Modified Bryan-Morrey Approach

- Preserving the integrity of the triceps insertion makes component insertion more difficult. An alternative approach for managing the triceps is to reflect it from the tip of the olecranon from medial to lateral, thereby improving exposure (**TECH FIG 3**).
- Define the medial triceps border and dissect the ulnar nerve free from its connections while protecting it in a vessel loop. The nerve is transposed into a subcutaneous pocket.
- The medial triceps is dissected to its ulnar attachment. Release the triceps from the medial condylar fragments, and transect the medial collateral ligament. Free the medial fragments from soft

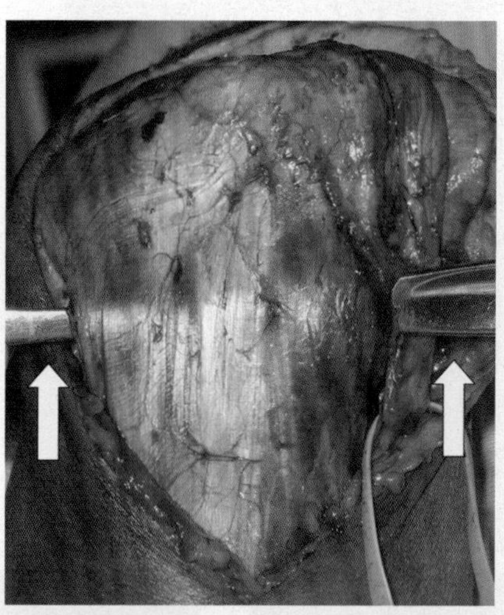

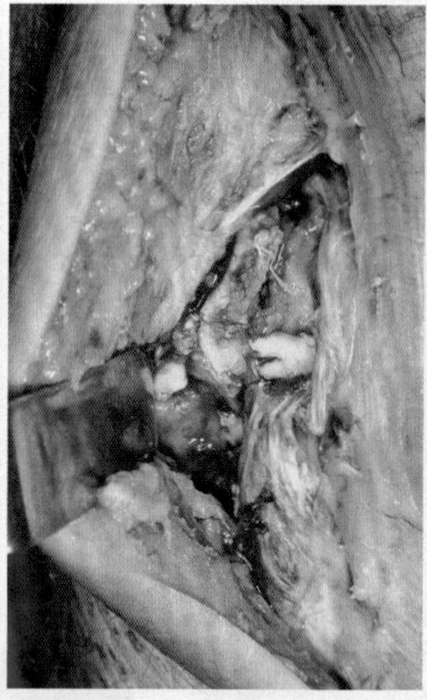

TECH FIG 2 • A. A periosteal elevator is introduced between the triceps and the humeral shaft, and the two structures are separated by sliding the elevator proximally and then distally to the level of the triceps insertion. **B.** The lateral corridor is defined, and lateral fragments are removed.

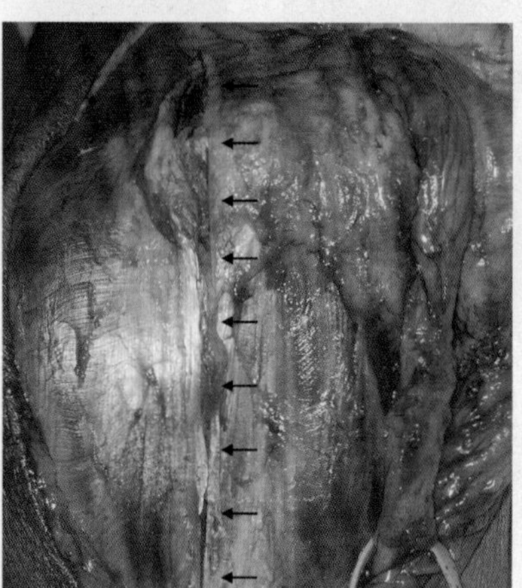

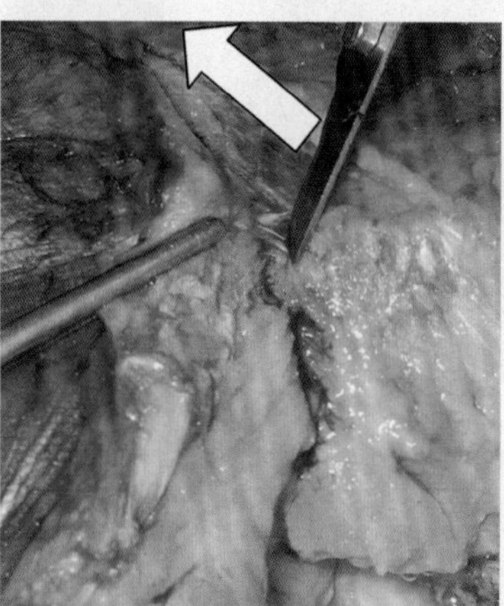

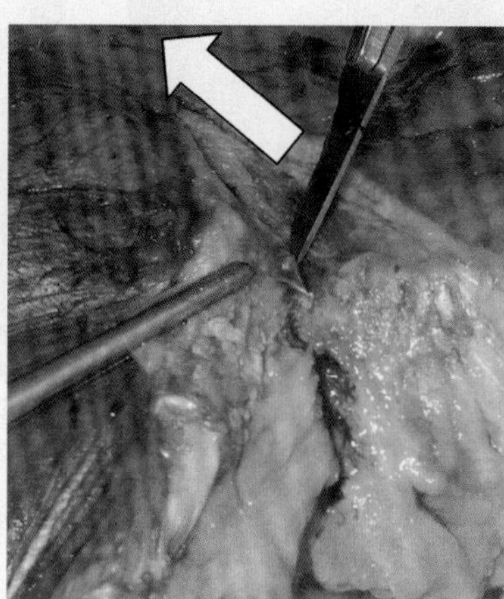

TECH FIG 3 • A. The triceps is split through its central tendon in line with the fibers. The tendinous portion is dissected from the olecranon to gain access to the ulna. **B,C.** To dissect the Sharpey fibers off the ulna, the surgeon uses the scalpel parallel to the ulna surface and maintains the release directly adjacent to the bone. *(continued)*

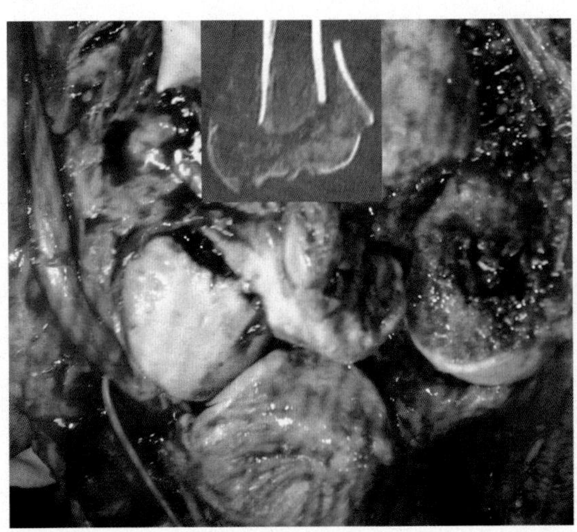

TECH FIG 3 • *(continued)* **D.** Comminuted distal humeral fracture in an osteoporotic elderly woman, with CT imaging confirming significant articular comminution. This is the view through the triceps split.

tissue attachments, and remove the medial fragments between the triceps and a gently anteriorly retracted ulnar nerve.

- Develop the interval between the anconeus and flexor carpi ulnaris along the subcutaneous border of the ulna.
- The triceps tendon is sharply elevated from the olecranon, in continuity with the anconeus, and subluxed laterally. Take care to release the Sharpey fibers adjacent to the bone in order to retain the flap thickness. Further access is afforded by raising the anconeus from its ulnar attachment while maintaining its attachment distally.
- As the triceps is reflected laterally, the lateral condylar fragments are identified and removed by releasing the common extensor tendon and lateral collateral ligament complex.

Bone Preparation

- Identify the olecranon fossa (if any part of it still exists). This landmark is the seating point for the base of the anterior flange of the Coonrad-Morrey humeral component (**TECH FIG 4A**). If the olecranon fossa is not present owing to a greater degree of comminution, an extended flange humeral component can be used.
- Release the anterior capsule and any soft tissue from the anterior surface of the distal humerus. This provides a site for the anterior humeral bone graft.
- The posterior flat surface of the humerus is identified because this plane approximates the axis of rotation of the distal humerus (**TECH FIG 4B**). Humeral canal preparation is completed with the canal broaches provided with the implant system being used.
- The ulnar canal preparation commences with removal of the tip of the olecranon. The intramedullary canal is entered at the base of the coronoid (**TECH FIG 4C,D**).
- The entry point is enlarged toward the coronoid with a burr to allow easier component insertion without cortical abutment, which leads to malalignment (**TECH FIG 4E**).
- During intramedullary preparation, the broaches must parallel the subcutaneous border of the ulna. This ensures that the track of insertion of the ulna parallels the intramedullary canal. This may require removal of bone from the greater sigmoid notch of the ulna.
- The tip of the coronoid is removed to avoid impingement during terminal flexion (**TECH FIG 4F,G**).
- The radial head does not need to be resected if there is no disease of the proximal radioulnar joint (**TECH FIG 4H**).
- During a distal humeral hemiarthroplasty (DHH), the bony preparation is focused on the medial and lateral columns. When these are not intact, reconstruction with temporary K-wire fixation to judge length and more definitively either wire or tension band fixation or plate and screw fixation should be attempted (**TECH FIG 4I–N**). The preservation and reconstruction of the columns are especially important when using an implant without an anterior flange.

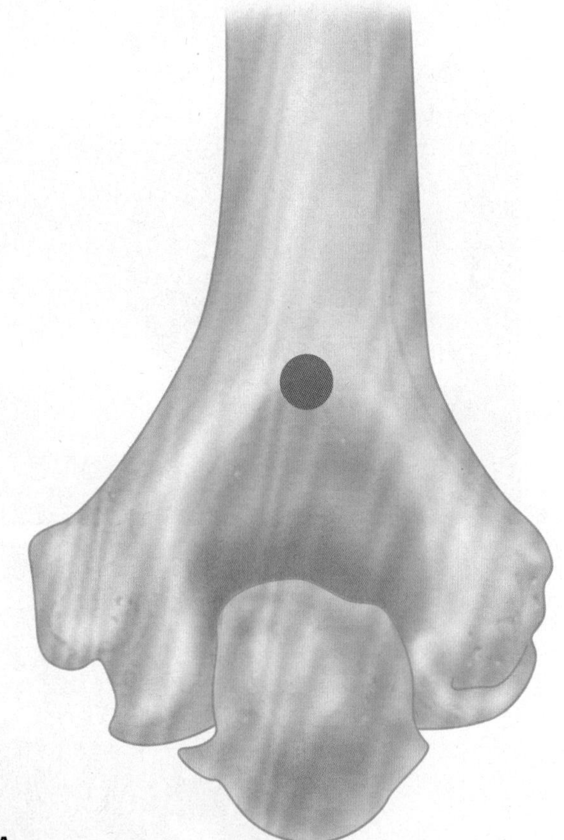

TECH FIG 4 • **A.** The humeral component entry point, the apex of the olecranon fossa, is identified, and humeral canal preparation is commenced by opening the canal with a bone nibbler or burr. *(continued)*

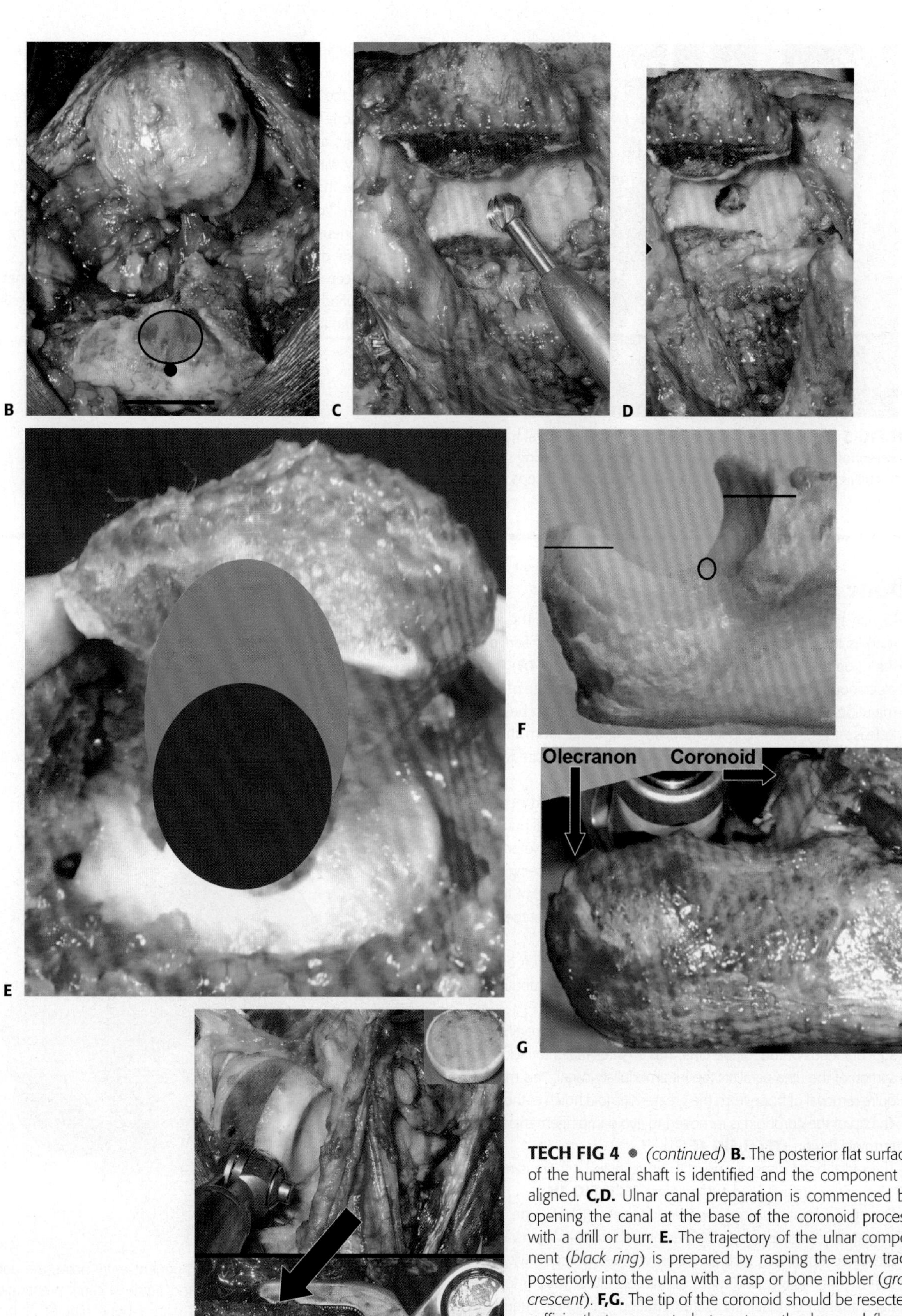

TECH FIG 4 • *(continued)* **B.** The posterior flat surface of the humeral shaft is identified and the component is aligned. **C,D.** Ulnar canal preparation is commenced by opening the canal at the base of the coronoid process with a drill or burr. **E.** The trajectory of the ulnar component (*black ring*) is prepared by rasping the entry track posteriorly into the ulna with a rasp or bone nibbler (*gray crescent*). **F,G.** The tip of the coronoid should be resected sufficiently to prevent abutment on the humeral flange during full flexion. Also shown are the resections of the olecranon and the entry point for the ulnar stem insertion. **H.** The partially resected radial head is used as a bone graft for incorporation behind the humeral flange.

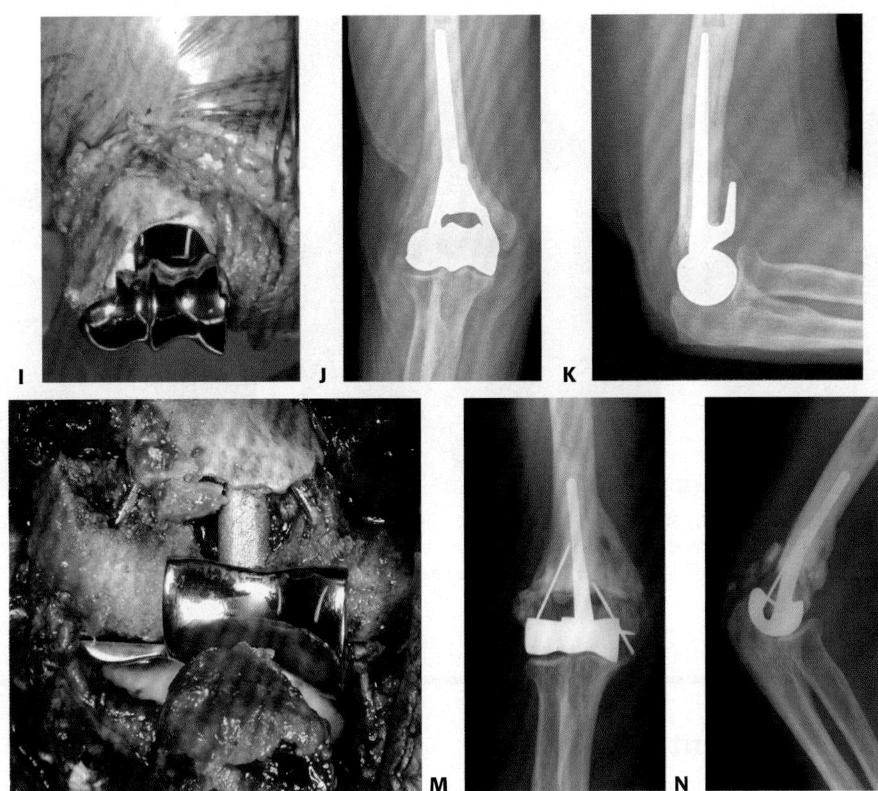

TECH FIG 4 • *(continued)* **I–K.** Latitude DHH. **I.** Intact medial and lateral humeral columns, with a red vessel loop loosely around the ulna nerve. **J.** AP radiograph demonstrating the trochlea and capitellum correctly sized for the host, greater sigmoid notch of the ulna, and the radial head. **K.** Lateral radiograph demonstrating a well-aligned radio capitellar joint and osseous integration of the anterior flange. **L–N.** Sorbie DHH. **L.** Fractured medial and lateral columns were reconstructed with K-wires, prior to implant insertion. **M.** AP radiograph demonstrating a well-seated Sorbie implant with healed medial and lateral columns. **N.** Lateral radiograph demonstrating a well-aligned radiocapitellar joint with posterior heterotopic ossification in the traumatically injured triceps muscle.

Implant Insertion and Soft Tissue Tensioning

- With the canal preparation completed (**TECH FIG 5A**), including pulse lavage of the medullary canals and cement restrictor placement, implant insertion can commence (**TECH FIG 5B,C**).
- Humeral insertion
  - When bone loss is at or below the level of the olecranon fossa, standard humeral insertion can occur. If bone loss occurs above the olecranon fossa (>2 cm), then humeral length must be restored.
  - Prepare a wedge-shaped bone "cookie" for placement behind the humeral flange.
  - Inject antibiotic cement into the humerus.
  - When inserting the humeral component, place the bone graft behind the anterior flange. Because the humeral condyles have been resected, the implant can be completely seated and coupled once the cement has hardened.
  - Maintain the component orientation relative to the posterior flat surface of the distal humerus.
  - Seat the component until the flange is completely engaged with the anterior cortex, and the bone graft is impacted and secured within the gap between flange and anterior cortex.
- Ulnar component insertion
  - Inject antibiotic cement into the ulnar canal.
  - The ulnar component is inserted such that the axis of rotation is recreated and the implant is perpendicular to the dorsal flat surface of the olecranon.
- DHH
  - When inserting a DHH, care should be focused on balancing soft tissues to allow radiocapitellar congruous articulation. The medial and lateral static restraints should either be repaired or reconstructed.

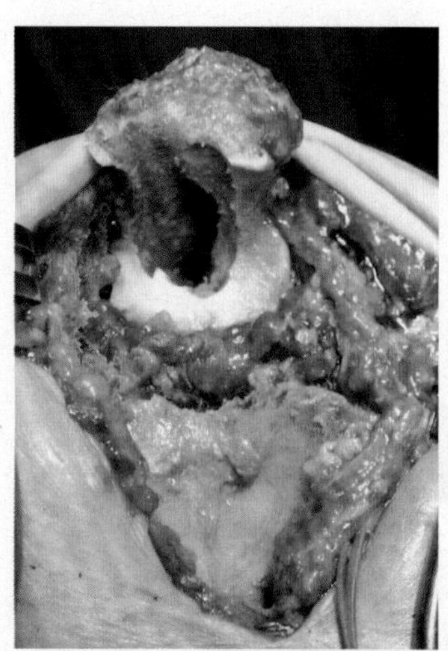

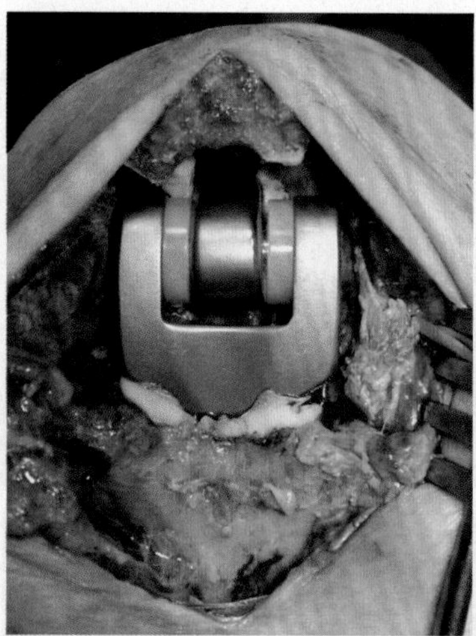

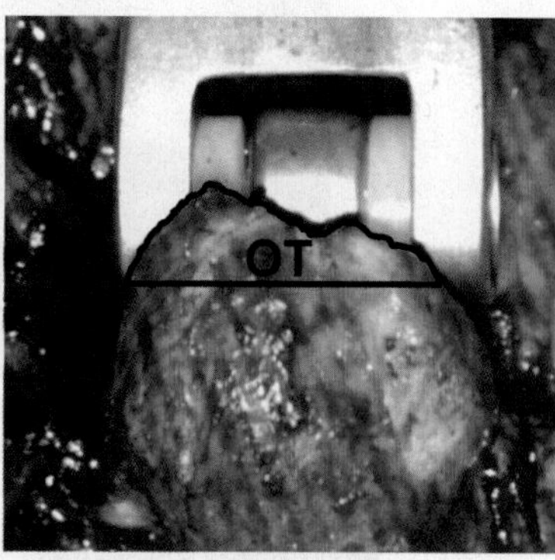

TECH FIG 5 • A. The prepared bony surfaces, with the fracture fragments removed, and just before implantation. **B.** The linked Coonrad-Morrey replacement is cemented and linked in situ. **C.** If in terminal extension there is abutment of the tip of the olecranon on the implant, the surgeon resects the olecranon tip (*OT*) but should not approach the triceps insertion footprint.

Triceps Reattachment

- The triceps is reattached using a nonabsorbable suture in a running locking mode (eg, running Krackow stitch) to achieve predictable purchase (**TECH FIG 6A,B**).
- Avoid capturing large amounts of triceps muscle fibers within the locking loops.
- The triceps tendon should be reattached to the flat of the olecranon process, not to the tip (**TECH FIG 6C,D**). Pass the sutures through bone tunnels (oblique crossing) that begin on the periphery of the flat reattachment area of the olecranon (**TECH FIG 6E**).
- Avoid tying the sutures directly over the midline of the proximal ulna, which is a source of painful symptoms and may require knot removal. Place the knot under the anconeus.
- When tensioning the triceps at reattachment, place the elbow at 30 to 45 degrees of flexion while tying the knot.
- Use a separate absorbable suture to "cinch" the triceps footprint onto the reattachment area (**TECH FIG 6F**).

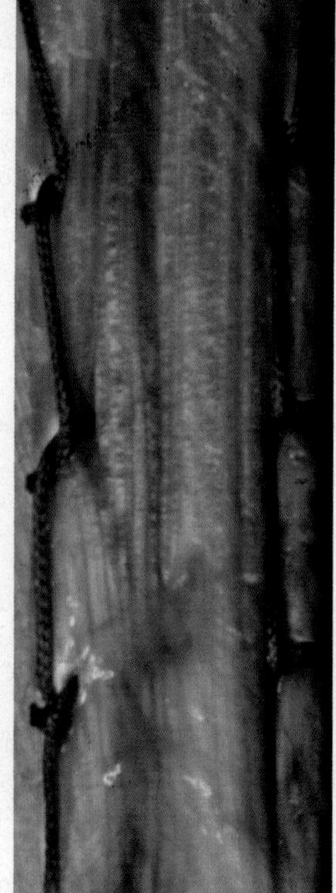

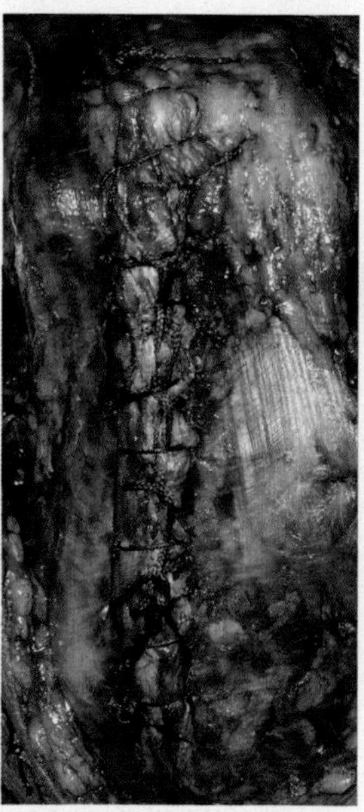

TECH FIG 6 • A,B. A running locking stitch is used to improve triceps purchase when reattaching the muscle to the ulna. **A.** An example of a running locking stitch on either side of the split tendon. **B.** A locking stitch that locks both sides of the split together with one continuous locking suture. It is then reinforced with a reversed across-split locking suture. *(continued)*

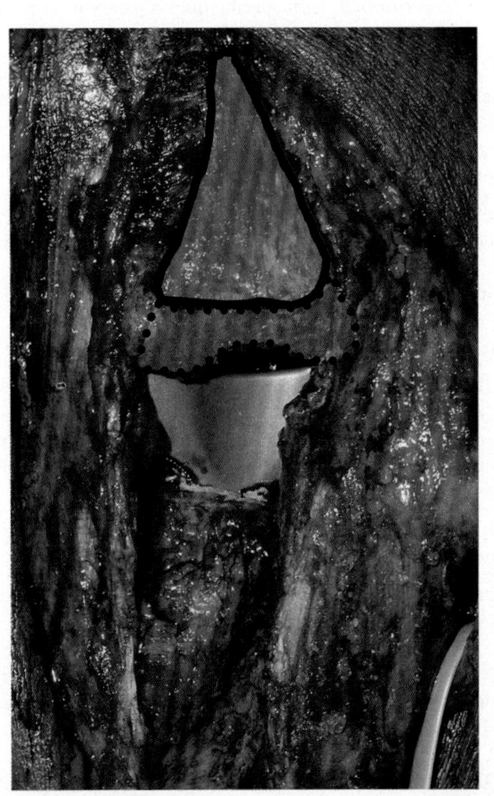

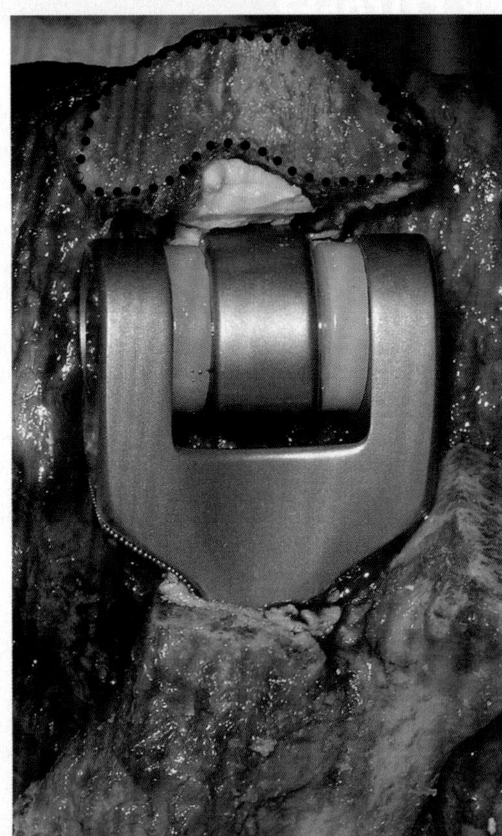

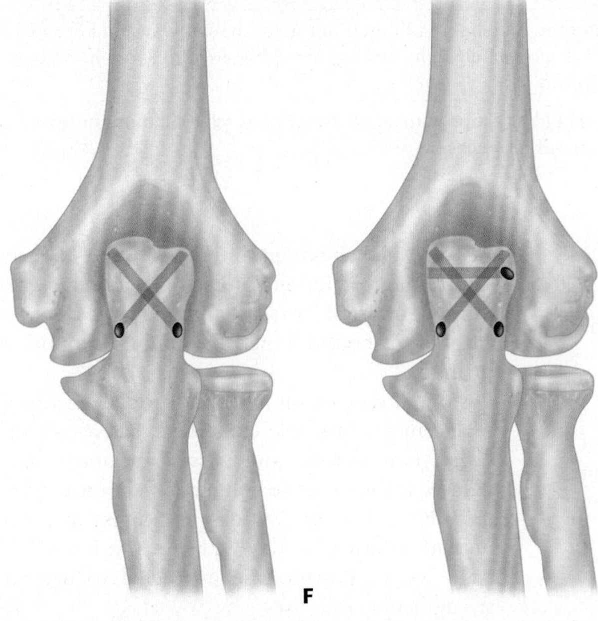

TECH FIG 6 • *(continued)* **C,D.** The triceps footprint to which reattachment should be attempted is predominantly on the flat part of the ulna or olecranon process, and not the tip, which is resected to prevent posterior abutment. **E.** Drill holes (1.5 to 2 mm) are oriented in a crossing fashion to secure the triceps to the footprint area. **F.** A separate cinch suture is used to increase the security and the area of contact between the triceps and the ulna, thereby improving healing potential.

Wound Closure

- The ulnar nerve is transposed into an anterior subcutaneous location.
- Reapproximate the flexor–pronator and common extensor masses to the triceps with absorbable suture. Do not overtighten this repair, as it will restrict motion.
- The use of a subcutaneous drain is a matter of surgeon preference. However, there is no literature demonstrating the efficacy of a postoperative drain in preventing hematoma.

PEARLS AND PITFALLS

Indications	▪ A complete history and physical examination should be performed, with specific questions about any bone mineral density problems and healing tendency. ▪ Care must be taken to address associated pathology at the elbow, wrist, and shoulder.
Planning	▪ The surgeon should consider fracture osteosynthesis when the patient has adequate bone stock and places high demand on the elbow. ▪ Arthroplasty should be available in the physiologically older and lower demand patient, with a view to converting to an acute arthroplasty if osteosynthesis is not possible intraoperatively.
Exposure	▪ Initial definition and protection of the ulnar nerve are important. Careful dissection of the nerve from the cubital tunnel restraints will allow freedom to move the nerve without risking traction injury during the remainder of the procedure. ▪ If the exposure involves removing the triceps from its ulnar attachment (Bryan-Morrey approach), the site of Sharpey fiber attachment should be marked and reattached anatomically. ▪ During a triceps sparing approach, the tendon attachment to the olecranon must be carefully preserved.
Inspection	▪ A thorough inspection of the ulna and radial articular surface should be performed to investigate the possibility of a hemiarthroplasty replacement in the appropriately selected younger patient. ▪ The surgeon should observe the state of the ulnar nerve and muscles around the elbow (especially triceps and brachialis); this will help to explain altered nerve function in the former and weakness and possible myositis ossificans and stiffness in the latter.
Bone preparation	▪ If the humeral columns are intact, then an attempt at preservation should be made, with their extensor and flexor mass attachments, during a total elbow replacement.
Implantation	▪ When planning length and implantation, the surgeon should pay careful attention to the tension of the brachialis and triceps. These muscles need appropriate tension to function well, but if overtensioned, the elbow will be stiff, and if undertensioned, the elbow will be weak. ▪ Hemiarthroplasty—plan to use an implant that is appropriate for the patient, for example, if younger and more active, may need to convert to a total replacement in the future, hence a "convertible" implant is an option. ▪ Hemiarthroplasty—avoid over- or understuffing or over- or undersizing the joint, with fluoroscopic examination after trial implantation. ▪ When an ulna osteotomy approach is chosen for DHH, prior to performing the osteotomy, place the plate onto the ulna, and predrill the screws. This saves time at the end of the case.
Wound closure	▪ Drains should be used at the discretion of the surgeon. If a drain is not used, the surgeon should pay close attention to hemostasis, and for the first 12 hours, a moderately tight bandage should be used to avoid hematoma formation. The dressing is removed on postoperative day 2.
Rehabilitation	▪ With triceps reattachment, the surgeon should be cautious to avoid overzealous rehabilitation for fear of compromising triceps healing, with subsequent avulsions or extension weakness.

POSTOPERATIVE CARE

- A volar plaster or thermoplastic splint is used to maintain the elbow in full extension for the first 24 to 48 hours. This avoids tension on the incision and on the triceps reattachment.
- The arm is elevated on pillows or with a Bradford sling overnight to prevent edema.
- Nonsteroidal anti-inflammatories are avoided because of their detrimental effects on tissue healing (bone to tendon and bone to bone). This is especially important when relying on ligamentous healing for a hemiarthroplasty.
- On the second day after surgery, the dressing is removed and the compliant patient should commence gentle active antigravity flexion, with passive gravity-assisted extension.
- A resting molded orthoplast splint with the elbow placed at 90 degrees of flexion is made to protect the triceps repair and wound.
- Graduated and targeted motion is prescribed, with greater than 90 degrees of elbow flexion attempted after 5 weeks. This allows sufficient time for the triceps to adhere and heal to the ulna. Aggressive flexion too early may result in triceps avulsion or pull-out. Triceps antigravity exercises can commence after 5 weeks.
- Always, at each patient interaction, the surgeon should reiterate the restrictions of use with an elbow arthroplasty: limited internal (varus) and external (valgus) rotatory torques, 2-pound repetitive and 10-pound single-event lifting.
- Postoperative care for a hemiarthroplasty varies from a total replacement. In stable constructs, active-assisted motion is begun immediately, and passive motion is avoided. Individuals with operative columnar fixation require additional immobilization for 2 weeks in a splint at night and intermittently during the day with the arm flexed at 90 degrees. At 6 weeks, patients are instructed to begin light elbow strengthening exercises.

COMPLICATIONS

- Triceps avulsion
- Stiffness
  - Overlengthened implantation
  - Overtensioned triceps reattachment
  - Overzealous closure of triceps to flexor–extensor compartments
  - Inadequate soft tissue release

- Impingement
  - Radial head on humeral component (distal yolk)
  - Coronoid on humeral component (anterior yolk)
  - Olecranon process on posterior humerus
- Deep venous thrombosis
- Infection
- Periprosthetic fracture
  - Osteoporotic bone
  - Stem–canal mismatched sizes
  - Stem–canal mismatched curvature
  - Inadequate opening for ulnar component at coronoid base
- Ulnar nerve neuropathy or injury

OUTCOMES

Total Elbow Arthroplasty

- Cobb and Morrey[6] reported 15 excellent and 5 good results, with one patient with inadequate data, in a cohort of patients with acute distal humeral fractures (average age of 72 years) at 3.3 years of follow-up.
- Ray et al[21] reported 5 excellent and 2 good functional results in a group of patients with an average age of 81 years at 2 to 4 years of follow-up.
- Gambirasio et al[11] reported excellent functional results in a cohort of 10 elderly patients with osteoporotic intra-articular fractures.
- Frankle et al[10] compared the outcomes of patients older than age 65 years with comminuted intra-articular distal humeral fractures treated with ORIF versus acute total elbow replacements. The ORIF group had 8 excellent results, 12 good results, 1 fair result, and 3 poor results, with 3 patients requiring conversion to elbow replacement. All 12 acute primary elbow replacements achieved excellent (n = 11) or good (n = 1) results.
- Kamineni and Morrey[15] reported an average Mayo Elbow Performance Score (MEPS) of 93/100 in a series of 49 acute distal humeral fractures (average patient age of 67 years) at 7 years of follow-up. The average arc of motion was 107 degrees.
- Lee et al[17] reported seven acute elbow replacements for distal humeral fractures in patients with an average age of 73 years. The average arc of motion was 89 degrees and the average MEPS was 94/100 at an average follow-up of 25 months.
- Abbas et al[1] reported 23 elbow replacements for complex and intra-articular fractures in patients with an average age of 75 years. MEPS was 93/100 with an average flexion arc of 93 degrees, at an average follow-up of 6 years.

Distal Humeral Hemiarthroplasty

- Smith and Hughes[22] have reported a large series of 26 patients (mean age of 62 years; range 29 to 92 years). Four patients required conversion to total joint replacement.
- Hughes et al[14] reviewed the early results and proposed a treatment algorithm incorporating the use of this technique in the overall management of distal humeral fractures.
  - DHH was performed on 30 patients (mean age of 65 years; range 29 to 91 years) for unreconstructable fractures of the distal humerus or salvage of failed internal fixation.
  - A triceps on approach was used in 6 patients and an olecranon osteotomy in 24 patients. A Sorbie Questor prosthesis (Wright Medical Technology, Arlington, TN) was used in 14 patients and a Latitude (Tornier Inc., Minneapolis, MN) in 16 patients.
  - Clinical review at a mean of 25 months (range 3 to 88 months) included the American Shoulder and Elbow Surgeons (ASES) elbow outcomes instrument, Mayo Elbow Performance Index (MEPI), and radiologic assessment.
  - At follow-up of 28 patients, mean flexion deformity was 25 degrees, flexion 128 degrees, range of prosupination 165 degrees, mean ASES 83, MEPI 77, and satisfaction 8/10. Acute cases scored better than salvage cases. Reoperation was required in 16 patients (53%); two revisions to a linked prosthesis for periprosthetic fracture and aseptic loosening at 16 and 53 months, 12 metalwork removals and four ulnar nerve procedures.
  - This is the largest reported experience of DHH. Early results of DHH show good outcomes after complex DHH, despite a technically demanding procedure. This series had metalware removal in 40%, symptomatic laxity in 12%, and column nonunion in 8%. Better results are obtained for treatment in the acute setting and with use of an olecranon osteotomy.
- Burkhart et al[5] reported on 9 good or excellent results and 1 "fair" result in a cohort of 10 females (average age of 75 years; acute hemiarthroplasty, n = 8; and hemiarthroplasty after failed osteosynthesis, n = 2), with a 12-month follow-up. The average range of motion was 17 degrees of extension deficit to 124 degrees of flexion, with 80 degrees of prosupination. No complications requiring revision surgery were reported.
- Adolfsson and Nestorson[3] reported eight excellent or good results, according to the Mayo elbow performance score, in eight females, average age of 79 years. The mean follow-up was 4 years, arc of motion was 31 degrees extension deficit to 126 degrees of flexion. Radiographic attrition of the ulna was observed, and one periprosthetic fracture at 3 years was reported.
- Argintar et al[4] reviewed the Tornier Latitude elbow hemiarthroplasty retrospectively in a small series of 10 patients and reported good to excellent results in short-term clinical outcomes. Unlike other hemiarthroplasty systems, the Latitude system is versatile with several stem lengths, a flange, and, perhaps most importantly, is convertible to a linked or unlinked total elbow arthroplasty.
- The Kudo prosthesis has shown good short-term clinical success. Adolfsson and Hammer[2] retrospectively reviewed four distal humerus hemiarthroplasties; with an average follow-up of 10 months, average extension was 20 degrees, flexion was 126 degrees, and pronation and supination were each 78 degrees. Three patients were deemed to have an excellent outcome and one patient had a good outcome, with the Mayo score. A longer term study by Adolfsson and Nestorson,[3] 4.5-year follow-up, eight patients who underwent distal humerus hemiarthroplasty demonstrated mean elbow motion arcs from 31 to 126 degrees. Of this group, five patients had an excellent outcome and three patients had a good outcome.

CONCLUSIONS

- Total elbow arthroplasty, in the setting of an acute unreconstructable distal humeral fracture, is a reliable option that provides pain relief and function compatible with a low-demand individual. The DHH has a potential niche in the younger, more active patient, but with limited experience, its use should be carefully considered.

REFERENCES

1. Abbas GA, Chutter GSJ, Williams JR. Retrospective review of primary total elbow replacement (TER) for osteoporotic fractures of distal humerus in the elderly over 10-year period. Injury Extra 2010;41:160.
2. Adolfsson L, Hammer R. Elbow hemiarthroplasty for acute reconstruction of intraarticular distal humerus fractures: a preliminary report involving 4 patients. Acta Orthop 2006;77:785–787.
3. Adolfsson L, Nestorson J. The Kudo humeral component as primary hemiarthroplasty in distal humeral fractures. J Shoulder Elbow Surg 2012;21:451–455.
4. Argintar E, Berry M, Narvy SJ, et al. Hemiarthroplasty for the treatment of distal humerus fractures: short-term clinical results. Orthopedics 2012;35:1042–1045.
5. Burkhart KJ, Nijs S, Mattyasovszky SG, et al. Distal humerus hemiarthroplasty of the elbow for comminuted distal humeral fractures in the elderly patient. J Trauma 2011;71:635–642.
6. Cobb TK, Morrey BF. Total elbow arthroplasty as primary treatment for distal humeral fractures in elderly patients. J Bone Joint Surg Am 1997;79:826–832.
7. Eastwood WJ. The T-shaped fracture of the lower end of the humerus. J Bone Joint Surg 1937;19:364–369
8. Faierman E, Wang J, Jupiter JB. Secondary ulnar nerve palsy in adults after elbow trauma: a report of two cases. J Hand Surg Am 2001;26:675–678.
9. Frankle MA, Herscovici D Jr, DiPasquale TG, et al. A comparison of open reduction and internal fixation and primary total elbow arthroplasty in the treatment of intraarticular fractures of the distal humerus in women older than 65 years. J Shoulder Elbow Surg 1999;9:455.
10. Frankle MA, Herscovici D Jr, DiPasquale TG, et al. A comparison of open reduction and internal fixation and primary total elbow arthroplasty in the treatment of intraarticular distal humerus fractures in women older than age 65. J Orthop Trauma 2003;17:473–480.
11. Gambirasio R, Riand N, Stern R, et al. Total elbow replacement for complex fractures of the distal humerus. An option for the elderly patient. J Bone Joint Surg Br 2001;83:974–978.
12. Holmes JC, Skolnick MD, Hall JE. Untreated median-nerve entrapment in bone after fracture of the distal end of the humerus: postmortem findings after forty-seven years. J Bone Joint Surg Am 1979;61:309–310.
13. Huang TL, Chiu FY, Chuang TY, et al. The results of open reduction and internal fixation in elderly patients with severe fractures of the distal humerus: a critical analysis of the results. J Trauma 2005;58:62–69.
14. Hughes J, Malone AA, Zarkadas P, et al. Distal humeral hemiarthroplasty (DHH) for intra-articular distal humeral fractures. J Bone Joint Surg Br 2012;94-B:162.
15. Kamineni S, Morrey BF. Distal humeral fractures treated with noncustom total elbow replacement. J Bone Joint Surg Am 2004;86-A(5):940–947.
16. Kamineni S, Morrey BF. Distal humeral fractures treated with noncustom total elbow replacement. Surgical technique. J Bone Joint Surg Am 2005;87(suppl 1):41–50.
17. Lee KT, Lai CH, Singh S. Results of total elbow arthroplasty in the treatment of distal humerus fractures in elderly Asian patients. J Trauma 2006;61:889–892.
18. Mohan K. Myositis ossificans traumatica of the elbow. Int Surg 1972;57:475–478.
19. Pajarinen J, Bjorkenheim JM. Operative treatment of type C intercondylar fractures of the distal humerus: results after a mean follow-up of 2 years in a series of 18 patients. J Shoulder Elbow Surg 2002;11:48–52.
20. Parsons M, O'Brien R, Hughes J. Elbow hemiarthroplasty for acute and salvage reconstruction of intra-articular distal humerus fractures. Tech Shoulder Elbow Surg 2005;6:87–97.
21. Ray PS, Kakarlapudi K, Rajsekhar C, et al. Total elbow arthroplasty as primary treatment for distal humeral fractures in elderly patients. Injury 2000;31:687–692.
22. Smith GC, Hughes JS. Unreconstructable acute distal humeral fractures and their sequelae treated with distal humeral hemiarthroplasty: a two-year to eleven-year. J Shoulder Elbow Surg 2013;22:1710–1723.
23. Thompson HC III, Garcia A. Myositis ossificans: aftermath of elbow injuries. Clin Orthop Relat Res 1967;50:129–134.
24. Zhao J, Wang X, Zhang Q. Surgical treatment of comminuted intra-articular fractures of the distal humerus with double tension band osteosynthesis. Orthopedics 2000;23:449–452.

Open Reduction and Internal Fixation of Radial Head and Neck Fractures

18

CHAPTER

Yung Han, George Frederick Hatch III, and John M. Itamura

DEFINITION

- Radial head and neck fractures are the most common elbow fractures in adults representing 33% of elbow fractures.
- They may occur in isolation or with concurrent osseous, osteochondral, and/or ligamentous injuries.
- Management (which involves nonoperative, open reduction internal fixation [ORIF], fragment excision, radial head excision, or radial head replacement) is aimed at restoring motion or both motion and stability to the elbow and forearm, depending on the pattern of injury. This chapter focuses on the decision-making principles and operative techniques for ORIF of radial head and neck fractures.

ANATOMY AND BIOMECHANICS

- The radial head is entirely intra-articular with two articulations: (1) radiocapitellar joint and (2) proximal radioulnar joint (PRUJ).
  - The radiocapitellar joint has a saddle-shaped articulation allowing flexion, extension, and forearm rotation.
  - The PRUJ, constrained by the annular ligament, allows rotation of the radial head in the lesser sigmoid notch of the proximal ulna.
    - To avoid creating a mechanical block to pronation and supination, implants must be limited to a 90-degree arc (the "safe zone") outside the PRUJ (**FIG 1**).[7]
- There is considerable variability in the shape of the radial head, from nearly round to elliptical, as well as variability in the offset of the head from the neck.[14]
- Blood supply to the radial head is tenuous with a major contribution from a single branch of the radial recurrent artery in the safe zone and minor contributions from both the radial and interosseous recurrent arteries which penetrate the capsule at its insertion into the neck (**FIG 2**).[26]
- The anterior band of the medial collateral ligament (MCL) is the primary stabilizer to valgus stress. The radial head, a secondary stabilizer, maintains up to 30% of valgus resistance in the native elbow. Therefore, in cases where the MCL is ruptured:
  - A radial head that is not reparable should be replaced with a prosthesis and not excised given its biomechanical importance.
  - It may be prudent to protect a repaired radial head from high valgus stress during early range of motion.
- The radial head also functions in the transmission of axial load, transmitting 60% of the load from the wrist to the elbow.[21] This is a crucial consideration when the interosseous membrane is disrupted in the Essex-Lopresti lesion.[9] Resection of the radial head in this setting results in devastating longitudinal radioulnar instability, proximal migration of the radius, and possible ulnar–carpal impingement.

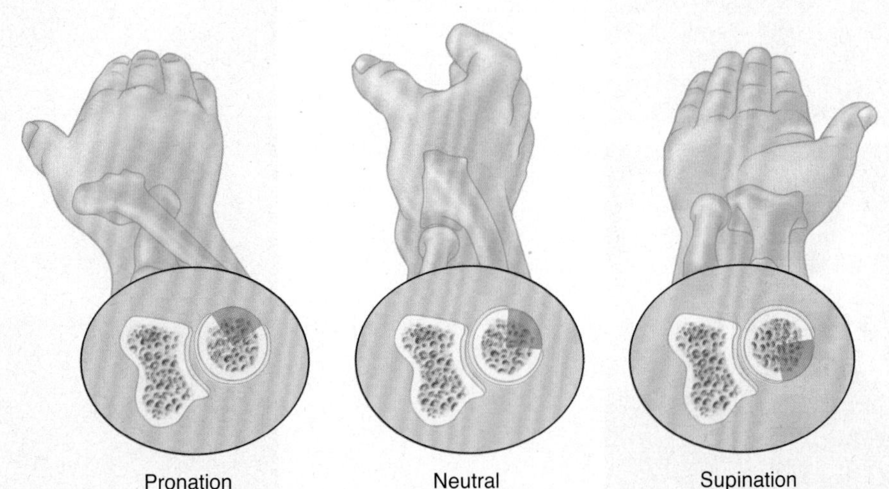

FIG 1 • The safe zone is a roughly 90-degree arc of the radial head that does not articulate with the ulna in the PRUJ with full supination and pronation. With the wrist in neutral rotation, the safe zone is anterolateral.

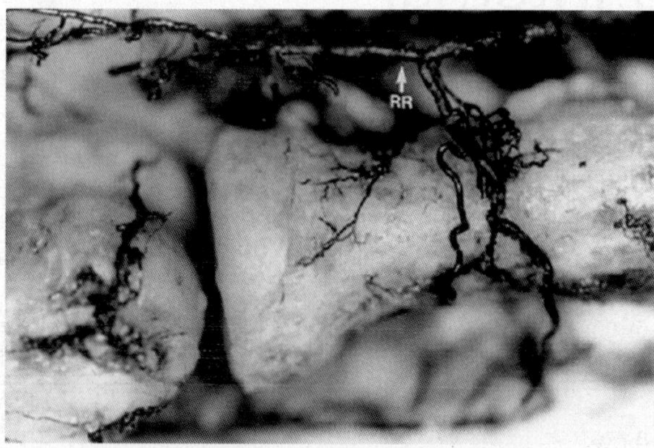

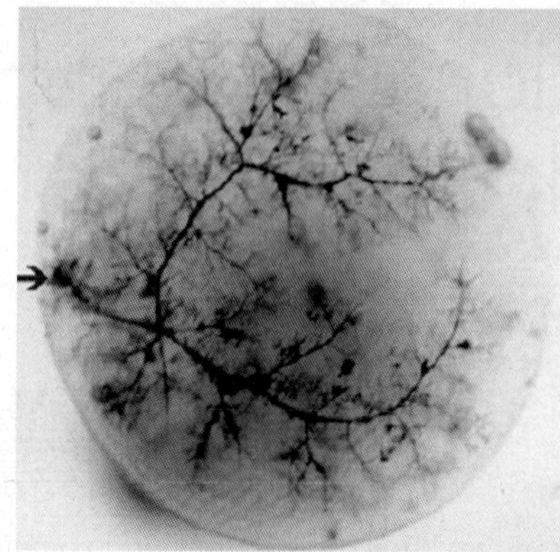

FIG 2 • **A.** The radial recurrent artery, a branch of the radial artery, provides the main blood supply to the radial head. **B.** In most cadaveric specimens, a branch of the radial recurrent penetrates the radial head in the safe zone. (From Yamaguchi K, Sweet FA, Bindra R, et al. The extraosseous and intraosseous arterial anatomy of the adult elbow. J Bone Joint Surg Am 1997;79[11]:1653–1662.)

PATHOGENESIS

- Radial head fractures result from trauma. A fall on an outstretched hand with the elbow in extension and the forearm in pronation produces an axial or valgus load (or both) driving the radial head into the capitellum, fracturing the relatively osteopenic radial head.[2]
- Nondisplaced or minimally displaced injuries do not usually have associated injuries. However, displaced, comminuted, or unstable fractures have a high association of soft tissue injuries (**FIG 3**) that can lead to considerable complications, including pain, arthrosis, instability, and disability:
  - Capitellar cartilage defects, capitellar bone bruises, and/or posterior dislocation can occur with radial head fractures.
- Axial loading may also rupture the interosseous membrane causing longitudinal radioulnar instability with dislocation of the distal radioulnar joint (DRUJ) (Essex-Lopresti fracture). An impacted radial neck or depressed radial head fracture should be highly suspicious of a concomitant interosseous membrane and DRUJ injury (**FIG 4**).
- The "terrible triad" injury results from valgus loading of the elbow, disrupting the MCL or lateral ulnar collateral ligament, and fracturing the radial head and coronoid process.
- Radial head fractures can also occur with proximal ulnar fractures (Monteggia fracture) (**FIG 5**).

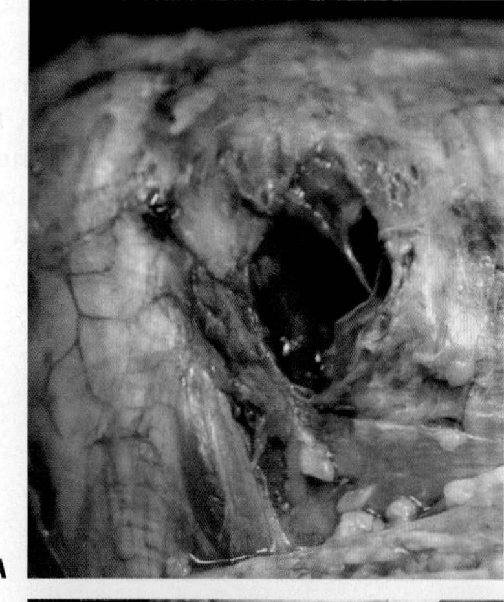

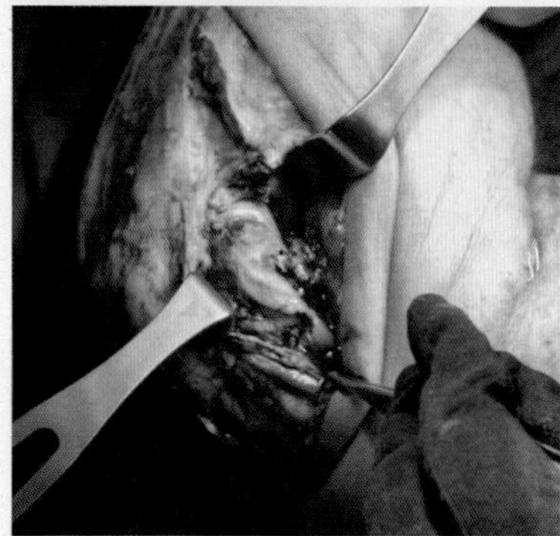

FIG 3 • Soft tissue injuries occur with unstable radial head fractures. Sample pictures showing (**A**) large capsular rupture and (**B**) avulsion of the lateral collateral ligament (LCL) and common extensor tendons from the lateral epicondyle.

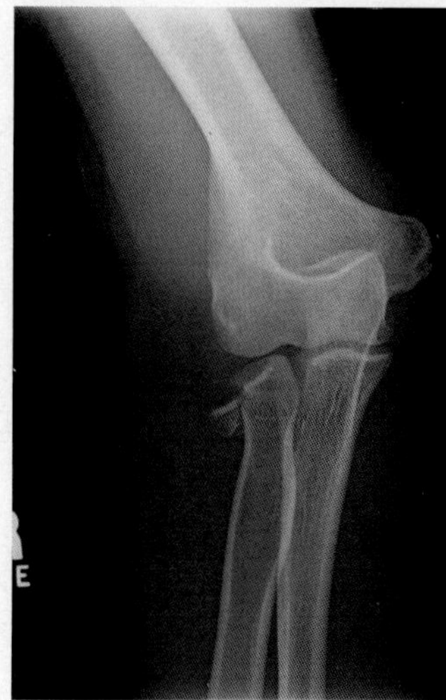

FIG 4 • AP x-ray showing a depressed articular fracture with impaction at the radial neck. This fracture pattern is highly suspicious for an Essex-Lopresti fracture. Radial head replacement is recommended. If ORIF is performed, the DRUJ should be stabilized to prevent instability.

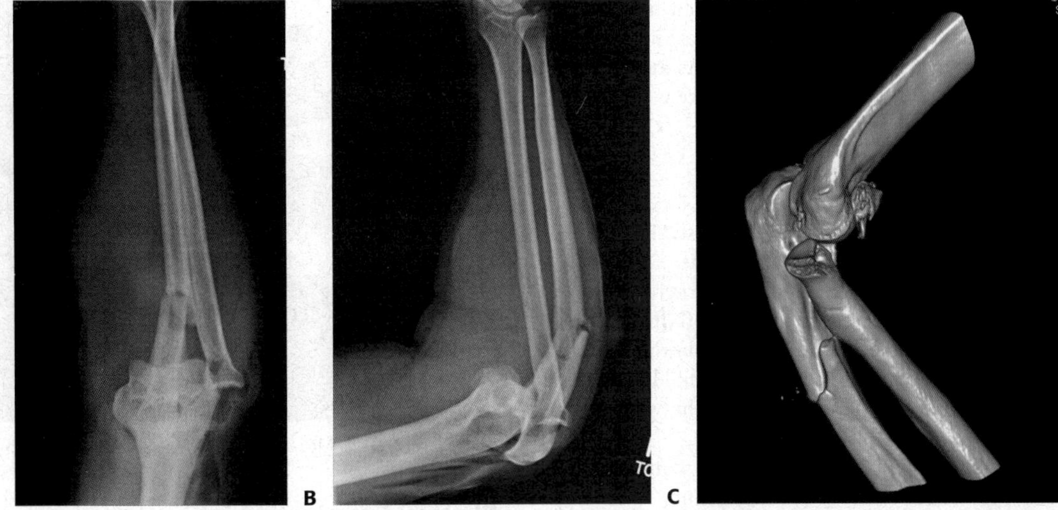

FIG 5 • A,B. AP and lateral x-ray showing a type II Monteggia fracture–posterior dislocation of radial head (or fracture) and proximal ulnar fracture with posterior angulation. **C.** CT scan clearly showing impaction fracture of the radial head that may not be appreciable on x-ray.

NATURAL HISTORY

- The original Mason classification was modified by Johnson, and then Morrey. Hotchkiss proposed that the classification system be used to provide guidance for treatment. It has poor intraobserver and interobserver reliability (**FIG 6**).[9]

Type I Fractures

- Nondisplaced and offer no block to pronation and supination on examination
- Represents approximately 82% of radial head fractures[18]
- Nonoperative treatment generally results in good to excellent outcomes with minimal loss of motion or resultant arthrosis.[1,3,8,12]
- Stiffness due to capsular contracture is the main reason for a poor outcome; however, it can often be managed successfully with physical therapy.

Type II Fractures

- Displaced marginal segments that can block normal forearm rotation. According to Broberg and Morrey,[6] the fragment should be greater than or equal to 30% of the articular surface and be displaced greater than or equal to 2 mm. We only include fractures with three or fewer articular fragments, which meet criteria for fractures that can be operatively reduced and fixed with reproducibly good results.
- Represents approximately 14% of radial head fractures[18]
- Earlier studies suggested nonoperative treatment or radial head excision as the standard treatment,[13,19,20,23] but as knowledge and technology advanced, optimal treatment has become more controversial.
- Greater than 2 mm of displacement has often been cited as an indication for ORIF, but good results have been obtained in studies treating 2 to 5 mm of displacement nonoperatively.[1,12]
- A mechanical block is the only clear indication for surgery.
- A recent meta-analysis[16] found successful nonoperative treatment in 80% compared to successful ORIF treatment in 93% for stable Mason type II fractures; however, the authors concluded that there was insufficient evidence to recommend optimal treatment.
- Complications from nonoperative treatment such as painful clicking, nonunion, and arthrosis can be treated with radial head excision or arthroplasty; however, it is considered with modest increase in function. It has shown 23% fair or poor results at 15 years of follow-up.[5]

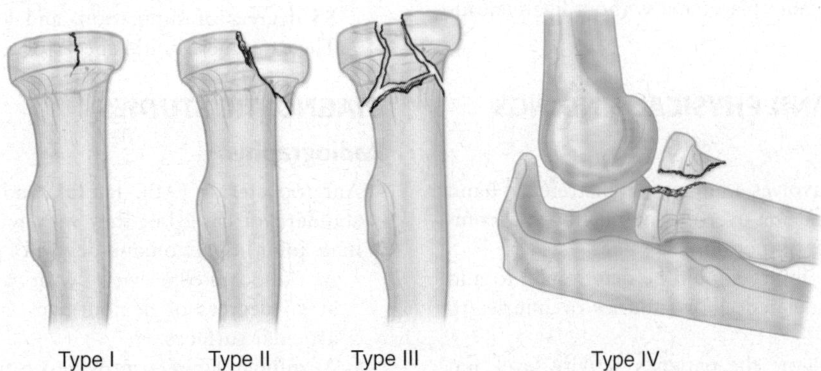

FIG 6 • The modified Mason classification for radial head fractures.

- Delayed excision of the radial head after failed nonoperative management may be considered with modest increase in function; it has shown 23% fair or poor results at 15 years of follow-up.[5] Other studies suggested that there is no difference between delayed and primary excision.[11]

Type III Fractures

- Comminuted or impacted articular fractures (see **FIG 4**) are optimally managed with prosthetic replacement.
- Represents approximately 3% of radial head fractures[18]
- Radial head arthroplasty or excision is considered when satisfactory reduction or stable fixation is not obtained or in comminuted fractures because fixation of a radial head with more than three articular fragments is fraught with poor results.[22]
- Results of excision are poor in patients with concomitant MCL, coronoid, or interosseous membrane injury.
- Radial head resection should be reserved for patients with low functional demands, limited life expectancy, or in the presence of infection, and when the surgeon has excluded elbow instability with a fluoroscopic examination.
- Radiographic, but usually clinically silent, degenerative changes such as cysts, sclerosis, and osteophytes occur radiographically in about 75% of elbows after radial head excision.
- There is also a demonstrable increase in ulnar variance at the wrist and increased carrying angle and a 10% to 20% loss of strength is expected.
- Radial head arthroplasty can provide radiocapitellar contact similar to the native radial head and thus resists valgus and posterior instability. Additionally, it resists proximal migration of the radius in response to axial loading. It facilitates uneventful healing of the MCL, interosseous ligaments, and DRUJ.

Type IV Fractures

- Radial head fractures associated with elbow instability. The radial head should never be resected in the acute setting.
- Represents approximately 1% of radial head fractures[18]
- Treatment involves immediate reduction of the elbow joint and treatment of the radial head fracture and associated bony injuries. Whether the radial head is fixed or replaced, it must be capable of bearing load immediately. If the radial head can be fixed, repair of the torn ligaments and application of a hinged fixator to protect the repaired radial head may be considered. Otherwise, satisfactory results have been obtained with radial head replacement without ligamentous repair.[10]

PATIENT HISTORY AND PHYSICAL FINDINGS

History

- The history typically involves a fall on an outstretched hand followed by pain and edema over the lateral elbow, accompanied by limited range of motion.
- The mechanism of the injury should be determined to add information about associated elbow injuries or injuries to the shoulder or hand.
- The examiner should note the patient's activity level and profession.

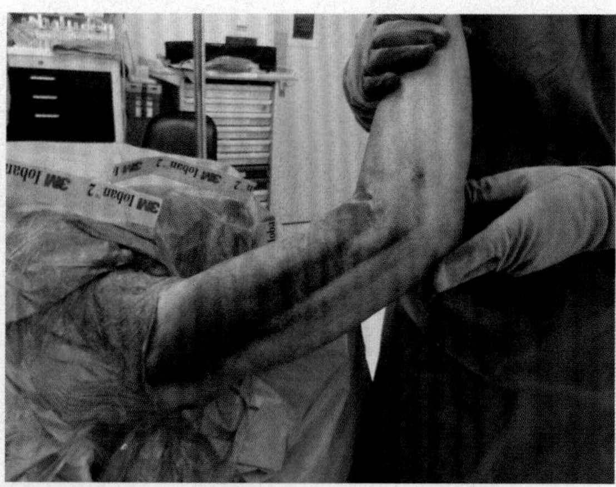

FIG 7 • MCL injury with extensive medial ecchymosis.

Physical Examination

- Physical examination should include neurovascular status, examination of the joint above (shoulder) and below (wrist), and examination of the skin to look for medial ecchymosis (**FIG 7**), which may suggest injury to the MCL.
  - A detailed examination of the elbow must include bony palpation of the medial and lateral epicondyles, olecranon process, DRUJ, and radial head as well as the squeeze test of the interosseous membrane and DRUJ to screen for potential longitudinal instability.
  - Varus and valgus stress testing, with or without fluoroscopy, can indicate injury to the anterior band of the MCL or to the lateral ulnar collateral ligament, respectively.
- Range-of-motion and stress examinations are vital to proper decision making and may obviate the need for advanced imaging if performed correctly with adequate anesthesia. If omitted, this will lead to undiagnosed associated injuries and may result in flawed decision making.
  - In the emergency department or office, adequate anesthesia may be obtained by aspirating hematoma, then injecting the elbow joint with 5 mL of local anesthetic and examining the elbow under fluoroscopy. This may be performed by the traditional lateral injection in the "soft spot" or posteriorly into the olecranon fossa (**FIG 8**).[25] A mechanical block is an indication for operative intervention.
  - If operative intervention is clearly indicated, this examination can be performed under a general anesthetic, provided the surgeon and patient are prepared for a change in operative plan as dictated by the examination.
  - Normal values are 0 to 145 degrees of flexion–extension, 85 degrees of supination, and 80 degrees of pronation. The examiner should check for a bony block to motion.

DIAGNOSTIC STUDIES

Radiography

- Anteroposterior (AP), lateral, and oblique views are the standard of care, but they may underestimate or overestimate joint impaction and degree of comminution.
  - A radiocapitellar view with forearm in neutral and at 45 degrees of flexion gives an improved view of the articular surfaces.
  - A sailboat sign can provide suspicion to an occult radial neck fracture.

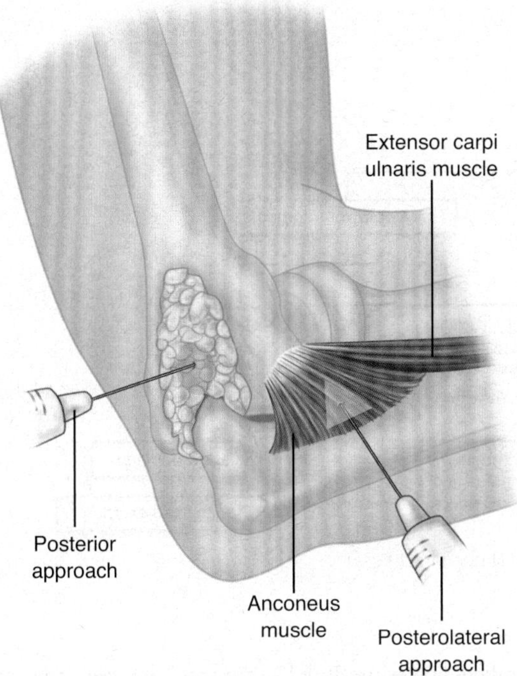

FIG 8 • The elbow joint can be aspirated and injected through the posterior and posterolateral approaches. They are equally effective and should be used based on soft tissue injury.

- If the examination reveals wrist or forearm tenderness, the examiner should have a low threshold for obtaining bilateral wrist posteroanterior (PA) views to rule out an Essex-Lopresti lesion. Alternatively, this can be done with a one cassette view to minimize radiation exposure (**FIG 9**).

Magnetic Resonance Imaging

- Magnetic resonance imaging (MRI) is a useful adjunct to physical examination for evaluating associated injuries such as collateral ligament tears, chondral defects, and loose bodies,[15] but it is not routinely indicated. Most of the associated injuries found on MRI at the time of injury have been found to be not clinically significant.[15,17]

Computed Tomography

- If decision is made for operative treatment, we routinely obtain a computed tomography (CT) scan to better understand the fracture pattern for preoperative planning, so that operative time is efficient and to minimize intraoperative surprises. Three-dimensional reconstructions provide further information not always easily appreciated on routine CT scans.

DIFFERENTIAL DIAGNOSIS

- Simple elbow dislocation
- Distal humerus fracture
- Olecranon fracture
- Septic elbow

NONOPERATIVE MANAGEMENT

- The standard protocol for treating radial head fractures is shown in **FIG 10**.
- Conservative management, with a week of sling immobilization followed by range of motion once the acute pain resolves, is the treatment of choice in nondisplaced radial head fractures, where universally good and excellent results have been reported.
- Nonoperative management is also the treatment of choice in fractures with less than 2 mm of displacement, with minor head involvement, and without bony blockage to range of motion.
  - A 7-day period of cast or splint immobilization is followed by aggressive motion after the inflammatory phase.
- Our current practice for fractures that are more than 2 mm displaced is to determine whether there is a blockage of motion on fluoroscopic examination.
  - If there is maintenance of at least 50 degrees of both pronation and supination, we typically recommend conservative treatment.

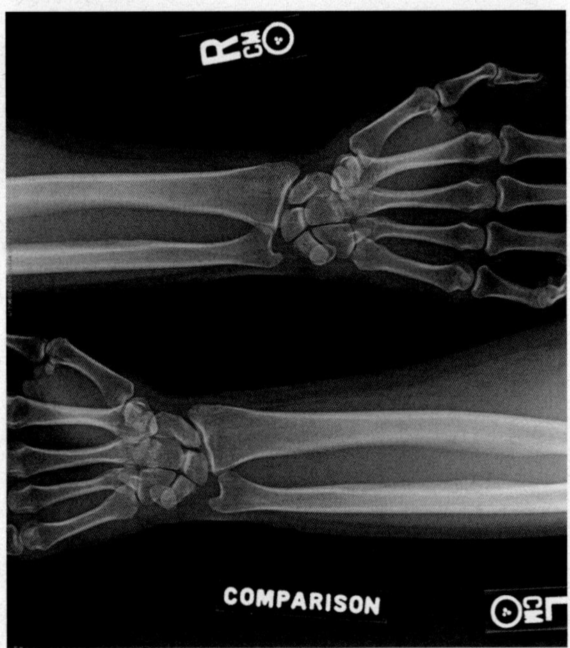

A

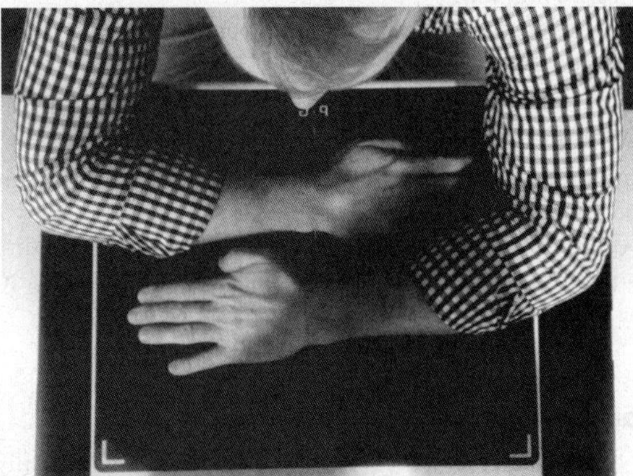

B

FIG 9 • **A.** A positive *Itamura simultaneous DRUJ view* showing negative ulnar variance of the uninjured left DRUJ compared with neutral ulnar variance of the right injured DRUJ suggesting interosseous membrane disruption. Patient had a right radial head fracture and proximal migration of the radius respective to the ulna (Essex-Lopresti fracture). **B.** Image is taken with 90-degree shoulder flexion, 90-degree elbow flexion, and 90-degree forearm pronation.

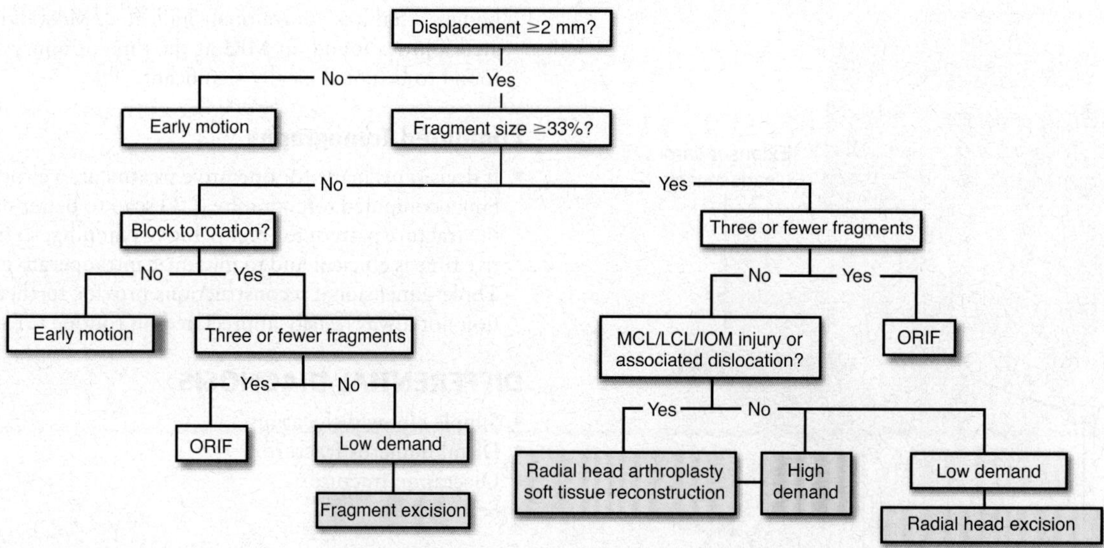

FIG 10 • Treatment algorithm for radial head fractures.

- If there is a blockage or instability, excision, fixation, or arthroplasty is recommended based on patient factors and instability.
- A recent report regarding the long-term results of nonoperative management (similar to that described) of 49 patients with radial head fractures encompassing over 30% of the joint surface and displaced 2 to 5 mm revealed that 81% of patients had no subjective complaints and minimal loss of motion versus the uninjured extremity. Only one patient had daily pain.[1]

SURGICAL MANAGEMENT

Preoperative Planning

- It is essential to review all imaging and perform thorough history, physical, and fluoroscopic examinations before making an incision.
  - The presence of instability or associated fractures warrants a more extensile approach.

Positioning

- Positioning depends on the planned approach and the surgeon's preference.
  - We prefer the patient supine with the affected extremity brought across the chest over a bump to allow access to the posterolateral elbow.
  - A sterile tourniquet is placed high on the arm.

Approach

- The posterolateral (Kocher) approach has traditionally been presented to approach radial head fractures; however, we prefer a modified Wrightington approach[24] which is a modified posterior (Boyd) approach[4] between the interval between the ulna and anconeus for the following reasons: (**FIG 11**).
  - It offers superior visualization of the radial head and neck which is important in ORIF.
  - It is also the only approach that allows visualization of the radioulnar, radiohumeral, and ulnohumeral joint spaces which is essential in selecting the appropriate radial head implant size if arthroplasty is warranted.
- The approach is extensile and can allow the surgeon to address ligamentous injuries in addition to the radial head fracture with less risk of neuroma formation and neurologic injury.

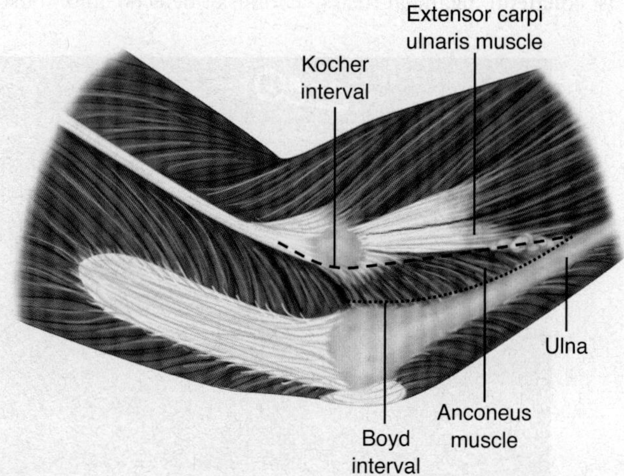

FIG 11 • Surgical intervals for the Boyd approach and the Kocher approach.

Kocher Approach

- The traditional posterolateral (Kocher) approach between the anconeus and extensor carpi ulnaris is cosmetic and spares the lateral ulnar collateral ligament.
  - We recommend not using an Esmarch tourniquet to allow visualization of penetrating veins that help identify the interval.
- A 5-cm oblique incision is made from the posterolateral aspect of the lateral epicondyle obliquely to a point three fingerbreadths below the tip of the olecranon in line with the radial neck (**TECH FIG 1A**).
- The radial head and epicondyle are palpated, and the fascia is divided in line with the skin incision.
- The Kocher interval is identified distally by small penetrating veins and bluntly developed, revealing the lateral ligament complex and joint capsule (**TECH FIG 1B**).
- The anconeus is reflected posteriorly and the extensor carpi ulnaris origin anteriorly. The capsule is incised obliquely anterior to the lateral ulnar collateral ligament (**TECH FIG 1C,D**).
- The proximal edge of the annular ligament may also be divided and tagged, with care taken not to proceed distally and damage the posterior interosseous nerve.

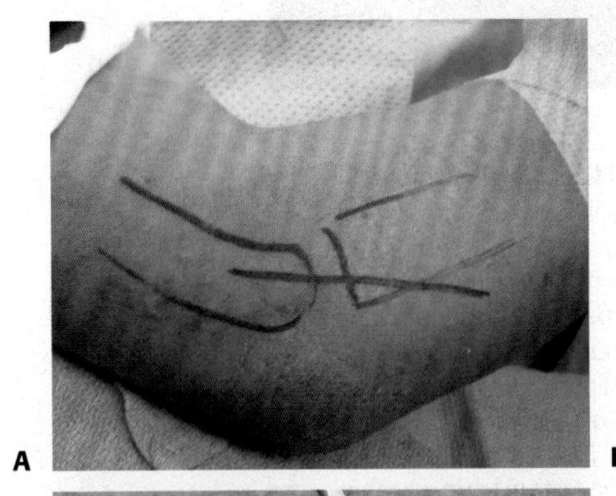

A

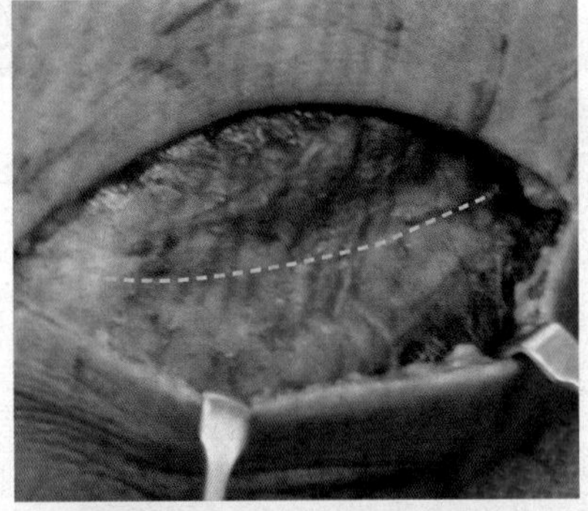

B

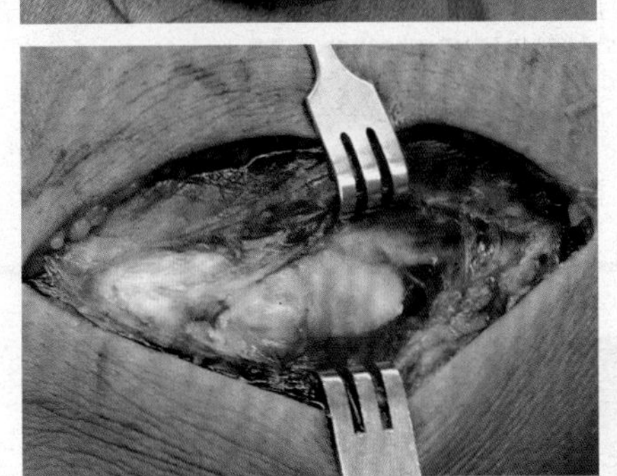

C

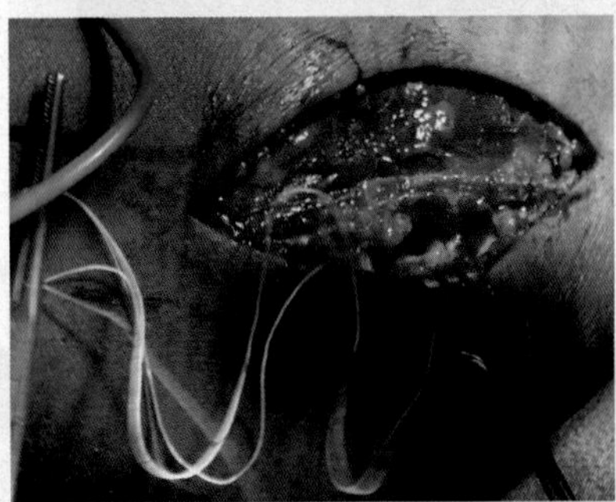

D

TECH FIG 1 • Kocher approach. **A.** The skin incision proceeds distally from the posterolateral aspect of the lateral epicondyle to the posterior aspect of the proximal radius. **B.** Full-thickness flaps are made and the fascial interval between the extensor carpi ulnaris and anconeus muscles is identified. **C.** With longitudinal incision of the fascia and blunt division of the muscles, the joint capsule is evident. **D.** The capsule is longitudinally incised, and the fascia is tagged with figure-8 stitches for later anatomic repair.

Modified Wrightington Approach

- An 8-cm straight longitudinal incision is made just lateral to the olecranon (**TECH FIG 2A**).
- Full-thickness skin flaps are developed bluntly over the fascia.
- The fascia is longitudinally incised in the interval between the anconeus and ulna (**TECH FIG 2B**).
- The anconeus is dissected off the ulna, elevating proximal to distal to preserve the distal vascular pedicle. Great care is taken not to violate the joint capsule or lateral ulnar collateral ligament by using blunt fashion (**TECH FIG 2C**).
- The lateral ulnar collateral ligament and annular ligament complex are sharply divided and tagged from their insertion on the crista supinatoris of the ulna. The radial head and its articulation with the capitellum are now evident (**TECH FIG 2D**).
- After repair or replacement, the ligaments are repaired to their insertion with suture anchors.

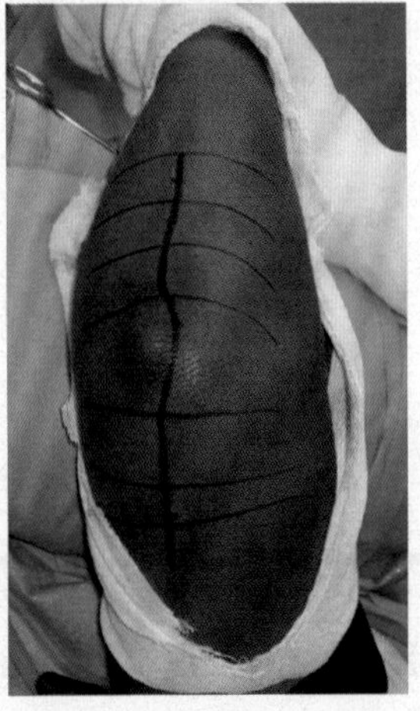

A

TECH FIG 2 • Modified Wrightington approach. **A.** Make an 8-cm longitudinal incision at the junction of the ulna and anconeus starting about four fingerbreadths distal to the olecranon and extending 2 cm proximal to the olecranon. *(continued)*

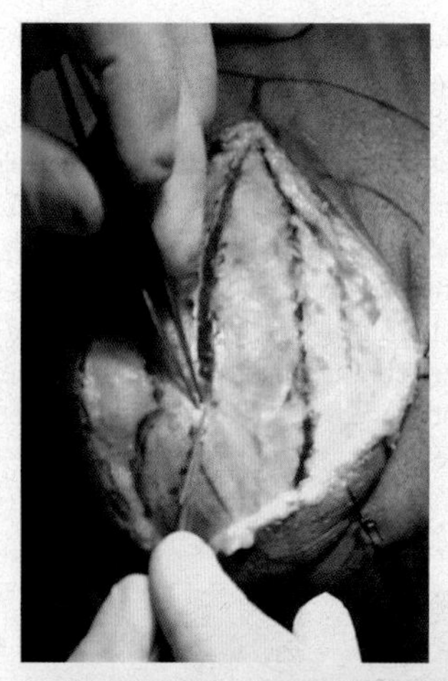

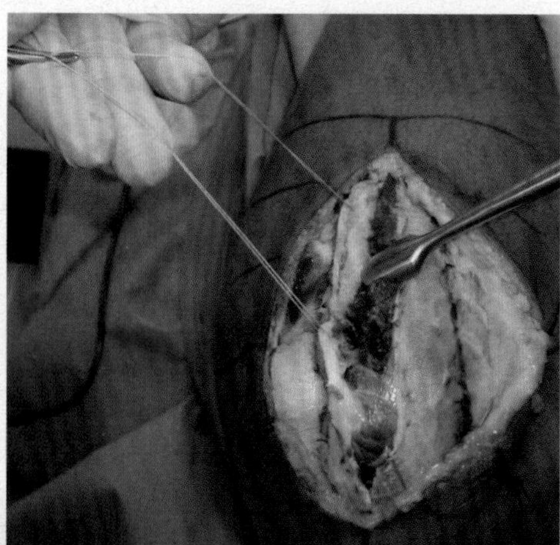

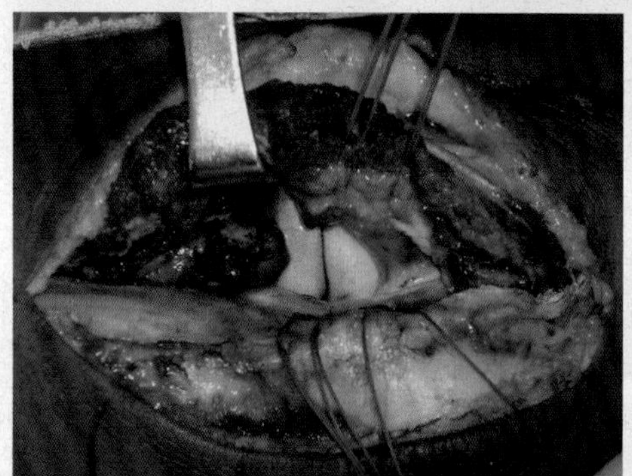

TECH FIG 2 • *(continued)* **B.** The interval between the ulna and anconeus is incised sharply, with care taken not to violate the periosteum or muscle to minimize the risk of proximal radioulnar synostosis. **C.** Blunt elevation of the anconeus is crucial to avoid damaging the capsule or lateral ligament complex. **D.** The capsule and lateral ligament complex are tagged during the approach to facilitate final repair with suture anchors.

Fracture Inspection and Preparation

- The fracture is now completely visible along with full visualization of the radial head by posteriorly subluxing the radial head out of the joint (**TECH FIG 3**).
- The wound is irrigated, and loose bodies are removed.
- The forearm is rotated to obtain a circumferential view of the fracture and appreciate the safe zone for hardware placement.
- If comminution (more than three pieces) is evident at this step or significant impaction with a DRUJ injury, we elect to replace the radial head.

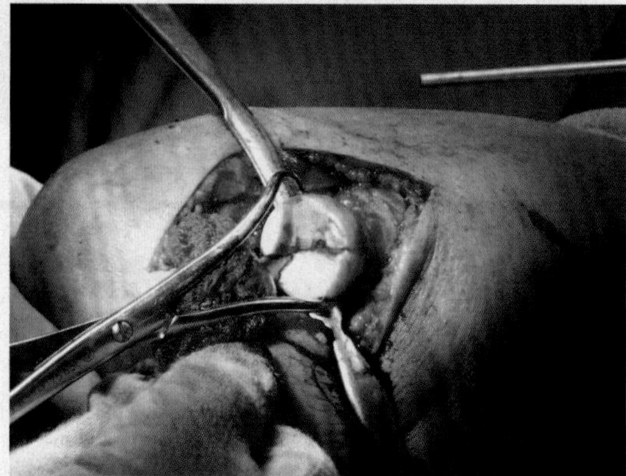

TECH FIG 3 • The modified Wrightington approach allows for full visualization of the radial head and fracture by subluxing the radial head posteriorly out of the joint.

Reduction and Provisional Fixation

- Any joint impaction is elevated and the void filed with local cancellous graft from the lateral epicondyle.
- The fragments are reduced provisionally with a tenaculum and held with small Kirschner wires placed out of the zone where definitive fixation is planned.
- It is acceptable to place this temporary fixation in the safe zone.

Fixation

- There are many options for definitive fixation[7]:
  - One or two countersunk 2.0- or 2.7-mm AO cortical screws perpendicular to the fracture
  - Mini-plates
  - Small headless screws
  - Polyglycolide pins
  - Poly-L-lactic acid screws
  - Small threaded wires
- We prefer to use two parallel Biotrak screws (Acumed, Hillsboro, Oregon), which are cannulated, headless, resorbable, and variable pitched for isolated head fractures (**TECH FIG 4**). For fractures with neck extension, we prefer AO 2.0- or 2.7-mm mini-plates along the safe zone.

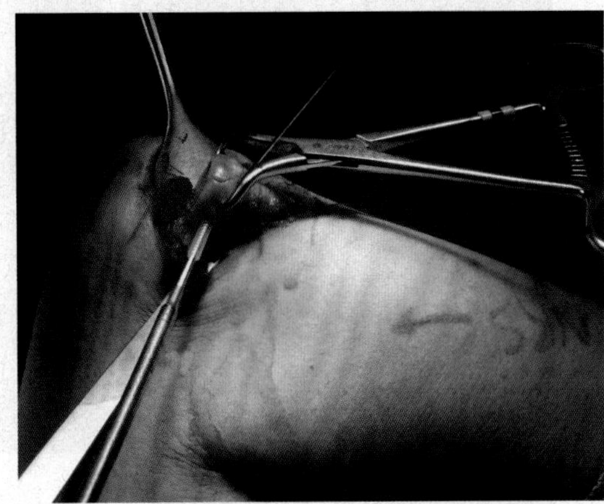

TECH FIG 4 • Tenaculum clamps and 0.062-inch Kirschner wires are placed outside the zone of planned definitive fixation to provisionally hold the reduction. Two Biotrak screws are inserted for definitive fixation while the fracture is held reduced.

Closure

- Any releases or injury to the annular ligament or lateral ulnar collateral ligament must be repaired anatomically. Drill holes with transosseous sutures are a proven method, but most authors now use suture anchors with reproducible results.
- Skin closure is performed in standard fashion with drains at the surgeon's discretion.

PEARLS AND PITFALLS

Protection of the posterior interosseous nerve	■ Pronation of the forearm moves the posterior interosseous nerve away from the operative field during posterior approaches. ■ Dissection should remain subperiosteally.
Comminution	■ We have a low threshold for excision or arthroplasty in the setting of comminution.
Fluoroscopy	■ A fluoroscopy unit should be available for examination under anesthesia before sterile preparation.
Hardware	■ Prosthetic radial head replacement should be discussed with the patient as an option and should be available in the room should the fracture prove to be comminuted. ■ A hinged external fixator should be available if instability may be an issue.
Examination	■ A thorough fluoroscopic examination is the most important factor in deciding what treatment is appropriate. To obtain a true lateral view, we recommend abducting the arm and externally rotating the shoulder while placing the elbow on the image intensifier.

POSTOPERATIVE CARE

- The elbow is immobilized in a splint for 7 to 10 days.
- Serial x-rays are obtained to detect any loss of reduction at immediate postoperative, 2 weeks, 6 weeks, and 3 months, until healing is achieved (**FIG 12**).
- Active range of motion is allowed as soon as tolerable. Supervised therapy may be considered if the patient is not making adequate progress.
- Associated injuries may call for more protected range of motion.
- Light activities of daily living are allowed at 2 weeks, with increased weight bearing at 6 weeks.

OUTCOMES

- The results of ORIF depend both on host factors such as the type of fracture, smoking, compliance, level of physical demand as well as surgical and rehabilitation protocols.
  - In uncomplicated fractures, over 90% satisfactory results can be expected.
  - Complications and resultant secondary procedures will be more likely in cases with undiagnosed instability and associated injury.

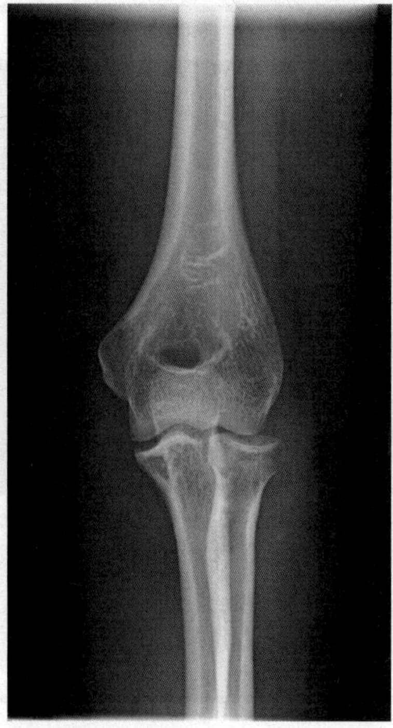

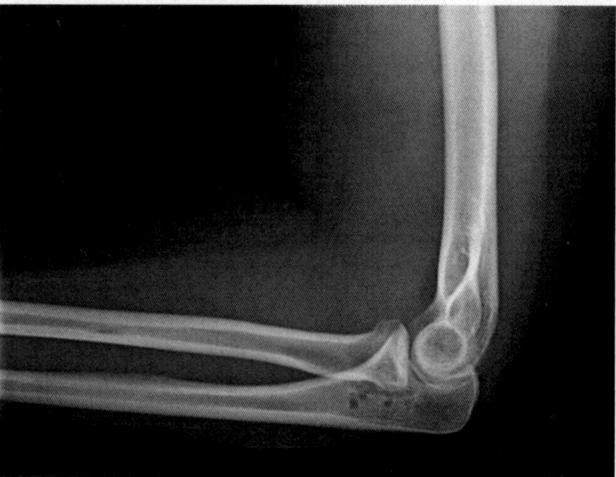

FIG 12 • Postoperative x-rays showing anatomic reduction of the radial head fracture. The Biotrak screws are radiolucent. Note that anchor holes are seen at the crista supinatoris where the lateral ulnar collateral ligament (LUCL) and annular ligament complex are repaired.

COMPLICATIONS

- Stiffness is the most common complication, with loss of terminal extension, supination, and pronation being most evident.
- Arthritis of the radiocapitellar joint or PRUJ
- Heterotopic ossification
- Symptomatic hardware may require secondary removal (**FIG 13**).
- Infection
- Early and late instability from missed or failed treatment of associated injuries
- The rate of avascular necrosis is about 10%, significantly higher in displaced fractures. This is expected given that the radial recurrent artery inserts in the safe zone where hardware is placed. This is generally clinically silent.
- Loss of reduction
- Nonunion (**FIG 14**)

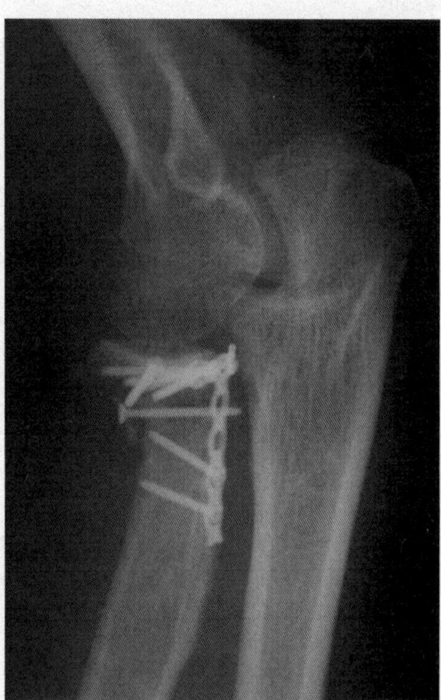

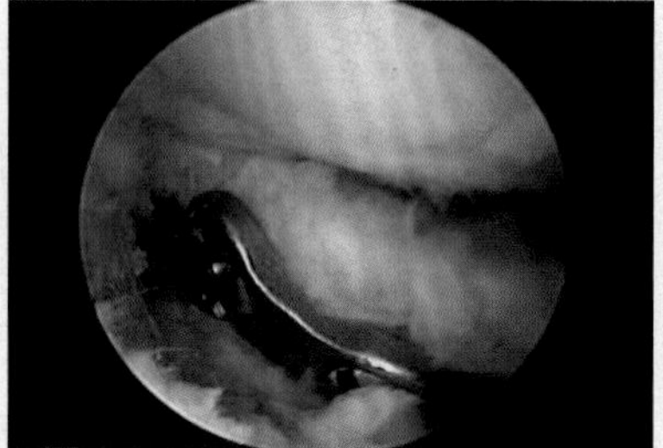

FIG 13 • A. Oblique radiograph demonstrating prominent hardware limiting forearm rotation. **B.** Arthroscopic view in the lateral gutter demonstrating hardware impingement at the PRUJ.

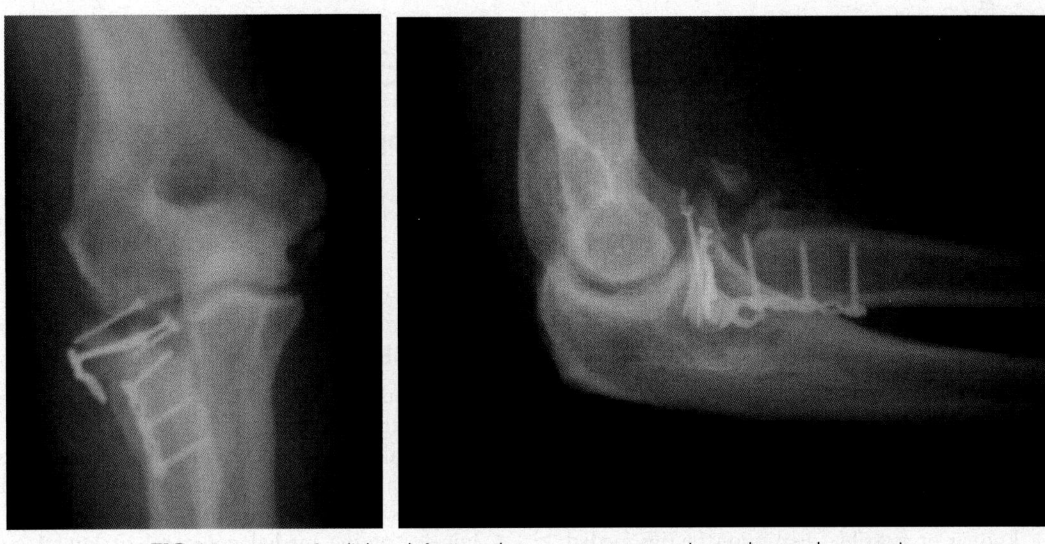

FIG 14 • ORIF of radial neck fracture that went on to nonunion and avascular necrosis.

REFERENCES

1. Akesson T, Herbertsson P, Josefsson PO, et al. Primary nonoperative treatment of moderately displaced two-part fractures of the radial head. J Bone Joint Surg Am 2006;88(9):1909–1914.
2. Amis AA, Miller JH. The mechanisms of elbow fractures: an investigation using impact tests in vitro. Injury 1995;26:163–168.
3. Antuna SA, Sánchez-Márquez JM, Barco R. Long-term results of radial head resection following isolated radial head fractures in patients younger than forty years old. J Bone Joint Surg Am 2010;92:558–566.
4. Boyd HB. Surgical exposure of the ulna and proximal third of the radius through one incision. Surg Gynecol Obstet 1940;71:86–88.
5. Broberg MA, Morrey BF. Results of delayed excision of the radial head after fracture. J Bone Joint Surg Am 1986;68(5):669–674.
6. Broberg MA, Morrey BF. Results of treatment of fracture-elbow dislocations of the elbow and intraarticular fractures. Clin Orthop Relat Res 1989;246:126–130.
7. Caputo AE, Mazzocca AD, Sontoro VM. The nonarticulating portion of the radial head: anatomic and clinical correlations for internal fixation. J Hand Surg Am 1998;23(6):1082–1090.
8. Esser RD, Davis S, Taavao T. Fractures of the radial head treated by internal fixation: late results in 26 cases. J Orthop Trauma 1995;9:318–323.
9. Essex-Lopresti P. Fractures of the radial head with distal radioulnar dislocation. J Bone Joint Surg Br 1951;33(2):244–250.
10. Harrington IJ, Tountas AA. Replacement of the radial head in the treatment of unstable elbow fractures. Injury 1981;12(5):405–412.
11. Herbertsson P, Josefsson PO, Hasserius R, et al. Fractures of the radial head and neck treated with radial head excision. J Bone Joint Surg Am 2004;86-A(9):1925–1930.
12. Herbertsson P, Josefsson PO, Hasserius R, et al. Uncomplicated Mason type-II and III fractures of the radial head and neck in adults. A long-term follow-up study. J Bone Joint Surg Am 2004;86-A(3):569–574.
13. Hotchkiss RN. Fractures and dislocations of the elbow. In: Rockwood CA Jr, Green DP, eds. Fractures in Adults, ed 4. Philadelphia: Lippincott-Raven, 1996:929–1024.
14. Itamura JM, Roidis NT, Chong AK, et al. Computed tomography study of radial head morphology. J Shoulder Elbow Surg 2008;17(2):347–354.
15. Itamura J, Roidis N, Mirzayan R, et al. Radial head fractures: MRI evaluation of associated injuries. J Shoulder Elbow Surg 2005;14(4):421–424.
16. Kaas L, Struijs PA, Ring D, et al. Treatment of Mason type II radial head fractures without associated fractures or elbow dislocation: a systematic review. J Hand Surg Am 2012;37(7):1416–1421.
17. Kaas L, van Riet RP, Turkenburg JL, et al. Magnetic resonance imaging in radial head fractures: most associated injuries are not clinically relevant. J Shoulder Elbow Surg 2011;20(8):1282–1288.
18. Kovar FM, Jaindl M, Thalhammer G, et al. Incidence and analysis of radial head and neck fractures. World J Orthop 2013;4(2):80–84.
19. McKee MD, Jupiter JB. Trauma to the adult elbow and fractures of the distal humerus. In: Browner BD, Jupiter JR, Levine AM, et al, eds. Skeletal Trauma, ed 2. Philadelphia: WB Saunders, 1998:1455–1522.
20. Morrey BF. Radial head fracture. In: Morrey BF, ed. The Elbow and Its Disorders, ed 3. Philadelphia: WB Saunders, 2000:341–364.
21. Morrey BF, An KN, Stormont TJ. Force transmission through the radial head. J Bone Joint Surg Am 1988;70(2):250–256.
22. Ring D, Quintero J, Jupiter JB. Open reduction and internal fixation of fractures of the radial head. J Bone Joint Surg Am 2002;84-A(10):1811–1815.
23. Roidis NT, Papadakis SA, Rigopoulos N, et al. Current concepts and controversies in the management of radial head fractures. Orthopedics 2006;29(10):904–916.
24. Stanley JK, Penn DS, Wasseem M. Exposure of the head of the radius using the Wrightington approach. J Bone Joint Surg Br 2006;88(9):1178–1182.
25. Tang CW, Skaggs DL, Kay RM. Elbow aspiration and arthrogram: an alternative method. Am J Orthop 2001;30:256.
26. Yamaguchi K, Sweet FA, Bindra R, et al. The extraosseous and intraosseous arterial anatomy of the adult elbow. J Bone Joint Surg Am 1997;79(11):1653–1662.

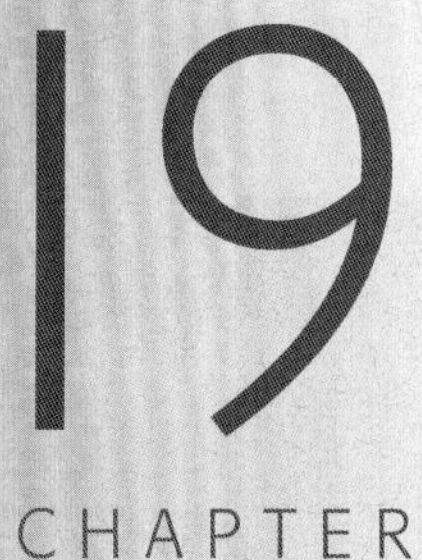

CHAPTER

Radial Head Replacement

Yishai Rosenblatt and Graham J. W. King

DEFINITION

- Radial head fractures are the most common fracture of the elbow and usually can be managed either nonoperatively or with open reduction and internal fixation (ORIF).[12]
- Radial head arthroplasty is indicated for unreconstructable displaced radial head fractures with an associated elbow dislocation or a known or possible disruption of the medial collateral, lateral collateral, or interosseous ligaments.[26]
- Most comminuted radial head fractures have an associated ligament injury, so radial head excision without replacement is uncommonly indicated in the setting of an acute radial head fracture.
- Biomechanical studies have shown that the kinematics and stability of the elbow are altered by radial head excision, even in the setting of intact collateral ligaments,[24] and are improved with a metallic radial head arthroplasty.[6,31,39]
- Radial head replacement is also indicated to treat posttraumatic conditions such as radial head nonunion and malunion and to manage elbow or forearm instability after radial head excision.[41]

ANATOMY

- The radial head has a circular concave dish that articulates with the spherical capitellum and an articular margin that articulates with the lesser sigmoid notch of the ulna.
- The articular dish has an elliptical shape that varies considerably in size and shape and is variably offset from the axis of the radial neck.[44]
- There is a poor correlation between the size of the radial head and the medullary canal of the radial neck, making a modular implant desirable for an optimal fit.[30]
- Elbow stability is maintained by joint congruity, capsuloligamentous integrity, and an intact balanced musculature.
- The radial head is an important valgus stabilizer of the elbow, particularly in the setting of an incompetent medial collateral ligament, which is the primary stabilizer against valgus force.
- The radial head is also important as an axial stabilizer of the forearm and resists varus and posterolateral rotatory instability by tensioning the lateral collateral ligament.[25]
- The lateral ulnar collateral ligament is an important stabilizer against varus and posterolateral rotational instability of the elbow[37] and should be preserved or repaired after radial head arthroplasty (**FIG 1**).
- The radial head accounts for up to 60% of the load transfer across the elbow.[19]

PATHOGENESIS

- Displaced radial head fractures typically result from a fall on the outstretched arm.
- Axial, valgus, and posterolateral rotational patterns of loading are all thought to be potentially responsible for these fractures.
- Injuries of the medial collateral or lateral collateral ligament or the interosseous ligament are typically associated with comminuted displaced unreconstructable radial head fractures.[9]
- In more severe injuries, dislocations of the elbow and forearm and fractures of the coronoid, olecranon, and capitellum can occur and further impair stability.

NATURAL HISTORY

- Long-term follow-up studies suggest a high incidence of radiographic arthritis with radial head excision, although the incidence of symptomatic arthritis varies widely between series.[7,22,23]
- Biomechanical data have demonstrated an alteration in the kinematics, load transfer, and stability of the elbow after radial head excision[6,24] that may lead to premature cartilage wear of the ulnohumeral joint and secondary pain due to arthritis.

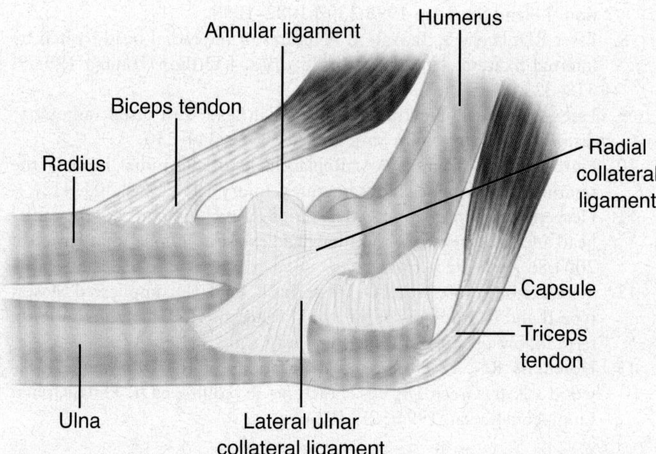

FIG 1 • The ligaments on the lateral aspect of the elbow include the lateral ulnar collateral ligament, the radial collateral ligament, and the annular ligament. The lateral ulnar collateral ligament is an important stabilizer against varus and posterolateral rotational instability of the elbow and should be preserved or repaired after radial head arthroplasty.

- Metallic radial head replacement in elbows with intact ligaments restores the kinematics and stability similar to that of a native radial head and has been shown to provide good clinical and radiographic outcome in most patients at medium-term follow-up; however, long-term outcome studies are lacking.[6]

PATIENT HISTORY AND PHYSICAL FINDINGS

- The mechanism of injury is typically a fall on the outstretched hand.
- The patient will complain of pain and limitation of elbow or forearm motion.
- A history of forearm or wrist pain should be sought.
- Inspection may reveal ecchymosis along the forearm or medial aspect of the elbow. Deformity may be evident if there is an associated dislocation.
- Careful palpation of the radial head, the medial and lateral collateral ligaments of the elbow, the interosseous ligament of the forearm, and the distal radioulnar joint should be performed. Local tenderness over one or all of these structures implies a possible derangement of the relevant structure.
- Because associated injuries of the shoulder, forearm, wrist, and hand are common, these areas should be carefully examined.
- Range of motion, including forearm rotation and elbow flexion–extension, should be evaluated. The presence of palpable and auditory crepitus should be noted.
- Loss of terminal elbow flexion and extension is expected as a consequence of a hemarthrosis in acute fractures, whereas loss of forearm rotation typically is caused by a mechanical impingement.
- A careful neurovascular assessment of all three major nerves that cross the elbow should be performed.
- The examiner should observe for localized or diffuse swelling in the elbow. Effusion represents hemarthrosis due to intra-articular fracture.
- The examiner should compare active and passive range of motion to the uninjured side. Reduced range of motion may be a result of hemarthrosis or mechanical block from a broken fragment. Intra-articular injection of a local anesthetic helps differentiate between reduced range of motion due to a mechanical block versus pain inhibition.
- The examiner should look for varus–valgus instability. Any gapping on the medial or lateral side beneath the examiner's hand is noted. Positive findings suggest medial or lateral collateral ligament insufficiency. Typically, this test is positive only when performed under a regional or general anesthetic, hence these injuries are easy to miss if an examination under anesthesia is not performed.
- The lateral pivot shift test is performed. Positive apprehension or a clunk that is seen or felt when the ulna and radius reduce on the humerus suggests posterolateral rotatory instability.

IMAGING AND OTHER DIAGNOSTIC STUDIES

- Anteroposterior (AP), lateral, and oblique elbow radiographs, with the x-ray beam centered on the radiocapitellar joint, usually provide sufficient information for the diagnosis and treatment of radial head fractures.
- Bilateral posteroanterior radiographs of both wrists in neutral rotation should be performed to evaluate ulnar variance in patients with wrist discomfort or a comminuted radial head fracture because there is a higher incidence of an associated interosseous ligament injury in these patients.[9]
- Computed tomography with sagittal, coronal, and three-dimensional (3-D) reconstructions may assist with preoperative planning and can help the surgeon predict whether a displaced radial head fracture can be repaired with ORIF or if an arthroplasty will likely be needed.

DIFFERENTIAL DIAGNOSIS

- Acute radial head fractures
- Other fractures or dislocations about the elbow (eg, supracondylar, capitellar, coronoid, osteochondral fractures)
- Radial head nonunion or malunion, posttraumatic arthritis
- Congenital dislocation of the radial head
- Forearm or elbow instability
- Lateral epicondylitis
- Rheumatoid arthritis or osteoarthritis
- Synovitis, inflammatory or infectious
- Tumors

NONOPERATIVE MANAGEMENT

- The indications for surgical management of radial head fractures are not well defined in the literature. Fragment size, number of fracture fragments, degree of displacement, and bone quality influence decision making regarding the optimal management.
- Nondisplaced fractures or small (<33% of the radial head) minimally displaced fractures (<2 mm of displacement) can be treated with early motion with an excellent outcome in the majority of patients.[21]
- Associated injuries and a block to motion are also important factors to consider when deciding between nonoperative and surgical management.

SURGICAL MANAGEMENT

- Small displaced fractures that cause painful crepitus or limited motion are managed with fragment excision if they are too small (typically, <25% of the diameter of the radial head) or osteopenic to be internally fixated.
- Larger displaced fractures are typically managed with ORIF with good outcomes in most patients.[35,46]
- Radial head fractures that are displaced but too comminuted to be anatomically reduced and stably fixed and that are too large to consider fragment excision (involve more than a quarter to a third of the radial head) should be managed by radial head excision with or without arthroplasty.[1,27]
- Patients who are known to have, or are likely to have, an associated ligamentous injury of the elbow or forearm should have a radial head arthroplasty because radial head excision is contraindicated (**FIG 2**).[29]
- The decision as to what fracture is reconstructable depends on surgeon factors (eg, experience), patient factors (eg, osteoporosis), and fracture factors (eg, fragment number and size, comminution, associated soft tissue injuries). The final decision is often made only at the time of surgery.
- Other indications for radial head arthroplasty include radial head nonunion or malunion, primary or secondary management of forearm or elbow instability (eg, Essex-Lopresti injury), rheumatoid arthritis or osteoarthritis, and tumors.

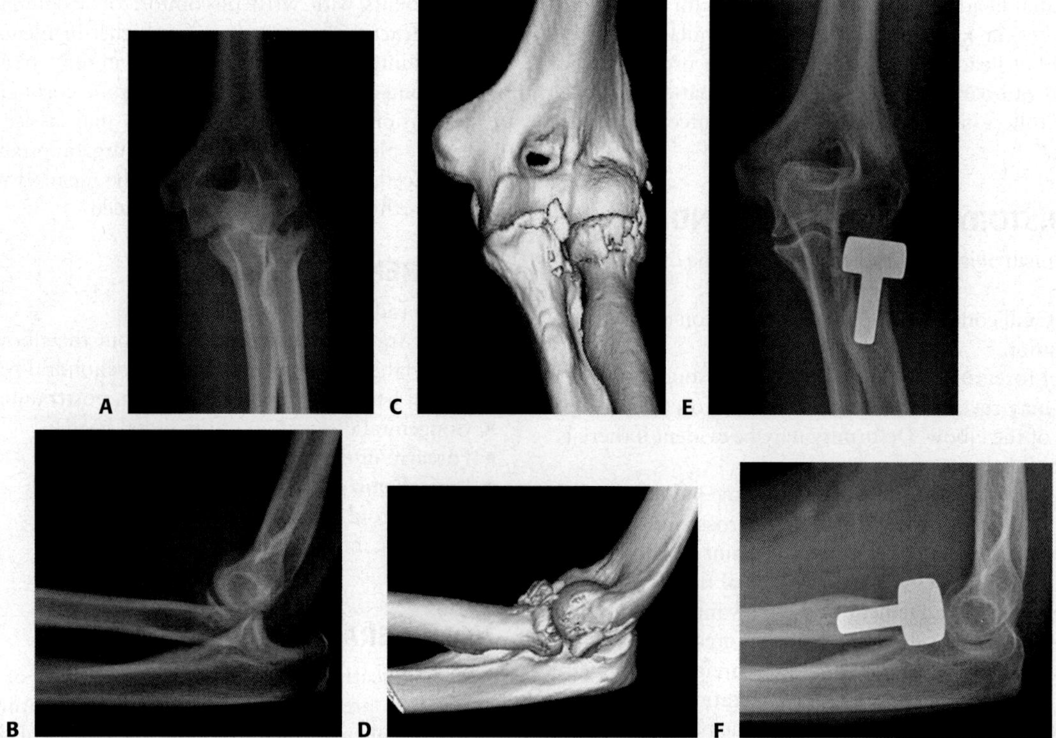

FIG 2 • A,B. AP and lateral radiographs of a 54-year-old woman who sustained a posterolateral elbow dislocation associated with a comminuted fracture of the radial head and coronoid—the "terrible triad." **C,D.** Preoperative 3-D reconstruction images demonstrating a comminuted radial head fracture with a small undisplaced coronoid fracture. **E,F.** Postoperative radiographs after modular radial head arthroplasty (Evolve, Wright Medical Technology, Arlington, TN) and repair of the lateral collateral ligament. Medial collateral ligament and coronoid repairs were not required because the elbow was sufficiently stable at the end of the procedure. A good functional outcome was achieved at the final follow-up.

Preoperative Planning

- Currently available devices include smooth stem spacer implants, press-fit ingrowth stems, monoblock and bipolar devices, and metallic or pyrolytic carbon articulations.
- Most implants have an axisymmetric circular design; however, one currently available device has a more anatomic nonaxisymmetric elliptical shape.[33,40,47]
- Silicone radial head implants offer little in the way of axial or valgus stability to the elbow and have been complicated by a high incidence of implant wear, fragmentation, and silicone synovitis leading to generalized joint damage. As a result, they have fallen out of favor and have been replaced by metallic implants.[18]
- Most metallic radial head implants that are currently available are modular with separate heads and stems, allowing improved size matching of the native radial head and neck relative to older monoblock designs.[17,28,30]
- Precise implant sizing and placement are critical with these devices to ensure correct capitellar tracking and to avoid a cam effect with forearm rotation, which may cause premature capitellar wear due to shearing of the cartilage and stem loosening due to increased loading of the stem–bone interface.[15]
- Preoperative radiographic templating of the contralateral normal radial head should be employed in the setting of a secondary radial head replacement but is not needed for acute fractures because the excised radial head is available for accurate implant sizing.

Positioning

- The patient is placed supine on the operating table and a sandbag is placed beneath the ipsilateral scapula to assist in positioning the arm across the chest.
- Alternatively, the patient can be positioned in a lateral position with the affected arm held over a bolster or in the supine position with the arm on a hand table.[5]
- Prophylactic intravenous antibiotics are administered.
- General or regional anesthesia is employed.
- A sterile tourniquet is applied.

Surgical Approach

- A midline posterior elbow incision is made just lateral to the tip of the olecranon (**TECH FIG 1A**).
- A full-thickness lateral fasciocutaneous flap is elevated on the deep fascia. This extensile incision decreases the risk of cutaneous nerve injury and provides access to the radial head, coronoid, and medial and lateral collateral ligaments for the management of more complex injuries (**TECH FIG 1B**).[11,38]
- Alternatively, a lateral skin incision centered over the lateral epicondyle and passing obliquely over the radial head can be used (see **TECH FIG 1A**).

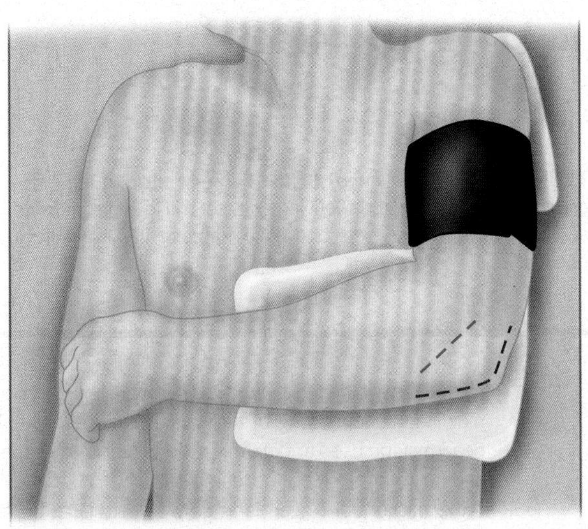

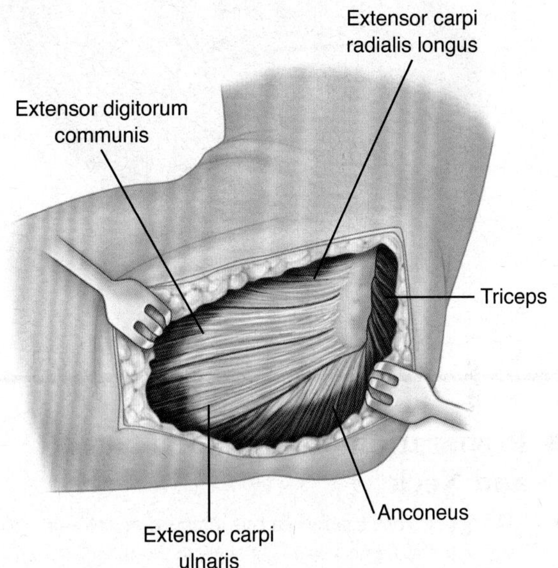

TECH FIG 1 • **A.** The patient is placed supine on the operating table and a sandbag is placed beneath the ipsilateral scapula to assist in positioning the arm across the chest. The posterior incision is indicated in *red*. Alternatively, a lateral skin incision centered over the lateral epicondyle and passing obliquely over the radial head can be used (*blue*). **B.** A midline posterior elbow incision made just lateral to the tip of the olecranon. A full-thickness lateral fasciocutaneous flap is elevated on the deep fascia. This extensile incision allows access to both the lateral and medial aspects of the elbow, in case of more complex injuries, and reduces the incidence of cutaneous nerve injury.

Common Extensor Split

- The common extensor tendon is identified.
  - The landmarks for this plane are a line joining the lateral epicondyle and the tubercle of Lister.
- The common extensor tendon is split longitudinally at the middle aspect of the radial head, and the underlying radial collateral and annular ligaments are incised (**TECH FIG 2A**).
  - Dissection should stay anterior to the lateral ulnar collateral ligament to prevent the development of posterolateral rotatory instability (see **FIG 1**).
  - The forearm is maintained in pronation to move the posterior interosseous nerve more distal and medial during the surgical approach.[10]
- If further exposure is required
  - The humeral origin of the radial collateral ligament and the overlying extensor muscles are elevated anteriorly off the lateral epicondyle to improve the exposure if needed (**TECH FIG 2B**).
  - Release of the posterior component of the lateral collateral ligament can be considered, but careful ligament repair is required at the end of the procedure in order to restore the varus and posterolateral rotatory stability of the elbow.[13]

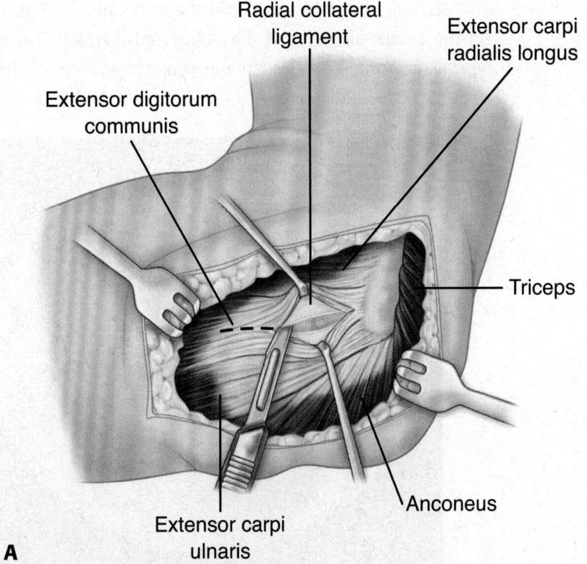

TECH FIG 2 • **A.** The common extensor tendon is split longitudinally at the middle aspect of the radial head, and the underlying radial collateral and annular ligaments are incised. The forearm is pronated to protect the posterior interosseous nerve. *(continued)*

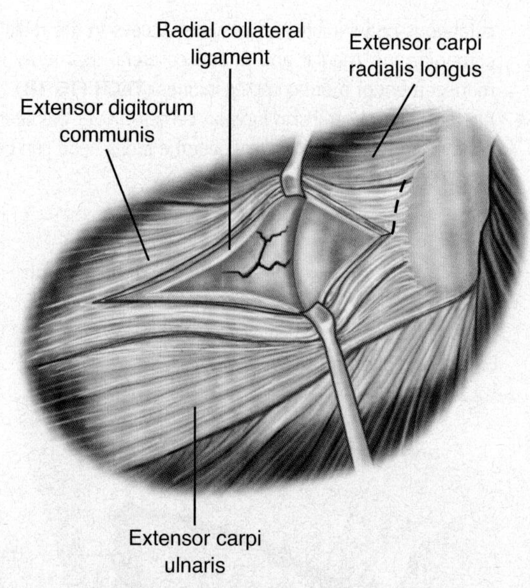

TECH FIG 2 • *(continued)* **B.** The humeral origin of the radial collateral ligament and the overlying extensor muscles are elevated anteriorly off the lateral epicondyle to improve the exposure if needed.

Preparation of the Radial Head and Neck

- All fragments of the radial head are removed, as well as a minimal amount of radial neck at a right angle to the medullary canal, to make a smooth surface for seating of the prosthetic radial head.
  - Complete fragment excision can be confirmed with the use of an image intensifier.
- The capitellum is evaluated for chondral injuries or osteochondral fractures.
- The radial head prosthesis is sized in one of several ways:
  - The resected radial head is reassembled in the provided sizing template to assist in the accurate sizing of the prosthesis (**TECH FIG 3A–C**).
  - The diameter of radial head prosthesis should be based on the minor diameter of the native radial head. This is typically 2 mm smaller than the major diameter of the elliptical native radial head.
  - Alternatively, if the radial head has been previously excised, radiographic templating of the contralateral normal radial head may be used to determine the appropriate diameter and height of the radial head implant.
  - If the native radial head is in between available implant sizes, the smaller implant diameter or thickness should be selected.
- The radial neck is delivered laterally using a Hohmann retractor carefully placed around the posterior aspect of the proximal radial neck (**TECH FIG 3D**).
  - An anteriorly based retractor should be avoided because of the risk of injury from pressure on the posterior interosseous nerve.
- The medullary canal of the radial neck is reamed using hand reamers until cortical contact is encountered.
  - A trial stem one size smaller than the rasp is inserted to achieve a loose press-fit.

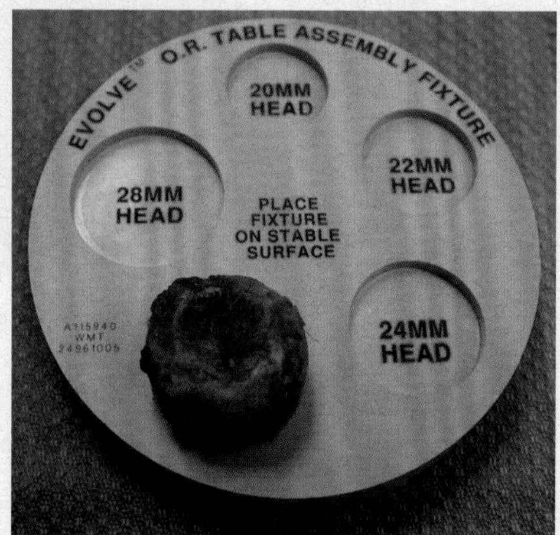

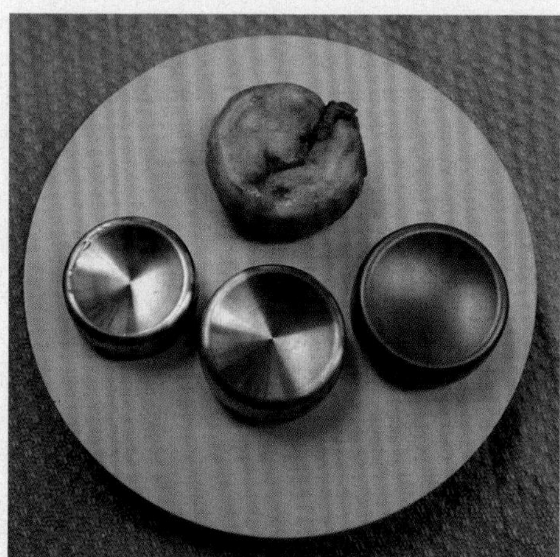

TECH FIG 3 • The resected radial head is reassembled in the provided sizing template (**A**) to assist in the accurate sizing of the prosthesis in terms of diameter (**B**) and height (**C**) and to ensure that all the fragments have been removed from the elbow. *(continued)*

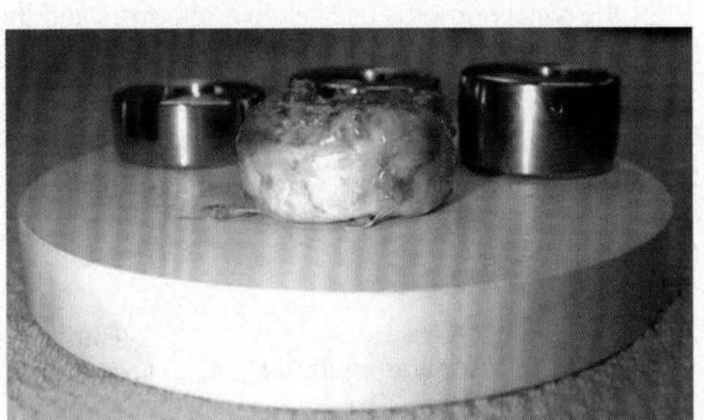

C

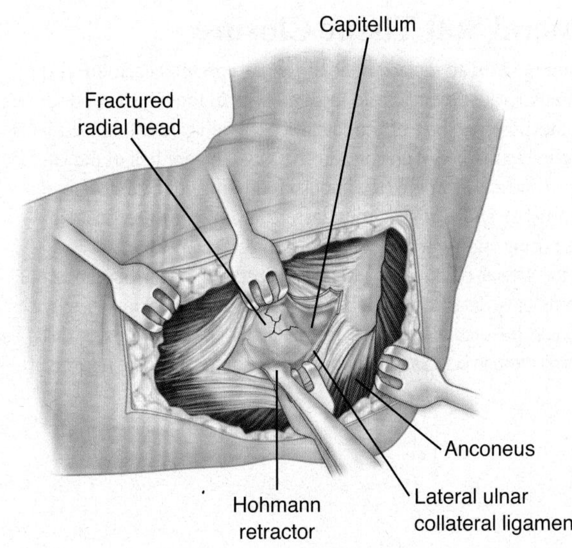

D

TECH FIG 3 • (continued) D. The radial neck is delivered laterally using a Hohmann retractor carefully placed around the posterior aspect of the proximal radial neck. An anteriorly based retractor should be avoided because of the risk of injury to the posterior interosseous nerve.

Radial Head Replacement

- A trial head is inserted onto the stem, and the diameter, height, tracking, and congruency of the prosthesis are evaluated both visually and with the aid of an image intensifier.
  - The radial head prosthesis should articulate at the same height as the radial notch of the ulna and about 1 to 2 mm distal to the tip of the coronoid (**TECH FIG 4A**).
  - The alignment of the distal radioulnar joint and ulnar variance, as well as the width of the lateral and medial portions of the ulnohumeral joint, are checked and compared to the contralateral wrist and elbow, respectively, under fluoroscopy.
- Overlengthening the radiocapitellar joint with a radial head implant that is too thick should be avoided to reduce the risk of cartilage wear on the capitellum from excessive pressure; a nonparallel medial ulnohumeral joint space that is wider laterally is suggestive of overstuffing.[4,16]
  - Some modular and bipolar implants allow insertion of the stem first, then placement of the head onto the stem with coupling in situ, which significantly reduces the surgical exposure needed (**TECH FIG 4B**).
- If the prosthesis is maltracking on the capitellum with forearm rotation, a smaller stem size should be trialed to ensure that the articulation of the radial head with the capitellum is controlled by the annular ligament and articular congruency and not dictated by the proximal radial shaft.

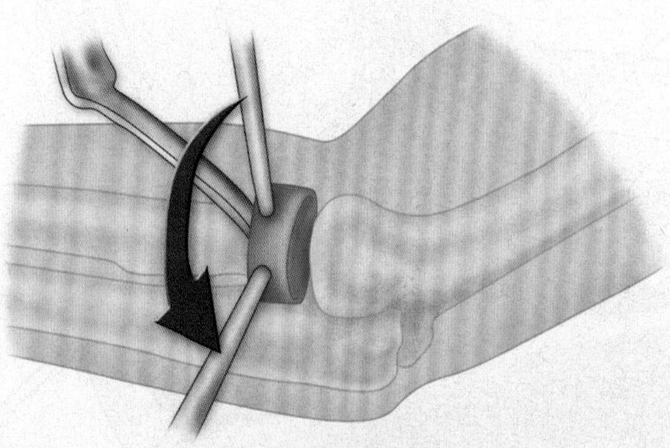

A

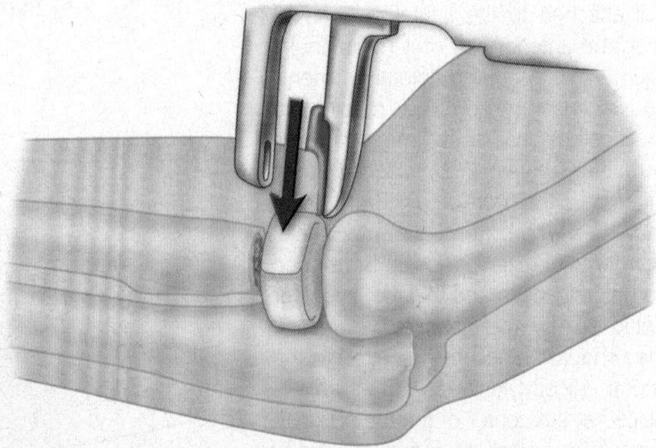

B

TECH FIG 4 • A. A trial stem is inserted. A trial head is inserted onto the stem and the diameter, height, tracking, and congruency of the prosthesis are evaluated both visually and with the aid of an image intensifier. **B.** Some modular and bipolar implants allow insertion of the stem first, then placement of the head onto the stem with coupling in situ, which significantly reduces the surgical exposure needed.

Lateral Soft Tissue Closure

- After radial head replacement, the lateral collateral ligament and extensor muscle origins are repaired back to the lateral condyle.
- If the posterior half of the lateral collateral ligament is still attached to the lateral epicondyle, then the anterior half of the lateral collateral ligament (the annular ligament and radial collateral ligament) and extensor muscles are repaired to the posterior half using interrupted absorbable sutures (**TECH FIG 5A**).
- If the lateral collateral ligament and extensor origin have been completely detached either by the injury or surgical exposure, they should be securely repaired to the lateral epicondyle using drill holes through bone and nonabsorbable sutures or suture anchors.
- A single drill hole is placed at the axis of motion (the center of the arc of curvature of the capitellum) and connected to two drill holes placed anterior and posterior to the lateral supracondylar ridge.
- A locking (Krackow) suture technique is employed to gain a secure hold of the lateral collateral ligament and common extensor muscle fascia (**TECH FIG 5B–D**).
- The ligament sutures are pulled into the holes drilled in the distal humerus using suture retrievers and the forearm is pronated, and varus forces are avoided, while tensioning the sutures before tying (**TECH FIG 5E**).
- The knots should be left anterior or posterior to the lateral supracondylar ridge to avoid prominence.

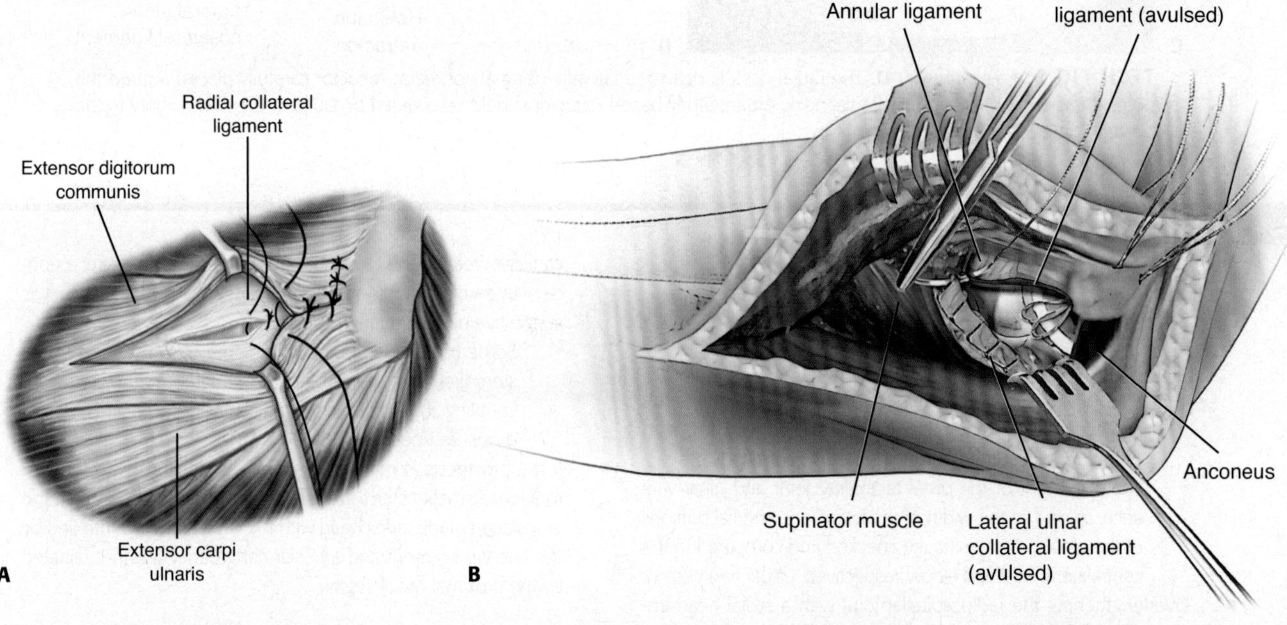

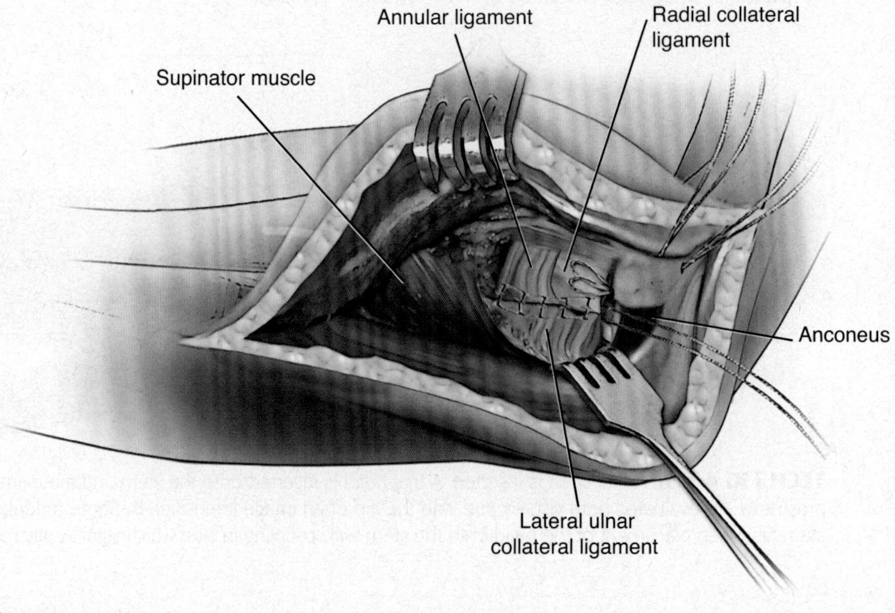

TECH FIG 5 • **A.** If the posterior half of the lateral collateral ligament is still attached to the lateral epicondyle, then the anterior half of it (the annular ligament and radial collateral ligament) and extensor muscles are repaired to the posterior half using interrupted absorbable sutures. *ECU*, extensor carpi ulnaris; *EDC*, extensor digitorum communis. **B–D.** If the lateral collateral ligament and extensor origin have been completely disrupted by the injury or detached by the surgical exposure, they should be securely repaired to the lateral epicondyle. A single drill hole is placed at the center of the arc of curvature of the capitellum and connected to two drill holes placed anterior and posterior to the lateral supracondylar ridge. A locking (Krackow) suture technique is employed to gain a secure hold of the lateral collateral ligament (**B**) as well as of the annular ligament (**C**). *(continued)*

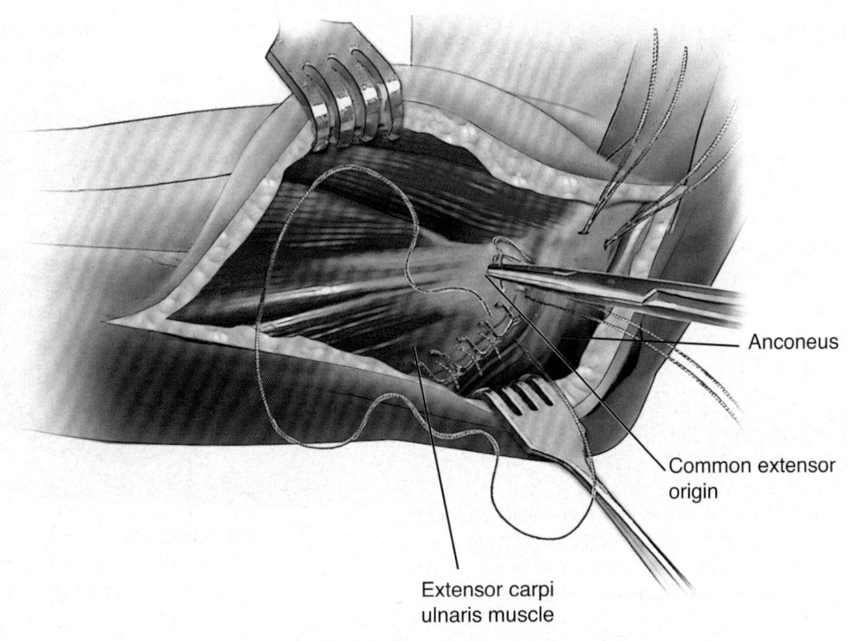

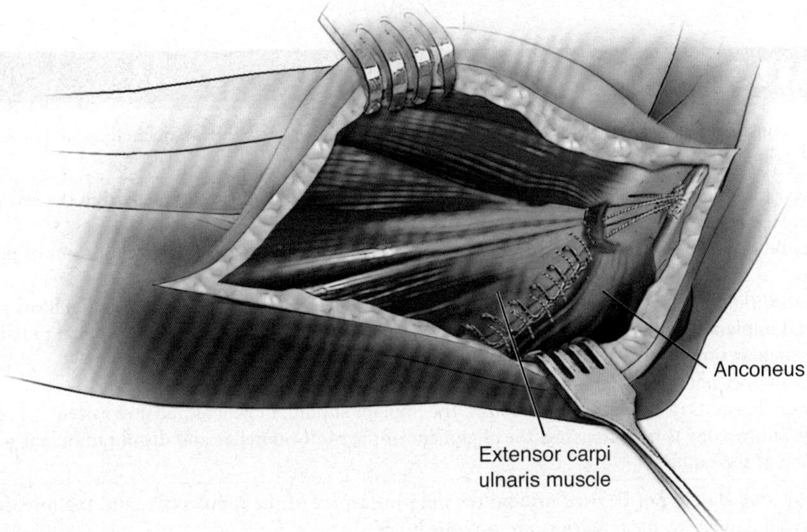

TECH FIG 5 • *(continued)* **D.** A second stitch is used in a similar manner to repair the common extensor muscle fascia. **E.** The sutures are pulled into the holes drilled in the distal humerus using suture retrievers, tensioned while keeping the forearm pronated and while avoiding varus forces, and eventually tied over the lateral supracondylar ridge.

Completion

- After replacement arthroplasty and lateral soft tissue closure, the elbow should be placed through an arc of flexion–extension while carefully evaluating for elbow stability in pronation, neutral, and supination.[5]
- Pronation is generally beneficial if the lateral ligaments are deficient,[13] supination if the medial ligaments are deficient,[2] and neutral position if both sides have been injured.
- In patients who have an associated elbow dislocation, additional repair of the medial collateral ligament and flexor–pronator origin should be performed if the elbow subluxates at 40 degrees or more of flexion.
- Tourniquet deflation and hemostasis should be secured before wound closure.

TECHNIQUES

Kocher Approach

- Alternatively, the radial head may be approached by using the Kocher interval[32] between the extensor carpi ulnaris and anconeus.
- The fascial interval between these muscles is identified by noting the diverging direction of the muscle groups and small vascular perforators that exit at this interval (**TECH FIG 6**).
- Care should be taken to preserve the lateral ulnar collateral ligament, which is vulnerable as the dissection is carried deeper through the capsule.

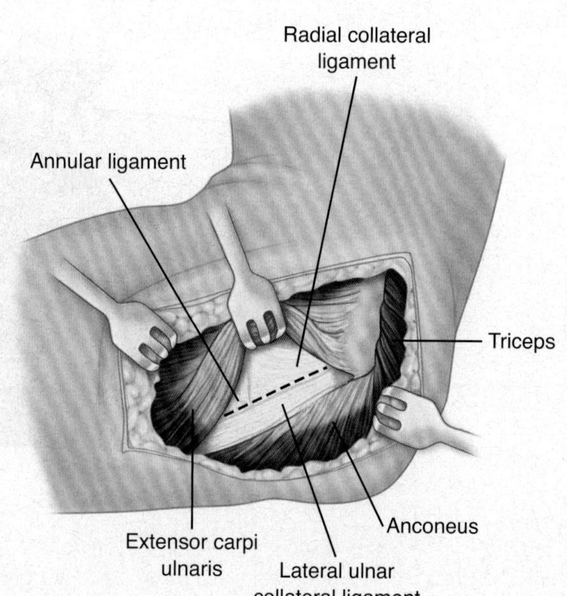

TECH FIG 6 • The extensor carpi ulnaris is elevated anteriorly, and an arthrotomy is performed at the midportion of the radial head. Care should be taken to preserve the lateral ulnar collateral ligament, which is vulnerable as the dissection is carried deeper through the capsule.

PEARLS AND PITFALLS

Indications	■ Displaced unreconstructable fracture of the radial head with known or probable associated medial or lateral collateral or interosseous ligament injury
Pearls	■ A preoperative radiographic template of the contralateral native radial head should be used in the setting of a secondary radial head replacement. ■ Dissection should stay anterior to the lateral ulnar collateral ligament to prevent the development of posterolateral rotatory instability. ■ The radial head should be sized based on the minor diameter and thickness of the excised radial head. ■ The radial head implant is typically 2 mm smaller than the major diameter of the native elliptical radial head. ■ Radial head articular surface height should be at the level of the proximal radioulnar joint. ■ If the radial head does not track well on the capitellum, the stem should be downsized. ■ If the native radial head is in between implant sizes, the implant should, in general, be downsized. ■ Intraoperative fluoroscopy is used to assess the alignment of the radiocapitellar and distal radioulnar joints and to avoid overlengthening of the radius.
Pitfalls	■ Hohmann retractors should not be used around the anterior aspect of the radial neck, and the forearm should be kept pronated to avoid damage to the posterior interosseous nerve. ■ The surgeon should avoid overstuffing the thickness or diameter of the radial head because of the risk of capitellar wear and pain. Filling the gap between the capitellum and radial neck is not a useful landmark for prosthesis thickness because lateral soft tissues are often deficient owing to the surgical exposure or initial injury.

POSTOPERATIVE CARE

- The elbow with stable ligaments should be splinted using anterior plaster slabs in extension and elevated for 24 to 48 hours to diminish swelling, decrease tension on the posterior wound, and minimize the tendency to develop a flexion contracture.
- In the setting of a more tenuous ligamentous repair or the presence of some residual instability at the end of the operative procedure, the elbow should initially be splinted in 60 to 90 degrees of flexion in the optimal position of forearm rotation to maintain stability.
- Perioperative antibiotics are continued for 24 hours postoperatively.
- Indomethacin 25 mg three times daily for 3 weeks may be considered in patients undergoing radial head arthroplasty to decrease postoperative pain, reduce swelling, and potentially lower the incidence of heterotopic ossification.
- Indomethacin should be avoided in elderly patients and those with a history of peptic ulcer disease, asthma, known allergy, or other contraindications to anti-inflammatory medications.
- For an isolated radial head replacement treated with a lateral ulnar collateral ligament–sparing approach, active range of motion should be initiated on the day after surgery.
  - A collar and cuff with the elbow maintained at 90 degrees is employed for comfort between exercises.

   - A static progressive extension splint is fabricated for nighttime use for patients without associated ligamentous disruptions and is employed for a period of 12 weeks. The splint is adjusted weekly as extension improves.
   - In patients with associated elbow dislocations or residual instability, extension splinting is not implemented until 6 weeks after surgery.
- Patients with associated fractures, dislocations, or ligamentous injuries should commence active flexion and extension motion within a safe arc 1 day postoperatively.
   - Active forearm rotation is performed with the elbow in flexion to minimize stress on the medial or lateral ligamentous injuries or repairs.
   - Extension is performed with the forearm in the appropriate rotational position—that is, pronation if the lateral ligaments are deficient,[13] supination if the medial ligaments are deficient,[2] and neutral position if both sides have been injured.
   - A resting splint with the elbow maintained at 90 degrees and the forearm in the appropriate position of forearm rotation is employed for 3 to 6 weeks.
- Passive stretching is not permitted for 6 weeks to reduce the incidence of heterotopic ossification.
- Strengthening exercises are initiated once the ligament injuries and any associated fractures have adequately healed, usually at 8 weeks postoperatively.

OUTCOMES

- Silicone radial head arthroplasty, although initially successful in many patients,[8,42] has fallen out of favor because of problems with residual instability and arthritis, implant fracture, and silicone synovitis due to particulate debris.[45]
- Although the short- and medium-term results of metallic radial head implants are encouraging, there is a paucity of literature demonstrating the long-term outcome with respect to loosening, capitellar wear, and arthritis.[14,17]
- Metallic radial head replacement in elbows with intact ligaments restores the kinematics and stability similar to that measured with a native radial head. Moreover, when the fractured radial head occurs in combination with ligamentous and soft tissue disruption, a metallic prosthesis restores elbow stability, with only mild residual deficits in strength and motion.
- Results appear to be better if surgery is performed early (<10 days from injury).[3,34]
- Moro et al[36] reported the functional outcome of 25 cases managed with a metallic radial head arthroplasty for unreconstructable fractures of the radial head at an average follow-up of 39 months. The results were rated as 17 good or excellent, 5 fair, and 3 poor.
   - The radial head prosthesis restored elbow stability when the fractured radial head occurred in combination with a dislocation of the elbow, rupture of the medial collateral ligament, fracture of the coronoid, or fracture of the proximal ulna.
   - There were mild residual deficits in strength and motion, and no patient required removal of the implant.
- Grewal et al[17] reported high satisfaction rate among 26 patients, 2 years following a modular, monopolar radial head arthroplasty with a loose press-fit stem for unreconstructable radial head fractures.
- Zunkiewicz et al[47] reported good functional outcome in 29 patients managed with a bipolar radial head prosthesis with a smooth unfixed telescoping stem with an average follow-up of 34 months. The prosthesis effectively restored stability and joint congruency to elbows with comminuted radial head fractures and valgus instability.
- Flinkkilä et al[15] reported high failure rate and early loosening of press-fit radial head implants which were used in acute unstable elbow injuries, 12 of 37 press-fit stems were radiographically loose at a mean follow-up of 11 months, with 9 of them necessitating implant removal.
- Harrington et al[20] reported their experience with metallic radial head arthroplasty in 20 patients at an average follow-up of 12 years. The results were excellent or good in 16 and fair or poor in 4.
- Improvements in radial head arthroplasty designs, sizing, and implantation techniques may lead to improved outcomes for unreconstructable radial head fractures.

COMPLICATIONS

- Posterior interosseous nerve injury can occur as a consequence of dissection distal to the radial tuberosity and placement of anterior retractors around the distal radial neck.
- Infection
- Loss of motion, mainly terminal extension due to capsular contracture, heterotopic ossification, or retained cartilaginous or osseous fragments
- Prosthetic loosening, failure or polyethylene wear[15,43]
- Capitellar wear and pain due to implant overstuffing
- Complex regional pain syndrome
- Instability or recurrent dislocations of the elbow due to an inadequate or failed ligament repair
- Osteoarthritis of the capitellum as a consequence of articular cartilage damage from the initial injury, from component insertion, from persistent instability, or due to loading from a radial head implant that is too thick

REFERENCES

1. Antuna SA, Sánchez-Márquez JM, Barco R. Long-term results of radial head resection following isolated radial head fractures in patients younger than forty years old. J Bone Joint Surg Am 2010;92(3):558–566.
2. Armstrong AD, Dunning CE, Faber KJ, et al. Rehabilitation of the medial collateral ligament-deficient elbow: an in vitro biomechanical study. J Hand Surg Am 2000;25(6):1051–1057.
3. Ashwood N, Bain GI, Unni R. Management of Mason type-III radial head fractures with a titanium prosthesis, ligament repair, and early mobilization. J Bone Joint Surg Am 2004;86-A(2):274–280.
4. Athwal GS, Rouleau DM, MacDermid JC, et al. Contralateral elbow radiographs can reliably diagnose radial head implant overlengthening. J Bone Joint Surg Am 2011;93(14):1339–1346.
5. Bain GI, Ashwood N, Baird R, et al. Management of Mason type III radial head fractures with a titanium prosthesis, ligament repair, and early mobilization. J Bone Joint Surg Am 2005;87(suppl, 1 pt 1):136–147.
6. Beingessner DM, Dunning CE, Gordon KD, et al. The effect of radial head excision and arthroplasty on elbow kinematics and stability. J Bone Joint Surg Am 2004;86-A(8):1730–1739.
7. Boulas HJ, Morrey BF. Biomechanical evaluation of the elbow following radial head fracture. Comparison of open reduction and internal fixation versus excision, silastic replacement, and non-operative management. Chir Main 1998;17:314–320.
8. Carn RM, Medige J, Curtain D, et al. Silicone rubber replacement of the severely fractured radial head. Clin Orthop Relat Res 1986;(209):259–269.

9. Davidson PA, Moseley JB Jr, Tullos HS. Radial head fracture. A potentially complex injury. Clin Orthop Relat Res 1993;(297):224–230.
10. Diliberti T, Botte MJ, Abrams RA. Anatomical considerations regarding the posterior interosseous nerve during posterolateral approaches to the proximal part of the radius. J Bone Joint Surg Am 2000;82(6):809–813.
11. Dowdy PA, Bain GI, King GJ, et al. The midline posterior elbow incision. An anatomical appraisal. J Bone Joint Surg Br 1995;77(5): 696–699
12. Duckworth AD, Clement ND, Jenkins PJ, et al. The epidemiology of radial head and neck fractures. J Hand Surg Am 2012;37(1):112–119.
13. Dunning CE, Zarzour ZD, Patterson SD, et al. Muscle forces and pronation stabilize the lateral ligament deficient elbow. Clin Orthop Relat Res 2001;(388):118–124.
14. El Sallakh S. Radial head replacement for radial head fractures. J Orthop Trauma 2013;27:e137–e140.
15. Flinkkilä T, Kaisto T, Sirniö K, et al. Short- to mid-term results of metallic press-fit radial head arthroplasty in unstable injuries of the elbow. J Bone Joint Surg Br 2012;94(6):805–810.
16. Frank SG, Grewal R, Johnson J, et al. Determination of correct implant size in radial head arthroplasty to avoid overlengthening. J Bone Joint Surg Am 2009;91(7):1738–1746.
17. Grewal R, MacDermid JC, Faber KJ, et al. Comminuted radial head fractures treated with a modular metallic radial head arthroplasty. Study of outcomes. J Bone Joint Surg Am 2006;88(10):2192–2200.
18. Gupta GG, Lucas G, Hahn DL. Biomechanical and computer analysis of radial head prostheses. J Shoulder Elbow Surg 1997;6:37–48.
19. Halls AA, Travill A. Transmission of pressures across the elbow joint. Anat Rec 1964;150:243–247.
20. Harrington IJ, Sekyi-Otu A, Barrington TW, et al. The functional outcome with metallic radial head implants in the treatment of unstable elbow fractures: a long-term review. J Trauma 2001;50:46–52.
21. Herbertsson P, Josefsson PO, Hasserius R, et al. Displaced Mason type I fractures of the radial head and neck in adults: a fifteen- to thirty-three-year follow-up study. J Shoulder Elbow Surg 2005;14:73–77.
22. Ikeda M, Oka Y. Function after early radial head resection for fracture: a retrospective evaluation of 15 patients followed for 3–18 years. Acta Orthop Scand 2000;71:191–194.
23. Janssen RP, Vegter J. Resection of the radial head after Mason type-III fracture of the elbow: follow-up at 16 to 30 years. J Bone Joint Surg Br 1998;80(2):231–233.
24. Jensen SL, Olsen BS, Søjbjerg JO. Elbow joint kinematics after excision of the radial head. J Shoulder Elbow Surg 1999;8:238–241.
25. Johnson JA, Beingessner DM, Gordon KD, et al. Kinematics and stability of the fractured and implant-reconstructed radial head. J Shoulder Elbow Surg 2005;14:195S–201S.
26. Johnston GW. A follow-up of one hundred cases of fracture of the head of the radius with a review of the literature. Ulster Med J 1962;31: 51–56.
27. Karlsson MK, Herbertsson P, Nordqvist A, et al. Long- term outcome of displaced radial neck fractures in adulthood: 16-21 year follow-up of 5 patients treated with radial head excision. Acta Orthop 2009;80:368–370.
28. King GJ. Management of radial head fractures with implant arthroplasty. J Am Soc Surg Hand 2004;4:11–26.
29. King GJ, Patterson SD. Metallic radial head arthroplasty. Tech Hand Up Extrem Surg 2001;5:196–203.
30. King GJ, Zarzour ZD, Patterson SD, et al. An anthropometric study of the radial head: implications in the design of a prosthesis. J Arthroplasty 2001;16:112–116.
31. King GJ, Zarzour ZD, Rath DA, et al. Metallic radial head arthroplasty improves valgus stability of the elbow. Clin Orthop Relat Res 1999;(368):114–125.
32. Kocher T. Textbook of Operative Surgery. London: Adam and Charles Black, 1911.
33. Lamas C, Castellanos J, Proubasta I, et al. Comminuted radial head fractures treated with pyrocarbon prosthetic replacement. Hand 2011;6:27–33.
34. Lapner M, King GJ. Radial head fractures. J Bone Joint Surg Am 2013;95(12):1136–1143.
35. Lindenhovius AL, Felsch Q, Doornberg JN, et al. Open reduction and internal fixation compared with excision for unstable displaced fractures of the radial head. J Hand Surg Am 2007;32(5):630–636.
36. Moro JK, Werier J, MacDermid JC, et al. Arthroplasty with a metal radial head for unreconstructible fractures of the radial head. J Bone Joint Surg Am 2001;83-A(8):1201–1211.
37. Morrey BF, An KN. Articular and ligamentous contributions to the stability of the elbow joint. Am J Sports Med 1983;11:315–319.
38. Patterson SD, Bain GI, Mehta JA. Surgical approaches to the elbow. Clin Orthop Relat Res 2000;(370):19–33.
39. Pomianowski S, Morrey BF, Neale PG, et al. Contribution of monoblock and bipolar radial head prostheses to valgus stability of the elbow. J Bone Joint Surg Am 2001;83-A(12):1829–1834.
40. Sarris IK, Kyrkos MJ, Galanis NN, et al. Radial head replacement with the MoPyC pyrocarbon prosthesis. J Shoulder Elbow Surg 2012;21:1222–1228.
41. Shore BJ, Mozzon JB, MacDermid JC, et al. Chronic posttraumatic elbow disorders treated with metallic radial head arthroplasty. J Bone Joint Surg Am 2008;90(2):271–280.
42. Swanson AB, Jaeger SH, La Rochelle D. Comminuted fractures of the radial head. The role of silicone-implant replacement arthroplasty. J Bone Joint Surg Am 1981;63(7):1039–1049.
43. van Riet RP, Sanchez-Sotelo J, Morrey BF. Failure of metal radial head replacement. J Bone Joint Surg Br 2010;92(5):661–667.
44. van Riet RP, Van Glabbeek F, Neale PG, et al. The noncircular shape of the radial head. J Hand Surg Am 2003;28(6):972–978.
45. Vanderwilde RS, Morrey BF, Melberg MW, et al. Inflammatory arthritis after failure of silicone rubber replacement of the radial head. J Bone Joint Surg Br 1994;76(1):78–81.
46. Zarattini G, Galli S, Marchese M, et al. The surgical treatment of isolated mason type 2 fractures of the radial head in adults: comparison between radial head resection and open reduction and internal fixation. J Orthop Trauma 2012;26:229–235.
47. Zunkiewicz MR, Clemente JS, Miller MC, et al. Radial head replacement with a bipolar system: a minimum 2-year follow-up. J Shoulder Elbow Surg 2012;21:98–104.

Open Reduction and Internal Fixation of Fractures of the Proximal Ulna

20

CHAPTER

David Ring

DEFINITION

- Fracture of the olecranon process is common, usually displaced, and nearly always treated operatively.
- Important injury characteristics include displacement, comminution, and subluxation or dislocation of the elbow, and all are accounted for in the Mayo classification (**FIG 1**).[6]
- Fracture-dislocations of the olecranon can be anterior (transolecranon) or posterior (the most proximal type of posterior Monteggia according to Jupiter and colleagues[3]) in direction.[2,3,9,10]
- The eponym Monteggia is best applied to metaphyseal or diaphyseal proximal ulnar fracture associated with dislocation of the proximal radioulnar joint.
- The Bado classification of Monteggia lesions with Jupiter subclassification of type II fractures is shown in Table 1.
- Equivalent injuries in adults
  - Variable pathology that is felt to be equivalent to injuries classified by the Bado system
  - Equivalent injuries do not always fall within the traditional definition of a Monteggia fracture in that they do not always have a concomitant radiocapitellar dislocation. Therefore, it can be argued that these injuries are not necessarily equivalent to Monteggia fractures.
  - Type I and type II injuries are the only ones that have equivalent injury patterns.

ANATOMY

- The greater sigmoid notch of the ulna is formed by the coronoid and olecranon processes and forms a nearly 180-degree arc capturing the trochlea.
- The region between the coronoid and olecranon articular facets is the nonarticular transverse groove of the olecranon, a common location of fracture and a place where precise articular reduction is not critical.
- The triceps has a broad and thick insertion from just superior to the point of the olecranon and the tip of the olecranon process that can be used to enhance fixation of small, osteoporotic, or fragmented fractures and can be split longitudinally, if needed, when applying a plate.
- The radioulnar articulation is stabilized by the triangular fibrocartilage complex (TFCC) at the distal radioulnar joint, the interosseous ligament in the midforearm, and the annular ligament at the proximal radioulnar joint (PRUJ). Fracture of the ulna with dislocation of the PRUJ disrupts the annular ligament, but typically, the other structures are spared.
- In a true Monteggia lesion (fracture-dislocation) of the forearm, the radial head dislocates anterolaterally from the PRUJ.

PATHOGENESIS

- Fractures of the olecranon and proximal ulna can result from a direct blow to the point of the elbow or indirect forces during a fall on the outstretched hand.

NATURAL HISTORY

- Stable nondisplaced or minimally displaced olecranon fractures are uncommon. The majority of olecranon fractures are displaced and benefit from operative treatment.
- The occasional untreated displaced simple olecranon fracture demonstrates a slight flexion contracture, some weakness of extension, no arthrosis, and little, if any, pain.

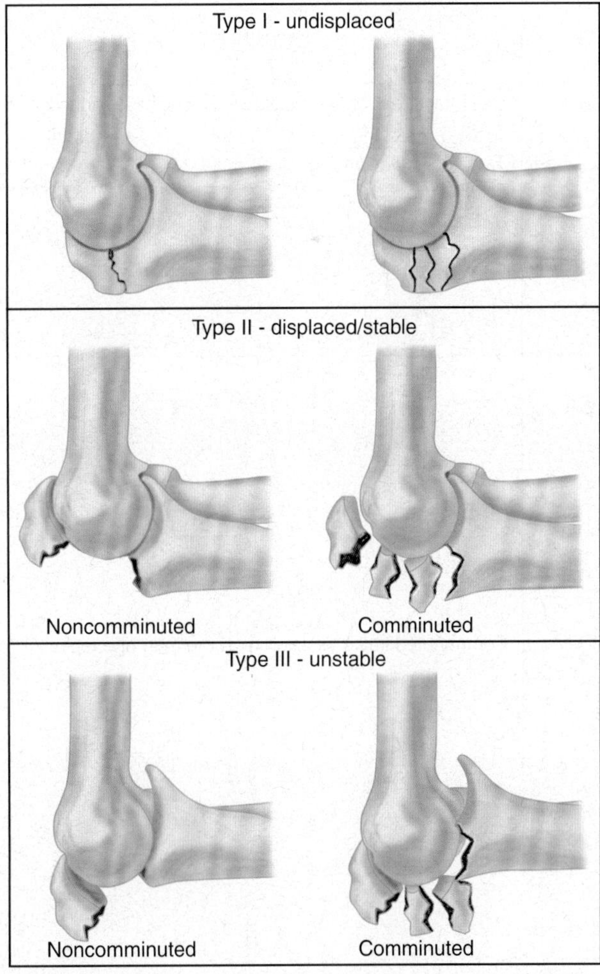

FIG 1 • The Mayo classification of olecranon fractures accounts for the factors that will influence treatment decisions: displacement, comminution, and dislocation or subluxation of the articulations.

Table 1 Bado Classification of Monteggia Lesions with Jupiter Subclassification of Type II Fractures

Type	Description	Illustration
I	Anterior dislocation of the radial head with fracture of the diaphysis of the ulna with anterior angulation of the ulnar fracture (most common type of lesion)	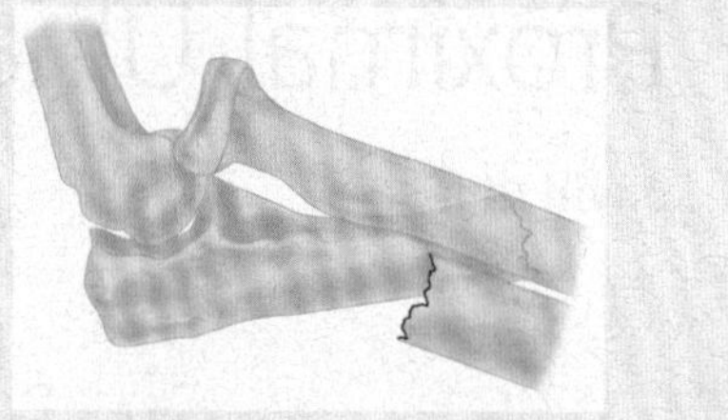
II	Posterior or posterolateral dislocation of the radial head with fracture of the ulnar diaphysis with posterior angulation of the ulnar fracture	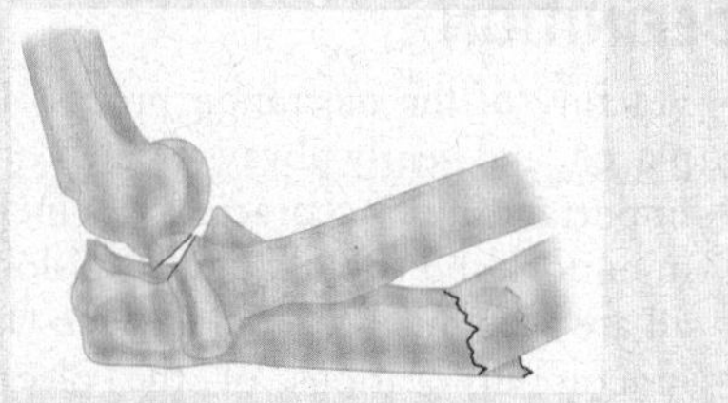
IIA	Fracture at the level of the trochlear notch (ulnar fracture involves the distal part of the olecranon and coronoid)	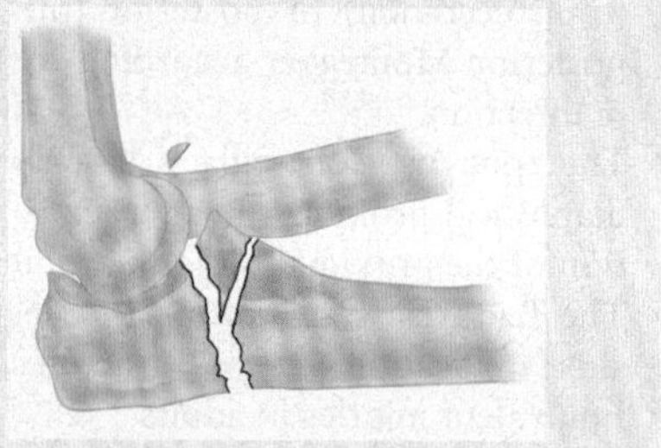
IIB	Ulnar fracture is at the metaphyseal–diaphyseal junction, distal to the coronoid.	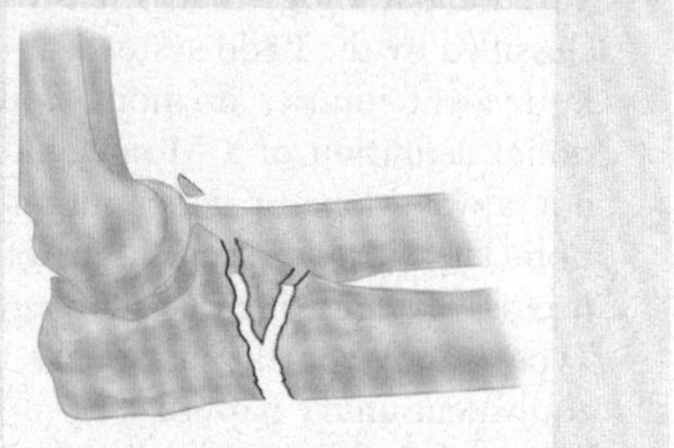
IIC	Ulnar fracture is diaphyseal.	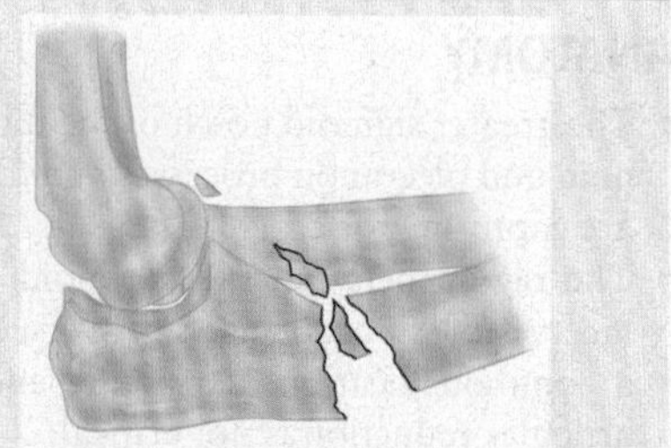
IID	Comminuted fractures involving more than one region	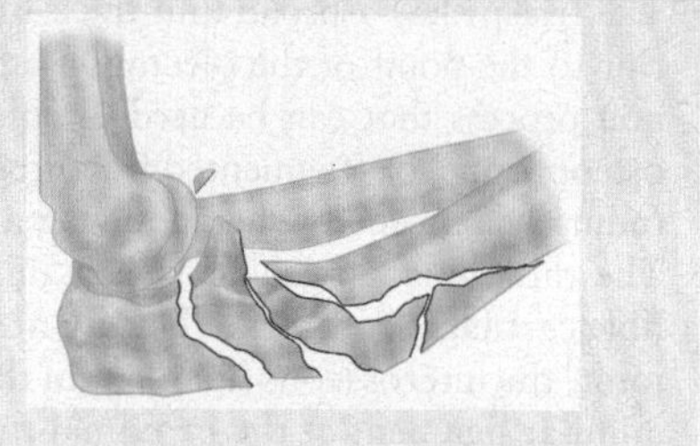

Table 1 *(continued)*

Type	Description	Illustration
III	Lateral or anterolateral dislocation of the radial head with fracture of the ulnar metaphysis	
IV	Anterior dislocation of the radial head with a fracture of the proximal third of the radius and ulna at the same level	

Adapted from Bado J. The Monteggia lesion. Clin Orthop Relat Res 1967;50:717; Jupiter JB, Leibovic SJ, Ribbans W, et al. The posterior Monteggia lesion. J Orthop Trauma 1991;5:395–402.

- In contrast, undertreated or poorly treated fracture-dislocations of the olecranon often lead to severe arthrosis and angulation of the arm under the influence of gravity.
- Even well-treated complex injuries are at risk for stiffness, heterotopic ossification, arthrosis, and occasionally nonunion.

PATIENT HISTORY AND PHYSICAL FINDINGS

- Knowledge of the characteristics of the patient (age, sex, medical health) and the injury (mechanism, energy) will help the surgeon understand the injury and determine optimal treatment.
- First, the patient is assessed for life-threatening injuries (Advanced Trauma Life Support [ATLS] protocol) and any medical problems that may have contributed to the injury.
- A secondary survey is performed to identify any other fractures, ipsilateral arm injuries in particular.
- The skin is inspected for any wounds associated with the fracture.
- The pulses are palpated, capillary refill inspected, and an Allen test performed if necessary.
- Peripheral nerve function is assessed.
- Patients with high-energy injuries, particularly those with ipsilateral wrist or forearm injuries, are at risk for compartment syndrome. If the clinical examination is suggestive or unreliable (owing to problems with mental status), compartment pressure monitoring should be performed.

IMAGING AND OTHER DIAGNOSTIC STUDIES

- Anteroposterior (AP) and lateral radiographs are used for initial characterization of the injury.
- Radiographs after reduction or splinting or oblique views can be useful.
- Computed tomography (CT) is useful for characterization of fracture-dislocations. In particular, three-dimensional (3-D) CT reconstructions can be useful for assessment of the coronoid and radial head.

DIFFERENTIAL DIAGNOSIS

- Elbow dislocation
- Essex-Lopresti fracture-dislocation of the forearm (disruption of the interosseous ligament and or TFCC usually with fracture of the radial head)
- Fracture-dislocations of the elbow ("terrible triad" injury)
- Distal humerus fracture

NONOPERATIVE MANAGEMENT

- Nonoperative management is appropriate for the rare fracture of the olecranon that is less than 2 mm displaced with the elbow flexed 90 degrees.
- Four weeks of splint immobilization followed by active-assisted mobilization of the elbow will usually result in a healed fracture and good elbow function.

SURGICAL MANAGEMENT

- The vast majority of olecranon fractures are displaced and merit operative treatment.
- Transverse, noncomminuted fractures not associated with fracture-dislocation are treated with tension band wiring.[4,8]
- Comminuted fractures and fracture-dislocations are treated with dorsal contoured plate and screw fixation.[1–3]
- The treatment of fracture-dislocations requires attention to the coronoid, radial head, and lateral collateral ligament.[2,9–11]
- Fracture-dislocations of the forearm (anterolateral Monteggia injuries) is treated with anatomic realignment of the ulna and plate and screw fixation.[10] Inadequate radiocapitellar alignment suggests residual ulnar angulation.

Preoperative Planning

- The fracture characteristics that determine treatment are defined on radiographs and CT.
- Templating the surgery with tracings of the radiographs is a useful way of running through the surgery in detail before

performing it, familiarizing oneself with the anatomy, anticipating problems, and ensuring that all of the implants and equipment that might be necessary are available.

Positioning

- In most patients, a lateral decubitus position with the arm over a bolster or support is best.
- Some patients with fracture-dislocations that require both medial and lateral access may be positioned supine with the arm supported on a hand table.
- A sterile pneumatic tourniquet is used.

Approach

- A dorsal longitudinal skin incision is used.

Tension Band Wiring

Reduction and Kirschner Wire Fixation

- Blood clot and periosteum are cleared from the fracture site to facilitate reduction.
- Limited periosteal elevation is performed at the fracture site to monitor reduction.
- A large tenaculum clamp is used to secure the fracture in a reduced position (**TECH FIG 1A,B**). A drill hole can be made in the dorsal cortex of the distal fragment to facilitate clamp application.
- Two 1.0-mm smooth Kirschner wires are drilled across the fracture site (**TECH FIG 1C**).
- If these are drilled obliquely from dorsal-proximal to volar-distal, they will exit the anterior ulnar cortex distal to the coronoid process, providing an anchoring point of cortical bone to limit the potential for pin migration.
- In anticipation of later impaction of the proximal ends of the wires, the Kirschner wires should be retracted 5 to 10 mm after drilling through the anterior ulnar cortex.

Wiring

- The apex of the ulnar diaphysis just distal to the flat portion of the proximal ulna is drilled with a 2.0-mm drill, with or without prior subperiosteal dissection.
- When two wires are used, a second drill hole is made a centimeter more distal.
- If one wire is used, it should be 18 gauge. My preference is to use two 22-gauge stainless steel wires to limit the size of the knots, which may diminish implant prominence. The wires are passed through the drill holes. A large-bore needle can be used to facilitate passage of the wire through the drill hole (**TECH FIG 2A**).
- The two tension wires are each passed over the dorsal ulna in a figure-of-eight fashion, then around the Kirschner wires, and underneath the insertion of the triceps tendon using a large-bore needle (**TECH FIG 2B**).

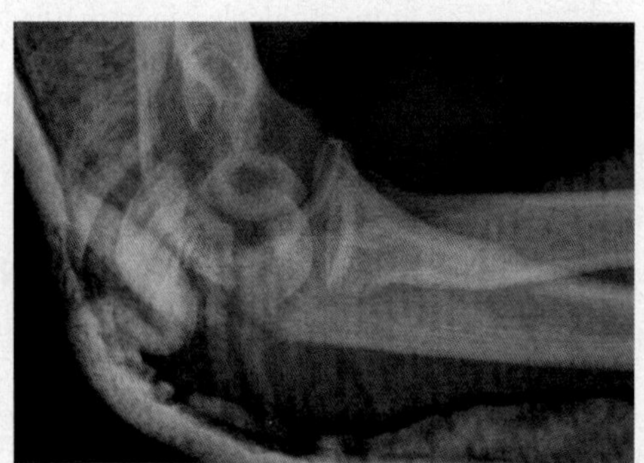

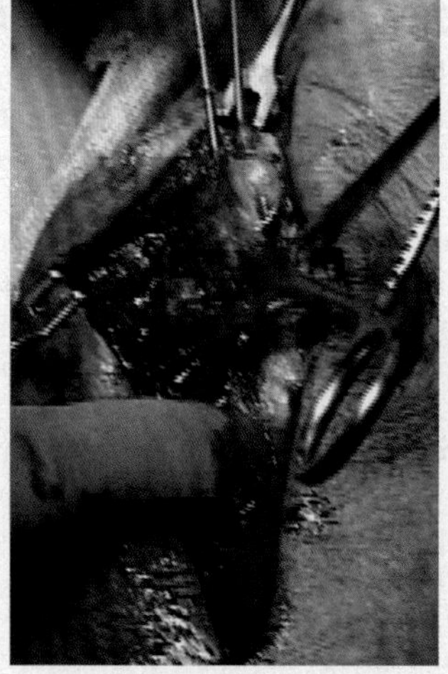

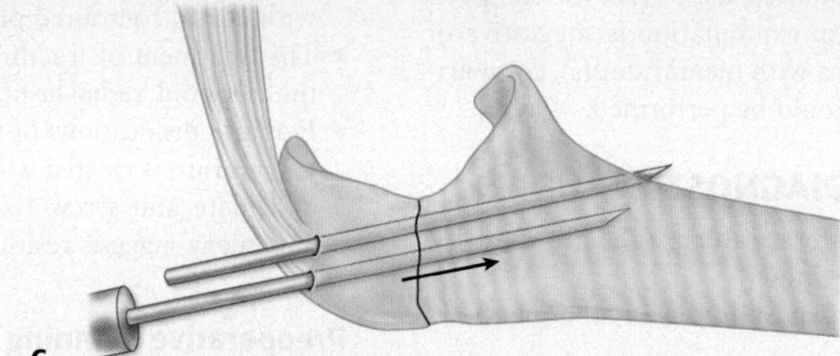

TECH FIG 1 • **A.** A lateral radiograph with the arm in plaster shows a transverse, noncomminuted fracture of the olecranon. **B.** An open reduction is held with a fracture reduction forceps. **C.** Two 1-mm Kirschner wires are drilled obliquely across the fracture site so that they exit the anterior ulnar cortex distal to the coronoid process. (**A,B:** Copyright David Ring, MD.)

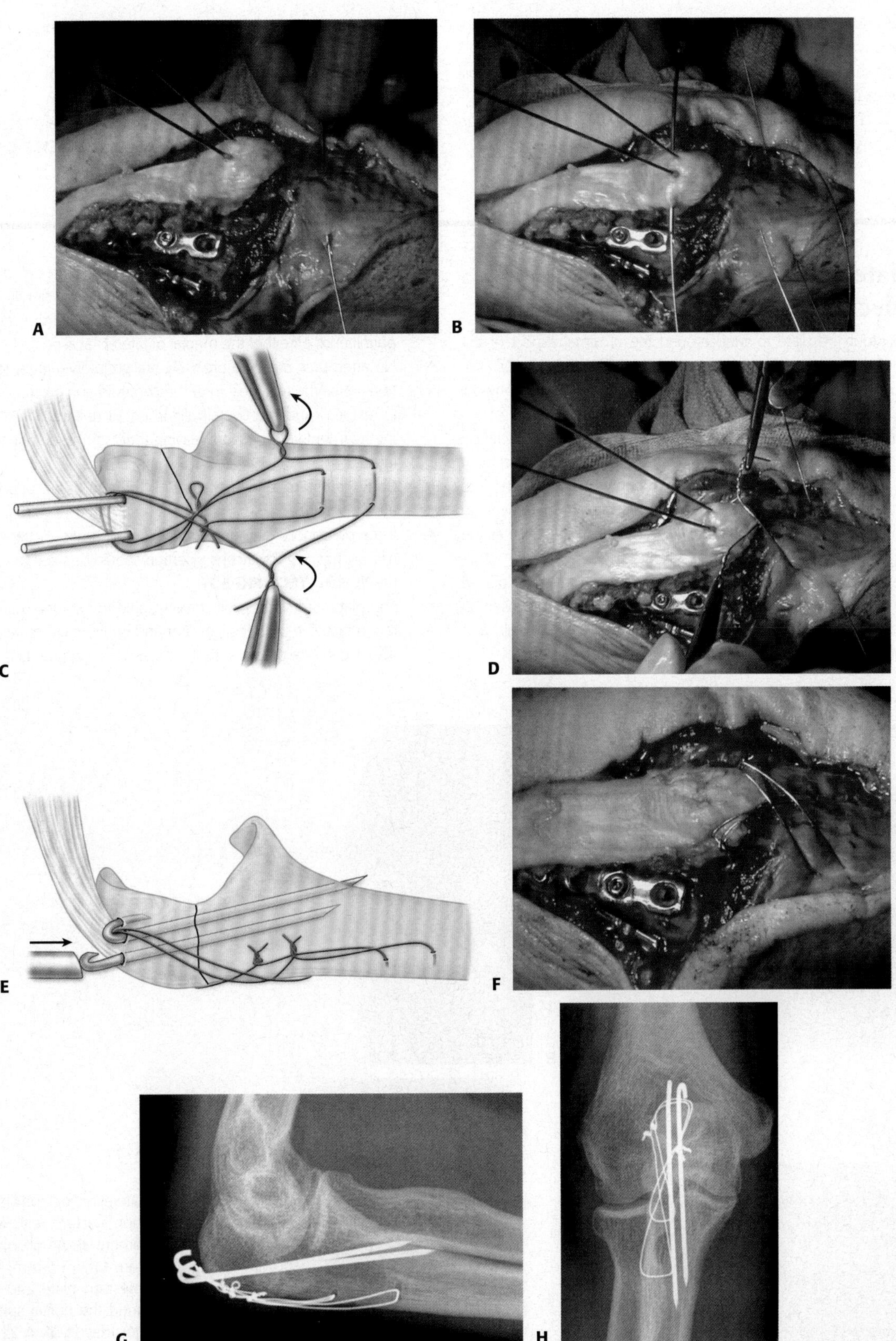

TECH FIG 2 • **A.** Two 22-gauge stainless steel tension wires are passed in a figure-of-eight fashion through drill holes in the ulnar shaft. **B.** They engage the triceps insertion proximally. **C,D.** The wires are tensioned on both sides. These do not need to be tight but simply snug, with all slack taken up. Attempts to tighten these smaller 22-gauge wires will break them. **E.** The proximal ends of the Kirschner wires are bent 180 degrees and impacted into the olecranon process, beneath the triceps insertion. **F.** The resulting fixation has a relatively low profile and is unlikely to migrate. **G,H.** Even these small wires are strong enough for active exercises to regain elbow motion. (**A,B,D,F–H:** Copyright David Ring, MD.)

- Each wire is tensioned both medially and laterally by twisting the wire with a needle holder (**TECH FIG 2C,D**).
- This should be done to take up slack only. These small wires will break if they are firmly tightened, which is not necessary.
  - The tightening should be done in a place that will make the wire knots less prominent.
  - After tightening, the knots are trimmed and bent into the soft tissues to either side.
  - The Kirschner wires are then bent 180 degrees and trimmed.
- These bent ends are then impacted into the proximal olecranon, beneath the triceps insertion, using a bone tamp (**TECH FIG 2E–H**).

Plate and Screw Fixation of Olecranon Fractures

- Contour the plate to wrap around the proximal aspect of the olecranon or use a precontoured plate (**TECH FIG 3A–C**).
- A straight plate will have only two or three screws in metaphyseal bone proximal to the fracture.
- Bending the plate around the proximal aspect of the olecranon provides additional screws in the proximal fragment. The most proximal screws can be very long, crossing the fracture line into the distal fragment. In some cases, these screws can be directed to engage one of the cortices of the distal fragment, such as the anterior ulnar cortex.
- A plate contoured to wrap around the proximal ulna can be placed on top of the triceps insertion. Alternatively, the triceps insertion can be incised longitudinally and partially elevated medially and laterally sufficiently to allow direct plate contact with bone.
- Distally, a dorsal plate will lie directly on the apex of the ulnar diaphysis. The muscle need only be split sufficiently to gain access to this apex—there is no need to elevate the muscle or periosteum off either the medial or lateral flat aspect of the ulna.
- No attempt is made to precisely realign intervening fragmentation—once the relationship of the coronoid and olecranon facets is restored and the overall alignment is restored, the remaining fragments are bridged, leaving their soft tissue attachments intact.
- Bone grafts are rarely necessary if the soft tissue attachments are preserved.
- If the olecranon fragment is small, osteoporotic, or fragmented, a wire engaging the triceps insertion should be used to reinforce the fixation (**TECH FIG 3D**).
- The plate and screws will serve to hold the coronoid and olecranon facets in proper alignment and bridge fragmentation, and the wire will help ensure fixation even if screw purchase is lost.

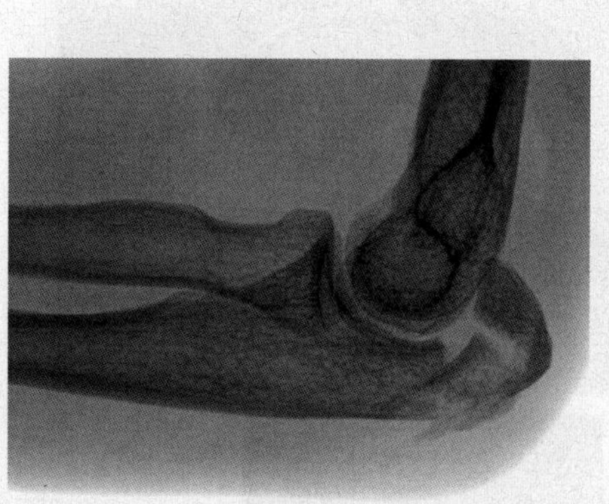
A

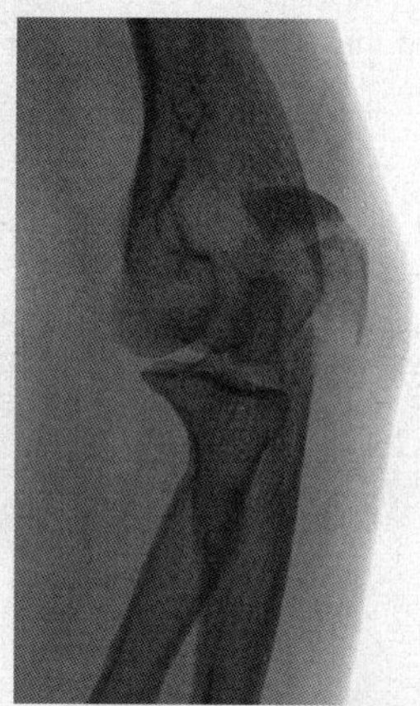
B

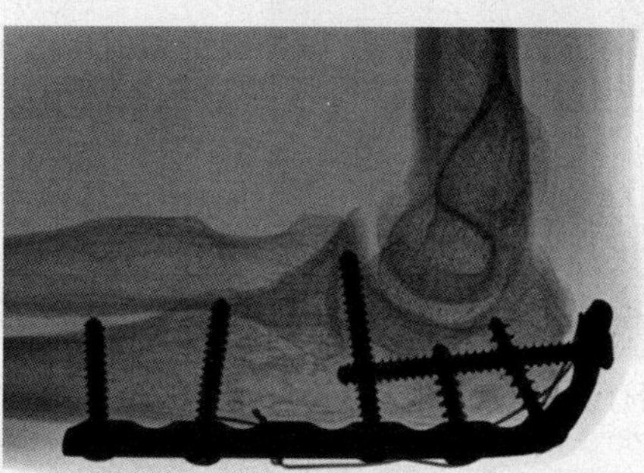
C

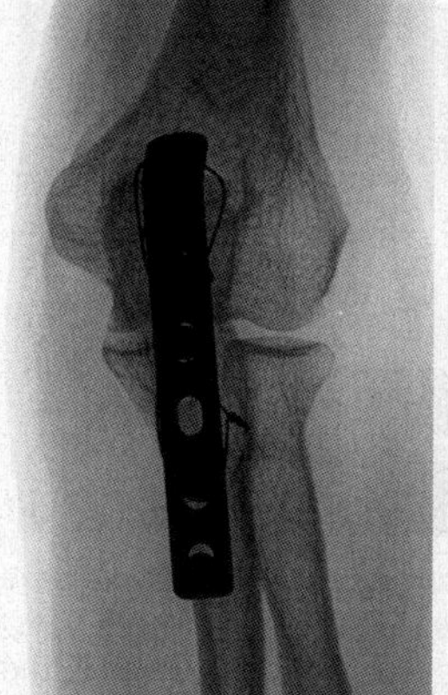
D

TECH FIG 3 • **A.** A lateral radiograph illustrates a comminuted olecranon fracture with a small proximal olecranon fragment. **B.** An oblique view shows the fragmentation. **C.** A 3.5-mm limited-contact dynamic compression plate and screws contoured to wrap around the dorsal surface of the olecranon is used for fixation. **D.** A 22-gauge stainless steel wire engages the triceps insertion—this is useful when the olecranon fragment is small, fragmented, or osteopenic. (Copyright David Ring, MD.)

Plate and Screw Fixation of the Fracture-Dislocations of the Olecranon

Exposure

- In the setting of a fracture-dislocation of the olecranon (**TECH FIG 4A**), fractures of the radial head and coronoid process can be evaluated and often definitively treated through the exposure provided by the fracture of the olecranon process.
  - With little additional dissection, the olecranon fragment can be mobilized proximally as one would do with an olecranon osteotomy, providing exposure of the coronoid through the ulnohumeral joint.
- If the exposure of the radial head through the posterior injury is inadequate, a separate muscle interval (eg, Kocher or Kaplan intervals) accessed by the elevation of a broad lateral skin flap can be used.
- If the exposure of the coronoid is inadequate through posterior injury and olecranon fracture, a separate medial or lateral exposure can be developed.
  - A medial exposure—between the two heads of the flexor carpi ulnaris, or by splitting the flexor–pronator mass more anteriorly, or by elevating the entire flexor–pronator mass from dorsal to volar—may be needed to address a complex fracture of the coronoid, particularly one that involves the anteromedial facet of the coronoid process.[7]
- When the lateral collateral ligament is injured, it is usually avulsed from the lateral epicondyle. This facilitates repair that can be performed using suture anchors or suture placed through drill holes in the bone.
- The fracture of the coronoid can often be reduced directly through the elbow joint using the limited access provided by the olecranon fracture (**TECH FIG 4B,C**).

Fixation

- Provisional fixation can be obtained using Kirschner wires to attach the fragments either to the metaphyseal or diaphyseal fragments of the ulna or to the trochlea of the distal humerus when there is extensive fragmentation of the proximal ulna.
- An alternative to keep in mind when there is extensive fragmentation of the proximal ulna is the use of a skeletal distractor (a temporary external fixator; **TECH FIG 5A**).
  - External fixation applied between a wire driven through the olecranon fragment and up into the trochlea and a second wire in the distal ulnar diaphysis can often obtain reduction indirectly when distraction is applied between the pins.
  - Definitive fixation can usually be obtained with screws applied under image intensifier guidance.
- The screws are placed through the plate when there is extensive fragmentation of the proximal ulna.
- A second, medial plate may be useful when the coronoid is fragmented.
- If the coronoid fracture is very comminuted and cannot be securely repaired, the ulnohumeral joint should be protected with temporary hinged or static external fixation or temporary pin fixation of the ulnohumeral joint, depending on the equipment and expertise available.
- A long plate is contoured to wrap around the proximal olecranon (**TECH FIG 5B**).
  - A very long plate should be considered (between 12 and 16 holes), particularly when there is extensive fragmentation or the bone quality is poor.
- When the olecranon is fragmented or osteoporotic, a plate and screws alone may not provide reliable fixation.
  - In this situation, it can be useful to use ancillary tension wire fixation to control the olecranon fragments through the triceps insertion (**TECH FIG 5C**).

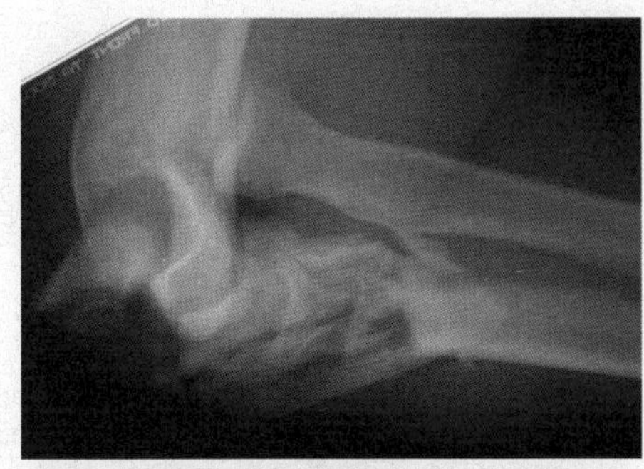

A

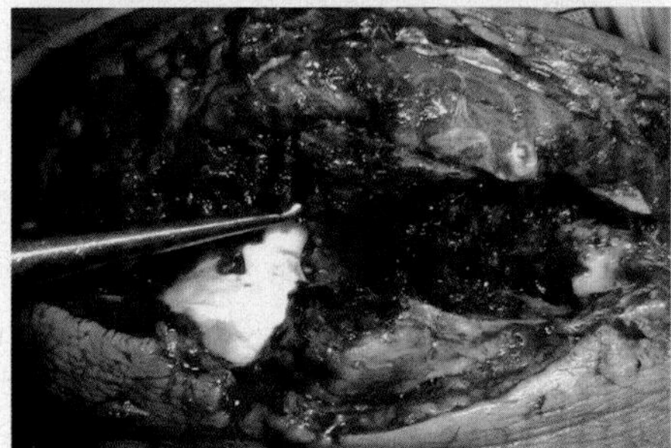

C

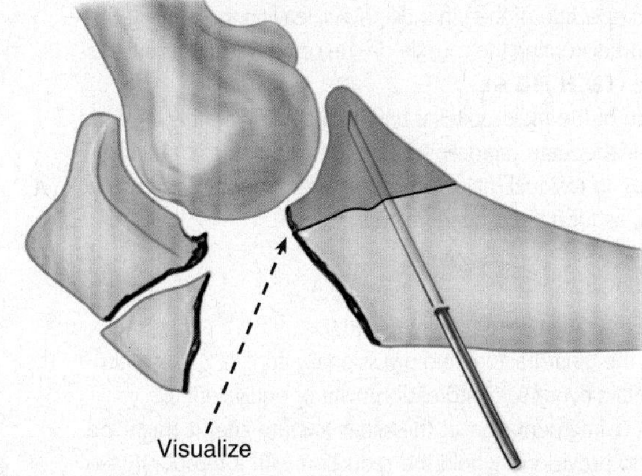

B

TECH FIG 4 • A. A complex anterior fracture-dislocation of the elbow. A lateral radiograph shows extensive comminution of the trochlear notch of the ulna, including the coronoid, and anterior displacement of the forearm. **B,C.** The coronoid fragments are connected to the dorsal metaphyseal fragments in this patient, which facilitates reduction and fixation. (**A,C:** Copyright David Ring, MD.)

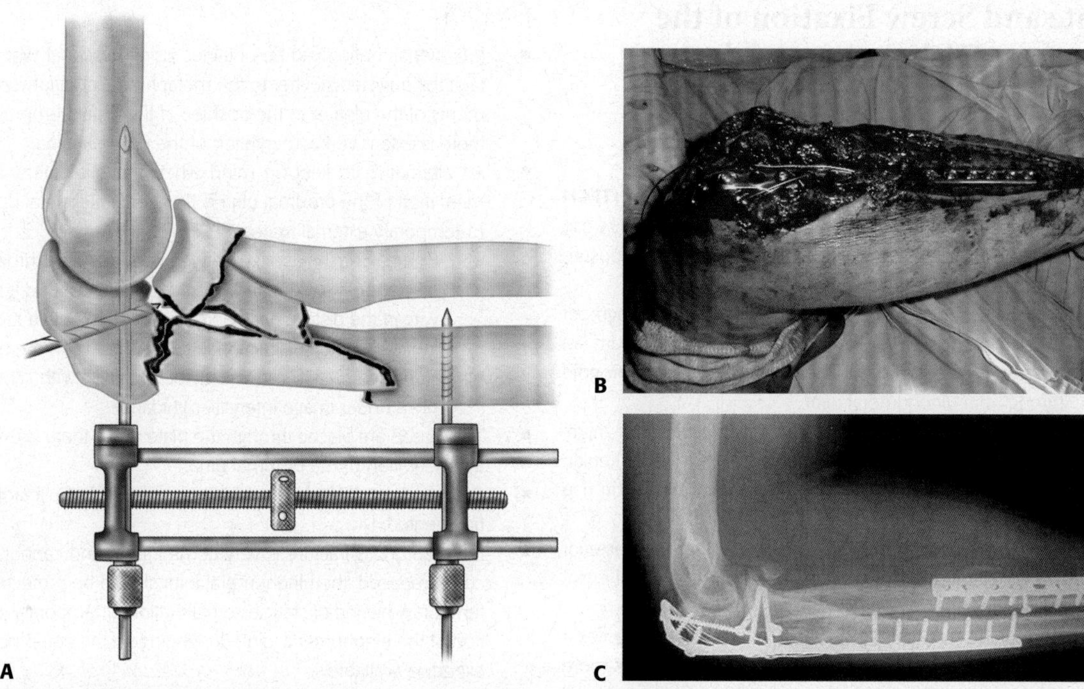

TECH FIG 5 • A. When there is diaphyseal comminution, a temporary external fixator may be useful. **B.** A long, 3.5-mm limited contact dynamic compression plate is used for fixation. A 22-gauge stainless steel wire is used to enhance fixation of the comminuted olecranon fragments. **C.** The comminution extending into the diaphysis heals with the bridging plate. The trochlear notch is restored with good elbow function. (**B,C:** Copyright David Ring, MD.)

Anterolateral Monteggia Fractures

Exposure

- The ulna is exposed through a dorsal incision elevating the muscle from one side of the ulnar diaphysis, leaving the periosteum intact and disrupting the muscle on the opposite side as little as possible (**TECH FIG 6**).
- Exposure of the radiocapitellar and PRUJs should rarely be necessary. Inadequate radiocapitellar/PRUJ alignment is nearly always due to residual malunion of the ulna. If necessary, expose the joint as for a radial head fracture.

Fixation

- Reduce the radiocapitellar joint or PRUJ.
- Realign the ulnar fracture and provisionally apply a 3.5-mm limited contact dynamic compression plate or equivalent.
- If there is fragmentation at the ulnar fracture site, it might be helpful to provisionally hold the reduction with a temporary external fixator (which the author has done) or temporary stabilization of the radiocapitellar articulation (which the author has not done) while getting provisional fixation of the ulna.
- Place two screws in each side of the plate proximal and distal to the fracture side and then check radiocapitellar/PRUJ alignment in several positions of elbow and forearm rotation and from several different radiographic angles under the image intensifier.

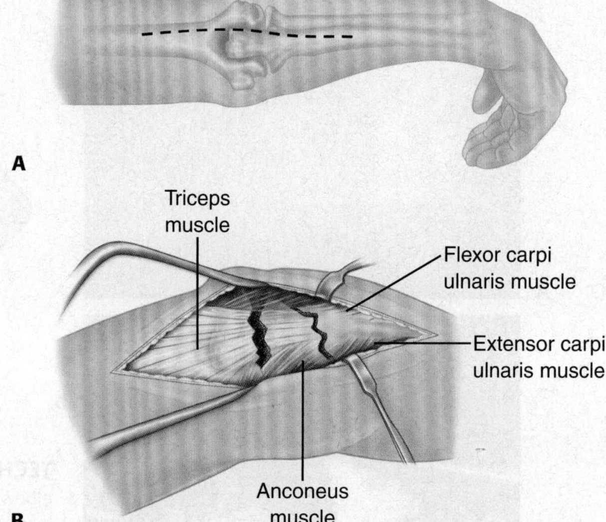

TECH FIG 6 • A. Posterior midline incision positioned just off the lateral aspect of the olecranon. **B.** Deep surgical interval uses the internervous plane between the anconeus and flexor carpi ulnaris.

- If the alignment is inadequate, revise your fixation of the ulna accordingly.
- Failure to obtain adequate length of the ulna can lead to persistent dislocation of the radial head (**TECH FIG 7**).
- Only enter the radiocapitellar joint if you can be 100% certain that the ulna is aligned properly. Interposition of the annular ligament is very uncommon.

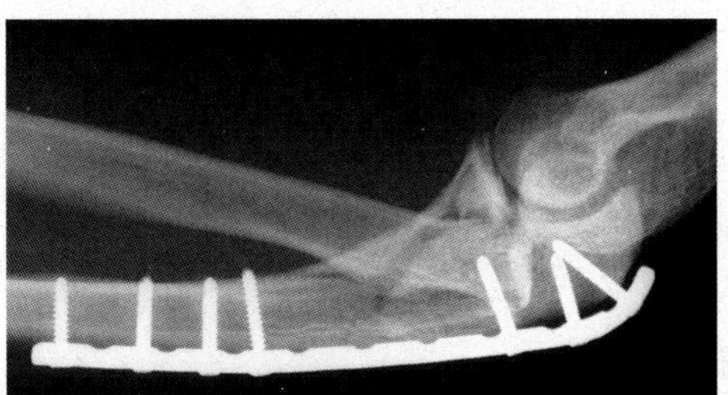

TECH FIG 7 • Malunion of the ulna with resulting apex dorsal angulation results in dislocation of the radial head.

PEARLS AND PITFALLS

Prominence of olecranon hardware	■ The use of two small (22-gauge) wires rather than one large one will result in smaller knots. Care taken to place the Kirschner wires below the triceps insertion and impacting them into bone will limit prominence and the potential for migration.[5,8]
Narrowing of trochlear notch	■ The surgeon should not use a tension wire alone on a comminuted fracture. An intact articular surface to absorb compressive forces with active motion is mandatory for tension band wiring to be effective.
Plate loosening	■ The surgeon should use a dorsal plate contoured to wrap around the olecranon, providing a greater number of screws and screws at different, nearly orthogonal angles. Use of a medial or lateral plate should be avoided.[10,11]
Loss of fixation of the proximal (olecranon) fragment	■ Screw fixation alone should not be trusted if the fragment is small, fragmented, or osteoporotic. A tension wire engaging the triceps insertion should be added.
Failure to recognize a complex injury	■ The surgeon should be vigilant for subluxation or dislocation of the elbow, fracture of the coronoid or radial head, and injury to the lateral collateral ligament. When identified, each injury is treated accordingly. The olecranon and proximal ulna are always secured with a plate and screws.

POSTOPERATIVE CARE

- When good fixation is obtained (which occurs in most patients), active-assisted and gravity-assisted elbow and forearm exercises can be initiated immediately after surgery. A delay of several days for comfort is reasonable.
- If the lateral collateral ligament was repaired, the patient must be instructed not to abduct the shoulder for the first month, as this imparts a varus moment across the elbow and stresses the ligament repair.
- If the fixation is tenuous, it is reasonable to immobilize the arm in a splint for a month or so before beginning exercises.

OUTCOMES

- Nonunion is nearly unheard of after simple olecranon fractures, and early implant failure is usually due to noncompliance.[6]
- The appeal of tension band wiring has been limited by prominence of the implants; however, if the techniques described herein are followed, few patients will request a second surgery specifically for implant removal.[8]
- Macko and Szabo[5] pointed out that it was initial implant prominence and not migration that led to implant-related problems after tension band wiring of olecranon fractures.
- In any case, a second surgery for implant removal is not unreasonable and it may not be appropriate to consider this a complication.
- Some surgeons have considered plate-and-screw fixation of simple, noncomminuted olecranon fractures.[1] However, plates can also cause symptoms, and if only a few screws can be placed in the olecranon fragment, particularly in the setting of fragmentation or osteoporosis, it may be preferable to use the soft tissue attachments to enhance fixation rather than relying on implant–bone purchase alone.
- Medial and lateral plates have been associated with early failure, malunion, and nonunion in the treatment of complex proximal ulnar fractures.[10,11]
- Dorsal plates perform better, but the elbow is often compromised in the setting of such complex injuries.

COMPLICATIONS

- Implant loosening
- Implant breakage
- Nonunion
- Malunion
- Instability
- Arthrosis

REFERENCES

1. Bailey CS, MacDermid J, Patterson SD, et al. Outcome of plate fixation of olecranon fractures. J Orthop Trauma 2001;15:542–548.
2. Doornberg J, Ring D, Jupiter JB. Effective treatment of fracture-dislocations of the olecranon requires a stable trochlear notch. Clin Orthop Relat Res 2004;(429):292–300.
3. Jupiter JB, Leibovic SJ, Ribbans W, et al. The posterior Monteggia lesion. J Orthop Trauma 1991;5:395–402.
4. Karlsson M, Hasserius R, Besjakov J, et al. Comparison of tension-band and figure-of-eight wiring techniques for treatment of olecranon fractures. J Shoulder Elbow Surg 2002;11:377–382.
5. Macko D, Szabo RM. Complications of tension-band wiring of olecranon fractures. J Bone Joint Surg Am 1985;67(9):1396–1401.
6. Morrey BF. Current concepts in the treatment of fractures of the radial head, the olecranon, and the coronoid. J Bone Joint Surg Am 1995;77A:316–327.
7. O'Driscoll SW, Jupiter JB, Cohen M, et al. Difficult elbow fractures: pearls and pitfalls. Instruct Course Lect 2003;52:113–134.
8. Ring D, Gulotta L, Chin K, et al. Olecranon osteotomy for exposure of fractures and nonunions of the distal humerus. J Orthop Trauma 2004;18:446–449.
9. Ring D, Jupiter JB, Sanders RW, et al. Transolecranon fracture-dislocation of the elbow. J Orthop Trauma 1997;11:545–550.
10. Ring D, Jupiter JB, Simpson NS. Monteggia fractures in adults. J Bone Joint Surg Am 1998;80(12):1733–1744.
11. Ring D, Tavakolian J, Kloen P, et al. Loss of alignment after surgical treatment of posterior Monteggia fractures: salvage with dorsal contoured plating. J Hand Surg Am 2004;29(4):694–702.

Open Reduction and Internal Fixation of Fracture-Dislocations of the Elbow with Complex Instability

21

CHAPTER

Niloofar Dehghan and Michael D. McKee

DEFINITION

- Simple dislocations of the elbow can most often be treated successfully with closed means: reduction and short-term immobilization followed by early motion.
- Fracture-dislocations of the elbow are more troublesome in that they often require operative intervention.
- Fractures associated with elbow dislocations often involve the radial head and coronoid. An elbow dislocation associated with fractures of the radial head and coronoid is termed the *terrible triad*.
- The principle of treating fracture-dislocations of the elbow is to provide sufficient stability through reconstruction of bony and ligamentous restraints such that early motion (within 2 weeks postoperatively) can be instituted without recurrent instability.
- Failure to achieve this will result in either recurrent instability or severe stiffness after prolonged immobilization.

ANATOMY

- Posterolateral dislocations of the elbow are associated with disruption of the medial collateral ligament (MCL) and lateral collateral ligament (LCL).
- The MCL is the primary stabilizer to valgus stress (**FIG 1**).
- The LCL is the primary stabilizer to posterolateral rotatory instability. Most often, the LCL disruption is proximally from the lateral epicondyle of the humerus, which creates a characteristic bare spot. Less commonly, the ligament may rupture midsubstance.[7] Secondary restraints on the lateral side that may also be disrupted are the common extensor origin and the posterolateral capsule.
- Radial head fractures have been classified by Mason:
  - Type I: small or marginal fracture with minimal displacement
  - Type II: marginal fracture with displacement
  - Type III: comminuted fractures of the head and neck[5]
  - Type IV: radial head fracture associated with elbow dislocation (Johnson modification)
- Coronoid fractures have been classified by Regan and Morrey[11] (**FIG 2**):
  - Type I: tip fractures (not avulsions)
  - Type II: less than 50% of the coronoid

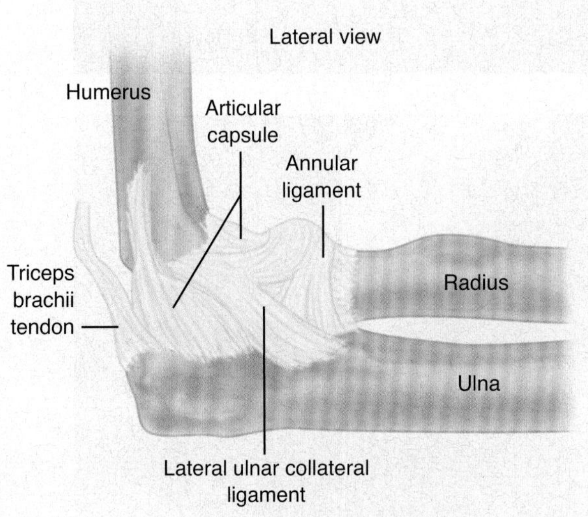

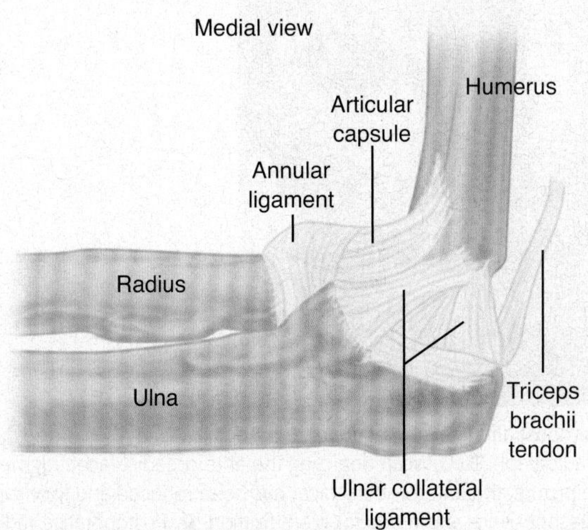

FIG 1 • The MCL and LCL complexes of the elbow. Note their points of attachment on the distal humerus and proximal ulna.

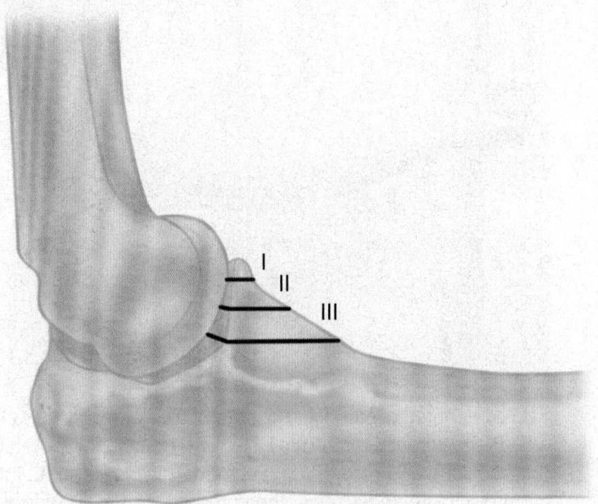

FIG 2 • Lateral view of the elbow depicting the different types of coronoid fractures.

- Type III: more than 50% of the coronoid
  - The insertion of the MCL is at the base of the coronoid and it may be involved in type III fractures.[1]
- Anteromedial facet fractures of the coronoid are a different entity and are caused by a primary varus force.[3]
  - The medial facet is important for varus stability of the elbow, just distal to this is the sublime tubercle, the insertion point of MCL.
  - Anteromedial facet fractures may lead to varus posteromedial instability, and disruption of the LCL (from the varus force) is often seen. However, there is also potential for valgus instability if the fractured fragment is large enough to include the MCL insertion.
  - These fractures are unstable and in general are best treated with open reduction internal fixation with use of a medial plate in a buttress fashion (**FIG 3**).

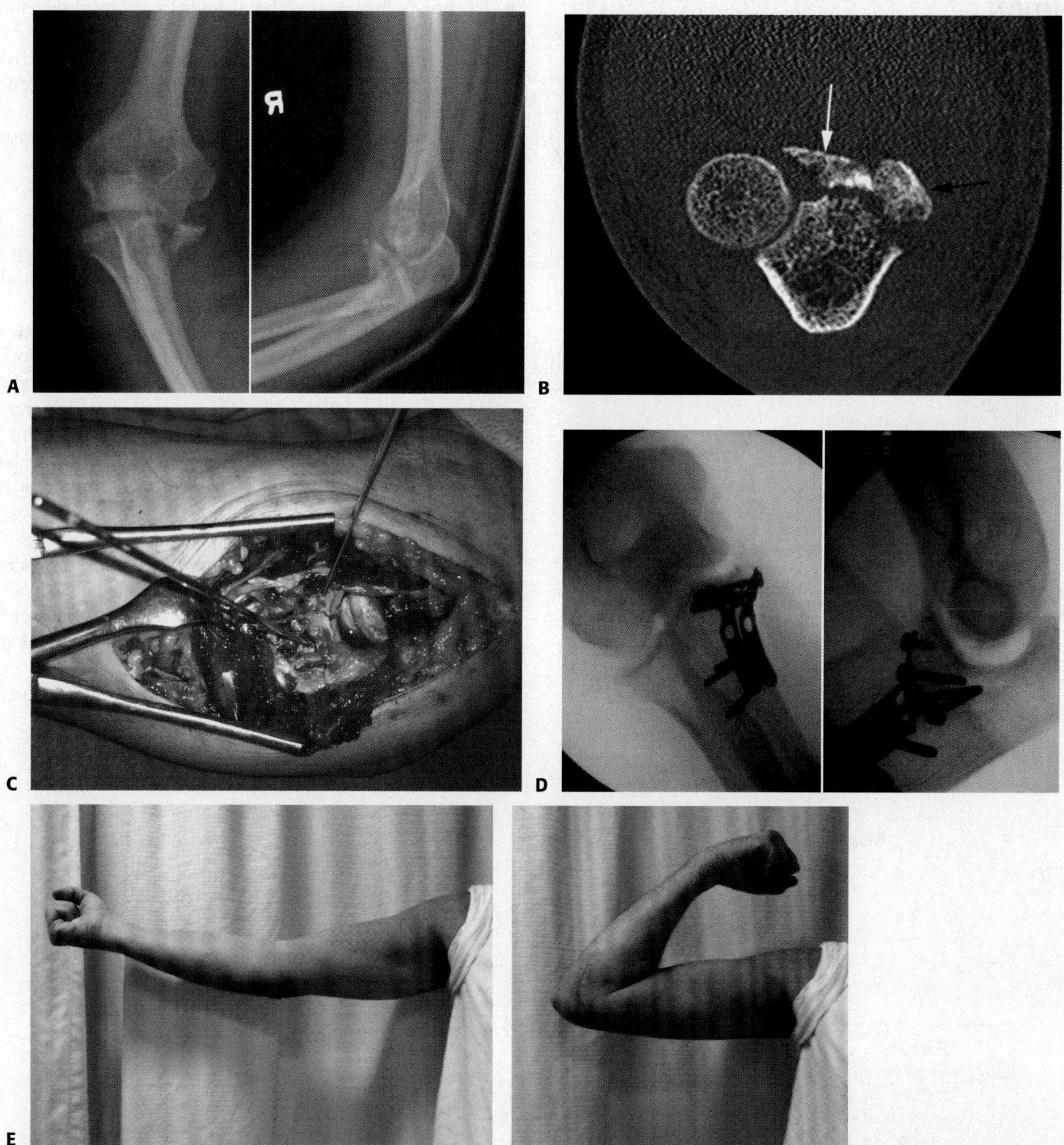

FIG 3 • Anteromedial facet fracture of the coronoid. **A.** Radiographs demonstrating fracture of the anteromedial facet of the coronoid as well as the coronoid tip. Varus instability can be appreciated on the AP radiograph. **B.** CT scan depicting the anteromedial facet fragment (*black arrow*) and coronoid tip fragment (*white arrow*). **C.** Intraoperative picture, the anteromedial facet has been reduced and fixed with a buttress plate and screws. The coronoid tip is held reduced with a Kirschner wire and ready for plate fixation. **D.** Postoperative radiograph demonstrating plate fixation of the coronoid tip as well as anteromedial facet with two separate plates. **E.** Clinical picture revealing medial-based incision and good postoperative range of motion.

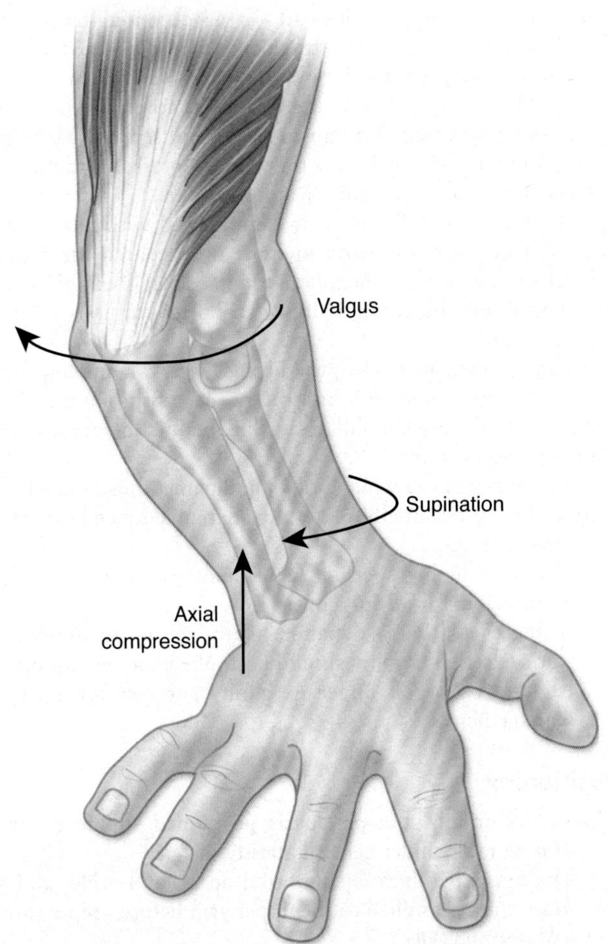

FIG 4 • Typical mechanism of elbow fracture-dislocation. Note the forces at play on the elbow.

PATHOGENESIS

- Fracture-dislocations of the elbow occur during falls onto an outstretched hand, falls from a height, motor vehicle accidents, or other high-energy trauma (**FIG 4**).
- Typically, there is a hyperextension and valgus or varus stress applied to the pronated arm.

NATURAL HISTORY

- Elbow dislocations with associated coronoid or radial head fractures have a poor natural history. These injuries are commonly treated with open reduction and surgical fixation, as redislocation or subluxation is likely with closed treatment.
- Treatment of the radial head fracture by excision alone in the context of an elbow dislocation has a high rate of failure due to recurrent instability and should be avoided.
- Problems of recurrent instability, arthrosis, and severe stiffness lead to poor functional results.[12]

PATIENT HISTORY AND PHYSICAL FINDINGS

- Fracture-dislocations of the elbow are acute and traumatic, so the history should be straightforward.
- It is not unusual for these injuries to occur with high-energy trauma, so a diligent search for other musculoskeletal and systemic injuries must accompany evaluation of the elbow. The ipsilateral shoulder and wrist should be evaluated.
- The evaluation and documentation of peripheral nerve and vascular function in the injured extremity is critical and should be performed before and after reduction maneuvers.

IMAGING AND OTHER DIAGNOSTIC STUDIES

- High-quality plain radiographs in the anteroposterior (AP) and lateral plane should be obtained before and after closed reduction.
  - Cast material can obscure bony detail after closed reduction.
- If there is any evidence of forearm or wrist pain associated with the elbow injury, these should be imaged as well.
- Computed tomography (CT) scans with reformatted images and three-dimensional (3-D) reconstructions are helpful in understanding the configuration of bony injuries (especially of the radial head and coronoid) and are helpful in treatment planning (**FIG 5**).

DIFFERENTIAL DIAGNOSIS

- Radial head or neck fractures without associated dislocation
- Coronoid fracture associated with posteromedial instability. The radial head is not fractured, making diagnosis more difficult.

NONOPERATIVE MANAGEMENT

- Initial treatment involves closed reduction and splinting with radiographs to confirm reduction (**FIG 6**).
- If reduction cannot be maintained because of bone or soft tissue injury, repeated attempts at closed reduction should not be attempted. This is thought to contribute to the formation of heterotopic ossification.
- In the setting of fracture-dislocation of the elbow with instability, the ability of nonoperative management to meet treatment goals is rare and surgery is indicated in almost all cases.

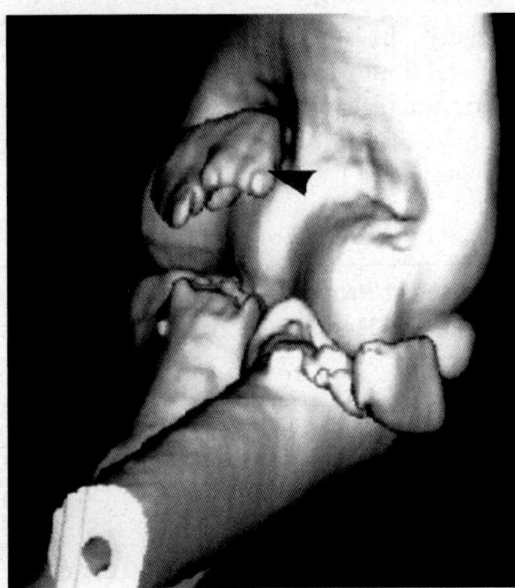

FIG 5 • 3-D CT reconstruction of "terrible triad" injury. The *arrow* represents the large coronoid fragment anterior to the elbow. (From Pugh DM, Wild LM, Schemitsch EH, et al. Standard surgical protocol to treat elbow dislocations with radial head and coronoid fractures. J Bone Joint Surg Am 2004;86A:1122–1130.)

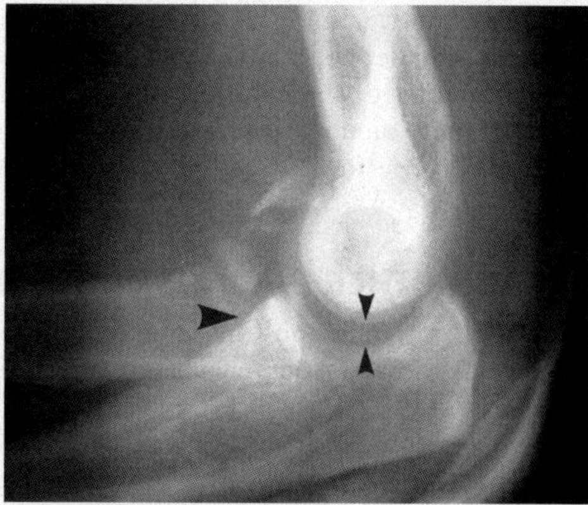

FIG 6 • Radiograph revealing nonconcentric reduction after closed reduction. The *small arrows* highlight the nonconcentric reduction of the ulnohumeral joint. (From Pugh DM, Wild LM, Schemitsch EH, et al. Standard surgical protocol to treat elbow dislocations with radial head and coronoid fractures. J Bone Joint Surg Am 2004;86A:1122–1130.)

SURGICAL MANAGEMENT

- The goals of surgery are to obtain and maintain a concentric and stable reduction of the ulnohumeral and radiocapitellar joint such that early motion within a flexion–extension arc of 30 to 130 degrees can be initiated. Early motion is key (within 2 weeks postoperatively) to avoid elbow stiffness and resultant poor function.
- Management of elbow dislocations with associated radial head and coronoid fractures should follow an established protocol (Table 1) that has produced reliable results.[10]
- The radial head is an important secondary stabilizer of the elbow to valgus stress and posterior instability.[9]
  - It is also a longitudinal stabilizer of the forearm to proximal translation.
  - If fractured in this setting, it must be fixed or replaced, as radial head excision leads to recurrent instability and unacceptable results.[12]

Preoperative Planning

- Before surgery, the surgeon must ensure that the proper equipment and implants are available.
- Coronoid tip fractures are fixed with small fragment or cannulated screws of appropriate size. In the setting of small fragments (ie, type 1) that are not amendable to screw fixation, sutures through the anterior capsule around the fragment can be used instead. Large coronoid fragments such as anteromedial facet fragments should be fixed with a minifragment plate and screws in buttress fashion.
- Radial head and neck fracture fixation is accomplished with screws alone or small fragment plates and screws. We often use countersunk Herbert screws or countersunk minifragment screws to fix articular head fragments.
- If the radial head fragment is comminuted with more than three fragments, the surgeon must be prepared for radial head replacement. A metallic, modular radial head implant system should be available if primary osteosynthesis cannot be achieved.
- An image intensifier is helpful during surgery. Films confirming concentric reduction and the proper positioning of implanted hardware should always be obtained before leaving the operating room.
- In rare instances in which bony and ligamentous repair fails to restore sufficient elbow stability, dynamic hinged external fixation is used.
  - This is a highly specialized technique that may not be appropriate for all surgeons.
  - In the event that a dynamic fixator is not an option, a static external fixation should be applied and patient must be referred to an upper extremity surgeon for further management.

Table 1 Treatment Protocol for Elbow Dislocation with Associated Radial Head and Coronoid Fractures

Step	Action
1	Fix the coronoid fracture.
2	Fix or replace the radial head.
3	Repair the LCL.
4	Assess elbow stability within 30–130 degrees of flexion–extension with the forearm in full pronation.
5	If the elbow remains unstable, consider fixing the MCL.
6	Failing this, apply a hinged external fixator to maintain concentric reduction and allow for early motion.

Positioning

- Most commonly, the patient is positioned supine on the operating table under general anesthesia.
  - The operative limb is supported on a hand table, and a tourniquet is applied to the upper arm before preparation and draping (**FIG 7**).
- Alternatively, the lateral decubitus position can be used with the operative limb supported by a padded bolster.
  - This position is used if hinged fixation is deemed likely.
  - A posterior skin incision can also be used in this position, with creation of full-thickness flaps to access both medial and lateral sides.

Approach

- The lateral approach is the workhorse for treatment of these injuries where the coronoid, radial head, and LCL can

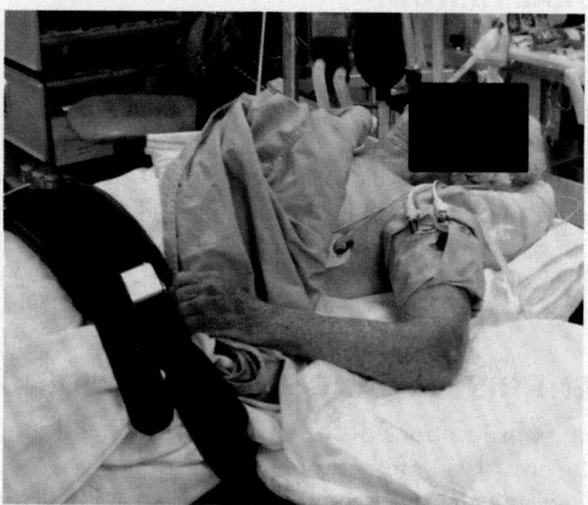

FIG 7 • Patient positioned supine with hand table.

be addressed. A direct lateral incision with the patient supine and the arm on a hand table is used.

- Landmarks and skin incision are shown in **FIG 8A**.
- The typical approach uses the Kocher interval between the anconeus and external carpi ulnaris. However, the surgeon should use the traumatic dissection that has occurred at the time of injury to gain exposure of the elbow.
- Typically, the LCL has been avulsed from the lateral distal humerus, leaving a bare spot (**FIG 8B**).[10]
- Some cases require a medial approach as well for either medial ligament reconstruction or plating of a coronoid fracture. This can be accomplished through a second medial incision.
  - The ulnar nerve is at risk in this approach and should be identified and protected. The common flexor origin is split distal to the medial epicondyle to expose the coronoid medially.
- Alternatively, a posterior skin incision can be used with elevation of full-thickness flaps at the fascial level to approach both laterally and medially.
  - The patient can be placed in the lateral decubitus position or supine with the arm across the chest for this approach.

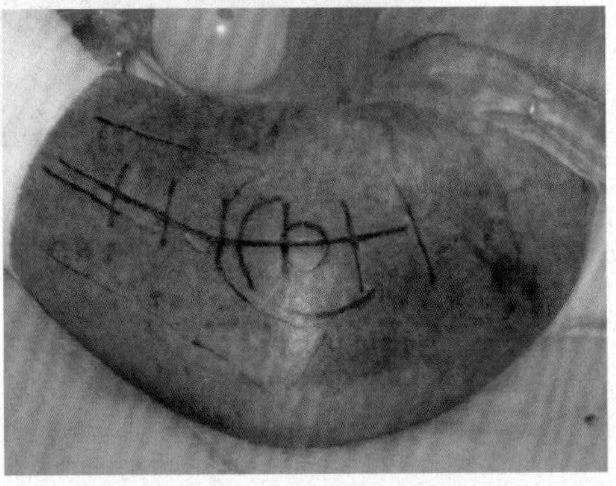

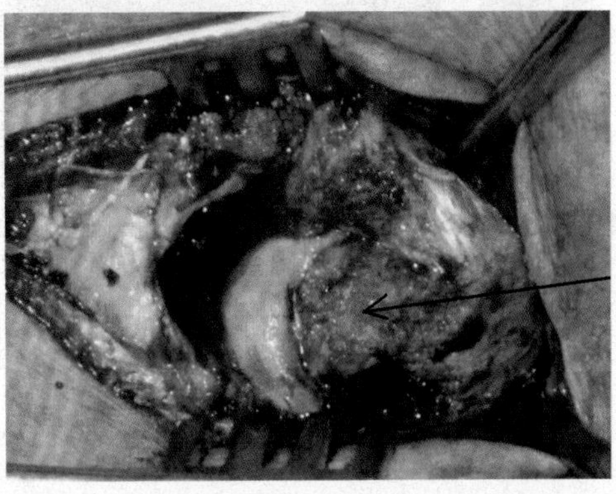

FIG 8 • **A.** Landmarks and skin incision. The underlying bones have been represented and the position of the lateral skin incision is marked with the *hashed line*. **B.** Avulsion of LCL. The *arrow* is pointing to the bare spot on the distal lateral humerus where the LCL complex has been avulsed.

TECHNIQUES

Lateral Exposure

- Make an incision along the lateral supracondylar ridge of the humerus curving at the lateral epicondyle toward the radial head and neck.
- At the fascial level, elevate full-thickness flaps and insert a self-retaining retractor (**TECH FIG 1**).
- Split the common extensor origin in line with its fibers.
- Make use of the traumatic dissection that occurred at the time of injury.
  - Most commonly, the LCL will have avulsed from the distal humerus, leaving a bare spot. The common extensor origin is avulsed as well two-thirds of the time.[9]
- Reconstruction occurs in an orderly fashion from deep to superficial (ie, coronoid first, then radial head, lastly LCL).
- If the radial head is to be replaced, its excision provides excellent exposure of the coronoid through the lateral approach.
  - If, on the other hand, the radial head is amendable to surgical fixation, set the free fragments aside to allow access for coronoid fixation first.

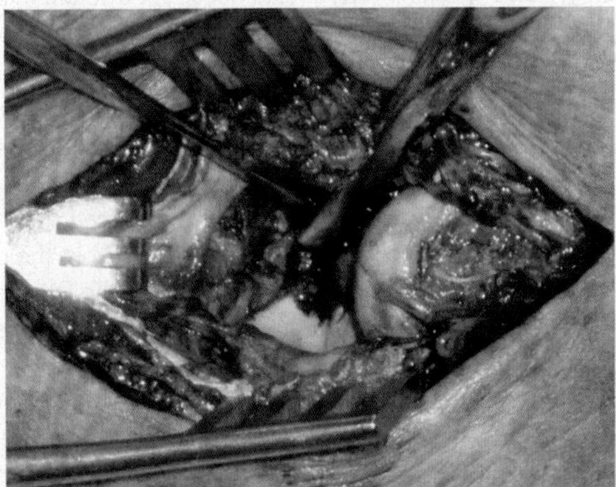

TECH FIG 1 • Lateral approach. In this case, the radial neck was fractured and the head has been removed. An excellent view of the coronoid is achieved. Here, a type I coronoid fracture is present.

Open Reduction and Internal Fixation of Coronoid Fracture

Type I Coronoid Fractures

- For type I fractures, we recommend fixation with a nonabsorbable (no. 2 braided) suture passed through the anterior elbow capsule just above the bony fragment (**TECH FIG 2**).
- Two parallel drill holes are made from the dorsal surface of the ulna through a separate small incision and directed toward the coronoid tip. These are made with a small drill or Kirschner wire. An anterior cruciate ligament (ACL) guide may be used to assist in tunnel placement.
- Once the suture is passed through the capsule, its ends are brought out each of the drill holes and tied over the ulna to

TECHNIQUES

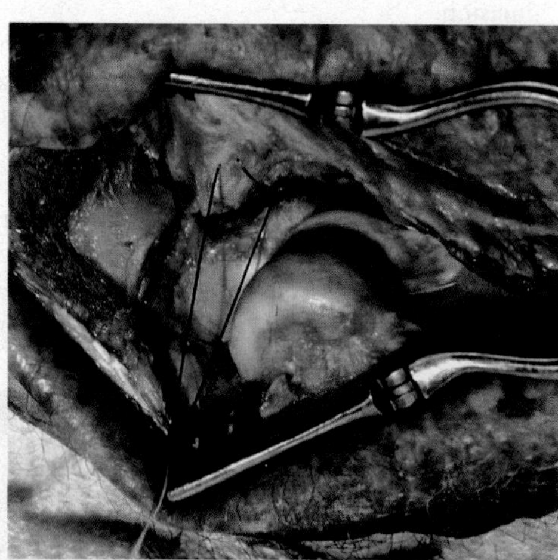

TECH FIG 2 • Suture fixation of a type I coronoid fracture. The suture is passed through the anterior capsule above the coronoid. Its ends will be passed through the proximal ulna and tied over the dorsal surface. This type of fixation is used if the coronoid fragment is too small to accept a screw. (From McKee MD, Pugh DM, Wild LM, et al. Standard surgical protocol to treat elbow dislocation with radial head and coronoid fractures. J Bone Joint Surg Am 2005;87[suppl 1, pt 1]:22–32.)

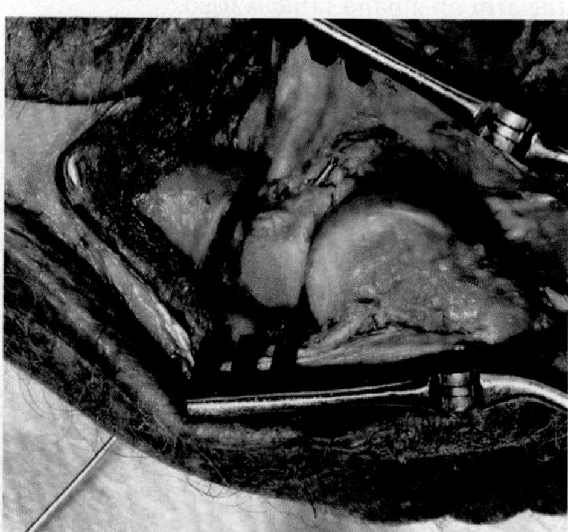

TECH FIG 3 • Coronoid fracture held reduced with Kirschner wire. (From McKee MD, Pugh DM, Wild LM, et al. Standard surgical protocol to treat elbow dislocation with radial head and coronoid fractures. J Bone Joint Surg Am 2005;87[suppl 1, pt1]:22–32.)

plicate the anterior elbow capsule and oppose the coronoid fracture fragment to the fracture site.

- The suture ends can be retrieved through the drill holes using an eyeleted Kirschner wire, a Keith needle, or a suture retriever.

Types II and III Coronoid Fractures

- Types II and III coronoid fractures can be fixed with one or two cannulated screws. Regular, partially threaded, cancellous screws can also be used.
- Once the fracture has been débrided and mobilized such that it can be anatomically reduced, pass a guidewire from the dorsal surface of the proximal ulna such that it exits at the fracture site.
  - Back the guidewire up until it is just buried and reduce the fracture.
- Hold the fragment reduced with a pointed instrument such as a dental pick and advance the wire across the fracture site into the fragment (**TECH FIG 3**). If there is enough space, insert a second wire across the fracture.
- Once one or two guidewires are in place, they are replaced with appropriate-length screws, cannulated or regular. It is critical to tap the fragment before screw placement to avoid splitting the fragment on screw insertion.
- Coronoid fractures that are comminuted may be difficult to treat. Typically, the largest fragment with articular cartilage is fixed.
- If screw fixation is not possible or access is difficult due to an intact radial head, the coronoid can be accessed through a medial approach, as described in the following text.

Medial Approach for Coronoid Fracture Fixation

- The medial approach can also be used in situations where surgical fixation of type II or type III coronoid is not possible due to an intact radial head.
- The medial approach can be used for surgical fixation of anteromedial facet fractures of the coronoid.
  - These fractures should be surgically fixed via a medial approach, by use of plate and screws. The plate is placed along the anterior aspect of the coronoid, buttressing the fragments from displacement.
- The medial approach is outlined in the following text.
  - A medial incision along the supracondylar ridge is used.
  - The ulnar nerve is identified and protected.
  - The common flexor origin is split to gain access to the coronoid on the proximal ulna.
  - From the medial side, a minifragment plate can be used in a buttress or spring fashion to secure a comminuted fracture.

Radial Head or Neck Fracture

- Radial head fracture is addressed after treatment of the coronoid injury because once the head is fixed or replaced, access to the coronoid from the lateral approach is limited.
- The decision to fix a radial head is largely based on the fracture configuration. If fracture comminution is limited such that the head is in two or three fragments, reduction and fixation is usually possible.
  - Fractures that are comminuted (with more than three fracture fragments) or with articular surface damage require replacement.
- Expose the head and neck as necessary for fracture reduction and fixation by extending the Kocher interval.

- The posterior interosseous nerve is at risk during more distal radial neck exposures. Its distance from the operative site can be maximized by keeping the forearm in full pronation. If fixation extending down the radial neck is planned, it is prudent to expose the posterior interosseous nerve and protect it.

Open Reduction and Internal Fixation of Radial Head Fractures

- For radial head fragments, reduce and hold the fragment to the intact head with a pointed reduction clamp.
- We secure the fragments with Herbert screws. The fragments can be held temporarily with a 2-mm Kirschner wire and then replaced with a Herbert screw. Similar countersunk minifragment screws may be used or headless differential pitch compression screws.
  - If the screw is inserted through articular cartilage, its head must be countersunk.
- Radial neck fractures, once reduced, can be held provisionally with a Kirschner wire.
- Definitive fixation is with a small fragment T-plate over the "safe zone" (**TECH FIG 4**).
  - Care is taken to not injure the posterior interosseous nerve while exposing the shaft or by trapping it under the plate distally.
- If the radial head cannot be reconstructed, it should be replaced (see in the following text).

Radial Head Replacement

- The replacement used must be metallic: Silicone implants are inadequate both biomechanically and biologically.[8]

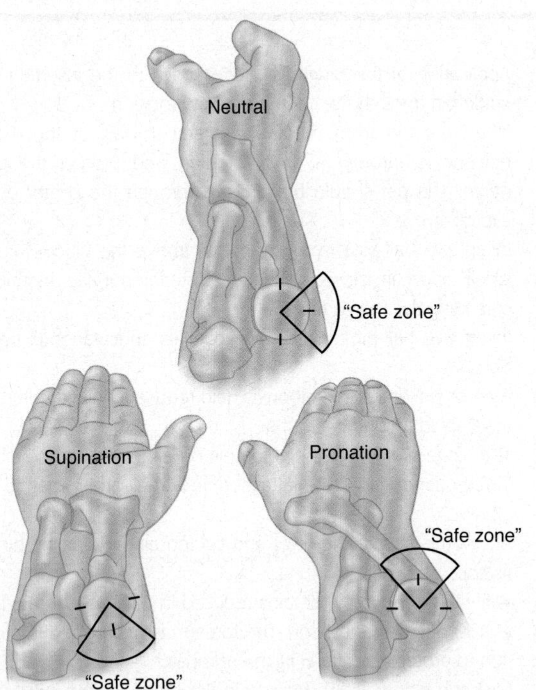

TECH FIG 4 • The safe zone for plating radial neck fractures. The 90-degree arc outlined does not articulate with the proximal ulna throughout the full range of forearm rotation. Plating a radial neck fracture in this zone will not interfere with rotation.

- The metal implant must also be modular, such that the stem diameter can be varied independent of the head diameter and thickness.
- Remove all the radial head fragments and save them on the back table. If required, cut the proximal radius at the level of the neck with a microsagittal saw.
- Ream the canal of the proximal radius to cortical bone with sequentially larger reamers.
- Radial head must be appropriately sized to prevent placement of a prosthesis that is too large:
  - Radial head size can be judged by reassembling the fractured fragments on the back table. One must measure the diameter as well as the length of the native radial head. In general, downsizing the head (diameter as well as length) slightly is recommended such that the elbow joint is not overstuffed.
  - View the articulation between the proximal radius and ulna to see if the diameter and length of the implant seems appropriate. Using the lesser sigmoid notch as a reference, the proximal aspect of the radial head components should be within 1 mm from the lateral aspect of the coronoid process. Extension of the component beyond this will lead to overstuffing the joint.[2]
  - Intraoperative radiographs may be taken, comparing to the contralateral side to assess the medial and lateral ulnohumeral joints. Gapping of the medial ulnohumeral joint is highly suggestive of overlengthening the radial component.[4]
  - Intraoperative assessment of range of motion should be performed with the trial component. Elbow range of motion, both flexion–extension and forearm rotation, should be checked. Stiffness and poor range of motion may be due to overstuffing the radiocapitellar joint. In case of instability, other elbow stabilizers such as LCL and coronoid must be assessed (see Persistent Instability in the following section). Use of an oversized component to gain stability must be avoided.
- Once satisfied with sizing, the definitive implant is inserted (**TECH FIG 5**).

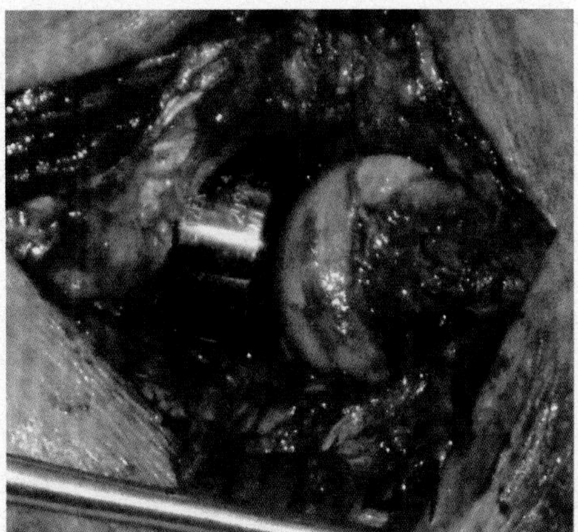

TECH FIG 5 • Radial head implant. An appropriately sized radial head implant has been inserted. It is held reduced with the forearm in full pronation. Note the anatomic alignment with the capitellum.

TECHNIQUES

Repair of the Lateral Collateral Ligament Complex

- Repair of the LCL complex is critical to reestablish elbow stability (**TECH FIG 6A**).
- It is most often avulsed from the distal humerus. Its anatomic attachment point is slightly posterior to the lateral epicondyle at the center of the arc of the capitellum.
- The LCL is a discrete structure that runs from the lateral epicondyle to the supinator crest of the ulna, deep to the common extensor origin (**TECH FIG 6B**).
- Use a no. 2 braided, nonabsorbable suture for the repair.
- The ligament can be reattached to the distal humerus through bone tunnels or using suture anchors. We prefer bony tunnels.
- Using a drill, Kirschner wire, or pointed towel clip, make holes in the distal lateral humerus above the epicondyle.
- Pass the suture through the holes and into the lateral ligament such that it will tighten on tying the sutures.
- At least two, preferably three, sutures through bone are required. Pass, cut, and snap all of the sutures (**TECH FIG 6C**).
  - Ensure that the elbow is now held in 90 degrees of flexion and full forearm pronation.
  - Incorporate the more superficial common extensor origin in the repair.
- Tie the sutures once they have all been passed and then close the lateral wound in layers.

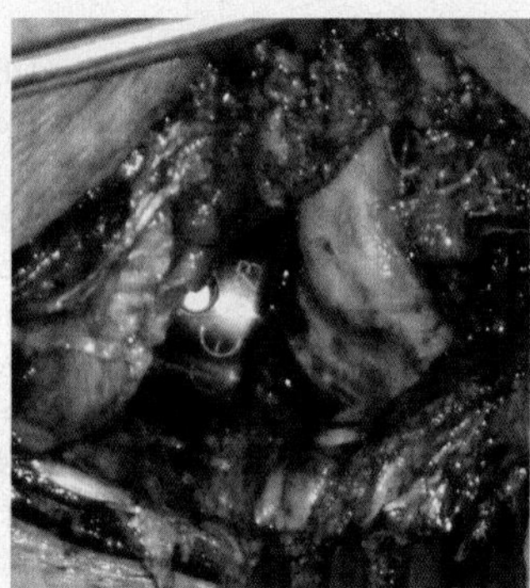
A

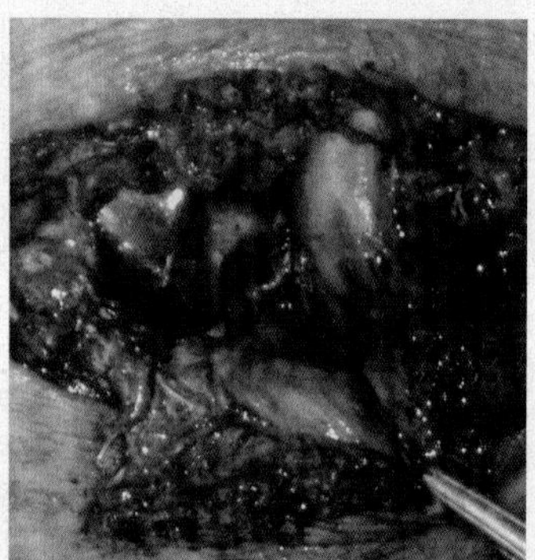
B

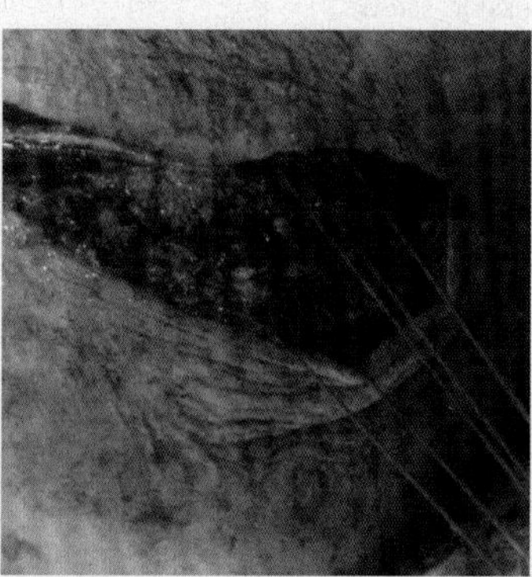
C

TECH FIG 6 • **A.** Elbow instability associated with deficient LCL. Without repair of the LCL, the radial head subluxes into a posterolateral position with forearm supination. Note that the radial head and capitellum are no longer in normal alignment. **B.** The LCL is held by the forceps. It is a distinct structure easily identified in this acutely injured elbow. **C.** Sutures passed for LCL repair.

Persistent Instability

- On occasion, repair of the coronoid, radial head, and LCL from the lateral approach is insufficient to restore elbow stability such that early motion may be initiated.
- In these cases, further efforts must be made to obtain such stability.
- Repair of the MCL through a separate medial incision is one option if a lateral approach has been used for coronoid and radial head fracture fixation.
- A deep approach to the medial aspect of the elbow puts the ulnar nerve at risk, and it must be identified and protected during the procedure.
- Usually, the MCL is torn in its midsubstance. Suture repair of this is often unsatisfying. Using a graft to replace the MCL is not recommended in the acute injury setting.
- If elbow stability remains insufficient, applying a hinged fixator is the final option.[6]
  - If the hinge is not available or the surgeon is not familiar with its use, a static fixator can be applied to maintain elbow reduction.

Hinged External Fixation

- The application of a hinged external fixator is not as commonly required now that the primary structures for elbow stability, and their repair, are more thoroughly understood.
- Application of the hinged fixator starts with the insertion of a guide pin through the center of elbow rotation.
- Insert the pin from medial to lateral starting at the medial epicondyle through a small incision and protect the ulnar nerve. The pin should be directed through the center of the capitellum.
- Insert two half-pins in the humerus above the elbow through small open incisions over the posterior surface by bluntly spreading the triceps fibers.
- Insert two half-pins in the ulna over its subcutaneous border dorsally.
- After pin insertion, the elbow is held reduced while the frame is assembled around it.
- The hinge slides over the guide pin on either side of the elbow. Three-quarter rings are attached proximal and distal to the elbow.
- Attach the pins to the rings and tighten all parts of the hinged fixator.
- Verify that the elbow remains reduced in the frame through 30 to 130 degrees of motion. The forearm is maintained in pronation to protect the lateral ligament repair.
- Lock the elbow at 90 degrees in the hinge for the initial postoperative course.
- Obtain plain radiographs in the operating room before the conclusion of the procedure.

PEARLS AND PITFALLS

Indications	■ Elbow dislocations with associated fractures of the coronoid or radial head must be recognized as complex dislocations. They usually require surgical treatment.
Goals of treatment	■ The goals are to obtain a concentric reduction with sufficient elbow stability such that early range of motion is possible and to avoid persistent instability, elbow stiffness, and arthritis.
Coronoid fractures	■ Repair of coronoid fractures is technically demanding but necessary for successful treatment.
Radial head	■ The surgeon should be prepared to replace the radial head if necessary with a metal, modular prosthesis. ■ Excision alone is not an option.
Lateral ligaments	■ Repair of the lateral ligaments is important to impart the necessary stability for early motion and to avoid late posterolateral rotatory instability.
Physiotherapy	■ It is important to emphasize to the patient the need to be diligent with rehabilitation and exercises, as this will have a great effect on the end result. ■ Immobilization beyond 2 weeks should be avoided.

POSTOPERATIVE CARE

- The injured elbow is placed in a well-padded plaster splint at 90 degrees of flexion and full pronation. The patient is given a sling for comfort.
- AP and lateral radiographs are obtained in the operating room to ensure congruent reduction and verify hardware placement.
- The patient may be discharged home on the same day after receiving adequate analgesia and prophylactic antibiotics.
- We do not routinely give prophylaxis for heterotopic ossification unless the patient has a concomitant head injury: In this case, indomethacin 25 mg three times a day is prescribed with a cytoprotective agent for 3 weeks.
- The patient returns to our clinic at 7 to 10 days postoperatively for staple removal. The splint is typically removed at this point.
  - Range-of-motion exercises are initiated at this time under the supervision of a physiotherapist.
  - Active and active-assisted flexion–extension between 30 and 130 degrees and forearm rotation with the elbow at 90 degrees of flexion is initiated.
  - A lightweight resting splint is made for the injured elbow that is removed for hygiene and physiotherapy.
- The patient returns at 4, 8, and 12 weeks after surgery for clinical review with plain radiographs. Thereafter, the interval of clinic visits is widened, but we follow our patients out to 2 years.
  - At 4 weeks, we allow unrestricted range of motion and at 8 weeks, unrestricted strengthening.
  - Evidence of fracture union is usually present between 6 and 8 weeks.
  - Progress with range of motion can be slow and frustrating for the patient but does not plateau until 1 year of follow-up.

OUTCOMES

- Following the protocol outlined for fracture-dislocations of the elbow should yield satisfactory functional results.
- Pugh et al[10] reported the results of this treatment protocol for 36 elbows at 34 months.
  - The flexion–extension arc averaged 112 degrees and rotation 136 degrees.
  - Fifteen patients had excellent results, 13 good, 7 fair, and 1 poor as measured by the Mayo Elbow Performance Score.
  - Eight patients had a complication requiring reoperation.

COMPLICATIONS

- The most likely complication after treatment is unacceptable elbow stiffness with a resultant nonfunctional range of motion.
  - An acceptable range is 30 to 130 degrees of flexion.
- At about 1 year after surgery, once motion has plateaued, patients are candidates for release with hardware removal if they are not happy with their range of motion and the flexion–extension arc is less than 100 degrees.
  - This is done through the lateral approach with an anterior and posterior capsulectomy plus manipulation under anesthesia.
  - A radial head implant in place can be downsized to improve motion, but it should not be simply removed. The lateral ligament complex is preserved.
  - In our series, this was necessary in 11% of cases.[10]
- Synostosis around the elbow is another possible cause of rotational forearm stiffness.
  - A resection can be planned to improve motion.
  - CT scanning preoperatively helps to define the extent of the lesion. Resection is technically demanding.
- Superficial and deep wound infection is possible after repair. Immediate and aggressive treatment is recommended with antibiotics initially and irrigation with débridement if rapid improvement is not seen.
- Persistent instability is rare but may occur despite best efforts at repair. Formal ligament reconstruction can be helpful in this setting.
- Posttraumatic arthritis may be a long-term problem.

REFERENCES

1. Cage DJ, Abrams RA, Callahan JJ, et al. Soft tissue attachments of the ulnar coronoid process. An anatomic study with radiographic correlation. Clin Orthop Relat Res 1995;(320):154–158.
2. Doornberg JN, Linzel DS, Zurakowski D, et al. Reference points for radial head prosthesis size. J Hand Surg 2006;31(1):53–57.
3. Doornberg JN, Ring DC. Fracture of the anteromedial facet of the coronoid process. J Bone Joint Surg Am 2006;88(10):2216–2224.

4. Frank SG, Grewal R, Johnson J, et al. Determination of correct implant size in radial head arthroplasty to avoid overlengthening. J Bone Joint Surg Am 2009;91:1738–1746.
5. Mason ML. Some observations on fractures of the head of the radius with a review of one hundred cases. Br J Surg 1954;42:123–132.
6. McKee MD, Bowden SH, King GJ, et al. Management of recurrent, complex instability of the elbow with a hinged external fixator. J Bone Joint Surg Br 1998;80(6):1031–1036.
7. McKee MD, Schemitsch EH, Sala MJ, et al. The pathoanatomy of lateral ligamentous disruption in complex elbow instability. J Shoulder Elbow Surg 2003;12:391–396.
8. Moro JK, Werier J, MacDermid JC, et al. Arthroplasty with a metal radial head for unreconstructable fractures of the radial head. J Bone Joint Surg Am 2001;83-A(8):1201–1211.
9. Morrey BF, Tanaka S, An KN. Valgus stability of the elbow. A definition of primary and secondary constraints. Clin Orthop Relat Res 1991;(265):187–195.
10. Pugh DM, Wild LM, Schemitsch EH, et al. Standard surgical protocol to treat elbow dislocations with radial head and coronoid fractures. J Bone Joint Surg Am 2004;86A:1122–1130.
11. Regan W, Morrey B. Fractures of the coronoid process of the ulna. J Bone Joint Surg Am 1989;71:1248–1254.
12. Ring D, Jupiter JB, Zilberfarb J. Posterior dislocation of the elbow with fractures of the radial head and coronoid. J Bone Joint Surg Am 2002;84-A(4):547–551.

Forearm and Wrist Fractures and Dislocations

22

CHAPTER

Open Reduction and Internal Fixation of Diaphyseal Forearm Fractures

Lee M. Reichel and John R. Dawson

DEFINITION

- Diaphyseal forearm fractures include isolated or combined radial and ulnar fractures ("both-bone fractures"). They occur distal to the elbow joint and proximal to the wrist joint.
- It is critical to evaluate the distal radioulnar joint (DRUJ) and radiocapitellar joint preoperatively, intraoperatively, and postoperatively to avoid missing Galeazzi- and Monteggia-type injuries.
- Fixation techniques should be tailored to the age of the patient and the location and pattern of fracture.
- Excellent functional results and union rates can be obtained when skeletal length and alignment are restored with stable internal fixation.

ANATOMY

- Complete knowledge of neural, vascular, and muscular anatomy is expected. Neural anatomy is particularly important, as a nerve injury in the forearm rarely completely recovers. Nerve injuries result in disabling, temporary or permanent, motor and sensory dysfunction in the hand.
- Injury
  - Radial, posterior interosseous (PIN), median, anterior interosseous (AIN), and ulnar nerve injuries can all occur, although their incidence is not frequent. Preoperative nerve assessment is best performed by measurement of static two-point discrimination. Acutely, motor examinations are difficult secondary to pain. If a nerve injury is suspected preoperatively, that nerve must be explored within the zone of injury. Although the majority of nerves are found to be in continuity, the surgeon should be prepared to repair the nerve either primarily or with nerve cable grafts following bony stabilization.
  - Unless injured preoperatively, the radial, median, and ulnar nerves are not typically encountered. If they are encountered, this should alert the surgeon that he or she might be in the wrong dissection interval.
  - Muscle injury may be significant following fracture. It is typically not clinically significant except for injury to the flexor pollicis longus, which may even be nonfunctioning in severe injuries. This can be difficult to differentiate preoperatively from a partial AIN injury.
- Approaches to the radius (**FIG 1**)
  - Five muscles cover the radius (supinator, flexor digitorum superficialis, pronator teres, flexor pollicis longus, pronator quadratus). When the soft tissue injury is significant, muscle size, fiber orientation, and tendinous insertions (particularly the pronator teres) help orient the surgeon. The supinator muscle is especially important to identify in both volar and posterior approaches to the radius to avoid injury to the PIN. Its fibers are obliquely oriented to the longitudinally oriented flexor and extensor muscles.
  - During the volar, or anterior, approach, the lateral antebrachial cutaneous nerve, superficial radial sensory nerve, AIN, and PIN are usually encountered. The lateral antebrachial cutaneous nerve is sometimes encountered during blunt scissor dissection through the subcutaneous fat following the skin incision. Proximally, the superficial radial nerve lies deep to the brachioradialis. One must avoid placing self-retaining retractors on it.
  - The radial artery is encountered in every anterior approach to the radius. It is found deep to the brachioradialis in the proximal one-third of the forearm and visualized just beneath the forearm fascia exiting near the divergence of the brachioradialis and flexor carpi radialis muscle bellies in the midforearm. In very proximal volar approaches, near the bicipital tuberosity, crossing veins and the recurrent radial artery can be visualized.
  - Superficial veins of the volar and dorsal forearm can be large and contribute to significant bleeding. Formal suture ligation may be needed for large veins.
  - During the dorsal, or posterior, approach to the radius, the PIN and possibly the superficial radial sensory nerve may be encountered.
- Approaches to the ulna (see **FIG 1**)
  - The dorsal ulnar cutaneous nerve is most commonly visualized passing in a volar to dorsal direction through the subcutaneous tissue, distal to the ulnar styloid. However, rarely, variations do exist where this nerve crosses the ulna more proximally. Therefore, blunt dissection through the subcutaneous fat in the distal one-third of the forearm is safest for preventing inadvertent nerve injury.
  - The entire ulna is a subcutaneous bone, and subperiosteal dissection provides extensile exposure. Flexor carpi ulnaris and flexor carpi radialis border the volar and dorsal sides of the ulna. These muscles converge in the middle third of the ulna, requiring only shallow intramuscular dissection to expose the ulnar shaft.
- Fixation
  - Both the AIN and PIN lay millimeters away from the radius in anterior and posterior approaches. Reduction clamps in-

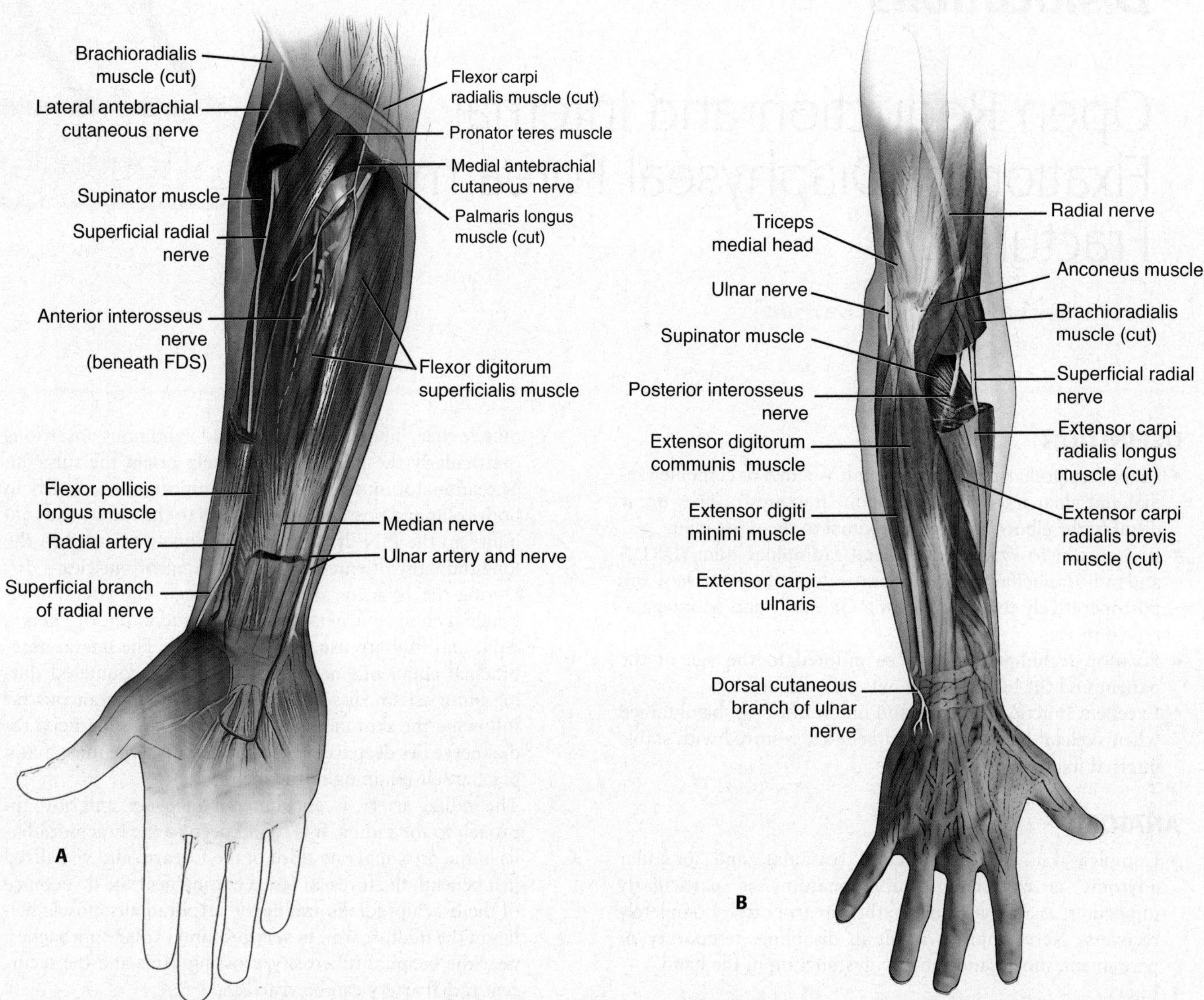

FIG 1 • Muscular and neurovascular anatomy of the forearm. **A.** During a volar approach to the forearm, the radial artery, superficial radial nerve, anterior interosseus neurovascular structures, and posterior interosseous nerve may all be encountered. Detailed knowledge of their location and ability to visually identify these structures are critical to avoiding injury when their anatomic location is disrupted by injury. **B.** Dorsal approaches must demand identification of the posterior interosseious nerve proximally and superficial radlal nerve branches distally. During distal third ulnar approaches, the dorsal cutaneous branch of the ulnar nerve may be encountered notably when anatomy is aberrant.

advertently placed around them when affixing a plate to the bone or reducing fracture fragments can damage them. Additionally, avoid using monopolar cautery on the ulnar aspect of the radius. When bleeding is encountered from the anterior interosseous vessels, they must be dissected away from the nerve prior to obtaining hemostasis to avoid nerve injury. Bleeding is stopped with bipolar cautery or small vascular clips.

- Osteology
  - The radius has a complex osteology with both a radial and sagittal bow. The radial bow has an arc of approximately 10 degrees and lies in the coronal midshaft, whereas the sagittal bow has an approximately 5 degree arc and lies in the proximal third of the radius.[9] Contouring of anteriorly placed plates on the proximal radius accommodates the sagittal bow. Anatomic plates are available to accommodate the radial bow.
  - The ulna is generally flat in the sagittal plane and curved in the coronal plane (with the exception of the proximal ulna which in some patients has a slight apex posterior curvature at the olecranon).[8] In the middle and distal thirds of the forearm, plate fixation can be placed anteriorly or posteriorly to avoid symptomatic hardware. In proximal ulnar shaft fractures, plate placement along the subcutaneous border, although possibly more symptomatic, obviates the need for plate contouring to the ulnar coronal bow. This placement also helps resist the forces generated during elbow flexion and extension from the long lever arm of the forearm.

PATHOGENESIS

- Direct trauma (guarding face against direct blow, gunshot wound)
- Indirect trauma (motor vehicle collision, falls)
- The incidence of associated injuries in patients presenting to a trauma center with a both-bone forearm fracture is significant. In one series of 87 patients presenting to a regional

trauma center, 40% had multiple injuries (25% with closed head injury, 26% associated major injuries in the same extremity).[3]

NATURAL HISTORY

- Closed treatment of radius or both-bone forearm fractures generally yields unacceptable results.[1]
- Plate fixation using 3.5-mm compression plates of radial and ulnar fractures is the standard of care yielding good or excellent functional results and union rates greater than 95%.[3]
- Restoration of forearm rotation depends on obtaining proper skeletal length and axial and rotational alignment.[11]

PATIENT HISTORY AND PHYSICAL FINDINGS

- Evaluate for life-threatening injuries first.
- When there is obvious injury to the forearm, it should be examined last so that satisfaction of search does not result in missed injuries.
- Examination begins at the neck and shoulder girdle away from the injured area. In an awake, cooperative patient, palpation of each bony structure will typically reveal injury for which imaging should be obtained. In an uncooperative or intubated patient, a very low threshold for obtaining imaging is needed.
- It is particularly important to palpate the radial head, collateral ligaments of the elbow, distal radius and ulna, and triangular fibrocartilage complex to avoid missing soft tissue, Monteggia, or Galeazzi injuries. If a ligamentous or tendinous injury is suspected in the setting of a stable joint, a magnetic resonance imaging (MRI) scan is ordered to make the diagnosis and allow for early repair if indicated.
- Usually, obvious gross deformity is present when both the radius and ulna are fractured, but isolated radius or ulna fractures are easily missed especially in a polytrauma, intubated, or noncommunicative patient.
- It is critical that the forearm compartments be visualized in their entirety and palpated to assess for compartment syndrome. All splints and dressings must be removed so the skin can be examined circumferentially. The signs and symptoms of compartment syndrome should be checked and documented even when they are "negative."
- The neurovascular examination at a minimum should include an assessment of radial and ulnar pulses and a detailed documented examination of the sensorimotor function of the median, radial, and ulnar nerves. Preoperative AIN function should be documented as well.

IMAGING AND OTHER DIAGNOSTIC STUDIES

- Anteroposterior and lateral radiographs of the forearm, wrist, and elbow generally suffice.
- Careful scrutiny of the DRUJ and radiocapitellar joint alignment are performed on wrist and elbow radiographs.
- In comminuted fractures, contralateral imaging of the uninjured forearm and wrist is helpful to determine the patient's native bony alignment and ulnar variance.

DIFFERENTIAL DIAGNOSIS

- Radial shaft fracture with DRUJ injury (Galeazzi fracture)
- Ulnar fracture with radiocapitellar dislocation (Monteggia fracture)
- Compartment syndrome

NONOPERATIVE MANAGEMENT

- Nonoperative care is reserved for middle or distal third isolated ulnar fractures with no associated injury to the proximal radioulnar joint (PRUJ) or DRUJ. Proximal fractures are rarely treated nonoperatively.
  - Generally, greater than 50% of bony overlap and less than 15 degrees of angulation are appropriate for nonoperative management.
  - Distal fractures can be maintained in a fracture brace or short-arm cast. Midshaft fractures can be immobilized in "Munster cast" as described earlier or in a fracture brace.
  - The duration of immobilization is until pain subsides and the patient can tolerate mobilization. Weight bearing through the extremity is avoided until there is clinical and radiographic evidence of fracture union. Early mobilization may lead to more rapid union.[2]
- Rarely, stable isolated nondisplaced radius shaft fractures can be treated in a cast or functional brace that allows elbow flexion and extension but no forearm rotation.
- Radiographic union can be expected between 8 and 10 weeks.

SURGICAL MANAGEMENT

- The two primary goals of treatment are to obtain union and restore function. The primary surgical aim is the stable restoration of length, angular alignment, and rotational alignment.
- Approach
  - Separate approaches are needed for the radius and ulna to minimize the risk of synostosis.
  - Radius fixation is performed through an anterior or a posterior approach. Anterior fixation minimizes but does not eliminate the possibility for symptomatic hardware. Anterior fixation is straightforward for middle-third and distal-third radius fractures but is more difficult in proximal-third fractures. The posterior approach has traditionally been recommended for the middle-third radius fracture but is rarely used. The posterior approach is most helpful during proximal radius exposure but care needs to be taken to protect the PIN.
  - The entire ulna can be exposed through a subcutaneous approach. Plate fixation can be on the subcutaneous surface, anterior surface, or dorsal surface.
- Internal fixation
  - The order of operation in both-bone forearm fractures depends on the degree of comminution of each bone. Typically, the less comminuted bone is fixed first so as to have the most precise restoration of length.
  - Radius fractures are stabilized with the arm extended, whereas the ulna is typically stabilized with elbow flexed 90 degrees. Therefore, if indicated, radius fixation first allows a stable forearm during elbow flexion for ulnar fixation.
  - 3.5-mm compression plates with six cortices of fixation on either side of the fracture are the standard of care. Anatomic and straight plates are available with locking and nonlocking screw options. Comminuted fractures may require bridge plating. Anatomic plates are very helpful for restoring the radial bow.
  - In osteoporotic fractures, the use of locking screws is indicated.

- Locked plates are also indicated when bridging a defect or when one segment is very short and six cortices of fixation cannot be achieved.
- Care must be taken to ensure plates and screws placed on the both the distal ulna and the proximal radius does not impinge in each respective radioulnar joint. Locked unicortical screws must sometimes be used to avoid screw tip prominence in the joint. Live intraoperative fluoroscopic examination is used to assessing screw placement near the DRUJ or PRUJ. Additionally, it is critical to pronosupinate the forearm to ensure there is no plate impingement in these joints.

- Bone grafting
  - Controversy exists regarding the role of acute autologous bone grafting. Use in the setting of comminuted segments of devascularized bone may be one indication.[6,7]
- Closure
  - The tourniquet must always be taken down and meticulous hemostasis obtained.
  - Fascia is left open and only skin and subcutaneous tissues are approximated.
  - When there is significant swelling that results in a tight closure, skin should be left open, and a delayed primary closure is usually obtainable after 72 hours.
  - Soft well-padded dressings with no tight circumferential wrapping minimize the risk of postoperative compartment syndrome.
- Special circumstances
  - If the patient presents with signs and symptoms of compartment syndrome, they should be taken STAT to the operating room for decompressive fasciotomy of the forearm and carpal tunnel at a minimum. Typically, a single volar incision fasciotomy with release of superficial and deep fascial structures will suffice in decompressing the forearm compartments. Mobile wad and dorsal extensor compartments and hand compartments need to be critically evaluated following volar fasciotomy. They should be released if any suspicion exists for compartment syndrome of these compartments.
  - When large areas of bone loss are present, bridge plating is useful to keep the forearm bones out to the proper length. Consider using stainless steel plates, rather than titanium, because of their greater strength.
    - Dissection should be kept at a minimum in anticipation of further reconstruction, and if a vascularized bone graft is anticipated, no unnecessary vascular dissection should be performed in order to protect recipient arteries and veins needed for final reconstruction.

Preoperative Planning

- Preoperatively, the surgeon needs to decide the approach and the type of fixation required.
- Approach
  - Middle- and distal-third radius fractures are stabilized through a volar approach.
  - Proximal-third fractures can be stabilized through either a volar or posterior approach. Proximal-third fractures requiring exposure of the radial neck are approached dorsally.
- Internal fixation
  - Plate selection for radius fractures depends on a variety of factors including the location of the fracture, fracture pattern, bone defects, quality of the bone, patient compliance, and size of the patient.
  - In proximal radius fractures, fixation of the proximal segment is frequently limited to two screws. The bone of the proximal radius near the radial tuberosity is more cancellous than cortical in nature, limiting screw purchase. Therefore, the use of locking plates and screws in the proximal segment can provide more reliable, stable internal fixation when the number of screws is limited. Additionally, when placed on the anterior radius surface, pronation must be evaluated for plate impingement between the ulna and biceps tendon at this level. A palpable clunk may be noted during pronation. If so, plate placement may need to be revised, but this can be difficult secondary to limited bone stock.
  - For simple pattern midshaft fractures, straight, small fragmentary 3.5-mm compression-type plates suffice with six cortices of fixation on each side of the fracture. A seven-hole plate is typically chosen with an open hole left over the fracture site (unless an interfragmentary screw can be placed through this hole).
  - Distal-third radius fractures can be stabilized with long periarticular volar locking plates, some of which incorporate a radial bow. Alternatively, small fragmentary 3.5-mm compression plates can be contoured distally to match the anterior metaphyseal curvature of the distal radius. Additionally, screw purchase in the cancellous distal radius may be poor, and placement of locking screws is sometimes helpful.

Positioning

- The patient is placed supine with the injured arm out on a radiolucent arm table. A nonsterile pneumatic tourniquet is placed on the upper arm protected by a stockinette or padding. If acute autologous bone grafting is considered, the ipsilateral anterior iliac crest should be included in the surgical field.

Approach

- For radius fractures, an anterior approach as described by Henry[5] or posterior approach as described by Thompson[10] may be used.
- All radius fractures, except those extending to the radial neck and head, can be stabilized through a volar approach. One should consider the following when choosing an approach to the proximal radius:
  - In proximal fractures, there is more depth in the volar approach than the posterior approach, sometimes limiting visualization.
  - The volar approach is between the flexor mass as it comes to its confluence at the medial humerus and the biceps tendon insertion on the radial tuberosity. This limits the soft tissue mobility significantly again, sometimes limiting visualization.
  - Large caliber vascular structures and a network of tortuous veins make wide exposure of the bone more difficult in the volar approach.
  - After identification and protection of the PIN, the posterior approach provides wide exposure of the tension side of the radius. Unfortunately, the PIN crosses the radius in proximal fractures, which make hardware placement more tedious and hardware removal, if needed, challenging.

Anterior (Volar) Approach to the Radius

- Light exsanguination is performed by elevation or loose wrapping with a sterile Ace wrap and the tourniquet is inflated.
- The incision is drawn centered on the fracture from the lateral edge of the biceps tendon to the radial styloid. Length depends on the degree of comminution but in general will comprise approximately one-third of the forearm length (**TECH FIG 1A**).
- An incision is made through the skin only, followed by blunt dissection down to the fascia. Attention is paid to visualization of the lateral antebrachial cutaneous nerve (**TECH FIG 1B**). (We generally score the skin with our knife blade then deepen the incision with a needle tip cautery through the dermis to aid in hemostasis at the skin level.)
  - Small branches of the lateral antebrachial cutaneous nerve if encountered are sacrificed to mobilize the main nerve out of the field of dissection.
- A sponge can be used to sweep away the deep fat off the fascia if needed.
- The fascia is incised and released with scissors.
- The radial artery and venae comitantes must be identified and mobilized. In the proximal third of the forearm, the radial artery lies deep to the brachioradialis muscle belly, which at this level nears the midline of the anterior forearm.
- Bipolar cauterization of perforators to the brachioradialis muscle allows mobilization of the radial artery medially.
- In the middle third of the forearm, the radial artery is more superficial—often in a layer of fat just beneath the fascia—as it exits the interval between brachioradialis muscle belly and flexor carpi radialis muscle belly (**TECH FIG 1C**). Again, the artery is mobilized medially.
- In the distal third of the forearm, it is sometimes safer to mobilize the radial artery laterally, and in the very distal forearm, the approach can be made through the floor of the flexor carpi radialis, thereby avoiding the radial artery completely.
- In the proximal forearm, the muscular envelope is deep, and dissection proceeds along the medial edge of brachioradialis.
- The superficial radial nerve is identified, and care is taken not to place retractors directly on the nerve.
- The supinator will be identified by the oblique muscle fiber orientation, and the surgeon must be mindful that the PIN runs proximal-medial to distal-lateral, entering 90 degrees to the orientation of the muscle fibers and fascia.
  - With the radius broken, it is difficult to effectively supinate the proximal forearm in order to protect the PIN.
  - If the bone is exposed distal to the supinator, a reduction forceps can be placed on the bone and the assistant can supinate the proximal radius. This allows the muscle to be peeled with a freer elevator or knife in a medial to lateral direction, safely keeping the PIN laterally.
  - Alternatively, the PIN can be identified, although this is usually not necessary.
- When dissecting near the biceps tuberosity, usually, a small amount of clear, thick fluid from the biceps bursae will be released as dissection nears the biceps insertion. This burst of fluid is helpful in orienting the surgeon to their location. Just proximal to this, there are typically multiple crossing vessels that need not be disturbed. They can be retracted en masse with a blunt retractor if necessary.

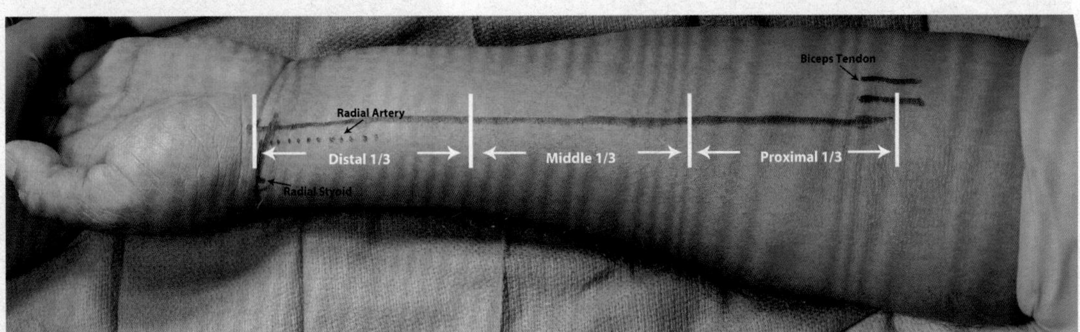

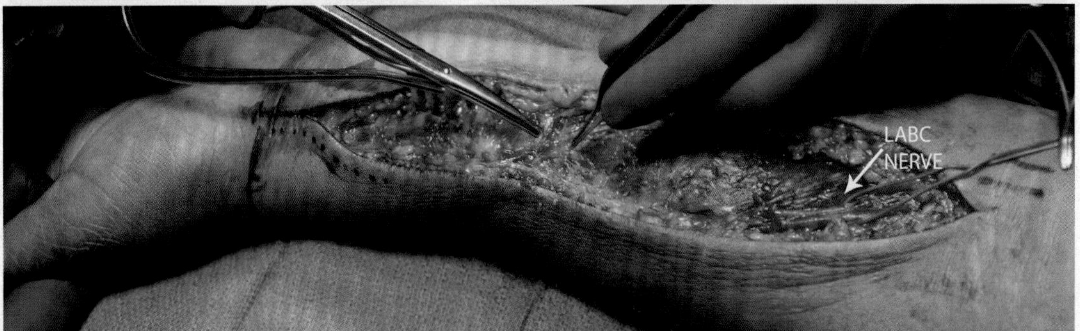

TECH FIG 1 • Anterior approach to the radius. **A.** The forearm is mentally divided in thirds. Each third has unique anatomic structures that must be recognized during the approach. Extensile exposure extends from the biceps tendon to the radial styloid. Distal-third fractures can alternatively be approached through the floor of the flexor carpi radialis (FCR) tendon. **B.** Blunt dissection is performed superficially, and the main trunk of the lateral antebrachial cutaneous nerve (LABC) is identified and protected. *(continued)*

- The most efficient dissection to the middle and distal thirds of the radius proceeds down to its lateral border. Proximally, where the supinator lies the dissection on the medial radius avoids the PIN.
  - In the middle third of the radius, the flexor digitorum profundus and pronator teres can be sharply released from lateral to medial.
  - The pronator teres can be Z-lengthened or taken off the bone in a subperiosteal fashion. Alternatively, if only a limited amount of exposure is needed, its muscle fibers can be dissected off the tendinous portion for a short distance, leaving the tendon intact. If taken off the radius, it can be sutured back down to the plate (**TECH FIG 1D**). Our preference is the latter during extensile exposures.
  - Distally, the flexor pollicis longus and pronator quadratus are taken off the radius laterally to medially with a knife.
- Bone fixation techniques are then performed as described in the following text (**TECH FIG 1G**).
- The tourniquet is always taken down. If a meticulous dissection has been performed with liberal use of bipolar cautery, little bleeding is encountered.
- Fascia is not closed, but inverted interrupted absorbable monofilament suture is used as needed to reapproximate the subcutaneous tissues followed by 3-0 nylon suture for the skin.

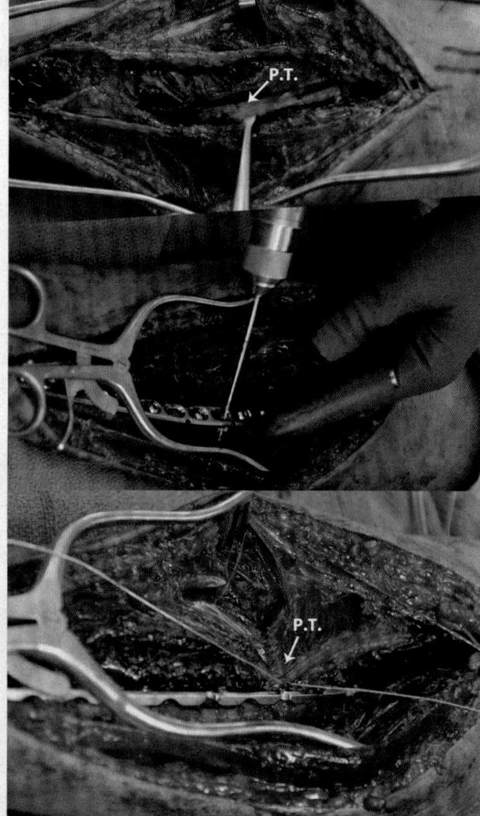

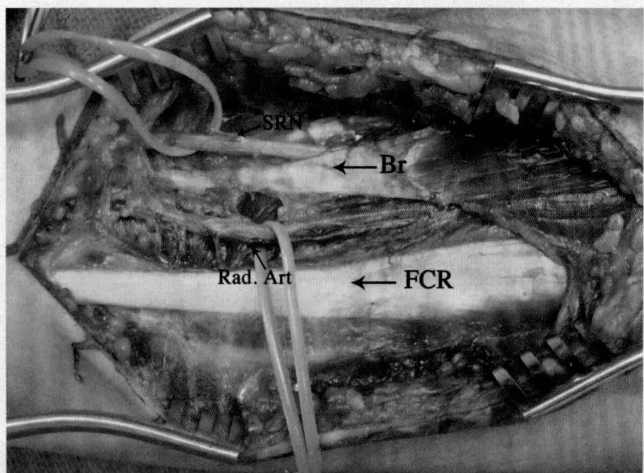

C D

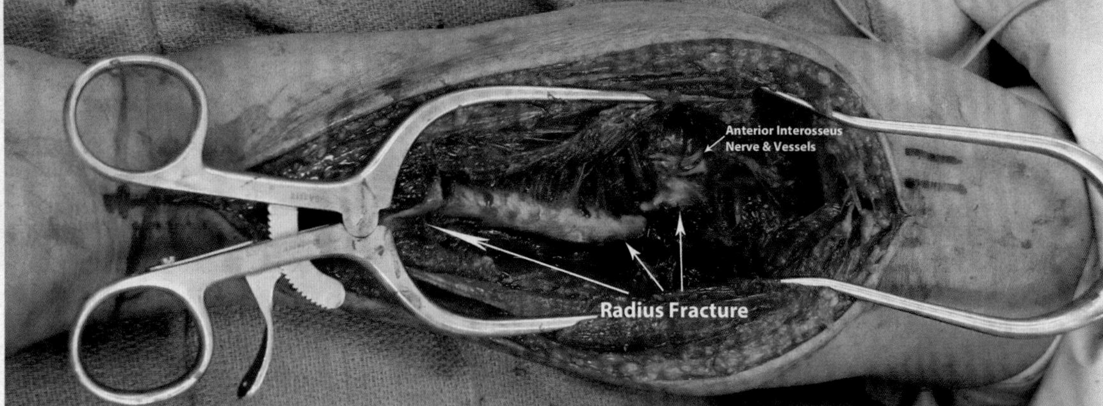

E

TECH FIG 1 • *(continued)* **C.** In the middle third, the radial artery (*Rad. Art*) and venae comitantes are identified exiting between brachioradialis (*Br*) and flexor carpi radialis (*FCR*). Light exsanguination assists in identifying vascular structures. The superficial radial nerve (*SRN*) is seen coursing between Br and FCR. **D.** The *upper* images demonstrate the pronator teres (*P.T.*) insertion on the radius. *Middle* image demonstrates drill hole placed through plate hole and radius for reattachment of P.T. (*lower* image). **E.** A segmental radius fracture and the AIN and vessel closely approximated to the proximal fragment. *(continued)*

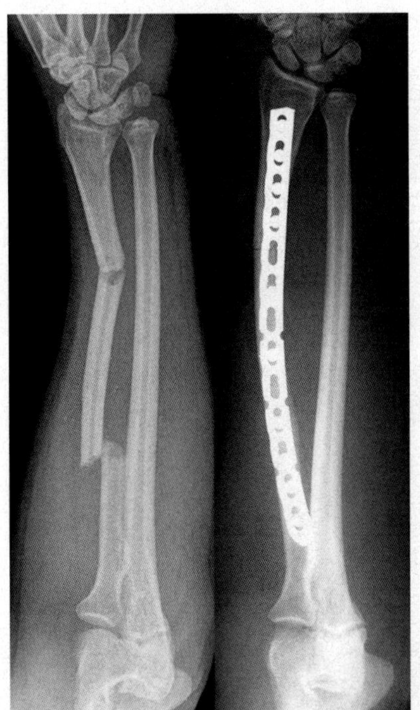

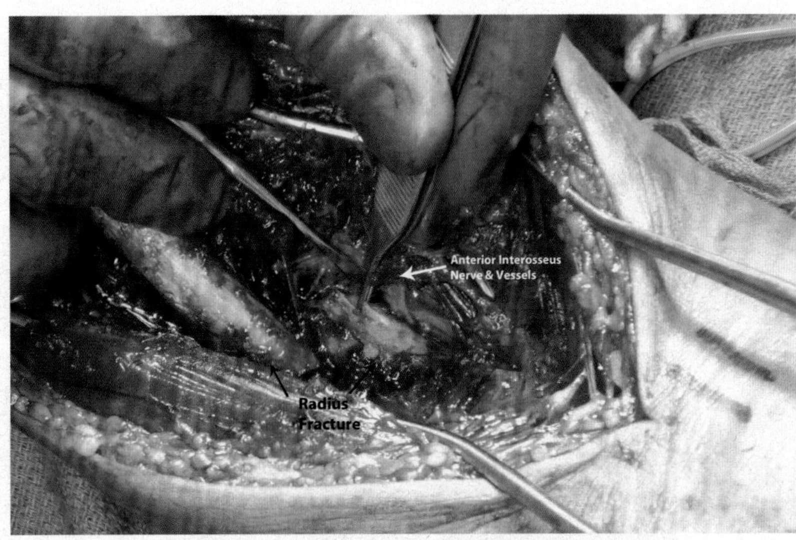

TECH FIG 1 • *(continued)* **F.** Retraction of vessels with a Freer, allowing safe exposure of radius. **G.** Anatomic plate fixation of the segmental radius fracture with restoration of the radial bow.

Posterior Approach to the Radius

- The posterior approach is typically used for proximal- or middle-third radius shaft fractures. Extensile exposure of the entire proximal and middle thirds of the radius is described in the following text.
- An incision is drawn from the lateral epicondyle of the humerus to Lister tubercle and centered on the fracture.
  - The incision length typically approximates one-third the length of the radius centered at the fracture (**TECH FIG 2A**).
  - Blunt dissection is performed down to the level of the fascia, and small fasciocutaneous flaps are elevated. Perforating fasciocutaneous vessels can usually be seen and cauterized with a needle-tip cautery.
  - Proximally, the interval lies between the white, thick tendinous band of the extensor digitorum communis tendon at the confluence of the extensor mass and the muscle belly of the extensor carpi radialis brevis just anterior to it (**TECH FIG 2B**).
  - It is important to identify the tendinous origin of the extensor digitorum communis, as the radial portion of the lateral collateral ligament complex of the elbow lies directly deep to it.
  - The fascia is incised just anterior to the white, thick tendinous band, and a Freer elevator is used to elevate the muscle fibers off the septum.
  - The deep facial layer is then carefully opened with scissors in a distal to proximal direction revealing the supinator muscle, identified by the changing direction of muscle fibers proximal/posterior to distal/anterior (**TECH FIG 2C**).
  - The PIN enters the supinator approximately 90 degrees to the orientation of its muscle fibers. By lifting the radial wrist extensors and brachioradialis off of the supinator with a blunt retractor, one can frequently identify the PIN entering the supinator.
  - Alternatively, the PIN is identified distally and traced proximally through the supinator (**TECH FIG 2D,E**).
- In the middle third of the radius, the abductor pollicis longus and extensor pollicis brevis are identified and elevated off the radius sharply for exposure.

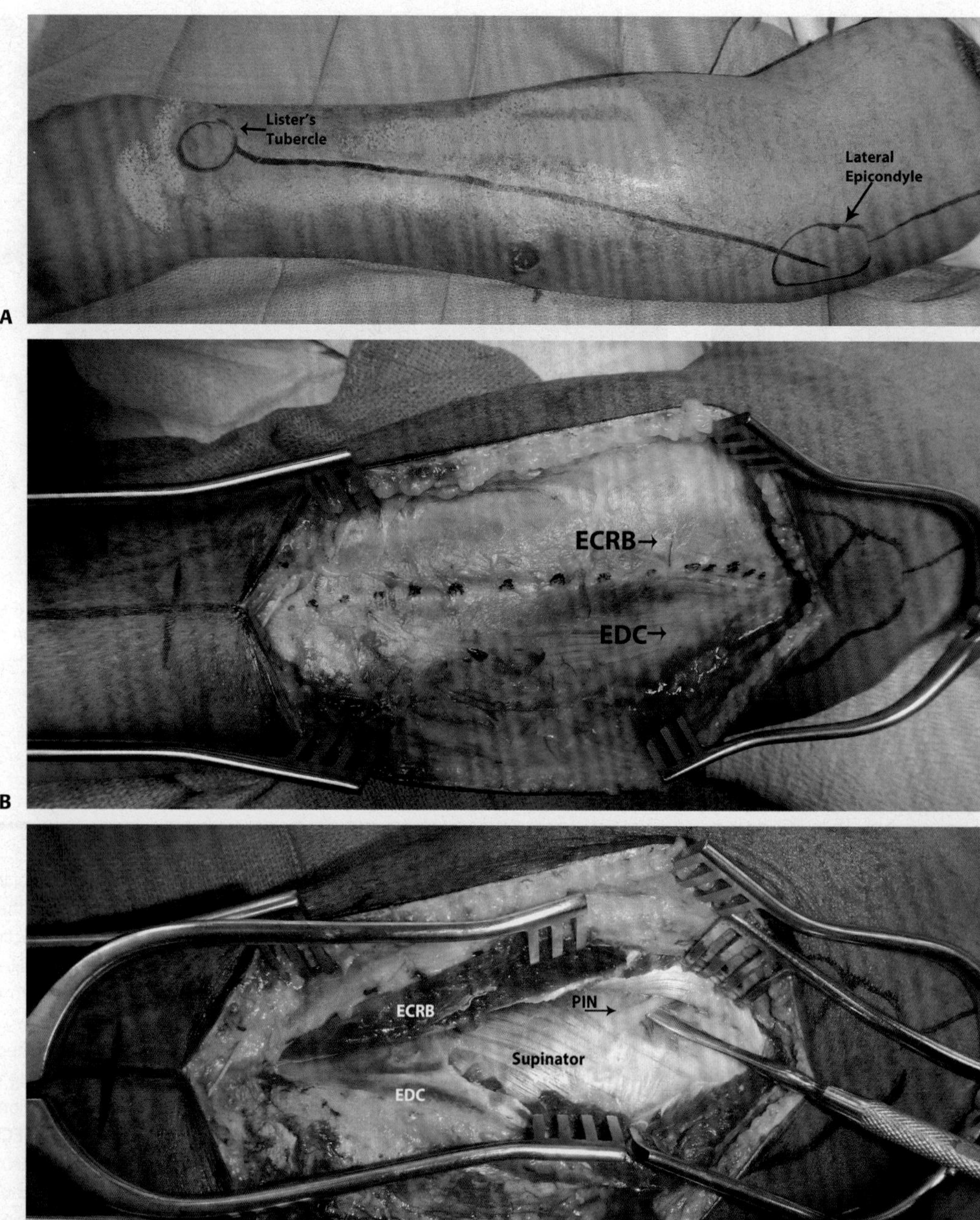

TECH FIG 2 • Posterior approach to the radius. **A.** Extensile exposure (lateral humeral epicondyle to Lister tubercle). **B.** Proximal interval is located between extensor digitorum communis (*EDC*) and extensor carpi radialis brevis (*ECRB*). **C.** The deep fascia of ECRB and EDC has been divided, and the oblique fibers of the supinator are now visualized. The posterior interosseous nerve (PIN) can be seen entering supinator perpendicular to its fibers. *(continued)*

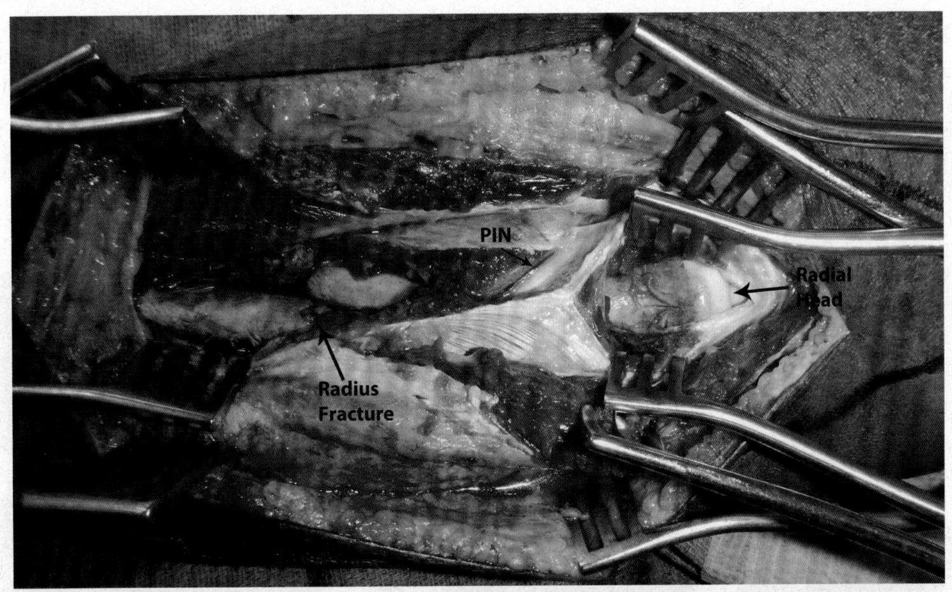

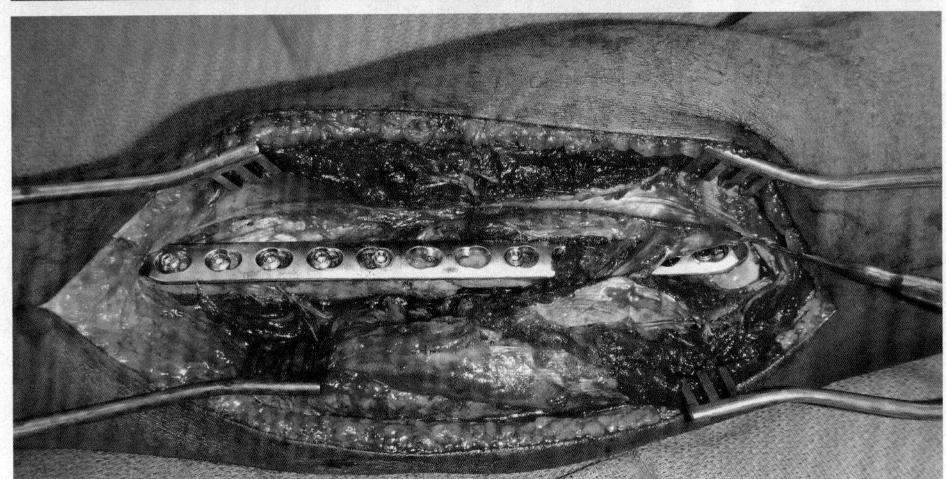

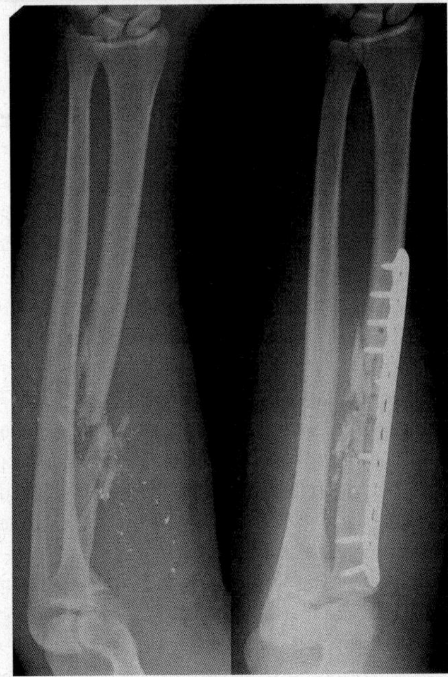

TECH FIG 2 • *(continued)* **D.** The supinator has been partially divided to reveal the PIN coursing through its substance. The radial head is seen proximally and the radius fracture is seen distally. **E.** A 3.5-mm locking compression plate has been applied to the proximal radius. In this case, only two screws of proximal fixation were available, therefore locking screws were used. **F.** Pre and postoperative radiographs demonstrating bridge plating of this comminuted proximal radius fracture. A 3.5-mm locking plate was utilized. Proximally, the plate placement must be scrutinized to avoid impingement during forearm pronosupination. In our experience, this fracture is at significant risk for infection and nonunion. Acute bone grafting was not performed secondary to concern for infection.

Approach to the Ulna

- The incision is drawn from the olecranon to the ulnar styloid centered on the fracture.
- After incision, blunt dissection down to the ulnar shaft is performed (**TECH FIG 3A**).
- In the distal third of the ulna, care must be taken not to injure the dorsal ulnar cutaneous nerve branch, which is typically found in the subcutaneous tissues just distal to the ulnar styloid, passing obliquely in a proximal-volar to distal-dorsal direction, obliquely to the dorsum of the hand. Rarely, it crosses the ulna more proximally.
- Once the ulna has been identified, sharp dissection readily exposes bone needed for fracture reduction and stabilization as previously described (**TECH FIG 3B,C**).

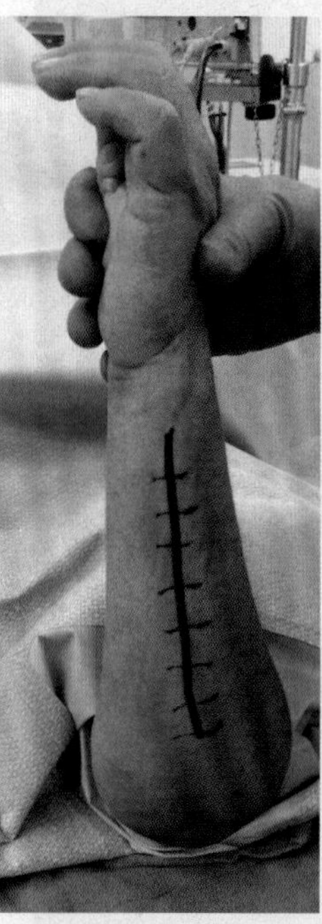

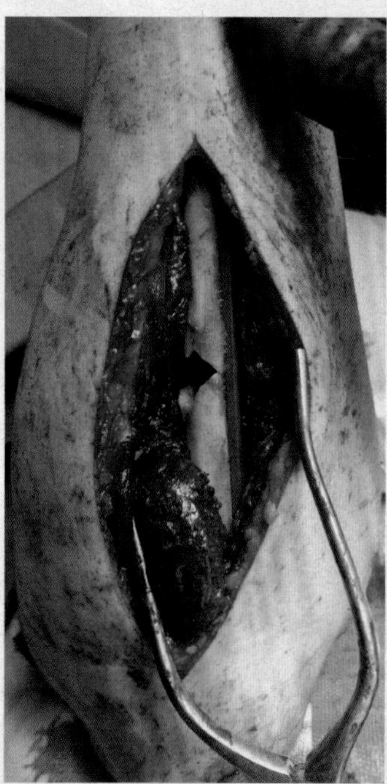

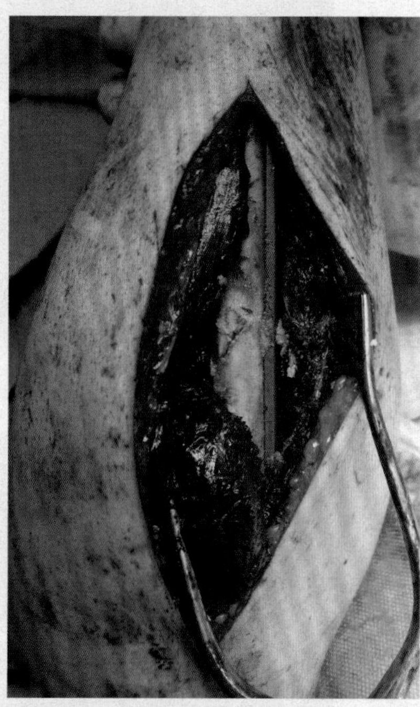

TECH FIG 3 • Approach to the ulna. **A.** Incision drawn along the ulnar subcutaneous border. **B.** Open reduction and internal fixation (ORIF) of the ulna with comminuted butterfly fragment with dorsal plate. **C.** Comminuted butterfly fragment and supplemental allograft bone graft fills the defect. (Autograft bone grafting for this type of defect may be preferred. This can be performed acutely in closed fractures if necessary.)

Fracture Reduction

- To stabilize transverse or short oblique fractures, the plate is applied on the distal fragment first affixing a far hole and then a near hole centered on the bony fragment.
  - Next, the proximal fragment is reduced and held reduced with reduction forceps while standard compression screws are placed.
  - A seven-hole, 3.5-mm compression plate with the open hole over the fracture site is typically used with three bicortical nonlocking screws placed on each side of the fracture.
  - Consider overbending the plate slightly into a concave configuration to compress the side of the fracture opposite the plate.
- For transverse fractures with a butterfly fragment, our preference is to reduce and stabilize the butterfly fragment with a free screw outside the plate. Often, this screw may be a 2.4-mm cortical screw.
  - Typically, a lag technique is not used unless the butterfly piece is large enough to accommodate two screws. The butterfly fragment is held reduced with a pointed reduction clamp and a bicortical screw is placed. A bicortical rather than lag screw is used to allow greater fixation in a small piece of bone that is already compressed using the clamp. If lag screw fixation is attempted and fails, it is usually impossible to affix the butterfly fragment.
  - This turns a three-part fracture into a two-part fracture, which is stabilized as earlier except aggressive compression is avoided so as to not displace the previously fixed butterfly fragment.
  - In our experience, even devascularized butterfly fragments typically unite when well fixed.
- Bridge plating using an anatomic plate is performed for comminuted fractures.
- Again, the plate is centered and fixed to the radius on one side of the comminuted segment. The assistant applies manual traction through the hand, and fluoroscopy is used until the desired length is achieved. The plate is then fixed to the other side of the comminuted segment.
  - If pulling the traction and affixing the plate is too cumbersome, the radius and ulna are pinned together with a 1.6-mm or 2-mm smooth stainless steel pin near the DRUJ to maintain the desired ulnar variance while plate fixation to the distal segment is applied.

- Full-length forearm or wrist films of the uninjured forearm in supination are very helpful in determining the correct bone length (intraoperative fluoroscopic imaging of the uninjured forearm and wrist can be used is preoperative imaging is not available). Ulnar variance is used a comparative marker of length.
- Long anatomic distal radius plates can be helpful for distal radial shaft fractures, particularly when bone quality is poor and more plate length is desired.
  - If 3.5-mm compression plates are used on the volar distal radial shaft, the distal segment of the plate should be contoured to match the slope of the distal radius.
  - Distally, the bone is cancellous in nature and cancellous-type screws may be preferred to gain better screw purchase.
- Despite the possibility of symptomatic hardware, proximal ulnar fractures are plated on the subcutaneous surface.
  - This surface has minimal sagittal bow and better resists angular stresses of elbow flexion and extension.
- Middle- and distal-third ulnar fractures can be plated anteriorly or posteriorly.
- Again, the plate is typically affixed first to the more narrow fragment of the fracture. Next, the fracture is reduced and the other fragment is fixed using compression technique.
- Combination plates (3.5-mm dynamic tubular plate [DCP]–one-third tubular) are helpful in balancing fixation plate strength and prominent hardware concerns in distal-third ulnar fractures. In very distal ulnar fractures, 90-90 fixation with locking hand modular plates, 2.5 mm or larger, may be helpful.
- When longer plate constructs are used on the radius (as in bridge plating or in the presence of a butterfly fragment), care must be taken to restore the radial bow to ensure the recovery of normal forearm rotation.
  - This may require either contouring of the plate chosen or use of an anatomic plate.

PEARLS AND PITFALLS

Compartment syndrome	■ Strictly avoid regional anesthetic when bony stabilization is done within the first several days from injury or when there is any significant swelling to avoid masking a compartment syndrome. ■ Never close the forearm fascia. Discuss preoperatively that the skin may need to be left open with planned delayed closure 2–3 days later. ■ If presenting with compartment syndrome, proceed with STAT decompressive fasciotomy, plating, primary closure of the ulnar wound, and delayed closure of the volar forearm wound.
Light exsanguination	■ Light exsanguination allows easy identification of vessels for mobilization and cauterization minimizing the risk of postoperative bleeding (see **TECH FIG 1C,E**).
Transverse fractures	■ This fracture pattern is difficult to hold reduced with clamps: First, fix plate to one side of the fracture using the hole farthest from the fracture and then fix the plate using the hole closest to the fracture. Last, reduce the other fractured segment and continue with compression plating.
Oblique fractures with butterfly fragments	■ Fix butterfly fragment to one side of fracture first to create a two-part fracture from a three-part fracture. If the fracture dictates that interfragmentary screws are best placed on the same surface of the bone as the plate, place them through the plate as to not interfere with plate placement on the bone.
Comminuted fractures	■ Obtain contralateral x-rays to evaluate "normal" bony architecture and ulnar variance. Strongly consider anatomic plates to aid in fracture reduction and restoration of radial bow.
Osteoporotic fractures	■ Consider longer than typical plate selection and liberal use of locking screws after compression is obtained.
Restoring radial bow in posterior approaches	■ If anatomic plating is needed during a posterior approach, a straight compression plate can be manually contoured to the edge of an unused anatomic anterior plate to prior to its placement to obtain the proper bow.

POSTOPERATIVE CARE

- Bulky, soft fan-folded dressings; loosely placed circumferential cast padding; and a sling are placed.
- Active range of motion of the shoulder, elbow, forearm, wrist, and hand is encouraged. Supervised therapy is recommended with a focus on pronosupination, which is the most difficult motion to recover.
- In patients with a lower pain tolerance, a long posterior splint that stabilizes the forearm in neutral but leaves the fingers free is placed. At the first postoperative visit, all immobilization is discontinued.
- Supervised therapy is recommended for patients not demonstrating improvement with self-directed range-of-motion exercises.

OUTCOMES

- Classically, Anderson and colleagues[1] defined an excellent result as fracture union with less than a 10 degree loss of wrist or elbow motion and less than 25% loss of forearm rotation. They reported 54% excellent results in compression plating of 106 both-bone fractures.[1] Using the same criteria, Chapman and colleagues[3] reported 86% excellent results in the treatment of both-bone fractures.

- Recently, Goldfarb and colleagues[4] used the Disability of the Arm, Shoulder, and Hand (DASH) and the musculoskeletal functional attachment (MFA) validated outcome measures to assess functional outcomes of both-bone forearm fractures treated with 3.5-mm compression plates.
  - They reported that pronation was significantly reduced compared to the uninjured limb.
  - Additionally, the outcome questionnaires found a subjective decrease in function when the range of motion of the forearm and wrist were less than the contralateral limb. Overall, outcomes based on DASH and MFA were considered good.[4]

COMPLICATIONS

- Larger series demonstrate an approximate 2% rate of postoperative infection.[3]
- Other postoperative complications include compartment syndrome, nerve injury, radioulnar synostosis, failure of fixation, and symptomatic hardware. Use of 4.5-mm compression plates has been associated with a higher incidence of refracture following plate removal presumable from the larger holes.[3]
- Nonunion is rare in simple pattern radius and ulnar shaft fracture. Those with segmental defects may go onto nonunion and need to be followed closely postoperatively. Smoking cessation and metabolic optimization may minimize nonunion development.
- Rotational malunion of radius fractures will significantly limit pronosupination, which is very difficult to correct.
- Superficial radial nerve parasthesias and dysthesias are not infrequent following radial shaft fracture fixation. These typically resolve and likely related to overretraction during anterior exposure.
- Iatrogenic AIN injury can occur with the use of monopolar cautery along the ulnar border of the radius (bipolar cautery should be used).
  - Additionally, the nerve can be injured by the placement of reduction clamps around the radius if care is not taken to stay close to bone with the clamp.
- Proximally placed volar radius plates can impinge between the radius, ulna, and biceps tendon. This may be discovered during intraoperative pronosupination testing.
  - Unfortunately, due to the limited bone stock, repositioning the plate once placed may not be possible. Planned hardware removal may be considered in these circumstances.
- When distal periarticular plates are used, especially long plates, it is imperative the plate fully contact the bone because it can irritate the flexor tendons if it is off bone.
- With no exceptions, the tourniquet must be taken down and meticulous hemostasis obtained.
  - Compartment syndrome can result from a bleeding subcutaneous vein even when the fascia is left open.

REFERENCES

1. Anderson LD, Sisk TD, Tooms RE, et al. Compression-plate fixation in acute diaphyseal fractures of the radius and ulna. J Bone Joint Surg Am 1975;57(3):287–297.
2. Cai XZ, Yan SG, Giddins G. A systematic review of the non-operative treatment of nightstick fractures of the ulna. J Bone Joint Surg Br 2013;95-B(7):952–959.
3. Chapman MW, Gordon JE, Zissimos AG. Compression-plate fixation of acute fractures of the diaphysis of the radius and ulna. J Bone Joint Surg Am 1989;71(2):159–169.
4. Goldfarb CA, Ricci WM, Tull F, et al. Functional outcome after fracture of both bones of the forearm. J Bone Joint Surg Br 2005;87(3):374–379.
5. Henry AK. Extensile Exposure, ed 2. Baltimore: Williams & Wilkins, 1970.
6. Moed BR, Kellam JF, Foster RJ, et al. Immediate internal fixation of open fractures of the diaphysis of the forearm. J Bone Joint Surg Am 1986;68(7):1008–1017.
7. Ring D, Rhim R, Carpenter C, et al. Comminuted diaphyseal fractures of the radius and ulna: does bone grafting affect nonunion rate? J Trauma 2005;59:438–441.
8. Rouleau DM, Faber KJ, Athwal GS. The proximal ulna dorsal angulation: a radiographic study. J Shoulder Elbow Surg 2010;19(1):26–30.
9. Rupasinghe SL, Poon PC. Radius morphology and its effects on rotation with contoured and noncontoured plating of the proximal radius. J Shoulder Elbow Surg 2012;21:568–573.
10. Thompson JE. Anatomical methods of approach in operations on the long bones of the extremities. Ann Surg 1918;68:309–329.
11. Trousdale RT, Linscheid RL. Operative treatment of malunited fractures of the forearm. J Bone Joint Surg Am 1995;77(6):894–902.

23

CHAPTER

Corrective Osteotomy for Radius and Ulna Diaphyseal Malunions

Vimala Ramachandran and Thomas F. Varecka

DEFINITION

- Malunion of the radial or ulnar shaft can lead to pain, loss of motion, loss of strength, and instability at the level of the wrist or elbow.
- Malrotation, angulation (with narrowing of the interosseous space between the radius and ulna), shortening, and loss of the radial bow have been shown in various studies to lead to decreased functional outcomes.[4,5,9,10,12]
- Arthritis has been reported at the level of the proximal radioulnar joint (PRUJ) with long-standing malunions, although the distal radioulnar joint (DRUJ) is most commonly affected by forearm malunions.[11]

ANATOMY

- The forearm can be thought of as a ring, connected at the PRUJ, the interosseous membrane, and the DRUJ (**FIG 1**).
- Force transmission occurs through the interosseous membrane from the radius distally to the ulna proximally.
- Radius
  - The radius lies parallel to the ulna in supination. With pronation, it rotates around the ulna while the ulna maintains its position throughout forearm rotation.
  - The radius shaft is triangular in cross-section, with the apex toward the attachment of the interosseous membrane.
  - It contains three surfaces: anterior, lateral, and posterior.
  - The shaft possesses a gentle bow, with the volar surface concave and the dorsal and lateral surfaces convex.[1]
  - Schemitsch and Richards[9] devised a formula that locates the apex and defines the magnitude of the radial bow for each individual (**FIG 2**).
- Ulna[1]
  - The ulna is a long bone that has a triangular cross-section in the proximal two-thirds and a circular cross-section distally.
  - It possesses three surfaces: anterior, posterior, and medial.
  - The proximal half of the shaft is slightly concave volarly. The distal half is relatively straight.
- The PRUJ consists of the radial head, the radial notch, the annular ligament, and the quadrate ligament.
- The DRUJ consists of the sigmoid notch, the ulnar head, the dorsal and volar radioulnar ligaments, the extensor carpi ulnaris (ECU) subsheath, and the triangular fibrocartilage complex (TFCC).

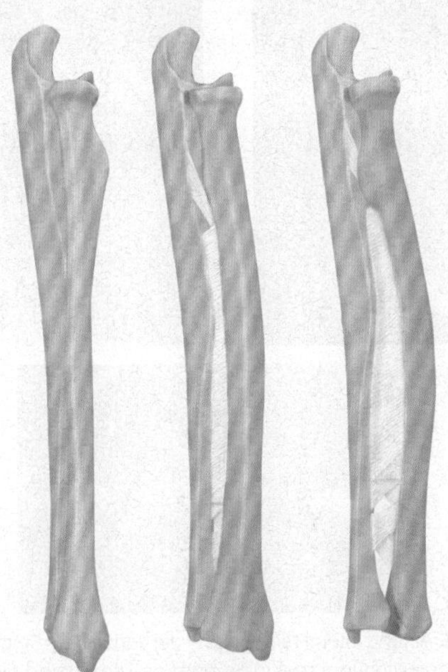

FIG 1 • Lateral projection of the radius and ulna. Relationship of the interosseous membrane to the radius and ulna during forearm rotation. The fibers of the interosseous membrane are longest with the forearm in neutral position and shorten in both pronation and supination.

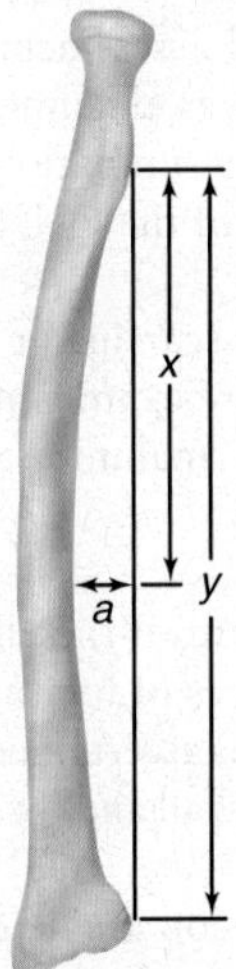

FIG 2 • Measurement of the location and magnitude of the radial bow. The distance y represents the length of the radius as measured from the bicipital tuberosity to the ulnar aspect of the radius. Line a, drawn perpendicular to y from the point of greatest curvature of the radius, represents the magnitude of the radial bow (expressed in millimeters). The distance x represents the length of the radius from the bicipital tuberosity to the point where a intersects y. The location of the radial bow is calculated by $x/y \times 100$. (Adapted from Schemitsch EH, Richards RR. The effect of malunion on functional outcome after plate fixation of fractures of both bones of the forearm in adults. J Bone Joint Surg Am 1992;74(7):1068–1078.)

PATHOGENESIS

- Both-bone forearm fractures occur through a variety of mechanisms, including indirect trauma (such as falls on an outstretched arm or motor vehicle accidents) and direct trauma (such as blows to the forearm).
- Acute fractures treated closed or with intramedullary nailing techniques are more likely to heal malunited.[7,8]
- Radius malunions have a greater effect on forearm rotation than ulna malunions.[10,12]
- A torsional deformity of greater than 30 degrees in the radius leads to significant loss of forearm motion.[4]
- Changes in the length–tension curve of the interosseous membrane may also account for loss of rotation.[12]

NATURAL HISTORY

- Fifty degrees of supination and 50 degrees of pronation are needed for activities of daily living.[6]
- Patients with untreated forearm malunions may experience loss of forearm rotation, PRUJ or DRUJ instability, wrist pain, loss of strength, and arthritis at the PRUJ.[11] The severity of the symptoms depends on the degree of malunion and the corresponding alteration in degree and location of the bow of the radius.
  - Malunions of 10 degrees or less lead to less than a 20-degree loss of forearm rotation and hence are clinically insignificant.[7]
  - Angular malalignment of more than 20 degrees in the radius or ulna results in clinically significant loss of motion. Greater than 15 degrees of malalignment leads to inability to perform activities of daily living.[5,7,10]
- Patients with greater than 15 degrees of malalignment or loss of the radial bow will have clinically significant loss of motion and strength if left untreated.

PATIENT HISTORY AND PHYSICAL FINDINGS

- The preoperative evaluation for patients with forearm malunions includes a detailed assessment of the patient's functional limitations as well as documentation of elbow and wrist range of motion, the supination–pronation arc of the forearm, and the stability of the PRUJ and DRUJ.
- Physical examination
  - The skin is inspected for scarring or previous incision sites.
  - Muscle bulk and tone are examined.
  - The wrist, elbow, and malunion site are palpated for tenderness.
- Range of motion
  - The flexion–extension arc of the elbow is measured with the shoulder at 30 degrees of forward flexion.
  - Rotation of the forearm is ascertained with the humerus stabilized against the chest wall and the elbow at 90 degrees of flexion.
  - Wrist flexion and extension are determined with the forearm in neutral rotation.
  - Joint loss of motion may indicate location of pathology.
  - A high degree of motion loss will lead to functional deficits.
- PRUJ and DRUJ
  - Stability of the PRUJ is assessed by palpation during passive pronation and supination.
  - The DRUJ is evaluated by stressing the ulna volarly and dorsally while stabilizing the radius.
  - Subluxation of the ulnar head or the ECU is evaluated during passive range of motion (ECU subluxation test).
  - The piano key test can also be used to assess for an unstable DRUJ. Patients with a positive piano key sign will have an ulnar head that shifts volarly with a minimal volarly directed force and then rebounds dorsally once that force is removed, much like a key in a piano.
  - Pain with compression of the radius and ulna at the level of the DRUJ may also be indicative of DRUJ instability or arthritis (DRUJ compression test).
- Neurovascular examination
  - The examiner should check for anterior interosseous nerve (OK sign), posterior interosseous nerve (PIN) (thumb extension), and ulnar nerve (abduction–adduction of fingers) function.
  - Inability to perform tasks identifies nerve injury.

IMAGING AND OTHER DIAGNOSTIC STUDIES

- Anteroposterior (AP) and lateral radiographs of both forearms should be obtained (**FIG 3A,B**).
  - Both the bicipital tuberosity and the radial styloid should be visualized for the film to be adequate.

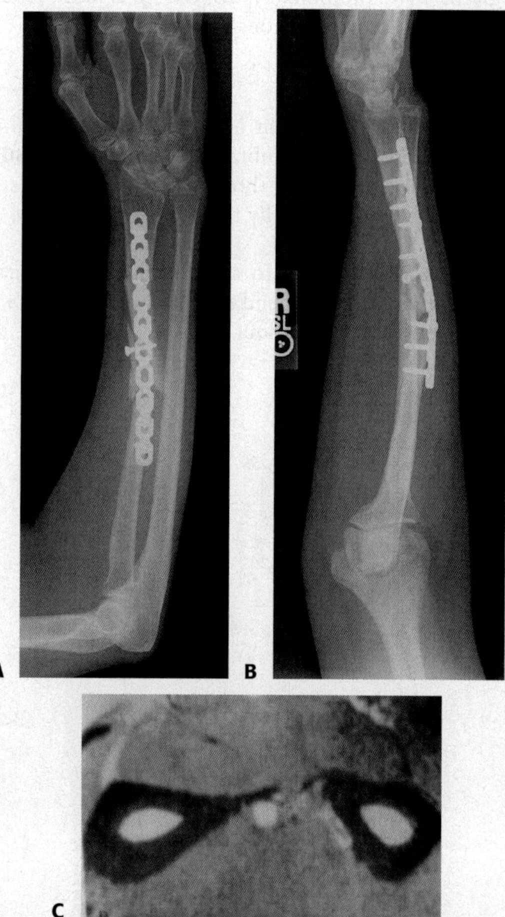

FIG 3 • **A,B.** AP and lateral radiographs demonstrate a segmental radius shaft fracture resulting in a malunion both proximally and distally despite open reduction and internal fixation. Note the loss of radial bow in both direction and magnitude, narrowing of the interosseous space between the radius and ulna, dorsal positioning of the distal ulna, and nonunion of the basilar ulnar styloid fracture. The patient was unable to supinate to neutral and demonstrated instability at the DRUJ. **C.** CT scan demonstrates narrowing of the interosseous space with heterotopic bone formation.

- The degree of angulation and comminution can be calculated from these films.
- Contralateral forearm films provide a comparison for the amount of shortening as well as for the location and angle of the radial bow.[9]
- A computed tomography (CT) (**FIG 3C**) scan or magnetic resonance imaging (MRI) can also be obtained to assess for malrotation.[2]

DIFFERENTIAL DIAGNOSIS

- DRUJ injury or instability
- PRUJ injury or instability
- Injury to the interosseous membrane
- Synostosis
- Nonunion

NONOPERATIVE MANAGEMENT

- Nonoperative treatment of malunions depends on the patient's symptoms and includes occupational therapy for strengthening and range of motion, removable off-the-shelf braces, non-narcotic medications, and custom-molded DRUJ orthoses.

SURGICAL MANAGEMENT

- Operative intervention for forearm malunions depends on the functional limitations of the patient, not the degree of deformity apparent on radiographs.
- Indications for surgery include loss of forearm rotation that leads to a functional deficit (rotational arc less than 100 degrees), DRUJ instability, unacceptable cosmesis, and painful nonunion.
- Risks to the patient include vascular injury, nerve injury or paresthesias (specifically the superficial radial nerve), infection, nonunion, delayed union, need for iliac crest bone graft, synostosis, loss of motion, and DRUJ instability.
- Patients treated within 1 year of the initial injury may be more likely to improve functionally and have a lower surgical complication rate.[11]
- Malunions of the radius and ulna are generally treated with an open approach, corrective osteotomy of one or both bones, compression plating, and bone grafting as necessary.
  - Generally, the more deformed bone is corrected first. If after correction of the first bone forearm rotation is still lacking, an osteotomy is performed on the second bone.
  - If both bones are equally deformed, the ulna is osteotomized and provisionally plated first to provide a working length for the radius.
- Restoration of the radial bow in large part determines functional outcome.
  - Patients whose radial bow is restored within 1.5 mm of magnitude and located within 4.3% of the contralateral forearm regain 80% of normal motion.
  - Eighty percent of grip strength is regained if the radial bow is located within 5% of the contralateral side.[9]
- Anatomic realignment of the radius and ulna will not improve functional deficits if a synostosis or significant scarring and contracture involving the soft tissues has occurred.
  - Occult injury to or contracture of the DRUJ and PRUJ must be identified and treated at the time of surgery.

Preoperative Planning

- Radiographs of the affected and contralateral extremity should be reviewed.
  - A CT scan is helpful to assess for rotational deformity.
- A corrective three-dimensional osteotomy is planned using standard AO technique (**FIG 4**).
- The need for corticocancellous iliac crest bone graft should be determined by the degree of shortening.
- The surgeon should be familiar with techniques for reconstruction or stabilization of the DRUJ should it remain unstable after correction of the malunion.

Positioning

- The patient is positioned supine on the operating table. A radiolucent hand board is attached to the table, centered on the patient's axilla. The affected extremity is then extended and can be positioned for either a volar or dorsal approach to the radius by rotating through the shoulder.
- The subcutaneous border of the ulna can be visualized by flexing the arm at the elbow or by placing the arm across the chest.
- A nonsterile tourniquet may be used on the arm.

Approach

- Radius shaft malunions may be approached either volarly or dorsally.
- The volar (Henry) approach is best suited for midshaft and distal radius shaft malunions.
  - The proximal radius shaft can be approached volarly in this manner; however, injury to the PIN can occur when dissecting the supinator muscle off the radius.

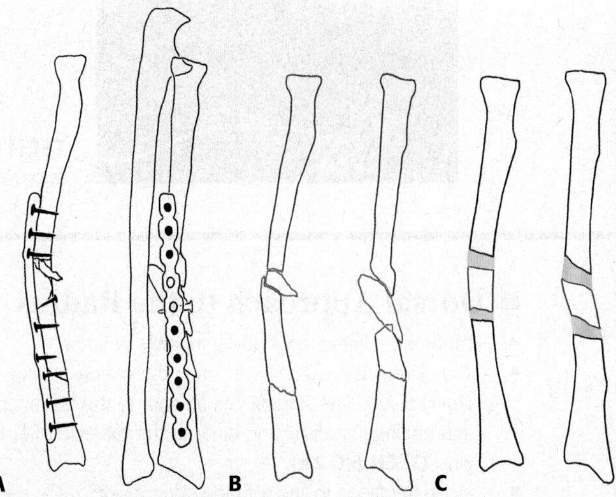

FIG 4 • Preoperative planning using AO technique for correction of the malunion of the case in **FIG 3**. **A.** The malunion is first sketched out from the preoperative radiographs. **B.** Each fragment is then drawn out separately. **C.** The osteotomy sites are noted on both the AP and lateral views. The radius is then realigned through the planned osteotomy sites and bone graft (*yellow*) is inserted to restore the normal magnitude and location of the radial bow.

- The approach is extensile and can be used to expose not only the entire length of the radius but also the wrist joint.[3]
- The dorsal (Thompson) approach to the radius is used most commonly for proximal malunions.
  - It provides access to the PIN, allowing the surgeon to isolate the nerve and retract it out of harm's way for the remainder of the procedure.
  - This approach may be of value for midshaft exposure of the radius, especially in the case of a midshaft segmental malunion (see **FIG 3A,B**).
  - The entire dorsal surface of the radius can be exposed through this approach.[3]
- The ulna is approached along its subcutaneous border.
  - The entire length of the ulna can easily be exposed through this approach.

Volar Approach to the Radius

- Landmarks: biceps tendon, brachioradialis (BR), radial styloid
- Center the skin incision over the malunion site and follow a line that begins lateral to the biceps tendon, continues over the medial edge of the BR, and ends distally at the level of the radial styloid.
  - The length of the incision depends on the amount of exposure needed to take down the malunion and plate the osteotomy.
- To expose the midshaft, dissect between the BR and the pronator teres (PT) proximally (**TECH FIG 1**).
  - The superficial radial nerve lies on the undersurface of the BR and must be protected.
- Ligate the recurrent radial artery to retract the BR laterally.
- Pronate the forearm and release the PT insertion.
- Dissect the PT muscle subperiosteally from a lateral to medial direction to expose the volar surface of the radius.
- To expose the distal radius, the surgical interval lies between the flexor carpi radialis (FCR) and the radial artery.
- Retract the FCR medially and the radial artery laterally to expose the flexor pollicis longus (FPL) and the pronator quadratus (PQ).
- Retract the FPL medially.
- Release the PQ from its radial insertion and dissect the muscle belly from the volar distal radius.

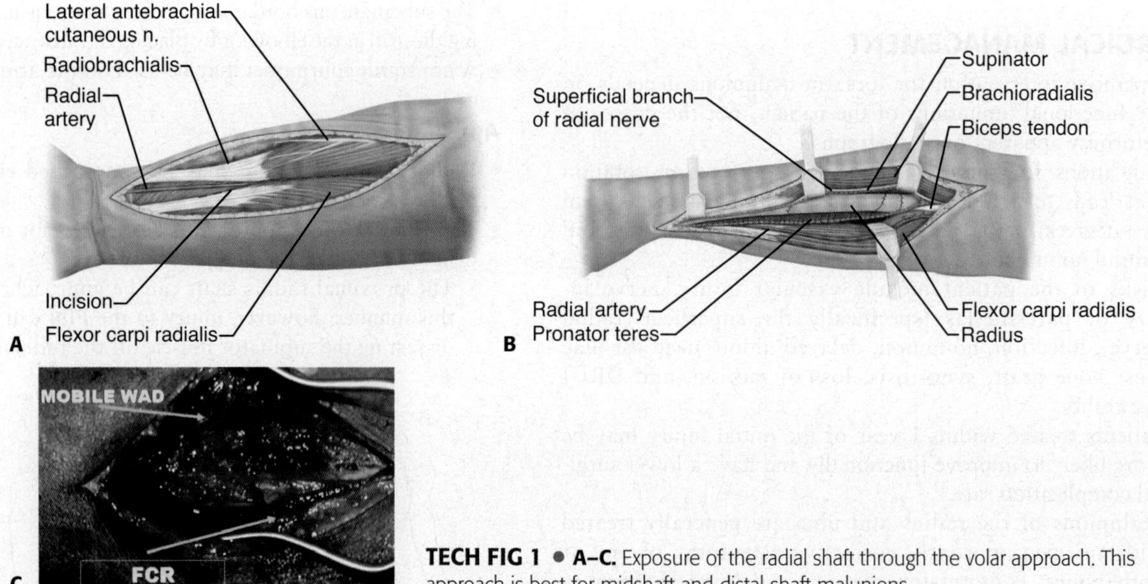

TECH FIG 1 • A–C. Exposure of the radial shaft through the volar approach. This approach is best for midshaft and distal shaft malunions.

Dorsal Approach to the Radius

- Landmarks: lateral epicondyle, tubercle of Lister
- The skin incision is centered over the malunion and follows a gently curved line starting just anterior to the lateral epicondyle and ending just distal and ulnar to the tubercle of Lister at the wrist (**TECH FIG 2A**).
- Incise the fascia in line with the skin incision.
- Dissect between the extensor digitorum communis (EDC) and the extensor carpi radialis brevis (ECRB) proximally.
- Pronate the forearm.
- Identify the PIN as it emerges from the supinator 1 cm proximal to the distal edge of the muscle (**TECH FIG 2B**).
  - Follow the nerve in a distal to proximal direction through the supinator, carefully preserving its motor branches.
- Once the nerve is fully mobilized and protected, supinate the arm and release the supinator from the anterior surface of the radius in a medial to lateral direction.
- To expose the midshaft of the radius dorsally, the abductor pollicis longus (APL) and the extensor pollicis brevis (EPB) must be mobilized as they cross radially over the dorsal shaft of the radius.
- Incise the fascia along the inferior and superior borders of the two muscles and lift them off the radius.
  - Retract them distally or proximally as needed for exposure of the malunion.

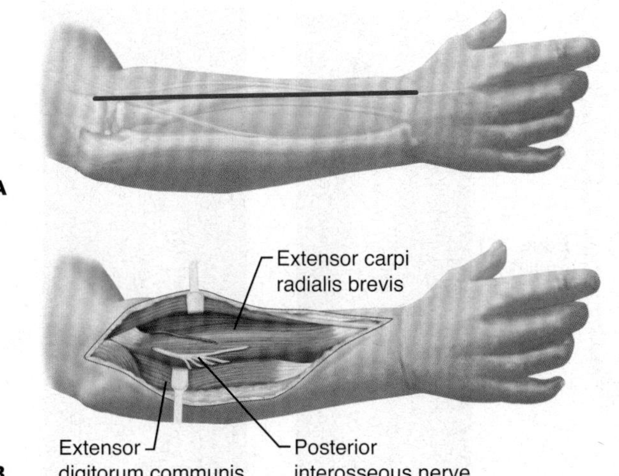

TECH FIG 2 • Exposure of the radius through the dorsal approach. This approach is best for proximal shaft malunions. **A.** Skin incision on dorsal surface, running from tip of lateral epicondyle toward radial styloid. **B.** The PIN is followed through the supinator, with its branches preserved.

Approach to the Ulna

- Landmark: subcutaneous border of the ulna
- Make a longitudinal incision along the subcutaneous border of the ulna (**TECH FIG 3A**).
- Incise the fascia in line with the skin incision.
- Dissect between the ECU dorsally and the flexor carpi ulnaris (FCU) volarly (**TECH FIG 3B**).
    - Take care to avoid disrupting the ECU subsheath distally over the ulnar head.

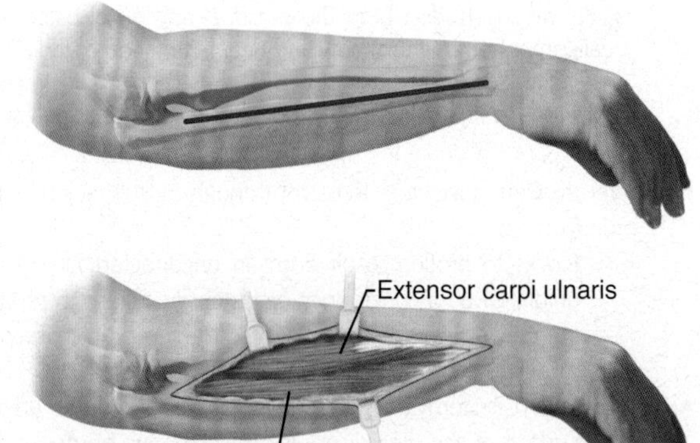

TECH FIG 3 • Exposure of the ulna. **A.** Skin incision along subcutaneous border of ulna. **B.** Dissection is performed between the ECU dorsally and the FCU volarly.

Reduction, Plating, and Bone Grafting

- Based on the preoperative scheme, perform the planned osteotomy at the site of malunion using a combination of a water-cooled saw and osteotomies.
- Bring the radius out to length and insert bone graft as necessary (**TECH FIG 4A**).
- Make a template for plate contouring so as to match the radial bow (**TECH FIG 4B,C**).
- Plate the malunion using a 3.5-mm compression plate and AO compression plating techniques (**TECH FIG 4D–G**).
    - Obtain a minimum of six cortices of fixation proximal and distal to the malunion.
    - In smaller patients, a 2.7-mm DC plate may be used instead.

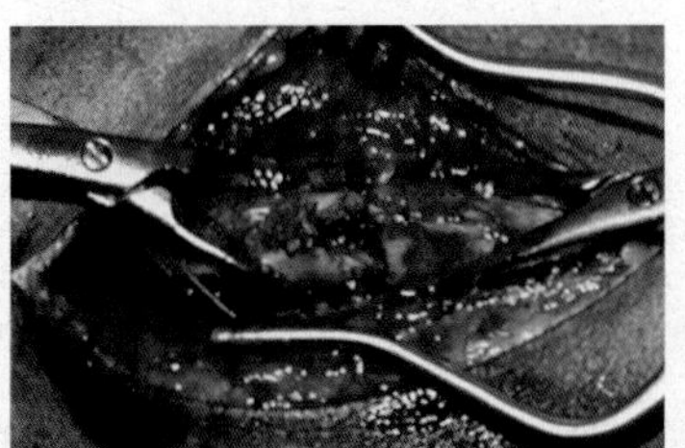

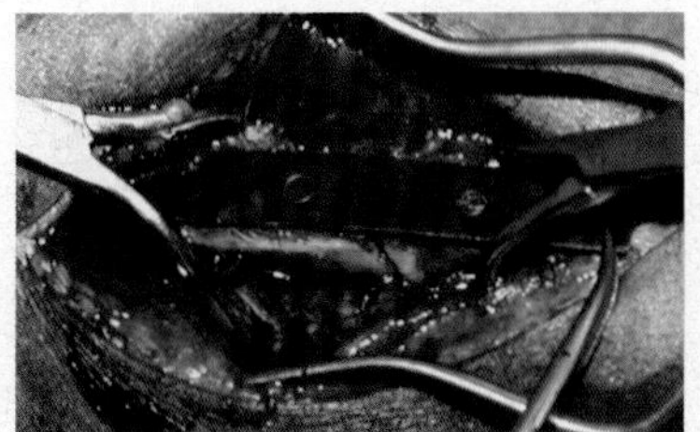

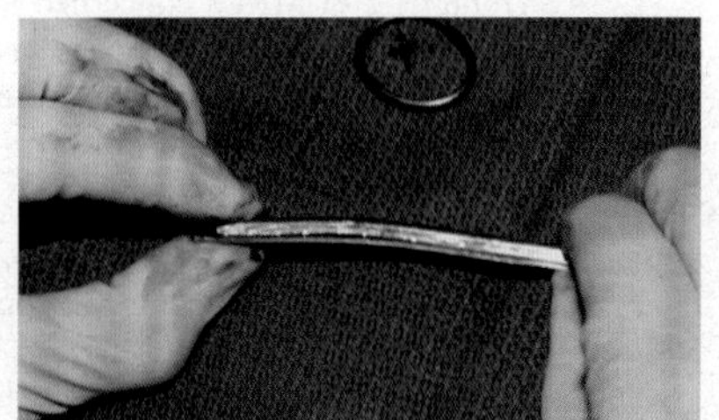

TECH FIG 4 • **A.** Reduction after osteotomy of the midshaft segmental radius malunion through a volar exposure in the patient in **FIGS 3** and **4**. Because of the segmental nature of this malunion, fixation was accomplished by plating both volarly and dorsally. **B.** A metal template is placed on the volar surface of the corrected radius. **C.** The template is used to precisely contour the plate so that when applied, the normal curvature of the radius is restored. *(continued)*

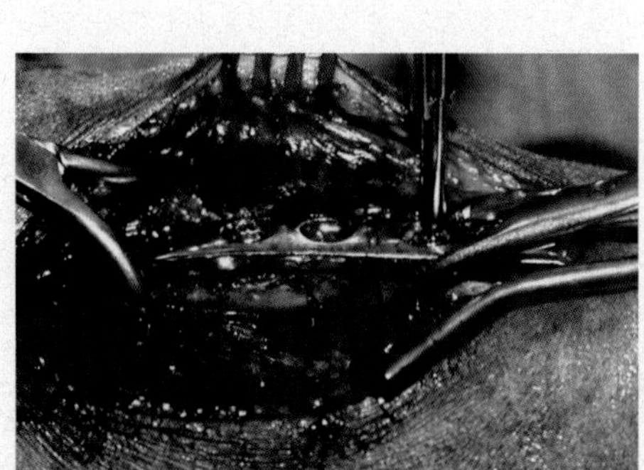

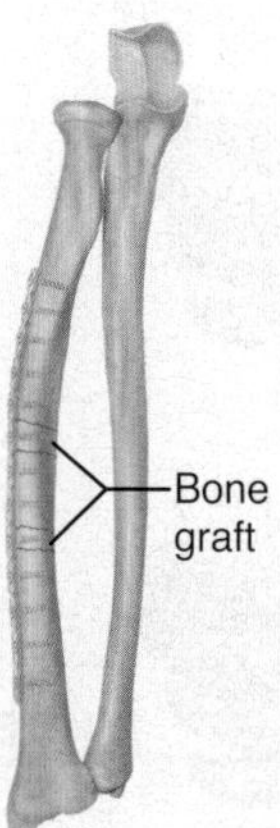

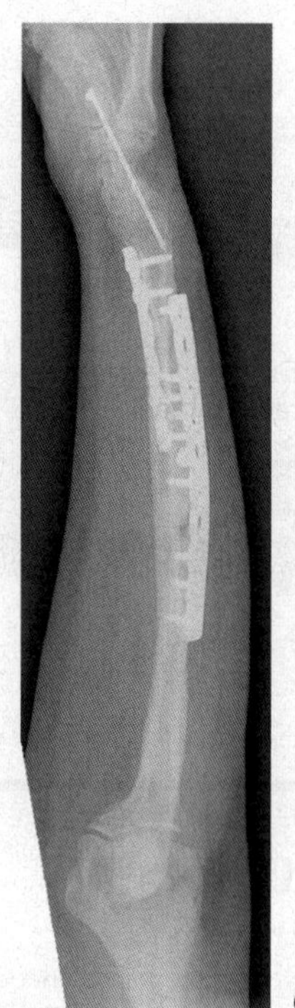

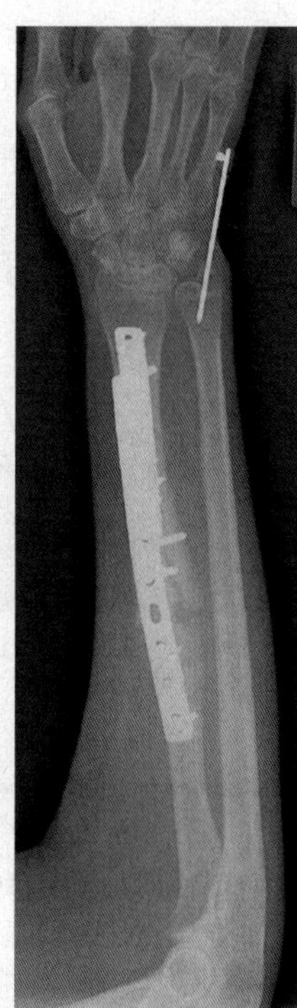

TECH FIG 4 • *(continued)* **D.** Plate fixation. **E.** Schematic depiction of plate and bone graft placement. **F,G.** Postoperative radiographs after dual plating of the segmental radial shaft malunion seen in **FIG 3**. Bone graft was inserted at both the proximal and distal osteotomy sites for realignment of the radial bow and near restoration of radial length. DRUJ instability was treated by fixation of the ulnar styloid fracture (using a 0.0620-inch K-wire) and postoperative immobilization in supination.

- After fixation, take the forearm through a full supination–pronation arc.
  - Blocks to motion result from an uncorrected ulnar malunion, DRUJ incongruency or instability, failure to restore the radial bow, synostosis, and soft tissue or interosseous membrane scarring and contracture.
- If an ulnar osteotomy is required, the plate can be placed on the volar surface of the ulna or on its subcutaneous border in the manner detailed earlier.
- If the DRUJ is unstable, consider palmar capsular reefing, reconstruction with tendon graft, fixation of an ulnar styloid base nonunion, or pinning of the joint in full supination.
- If the joint is incongruent or arthritic, consider ulnar shortening, matched resection arthroplasty, Darrach resection, or the Sauvé-Kapandji procedure.
- Reapproximate tendon insertions. For example, in the case of a volar exposure to the distal radius, repair the PQ to its radial insertion using absorbable suture.
- Close the subcutaneous tissues and skin.
  - To minimize the risk of compartment syndrome, do not close the fascia.
- Apply a volar splint.
  - In patients with concomitant DRUJ instability, a sugar-tong splint with the forearm in full supination is placed.

PEARLS AND PITFALLS

Indications	■ Assess DRUJ stability. ■ Determine that lack of motion is not due to soft tissue contracture, synostosis, or interosseous membrane scarring, for which realignment of the malunion would not improve motion.
Osteotomy	■ Obtain contralateral forearm films to determine location and magnitude of radial bow. ■ Obtain CT or MRI if concerned for rotational malunion. ■ Perform detailed preoperative drawings to determine the ideal location for the osteotomy, the degree and direction of correction required, and the need for bone graft. ■ Obtain consent for bone graft.
Approach	■ If a volar approach to the proximal radius is chosen, avoid injury to the PIN by careful subperiosteal stripping of the supinator from the radius and gentle retraction of the supinator laterally to prevent a traction neurapraxia. Avoid placing a retractor around radial neck, as this can compress the PIN (or cause a traction injury of the nerve). Gently retract the superficial radial nerve and radial artery. ■ Protect the PIN during dissection when approaching the proximal radius dorsally. The nerve lies directly on bone dorsally, opposite of the bicipital tuberosity in 25% of patients. Avoid trapping the nerve between the plate and bone when placing a plate proximally.
DRUJ	■ Determine the cause of instability of the DRUJ once malalignment is restored. ■ Perform a procedure that addresses the precise cause of the DRUJ instability.

POSTOPERATIVE CARE

- In a compliant patient with secure fixation, the splint may be removed 5 to 7 days after surgery and range-of-motion exercises initiated.
  - A removable orthosis is worn for the next 4 to 5 weeks.
- Strengthening exercises are begun 6 weeks after surgery.
  - Resistive strength training is delayed until radiographic evidence of healing is present (usually 8 to 12 weeks postoperatively).
- Normal activities are resumed when a solid union is present.
- Plates are generally not removed in adults.
- If concomitant DRUJ instability is present:
  - A Munster cast is applied at the first postoperative visit. The forearm is held in full supination for 6 weeks.
  - Finger range-of-motion and elbow flexion–extension exercises are begun at the first postoperative visit.
  - At 6 weeks, any pins in the DRUJ are removed and supination–pronation exercises are initiated.

OUTCOMES

- Trousdale and Linscheid[11] retrospectively reviewed 27 patients with corrective osteotomies for forearm malunions. Indications for surgery included loss of rotation (20 patients), unstable DRUJ (6 patients), and cosmesis (1 patient).[11]
  - Of the 6 patients with DRUJ instability, 5 had stable wrist joints at follow-up. Three patients were stabilized with correction of the deformity alone and 3 required reefing of the palmar capsule and temporary pinning of the DRUJ with Kirschner wires (K-wires).
  - The patient who underwent the procedure for cosmesis lost 10 degrees of rotation but was happy with the overall appearance and function.
  - The age of the patient at the time of injury, location of the malunion, and involvement of one or both bones were not associated with the final outcome.
  - Shorter time from injury to corrective surgery (<12 months) was associated with improved forearm rotation and a lower complication rate.

COMPLICATIONS

- A 48% complication rate was noted in Trousdale and Linscheid's[11] study.
- Infection
- Wrist pain
- Loss of motion
- Heterotopic ossification
- DRUJ instability
- Delayed union or nonunion
- Superficial radial nerve paresthesias

REFERENCES

1. Botte M. Skeletal anatomy. In: Doyle J, Botte M, eds. Surgical Anatomy of the Hand and Upper Extremity. Philadelphia: Lippincott Williams & Wilkins, 2003:3–91.
2. Dumont CE, Pfirrmann CW, Ziegler D, et al. Assessment of radial and ulnar torsion profiles with cross-sectional magnetic resonance imaging. J Bone Joint Surg Am 2006;88(7):1582–1588.
3. Hoppenfeld S, deBoer P. The forearm. In: Hoppenfeld S, deBoer P, eds. Surgical Exposures in Orthopaedics, ed 2. Philadelphia: Lippincott Williams & Wilkins, 1994:117–146.
4. Kasten P, Krefft M, Hesselbach J, et al. How does torsional deformity of the radial shaft influence the rotation of the forearm? A biomechanical study. J Orthop Trauma 2003;17:57–60.
5. Matthews LS, Kaufer H, Garver DF, et al. The effect on supination-pronation of angular malalignment of fractures of both bones of the forearm. J Bone Joint Surg Am 1982;64(1):14–17.
6. Morrey BF, Askew LJ, Chao EY. A biomechanical study of normal functional elbow motion. J Bone Joint Surg Am 1981;63(6):872–877.
7. Sarmiento A, Ebramzadeh E, Brys D, et al. Angular deformities and forearm function. J Orthop Res 1992;10:121–133.
8. Schemitsch EH, Jones D, Henley MB, et al. A comparison of malreduction after plate and intramedullary nail fixation of forearm fractures. J Orthop Trauma 1995;9:8–16.
9. Schemitsch EH, Richards RR. The effect of malunion on functional outcome after plate fixation of fractures of both bones of the forearm in adults. J Bone Joint Surg Am 1992;74(7):1068–1078.
10. Tarr RR, Garfinkel AI, Sarmiento A. The effects of angular and rotational deformities of both bones of the forearm. An in vitro study. J Bone Joint Surg Am 1984;66(1):65–70.
11. Trousdale RT, Linscheid RL. Operative treatment of malunited fractures of the forearm. J Bone Joint Surg Am 1995;77(6):894–902.
12. Tynan MC, Fornalski S, McMahon PJ, et al. The effects of ulnar axial malalignment on supination and pronation. J Bone Joint Surg Am 2000;82-A(12):1726–1731.

24 CHAPTER

Operative Treatment of Radius and Ulna Diaphyseal Nonunions

John R. Dawson and Lee M. Reichel

DEFINITION

- A diaphyseal forearm fracture should be treated as a nonunion if there is either no likelihood that the fracture will go on to union (ie, large segmental defect) or if the fracture has ceased to demonstrate any progression of healing.
- Secondary to the advent of compression plating, the incidence of forearm nonunions is low, with rates in the radius of 2% and the ulna of 4%.[7]

ANATOMY

- The ulna functions as a straight, stable axis around which the bowed radius rotates. The bow of the radius is apex radial and apex dorsal.
- The distal radioulnar joint (DRUJ), the interosseous membrane (IOM), and the proximal radioulnar joint (PRUJ) are the ties that bind the two bones together (**FIG 1**).
- There is length variability built into the relationship between the radius and ulna: the radius is at its relative longest in full supination and relative shortest during full pronation.
- Despite this, there is a very close coordination of length between the two bones that is important to normal forearm function. The forearm itself can be thought of as a joint.

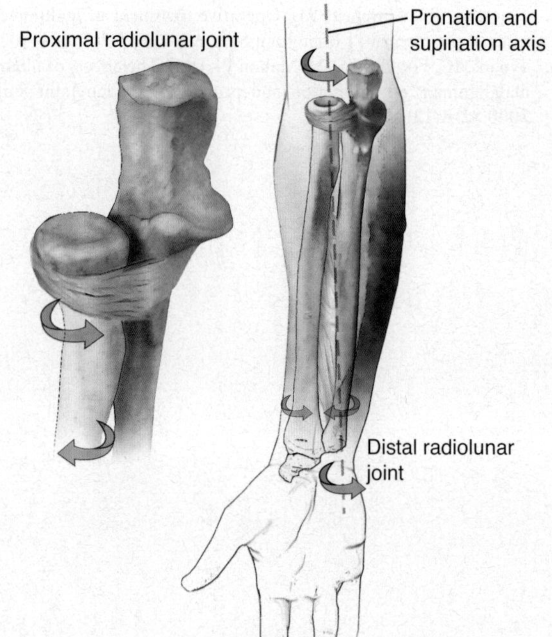

FIG 1 • The two bones of the forearm form a functional unit, with the axis of rotation extending from the radiocapitellar joint to the DRUJ.

- Extrinsic and intrinsic hand extensors and flexors originate in the forearm as well as do the wrist flexors. Additionally, the forearm provides passage to the neural and vascular elements that give the hand its intricate function. Forearm nonunions, depending on their etiology, can result in a considerable amount of scarring that obliterates normal tissue planes and complicates surgical dissection.

PATHOGENESIS

- In the case of a single-bone injury, radius or ulna, if there is any bone deficit at the fracture site, there is an increased risk of nonunion because the length stability of the uninjured bone acts as a distracting force.
- Diaphyseal comminution at the fracture site increases the incidence of nonunion to 12% despite plate fixation.[8] Gunshot blasts are a common mechanism which results in comminution.
- Although isolated radius fractures are treated operatively to ensure reestablishment of the radial bow that is so vital to forearm rotation, isolated ulnar shaft fractures are frequently treated nonoperatively.
  - Even with nonoperative treatment, most ulnar fractures go on to union: Nonunion rates are around 3%.[1]
- Internal fixation must be able to withstand the torsional stresses involved in forearm rotation. Inadequate fixation and poor surgical technique are a frequent cause of hypertrophic nonunion (**FIG 2A**).

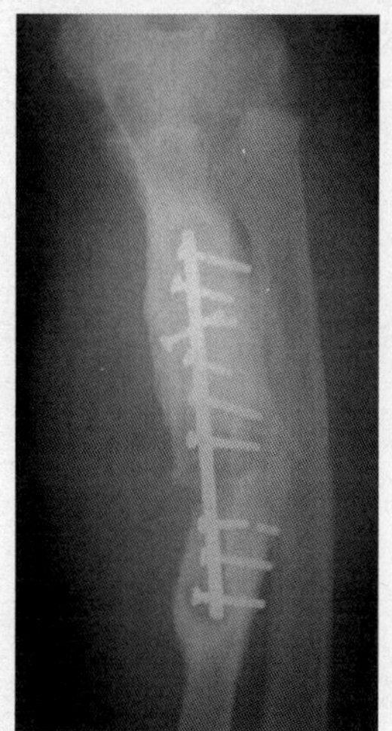

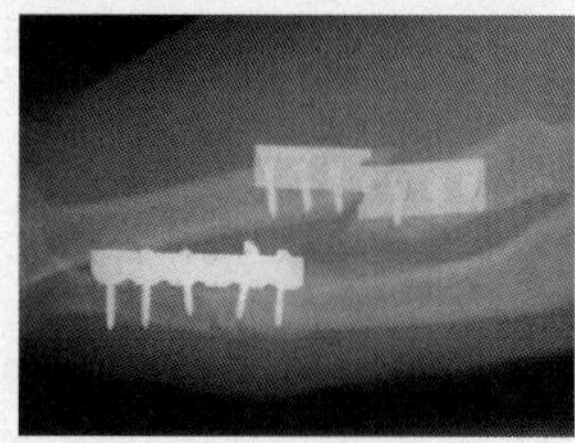

A B

FIG 2 • **A.** Radiograph showing an infected, hypertrophic nonunion. The abundant callus formation indicates a biologically active nonunion. **B.** Radiograph showing an atrophic nonunion. There is complete absence of callus at the fracture site. The problem in an atrophic nonunion is lack of biologic activity. (Courtesy of Thomas R. Hunt III, MD.)

- Many of the injuries that result in nonunion involve a defect; thus, most diaphyseal nonunions of the forearm are atrophic in nature (**FIG 2B**).[7]
- Open both-bone forearm fractures and ballistic injuries are frequently associated with bone loss at the fracture site.
  - Periosteal stripping, loss of the fracture hematoma, soft tissue and bone loss, and increased infection rate all increase the rate of nonunion.
  - Comminuted open fractures with loss of bone have the highest rates of nonunion.[4]

NATURAL HISTORY

- Nonunions of the forearm do not heal without surgical intervention.
- The resultant loss of stability of one or both bones unhinges the entire mechanism of forearm motion with subsequent loss of pronation and supination.
- Because the movement of the PRUJ and DRUJ are intricately related to the normal length and rotational relationships between the radius and ulna, motion at these joints is affected by a forearm nonunion.
- Without treatment, the deformity that results from forearm nonunion can become permanent.

PATIENT HISTORY AND PHYSICAL FINDINGS

- Although some nonunion patients present with clear deformity, there are others whose only complaint is pain. Frequently, there is also a limitation in forearm rotation.
  - Additionally, limitations in wrist and finger motion are frequently present when there is significant change in ulnar variance secondary to bone shortening.
- Pain may be exacerbated by use of the extremity for lifting and pushing and strength is severely impaired.
- Pain may be caused by torsional stressing of the forearm.
- Physical examination
  - Evaluate the skin and soft tissue envelope. Long-standing infected nonunions may develop draining sinuses.
  - Thorough vascular examination to look for any vasculopathy
  - Palpate the nonunion site for pain.
  - Stress the forearm by resisting flexion, extension, pronation, and supination.
  - Look for loss of motion at the elbow or wrist.
  - Look for a loss of pronation or supination.
- Infection is always considered as a cause of nonunion, especially if the initial fracture was open or if the patient has had surgery on the affected arm.
  - If the patient was previously treated at another facility, be sure to clarify if there was any postoperative drainage or if antibiotics were required. Obtain the previous records if possible.
- As is the case for any nonunion patient, look for host factors that affect bone healing such as tobacco use. A detailed metabolic workup should be performed that includes tests for vitamin D, albumin, pre-albumin, calcium, alkaline phosphatase (ALP), hemoglobin A1c (for diabetics), thyroid-stimulating hormone (TSH), and testosterone.

IMAGING AND OTHER DIAGNOSTIC STUDIES

- Anteroposterior (AP) and lateral radiographs in neutral forearm rotation should be obtained of both the affected forearm as well as of the uninjured forearm. This provides a comparison view for a full evaluation of the deformity.
- In the event of a questionable nonunion, computed tomography (CT) can be used to evaluate bone healing at the site in question.
  - CT also helps elucidate rotational deformities, the presence and extent of a synostosis, and the bony relationships of the DRUJ and PRUJ.
- An infection workup should be performed in all patients. This includes an erythrocyte sedimentation rate (ESR), C-reactive protein (CRP), and a complete blood count (CBC).
  - If laboratory tests are normal, but infection is seriously suspected, consider a technetium 99m bone scan followed by an indium 111–labeled leukocyte scan.
  - Magnetic resonance imaging (MRI) or a biopsy of the nonunion site can also be used to evaluate for infection.

DIFFERENTIAL DIAGNOSIS

- Infection
- Forearm malunion
- Undiagnosed PRUJ or DRUJ injury
- Symptomatic implants
- IOM injury

NONOPERATIVE MANAGEMENT

- Nonoperative management of a symptomatic nonunion should be reserved for patients who are poor operative candidates or noncompliant with treatment efforts. As with any nonunion, the treatment course is long and complicated and requires patience on the part of both the patient as well as the surgeon.
  - Patient participation is essential, and smoking cessation is required prior to repair of the nonunion. Smoking cessation should be stopped 4 weeks prior to surgery to negate the anti-inflammatory effects.
  - Typically, two nicotine tests 2 weeks apart prior to surgery confirms smoking cession.
- Rarely, a patient will develop a stable, fibrous union that allows for pain-free function. These patients do not require an operation.

SURGICAL MANAGEMENT

- The primary goal of treatment is to obtain union. Significant improvements in range of motion are not always realized. In some cases where forearm motion is taking place through the nonunion site, obtaining union can even result in loss of motion. The patient should be aware of this preoperatively.
  - Surgery focused on the PRUJ or DRUJ may be required to improve motion.
- Previously operated wound beds have severe scarring, and there is an increased risk of neurovascular injury during surgery.

Preoperative Planning

- Full-length multiplanar radiographs of both forearms should be obtained to assess for any deformity. The normal variance of the uninjured wrist should be noted in full supination.
- Determination of nonunion type should be made—either hypertrophic or atrophic. This will determine what type of treatment is necessary to gain union.

- If the patient is infected, a staged treatment course should be considered as well as intraoperative plans for the evaluation of the infection.
  - Preoperative antibiotics may be held until cultures are taken intraoperatively.
  - Tissue from the nonunion site should be sent for aerobic, anaerobic, fungus, and acid-fast bacillus (AFB) cultures.
  - Consider sending samples for stat sectioning and examination under high-powered field for the presence of white blood cell (WBC).
  - The patient should be warned that if gross purulence is encountered during the operation, surgery may be abandoned or changed to a débridement procedure that possibly uses antibiotic cement beads or a spacer.
- Plates should be templated preoperatively. Dynamic compression plates (DCP), limited contact dynamic compression plates (LC-DCP), combination locking plates, and anatomic plates may all be used.
  - For most fractures, six cortices of fixation on either side of the fracture should be a goal.
  - Frequently, poor bone quality secondary to disuse osteopenia is present. For these patients, longer plates with locking options should be considered.
- If bone graft is planned, the source should be identified preoperatively and the side effect and complication profiles discussed with the patient.
  - If cancellous graft alone is required, the patient may be allowed to participate in the choosing of the graft source (distal radius, anterior iliac crest, posterior iliac crest, and Reamer/Irrigator/Aspirator [RIA, Synthes, West Chester, PA]).
  - If a defect is present or expected, the need for tricortical iliac crest autograft, an allograft fibula, or a vascularized autograft should be mentioned to the patient.
  - The morbidity associated with each graft option should be discussed in detail.
- A complete examination of both forearms should be performed under anesthesia prior to starting the surgical portion of the procedure.
- Ensure that all potentially necessary surgical instruments are available. This could include such specialty items as full-length anatomic plates, curved curettes, osteotomes, and a high-speed burr.
- We do not use allograft bone chips as a cancellous graft expander unless our harvest provided an extraordinarily poor yield.
- When using cancellous grafting or the Masquelet technique, consider using bone morphogenic protein (BMP), as it has been shown to have a higher incidence of healing in those instances.[2]

Positioning

- Supine positioning on the radiolucent table with a radiolucent hand table
- C-arm imaging should be tested prior to starting the case to ensure that full-length images of the forearm can be obtained without difficulty.
  - Consider saving rotational profile images of the contralateral forearm for intraoperative referral.
- If anterior iliac crest grafting is planned, then the ipsilateral iliac crest should be prepped appropriately.
- If a large amount of graft is required, the authors recommend the RIA for harvesting from the contralateral femur, as harvesting posterior iliac crest bone graft (PICBG) requires a significant positioning change.

Approach

- If there has previously been surgery on the forearm, these incisions should be used if possible.
- In general, one should adhere to careful dissection techniques with minimal periosteal stripping and minimal muscle elevation. The available blood supply to the nonunion site should be compromised as little as possible.
  - The medullary canals should be recannulated using a drill until bleeding emanates from the canal (**FIG 3**).
  - To increase blood flow, the cortex of the bone on either side of the nonunion may be feathered with an

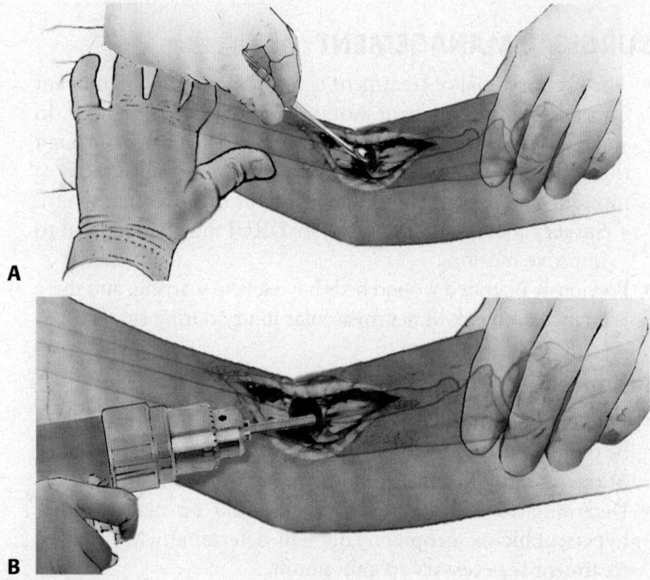

FIG 3 • **A.** Complete débridement of the nonunion site is the essential first step. Any fibrous or necrotic material must be removed and the bone ends delivered. **B.** Medullary canals are opened using increasing diameter drill bits to allow vascular ingrowth.

osteotome or fenestrated with a small-diameter drill or K-wire.

- For access to the mid and distal radius, the volar approach of Henry provides excellent exposure. (Refer to the chapter in this book entitled, "Diaphyseal Forearm Fractures," for a complete description.)
- Proximal radius nonunions may be best accessed using the dorsal approach of Thompson.
- The ulna is accessed along its entire length using the subcutaneous approach. The dorsal ulnar cutaneous branch of the ulnar nerve should be identified distally.

Direct Compression

- In the event of a hypertrophic nonunion, improved stability with compression across the nonunion is the goal of treatment.
- To make room for the footprint of the plate, the hypertrophic bone is elevated with an osteotome with minimal subperiosteal dissection, effectively creating vascularized local graft.
- A small cortical window allows access to both the medullary canal as well as to the nonunion site and both can be drilled or curetted if necessary. Usually, only a small amount of autograft is required, and this can be packed into the nonunion site through the cortical window. The distal radius is an excellent source of autograft for this purpose.
  - If the orientation on the nonunion allows, a lag screw can be placed followed by a neutralization plate.
  - Compression may also be achieved using the plate and placing screws obliquely in the holes away from the nonunion site.
- When a nonunion of the both the radius and ulna exists, both bones can be shortened the same amount to allow for direct compression of the bone ends.
  - If necessary, an uninjured bone can be considered for osteotomy, shortening to match the nonunited bone and compressive fixation. This should be considered with caution and not without a long conversation with the patient preoperatively that includes the risks of a potential second nonunion site and tendon dysfunction.
- In the case of a long-standing distal nonunion with DRUJ dislocation, distal ulnar excision and radius shortening can be performed (**TECH FIG 1A,B**).

A
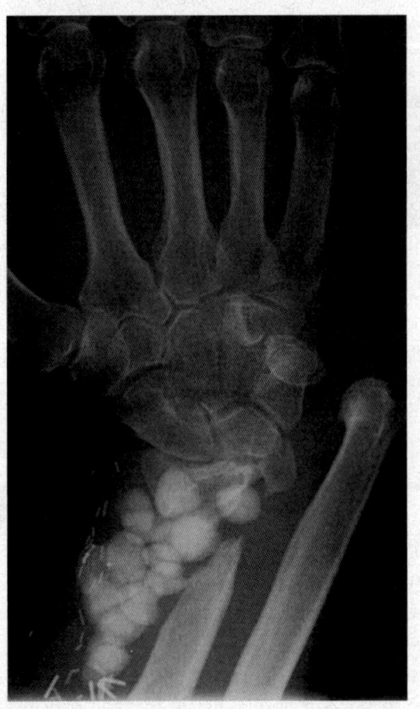

B
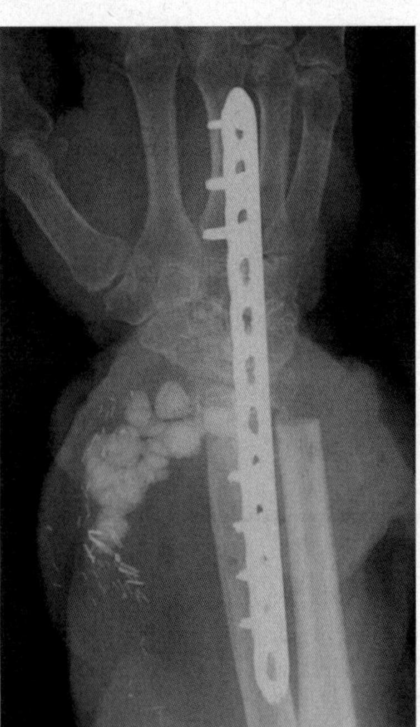

TECH FIG 1 • **A.** An extreme example of a distal-third radius shaft fracture with a significant bone defect and DRUJ injury. **B.** The ulna was shortened, and the radius nonunion was compression-plated in addition to the wrist being fused.

Cancellous Autograft

- For the repair of nonunions that are atrophic or otherwise have a defect
- The nonunion site is excised back to bleeding bone.
- A bridge plate is placed, generally using at least one or two locking screws proximally and distally for fixation.
  - The plate will need to function in place of the bone for an extended period of time, and adding locking screws increases the torsional strength of the construct and thus its longevity.
  - Consider using a stainless steel plate for its greater strength.
  - Care must particularly be taken when plating two parts of a bone separated by a defect. Matching the rotation of each piece as well as establishing overall length can be difficult. The contralateral forearm is an excellent template. A bone model can also be very helpful in understanding the osteology of the bone in question, particularly the radius.

- An external fixator, laminar spreader, or articulated tensioner can be useful in reestablishing length.
- The entire defect is filled with cancellous autograft. Typically, no bone substitutes are used (**TECH FIG 2A,B**).
- Ensure that cancellous graft does not lie on the IOM for risk of synostosis formation.
- This has been successfully used for defects up to 6 cm in length, but it would more generally be used for a smaller defect, less than 3 cm.[7]

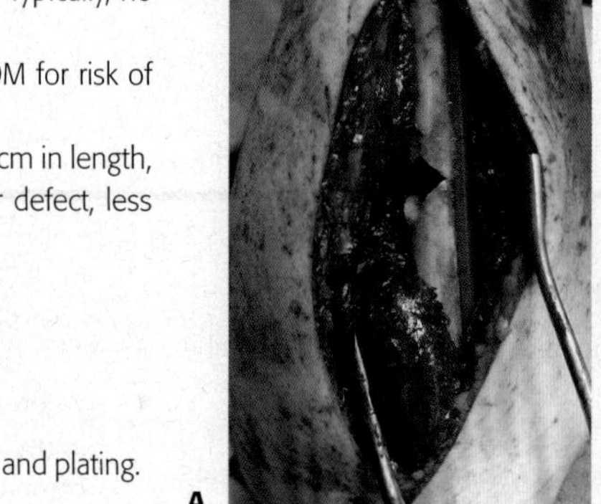
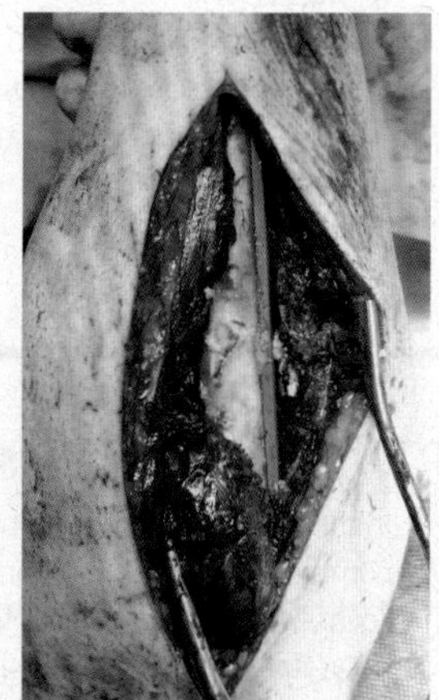

TECH FIG 2 • **A.** A partial defect after débridement and plating. **B.** Cancellous autograft packed into the defect.

Tricortical Iliac Crest Autograft

- For the repair of nonunions that are atrophic or otherwise have a defect
- The nonunion site is excised back to bleeding bone. Osteotomies proximal and distal to the nonunion site are made perpendicular to the long axis of the bone using an irrigation-cooled saw to protect against thermal necrosis of the freshly cut bone.
- The intramedullary canals are cannulated.
- The defect is measured.
- A tricortical iliac crest graft of larger than necessary dimensions is harvested and cut to size to fill the defect.
- A plate is placed on the bone with at least three holes proximal and distal to the defect. The crest graft can be secured to the plate with one or two unicortical locking screws if necessary, although ideally this is avoided.
- Each of the two graft/bone interfaces can then be compressed by technique using the plate or an articulated tensioner. The structural graft is held in place by the compression (**TECH FIG 3**).
- The wound is then irrigated and closed.

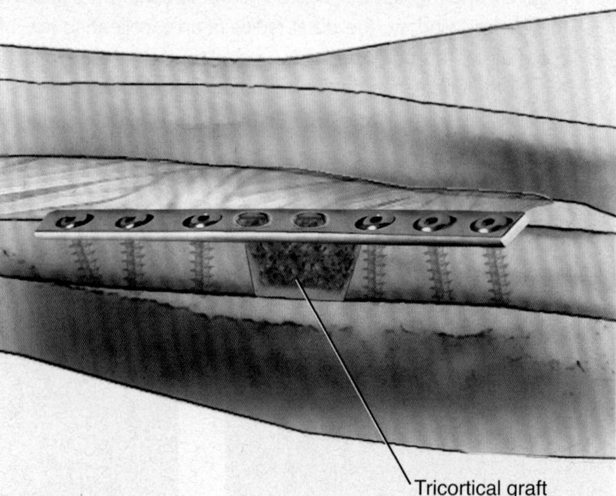

TECH FIG 3 • Modified Nicoll technique with tricortical iliac crest graft. The graft is chamfered, allowing the graft to be compressed as the plate is applied.

Masquelet Technique

- In cases of partial or segmental defect, antibiotic-containing methylmethacrylate cement is used to fill the defect, and a bridge plate can applied to span the zone of injury. Length and rotation must be verified against the opposite side and with assessment of pronation and supination range of motion.
- All of the necrotic bone and fibrous tissue in the nonunion site is débrided.
- Similar to the technique for cancellous grafting, a bridge plate must be carefully applied.
- The cement should be packed in the defect in a manner that will make the extraction process easier.
  - Prescoring the cement makes extracting the cement in pieces easier.
  - The cement should overlap the cut bone ends by a millimeter or two to prevent fibrous tissue forming over the freshly cut bone.
- After a 6-week interval, through the original incision, the pseudomembrane is incised longitudinally, and the cement spacer is removed. Cancellous autograft with or without BMP is used to fill the void. Again, the volume of graft required should be estimated preoperatively and a graft source chosen that best facilitates that volume.

Vascularized Bone Grafting

- A donor graft is chosen based on the grafting requirements.
- The distal ulna can be grafted using a distal radius bone graft based on the fourth extensor compartment artery (ECA). Although this form of grafting may only be used to graft defects less than 2 cm in length, it has a wide arc of mobilization and can be used for much of the distal third of the ulna.[6]
- Nonunions of the radius and/or ulna with bone defects greater than 6 to 8 cm may be grafted using a vascularized fibula with or without an associated skin island for flap monitoring (**TECH FIG 4A–D**). The associated skin island is helpful not only for monitoring but also for tension-free wound closure. The fibula can be compression-grafted in place as previously described for tricortical grafts. For defects in both bones, the graft can be butterflied on a singular vascular pedicle and used for both defects.[1]

A 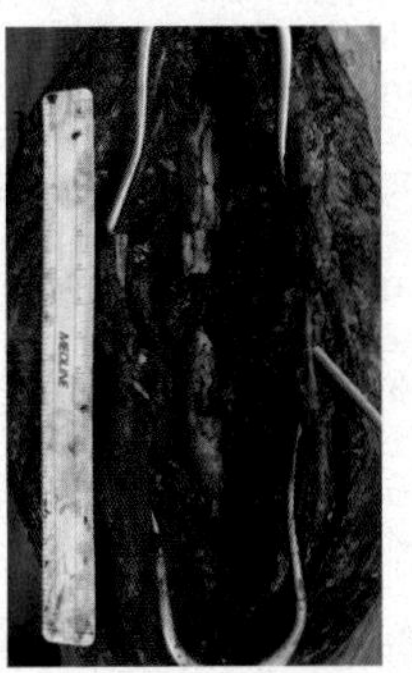
B 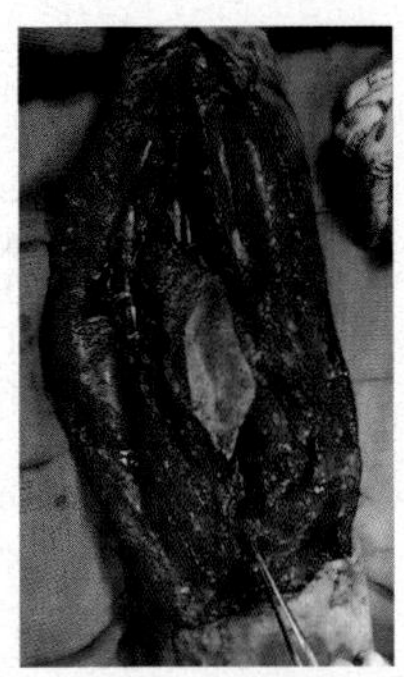
C 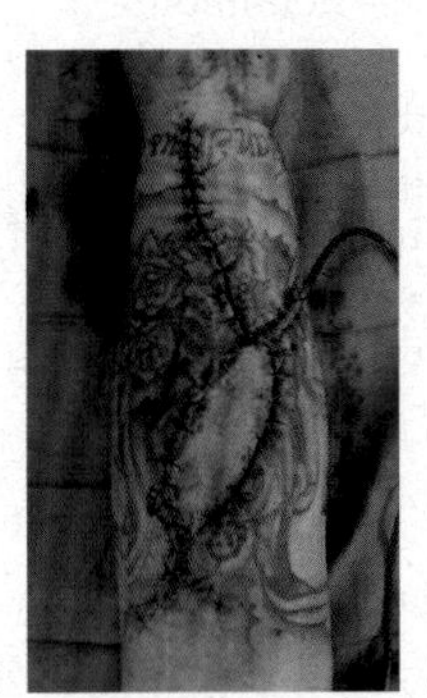
D 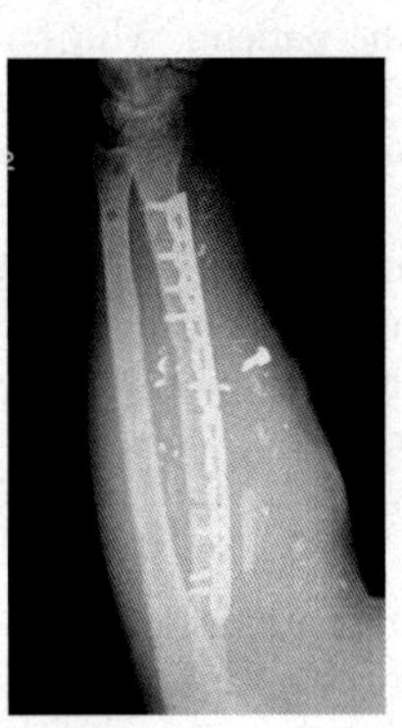

TECH FIG 4 • **A.** A 6-cm defect in the radius. **B.** An appropriately sized free fibula graft was compression-plated in the defect. The associated skin island is seen. **C.** At case end, with the skin island incorporated into the initial incision. **D.** At 6 weeks follow-up. The patient eventually went on to union.

PEARLS AND PITFALLS

Patient preparation	▪ Demand smoking cessation prior to operative intervention. Perform a metabolic workup on all patients.
Patient decision making	▪ Ensure that the patient understands the risk and morbidity associated with nonunion surgery and autologous bone grafting. Explain that functional outcomes are frequently not as good as surgical outcomes.
Abnormal operative anatomy	▪ Start tissue dissection outside the zone of previous surgery to establish and define normal tissue planes. ▪ Take time and care during dissection, as scarring and muscle contractions can significantly alter the relevant neurovascular anatomy.
Establish blood flow at the nonunion site	▪ Cannulate the intramedullary canals with a 3.5- or 4.0-mm drill bit. Feather or fenestrate the surrounding cortical bone.
Reestablish normal anatomy	▪ Take contralateral forearm images in the operating room prior to starting surgery. Have a forearm bone model available if possible. ▪ Consider using anatomic plates.
Regain length	▪ Use a temporary external fixator or the articulating tensioner to lengthen the bone in question.
Disuse osteopenia at nonunion site	▪ Use long, locking plates to distribute the load more evenly.
Defect management	▪ Cut cortical grafts longer than the measured defect. ▪ Use stainless steel plates with locking secures for longer lasting bridge constructs. ▪ Consider spacer placement and using the Masquelet technique.

POSTOPERATIVE CARE

- Postoperative splints are typically used to facilitate wound healing; however, these are removed at the first postoperative visit and active range-of-motion exercises are begun.
  - Lifting is restricted to less than 2 to 5 pounds—patients should be able to do many of their normal activities of daily living, and this is encouraged.
- Advancement of lifting restrictions is usually delayed for 3 to 4 months or until there is radiographic evidence of bony union.
- If there is a delay in motion recovery postoperatively, static-progressive night splinting is instituted to regain motion. Manipulations of the forearm should be avoided.

OUTCOMES

- As in forearm fractures, forearm nonunions have high rates of nonunion after operative treatment. The aforementioned methods cite healing rates between 95% and 100%.[3,5,7]
- In the cases of forearm nonunions that are related to either poor initial operative technique or to bone loss, solving the causal problem during the nonunion surgery usually leads to success in treating the nonunion.
  - In those patients whose nonunion was caused by infection, recurrence of the infection is a poor prognostic indicator. Almost all the patients who fail their nonunion repair have a recurrence of a deep infection.
- Overall, patient satisfaction does not mirror the success of achieving bony union. Roughly only two-thirds of patients report good or excellent results.[3,5,7] This likely represents the high demands that patients require of their upper extremities as well as the limitations of motion that frequently occur in revision forearm surgery.

COMPLICATIONS

- New onset infection or resurgence of the organism(s) of a previously infected nonunion can both occur.
- Frequently, the nonunion has already altered the normal range of motion of the forearm through scar tissue and contracture formation. Repair of the nonunion unfortunately can add to scar tissue and contracture formation and result in even more loss of motion. (Fortunately, pain and subjective feeling of stability of the limb improve.)
- Secondary to extensive scar tissue formation associated with nonunions and the extensile exposure needed for repair, the propensity of neurovascular injury is greater secondary to the loss of "normal" tissue planes.
- Recurrent nonunion and hardware failure
- In the event of extensive dissection in the area of the IOM, synostosis may occur.
- Donor site pain or dysesthesias

REFERENCES

1. Cai XZ, Yan SG, Giddins G. A systematic review of the non-operative treatment of nightstick fractures of the ulna. Bone Joint J 2013; 95(7): 952–959.
2. Calori GM, Colombo M, Mazza E, et al. Monotherapy vs. polytherapy in the treatment of forearm non-unions and bone defects. Injury 2013;44(suppl 1):S63–S69. doi:10.1016/S0020-1383(13)70015-9.
3. Kamrani RS, Mehrpour SR, Sorbi R, et al. Treatment of nonunion of the forearm bones with posterior interosseous bone flap. J Orthop Sci 2013;18(4):563–568. doi:10.1007/s00776-013-0395-0.
4. Moed BR, Kellam JF, Foster RJ, et al. Immediate internal fixation of open fractures of the diaphysis of the forearm. J Bone Joint Surg Am 1986;68(7):1008–1017.
5. Moroni A, Rollo G, Guzzardella M, et al. Surgical treatment of isolated forearm non-union with segmental bone loss. Injury 1997;28(8): 497–504.
6. Pagnotta A, Taglieri E, Molayem I, et al. Posterior interosseous artery distal radius graft for ulnar nonunion treatment. J Hand Surg Am 2012;37(12):2605–2610. doi:10.1016/j.jhsa.2012.09.004.
7. Ring D, Allende C, Jafarnia K, et al. Ununited diaphyseal forearm fractures with segmental defects: plate fixation and autogenous cancellous bone-grafting. J Bone Joint Surg Am 2004;86-A(11): 2440–2445.
8. Ring D, Rhim R, Carpenter C, et al. Comminuted diaphyseal fractures of the radius and ulna: does bone grafting affect union rate? J Trauma 2005;59(2):438–441. doi:10.1097/01.ta.0000174839.23348.43.

Open Reduction and Internal Fixation of Ulnar Styloid, Head, and Metadiaphyseal Fractures

CHAPTER 25

Eon K. Shin and Peter Goljan

DEFINITION

- The distal ulna is the fixed point[7] around which the radius and the hand function (**FIG 1A**).
- Fractures of the distal ulna are often inadequately treated in comparison to its larger counterpart, the radius (**FIG 1B,C**).
- Recent literature has devoted increased attention to the treatment and outcomes of these fractures and associated injuries.[3,10,16,19,20]

ANATOMY

- The ulnar head forms the fixed point on which the hand and radius rest[7] (**FIG 2A**).
- The radius rotates around the ulnar head through the distal radioulnar joint (DRUJ) during forearm pronation and supination.[6,7]
- This joint is connected to the carpus by a complicated ligament apparatus, the triangular fibrocartilage complex (TFCC).
- The stability of the DRUJ is achieved through bony congruity between the sigmoid notch of the radius and the ulnar head supported by the radioulnar ligaments[1,6] (**FIG 2B**).
  - The spheres of the two articular surfaces differ (**FIG 2C**).
  - Sixty percent of the joint surfaces are in contact in neutral forearm position.[1]
  - In full pronation and supination, there is only 10% bony contact.[1]
  - The ligaments run from the fovea of the ulnar head and the base of the ulnar styloid to the dorsal and palmar edges of the sigmoid notch on the distal radius[1,15] (see **FIG 2B**).

PATHOGENESIS

- Isolated ulnar fractures most commonly occur when the forearm is struck by an object, explaining the eponym "nightstick fracture."
- Distal ulnar fractures are most often due to a fall on an outstretched hand.
- It is a common understanding that ulnar-sided injuries are more often caused by falls backward in which the forearm is in supination, loading the ulnar side of the distal forearm and wrist and causing distal ulnar fractures, triquetral chip fractures, TFCC injuries, and so forth.
  - In contrast, radial-sided injuries are more often caused by falls forward, loading the radial side of the forearm and wrist and causing scaphoid fractures, distal radius fractures, and so forth.

NATURAL HISTORY

- Many distal ulnar fractures leave only marginal long-term problems.
- Some distal ulnar malunions cause DRUJ incongruency with subsequent instability or blocked forearm rotation (**FIG 3**).

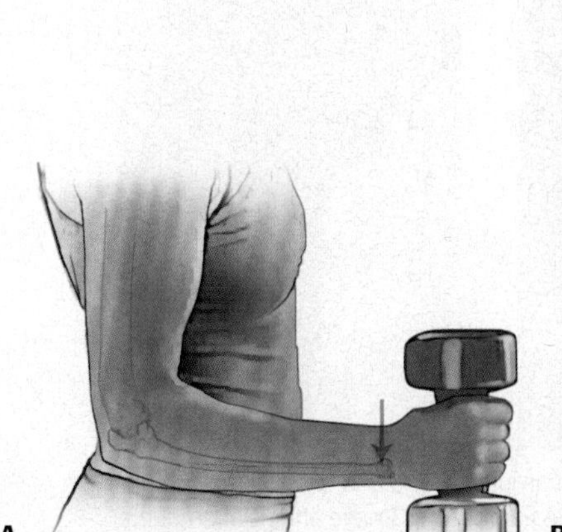
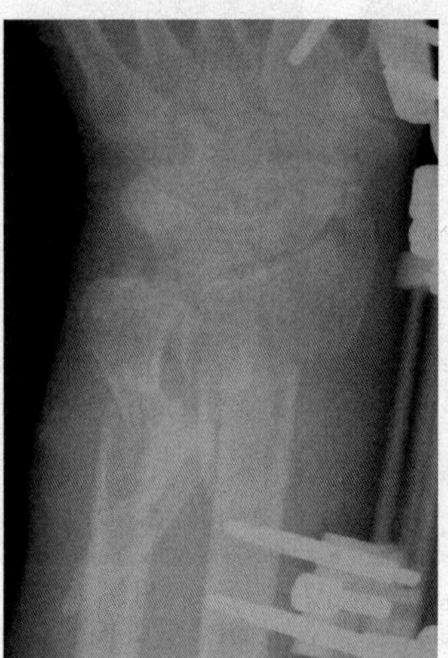
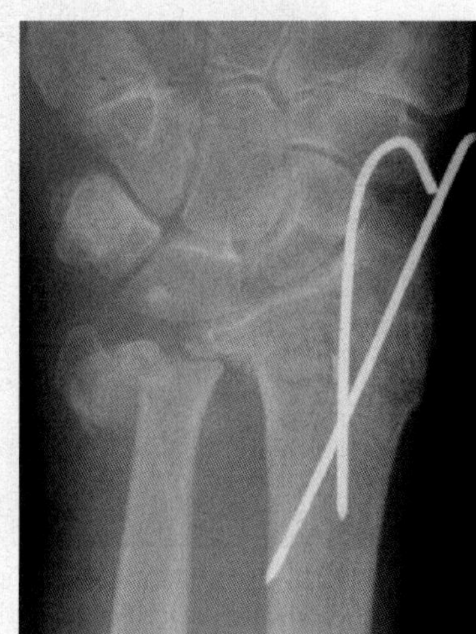

FIG 1 • **A.** The distal ulna is the fixed point on which performance of most daily hand activities depends. **B,C.** Fractures of the distal ulna are often neglected in comparison to those of its larger counterpart, the radius, which always attracts attention and treatment efforts. The outcome after distal forearm fractures could be improved if the fixed point—the distal ulna—is addressed surgically at the same time as the radius is operated on.

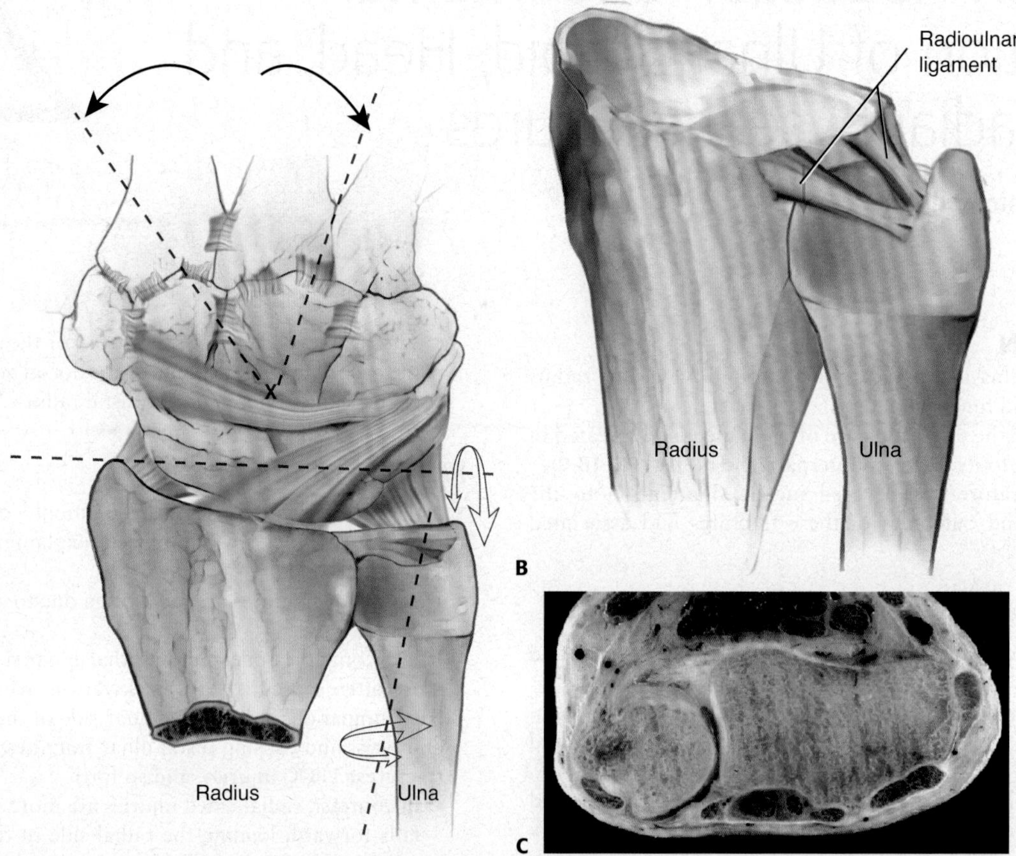

FIG 2 • **A.** The distal ulna is the fixed point around which the radius rotates in pronation and supination. Through the ulnocarpal ligaments, the distal ulna relates to the hand, allowing daily hand activities. **B.** The DRUJ is stabilized through the bony congruity between the ulnar head and the sigmoid notch on the radius as well as the dorsal and volar radioulnar ligaments. The radioulnar ligaments include dorsal and volar components that originate on the margins of the sigmoid notch and insert into the fovea and at the base of the ulnar styloid. These ligaments act as reins in the pronation and supination. **C.** The spheres of the two articular surfaces differ: the ulnar head has a shorter radius of curvature compared with the sigmoid notch.

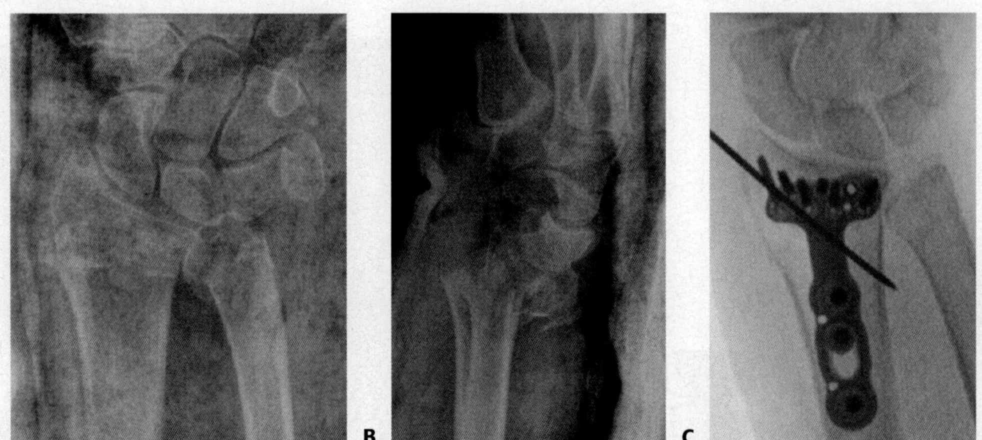

FIG 3 • **A,B.** Radiographs showing a distal radius fracture together with an ulnar head and styloid fracture. The complexity of the ulnar-sided injury was underappreciated. **C.** Intraoperative fluoroscopic image after fixation of the distal radius fracture, revealing displaced and unstable ulnar fractures. *(continued)*

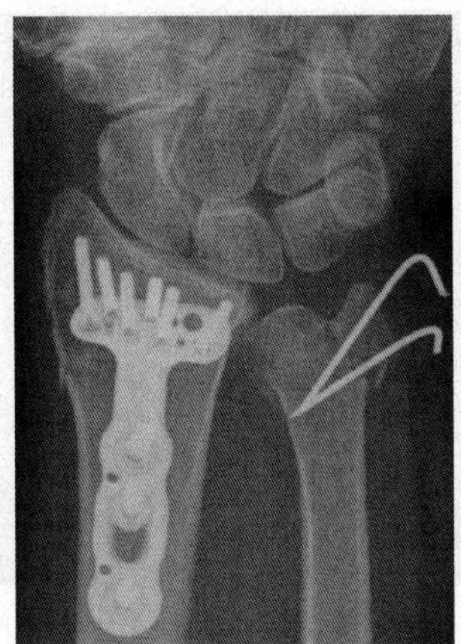
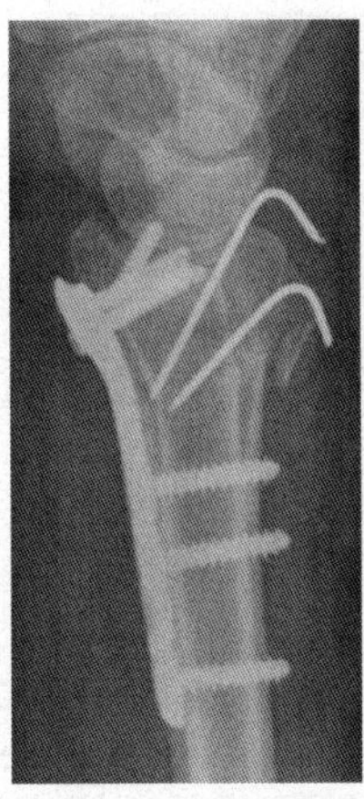
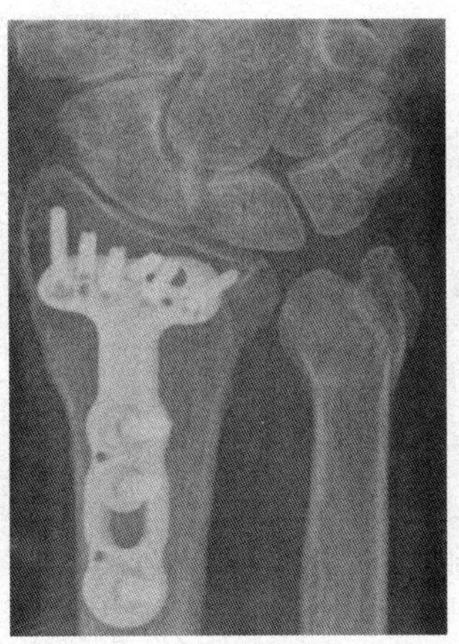
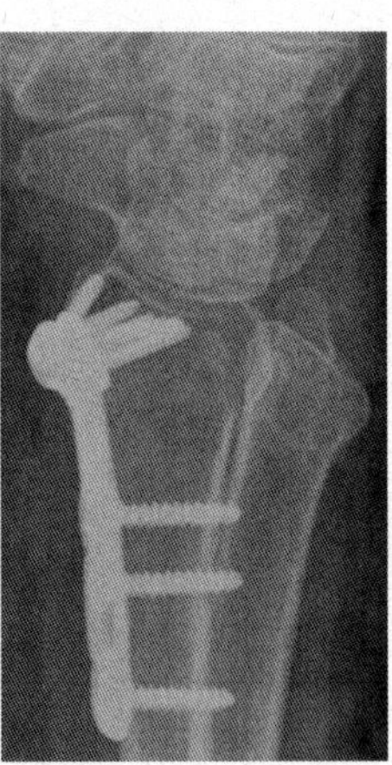

FIG 3 • *(continued)* **D,E.** The distal radius fracture was stabilized using a volar locking plate. The ulnar head and styloid fractures were partially reduced and fixed with two Kirschner wires. The surgeon adequately secured the ulnar styloid fracture but not the ulnar head fracture and postoperatively did not restrict forearm rotation. **F,G.** These radiographs reveal the eventual ulnar head malunion that resulted in DRUJ instability and diminished forearm rotation. The situation was salvaged using an ulnar head replacement prosthesis.

This is why management of these deceptive fractures is important.
- DRUJ stability is an important treatment goal.

IMAGING AND OTHER DIAGNOSTIC STUDIES

- Posteroanterior, lateral, and oblique radiographs typically reveal the pathology.
- Computed tomography (CT) is useful in examining articular fractures of the ulnar head.
- Magnetic resonance imaging (MRI) can be used to evaluate the integrity of the TFCC.
- Arthroscopy should be considered if a radiograph leads the physician to suspect DRUJ dissociation without radiographic explanations, such as a displaced ulnar styloid base fracture.
  - Diagnostic arthroscopy prior to excision of an ulnar styloid nonunion can be useful to evaluate TFCC integrity.[16]

SURGICAL MANAGEMENT

Findings and Indications

Distal Radioulnar Joint Dissociation

- Radiographs occasionally reveal DRUJ dissociation in the absence of an ulnar-sided fracture (**FIG 4**). This results from detachment of the radioulnar ligament[12] (**FIG 5A**).
  - Such radioulnar ligament injuries have been found to cause DRUJ laxity and a worse outcome after distal radius fractures in patients without osteoporosis[11] (**FIG 5B**).
  - Arthroscopically assisted repair or open repair and reattachment of the radioulnar ligament to the fovea of the ulnar head are required to restore stability in the DRUJ (**FIG 5C**) (see Chap. 63).
  - Satisfactory DRUJ stability has been demonstrated to improve outcome scores.[3,10,20]

Ulnar Styloid Fractures

- The importance of ulnar styloid fractures and the need for operative intervention depends on the involvement of the radioulnar ligament insertion site around the fovea of the ulnar head at the base of the styloid (**FIG 6A**).
  - Recent literature has demonstrated satisfactory outcomes of distal radius and ulna fractures in which the ulna was left unaddressed following radius fixation.[3,10,20]
    - An ulnar styloid nonunion was not demonstrated to cause postoperative ulnar-sided wrist pain.[20]
  - Adequate demonstration of DRUJ stability is essential during treatment.
  - If a fracture at the base of the ulnar styloid is displaced more than 2 mm, careful assessment of DRUJ stability is necessary and operative treatment may be required[13] (**FIG 6B,C**).
  - Radial translation of the fractured ulnar styloid is caused by the detachment of the radioulnar ligament. This increases the indication (**FIG 6D**) more than axial, distal fracture displacement (detaching the ulnotriquetral collateral ligament).
  - Ulnar styloid fractures at the tip are likely to be stable and do not require fixation, as the radioulnar ligament remains attached to the ulnar head at the base of the styloid (**FIG 6E,F**).

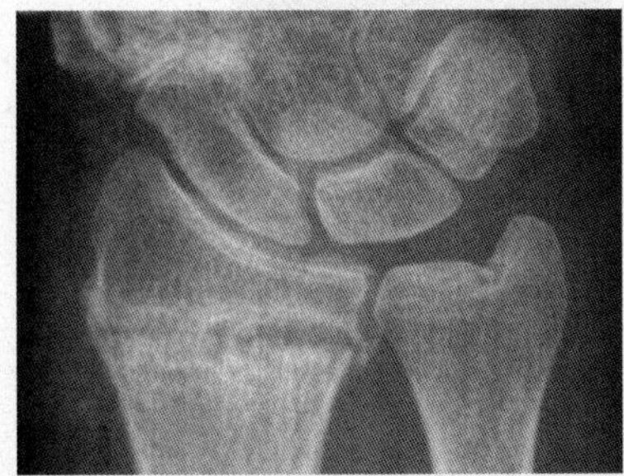
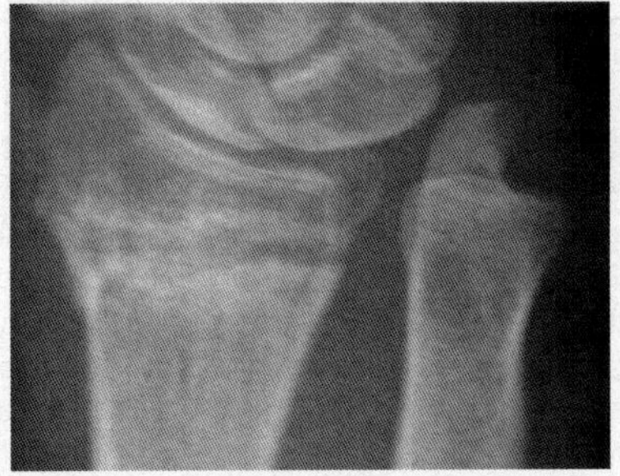

FIG 4 • **A.** An undisplaced distal radius fracture with no obvious distal ulna pathology. **B.** The same fracture with a stress test to the DRUJ, and an obvious DRUJ dissociation is seen as a sign of a complete radioulnar ligament detachment in the absence of an ulnar styloid fracture.

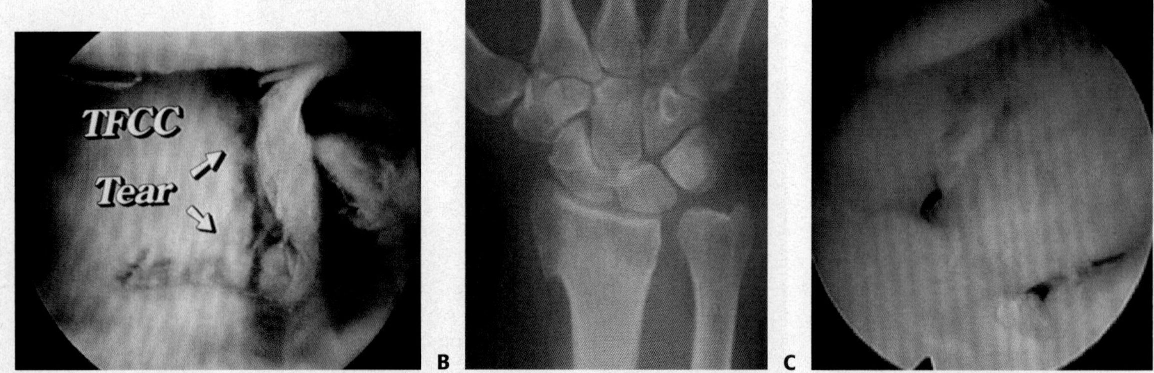

FIG 5 • **A.** Arthroscopic view of an radioulnar (peripheral TFCC) detachment. The lunate is seen at the *top*, the radius *below*, and the detached surface with bleeding at the *right* side. **B.** DRUJ dissociation after a distal radius fracture with a complete detachment of the radioulnar ligament in the absence of any ulnar-sided fracture. **C.** Arthroscopic view of an arthroscopically assisted repair and reattachment of an avulsed radioulnar ligament. The lunotriquetral interval is seen on *top*, the radius joint surface is seen in the *lower left* corner, and the *blue sutures* are bringing down the ligament toward the fovea of the ulnar head, which is not seen arthroscopically.

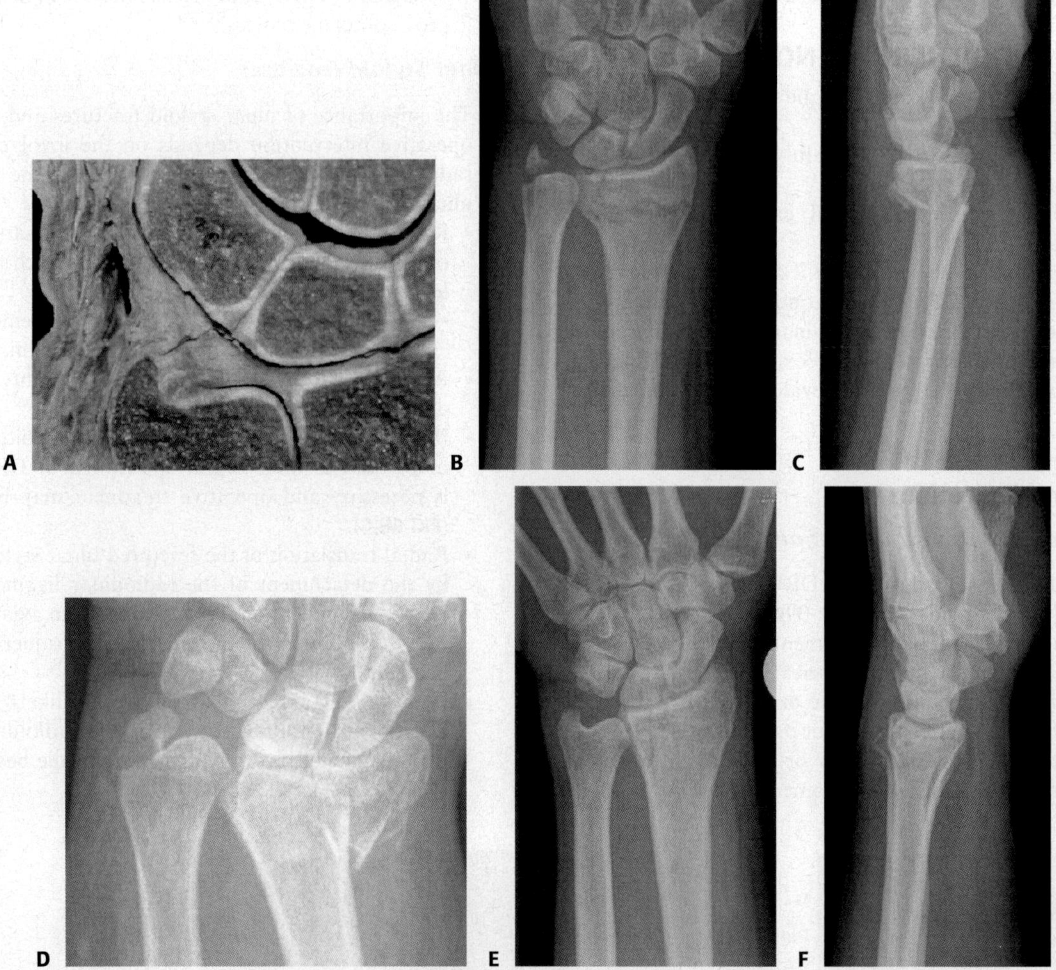

FIG 6 • **A.** The radioulnar ligament has superficial and deeper components, which insert at the fovea of the ulnar head and partly attach to the base of the ulnar styloid. Consequently, a fracture at the base of the ulnar styloid may or may not detach the main DRUJ-stabilizing ligament. **B,C.** Ulnar styloid fractures at the base may detach the radioulnar ligament and in the presence of DRUJ instability may require operative intervention. **D.** Radial displacement (detaching the radioulnar ligament) increases the indication for surgical treatment. **E,F.** Ulnar styloid tip fractures represent avulsion fractures from the ulnotriquetral collateral ligament. Treatment may not be required in an otherwise stable wrist.

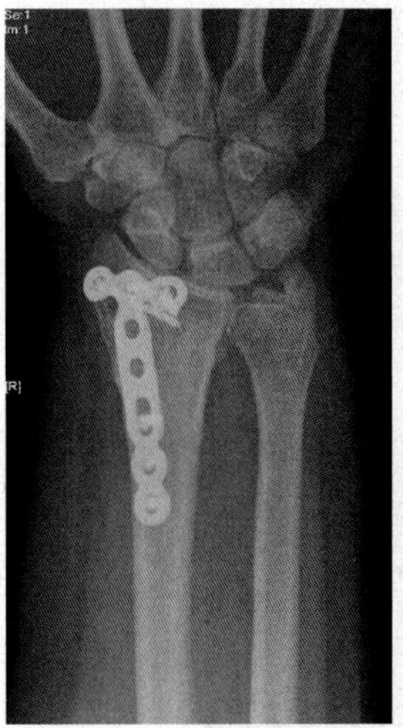
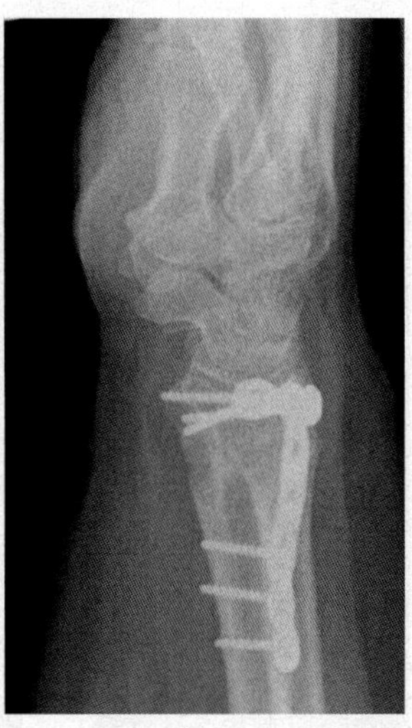
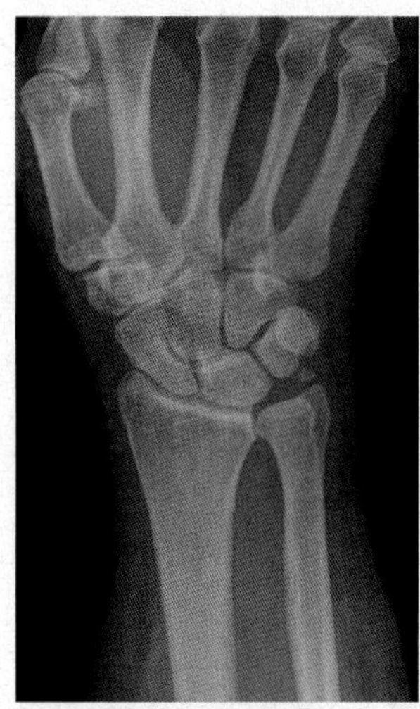
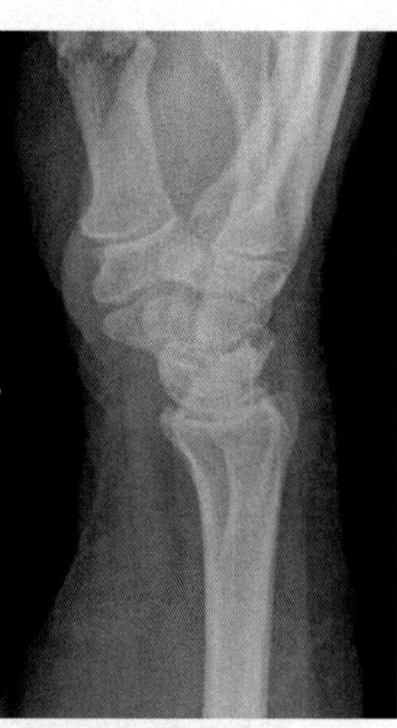

FIG 7 • **A,B.** Abutment of the ulnar styloid into the triquetrum on the ulnar side of the carpus. **C,D.** An ulnar styloid nonunion causing problems as a loose body.

- Ulnar-sided injuries associated with distal radius fractures should be carefully assessed radiographically and clinically after open reduction and internal fixation (ORIF) of the radius fracture.
  - Ulnar fracture reduction and DRUJ joint stability are often improved after treatment of the radius fracture.
  - Stable DRUJ means that the radioulnar ligament is not attached to the fractured ulnar styloid and therefore can be treated nonoperatively.
  - Unstable DRUJ indicates that the radioulnar ligament is detached *with* the styloid fracture. The styloid should be reduced and stabilized or the ligament reattached.

Ulnar Styloid Nonunion

- Recent literature has evaluated the effect of ulnar styloid nonunion on clinical outcomes.
  - No differences have been reported between patients with and without ulnar styloid nonunions.[3,10,20]
  - Symptomatic ulnar styloid nonunions have been associated with TFCC tears.[16] Diagnostic arthroscopy at the time of surgical excision of a nonunion may help to identify and repair possible concomitant TFCC pathology.
- Physical findings of ulnar styloid nonunion may include ulnar-sided wrist pain worse with loading in rotation and tenderness over the ulnar styloid.[3,8] Symptoms from an ulnar styloid nonunion could be related to the following:
  - DRUJ instability from a malfunctioning radioulnar ligament (peripheral TFCC detachment)[8] (see **FIG 5B**)
  - Impingement of the overlying extensor carpi ulnaris (ECU) tendon
  - Abutment on the carpus[8] (**FIG 7A,B**)
  - Soft tissue irritation from the loose body (**FIG 7C,D**)

Ulnar Head Fractures

- Ulnar head fractures are most often associated with distal radius fractures, and the pattern of the distal radius fracture will have a strong influence on the overall functional outcome.
- Ulnar head fractures are seen either alone or with involvement of extra-articular portions of the distal ulna, proximally toward the diaphysis or distally including the styloid (see **FIG 3A,B**).

Distal Ulnar Neck and Shaft Fractures

- A distal ulnar neck or distal shaft fracture is a fracture that occurs within 4 cm of the distal dome of the ulnar head (**FIG 8A–D**).
- Some distal ulnar fractures in association with distal radius fractures realign after manipulation and are considered to be stable once the radius is reduced.[17,18]
- It is difficult to immobilize unstable fractures with a cast alone. Three-point fixation, even in an above-elbow cast, is not effective (**FIG 8E,F**).

Comminuted Intra-articular Distal Ulnar Fractures

- Comminuted distal ulnar fractures that are irreducible and cannot be reconstructed present a challenge to the treating surgeon.[2,5,14,19]
  - Salvage procedures such as the Darrach procedure and Sauvé-Kapandji procedure (**FIG 9A,B**) have been used as primary options with success.[2,19]
  - These surgeries may be effective with appropriate patient selection, such as low-demand or elderly patients.[2]
- In cases of severe ulnar fractures in elderly patients, fixing the radius and leaving the ulna unfixed has even been demonstrated as effective.[14]
- If primary fixation is performed, it is generally recommended that the initial approach be geared toward restoring the anatomy and maintaining the overall alignment of the ulna and DRUJ.

Approach

- The described approach is used for all distal ulnar fractures, including the ones extending into the neck of the ulna and into the distal shaft.
- This approach can, for instance, access an ulnar styloid fracture or nonunion and at the same time visualize, assess, and allow treatment of any associated TFCC pathology.

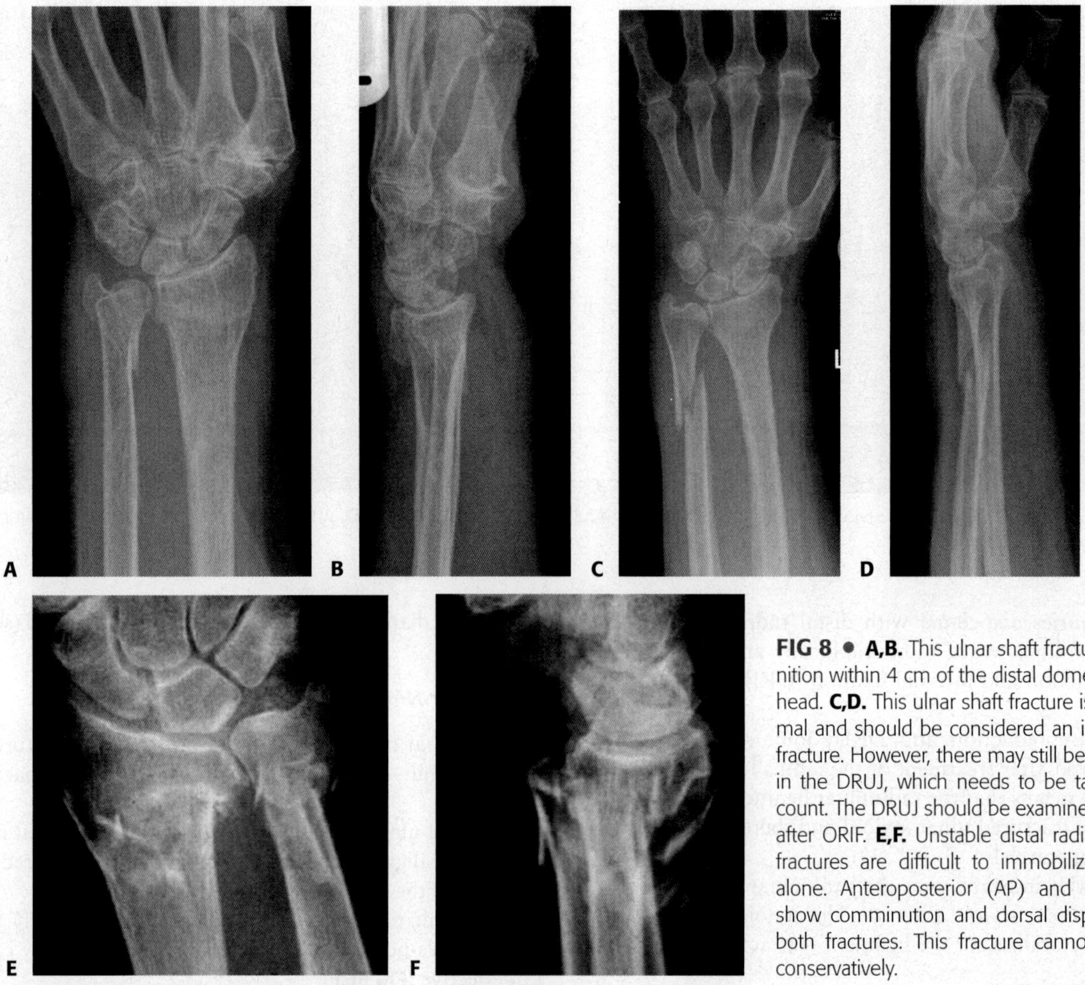

FIG 8 • A,B. This ulnar shaft fracture is by definition within 4 cm of the distal dome of the ulnar head. **C,D.** This ulnar shaft fracture is more proximal and should be considered an isolated ulnar fracture. However, there may still be involvement in the DRUJ, which needs to be taken into account. The DRUJ should be examined for stability after ORIF. **E,F.** Unstable distal radius and ulnar fractures are difficult to immobilize with casts alone. Anteroposterior (AP) and lateral views show comminution and dorsal displacement in both fractures. This fracture cannot be treated conservatively.

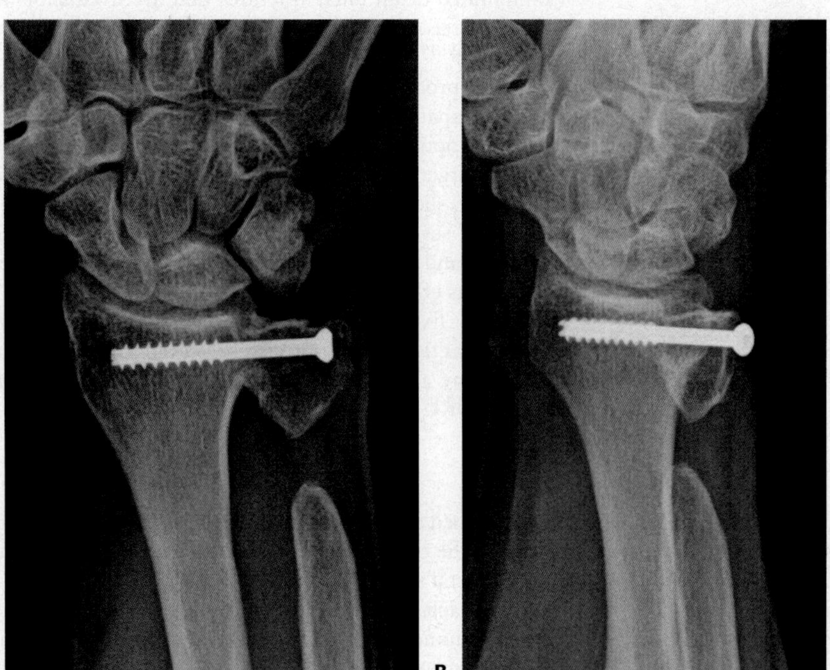

FIG 9 • A,B. AP and lateral radiographs of a Sauvé-Kapandji procedure following traumatic distal ulnar fracture.

Incision and Exposure

- Approach the distal ulna through a dorsal zigzag incision centered over the DRUJ (**TECH FIG 1A,B**).
  - This approach allows reattachment of all crucial stabilizing structures at the time of wound closure.
  - Carefully protect the dorsal sensory branches of the ulnar nerve (**TECH FIG 1C**).
- Incise the retinaculum overlying the fifth extensor compartment (**TECH FIG 1D**).
- Elevate the ulnar retinacular flap in the interval between the extensor retinaculum and the separate dorsal sheet for the ECU tendon.
  - Preserve the integrity of the separate ECU compartment (**TECH FIG 1E**).
- Open the dorsal capsule of the DRUJ using an ulnarly based flap raised from the 4–5 septum (**TECH FIG 1F**).
- Identify the 4,5 intercompartmental artery.
- Begin the capsular incision at the neck of the ulna and extend it to the 4,5 intercompartmental artery, which is diathermied.
- The incision continues along this line to the level of the radiocarpal joint, where it then extends distally and ulnarly along the dorsal radiotriquetral ligament to the triquetrum.
  - By staying in a flat layer along the dorsal cortex of the radius, the dorsal radioulnar ligament attachment is not violated.
- The DRUJ and the spanning TFCC are then readily visualized. The ulnocarpal joint is often hidden behind the synovium over the meniscus homolog (**TECH FIG 1G**).
  - If required, remove the synovium dorsal to the radioulnar ligament to gain access to the ulnar styloid and the ulnocarpal joint.
- In cases of a distal neck fracture without any intra-articular involvement or soft tissue components, the approach stays proximal to the capsular flap. However, the retinacular flap needs to be raised to address the distal metaphyseal fractures.

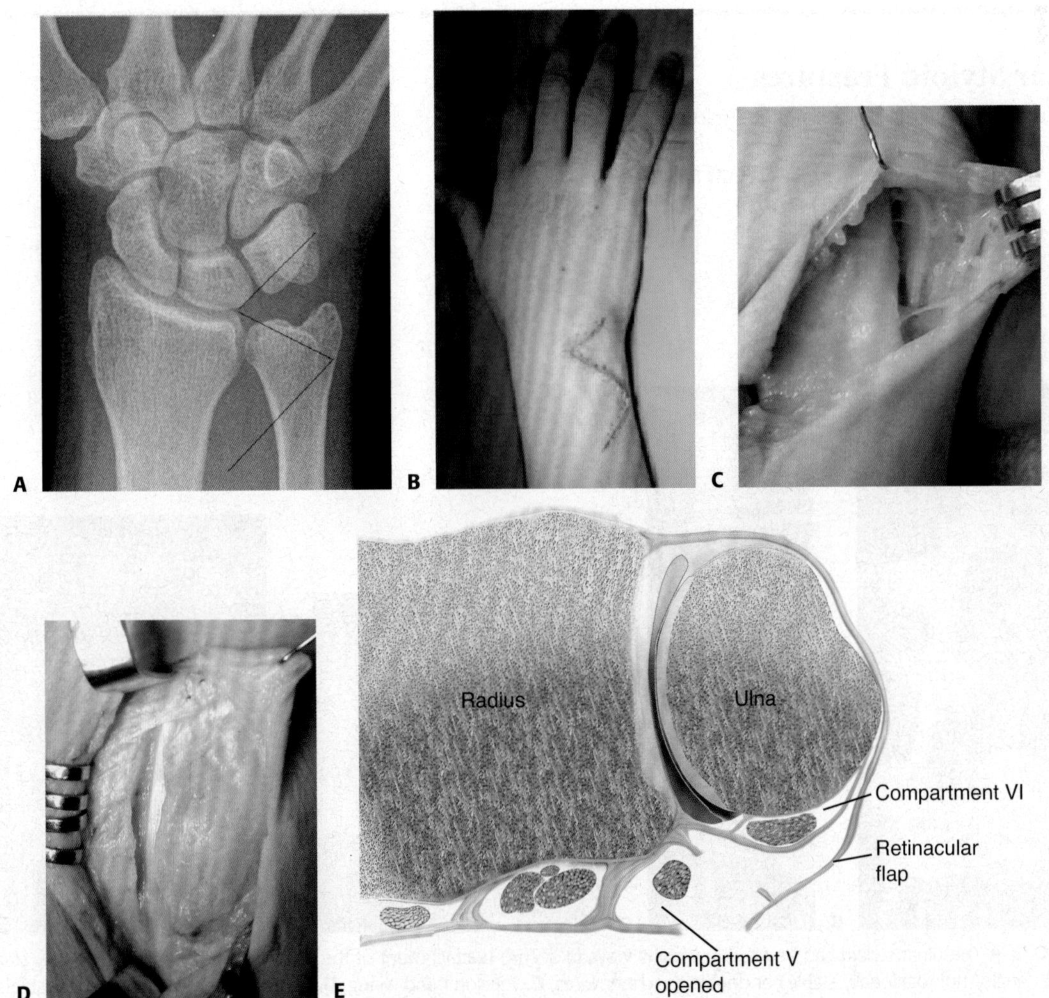

TECH FIG 1 • Surgical approach to all distal ulnar fractures. **A,B.** A dorsal zigzag incision is made with the center directed toward the DRUJ. **C.** Subcutaneous dissection should be performed so that the dorsal cutaneous branch from the ulnar nerve is protected. **D.** The retinaculum is identified and an approach through the fifth extensor compartment is done. **E.** The retinaculum is elevated as an ulnarly based flap between the true retinaculum and the separate dorsal sheet for the ECU tendon (which should be preserved). The ECU is thereby kept in its tendon sheath. *(continued)*

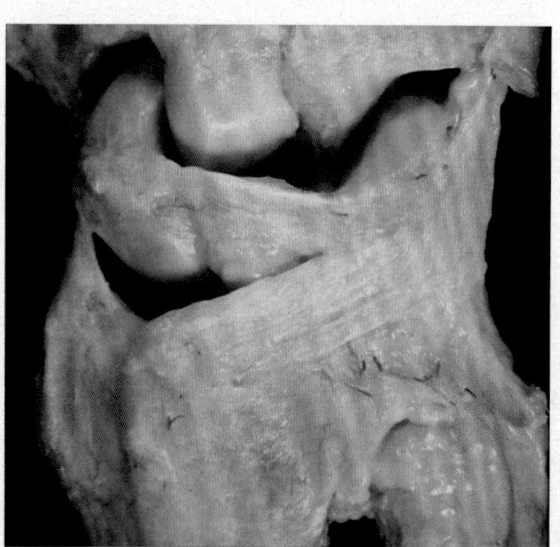

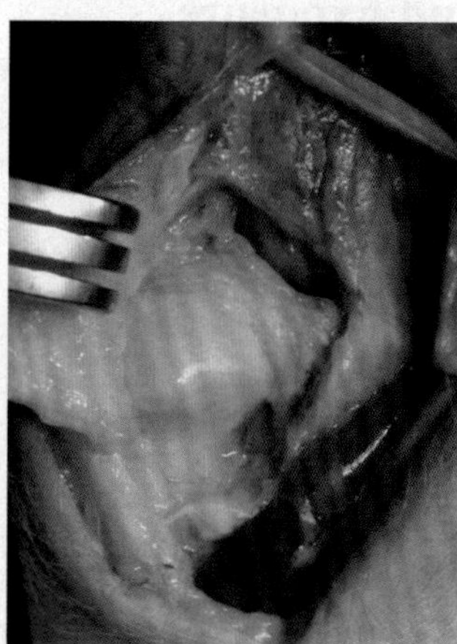

TECH FIG 1 • *(continued)* **F.** An ulnarly based capsular flap is raised from the 4–5 septum to gain access to the distal ulna. **G.** As shown in this dissected specimen, the ulnocarpal joint is often hidden behind the synovium over the meniscus homolog. (**C,D:** Courtesy of M. Garcia-Elias, Spain.)

Ulnar Styloid Fractures

- Options for fixation of ulnar styloid base fractures include the following:
  - Single or double Kirschner wires (**TECH FIG 2A,B**)
  - Tension band wiring (**TECH FIG 2C**)
  - Wire loop or suture
  - Screw fixation (**TECH FIG 2D**)

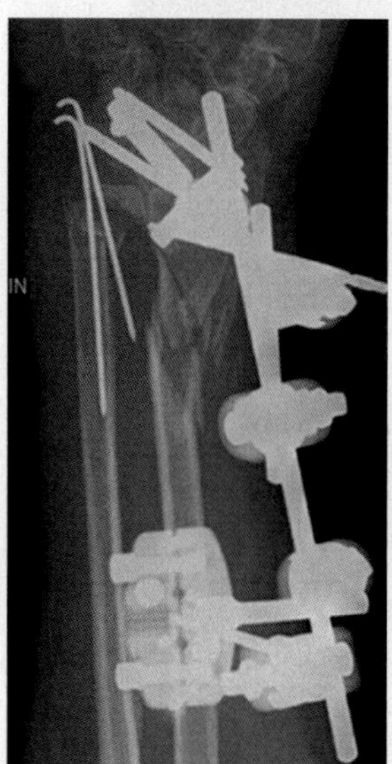

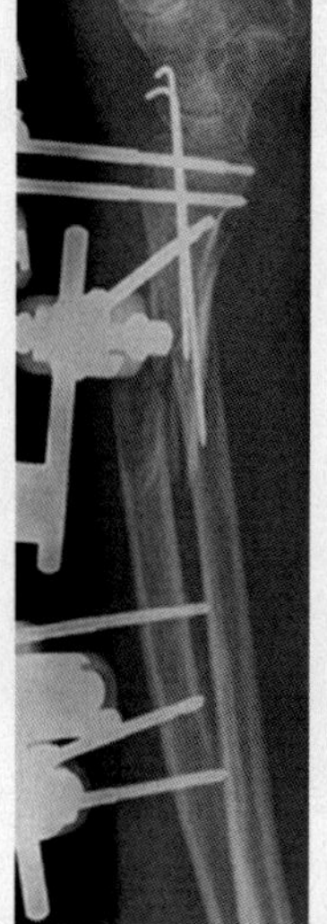

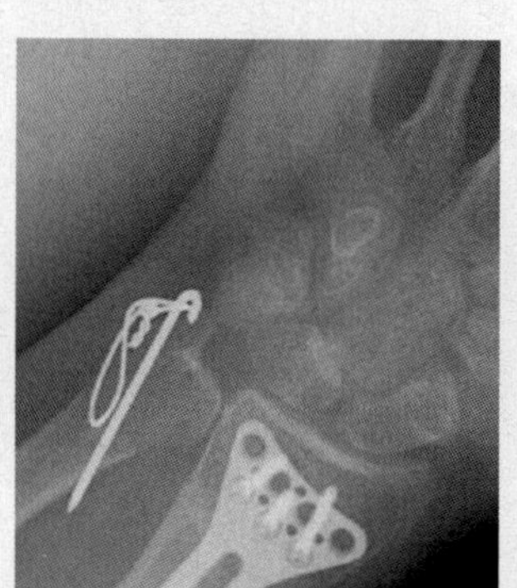

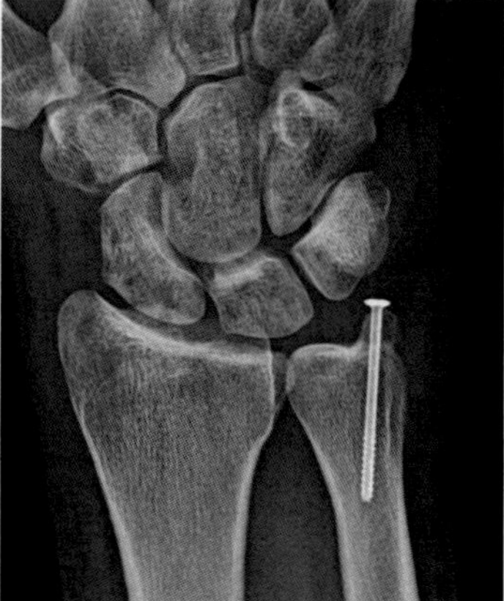

TECH FIG 2 • The ulnar styloid can be fixed in various ways to secure reattachment of the radioulnar ligament and thereby stabilize the DRUJ. **A,B.** Single (not rotationally stable) or double Kirschner wires. **C.** Tension band wiring. **D.** Screw fixation (not rotationally stable).

Ulnar Styloid Nonunions

- Reattachment of the nonunited fragment to the ulnar head is indicated if the fragment is large.[8]
- If the fragment is small, it should be excised and the radioulnar ligament reattached directly to the fovea of the ulnar head.[8]
- If the fragment is small and located distally and there is no DRUJ instability, the ulnar styloid can be excised without any associated ligament procedure.[8]
- Consider wrist arthroscopy prior to styloid excision in order to evaluate for potential concomitant TFCC pathology (**TECH FIG 3A,B**).

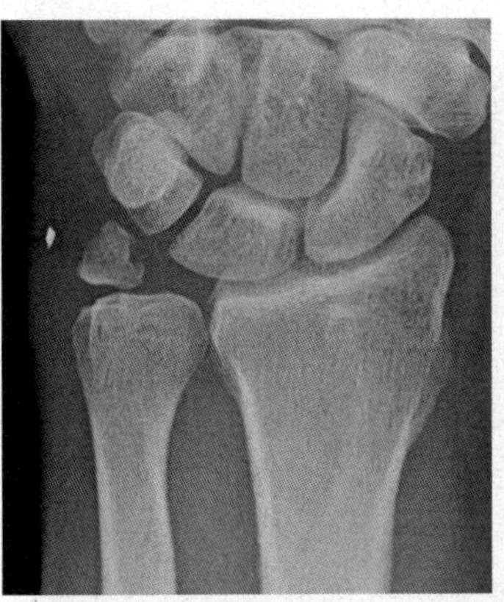

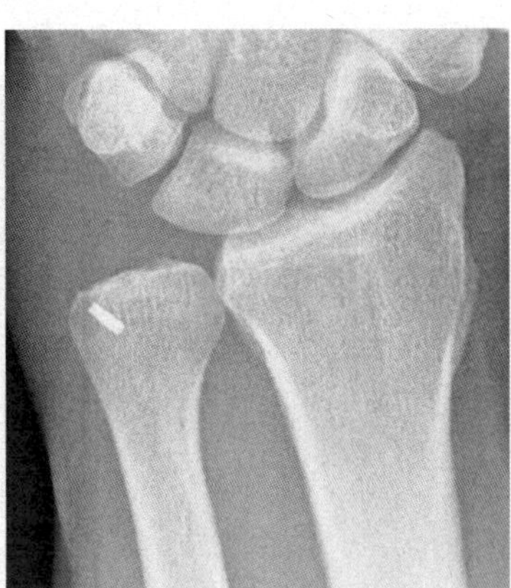

TECH FIG 3 • Intraoperative evaluation of the TFCC is essential when performing styloidectomy for ulnar styloid nonunion. **A.** Preoperative ulnar styloid nonunion. **B.** Following ulnar styloid excision, the TFCC was repaired using a suture anchor.

Ulnar Head Fractures

- Ulnar head fractures without a proximal extra-articular component
  - Fractures that are displaced (with an intra-articular step-off) or unstable are treated with ORIF using buried headless compression screws[9] or Kirschner wires.
  - Immobilization after fixation depends on the stability of the fracture and its fixation.
- Ulnar head fractures with a proximal extra-articular component
  - The intra-articular component is reduced and stabilized.
  - If the extra-articular component extends proximally toward the neck of the distal ulna, a condylar blade plate is recommended (**TECH FIG 4**), whereas tension band wiring is recommended if the extra-articular component involves the ulnar styloid (see **TECH FIG 2C**).
  - Immobilization after fixation depends on the stability of the fracture and its fixation.

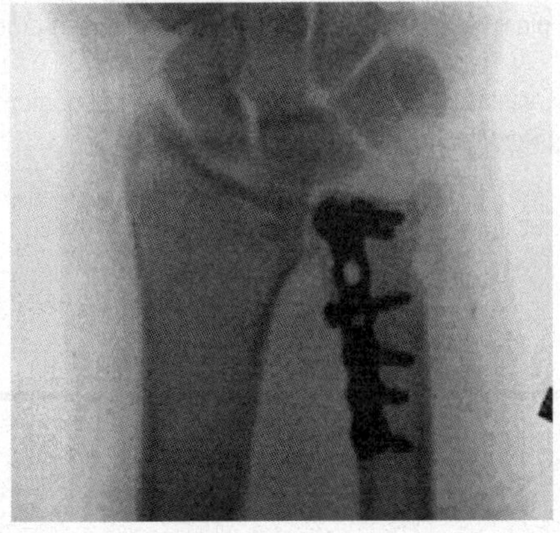

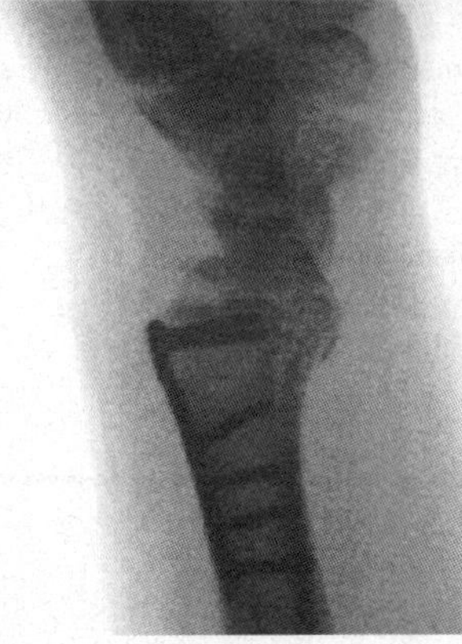

TECH FIG 4 • **A,B.** Irreducible or unstable distal forearm fractures require ORIF.[18] AP and lateral radiographs show a dorsally displaced distal forearm fracture fixed with a blade plate.

Distal Ulnar Neck and Shaft Fractures

- Irreducible or unstable fractures require ORIF.[18]
- This can be achieved using either a condylar blade plate[18] (see **TECH FIG 3**) or tension band wiring supplemented by intrafragmentary screws (**TECH FIG 5**).

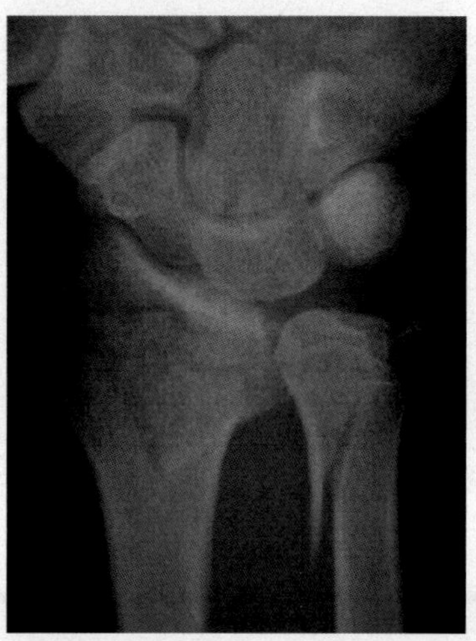
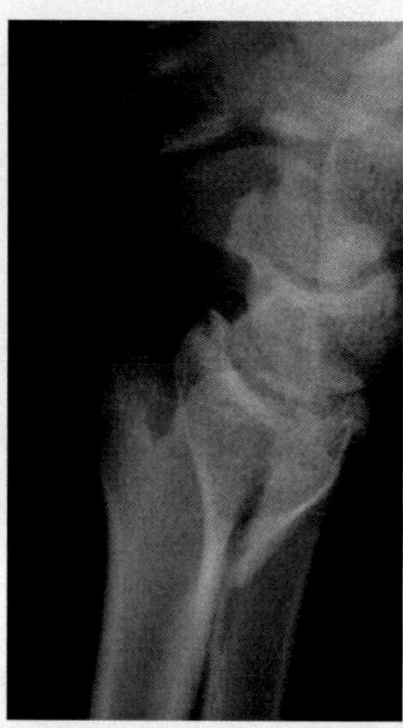
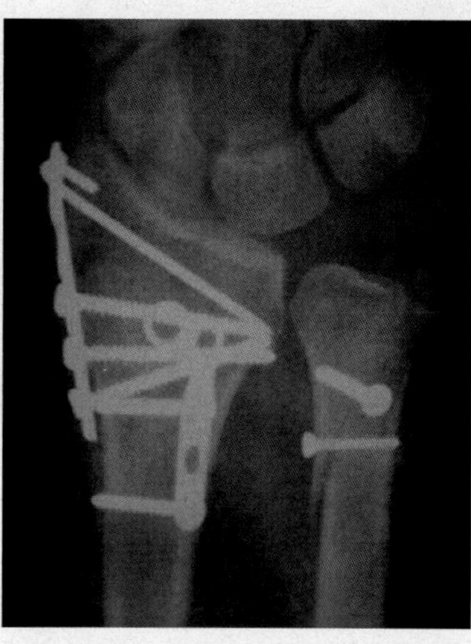

TECH FIG 5 • **A,B.** AP and lateral radiographs show a dorsally displaced distal forearm fracture. ORIF was performed using both a dorsoradial and a dorsoulnar approach to stabilize the fractures. **C.** Because of the comminution around the ulnar styloid base, fixation was achieved with a suture loop.

Comminuted Intra-articular Distal Ulnar Fractures

- Treatment options exist for comminuted intra-articular distal ulnar fractures:
  - Restoration of the anatomy and overall alignment of the ulna and DRUJ as mentioned earlier
    - This can be accomplished with manipulation and above-elbow cast immobilization alone or alternatively by surgical means with temporary wiring or external fixation.
    - The potential problems with this management technique are wrist stiffness and reduced forearm rotation that may not be corrected with a late salvage procedure.
  - Primary distal ulnar head replacement[5]
    - The theoretical advantage is reduced stiffness (from having early movement) and less DRUJ pain.
  - Total or partial excision of the ulnar head as well as DRUJ arthrodesis with distal ulnar neck resection (Sauvé-Kapandji procedure)
  - Distal ulnar resection with ECU tenodesis (Darrach procedure)[4]
  - Care is taken not to resect beyond the proximal portion of the sigmoid notch.

POSTOPERATIVE CARE

- Stable fixation of the distal ulnar complex still requires protection postoperatively with a below-elbow splint.
- Intermediate stable fixation requires 4 weeks of protection using a sugar-tong–type splint to allow flexion and extension of the elbow but protect against uncontrolled pronation and supination.
- Unstable fixation after internal, external, or nonoperative treatment requires above-elbow protection in neutral forearm rotation to limit movement for the first 6 weeks. There is otherwise a risk that rotational forces will cause a nonunion or malunion.

OUTCOMES

- Increased attention to the outcomes of ulnar-sided fractures has demonstrated a trend of equivalent outcomes regardless of treatment or presence of styloid nonunion.
- DRUJ stability is cited as the most important factor for postoperative satisfaction.
- With greater understanding of the relationship between the ulnar styloid, the radioulnar ligament, and the TFCC, improved outcomes can be achieved.

COMPLICATIONS

- Stiffness of the DRUJ with limited pronation and supination
- Prominent hardware with operative fixation
- Infection
- Nonunion
- Malunion

REFERENCES

1. af Ekenstam F, Hagert CG. Anatomical studies on the geometry and stability of the distal radio ulnar joint. Scand J Plast Reconstr Surg 1985;19:17–25.
2. Arora R, Gabl M, Pechlaner S, et al. Initial shortening and internal fixation in combination with a Sauvé-Kapandji procedure for severely comminuted fractures of the distal radius in elderly patients. J Bone Joint Surg Br 2010;92:1158–1562.
3. Buijze GA, Ring D. Clinical impact of united versus nonunited fractures of the proximal half of the ulnar styloid following volar plate fixation of the distal radius. J Hand Surg Am 2010;35:223–227.
4. Darrach W. Partial excision of lower shaft of ulna for deformity following Colles's fracture. 1913. Clin Orthop Relat Res 1992;(275):3–4.
5. Grechenig W, Peicha G, Fellinger M. Primary ulnar head prosthesis for the treatment of an irreparable ulnar head fracture dislocation. J Hand Surg Br 2001;26(3):269–271.
6. Hagert CG. Current concepts of the functional anatomy of the distal radioulnar joint, including the ulnocarpal junction. In: Büchler U, ed. Wrist Instability. Berlin: Martin Dunitz, 1996:15–21.
7. Hagert CG. The distal radioulnar joint in relation to the whole forearm. Clin Orthop Relat Res 1992;(275):56–64.
8. Hauck RM, Skahen J III, Palmer AK. Classification and treatment of ulnar styloid nonunion. J Hand Surg Am 1996;21(3):418–422.
9. Jakab E, Ganos DL, Gagnon S. Isolated intra-articular fractures of the ulnar head. J Orthop Trauma 1993;7:290–292.
10. Kim JK, Koh YD, Do NH. Should an ulnar styloid fracture be fixed following volar plate fixation of a distal radial fracture? J Bone Joint Surg Am 2010;92:1–6.
11. Lindau T, Adlercreutz C, Aspenberg P. Peripheral tears of the triangular fibrocartilage complex cause distal radioulnar instability after distal radius fractures. J Hand Surg Am 2000;25(3):464–468.
12. Lindau T, Arner M, Hagberg L. Intraarticular lesions in distal fractures of the radius in young adults: a descriptive arthroscopic study in 50 patients. J Hand Surg Br 1997;22(5):638–643.
13. May MM, Lawton JN, Blazar PE. Ulnar styloid fractures associated with distal radius fractures: incidence and implications for distal radioulnar joint instability. J Hand Surg Am 2002;27(6): 965–971.
14. Namba J, Fujiwara T, Murase T, et al. Intra-articular distal ulnar fractures associated with distal radial fractures in older adults: early experience in fixation of the radius and leaving the ulna unfixed. J Hand Surg Eur Vol 2009;34:592–597.
15. Palmer AK, Werner FW. The triangular fibrocartilage complex of the wrist—anatomy and function. J Hand Surg Am 1981;6(2):153–162.
16. Protopsaltis TS, Ruch DS. Triangular fibrocartilage complex tears associated with symptomatic ulnar styloid nonunions. J Hand Surg Am 2010;35:1251–1255.
17. Richards TA, Deal DN. Distal ulna fractures. J Hand Surg Am 2014;39:385–391.
18. Ring D, McCarty PL, Campbell D, et al. Condylar blade plate fixation of unstable fractures of the distal ulna associated with fractures of the distal radius. J Hand Surg Am 2004;29(1):103–109.
19. Ruchelsman DE, Raski KB, Rettig ME. Outcome following acute primary distal ulna resection for comminuted distal ulna fractures at the time of operative fixation of unstable fractures of the distal radius. Hand 2009;4:391–396.
20. Zenke Y, Sakai A, Oshige T, et al. The effect of an associated ulnar styloid fracture on the outcome after fixation of a fracture of the distal radius. J Bone Joint Surg Br 2009;91:102–107.

CHAPTER

Reduction and Stabilization of the Distal Radioulnar Joint following Galeazzi Fractures

Benjamin S. Zellner, John R. Dawson and Lee M. Reichel

DEFINITION

- Fracture of the radial shaft with an associated distal radioulnar joint (DRUJ) dislocation (**FIG 1A,B**)
- It is well established that anatomic stabilization of the radial shaft fracture typically results in a stable DRUJ that can be treated nonoperatively with a period of immobilization.
- When the DRUJ is either irreducible or unstable, following anatomic reduction and compression plating of the radius fracture, operative stabilization of the DRUJ is required.
- Pediatric injury is not discussed in this chapter.

ANATOMY

- DRUJ
  - Stability to the DRUJ is conferred through the bony articulation between the sigmoid notch of the radius and the ulnar head, ligamentous attachments, and muscular stabilizers.[5]
  - The radius of curvature of the ulnar head is smaller than the sigmoid notch, resulting in a loosely constrained bony articulation. This allows both rotational and translational movements between the radius and ulna with pronosupination. In addition, this loose bony articulation must depend on soft tissue components to be the primary joint stabilizers.[5]

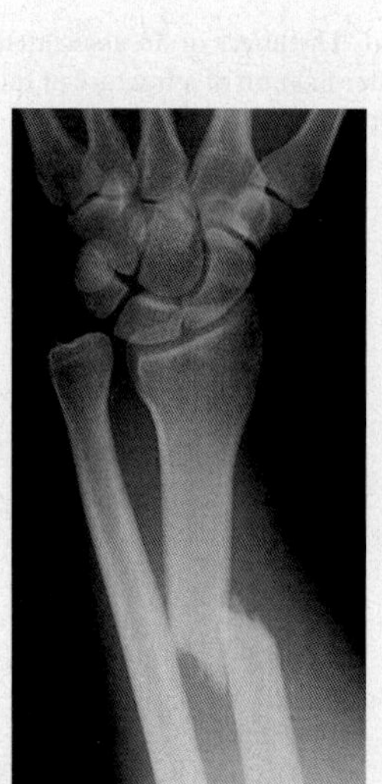

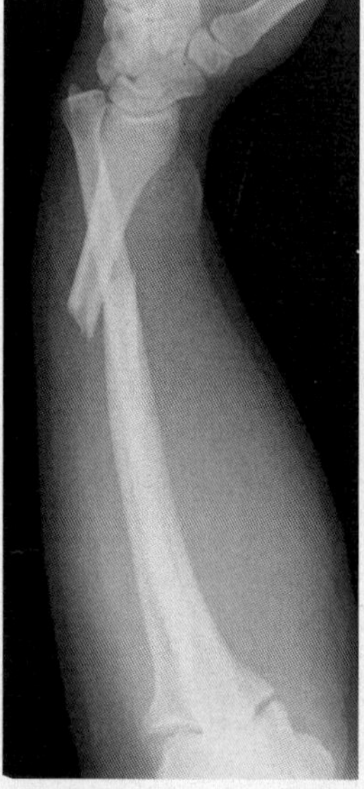

FIG 1 • Classic Galeazzi injury. **A.** A distal-third radial shaft fracture with ulnar angulation of the distal fragment, radial shortening, and DRUJ widening. **B.** Apex dorsal angulation of radial shaft fracture with dorsal dislocation of ulnar head.

- Triangular fibrocartilage complex (TFCC)
  - The dorsal and volar radioulnar ligaments of the TFCC are considered the primary stabilizers of the DRUJ.[18]
  - The deep fibers of the radioulnar ligaments attached at the fovea are located at the base of the ulnar styloid.
  - For this reason, in the less common instance when an ulnar styloid base fracture accompanies a Galeazzi fracture-dislocation, fixation of ulnar styloid fracture may restore DRUJ stability.
- Distal interosseous membrane (DIOM) and distal oblique bundle (DOB)
  - The DIOM lies deep to the pronator quadratus and connects the radius and ulna (**FIG 2A**).
  - Biomechanical studies demonstrate that the distal membranous portion of the interosseous membrane functions as a secondary stabilizer of the DRUJ.[14,20]
  - When present, the DOB originates at the distal ulna and inserts at the inferior rim of the sigmoid notch of the radius blending with the capsular tissue of the DRUJ.[18] Cadaveric studies report the DOB is present in 40% of specimens (**FIG 2B**).[15]
  - Moritomo[14] has hypothesized that in Galeazzi fracture-dislocations, when there is loosening but not rupture of the DOB, instability can be managed by anatomic reduction of the radius.
  - Radius reduction and the subsequent retensioning of the DOB restore stability even when a TFCC injury is present. Persistent DRUJ instability after radial fracture restoration may be the result of DOB disruption.[14]
- Radius
  - The majority of Galeazzi fracture-dislocations occurs in distal third of the radius but can occur anywhere along the radius.[12]
    - Greater than 50% of radial shaft fractures less than 7.5 cm from the distal radial articular surface are associated with injury to the DRUJ compared to 6% of more proximal radial shaft fractures.[17]

PATHOGENESIS

- Mechanism of injury
  - Axial loading of an outstretched arm with forceful hyperpronation of the forearm. Direct trauma to the dorsal radial forearm has also been reported.[12]
  - More common in higher energy injuries with a high incidence of associated injuries (30% to 50%)[13]
  - The radius fractures and shortens. This shortening results in tearing of the TFCC from its foveal attachment (or an ulnar styloid base fracture with TFCC remaining attached) and subsequent dislocation of the DRUJ.

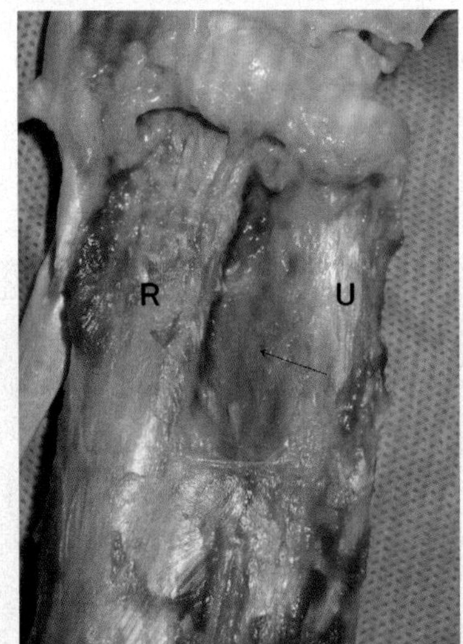

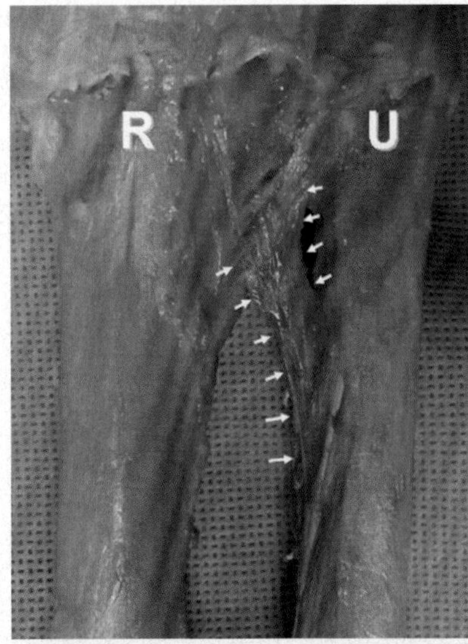

FIG 2 • DOB. **A.** DIOM with no DOB present. **B.** DOB is the thick fibrous band from the proximal ulna to the distal radius (*white arrows*). *R*, radius; *U*, ulna. (From Moritomo H. The distal interosseous membrane: current concepts in wrist anatomy and biomechanics. J Hand Surg Am 2012;37(7):1501–1507. Reprinted with permission from Elsevier.)

- Galeazzi and irreducible DRUJ (following radius fixation)
  - When the DRUJ cannot be reduced, soft tissue interposition should be suspected. In these instances, the joint capsule, TFCC, and/or the extensor tendons are frequently interposed (extensor carpi ulnaris [ECU], extensor digiti minimi, extensor digitorum communis).[2,4]
- Galeazzi and unstable DRUJ (following radius fixation)
  - It is established that a TFCC (Palmar 1B) injury (or ulnar styloid base fracture with the TFCC attached) occurs in a Galeazzi fracture-dislocation.[17] TFCC injury, in addition to DIOM and DOB injury (as described earlier), likely results in continued, significant instability after radius fixation.

NATURAL HISTORY

- Galeazzi fracture-dislocations account for approximately 6% of all closed forearm fractures in adults with a male predominance.[13]
- Nonoperative management results in an apex dorsal radius malunion with a dorsally prominent ulnar head. Limitations in pronation, supination, wrist flexion, and wrist extension are common. Pain occurs at the ulnar side of the wrist over the prominent ulnar head.
- In contrast, early operative management typically results in excellent or satisfactory results following anatomic reduction and stabilization of radius fracture and DRUJ.

PATIENT HISTORY AND PHYSICAL FINDINGS

- A high percentage of associated injuries occur, and life-threatening injuries should be assessed first.
- Patients report severe forearm and wrist pain. Deformity is typically present with a prominent ulnar head.
- Open injuries of the radius and ulna can occur, and close evaluation of the skin should be performed.
- Neurovascular injuries and compartment syndrome have not been widely reported with a Galeazzi injury but should be assessed for completeness and documented even when "negative." Therefore, all splints, dressings, and clothing need to be removed for proper inspection and palpation and neurovascular examination.
- Examination of the DRUJ of the noninjured contralateral extremity is helpful prior to surgical management of the Galeazzi injury to understand the patient's native DRUJ laxity, especially at the limits of pronation and supination.

IMAGING AND OTHER DIAGNOSTIC STUDIES

- Anteroposterior and lateral radiographs of the wrist, forearm, and elbow suffice for diagnosing Galeazzi fracture-dislocations.
- At presentation, radiographs typically demonstrate the following:
  - Shortening of the radius on the anteroposterior view with a widened DRUJ
  - Apex medial angulation of the distal radial segment (toward the ulna)
  - An apex dorsal angulation of the radius on the lateral radiograph with a dorsal dislocation of the DRUJ
  - An ulnar styloid base fracture may also be present.
- DRUJ subluxation is notoriously difficult to identify.
  - Postoperatively, if there is any concern whether the DRUJ is reduced, computed tomography (CT) or magnetic resonance imaging (MRI) should be obtained.
  - The DRUJ is well visualized in the axial plane to determine subluxation or dislocation.
  - Multiple methods have been devised to identify and quantify DRUJ subluxation using CT (Mino's criteria, congruency method, epicenter method, and radioulnar ratio).[11] Unfortunately, no reference standard exists (**FIG 3A–C**).
  - Despite the advantages of advanced imaging, it is not typically necessary at presentation as soft tissue injury is implied based on radiographic findings in a Galeazzi injury pattern.

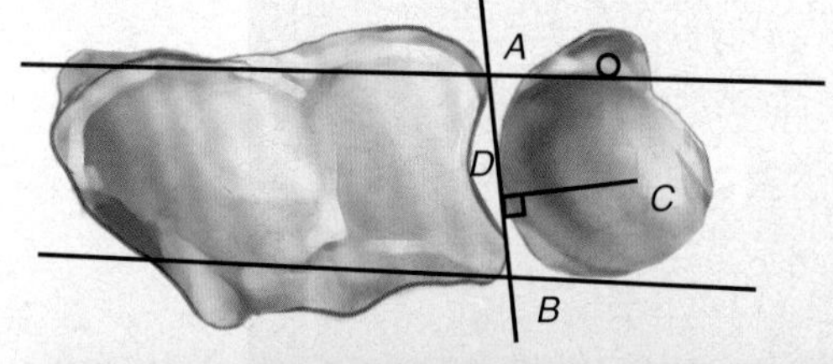

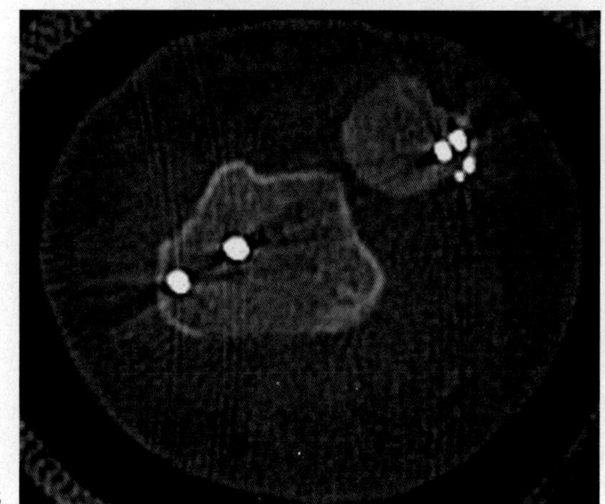

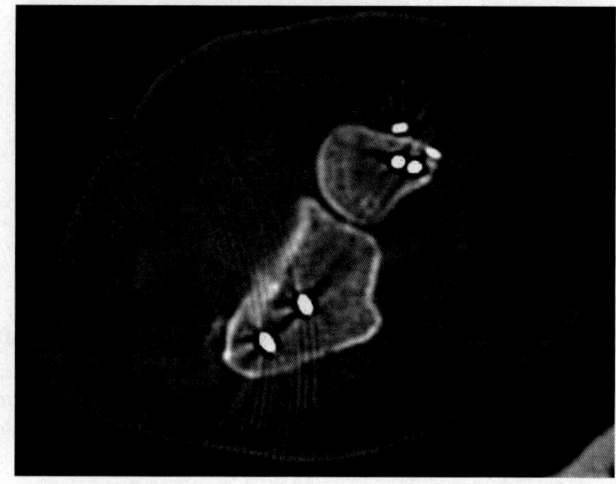

FIG 3 • A. Radioulnar ratio method to measure DRUJ subluxation on a CT scan. See text for details. **B.** Axial CT scan demonstrating dorsally dislocated ulna following ulnar styloid open reduction internal fixation (ORIF). **C.** Axial CT scan following reduction and pinning of the dislocated DRUJ. (**A:** Adapted from Lo IK, MacDermid JC, Bennett JD, et al. The radioulnar ratio: a new method of quantifying DRUJ subluxation. J Hand Surg Am 2001;26:236–243.)

DIFFERENTIAL DIAGNOSIS

- Isolated radial shaft fracture
- Radial head or neck fracture with DRUJ injury (Essex-Lopresti lesion)
- Distal radius fracture with DRUJ injury
- Ulnar-sided carpal or ligamentous injuries

NONOPERATIVE MANAGEMENT

- No role exists for nonoperative care of a Galeazzi injury in a patient who is medically able to have surgery. Hughston's[7] classic series demonstrated that 35 of 38 patients treated without surgery resulted in failure.

SURGICAL MANAGEMENT

- Galeazzi fracture-dislocations need to be treated expeditiously. Delay in treatment more than 10 days may negatively impact final range of motion of the forearm.[13]
- The need for operative stabilization of the DRUJ can only be determined intraoperatively after the radius fracture has been stabilized, and the DRUJ is examined for instability.

Preoperative Planning

- Preoperatively, the surgeon decides the surgical approach and method of fixation of the radius fracture. It is presumed that at a minimum, the TFCC is injured and the DRUJ will be evaluated intraoperatively.
  - Decision making and technique regarding approach and fixation of the radius has been described in detail in the chapter entitled Open Reduction Internal Fixation of Diaphyseal Forearm Fractures (also in Chap. 1).
- Examination under anesthesia of the uninjured wrist is performed.
- Depending on intraoperative findings, the surgeon must be prepared to pin the radius to the ulna, explore the dorsal DRUJ, and possibly repair the TFCC using either open or an arthroscopic technique.
- *Evaluation of DRUJ instability following radial fixation*
  - The decision to proceed with operative stabilization of the DRUJ for residual instability following radius fixation is not straightforward. Unfortunately, there is no reference standard for evaluating DRUJ stability.
  - DRUJ instability should always be evaluated after radius stabilization.
  - Classically, the elbow is flexed to 90 degrees, and the ulna is stressed both volarly and dorsally in supination, neutral, and pronation while laxity, subluxation, or dislocation is assessed. Any laxity less than full dislocation is difficult to quantify even when measured against the examination of the uninjured wrist.
  - Giannoulis and Sotereanos[4] suggested that instability is confirmed following fixation of the radius if the ulnar head can be translated dorsally out of the sigmoid notch (with the forearm fully supinated).
  - Jupiter[8] has suggested that laxity at the DRUJ should be expected (in displaced distal radius fractures) and that the traditional method of stressing the ulna dorsally and volarly is subjective and lacks interobserver validity. He recommends that the surgeon compress the ulna to the radius after bony fixation and rotate the hand and wrist. Only when a palpable "clunk" is present is true instability present. This implies that the distal oblique band of the interosseous membrane has been disrupted.

Positioning

- The patient is placed supine with the injured arm out on a radiolucent arm table. A nonsterile padded pneumatic tourniquet is placed on the upper arm.
- If arthroscopy is planned to address an unstable DRUJ, the upper arm should be stabilized to the arm table or a distraction device be made available.

Approach

- Reduction or stabilization of the radius fracture is typically performed with a 3.5-mm compression plate through an anterior approach as described by Henry.[6]
  - Anatomic restoration of length, alignment, and rotation of the radius must be achieved to assist in restoring stability of the DRUJ.
  - Radial shaft fixation is described in detail in the chapter entitled Open Reduction Internal Fixation of Diaphyseal Forearm Fractures.
- Although the preoperative images may demonstrate DRUJ injury (ie, ulnar styloid fracture, DRUJ subluxation/dislocation, or a widened DRUJ), final consideration of fixation is based on the intraoperative findings (**FIG 4**).
- *Treatment of the unstable DRUJ after radial fixation with no ulnar fracture*
  - No reference standard exists for the specific treatment of the unstable DRUJ noted after radius fixation.
  - Pinning the radius to the ulna in a position of DRUJ reduction is the most commonly reported procedure in larger cases series, with excellent results reported.[6,12] A recent study evaluated 40 patients who had a single 1.2- or 1.6-mm smooth stainless steel pin placed proximal to the sigmoid notch with the forearm in supination for 4–6 weeks for DRUJ instability after radial fixation. At 6.8-year follow-up, none of these patients required more DRUJ surgery or had persistent DRUJ instability. Consideration may also be given to splinting in forearm supination for 4–6 weeks.
- *Treatment of the unstable DRUJ after radial fixation with large ulnar styloid base fracture*
  - Instability with an associated ulnar styloid fracture is less frequent in Galleazi injuries. Maintenance of stability has been reported with operative fixation of the ulnar styloid base.[10] Screw or tension band fixation is commonly performed.
- *Treatment of the irreducible DRUJ after radial fixation*
  - If the DRUJ remains irreducible after anatomic reduction of the radial shaft fracture, soft tissue interposition is suspected. Open reduction to remove soft tissue and TFCC repair should be performed.[10]

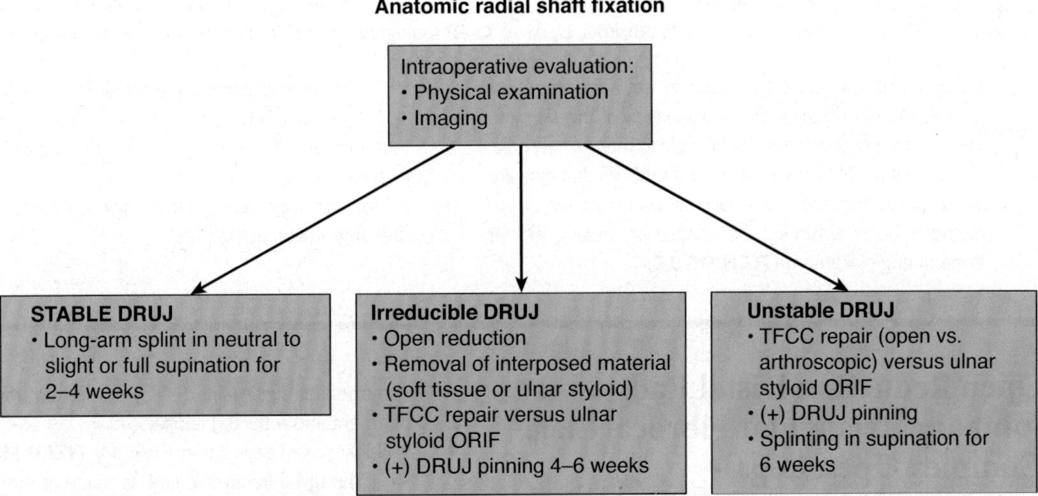

FIG 4 • Algorithm for management of DRUJ stability.

TECHNIQUES

Radius and Ulna Transfixation Pinning

- Indicated for treatment of the unstable DRUJ after radius fixation and no ulna fracture
- Following radius shaft fixation, the elbow is flexed to 90 degrees, and the forearm is brought to full supination. The radius is manually stabilized through the wound. Subluxation or dislocation with attempted palmar or dorsal translation is considered instability. Alternatively, the method described by Jupiter[8] is performed to assess stability.
- The elbow is extended, and using intraoperative fluoroscopy, the skin is marked at the position of planned smooth stainless steel pin insertion. Transfixation pins should be placed proximal to the sigmoid notch. A skin incision is made directly over the radius with blunt dissection to the bone.
- A drill guide is then placed under direct visualization to the radius, and a smooth pin is driven through the radius and stopped prior to entering the ulna.
- The forearm is placed in approximately 20 degrees of supination, and the assistant squeezes the radius and ulna together manually while the pin is then driven into the ulna. (Alternatively, depending on the subjective degree of instability, this procedure can be performed in full supination.)
- Under oscillation, the smooth pin can be driven through the ulna and out the skin.
- The same procedure is repeated with a second pin.
- Pins are cut and bent outside the skin on both the radial and ulnar side allowing easy retrieval in the event of pin breakage (**TECH FIG 1A**).
- Alternatively, the pins may be driven through the ulna into the radius.
  - In this case, prior to having the pins exit the far cortex of the radius, an incision is made, and the superficial radial nerve (SRN) is identified and protected as the pins are visualized passing radially out of the skin (**TECH FIG 1B**).

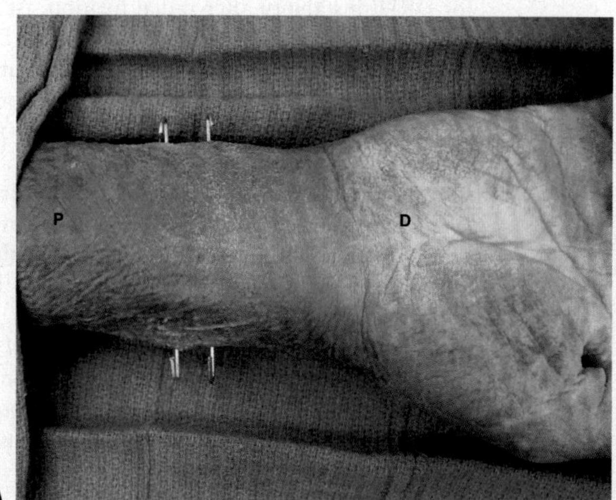

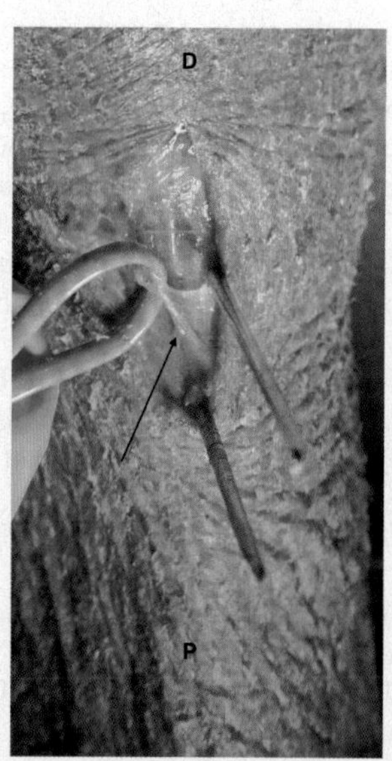

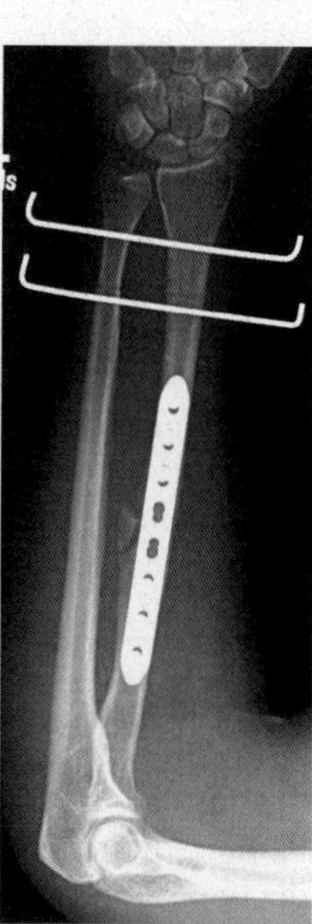

TECH FIG 1 • DRUJ Pinning. **A.** Placement of pins on an anteroposterior (AP) view. Pins (1.6 mm or 2.0 mm) are brought out of the skin on both the radial and ulna sides (allowing easy retrieval in the event of breakage). **B.** SRN is located near pin sites on the radial side. SRN (*arrow* and vessel loop). *P*, proximal; *D*, distal. **C.** AP radiograph demonstrating pins placed proximal to the DRUJ.

  - If the surgeon prefers the pins not to exit an incision, just prior to the pin reaching the undersurface of the skin, the skin can be pulled over the tip of the pin to make a new hole.
  - The advantage of ulna to radius pin fixation is that pins are being driven from the small-diameter bone into the bigger diameter bone, lessening the chance of missing the far bone during placement (**TECH FIG 1C**).
  - The disadvantage is that the SRN is at risk of being injured by exiting pins.
- Intraoperative fluoroscopy is used to confirm DRUJ reduction prior to leaving the operating room.
- A long-arm posterior splint is applied after application of soft dressings covering the pins.

Open Reduction Distal Radioulnar Joint and Triangular Fibrocartilage Complex Open Repair

- *Indicated in the treatment of the irreducible DRUJ following radial fixation*
- If the DRUJ remains irreducible after anatomic reduction of the radial shaft fracture, soft tissue interposition is suspected. Open reduction to remove interposed soft tissue and TFCC repair should be performed.[10]
- The following description assumes the native anatomy is not disrupted. Unfortunately, if this approach is being made for an irreducible DRUJ, there will be disrupted tissue planes as a result of interposed structures, capsular tears, etc. It is important to be able to identify the structures and attempt to restore them to their native positions, stabilizing them with tissue repair after joint reduction.
- A 2- to 3-cm gently curved dorsal longitudinal incision is made over the distal ulna, and blunt dissection is performed through the subcutaneous tissue, cauterizing small vessels with bipolar cautery (**TECH FIG 2A**).
- The dorsal cutaneous branch of the ulnar nerve is identified and care is taken throughout the procedure to protect it.
- A longitudinal incision is made through the thin extensor retinaculum between the fourth and fifth extensor compartments (**TECH FIG 2B**).[3]
  - Avoid amputating the flap during radial to ulnar elevation.
  - Avoid violation of the ECU subsheath.
- The extensor digiti quinti (EDQ) is released from the fifth compartment and retracted radially.
- An ulnar-based capsulotomy is made (**TECH FIG 2C**).
  - The distal transverse limb is made at the level of the palpable triquetrum, proceeding in an ulnar to radial direction along the dorsal radiocarpal ligament, from the ECU tendon to the floor of the fifth compartment.
  - The capsulotomy is then continued proximally in a longitudinal fashion through the floor of the fifth compartment to the level of the ulnar neck.
  - Care needs to be taken not to cut through the dorsal radioulnar ligament of the triangular fibrocartilage (TFC).
  - Small double skin hooks placing tension on the capsular flap will assists in avoiding injury to the underlying TFC.
  - Finally, the proximal transverse capsulotomy is made across the ulnar neck to ECU tendon.
- If needed for visualization and working space, the ulnomeniscal homolog, which extends distal from the TFC into the ulnocarpal joint, can be excised.
  - Bipolar cautery may be needed for hemostasis following its excision.[3]
- The key to the entire dissection is to create clean planes that sharply define the structures, allowing them to be repaired during layered closure.
- Next, a small curette is used to create a small trough in the ulna fovea exposing cancellous bone.

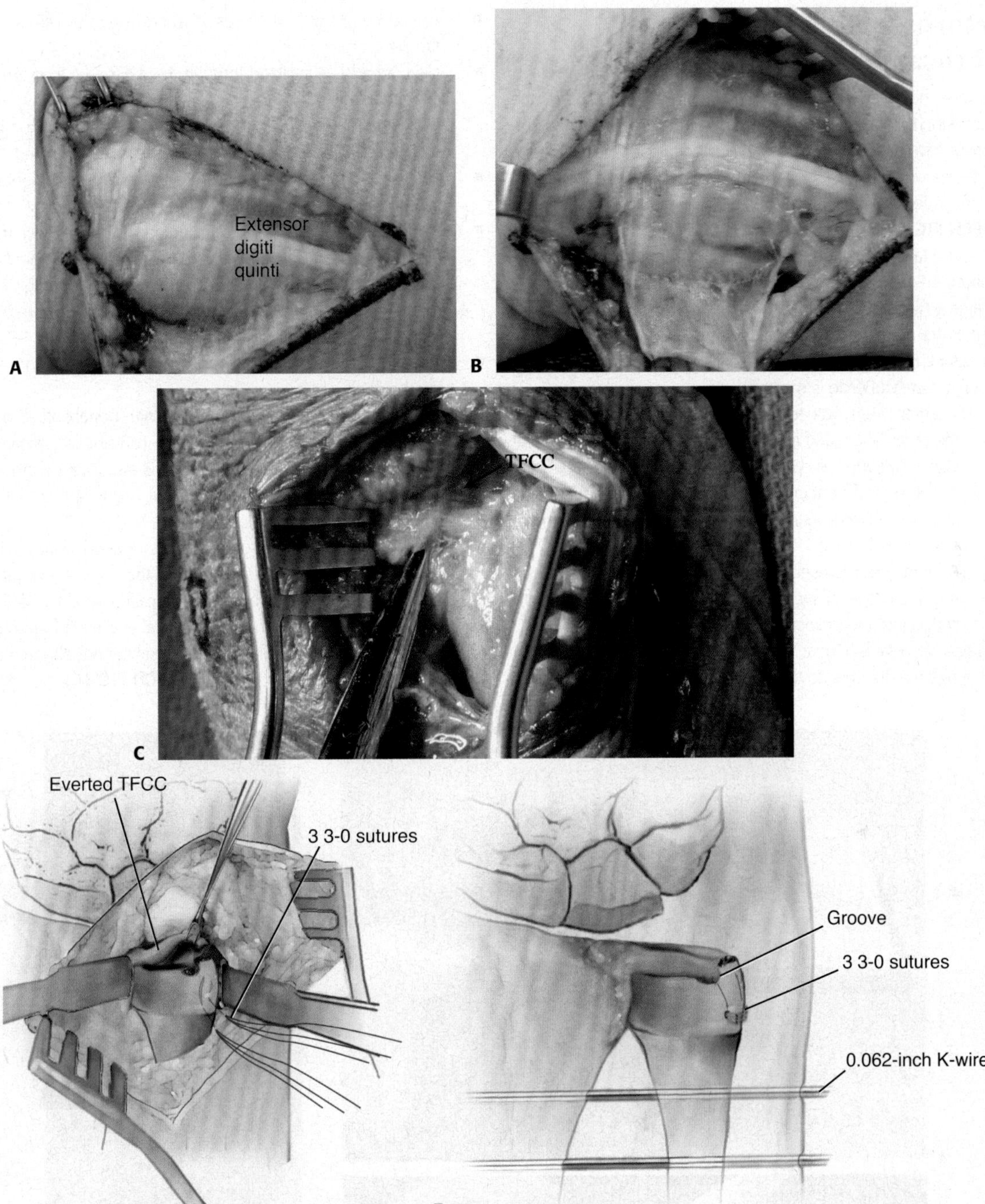

TECH FIG 2 • Open DRUJ/TFCC exposure and repair. **A.** Incision. **B.** Extensor retinaculum opened exposing fifth compartment. **C.** TFCC and DRUJ exposed. **D.** 3-0 nonabsorbable sutures placed through TFCC and ulna bone tunnels. **E.** Final construct demonstrating transfixation with 0.062-inch K-wires and TFCC repair.

- A 0.045-inch smooth stainless steel pin is used to drill two bone tunnels, separated by a 1-cm bony bridge, from the medial ulna to the ulnar fovea.
  - Next, three 3-0 braided nonabsorbable suture are passed one at time through one of the bone tunnels, through the TFC, and back out the other bone tunnel (outside-in to inside-out) (**TECH FIG 2D**).[9]
- Prior to tying the sutures, the DRUJ is reduced and pinned with two 1.6- or 2-mm smooth stainless steel pins as previously described.
- Finally, the sutures are tied down over the ulna.
- A layer-by-layer closure is performed. The dorsal radioulnar ligament of the TFC can be sutured back to the capsule during closure (**TECH FIG 2E**).

Arthroscopic Triangular Fibrocartilage Complex Repair

- It should be noted that while this procedure can be used for the treatment of Galeazzi fracture-dislocations, the procedure and outcomes have not been rigorously evaluated in published literature.
- The surgeon is seated facing the monitor. Finger traps are placed on the index and long fingers, and a 15-pound traction is applied (**TECH FIG 3A,B**).
- Three portals are needed for arthroscopic TFCC repair (3-4 visualization, 4-5 working, and 6U outflow). Skin markings of the bony anatomy (radial styloid, ulnar styloid, Lister tubercle) and planned portals are made prior to inflating tourniquet.
- To establish the 3-4 portal, the soft spot approximately 1 cm distal to Lister tubercle is marked.
  - Insert an 18-gauge needle, angled to match the sagittal tilt of the distal radius, and inject 4 mL of saline (or 1% lidocaine with 1:100,000 epinephrine) to insufflate the radiocarpal joint.
  - A 4-mm skin incision is made at the planned portal site, and blunt dissection to the level of the capsule with a mosquito is performed.
  - A blunt trocar is used to penetrate the joint capsule and avoid cartilage injury, and a 1.9-mm camera is then inserted into the radiocarpal joint.
- Outflow is established at the 6U portal with insertion of an 18-gauge needle ulnar to the ECU into the ulnocarpal joint.
- The 4-5 working portal is established using the same steps as the 3-4 portal.
- Next, a probe is inserted through the 4-5 portal to examine the integrity of the TFCC.
  - In a Galeazzi fracture-dislocation, a foveal avulsion is present (Palmer 1B), and the tear is easily recognized.
- To begin TFCC repair, a 2-mm shaver is placed through the 4-5 portal, and unstable tear edges are débrided.
- Next, a 2-cm longitudinal skin incision is made over the medial distal ulna and blunt dissection proceeds to the bone. A 0.062-inch smooth stainless steel pin is placed obliquely from medial ulna to fovea and directly visualized arthroscopically entering the fovea.
- The pin is then overdrilled (outside-in) with a 3.0-mm cannulated drill bit.
- A sharp-tipped suture passer loaded with nonabsorbable suture is passed through the bone tunnel (outside-in), piercing the TFCC at the desired location. Suture is then passed around the TFCC into the joint and retrieved out of the 4-5 portal with a suture grasper.
- Another sharp-tipped suture passer loaded with a looped Nitinol wire is then passed through the ulnar bone tunnel to penetrate the TFCC at a different location. The looped Nitinol wire is retrieved through the 4-5 portal and used to retrieve the previously passed suture out the bone tunnel, thus creating a mattress stitch through the TFCC (**TECH FIG 3C**).

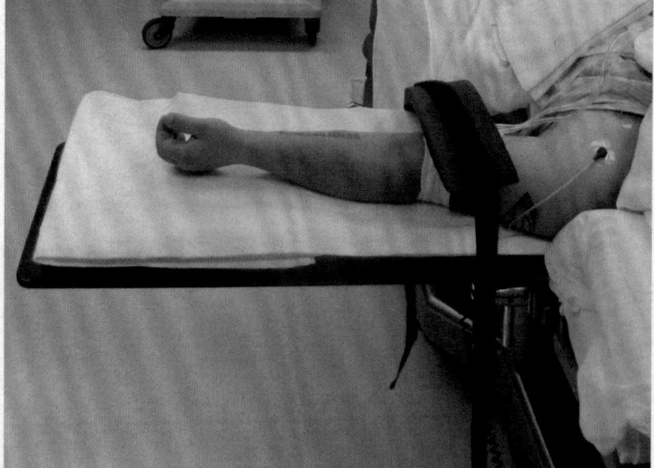

A

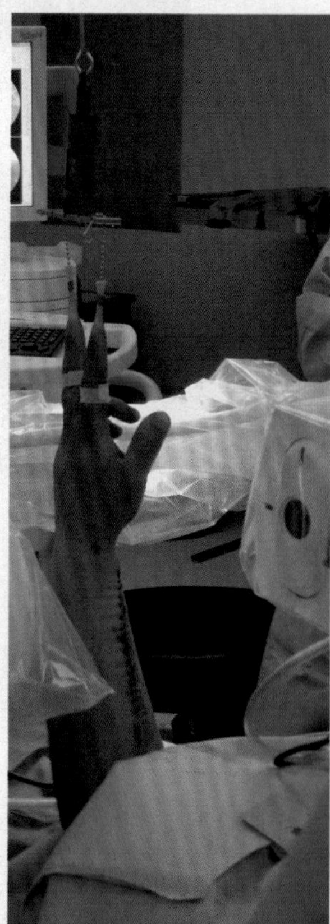

B

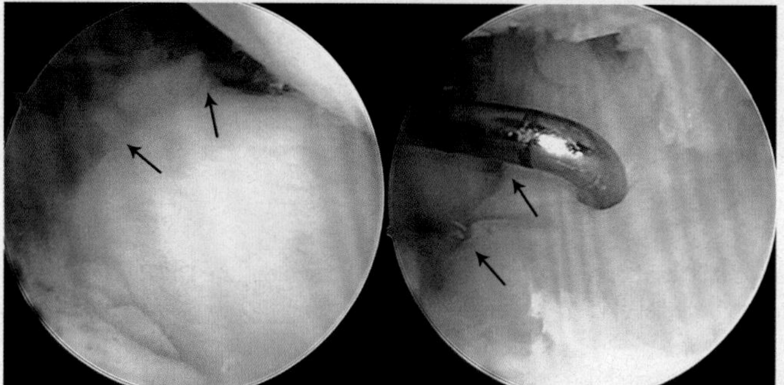

C

TECH FIG 3 • Wrist arthroscopy to address TFCC injury. **A.** The patient is placed supine with an arm board; a strap is used to securely fashion the arm to the table. A boom is placed on the contralateral side. **B.** Finger traps are positioned, the weight is attached. Fluoroscopy is used to access DRUJ reduction. **C.** TFCC Palmer 1B injury is present and repaired in this case with two horizontal mattress sutures.

- Traction is placed on the suture to evaluate the repair. Additional sutures may be passed as needed.
- Prior to tying down the sutures, two 1.6- or 2.0-mm smooth stainless steel pins are placed across the radioulnar joint as previously described.
- Finally, a drill hole for a bioabsorbable suture anchor is created proximal to the bone tunnel on the medial edge of the ulna.
  - The sutures are placed through the anchor, and tension is placed while directly visualizing the TFCC.
  - The suture anchor is then inserted.
- Wound closure, sterile dressings, and long posterior splint are applied.

Open Reduction Internal Fixation of Ulnar Styloid Fracture

- Indicated in the *treatment of the unstable DRUJ after radius fixation with large ulnar styloid base fracture*
- Two different approaches can be used:
  - An extensile approach is described for open TFCC repair. This has the advantage of assessing whether the TFCC has torn off the ulnar styloid fragment.
  - Alternatively, while offering less visualization, an incision can be made immediately over the ulnar styloid, resulting in less disruption to stabilizing soft tissue structures of the DRUJ.
    - This incision is begun 1 cm distal to the styloid and carried proximally to the ulnar neck.
    - Blunt dissection distal to the ulna styloid is performed to identify the dorsal ulnar cutaneous branch, which passes volar to dorsal, most often immediately distal to the ulnar styloid.
- Typically, there is soft tissue interposed at the fracture site and this is cleared with a hemostat or dental pick. The forearm is then rotated through pronosupination until the styloid fracture reduces to the fracture footprint.
- A 3.5-mm toothed drill guide fits nicely over the styloid tip and can be used to compress the styloid, whereas two 0.045 or 0.054-inch smooth stainless steel pins are driven through both the styloid and the far ulnar cortex. The pins are then backed out of the far ulnar cortex slightly. (**TECH FIG 4A**).
- A transverse (dorsal to volar) 2-mm drill hold is made proximally through the ulnar neck, and a 27-gauge wire is placed through the TFCC at its insertion on the ulnar styloid.
  - A figure-of-eight bend is made, and one limb is passed volar to dorsal through the transverse bone hole, whereas the other is passed dorsal to volar.
  - The wire is then twisted to tension, and the pins are bent and cut. The bent tips are pointed radially and driven into the styloid with a small bone tamp, capturing the wire (**TECH FIG 4B**).
- Alternatively, after placing the pins through the ulnar styloid, a 2-0 suture anchor can be placed in the ulnar neck and the sutures passed in opposite directions around the styloid. The limbs are tied down to the medial ulnar shaft, and the pins are bent and cut as previously discussed (**TECH FIG 4C**).
- Plate and screw construct may also be used for buttress effect, but implant prominence must be considered (**TECH FIG 4D**).
- Headless compression screw fixation is advocated by some. We have noted frequent failure and malreduction with this technique. If screw fixation is used, bicortical fixation is recommended (**TECH FIG 4E**).
- If the DRUJ is still unstable, proceed with radioulnar transfixation pinning.
- Wound closure, sterile dressings, and long posterior splint are applied.

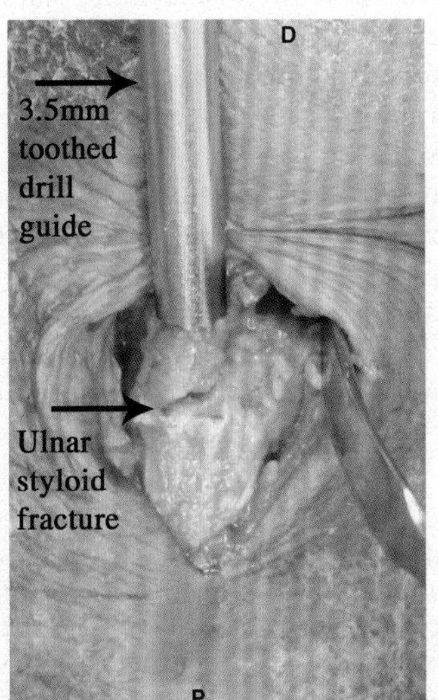

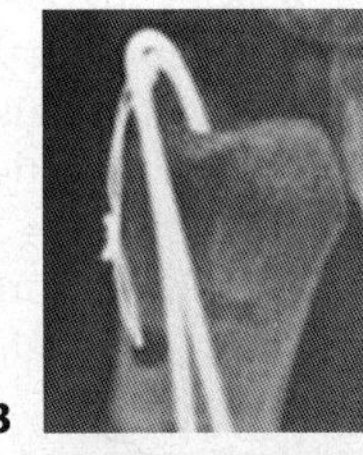

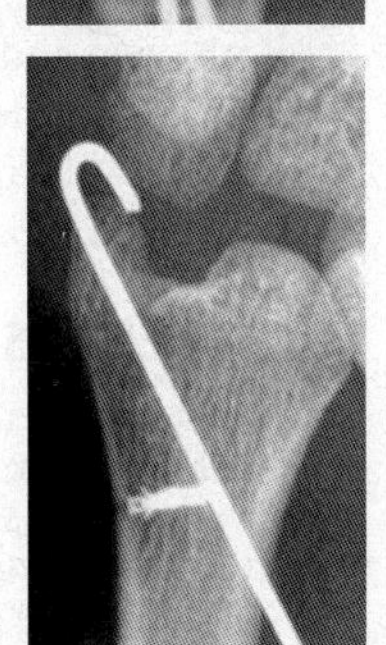

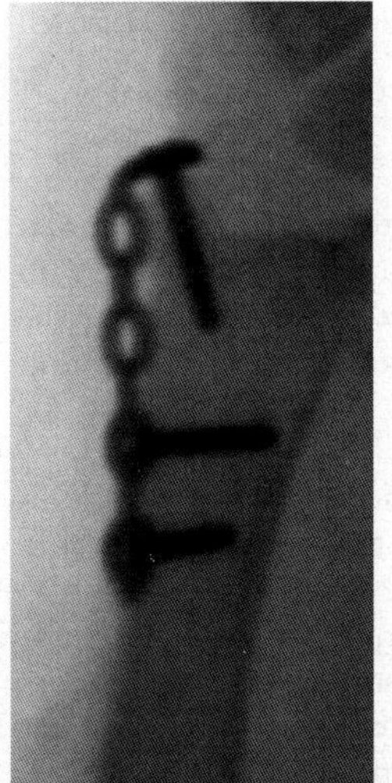

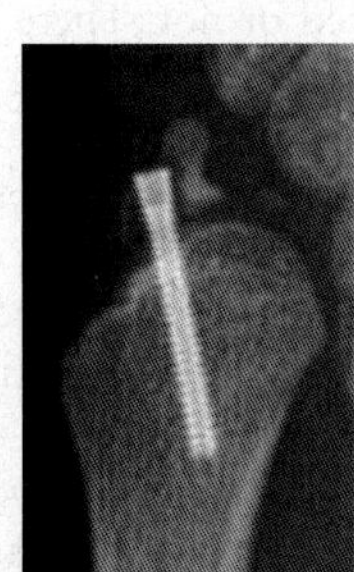

TECH FIG 4 • Ulnar styloid fracture fixation. **A.** The distal ulna is exposed at the ulnar styloid and a 3.5-mm drill guide is used to reduce the fracture and to pass K-wires. **B.** Anteroposterior (AP) radiograph of a tension band open reduction internal fixation (ORIF). **C.** Tension band construct with a suture anchor. **D.** ORIF with plate and screw construct. **E.** Loss of fixation using headless compression screw.

PEARLS AND PITFALLS

Radius is stabilized and DRUJ is stable.	■ Confirm reduction with intraoperative radiographs. Immobilize forearm in neutral to slight supination in long-arm cast or splint in neutral for 2–4 weeks to allow for TFCC healing.
Radius is anatomically reduced and DRUJ is irreducible.	■ Proceed with open reduction to removed interposed soft tissue structures and open repair of TFCC (with radioulnar pinning).
Radius is anatomically reduced and DRUJ is grossly unstable.	■ Proceed with radioulnar pinning (4–6 weeks) verses supination splinting for 6 weeks. ■ Consideration can be giving to open verses arthroscopic TFCC repair (with radioulnar pinning).
Follow-up examination	■ Confirm at each follow-up DRUJ reduction radiographically. If there is any question of subluxation, evaluate axial imaging with CT scan.

POSTOPERATIVE CARE

- *Stable internal fixation of the radius and stable DRUJ*
  - Long-arm splint with forearm in neutral for 2 weeks.
  - A retrospective review of patients with a stable DRUJ following radial fixation found that immobilization in supination for 4 weeks has no advantage over immobilization in neutral for a shorter time.[16]
- *Internal fixation of radius and DRUJ stabilization (pinning or open TFCC repair)*
  - Long-arm splint with forearm in neutral to slight supination for 4 to 6 weeks.
  - If the radius and ulna have been pinned together, the patient is seen every 2 to 3 weeks to evaluate pin sites when they are left out of the skin.
  - Full range of motion of the shoulder as allowed with long-arm immobilization. At minimum, patients are encouraged to do shoulder pendulum exercises. Finger range of motion is encouraged as well.
  - At each postoperative visit, radiographs must confirm reduction of the DRUJ. If there is any concern that the DRUJ is not reduced, CT scan is obtained.
  - Pins are removed at 4–6 weeks. Following pin removal, pronosupination exercises are encouraged. Supervised therapy is recommended.

OUTCOMES

- A study of 17 patients with near-anatomically reduced radial shaft fractures, 10 without a DRUJ dislocation and 7 with a DRUJ dislocation, found comparable results whether the DRUJ was injured or not. There was an average follow-up of 19 years, and neither pinning of the radius to ulna nor TFCC repair was performed.[19]
  - Specifically, no significant differences in the Mayo Modified Wrist Score or Disabilities of the Arm, Shoulder, and Hand questionnaire were found. No differences in DRUJ laxity compared to the contralateral wrist were present.[16]
- Pinning the radius to the ulna in a position of DRUJ reduction is the most commonly reported procedure in larger cases series, with excellent results reported.[10,17]
  - A recent study evaluated 40 patients who had a single 1.2- or 1.6-mm smooth stainless steel pin placed proximal to the sigmoid notch with the forearm in supination for 6 weeks for DRUJ instability after radial fixation. At 6.8-year follow-up, none of these patients required more DRUJ surgery or had persistent DRUJ instability.[10]
- Instability with an associated ulnar styloid fracture is less frequent in Galleazi injuries. Maintenance of stability has been reported with operative fixation of the ulnar styloid base.[16] Screw or tension band fixation is commonly performed.
- Classically, Mikić[12] defined an excellent result as radius union, perfect alignment, no loss of length, no subluxation of the DRUJ, and no limitation of supination or pronation. Using this criteria, Rettig and Raskin[17] reported 95% excellent results in 40 Galeazzi fracture-dislocations. Twenty-seven patients demonstrated DRUJ stability after radial fixation only. Ten patients demonstrated DRUJ instability and were treated with radioulnar pinning with two 1.6-mm smooth stainless steel pins only. Three patients had irreducible DRUJs and required open reduction, TFCC repair, and pinning of the DRUJ. None of the patients treated for an unstable or irreducible DRUJ had a poor result.
- Loss of pronosupination and wrist flexion are commonly reported, although the amount reported varies significantly in published literature.

COMPLICATIONS

- Specific to Galeazzi fracture-dislocations, subluxation or dislocation of the DRUJ can occur. This is most commonly a result of nonanatomic alignment of the radius.
- Pin site infection and pin breakage of radioulnar transfixation pins can also occur.
- As with all forearm fractures, malunion and nonunion can occur, although rare with appropriately applied compression plating.
- Both open and arthroscopic TFCC repair are associated with dorsal ulnar nerve cutaneous branch postoperative neuropathy. Notably, there is some evidence that the risk is increased with open repair.[1]

REFERENCES

1. Anderson ML, Larson AN, Moran SL, et al. Clinical comparison of arthroscopic versus open repair of triangular fibrocartilage complex tears. J Hand Surg Am 2008;33(5):675–682.
2. Cetti NE. An unusual cause of blocked reduction of the Galeazzi injury. Injury 1977;9(1):59–61.
3. Garcia-Elias M, Hagert E. Surgical approaches to the distal radioulnar joint. Hand Clin 2010;26(4):477–483.
4. Giannoulis FS, Sotereanos DG. Galeazzi fractures and dislocations. Hand Clin 2007;23(2):153–163.
5. Hagert E, Hagert CG. Understanding stability of the distal radioulnar joint through an understanding of its anatomy. Hand Clin 2010;26(4):459–466.

6. Henry AK. Extensile Exposure, ed 2. Baltimore: Williams & Wilkins, 1970.
7. Hughston JC. Fracture of the distal radial shaft; mistakes in management. J Bone Joint Surg Am 1957;39-A(2):249–264.
8. Jupiter JB. Commentary: the effect of ulnar styloid fractures on patient-rated outcomes after volar locking plating of distal radius fractures. J Hand Surg Am 2009;34(9):1603–1604.
9. Kleinman WB. Repairs of chronic peripheral tears/avulsions of the triangular fibrocartilage. In: Blair WF, ed. Techniques in Hand Surgery. Baltimore: Williams & Wilkins, 1996.
10. Korompilias AV, Lykissas MG, Kostas-Agnantis IP, et al. Distal radioulnar joint instability (Galeazzi type injury) after internal fixation in relation to the radius fracture pattern. J Hand Surg Am 2011;36(5):847–852.
11. Lo IK, MacDermid JC, Bennett JD, et al. The radioulnar ratio: a new method of quantifying distal radioulnar joint subluxation. J Hand Surg Am 2001;26(2):236–243.
12. Mikić ZD. Galeazzi fracture-dislocations. J Bone Joint Surg Am 1975;57(8):1071–1080.
13. Moore TM, Klein JP, Patzakis MJ, et al. Results of compression-plating of closed Galeazzi fractures. J Bone Joint Surg Am 1985;67(7):1015–1021.
14. Moritomo H. The distal interosseous membrane: current concepts in wrist anatomy and biomechanics. J Hand Surg Am 2012;37(7):1501–1507.
15. Noda K, Goto A, Murase T, et al. Interosseous membrane of the forearm: an anatomical study of ligament attachment locations. J Hand Surg Am 2009;34(3):415–422.
16. Park MJ, Pappas N, Steinberg DR, et al. Immobilization in supination versus neutral following surgical treatment of Galeazzi fracture-dislocations in adults: case series. J Hand Surg Am 2012;37(3):528–531.
17. Rettig ME, Raskin KB. Galeazzi fracture-dislocation: a new treatment-oriented classification. J Hand Surg Am 2001;26(2):228–235.
18. Thomas BP, Sreekanth R. Distal radioulnar joint injuries. Indian J Orthop 2012;46(5):493–504.
19. van Duijvenbode DC, Guitton TG, Raaymakers EL, et al. Long-term outcome of isolated diaphyseal radius fractures with and without dislocation of the distal radioulnar joint. J Hand Surg Am 2012;37(3):523–527.
20. Watanabe H, Berger RA, Berglund LJ, et al. Contribution of the interosseous membrane to the distal radioulnar joint constraint. J Hand Surg Am 2005;30(6):1164–1171.

27

CHAPTER

K-Wire Fixation of Distal Radius Fractures with and without External Fixation

Christopher Doumas, Owen L. Ala, and David J. Bozentka

DEFINITION

- Distal radius fractures occur at the distal end of the bone, originating in the metaphyseal region and often extending to the radiocarpal and distal radioulnar joints (DRUJ).
- Distal radius fractures can be classified as stable or unstable and extra- or intra-articular to assist in treatment decisions.
- Fractures may angulate dorsally or volarly and may have significant comminution depending on the energy of the injury and the quality of the bone.
- Percutaneous pins or K-wires, typically 0.062 or 0.045 inches, can be used for treatment of simple intra-articular or extra-articular fractures with mild comminution and no osteoporosis.
- Percutaneous pins can aid reduction and stabilize the fragments in a minimally invasive manner.
- Percutaneous pins can support the subchondral area of the distal radius and maintain the articular reduction in highly comminuted fractures, which is useful when combined with other fixation methods.
- Smooth percutaneous pins may also be placed across the physis to maintain a reduction in children with minimal risk of a growth arrest.
- Highly comminuted fractures are more difficult to fix rigidly and often require external and/or internal fixation to maintain alignment during healing.
- External fixators can be hinged or static and may or may not bridge the wrist joint.
- K-wire fixation of extra-articular and simple intra-articular fractures has received more support over the last few years after several prospective randomized trials comparing K-wire fixation to volar plating has shown no difference in outcome at 1 year.

ANATOMY

- The distal radius consists of three articular surfaces: the scaphoid fossa, the lunate fossa, and the sigmoid notch.
- Ligamentotaxis aids in the reduction of intra-articular and comminuted fractures.
  - Volar extrinsic ligamentous attachments include the radioscaphocapitate, long radiolunate, and short radiolunate ligaments.
  - Dorsal extrinsic ligamentous attachments include the radiotriquetral ligament.
- Dorsal and radial to the second metacarpal lie the first dorsal interosseous muscle and the terminal branches of the radial sensory nerve.
- The distal radial sensory nerve branches lie superficial to the distal radius and should be protected during dissection and pin placement.
- The radial sensory nerve emerges between the brachioradialis and the extensor carpi radialis longus (ECRL) muscle bellies (**FIG 1**).
- The terminal branches of the lateral antebrachial cutaneous nerve lie superficial to the forearm fascia at the radial wrist.
- There is a bare spot of bone between the first and second dorsal compartments in the region of the radial styloid.
- The brachioradialis tendon inserts onto the radial styloid deep to the first dorsal compartment.
- The ECRL and the extensor carpi radialis brevis (ECRB) lie dorsal to the brachioradialis in the second dorsal compartment.
- Lister tubercle is dorsal, with the extensor pollicis longus (EPL) tendon on its ulnar side, in the third dorsal compartment.

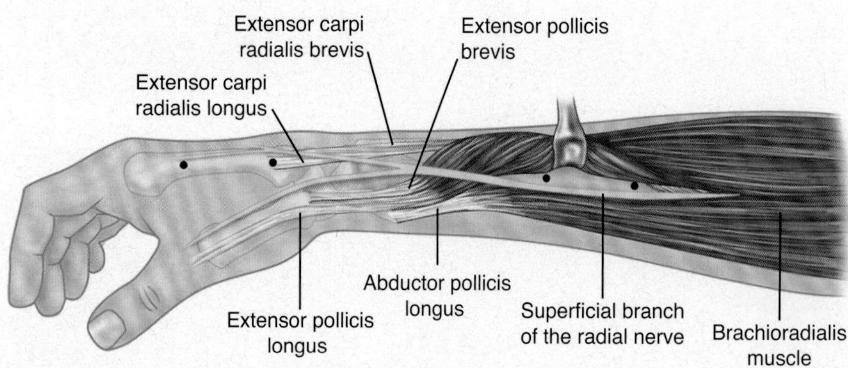

FIG 1 • Anatomy surrounding the radial sensory nerve branch in the forearm.

- The extensor digitorum communis tendons lie over the dorsal ulnar half of the distal radius in the fourth dorsal compartment.
- The extensor digiti minimi lies over the DRUJ in the fifth dorsal compartment.

PATHOGENESIS

- Distal radius fractures are the most common fractures of the upper extremity in adults, representing about 20% of all fractures seen in the emergency room.[22]
- Mechanism of injury typically is a fall on an outstretched hand with axial loading, but other common histories include motor vehicle accidents or pathologic fractures.
- Higher energy injuries cause increased comminution, angulation, and displacement.
- Osteoporosis, tumors, and metabolic bone diseases are risk factors for sustaining pathologic distal radius fractures.
- In children, fractures typically occur along the physis due to its relative weakness compared to the surrounding ligaments.

NATURAL HISTORY

- Distal radius fractures needing no reduction and those that are stable after reduction typically recover functional range of motion with minimal long-term sequelae.
- Three parameters that affect outcome include articular congruity, angulation, and shortening.[21,26]
  - Two millimeters or more of articular surface incongruity of the distal radius can lead to degenerative changes, pain and stiffness.
  - Dorsal angulation can lead to decreased range of motion and increased load transfer to the ulna.
  - Radial shortening can lead to decreased range of motion, pain, and ulnar impaction of the carpus.

PATIENT HISTORY AND PHYSICAL FINDINGS

- The history of a fall on an outstretched hand is the most common presentation for a patient with a distal radius fracture.
- Motor vehicle or motorcycle accidents and osteoporosis account for most comminuted fractures.
- It may be clinically indicated to implement a workup for osteoporosis.
- Pain, tenderness, swelling, crepitus, deformity, ecchymosis, and decreased range of motion at the wrist are typical symptoms and warrant radiographic evaluation.
- Physical examination should include the following:
  - Inspection: Evaluate the integrity of the skin, cascade of the digits, direction of displacement, and presence of any swelling.
  - Identify points of maximal tenderness to differentiate between distal radius injuries and carpal or ligamentous injuries.
  - Palpate specific areas of the wrist and hand to differentiate distal intra-articular, DRUJ, and carpal injuries.
  - Two-point discrimination: Higher than normal (5 mm) results in the form of progressive neurologic deficit may signify an acute carpal tunnel syndrome or ulnar neuropathy.
  - Passive finger stretch test to assist with diagnosis of compartment syndrome.
  - EPL tendon function should be evaluated.
    - EPL assessment: Assess the resting position of the thumb interphalangeal joint and the patient's ability to lift the thumb off of a flat surface to determine the continuity of the EPL tendon.
  - Palpation of forearm and elbow to assess for concomitant injury proximally
  - The DRUJ must be assessed for displacement and instability.
  - The bony anatomy must be carefully evaluated to avoid missing minimally displaced fractures, which may displace without treatment.
  - Skin should be assessed to avoid missing an open fracture.
  - Swelling should be monitored to allow for early diagnosis of compartment syndrome.
  - Sensory examination should be monitored for progressive changes, which may represent acute carpal tunnel syndrome.

IMAGING AND OTHER DIAGNOSTIC STUDIES

- Radiographic evaluation should include posteroanterior (PA), lateral, and oblique views to assess displacement, angulation, comminution, and intra-articular involvement and allow for radiologic measurements.[18,22] Often, comparison x-rays of the uninjured wrist are helpful.
  - Lateral articular (volar) tilt is the angle between the radial shaft and a tangential line parallel to the articular margin as seen on the lateral view (**FIG 2A**). The normal angle is 11 degrees.
  - Radial inclination, measured on the PA view (**FIG 2B**), is the angle between a line perpendicular to the shaft of the radius at the ulnar articular margin and the tangential line along the radial styloid to the ulnar articular margin. The normal angle is 22 degrees.
  - Ulnar variance, also measured on the PA view (see **FIG 2B**), is the distance between the radial and ulnar articular surfaces. Ulnar variance is compared to the contralateral side.

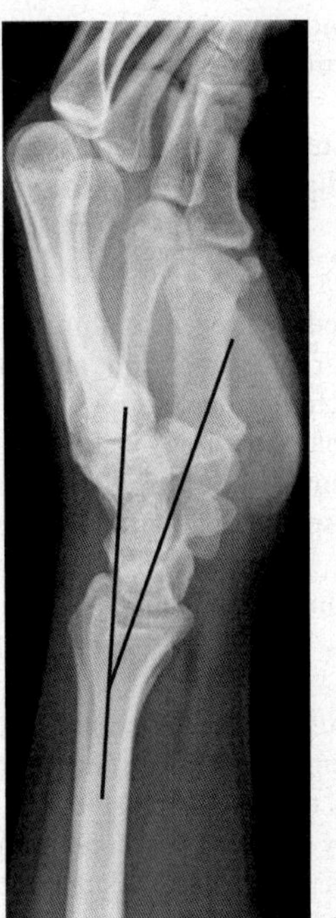

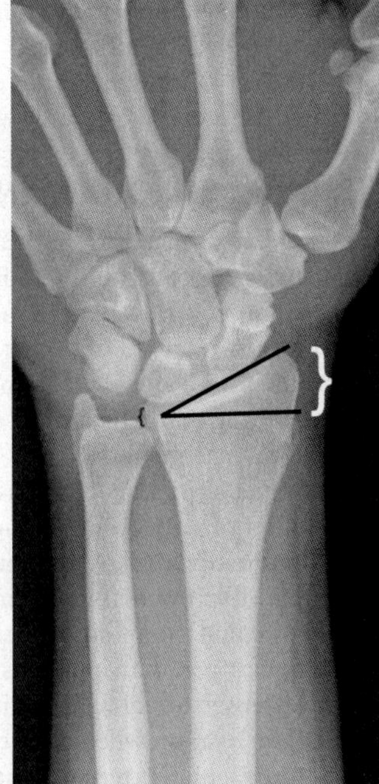

FIG 2 • A. Lateral radiograph of the wrist demonstrating volar tilt (*black lines*). **B.** PA radiograph demonstrating radial inclination (*black lines*), ulnar variance (*red bracket*), and radial height (*white bracket*).

- Traction radiographs help assess intra-articular involvement, intercarpal ligamentous injury, and potential fracture reduction through ligamentotaxis.
- Computed tomography (CT) scans are useful in fully elucidating the anatomy of the fracture, including impaction, comminution, and size of the fragments.
  - CT scans often significantly alter the original treatment plan.[14]
- Magnetic resonance imaging (MRI) is rarely performed acutely but can diagnose concomitant ligamentous injuries, triangular fibrocartilage complex injuries, and occult carpal fractures.

DIFFERENTIAL DIAGNOSIS

- Bony contusion
- Radiocarpal dislocation
- Scaphoid or other carpal fracture
- Perilunate or lunate fracture-dislocation
- Distal ulnar fracture
- Wrist ligament or triangular fibrocartilage complex injury
- DRUJ injury

NONOPERATIVE MANAGEMENT

- Nonoperative treatment consists of splinting or casting for stable fracture patterns using a three-point mold.
- Fractures amenable to nonoperative treatment include fractures that are stable after reduction with minimal metaphyseal comminution, shortening, angulation, and displacement.
  - Evaluation for secondary displacement weekly for 2 to 3 weeks is critical as the swelling subsides.
- Unstable patterns will displace if not surgically stabilized.
  - There is little role for nonoperative treatment in highly comminuted fractures.
- The physiologic age, medical comorbidities, and functional level of the patient should be considered in determining the need for surgical treatment.
- Early range of motion of the nonimmobilized joints is essential in the nonoperative treatment of all fractures near the wrist to prevent contracture.
  - The cast or splint must not extend past the metacarpophalangeal joints so as to allow digital motion.

SURGICAL MANAGEMENT

- Surgical treatments are indicated to prevent malunion and improve pain control, function, range of motion, and to decrease the time of return to function.
- Surgery is reserved for unstable fractures, including displaced, intra-articular, comminuted, or severely angulated injuries and fractures that displace following attempted closed management.
- Percutaneous pinning can assist in obtaining and maintaining reduction of displaced fractures with limited comminution in a minimally invasive manner.
- External fixators maintain radius length but cannot always control angulation and displacement; therefore, supplementation with percutaneous pins is typically performed.[2]
- Conversely, external fixators may augment percutaneous pins and plate fixation when extensive comminution is present.
  - Supplemental external fixation should be considered for fractures with comminution of over 50% of the diameter of the radius on a lateral view or when significant volar cortical comminution is present.
- External fixation may be used as a neutralization device because the distraction forces decrease soon after fracture reduction.
- External fixators also are useful for "damage control orthopaedics" to temporarily stabilize wrist fractures, especially for complex, combined, open injuries.
- For nonbridging external fixation, there must be at least 1 cm of volar cortex intact and adequate fragment sizes to allow proper pin placement.
- A relative contraindication to pin fixation with or without external fixation is a volar shear injury, which should be reduced and stabilized using a volar plate and screws.

Preoperative Planning

- All radiographs should be reviewed before surgery and brought into the operating room.
- Analysis of the pattern and presumed stability of the fracture fragments determines whether percutaneous fixation, with or without external fixation, is suitable.
- For intra-articular fractures, the specific fragments to be reduced and fixed must be identified preoperatively to avoid incomplete reduction of the joint surface.
- The surgeon must be prepared to change his or her management decision intraoperatively if the fracture behavior is different from anticipated. A variety of fixation devices should be available in the operating room.

Positioning

- The patient is positioned supine on the operating table with a radiolucent arm board.
- A tourniquet is applied near the axilla with the splint still in place (**FIG 3**).
- Fluoroscopy should be used for confirmation of reduction and fixation throughout the procedure.
- There must be enough range of motion of the shoulder and elbow to allow standard anteroposterior (AP), lateral, and oblique images.

Approach

- Various approaches can be used in the application of external fixators and the insertion of percutaneous pins.
- Distal external fixator half-pins may be placed directly into the second metacarpal or into other carpal bones (for injuries

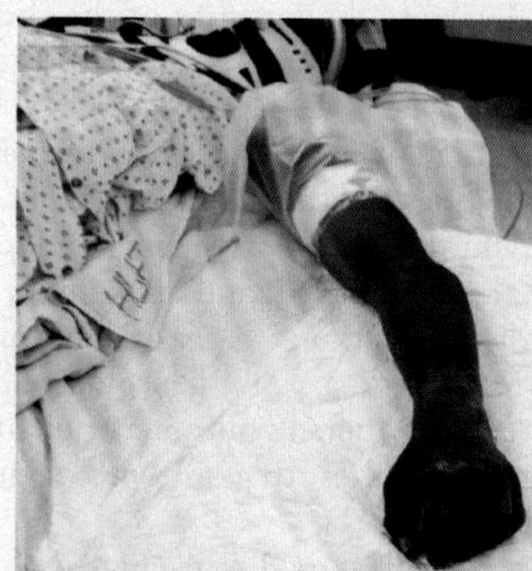

FIG 3 • Positioning of patient supine on the hand table with tourniquet in place.

including the second metacarpal). Wires and half-pins from nonbridging fixators may be placed in the distal radius itself.

- Percutaneous pins can be inserted through the radial styloid between the first and second dorsal compartments, through Lister tubercle, through the interval between the fourth and fifth dorsal compartments, and across the DRUJ (**FIG 4**).
  - Caution is taken to avoid skewering tendons and nerves and to avoid penetrating the articular surface.

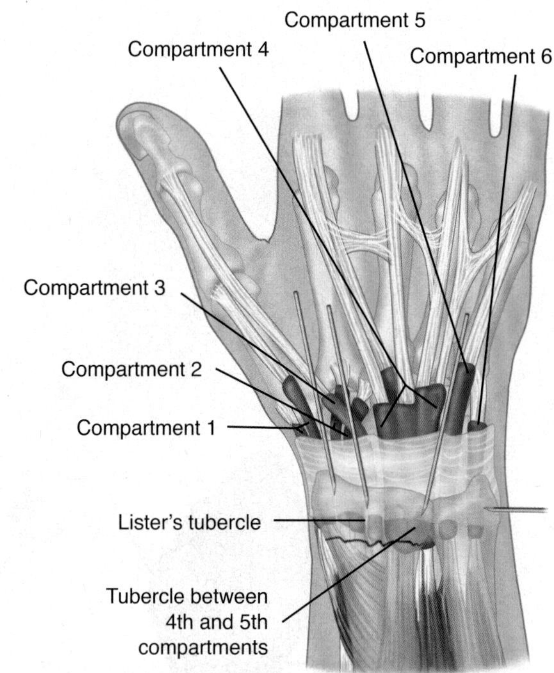

FIG 4 • Areas for K-wire insertion at the distal radius.

TECHNIQUES

Closed Reduction of a Distal Radius Fracture

- Closed reduction should be performed before fixation using a combination of distraction and palmar translation of the distal radius fragment and carpus.[1]
- Use of a padded bump or towel roll will aid in the reduction (**TECH FIG 1**).
- Overdistraction will cause increased dorsal angulation due to the intact short, stout volar ligaments.[1]
- Excessive palmar flexion of the wrist can restore volar tilt but leads to an increased incidence of stiffness and carpal tunnel syndrome.[7,8]
- Overdistraction can be assessed by measuring the carpal height index, measuring the radioscaphoid and midcarpal joint spaces, checking full finger flexion into the palm, or evaluating index finger extrinsic extensor tightness.[9]

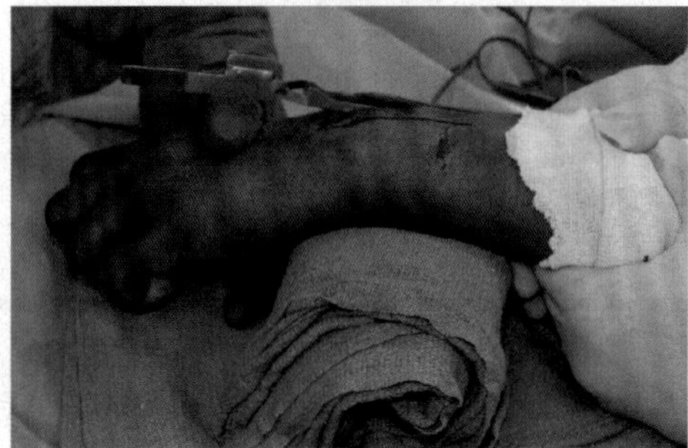

TECH FIG 1 • Closed reduction over a towel bump using traction and palmar translation.

Kapandji Technique for Percutaneous Pinning

- Closed reduction is obtained using a bump, and the reduction is confirmed using fluoroscopy.
- This technique should be employed in patients younger than 55 years of age with minimal comminution. It should not be used in osteoporotic, elderly patients or those with comminution secondary to a higher risk of reduction loss. External fixation should be used to supplement pinning in these patient populations.[27]
- An incision is made radially and a 0.062-inch pin is manually inserted into the fracture site, taking care to protect the sensory nerve branches and the first dorsal compartment tendons (**TECH FIG 2A**).
  - The pin is angled distally, levering the bone back into its normal position and restoring the radial inclination (**TECH FIG 2B**). The pin is advanced proximally and ulnarly through the far cortex using power. This pin act as a buttress to maintain radial inclination (**TECH FIG 2C**).
- A second incision is placed dorsally, and a second pin is manually inserted into the fracture (**TECH FIG 2D**).
  - The pin is angled distally, levering the bone back into its normal position and restoring the volar tilt (**TECH FIG 2E**). This pin act as a buttress to maintain volar tilt (**TECH FIG 2F**).
- Using the modified technique, a third pin is inserted retrograde using power, starting at the radial styloid and proceeding into the ulnar cortex of the radius, proximal to the fracture line.
- The pins are buried and cut just below the skin, and the skin is sutured.
  - Alternatively, the pins may be bent using two needle drivers and left outside the skin.
- The pins are then cut and covered with pin caps or antibiotic gauze.
- A sterile dressing is applied, followed by a splint.

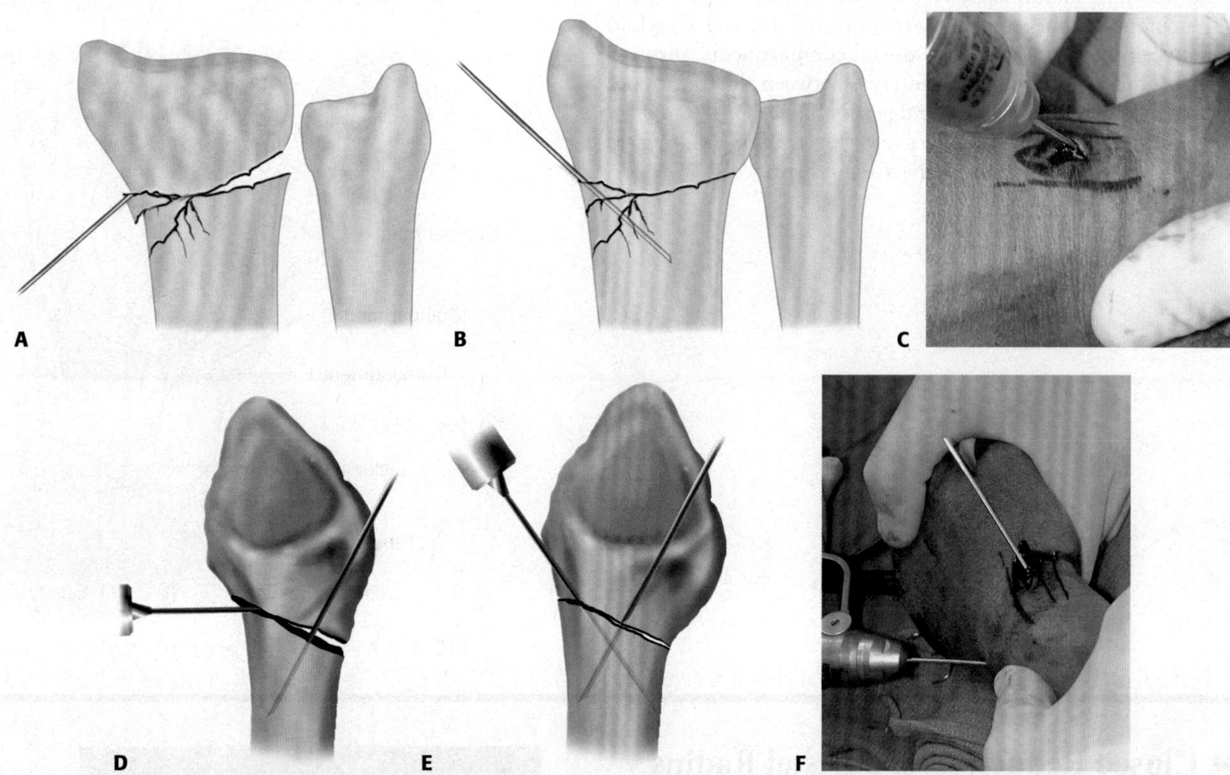

TECH FIG 2 • A. An incision is made over the radial styloid, and a K-wire is manually inserted into the fracture site. **B.** The wire is levered distally to correct the radial inclination. **C.** The wire is advanced proximally, using power, into cortical bone. **D.** An incision is made over Lister tubercle, and a wire is inserted into the fracture site. **E,F.** The wire is levered distally to correct the dorsal angulation and advanced proximally using power into cortical bone.

Author's Preferred Technique for Percutaneous Pinning

- Closed reduction is obtained using a bump, and the reduction is confirmed using fluoroscopy (**TECH FIG 3A,B**).
- A small incision is placed over the bare spot on the radial styloid between the first and second dorsal compartments (**TECH FIG 3C**).

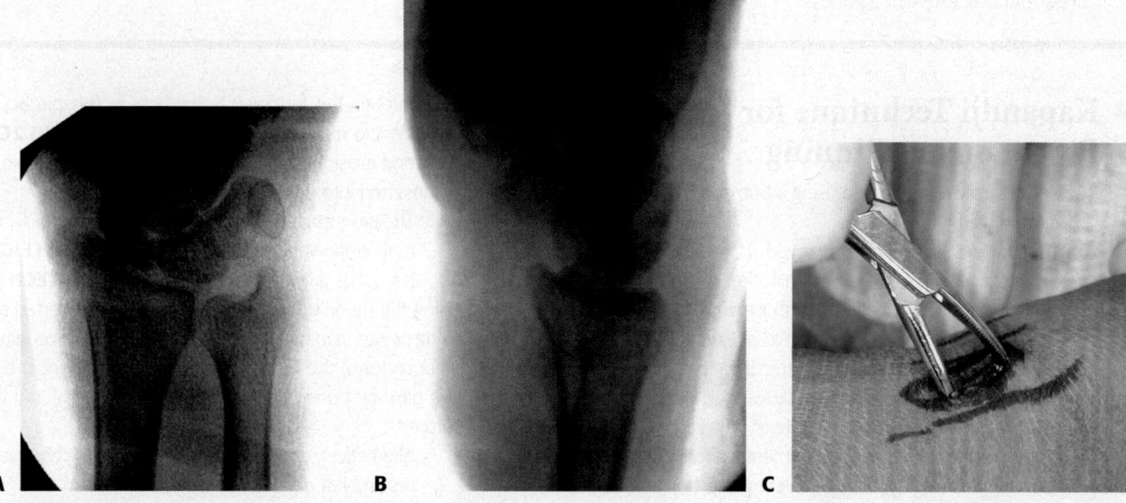

TECH FIG 3 • A,B. PA and lateral views demonstrating reduction of distal radius fracture. **C.** The incision is made over the radial styloid. *(continued)*

- Two 0.062-inch smooth K-wires are placed retrograde from the radial styloid across the reduced fracture, engaging the opposite cortex in a divergent fashion (**TECH FIG 3D,E**).
- A small incision is placed over the interval between the fourth and fifth dorsal compartments.
- One or two K-wires are placed retrograde from the dorsoulnar corner of the distal radius across the reduced fracture, engaging the opposite cortex in a divergent fashion (**TECH FIG 3F–H**).
- The pins are cut just beneath the skin, which is closed with a 5-0 nylon suture.
- Alternatively, the pins are bent and cut and left outside the skin (**TECH FIG 3I**).
- A dressing and splint are then applied.

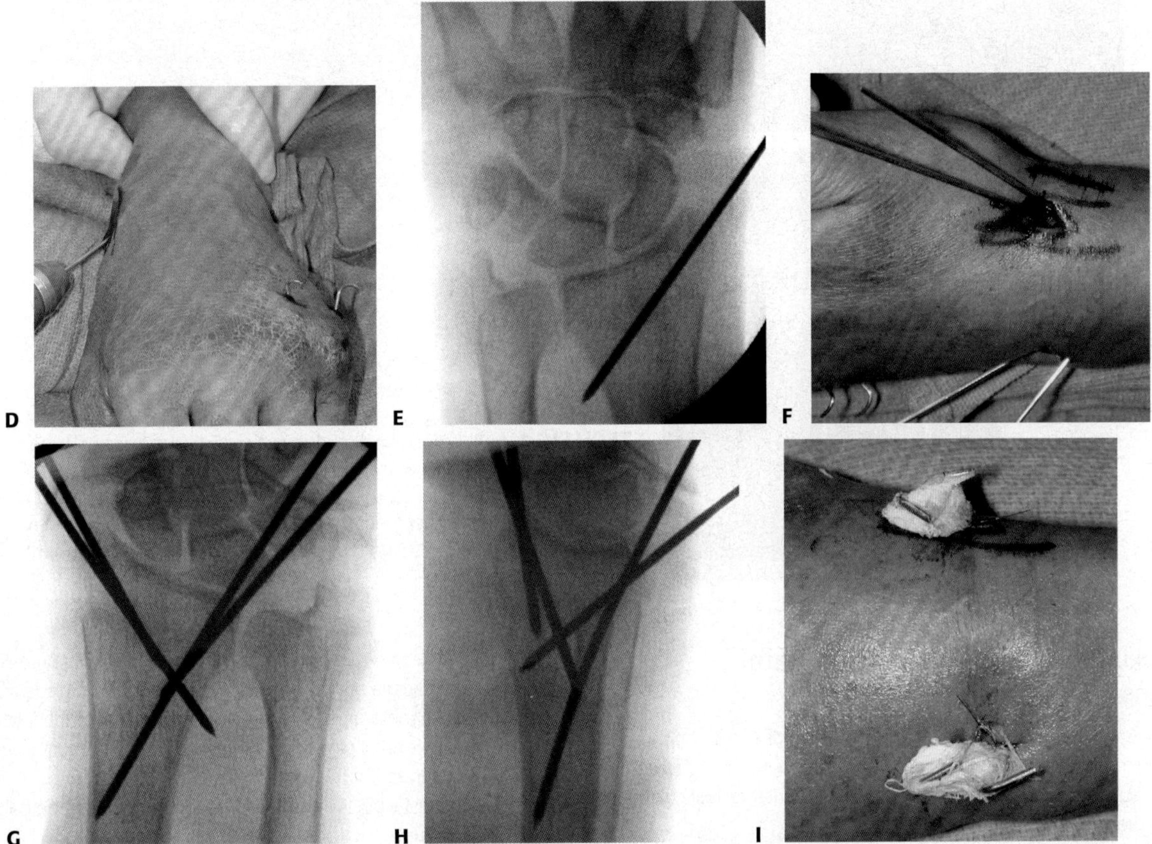

TECH FIG 3 • *(continued)* **D.** A pin is inserted retrograde into the radial styloid. **E.** PA radiograph demonstrating the course of the radial styloid wire. **F.** Two radial styloid wires and two dorsoulnar wires are in place. **G.** PA view showing fixation and the path of the wires. **H.** Lateral view showing fixation and path of wires. **I.** Pins are bent, cut, and covered above the skin.

Bridging External Fixator Application

Distal Pin Placement

- A 3-cm incision is made over the dorsal index metacarpal, exposing the proximal two-thirds.
- The distal sensory nerve branches are retracted, and the first dorsal interosseous muscle is elevated from the metacarpal to identify the insertion of the ECRL (**TECH FIG 4A**).
- The index metacarpophalangeal joint is flexed to protect the sagittal band and first dorsal interosseous aponeurosis.
- The metacarpal drill guide is placed on the radial base of the index metacarpal at the flare of the metaphysis. Partially threaded 3- to 4-mm pins are used, with or without predrilling.
- A long-threaded pin is placed through the index and long metacarpal bases, obtaining three cortices of fixation.
- Care is taken not to enter the carpometacarpal joint.
- The double drill guide is then placed over the first pin, and the distal short-threaded pin is placed through both cortices of the index metacarpal shaft (**TECH FIG 4B,C**).
- Fluoroscopy confirms placement and length of the pins.

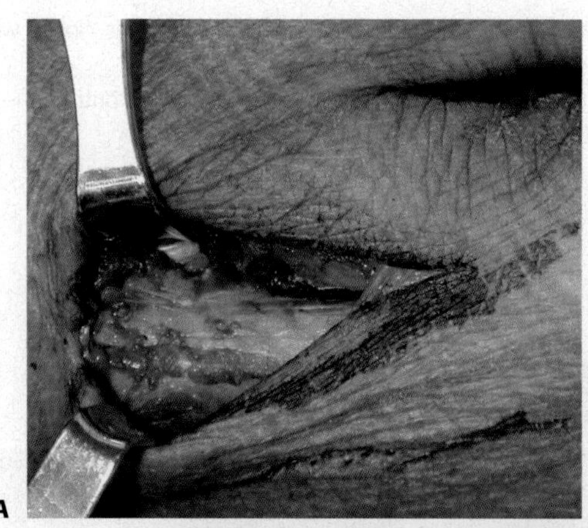

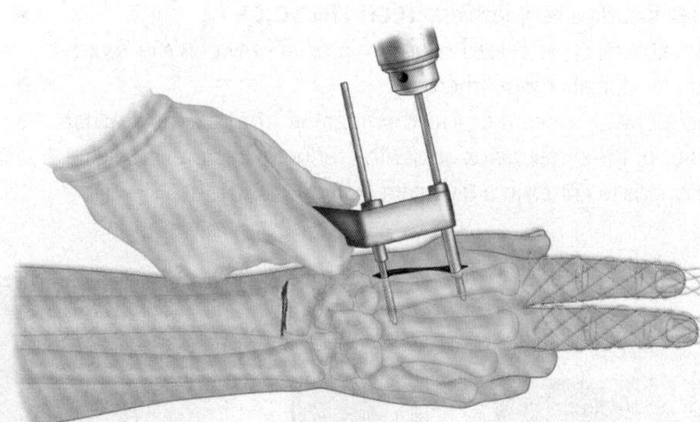

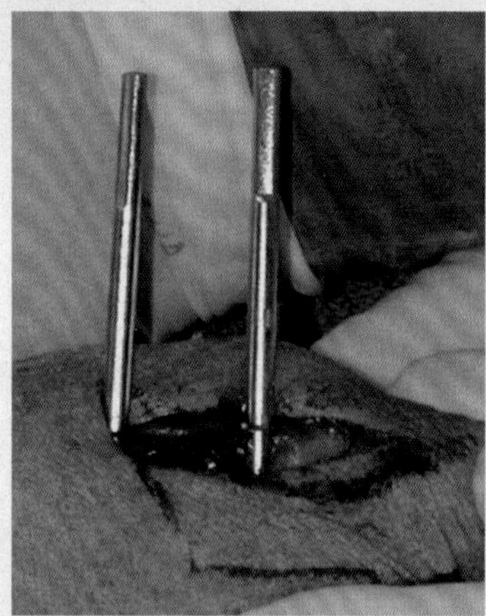

TECH FIG 4 • **A.** An incision is made over the second metacarpal base, with reflection of the first dorsal interosseous muscle and radial sensory nerve terminal branches. (The thumb is at the top of the photograph.) **B.** Diagram showing placement of fixator pins in the shaft of the index and the base of the index and long metacarpals. **C.** Parallel placement of two metacarpal pins.

Proximal Pin Placement and Frame Construction

- A 4- to 5-cm incision is made over the radial forearm, proximal to the first dorsal compartment musculature, through skin and subcutaneous tissue, avoiding the lateral antebrachial cutaneous nerve branches.
- The fascia overlying the interval between the brachioradialis and the ECRL is divided, and the radial sensory nerve is identified and retracted (**TECH FIG 5A**).
  - The interval between the ECRL and ECRB may also be used to avoid the radial sensory branch.
- The double drill guide is placed onto the diaphysis of the radius between the brachioradialis and the radial wrist extensors or between the ECRL and ECRB (**TECH FIG 5B**).
- Threaded 3- to 4-mm pins are placed, with or without predrilling.
  - The fracture should be reduced, and the pins placed parallel to the metacarpal pins to facilitate alignment of the fracture.
  - The proximal pin should be placed bicortically, just distal to the tendon of the pronator teres.
  - The distal pin is then drilled bicortically through the double drill guide.
- Pin placement is confirmed using fluoroscopy.
- The incisions are closed using nylon suture, ensuring no tension is on the skin at the pin sites.
- Clamps and rods or adjustable fixators may then be applied to the pins to achieve and maintain final reduction (**TECH FIG 5C**).
- Supplementary K-wire fixation is added before or after external fixation (**TECH FIG 5D**).

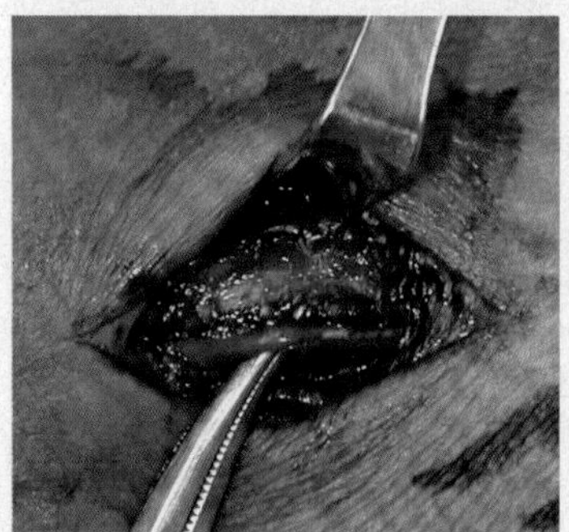

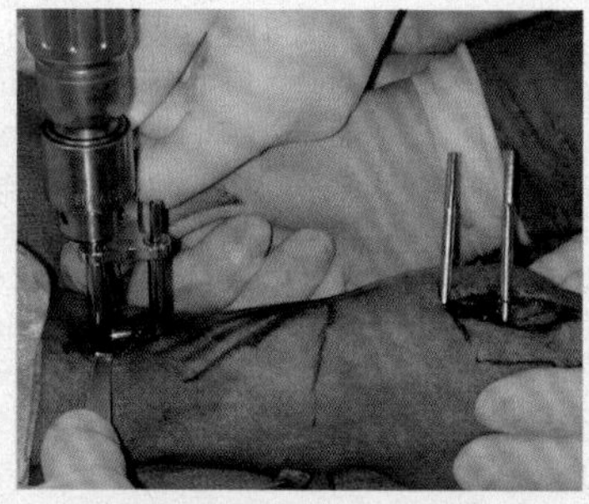

TECH FIG 5 • **A.** Incision over the radial forearm demonstrating the radial sensory nerve branch deep to the fascia. (The hand is to the right.) **B.** The double drill guide is placed onto the radius. *(continued)*

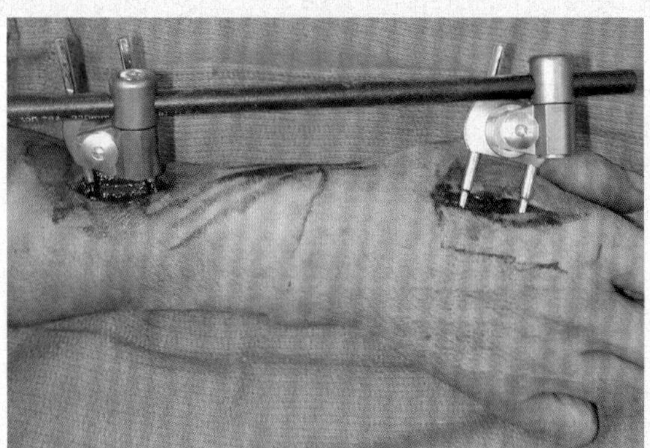

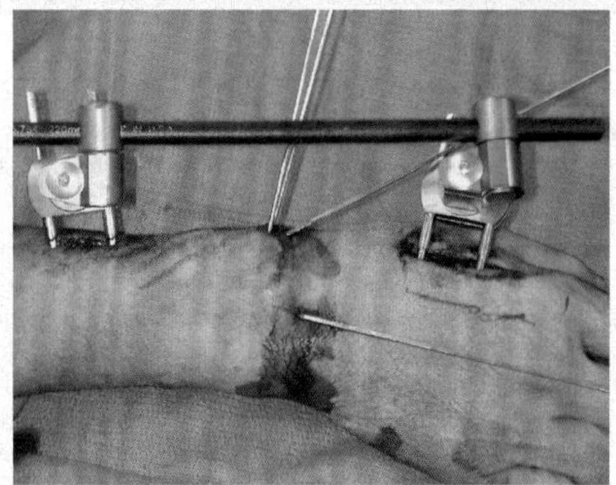

TECH FIG 5 • *(continued)* **C.** Final reduction is maintained by the addition of clamps and rods. **D.** K-wires are used for supplemental fixation when necessary.

Nonbridging External Fixator Application

- Fracture reduction can be performed after insertion of the distal pins, allowing direct control of the distal fragment.
- The wrist is placed for a lateral fluoroscopic view, and a marker is used to determine the level of incision halfway between the radiocarpal joint and the fracture. A short transverse skin incision is made just proximal to the radiocarpal joint.
- A longitudinal incision is then made through the retinaculum on either side of Lister tubercle, and the EPL is protected.
- The first distal pin is drilled using power, parallel to the radiocarpal joint on the lateral view, halfway between the fracture and the joint surface (**TECH FIG 6A**).
- The second distal pin is placed between the second and third dorsal compartments, between the radial wrist extensors and the EPL tendon.
- This pin should be placed parallel to the first pin in both planes, with the starting point halfway between the radiocarpal joint and the fracture.
- The two proximal radius pins are placed using the technique described for placement of a bridging external fixator.
- The incisions are closed, after which the clamps are applied but not tightened.
- Reduction is achieved by manipulation of the distal pins and clamps.
  - Pushing the pins in the dorsal/volar plane corrects dorsal tilt.
  - Adjusting the pin clamp can correct radial inclination.
- Reduction is confirmed using fluoroscopy, and the clamps are tightened (**TECH FIG 6B**).

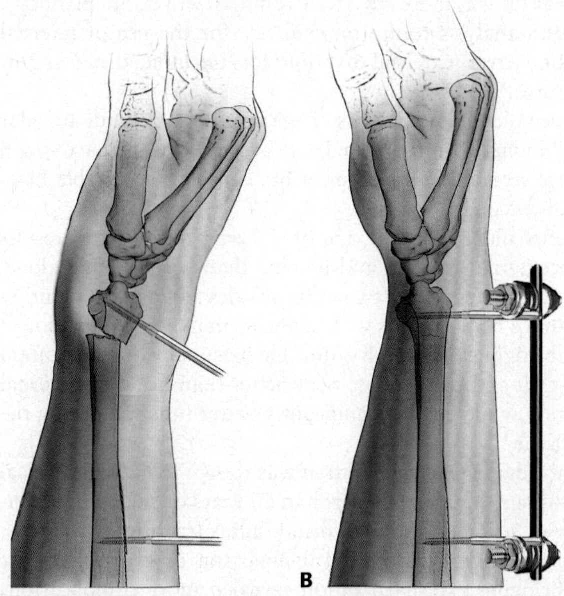

TECH FIG 6 • **A.** Distal pin placement. **B.** Final reduction with nonbridged external fixator in place.

PEARLS AND PITFALLS

Indications	■ Determine stability ■ Determine comminution and supplement fixation with external or internal fixation as necessary.
Surgical approach	■ Make skin incisions for pin placement to avoid sensory nerves, tendons, and crossing veins. ■ Obtain adequate exposure of the radial sensory branch at forearm and hand to avoid injury.
Hardware placement	■ Choose pins of appropriate diameter. ■ Supplement fixation with pins using external or internal fixation as necessary. ■ Do not leave pins more than 1 to 2 mm out of the cortex, and keep all pins extra-articular. ■ If placing the proximal metacarpal pin in metaphyseal bone, ensure that three cortices are penetrated. ■ Do not back out conical pins because fixation will be lost. ■ Evaluate the DRUJ after fixation to determine stability. ■ Subcutaneous pins are more costly to remove because that requires a second procedure, but they have a lower infection rate. Therefore, if fixation is needed for an extended period, bury the pins. ■ Overdistraction of the carpus must be avoided because it is associated with chronic pain–mediated syndromes and nonunion.
Postoperative management	■ Allow for adequate immobilization. ■ Encourage early range of motion of the fingers, elbow, and shoulder whenever possible. ■ Educate the patient regarding appropriate pin care. ■ Begin strengthening only after healing is complete and range of motion is maximized.

POSTOPERATIVE CARE

- After fixation with percutaneous pins, the wrist is immobilized alone in a short-arm splint to allow for swelling but provide stability. A cast is applied after the swelling goes down.
- Isolated radial styloid fractures fixed with pins can be placed in a volar wrist splint.
- External fixation devices typically require no additional immobilization, although a volar forearm–based Orthoplast (Johnson & Johnson, Langhorne, PA) splint may be used for support and patient comfort.
- The splint or cast is continued for 4 to 8 weeks until healing occurs and the pins are removed.
- K-wires and half-pins should be inspected and cleaned regularly using either soap and water or half-strength hydrogen peroxide and water.
- Finger, elbow, and shoulder range of motion are begun immediately, and wrist range of motion is begun as the fracture heals.

OUTCOMES

- Multiple prospective randomized trials comparing volar plate fixation to closed reduction and percutaneous pinning have demonstrated quicker return to functional recovery with volar plate fixation but no difference in function at 1 year.[12,13,20,28]
- Functional and cost comparison of extra-articular and simple intra-articular fractures treated with volar plate fixation versus closed reduction and percutaneous fixation showed only a significant cost increase with volar plate fixation and no difference in function. This study calls into question the extra cost associated with volar plate fixation. No external fixation was used to augment the percutaneous fixation which would increase the cost of this treatment method and may negate the cost benefit of percutaneous fixation.[5]
- A prospective randomized trial comparing percutaneous pinning and casting versus external fixation with augmentation (eg, pins, screws, bone graft) found no difference in clinical outcomes for fractures with minimal articular displacement.[10]
- In patients older than 60 years of age, percutaneous pinning has been shown to provide only marginal radiographic improvement over cast immobilization alone, with no correlation with clinical outcome.[4]
- Ebraheim et al[6] reported excellent outcomes for restoration of radiographic parameters and functional outcomes with intrafocal pinning and trans-styloid augmentation.
- An evaluation of percutaneous pinning outcomes found the best results for metaphyseal fractures. Good results were found for intra-articular fractures. The worst results were seen in fractures with associated ulnar styloid fractures and fractures in elderly persons.[19]
- A retrospective review of radiographic and clinical outcomes of open reduction internal fixation (volar and dorsal) versus external fixation revealed no significant differences, except that palmar tilt was more effectively restored with dorsal plating.[29]
- A meta-analysis found no evidence for the use of internal fixation over external fixation for unstable distal radius fractures.[16]
- Women older than 55 years of age with unstable intra-articular distal radius fractures treated with external fixation have a high rate of secondary displacement but can have acceptable functional outcomes.[11]
- Patients older than the age of 55 years have better results with external fixation and pinning than with pinning alone. Younger patients with two or more sides having comminution also have better results with supplemental external fixation.[27]
- Nonbridging external fixation has been shown to maintain volar tilt and carpal alignment better than bridging external fixation while having significantly better function during the first year.[17]
- Nonbridging external fixation was shown to have no clinical advantage in patients older than 60 years of age with moderately or severely displaced distal radius fractures.[3]
- A prospective, randomized comparison of bridging versus nonbridging external fixation revealed more complications in the nonbridging fixators and better outcomes in the bridged fixator group.[23]

- A prospective study compared unrepaired ulnar styloid fractures to those without ulnar styloid fractures and found no significant differences in clinical outcome. However, DRUJ instability was not evaluated.[24]

COMPLICATIONS

- Infection (pin tract or deep). Pin tract infections occur in 10% to 30% of patients and historically have been a major problem with this treatment method.[9,10]
- Pin tract infections can be minimized by reducing the time pins are left in place or by burying the pins beneath the skin.[15,25]
- One study showed that pin tract infections can be reduced to a 2% incidence if they are only left in place for 30 days, then removed in the office, and the wrist then casted for another 2 weeks without the pins in place.
- If K-wires are going to be left in place for longer than 30 days, they should be buried under the skin at the time of surgery to help prevent pin tract infections.
- Injury to tendons, vessels, and nerves due to percutaneous technique. Stiffness may result if tendons are inadvertently skewered, and the radial sensory branch can be injured.
- Injury to the radial sensory branch can cause a painful neuroma and should be avoided.
- Loss of range of motion
- Posttraumatic arthritis
- Weakness in grip or pinch
- Tenosynovitis and tendon rupture
- Malunion or nonunion
- Compartment syndrome
- Carpal tunnel syndrome
- Hardware failure
- Nonunion (associated with overdistraction with an external fixator)
- Complex regional pain syndrome (CRPS)[30]
- Vitamin C should be prescribed to prevent CRPS (500 mg once a day for 50 days)

REFERENCES

1. Agee JM. Distal radius fractures. Multiplanar ligamentotaxis. Hand Clin 1993;9(4):577–585.
2. Anderson JT, Lucas GL, Buhr BR. Complications of treating distal radius fractures with external fixation: a community experience. Iowa Orthop J 2004;24:53–59.
3. Atroshi I, Brogren E, Larsson GU, et al. Wrist-bridging versus non-bridging external fixation for displaced distal radius fractures: a randomized assessor-blind clinical trial of 38 patients followed for 1 year. Acta Orthop 2006;77(3):445–453.
4. Azzopardi T, Ehrendorfer S, Coulton T, et al. Unstable extra-articular fractures of the distal radius: a prospective, randomised study of immobilisation in a cast versus supplementary percutaneous pinning. J Bone Joint Surg Br 2005;87(6):837–840.
5. Dzaja I, MacDermind JC, Roth J, et al. Functional outcomes and cost estimation for extra-articular and simple intra-articular distal radius fractures treated with open reduction and internal fixation versus closed reduction and percutaneous Kirschner wire fixation. Can J Surg 2013;56(6):378–384.
6. Ebraheim NA, Ali SS, Gove NK. Fixation of unstable distal radius fractures with intrafocal pins and trans-styloid augmentation: a retrospective review and radiographic analysis. Am J Orthop 2006;35(8):362–368.
7. Gupta A. The treatment of Colles' fracture. Immobilisation with the wrist dorsiflexed. J Bone Joint Surg Br 1991;73(2):312–315.
8. Gupta R, Bozentka DJ, Bora FW. The evaluation of tension in an experimental model of external fixation of distal radius fractures. J Hand Surg Am 1999;24:108–112.
9. Hargreaves DG, Drew SJ, Eckersley R. Kirschner wire pin tract infection rates: a randomized controlled trial between percutaneous and buried wires. J Hand Surg Br 2004;29(4):374–376.
10. Harley BJ, Scharfenberger A, Beaupre LA, et al. Augmented external fixation versus percutaneous pinning and casting for unstable fractures of the distal radius—a prospective randomized trial. J Hand Surg Am 2004;29(5):815–824.
11. Hegeman JH, Oskam J, Vierhout PA, et al. External fixation for unstable intra-articular distal radial fractures in women older than 55 years. Acceptable functional end results in the majority of the patients despite significant secondary displacement. Injury 2005;36(2):339–344.
12. Jeudy J, Steiger V, Boyer P, et al. Treatment of complex fractures of the distal radius: a prospective randomized comparison of external fixation "versus" locked volar plating. Injury 2012;43(2):174–179.
13. Karantana A, Downing ND, Forward DP, et al. Surgical treatment of distal radial fractures with a volar locking plate versus conventional percutaneous methods: a randomized controlled trial. J Bone Joint Surg Am 2013;95(19):1737–1744.
14. Katz MA, Beredjiklian PK, Bozentka DJ, et al. Computed tomography scanning of intra-articular distal radius fractures: does it influence treatment? J Hand Surg Am 2001;26(3):415–421.
15. Lakshmanan P, Dixit V, Reed MR, et al. Infection rate of percutaneous Kirschner wire fixation for distal radius fractures. J Orthop Surg 2010;18:85–86.
16. Margaliot Z, Haase SC, Kotsis SV, et al. A meta-analysis of outcomes of external fixation versus plate osteosynthesis for unstable distal radius fractures. J Hand Surg Am 2005;30(6):1185–1199.
17. McQueen MM. Redisplaced unstable fractures of the distal radius. A randomised, prospective study of bridging versus nonbridging external fixation. J Bone Joint Surg Br 1998;80(4):665–669.
18. Nana AD, Joshi A, Lichtman DM. Plating of the distal radius. J Am Acad Orthop Surg 2005;13(3):159–171.
19. Rosati M, Bertagnini S, Digrandi G, et al. Percutaneous pinning for fractures of the distal radius. Acta Orthop Belg 2006;72(2):138–146.
20. Rozental TD, Blazar PE, Franko OI, et al. Functional outcomes for unstable distal radial fractures treated with open reduction and internal fixation or closed reduction and percutaneous fixation. A prospective randomized trial. J Bone Joint Surg Am 2009;91(8):1837–1846.
21. Short WH, Palmer AK, Werner FW, et al. A biomechanical study of distal radial fractures. J Hand Surg Am 1987;12(4):529–534.
22. Simic PM, Weiland AJ. Fractures of the distal aspect of the radius: changes in treatment over the past two decades. Instr Course Lect 2003;52:185–195.
23. Sommerkamp TG, Seeman M, Silliman J, et al. Dynamic external fixation of unstable fractures of the distal part of the radius. A prospective, randomized comparison with static external fixation. J Bone Joint Surg Am 1994;76(8):1149–1161.
24. Souer JS, Ring D, Matschke S, et al. Effect of an unrepaired fracture of the ulnar styloid base on outcome after plate and screw fixation of a distal radius fracture. J Bone Joint Surg Am 2009;91(4): 830–838.
25. Subramanian P, Kantharuban S, Shilston S, et al. Complications of Kirschner-wire fixation in distal radius fractures. Tech Hand Up Extrem Surg 2012;16(3):120–123.
26. Trumble TE, Schmitt SR, Vedder NB. Factors affecting functional outcome of displaced intra-articular distal radius fractures. J Hand Surg Am 1994;19(2):325–340.
27. Trumble TE, Wagner W, Hanel DP, et al. Intrafocal (Kapandji) pinning of distal radius fractures with and without external fixation. J Hand Surg Am 1998;23(3):381–394.
28. Wei DH, Raizman NM, Bottino CJ, et al. Unstable distal radial fractures treated with external fixation, a radial column plate, or a volar plate. A prospective randomized trial. J Bone Joint Surg Am 2009;81(7):1568–1577.
29. Westphal T, Piatek S, Schubert S, et al. Outcome after surgery of distal radius fractures: no differences between external fixation and ORIF. Arch Orthop Trauma Surg 2005;125(8):507–514.
30. Zollinger PE, Tuinebreijer WE, Breederveld RS, et al. Can vitamin C prevent complex regional pain syndrome in patients with wrist fractures? A randomized, controlled, multicenter dose-response study. J Bone Joint Surg Am 2007;89(7):1424–1431.

28 CHAPTER

Arthroscopic Reduction and Fixation of Distal Radius and Ulnar Styloid Fractures

William B. Geissler and Jason M. Clark

DEFINITION

- A bimodal age distribution exists for patients with distal radius fractures (ie, young adults vs. elderly persons), and they frequently have a different mechanism of injury.
- Patients 65 years of age or older have an annual incidence of 8 to 10 fractures of the distal radius per 1000 person-years.
  - The incidence is seven times higher in women than in men.
  - Sixteen percent of white women and 23% of white men will sustain a fracture of the distal radius after the age of 50 years.
- Fractures of the distal radius are one of the most common skeletal injuries treated by orthopaedic surgeons.
- These injuries account for one-sixth of all fractures that are evaluated in the emergency department.
- Displaced intra-articular fractures of the distal radius are a unique subset of radius fractures.[25]
  - These fractures are a high-energy injury.
  - This high-energy injury results in comminuted fracture patterns.
  - These fractures are less amenable to traditional closed manipulation and casting.
- The prognosis for these fractures depends on the amount of residual radius shortening, both radiocarpal and radioulnar articular congruity, and associated soft tissue injuries.[31]

ANATOMY

- The distal radius serves as a plateau to support the carpus.
- The distal radius has three concave articular surfaces: the scaphoid fossa, the lunate fossa, and the sigmoid notch.
- The distal articular surface of the radius has a radial inclination averaging 22 degrees and palmar tilt averaging 11 degrees.
- Radial-based volar and dorsal ligaments arise from the distal radius to support the wrist.
- The sigmoid notch of the distal radius articulates with the ulnar head about which it rotates.
  - The distal radioulnar joint (DRUJ) is primarily stabilized by the triangular fibrocartilage complex (TFCC).
- The sigmoid notch angles distally and medially at an average of 22 degrees.

PATHOGENESIS

- The biomechanical characteristics of each fracture type depend on the mechanism of injury.
- Fernandez and Geissler[11] developed a classification based on the mechanism of injury. They noted that the associated ligamentous lesions, subluxations, and associated carpal fractures are related directly to the degree of energy absorbed by the distal radius.
  - Type I fractures are bending fractures of the metaphysis in which one cortex fails due to tensile stress and the opposite one undergoes a certain degree of comminution (eg, extra-articular Smith or Colles fractures).
  - Type II fractures are shearing fractures of the joint surface (eg, radial styloid fractures, Barton fracture).
  - Type III fractures are compression fractures of the joint surface with impaction of the subchondral and metaphyseal cancellous bone (ie, intra-articular comminuted fractures).
  - Type IV fractures are avulsion fractures of ligamentous attachments, including radial styloid and ulnar styloid fractures, and are associated with radiocarpal fracture-dislocations.
  - Type V fractures are high-energy injuries that involve a combination of bending, compression, shearing, and avulsion mechanisms or bone loss.
- Several studies have shown that a high incidence of associated soft tissue injuries is seen with displaced intra-articular distal radius fractures.[16,18–20,24,26,29]
  - Arthroscopic studies demonstrate a high incidence of injury to the TFCC, followed by the scapholunate interosseous ligament (SLIL), and then the lunotriquetral interosseous ligament (LTIL) (which is the least injured).
  - A spectrum of injury occurs to the interosseous ligament in which it attenuates and eventually tears and the degree of rotation between the carpal bones increases.
  - Geissler et al[15] defined an arthroscopic classification of interosseous ligament tears that helps define the degree of ligament injury and secondary instability as well as proposes treatment (Table 1; see also Chap. 67).

NATURAL HISTORY

- Intra-articular fractures of the distal radius have two pathologies: the associated global injury to the soft tissues and the injury to the bone itself.
- The natural history for an intra-articular fracture of the distal radius depends on restoration of anatomy as well as detection and management of any associated soft tissue injuries.[4,11]
- Knirk and Jupiter[20] documented the importance of articular restoration over extra-articular orientation in predicting outcomes for fractures of the distal radius.
  - They showed solid evidence that the largest tolerable articular step-off is 2 mm.
  - They demonstrate that the better the restoration of the articular surface, the better the outcome.
- A loss in radius length of 2.5 mm will shift the normal load transmitted across the ulna from 20% to 42%, which may lead to various stages of ulnar impaction syndrome.
- SLIL and TFCC injuries are often associated with distal radius fractures and may be missed on plain x-ray.
  - In one study, nearly one-third of fractures had an associated SLIL injury and greater than 60% had a TFCC injury.[1]

Table 1 Geissler Arthroscopic Classification of Carpal Instability

Grade	Definition	Arthroscopic Findings	Management
I	Attenuation/hemorrhage of interosseous ligament as seen from the radiocarpal joint. No incongruency of carpal alignment in the midcarpal space.	There is a loss of the normal concave appearance between the carpal bones, and the interosseous ligament attenuates and becomes convex as seen from the radiocarpal space. In midcarpal space, the interval between the carpal bones will still be tight and congruent, with no step-off.	Immobilization
II	Attenuation/hemorrhage of the interosseous ligament as seen from the radiocarpal joint. Incongruency/step-off as seen from the midcarpal space. A slight gap between the carpal bones may be present.	A slight gap (less than the width of a probe) between the carpal bones may be present. The interosseous ligament continues to become attenuated and is convex as seen from the radial carpal space. In the midcarpal space, the interval between the involved carpal bones is no longer congruent, and a step-off is present. In scapholunate instability, palmar flexion of the dorsal lip of the scaphoid will be seen as compared to the lunate. In lunotriquetral instability, increased translation between the triquetrum and lunate will be seen when palpated with a probe.	Arthroscopic reduction and pinning
III	Incongruency/step-off of carpal alignment is seen in both the radiocarpal and midcarpal spaces.	The interosseous ligament has started to tear, usually from volar to dorsal, and a gap is seen between the carpal bones in the radiocarpal space. A probe often is helpful to separate the involved carpal bones in the radiocarpal space. In the midcarpal space, a 2-mm probe may be placed between the carpal bones and twisted.	Arthroscopic/open reduction and pinning
IV	Incongruency/step-off of carpal alignment is seen in both the radiocarpal and midcarpal spaces. Gross instability with manipulation is noted.	A 2.7-mm arthroscope may be passed through the gap between the carpal bones. The interosseous ligament is completely detached between the involved carpal bones. This is the "drive-through" sign, when the arthroscope may be freely passed from the radiocarpal space through the tear to the midcarpal space.	Open reduction and repair

- In another study, SLIL injuries were found in more than half, LTIL injuries in one-third, and TFCC in 60%. Only 17% of patients were free of any of the three injuries.[28]
- Untreated complete tears of the SLIL, which are highly associated with radial styloid fractures, may progress to a wrist with scapholunate advanced collapse.

PATIENT HISTORY AND PHYSICAL FINDINGS

- A thorough history should be obtained, including the circumstances surrounding the injury as well as any additional injuries.
  - Neurologic basis
  - Cardiac basis
  - Patients' level of independence, dominant hand, status with assisted devices, work, activity level, and support structure should be determined.
- Physical examination, while concentrating on the wrist, should also include the hand, elbow, and shoulder to check for concomitant injuries.
  - The hand, wrist, forearm, arm, and shoulder must be carefully inspected for open injury so that tetanus and antibiotic prophylaxis may be initiated if necessary.
  - A thorough distal sensory and motor function examination should be carried out in an organized manner.
  - Vascular examination should include palpation of both the radial and ulnar pulses and determination of capillary refill time.
  - Precise palpation is used to define areas of potential trauma.
- Diminished sensibility, pallor, altered capillary refill, increased tenseness of the soft tissues, and pain out of proportion should raise suspicion for significant soft tissue injury, including compartment syndrome.

IMAGING AND OTHER DIAGNOSTIC STUDIES

- Posteroanterior (PA), oblique, and lateral radiographs are the primary radiographic studies used to workup distal radius fractures.
  - Radiographs of the uninvolved contralateral extremity are useful to compare radial inclination, ulnar variance, and sigmoid notch anatomy.
  - PA projections are useful to evaluate the radial inclination, radius height, presence of ulnar styloid fractures, widening of the DRUJ, widening of intercarpal spaces, and intra-articular involvement (**FIG 1A**).
    - Standard radiographic parameters of the distal radius include radial inclination of 22 degrees (range 13 to 30 degrees), radius length of 12 mm (range 8 to 18 mm), and volar tilt of 11 degrees (range 1 to 21 degrees).
    - Ulnar variance should be measured with the shoulder in 90 degrees of abduction, the elbow at 90 degrees of flexion, and the wrist in neutral pronation–supination.
  - A lateral projection is used to assess volar and dorsal tilt of the distal fragment, dislocation or subluxation of the DRUJ or carpus, lunate angulation, and dorsal comminution (**FIG 1B**).

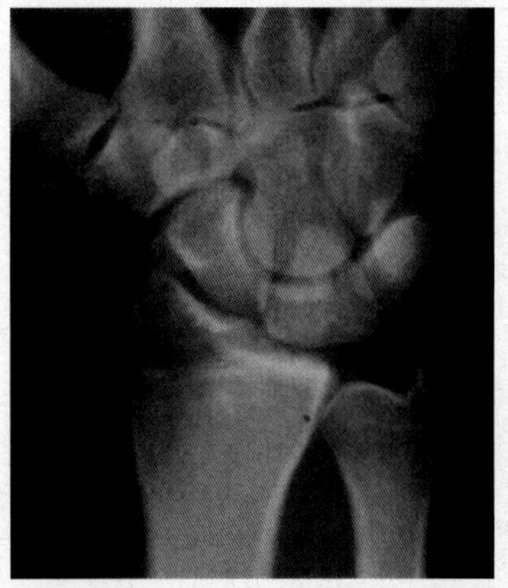
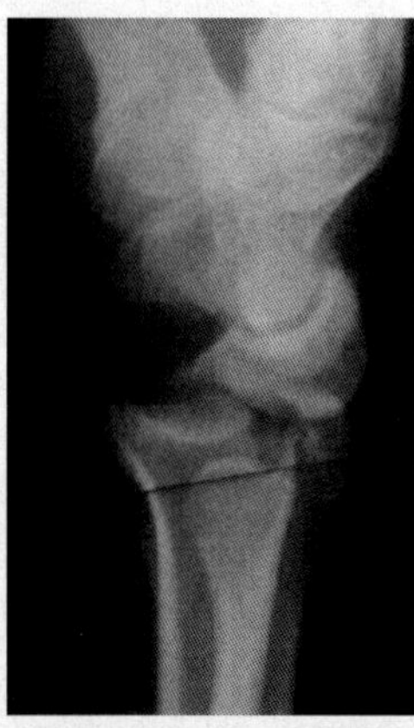

FIG 1 • **A.** PA radiographic view showing a minimally displaced radial styloid fracture fragment. **B.** The lateral view shows a complete fracture-dislocation of the wrist.

- A modified lateral radiograph with the beam angulating 10 to 30 degrees proximally improves visualization of the articular surface and evaluation of the volar rim of the lunate facet represented by the anterior teardrop.
- An additional 30-degree anteroposterior (AP) cephalic projection is useful to evaluate the dorsal ulnar margin of the distal radius.
- Oblique radiographs are very helpful because major fracture fragments may be rotated out of their anatomic planes.
- Computed tomography (CT) evaluation, particularly three-dimensional CT, can further delineate fragment location, joint compression, and rotation.
- Magnetic resonance imaging (MRI) evaluation is useful in assessing for associated soft tissue injuries such as TFCC tears, interosseous ligament injuries, and carpal fractures.
- Radiographic signs that demonstrate that the distal radius fracture is likely unstable and closed reduction would be insufficient include the following[21]:
  - Lateral tilt greater than 20 degrees dorsal
  - Dorsal comminution greater than 50% of the lateral width
  - Initial fragment displacement greater than 1 cm
  - Volar translation greater than 2 mm
  - Initial radius shortening more than 5 mm
  - Intra-articular step-off greater than 2 mm
  - Associated ulnar fracture
  - Severe osteoporosis
  - Age older than 60 years

DIFFERENTIAL DIAGNOSIS

- Carpal bone fracture
- Metacarpal or phalangeal fracture
- DRUJ disruption
- Essex-Lopresti lesion
- Interosseous ligament tear
- Carpal dislocation (perilunate)

NONOPERATIVE MANAGEMENT

- Displaced fractures of the distal radius are reduced using an adequate anesthetic agent.
  - Knowledge of the mechanisms of injury helps facilitate manual reduction. Force is applied opposite the force that caused the fracture.
  - Gentle traction is necessary to disimpact the fracture fragments, followed by palmar translation of the hand and carpus in respect to the radius.
  - The radius articular surface will rotate around the intact volar cortical lip to restore volar inclination with palmar translation.
  - Care must be taken to avoid trauma to the skin during the reduction maneuver, particularly in elderly patients where the skin may be fragile.
- A splint is supplied following the reduction. No consensus has been established regarding wrist or forearm position, long-arm versus short-arm immobilization, or splint versus cast.
  - Extreme positions of wrist flexion and ulnar deviation should be avoided.
  - Postreduction radiographs are taken in plaster.
- Depending on stability of the fracture, most patients treated nonoperatively require weekly visits for the first 3 weeks to monitor fracture reduction.
  - In patients older than 65 years, one-third of initially undisplaced fractures subsequently collapsed to some degree.
  - One study of elderly patients with moderately displaced fractures of the distal radius found that two-thirds of the correction obtained by closed manipulation was lost at 5 weeks.
- Patients with minimally displaced or nondisplaced fractures of the distal radius treated nonoperatively must be made aware of possible complications, including rupture of the extensor pollicis longus tendon, carpal tunnel syndrome, and compartment syndrome.
- Elderly patients typically tolerate nonoperative management well.
  - Patients older than 65 years undergoing nonoperative results have comparable results to those that undergo operative treatment despite unsatisfactory radiographic outcomes.[2,3]

SURGICAL MANAGEMENT

- Distal radius fractures without extensive metaphyseal comminution are ideal candidates for arthroscopic-assisted fixation with K-wires or cannulated screws.[14,15,22]
  - Radial styloid fractures
  - Impacted fractures
  - Die-punch fractures
- Three-part T-type fractures and four-part fractures with metaphyseal comminution are best treated with a combination of volar plate stabilization. Wrist arthroscopy is used as an adjunct to fine-tune the articular reduction and evaluate for associated soft tissue lesions.
- Distal radius fractures that may be minimally displaced, and fractures with strongly suspected associated soft tissue injury, also are candidates for arthroscopic-assisted fixation to stabilize the fracture but, more importantly, to evaluate and treat the acute associated soft tissue injury.
- Stabilization of associated ulnar styloid fragments is controversial.[20] Wrist arthroscopy provides a rationale as to when to stabilize an ulnar styloid fragment.

Preoperative Planning

- All radiographic studies are reviewed.
- Equipment needed for arthroscopic treatment and for open stabilization is made available.
  - Small joint instrumentation is essential for arthroscopic-assisted fixation of distal radius fractures. The small joint

arthroscope is approximately 2.7 mm in diameter, and even smaller scopes may be used if desired. In addition, a small joint shaver (3.5 mm or less) is useful to clear fracture debris and hematoma.

- The ideal timing for arthroscopic-assisted fixation of distal radius fractures is 3 to 10 days following injury.[13]
  - Earlier attempts at fixation may be complicated by soft tissue swelling and troublesome bleeding, obscuring visualization.
  - After 10 days, the fracture fragments start to become sticky and more difficult to percutaneously elevate and reduce.

Positioning

- Arthroscopic-assisted fixation of distal radius fractures may be performed with the arm suspended vertically in a traction tower, horizontally in a traction tower, or with finger traps applied attached to weights hanging over the edge of the hand table.
  - Wrist arthroscopy in the horizontal position may make it easier to simultaneously monitor the reduction fluoroscopically and place hardware. However, it does not allow for simultaneous volar access to the wrist.
  - Suspending the wrist in a vertical position with a traction tower allows simultaneous access to both the volar and dorsal aspects of the wrist. This is particularly useful when wrist arthroscopy is used as an adjunct to volar plate fixation of the distal radius fracture.
- A new traction tower has been designed to allow simultaneous evaluation of the intra-articular reduction of the distal radius arthroscopically and fluoroscopically (**FIG 2A**).
  - The surgeon may stabilize a comminuted fracture of the distal radius with a plate, and simultaneously evaluate the articular reduction arthroscopically.
  - The traction tower allows for traction of the wrist in either the vertical or horizontal planes, depending on the surgeon's preference (**FIG 2B**).

Approach

- The wrist is suspended in a traction tower, and the standard dorsal 3-4 viewing portal, 4-5 or 6R working portal, and 6U inflow portal are made.
- It is difficult to palpate the normal extensor tendon landmarks for traditional wrist arthroscopy in patients who sustain a fracture of the distal radius because of swelling.[17] However, the bony landmarks usually can still be palpated. These bony landmarks include the bases of the metacarpals, the dorsal lip of the radius, and the ulnar head.
- The 3-4 portal is made in line with the radial border of the long finger. It is very useful to place an 18-gauge needle into the proposed location of the 3-4 portal before making a skin incision.
  - If the portal is placed too proximal, the arthroscope may be placed within the fracture pattern itself. If it is placed too distal, it can injure the articular surface of the carpus.
- Once the precise ideal location of the portal is located, the portal is made by pulling the skin with the surgeon's thumb against the tip of a no. 11 blade. Blunt dissection is carried down with a hemostat, and the arthroscope, with a blunt trocar, is introduced into the dorsal 3-4 portal.
  - This technique decreases potential injury to cutaneous nerves.
- Thorough irrigation of the joint is necessary to wash out fracture hematoma and debris and improve visualization. Inflow may be provided through the arthroscope cannula or separately through a 14-gauge needle into the 6U portal.
  - Use of a separate 6U inflow portal is recommended. The small joint arthroscopy cannula does not allow as much space between the cannula and the arthroscope, limiting the amount of flow through the cannula.
  - Outflow to the wrist is provided through intravenous extension tubing connected to the arthroscope cannula.
- The 4-5 working portal is made in line with the mid-axis of the ring metacarpal. Alternatively, the 6R working portal is made just radial to the palpable extensor carpi ulnaris tendon.
  - An 18-gauge needle is placed into the joint and should lie just distal to the articular disc.
  - A 4-5 or 6R portal usually is located just proximal to the 3-4 portal because of the natural radial slope of the distal radius.

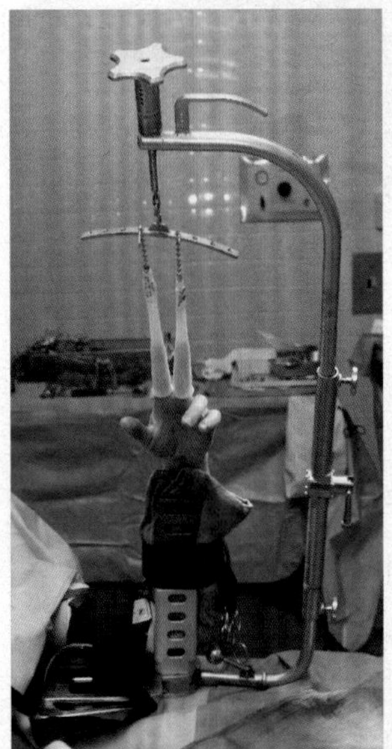
A

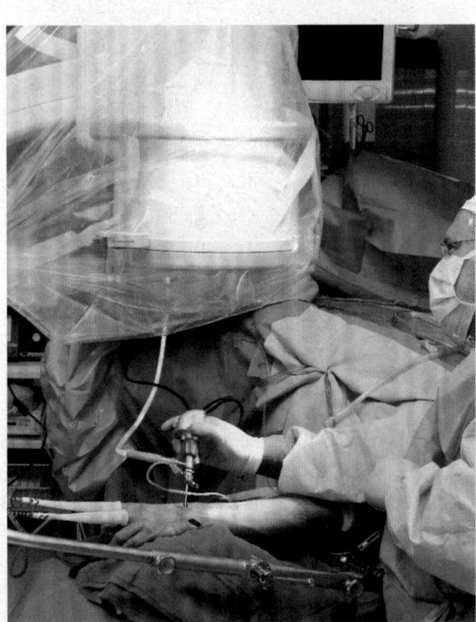
B

FIG 2 • **A.** This traction tower uses a suspension bar at the side rather than at the center of the wrist. This allows easy fluoroscopic evaluation of the fracture reduction, with simultaneous full access to the volar and dorsal aspects of the wrist. **B.** The tower can be flexed into a horizontal position for surgeons who prefer to treat distal radius fractures in that position.

- More recently, del Piñal et al[7] described a dry arthroscopy technique in order to avoid the risk of compartment syndrome from fluid infusion.
  - Although the setup is similar, there have been a few notable difficulties that are associated with the lack of fluid infusion.
  - To avoid fogging of the arthroscope, the scope should be warmed in warm saline prior to placing it in the wrist or by adding anti-fog drops to the end of the scope.
  - The arthroscope valve is left in the open position to prevent collapse of the capsule, and a shaver is placed in the 6R portal on suction to help clear debris and blood.
  - Hematoma and debris will still need to be occasionally flushed through the joint with saline for adequate visualization.

TECHNIQUES

Radial Styloid Fractures

- An isolated fracture of the radial styloid is an ideal fracture pattern to manage arthroscopically, especially for the surgeon beginning to gain experience in arthroscope-assisted fixation of distal radius fractures.
- In addition, radial styloid fractures have a high incidence of associated injury to the SLIL, which is best assessed arthroscopically.
- Insert one or two guidewires from a cannulated screw system percutaneously into the radial styloid—not across the fracture site—using a wire driver in oscillation mode.
  - Evaluate the position of the wires under fluoroscopy to ensure they are centered in the radial styloid fragment.
- Suspend the wrist in a traction tower and establish the standard arthroscopic portals.
- Insert the scope in the dorsal 3-4 portal and clear the joint of debris and hematoma.
- Transfer the arthroscope to the 6R or 4-5 portal to look across the wrist and effectively judge rotation and reduction of the radial styloid fragment.
- Using the previously placed guidewires as joysticks, manipulate and anatomically reduce the fracture fragment under direct arthroscopic observation.
  - A trocar can be inserted through the 3-4 portal to help further guide the reduction of the radial styloid fragment (**TECH FIG 1A,B**).

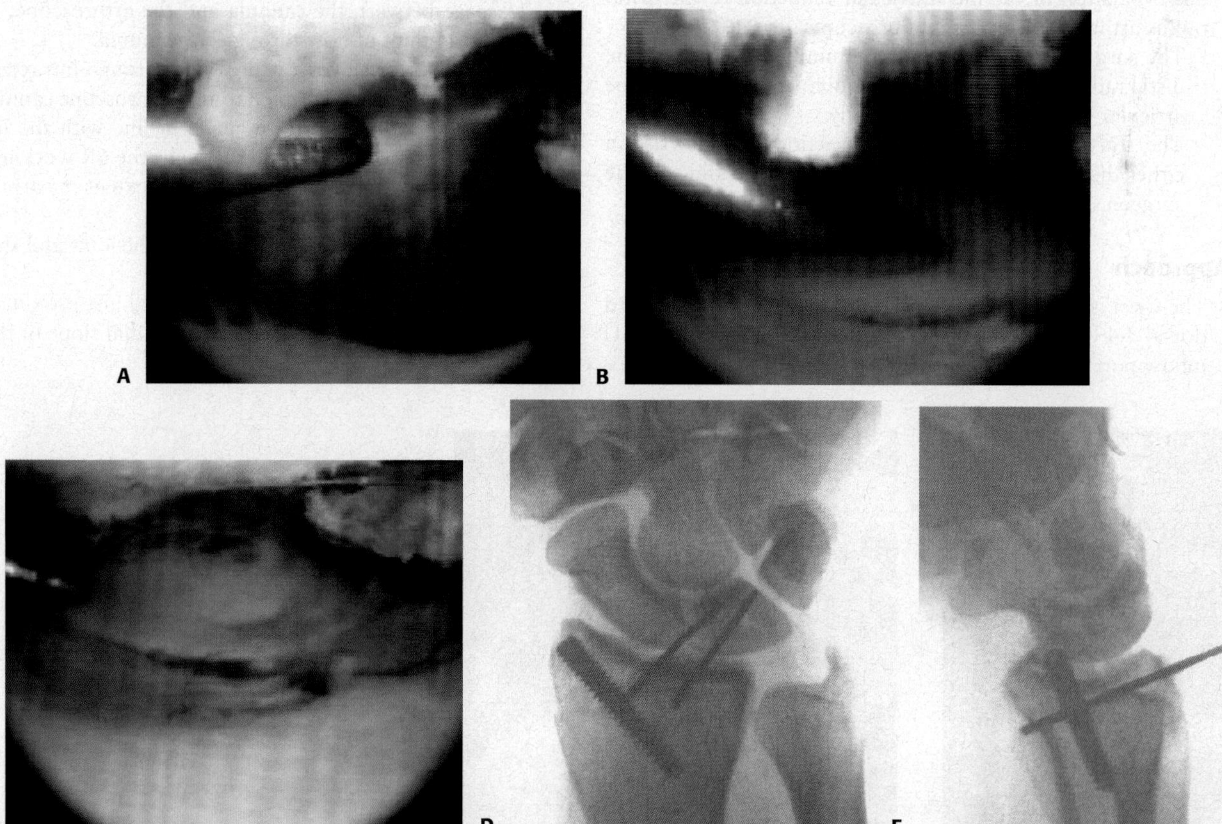

TECH FIG 1 • **A.** Arthroscopic view of the patient whose radiographs are seen in **FIG 1**. The arthroscope is in the 6R portal looking across the wrist, and a blunt trocar is in the 3-4 portal. The displaced radial styloid fragment is well visualized. **B.** A combination of joysticks inserted into the radial styloid fragment and a trocar inserted into the 3-4 portal allows anatomic reduction of the displaced radial styloid fragment and radiocarpal joint. **C.** The radial styloid fragment is anatomically reduced (with no residual rotation) and stabilized. **D.** PA view demonstrating anatomic reduction to the radial styloid fragment. Headless cannulated screws are used, if possible, to avoid soft tissue irritation. **E.** Lateral view showing anatomic restoration to the radial styloid fragment and restoration of the carpus in line with the radius.

- Once the fracture is judged to be absolutely anatomic, the guidewires are advanced across the fracture site into the radius shaft and evaluated under fluoroscopy (**TECH FIG 1C**).
  - In many cases, the fracture reduction may look anatomic under fluoroscopy, but when viewed arthroscopically, the radial styloid fragment is seen to be slightly rotated.[2]
- Guidewires alone can be used to stabilize the fracture, but cannulated screws (with or without heads) are recommended (**TECH FIG 1D,E**).
  - Cannulated screws decrease soft tissue irritation and potential pin tract infection as compared with K-wires.

Three-Part Fractures

- Three-part fractures that involve a displaced fracture of the radial styloid and a lunate facet fragment without metaphyseal comminution are ideal for arthroscopic-assisted reduction (**TECH FIG 2A,B**).
- Reduce and provisionally stabilize the radial styloid fragment with guidewires under fluoroscopic guidance.
  - The radial styloid serves as a landmark to which the depressed lunate facet fragment is reduced.
- Suspend the wrist in the traction tower, establish portals, and evacuate the fracture debris and hematoma.
  - The depressed lunate facet fragment is best seen with the arthroscope in the 3-4 portal (**TECH FIG 2C,D**).
- Percutaneously place an 18-gauge needle directly over the depressed fragment as viewed arthroscopically.
- Insert a large K-wire about 2 cm proximal to the previously placed 18-gauge needle to percutaneously elevate the depressed lunate facet fragment.

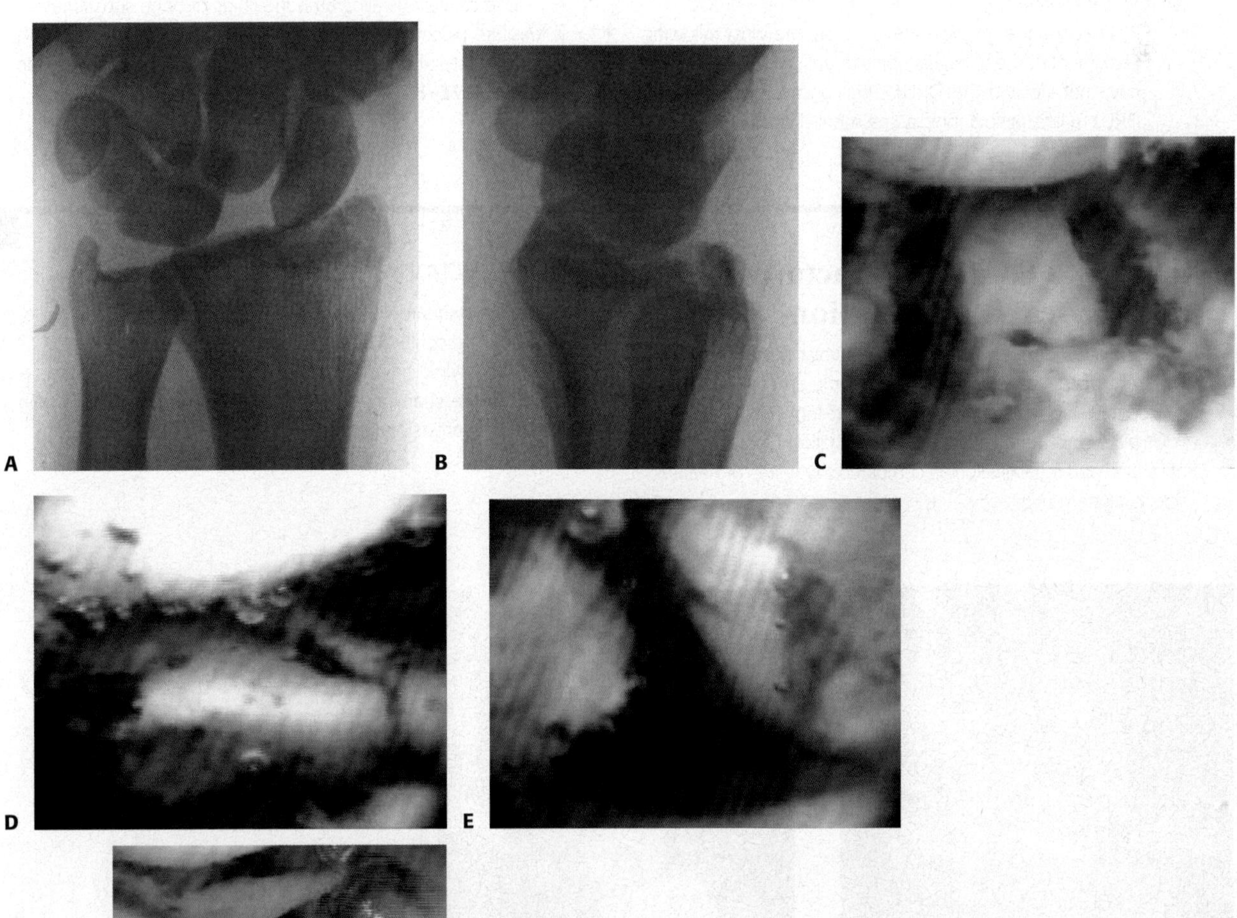

TECH FIG 2 • **A.** PA view showing an impacted scaphoid facet fracture fragment with an obvious injury to the SLIL. **B.** Lateral view showing a dorsal rim fracture fragment. **C.** The arthroscope is in the 6R portal, demonstrating the impacted scaphoid facet fracture fragment. This would be quite difficult to view through an open arthrotomy but is well visualized arthroscopically under bright light and magnified conditions. **D.** The impacted scaphoid facet fragment is elevated back to the volar rim, using the rim as a landmark to judge rotation. **E,F.** Geissler grade III tear involving the SLIL as seen through the 3-4 portal (**E**) and the radial midcarpal portal (**F**). *(continued)*

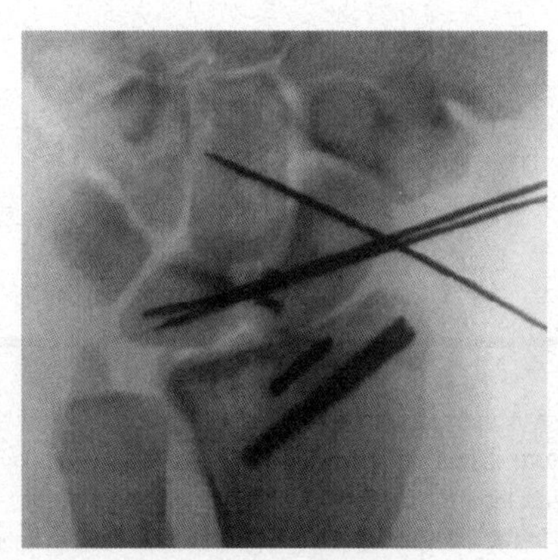

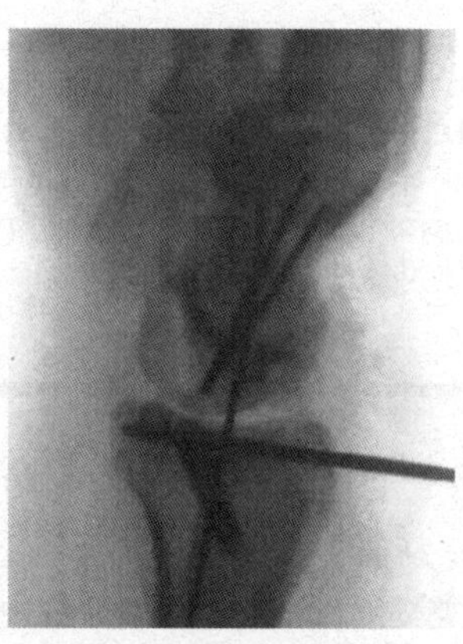

TECH FIG 2 • *(continued)* **G,H.** PA and lateral radiographs showing anatomic reduction to the impacted scaphoid facet fracture. (The tear of the SLIL also was acutely repaired.)

- Use a bone tenaculum to further diminish the gap between the radial styloid and lunate facet fragments.
- Place guidewires transversely under the subchondral surface of the radius from the radial styloid into the anatomically reduced lunate facet fragment.
  - It is important to pronate and supinate the wrist following placement of the transverse pins to ensure the guidewires have not violated the DRUJ. The concave nature of the DRUJ makes radiographic assessment difficult.
- Consider insertion of bone graft to support the reduced lunate fragment and avoid late settling.
  - Make a small incision between the fourth and fifth dorsal compartments.
  - Use cancellous allograft bone chips or bone substitutes.
- If feasible, place headless cannulated screws to stabilize both the radial styloid and the impacted lunate facet fragments (**TECH FIG 2E–H**).

Three-and Four-Part Fractures with Metaphyseal Comminution

- A combination of open surgery, using a volar plate for stability, and arthroscopy, as an adjunct to assist the articular reduction, is used if metaphyseal comminution is present (**TECH FIG 3**).
- Volar plate stabilization is very stable and allows for early range of motion and rehabilitation as compared to K-wires or headless screws alone.

Open Reduction and Stabilization

- Perform a standard volar approach, and do not open the radiocarpal joint capsule (**TECH FIG 4A**).
- The radial styloid fragment and the volar ulnar fragment are reduced to the shaft under direct visualization. The radial styloid fragment is provisionally pinned.

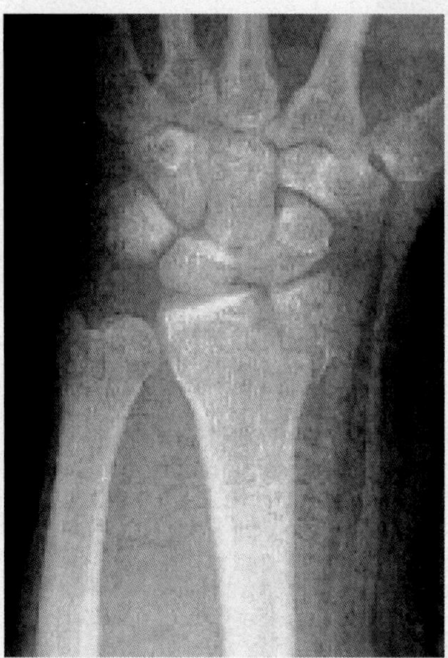

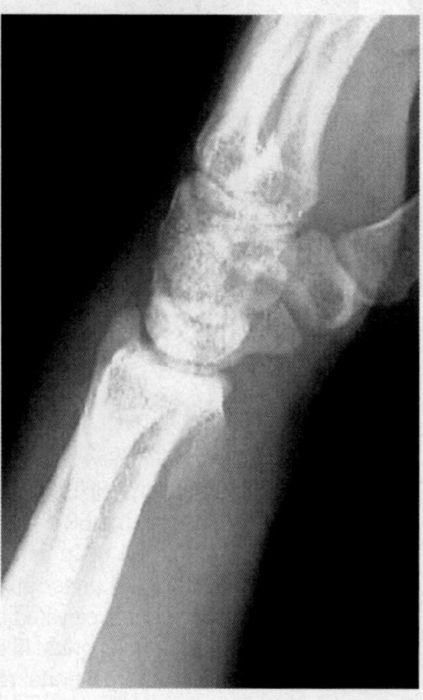

TECH FIG 3 • **A.** The PA radiograph shows a displaced fracture of the radial styloid. **B.** This lateral radiograph shows metaphyseal comminution associated with the displaced radial styloid fragment. Because of the metaphyseal comminution, it was decided to stabilize the fracture using a volar plate.

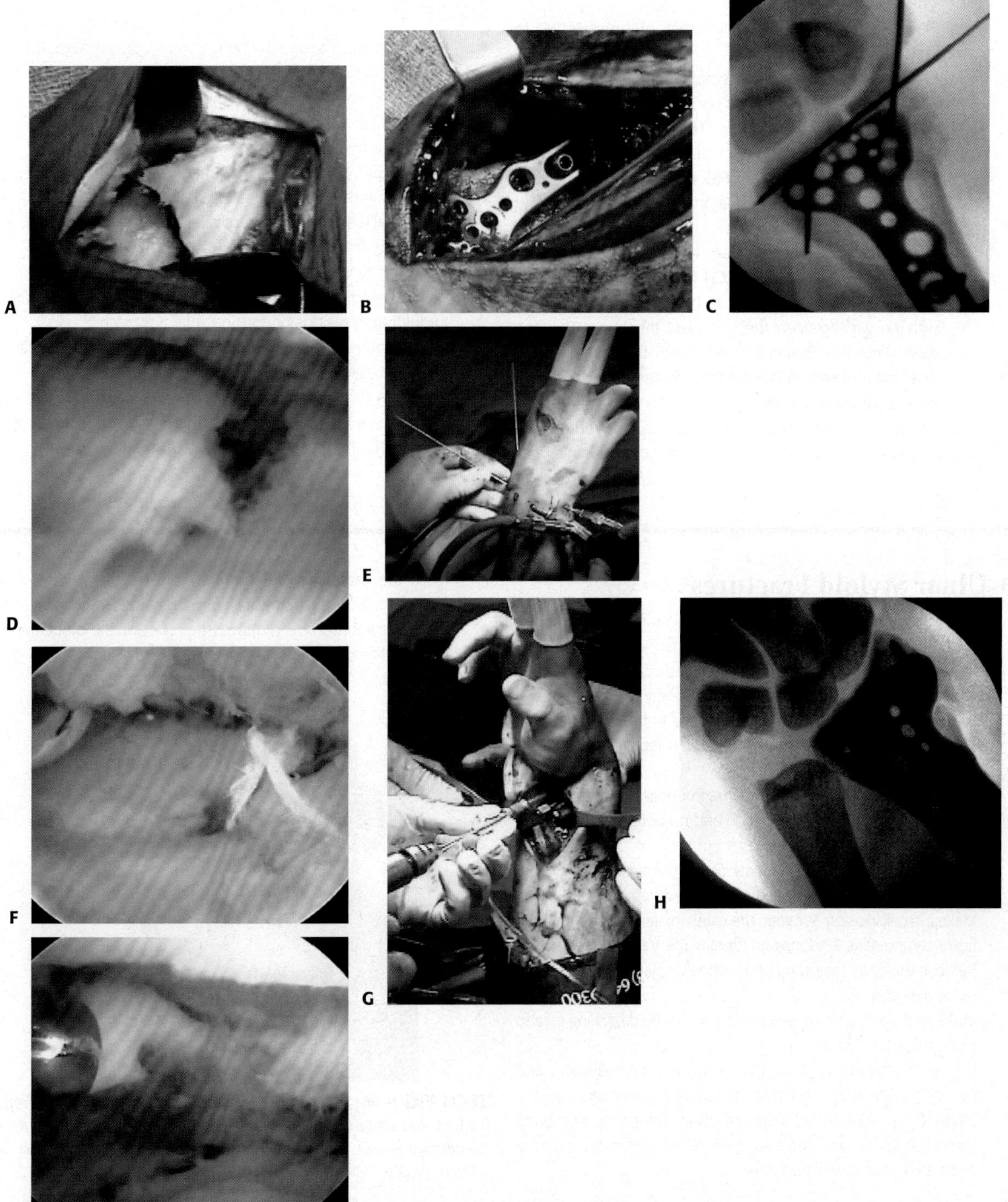

TECH FIG 4 • **A.** A standard volar approach is made, centered over the flexor carpi radialis tendon, and the fracture site is exposed. **B.** A volar distal radius locking plate is applied. The initial screw is placed through the proximal plate to secure the plate to the shaft. **C.** The intra-articular reduction is viewed under fluoroscopy and provisionally pinned. A displaced intra-articular fracture fragment can still be identified. **D.** The arthroscope is in the 3-4 portal, showing the volar capsule blocking reduction of the radial styloid fragment. **E.** Joysticks previously inserted into the radial styloid fragment are then used to control and anatomically reduce the radial styloid fragment. **F.** The arthroscope is in the 6R portal looking across the wrist. Anatomic reduction of the radial styloid fragment is documented. **G.** Once the anatomic restoration of the articular surface is evaluated both arthroscopically and fluoroscopically, the distal screws are placed in the plate. **H.** Fluoroscopic view showing anatomic restoration to the articular surface of the distal radius. **I.** The patient had an associated osteochondral fracture of the lunate, not visible on plain radiographs. The displaced fragment is arthroscopically removed.

- Apply a volar distal radius locking plate to stabilize the volar bone fragments (**TECH FIG 4B**).
  - Place a screw in the proximal portion of the plate first to reduce the plate to the shaft.
  - Provisionally pin the distal fragments through the plate.
- Manipulate the articular fragments under fluoroscopy to obtain as anatomic a reduction as possible (**TECH FIG 4C,D**).
- Suspend the wrist in the traction tower and reduce the articular fragments arthroscopically (**TECH FIG 4E,F**).
  - If articular reduction is not anatomic, remove the pins and fine-tune the reduction.
- Once the fracture reduction is thought to be anatomic, place the distal screws through the plate (**TECH FIG 4G–I**).
  - It is important that the fracture be reduced to the plate, with no gap between the plate and the bone. This can be achieved by flexion of the wrist in the tower and by insertion of a nonlocking screw first, before the insertion of standard locking screws.
- Place the remaining proximal and distal screws if the reduction is anatomic under both fluoroscopy and arthroscopy.

Reduction and Stabilization of a Dorsal Die-Punch Fragment

- It is not possible to see the reduction of a dorsal die-punch fragment through the volar approach when stabilized with a plate. Arthroscopy can be helpful in this scenario.
- Insert the volar plate as previously described and provisionally fix the device to the radius.
  - Frequently, the dorsal fragment may still be slightly proximal in relation to the radial shaft.
- The dorsal die-punch fragment is best seen with the arthroscope in the 6R portal.
- Establish the volar radial portal between the radioscaphocapitate ligament and the long radiolunate ligament, as viewed directly through the previous performed volar approach.[23]
- Percutaneously elevate and anatomically reduce the dorsal die-punch fragment as viewed arthroscopically.
- Once this has been achieved, place the screws into the plate and observe their path arthroscopically to ensure adequate stabilization of the dorsal die-punch fragment.

Ulnar Styloid Fractures

- Following anatomic reduction of the distal radius fracture, insert the arthroscope in the dorsal 3-4 portal and the probe in the 6R portal. Palpate the tension of the articular disc.
  - Good tension indicates that the majority of the peripheral TFCC fibers are intact or still attached to the proximal ulna.
  - A peripheral tear of the articular disc is repaired arthroscopically when detected.[30]
- Stabilization of a large ulnar styloid fragment is considered when the articular disc is lax by palpation and no peripheral TFCC tear is identified (**TECH FIG 5**).
  - In this instance, the majority of the fibers of the TFCC are attached to the displaced ulnar styloid fragment.
- Make a small incision between the extensor carpi ulnaris and the flexor carpi ulnaris tendons and identify the fracture site.
- Retrieve the distal fragment, which often displaces in a distal and radial direction.
- Mobilize the styloid fragment using a no. 15 blade, taking care to protect the TFCC insertion.
- Reduce the fragment anatomically, under direct visualization, and insert a guidewire in a retrograde manner for provisional stability.
- Stabilize the ulnar styloid fragment using either a tension band technique (with wire and two K-wires) or, preferably, using a micro headless cannulated screw.
- Place the cannulated headless screw over the guidewire and verify fracture reduction with fluoroscopy.
- Insert the arthroscope into the 3-4 portal and the probe into the 6R portal to document restoration of TFCC tension.

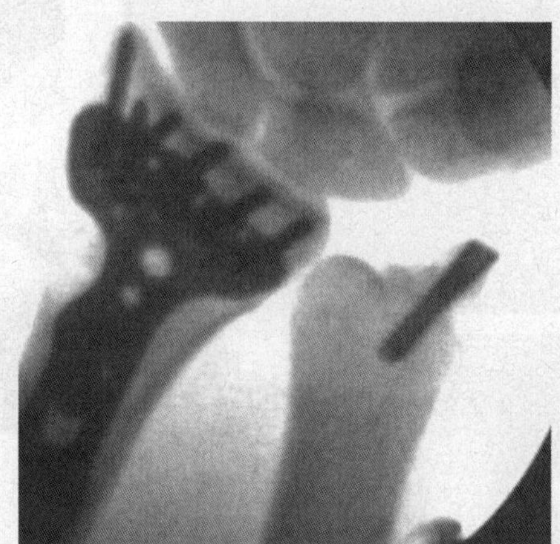

TECH FIG 5 • In this case, following reduction to the distal radius fracture, the articular disc was palpated and found to be lax but with no peripheral tear. The large ulnar styloid fragment was reduced with a micro Acutrak screw.

Intra-articular Distal Radius Fracture Malunion

- Malunion of a distal radius fracture can rapidly lead to a degenerative joint in active individuals.
- Immediate correction of the malunion is needed for any chance of stopping degeneration of the articular surface.
- Correction of the malunion under arthroscopy allows both the ability to access the current state of the joint surface and assures adequate alignment of the fractures while providing good long-term results. Recently, this is has been described by del Piñal et al.[5,6]
- The hand is placed into traction, and standard 3-4 and 6R portals are developed as previously described.

- Place the arthroscope into the 3-4 portal to visualize the joint surface.
  - If severe chondral defects are noted, then either an arthroplasty or arthrodesis should be considered.
  - The joint will often be filled with synovitis and fibrin debris. A shaver is placed into the 6R position, and the joint is cleared of the debris to obtain adequate visualization.
- The hand is removed from traction and a volar plate is placed as previously described through a volar approach and attached to the shaft.
- Next place the hand back into traction and place the arthroscope back into the 6R portal to visualize the malunited fragments. A volar radial portal may be placed at this time to be used for instruments along with the 3-4 portal.
- Osteotomes are then introduced for cutting the fragments through the 3-4 and volar radial portal by introducing the blade parallel to the tendons and then rotating it into the joint.
- The osteotomes are then advanced over the external callus to free up the individual fragments.
  - Care should be taken to not overshoot the joint and plunge the osteotome volarly or dorsally potentially severing tendons.
- The fragments are then elevated either with a probe or percutaneously.
- After the fragments have been elevated, the locking pegs of the plate are then advanced as previously described.

Arthroscopic Resection Arthroplasty

- Patients with severe loss of cartilage of the carpus should be considered for salvage procedures such as total wrist arthrodesis or arthroplasty.
- Although results are early, del Piñal et al[8] demonstrated that good pain relief and return of motion could be obtained by resecting the fragments and creating a smoother joint surface. This could provide a temporary treatment for active patients and possibly a definitive treatment for low-demand patients.[8]
- Diagnostic arthroscopy is first performed. Evaluation of the midcarpus must be performed to exclude pathology at this site.
- Typically, there is significant amount of debris and synovitis that must be débrided with a shaver to visualize the radiocarpal joint.
- A burr is then placed in the radiocarpal joint to smooth the raised malunited cancellous surface of the radius to a level slightly below the normal cartilaginous surface.
- The injured area of carpus is then likewise débrided with a shaver to obtain a smooth surface.
- Patients are started on range-of-motion exercises immediately unless excluded by other concomitant procedures.

PEARLS AND PITFALLS

Timing of reduction	■ Arthroscopically assisted reduction of distal radius fractures is most ideal between 3 and 10 days following injury. Assisted fixation before 3 days usually is complicated by bleeding that can obscure visualization. Percutaneous fracture reduction more than 10 days after the injury is exceedingly difficult and often unsuccessful due to early bony healing.
Arthroscopic visualization	■ It is important to take the time to thoroughly irrigate and débride the joint of hematoma and debris. This especially helps visualization of fragment rotation. Irrigation through a separate 6U inflow portal is helpful. A Coban wrap (3M, St. Paul, MN) may be placed around the forearm to limit fluid extravasation into the soft tissues.
Instrumentation	■ Large joint instrumentation will damage the articular cartilage and is not appropriate. A mobile traction tower is extremely helpful in arthroscopic-assisted management of distal radius fractures.
Fixation	■ Do not accept poor fixation just to treat the patient arthroscopically. Fixation should be chosen to fit the personality of the fracture. For example, K-wires should not be used to stabilize a volar Barton fracture when volar plate stabilization is the obvious superior choice. Although K-wires are easy to insert, they hinder rehabilitation and have the potential for pin tract infections. ■ Cannulated screws are recommended when arthroscopically stabilizing a fracture of the distal radius without metaphyseal comminution. ■ Multiple carpal fractures and ligamentous injuries may be treated during the same procedure (**FIG 3A,B**). ■ Volar plate fixation is recommended when metaphyseal comminution is present. ■ Arthroscopic evaluation of the wrist while the distal screws of the volar plate are being placed offers the advantage of seeing the screws penetrate into the fracture fragments, thereby ensuring stability. Arthroscopic evaluation is helpful in variable-angle volar locking plates to ensure the screws do not violate the joint.
Observation	■ It is imperative following arthroscopically assisted reduction of the distal radius in the radiocarpal space to evaluate the midcarpal space. The midcarpal space is the most sensitive and ideal location to evaluate intercarpal stability. In addition, loose bodies from the capitate or hamate occasionally are seen, particularly in association with lunate die-punch fractures. Arthroscopic evaluation also aids in determining when to fix the ulnar styloid.

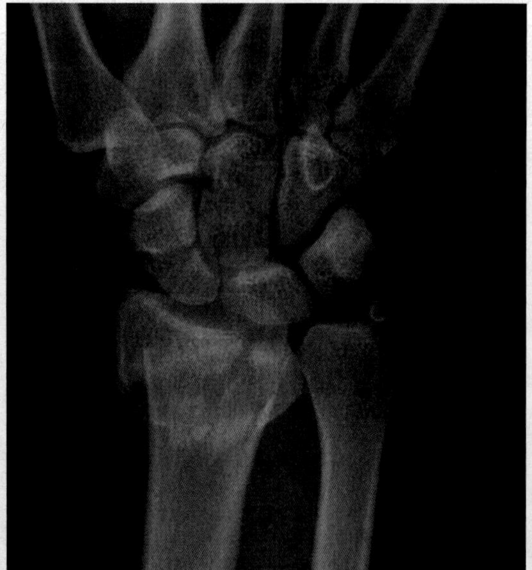
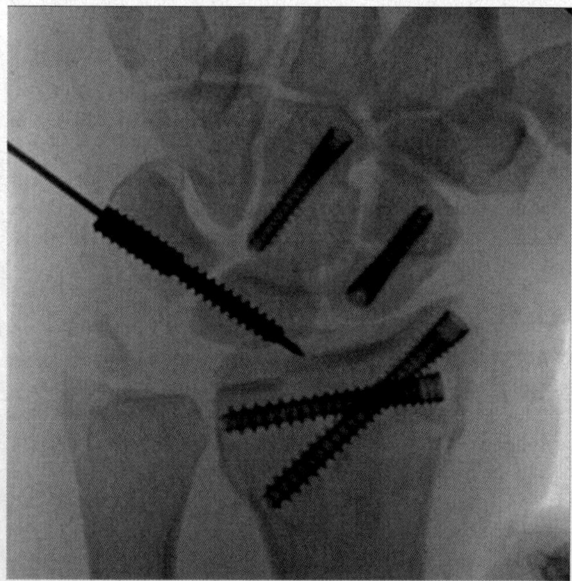

FIG 3 • **A.** AP radiographic view showing three-part intra-articular distal radius fracture along with an obvious transverse scaphoid fracture. A more subtle capitate fracture is also seen. **B.** An intraoperative PA radiographic view is seen. The patient required two Acutrack (Acumed, Hillsboro, OR) cannulated compression screws for repair of the distal radius fracture. The capitate and scaphoid were likewise repaired using Acutrack cannulated screws. Intraoperatively, a lunotriquetral ligament tear was seen and the interval stabilized with an Acumed Scapholunate Intercarpal (SLIC) screw (Acumed).

POSTOPERATIVE CARE

- The degree of postoperative immobilization depends on numerous factors, including the mode of fracture stabilization, the quality of the bone for internal fixation, the stability of the fixation, and the management of any associated soft tissue injuries that were addressed during the arthroscopic evaluation.
- Immediate range of motion of the digits and wrist is initiated in patients with volar plate fixation with good bone stock and solid fixation.
- In patients with soft osteopenic bone with volar plate fixation, digital range-of-motion exercises are initiated immediately, but wrist range of motion is delayed approximately 3 to 4 weeks to permit some fracture healing.
  - Soft bone may collapse around the rigid plate.
- In patients without metaphyseal comminution treated by arthroscopically assisted stabilization with cannulated screws, range of motion is initiated as the patient tolerates.
- In patients treated with percutaneous K-wires, the wrist is immobilized until the wires are removed, usually 4 to 6 weeks after surgery.
- A patient with an unstable DRUJ is treated by TFCC repair or ulnar styloid reduction and fixation is restricted from pronation and supination for 2 to 4 weeks.

OUTCOMES

- The literature is relatively sparse regarding the results of arthroscopically assisted fixation of displaced intra-articular distal radius fractures.[9,10,12,13,22,27,30]
- A comparison study of 12 open and 12 arthroscopic reductions of comminuted AO types VII and VIII fractures of the distal radius found that the arthroscopic group had increased range of motion as compared to the open stabilization group.[32]
- A second comparison study of 38 patients who underwent arthroscopically assisted fixation compared to open reduction found the arthroscopically assisted group had better results and improved range of motion.[3]
- One study compared 15 patients with arthroscopically assisted fixation to 15 patients who underwent closed reduction and external fixation.[30] In this study, there were 10 tears of the TFCC in the group that underwent arthroscopic reduction, of which 7 were peripheral and repaired. There were no signs of DRUJ instability at final follow-up visit. In the 15 patients who underwent stabilization by external fixation alone, 4 patients had continued complaints of instability of the distal radial joint, very possibly the result of undiagnosed and untreated TFCC tears.
- Ono et al[27] evaluated articular gaps and step-offs following open reduction and plating for intra-articular distal radius fractures without arthroscopic assistance. They evaluated 70 patients prospectively, recording both gaps and step-offs from CT preoperatively and the arthroscope postoperatively. The authors noted 40 patients had a gap of greater than or equal to 1 mm and 15 had a step-off of greater than or equal to 1 mm postoperatively.[27]

COMPLICATIONS

- Failure of fixation
- Late settling of the fracture despite fixation
- Flexor and extensor tendon irritation
- Painful metal requiring removal

- Neuromas of the dorsal sensory branch of the radial and ulnar nerves
- Carpal tunnel syndrome
- Reflex sympathetic dystrophy
- Wrist and hand stiffness

REFERENCES

1. Abe Y, Yoshida K, Tominaga Y. Less invasive surgery with wrist arthroscopy for distal radius fractures. J Orthop Sci 2013;18:398–404.
2. Arora R, Gabl M, Gschwentner M, et al. A comparative study of clinical and radiologic outcomes of unstable colles type distal radius fractures in patients older than 70 years: nonoperative treatment versus volar locking plating. J Orthop Trauma 2009;23(4):237–242.
3. Arora R, Lutz M, Deml C, et al. A prospective randomized trial comparing nonoperative treatment with volar locking plate fixation for displaced and unstable distal radial fractures in patients sixty-five years of age and older. J Bone Joint Surg Am 2011;93(23):2146–2453.
4. Bradway JK, Amadio PC, Cooney WP. Open reduction and internal fixation of displaced comminuted intra-articular fractures of the distal end of the radius. J Bone Joint Surg Am 1989;71(6):839–847.
5. del Piñal F, Cagigal L, García-Bernal FJ, et al. Arthroscopically guided osteotomy for management of intra-articular distal radius malunions. J Hand Surg Am 2010;35(3):392–397.
6. del Piñal F, García-Bernal FJ, Delgado J, et al. Correction of malunited intra-articular distal radius fractures with an inside-out osteotomy technique. J Hand Surg Am 2006;31(6):1029–1034.
7. del Piñal F, García-Bernal FJ, Pisani D, et al. Dry arthroscopy of the wrist: surgical technique. J Hand Surg Am 2007;32(1):119–123.
8. del Piñal F, Klausmeyer M, Thams C, et al. Arthroscopic resection arthroplasty for malunited intra-articular distal radius fractures. J Hand Surg Am 2012;37(12):2447–2455.
9. Doi K, Hattori T, Otsuka K, et al. Intra-articular fractures of the distal aspect of the radius arthroscopically assisted reduction compared with open reduction and internal fixation. J Bone Joint Surg Am 1999;81(8):1093–1110.
10. Edwards CC II, Haraszti CJ, McGillivary GR, et al. Intra-articular distal radius fractures: arthroscopic assessment of radiographically assisted reduction. J Hand Surg Am 2001;26(6):1036–1041.
11. Fernandez DL, Geissler WB. Treatment of displaced articular fractures of the radius. J Hand Surg Am 1991;16:375–384.
12. Geissler WB. Arthroscopically assisted reduction of intra-articular fractures of the distal radius. Hand Clin 1995;11:19–29.
13. Geissler WB. Intra-articular distal radius fractures: the role of arthroscopy? Hand Clin 2005;21:407–416.
14. Geissler WB, Freeland AE. Arthroscopically assisted reduction of intraarticular distal radial fractures. Clin Orthop Relat Res 1996;(327):125–134.
15. Geissler WB, Freeland AE, Savoie FH, et al. Intracarpal soft-tissue lesions associated with an intra-articular fracture of the distal end of the radius. J Bone Joint Surg Am 1996;78(3):357–365.
16. Geissler WB, Savoie FH. Arthroscopic techniques of the wrist. Mediguide Orthop 1992;11:1–8.
17. Hanker GJ. Wrist arthroscopy in distal radius fractures. Proceedings of the Arthroscopy Association North America Annual Meeting, Albuquerque, NM, October 7–9, 1993.
18. Hixon ML, Fitzrandolph R, McAndrew M, et al. Acute ligamentous tears of the wrist associated with Colles fractures. Proceedings of the Annual Meeting of the American Society for Surgery of the Hand, Baltimore, 1989.
19. Hollingworth R, Morris J. The importance of the ulnar side of the wrist in fractures of the distal end of the radius. Injury 1976;7:263–266.
20. Knirk JL, Jupiter JB. Intra-articular fractures of the distal end of the radius in young adults. J Bone Joint Surg Am 1986;68(5):647–659.
21. Lafontaine M, Hardy D, Delince P. Stability assessment of distal radius fractures. Injury 1989;20:208–210.
22. Levy HJ, Glickel SZ. Arthroscopic assisted internal fixation of intraarticular wrist fractures. Arthroscopy 1993;9:122–124.
23. Lindau T. Treatment of injuries to the ulnar side of the wrist occurring with distal radial fractures. Hand Clin 2005;21:417–425.
24. Melone CP Jr. Articular fractures of the distal radius. Orthop Clin North Am 1984;15:217–236.
25. Mohanti RC, Kar N. Study of triangular fibrocartilage of the wrist joint in Colles fracture. Injury 1979;11:321–324.
26. Mudgal CS, Jones WA. Scapholunate diastasis: a component of fractures of the distal radius. J Hand Surg Br 1990;15:503–505.
27. Ono H, Katayama T, Furuta K, et al. Distal radial fracture arthroscopic intraarticular gap and step-off measurement after open reduction and internal fixation with a volar locked plate. J Orthop Sci 2012;17(4):443–449.
28. Oqawa T, Tanaka T, Yanai T, et al. Analysis of soft tissue injuries associated with distal radius fractures. BMC Sports Sci Med Rehabil 2013;5(1):19.
29. Ruch DS, Vallee J, Poehling GG, et al. Arthroscopic reduction versus fluoroscopic reduction in the management of intra-articular distal radius fractures. Arthroscopy 2004;20:225–230.
30. Short WH, Palmer AK, Werner FW, et al. A biomechanical study of distal radial fractures. J Hand Surg Am 1987;12:529–534.
31. Stewart NJ, Berger RA. Comparison study of arthroscopic as open reduction of comminuted distal radius fractures. Abstract. Presented at the 53rd Annual Meeting of the American Society for Surgery of the Hand, January 11, 1998, Scottsdale, AZ.
32. Trumble TE, Schmitt SR, Vedder NB. Factors affecting functional outcome of displaced intra-articular distal radius fractures. J Hand Surg Am 1994;19:325–340.

Fragment-Specific Fixation of Distal Radius Fractures

Robert J. Medoff

DEFINITION

- Fragment-specific fixation is a treatment approach for complex articular fracture patterns characterized by independent fixation of each major fracture component with an implant specific for that particular fragment (**FIG 1**).
- Fragment-specific implants are usually low profile and have a certain degree of "spring-like" elasticity; the combination of independent fixation of multiple fragments in different planes can restore articular anatomy without the need for effective thread purchase in small periarticular fragments.
- Surgical planning is extremely important to determine whether a single approach or a combination of surgical approaches is needed to visualize and fix each of the main fracture components that make up a particular injury. For distal radius fixation, a complete set of implants should be available to address any of the five primary fracture elements: the radial column, ulnar corner, volar rim, dorsal wall, and/or impacted articular fragments. In addition, identification and treatment of distal radioulnar joint (DRUJ) disruption and injuries of the ulnar column should be included.
- As a general rule, this technique avoids creation of large holes in small distal fragments, with fixation based and often triangulated to the stable ipsilateral cortex of the proximal fragment.
- The goal of fragment-specific fixation is creation of a multiplanar, load-sharing construct that restores an anatomic articular surface with enough stability to initiate motion postoperatively.[2,7,11]

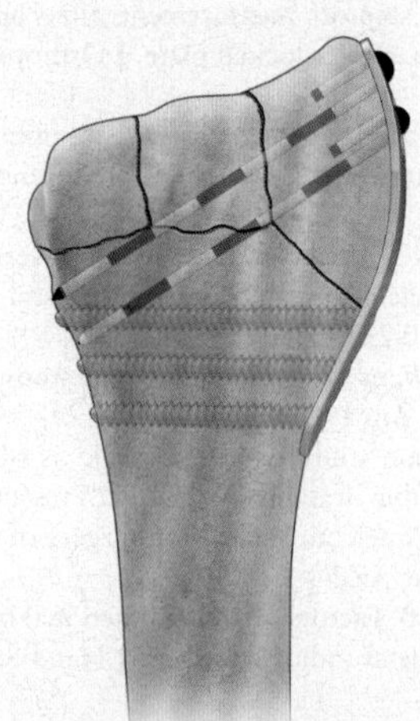

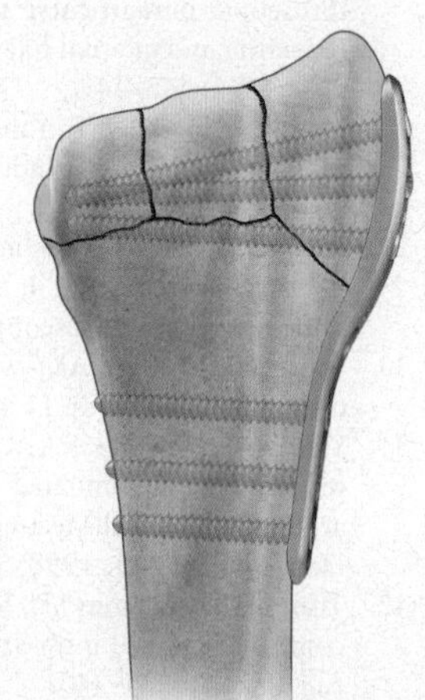

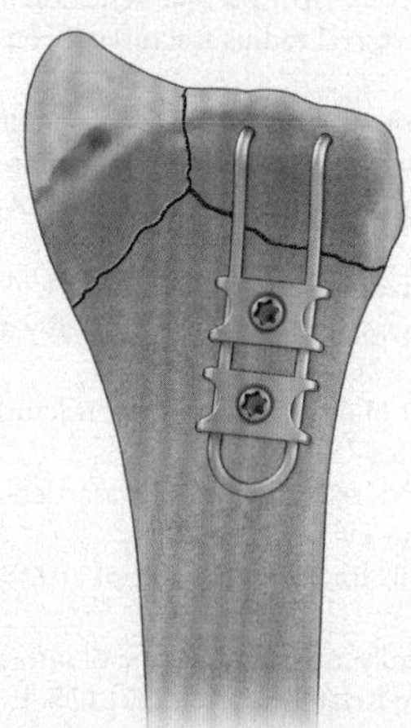

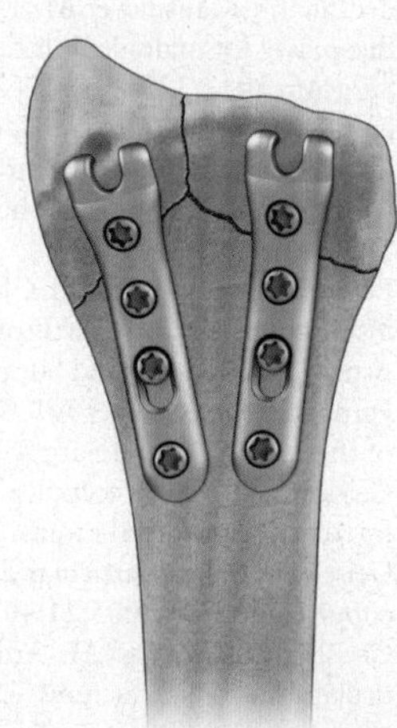

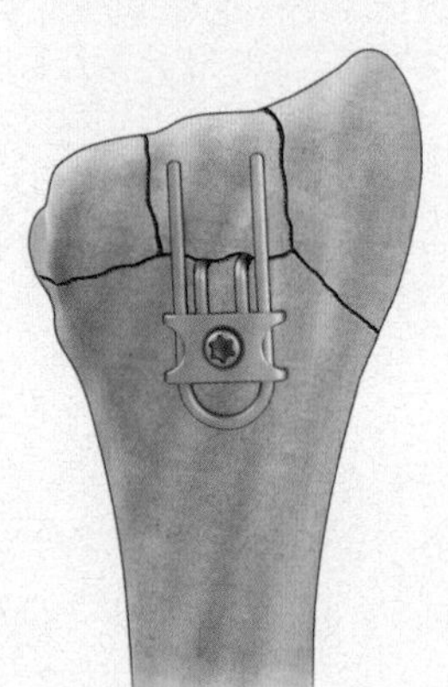

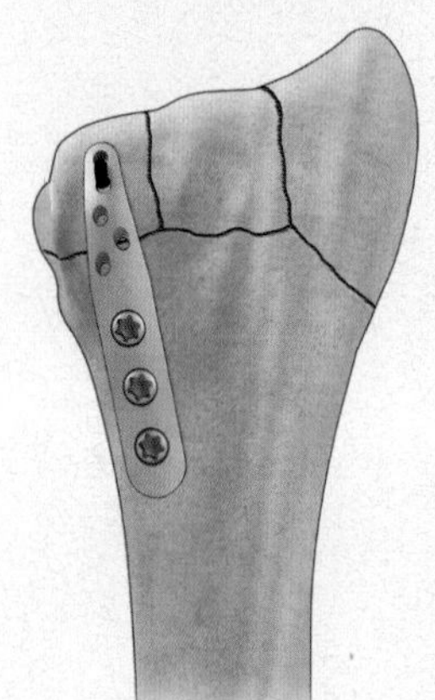

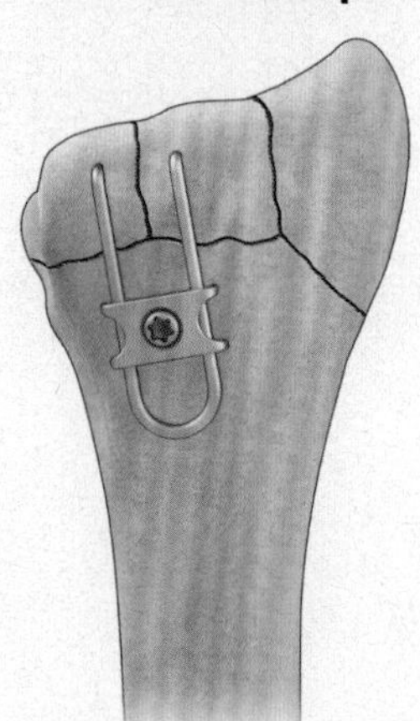

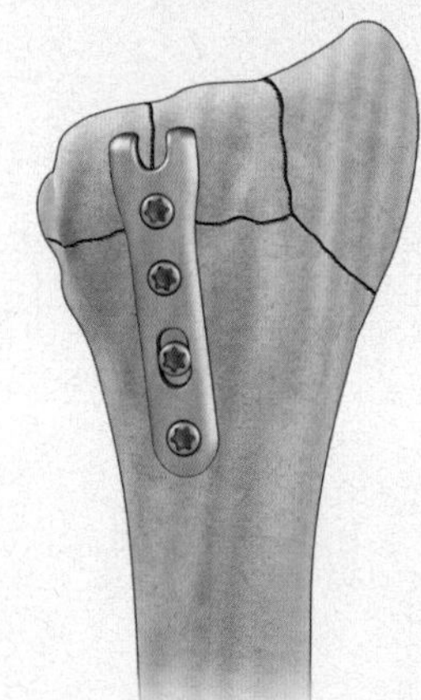

FIG 1 • Fragment-specific implants.

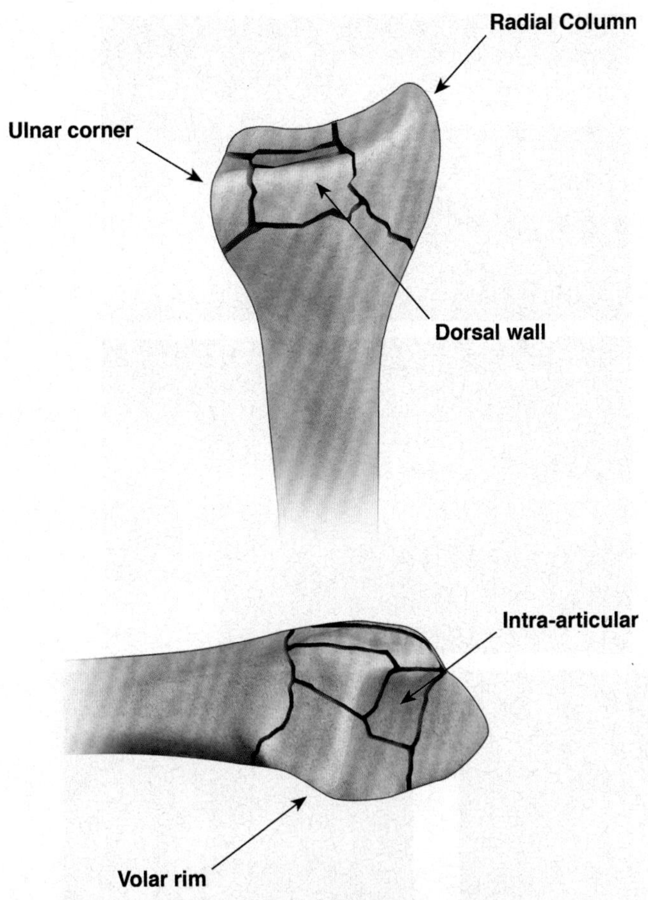

FIG 2 • Articular fracture components.

ANATOMY

Essential Basic Anatomy

- The palmar cutaneous branch of the median nerve typically lies in the subcutaneous tissue between the tendons of the flexor carpi radialis (FCR) and palmaris longus; radial-based incisions should *not* extend distally into a carpal tunnel approach in order to avoid injury to this nerve.
- The terminal branches of the lateral antebrachial cutaneous nerve and dorsal sensory branch of the radial nerve run in the subcutaneous tissue radial to the course of the radial artery. Exposure of the radial column by elevating a radial skin and subcutaneous flap using blunt dissection from a proximal to distal direction along the surface of the first dorsal compartment tendons helps avoid injury to these structures.
- The pronator quadratus inserts along the ridge at the distal flare of the radius; dissection distally should be limited to no more than 1 to 2 mm distal to the ridge to avoid compromise of the important volar carpal ligaments.

Essential Osseous Anatomy

- Structurally, the wrist can be thought of in terms of three basic support columns: a radial column that includes the radial border of the distal radius and scaphoid facet, a middle column consisting of the central and ulnar part of the radial shaft and lunate facet, and an ulnar column that includes the DRUJ, the triangular fibrocartilage complex (TFCC), and the ulnar head.
- The radial column fragment involves the pillar of bone along the radial border of the distal radius (**FIG 2**). Restoration of radial length is important to correct the axial position of the carpus, unloading deforming compressive forces that can interfere with reduction of middle column injuries. Typically, the terminal portion of the brachioradialis inserts on the base of the radial column fragment and may be a deforming force that contributes to proximal displacement of the radial column fragment. Metaphyseal comminution along the base of the radial column fragment may also contribute to radial column instability. Although not common, radial column injuries with secondary coronal fracture page or segmental comminution into the shaft proximally can be particularly unstable fracture patterns.
- The volar rim of the lunate facet is a primary load-bearing structure of the articular surface. Instability of the volar rim occurs in two patterns:
  - In the volar instability pattern, the volar rim migrates in a proximal and volar direction resulting in secondary palmar translation of the carpus.
  - In the axial instability pattern of the volar rim, axial impaction of the carpus drives the volar rim into dorsiflexion, resulting in secondary axial and dorsal subluxation of the carpus.
- The ulnar corner fragment involves the dorsal half of the sigmoid notch and usually includes a small dorsal ulnar corner of the articular surface of the lunate facet. This fracture component is the result of impaction of the lunate into the articular surface, causing the fragment to migrate dorsally and shorten proximally. Residual displacement of the ulnar corner may result in instability of the DRUJ as well as restriction of forearm rotation.
- Dorsal wall fragmentation may be a typical finding in either dorsal bending or axial loading injuries. If displaced, this fracture component is often associated with dorsal subluxation of the carpus in addition to the typical dorsal angulation of the articular surface.
- Free articular fragments may be impacted within the metaphyseal cavity and result in incongruity of the articular surface. Elevation of dorsal wall fragments allows direct access to reduction of free articular fragments.

PATHOGENESIS

- Distal radius fractures are not all the same; it is a mistake to expect that a single method of treatment is uniformly effective. Careful analysis of the fragmentation pattern and the principle directions of fracture displacement can often provide useful information about the mechanism of injury and type of instability.[4]
- Dorsal bending injuries result in extra-articular fractures with dorsal displacement (**FIG 3A**). Comminution of the dorsal wall and compression into metaphyseal cavity can result in dorsal instability.
- Volar bending injuries result in extra-articular fractures with volar displacement (**FIG 3B**). Fractures with significant volar displacement are nearly always unstable and require some type of intervention to obtain and hold a reduction until union.

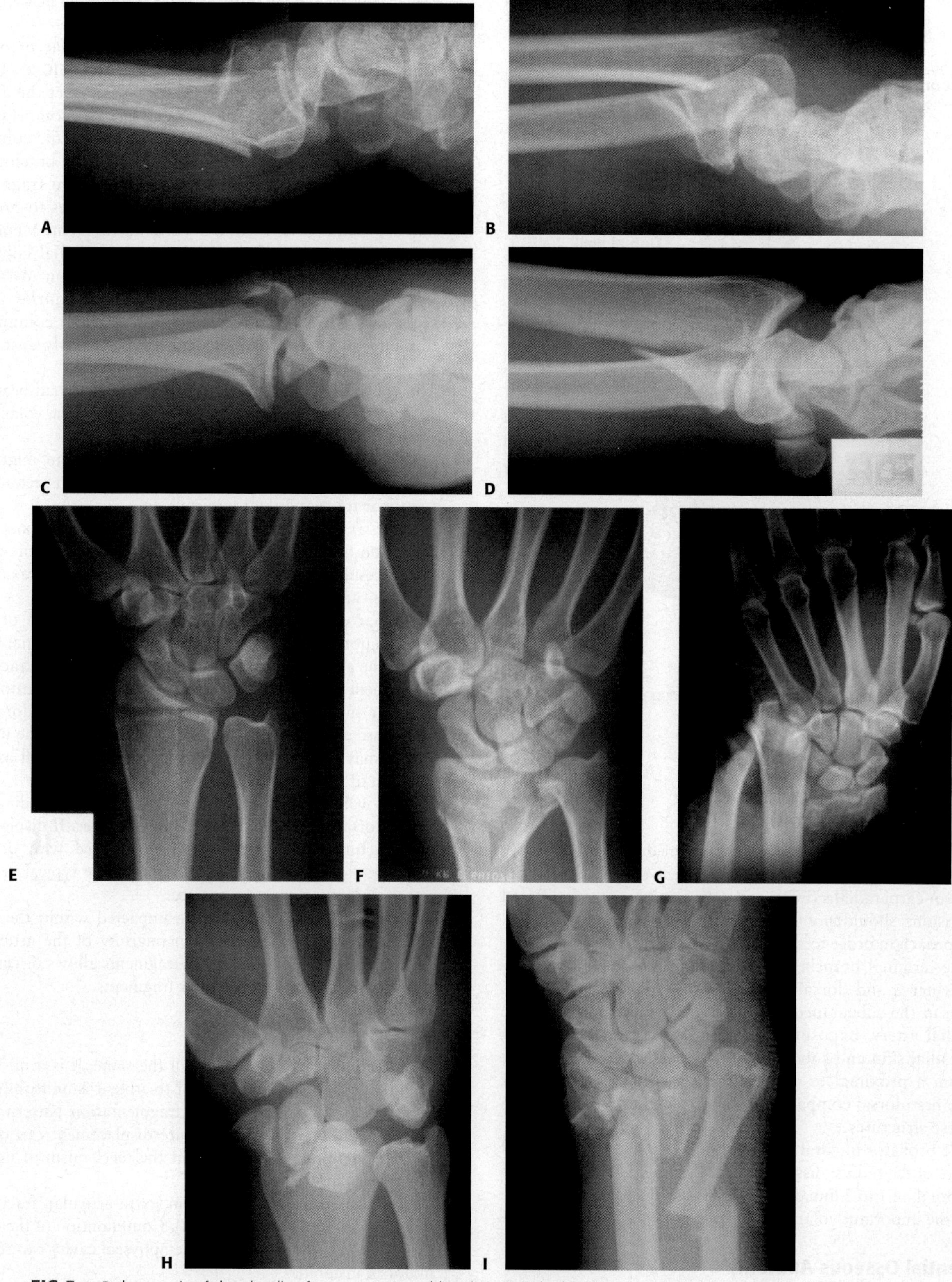

FIG 3 • Pathogenesis of dorsal radius fractures. **A.** Dorsal bending. **B.** Volar bending. **C.** Dorsal shear. **D.** Volar shear. **E.** Radial shear. **F.** Three-part articular. **G.** Comminuted articular. **H.** Carpal avulsion. **I.** High energy.

- Dorsal shearing injuries present as fractures of the dorsal rim and are often associated with dorsal instability of the carpus (**FIG 3C**). These injuries often have a depressed articular fragment and may have additional radial column involvement.
- Volar shearing injuries present as displaced fractures of the volar rim and result in volar instability of the carpus (**FIG 3D**). This pattern often has multiple articular fragments and is highly unstable. It is not usually amenable to closed methods of treatment.
- Radial shearing fractures (chauffeur's fracture) are identified by a characteristic transverse fracture line across the radial styloid that extends into the radiocarpal joint. These injuries often have more extensive chondral disruption than may be appreciated from the radiographic findings (**FIG 3E**).
- Simple three-part fractures are usually the result of low-energy injuries that combine a dorsal bending mechanism with some axial loading across the carpus (**FIG 3F**). This pattern is characterized by the presence of an ulnar corner fragment involving the dorsal portion of the sigmoid notch, a main articular fragment, and a proximal shaft fragment.
- Complex articular fractures are usually the result of axial loading injuries from moderate to high-energy trauma. In addition to articular comminution, this pattern may often generate a significant defect in the metaphyseal cavity or complete disruption of the DRUJ (**FIG 3G**).
- The avulsion/carpal instability pattern is primarily a ligamentous injury of the carpus with associated osseous avulsions of the distal radius. Bone fragments are typically small and very distal (**FIG 3H**).
- Injuries from a high-energy mechanism present as complex comminuted fractures of the articular surface with extension into the radial/ulnar shaft (**FIG 3I**).

IMAGING AND OTHER DIAGNOSTIC STUDIES

- Posteroanterior (PA), standard lateral (**FIG 4A,B**), and 10-degree lateral views are routine views for radiographic evaluation of the distal radius. The 10-degree lateral view (**FIG 4C,D**) clearly visualizes the ulnar two-thirds of the articular surface from the base of the scaphoid facet through the entire lunate facet. Oblique views may also be helpful for evaluating the injury.
- The radiographic features of distal radius fractures include the following[8]:
  - Carpal facet horizon (**FIG 5A,B**). This is the radiodense horizontal landmark that is used to identify the volar and dorsal rim on the PA view. If the articular surface has palmar tilt, the x-ray beam is tangential to the subchondral bone of the volar portion of the lunate facet, with the result that the carpal facet horizon identifies the volar rim. However, if the articular surface has displaced into dorsal tilt, the x-ray beam becomes tangential to the subchondral bone of the dorsal portion of the lunate facet instead, and the carpal facet horizon identifies the dorsal rim (not shown). The carpal facet horizon corresponds to the portion of the articular surface visualized on the 10-degree lateral x-ray projection.
  - Teardrop angle (normal 70 ± 5 degrees; **FIG 5C,D**). The teardrop angle is used to identify dorsiflexion of the volar

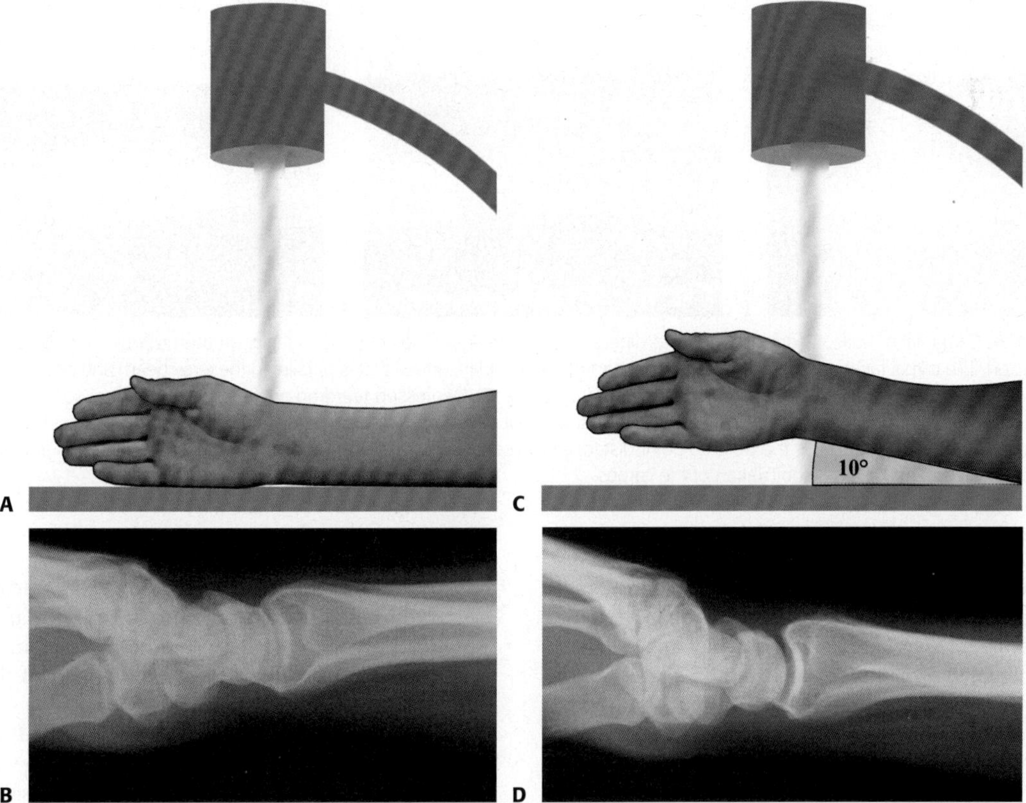

FIG 4 • **A.** Positioning for standard lateral radiography. **B.** Standard lateral radiograph. **C.** Positioning for 10-degree lateral radiography. **D.** Ten-degree lateral radiograph. Note the improved visualization of the articular surface of the base of the scaphoid facet and the entire lunate facet.

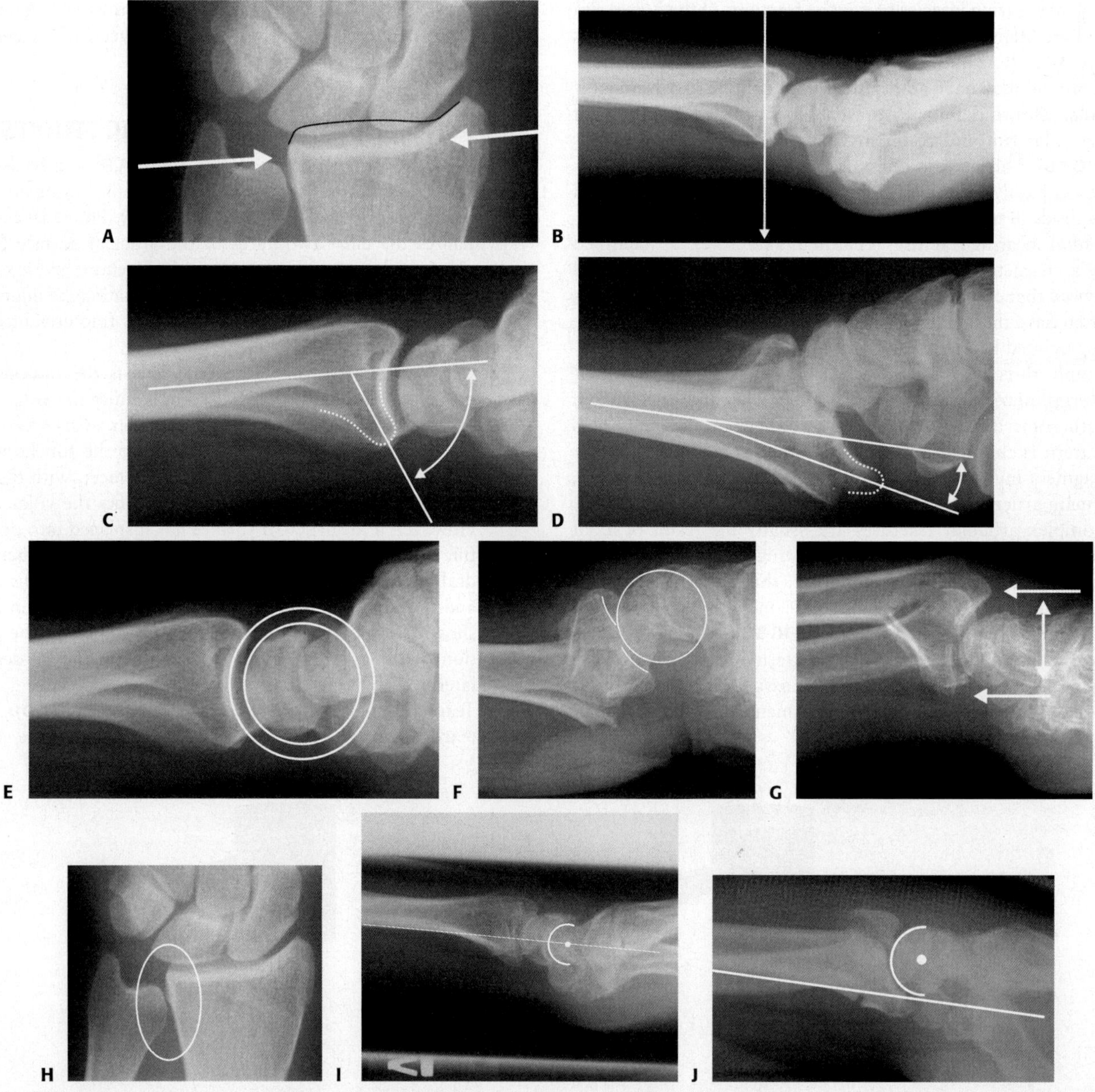

FIG 5 • **A.** Carpal facet horizon (*arrows*). Used to differentiate between the volar and dorsal rim on the PA projection. **B.** Origin of carpal facet horizon. The carpal facet horizon is formed by that part of the articular surface that is parallel to the x-ray beam and depends on whether the articular surface is in volar or dorsal tilt. **C.** Normal teardrop angle. **D.** Depressed teardrop angle in this case is caused by axial instability of the volar rim. **E.** Normal articular congruency. **F.** Abnormal articular congruency, indicating disruption across the volar and dorsal surfaces of the lunate facet. **G.** AP interval is the point-to-point distance between the corners of the dorsal and volar rim. **H.** DRUJ interval. **I.** Normal lateral carpal alignment. **J.** Dorsal subluxation of the carpus.

rim of the lunate facet. Depression of the teardrop angle to a value less than 45 degrees indicates that the volar rim of the lunate facet has rotated dorsally and impacted into the metaphyseal cavity (axial instability pattern of the volar rim). This may be associated with axial and dorsal subluxation of the carpus. Restoration of the teardrop angle is necessary to correct this type of malreduction.

- Congruency of the articular surface (**FIG 5E,F**). The subchondral outline of the articular surface of the distal radius is normally both congruent and concentric with the subchondral outline of the base of the lunate; a uniform joint interval should be present between the radius and lunate along the entire articular surface. When the joint interval between these articular surfaces is not uniform, discontinuity and disruption of the lunate facet has occurred.
- Anteroposterior (AP) distance (normal: females 18 ± 1 mm, males 20 ± 1 mm; **FIG 5G**). The AP distance is the point-to-point distance from the dorsal to palmar rim of the lunate facet. It is best evaluated on the 10-degree lateral view. Widening of the AP distance implies discontinuity of the volar and dorsal portion of the lunate facet.

- DRUJ interval (**FIG 5H**). The DRUJ interval measures the degree of apposition between the head of the ulna and the sigmoid notch (normal: 2 mm or less). This parameter is best measured with the forearm in neutral rotation. Significant widening of the DRUJ interval implies disruption of the DRUJ capsule and TFCC. Coronal malalignment of the distal radial fragment is often suggested by widening of the DRUJ interval.
- Lateral carpal alignment (**FIG 5I,J**). On the 10-degree lateral view and with the wrist in neutral position, the rotational center of the capitate normally aligns with a line extended from the volar surface of the radial shaft. Dorsal rotation of the volar rim results in a dorsal shift of lateral carpal alignment as the carpus subluxes dorsally. This may place the flexor tendons at a mechanical disadvantage, affecting grip strength.

- In addition to injury films, reassessing radiographs after reduction can be very helpful in determining the personality and specific components of a particular fracture.
- Computed tomography (CT) scans allow higher resolution and definition of fracture characteristics, particularly for highly comminuted fractures. Preferably, an attempt at closed reduction before obtaining a CT scan will help limit distortion of the image. CT scans are particularly helpful for visualizing intra-articular fragments as well as DRUJ disruption and incongruity of the sigmoid notch.
- Clinical evaluation of the carpus, interosseous membrane, and elbow, combined with radiographic studies when needed, should be included to identify the presence of other injuries that may affect the decision for a particular treatment.

SURGICAL MANAGEMENT

Operative Indications

- General parameters
  - Shortening of more than 5 mm
  - Radial inclination of less than 15 degrees
  - Dorsal angulation of more than 10 degrees
  - Articular step-off of more than 1 to 2 mm
  - Depression of teardrop angle to less than 45 degrees
- Volar instability
- DRUJ instability
- Displaced articular fractures
- Young, active patients are generally less tolerant of residual deformity and malposition.

Preoperative Planning

- Extra-articular fractures: multiple options
  - Volar plating through a volar approach
  - Dorsal plating through a dorsal approach
  - Fragment-specific fixation
    - Radial pin plate (TriMed, Inc., Valencia, CA) and volar buttress pin (TriMed, Inc.) fixation through a limited incision volar or standard volar approach
    - Radial pin plate and either an ulnar pin plate dorsally or a dorsal buttress pin through a dorsal or combined approach
    - Fixed-angle radial column plate using either a volar or dorsal radial column exposure
    - Volar hook plates with or without radial column plate using a volar approach
- Intra-articular fractures: Surgical approach is based on the fragmentation pattern.
  - Unstable volar rim fragments require a standard volar or rarely an ulnar-based volar approach for adequate visualization.
  - Fixation of the radial column can be done either through a limited-incision volar radial approach (Henry), a volar approach with radial extension combined with pronation of the forearm, or a dorsal approach with radial extension combined with supination of the forearm.
  - Fixation of dorsal, ulnar corner, and free intra-articular fragments can be done through a dorsal approach.

Positioning

- The patient is supine.
- The affected arm is placed on an arm board out to the side.
- C-arm
  - If the arm board is radiolucent, the C-arm can be brought in from the end of the arm board and images taken directly with the wrist on the arm board.
  - If the arm board is not radiolucent, the C-arm is brought in along the side of the table from the foot, and the arm is brought off the arm board for each image.

Operative Sequence

- Initial restoration of radial column length with traction and provisional trans-styloid pin fixation can be helpful to hold the carpus out to length and unload the lunate facet.
- The volar rim is reduced and fixed. For complex injuries, this is usually the keystone on which to build stable fixation.
- The dorsal ulnar corner is reduced and fixed if necessary.
- Free intra-articular fragments and the dorsal wall fragments are reduced and stabilized as necessary.
- Bone graft is applied if the metaphyseal defect is large.
- Fixation is completed with a radial column plate.
- Depending on the nature of the fracture, fixation may be a subset of these steps.

Approach

- The repair is undertaken by means of one of the following approaches:
  - Limited-incision volar approach (distal limb of Henry approach)
  - Dorsal approach
  - Extensile volar approach (FCR approach)
  - Volar ulnar approach

Limited-Incision Volar Approach

- Make a longitudinal incision along the radial side of the radial artery.
- Proximally, insert the tip of a tenotomy scissors over the surface of the first dorsal compartment sheath and sweep distally to elevate a radial skin flap.
- Pronate the forearm and sharply expose the bare area of bone over the radial styloid situated in the interval between the first and second dorsal compartments (**TECH FIG 1A**).
- Leaving the distal 1 cm of sheath intact, open the first dorsal compartment proximally and mobilize the tendons. Reflect the insertion of brachioradialis to complete exposure of the radial column (**TECH FIG 1B**).
- If needed, the dissection can be continued through the floor of the incision to expose the volar surface. Detach the insertion of the pronator quadratus radially and distally and reflect to the ulnar side. Alternatively, create an ulnar skin flap superficial to the artery and continue the exposure through a standard volar approach.
- Exposure of the ulnar side of the volar rim may be difficult with this approach, particularly with large patients or in the presence of significant swelling.

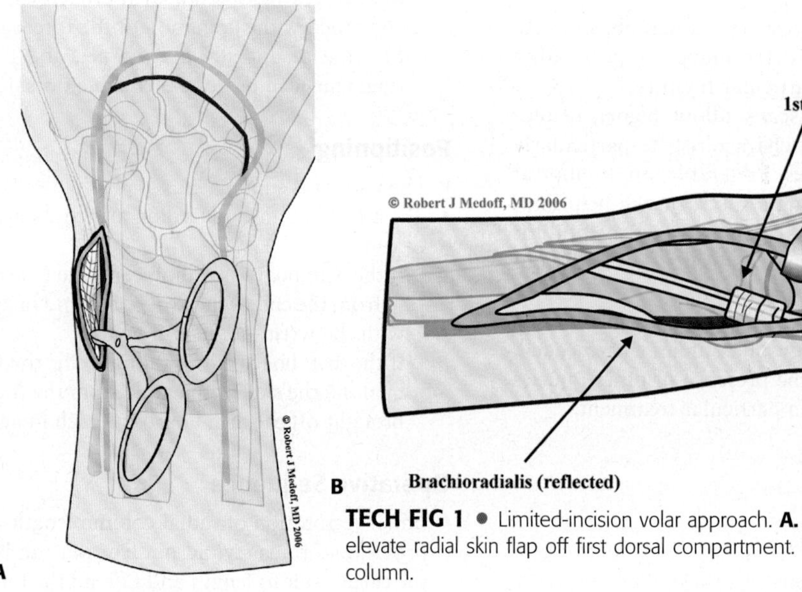

TECH FIG 1 • Limited-incision volar approach. **A.** Sweeping tenotomy scissors to elevate radial skin flap off first dorsal compartment. **B.** Deep exposure of the radial column.

Dorsal Approach

- Make a longitudinal skin incision dorsally along the ulnar side of the tubercle of Lister (**TECH FIG 2A**).
- Identify the extensor digitorum communis (EDC) tendons visible proximally through the translucent extensor sheath. Incise the dorsal retinacular sheath.
- Develop the interval between the third and fourth compartment tendons for access to dorsal wall and free, impacted articular fragments. Resect a segment of the terminal branch of the posterior interosseous nerve (**TECH FIG 2B**).
- Transpose the extensor pollicis longus (EPL) from the tubercle of Lister if required for additional exposure.
- Develop the interval between the fourth and fifth extensor compartments to gain access to the ulnar corner fragment.
- A dorsal capsulotomy can be done to visualize the articular surface and carpus as needed.
- To gain access to the radial column through a dorsal exposure, extend the incision distally and elevate a radial subcutaneous flap and supinate the wrist.
- To gain access to the distal ulna, the incision can be extended as needed to elevate an ulnar subcutaneous flap.

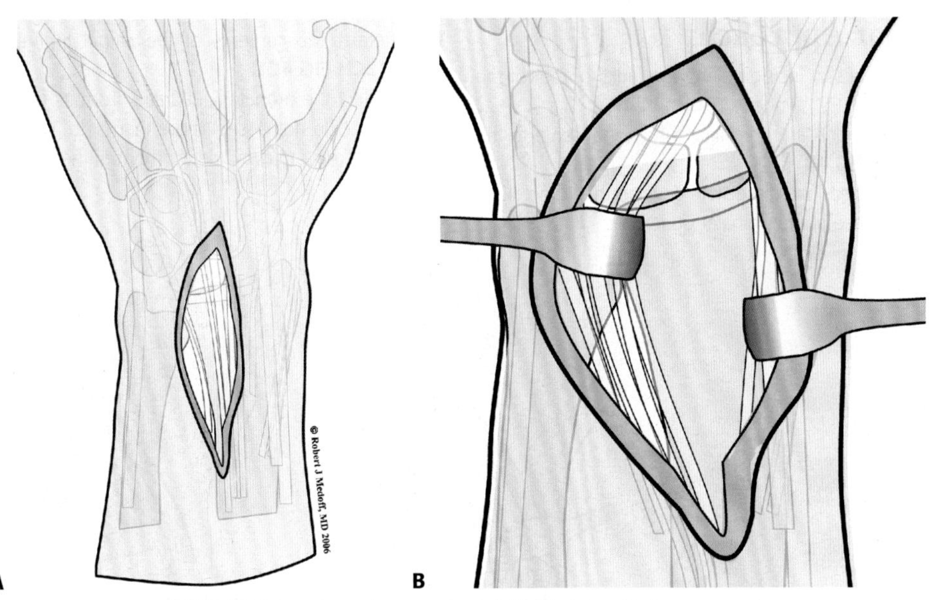

TECH FIG 2 • Dorsal approach. **A.** Initial incision. **B.** Deep exposure.

Extensile Volar Approach

- Start the skin incision at the distal pole of the scaphoid and angle it toward the radial border of the flexor wrist crease. Continue the incision proximally along the FCR tendon (**TECH FIG 3A**).
- Continue the exposure with deeper dissection in the plane between the FCR tendon and the radial artery.
- Separate the interval between the contents of the carpal tunnel and the surface of the pronator quadratus with blunt dissection with a finger or sponge. Retract the FCR, median nerve, and flexor tendons to the ulnar side (**TECH FIG 3B**).
- Divide the radial and distal attachment of the pronator quadratus and reflect it to the ulnar side. Limit the distal dissection to no more than 1 or 2 mm beyond the distal radial ridge to avoid detachment of the volar wrist capsular ligaments (**TECH FIG 3C**).
- Reflect the brachioradialis from its insertion on the distal fragment if needed. Bone graft can be applied through the radial fracture defect.
- If access to the radial column is needed, elevate a radial subcutaneous flap superficial to the radial artery and continue the exposure along the superficial surface of the first dorsal compartment tendon sheath as described with the limited incision volar approach. Pronate the wrist, and retract the radial skin flap to expose the radial column.

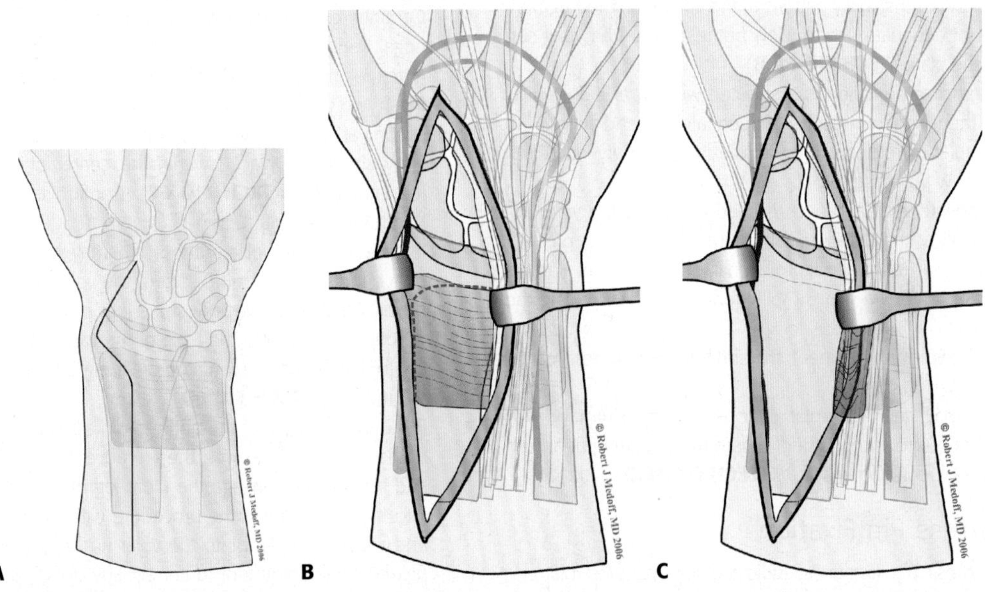

TECH FIG 3 • Extensile volar approach. **A.** Initial incision. **B.** Line of incision in pronator quadratus. **C.** Deep exposure.

Volar Ulnar Approach

- Make a longitudinal skin incision along the radial border of the flexor carpi ulnaris (FCU) tendon (**TECH FIG 4A**).
- Reflect the FCU tendon and the ulnar artery and nerve to the ulnar side (**TECH FIG 4B**).
- With blunt finger or sponge dissection, develop the plane along the superficial surface of the pronator quadratus.
- Retract the contents of the carpal tunnel to the radial side (**TECH FIG 4C**).
- Reflect the pronator quadratus from its ulnar and distal attachment. Do not dissect more than 1 to 2 mm beyond the distal radial ridge to avoid detachment of the volar wrist capsule.

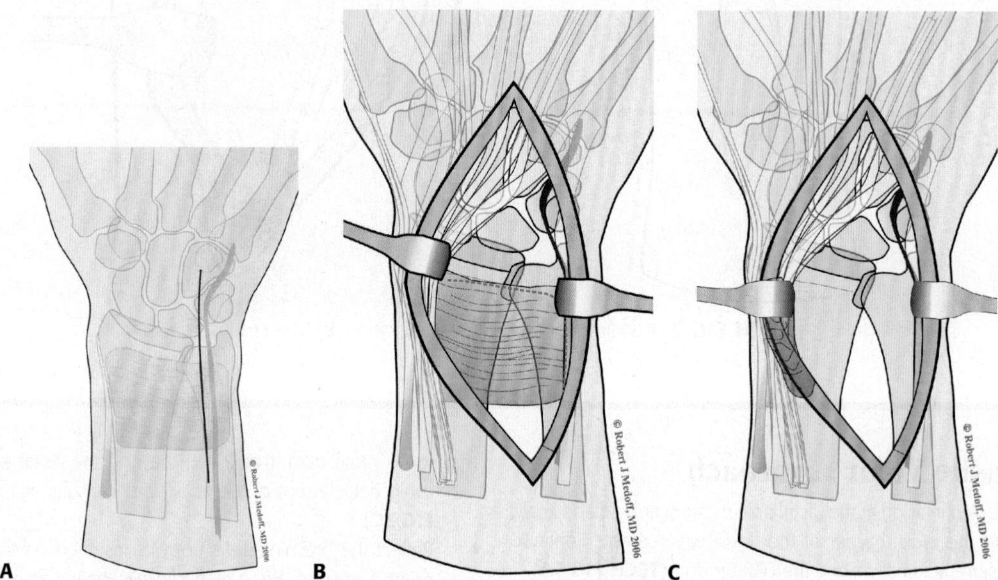

TECH FIG 4 • Volar ulnar approach. **A.** Incision. **B.** Initial exposure. **C.** Completed exposure.

Volar Rim Fragment

Small Fragment Plate Fixation

- Small fragment volar plate fixation may be indicated for treatment of a volar instability pattern of the volar rim. The fragment must be of adequate size to allow buttressing on the volar surface by the plate (**TECH FIG 5A,B**).
- If volar rim fragmentation is associated with an axial instability pattern, the fragment must be of adequate size and strength to allow angular correction of the dorsiflexion deformity with distal locked screw purchase.
- An appropriate volar approach is used to expose the volar rim fragment. If a shortened radial column fragment is present, restoring radial length and provisionally holding with a trans-styloid Kirschner wire may simplify reduction by unloading the lunate facet.
- Reduce the volar rim fragment; this should restore normal carpal alignment.
- Apply a small fragment volar plate and fix it proximally with cortical bone screws. If needed, secure the distal fragment with standard or locking bone screws (**TECH FIG 5C,D**).

Volar Buttress Pin Fixation

- Volar buttress pin fixation is indicated for unstable volar rim fragments and can be a particularly effective technique when faced with small distal fragments or axial instability patterns of the volar rim (depressed teardrop angle; **TECH FIG 6A,B**).
- Use an appropriate volar approach to expose the volar rim fragment. If necessary, restore radial length and provisionally hold it with a trans-styloid Kirschner wire to unload the lunate facet.
- Continue exposure for up to 1 to 2 mm beyond the distal radial ridge. Reduce the volar rim fragment as much as possible and note the orientation of the teardrop on the 10-degree lateral view.
- Insert two 0.045-inch Kirschner wires transverse to one another starting at an entry site 1 to 2 mm beyond the distal radial ridge. They should be placed within the center of the teardrop on the lateral view (**TECH FIG 6C**). Confirm the position of the Kirschner wires with C-arm.
- If necessary, the volar buttress pin may be contoured with a wire bender to match the flare of the volar surface of the distal radius. Adjust the trajectory of the legs of the implant to make a 70-degree angle with the base of the wire form. Cut the legs to appropriate length, leaving the ulnar leg 2 to 3 mm longer than the radial leg (**TECH FIG 6D**).
- Place the ulnar leg of the buttress pin adjacent to the entry site of the ulnar Kirschner wire, then remove the ulnar Kirschner wire and immediately engage the ulnar leg of the volar buttress pin into the hole. Repeat the procedure with the radial leg. Impact and seat the implant into the volar rim fragment. Apply to the proximal shaft fragment to correct any dorsiflexion of the volar rim (**TECH FIG 6E**).

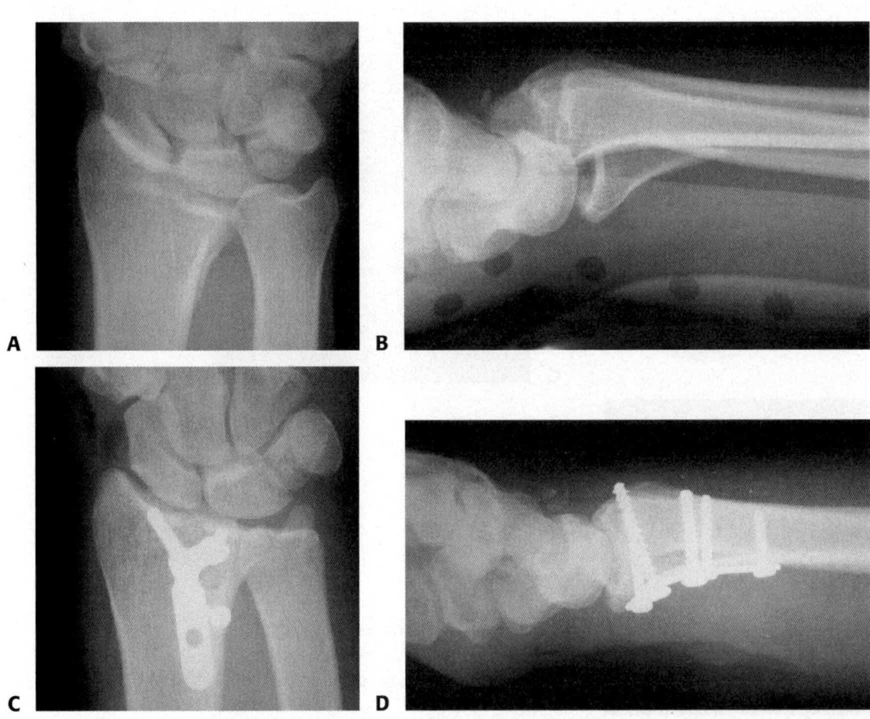

TECH FIG 5 • Volar rim fixation with small fragment plate. **A,B.** Shear fracture of volar rim with volar instability pattern. **C,D.** Fixation with small fragment plate.

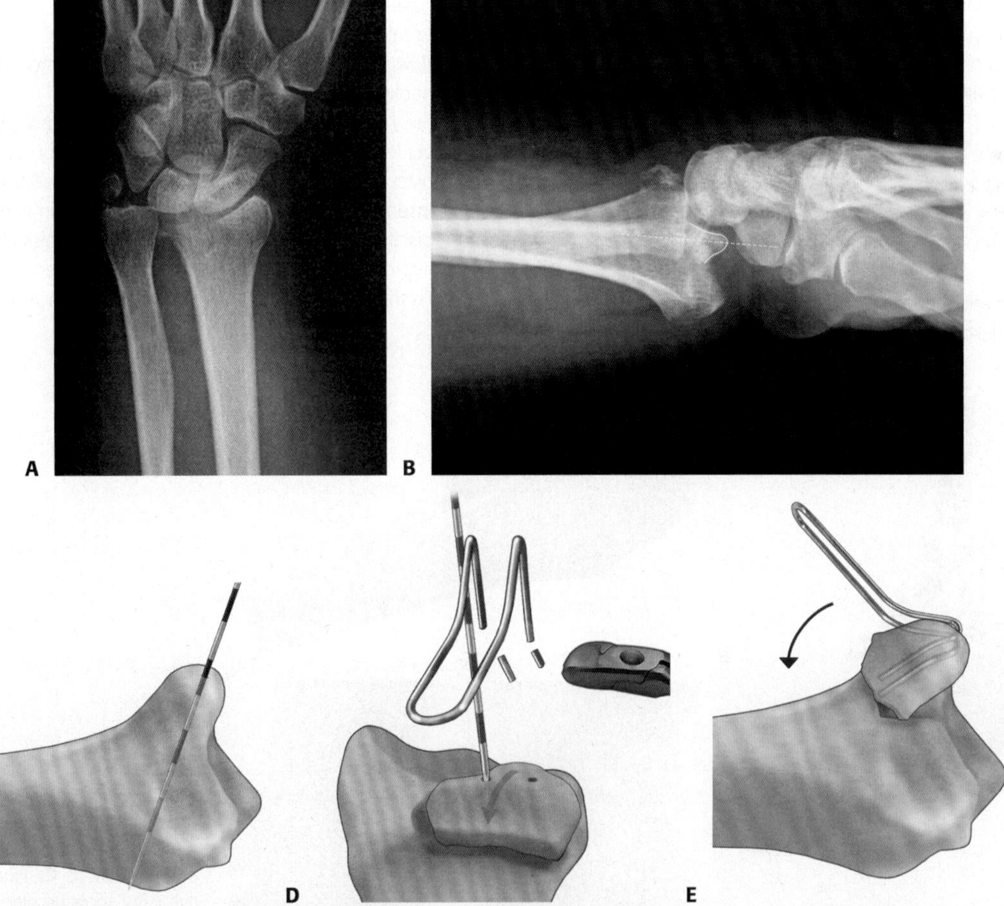

TECH FIG 6 • Volar rim fixation with a volar buttress pin. **A,B.** Articular fracture with axial instability pattern of volar rim. **C.** Insertion of Kirschner wires. **D.** Cutting and inserting legs. **E.** Reduction of teardrop. *(continued)*

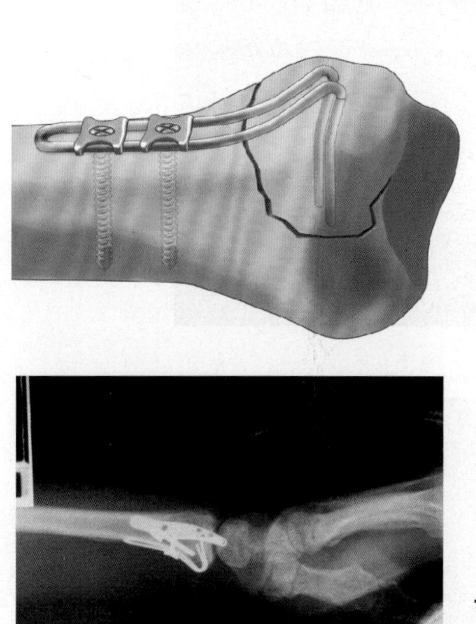

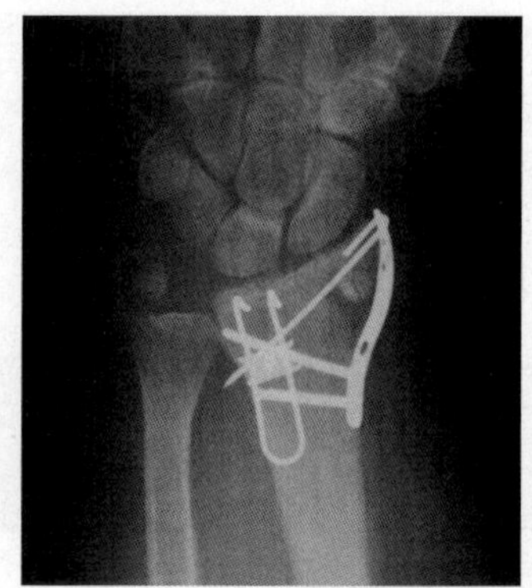

TECH FIG 6 • *(continued)* **F.** Completed fixation. **G,H.** Volar buttress pin fixation to control rotational alignment of volar rim fragment.

- Fine-tune the reduction and fix it proximally with a minimum of two screws and washers (**TECH FIG 6F–H**). If needed, a blocking screw can be placed just proximal to the end of the buttress pin to prevent shortening of the fragment. Alternatively, a wire plate can be used to secure the implant proximally.

Volar Hook Plate Fixation

- Volar hook plates are useful alternative to volar buttress pins for fixation of unstable volar rim fragments, particularly for small distal fragments associated with axial instability patterns of the volar rim or volar instability patterns associated with volar shear fractures.
- Expose and reduce the volar rim fragment according to the technique described for the volar buttress pin. If possible, provisionally hold the reduction with a Kirschner wire in the radial and ulnar border.
- Position and insert a 0.045-inch Kirschner guidewire distally down the center of the teardrop along the intended path of the hooks of the plate. Confirm the position with the C-arm.
- For hard bone, place a volar hook plate drill guide over the guidewire, and predrill the cortex for insertion of the hooks. In osteoporotic bone, this step may not be necessary.
- Insert the volar hook plate over the guide pin and seat into the distal fragment (**TECH FIG 7A–C**). Place a distal locking peg of appropriate length after predrilling with a fixed-angle peg guide. Fix the plate proximally with standard bone screws.

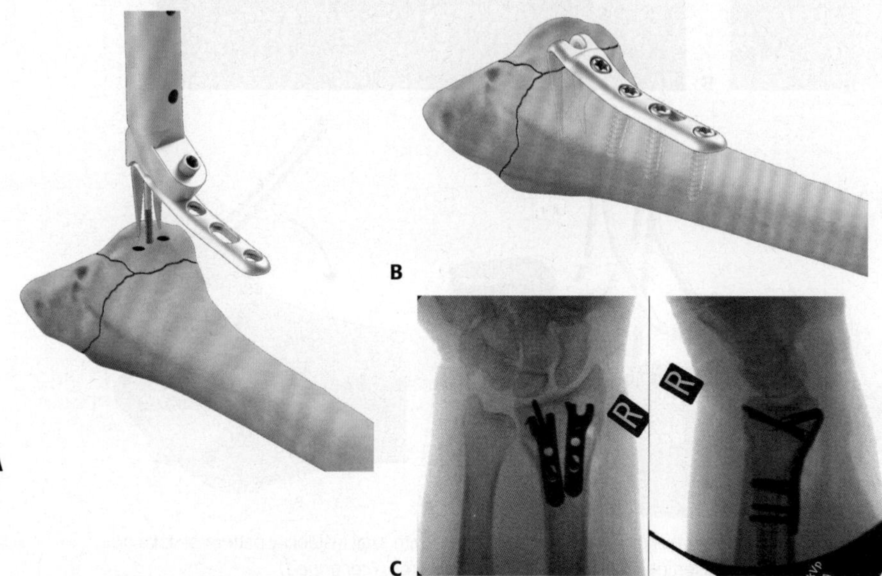

TECH FIG 7 • Volar rim fixation with a volar hook plate. **A.** Insertion of volar hook plate over guide pin through predrilled holes. **B.** Completed fixation. **C.** Final intraoperative x-ray showing placement of two volar hook plates into separate distal rim fragments.

Radial Column Fixation with Radial Plate

- Expose the radial column with any of the approaches previously described. Sharply expose the interval between the first and second dorsal compartments over the tip of the radial styloid. Release the tendon sheath of the first dorsal compartment proximally, leaving the last 1 cm of tendon sheath intact.
- Retract the tendons of the first dorsal compartment volarly for distal exposure and dorsally for proximal exposure along the shaft. Release the terminal insertion of the brachioradialis to complete exposure of the radial column.
- After the initial fracture exposure, restore radial length with traction and ulnar deviation of the wrist. If needed, structural bone graft can be inserted through the radial fracture defect.
- Insert a 0.045-inch trans-styloid Kirschner wire angled to engage the far cortex of the proximal fragment (**TECH FIG 8A**). When the advancing tip of the Kirschner wire hits the far cortex, place a drill sleeve over the Kirschner wire and use as a drill stop to limit penetration of the far cortex to 1 to 2 mm.
- Once the radial column is temporarily fixed with a trans-styloid Kirschner wire, reduce and stabilize other volar, dorsal, and articular fracture elements before completing fixation of the radial column.
- Select a distal pin hole and slide a radial pin plate over the trans-styloid Kirschner wire. Proximally, guide the plate under the tendons of the first dorsal compartment and secure it initially with a single 2.3-mm bone screw.
- Insert a second trans-styloid Kirschner wire through a nonadjacent distal pin hole. Use the previous technique to limit penetration of the Kirschner wire through the far cortex to 1 to 2 mm.
- Mark a reference point where the Kirschner wire crosses the surface of the plate. Withdraw the Kirschner wire 1 cm and cut it 1 cm or more above the reference mark (**TECH FIG 8B**).
- Position the reference mark between the lower two posts of a wire bender and create a hook (**TECH FIG 8C**). By starting the bend at the reference mark, this ensures that a Kirschner wire of proper length that extends 1 to 2 mm beyond the far cortex is created.
- Complete the bend with a pin clamp, overbending slightly to allow the hook to snap into an adjacent pin hole or over the edge of the plate (**TECH FIG 8D**). With a free 0.045-inch Kirschner wire, predrill a hole to accept the end of the hook.
- Impact the Kirschner wire with a pin impactor and fully seat the hook (**TECH FIG 8E**). Repeat the procedure with the second Kirschner wire.
- Complete proximal fixation with 2.3-mm cortical bone screws (**TECH FIG 8F,G**).

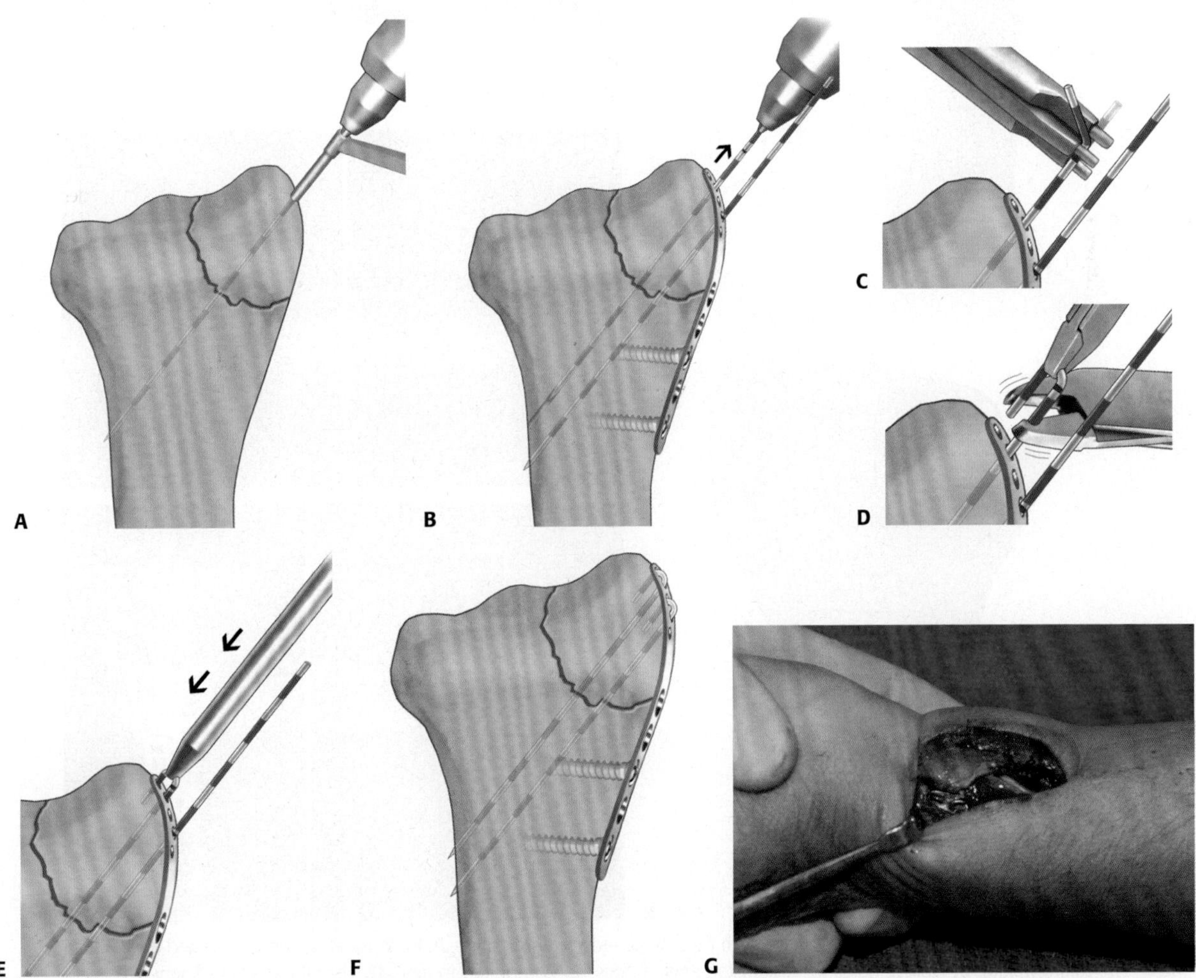

TECH FIG 8 • Radial column fixation with radial pin plate. **A.** Insertion of trans-styloid Kirschner wire. **B,C.** Creation of pin hook. **D,E.** Completion and impaction of pin hook. **F,G.** Completed radial column fixation.

Radial Column Fixation with Fixed-Angle Radial Column Plate

- Expose and reduce the radial column with the technique described previously.
- Position the fixed-angle radial column plate and temporarily fix with a Kirschner wire both proximally and distally (**TECH FIG 9A**). Confirm reduction of the radial column and plate position with the C-arm.
- Using fixed-angle drill guides, drill, measure, and insert locking fixation pegs of appropriate length into the distal fixed-angle holes in the plate and standard bone screws proximally into the shaft (**TECH FIG 9B–E**).

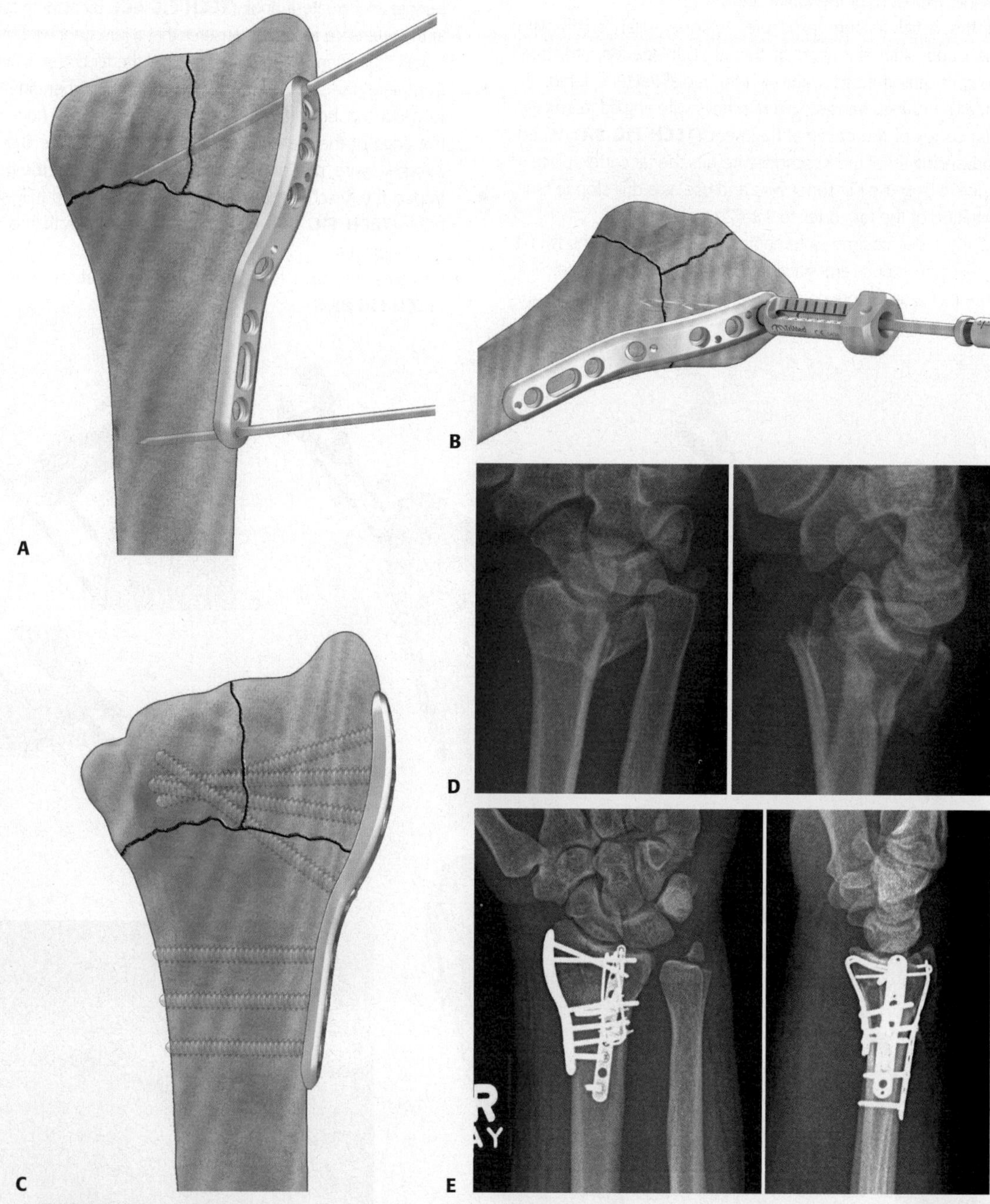

TECH FIG 9 • Radial column fixation with fixed-angle radial column plate. **A.** Provisional placement of fixed-angle radial column plate. **B.** Drilling holes for distal fixed-angled pegs. **C.** Completed fixation. **D.** Unstable fracture injury films with segmental radial column comminution. **E.** Films 2 months postoperatively. Fixed-angle radial column support is used to avoid radial column shortening.

Ulnar Corner and Dorsal Wall Fixation

Ulnar Pin Plate

- Through a dorsal approach, expose and reduce the dorsal ulnar corner fragment, dorsal wall fragment, or both.
- Insert a 0.045-inch Kirschner wire through the fragment (**TECH FIG 10A**), angled proximally and slightly radially to purchase the far cortex of the proximal fragment.
- Insert structural bone graft into the metaphyseal defect if present to support the subarticular surface.
- If the plate is aligned along the pulnar border of the shaft, add a 15-degree torsional bend to the plate (twist the proximal end of the plate into slight supination). Often, a little extra extension can be contoured at the distal end of the plate (**TECH FIG 10B**).
- Slide the plate over the Kirschner wire and fix it proximally with a 2.3-mm bone screw (**TECH FIG 10C**).
- Insert a second Kirschner wire if the fragment is large enough. Create and impact hooks as described for the radial pin plate (**TECH FIG 10D–F**).
- If the Kirschner wire tips protrude beyond the volar cortex, they can be cut flush to the bone surface through a volar incision.

Dorsal Buttress Pin

- Through a dorsal approach, expose and reduce the dorsal ulnar corner fragment, dorsal wall fragment, or both.
- Insert structural bone graft into the metaphyseal defect if present to support the subarticular surface.
- Insert two 0.045-inch Kirschner wires through the dorsal cortex and behind the subchondral bone; check the position with

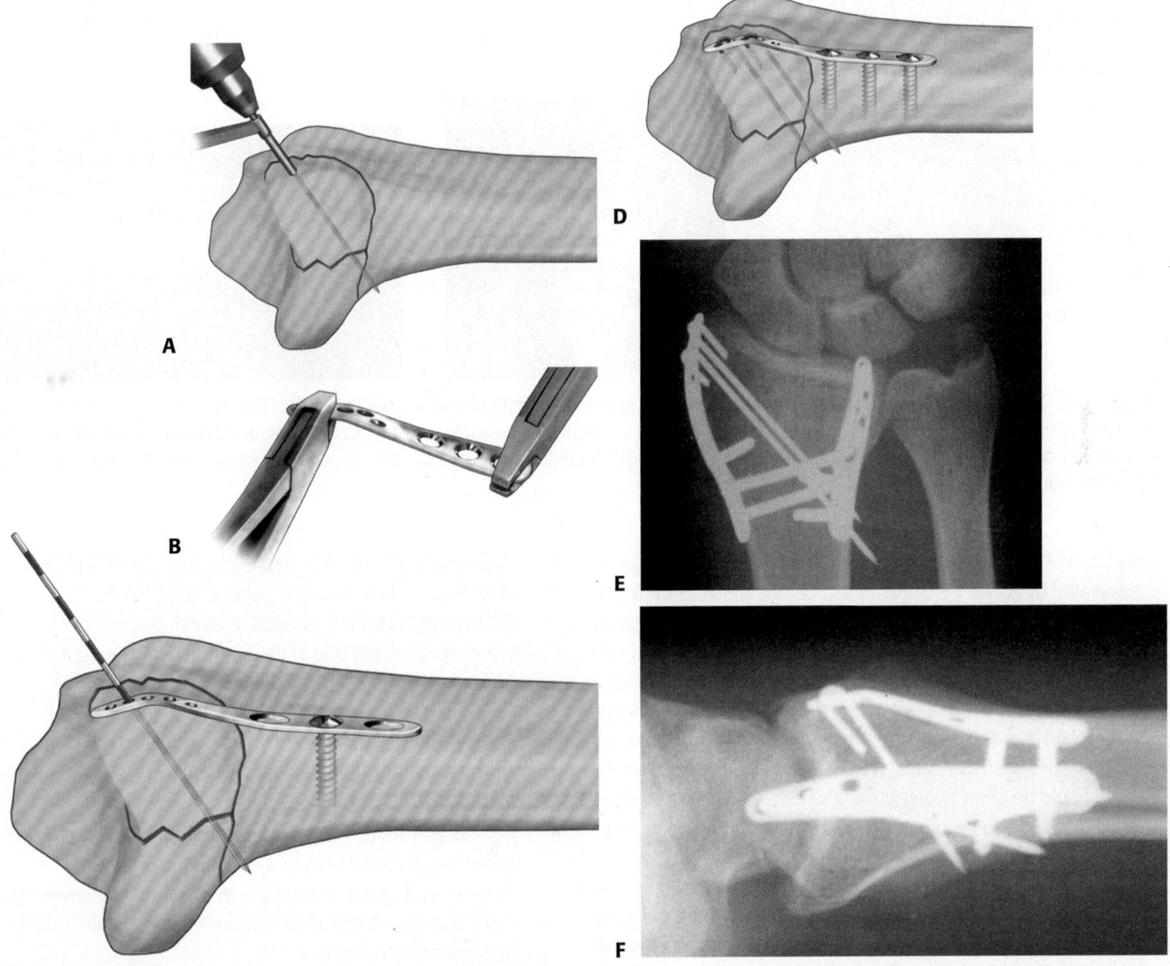

TECH FIG 10 • Ulnar corner fixation with an ulnar pin plate. **A.** Insertion of the interfragmentary Kirschner wire. **B.** Contouring the plate. **C.** Application of the plate and insertion of the initial fixation screw. **D.** Fixation completed. **E,F.** Radial and ulnar pin plate fixation of a three-part articular pattern (radial column and ulnar corner fragment).

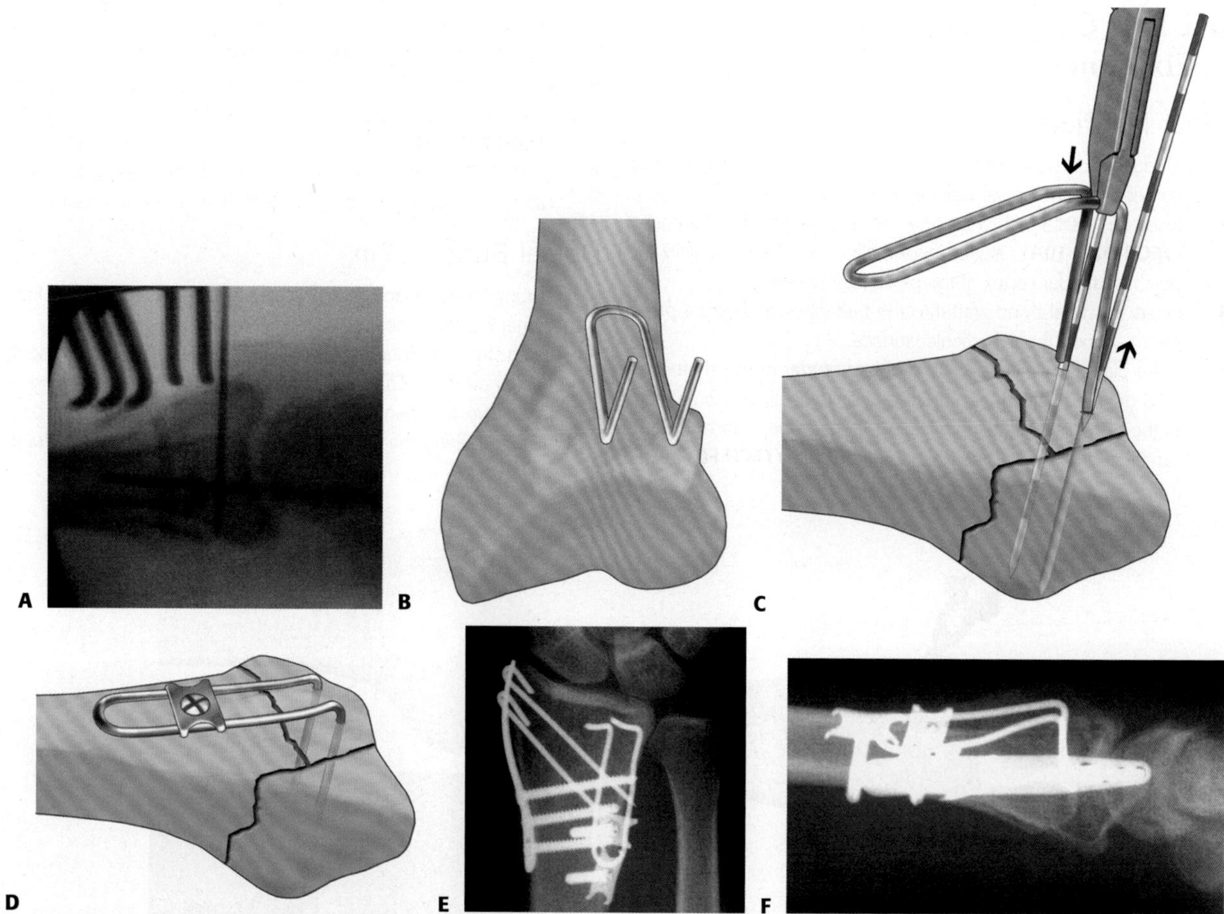

TECH FIG 11 • Dorsal buttress pin fixation. **A.** The position of the Kirschner wires is checked with a C-arm before inserting the implant. **B.** Placing an implant upside-down on bone to template the trajectory of the Kirschner wires. **C.** Inserting the dorsal buttress pin. **D.** Buttress pin fixation completed. **E,F.** Fixation of a three-part articular fracture with radial column and ulnar corner fragment with radial column plate and dorsal buttress pin.

the C-arm (**TECH FIG 11A**). The Kirschner wires should be separated by about 1 cm and should be transverse to the longitudinal axis of the shaft; on the lateral view, it may be necessary to angle the Kirschner wires proximally to avoid penetration into the joint if the entry site is near the dorsal rim. Initially placing a dorsal buttress pin upside-down on the bone can be helpful as a template in order to visualize the proper position and insertion angle of the Kirschner wires (**TECH FIG 11B**). Particular attention should be given to determining whether the insertion angle should include some pronation or supination in order to avoid torsion of the wire form as it is secured proximally.

- Ensure that the leading tips of the legs of the dorsal buttress pin are straight and cut to the required length. Leave the ulnar leg 2 to 3 mm longer than the radial leg so one leg can be engaged at a time. Direct the legs proximally if needed to match the insertion angle of the Kirschner wires.
- Place the ulnar leg of the buttress pin adjacent to the insertion site of the ulnar Kirschner wire, and then withdraw the Kirschner wire and immediately engage the leg in the hole (**TECH FIG 11C**). Repeat with the radial Kirschner wire to engage the radial leg of the buttress pin. Impact and seat the buttress pin (**TECH FIG 11D**).
- Fine-tune the reduction and complete the fixation proximally with one or two 2.3-mm cortical bone screws and washers (**TECH FIG 11E,F**). If needed, a blocking screw can be placed just proximal to the end of the buttress pin to prevent shortening of the fragment.

Dorsal Hook Plate Fixation

- Dorsal hook plates are another alternative for fixation of dorsal fragments.
- Expose and reduce ulnar corner and/or dorsal wall fragments according to the technique described previously.
- Position and insert a 0.045-inch Kirschner guidewire distally along the intended path of the hooks of the plate. Confirm the position with the C-arm.
- If needed, predrill the holes for insertion of the hooks. In osteoporotic bone, the hooks can be simply pushed into the fragment (**TECH FIG 12A**).
- Verify the position and reduction with C-arm and complete fixation with proximal bone screws (**TECH FIG 12B**).

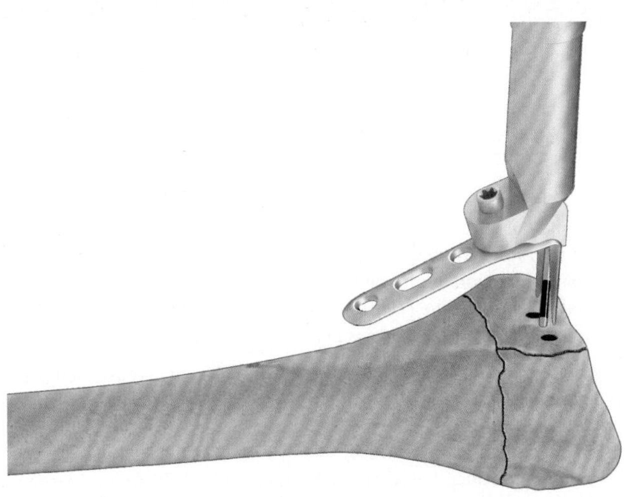

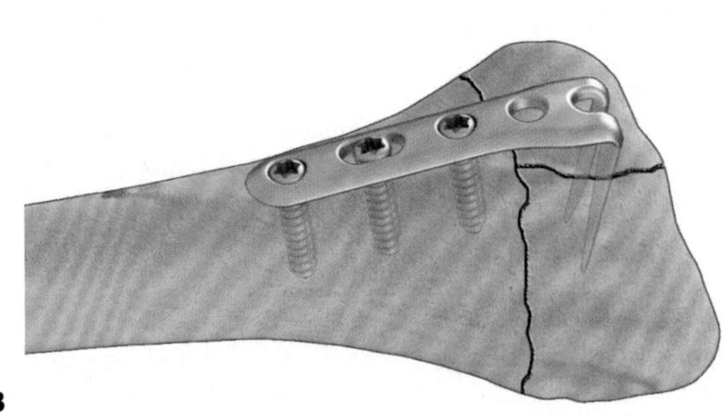

TECH FIG 12 • Dorsal hook plate fixation. **A.** Placement of dorsal hook plate. **B.** Completed fixation.

Free Articular Fragment Support with a Buttress Pin

- Free articular fragments impacted into the metaphyseal cavity can be reduced and stabilized by providing support to the subchondral surface of the fragment, in combination with peripheral cortical stabilization circumferentially around the articular fragment.
- In some cases, impacted free articular fragments may be adequately supported by a properly applied locking plate to provide subchondral support.
- An alternative method is to use structural bone graft to support the free articular fragment in combination with fragment-specific fixation of the surrounding cortical shell, resulting in containment of the graft within the metaphysis.
- A dorsal buttress pin can also be used for direct subchondral support of impacted articular fragments. The legs of the implant are cut to length and inserted through the dorsal defect, slid distally directly behind the articular fragment, and then fixed proximally with a screw and washer. The articular fragment is sandwiched between the base of the lunate and the legs of the implant (**TECH FIG 13A–C**).

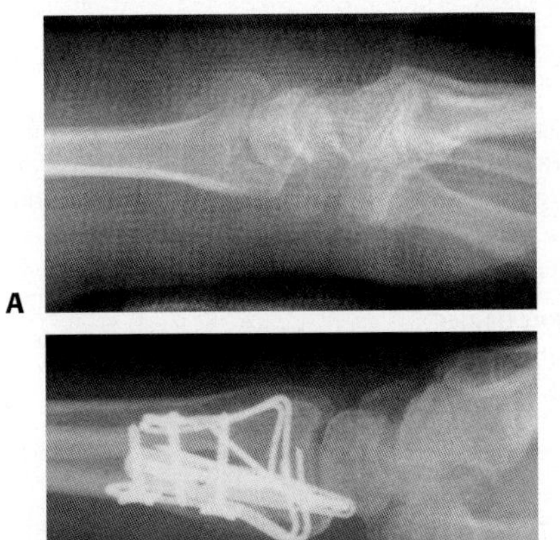

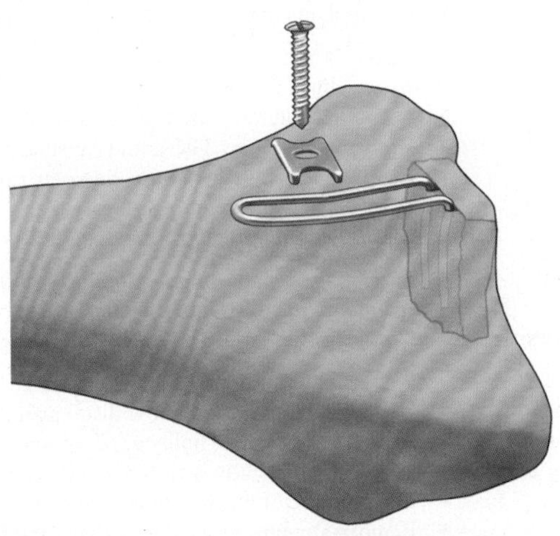

TECH FIG 13 • **A.** Depressed articular fragment. **B.** Support of free articular fragment with a buttress pin. **C.** Dorsal buttress pin to support fragment from endosteal surface.

PEARLS AND PITFALLS

Determining whether a fragment is on the volar or dorsal side of the distal radius on the PA view	■ Correlation of the carpal facet horizon with the lateral view allows identification whether a fragment is dorsal or volar. ■ If the articular surface is tilted dorsally, the carpal facet horizon identifies the dorsal rim. ■ If the articular surface is tilted volarly, the carpal facet horizon identifies the volar rim.
Reduction of unstable fracture pattern	■ Identify and initiate reduction with the fragment that best stabilizes the carpus to its normal spatial relationship. Reduction of the volar rim of the lunate facet, paying particular attention to restoration of length and correction of the teardrop angle, is often the keystone to management of complex articular injuries. In addition, initial reduction of the radial column with a provisional trans-styloid Kirschner wire can help restore carpal length and unload impaction along the lunate facet. ■ The addition of structural bone graft, either through the fracture line at the base of the radial column or through a dorsal defect, can help stabilize the reduction during operative fixation.
Coronal malalignment of the distal fragment with widening of the DRUJ	■ Correction of coronal malalignment by reducing radial translation of distal fragments before completing volar fixation both proximally and distally. ■ An elastic, slightly overcontoured radial column plate such as a radial pin plate can help close sagittal fracture gaps and seat the sigmoid notch against the ulnar head. ■ Assess the clinical stability of the DRUJ and consider TFCC repair or ulnar styloid fixation as needed.
Small or dorsally rotated volar rim fragment; loss of fixation of small volar ulnar fragment	■ Ensure adequate fixation of volar ulnar corner fragment. ■ Consider volar buttress pin or volar hook plate fixation for extremely distal or dorsally rotated volar rim fragments. ■ Avoid release of the volar wrist capsule. When necessary, the legs of an implant can be inserted through the capsule. ■ Larger fragments may have adequate support with a standard volar plate.
Unrecognized carpal ligament injury	■ Maintain a high index of suspicion for ligamentous injuries of the carpus. Consider arthroscopic evaluation, particularly in the context of radial or dorsal shear fractures, carpal avulsion/instability patterns, or articular fractures associated with a significant longitudinal step-off between the scaphoid and lunate facets.
Complications	
Missed fragment: fracture displacement after surgery	■ Careful analysis of radiographic features both before and during reduction; CT scan when needed. ■ Preoperative planning to select approaches that allow complete visualization of all major fragments. ■ Complete set of implants and instruments available before surgery. ■ Evaluate stability of fixation with range of motion under observation before closing operative incision.
Loss of radial length: proximal migration of articular surface	■ Graft the metaphyseal defect when needed with structural bone graft. ■ Use implants that buttress the subchondral bone.
DRUJ dysfunction: pain, instability, or limitation of forearm rotation	■ Assess clinical stability of DRUJ at the end of procedure. ■ Use radial column plate to push distal fragment against ulna to seat sigmoid notch against ulnar head. ■ Evaluate and repair TFCC and capsular tears when necessary. ■ Reduce and fix ulnar corner and volar rim fragments to restore congruity of sigmoid notch. ■ Ensure that radial length is restored. ■ Mild, uncomplicated postoperative ulnar-sided wrist pain often spontaneously resolves over 6–12 months.
Stiffness: slow, restricted return of movement of wrist, forearm, and fingers; associated with pain	■ Early range of motion and mobilization of soft tissues ■ Avoidance of constricting bandages and postoperative swelling ■ Consider occupational therapy when needed.
Tendinitis or rupture: pain with resisted motion, loss of tendon function, clicking and pain	■ Use implants that have a low distal profile. ■ Avoid placing sharp, bulky edges of hardware in proximity to tendons. ■ Cover plates distally with retinacular flap when needed. ■ Consider use of buttress pins (which have a very low profile) when possible. ■ Remove any pins or hardware that back out or become prominent postoperatively. ■ Ensure that volar plates do not extend up beyond distal volar ridge into soft tissues. ■ Avoid long screws or pins, particularly when placed from volar to dorsal. Distal screws should normally be 2–4 mm shy of the dorsal cortical margin.

POSTOPERATIVE CARE

- At the end of the surgical procedure, confirm the stability of fixation as well as the stability of the DRUJ.
- If stable, apply a removable wrist brace and instruct the patient to initiate gentle range-of-motion exercises of the fingers, wrist, and forearm twice or more daily as tolerated. For noncompliant patients or injuries with tenuous fixation, use a cast for 2 to 3 weeks postoperatively or until radiographic evidence of healing is identified.
- Avoid resistive loading across the wrist until signs of radiographic healing are present; typically, this occurs by 4 weeks postoperatively. Specifically instruct older patients not to push up out of a chair or lift heavy objects after surgery.
- If there is persistent stiffness after 4 weeks, initiate physical and occupational therapy.

OUTCOMES

- Konrath and Bahler[5] reported 27 patients with at least 2 years of follow-up:
  - One fracture lost reduction.
  - Patient satisfaction was high (average Disabilities of the Arm, Shoulder, and Hand [DASH] scores 17 and Patient-Rated Wrist Evaluation [PRWE] scores 19 at follow-up).
  - In only three cases was hardware removed; no tendon ruptures occurred.
- Schnall et al[10] reported on two groups of patients: group I had sustained high-energy trauma and group II had lower energy injuries.
  - Group I patients averaged return to work in 6 weeks, with all fractures uniting without loss of position or deformity.
  - Two patients in group I required removal of painful hardware.
  - Group II patients averaged 2 degrees of loss of volar tilt, a 0.3-mm change in ulnar variance, and no loss of joint congruity at follow-up.
  - Grip strength in group II patients was 67% of the contralateral side.
- Benson et al[3] reported on 85 intra-articular fractures in 81 patients with a mean follow-up of 32 months.
  - There were 64 excellent and 24 good results, with an average DASH score of 9 at final follow-up.
  - Flexion and extension motion was 85% and 91% of the opposite side at final follow-up.
  - Grip strength was 92% of the opposite side at final follow-up.
  - Sixty-two percent of patients had a 100-degree arc of flexion–extension and normal forearm rotation by 6 weeks postoperatively.
  - Postoperative radiographic alignment was maintained at follow-up.
  - There were no cases of symptomatic arthritis.
- Abramo et al[1] reported a randomized, prospective study on 50 unstable fractures too unstable for closed methods of management, with fractures randomized to either external fixation or fragment-specific fixation and with follow-up at 1 year[1] and 5 years.[6]
  - At 1 year, internal fixation resulted in better grip strength and range of motion.
  - No difference in subjective outcome was observed at 5 years.
  - There were five malunions in the external fixation group, compared to only one malunion in the fragment-specific group.
  - Differences in grip strength tended to equalize at 5-year follow-up.
- Saw et al[9] reported on 22 unstable C2 and C3 fractures of the distal radius treated with fragment-specific fixation with a minimum of 6 months follow-up.
  - At follow-up, radial inclination was restored to an average of 25 degrees and volar tilt to 8 degrees.
  - Twenty of 22 fractures had restoration of articular congruity to less than 2 mm.
  - Mean flexion/extension was 50 to 63 degrees, and mean pronation/supination arc of 149 degrees.
  - Mean subjective PRWE score at follow-up was 20.
  - Treatment approach was felt to be a powerful tool for difficult fractures, but acknowledge a significant learning curve.

COMPLICATIONS

- Stiffness: common early, uncommon at follow-up
  - Recovery can be accelerated by anatomic fixation that is stable enough to start motion immediately after surgery. The relative degree of trauma to the bone and soft tissues, combined with underlying physiologic factors, is also a critical factor that can lead to slow recovery of motion or residual stiffness.
- Malunion or nonunion: rare
  - Loss of reduction may occur, particularly if a major fracture component is missed and left untreated. In addition, osteoporosis, failure to graft the metaphyseal defect, and associated DRUJ injuries may contribute to loss of reduction or malunion.
  - Pin plates are able to resist translational displacements but are less effective for preventing loss of length; they require osseous contact between the proximal and distal fragments or additional support by bone graft or a secondary implant that will buttress the subchondral surface.
  - Nonunions are extremely rare.
- Tendinitis or tendon rupture: uncommon
  - If pins are noted postoperatively to back out, they should be removed. Leaving the distal 1 cm of tendon sheath of the first dorsal compartment intact helps avoid tendon contact with hardware.
  - Using low-profile implants dorsally, covering the distal ends with a strip of retinacular sheath or both is also helpful.
  - The surgeon should avoid leaving screws or pins protruding from the dorsal or volar surfaces of the bone.
- Painful hardware: rare
  - Painful hardware can be related to migration of a pin or settling of the fracture proximally. Overbending pin hooks and using bone graft or buttressing implants can help avoid this problem.
  - Remove hardware when painful.
- Late arthritis is uncommon and related to the articular damage at the time of injury as well as the quality of the articular restoration.
- Infections, bleeding, carpal tunnel syndrome, and other nerve injuries are uncommon and often related to the primary injury.
- Complex regional pain syndrome is uncommon.

REFERENCES

1. Abramo A, Kopylov P, Geijer M, et al. Open reduction and internal fixation compared to closed reduction and external fixation in distal radial fractures. Acta Orthop 2009;80(4):478–485.
2. Barrie K, Wolfe S. Internal fixation for intraarticular distal radius fractures. Tech Hand Up Extrem Surg 2002;6:10–20.
3. Benson LS, Minihane KP, Stern LD, et al. The outcome of intra-articular distal radius fractures treated with fragment-specific fixation. J Hand Surg Am 2006;31(8):1333–1339.
4. Fernandez DL, Jupiter JB. Fractures of the Distal Radius, ed 2. New York: Springer, 2002:42–50.
5. Konrath G, Bahler S. Open reduction and internal fixation of unstable distal radius fractures: results using the trimed fixation system. J Orthop Trauma 2002;16:578–585.
6. Landgren M, Jerrhag D, Tägil M, et al. External or internal fixation in the treatment of non-reducible distal radial fractures? Acta Orthop 2011;82(5):610–613.
7. Leslie BM, Medoff RJ. Fracture-specific fixation of distal radius fractures. Tech Orthop 2000;15:336–352.
8. Medoff R. Essential radiographic evaluation for distal radius fractures. Hand Clin 2005;21:279–288.
9. Saw N, Roberts C, Cutbush K, et al. Early experience with the TriMed fragment-specific fracture fixation system in intraarticular distal radius fractures. J Hand Surg Eur Vol 2008;33(1):53–58.
10. Schnall SB, Kim BJ, Abramo A, et al. Fixation of distal radius fractures using a fragment specific system. Clin Orthop Relat Res 2006;445:51–57.
11. Swigart C, Wolfe S. Limited incision open techniques for distal radius fracture management. Orthop Clin North Am 2001;32:317–327.

Intramedullary and Dorsal Plate Fixation of Distal Radius Fractures

30

CHAPTER

Nayoung Kim, Fred Liss, Christopher Doumas, and Pedro K. Beredjiklian

DEFINITION

- Distal radius fractures typically originate in the radial metaphysis and occasionally enter the radiocarpal joint and distal radioulnar joint (DRUJ).
- These fractures may be stable or unstable, intra-articular or extra-articular, and have significant incidences of associated bony and soft tissue injuries about the wrist.
- Distal radius fractures are most commonly dorsally displaced or angulated (apex volar).
- Treatment is based on fracture stability, comminution, articular segment displacement, articular surface displacement, and the functional demand of the patient.
- Stability is related to initial fracture displacement, residual dorsal angulation after closed reduction, dorsal comminution, age of the patient, and associated distal ulnar fracture and intra-articular fracture extension.[9,11]

ANATOMY

- The distal radius has articulations at the scaphoid fossa, lunate fossa, and sigmoid notch.
- The normal bony anatomy includes volar tilt of 10 degrees, radial height of 11 mm, and radial inclination of 22 degrees.
- Ulnar variance (the length of the radius relative to the ulnar head at the sigmoid notch) is variable and patient dependent.
- Dorsal ligamentous structures include the dorsal intercarpal ligament and the dorsal radiocarpal ligament.
- The dorsal radiocarpal ligament originates from the dorsal lip of the radius and attaches on the ulnar carpus.
- The dorsal intercarpal ligament represents a capsular thickening on the dorsum of the carpus, of which the fiber alignment is perpendicular to the long axis of the radius.
- Volar ligamentous origins include the radioscaphocapitate ligament, the long radiolunate ligament, and the short radiolunate ligament, among others.
- The triangular fibrocartilage complex (TFCC) consists of the triangular fibrocartilage and volar radioulnar and dorsal radioulnar ligaments.
- The volar radioulnar and dorsal radioulnar ligaments originate from the volar and dorsal edges of the sigmoid notch, respectively, become confluent, and then insert together at the base of the ulnar styloid.
- The extensor retinaculum lies superficial to the extensor tendons and deep to the subcutaneous tissues. It has septations creating six dorsal compartments (**FIG 1**).
  - The first compartment lies over the radial styloid and contains the abductor pollicis longus and the extensor pollicis brevis tendons (each may have multiple slips).
  - The second compartment, containing the extensor carpi radialis longus and extensor carpi radialis brevis, lies radial to the tubercle of Lister.
  - The third compartment, containing the extensor pollicis longus (EPL), lies ulnar to the tubercle of Lister.
  - The fourth compartment, containing the extensor indicis proprius and extensor digitorum communis, lies over the dorsoulnar distal radius.
  - The fifth compartment, containing the extensor digiti minimi, lies over the DRUJ.
  - The sixth compartment, containing the extensor carpi ulnaris, lies over the distal ulna.

PATHOGENESIS

- Distal radius fractures typically occur due to a fall on an outstretched hand.
- Fractures occur when the force of axial loading exceeds the failure strength of cortical and trabecular bone.[14]
- The fracture pattern is determined by the magnitude and direction of the force applied and the position of the hand during impact.[5,13]
- Dorsally displaced or angulated fractures occur when the wrist is neutral or extended and an axially or dorsally directed force is applied to the carpus.
- Osteoporosis, metabolic bone diseases, and bone tumors increase the risk of fracture.

NATURAL HISTORY

- Distal radius fractures are either stable or unstable.
- Satisfactorily positioned stable fractures, when treated nonoperatively, historically have excellent outcomes in terms of range of motion, pain, strength, and function.[1]
  - Nonoperative management consists of immobilization with either a cast or a splint molded to prevent dorsal displacement.

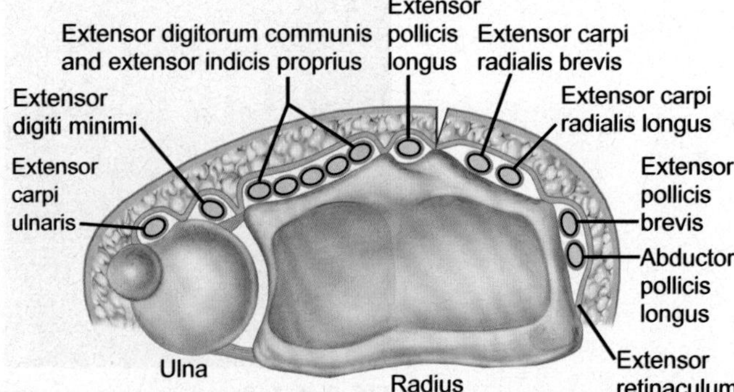

FIG 1 • Anatomy of the distal radius. The six dorsal extensor compartments at the level of the extensor retinaculum.

- Displaced, unstable, and comminuted fractures often require operative treatment.
- The goals of surgical treatment are to provide stability and improve bony alignment in order to achieve pain control, improve range of motion, and increase function.[1,8]
- Two millimeter or more of the articular surface displacement of the distal radius leads to degenerative changes in young adults.[8,12]
- Ten degrees of dorsal tilt (dorsal fracture angulation of 20 or more degrees) is considered unacceptable and may lead to pain, decreased motion, and grip strength.
- Postreduction radial shortening of more than 3 degrees is considered unsatisfactory because it results in increase load across the ulnocarpal joints, leading to painful impaction syndrome.[10,12]

PATIENT HISTORY AND PHYSICAL FINDINGS

- A history of trauma is the most common patient presentation, but pathologic fractures may occur with minimal stress or trauma.
- Patients complain of localized pain and present with swelling, decreased range of motion, and ecchymosis about the fracture.
- A history of previous fractures in an older patient should alert the physician to the possibility of underlying osteoporosis.
- The skin should be carefully examined to rule out the presence of an open fracture and to assess swelling before surgery or casting. If the wrist is markedly swollen or if swelling is anticipated, casting should be delayed and a splint should be placed.
- Neurologic symptoms in the form of numbness, tingling, and radiating pain into the digits should alert the physician to the possibility of acute carpal tunnel syndrome (which is considered a surgical emergency). Careful neurologic assessments should be performed to rule out the presence of a progressive neurologic deficit.
- If acute carpal tunnel syndrome is suspected, then immediate examination should include the following:
  - Remove splints and dressings to visualize all areas of skin.
  - Palpate for areas of tenderness or deformity. Palpate anatomic snuffbox.
  - Visualize and palpate the elbow for swelling, ecchymosis, tenderness, crepitus, and deformity.
  - Visualize and palpate the hand and fingers for swelling, ecchymosis, tenderness, crepitus, and deformity.
  - Use two-point tool or paper clip bent to 5 mm and touch radial and ulnar aspects of all fingers with one or two points. Greater than normal (5 mm) two-point testing in the form of progressive neurologic deficit may signify an acute or chronic carpal tunnel syndrome.

IMAGING AND OTHER DIAGNOSTIC STUDIES

- Posteroanterior (PA), lateral, and oblique radiographic views are critical in evaluating all suspected distal radius fractures.
  - Consider imaging the uninjured wrist for comparison and to serve as a template for surgical reconstruction.
  - Radiographs of the elbow should be obtained in almost all cases, especially if any tenderness, swelling, or deformity is detected clinically.
- Radiographic measurements taken from the PA view (**FIG 2A**) include the following[14,24]:
  - Radial inclination, which is the angle between a line perpendicular to the shaft of the radius at the articular margin and a line along the radial articular margin
    - Normal angle: 21 degrees
  - Radial length, which is the distance from a line tangential to the ulnar articular margin to a line drawn perpendicular to the long axis of the radius at the radial styloid tip
    - Normal length[4]: 9 to 11 mm
  - Ulnar variance, which is the distance from a line perpendicular to the long axis of the radius at the sigmoid notch and a line tangential to the ulnar articular surface
    - Normal length[4]: 0 mm
- Lateral articular (volar) tilt is the angle between a line for the articular surface of the radius and a perpendicular line to the long axis of the radius.
  - Normal angle: 11 degrees volar tilt (**FIG 2B**)[4,14,24]
- Computed tomography (CT) scans can fully elucidate the anatomy of the fracture, particularly articular disruption or incongruity. They also help to determine the necessary surgical approach by defining the location and extent of comminution.
  - CT scans increase the interobserver reliability of treatment plans and may actually alter the initial treatment plan based on plain radiographs.[7]

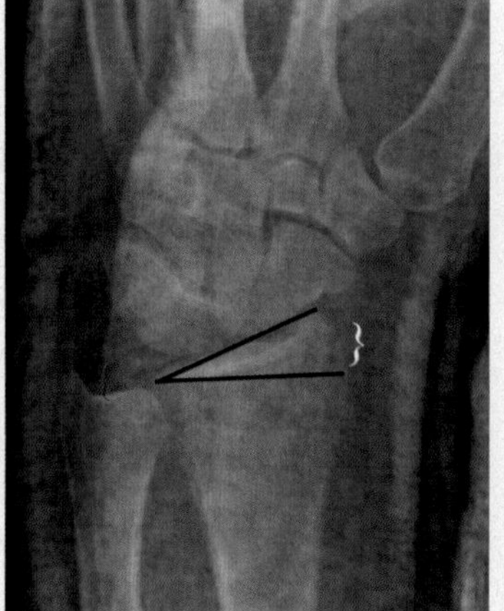

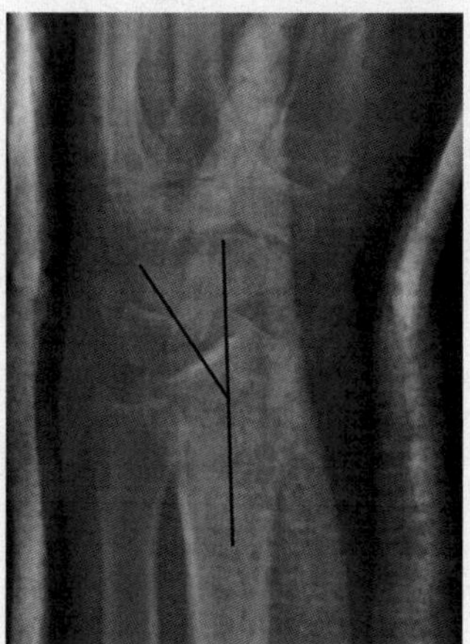

FIG 2 • **A.** PA radiograph demonstrating radial inclination *(black lines)*, ulnar variance *(red)*, and radial height *(white bracket)*. **B.** Lateral radiograph of the wrist demonstrating volar tilt *(black lines)*.

- Axial views provide a clear view of the DRUJ, which aids to identify subluxation, dislocation, bony fragments, and radioulnar ligament avulsions.[19]
- Magnetic resonance imaging (MRI) is used in cases when the presence of a fracture is uncertain.[19]
  - MRI can be useful in evaluating for concomitant ligamentous injuries, TFCC injuries, stress fractures, and occult carpal fractures.

DIFFERENTIAL DIAGNOSIS

- Bony contusion
- Wrist dislocation
- Scaphoid or other carpal fracture
- Carpal instability or dislocation
- Distal ulnar fracture
- Wrist ligament or TFCC sprain or tear

NONOPERATIVE MANAGEMENT

- Closed reduction can be performed in the emergency department (after hematoma block with 1% plain lidocaine) with longitudinal axial traction followed by volar displacement of the carpus. A bivalved, short-arm, well-molded cast or sugar-tong splint should be applied. It is appropriate to offer patients the option of reduction under intravenous (IV) sedation or general anesthesia.
- Casting is the most commonly used method to definitively treat distal radius fractures and is preferred for nondisplaced or minimally displaced fractures and those that are stable after a reduction maneuver (ie, restored volar tilt with minimal dorsal comminution). A precise three-point mold is required to maintain fracture reduction.
- Removable splinting can be considered when treating completely nondisplaced stable fractures in young adults.
- If nonoperative treatment is chosen, repeat radiographs should be taken on a weekly basis for the first 3 weeks to ensure that the reduction is maintained. The physician should have a low threshold for changing the cast.
- Any sign of dorsal migration indicates instability, and operative stabilization should be considered.
- Finger range of motion is begun immediately, and wrist range of motion can be started as the fracture heals and is managed in a removable splint.

SURGICAL MANAGEMENT

- Open reduction and internal fixation with a dorsal plate can be used successfully in the treatment of displaced, unstable, comminuted fractures of the distal radius that fail to respond to closed treatment.
  - Dorsal plating buttresses the fracture to correct deformity and maintain fracture reduction.
  - New intramedullary implants have been designed to alleviate some of the complications associated with traditional dorsal plates and allow a less invasive option for fixation of dorsally displaced fractures (**FIG 3A,B**).
- Indications for plating include the following:
  - Severe initial dorsal displacement (>20 degrees from normal, ≥10 degrees dorsal tilt)[10]
  - Marked dorsal comminution (≥50% of the diameter of the radius shaft on the lateral radiograph)
  - Residual (after reduction) dorsal tilt greater than 10 degrees past neutral
  - Postreduction greater than 3 mm of radius shortening[10]
  - Dorsal intra-articular fragment displacement or step-off of more than 2 mm[10]
- Stabilization using an intramedullary device is indicated for distal radius fractures without extensive articular involvement in which a limited incision and shorter procedure are desired (see **TECH FIG 4E**).[3]
  - Comminution of the volar metaphysis is a relative contraindication for the use of a dorsal intramedullary implant.
  - Intramedullary fixation should not be used to treat marginal or sagittal shear-type intra-articular fractures or displaced fragments from intra-articular fractures.[3,15]
- The surgeon should be prepared to change management intraoperatively and therefore, in advance of the procedure, must have additional stabilization options available such as percutaneous pins or an external fixator.

Preoperative Planning

- All radiographic imaging must be reviewed before surgery.
- It is helpful to compare radiographs of the injured wrist to the uninjured wrist.
- Displaced intra-articular fragments must be identified and consideration given to the value of obtaining CT.

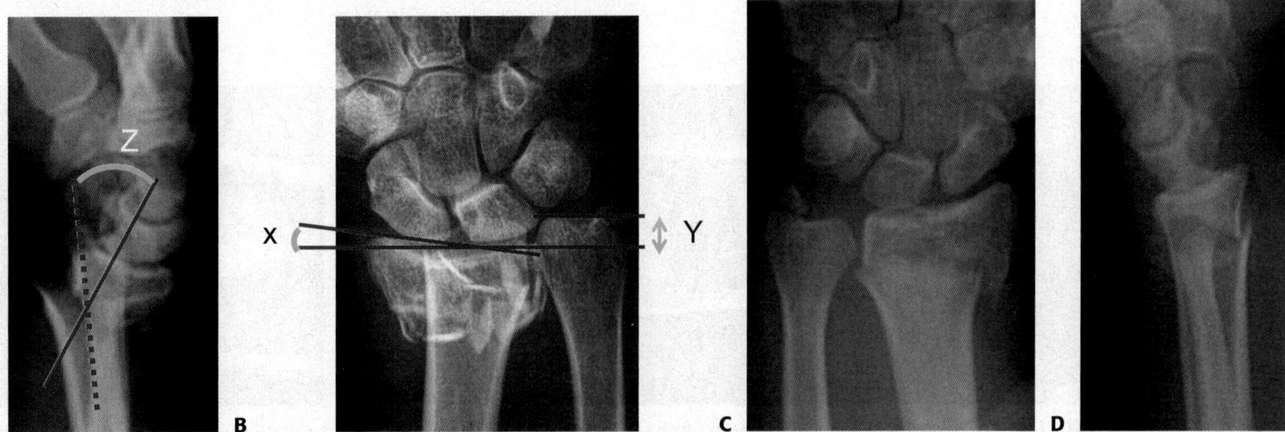

FIG 3 • A. PA radiograph (**A**) and lateral radiograph (**B**) of a healed distal radius fracture fixed with an intramedullary plate. **C,D.** PA and lateral radiographs showing an unstable metaphyseal distal radius fracture. (**C,D:** Copyright Thomas R. Hunt III, MD.)

- Dorsal comminution must be evaluated to determine fracture stability and the need for bone grafting.
- The distal extent of the fracture must be determined to enable the buttress plate to function properly.
- Bone should be evaluated for osteopenia, osteoporosis, and tumors.

Positioning

- The patient is placed supine on a regular operating table.
- A tourniquet is placed near the axilla with the splint in place.
- After anesthesia has been administered, the arm is placed on a radiolucent hand table (**FIG 4**).
- Motion of the shoulder and elbow should be adequate to allow adequate reduction and positioning.
- Image intensification using fluoroscopy should be performed throughout the procedure to assess fracture reduction and the position of the hardware.

Approach

- The dorsal approach to the distal radius through the third dorsal compartment with subperiosteal elevation of the adjacent compartments provides the exposure needed to place a dorsal plate while protecting the extensor tendons from the potential abrasive effects of the plate and screws, therefore minimizing the risks of tendon adhesions, tenosynovitis, and tendon rupture.
- The approach used to place an intramedullary device depends on the nature of the implant and the location and extent of the fracture.
  - Dorsal intramedullary implants are placed through a limited dorsal approach through the third extensor compartment.
  - Radial intramedullary implants are placed through a small radial incision with careful protection of the radial sensory nerve.

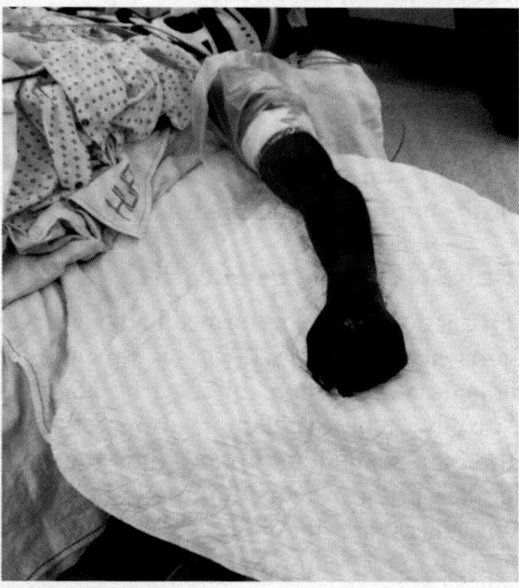

FIG 4 • Patient is positioned supine with arm on a hand table and tourniquet applied on proximal arm.

TECHNIQUES

Dorsal Plate Fixation of Distal Radius Fractures

Incision and Dissection

- The skin incision is centered over the tubercle of Lister (**TECH FIG 1A**).
- The subcutaneous tissues are dissected down to extensor retinaculum, with care to preserve any sensory nerve branches while obtaining hemostasis with bipolar electrocautery (**TECH FIG 1B**).
- The extensor retinaculum is incised just ulnar to the tubercle of Lister, exposing the EPL tendon (**TECH FIG 1C**).
- The hematoma is evacuated and the EPL tendon is freed proximally and distally by incising the septa of the third compartment (**TECH FIG 1D**).
- The EPL tendon can then be removed from the third compartment and protected for the rest of the surgical procedure.
- The extensor compartments are subperiosteally elevated using a scalpel in radial and ulnar directions in order to expose the dorsal cortex of the distal radius (**TECH FIG 1E,F**).
  - If properly maintained, the periosteum of the extensor compartments can be repaired after placement of the fixation device and will serve as a barrier between the dorsal plate and the extensor tendons.

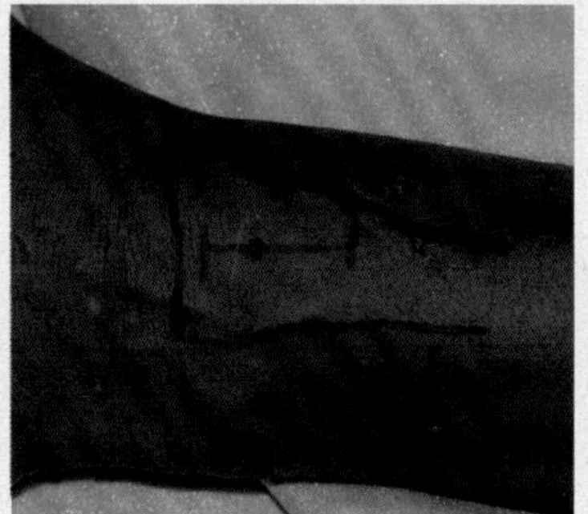

A

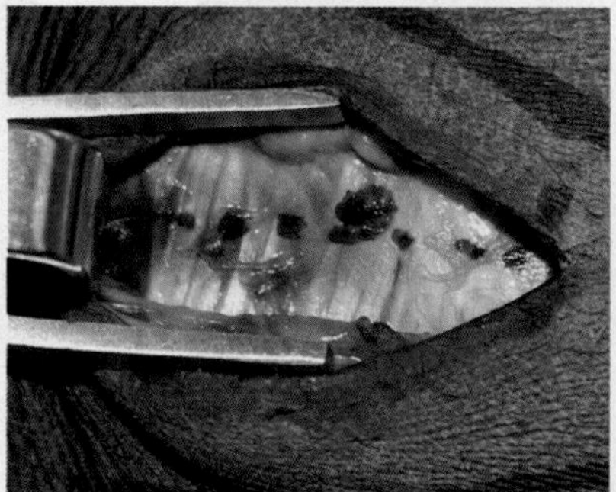

B

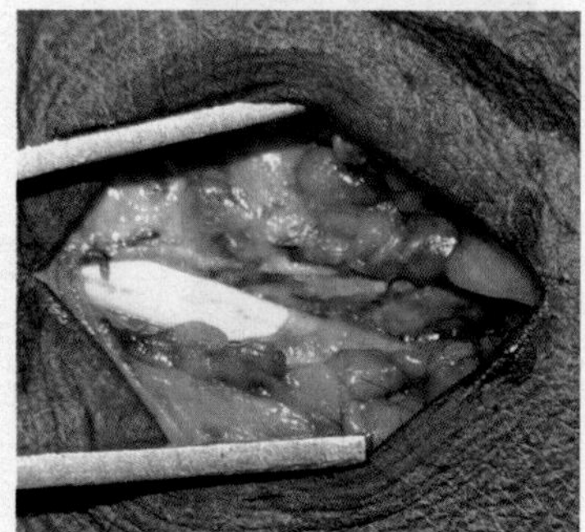

C

TECH FIG 1 • **A.** Skin incision is drawn in relation to the tubercle of Lister. **B.** Skin incision is carried down to extensor retinaculum. Tubercle of Lister and retinacular incision are drawn. **C.** The retinaculum is incised and the EPL tendon is exposed. Hematoma has already been evacuated. *(continued)*

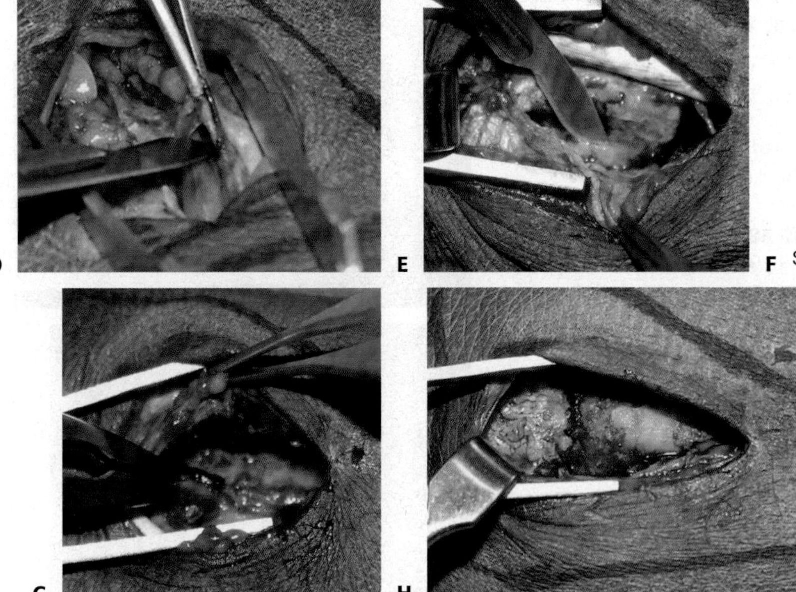

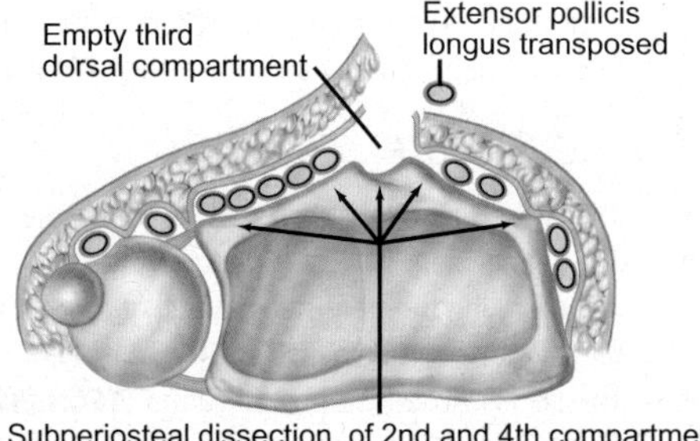

TECH FIG 1 • *(continued)* **D.** Exposing EPL by incising the septa of the third dorsal compartment. **E.** Subperiosteal elevation of the second and fourth dorsal compartments. **F.** Diagram demonstrating the transposition of EPL and dissection deep to the extensor compartments. **G.** Removal of tubercle of Lister. **H.** Exposing the radial shaft with a periosteal elevator.

- The tubercle of Lister is almost always involved in the fracture and should be completely removed using a rongeur (**TECH FIG 1G**).
- The radius shaft is exposed with a periosteal elevator (**TECH FIG 1H**).

Reduction and Plate Fixation

- Reduction is obtained and confirmed using axial traction and palmar translation of the hand (**TECH FIG 2A**).
- If reduction of articular fragments is needed, the radial portion of the origin of the dorsal radiocarpal ligament can be elevated sharply off the radius, allowing direct visualization of the articular surfaces.
- Kirschner wires can be used for temporary fixation.
- Bone graft is inserted to support reduced articular fragments and then the dorsal plate is applied directly on the radius (**TECH FIG 2B**).
- The plate is first secured with a bicortical screw inserted through the oval sliding hole.
- Fracture reduction and placement of the plate are confirmed using fluoroscopy.
- The plate is secured to the distal fragment with one or two cancellous screws. Depending on the implant used, the surgeon should avoid placing the distal ulnar screw through the plate as the prominence of the screw head may irritate the overlying digital extensor tendons in the fourth dorsal compartment.

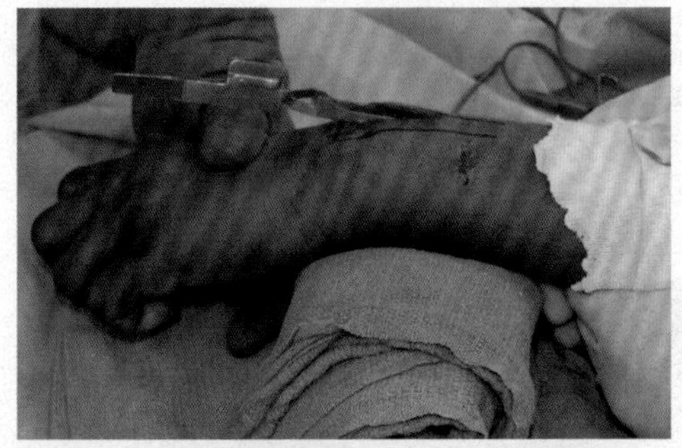

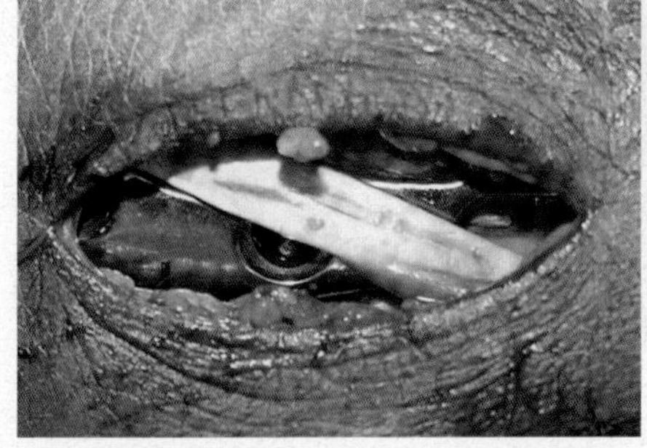

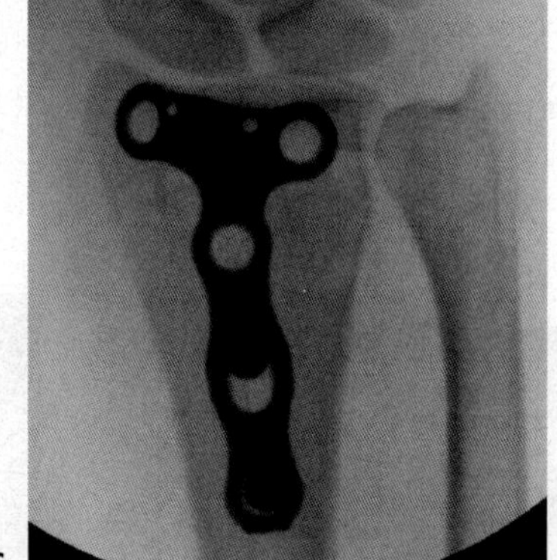

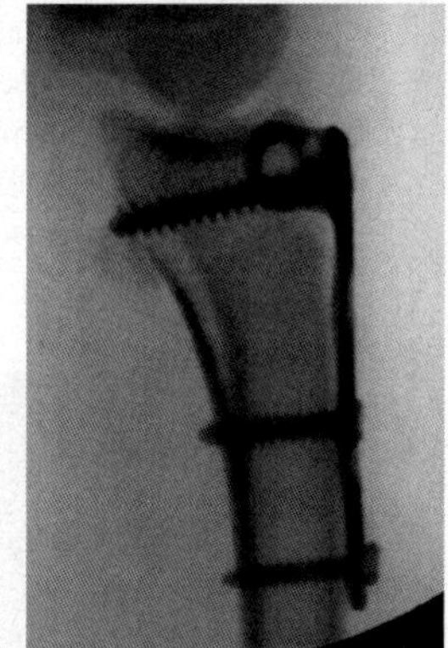

TECH FIG 2 • **A.** Reduction maneuver. The distal radius is reduced over a bump of towels using traction and palmar displacement of the carpus. **B.** Plate placement. The plate is placed deep to the EPL and aligned distally over the distal radius. **C,D.** Reduction imaging. **C.** PA fluoroscopic view demonstrating final reduction with well-aligned plate. **D.** Lateral fluoroscopic view demonstrating final reduction with appropriate-length screws and good distal buttressing of the fracture. Volar tilt has been restored.

- Additional cortical screws are added in the radius shaft.
- Reduction and stability are confirmed (**TECH FIG 2C,D**).

Wound Closure

- The wound must always be copiously irrigated.
- The retinaculum is closed deep to the transposed EPL tendon, incorporating the periosteal layer that forms the floor of the extensor compartments (**TECH FIG 3A**).
- The skin is closed with nylon suture (**TECH FIG 3B**).
- Finally, a short-arm volar splint is applied over a sterile dressing. Care should be taken to extend the splint to, but not across the distal transverse palmar flexion crease, in order to reduce the risk of postoperative intrinsic muscle and finger joint contractures.

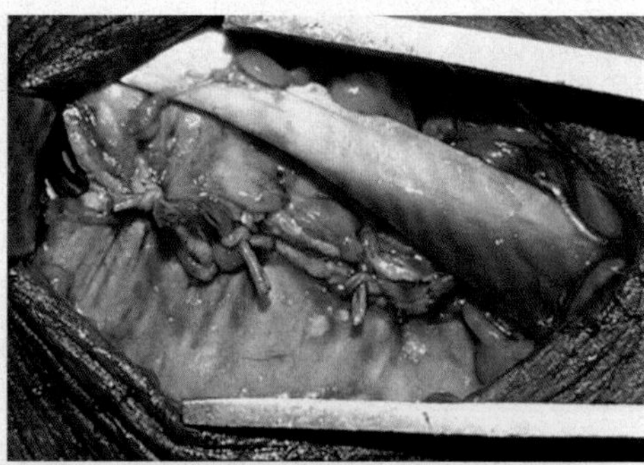

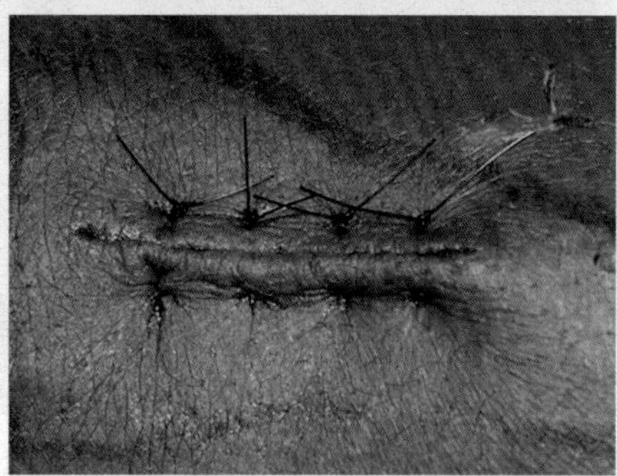

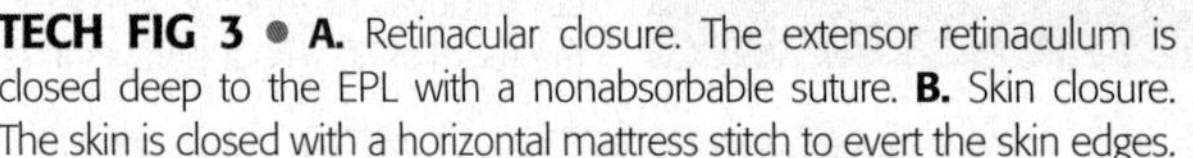

TECH FIG 3 • **A.** Retinacular closure. The extensor retinaculum is closed deep to the EPL with a nonabsorbable suture. **B.** Skin closure. The skin is closed with a horizontal mattress stitch to evert the skin edges.

Fixation of Distal Radius Fractures using a Dorsal Intramedullary Device (Tornier)

- The fracture is exposed using a limited version of the incision detailed for placement of a dorsal plate (**TECH FIG 4A**).
  - The extensor retinaculum is incised just ulnar to the tubercle of Lister, exposing the EPL tendon.
  - The EPL tendon is freed proximally and distally by incising the septum of the third dorsal compartment.
  - The EPL tendon should then be transposed and protected for the rest of the surgical procedure.
- A scalpel is used to subperiosteally elevate the fourth and portions of the second extensor compartment in radial and ulnar directions.
  - The dorsal cortex of the distal radius is exposed and room is created for seating of the extramedullary portion of the device.
- The tubercle of Lister is removed, and an awl is used to create an entry point in the dorsal cortex (**TECH FIG 4B**).
  - This usually involves a portion of the fracture line.
- The canal is rasped until the rasp may be fully seated (**TECH FIG 4C**).
- The implant is placed using the insertion device to control rotation (**TECH FIG 4D**).
  - Typically, the fracture reduces as the device is inserted and seated due to the buttress effect and three-point fixation of the implant within the canal.
- Lag screws are inserted as required, followed by a cover lock to create fixed-angle stability.
- Reduction and stabilization are confirmed radiographically (**TECH FIG 4E,F**).
- Wound closure and splinting are as described earlier.

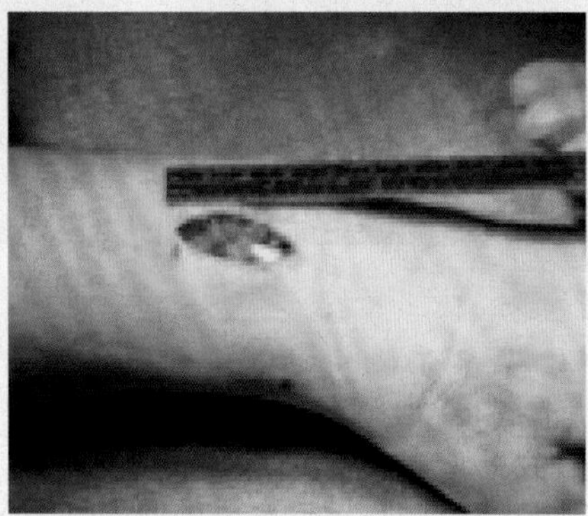

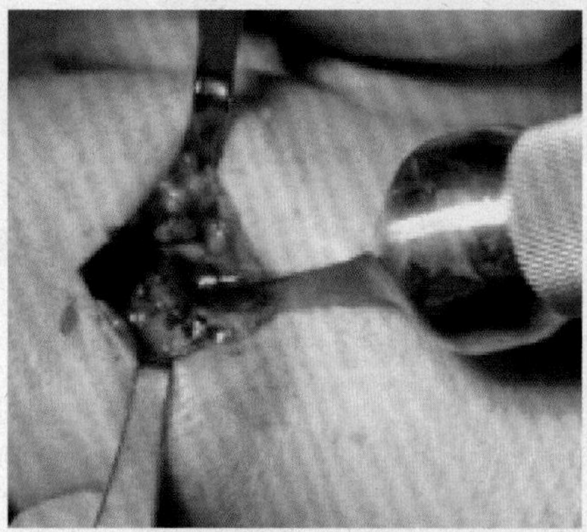

TECH FIG 4 • **A.** A 2.5-cm dorsal incision is used for exposure. **B.** The awl is inserted through the fracture site after removal of the tubercle of Lister. *(continued)*

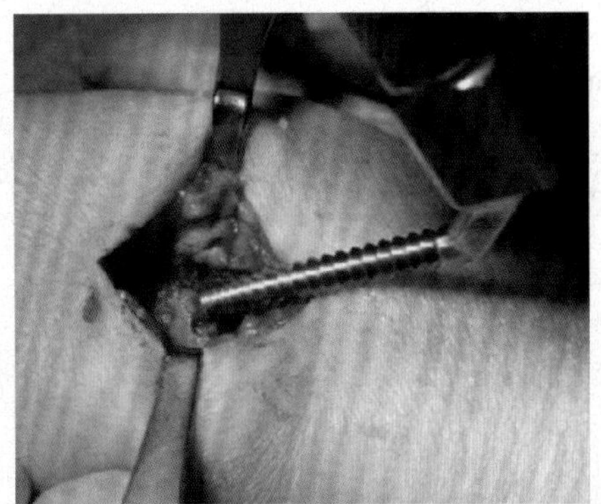

C

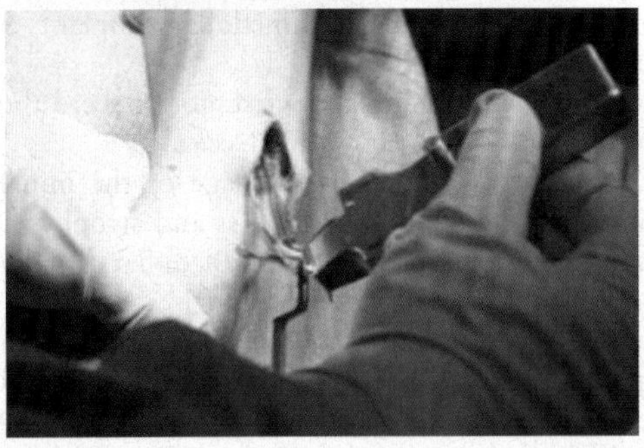

D

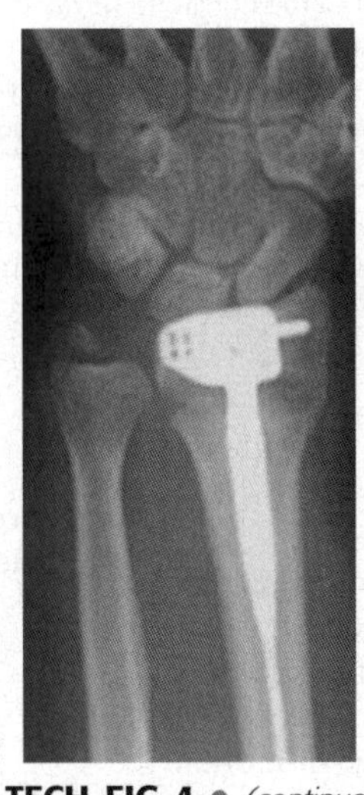

E

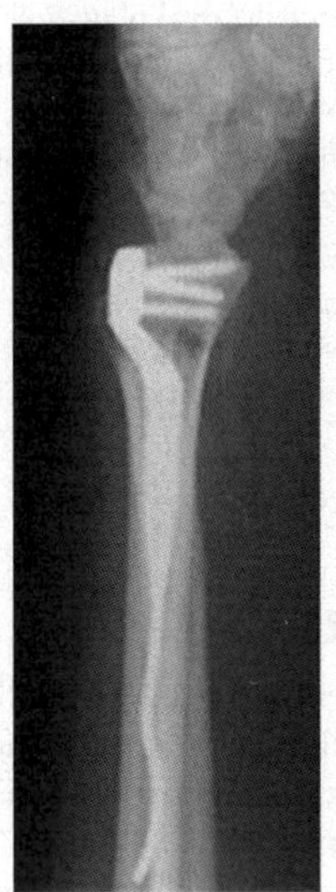

F

TECH FIG 4 • *(continued)* **C.** A rasp is used to create a path for the implant. **D.** The implant is placed using the insertion device so as to control rotation during seating. **E,F.** An unstable metaphyseal distal radius fracture has been reduced and stabilized using a dorsal intramedullary device (Tornier Corp). (**E,F:** Copyright Thomas R. Hunt III, MD.)

Fixation of Distal Radius Fractures using a Radial Intramedullary Device (Wright Medical)

- A 2- to 3-cm incision is made over the radial styloid between the first and second extensor compartments.
- Care is taken to protect branches of the radial sensory nerve.
- A cannulated drill is used to penetrate the cortex 2 to 3 mm proximal to the radiocarpal joint line to create the entry point.
- After insertion of a starter awl, the canal is broached sequentially under fluoroscopic guidance to fit the medullary canal.
- The implant is then inserted with the insertion jig, making sure the implant is countersunk into the radial styloid.
- The proximal interlocking screws are then placed using the insertion jig, using small incisions of the dorsal aspect of the forearm.
- The distal interlocking screws are placed last using the insertion jig.
  - Small adjustments to radial height and tilt can be made at this time.
- Reduction and stabilization are confirmed radiographically.
- Wound closure and splinting are as described earlier.

PEARLS AND PITFALLS

Indications	■ Determine the direction of fracture stability. ■ Determine the area and extent of comminution. ■ Ensure that an acute carpal tunnel syndrome does not exist.
Surgical approach	■ Incise the extensor retinaculum sharply to allow easier repair. ■ Expose only the third dorsal compartment. ■ Remove the tubercle of Lister to allow better plate contouring.

Hardware choice and placement	■ Choose a low-profile implant system that offers the flexibility needed to stabilize the fracture. ■ Place the plate distally to ensure buttress effect. ■ Place the oval plate hole screw initially. ■ Do not place the plate distal to the dorsal lip of the distal radius. ■ Avoid placing the distal ulnar screw. ■ Although titanium implants and their particulate debris have been implicated in the development of tenosynovitis and other tendon pathology, there is no clear scientific evidence to substantiate these claims.
Postoperative management	■ Avoid casting for long periods. ■ Encourage early active range of motion of the wrist and fingers. ■ Avoid using a sling to prevent unnecessary shoulder and elbow stiffness. ■ Do not begin strengthening until range of motion is restored.

POSTOPERATIVE CARE

- Postoperatively, the patient is placed in a bulky dressing that allows motion of the digits, elbow, and shoulder. A volar resting splint may be used to support the wrist if there is any concern about fixation strength.
- The patient is encouraged to begin finger range-of-motion exercises immediately after surgery.
- Seven to 10 days after surgery, the sutures are removed, Steri-Strips are applied, and the incision is allowed to get wet.
- The patient is evaluated by an occupational therapist, who provides a thermoplastic splint, and can start active and active-assisted range-of-motion exercises depending on fracture stability.
- When the fracture heals at about 6 weeks, gentle passive range of motion and strengthening may be started.
- There is evidence that vitamin C 500 mg/day for 50 days after distal radius fracture may have a preventative effect on complex regional pain syndrome.[27]

OUTCOMES

- Dorsal plating has recently been shown biomechanically to be stronger and stiffer than volar plating for dorsally unstable fractures.[23]
- Dorsal plating has been associated with a higher complication rate than other means of stabilization.[2,14,18]
- Extensor tenosynovitis and tendon rupture have been prevalent in the past, mainly due to bulky implants.
- There has been renewed interest in dorsal plating of the distal radius as it has been shown to have a low rate of tendon-related complications with the use of low-profile, anatomic implants.[6,18,20]
- Recent studies show no statistically significant difference between dorsal or volar fixation in the overall risk of complications.[16,25,26]
  - Volar locking plates are associated with a higher rate of neuropathic complications than dorsal low-profile plates.[26]
  - It has been reported that after a 1-year follow up, there was a 21% complication rate with volar plates and a 14% complication rate with dorsal plates.[26]
- Clinical reports have suggested that low-profile systems are more important in satisfactory outcomes for dorsal plating, with a much lower rate of complications.[18,26]
- Fixation with low-profile dorsal plates can result in at least 80% of contralateral wrist range of motion, about 80% to 90% of grip strength, and over 90% pinch strength, with minimal risk of tendon rupture.[6,20]
- Present studies show that intramedullary implants offer stable fixation[15,17,22]:
  - The mean grip strength and wrist motion were about 76% after 3 months and 91% after 1 year.[15]
  - This stability indicates early usage of the injured wrist which helps avoid muscle stiffness and atrophy.[22]
- It has been demonstrated that intramedullary implants have less complications than plate fixation[15,17,21]:
  - There are fewer soft tissue complications because the implant does not have contact with surrounding tissues because the device is entirely within the medullary canal.[15,17,21]
  - Intramedullary fixation does not devascularize the fracture fragments and therefore does not need a section of periosteum to surround the fracture.[22]

COMPLICATIONS

- Infection (pin tract or deep)
- Injury to tendons, vessels, and nerves
- Stiffness
- Posttraumatic arthritis
- Weakness in grip or pinch
- Tenosynovitis and tendon ruptures
- Malunion or nonunion
- Compartment syndrome
- Carpal tunnel syndrome
- Late tendon rupture, potentially related to implant design and material
- Hardware failure
- Complex regional pain syndrome type I
- TFCC injuries
- Radial shortening
- DRUJ instability
- Loss of reduction
- Loss of motion

DISCLOSURE

Dr. Beredjiklian owns shares of stock on Tornier, Inc.

REFERENCES

1. Glowacki KA, Weiss AP, Akelman E. Distal radius fractures: concepts and complications. Orthopedics 1996;19:601–608.
2. Grewal R, Perey B, Wilmink M, et al. A randomized prospective study on the treatment of intra-articular distal radius fractures: open reduction and internal fixation with dorsal plating versus mini open reduction, percutaneous fixation, and external fixation. J Hand Surg Am 2005;30(4):764–772.

3. Ilyas AM. Intramedullary fixation of distal radius fractures. J Hand Surg Am 2009;34(2):341–346.
4. Ipaktchi K, Livermore M, Lyons C, et al. Current concepts in the treatment of distal radial fractures. Orthopedics 2013;36:778–784.
5. Jupiter JB, Fernandez DL. Comparative classification for fractures of the distal end of the radius. J Hand Surg Am 1997;22(4):563–571.
6. Kamath AF, Zurakowski D, Day CS. Low-profile dorsal plating for dorsally angulated distal radius fractures: an outcomes study. J Hand Surg Am 2006;31(7):1061–1067.
7. Katz MA, Beredjiklian PK, Bozentka DJ, et al. Computed tomography scanning of intra-articular distal radius fractures: does it influence treatment? J Hand Surg Am 2001;26(3):415–421.
8. Knirk JL, Jupiter JB. Intra-articular fractures of the distal end of the radius in young adults. J Bone Joint Surg Am 1986;68(5):647–659.
9. Lafontaine M, Hardy D, Delince P. Stability assessment of distal radial fractures. Injury 1989;20:208–210.
10. Lichtman DM, Bindra RR, Boyer MI, et al. Treatment of distal radius fractures. J Am Acad Orthop Surg 2010;18:180–189.
11. Mackenney PJ, McQueen MM, Elton R. Prediction of instability in distal radial fractures. J Bone Joint Surg Am 2006;88(9):1944–1951.
12. Meyer C, Chang J, Stern P, et al. Complications of distal radial and scaphoid fracture treatment. J Bone Joint Surg Am 2013;95(16):1517–1526.
13. Murray J, Gross L. Treatment of distal radius fractures. J Am Acad Orthop Surg 2013;21:502–505.
14. Nana AD, Joshi A, Lichtman DM. Plating of the distal radius. J Am Acad Orthop Surg 2005;13:159–171.
15. Nishiwaki M, Tazaki K, Shimizu H, et al. Prospective study of distal radial fractures treated with an intramedullary nail. J Bone Joint Surg Am 2011;93(15):1436–1441.
16. Rausch S, Schlonski O, Klos K, et al. Volar versus dorsal latest-generation variable-angle locking plates for the fixation of AO type 23C 2.1 distal radius fractures: a biomechanical study in cadavers. Injury 2013;44:523–526.
17. Rhee PC, Shin AY. Minimally invasive flexible insertion and rigid intramedullary nail fixation for distal radius fractures. Tech Hand Up Extrem Surg 2012;16:159–165.
18. Rozental TD, Beredjiklian PK, Bozentka DJ. Functional outcome and complications following two types of dorsal plating for fractures of the distal part of the radius. J Bone Joint Surg Am 2003;85-A(10): 1956–1960.
19. Schneppendahl J, Windolf J, Kaufmann RA. Distal radius fractures: current concepts. J Hand Surg Am 2012;37:1718–1725.
20. Simic PM, Robison J, Gardner MJ, et al. Treatment of distal radius fractures with a low-profile dorsal plating system: an outcomes assessment. J Hand Surg Am 2006;31(3):382–386.
21. Tan V, Bratchenko W, Nourbakhsh A, et al. Comparative analysis of intramedullary nail fixation versus casting for treatment of distal radius fractures. J Hand Surg Am 2012;37(3):460–468.
22. Tan V, Capo J, Warburton M. Distal radius fracture fixation with an intramedullary nail. Tech Hand Up Extrem Surg 2005;9:195–201.
23. Trease C, McIff T, Toby EB. Locking versus nonlocking T-plates for dorsal and volar fixation of dorsally comminuted distal radius fractures: a biomechanical study. J Hand Surg Am 2005;30(4): 756–763.
24. Trumble TE, Culp RW, Hanel DP, et al. Intra-articular fractures of the distal aspect of the radius. Instr Course Lect 1999;48:465–480.
25. Wei J, Yang TB, Luo W, et al. Complications following dorsal versus volar plate fixation of distal radius fracture: a meta-analysis. J of Int Med Res 2013;41:265–275.
26. Yu YR, Makhni MC, Tabrizi S, et al. Complications of low-profile dorsal versus volar locking plates in the distal radius: a comparative study. J Hand Surg Am 2011;36(7):1135–1141.
27. Zollinger PE, Tuinebreijer WE, Breederveld RS, et al. Can vitamin C prevent complex regional pain syndrome in patients with wrist fractures? A randomized, controlled, multicenter dose-response study. J Bone Joint Surg Am 2007;89(7):1424–1431.

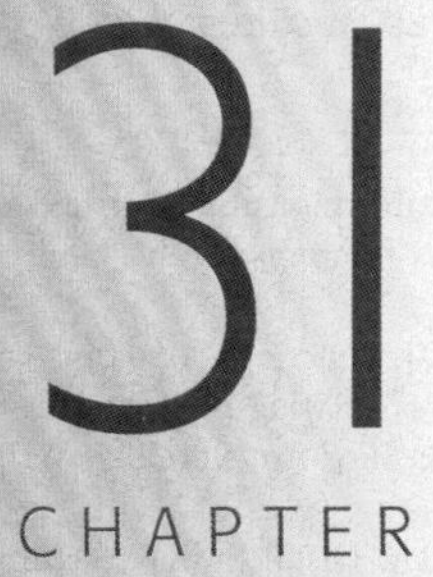

CHAPTER

Volar Plating of Distal Radius Fractures

John J. Fernandez and Philipp N. Streubel

DEFINITION

- Distal radius fractures are defined by their involvement of the metaphysis of the distal radius.
- They are assessed on the basis of fracture pattern, alignment, and stability:
  - Articular versus nonarticular
  - Reducible versus irreducible
  - Stable versus unstable
- Irreducible or unstable fractures require surgical reduction and stable fixation.
- Volar plating historically has been the method of choice for volar shear-type fractures.
  - Fixed-angle plates have become the preferred method of fixation for most types of distal radius fractures.

ANATOMY

- The distal radius serves as a buttress for the proximal carpus, transmitting 75% to 80% of its forces into the forearm.
  - The remaining 20% to 25% of force is transmitted through the distal ulna and the triangular fibrocartilage complex (TFCC).
- Thickness of distal radius articular cartilage is 1 mm or less.[16]
- Dorsally
  - The distal radius is the origin for the dorsal radiocarpal ligament.
  - It is the floor of the fibro-osseous extensor tendon compartments and includes Lister tubercle, assisting in extensor pollicis longus function (**FIG 1A**).
  - The extensor tendons are in immediate contact with the dorsal surface of the distal radius.
- Volarly
  - The distal radius is the origin for volar extrinsic ligaments of the wrist, including the radioscaphocapitate ligament and long and short radiolunate ligaments.
  - It also is the origin of the pronator quadratus.
  - The flexor tendons are separated from the distal radius by the pronator quadratus.
- Ulnarly
  - The distal radius is the origin for the triangular fibrocartilage (see **FIG 1A**).
  - It also contains the sigmoid notch, which articulates with the head of the distal ulna, allowing forearm rotation.
- Distally
  - The surface is divided into a triangular scaphoid fossa and a square lunate fossa articulating with each respective carpal bone (**FIG 1B**).
- The distal articular surface is inclined approximately 22 degrees ulnarly in the coronal plane and 11 degrees volarly in the sagittal plane (**FIG 1C,D**).
- The metaphysis is defined by the distal radius within a length of the articular surface that is equivalent to the widest portion of the entire wrist.
- The dorsal cortical bone is less substantial than the volar cortical bone, contributing to the characteristic dorsal bending fracture pattern of distal radius fractures.

PATHOGENESIS

- The mechanism of injury in a distal radius fracture is an axial force across the wrist, with the pattern of injury determined by bone density, the position of the wrist, and the magnitude and direction of force.
- Most distal radius fractures result from falls with the wrist extended and pronated, which places a dorsal bending moment across the distal radius.
  - Relatively weaker, thinner dorsal bone collapses under compression, whereas stronger volar bone fails under tension, resulting in a characteristic "triangle" of bone comminution with the apex volar and greater comminution dorsal.
- Other possible mechanisms form a basis for some fracture classifications such as the one proposed by Jupiter and Fernandez.[6]
  - Bending
  - Axial compression
  - Shear
  - Avulsion
  - Combinations
- Articular involvement and its severity are the basis of some fracture classifications, such as the AO Orthopaedic Trauma Association (AO/OTA)[10] and Melone[12] classifications.
- Articular involvement splits the distal radius into distinct fragments separate from the radius shaft (**FIG 2**):
  - Scaphoid fossa fragment
  - Lunate fossa fragment. With comminution of this fragment may be separated into two impacted articular fragments, involving the dorsal ulnar corner and the volar rim.[11]

NATURAL HISTORY

- Clinical outcome usually, but not always, correlates with deformity.
  - Variable residual deformity can be tolerated best by individuals with fewer functional demands.
- As wrist deformity increases, physiologic function is progressively altered.
  - Intra-articular displacement of 1 to 2 mm results in an increased risk of osteoarthritis.[3,7]
  - Radial shortening of 3 to 5 mm or more results in increased loading of the ulnar complex.[1,15]

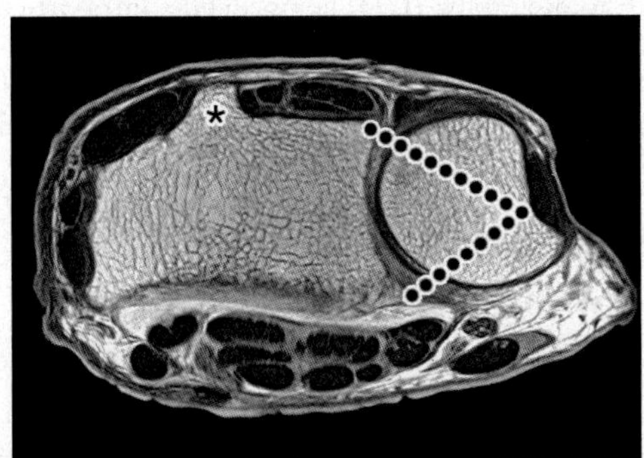

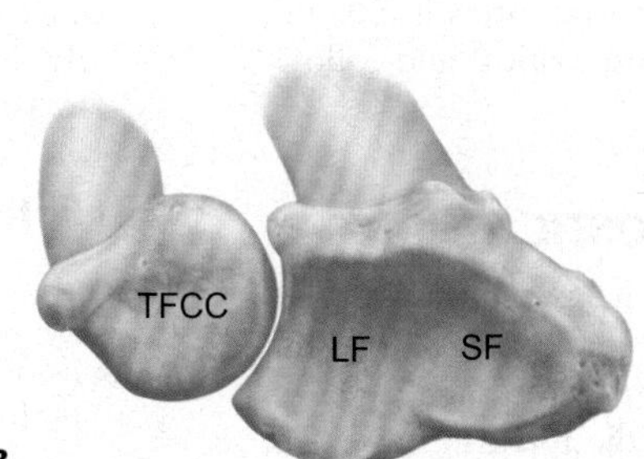

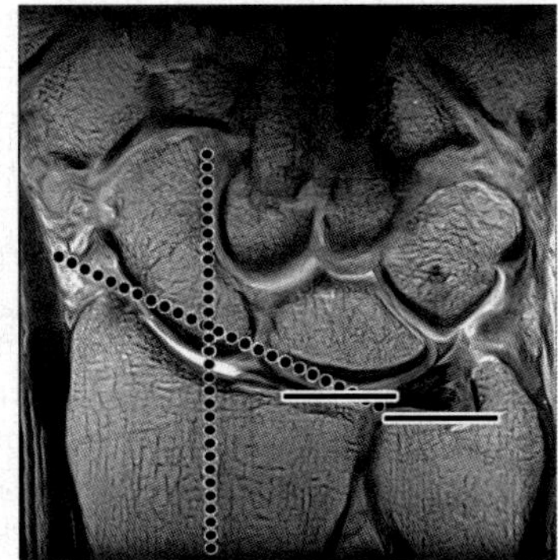

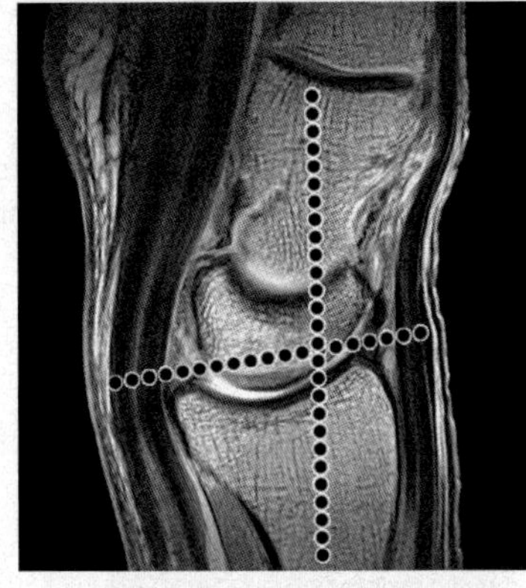

FIG 1 • **A.** Axial magnetic resonance (MR) image of the wrist at the level of the distal radius. Lister tubercle is marked with an *asterisk*. *Dotted lines* represent dorsal and volar borders of the triangular fibrocartilage that helps stabilize the distal radioulnar joint. The dorsal distal radius acts as an attachment for dorsal extensor compartment sheaths. **B.** The distal articular surface of the radius is divided into a triangularly shaped scaphoid fossa (*SF*) and a square-shaped lunate fossa (*LF*). The distal ulna and the *TFCC* act as ulnar buttresses for the wrist. **C.** MR coronal cut of the distal radius. The articular surface of the distal radius is inclined about 22 degrees relative to the forearm axis (*dotted lines*). The ulnar aspect of the distal radius (ie, the lunate fossa) usually is distal to the end of the distal ulna (ie, negative ulnar variance). Note the *solid lines* marking ulnar variance. **D.** MR sagittal cut of the distal radius. The articular surface of the distal radius is inclined approximately 11-degree palmar relative to the forearm axis (*dotted lines*). Proximally, there exists relatively thinner dorsal cortical bone versus the thicker volar bone.

  - Dorsal angulation greater than 10 degrees shifts contact forces to the dorsal scaphoid fossa and the ulnar complex, causing increased disability.[17,20]
- The incidence of associated intracarpal injuries increases with fracture severity. Such injuries can account for poor outcomes. These injuries often are not recognized at first, leading to delayed treatment.[4,18]
  - TFCC tears
  - Scapholunate and lunotriquetral ligament tears
  - Chondral injuries involving the carpal surfaces
  - Distal radioulnar joint injury
  - Distal ulnar fractures

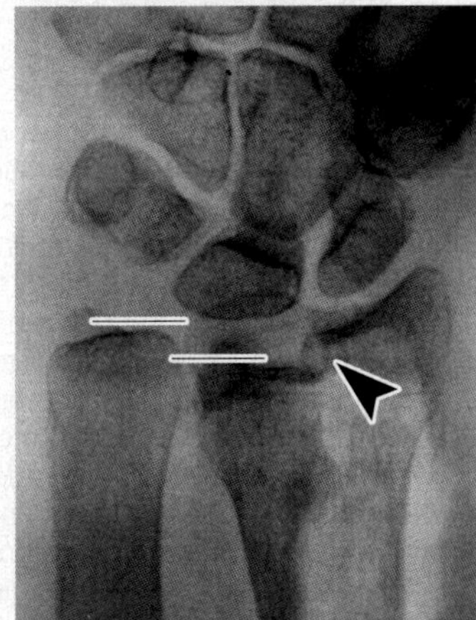

FIG 2 • The *arrowhead* points to the articular split. Articular displacement of the scaphoid fossa fragment radially and the lunate fossa fragment ulnarly is apparent, as is significant shortening (ulnar positive variance) as outlined by the *lines*.

- By predicting the stability of a distal radius fracture, deformity and its complications can be minimized. Several risk factors have been suggested by LaFontaine et al[8] and others. The presence of three or more indicates instability:
  - Dorsal (or volar apex) angulation greater than 20 degrees
  - Dorsal comminution
  - Intra-articular extension
  - Associated ulnar fracture
  - Patient age older than 60 years

PATIENT HISTORY AND PHYSICAL FINDINGS

- The mechanism of injury should be sought to assist in assessing the energy and level of trauma.
- Associated injuries are not uncommon and should be carefully ruled out.
  - Injuries to the hand, carpus, and proximal arm, including other fractures or dislocations
  - Injuries to other extremities or the head, neck, and torso
- Establish the patient's functional and occupational demands.
- Document coexisting medical conditions that may affect healing such as smoking or diabetes.
- Determine possible risk factors for anesthesia and surgery, such as cardiac disease.
- The physical examination should document the following:
  - Condition of surrounding soft tissues (ie, skin and subcutaneous tissues)
  - Quality of vascular perfusion and pulses
  - Integrity of nerve function
  - Sensory two-point discrimination or threshold sensory testing
  - Motor function of intrinsic muscles, including thenar and hypothenar muscles, of the hand

- Examination of the distal ulna, TFCC, and distal radioulnar joint should rule out disruption and instability.
- Reliable physical examination of the carpus often is difficult, making radiographic review even more critical and follow-up examinations important.

IMAGING AND OTHER DIAGNOSTIC STUDIES

- Imaging establishes fracture severity, helps determine stability, and guides the operative approach and choice of fixation.
- Plain radiographs should be obtained before and after reduction: posteroanterior (PA) (with the forearm in neutral rotation), lateral, and two separate oblique views.
  - Oblique views, in particular, help evaluate articular involvement, particularly the lunate fossa fragment (**FIG 3A,B**).
  - The lateral view should be modified with the forearm inclined 15 to 20 degrees to best visualize the articular surface (**FIG 3C**; see **TECH FIG 5B,C**).
- Fluoroscopic evaluation can be useful because it gives a complete circumferential view of the wrist and, with traction applied, can help evaluate injuries of the carpus.
- Computed tomography (CT) helps define intra-articular involvement and helps detect small or impacted fragments, which may not be apparent on plain radiographs, particularly those involving the central portion of the distal radius (**FIG 3D,E**).

DIFFERENTIAL DIAGNOSIS

- Diagnosis is directly confirmed by radiographs.
- Associated and contributory injuries should always be considered.
  - Pathologic fracture (eg, related to tumor, infection)
  - Associated injuries to the carpus (eg, scaphoid fracture, scapholunate ligament injury)

NONOPERATIVE MANAGEMENT

- Nonoperative treatment is reserved for distal radius fractures that are reducible and stable based on the criteria previously discussed.
- The goal of nonoperative treatment is to immobilize the wrist while maintaining acceptable alignment until the fracture is healed.

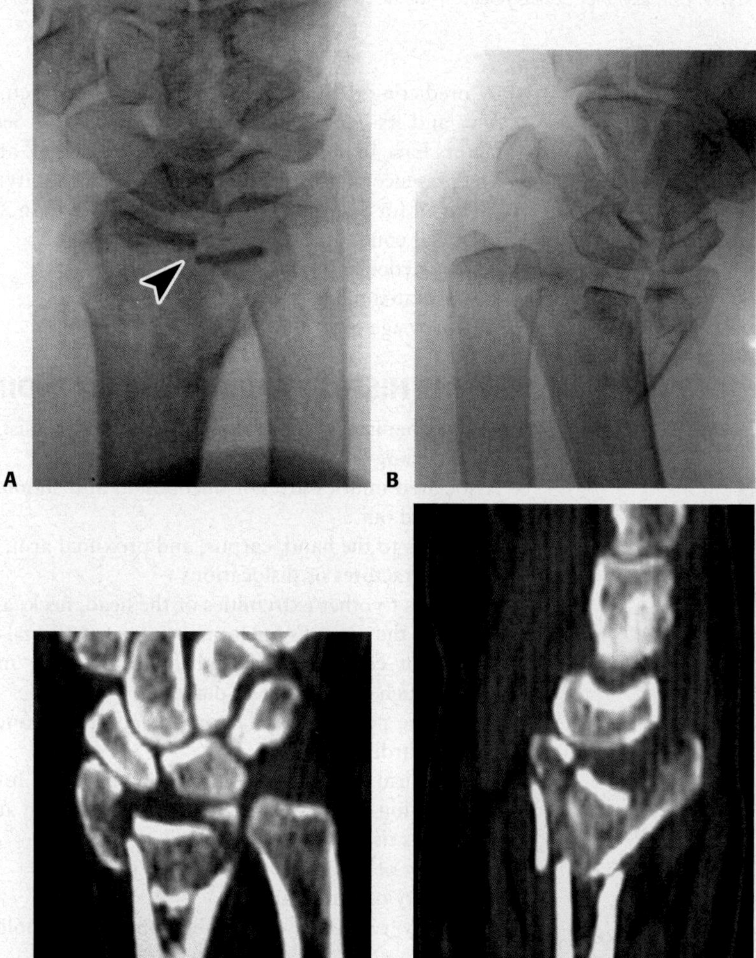

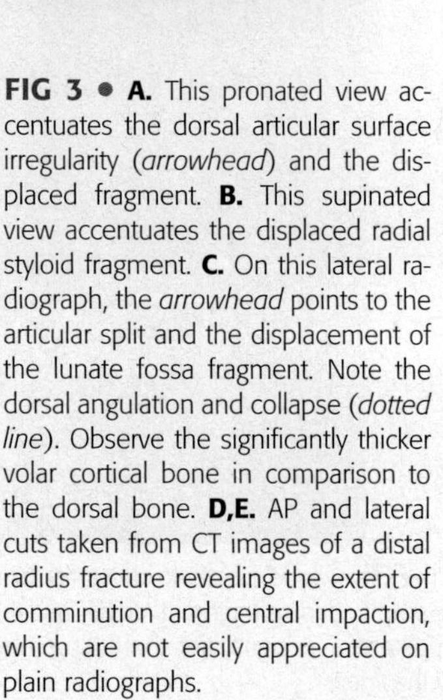

FIG 3 • **A.** This pronated view accentuates the dorsal articular surface irregularity (*arrowhead*) and the displaced fragment. **B.** This supinated view accentuates the displaced radial styloid fragment. **C.** On this lateral radiograph, the *arrowhead* points to the articular split and the displacement of the lunate fossa fragment. Note the dorsal angulation and collapse (*dotted line*). Observe the significantly thicker volar cortical bone in comparison to the dorsal bone. **D,E.** AP and lateral cuts taken from CT images of a distal radius fracture revealing the extent of comminution and central impaction, which are not easily appreciated on plain radiographs.

- Goals for treatment[9]
  - Radial inclination greater than 10 degrees
  - Ulnar variance less than 3-mm positive
  - Palmar tilt less than 10 degrees dorsal or 20 degrees volar
  - Articular congruity with less than a 2-mm gap or step-off
- Patients are immobilized in a short-arm cast for 6 weeks. Radiographic follow-up is performed on a weekly basis for the first 2 to 3 weeks to identify fracture displacement that may warrant reduction.

SURGICAL MANAGEMENT

- The goal of operative treatment is to achieve acceptable alignment and stable fixation.
- Various methods of fixation are available: pins, external fixators, intramedullary devices, and plates (volar, dorsal, fragment specific).

Preoperative Planning

- Preoperative medical and anesthesia evaluation are performed as required.
- Discontinue blood-thinning medications (anticoagulants and nonsteroidal anti-inflammatory drugs, especially acetylsalicylic acid).
- Request necessary equipment, including fluoroscopic and power equipment.
- Confirm the plate fixation system to be used, and check the equipment before beginning surgery for completeness (ie, all appropriate drills, plates, and screws).
- Have a contingency plan or additional fixation (external fixator, bone graft, or bone graft substitute).
- Review and have previous radiographic studies available.
- Consider use of a regional anesthetic for postoperative pain control.

Positioning

- Place the patient in the supine position with the affected extremity on an arm table.
- Apply an upper arm tourniquet, preferably within the sterile field.
- Incorporate weights or a traction system to apply distraction across the fracture (**FIG 4**).
- The surgeon is seated so that the elbow is pointing toward the patient's torso and the dominant hand works toward the fingers of the patients.
- The assistant is seated opposite the surgeon.
- The fluoroscopy unit is brought in from the end or corner of the table.

Approach

- Dorsal exposure allows for direct visualization of the articular surface when necessary.

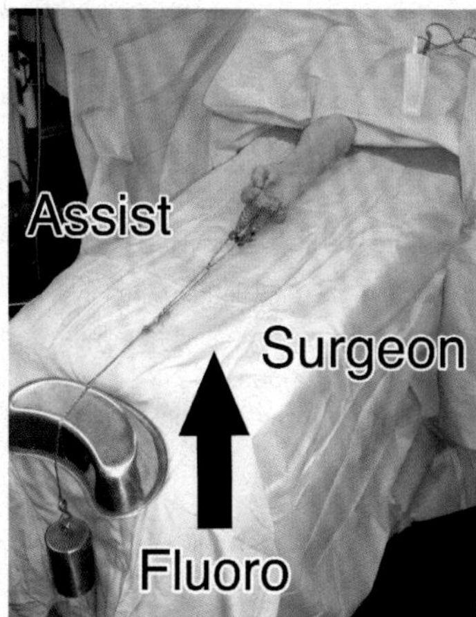

FIG 4 • Traction is applied over the arm table with finger traps and hanging weights. The surgeon sits on the volar side and the assistant on the dorsal side. Fluoroscopy can be brought in from any direction but preferably from the side adjacent or the opposite surgeon.

- Fracture comminution is more severe dorsally, making overall alignment more difficult to judge.
- The thicker volar cortex is less comminuted, allowing for more precise reduction and buttressing of bone fragments.
- Sometimes, both dorsal and volar exposures may be necessary to achieve articular congruency and volar reduction and fixation, respectively.
- An extended volar ulnar exposure may be necessary to manage isolated volar fractures of the lunate facet or to perform a simultaneous carpal tunnel release if indicated.
- The techniques described in this chapter use the volar approach to distal radius, as described by Henry (**FIG 5**).

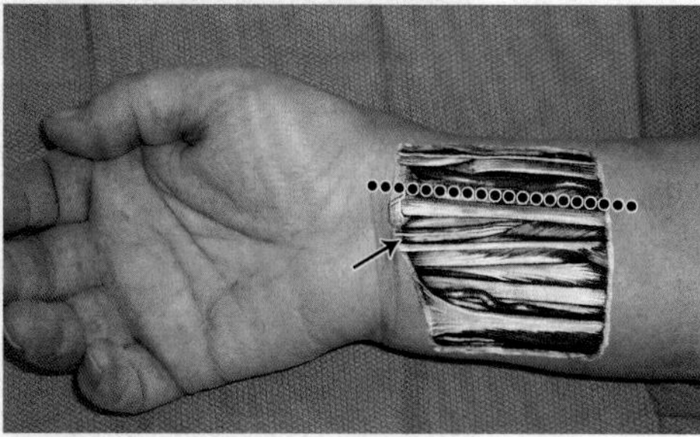

FIG 5 • The volar incision is represented by the *dotted line* just proximal to the wrist flexion creases and radial to the flexor carpi radialis longus. Care is exercised to avoid dissection from ulnar to the flexor carpi radialis because the palmar cutaneous nerve branch of the median nerve (*arrow*) is at risk.

Volar Fixed-Angle Plate Fixation of the Distal Radius

Incision and Dissection

- Make a 4- to 8-cm longitudinal incision from the proximal wrist flexion crease proximally, along the radial border of the flexor carpi radialis tendon.
  - Use a zigzag incision to cross the wrist flexion creases if required.
- Carefully avoid the palmar cutaneous branch of the median nerve which arises within 10 cm of the wrist flexion crease and travels along the ulnar side of the flexor carpi radialis tendon.
  - Branches of the dorsal radial sensory nerve and lateral antebrachial cutaneous nerve may appear along the path of the incision and also need to be protected.
- At the distal end of the incision, protect the palmar branch of the radial artery to the deep palmar arch.
  - It usually is not necessary to dissect out the radial artery (**TECH FIG 1A**).
- Incise the anterior sheath of the flexor carpi radialis tendon and retract the tendon ulnarly to help protect the median nerve (**TECH FIG 1B**).
- Incise the posterior sheath of the flexor carpi radialis tendon.
  - The deep tissues likely will bulge out from the pressure of swelling and fracture hematoma.
  - The median nerve is at risk lying within the subcutaneous tissues along the ulnar portion of the wound (**TECH FIG 1C,D**).
  - The flexor pollicis longus tendon sits along the radial margin of the wound.
- Using blunt dissection with a gauze-covered finger, sweep the tendons and the nerve ulnarly.
  - A self-retaining retractor is carefully placed just deep to the radial artery radially and the tendons and median nerve ulnarly.
  - The pronator quadratus is now visualized on the floor of the wound.
- Incise the pronator quadratus at its radial insertion, leaving fascial tissue on either side to aid in closure. Also, determine the proximal and distal extent of the muscle, and make horizontal incisions at both of those points (**TECH FIG 1E**).
  - The distal margin of the pronator quadratus attaches along the distal volar lip of the distal radius, along the "teardrop" and the watershed line.
  - The radial margin is in proximity to the tendons of the first dorsal compartment and the brachioradialis.

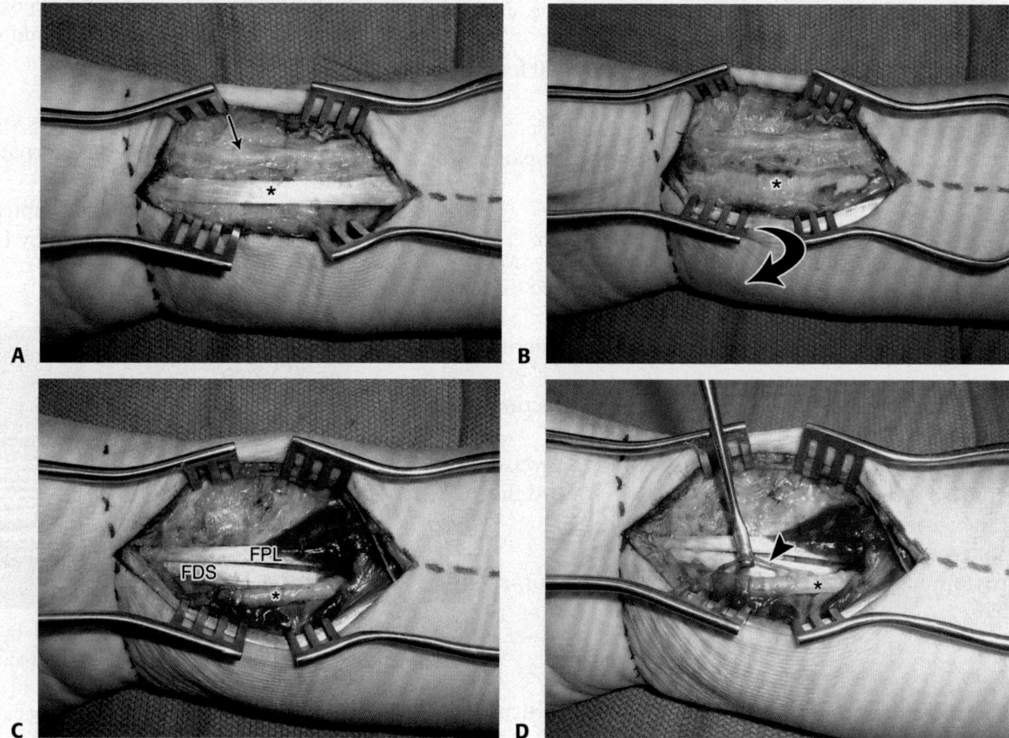

TECH FIG 1 • **A.** The interval between the radial artery (*arrow*) and the flexor carpi radialis tendon (*asterisk*) is seen. **B.** The posterior sheath (*asterisk*) of the flexor carpi radialis is visible after retracting the flexor carpi radialis ulnarly (*arrow*). Be careful during deeper dissection because swelling and hematoma may distort the position of the median nerve beneath the sheath. **C.** Following incision in the flexor carpi radialis posterior sheath, the deep tendons are visible, including the flexor pollicis longus (*FPL*) and the flexor digitorum superficialis (*FDS*) of the index finger. The median nerve also is visible (*asterisk*). **D.** The palmar cutaneous nerve branches of the median nerve (*arrowhead*) and median nerve (*asterisk*) are both at risk for injury during this approach. Be careful regarding placement of retractors and during dissection and plate placement. *(continued)*

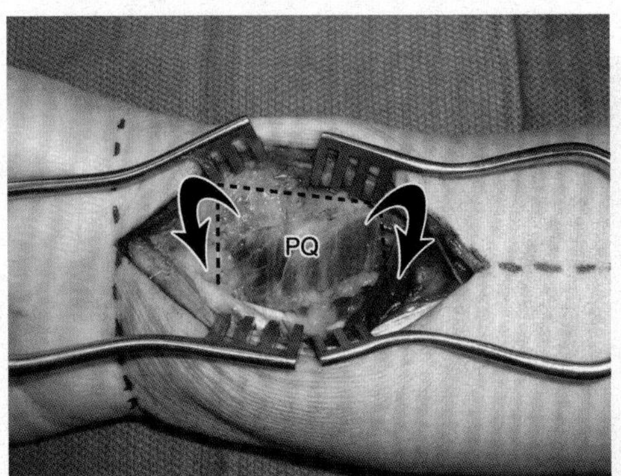

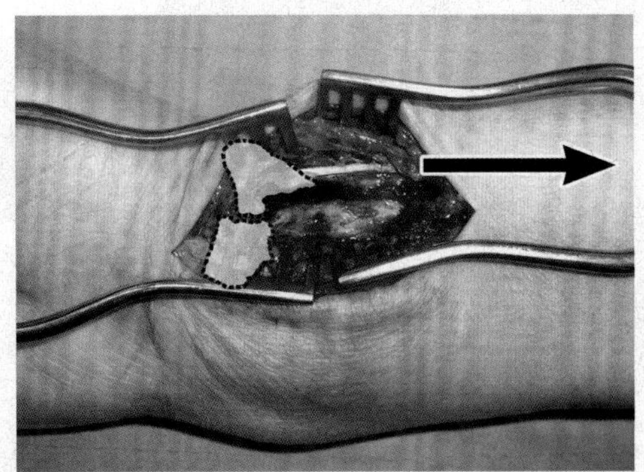

E F

TECH FIG 1 • *(continued)* **E.** The pronator quadratus (*PQ*) is incised distally, radially, and proximally and then reflected ulnarly after dissection off the volar distal radius. **F.** The brachioradialis (*arrow*) can be a deforming force, especially in comminuted fractures and in those for which treatment has been delayed. This tendon can be released if necessary.

- Subperiosteally, dissect the pronator quadratus off the volar surface of the distal radius as an ulnarly based flap with a knife or elevator.
- Retract the pronator ulnarly with the flexor tendons and median nerve.
- Particularly, if significant shortening of radial-sided fracture fragments has occurred, incise the broad insertion of the brachioradialis to eliminate the deforming force (**TECH FIG 1F**).
  - Release the first dorsal compartment and retract the tendons before releasing the brachioradialis.
  - Alternatively, Z-lengthen the brachioradialis tendon to allow for repair at the completion of the case.

Fracture Reduction and Provisional Fixation

- Apply a lobster claw clamp around the radius shaft at a perpendicular angle to the volar surface at the most proximal portion of the wound (**TECH FIG 2A**).
  - This allows for excellent control of the proximal shaft for rotation and translation, providing an excellent counterforce when correcting the dorsal angulation collapse.
  - It also aids in soft tissue retraction.
- With the fracture now exposed, apply traction distally to distract and disimpact the fragments.
- Carefully clean the fracture of any interposed muscle, fascia, hematoma, or callus while maintaining the bony contours.
- In the case of significant volar comminution, reduce and provisionally stabilize the fragments with K-wires.
  - Take plate positioning into account when placing these K-wires.
- The articular surface is first reduced, if necessary.
- Under fluoroscopic guidance, manipulate the articular fragments through the fracture with a periosteal elevator, osteotome, or K-wires (**TECH FIG 2B,C**).
  - Longitudinal traction is important during this reduction phase. It can be performed by an assistant or using cross-table weights and finger traps.
  - A dorsal exposure is performed at this stage if there is significant articular impaction, particularly centrally, that cannot be corrected using the extra-articular technique described here.
- Place K-wires from the radial styloid fragment into the lunate fossa fragment to maintain the articular reduction (**TECH FIG 2D**).
  - The K-wires should be placed as close as possible to subchondral bone (**TECH FIG 2E,F**).
- Once the distal articular reduction is complete, reduce the distal radius as a single unit to the radius shaft.
- Insert K-wires as required to maintain the provisional reduction between the distal fragments and the proximal shaft fragment.
  - If radial collapse and translation are prominent, a large K-wire can be introduced into the radial portion of the fracture. By advancing it proximally and ulnarly, it behaves like an intrafocal pin, providing a radial buttress by pushing the distal fragment ulnarly.
  - A similar technique can be applied through the dorsal fracture to assist in maintaining palmar tilt correction.

Plate Application

- Apply a fixed-angle volar plate to the volar surface of the distal radius and shaft. Position the plate to accommodate for the unique design characteristics of the plating system as well as the location of the fracture fragments.
  - Each plating system has unique characteristics that determine its optimal placement.
  - Ideally, the plate should be placed as close to the articular margin as possible without the distal locking pegs or screws penetrating the joint.
  - If the fracture has not yet been fully reduced, this must be taken into account when placing the device.
  - Plate placement distal to the watershed line should be avoided as this increases the risk for flexor tendon rupture.
- Clamp the previously applied lobster claw to the proximal portion of the plate to keep the plate centralized on the radius shaft.
- Place provisional K-wires through the plate to maintain position (**TECH FIG 3**). Then fluoroscopically confirm proper plate position in both the distal proximal and radioulnar directions.
  - Proper alignment of the plate can be determined only using a true anteroposterior (AP) image in which the distal radioulnar joint is well visualized.
  - The K-wires allow for fine adjustment in plate position before committing to insertion of a screw.

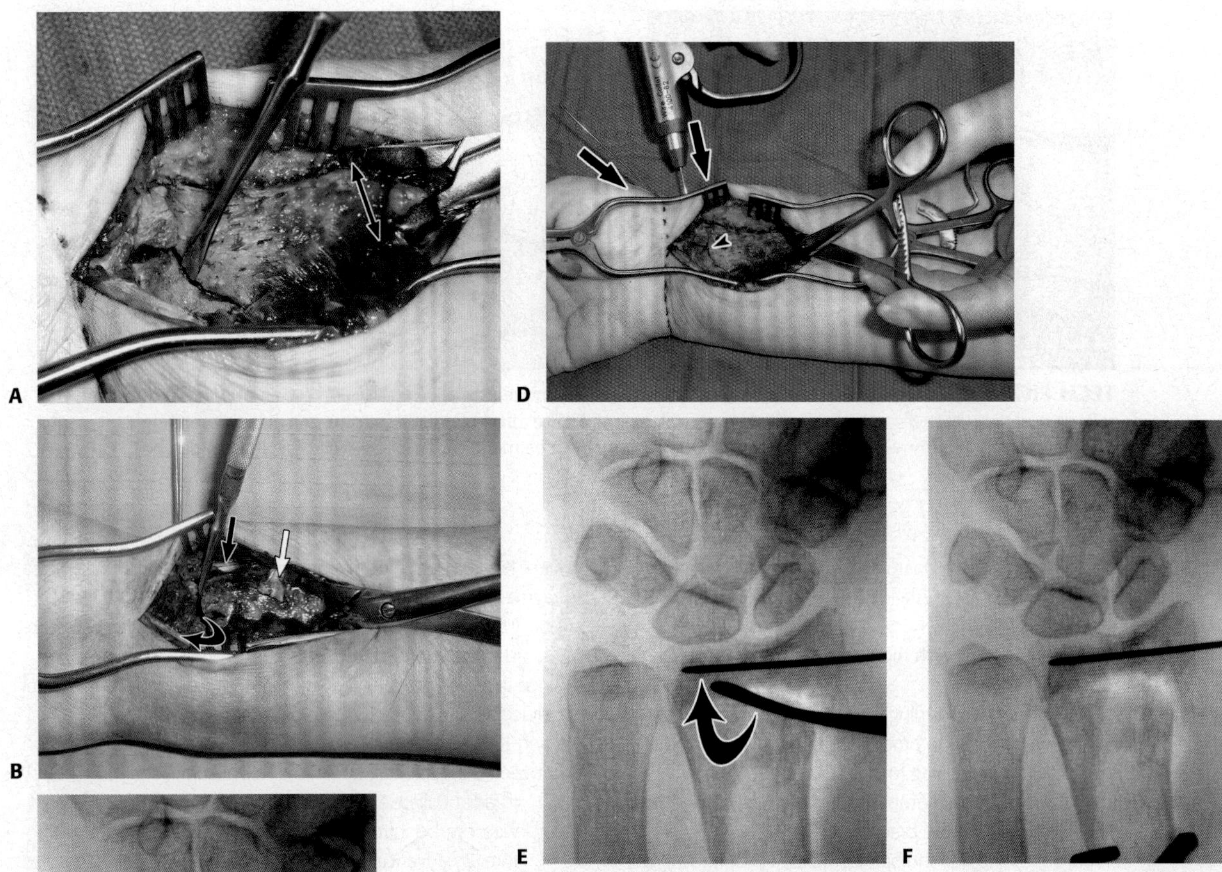

TECH FIG 2 • **A.** A lobster claw clamp (*double arrow*) is applied to the radius shaft well proximal to the fracture. This instrument helps the surgeon control the radius during reduction and define the lateral margins of the radius. A Freer elevator is inserted into the fracture to help disimpact the fragments and assist in their reduction. **B.** The brachioradialis (*white arrow*) is released, and the first compartment extensor tendons are visible in the background (*black arrow*). An instrument can now be placed to assist in the reduction (*arrow*). **C.** The Freer elevator is used to reduce the fragments. In this case, the intra-articular step-off is being corrected, and the radial length and inclination are being restored. **D.** K-wires are placed across the radial styloid into the reduced ulna fossa fragment. An assistant usually applies traction, and the lobster claw clamp can be used for powerful leverage. If there is no articular involvement, this K-wire can be placed into the radius metaphysis or diaphysis proximally. **E.** The K-wire should be placed as close as possible to the subchondral bone, avoiding areas of comminution. **F.** The K-wire should maintain the articular reduction without any support.

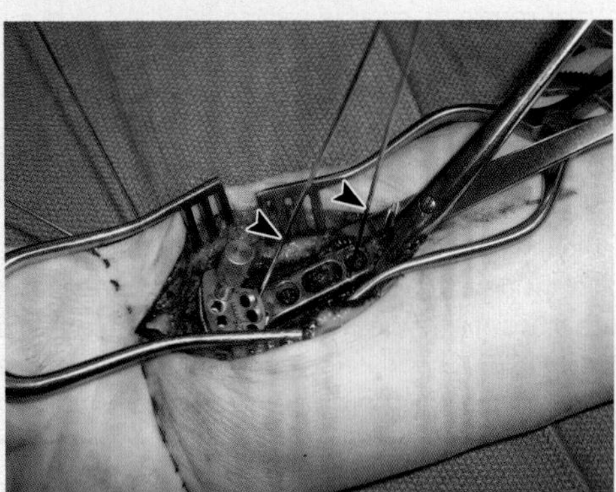

TECH FIG 3 • Keep the plate centered on the radius and as distal as possible. The lobster claw clamp helps keep the plate centered. K-wires (*arrowheads*) are helpful as provision fixation until alignment can be confirmed radiographically and screws placed.

- Drill and insert a provisional screw in the oblong hole in the plate.
  - If the bone is osteopenic, a screw longer than the initial measurement should be placed to ensure that both cortices are engaged. Otherwise, the plate may not be held securely, and reduction will be compromised. After the remaining screws have been secured, this screw can be replaced with one of appropriate length.
- Insert at least one additional proximal screw and remove the provisional K-wires holding the plate in place.

Distal Fragment Reduction

- Once the plate has been secured proximally, execute any additionally needed reduction.
  - A well-designed plate serves as an excellent buttress for correction of palmar tilt (**TECH FIG 4A**).

- Apply counterforce through the lobster claw clamp in a dorsal direction while the distal hand and wrist are translated palmarly and flexed (**TECH FIG 4B**).
  - This maneuver reduces the distal radius to the plate, effectively restoring volar tilt by pushing the lunate against the volar lip of the distal radius (**TECH FIG 4C,D**).
- Additional distraction and ulnar deviation correct radial collapse and loss of radial inclination.

Plate Fixation

- While the reduction is held, drill the holes in the distal plate segment (**TECH FIG 5A**).
  - Some plate systems allow for provisional fixation using K-wires placed through the distal plate segment.
  - Do not penetrate the dorsal distal radius with the drill, thereby avoiding injury to the dorsal extensor tendons.
- Drill and place the distal ulnar screws first and then proceed radially and proximally.
- Accurate screw placement using the same inclination of the drill is required to avoid cross-threading into the plate and lessening stability.
- Judge the placement of all distal screws or pegs precisely using fluoroscopic imaging in multiple planes.
  - In order to confirm extra-articular placement of distal screws, perform a "true" lateral view of the wrist with the x-ray beam at a 20-degree angle to the radius shaft (**TECH FIG 5B,C**). This is facilitated by lifting the wrist off the table with the elbow maintained on the table and the forearm at a 20-degree angle to the table (**TECH FIG 5D,E**).
  - The extensor pollicis longus is at greatest risk of injury from a protruding screw.
  - Because of the prominence of Lister tubercle and the triangular configuration of the distal radius, the lateral view of the wrist may not accurately rule out dorsal screw protrusion.
  - The dorsal horizon view can aid in assessing adequate screw length dorsally. It is obtained by wrist hyperflexion and aiming the beam of the image intensifier along the long axis of the radius.[5]
- Sequentially insert the remaining distal screws or pegs, followed by the remaining proximal plate screws (**TECH FIG 5F**).
- If necessary, add bone graft or bone graft substitute around the plate into the fracture site or through a small dorsal incision.
- Precisely assess the stability of the construct after the plate has been applied. If appropriate, remove the provisional K-wires.
  - If the K-wires are deemed critical for fracture stability, they can be left in place and removed 4 to 8 weeks later.
  - If residual instability exists, add additional fixation with K-wires, an external fixator, a dorsal plate, or a combination.

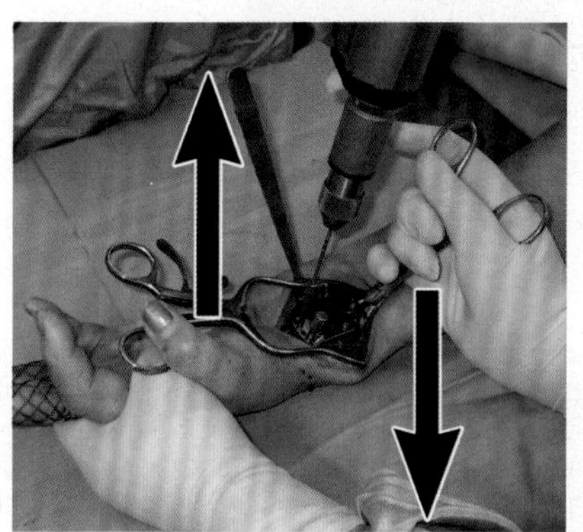
A

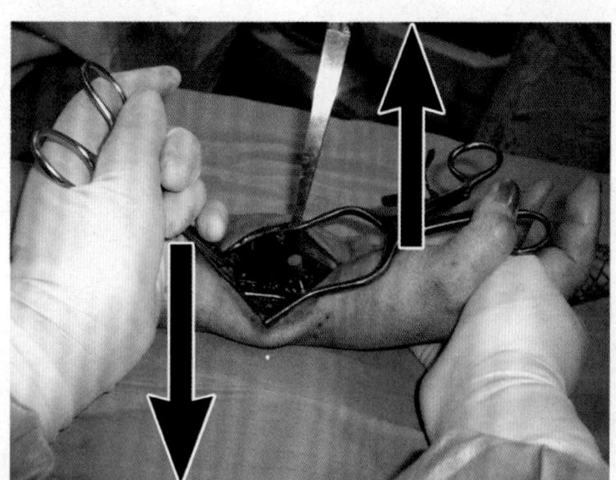
B

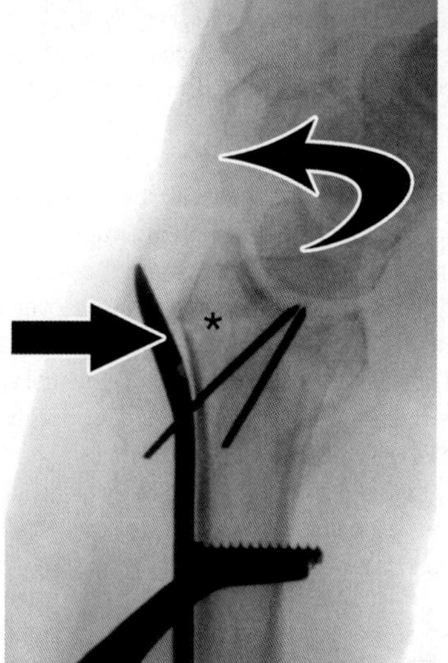

C

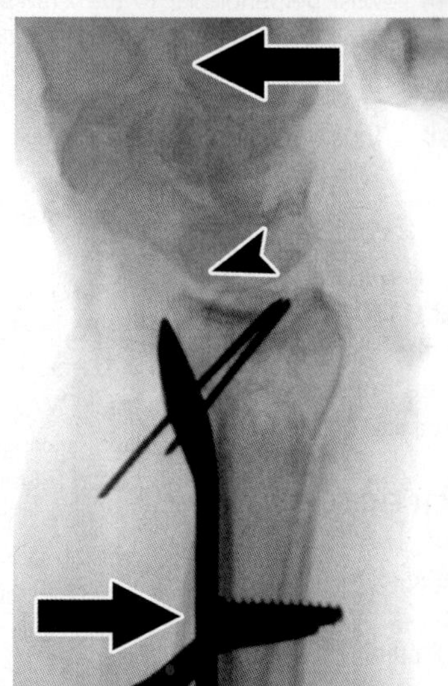
D

TECH FIG 4 • **A.** The final reduction is performed with traction on the hand and with the radius held proximally with a clamp. Once the reduction is confirmed radiographically, the assistant places the distal screws or K-wires. **B.** The hand is translated (not appreciably flexed) palmarly while the radius shaft is held with the clamp. Prereduction (**C**) and postreduction (**D**) radiographs demonstrating the palmar translation reduction maneuver. The volar plate acts as a strong buttress (*arrows*), allowing the translated lunate to push on the volar radius (*asterisk*) and correct the dorsal angulation deformity.

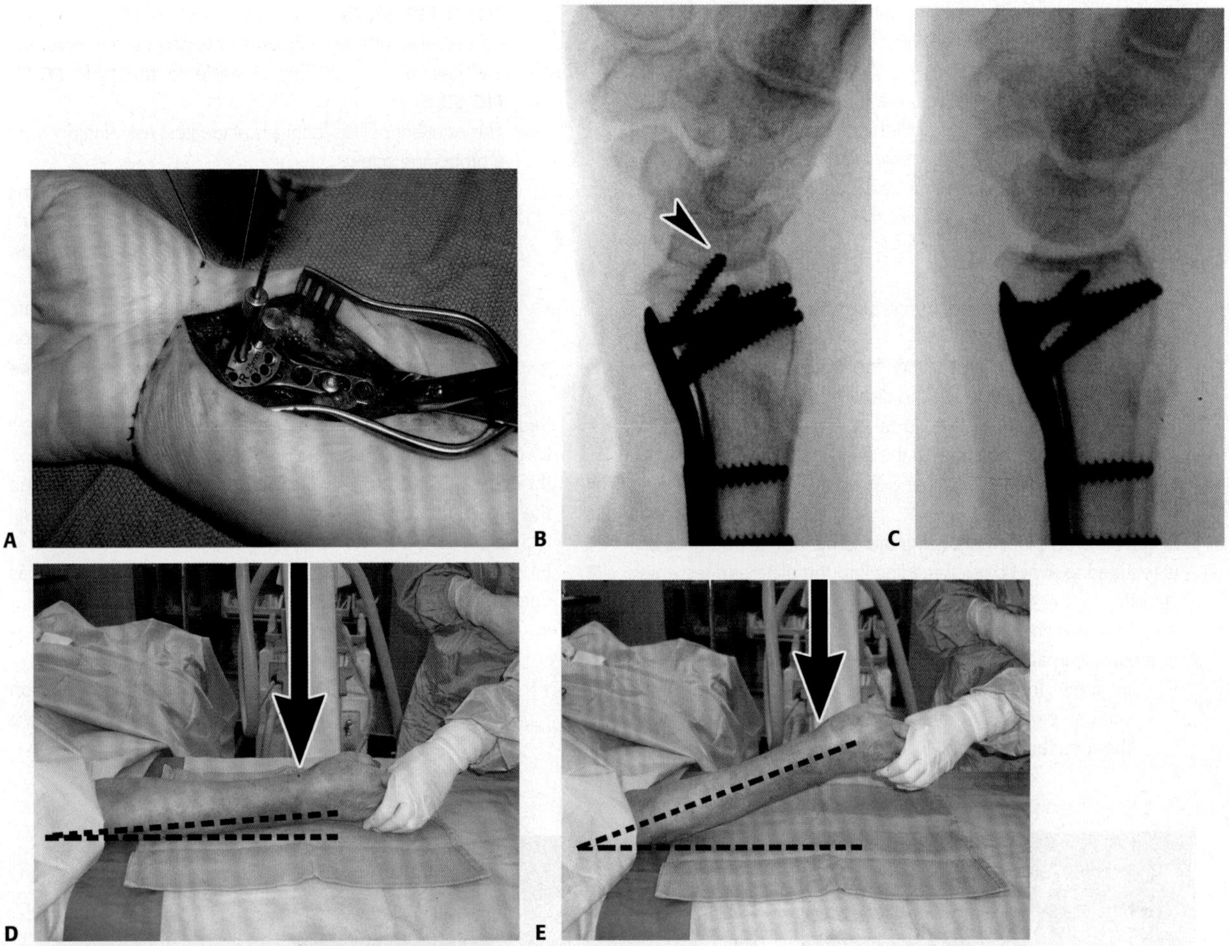

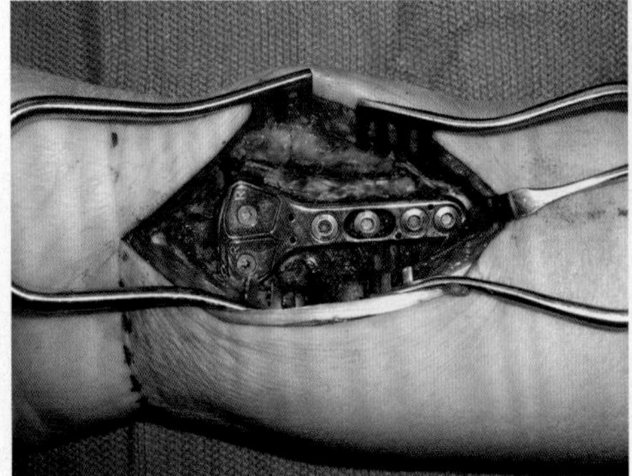

TECH FIG 5 • A. The remaining holes can now be drilled and screws placed where needed. **B.** This screw (*arrowhead*) looks as though it has penetrated the joint, when in reality, it is simply the angle of the radiographic beam that throws its projection into the joint. **C.** A true lateral view of the distal radius is necessary to judge placement of the radial screws. **D.** A radiograph is being taken with the wrist perpendicular to the x-ray beam (*arrow*). This is not a true lateral image because the distal surface of the radius is inclined 20 degrees radially. **E.** By lifting the hand and wrist 20 degrees off the table, a true lateral image can be achieved. The x-ray beam is now perpendicular to the joint (*arrow*). **F.** The remaining screws have been placed.

Closure

- Repair the pronator quadratus to its insertion site with a series of 3-0 absorbable horizontal mattress sutures (**TECH FIG 6A**).
  - In many cases, it is impossible to repair the pronator quadratus because the muscle and fascia are extremely thin or the muscle is damaged. In this situation, the muscle can be débrided or simply left in place.
- Before skin closure, obtain final radiographs (**TECH FIG 6B,C**) and assess the stability of the distal radioulnar joint.
- Place a drain only if excessive bleeding is anticipated.
- Consider methods to minimize postoperative pain.
  - Percutaneous placement of a pain pump catheter
  - Injection of a long-acting local anesthetic
- Close the subcutaneous tissues with a 4-0 braided absorbable suture and reapproximate the skin with interrupted 4-0 or 5-0 nylon sutures or a running subcuticular stitch.
- Place two layers of gauze and a nonadherent gauze over the wound, wrap the wrist and forearm with thick Webril (Kendall, Mansfield, MA), and apply a below-elbow splint in a neutral wrist position, leaving the metacarpophalangeal joints free for range of motion (ROM) (**TECH FIG 6D**).
  - If there is injury to the ulnar wrist (eg, ulnar styloid fracture, distal radioulnar joint injury), immobilize the forearm in slight supination with an above-elbow or sugar-tong (Munster) splint.

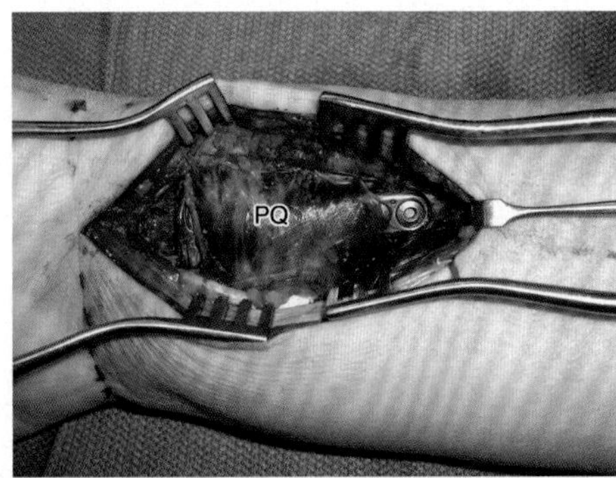

A

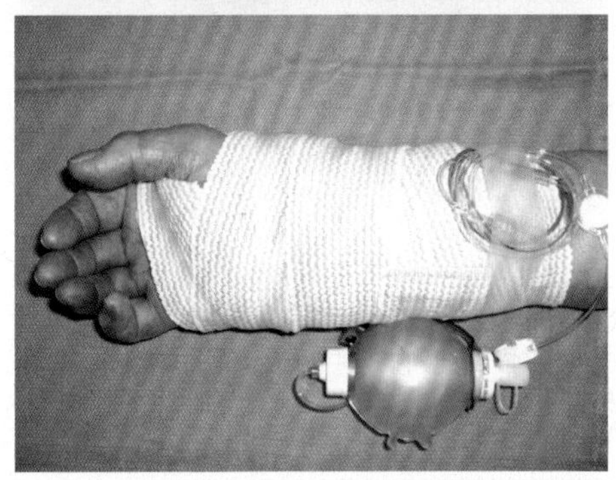

D

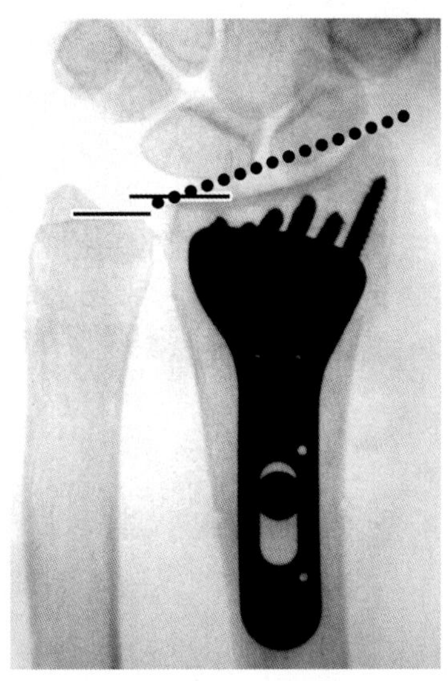

B

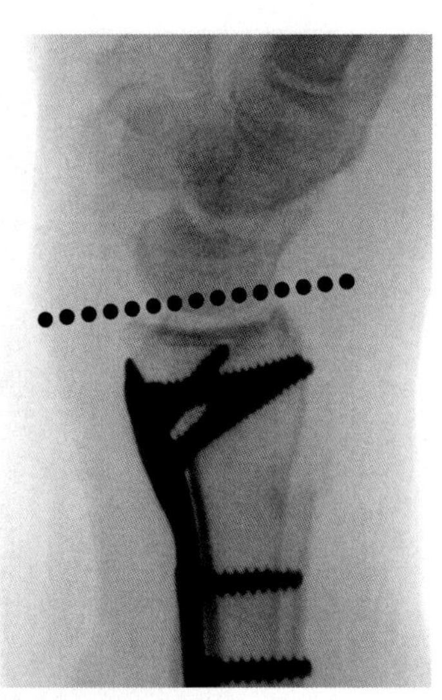

C

TECH FIG 6 • A. The pronator quadratus (*PQ*) has been repaired. **B.** AP radiograph demonstrating correction of the articular surface, radial height (*lines*), and radial inclination (*dotted line*). **C.** Lateral radiograph demonstrating correction of the palmar tilt (*dotted line*). **D.** A bulky dressing is applied with a volar splint holding the wrist in a neutral position. A pain pump catheter has been inserted for additional pain control.

Volar Fixed-Angle Plate Using the Plate as Reduction Tool

- We do not recommend use of the volar fixed-angle plate as a reduction tool in the acute setting. It is best employed (if at all) for a malunion or perhaps for a fracture with minimal articular comminution.
  - This technique is difficult because the plate must be applied accounting for the coronal, sagittal, and translational deformities associated with the fracture fragments before the reduction has been achieved.
- Perform the surgical approach as previously described.
- Address first any distal articular involvement with reduction and K-wire fixation.
- Affix the plate to the distal fragment, accounting for where the plate will sit on the radius shaft once the reduction is completed.
- Place the screws so that they are parallel to the articular surface on the lateral x-ray view (**TECH FIG 7A,B**).
- On the AP radiograph, align the plate with the perpendicular of the radial inclination of the distal radius (20 degrees; **TECH FIG 7C,D**).
- Once distal fixation is complete, secure the proximal plate to the radius shaft, thereby completing the reduction.
- Close and splint as described previously.

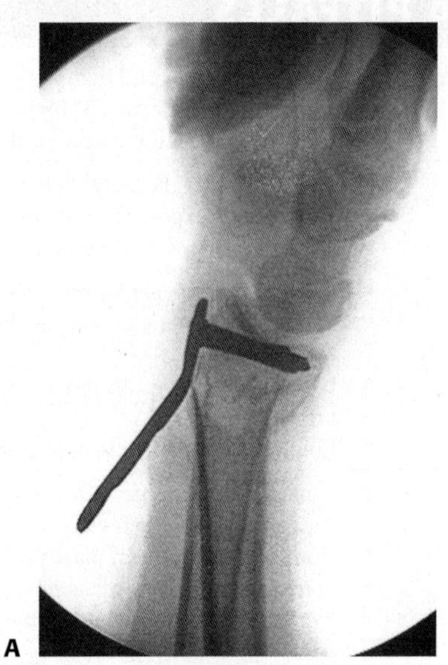

A

TECH FIG 7 • A. The volar plate is applied with the distal screws placed first (parallel to distal articular surface). *(continued)*

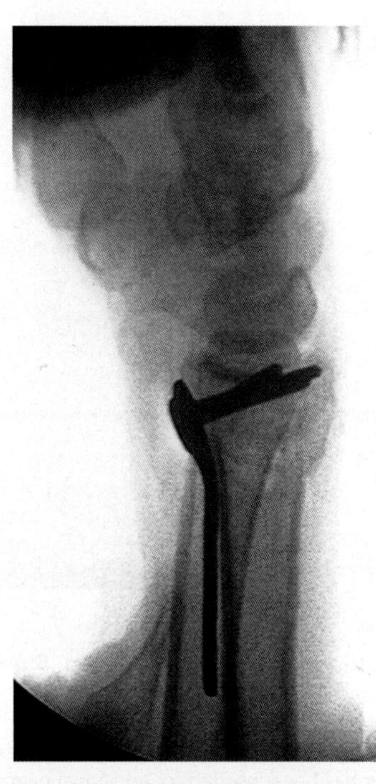

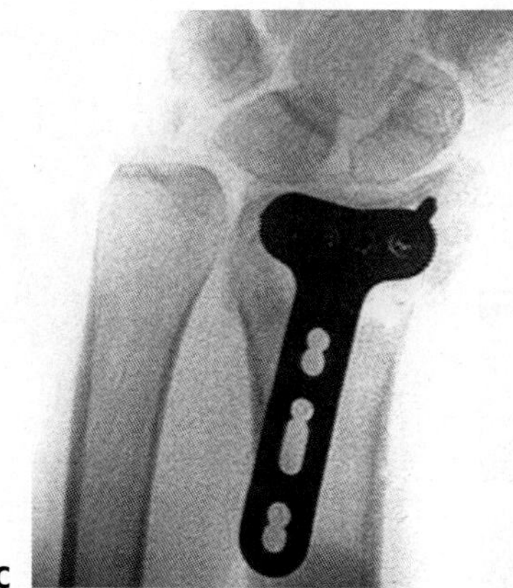

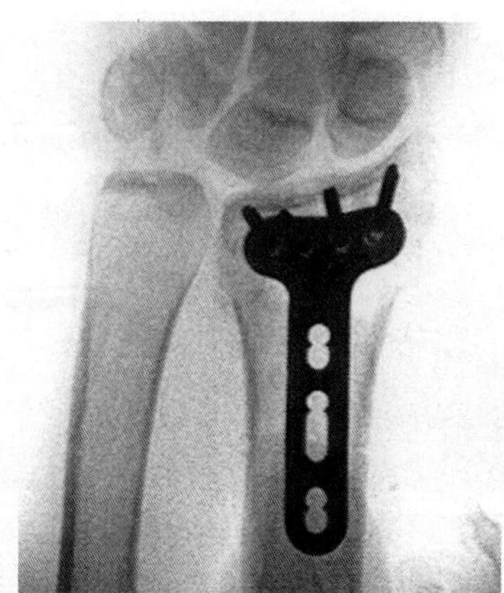

TECH FIG 7 • *(continued)* **B.** Reducing the plate to the diaphysis proximally accomplishes the reduction. **C.** The plate is applied at approximately a 20-degree angle relative to the distal articular surface or to the amount of angulation that is estimated. **D.** By reducing the plate to the diaphysis, the distal angulation is corrected.

PEARLS AND PITFALLS

Preoperative planning	▪ Obtain multiple radiographs in different positions (eg, several oblique views), especially in the setting of comminution or articular involvement. ▪ Obtain a CT scan if assessing the pattern of fracture when radiographs alone are difficult or uncertain.
Surgical approach	▪ Avoid crossing the distal flexion creases of the wrist. ▪ Avoid ulnar exposure to the midline of the flexor carpi radialis. ▪ Use extra care with deep dissection in the presence of hematoma or significant swelling.
Fracture reduction	▪ Employ traction across the wrist with a device or weights. ▪ Use a lobster claw clamp on the proximal radius shaft for control of the forearm and as a reference for the lateral margins. ▪ Use instruments to disimpact and reduce articular fragments through the fracture itself, either volarly, dorsally, or both. ▪ Employ a temporary K-wire to stabilize the reduction before placement of the plate.
Plate alignment	▪ Confirm appropriate radial–ulnar positioning of the proximal plate using a true AP radiograph (ie, forearm in supination with open view of the distal radioulnar joint). ▪ Confirm proper distal plate position on a true lateral view (ie, forearm 20 degrees off the table). ▪ Place the plate as distal as possible, up to the volar teardrop (watershed line) of the distal radius, if possible. ▪ Evaluate the screws for possible joint penetration using 360-degree fluoroscopic images.
Plate fixation	▪ Use K-wires to fix the plate provisionally to the proximal radius. ▪ The initial "oblong hole" screw should be slightly longer than the measured length to ensure better initial fixation.
Postoperative	▪ Closure of the pronator quadratus is not critical and should be reserved for more substantial muscles with limited trauma. ▪ Begin immediate ROM to digits with edema.

POSTOPERATIVE CARE

- The wrist is splinted in a neutral position, leaving the digits free.
  - If the fracture is particularly tenuous or there is injury to the ulnar wrist, a long-arm or sugar-tong (Munster) splint is applied.
- Vitamin C 500 to 1500 mg per day for 6 weeks is recommended to reduce the incidence of complex regional pain syndrome.[22]
- The patient is instructed to perform active ROM exercises for the digits every hour and to engage in strict elevation for at least 3 days.
  - It is critical to emphasize edema prevention and immediate ROM of the digits.
- At 1 week postoperatively, the splint is removed and the wound is examined.
- If swelling permits, the therapist fabricates a molded Orthoplast splint (Johnson & Johnson Orthopedics, New Brunswick, NJ) to be worn at all times.
- Active ROM exercises of the wrist are implemented 1 week postoperatively.
- At 4 to 6 weeks, putty and grip exercises are added.
- At 6 to 8 weeks, the splint is discontinued, and progressive strengthening exercises are advanced.
- If necessary, progressive passive ROM can begin, including use of dynamic splints.
- At 10 to 12 weeks, the patient usually can be discharged to all activities as tolerated.
- Elderly patients with distal radius fractures are at increased risk of sustaining other osteoporosis-related fractures. A referral to an osteoporosis clinic is advised.

OUTCOMES

- Overall good to excellent results can be expected in over 80% of patients with ROM, strength, and outcomes scoring.[13,14,19,21]
- Studies comparing volar fixation to other forms of fixation (eg, external fixators, pins, and dorsal plating) have revealed similar if not superior results.
  - Results appear to be superior in the early recovery period, with the final outcome yielding equivalent results among all fixation groups.
  - Some studies suggest better maintenance in overall reduction compared to other forms of fixation.

COMPLICATIONS

- Complication rates as high as 27% have been reported.
- Complications can be categorized into those involving hardware, fracture, soft tissues, nerves, and tendons.[2]
- Failures of hardware, such as plate or screw breakage, can occur but are rare. Usually, such failures are an indication of other problems, such as nonunion.
- The hardware becomes unacceptably prominent in a minority of patients.
  - This complication may become evident only after some time has elapsed, as swelling of fibrous tissue subsides and bone remodels.
  - The most common sites include the dorsal wrist, when screws have been inserted, and the radial wrist, when a plate has been used.
  - It can be avoided with careful screw and plate placement and radiographic verification of their position.
- Nonunion and delayed union are unusual. Consider a diagnosis of osteomyelitis or other risk factors such as smoking.
- Loss of fracture reduction and fixation can occur and is most common in patients with osteopenic bone or comminuted and articular fractures.
  - This can be avoided with frequent and early follow-up with repeat radiographs.
  - If instability is suspected, the fracture can be casted.
  - In the operating room, if instability is suspected, additional fixation should be considered (eg, external fixator, pins, bone graft).
- Soft tissue complications are proportional to the energy of the initial injury.
- Open wounds usually can be addressed with local measures.
- Significant swelling must be addressed with early and aggressive modalities. Swelling can lead to other complications, such as joint stiffness and tendon adhesions.
- Nerve injuries can be the result of initial trauma or subsequent surgical trauma.
  - Assess and document neurologic status before surgery.
  - Avoid further injury to nerves with careful placement of retractors.
  - The palmar cutaneous branch of the median nerve can be injured during incision and exposure.
  - Postoperative neuromas can cause pain and sensitivity along scar.
  - Avoid the nerve with a well-placed incision radial to the flexor carpi radialis and careful deep dissection.
- Postoperative swelling also can lead to median neuropathy. Carpal tunnel release should be performed if there is any suspected compression neuropathy or if this is to be anticipated as a result of postoperative swelling.
- Tendon complications include adhesions and ruptures.
- Most tendon adhesions involve the dorsal extensor tendons resulting in extrinsic extensor tightness.
- Flexor tendon adhesions are uncommon and involve primarily the flexor pollicis longus.
- Tendon ruptures have been described, especially involving the flexor pollicis longus and the extensor pollicis longus, as a result of plate and screw prominence, respectively.
  - The distal screws must not be left prominent, and caution must be applied when drilling.
  - The sagittal and coronal profiles of the plate being used must be taken into consideration—some plates are very prominent and extend far radially.

REFERENCES

1. Aro HT, Koivunen T. Minor axial shortening of the radius affects outcome of Colles' fracture treatment. J Hand Surg Am 1991;16(3):392–398.
2. Arora R, Lutz M, Hennerbichler A, et al. Complications following internal fixation of unstable distal radius fracture with a palmar locking-plate. J Orthop Trauma 2007;21(5):316–322.
3. Fernandez JJ, Gruen GS, Herndon JH. Outcome of distal radius fractures using the short form 36 health survey. Clin Orthop Relat Res 1997;(341):36–41.
4. Geissler WB, Freeland AE, Savoie FH, et al. Intracarpal soft-tissue lesions associated with an intra-articular fracture of the distal end of the radius. J Bone Joint Surg Am 1996;78(3):357–365.
5. Joseph SJ, Harvey JN. The dorsal horizon view: detecting screw protrusion at the distal radius. J Hand Surg Am 2011;36(10):1691–1693.
6. Jupiter JB, Fernandez DL. Comparative classification for fractures of the distal end of the radius. J Hand Surg Am 1997;22(4):563–571.

7. Knirk JL, Jupiter JB. Intra-articular fractures of the distal end of the radius in young adults. J Bone Joint Surg Am 1986;68(5):647–659.
8. Lafontaine M, Hardy D, Delince P. Stability assessment of distal radius fractures. Injury 1989;20(4):208–210.
9. Lichtman DM, Bindra RR, Boyer MI, et al. American Academy of Orthopaedic Surgeons clinical practice guideline on: the treatment of distal radius fractures. J Bone Joint Surg Am 2011;93(8):775–778.
10. Marsh JL, Slongo TF, Agel J, et al. Fracture and dislocation classification compendium–2007: Orthopaedic Trauma Association classification, database and outcomes committee. J Orthop Trauma 2007;21 (10 suppl):S1–S133.
11. Medoff RJ. Essential radiographic evaluation for distal radius fractures. Hand Clin 2005;21(3):279–288.
12. Melone CP Jr. Articular fractures of the distal radius. Orthop Clin North Am 1984;15(2):217–236.
13. Musgrave DS, Idler RS. Volar fixation of dorsally displaced distal radius fractures using the 2.4-mm locking compression plates. J Hand Surg Am 2005;30(4):743–749.
14. Orbay JL, Fernandez DL. Volar fixed-angle plate fixation for unstable distal radius fractures in the elderly patient. J Hand Surg Am 2004;29(1):96–102.
15. Pogue DJ, Viegas SF, Patterson RM, et al. Effects of distal radius fracture malunion on wrist joint mechanics. J Hand Surg Am 1990;15(5):721–727.
16. Pollock J, O'Toole RV, Nowicki SD, et al. Articular cartilage thickness at the distal radius: a cadaveric study. J Hand Surg Am 2013;38(8):1477–1481.
17. Porter M, Stockley I. Fractures of the distal radius. Intermediate and end results in relation to radiologic parameters. Clin Orthop Relat Res 1987;(220):241–252.
18. Richards RS, Bennett JD, Roth JH, et al. Arthroscopic diagnosis of intra-articular soft tissue injuries associated with distal radial fractures. J Hand Surg Am 1997;22(5):772–776.
19. Rozental TD, Blazar PE, Franko OI, et al. Functional outcomes for unstable distal radial fractures treated with open reduction and internal fixation or closed reduction and percutaneous fixation. A prospective randomized trial. J Bone Joint Surg Am 2009;91(8): 1837–1846.
20. Short WH, Palmer AK, Werner FW, et al. A biomechanical study of distal radial fractures. J Hand Surg Am 1987;12(4): 529–534.
21. Wright TW, Horodyski M, Smith DW. Functional outcome of unstable distal radius fractures: ORIF with a volar fixed-angle tine plate versus external fixation. J Hand Surg Am 2005;30(2):289–299.
22. Zollinger PE, Tuinebreijer WE, Breederveld RS, et al. Can vitamin C prevent complex regional pain syndrome in patients with wrist fractures? A randomized, controlled, multicenter dose-response study. J Bone Joint Surg Am 2007;89(7):1424–1431.

Bridge Plating of Distal Radius Fractures

32

CHAPTER

Paul A. Martineau, Kevin J. Malone, and Douglas P. Hanel

DEFINITION

- High-energy fractures of the distal aspect of the radius with extensive comminution of the articular surface and extension into the diaphysis represent a major treatment challenge. Standard plates and techniques may be inadequate for the management of such fractures.
- Before the introduction of the bridge plating technique, treatment of these injuries was limited to cast immobilization or external fixation with or without Kirschner wire augmentation. Both of these methods are associated with unacceptably high complication rates.

ANATOMY

- The articular surface of the distal radius is tilted 21 degrees in the anteroposterior plane and 5 to 11 degrees in the lateral plane.
- The dorsal cortex surface of the radius thickens to form the tubercle of Lister.
- A central ridge divides the articular surface of the radius into a scaphoid facet and a lunate facet.
- Because of the different areas of bone thickness and density, fractures tend to occur in the relatively weaker metaphyseal bone and propagate intra-articularly between the scaphoid and lunate facets.
- The degree, direction, and magnitude of applied load may cause coronal or sagittal splits within the lunate or scaphoid facets.

PATHOGENESIS

- Two subsets of patients with distal radius fractures continue to represent unique treatment challenges:
  - Patients with high-energy wrist injuries with fracture extension into the radial diaphysis
  - Patients with multiple injuries who require load bearing through the injured wrist to assist with mobilization and nursing care

NATURAL HISTORY

- Lafontaine et al[13] showed that the end results of comminuted distal radius fractures treated by closed methods resembled the prereduction radiographs more than any other radiographs during treatment, even when the reduction successfully restored wrist anatomy.
- A number of studies clearly show that restoration of normal anatomy after distal radius fracture provides better function.[4,6–8,10–12,14]
- Functional outcome scores in patients without anatomic reduction are poor.[4,15]
- Malunion of the distal radius has been associated with pain, stiffness, weak grip strength, and carpal instability in a substantial percentage of patients.[8] Long-term consequences include degenerative arthritis in up to 50% of patients with even minimal displacement in the young adult population.[16]
- As surgical treatment (plating in particular) ensures more consistent correction of displacement and maintenance of reduction, there has been a trend toward operative treatment in both the elderly and the young population.

PATIENT HISTORY AND PHYSICAL FINDINGS

- In the management of high-energy distal radius fractures, a complete history should include the mechanism of injury. These fractures are commonly the result of axial loading as opposed to the bending forces, which are all low-velocity fractures.
- Examination of the soft tissue envelope of the wrist should be performed to rule out open fractures.
- Because of the high-energy nature of these fractures, patients are at increased risk of neurovascular compromise. Careful examination for signs of impending compartment syndrome as well as median nerve dysfunction from an acute carpal tunnel syndrome should be clearly documented.
- Associated injuries should be ruled out, and appropriate patient clearance according to advanced trauma life support guidelines should be obtained.

IMAGING AND OTHER DIAGNOSTIC STUDIES

- Good-quality pre- and postreduction wrist radiographs should be obtained preoperatively to assess the fracture pattern and rule out associated injuries to the carpus or distal radioulnar joint (DRUJ).
- Computed tomography (CT) scans may be helpful to assess complex intra-articular distal radius fractures.

NONOPERATIVE MANAGEMENT

- There is no acceptable nonoperative management for high-energy comminuted distal radius fractures.

SURGICAL MANAGEMENT

- The use of internal distraction plating or bridge plating for distal radius fractures was introduced by Burke and Singer.[3] The technique was expanded by Ruch et al,[17] who described the use of a 12- to 16-hole 3.5-mm dynamic compression plate (DCP) (Synthes, Paoli, PA) placed in the floor of the fourth dorsal extensor compartment to span from the intact radius diaphysis to the third metacarpal.[5,17]
- The bridge plating technique provides strong fixation and allows for distraction across impacted articular segments.
- The technique can be combined with a limited articular fixation approach for fracture patterns with intra-articular extension.
- Bridge plating of the distal radius was further refined by Hanel et al.[9] The authors described a variant of the bridge

Table 1 Indications for Bridge Plating of Distal Radius Fractures

Indication	Explanation
Metadiaphyseal comminution of the radius	Extensive comminution in metadiaphyseal region is difficult to treat with standard implants used for distal radius fractures.
Need for weight bearing through the upper extremity	Patients with associated lower limb injuries may require the need for early weight bearing through the upper extremities.
Polytrauma	Nursing care of the multiply injured patient may be easier with spanning internal fixation than with external fixation.
Augmented fixation	In osteoporotic bone, bridge plating can be used to augment tenuous fixation.
Carpal instability	Carpal instability, particularly radiocarpal, isolated or in combination with a distal radius fracture, may be held in a reduced position with the help of spanning internal fixation.

plating technique using 2.4-mm AO plates passed extra-articularly through the second dorsal compartment and secured onto the dorsal radial aspect of the radius diaphysis and the second metacarpal (Table 1).

Preoperative Planning

- A 22-hole 2.4-mm titanium mandibular reconstruction plate (Synthes) or a 2.4-mm stainless steel plate specifically designed for use as a distal radius bridge (DRB) plate (Synthes) is used for DRB plating.
- The mandibular reconstruction plate is made of titanium and has square ends and scalloped edges and threaded holes to accept locking screws. The DRB plate that the authors currently use is made of stainless steel and has tapered ends to facilitate sliding the plate within the extensor compartment; it also has locking screws.

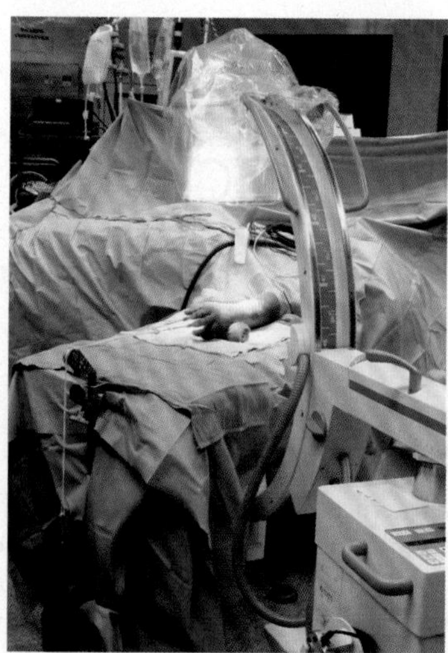

FIG 1 ● Setup for this procedure, with longitudinal traction applied through finger traps and the C-arm coming in from above or below the hand table.

Positioning

- With the patient anesthetized and supine on the operating table, the involved extremity is draped free and centered on a radiolucent hand table.
- Finger traps are applied to the index and middle fingers and 4.5 kg of longitudinal traction is applied through a rope and pulley system.
- A C-arm comes in from above or below the hand table (**FIG 1**).

Approach

- Under image intensification, the closed reduction maneuver described by Agee[1] is performed.
- Plates are passed extra-articularly through the second dorsal compartment and secured onto the dorsal radial aspect of the radius diaphysis and the second metacarpal.
- The interval between the extensor carpi radialis longus (ECRL) and extensor carpi radialis brevis (ECRB) is developed and the diaphysis of the radius exposed.
- The DRB plate is introduced beneath the muscle bellies of the outcroppers extraperiosteally and advanced distally between the ECRL and ECRB tendons.

Closed Reduction Maneuver of Agee

- Longitudinal traction is first used to restore length and to assess the benefit of ligamentotaxis for the restoration of articular step-off (**TECH FIG 1A,B**).
- Next, the hand is translated palmarly relative to the forearm to restore sagittal tilt and to assess the integrity of the volar lip of the radius (**TECH FIG 1C–F**).
- Finally, pronation of the hand relative to the forearm is performed to correct the supination deformity.
- Once the initial reduction maneuver is completed, the bridge plate is then applied.

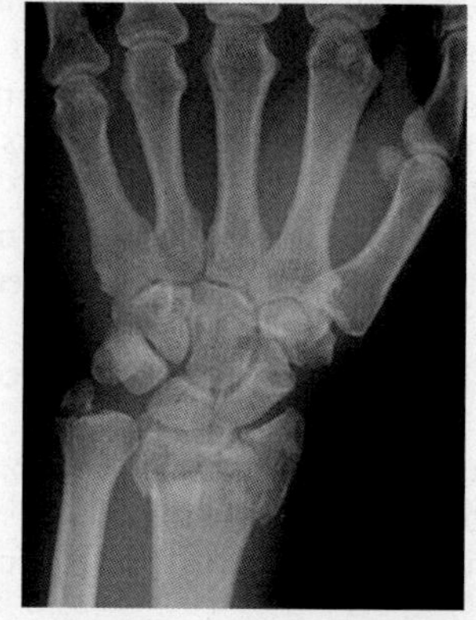

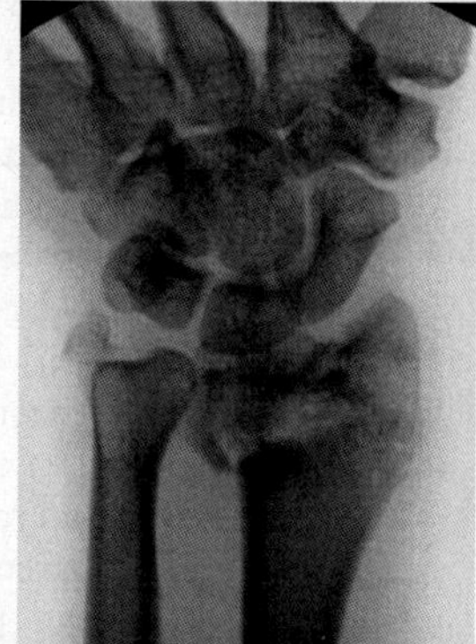

TECH FIG 1 ● Radiographs show an anteroposterior (AP) projection of the wrist injury before (**A**) and after (**B**) distraction is applied. *(continued)*

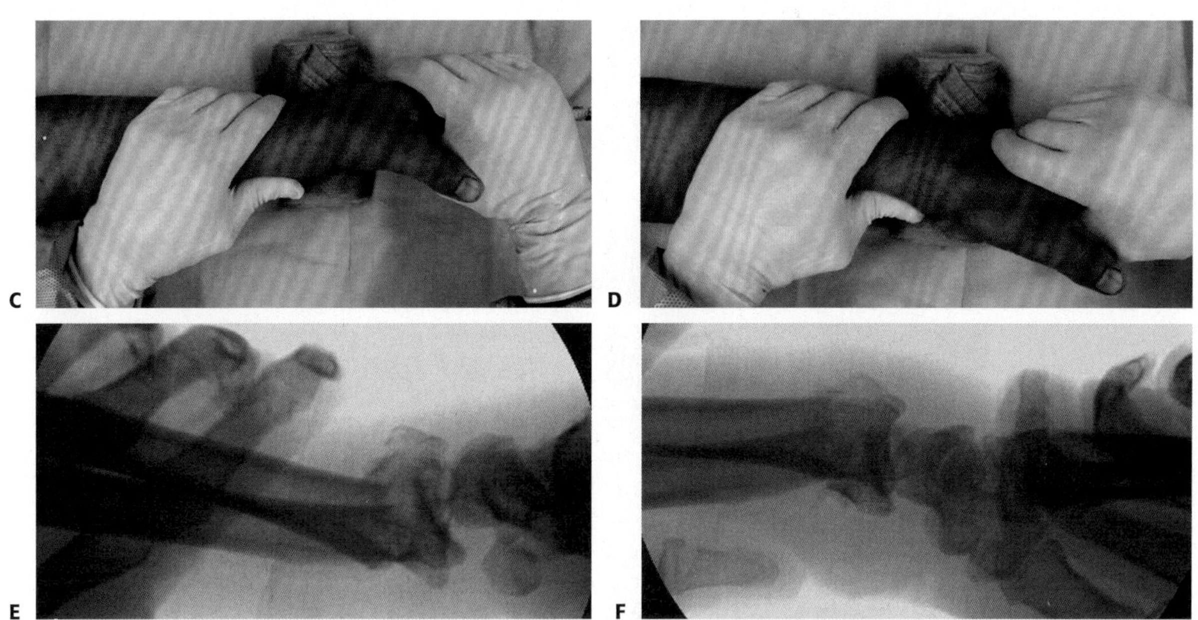

TECH FIG 1 • *(continued)* Clinical pictures show the wrist deformity before (**C**) and after (**D**) application of the Agee reduction maneuver, which is a combination of longitudinal traction and volar translation of the carpus. Radiographs show the wrist deformity before (**E**) and after (**F**) application of the Agee reduction maneuver.

Approach and Plate Insertion

- The DRB plate is superimposed on the skin from the radial diaphysis to the distal metadiaphysis of the second metacarpal. The position of the plate is verified with image intensification and markings are placed on the skin at the level of the proximal and distal four screw holes of the plate (**TECH FIG 2A–C**).
- The subcutaneous tissues are infiltrated with 0.25% bupivacaine with epinephrine to promote hemostasis.
- A 5-cm incision is made at the base of the second metacarpal and continued along the second metacarpal shaft. In the depths of this incision, the insertions of the ECRL and ECRB are identified as they pass beneath the distal edge of the second dorsal wrist compartment to insert on the second and third metacarpal bases, respectively.
- A second incision is made just proximal to the outcropper muscle bellies (abductor pollicis longus and extensor pollicis brevis), in line with ECRL and ECRB tendons. The interval between the ECRL and ECRB is developed and the diaphysis of the radius exposed (**TECH FIG 2D,E**).
- The DRB plate is introduced beneath the muscle bellies of the outcroppers extraperiosteally and advanced distally between the ECRL and ECRB tendons (**TECH FIG 2F**).

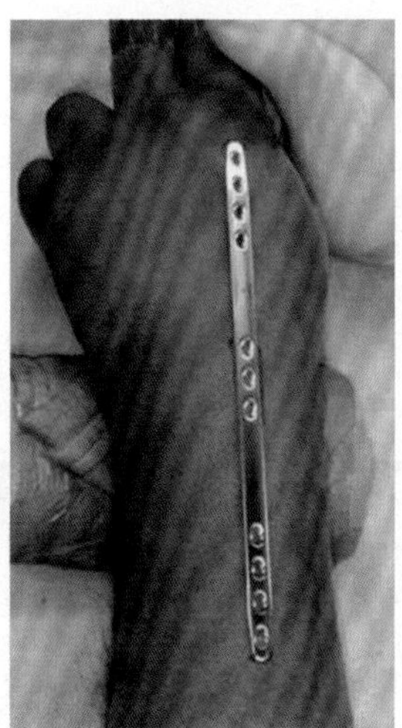

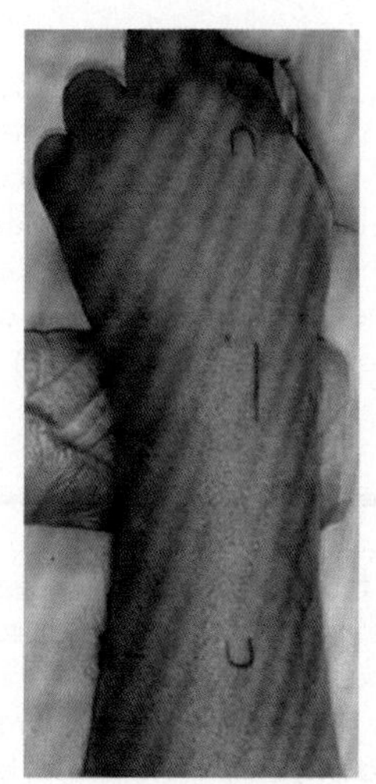

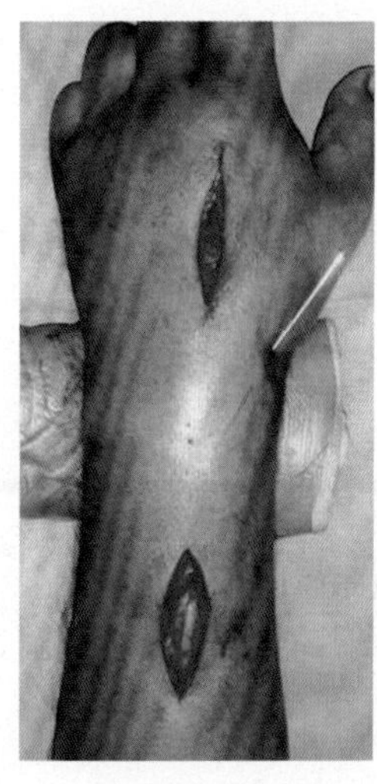

TECH FIG 2 • **A.** The plate is placed over the forearm and hand. Radiographs can be taken to confirm the position of the plate. The plate should be centered over the second metacarpal distally and the radius proximally. This will be along the course of the ECRL. **B.** Outline of the plate. **C.** Incisions are made over the second metacarpal and the radius. *(continued)*

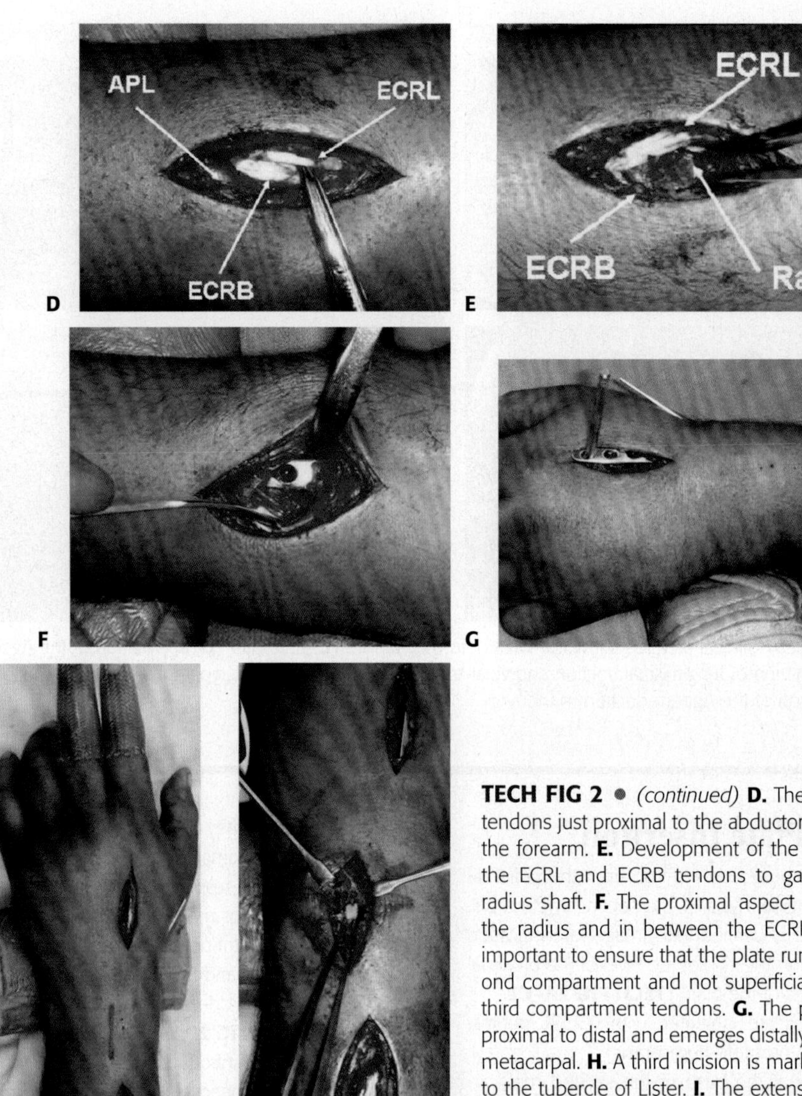

TECH FIG 2 • *(continued)* **D.** The ECRL and ECRB tendons just proximal to the abductor pollicis longus in the forearm. **E.** Development of the interval between the ECRL and ECRB tendons to gain access to the radius shaft. **F.** The proximal aspect of the plate over the radius and in between the ECRL and ECRB. It is important to ensure that the plate runs within the second compartment and not superficial to the first and third compartment tendons. **G.** The plate is advanced proximal to distal and emerges distally over the second metacarpal. **H.** A third incision is marked out just ulnar to the tubercle of Lister. **I.** The extensor pollicis longus tendon has been released from its compartment, and bone graft is inserted through the dorsal fracture line just ulnar to the bridge plate.

- Some resistance may be encountered as the plate emerges distally but can usually be easily overcome with gentle manipulation of the plate (**TECH FIG 2G**).
  - Occasionally, the plate will not pass through the compartment. In these cases, a guidewire or stout suture retriever is passed along the compartment from distal to proximal. The plate is secured to the distal end of the wire and delivered into the hand.
  - In the rare instance that these measures fail, a third incision is made directly over the metaphysis of the radius, the proximal half of the second compartment is incised, and the plate is passed under direct vision.
- The third, or periarticular, incision may also be used to assess the articular surface, reduce die-punch fragments, and introduce bone graft (**TECH FIG 2H,I**).

■ Plate Fixation and Articular Fixation

- After the bridge plate is passed, it is then secured to the second metacarpal by placing a nonlocking fully threaded 2.4-mm cortical screw through the most distal plate hole. The proximal end of the plate is then identified in the forearm.
- If the radial length has not been restored, then the plate, secured to the second metacarpal, is pushed distally until the length is reestablished and a fully threaded 2.4-mm nonlocking screw is placed in the most proximal plate hole. By using nonlocking screws, the plate is effectively lagged onto the intact bone.

- Plate alignment along the longitudinal axis of the radius is guaranteed by securing the most distal and most proximal screw holes first.
- The remaining holes are secured with fully threaded locking screws inserted with bicortical purchase.
- It has been our experience that as the plate is passed along the radial diaphysis, through the second compartment and along the second metacarpal, extra-articular alignment, radial inclination, volar tilt, and radial length are restored.
- Intra-articular reduction may be further adjusted by using limited periarticular incisions to allow for direct manipulation of articular fragments, placement of subchondral bone grafts, repair of intercarpal ligament injuries, and augmentation of fracture fixation with Kirschner wires and periarticular plates.
- Displaced volar medial fracture fragments that are not reduced with this technique require a separate volar incision and appropriate buttress support.
- The biomechanical stability of spanning plates is strong and predictable. Behrens and Johnson,[2] studying the rigidity of external fixator configurations, demonstrated that rigidity is directly proportional to how close the longitudinal fixator bar is to the bone and the fracture. A bridge plate, resting directly against the radius proximally and metacarpals distally, therefore optimizes the conditions to obtain the strongest possible fixator construct.
- A DRB plate fixed with a minimum of three screws at either end of the plate confers significantly more stability than would an external fixator used to stabilize a comparable fracture (**TECH FIG 3**).[18]

A 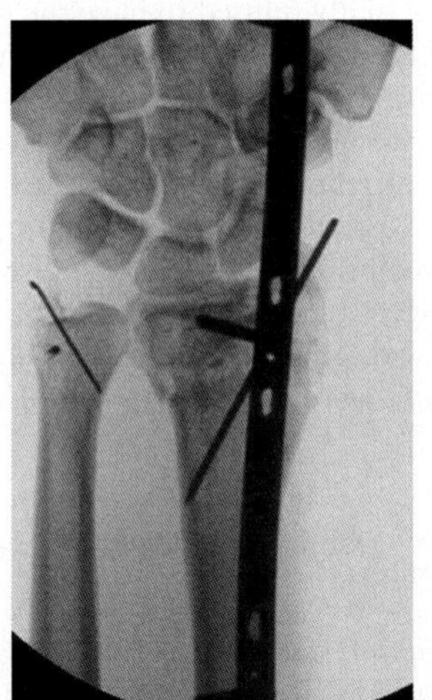
B 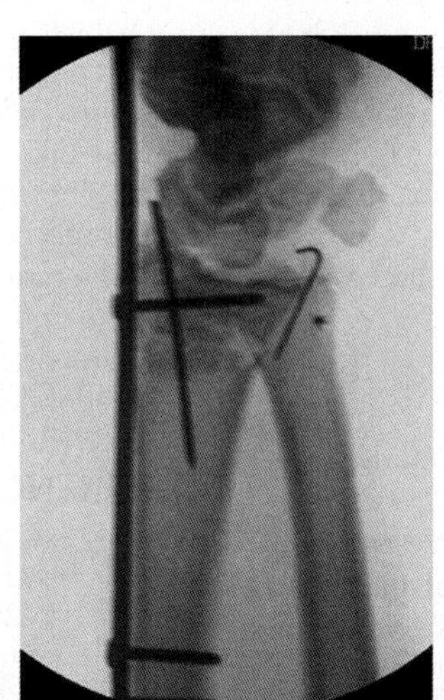
C 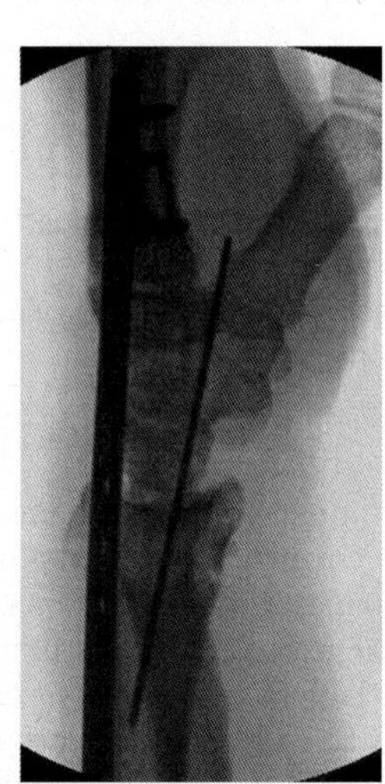

TECH FIG 3 • Final AP (**A**), oblique (**B**), and lateral (**C**) radiographic images.

Distal Radioulnar Joint Management

- DRUJ stability is assessed after radius reconstruction. If the DRUJ is stable, the limb is immobilized in a long-arm splint with the forearm in supination for the first 10 to 14 days postoperatively.
- If the DRUJ is unstable, and there are no contraindications to prolonging the operation, repair or reconstruction of DRUJ and triangular fibrocartilage complex is undertaken.
- If, however, the patient's condition does not allow the operation to be prolonged, the ulnar head is reduced manually into the sigmoid notch and the ulna is transfixed to the radius with a minimum of two 1.6-mm Kirschner wires passed proximal to the DRUJ.

PEARLS AND PITFALLS

Hardware removal	■ At the time of hardware extraction, if a mandibular reconstruction plate was used, the screws are removed and the plate is twisted axially 720 degrees to break up the soft tissue adhesions and callus that tend to grow around and onto the scalloped edges of the titanium plate. This maneuver is not usually required when the smooth-edged stainless steel DRB is used. ■ A removable short-arm splint is worn for 2–3 weeks after plate removal. Hand therapy at this point is directed at regaining motion and strength.

POSTOPERATIVE CARE

- Digit range-of-motion exercises start within 24 hours of surgery. Load bearing through the forearm and elbow is allowed immediately as well as the use of a platform crutch when the patient is physiologically stable. One month postoperatively, the platform is removed and weight bearing is allowed through the hand grip of regular crutches. Lifting and carrying are restricted to about 4.5 kg until fracture healing.
- DRUJ stability and forearm motion are assessed 2 weeks after reduction. If the patient can supinate the forearm with little effort and the DRUJ is stable, then splinting is discontinued and axial loading through the extremity is allowed at this point.
- If the patient has difficulty maintaining supination, or if the DRUJ was reconstructed acutely, a removable long-arm splint is fabricated.
- If the DRUJ was transfixed with Kirschner wires, then the wires are removed on the third postoperative week and DRUJ stability is reassessed.
- Supplemental Kirschner wires for articular fixation are removed 6 weeks postoperatively.
- The DRB plate and screws are removed usually no earlier than 12 weeks after injury.

OUTCOMES

- The bridge plating technique for distal radius fractures was reviewed in a retrospective study consisting of 62 consecutive patients treated in this fashion.[9] The series represents the senior author's 10-year experience with the technique at a level 1 trauma center. Patients managed with bridge plating either for distal radius fractures with extensive metadiaphyseal comminution or for distal radius fractures associated with other injuries requiring weight bearing through the affected extremity represented 13% of distal radius fractures treated with operative fixation during this period. Fracture healing occurred in all 62 patients.
  - In each case, radial length was within 5 mm of neutral ulnar variance, radial inclination was greater than 5 degrees, and palmar tilt was at least neutral.
  - There were also no articular gaps or step-offs greater than 2 mm and the DRUJ was stable in all cases.
  - The plates were removed on average 112 days after placement.
  - Forty-one of the 62 patients have returned to their previous levels of employment. Of the remaining 21 patients, 8 were unemployed at the time of injury and remain so.
  - Thirteen patients sustained multiple injuries requiring considerable changes in occupation and lifestyle. Only 1 of these 13 patients considers the wrist fracture to be the limiting factor in failing to return to work.
  - Overall, these results compare favorably with the findings of Burke and Singer[3] and Ruch et al.[17]
- Similarly, Ruch et al[17] showed that 64% of patients obtained excellent radiographic and functional results and another 27% of patients obtained good results in their prospective cohort of patients with comparable pathology.
- The authors of each of these studies propose that distraction plating allows fracture reduction and fixation over a broad metadiaphyseal area while effectively diverting compression forces away from the fracture site.
- The use of bridge plating in the treatment of distal radius fractures avoids the complications of external fixation. A bridge plate can remain implanted for extended periods without deleterious effects on functional outcome. All patients in our series went on to heal with acceptable metadiaphyseal and intra-articular alignment. In patients with multiple traumatic injuries, bridge plating allowed earlier postoperative load bearing across the affected wrist. This enabled independent transfers and the use of ambulatory aids. Application of bridge plates is simple and surgical time is comparable with the application of an external fixator.

COMPLICATIONS

- There was one documented hardware failure in the series in a patient who initially refused to have the implant taken out and continued to work in heavy manual labor for 19 months before the bridge plate failed.
- In addition, there were no cases of excessive postoperative finger stiffness or reflex sympathetic dystrophy.
- This reflects the overall infrequent complications reported in the literature for bridge plating of the distal radius. In fact, Burke and Singer[3] reported no complications and Ruch et al[17] reported no hardware failures and only three patients who developed long finger extensor lag of 10 to 15 degrees.

REFERENCES

1. Agee JM. Distal radius fractures. Multiplanar ligamentotaxis. Hand Clin 1993;9:577–585.
2. Behrens F, Johnson W. Unilateral external fixation. Methods to increase and reduce frame stiffness. Clin Orthop Relat Res 1989;(241):48–56.
3. Burke EF, Singer RM. Treatment of comminuted distal radius with the use of an internal distraction plate. Tech Hand Up Extrem Surg 1998;2:248–252.
4. Drobetz H, Bryant AL, Pokorny T, et al. Volar fixed-angle plating of distal radius extension fractures: influence of plate position on secondary loss of reduction: a biomechanic study in a cadaveric model. J Hand Surg Am 2006;31(4):615–622.
5. Ginn TA, Ruch DS, Yang CC, et al. Use of a distraction plate for distal radial fractures with metaphyseal and diaphyseal comminution. Surgical technique. J Bone Joint Surg Am 2006;88(suppl 1, pt 1):29–36.
6. Gradl G, Jupiter JB, Gierer P, et al. Fractures of the distal radius treated with a nonbridging external fixation technique using multiplanar K-wires. J Hand Surg Am 2005;30(5):960–968.
7. Graff S, Jupiter J. Fracture of the distal radius: classification of treatment and indications for external fixation. Injury 1994;25(suppl 4): S14–S25.
8. Handoll HH, Madhok R. Surgical interventions for treating distal radial fractures in adults. Cochrane Database Syst Rev 2003;(3):CD003209.
9. Hanel DP, Lu TS, Weil WM. Bridge plating of distal radius fractures: the Harborview method. Clin Orthop Relat Res 2006;445:91–99.
10. Hastings H II, Leibovic SJ. Indications and techniques of open reduction. Internal fixation of distal radius fractures. Orthop Clin North Am 1993;24:309–326.
11. Kamath AF, Zurakowski D, Day CS. Low-profile dorsal plating for dorsally angulated distal radius fractures: an outcomes study. J Hand Surg Am 2006;31:1061–1067.
12. Konrath GA, Bahler S. Open reduction and internal fixation of unstable distal radius fractures: results using the Trimed fixation system. J Orthop Trauma 2002;16:578–585.
13. Lafontaine M, Hardy D, Delince P. Stability assessment of distal radius fractures. Injury 1989;20:208–210.
14. McQueen MM. Non-spanning external fixation of the distal radius. Hand Clin 2005;21:375–380.

15. McQueen MM, Simpson D, Court-Brown CM. Use of the Hoffman 2 compact external fixator in the treatment of redisplaced unstable distal radial fractures. J Orthop Trauma 1999;13:501–505.
16. Orbay JL, Touhami A. Current concepts in volar fixed-angle fixation of unstable distal radius fractures. Clin Orthop Relat Res 2006;445: 58–67.
17. Ruch DS, Ginn TA, Yang CC, et al. Use of a distraction plate for distal radial fractures with metaphyseal and diaphyseal comminution. J Bone Joint Surg Am 2005;87(5):945–954.
18. Wolf JC, Weil WM, Hanel DP, et al. A biomechanic comparison of an internal radiocarpal-spanning 2.4-mm locking plate and external fixation in a model of distal radius fractures. J Hand Surg Am 2006;31:1578–1586.

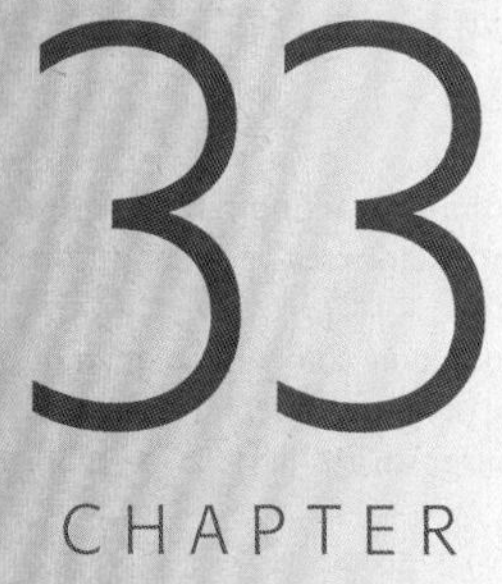

CHAPTER 33

Corrective Osteotomy for Distal Radius Malunion

David Ring, Diego Fernandez, and Jesse B. Jupiter

DEFINITION

- Distal radius malunion is best defined as malalignment associated with dysfunction.
  - Malalignment does not always result in dysfunction. In particular, the vast majority of older, low-demand patients function very well with deformity.
- Dysfunction can include loss of motion, loss of strength, or pain.[1,2,5]
- Pain can be the most difficult to associate with deformity. Osteotomy for pain—as with any surgery for pain—is relatively unpredictable and should be undertaken with caution. Carpal malalignment, ulnocarpal impaction, and distal radioulnar joint (DRUJ) malalignment are all potentially painful and can be variably addressed.
- The relationship between distal radius malunion and carpal tunnel syndrome is debated. Some surgeons claim a direct causal relationship as well as the ability to improve carpal tunnel syndrome with osteotomy alone.

ANATOMY

- Loss of alignment can be measured on radiographs.
- Angulation of the articular surface on the lateral view is measured as the angle between a line connecting the dorsal and palmar lips of the distal radius articular surface on the lateral view and a line perpendicular to the radius shaft.
- Ulnarward inclination (often called *radial inclination*, a misnomer because the articular surface tilts toward the ulna) is measured as the angle between a line connecting the ulnar limit and the radial limit of the distal radius articular surface on the posteroanterior (PA) view and a line perpendicular to the radial shaft.
- Ulnar variance is a better measure of shortening of the radius than radial length. It is measured as the distance between two lines drawn perpendicular to the radial shaft on the PA view, one at the level of the most ulnar corner of the lunate facet and the other at the distal limit of the ulnar head.
  - Positive ulnar variance means that the ulna is longer than the radius. Negative means the ulna is shorter.
- Loss of articular surface alignment can be measured on radiographs as gap, step, or subluxation.
  - This is most accurately measured using computed tomography (CT) images (**FIG 1**).
- Sources of variability in radiographic measurements include variation in the radiographs, imprecision in the measurement techniques, and imprecision in the selection of the points of reference.

PATHOGENESIS

- Fractures of the distal radius heal rapidly. A malaligned healing fracture can be considered a malunion within 4 to 6 weeks of injury.
- Risk factors for fracture instability, loss of reduction, and malunion include age older than 60 years, more than 20 degrees of dorsal angulation, dorsal metaphyseal comminution, comminution extending to the volar metaphyseal cortex, associated fracture of the ulna, and displaced articular fracture.
- Risk factors for fracture instability include age, metaphyseal comminution, dorsal tilt, ulnar variance, and lack of functional independence.
- Manipulation of previously reduced fractures that redisplace in a cast or splint signifies instability and is not worthwhile.
- Limitations of various treatment techniques may contribute to creation of a malunion.
  - Percutaneous pins alone may not be sufficient to maintain alignment when there is substantial metaphyseal comminution.
  - External fixation alone without ancillary percutaneous pin fixation of the fracture

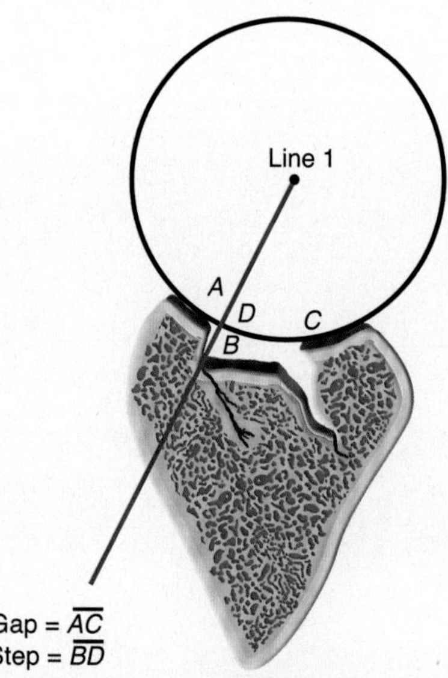

FIG 1 • The arc method for measuring articular malalignment of the distal radius. The distance between *B* and *D* is the articular step, and the distance between *A* and *C* is the maximum articular gap. (After Catalano LW III, Cole RJ, Gelberman RH, et al. Displaced intra-articular fractures of the distal aspect of the radius: long-term results in young adults after open reduction and internal fixation. J Bone Joint Surg Am 1997;79[9]:1290–1302.)

- Early removal of pins or an external fixator. Settling of the fracture can also be observed after implant removal more than 6 weeks after injury, particularly when there is substantial metaphyseal comminution.
- Nonlocked plates may loosen in osteopenic metaphyseal bone.
- Complacence must be avoided. Many older patients desire optimal wrist alignment and function, and treatment decisions should not be made on chronologic age alone.

NATURAL HISTORY

- Ulnar-sided wrist pain can improve for a year or more after fracture of the distal radius, so patience is warranted.
- Lack of forearm rotation may be related to capsular contracture or bony malalignment. For slight malunions, patience with exercises and rehabilitation is advisable.
- Although it is often stated that an extra-articular distal radius malunion leads to future arthrosis, there are no data to support this contention.
  - After a recovery period of 1 to 2 years from fracture, the functional deficits seem fairly stable.
- Articular incongruity or subluxation in relatively nonarticular areas can be reasonably well tolerated, but in most cases, intra-articular incongruity will lead to arthrosis, pain, and dysfunction. There is no clear time frame for these changes—indeed, symptoms do not correlate well with radiographic anatomy or arthrosis and the predictors of arthrosis are not well established.

PATIENT HISTORY AND PHYSICAL FINDINGS

- Pain should be very discrete and specific. It is important that there be a direct correlation of the pain with a clear operative target. Vague, diffuse, or disproportionate pain should not be treated with osteotomy. Pain alone is not a good indication for osteotomy, so the interview should elicit specific aspects of the pain for which there is a good operative target and the risks of surgery are justified.
- Lack of motion should be clearly due to malalignment and not due to pain or protectiveness—likewise for instability of the DRUJ.
- Range of motion: A goniometer is used to measure wrist flexion, extension, radial and ulnar deviation, supination, and pronation.
- Ulnocarpal compression: The carpus is forcefully ulnarly deviated toward the ulna.
  - Consistent reproduction of usual pain with ulnar deviation tasks is consistent with ulnocarpal impaction.
- The examiner can test for DRUJ instability by stabilizing the radius and trying to subluxate the distal ulna dorsal and volar from the sigmoid notch of the radius.
  - Substantially, less stability than the opposite side may correlate with symptomatic DRUJ instability, but this is a very difficult and subjective test.
- Scaphoid shift test: Instability compared to the opposite wrist would indicate a possible scapholunate interosseous ligament tear, indicating a potential dissociative rather than the typical nondissociative carpal malalignment usually associated with distal radius malunion.
- Grip strength is one of the measure of wrist dysfunction, but it is largely determined by pain and effort—both strongly influenced by psychosocial factors.

IMAGING AND OTHER DIAGNOSTIC STUDIES

- PA and lateral radiographs of the wrist (**FIG 2A–D**) can be supplemented by specific radiographs for evaluation of the joint surface, particularly for potential articular malunions.
  - Comparison with the opposite, uninjured wrist is useful and serves as a template for surgical correction.
- CT, particularly three-dimensional CT, is useful to precisely evaluate the joint surfaces (**FIG 2E**).

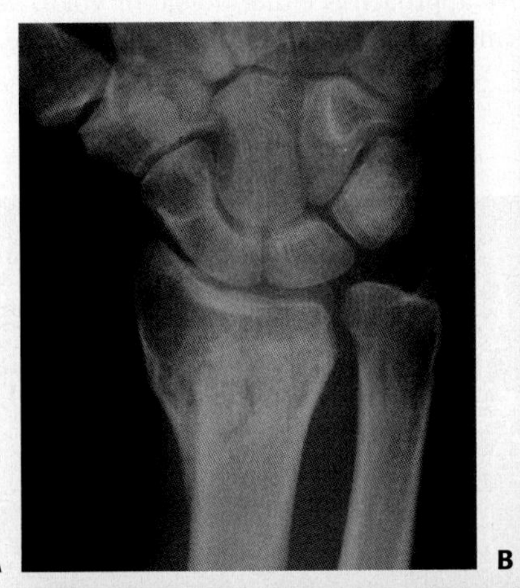

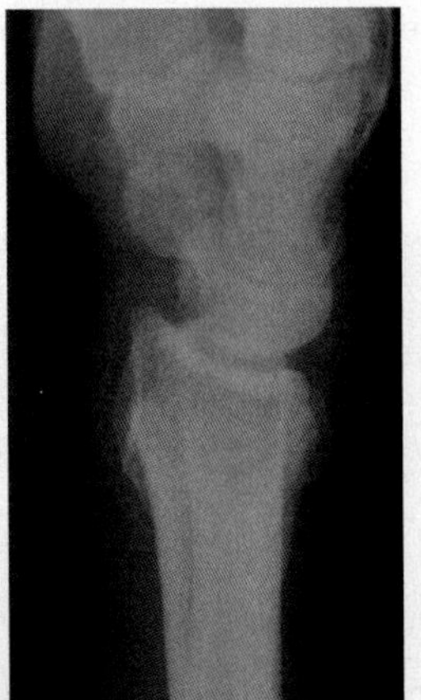

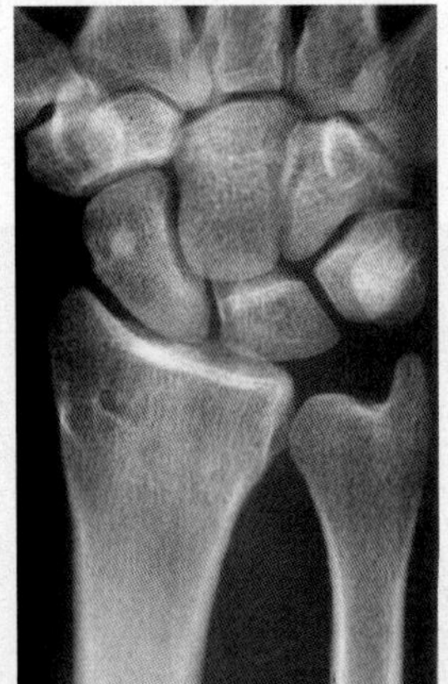

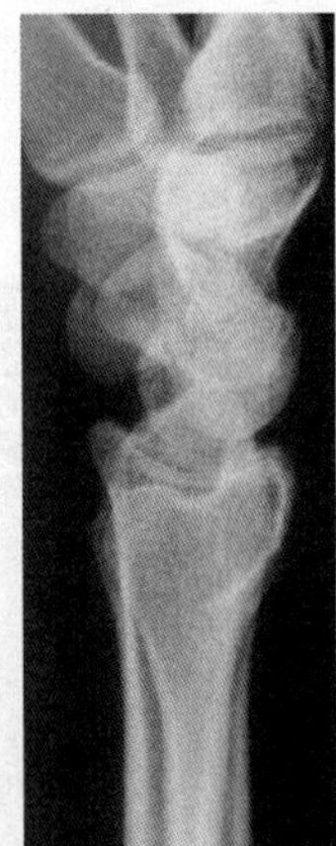

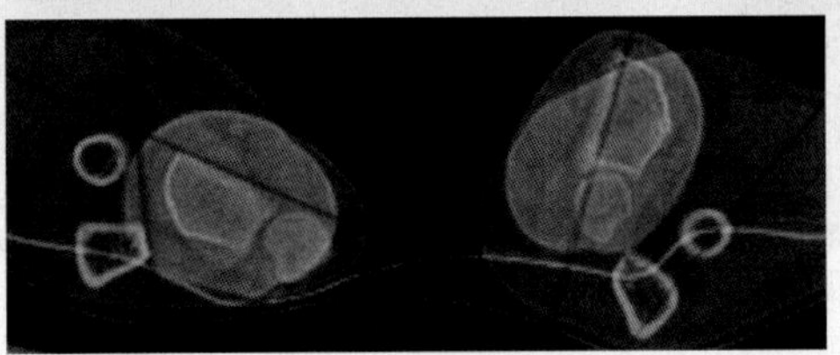

FIG 2 • **A,B.** Anteroposterior (AP) and lateral radiographs of extra-articular dorsally angulated malunion. **C,D.** PA and lateral radiographs of an extra-articular dorsally displaced malunion. **E.** CT shows rotational deformity associated with a volarly displaced extra-articular fracture. (Copyright Diego Fernandez, MD, PhD.)

- Neurophysiologic tests (nerve conduction velocity and electromyography) are ordered to evaluate any symptoms or signs of carpal tunnel syndrome that may need to be addressed.

DIFFERENTIAL DIAGNOSIS

- Stiffness: capsular stiffness and tendon adhesions
- Numbness: idiopathic carpal tunnel syndrome
- Pain: another discrete source of pain or even nonspecific pain

NONOPERATIVE MANAGEMENT

- Nonoperative management is appropriate for low-demand and infirm individuals. Splints are weaned after 6 weeks of cast immobilization. Patients who struggle to regain motion may benefit from working with an occupational therapist or a certified hand therapist. Normal activities are resumed in 3 or 4 months. The patient may return every 2 or 4 months or so until satisfied with the result.
- Patience is warranted in many situations, particularly for patients with ulnar-sided wrist pain thought to be due to an extra-articular malunion.
  - This discomfort is the last pain to go away after a distal radius fracture and can last up to a year.

SURGICAL MANAGEMENT

- Surgery is appropriate when a radiographic deformity correlates with a specific anatomically correctable problem and the deformity is associated with a substantial risk of dysfunction or arthrosis.
  - The patient must understand the risks and benefits of intervening.
  - The surgeon should be wary of pain as the primary complaint because pain is strongly influenced by psychosocial factors, and pain relief is an achievable goal only when consistent with an objective, correctable anatomic deformity such as discomfort clearly associated with a substantial ulnocarpal impingement.
  - When the issue is restriction of motion and there is less than 20 degrees of dorsal tilt or less than 5 mm of ulnar positive variance, a nonoperative approach may be warranted.
- There are no fixed rules or thresholds for acceptable alignment. The correlation with symptoms and disability is more important.
- Intra-articular osteotomies should be considered only when the malalignment is simple and the planned correction is straightforward.
  - For instance, osteotomy of a volar shearing fracture would be considered when the fragment is large, there is little or no articular comminution or impaction, and the dorsal fragments are not healed in a malaligned position.
- Distal radius osteotomy need not be performed urgently. The patient should have demonstrated excellent exercise skills and full finger motion and there should be no significant nerve or tendon dysfunction or edema.
  - In the case of an intra-articular malunion, intervening early (optimally within 10 weeks) when the fracture is not completely healed may take precedence over these concerns.

Preoperative Planning

- The desired angular, rotational, and length corrections are planned based on preoperative radiologic studies, including a radiograph of the opposite wrist if uninjured (**FIG 3A,B**).
- It can be useful to draw and write out a reconstruction plan, particularly for complex malunions (**FIG 3C–E**). In that way, every contingency is anticipated and the surgery is likely to go more smoothly.

Positioning

- The patient is positioned supine with the arm supported on a hand table.
- A nonsterile pneumatic tourniquet is used and inflated after exsanguination and before the skin incision.

Approach

- The operative approach is either dorsal or volar, depending on the deformity and the chosen surgical technique.

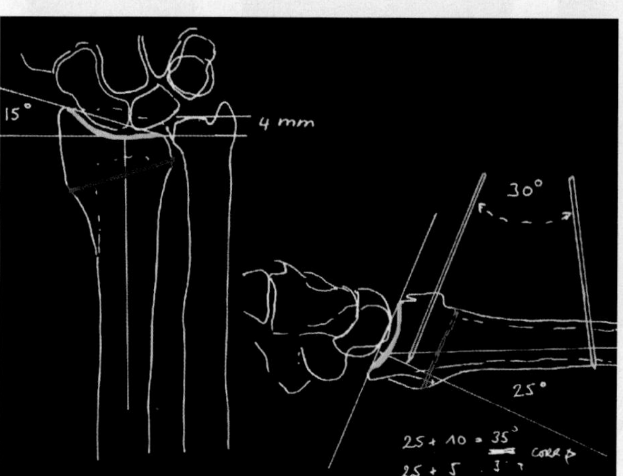

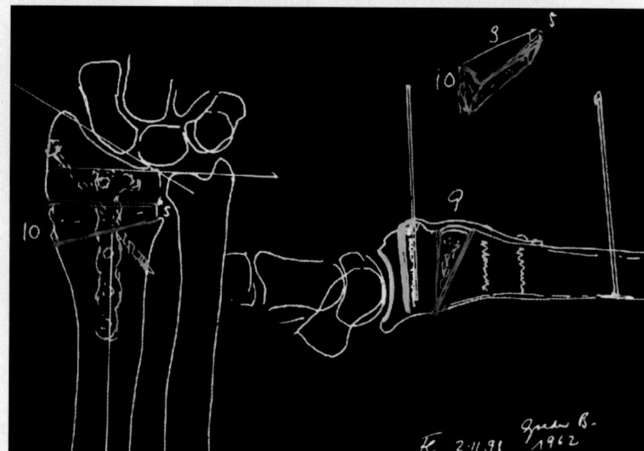

FIG 3 • A,B. Preoperative plans for dorsal osteotomy in the patient in **TECH FIGS 1** to **3**: preosteotomy plan (**A**) and postosteotomy and corticocancellous bone grafting plan (**B**). *(continued)*

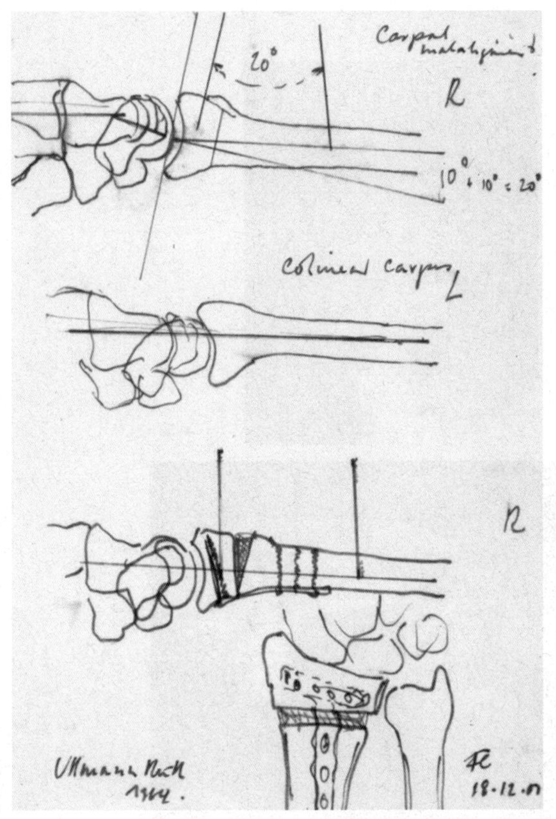

C

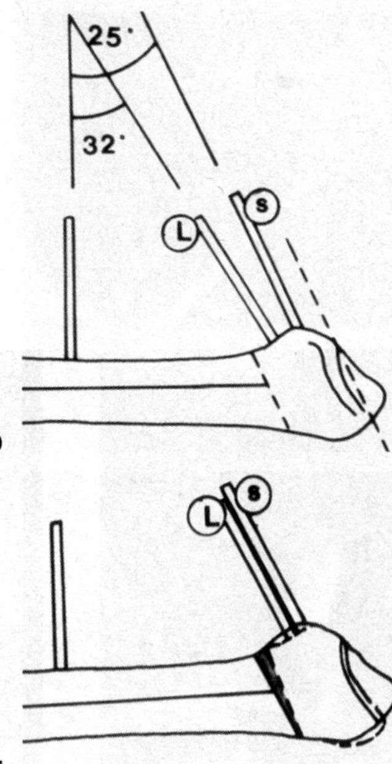

FIG 3 • *(continued)* **C.** Preoperative plan for an extra-articular osteotomy through a volar approach in the patient in **TECH FIGS 4** and **5**. **D,E.** Preoperative plans for an intra-articular dorsally angulated malunion in the patient in **TECH FIG 6**. (Copyright Diego Fernandez, MD, PhD.)

Dorsal Extra-articular Distal Radius Osteotomy: Corticocancellous Graft

Exposure

- Make a longitudinal incision centered over the tubercle of Lister, in line with the third metacarpal (**TECH FIG 1A**).
- Elevate skin flaps, taking care to protect the branches of the superficial radial nerve in the radial skin flap.
- Incise the retinaculum over the third extensor compartment. Remove the tendon of the extensor pollicis longus (EPL) and transpose it radialward (**TECH FIG 1B**).
  - The EPL tendon will be left in the subcutaneous tissues at the completion of the procedure.
- Elevate the fourth dorsal compartment and its tendons subperiosteally.
  - Preserve the integrity of this compartment.
- It is usually not possible to elevate the second dorsal compartment subperiosteally, so simply retract the extensor carpi radialis brevis and longus tendons radialward after opening the compartment.

Osteotomy and Realignment

- Kirschner wires drilled parallel to the articular surface can facilitate monitoring of realignment (**TECH FIG 2A**).

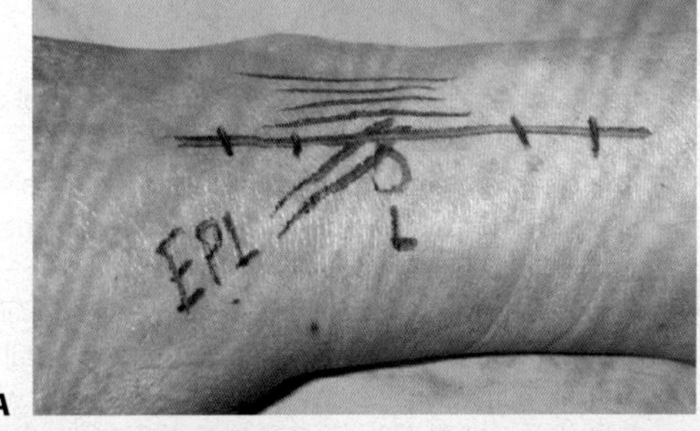

A

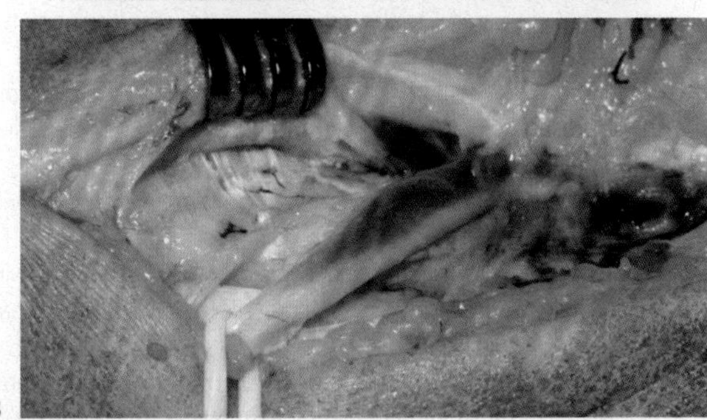

B

TECH FIG 1 • Correction of extra-articular dorsally angulated malunion in the patient in **FIG 2A,B**. **A.** Straight longitudinal skin incision. **B.** The EPL is mobilized and transposed dorsoradially into the subcutaneous tissues. (Copyright Diego Fernandez, MD, PhD.)

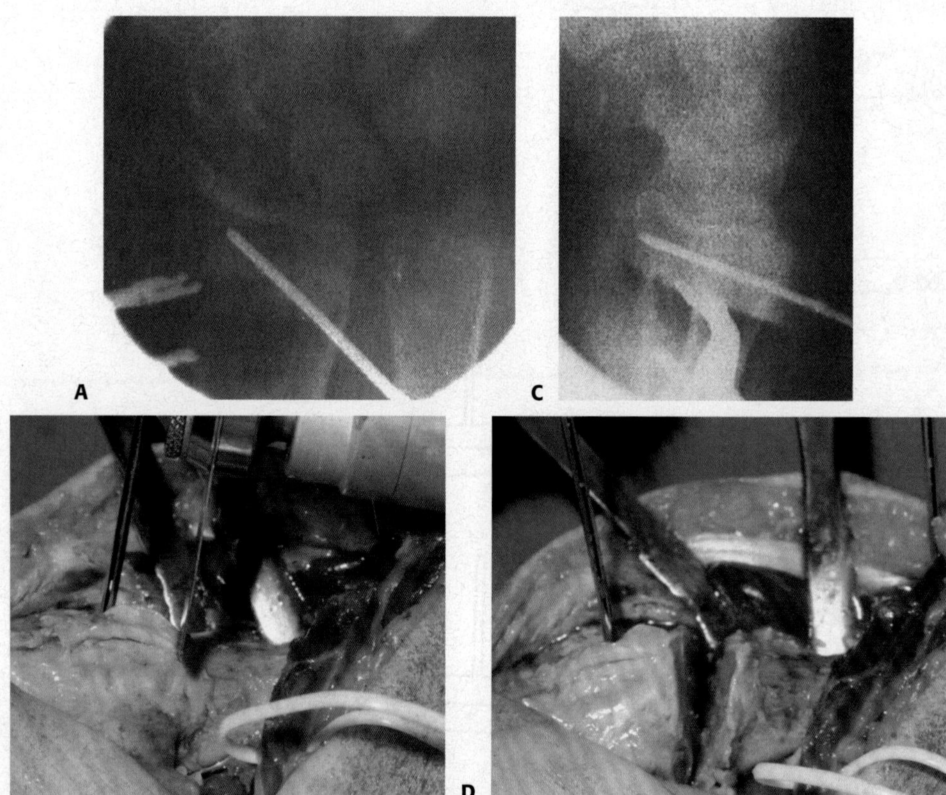

TECH FIG 2 • A. Kirschner wires are placed parallel to the articular surface. Fluoroscopic image showing pin placement. **B.** The osteotomy is made with a saw as close as possible to the original fracture site. **C.** Lateral fluoroscopic image showing use of a lamina spreader to realign the distal fragment. **D.** The osteotomy has been opened and is ready for graft placement. (Copyright Diego Fernandez, MD, PhD.)

- A distractor or small external fixator may facilitate realignment and provisionally stabilize the fracture.
  - The proximal threaded pin is drilled into the radial diaphysis perpendicularly in a position that will not interfere with implant application.
  - The distal threaded pin is drilled at an angle equal to the desired correction of the lateral tilt of the distal radius articular surface so that distraction of the two pins will bring this pin parallel to the proximal pin (perpendicular to the radius), thereby restoring alignment.
  - The pins should be drilled so that they also help restore the appropriate ulnarward inclination of the distal radius articular surface when distracted.
  - Planned angular corrections can be monitored with sterile geometric templates.
- The osteotomy is made parallel with the distal Kirschner wire and as close to the original fracture site as possible using an oscillating saw (**TECH FIG 2B**).
- If the fracture is not yet completely healed (nascent malunion—usually within 4 months of injury), recreate the original fracture line by carefully removing fracture callus at the fracture site.
  - This callus can be saved and used as bone graft.
- If the fracture is solidly healed, attempt to identify the prior fracture site. If this is uncertain, choose a site that creates a distal fragment large enough to facilitate manipulation and internal fixation while trying to stay distal enough to take advantage of the healing capacity of metaphyseal bone.
- A lamina spreader can be used to help realign the distal fragment as well (**TECH FIG 2C,D**).
  - Care must be taken when operating on osteoporotic bone.
- Additional provisional stability can be provided by placing 1.6-mm smooth Kirschner wires.
- If the ulnar variance can be restored with angular realignment alone, the volar cortex can be cracked and hinged open in an attempt to maintain some stability of the osteotomy. If lengthening of the volar cortex is required to restore ulnar variance, a second distractor in another plane (eg, direct radial) may prove useful for obtaining and maintaining alignment.

Graft Insertion and Fixation

- Once the osteotomy is created and the radius realigned, bone graft is inserted.
- Harvest bone graft (**TECH FIG 3A**). Either a corticocancellous (structural) bone graft or cancellous bone graft can be used.
  - Potential advantages of a structural graft include immediate structural support (**TECH FIG 3B**) and the possibility of using a smaller implant and thereby avoiding tendon irritation.
  - A cancellous (nonstructural) bone graft can be harvested using trephines (**TECH FIG 3C**). This avoids tedious, difficult, and unpredictable harvest and contouring of corticocancellous grafts as well as the morbidity associated with harvest of a standard iliac crest bone graft.
- Apply a single T- or Pi-shaped plate or two 2.0- or 2.4-mm plates (one applied dorsally, ulnar to the tubercle of Lister, and

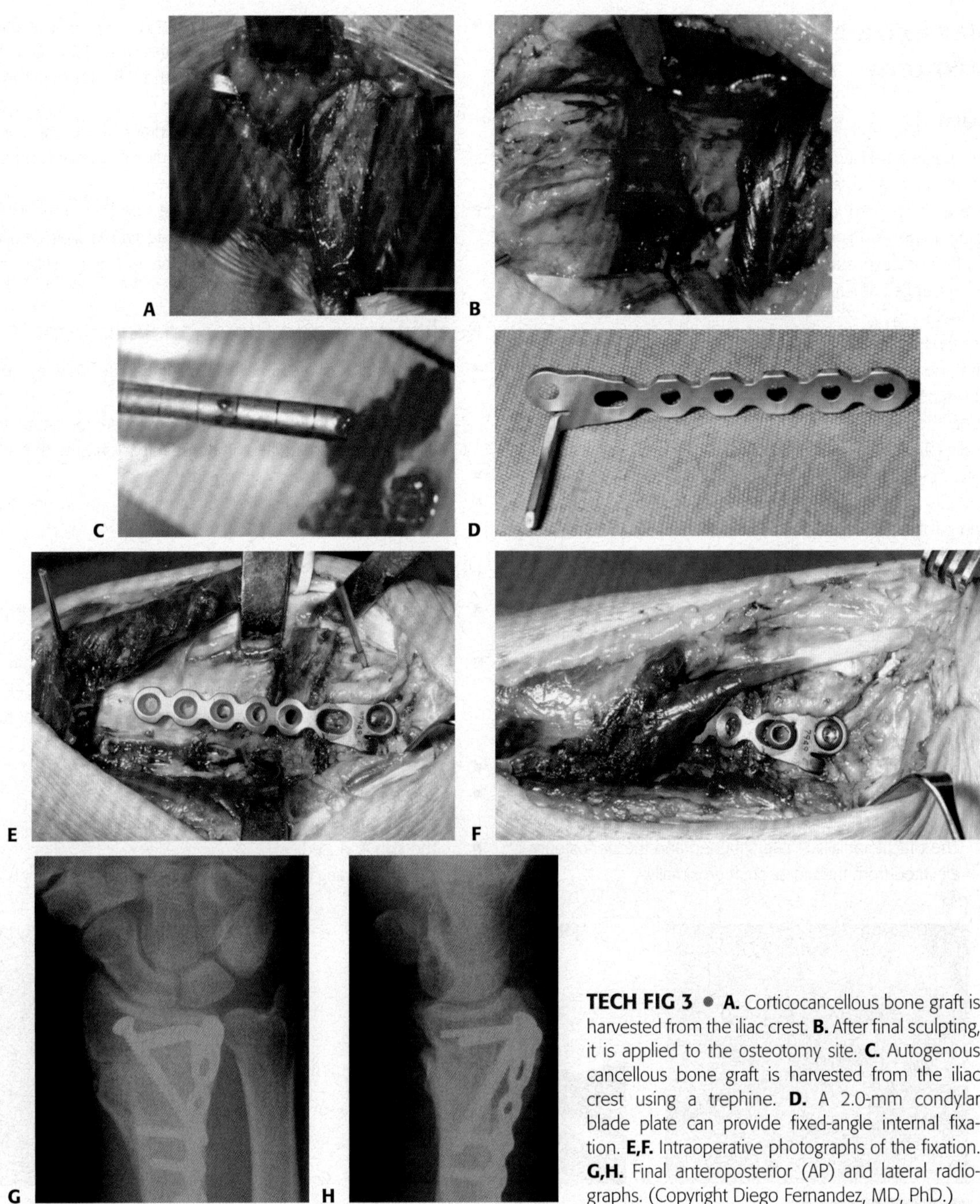

TECH FIG 3 • **A.** Corticocancellous bone graft is harvested from the iliac crest. **B.** After final sculpting, it is applied to the osteotomy site. **C.** Autogenous cancellous bone graft is harvested from the iliac crest using a trephine. **D.** A 2.0-mm condylar blade plate can provide fixed-angle internal fixation. **E,F.** Intraoperative photographs of the fixation. **G,H.** Final anteroposterior (AP) and lateral radiographs. (Copyright Diego Fernandez, MD, PhD.)

the other applied radially between the first and second dorsal compartments).
- When a structural, corticocancellous bone graft is used, a single plate or a plate and separate screw may be adequate (**TECH FIG 3D–H**).
- Plates with angular stable screws or blades in the distal fragment may be more reliable than standard screws, particularly if the bone is of poor quality and if nonstructural graft is chosen.

- Once implants are placed and stability is ensured, remove all provisional fixation devices.
- This entire process is monitored using image intensification to confirm appropriate osteotomy site, correction of alignment, and implant placement.
- Repair the extensor retinaculum with absorbable suture.
  - In some cases, a flap of retinaculum is brought deep to the tendons to add a layer of protection between the implants and extensor tendons.
  - We usually do not close the retinaculum, and we no longer make retinacular flaps.
- The tourniquet is deflated and hemostasis ensured.
- The skin is closed.
- A bulky dressing incorporating a volar plaster wrist splint is applied.

Volar Extra-articular Distal Radius Osteotomy

Exposure

- Use a volar-radial Henry (flexor carpi radialis [FCR]) approach for both dorsally and volarly angulated malunions (see **FIG 2C,D**).
- Make a 5- to 7-cm longitudinal incision over the FCR tendon ending at the wrist flexion crease.
  - If more exposure is required, the incision is angled or zigzagged at least 45 degrees toward the scaphoid distal pole.
- Incise the FCR sheath, retract the tendon ulnarly, and incise the floor.
- Leave the radial artery undissected and protected in the radial soft tissues.
- Sweep the fat overlying the pronator quadratus together with the digital flexors and median nerve ulnarward with a sponge or blunt elevator.
- Proximally in the incision, elevate the most distal aspect of the origin of the flexor pollicis longus from the volar distal radius (taking care to cauterize a consistent artery in this region) and retract it ulnarly with a small Hohmann retractor placed around the ulnar border of the radius.
- Expose the radial border of the radius using a blunt elevator and Hohmann retractors.
- Incise the pronator quadratus over its most radial and distal limits (L-shaped incision) and elevate it subperiosteally.
  - Leaving the periosteum with the muscle can facilitate later repair.
- For dorsally angulated malunions, release of the radial and dorsal soft tissues facilitates realignment.
  - The brachioradialis is Z-lengthened and the periosteum is elevated from the radius shaft proximally.
- After osteotomy in the manner detailed earlier (for the dorsal approach to malunions), pronate the proximal radius shaft out of the wound, providing access to the dorsal periosteum, which can be isolated and divided.
  - With the release of the brachioradialis and the dorsal periosteum, realignment of the radius is usually comparable to an acute fracture.
- Volarly angulated malunions do not need an extensive soft tissue release in most cases. The plate can facilitate realignment by pushing the distal fragments into position as the proximal screws are tightened.

Realignment and Provisional Fixation

- The fragments are realigned using the techniques described earlier (**TECH FIG 4**).
  - The techniques are similar to those for acute fractures once an adequate soft tissue release has been performed.
- Apply a fixed-angle volar implant.
- Insert provisional Kirschner wires either through or adjacent to the plate (see **TECH FIG 4**).

Plate Fixation

- Placement of the plate will frequently help reduce the proximal and distal fragments (**TECH FIG 5A,B**).
- After final plate fixation and removal of provisional fixation, apply cancellous graft to the osteotomy site (**TECH FIG 5C–F**).
  - Excellent access is available radially for placement of the bone graft.
- The tourniquet is deflated and hemostasis ensured.
- Repair the pronator quadratus if possible.
  - It can be sutured to the brachioradialis tendon.
- The skin is closed.
- A bulky dressing incorporating a volar plaster wrist splint is applied.

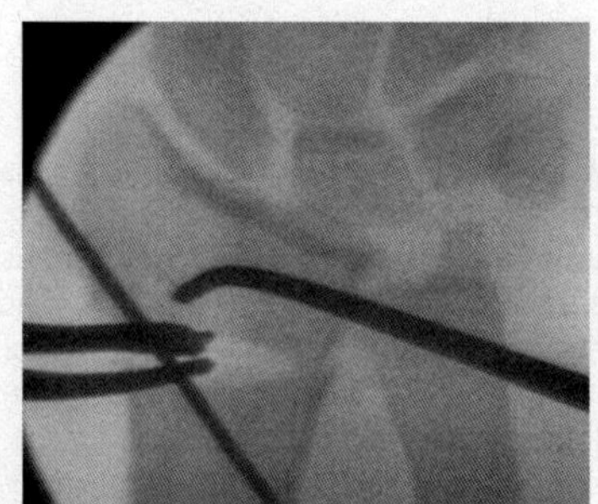
A

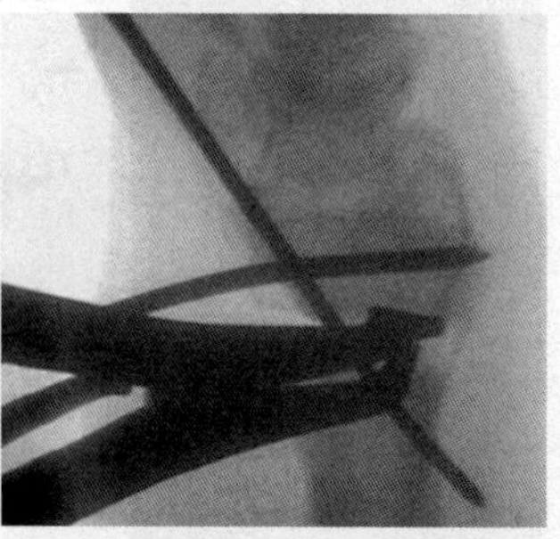
B

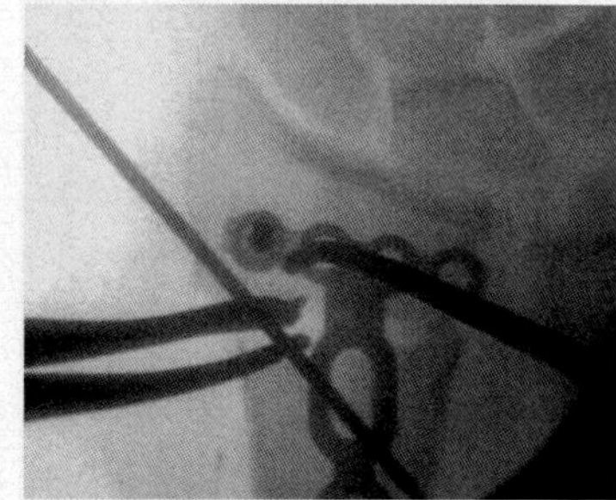
C

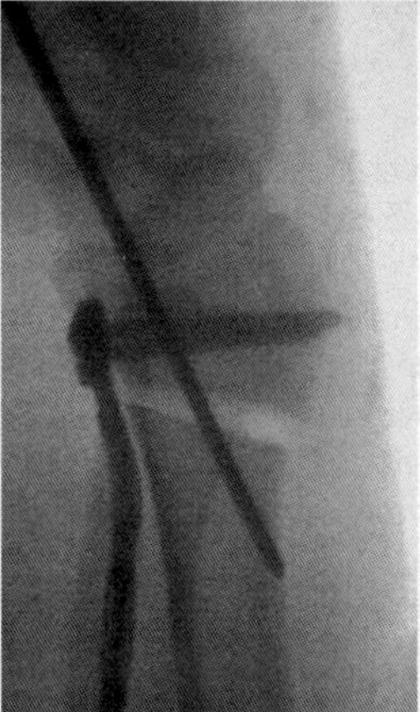
D

TECH FIG 4 • A–D. Realignment and provisional fixation of an extra-articular dorsally displaced malunion in the patient in **FIG 2C,D**.

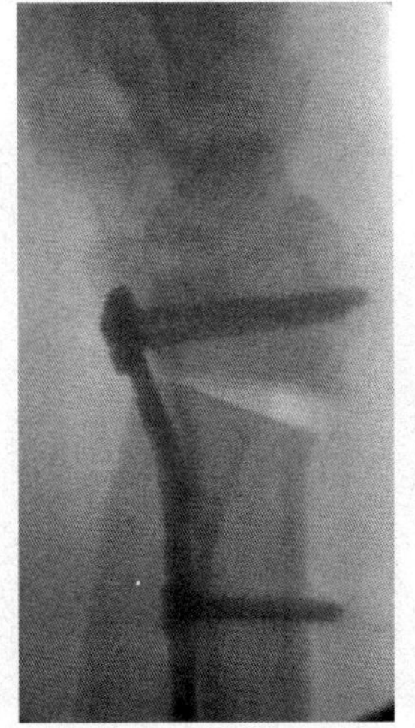
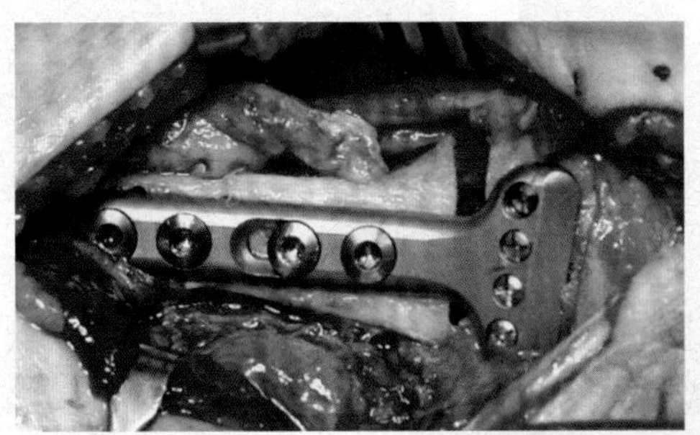
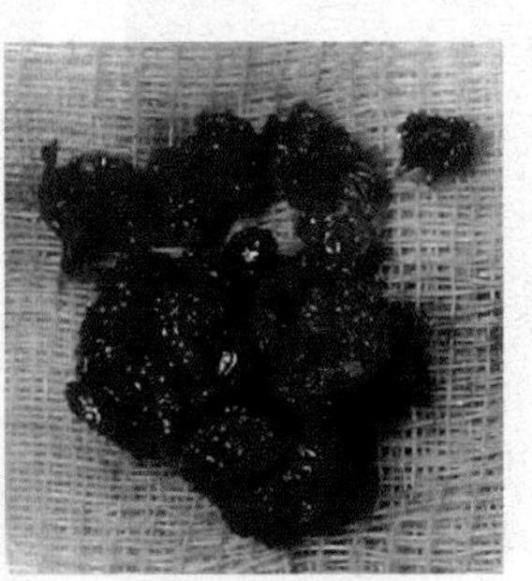
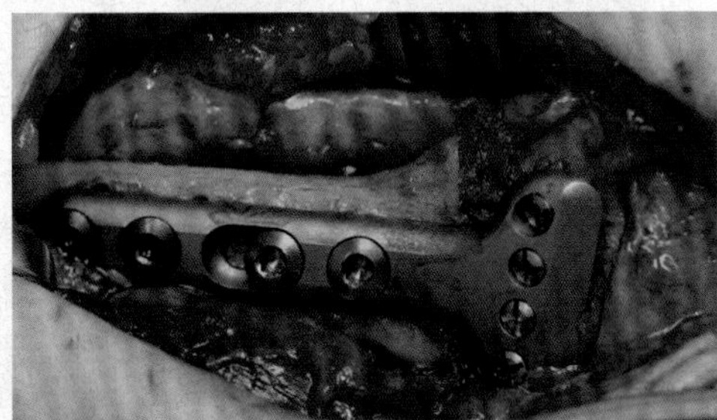
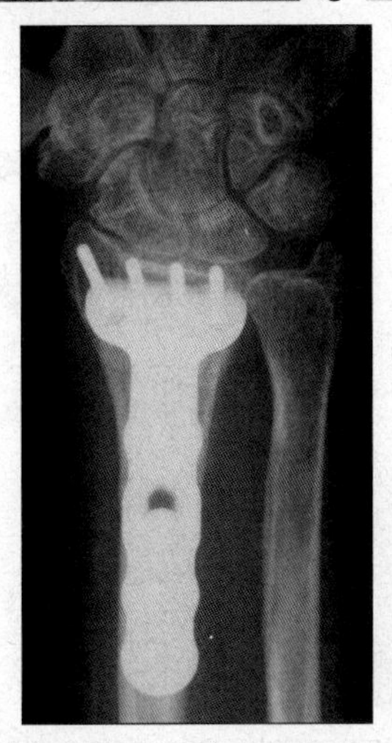
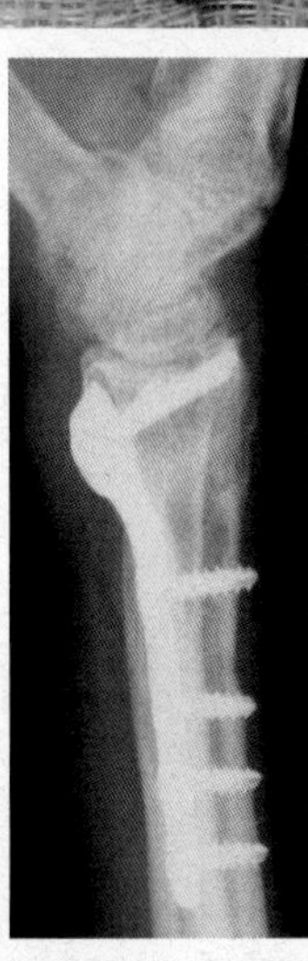

TECH FIG 5 • **A.** Fluoroscopic image of plate fixation and realignment. **B.** Defect after correction. Autogenous cancellous graft (**C**) and graft placement (**D**), showing final clinical appearance. **E,F.** Final PA and lateral radiographs. (Copyright Diego Fernandez, MD, PhD.)

Intra-articular Distal Radius Osteotomy

- Intra-articular osteotomy should be attempted only when there is a simple fracture line that can be clearly identified by direct visualization as well as under image intensification (**TECH FIG 6A–C**).
  - Incompletely healed fractures (fewer than 3 to 4 months since injury) are ideal.
- Depending on the locations of the malunited articular fragments, perform either a dorsal or a volar exposure in the manner detailed earlier.
  - When a dorsal exposure is used, a transverse capsulotomy allows access to the joint and monitoring of the articular osteotomy and realignment.
  - In the case of a volar exposure, the capsule is not incised, but articular exposure may be possible through the osteotomy site.
- The osteotomy should recreate the original fracture line. This is monitored directly and under image intensification.
- Reduction is accomplished by soft tissue release and direct fragment manipulation. For many malunions, it is necessary to remove bone or callus from the fracture site to realign the fracture fragment. Callus or bone is removed until the fracture fragment fits properly (**TECH FIG 6D**).
- Provisional Kirschner wires are used to hold the reduction (**TECH FIG 6E,F**).
- The implants are then applied.
  - Dorsally, a single T- or Pi-shaped plate or two 2.0- or 2.4-mm plates (one applied dorsally, ulnar to the tubercle of Lister, and the other applied radially between the first and second dorsal compartments) can be used (**TECH FIG 6G,H**).
  - Volarly, a T-shaped plate is usually used.
  - After final plate fixation, provisional fixation is removed.
- This entire process is monitored using image intensification to confirm appropriate osteotomy site, correction of alignment, and implant placement.
- Deflate the tourniquet, close the wound, and apply the splint in the manner detailed earlier.

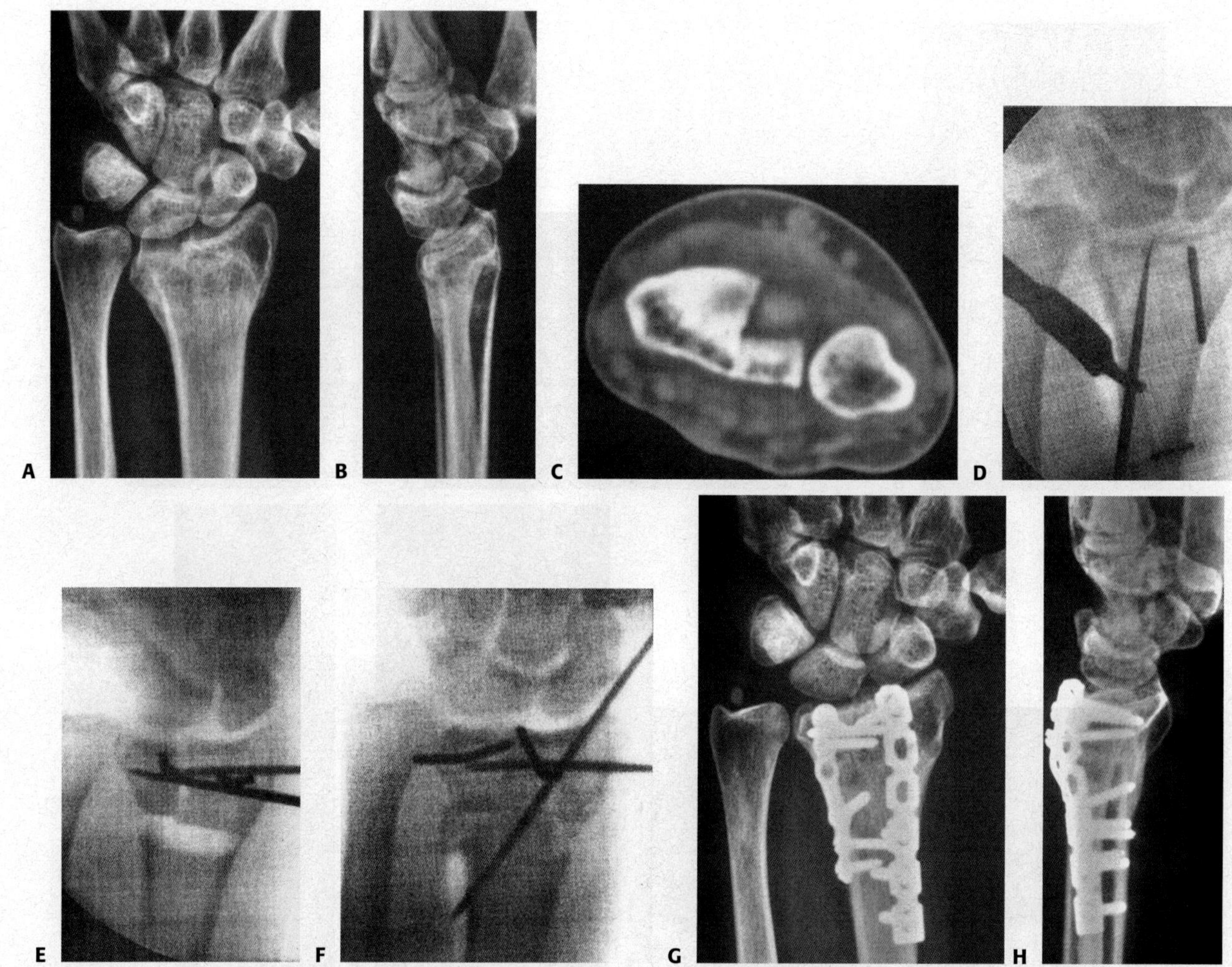

TECH FIG 6 • A–C. PA and lateral radiographs and CT of an intra-articular dorsally angulated malunion. **D.** A Freer elevator is used under fluoroscopy to reposition the articular fragment. **E,F.** Intraoperative fluoroscopic views showing provisional correction and fixation. **G,H.** Final plate and screw fixation. (Copyright Diego Fernandez, MD, PhD.)

PEARLS AND PITFALLS

Preoperative plan	■ A poor or incomplete preoperative plan will increase the amount of uncertainty and hesitation during surgery. This will increase the operative time and the frustration level and will decrease the satisfaction with the surgery. ■ Making a detailed preoperative plan will improve the efficiency and efficacy of the procedure.
Extra-articular malunions	■ Manipulating the distal fragment can be much more difficult with poor-quality bone. ■ The use of a distractor or small external fixator greatly facilitates realignment and provisional stabilization of the fragments. ■ Consider using two distractors in perpendicular planes (eg, one dorsal and one direct radial) to help obtain and maintain alignment. ■ Restoration of length in addition to that gained with angular realignment (ie, lengthening of both the dorsal and volar cortices) is much more difficult. ■ The most difficult part of performing an osteotomy for a dorsal angulated malunion from a volar approach is realignment of the bone. ■ An extended FCR exposure allows release of the dorsal periosteum and Z-lengthening of the brachioradialis, both of which facilitate realignment of the radius.
Intra-articular malunions	■ Handling small articular fracture fragments can be difficult. ■ Each fragment can be realigned using a Kirschner wire as a joystick. ■ The articular osteotomy is easiest when the original fracture lines can be identified. ■ Try to intervene within 3 months of injury when articular malunion is identified.

POSTOPERATIVE CARE

- Active and active-assisted exercise of the fingers and forearm, finger exercises to reduce swelling, and active functional use of the limb for light tasks are encouraged immediately.
- The initial plaster splint is exchanged for a custom Orthoplast removable splint 2 weeks after the surgery.
- The patient gradually weans out of the splint between 4 and 6 weeks after surgery and initiates active and active-assisted wrist exercises.
- Strengthening and forceful use of the arm are restricted until early radiographic union is apparent.
- Unrestricted use of the limb is allowed when solid union is present clinically and radiographically.

OUTCOMES

- Fernandez'[1,2] articles describing dorsal osteotomy with corticocancellous bone graft with and without Bowers arthroplasty of the DRUJ established the value of the technique for improving function in patients with symptomatic distal radius malunions.
  - He documented good or excellent results in 75% and 80% of patients, respectively, noting that satisfactory results depend on the absence of degenerative changes in the radiocarpal and intercarpal joints, and the presence of adequate preoperative range of motion of the wrist.
  - Corrective osteotomy with carefully preoperatively planned structural corticocancellous bone graft does not reliably achieve the planned correction.[12]
  - Nonunions, loss of alignment, and major complications were not reported in these series.
- Jupiter and Ring[5] demonstrated that early correction of distal radius deformity shortened the period of disability without increasing complications and that the combination of cancellous autograft and locking plates was as reliable as corticocancellous bone grafting.[9]
  - Nonunions, loss of alignment, and major complications were not reported in these series.
- Several small articles have established the safety and efficacy of volar osteotomy for a dorsally displaced fracture.[4,6]
- Shea et al[10] established the safety and efficacy of osteotomy for volar extra-articular malunions in a case series.
- Fernandez et al[3] established the safety and efficacy of osteotomy for a radially deviated extra-articular malunion in a case series.
- Several case series have documented the safety and efficacy of intra-articular osteotomy.[7,8,11]

COMPLICATIONS

- Nonunion
- Loss of alignment
- Loss of fixation
- Infection
- Wound problems
- Nerve injury

REFERENCES

1. Fernandez DL. Correction of post-traumatic wrist deformity in adults by osteotomy, bone grafting, and internal fixation. J Bone Joint Surg Am 1982;64(8):1164–1178.
2. Fernandez DL. Radial osteotomy and Bowers arthroplasty for malunited fractures of the distal end of the radius. J Bone Joint Surg 1988;70(10):1538–1551.
3. Fernandez DL, Capo JT, Gonzalez E. Corrective osteotomy for symptomatic increased ulnar tilt of the distal end of the radius. J Hand Surg Am 2001;26(4):722–732.
4. Henry M. Immediate mobilisation following corrective osteotomy of distal radius malunions with cancellous graft and volar fixed angle plates. J Hand Surg Eur Vol 2007;32:88–92.
5. Jupiter JB, Ring D. A comparison of early and late reconstruction of the distal end of the radius. J Bone Joint Surg 1996;78(5):739–748.
6. Malone KJ, Magnell TD, Freeman DC, et al. Surgical correction of dorsally angulated distal radius malunions with fixed angle volar plating: a case series. J Hand Surg Am 2006;31(3):366–372.
7. Marx RG, Axelrod TS. Intraarticular osteotomy of distal radial malunions. Clin Orthop Relat Res 1996;(327):152–157.
8. Ring D, Prommersberger KJ, Gonzalez del Pino J, et al. Corrective osteotomy for intra-articular malunion of the distal part of the radius. J Bone Joint Surg Am 2005;87(7):1503–1509.
9. Ring D, Roberge C, Morgan T, et al. Osteotomy for malunited fractures of the distal radius: a comparison of structural and structural autogenous bone grafts. J Hand Surg Am 2002;27(2):216–222.
10. Shea K, Fernandez DL, Jupiter JB, et al. Corrective osteotomy for malunited, volarly displaced fractures of the distal end of the radius. J Bone Joint Surg Am 1997;79(12):1816–1826.
11. Thivaios GC, McKee MD. Sliding osteotomy for deformity correction following malunion of volarly displaced distal radial fractures. J Orthop Trauma 2003;17:326–333.
12. von Campe A, Nagy L, Arbab D, et al. Corrective osteotomies in malunions of the distal radius: do we get what we planned? Clin Orthop Relat Res 2006;450:179–185.

Carpal Fractures and Avascular Necrosis

Percutaneous Fixation of Acute Scaphoid Fractures

Peter J.L. Jebson, Jane S. Tan, and Andrew Wong

DEFINITION

- Located in the proximal carpal row, the scaphoid serves as an important link between the proximal and distal carpal rows. It is the most commonly fractured carpal bone, accounting for about 1 in every 100,000 emergency room visits.[17]
- Scaphoid fractures typically result from a fall on an outstretched hand or less commonly following forced palmar flexion of the wrist[16] or axial loading of the flexed wrist such as in punching.[14,26]
  - There are about 345,000 scaphoid fractures annually in the United States.

ANATOMY

- The scaphoid has a complex three-dimensional geometry that has been described as a "twisted peanut."[8] Anatomically, the scaphoid is organized into proximal pole, waist, and distal pole regions.
- Scaphoid dimensions vary between genders; the male scaphoid is usually longer and wider than the females. In addition, the diameter of most commercially available standard screws are larger than the proximal pole of the female scaphoid.[13]
- The scaphoid articulates with the radius, lunate, capitate, trapezium, and trapezoid; thus, its surface is almost completely covered with hyaline cartilage. This feature has several important implications, including articular disruption during wire or screw insertion, paucity of vascular supply, and the absence of periosteum.
  - Lacking periosteum, the scaphoid heals almost completely by primary bone healing, resulting in minimal callus and a biomechanically weak early union.[23]
  - Blood supply comes from branches of the radial artery that enter the scaphoid via two main routes[7]:
    - A dorsal branch, which enters the scaphoid via the dorsal ridge, provides the primary supply and 70% to 80% of the overall vascularity, including the entire proximal pole (via retrograde endosteal branches).
    - A volar branch, which enters through the tubercle, supplies 20% to 30% of the internal vascularity, all in the distal pole.
- The precarious blood supply contributes to the high incidence of nonunion after a fracture at the scaphoid waist or proximal pole. It also places the proximal pole at risk for the development of avascular necrosis.

PATHOGENESIS

- A scaphoid fracture classically occurs in a young, active adult most commonly following a fall onto an outstretched hand.
  - Studies have demonstrated that wrist extension of more than 95 degrees combined with more than 10 degrees of radial deviation is required for a scaphoid fracture to occur. In this position, the scaphoid abuts the distal radius, resulting in fracture.
  - The scaphoid can also be fractured following a forced palmar flexion of the wrist injury such as punching an object.[14,26]
- Seventy percent to 80% of scaphoid fractures occur at the waist region, whereas 10% to 20% involve the proximal pole and 5% occur at the distal pole and tuberosity.
- In children, the most common location for a scaphoid fracture is the distal pole.[2]
  - Although rare, scapholunate ligament injuries can occur in association with a scaphoid fracture.[15,22,28,31]

NATURAL HISTORY

- The true natural history of an untreated scaphoid fracture is unknown due to limitations in the existing literature, particularly with respect to study design.[16] However, several retrospective studies have suggested that if a nonunion occurs, a predictable pattern of wrist arthritis develops, usually within 10 years of the injury.[19,21]
- Unrecognized, untreated, or inadequately treated scaphoid fractures have an increased likelihood of nonunion and secondary carpal instability.
- A fracture through the proximal pole has the highest likelihood of nonunion, followed by a fracture of the scaphoid waist.
- If the scaphoid fracture is unstable, extension forces exerted on the proximal fragment (via the long radiolunate and the radioscaphocapitate ligaments) and flexion forces at the distal fragment result in a flexion ("humpback") deformity of the scaphoid.
  - This deformity and loss of scaphoid support results in carpal instability, most frequently a dorsal intercalated segment instability (DISI) pattern, which eventually leads to arthritis as previously described.
- The overall incidence of nonunion after fracture at the scaphoid waist region is about 5% to 10%.[18]

PATIENT HISTORY AND PHYSICAL FINDINGS

- A patient with an acute or subacute scaphoid fracture presents with radial-sided wrist pain, swelling, and loss of motion, particularly with dorsiflexion.
- Classic physical examination findings include the following:
  - Edema over the dorsoradial aspect of the wrist
  - Tenderness to palpation between the first and third dorsal compartments (the "anatomic snuffbox")
  - Tenderness with palpation volarly over the distal tubercle

- Pain with axial compression of the wrist (scaphoid compression test)
- Acutely, swelling and ecchymosis over the volar radial wrist

IMAGING AND OTHER DIAGNOSTIC STUDIES

- The following plain radiographs should routinely be ordered in the patient with a suspected scaphoid fracture: posteroanterior (PA), oblique, lateral, and dedicated scaphoid views.
  - The PA view allows visualization of the proximal pole of the scaphoid.
  - The semipronated oblique view provides the best visualization of the waist and distal pole regions.
  - The semisupinated oblique view provides the best visualization of the dorsal ridge.
  - The lateral view permits an assessment of fracture angulation, carpal alignment, and carpal instability.
  - The dedicated scaphoid view is a PA view with the wrist in ulnar deviation. This results in scaphoid extension, allowing visualization of the scaphoid in profile.
- Displaced and unstable fractures are defined by the following criteria:
  - At least 1 mm of displacement
  - More than 10 degrees of angular displacement
  - Fracture comminution
  - Radiolunate angle of more than 15 degrees
  - Scapholunate angle of more than 60 degrees
  - Intrascaphoid angle of more than 35 degrees
- Computed tomography (CT) scan is helpful in identifying and characterizing an acute fracture and evaluating for a nonunion. Thin 1-mm cuts are obtained in the sagittal and coronal planes.
- Magnetic resonance imaging (MRI) is useful for diagnosing an occult fracture and, when combined with gadolinium administration, can be used to assess the vascularity of the proximal pole and the presence of avascular necrosis. Bone bruising without a fracture detected on MRI may eventually be found to be the result of an occult fracture in 2% of cases.[27]
- Technetium bone scan has been shown to be up to 100% sensitive in identifying occult fractures but lacks specificity. It is optimally used 48 hours after injury.

DIFFERENTIAL DIAGNOSIS

- Scapholunate injury
- Wrist sprain
- Wrist contusion
- Fracture of other carpal bones
- Distal radius fracture

NONOPERATIVE MANAGEMENT

- Nonoperative management, specifically cast immobilization, is indicated for a nondisplaced, acute (<4 weeks from injury) fracture of the distal pole. For a nondisplaced, acute waist fracture, there is debate regarding the preferred treatment approach—cast immobilization or surgical stabilization.
- With cast immobilization, there is no consensus regarding the preferred position of the wrist, the need to immobilize other joints besides the wrist, and the duration of immobilization.[4]
  - Clinical studies have demonstrated no benefit with thumb immobilization nor any influence of wrist position on the rate of union.
  - Studies have also demonstrated no difference in union rates with use of a long-arm versus short-arm cast; however, a small randomized prospective study by Gellman et al[9] demonstrated a shorter time to union and fewer nonunions and delayed unions with the initial use of a long-arm cast.
- In general, cast immobilization is required for 6 weeks after a distal pole fracture and 10 to 12 weeks following a nondisplaced waist fracture.
  - Confirmation of fracture union requires serial plain radiographs demonstrating progressive obliteration of the fracture line and clear trabeculation across the fracture site.[6]
- If there is any question regarding fracture union, particularly if the patient is returning to a contact sport, a CT scan should be obtained.

SURGICAL MANAGEMENT

- Operative treatment is advocated for fractures that are unstable or displaced (see previously mentioned criteria) and following a significant treatment delay.[20]
- Percutaneous fixation is indicated for the following:
  - Nondisplaced fractures of the scaphoid waist
  - Displaced fractures of the scaphoid waist
  - Proximal pole fractures
- Percutaneous stabilization of scaphoid fractures may be performed using either a volar or dorsal approach under fluoroscopic guidance.[3,11,12] If desired, a dorsal arthroscopically assisted reduction and fixation (AARF) technique can be used, which allows direct visualization after fracture reduction and stabilization.[23–25]
  - Regardless of the technique used, the screw must be inserted in the middle third or central axis of the scaphoid, as this provides the greatest stability and stiffness, and decreases time to union.[1,29,30]

Preoperative Planning

- All imaging studies should be reviewed to identify the location of the fracture and the size of the scaphoid, both of which influence implant selection.
- Plain radiographs should be templated to determine the approximate screw length.
  - The smaller size of the female scaphoid must be taken into consideration when planning internal fixation, as the diameters of most commercially available headless screws are larger than the proximal pole.[13]
- Required equipment
  - Portable mini-fluoroscopy unit
  - Kirschner wires
  - Cannulated headless compression screw system
  - Wrist arthroscopy equipment and traction tower for AARF

Positioning

- The patient is positioned supine on the operating table, with the shoulder abducted 90 degrees and the arm on a radiolucent hand table.
- A pneumatic tourniquet is applied to the upper arm.
- The portable fluoroscopy unit is positioned at the end of the hand table.

Dorsal Arthroscopy-Assisted Reduction and Fixation

Nondisplaced Fracture of the Scaphoid Waist or Proximal Pole

- Position the wrist to obtain a PA view of the wrist.
- Under fluoroscopic guidance, gently pronate the wrist until the scaphoid appears as an oblong cylinder, indicating that the proximal and distal poles are aligned.
- Flex the wrist about 45 degrees until the cylinder rotates into the plane of imaging, forming a "ring" sign. The center of the ring indicates the central axis of the scaphoid (**TECH FIG 1**).
- Using a 14-gauge angiocatheter as a guide for wire insertion, place the tip of a 0.045-inch guidewire through the catheter and onto the proximal pole of the scaphoid, at the center of the scaphoid ring. Confirm correct positioning with fluoroscopy.[24,25]
- Insert the guidewire down the central axis of the scaphoid using a wire driver. Keep the wrist flexed to avoid bending the wire.
- Insert the guidewire through the trapezium and advance it until the proximal tip of the guidewire clears the radiocarpal joint such that the wrist can be extended for arthroscopic examination.
- Confirm correct wire position with fluoroscopy.
- Perform a diagnostic arthroscopy to assess for any associated injuries and to evaluate the fracture reduction.[24,25]
  - The radial midcarpal portal is used to evaluate the accuracy of fracture reduction.
  - The 3-4 and 4-5 portals are used assess the integrity of the radiocarpal and intercarpal ligaments.
- Create a small longitudinal incision over each portal site, and bluntly dissect down to the capsule with a hemostat. Enter the capsule with a blunt trocar.
- Confirm accurate fracture reduction and assess for other intra-articular injuries.
- Remove the hand from traction for screw insertion.
- The radial midcarpal portal is used to evaluate the accuracy of fracture reduction.
- The 3-4 and 4-5 portals are used to assess the integrity of the radiocarpal and intercarpal ligaments.
- Suspend the hand vertically in finger traps and apply 10 pounds of traction to the upper arm to distract the radiocarpal and midcarpal articulations.
- Create a small longitudinal incision over each portal site and bluntly dissect down to the capsule with a hemostat. Enter the capsule with a blunt trocar.
- Remove the hand from traction for screw insertion.
- Position the wrist again to obtain the ring sign, and maintain the wrist in flexion.
- Drive the guidewire from volar to dorsal, perpendicular to the fracture line, until the distal tip lies just within the distal pole of the scaphoid (**TECH FIG 2A–C**).
- Place a second guidewire of equal length against the tip of the proximal pole, parallel and next to the first guidewire. The difference between lengths of the protruding wires represents the length of the scaphoid.
- Subtract at least 4 mm from the length of the scaphoid to obtain the desired screw length.
- Make a small longitudinal incision around the guidewire and bluntly dissect down to the joint capsule. Carefully retract the extensor pollicis longus and extensor digitorum communis tendons away from the surgical site.
- Use the cannulated reamer to ream the near cortex only.
- Insert an Acutrak 2, mini-Acutrak 2 screw (Acumed, Beaverton, OR), or other cannulated headless compression screw of appropriate length (at least 4 mm shorter than the measured scaphoid length) to within 1 to 2 mm of the distal surface.
  - The tip of the screw should not penetrate the distal surface, and the proximal end of the screw should rest 2 mm deep to the proximal articular cartilage (**TECH FIG 2D,E**).
- Confirm satisfactory screw position and fracture reduction with fluoroscopy. The screw should be inserted down the central axis of the scaphoid. If any doubt exists, use the arthroscopic portals to confirm that the screw is buried in the scaphoid.
  - The 3-4 portal and the radial midcarpal portals provide the best view to ensure that the fracture is adequately reduced and that there is no violation of the midcarpal joint.

Displaced Scaphoid Waist Fracture

- Insert two percutaneous 0.062-inch smooth Kirschner wires dorsally into each fragment perpendicular to the long axis of the scaphoid to be used as joysticks to reduce the fracture (**TECH FIG 3A,B**).
- Position the wrist as previously described.
- The guidewire from the Acutrak 2 system (or the surgeon's chosen system) is inserted from proximal to distal, starting dorsally and aiming for the central axis of the distal fragment.
  - The guidewire is driven through the distal fragment and out through the volar skin of the hand. The protruding tip is then pulled volarly until the wire is only in the distal fragment (**TECH FIG 3C**).[24,25]

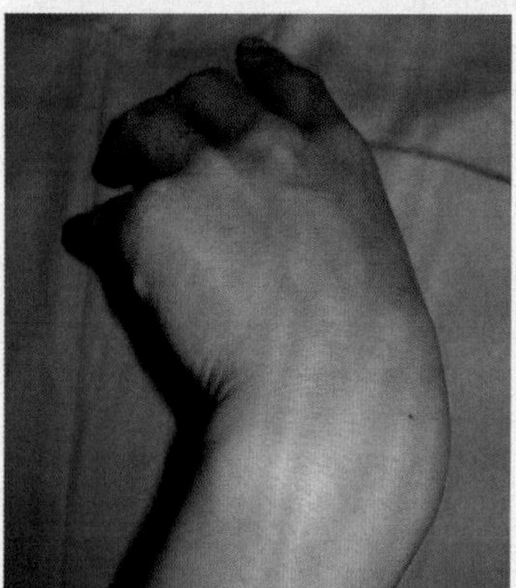

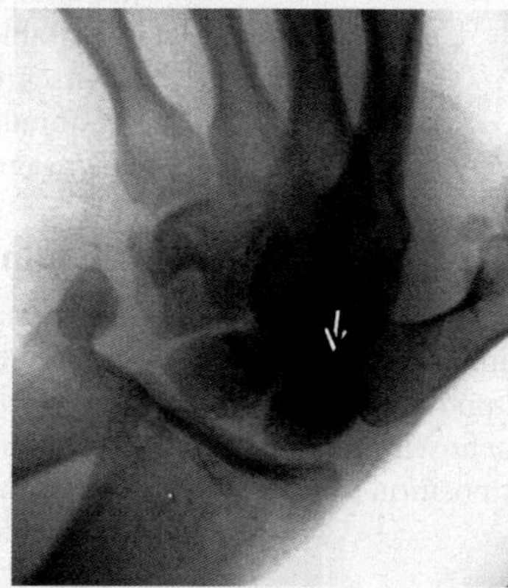

TECH FIG 1 • The scaphoid ring sign indicates the central axis of the scaphoid, which is critical for accurate insertion of the cannulated compression screw. **A,B.** The wrist is positioned in flexion and pronation until the scaphoid appears as a ring (*arrow*) on fluoroscopic imaging. A 0.045-inch guidewire is inserted through the center of the ring.

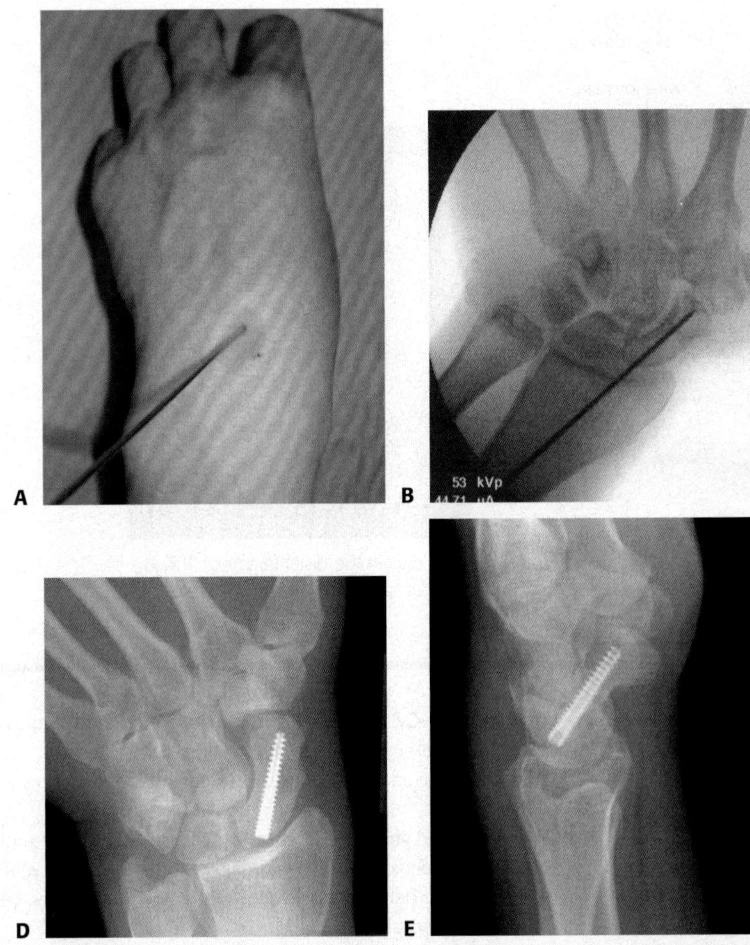

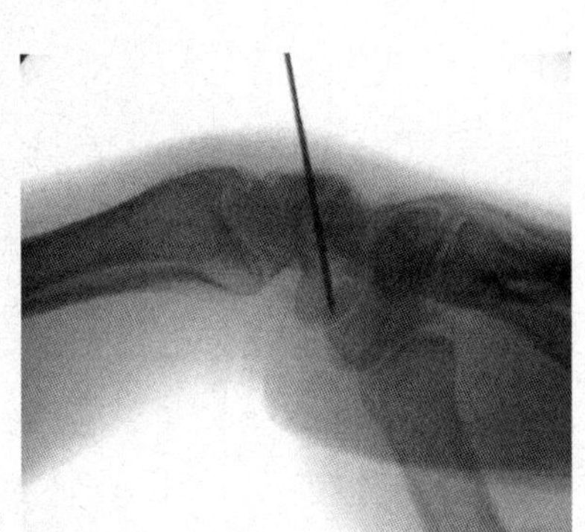

TECH FIG 2 • **A–C.** Before screw insertion, the position of the Kirschner wire must be changed from its position used for arthroscopy. The Kirschner wire should be driven from volar to dorsal until the distal end lies just beneath the articular surface of the scaphoid. **D,E.** Screw fixation of minimally displaced scaphoid fracture via the dorsal percutaneous technique. The screw tip should rest within 1 to 2 mm of the distal cortex. Excellent compression should be obtained with this technique.

- The proximal fragment, which is now freely mobile, is reduced manually using the Kirschner wire joysticks.
  - Once the fracture is reduced, the central guidewire is driven from volar to dorsal into the proximal fragment, securing it in place (**TECH FIG 3D**).[24,25]
- The guidewire is further advanced from volar to dorsal until its distal tip is just within the subchondral bone of the distal articular surface. This allows for measurement of the screw length as previously described.
- An additional 0.045-inch Kirschner wire is inserted parallel to the guidewire to prevent rotation of the scaphoid fragments during reaming and screw implantation.
  - Maintenance of reduction during and after screw insertion is confirmed with fluoroscopy, and all wires are subsequently removed.

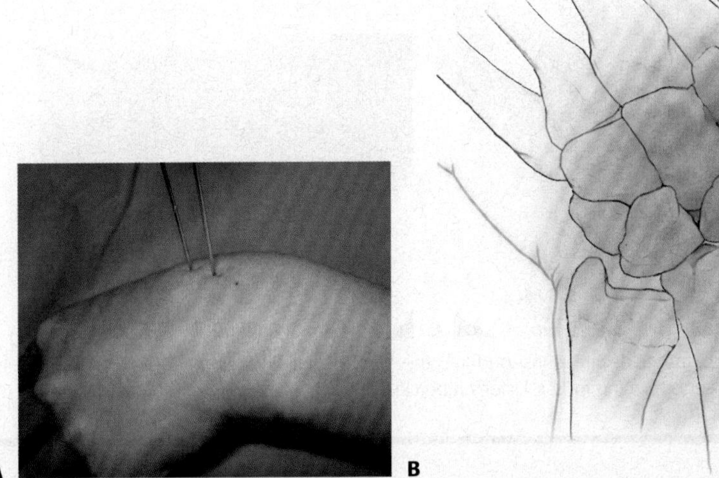

TECH FIG 3 • **A.** Reduction of a displaced scaphoid waist fracture using Kirschner wire joysticks. **B.** The Kirschner wire joystick technique for fracture reduction. *(continued)*

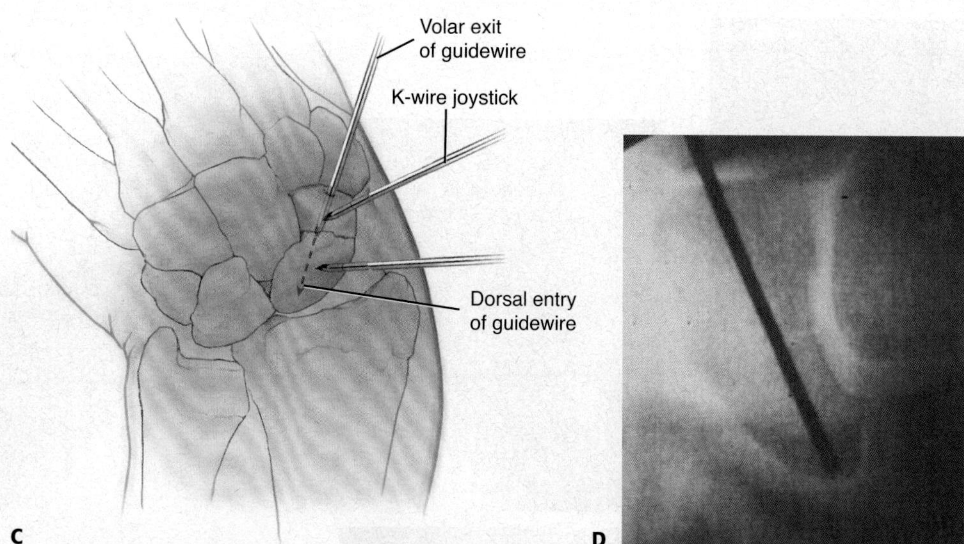

TECH FIG 3 • *(continued)* **C.** The guidewire is pulled volarly until it remains only in the distal fragment. The joysticks are then utilized to reduce the fracture. **D.** The guidewire is driven from volar to dorsal, transfixing the proximal fragment.

Volar Percutaneous Approach

- Position the patient in a supine position with the shoulder abducted and the forearm in supination. The wrist is placed into an extended and ulnarly deviated position over a rolled towel to gain access to the distal pole of the scaphoid.[12]
- Position the portable fluoroscopy unit such that PA and lateral views of the wrist can be obtained. Image intensification is used to locate the distal scaphoid tuberosity.
- A small longitudinal stab incision is made at this point, and the soft tissues are bluntly dissected down to the scaphotrapezial articulation.
- Introduce the guidewire on the distal scaphoid tuberosity. Under image guidance, the wire is advanced toward the center of the proximal pole, aiming for the Lister's tubercle (**TECH FIG 4**).
  - The volar prominence of the trapezium may be partially excised to facilitate the correct starting point and trajectory for the guidewire.
  - Alternatively, the guidewire may be placed directly through the trapezium into the scaphoid distal pole.[11]
- Advance the guidewire to the subchondral bone of the proximal pole.
- Place a second guidewire of equal length against the surface of the distal scaphoid, adjacent and parallel to the first guidewire. The difference between the lengths of the wires represents the length of the scaphoid.
- Subtract 4 mm from the length of the scaphoid to obtain the desired screw length.
- Use the cannulated reamer to ream the near cortex.
- Insert an Acutrak 2 or mini-Acutrak 2 screw (or a screw from the surgeon's chosen system) of appropriate length, remove the guidewire, and confirm satisfactory screw position and fracture reduction with fluoroscopy.

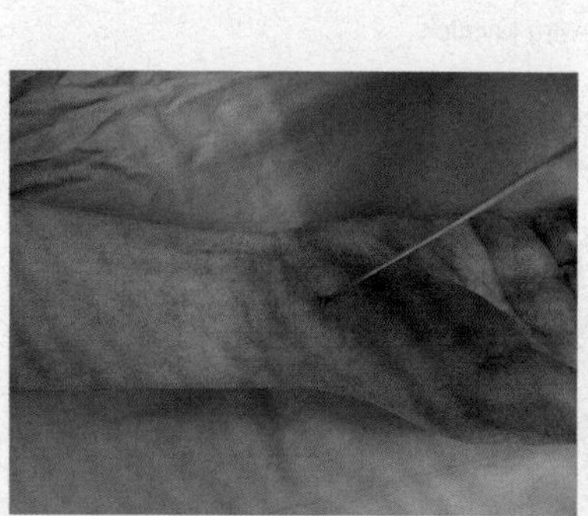

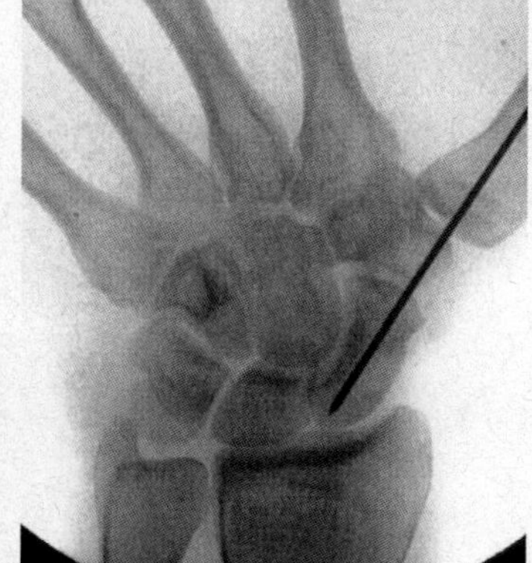

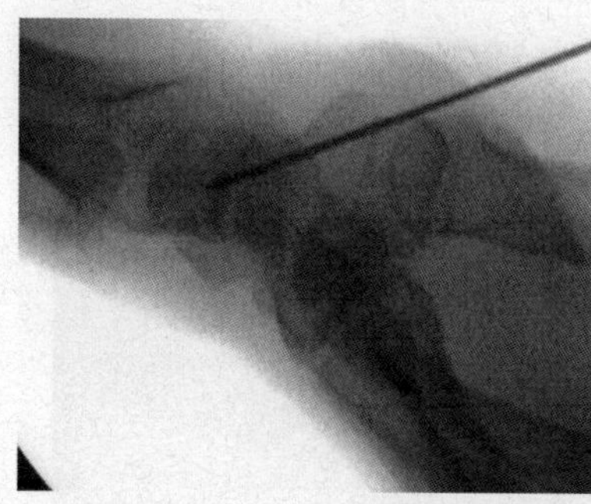

TECH FIG 4 • A–C. In the percutaneous volar approach, the guidewire is inserted into the scaphoid at the scaphotrapezial joint and into the center of the proximal pole. The wire should be inserted aiming for the Lister's tubercle.

PEARLS AND PITFALLS

Dorsal Technique

Injury to dorsal structures	▪ Blunt dissection through the capsule minimizes the risk of injury.
Malpositioning of guidewire	▪ Pronate and flex the wrist until the ring sign is noted; the center of the ring is the insertion point for the guidewire.
Screw penetration	▪ Select a screw that is at least 4 mm shorter than the measured length of the scaphoid. ▪ A common mistake is to place a screw that ends up too long once the screw compresses the fragments. ▪ Confirm central position of guidewire via fluoroscopy.
Reduction of unstable fracture	▪ Kirschner wires may be used as joysticks for reduction. ▪ A derotational Kirschner wire should be placed before reaming and screw insertion if the fragments are unstable.
Extremely small proximal pole fractures	▪ Use a mini-Acutrak 2 screw to prevent comminution of the proximal fracture fragment.

Volar Technique

Injury to volar structures	▪ Blunt dissection to the scaphoid minimizes the risk of injury.
Malpositioning of guidewire	▪ A central starting point on the distal scaphoid tuberosity can be hindered by the trapezium. ▪ Part of the volar trapezium can be resected to achieve a correct starting point for trajectory of the guidewire, or the wire may be inserted through the trapezium.
Screw penetration	▪ Select a screw that is at least 4 mm shorter than the measured length of the scaphoid. ▪ Confirm central position of guidewire via fluoroscopy.

POSTOPERATIVE CARE

- Dressings are applied, and the limb is immobilized in a forearm-based splint, immobilizing only the wrist. The thumb and fingers remain free for range-of-motion exercises.
- The patient is instructed in the importance of limb elevation and finger range-of-motion exercises.
- At 2 weeks postoperatively, the sutures are removed, a removable wrist splint is applied, and a wrist range-of-motion exercise program is initiated if fixation is rigid, the fracture is stable, and bone quality is good.
  - If the patient is noncompliant, the fracture is deemed unstable, the fixation is less than ideal, or bone quality is poor, then a short-arm cast is applied for at least 6 weeks.
- Plain radiographs are obtained at 2, 6, 12, and 24 weeks postoperatively.
- The splint (or cast) is discontinued when union is confirmed on serial plain radiographs. If there is any question regarding fracture union, a CT scan is obtained.
- Unprotected strenuous activity or contact sports are not permitted until 3 months postoperatively.
  - Contact sports may be permitted sooner in a brace depending on the type of sport, player position, and quality of fixation.

OUTCOMES

- Results of contemporary techniques of percutaneous fixation are excellent; it has been shown to allow for earlier mobilization and return to activity and high satisfaction rates compared to nonoperative measures.[3,5,11,12,23,24,32]
  - The surgical approach (dorsal vs. volar percutaneous) does not affect the clinical and functional outcome.[11] Use of the transtrapezial approach does not lead to symptomatic scaphotrapezial arthritis at the short- to medium-term follow-up.[10]
- Earlier mobilization avoids complications such as muscle atrophy and joint stiffness.
- Percutaneous techniques result in decreased soft tissue damage compared to conventional open techniques.[32]
- In a series of 27 consecutive patients, the union rate (confirmed by CT) was 100%. The average time to union was 12 weeks, with a prolonged time to union noted in patients with a proximal pole fracture.[24]

COMPLICATIONS

- The risks associated with open reduction and internal fixation, such as damage to the ligamentous support of the carpus and disruption of the dorsal blood supply, are minimized.
- Possible complications include the following[25]:
  - Nonunion
  - Malunion
  - Injury to the dorsal sensory branch of the radial nerve
  - Extensor tendon injury
  - Infection
  - Technical problems: screw protrusion, screw malposition, bending or breakage of guidewire.
  - Erosion of the trapezium and discomfort from the head of the screw has been reported with the use of a percutaneous cannulated screw inserted via the volar approach.[32]

REFERENCES

1. Adams BD, Blair WF, Reagan DS, et al. Technical factors related to Herbert screw fixation. J Hand Surg Am 1988;13(6):893–899.
2. Amadio PC, Moran SL. Fractures of the carpal bones. In: Green D, Hotchkiss R, Pederson WC, eds. Green's Operative Hand Surgery, ed 5. Philadelphia: Churchill Livingstone, 2005:711–740.
3. Bond CD, Shin CA. Percutaneous cannulated screw fixation of acute scaphoid fractures. Tech Hand Up Extrem Surg 2000;4:81–87.
4. Burge P. Closed cast treatment of scaphoid fractures. Hand Clin 2001;17:541–552.
5. Chen AC, Chao EK, Hung SS, et al. Percutaneous screw fixation for unstable scaphoid fractures. J Trauma 2005;59:184–187.

6. Dias JJ, Taylor M, Thompson J, et al. Radiographic signs of union of scaphoid fractures: an analysis of inter-observer agreement and reproducibility. J Bone Joint Surg Br 1988;70:299–301.
7. Gelberman RH, Menon J. The vascularity of the scaphoid bone. J Hand Surg Am 1980;5:508–513.
8. Gelberman RH, Wolock BS, Siegel DB. Fractures and non-unions of the carpal scaphoid. J Bone Joint Surg Am 1989;71A:1560–1565.
9. Gellman H, Caputo RJ, Carter V, et al. Comparison of short and long thumb-spica casts for non-displaced fractures of the carpal scaphoid. J Bone Joint Surg Am 1989;71(3):354–357.
10. Geurts G, van Riet R, Meermans G, et al. Incidence of scaphotrapezial arthritis following volar percutaneous fixation of nondisplaced scaphoid waist fractures using a transtrapezial approach. J Hand Surg Am 2011;36(11):1753–1758.
11. Gürbüz Y, Kayalar M, Bal E, et al. Comparison of dorsal and volar percutaneous screw fixation methods in acute Type B scaphoid fractures. Acta Orthop Trauma Tur 2012;46(5):339–345.
12. Haddad FS, Goddard NJ. Acute percutaneous scaphoid fixation. A pilot study. J Bone Joint Surg Br 1998;80(1):95–99.
13. Heinzelmann AD, Archer G, Bindra RR. Anthropometry of the human scaphoid. J Hand Surg 2007;32(7):1005–1008.
14. Horii E, Nakamura R, Watanabe K, et al. Scaphoid fracture as a "puncher's fracture." J Ortho Trauma 1994;8:107–110.
15. Jørgsholm P, Thomsen NO, Björkman A, et al. The incidence of intrinsic and extrinsic ligament injuries in scaphoid waist fractures. J Hand Surg 2010;35(3):368–374.
16. Kerluke L, McCabe SJ. Nonunion of the scaphoid: a critical analysis of recent natural history studies. J Hand Surg Am 1993;18(1):1–3.
17. Kozin SH. Incidence, mechanism, and natural history of scaphoid fractures. Hand Clin 2001;17:515–524.
18. Leslie IJ, Dickson RA. The fractured carpal scaphoid. Natural history and factors influencing outcome. J Bone Joint Surg Br 1981;63-B(2): 225–230.
19. Mack GR, Bosse MJ, Gelberman RH, et al. The natural history of scaphoid nonunion. J Bone Joint Surg Am 1984;66(4):504–509.
20. Martus JE, Bedi A, Jebson PJ. Cannulated variable pitch compression screw fixation of scaphoid fractures using a limited dorsal approach. Tech Hand Upper Ext Surg 2005;9:202–206.
21. Ruby LK, Stinson J, Belsky MR. The natural history of scaphoid non-union: a review of fifty-five cases. J Bone Joint Surg Am 1985;67(3):428–432.
22. Schädel-Höpfner M, Junge A, Böhringer G. Scapholunate ligament injury occurring with scaphoid fracture—a rare coincidence? J Hand Surg Br 2005;30:137–142.
23. Slade JF III, Dodds SD. Minimally invasive management of scaphoid nonunions. Clin Orthop 2006;445:108–119.
24. Slade JF III, Gutow AP, Geissler WB. Percutaneous internal fixation of scaphoid fractures via an arthroscopically assisted dorsal approach. J Bone Joint Surg Am 2002;84:21–36.
25. Slade JF III, Jaskwhich D. Percutaneous fixation of scaphoid fractures. Hand Clin 2001;17:553–574.
26. Sutton PA, Clifford O, Davis TRC. A new mechanism of injury for scaphoid fractures: 'test your strength' punch-bag machines. J Hand Surg Eur Vol 2010;35(5):419–420.
27. Thavarajah D, Syed T, Shah Y, et al. Does scaphoid bone bruising lead to occult fractures? A prospective study of 50 patients. Injury 2011;42:1303–1306.
28. Thomsen L, Falcone MO. Lesions of the scapholunate ligament associated with minimally displaced or non-displaced fractures of the scaphoid waist. Which incidence? Chir Main 2012;31:234–238.
29. Trumble TE, Clarke T, Kreder HJ. Non-union of the scaphoid. Treatment with cannulated screws compared with treatment with Herbert screws. J Bone Joint Surg Am 1996;78(12):1829–1837.
30. Trumble TE, Gilbert M, Murray LW, et al. Displaced scaphoid fractures treated with open reduction and internal fixation with a cannulated screw. J Bone Joint Surg Am 2000;82(5):633–641.
31. Wong TC, Yip TH, Wu WC. Carpal ligament injuries with acute scaphoid fractures: a combined wrist injury. J Hand Surg Br 2005;30:415–418.
32. Yip HS, Wu WC, Chang RY, et al. Percutaneous cannulated screw fixation of acute scaphoid waist fracture. J Hand Surg Br 2002;27(1):42–46.

Open Reduction and Internal Fixation of Scaphoid Fractures

35 CHAPTER

Asheesh Bedi, Peter J.L. Jebson, and Levi Hinkelman

DEFINITION

- The scaphoid is the most commonly fractured carpal bone, accounting for 1 in every 100,000 emergency department visits.[15]
- Scaphoid fractures typically result from a fall on an outstretched hand or less commonly following forced palmar flexion of the wrist[20] or axial loading of the flexed wrist such as in punching.[12]
- Scaphoid nonunion or proximal pole avascular necrosis (AVN) after a fracture has been associated with considerable morbidity and a predictable pattern of wrist arthritis.[18,21,25]
- The complex anatomy and tenuous blood supply to the scaphoid make operative management of these fractures technically challenging.[25]

ANATOMY

- The scaphoid has a complex three-dimensional geometry that has been likened to a "twisted peanut." It can be divided into three regions: proximal pole, waist, and distal pole.
- The scaphoid functions as the primary link between the forearm and the distal carpal row and therefore plays a critical role in maintaining normal carpal kinematics.
- Articulating with the scaphoid fossa of the radius, the lunate, capitate, trapezium, and trapezoid, more than 70% of the scaphoid is covered with articular cartilage.
- Gelberman and Menon[8] have described the vascular supply of the scaphoid. The main arterial supply is from the radial artery; it enters the scaphoid via two main branches:
  - A dorsal branch, entering through the dorsal ridge, is the primary supply and provides 70% to 80% of the vascularity, including the entire proximal pole via retrograde endosteal branches.
  - A volar branch, entering through the tubercle, supplies the remaining 20% to 30%, predominantly the distal pole and tuberosity.
- The proximal pole is at increased risk for AVN secondary to disruption of its tenuous retrograde blood supply after a fracture of the scaphoid waist or proximal pole.
- Due to its tenuous vascular supply, the scaphoid heals almost entirely by primary bone healing, resulting in minimal callus formation.
- The size and shape of the scaphoid, in combination with its precarious blood supply, demands attention to detail and accurate implantation of fixation devices during fracture fixation. Scaphoid dimensions vary between genders; the male scaphoid is usually longer and wider than the females. In addition, the diameter of most commercially available standard screws are larger than the proximal pole of the female scaphoid.[11]

PATHOGENESIS

- Scaphoid fractures are most commonly seen in young, active males.[15]
- With the wrist dorsiflexed greater than 95 degrees, in combination with 10 degrees or more of radial deviation, the distal radius abuts the scaphoid and precipitates a fracture.[15]
- The scaphoid can also be fractured with forced palmar flexion of the wrist[20] or axial loading of the flexed wrist.[12]
- Most of these fractures occur at the waist region, although 10% to 20% occur in the proximal pole.
- Proximal pole fractures are associated with an increased risk of nonunion, delayed union, and AVN.
- In children, scaphoid fractures are less common and are most frequently seen in the distal pole.

NATURAL HISTORY

- An untreated or inadequately treated scaphoid fracture has a higher likelihood of nonunion. The overall incidence of nonunion is estimated at 5% to 10%, but the risk is significantly increased with nonoperative treatment of a displaced waist or proximal pole fracture.
- The natural history of scaphoid nonunions is controversial, but they are believed to result in a predictable pattern of progressive radiocarpal and midcarpal arthritis.[8,9,14,17,18,21,25]
- In an established scaphoid nonunion, the distal portion of the scaphoid may flex, producing a "humpback" deformity of the scaphoid. The loss of scaphoid integrity can result in carpal instability and abnormal carpal kinematics, most frequently manifesting as a dorsal intercalated segment instability (DISI) pattern.
  - The pattern of carpal instability and secondary arthrosis due to an unstable scaphoid nonunion has been termed an *SNAC wrist* (scaphoid nonunion advanced collapse pattern of wrist arthritis).[14,21]
  - In the SNAC wrist, there is a loss of carpal height with proximal capitate migration, flexion and pronation of the scaphoid, and secondary midcarpal arthritis.[21]
- Factors associated with the development of a scaphoid fracture nonunion include the following[17]:
  - Delayed diagnosis or treatment
  - Inadequate immobilization

- Proximal fracture
- Initial and progressive fracture displacement
- Fracture comminution
- Presence of associated carpal injuries (ie, perilunate injury)

PATIENT HISTORY AND PHYSICAL FINDINGS

- Scaphoid fractures classically occur in the active, young adult population. Patients present with radial-sided wrist pain.
- Classic physical examination findings include the following:
  - Swelling over the dorsoradial aspect of the wrist
  - Tenderness to palpation in the "anatomic snuffbox"
  - Tenderness with palpation volarly over the distal tubercle
  - Pain with axial compression of the wrist (scaphoid compression test)
- Scaphoid fractures can be part of a greater arc injury.
  - The physician should examine the entire wrist carefully for areas of tenderness and swelling.
  - Plain radiographs are scrutinized for an associated ligamentous injury or disruption of the midcarpal joint as seen in the transscaphoid perilunate fracture-dislocation.

IMAGING AND OTHER DIAGNOSTIC STUDIES

- The following plain radiographs should routinely be ordered in the patient with a suspected scaphoid fracture: posteroanterior (PA), oblique, lateral, and dedicated scaphoid views.
  - The PA view allows visualization of the proximal pole of the scaphoid.
  - The semipronated oblique view provides the best visualization of the waist and distal pole regions.
  - The semisupinated oblique view provides the best visualization of the dorsal ridge.
  - The lateral view permits an assessment of fracture angulation, carpal alignment, and carpal instability.
  - The dedicated scaphoid view is a PA view with the wrist in ulnar deviation. This results in scaphoid extension, allowing visualization of the scaphoid in profile (**FIG 1A**).
- The following criteria define a displaced or unstable fracture as noted on plain radiographs[2,9,17]:
  - At least 1 mm of displacement
  - More than 10 degrees of angular displacement
  - Fracture comminution
  - Radiolunate angle of more than 15 degrees
  - Scapholunate angle of more than 60 degrees
  - Intrascaphoid angle of more than 35 degrees
- Computed tomography (CT) with reconstruction images in multiple planes is used to identify an acute fracture not detected on plain radiographs and to determine the amount of displacement and comminution (**FIG 1B,C**).
  - CT is most useful in evaluating an established scaphoid nonunion or malunion.[6]
  - Because plain radiographs are often unreliable, CT is preferred for confirming union after a scaphoid fracture particularly before permitting a return to contact sports.
- Magnetic resonance imaging (MRI) may be indicated in the evaluation of a suspected scaphoid fracture not detected on plain radiographs (**FIG 1D,E**). MRI is highly sensitive, with

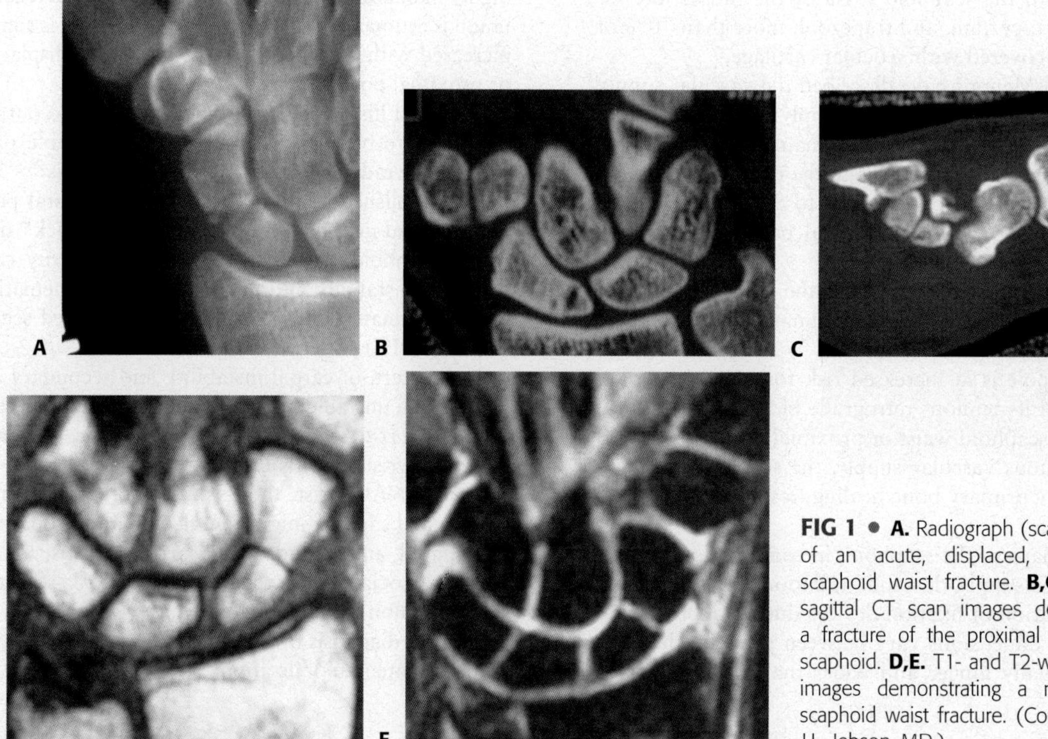

FIG 1 • **A.** Radiograph (scaphoid view) of an acute, displaced, comminuted scaphoid waist fracture. **B,C.** Axial and sagittal CT scan images demonstrating a fracture of the proximal pole of the scaphoid. **D,E.** T1- and T2-weighted MRI images demonstrating a nondisplaced scaphoid waist fracture. (Copyright Peter J.L. Jebson, MD.)

a specificity approaching 100% when performed within 48 hours of injury.[16]

- Bone bruising without a fracture detected on MRI can lead to an occult fracture in 2% of cases.[23]
- MRI with intravenous gadolinium contrast is helpful in assessing the vascularity of the proximal pole, particularly in the patient with an established nonunion.

- A technetium bone scan has been shown to be up to 100% sensitive in identifying an occult fracture.[27] Unfortunately, it is also associated with a low specificity and often will not be positive immediately after the fracture.

DIFFERENTIAL DIAGNOSIS

- Scapholunate injury
- Wrist sprain
- Wrist contusion
- Fracture of other carpal bone
- Greater arc injury
- Distal radius fracture

NONOPERATIVE MANAGEMENT

- Nonoperative management is indicated for a nondisplaced, stable scaphoid waist or distal pole fracture.
  - Unstable fractures and nondisplaced fractures of the proximal pole are indications for internal fixation based on studies that have demonstrated a poor outcome with nonoperative treatment.[2,4,17]
- The appropriate type and duration of cast immobilization remain controversial and none has proven to be superior. Our preference is a short-arm thumb spica cast until the clinical examination and radiologic studies (usually a CT scan) confirm fracture union. If there are concerns for patient compliance, we prefer an initial period (4 to 6 weeks) of long-arm thumb spica cast immobilization.
  - Clinical studies have failed to demonstrate any benefit from including the thumb or fingers in the cast.[2,4]
  - Similarly, wrist position has not been proven to improve scaphoid fracture healing.
  - Numerous studies have revealed no difference in union rates for a long-arm versus short-arm cast; however, a randomized prospective study by Gellman et al[10] documented a shorter time to union and fewer nonunions and delayed unions with initial use of a long-arm cast.
- The morbidity of a nonoperative approach, specifically cast immobilization, has become of increasing concern. A prolonged duration of immobilization is often required for waist fractures, and this can be accompanied by muscle atrophy, stiffness, reduced grip strength, and residual pain. In addition, cast immobilization can cause significant inconvenience for the patient and interference with activities of daily living. The prolonged duration of immobilization is of particular concern in the young laborer, athlete, or military personnel, who typically desire expedient functional recovery.[5,19,29]
- If the clinical history and physical examination are suggestive of a scaphoid fracture but initial radiographs are negative, the wrist should be immobilized for 2 weeks. Repeat radiographs are then obtained. If a fracture is present, resorption at the fracture may be noted. If wrist pain and "snuffbox" tenderness persist but radiographs are negative, an MRI or CT scan may be obtained.[16,27]
- Alternatively, if there is a high index of suspicion at initial presentation with "normal" radiographs or if there is a need to know the status of the scaphoid, such as in the elite athlete, we prefer MRI.

SURGICAL MANAGEMENT

- Indications for open reduction and internal fixation (ORIF) of scaphoid fractures include the following[2,17]:
  - Proximal pole fracture
  - A displaced, unstable fracture of the scaphoid waist
  - Associated carpal instability or perilunate instability
  - Associated distal radius fracture
  - Delayed presentation (more than 3 to 4 weeks) with no prior treatment
  - A nondisplaced, stable scaphoid waist fracture in a patient who wishes to avoid the morbidity of cast immobilization. In this clinical scenario, operative treatment should occur only after an explanation of the rationale for, and the risks and benefits of, operative treatment versus cast immobilization.

Preoperative Planning

- All imaging studies should be reviewed to accurately define the fracture pattern.
- Required equipment are as follows:
  - Portable mini-fluoroscopy unit
  - Kirschner wires
  - Cannulated headless compression screw system. We prefer to use the Acutrak 2 or mini-Acutrak 2 screw system (Acumed, Beaverton, OR), but any cannulated screw system that permits screw insertion beneath the articular surface may be used.

Positioning

- General or regional anesthesia may be used.
- The patient is positioned supine on the operating table with a radiolucent hand table at the shoulder level.
- The fluoroscopy unit is draped and positioned at the end of the hand table.
- A pneumatic tourniquet is carefully applied to the proximal arm.
- An intravenous antibiotic is provided before inflation of the tourniquet as prophylaxis for infection.
- The limb is prepared and draped, followed by exsanguination of the limb with an Esmarch bandage and tourniquet inflation, usually to a pressure of 250 mm Hg.

Approach

- ORIF of scaphoid fractures can be performed through either a dorsal or volar approach.
- The specific approaches that will be described include the following:
  - Open dorsal approach[19]
  - Open volar approach

Open Dorsal Approach (Authors' Preferred Approach)

Exposure

- Pronate the forearm and make a longitudinal skin incision, about 2 to 3 cm long, beginning at the proximal aspect of the tubercle of Lister and extending distally along the axis of the third metacarpal (**TECH FIG 1A**).
  - If the fracture is nondisplaced, a smaller skin incision and limited capsulotomy may be used.
- Raise skin flaps at the level of the extensor retinaculum.
- Incise the extensor retinaculum overlying the third compartment immediately distal to the tubercle of Lister and carefully release the fascia overlying the extensor pollicis longus (EPL) tendon, permitting gentle retraction of the EPL radially. Similarly, incise the dorsal hand fascia longitudinally.
  - Gently retract the extensor digitorum communis (EDC) tendons ulnarly while retracting the extensor carpi radialis brevis (ECRB) and extensor carpi radialis longus (ECRL) tendons radially with the EPL, thus exposing the underlying radiocarpal joint capsule (**TECH FIG 1B**).
- For nondisplaced fractures, make a limited transverse capsulotomy just distal to the dorsal rim of the radius.
  - Evacuate fracture hematoma.
  - Inspect the scapholunate ligament complex for associated injury.[13,22,24,28]
- If the fracture is displaced, it is often helpful to create an inverted T-shaped capsulotomy with the longitudinal limb directly over the scapholunate ligament complex (**TECH FIG 1C**). Extend the longitudinal limb of the capsulotomy to expose the scaphocapitate articulation and the radial aspect of the midcarpal joint.
  - The tubercle of Lister is helpful in locating the scapholunate articulation.
- Carefully elevate the capsular flaps from the proximal pole of the scaphoid and lunate. Avoid damaging the important dorsal component of the scapholunate ligament.
  - Especially when elevating the radial flap, take care to avoid stripping the dorsal ridge vessels entering at the scaphoid waist region.

Fracture Reduction and Provisional Fixation

- Distract the carpus manually via longitudinal traction on the index and long fingers.
- If the fracture is displaced, insert 0.045-inch Kirschner wire joysticks perpendicularly into the proximal and distal scaphoid fragments to assist in the reduction (**TECH FIG 2A**).
  - The accuracy of the reduction can be determined by assessing congruency of the radioscaphoid and scaphocapitate articulations.
- When a satisfactory reduction has been achieved, obtain provisional fixation with parallel derotational 0.045-inch Kirschner wires.
  - The first wire is inserted dorsal and ulnar to the central axis of the scaphoid, into the trapezium for enhanced stability.
  - The second derotational wire may be inserted volar and radial to the anticipated central axis insertion site if more fixation is needed.
  - The derotational wires must be placed such that they will not interfere with central axis guidewire placement, reaming, and screw insertion (**TECH FIG 2B**).

Guidewire Placement

- The starting position for guidewire is at the membranous portion of the scapholunate ligament origin (**TECH FIG 3A,B**).
  - In very proximal fractures, the starting point for the guidewire is as far proximally in the scaphoid as possible, at the mid-aspect of the membranous portion of the scapholunate ligament complex. This point is critical to avoid propagation of the fracture into the proximal scaphoid during insertion of the screw.
- With the wrist flexed over a bolster, insert the guidewire down the central axis of the scaphoid in line with the thumb metacarpal.
  - Be very patient with this important step; proceed with reaming and screw insertion only after central placement has been confirmed on the PA, lateral, and 30-degree pronated lateral views (**TECH FIG 3C**).
  - It is critical to insert the wire in the optimal position in all three views to avoid violating the midcarpal joint or the volar surface of the scaphoid.
  - Take care to avoid bending the guidewire.
- Advance the wire up to but not into the scaphotrapezial joint.

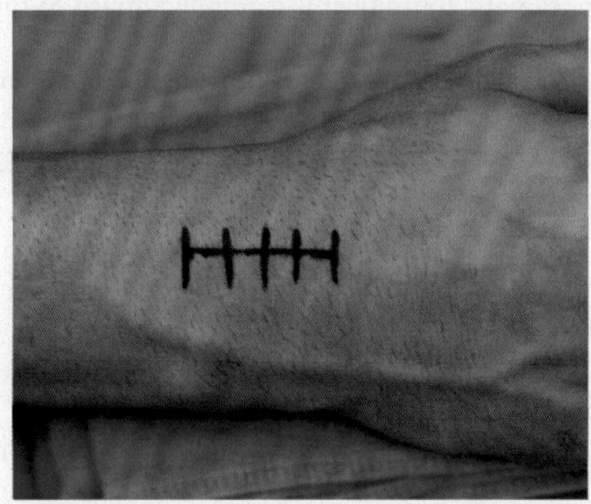
A

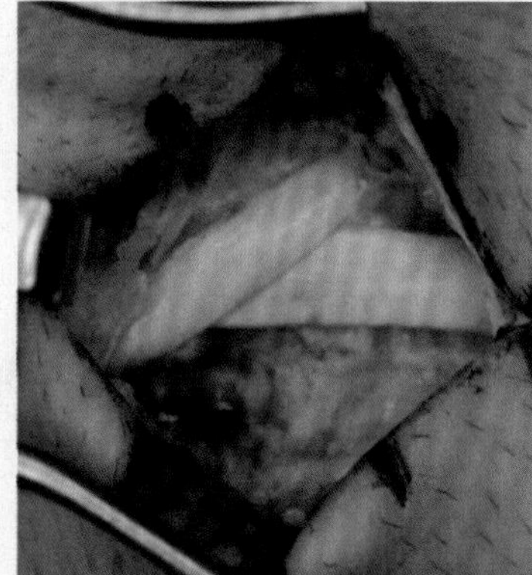
B

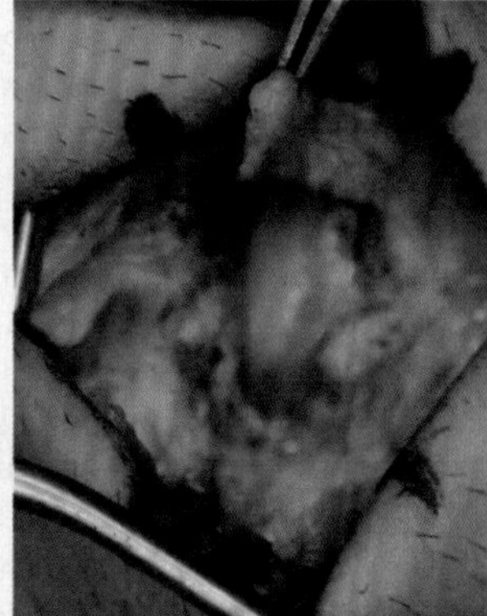
C

TECH FIG 1 • **A.** Skin incision used for ORIF of scaphoid fractures via the dorsal approach. **B.** Retracting the thumb and wrist extensor tendons radially and the finger extensor tendons ulnarly facilitates exposure of the underlying capsule. **C.** A limited capsulotomy should be performed to expose the proximal scaphoid and scapholunate ligament. (Copyright of Peter J.L. Jebson, MD.)

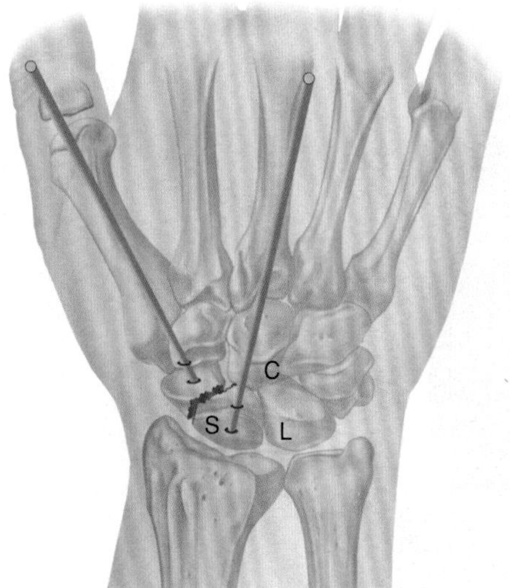

A

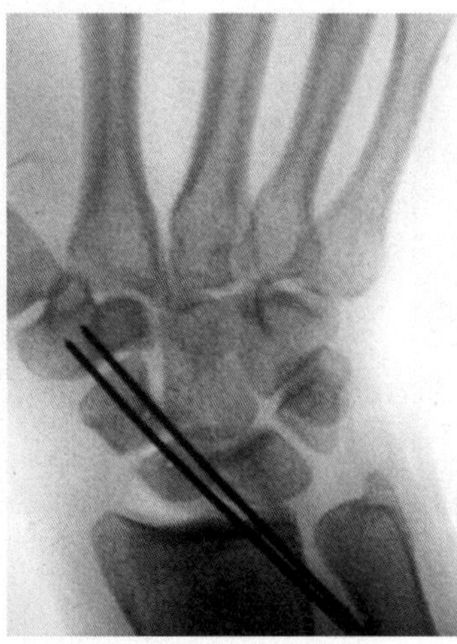

B

TECH FIG 2 • A. Percutaneous insertion of Kirschner wires into the proximal and distal scaphoid (*S*) fragments is helpful to facilitate manual reduction of a displaced fracture. *C*, capitate; *L*, lunate. **B.** A displaced scaphoid waist fracture has been stabilized with a derotational Kirschner wire placed dorsally and ulnarly to the guidewire. The derotational Kirschner wire does not interfere with insertion of the screw in the central axis. (Radiograph Copyright Peter J.L. Jebson, MD.)

Screw Insertion

- Determine screw length by measuring the guidewire (**TECH FIG 4A**).
  - In the case of minimal fragment separation, subtract 4 mm from the measured length of the wire to allow recession of the proximal screw beneath the articular surface.
  - If fragments are more displaced, consider compression and choose an even shorter screw. The common mistake is placement of a screw that is too long.
- Advance the wire into the trapezium to avoid loss of position during drilling.
- Use the cannulated drill to open up the proximal cortex (**TECH FIG 4B**) and manually insert the screw (**TECH FIG 4C,D**).
  - We use the larger Acutrak 2 screw when feasible, but the mini-Acutrak 2 system may be necessary in patients with a small scaphoid or if the fracture is located proximally such that insertion of an Acutrak 2 screw may result in inadvertent propagation of the fracture to the insertion site with fragmentation of the proximal scaphoid. Any cannulated, headless compression screw may be used but size is critical.
- Remove the guidewire and assess screw position via fluoroscopy using the same views.
  - If the fracture is highly unstable or the quality of fixation is less than ideal, two micro-Acutrak 2 screws (or equivalent screws) may be carefully inserted for enhanced stability.
  - If a limited capsulotomy is used, it does not need to be repaired. Capsule repair is recommended with the larger T-shaped capsulotomy.

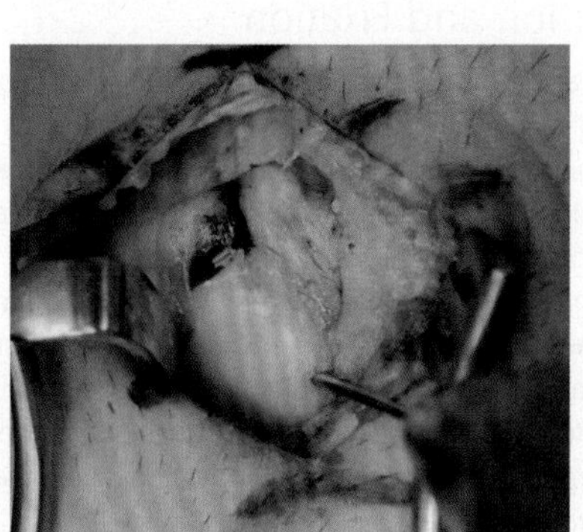

A

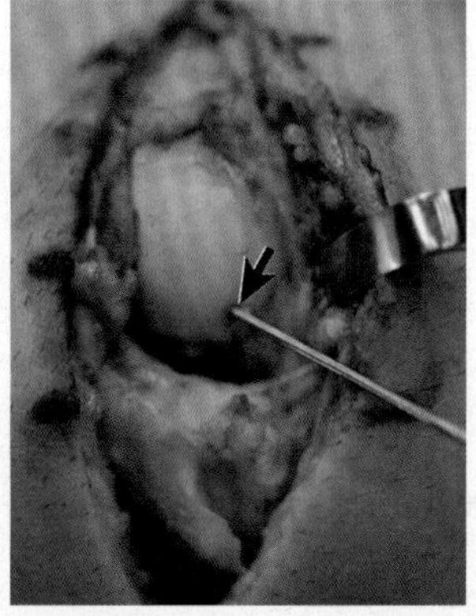

B

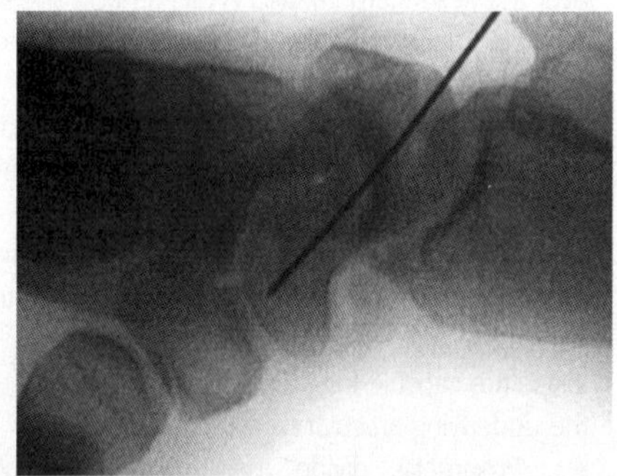

C

TECH FIG 3 • A,B. Note the starting point at the membranous portion of the scapholunate ligament (*arrow*). **C.** The 30-degree pronated oblique view demonstrating guidewire placement down the central axis of the scaphoid. **A:** Top is distal, bottom is proximal, left is radial, and right is ulnar. (Copyright Peter J.L. Jebson, MD.)

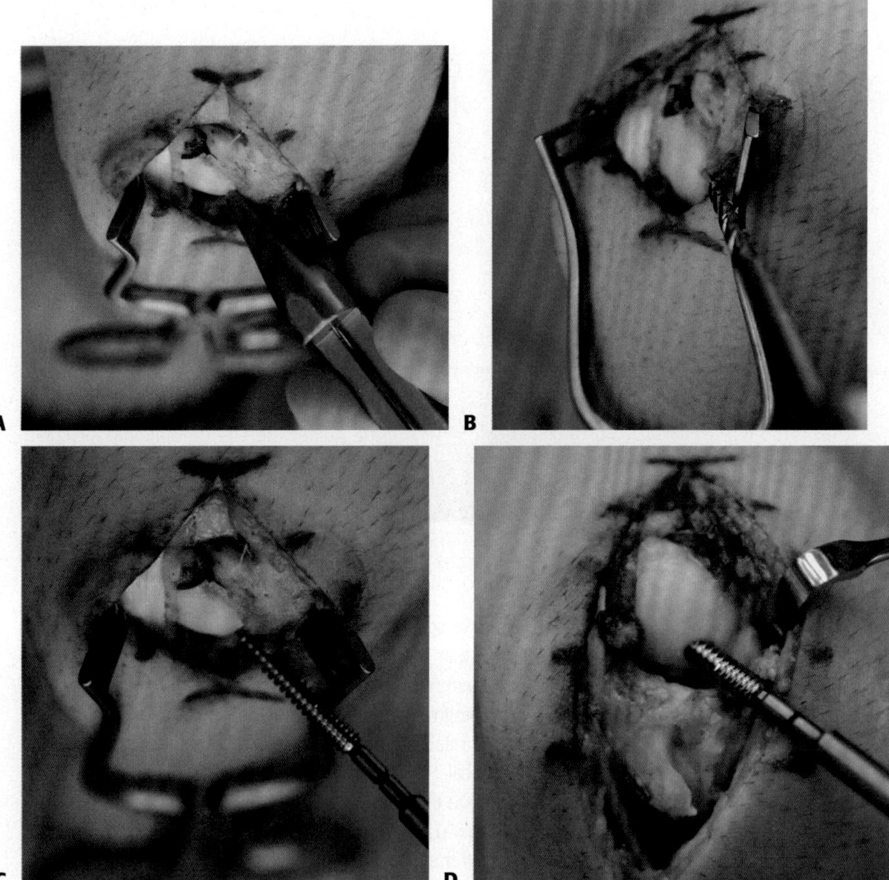

TECH FIG 4 • **A.** Determining the appropriate screw length. **B.** Reaming with the cannulated reamer. **C,D.** Insertion of the screw. **A–D:** Top is distal, bottom is proximal, left is radial, and right is ulnar. (Copyright Peter J.L. Jebson, MD.)

Open Volar Approach

Exposure

- Radially, deviate the wrist and palpate the scaphoid tubercle.
- Make a 3- to 4-cm incision centered over the scaphoid tubercle, directed distally toward the base of the thumb and proximally over the flexor carpi radialis (FCR) tendon sheath. If the superficial volar branch of the radial artery is encountered, cauterize it at the level of the wrist flexion crease.
- Open the FCR sheath, and retract the tendon ulnarly. Open the floor of the sheath distally to expose the underlying volar wrist capsule.
- Distally, develop the interval by splitting the origin of the thenar muscles in line with their fibers over the distal scaphoid and trapezium.
- Incise the capsule longitudinally, taking care to avoid damage to the underlying articular cartilage.
  - Proximally, divide the thickened radiolunate and radioscaphocapitate ligaments to allow exposure of the proximal scaphoid pole.
- Identify the scaphotrapezial joint with a Freer elevator and bluntly expose it.
  - Dissection over the radial aspect of the scaphoid is limited to avoid injury to the dorsal ridge vessel.
- Define and clear the fracture site by irrigation, sharp excision of periosteal flaps, and curetting of debris and hematoma.
  - Assess the instability of the fracture by wrist manipulation.
  - It is critical to identify any bone loss, as compression during screw placement can result in an iatrogenic malunion.

Fracture Reduction and Fixation

- Obtain correct fracture alignment through longitudinal traction, followed by wrist manipulation.
  - An anatomic reduction may also be achieved by direct manipulation of the fragments with a dental pick, pointed reduction forceps, or joystick Kirschner wires.
- Place a provisional 0.045-inch Kirschner wire to secure the reduction. Insert the wire in a retrograde manner from volar distal to dorsal proximal, gaining fixation in the proximal pole.
  - It is critical to place this wire such that it does not interfere with subsequent screw placement which should be placed in the central axis of the scaphoid.
- The central axis guidewire is placed, taking into consideration all the factors detailed previously.
- To gain the needed dorsal starting position in the distal scaphoid pole, displace the trapezium dorsally with an elevator or resect a small portion of the proximal volar trapezium with a rongeur (**TECH FIG 5**).

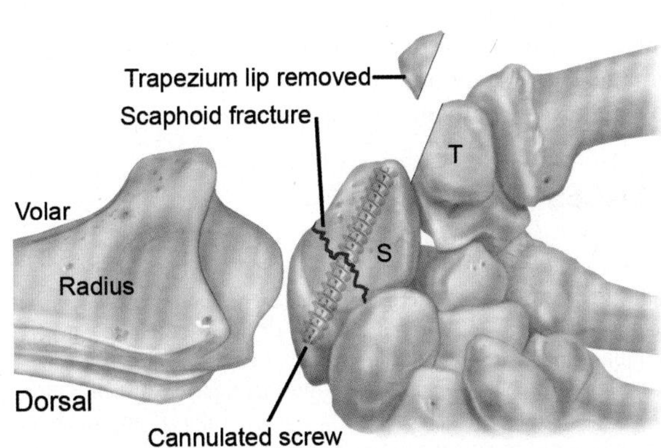

- The cannulated compression screw may be inserted using a freehand technique or a commercial device, which simultaneously facilitates fracture reduction and guidewire positioning.
  - Fluoroscopy is invaluable during wire and screw insertion and to confirm accurate placement and fracture reduction as described earlier.
- Precisely repair the volar wrist capsule and radiolunate and radioscaphocapitate ligaments with permanent suture.

TECH FIG 5 • Accurate insertion of a screw via the volar approach usually requires partial resection or dorsal displacement of the volar trapezium to expose the distal scaphoid.

PEARLS AND PITFALLS

Injury to the scaphoid blood supply	■ Meticulous limited dissection of the capsule. Avoid any dissection on the dorsal ridge of the scaphoid.
Malpositioning of guidewire	■ Pronate and flex wrist during the dorsal approach to allow appropriate trajectory. Confirm position on multiple views to ensure insertion in the central axis of the scaphoid.
Screw position	■ Select a screw that is 4 mm shorter than measured length unless fracture fragments are separated; in that case, choose a shorter screw.
Reduction of an unstable fracture	■ Perpendicular Kirschner wire joysticks inserted into the proximal and distal scaphoid fragments are useful to obtain a reduction. ■ Provisional derotational Kirschner wires placed before screw insertion can be used to stabilize fragments during screw insertion. ■ Recognize comminution and bone loss to avoid inadvertent shortening or malreduction with screw compression.
Small proximal pole fracture	■ Use of a small screw (ie, mini-Acutrak 2) may be necessary to prevent comminution of the proximal fragment. ■ Confirm central axis screw position, especially in the proximal pole.

POSTOPERATIVE CARE

- The patient is immobilized in a below-elbow volar splint and discharged to home with instructions on strict limb elevation and frequent digital range-of-motion exercises.
- At 2 weeks, the patient returns for suture removal. Range-of-motion exercises are begun, and a removable forearm-based thumb splint is worn. The splint is discontinued at 6 weeks postoperatively.
  - If the fracture involves the proximal pole or if significant comminution was noted at surgery and there is concern regarding stability of the fixation, immobilization in a short-arm cast for 6 to 10 weeks is indicated. Typically, such fractures take longer to achieve union.
- After cast removal, a formal supervised therapy program is initiated to achieve satisfactory range of motion, strength, and function.
- Fracture healing is assessed at 2, 6, and 12 weeks postoperatively with plain radiography. Fracture union is defined as progressive obliteration of the fracture and clear trabeculation across the fracture site (**FIG 2**).
- If there is any question regarding fracture union, a CT scan is obtained at 3 months postoperatively or before the patient is allowed to return to unrestricted sporting activities.

OUTCOMES

- Surgical fixation of unstable, displaced scaphoid fractures has been increasingly advocated, given the unsatisfactory outcomes that have been reported with nonoperative management.[2,4,17] Rigid internal fixation allows for early physiotherapy throughout the healing phase, a more rapid time to union, improved range of motion, and rapid functional recovery.[5,10,19,29] Several studies have reported a high rate of union and excellent clinical outcome with minimal morbidity using both limited open and percutaneous techniques.[1,3,5,10,26,29]
- Clinical and biomechanical studies have also recently documented the importance of screw position after fixation of

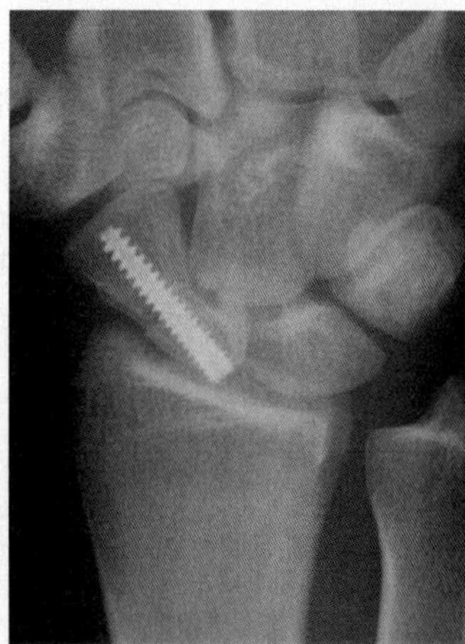

FIG 2 • A healed scaphoid waist fracture after ORIF via the dorsal approach. Although the screw may appear slightly long, both the proximal scaphoid and distal scaphoid are covered with hyaline cartilage not detected on diagnostic imaging. (Copyright Peter J.L. Jebson, MD.)

scaphoid fractures.[7,25] Central placement of the screw is biomechanically advantageous, with greater stiffness and load to failure.[7] Trumble et al[25] demonstrated more rapid progression to union with central screw position in cases of scaphoid nonunion.

- A volar approach has traditionally been used for screw insertion. However, recent studies have raised potential concerns regarding eccentric screw placement and damage to the scaphotrapezial articulation with this approach.[29]
- Our preferred technique for fixation of a scaphoid proximal pole or waist region fracture involves a limited dorsal approach with compression screw fixation.[19] The technique is simple and permits visualization of a reliable starting point for screw placement within the central axis of the scaphoid, offering a significant potential advantage over the volar approach. We recently reported our clinical experience in a consecutive series of nondisplaced scaphoid waist fractures.[3]

COMPLICATIONS

- Postoperative wound infections are rare and can be prevented with routine preoperative antibiotic prophylaxis, thorough wound irrigation, and appropriate soft tissue management.
- Intraoperative technical problems
  - Inadvertent bending or breakage of the guidewire can occur if the wrist is dorsiflexed with the wire in position or during drilling before screw insertion.
  - Care should be taken to confirm that the screw is fully seated beneath the articular cartilage to avoid prominence and erosion of the distal radius articular surface. Similarly, failure to carefully judge accurate screw length intraoperatively can result in prominence within the scaphotrapezial articulation.
- Nonunion with or without AVN can occur despite compression screw fixation, particularly with a proximal pole or displaced waist fracture. Stripping of the dorsal ridge vasculature should be avoided. Supplemental cancellous bone graft from the distal radius may be used at the time of fixation of a displaced or comminuted fracture if desired.
- Other potential but rare complications
  - Hypertrophic scar
  - Injury to the dorsal branches of the superficial radial nerve
  - Damage to the scaphotrapezial articulation
  - Proximal pole fragment comminution

REFERENCES

1. Adams BD, Blair WF, Reagan DS, et al. Technical factors related to Herbert screw fixation. J Hand Surg Am 1988;13(6):893–899.
2. Amadio PC, Moran SL. Fractures of the carpal bones. In: Green D, Hotchkiss R, Pederson WC, eds. Green's Operative Hand Surgery, ed 5. Philadelphia: Churchill Livingstone, 2005:711–740.
3. Bedi A, Jebson PJ, Hayden RJ, et al. Internal fixation of acute, nondisplaced scaphoid waist fractures via a limited dorsal approach: an assessment of radiographic and functional outcomes. J Hand Surg Am 2007;32(3):326–333.
4. Burge P. Closed cast treatment of scaphoid fractures. Hand Clin 2001;17:541–552.
5. Chen AC, Chao EK, Hung SS, et al. Percutaneous screw fixation for unstable scaphoid fractures. J Trauma 2005;59:184–187.
6. Dias JJ, Taylor M, Thompson J, et al. Radiographic signs of union of scaphoid fractures. An analysis of inter-observer agreement and reproducibility. J Bone Joint Surg Br 1988;70(2):299–301.
7. Dodds SD, Panjabi MM, Slade JF III. Screw fixation of scaphoid fractures: a biomechanical assessment of screw length and screw augmentation. J Hand Surg Am 2006;31(3):405–413.
8. Gelberman RH, Menon J. The vascularity of the scaphoid bone. J Hand Surg Am 1980;5(5):508–513.
9. Gelberman RH, Wolock BS, Siegel DB. Fractures and non-unions of the carpal scaphoid. J Bone Joint Surg Am 1989;71A:1560–1565.
10. Gellman H, Caputo RJ, Carter V, et al. Comparison of short and long thumb-spica casts for non-displaced fractures of the carpal scaphoid. J Bone Joint Surg Am 1989;71(3):354–357.
11. Heinzelmann AD, Archer G, Bindra RR. Anthropometry of the human scaphoid. J Hand Surg Am 2007;32(7):1005–1008.
12. Horii E, Nakamura R, Watanabe K, et al. Scaphoid fracture as a "puncher's fracture." J Orthop Trauma 1994;8:107–110.
13. Jørgsholm P, Thomsen NO, Björkman A, et al. The incidence of intrinsic and extrinsic ligament injuries in scaphoid waist fractures. J Hand Surg Am 2010;35(3):368–374.
14. Kerluke L, McCabe SJ. Nonunion of the scaphoid: a critical analysis of recent natural history studies. J Hand Surg Am 1993;18(1):1–3.
15. Kozin SH. Incidence, mechanism, and natural history of scaphoid fractures. Hand Clin 2001;17:515–524.
16. Kukla C, Gaebler C, Breitenseher MJ, et al. Occult fractures of the scaphoid. The diagnostic usefulness and indirect economic repercussions of radiography versus magnetic resonance scanning. J Hand Surg Br 1997;22(6):810–813.
17. Leslie IJ, Dickson RA. The fractured carpal scaphoid. Natural history and factors influencing outcome. J Bone Joint Surg Br 1981; 63-B(2):225–230.
18. Mack GR, Bosse MJ, Gelberman RH, et al. The natural history of scaphoid nonunion. J Bone Joint Surg Am 1984;66(4):504–509.
19. Martus J, Bedi A, Jebson PJL. Cannulated variable pitch compression screw fixation of scaphoid fractures using a limited dorsal approach. Tech Hand Up Extrem Surg 2005;9:202–206.
20. Ritchie JV, Munter DW. Emergency department evaluation and treatment of wrist injuries. Emerg Med Clin North Am 1999;17: 823–842.
21. Ruby LK, Stinson J, Belsky MR. The natural history of scaphoid non-union. A review of fifty-five cases. J Bone Joint Surg Am 1985;67(3):428–432.
22. Schädel-Höpfner M, Junge A, Böhringer G. Scapholunate ligament injury occurring with scaphoid fracture—a rare coincidence? J Hand Surg Br 2005;30:137–142.
23. Thavarajah D, Syed T, Shah Y, et al. Does scaphoid bone bruising lead to occult fractures? A prospective study of 50 patients. Injury 2011;42:1303–1306.

24. Thomsen L, Falcone MO. Lesions of the scapholunate ligament associated with minimally displaced or non-displaced fractures of the scaphoid waist. Which incidence? Chir Main 2012;31:234–238.
25. Trumble TE, Clarke T, Kreder HJ. Non-union of the scaphoid: treatment with cannulated screws compared with treatment with Herbert screws. J Bone Joint Surg Am 1996;78(12):1829–1837.
26. Trumble TE, Gilbert M, Murray LW, et al. Displaced scaphoid fractures treated with open reduction and internal fixation with a cannulated screw. J Bone Joint Surg Am 2000;82(5):633–641.
27. Waizenegger M, Wastie ML, Barton NJ, et al. Scintigraphy in the evaluation of the "clinical" scaphoid fracture. J Hand Surg Br 1994;19(6):750–753.
28. Wong TC, Yip TH, Wu WC. Carpal ligament injuries with acute scaphoid fractures: a combined wrist injury. J Hand Surg Br 2005;30:415–418.
29. Yip HS, Wu WC, Chang RY, et al. Percutaneous cannulated screw fixation of acute scaphoid waist fracture. J Hand Surg Br 2002;27(1):42–46.

Volar Wedge Bone Grafting and Internal Fixation of Scaphoid Nonunions

Evan D. Collins

DEFINITION

- The scaphoid is the most commonly fractured carpal bone in the wrist. Scaphoid fractures that fail to heal after 6 months of treatment are categorized as nonunions and represent about 5% to 10% of all scaphoid fractures.
- Untreated nonunions reportedly lead to progressive arthrosis and wrist pain.[6]
- Volar wedge bone grafting is an effective surgical technique in the treatment of certain scaphoid nonunions based on the following:
  - Location of the fracture
  - Degree of the deformity
  - Vascularity of the scaphoid
- This general technique can also be adapted to increase its versatility.

ANATOMY

- Nearly 80% of the scaphoid's surface is covered by articular cartilage.[6]
- Through ligamentous connections, the scaphoid serves as the bridge or link between the proximal and distal rows (**FIG 1**). Due to these strong tethers proximally and distally, it is highly susceptible to an acute fracture after a fall on an outstretched hand.[18]
- Other key factors that influence scaphoid fracture healing are its tenuous vascular supply and its unique bony architecture.
  - The vulnerable vascularity of the scaphoid, especially the proximal pole, is well described in the literature.[8,14–16,20] This is the result of the scaphoid's retrograde blood supply, with approximately 70% of the vascular supply provided through the dorsal ridge vessel and 30% through branches to the scaphoid tubercle (at the level of the radiocarpal joint via superficial palmar branch perforators off the radial artery).
  - The complex geometry of the bone makes it difficult to anatomically reduce the bone fragments.

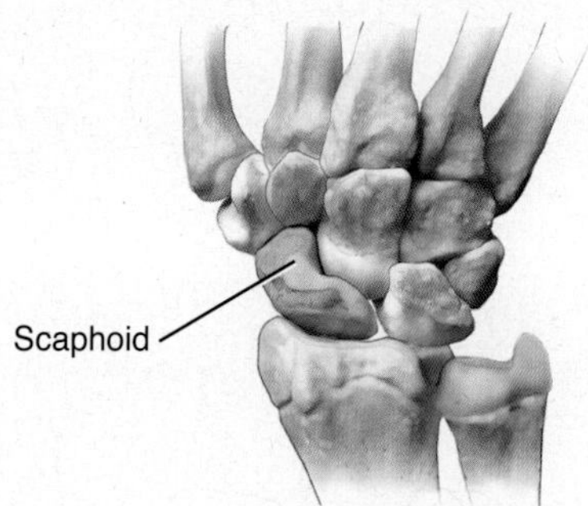

FIG 1 • Anatomy of the wrist joint. The scaphoid bridges the proximal and distal carpal rows and is largely covered by articular cartilage.

PATHOGENESIS

- Although there may be a variety of reasons for the development of a scaphoid nonunion, a fractured scaphoid usually fails to heal for three primary reasons:
  - The fracture is either undetected or untreated within the first 4 weeks after the injury.
  - The location of the fracture is proximal, resulting in poor vascularity of the most proximal fragment.
  - The fracture is displaced more than 1 mm.

NATURAL HISTORY

- Scaphoid nonunion advanced collapse (SNAC), described in the literature, is a predictable sequence of changes that occurs as a result of scaphoid nonunion leading to wrist arthrosis, often associated with pain and limitation of motion.[4,5]
- In studying patients with painful wrists over a 15-year period to determine who will develop symptoms, it is evident that the incidence of symptomatic wrist pathology requiring reconstruction is significantly higher for scaphoid nonunions that have gone untreated.[1]
- Techniques used to detect an acute scaphoid fracture and its susceptibility to nonunion, wrist pain, and corresponding arthrosis have been discussed in great detail in the literature.[14,15,20]

PATIENT HISTORY AND PHYSICAL FINDINGS

- The patient who presents with a scaphoid nonunion is usually a man between the ages of 18 and 35 years.
- Unrecognized injuries in adolescence may present with pain related to early SNAC wrist arthrosis in the middle-aged adult.
- Patients generally complain of wrist pain that limits range of motion or hinders activities such as push-ups, weightlifting, or simple daily tasks such as opening a door. Moderate to heavy pinch and grip pain have also been described.
- A specific event resulting in the original scaphoid fracture years before is rarely cited by the patient on presentation.
- Consistent physical examination findings include subtle tenderness in the region of the scaphoid tubercle or the anatomic snuffbox, limited wrist extension compared to the contralateral side, and localized pain on the radial side along the radiostyloid or scaphoid with loaded wrist extension. If arthrosis has developed, soft tissue swelling may be noted over the dorsal and radial wrist.

IMAGING AND OTHER DIAGNOSTIC STUDIES

- Standard radiographs include posteroanterior (PA), lateral, and scaphoid oblique 45- and 60-degree pronated views (**FIG 2**). Such views
  - Confirm the diagnosis
  - Provide information regarding displacement, angulation, shortening, and the presence of a "humpback deformity"
  - Reveal compensatory carpal instability, dorsal intercalated segment instability (DISI)
- As part of a treatment algorithm, dividing scaphoid fracture nonunions into either proximal, middle, or distal is very helpful.
- Other factors considered in diagnostic assessment include previous wrist fracture or sprain later becoming symptomatic; tenderness on the scaphoid tubercle or in the anatomic snuffbox; localized pain to the radial side of the wrist along the radiostyloid or scaphoid itself, with a loaded dorsiflexed wrist; and pinching and heavy grip pain.
- Once the scaphoid nonunion is diagnosed, a computed tomography (CT) scan performed in the plane of the scaphoid helps define bony architecture. Sagittal and coronal images are particularly helpful in characterizing the nonunion site and its orientation, displacement, and degree of bone loss.
  - Scaphoid collapse (or humpback deformity) is most clearly determined by measuring the lateral intrascaphoid angle on the sagittal CT views.
- Magnetic resonance imaging (MRI), especially when combined with intravenous gadolinium, is helpful in defining the presence or absence of osteonecrosis and any associated ligamentous or cartilaginous injuries. If osteonecrosis of the proximal fragment is seen, the surgeon should consider a vascularized bone graft[10] (see Chap. 38) rather than the nonvascularized grafting procedure described in this chapter.

DIFFERENTIAL DIAGNOSIS

- De Quervain tendinitis
- Scaphotrapeziotrapezoidal arthritis
- Scaphoid lunate instability, static, and dynamic
- Radial styloid fracture
- Trapezial ridge fracture

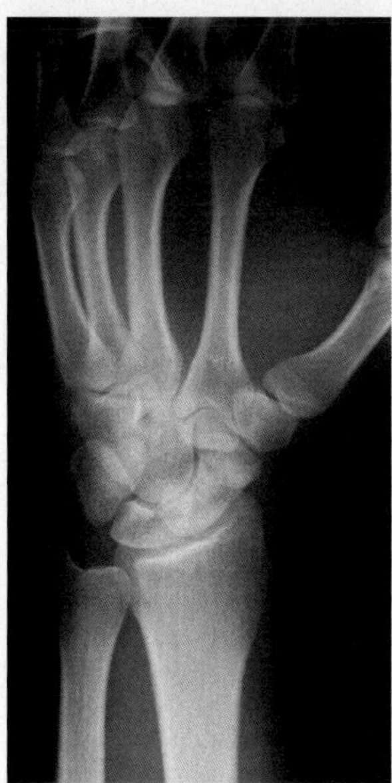

FIG 2 • An oblique view of a scaphoid that has not healed.

NONOPERATIVE MANAGEMENT

- Surgery is generally indicated for established scaphoid nonunions that are displaced and symptomatic because of the strong likelihood that radiocarpal arthrosis may develop with this type of persistent nonunion.[18,20]
- Nonoperative management may be appropriate for minimally symptomatic scaphoid nonunions. All factors should be taken into consideration when determining the most appropriate treatment: Scaphoid nonunion alone is not an absolute reason for surgery.[12]

SURGICAL MANAGEMENT

- Volar wedge bone grafting is the preferred surgical technique for treatment of a scaphoid nonunion without osteonecrosis but with shortening, an increased intrascaphoid angle causing a humpback deformity, and concomitant carpal collapse. Although many scaphoid nonunions without deformity can be effectively treated with the described procedure, other approaches and grafting techniques that are less invasive may be an option, especially for proximal pole nonunions.[2]
- Determining which bone graft is necessary depends on how much shortening is anticipated.[3]
  - The benefits of distal radius bone grafting include its location within the same surgical field and can be harvested as a vascularized or nonvascularized graft. One important disadvantage is the creation of a relatively large defect and stress riser within the distal radius. Also, it is not possible to obtain a bicortical or a tricortical piece of bone for a more structural bone graft.
  - Iliac crest bone graft may be harvested in large quantities and as a bicortical or tricortical piece of bone. It is relatively simple to procure and has a long history of success in such cases, a standard by which all others are currently measured. The disadvantages of this type of bone graft include a separate incision with associated morbidity as well as a reported risk of cutaneous nerve injuries. Also, it cannot be converted to a vascularized pedicle bone graft.
- When an MRI reveals the presence of osteonecrosis, a vascularized procedure should be considered (see Chap. 38).[14,15,20]

Preoperative Planning

- After assessing all diagnostic studies, including plain films, MRI and CT scans, the type of bone graft is determined.
- Two types of fixation screws can be used.
  - One type of screw has a smooth shank and two threaded heads. This screw is strong and creates high compression but may not be appropriate for all nonunions. The scaphoid nonunion fragments must be large enough to ensure that no threads of the screw cross into the bone graft site and yet the screw can be completely buried within the bone.
  - The other type of compression screw uses a deferential pitch between the proximal and distal portion of the screw. This screw may be more versatile, although it lacks compression strength compared to the above mentioned screw.
  - If compression screws are not deemed appropriate for the type of nonunion that exists, multiple K-wires can be used.

- A regional anesthetic block is used for most patients and is helpful for alleviating postoperative pain. When iliac crest grafting is chosen, additional general anesthesia is needed.
- All radiographic studies are reviewed and brought to the operating room for reevaluation during the case.

Positioning

- The patient is placed in the supine position with the upper extremity positioned on a hand table.
- If an ipsilateral iliac crest bone graft is used, the hip on the same side as the affected hand is prepared and draped. A small bump is placed under the hip for patients with significant adipose tissue.
- A tourniquet is applied to the proximal arm.

Approach

- The location of the scaphoid nonunion helps determine the surgical approach. Wedge bone grafting of a waist nonunion is performed using a standard volar approach.
- For proximal pole fractures with evidence of osteonecrosis, a dorsal or dorsal radial approach with use of a vascularized bone graft should be considered.[13,19]

Volar Wedge Bone Grafting Using Distal Radius Bone Graft and Intraosseous Compression Screw Fixation

Incision and Initial Dissection

- An incision is drawn over the flexor carpi radialis (FCR) tendon and extended distally between the glabrous skin of the thenar eminence toward the distal pole of the scaphoid. The incision should be angled across the wrist flexion crease (**TECH FIG 1A**).
- After exsanguination, the skin is incised, and the FCR tendon is identified. Distally in the wound, a volar branch of the radial artery is often sacrificed to gain exposure (**TECH FIG 1B**).
- The floor of the FCR tendon is sharply incised over the entire course of the incision, and the digital flexors and median nerve are swept ulnarly. They are carefully protected throughout the case. A blunt Wheatlander is used to maintain visualization of this interval between the radial artery and the FCR tendon.
  - The volar extrinsic ligaments, the radioscaphocapitate (RSC) and long radiolunate (LRL), are identified and precisely incised in line with the incision. Much of the LRL and a portion of the RSC are left intact, helping to stabilize the proximal pole (**TECH FIG 1C**).
    - This stability facilitates the reduction of the distal fragment to the proximal fragment.
    - Preserving this ligamentous support also helps maintain fracture reduction during the placement of an intraosseous compression screw by counteracting the torque created during screw insertion.
- Deep dissection proceeds to the scaphotrapezial joint. This interval is exposed using a transverse capsular incision allowing for later insertion of the intraosseous screw.
- The articulation between the scaphoid and capitate is carefully exposed. This visualization is important to confirm reduction of the scaphoid fragments.
- During exposure, it is critical to avoid dissection over the distal dorsoradial scaphoid to avoid interrupting the contribution by the dorsal ridge vessel.

Nonunion Exposure and Preparation

- A no. 64 Beaver blade and Freer elevator are used to define the location of the nonunion and the borders of the scaphoid itself. Time spent here makes eventual reduction and bone graft placement simpler (**TECH FIG 2A,B**).

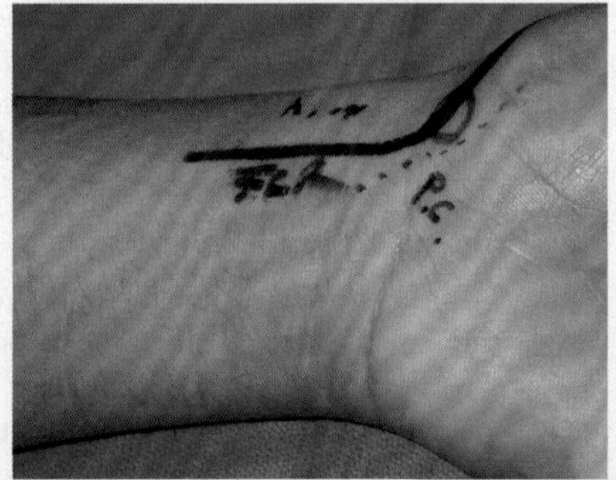
A

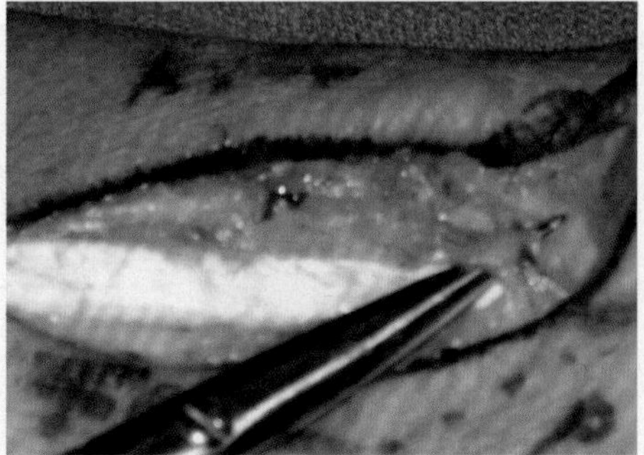
B

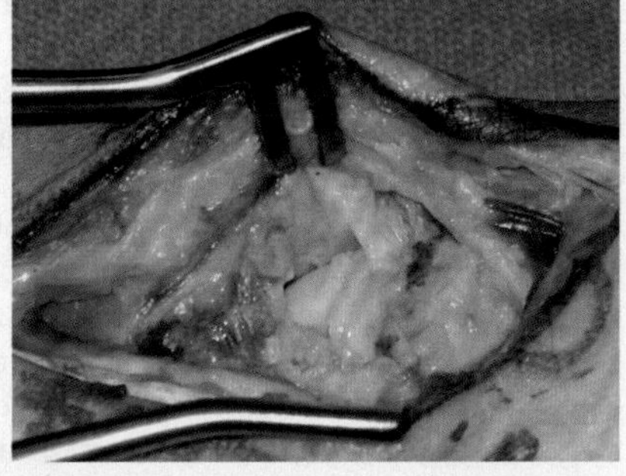
C

TECH FIG 1 • **A.** The skin incision is marked out. **B.** The volar branch of the radial artery is often sacrificed to gain exposure. **C.** After the floor of the FCR is longitudinally divided, a portion of the RSC ligament is visualized.

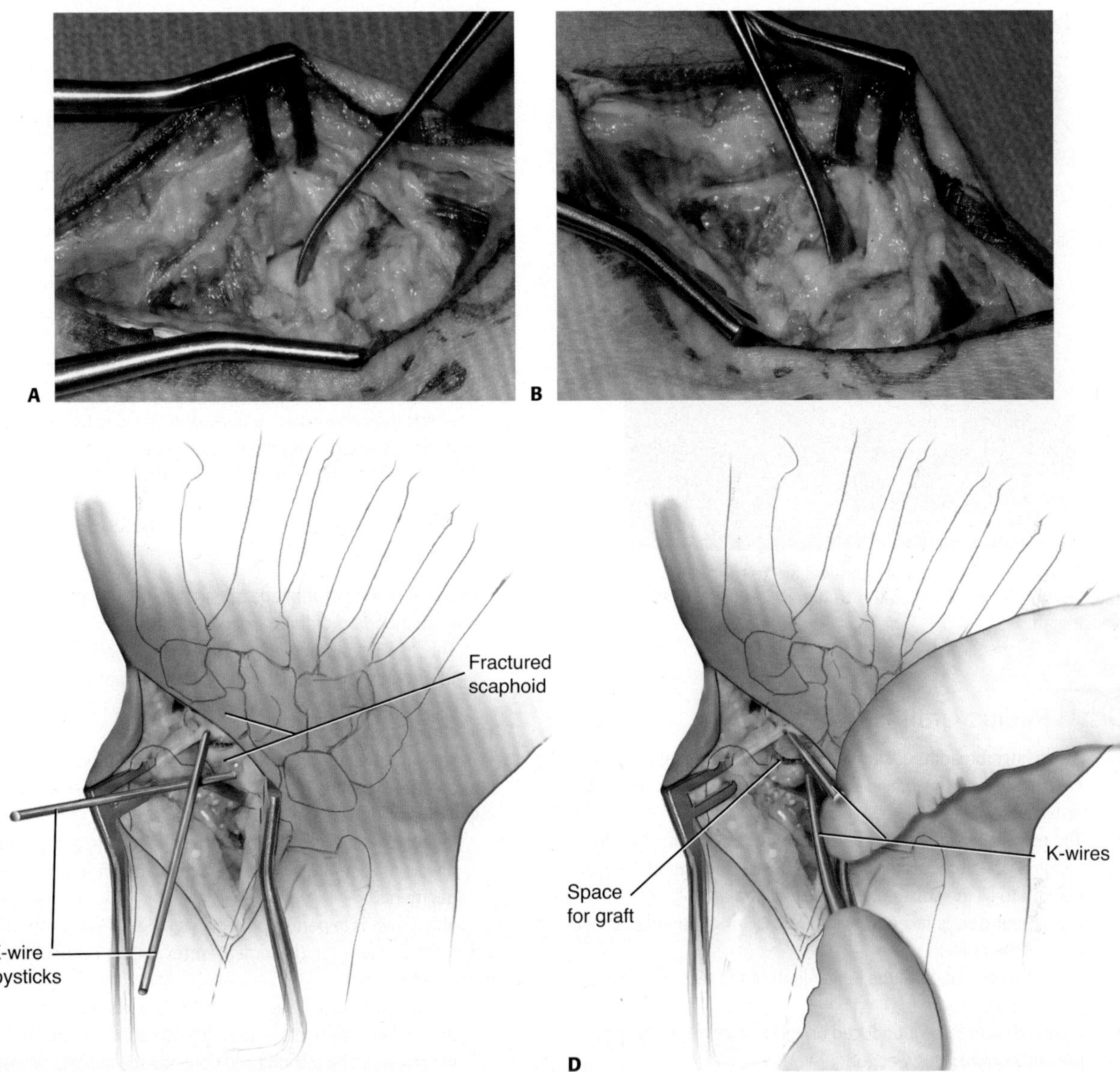

TECH FIG 2 • **A,B.** A Freer elevator identifies the nonunion site. **C.** K-wires are used as joysticks to control the scaphoid proximal and distal fragments. **D.** Manipulation of the K-wires allows for access to the nonunion site for débridement and then graft placement.

- Two joystick K-wires are placed, one angled proximally in the proximal fragment and one angled distally in the distal fragment (**TECH FIG 2C**).
  - These K-wires facilitate manipulation of the fragments and therefore access to the nonunion site for débridement (**TECH FIG 2D**).
- The proximal and distal poles are examined carefully for osteolysis and sclerosis. A small curette or rongeur is used for débridement and removal of intervening fibrous tissue. Débridement is complete once good punctate bleeding is noted. In some situations, deflating the tourniquet temporarily can be of value in assessing viability of the fragments.

Fracture Reduction and Preliminary Stabilization

- By bringing the joysticks/crossed K-wires into a more parallel position (relative to one another) and rotating the distal K-wire into slight supination, the humpback deformity is improved, and the initial fracture reduction is accomplished (**TECH FIG 3**).
- A retrograde K-wire may be inserted along the longitudinal axis of the scaphoid to temporarily hold the reduction.
  - If placed in an appropriately eccentric position, this K-wire may serve effectively as a derotation K-wire during screw insertion and yet remain out of the path of the screw.
- Restoration of scaphoid length and anatomic reduction of the fragments are best assessed by direct visualization and fluoroscopy.
  - Lateral images will reveal correction of the DISI deformity.
  - PA images document proper length of the scaphoid and determine if the Gilula lines are reestablished.[9]
- The size of the volar wedge graft needed to maintain the reduction is now determined based on the volar defect noted after the reduction is accomplished.

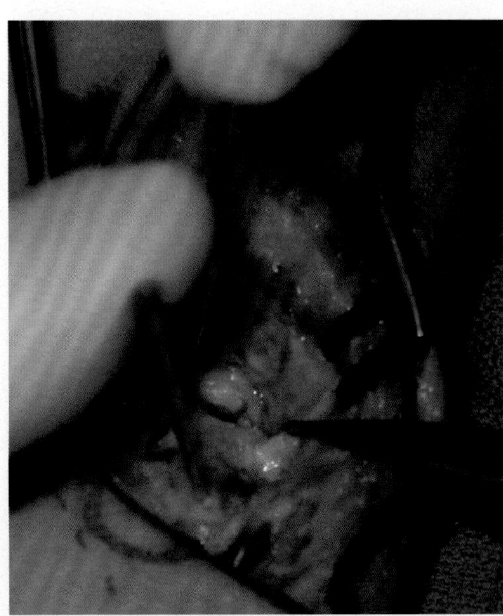

TECH FIG 3 • The scaphoid joysticks are used to reduce the fracture, and the length is estimated to determine the size of the volar wedge graft.

Distal Radius Graft Harvest

- A two-fingerbreadth incision is made more proximally than initially described. This provides the necessary access to the volar distal radius.
- The pronator quadratus is elevated using cautery, and the distal radius is perforated using K-wires to outline the size of the graft needed to fill the volar defect in the scaphoid.
  - Great care is taken to avoid destabilizing the radial cortex of the radius.
  - The orientation of the longer limb of the rectangular graph is distal proximal.
- A curved osteotome introduced on three sides allows harvest of the corticocancellous wedge.
- A curette is then used to harvest as much cancellous bone as necessary.

Graft Contouring and Insertion

- The volar cortical defect in the reduced scaphoid is "regularized" using a small water-cooled sagittal saw or a fine rongeur.
  - Very little bone is removed from the fracture fragments to create a standard-shaped trough.
  - Creating such a "regular" defect makes insertion of the wedge graft easier and more secure.
- The same saw or rongeur is used to shape the corticocancellous graft to match the regularized defect.
- The prepared proximal and distal fragments are packed with cancellous bone, and the corticocancellous graft is tapped into place (**TECH FIG 4A**).
  - Before graft insertion, the longitudinal K-wire, whether it is the K-wire placed to maintain reduction or the K-wire over which the cannulated compression screw is to be placed, is withdrawn into the distal pole and then reinserted after placement of the graft into the trough.

Cannulated Intraosseous Compression Screw Fixation

- At the level of the scaphotrapezial joint, a small rongeur is used to remove a portion of the trapezial lip.[20]
  - This facilitates placement of the K-wire and screw down the center longitudinal access of the scaphoid. A center screw position on all fluoroscopic views has been demonstrated to lead to increased healing rates.
- A K-wire from the compression screw system is then inserted in a retrograde direction (distal to proximal) into the center of the scaphoid, perpendicular to the fracture line.
  - If the K-wire is not perpendicular to the fracture, compression generated from the screw may malreduce the fragments.
- Once the K-wire is in perfect position, as judged fluoroscopically, and is fixed in the far (proximal) cortex of the scaphoid, the length is measured.
  - Factors such as cartilage thickness and distance between the fracture fragments is taken into account. It is critical that the screw not be too long and not enter the radiocarpal joint.
- Although some surgeons advocate advancing the K-wire into the distal radius after the measurement is taken so that the wire

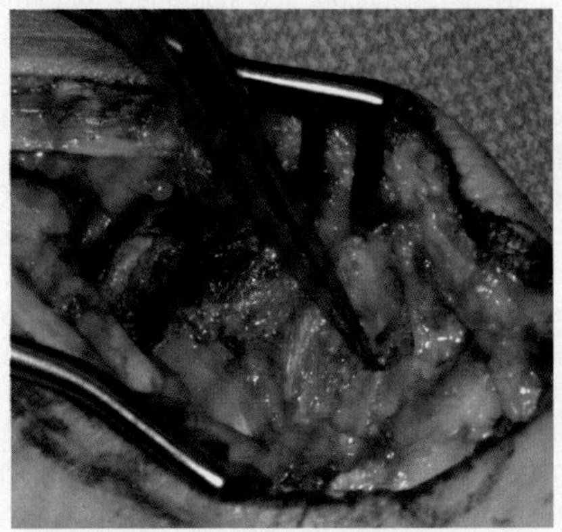

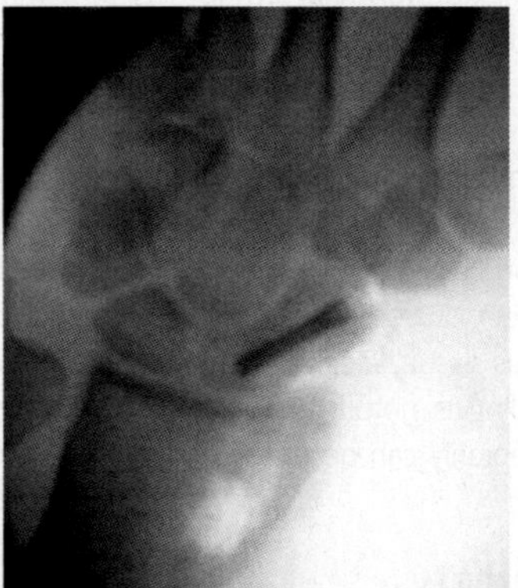

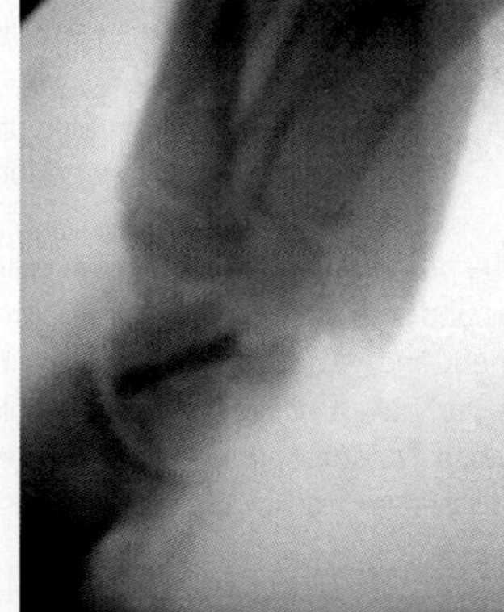

TECH FIG 4 • **A.** The wedge placement is complete. **B,C.** PA and lateral views of the compression bone screw after harvesting the bone graft from the distal radius.

remains in position during drilling, that practice is dangerous. It is preferable to leave the K-wire in the scaphoid.
  - Advancing the K-wire can result in cutting the guidewire during drilling or screw placement (particularly with a second-generation compression screw that has cutting flutes at the distal end).
- If not already present, an eccentric K-wire is placed to maintain the reduction during screw insertion.
- Under fluoroscopic guidance, a cannulated drill is used followed, in some cases, by a cannulated bone tap.
  - Especially during drilling, the surgeon must be careful to remain parallel with the wire.
  - The corticocancellous bone graft must be visualized at all times during these procedures to make certain position is maintained. Maintaining finger pressure over the graft during screw insertion is helpful.
- Imaging confirms proper screw location, fracture reduction, and construct stability. The K-wire is removed from the cannulated screw, and the eccentric K-wire is removed (**TECH FIG 4B,C**).
- The wound is then irrigated, and the volar extrinsic ligaments are repaired precisely with permanent suture. The remainder of the joint capsule may be closed with an absorbable suture.
- Bone filler, preferably cadaver dried cancellous bone chips, can be inserted into the distal radius harvest site with a small tamp to compress and fill the defect. This potentially decreases the risk of hematoma formation. The periosteal sleeve is then closed over the distal radius with absorbable suture.
- Skin is closed using nylon suture, and the tourniquet is then deflated after placement of a thumb spica splint.

K-Wire Fixation

- If compression screw fixation is not feasible, then retrograde, nonthreaded K-wires are recommended and placed in the same manner as described earlier for the bone screw.
  - The wires should be left under the skin and removed once the bone has healed.
- K-wires provide adequate stability and may be a better fixation choice with large bone grafts as well as small proximal or distal fragments.

Iliac Crest Graft Harvest

- Rather than obtaining bone graft from the distal radius, a standard technique of harvesting bone from the iliac crest may be used.[16,20]
- A 2- to 3-cm incision is made just inferior to the superior border of the iliac crest just posterior to the anterior superior iliac spine (ASIS).
  - The incision is kept below the belt line to minimize postoperative incisional tenderness.
  - The incision is posterior to the ASIS to avoid iatrogenic nerve injury and subsequent numbness and pain over the proximal lateral thigh.
- Dissection is accomplished using cautery through the deep fascia down to the crest. The superior crest is exposed and muscles are released from a portion of the outer table using cautery and an elevator.
- A water-cooled sagittal saw and a curved osteotome are used to harvest a bicortical segment of corticocancellous graft.
  - The graft is slightly larger than the measured defect in the scaphoid.
  - The inner table is left intact.
  - The harvested outer table will be volar when the graft is placed in the scaphoid and the superior crest will be radial.
- A curette is used to harvest cancellous bone graft.
- The wound is copiously irrigated and temporarily packed with thrombin-soaked Gelfoam while attention is redirected to the scaphoid.
- After the scaphoid is reconstructed, the Gelfoam is removed and the wound is again irrigated.
- If indicated, a small suction drain is placed below the fascia.
- The wound is closed in layers with a running locking stitch used for the fascia.
- A local anesthetic with epinephrine may be injected before harvest of the graft or after closure.

PEARLS AND PITFALLS

When MRI reveals osteonecrosis in a scaphoid nonunion	■ Volar wedge bone grafting and internal fixation is the treatment option that is most effective when applied to scaphoid waist fractures, distal-third fractures of the scaphoid without osteonecrosis, or scaphoid waist fractures with concomitant carpal collapse and a nondissociated DISI pattern. When osteonecrosis is present, a vascularized procedure may be preferable.
Surgeon prefers an adaptable graft should physical findings during the procedure reveal osteonecrosis not revealed on MRI	■ The advantage of harvesting from the distal radius rather than the iliac crest exists when the MRI is inconsistent with physical examination findings during the procedure. Harvesting from the distal radius allows the surgeon to use a modified pedicle technique using the pronator quadratus and the periosteum of the distal radius and place it into the volar defect as a vascularized bone graft if necessary.[20]
Fixation for greatest chance of bone healing	■ Although either compression bone screws or K-wires can be used as effective fixation in this procedure, compression screws are believed to improve chances of overall bone healing.[7,11,18]

POSTOPERATIVE CARE

- When a screw is placed for internal fixation, a thumb spica splint is applied after the procedure.
- The patient returns for a follow-up visit 10 days after surgery. During this visit, the hand is examined for swelling and sutures may be removed.
- A thumb spica, short-arm cast is applied, leaving the interphalangeal joint free. The patient is followed radiographically at intervals of 3 to 4 weeks.
- CT scans are the most predictable way to determine if the scaphoid has healed. This evaluation is recommended before allowing the patient to resume vigorous activities.

OUTCOMES

- Symptomatic scaphoid nonunions with shortening respond well to volar wedge bone grafting with internal fixation, particularly when scaphoid length is restored and when any bony union is achieved.
- A higher rate of bone healing is achieved when a compression bone screw is used as the internal fixation. Reported results show that internal fixation leads to better functional results than standard techniques of bone grafting.[7,11,16–18]
- Bones failing to heal after the procedure have been shown to respond well to vascularized grafts. Other options for failure to heal include partial scaphoid excision, complete scaphoid excision with four-corner fusion, proximal row carpectomy, radial styloidectomy, and complete wrist fusion.

COMPLICATIONS

- Radiographic findings may not match the findings at surgery. This affects the outcome to varying degrees, depending on the type of graft harvested.
- Persistent nonunion and osteonecrosis resulting in wrist arthrosis
- Scarring associated with repair of the capsule, causing some postoperative stiffness

REFERENCES

1. Allende BT. Osteoarthritis of the wrist secondary to non-union of the scaphoid. Int Orthop 1988;12:201–211.
2. Amadio PC, Berquist TH, Smith DK, et al. Scaphoid malunion. J Hand Surg Am 1989;14(4):679–687.
3. Barton N. Experience with scaphoid grafting. J Hand Surg Br 1997; 22(2):153–160.
4. Cooney WP III, Dobyns JH, Linscheid RL. Nonunion of the scaphoid: analysis of the results from bone grafting. J Hand Surg Am 1980;5:343–354.
5. Cooney WP, Linscheid RL, Dobyns JH. Scaphoid fractures. Problems associated with nonunion and avascular necrosis. Orthop Clin North Am 1984;15:381–391.
6. Düppe H, Johnell O, Lundborg G, et al. Long-term results of fracture of the scaphoid. A follow-up study of more than thirty years. J Bone Joint Surg Am 1994;76(2):249–252.
7. Filan SL, Herbert TJ. Herbert screw fixation of scaphoid fractures. J Bone Joint Surg Br 1996;78(4):519–529.
8. Gelberman RH, Menon J. The vascularity of the scaphoid bone. J Hand Surg Am 1980;5:508–513.
9. Gilula LA, Destouet JM, Weeks PM, et al. Roentgenographic diagnosis of the painful wrist. Clin Orthop Relat Res 1984;(187):52–64.
10. Hunter JC, Escobedo EM, Wilson AJ, et al. MR imaging of clinically suspected scaphoid fractures. AJR Am J Roentgenol 1997;168:1287–1293.
11. Inoue G, Shionoya K, Kuwahata Y. Herbert screw fixation for scaphoid nonunions. An analysis of factors influencing outcome. Clin Orthop Relat Res 1997;(343):99–106.
12. Kerluke L, McCabe SJ. Nonunion of the scaphoid: a critical analysis of recent natural history studies. J Hand Surg Am 1993;18:1–3.
13. Kuhlmann JN, Mimoun M, Boabighl A, et al. Vascularized bone graft pedicled on the volar carpal artery for non-union of the scaphoid. J Hand Surg Br 1987;12:203–210.
14. Lindström G, Nyström A. Natural history of scaphoid non-union with special reference to "asymptomatic" cases. J Hand Surg Br 1992;17:697–700.
15. Moreno R, Gupta A. Scaphoid fractures. First Hand News, a publication of the Christine M. Kleinert Institute for Hand and Microsurgery, Inc., Summer 2004.
16. Mulier T, Adrianssens N, Nijs S, et al. Scaphoid delayed unions and nonunions: a prospective study comparing different treatment methods. Folia Traumatologica Lovanienia 2003;84–93.
17. Rajagopalan BM, Squire DS, Samuels LO. Results of Herbert-screw fixation with bone-grafting for the treatment of nonunion of the scaphoid. J Bone Joint Surg Am 1999;81:48–52.
18. Ring D, Jupiter JB, Herndon JH. Acute fractures of the scaphoid. J Am Acad Orthop Surg 2000;8:225–231.
19. Sawaizumi T, Nanno M, Nanbu A, et al. Vascularised bone graft from the base of the second metacarpal for refractory nonunion of the scaphoid. J Bone Joint Surg Br 2004;86(7):1007–1012.
20. Trumble TE, Salas P, Barthel T, et al. Management of scaphoid nonunions. J Am Acad Orthop Surg 2003;11:380–391.

Vascularized Bone Grafting of Avascular Scaphoid Nonunions

37 CHAPTER

Alexander D. Mih

DEFINITION

- Scaphoid fractures account for 60% of carpal bone fractures.
- Nonunions occur in up to 15% of scaphoid fractures and often result from delayed treatment, inadequate immobilization, displacement of the fracture, or proximal pole involvement or in the setting of avascular necrosis (AVN).

ANATOMY

- The blood supply to the scaphoid travels in a distal to proximal direction and emanates from the radial artery. Intraosseous vessels traverse the scaphoid to supply the proximal pole.
- In about 30% of scaphoids, there is either a single or no vascular channel found reaching the proximal pole.
- Studies of vascularity of the distal radius have identified several sources of vascularized bone graft available for nonunion treatment.
- Animal studies of vascularized bone grafts have documented a significant increase in blood flow present when compared to nonvascularized grafts.

PATHOGENESIS

- Without adequate blood flow, the normal bone healing response cannot be completed. The scaphoid fracture site fills with fibrous connective tissue and motion persists at the site of the fracture.
- In some cases, the bone undergoes changes of AVN with cellular death, edema, and the eventual loss of trabecular architecture.
- Studies have shown that in cases in which the trabecular bone pattern has been lost, union may be difficult if not impossible to achieve.

NATURAL HISTORY

- Nonunion of the scaphoid severely alters the normal carpal biomechanics and subjects the cartilage to shear forces detrimental to its survival.

PATIENT HISTORY AND PHYSICAL FINDINGS

- Often, patients recall injuring their wrists several years before developing pain severe enough to seek medical attention.
- Patients usually complain of limited range of wrist motion and pain, often with grip or weight bearing. The patients have often significantly reduced their activity level due to persistent pain.
- In most cases, the patient will experience tenderness to palpation at the anatomic snuffbox (**FIG 1A**), the radial styloid–scaphoid joint (**FIG 1B**), or the distal pole of the scaphoid (**FIG 1C**), which is palpable on the palmar side of the wrist.
- Wrists with established scaphoid nonunions have an arc of motion that is significantly reduced from the uninvolved side, primarily in extension.

IMAGING AND OTHER DIAGNOSTIC STUDIES

- Standard radiographic studies include posteroanterior (PA), lateral, and scaphoid (ulnar deviation) views (**FIG 2**).
- Classic radiographic findings begin at the radial styloid distal pole of scaphoid interface and proceed to involve the entire scaphoid fossa, the midcarpal joint, and eventually, the entire radiocarpal articulation.
- Computed tomography (CT) is essential for determining union as well as for identifying patients in whom the normal trabecular bone pattern has been lost. Proximal pole sclerosis and absence of converging trabecular bone at the fracture site correlate to AVN.

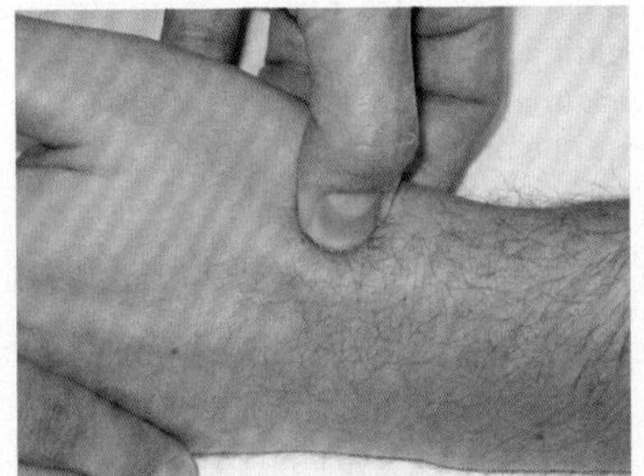

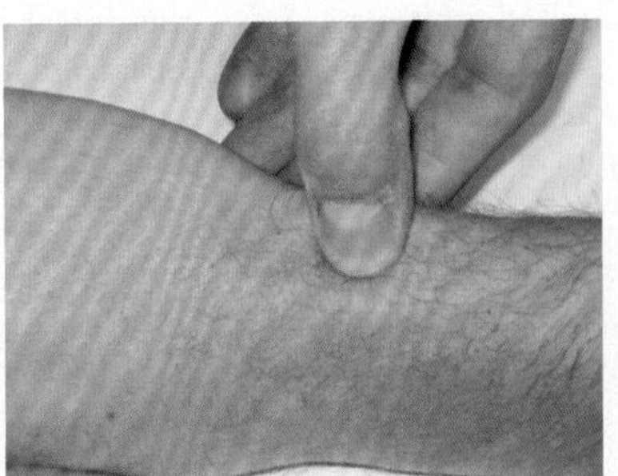

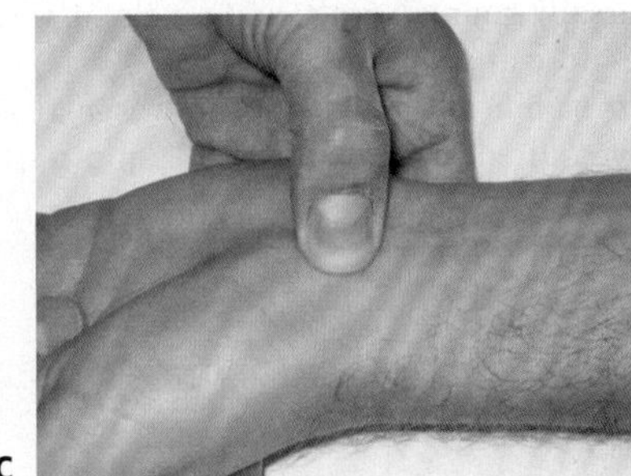

FIG 1 • **A.** Tenderness at the anatomic snuffbox is a classic finding of scaphoid nonunion. **B.** The radial styloid–scaphoid interface is the earliest site of degenerative change in scaphoid nonunions, and patients will often display tenderness at that location. **C.** The distal pole of the scaphoid is palpable at the base of the thumb on the palmar aspect of the wrist. Tenderness at this region is usually found in cases of scaphoid nonunion.

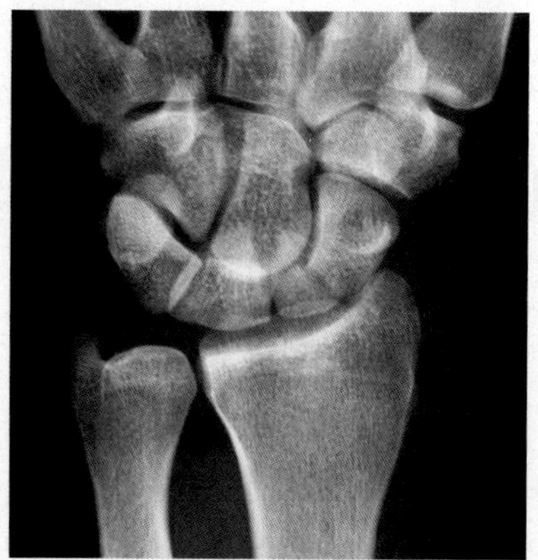
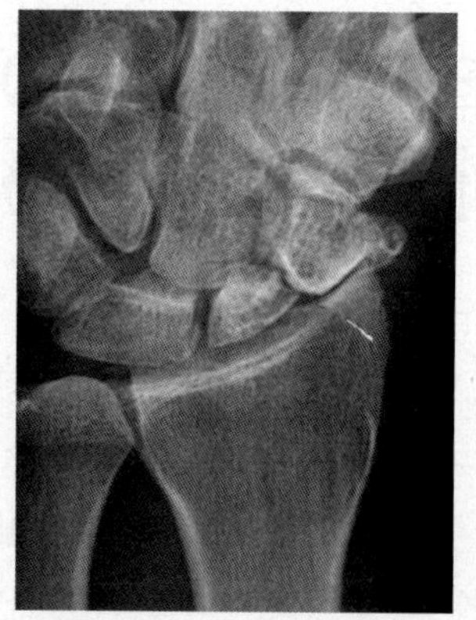
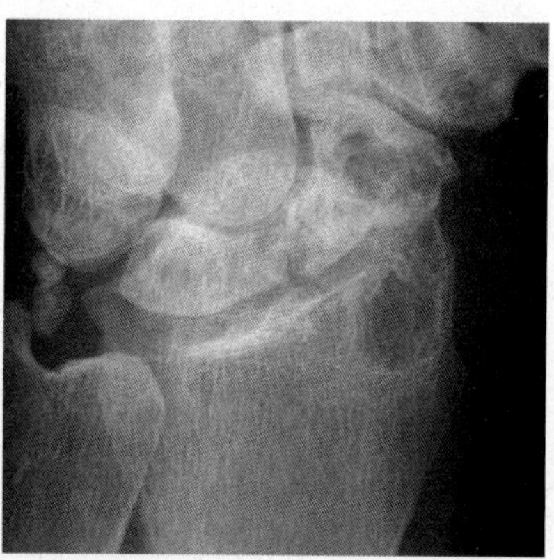

FIG 2 • **A.** Early radiographic appearance of scaphoid nonunion before degenerative change. **B.** Development of degenerative changes at the radial styloid–scaphoid interface. **C.** Advanced changes involving the entire scaphoid fossa.

- Magnetic resonance imaging (MRI) is useful in evaluating the scaphoid for vascularity, although definitive determination of avascularity may be difficult. Although contrast-enhanced MRI has shown improved sensitivity over noncontrast studies in detecting AVN, it may not be effective in detected AVN in up to 25% of cases.

DIFFERENTIAL DIAGNOSIS

- Ligamentous injury to the wrist
- Wrist synovitis
- Intraosseous ganglia
- Primary AVN of the scaphoid

NONOPERATIVE MANAGEMENT

- Nonoperative treatment is of limited usefulness for established nonunions.
- Investigators have attempted the use of bone stimulators, which use either electrical stimulation or ultrasound.
- There is little evidence in the literature supporting the use of these units for treatment of established scaphoid nonunions with AVN.

SURGICAL MANAGEMENT

- A vascularized distal radial bone graft is indicated for scaphoid nonunions with and without evidence of avascularity.
- Correction of a "humpback deformity" requires extensive mobilization of the pedicle when attempting the use of a dorsally sourced graft, and a palmar vascularized graft may be more appropriate.
- For significant collapse, a nonvascular iliac crest graft may be required to create a compression-resistant construct.
- When early degenerative changes are present, a radial styloidectomy should accompany the use of a vascularized distal radial graft.
- The presence of more advanced degenerative joint disease or carpal malalignment is a contraindication to performing surgery to obtain bony union.
- Although the use of a vascularized graft distal radius has been shown to achieve union in 71% to 96% of scaphoid nonunions, the success rate in patients with AVN has been reported in the 50% to 60% range.[1,6,9]

Preoperative Planning

- Radiographs must be evaluated to rule out carpal instability or the degenerative changes frequently found in established nonunions. When there has been the development of dorsal intercalary segmental instability (DISI), over 50% of patients undergoing vascularized grafting will suffer failure to achieve union.

Positioning

- The patient is placed supine on the operating table with the arm placed on an arm board.
- Surgery is performed under tourniquet control.

Approach

- Vascularized grafting may be carried out through a dorsal or palmar approach. Anatomic studies have shown that the dorsal irrigating vessels are further from the articular surface than irrigating vessels on the palmar surface of the radius.[5,8,10] The palmar vessels have been shown in some anatomic studies to be of greater diameter.[3]

Vascularized Radius Bone Grafting Using the 1,2 Intercompartmental Supraretinacular Artery

Exposure

- A curvilinear incision is made over the dorsoradial aspect of the wrist, centered between the first and second extensor compartments (**TECH FIG 1A**).[7]
- The 1,2 intercompartmental supraretinacular artery (1,2 IC SRA) lies on the surface of the retinaculum between the first and second compartments (**TECH FIG 1B**).
  - The irrigating branch enters the distal radius and supplies bone distal and dorsal to the brachioradialis insertion.
  - Avoidance of exsanguination before tourniquet inflation facilitates its identification.
- The first and second compartments are unroofed on their radial and ulnar aspects, respectively, to avoid damage to this irrigating vessel.

Graft Harvest

- The periosteum is scored with a scalpel to outline the graft shape, which measures 1.5 cm in the longitudinal dimension and 0.5 to 0.75 cm in the transverse dimensions (**TECH FIG 2A**). The distal graft margin extends to a point 0.5 to 1 cm from the articular surface.
- Osteotomes are used to elevate the cortical cancellous graft.
- The soft tissue envelope containing the vessel is elevated from the radial periosteum distal to the site of graft harvest

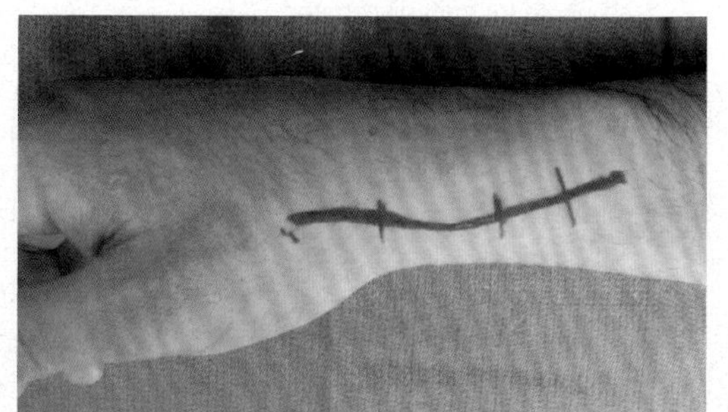

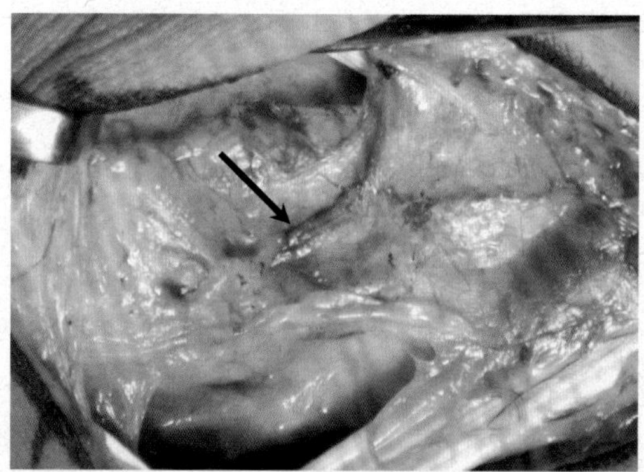

TECH FIG 1 • **A.** The incision is made over the dorsoradial aspect of the distal radius. **B.** The 1,2 IC SRA is visible between the first and second compartments (*arrow*).

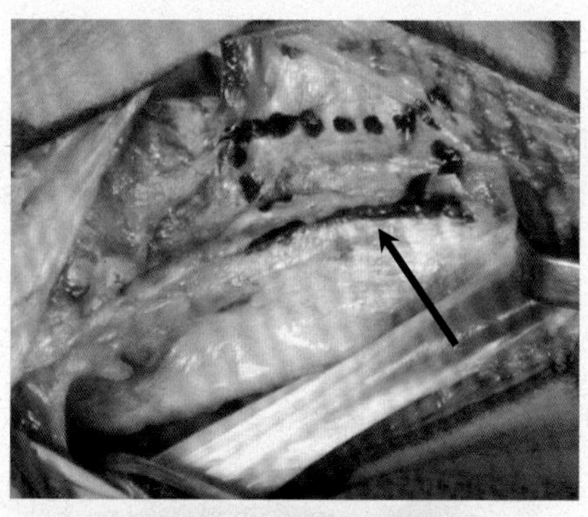

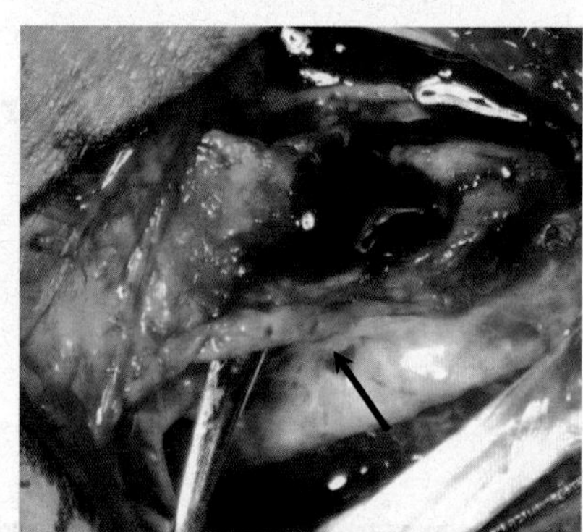

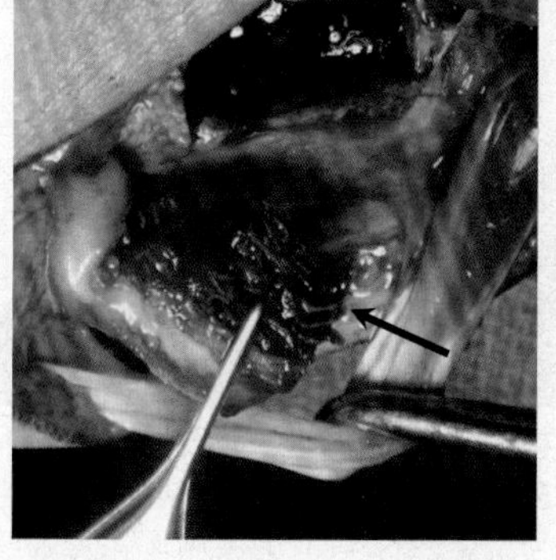

TECH FIG 2 • **A.** The site of the graft is scored and elevated with an osteotome. (Carpus is to the left in all parts.) **B.** Soft tissue sleeve containing irrigating artery is elevated from the distal radius (*arrow*). **C.** Vascularized graft is evaluated for bleeding with tourniquet deflation (*arrow* is at cancellous surface).

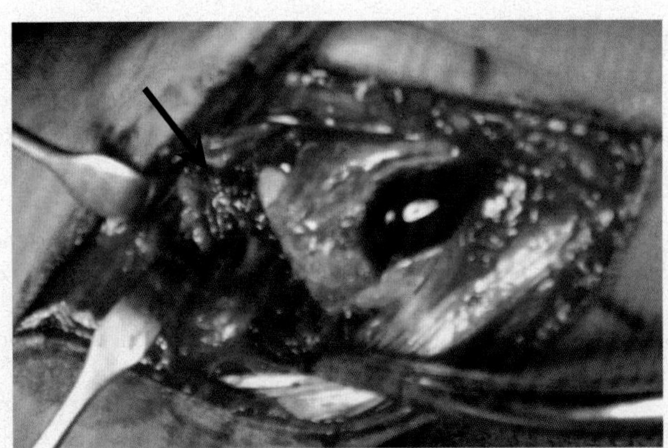

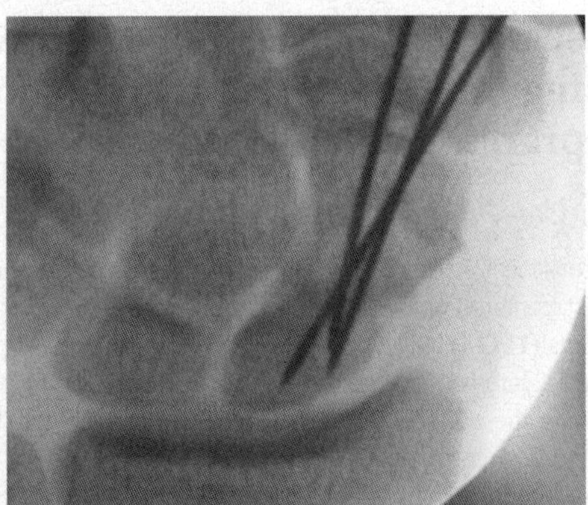

TECH FIG 3 • **A.** The vascularized graft is rotated into the nonunion site (*arrow*) and press-fit into position. **B.** Kirschner wire placement is percutaneous, from distal to proximal.

(**TECH FIG 2B**). This can usually be accomplished with a scalpel or Freer elevator.
  - The 1,2 IC SRA is not dissected free; rather, it is left as part of the retinacular septum.
- The tourniquet is deflated, and perfusion of the vascularized bone graft is evaluated (**TECH FIG 2C**).

Graft Placement

- The joint capsule is incised in the distal portion of the incision, and the scaphoid nonunion is identified.
  - A radial styloidectomy greatly increases the exposure of the scaphoid and reduces the possibility of bone graft impingement.
- Intervening fibrous tissue and sclerotic bone are removed from the nonunion site using rongeurs and curettes to prepare the scaphoid for graft placement.
- Cancellous bone graft from the distal radius is packed proximally and distally to fill voids created by débriding sclerotic bone.
- The carefully contoured vascularized graft is then rotated into the nonunion site and press-fit into position, taking care to avoid torsion of the vascular pedicle (**TECH FIG 3A**).
- Kirschner wires are advanced from the distal pole of the scaphoid to the proximal pole to secure the graft in place (**TECH FIG 3B**).
- The radial capsule is closed loosely with absorbable suture, and the skin is closed in a routine fashion.
  - The pedicle must not be compressed.
- The patient is placed in a short-arm thumb spica splint.

Vascularized Distal Radial Bone Graft Using the Palmar Carpal Artery

Exposure

- The distal palmar forearm is approached through a Henry approach extended distally and laterally toward the scaphoid tubercle (**TECH FIG 4A**).[2]
- The palmar carpal artery lies between the distal radius periosteum and the most distal portion of the superficial aponeurosis of the pronator quadratus just proximal to the radiocarpal joint articular surface.
- Proximal retraction of the superficial aponeurosis of the pronator quadratus allows for exposure of the palmar carpal artery (**TECH FIG 4B**).

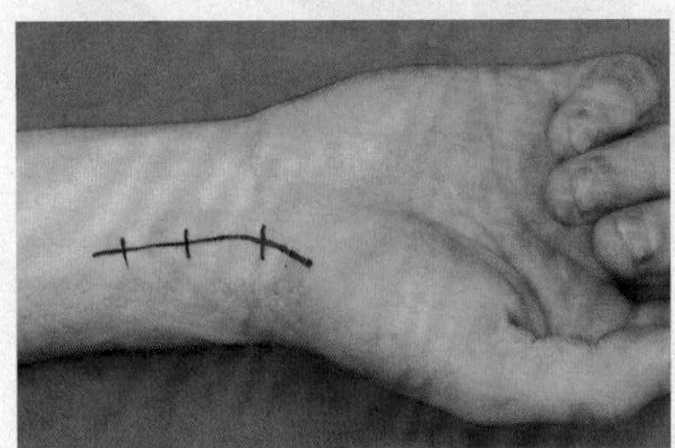

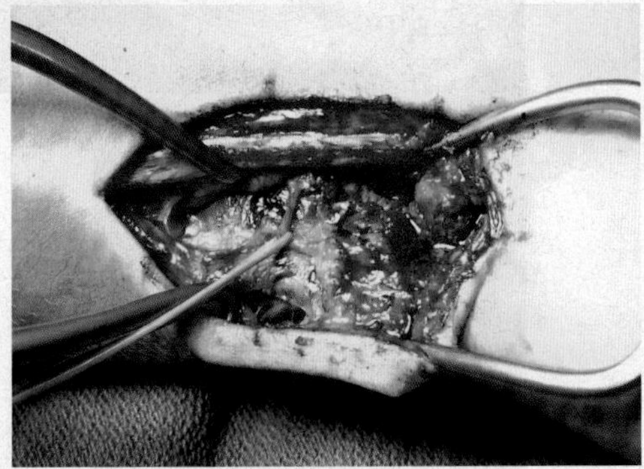

TECH FIG 4 • **A.** The palmar distal radius graft is harvested through the distal portion of the Henry approach to the distal forearm. **B.** The palmar carpal artery is exposed distal to superficial aponeurosis of the pronator quadratus. *(continued)*

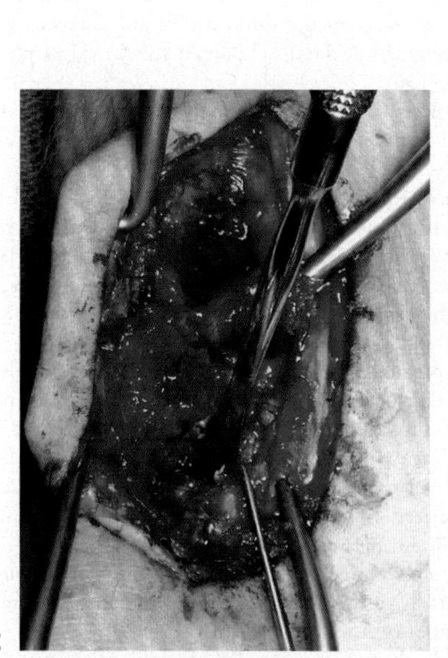
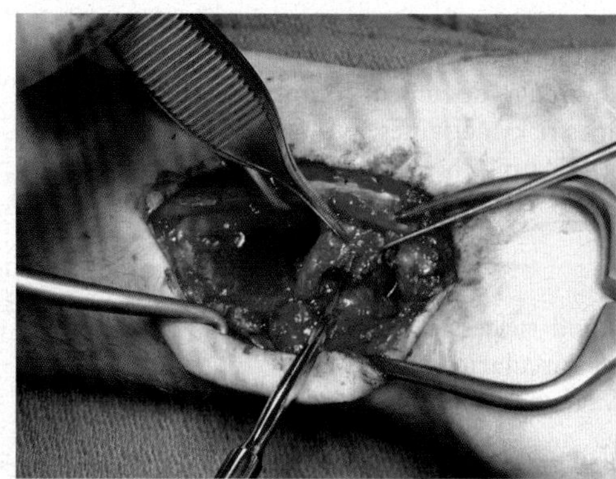
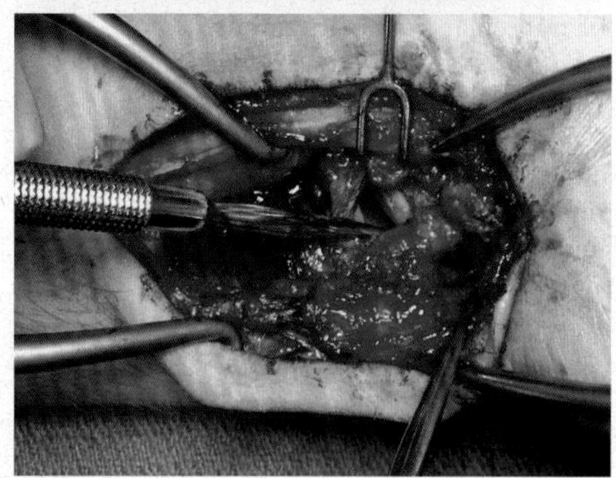

TECH FIG 4 • *(continued)* **C.** The scaphoid nonunion site (at tip of Freer elevator) is débrided to remove fibrous tissue. **D.** The palmar corticocancellous graft (in forceps) is rotated into the nonunion site. **E.** The graft is press-fit into the nonunion site and secured with internal fixation.

Graft Harvest

- Periosteum on either side of the palmar carpal artery is incised, and the artery is gently mobilized laterally to the radial artery.
- Bone graft harvest from the ulnar half of the distal radius is initiated by periosteal incision with a scalpel, followed by osteotomy and elevation with small osteotomes.
- Incision through the radioscaphocapitate ligament exposes the scaphoid nonunion site and allow for removal of fibrous tissue (**TECH FIG 4C**).

Graft Placement

- The graft is rotated and fitted into the nonunion site placing the cortical bone along the palmar surface (**TECH FIG 4D**).
- The graft is press-fit between the scaphoid proximal and distal portions while avoiding the vascular pedicle. Internal fixation is used to secure the bony elements (**TECH FIG 4E**).
- Repair of the radioscaphocapitate ligament is performed prior to final soft tissue closure.

PEARLS AND PITFALLS

Avoid compression screw fixation.	■ Graft fracture often will occur. ■ Kirschner wire removal facilitates imaging studies.
Perform a radial styloidectomy with the dorsal approach.	■ Improves exposure and reduces the chance of graft impingement
Do not exsanguinate before tourniquet inflation.	■ Visibility of the irrigating artery is enhanced with blood present in the vessels.
The retinaculum should be opened over the radial side of the first compartment and the ulnar side of the second compartment when using the 1,2 IC SRA.	■ This diminishes chances of damaging the irrigating artery. ■ Graft is harvested from the radius just distal and dorsal to the brachioradialis insertion.
The palmar carpal artery lies close to the articular surface of the distal radius.	■ Care must be taken to avoid joint violation with graft harvest.

POSTOPERATIVE CARE

- Kirschner wires are removed when healing is observed, usually 4 to 6 weeks after surgery.
- CT scanning may be required to document complete healing before the patient resumes risky activities.
- MRI may be useful in evaluating the scaphoid for vascularity and may be done after Kirschner wire removal.

OUTCOMES

- Recent reports have found successful union rates of 71% to 96% with the use of vascularized grafts from the distal radius. In cases with AVN, union rates have been reported in the 50% to 60% range.
- Previous reports have shown that patients with MRI evidence of AVN or loss of trabecular bone pattern noted on CT have a decreased level of success with reconstructive surgery. Treatment is rarely successful when both findings are present.
- A recent study has identified risk factors for failure: proximal pole AVN, radiographic degenerative changes, loss of carpal alignment, inadequate fracture fixation, tobacco use, advanced age, and female gender.[4]

COMPLICATIONS

- Failure to gain union
- Progressive degenerative changes
- Impingement of bone on radial styloid
- Infection

REFERENCES

1. Chang MA, Bishop AT, Moran SL, et al. The outcomes and complications of 1,2-intercompartmental supraretinacular artery pedicled vascularized bone grafting of scaphoid nonunions. J Hand Surg 2006;31(3):387–396.
2. Gras M, Mathoulin C. Vascularized bone graft pedicled on the volar carpal artery from the volar distal radius as primary procedure for scaphoid non-union. Orthop Traumatol Surg Res 2011;97:800–806.
3. Haerle M, Schaller HE, Mathoulin C. Vascular anatomy of the palmar surfaces of the distal radius and ulna: its relevance to pedicled bone grafts at the distal palmar forearm. J Hand Surg Br 2003;28(2):131–136.
4. Hankins CL, Budoff JE. Analysis of wrist motion following vascularized bone graft to the proximal scaphoid. J Hand Surg 2011;36(4):583–586.
5. Sheetz KK, Bishop AT, Berger RA. The arterial blood supply of the distal radius and ulna and its potential use in vascularized pedicled bone grafts. J Hand Surg Am 1995;20(6):902–914.
6. Shin AY, Bishop AT. Pedicled vascularized bone grafts for disorders of the carpus: scaphoid nonunion and Kienbock's disease. J Am Acad Orthop Surg 2002;10:210–216.
7. Steinmann SP, Bishop AT, Berger RA. Use of the 1,2 intercompartmental supraretinacular artery as a vascularized pedicle bone graft for difficult scaphoid nonunion. J Hand Surg 2002;27(3):391–401.
8. Waitayawinyu T, Robertson C, Chin SH, et al. The detailed anatomy of the 1,2 intercompartmental supraretinacular artery for vascularized bone grafting of scaphoid nonunions. J Hand Surg Am 2008;33(2):168–174.
9. Waters PM, Stewart SL. Surgical treatment of nonunion and avascular necrosis of the proximal part of the scaphoid in adolescents. J Bone Joint Surg Am 2002;84-A(6):915–920.
10. Zaidemberg C, Siebert JW, Angrigiani C. A new vascularized bone graft for scaphoid nonunion. J Hand Surg 1991;16(3):474–478.

38 CHAPTER

Partial Scaphoid Excision of Scaphoid Nonunions

Rafael J. Diaz-Garcia and Joseph E. Imbriglia

DEFINITION

- Scaphoid fractures are quite commonplace, representing the most frequently fractured carpal bone with an annual incidence of approximately 29 per 100,000.[5] Fractures of the scaphoid, when treated acutely and appropriately, have union rates greater than 90%.[3,9] However, without proper diagnosis and treatment, scaphoid fractures frequently result in nonunion.
- Initial treatment for a scaphoid nonunion is typically open reduction and internal fixation (ORIF) with bone graft, be it a corticocancellous wedge or a vascularized graft.
  - Despite appropriate internal fixation and bone grafting, failure rates are approximately 15% in waist fractures and 33% in proximal pole fractures.[12]
- If ORIF and bone grafting fails, the surgeon is then left with difficult choices.
  - Revision ORIF with bone grafting (failure rate of 50%)[2,16]
  - Salvage procedure which may have a higher rate of satisfactory results
  - Silicone prostheses previously described have had poor results due to silicone synovitis and implant loosening, dislocation, and breakage.[13]
  - When a patient has pain caused by a chronic scaphoid nonunion (**FIG 1**) with posttraumatic arthritis limited to the distal pole of the scaphoid and radial styloid, partial scaphoid excision (distal fragment) provides a reasonable, low-morbidity alternative treatment option.[4,11,15]

ANATOMY

- The scaphoid bone represents the bridge between the proximal and distal rows of the carpus. It is tilted in both the volar and radial planes in respect to the central axis of the forearm, articulating with both rows.

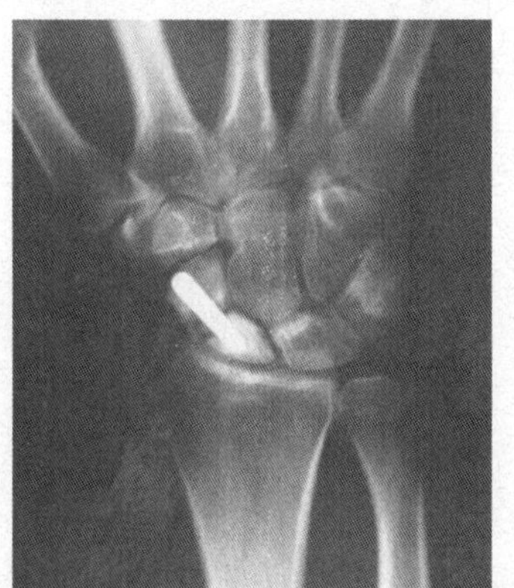
A

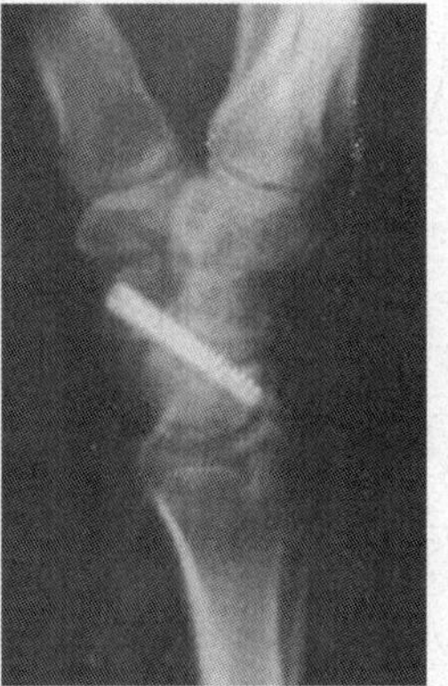
B

FIG 1 • Failed ORIF of a scaphoid nonunion (PA and lateral views).

- The scaphoid is mostly covered in articular cartilage and has important intrinsic and extrinsic ligamentous attachments.
- Most of the vascular supply to the scaphoid enters the bone distal to the waist and perfuses in a retrograde fashion (**FIG 2**).[6,17]
  - The proximal pole is most at risk secondary due to its tenuous blood supply.
- All of these anatomic features make surgical management complex.

PATHOGENESIS

- Patients with scaphoid fractures who present with delays (>4 weeks) in both diagnosis and treatment can develop a nonunion. Other risk factors for nonunion include proximal fracture location, comminution, fragment displacement or angulation, and associated carpal instability. As with other fractures, smokers are at increased risk for nonunion.
  - Acute scaphoid fractures with fracture fragment displacement more than 1.0 mm, an intrascaphoid angle more than 45 degrees, or a height-to-length ratio more than 0.65 have a higher incidence of nonunion.[18]
- Because the scaphoid serves as a bridge between the proximal and distal carpal rows, a scaphoid fracture can severely disrupt wrist biomechanics and normal loading patterns.
  - Scaphoid fractures disrupt the normal linkage between the two rows, and thus the proximal fragment remains with the lunate via the scapholunate ligament and the distal fragment flexes unimpeded.
    - Scaphoid collapse reduces the carpal height and allows the lunate to rotate in a dorsal intercalated segmental instability (DISI) pattern.
    - Scaphoid nonunion advanced collapse (SNAC) arthritis develops from the altered biomechanics.

NATURAL HISTORY

- Most patients with scaphoid fractures, and thus nonunions, are young males between the ages of 20 and 30 years.[5,7]
- There is controversy regarding the true natural history of patients with scaphoid nonunions given that most studies are biased toward symptomatic patients.[8] However, it is widely believed that radiographic signs of posttraumatic arthritis will develop in almost 100% of patients with a scaphoid nonunion. These degenerative changes occur in a predictable pattern, and the process may take 5 to 20 years.[8,10,14]
- Arthritis first develops between the distal pole of the scaphoid and the radial styloid (SNAC wrist stage I; **FIG 3A**).
- Left untreated, stage I SNAC will progress to involve the midcarpal joint (SNAC stages II and III; **FIG 3B,C**).

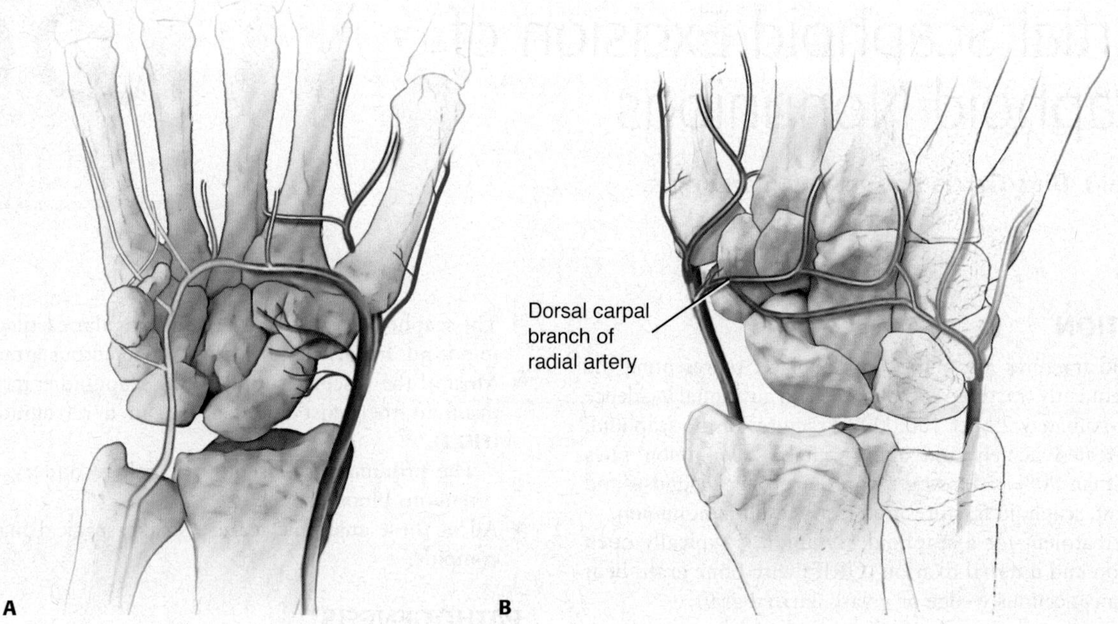

FIG 2 • **A.** Volar intraosseous blood supply to the scaphoid with laterovolar and distal vessels visualized. **B.** Dorsal intraosseous blood supply to the scaphoid.

- Many patients present once pain and decreased range of motion in the wrist has become increasingly severe. In these cases, salvage procedures requiring arthrodesis are often the only options left.

PATIENT HISTORY AND PHYSICAL FINDINGS

- Most patients present having previously sustained a dorsiflexion injury, although not all patients will remember specific trauma. Some patients will present with no previous treatment and a chronic nonunion (**FIG 4**), and others will have failed to respond to either operative or nonoperative therapy.
  - Slow progression over the preceding years of pain aggravated by use, loss of motion, and loss of grip strength are consistent presenting complaints.
  - It is critical to know the patient's smoking history, occupation, and previous operations, as these will dictate future interventions.
- The examiner should palpate the anatomic snuffbox, which lies between the extensor pollicis longus and extensor pollicis brevis tendons. Pain in this region may be indicative of a fracture. As arthritis develops, there may be tenderness and soft tissue fullness along the entire radiocarpal joint due to synovitis.

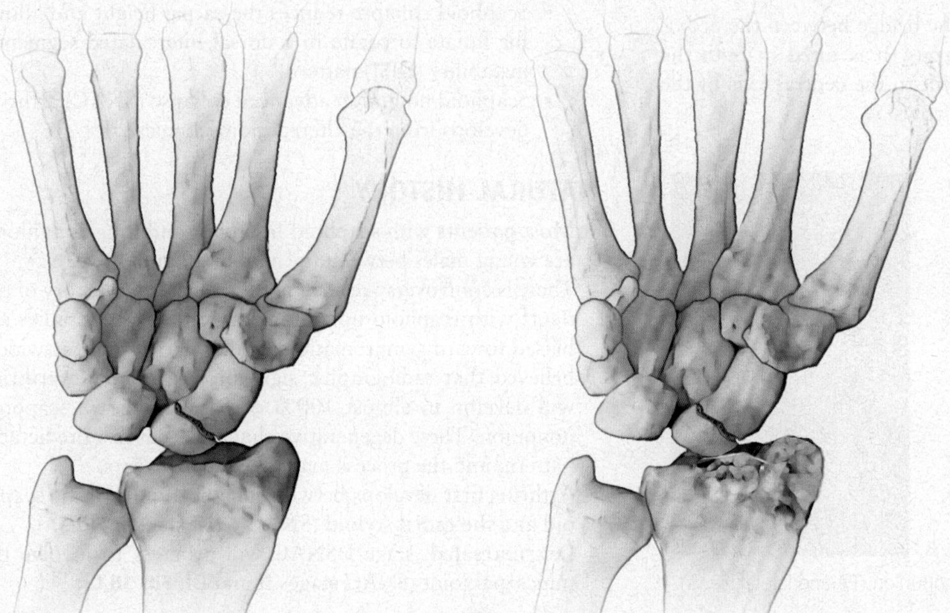

FIG 3 • **A.** Arthritis observed between the distal pole of the scaphoid and the radial styloid (SNAC grade I). *(continued)*

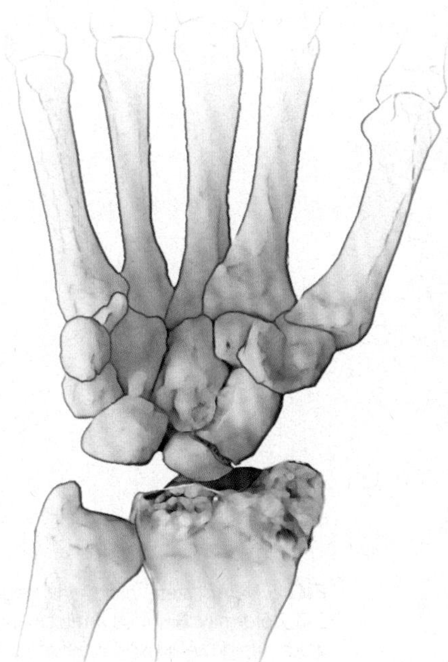

FIG 3 • *(continued)* **B,C.** Stage I SNAC can progress to involve the scaphocapitate articulation (SNAC grade II) with eventual diffuse arthritis in the midcarpal joint (SNAC grade III).

- Measurements of grip strength and range of motion (ROM) need to be ascertained.
  - Strength is often decreased by as much as 30% to 40% if the patient is experiencing pain.
- There will often be a decrease in dorsiflexion of the wrist relative to the contralateral unaffected side.

IMAGING AND OTHER DIAGNOSTIC STUDIES

- Posteroanterior (PA), lateral, and ulnar and radial deviation views of the wrist are required. These views are usually enough to determine if a partial scaphoid excision is indicated.
  - The lateral plain radiograph allows one to determine the degree of DISI (**FIG 5A**).

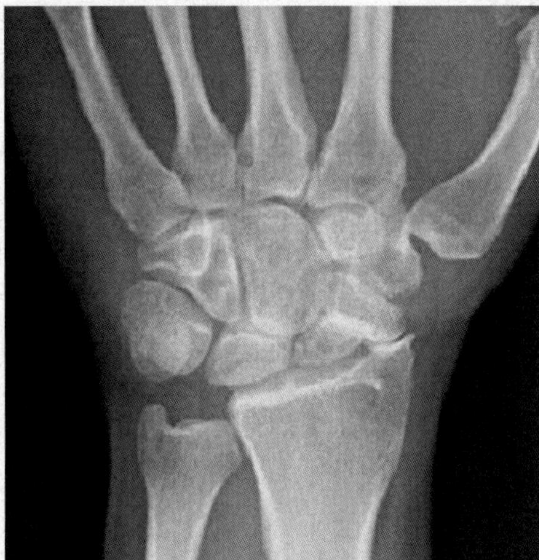

FIG 4 • Chronic nonunion of the scaphoid with SNAC in a patient with no previous treatment.

  - If the radiographs reveal intercarpal arthritis (**FIG 5B**) or a small avascular proximal pole fragment, partial scaphoid excision may be contraindicated.
  - If minimal radioscaphoid arthritis is observed, ORIF (with nonvascularized or vascularized bone graft) to reconstruct the nonunited scaphoid might be the best option.
- A magnetic resonance imaging (MRI) is often ordered by physicians in the management of scaphoid nonunions to evaluate the blood supply of the proximal pole. However, these studies have little influence in patients who are candidates for a distal fragment excision.
- From a radiographic perspective, the ideal candidate for distal pole excision of the scaphoid has a nonunion of the scaphoid fracture at the level of the waist or distal pole with concomitant degenerative joint disease between the distal radius and distal pole only (SNAC stage I).

DIFFERENTIAL DIAGNOSIS

- Acute scaphoid fracture
- First or second extensor compartment tendonitis
- Scapholunate ligament injury
- Basilar thumb arthritis
- Scaphotrapeziotrapezoid arthritis
- Inflammatory arthritis

NONOPERATIVE MANAGEMENT

- Nonoperative management of chronic wrist pain should always be considered in discussion with patients about treatment options. The symptoms may be months or even years old, so there is little rush to intervene if the patient desires further delay.
- The treatment of any painful joint begins with intermittent immobilization (wrist splinting), activity modification, and nonsteroidal anti-inflammatory drugs (NSAIDs).
- If immobilization and NSAIDs are ineffective, temporary pain relief can almost always be gained with a steroid injection. These temporizing treatments also put the pain in perspective for the patient. The patient may conclude that medication and splinting is all that is necessary.
- During the nonoperative management period, the surgeon gains a perspective on the degree of patient discomfort and simultaneously gauges the patient's expectations.
  - The operation will work better and the patient will be more satisfied if the patient's and surgeon's expectations are similar.

SURGICAL MANAGEMENT

- Surgical options to treat persistent pain resulting in compromised function in a patient with a scaphoid nonunion and arthritis limited to the area between the distal fragment of the scaphoid and the radial styloid (stage I SNAC wrist arthritis) include the following:
  - ORIF of the scaphoid nonunion combined with radial styloidectomy
  - Resection of the distal scaphoid fragment
  - Partial wrist arthrodesis
  - Proximal row carpectomy
  - Wrist denervation

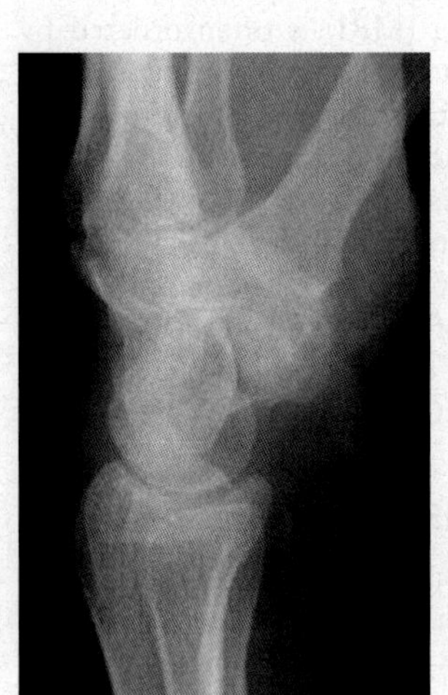

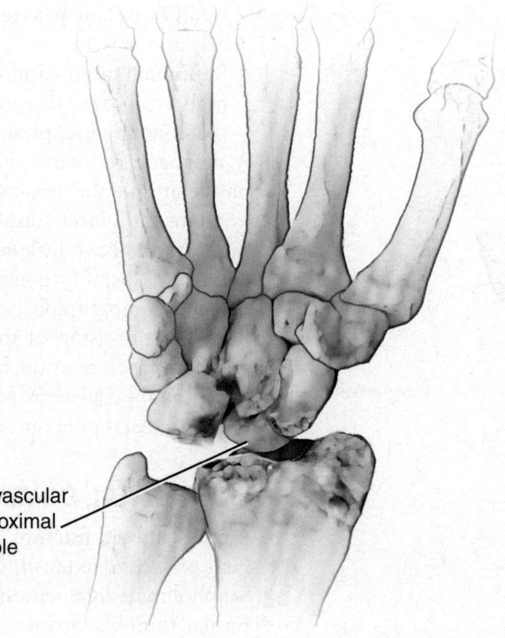

A B

FIG 5 • A. Lateral plain radiograph displaying a DISI deformity. **B.** When intercarpal arthritis (SNAC grade III) or an avascular proximal pole is found, partial scaphoid excision may be contraindicated.

- A patient with an untreated scaphoid nonunion and no arthritis is best treated by ORIF of the scaphoid with bone grafting. In a patient with SNAC wrist stage II, it is too late for a distal pole excision; this patient may require a proximal row carpectomy or scaphoid excision with intercarpal fusion.
- Most patients requiring excision of the distal pole have undergone prior treatment that has failed, and both the surgeon and the patient are searching for a reliable procedure with low morbidity to help alleviate the patient's pain and improve function.
- Distal scaphoid excision requires robust and taut radioscaphocapitate and long radiolunate ligaments in order to support the remaining proximal carpus and prevent collapse (DISI) of the wrist.
- Contraindications to distal pole excision include the following:
  - Preexisting significant DISI deformity. The DISI deformity may indeed get worse with distal pole excision in an individual with poor ligamentous support.
  - Proximal pole that is less than half the entire size of the scaphoid. If the distal fragment is greater than 50% of the size of the scaphoid, resultant collapse of the carpus may occur with severe morbidity.

Preoperative Planning

- Preoperative planning is done based on a thorough review of the patient's plain radiographs.
  - If the distal pole is to be excised, there must be enough proximal pole (>½) left to support the distal row of the carpus. If only a very small (and possibly an avascular) proximal pole remains, the carpus is likely to collapse, resulting in failure of the procedure.

Positioning

- The patient is placed in the supine position with the extremity on an arm board.
- A proximal arm pneumatic tourniquet is applied.

Approach

- The distal pole of the scaphoid can be excised through either a dorsal or palmar approach. The approach may be dictated by existing scars.
  - The palmar approach is the preferred method due to the relatively accessible palmar position of the distal fragment.
  - An advantage of the dorsal approach is the ease of excision of the posterior interosseous nerve for wrist denervation.
  - A radial styloidectomy can be performed through either approach.

Volar Approach for Excision of the Distal Scaphoid Fragment

Incision and Scaphoid Excision

- An incision is made directly over the flexor carpi radialis (FCR) tendon, incorporating any previous incisions (**TECH FIG 1A,B**).
- The tendon is retracted ulnarly and the subsheath of the tendon is incised longitudinally (**TECH FIG 1C**).
- The radiocarpal joint capsule is opened longitudinally and the distal pole of the scaphoid is excised with osteotomes and rongeurs (**TECH FIG 1D–G**).

Radial Styloidectomy

- If indicated, an oblique radial styloidectomy can be performed at this point using an osteotome.
- In this situation, the distal pole may be too large to excise and a radial styloidectomy can accomplish the same purpose.
- The styloidectomy should be large enough so that the arthritic distal pole no longer touches the radius in radial deviation but not so large as to disrupt the origin of the radioscapholunate ligament, as this may preclude later proximal row carpectomy.

Wound Closure

- The capsule and volar extrinsic ligaments are closed with interrupted permanent sutures.
- The skin is closed with interrupted nonabsorbable sutures.

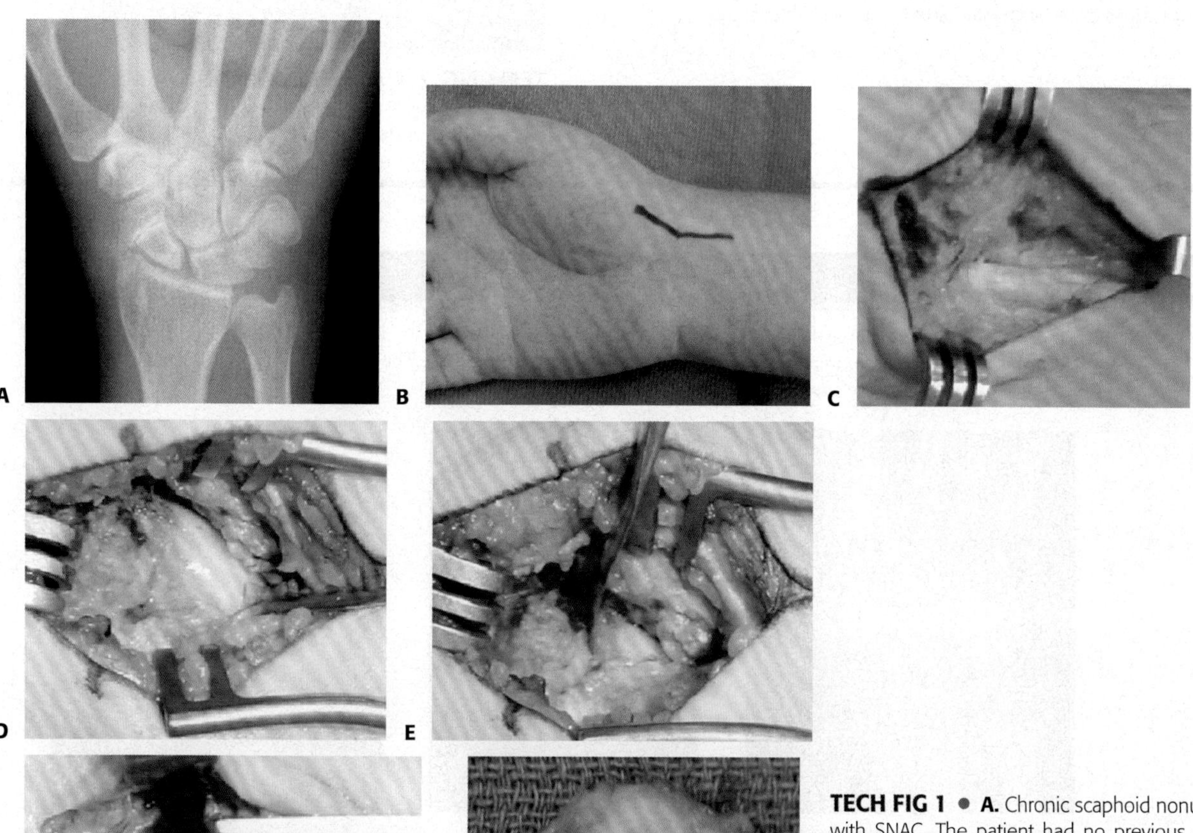

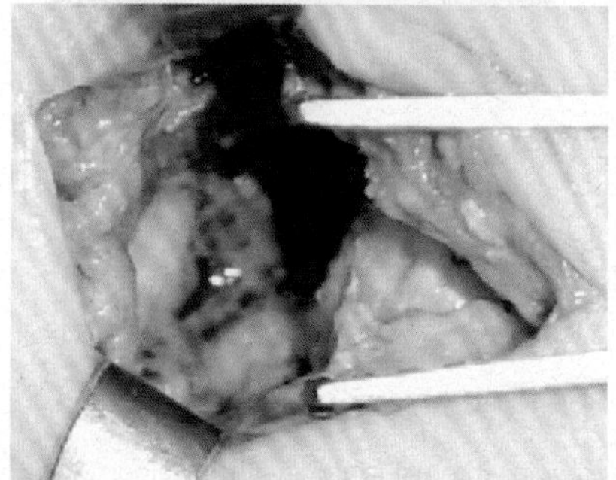

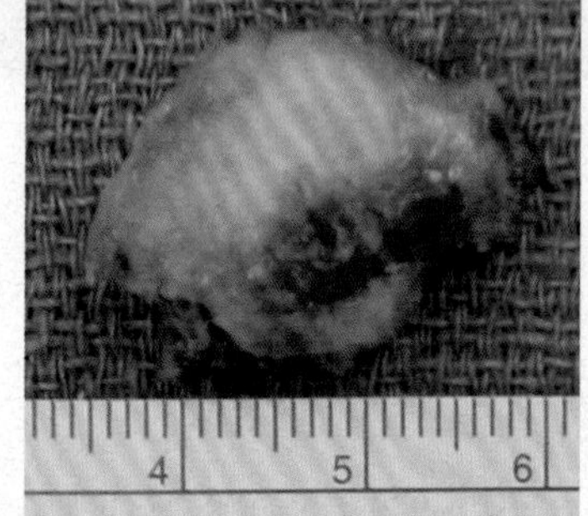

TECH FIG 1 • **A.** Chronic scaphoid nonunion with SNAC. The patient had no previous treatment. **B.** An incision is made directly over the FCR tendon. **C.** The tendon is retracted and its subsheath opened longitudinally. **D.** The radiocarpal joint is opened longitudinally and the scaphoid is visualized. **E,F.** The distal pole of the scaphoid is excised with osteotomes and rongeurs. If indicated, a radial styloidectomy can be performed at this point. **G.** Excised distal pole of the scaphoid.

TECHNIQUES

Dorsal Approach for Excision of the Distal Scaphoid Fragment

- An incision is made over the radial aspect of the carpus, incorporating any old incisions (**TECH FIG 2**).
- The radial sensory nerve is identified and retracted.
- The interval between the extensor pollicis longus and the radial wrist extensors is entered.
- The radial artery and its branches are retracted and protected, and then the joint capsule is incised.
- The distal scaphoid fragment will be deep and is best removed using rongeurs after defining its borders with a no. 15 blade.
- A radial styloidectomy can be performed if necessary as mentioned earlier.
- The capsule is closed with absorbable suture.
- The skin is closed with interrupted nonabsorbable sutures.
- The patient is placed in a well-padded forearm-based splint, leaving the finger metacarpophalangeal joints and thumb interphalangeal joint free. This volar thumb spica splint is placed after either the volar or dorsal approach.

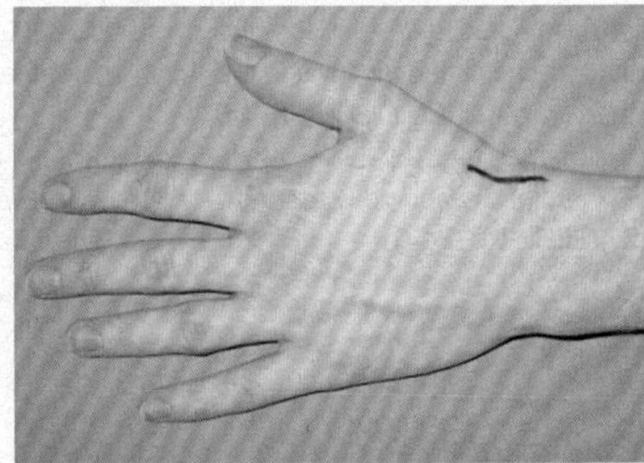

TECH FIG 2 • An incision over the dorsoradial aspect of the wrist may be used when prior surgery has been performed.

PEARLS AND PITFALLS

Indications

- It is critical to observe that arthritis does not involve the midcarpal joint.
- There must be enough proximal scaphoid remaining to support the carpus. The proximal 50% of the scaphoid should be sufficient to support the capitate and the remaining carpus (**FIG 6**).

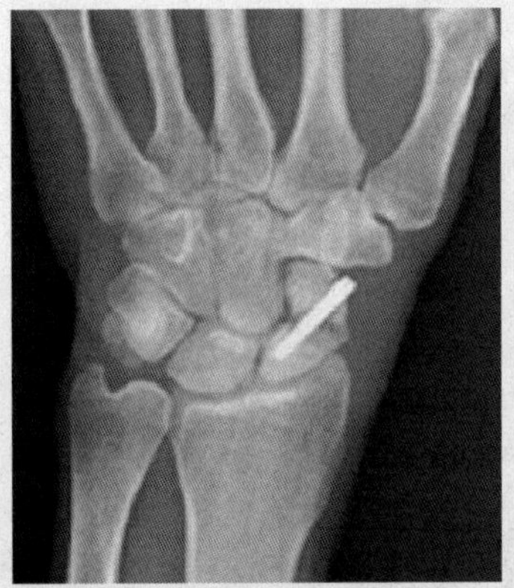

A

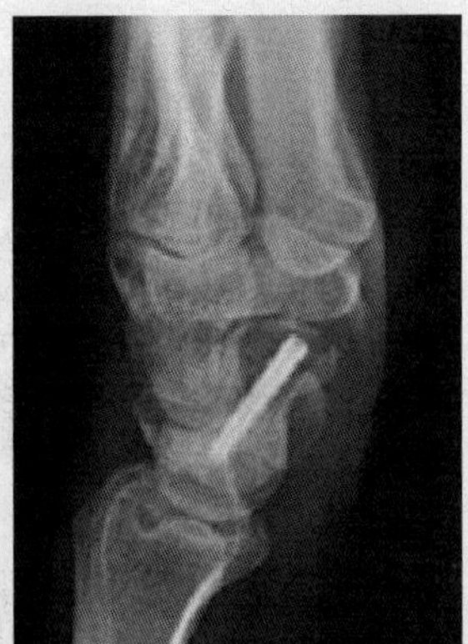

B

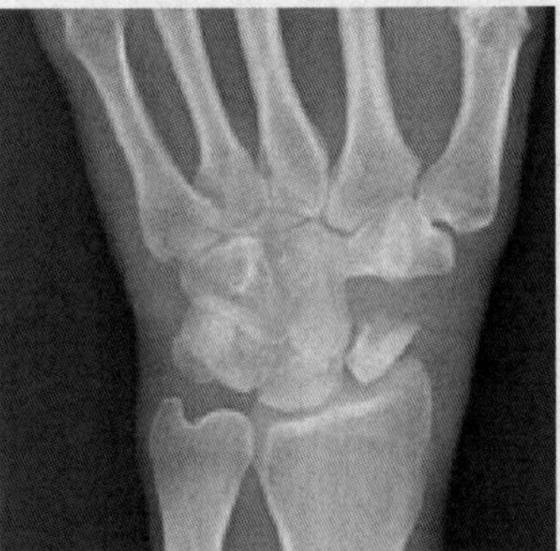

C

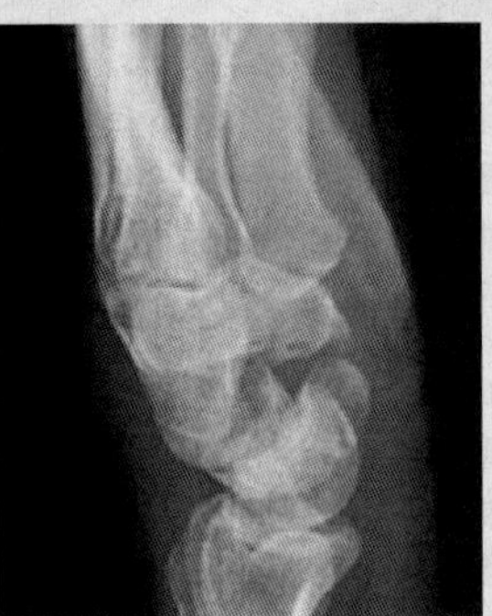

D

FIG 6 • **A,B.** Scaphoid nonunion after previous internal fixation with development of SNAC wrist arthritis. **C,D.** Collapse of the scaphoid resulting from too much resection (more than two-thirds) of the distal pole of the scaphoid, with evidence of DISI deformity on postoperative radiographs.

Approach and technique

- The procedure is simpler to perform through a palmar approach.
- Avoid injury to either the radial sensory nerve or radial artery.
- Interpositional material in the space left by the resected distal pole of the scaphoid is not necessary.

POSTOPERATIVE CARE

- Patients are immobilized for 2 weeks in a well-padded volar splint.
- The splint and sutures are removed 2 weeks after the procedure.
- A removable orthosis is applied and the patient is instructed on active and passive ROM exercises.
- Once active and passive ROM has been achieved, strength exercises are started (usually at 4 weeks postoperatively).
- Regaining full ROM and strength typically takes about 3 months.
- Pain relief is noticeable within 2 to 4 weeks of surgery.

OUTCOMES

- Review of outcomes in the literature suggest that both ROM and grip strength improve postoperatively.[3–5]
- Pain relief can be expected if the proper indications for surgery are followed.
- All patients have some degree of DISI preoperatively, and this pattern of deformity may worsen after excision of the distal pole of the scaphoid. DISI deformities that are severe can result in both loss of motion and pain. This problem is not well documented in the literature but certainly exists.[5]
- In the patient undergoing multiple procedures, outcomes of distal pole excision are better than attempting another bone graft and internal fixation, where the failure rate can approach 50%.[1]

COMPLICATIONS

- The presence of midcarpal arthritis undiagnosed before distal pole excision can lead to persistent pain.
- Resection of too large a distal pole (>50%) can result in collapse of the scaphoid.
- If the procedure is performed in a very loose-jointed individual, the DISI pattern may significantly worsen, leading to persistent pain.

REFERENCES

1. Bishop AT. Vascularized bone grafts. In: Green DG, Hotchkiss R, Pederson W, eds. Green's Operative Hand Surgery. New York: Churchill Livingstone, 1999.
2. Chang MA, Bishop AT, Moran SL, et al. The outcomes and complications of 1,2 intercompartmental supraretinacular artery pedicled vascularized bone grafting of scaphoid nonunions. J Hand Surg Am 2006;31(3):387–396.
3. Dias JJ, Wildin CJ, Bhowal B, et al. Should acute scaphoid fractures be fixed? A randomized controlled trial. J Bone Joint Surg Am 2005;87(10):2160–2168.
4. Drac P, Manak P, Pieranova L. Distal scaphoid resection arthroplasty for scaphoid nonunion with radioscaphoid arthritis. Biomed Pap Med Fac Univ Palacky Olomouc Czech Repub 2006;150: 143–145.
5. Duckworth AD, Jenkins PJ, Aitken SA, et al. Scaphoid fracture epidemiology. J Trauma Acute Care Surg 2012;72(2):E41–E45.
6. Gelberman RH, Menon J. The vascularity of the scaphoid bone. J Hand Surg Am 1980;5(5):508–513.
7. Hove LM. Epidemiology of scaphoid fractures in Bergen, Norway. Scand J Plast Reconstr Surg Hand Surg 1999;33:423–426.
8. Kerluke L, McCabe SJ. Nonunion of the scaphoid: a critical analysis of recent natural history studies. J Hand Surg Am 1993;18:1–3.
9. Kuschner SH, Lane CS, Brien WW, et al. Scaphoid fractures and scaphoid nonunion. Diagnosis and treatment. Orthop Rev 1994; 23:861–871.
10. Lindström G, Nyström A. Natural history of scaphoid non-union, with special reference to "asymptomatic" cases. J Hand Surg Br 1992;17:697–700.
11. Malerich MM, Clifford J, Eaton B, et al. Distal scaphoid resection arthroplasty for the treatment of degenerative arthritis secondary to scaphoid nonunion. J Hand Surg Am 1999;24:1196–1205.
12. Merrell GA, Wolfe SW, Slade JF III. Treatment of scaphoid nonunions: quantitative meta-analysis of the literature. J Hand Surg Am 2002;27(4):685–691.
13. Peimer CA, Medige J, Eckert BS, et al. Reactive synovitis after silicone arthroplasty. J Hand Surg Am 1986;11:624–638.
14. Ruby LK, Stinson J, Belsky MR. The natural history of scaphoid non-union: a review of 55 cases. J Bone Joint Surg Am 1985;67: 428–432.
15. Ruch DS, Papadonikolakis A. Resection of the scaphoid distal pole for symptomatic scaphoid nonunion after failed previous surgical treatment. J Hand Surg Am 2006;31:588–593.
16. Smith BS, Cooney WP. Revision of failed bone grafting for nonunion of the scaphoid. Treatment options and results. Clin Orthop Relat Res 1996;(327):98–109.
17. Taleisnik J, Kelly PJ. The extraosseous and intraosseous blood supply of the scaphoid bone. J Bone Joint Surg Am 1966;48:1125–1137.
18. Trumble TE, Salas P, Barthel T, et al. Management of scaphoid nonunions. J Am Acad Orthop Surg 2003;11:380–391.

39 CHAPTER

Surgical Treatment of Carpal Bone Fractures Excluding the Scaphoid

Kenneth R. Means, Jr. and Thomas J. Graham

DEFINITION

- These injuries include fractures of the lunate, triquetrum, pisiform, hamate body or hook, capitate, trapezoid, and trapezial body or ridge.
- Any fracture involving the carpal bones should raise suspicion of associated carpal instability.

ANATOMY

- Certain anatomic features of the carpal bones make them more susceptible to injury. These include the unique osteologic regions of some of the carpal bones, such as the hook of the hamate, the ridge or tubercle of the trapezium, and the neck of the capitate.
- The slender shape and projection of the hamate hook make it an obvious injury target for direct trauma to the palmar–ulnar surface of the wrist (**FIG 1A**). Surgeons can identify the hook by placing their thumb interphalangeal joint on the patient's pisiform and flexing their thumb toward the patient's first web space. The surgeon's thumb tip will land directly on top of the patient's hamate hook.
- The trapezial ridge may be considered a radial-sided analogue to the hamate hook in that it is a relatively prominent volar projection, further accentuated by the deep groove for the flexor carpi radialis (FCR) tendon that runs along its ulnar side (**FIG 1B**).
- The strong, inelastic transverse carpal ligament attaches to the hamate hook ulnarly and the trapezial tubercle radially.
- These facts make the ridge of the trapezium more susceptible to fracture after direct trauma to the thenar region of the hand.
- The constricted neck portion of the capitate lies between the dense head proximally and the body distally. The body, which accounts for the distal half of the capitate, is rigidly constrained by its associations with the index, middle, and ring finger metacarpal bases; the trapezoid; and the hamate. As a result the capitate neck is a biomechanically vulnerable area.
- Transverse plane fractures through the capitate neck are reported as being the most common.
- Fractures across the neck place the capitate head at risk for avascular necrosis because the blood supply to the capitate flows retrograde toward the head proximally.

PATHOGENESIS

- Traumatic fractures of the carpal bones may occur via direct or indirect mechanisms.
- Direct mechanisms include crush injuries, which should alert the physician to the possible development of compartment syndrome of the hand. Compressive trauma to the hand in the anteroposterior (AP) plane will flatten the palmarly directed concave longitudinal and horizontal arches of the carpus and should raise suspicion for potential carpal body fractures and axial disruptions.
  - The presence of a seemingly unusual carpal bone fracture may be a herald of a globally destructive injury to the hand and other associated injuries, such as carpometacarpal (CMC) fracture-dislocations, longitudinal fractures of the metacarpals, severe thumb damage, and significant soft tissue injuries. This constellation of pathologies has been referred to as the "exploded hand" (**FIG 2**).

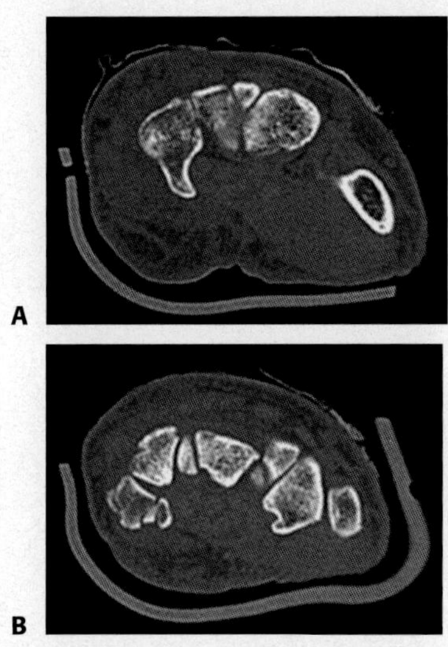

FIG 1 • **A.** CT scan showing hamate hook. **B.** CT scan showing trapezial ridge.

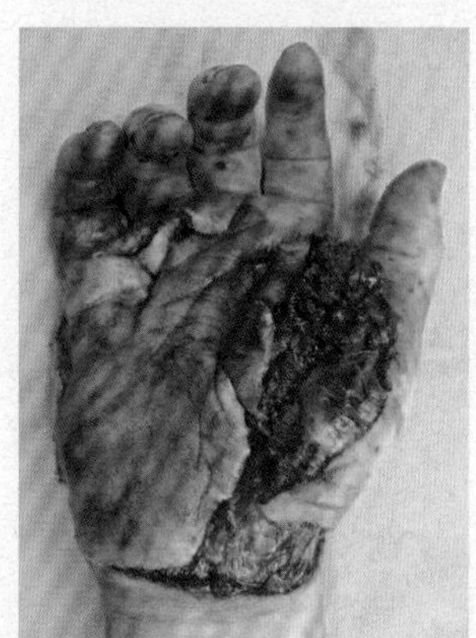

FIG 2 • Exploded hand is a constellation of injuries that can include CMC fracture-dislocations, longitudinal fractures of the metacarpals, severe thumb damage, and significant soft tissue damage. (Reprinted from Graham TJ. The exploded hand syndrome: logical evaluation and comprehensive treatment of the severely crushed hand. J Hand Surg Am 2006;31[6]:1012–1023; copyright 2006, with permission from Elsevier.)

- More focused direct trauma to individual carpal bones may also cause a fracture. Examples of this include direct blows to the dorsum of the hand, typically causing capitate, hamate body, triquetrum, or trapezium fractures, or direct injury to the palmar surface of the hand usually from a racquet or club, often causing a hamate hook or trapezial ridge fracture.
- Indirect trauma includes the progressive perilunate instability patterns that are well described and may lead to fractures of the lunate, capitate, triquetrum, or other carpal bones.
  - Scaphocapitate syndrome involves a dorsiflexion and radial deviation mechanism by which the scaphoid bone fractures and is followed by a fracture of the capitate through the neck in the coronal plane. The capitate head may rotate up to 180 degrees from its anatomic position.
  - A progressive perilunate instability pattern can produce a similar coronal fracture through the capitate neck but normally without such a severe degree of capitate head rotation.
- Minor indirect trauma can cause isolated carpal bone fractures.
  - The commonly seen avulsion fractures from the dorsum of the triquetrum may occur when a fall onto the palmar flexed wrist causes the dorsal radiotriquetral (also known as *dorsal radiocarpal*) ligament to avulse a portion of the dorsal cortex. However, this seemingly innocuous injury can be associated with significant radiocarpal and/or intracarpal instability patterns and the practitioner should carefully exclude these more severe injuries whenever treating a dorsal triquetral avulsion fracture.
  - An impaction type of fracture of the triquetrum body may be seen more often in patients with an elongated ulnar styloid.

NATURAL HISTORY

- The natural history of carpal bone fractures depends both on the specific bone in question as well as associated impairment of other structures.
- All of the carpal bones have at least three articular surfaces, except the pisiform, which articulates only with the triquetrum. Anatomic reduction of articular facets is a primary surgical goal in an effort to decrease the incidence and severity of posttraumatic arthritis.
- Avascular necrosis can have a profoundly negative impact on final outcome after carpal bone fracture.
  - Concerns of vascular disruption arise when lunate and capitate fractures occur, although generally, fractures of the lunate are not associated with avascularity.
- The potential for nonunion is most often seen with hamate hook fractures, capitate neck fractures, and trapezial ridge fractures, especially Palmer type II fractures that involve the tip and not the base of the ridge.
- Barring nonunion, the related instabilities and involvement of other hand components in association with carpal fractures excluding the scaphoid are the most troublesome issues and will most significantly affect patient outcome.

PATIENT HISTORY AND PHYSICAL FINDINGS

- Determining the mechanism of injury is the most important component of taking the patient's history.
- Neurovascular symptoms should be explored, especially when a severe crush or high-energy mechanism is involved, or in cases of hamate hook or pisiform fractures, with special attention to the ulnar neurovascular structures within Guyon's canal.
  - A complete evaluation of the median, radial, ulnar, and digital nerves is warranted. Assessment of capillary refill, color, temperature, and Doppler signal determines the vascular status. Clinical or Doppler Allen examination may be warranted if radial and/or ulnar artery thrombosis or disruption is suspected.
- The examiner should observe the patient's hand and wrist for swelling, deformity, and skin and soft tissue injuries, including possible open fractures or fracture-dislocations.
  - Swelling and soft tissue damage give an indication as to the severity of the injury. The presence of deformity alerts the examiner to possible carpal dislocations that require emergent reduction. Open fractures and fracture-dislocations will guide surgical management.
- The examiner should ask the patient where the pain is most significant. The examination should start away from, and progress toward, this point. The hand, forearm, and elbow should also be palpated to assess for possible associated injuries.
  - The most obvious area of pain and tenderness is usually the most structurally significant. However, it may mask other more subtle injuries that should be detected by a more thorough global examination.

IMAGING AND OTHER DIAGNOSTIC STUDIES

- Routine AP, lateral, and oblique views of the wrist and hand are obtained (**FIG 3A**).
  - Radiographs of the elbow and forearm are ordered if indicated.
- Dynamic radiographic images, including stress and distraction views, help to rule out carpal instability and may determine the ability to obtain closed reduction.
- Special views, often best performed with fluoroscopy, help to profile difficult-to-see structures.
  - The hook of the hamate is evaluated with the carpal tunnel view or the supinated/oblique/radial deviation view with the thumb abducted (referred to as the *papillon view*) (**FIG 3B**).
  - The trapezial ridge is visualized on the carpal tunnel view (**FIG 3C**).
  - The pisotriquetral joint is best seen on a 45-degree supinated lateral view of the wrist.
- Computed tomography (CT) scans effectively assess osseous detail and will often detect more subtle associated carpal fractures that may be missed on routine radiographs.
  - CT is considered the imaging modality of choice for confirming a hamate hook fracture if plain films are nondiagnostic.

NONOPERATIVE MANAGEMENT

- Isolated carpal bone fractures without associated carpal instability, significant displacement, or intra-articular step-off may be managed nonoperatively.
  - This usually includes use of a cast or brace for several weeks (usually 4 to 6 weeks) until symptoms have improved, tenderness is resolving, and radiographs are stable.
  - Short-arm thumb spica casts or splints have been recommended for isolated trapezium and capitate fractures.

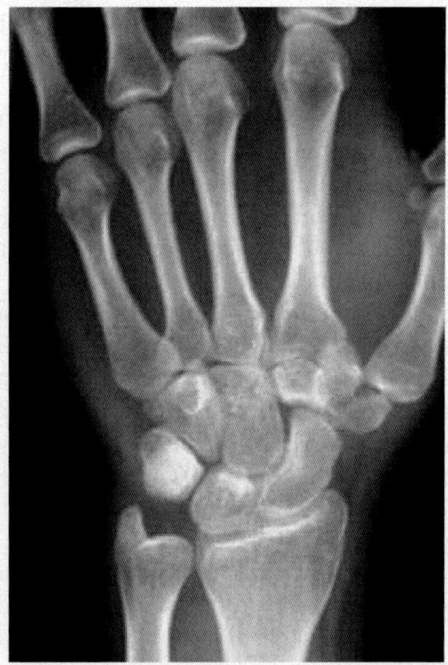

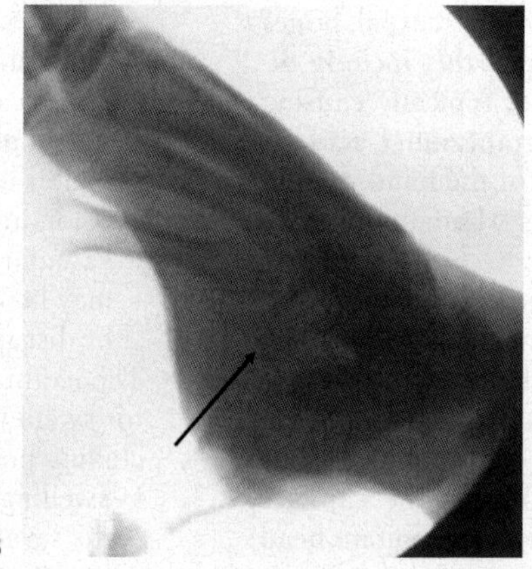

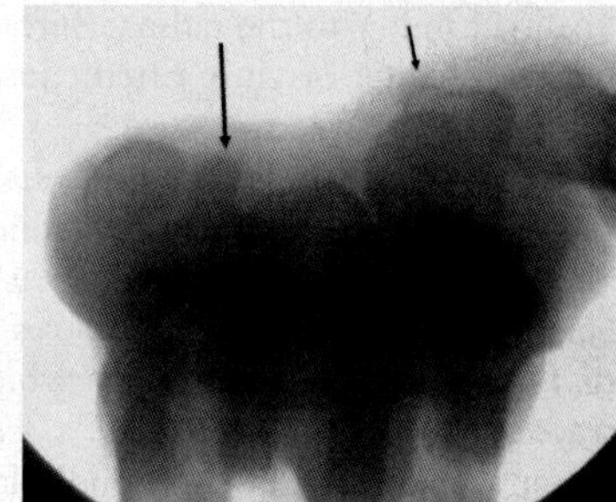

FIG 3 • **A.** AP radiograph of wrist showing trapezial body fracture. **B.** Supination, oblique, radial deviation radiograph showing normal hamate hook (*arrow*). **C.** Carpal tunnel view showing normal hamate hook (*large arrow*) and trapezial ridge (*small arrow*).

The fingers should be left free for gentle range of motion but nothing more than light activities of daily living.

- A specific fracture of note is the hamate hook.
  - These fractures can be treated with cast immobilization if nondisplaced and acute (<1 month).
  - There is a relatively high rate of symptomatic nonunion, and surgical intervention may eventually be necessary. Close follow-up to determine whether union has occurred is warranted because nonunions may lead to flexor tendon rupture.
- Similar to the treatment of the hamate hook, trapezial ridge fractures may be initially immobilized and later excised if symptomatic nonunion develops.

SURGICAL MANAGEMENT

Indications

- Indications for surgical management of these fractures include those that significantly involve an articular surface or are structurally destabilizing to the remainder of the carpus, such as a displaced or unstable capitate body fracture.
  - Other operative indications include those that are true for most fractures, such as open injuries and those requiring nerve, vessel, tendon, ligament, or soft tissue repair.
  - If stable and near-anatomic reduction of carpal fractures is not possible, primary limited arthrodesis or carpectomy may be indicated.
- Because of the unique nature of each carpal bone, more specific indications will be considered for each fracture.
- Late reconstructive options include partial or total wrist arthrodesis or proximal row carpectomy for symptomatic arthritic changes.
  - Trapezial excision with or without thumb metacarpal suspensionplasty may be used for posttraumatic arthritis after trapezial body fractures. Thumb trapeziometacarpal fusion is also an option in these situations but is usually reserved for young heavy laborers.
  - Total or hemi-wrist arthroplasty for select cases may become a more popular option as techniques improve.

Lunate Fractures

- In general, fractures that are of sufficient size and displacement should be reduced and internally fixed.
- Fractures that involve the palmar surface of the lunate where stout volar extrinsic wrist ligaments (long and short radiolunate) and vascular conduits (radioscapholunate ligament of Testut) attach should be stabilized.
- If the capitate is subluxated volarly relative to the lunate and radius, such as when there is a lunate palmar lip fracture, this must be corrected with reduction and fixation of the lunate palmar fragment.
  - These fractures are routinely approached palmarly as described in Techniques.
  - Alternatively, a standard third and fourth interval dorsal exposure (described under Capitate Fractures) can be used if the fracture pattern dictates a dorsal approach and fixation.
  - Dorsal lip fractures of the lunate typically involve the scapholunate ligament, and if they are displaced, they should be reduced and stabilized to try to prevent scapholunate advanced collapse (SLAC). This is usually performed with small interfragment screw fixation.

Triquetral Fractures

- In general, displaced fractures of the triquetral body that are of sufficient size are best treated by open reduction and internal fixation (ORIF).
  - This can be accomplished through use of pins or screws into the triquetrum alone or in combination with pinning to the lunate or to the hamate as dictated by the fracture.
- The triquetrum may be removed in its entirety if it is not amenable to repair, although a volar intercalated segment instability (VISI) pattern may occur if performed in isolation.
- An apparently isolated fracture of the triquetrum may in fact be part of a reverse perilunate instability pattern (in which the portal of energy entry is at the ulnar wrist) and may be associated with other fractures and ligament disruptions.

Pisiform Fractures

- The pisiform, similar to another sesamoid bone, the patella, most often fractures in a transverse pattern via an indirect avulsion mechanism through the flexor carpi ulnaris (FCU) or in a pattern of comminution from a direct blow.
- Virtually all pisiform fractures are treated nonoperatively initially and then excised late if immobilization of the fracture fails to relieve symptoms after 2 or 3 months.
  - Fractures that are of sufficient size and displacement can be reduced and internally fixed, although this is rarely indicated.
  - The approach described in Techniques can be used for fixation or excision of the pisiform.
- The pisiform is the last carpal bone to ossify, usually by age 12 years, and may have a nonpathologic fragmented appearance before complete ossification.

Hook of Hamate Fractures

- If an acute hamate hook fracture is truly nondisplaced, it can be treated nonoperatively initially. If the fracture is displaced or remains persistently symptomatic or nonunited, excision is indicated, even for base fractures (**FIG 4A**).
- ORIF is associated with relatively high complication rates and provides little or no advantage over simple fragment excision.
  - If ORIF is desired, the hook is exposed as described in Techniques and standard internal screw fixation principles are used.

Hamate Body Fractures

- Fractures of the hamate body are often associated with fourth and/or fifth CMC dislocations (**FIG 4B,C**). ORIF is recommended to reduce the articular surfaces and stabilize the CMC joints.
- These injuries most often result from a dorsal shear mechanism with fracture of the hamate body in the frontal plane. The metacarpals displace dorsally and proximally with the dorsal hamate fracture fragment.

Capitate Fractures

- Capitate fractures are by and large associated with high-energy trauma to the wrist.
  - In addition to fractures associated with progressive perilunate instability patterns and the scaphocapitate syndrome, capitate fractures may also occur due to axial loading along the middle finger ray or via direct trauma.
  - If caused by axially directed forces, the fracture line is often in the frontal plane and involves the long finger CMC joint, similar to the hamate dorsal shear fractures described earlier. The capitate may be essentially divided in half in this frontal plane.
  - In these cases, ORIF is performed through a dorsal approach.
- Truly isolated capitate fractures with minimal displacement heal by immobilization, but this often takes time.

Trapezoid Fractures

- The trapezoid is believed to be the least frequently fractured carpal bone.
- As with the other bones of the distal carpal row, assessment of the associated index CMC joint is necessary to rule out a fracture-dislocation.
  - Frontal plane dorsal shear fractures of the trapezoid can destabilize the index CMC.
- These fractures and fracture-dislocations can often be treated by closed reduction and pinning.
- If an open approach is required to reduce the articular surface and CMC joint, a standard third and fourth extensor compartment interval dorsal approach may be used. Fixation can be accomplished with pins or screws.
- A limited exposure (as described in the following text) is an alternative.

Trapezium Fractures

- Fractures of the body of the trapezium nearly always involve one of its four articular facets and frequently lead to subluxation of the thumb CMC joint (**FIG 5**).

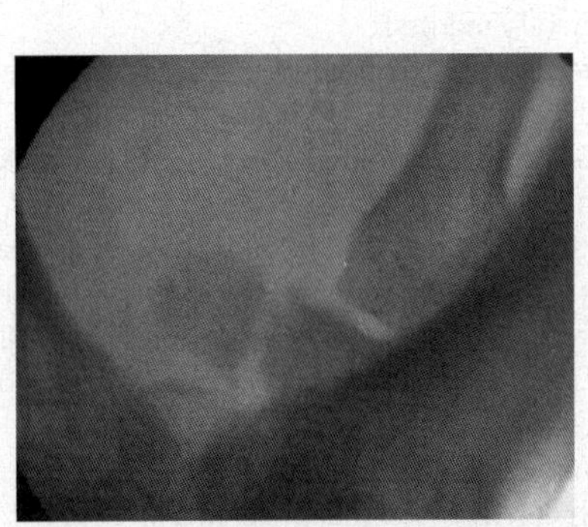
A

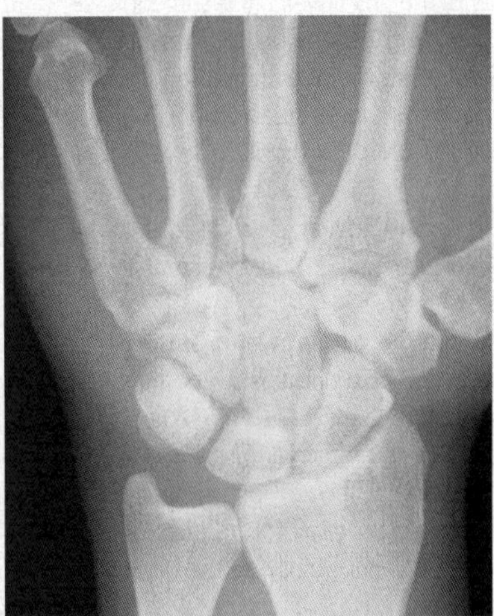
B

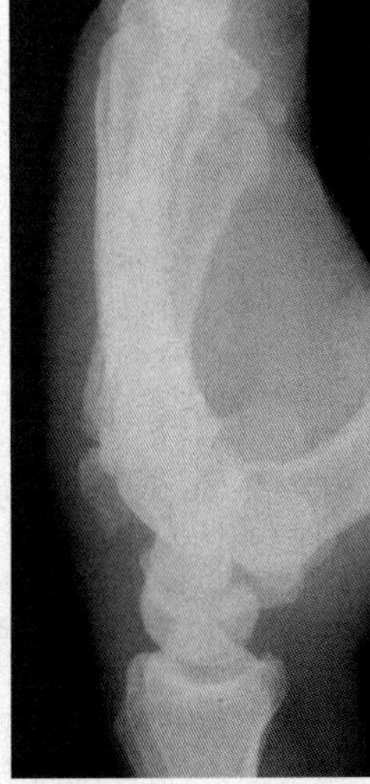
C

FIG 4 • Hamate fractures. **A.** Supination, oblique, radial deviation radiograph showing hamate hook fracture. **B,C.** AP and lateral radiographs of a hamate body dorsal shear fracture associated with the small finger and ring finger CMC articulation as well as a fracture of the base of the ring finger metacarpal.

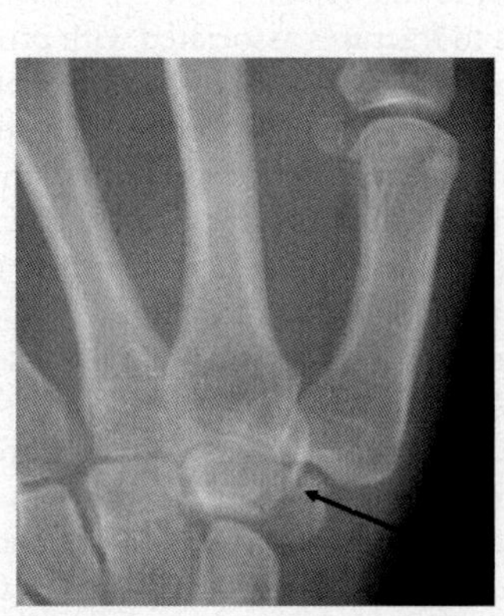
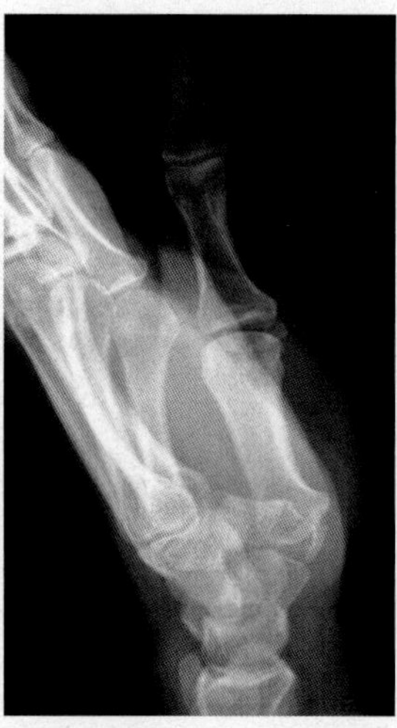

FIG 5 • **A,B.** Trapezial body fractures.

- If internal fixation is not possible, trapezial excision and palmar oblique ligament reconstruction, or the surgeon's preferred alternative procedure used for routine thumb CMC osteoarthritis, is performed.

Preoperative Planning

- Examination under anesthesia, possibly with concomitant fluoroscopic imaging, helps confirm whether carpal instability coexists.
- The surgeon should ensure that all needed fixation implants and systems are available before bringing the patient to the operating room.
- A hand table, a well-padded upper arm tourniquet, and a mobile mini-fluoroscopy unit are used.
- Anesthesia and analgesia may be obtained through regional or general methods.

Approach

- Carpal fractures may be approached dorsally, palmarly, radially, or ulnarly depending on the reduction needs, implants used, and location and characteristics of the fracture(s).
- Some surgeons use wrist or small joint arthroscopy as an aid to fracture reduction and management.

TECHNIQUES

Open Reduction and Internal Fixation of Lunate Fractures

Incision and Dissection

- An extended carpal tunnel approach is used for palmar exposure.
- The incision begins in the palm, just ulnar to the thenar crease and in line with the radial border of the ring finger. If the surgeon is comfortable with the deep anatomy, especially the possible anatomic variations involving the thenar motor branch, the incision in the palm may also be along the thenar crease itself.
- The incision is extended proximally until the distal volar wrist crease is reached.
- A curved or zigzag continuation of the incision is made at the crease to avoid crossing perpendicular to the wrist crease and associated scarring and flexion contracture.
- The incision may be continued into the distal forearm, staying ulnar to the palmaris longus so as to avoid damage to the palmar cutaneous branch of the median nerve (**TECH FIG 1A**).
- The exposure is deepened distally until the palmar fascia is encountered (**TECH FIG 1B**). This fascia is incised longitudinally just radial to the hamate hook. Dissection distal to the level of the hamate hook must be performed very carefully, as the ulnar neurovascular bundle is in this region.
- The transverse carpal ligament is opened longitudinally, staying just radial to the hamate hook and again being very cautious at the distal aspect of the exposure.
- The incision is continued proximally, releasing the distal volar forearm fascia, again staying ulnar to the palmaris longus.
    - The contents of the carpal canal are now visualized (**TECH FIG 1C**).
- The digital flexors and median nerve are gently and bluntly retracted radially, revealing the floor of the canal that overlies the volar carpus (**TECH FIG 1D**).
- The volar capsule of the wrist joint is incised longitudinally, providing exposure of the volar carpus and radiocarpal joint.

Reduction and Fixation

- The palmar lip fracture of the lunate is identified, cleaned, and anatomically reduced.
- The fracture may be fixed with small interfragment screws or buried Kirschner wires (**TECH FIG 2**).
    - Screws are favored, if at all possible, to minimize chances of hardware migration into the carpal tunnel.
- Fluoroscopic images are necessary to confirm that any carpal subluxation has been corrected by stabilizing the lunate fracture.
- The volar wrist capsule is repaired and the median nerve and digital flexors are allowed to return to their normal resting position.
- The transverse carpal ligament may be repaired in a lengthened fashion or left divided (our preference).
- Subcutaneous tissue and skin closure is performed according to the surgeon's routine.

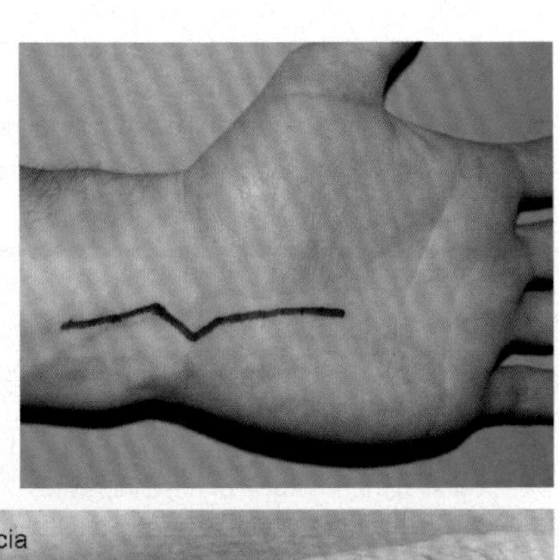

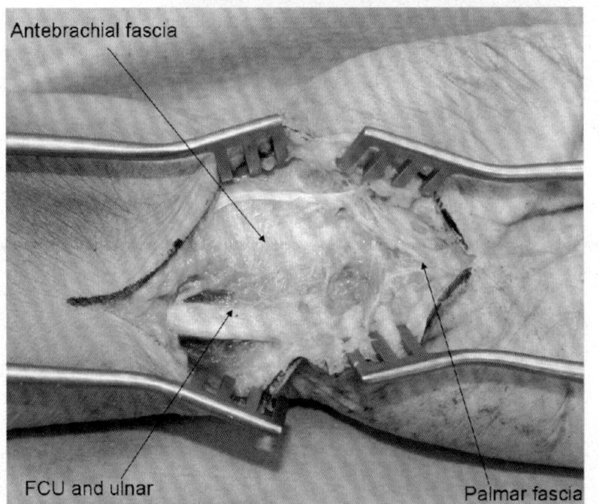

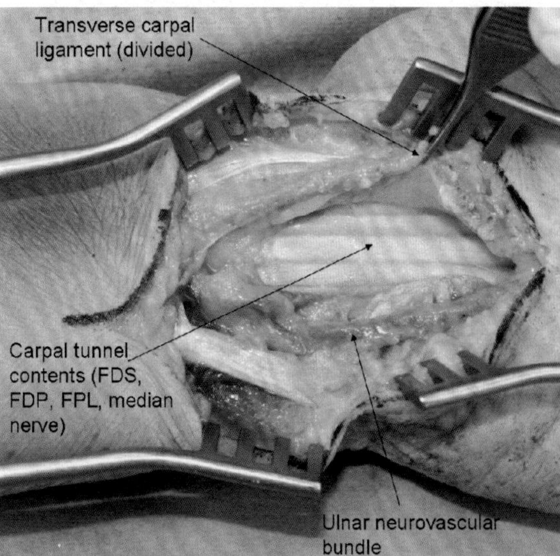

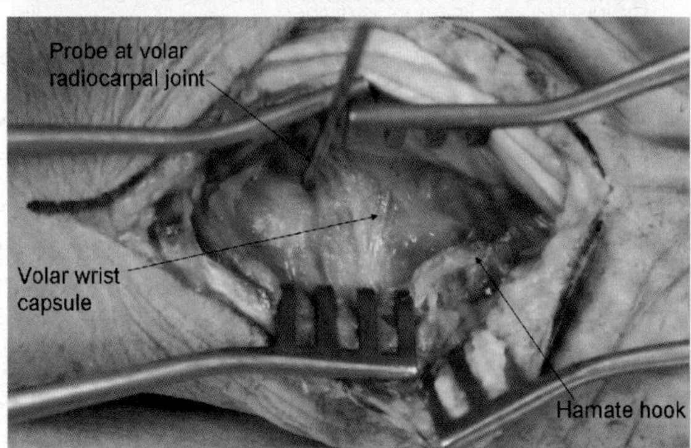

TECH FIG 1 • Fixation of lunate palmar lip fractures. **A.** Carpal tunnel approach. The incision can be continued into the distal forearm, staying ulnar to the palmaris longus to avoid damage to the palmar cutaneous branch of the median nerve. **B.** Palmar fascia and antebrachial fascia exposed. **C.** Transverse carpal ligament released from hamate hook. **D.** Volar wrist capsule exposed.

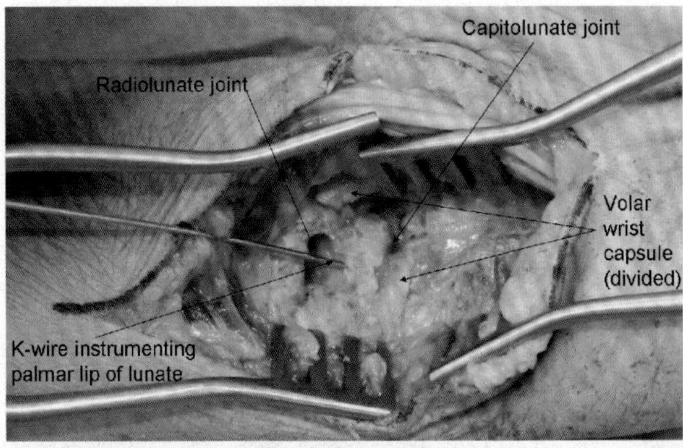

TECH FIG 2 • Palmar lunate lip exposed and instrumented.

Open Reduction and Internal Fixation of Triquetral Fractures

- Access to the triquetrum is usually achieved through the standard dorsal approach to the wrist that is described for capitate fractures.
- If there is truly isolated triquetral pathology, a more limited dorsal approach between the fifth and sixth extensor compartments is used.
  - This incision is centered distal to that which would be used for distal radioulnar joint (DRUJ) exposure.

- The fifth compartment (extensor digiti minimi [EDM]) is retracted radially, whereas the sixth compartment (extensor carpi ulnaris [ECU]) is retracted ulnarly.
- The carpal capsule is incised longitudinally or obliquely depending on the fracture and the integrity of the dorsal radiotriquetral ligament.
- The triquetral fracture may now be cleaned, reduced, and fixed with mini-screws or Kirschner wires as the fracture pattern prescribes.
- Supplemental pinning to the lunate or hamate is performed as needed.
- The capsule is closed, followed by routine subcutaneous tissue and skin closure all according to surgeon preference.

Excision or Open Reduction and Internal Fixation of Pisiform Fractures

- A curvilinear incision is made with special care not to cross the distal volar wrist crease perpendicularly. The incision is made centered on or just radial to the pisiform.
- The ulnar neurovascular bundle is identified proximally and traced distally just past the pisiform body.
- The pisohamate ligament is divided.
- The FCU tendon, if intact, is divided longitudinally directly over the pisiform and the FCU and pisiform periosteum are elevated radially and ulnarly.
- At this point, the pisiform can be excised or internally fixed with minifragment screws or Kirschner wires.
  - The risk for hardware migration, penetration into the pisotriquetral joint, and other complications in the region of the ulnar neurovascular bundle must be weighed against the good results expected with simple excision.
- The split FCU is closed with a nonabsorbable suture, and the subcutaneous tissue and skin are sutured in routine fashion.

Hook of Hamate Excision

- The hamate hook can be approached through a volar incision (our preferred method) or directly ulnar, proceeding palmar to the small finger metacarpal and dorsal to the abductor digiti minimi.
- A volar longitudinal or curvilinear skin incision is made, centered over the hook (**TECH FIG 3A**).
- The ulnar nerve and artery are identified proximally first and then traced distally, ulnar and superficial to the hamate hook (**TECH FIG 3B–D**).
- Once the level of the hook is reached distally, the ulnar neurovascular bundle is gently retracted ulnarly.
- Soft tissue attachments to the tip of the hook are incised longitudinally, including the transverse carpal ligament radially and the pisohamate ligament ulnarly and proximally.
- The deep motor branch of the ulnar nerve should be identified as it passes distally around the base of the hamate hook in an ulnar to radial direction and must be protected during excision (**TECH FIG 3E**).
- The digital flexors within the carpal canal are identified. The ring and small finger flexors, especially the profundus tendons, are

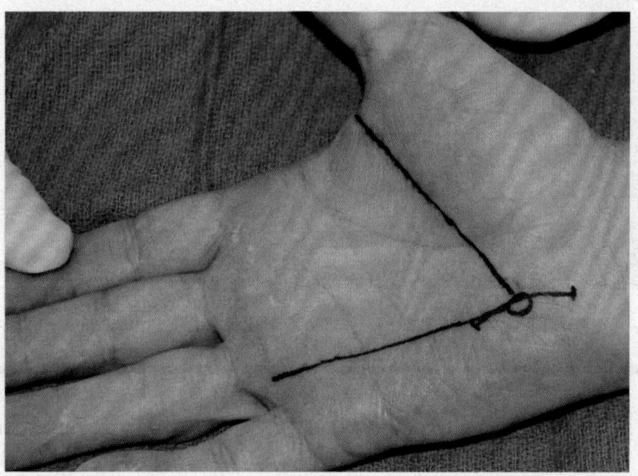

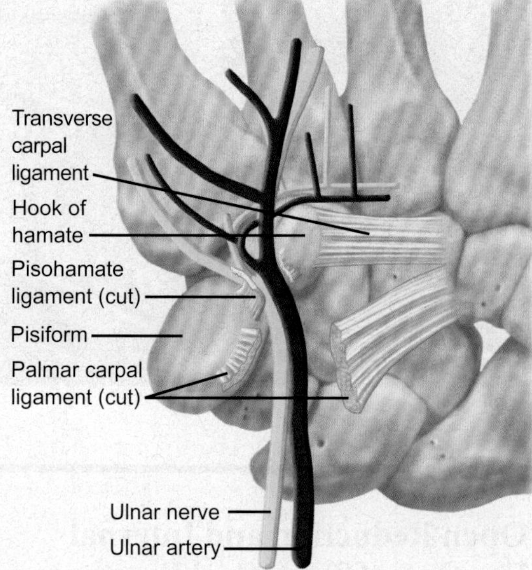

TECH FIG 3 • Excision of hamate hook fractures. **A.** The cardinal line of Kaplan, drawn from the apex of the first web space to the ulnar border of the hand, intersects a second line drawn along the ulnar margin of the ring digit at the hamate hook (*circle*). A 3-cm incision is centered over the hamate hook, gently curving with the radial border of the hypothenar eminence. **B.** The ulnar nerve and artery can be found proximally first and then traced distally, ulnar and superficial to the hamate hook. *(continued)*

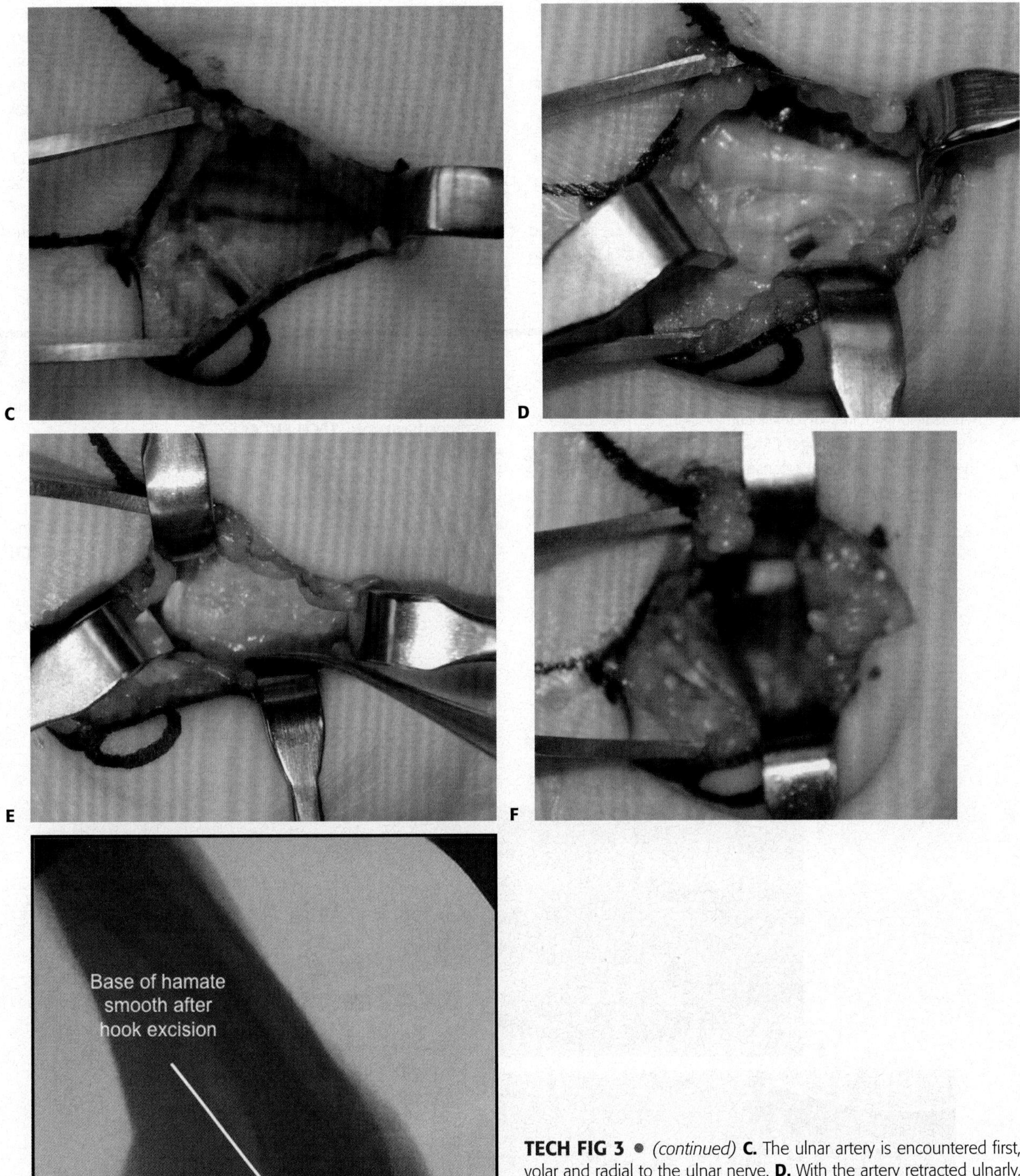

TECH FIG 3 • *(continued)* **C.** The ulnar artery is encountered first, volar and radial to the ulnar nerve. **D.** With the artery retracted ulnarly, the common digital nerve to the fourth web space and the small digit ulnar sensory nerve are visualized. The deep motor branch and the hypothenar motor branch have already been given off. **E.** The hamate hook is subperiosteally exposed and its margins are palpated with an elevator. The deep motor branch curves radially, closely associated with the distal surface of the hook. **F.** Care is also taken to protect the flexor tendons during exposure and resection, seen here on the radial margin of the hook. **G.** Fluoroscopy after hook excision can be helpful to ensure that the hook has been removed in its entirety and that no significant prominences remain.

inspected to ensure integrity and should be débrided or repaired or reconstructed as needed (**TECH FIG 3F**).
  - The tendons are then gently retracted radially.
- The hook is cleared of all soft tissue attachments down to the level of the fracture site.
  - Use of a no. 69 Beaver blade eases this exposure.
- Using a rongeur or similar tool, the fractured hook is removed piecemeal, again with care to protect the deep ulnar motor branch and other structures.
- Once the fragment is removed, the remaining base is inspected and smoothed with a rongeur, curette, or similar tool until there are no sharp bony prominences (**TECH FIG 3G**).
- The surrounding periosteum is closed if possible. The fingers are ranged in flexion/extension to make sure that the flexor tendons are not running over any sharp edges following the hamate hook excision. If there is a complete rupture of one of the profundus tendons due to attritional wear against the hamate hook fracture, we prefer side transfer to one of the intact profundus tendons. This typically necessitates lengthening of the exposure distally, and the neurovascular structures should be dissected and protected before performing the tendon work.
- Subcutaneous tissue and skin closure is performed in a routine manner.

Hamate Body Fractures

- A dorsal longitudinal or curvilinear incision is made centered over the ring or small finger CMC joints (**TECH FIG 4A**).
- The ring and small finger extensor tendons are retracted radially or ulnarly together or individually as needed.
  - There can be significant variation in the anatomic appearance and interconnections of the extensor digitorum communis tendons to the ring and small fingers as well as the EDM (**TECH FIG 4B**). These variations usually dictate which direction to retract the tendons and whether to retract them together or individually to give the best access to the CMC joints.
- The CMC joint capsule and dorsal CMC ligaments are incised longitudinally. The CMC joint is cleared of any hematoma and bone fragments (**TECH FIG 4C**).
- The fracture site is cleared of hematoma and reduced while directly visualizing the distal articular surface.
  - A dental pick is useful to reduce small fragments.
- The fracture is temporarily stabilized with Kirschner wires, and fluoroscopic images are taken to confirm reduction (**TECH FIG 4D,E**).
- If there is a large dorsal fragment, two or more dorsal to volar lag screws (usually 2.0-mm screws or smaller) are placed

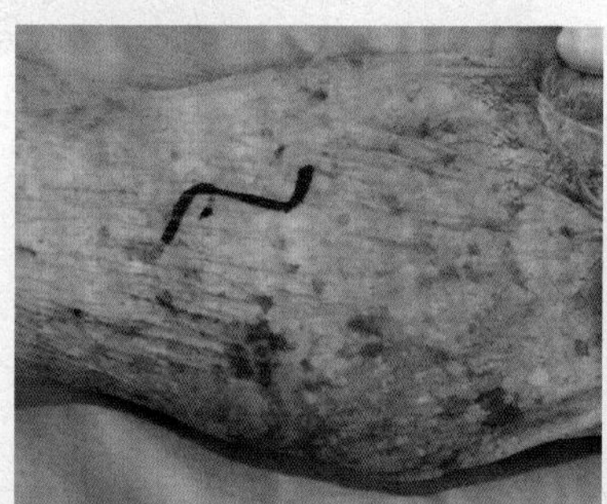
A

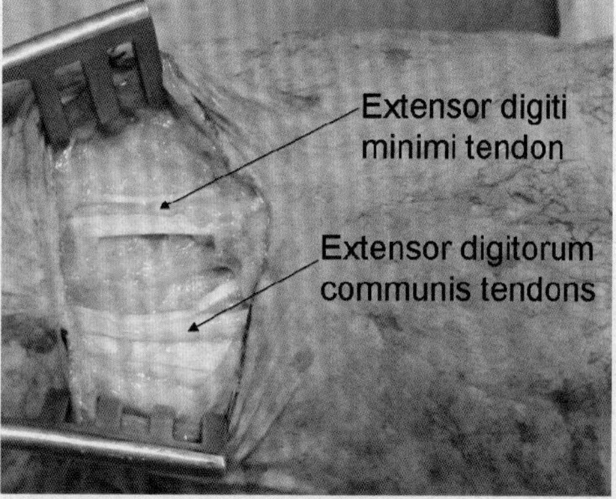

B

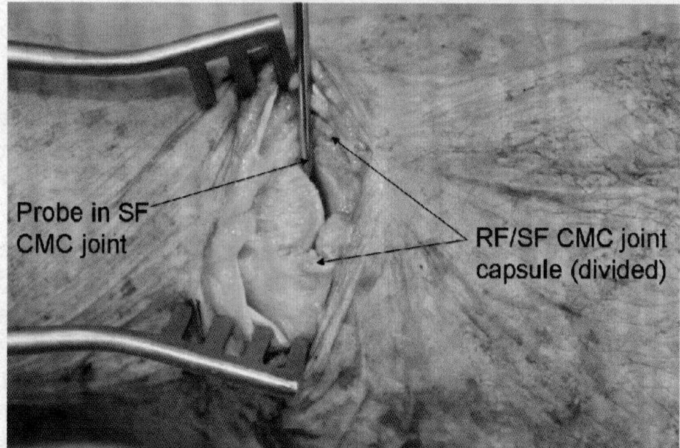

C

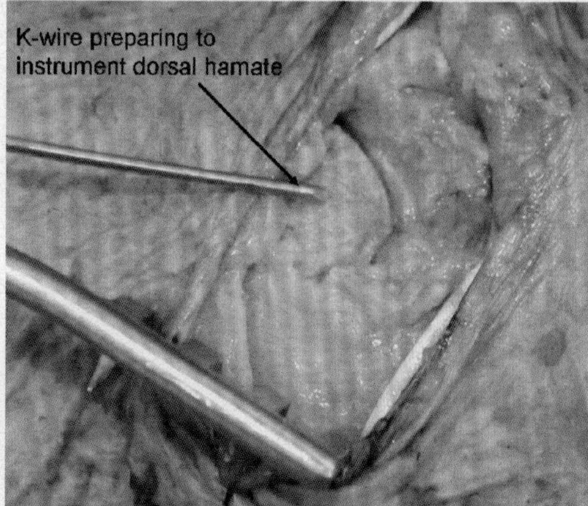

D

TECH FIG 4 • Fixation of hamate dorsal shear fractures. **A.** Dorsal curvilinear incision centered on ring finger–small finger CMC joint. **B.** Extensor tendons exposed. **C.** Ring finger–small finger CMC joint exposed. **D.** Dorsal hamate reduced and instrumented. *(continued)*

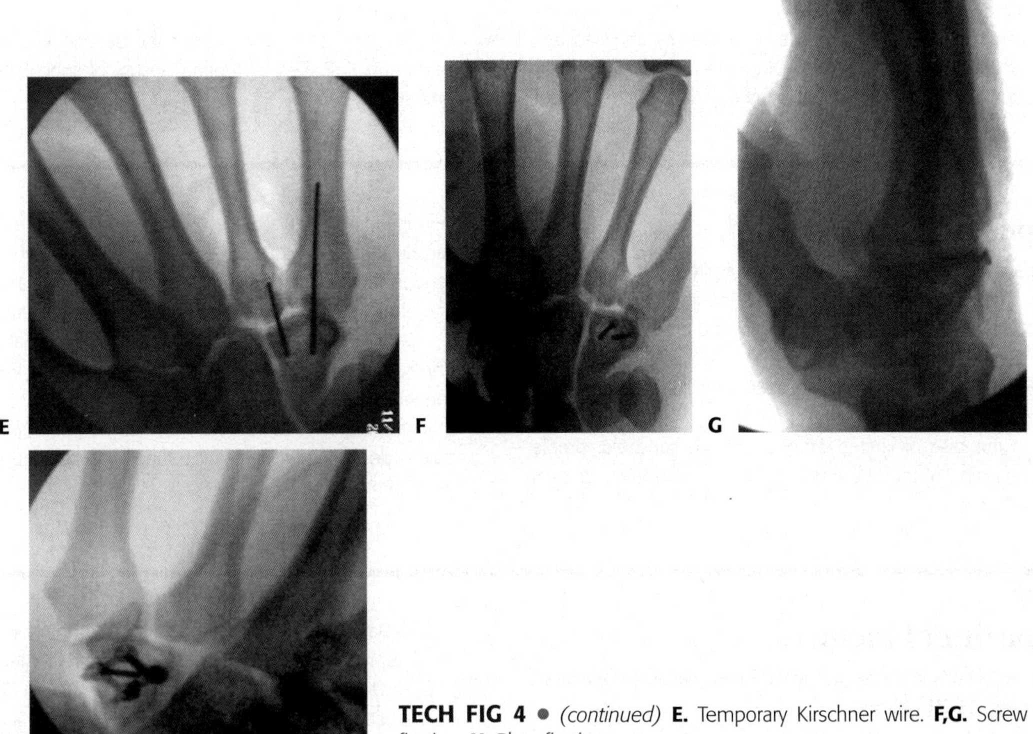

TECH FIG 4 • *(continued)* **E.** Temporary Kirschner wire. **F,G.** Screw fixation. **H.** Plate fixation.

perpendicular to the fracture line into the hamate body (**TECH FIG 4F,G**).

- If there are several small fragments, individual screws may be used for each piece or a dorsal plate may be more effective (**TECH FIG 4H**).
- Fluoroscopic images are necessary to confirm that the screws do not protrude outside of the palmar hamate cortex which could potentially damage the ulnar neurovascular structures or flexor tendons.
- The dorsal capsuloligamentous sleeve is closed if possible, thus providing a smooth gliding surface between the extensor tendons and the CMC joint and hardware.
- The CMC joints may be pinned temporarily if still unstable.
  - In the acute setting, if the dorsal hamate fracture is of sufficient size and securely stabilized and the joint capsule is closed, this is usually not necessary.
- Soft tissues and skin are closed in a routine manner.

Capitate Fractures

- Often, a standard approach to the dorsal carpus is required and is carried out through the routine third and fourth extensor compartment interval.
- A dorsal midline longitudinal or curvilinear skin incision is made, in line with the middle finger ray and centered on the capitate.
- Full-thickness skin flaps are elevated radially and ulnarly.
- The extensor pollicis longus (EPL) is identified, released from its third extensor compartment, and transposed radially.
- The plane between the extensor tendons and the wrist capsule is developed by elevating the second and fourth compartments radially and ulnarly, respectively.
- The joint capsule and dorsal intercarpal ligament are usually divided longitudinally for access to the capitate body.
  - Alternatively, the capsule can be opened longitudinally distal to the dorsal intercarpal ligament (**TECH FIG 5**).
  - The capsule can also be incised transversely distal to the ligament and in line with its fibers, provided that exposure

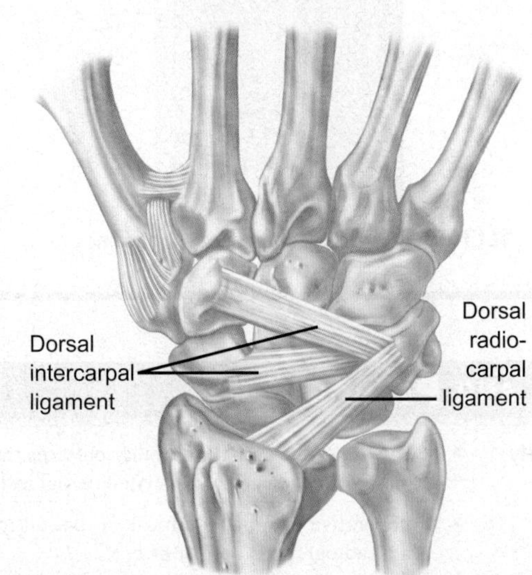

TECH FIG 5 • Dorsal intercarpal ligament anatomy.

of the capitate is adequate for reduction and fixation of the fracture.

- The fracture site is explored, cleaned as necessary, and stabilized with mini-screws, plates, or pins as indicated.
- The capsule and dorsal intercarpal ligament, if divided, are repaired.
- The EPL tendon is left transposed, superficial to the extensor retinaculum.
- The retinaculum is closed over the second and fourth compartments, followed by routine closure of subcutaneous tissue and skin.

Trapezoid Fractures

- The trapezoid is approached through a limited dorsal longitudinal or curvilinear incision centered over the index CMC.
  - Care must be exercised to identify and protect dorsoradial sensory nerve branches.
- The EPL tendon is identified, released, and transposed radially if needed.
  - In the case of limited exposure of the trapezoid, simple retraction of the EPL distal to the extensor retinaculum is effective.
- A longitudinal interval is developed between the extensor carpi radialis longus (ECRL) and extensor carpi radialis brevis (ECRB) tendons with radial and ulnar retraction, respectively.
  - It is important to stay ulnar to the ECRL to avoid inadvertent damage to the dorsal branch of the radial artery.
- The capsule is divided longitudinally, exposing the trapezoid and the index CMC joint.
- Fracture fixation is carried out with mini-screws or pins, the capsule is closed, and routine subcutaneous tissue and skin closure is performed.

Trapezium Fractures

- Fractures of sufficient size and significant displacement are internally fixed (**TECH FIG 6**).
  - Excision rather than internal fixation may be warranted based on preoperative and intraoperative considerations.
- Unless the fracture planes dictate a specific approach for fixation, the surgeon has the option of using whichever approach he or she is most comfortable with for routine surgical treatment of thumb CMC arthritis (see Chap. 117).
  - The Wagner approach (described in the following) is one such approach frequently used for surgical reconstruction of thumb CMC arthritis and is an effective exposure for internal fixation of body fractures.

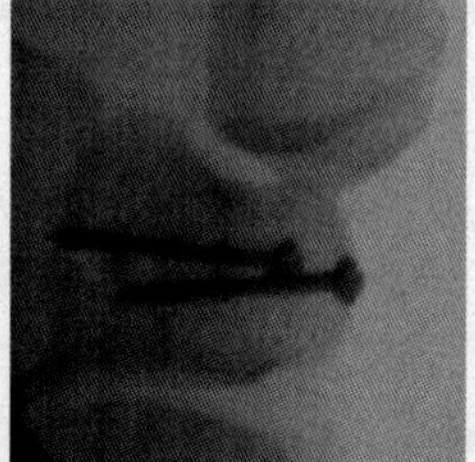

TECH FIG 6 • ORIF of a trapezial body fracture.

  - Isolated trapezial ridge fractures and nonunions are best approached using the FCR approach centered on the scaphotrapezial joint, with retraction of the FCR ulnarly or radially out of its trapezial groove to gain access to the ridge. The Wagner approach is also effective.
- For the Wagner approach, an incision is made along the radial border of the thumb metacarpal at the glabrous skin border.
- At the distal volar wrist crease, the incision is continued ulnarly to the level of the FCR tendon.
  - Superficial radial sensory nerve and lateral antebrachial cutaneous nerve branches may be encountered and should be carefully preserved.
- The thenar musculature is elevated in a radial to ulnar direction off the thumb metacarpal base.
- Once the FCR tendon sheath is reached, it is incised longitudinally and the tendon is retracted ulnarly if necessary.
- The capsule overlying the trapeziometacarpal and scaphotrapezial joints is opened and the joints are visualized.
- The entire length of the trapezium may be exposed if needed, but we avoid excessive subperiosteal dissection, doing so only where necessary for accurate fracture reduction.
  - Extensive exposure may result in delayed union or nonunion.
- At this point, internal fixation is performed if technically feasible, usually using lag screw fixation.
- The capsule is carefully reapproximated, and the subcutaneous tissues and skin are closed.

PEARLS AND PITFALLS

Carpal instability	■ Be aware of the carpal instability patterns that can accompany these fractures and treat accordingly. ■ Failure to recognize an associated carpal instability pattern can lead to progressive carpal collapse and degeneration.
Fracture identification	■ Preoperative imaging is critical so that all fractures that require stabilization are identified; consider CT scanning if plain radiographs are insufficient. ■ Failing to identify all unstable fractures before or during surgery can necessitate a return to the operating room.

Screw size	■ Use small interfragmentary screws or even small plates for fracture fixation whenever possible to decrease chances for hardware migration and to increase stability and possibly allow earlier range of motion.
Excision versus fixation	■ We recommend hamate hook excision as opposed to fixation due to the minimal, if any, added benefit with fixation and the concern for significant nerve and tendon injuries with internal fixation.
Future surgery	■ Be sure the patient is aware of the possible need for further surgery in the future, such as for hamate hook excision, addressing capitate avascular necrosis, excisional arthroplasty or arthrodesis for posttraumatic articular degeneration of any joints involved with the initial trauma, and so forth.

POSTOPERATIVE CARE

- Patients are placed in a well-padded volar plaster wrist splint postoperatively.
  - The digits, including the metacarpophalangeal (MCP) joints, are left free unless there is some contraindication, such as a dorsal hamate fracture with CMC dislocation, which may require inclusion of MCP joints.
  - If there is no contraindication, we encourage early digital range of motion and elevation.
  - Following ORIF of a trapezial fracture, a short-arm thumb spica splint is applied.
- One to 2 weeks postoperatively, the patient is placed in a custom-fabricated splint (assuming there is no associated carpal instability).
  - If pins were used and are left outside of the skin, pin care is initiated at this time. Pins are usually removed 4 to 8 weeks postoperatively.
- In the case of a CMC joint fracture in which relatively large fracture fragments are anatomically stabilized with rigid internal fixation, near-immediate postoperative range of motion is initiated.
- For most other fractures, a total of about 6 weeks of wrist immobilization is followed by progressive range of motion.

OUTCOMES

- Most isolated carpal bone body fractures unite, and it is generally thought that these patients do quite well with regard to symptomatic and functional recovery.
- The potentially symptomatic exceptions involving the hamate hook and trapezial ridge are easily treated by excision. Posttraumatic symptoms from other fractures, such as of the pisiform, trapezium, or triquetrum, may usually be addressed with isolated carpal bone excision with or without reconstruction, depending on the bone in question and other soft tissue and ligamentous considerations. For those carpal bones that cannot typically be simply excised, such as the hamate body and capitate, symptomatic posttraumatic changes may require partial or total wrist arthrodesis or other reconstructive options.
- Associated injuries are often the most problematic, and patients must understand the guarded prognosis for severe destabilizing carpal injuries.

COMPLICATIONS

- Those complications common to all surgical procedures may occur, including but not limited to bleeding, infection, damage to structures, failure of surgery, potential need for more surgery, and untoward effects of anesthesia.
  - Patients must also understand the relative severity of their injuries and risk for pain, stiffness, and loss of function.
- Capitate neck fractures are sometimes associated with nonunion or delayed union (up to 50% or more of isolated fractures) and may be analogous to scaphoid proximal pole fractures.
  - Treatment of such nonunions is similar for both entities.
- Although rare, avascular necrosis of the capitate head may follow a capitate neck fracture that disrupts the vascular supply.
  - The capitate head may be excised with or without interpositional arthroplasty if attaining union is not likely because of avascularity or other issues.
- Intra-articular fractures of the carpal bones are often complicated by posttraumatic arthritis. When symptomatic, treatment with traditional arthritis remedies, such as activity modification, anti-inflammatory medications, immobilization, or steroid injection, can be tried. If these fail to relieve the patient's symptoms to his or her satisfaction, the patient may elect to proceed with partial or total wrist arthrodesis, partial carpectomy, whether of the proximal row or otherwise, or selective arthroplasties as indicated.

SUGGESTED READINGS

1. Adler JB, Shaftan GW. Fractures of the capitate. J Bone Joint Surg Am 1962;44-A:1537–1547.
2. Amadio PC, Moran SL. Fractures of the carpal bones. In: Green DP, Hotchkiss DP, Pederson RN, et al, eds. Operative Hand Surgery, ed 5. Philadelphia: Elsevier, 2005;771–768.
3. Cohen MS. Fractures of the carpal bones. Hand Clin 1997;13:587–599.
4. Gelberman RH, Gross MS. The vascularity of the wrist: identification of arterial patterns at risk. Clin Orthop Relat Res 1986;(202):40–49.
5. Hoppenfeld S, deBoer P. Surgical Exposures in Orthopaedics: The Anatomic Approach, ed 2. Philadelphia: Lippincott Williams & Wilkins, 1994.
6. Vigler M, Aviles A, Lee SK. Carpal fractures excluding the scaphoid. Hand Clin 2006;22:501–516.
7. Yu HL, Chase RA, Strauch B. Atlas of Hand Anatomy and Clinical Implications. St. Louis: Mosby, 2004.

40
CHAPTER

Osteotomy of the Radius for Treatment of Kienböck Disease

Cameron T. Atkinson, Jeffrey E. Budoff, and David S. Zelouf

DEFINITION

- Kienböck disease is a disorder of undetermined etiology that results in avascular necrosis (AVN) of the lunate.[7]

ANATOMY

Lunate Vascularity

- The extraosseous blood supply of the lunate is extensive: Branches of the radial and anterior interosseous arteries form a dorsal lunate plexus and branches of the radial, ulnar, and anterior interosseous arteries as well as the recurrent deep palmar arch form a volar plexus.
- The intraosseous blood supply is variable. Because the lunate is covered by cartilage proximally and distally, vessels can enter the bone only at its dorsal and volar poles.[2,16]
  - Three studies have identified "lunates at risk" from a vascular standpoint. The vulnerable lunate is one that has large areas of bone dependent on a single intraosseous vessel, which occurs in 7% to 20%. In addition, 31% of lunates have no internal arterial branching.[8,9,19] These internal vascular arrangements may render the lunate more vulnerable to AVN, as injury to the single vessel could not be compensated for by collateral flow.

Ulnar Variance

- The standard posteroanterior (PA) wrist radiograph is taken with the shoulder and elbow at 90 degrees and the forearm in neutral rotation.
- In this view, the length of the distal ulna with respect to the distal radius is called *ulnar variance* (**FIG 1**).
  - When the ulna is the same length as the radius, it is said to have neutral ulnar variance. When the ulna is shorter than the radius, it is referred to as *negative ulnar variance*, and when the ulna is longer than the radius, it is referred to as *positive ulnar variance*.
- Theoretically, a negative ulnar variance increases shear forces on the lunate.
  - The triangular fibrocartilage complex (TFCC) is thicker in these patients and the difference in compliance between it and the ulnar edge of the radius is accentuated, leading to greater shear force.
  - In addition, loads across the radiocarpal joint are borne disproportionately by the radius.[7]
- In the North American population, Kienböck disease is associated with a negative ulnar variance.
  - This relationship does not hold true in the Japanese literature.[2]
  - There is no evidence that the relationship between negative ulnar variance and Kienböck disease is causal.[6,26]
- Other authors have noted a tendency toward smaller lunates in patients with Kienböck disease.[3]

PATHOGENESIS

- The cause of Kienböck disease is incompletely understood. Current thinking is that acute or repetitive trauma causes excessive shear forces on a lunate at risk, interrupting its intraosseous vascularity and leading to AVN.[1,2]
- Although a history of injury is elicited in over 50% of cases, the absence of a single traumatic event is still very common.
  - Fracture of the lunate has been reported in up to 82% of lunates with Kienböck disease.[2] However, it remains unclear whether these fractures are the cause or the result of AVN.
  - Kienböck disease is not seen after lunate or perilunate dislocations.[7,16]
    - Although transient ischemia may be seen after carpal fracture-dislocations, this spontaneously resolves after 5 to 32 months and should be treated expectantly.[1,2]

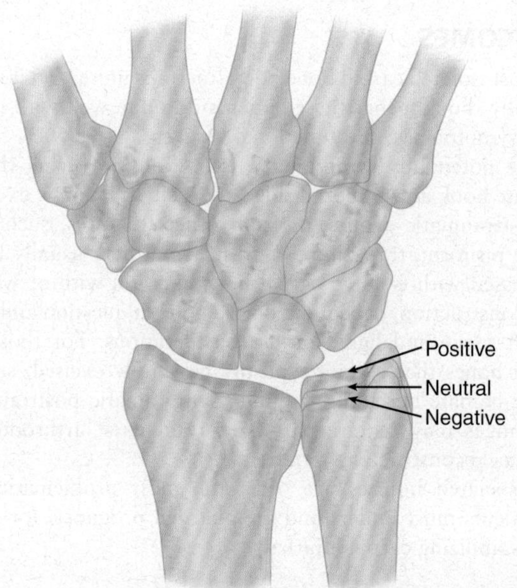

FIG 1 • Measurement of ulnar variance. Ulnar variance is determined by extending a line from the radius' articular surface ulnarward and measuring the distance between this line and the distal surface of the ulnar head. Neutral ulnar variance occurs when the carpal surface of the radius and ulna are equal in height. If the ulna is shorter than the radius, negative ulnar variance exists; if the ulna is longer than the radius, positive ulnar variance exists.

- The key feature of transient ischemia is that no progressive radiographic collapse occurs, as opposed to Kienböck disease, where radiographic changes and collapse are predictable.
- It has been suggested that Kienböck disease may be due to venous outflow obstruction with intraosseous vascular congestion rather than arterial insufficiency. Increased intraosseous pressure has been shown in lunates with Kienböck disease as well as in femoral heads with AVN.
  - This is more consistent with venous stasis than arterial compromise.
  - This increased pressure could also be due to bony collapse.[3,7]
- Once the lunate becomes avascular, stress fractures occur first in the proximal lunate adjacent to the radial articular surface, where the blood supply is poorest.[2,8,16] Consequently, the proximal lunate is usually more involved and more flattened than the distal lunate. In addition, the radial lunate that articulates with the distal radius is usually more involved than the ulnar lunate that overlies the triangular fibrocartilage, probably because of the difference in compliance between the two supporting surfaces. This difference is accentuated in patients with negative ulnar variance.[16]
- Lunate collapse leads to loss of carpal height. If a coronal plane fracture is present, the compressive forces of the capitate displace these two fragments volarly and dorsally.[16]

NATURAL HISTORY

- The natural history of Kienböck disease is one of progressive fragmentation and collapse of the lunate, loss of carpal height with scaphoid flexion, and proximal capitate migration leading to perilunate arthritis. However, these changes do not universally lead to a poor clinical outcome.[7]
- A follow-up study of 49 patients compared 23 wrists treated with mean 8 weeks of immobilization and 26 without treatment.[14]
  - In both groups, the majority reported a gradual decrease in symptoms over time.
  - At mean 20.5 years of follow-up, 83% of the wrists in the immobilized group were pain-free or were painful only with heavy work.
  - In the nontreated group, this was true for 77%.
  - In all wrists, the lunate was deformed and 67% developed radiocarpal arthritis on radiographs.
  - The authors concluded that Kienböck disease has a naturally benign course.
  - There was no correlation between residual symptoms and the radiographic appearance, including the appearance of arthritis.
  - In this study, immobilization did not lead to any long-term benefit.

PATIENT HISTORY AND PHYSICAL FINDINGS

- Most patients with Kienböck disease are young, active patients between 20 to 40 years of age.
  - This has led to significant concerns about the long-term effects of this disorder.
- The male–female ratio is approximately 3:1 to 7:1. It is rarely bilateral.[3,27]
  - Regardless of gender, more than 95% of patients are engaged in heavy manual labor.[27]
- The most common complaints are dorsal central wrist pain, stiffness, and significant weakness of grip, which is often reduced to 50% of the opposite hand.[2,7,16]
  - There may be a long history of symptoms before presentation.
  - The pain may vary in intensity from mild discomfort to constant, debilitating pain. It is often activity related and improves with rest and immobilization.
  - A history of trauma is variable.[2,7]
- The wrist is typically mildly swollen dorsally, consistent with synovitis, and is tender over the lunate.
- Flexion and extension are predictably diminished.
  - Wrist flexion is more likely to be limited than extension because the volar pole of the lunate often extrudes so that it impinges against the volar rim of the distal radius.
  - Forearm rotation is not affected.[16]
- Although Kienböck disease has been reported in association with steroid use, septic emboli, sickle cell disease, gout, carpal coalition, and cerebral palsy, there is no well-defined correlation with any systemic or neuromuscular process that warrants screening when considering the diagnosis.[3]

IMAGING AND OTHER DIAGNOSTIC STUDIES

Radiographic Classification

- Kienböck disease is diagnosed radiographically, and staging is based on plain radiographs.
- In 1977, Lichtman and Degnan[15] modified Stahle's original radiographic classification in an attempt to help guide treatment decisions (**FIG 2**).
- Stage I
  - Radiographs are normal, although a linear fracture without sclerosis or lunate collapse is occasionally present.
  - Magnetic resonance imaging (MRI) shows the characteristic changes of AVN (**FIG 3A**).[7,27]
- Stage II
  - The lunate becomes sclerotic and radiodense, similar to the radiologic appearance of other bones with AVN (**FIG 3B**). A coronal fracture splitting the lunate into dorsal and volar fragments may be noted.
  - Late in stage II, some loss of lunate height on the radial side may be evident.
  - The lunate retains its overall shape, and its anatomic relationship to the other carpal bones is not significantly altered.[15,27]
- Stage III
  - The lunate collapses in the coronal plane and elongates in the sagittal plane. The carpal architecture is altered and the capitate begins to migrate proximally.
  - Stage IIIA
    - Lunate collapse has occurred, but carpal height is relatively unchanged and carpal collapse has not yet led to proximal migration of the capitate or scaphoid flexion. Therefore, the carpal kinematics have not yet been significantly altered.
  - Stage IIIB
    - The carpal collapse with proximal capitate migration has led to fixed scaphoid flexion, which may be noted on the anteroposterior (AP) radiograph as the "cortical ring sign."[3,5,27]

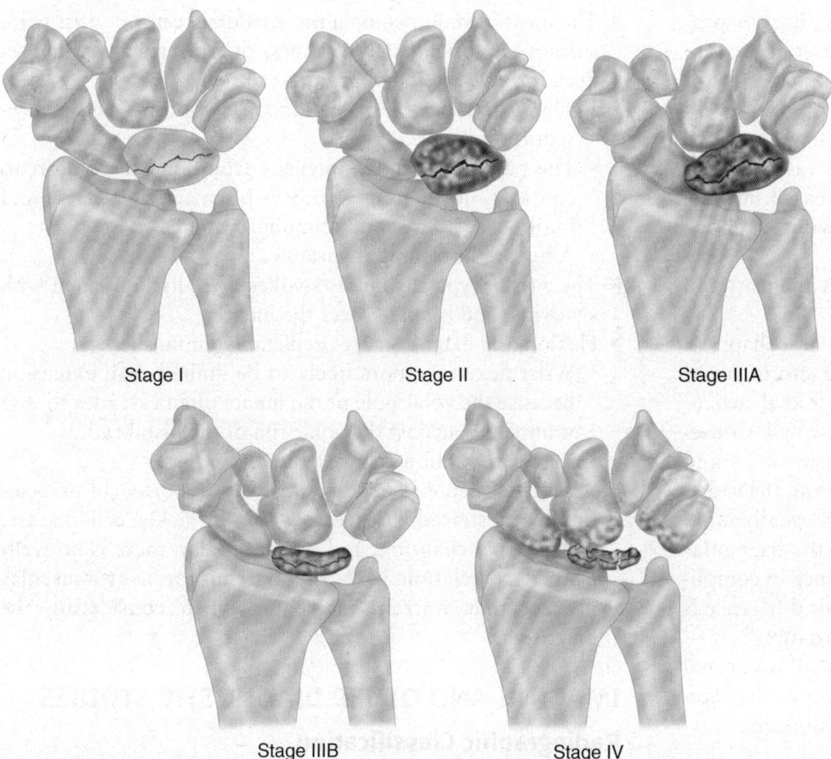

FIG 2 • Kienböck disease stage classification based on radiographic appearance.

- Stage IV
  - Arthritis of the radiocarpal or midcarpal joint has resulted from the collapse, fractures, and altered carpal kinematics, leading to joint space narrowing, osteophyte formation, subchondral sclerosis, and degenerative cysts.[3,27]

Magnetic Resonance Imaging and Computed Tomography

- MRI is extremely sensitive in detecting changes in marrow fat that are consistent with, but not diagnostic of, AVN.
- Decreased signal on T1 sequences represents replacement of the normal fatty marrow by dead bone or fibrous tissue.[27]
  - Because MRI detects only the loss of marrow fat and not AVN specifically, to consider an MRI diagnostic for Kienböck disease, over 50% of the lunate should be hypointense on T1 because the changes of Kienböck disease are diffuse, as opposed to other conditions such as ulnocarpal impaction, fractures, and intraosseous tumors, which cause more focal MRI changes.[4,25,28]
  - It is possible that a large enchondroma, interosseous ganglion, or other marrow-replacing lesion could lead to MRI changes in over 50% of the lunate. Thus, there is currently no truly pathognomonic imaging sign for Kienböck disease.[4]
- T2 images typically show low signal intensity, which represents replacement of the normal fatty marrow by fibrosis.[27]
  - An increased T2 signal may occur if intramedullary edema is present or if revascularization is occurring.[3,4,25] Thus, when the T2 images show normal or increased signal intensity, an earlier stage of disease with a better prognosis can be inferred.[25,27]

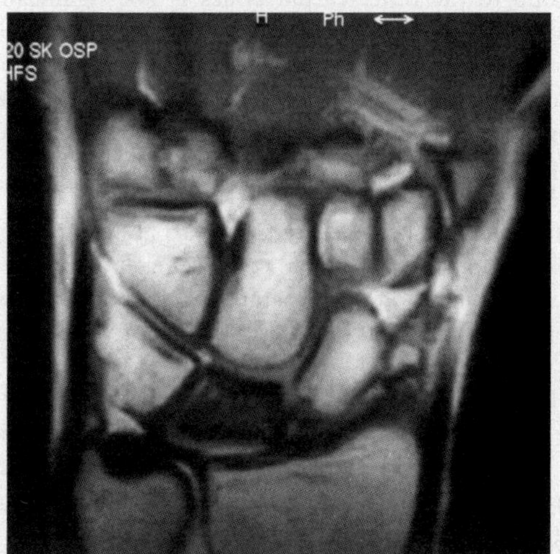

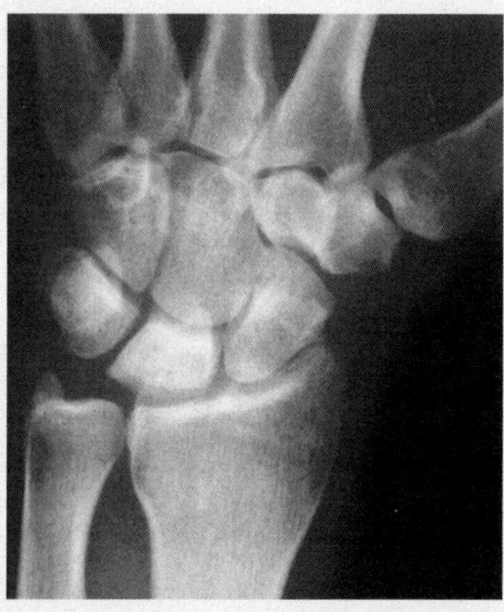

FIG 3 • **A.** MR image of wrist with Kienböck disease demonstrates diminished signal intensity of the lunate. **B.** Radiograph showing density changes in the lunate in Kienböck disease. (From Bishop AT, Pelzer M. Avascular necrosis. In: Berger RA, Weiss AP, eds. Hand surgery, vol 2. Philadelphia: Lippincott Williams & Wilkins, 2004:554.)

- Although it cannot diagnose AVN directly, MRI is still the optimal imaging modality and gold standard for diagnosing Kienböck disease, especially before trabecular bone has been destroyed.
- Gadolinium-enhanced MRI may provide a more sensitive means of evaluating lunate vascularity.
- Computed tomography (CT) may upstage the disease compared with radiographs in 89% of those originally considered to have stage I, 71% with apparent stage II, and 9% with apparent stage III disease on radiographs.[3]
  - Once lunate collapse has occurred, CT best reveals the extent of necrosis and trabecular destruction.

DIFFERENTIAL DIAGNOSIS

- Ulnocarpal impaction
- Rheumatoid arthritis
- Radial-sided triangular fibrocartilage tears
- Posttraumatic arthritis
- Acute fracture
- Carpal instability
- Lunate fracture
- Enchondroma
- Osteoid osteoma
- Bone island
- Occult or intraosseous ganglion
- Intraosseous cyst
- Transient ischemia
- "Bone bruise"
- Paget disease
- Gaucher disease[4]

NONOPERATIVE MANAGEMENT

- A trial of 2 weeks to 3 months of immobilization may be attempted for patients with stage I Kienböck disease, especially young patients with hyperintense lunates on T2 magnetic resonance (MR) images.
  - The theory behind the use of immobilization is that by decreasing the forces across the carpus, the lunate may be able to revascularize.[15]
  - Most series report poor results with immobilization, and progressive collapse is common.
  - There is no study of immobilization consisting of patients with only stage I Kienböck disease. Consequently, the efficacy of immobilization in patients with stage I disease is anecdotal.
- Immobilization does not decrease compressive forces across the lunate, which are imparted by the capitate. The capitate may still force any fracture fragments apart, leading to collapse and displacement.
  - Immobilization leads to stiffness.
  - The earlier the lunate is unloaded, the less collapse is anticipated. For this reason, early surgical decompression may be considered rather than immobilization, and many clinicians treat stage I disease surgically.[16]
- In Trumble and Irving's[28] series of 22 patients with various stages of Kienböck disease treated with immobilization, 17 showed disease progression with continued collapse of the lunate and 5 showed no improvement.
  - In Lichtman et al's series, 19 of 22 had unsatisfactory results.[1,3]
- When immobilization fails to reverse the avascular changes, the process will almost always advance to stage II, where surgical management is strongly recommended.[1,3]
  - In a series of patients with stage II or more advanced disease treated with immobilization, 76% (19 out of 25) had either undergone total wrist arthrodesis or experienced daily problems with their wrists at mean 8-year (1 to 11 years) follow-up.[18]
- A study of 18 patients with stage II or III disease treated nonoperatively were compared with those treated by radius shortening.
  - Patients treated surgically had less pain and better grip strength.
  - In some patients with stage III disease treated nonoperatively, there was rapid deterioration to carpal collapse.
  - Although radius shortening did not reverse or prevent carpal collapse, it slowed the process.[22]

SURGICAL MANAGEMENT

- There is no agreement on the optimal way to treat Kienböck disease.[7] Multiple options for surgical management exist and the results do not vary significantly between the different procedures.
  - The mainstays of treatment are radius shortening osteotomy and proximal row carpectomy.[7]
  - Two major radiographic features influence treatment choice: the stage of the disease and ulnar variance.[15]
- Radius shortening osteotomy is currently the benchmark against which other treatments are judged.[16]
  - For stages I to IIIB, radius shortening osteotomy is a very popular option in patients who are ulnar negative. Although the use of radius shortening in stage IIIB is controversial because lunate height and normal carpal kinematics will not be reestablished, potentially leading to progressive degenerative changes, very good results have been demonstrated in these patients with this procedure.[1,30,31] Radius shortening is contraindicated for stage IV disease unless symptoms are severe and salvage procedures are not desired.[30]
  - Radius shortening decreases joint compression forces at the radiolunate joint by redistributing them to the radioscaphoid and ulnolunate joints. In addition, it relatively lengthens the tendons crossing the wrist, diminishing overall joint compressive forces.[20]
    - As opposed to ulnar lengthening, no intercalary bone graft is required and only one interface needs to heal, instead of two.
    - In addition, radius shortening leads to a relative lengthening of the musculotendinous units crossing the wrist, resulting in less force transmission across the carpus. Ulnar lengthening does not provide this particular advantage.[20]
    - After radius shortening, the ulnar head and TFCC support more of the wrist's compressive load through the triquetrum and the ulnar aspect of the lunate. The TFCC is thicker in patients with negative ulnar variance, which provides a compliant pad to support the ulnar carpus.
  - Because radius shortening osteotomy is an extra-articular procedure, it does not alter normal carpal joints or interfere with intracarpal relationships. It "burns no bridges,"

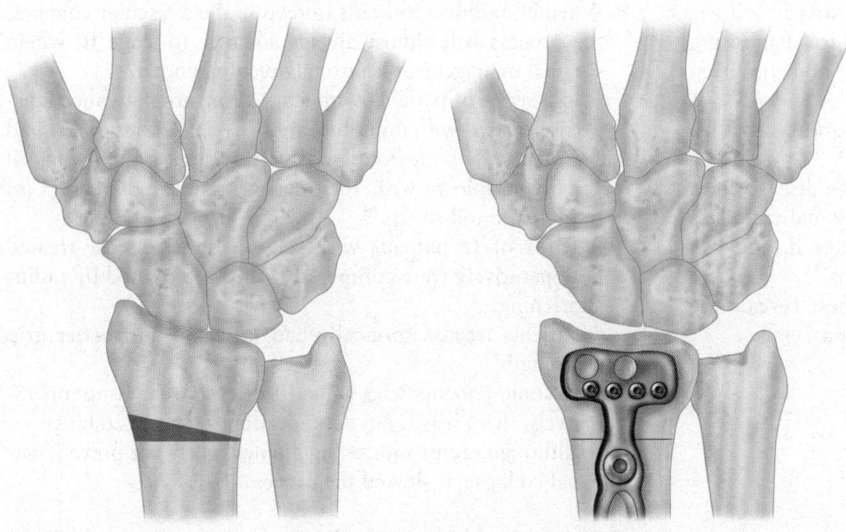

FIG 4 • Lateral closing wedge osteotomy. (Adapted from Soejima O, Iida H, Komine S, et al. Lateral closing wedge osteotomy of the distal radius for advanced stages of Kienbock's disease. J Hand Surg Am 2002;27[1]:31–36.)

and intracarpal procedures can always be undertaken at a later date if the radius shortening is ineffective and disease progression occurs.[30]

- In patients who are ulnar neutral or ulnar positive, a radial closing wedge osteotomy (**FIG 4**) or capitate shortening with or without capitohamate fusion can be performed.
  - Although radius shortening in patients with neutral or positive ulnar variance is not advised, good results have been reported even in these patients.[2,30]
- For stages I to IIIA, revascularization using a vascularized pedicle or bone graft may be performed and may be combined with radius shortening or another unloading procedure (see Chap. 41).
- In patients with stage IIIB disease, proximal row carpectomy, scaphotrapeziotrapezoid fusion, or scaphocapitate fusion may be performed with or without lunate excision and soft tissue interposition.
  - There is data to suggest that even in patients with static carpal malalignment, radius shortening osteotomy can result in a successful clinical result.[5]
- For stage IV disease, proximal row carpectomy or total wrist fusion may be indicated. A study of arthroscopic débridement for stage III or IV disease showed some pain relief at 19 months of follow-up.[17]
- Based on the hypothesis that Kienböck disease is due to venous obstruction, "metaphyseal core decompression" of the distal radius has also been reported with good results.[10]
- Wrist denervation may also be considered and can be used as an adjunct at any stage.[3]
- Lateral closing wedge osteotomies increase lunate coverage (joint contact area) in proportion to the decrease in radial inclination.
  - This transfers the compressive forces of the capitate from the lunate to the scaphoid, decreasing pressure at the radiolunate joint.[20,29]
  - To keep the wrist straight in relation to the forearm, the patient is forced to ulnarly deviate the wrist, extending the scaphoid, which may further transfer forces from the capitate to the scaphoid and decrease forces on the lunate.[23]

Preoperative Planning

- Good-quality, standard preoperative PA radiographs should be taken with the shoulder and elbow flexed 90 degrees and the forearm in neutral rotation.
- Although many authors have recommended removing sufficient bone during radius shortening to result in an ulnar neutral to 1-mm positive variance, 90% of the strain reduction occurs within the first 2 mm of shortening.[2,3,7]
  - Good results with excellent relief of symptoms have been reported removing only 2 mm of bone, regardless of variance. This has the advantages of technical ease and decreases the risk of distal radioulnar joint (DRUJ) incongruity and ulnocarpal impaction, which may occur with excessive shortening.
  - In patients with significant obliquity of the sigmoid notch, radius shortening should be limited to 2 mm to avoid overcompressing the DRUJ.
- Postoperative ulnocarpal impaction and DRUJ incongruity are especially likely with shortenings of 4 mm or more, leading to pain with forearm rotation or limitation of forearm rotation.[30] Therefore, shortening of the radius by over 4 mm is not recommended.
  - Patients with more than 4 mm of shortening and age older than 30 years were found to be more likely to have poor results.[2]

Positioning

- The patient is positioned supine with the arm on a radiolucent hand table.

Approach

- A volar approach to the radius is performed.

Volar Approach

- A longitudinal incision is made over the flexor carpi radialis (FCR) tendon, ending distally at the distal volar wrist crease (**TECH FIG 1B**).
- The approach is continued through the FCR sheath with the FCR tendon retracted ulnarly to protect the palmar cutaneous branch of the median nerve.
- The plane between the FCR and deep muscles of the radius (pronator quadratus and FPL) is bluntly dissected (**TECH FIG 1C**).
- The distal border of the pronator quadratus and the radial insertions of the pronator quadratus and flexor pollicis longus muscles are incised with a knife, with care taken to retract and protect the radial artery, which does not need to be formally identified.
- The volar surface of the radius is then subperiosteally exposed in a radial to ulnar direction (**TECH FIG 1D**).
- Circumferential subperiosteal dissection should be avoided to preserve maximal blood supply to the osteotomy.

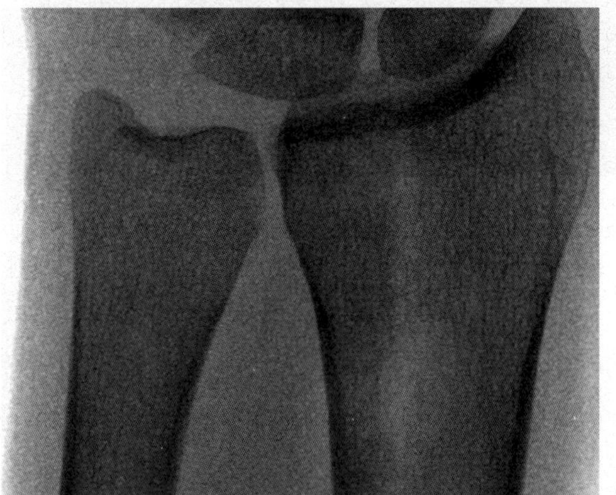
A

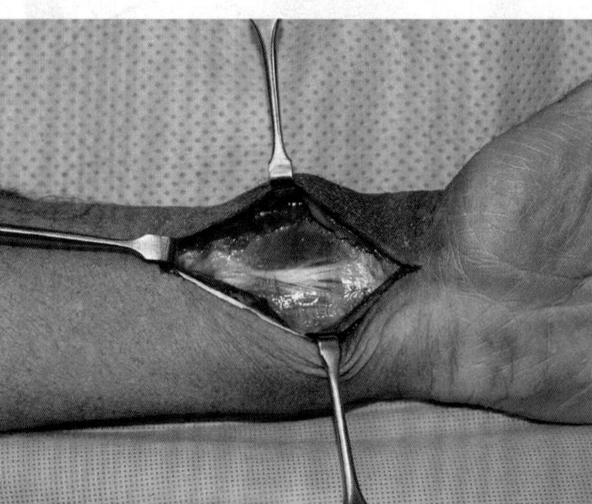
C

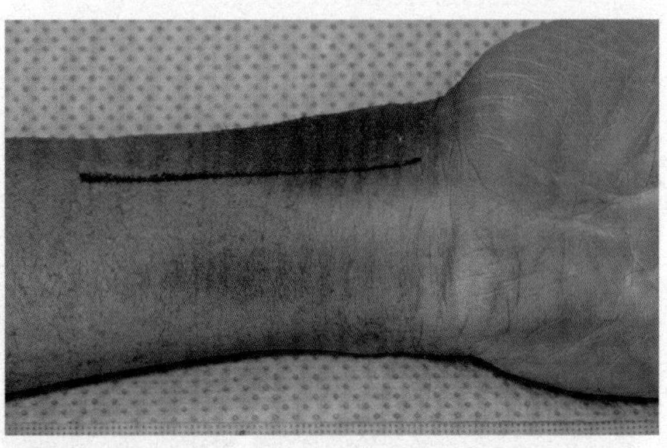
B

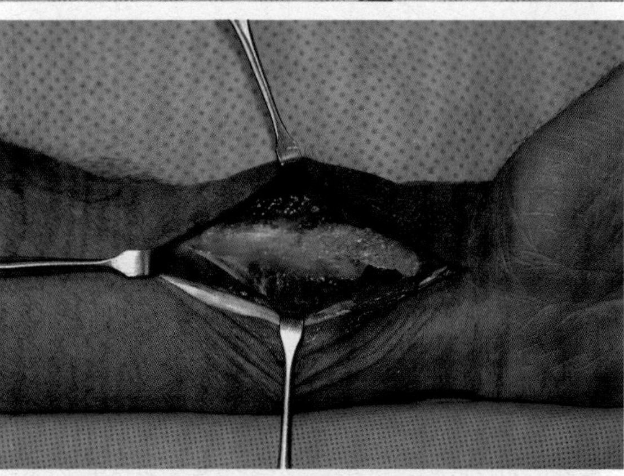
D

TECH FIG 1 • **A.** Preoperative radiograph demonstrating negative ulnar variance. **B.** Incision. **C.** The pronator quadratus is exposed. **D.** The volar distal radius is subperiosteally exposed.

Radius Shortening Osteotomy

Initial Plate Application

- Traditionally, a seven-hole 3.5-mm dynamic compression plate was placed as far distally as possible without riding up the volar lip of the distal radius.[30]
  - However, the newer fixed-angle volar plates used for fixation of distal radius fractures work very well and allow the osteotomy to be placed in metaphyseal bone.
- To decrease the risk of nonunion, the osteotomy should be performed as distal as possible to be through metaphyseal cancellous bone, staying proximal to the DRUJ.
- The plate is placed over the distal radius and provisionally fixed with Kirschner wires (**TECH FIG 2A**).
  - Care should be taken to place the plate distal enough to ensure distal screws are as close to the subchondral bone as possible without intra-articular screw penetration.
  - It is, however, possible to place the plate too distal depending on the design of the plate, putting the flexor tendons at risk of attritional injury. The most distal aspect of the plate should not be distal to the watershed line of the distal radius.[12,24]

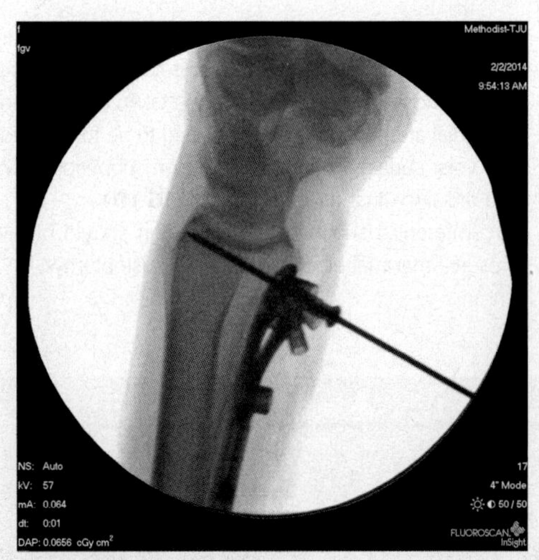

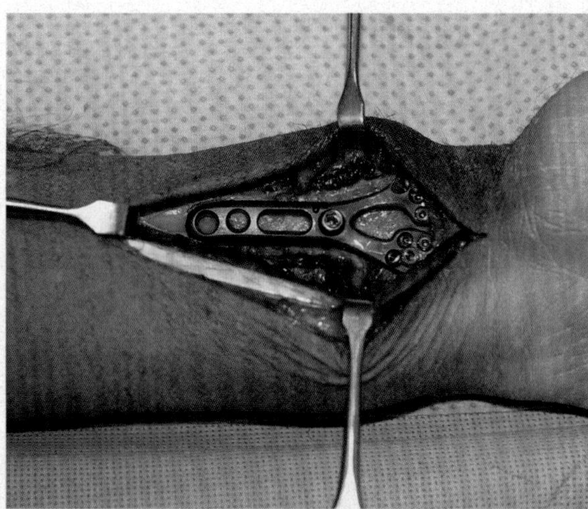

TECH FIG 2 • **A,B.** The volar locking plate is placed so that its distal fixation (represented radiographically by a Kirschner wire) travels just proximal to the subchondral surface. Distal locking screw fixation is placed.

- Following fluoroscopic confirmation of appropriate placement, fixed-angle screws are placed through the distal rows of the plate (**TECH FIG 2B**).
- A bicortical screw is placed 1 cm proximal to (not through) the plate for use later as a means to reduce and compress the osteotomy. It should be longer than measured to allow bicortical purchase but also to allow the head to sit several milimeters up from the volar cortex for later use in compressing the osteotomy.

Radius Osteotomy

- The osteotomy is marked proximal to the distal fixation and proximal to the DRUJ (**TECH FIG 3A**).
- The plate is removed and a transverse osteotomy is made volar to dorsal (**TECH FIG 3B**).
  - An oblique osteotomy provides a larger surface area for healing and can allow for placement of an interfragmentary compression screw.[2]

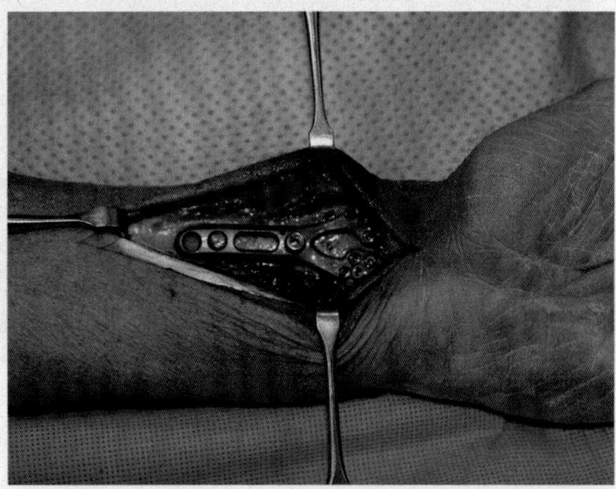

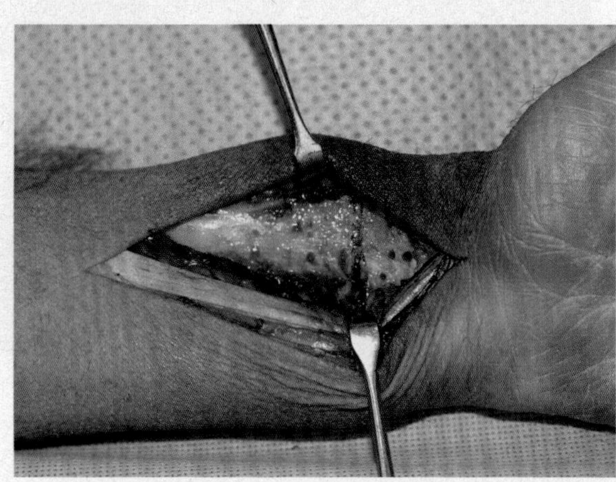

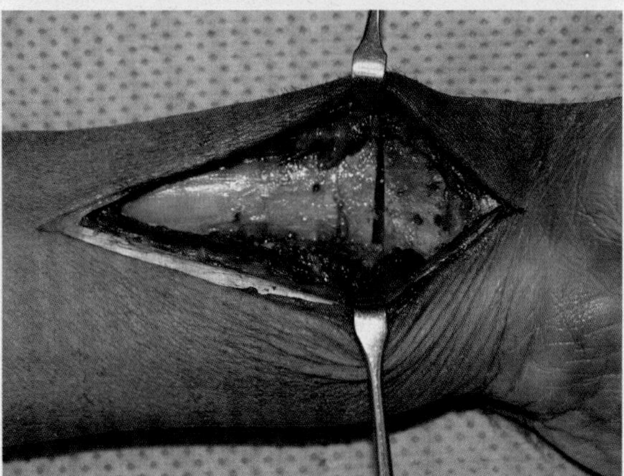

TECH FIG 3 • **A,B.** The osteotomy site is marked between the plate's proximal and distal fixation. When using a plate specifically designed for the fixation of distal radius fractures, this places the osteotomy proximal to the distal radioulnar joint. **C.** The osteotomy is created with a saw transversely taking 2 to 3 mm of bone leaving the dorsal cortex to be removed last.

- An oblique osteotomy, however, is more technically demanding than a transverse osteotomy, and the purchase obtained with the interfragmentary screw used for additional fixation with an oblique osteotomy can be poor.
- A longitudinal line may be marked across the osteotomy site to allow rotational assessment. However, the flat surface of the volar cortex allows for easy assessment of rotation.
- An elevator can be placed on the dorsal surface of the osteotomy to protect the extensor tendons from the saw. Care should, however, be taken to avoid stripping the periosteum from the dorsal cortex of the radius at the level of or near the eventual osteotomy.
- Two to 3 mm of shortening may be appropriate regardless of the amount of negative ulnar variance present.
  - Excellent results have been reported with osteotomies that do not fully correct the radius length to neutral variance.[30,31]
- The 2 to 3 mm to be taken is measured out and marked and the full amount of bone to be taken is removed from volar to dorsal so that the dorsal cortex remains intact to stabilize the bone during bone removal.
- The dorsal cortex is then removed last leaving a completed osteotomy (**TECH FIG 3C**).
  - While performing the osteotomy, constant cool irrigant is used to avoid thermal osteonecrosis.
- Although a slight (1 mm) concave bend in the plate over the osteotomy site may occasionally be needed to achieve compression of the dorsal osteotomy surface, this is not usually necessary.

Final Plate Application and Osteotomy Fixation

- The plate and its distal fixation are then replaced.
- Approximation of the two bone ends may also be facilitated by radial deviation of the wrist[30] and use of a bone-holding clamp.
  - A locking tower is secured into the most proximal hole of the plate (**TECH FIG 4A**).
    - The clamp is placed around the locking tower and the screw proximal to the plate.
    - The clamp is closed to compress the osteotomy taking care not to overcompress it and cause malalignment.
  - Alternatively, a Verbrugge clamp can be used to compress the osteotomy.
    - The hooked end of the Verbrugge is placed in the plate's most proximal screw hole and the bifid end is placed around the screw proximal to the plate.
  - One final option for compression is an articulated tension device.
    - The device is secured to the radial shaft using the previously metioned bicortical screw proximal to the plate.
    - The other end of the device is then hooked into the proximal aspect of the plate and the device is tightened using the T-handle wrench.
- With the clamp applied, the reduction is evaluted fluoroscopically and adjustments made as necessary.
  - An additional clamp from the proximal ulnar aspect of the radial shaft to the distal aspect of the radius or the plate itself may be needed to correct excessive radial translation of the distal fragment (**TECH FIG 4B**). Care should be taken, however, to not overcorrect the translation of the distal fragment, as this can result in loss of forearm rotation.
- The first screw is placed in a compression mode eccentrically in the plate hole in the oblong hole (**TECH FIG 4C**).
- After again assuring adequate reduction and alignment fluoroscopically, the remaining proximal screws are placed (**TECH FIG 4D**).
- Forearm rotation should be checked to ensure that it is full.
  - If forearm rotation is limited after osteotomy, the distal fragment of the radius should be allowed to translate radially or a lateral closing wedge component added.[20]
- Radiographs can show some mild residual gap at the osteotomy site, even with full compression under direct vision (**TECH FIG 4E,F**).[30]
- Intraoperative radiographs may not demonstrate the eventual ulnar variance (amount of radius shortening) because of soft tissue restraints at the DRUJ. In these cases, postoperative radiographs will demonstrate the anticipated correction.[20]

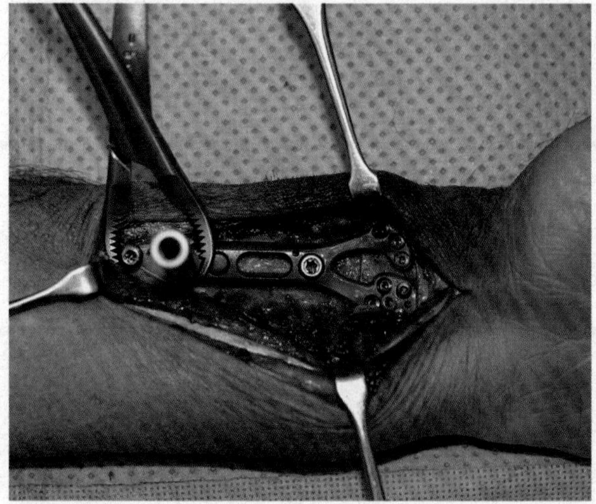

A

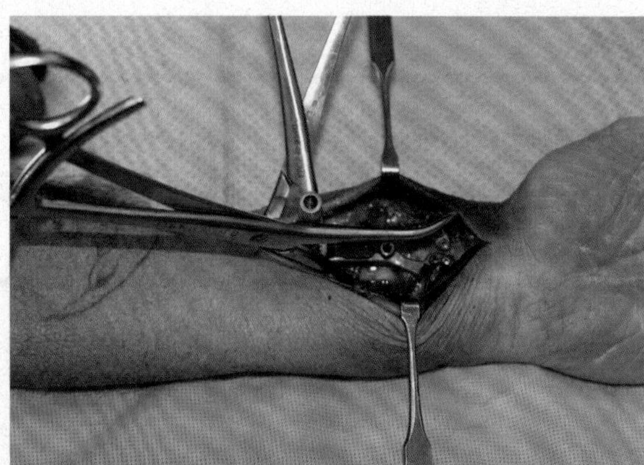

B

TECH FIG 4 • **A.** The plate and its distal fixation are replaced. The bicortical screw a few millimeters longer than the bone width placed 1 to 2 cm proximal to the plate and left proud can be seen proximally in the incision. A bone-holding clamp is placed around a locking tower and around the proximal screw. Squeezing the clamp provides a tremendous mechanical advantage to facilitate osteotomy closure. **B.** An additional clamp from the proximal ulnar aspect of the radius shaft to the distal aspect of the radius radially or the plate itself may be needed to correct excessive radial translation of the distal fragment. *(continued)*

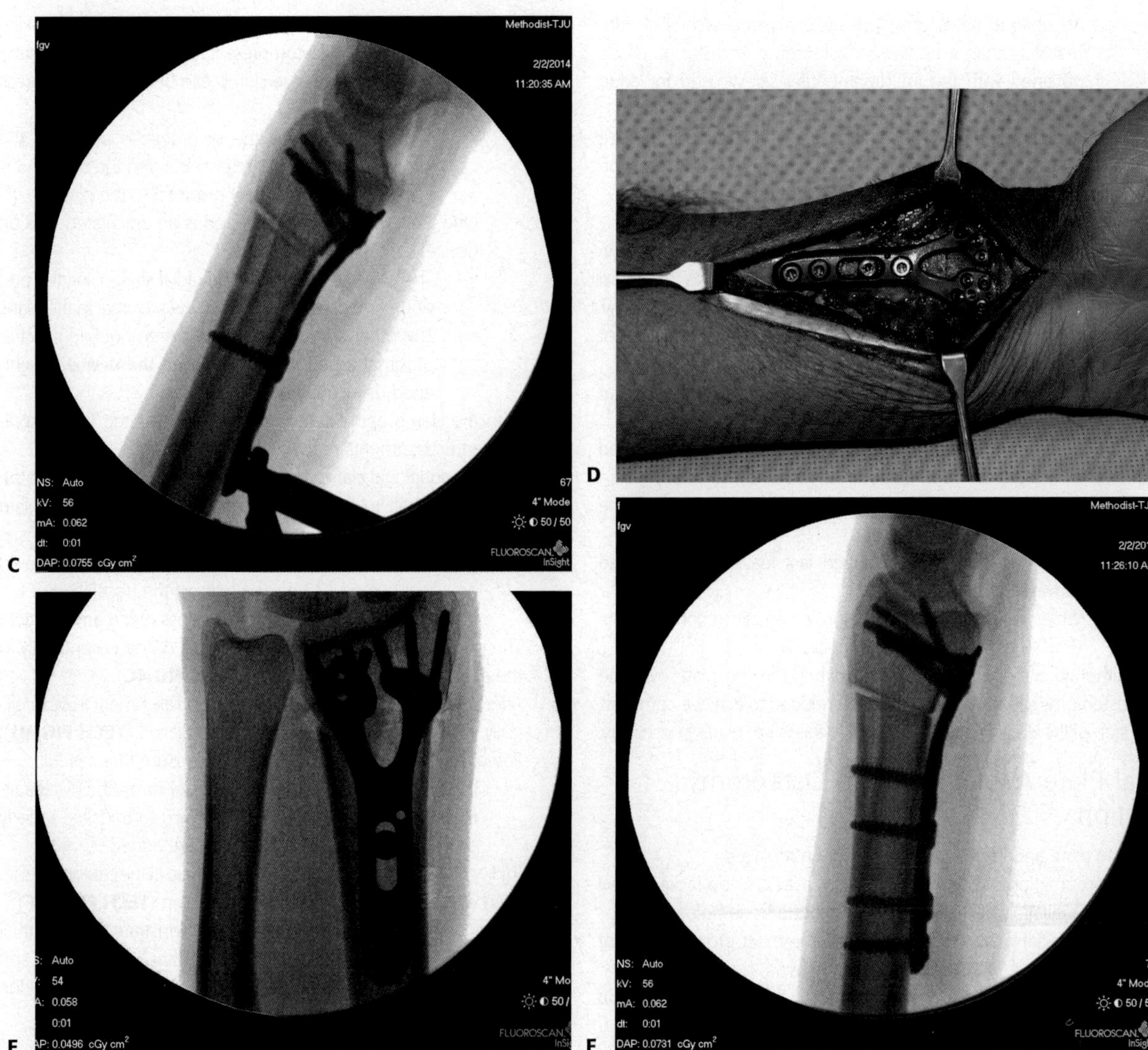

TECH FIG 4 • *(continued)* **C.** With the clamp compressing the osteotomy, the first proximal screw is drilled eccentrically through the most proximal aspect of a plate hole to provide additional compression. **D.** Three more proximal bicortical screws are placed to result in a stable and well-compressed osteotomy. **E,F.** Intraoperative PA and lateral radiographs.

Radial Closing Wedge Osteotomy

- A radial closing wedge osteotomy may be performed through the same approach with the same fixation.
- A 15-degree radial closing wedge osteotomy is performed 4 to 5 cm proximal to the tip of the radial styloid and proximal to the DRUJ.[29]

PEARLS AND PITFALLS

Radius shortening	▪ Two to 3 mm of shortening is all that is needed in the vast majority of cases. Shortening the radius by only 2–3 mm makes compression of the osteotomy easier. ▪ In cases of significant DRUJ obliquity, shortening the radius greater than 2 mm may lead to DRUJ problems.
Fragment handling	▪ If rotation is not full or the DRUJ is compromised after osteotomy, radial translation of the distal fragment should be considered.
Bone-holding clamp	▪ Use of a clamp compressing against a screw proximal to the plate gives the surgeon a tremendous mechanical advantage in shortening the osteotomy.

POSTOPERATIVE CARE

- The extra-articular nature of this procedure combined with stable internal fixation allows for quick postoperative rehabilitation.
- The wrist is splinted for 2 weeks, after which a removable splint may be used and gentle motion started.
- The osteotomy usually heals in 2 to 3 months, although 4 or 5 months is occasionally required.

OUTCOMES

- A review of the reported series by Weiss[30] in 1993 included 121 patients treated with radius shortening, with about 85% good or excellent results at just over 4 years of follow-up.
- One study reviewed 30 wrists after radius shortening osteotomy for stages I to IIIB Kienböck disease at mean 3.8 years of follow-up.[31]
  - Pain decreased in 87% and grip strength improved in 49%. However, the radiographic appearance of the lunate changed little if at all.
  - The authors noted that good results could be obtained by shortening less than that required to attain neutral ulnar variance.
  - The exact amount of radius shortening may not be as important as the relative unloading of the lunate resulting from the shortening of the radius. The amount of shortening needed to be effective may be only about 2 mm. Radius shortening may therefore be used in ulnar neutral wrists.
  - In addition, excellent results were realized in patients with stage IIIA and IIIB disease. There was one nonunion. Only 10 of 30 wrists had evidence of possible lunate revascularization, as indicated by decreased sclerosis and a more normal trabecular pattern.
- Clinical improvement after radius shortening or radial wedge osteotomy does not necessarily correlate with the radiographic results.[2,7,23] It appears that the lunate "stands still in time" after radius shortening, with no significant further deterioration or improvement in the lunate architecture or height.[30]
- Another study reviewed 68 radius shortening osteotomies at a mean of 52 months of follow-up.[20]
  - Pain was diminished in 93%, grip strength was improved in 74%, and motion was improved in 52% and worsened in 19%.
  - Twenty-five patients had undergone one or more additional procedures concurrently, which did not lead to a significant difference in clinical outcomes.
  - Complications were uncommon; there were no nonunions, but ulnocarpal impaction developed in two patients.
  - Lunate density was improved in 40%, unchanged in 46%, and increased (worsened) in 14%.
  - Fifty-five percent of wrists that underwent concurrent vascularized bone grafting of the lunate had an improved radiographic appearance, compared to only 20% that underwent isolated radius shortening.
- It has been suggested that prognosis is improved in younger patients due to increased remodeling potential.[15]
  - Teenage patients (aged 11 to 19 years) were treated by radius shortening or lateral closing wedge osteotomy. Two had neutral or positive ulnar variance. At a mean 50 months of follow-up, 10 of 11 were pain-free. Five of 6 with stage IIIB disease had excellent outcomes.
  - The other patient had moderate wrist pain during strenuous activity, leading to only a fair result after lateral closing wedge osteotomy for stage IIIB disease.
  - Radiographic improvement, indicating possible lunate revascularization, was seen in 8 of 11 patients.
  - There were no complications of radial overgrowth or growth abnormalities in these patients.
- Radiographic stage does correlate with clinical outcome postoperatively,[21] but even advanced Kienböck disease can be treated with radius shortening osteotomy with good results.[5]
  - Fourteen patients with stage IIIB and 17 with stage II and IIIA disease were compared retrospectively at a mean of 74 months.
  - Disability of Arm, Shoulder, and Hand (DASH) scores averaged 15 in the IIIB group as compared to 12 in the II and IIIA group. Grip strength was 77% of the opposite side for stage IIIB wrists versus 85% for stage II and IIIA. Only one patient in the stage IIIB group went on to wrist arthrodesis.
- Twenty-five patients were followed for a minimum of 10 years (mean 14.5 years) after radius osteotomy.[13]
  - Ninety-six percent had good or excellent results.
  - Pain, motion, and grip strength were all significantly improved after surgery and the results were maintained.
  - Although radiologic improvement was not drastic and carpal height did not significantly improve, sclerosis and bone cysts improved and there was evidence of improved lunate revascularization over time.
  - Osteoarthritic changes were observed in 54% at 5 years and in 73% at the time of final follow-up, but the arthrosis was generally mild and did not affect the clinical results.
  - Severe osteoarthritis and proximal migration of the capitate were avoided.

- Radius shortening was used for patients with negative ulnar variance and closing wedge osteotomy for those with positive ulnar variance. These procedures gave identical outcomes.
- Iwasaki et al[11] also noted that both radius shortening and lateral closing wedge osteotomies gave equally acceptable results in adult patients.
- Good long-term results were reported in 100% of 13 patients at a mean of 14 years after radial closing wedge osteotomy.[29]
  - Pain relief was good, and improvements in grip strength and range of motion were seen.
  - Radiographic changes improved in 1, did not change in 4, and advanced in 8.

COMPLICATIONS

- Nonunion has been reported in up to 6% of cases.[7]
  - If the fixation remains stable, treatment should consist of autogenous cancellous bone grafting if healing has not occurred by 5 or 6 months.
- A second operation may occasionally be necessary for plate removal, but this is uncommon.
- Care must be taken not to overshorten the radius, or DRUJ incongruity or ulnocarpal impaction may occur.[30]

REFERENCES

1. Alexander AH, Lichtman DM. Kienbock's disease. Orthop Clin North Am 1986;17:461–472.
2. Alexander CE, Alexander AH, Lichtman DM. Kienbock's disease and idiopathic necrosis of carpal bones. In: Lichtman DM, Alexander AH, eds. The Wrist and Its Disorders, ed 2. Philadelphia: WB Saunders, 1997:329–346.
3. Allan CH, Joshi A, Lichtman DM. Kienbock's disease: diagnosis and treatment. J Am Acad Orthop Surg 2001;9:128–136.
4. Budoff JE, Lichtman DM. Spontaneous wrist fusion: an unusual complication of Kienbock's disease. J Hand Surg Am 2005;30(1): 59–64.
5. Calfee RP, Van Steyn MO, Gyuricza C, et al. Joint leveling for advanced Kienböck's disease. J Hand Surg Am 2010;35(12):1947–1954.
6. Chung KC, Spilson MS, Kim MH. Is negative ulnar variance a risk factor for Kienböck's disease? A meta-analysis. Ann Plast Surg 2001;47:494–499.
7. Divelbiss B, Baratz ME. Kienbock's disease. J Am Soc Surg Hand 2001;1:61–72.
8. Gelberman RH, Bauman TD, Menon J, et al. The vascularity of the lunate bone and Kienbock's disease. J Hand Surg Am 1980;5(3): 272–278.
9. Gelberman RH, Szabo RM. Kienbock's disease. Orthop Clin North Am 1984;15:355–367.
10. Illarramendi AA, Schulz C, De Carli P. The surgical treatment of Kienbock's disease by radius and ulna metaphyseal core decompression. J Hand Surg Am 2001;26(2):252–260.
11. Iwasaki N, Minami A, Ishikawa J, et al. Radial osteotomies for teenage patients with Kienbock disease. Clin Orthop Relat Res 2005;439: 116–122.
12. Kitay A, Swanstrom M, Schreiber JJ, et al. Volar plate position and flexor tendon rupture following distal radius fracture fixation. J Hand Surg Am 2013;38(6):1091–1096.
13. Koh S, Nakamura R, Horii E, et al. Surgical outcome of radial osteotomy for Kienbock's disease: minimum 10 years of follow-up. J Hand Surg Am 2003;28(6):910–916.
14. Kristensen SS, Thomassen E, Christensen F. Kienbock's disease—late results by non-surgical treatment. A follow-up study. J Hand Surg Br 1986;11(3):422–425.
15. Lichtman DM, Degnan GG. Staging and its use in the determination of treatment modalities for Kienbock's disease. Hand Clin 1993;9: 409–416.
16. Linscheid RL. Kienbock's disease. Instr Course Lect 1992;41:45–53.
17. Menth-Chiari WA, Poehling GG, Wiesler ER, et al. Arthroscopic debridement for the treatment of Kienbock's disease. Arthroscopy 1999;15:12–19.
18. Mikkelsen SS, Gelineck J. Poor function after nonoperative treatment of Kienbock's disease. Acta Orthop Scand 1987;58:241–243.
19. Panagis JS, Gelberman RH, Taleisnik J, et al. The arterial anatomy of the human carpus. Part II: the intraosseous vascularity. J Hand Surg Am 1983;8(4):375–382.
20. Quenzer DE, Dobyns JH, Linscheid RL, et al. Radial recession osteotomy for Kienbock's disease. J Hand Surg Am 1997;22(3):386–395.
21. Rodrigues-Pinto R, Freitas D, Costa LD, et al. Clinical and radiological results following radial osteotomy in patients with Kienböck's disease: four- to 18-year follow-up. J Bone Joint Surg Br 2012;94(2): 222–226.
22. Salmon J, Stanley JK, Trail IA. Kienbock's disease: conservative management versus radial shortening. J Bone Joint Surg Br 2000;82(6):820–823.
23. Soejima O, Iida H, Komine S, et al. Lateral closing wedge osteotomy of the distal radius for advanced stages of Kienbock's disease. J Hand Surg Am 2002;27(1):31–36.
24. Soong M, Earp BE, Bishop G, et al. Volar locking plate implant prominence and flexor tendon rupture. J Bone Joint Surg Am 2011;93(4):328–335.
25. Sowa DT, Holder LE, Patt PG, et al. Application of magnetic resonance imaging to ischemic necrosis of the lunate. J Hand Surg Am 1989;14(6):1008–1016.
26. Stahl S, Stahl AS, Meisner C, et al. Critical analysis of causality between negative ulnar variance and Kienböck disease. Plast Reconstr Surg 2013;132:899–909.
27. Szabo RM, Greenspan A. Diagnosis and clinical findings of Kienbock's disease. Hand Clin 1993;9:399–408.
28. Trumble TE, Irving J. Histologic and magnetic resonance imaging correlations in Kienbock's disease. J Hand Surg Am 1990;15(6):879–884.
29. Wada A, Miura H, Kubota H, et al. Radial closing wedge osteotomy for Kienbock's disease: an over-10-year clinical and radiographic follow-up. J Hand Surg Br 2002;27(2):175–179.
30. Weiss AP. Radial shortening. Hand Clin 1993;9:475–482.
31. Weiss AP, Weiland AJ, Moore JR, et al. Radial shortening for Kienböck disease. J Bone Joint Surg Am 1991;73(3):384–391.

Vascularized Bone Grafting and Capitate Shortening Osteotomy for Treatment of Kienböck Disease

41

CHAPTER

Nilesh M. Chaudhari, Mohamed Khalid, and Thomas R. Hunt III

DEFINITION

- Lunate revascularization for Kienböck disease involves transfer of either a vessel or a pedicled bone graft to the lunate in an attempt to reverse avascular necrosis.
- Vascularized bone grafts from the pisiform, volar and dorsal radius metaphysis, second metacarpal head,[6] and iliac crest (via free microvascular graft)[2] have all been reported.
- Unloading procedures, such as a capitate shortening osteotomy, are often combined with a revascularization procedure to protect the graft and to alter forces through the lunate.

ANATOMY

Vascular Anatomy of the Dorsal Distal Radius

- The dorsal distal radius is primarily supplied by the branches of the radial artery and the posterior division of the anterior interosseous artery (pAIA) (**FIG 1**).
- The 2,3 intercompartmental supraretinacular artery (2,3 IC SRA) is superficial to the extensor retinaculum and passes between the second and third extensor compartments (see **FIG 1**).
- The fourth extensor compartment artery (ECA) is located deep to the extensor retinaculum in the fourth extensor compartment (see **FIG 1**).
  - It lies directly adjacent to the posterior interosseous nerve on the radial floor of that compartment.
  - It originates from the pAIA or the fifth ECA.
  - It anastomoses with the dorsal intercarpal arch and the dorsal radiocarpal arch.
  - The fourth ECA is a source of numerous small nutrient arteries to the dorsal radius at the level of the fourth extensor compartment that penetrate deeply into cancellous bone.
- The fifth ECA is located deep to the extensor retinaculum in the fifth extensor compartment or within the septum between the fourth and fifth extensor compartments (see **FIG 1**).
  - It is the largest of the four dorsal vessels.
  - It originates from the pAIA and anastomoses distally with the fourth ECA, the dorsal intercarpal arch, the radiocarpal arch, the 2,3 IC SRA, and/or the oblique dorsal artery of the distal ulna.
- The fourth and fifth ECA pedicle is ideal for use in grafting the lunate because of the large diameter of the fifth ECA, the length of combined pedicle, the ulnar location of the fifth ECA (away from necessary incisions), and the multiple anastomoses, which provide retrograde flow.
  - The fifth ECA by itself seldom provides direct nutrient branches to the radius.
  - A 2,3 IC SRA graft based on antegrade flow through the fifth ECA can be used if the fourth ECA is damaged or not present.

Vascular Anatomy of the Dorsal Hand

- The blood supply to the hand consists of a series of anastomotic arches over the carpus that form the dorsal carpal arch, usually with contributions from both the radial and ulnar arteries (see **FIG 1**).[3,8]
- The dorsal carpal arch lies distal and deep to the extensor retinaculum.
- The dorsal metacarpal arteries lie just deep to the fascia overlying the interossei muscles.
- The second, third, and fourth dorsal metacarpal arteries arise from the dorsal carpal arch. They terminate by dividing into digital arteries.
  - The digital arteries are also supplied by perforating branches from the deep palmar arch.
- The first and fifth dorsal metacarpal arteries are direct branches from the radial and ulnar arteries, respectively.

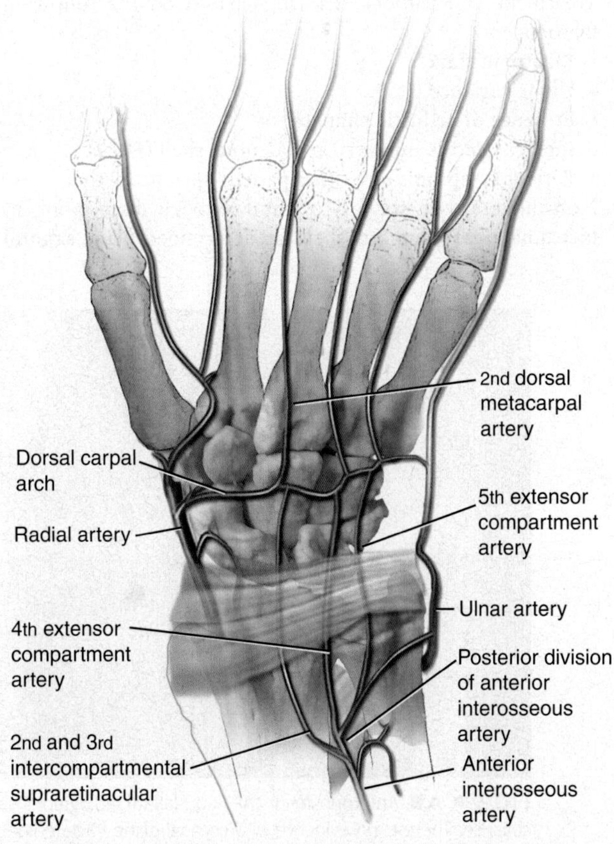

FIG 1 • Arterial anatomy of the dorsal distal radius and wrist.

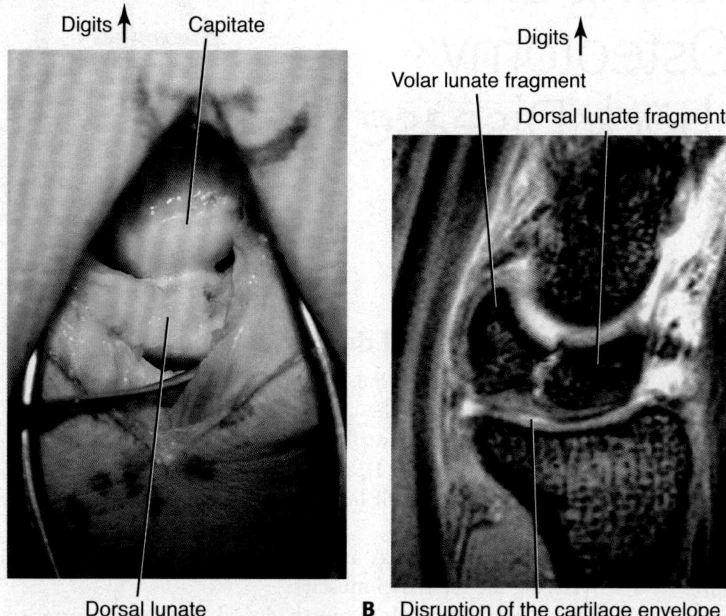

FIG 2 • **A.** At the time of surgery, the articular surfaces are carefully evaluated. **B.** T2-weighted MRI sagittal image of the lunate revealing a coronal plane fracture line, separation of volar and dorsal fragments, and interruption in the cartilaginous envelope. (Copyright Thomas R. Hunt, III, MD.)

- The second dorsal metacarpal artery is the preferred vascular source for vessel implantation due to its size and predictable presence.
  - If this vessel is damaged or cannot be found, the third dorsal metacarpal artery may be used.

SURGICAL MANAGEMENT

- Treatment of Kienböck disease is based on the following factors:
  - Lichtman stage
  - Ulnar variance
  - Presence of arthritic changes
  - Integrity of the lunate's cartilaginous shell (**FIG 2**)
  - Patient symptoms and other patient-specific factors
- Nonsmokers with stage I to IIIA Kienböck disease, an intact lunate cartilaginous shell (as determined using sagittal images and at surgery), and limited arthritic changes are suitable candidates for treatment using a vascularized grafting procedure (**FIG 3**).
- Relative contraindications to vascularized grafting include the following:
  - Previous surgery with exposure of the dorsal aspect of the hand and wrist
  - Age older than 60 years
  - History of peripheral vascular diseases or poorly controlled diabetes
- Vascular grafting is accompanied by a lunate unloading procedure.
  - Unloading has been shown to improve symptoms related to Kienböck disease (see Chap. 40).
  - Altering force distribution through the lunate serves to protect the vascular grafts and to encourage revascularization.

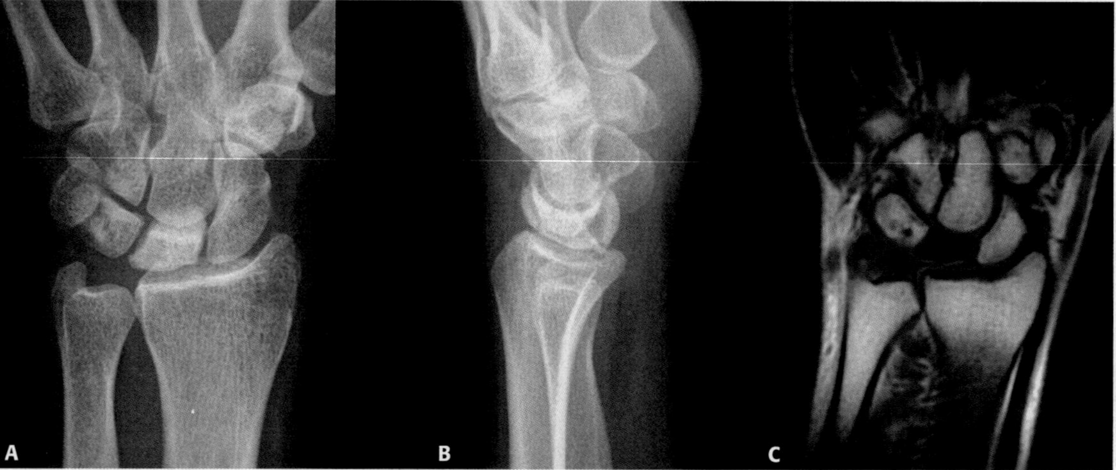

FIG 3 • **A,B.** Anteroposterior (AP) and lateral radiographs showing stage II to III Kienböck disease with sclerosis and subtle, early collapse. There is no evidence of a coronal plane fracture line. **C.** T1-weighted MRI coronal image showing loss of marrow signal of the lunate. (Copyright Thomas R. Hunt, III, MD.)

- Unloading procedures commonly used in conjunction with a vascular procedure include the following:
  - Capitate shortening osteotomy is our preferred choice in patients with positive or neutral ulnar variance. This procedure is completed before inserting the vascular graft or vessel.
  - Scaphocapitate pinning or external fixation (4 to 6 weeks) is used when ulnar variance is positive and a contraindication to capitate shortening osteotomy exists.
  - Radius shortening and angular osteotomy is used when ulnar variance is negative (see Chap. 40).
  - Intercarpal arthrodesis (see Chap. 108)

Preoperative Planning

- The surgeon should review all imaging studies to determine the stage of the disease, ulnar variance, and the status of the lunate's articular shell.

Positioning

- The patient is positioned supine with the arm on a radiolucent arm board.
- A proximal arm tourniquet is applied. Gravity exsanguination of the limb before tourniquet inflation allows visualization of the vessels.

Approach

- The surgeon should consider arthroscopic assessment before the open approach if the status of the lunate articular shell is in question.
  - The 4-5 portal and ulnar midcarpal portal should be avoided, as they may damage the fourth and fifth ECA.
- Dorsal approaches to the hand and the wrist are used.
- Specific incision placement varies based on the graft choice and associated lunate unloading procedure.

TECHNIQUES

Vascularized Bone Grafting

Exposure and Identification of the Fourth and Fifth Extensor Compartment Arteries

- Make a 5- to 6-cm longitudinal skin incision between fourth and fifth extensor compartments, ending distally between the third and fourth metacarpal bases.
- Incise the fifth extensor compartment.
- Identify the fifth ECA and its venae comitantes on the radial aspect of the compartment lying adjacent to or partially within the septum and separating the fourth and fifth extensor compartments (**TECH FIG 1**).
- Trace the fifth ECA proximally to its origin from the pAIA as it emerges from the interosseous membrane.
- Identify the fourth ECA arising from the same feeding vessel.
- Trace the fourth ECA distally and identify the area of greatest vascular penetration into bone, typically 1 cm proximal to the radiocarpal joint.

Lunate Preparation

- Elevate the extensor retinaculum as a radial-based flap from the fifth through the second extensor compartments to allow joint capsulotomy.
  - Carefully protect the dorsal carpal arch.
- Perform a ligament-splitting capsulotomy and protect the scapholunate and lunotriquetral ligaments.
- Inspect the lunate, its cartilage shell, and surrounding articular surfaces.
  - Consider vascularized bone grafting only if the shell is not compromised, the bone is not fragmented, and the joint is not arthritic.

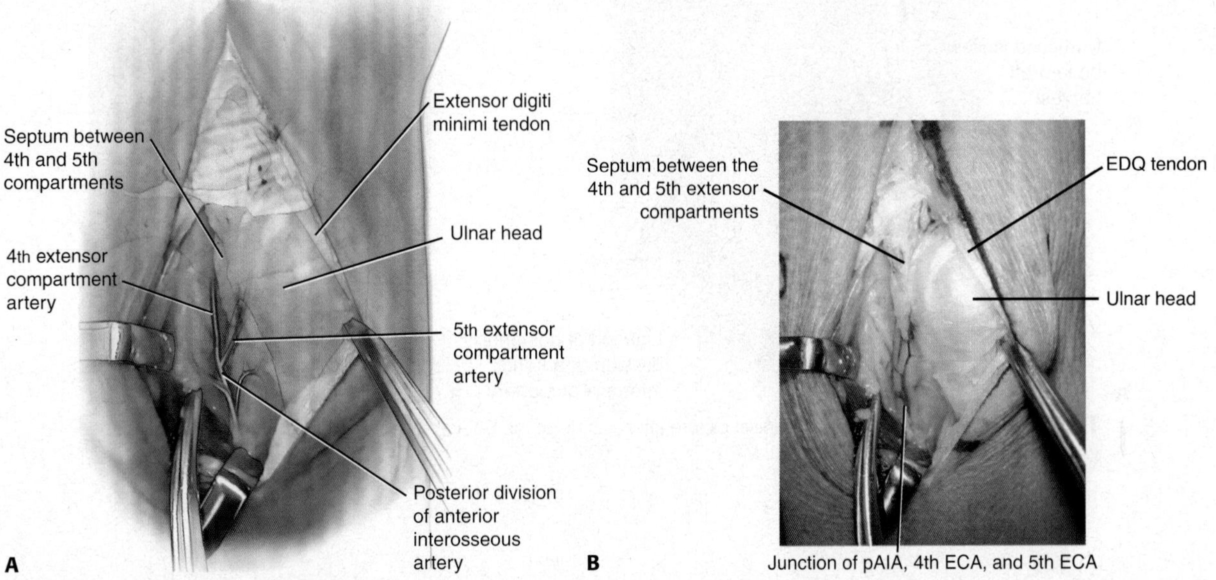

TECH FIG 1 • **A.** The fifth ECA is identified and carefully traced proximally to its origin from the pAIA. **B.** Matching clinical photograph showing fourth and fifth extensor compartment arteries. (**B:** Copyright Thomas R. Hunt, III, MD.)

- Enter the noncartilaginous portion of the dorsal lunate cortex using a small curette or a 2- to 3-mm round burr.
- Through this dorsal cortical window and under direct visualization and fluoroscopic guidance, carefully remove necrotic bone from the lunate by hand with curved and straight curettes.
  - Leave a shell of intact subchondral bone.
- If the lunate is collapsed, expand it gently using a small blunt-ended lamina spreader.
  - The amount of expansion obtained is highly variable.
  - Use of a lamina spreader in this manner is not suggested in cases with bone fragmentation.
- Determine the graft size required by measuring the dorsal excavated area of the lunate.

Elevation of the Vascularized Bone Graft

- Using a smooth 0.045-inch Kirschner wire, outline the area of the distal radius most infiltrated by nutrient vessels from the fourth ECA.
  - The size of the graft is influenced by the nutrient vessels and the earlier measurement.
- Ligate the pAIA proximal to the fourth and fifth ECA branches (**TECH FIG 2**).
- Sharply elevate the vascular pedicle from the bone while protecting the nutrient vessels at the graft site.
- Complete elevation of the corticocancellous graft using sharp osteotomes, with judicious handling of the vascularized pedicle (see **TECH FIG 2**).
- Deflate the tourniquet to verify blood flow to the graft.
- Protect the pedicle graft in a moist sponge.

Placement of the Vascularized Bone Graft into the Lunate

- Obtain cancellous bone graft from the donor site in the distal radius and pack this graft into the lunate cavity using fluoroscopic images for guidance.
- Using small, precise rongeurs, contour the corticocancellous pedicle graft to the size needed.
- Insert the vascularized bone graft with the cortical surface arranged in a proximal–distal orientation and without tension on the vascular leash (**TECH FIG 3**).
  - This allows the graft to serve as a strut to help maintain lunate height during revascularization.
  - No internal fixation is necessary to secure the graft in the lunate.

Closure

- Repair the capsule using absorbable suture, taking great care to avoid pressure on the vascular pedicle.
- Close the extensor retinaculum with absorbable suture and the skin with Prolene.
- Apply a nonocclusive dressing and a volar, below-elbow splint.

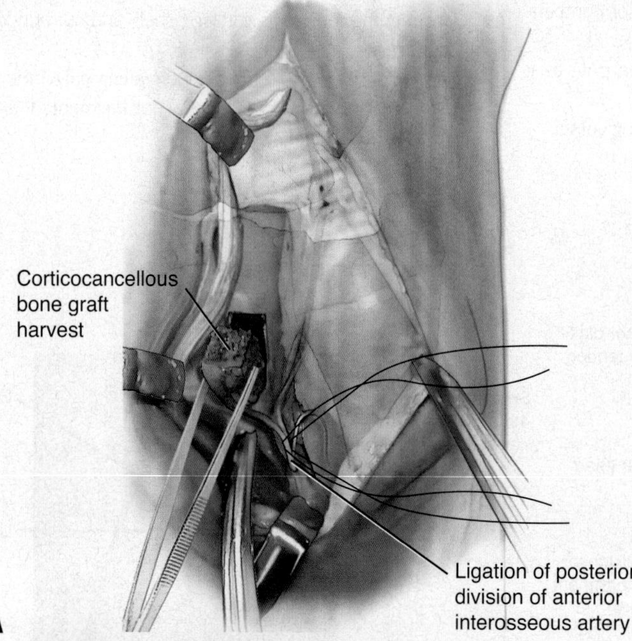

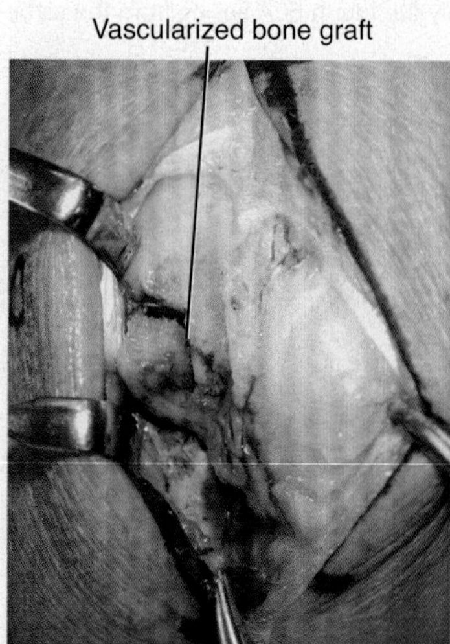

TECH FIG 2 • **A,B.** Drawing and clinical picture after ligation of the pAIA and harvest of the corticocancellous bone graft. (**B:** Copyright Thomas R. Hunt, III, MD.)

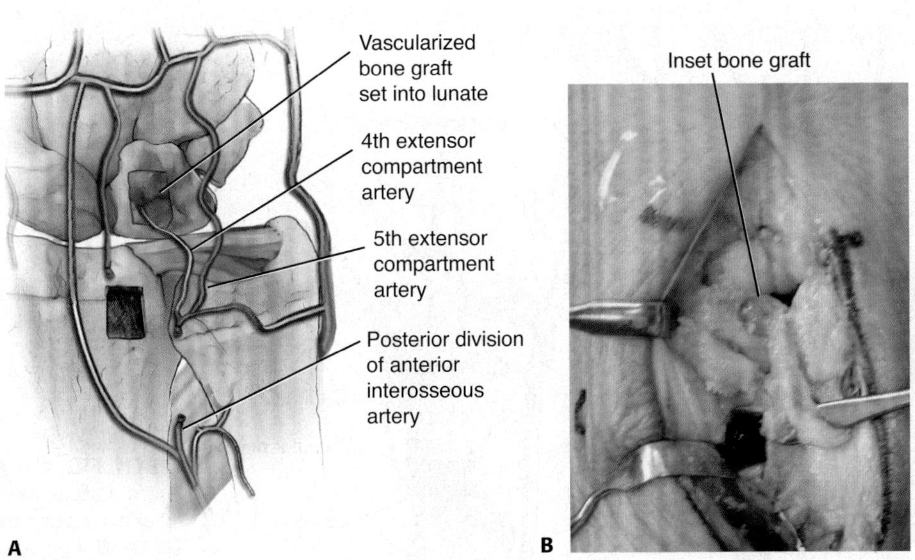

TECH FIG 3 • A,B. Drawing and corresponding clinical picture showing inset of the vascularized bone graft into the prepared lunate. Note the proximal–distal orientation of the cortex. (**B:** Copyright Thomas R. Hunt, III, MD.)

Vascular Bundle Implantation

Incision and Approach

- Make an extensive dorsoradial incision extending from the second metacarpophalangeal joint to a point about 4 cm proximal to the wrist, which gently slopes ulnarly around the tubercle of Lister.
  - Visualize and protect the dorsal sensory branch of the radial nerve.
- Incise the extensor retinaculum over the third compartment and transpose the extensor pollicis longus into a subcutaneous position.
- Retract the contents of the fourth extensor compartment ulnarly and the second extensor compartment radially.
- Use fluoroscopy to confirm the lunate's location.
- Perform a standard ligament-splitting capsulotomy.
  - Take care to avoid injury to the transverse basal dorsal metacarpal arch from which the vascular pedicle arises.
- Inspect the lunate and surrounding joints. Perform a synovectomy as required.

Elevation of the Second Dorsal Metacarpal Vascular Pedicle

- In the interval between the second and third metacarpals, incise the interosseous muscle fascia from proximal to distal.
  - The vessels lie underneath the aponeurosis that covers the interosseous muscles.
- Elevate the artery and venae comitantes along with a thin layer of surrounding perivascular areolar tissue from the second dorsal web space to the dorsal carpal arch (**TECH FIG 4A**).
  - Identify and coagulate all branches off this main metacarpal artery.
- Ligate the vessel at its most distal location.
  - This should provide a 5- to 6-cm vessel of adequate length to reach the dorsal lunate.

Lunate Preparation and Implantation of the Vascular Bundle

- Curette and expand the lunate as discussed earlier.
- Pack autogenous cancellous bone graft into the lunate.
- Use a 2.7-mm bit and drill from dorsal to volar through the body of the lunate.
- Sew a 5-0 monofilament suture to the end of the mobilized vessel, then place the suture ends through the eye of a straight needle.
- Feed the vessel into the avascular portion of the lunate by passing the needle from dorsal to volar through the previously drilled hole, exiting the palmar skin just ulnar to the flexor carpi radialis tendon (**TECH FIG 4B**).
- Make a small skin incision over the needle and tie the suture over the palmar antebrachial fascia.
- Release the tourniquet to assess vessel patency.
- Achieve hemostasis and close the capsule, retinaculum, and skin in the manner described earlier.
- Apply a nonocclusive dressing and a volar, below-elbow splint.

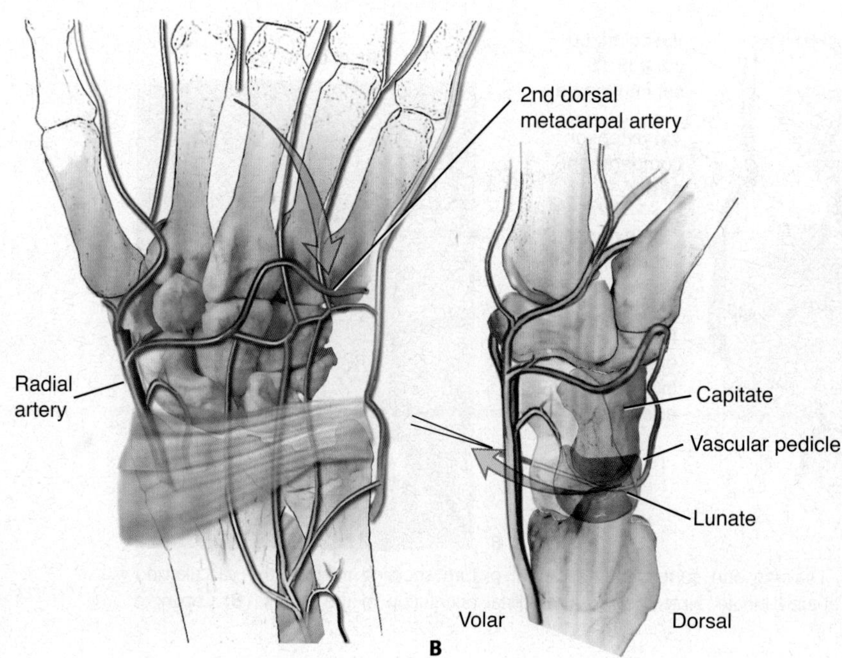

TECH FIG 4 • A. The artery has been ligated distally and mobilized proximally along with its perivascular tissue. **B.** Fine suture is sewn to the edge of the vessel lumen and placed into a straight Keith needle for insertion into the lunate from a dorsal to volar direction.

Capitate Shortening Osteotomy

Capitate Osteotomy

- After the capsular-sparing incision is performed for the vascular procedure but before the graft or vessel is inset into the lunate, identify the waist of the capitate and confirm the osteotomy site with fluoroscopic imaging.
  - The osteotomy should correspond to the level of the scaphotrapeziotrapezoidal joints (**TECH FIG 5A**).
- Use a sharp osteotome, a fine water-cooled saw, or both to resect a 2.0-mm wafer bone from the capitate (**TECH FIG 5B**).
  - Complete the proximal cut before the distal cut.
- Perform a trial reduction using a Freer elevator in the midcarpal joint to control and compress the proximal capitate fragment.
- If this trial reduction reveals that the proximal hamate is prominent in the midcarpal joint or the hamate–lunate articulation is incongruous, perform a hamate osteotomy in the same manner and at the same level as the capitate osteotomy.

Osteotomy Fixation

- Compress the two cut surfaces of the capitate manually as discussed earlier in preparation for placement of a cannulated, headless compression screw.

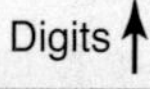

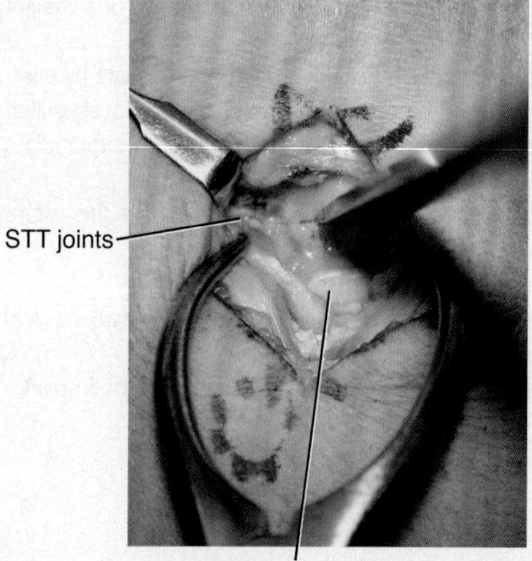

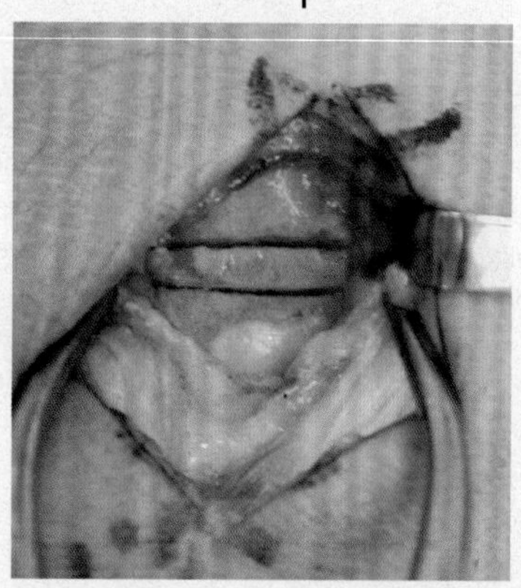

TECH FIG 5 • A. The capitate osteotomy is performed at the waist, which corresponds to the level of the scaphotrapeziotrapezoidal joints. **B.** A 2-mm wafer of bone is removed from the capitate. The proximal cut is completed first. The cuts must be parallel to ensure precise reduction. (Copyright Thomas R. Hunt, III, MD.)

- Place the guidewire across the osteotomy site of the capitate from proximal to distal.
  - Wrist flexion helps present the capitate head into the field. Be careful to avoid distraction of the osteotomy with this maneuver.
  - Confirm the placement of the guidewire with fluoroscopy.
- Insert the headless compression screw over the guidewire and achieve compression across the osteotomy site (**TECH FIG 6A**).
- Complete the vascular procedure as indicated and close the wrist capsule, the extensor retinaculum, and the skin (**TECH FIG 6B**).
- Apply a bulky hand dressing with a volar splint.

A

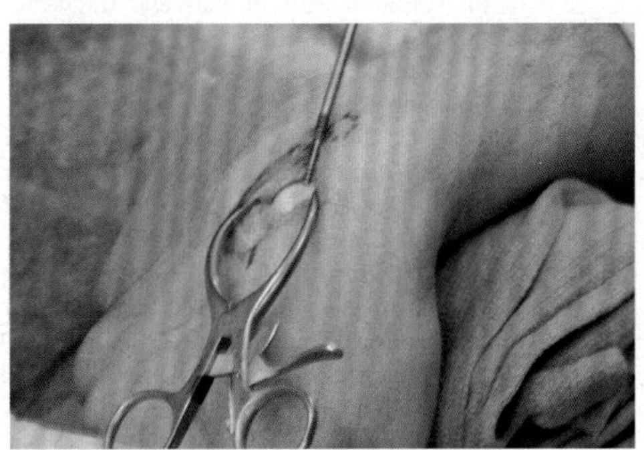

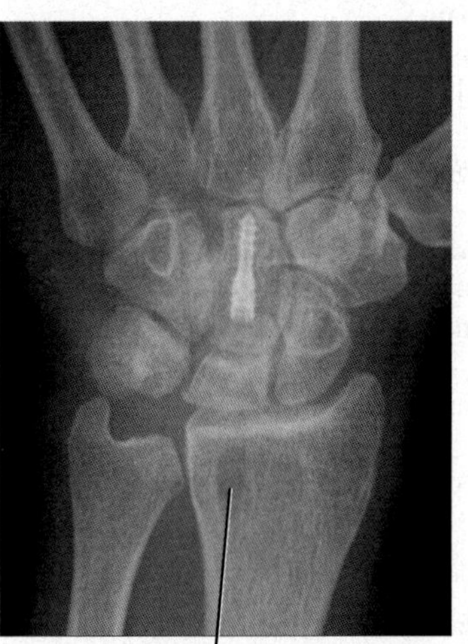

B

TECH FIG 6 • A. A headless compression screw is inserted antegrade. Wrist flexion provides access to the capitate head. **B.** Posteroanterior radiograph after vascularized bone grafting and capitate shortening osteotomy. (Copyright Thomas R. Hunt, III, MD.)

PEARLS AND PITFALLS

Tourniquet	■ Gravity exsanguination allows visualization of the vessels, simplifying exposure and harvest.
Lunate preparation	■ Examine the cartilage shell of the lunate before harvesting the vascularized graft. Separation of dorsal and volar fragments can take place during débridement and bone expansion if performed in patients with a fracture line noted on the sagittal magnetic resonance imaging (MRI) views.
Elevation of vascularized bone graft	■ Elevate the vascular pedicle with its perivascular tissue sufficiently to allow tension-free placement of the graft.
Capitate osteotomy	■ Evaluate the prominence of the hamate at the midcarpal joint. If present, consider performing a hamate shortening osteotomy as well.

POSTOPERATIVE CARE

- Remove the dressing 10 to 14 days postoperatively and apply a below-elbow cast for 3 weeks.
- Remove the cast 4 to 5 weeks after surgery and initiate supervised therapy emphasizing active wrist motion. Over the next 4 weeks, the patient can progress to active-assisted and then passive range-of-motion exercises.
  - A removable splint is used for 3 to 4 weeks.
- Evaluate the progress of healing using serial radiographs.
- Strengthening is initiated at 3 months after surgery and slowly progressed.
- Patients undergoing revascularization of the lunate are followed for 1 to 3 years.

OUTCOMES

- Lunate revascularization techniques have demonstrated promising clinical results for Kienböck disease.[1,7]
- Mazur et al[4] described the results of nine reverse flow pedicle grafts obtained from the radius metaphysis in patients with stage IIIA Kienböck disease.
  - Grip strength was improved by 25%, ultimately measuring 60% to 100% of the opposite side.
  - Range of motion of the wrist joint was not significantly different from the preoperative status.
  - Radiographic measurements demonstrated no change in the modified carpal height ratio, lunate index, or scapholunate angle.

- MRI data demonstrated progressive signs of revascularization over time. Normalization of T2 values was seen initially by 18 months, followed by normalization of T1 values by 36 months.
- Moran et al[5] retrospectively reviewed the results of 24 patients treated with vascularized bone graft using fourth and fifth ECA.
  - Grip strength improved from 50% to 89% of the unaffected side.
  - Ninety-two percent of the patients had significant improvement in their pain.
  - Seventy-seven percent of patients showed no further collapse on postsurgical radiographs.
  - Seventy-one percent of the patients showed evidence of revascularization with improvement in the T2 signal, T1 signal, or both.
- Waitayawinyu et al[9] described the results of 14 patients who had capitate shortening osteotomy with vascularized bone grafting for Kienböck disease; all had positive ulnar variance.
  - Grip strength was improved from 58% to 78% of the normal side.
  - Average time to osteotomy healing was 48 days.

COMPLICATIONS

- Failure of revascularization of the lunate or progression of disease may necessitate a second procedure such as intercarpal arthrodesis, proximal row carpectomy, total wrist arthrodesis, or wrist denervation.
- Continued inflammation or disease progression may cause persistent pain, which may require brief periods of splinting during symptomatic flares.

REFERENCES

1. Bochud RC, Büchler U. Kienböck's disease, early stage 3—height reconstruction and core revascularization of the lunate. J Hand Surg Br 1994;19(4):466–478.
2. Galb M, Reinhart C, Lutz M, et al. Vascularized bone graft from the iliac crest for the treatment of nonunion of the proximal part of the scaphoid with an avascular fragment. J Bone Joint Surg Am 1999;81(10):1414–1428.
3. Hori Y, Tamai S, Okuda H, et al. Blood vessel transplantation to bone. J Hand Surg Am 1979;4(1):23–33.
4. Mazur KU, Bishop AT, Berger RA. Vascularized bone grafting for Kienböck's disease: method and results of retrograde-flow metaphyseal grafts. Presented at the American Society for Surgery of the Hand 51st Annual Meeting, Nashville, TN, 1996.
5. Moran SL, Cooney WP, Berger RA, et al. The use of the 4+5 extensor compartmental vascularized bone graft for the treatment of Kienböck's disease. J Hand Surg Am 2005;30(1):50–58.
6. Sheetz KK, Bishop AT, Berger RA. The arterial blood supply of the distal radius and ulna and its potential use in vascularized pedicle bone grafts. J Hand Surg Am 1995;20(6):902–914.
7. Shin AY, Bishop AT. Vascularized bone grafts for scaphoid non-unions and Kienböck's disease. Orthop Clin North Am 2001;32:263–277.
8. Tamai SH, Yajima H, Mizumoto S, et al. Treatment of Kienböck's disease with vascular bundle implantation. Transaction of the American Society of Surgery of the Hand 1980;3:69.
9. Waitayawinyu T, Chin SH, Luria S, et al. Capitate shortening osteotomy with vascularized bone grafting for the treatment of Kienböck's disease in the ulnar positive wrist. J Hand Surg Am 2008;33(8):1267–1273.

Ligament Stabilization of the Unstable Thumb Carpometacarpal Joint

42 CHAPTER

Richard Y. Kim and Robert J. Strauch

DEFINITION

- Thumb carpometacarpal (CMC) joint instability can occur as a result of ligament laxity or trauma.
- Regardless of the cause, injury to the stabilizing ligaments surrounding the CMC joint leads to instability and dorsoradial subluxation or dislocation of the thumb metacarpal.

ANATOMY

- The thumb CMC joint is a biconcave–convex joint similar to a horseback rider's saddle.[5]
- The base of the thumb metacarpal has a prominent volar styloid process (beak) that articulates with a recess in the volar trapezium when in flexion.
- There are 16 ligaments that provide stability to the thumb CMC joint.[1] Of these ligaments, the two that provide the most restraint against dorsoradial subluxation of the thumb metacarpal are the dorsoradial and volar beak ligaments (**FIG 1**).[1,5,11,15,18] A recent systematic review of the literature demonstrates that the dorsal ligaments are the primary stabilizers of the thumb CMC joint.[10]
  - The volar beak ligament (deep anterior oblique ligament, palmar ligament, ulnar ligament) originates from the volar central apex of the trapezium and inserts onto the volar beak of the thumb metacarpal.[1] It lies immediately under a more widely based superficial anterior oblique ligament, which is located immediately deep to the thenar musculature and has a broad insertion across the base of the thumb metacarpal. More recent studies indicate that the beak ligament may not be as substantial as once thought.
  - The dorsoradial ligament originates from the dorsoradial tubercle of the trapezium and inserts onto the dorsal base of the thumb metacarpal. It is the thickest, widest, shortest, and strongest of the CMC ligaments.[5]

PATHOGENESIS

- The biconcave–convex nature of the thumb CMC joint allows for a wide range of thumb motion but is inherently unstable.[8] Laxity or incompetence of the supporting ligaments, especially the dorsoradial ligaments, will cause instability of the thumb CMC joint.[12,15] Especially in middle-aged women, the cause of the laxity is often idiopathic.
- In addition, there is a population of patients who have inherent ligament laxity, such as those with collagen disorders such as Ehlers-Danlos syndrome.
- In the setting of trauma, acute thumb CMC joint dislocation occurs with axial loading and flexion of the thumb metacarpal. In all reported cases, the dislocation occurs in a dorsoradial direction.[14,15]

NATURAL HISTORY

- Ligamentous laxity at the thumb CMC joint may cause degenerative changes to the joint cartilage and lead to arthritis,

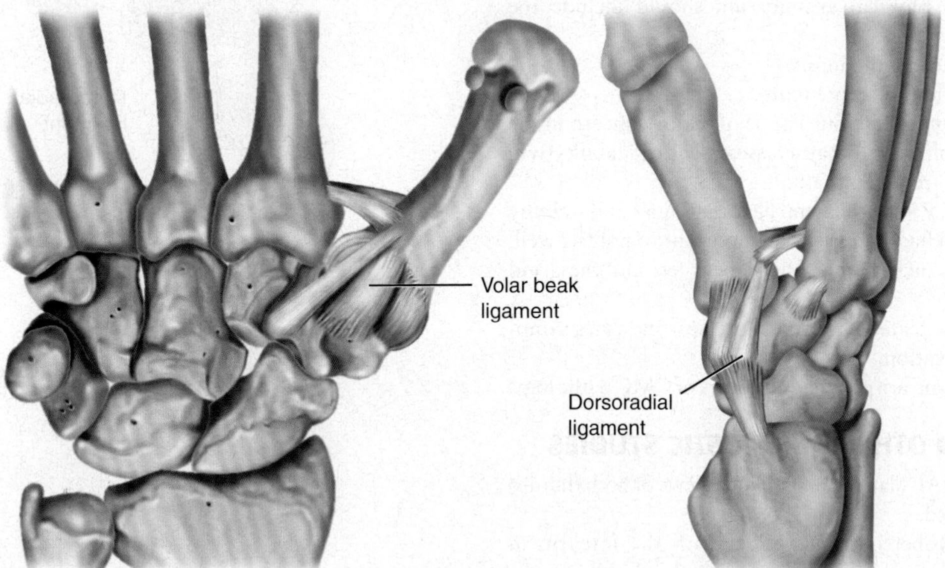

FIG 1 • The stabilizing ligaments of the thumb CMC joint. Of these, the dorsoradial and volar beak ligaments are the most important in preventing dorsoradial subluxation of the thumb metacarpal.

corresponding to higher stages in the Eaton-Littler staging system.[3]

- If the ligamentous laxity is symptomatic and causing pain, ligament reconstruction can be successful in reducing pain in over 90% of patients. Ligament reconstruction has also been shown to potentially halt the progression of arthritis.[6]
- For traumatic dislocations, a stable reduction is important for thumb function. If the thumb CMC joint remains unstable, functions such as key pinch and grasp may be compromised.
  - Open ligament reconstruction of these unstable thumb CMC joint dislocations may decrease the incidence of recurrent instability and joint degeneration compared to closed reduction and pinning.[14]

PATIENT HISTORY AND PHYSICAL FINDINGS

Nontraumatic Ligamentous Laxity

- The history should include questions about ligament laxity involving other joints. Metabolic diseases such as Ehlers-Danlos syndrome are notable.
- Radiographic findings often do not correlate with symptomatology. Therefore, it is important to elicit from the patient the exact symptoms and their severity.
- Any history of previous nonoperative treatments should be noted. If splinting and steroid injections have not been attempted, it may be beneficial to attempt these treatment modalities before discussing surgery.
- The physical examination should determine the degree of subluxation and reducibility of the thumb CMC joint.
- The thumb metacarpophalangeal (MCP) joint should also be examined for possible hyperextension laxity.
- Pinch strength and opposition should be tested and compared to the contralateral side.
- The hand should also be evaluated for concomitant carpal tunnel syndrome, flexor carpi radialis tunnel syndrome, and de Quervain tenosynovitis, as these may also need to be addressed.

Traumatic Injuries

- In addition to the evaluation cited for nontraumatic laxity, the history and physical examination should include the following:
  - Time and nature of the injury
  - Status of the thumb before injury
  - Stability of joint reduction: This is of major concern in the physical examination because assessment of stability will determine the treatment path.
  - Associated MCP joint collateral ligament injury and stability
- Other associated hand injuries are important to note as well.
- Tests to perform include the ballottement test and the grind test.
  - Tenderness associated with dorsal pressure indicates symptomatic subluxation.
- Crepitance and pain are positive indicators of CMC pathology.

IMAGING AND OTHER DIAGNOSTIC STUDIES

- Anteroposterior (AP), lateral, and oblique views of both thumbs should be obtained.
  - A true AP (Robert) view is taken with the forearm in maximal pronation and the dorsum of the thumb resting on the imaging table. The beam is then angled 15 degrees from distal to proximal.[5]
  - A true lateral film of the thumb is one in which the sesamoids volar to the thumb MCP joint overlap each other.
  - A 30-degree oblique stress view of the thumb CMC joint is performed by pressing the radial side of the thumb tips together. This maneuver will subluxate the thumb metacarpal base radially, thereby demonstrating the degree of laxity in the radial direction.[17]

DIFFERENTIAL DIAGNOSIS

- de Quervain tenosynovitis
- Flexor carpi radialis tunnel syndrome
- C6 radiculopathy
- Trigger thumb

NONOPERATIVE MANAGEMENT

- For symptomatic ligament laxity and stage I or II basal joint disease, conservative management should first be attempted. This includes thumb spica splint immobilization and anti-inflammatory medications.[7,16]
- If the symptoms do not improve, a steroid injection into the CMC joint can be attempted. The number of injections should be limited to a maximum of three; theoretically, more than three injections increases joint morbidity.
- In the scenario of acute trauma, reduction of the CMC joint should be performed by applying axial traction and palmar-directed pressure to the base of the thumb metacarpal, along with pronation of the thumb metacarpal. After reduction, if the joint remains reduced and is stable, the injury can be treated with cast immobilization.
- If the joint is unstable at all after an attempt at closed reduction, surgical management is indicated.[14]

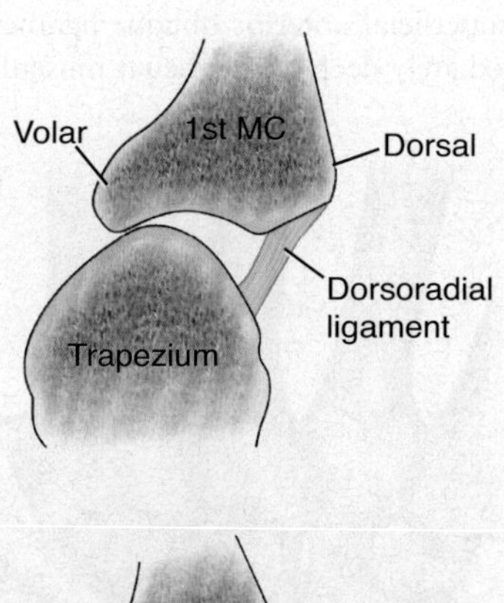

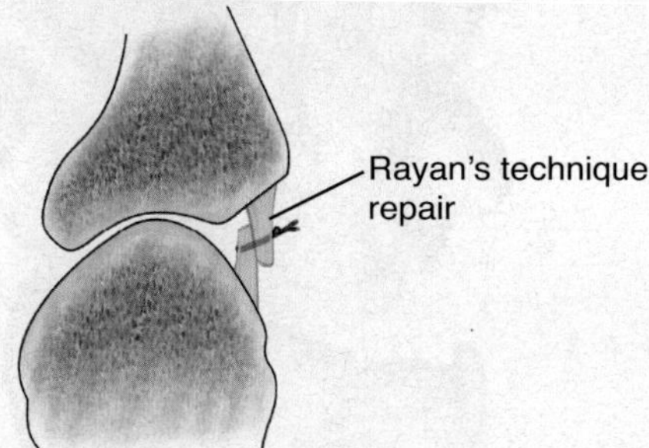

FIG 2 • Rayan's technique for thumb CMC stabilization: the dorsoradial ligament is imbricated and tightened and the CMC joint is pinned with a .045 K-wire for 4 weeks.[13]

SURGICAL MANAGEMENT

- Freedman et al[6] have demonstrated that open ligament reconstruction for symptomatic thumb CMC joint laxity can potentially halt or slow the progression to degenerative arthritis. By providing joint stability, shear forces on the CMC joint and translation of the metacarpal on the trapezium can be minimized.
- In the presence of articular pathology, arthroplasty may be the treatment of choice, depending on the degree of chondromalacia.
- If greater than 30 degrees of MCP hyperextension is present with lateral pinch, MCP capsulodesis or arthrodesis may also need to be considered.[17]
- If carpal tunnel syndrome or de Quervain tenosynovitis is present, carpal tunnel release or first dorsal compartment release may be need to be addressed at the time of surgery.
- For traumatic thumb CMC joint dislocations, Simonian and Trumble[14] have shown that ligament reconstruction was superior to percutaneous pinning of unstable joints.
- Rayan[13] has described a method for capsulodesis of the important dorsoradial ligament in the setting of either traumatic CMC joint instability or early Eaton stage I disease ligament laxity. This is described in **FIG 2**. Rayan's technique is an imbrication of the dorsoradial ligament followed by trapeziometacarpal (TMC) joint pinning. Rosenwasser has described an alternative technique described in **FIG 3** which involves advancement of the dorsoradial ligament either distally or proximally by means of a suture anchor placed into either the metacarpal insertion or the trapezial origin of the dorsoradial ligament, respectively. The senior author (RJS) similarly tightens and advances the dorsoradial ligament by means of a suture anchor placed into its metacarpal insertion. This is a promising technique compared to open ligament reconstruction though long term outcomes are not yet reported.[2]
- When the injury pattern results in fracture-dislocations such as unstable Bennett and Rolando fractures, percutaneous pinning or open reduction and internal fixation may be the treatment of choice.

Preoperative Planning

- Plain films should be reviewed.
- In the case of acute trauma, associated fractures and hand injuries should be addressed.
- A preoperative Allen test should be performed because all procedures involving the thumb CMC joint are in close vicinity to the radial artery and iatrogenic injury may occur.

Positioning

- The procedure is performed with the patient supine and the arm on a standard hand table.
- The operating table should be turned away from the anesthesia machines to allow the surgeon and assistant to sit across from each other at the hand table.

Approach

- A number of techniques have been described for ligament reconstruction of the thumb CMC joint using a variety of different tendons, including the flexor carpi radialis, palmaris longus, extensor carpi radialis longus, extensor pollicis brevis, and abductor pollicis longus (APL).
- The technique presented here is the classic volar ligament reconstruction described by Eaton and Littler.[4] This method effectively reconstructs both the volar and dorsal ligaments using the flexor carpi radialis.

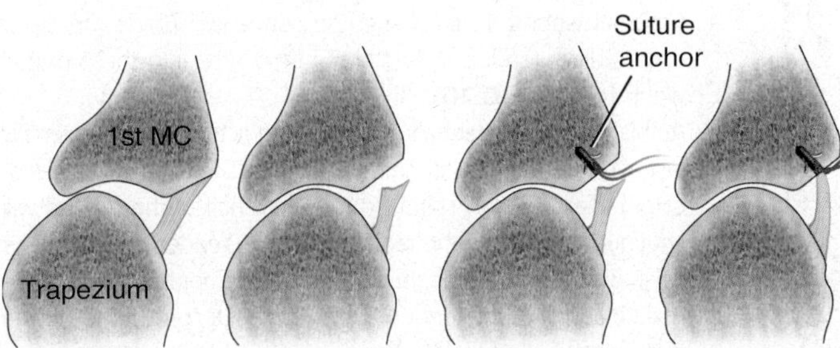

FIG 3 • The technique favored by Rosenwasser: the dorsoradial ligament is advanced into a suture anchor placed into the thumb metacarpal base in order to stabilize the CMC joint. The joint is immobilized in a thumb spica splint for 4 weeks, no pin is used.

Modified Wagner Approach to the Thumb Carpometacarpal Joint

- The incision is started longitudinally along the radial side of the thenar mass, at the junction between the glabrous and nonglabrous skin. The distal extent of the incision is near the midportion of the thumb metacarpal (**TECH FIG 1A**).
- Proximally at the wrist crease, the incision is brought transversely across the wrist to the ulnar side of the flexor carpi radialis tendon.
- Once through the skin, care should be taken to avoid transection of superficial radial sensory nerve branches that may be crossing the operative field.
- The soft tissue is bluntly dissected until the thenar musculature is identified (**TECH FIG 1B**). The radial border of the thenar muscle mass is incised and the muscles are elevated extraperiosteally to expose the CMC joint capsule. The capsule is incised and the thumb metacarpal base, the CMC joint, and the trapezium exposed (**TECH FIG 1C**).
- Blunt dissection is continued dorsally toward the extensor pollicis longus and brevis tendons. The dorsal metacarpal cortex is exposed between these tendons.

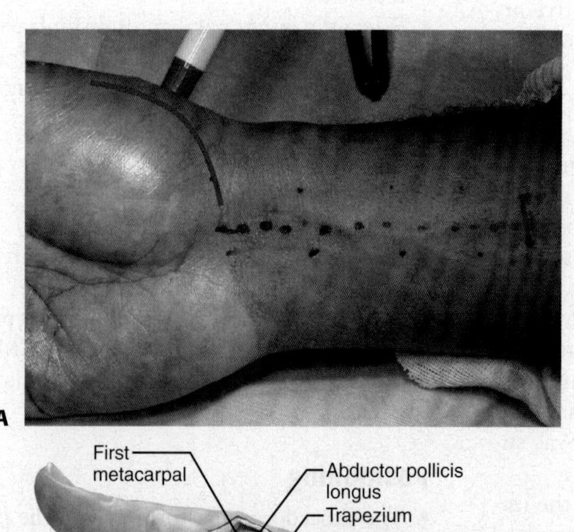

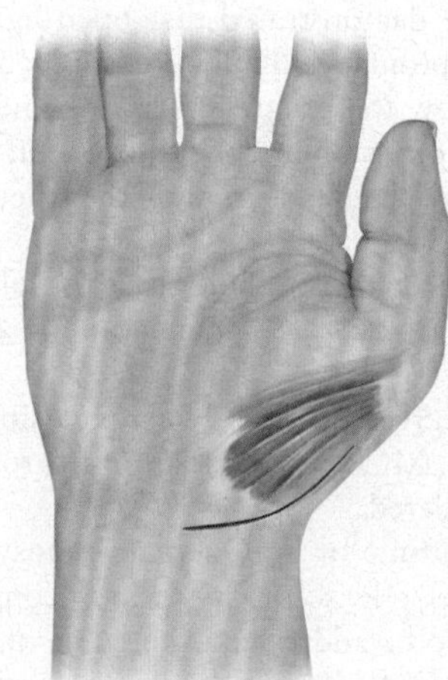

TECH FIG 1 • **A.** Modified Wagner incision (*red line*). **B.** Thenar musculature. **C.** The radial border of the thenar muscles is incised and elevated, exposing the thumb CMC joint.

Flexor Carpi Radialis Graft Harvest

- The flexor carpi radialis tendon is identified just radial to the palmaris longus tendon at the wrist crease. The tendon sheath is then opened.
- A transverse incision is made proximally in the forearm overlying the flexor carpi radialis musculotendinous junction, about 8 to 10 cm proximal to the wrist crease (**TECH FIG 2A,B**).
- The soft tissue is bluntly dissected until the tendon sheath is identified and opened. The flexor carpi radialis tendon is then exposed.
- A longitudinal split is made in the midline of the tendon just proximal to its insertion onto the trapezium. A 0 Prolene suture is then passed through the longitudinal split (**TECH FIG 2C**).
- A pediatric feeding tube is now passed from the proximal wound into the distal wound, just underneath the flexor carpi radialis tendon sheath but superficial to the flexor carpi radialis tendon fibers. The tip of the feeding tube is cut off, and the two ends of the Prolene suture are passed through the end of the feeding tube from distal to proximal. Once the suture is seen in the proximal wound, the feeding tube can be removed, leaving the ends of the Prolene suture in the proximal wound site (**TECH FIG 2D–F**).
- The two suture ends in the proximal wound are now pulled so that the rest of the suture is delivered from the distal to the proximal wound. In so doing, the suture will divide the flexor carpi radialis tendon in half along its course into the proximal wound (**TECH FIG 2G**).
- At this time, the ulnar half of the tendon is transected proximally just after the musculotendinous junction. The fibers of the flexor carpi radialis tendon spiral, so the ulnar half of the tendon will continue to become the radial half of the tendon distally at the wrist. Before transection, traction should be applied to the proximal ulnar half of the tendon to ensure that it corresponds to the distal radial half of the tendon.
- The split flexor carpi radialis tendon is finally delivered into the distal wound (**TECH FIG 2H**).

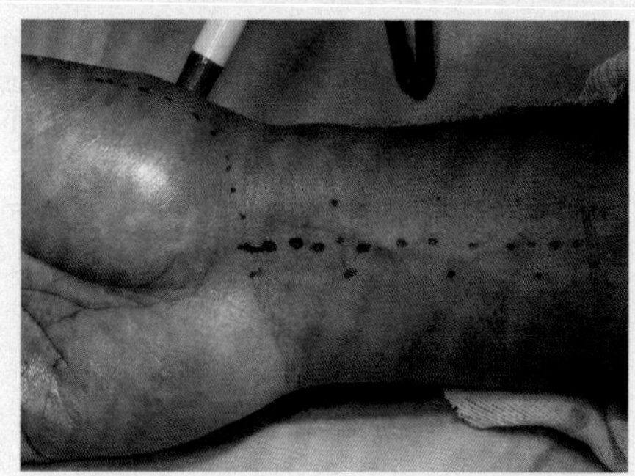

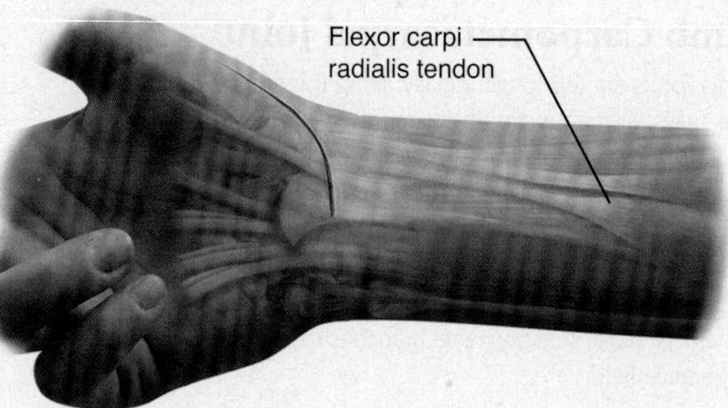

TECH FIG 2 • **A.** Flexor carpi radialis harvest incision is made 8 to 10 cm proximal to the wrist crease (*red line*). **B.** Flexor carpi radialis musculotendinous junction. *(continued)*

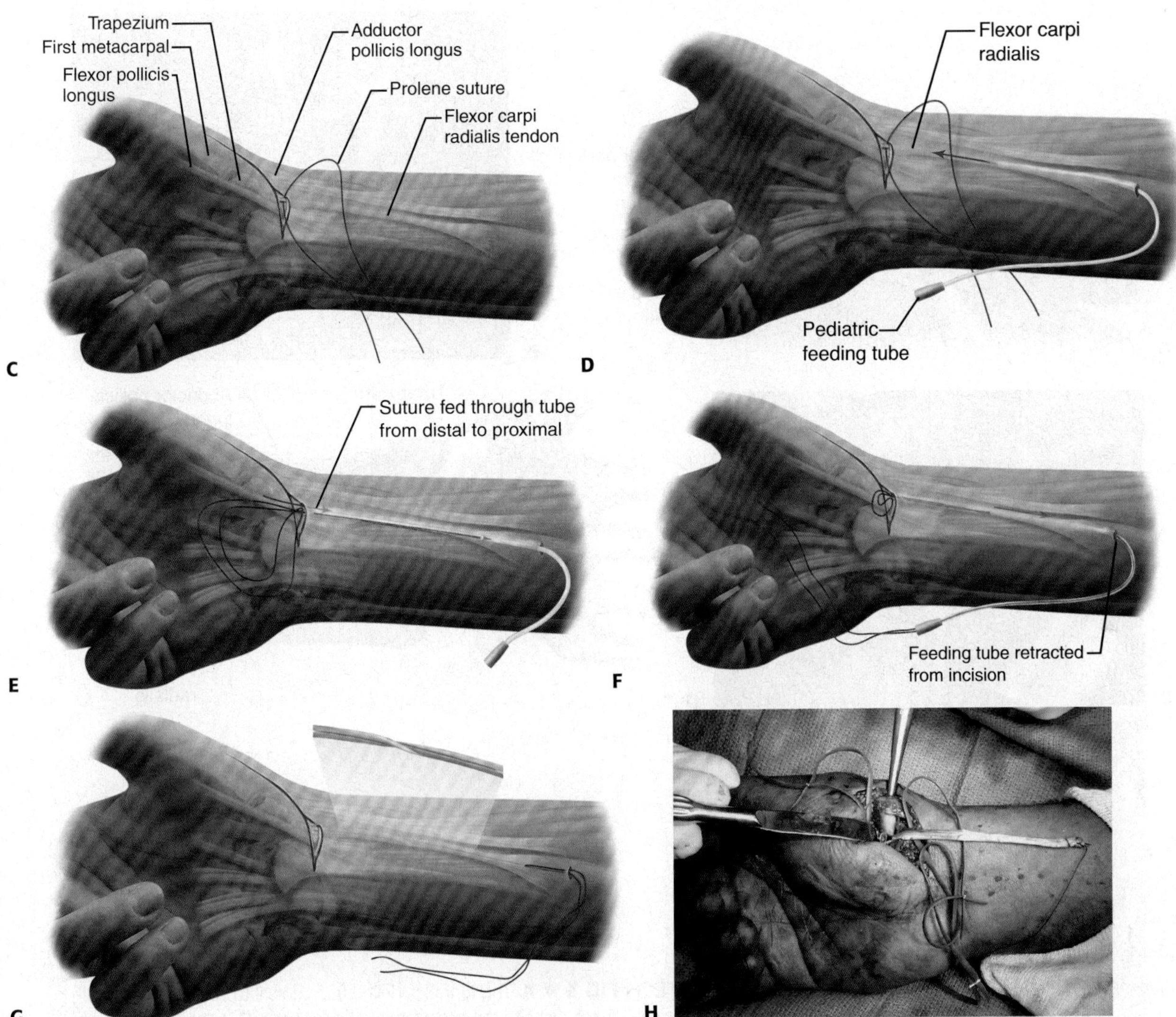

TECH FIG 2 • *(continued)* **C.** A longitudinal split is made through the flexor carpi radialis distally and a 0 Prolene suture is passed through it. **D.** A pediatric feeding tube is passed from the proximal to the distal wound. **E.** The Prolene suture is then passed through the feeding tube from distal to proximal. **F.** The feeding tube is removed, leaving the Prolene suture ends in the proximal wound. **G.** The two suture ends are pulled, thereby dividing the flexor carpi radialis tendon in half until the proximal wound is reached. The flexor carpi radialis tendon spirals, so the distal radial half corresponds to the proximal ulnar half of the tendon. **H.** The split flexor carpi radialis tendon is delivered into the distal wound.

Metacarpal Tunnel Placement and Flexor Carpi Radialis Graft Passage and Fixation

- A tunnel is made from dorsal to volar in the thumb metacarpal, 1 cm distal to the articular base. The tunnel should start dorsal to the APL insertion and then course parallel to the articular surface, exiting volarly just distal to the insertion of the volar beak ligament onto the metacarpal base.
  - The tunnel is started by first drilling a 0.045 Kirschner wire from dorsal to volar in the manner described. The tunnel is enlarged by drilling a 0.062 Kirschner wire, followed by a 3.5-mm drill (**TECH FIG 3A,B**).
- Once completed, a nylon whipstitch is placed in the end of the flexor carpi radialis graft. The ends of the stitch are passed through the metacarpal tunnel from a volar to dorsal direction. The stitch is pulled dorsally, delivering the flexor carpi radialis graft through the metacarpal tunnel to the dorsum (**TECH FIG 3C**).
- As the graft exits the dorsal hole in the metacarpal, the thumb is extended and abducted. The graft is pulled tightly and then allowed to relax 2 to 3 mm to set the appropriate tension.

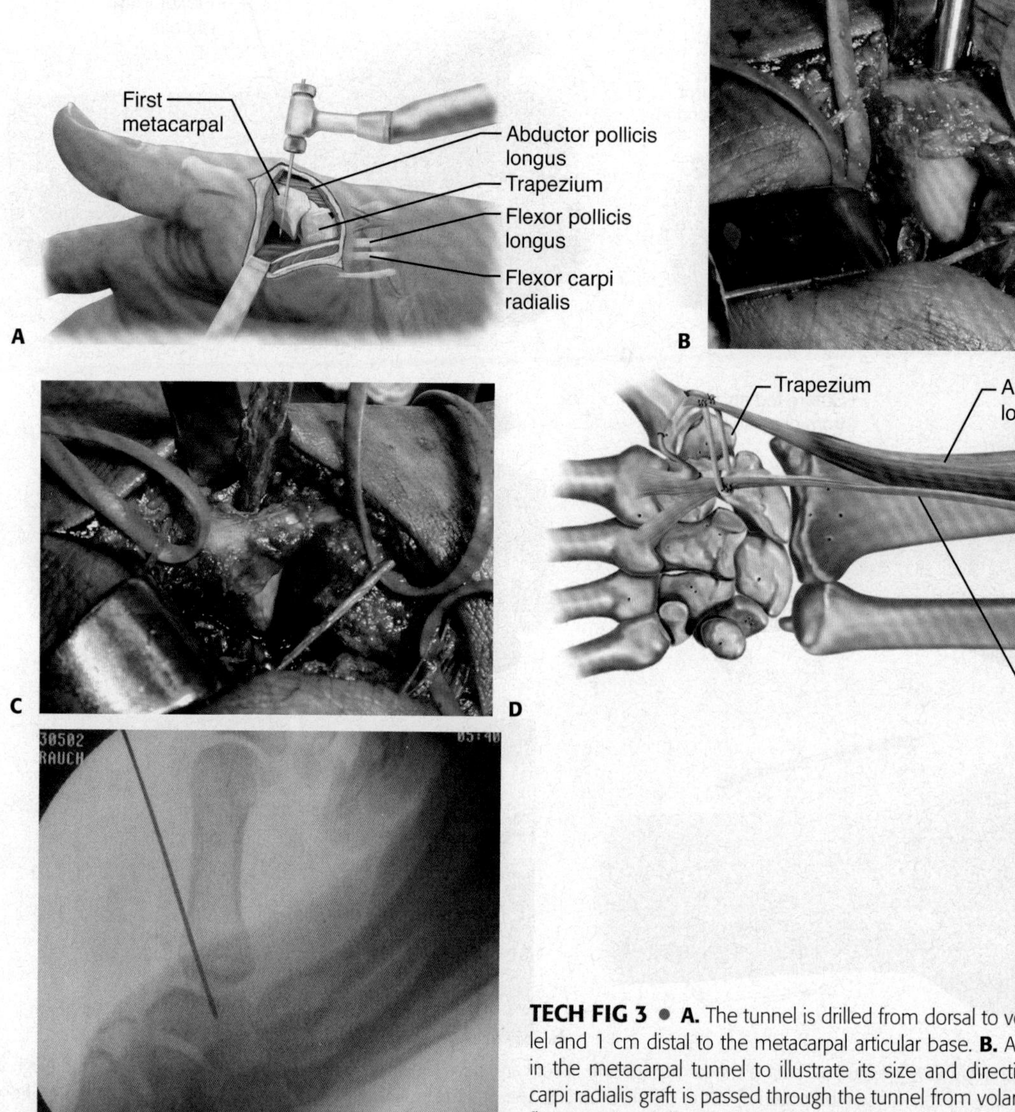

TECH FIG 3 • **A.** The tunnel is drilled from dorsal to volar, staying parallel and 1 cm distal to the metacarpal articular base. **B.** A curette is shown in the metacarpal tunnel to illustrate its size and direction. **C.** The flexor carpi radialis graft is passed through the tunnel from volar to dorsal. **D.** The flexor carpi radialis graft is passed underneath and sutured to the APL, the remaining flexor carpi radialis, and back dorsally to the APL if the graft length permits. **E.** A 0.045 Kirschner wire is drilled from the thumb metacarpal into the trapezium to protect the ligament repair.

- Once the graft tension is set, the graft is sutured to the metacarpal periosteum where it exits the dorsal hole using nonabsorbable 3-0 suture material.
- The flexor carpi radialis graft is then passed under the APL tendon radially toward the volar side of the wrist. The graft is sutured to the APL with similar nonabsorbable 3-0 suture material as it is passed underneath it.
- The graft is then passed underneath and around the ulnar portion of the flexor carpi radialis tendon that has remained intact. The graft is also sutured to the flexor carpi radialis tendon as it is looped around it.
- If there is additional length to the graft, it is brought back dorsally and again passed underneath and sutured to the APL (**TECH FIG 3D**).
- A 0.045-inch Kirschner wire is drilled from the radial thumb metacarpal base into the trapezium to immobilize the CMC joint. The wire is removed after 5 weeks once adequate soft tissue healing has occurred (**TECH FIG 3E**).

Wound Closure

- The thenar muscle mass is reapproximated and sutured using synthetic absorbable 3-0 suture material.
- The proximal and distal skin incisions are closed with 5-0 nylon sutures (**TECH FIG 4**).
- The hand is then placed in a short-arm thumb spica splint.

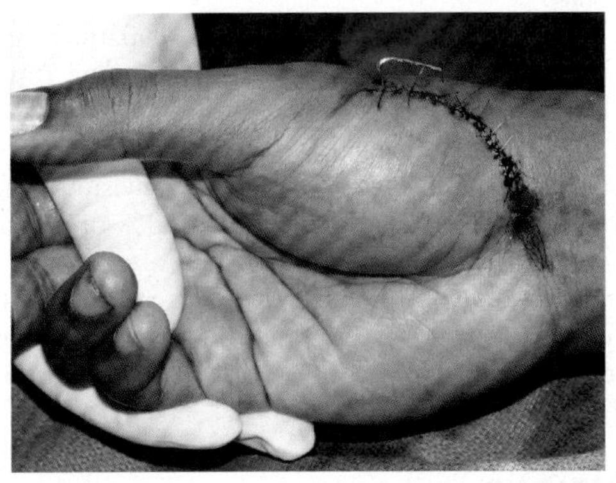

TECH FIG 4 • Final wound closure with nylon sutures.

PEARLS AND PITFALLS

Indications	■ In the setting of stage I or II basal joint disease and ligament laxity, the status of the articular cartilage must be carefully assessed intraoperatively. If significant cartilage damage is present, arthroplasty may be preferred.
Approach	■ Care must be taken to identify and preserve the superficial radial sensory nerve and lateral antebrachial cutaneous nerve branches to prevent neuroma formation.
Flexor carpi radials graft harvest	■ The entire insertion of the flexor carpi radialis onto the second metacarpal base must be left intact. ■ Transect the proximal portion of the graft near the musculotendinous junction to ensure that adequate graft length will be obtained. ■ Once the graft harvest is completed, the graft should occasionally be moistened through the remainder of the procedure to prevent desiccation and tenocyte injury.
Metacarpal tunnel placement	■ Start with a small-diameter tunnel. Gradually increase the diameter of the tunnel until the graft fits snugly through it. ■ When creating the tunnel, be careful not to injure the insertion of the APL onto the radial base of the thumb metacarpal.
Flexor carpi radialis graft passage and fixation	■ It is important to set the appropriate graft tension. After placing a few periosteal sutures to hold the graft, make sure that the thumb can still be brought back into a neutral position. ■ Before weaving the graft under the APL and around the intact flexor carpi radialis tendons, check an image to ensure that the CMC is adequately reduced. ■ Braided synthetic suture such as Ethibond is soft and may be less palpable than stiffer suture such as Prolene.

POSTOPERATIVE CARE

- AP, lateral, and oblique films or fluoroscopic mini C-arm views are obtained intraoperatively to evaluate CMC joint congruency and Kirschner wire placement.
- The thumb spica splint is left in place for 2 weeks. At 2 weeks of follow-up, the dressings are taken down, sutures are removed, and a new thumb spica splint is applied.
- At 5 weeks of follow-up, the Kirschner wire is removed and a removable thumb splint is used for protection. The splint can be removed for therapy, which can be started at this time.
- Therapy should start with active range-of-motion exercises of the wrist, thumb CMC, MCP, and interphalangeal joints. Thumb abduction, flexion, and opposition are emphasized.
- Strengthening exercises can be started at 2 months after surgery, and full activity without restrictions can begin at 3 months.

OUTCOMES

- When performed for stage I basal joint disease, ligament reconstruction has been shown to improve pain and establish joint stability.
  - In a number of long-term follow-up studies of over 5 years, 87% to 100% of patients demonstrated joint stability against stress testing, 29% to 67% of patients reported no pain, and 83% to 100% reported marked improvement in pain. Interestingly, only 0% to 37% of patients progressed to a higher stage of arthritis.[6,9]
  - Freedman et al[6] reviewed their long-term results of 24 thumbs that underwent ligament reconstruction for stage I or II disease. After a minimum of 10 years of follow-up, 29% of patients reported no pain, 54% reported pain with strenuous activity only, and 17% of patients had pain during activities

of daily living. When tested against stress, 87% demonstrated joint stability.

- Simonian and Trumble[14] found that 89% of patients who underwent ligament reconstruction after traumatic thumb CMC dislocation had no pain with work at 2 years of follow-up. Also, none of the patients in this treatment group had any evidence of joint instability, and no revision procedures were required. This is in contrast to 50% of patients who had residual joint instability and pain after closed reduction and percutaneous pinning. Of this treatment group, 38% required revision surgery and underwent ligament reconstruction. Twelve percent of these patients required CMC arthrodesis.

COMPLICATIONS

- Residual joint instability
- Residual pain, likely due to untreated arthritis involving surrounding joint articulations, such as the scaphotrapezial joint
- Radial artery injury
- Superficial radial nerve or lateral antebrachial cutaneous nerve injury
- Pin tract infection

REFERENCES

1. Bettinger PC, Linscheid RL, Berger RA, et al. An anatomic study of the stabilizing ligaments of the trapezium and trapeziometacarpal joint. J Hand Surg Am 1999;24(4):786–798.
2. Birman MV, Danoff JR, Yemul KS, et al. Dorsoradial ligament imbrication for thumb carpometacarpal joint instability. Tech Hand Up Extrem Surg 2014;18(2):66–71. doi:10.1097/BTH.0000000000000035.
3. Eaton RG, Glickel SZ, Littler JW. Tendon interposition arthroplasty for degenerative arthritis of the trapeziometacarpal joint of the thumb. J Hand Surg Am 1985;10(5):645–654.
4. Eaton RG, Littler JW. Ligament reconstruction for the painful thumb carpometacarpal joint. J Bone Joint Surg Am 1973;55(8):1655–1666.
5. Edmunds JO. Traumatic dislocations and instability of the trapeziometacarpal joint of the thumb. Hand Clin 2006;22:365–392.
6. Freedman DM, Eaton RG, Glickel SZ. Long-term results of volar ligament reconstruction for symptomatic basal joint laxity. J Hand Surg Am 2000;25:297–304.
7. Glickel SZ, Gupta S. Ligament reconstruction. Hand Clin 2006;22:143–151.
8. Imaeda T, An KN, Cooney WP III. Functional anatomy and biomechanics of the thumb. Hand Clin 1992;8:9–15.
9. Lane LB, Eaton RG. Ligament reconstruction for the painful "prearthritic" thumb carpometacarpal joint. Clin Orthop Relat Res 1987;(220):52–57.
10. Lin JD, Karl JW, Strauch RJ. Trapeziometacarpal joint stability: the evolving importance of the dorsal ligaments. Clin Orthop Relat Res 2014;472:1138–1145.
11. Pellegrini VD Jr. Osteoarthritis of the trapeziometacarpal joint: the pathophysiology of articular cartilage degeneration. I. Anatomy and pathology of the aging joint. J Hand Surg Am 1991;16:967–974.
12. Pellegrini VD Jr. Pathomechanics of the thumb trapeziometacarpal joint. Hand Clin 2001;17:175–184.
13. Rayan G, Do V. Dorsoradial capsulodesis for trapeziometacarpal joint instability. J Hand Surg Am 2013;38:382–387.
14. Simonian PT, Trumble TE. Traumatic dislocation of the thumb carpometacarpal joint: early ligamentous reconstruction versus closed reduction and pinning. J Hand Surg Am 1996;21:802–806.
15. Strauch RJ, Behrman MJ, Rosenwasser MP. Acute dislocation of the carpometacarpal joint of the thumb: an anatomic and cadaver study. J Hand Surg Am 1994;19:93–98.
16. Swigart CR, Eaton RG, Glickel SZ, et al. Splinting in the treatment of arthritis of the first carpometacarpal joint. J Hand Surg Am 1999;24:86–91.
17. Tomaino MM, King J, Leit M. Thumb basal joint arthritis. In: Green DP, ed. Green's Operative Hand Surgery, ed 5. Philadelphia: Elsevier/Churchill Livingstone, 2005:461–485.
18. Van Brenk B, Richards RR, Mackay MB, et al. A biomechanical assessment of ligaments preventing dorsoradial subluxation of the trapeziometacarpal joint. J Hand Surg Am 1998;23:607–611.

43

CHAPTER

Operative Treatment of Thumb Carpometacarpal Joint Fractures

John T. Capo, Joshua T. Mitgang, and Colin Harris

DEFINITION

- The first carpometacarpal (CMC) joint comprises the thumb metacarpal base and the trapezium.
- The thumb CMC joint is vital to the function of the hand, and injuries can result in pain, weakness, and loss of grip or pinch strength.
- Two fracture-dislocation patterns commonly result from trauma to the thumb CMC joint: *Bennett* and *Rolando* fractures.
  - Bennett fractures are intra-articular fractures in which the metacarpal shaft is radially displaced by the pull of the abductor pollicis longus (APL) tendon, leaving an intact ulnar fragment at the base of the thumb metacarpal that is held reduced by the strong volar beak ligament (**FIG 1A**).
  - Rolando fractures are complex intra-articular fractures involving the base of the thumb metacarpal that often have a T- or Y-type pattern. These fractures are classically described as being three-part; however, the name also applies to more comminuted fracture variants (**FIG 1B**).[10]

ANATOMY

- Understanding the deforming forces in these fracture-dislocations is important when deciding on treatment options and determining prognosis.

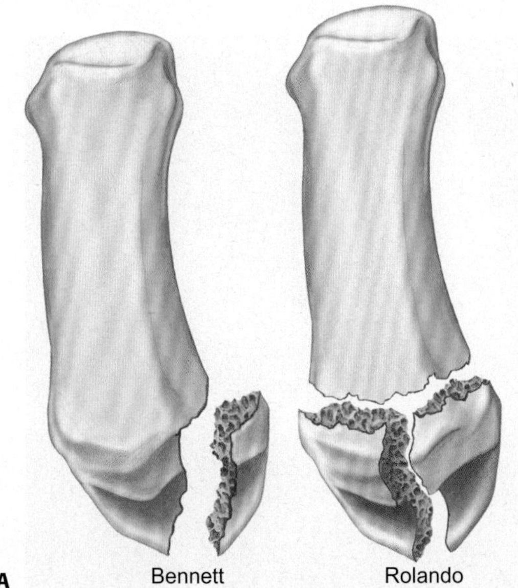

FIG 1 • **A.** A typical Bennett fracture is a unicondylar fracture of the base of the first metacarpal with the fracture fragment consisting of the volar ulnar corner of the proximal metacarpal. **B.** A Rolando fracture is multifragmentary, with the entire articular base of the metacarpal being involved. By definition, no portion of the metacarpal shaft is in continuity with the CMC joint.

- The thumb metacarpal serves as the site of attachment for several tendons, including the APL at the proximal base, the adductor pollicis distally, and the thenar muscles volarly.[15]
- The articular surfaces of the thumb metacarpal base and trapezium resemble reciprocally interlocking saddles and allow motion in many planes.[11,15]
- Joint stability is maintained by five primary ligaments: the anterior volar (beak), the posterior oblique, the dorsoradial, and the anterior and posterior intermetacarpal ligaments (**FIG 2**).[7]
- Buchler et al[2] described three zones at the base of the thumb metacarpal (**FIG 3**):
  - Zone 2 represents the central portion of the joint that is normally loaded.
  - Zone 1 includes the volar aspect of the joint.
  - Zone 3 involves the dorsal aspect of the joint.
- The trapezium has several important adjacent articulations. These include the first metacarpal base, the radial aspect of the second metacarpal base, the scaphoid, and the trapezoid (along with the trapezium, these last two make up the scaphotrapeziotrapezoid [STT] joint) (**FIG 4**).

PATHOGENESIS

- Bennett fractures occur when the partially flexed thumb metacarpal is axially loaded, resulting in a Bennett articular fragment (the volar ulnar portion of the metacarpal base) and the remainder of the metacarpal that displaces dorsally, proximally, and radially.
- Rolando fractures result from a similar injury mechanism and may have a variable degree of comminution at the base of the thumb metacarpal.
- In Bennett-type fractures, the thumb metacarpal shaft is displaced dorsally and proximally by the pull of the APL at the metacarpal base, the extensor pollicis longus (EPL) which inserts more distally, and angulated ulnarly by the APL (**FIG 5A**).[15]
- Rolando-type fractures are subject to the same deforming forces, except that the APL can sometimes displace both the shaft and the dorsoradial basilar articular fragment.
- Due to the deforming forces that act on the fracture fragments, both injury patterns are usually unstable and difficult to reduce and stabilize by closed means.

NATURAL HISTORY

- Injuries to the thumb metacarpal base represent 80% of all thumb fractures.[5,9]
- Nonoperative treatment is generally reserved for nondisplaced fractures. There is a low likelihood of maintaining reduction using closed means in displaced fractures.
- Residual subluxation of the metacarpal shaft leads to basal joint incongruity and the potential for developing

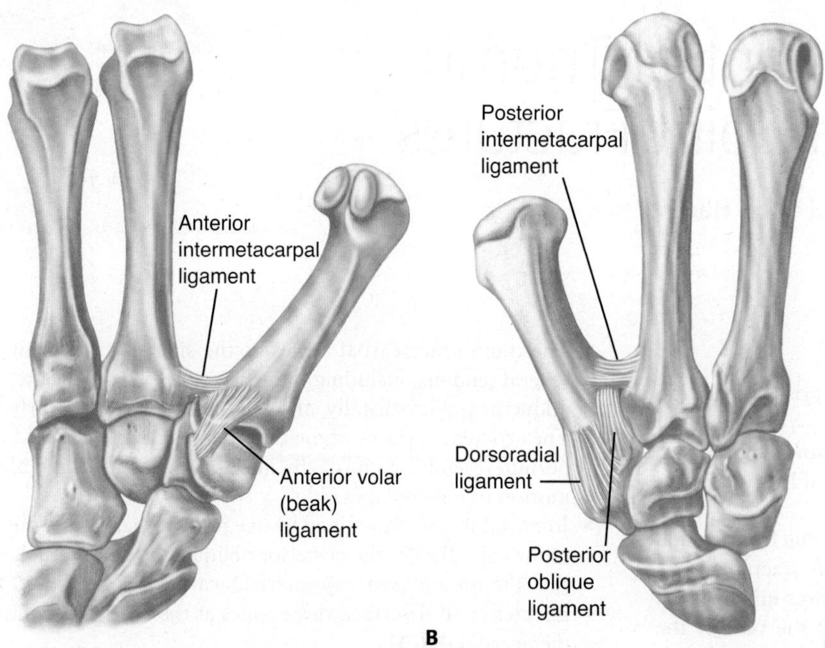

FIG 2 • **A,B.** Anterior and posterior views of the thumb basal joint stabilizing ligamentous structures. The crucial anterior volar oblique (beak) ligament is often attached to the displaced Bennett fragment.

posttraumatic arthrosis.[3] In addition, residual intra-articular step-off greater than 1 mm may predispose the patient to the development of arthrosis.[6,18]

PATIENT HISTORY AND PHYSICAL FINDINGS

- Most of these fractures occur with direct trauma to the thumb tip, often from a fall or sports-related injury.
- The injury is most common in young males, and two-thirds occur in the dominant hand.[9,15]
- The history should reveal whether the patient had preexisting basal joint arthritis, which is common and will affect treatment options and expected results.
- Common physical examination findings include tenderness and ecchymosis surrounding the thumb CMC joint, crepitus with attempted motion, instability, and a "shelf" deformity resulting from displacement of the metacarpal shaft dorsally (**FIG 5B**).[16]
  - Metacarpal subluxation or dislocation represents an unstable fracture.
- Range of motion is decreased and may be associated with crepitus. Adjacent joints may also have arthrosis and decreased range of motion.
- It is important to perform a complete neurovascular examination and to search for associated pathology such as wrist ligamentous injuries.
  - Neurovascular injuries are uncommon, but compartment syndrome should be suspected in higher energy injuries. A recent case study described the first documented case of

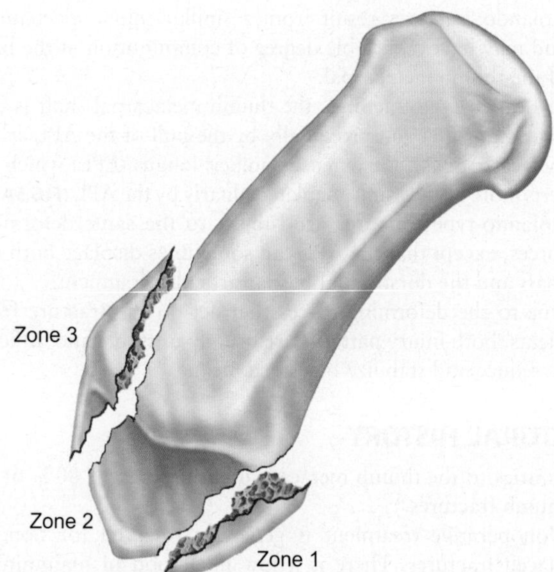

FIG 3 • The three zones found in fractures of the first metacarpal base. The central zone 2 is critical for joint stability and if involved usually requires open reduction and internal fixation.

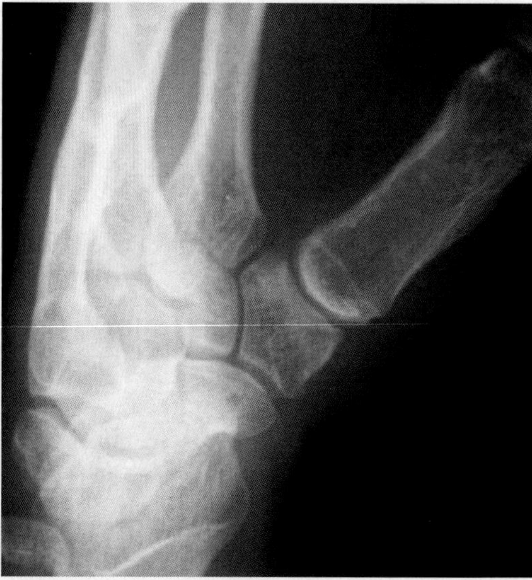

FIG 4 • A radiographic view of the trapezium and its articulations including the basal joint. The view is taken with the patient's arm abducted 45 degrees with the hand pronated 45 degrees with the x-ray beam vertically oriented. This evaluates both sides of the basal joint and associated trapezial joint fractures. (Copyright Joshua Mitgang, MD.)

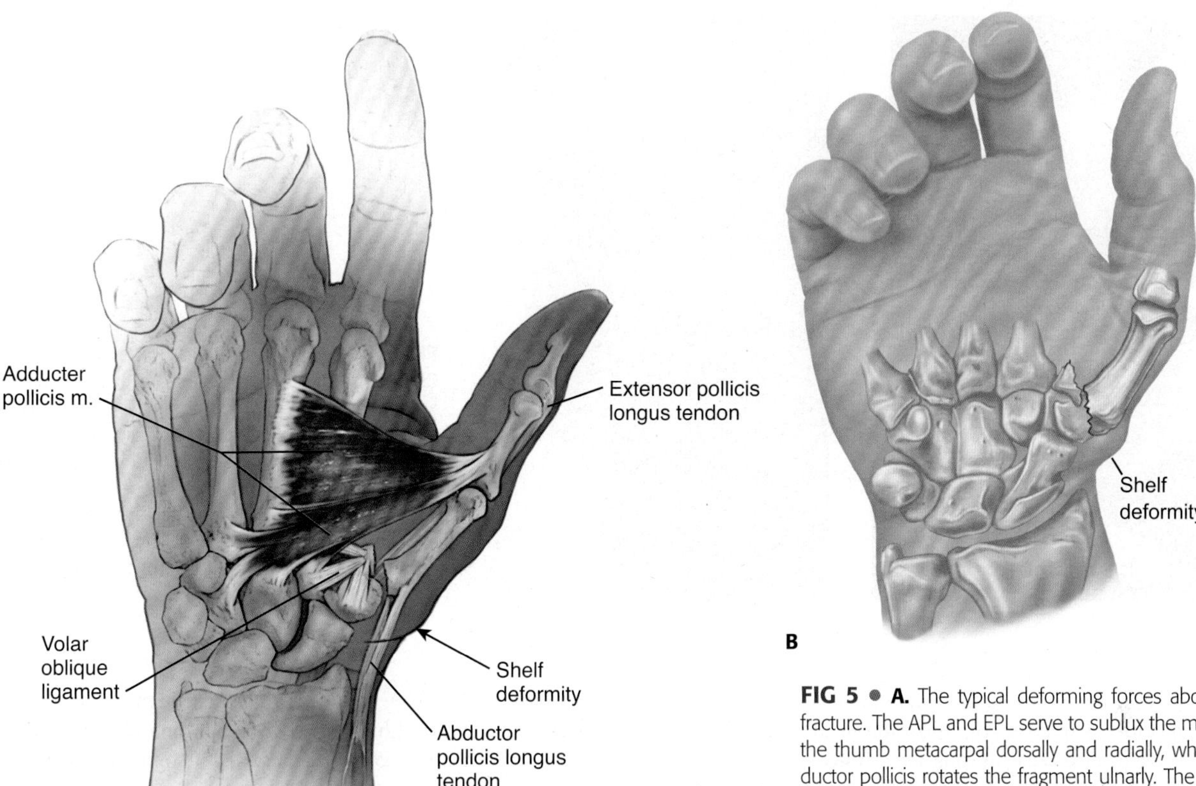

FIG 5 • **A.** The typical deforming forces about a Bennett fracture. The APL and EPL serve to sublux the main portion of the thumb metacarpal dorsally and radially, whereas the adductor pollicis rotates the fragment ulnarly. The volar oblique ligament holds the volar ulnar fragment of the thumb metacarpal in place. **B.** A typical shelf deformity is depicted in a Bennett fracture. When viewing the thumb from the lateral perspective, the thumb metacarpal shaft can be seen riding dorsally as it displaces from the unstable CMC joint.

thenar compartment syndrome from a thumb metacarpal base fracture.[20]

- Function of the EPL, flexor pollicis longus (FPL), and extensor pollicis brevis (EPB) should be confirmed.

IMAGING AND OTHER DIAGNOSTIC STUDIES

- Anteroposterior (AP), lateral, and oblique images of the hand should be obtained, although the oblique plane of the thumb in relation to the hand may make these images difficult to interpret.
  - A true AP view of the thumb CMC joint, known as the *Roberts view*, can be obtained with the forearm maximally pronated with the dorsum of the thumb placed on the cassette (**FIG 6A**).[17]
- A true lateral view, advocated by Billing and Gedda,[1] is obtained with the hand pronated 20 degrees and the thumb positioned flat on the cassette. The x-ray beam is tilted 10 degrees from vertical in a distal to proximal direction (**FIG 6B**).
- Radiographs of the contralateral, uninjured basal joint are helpful in certain cases as a template for reconstruction.
- Computed tomography may be indicated if a significant amount of articular comminution is present or when plain films inadequately demonstrate the pathology.
- A traction view may be helpful in Rolando-type fractures (**FIG 6C**).
- Fluoroscopy alone should be used with caution in ensuring anatomic reduction, as this has recently been shown to be less accurate than plain x-rays or direct visualization.[4]

DIFFERENTIAL DIAGNOSIS

- Bennett-type fracture
- Rolando-type fracture
- Basal joint degenerative joint disease
- STT joint arthrosis
- Thumb CMC joint ligamentous injury
- Trapezial body fracture
- De Quervain tenosynovitis

NONOPERATIVE MANAGEMENT

- Nondisplaced, minimally comminuted fractures may be treated with closed reduction and thumb spica casting, but precise molding of the cast and close observation for fracture displacement are necessary.
- In a Bennett fracture, closed treatment may be indicated if there is minimal displacement between the volar ulnar fragment and the metacarpal shaft. Most importantly, a concentric reduction of the metacarpal base and the CMC joint in Bennett fractures must be maintained.[6]
- Several factors make closed treatment of these intra-articular fractures problematic and worsen results:
  - Difficulty in providing accurate three-point molding of the thumb metacarpal
  - Treatment of patients 4 or more days after the initial injury
  - Difficulty assessing the adequacy of reduction with radiographs taken through the cast[5,10]

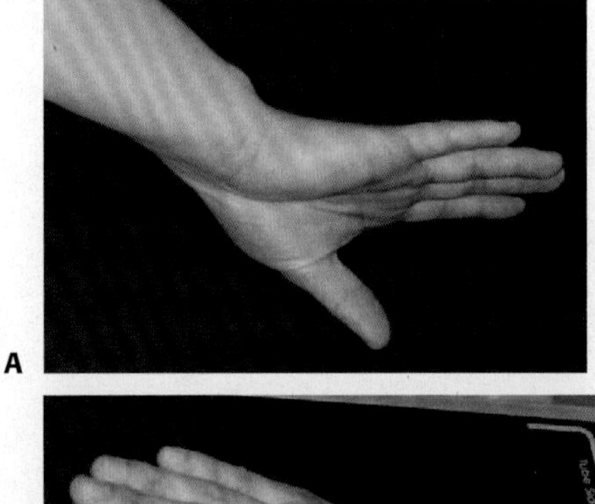

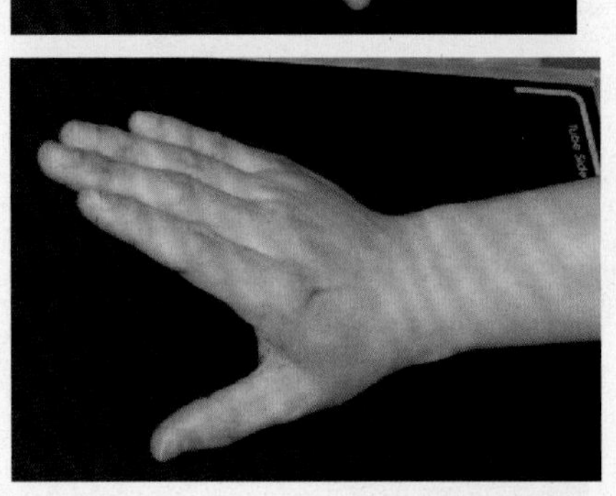

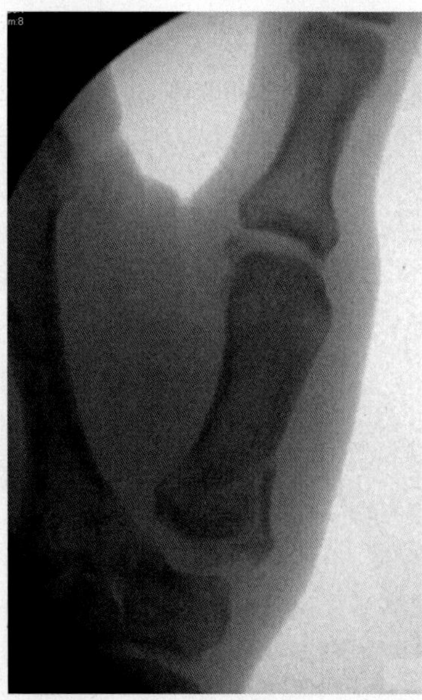

FIG 6 • **A.** An ideal AP view of the thumb and CMC joint is taken with the forearm hyperpronated and the dorsum of the thumb on the cassette. **B.** A true lateral view of the CMC joint is obtained with the radial aspect of the thumb on the cassette and the other fingers clear of the x-ray beam. **C.** A fluoroscopic view of a Rolando fracture with traction applied. Distraction at the CMC joint helps to delineate the fragments at the base of the metacarpal. (Copyright John Capo, MD.)

- Some studies looking at closed treatment have demonstrated decreased motion, grip strength, and radiographic evidence of degenerative joint disease at long-term follow-up.[14]
- Development of degenerative changes may occur if there is any residual subluxation of the thumb metacarpal shaft.[3,9]

SURGICAL MANAGEMENT

- The majority of displaced Bennett fractures and almost all Rolando fractures require percutaneous Kirschner wire fixation or open reduction and internal fixation.
- The goals of surgery are to restore the articular congruity of the thumb CMC joint and to align the first metacarpal base articular surface with the trapezium.
- In thumb CMC joint fractures associated with trapezial body fractures, the trapezial articular surface should first be reduced anatomically before proceeding to the thumb metacarpal fracture.[16]

Bennett Fractures

- Closed reduction and percutaneous pinning is the preferred treatment for most Bennett fractures with displaced fracture fragments representing less than 25% to 30% of the articular surface.[7,16]
- The metacarpal base often needs to be pinned to the unfractured second metacarpal, trapezoid, or trapezium to lessen the deforming forces on the fracture.
- Open reduction is necessary when there is residual displacement of the joint surface greater than 2 mm after attempted closed reduction and percutaneous pinning or impaction in the force-bearing aspect of the joint surface (Buchler zone 2).[15]

Rolando Fractures

- Closed reduction with longitudinal traction and percutaneous pinning is indicated if successful reduction can be achieved under fluoroscopic guidance; this is usually successful only when large T- or Y-type fragments are present.
- If the joint cannot be reduced by closed methods, open reduction and internal fixation with a combination of smooth wires; screws; and 1.5- to 2.7-mm L, T, or blade plates is indicated.
- Significant comminution may require either external fixation or a combination of external fixation, limited internal fixation with Kirschner wires and small (1.3 or 1.5 mm) screws, and cancellous bone grafting as advocated by Buchler et al.[2]

Preoperative Planning

- A thorough history and physical examination are mandatory to choose the appropriate treatment and rule out associated injuries.
- True AP, lateral, and oblique radiographs of the thumb should be obtained in all cases. Traction radiographs help assess the effects of ligamentotaxis on fracture reduction.
- Surgery may be performed acutely, but if significant soft tissue swelling is present, elevation in a well-padded thumb spica splint for 2 to 5 days may be necessary before undergoing operative fixation.[16]

Positioning

- The patient is placed supine on the operating room table.
- A radiolucent hand table is used to allow for intraoperative fluoroscopy.
- The patient is moved toward the operative side to center the hand on the table.
- A nonsterile tourniquet is placed on the upper arm.
- General, regional (axillary or infraclavicular), or local (wrist block with local infiltration) anesthesia can be used, although muscle relaxation is often necessary to obtain proper reduction.[7,16]

Approach

- The Wagner approach can be used for both Bennett and Rolando fractures in which open reduction is necessary.

Closed Reduction and Percutaneous Pinning of Bennett and Rolando Fractures

- Longitudinal traction, abduction, and pronation of the thumb is performed while applying direct manual pressure over the metacarpal base.[16]
- Traction is maintained and the reduction is held while fluoroscopy is used to verify acceptable fracture reduction and alignment of the articular surface (**TECH FIG 1A,B**).
- Fine-tuning the amount of traction, abduction, and pronation can be done using fluoroscopic guidance.
- Smooth 0.045-inch Kirschner wires are inserted from the proximal thumb metacarpal shaft into the uninjured index metacarpal base or trapezium. These wires stabilize the concentrically reduced metacarpal shaft and CMC joint (**TECH FIG 1C**).
- If the Bennett fracture fragment is of ample size, fixation to the fragment may be used in addition (**TECH FIG 1D**).
- Large fragments may be manipulated percutaneously with Kirschner wire "joysticks" and then stabilized.
- The wires are bent and cut outside of the skin, followed by application of a well-padded thumb spica splint with the thumb in abduction and wrist in extension.
- If less than 2 mm of step-off cannot be obtained by closed reduction, the surgeon should consider abandoning this technique for an open reduction and internal fixation.[7,16]
- In rare instances, a similar technique can be used for Rolando fractures, with large T- or Y-type fracture patterns with minimal comminution.

A
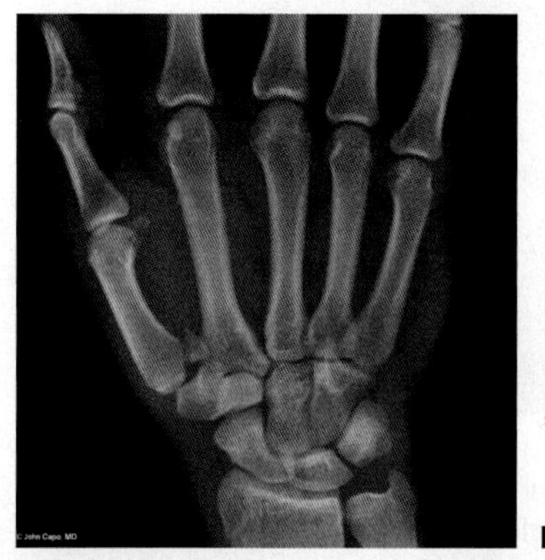
B
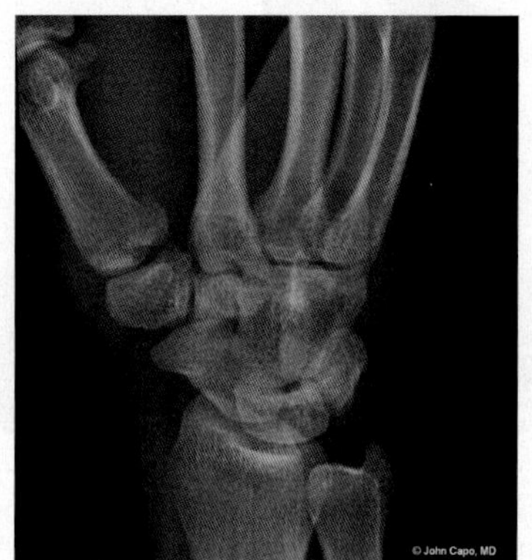
C
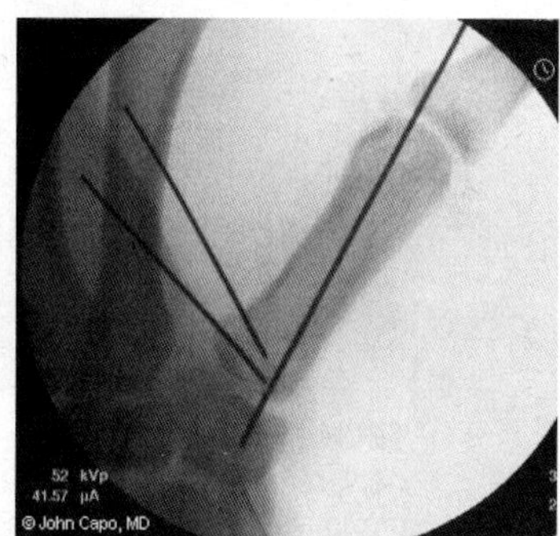

D
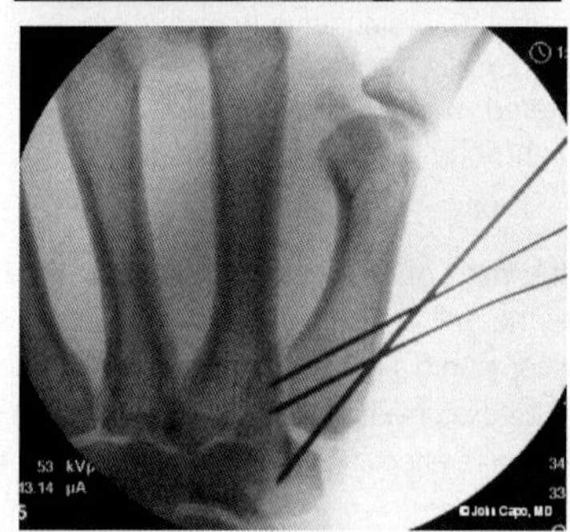

TECH FIG 1 • **A,B.** Lateral and posteroanterior (PA) views of a Bennett fracture with intra-articular displacement. **C.** The metacarpal base is first reduced to the trapezium and then a pin (0.045) is placed across the CMC joint. Two additional pins are provisionally placed and readied to stabilize the Bennett fracture fragment. **D.** The two smaller pins (0.035) are then advanced across into the Bennett fragment. (Copyright John Capo, MD.)

Open Reduction and Internal Fixation of Bennett Fractures

Incision and Dissection

- A Wagner approach is used for open reduction of a Bennett fracture (**TECH FIG 2A**).
- An incision is made on the dorsoradial aspect of the thumb CMC joint at the junction of the glabrous and nonglabrous skin and curved in a volar direction toward the distal wrist crease to the flexor carpi radialis (FCR) tendon sheath (**TECH FIG 2B**).
  - The palmar cutaneous branch of the median nerve, the superficial radial nerve, and distal branches of the lateral antebrachial cutaneous nerve are at risk in this approach and should be carefully protected (**TECH FIG 2C**).
- The thenar muscles are elevated extraperiosteally from the CMC joint and a longitudinal capsulotomy is made to expose the joint and the fracture fragments.
- An effort should be made to preserve all soft tissue attachments to the fracture fragments (**TECH FIG 2D**).
- The fracture line is exposed and cleaned of all hematoma and early callus.
  - This often requires abduction, supination, and dorsal displacement of the metacarpal shaft to expose the volar ulnar Bennett fragment.

Reduction and Fixation

- The displaced thumb metacarpal shaft should be reduced to the volar ulnar fragment under direct visualization and secured with fine reduction clamps or Kirschner wires (**TECH FIG 3A**).

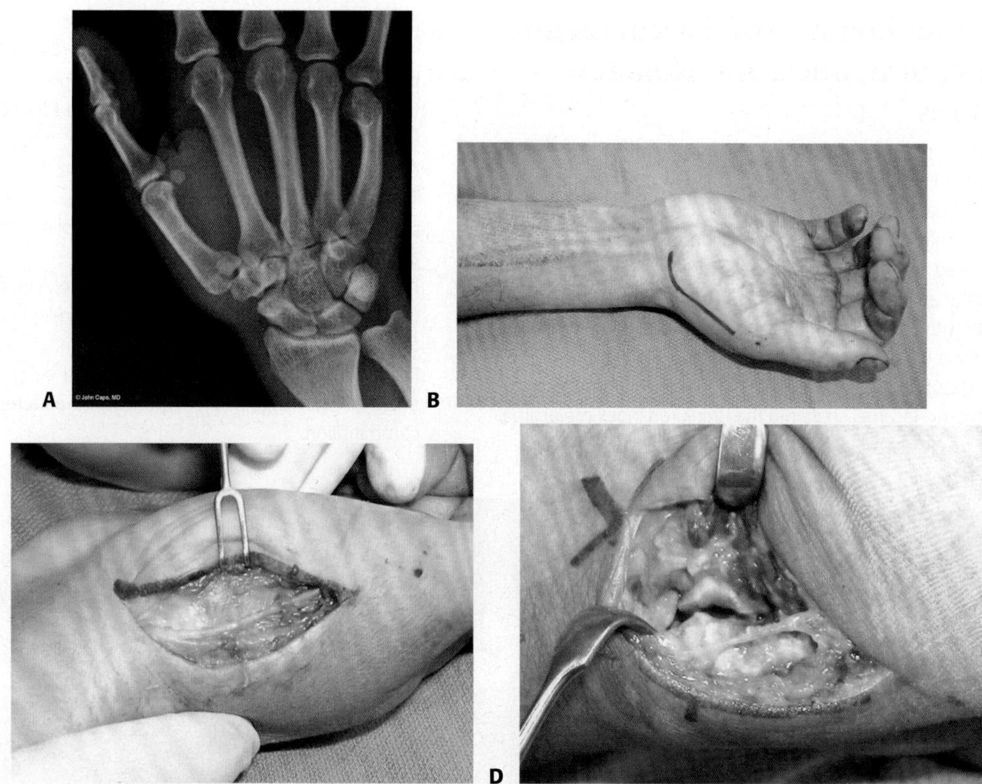

TECH FIG 2 • A. A preoperative radiograph demonstrating a large (~40%) Bennett fracture with intra-articular displacement. **B.** The typical incision for open reduction and internal fixation of a Bennett or Rolando fracture. The proximal aspect starts at the FCR tendon sheath. In the case of a Rolando fracture, especially one treated by plate fixation, the distal portion of the incision should extend along the thumb metacarpal. **C.** Distal nerve branches are seen during the exposure of these fractures. The nerves can usually be retracted dorsally to allow exposure of the CMC joint. **D.** The thenar muscles are reflected volarly and the CMC joint is entered. The volar oblique fracture is now clearly visualized. Care is taken to maintain soft tissue attachments. (Copyright John Capo, MD.)

- One or two 0.045-inch smooth Kirschner wires are used to provisionally hold the reduction, or in certain fracture patterns, they can serve as the definitive means of fixation.
- Alternatively, 1.3- to 2.0-mm screws can be placed in an interfragmentary compression fashion for added stability (**TECH FIG 3B**).[8]
  - One Kirschner wire is removed at a time and replaced with a screw.
  - Generally, the path of the removed Kirschner wire effectively guides the drill in the appropriate direction. Use of a mini-fluoroscopy unit is helpful.
  - Care should be exercised to avoid overcompression, which may cause an alteration in the arc of curvature of the articular surface.

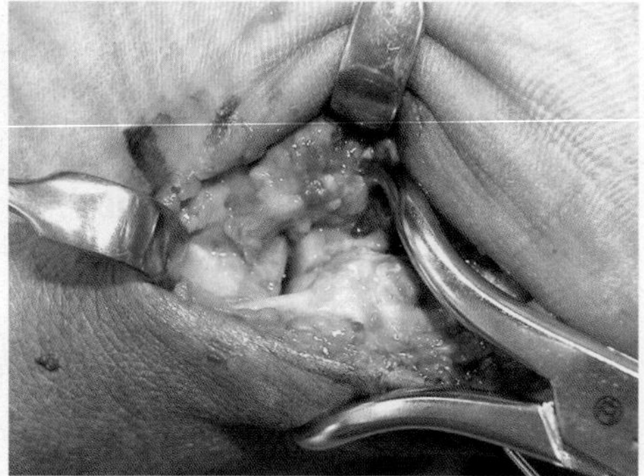

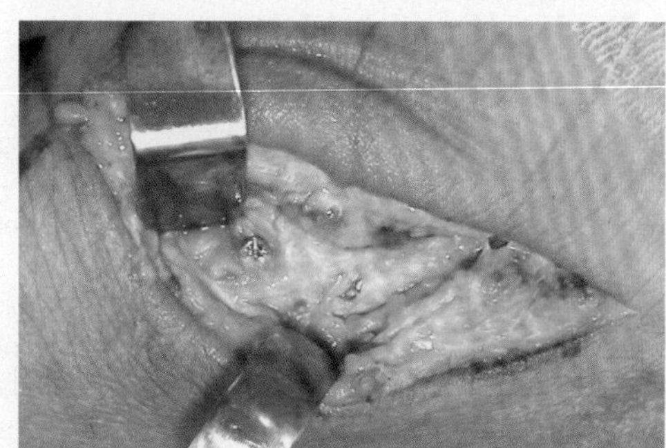

TECH FIG 3 • A. The fracture is cleared of hematoma and then reduced with a pointed reduction forceps. A provisional Kirschner wire is placed percutaneously from the dorsal metacarpal shaft into the fragment. **B.** Two screws of 1.3 mm diameter are placed in a lag fashion from the metacarpal shaft into the fracture fragment. *(continued)*

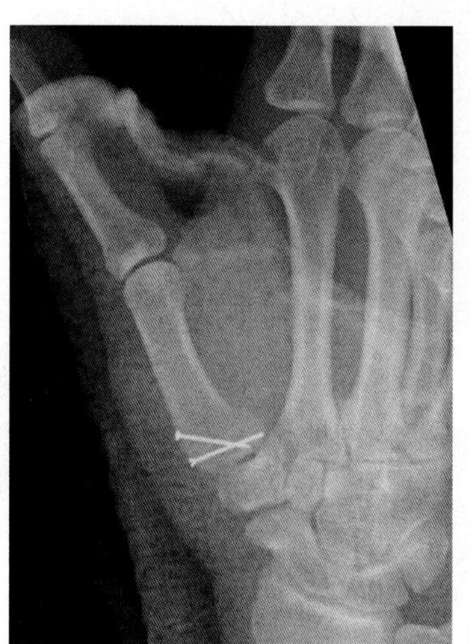

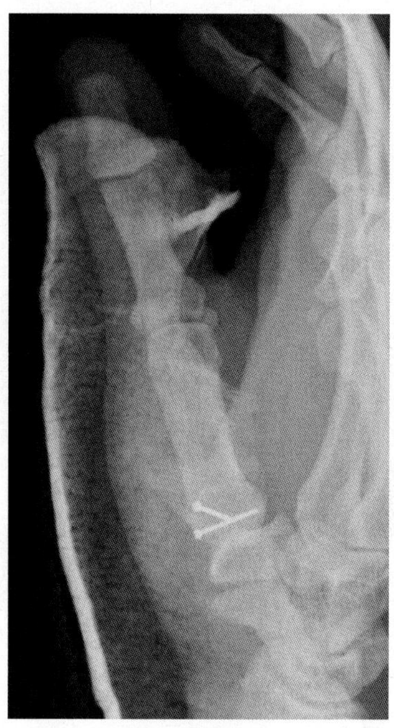

TECH FIG 3 • *(continued)* **C,D.** Lateral and AP postoperative views showing reduction of the fracture and articular surface with two screws inserted in different planes. (Copyright John Capo, MD.)

- Screws should be precisely evaluated radiographically to be certain they are not in the CMC joint or adjacent second metacarpal base (**TECH FIG 3C,D**).
- If fixation is tenuous, the metacarpal base can be pinned to the second metacarpal or to the carpus for added stability.
- Anatomic reduction of the articular surface is verified under direct visualization.
- The wound is closed in layers with absorbable sutures in the joint capsule, followed by nylon sutures in the skin. A thumb spica splint is applied.

Open Reduction and Internal Fixation of Rolando Fractures

Incision and Dissection

- The previously described Wagner approach is used to expose the thumb CMC joint (**TECH FIG 4A,B**).
- The radial portion of the incision is extended distally to expose the diaphysis of the thumb metacarpal. Branches of the radial sensory nerve must be protected at this stage (**TECH FIG 4C**).

Reduction and Fixation

- The basilar articular fragments are then reduced under direct visualization, and provisional fixation is performed with Kirschner wires or bone reduction clamps (**TECH FIG 5A**).
- A lag screw can be placed in a transverse direction by overdrilling the proximal cortex to compress the basilar fragments together, followed by application of a minifragment neutralization plate or by additional Kirschner wires to stabilize the shaft (**TECH FIG 5B,C**).[6,16]

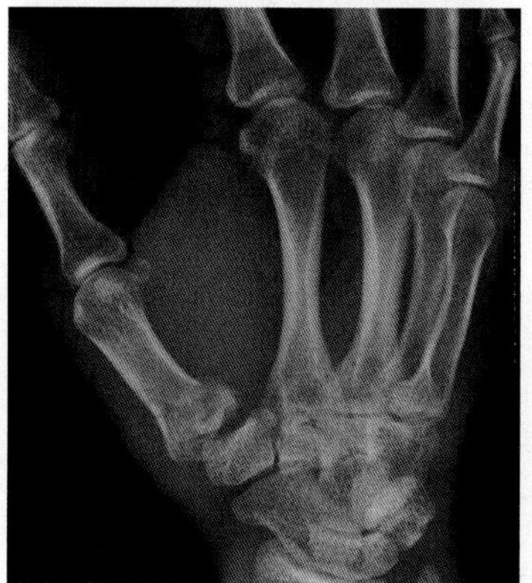

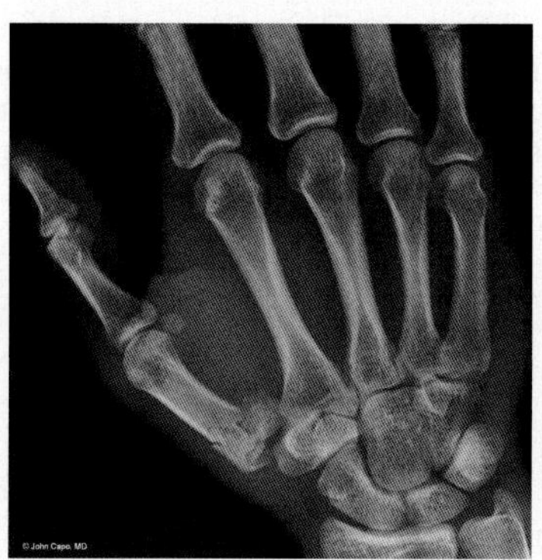

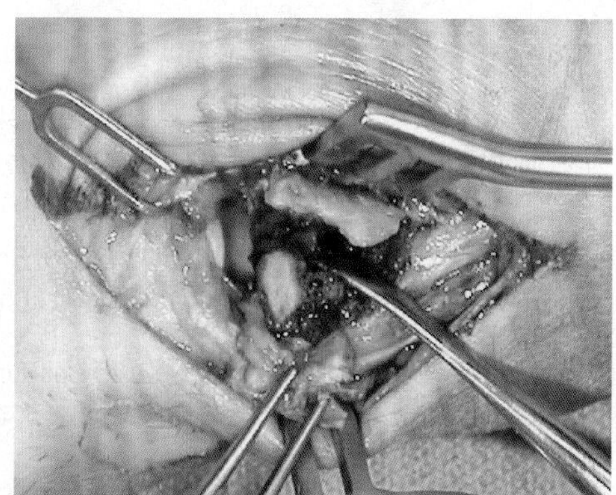

TECH FIG 4 • **A,B.** Preoperative radiographs of a Rolando fracture demonstrating severe intra-articular comminution. **C.** The thumb thenar muscles have been elevated from the CMC joint and a capsulotomy has been performed. The fracture fragments are identified and cleared of hematoma. (Copyright John Capo, MD.)

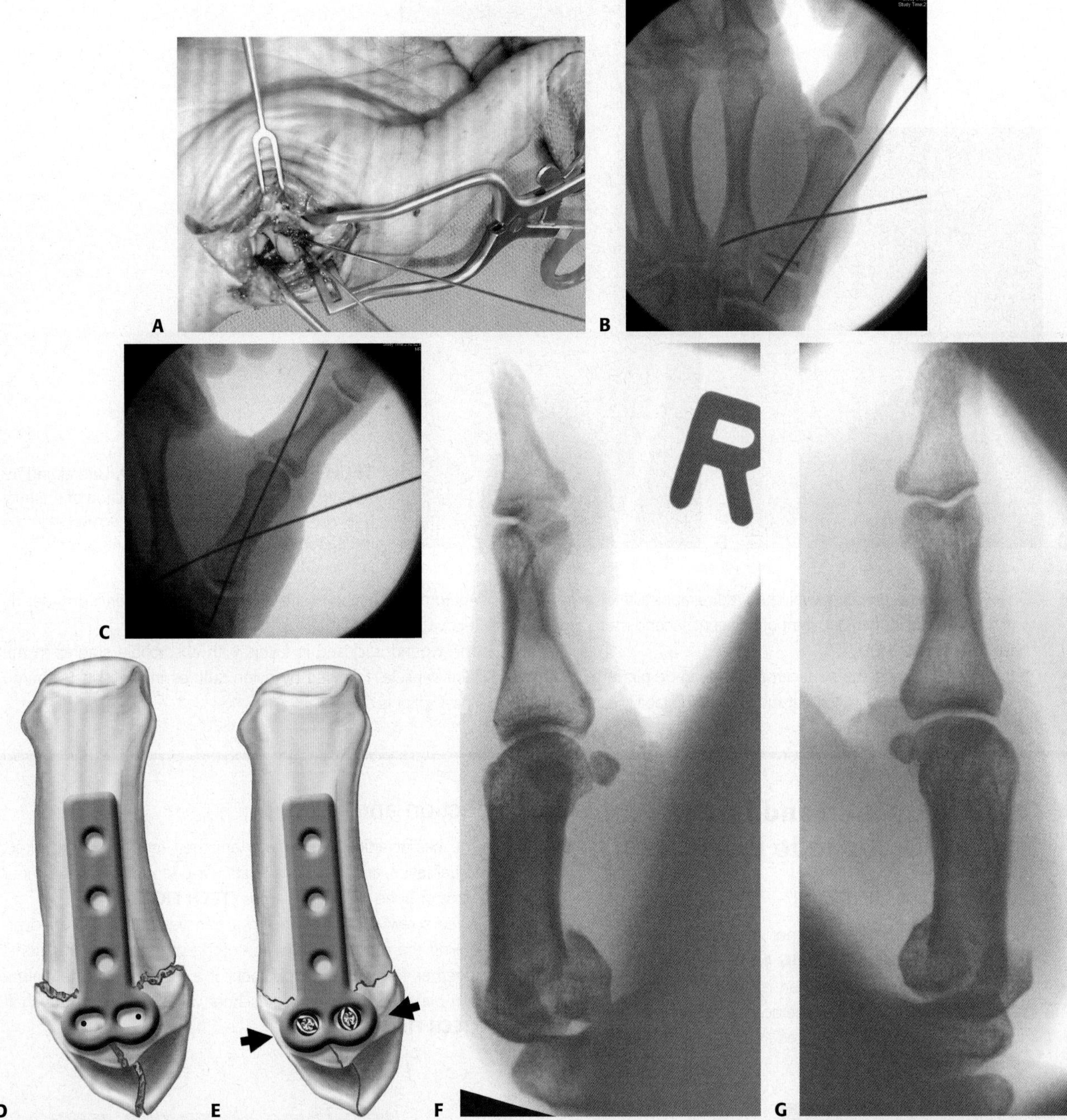

TECH FIG 5 • A. The articular surface is first reduced and provisionally stabilized with multiple small Kirschner wires. **B,C.** Intraoperative fluoroscopic lateral and AP views demonstrate excellent restoration of the joint surface. Kirschner wires have been placed from the thumb metacarpal into the trapezium and second metacarpal to stabilize the construct. **D.** The two proximal holes of the T plate are drilled offset for articular fragment reduction. **E.** The two proximal screws are tightened to compress the proximal fragments. **F,G.** AP and lateral views of a comminuted, displaced Rolando fracture. *(continued)*

- If greater fracture stability is desired, a small (1.5 to 2.7 mm) T, L, or blade plate can be used.
  - The palmar radial incision is extended further distally to expose the thumb metacarpal shaft to accommodate the plate.
  - Reduction is obtained using the earlier techniques, with axial traction to maintain appropriate length and bone reduction forceps or smooth Kirschner wires to provisionally hold the articular reduction.
  - Once the fracture fragments are aligned, the plate is secured to the thumb metacarpal, with the transverse portion of the plate placed over the basilar fracture fragments.[16]
  - The most palmar and dorsal proximal holes of the T portion of the plate can be drilled eccentrically to allow for compression at the fracture site between the basilar fragments,[8,13] followed by fixation of the plate to the metacarpal shaft with cortical screws (**TECH FIG 5D,E**).

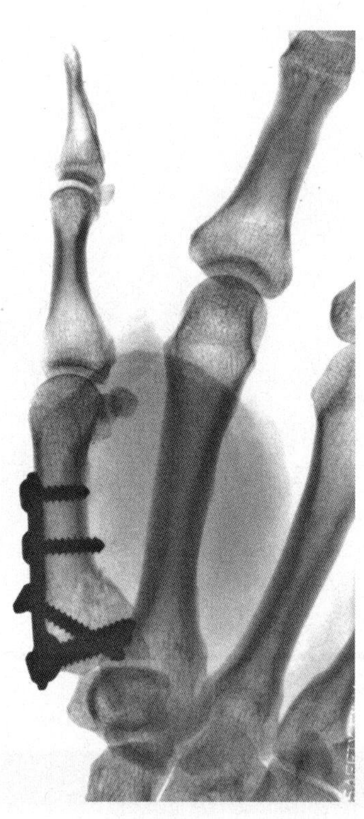

H

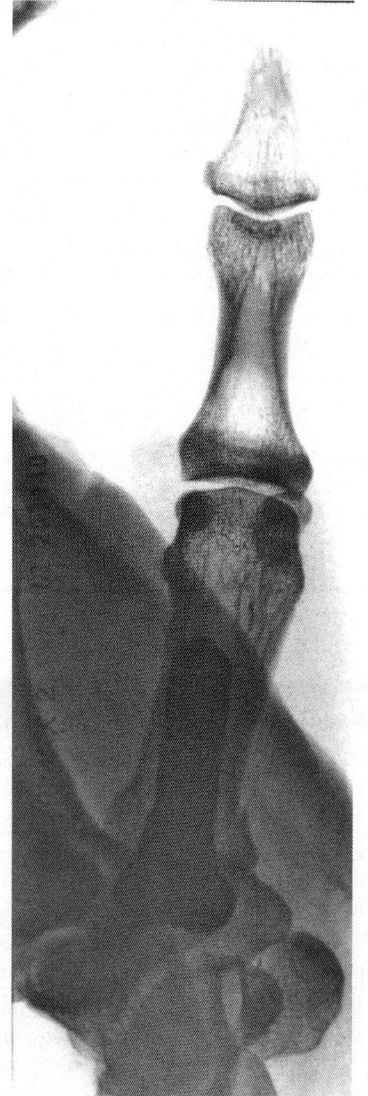

I

TECH FIG 5 • *(continued)* **H,I.** Postoperative radiographs demonstrating excellent articular reduction using a 2-mm T plate. (**A–C:** Copyright John Capo, MD; **D,E:** Adapted from Howard F. Fractures of the basal joint of the thumb. Clin Orthop Relat Res 1987;[220]:46–51; **F–I:** Courtesy of Dominik Heim, MD.)

- Additionally, a lag screw can be placed between the shaft and the basilar fragment either within or outside of the plate. An appropriate bit is used for overdrilling of the shaft fragment, followed by core drilling of the distal basilar fragment. This interfragmentary screw increases the stability of the construct and may allow for earlier functional range of motion (**TECH FIG 5F–I**).
- The joint surface reduction is visualized directly with distal traction of the thumb and ensured to be anatomic.
- The wound is then irrigated and closed in layers, followed by immobilization in a well-padded thumb spica splint.

Application of an External Fixator for Comminuted Rolando Fractures

- Before this procedure, a radiograph of the contralateral thumb CMC joint is advised for templating and to judge postreduction length.
- A mini-external fixator (2.0- to 2.5-mm pins) is applied to the thumb and index metacarpals using standard technique with a quadrilateral frame configuration.[2,12]
- Exposure and open reduction are then performed as discussed previously.
- Distraction is maintained using the external fixator, and the depressed joint fragments are elevated and aligned using the preoperative radiograph of the opposite side as a guide.
  - A sharp dental pick is an excellent tool to manipulate small fragments.

- 0.045-inch smooth Kirschner wires or interfragmentary screws can then be used to secure the fracture fragments.
- The external fixator is loosened to decrease the flexion deformity of the thumb metacarpal shaft and to ensure the base of the thumb is maintained in the proper position. It should be colinear with the base of the second metacarpal base.
- At the end of the procedure, the thumb should be in 45 degrees of palmar and radial abduction and about 120 degrees of pronation in relation to the plane of the hand (**TECH FIG 6**).
- The incision is irrigated and closed in layers.

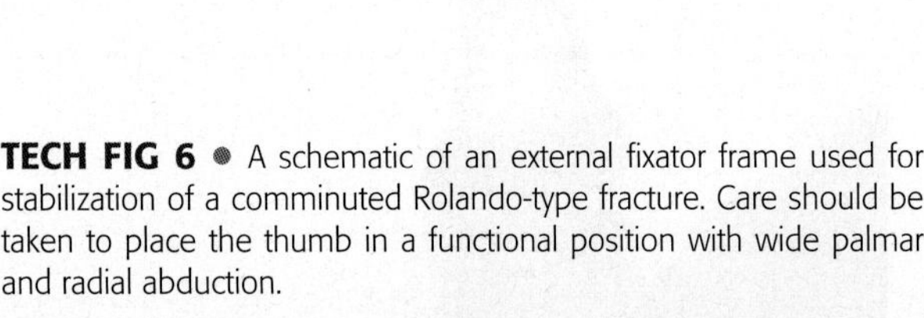

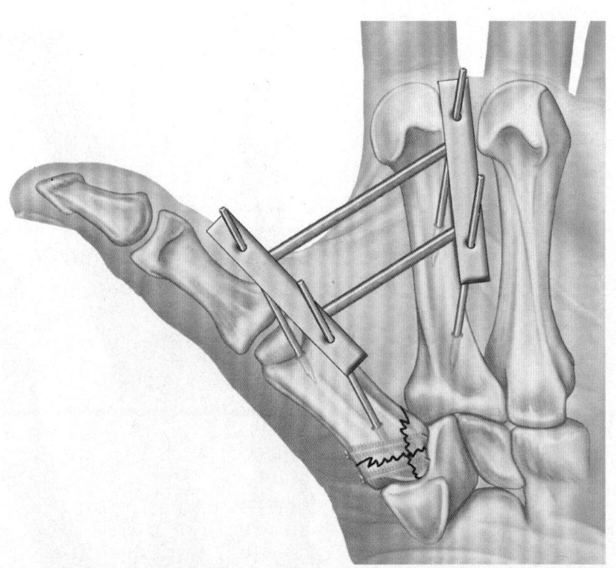

TECH FIG 6 • A schematic of an external fixator frame used for stabilization of a comminuted Rolando-type fracture. Care should be taken to place the thumb in a functional position with wide palmar and radial abduction.

PEARLS AND PITFALLS

Indications	▪ Operative treatment should be considered if greater than 2 mm of step-off persists after closed reduction. Displaced Bennett fractures greater than 20%–25% of joint surface usually require open reduction and internal fixation for optimal reduction.
Preoperative evaluation	▪ Proper radiographs, including a true lateral view and an AP hyperpronated view, must be obtained before operative treatment. CT scanning is usually indicated only if significant comminution is present or if plain radiographs are difficult to interpret.
Thumb position	▪ The thumb should be placed in a position of function with pinning and postoperative splinting. This position is palmar and radial abduction of 45 degrees and pronation of 120 degrees.
Joint reduction	▪ Joint reduction must be obtained because residual displacement leads to poor outcomes. If adequate joint reduction cannot be verified by fluoroscopy, then open treatment and direct visualization is mandatory. Percutaneous methods may be inadequate for fractures involving more than 25%–30% of the joint surface.[15]
Postoperative management	▪ Thumb spica casting for 4–6 weeks is necessary if percutaneous Kirschner wire fixation is used. Premature early motion may break Kirschner wires that span the adjacent joints. Range-of-motion exercises can be begun 1–2 weeks postoperatively if stable plate fixation is used.

POSTOPERATIVE CARE

Bennett Fractures

- A thumb spica splint is applied in the operating room. Pin sites are inspected at 1 week and a thumb spica cast is applied for 4 to 6 weeks, until fracture union.
- Hand therapy is begun at 2 to 3 weeks for thumb interphalangeal (IP) and metacarpophalangeal (MP) joint motion and index through small finger range of motion.
- Pins are removed at 4 to 6 weeks and therapy is advanced to the CMC joint along with intermittent immobilization using a removable thumb spica splint.[16]
- In patients treated with interfragmentary compression screws and therefore more stable fixation, active range-of-motion exercises can be started at 1 to 2 weeks postoperatively with a removable splint for protection.[20]

Rolando Fractures

- Patients treated with closed reduction and percutaneous pinning are placed in a thumb spica splint, which is removed at 1 week for pin inspection. A thumb spica cast is applied for an additional 4 to 5 weeks.
- The pins are removed in the outpatient office at 6 weeks after surgery. A removable splint may be continued for 2 to 4 additional weeks while active range-of-motion exercises are advanced.[16]
- In patients treated with stable plate fixation, active range-of-motion exercises may be instituted at 1 to 2 weeks after surgery. Patients typically wear a removable splint for 2 to 4 weeks.[20]
- If a severe injury dictated the use of external fixation, the pins and frame should remain in place for about 6 weeks or until fracture stability is adequate based on interval

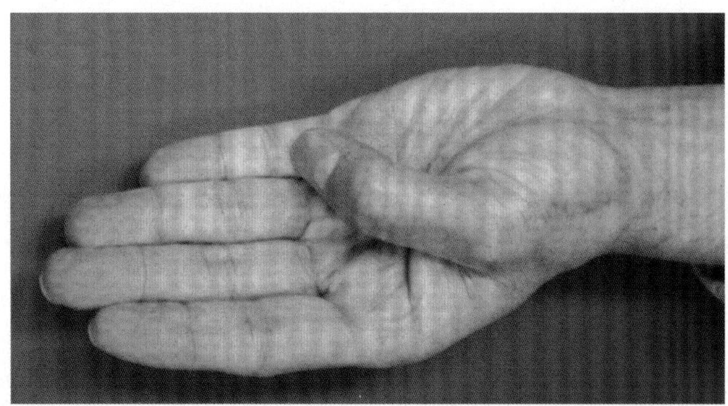

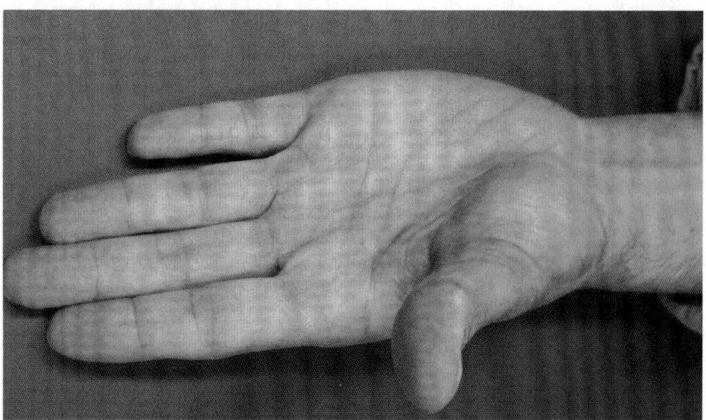

FIG 7 • Clinical photographs of a patient with a Rolando fracture who had undergone open reduction and internal fixation 8 months previously, demonstrating a functional range of flexion (**A**) and extension (**B**). (Copyright John Capo, MD.)

radiographs. A removable thumb spica splint can then be worn for an additional 4 to 6 weeks.

OUTCOMES

- The majority of patients can expect a successful recovery after operative treatment of Bennett or Rolando fractures[19] (**FIG 7**).
- Superior results are seen in operatively treated fractures in which there is no residual subluxation of the thumb metacarpal shaft and less than 2 mm of intra-articular displacement.[3,15]
- It is generally agreed that if pain and articular incongruity persist after 6 months following closed or open treatment, arthrodesis of the thumb metacarpal to the trapezium or basal joint arthroplasty may be indicated.
  - CMC joint fusion is durable, but patients have difficulty with placing their hand on a flat surface and getting the hand into a pants pocket.
  - Basal joint arthroplasty for acute fractures should be reserved for older, lower demand patients.

COMPLICATIONS

- Malunion and subsequent arthrosis resulting from inadequate articular reduction
- Pin tract infection
- Injury to the superficial cutaneous nerves during open dissection and percutaneous fixation
- Contracture of the first web space from immobilization or pinning of the thumb in an adducted position

REFERENCES

1. Billing L, Gedda KO. Roentgen examination of Bennett's fracture. Acta Radiol 1952;38:471–476.
2. Buchler U, McCollam SM, Oppikofer C. Comminuted fractures of the basilar joint of the thumb: combined treatment by external fixation, limited internal fixation, and bone grafting. J Hand Surg Am 1991;16(3):556–560.
3. Cannon SR, Dowd GS, Williams DH, et al. A long-term study following Bennett's fracture. J Hand Surg Br 1986;11:426–431.
4. Capo JT, Kinchelow T, Orillaza NS, et al. Accuracy of fluoroscopy in closed reduction and percutaneous fixation of simulated Bennett's fracture. J Hand Surg Am 2009;34(4):637–641.
5. Charnley J. Finger fractures. The Closed Treatment of Common Fractures, ed 3. Edinburgh: Churchill Livingstone, 1981:150.
6. Cullen JP, Parentis MA, Chinchilli VM, et al. Simulated Bennett fracture treated with closed reduction and percutaneous pinning. A biomechanical analysis of residual incongruity of the joint. J Bone Joint Surg Am 1997;79:413–420.
7. Day S, Stern P. Fractures of the metacarpals and phalanges. In: Wolfe S, Hotchkiss R, Pederson W, et al, eds. Green's Operative Hand Surgery, ed 6. Philadelphia: Elsevier, 2011:283–287.
8. Foster RJ, Hastings H II. Treatment of Bennett, Rolando, and vertical intra-articular trapezial fractures. Clin Orthop Relat Res 1987;(214): 121–129.
9. Gedda KO. Studies on Bennett fractures: anatomy, roentgenology, and therapy. Acta Chir Scand Suppl 1954;193:1–114.
10. Griffiths JC. Fractures of the base of the first metacarpal bone. J Bone Joint Surg Br 1964;46:712–719.
11. Haines R. The mechanism of rotation at the first carpometacarpal joint. J Anat 1944;78:44–46.
12. Jobe M, Calandruccio J. The hand: fractures, dislocations, and ligamentous injuries. In: Canale T, ed. Campbell's Operative Orthopedics, ed 10. Philadelphia: Elsevier, 2003:3489.
13. Jupiter J, Axelrod T, Belsky M. Fractures and dislocations of the hand. In: Browner B, Jupiter J, Levine A, et al, eds. Skeletal Trauma: Basic Science, Management, and Reconstruction, ed 4. Philadelphia: Elsevier, 2009:1221–1341.
14. Livesley J. The conservative management of Bennett's fracture-dislocation: a 26-year follow-up. J Bone Joint Surg Br 1990;15(3):291–294.
15. Pellegrini VD Jr. Fractures at the base of the thumb. Hand Clin 1988;4: 87–102.
16. Raskin K, Shin S. Surgical treatment of fractures of the thumb metacarpal base: Bennett's and Rolando's fractures. In: Strickland J, Graham T, eds. The Hand (Master's Techniques in Orthopaedic Surgery). Philadelphia: Lippincott Williams & Wilkins, 2005:125–135.
17. Roberts P. Bulletins et memoires de la Societe de Radiologie Medicale de France, 1936;24:687.
18. Thurston AJ, Dempsey SM. Bennett's fracture: a medium to long-term review. Aust N Z J Surg 1993;63:120–123.
19. Uludag S, Ataker Y, Seyahi A, et al. Early rehabilitation after stable osteosynthesis of intra-articular fractures of the metacarpal base of the thumb [published online ahead of print June 21, 2013]. J Hand Surg Eur Vol.
20. Werman H, Rancour S, Nelson R. Two cases of thenar compartment syndrome from blunt trauma. J Emerg Med 2013;44(1):85–88.

Dislocations and Chronic Volar Instability of the Thumb Metacarpophalangeal Joint

Robert R. Slater, Jr.

DEFINITION

- Disruption of the restraining structures on the volar surface of the joint between the metacarpal and proximal phalanx of the thumb may result in excessive joint motion and abnormal hyperextension.
- Often painful, this instability frequently causes significant functional deficits because so much of what humans do with their hands depends on having a stable, pain-free thumb to oppose the other digits.
- Acute injuries, including joint dislocations, must be treated correctly and promptly to afford the best chance for successful outcomes.
- Chronic volar instability is seen less often than is collateral ligament incompetence, but it should not be overlooked. It can be treated effectively with a variety of techniques which will be discussed in this chapter.

ANATOMY

- The thumb metacarpophalangeal (MP) joint has features of both a ginglymus (hinge) joint and a condyloid joint. The joint moves mostly in a flexion–extension mode (ginglymus style), but there are also elements of rotation and abduction–adduction in the normal joint (condyloid).
- Thumb MP joint motion varies widely from individual to individual because of the spectrum of metacarpal head geometry seen in "normal" hands.
  - Some metacarpal heads are more rounded and allow greater flexion, extension, and rotation, whereas others are flatter and allow relatively less range of motion (ROM).
- The joint derives its stability mostly from soft tissue constraints not bony architecture (**FIG 1**).
- The proper collateral ligaments originate from the region of the lateral condyles of the metacarpal and pass palmarly and obliquely to insert on the palmar portion of the proximal phalanx.
- The accessory collateral ligaments originate from the same region but slightly more proximal and traverse distally and palmarly in an oblique fashion to insert on the volar plate and sesamoids.
- The volar plate serves as the floor of the MP joint. The adductor pollicis (AdP) inserting into the ulnar sesamoid at the distal edge of the volar plate and the insertions of the flexor pollicis brevis (FPB) and abductor pollicis brevis (APB) into the radial sesamoid at the radial distal edge of the volar plate provide additional volar support.
  - The AdP, FPB, and APB also contribute fibers to the extensor mechanism by way of the adductor and abductor aponeuroses and thus provide a modicum of lateral joint stability.

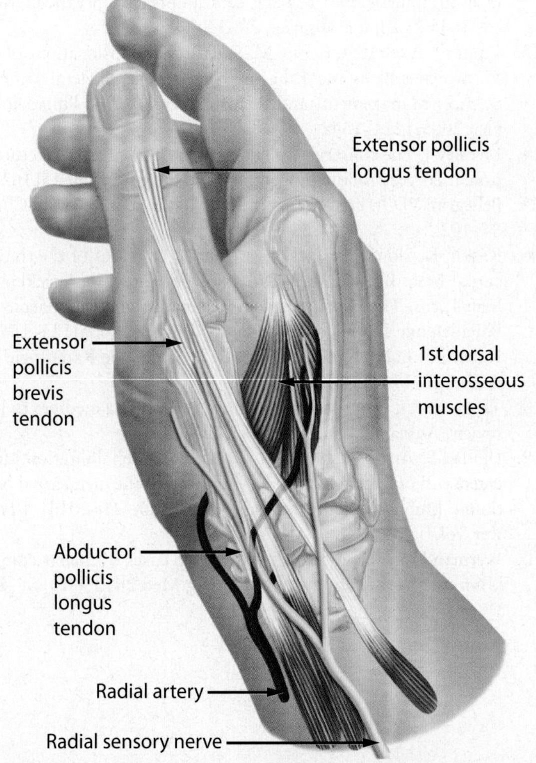

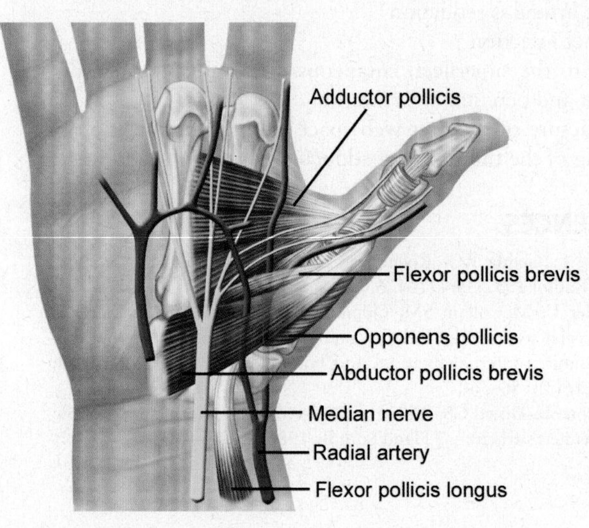

FIG 1 • Anatomy of the thumb MP joint.

- Dorsally, the extensor pollicis brevis inserts onto the base of the thumb proximal phalanx and the extensor pollicis longus inserts at the base of the thumb distal phalanx; both traverse the MP joint and add to the stabilizing forces surrounding the joint.
- The MP joint capsule itself surrounds the joint and contributes slightly to stability.

PATHOGENESIS

- Dorsal dislocations of the thumb MP joint are much more common than are volar dislocations.[4,5]
- The typical mechanism is a hyperextension force strong enough to rupture the volar plate and joint capsule.
  - For example, dislocations may occur when a ball strikes a player's thumb or when there is a direct blow or fall that drives the proximal phalanx into sudden hyperextension.
- Occasionally, the radial or ulnar collateral ligaments (or both) of the MP joint are ruptured along with the volar plate. Their treatment is addressed in other chapters.
- Sometimes, the instability occurs in the setting of a patient with generalized ligamentous laxity such as Ehlers-Danlos syndrome (or other collagen disorders), but in those situations, symptoms are less common and patients typically learn to compensate for the joint laxity.

NATURAL HISTORY

- Posttraumatic instability left untreated may result in weakness of pinch and grip and progress to painful arthrosis due to the abnormal biomechanics of the damaged joint.

HISTORY AND PHYSICAL EXAMINATION

- In traumatic cases, it is important to inquire about the mechanism of injury.
  - If patients recall which way the thumb was "pointing" at the time of injury, it helps the examiner determine which structures were likely injured.
  - With the ubiquitous presence of cell phone cameras and digital cameras, photos of the deformity right after the injury are often available and can be helpful in confirming the suspected injury.
  - Was the joint dislocated and did it reduce spontaneously or with assistance from a coach, trainer, or the patient?
  - How difficult was the reduction?
- Physical examination should include an assessment of ROM and grip and pinch strength, particularly in comparison with the contralateral thumb. Focal areas of tenderness should be ascertained. Residual tenderness along the volar plate may persist long after the injury.
  - The examiner should observe the resting joint posture; dislocated joints exhibit obvious deformity.
  - The examiner should check for open wounds and assess the vascular status. Open wounds or vascular compromise mandate emergent treatment.
  - Limited or absent interphalangeal joint ROM suggests flexor pollicis longus tendon entrapment.
  - Dislocated or painful MP joints will have limited ROM.
  - Volar plate stability is assessed because instability must be recognized and treated appropriately to maximize outcomes.
  - Severe collateral ligament injury is uncommon in conjunction with volar plate instability but must be recognized and treated where indicated.
  - An acute dislocation is rarely subtle, but when patients present with chronic instability symptoms, there may be guarding against full joint extension and soft tissue thickening in areas of chronic pathology.

IMAGING AND DIAGNOSTIC STUDIES

- Plain radiographs of the thumb in three views (anteroposterior [AP], lateral, and oblique) are requisite.
  - Injury films will reveal the direction of joint dislocation and any associated fractures (**FIG 2A–C**).

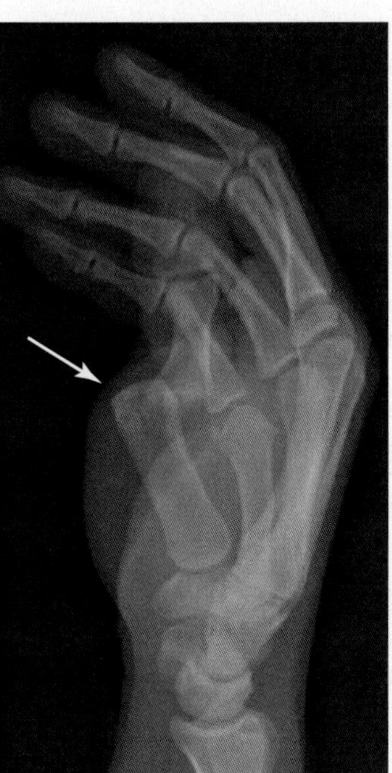

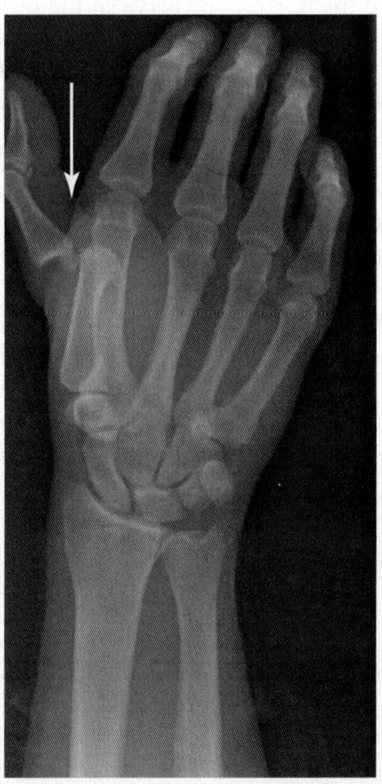

FIG 2 • X-rays showing MP joint dislocation on AP (**A**) and lateral (**B**) films. *(continued)*

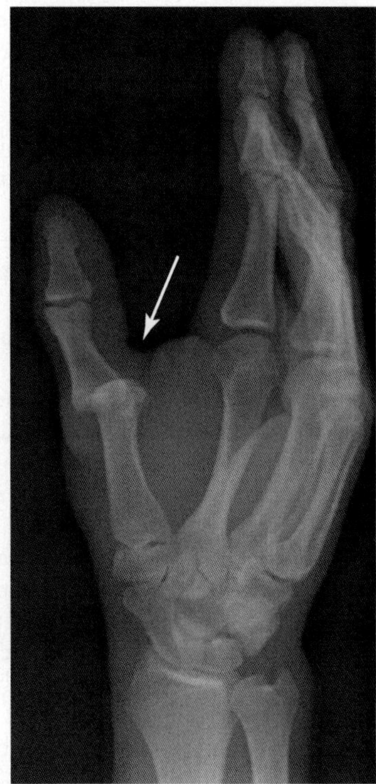

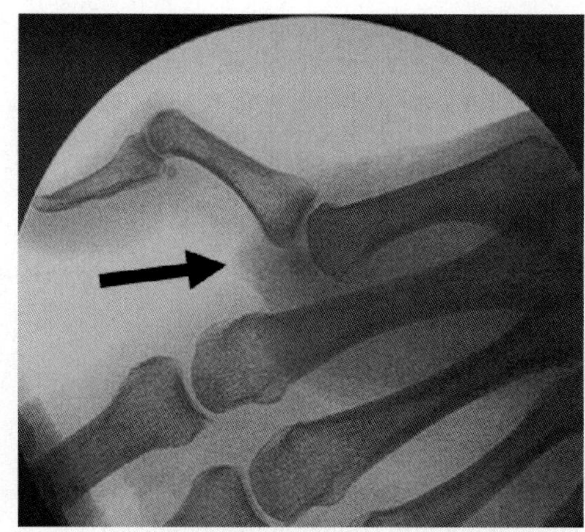

FIG 2 • *(continued)* **C.** Oblique injury film of the thumb (vs. hand) shows a dorsal MP joint dislocation (*arrow*). **D.** Fluoroscopic imaging shows joint instability.

- In the chronic setting, films may show evidence of prior fractures or bony injuries as well as the positions of the sesamoid bones relative to the joint space. In cases of chronic volar plate instability, the proximal phalanx may show subtle dorsal subluxation on the metacarpal head (that is more commonly noted when there has been injury to the dorsal capsule in association with collateral ligament damage).
- Arthritic changes at the MP joint seen on the plain films will alter the treatment options. If the chronically unstable joint is already arthritic at the time of presentation, then an arthrodesis will be a better option than a soft tissue reconstruction.

- Fluoroscopic real-time imaging and stress testing may confirm the suspected joint instability (**FIG 2D**).
  - A digital block may be placed to facilitate an adequate examination.
- Ultrasound, magnetic resonance (MR) imaging, and arthrography[7,8,10] are advocated by some, but these studies are rarely of additional value in the assessment of thumb MP joint stability.

DIFFERENTIAL DIAGNOSIS

- Fracture
- Collateral ligament injury
- Ligament laxity, generalized (eg, Ehlers-Danlos syndrome)
- Arthritis
- Locked trigger thumb (stenosing tenosynovitis)

NONOPERATIVE MANAGEMENT

- Most acute thumb MP dislocations can be reduced via closed means, avoiding surgery.
- The reduction maneuver for a dorsal dislocation usually requires only slight hyperextension to gently "unlock" the proximal phalanx from its perch on the metacarpal head, followed by direct volarly and distally directed pressure on the base of the proximal phalanx to gently slide it over the metacarpal head to achieve reduction.
  - Subtle, slight rotation (pronation and supination) at the same time may help ease any interposed soft tissue out of the way as the phalanx reduces.
  - Longitudinal traction and excessive hyperextension should be avoided because the soft tissue tension generated may cause one or more structures surrounding the joint to slip between the metacarpal head and the proximal phalanx, blocking reduction.
    - The volar plate, the flexor pollicis longus, and one or both sesamoid bones have all been described as culprits that have become incarcerated in the joint space, preventing reduction.[2,3,5,9]
- Once the joint is reduced, the patient should be able to flex and extend the thumb joints and the radiographs should show concentrically reduced and congruent joint surfaces (**FIG 3**).
  - If either of those conditions is not met, it suggests there may be residual soft tissue interposed in the joint, an indication for open reduction.
- After successful closed reduction, the thumb should be splinted in flexion to relax the injured volar structures.
- After a few days, when the acute swelling has dissipated, the splint may be changed to a thumb spica cast, again with the MP joint flexed, for an additional 2 to 3 weeks. Rehabilitation can commence thereafter, emphasizing ROM exercises within a safe zone of motion from full flexion to just short of neutral extension and then increasing gradually to unrestricted ROM and hand use by 6 weeks after injury.
  - For patients engaged in activities that risk forced hyperextension of the thumb such as ball sports, taping or splinting

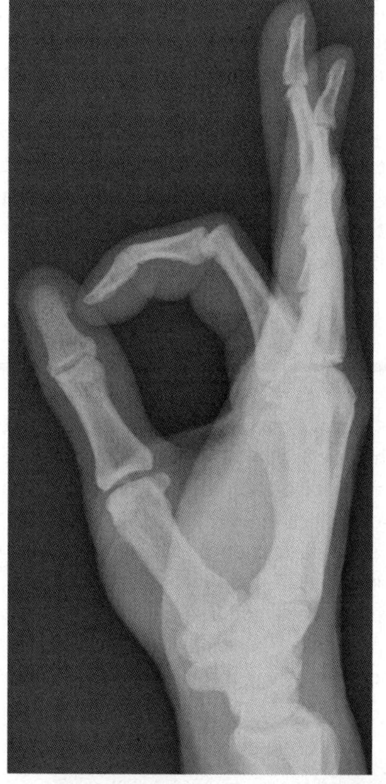
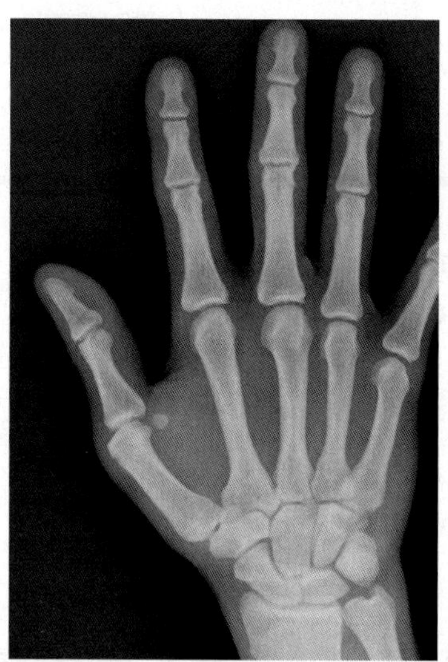
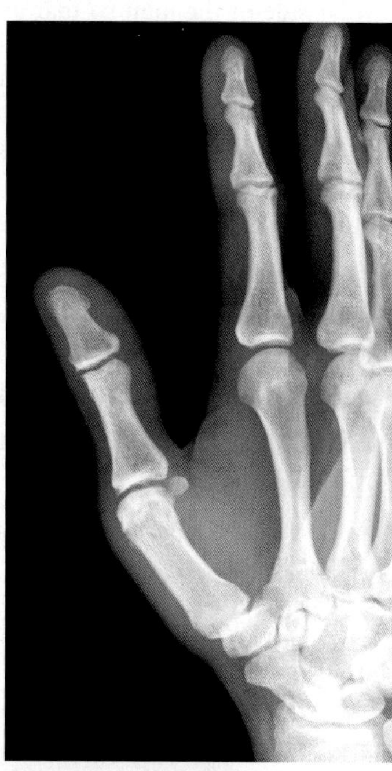

FIG 3 • **A–C.** Postreduction views of the patient in **FIG 2** confirm congruent joint surfaces and satisfactory alignment, including the sesamoid bone positions.

may be required during these activities for several additional weeks.

- Failure to recognize or treat the acute instability or overly aggressive progression to full, unlimited hand use may result in chronic volar instability.
  - Nonoperative management then is limited to providing the patient with a custom-molded splint to prevent hyperextension of the MP joint.
  - A properly trained hand therapist is invaluable in assisting patients who prefer to manage the problem nonoperatively and use a protective splint rather than proceeding with surgical treatment for their chronic instability.
- Volar dislocation is very rare. There are only a few cases reported in the literature and all required open reduction.[4,5]

SURGICAL MANAGEMENT

- Open reduction is required when attempts at closed manipulation and reduction of acute dislocations fail.
  - Failure is typically the result of soft tissue interposition in the joint that blocks reduction. Tissue interposition may have happened at the time of the original injury or as a result of a well-meaning coach, friend, or medical colleague trying to reduce the dislocation by applying vigorous traction, which can cause the soft tissues to become incarcerated.
- Chronic instability, which is persistently symptomatic despite nonoperative treatment, is best treated with a soft tissue stabilization technique unless moderate to severe arthrosis is present or the instability is global and exceedingly severe. In those cases, arthrodesis is the treatment of choice.

Preoperative Planning

- The physician should review all imaging studies. In most cases, those will be limited to plain radiographs and perhaps spot films from fluoroscopic evaluations.
  - Films should be reviewed for any bony abnormalities, especially nondisplaced fractures. One should avoid fracture displacement during intraoperative manipulation of the thumb.
  - In fracture-dislocations of the MP joint, larger fragments are stabilized using Kirschner wires or screws and smaller avulsion-type fragments are excised and the ligament is secured to the bone.
  - For chronic cases, it is important to review the films and rule out osteoarthrosis, which would warrant different treatment strategies.
- Examination under anesthesia with the assistance of fluoroscopy can be useful to confirm the degree and direction of joint instability.
  - Spot films obtained before and after surgical stabilization can be helpful visual aids for use in postoperative discussions with the patient and his or her family to explain again the nature of the problem and how it was treated.

Positioning

- The patient should be supine on the operating table with a standard hand table attached and projecting out from the operating table to support the operative hand.
- A tourniquet should be placed on the operative arm and checked for proper function and pressure before initiation of the surgery (typically 250 or 100 mm Hg greater than systolic blood pressure).

Approach

- Acute, irreducible MP joint dislocations are best approached from the volar side of the joint so that any soft tissues that may be trapped in the joint can be identified and carefully protected, *before* they are injured by approaching them "blindly" from the dorsal side.
  - If there is an open wound, it can be incorporated into the surgical incision.
  - A lateral approach is also possible but less often used.
- Chronic MP joint volar instability that is amenable to soft tissue stabilization should also be approached from the volar aspect of the joint so the pathology can be visualized and addressed directly.
- If chronic MP joint instability has resulted in arthritis, arthrodesis is a better solution. This may be accomplished in a variety of ways using a variety of hardware options, including screws, plates, and wires. All are best placed through a dorsal approach.

Open Reduction of Acute Metacarpophalangeal Joint Dislocations

- Make a zigzag (Bruner-type) incision, centered at the level of the MP joint.
- Gently elevate the skin flaps to expose the underlying soft tissues, which will by definition be displaced from their usual locations (**TECH FIG 1**).
- Identify the neurovascular bundles and mobilize them enough to ensure their protection.
  - Small rubber loops can be placed around them if desired both for protection and for easy identification.
- Retract the soft tissues enough to identify whatever structure is interposed into the MP joint and reflect it out of the joint.
  - Most often, that is the flexor pollicis longus tendon or the volar plate. The volar plate may have the sesamoids still attached to its distal edge if it has failed proximally.

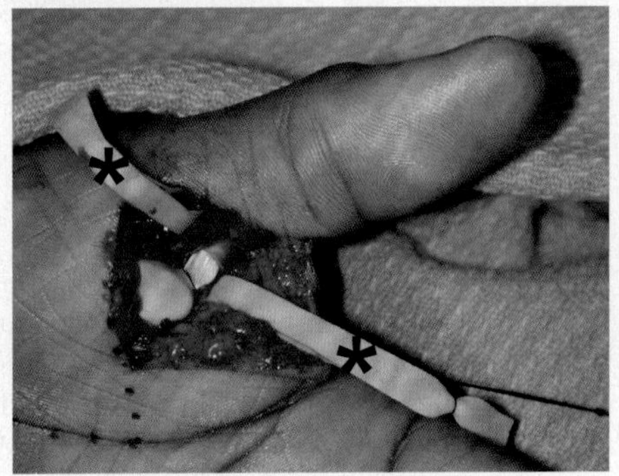

A

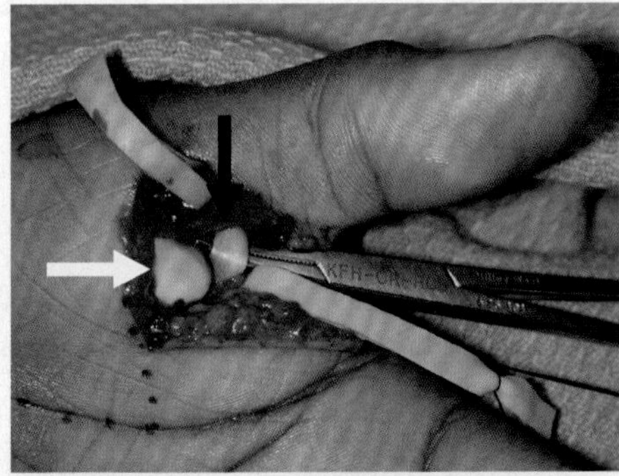

B

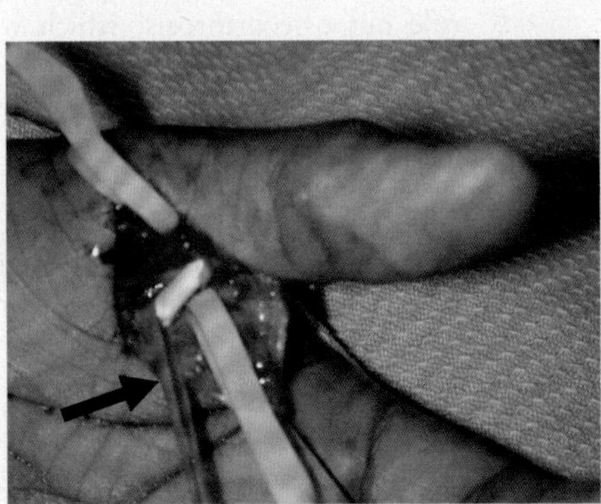

C

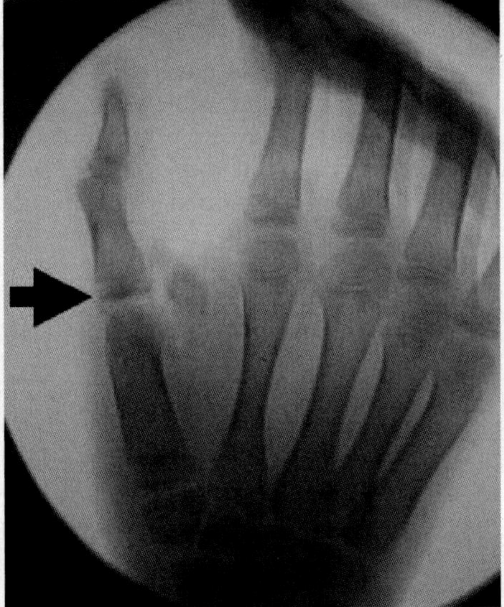

D

TECH FIG 1 • Open reduction of dorsal thumb MP joint dislocation. **A.** Make a volar surgical approach and carefully identify the neurovascular bundles; tag and protect them with soft rubber loops (*asterisks*). **B.** The flexor pollicis longus (*black arrow*) is interposed and trapped behind the metacarpal head (*white arrow*). **C.** Umbilical tape (*arrow*) passed around the flexor pollicis longus delivers the tendon safely out of harm's way, allowing the joint to be reduced. **D.** Intraoperative fluoroscopy is helpful for verifying anatomic reduction (*arrow*) with congruent joint surfaces and smooth gliding through a safe ROM.

- Reduce the joint and check for smooth, congruent joint motion.
- Check the stability of the collateral ligaments. Providing the joint does not gap open more than 25 degrees due to collateral ligament damage (rare), no further treatment for that component of the joint injury is needed.
- In some cases, it may be possible to place sutures through the volar plate at its torn proximal or distal edge and tack that back to its normal insertion point. Otherwise, simply replacing the plate in normal alignment will be adequate when combined with proper rehabilitation (discussed later in the chapter).
- Replace the neurovascular bundles and flexor pollicis longus into their proper locations and close the wound in routine fashion.

Chronic Volar Instability

Volar Plate Advancement and Sesamoid Arthrodesis

- The Tonkin procedure[13] was originally described to treat MP instability resulting secondarily from osteoarthrosis of the thumb carpometacarpal joint or in patients with cerebral palsy, but it is now considered a valuable technique or treating posttraumatic instability of the MP joint.
- Approach the MP joint through a volar or volar radial incision (**TECH FIG 2A**).
- Divide the accessory radial collateral ligament at its insertion into the volar plate and mobilize the plate to advance it proximally (**TECH FIG 2B**).
- Denude the articular surface of the sesamoid bones. A Beaver blade works well.
- Decorticate a trough along the retrocondylar fossa of the metacarpal neck to accept the sesamoids.
- Drill Keith needles through that area of the retrocondylar fossa using a wire driver. The needles should exit the metacarpal dorsally (**TECH FIG 2C**).
- Advance the sesamoids and volar plate into the prepared trough and secure the sutures dorsally (**TECH FIG 2D**).

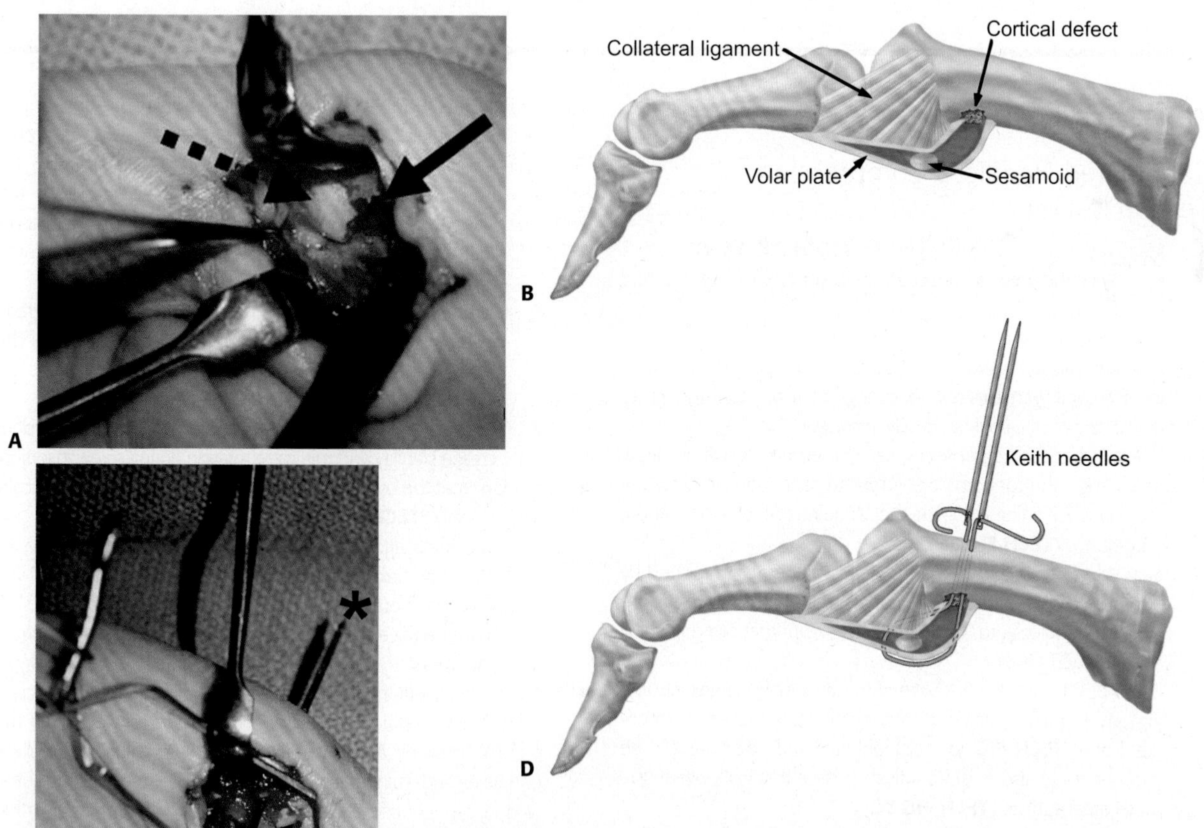

TECH FIG 2 • Sesamoid arthrodesis in the manner of Tonkin. **A,B.** Through a volar or radial lateral approach, create a cortical defect in the metacarpal retrocondylar fossa (*solid arrow*), which will accept the denuded sesamoids while preserving the articular surface of the metacarpal head (*dashed arrow*). **C.** Advance and secure the volar construct including the sesamoids into the prepared trough (*arrow*), using sutures in the volar plate that are brought through the metacarpal neck via Keith needles drilled through the bone. **D.** The sutures are tensioned and tied over the dorsal metacarpal (*asterisk*). *(continued)*

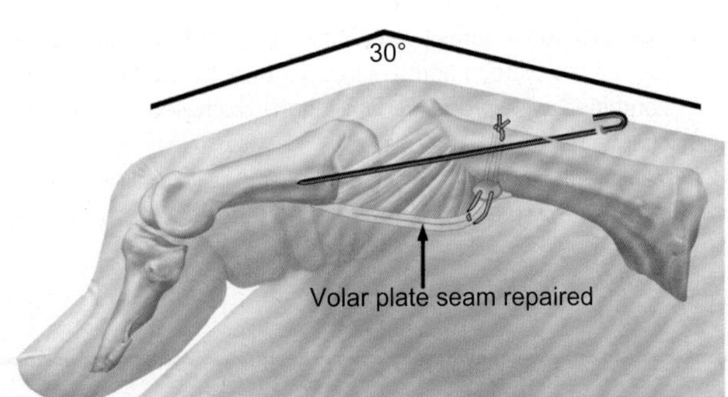

TECH FIG 2 • *(continued)* **E.** A Kirschner wire is drilled across the MP joint to keep it flexed 30 degrees, protecting the repaired volar structures during initial healing.

- Variations
  - Schuurman and Bos[12]: Place sutures through the proximal edge of the volar plate and pass them through the metacarpal via the Keith needles. Reinforce the construct with nonabsorbable sutures to local tissue where possible.
  - Eaton and Floyd[1]: Place sutures in the proximal corner of the volar plate and pass them subperiosteally from volar to dorsal around the metacarpal and secure them to advance the volar plate snugly into the prepared retrocondylar fossa.
- Pin the MP joint in about 30 degrees of flexion using a Kirschner wire (**TECH FIG 2E**).
- Close the wound in routine fashion and apply dressings and a thumb spica splint.
- Remove the sutures at 10 to 14 days as usual and apply a thumb spica cast.
- Remove the Kirschner wire and cast at 4 weeks and begin active flexion exercises using a removable protective splint for an additional 2 weeks.

Tendon Graft Tenodesis

- A procedure used by Littler and cited by Glickel et al[3] has been described whereby a free tendon graft (usually the palmaris longus) is woven through drill holes in the proximal phalanx and metacarpal and secured in place to provide a passive restraint against MP joint hyperextension.
  - However, the bulk of soft tissue that results from this procedure and the amount of dissection needed to perform it have caused this operation to fall out of favor.
  - Local tissue mobilization in conjunction with suture anchors provides a better solution.

Arthrodesis

Cannulated Headless Compression Screw Fixation

- Make a dorsal longitudinal approach (**TECH FIG 3A–D**).
  - Split the interval between extensor pollicis longus and brevis.
  - Split the joint capsule longitudinally.
- Mobilize the joint adequately. That requires releasing the remaining collateral ligaments and recessing the volar plate enough to deliver the metacarpal head fully into view.
- Use a water-cooled oscillating saw to remove the metacarpal head. Angle the cut from dorsal-distal to palmar-proximal so that the final positioning will leave the MP joint surface flexed about 15 degrees (**TECH FIG 3E**).
  - All the flexion for the arthrodesis will be accomplished by this cut. Preparation of the proximal phalanx base will be perpendicular to the longitudinal axis of that bone and will not add flexion.
- Use a burr to prepare the base of the proximal phalanx, removing any remaining articular cartilage and eburnated subchondral bone (**TECH FIG 3F**). Osteophytes and ridges should be trimmed away also to make a flush surface that will oppose the metacarpal surface (**TECH FIG 3G**).
  - Alternatively, carefully protect the underlying flexor pollicis longus and use a water-cooled oscillating saw to remove the needed bone.
- Avoid excessive bone resection that will shorten the thumb. Cup and cone reamers are an alternative to straight bone cuts and may minimize shortening and maximize flexibility in positioning the arthrodesis.
- Reduce the fusion surfaces and drive a guidewire for the selected cannulated screw set from the metacarpal into the medullary cavity of the proximal phalanx (**TECH FIG 3H**).
  - Be certain that the starting point for the guidewire is sufficiently proximal on the dorsal surface of the metacarpal that the screw does not fracture the cortical bridge when inserted.
  - Alternatively, the guidewire may be drilled in a retrograde fashion starting at the cut end of the metacarpal head. The fusion surfaces are then reduced and the guidewire is advanced into the phalanx in an antegrade manner.
  - Consider placing a second temporary Kirschner wire to increase stability and minimize rotation during screw insertion.
- Confirm that the overall alignment is satisfactory radiographically and clinically (**TECH FIG 3I**).
  - The metacarpal and phalanx should be colinear in the AP plane and flexed about 15 to 20 degrees in the lateral plane. Rotation should be neutral or slight pronation for pinch.
  - Intraoperative fluoroscopy is helpful to confirm correct alignment.
- Adjust the position of the guidewire for the cannulated screw such that its distal tip is just past the narrowest portion of the proximal phalanx. A screw ending at this level will have excellent purchase and gain maximum stability. Measure the Kirschner wire length, choose the proper length screw (keeping in mind the likelihood of compression at the arthrodesis site), and then advance the guidewire distally into the cortex.
- Drill, tap, and place the selected screw, avoiding any prominence over the dorsal metacarpal. Tighten securely while the reduction is compressed manually (**TECH FIG 3J**).

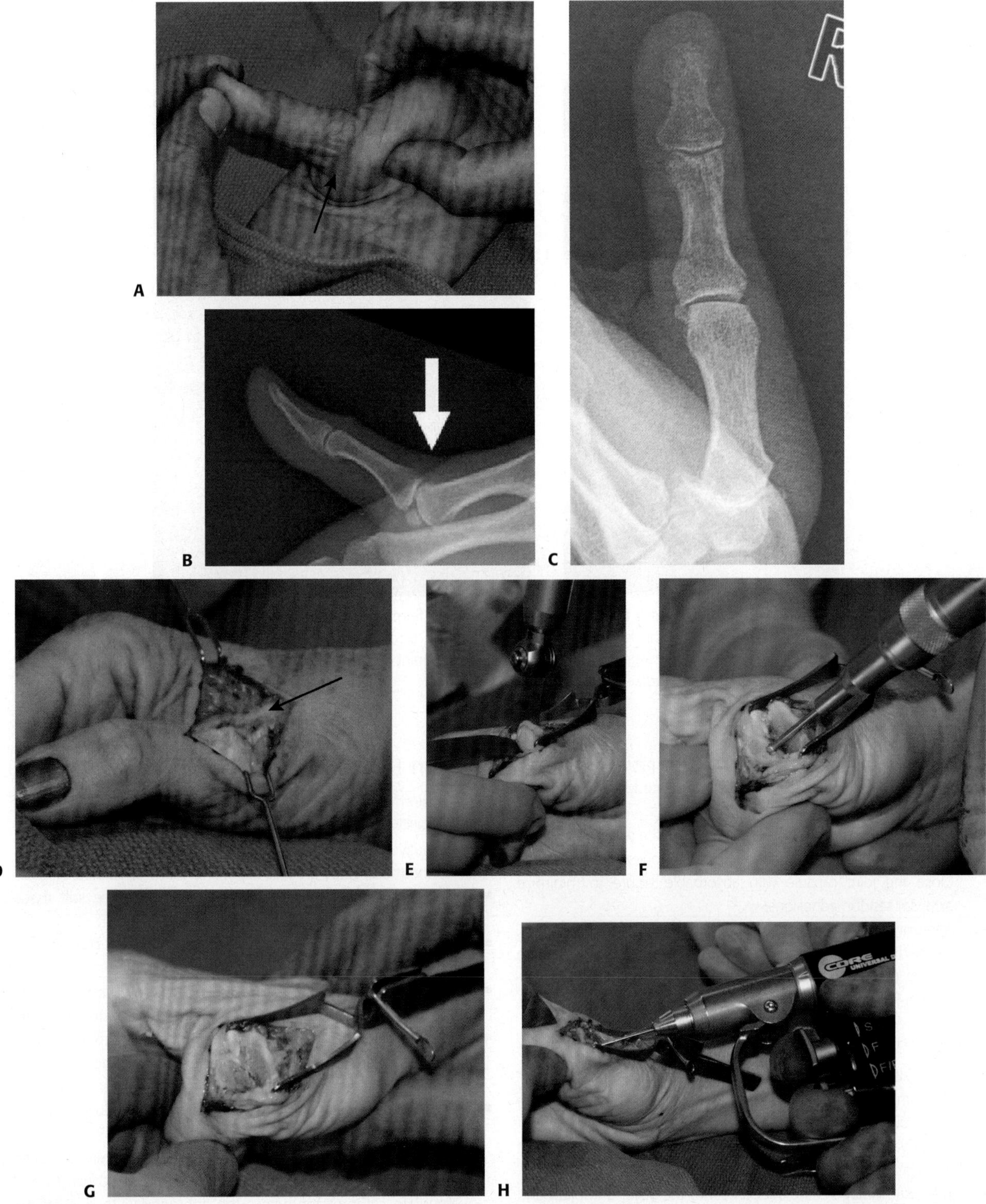

TECH FIG 3 • Clinical examination (**A**) shows MP joint hyperextension (*arrow*), but in this case, it is chronic and associated with joint space narrowing and asymmetry indicative of osteoarthrosis, as seen on radiographs (**B,C**), as well as hyperextension (*arrow* in **B**). **D.** Through a dorsal approach, the interval between the extensor pollicis brevis and longus (*arrow*) is developed and the joint is entered. **E.** Remove the metacarpal head with an oscillating saw. **F.** Prepare the base of the proximal phalanx with a burr. **G.** The opposing bone surfaces should be flush-cut and angled slightly so the final arthrodesis position is 15 to 20 degrees of flexion. **H.** The guidewire for the chosen cannulated screw is drilled across from metacarpal into the medullary canal of the proximal phalanx. *(continued)*

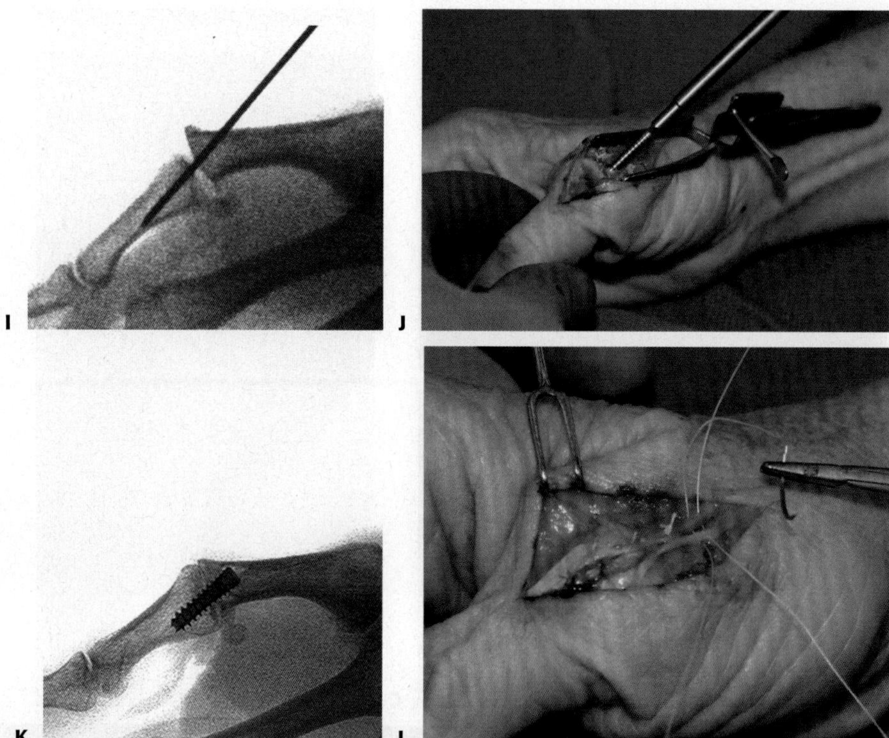

TECH FIG 3 • *(continued)* **I.** Its position is checked with fluoroscopy. **J.** After the proper implant length is measured and the leading cortex overdrilled, the screw is inserted over the guidewire. **K.** Confirm correct final positioning with fluoroscopy. **L.** The joint capsule is closed and the extensor mechanism reapproximated.

- Reconfirm correct alignment in all planes, paying particular attention to rotation. Confirm satisfactory hardware positioning (**TECH FIG 3K**).
- Morselized bone graft can be harvested from the resected metacarpal head and packed in and around the arthrodesis site if needed.
- Close the joint capsule with absorbable suture to minimize extensor tendon adhesions.
- Approximate the extensor tendon interval with interrupted, inverted permanent suture and close the wound in a routine fashion (**TECH FIG 3L**).
- Place a forearm-based thumb spica splint.

Dual Cannulated Compression Screws

- As an alternative to the technique described earlier using a single compression screw, dual parallel cannulated screws is an alternative (**TECH FIG 4A–E**).
- The advantage of using two screws is to better resist rotation and provide additional stability to the construct.
- The disadvantage is the added cost of the second implant and the increased technical challenge.
- The surgical steps are the same as those for a single screw, but care is necessary to place the first guidewire to one side of midline so there is sufficient space to place the second screw in parallel fashion (see **TECH FIG 4A–E**).

Tension Band Wiring

- Tension band wiring (**TECH FIG 5A,B**) has the advantages of versatility if there is more arthritic deformity than anticipated preoperatively and it does not require special implants.
- Furthermore, wires are less expensive than cannulated screws.
- The disadvantage is the buried wires may cause soft tissue irritation or back out and require removal.
- Prepare the joint surfaces as described for the compression screw technique.
- Drill two Kirschner wires (0.045 inch) in parallel fashion across the arthrodesis site and leave them prominent until the next step.
- Drill a small hole across the proximal phalanx perpendicular to the axis of the Kirschner wires, which can be performed using another Kirschner wire.
- Pass a small gauge stainless steel wire (eg, 24-gauge) through the prepared hole in the phalanx and around the protruding Kirschner wires in the metacarpal in a figure-8 pattern, and then twist the ends of the wire to tighten down the construct and generate compression across the arthrodesis site. Clip off the excess compression wire.
- Bend the Kirschner wires and clip them off with just enough remaining to capture the wire. Be sure the ends of all wires are buried to minimize the soft tissue irritation.

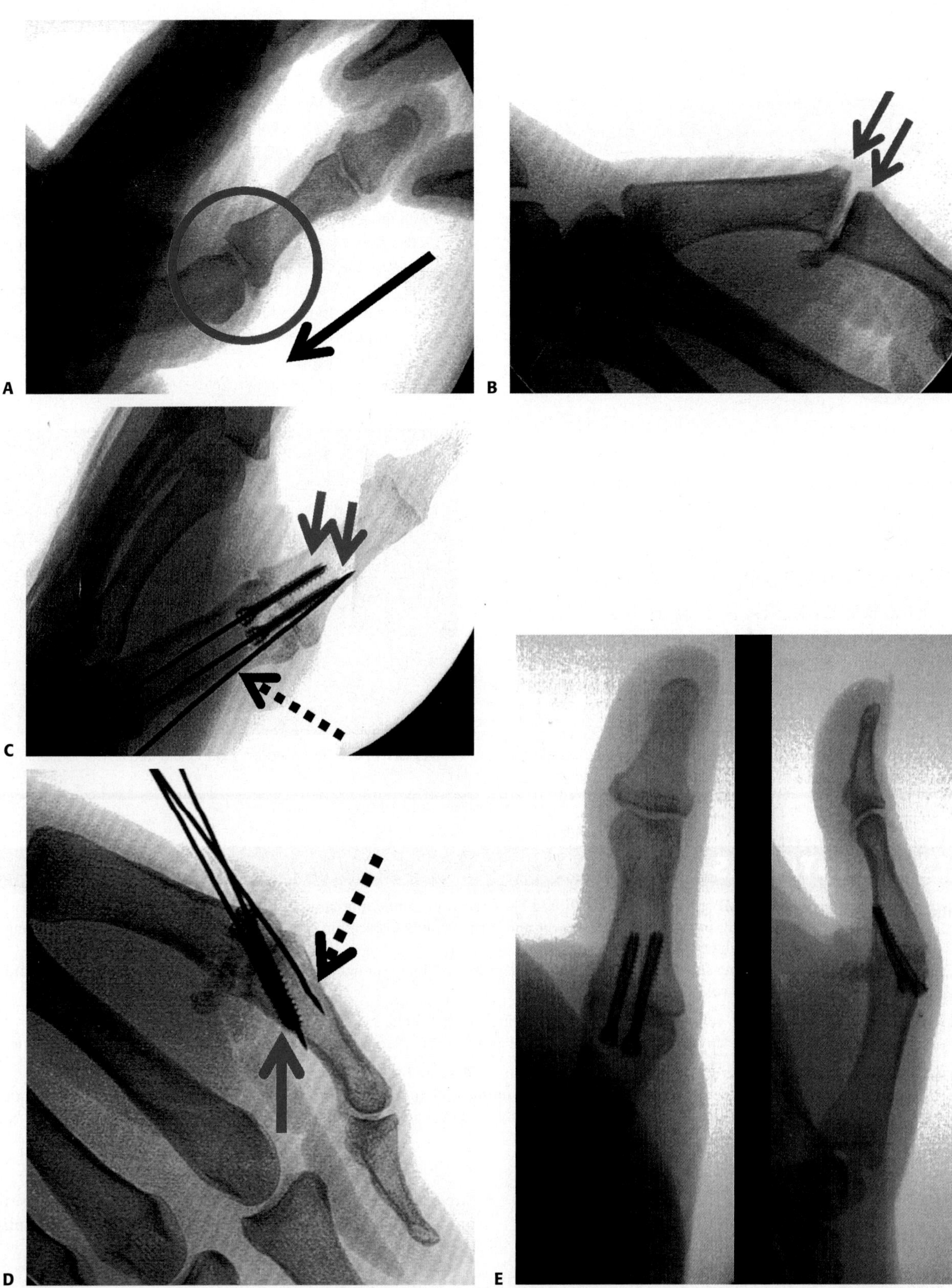

TECH FIG 4 • Double cannulated screw arthrodesis technique. **A.** Axial load applied across the chronically unstable MP joint (direction of *arrow*) produces pain due to the arthritic joint surfaces (also note secondary problem of radial collateral ligament attenuation in this case). **B.** Flush-cut joint surfaces to prepare fusion site (*arrows*). **C,D.** Place two parallel guidewires first (*solid arrows*) and then drive in cannulated screws of appropriate length. A temporary third Kirschner wire can be used (*dashed arrow*) to provisionally hold construct and prevent rotation while guidewires and screws placed. **E.** Final appearance of solid arthrodesis, shown 1 year postoperative.

TECHNIQUES

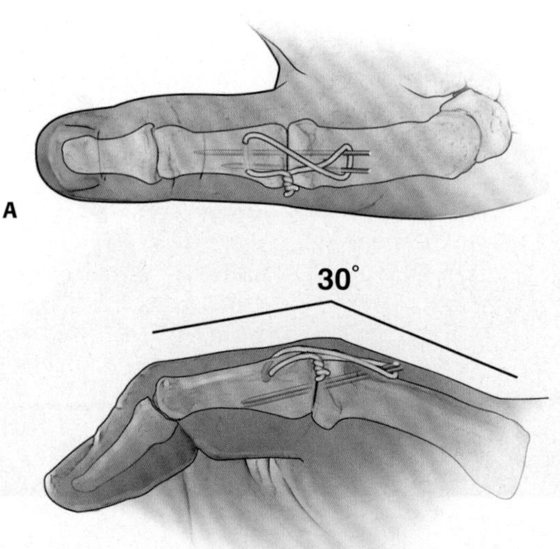

TECH FIG 5 • Tension band wire technique of arthrodesis in AP (**A**) and lateral (**B**) projections. Note the presence of the two parallel Kirschner wires, bent over at ends, and the stainless steel wire figure-8 construct.

Plate and Screw Fixation

- It may be desirable to use plate and screw fixation rather than cannulated screws in such cases as nonunion after attempted arthrodesis; failure of implant arthroplasty; and traumatic injuries with severe deformity, bone loss, or segmental defects (**TECH FIG 6**).
  - The advantage of plates and screws is that more rigid, secure fixation can be achieved immediately, avoiding the concern for rotation or loosening around a single cannulated screw.
  - The disadvantage of that technique is that hardware prominence and tendon irritation and adhesions are more often a source of subsequent trouble.
- If plate and screw fixation is chosen as the desired technique, then the overall approach and bone preparation are similar to that described for the cannulated screw technique.
- With the arthrodesis site reduced and temporarily stabilized with a Kirschner wire, a 2.0-mm, five-hole compression plate is contoured to the dorsal surface of the bones.
- The plate is first secured distally and then applied proximally using compression technique principles.
  - It is critical to avoid long screws and irritation of the flexor pollicis longus.
- Closure and postoperative care are similar to that described earlier.

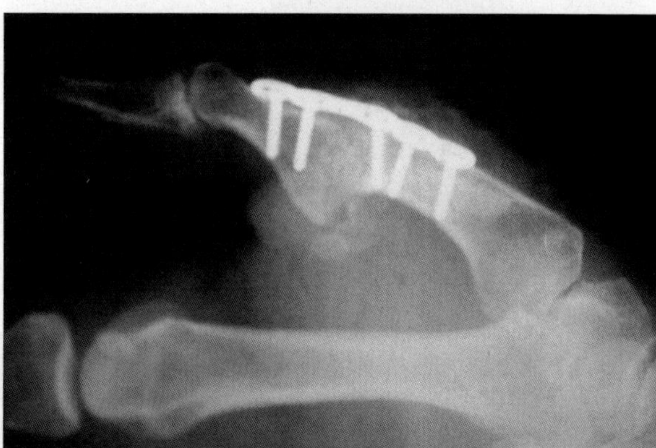

TECH FIG 6 • Arthrodesis with plate and screw fixation.

PEARLS AND PITFALLS

Initial treatment	▪ Acute MP joint dislocations should be reduced promptly, but straight traction should be avoided because it can result in soft tissue entrapment and turn a simple dislocation into a complex, irreducible injury requiring open reduction. ▪ The joint should be immobilized and protected long enough and rehabilitated carefully enough to avoid chronic volar instability.
Treatment indications	▪ Chronic volar instability without arthritic change can be treated with a variety of capsulodesis procedures. ▪ When arthritic changes have developed as a result of chronic instability, MP joint arthrodesis should be done.
Hardware problems	▪ Cannulated screws work well for MP arthrodesis and leave the hardware buried. ▪ Plates and screws, Kirschner wire fixation, and transosseous wiring techniques can be effective ways of achieving arthrodesis but are more likely to cause hardware problems requiring subsequent treatment.

POSTOPERATIVE CARE

Acute Dislocation

- The MP joint is generally stable once a dislocation is reduced acutely, whether by closed or open methods.
- The MP joint should be held in about 30 degrees of flexion in a short-arm thumb spica splint or cast for 2 weeks.
- ROM exercises can begin thereafter, using a removable thumb spica splint for an additional 4 weeks, gradually weaning out of the splint and advancing activities as symptoms allow.
- Supervised hand therapy is often helpful for patients to guide their recovery of motion and strength and optimize their outcomes.

Chronic Instability

- Volar plate advancement procedures and the Tonkin sesamoid arthrodesis procedure should be protected with the thumb MP joint flexed in a cast for 4 to 6 weeks, depending on the surgeon's assessment of tissue quality and patient compliance. Then, supervised ROM can begin, but MP joint hyperextension forces should be avoided for 8 to 12 weeks.

- MP joint arthrodesis procedures require longer protection so that the fusion site is not stressed or disrupted before final bony union.
  - Generally, it is best to use a thumb spica splint (plaster) for the first 10 to 14 days after surgery until the swelling decreases and the sutures are removed.
  - Then a thumb spica cast can be used for an additional 3.5 to 4 weeks, at which time a custom-molded, removable splint can be used to protect the arthrodesis site but allow ROM of the uninvolved adjacent joints of the hand to prevent undue stiffness.
  - By 12 weeks, most arthrodeses are healed solidly enough to allow unrestricted hand use.

OUTCOMES

- Acute volar instability and dorsal dislocations of the MP joint that are treated appropriately can be expected to have a good prognosis.[2,3,11] Whether the dislocation is reduced closed or open reduction is required, once the joint is reduced it is usually stable.
- Following rehabilitation as outlined earlier, there may be some residual joint stiffness. Although that may continue to improve for up to 1 year after injury, the lost ROM is rarely a functional problem.
- Tonkin et al[13] reported successful outcomes in 38 of 42 cases (90%) of sesamoid arthrodeses for chronic MP joint volar instability. Those results compare favorably with outcomes following other capsulodesis and volar plate reinforcing procedures.[6] The advantage of all such procedures is that hyperextension is blocked, restoring stability to the joint, while still allowing the MP joint to flex. Mean loss of flexion compared with the preoperative condition was 8 degrees in the series reported by Tonkin et al.[13]
- More recently, Kim et al[9] reported excellent results and improved Disability of the Arm, Shoulder, and Hand (DASH) scores in patients treated with sesamoidectomy and volar plate repair using suture anchors.
- Outcomes after arthrodesis for chronic volar instability must be viewed with the proper surgical goal in mind. The goal is to relieve pain (from instability and arthritic change) and provide stability to the thumb ray. Success rates are high, barring any unfortunate complications as discussed next.

COMPLICATIONS

- Complications following MP joint dislocations are uncommon and mostly limited to the sequelae of concomitant soft tissue injuries.
  - Damage to the adjacent neurovascular structures can result from the initial traumatic injury or careless surgical technique at the time of open reduction.
  - Damage to the flexor pollicis longus tendon may occur when it gets trapped in the joint or again when it is manipulated surgically during an open reduction.
- A complication encountered more often is persistent, chronic instability of the MP joint that results from failure to recognize the nature of the original injury or rehabilitate it properly.
- Complications after treatment for chronic MP joint volar instability are likewise uncommon and generally related to failure of the chosen procedure.
- Volar plate advancement can fail due to stretching out over time or a second trauma that causes acute rupture of the repair or sutures.
- Nonunion of attempted arthrodesis is always a risk, but fortunately, in the small joints of the hand, including thumb MP joints, it is uncommon. Nonunion rates range from 0% to 12% in several reported series.[14]
- Hardware causing soft tissue irritation is a potential complication. That can be from superficial pin tract infections in cases where Kirschner wires are used to maintain joint reduction to extensor tendon irritation when fusions are done using plates and screws.

REFERENCES

1. Eaton RG, Floyd WE III. Thumb metacarpophalangeal capsulodesis: an adjunct procedure to basal joint arthroplasty for collapse deformity of the first ray. J Hand Surg Am 1988;13(3):449–453.
2. Glickel SZ. Metacarpophalangeal and interphalangeal joint injuries and instabilities. In: Peimer CA, ed. Surgery of the Hand and Upper Extremity. New York: McGraw-Hill, 1996:1043–1067.
3. Glickel SZ, Barron OA, Catalano LW. Dislocations and ligament injuries in the digits. In: Green DP, Hotchkiss RN, Pederson WC, et al, eds. Green's Operative Hand Surgery, ed 5. Philadelphia: Elsevier, 2005: 343–388.
4. Gunther SF, Zielinski CJ. Irreducible palmar dislocation of the proximal phalanx of the thumb: case report. J Hand Surg Am 1982;7(5): 515–517.
5. Hirata H, Takegami K, Nagakura T, et al. Irreducible volar subluxation of the metacarpophalangeal joint of the thumb. J Hand Surg Am 2004;29(5):921–924.
6. Jones DM, Jebsen PJ, Blair WF. Chronic post-traumatic hyperextension instability of the thumb MP joint: results of the volar capsulodesis procedure. Iowa Orthop J 1996;16:122–125.
7. Kahler DM, McCue FC III. Metacarpophalangeal and proximal interphalangeal joint injuries of the hand, including the thumb. Clin Sports Med 1992;11:57–76.
8. Kijowski R, De Smet AA. The role of ultrasound in the evaluation of sports medicine injuries of the upper extremity. Clin Sports Med 2006;25:569–590.
9. Kim BS, Yoon HG, Park KH, et al. Sesamoidectomy and volar plate repair using suture anchor for hyperextension injury of the MP joint of the thumb. Hand Surg 2013;18:287–295.
10. Masson JA, Golimbu CN, Grossman JA. MR imaging of the metacarpophalangeal joints. Magn Reson Imaging Clin North Am 1995;3: 313–325.
11. Posner MA, Retaillaud JL. Metacarpophalangeal joint injuries of the thumb. Hand Clin 1992;8:713–732.
12. Schuurman AH, Bos KE. Treatment of volar instability of the metacarpophalangeal joint of the thumb by volar capsulodesis. J Hand Surg Br 1993;18(3):346–349.
13. Tonkin MA, Beard AJ, Kemp SJ, et al. Sesamoid arthrodesis for hyperextension of the thumb metacarpophalangeal joint. J Hand Surg Am 1995;20(2):334–338.
14. Weiland AJ. Small joint arthrodesis. In: Green DP, Hotchkiss RN, Pederson WC, eds. Green's Operative Hand Surgery. Philadelphia: Churchill Livingstone, 1999:95–107.

Arthroscopic and Open Primary Repair of Acute Thumb Metacarpophalangeal Joint Radial and Ulnar Collateral Ligament Disruptions

Alejandro Badia and Prakash Khanchandani

DEFINITION

- Ulnar collateral ligament (UCL) and radial collateral ligament (RCL) tears of the thumb metacarpophalangeal joint (MCP) are common injuries resulting from disruption of the continuity of these ligaments.
- These disruptions are frequently the result of an athletic injury, a fall, or a motor vehicle accident.

ANATOMY

- The MCP joint of the thumb is transitional between a condyloid and ginglymus joint. The articulating surface of the base of the proximal phalanx is a shallow concavity that provides relatively little intrinsic stability. Hence, most of the joint's stability is afforded by its ligament and capsular supports.
- The RCL and UCL are both structurally similar, composed of both proper and accessory components, and are the main stabilizers of the thumb MCP joint.[27]
- The proper collateral ligaments, which originate from a fossa in the metacarpal neck dorsal to the axis of rotation, are the primary ligamentous supports. They fan out from their proximal origins to distal insertions on the lateral and volar aspects of the base of proximal phalanx.
- The accessory collateral ligaments act as supplementary supports originating from the palmar aspect of the metacarpal neck fossa and inserting into the volar plate and the sesamoid on respective sides of the joint.[27]
- The collateral ligaments provide not only medial and lateral stability but also stability in the dorsovolar plane by virtue of their dorsal origin and their volar insertion.[26]
- The volar plate is a central fibrocartilaginous structure extending from the neck of the metacarpal proximally to the base of the proximal phalanx distally.
- One difference between the ulnar and radial sides of the MCP joint is related to the aponeurosis. The broad abductor aponeurosis covers the entire radial side of the MCP joint, whereas the much narrower adductor aponeurotic sheath spans the ulnar side of the joint.

PATHOGENESIS

- Acute injury of the UCL usually results from sudden forceful abduction and extension at the thumb MCP joint.[21,25]
  - This can take place during a fall on an outstretched hand with the thumb abducted, as seen in skiers,[8] or in baseball players when the glove strikes the ground while fielding.
  - The extent of the injury and the grade of the injury depend on the loading force at the time of impact. The most common injury of the thumb MCP joint is a partial disruption or sprain of the UCL.
  - Tears of the UCL can occur anywhere within the ligament's substance, although most take place at or near the site of insertion into the proximal phalanx, sometimes with an avulsion fracture (**FIG 1A**).[4,9,28]
  - The narrower adductor sheath on the ulnar aspect of the joint allows superficial displacement and entrapment of the torn proximal end of UCL, termed a *Stener lesion* (**FIG 1B**).[28] Because of the broader abductor aponeurosis, however, such a lesion is not seen on the radial side.[11]
- RCL injuries are generally caused by sudden adduction and extension of the MCP joint, commonly occurring during athletic injuries.[5] They can also occur by direct blunt impact to the lateral side of the thumb.
  - The RCL is more often injured close to its origin on the dorsoradial metacarpal head. It may also be disrupted in its midsubstance.

NATURAL HISTORY

- Untreated UCL injuries are relatively common. Patients are often sent away being told they simply have a "sprain." If instability is present and not corrected, the patient may experience pinch weakness and eventually chronic pain.
- Untreated RCL tears are even more common and often result in late degenerative arthritis, commonly requiring MCP arthrodesis.
  - Less severe avulsions may lead to prominent osteophytes on the dorsoradial aspect of the metacarpal neck, suggesting the prior injury.
- Mondry[19] first described the unstable thumb MCP joint in 1940, whereas Watson-Jones[30] mentioned the importance of the UCL in relation to stability of the MCP joint of the thumb.
  - Campbell[6] described gamekeeper's thumb as a chronic instability of the UCL in Scottish gamekeepers.
  - Gerber et al[13] popularized the term *skier's thumb* to refer to acute UCL injuries.
  - Stener[28] outlined the ligamentous anatomy of the thumb MCP joint and subsequent pathoanatomy of the lesion now termed the Stener lesion. Stener also described

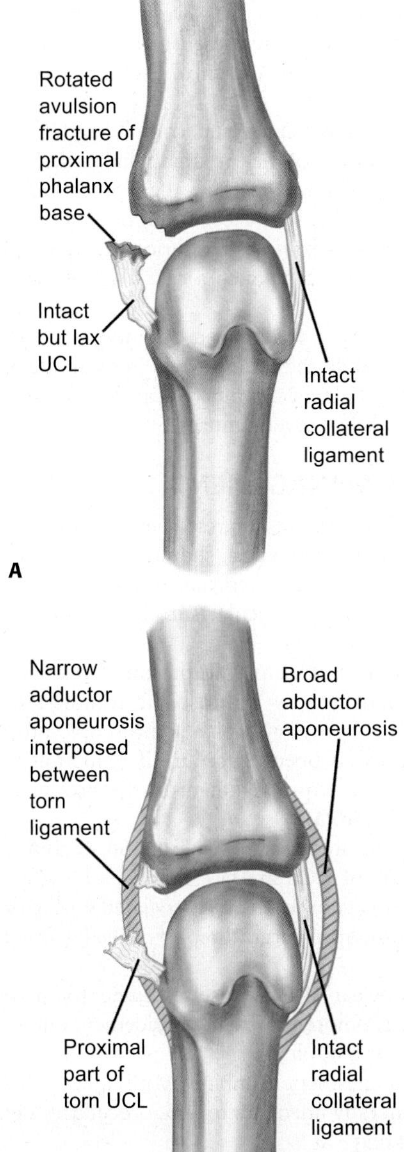

FIG 1 • **A.** A bony gamekeeper's thumb. **B.** The narrow adductor aponeurosis is interposed between the avulsed ligament–bone and the site of attachment.

avulsion of the UCL leading to articular fracture of the proximal phalanx, now popularly referred to as a *bony gamekeeper's thumb*.[29]

- Moberg and Stener[18] reported that UCL disruption is 10 times more common than RCL disruption. This frequency has been widely confirmed.[9,23,26]

- Frank and Dobyns[12] reported that RCL injuries are somewhat more common than initially thought, with incidences ranging from 23% to 35% of collateral ligament injuries.
  - This has echoed our experiences with the more subtle RCL injuries often being neglected, causing late morbidity.

PATIENT HISTORY AND PHYSICAL FINDINGS

Ulnar Collateral Ligament Tears

- Patients with UCL tears present with pain, stiffness, tenderness, and swelling of the MCP joint. The defining symptom, however, may be marked pinch weakness.
- On examination, there is discrete tenderness over the ulnar joint line, at the ulnar side of the metacarpal neck, and most classically at the volar ulnar base of the proximal phalanx.[2]
- Physical examination is critical in establishing the need for surgical treatment by distinguishing between a partial and a complete ligament tear.
- A valgus stress examination comparing the stability of the injured versus the uninjured UCL is the best method to detect a complete tear.
  - The stress test may be aided by live fluoroscopy and the use of a local anesthetic block.
  - The presence of an associated fracture should not deter the examiner from performing a stress test. Nondisplaced avulsion fractures at the insertion site of the proper collateral ligament may coexist with a complete ligament tear.
  - The results of the stress test are based on angular instability of the joint and the quality of the "end point."
  - Laxity of more than 30 degrees in extension and 15 degrees in flexion as compared to the contralateral side should be highly suggestive of a complete tear of the UCL.[15]
- The presence of fullness or a palpable mass on the ulnar aspect of the metacarpal head and neck, representing a Stener lesion,[1] is strongly suggestive of a completely disrupted and retracted UCL.
- Volar subluxation of the MCP joint signifies loss of the dorsal volar stabilizing effect of the collateral ligament and is also consistent with a complete tear.

Radial Collateral Ligament Tears

- RCL tears present as localized tenderness over the radial base of the proximal phalanx but more commonly over the metacarpal head.
- The dorsoradial aspect of the metacarpal head may be prominent due to soft tissue swelling.
- Acute RCL injuries are assessed in the same manner as discussed for UCL injuries.
  - For the stress test of the RCL in extension and 30 degrees of flexion, laxity of the joint greater than 30 degrees as compared to the uninjured side suggests a complete tear of the RCL.
- The emphasis on distinguishing partial tears from complete tears does not directly affect treatment and therefore is less important than for UCL injuries. Even complete RCL tears are not capable of retracting behind the aponeurosis and therefore may be treated nonoperatively.
- RCL injuries are more common than often thought. Significant radial-sided pain with laxity or subtle radiographic signs of dorsal capsule avulsion necessitate treatment (**FIG 2**).

IMAGING AND OTHER DIAGNOSTIC STUDIES

- Radiographs include posteroanterior, lateral, and oblique views of the thumb. Images of the contralateral thumb are used for comparison and may reveal subtle joint subluxation.

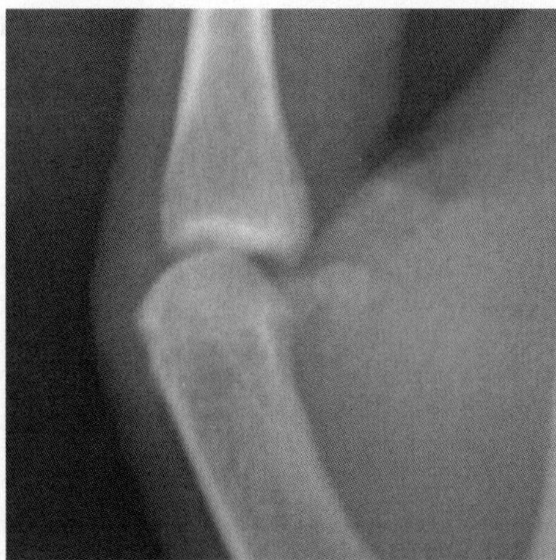

FIG 2 • Radiograph showing a chronic neglected RCL tear. There is subtle volar subluxation of the proximal phalanx. Oblique views often demonstrate a small bony prominence on the metacarpal neck dorsum.

- Stress radiographs of the MCP joint in full extension and in 30 degrees of flexion are rarely required, although occasionally can help distinguish between a partial and complete ligament injury.[4,12]
- MCP joint arthrography, magnetic resonance imaging (MRI), and ultrasound have all been used to determine the degree of ligament injury and displacement but are almost never required.
  - On MRI, a Stener lesion is characterized by a "yo-yo on a string" sign.

DIFFERENTIAL DIAGNOSIS

- Diffuse capsular injury without discrete ligament tear
- Fracture or articular cartilage injury
  - The articular surface is best assessed via arthroscopy or perhaps MRI.
- Arthritis
  - Diffuse soft tissue injury involving a previously asymptomatic but arthritic joint can result in persistent pain.

NONOPERATIVE MANAGEMENT

- Treatment depends on the severity of injury, the type of tear,[7,14,16,17,20,22] and the presence of an avulsion fracture involving a significant portion of the articular surface or an open physis.
- Partial UCL and partial and complete RCL tears without volar subluxation of the proximal phalanx can be effectively managed by immobilization, then protected mobilization using a removable splint for a total of 4 to 6 weeks.
  - Initial immobilization is traditionally accomplished using a thumb spica cast. Such a cast allowing wrist motion is preferable.
  - Alternatively, a customized thermoplastic splint that immobilizes only the thumb MCP joint and leaves the wrist and interphalangeal joint free can be used for reliable patients with less severe injuries.

SURGICAL MANAGEMENT

- Complete UCL disruption, especially if denoted by a Stener lesion or joint subluxation, should be treated surgically. Additionally, a displaced avulsion fracture involving a significant portion of the articular surface should be reduced and stabilized operatively.
- An avulsion fracture of the proximal phalanx can be effectively managed by arthroscopic techniques.[3,23,24] Occasionally, it is necessary for an arthroscopic procedure to be converted to an open procedure if reduction of a large or comminuted fracture fragment in the proximal phalanx is not feasible (**FIG 3**).
- Injuries associated with a Stener lesion warrant open repair.
- Partial tears of RCL are best managed by cast immobilization, whereas complete tears associated with palmar subluxation require open surgical repair of the ligament and dorsal capsule.[10]
- Arthroscopy can also be a useful adjunct to open procedures, as it allows a more thorough débridement and evaluation of concomitant pathology.
- A regional anesthetic combined with light intravenous sedation is generally adequate for the procedures detailed in the following text.

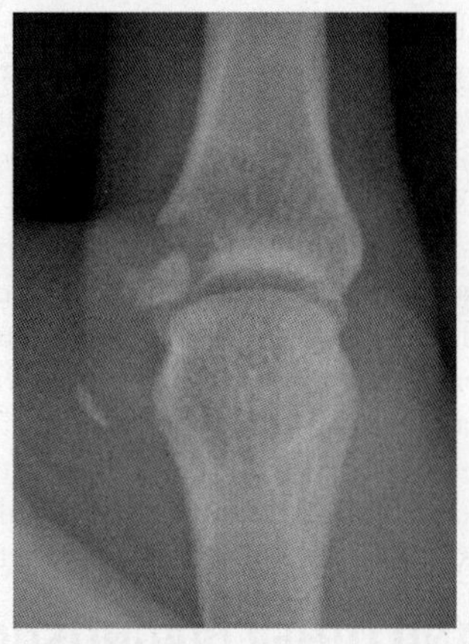

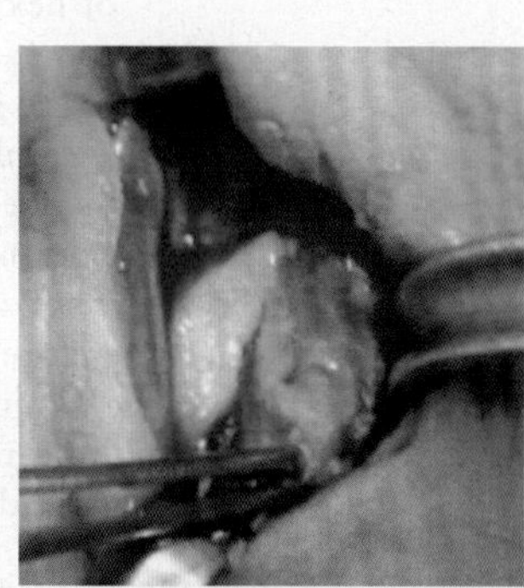

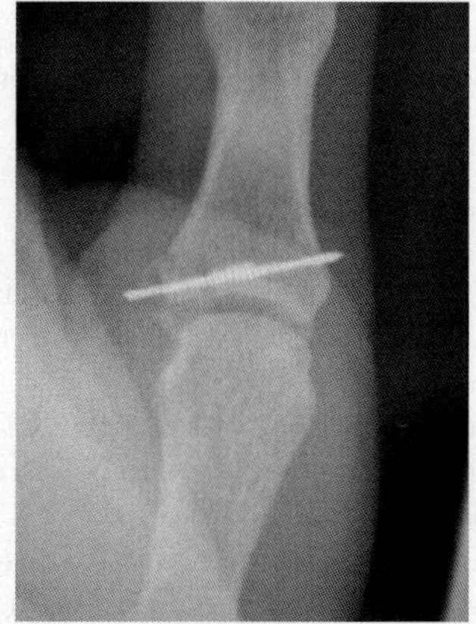

A B C

FIG 3 • **A.** Preoperative radiograph showing an avulsion fracture at the UCL insertion site. **B.** Arthroscopic reduction failed and an open procedure was performed because of the interposition of the adductor aponeurosis at the fracture site and unrecognized fracture comminution. **C.** Postoperative radiograph showing fixation of the fragment and attachment of the ligament using a Kirschner wire and a bone anchor.

Acute Ulnar Collateral Ligament Disruptions

Arthroscopic Treatment of Ulnar Collateral Ligament Avulsion Fractures

- Traction is applied using a finger trap placed on the thumb with 5 pounds of counterforce.
  - A traction tower is not used in order to facilitate fluoroscopy.
- Palpate the joint and then inject 1 to 2 mL of lidocaine using an 18-gauge needle.
  - Take care to avoid injuring the articular cartilage.
- Insert a 1.9-mm 30-degree arthroscope via a longitudinal portal stab wound on the radial side of the extensor pollicis longus tendon.
  - This allows the best visualization of the ulnar-sided pathology.
- Insert a 2-mm full-radius shaver in the ulnar portal and evacuate the hematoma and any minute bone fragments that may prevent visualization.
- Perform a synovectomy, with emphasis on the ulnar side. This allows clear delineation of the avulsed fracture fragment (**TECH FIG 1A**).
- Insert a small probe through the ulnar portal and hook the fragment on its radial side, within the fracture site. Gentle proximal and radial traction on the ulnar fragment typically accomplishes the reduction.
  - Preoperative radiographs help to plan the specific maneuver necessary for fracture reduction, but the arthroscopic picture will ultimately determine the direction of fragment derotation required to achieve anatomic reduction of the joint.
- Reintroduce the shaver as needed for débridement and to assist fracture reduction.
- Insert a 0.035-inch Kirschner wire percutaneously into the joint just proximal and ulnar to the reduced bony fragment (**TECH FIG 1B**).
- Arthroscopic visualization aids in placement and orientation of the transfixing Kirschner wire using the wire driver (**TECH FIG 1C**).
- Using the wire driver, engage the radial cortex to stabilize the fracture fragment.
- Use both fluoroscopy and arthroscopy to determine the adequacy of fragment reduction as well as to confirm proper wire placement and fracture stability (**TECH FIG 1D,E**).
- Cut the wire just underneath the skin (**TECH FIG 1F**).
- Close the skin and apply a bulky thumb spica plaster splint while the thumb is still suspended.
- Final fluoroscopic pictures are taken and the tourniquet is released.

Open Repair of Complete Ulnar Collateral Ligament Disruptions

- Make a curvilinear or a longitudinal lazy Z incision with the superior or dorsal portion proximal.
  - The UCL origin is more dorsal and fans out in volar fashion.

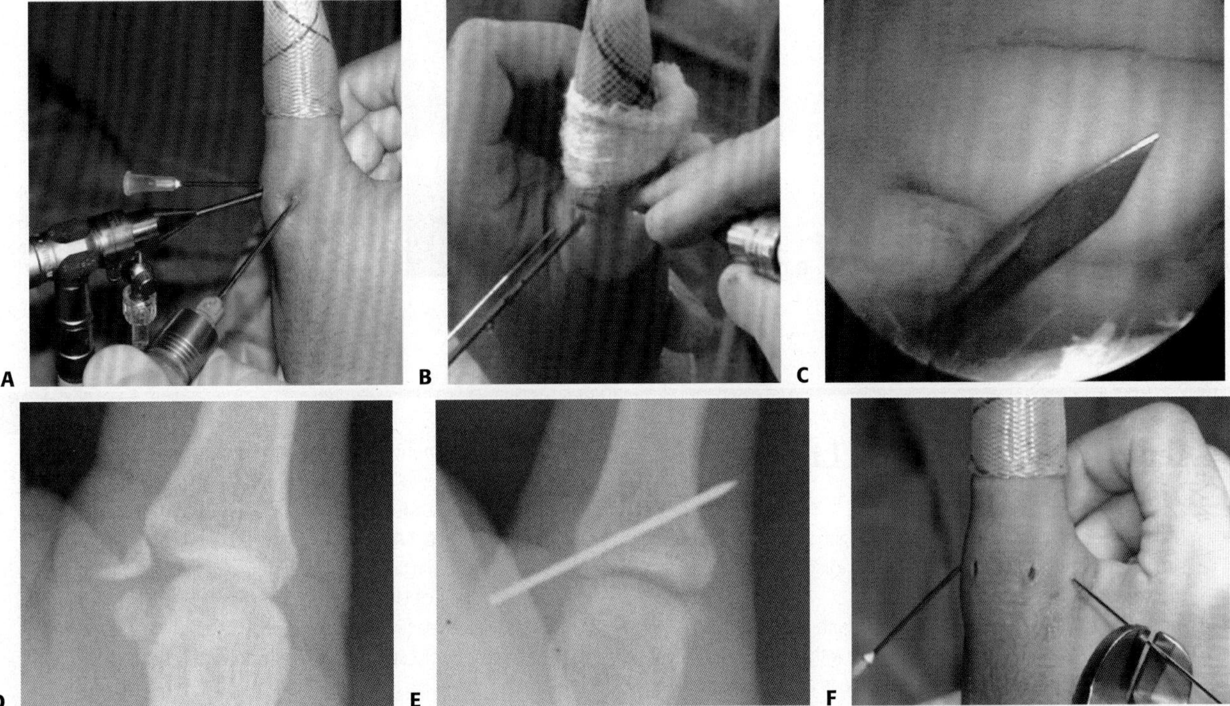

TECH FIG 1 • **A.** With the arthroscope in the dorsoradial portal and the shaver in the dorsoulnar portal, arthroscopic débridement is performed before reduction of the fragment. **B.** The fragment is reduced arthroscopically and stabilized with a Kirschner wire. **C.** Arthroscopic view showing the Kirschner wire and the fracture fragment before reduction. **D.** This displaced and rotated bony avulsion fracture at the attachment of the UCL is reduced arthroscopically and stabilized. **E.** Radiograph showing anatomic arthroscopic reduction and pinning. **F.** The Kirschner wire, fixing the avulsed fragment, is cut beneath the skin.

- Dissect the subcutaneous tissues with small tenotomy scissors, taking care to maintain hemostasis using a bipolar cautery.
  - Identify the dorsoradial sensory nerve branches and gently retract them dorsally.
- Take note of the oblique transverse fibers of the adductor aponeurosis. In more severe injuries, the aponeurosis may be torn, revealing the underlying UCL.
- Divide the adductor aponeurosis longitudinally, allowing the muscular origin of the adductor pollicis to pull back the fascia and facilitate posterior retraction of the aponeurosis.
  - The torn UCL is seen directly under the incised adductor aponeurosis (**TECH FIG 2A**).
  - In the case of a Stener lesion, the retracted and displaced stump of the UCL is visualized just superficial to the proximal edge of the adductor aponeurosis before incision.
- Determine the direction of the UCL fibers and incise the joint capsule on the ligament's dorsal margin.
- Inspect the joint and perform a limited débridement and synovectomy as indicated.
- Precisely determine the location and degree of UCL injury.
  - Less common intrasubstance tears are repaired primarily with 3-0 or 4-0 permanent suture in a mattress or figure-of-eight configuration.
  - Avulsion of the ligament attachment from the base of the proximal phalanx is most frequently encountered and is treated by reattaching the ligament's insertion.
- Isolate the anatomic insertion site for the proper collateral ligament on the volar ulnar base of the proximal phalanx and prepare the site for ligament attachment by débriding the remaining soft tissue down to bleeding bone.
  - Creating a small bony trough at the insertion site helps stimulate bleeding and ligament attachment (**TECH FIG 2B**).
- Prepare the UCL stump by mobilizing it on its margins and freshening the distal end with a no. 15 blade.
- Insert a 2-mm or smaller suture anchor into the prepared bony site and verify its position with fluoroscopy.
- While the thumb is deviated in an ulnar direction, reattach the ligament stump to the proximal phalanx by placing a horizontal mattress stitch using the suture from the anchor.
- Repair the accessory portion of the UCL by placing 3-0 or 4-0 permanent suture from the ligament into the ulnar margin of the volar plate.
- Additional permanent sutures may be placed to secure the repaired UCL to surrounding soft tissues.
- Close the capsule to the dorsal margin of the ligament using 4-0 absorbable suture.
- Precisely reconstruct the adductor aponeurosis with 4-0 inverted interrupted permanent suture and close the skin.
- Ensure restoration of stability and maintenance of full MCP joint flexion.
- Place a forearm-based thumb spica splint.
- Very severe injuries with extensive disruption of soft tissue stabilizers may rarely require augmentation with a temporary Kirschner wire.

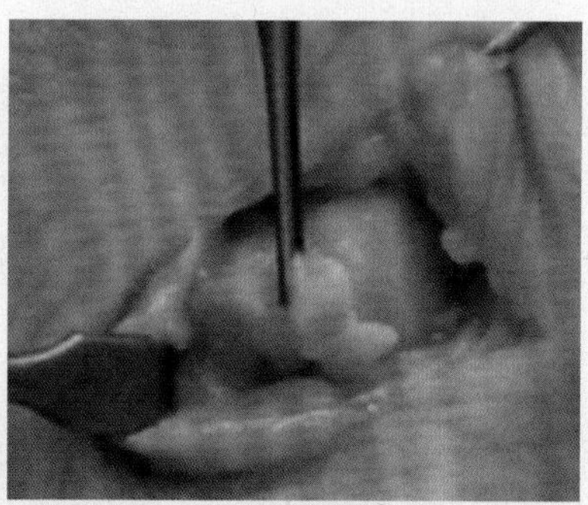

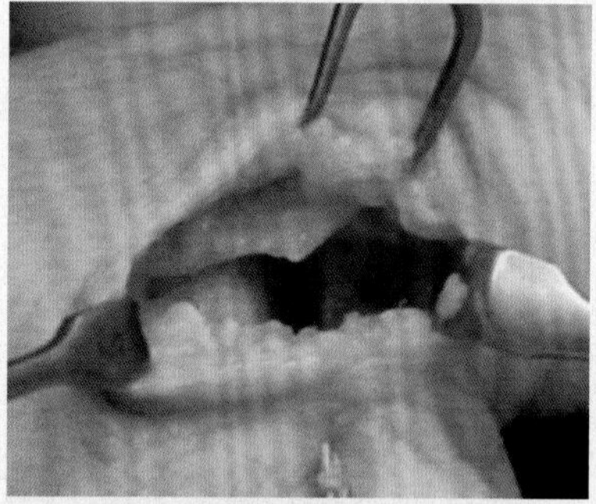

TECH FIG 2 • **A.** Avulsed UCL (Stener lesion) is well visualized after division of the adductor aponeurosis. **B.** At the anatomic site of UCL insertion, the bone is prepared and a bone anchor inserted.

Acute Radial Collateral Ligament Disruptions

- Make a dorsoradial curvilinear or a longitudinal lazy Z incision similar to that used for the repair of UCL disruptions and dissect the soft tissues as detailed earlier.
- Incise the abductor aponeurosis in line with the RCL.
- Radial-sided lesions are often coupled with concomitant avulsions of the dorsal capsule. If the capsule is intact, incise it along the dorsal margin of the RCL to inspect the joint.
- Isolate the ligament and its point of disruption, and then mobilize the structure to allow for anatomic repair.
  - Typically, disruptions take place at the proximal origin (**TECH FIG 3A**).
- Débride the bone and ligament stump in the manner detailed for open repair of UCL avulsions.
  - Remove reactive bone and early osteophytes at the site of ligament or capsule avulsion with a rongeur.

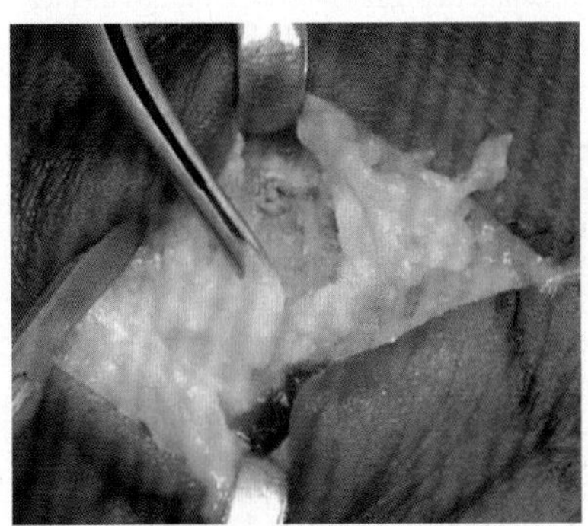
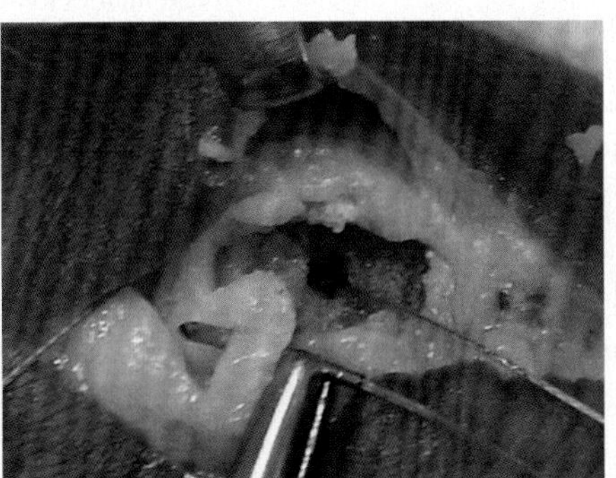
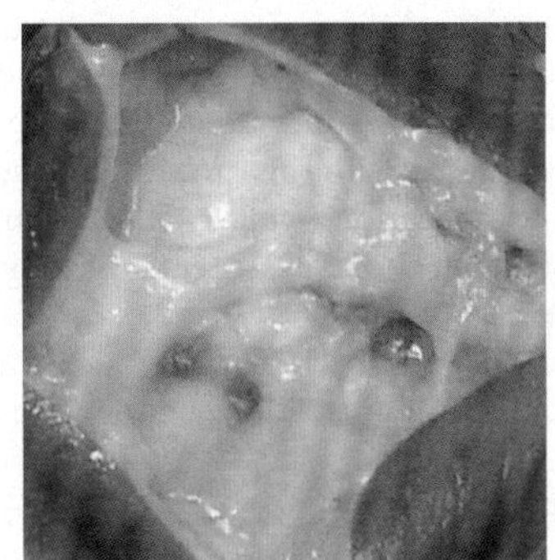

TECH FIG 3 • **A.** Dorsal capsule to be repaired to the metacarpal head with decortication in a chronic RCL injury. **B.** Anchors placed in the bone with the ligament ready to be sutured. **C.** Completed reconstruction of the RCL with repaired abductor aponeurosis and demonstrated course of the radial sensory nerve, which is protected throughout the procedure.

- Place a 2.0-mm or smaller suture anchor in the collateral recess, the dorsoradial distal metacarpal.
  - Ensure proper placement radiographically.
- Reattach the ligament to its anatomic point of origin using the suture from the anchor (**TECH FIG 3B**).
- Repair the capsule and further secure the RCL to surrounding soft tissue with 3-0 or 4-0 permanent suture (**TECH FIG 3C**).
- Repair the abductor aponeurosis and skin as described earlier.
- Ensure restoration of stability and maintenance of full MCP joint flexion.
- Place a forearm-based thumb spica splint.
- Very severe injuries with extensive disruption of soft tissue stabilizers may rarely require augmentation with a temporary Kirschner wire.

PEARLS AND PITFALLS

- MCP ligamentous lesions require a high index of suspicion.
- The obvious lesions with instability will likely get appropriate repairs with subsequent rehabilitation programs.
- Missing a significant ligament tear may cause few physical problems short term but may become a chronic painful lesion long term.
  - This is where arthroscopy may also play a good role. The chronically painful lesions may not demonstrate laxity or even a gross physical problem. Nevertheless, the pain is present and repeat corticosteroid injections are certainly not a solution. Arthroscopic synovectomy or capsular or ligamentous débridement will alter the articular milieu enough to allow for resolution of chronic pain and swelling. All this is coupled with rapid resolution of symptoms and recovery of range of motion.

POSTOPERATIVE MANAGEMENT

- Bony gamekeeper's thumb
  - A fiberglass thumb spica cast is applied at 1 week postoperatively and the pin is removed under local anesthesia at about 5 weeks postoperatively.
  - A brief course of physical therapy is initiated. The patient is given a hand-based thumb–carpometacarpal type of removable splint to be used during strenuous activities.
  - Therapy is usually short term, owing to less swelling and stiffness as compared with open approaches.
  - All unrestricted activities are permitted at 8 weeks.
- UCL and RCL injuries: True ligament-to-bone healing is necessary, so 6 weeks of postoperative thumb spica immobilization is critical to success.

OUTCOMES

- Clinical results after a combined arthroscopic and open procedure can be excellent.
- Functional outcome after repair of either UCL or RCL injuries tends to be excellent. Perhaps this is because thumb stability, not MCP motion, is critical to hand function.
  - Although the MCP joint often remains fairly stiff long after immobilization is discontinued, the resultant disability is minimal, considering that people demonstrate a wide range of normal MCP arc of motion.
  - Many contralateral thumbs display a flexion arc of less than 20%; therefore, the normal restoration of full motion is not the goal. Good stability without pain should be the aim.
- RCL injuries of the thumb tend to have a higher tendency to develop posttraumatic arthritis.
  - Our long-term experience has shown the need for late arthrodesis on only two occasions. These are cases in which significant volar subluxation is present, and the articular wear at time of surgery was likely predictive of this long-term outcome.
  - A chronically painful thumb, with any degenerative changes on radiographs, coupled with volar posturing of the phalanx, should likely be considered straightaway for fusion.
  - Thorough counseling of the patient indicating the minimal deficit produced by arthrodesis is helpful.

COMPLICATIONS

- Careful surgical dissection should avoid the most common complication, which would be iatrogenic trauma to the dorsal sensory nerve. Once done, there are minimal complications associated with this area of hand surgery.
- Other complications can include stiffness, as previously discussed, infection, persistent instability, or chronic pain syndromes.
- Recalcitrant pain or instability can simply be managed by arthrodesis, still portending a good functional outcome.

REFERENCES

1. Abrahamsson S, Sollerman C, Lundborg G, et al. Diagnosis of displaced ulnar collateral ligament of the metacarpophalangeal joint of the thumb. J Hand Surg Am 1990;15(3):457–460.
2. Arnold DM, Cooney WP, Wood ME. Surgical management of chronic ulnar collateral ligament injury of the thumb metacarpophalangeal joint. Orthop Rev 1992;21:583–588.
3. Badia A. Arthroscopic reduction and internal fixation of bony gamekeepers thumb. Orthopedics 2006;29:675–678.
4. Bowers WH, Hurst LC. Gamekeeper's thumb. Evaluation by arthrography and stress roentgenography. J Bone Joint Surg Am 1977;59(4):519–524.
5. Camp RA, Weatherwax RJ, Miller EB. Chronic posttraumatic radial instability of the thumb metacarpophalangeal joint. J Hand Surg Am 1980;5(3):221–225.
6. Campbell CS. Gamekeeper's thumb. J Bone Joint Surg Br 1955; 37-B(1):148–149.
7. Campbell JD, Feagin JA, King P, et al. Ulnar collateral ligament injury of the thumb: treatment with glove spica cast. Am J Sports Med 1992;20:29–30.
8. Carr D, Johnson RJ, Pope MH. Upper extremity injuries in skiing. Am J Sports Med 1981;9:378–383.
9. Coonrad RW, Goldner JL. A study of the pathological findings and treatment in soft tissue injuries of the thumb metacarpophalangeal joint. J Bone Joint Surg Am 1968;50(3):439–451.
10. Dray GJ, Eaton RG. Dislocations and ligament injuries in the digits. In: Green DP, ed. Green's Operative Hand Surgery, ed 2. New York: Churchill Livingstone, 1988:777–811.
11. Durham JW, Khuri S, Kim MH. Acute and late radial collateral ligament injuries of the thumb metacarpophalangeal joint. J Hand Surg Am 1993;18(2):232–237.
12. Frank WE, Dobyns J. Surgical pathology of collateral ligamentous injuries of thumb. Clin Orthop Relat Res 1972;83:102–114.
13. Gerber C, Senn E, Matter P. Skier's thumb. Surgical treatment of the recent injuries to the ulnar collateral ligament of the thumbs metacarpophalangeal joint. Am J Sports Med 1981;93:171–177.
14. Glickel SZ, Malerich M, Pearce SM, et al. Ligament replacement for chronic instability of the ulnar collateral ligament of the metacarpophalangeal joint of the thumb. J Hand Surg Am 1993;18:930–941.
15. Heyman P, Gelberman RH, Duncan K, et al. Injuries of the ulnar collateral ligament of the thumb metacarpophalangeal joint. Biomechanical and the prospective clinical studies on the usefulness of the valgus stress testing. Clin Orthop Relat Res 1993;(292):165–171.
16. Kozin SH. Treatment of thumb ulnar collateral ligament ruptures with the Mitek bone anchor. Ann Plast Surg 1995;35:1–5.
17. Kozin SH, Bishop AT. Tension wire fixation of avulsion fractures at the thumb metacarpophalangeal joint. J Hand Surg Am 1994;19(6):1027–1031.
18. Moberg E, Stener B. Injuries to the ligaments of the thumb and fingers: diagnosis, treatment and prognosis. Acta Chir Scand 1953;106: 166–186.
19. Mondry F. Beitrag fur Operative Behandlung des Wackeldaumens. Zentralbl Chir 1940;67:1532.
20. Neviaser RJ, Wilson JN, Lievano A. Rupture of the ulnar collateral ligament of the thumb (gamekeeper's thumb). Correction by dynamic repair. J Bone Joint Surg Am 1971;53(7):1357–1364.
21. Parikh M, Nahigian S, Froimson A. Gamekeeper's thumb. Plast Reconstr Surg 1980;58:24–31.
22. Pichora DR, McMurtry RY, Bell MJ. Gamekeeper's thumb: a prospective study of functional bracing. J Hand Surg Am 1989;14(3): 567–573.
23. Rozmaryn LM, Wei N. Metacarpophalangeal arthroscopy. Arthroscopy 1999;15:333–337.
24. Ryu J, Fagan R. Arthroscopic treatment of acute complete thumb metacarpophalangeal ulnar collateral ligament tears. J Hand Surg Am 1995;20(6):1037–1042.
25. Smith MA. The mechanism of acute ulnar stability of the metacarpophalangeal joint of the thumb. Hand 1980;12:225–230.
26. Smith RJ. Posttraumatic instability of the metacarpal joint of the thumb. J Bone Joint Surg Am 1977;59(1):14–21.
27. Smith RJ, Desantolo A. Lateral instability at the metacarpophalangeal joint of the thumb. Handchirurgie 1972;4:95–98.
28. Stener B. Displacement of the ruptured ulnar collateral ligament of the metacarpophalangeal joint of the thumb: a clinical and anatomical study. J Bone Joint Surg Br 1962;44B:869–879.
29. Stener B. Hyperextension injuries of the metacarpophalangeal joint of the thumb-rupture of flexor pollicis brevis: an anatomic and clinical study. Acta Chir Scand 1963;125:275–293.
30. Watson-Jones R. Fractures and Joint Injuries, ed 4. Baltimore: Williams & Wilkins, 1955.

Reconstruction of Chronic Radial and Ulnar Instability of the Thumb Metacarpophalangeal Joint

46

CHAPTER

Steven Z. Glickel

DEFINITION

- Chronic instability of the ulnar collateral ligament (UCL) and the radial collateral ligament (RCL) of the metacarpophalangeal (MCP) joint of the thumb usually results from unrecognized or untreated acute tears of the ligament. Much less commonly, it results from chronic, repetitive trauma which, over time, renders the ligament incompetent.
- Persistent laxity may cause pain and weakness and, eventually, osteoarthritis resulting from asymmetric wear of the articular cartilage.

ANATOMY

- The MCP joint of the thumb has characteristics of both a condyloid and a ginglymus joint. The radial condyle is taller in the dorsovolar dimension than the ulnar condyle.
- The dorsoulnar and dorsoradial digital nerves are terminal branches of the superficial sensory branch of the radial nerve and invariably cross the operative field in the plane immediately superficial to the adductor and abductor aponeuroses, respectively.
  - They are at risk during reconstruction of the collateral ligaments. During the exposure of the joint, the nerve should be mobilized and gently retracted. Forceful retraction may cause a neurapraxia and hypesthesia distal to the nerve on the dorsum of the thumb on the involved side.
- The adductor aponeurosis is an extension of the tendon of the adductor pollicis muscle, which contributes obliquely oriented fibers to the extensor mechanism distal to the vertical fibers.
- The abductor aponeurosis is an extension of the tendon of the abductor pollicis brevis muscle, which contributes obliquely oriented fibers to the extensor mechanism distal to the vertical fibers.
- The proper UCL and RCL originate from fossae of the condyle of the metacarpal head on the radial and ulnar sides and pass obliquely from dorsal-proximal to volar-distal to insert on the volar third of the base of the proximal phalanx. The ligament widens as it goes from its metacarpal origin to its proximal phalangeal insertion.
  - The proper collateral ligaments are tight in MCP joint flexion and lax in extension.
- The accessory collateral ligaments originate on the metacarpal head contiguous with but just volar to the proper collateral ligament and extend obliquely across the MCP joint, inserting on the sesamoid and volar plate.
  - The accessory collateral ligaments are tight in extension and lax in flexion.
- By definition, to have a complete ligament rupture, both the proper and the accessory collateral ligaments must be torn.
- The Stener lesion is a palpable soft tissue mass on the ulnar aspect of an injured MCP joint. It results from a tear of the UCL caused by forceful radial deviation of the proximal phalanx, angulating the MCP joint 70 degrees or more. The ligament tears distally at or near its insertion on the volar ulnar base of the proximal phalanx. As the proximal phalanx deviates radially, the ruptured UCL remains attached to its metacarpal origin. As the proximal phalanx returns to its resting, neutral position, the UCL stump comes to lie proximal and superficial to the adductor aponeurosis. Hence, the avulsed ligament is separated from its deep insertion by the aponeurosis, preventing ligament healing.
- The abductor aponeurosis is wider than the adductor aponeurosis. When the RCL tears, the ends of the torn ligament remain deep to the abductor aponeurosis. Hence, a Stener type of lesion rarely occurs on the radial side.
- Tears of the collateral ligaments result in rotatory deformities of the MCP joint. When one ligament is torn and the other is intact, the metacarpal head subluxates volarly on the injured side, rotating around the axis of the intact ligament. The metacarpal head on the injured side appears to be prominent due to the volar translation of the base of the proximal phalanx on that side.

PATHOGENESIS

- The UCL of the MCP joint of the thumb is usually torn by forceful abduction and extension of the thumb, as in a fall on the outstretched hand with the thumb abducted. The proximal phalanx deviates radially and, if there is sufficient force, the UCL either avulses from its insertion on the base of the proximal phalanx or, less commonly, tears in its midsubstance or from its origin on the metacarpal head.[19]
- There are four primary causes of chronic instability of the UCL.
  - Failure to diagnose an acute, complete tear resulting in no treatment
  - Failure to diagnose a Stener lesion resulting in inadequate, nonoperative treatment of a recognized acute, complete, and displaced tear
  - Inadequate treatment or insufficient immobilization of a recognized, acute tear without a Stener lesion
  - Progressive attenuation of the ligament due to repetitive trauma
- Tears of the RCL typically result from forceful ulnar deviation and extension of the MCP joint.
  - Proximal and distal avulsions of the ligament occur with roughly equal frequency.
  - Intrasubstance tears occur infrequently.

- Chronic instability of the RCL has three primary causes.
  - Most commonly, chronic laxity is due to failure to recognize an acute tear resulting in no treatment or inadequate or late treatment.
  - Even when the pathology is recognized, conservative management may fail because surgeons tend to be less aggressive about treatment of radial compared to ulnar-sided collateral ligament injuries.
  - Chronic attenuation due to repetitive trauma is uncommon but does occur.

NATURAL HISTORY

- Over time, chronic tears of the collateral ligaments of the thumb MCP joints cause progressive weakness of pinch and grip due to instability and pain. There may also be increasing deformity as the proximal phalanx on the injured side translates volarly causing dorsal prominence of the metacarpal head on that side. Occasionally, the proximal phalanx deviates in the coronal plane away from the side of the injured ligament resulting in a static deformity.
  - Incompetence of the UCL diminishes the thumb's ability to act as a stable post against which to pinch with the index finger. Patients often have difficulty holding large objects that require counterpressure by a stable thumb.
  - Patients with chronic RCL instability often have pain with torsional motions such as unscrewing jar tops.
- Chronic laxity may cause incongruity and asymmetric wear of the MCP joint, which may progress to posttraumatic osteoarthritis of the joint.
  - Arthritis of the joint causes increasing pain, stiffness, and weakness.

PATIENT HISTORY AND PHYSICAL FINDINGS

- Obtaining a relevant history from patients with chronic instability of the thumb MCP joint includes eliciting a history of trauma to the thumb in the recent or distant past.
- Patients are questioned about pain in the thumb, particularly if it is exacerbated by forceful pinch and grasp and torsional activities such as turning keys in locks, turning doorknobs, or unscrewing jar tops.
  - The examiner should establish the chronicity of the symptoms and whether they are increasing in severity.
- Assessment of instability of the thumb MCP collateral ligaments is primarily clinical.
- Clinical examination begins with observation.
  - The resting posture of the thumb at the MCP joint is occasionally indicative of pathology. The joint may be angulated or rotated in its resting posture if the collateral ligament is grossly incompetent and the instability is chronic.
  - In thumbs with chronic RCL instability, there is often a dorsal prominence on the radial aspect of the metacarpal head. Such a prominence is generally less apparent in cases of chronic UCL instability.
- The involved side of the joint is often tender to palpation.
- Palpation of a fullness or soft tissue mass on the ulnar side of the metacarpal head is strongly suggestive of a Stener lesion.
- Stability of the collateral ligament is tested in extension and 30 degrees of MCP joint flexion (under local anesthesia if needed but that is rarely required). There is no consensus in the literature concerning the degree of instability that is diagnostic of a complete tear.
  - Valgus stress of the MCP joint in flexion is used to assess the stability of the proper UCL, whereas stress with the joint in extension is used to assess the accessory UCL as well.
  - The criteria for diagnosis of a complete ligament disruption that are most accurate were described by Heyman et al[3] and include 30 to 35 degrees of laxity of the ulnar side of the MCP joint when stressed in extension and 15 degrees more laxity than the contralateral thumb when stressed in 30 degrees of flexion.
  - Laxity in extension suggests that the accessory and proper collateral ligaments are both torn.
  - A more subtle, but often very helpful, finding is the presence or absence of a discrete end point to joint opening when stressed. Absence of a solid end point is strongly suggestive of a complete ligament tear.
- To test for joint degeneration, the MCP joint is passively moved in extension and flexion radially and ulnarly deviated. The joint is axially loaded as it is moved. Crepitus and pain strongly suggest the presence of osteoarthritis, a contraindication to reconstruction of an unstable MCP joint.

IMAGING AND OTHER DIAGNOSTIC STUDIES

- Radiographic evaluation includes posteroanterior (PA), lateral, and oblique radiographs of both thumbs.
  - Fractures should be ruled out.
  - The lateral view may show volar subluxation of the MCP joint, which is fairly common and may be the result of extension of the collateral ligament tear to involve the dorsal capsule. This may occur with both UCL and RCL tears. An isolated tear of the dorsal joint capsule very rarely causes volar subluxation without an associated collateral ligament injury.
  - A comparison lateral radiograph of the contralateral thumb is very helpful if volar subluxation is suspected.
- Stress views of the MCP joint have been recommended to demonstrate instability radiographically.
  - Most experienced clinicians rely almost exclusively on physical examination and static plain radiographs to make the diagnosis. Stress views done by the treating surgeon can be used to confirm the diagnosis and provide documentation for the medical record.
- Magnetic resonance imaging (MRI), ultrasound, and arthrography are rarely indicated to assess completeness of the UCL tear, particularly in the setting of a chronic injury. MRI and ultrasound can show the presence of a Stener lesion, but in the setting of a chronic injury, the presence or absence of a Stener lesion does not substantially alter the treatment plan.
- The use of arthroscopy as a diagnostic and treatment modality in the setting of chronic UCL instability remains investigational. Although the ligament and joint pathology may be able to be visualized, reconstruction using the arthroscope is a challenge, which has not yet yielded reportable results.

DIFFERENTIAL DIAGNOSIS

- Fracture of the thumb metacarpal head or base of the proximal phalanx
- Synovitis of the MCP joint

- Chronic partial tear of the UCL or RCL
- MCP joint arthrosis

NONOPERATIVE MANAGEMENT

- Customized hand-based thermoplastic splints, nonsteroidal anti-inflammatory medication, and corticosteroid injections may improve the synovitis and pain resulting from chronic instability and early degenerative arthritis. The duration of pain relief is unpredictable but usually in the range of a few weeks to months.

SURGICAL MANAGEMENT

- The indication for reconstruction of chronic UCL or RCL disruption is failure of conservative treatment, with persistent pain and instability of the MCP joint.
- Instability alone is a soft indication for surgery.
  - Theoretically, the asymmetric wear of the articular cartilage resulting from chronic laxity causes degeneration of the articular cartilage. This can be used as an argument for prophylactic reconstruction.
  - However, most patients without pain are hesitant to consider surgery and the prolonged rehabilitation required thereafter.
- Contraindications to reconstruction of UCL or RCL tears include osteoarthritis, "multidirectional" instability, and fixed subluxation of the joint.
  - Mild chondromalacia is not a contraindication to reconstruction but more significant cartilage degeneration is better treated by MCP arthrodesis.
    - If an arthritic joint is stabilized by reconstruction, pain is likely to persist and increase over time, necessitating conversion to an arthrodesis.
  - Fixed instability of the MCP joint is an uncommon contraindication to ligament reconstruction.
  - Reconstruction of the incompetent ligament in this scenario would require an extensive joint release, creating multidirectional instability.
  - Failure to release the joint adequately would preclude anatomic realignment or result in rapid recurrence of the preoperative deformity and instability.
- Reconstruction of chronic instability may involve mobilization of the disrupted ligament, mobilization of local tissues, or ligament replacement using a tendon graft.
  - The decision is made at the time of surgery.
  - The more chronic the injury and the more dramatic the laxity and deformity, the more likely the need for replacement of the ligament with a graft. The prevailing wisdom is that if an MCP collateral ligament has been torn for more than 6 weeks, it cannot be used for secondary repair or reconstruction. I have not found that to be the case. I have used ligaments torn for as much as several months for secondary repair but the tissue has to be supple and able to be mobilized. Significantly, fibrotic ligament should be excised and reconstructed.

Preoperative Planning

- The patient is asked to actively bring all five digits together and simultaneously flex the wrist against resistance. The volar wrist is inspected for the presence of a palmaris longus (PL) tendon.
- Examination under anesthesia may show even greater joint laxity than anticipated based on an awake examination with the patient guarding.

Positioning

- The patient is supine on the operating room table with the arm on a hand table at an angle slightly less than perpendicular to the torso.

Approach

- Lazy S incision centered over the MCP joint
- Midaxial incision
- Chevron-shaped incision centered over the midaxial point of the MCP joint

TECHNIQUES

Reconstruction of Chronic Ulnar Collateral Ligament Disruptions Using Tendon Graft

Exposure

- Incise the skin over the ulnar joint line (**TECH FIG 1A,B**).
- Elevate skin flaps and retract them with 4-0 silk sutures.
- Identify and protect the branch of the dorsoulnar digital nerve that invariably crosses the wound (**TECH FIG 1C**).
- Identify the frequently fibrotic adductor aponeurosis.
  - The proximal stump of the torn UCL may be visualized at the proximal margin of the adductor aponeurosis if a Stener lesion is present.
- Incise the adductor aponeurosis longitudinally, exposing the underlying torn UCL (**TECH FIG 1D**).
- If the ligament cannot be defined and mobilized sufficiently for direct repair or reinsertion, the remnant of the ligament is excised, exposing the ulnar side of the distal metacarpal head, the base of the proximal phalanx, and the MCP joint (**TECH FIG 1E**).
- The MCP joint is "booked open" to visualize the articular cartilage.
  - Significant degenerative disease is a contraindication to reconstruction. Mild chondromalacia can be tolerated and is not necessarily a contraindication to reconstruction (**TECH FIG 1F**).

Bone Preparation

- Make two holes in the ulnar base of the proximal phalanx using handheld gouges of increasing diameter (**TECH FIG 2A**). Alternatively, a drill can be used to make the holes using a drill guide or tissue protector to prevent wrapping up adjacent tissue.
  - The diameter of the hole required depends on the size of the tendon graft to be used for reconstruction.
  - The preferred donor is the PL, which is usually fairly thin and can fit in a relatively small hole.
- The gouge holes must be made far enough apart to preserve a substantial bony bridge between the holes.
  - A bridge that is too narrow can fracture during passage of the tendon graft.

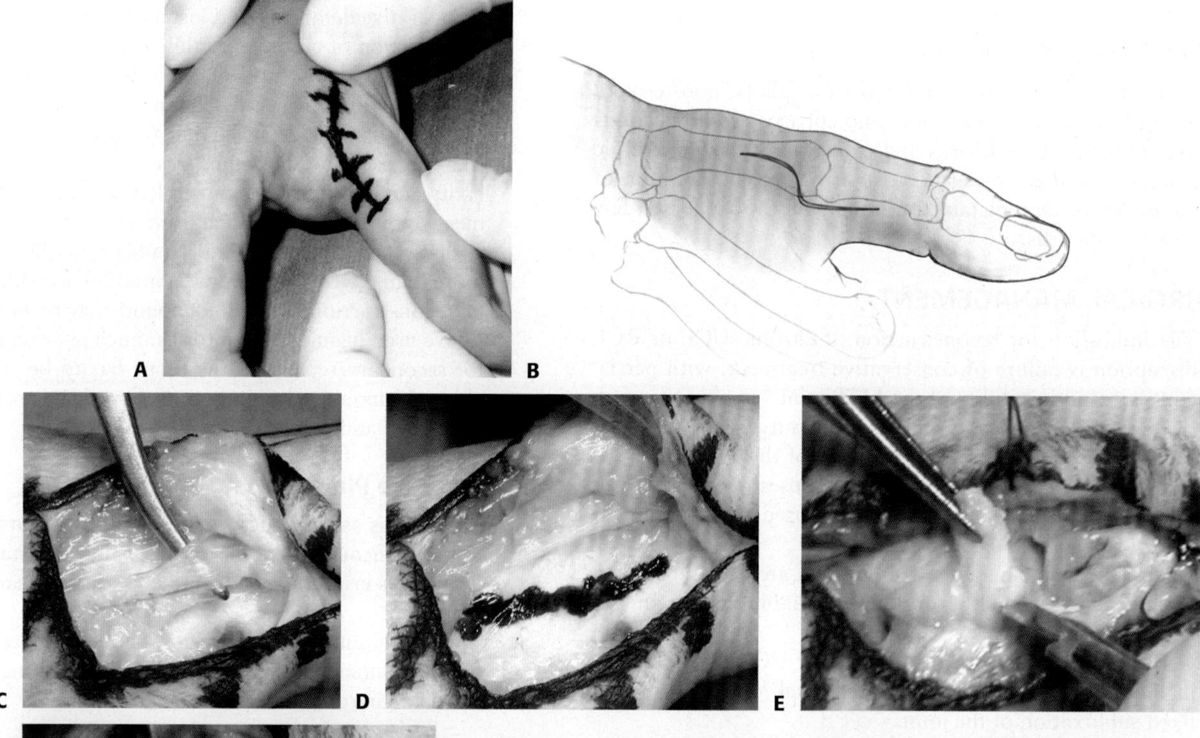

TECH FIG 1 • **A.** The lazy S incision used for UCL reconstruction. The proximal incision is dorsal and the distal incision is midaxial. **B.** A chevron-shaped incision is made centered over the ulnar side of the MCP joint. **C.** A dorsal ulnar sensory nerve branch is identified and protected throughout the surgery. **D.** The adductor aponeurosis is incised longitudinally about 2 mm from the extensor expansion, providing a cuff of tissue dorsally to facilitate an adequate repair at the end of the procedure. **E.** Excision of the UCL remnants exposes the MCP joint, the metacarpal head, and the base of the proximal phalanx. **F.** The MCP joint is inspected for degenerative changes. Extensive degenerative disease is a contraindication to reconstruction. Arthrodesis is appropriate in the setting of an arthritic MCP joint. This joint shows no evidence of arthritis.

- Place the holes at the 7 o'clock and 11 o'clock positions in the base of the proximal phalanx if looking at the right thumb end on. Make the holes at an angle of about 45 degrees to the bone surface and direct them toward each other in order to converge within the medullary canal and create a bone tunnel.
- Prebend a 28-gauge stainless steel wire into the approximate arc of curvature of the bone tunnel to facilitate its passage. An alternative to wire is a 0 polypropylene nonbraided synthetic suture. Leave the needle on the suture and pass the back end of the needle through the bone tunnel. The sharp end of the needle tends to get caught up by the trabecule in the medullary canal more readily.
- Pass the wire through the bone tunnel and secure the ends with a hemostat.
- Create a second bone tunnel in the metacarpal neck. Use the gouges beginning at the fossa from which the UCL normally originates on the ulnar side of the metacarpal neck and extending slightly obliquely, from distal to proximal, across the metacarpal, exiting radially (**TECH FIG 2B,C**). A 1-cm longitudinal incision is made over the tip of the gouge to provide access to the gouge hole and periosteum adjacent to it.
  - Most often, the small, medium, and large gouges are used to create one large hole because both ends of the tendon graft are passed through this hole.
- A second 28-gauge stainless steel wire is placed through this bone tunnel and the ends are secured with another hemostat.
- Preset a 0.045-inch Kirschner wire (sharp at both ends) in the metacarpal head for later advancement across the MCP joint.
  - Radially deviate the proximal phalanx to expose the metacarpal head.
  - Starting in the center of the metacarpal head and aiming at an angle of about 45 degrees, advance the wire retrograde through the radial cortex of the metacarpal shaft and then withdraw it proximally until it is just below the articular surface of the metacarpal head.

Tendon Graft Harvest and Passage

- Harvest the PL for use as a graft.
  - If the palmaris is absent, use half of the flexor carpi radialis (FCR) tendon or the plantaris tendon.
  - The obvious advantage of the FCR is its availability without requiring a second surgical site.
- Make a short transverse incision over the PL tendon at the distal wrist flexion crease (**TECH FIG 3A**) and mobilize the tendon distally.

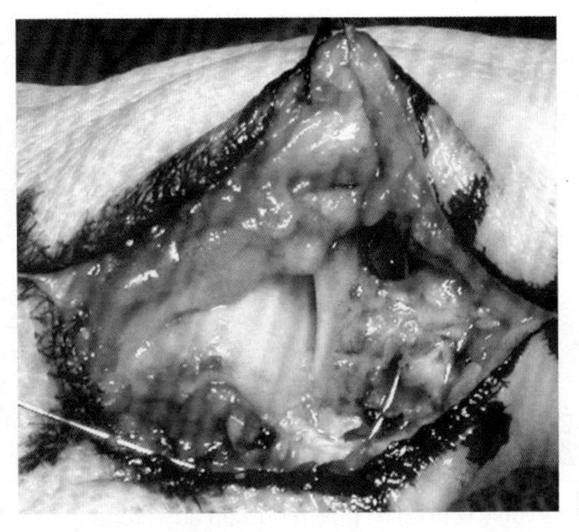

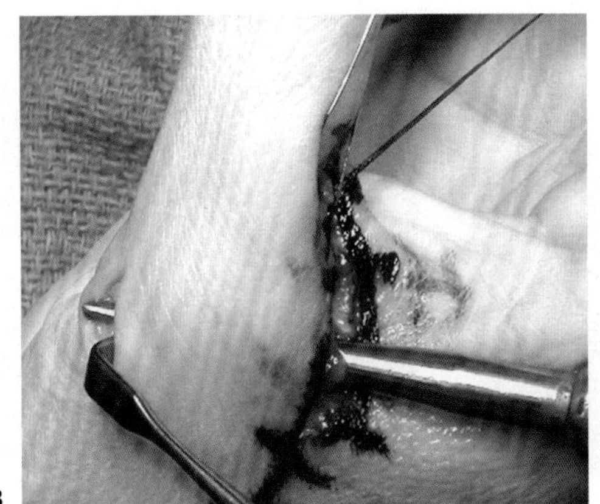

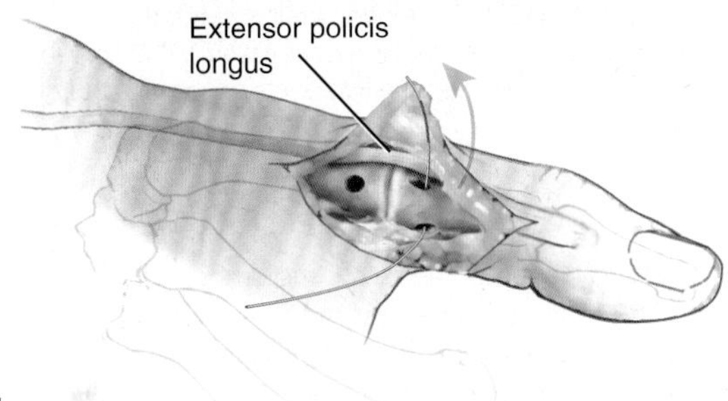

TECH FIG 2 • **A.** The proximal phalangeal holes are made at the 7 o'clock and 11 o'clock position; the surgeon must be careful to make a wide bone bridge to avoid fracture. A 28-gauge wire is placed into the bone tunnel to assist with passage of the tendon graft. **B.** A large gouge is used to create a single hole in the metacarpal head. An incision is made radially over the end of the gouge to allow for fixation of the graft. **C.** The adductor aponeurosis has been divided and the collateral ligament remnants have been excised. Gouge holes have been made in the base of the proximal metacarpal head.

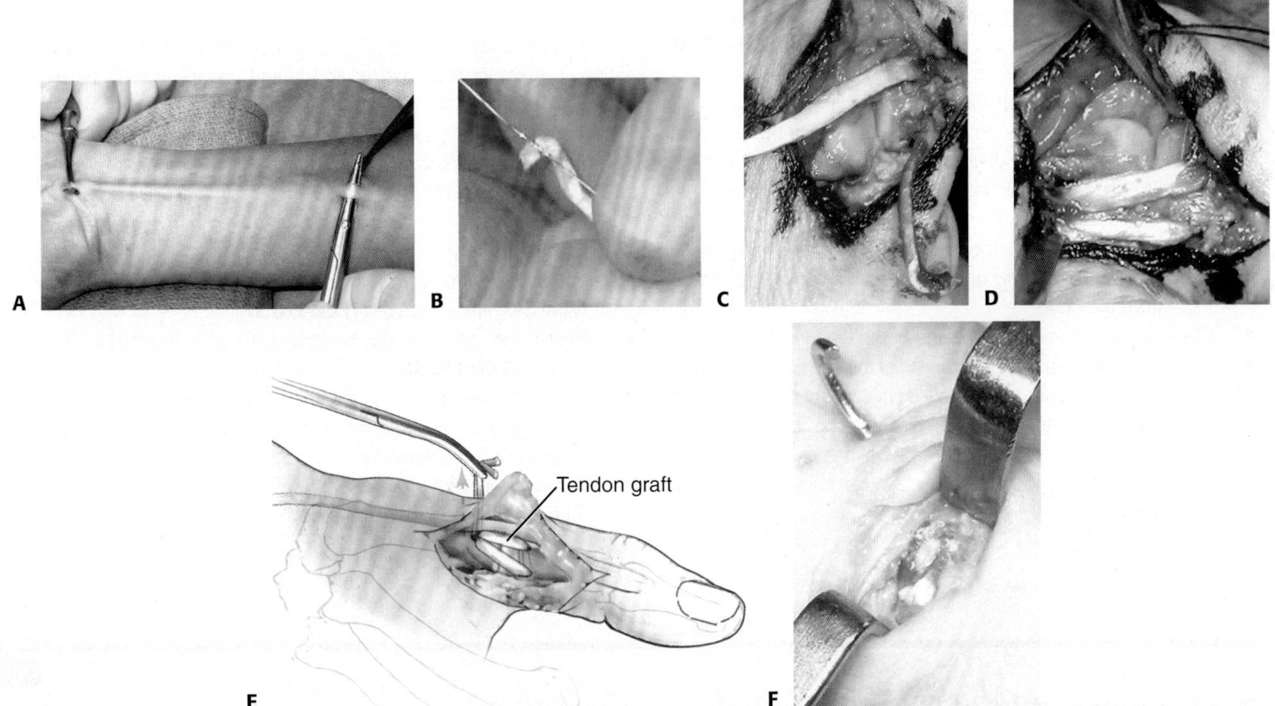

TECH FIG 3 • **A.** If it is present, the PL tendon is harvested with two small transverse incisions. Great care is taken to protect the median nerve during harvest. **B.** The wire is tied over the end of the tendon graft and is used to pull the graft through the bone tunnel in the proximal phalanx for reconstruction of the RCL in this case. **C.** The PL tendon is placed through the proximal phalangeal holes using the previously placed wire. Care is taken not to pull against the bone bridge during graft placement. **D.** Both ends of the tendon graft are passed together through the hole in the metacarpal head. **E.** The graft has been passed through the gouge holes and is secured on the radial side of the thump MCP joint by tying the ends into a knot; it is further secured with sutures to local tissue. **F.** The graft ends are tied into a knot and secured to the local periosteum with 3-0 nonabsorbable suture. *(continued)*

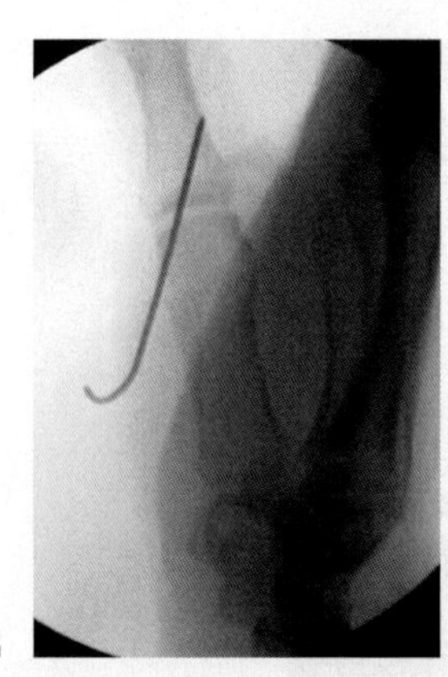

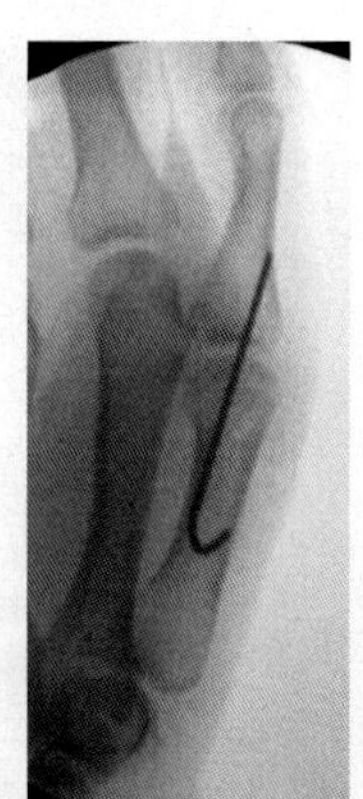

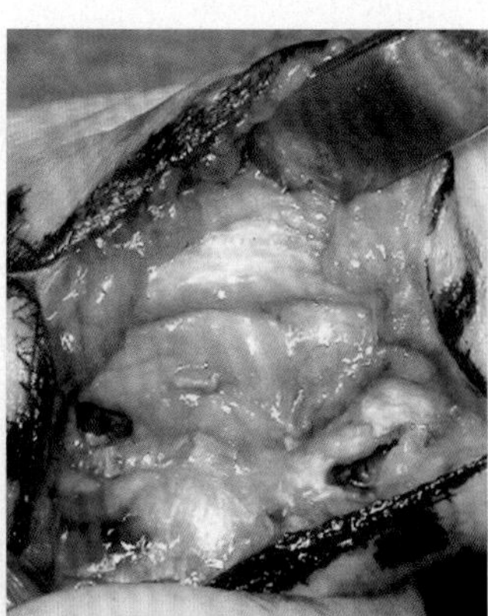

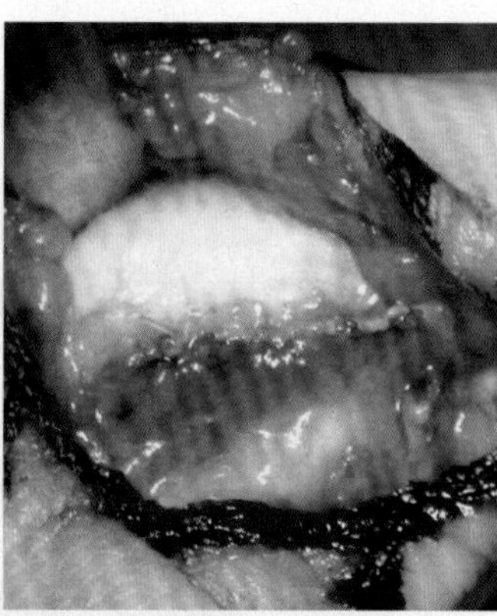

TECH FIG 3 • *(continued)* **G,H.** Anteroposterior (AP) and lateral radiographs verify concentric joint reduction and proper placement of the transfixing 0.045-inch Kirschner wire. The Kirschner wire is left in place for 6 weeks. **I.** The tendon graft is sutured to the dorsal and volar remnants of the native collateral ligament for additional fixation. **J.** The adductor aponeurosis is repaired with 5-0 absorbable suture. This layer must be repaired separately from the collateral ligament as differential gliding between the two layers occurs with thumb motion.

- Make a second, proximal incision over the PL musculotendinous junction and mobilize the tendon at this level and under the skin bridge.
  - Use of a tendon stripper is an alternative method of harvest.
- After incising the PL as distal as possible, apply firm traction and withdraw the tendon through the proximal incision, and then divide the tendon at the musculotendinous junction.
- Secure the tendon graft to the limb of the stainless steel wire emerging from the more volar of the two proximal phalangeal gouge holes by tying a knot around one end of the tendon graft (**TECH FIG 3B**) or by using a grasping suture placed through the graft.
- Moisten the tendon graft with saline.
- Pull the wire to draw the tendon into and through the bone tunnel, emerging from the dorsal hole (**TECH FIG 3C**).
  - The tendon is pulled using moderately firm traction and a circular motion of the wire.
  - Avoid fracturing the bony bridge between the gouge holes by pulling too firmly on the wire with a vector of pull away from the bone.
- The wire is removed from the end of the tendon.
- Remove this wire and tie the ulnar end of the wire previously placed in the metacarpal bone tunnel around both ends of the tendon graft.
- Using the same technique combining saline lubrication, traction, and rotation of the wire, bring the two ends of the graft together and through the metacarpal gouge hole, exiting radially (**TECH FIG 3D,E**).
- Set the tension of the reconstruction by pulling on both limbs of the graft simultaneously and stressing the joint with radially directed force on the proximal phalanx.
  - Flexion and extension should not be limited significantly and the joint should open minimally with stress.
- When the desired tension is achieved, tie the ends of the graft in a knot (**TECH FIG 3F**).
- Suture the knot to the adjacent periosteum with two mattress sutures stitches of 3-0 braided synthetic suture.
  - Alternatively, place a bone anchor adjacent to the metacarpal tunnel on the radial side and use the loaded sutures to secure the knot.
- Transfix the MCP joint by driving the previously placed Kirschner wire antegrade, across the joint into the proximal phalanx (**TECH FIG 3G,H**).
- Bend and cut the proximal end of the Kirschner wire superficial to the skin.
- Suture the tendon graft to the native collateral ligament remnants using 3-0 braided suture (**TECH FIG 3I**).
- Repair the adductor aponeurosis with 5-0 absorbable PDS suture (**TECH FIG 3J**).
- Reapproximate the skin with either subcuticular 4-0 absorbable nonbraided synthetic suture such as Monocryl or interrupted, absorbable 5-0 plain suture.
- A forearm-based thumb spica splint is applied, leaving the thumb interphalangeal joint free.

Reconstruction of Chronic Radial Collateral Ligament Disruptions Using Tendon Graft

- The steps used to stabilize the radial MCP joint using a tendon graft are much the same as those detailed for reconstruction of chronic UCL disruptions.

Exposure

- Center the skin incision over the radial MCP joint line (**TECH FIG 4A**).
  - Identify and protect the branch of the dorsoradial digital nerve (**TECH FIG 4B**).

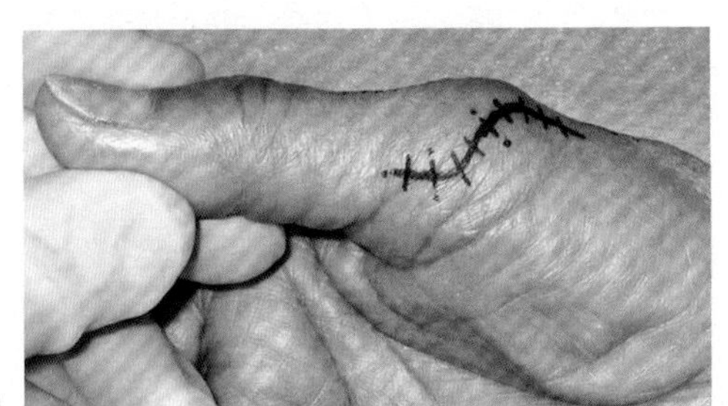

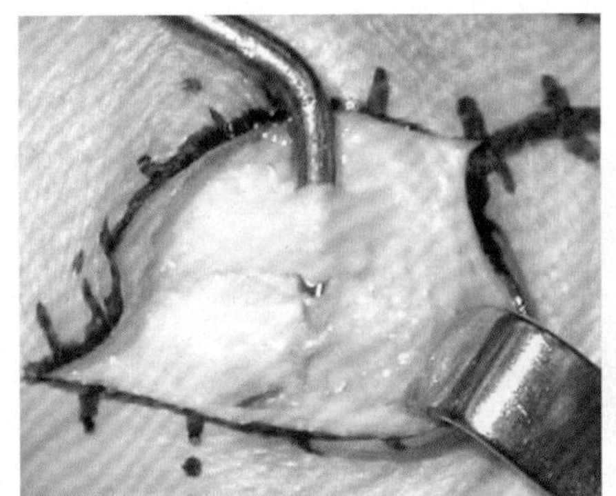

TECH FIG 4 • **A.** A lazy S incision is used for RCL reconstruction. **B.** A dorsal radial sensory nerve branch is identified and protected.

- Incise the abductor aponeurosis longitudinally, exposing the underlying torn RCL.
  - In thumbs with chronic instability, the RCL may be densely fibrotic and adherent to the overlying aponeurosis.
- Excise the remnant of the RCL, exposing the radial side of the metacarpal head, base of the proximal phalanx, and MCP joint.
- Deviate the MCP joint to visualize the articular cartilage and ensure the absence of significant arthrosis.

Bone Preparation

- Using handheld gouges of increasing diameter in the manner previously detailed, make two holes in the radial base of the proximal phalanx.
  - The holes are made at the 1 o' clock and 5 o'clock positions in the base of the proximal phalanx if looking at the right thumb end on (**TECH FIG 5A,B**).
  - The holes are made at an angle of about 45 degrees directed toward each other to create a continuous bone tunnel within the medullary canal.
  - The holes must be spaced far enough apart to maintain a substantial bony bridge.
  - A 28-gauge stainless steel wire is passed from one hole to the other through the tunnel created in the medullary canal to be used for later passage of the tendon graft in the manner described earlier for UCL reconstruction.
- Create a bone tunnel in the metacarpal neck beginning at the fossa from which the RCL normally originates on the radial side of the metacarpal head and extending slightly obliquely, from distal to proximal, across the metacarpal, exiting ulnarly (**TECH FIG 5C**).
  - A second 28-gauge stainless steel wire is placed through this hole and the ends are secured with a second hemostat.
- Preset a 0.045-inch Kirschner wire in the metacarpal head to be used later for transfixing the MCP joint. The pin can be passed from distal to proximal and then withdrawn into the metacarpal head proximally.

Tendon Graft Passage

- Introduce the tendon graft into the prepared bone tunnels using the techniques described for UCL reconstruction (**TECH FIG 6A,B**).
- The tension of the reconstruction is set and the graft secured in the manner reviewed.
- The MCP joint is transfixed and the wound closed (**TECH FIG 6C**).
- A forearm-based thumb spica splint is applied, leaving the thumb interphalangeal joint free.

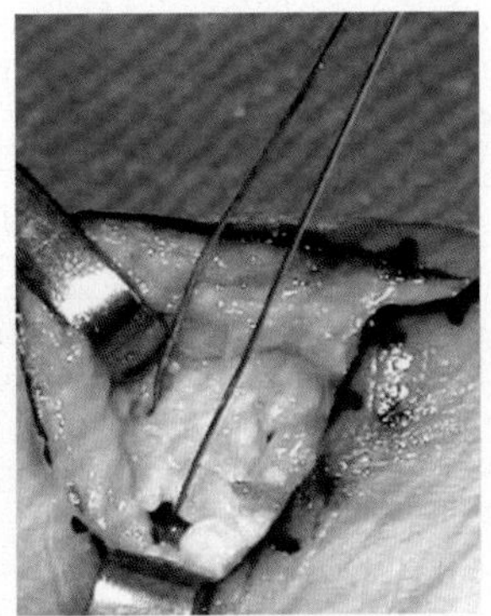

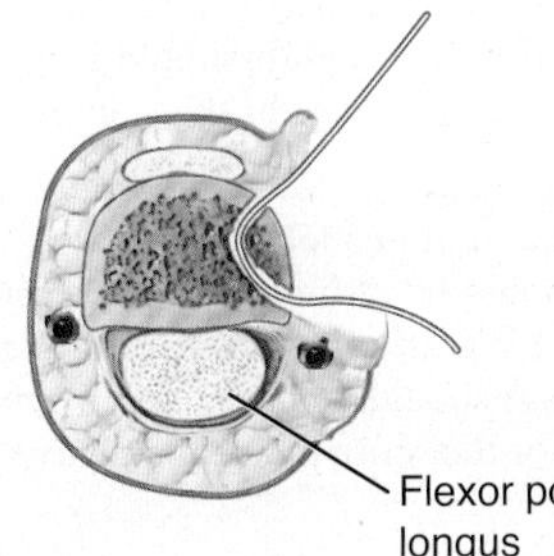

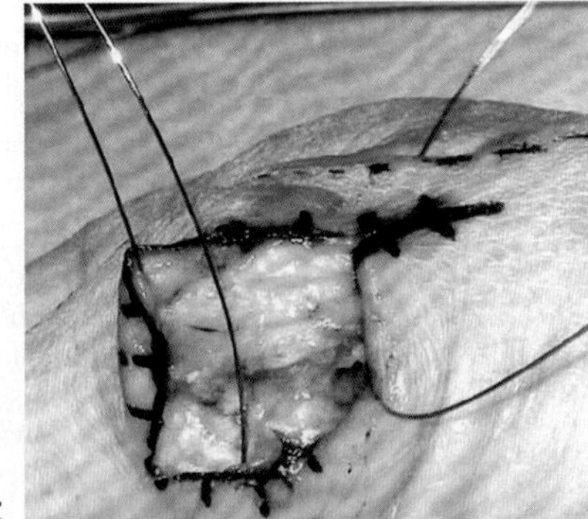

TECH FIG 5 • **A.** Two holes are made in the base of the proximal phalanx using a small then a medium gouge. A 28-gauge wire is placed through the bone tunnel to be used later for passage of the graft. **B.** An axial view of the proximal phalanx of a right thumb demonstrating the 1 o'clock and 5 o'clock positions of the gouge holes when viewed from the side. **C.** A single large hole is made in the metacarpal neck and another 28-gauge wire is placed through this hole, exiting ulnarly.

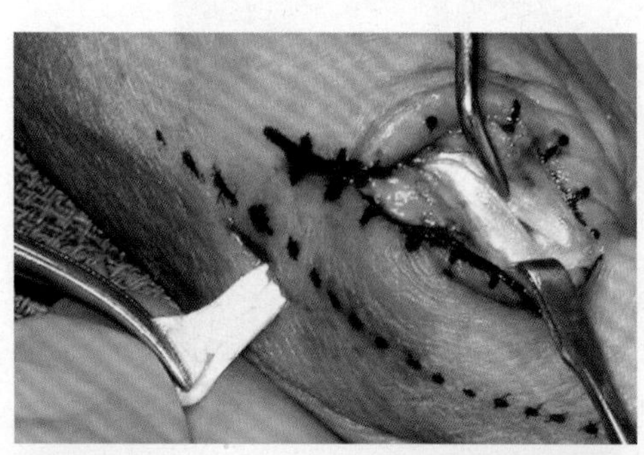

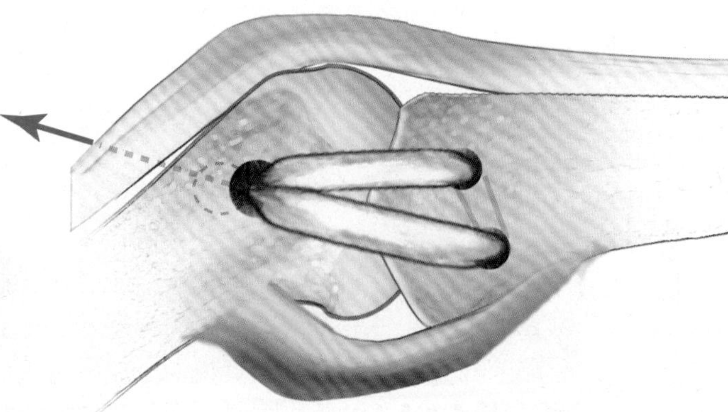

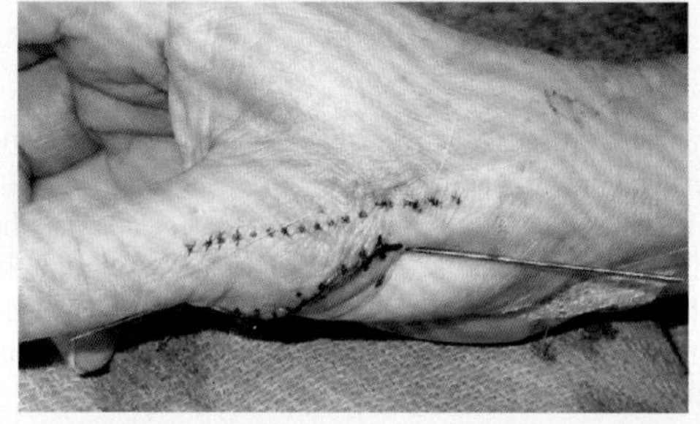

TECH FIG 6 • **A.** Both tendon ends are pulled together through the metacarpal head, exiting ulnarly. **B.** Converging gouge holes are made at the base of the proximal phalanx and an oblique hole is made in the metacarpal head. Subsequently, the graft is passed through these holes. **C.** The final photograph after wound closure and pin placement.

PEARLS AND PITFALLS

Traction on the dorsoulnar digital nerve	▪ Excessive traction on the dorsoulnar digital nerve may cause numbness, paresthesias, and dysesthesia on the dorsoulnar aspect of the thumb distal to the incision.
Tools	▪ Using handheld gouges gives the operator good control of the direction and progressive enlargement of the holes in the proximal phalanx and metacarpal. ▪ If power tools are used to make the holes, soft tissue adjacent to the holes can be inadvertently wrapped up in the spinning instrument. This can be obviated by using a tissue protector (drill guide) if a drill is used. Alternatively, the holes can be made with a burr. The heat generated by a burr may also burn the bone.
Making holes in the proximal phalanx	▪ The most important aspect of making the holes in the base of the proximal phalanx is to make them wide enough apart to maintain a substantial bone bridge. ▪ The greatest risk is making the holes too close together. The consequence is that the bridge fractures when the tendon graft is pulled through the holes. When the tendon is pulled through the bone tunnel, the wire should be pulled longitudinally more or less parallel to the axis of the bone tunnel using longitudinal traction and a twisting motion. It should not be pulled up and away from the bone in a direction more perpendicular to the axis of the bone tunnel. Pulling the wire perpendicular to the axis of the bone tunnel will increase the likelihood of fracture of the bone bridge.
Tying the wire	▪ The wire used for passage of the tendon graft should be tied in a knot around the end of the tendon graft using hemostats, not manually; it can cut the skin of the surgeon's fingers if done manually with too much force.
Graft tension	▪ The graft can be made too tight, limiting motion of the MCP joint and possibly causing pain postoperatively. The knot in the graft should be sutured after the tension has been set and felt to be appropriate. A less likely possibility is that the graft is too loose, resulting in persistent laxity of the joint. ▪ After the tension is set, the joint should be flexed and extended to ascertain that the reconstruction is not too tight to allow motion or too loose to adequately correct the instability.

POSTOPERATIVE CARE

- The thumb is immobilized in a thumb spica splint or cast for 6 weeks postoperatively.
- At 6 weeks after surgery, the splint or cast and pin are removed.
  - The thumb is immobilized after cast removal in a customized, thermoplastic short opponens splint fashioned by the hand therapist.
  - The splint is worn most of the time except when the patient is exercising the thumb or is sedentary for a period of 2 weeks.
- Therapeutic exercise is done with the therapist and at home and includes active and active-assisted range of motion in flexion and extension, avoiding laterally directed force on the proximal phalanx opposite the direction of the reconstruction, which would stress the reconstruction.
  - Patients are instructed to do 12 repetitions of range-of-motion exercise four or more times per day.
- After 2 weeks, the thermoplastic splint is eliminated except for strenuous activity.
- Patients continue range-of-motion exercises and begin strengthening with soft putty and light gripping.
- At 12 weeks after surgery, pinch and grip strengthening and light free weights are initiated.
- Full, unrestricted activity is allowed 16 weeks postoperatively.
- Patients are expected to regain about 80% of the range of motion of the contralateral thumb MCP joint and nearly full range of motion of the interphalangeal joint.
  - Key pinch strength should be more than 90% of the contralateral, uninjured thumb at final follow-up.

OUTCOMES

- Reconstruction of the UCL using the technique described in this chapter produces results only slightly less favorable than UCL repair.
- Range of motion of the MCP joint averaged 80% of the uninjured side. Motion of the interphalangeal joint is often limited initially after reconstruction but at final follow-up was 94% of the unoperated thumb.[2]
- Key pinch strength averaged 95% and grip strength averaged 103% of the unoperated thumb not corrected for handedness.[2]
- Sixty-nine percent of patients had no pain postoperatively and the remainder had mild or intermittent pain. Eighty-eight percent of patients had no functional limitations, 8% had minimal limitations, and 2% had moderate functional limitation.[2]
- None of the reconstructions that had normal or minimally degenerated cartilage required revision due to development or progression of degenerative disease.[2]
- Results of RCL reconstruction in the hands of the same authors were similar to those of UCL reconstruction, although range of motion of the MCP joint was 20% less than for UCL.[1]
- Range of motion of the MCP joint on the operated side was 59% of the unoperated side and interphalangeal range of motion was 94% of the unoperated thumb.[1]
- Both grip and key pinch strength were equal in the operated and unoperated thumbs.[1]
- The MCP joints were equally stable to stress in operated and unoperated thumbs.[1]
- Patients had minimal pain and no significant functional limitations. All returned to their preoperative occupations.[1]

COMPLICATIONS

- Some patients develop transient hypesthesia on the dorsal aspect of the thumb distal to the incision due to intraoperative traction on a branch of the radial sensory nerve.
  - This generally resolves over several weeks.
- Occasionally, patients develop stiffness of the MCP joint that is persistent. This may be the result of the reconstruction being too tight.
- The MCP joint occasionally develops some laxity postoperatively, which may be a consequence of the reconstruction being too loose or the patient being too aggressive during rehabilitation. Therapists should be cautioned about beginning key pinch strengthening too early or too aggressively.
- The bony bridge between the proximal phalangeal gouge holes can theoretically crack intraoperatively, but this has not happened to the authors or their colleagues in practice.
  - If it did occur, an alternative form of fixation of the graft to the proximal phalanx would have to be used, such as suturing the graft to the adjacent periosteum, pulling it out through a gouge hole on the opposite side of the phalanx, or employing a suture anchor.

REFERENCES

1. Catalano LW III, Cardon L, Patenaude N, et al. Results of surgical treatment of acute and chronic grade III tears of the radial collateral ligament of the thumb metacarpophalangeal joint. J Hand Surg Am 2006;31(1):68–75.
2. Glickel SZ, Malerich M, Pearce SM, et al. Ligament replacement for chronic instability of the ulnar collateral ligament of the metacarpophalangeal joint of the thumb. J Hand Surg Am 1993;18(5):930–941.
3. Heyman P, Gelberman RH, Duncan K, et al. Injuries of the ulnar collateral ligament of the thumb metacarpophalangeal joint—biomechanical and prospective clinical studies on the usefulness of valgus stress testing. Clin Orthop Relat Res 1993;(292):165–171.

SUGGESTED READINGS

Alldred AJ. Rupture of the collateral ligament of the metacarpophalangeal joint of the thumb. J Bone Joint Surg Br 1955;37-B(3):443–445.

Bean CH, Tencer AF, Trumble TE. The effect of thumb metacarpophalangeal ulnar collateral ligament attachment site on joint range of motion: an in vitro study. J Hand Surg Am 1999;24(2):283–287.

Breek JC, Tan AM, van Thiel TP, et al. Free tendon grafting to repair the metacarpophalangeal joint of the thumb. J Bone Joint Surg Br 1989;71(3):383–387.

Camp RA, Weatherwax RJ, Miller EB. Chronic posttraumatic radial instability of the thumb metacarpophalangeal joint. J Hand Surg Am 1980;5(3):221–225.

Campbell CS. Gamekeeper's thumb. J Bone Joint Surg Br 1955;37-B(1):148–149.

Coonrad RN, Goldner JL. A study of the pathological findings and treatment in soft-tissue injury of the thumb metacarpophalangeal joint. With a clinical study of the normal range of motion in one thousand thumbs and a study of post mortem findings of ligamentous structures in relation to function. J Bone Joint Surg Am 1968;50(3):439–451.

Coyle MP Jr. Grade III radial collateral ligament injuries of the thumb metacarpophalangeal joint: treatment by soft tissue advancement and bony reattachment. J Hand Surg Am 2003;28(1):14–20.

Durham JW, Khuri S, Kim MH. Acute and late radial collateral ligament injuries of the thumb metacarpophalangeal joint. J Hand Surg Am 1993;18(2):232–237.

Glickel SZ. Metacarpophalangeal and interphalangeal joint injuries and instabilities. In: Peimer CA, ed. Surgery of the Hand and Upper Extremity. New York: McGraw-Hill, 1996:1043–1068.

Kaplan EB, Riordan DC. The thumb. In: Spinner M, ed. Kaplan's Functional and Surgical Anatomy of the Hand, ed 3. Philadelphia: JB Lippincott, 1984:116–117.

Lyons RP, Kozin SH, Failla JM. The anatomy of the radial side of the thumb static restraints in preventing subluxation and rotation after injury. Am J Orthop 1998;27:759–763.

Melone CP Jr, Beldner S, Basuk RS. Thumb collateral ligament injuries. An anatomic basis for treatment. Hand Clin 2000;16:345–357.

Mitsionis GI, Varitimidis SE, Sotereanos GG. Treatment of chronic injuries of the ulnar collateral ligament of the thumb using a free tendon graft and bone suture anchors. J Hand Surg Br 2000;25(2):208–211.

Osterman AL, Hayken GD, Bora FW. A quantitative evaluation of thumb function after ulnar collateral ligament repair and reconstruction. J Trauma 1981;21:854–861.

Smith RJ. Post-traumatic instability of the metacarpophalangeal joint of the thumb. J Bone Joint Surg Am 1977;59(1):14–21.

Stener B. Displacement of the ruptured ulnar collateral ligament of the metacarpo-phalangeal joint of the thumb: a clinical and anatomical study. J Bone Joint Surg Br 1962;44-B(4):869–879.

Operative Treatment of Finger Carpometacarpal Joint Fracture-Dislocations

CHAPTER 47

John J. Walsh IV

DEFINITION

- Fractures and dislocations of the carpometacarpal (CMC) joints of the index through small fingers involve intra-articular fractures at the base of the metacarpals or pure dislocations between the metacarpals and carpus. The fracture can involve the base of the metacarpal or the trapezoid, capitate, or hamate articular surface.
- These fractures and dislocations can result in instability and articular incongruity (**FIG 1**).

ANATOMY

- The CMC joints connect the metacarpals and the distal carpal row.
- The shape and degree of constraint present in the joints differ from finger to finger.
  - The index and middle fingers have highly constrained articulations due to the shape of the index CMC articulation and supporting soft tissues.[4] These include the flexor carpi radialis tendon, extensor carpi radialis longus and brevis tendons, and very strong capsular insertions. This provides for a strong radial column for the hand and efficient force transfer to the radius (**FIG 2A**).
  - The ring and small fingers have a gliding articulation on the hamate, which allows for the closure of the hand around objects and is very important in power grip. This mobility makes them more susceptible to injury. The extensor carpi ulnaris tendon attaches to the dorsal base of the small finger metacarpal.[4]
- The deep motor branch of the ulnar nerve crosses around the base of the hamate hook from ulnar to radial and runs along the volar surface of the CMC joints (**FIG 2B**). It is vulnerable at the time of injury or during fixation.

PATHOGENESIS

- Injuries of the CMC joints may be divided into two broad categories.
  - The first, involving a load applied to a flexed metacarpal, is by far the most common mechanism. This injury usually involves the ring and small fingers displacing dorsally as a unit relative to the hamate. This may occur as a dislocation only or include a marginal fracture of the hamate.[8]
  - The second mechanism involves an axially directed force that creates a comminuted fracture of the articular surface (**FIG 3A**). Severe crushing injuries can cause multiple dislocations and fractures diffusely throughout the CMC region[1,7] (**FIG 3B,C**).

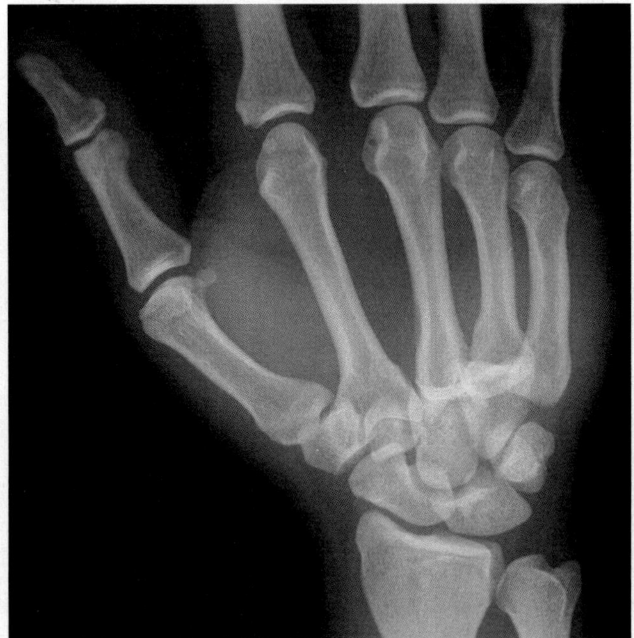

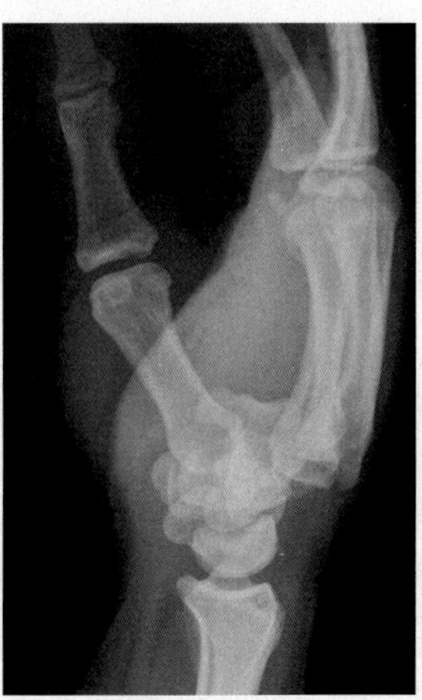

FIG 1 • **A,B.** Multiple dorsal CMC dislocations involving the index through small fingers.

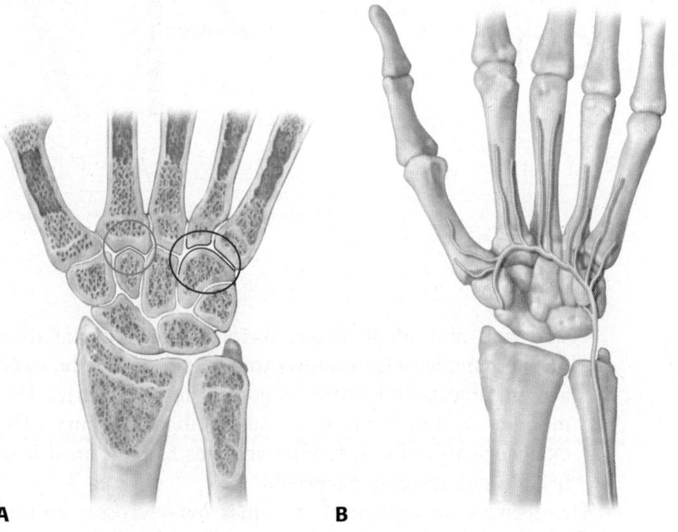

FIG 2 • **A.** Variable articular congruity of the various CMC joints. **B.** Deep motor branch of the ulnar nerve adjacent to the metacarpal bases.

NATURAL HISTORY

- The natural result of an untreated fracture-dislocation is progressive arthritis of the involved joints. This occurs due to progressive subluxation of the joint(s) and articular incongruity (**FIG 4A–D**).

PATIENT HISTORY AND PHYSICAL FINDINGS

- The patient's history is important to assess the mechanism of injury, which provides further clues regarding concomitant injuries in the extremity.
- Examine the hand for tenderness and local swelling.
- Assess neurovascular integrity, especially function of the deep motor branch of the ulnar nerve (first dorsal interosseous contraction).
- Examine the limb for other injuries.
- Associated injuries should be detected by examination and verified by radiographs.
- Preoperative notation of nerve function is important when comparing function following reduction and fixation.

IMAGING AND OTHER DIAGNOSTIC STUDIES

- Radiographs of the CMC joints require careful positioning to assess each joint.
  - The transverse metacarpal arch causes the CMC joints of the index and middle fingers to appear in an oblique projection when a standard posteroanterior (PA) radiograph is obtained of the ring and small finger CMC joints and vice versa (**FIG 5A**).

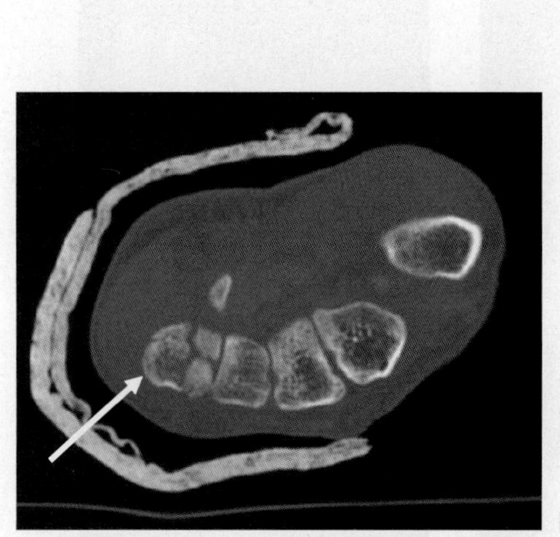

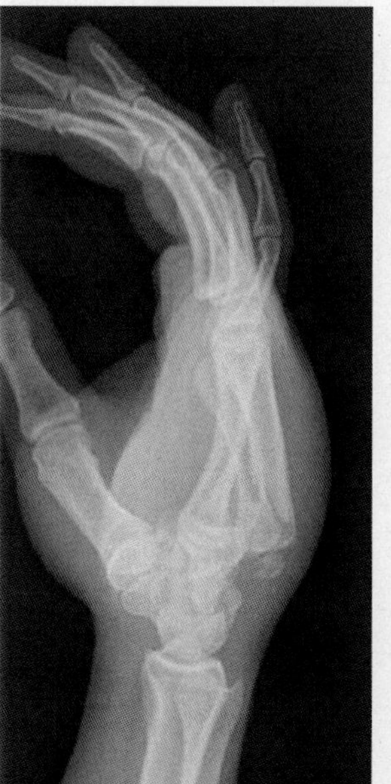

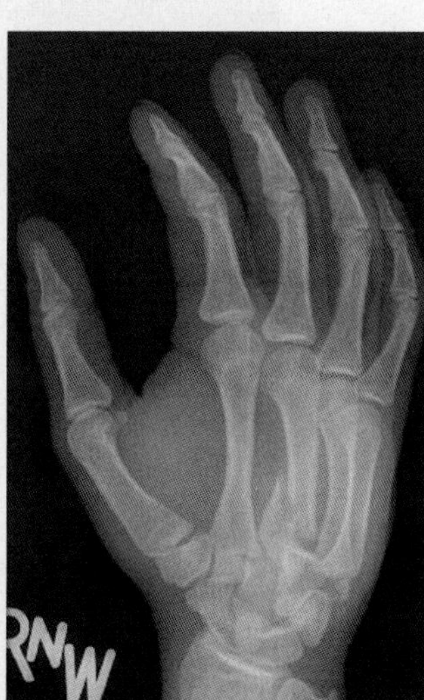

FIG 3 • **A.** Comminuted fracture of the fifth metacarpal base. *Arrow* indicates comminution of small finger metacarpal base. **B,C.** Multiple fractures and dislocations involving the ulnar side of the hand.

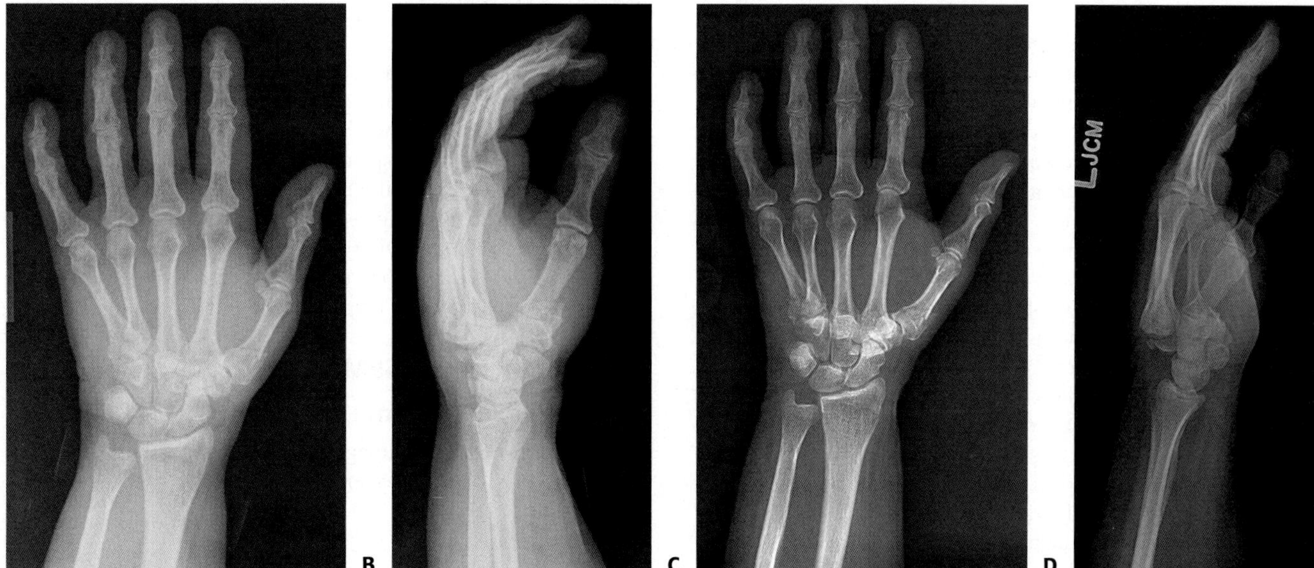

FIG 4 • **A.** PA radiograph demonstrating subluxation of index through small finger metacarpal bases and thumb metacarpal fracture. **B.** Lateral radiograph of subluxated metacarpals. **C.** PA radiograph of same patient demonstrating complete dislocation 2 weeks after injury. **D.** Lateral view demonstrating dislocation.

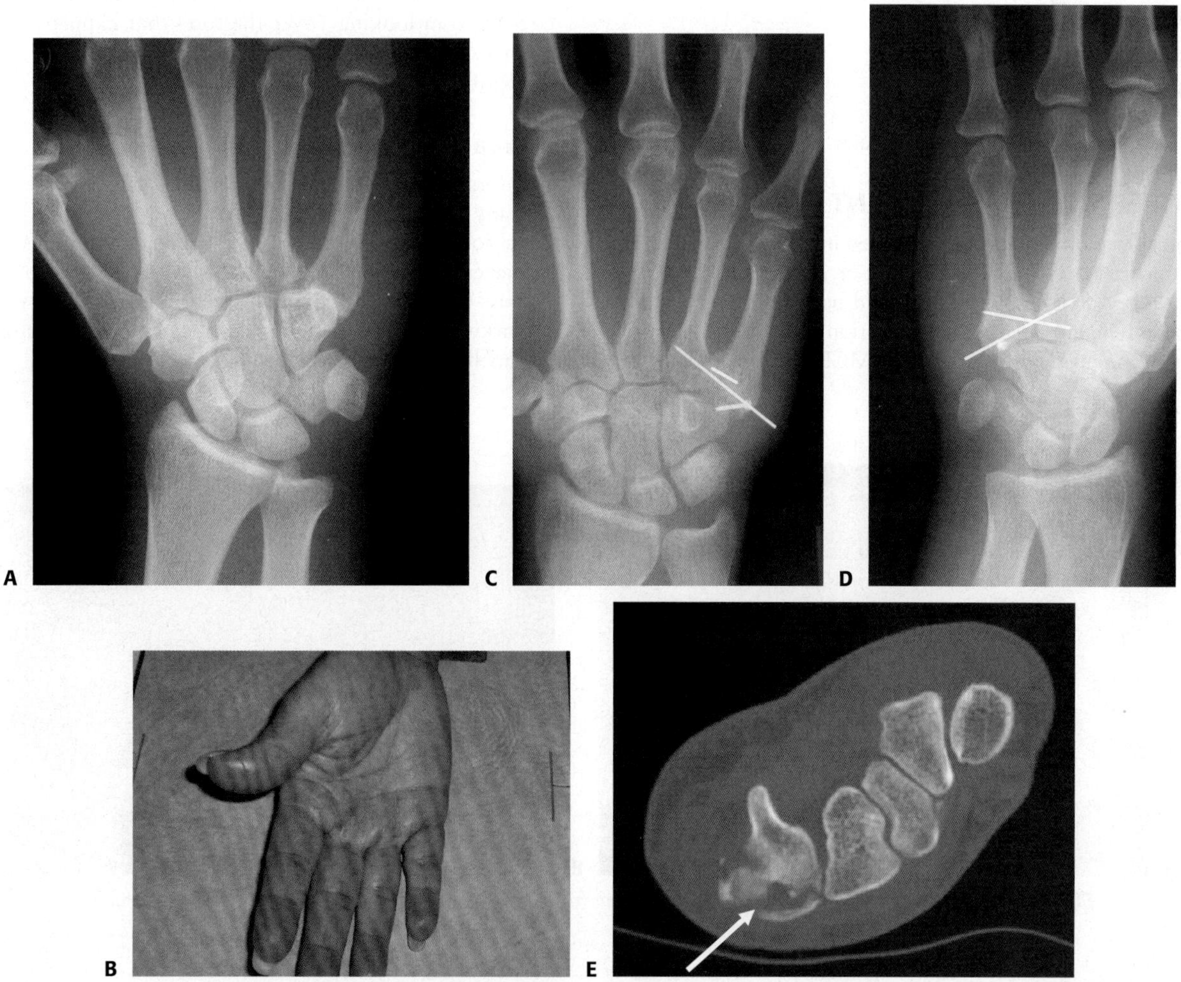

FIG 5 • **A.** A conventional PA view of the hand creates an oblique view of the ring and small finger bases. **B.** Hand properly positioned for AP view of the ring and small finger CMC joints. **C.** Postoperative PA film after open reduction with internal fixation of the ring and small finger CMC joints. **D.** AP projection clearly shows the joint reduction in the same patient shown in **C**. **E.** CT scan of the fracture of the dorsal lip of the hamate. *Arrow* indicates hamate comminution and displacement of dorsal lip fragment.

- A true frontal radiograph is most easily obtained by positioning the hand in an anteroposterior (AP) projection with the dorsum of the hand placed flat on the cassette (or image intensifier, if using fluoroscopy). The base of the affected metacarpal should lie on the cassette (**FIG 5B**). This will result in a far more accurate portrayal of the joint, essential for assessing the fracture as well as checking hardware position after fixation.
- Visualization of the joint surfaces at the base of the ring and small fingers differs in a typical PA projection (**FIG 5C**) and a properly positioned film of the same patient (**FIG 5D**).
  - The same principle holds for obtaining lateral radiographs. A semisupinated lateral view will best visualize the base of the index and middle CMC joints,[5] and a semipronated lateral view will best show the bases of the ring and small finger CMC joints.[2]
- A computed tomography (CT) scan should be obtained in most cases to assess for articular injury. CT also is especially helpful for visualizing impacted articular surface fragments. The best visualization and determination of fracture patterns will be possible if the scan is obtained after preliminary reduction of any displaced fractures or dislocations associated with a fracture (**FIG 5E**).[10]

DIFFERENTIAL DIAGNOSIS

- Metacarpal fracture
- Carpal bone fracture
- CMC fracture-dislocation
- Fracture associated with neurovascular injury

NONOPERATIVE MANAGEMENT

- Nondisplaced fractures can be treated in a below-elbow cast that incorporates the affected digit or digits and one adjacent digit.[5,9] Special attention should be paid to positioning the hand in an intrinsic-plus position. Capsular contractures of the metacarpophalangeal (MCP) joints can develop relatively rapidly in hands with the MCP joints immobilized in extension.
- Radiographs following cast immobilization should be checked carefully to ensure that no dorsal subluxation is present and should be repeated at weekly intervals for the first 2 weeks to prevent healing in a displaced position.
- These injuries, especially those involving a dislocation, have a known propensity for recurrent dorsal subluxation following reduction. Most will require operative fixation.[2,4,9] Some authors believe nonoperative management does have a role despite intra-articular displacement and shortening.[4,12]

SURGICAL MANAGEMENT

Preoperative Planning

- Careful review of all imaging studies will facilitate planning of fracture fragment exposure and identify sites for internal fixation.

Positioning

- The patient is positioned supine on the operating table with a standard arm table.
- The surgeon often is more comfortable seated on the head side of the arm table. This avoids the neck strain that may result from looking "over the top" that happens when the arm externally rotates and the surgeon is seated on the axilla side of the table (**FIG 6A**).

Approach

- A dorsal extensile approach provides satisfactory exposure of any of the CMC joints.
- Incisions placed between metacarpals allow access to two adjacent joints.
- Cross the wrist with oblique extensions if necessary.
- Marking out the anticipated locations of nearby nerve branches can be helpful (**FIG 6B**).

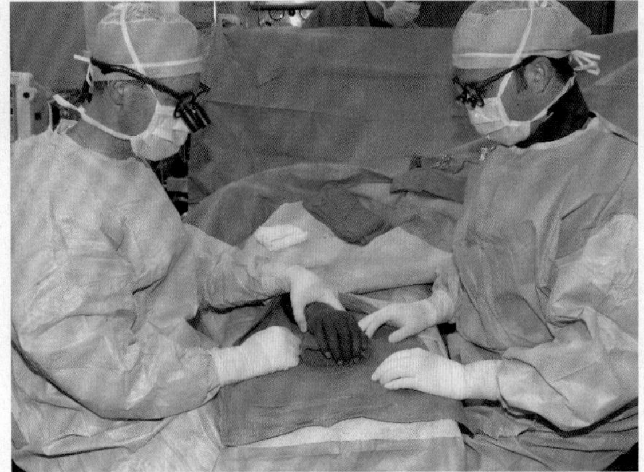

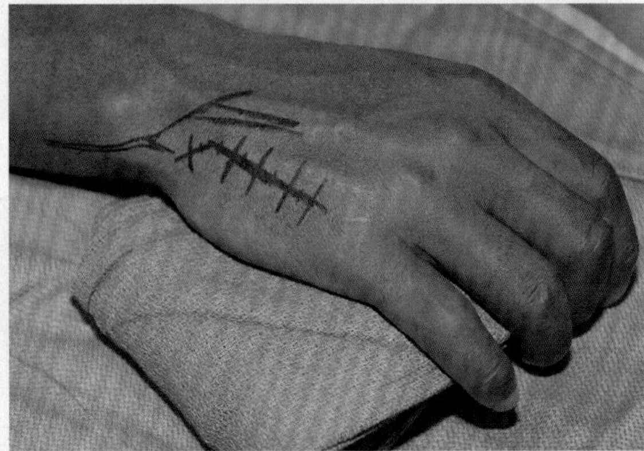

FIG 6 • **A.** Positioning of the surgeon (*left*) and assistant (*right*). **B.** Skin incision marked with probable course of nerve.

Dorsal Exposure

- Following incision of the skin, careful spreading dissection should be used to locate and protect the dorsal cutaneous nerve branches in the operative field.
  - Ulnar sensory nerves are most commonly encountered during exposure of the CMC joints of the ring and small fingers (**TECH FIG 1**) and radial sensory nerves during exposure of the index and middle finger CMC joints.
- Extensor tendons are mobilized and retracted.

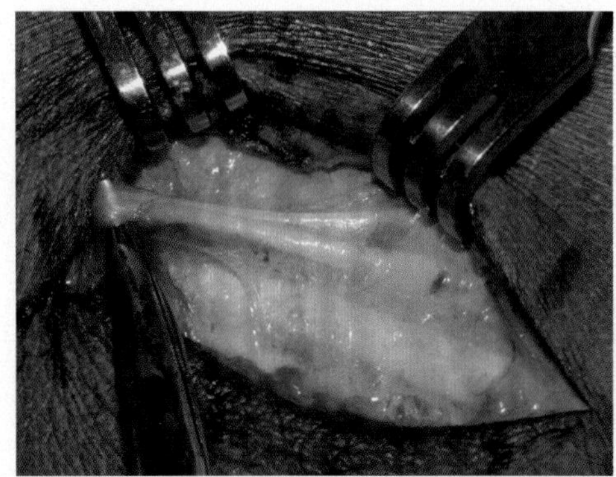

TECH FIG 1 • Dorsal cutaneous branch of the ulnar nerve crossing the incision.

Fracture Exposure

- Careful mobilization of the fracture fragments with minimal soft tissue stripping is important.
- This can be facilitated by the use of a Beaver blade, a dental pick, and a fine synovial rongeur.
  - The rongeur is useful because it is helpful to débride fracture callus and hematoma.

Fracture Reduction

- The fracture is then reduced and held provisionally using fine Kirschner wires (K-wires) (**TECH FIG 2A**). The surgeon must be aware of the planned location for definitive hardware placement, given the limited room available.
  - Pins temporarily driven across the base of an articular fragment into the corresponding carpal bone can be helpful in stabilizing any mobile pieces of bone (**TECH FIG 2B**).
- The conventional technique of first reconstructing the articular surface, followed by securing the shaft to the reassembled joint surface, is useful.
  - Confirmation of the provisional reduction should be obtained with fluoroscopy before any definitive screw placement (**TECH FIG 2C**).
- The corresponding articular surface on the uninjured bone is used as a mold for the fragments, serving as a guide to reassembly of the injured bone.
  - This technique works regardless of whether the injury is in the metacarpal base, as pictured in these figures, or in a distal articular injury of one of the carpal bones (**TECH FIG 2D**).

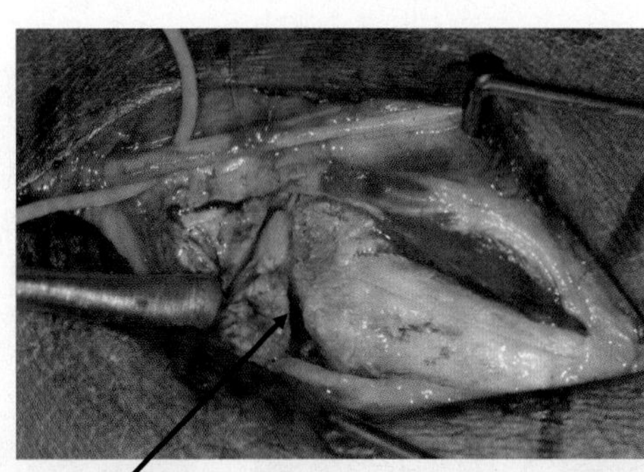

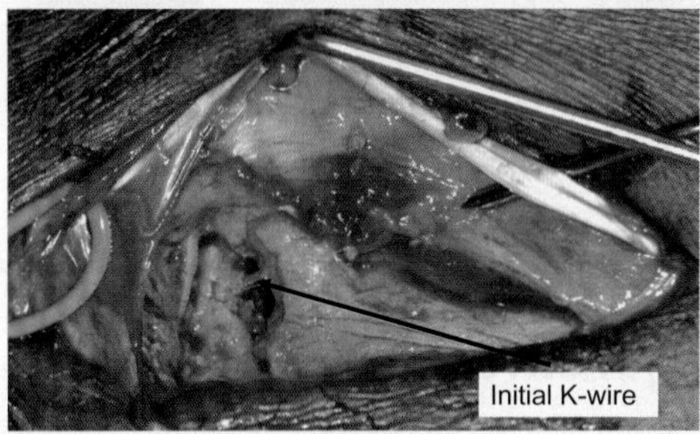

TECH FIG 2 • **A.** Provisional fracture reduction using the hamate surface as a mold for articular reduction of the metacarpal base. **B.** Initial reduction of the shaft and stabilization of the articular surface. *(continued)*

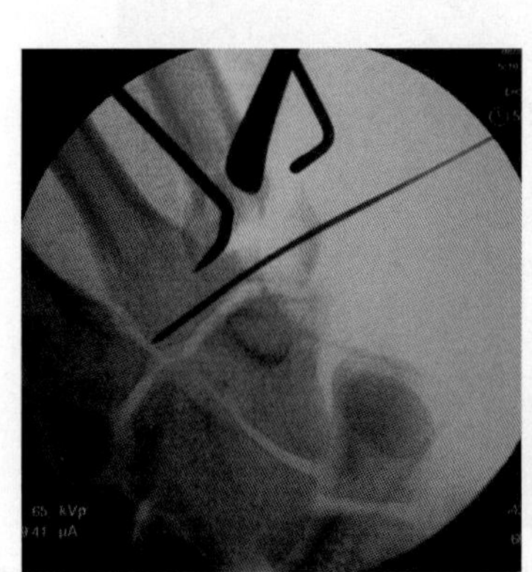

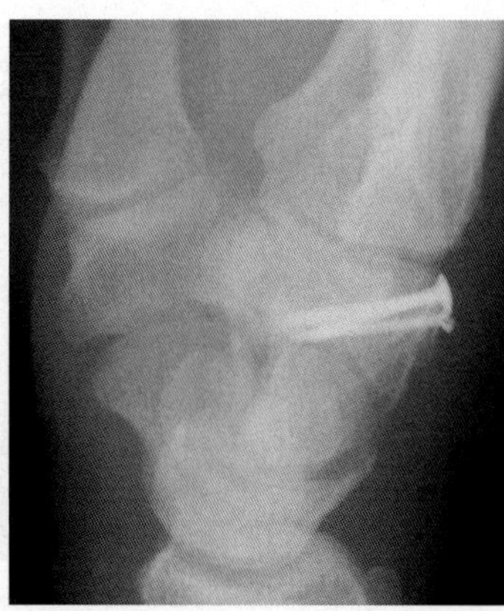

TECH FIG 2 • *(continued)* **C.** Fluoroscopic view of articular reduction. **D.** Dorsal hamate lip fixation with three screws.

Definitive Fixation

- Wires can be replaced by screws if fragment size permits (**TECH FIG 3A**).
  - Placing the fragments under compression manually and inserting screws sometimes is preferable to using the lag screw technique, which requires overdrilling the near side and may risk iatrogenic comminution.
- Simple K-wire fixation is satisfactory for isolated dislocations with fracture (**TECH FIG 3B**).
  - The insertion point for a percutaneous wire often is quite distant from the dislocation site in crushed and severely swollen hands.

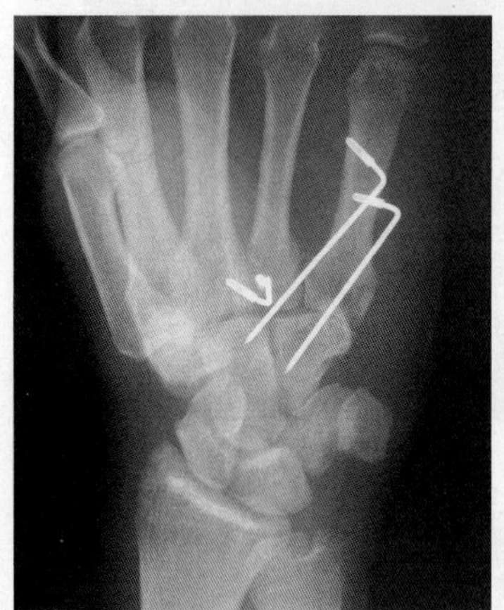

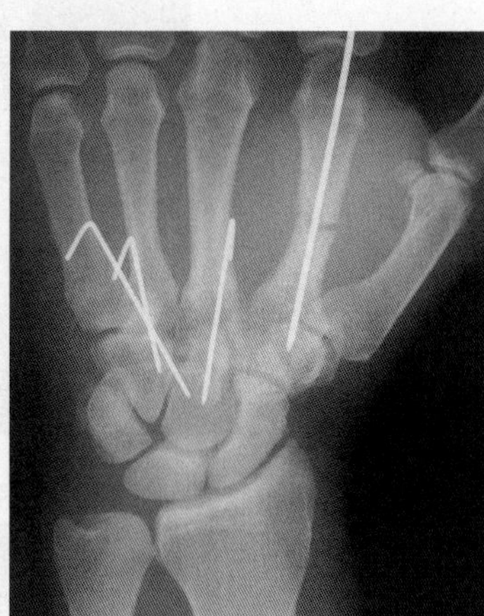

TECH FIG 3 • **A.** Fracture-dislocation of the ring and small finger metacarpal bases using pins and a screw. **B.** Percutaneous K-wire fixation of a metacarpal shaft fracture and CMC dislocation.

Adjunctive Techniques

- The construct can be protected by placing the affected metacarpal under slight distraction and pinning it to the adjacent metacarpal.
- Alternatively, the proximally directed deforming force of the extensor carpi ulnaris can be reduced by detaching it from the base of the small finger metacarpal at the beginning of the procedure and securing it to the hamate at the close, thereby avoiding proximal pull on the base of the small finger metacarpal.
  - I have never found it necessary to use this alternative approach, but it may be helpful in a delayed presentation, where myostatic contractures due to shortening are present.

PEARLS AND PITFALLS

Imaging	■ Ensure that adequate radiographs are available for intraoperative review. ■ If necessary, obtain a CT scan.
Positioning	■ It is often easier for the surgeon to be seated on the outside of the hand table, instead of in the axilla between the table and patient, due to the limited internal rotation present in the shoulder, which can make visualization difficult from the usual seating position.
Exposure	■ The dorsal cutaneous branch of the ulnar nerve crosses the incision obliquely and lies immediately across the operative field for exposure of the fourth and fifth CMC joints. Cutting this nerve often is associated with very symptomatic neuromas, although the sensory deficit is well tolerated.
Fracture management	■ Fragments can be small, and periosteal stripping can result in devitalization. Use fracture lines for visualization of the articular surface as much as possible. A dental pick, fine K-wire joysticks, and provisional fixation before final screw insertion can be helpful. Provisional fixation should be done with careful attention to the anticipated location of definitive fixation. Avoid malrotation of the shaft during reduction by grasping it together with one or two adjacent metacarpals when aligning it relative to the joint. Small degrees of malrotation at the base of the metacarpal can result in substantial distal overlap of the digits.
Postoperative protection	■ Consider placing a temporary distraction K-wire between adjacent metacarpals to limit the load placed on the articular surface before it has healed.

POSTOPERATIVE CARE

- Aftercare following operative fixation falls into three general phases: acute swelling control and wound healing (10 to 14 days), fracture consolidation and maintenance of digit range of motion (4 to 6 weeks), and restoration of global hand function and strength (2 to 6 months).
- Immediate measures following surgery include strict elevation and range-of-motion exercises through a full arc of motion.[4] This limits swelling, reduces pain, and prevents accumulation of protein-rich edema fluid that will slow rehabilitation.
- The relative speed at which the hand can be mobilized during the weeks after surgery depends on a number of factors, including the magnitude of the original injury, stability of fixation, reliability of the patient, and specific occupational or athletic needs.
- The radiograph in **TECH FIG 2D** shows the hand of a physician with stable fixation of a dorsal hamate injury who was mobilized and given a 1-pound lifting restriction shortly after surgery to allow continuation of his residency training.
  - In contrast, unreliable patients require immobilization for 6 weeks in a cast (see **TECH FIG 3B**).
- Patients should be warned that full grip strength is the last thing that will recover and may take months.[2] It is not uncommon for patients to report pain with a handshake for an extended period of time.

OUTCOMES

- Opinions on outcomes vary with regard to overall success. A dichotomy exists between recommendation for operative and nonsurgical treatment. Kjaer-Petersen and colleagues[6] found that, regardless of treatment, long-term symptoms were present in 38% of patients at 4.3 years of follow-up.
- Petrie and Lamb,[12] who used immediate, unrestricted motion, reported on results at 4.5 years. Even with metacarpal shortening and irregularities in the articular surface, only one patient had work limitations.
- Another study found that pain was related to the degree of posttraumatic arthritis secondary to articular incongruity and advocated anatomic reduction and internal fixation.[11]
- Multiple CMC dislocations were reviewed by Lawliss and Gunther,[7] and poor results were noted in dislocations of the second and third CMC joints (which require higher energy for dislocation) and in those patients with an ulnar nerve injury.

COMPLICATIONS

- Complications include those common to any periarticular surgery:
  - Failure of wound healing
  - Hematoma formation
  - Neurovascular injury
  - Neuroma formation
  - Tendon adhesions
  - Posttraumatic arthritis
  - Nonunion or malunion
  - Joint stiffness
  - Weakness
- Occasionally, small fragments may resorb, leading to collapse and articular incongruity (**FIG 7**).
- Long-term arthritis can be treated with fusion of the affected joint.[4]

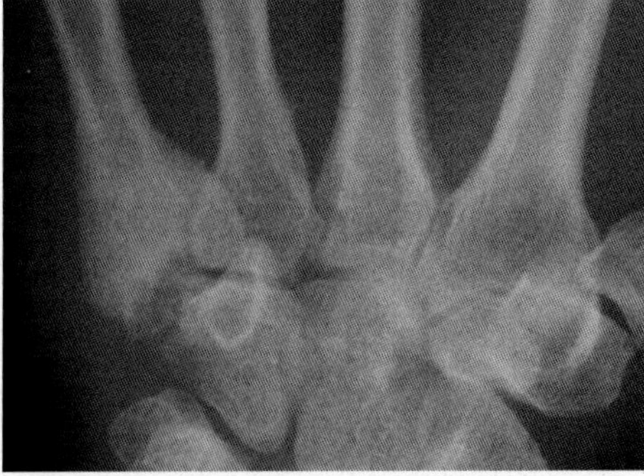

FIG 7 • Radiograph taken several months following K-wire fixation of a fracture-dislocation of the fifth CMC joint. Fragments were too small for screw fixation and were resorbed.

- Alternatively, an interposition "anchovy" using the palmaris longus as a biologic spacer can be inserted after resection of the arthritic joint surfaces, analogous to that performed for thumb basal joint arthritis.[3]
- A recent report described using a proximal interphalangeal (PIP) joint silicone implant as an interposition spacer in the fifth metacarpal–hamate interspace for three patients with chronic arthritis of the fifth CMC–hamate joint.[13] The follow-up was extremely short (mean 20 months), and the known propensity for silicone implant fracture over time will determine whether this is a satisfactory long-term solution for patients with this form of arthritis.

REFERENCES

1. Bergfield TG, DuPuy TE, Aulicino PL. Fracture-dislocations of all five carpometacarpal joints: a case report. J Hand Surg Am 1985;10:76–78.
2. Bora FW Jr, Didizian NH. The treatment of injuries to the carpometacarpal joint of the little finger. J Bone Joint Surg Am 1974;56:1459–1463.
3. Gainor BJ, Stark HH, Ashworth CR, et al. Tendon arthroplasty of the fifth carpometacarpal joint for treatment of posttraumatic arthritis. J Hand Surg Am 1991;16:520–524.
4. Glickel SZ, Barron OA, Catalano LW. Dislocations and ligament injuries in the digits. In: Green DP, Hotchkiss RN, Pederson WC, et al, eds. Green's Operative Hand Surgery, ed 5. Philadelphia: Churchill Livingstone, 2005:364–366.
5. Hsu JD, Curtis RM. Carpometacarpal dislocations on the ulnar side of the hand. J Bone Joint Surg Am 1970;52:927–930.
6. Kjaer-Petersen K, Jurik AG, Petersen LK. Intra-articular fractures at the base of the fifth metacarpal: a clinical and radiographical study of 64 cases. J Hand Surg Br 1992;17:144–147.
7. Lawliss JF III, Gunther SF. Carpometacarpal dislocations. J Bone Joint Surg Am 1991;73:52–59.
8. Lilling M, Weinberg H. The mechanism of dorsal fracture dislocation of the fifth carpometacarpal joint. J Hand Surg Am 1979;4:340–342.
9. Lundeen JM, Shin AY. Clinical results of intraarticular fractures of the base of the fifth metacarpal treated by closed reduction and cast immobilization. J Hand Surg Br 2000;25:258–261.
10. Marck KW, Klasen HJ. Fracture-dislocation of the hamatometacarpal joint: a case report. J Hand Surg Am 1986;11:128–130.
11. Papaloizos MY, Le Moine PH, Prues-Latour V, et al. Proximal fractures of the fifth metacarpal: a retrospective analysis of 25 operated cases. J Hand Surg Br 2000;25:253–257.
12. Petrie PW, Lamb DW. Fracture-subluxation of the base of the fifth metacarpal. Hand 1974;6:82–86.
13. Proubasta IR, Lamas CG, Ibañez NA, et al. Treatment of little finger carpometacarpal posttraumatic arthritis with a silicone implant. J Hand Surg Am 2013;38(10):1960–1964.

Operative Treatment of Metacarpal Fractures

48

CHAPTER

José M. Nolla

DEFINITION

- Hand metacarpals can fracture at their base, shaft, neck, or head. Such fractures can lead to shortening, rotation, or angulation.
- Metacarpals provide a base for each finger and injury to a metacarpal can severely compromise independent digital function.
- Treatment strategy for metacarpal injuries must consider the ability of the human hand to compensate for such injuries.

ANATOMY

- The thumb metacarpal (first) is highly independent and is stabilized by its carpometacarpal (CMC) joint and supporting muscles.
- The other four metacarpals (second to fifth) are tightly connected through the CMC joints proximally and the deep transverse metacarpal ligaments distally. These ligaments connect the volar plate and head of each metacarpal to the adjacent metacarpal. The ligaments also have a significant role in preventing shortening and rotation of fractures of the central (third to fourth) metacarpals (**FIG 1**).
- The thumb metacarpal has a round cross-sectional shape, whereas the other metacarpals tend to have a triangular shape with a dorsal, anterolateral, and anteromedial facets (**FIG 2A**).
- The dorsal and volar interosseous muscles cover the ulnar and radial surfaces of each metacarpal (see **FIG 2A**). These muscles provide blood supply to the metacarpals but are also at risk of contracture in cases of injury leading to severe hand edema and compartment syndrome.
- The deep palmar arch and the deep branch of the ulnar nerve lie just volar to the metacarpals and are at risk during fracture and surgery.
- On either side of the metacarpal head, there are fossae and tubercles that create a recess from which the collateral ligaments of the metacarpophalangeal (MP) joint arise (**FIG 2B**).
- The extensor tendons lie just superficial to the base and shaft of each metacarpal. At the level of the metacarpal head, they contribute to the dorsal extensor apparatus of each finger (see **FIG 2B**).

PATHOGENESIS

- Axial load is the most common injury mechanism for a metacarpal fracture. Due to the normal curvature of the fifth metacarpal, such an axial load will include a bending

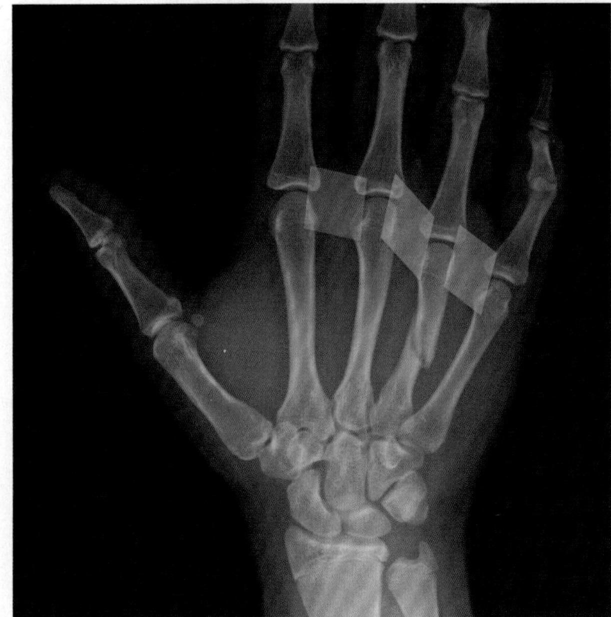

FIG 1 • The deep transverse metacarpal ligaments (*shaded yellow*) protect the fractured metacarpal from excessive shortening and rotation.

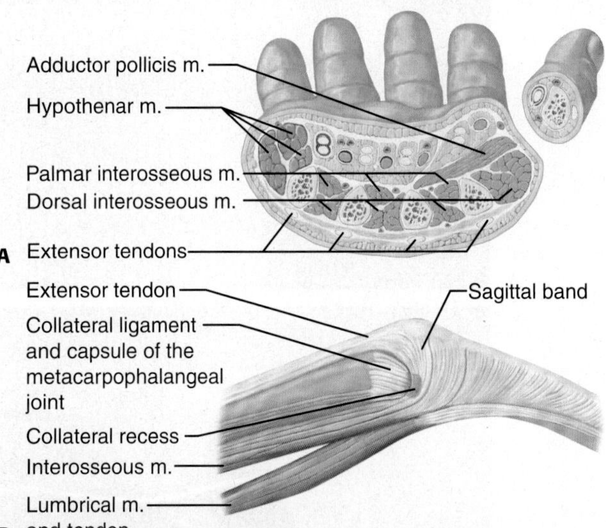

FIG 2 • **A.** The metacarpals have a triangular shape. The interosseous muscles cover the radial and ulnar surfaces of the metacarpals. The extensor tendons are in close proximity to the dorsal surface. **B.** The dorsal apparatus covers the MP joint. The extrinsic extensor tendons extend the MP joint and the intrinsic tendons flex it.

component and lead to an apex dorsal fracture at the neck, also known as a *boxer's fracture* (**FIG 3A**).

- Axial loads may also be transmitted proximally on the metacarpal and lead to a CMC fracture-dislocation.
- Torsional injuries will lead to spiral oblique fractures (**FIG 3B**).
- Bending injuries from direct impact may lead to short oblique or transverse metacarpal fractures (**FIG 3C**). The addition of butterfly fragments and comminution is dependent on a combination of additional loads.
- Crush injuries can lead to comminuted fractures with significant soft tissue injuries and a heightened risk of compartment syndrome (**FIG 3D**).

NATURAL HISTORY

- Metacarpal fractures are mainly affected by shortening and rotation. The effect of these two components is minimized in the central metacarpals due to the stabilizing effect of

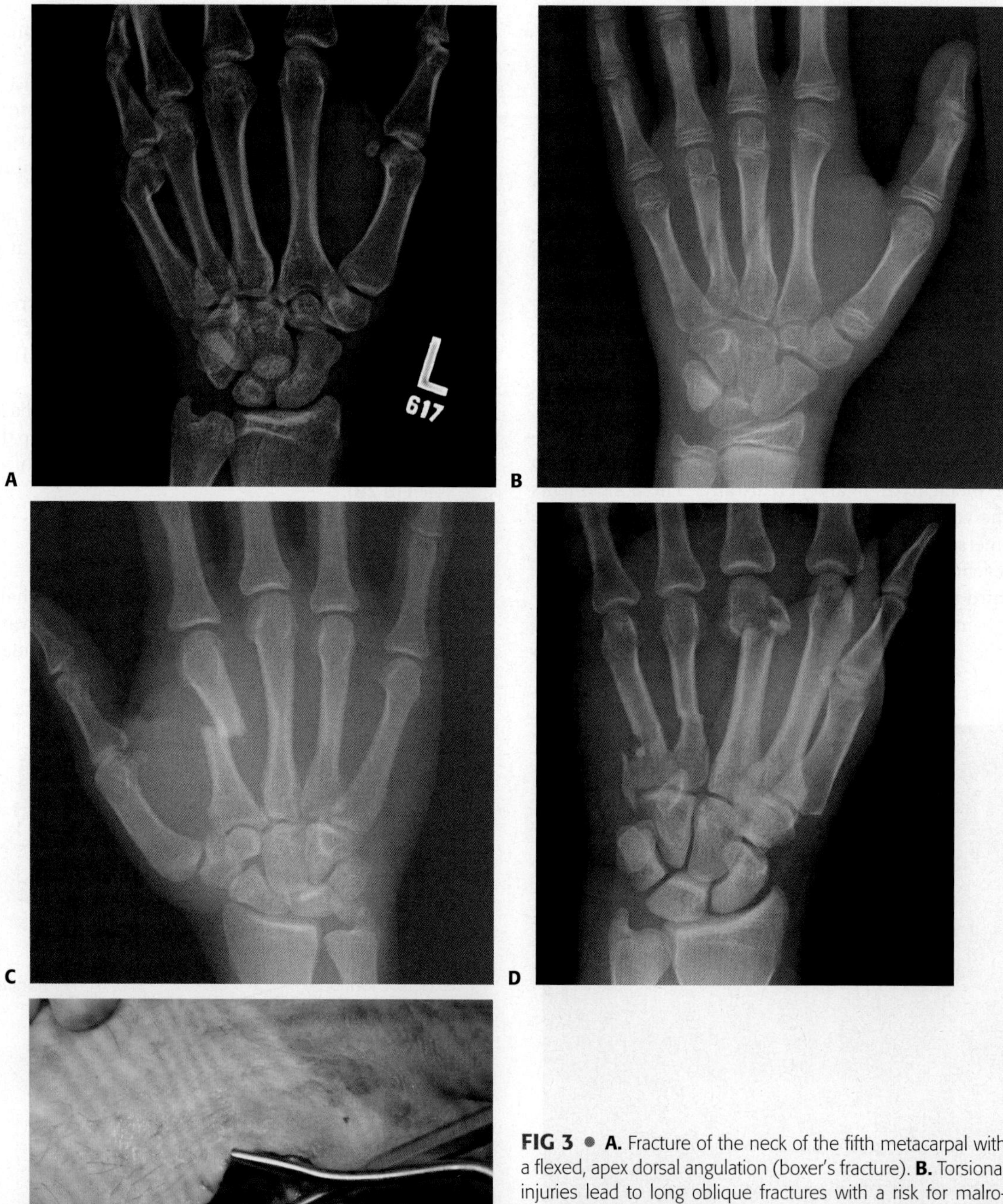

FIG 3 • **A.** Fracture of the neck of the fifth metacarpal with a flexed, apex dorsal angulation (boxer's fracture). **B.** Torsional injuries lead to long oblique fractures with a risk for malrotation. **C.** Short transverse fracture from a direct impact. **D.** Crush injuries can lead to a combination of injuries with an increased risk of compartment syndrome and significant stiffness. The shortened fourth metacarpal pulls the head of third metacarpal in a proximal and ulnar direction through deep transverse metacarpal ligament. **E.** Neglected fight bite injury ultimately leading to loss of the metacarpal head.

the deep transverse metacarpal ligaments and the bordering intact metacarpals. This stabilizing effect is lost in cases of multiple metacarpal fractures and more severe injuries (see **FIG 3D**).
  - Shaft fractures of the third and fourth metacarpals tend to do well with minimal intervention. Border metacarpals are more prone to shortening and rotation.
- Every 2 mm of shortening of the metacarpal can lead to a 7-degree lag at the MP joint.[12]
- Fractures of the metacarpal neck typically result in apex dorsal angulation, which may lead to significant shortening. The increased mobility afforded by the ulnar CMC joints allows more tolerance of angulation in the ulnar metacarpals (fourth and fifth). Whereas some have accepted up to 70 degrees, most authors have recommended intervention if the angulation exceeds 30 to 40 degrees.[4,6,9] The radial metacarpals (second to third) have stiffer CMC joints, and correspondingly, the tolerance for angulation is reduced to only 10 to 15 degrees.[7]
- Thumb metacarpal extra-articular base and shaft fractures can easily tolerate 30 degrees of angulation due to its highly mobile CMC joint.[1]
- Fractures of the metacarpal head with a significant gap or step-off, or fractures that involve a significant portion of the articular surface, should be considered for open reduction and stabilization.[2]

PATIENT HISTORY AND PHYSICAL FINDINGS

- History: Note the mechanism of injury, time since injury, and any treatment received so far. Also, note the age, vocation, and hobbies of the patient. Comorbidities should also be recorded.
- Inspection: The skin needs to be checked for any signs of an open fracture. A small laceration near the MP joint may be the only sign of a "fight bite" injury which requires urgent débridement to prevent joint and bone infection (**FIG 3E**). Also, note digit malrotation and extension lag at the MP and proximal interphalangeal (PIP) joints. A severely edematous hand may signal compartment syndrome or an internal degloving injury.
- Palpation: The neurovascular examination should include checking activation of the first dorsal interosseous muscle to confirm activity of the motor branch of the ulnar nerve. Tense compartments and pain with passive motion may signal a developing compartment syndrome.

IMAGING AND OTHER DIAGNOSTIC STUDIES

- The posteroanterior (PA) view can show shortening, especially relative to the adjacent metacarpals. Fracture angulation can be seen on the lateral view but is often best seen on the oblique view. Fractures of the base of the fifth metacarpal are best seen on the pronated oblique view.
- Specialized views of the metacarpal head can show the volar aspect (Brewerton) or the dorsal aspect (skyline).
- Traction views in the anesthetized patient may help elucidate pattern and extent of injury.
- Computed tomography (CT) scan can help in extensively comminuted fractures or articular injuries.

DIFFERENTIAL DIAGNOSIS

- Open fractures
- Fight bite with bacterial inoculation of the MP joint
- Pathologic fractures

NONOPERATIVE MANAGEMENT

- Shaft fractures that are not displaced and not angulated can be treated with a brief period of immobilization followed by protected activities. Those with angulation of greater than 20 degrees (30 on the small finger) deserve an attempt at closed reduction (**FIG 4A**).
- Acute (<7 to 10 days), isolated fourth or fifth metacarpal neck fractures angled more than 30 to 40 degrees benefit from reduction and immobilization. Only 15 degrees should be accepted for the second or third metacarpals. A dorsally directed force can be applied to the head of the metacarpal through the Jahss maneuver (**FIG 4B**) or directly on the metacarpal head (**FIG 4C**).
- The position of the MP joint during immobilization for treatment of fifth metacarpal neck fractures has not been

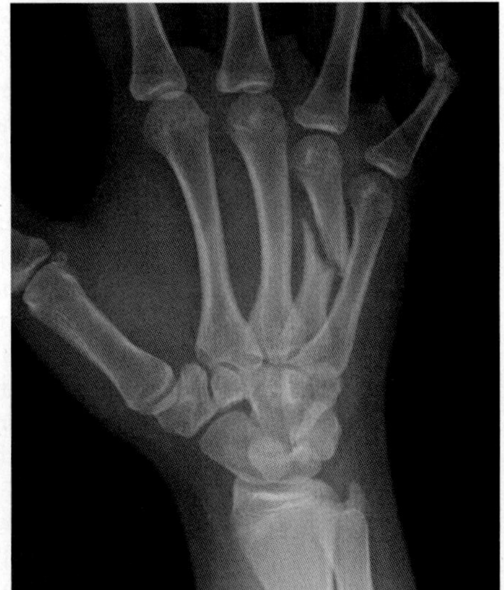

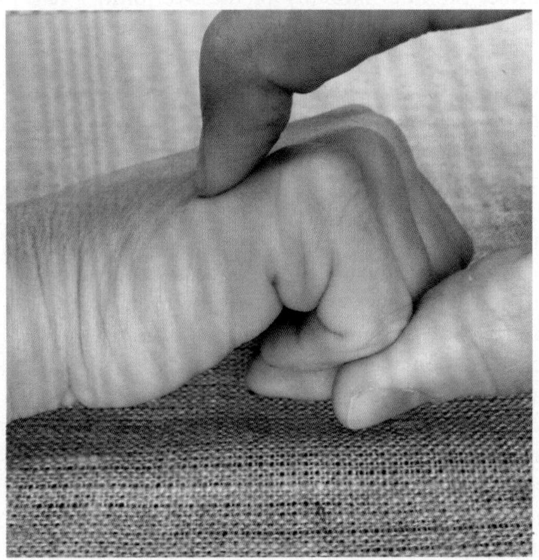

FIG 4 • **A.** Angled metacarpal shaft fractures deserve an attempt at closed reduction. **B.** Jahss maneuver. A dorsally directed force is applied to the flexed PIP joint while the metacarpal is stabilized proximally. *(continued)*

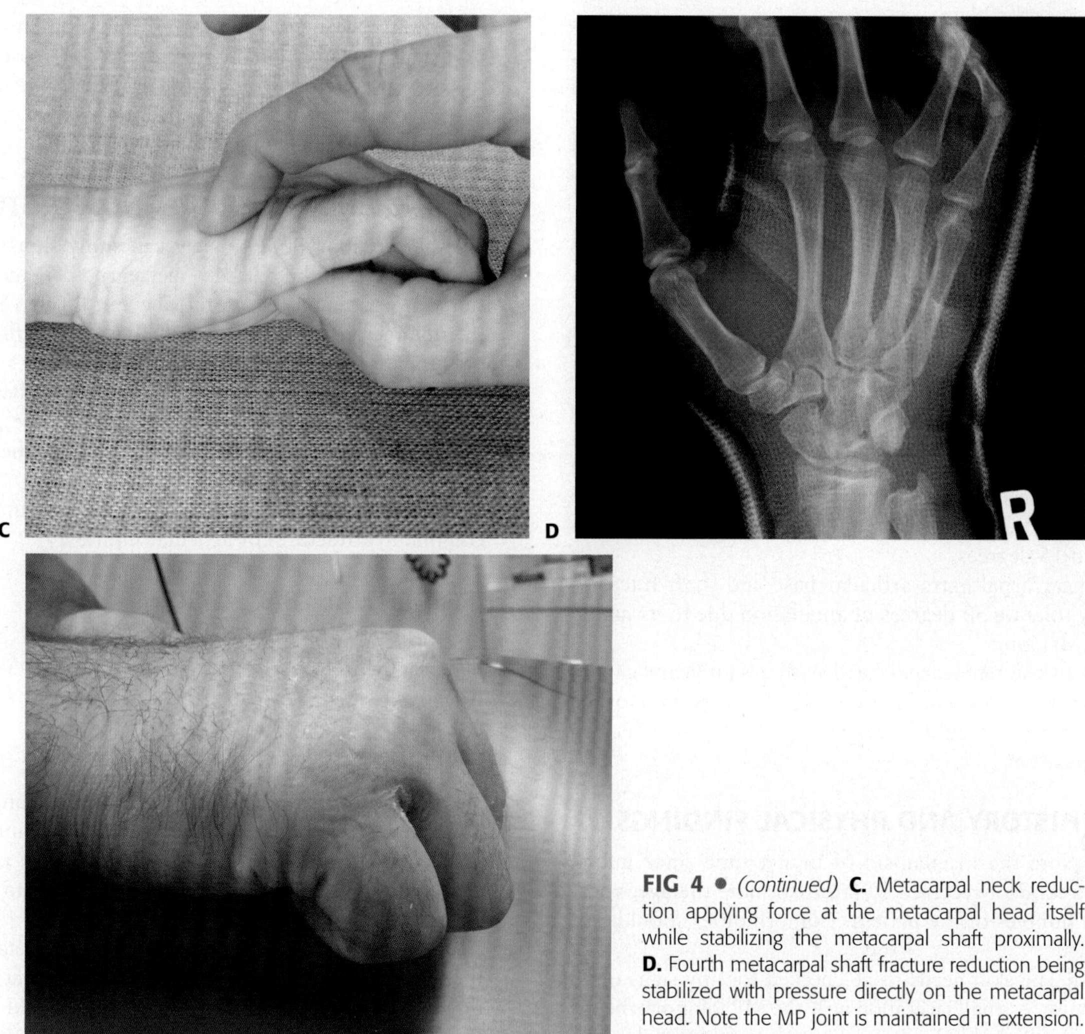

FIG 4 • *(continued)* **C.** Metacarpal neck reduction applying force at the metacarpal head itself while stabilizing the metacarpal shaft proximally. **D.** Fourth metacarpal shaft fracture reduction being stabilized with pressure directly on the metacarpal head. Note the MP joint is maintained in extension. **E.** MP flexion on the day of cast removal after being casted for 4 weeks.

shown to affect the final mobility of the MP joint.[14] It is often easier to immobilize the MP joint in extension while applying direct pressure on the metacarpal head (**FIG 4D,E**).[5]

- Be aware that prolonged immobilization of MP joints in extension may lead to collateral ligament contracture and result in difficulty regaining MP flexion.

SURGICAL MANAGEMENT

- Indications for surgery include open fractures, open joint injuries (such as fight bites), malrotated fractures, unstable fractures, and those associated with other injuries that need surgery such as tendon or nerve lacerations.
- Relative indications for surgery include extensor tendon lag, metacarpal shortening, prominence of the metacarpal head in the palm, multiple metacarpal fractures, and intra-articular fractures.
- Contraindications for internal fixation include grossly contaminated fractures and infirmed patients.
  - Contaminated fractures should be débrided and temporarily stabilized until definitive fixation can be performed.
- Percutaneous pins have the advantage of minimizing soft tissue injury. However, the fracture must be reducible through closed means.
- Percutaneous pins can be placed in a retrograde direction from distal to proximal entering the metacarpal through the collateral recesses. This technique allows stabilization of proximal neck or shaft fractures. Flexion of the MP joint facilitates access to the collateral ligament recesses.
- Antegrade pin fixation (bouquet pinning) from proximal to distal can provide stability to shaft and neck fractures. This technique has the advantage of avoiding the MP joints altogether, which, if enough stability is present, may even permit early motion. In the treatment of neck fractures, it may lead to less MP stiffness compared to retrograde (collateral recess) pinning.[10] However, placement of the antegrade wires can be more challenging technically.
- There are many occasions when the fracture cannot be easily reduced through closed techniques and open approach is required. Such an approach allows for an anatomic reduction and placement of stable fixation. However, it also introduces a degree of soft tissue insult.

- Screws provide rigid fixation while at the same time minimizing implant bulk. However, they are appropriate only for long oblique or spiral fractures whose lengths are at least twice the diameter of the bone at the level of the fracture.
- Plates provide rigid fixation in short oblique and transverse fractures but require significant soft tissue dissection. Rarely, the hardware will have to be removed once the fracture is healed.
- External fixators allow treatment of more complex fractures while minimizing soft tissue injury but do not allow precise control of the fracture fragments. External fixation may be desirable in the treatment of injuries with massive soft tissue disruption.

Preoperative Planning

- The fracture itself and its character will dictate much of the approach to the fracture. However, respect of the soft tissue is of utmost importance.
- Crush injuries with significant degloving of the soft tissues may be best managed with limited or percutaneous approaches to limit further embarrassment of the tissue envelope.
- Grossly contaminated wounds, or those with tenuous soft tissues, may be best managed initially with limited fixation until more definitive fixation can be performed (**FIG 5A**).
- Bone grafting may also need to wait until the soft tissues have stabilized (**FIG 5B**).
- The need to address nerve, vessel, or tendon injuries may also affect the approach (**FIG 5C**).

Positioning

- Most hand fractures are addressed with the patient supine and the hand on a hand table. Concomitant injuries or conditions may affect access to the hand.
- Regional or general anesthesia is most commonly used for metacarpal fractures. Local anesthesia may be appropriate in some circumstances.

Approach

- Most fractures are approached dorsally due to the proximity of the bone to the skin and the ease of handling the extensor tendons and dorsal sensory nerves. The border metacarpals may also be approached through their respective subcutaneous borders to further minimize soft tissue insult.

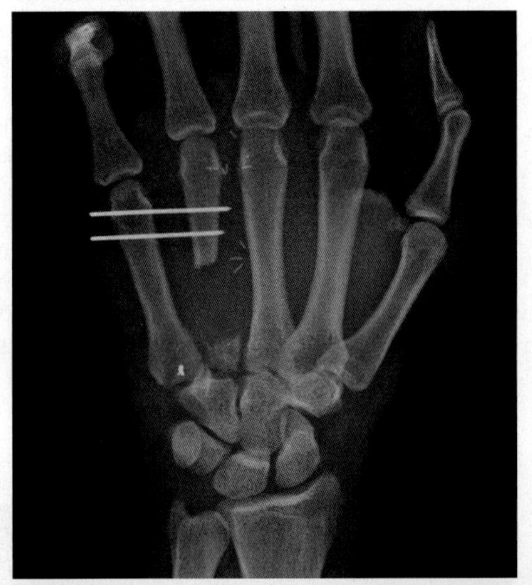

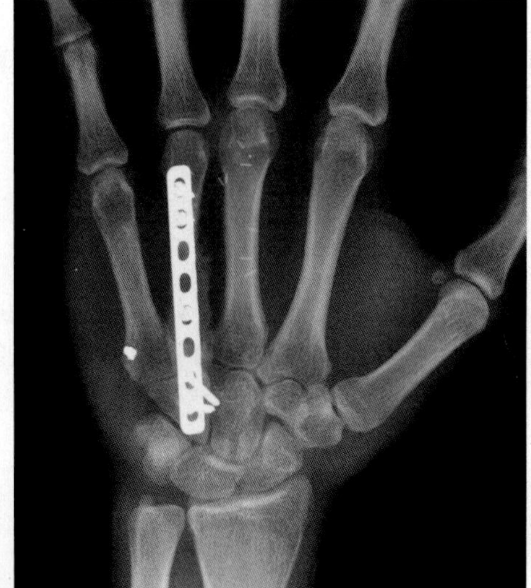

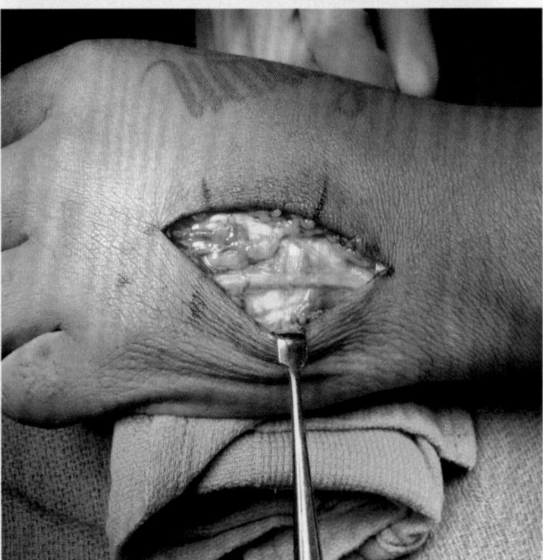

FIG 5 • **A.** Missing fourth metacarpal shaft and base after gunshot wound. Patient had tenuous dorsal skin. Metacarpal head temporarily stabilized with buried pins from fifth metacarpal. **B.** Once the soft tissues stabilized, the metacarpal was grafted from the iliac crest and stabilized with plate and screws to the hamate. **C.** Dorsal sensory branch of the ulnar nerve travelling through the center of the wound on a different patient.

- Dorsal incisions provide excellent exposure of the dorsal aspect of the metacarpals. The incision is best made to the side of the metacarpal, on its border, to minimize extensor tendon irritation. In case of adjacent fractures, the incision is made between the metacarpals. A proximal incision provides access to the base of the metacarpal for percutaneous pinning and a distal incision can give access to the head of the metacarpal. The extensor tendons are retracted to either side for base and shaft fractures.
- A dorsal approach to the head and neck will often require division of the juncturae tendinum, which should be repaired at the end of the procedure. If the MP joint must be exposed, the extensor tendon is best split longitudinally. In the case of the index finger, the split is made between the extensor digitorum communis (EDC) and extensor indicis proprius (EIP). For the small finger, the exposure will be between the EDC and extensor digitorum minimi (EDM) (**FIG 6**).
- Coronal shear fractures of the head and neck may require a volar approach. A volar longitudinal incision is made similar to a trigger finger incision. The A1 pulley is opened. The approach is extended proximally and the flexor tendons are retracted to reveal the neck of the metacarpal.

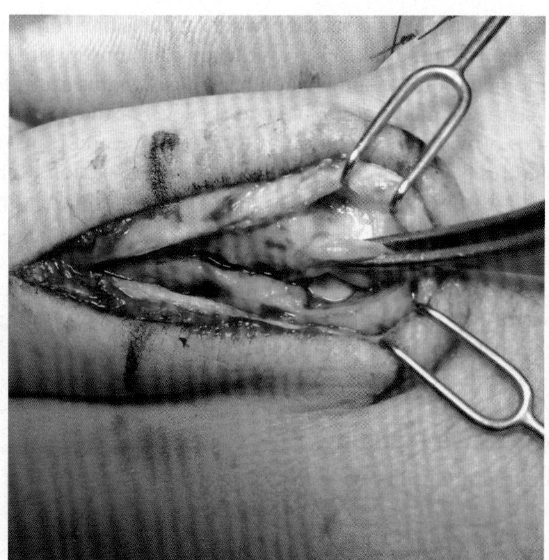

FIG 6 • Dorsal approach to the MP joint of an index finger. Extensor tendon beneath top retractor. Capsule grabbed by pickup forceps. Articular cartilage seen deep to capsule.

TECHNIQUES

Closed Reduction and Pin Fixation of Metacarpal Fractures

Retrograde Collateral Recess Pinning

- Retrograde fixation (**TECH FIG 1A**) can be used in proximal and some distal metacarpal shaft fractures (**TECH FIG 1B,C**).
- The MP joint is flexed 70 to 90 degrees, and a 0.035 to 0.045 smooth Kirschner wire (K-wire) is inserted through the skin and the collateral recess into the distal metacarpal. The position of the wire is confirmed with fluoroscopy.
- The fracture is anatomically reduced using closed means which can include three-point bend, traction, and rotation.
- The wire is advanced into the neck, across the fracture, to the base of the metacarpal while maintaining the reduction. A second wire is placed through the opposite recess in a similar manner (**TECH FIG 1D,E**).
- The K-wires are either cut below the skin (author's preference) or left external, and the hand is immobilized with a forearm-based splint with the MP joint in 70 to 90 degrees of flexion while allowing motion of the interphalangeal (IP) joints.
- The pins are removed at 4 weeks and a motion program is instituted. A removable splint is used for an additional 2 weeks.

A

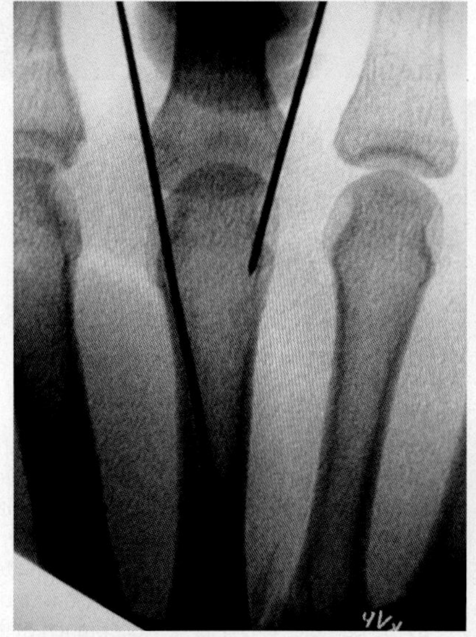

B

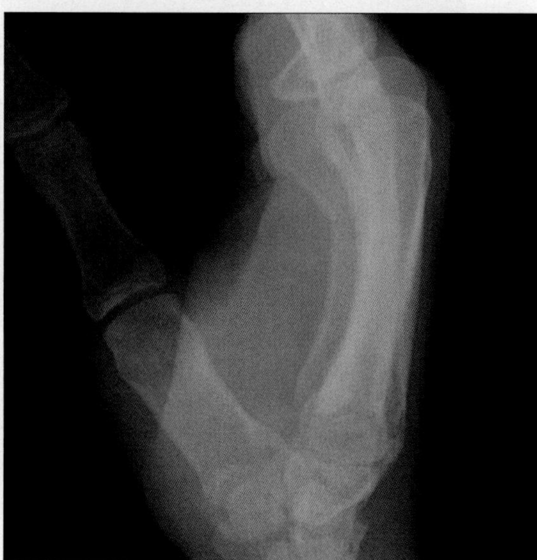

TECH FIG 1 • **A.** Retrograde (collateral recess) pinning. **B,C.** Angled distal metacarpal fracture. *(continued)*

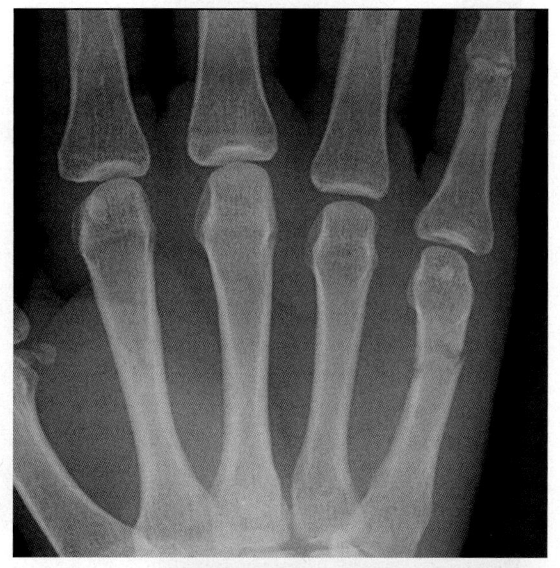
C

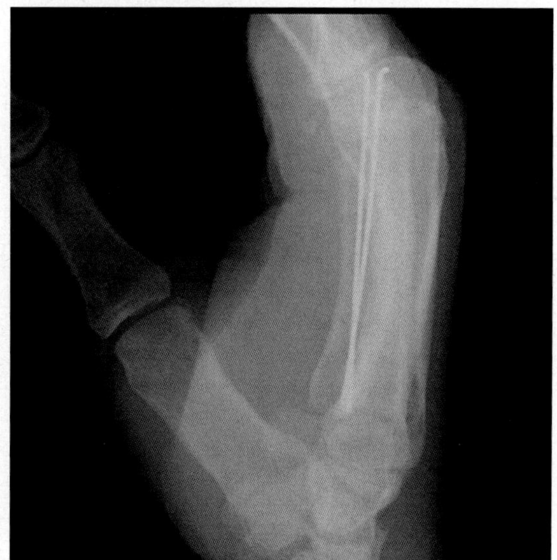
D

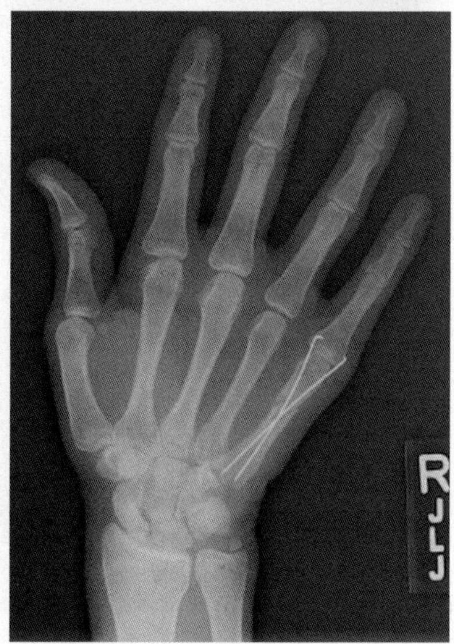

E

TECH FIG 1 • *(continued)* **D,E.** Fracture stabilized with two pins that have been advanced to the base of the metacarpal. (Copyright Thomas R. Hunt III, MD, DSc.)

Antegrade Bouquet Pinning

- This technique requires a rotationally stable fracture that can be reduced through closed means (**TECH FIG 2A**).
- An incision is made at the base of the metacarpal. Careful dissection is carried through the soft tissues protecting the cutaneous nerve branches. The extensor tendons are retracted and the metaphysis of the base of the metacarpal is exposed.
  - In the case of a fifth metacarpal, it is easier to make this approach straight ulnar as opposed to dorsal (**TECH FIG 2B**).
- A unicortical 2.7- or 3.5-mm tunnel is made with a drill. This tunnel is created angled in a proximal to distal direction (**TECH FIG 2C**).
  - Commercially available sets include an awl that helps in establishing the tunnel through which the definitive fixation is placed.
- Two or three prebent wires (**TECH FIG 2D**) are then advanced through the tunnel, across the fracture, and lodged into the metacarpal head subchondral bone (**TECH FIG 2E**).
  - Great care must be exercised advancing the wires to prevent them from penetrating through the opposite cortex.
  - The wires can be advanced with a needle holder or a pin holder using some gentle oscillation.
- The hand is initially immobilized in a forearm-based splint with the MP joint in 70 to 90 degrees of flexion while allowing some motion of the IP joints.
  - If stable fixation is accomplished early, MP joint motion is initiated. The affected finger can be buddy taped to the adjacent finger to avoid rotational forces across the fracture.
- The wires may be removed after 4 weeks or, if cut at the level of the bone, they may be left in place indefinitely.

Transverse Pinning

- Transverse wires are sometimes necessary because the medullary canal of the metacarpal is too small to accommodate intramedullary wires (**TECH FIG 3A**).
- This technique can be used to stabilize distal metacarpal base and shaft fractures that have an adjacent intact metacarpal. It

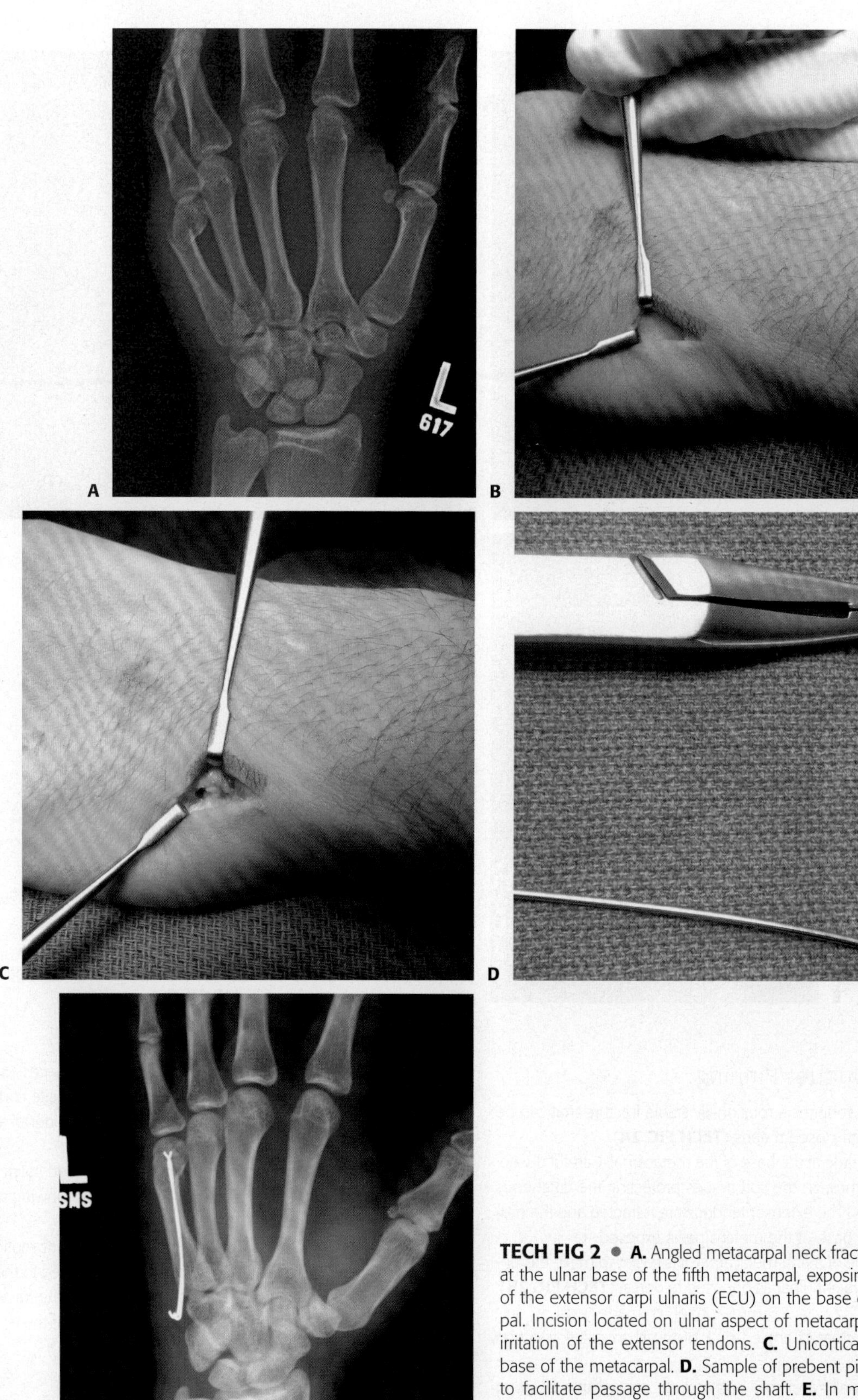

TECH FIG 2 • **A.** Angled metacarpal neck fracture. **B.** Incision at the ulnar base of the fifth metacarpal, exposing the insertion of the extensor carpi ulnaris (ECU) on the base of the metacarpal. Incision located on ulnar aspect of metacarpal to minimize irritation of the extensor tendons. **C.** Unicortical tunnel at the base of the metacarpal. **D.** Sample of prebent pin. Tip is angled to facilitate passage through the shaft. **E.** In metacarpal neck fractures or those at risk of shortening, it is important to bring the pins to the subchondral bone of the metacarpal head but not violate the head.

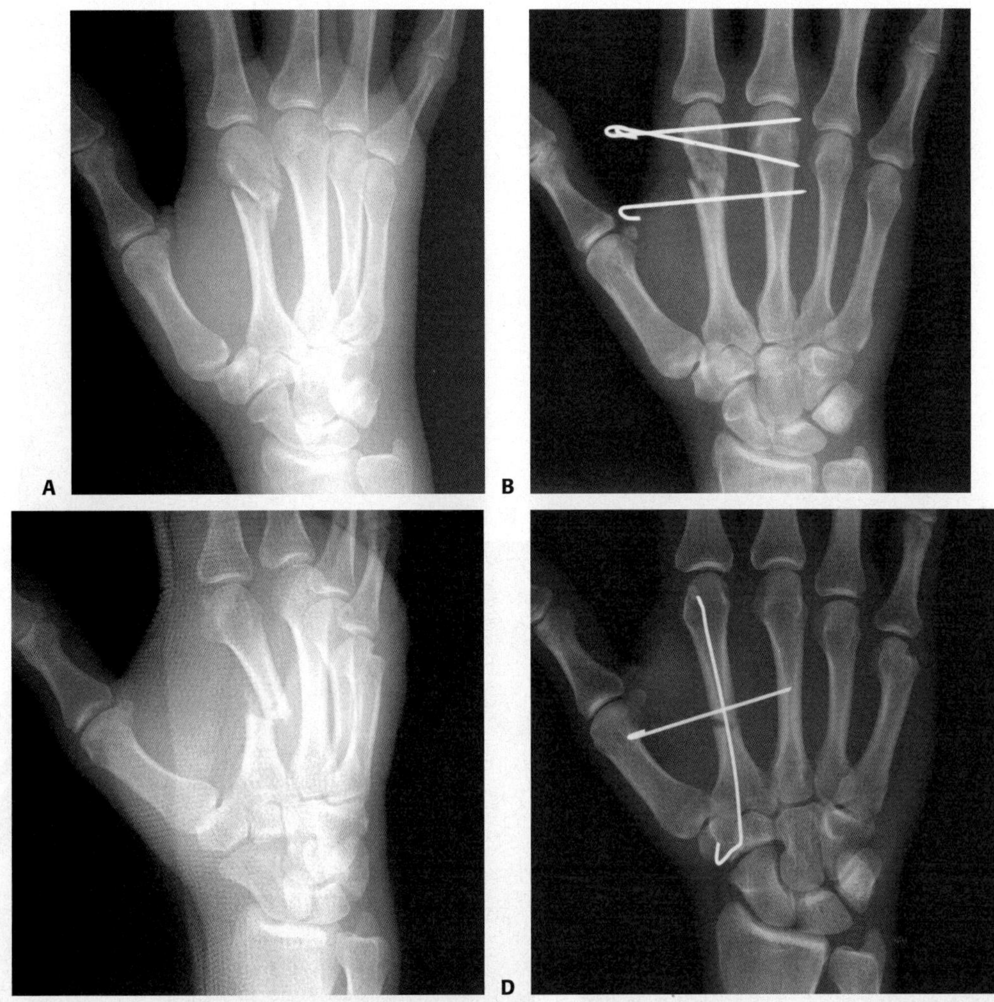

TECH FIG 3 • **A.** Second metacarpal fracture with an intact adjacent metacarpal and a narrow medullary canal. **B.** Fixation using one proximal pin to secure the shaft and two distal pins to secure the distal fragment. **C,D.** Fracture where the narrow medullary space made it difficult to pass a second wire through the canal. Supplemental fixation achieved through a transverse pin on the distal fragment.

is appropriate for border metacarpals with enough intact distal (or proximal) metacarpal to accommodate two distal wires.

- The fracture is anatomically reduced through closed means.
- The proximal fragment is first stabilized by pinning it to the adjacent intact metacarpal.
  - Use the nick and spread technique while placing the wires to minimize the risk of iatrogenic cutaneous nerve injury.
  - Keep pressure between the adjacent metacarpals to prevent convergence between the metacarpals as the wire is advanced.
  - Be mindful of the arch-like arrangement of the metacarpals.
- The distal fragment is stabilized by placing two wires through the distal fragment into the adjacent intact metacarpal (**TECH FIG 3B**).
- The hand is immobilized in a forearm-based splint with the MP joints flexed 70 to 90 degrees while the pins are in place. The pins are kept for 3 to 4 weeks. The IP joints are left free to move.
- The pins are removed at 3 to 4 weeks, and the hand is placed in a removable splint for an additional 2 weeks.
- Alternatively, transverse pins can be used to augment other forms of fixation or control rotation (**TECH FIG 3C,D**).

Open Reduction and Plate/Screw Stabilization of Metacarpal Fractures

Dorsal Approach for Fixation

- Fractures that cannot be reduced through closed means require an open approach (**TECH FIG 4A–C**).
- A longitudinal incision is made parallel and adjacent to the metacarpal. If two metacarpals are fractured, the incision can be made between the metacarpals.
- The sensory nerve branches are protected. The extensor tendons are retracted. If a junctura tendinum is in the area of the fracture, it can be divided but should be repaired at the end of the procedure.

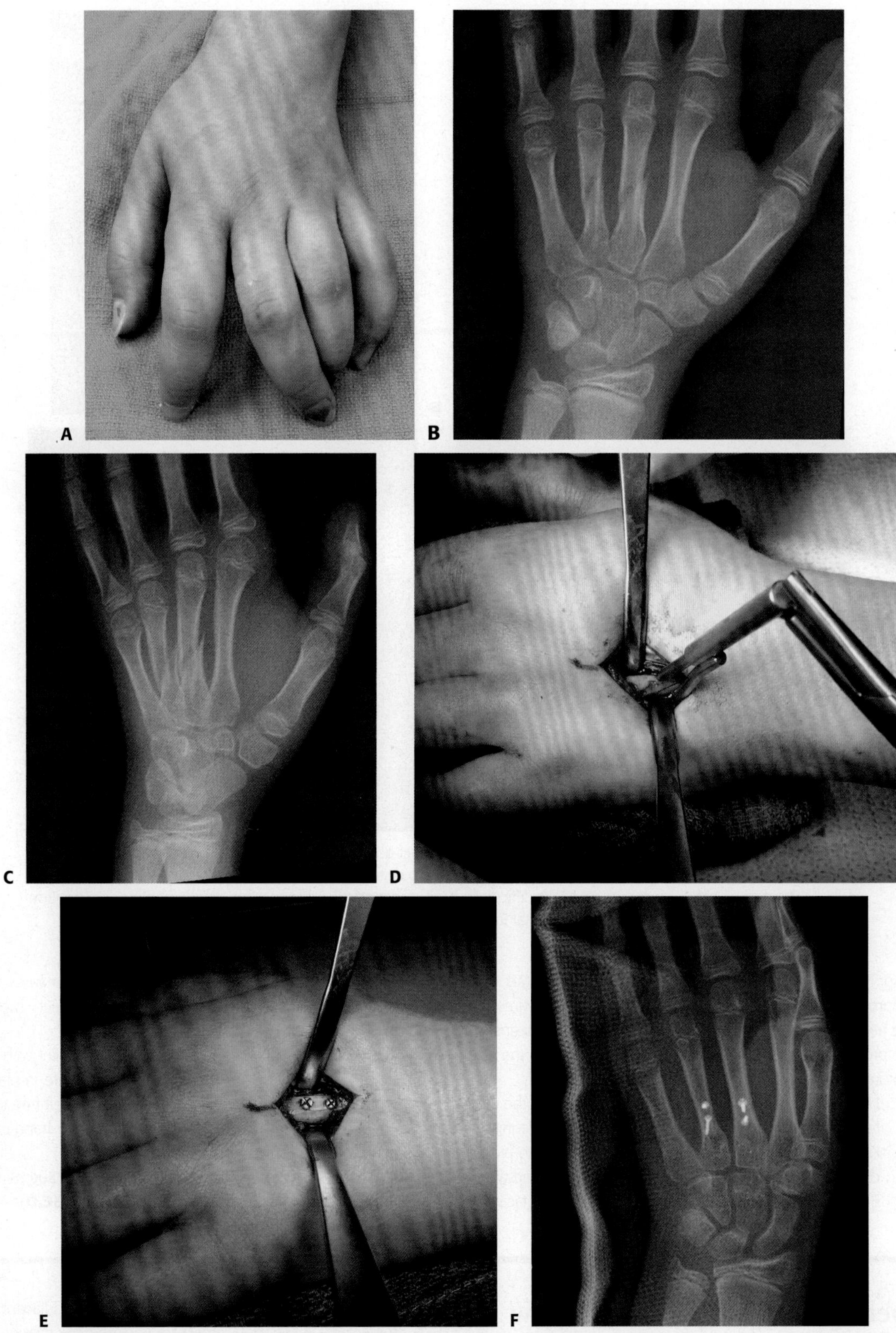

TECH FIG 4 • A–C. Patient with torsional injury to long and ring fingers leading to spiral fractures of the third and fourth metacarpals. The combined injury made it possible for malrotation to develop. **D.** Reduction is maintained with a reduction clamp. **E,F.** Fracture stabilized with 1.5-mm screws. One screw is perpendicular to the fracture to compress fracture and the other is perpendicular to the metacarpal to stabilize axial loads. *(continued)*

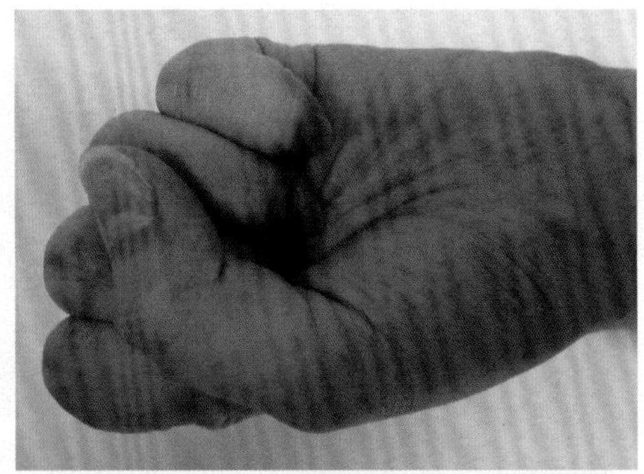

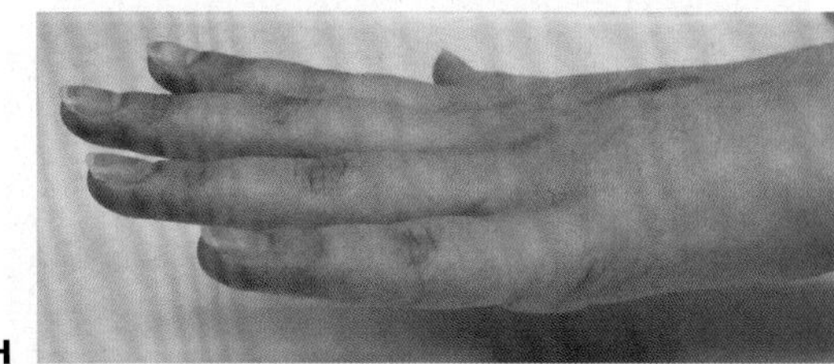

TECH FIG 4 • *(continued)* **G,H.** Motion at 6 weeks after surgery.

- The periosteum is elevated at the fracture site to assist with assessment of fracture reduction. As much of the interosseous muscle is left attached to the metacarpal as feasible to preserve blood supply to the bone.
- The fracture is reduced and provisionally stabilized with reduction clamps (**TECH FIG 4D**).

Lag Screw Fixation

- Long oblique and spiral fractures whose lengths are at least twice the diameter of the bone at the level of the fracture are amenable to limited fixation with screws only (see **TECH FIG 4A–C**).
- Appropriately sized lag screws (1.4 to 2.7 mm) are placed. Typically, two or three screws are used (**TECH FIG 4E,F**).
- The first screw is placed perpendicular to the fracture in order to compress it and the second screw is placed perpendicular to the bone to resist longitudinal forces.
- In order to get proper compression with a lag screw construct, it is important to overdrill the near cortex.
  - When using a 2.0-mm screw system, a 1.5-mm drill bit is used to drill both cortices.
  - The near cortex is then overdrilled with a 2-mm drill bit.
  - A countersink is used to maximize contact between the head of the screw and the bone.
  - The size of the screw is measured and an appropriately sized screw is placed.
- The periosteum and interosseous muscle fascia are reapproximated to cover the screws.
- The juncturae tendinum are repaired and the skin is closed in standard fashion.
- The hand is then immobilized with the MP joints flexed 70 to 90 degrees with a forearm-based splint. Early motion can be started as early as 4 to 7 days, depending on fracture stability (**TECH FIG 4G,H**).

Plate and Screw Fixation

- Short oblique and transverse fractures that require an open reduction are well stabilized with plates and screws.
  - Short oblique fractures are most often treated using a neutralization plate combined with lag screws (**TECH FIG 5A–D**).
  - Transverse fractures benefit from compression plating (**TECH FIG 5E,F**).
- Using the approach detailed earlier, the fracture is exposed and the periosteum is elevated at the fracture site to assist with the fracture reduction.
- The fracture is then provisionally stabilized with a reduction clamp or wires.

Short Oblique Fractures

- In the case of a short oblique fracture, the fracture is stabilized using the lag screw technique mentioned earlier. A neutralization plate is added for additional stability (see **TECH FIG 5C,D**).
  - Typically, 2.0- to 2.7-mm plates and screws are used (see **TECH FIG 5D**).
  - The plate should be prebent into a slight concave configuration to accommodate the normal curvature of the metacarpal and to provide mild compression when indicated.
  - The fixation should include at least two bicortical screws on either side of the fracture.
  - When drilling in a dorsal to volar direction at the base of metacarpals, it is important to very carefully drill the opposite cortex. The motor branch of the ulnar nerve is in the vicinity and can be injured. Using the drill in the oscillating mode can help prevent such injuries.
  - In some cases, the lag screw may be placed through a hole in the plate depending on fracture configuration and plate placement.
- The plate is first secured to one fragment with one or two centrally drilled bicortical screws.
- Two additional screws are then placed in the opposite fragment.
  - If the fracture has already been compressed through a lag screw, these final screws can be placed centrally in the plate holes in a static mode (see **TECH FIG 5C,D**).
- Fracture fixation is completed once at least two bicortical screws are placed on either side of the fracture.

Transverse Fractures

- Transverse fractures do not provide the opportunity to compress the fracture through lag screws. In such situations, the fracture is compressed using the compression plate technique (see **TECH FIG 5E,F**).
- The plate is bent into a slight concave configuration to allow compression of the far cortex once the plate is secured to

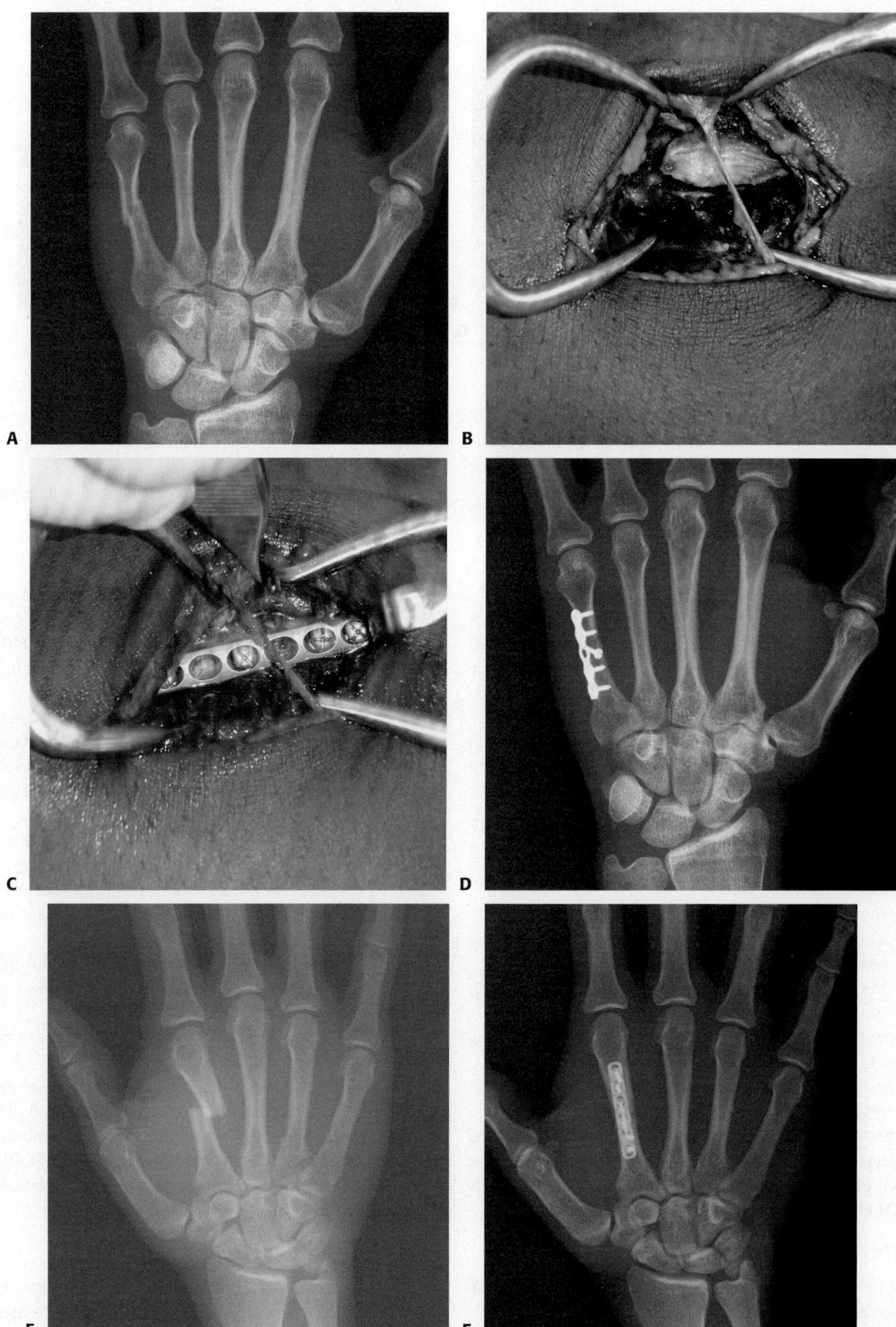

TECH FIG 5 • A,B. Short oblique fracture of the metacarpal. **C,D.** Fracture stabilized with a lag screw and a neutralization plate. **E,F.** Short transverse fracture of the second metacarpal stabilized with a compression plate. (**C,D:** Copyright Thomas R. Hunt III, MD, DSc.)

the bone. It is positioned about the fracture such that at least four cortices of fixation can be obtained both proximal and distal to the fracture.

- The first bicortical screw is placed in one of the screw holes closest to the fracture.
- The second screw is placed on the opposite side of the fracture in the screw hole on that side that is closest to the fracture. This screw is placed in a compression mode.
  - The screw hole is drilled eccentrically in the hole, as far from the fracture as possible.
- The remaining screws may be placed in either a compression or static mode.
- In cases of simple fractures with minimal comminution, nonlocking plates are appropriate, but locking plates may be considered in fractures with osteopenic or missing bone.
- The periosteum is closed over the plate to protect the overlying tendons. The juncturae tendinum are repaired. The skin is closed in a standard fashion.
- A splint in the functional position is applied to maintain the MP joints flexed 70 to 90 degrees for 4 to 7 days. The patient is then able to start a motion program.
- Radiographic confirmation of consolidation of transverse fractures can be delayed in which case clinical judgment has to be made as to when to allow unrestricted activities.

Dorsal Approach with Stabilization of Metacarpal Head Fractures

- Displaced intra-articular fractures can benefit from an open reduction and fixation (**TECH FIG 6A,B**).
- A dorsal approach is performed with a longitudinal incision over the metacarpal head.
  - In the case of the third and fourth metacarpals, the extensor digitorum is split longitudinally.
  - In the case of the second metacarpal, the extensor tendon is split between the fibers of the EDC and EIP.
  - In the case of the fifth metacarpal, the extensor is split between the fibers of the EDC and the EDM.
- The tendon fibers are separated from the underlying capsule. The capsule is split longitudinally and the fracture is exposed (**TECH FIG 6C**).
- The fracture is then visualized and disimpacted.

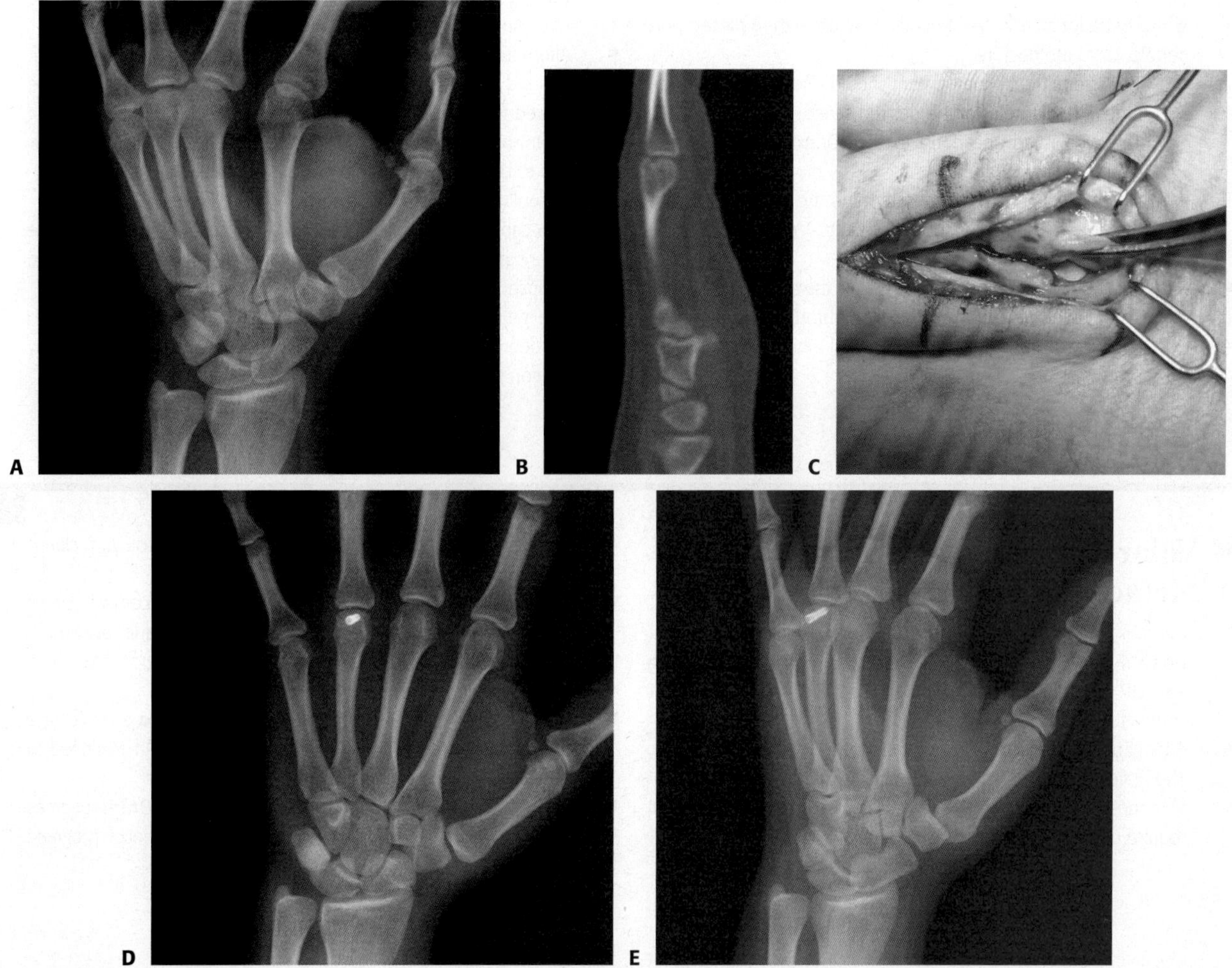

TECH FIG 6 • **A,B.** Intra-articular head fracture of the fourth metacarpal. **C.** Dorsal approach to an MP joint. Extensor tendon beneath top retractor. Capsule grabbed by pickup forceps. Articular cartilage seen deep to capsule. **D,E.** Intra-articular fracture stabilized with headless screws. *(continued)*

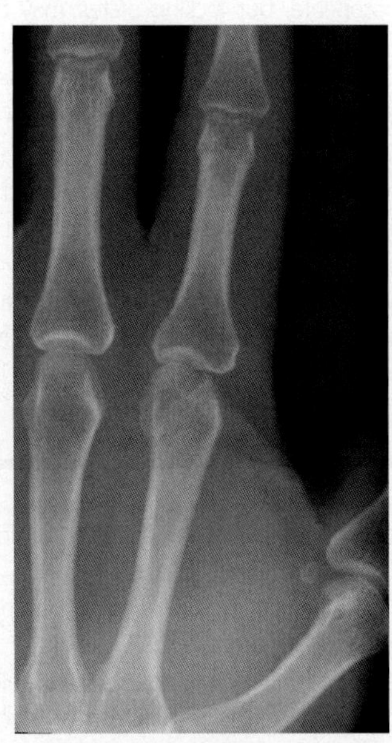
F

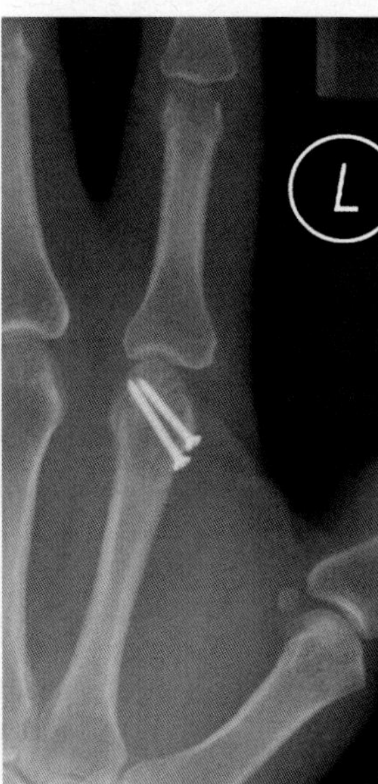

G

TECH FIG 6 • *(continued)* **F,G.** Intra-articular head fracture stabilized with extra-articular screws.

- Once reduction is attained, it is maintained with a reduction clamp.
- A guidewire for a cannulated headless screw is then placed perpendicular to the fracture.
  - The size of the bony fragment should also be at least three times the diameter of the desired screw.
  - The wire is advanced up to the cortex in the opposite fragment.
  - A depth gauge is used to determine the proper length of the screw. The screw should be 2 to 4 mm shorter than the measured length.
- A cannulated drill bit is then used to prepare the track for the screw.
  - The guidewire can be advanced through the opposite cortex to prevent accidental removal while drilling for the screw.
- A properly sized screw is placed across the fracture and advanced beneath the articular surface (**TECH FIG 6D,E**).
  - An additional screw can be placed for increased stability.
- Alternatively, the fracture can be stabilized with traditional-headed screws (1.5 to 2.4 mm) (**TECH FIG 6F,G**). These are placed from the nonarticular portion of the fracture after drilling up to, but not through, the articular surface. If a headed screw has to be placed through the articular surface, it must be countersunk beneath the cartilage.
- The capsule is closed with absorbable suture. The split in the extensor tendon is repaired with nonabsorbable suture. The skin is closed in standard fashion.
- The patient is then splinted with the MP joints flexed 70 to 90 degrees for 4 to 7 days. The patient may then begin an early motion program.

Volar Approach with Stabilization of Metacarpal Head Fractures

- Coronal fractures that extend into the metacarpal neck provide the opportunity to address the fracture without opening the MP joint and therefore minimizing the risk of MP joint contracture (**TECH FIG 7A,B**).
- A longitudinal incision is made on volar aspect of the A1 pulley. The pulley is opened and the flexor tendons are retracted.
- The metacarpal neck and the fracture are exposed. This will require division of the periosteum and volar plate.
- The fracture is reduced and held in place with a reduction clamp or temporary K-wires.
- The fracture is then stabilized with at least two bicortical screws (1.5 to 2.0 mm) using the lag screw technique previously discussed (**TECH FIG 7C,D**).
  - The screws must be countersunk.
- The volar plate and periosteum are then repaired to cover the screw heads. The A1 pulley is left open. The skin is closed in standard fashion.
- The patient is then splinted with the MP joints flexed 70 to 90 degrees for 4 to 7 days. The patient may then begin an early motion program.

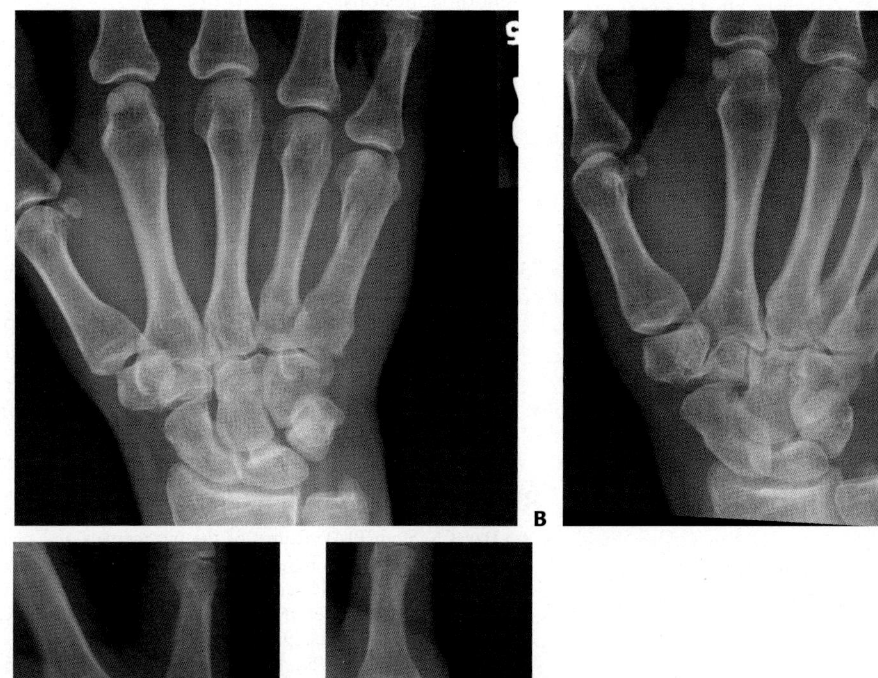

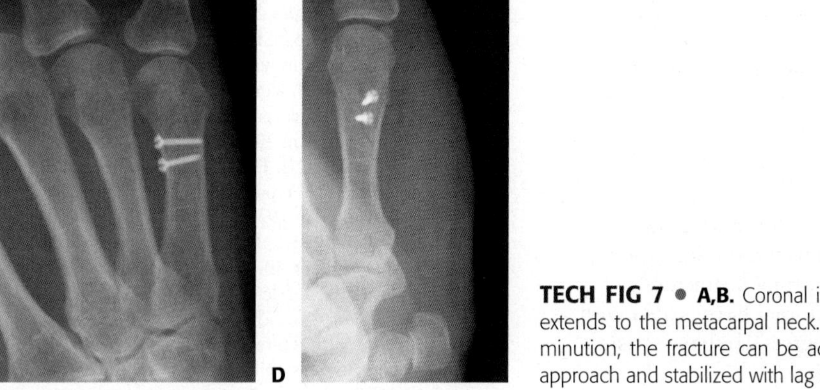

TECH FIG 7 • A,B. Coronal intra-articular fracture that extends to the metacarpal neck. **C,D.** If there is no comminution, the fracture can be addressed through a volar approach and stabilized with lag screws.

PEARLS AND PITFALLS

Natural history	■ Many metacarpal fractures can do exceedingly well with minimal intervention.
Fight bites	■ Be vigilant of small lacerations near the MP joint, which may be the only sign of a fight bite that needs urgent débridement to prevent a devastating infection.
Severe trauma	■ Polytrauma patients with severe hand injuries are at risk of missed injuries, open fractures, compartment syndrome, and intrinsic contracture.
Fracture reduction	■ Pins can be used to manipulate the fracture to a reduced position. ■ Sometimes, it is easier to apply the plate to one side of the fracture and then perform the reduction and fixation to the opposite side of the fracture. ■ Always check finger rotation prior to completing fixation.
Drilling	■ Critical structures can be protected during drilling by using the oscillation mode.
Mobilization	■ Allow tendon-gliding exercises as early as possible to minimize scar formation.

POSTOPERATIVE CARE

- Immobilization in the postoperative period will depend on the stability of the reconstruction and the status of the soft tissues.
- Fractures stabilized with retrograde (collateral recess) or transverse pins should be immobilized with the MP joints flexed 70 to 90 degrees for 3 to 4 weeks while the pins are in place. The IP joints should be allowed to move to minimize stiffness.
- Fractures stabilized with antegrade (bouquet) pins should be immobilized with the MP joints flexed 70 to 90 degrees for 3 to 4 weeks. Some authors allow early motion of the MP joint with bouquet pinning, understanding that there may be some loss of reduction.[3]
- Fractures that have been stabilized with rigid fixation such as plates or screws should be immobilized in a splint with the MP joints flexed 70 to 90 degrees for 4 to 7 days. An early motion program can then be instituted. A removable splint in the functional position should be used for protection until fracture stability.
- A hand therapist can be consulted if significant stiffness or lack of progress is noted during the early recovery period. However, in patients with severe injuries, it is often best to start therapy early.
- Protected activities should continue until fracture stability, which is often at least 4 to 6 weeks.
- In cases of delayed union, bone grafting can be considered.
- If plates are bothersome, they can be removed as early as 4 to 6 months after fracture consolidation.

OUTCOMES

- Metacarpal shaft fractures with limited shortening (2 to 5 mm) do well without surgery due to the stabilizing effect of the adjacent metacarpal and supporting ligaments.[8]
- Fractures of the fifth metacarpal neck that have healed with significant angulation of up to 70 degrees can have satisfactory outcomes.[6,15]
- Percutaneous pins can stabilize the reduction of many distal and proximal metacarpal shaft fractures.
- In the treatment of metacarpal neck fractures, antegrade (bouquet) pinning may lead to less stiffness of the MP joint compared to retrograde (collateral recess) and transverse pinning.[10,16]
- Plate fixation of short oblique, transverse, or multiple metacarpal fractures can provide the necessary stability to start an early motion program but on occasion will require hardware removal.[11]
- Screw fixation of articular head fractures can stabilize the fracture, but a degree of stiffness of the MP joint is expected.[13]

COMPLICATIONS

- Some degree of stiffness affects the surgical treatment of most metacarpal fractures.
- Stiffness of the MP joint can originate from contracture of the collateral ligaments and capsule after a period of immobilization. It may also occur from adhesions of the extensor tendons, especially after an open approach. Early mobilization as tolerated by the fixation can minimize it.
- Extension lag may develop from fracture shortening or tendon adhesions.
- Loss of articular congruity of the metacarpal head may block motion.
- Malrotation is poorly tolerated by most patients and should be addressed surgically.
- The dorsal sensory branches of the ulnar and radial nerve are very sensitive to manipulation.
- The deep motor branch of the ulnar nerve can be caught in the cutting tips of an inadvertent drill passage.
- Even though nonunions of metacarpal are rare, delayed unions can be seen, especially in short transverse fractures treated with a plate. If a nonunion does develop and the plate breaks, consideration should be given to bone grafting and revision fixation.
- Pin site infections can often be treated with oral antibiotics until the pins can be safely removed.

REFERENCES

1. Day CS, Stern PJ. Fractures of the metacarpals and phalanges. In: Wolfe SW, Hotchkiss RN, Pederson WC, et al, eds. Green's Operative Hand Surgery, ed 6. Philadelphia: Elsevier, 2011:239–258.
2. Diaz-Garcia R, Waljee JF. Current management of metacarpal fractures. Hand Clin 2013;29(4):507–518.
3. Downing ND, Davis TR. Intramedullary fixation of unstable metacarpal fractures. Hand Clin 2006;22:269–277.
4. Eichenholtz SN, Rizzo PC III. Fracture of the neck of the fifth metacarpal bone—is overtreatment justified? JAMA 1961;178:425–426.
5. Hofmeister EP, Kim J, Shin AY. Comparison of 2 methods of immobilization of fifth metacarpal neck fractures: a prospective randomized study. J Hand Surg Am 2008;33(8):1362–1368.
6. Hunter JM, Cowen NJ. Fifth metacarpal fractures in a compensation clinic population. A report on one hundred and thirty-three cases. J Bone Joint Surg Am 1970;52:1159–1165.
7. Jupiter JB, Belsky MR. Fracture and dislocations of the hand. In: Browner BD, Jupiter JB, Levine AM, et al, eds. Skeletal Trauma. Philadelphia: WB Saunders, 1992:925–1024.
8. Khan A, Giddins G. The outcome of conservative treatment of spiral metacarpal fractures and the role of the deep transverse metacarpal ligaments in stabilizing these injuries. J Hand Surg Eur Vol 2015;40(1):59–62.
9. Manueddu CA, Della Santa D. Fasciculated intramedullary pinning of metacarpal fractures. J Hand Surg Br 1996;21(2):230–236.
10. Schädel-Höpfner M, Wild M, Windolf J, et al. Antegrade intramedullary splinting or percutaneous retrograde crossed pinning for displaced neck fractures of the fifth metacarpal? Arch Orthop Trauma Surg 2007;127:435–440.
11. Souer JS, Mudgal CS. Plate fixation in closed ipsilateral multiple metacarpal fractures. J Hand Surg Eur Vol 2008;33(6):740–744.
12. Strauch RJ, Rosenwasser MP, Lunt JG. Metacarpal shaft fractures: the effect of shortening on the extensor tendon mechanism. J Hand Surg Am 1998;23(3):519–523.
13. Tan JS, Foo AT, Chew WC, et al. Articularly placed interfragmentary screw fixation of difficult condylar fractures of the hand. J Hand Surg Am 2011;36:604–609.
14. Tavassoli J, Ruland RT, Hogan CJ, et al. Three cast techniques for the treatment of extra-articular metacarpal fractures: comparison of short-term outcomes and final fracture alignments. J Bone Joint Surg Am 2005;87:2196–2201.
15. van Aaken J, Kämpfen S, Berli M, et al. Outcome of boxer's fractures treated by a soft wrap and buddy taping: a prospective study. Hand 2007;2(4):212–217.
16. Winter M, Balaguer T, Bessière C, et al. Surgical treatment of the boxer's fracture: transverse pinning versus intramedullary pinning. J Hand Surg Eur Vol 2007;32:709–713.

CHAPTER 49

Operative Treatment of Extra-articular Phalangeal Fractures

Richard L. Uhl and Michael T. Mulligan

DEFINITION

- Extra-articular fractures of the phalanges include metaphyseal and diaphyseal fractures of the proximal, middle, and distal phalanges.
- Extra-articular fractures of the phalanx can range from an isolated bony injury to injuries that affect the entire soft tissue envelope, flexor and extensor tendons, and the neurovascular structures.

ANATOMY

- The phalanges are the long, tubular bones of the hand that enable a functional arc of motion.
- The extensor mechanism of the finger glides directly on top of the phalanges, with only a thin layer of periosteum and peritenon between bone and tendon in adults.
  - Fractures of the phalanges and the resultant bleeding, swelling, and scarring can greatly inhibit extensor function.
  - Early motion of the extensor mechanism can help minimize adhesions between bone and tendon. This is an essential principle that must be kept in mind when treating these injuries.
  - Hardware, particularly a plate, placed dorsally beneath the tendon may interfere with extensor tendon function. This has led many to recommend alternate fixation methods as well as advocate plate placement on the lateral aspect of the bone.
  - Even a low-profile dorsal plate can lead to extensor imbalance. A plate on the proximal phalanx effectively shortens and tightens the central slip tendon, leading to limited proximal interphalangeal flexion (**FIG 1**).
  - There is even less room to place a dorsal plate under the triangular ligament and terminal tendon over the middle phalanx (**FIG 2**).

PATHOGENESIS

- Because the fingers project from the hand, they are subject to bending and twisting forces in a wide variety of situations.
- The fracture pattern depends on the position of the digit at the time of injury and the direction and degree of force applied.
  - Long spiral fractures tend to result from torsional forces.
  - Transverse fractures tend to occur after angular and three-point bending forces.
- Fingers are also subject to direct trauma, such as a blow from a hammer, crush injury from a window or door, or a gunshot.
  - These injuries are often associated with skin, tendon, nerve, and artery injuries, all of which worsen the prognosis for recovery of function.
  - Most distal phalanx fractures are comminuted in nature and result from a crush mechanism. Significant displacement of the fragments is associated with a nail bed disruption (**FIG 3**).
- Fractures of the proximal phalanx will generally assume a position of apex volar angulation.
  - The portion of the intrinsic muscle tendons that insert on the base of the proximal phalanx pull the proximal fragment into flexion. The central slip pulls the distal fragment into extension (**FIG 4**).

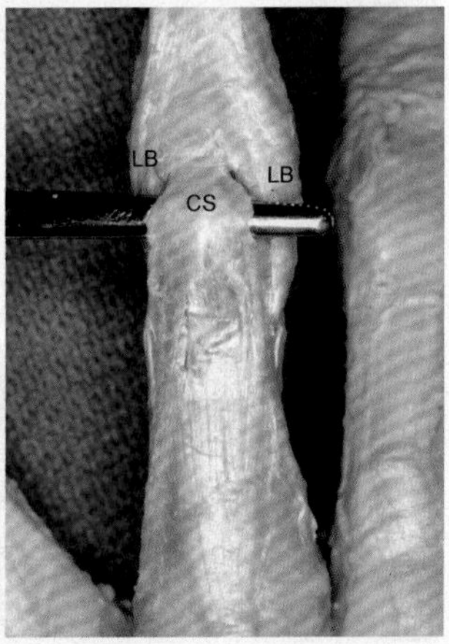

FIG 1 • Anatomic dissection of a digit showing the relationship and position of the lateral bands (*LB*) and the central slip (*CS*) at the proximal interphalangeal (PIP) joint. The forceps demonstrate the effect of a bulky plate inserted under the extensor tendon.

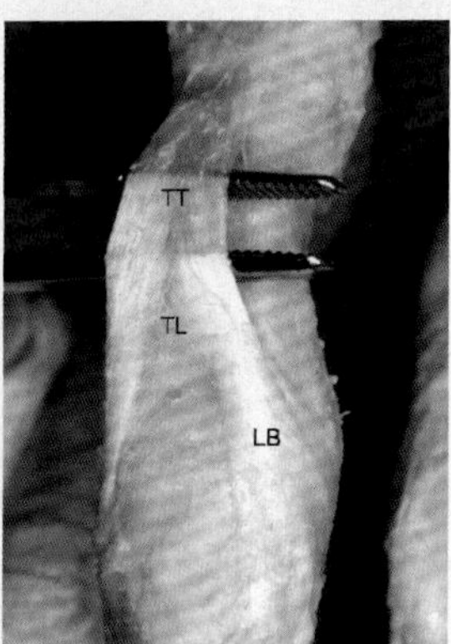

FIG 2 • The terminal tendon (*TT*) is formed by a confluence of the lateral bands (*LB*). The triangular ligament (*TL*) keeps the tendons on the dorsal aspect of the finger. The terminal tendon is intimately associated with the middle phalanx.

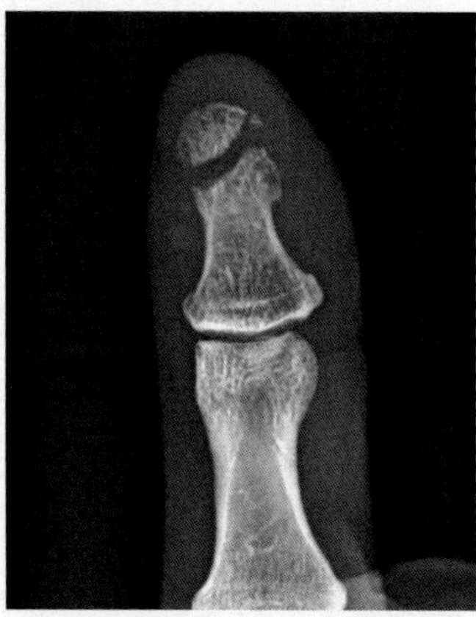

FIG 3 • Displacement of the tuft of the distal phalanx usually indicates disruption of the nail bed.

- Fractures of the middle phalanx deform less predictably but often assume an apex volar angulation due to the pull of the flexor digitorum superficialis tendon on the volar base of the middle phalanx proximal fragment and the force exerted by the terminal extensor tendon on the distal fragment.
- Both the extensor and flexor tendons insert on the distal phalanx at the base only. The flexor tendon insertion is more distal than the extensor tendon insertion. It is possible to have an extra-articular fracture between the two insertion sites, a so-called Seymour fracture in adults, which angulates in a dorsal apex direction.

NATURAL HISTORY

- Extra-articular fractures of the phalanges typically will heal in patients who do not seek clinical treatment but often with residual deformity.
- There is a linear relationship between the degree of proximal phalanx angulation and the extensor lag, which occurs because of the relative lengthening of the extensor mechanism.[22]
  - The operative correction of such deformity must be balanced with the potential for stiffness after surgical intervention as well as other potential surgical complications.

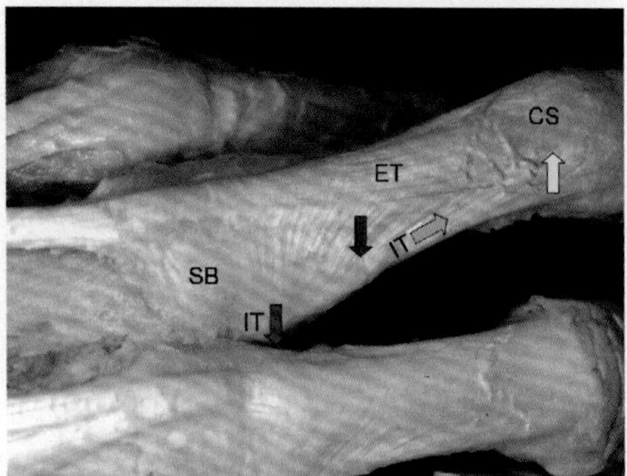

FIG 4 • Most proximal phalanx fractures assume an apex volar angulation (*red arrow*). This is due to a combination of tendon forces. The portion of the intrinsic tendon (*IT*) that inserts at the base of the proximal phalanx pulls the proximal fragment into flexion (*blue arrow*). The central slip (*CS*) is formed from the common extensor tendon (*ET*) and a contribution from the intrinsic tendon as they cross dorsally (*green arrow*). The central slip pulls the distal fragment into extension (*yellow arrow*), resulting in an apex volar angulation. The sagittal band (*SB*) should always be preserved.

PATIENT HISTORY AND PHYSICAL FINDINGS

- A thorough history including the date and mechanism of injury, the patient's handedness, occupation, hobbies, and treatment rendered to date must be obtained.
- As part of the history, it is important to know any previous injuries and functional limitations of the hand being evaluated.
- The clinician should evaluate the cascade of the digits, looking for subtle changes in the attitude and position of the fingers. This may help to localize areas of injury.
- Pain with palpation helps to localize the area of injury if there is no clear deformity of the digit. Palpation can also be useful to assess clinical fracture healing.
- Phalangeal fractures can be displaced in the anteroposterior (AP) or lateral plane, rotated, shortened, or can exhibit a combination of these deformities.
  - Resultant hand function will depend on the specific deformity and its location along the skeleton.
  - The more proximal the fracture, the greater the potential for angular or rotational deformity at the fingertip.
  - Rotational deformity affects ultimate function the greatest, especially if the rotation causes the fingers to scissor (**FIG 5A**).
    - Rotation can be evaluated by asking the patient to flex and extend the digits as a unit. The clinician should compare the relative position of the injured digit to adjacent digits on both the injured and uninjured hands.
    - A digital anesthetic block can facilitate the examination.
    - The digits should generally point toward the distal pole of the scaphoid during flexion.
    - It is often difficult for the patient to make a fist at the initial assessment due to pain and swelling. In these cases, comparing the plane of the nail bed of the injured finger to the adjacent nail beds can provide a valuable clue to the presence of a rotational deformity (**FIG 5B**).

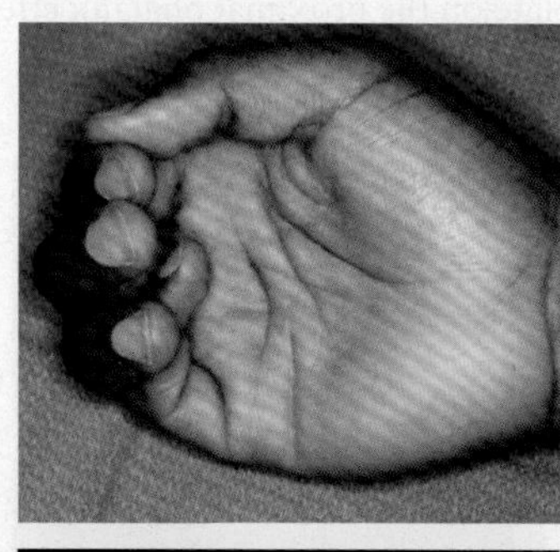

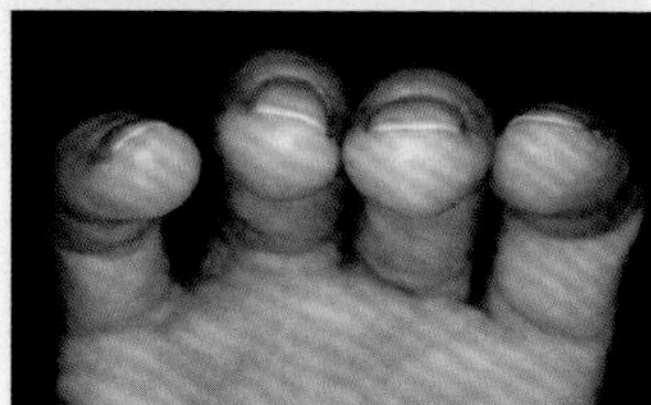

FIG 5 • A. Rotational deformity is the least tolerated deformity in the fingers. Assessment can be difficult, however, if the patient cannot make a fist. **B.** Rotation can be assessed by observing the planes of the fingernails to each other. The nail that is rotated out of the plane of the others (in this case, the ring finger) indicates a rotational deformity of that digit.

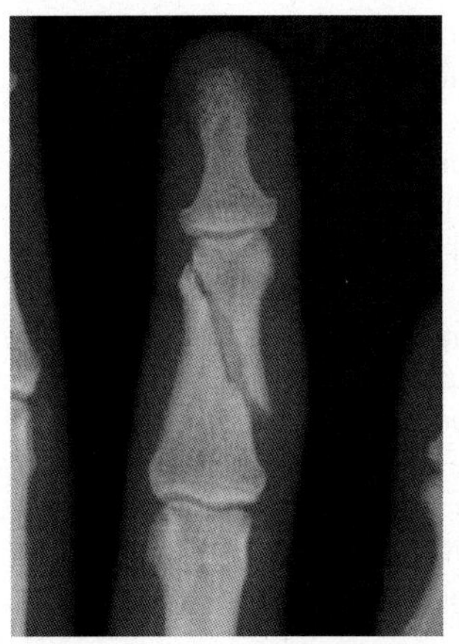

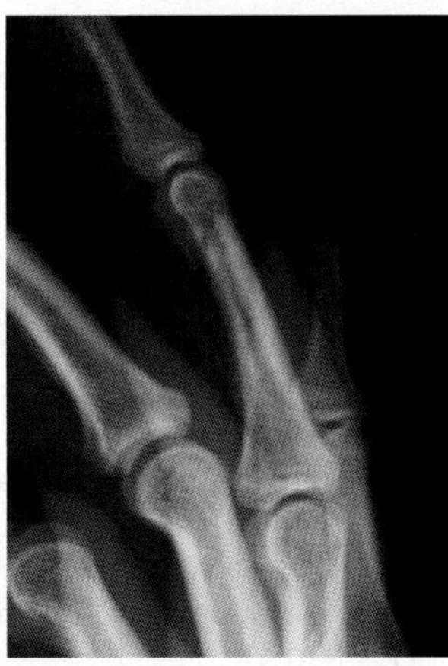

FIG 6 • Posteroanterior (**A**) and lateral (**B**) radiographs showing an unstable spiral fracture of the middle phalanx. This fracture pattern is prone to shortening and rotational deformity.

- Neurovascular status
  - Altered skin color and diminished turgor and capillary refill of the digit are clear indicators of vascular compromise.
  - Two-point discrimination can be used to assess innervation density and is an excellent method for evaluating the integrity of digital nerves in adults.
- Condition of the soft tissue envelope
  - The skin may be visibly damaged with lacerations, degloving, or burns. Its condition will influence treatment.
  - A subungual hematoma is common with a distal phalanx fracture.

IMAGING AND OTHER DIAGNOSTIC STUDIES

- PA, oblique, and lateral radiographs will provide sufficient imaging for the majority of extra-articular phalangeal fractures.
  - Critical evaluation may show subtle rotational malalignment if a true lateral view of either the base or the condyles of a phalanx does not match up across its corresponding joint.
  - Slightly oblique lateral views are useful for imaging fractures at the base of the proximal phalanx, where the overlap on a true lateral view makes evaluation difficult.
- Unstable fracture patterns, such as spiral fractures with rotation and shortening, or midshaft transverse or short oblique fractures with angulation, should be recognized on the plain radiographs (**FIG 6A,B**).
- A mobile, small fluoroscopy unit allows magnification to help characterize subtle injuries and dynamic evaluation to gauge fragment stability.
- More sophisticated imaging (magnetic resonance imaging [MRI], computed tomography [CT], ultrasound) is rarely needed to make the diagnosis of a phalangeal fracture or to guide treatment.

DIFFERENTIAL DIAGNOSIS

- Although there are other causes of hand pain and deformity (eg, osteoarthritis, congenital deformity, tumor, infection), the patient history and plain radiographs should leave little doubt that the patient has a phalanx fracture.
- If a fracture is not evident, all the following diagnoses should be considered:
  - Acute sprains (collateral ligament or volar plate injury)
  - Tendon injury (mallet finger, boutonnière injury, sagittal band injury, flexor tendon avulsion, or pulley rupture)
  - Nondisplaced fracture or bony contusion
  - Stenosing tenosynovitis or trigger finger
  - Acute infection
  - Benign and malignant lesions of the digits

NONOPERATIVE MANAGEMENT

- Many phalangeal fractures are stable and can be treated effectively by closed means.[4,9–11] Each fracture must be addressed individually, taking into account the condition of the soft tissue envelope, the fracture characteristics, and the functional needs of the patient.
  - Mild (nonrotational) deformities do well with immobilization and protection while the fractures heal, but unstable or malrotated fractures benefit from surgical intervention.
  - Distal phalanx fractures are most commonly amenable to nonoperative treatment.
  - Results are good or excellent in more than 70% of extra-articular phalangeal fractures treated nonoperatively.[2,7,16,19]
- Early motion is always desirable, but it is somewhat less important with closed treatment.
  - Immobilization beyond 3 weeks increases stiffness and leads to worse outcomes.[21]
- Closed treatment
  - Less scarring to the extensor mechanism
  - Less ability to move early, unless the fracture is very stable
  - Less ability to hold a fracture that required reduction
- Internal fixation
  - Greater scarring of the extensors, especially with a dorsal approach and a dorsal implant
  - Early motion is essential
  - Greatest ability to hold the fracture in a stable, corrected position
- If a fracture is incomplete, complete but nondisplaced, or impacted (such as the metaphysis at the base of the proximal phalanx), a short period (1 to 2 weeks) of splinting followed by buddy taping to the adjacent digit is appropriate (**FIG 7**).

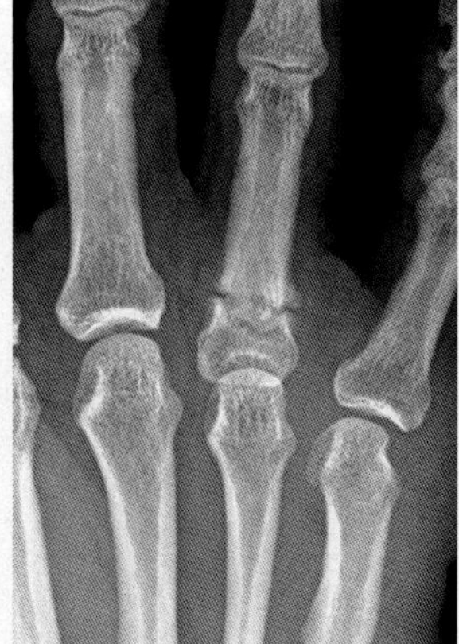

FIG 7 • This fracture is stable because it is well aligned (on the PA and lateral radiographs) and that alignment does not change with motion. This fracture was treated with splinting for 2 weeks and buddy taping for 2 more weeks.

- A fracture that can be adequately reduced but is relatively unstable can occasionally be held reduced with a splint.
  - This has the advantage of avoiding a trip to the operating room and the possible complications of surgical fixation but requires close follow-up and serial radiographs to ensure that reduction is maintained (**FIG 8**).

SURGICAL MANAGEMENT

- When considering any surgery, it is necessary to balance the potential benefits of surgery with the risks of the procedure.
  - The goal of surgery is to restore alignment and to stabilize the fracture to a degree sufficient to begin early motion.
- Any phalangeal fracture with a significant injury to the soft tissue envelope has a worse prognosis.
  - Stable fixation (to the degree that it does not further compromise the soft tissues) and early motion assume a greater importance in phalangeal fractures with associated soft tissue injuries.
  - Patients with open fractures are treated with the appropriate intravenous antibiotic therapy.[20]
- Once the decision is made to surgically intervene, the surgeon must decide which mode of fixation will best suit the fracture pattern.
  - This decision is often made intraoperatively and is frequently based on the ability of the fracture to be adequately reduced closed.
- Fractures that are reduced closed are stabilized externally with a cast or fixator or are held with Kirschner wires placed percutaneously.
  - Kirschner wiring and external fixation are techniques that, when appropriately applied, will result in acceptable outcomes without potential soft tissue surgical interruption and scarring.[6]
- Open reduction and internal fixation with plates and screws will potentially provide more stable fixation but, without early mobilization, could result in decreased range of motion.[12]
  - Overly aggressive soft tissue stripping will cause extensor tendon adhesions and bulky implants will affect extensor tendon balance and function.[18]
- An algorithm can be used to aid in the decision-making process (**FIG 9**).

Methods

Percutaneous Wire Fixation

- Closed reduction with percutaneous fixation can be used to treat the majority of unstable spiral fractures of the phalanges.
- The technique is also suitable for transverse metaphyseal fractures, but it may be less suited for transverse diaphyseal fractures.
- When the wires are inserted radial and ulnar to the extensor mechanism, percutaneous wire fixation offers the advantage

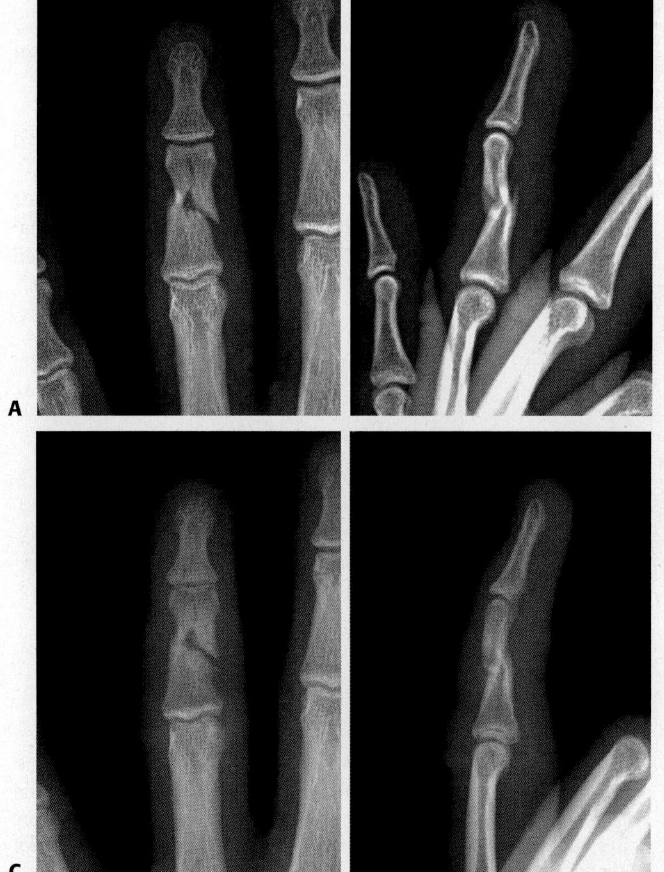
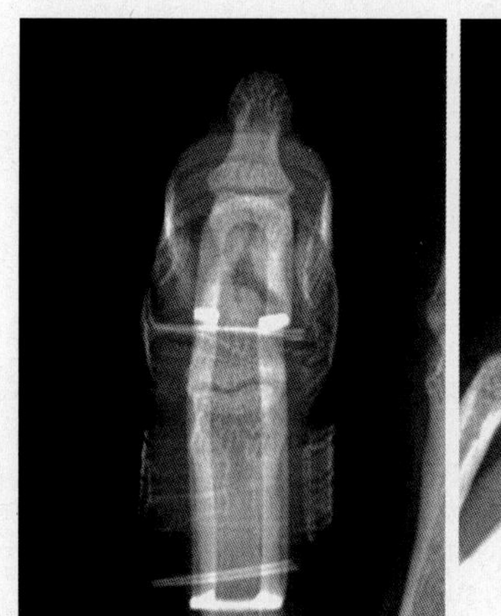
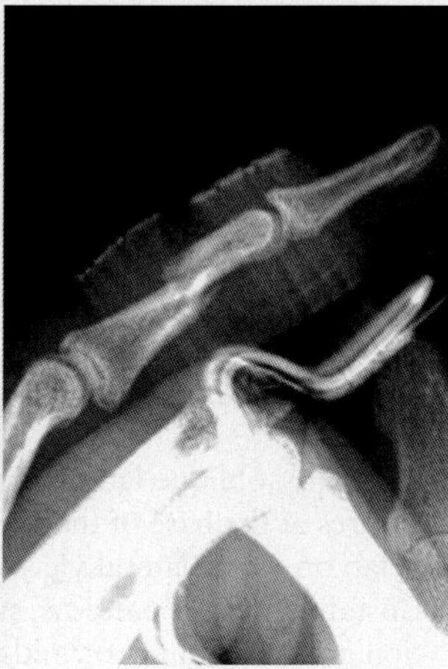

FIG 8 • **A.** This middle phalanx fracture shows apex volar angulation, which was easily reducible under digital block anesthesia, but the reduction was unstable and the deformity quickly recurred. **B.** A padded aluminum splint was fabricated to apply a three-point force to hold the fracture reduced. **C.** After 4 weeks of splinting, the fracture had healed and the splint was removed. By 6 weeks, motion was full, with mild discomfort with gripping.

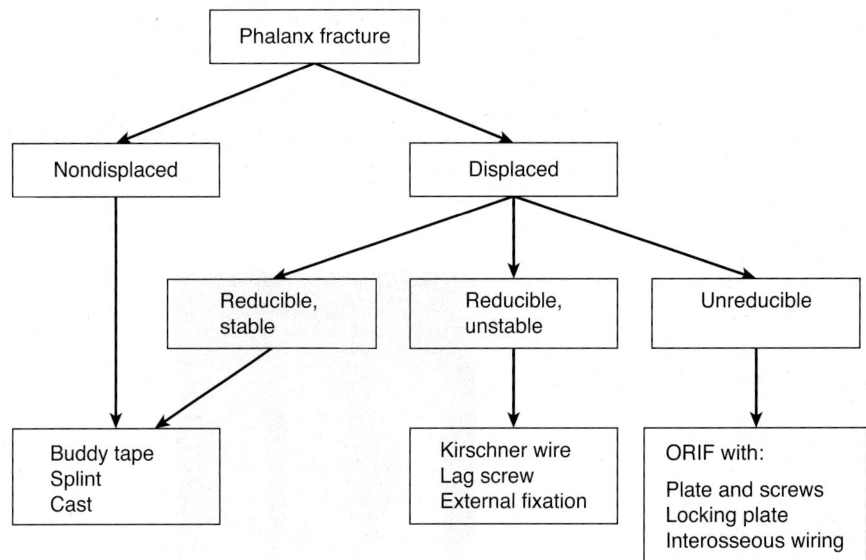

FIG 9 • Decision algorithm for the progression to open surgical treatment for phalangeal fractures and the subsequent treatment options for fixation.

of minimal disruption of the soft tissues in general and the extensor mechanism in particular.

- This technique is best suited for fractures less than 10 days old. After that time, early healing makes accurate closed reduction more difficult.
- Kirschner wires provide less stable fixation than plates and screws and may restrict soft tissue gliding due to their prominence. This restriction of early motion may lead to increased stiffness. They may also irritate or abrade adjacent fingers.

Interosseous Wire Fixation

- Interosseous wire fixation is more rigid than Kirschner wire fixation but requires open reduction and additional dissection to expose the bone surfaces.
  - This method of fixation is less bulky than a plate and, as such, is particularly well suited for fractures of the middle phalanx when percutaneous pinning is not possible.
- Interosseous wiring works best with a transverse fracture. The wires provide compression to stabilize the fracture. Interosseous wiring will not work if the fracture is comminuted. Interosseous wiring is made more stable when it is combined with pin fixation and placed in a 90-degree configuration.

Lag Screw Fixation

- Lag screw fixation is best suited for oblique and simple spiral fractures.
  - Lag screws can be used alone if the length of the fracture is greater than twice the diameter of the bone at the level of the fracture.[13]
  - If the obliquity is less, a neutralization plate should be added.
- Comminuted and transverse fractures are not amenable to lag screw fixation.
- Contemporary lag screws are extremely low profile, making them an excellent fixation option in the phalanx, especially the middle phalanx.
- Lag screw fixation is more rigid than Kirschner wire fixation, and unlike wires, the screws do not need to be removed.
- Lag screws can be inserted percutaneously, but the procedure can be technically challenging.
- Usually, an oblique fracture will be visualized best in the AP plane and the screws inserted from the lateral aspects.
  - Spiral fractures frequently require the screws to be placed in two planes.
  - Multiplanar screw fixation greatly increases the biomechanical stability.

Plate Fixation

- Plate fixation is best suited for transverse fractures, short oblique fractures, periarticular metaphyseal fractures, and comminuted fractures, in which the plate serves as a bridge to maintain phalangeal length.
  - Midshaft, transverse fractures are fixed with a straight plate. At least two screws should be placed in either side of the fracture site with fixation of four cortices.
  - If close to the metaphysis, a T plate or a Y plate will allow improved fixation compared with a straight plate.
  - Adding a lag screw across an oblique fracture, either through the plate or as an adjunct to plate fixation, will add to the rigidity of the construct.
  - Compression, obtained by eccentrically drilling one or more of the screws in the plate, will increase fracture stability.
  - Locked plates provide greater stability for periarticular and comminuted fractures.
- Plate fixation requires more extensive soft tissue dissection and increases the risk of postoperative extensor scarring. Immediate motion of the digits is essential to minimize the scarring.

Preoperative Planning

- Preoperative posteroanterior, lateral, and oblique radiographs are essential.
  - Evaluation of these studies helps determine the plane of the fracture and the size of the fracture fragments, allowing the surgeon to choose the best surgical approach and the ideal fixation technique.

- The surgeon must be certain that all potential implants are available. Surgical error can frequently be traced to implant availability problems.
  - Many sets include only one or two plates of a given size and shape. In the case of multiple digit involvement, extra plates and screws are helpful.
- Intraoperative imaging using a fluoroscopy unit is imperative.
- The surgeon should plan for alternative approaches and means of fixation should comminution or soft tissue problems preclude the original plan.

Positioning

- The patient is placed supine on the operating table with a radiolucent hand table attached.
- A padded arm or forearm tourniquet is used for all cases.

Approach

- The phalanx is most commonly approached laterally or dorsally. The exact approach used for open reduction is often based on the location of the fracture as it relates to the extensor mechanism (**FIG 10**).
- The sagittal bands at the metacarpophalangeal (MP) joint, the central slip insertion, and the triangular ligament should be preserved whenever possible.
  - Motion is necessarily delayed after surgery if these structures are incised and subsequently repaired.
  - A portion of the lateral band may be excised rather than repaired as part of the midaxial approach.
  - Longitudinal incisions in the midportion of the extensor tendon and in the midaxial interval between the central extensor and the lateral band allow early motion (see **FIG 10**).
- At the middle phalanx level, a midaxial approach on the edge of the terminal tendon is preferred so that the tendon can be pulled to the side, exposing the bone (see **FIG 2**).
  - The midaxial approach is also useful when using lag screw fixation, as the screws are usually inserted on the lateral aspect of the bone.

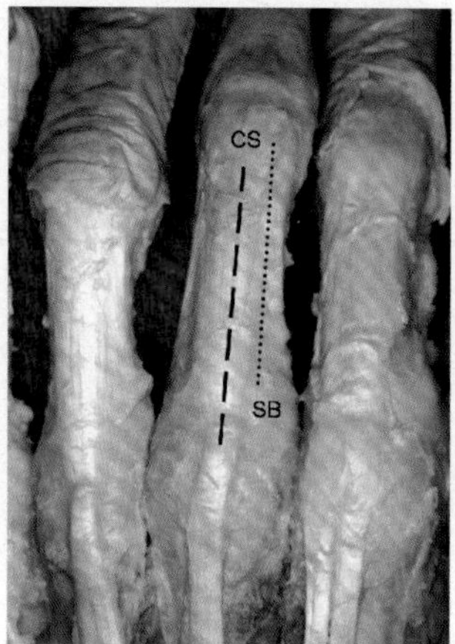

FIG 10 • The surgical approach to the proximal phalanx can be straight dorsal, through the extensor tendon (*dashed line*), or midaxial (*dotted line*), between the dorsal tendon and the intrinsic contribution. Care must be taken not to disrupt the central slip (*CS*) with the dorsal approach and not to disrupt the sagittal bands (*SB*) with the midaxial approach. Thus, the dorsal approach is better suited for the more proximal fractures and the midaxial approach is better for the more distal fractures.

TECHNIQUES

Percutaneous Kirschner Wire Fixation

Fracture Reduction

- Before performing any reduction maneuver, obtain posteroanterior and lateral C-arm images for reference.
  - If the fracture is very close to the MP joint, a slightly oblique lateral view will show the fracture better by avoiding some of the overlap of the other MP joints.
- Unstable spiral fractures of the phalanges are usually shortened, rotated, and angulated (**TECH FIG 1A**).
- Begin the reduction by applying longitudinal traction.
  - This can be accomplished with direct traction on the digit. Use a moist gauze, finger traps, or a pointed towel clip applied distal to the fracture.
- While traction is applied, correct the rotational deformity (**TECH FIG 1B**). Any angular deformity is then corrected before placing a reduction clamp across the fracture.
  - Flexing the MP joint stabilizes the proximal P1 fragment by tightening the collateral ligaments.
- Apply a reduction clamp (a towel clip-like device with sharp points) across the fracture percutaneously to hold the reduction.
  - When considering the cross-sectional anatomy of the finger, remember that the bone lies in the dorsal two-thirds not in the midline (**TECH FIG 1C**). Thus, the clamp tips should enter the skin dorsal to the midlateral line.
  - Placing the clamp at a slight angle so that it is more perpendicular to the fracture will improve the stability of the reduction through fracture compression.
  - Reduction can further be fine-tuned by twisting the clamp slightly when tightening.

Fracture Stabilization

- After checking the reduction with the fluoroscope, drill the Kirschner wires across the fracture site until they gain purchase in the far cortex (**TECH FIG 1D**).
  - Usually, 0.045-inch Kirschner wires are used in the proximal phalanx. Fixation in the small finger and in the more distal phalanges may require a smaller 0.035-inch Kirschner wire size (**TECH FIG 2**).
  - Diamond-tipped smooth Kirschner wires are preferred.
- Crossed wires can be used to secure transverse fractures.
  - This method is useful for metaphyseal fractures (**TECH FIG 3**) and to stabilize middle phalanx fractures to avoid the need for plate fixation (**TECH FIG 4**).
  - Avoid distraction at the fracture site when using crossed wires.

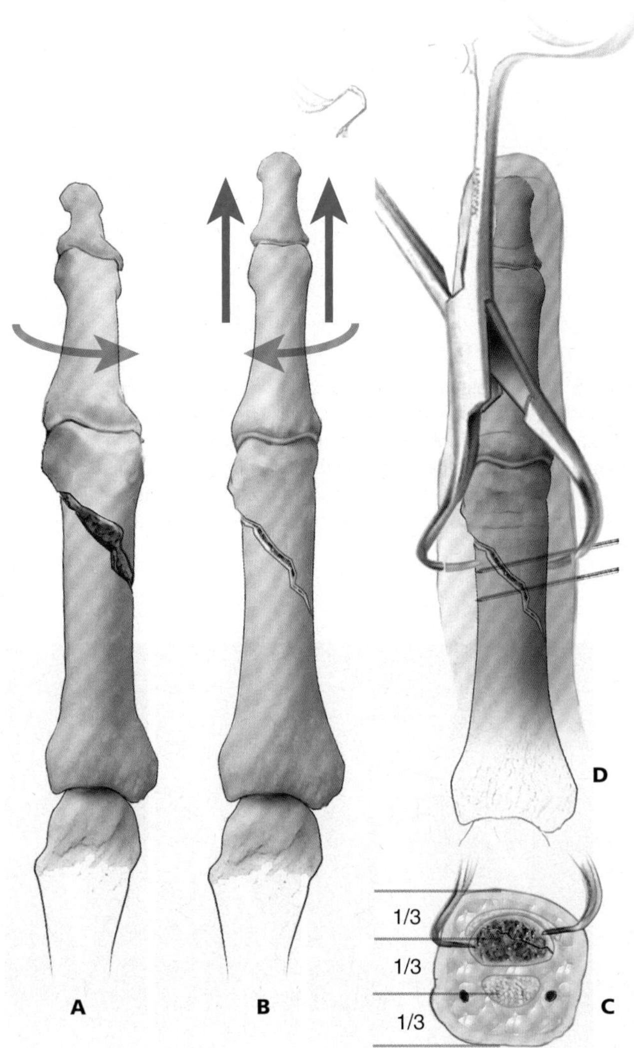

TECH FIG 1 • **A.** Unstable phalangeal fractures deform with shortening, rotation, and angulation. **B.** Longitudinal traction is applied first, and then the rotation and angulation are corrected. **C.** The bone is in the dorsal two-thirds of the finger rather than in the middle. The neurovascular bundles are in the volar third and should, of course, be avoided when the reduction clamp is applied. **D.** When the fracture is reduced and compressed with the reduction clamp, the wires are drilled across the fracture site.

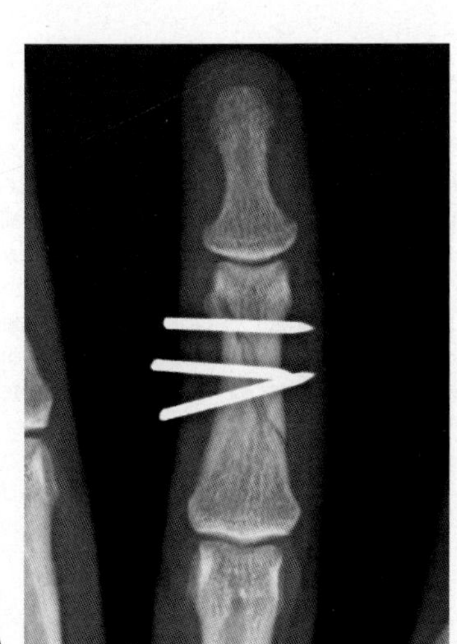

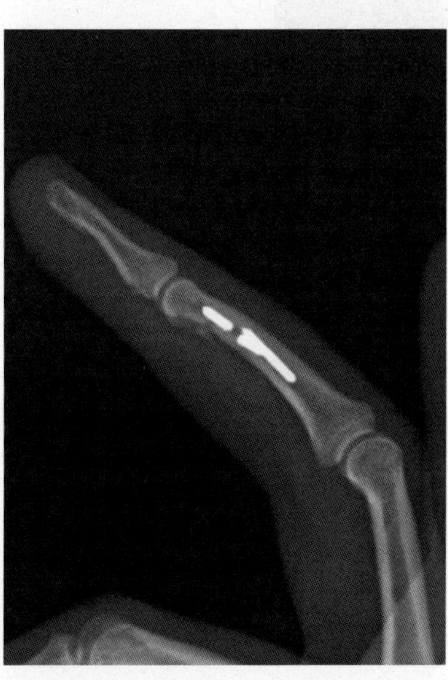

TECH FIG 2 • Postoperative posteroanterior (**A**) and lateral (**B**) radiographs showing an unstable spiral middle phalanx fracture (seen in **FIG 6**) treated with percutaneous pinning using the method described.

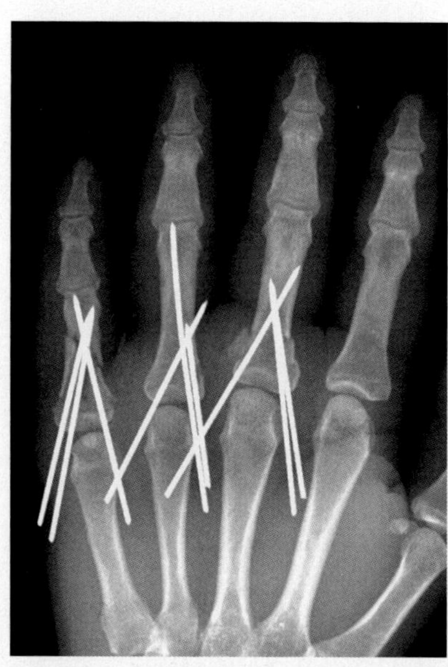

TECH FIG 3 • This patient sustained a crush injury to the hand resulting in fractures of the middle, ring, and small fingers. The fingers were reduced by flexing the MP joints. The pins were passed between the metacarpal heads rather than spearing the extensor tendons. This helps to hold the MP joints in a flexed position once pinned. Active motion of the proximal and distal interphalangeal joints was started in the immediate postoperative period.

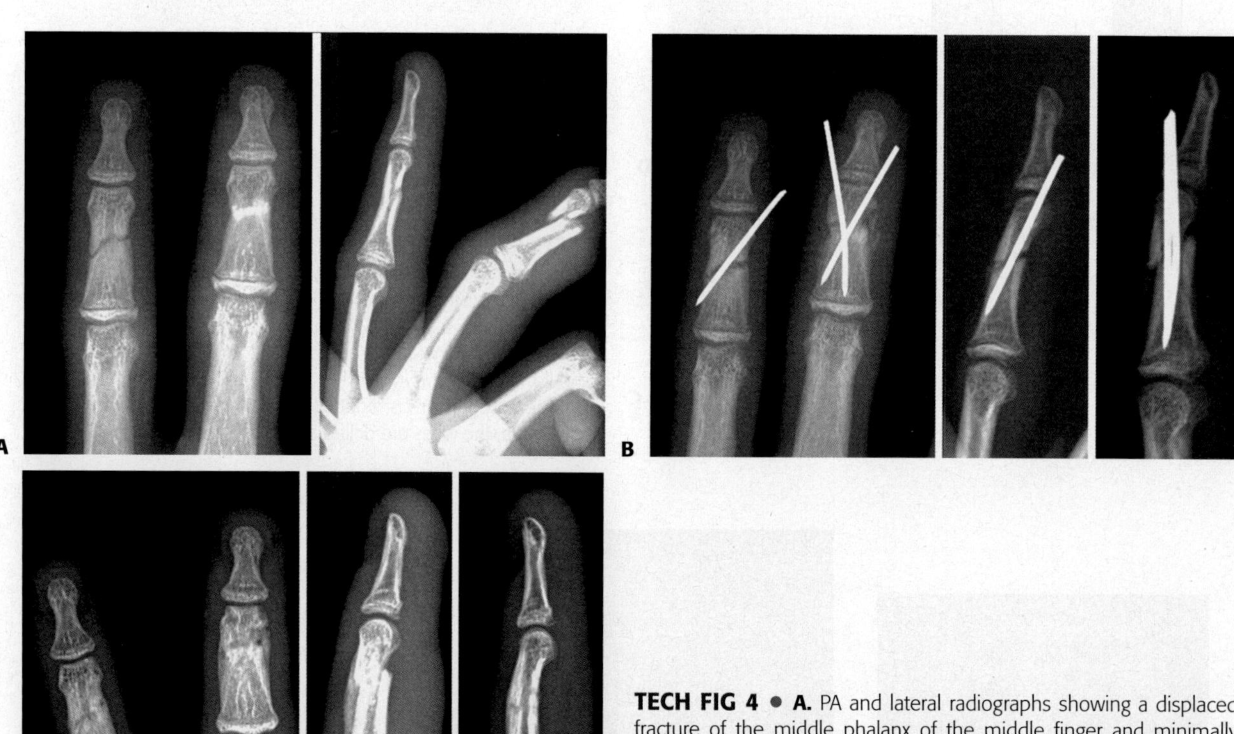

TECH FIG 4 • **A.** PA and lateral radiographs showing a displaced fracture of the middle phalanx of the middle finger and minimally displaced middle phalanx fracture of the ring finger. Note the importance of the lateral radiograph to assess the displacement of the middle finger fracture. **B.** The middle finger fracture was stabilized with crossed pins. The ring finger was fixed with a single pin to avoid displacement after early motion was started. **C.** The healed fractures after pin removal.

Interosseous Wire Fixation

Exposure

- Open reduction and fairly extensive fracture exposure is required for placement of the intraosseous wires, especially when using a dorsovolar wire.[1]
- Expose the fracture using either a dorsal or midaxial approach.
- Place the bone in the "shotgun" position (apex dorsal) and gently elevate the soft tissues from the proximal and distal fragments 3 to 5 mm at the fracture site.
- Drill transverse and AP holes 2 to 5 mm away from the fracture site using a 0.045 smooth Kirschner wire.

Fracture Reduction and Stabilization

- Reduce the fracture and verify reduction through direct observation and with a fluoroscopy image.
- Pass a 24-gauge steel wire through the transverse hole and a second wire through the AP holes.
- Tighten the wire loops sequentially by pulling the wire away from the fracture and twisting slowly to stabilize and compress the fracture (**TECH FIG 5**).
  - Do not fully tighten the first wire until the second wire has been at least partially tightened.
  - Plan placement of the wire loops so as to lay them flat against bone and minimize soft tissue irritation.
- If greater stability is required, drill a 0.035 to 0.045 smooth Kirschner wire obliquely across the fracture.

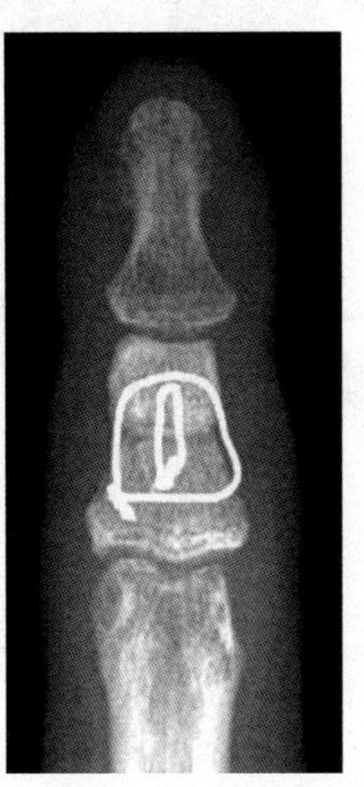

TECH FIG 5 • Posteroanterior radiograph of an infected nonunion of the middle phalanx treated by débridement, squaring of the nonunion ends, and 90-90 interosseous wiring.

Lag Screw Fixation

- Lag screws can be inserted percutaneously, but the procedure is technically challenging. Precise reduction of the fracture is the first priority and should not be sacrificed in an attempt to limit incision length.
- Most often, the midaxial approach will provide the best exposure with the least amount of soft tissue stripping.
- Screw size and number are determined based on fracture location, fracture characteristics, and the size of the bone fragments (**TECH FIG 6**).
  - When considering the use of multiple screws and screw location within the fragment, screws should be placed at least two screw diameters from the tip of the fracture and centered within the fragment.
  - The distance between screws should also be at least two screw diameters.
  - The screws' orientation should be between perpendicular to the fracture line and perpendicular to the bone itself.
    - Screws placed perpendicular to the fracture provide maximal compression.
    - Screws placed more perpendicular to the bone provide axial stability.
  - Screws should always be drilled along a diameter (ie, crossing through the middle of the bone).

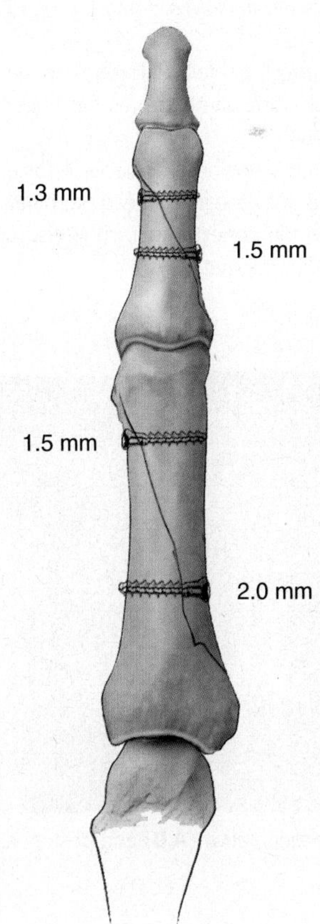

TECH FIG 6 • Screw size is determined by the bone size. Usually, 1.5- or 2.0-mm screws are used in the proximal phalanx and 1.3- or 1.5-mm screws in the middle phalanx.

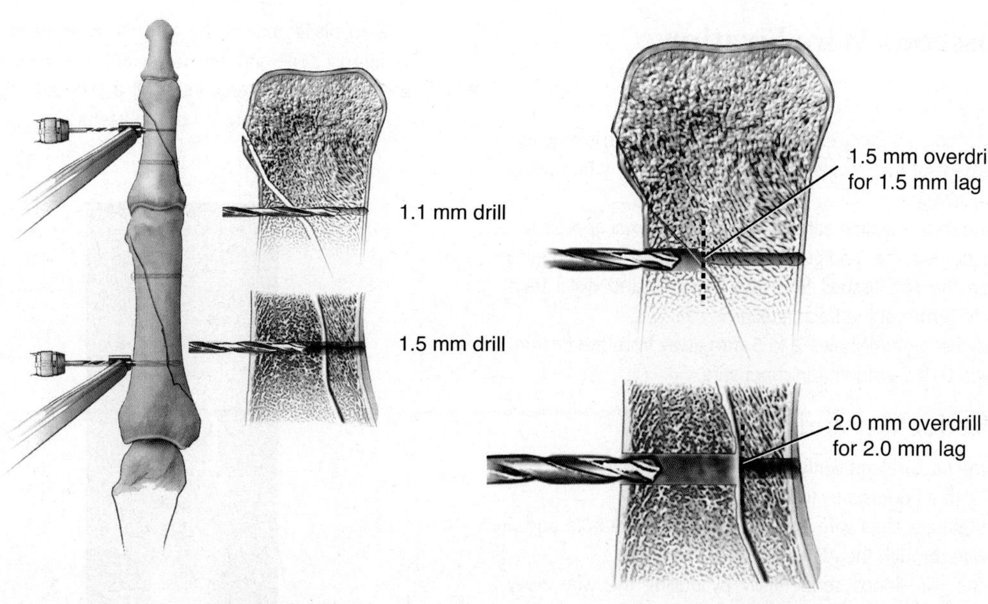

TECH FIG 7 • A. The tap drill for the chosen screw size is drilled from the near cortex, across the fracture, and into the far cortex. The hole should be oriented so the drill crosses through the center of the bone and is centered in the far fragment as well. **B.** To gain a lag effect, the near cortex is opened to the outer diameter of the screw (overdrilled) so the screw threads will engage only in the far cortex, compressing the fractures as the screw is tightened.

- Reduce and hold the fracture with a clamp while the drill is advanced across the fracture site into the opposite cortex (**TECH FIG 7A**).
- To gain a lag effect, create a gliding hole in the near cortex using a drill bit that is the same size as the screw's outer diameter (**TECH FIG 7B**).
- Countersink the screw head to disperse forces as compression is applied and decrease screw head prominence.
  - Because the cortex is thin, countersinking is not recommended in the metaphysis.
- Insert a self-tapping screw through the gliding hole and into the far cortex.
- When the screw is tightened, the fracture is compressed.
  - During final tightening, exert steady forward pressure and turn the screw slowly to avoid stripping the far cortex.
- Repeat the procedure for additional screws (**TECH FIG 8**).
- Alternatively, reduce the fracture with a clamp, then stabilize it with a Kirschner wire smaller than the core diameter of the screw. Place the first lag screw as described, then remove the Kirschner wire and insert the second screw through the predrilled Kirschner wire hole.

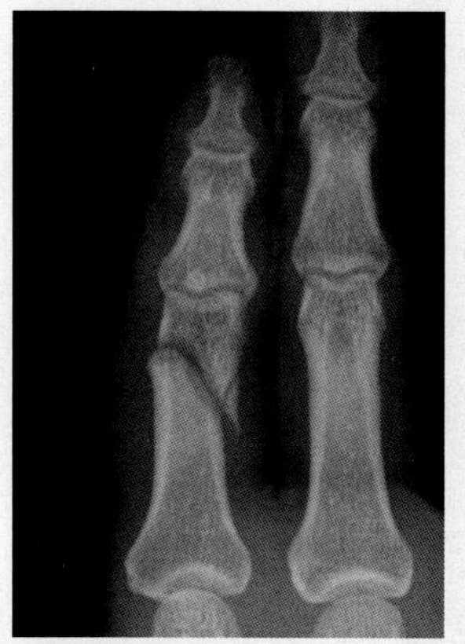
A
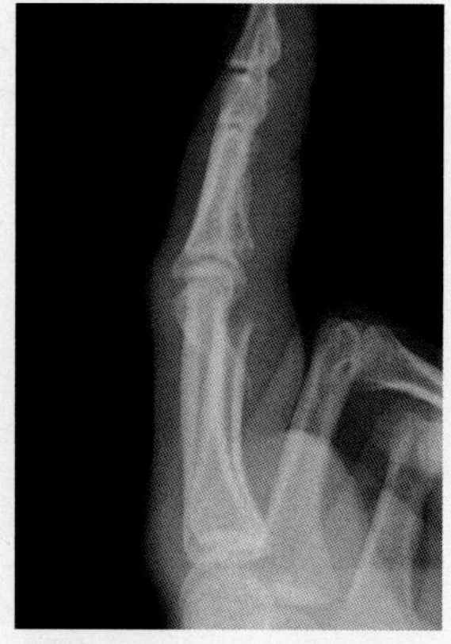
B
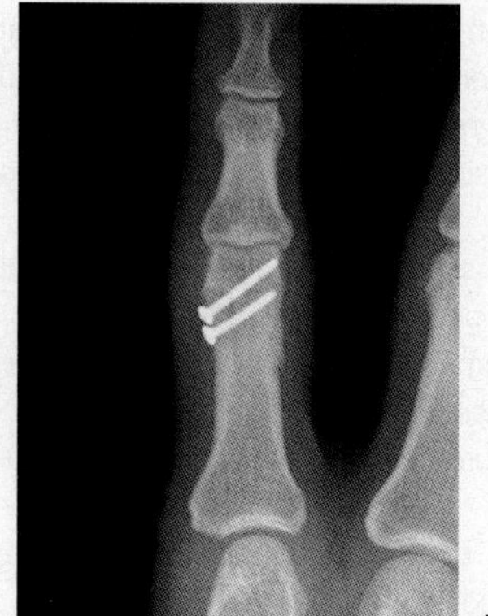
C
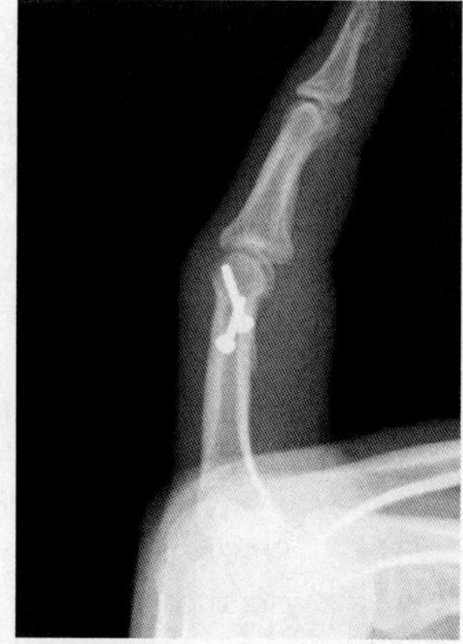
D

TECH FIG 8 • Preoperative (**A,B**) and postoperative (**C,D**) radiographs of a distal oblique fracture of the proximal phalanx fixed with two lag screws.

Plate Fixation

- Plates can be placed either dorsally or laterally on the bone.
- Lateral placement via the midaxial approach has the advantage of less extensor disruption and potentially fewer adhesions.[15]
- If the plate is applied to the dorsal surface, drilling beyond the volar cortex or inserting a screw that extends beyond the volar cortex may damage the flexor tendons.
- Once exposed, clear the fracture site of soft tissue and reduce the fracture.

Fixation of Metaphyseal Fractures: T-Plate Technique

- Provisionally place the plate on the bone using a pointed reduction clamp, a specialized plate-holding clamp, or by having an assistant hold the plate on the bone.
- Insert the screw in the middle of the T plate first, but before screw tightening, align the plate perpendicular to the adjacent joint (**TECH FIG 9A**).
- Perform the final fracture reduction and insert a screw on the other side of the fracture (**TECH FIG 9B**).
- Assess the length, angulation, and, most importantly, the rotation clinically and radiographically.
- Insert the remaining screws (**TECH FIG 9C**).
- Stable fixation will allow early motion, which is essential to regain function (**TECH FIG 10**).

Fixation of a Comminuted Shaft Fractures: Locking Plate Technique

- Conventional plates may not provide sufficient fixation if the phalanx shaft is comminuted.
  - Plates with locked screws can be used to gain secure fixation of a fragment with as few as two screws.
  - Locking plates with preattached short drill guides allow temporary fixation using small wires through the guides. These wires are later replaced with locking screws.
- Center the proximal end of the plate just distal to the joint surface and insert a wire through the guide (**TECH FIG 11A**).
- Align the plate with the longitudinal axis, perpendicular to the joint surface and insert a second wire (**TECH FIG 11B**).
- Apply traction and correct rotation. Center the distal end of the plate on the bone and insert an additional wire (**TECH FIG 11C**).
- Correct any residual angulation and insert an additional wire, if needed.
- Drill and insert locking screws in any remaining viable holes (**TECH FIG 11D**).
- Replace the wires with locking screws (**TECH FIGURE 12**).

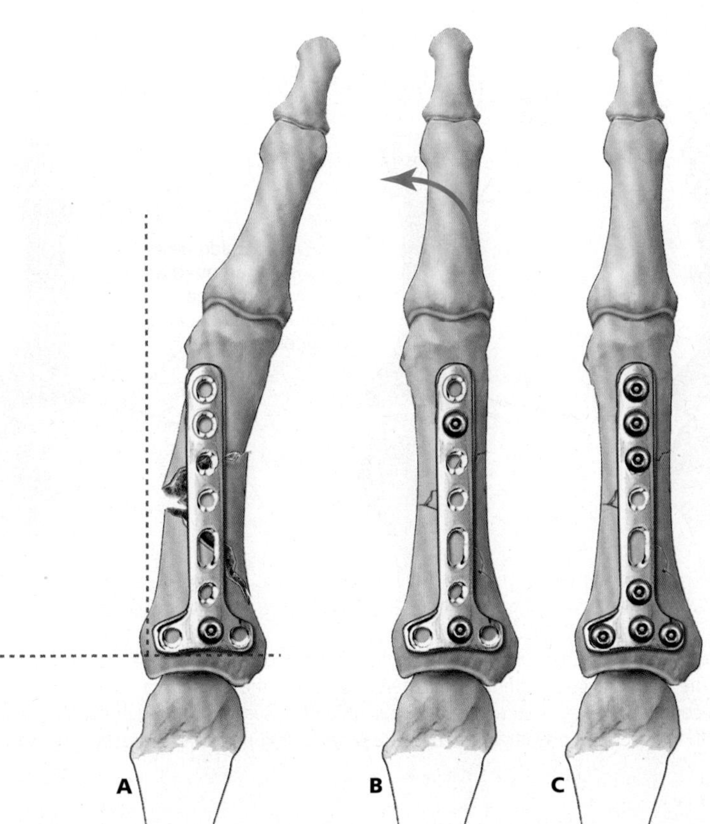

TECH FIG 9 • **A.** The T plate is aligned perpendicular to the joint line and secured with a single screw. **B.** The distal portion of the fracture is brought into alignment and secured with one additional screw. **C.** Length, angulation, and rotational correction are all confirmed before insertion of the remaining screws.

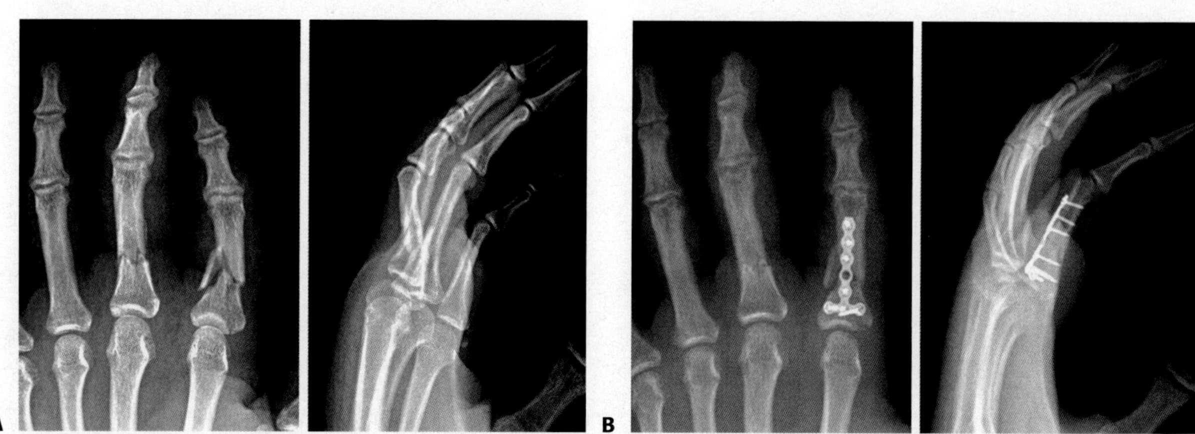

TECH FIG 10 • A. Preoperative posteroanterior and lateral radiographs showing a comminuted index finger proximal phalanx fracture with significant shortening, angulation, and rotation and a middle finger proximal phalanx fracture with reasonable alignment. The middle finger had a significant crush injury and a large volar wound. **B.** The index finger proximal phalanx fracture is fixed with a T plate, which is used to restore alignment, length, and rotation while bridging the fracture. Rather than risking additional vascular compromise to the middle finger with pins or open reduction, the relatively stable fracture of the middle proximal phalanx was treated by closed means. Active motion of both fingers was started 1 week after open reduction and internal fixation.

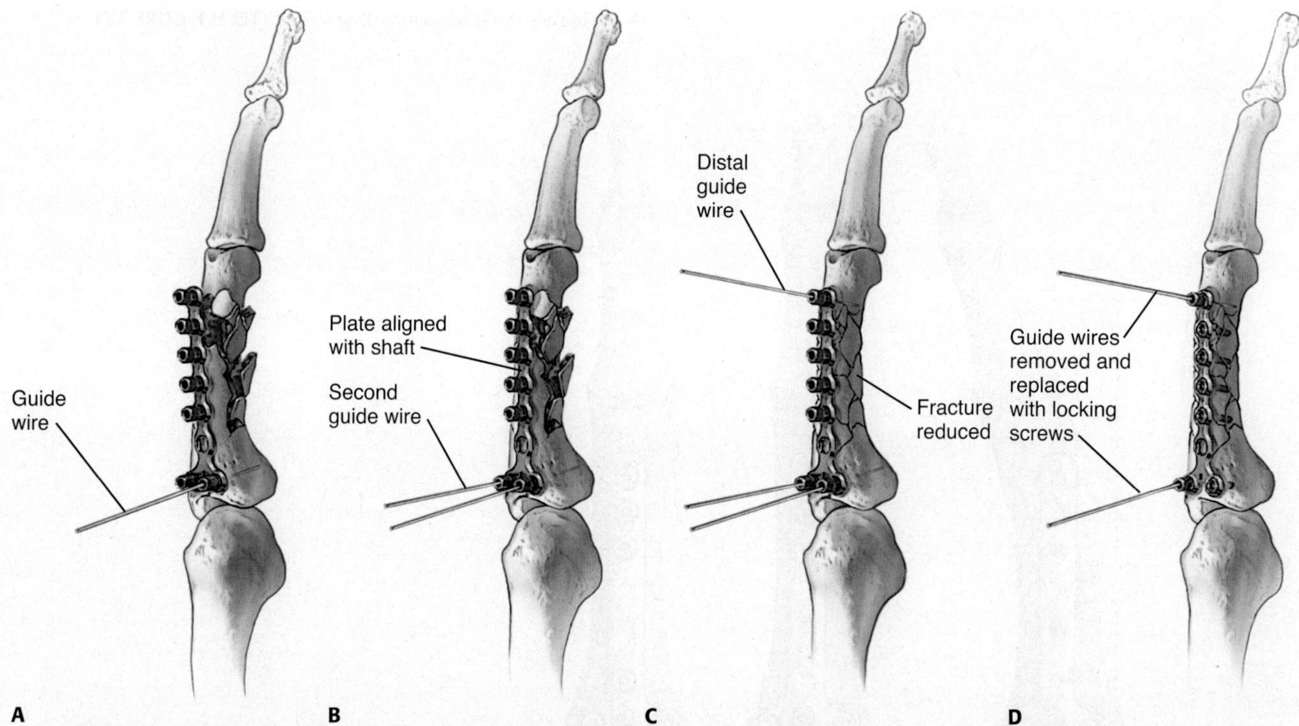

TECH FIG 11 • A. The proximal end of the locking plate is center on the bone as close to the joint as possible. A wire is inserted in the short drill guide to secure the proximal end of the plate. **B.** The plate is aligned with the shaft, perpendicular to the joint and a second proximal wire inserted. **C.** The fracture is reduced, and with the plate centered on the distal end of the phalanx, a wire is inserted through the short drill guide. **D.** Locking screws are inserted in remaining holes with intact bone beneath. Holes over areas of comminution are bypassed. The wires are replaced with locking screws to complete the fixation.

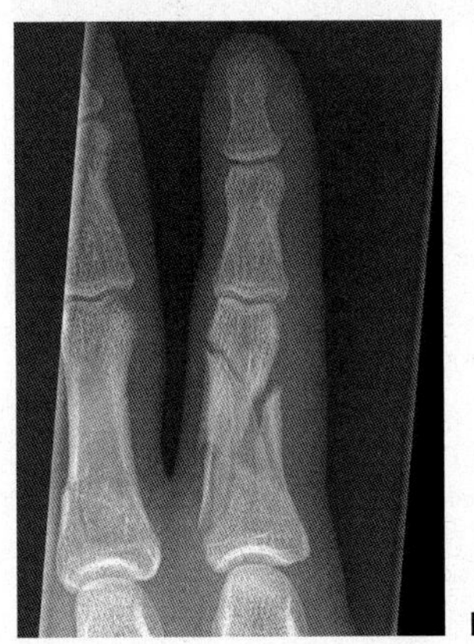

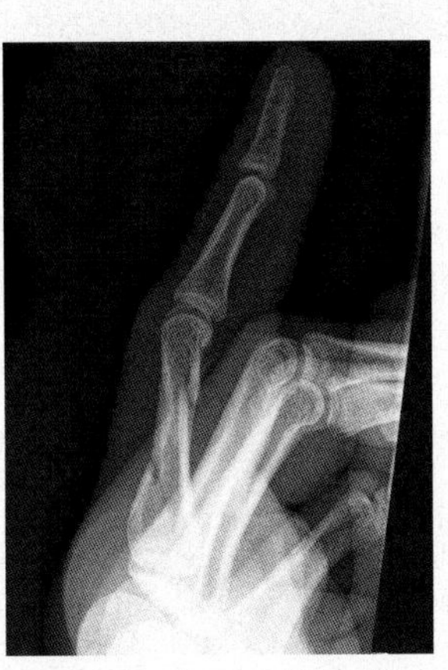

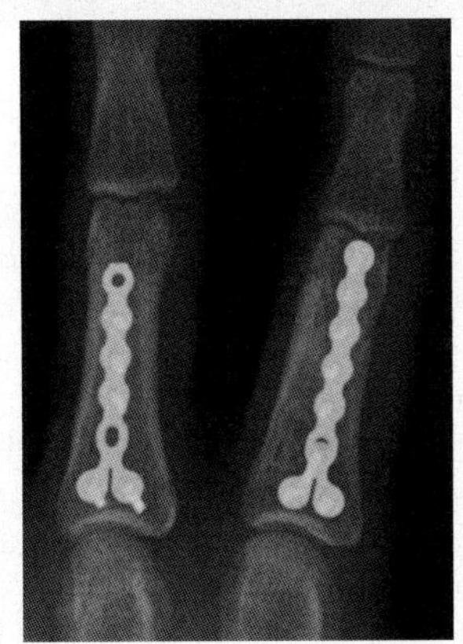

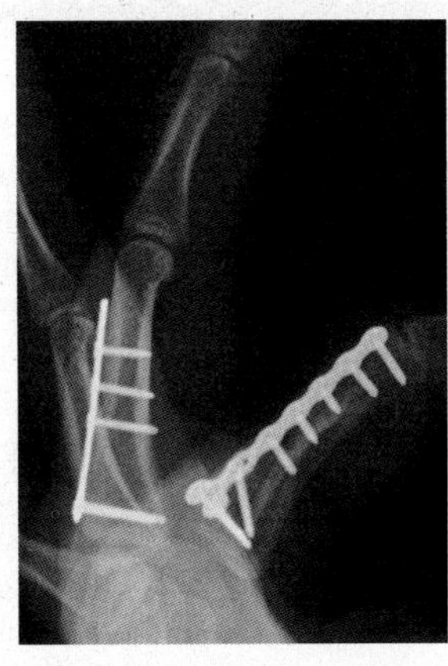

TECH FIG 12 • Posteroanterior (**A**) and lateral (**B**) radiographs of a patient with a comminuted index finger proximal phalanx fracture and less comminuted middle finger proximal phalanx fracture. Postoperative posteroanterior (**C**) and lateral (**D**) radiographs of the fixed fractures using the method described in the text.

Other Methods

- Some authors have described using Kirschner wires as stacked intramedullary nails to secure phalangeal fractures. Intrafocal pinning is an excellent way to stabilize juxta-articular fractures of the proximal phalanx.[5]
  - By placing several wires along the canal, the fracture can be stabilized sufficiently to allow early motion.
  - Inserting the wires from the side of the finger minimizes extensor tendon injury (**TECH FIG 13A**).
- Other methods of fixation not commonly used for extra-articular phalangeal fractures include external fixation and bridging Kirschner wire fixation (**TECH FIG 13B**).
  - These rarely used methods are most useful for temporary fixation while allowing the soft tissue injuries to heal.
  - External fixation is more advantageous for border digits. For treatment of extra-articular phalangeal fractures, these fixators should not be placed across a joint if at all possible.[17]

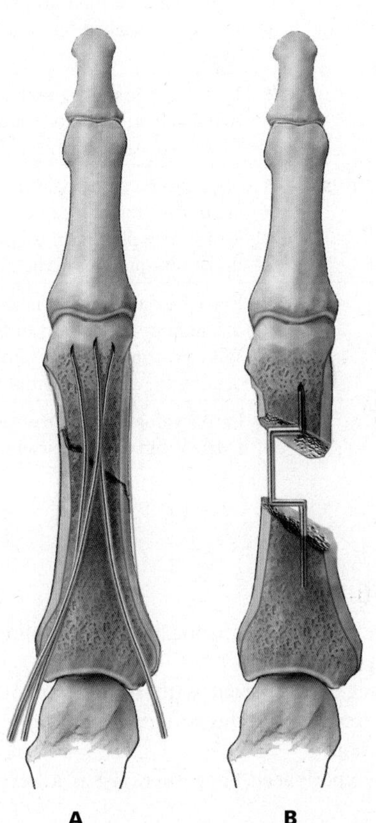

TECH FIG 13 • **A.** Intramedullary Kirschner wires can be stacked in the canal to provide intramedullary support to a phalangeal fracture. Wires are inserted from the sides to minimize extensor tendon damage. **B.** In the case of soft tissue damage with bone loss, a square U-shaped bend in a Kirschner wire can be used to temporarily maintain length while the soft tissue heals.

PEARLS AND PITFALLS

Indications	■ Thorough history and physical assessment must be obtained. ■ Recognizing malalignment, especially in the rotational plane, is crucial.
Choice of technique	■ Preoperative planning is critical. ■ Choose the least invasive method that will align and stabilize the fracture. ■ If open reduction is planned, and especially if plate fixation is chosen, stable fixation must be obtained to allow early motion.
Kirschner wiring	■ Avoid placing crossed pins with their intersection at the level of the fracture, as this may cause distraction at the fracture site. ■ Smooth pin wiring is not without complications.[3]
Plate fixation	■ Placing the plate laterally or dorsolaterally may minimize the negative effects on the extensor mechanism. ■ Do not detach the insertion of the central slip at the dorsal base of the middle phalanx. ■ Augmenting fixation with a lag screw either through or adjacent to the plate markedly increases fracture stability. ■ If plating dorsally, avoid placing overly long screws, which may damage flexor tendons. ■ Always check plate placement and length fluoroscopically. ■ Thoughtful placement of temporary Kirschner wires will avoid frustration with simultaneous fracture reduction and plate placement. ■ Temporary Kirschner wire placement can maintain fracture reduction as well as take the place of predrilling for screws; replace the Kirschner wire with an appropriately sized screw. ■ After a midaxial approach and placement of a plate on the proximal phalanx, excise rather than repair the lateral band to minimize scarring and maximize motion. ■ Plates with locked screws can be used to gain secure fixation of a comminuted fracture segment with a single screw.
External fixation	■ Useful in markedly comminuted fractures with bone loss ■ Avoid spanning joints if possible. ■ Most applicable for border digits
Distal phalanx fractures	■ Nonunions can be painful. ■ Support of the nail bed can help prevent later nail deformities. ■ Temporary pinning through the distal interphalangeal joint can provide stability and is an easier technique than cross-pinning in the distal phalanx.
Problems	■ Recognize and correct malalignment in the operating room. Clinical and radiographic assessment is required throughout the process of fracture reduction and stabilization. Always compare with the contralateral hand. ■ With postoperative swelling, it is our practice to always include more than one digit in the postoperative dressing to avoid potential vascular complications.
Postoperative care	■ Early evaluation and treatment by an experienced hand therapist will improve outcome. ■ Diligent pin care in Kirschner wire and external fixator constructs is necessary to avoid infection.

POSTOPERATIVE CARE

- Postoperative care depends on the location of the injury and the bony fixation.
- The best outcomes are achieved with restoration of anatomic alignment, respect for the soft tissue envelope, and early range of motion.
- Treatment by an experienced hand therapist is a key component.
  - In the early phases, therapy consists of edema control and mobilization of adjacent digits and joints.
  - If adequate fracture stabilization is obtained, then active mobilization of the involved digit is started almost immediately.
  - If fracture fixation is not ideal, active motion of the involved segment should be started no later than 3 to 4 weeks after surgery regardless of the radiographic appearance.
  - Protected mobilization should include removable splints that allow motion of adjacent digits and joints. As healing progresses, these splints are eliminated and buddy taping is employed.
- Return to full activity is usually possible by 8 weeks.

OUTCOMES

- Virtually all phalangeal fractures will heal in 4 to 6 weeks. Malalignment, especially rotation, and stiffness will diminish the outcome.
- Most simple fractures treated with splinting, percutaneous pinning, or open reduction and internal fixation will regain near-full motion in 2 to 6 months, if the principles are followed and the proper intraoperative and postoperative techniques are employed.
- In complex injuries where early motion is delayed because of concomitant soft tissue injury or prolonged splinting, the final outcome will be worse.

- Sometimes, hardware removal, tenolysis, and joint release are needed to improve motion.
  - Such procedures should be attempted only after tissue equilibrium has been reached (usually at least 4 months after the initial injury or surgery).

COMPLICATIONS

- Loss of motion
  - Surgical: careful soft tissue handling with avoidance of prominent hardware
  - Postoperative: Elevation, ice, early motion of all non-injured joints, and controlled mobilization of injured segments as soon as possible are the best preventive measures.
  - If the problem persists and, despite a period of hand therapy, passive motion greatly exceeds active motion, tenolysis is a reliable method of treatment.[8,14]
- Malunion
  - Malreduction is common and, once secured with a plate and screws, difficult to correct. It is important to assess rotation on all phalangeal fractures before final fixation.
  - Accurate assessment is often difficult because the patient cannot make a full fist. Therefore, a reduction that was thought to be adequate in the face of restricted motion may prove inadequate once full motion is regained.
  - If significant enough, osteotomy should be considered.
- Neurovascular injury while pinning a fracture
  - By observing the cross-sectional anatomy of the digit, damage to the neurovascular bundle can usually be avoided when inserting the wires.
  - Care must be taken when the wire passes through the second cortex, as it will usually be heading directly toward the neurovascular bundle.
  - Inserting the wires initially by hand until bone contact is made and using small open incisions may decrease the chance of injury when inserting the wire close to the neurovascular bundle.
- Complex regional pain syndrome
  - Early recognition and treatment are essential.
  - A high index of suspicion is needed to identify key symptoms:
    - Swelling despite elevation and other edema control efforts
    - Stiffness, especially in adjacent digits, despite efforts toward early mobilization
    - Color changes in the hand
    - Mottling or shiny appearance of the skin
    - Abnormal hair growth
    - Burning pain in the hand
- Tendon rupture
- Nonunion
- Infection
- Pin loosening and migration
- Implant failure
- Pain and symptoms from retained hardware

REFERENCES

1. Al-Qattan MM, Al-Zahrani K. Open reduction and cerclage wire fixation for long oblique/spiral fractures of the proximal phalanx of the fingers. J Hand Surg Eur 2008;33:170-173.
2. Barton NJ. Fractures of the shafts of the phalanxes of the hand. Hand 1979;11:119–133.
3. Botte MJ, Davis JL, Rose BA, et al. Complications of smooth pin fixation of fractures and dislocations in the hand and wrist. Clin Orthop Relat Res 1992;(276):194–201.
4. Carpenter S, Rohde RS. Treatment of phalangeal fractures. Hand Clin 2013;29:519–534.
5. Crofoot CD, Saing M, Raphael J. Intrafocal pinning for juxta-articular phalanx fractures. Tech Hand Up Extrem Surg 2005;9:164–168.
6. Eaton RG, Hastings HH. Point/counterpoint: closed reduction and internal fixation versus open reduction and internal fixation for displaced oblique proximal phalangeal fractures. Orthopedics 1989;12:911–916.
7. Ebinger T, Erhard N, Kinzl L, et al. Dynamic treatment of displaced proximal phalangeal fractures. J Hand Surg Am 1999;24:1254–1262.
8. Faruqui S, Stern PJ, Kiefhaber TR. Percutaneous pinning of fractures in the proximal third of the proximal phalanx: complications and outcomes. J Hand Surg Am 2012;37:1342–1348.
9. Franz T, von Wartburg U, Schibli-Beer S, et al. Extra-articular fractures of the proximal phalanges of the fingers: a comparison of 2 methods of functional, conservative treatment. J Hand Surg Am 2012;37: 889–898.
10. Gaston RG, Chadderdon C. Phalangeal fractures: displaced/nondisplaced. Hand Clin 2012;28:395–401.
11. Held M, Jordaan P, Laubscher M, et al. Conservative treatment of fractures of the proximal phalanx: an option even for unstable fracture patterns. Hand Surg 2013;18:229–234.
12. Henry MH. Fractures of the proximal phalanx and metacarpals in the hand: preferred methods of stabilization. J Am Acad Orthop Surg 2008;16:586–595.
13. Horton TC, Hatton M, Davis TR. A prospective randomized controlled study of fixation of long oblique and spiral shaft fractures of the proximal phalanx: closed recuction and percutaneous Kirschner wiring versus open reduction and lag screw fixation. J Hand Surg Br 2003;28:5–9.
14. Kurzen P, Fusetti C, Bonaccio M, et al. Complications after plate fixation of phalangeal fractures. J Trauma 2006;60:841–843.
15. Lins RE, Myers BS, Spinner RJ, et al. A comparative mechanical analysis of plate fixation in a proximal phalangeal fracture model. J Hand Surg Am 1996;21:1059–1064.
16. Maitra A, Burdett-Smith P. The conservative management of proximal phalanx fractures of the hand in an accident and emergency department. J Hand Surg Br 1992;17(3):332–336.
17. Margić K. External fixation of closed metacarpal and phalangeal fractures of digits: a prospective study of one hundred consecutive patients. J Hand Surg Br 2006;31(1):30–40.
18. Pehlivan O, Kiral A, Solakoglu C, et al. Tension band wiring of unstable transverse fractures of the proximal and middle phalanges of the hand. J Hand Surg Br 2004;29:130–141.
19. Reyes FA, Latta LL. Conservative management of difficult phalangeal fractures. Clin Orthop Relat Res 1987;(214):23–30.
20. Sloan JP, Dove AF, Maheson M, et al. Antibiotics in open fractures of the distal phalanx? J Hand Surg Br 1987;12(1):123–124.
21. Strickland JW, Steichen JB, Kleinman WB, et al. Phalangeal fractures: factors influencing digital performance. Orthop Rev 1982;11:39–50.
22. Vahey JW, Wegner DA, Hastings H III. Effect of proximal phalangeal fracture deformity on extensor tendon function. J Hand Surg Am 1998;23(4):673–681.

Open Reduction and Internal Fixation of Phalangeal Condylar Fractures

Greg Merrell, Barrett Weiss, and Arnold-Peter Weiss

DEFINITION

- Phalangeal condylar fractures include unicondylar and bicondylar intra-articular fracture of the distal ends of the proximal and middle phalanx.
  - Proximal phalangeal condylar fractures are more common and, due to the propensity of stiffness at the proximal interphalangeal (PIP) joint regardless of treatment, require careful attention.
  - Condylar fractures of the distal middle phalanx, although still frequently requiring treatment, have some degree of forgiveness regarding range of motion (ROM) issues.
- Table 1 demonstrates the variety of condylar fracture patterns typically observed.

ANATOMY

- Collateral ligaments, finger position, and direction of force play a role in both fracture pattern and the direction of displacement (**FIG 1**).
- Blood is supplied to the condyles by a branch of the digital artery and vein that travels with the collateral ligaments.
  - Care must be taken not to disrupt this blood supply or to strip small fragments of their soft tissue attachments.

Table 1 Condylar Fracture Patterns

Fracture Configuration	Illustration	Characteristics	Fixation: Nondisplaced Fracture	Fixation: Displaced Fracture
Type I: unicondylar short oblique		Unstable	Could consider nonoperative treatment but must follow closely. Otherwise, two percutaneous K-wires	Joystick closed reduction and K-wires, open reduction and screws, or K-wires
Type II: unicondylar long oblique		Unstable but fixation is a little easier than type I	Could consider nonoperative treatment but must follow closely. Otherwise, two or three percutaneous K-wires	Joystick closed reduction and K-wires, open reduction and screws, or K-wires

(continued)

Table 1 *(continued)*

Fracture Configuration	Illustration	Characteristics	Fixation	
			Nondisplaced Fracture	**Displaced Fracture**
Type III: dorsal coronal	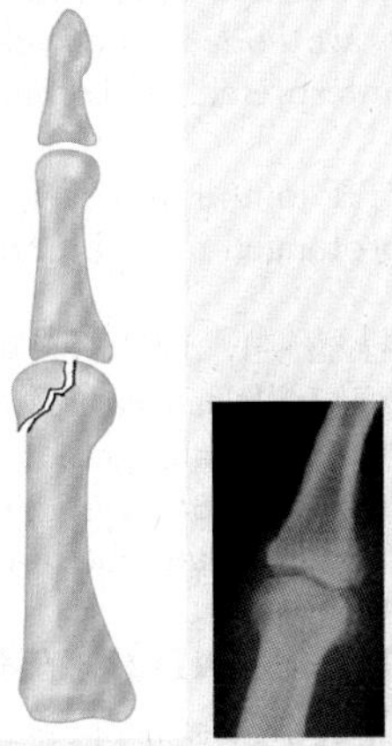	Often stable	<25% and stable joint: consider nonoperative treatment or excision. >25% and nondisplaced: could consider nonoperative treatment but must follow closely. Otherwise, two percutaneous K-wires	>25% and displaced or <25% with subluxed joint: joystick closed reduction and K-wires or open reduction and K-wires (rarely screws)
Type IV: volar coronal	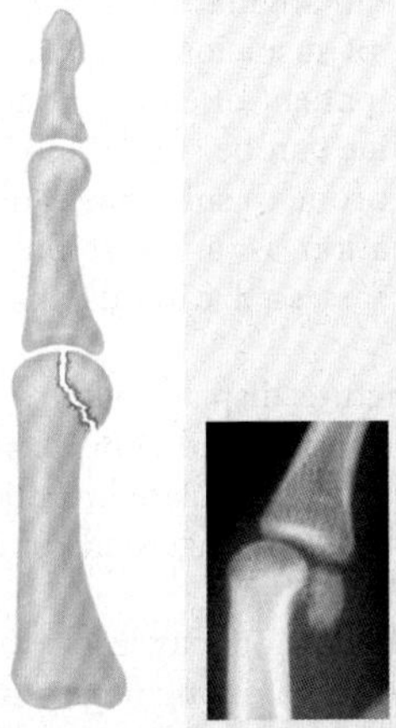	Unstable	<25% and stable joint: consider nonoperative treatment or excision. >25% and nondisplaced: could consider nonoperative treatment but must follow closely. Otherwise, two percutaneous K-wires	>25% and displaced or <25% with subluxed joint: joystick closed reduction and K-wires or open reduction and K-wires (rarely screws)
Type V: bicondylar	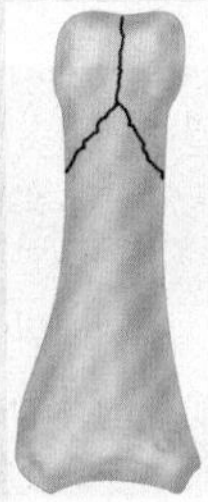	Unstable	A nondisplaced fracture: could consider K-wires	Usually requires open reduction and screws, plates, or K-wires
Type VI: triplane-type bicondylar	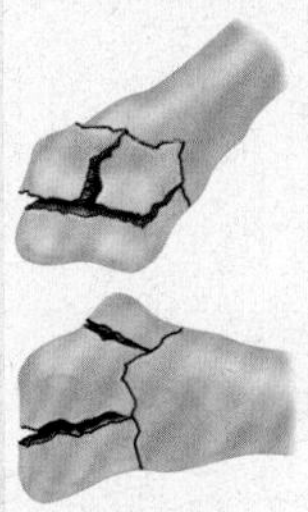	Unstable	Percutaneous K-wires	Usually requires open reduction with dorsal to volar screws

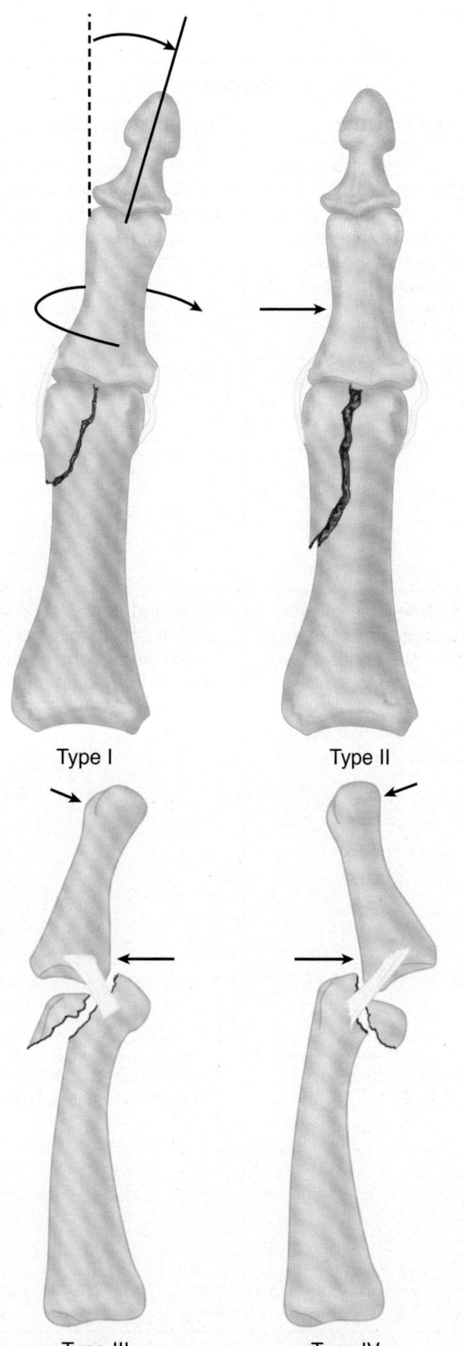

FIG 1 • Direction of applied force determines the fracture type.

PATHOGENESIS

- These fractures often are sports-related injuries.
- The mechanism is hypothesized to be tension or rotation force through the collateral ligaments for an oblique fracture and compression and subluxation in the case of a coronal fracture.[1,6]
- Fractures often are unstable because there is a minimal periosteal sleeve, forces seen at the joint are substantial, and the oblique nature of the fracture line is inherently unstable.
- Most commonly, the condyle toward the midline of the hand (ie, the middle finger axis) is fractured: the ulnar condyle in the index finger and thumb and the radial condyle in the ring and small fingers.

NATURAL HISTORY

- In developed countries, these fractures rarely go untreated, but they often are *undertreated*, given that their presentation may be interpreted as a "minimally displaced finger fracture."
- Similar to any PIP joint injury, lack of immobilization in full extension or prolonged immobilization will likely lead to a stiff finger.
- If treated conservatively, displacement of the fracture, a common occurrence, will lead either to early painful arthritic changes or rotational malalignment on full flexion or both. The only potential exception is in children with significant growth potential remaining due to remodeling.[5]

PATIENT HISTORY AND PHYSICAL FINDINGS

- A typical patient is a 24-year-old male basketball player who has sustained an angular impact to the finger from the ball.
- A high index of suspicion is required when evaluating these patients. The patient often is still able to flex the finger, and the fracture line can be subtle. However, even nondisplaced fractures are prone to subsequent displacement.
- Joint subluxation is an absolute indication for surgery and must be assessed carefully both radiographically and clinically.
- With any fracture displacement, a rotational deformity of the finger may occur and is best assessed by either looking end on at the digit for isolated rotation of the nail plate compared to the adjacent fingernails or evaluating position with PIP flexion (**FIG 2A**).
- Subtle joint depression may lead to angular deformity; this is best assessed by examining fingers in full extension (**FIG 2B**).

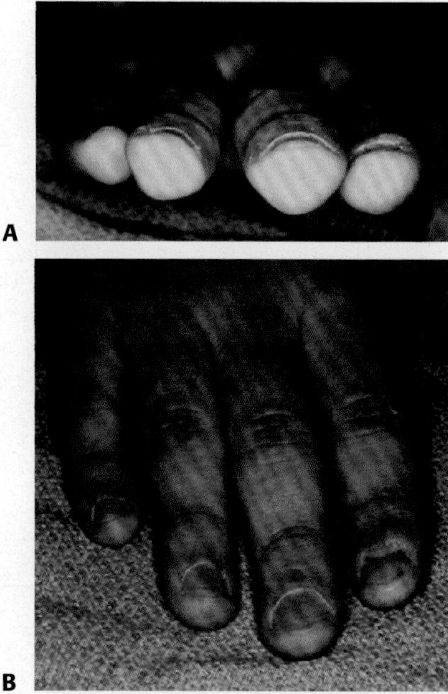

FIG 2 • **A.** End-on observation of the fingers can demonstrate subtle rotational deformities. **B.** Observation of the fingers in full extension can demonstrate subtle angular deformities caused by a displaced condyle.

IMAGING AND OTHER DIAGNOSTIC STUDIES

- The fracture pattern dictates the type of fixation or treatment.
- Multiple views should be obtained as needed to understand the geometry. Fluoroscopy often is helpful in obtaining precise views.
  - Osteochondral fragments are often larger than they appear because the cartilage is radiolucent.
  - Hidden fracture lines are common and are often not visualized until exposed at surgery.
- Computed tomography (CT) is occasionally helpful.

DIFFERENTIAL DIAGNOSIS

- Collateral ligament or volar plate avulsion
- PIP dislocation
- Distal phalangeal shaft fracture

NONOPERATIVE MANAGEMENT

- Reports regarding the results of nonoperative treatment present conflicting results.
  - Weiss and Hastings[6] found five of seven nondisplaced fractures treated conservatively went on to displace and required surgery.
  - In an 11-year follow-up study, using a functional outcome score, O'Rourke et al[4] demonstrated several interesting points:
    - Twenty-seven percent of patients experienced joint aching in cold weather.
    - Four patients at 1-year follow-up had moderate pain and considered arthrodesis. However, by the time they got off the waiting list, their symptoms had subsided to the point that they declined surgery.
    - No patient had less movement in the joint at year 11 than at year 1.
    - Twenty-five percent of patients had continued improvement in ROM after 12 months follow-up.
    - Three patients with displaced bicondylar fractures treated conservatively had outcomes of good, fair, and poor, respectively.
    - Three patients with displaced unicondylar fractures treated conservatively had a good outcome; however, in O'Rourke et al's[4] discussion, they conclude that these fractures should be treated with reduction and fixation.
- Operating on nondisplaced or minimally displaced fractures can be viewed in two ways:
  - On the one hand, a percentage of patients would be subjected to a procedure that they did not need. Also, with close follow-up, if a fracture were to displace later, it could be addressed at that point, although it would require slightly more work to regain reduction and functional restoration.
  - On the other hand, there is minimal morbidity in percutaneous pinning and that would minimize the likelihood of displacement in a fracture that often is unstable.
  - Given the propensity for displacement and the potential functional difficulties with malunion, we recommend, at a minimum, percutaneous stabilization of most condylar fractures.
- Several review texts suggest that coronal fractures of less than 25% of the joint surface with a stable congruent joint can be treated nonoperatively or with fragment excision. Although this may be true, there are few biomechanical or clinical outcomes data to support the statement.
- A recent study examining the remodeling potential of distal condylar malunions in children demonstrated a substantial remodeling potential and functional ROM without pain. Although the series was small, malunions of unicondylar phalangeal fractures in children are likely best treated nonoperatively.[6]

SURGICAL MANAGEMENT

Preoperative Planning

- Preoperative planning should be mindful of the goals of treatment of any articular fracture established by the AO:
  - Anatomic reduction of the articular surface
  - Restoration of stability
  - Minimizing soft tissue injury
  - Early mobilization
- Access to a mini C-arm is highly advantageous.
  - Fluoroscopic examination under anesthesia provides a good sense of joint stability and fracture fragment orientation.
  - Fracture reduction, implant placement, and fracture stability are effectively evaluated fluoroscopically.

Positioning

- The patient is positioned supine with a hand table.
- If an assistant is unavailable, finger-trap traction also may be helpful.

Approach

- A unicondylar fracture typically is approached either between the central slip and lateral band (**FIG 3**) or via a midaxial approach.
  - The lateral (midaxial) approach is suggested as a means to minimize extensor mechanism scarring but only if significant joint incongruity or comminution is absent.
  - If more extensive joint visualization is needed, the extensor mechanism can be incised and repaired later.
- A bicondylar or triplane fracture requires a more global joint and fragment exposure (**FIG 4**).
  - A dorsal, slightly curvilinear incision is made.
  - The extensor tendon may be split longitudinally, but preferably, incisions are made on its borders, allowing mobilization and excellent joint exposure.
- A palmar approach is rarely used except for volar coronal shear fractures.
  - If necessary, make a Brunner-style volar incision, and retract the flexor tendons to expose the volar plate.
  - If possible, reflect the volar plate on one side and up the lateral edge for exposure via a triangle-shaped flap.
  - If more complete exposure is needed, make a transverse incision along the proximal edge of the volar plate, leaving enough proximal cuff to reattach the volar plate.
  - Elevate the volar plate on a distal hinge, repair the fracture, and then reattach the volar plate.
- The PIP joint is prone to stiffness from injury, so every effort should be made to minimize surgical disruption of the soft tissues.
- Avoid at all costs stripping soft tissue attachments from small fracture fragments.

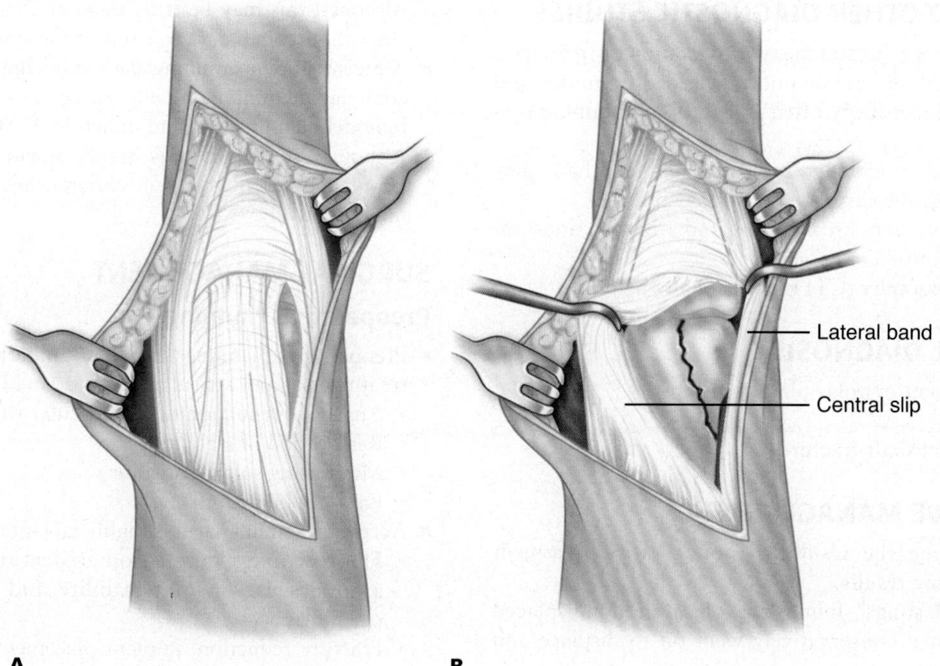

FIG 3 • A dorsolateral incision (**A**) with dissection between the lateral band and extensor mechanism (**B**) provides excellent exposure.

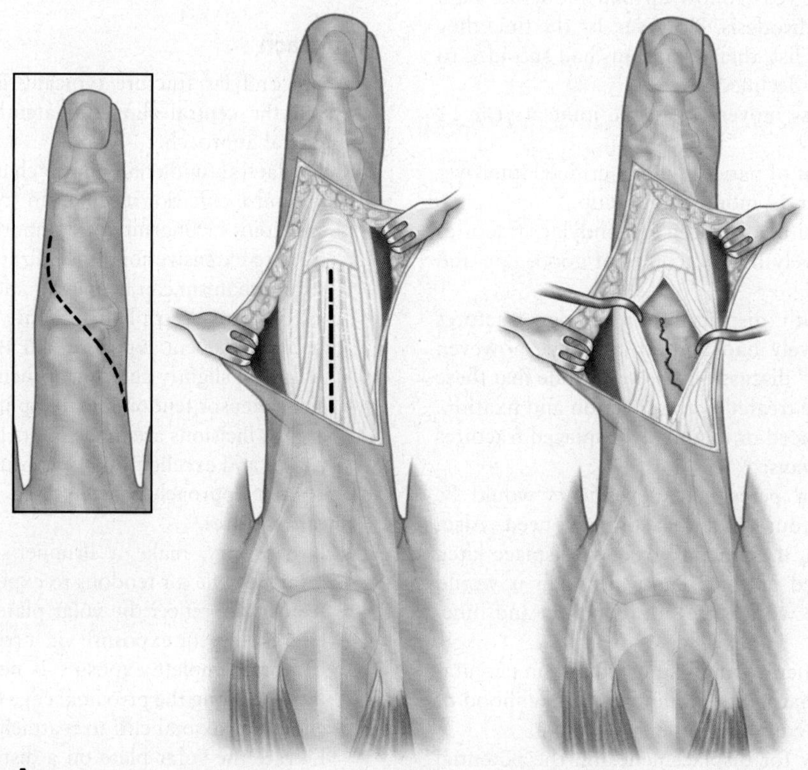

FIG 4 • A dorsolateral incision (**A**) with midline incision in the extensor mechanism (**B**) can provide additional exposure if needed.

Percutaneous Reduction of Short and Long Oblique Fractures Using K-Wires, Minifragment Screws, or Cannulated Headless Compression Screws

Tips for Achieving Fixation

- Visualize the fracture well using live fluoroscopy.
  - Fracture displacement typically is in an oblique plane, sometimes not well appreciated on the straight anteroposterior or lateral views.
  - Use of the view on live fluoroscopy that best shows the displacement will make it possible to determine when reduction has truly been achieved.
- Apply traction and rotation to the distal aspect of the finger to assist reduction through ligamentotaxis (**TECH FIG 1A**).
- Try percutaneous manipulation of the fragment with a dental pick.
  - If reduction is achieved, place either a pointed reduction clamp or the first K-wire to hold the position.
- If the dental pick does not work, place one prong of a pointed reduction clamp through the skin into the stable condyle, then place the other prong into the fragment and try to reduce the fragment with a slight rotation of the clamp (**TECH FIG 1B**).
  - Resist the urge to use clamp compression to force a reduction because the small fragments shatter easily.
  - Avoid placing the clamp volar to the midaxial line to avoid iatrogenic injury to the neurovascular bundle.
- If the earlier techniques are not effective, try a 0.035-inch K-wire joystick or proceed with an open reduction.

Fixation Choices

- If a percutaneous reduction is achieved, we prefer the use of multiple 0.028-inch K-wires.
- If open reduction is necessary, we prefer the stability of screw fixation.
  - Occasionally, fragments are too small or comminuted for screw fixation, necessitating the use of K-wires.

K-Wire Fixation

- A single K-wire is not sufficient fixation and may allow subsequent displacement (the fracture can "rotate" on the single fixation point).
- Drive two K-wires from the fragment into the shaft either transversely or obliquely depending on the fracture orientation (**TECH FIG 2**).
  - The first wire should be placed perpendicular to the fracture line to maximize fixation and minimize displacement while capturing the reduction.
  - Additional wires should be placed slightly oblique to the first wire so that the fracture fragment cannot displace along the axis of two parallel wires.
  - The best bone quality is found distal and volar; therefore, to avoid injury, insert wires from the dorsal side of the intact condyle and advance them distally and volarly.
- Hold the PIP joint in extension while driving wires.
  - This position keeps the lateral bands dorsal, and the entry of the K-wire can be just volar to the lateral bands.
  - The condyle, as viewed on a lateral image, is the area with the least excursion of the collateral ligaments; therefore, K-wires in the volar position cause the least restriction of motion.
- The use of 0.028-inch K-wires avoids further fragmentation of fragments and usually provides sufficient fixation.

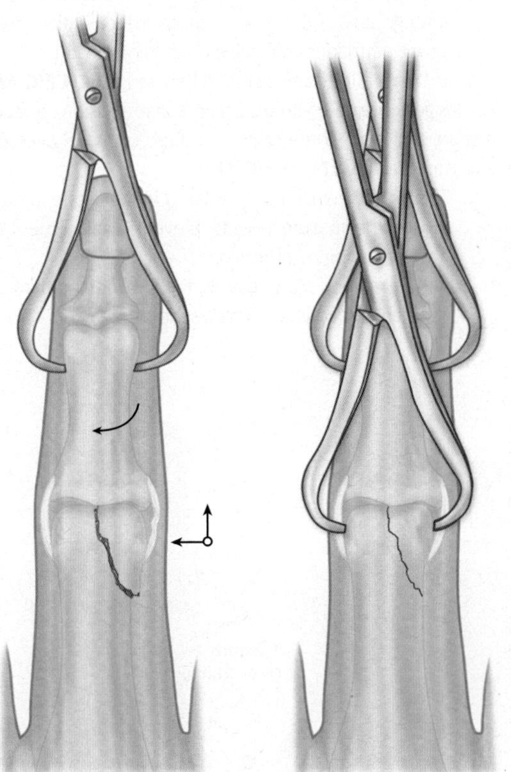

TECH FIG 1 • Percutaneous fracture reduction with traction and rotational correction (**A**), followed by percutaneous clamping (**B**).

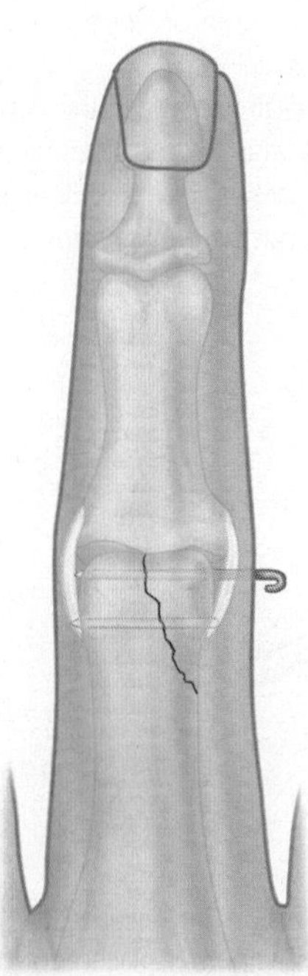

TECH FIG 2 • Pinning with K-wires.

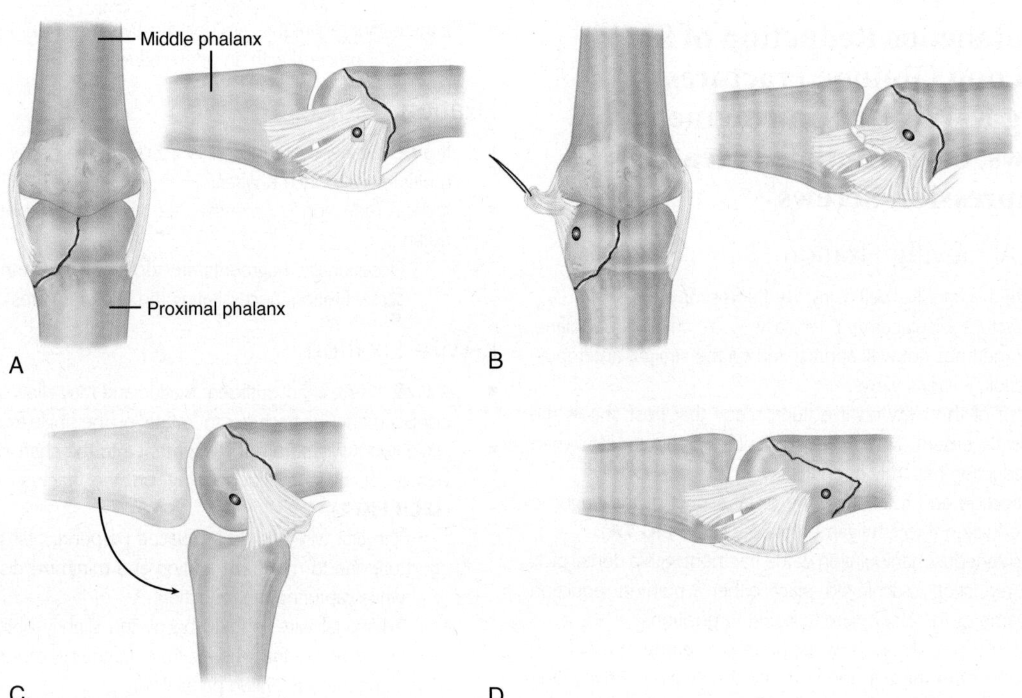

TECH FIG 3 • The four methods for screw placement to minimize impingement on collaterals. Methods **A** and **C** require seating the screw head almost flush with the bone. **A.** Creation of a small window in the collateral for screw placement. **B.** Reflection of the proximal part of the collateral ligament for screw placement. **C.** Flexion to allow exposure of the condyle for screw placement. **D.** In a longer fracture, placement of the screw proximal to collateral insertion.

Screw Fixation

- Screw fixation should avoid the collateral ligaments by one of four methods (**TECH FIG 3**):
  - Flexing the joint and passing the screw distal and dorsal to the collateral ligaments
  - Keeping the joint in extension, with subperiosteal stripping of a limited portion of the collateral ligament origin from proximal to distal
  - Excising a small window in the collateral ligament for the screw head, which is gently countersunk
  - Placing the screw proximal to the collateral ligament if the fracture extends far enough proximally
  - Screw fixation must not impinge on the collateral ligaments through any of the four methods listed, or the screw will cause permanent difficulties with joint motion.
- 1.0- or 1.3-mm lag screws should be used (**TECH FIG 4A–E**).
- For longer oblique fractures, make a stab incision, spread with a snap, and place three screws or three or more wires spaced along the fracture (**TECH FIG 4F**).
  - The first screw should be placed in lag mode, perpendicular to the fracture line, to prevent displacement of the fracture during compression.
  - If there is good compression, the second and third screws can be inserted in a neutralization mode.

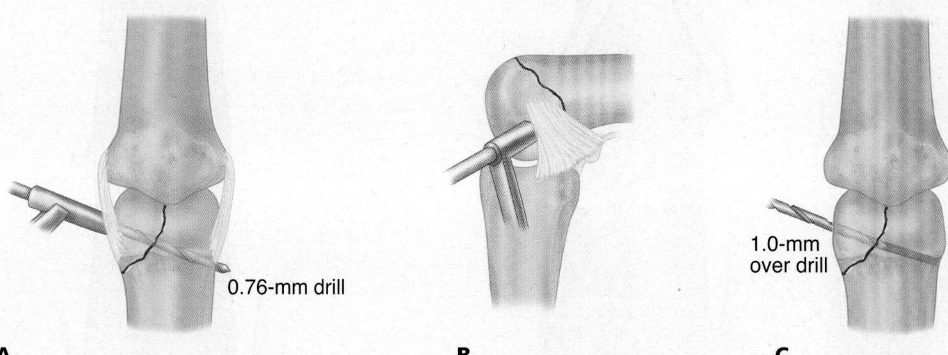

TECH FIG 4 • Placement of a lag screw. **A.** A 0.076-inch drilling is done through both cortices. **B.** The joint is flexed to permit placement of the screw out of the way of the collateral ligaments. **C.** Overdrilling only the proximal cortex with a 1.0-mm drill. *(continued)*

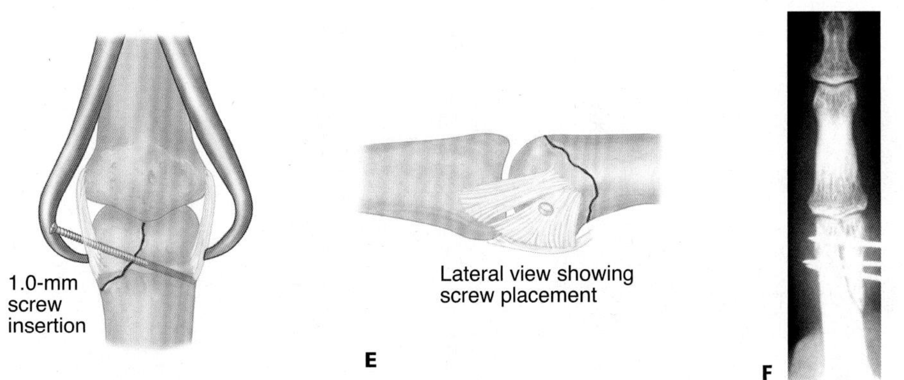

TECH FIG 4 • *(continued)* **D.** Compression of fragments by a reduction clamp while placing the lag screw. **E.** Position of the screw head after extension of the joint. **F.** Long oblique fracture maintained with three 0.028-inch K-wires.

- If compression from the first screw is poor, additional screws can be placed in the lag mode.
- Consider placing one screw more perpendicular to the long axis of the phalanx to resist axial forces.
- While screws are being placed, the reduction can be held either by a reduction clamp or with a temporary K-wire. The hole made by the temporary K-wire, after removal, can be used for the last screw.

Dorsal and Volar Coronal Shear Fracture Treated with Screws or K-Wires

- A dorsal approach typically is used for dorsal fractures and a volar approach for volar fractures.
- Dental picks are used for all fragment manipulation and reduction.
- Traction generally does not help reduction.
- Because fragments usually are very small, fixation with 0.028-inch K-wires may involve crossing the joint surface.
- Typically, a trade-off must be made in terms of implant position.
  - For example, in a dorsal shear fragment, it may be necessary for a K-wire to pass through the dorsal articular surface of the fragment into the condyle below. Try to stay as dorsal as possible to minimize impingement in extension while still securing the fragment adequately. It is possible to bury a screw beneath the articular surface, but if it is possible to use K-wires, they are preferred for their small and temporary footprint. A dorsal shear fracture with a nonarticular component would be a better choice for screw fixation than an all-articular fragment.
- We do not have experience with absorbable implants but would be concerned about their use due to the small size of the fragments and potential resorption osteolysis.

Bicondylar Fracture Treated with Open Reduction and Internal Fixation

- Use a dental pick to align the condylar fragments and secure with a K-wire or screw.
- Similar to previous discussion, if reduction is achieved percutaneously, one or two K-wires may be used to secure the condyles to each other
- Typically, open reduction is required, in which case screws are preferred whenever possible.
- Occasionally, if it is difficult to secure the two condylar fragments to each other, try reducing the largest condylar piece to the shaft and hold it with a K-wire. Then, reduce the smaller condylar piece or pieces to the main construct. Once the entire reduction is achieved and held with clamps or K-wires, a screw can be placed transversely across the condyles.
- If minimal metaphyseal comminution is present, the condylar fragments are secured to the shaft using K-wires (**TECH FIG 5**).

Condylar Plate

- If metaphyseal comminution is present, consider a condylar plate (**TECH FIG 6**).
- The reduction starts with the condylar fragments, ignoring any proximal comminution.
- These fragments are held temporarily while the condylar plate is drilled and placed into just the distal fragment.
- Care must be taken to align the plate on the condyles so that the plate aligns with the shaft, once the condylar/plate construct is reduced to the shaft, bypassing the comminution.

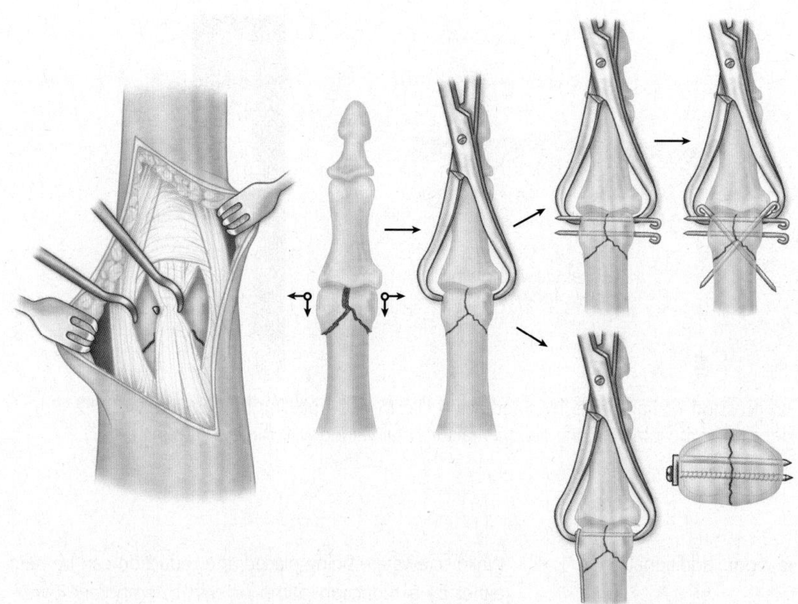

TECH FIG 5 • Reduction of bicondylar fractures begins with reduction of the condyles to each other. The condyles are then secured to the shaft.

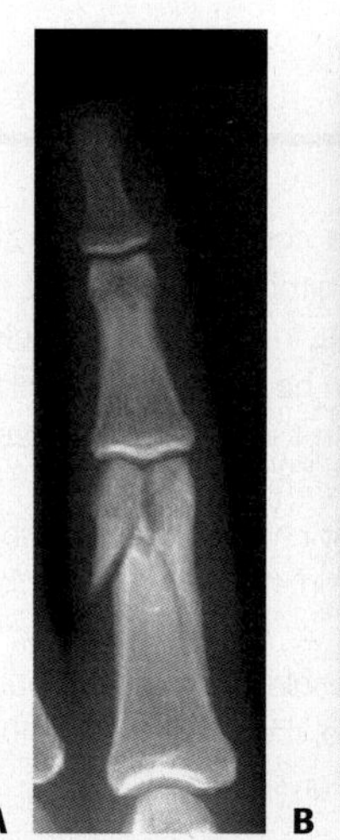

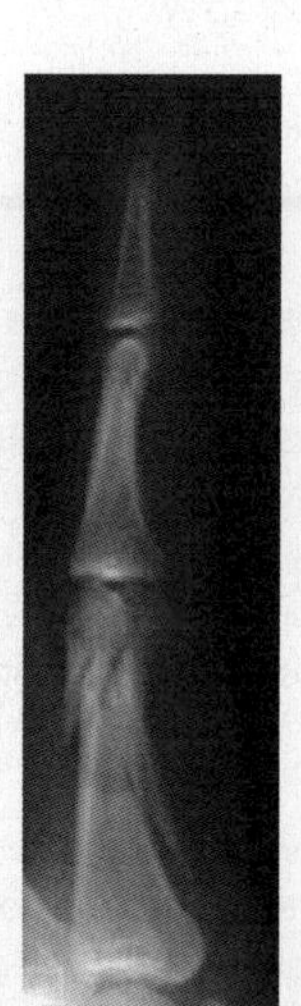

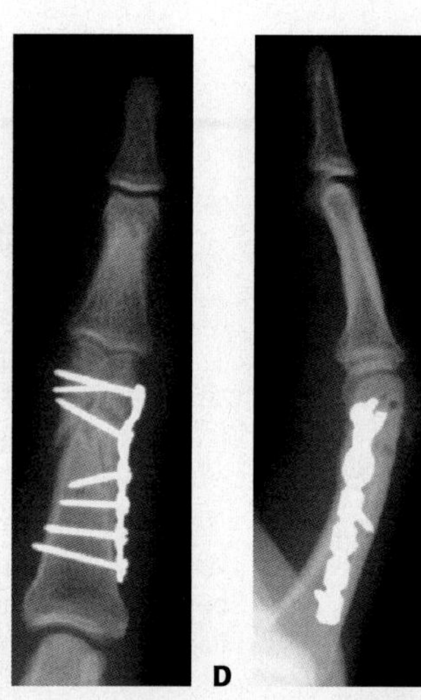

TECH FIG 6 • A,B. Radiographs of a bicondylar fracture. **C,D.** Postoperative radiographs after reduction and application of a condylar plate fixation. (Courtesy of Alan Freeland, MD.)

Triplane Fracture Treated with Open Reduction and Fixation Using Lag Screws and K-Wires

- An extensile dorsal approach is used.
- **TECH FIG 7** shows a triplane fracture in a 42-year-old carpenter with a table saw injury, who was treated as follows:
  - The collateral ligaments were attached to the two volar condylar pieces.
  - Lag screws were placed into each condyle from dorsal to volar.
  - A K-wire was used to secure the condyles to the shaft and keep the joint reduced.
- Metaphyseal comminution has been treated with bone grafting and, in some cases, distraction external fixation for 3 weeks, after which motion is commenced.[1]

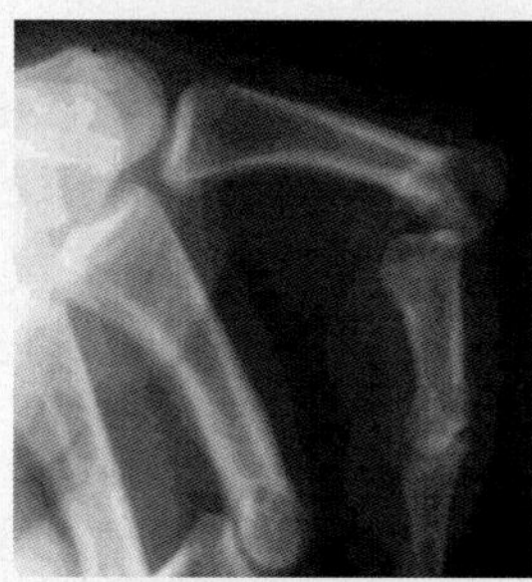

TECH FIG 7 • Triplane fracture in a 42-year-old carpenter with a table saw injury. **A.** Lateral radiograph shows the injury. *(continued)*

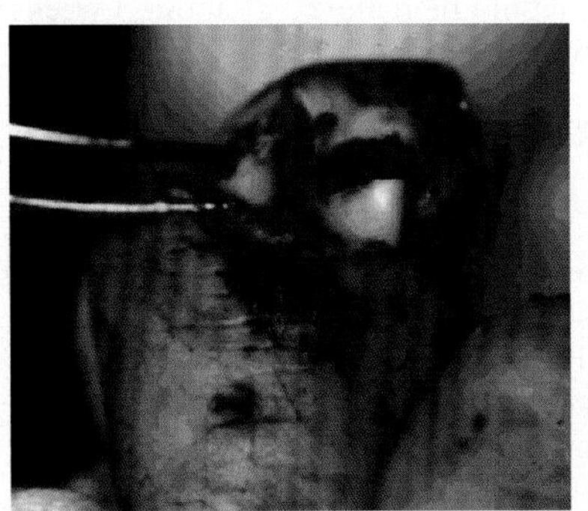
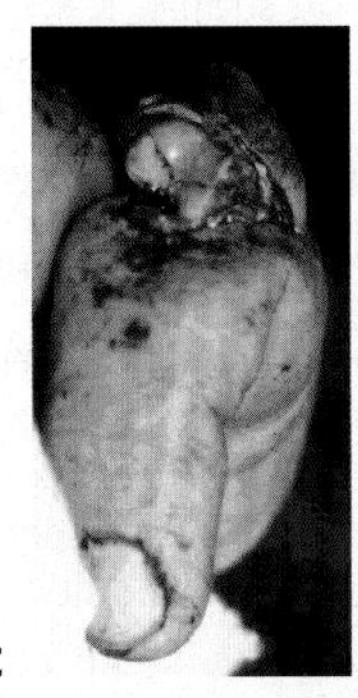
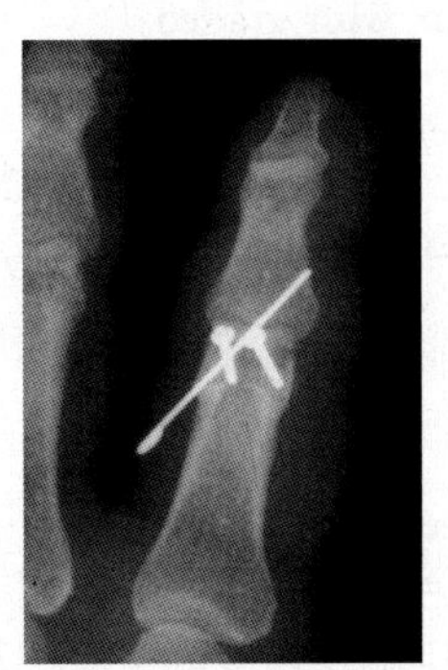
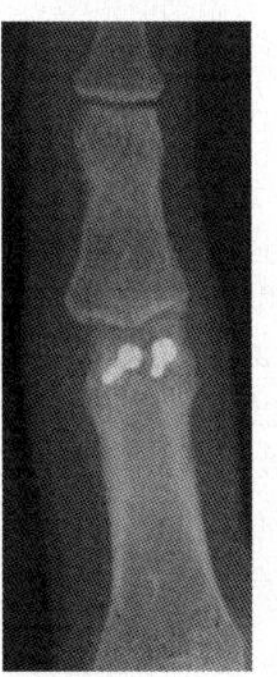
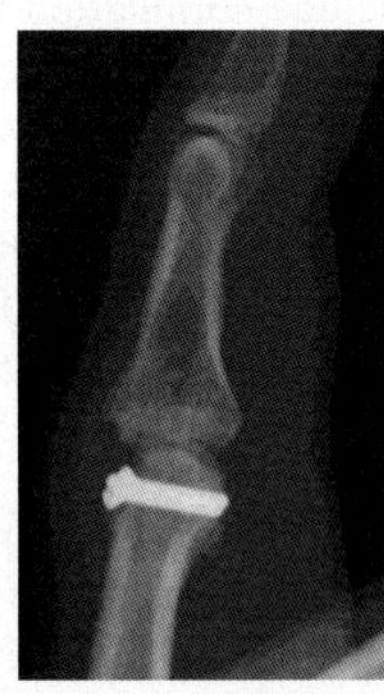

B C D E F

TECH FIG 7 • *(continued)* **B.** Clinical photograph of the injury with the collateral ligaments attached to the two volar condylar pieces. **C,D.** Postreduction photograph and radiograph demonstrating lag screws placed into each condyle from dorsal to volar. A K-wire was used to secure the condyles to the shaft and keep the joint reduced. **E,F.** AP and lateral radiographs 1 year postoperatively. (Courtesy of Jesse Jupiter, MD.)

PEARLS AND PITFALLS

Difficulties with closed reduction and pinning	■ Try using traction with rotation, a dental pick, pointed reduction clamp, or a K-wire as a joystick into the displaced fragment.
Preventing fracture of a small fragment	■ Make sure the screw diameter is no more than one-third the size of the fragment and is placed one screw diameter from the edge of the fragment.
Maintaining reduction and pinning small fragments	■ Use a cannulated reduction forceps.
Obtaining maximum mechanical stability	■ Place the screw from the fragment into the phalanx, "from the island to the mainland."
Maximizing reduction with small intra-articular fragments	■ Reduce the large fragments first. Often, the smaller pieces then fall into place with soft tissue tensioning or can be excised: "rule of vassals or majority rule."
Minimizing postoperative adhesions	■ Avoid plating the phalanges whenever possible. Meticulous handling of soft tissue and sharp dissection where possible rather than blunt spreading minimizes tissue trauma and permits early AROM.

POSTOPERATIVE CARE

- Fracture stability dictates the protocol, but most patients should be started on active range of motion (AROM) within 1 week, with extension splinting of the PIP joint while at rest.
  - It is important for the surgeon and therapist to communicate regarding the extent of injuries, type of fracture fixation used, and coexisting conditions because these variables will affect the rate of healing and progression of therapy.
  - Exercises should be performed at least six times per day.
  - When immobilization is involved, it is extremely important for the patient to perform AROM to all noninvolved joints to prevent secondary weakness and stiff joints in the involved extremity as well as to aid edema control.
- One to 7 days after surgery
  - Control edema with Coban wraps (3M, St. Paul, MN), compressive digit sleeves, elevation and AROM, and contrast baths (if no pin or sutures are present).
  - A hand-based safe-position splint including the involved digit and an adjacent digit is worn between exercises and at night. Use a forearm-based splint including all digits if multiple digits are involved.
- AROM exercises are used based on the stability of fracture:
  - Composite flexion and extension of the digits
  - Blocking of the PIP and distal interphalangeal (DIP) joints to provide differential gliding of the flexor digitorum superficialis and profundus tendons (especially important following a volar exposure)
  - Reverse blocking (metaphalangeal [MP] joints passively flexed with active interphalangeal [IP] joint extension), flexor and extensor tendon glides
- Seven to 14 days postsurgery
  - Gentle assisted AROM and passive ROM may begin as tolerated, again based on fracture stability. Passive ROM should not begin with K-wires in place.
  - Avoid painful ROM and monitor splints closely for excessive forces on the PIP joint. This can result in a counterproductive inflammatory and fibroblastic response.
- Early scar management (approximately 10 to 14 days)
  - When the incision or pin site has healed, begin scar massage with lotion.
  - Superficial heat application applied before scar massage helps increase scar pliability.

- If scar sensitivity develops, introduce scar desensitization to include stimulation of the sensitive scar with graded textures and tactile pressure and tapping of scar, progressing as the patient develops increased tolerance to each stimulus.
- If scar adherence persists, use iontophoresis with Iodex (Baar Products, Inc., Downingtown, PA) to soften the scar.
- For a raised scar, encourage scar remodeling by use of a nocturnal scar pad, such as elastomer or Otoform K (AliMed, Inc., Dedham, MA).

- After initial fracture healing (about 4 to 6 weeks)
  - Assisted and passive ROM should be started if they have not been initiated earlier.
  - Continue the "safe position" splint between exercises and at night.
  - As the patient's pain level decreases and functional use of the involved digit increases, reduce the splint to a gutter splint worn at night to prevent PIP flexion contracture.
  - If a flexion contracture develops at the PIP joint, consider serial extension casting of the involved digit. The contracture should be no more than 45 degrees because the patient will have difficulty donning the serial cast with any greater degree of joint contracture. Dynamic splinting or static progressive splinting by day may be used as needed.
  - Progressively wean splints as passive ROM improves and encourage active ROM.
- Strengthening (about 8 weeks)
  - Progressive strengthening can be initiated with light putty and further progressed with activities appropriate for the patient's occupation.
- About 10 weeks
  - Discharge all splinting.
  - Encourage unrestricted use of the involved digit and hand.
  - In closed fractures, with a good soft tissue envelope and blood supply, K-wires should be removed at about 3 weeks to facilitate rehabilitation.

Overcoming Issues Related to Rehabilitation

Decreased PIP Joint Flexion

- The reason for decreased flexion at the PIP joint must be determined. If the joint has full PIP joint flexion on passive ROM and decreased PIP joint flexion on active ROM, the problem most likely is caused by adhesions.
- Treatment should attempt to regain ROM through active exercise:
  - Before treatments, application of heat is useful to increase tissue extensibility for increased ROM gains and assist the patient with increased tolerance to exercise.
  - Superficial modalities such as moist hot pack, paraffin, and Fluidotherapy may be used. Benefits of Fluidotherapy include the ability to actively stretch with application of heat.
  - Ultrasound may be used to heat deeper tissues.
- Exercises
  - Tendon glides
  - Isolated blocking of the flexor digitorum superficialis and profundus tendons to maximize differential tendon gliding
  - Active flexion of the digit against resistance, such as hook fist exercises performed with therapeutic putty or raking the digits through putty
  - Blocking splint for exercise: The MP joints are blocked in extension by a splint with the PIP joints free. The patient performs active PIP flexion and extension to increase differential glide of the tendons (**FIG 5A**).
  - Neuromuscular electrostimulation of the flexor digitorum superficialis and profundus may be used to assist active ROM and tendon glide.

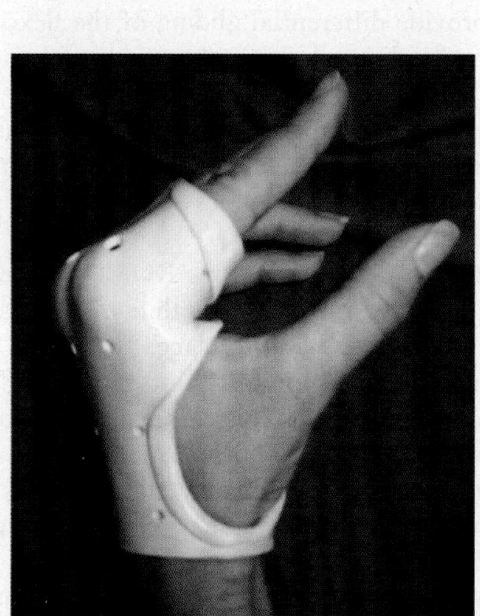
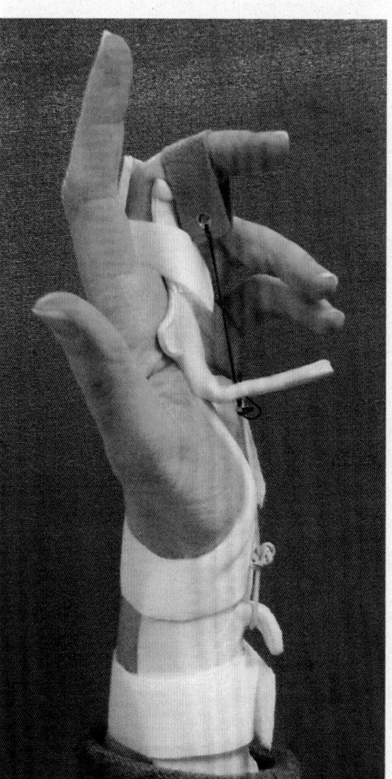
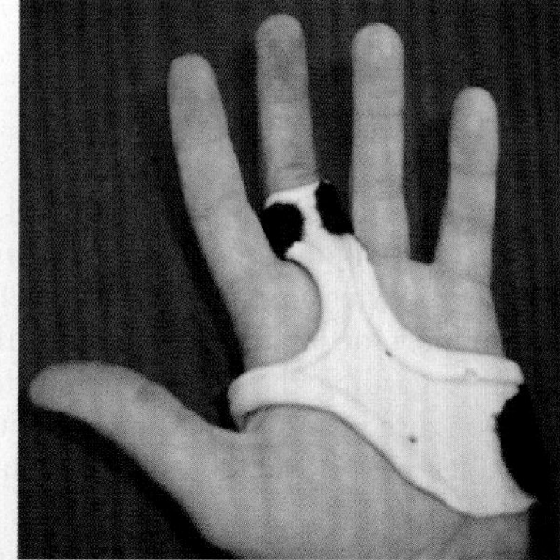
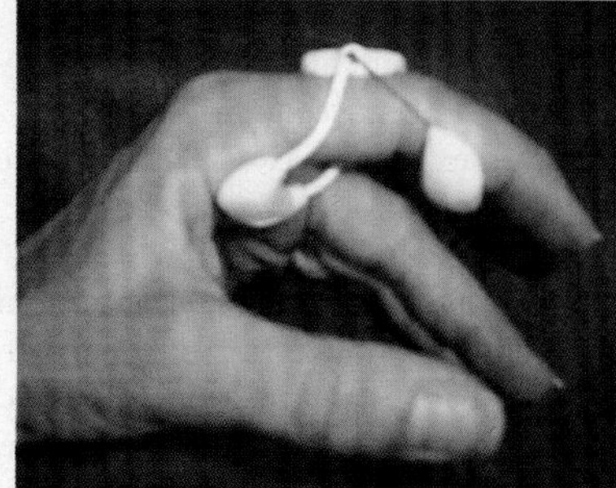

FIG 5 • **A.** MP blocking splint. **B.** Dynamic flexion splint. **C.** Reverse blocking splint. **D.** Finger-based dynamic PIP extension splint.

- If the fracture is healed and passive ROM of the joint is limited in flexion, passive ROM exercises and splinting alternatives will assist to progressively stretch a tight joint capsule and elongate shortened ligaments. Splinting options include the following:
  - Static progressive splinting
  - Use of a dynamic flexion splint (**FIG 5B**)
- Passive ROM and joint mobilizations are appropriate if the fracture is healed.
  - Use of heat (as discussed earlier) to increase tissue extensibility will make the patient more comfortable and help increase ROM. To assist stretch into flexion with heat, try wrapping the digit(s) in flexion with Coban and dipping them in paraffin.

Decreased PIP Joint Extension

- The appropriate treatment approach depends on the structures involved. If the PIP joint can be passively placed into full extension but is unable to actively extend, the extensor apparatus may be scarred down.
- The following treatments are beneficial to increase active extension of the PIP joint.
  - Before beginning the exercises, use of superficial heat modalities and ultrasound will assist to increase tissue extensibility, ROM gains, and the patient's tolerance to exercises.
  - Active exercises include the following:
    - Active reverse blocking (passively flex the MP joints while actively extending the IP joints to transmit the extension force to the IP joints)
    - A reverse blocking splint is helpful to assist the patient with reverse blocking (**FIG 5C**).
    - Block the MP joint in flexion while actively extending the PIP joint into extension with simultaneous neuromuscular electrostimulation of the extensor digitorum communis muscle and the intrinsic muscles.
    - Active extension against resistance, such as Theraputty
- If the fracture is healed and passive ROM of the PIP is limited with extension, exercises and splinting can assist with improving passive ROM.
  - Serial casting PIP into extension
  - Finger-based dynamic PIP extension splint (**FIG 5D**)
  - Dynamic extension splint with MP block in flexion
- Passive ROM and joint mobilizations with heat applied before these manual activities are appropriate if the fracture is healed.

Scar Adhesions Limiting Tendon Glide

- Active ROM, including extensor/flexor tendon glides, and scar massage and reverse scar massage (opposite the direction of the adhesion with active ROM) are key to decreasing adhesions of the tendon.
- These modalities work well in conjunction and may be used individually or in combination based on the patient's individual needs.
  - Superficial heat (eg, Fluidotherapy, moist heat, paraffin)
  - Ultrasound
  - Scar pad (eg, elastomere, Otoform K)
  - Iontophoresis with Iodex to soften scar

OUTCOMES

- In one series of 36 patients, the arc of motion of the PIP joint averaged 72 degrees with a 13-degree extensor lag. Patients with volar coronal fractures fared worse, with an average arc of 57 degrees.[6]
- In the McCue series of 32 patients treated with open reduction and two K-wires, flexion averaged greater than 93 degrees and extensor lag averaged less than 5 degrees.[3]

COMPLICATIONS

- Loss of PIP joint motion is the most common complication.
  - Fixation must be secure enough to allow early motion.
  - Delay of motion of the hand by more than a few weeks significantly decreases final outcome.[2] Ideally, motion should be initiated in the immediate postoperative period.
  - Increases in motion may be obtained up to 1 year after the injury, although opportunity does decrease with time.[2]
  - Dorsal capsulotomies and extensor tenolysis are options for patients lacking flexion.
- Loss of reduction is common if fractures are not stabilized or are stabilized with only one point of fixation.[6]

REFERENCES

1. Chin KR, Jupiter JB. Treatment of triplane fractures of the head of the proximal phalanx. J Hand Surg Am 1999;24:1263–1268.
2. Freeland AE, Benoist LA. Open reduction and internal fixation method for fractures at the proximal interphalangeal joint. Hand Clin 1994;10:239–250.
3. McCue FC, Honner R, Johnson MC, et al. Athletic injuries of the proximal interphalangeal joint requiring surgical treatment. J Bone Joint Surg Am 1970;52(5):937–956.
4. O'Rourke SK, Gaur S, Barton NJ. Long-term outcome of articular fractures of the phalanges: an eleven year follow-up. J Hand Surg Br 1989;14:183–193.
5. Puckett BN, Gaston RG, Peljovich AE, et al. Remodeling potential of phalangeal distal condylar malunions in children. J Hand Surg Am 2012;37:34–41.
6. Weiss AP, Hastings H II. Distal unicondylar fractures of the proximal phalanx. J Hand Surg Am 1993;18:594–599.

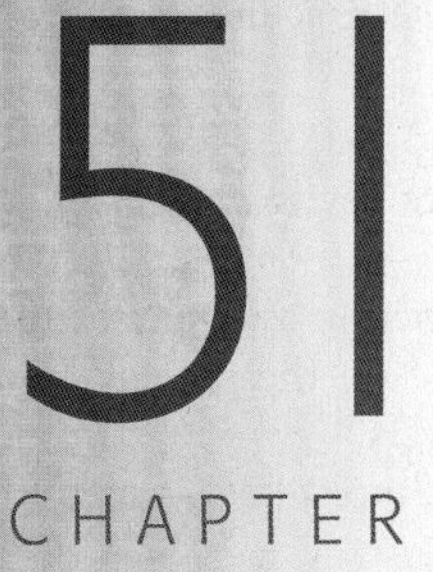

CHAPTER

Dorsal Block Pinning of Proximal Interphalangeal Joint Fracture-Dislocations

Elizabeth King, Mark Goleski, and Jeffrey Lawton

DEFINITION

- The laymen's term "jammed finger" often is used to indicate an injury sustained to the proximal interphalangeal (PIP) joint. If the injury occurs with sufficient force, the joint may suffer a fracture-dislocation, which can be a challenging injury to treat.
- PIP fracture-dislocations, with a dorsal displacement of the middle phalanx are caused by disruption of the volar fibrocartilaginous plate, fragmentation of the middle phalanx where it attaches to this plate, and damage to the collateral ligaments on each side of the joint. Instability with dorsal displacement of the middle phalanx may result, accentuated by the unbalanced pull of the central slip.
- Stiffness, pain, persistent subluxation, degenerative arthritis, and long-term dysfunction are common sequelae, even with appropriate treatment in the best of circumstances.
- Dynamic external skeletal traction, extension block splinting or pinning, transarticular pinning, open reduction with internal fixation (ORIF), and volar plate arthroplasty are the techniques most commonly used to treat these injuries.
  - None of these techniques have proven to be satisfactory for all patients in all instances.
- Extension block pinning has been used with reasonable success to stabilize unstable PIP fracture-dislocations. The use of this technique is predicated upon first obtaining the reduction and then allowing the extension block pin to maintain the reduction.
  - A retrograde K-wire is placed into the head of the proximal phalanx, mechanically blocking full extension of the joint and thereby preventing dorsal subluxation of the middle phalanx.
  - The advantages of this technique include its simplicity and the early mobility it affords an injured joint. It can be used alone or in combination with volar plate arthroplasty or ORIF.

ANATOMY

- The PIP joint acts primarily as a hinge joint in the sagittal plane, although it does possess a few additional degrees of motion in the coronal and axial planes.[17] It has an average range of flexion–extension of 105 degrees.[16]
- The joint has a great deal of stability throughout its range of motion (ROM).[16]
- When healthy, the joint is most stable in full extension.
  - A tongue-and-groove structure, formed by the bicondylar head of the proximal phalanx and the reciprocal concave surfaces of the middle phalanx, contours closely in this position.[16]
- In the pathologic setting of a dorsal fracture-dislocation, some flexion confers PIP stability. As the joint flexes, the ligamentous elements lying volarly to the axis of rotation are primarily responsible for maintaining stability.[16]
  - The volar plate, a structure that is ligamentous at its origin on the proximal phalanx and cartilaginous at its insertion on the middle phalanx, and the two collateral ligaments, one on the radial and one on the ulnar side of the joint, are the most important structures for stability (**FIG 1**).
  - Two out of three of these structures must be impaired for displacement of the middle phalanx to occur.

PATHOGENESIS

- Although the PIP joint may become dislocated in any direction, dorsal displacement of the middle phalanx is the most common.
- Simultaneous hyperextension and axial compression forces—such as those seen when a ball strikes the tip of the finger—stress the volar plate and the collateral ligaments.
- Type I injury
  - If the force of injury is mild, it will result in only partial disruption of the collateral ligaments and the volar plate at its distal insertion on the middle phalanx.
  - The articular surfaces remain intact and the joint is stable.
  - If appropriate treatment is initiated promptly, an excellent long-term result is anticipated.[13]
- Type II injury
  - If the force of injury is more substantial, bilateral longitudinal splitting of the collateral ligaments may occur in addition to rupture of the volar plate. Complete dorsal displacement of the middle phalanx is then possible due to the unopposed pull of the central slip.
  - The joint can be readily reduced and usually is stable following reduction.

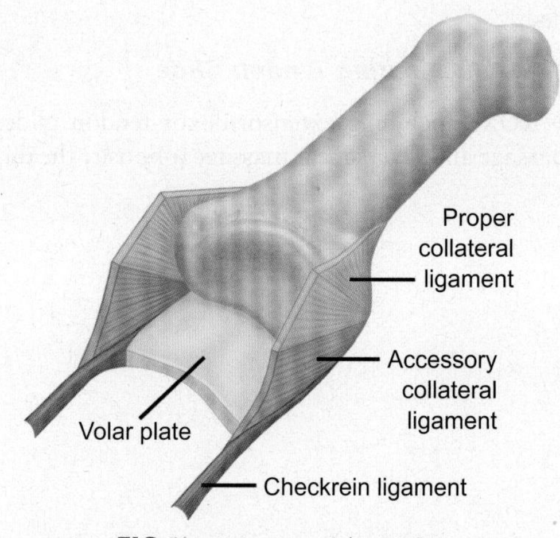

FIG 1 • Anatomy of the PIP joint.

- Type III injury—stable
  - If an avulsion fracture of the middle phalanx occurs at the attachment of the volar plate, the joint may still remain stable. When less than 30% to 40% of the joint surface is involved, the joint remains stable following reduction because collateral ligament integrity is maintained.[4,15]
- Type III injury—unstable
  - If the fracture at the base of the middle phalanx involves greater than 40% to 50% of the articular surface, collateral ligament support is lost. The joint exhibits persistent dorsal subluxation of the middle phalanx due to unopposed pull of the extensor tendon and lack of volar restraints.
  - Closed reduction, although often possible, cannot be maintained often leading to unsatisfactory overall results.[19]
- A cadaveric biomechanical study of PIP joint fracture-dislocations reported that joints with simulated bony articular defects of the middle phalanx of 20% were stable through digit ROM. Simulated volar articular defects greater than 40% led to greater than 1 mm of dorsal subluxation.[21]

NATURAL HISTORY

- The outcome following even a minor injury is often less satisfactory than the patient anticipates (ie, not "back to normal" in terms of appearance, ROM, and comfort). Although it is possible for a PIP joint that has suffered a fracture-dislocation to regain excellent function, persistence of a slightly stiff joint with a cosmetically thickened outline is common.
  - Delay in treatment or lack of vigilant care negatively affects outcome.[10]
  - Prolonged immobilization of the joint following reduction leads to stiffness. Early mobilization can avoid stiffness and may benefit the damaged articular cartilage.[18]
- Patients should be reassured, however, that carefully planned treatment and compliance with the postoperative therapy regimen leads to long-term satisfactory results in most cases.[10]

PATIENT HISTORY AND PHYSICAL FINDINGS

- The history should elicit the mechanism of injury, nature of any medical treatment or manipulation of the digit before the current visit, and time elapsed since the injury.
  - The likelihood of a favorable result diminishes with increased time from injury, particularly beyond 6 weeks.[9]
- The digit will look surprisingly normal at presentation in many cases, particularly if it has already been reduced.
- The neurovascular status should be documented on examination before performing digital anesthetic block and reduction.
- With the forearm supinated and the hand relaxed, observe the position of the patient's fingers. Note the axial and rotational alignment of the digit.
  - The uninjured, quiescent hand has increasing flexion tone in the digits from the radial to the ulnar side,[2] a phenomenon known as the *flexion or resting cascade* (**FIG 2A**).
- Observe the patient's fingers directly and fluoroscopically as he or she attempts to move them through a normal ROM. Dorsal subluxation often can be detected visually and through palpation.
  - Digital or wrist block anesthesia can be used to relieve discomfort associated with motion (**FIG 2B**).
  - If the joint can be moved through a full arc of motion without subluxation, adequate joint stability remains, and only brief immobilization will be required.
  - If redisplacement occurs, significant instability will result. The position of redisplacement is a clue both to the specific site of ligament injury and the optimal position for joint immobilization.[8] Loss of active extension implies central slip injury.
- For grossly stable digits, manipulate the joint passively through the normal ROM. Gentle lateral and dorsovolar shearing stresses are applied at full extension and at 30 degrees of flexion. The findings are compared to those of the contralateral uninjured digit (**FIG 2C**).
  - The position of the PIP joint at the point of instability suggests which of the soft tissue supports has been injured. Instability at more than 70 degrees of flexion indicates damage to the collateral ligaments. Instability in extension indicates disruption of both the collateral ligaments and the volar plate. The degree of joint laxity suggests the extent of injury to the ligaments, from microscopic tearing to complete rupture.
- Palpate the PIP joint from all sides to determine point tenderness. Point tenderness often is valuable in localizing the injured structure.
  - Absence of point tenderness on the condyles may rule out significant injury to these structures. If the volar lip of the middle phalanx has been fractured, minor tenderness over the dorsum of the middle phalanx and greater tenderness volarly and laterally will be present.[5]

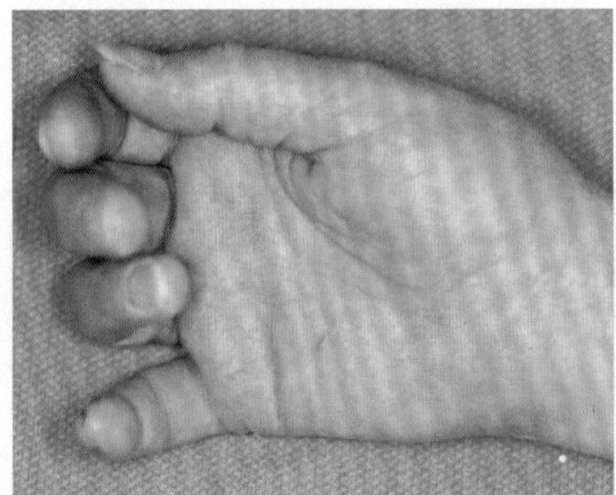
A

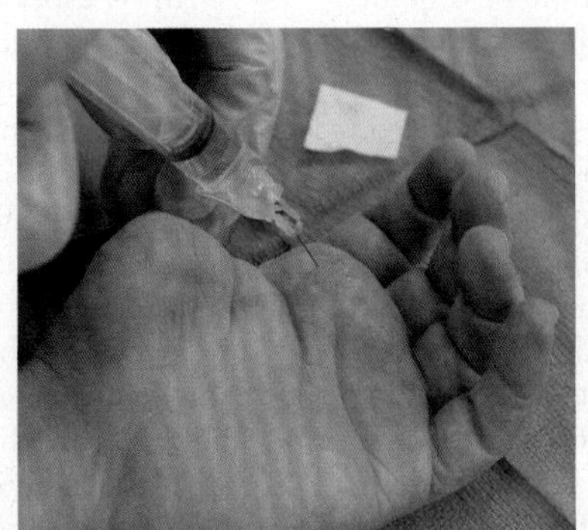
B

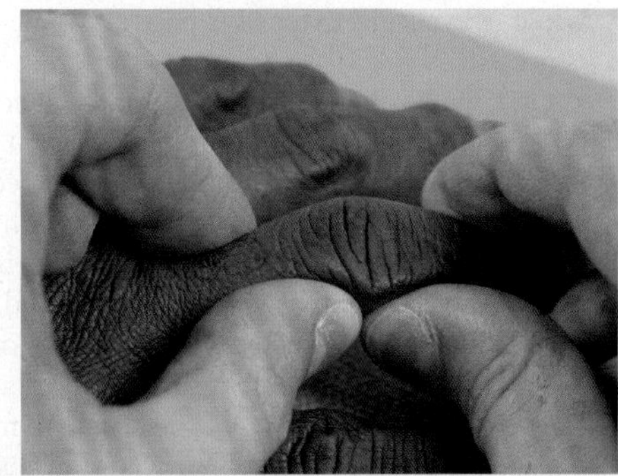
C

FIG 2 • **A.** Disruption of resting flexor cascade. **B.** Digital block technique. **C.** Passive stability evaluation.

IMAGING AND OTHER DIAGNOSTIC STUDIES

- Obtain anteroposterior, lateral, and oblique radiographs of the injured digit. Assess the digit for joint dislocation, subluxation, and fracture.
  - Evaluate the radiographs before performing the physical examination to detect potentially unstable fractures or dislocations before they are manipulated.
  - Radiographs of the hand as a whole (eg, the "fanned four-finger lateral" view) are not adequate. Subtle fracture-dislocations may be missed due to poor depiction of the areas of suspected pathology.[22]
- Fluoroscopy is extremely valuable in defining the pathoanatomy and determining stability.
- Computed tomography (CT) scanning may occasionally be indicated, particularly to assess suspected articular depression.[10]

DIFFERENTIAL DIAGNOSIS

- Fracture
- Fracture-dislocation
- PIP dislocation
- Collateral ligament and PIP joint sprain
- PIP volar plate injury
- PIP joint infection
- Localized soft tissue infection
- Flexor digitorum profundus tendon rupture
- Extensor tendon central slip injury
- Closed pulley rupture (flexor sheath)
- Swan neck/boutonnière deformity

NONOPERATIVE MANAGEMENT

- Most type I, type II, and type III stable injuries (and some type III unstable injuries) are amenable to nonoperative treatment.
- The joint can be immobilized for a short time to afford the patient comfort and to allow soft tissue recovery.
  - A dorsal splint is applied to the digit at 20 to 30 degrees of flexion, avoiding immobilization beyond 30 degrees to decrease the risk of flexion contracture.
  - The duration of immobilization reflects the minimum amount of time needed to allow for healing and obtain joint stability. Type I injuries are immobilized for a few days, whereas type III injuries may be immobilized (complete vs. extension blocking) for 2 to 3 weeks.
  - Avoidance of prolonged immobilization and patient education about early mobility are the most important aspects of this treatment, as stiffness and contracture are very common sequelae.
- Extension block splinting allows early motion of a joint while preventing extension past an angle where instability is present.[7,12,13,20]
  - First, the position in which the joint subluxates is determined.
  - A length of aluminum splint is then bent to an angle 10 or 15 degrees greater than this point of redisplacement and secured to the dorsum of the hand with adhesive tape or as part of a short-arm cast. The hand is positioned with 25 degrees of extension at the wrist and 45 to 60 degrees of flexion at the metacarpophalangeal joint[7] (**FIG 3A,B**).
    - If the angle of the splint is greater than 60 degrees, the arc of motion may be insufficient for the patient to achieve adequate flexibility, and it may be necessary to consider another treatment regimen.
  - An extension block splint made from two pieces of AlumaFoam (Hartmann International, Rock Hill, SC) and spanning only the finger itself is another option (**FIG 3C,D**).
    - The two Alumafoam pieces are held to each side of the PIP joint with adhesive tape and are bent such that they come into contact with each other at a particular degree of extension, thus preventing motion beyond that point.[20]
  - In general, extension block splinting is recommended for fractures involving less than 40% of the articular surface. Successful results have been noted, however, with fractures involving up to 75% of the joint.[12]
  - Following application of the splint, radiographs are taken to confirm satisfactory reduction, and the patient is encouraged to flex the finger as much as the swelling allows.
  - As the fracture-dislocation heals, the extension block splint is progressively adjusted toward full extension, usually during a period of 3 to 8 weeks.[7] Weekly radiographs and splint adjustments are required.
  - In certain instances, the digit may be too short, stocky, or swollen for such treatment, or patient compliance and sophistication for such a regimen may be in question. In such a case, extension block pinning may be the better option.
- Because of the possibility of recurrent subluxation, the use of conservative treatment must be matched with frequent and careful assessment of the joint. Serial radiographs should be obtained weekly to document continued reduction of the joint and progressive healing of any fractures.[7]

SURGICAL MANAGEMENT

- Operative treatment is indicated for unstable fracture-dislocations in which closed treatment does not provide a congruent reduction of the joint. This includes most type III unstable injuries with fractures that involve more than 40% to 50% of the volar articular surface.
- As noted earlier, many surgical options are available. The choice of procedure is based on the exact nature of the injury and the surgeon's comfort with each option.
- Extension block pinning can serve as a stand-alone procedure or can augment other techniques.
- Dynamic skeletal traction methods, which use the principles of ligamentotaxis to maintain concentric joint reduction, are especially useful when the fracture is significantly comminuted.[1]
  - These methods allow early active ROM.
  - Drawbacks include the following:
    - Significant skill on the part of the surgeon is required, along with close postoperative supervision and adjustment.
    - The external device may be cumbersome for the patient.
- ORIF is especially useful when the avulsed volar fragment is large and minimally comminuted.[11] However, if the joint is stabilized with transarticular pinning as part of the ORIF procedure, stiffness usually results and extension block pinning might be of benefit.
- Volar plate arthroplasty, the use of the distal aspect of the fibrocartilaginous volar plate to resurface the comminuted volar articular surface of the middle phalanx, is another option that can be employed when comminution of the volar fragment makes other techniques infeasible.[3] Most authors have reported reasonably favorable results, but residual stiffness and contracture have been reported as well.[6]
- Simple reduction with transarticular pinning (with no attempt at articular reconstruction) may be useful in injuries

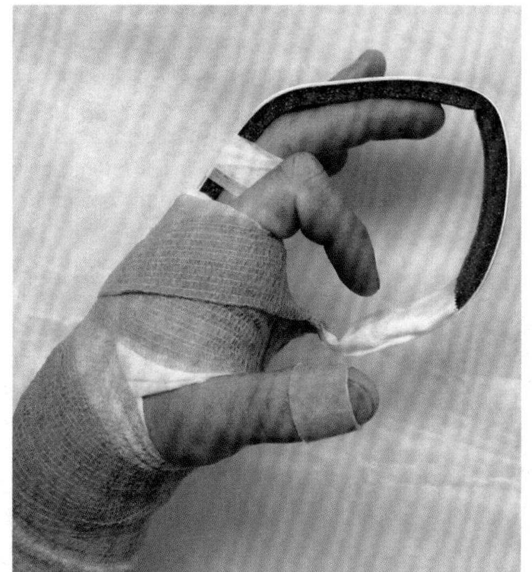

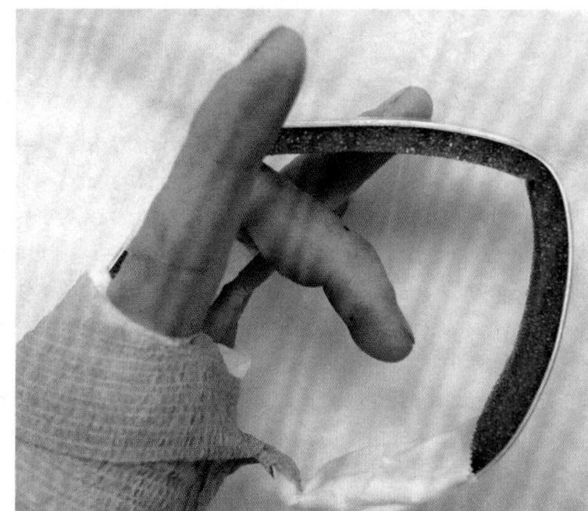

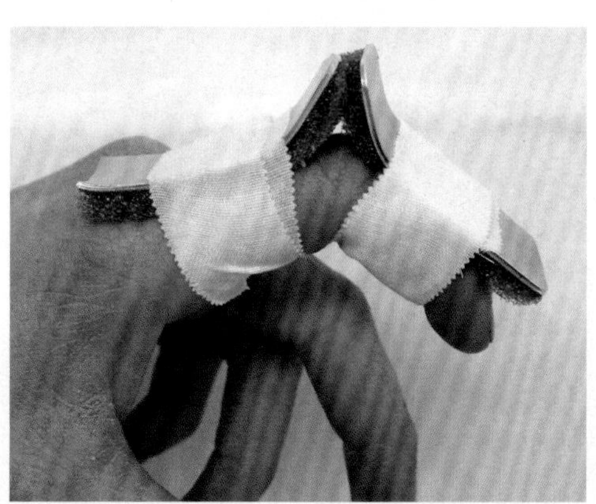

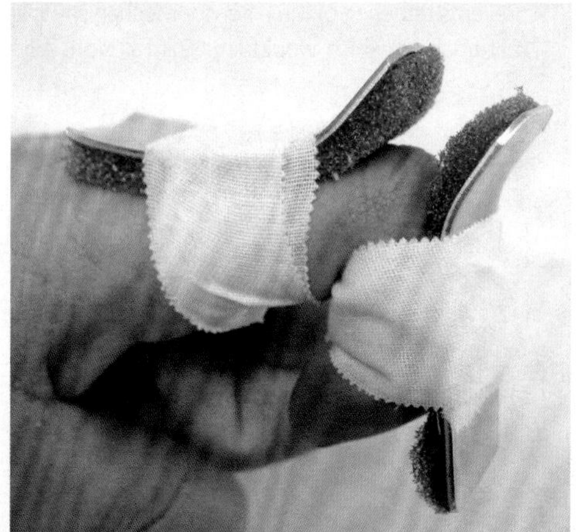

FIG 3 • **A,B.** Extension blocking splint. **C,D.** Alternative aluminum and foam extension blocking splint.

with less than 40% articular involvement. Extension block splinting may be equally effective in these milder instances and confers a lower risk of joint contracture.[10]

- Extension block pinning is a viable alternative for mild to moderately unstable PIP fracture-dislocations under the following circumstances:
  - The fracture-dislocation can be reduced but not stabilized effectively with an extension block splint.[14,22,23]
  - Patient compliance is uncertain.
  - The finger is too short or swollen to fit appropriately into an extension block splint.
  - May be used alone or in combination with an ORIF or a volar plate arthroplasty procedure.[3] As a stand-alone procedure, the ability to achieve and document a concentric reduction in a closed fashion is mandatory.

Preoperative Planning

- Before the operation, the patient should be provided realistic expectations regarding outcome.
  - He or she should be aware of the possibility that immobilization, splinting, and long-term rehabilitation may be necessary.
- The patient should be instructed to keep the injured hand clean before the procedure and to avoid additional skin injury to minimize the potential for infection. Fingernails should be trimmed and cleaned and the hands thoroughly scrubbed with antiseptic soap before the operation.
- Intraoperative decision making often is necessary. The surgeon should be comfortable performing alternative procedures and should have the necessary equipment available if operative findings require an alteration in the original surgical plan.

Positioning

- The method of preparing, draping, and positioning the upper extremity is the same as for most hand surgeries.
- A well-padded, proximal upper extremity tourniquet is applied.

Approach

- Extension block pinning is a percutaneous technique; no approach is required.

Extension Block Pinning

- The PIP joint is reduced by flexing the joint to 90 degrees and applying axial traction.
  - Concentric reduction of the joint is confirmed with fluoroscopy (**TECH FIG 1A**).
  - If an open wound is present or the joint cannot be manipulated into an acceptable reduction, such as may occur with soft tissue entrapment, open reduction becomes necessary.
- Following reduction through either open or closed methods, and with the joint flexed 90 degrees or more, a smooth 0.035- to 0.045-inch K-wire is placed percutaneously into the distal, dorsal aspect of the proximal phalanx tangentially skiving across the dorsal lip of the base of the middle phalanx[14,23] (**TECH FIG 1B**).
  - The wire is inserted in a retrograde direction, approximately 30 degrees off the long axis of the proximal phalanx.
  - When placing the K-wire centrally, hyperflexing the PIP joint prevents tethering of the extensor mechanism to the proximal phalanx, which would limit joint flexion. Alternatively, the K-wire can be placed to one side of the central tendon to avoid tethering the extensor mechanism.
- The wire is guided with fluoroscopy through the shaft of the proximal phalanx and is left protruding from the head of the bone. Fluoroscopy is used to confirm a congruous joint reduction following the procedure.
- The joint is then passively extended to the limit of the K-wire, and the reduction of the joint is again evaluated fluoroscopically (**TECH FIG 1C**).
  - If the joint continues to subluxate dorsally in extension, a V-shaped gap between the articular surfaces of the head of the proximal phalanx and the dorsal lip of the middle phalanx will be seen on radiographs.[16]
- With the pin in this position (**TECH FIG 1D**), the patient will maintain full active flexion of the finger, but extension of the digit beyond the point where subluxation is possible will be mechanically blocked by the pin (**TECH FIG 1E,F**).
  - An arc of motion greater than 60 degrees is ideal with this technique.

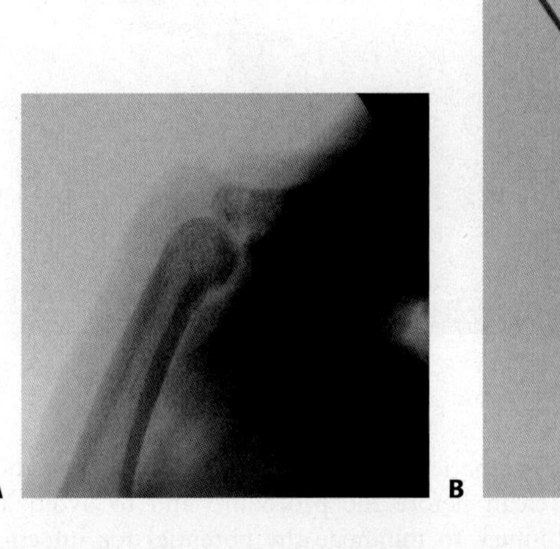
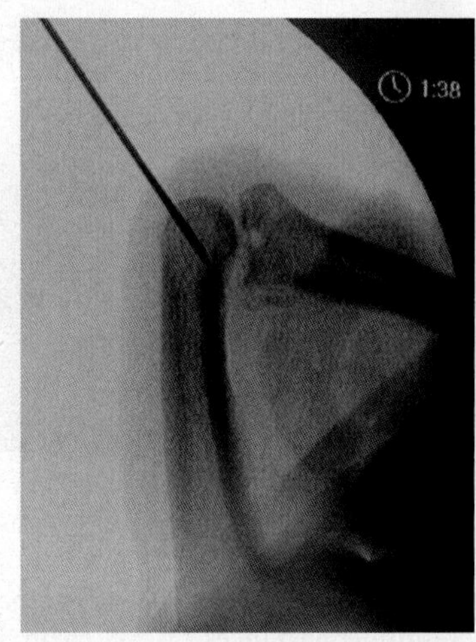

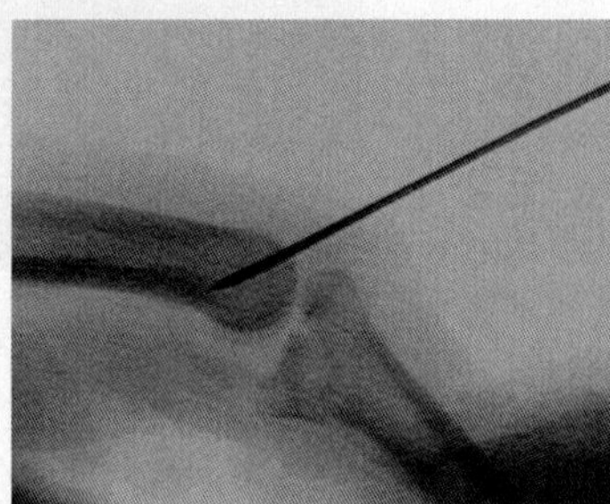
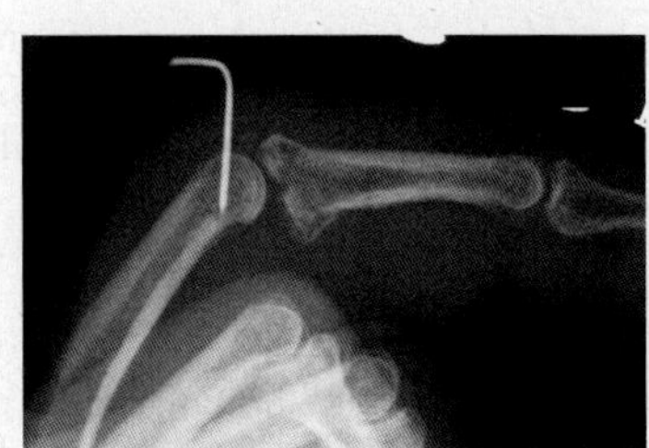
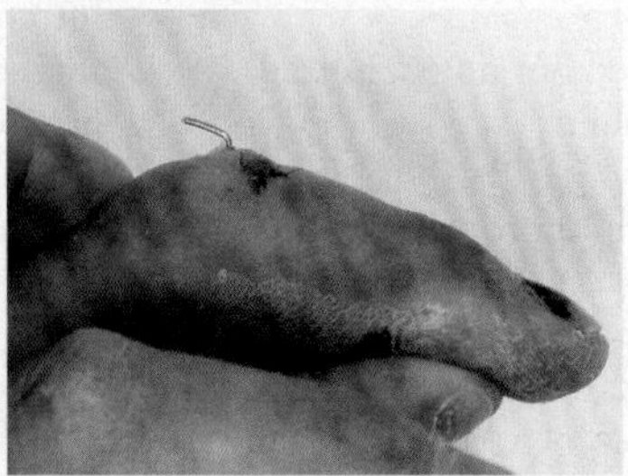
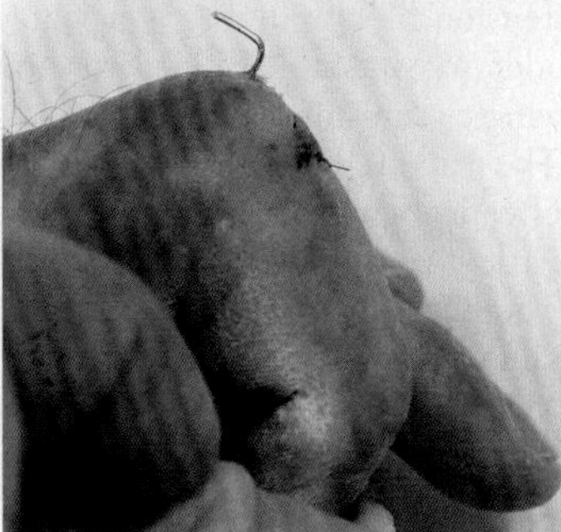

TECH FIG 1 • Dorsal block pinning. **A.** Fluoroscopic view confirms adequate joint reduction. Note that fracture reduction is not anatomic but is considered acceptable in this clinical scenario. **B.** Insertion of the retrograde K-wire with the joint hyperflexed to avoid tethering the extensor mechanism. **C.** Passive intraoperative extension of the joint to the level of the K-wire. The dorsal joint remains concentrically reduced. **D.** The K-wire is left protruding through the bone, and its placement is confirmed by fluoroscopy. **E,F.** The patient should be able to move the finger through an arc of about 60 degrees.

PEARLS AND PITFALLS

- The patient's ability to comply with fairly complex and intensive hand therapy should be confirmed before surgery.
- The insertion point for the K-wire can be located by a freehand technique and then confirmed with fluoroscopy.
- Easy passive flexion of the joint through an arc of 60 degrees or greater should be confirmed following pin insertion (eg, 30–95 degrees ROM).
- The surgeon should remain hypervigilant for the presence of a V sign in full passive extension.
- The surgeon should ensure that the skin is not tented by the K-wire.

POSTOPERATIVE CARE

- The patient should have a thermoplastic splint fabricated for protection and should begin a supervised program with a hand therapist 3 to 5 days after surgery.
  - Gentle active ROM exercises are allowed immediately and should be encouraged in most cases.
    - If the injury is especially serious—for example, injuries that required volar plate arthroplasty or that contained significant comminution—immobilization for up to 2 weeks may be indicated.[14]
- Pin care must be explained carefully and performed regularly.
- Remember that pin tract infection, although always a complication to be addressed, is potentially quite serious as the pin is either intra-articular or juxta-articular.
- The pin is removed 3 weeks after surgery, and vigorous active flexion and extension are encouraged. Reverse blocking is initiated with metacarpophalangeal (MP) flexion.
  - Full extension should be limited for 1 additional week.[14]
- Active and passive joint exercises, including dynamic extension splinting, is initiated after 6 to 8 weeks of therapy, until full motion is achieved.
- Buddy taping or wrapping can be used if additional, longer term protection is needed.

OUTCOMES

- The outcome for intervention into PIP fracture-dislocations depends heavily on the severity of the initial injury.
- Because few cases of extension block pinning used as the sole intervention are described in the literature, it is difficult to assess the long-term outcome of the procedure.
- Inoue and Tamura[14] reported the use of extension block pinning in 14 cases of fracture-dislocation of the PIP joint with an average fracture fragment size of 38% of the articular surface (range 25% to 60%). Ten patients regained full ROM, and four patients regained a more limited ROM (89, 65, 64, and 40 degrees, respectively). The average ROM for all patients was 94.4 degrees.
  - The authors attributed the four cases with less satisfactory results to the use of a 60-degree extension block splint postoperatively in one patient and significant comminution in the other three patients.
- Viegas[23] reported the use of this technique in three cases of fracture-dislocation of the PIP joint. One case involved a 45% single fragment fracture seen 1 day postinjury and another 35% comminuted fracture seen 17 days postinjury. Following pin removal and 1 month of passive and active exercises, both patients regained full ROM. A third case involved a 75% comminuted fracture seen 2 days postinjury. The patient's ROM after pin removal was 30 to 65 degrees. Because the patient did not return for further care, no final outcome was available.
- Extension block pinning has been described in combination with other percutaneous techniques with good results:
  - Vitale et al[24] reported a series of six unstable dorsal fracture-dislocations of the PIP joint treated with a combined technique of percutaneous fracture reduction, volar pinning of the fracture fragment, and dorsal block pinning. At mean 18 months follow-up, there were no redislocation events, and average ROM was 4 degrees extension to 93 degrees in flexion. All fractures healed and there were no complications in this series.[24]
  - Waris and Alanen[25] describe a technique for percutaneous intramedullary fracture reduction used in conjunction with dorsal block pinning. In their series of 18 dorsal PIP fracture-dislocations, reduction of the joint was achieved with extension block splinting, and impacted volar fragments were then reduced using a percutaneous technique. At a mean follow-up of 5 years, the average active ROM at the PIP joint was 83 degrees and mean Disability of the Arm, Shoulder, and Hand (DASH) scores indicated little functional impairment.[25]

COMPLICATIONS

- Persistent pain and swelling
- Stiffness
- Flexion contracture/extensor lag
- Redisplacement of the joint and persistent subluxation
- Angulation and rotation of the middle phalanx
- Weakness
- Boutonnière deformity
- Posttraumatic arthritis (not necessarily symptomatic)

REFERENCES

1. Agee JM. Unstable fracture dislocations of the proximal interphalangeal joint. Treatment with the force couple splint. Clin Orthop Relat Res 1987;(214):101–112.
2. American Society for Surgery of the Hand. General principles of management. In: The Hand: Primary Care of Common Problems. New York: Churchill Livingstone, 1985:1–17.
3. Blazar PE, Robbe R, Lawton JN. Treatment of dorsal fracture/dislocations of the proximal interphalangeal joint by volar plate arthroplasty. Tech Hand Up Extrem Surg 2001;5:148–152.
4. Deitch MA, Kiefhaber TR, Comisar BR, et al. Dorsal fracture dislocations of the proximal interphalangeal joint: surgical complications and long-term results. J Hand Surg Am 1999;24(5):914–923.
5. Dias JJ. Intraarticular injuries of the distal and proximal interphalangeal joints. In: Berger RA, Weiss AC, eds. Hand Surgery. Baltimore: Lippincott Williams & Wilkins, 2004:153–174.
6. Dionysian E, Eaton RG. The long-term outcome of volar plate arthroplasty of the proximal interphalangeal joint. J Hand Surg Am 2000;25:429–437.
7. Dobyns JH, McElfresh EC. Extension block splinting. Hand Clin 1994;10:229–237.
8. Eaton RG, Littler JW. Joint injuries and their sequelae. Clin Plast Surg 1976;3:85–98.

9. Eaton RG, Malerich MM. Volar plate arthroplasty for the proximal interphalangeal joint: a review of ten years' experience. J Hand Surg Am 1980;5:260–268.
10. Glickel SZ, Barron OA, Catalano LW III. Dislocations and ligament injuries in the digits. In: Green DP, Hotchkiss RN, Pederson WC, et al, eds. Green's Operative Hand Surgery, ed 5. Philadelphia: Elsevier, 2005:343–388.
11. Green A, Smith J, Redding M, et al. Acute open reduction and rigid internal fixation of proximal interphalangeal joint fracture dislocation. J Hand Surg Am 1992;17:512–517.
12. Hamer DW, Quinton DN. Dorsal fracture subluxation of the proximal interphalangeal joints treated by extension block splintage. J Hand Surg Br 1992;17:586–590.
13. Incavo SJ, Mogan JV, Hilfrank BC. Extension splinting of palmar plate avulsion injuries of the proximal interphalangeal joint. J Hand Surg Am 1989;14:659–661.
14. Inoue G, Tamura Y. Treatment of fracture-dislocation of the proximal interphalangeal joint using extension-block Kirschner wire. Ann Chir Main Memb Super 1991;10:564–568.
15. Kiefhaber TR, Stern PJ. Fracture dislocations of the proximal interphalangeal joint. J Hand Surg Am 1998;23:368–380.
16. Kraemer BA, Gilula LA. Phalangeal fractures and dislocations. In: Gilula LA, ed. The Traumatized Hand and Wrist: Radiographic and Anatomic Correlation. Philadelphia: WB Saunders, 1992: 105–170.
17. Leibovic SJ, Bowers WH. Anatomy of the proximal interphalangeal joint. Hand Clin 1994;10:169–178.
18. Salter RB, Simmonds DF, Malcolm BW, et al. The biological effect of continuous passive motion on the healing of full-thickness defects in articular cartilage. An experimental investigation in the rabbit. J Bone Joint Surg Am 1980;62(8):1232–1251.
19. Schenck RR. Classification of fractures and dislocations of the proximal interphalangeal joint. Hand Clin 1994;10:179–185.
20. Strong ML. A new method of extension-block splinting for the proximal interphalangeal joint—preliminary report. J Hand Surg Am 1980; 5:606–607.
21. Tyser AR, Tsai MA, Parks BG, et al. Stability of acute dorsal fracture dislocations of the proximal interphalangeal joint. A biomechanical study. J Hand Surg 2014;39:13–18.
22. Vercillo AP, Squier RC, Ritland GD, et al. Finger dislocations in alcoholics. Conn Med 1987;51:293–295.
23. Viegas SF. Extension block pinning for proximal interphalangeal joint fracture dislocations: preliminary report of a new technique. J Hand Surg Am 1992;17:896–901.
24. Vitale MA, White NJ, Strauch RJ. A percutaneous technique to treat unstable dorsal fracture-dislocations of the proximal interphalangeal joint. J Hand Surg Am 2011;36(9):1453–1459.
25. Waris E, Alanen V. Percutaneous, intramedullary fracture reduction and extension block pinning for dorsal proximal interphalangeal fracture-dislocations. J Hand Surg Am 2010;35(12):2046–2052.

Dynamic External Fixation of Proximal Interphalangeal Joint Fracture-Dislocations

CHAPTER 52

Grey Giddins and Alex Cowey

DEFINITION

- Proximal interphalangeal (PIP) joint bone injuries may affect the convex side of the joint (end of the proximal phalanx) or the concave side of the joint (base of the middle phalanx).
- Convex-side injuries are typically simple (two fragment) injuries best treated conservatively or with open reduction and internal fixation if displaced.
- Concave-side injuries tend to be comminuted (multifragmented), presenting either as fracture-subluxations/dislocations or a pilon-type fracture.
- Fracture-subluxations/dislocations typically involve dorsal displacement of the main fragment of the middle phalanx (**FIG 1A**), although volar and lateral subluxations and dislocations do occur (**FIG 1B,C**).
- Dorsal fracture-dislocations typically occur after a hyperextension injury of the PIP joint.
- Pilon-type fractures are compression fractures of the base of the middle phalanx and are characterized by depression of the central articular component and splaying of the articular margins, typically highly comminuted (**FIG 1D,E**) and there maybe longitudinal extension along the length of the middle phalanx. The classic mechanism is a longitudinal (end-on) force, crushing the base of the middle phalanx, such as fall or miscatching a ball.

ANATOMY

- The distal end of the proximal phalanx is a convex surface made up of two condyles. The proximal end of the middle phalanx is a concave surface (**FIG 2A**).

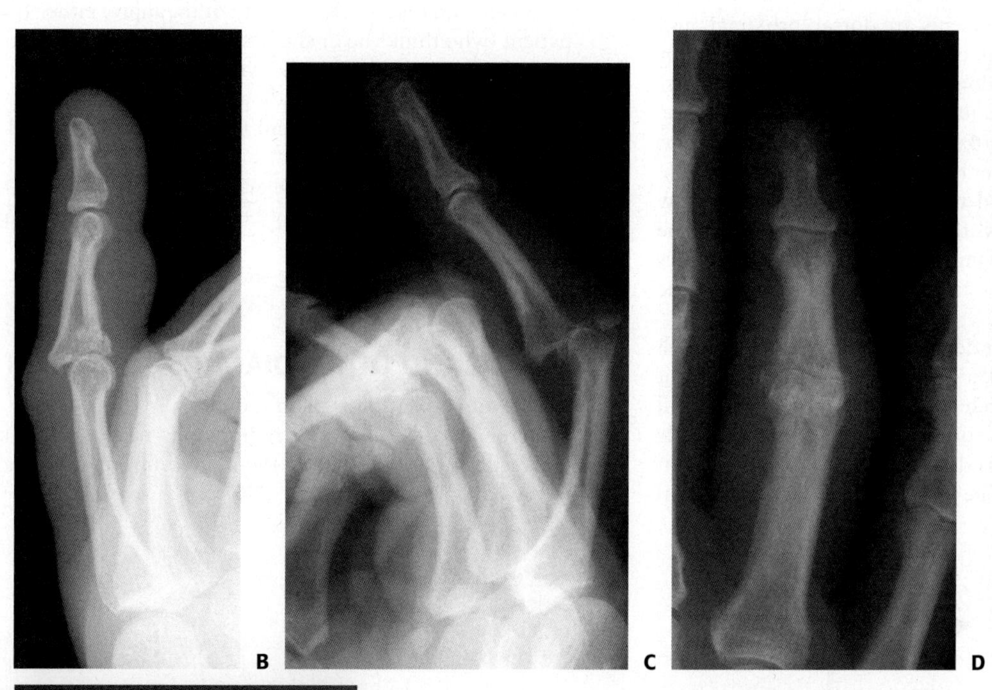
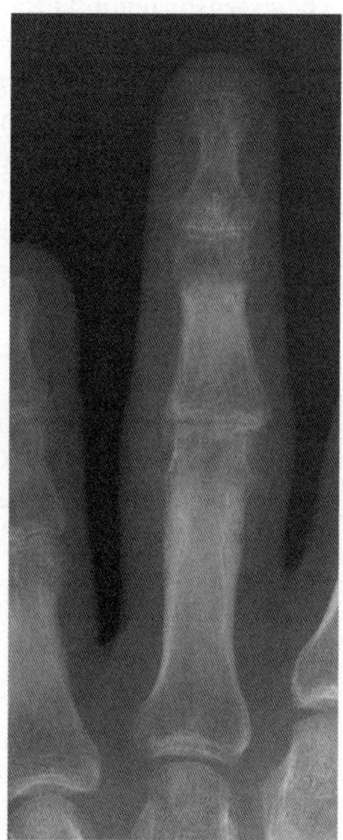
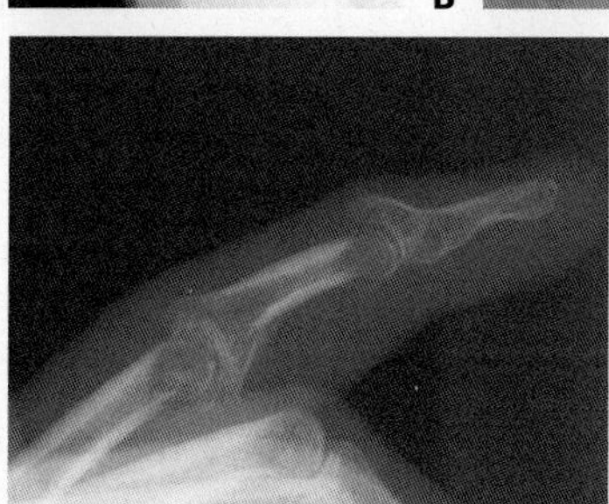

FIG 1 • **A.** A typical (more severe) dorsal fracture-dislocation with involvement of about 65% of the volar articular surface. **B,C.** PIP joint volar dislocation. **D,E.** PIP joint pilon fracture.

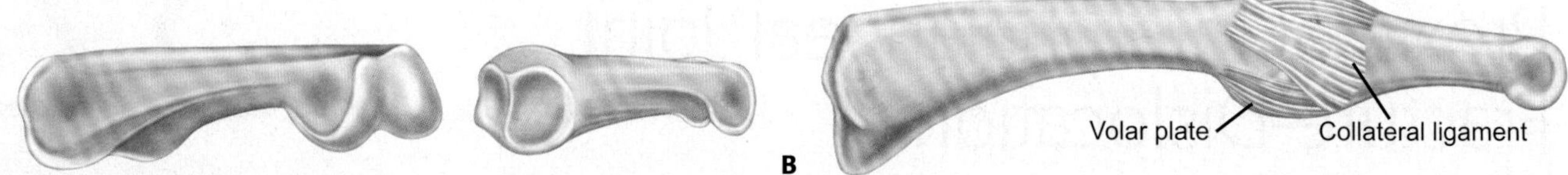

FIG 2 • **A.** The distal end of the proximal phalanx is a convex surface made up of two condyles. The proximal end of the middle phalanx is a concave surface. The two are linked by ligaments. **B.** The strongest is the volar plate and the volar part of the lateral collateral ligaments. These resist dorsal subluxation of the PIP joint when loaded.

- The stability of the PIP joint is secondary to the bony congruency, the tendons that cross the joint (flexor and extensors) plus a series of ligaments (**FIG 2B**):
  - Volar plate—a very strong concave structure, such as the roof of a tunnel, running from the volar surface of the proximal phalanx to the volar surface of the middle phalanx
  - Radial and ulnar collateral ligaments
    - True collaterals—run from the proximal phalanx to the volar 50% of the middle phalanx
    - Accessory collaterals—run from the proximal phalanx into the volar plate
    - These ligaments work together to resist dorsal subluxation of the PIP joint when loaded and are said to act as three sides of a box with joint instability being inevitable if two of the three sides are injured.

PATHOGENESIS

- The extensor tendon attachments are dorsal, proximal, and relatively weak through the central slip, whereas the flexor digitorum superficialis tendon slips insert volarly, more distally, and are stronger. The joint center of rotation is in the middle of the head of the proximal phalanx. Thus, the flexor moment arm is much greater than the extensor moment arm.
- The shape of the joint and the soft tissue restraints allow a powerful lever arm to work for flexion. If, however, the volar restraints fail following trauma, the resultant forces lead to dorsal subluxation and proximal migration of the middle phalanx (**FIG 3A**).
- In practice, it is possible for dorsal subluxation to occur with an injury to as little as 10% of the volar joint surface, but this is uncommon. Research has shown that the joint will be stable if less than 42% of the volar half of the middle phalanx articular surface is damaged as measured on a lateral radiograph (**FIG 3B**). The reason for this is the collateral ligaments remain functional despite the incompetence of the volar plate, hence two sides of the box are competent. Once more than 42% of the volar joint surface is involved, the collaterals become incompetent and all three sides of the box are lost.
- For pilon-type fractures, the condyles of the proximal phalanx are driven up into the base of the middle phalanx, displacing the central part of the articular surface distally and splaying the dorsovolar and lateral margins of the middle phalanx joint surface. This injury is longitudinally unstable and results in proximal migration and diminution or obliteration of the joint space, usually with significant articular incongruity.

PATIENT HISTORY AND PHYSICAL FINDINGS

- The majority of patients present acutely within a few days of the injury, although presentation after 2 weeks and even after 6 weeks is not unheard of. The delays are usually due to underestimation of the severity of the injury either by the patient (who thinks he or she has a sprain and it will resolve) or medical/paramedical staff (who fail to perform or interpret properly an adequate radiograph).
- The finger will be swollen and tender, centered around the PIP joint.
- An angular deformity may be evident.
- Subluxation of the joint may be clinically evident, visually or by palpation.
- There will be reduced range of movement throughout the finger and particularly in the PIP joint.

IMAGING AND OTHER DIAGNOSTIC STUDIES

- The key investigation is plain radiology.
- Posteroanterior and lateral radiographs need to be taken, centered on the PIP joint of the injured finger; radiographs of the hand are not adequate (**FIG 4**).

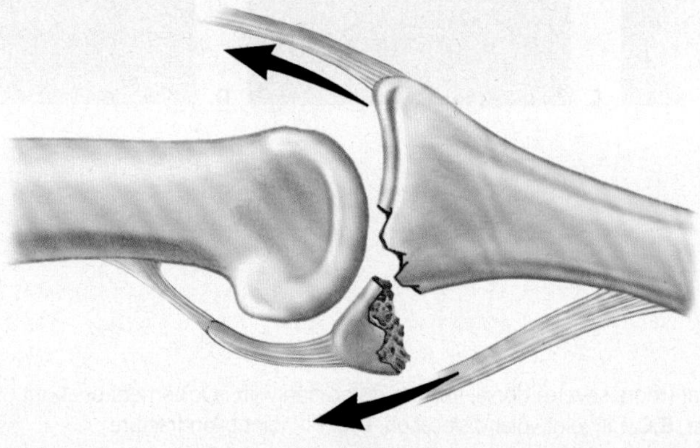

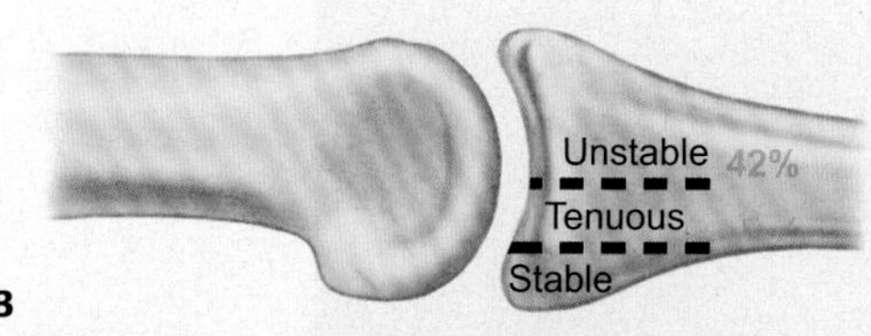

FIG 3 • **A.** Diagram of fracture-dislocation. **B.** Diagram showing volar loss, which may lead to instability.

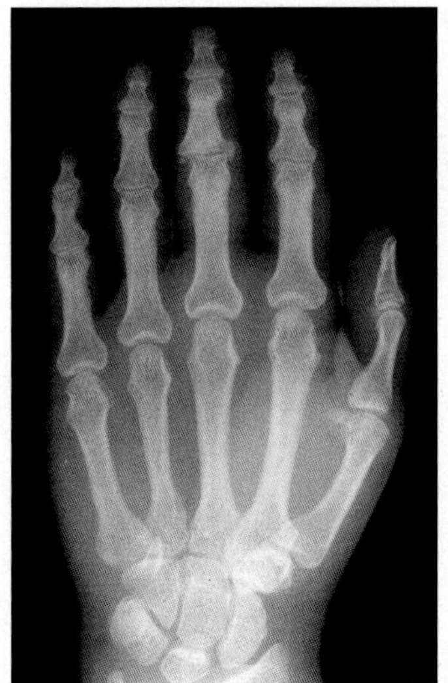
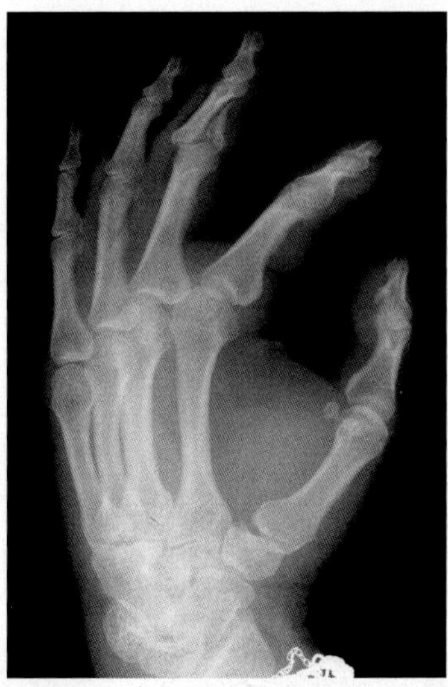
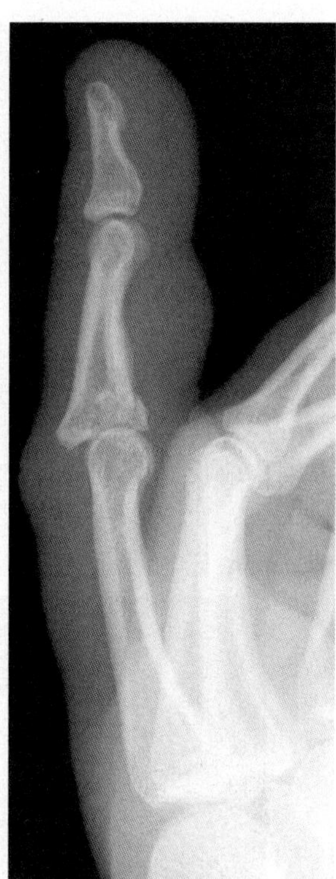

FIG 4 • A–C. Hand radiographs are interpretable only with a true lateral radiograph of the PIP joint.

- Subluxation and dislocation are best visualized on the lateral radiograph and may be quite subtle, appearing as joint incongruity at the dorsum of the joint (the triangle sign, due to dorsal overhang of the base of the middle phalanx) (**FIG 5E**).
- The key information obtained from the radiographs (supplemented by physical examination) can be used to differentiate stable from unstable injuries, either of fracture-subluxations or dislocations or pilon fractures.
- Fluoroscopy can be of great value in assessing the injury and joint stability.

DIFFERENTIAL DIAGNOSIS

- Soft tissue
  - Volar plate injury
  - Collateral ligament injury
  - Central slip injury
- Bone
  - Proximal phalanx condylar injury
  - Proximal phalanx distal diaphyseal injury
  - Middle phalanx proximal diaphyseal injury

NONOPERATIVE MANAGEMENT

- If the injury is stable, early protected mobilization can start within 1 week of injury.

Fracture-Dislocation

- Mild injuries with limited volar plate avulsion reduce either spontaneously or with assistance, usually under local anesthesia, radiographs may reveal a small volar bone avulsion from the base of the middle phalanx (**FIG 5A–D**). These injuries are longitudinally stable and can be treated with early mobilization concentrating on regaining extension, which is commonly lost.
  - Only if there is significant preexisting volar plate laxity (often occurs in young women) is there a need for an extension block splint for up to 6 weeks.
- Most patients regain full or nearly full movement but may be left with minor swelling and stiffness and mild cold discomfort.
  - Heavy activity may cause discomfort.
  - In approximately 5% of patients, the joint remains significantly swollen and uncomfortable beyond 6 weeks. This is probably due to persistent joint synovitis, which usually resolves with a steroid injection.
- If the joint is unstable but there is limited volar joint damage (less than about 30%), it may reduce when held in flexion with a dorsal block splint.
  - Joint reduction and congruity must be documented radiologically and should not require more than about 50 degrees of joint flexion, or unacceptable PIP joint stiffness may result.
  - Patients should be encouraged to flex and extend to the splint. They should be seen weekly for 4 weeks. Flexion of the splint is reduced by about 10 degrees each week. At each increase in extension, the reduction needs to be precisely checked radiologically.
  - A reasonable range of movement with only a mild flexion contracture and loss of flexion is anticipated.

Pilon Fractures

- The majority of pilon-type fractures have significant displacement and surgical stabilization is required to achieve longitudinal stability and early movement, but in a small number of cases, there is minimal displacement (<1 mm)

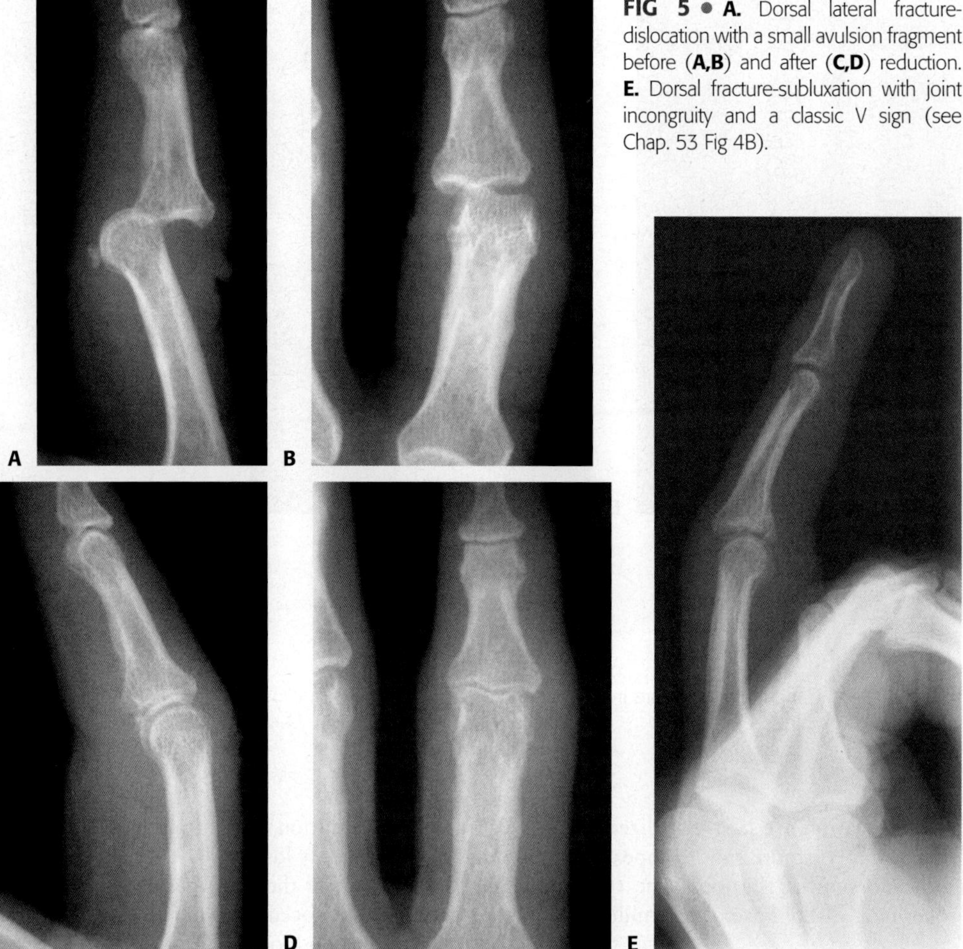

FIG 5 • A. Dorsal lateral fracture-dislocation with a small avulsion fragment before (**A,B**) and after (**C,D**) reduction. **E.** Dorsal fracture-subluxation with joint incongruity and a classic V sign (see Chap. 53 Fig 4B).

and a reasonable joint space (**FIG 6**). These are usually stable injuries but must be carefully assessed clinically.

- Most of these patients can achieve a range of movement from 10 to 20 degrees short of full extension to 70 to 80 degrees of flexion with only mild discomfort.
- Patients can start early gentle mobilization with part-time protection in a splint at night and outdoors for 4 weeks.
- Patients treated with early, protected mobilization need clinical and radiologic review weekly for at least 2 to 3 weeks.
- Most patients will achieve a nearly full range of motion with minimal pain, stiffness, or swelling.

SURGICAL MANAGEMENT

- There are a variety of surgical techniques described for the stabilization of PIP joint fracture dislocations and pilon-type fractures ranging from percutaneous wires, open reduction and internal fixation as well as external fixation. Each case should be judged on its own merits and the advantages and disadvantages of the various techniques considered fully. The surgical technique described in the following text is that of dynamic external fixation, a well-recognized technique for such injuries designed to allow early mobilization.

Preoperative Planning

- The proximal wire is always placed at or near the center of rotation of the injured joint.

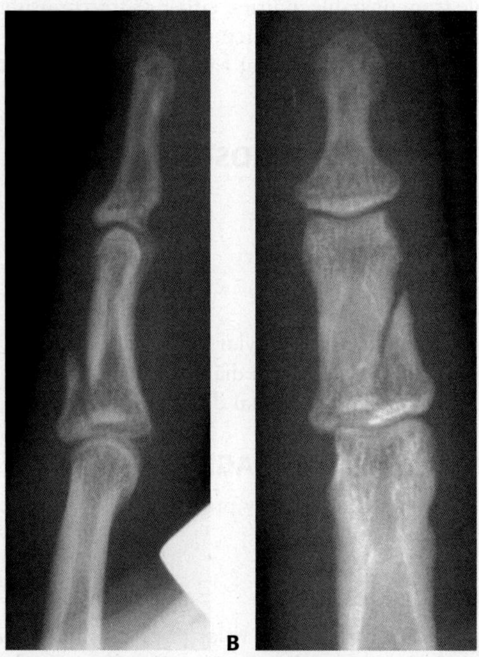

FIG 6 • A,B. Pilon fracture that was sufficiently congruent and comfortable to respond to early mobilization with a good long-term result. This could not have been predicted radiologically, and all cases require clinical assessment.

- Distal wire placement needs to be planned.
  - For fractures localized to the base of the middle phalanx, the distal wire can be anywhere from the midpart of the middle phalanx or more distal. In fact, the middle phalanx is narrowest at this point, so the wire is more easily placed distally.
  - If the fracture extends distally, as can easily occur with pilon fractures, the distal wire should be distal to that extension to ensure adequate fixation and stability. The distal wire can be placed as far distal as the head of the middle phalanx.
- The procedure is best performed under local anesthesia. This allows the patient to participate during the operation. The patient also understands what has happened and is often clearer about the postoperative regimen.

Positioning

- Informed consent is needed, with a discussion of the risks and benefits of the various conservative (nonoperative) and surgical options.
  - Risks include infection, nerve injury, stiffness, scar tenderness, nonunion, malunion, the need for revision procedures, and the risk associated with any operation (ie, making the patient worse).
- The digit needs to be marked very clearly, especially if the patient is receiving general anesthesia (the minority of patients).
- Preoperative antibiotics are recommended in line with the local hospital policy.
- The patient lies supine with the affected hand out on an arm board at 90 degrees to the table (ie, standard position for hand surgery).
- A proximal arm tourniquet is applied as a backup to the digital tourniquet.
- The skin is prepared with chlorhexidine in an alcohol solution with a pink dye to ensure that all the fingers have been fully painted. If the finger has had adhesive dressings on it or has not been well cleaned, the anesthetized finger is scrubbed before skin preparation.
- The operated arm is draped sterilely.

Approach

- The operation is performed closed with insertion of percutaneous wires.

TECHNIQUES

Inserting the Wires

- 1.1-mm K-wires are used routinely: 0.9-mm wires are too flexible and 1.6-mm wires are too rigid. 1.2-mm wires have been used successfully, but 1.1-mm wires are recommended.
- Identify the level of the center of rotation of the PIP joint with the image intensifier and mark this level on the skin (**TECH FIG 1A,B**).
- Insert the wire partially through the proximal phalanx and check carefully on the image intensifier with true posteroanterior and lateral projections (**TECH FIG 1C**).
  - *This is the most important part of the operation and must be right.* If you place the wire too distally, it will be intracapsular, risking joint infection if pin tract sepsis develops; but if you are too proximal, it will prevent fully joint movement, so aim for 1 to 2 mm proximal of the center of the proximal phalanx head. Insert the wire all the way through the proximal phalanx so equal lengths are visible both sides.
- Identify an appropriate level in the distal half to two-thirds of the middle phalanx, distal to any fracture extension in the shaft of the middle phalanx, with the image intensifier.
  - Mark this level on the skin.
  - This wire may be inserted near the center of rotation of the distal interphalangeal (DIP) joint, in the distal middle

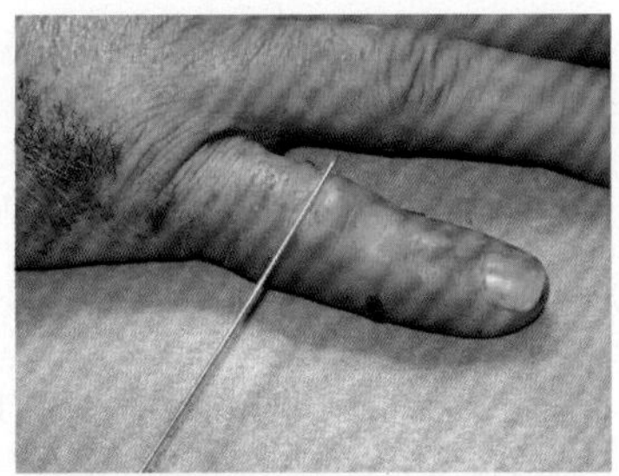
A

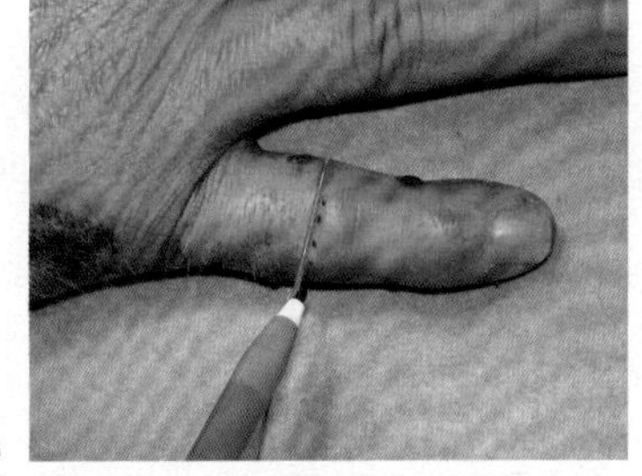
B

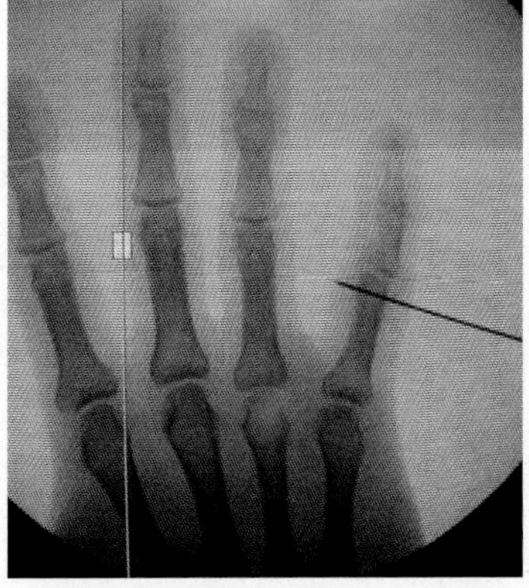
C

TECH FIG 1 • **A,B.** Checking the position for the first wire at the level of the center of rotation of the PIP joint with the image intensifier and marking it on the skin. **C.** Wire inserted across the head of the proximal phalanx and confirmed on the image intensifier before advancing further. *(continued)*

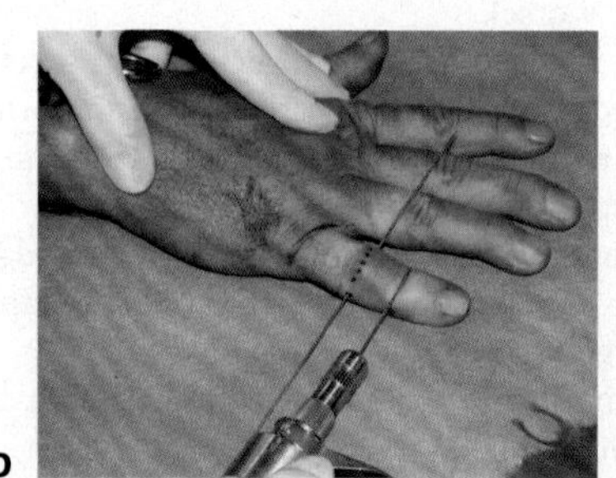
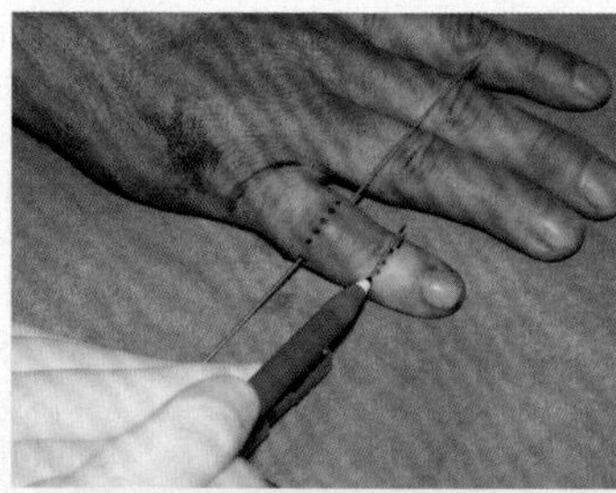
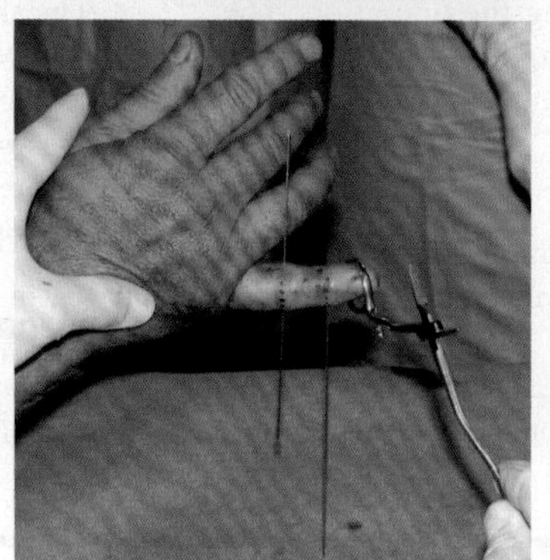
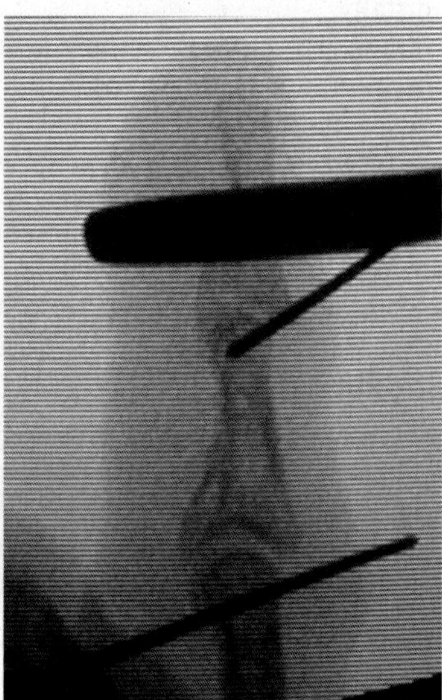

TECH FIG 1 • *(continued)* **D,E.** Finding and marking the position of the distal wire as for the proximal wire. This placement is more distal in the head of the middle phalanx than average because the DIP joint was also injured. **F,G.** Inserting the distal wire and confirming its position on the image intensifier.

phalanx. This is acceptable because the bone is wider and provides more margin for error (**TECH FIG 1D,E**).

- Insert the wire partially through the middle phalanx and check carefully (posteroanterior and lateral) on the image intensifier (**TECH FIG 1F,G**).
  - The wire should be perpendicular to the long axis of the finger and parallel to both the plane of rotation and the first wire (which should also be in the plane of rotation).
  - Insert the wire so equal lengths are present on either side of the finger. This helps in the wire bending. If one end is too short, it can become difficult to bend, especially in patients with long fingers.

Bending the Wire

- Wire bending is the more technically demanding part of the procedure. It is important to understand and follow the steps carefully.
  - One may create the construct in reverse of that described in the following text, but this results in motion on the proximal wire rather than the distal wire, which in theory increases the risk of pin tract and PIP joint sepsis.
- A medium needle holder is recommended to bend the wires as it allows adequate clearance from the finger, is robust enough to allow wire bending, yet fine enough to undertake the task.
- First, place the needle holder against the skin and bend the distal wire on each side to 90 degrees; in fact, bend it to just beyond 90 degrees and it will spring back (**TECH FIG 2A,B**).
- Rotate the distal wire so it lies on the proximal wire and then bend each end of the distal wire to make the linkage between the wires (**TECH FIG 2C,D**).
  - It is *critical* that this bend is sufficiently distal in the wire (proximal relative to the finger) to ensure that the construct is long enough and provides adequate joint distraction.
  - If the bend is not distal enough, it is difficult to salvage, and you will probably need to remove the distal wire and insert a new wire.
- Grip the distal wires with the medium needle holder just after the second bend and bend the distal end back up about 135 degrees, creating a Z shape (**TECH FIG 2E**).
  - The proximal wire will sit in the distal narrow angle of the Z.
  - It important to put the Zs at the same level, although the construct can tolerate some mismatch.
  - If the Zs are at different levels, careful unbending or further bending of the wires should help.
- The proximal wire is flicked into place in the distal angle of the Z (**TECH FIG 2F**).
  - It should bow, showing that tension has been applied across the construct and thus traction across the joint.
  - Improved fracture and joint alignment can be visualized on the image intensifier.

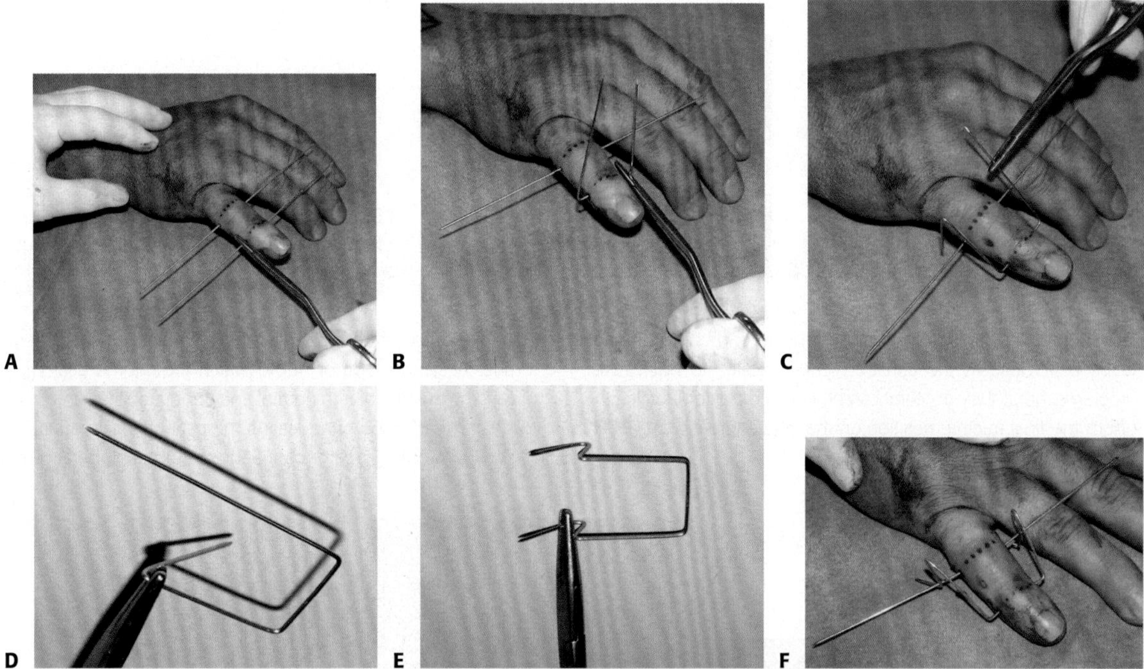

TECH FIG 2 • **A,B.** Grasping the distal wire with the needle holder and making the first bend. **C,D.** Start and completion of the second wire bend. **E.** Third wire bend shown on a freestanding wire. **F.** The properly bent distal wire is placed around the proximal wire distracting the joint.

Tidying Up and Ensuring the Construct Does Not Disengage

Proximal Wire

- Bend the proximal wire down. Place the medium needle holder on the wire, pushing the Z construct of the distal wire against the skin (**TECH FIG 3A,B**).
  - This ensures that the construct is neither too bulky nor too close to the finger, allowing for some swelling.
  - A distance of about 3 to 4 mm is effective.
- Bend the proximal wire down about 135 degrees (**TECH FIG 3C**).
- Cut the proximal wire with wire cutters about 3 mm after the bend and crimp the cut ends (**TECH FIG 3D,E**).
  - If too short, it cannot be bent; if too long, it will abut the finger.

Distal Wire

- Crimp the distal point of the wire and the part of the proximal wire just outside the skin down together with the medium needle holders (**TECH FIG 4A**).
  - Do not crimp too far or the middle phalanx wire will be gripped and not allow full rotation.
  - The wire has to be bent enough to ensure that the construct cannot disengage.
- Bend the distal tail of each Z over to ensure that the proximal wire cannot disengage (**TECH FIG 4B**).

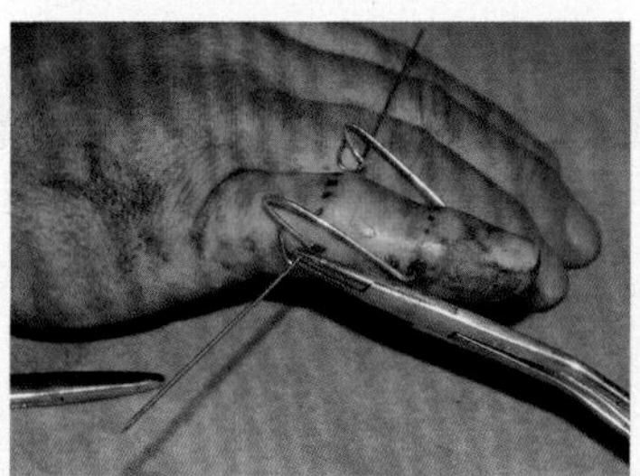

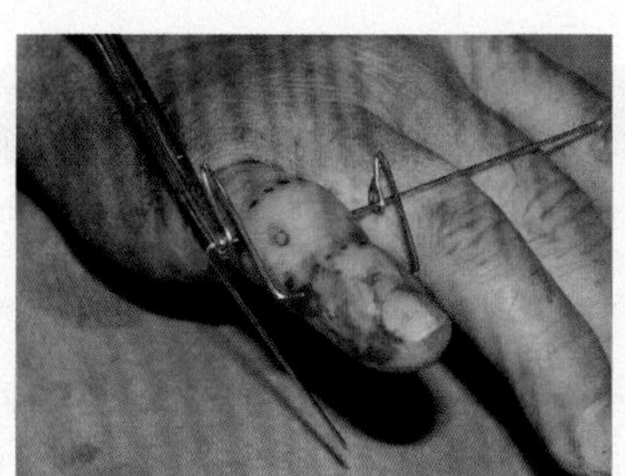

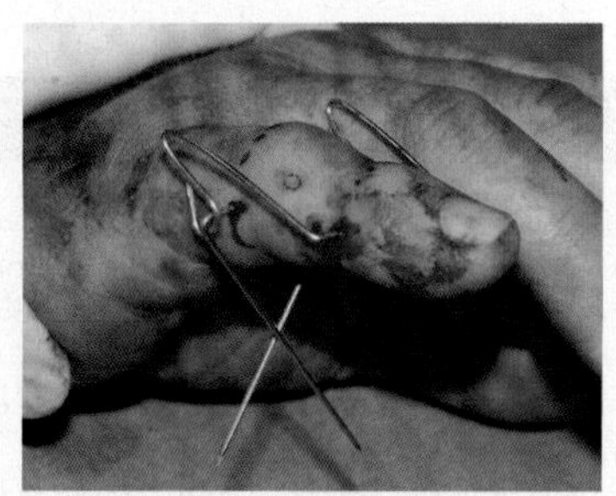

TECH FIG 3 • **A,B.** Grasping the proximal wire and making the first bend on the proximal wire shown on a patient. **C.** Bend the wire approximately 135 degrees. *(continued)*

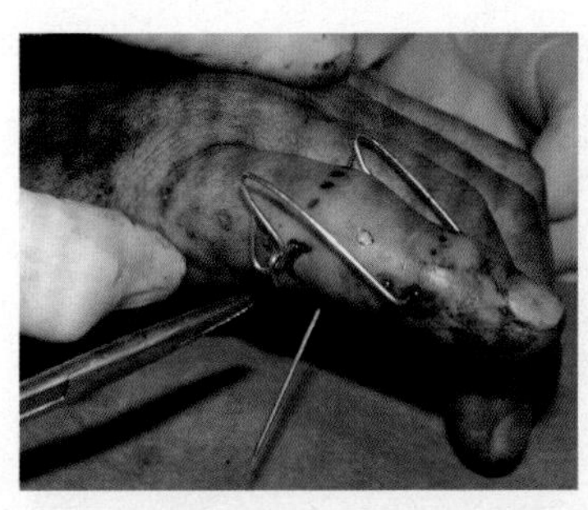

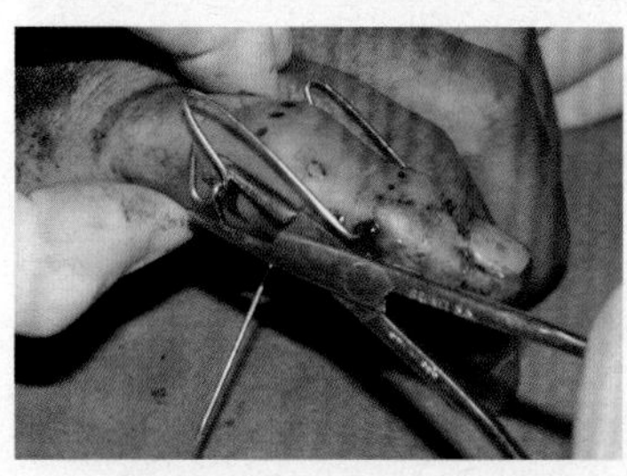

TECH FIG 3 • *(continued)* **D.** Cut the proximal wire 3 mm after the bend. **E.** Crimping cut ends of proximal wires.

- This process leaves slightly irregular cut wire ends. These need to be kept close to the construct and typically do not cause problems, but if they do, they can be covered postoperatively.
- Check the final fracture position on the image intensifier (**TECH FIG 4C,D**).
- At the end of the operation, if the patient is under local anesthesia, ask him or her to watch the injured digit while extending the PIP joint to neutral and flexing to at least 90 degrees.
  - This method of educating the patient is painless and gives him or her greater confidence in the postoperative period.

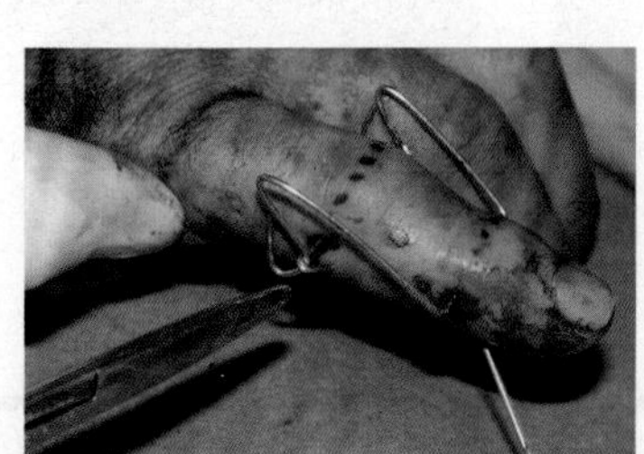

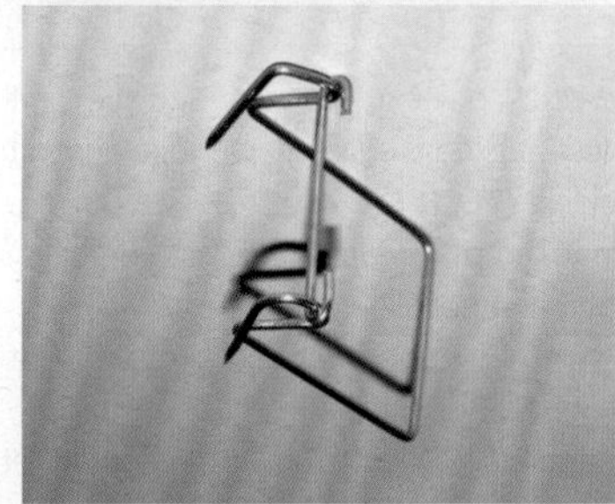

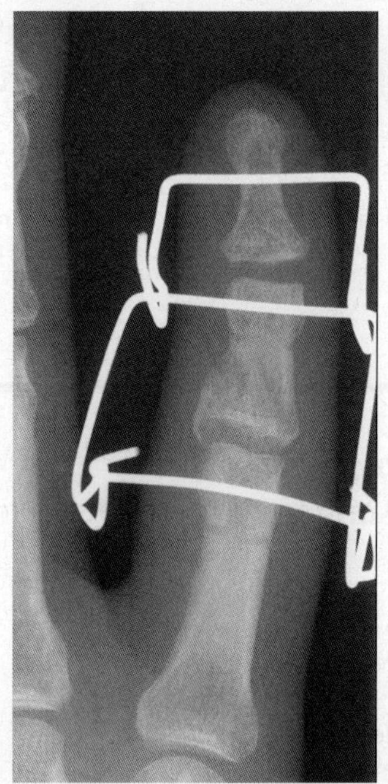

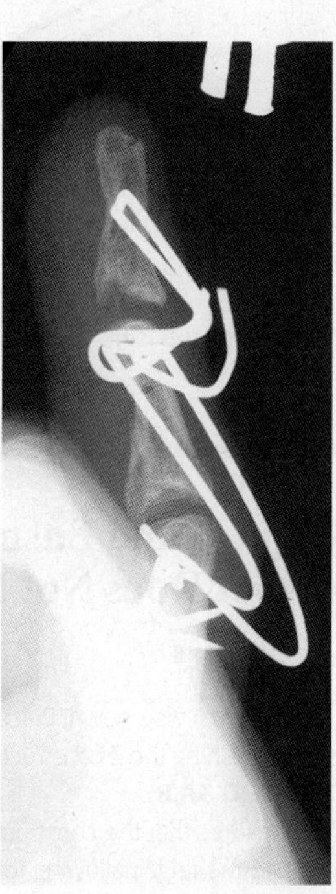

TECH FIG 4 • **A,B.** Distal wire bends completed. The fourth bend is just to prevent disengagement of the construct. **C,D.** The position of the final construct on a patient on whom, for the only time in the authors' practice, we used a double fixator on one finger. The PIP joint had a pilon fracture, which is well but not perfectly reduced. The DIP joint had a fracture-dislocation that is also well but not perfectly reduced.

PEARLS AND PITFALLS

- External fixation is typically very reliable and flexible in the treatment of PIP fractures and dislocations, as long as the patient understands the importance of moving their finger with the fixator in place; thus, patient selection is key.
- At the operation, the key is to place the proximal wire at or just proximal to the center of rotation of the PIP joint in the head of the proximal phalanx.
- Bending of the wires requires practice but with experience becomes easy. It is important to avoid putting twist into the wires to optimize motion in the construct.
- Sufficient tension in the construct and across the joint is critical.
- If inadequate, the wire bends may be adjusted, but probably, the distal wire will need to be replaced.

POSTOPERATIVE CARE

- The construct should not disimpact if made properly. If it does, it can usually be adjusted in clinic with further wire bending. Local anesthesia may be needed.
- The hand is elevated maximally for 3 to 5 days, and movement is started once the patient is comfortable.
- The use of a long-acting local anesthetic means that the patient can go home and start taking simple nonsteroidal oral analgesics. It is important that pain is sufficiently controlled to allow finger movement; that said, significant pain is rare and analgesics are not usually required after the first week.
- Long, slow stretches both into extension and into flexion are emphasized. They should be performed hourly.
  - The stretches should be held for 5 minutes at a time. They should not be painful, although they need to be at least on the edge of discomfort or in the mildly uncomfortable range. Painful stretches will lead to more swelling, increase the risk of complex regional pain syndrome type I, and discourage the patient from performing exercises.
  - Formal therapy visits begin the second postoperative week. In addition to PIP motion, DIP motion is emphasized. The therapist works with these patients at least weekly.
- The patient is checked after 5 to 7 days.
  - The dressing is removed and radiographs are performed to ensure that the reduction has been maintained.
  - The dressings are left off and the patient is instructed in pin tract care (see in the following text), care of the sharp wire points (ie, covering them with tape if necessary), and stretching exercises, supported by a hand therapist.
- The pins are cleaned and dried as one would for their hand day to day.
  - Assuming that the pin tracts stay dry, nothing more needs to be done.
  - If the pin tracts start oozing, clean with preboiled water four times a day.
  - If the pin sites do not improve within 24 hours, the patient should seek medical help for antibiotics.
  - The redness and oozing should resolve within 2 to 3 days. If not, the patient may require intravenous antibiotics and early pin removal, but this is extremely rare.
- The patient is checked again about 2 weeks postoperatively.
  - At this stage, the finger will still be mildly swollen.
  - There should be minimal or no pain except with stretches.
  - The pin tracts should be clean and dry.
  - The range of movement should be in the PIP joint a fixed flexion deformity of no more than 10 degrees and flexion to at least 50 degrees and in the DIP joint full extension and flexion to at least 50 degrees.
- If this has been achieved, the patient returns to the office 4 to 5 weeks postoperatively for wire removal. There appears no good reason to leave the wires longer, and the incidence of pin tract sepsis increases after 4 weeks.
- Final review takes place 10 to 12 weeks after surgery.

OUTCOMES

- The finger will still be mildly swollen; this will never resolve fully.
- The expected final range of movement should be about 10 to 90 degrees in the PIP joint and full (0 to 70 degrees) in the DIP joint. There should be no rest pain, but there will probably be some achiness with heavy use. The pin tracts should have healed with minimal, if any, tenderness or cosmetic abnormality.
- Pilon-type fractures typically reduce only in part, with at least one impacted fragment remaining in the middle phalanx.
  - Because the concave side of the joint seems to tolerate some incongruity well, this fragment is not routinely disimpacted.
- Fracture-dislocations also tend to reduce incompletely, with some mild residual dorsal subluxation of the joint surface (ie, widening of the joint on the lateral view). If mild, this too is well tolerated.
- Traction devices generally give reliable results, with range of motion of about 89 degrees and only 2% poor results compared with open reduction and internal fixation which typically give a range of motion of 79 degrees and 10% to 12% poor results.

COMPLICATIONS

- Pin tract infection is the most common risk, but if the wires are removed between 4 and 5 weeks, it is uncommon (<10% of cases). It typically resolves with cleaning, elevation, and 2 to 3 days of oral antibiotics.
- Mild malunion is not uncommon but often accepted and well tolerated.
- Nonunion has not occurred as a functional problem, although radiographs may show odd ununited peripheral fragments of bone.
- Nerve injury may occur but is rare.
- Significant poor results and persistent rest pain occur in only about 3% to 5% of patients and is often seen in noncompliant patients so careful patient selection is important.

SUGGESTED READINGS

1. Agee JM. Unstable fracture dislocation of the proximal interphalangeal joint. Treatment with the force couple splint. Clin Orthop Relat Res 1987;(214):101–112.
2. Aladin A, Davis TR. Dorsal fracture-dislocation of the proximal interphalangeal joint: a comparative study of percutaneous Kirschner wire fixation versus open reduction and internal fixation. J Hand Surg Br 2005;30(2):120–128.
3. Allison DM. Fractures of the base of the middle phalanx treated by dynamic external fixation. J Hand Surg Br 1996;21(3):305–310.
4. Badia A, Riano F, Ravikoff J, et al. Dynamic intradigital external fixation for proximal interphalangeal joint fracture dislocations. J Hand Surg Am 2005;30(1):154–160.
5. Deitch MA, Kiefhaber TR, Comisar RB, et al. Dorsal fracture dislocations of the proximal interphalangeal joint: surgical complications and long-term results. J Hand Surg Am 1999;24(5):914–923.
6. Deshmukh SC, Kumar D, Mathur K, et al. Complex fracture-dislocation of the proximal interphalangeal joint of the hand. Results of a modified pins and rubbers traction system. J Bone Joint Surg 2004;86B:406–412.
7. De Smet L, Boone P. Treatment of fracture-dislocation of the proximal interphalangeal joint using the Suzuki external fixator. J Orthop Trauma 2002;16(9):668–671.
8. de Soras X, de Mourgues P, Guinard D, et al. Pins and rubbers traction system. J Hand Surg Br 1997;22(6):730–735.
9. Duteille F, Pasquier P, Lim A, et al. Treatment of complex interphalangeal joint fractures with dynamic external traction: a series of 20 cases. Plast Reconstr Surg 2003;111(5):1623–1629.
10. Fahmy NRM. The Stockport Serpentine Spring System for the treatment of displaced comminuted intra-articular phalangeal fractures. J Hand Surg Br 1990;15(3):303–311.

11. Grant I, Berger AC, Tham SK. Internal fixation of unstable fracture dislocations of the proximal interphalangeal joint. J Hand Surg Br 2005;30(5):492–498.
12. Hamilton SC, Stern PJ, Fassler PR, et al. Mini-screw fixation for the treatment of proximal interphalangeal joint dorsal fracture-dislocations. J Hand Surg Am 2006;31(8):1349–1354.
13. Hastings H II, Carroll C IV. Treatment of closed articular fractures of the metacarpophalangeal and proximal interphalangeal joints. Hand Clin 1988;4(3):503–527.
14. Inanami H, Ninomiya S, Okutsu I, et al. Dynamic external finger fixator for fracture dislocation of the proximal interphalangeal joint. J Hand Surg Am 1993;18A:160–164.
15. Kiefhaber T, Stern PJ. Fracture-dislocations of the proximal interphalangeal joint. J Hand Surg Am 1998;23(3):368–380.
16. Krakauer JD, Stern PJ. Hinged device for fractures involving the proximal interphalangeal joint. Clin Orthop Relat Res 1996;(327):29–37.
17. Schenk RR. The dynamic traction method. Combining movement and traction for intra-articular fractures of the phalanges. Hand Clin 1994;10:187–198.
18. Seno N, Hashizume H, Inoue H, et al. Fractures of the base of the middle phalanx of the finger: classification, management and long-term results. J Bone Joint Surg Br 1997;79(5):758–763.
19. Weiss AP. Cerclage fixation for fracture dislocation of the proximal interphalangeal joint. Clin Orthop Relat Res 1996;(327):21–28.

Open Reduction and Internal Fixation of Proximal Interphalangeal Joint Fracture-Dislocations

53

CHAPTER

Nikhil Oak, Brian Najarian, and Jeffrey Lawton

DEFINITION

- Proximal interphalangeal (PIP) joint fracture-dislocations are intra-articular injuries that include a concomitant soft tissue injury to the surrounding capsular and ligamentous structures.
- The injury can result from axial, bending, and torsional loads, or a combined mechanism.
- These injuries are relatively common and potentially disabling and may result in the following:
  - Joint stiffness/swelling
  - Persistent subluxation
  - Posttraumatic arthritis
  - Chronic pain
- Stability, a concentric joint reduction and alignment are more important goals than articular congruency in determining a successful outcome.
- Evaluation and treatment may be delayed, with the injury dismissed as a "jammed finger."[32]

ANATOMY

- The PIP joint acts as a bicondylar sloppy hinge joint, consisting of radial and ulnar condyles on the proximal phalanx with matching concavities on the middle phalangeal base. This allows for a wide range of motion (ROM) in flexion and extension but relative rigidity in abduction and adduction.[19]
  - The PIP joint has an arc of motion of approximately 120 degrees and accounts for 85% of the motion required to grasp an object.[2]
  - The heads of the proximal phalanx are trapezoidal in shape tapering toward the ring finger; this allows for a normal finger flexion cascade toward the distal pole of the scaphoid.[19]
- The joint derives its stability from its bony articular congruence and its soft tissue restraints and allows for lateral as well as rotational stability with loading (**FIG 1**).
  - The volar plate resists dorsal (hyperextension) stresses, is taut in extension, and most often fails distally.
    - Checkrein ligaments are slender proximal extensions of the volar plate under which transverse branches of the digital arteries pass supplying the joint, vincula, and the flexor tendons.
  - Collateral ligaments, the primary soft tissue restraints, have two components:
    - The proper collateral ligaments (radial and ulnar), which insert on the middle phalanx, provide the principal resistance to abduction/adduction stress. These ligaments are commonly injured in dorsal dislocations. Injury to the radial collateral ligament is more common than injury to the ulnar collateral ligament.
    - The accessory collateral ligaments arise from a conjoined origin just volar to the proper collateral ligament and insert onto the volar plate.
- The extensor complex limits volarly directed stress.
  - The central slip attaches to the dorsal tubercle on the base of the middle phalanx.
  - The conjoint lateral tendons run obliquely on each side of the joint.
  - The transverse retinacular ligament connects the central slip and the conjoint lateral bands and extends laterally.
- For a dislocation to occur, at least one, often two, and sometimes all three of these structures must be significantly disrupted.

PATHOGENESIS AND CLASSIFICATION

- The PIP joint is uniquely susceptible to injury.
- The pattern of joint injury depends on the direction, degree, and rate of force application as well as the position of the joint at the time of injury.
- The three main groups of PIP fracture-dislocations are defined by the mechanism of injury force and the direction of deformity (**FIG 2**).
  - *Dorsal* subluxation or dislocation of the middle phalanx, the most common type, is caused by hyperextension and axial loading of the middle phalanx against the head of the proximal phalanx. The result is a fracture involving the volar base of the middle phalanx and dorsal positioning of the middle phalanx.

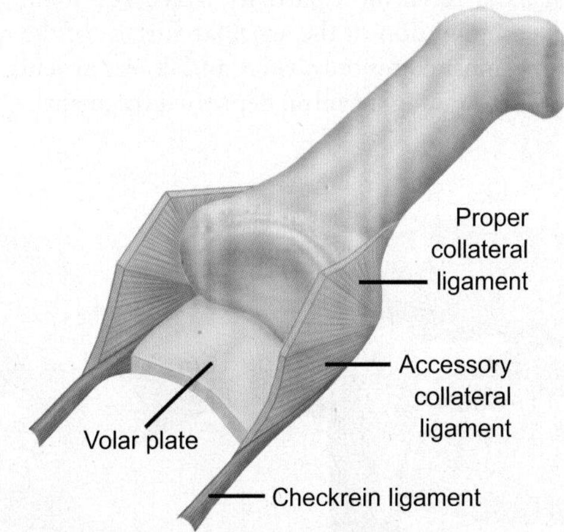

FIG 1 • Diagram of PIP joint anatomy. The PIP joint is a hinge joint that derives its stability from bony articular congruence of the proximal and middle phalanx and soft tissue restraints: the volar plate and its checkrein ligament extensions, the proper and accessory collateral ligaments, and the extensor complex (not shown).

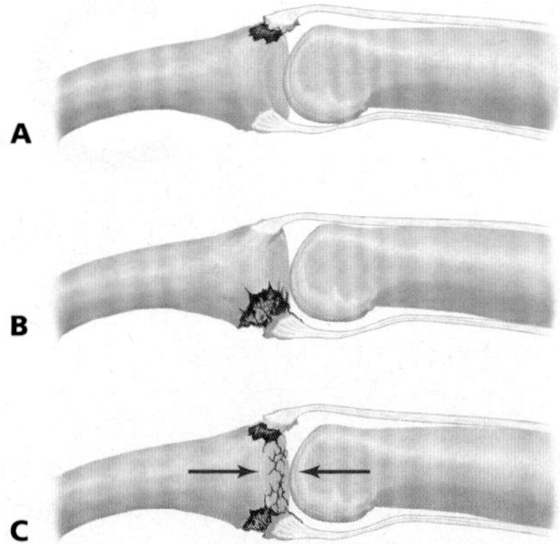

FIG 2 • PIP fracture-dislocation classifications. The three main groups of PIP fracture-dislocations are volar (**A**), dorsal (**B**), and pilon (**C**).

- This injury can be subclassified into three types based on the amount of volar middle phalanx articular surface involved, as determined on a lateral radiograph.[8,15] The degree of instability is directly proportional to volar lip fragment size due to the loss of collateral ligament support and the articular buttress (see Fig 3B in Chap. 52).[17,29,32]
  - *Stable:* less than 30% of the articular surface, reduced even in extension
  - *Tenuous:* 30% to 50% of the articular surface, reduction is maintained with less than 30 degrees of flexion
  - *Unstable:* either more than 50% of the articular surface *or* 30% to 50% of the articular surface but requiring more than 30 degrees of flexion to maintain reduction
- *Volar* subluxation, or dislocation of the middle phalanx, is less common and is thought to be caused by forced flexion of an extended joint.
  - *Stable:* joint reduction in extension
  - *Unstable:* palmar subluxation of middle phalanx with the joint extended
- *Pilon injuries* are almost always unstable. They are caused by an axial force on a partially flexed PIP joint, resulting in comminution of the articular surface of the middle phalanx (most commonly, volar and dorsal articular fragments surrounding a central depressed fragment).
- Unicondylar fractures of the head of the proximal phalanx are included in a classification system proposed by Weiss and Hastings[31] (see Chap. 50).
  - These injuries can also be accompanied by a dislocation of the PIP joint and are nearly always unstable. They often are amenable to the same approaches and fixation methods presented here.

NATURAL HISTORY

- Following injury, the PIP joint quickly stiffens. Pain and instability limit motion initially, followed by fibrosis of the joint capsule and ligaments.
- Over time, the unreduced PIP joint will become arthritic and painful.

HISTORY AND PHYSICAL FINDINGS

- Patients present following a traumatic event to the digit, frequently one that occurred some time ago.
  - In the acute setting, the primary complaints are pain and swelling of the joint and digit.
  - Patients with subacute and chronic injuries are focused primarily on stiffness, loss of function, and persistent swelling, and secondarily on pain.
  - The history must include a detailed description of the mechanism of injury and any previous treatment.
- Inspection
  - Evaluate the skin and soft tissues for swelling and for any open or healed wounds that could indicate an open fracture-dislocation.
  - Deformity in extension or flexion indicates whether the dislocation is volar or dorsal, respectively.
  - Axial or rotational malalignment may result from articular depression of a condyle. This can be recognized clinically as subtle angulation when full digital extension and flexion is attempted.
- Tenderness
  - The location of greatest tenderness on palpation may indicate which soft tissue structures are injured.
- ROM
  - Adequate evaluation may be difficult in the acute setting due to pain. After neurologic examination, a digital block may be necessary.
  - Elson test (**FIG 3**)

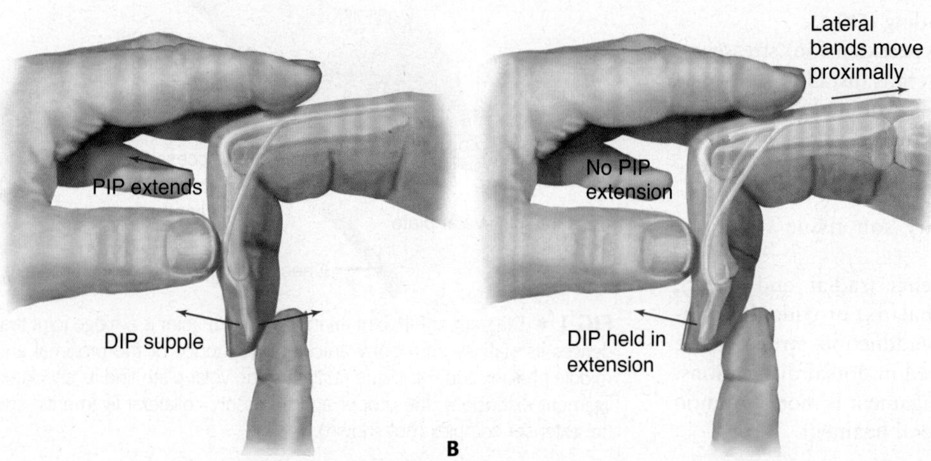

FIG 3 • Elson test. **A.** Intact central slip. From a 90-degree flexed position, the patient can actively extend the PIP joint of the involved finger against resistance. The DIP joint is supple. **B.** Ruptured central slip. The patient cannot actively extend the PIP joint against resistance and has fixed extension at the DIP joint, due to the extensor action of the lateral bands alone.

- From a 90-degree flexed position over the edge of a table, ask the patient to actively extend the PIP joint of the involved finger against resistance. If the central slip is intact, the examiner will feel an extension force from the middle phalanx. In addition, the distal interphalangeal (DIP) joint remains flail during this effort because the competent central slip prevents the lateral bands from acting distally.
- An *absence* of extension force at the PIP joint and fixed/rigid extension at the DIP joint (due to the extensor action of the lateral bands alone) is diagnostic of a complete rupture of the central slip. In the acute setting, the patient may be reluctant to perform this test due to pain, but this can be relieved by proximal infiltration with local anesthetic around the dorsal sensory nerves of the digit.[9]
- Note the ROM through which the joint remains reduced. In the case of a dorsal dislocation, the degree of extension that results in instability or redislocation determines the angle for the extension block splint.
- An irreducible joint is consistent with entrapment of a soft tissue structure (eg, volar plate, collateral ligament, flexor or extensor tendon) in the joint, which usually necessitates surgery.

- The neurovascular examination is usually normal.
  - Subjective complaints of paresthesias and objective measure of capillary refill should be noted, both pre- and postreduction.

IMAGING AND OTHER DIAGNOSTIC STUDIES

- Posteroanterior (PA) and lateral radiographs of the involved digit(s) are required.
  - Partially supinated and pronated oblique views may help to identify fracture planes, determine the extent of comminution, and may be valuable for surgical planning.
  - It is critical to determine the amount of articular involvement on a true lateral film in full PIP joint extension to evaluate stability of the joint.
  - Radiographs can be misleading, suggesting that a very simple fracture involving only a small fragment of the bone has occurred. This fragment is potentially the major attachment of a collateral ligament, the volar plate, or a tendon. The resultant incompetence of these structures can render the joint grossly or potentially unstable (**FIG 4A**).
- V sign[17,20] (**FIG 4B**)
  - On a postreduction true lateral radiograph of the digit, divergence of the dorsal articular surfaces from the central portion of the joint creates a V-shaped gap between the articular surfaces of the head of the proximal phalanx and the undamaged portion of the middle phalanx base.
  - The presence of this sign indicates an incompletely reduced joint.
- Dynamic fluoroscopy is extremely valuable in evaluating the reduction and its stability.
  - Hinged flexion is a variant of the V sign in which congruent rotation of the joint is replaced by abnormal translation, as the joint is actively flexed and extended across the flattened fracture segments.
  - The joint position that results in instability or redislocation is best determined fluoroscopically.

DIFFERENTIAL DIAGNOSIS

- Pure dislocation (simple or complex)
- Extra-articular fractures
- Jammed finger—collateral sprain[11,18,34]
- Volar plate injury
- Central slip injury

GOALS OF TREATMENT

- Correction of joint subluxation and concentric reduction
- Early motion to minimize adhesions and joint contracture
- Anatomic restoration desirable but less important than above goals[1,25–27]

NONOPERATIVE MANAGEMENT

- Prompt recognition of the complexity of injury and an understanding of the appropriate treatment options are essential for optimal management of these fractures.[22]
- Although fractures and dislocations of the PIP joint have the potential to be disabling, most can be treated with closed reduction, splinting, early motion, and close follow-up.
- Closed reduction is almost always successful for acute dorsal PIP dislocations. Volar dislocations are more problematic, especially if the deformity has a rotary component.
  - Reductions performed immediately after the injury, such as coming to the sideline, often can be accomplished without

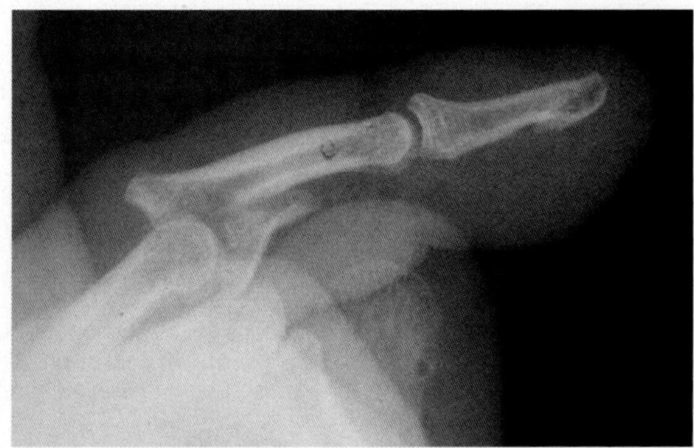

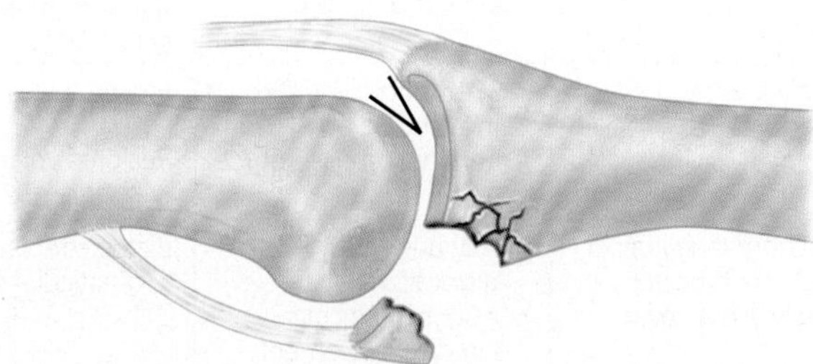

FIG 4 • **A.** Unstable dorsal PIP fracture-dislocation. This lateral radiograph of a typical PIP joint fracture demonstrates dorsal dislocation of the middle phalanx on the proximal phalanx due to the large amount of volar articular surface involved (over 50%). **B.** The V sign in an incompletely reduced dorsal fracture-dislocation. Divergence of the dorsal articular surfaces from the central portion of the joint creates a V-shaped gap, which can be demonstrated on a lateral radiograph.

anesthesia. If reduction is delayed, a digital block with 1% lidocaine (without epinephrine) is helpful.
- Always make sure to complete a careful neurologic examination of the digit before performing an anesthetic block. Confirm adequate anesthesia before manipulation.
- Be gentle and limit the number of attempts. Irreducible dislocations usually are caused by soft tissue interposition.

- Dorsal dislocations can be reduced with gentle traction on the finger with the wrist in the neutral position, followed by pressing the base of the middle phalanx in a volar direction while holding the proximal phalanx steady.
- Volar dislocations *without* a rotatory component are usually reducible with gentle traction.
  - Place the wrist in the neutral position, and, with longitudinal traction, apply a dorsally directed force to the middle phalanx and a volarly directed force on the proximal phalanx.
  - These dislocations, which usually can be treated with closed reduction, commonly involve an avulsion of the central slip.
- Volar dislocations *with* a rotatory component often are difficult to reduce by closed means. The head of the proximal phalanx becomes entrapped between the central slip and one of the lateral bands of the extensor mechanism.
  - These injuries occasionally can be reduced closed by placing the metacarpophalangeal (MCP) and PIP joints in 90 degrees of flexion with the wrist extended, applying light traction, and rotating the middle phalanx in the direction opposite to the deformity.

SURGICAL MANAGEMENT

- Surgical management can be difficult:
  - The fracture fragments can be small and comminuted, making anatomic reduction and stabilization with implants difficult.
  - The need for early mobilization of the joint to prevent stiffness requires rigid fixation of these fragments.
- These fractures have a high risk of redisplacement, and patients must be warned of the possibility that repeat surgical treatment of the fracture may be necessary.
- The specific injury and fracture pattern often dictates the most appropriate method of treatment. Some methods can be used in combination.
  - For stable, reducible fractures, typically involving less than 30% of the articular surface, treatment includes the following:
    - Extension block splinting and pinning[24]
    - Traction, dynamic or static[1,26,16] (see Chap. 52)
- Unstable, irreducible fractures, typically involving more than 30% to 50% of the joint, require the following:
  - External fixation
  - Percutaneous fixation
  - Open reduction with internal fixation (ORIF) using K-wires, screws, cerclage wires
- When dorsal fracture-dislocations are associated with bone loss or fracture comminution to such a degree that a stable reduction is unobtainable using the methods listed earlier, two salvage procedures are commonly employed:
  - *Volar plate arthroplasty.* The volar plate is advanced into the middle phalangeal defect, simultaneously restoring stability and resurfacing the damaged articular surface[7,21] (see Chap. 54).
  - *Hemi-hamate autograft reconstruction.* The fractured middle phalangeal base is débrided, and the defect is replaced using a size-matched portion of the dorsal/distal hamate osteoarticular surface and secured with minifragment screws[33] (see Chap. 55).
- Table 1 illustrates some of the indications, advantages, and disadvantages of ORIF and some of the salvage options discussed in this chapter.[10]

Indications

- Unstable and tenuous fractures requiring more than 30 degrees of flexion to maintain reduction
  - Closed management of these fractures, requiring extreme flexion to prevent redislocation, is likely to result in a significant flexion contracture.

Table 1 Advantages and Disadvantages of Techniques for Repair of Proximal Interphalangeal Joint Fracture-Dislocation

Technique	Indications	Advantages	Disadvantages	Pearls
ORIF	Minimal comminution Intact dorsal cortex	Anatomic reduction Can use bone graft Early ROM	Technically difficult if multiple fragments Increased risk of infection	Consider other options in older patients (older than 60 yo), for example, dorsal block pinning.
Volar plate arthroplasty	<50% articular surface involved Comminution base of P2	Proven track record Restores volar buttress	Redislocation (especially if >50% P2 base fractured) Stiffness Arthritis	Careful patient selection
Osteochondral autograft (ie, hemi-hamate, radial styloid, toes)	Highly unstable dislocations: • >60% of articular surface involvement • Acute or chronic dislocation	Biologic replacement of articular surface	Donor morbidity Technically demanding	Consider osteochondral autograft if >50% is involved. Short-term results are promising.

ORIF, open reduction with internal fixation; ROM, range of motion; P2, middle phalanx.

- Fractures with fragments that are irreducible by closed methods and amenable to internal fixation with available hardware
- Significant articular depression, displacement, or incongruity

Preoperative Planning

- Radiographic evaluation, as discussed earlier
- The surgeon must be adept at various techniques, and the patient should be counseled that intraoperative observations will dictate the definitive method of fixation.

Positioning

- The patient is placed supine with a radiolucent hand table.
- A brachial tourniquet is placed on the upper arm before draping and is inflated to 250 mm Hg just before the incision is made.
- Although surgery can be performed under a wrist or digital block, an axillary block is preferred to obtain adequate sensory anesthesia and motor relaxation of the flexors and extensors and to allow a generous tourniquet time as is sometimes required in these cases.
- The operative hand is supinated, and a "lead hand" positioner can be used to hold it in place.

Operative Equipment

- A mini C-arm fluoroscopy unit is necessary to confirm fracture reduction, joint reduction, and correct placement of implants.
- Minifragment plate and screw set
- A 24-gauge wire
- Kirschner wires (K-wires)

Approach

- The volar (Bruner) approach, the dorsal (Chamay) approach, and the midaxial approach are all useful.
- An approach is chosen based on the fracture pattern and the direction of instability.
  - When most of the fracture comminution is dorsal, a dorsal Chamay or midaxial approach is selected.
  - When most of the comminution is central or volar, as is more common with dorsal fracture-dislocations, a volar Bruner incision is employed.

TECHNIQUES

Exposure

Volar Approach (Bruner)

- A palmar zigzag skin incision is made from the MCP joint crease across the PIP joint to the DIP flexion crease. In a larger or longer digit, two limbs of a Bruner[3,13] incision may be necessary between the flexion creases (**TECH FIG 1A,B**).
- An ulnarly based, thick subcutaneous flap is mobilized at the level of the flexor sheath.
- The digital neurovascular structures are mobilized from the flexor sheath apparatus.
  - Untethering the neurovascular bundles from the flexor sheath is necessary to avoid traction on the associated structures if the joint is dorsally displaced during exposure and fixation.

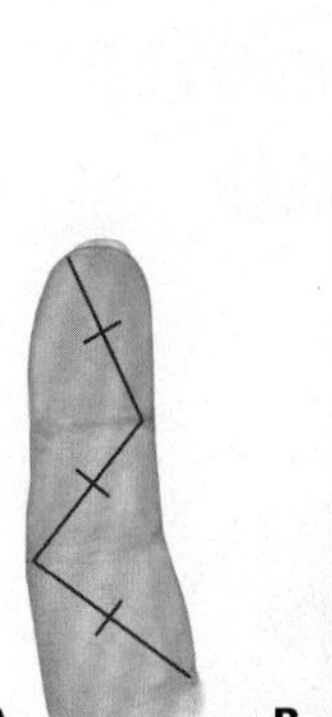
A

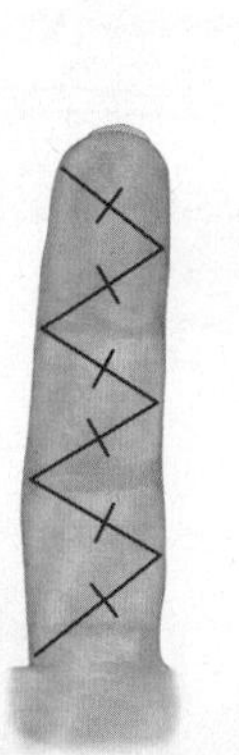
B

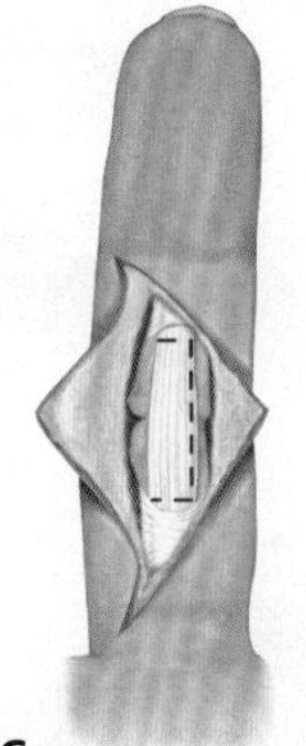
C

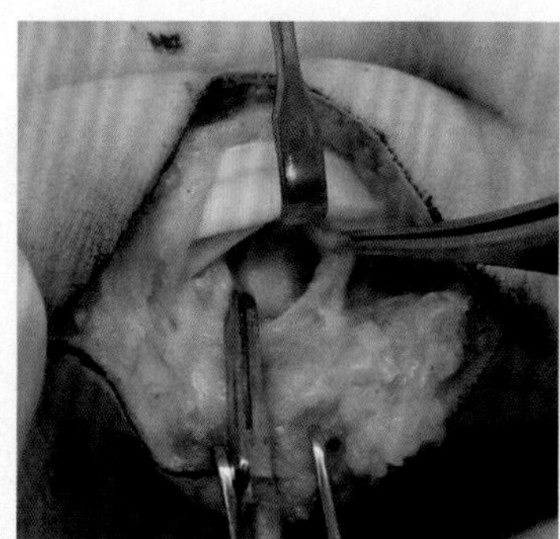
D

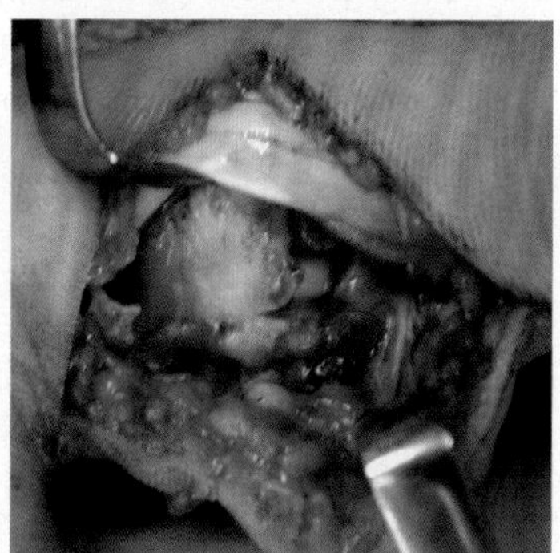
E

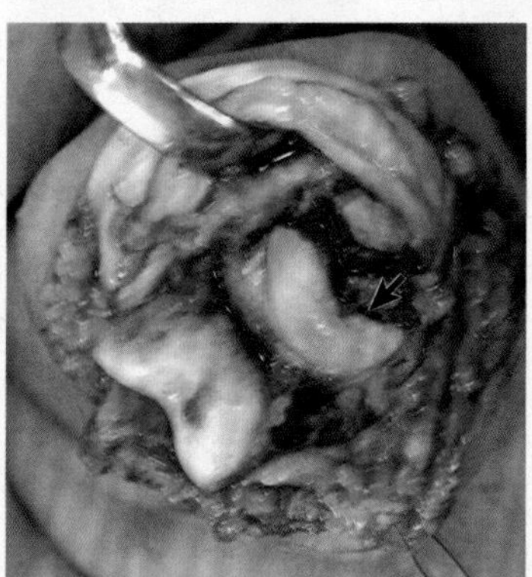
F

TECH FIG 1 • **A.** The Bruner approach uses a palmar zigzag skin incision from the MCP flexion crease across the PIP joint level to the DIP flexion crease. **B.** In larger digits, two limbs may be necessary between flexion creases. **C.** Once the flexor sheath is exposed, it can be incised on three sides between the A2 and A4 pulleys and the flap retracted laterally. Alternatively, the sheath can be split down its center longitudinally to expose the flexor tendons. The pathways of the incisions are demonstrated by the *dotted line*. **D.** After retraction of the incised flexor sheath, the flexor digitorum profundus (FDP) and flexor digitorum sublimis (FDS) tendons are exposed. Gently retract them to one side with a blunt retractor to expose the volar plate and the base of the middle phalanx. Not uncommonly, the volar plate is still attached to the volar lip of the middle phalangeal fracture fragment. **E,F.** Shotgun exposure of the PIP joint. **E.** The PIP joint is distracted while the flexor tendons are retracted laterally. **F.** The joint is then gently hyperextended until it maintains this shotgun alignment of its own accord (~130 degrees), exposing the articular surfaces (*arrow*, fractured volar middle phalanx base). (**D–F:** Hand is to the left and the finger is to the right).

- The flexor sheath over the PIP joint (including the A3 pulley) is incised on three sides, creating a rectangular flap between the A2 and A4 pulleys (**TECH FIG 1C**).
  - Alternatively, the flexor sheath may be split longitudinally to expose the underlying flexor tendons.
- The flexor digitorum profundus and flexor digitorum superficialis tendons are retracted to the side to expose the volar plate (**TECH FIG 1D**).
  - A Penrose drain placed around the tendons permits atraumatic retraction.
- The PIP joint and bare surface of the volar fragment are exposed by dividing the volar plate in the transverse plane just proximal to its distal insertion.
  - Make sure to leave a small amount of the distal portion attached to the bony fragment of the middle phalanx for later repair.
  - Retract the main portion of the volar plate proximally, creating a proximally based flap. The volar plate is *not* excised.
- Sharp recession of the collateral ligaments at their proximal or distal volar attachments may be required to access fragments that are more dorsal than the volar third of the middle phalangeal base or to reduce chronic subluxations.
  - Most often, the collateral ligaments are elevated only from their middle phalangeal insertion.
- If a comprehensive exposure of the PIP joint is required, the collateral ligaments are released from their site of insertion, and the PIP joint is distracted and then gently hyperextended until it maintains this alignment of its own accord (about 130 degrees). This has been referred to as *shotgun* exposure of the joint[7] (**TECH FIG 1E,F**).
  - Watch the neurovascular bundles closely during this hyperextension maneuver to ensure they can easily subluxate dorsally.

Dorsal Approach (Chamay)

- A longitudinal skin incision is made over the dorsal aspect of the PIP joint centered along the midline over the proximal and middle phalanx curving around the dorsal aspect of the PIP joint, exposing the extensor mechanism[4] (**TECH FIG 2A**).
- A distally based, extended V-shaped flap of central slip with the apex extending as far as the proximal third of the proximal phalanx is made (**TECH FIG 2B**).
- The extensor flap is reflected distally, allowing the intact lateral bands to slip palmarly and laterally, providing a wide exposure of the PIP joint.
- On completion of the surgery, the central slip is securely sutured in place with 4-0 nonabsorbable suture.
- This long zone of tendon reapproximation creates a repair that is strong and will allow early active motion within the first 48 hours.

Midaxial Approach

- Identify the midaxial line by marking the axes of the interphalangeal (IP) joints and drawing a line through these points proximally and distally (**TECH FIG 3A**).
  - Make the skin incision on this midaxial line. The digital nerve and artery lie about 2 mm volar to the margin of the incision (**TECH FIG 3B**).
  - Avoid a radial-sided incision on the index finger and an ulnar-sided incision on the small finger. These surfaces are important for contact and should be protected from potential scar sensitivity.
- The first structure encountered in the subcutaneous fat is Cleland ligament, which contains fibers that run volar to dorsal and consist of thin fascial layers surrounding the digital nerve and artery. It can be isolated from adjacent fat at the level of the PIP joint.

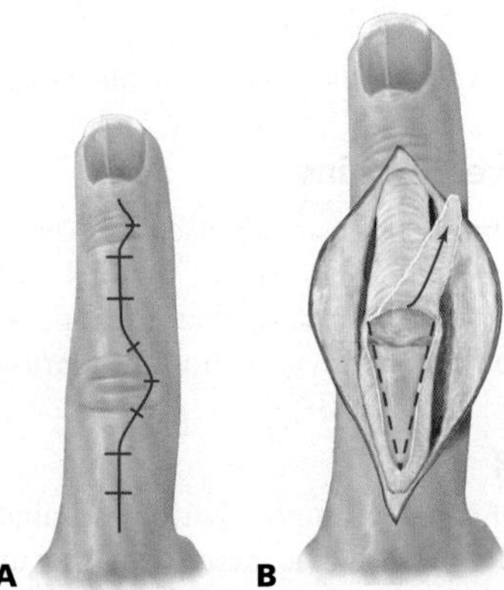

TECH FIG 2 • Dorsal (Chamay) approach. **A.** A longitudinal skin incision is made midline over the dorsal aspect of the proximal phalanx proximally and then is curved laterally and distally around the dorsal aspect of the PIP joint. **B.** After superficial dissection is carried down to expose the extensor mechanism, a distally based, V-shaped flap of central slip is created, with the apex of the flap extending to the proximal third of the proximal phalanx. This pedicle flap of central slip is then pulled distally with a hooked retractor to expose the PIP joint.

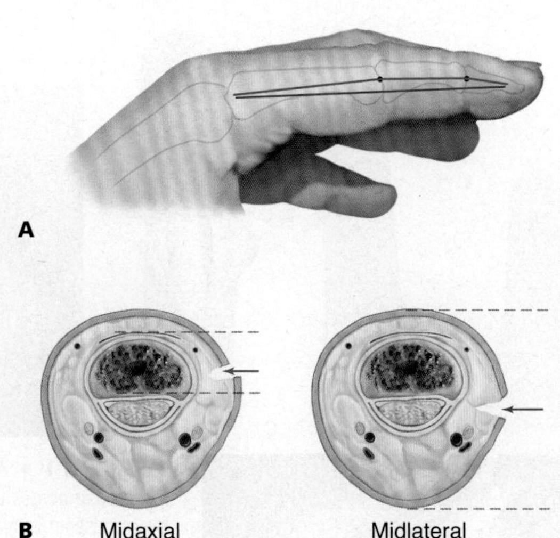

TECH FIG 3 • **A.** Diagrams demonstrating the midaxial (*blue line*) and midlateral (*red line*) approaches. The midlateral approach is shown for reference, but the midaxial approach is the one most often used clinically. Midaxial approach (*blue*): Flex the finger and mark the motion axes of the IP joints by marking the points at the IP joints where the flexion creases end dorsally. Draw a line through these points proximally and distally (*blue line*). **B.** In a cross-sectional diagram of these approaches, the midaxial dissection will be dorsal to the neurovascular bundle and the midlateral dissection will be at the level of the neurovascular bundle.

- Once Cleland ligament is divided, carry the dissection slightly volarly, deep to the neurovascular bundle, and expose the lateral aspect of the middle phalanx and lateral margin of the flexor sheath.
  - The neurovascular bundle remains in the volar flap.
- Enter the joint between the volar plate and the accessory collateral ligament to inspect the joint.
- Additional exposure is gained by elevating the collateral ligament at the origin or the insertion.

Fracture and Joint Reduction

- The joint and fractures are exposed, cleansed of hematoma, and fully evaluated.
  - If soft tissues are interposed, a fine curved hemostat or dental pick may be introduced to clear the fracture site.
- A dental pick or Freer elevator may be used to carefully manipulate and elevate depressed articular fragments, restoring articular congruity.
  - Maintain cancellous and subchondral bone on the articular cartilage-bearing fragments.
- Cancellous bone grafting may be required to prevent articular surface collapse in highly comminuted fractures.
  - Allograft or autograft (often harvested from the dorsal distal radius) can be used. The graft material is packed into the metaphysis through either direct application or a cortical window.
- Small 0.045- or 0.030-inch K-wires may be used to provisionally stabilize the reduction.
- Preliminary joint reduction, fracture reduction, and articular restoration are confirmed under direct vision and with fluoroscopy.
- Fracture fixation may proceed through various methods, depending on fracture pattern and surgeon's preference.
- Following definitive fixation, the digit is put through full ROM under fluoroscopy to ensure a stable concentric reduction has been achieved without sign of abnormal joint motion.
  - Close evaluation of lateral fluoroscopic images is critical to ensure that the PIP joint does not remain dorsally subluxated.
  - If the joint is not concentrically reduced or the internal fixation of the fracture is tenuous, it may be augmented with dynamic external fixation,[17] extension block pinning, or a transarticular K-wire.[6]

Minifragment Fixation

- Screw fixation, if attainable, provides excellent stability and may allow earlier ROM and improved functional restoration. This form of stabilization is indicated for larger and fewer fragments (**TECH FIG 4A–D**).[12,14]
  - Be aware that these fragments are often more comminuted than expected, and screws may further fragment the bone, making ultimate fixation difficult.[10]
- After anatomic reduction of the fragments is achieved by careful manipulation and the fragments are stabilized with clamps or K-wires (as needed), appropriately sized screws, typically in the 1.0- to 1.7-mm range, are chosen.
- The screw hole is drilled as perpendicular to the fracture plane as possible, and the depth is measured.

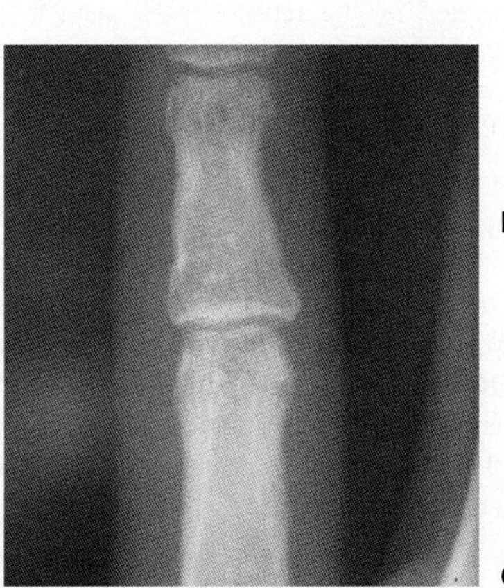
A

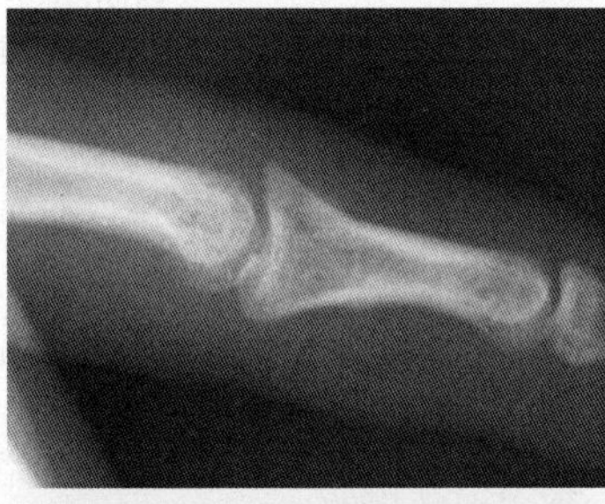
B

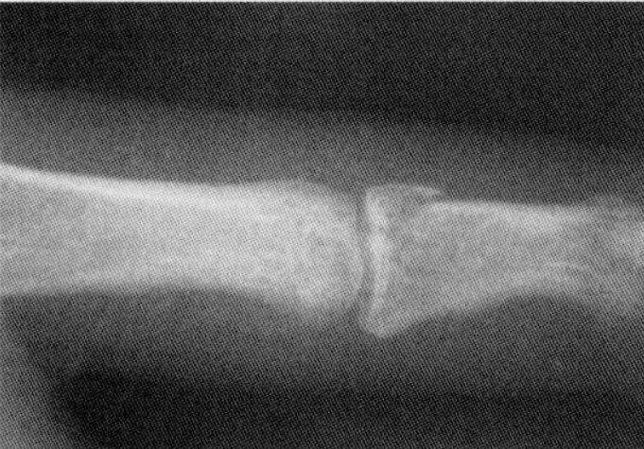
C

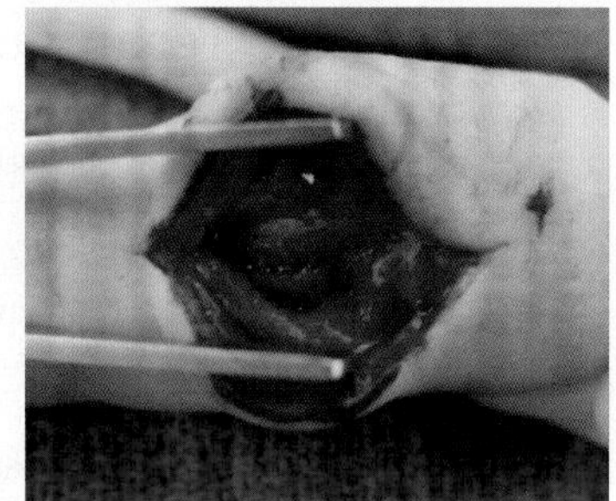
D

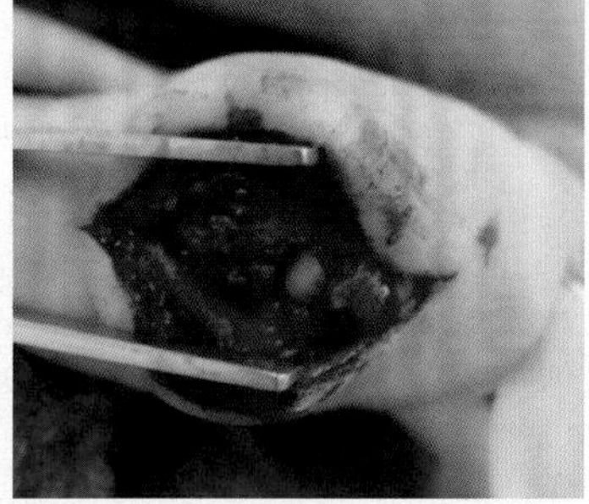
E

TECH FIG 4 • A–C. Preoperative anteroposterior (AP), lateral, and oblique radiographs demonstrating a displaced small finger PIP intra-articular fracture with a large dorsal/ulnar fragment. **D,E.** Intraoperative photos show the dorsal approach to the PIP joint. **D.** The fragment was large enough to be amenable to microscrew fixation. **E.** Using standard AO technique, a 1.7-mm screw was placed to achieve stable fixation of the fragment. The head of the screw has been countersunk. *(continued)*

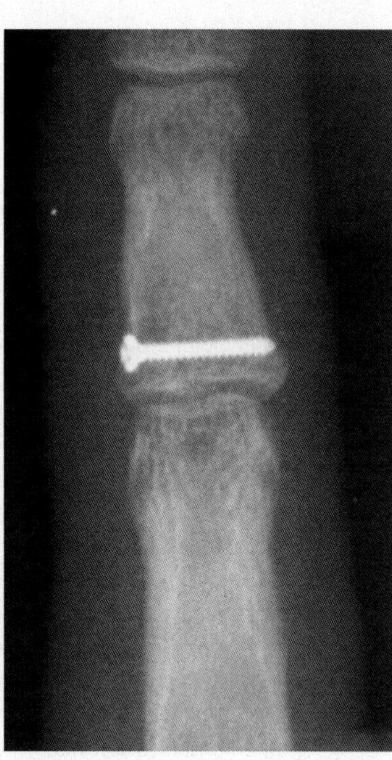

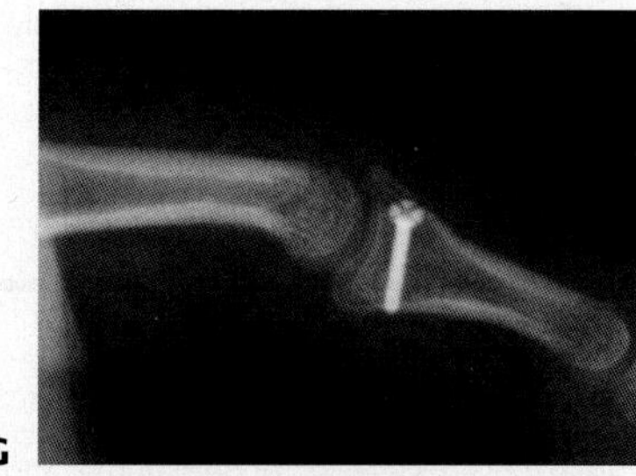

TECH FIG 4 • *(continued)* **F,G.** Postoperative AP and lateral radiographs demonstrate the screw in position and a reduced joint surface.

- If possible, an interfragmentary lag technique is preferred. This is done by overdrilling the near fragment cortex with a drill equal to the screw's outer diameter.
- A self-tapping, minifragment cortical screw is placed.
  - Countersinking of screws or use of headless screws may be helpful to avoid soft tissue tethering and tendon irritation (**TECH FIG 4E**).
- If the fragment is large enough, two screws, or a screw and a supplementary threaded K-wire (0.028 inch), can be used to prevent rotation of the fragment (**TECH FIG 4F,G**).
- After the procedure, PIP joint ROM can be compromised, with a residual flexion contracture occurring in more than 80% of cases of volar fracture and dorsal instability.[14,28]

Cerclage Wire Technique

- The cerclage wire technique[30] allows reduction of multiple small articular fragments and provides adequate fixation to allow early ROM exercises (**TECH FIG 5A**).
  - A thorough joint release is required, which carries the risk of increased fibrosis and stiffness postoperatively.
- A volar incision with a shotgun exposure of the PIP joint is used (**TECH FIG 5B**).
- Careful elevation of the central slip is performed.
- A thin ring of periosteum around the bony fragments of the middle phalanx is cleared by sharp dissection.
  - This allows the wire loop to seat directly against bone, providing firm fixation of the fracture fragments.
  - The normal shape of the base of the middle phalanx (reverse funnel contour) also aids in fixation of the wire and prevents postoperative slippage, even with early ROM.
- A 24-gauge steel wire is formed into a loop and twisted on itself until the loop is partially closed, just larger than the base of the middle phalanx.
- After fracture reduction, the loop of wire is seated and gently tightened, allowing circumferential compression of the fracture fragments (**TECH FIG 5C**).
- Final confirmation of articular reduction is made, with careful attention to the correction of central depression and joint subluxation (**TECH FIG 5D**).
- The twisted portion of the loop is placed on the volar or volar lateral surface of the middle phalanx base, flush to the cortex, at the edge of the volar plate.
- The wire is covered by the repaired volar plate to prevent mechanical irritation of the flexor tendons.

Supplementary K-Wire Addition

- A supplementary K-wire may be necessary, depending on fracture configuration (**TECH FIG 6A,B**).
- The cerclage wire is loosely twisted around the base of the middle phalanx, maintaining the position of the articular fragments prior to the replacement of the central and volar depressed fragment (**TECH FIG 6C**).
- After replacement of the central fragment and further fixation with a K-wire, the cerclage wire is tightened (**TECH FIG 6D,E**) and the excess tail end can be cut.

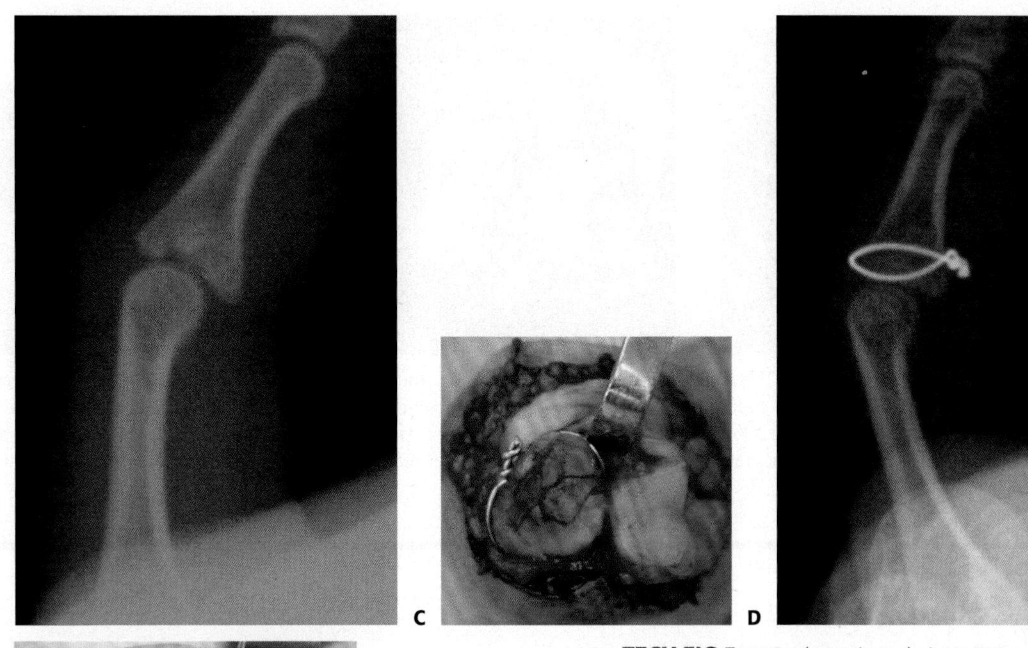

TECH FIG 5 • Cerclage wire technique. **A.** Lateral radiograph demonstrates a pilon-type fracture pattern of the middle phalanx, with depressed central articular fragments. **B.** After shotgun exposure, central articular impaction is evident in addition to marginal comminution. This fracture is a good candidate for cerclage wiring because this pattern would be difficult to reduce and maintain with screw or K-wire fixation. **C.** The central fragment has been reduced, and a 24-gauge steel wire was formed into a loop and gently placed, allowing circumferential compression of the fracture fragments. **D.** A postoperative lateral radiograph confirms correction of the central articular depression.

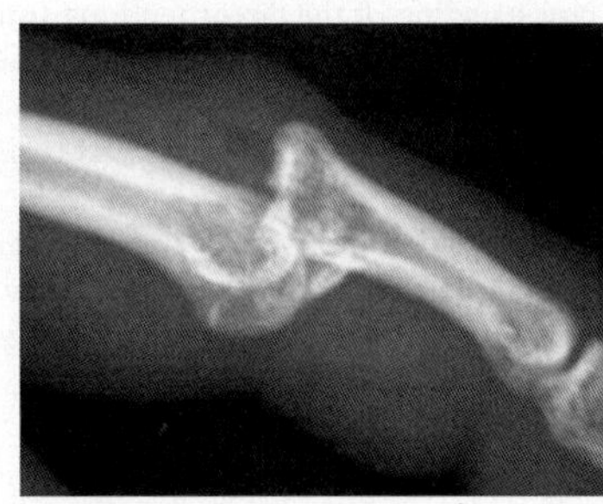

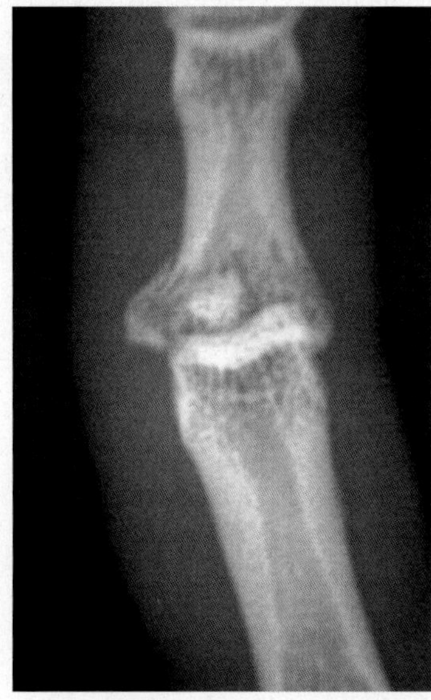

TECH FIG 6 • Cerclage wire technique with K-wire supplementation. **A,B.** Preoperative lateral and AP injury radiographs demonstrating a dorsal fracture-dislocation with central and volar articular depression and comminution. *(continued)*

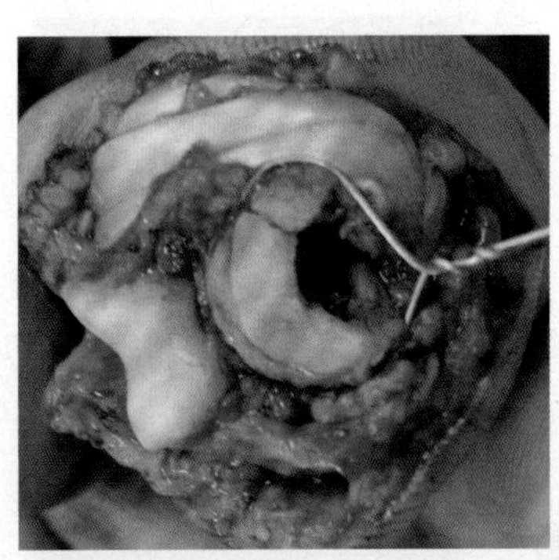
C

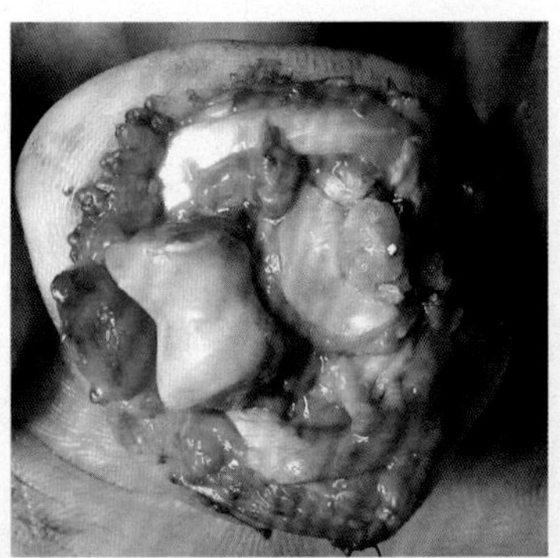
D

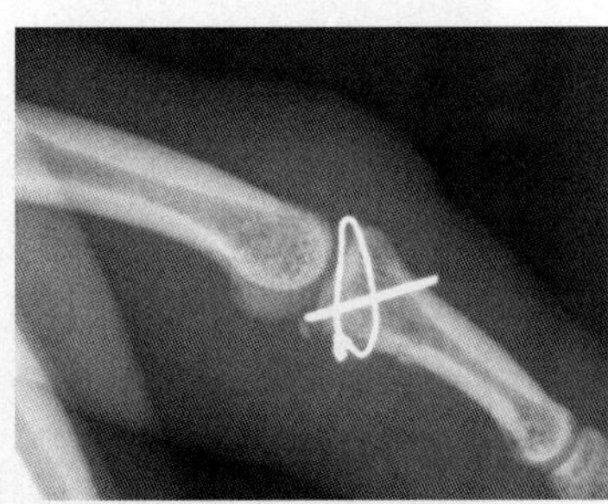
E

TECH FIG 6 • *(continued)* **C.** The cerclage wire is twisted loosely to around the base of the middle phalanx, maintaining the position of the articular fragments before reduction of the central and volar depressed fragment. **D.** After reduction of the central fragment and further fixation with a K-wire, the cerclage wire is tightened. The "tail" is then turned 90 degrees so that it is flush with the bone and cut. **E.** A postoperative lateral radiograph demonstrates restoration of the articular surface and reduction of the dislocation.

Closure and Splinting

- The volar plate or central slip flaps are closed with a 4-0 nonabsorbable suture.
- The flexor tendon sheath is closed using either absorbable or nonabsorbable 5-0 or 6-0 suture.
- The tourniquet is deflated, and hemostasis is achieved with bipolar cautery.
- The skin is closed with 5-0 nylon suture.
- The patient is placed into an intrinsic-plus volar splint. Usually, the MCP joints are flexed 70 to 90 degrees, and the IP joints are extended based on the stability of fixation and joint reduction.

PEARLS AND PITFALLS

- PIP fracture-dislocations often are missed by athletic trainers and patients, dismissed as a jammed finger.[11,18,32,34]
- Avoid forceful passive testing for stability, which can convert a partial tear to a complete one. Instability of any of these structures to passive stress is unlikely to change the management of an injury that is stable with active ROM. The one potential exception to this is complete rupture of the radial collateral ligament of the index finger PIP joint in a young active patient. This injury may be surgically repaired primarily because stability at this joint (required for a normal pinch grip) may be more important than full ROM.[13]
- Make sure to preserve the A2 and A4 pulleys. Failure to do so will result in bowstringing of the flexor tendons and a compromised outcome.
- Screw fixation should not be attempted for fracture fragments that are too small or too comminuted (eg, more than three fragments).
- Make sure to angle the K-wire or screw toward the distal dorsal cortex to maximize screw length and purchase.
- Fracture fragments are delicate. Take your time and select the correct starting location and track of the screws and K-wires. Multiple passes will result in poor fixation and further fracture fragmentation.
- After screw or K-wire insertion, check a lateral radiograph to ensure that the implant does not violate the extensor mechanism.
- To avoid recurrent dislocation, any bony defect remaining behind the repaired volar plate complex should be filled with bone graft. Otherwise, the head of the proximal phalanx will fall into the defect, resulting in recurrent dorsal subluxation of the middle phalanx.

POSTOPERATIVE CARE

- Progressive active and active-assisted ROM begins on postoperative day 2 or 5, depending on initial patient comfort.
  - A thermoplastic splint provides protected mobilization.
  - Relatively, more aggressive flexion than extension (<30 degrees) is pursued with the therapist.
- Close clinical and radiographic follow-up for the first few weeks is necessary to monitor for any loss of reduction.
- All restrictions on motion are removed at 5 to 6 weeks, and radiographic signs of healing are followed.
- Therapy is continued for 1 to 2 months after removal of the splint, initially to recover motion and subsequently to strengthen the hand.

OUTCOMES

- Green et al[13] reported on two patients with dorsal fracture-dislocations who underwent ORIF and reported an average active ROM of 95 degrees at 1-year follow-up, with neither patient demonstrating any evidence of subluxation.[17]
- Hastings and Carroll[15] reported on 15 patients treated with ORIF using various combinations of K-wire fixation, tension

band wire fixation, and screw fixation. Eventual average postoperative ROM was 17 to 90 degrees.

- Grant et al[12] noted on 14 patients that the average total active ROM of the PIP was 100 degrees (65 to 115 range), whereas Cheah et al[5] on 13 patients noted an average PIP motion of 75 degrees after internal mini-screw or mini-plate fixation of fracture fragments.
- Deitch et al[6] reported on 24 patients with unstable dorsal fracture-dislocations of the PIP joint treated with two methods, volar plate arthroplasty and ORIF. At an average follow-up of 46 months, results indicated that if reduction of the joint is maintained, patients could expect few functional deficits despite radiographic degenerative changes and loss of mobility.
- Weiss[30] reported on 12 patients with dorsal fracture-dislocations treated with cerclage wire fixation and reported an average ROM of 89 degrees at 2 years follow-up, with no complications and only 1 patient with evidence of radiographic degenerative changes.
- Stern et al[27] reported on 20 patients with pilon fracture-dislocations of the PIP joint. They used three treatment methods: splinting, skeletal traction, and open reduction with K-wire fixation. After a clinical and radiographic follow-up of 25 months, skeletal traction led to fewer complications and clinically comparable outcomes to open reduction (achieving an average ROM of 80 degrees vs. 70 degrees, respectively).
- Although clinical experience supports anatomic reduction of intra-articular fractures in weight-bearing joints such as the hip or knee, most laboratory and clinical reports support the theory that anatomic surface restoration is unnecessary if subluxation is corrected and motion is instituted shortly after injury.[1,14,23,25]

COMPLICATIONS

- Degenerative arthritis
- Loss of PIP joint motion, stiffness, flexion contracture, and extensor lag
- Loss of fixation or redisplacement
- Persistent subluxation or dislocation
- Infection
- Malunion
- Boutonnière deformity
- Pain

REFERENCES

1. Agee JM. Unstable fracture dislocations of the proximal interphalangeal joint. Treatment with the force couple splint. Clin Orthop Relat Res 1987;(214):101–112.
2. Blazar PE, Steinberg DR. Fractures of the proximal interphalangeal joint. J Am Acad Orthop Surg 2000;8:383–890.
3. Bruner JM. Surgical exposure of flexor tendons in the hand. Ann R Coll Surg Engl 1973;53:84–94.
4. Chamay A. A distally based dorsal and triangular tendinous flap for direct access to the proximal interphalangeal joint [in French]. Ann Chir Main 1988;7:179–183.
5. Cheah AE, Tan DM, Chong AK, et al. Volar plating for unstable proximal interphalangeal joint dorsal fracture-dislocations. J Hand Surg Am 2012;37:28–33.
6. Deitch MA, Kiefhaber TR, Comisar BR, et al. Dorsal fracture dislocations of the proximal interphalangeal joint: surgical complications and long-term results. J Hand Surg Am 1999;24:914–923.
7. Eaton RG, Malerich MM. Volar plate arthroplasty of the proximal interphalangeal joint: a review of ten years' experience. J Hand Surg Am 1980;5:260–268.
8. Elfar J, Mann T. Fracture-dislocations of the proximal interphalangeal joint. J Am Acad Orthop Surg 2013;21:88–98.
9. Elson RA. Rupture of the central slip of the extensor hood of the finger. A test for early diagnosis. J Bone Joint Surg Br 1986;68:229–231.
10. Freeland AE, Benoist LA. Open reduction and internal fixation method for fractures at the proximal interphalangeal joint. Hand Clin 1994;10:239–250.
11. Glickel SZ, Barron OA. Proximal interphalangeal joint fracture dislocations. Hand Clin 2000;16:333–344.
12. Grant I, Berger AC, Tham SK. Internal fixation of unstable fracture dislocations of the proximal interphalangeal joint. J Hand Surg Br 2005;30:492–498.
13. Green A, Smith J, Redding M, et al. Acute open reduction and rigid internal fixation of proximal interphalangeal joint fracture dislocation. J Hand Surg Am 1992;17:512–517.
14. Hamilton SC, Stern PJ, Fassler PR, et al. Mini-screw fixation for the treatment of proximal interphalangeal joint dorsal fracture-dislocations. J Hand Surg Am 2006;31:1349–1354.
15. Hastings H II, Carroll C IV. Treatment of closed articular fractures of the metacarpophalangeal and proximal interphalangeal joints. Hand Clin 1988;4:503–527.
16. Hastings H II, Ernst JM. Dynamic external fixation for fractures of the proximal interphalangeal joint. Hand Clin 1993;9:659–674.
17. Kiefhaber TR, Stern PJ. Fracture dislocations of the proximal interphalangeal joint. J Hand Surg Am 1998;23:368–380.
18. Kiefhaber TR, Stern PJ, Grood ES. Lateral stability of the proximal interphalangeal joint. J Hand Surg Am 1986;11:661–669.
19. Leibovic SJ, Bowers WH. Anatomy of the proximal interphalangeal joint. Hand Clin 1994;10:169–178.
20. Light TR. Buttress pinning techniques. Orthop Rev 1981;10:49–55.
21. Malerich MM, Eaton RG. The volar plate reconstruction for fracture-dislocation of the proximal interphalangeal joint. Hand Clin 1994;10:251–260.
22. McCue FC, Honner R, Johnson MC, et al. Athletic injuries of the proximal interphalangeal joint requiring surgical treatment. J Bone Joint Surg Am 1970;52:937–956.
23. Morgan JP, Gordon DA, Klug MS, et al. Dynamic digital traction for unstable comminuted intra-articular fracture-dislocations of the proximal interphalangeal joint. J Hand Surg Am 1995;20:565–573.
24. Phair IC, Quinton DN, Allen MJ. The conservative management of volar avulsion fractures of the P.I.P. joint. J Hand Surg Br 1989;14:168–170.
25. Salter RB. The physiologic basis of continuous passive motion for articular cartilage healing and regeneration. Hand Clin 1994;10:211–219.
26. Schenck RR. Dynamic traction and early passive movement for fractures of the proximal interphalangeal joint. J Hand Surg Am 1986;11:850–858.
27. Stern PJ, Roman RJ, Kiefhaber TR, et al. Pilon fractures of the proximal interphalangeal joint. J Hand Surg Am 1991;16:844–850.
28. Tan JS, Foo AT, Chew WC, et al. Articularly placed interfragmentary screw fixation of difficult condylar fractures of the hand. J Hand Surg Am 2011;36:604–609.
29. Tyser AR, Tsai MA, Parks BG, et al. Stability of acute dorsal fracture dislocations of the proximal interphalangeal joint: a biomechanical study. J Hand Surg Am 2014;39(1):13–8.
30. Weiss AP. Cerclage fixation for fracture dislocation of the proximal interphalangeal joint. Clin Orthop Relat Res 1996;(327):21–28.
31. Weiss AP, Hastings H II. Distal unicondylar fractures of the proximal phalanx. J Hand Surg Am 1993;18:594–599.
32. Williams CS IV. Proximal interphalangeal joint fracture dislocations: stable and unstable. Hand Clin 2012;28:409–416.
33. Williams RM, Kiefhaber TR, Sommerkamp TG, et al. Treatment of unstable dorsal proximal interphalangeal fracture/dislocations using a hemi-hamate autograft. J Hand Surg Am 2003;28:856–865.
34. Wolfe SW, Katz LD. Intra-articular impaction fractures of the phalanges. J Hand Surg Am 1995;20:327–333.

54 CHAPTER

Volar Plate Arthroplasty

Beverlie L. Ting and Philip E. Blazar

DEFINITION

- Volar plate arthroplasty (VPA) is used in the treatment of both acute and chronic dorsal fracture-dislocations of the proximal interphalangeal (PIP) or distal interphalangeal (DIP) joint.[8]
- In VPA, local tissue (volar plate) is advanced to recreate a volar restraint to dorsal subluxation/dislocation and maintain concentric reduction of the PIP or DIP joint.
- VPA has also been used to treat osteoarthritis, as advanced volar plate tissue resurfaces part of the degenerative volar portion of the joint.[3]

ANATOMY

- The volar plate is a fibrocartilaginous structure that lies palmar to both the PIP and DIP joints and is the primary restraint to hyperextension and dorsal subluxation/dislocation of these joints.[2,7,9]
  - Proximally, the volar plate of the PIP joint is "swallowtail" shaped with two thickened lateral checkrein ligaments that attach to the volar periosteum of the proximal phalanx and the flexor tendon sheath (**FIG 1A**). A nutrient artery supplying the PIP joint emerges from the hiatus formed between the two checkrein ligaments.
  - Distally, the volar plate inserts centrally onto the volar periosteum and converges laterally with the collateral ligaments to form more robust attachments (**FIG 1B**).
  - The volar plate glides proximally and distally with joint motion.
- The collateral ligaments originate dorsal to the interphalangeal joints and pass obliquely and volarly to their distal insertions: The proper collateral ligaments insert on the volar third of the base of the phalanx, whereas the accessory collateral ligaments insert on the lateral margin of the volar plate (see **FIG 1B**).
  - In subacute or chronic cases of dorsal joint subluxation or dislocation, these ligaments contract, thereby accentuating the deformity by virtue of their oblique orientation.
- The flexor digitorum superficialis (FDS) inserts just distal to the volar plate on the middle phalanx, which flexes the middle phalanx while the central slip dorsally subluxates the middle phalanx when volar restraints are lost.

PATHOGENESIS

- Dorsal fracture-dislocations of the PIP and DIP are caused by hypertension or axial compression mechanisms. With hyperextension, rupture or avulsion-type injuries of the volar base of the middle phalanx occurs, whereas axial compression results in impaction or comminuted fracture patterns.
- Dorsal fracture-dislocations of the PIP occur when an axial load drives the partially flexed middle phalanx into the head of the proximal phalanx, shearing the volar articular surface of the base of the middle phalanx.
- Late presentation with chronic subluxation or dislocation (>6 weeks) is common, as these injuries are often misperceived as minor "sprains."

NATURAL HISTORY

- Chronic subluxation of the PIP joint leads to poor function and degenerative arthritis.
  - Flexion of the joint is limited and painful.

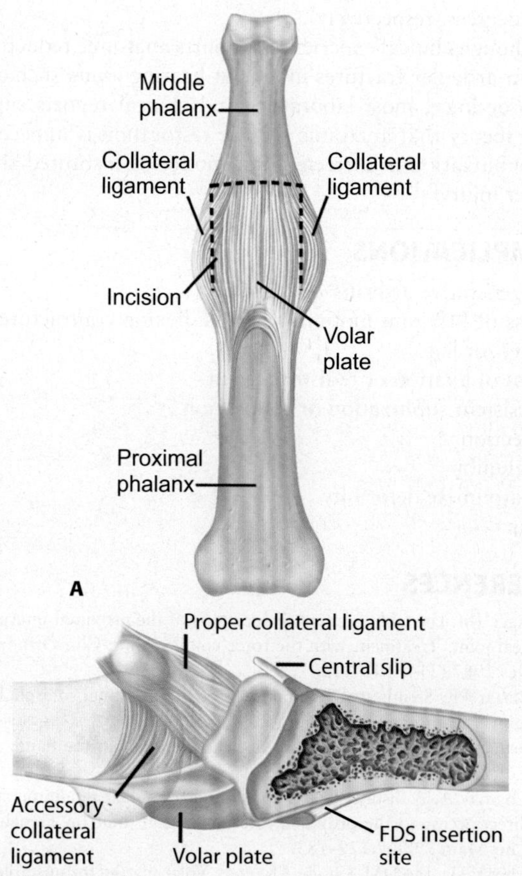

FIG 1 • A. Volar view of the PIP joint. The PIP joint is supported by ligamentous structures that include the collateral ligaments on each side, with the volar plate and flexor tendons underneath. **B.** Sagittal view of the PIP joint showing the relative positions of the central slip, volar plate, collateral ligaments, and accessory collateral ligaments.

- Despite optimal surgical treatment, PIP joint fracture-dislocations often result in some loss of PIP and/or DIP joint motion.
- PIP joint injuries, even those that do not require surgical treatment, commonly result in a protracted period of symptoms (eg, swelling, stiffness, pain) beyond what patients expect from a "minor" injury.

PATIENT HISTORY AND PHYSICAL FINDINGS

- When taking the patient's history, ask about the mechanism of injury, time since injury, any prior injuries, and the direction of deformity. Time since injury and mechanism of injury help determine the most appropriate treatment.
- Inspect the finger for any swelling or deformity. Clinical deformity may be subtle, even with significant subluxation.
- Examine range of motion, noting degrees of PIP motion. With joint subluxation, patients will have painful and limited flexion.
- Examine joint stability; joints that are unstable will need intervention to restore stability (eg, extension block splinting, VPA).

IMAGING AND OTHER DIAGNOSTIC STUDIES

- Every patient with a PIP injury must have anteroposterior, lateral, and oblique radiographs to evaluate for a PIP joint fracture or subluxation (**FIG 2A**).
  - The severity of the fracture and degree of involvement of the middle phalanx often are much greater than they appear on these radiographs.
- In evaluating for a subluxation by radiographs, a true lateral view of the PIP joint is mandatory. A dorsal V sign at the joint indicates that the articular surfaces are neither congruent nor parallel (**FIG 2B**).
  - A lateral view is used to evaluate the percentage of articular surface involved.
  - Lateral views in both flexion and extension can be useful to detect hinging on the fracture margin, which can appear as normal motion on clinical examination.[9]
- Fluoroscopy allows dynamic evaluation of the joint and its stability and often is also the best way to obtain magnified images and a perfect lateral view.
- Computed tomography (CT) scans rarely are needed but can effectively evaluate the articular surfaces and define the bone loss.

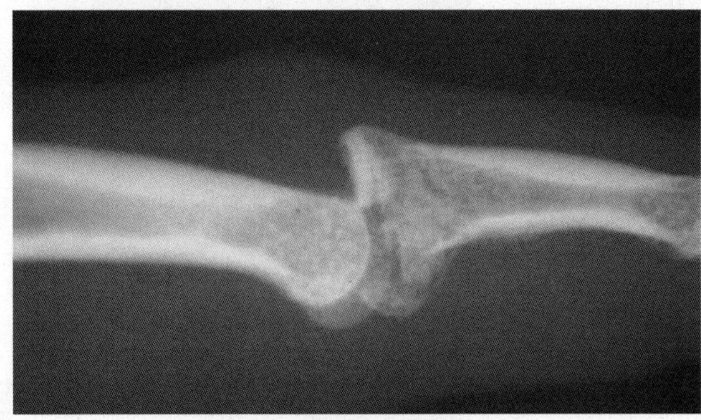

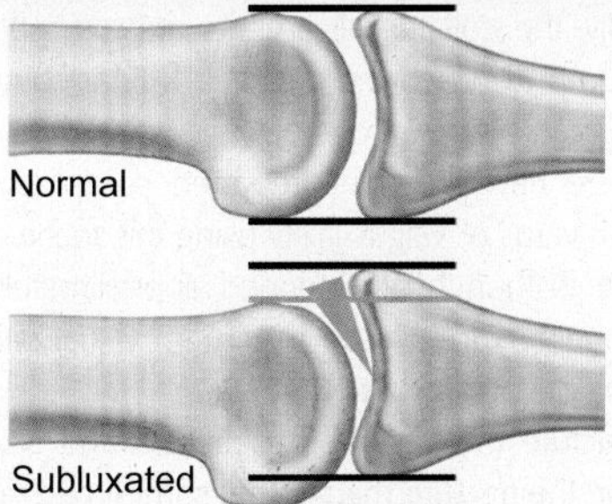

FIG 2 • **A.** Lateral radiograph of subluxation of the PIP joint. **B.** PIP joint subluxations typically display a signature dorsal V sign on the lateral radiograph, as described by Light[11] (as depicted by the shaded triangle).

DIFFERENTIAL DIAGNOSIS

- Acute central slip injury (ie, boutonnière deformity)
- PIP joint fracture
- PIP dislocation
- Volar plate or collateral ligament sprain without instability

NONOPERATIVE MANAGEMENT

- Closed reduction and extension block splinting are appropriate for PIP fracture-subluxations when a stable concentric joint reduction is maintained without evidence of hinging.
  - If more than 60 degrees of flexion is required to maintain reduction, surgical reconstruction should be strongly considered.
- Articular defects will often dramatically remodel in a concentrically reduced, mobilized joint.

SURGICAL MANAGEMENT

- For simplicity, the techniques here describe VPA for the PIP joint, but the same principles may apply to the DIP joint. The primary difference is that the flexor digitorum profundus (FDP) insertion on the volar base of the distal phalanx makes exposure of the volar plate more complicated.
- Indications
  - Acute fracture-dislocations that are unstable after closed reduction of the PIP joint in cases in which the volar base of the middle phalanx is not reconstructable or if surgical reconstruction is less likely to achieve a functional result.
  - Chronic subluxations or dislocations up to 2 years following trauma
  - A normal articular contour of the proximal phalanx is a prerequisite.
  - An intact dorsal cortex and dorsal articular surface are required.
  - Some authors used VPA for chronic osteoarthritis in select situations.[3]

Preoperative Planning

- Fractures typically involve over 30% of the surface of the middle phalanx base, and the joint is subluxated or dislocated. If the fracture involves under 30% of the joint surface, it typically can be managed either in a closed manner or with less invasive techniques for the acute scenario.[1,4,9]

- The literature is unclear whether a specific degree of involvement of the articular surface precludes VPA (ie, is too large), but involvement of the dorsal cortex is a contraindication.
  - VPA for injuries involving over 50% of the middle phalanx articular surface results in a higher likelihood of recurrent subluxation.[5]
- In chronic dislocations, soft tissue contracture and heterotopic bone may make dissection and relocation more complex.

Positioning

- The patient is positioned supine on the operating table with the affected arm on a hand table.
- Intraoperative fluoroscopy is critical to this procedure, and it is important to position the hand relative to the fluoroscopy unit so that a true lateral view of the injured PIP joint may easily be obtained.
- The surgery is performed under tourniquet control.

TECHNIQUES

Primary Incisions and Excisions on the Volar Side

- The joint is exposed using two limbs of a Bruner incision centered at the PIP flexion crease, elevating a radially based flap (**TECH FIG 1A**).
- The radial and ulnar neurovascular bundles are identified and mobilized throughout the field to prevent a traction injury when the PIP joint is hyperextended to achieve optimal visualization (**TECH FIG 1B**).
- The flexor sheath is incised as a rectangular flap between the A2 and A4 pulleys and protected for later repair.
- The flexor tendons are atraumatically retracted radially or ulnarly, as needed to visualize the volar plate (**TECH FIG 1C,D**). Use of blunt retractors or a 1/4-inch Penrose drain can be helpful.

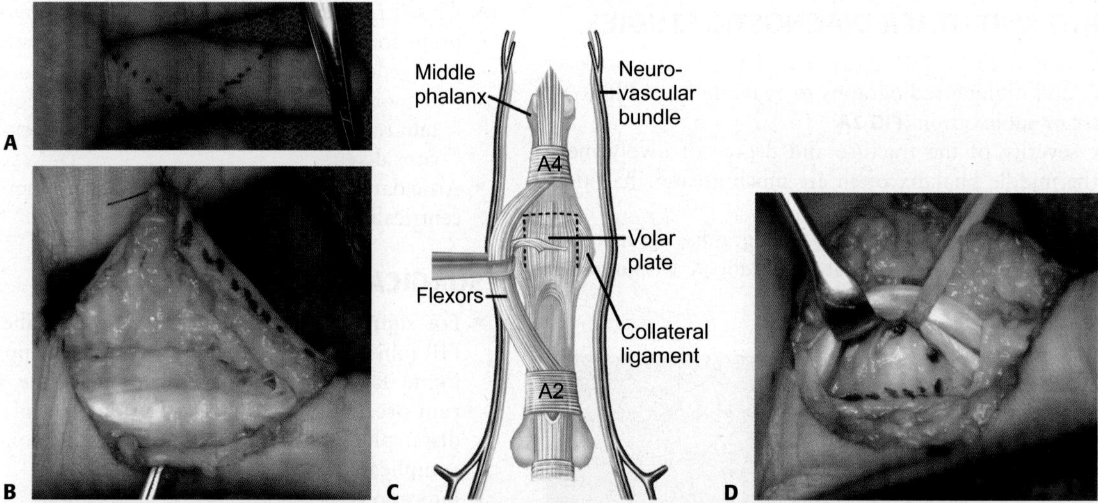

TECH FIG 1 • **A.** The Bruner incision is centered over the PIP flexion crease, with the vertex on the ulnar side. **B.** To prevent traction injuries, mobilization of the neurovascular bundles is necessary. **C.** Illustration of retraction of the flexor tendons and neurovascular bundles relative to the volar plate. **D.** The flexor tendons must be retracted radially and ulnarly to access the volar plate. The proposed incision to detach and mobilize the volar plate is outlined in pen.

Detachment and Preparation of the Volar Plate

- The volar plate is detached from the middle phalanx along with any attached fracture fragments.
- The volar plate is incised from the proper and accessory collateral ligaments through an incision along its radial and ulnar most margins (**TECH FIG 1D**).
  - Care must be taken to preserve length and width of the volar plate flap to maximize the stability of the arthroplasty and minimize flexion contracture.
  - The flap should be symmetric in the coronal plane to avoid angular deformity.
- Classically, the collateral ligaments are excised, leaving only a distal stump to which the radial and ulnar corners of the volar plate flap can be secured.[6,8]
  - There have been no reported complications associated with varus or valgus laxity using this technique.
- The joint is then hyperextended approximately 180 degrees ("shotgunning") to achieve maximum visualization of the base of the middle phalanx (**TECH FIG 2**).
- Small fracture fragments are débrided and saved to fill bony defects at the fracture margin that sometimes result in hinging.[5]
- Care is taken to avoid overresection and loss of the dorsal articular support.

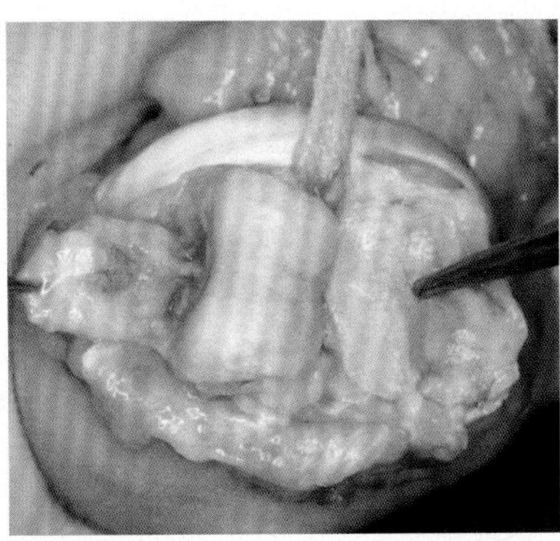

TECH FIG 2 • Shotgunning. Hyperextending the joint allows clear visualization of the volar plate to the *left*, the avulsed bone, and the articular surface of each phalanx. The trough is fashioned symmetrically in the coronal plane, at the dorsal most aspect of the articular defect to the *right* as shown by the forceps.

Shaping the Articular Surface of the Middle Phalanx

- A transverse trough is fashioned with an osteotome or a rongeur across the middle phalanx and finished with a small curette, at the junction between the intact articular surface and the fracture defect (see **TECH FIG 2**).
- This trough must be symmetric in the coronal plane to avoid angular deformity. The depth of the trough at its dorsal side should be the thickness of the volar plate, thereby allowing a smooth transition from articular cartilage to transposed volar plate.

Transposing the Volar Plate

- Two 3-0 nonabsorbable grasping sutures (eg, Bunnell fashion) are placed along both the ulnar and radial most margins of the volar plate flap (**TECH FIG 3A**).
- Two straight Keith needles are passed through each side of the base of the middle phalanx using a wire driver. They are placed as far radially (or ulnarly) and distally in the bone defect as possible and directed centrally to penetrate the cortex distal to the central slip insertion (**TECH FIG 3B**).
  - The sutures are tensioned as the middle phalanx is flexed, bringing the volar plate into the defect at a level that produces a smooth transition from the intact dorsal base of the middle phalanx to the volar plate.
- Examine the reduction with a true lateral fluoroscopic view on a mini C-arm (**TECH FIG 3C**).
  - The base of the middle phalanx should glide over the head of the proximal phalanx and should not hinge open dorsally.
  - The fingertip should be able to touch the distal palmar crease (110 degrees of flexion).
- If the PIP joint lacks substantial extension or has inadequate flexion, it may be necessary to advance the volar plate distally by teasing the checkrein ligaments from their origin or by fractional lengthening through step cutting (see **TECH FIG 3A**).

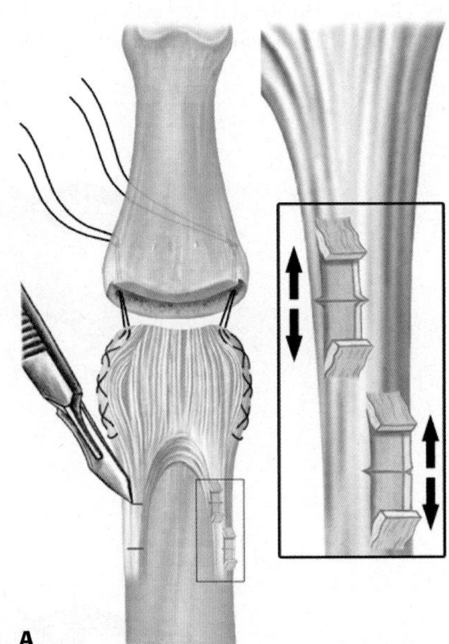

TECH FIG 3 • **A.** Suturing the volar plate. Sutures are passed through the margins of the volar plate and through the base of the middle phalanx using straight Keith needles. The volar plate is advanced into the trough, resurfacing the PIP joint. It may be necessary to advance the volar plate by step cut lengthening of the checkrein ligaments. *(continued)*

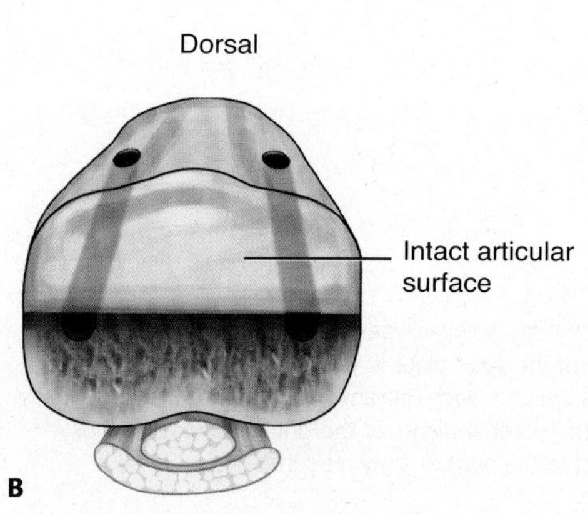

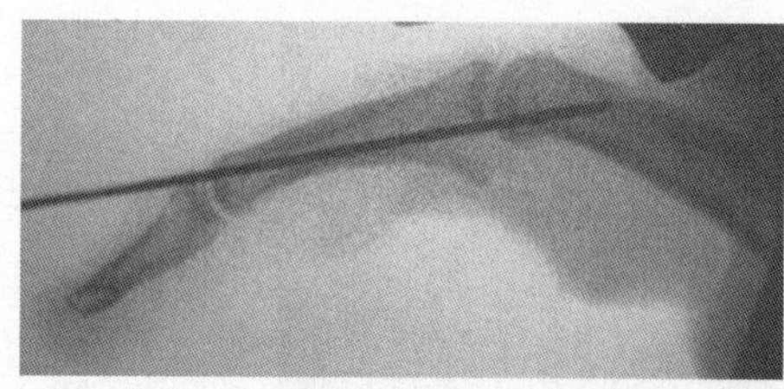

TECH FIG 3 • *(continued)* **B.** This diagram shows the needle holes in relation to the transverse bone trough created at the volar base of the middle phalanx. The holes should be placed as far dorsal and lateral as possible in the prepared bone trough for maximum stability. **C.** The PIP joint has now been reduced and stabilized as shown.

Securing the Volar Plate

- The sutures may be tied over a button dorsally.
  - Alternatively, the sutures may be tied directly onto periosteum via a small incision distal to the central slip insertion, which avoids the risk of skin necrosis. Care must be taken to ensure the sutures do not entrap the lateral bands or injure the central slip.
  - More recently, a study demonstrated acceptable short-term results using a suture anchor inserted at a 45-degree angle along with 4-0 nonabsorbable, braided polyester suture in a Kessler fashion to secure the volar plate.[10]
- Additional lateral stability can be achieved by suturing the volar plate to the distal stumps of the collateral ligaments with 4-0 braided, nonabsorbable suture, although this is not routinely performed.
- In the acute setting, fractured bone fragments collected during the volar plate detachment may be placed in the defect of the middle phalanx, distal to the advanced volar plate. This provides support to the base of the phalanx.
  - A slip of FDS can also be used to restore the palmar buttress and add to volar stability via dynamic tenodesis.[5]
- A Kirschner wire (K-wire) is used with the joint in slight flexion (10 to 15 degrees) to maintain reduction for 3 weeks (**TECH FIG 4**).
  - Alternatively, the joint reduction can be maintained with an articulated external fixator to allow for early motion.

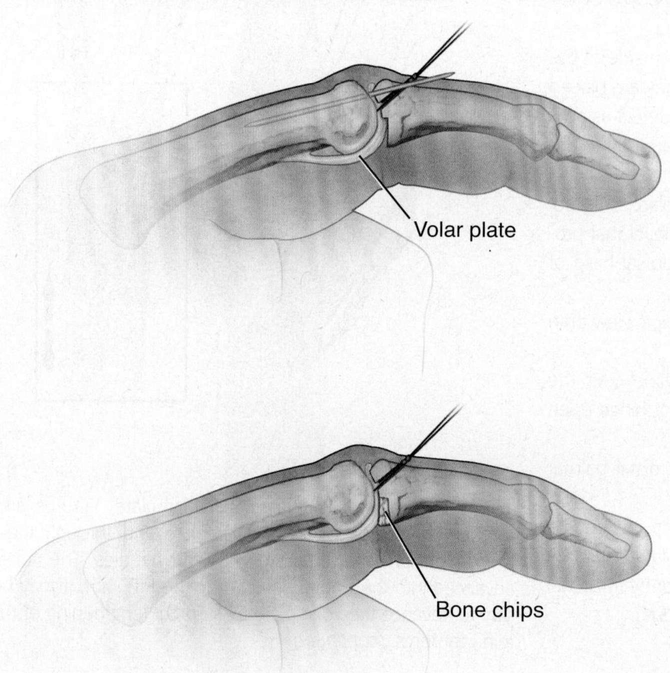

TECH FIG 4 • Lateral diagram of VPA. The overall diagram of this procedure illustrates the joint with a double-ended K-wire for stability and the volar plate secured by sutures.

PEARLS AND PITFALLS

Angular deformity	▪ The trough must be transverse, and tension of the volar plate flap must be symmetric in the coronal plane.
Recurrent subluxation	▪ Fixation with a K-wire or articulated fixator for 2–3 weeks is recommended.
Loss of flexion	▪ Aggressive range of motion to restore flexion at both the PIP and DIP joints is essential and safe because these injuries typically are more stable in flexion.
Neurologic injury	▪ Meticulous dissection of both neurovascular bundles is required before shotgunning the joint open.
Loss of extension	▪ Some loss of extension is expected. Failure to lengthen the checkrein ligaments may lead to an unacceptable contracture.

POSTOPERATIVE CARE

- The K-wire is removed at 2 to 3 weeks, when active flexion and extension are begun.
- An extension block splint is used during weeks 3 to 6 after the operation.
- Motion of the DIP is encouraged before K-wire removal, as deficits in DIP motion have been reported after VPA.
- After 6 weeks, the pullout suture, if one was used, is removed.
- A dynamic extension splint may be used at 6 weeks if the achieved extension is not as expected based on intraoperative range of motion.

OUTCOMES

- Long-term studies have demonstrated that more PIP motion is restored in acute injuries than in chronic injuries: 85 degrees of active PIP motion versus 60 degrees.[6]
- Patients can expect to see continued improvement in range of motion up to 1 year after VPA.
- Mild contractures of the DIP joint (10 to 20 degrees) are common. Patients are encouraged in DIP motion during rehabilitation.

COMPLICATIONS

- Resubluxation or dislocation
- Flexion contracture of the PIP or DIP joint
- Angular deformities
- Pin and wire tract infections
- Pain
- Stiffness
- Degenerative arthrosis

REFERENCES

1. Blazar PE, Robbe R, Lawton JN. Treatment of dorsal fracture/dislocations of the proximal interphalangeal joint by volar plate arthroplasty. Tech Hand Up Extrem Surg 2001;5(3):148–152.
2. Bowers WH, Wolf JW Jr, Nehil JL, et al. The proximal interphalangeal joint volar plate. I. An anatomical and biomechanical study. J Hand Surg Am 1980;5(1):79–88.
3. Burton RI, Campolattaro RM, Ronchetti PJ. Volar plate arthroplasty for osteoarthritis of the proximal interphalangeal joint: a preliminary report. J Hand Surg Am 2002;27(6):1065–1072.
4. Calfee RP, Sommerkamp TG. Fracture-dislocation about the finger joints. J Hand Surg Am 2009;34(6):1140–1147.
5. Deitch MA, Kiefhaber TR, Comisar BR, et al. Dorsal fracture dislocations of the proximal interphalangeal joint: surgical complications and long-term results. J Hand Surg Am 1999;24(5):914–923.
6. Dionysian E, Eaton RG. The long-term outcome of volar plate arthroplasty of the proximal interphalangeal joint. J Hand Surg Am 2000;25(3):429–437.
7. Durham-Smith G, McCarten GM. Volar plate arthroplasty for closed proximal interphalangeal joint injuries. J Hand Surg Br 1992;17(4):422–428.
8. Eaton RG, Malerich MM. Volar plate arthroplasty of the proximal interphalangeal joint: a review of ten years' experience. J Hand Surg Am 1980;5(3):260–268.
9. Elfar J, Mann T. Fracture-dislocations of the proximal interphalangeal joint. J Am Acad Orthop Surg 2013;21(2):88–98.
10. Lee LS, Lee HM, Hou YT, et al. Surgical outcome of volar plate arthroplasty of the proximal interphalangeal joint using the Mitek micro GII suture anchor. J Trauma 2008;65(1):116–122.
11. Light TR. Buttress pinning techniques. Orthop Rev 1981;10:49–55.

Hemi-Hamate Autograft Reconstruction of Unstable Dorsal Proximal Interphalangeal Joint Fracture-Dislocations

Thomas R. Kiefhaber, Rafael M. M. Williams, and Meredith N. Osterman

DEFINITION

- Proximal interphalangeal (PIP) joint fracture-dislocations occur with the following fracture patterns[11]:
  - Palmar lip fracture-dislocations: fracture of the middle phalanx palmar lip with dorsal subluxation of the middle phalanx on the head of the proximal phalanx
  - Dorsal lip fracture-dislocations: fracture of the dorsal lip of the middle phalanx with palmar subluxation of the middle phalanx
  - Pilon fractures: Pilon fractures include a loss of continuity of both the dorsal and palmar cortical margins of the middle phalangeal articular surface. The base of the middle phalanx usually is highly comminuted, and the articular fragments may be significantly impacted.
- PIP fractures are further classified as "stable" or "unstable."
  - Stable fractures maintain concentric joint reduction throughout the range of motion (ROM).
  - Unstable fractures sublux or dislocate during parts of the motion arc.
- Dorsal lip fracture treatment is complicated by the need to reestablish continuity of the extensor tendon insertion onto the middle phalanx.
- Pilon fractures are best treated with some form of traction and early motion.
- Unstable palmar lip fractures are amenable to treatment with hemi-hamate autograft and are the focus of this chapter.

ANATOMY

- The PIP joint is a complex hinge articulation that provides more than 95 degrees of flexion while maintaining stable, concentric reduction of the joint surfaces.
- Several forces encourage dorsal migration of the middle phalanx: The extensor tendon lifts the middle phalanx and the mid-middle phalanx superficialis insertion levers the middle phalanx dorsally[7] (**FIG 1A**).
- The only restraints on middle phalangeal dorsal translation are the palmar plate and the cup-shaped geometry of the middle phalanx articular surface. The middle phalangeal palmar lip wraps around the proximal phalanx head and acts as a hook, preventing dorsal translation.
- Palmar lip fractures disrupt both of the restraints to dorsal subluxation. The palmar plate is no longer attached, and the middle phalangeal palmar lip is disrupted. The slope of the remaining middle phalangeal articular surface encourages the middle phalanx to travel up and over the proximal phalangeal head.
- A direct relation exists between the amount of palmar articular surface disrupted and stability (**FIG 1B**).
  - Hastings and Hamlet[8] has shown that when 42% of the palmar articular surface is damaged, the joint always exhibits dorsal instability.
  - In the clinical setting, fractures with as little as 30% articular surface involvement can be unstable.
- Hemi-hamate arthroplasty restores stability by rebuilding the cup-shaped geometry of the middle phalangeal base and restoring the palmar plate attachment.

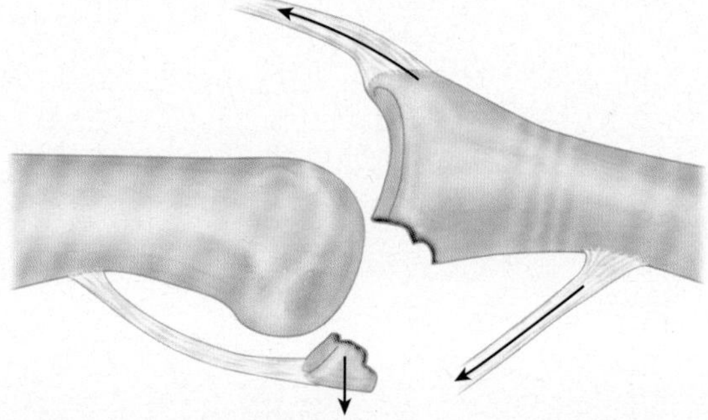

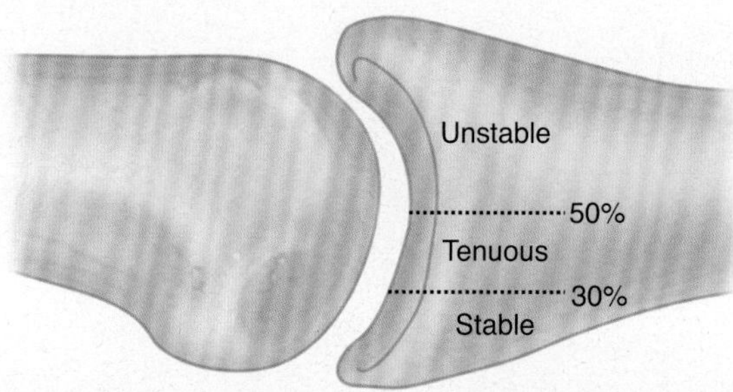

FIG 1 • **A.** Unstable PIP fracture-dislocation. The upward pull of the central tendon insertion and the distal superficialis insertion pull and push the middle phalanx up and over the proximal phalangeal head. The only forces preventing dorsal subluxation are the middle phalanx palmar lip and the palmar plate, both of which are lost in an unstable PIP palmar lip fracture. **B.** PIP instability after a fracture. A direct relation exists between the amount of middle phalanx palmar lip destroyed by the fracture and the resultant PIP joint stability. Articular damage in excess of 50% of the joint surface always renders the joint unstable, whereas fractures involving less than 30% usually are stable. Tenuous fractures (ie, those with articular damage of 30% to 50% of the joint surface) must be assessed with lateral radiographs. If the joint will not stay reduced with less than 30 degrees of flexion, it must be classified as "unstable."

PATHOGENESIS

- The middle phalangeal palmar lip fracture that is associated with unstable dorsal PIP fracture-dislocations is created by either avulsion of the fracture fragment or an impaction shear mechanism.
- Avulsion fractures result from PIP joint hyperextension and traction through the palmar plate attachment (**FIG 2A**).
  - The fracture fragment is not comminuted and represents less than 30% of the articular surface.
  - These injuries usually are stable and rarely require surgical intervention. If the joint is unstable, osteosynthesis with lag screws often is possible because of the lack of comminution and the substantial size of the fragment.
- Impaction shear PIP fracture-dislocations result from a longitudinally applied load to the tip of the finger with the PIP joint slightly flexed, such as in a mishandled ball catch. The force drives the middle phalanx into and over the proximal phalanx head, resulting in a middle phalangeal palmar lip fracture that is highly comminuted (**FIG 2B**).
  - Up to 80% of the joint surface can be involved, and the articular fragments are often deeply impacted into the soft metaphyseal bone.
- Disruption of the terminal extensor tendon (mallet finger) often occurs in association with unstable dorsal PIP fracture-dislocations.

NATURAL HISTORY

- The long-term prognosis for PIP fracture-dislocations is theoretically affected by the quality of the joint surface restoration and the maintenance of concentric reduction of the middle phalanx on the proximal phalangeal head.
  - The PIP joint seems to tolerate less than perfect restoration of a smooth joint surface. As long as motion is initiated quickly, small gaps and step-offs seem to be tolerated.

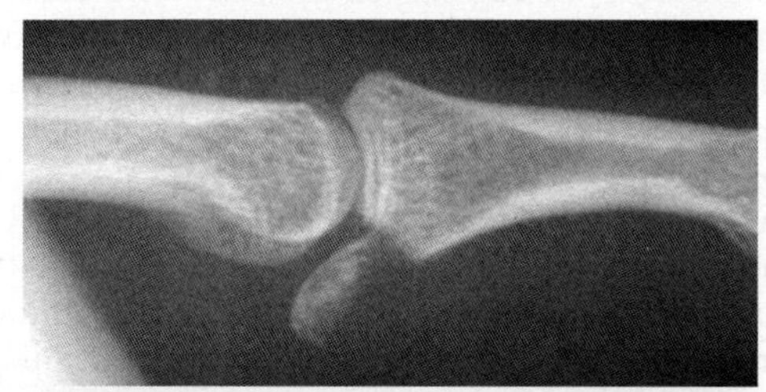

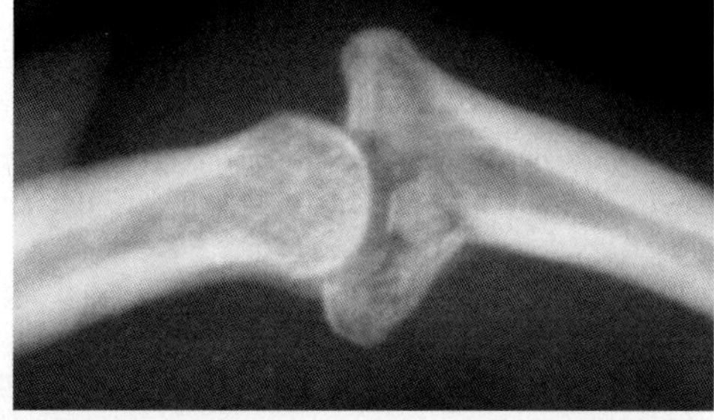

FIG 2 • Fracture types. **A.** Avulsion fracture. Avulsion fractures usually are caused by a forced PIP joint hyperextension. The fragment is not comminuted and involves less than 30% of the joint surface. The PIP joint is most often stable. **B.** Impaction shear fracture. This type of PIP fracture-dislocation is caused by a longitudinal load to the joint. The fracture fragments are comminuted and impacted into the middle phalanx. The joint reduction often is unstable.

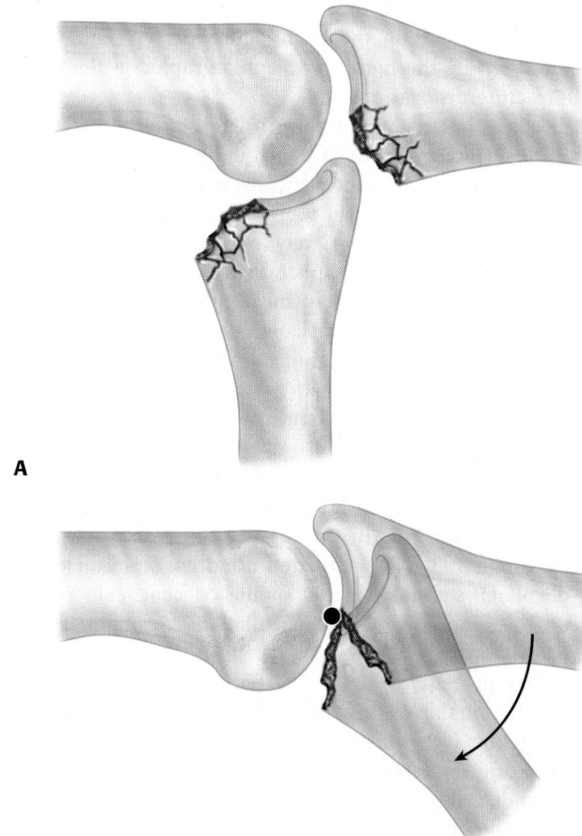

FIG 3 • Gliding or hinging. **A.** Normal PIP flexion occurs as the middle phalanx glides around the proximal phalanx head. **B.** When the middle phalanx palmar lip is lost, PIP flexion can occur by hinging at the fracture margin. Treatment of unstable PIP fracture-dislocations must rebuild the cup-shaped middle phalanx base and restore a normal gliding motion.

  Long term, some remodeling occurs, and most patients do not need to be treated for symptomatic posttraumatic degenerative arthritis.
  - Joint reduction that is less than perfect is not well tolerated. When the middle phalanx rides dorsally on the proximal phalangeal head, PIP flexion occurs by "hinging" at the fracture margin.[11] The joint pivots on the palmar edge of the fracture, and the proximal phalanx falls into the fracture defect at the palmar base of the middle phalanx. The proximal phalangeal articular cartilage suffers accelerated wear, whereas the remaining undamaged middle phalangeal articular surface remains unused throughout the motion arc (**FIG 3**).
- Treatment of unstable PIP palmar lip fractures is directed toward reestablishing joint stability so that flexion occurs by "gliding" of the remaining middle phalangeal articular cartilage on the head of the proximal phalanx.

PATIENT HISTORY AND PHYSICAL FINDINGS

- Assess alignment in the coronal plane. Lateral deviation suggests asymmetric compression of articular fragments.
- Assess alignment in the sagittal plane. Lack of colinearity of the middle and proximal phalanx suggests persistent joint subluxation or dislocation.
- Associated mallet injuries must be treated concurrently with a distal interphalangeal (DIP) joint extension splint.

IMAGING AND OTHER DIAGNOSTIC STUDIES

- Plain radiographs in the posteroanterior (PA) and lateral planes provide the mainstay of radiographic evaluation of PIP fracture-dislocations.
- Inspect the lateral radiograph to determine the percentage of joint surface fractured and the quality of the reduction.
  - If the joint is not concentrically reduced with less than 30 degrees of flexion, the joint is classified as unstable and must be treated appropriately (see **FIG 1B**).
- On every lateral radiograph taken throughout the treatment course, carefully scrutinize the quality of the reduction. The remaining articular cartilage on the middle phalanx base must be in full contact with the proximal phalanx head. Any dorsal gap between the two surfaces—a "V" sign—indicates persistent instability and must be corrected (**FIG 4**).
- The percentage of the middle phalanx articular surface consumed by the fracture can be used to predict joint reduction stability[7,8,11] (see **FIG 1B**):
  - Less than 30%: The reduction usually is stable. The middle phalanx almost always remains concentrically reduced on the head of the proximal phalanx throughout a full ROM.
  - Thirty percent to 50%: The reduction is tenuous. The middle phalanx may or may not subluxate dorsally when the PIP joint is extended. If any subluxation is noted on the lateral radiograph with the PIP joint fully extended, flex the joint to 30 degrees and repeat the lateral radiograph.
    - If concentric reduction is achieved and the palmar fragments are sitting where they will reconstitute a palmar lip, some form of extension block treatment may be employed.
    - If the joint will not stay reduced with less than 30 degrees of flexion, the joint is unstable and must be treated accordingly.
  - Over 50%: The PIP joint is unstable, and surgical intervention usually is required to rebuild the cup-shaped geometry of the middle phalanx base and to reattach the palmar plate.
- Inspect the PA view to determine asymmetric compression of middle phalanx articular fragments leading to varus or valgus angulation.
- Computed tomography (CT) or magnetic resonance imaging (MRI) evaluation rarely is necessary.

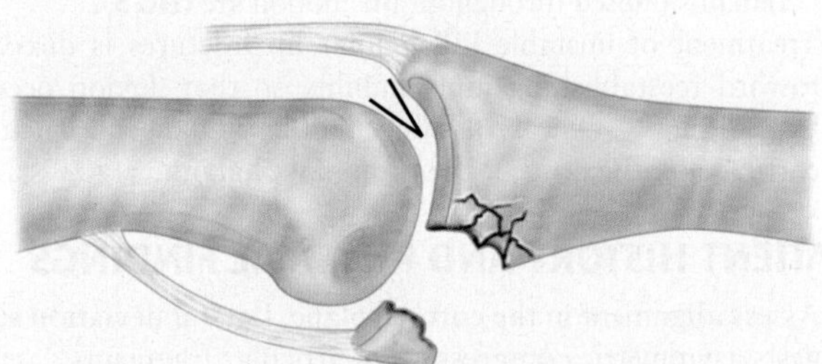

FIG 4 • Unstable PIP palmar lip fracture-dislocation. Extensive damage has occurred to the palmar lip of the middle phalanx, but the dorsal cortical margin and a small amount of dorsal articular cartilage remain intact. Even slight dorsal subluxation can be detected by looking for a V-shaped gap between the middle and proximal phalanges.

DIFFERENTIAL DIAGNOSIS

- In patients with a history of recent trauma and radiographic confirmation of a large PIP palmar lip fracture associated with dorsal subluxation, the diagnosis of an unstable PIP dorsal fracture-dislocation is obvious.
- Dorsal dislocation and disruption of the middle phalanx palmar lip also may be seen in chronic PIP fracture-dislocations and occasionally in association with various forms of arthritis.

NONOPERATIVE MANAGEMENT

- Unstable PIP fracture-dislocations rarely can be managed nonoperatively. When over 50% of the middle phalanx articular surface is consumed by fracture, all restraints to dorsal subluxation are lost. The cup-shaped geometry of the middle phalanx base must be restored and the palmar plate reattached. Both goals can be accomplished with osteosynthesis of a single large fragment,[4,5,10] palmar plate arthroplasty,[3] or a hemi-hamate osteochondral autograft.[6,17,18]
- Stable PIP fracture-dislocations are treated nonoperatively. If the joint does not hyperextend and the lateral radiograph in full extension confirms concentric reduction, buddy tape the fingers and allow early ROM. If the joint hyperextends, some flexion must be maintained for 3 weeks while the fracture fragments consolidate enough to restore functional palmar plate continuity. Apply a dorsal blocking splint that prevents PIP hyperextension but allows full active flexion.
- Nonoperative treatment of tenuous PIP fracture-dislocations requires careful thought, patient cooperation, and meticulous follow-up.
  - The primary treatment goal is to maintain joint reduction while the middle phalanx palmar fragments consolidate and restore the cup-shaped geometry of the middle phalanx base. Joint reduction must be achievable with less than 30 degrees of flexion, and the palmar fragments must fall into a position that will restore the middle phalanx palmar lip.
  - A secondary goal is to provide immediate active ROM. Any treatment method that prevents extension past 30 degrees and allows full flexion can be employed. Options range from simple extension block splints[13] or pins[16] to external traction[14,15] or complex frame constructions.[9,12]

SURGICAL MANAGEMENT

- Hemi-hamate osteochondral autograft is indicated for the treatment of unstable PIP fracture-dislocations. The middle phalanx dorsal cortex must be intact.
- Hemi-hamate arthroplasty is a valuable salvage procedure for treatment that has failed with traction, external fixation devices, extension block splinting, or palmar plate arthroplasty.
- Chronic PIP dorsal dislocations also are amenable to treatment with hemi-hamate autograft if enough intact cartilage remains on both sides of the joint. Undamaged cartilage must be present on the palmar 50% of the proximal phalanx head and on at least a small rim of the middle phalanx dorsal articular surface.

Preoperative Planning

- Review the radiographs to determine the extent of articular surface damaged by the fracture, joint stability, and the quality of the remaining articular surface.
- Patients with extensive preexisting degenerative arthritis may be better served with a PIP arthrodesis or total joint arthroplasty than with hemi-hamate arthroplasty.
- Assess the finger for radial or ulnar deviation. If coronal plane angulation is observed, it will be necessary to level the middle phalangeal joint surface during fracture site preparation and graft placement.
- Examine the patient for a mallet finger. If the terminal extensor tendon has been damaged, plan to include a mallet splint in the postoperative regimen.

Positioning

- Position the patient supine with the arm extended onto a radiolucent hand table.
- A mini C-arm is required for the procedure.
- Either regional or general anesthesia may be used, depending on the patient's or surgeon's preference.
- Perioperative antibiotics are provided.
- An upper arm tourniquet is applied. This is preferred over a forearm tourniquet, which puts pressure on the flexor muscles and causes excessive finger flexion.
- If necessary, the dorsum of the hand is shaved at the fourth and fifth carpometacarpal (CMC) joints to facilitate harvesting of the graft.

Approach

- We recommend performing the PIP portion of the procedure through a Brunner incision because this incision provides excellent visualization of the fracture, the pulley system, and the neurovascular bundles.
- The hamate graft is harvested through a transverse incision at the level of the fourth and fifth CMC joints.

TECHNIQUES

Fracture Site Preparation

- Use a lead hand to position the hand palm up with the fingers extended. It will be necessary to remove the lead hand intermittently to facilitate use of fluoroscopy.
- Make a Brunner incision from the base of the finger to the DIP flexor crease (**TECH FIG 1A**).
- Coagulate intervening vessels with bipolar cautery as the full-thickness flaps are elevated.
- Identify the neurovascular bundles proximally and mobilize them away from the flexor sheath throughout the length of the dissection.
- Divide Cleland ligaments dorsal to the neurovascular bundles. This allows full visualization of the collateral ligaments and facilitates retraction of the neurovascular bundles without excessive traction.
- Retract skin flaps with 5-0 nylon suture.
- Open the flexor tendon sheath from the distal end of the A2 pulley to the proximal edge of the A4 pulley. Start the dissection with a longitudinal incision along the edge of the flexor tendon sheath that is closest to the surgeon.
  - Create a flexor tendon sheath flap by making transverse incisions at the proximal end of A4 and the distal margin of A2. Elevate the flexor tendon sheath flap away from the surgeon (**TECH FIG 1B**).
  - Take care to prevent superficial damage to the flexor tendons while incising the flexor sheath.
- With the flexor tendons retracted away from the midline, make longitudinal incisions down the lateral margins of the palmar plate to separate the palmar plate from the accessory collateral ligaments. The distal attachment of the palmar plate will already be detached (ie, avulsed) as a result of the injury, but it still may need to be gently mobilized. Leave any remaining bone fragments attached to the distal edge of the palmar plate.
  - If the fragments are large enough to accept interfragmentary screws, consider open reduction and internal fixation instead of proceeding with the hemi-hamate autograft.
- Release the collateral ligaments distally. Leave a small stump on the middle phalanx to facilitate repair at the end of the procedure.
- "Shotgun" the joint open (**TECH FIG 1C**).
  - Retract the flexor tendons away from the midline.
  - Hyperextend the PIP joint to expose the base of the middle phalanx and the head of the proximal phalanx.
  - If necessary, use a Freer elevator to prevent impingement of the intact dorsal base of the middle phalanx against the head of the proximal phalanx.
    - Caution: Forceful hyperextension may lead to fracture of the dorsal articular fragment.
  - Only if absolutely necessary, release 1 to 2 mm of the A4 pulley to facilitate adequate mobilization of the flexor tendons. The A4 pulley is essential for finger function and must not be released completely.
- Assess the damage to the articular surfaces of the middle phalanx and the head of the proximal phalanx.
- Prepare the middle phalanx to receive the autograft (see **TECH FIG 1C**).
  - Elevate and excise impacted fragments of articular cartilage.
  - Use an oscillating saw to level the surface of the bony defect and to remove sufficient bone to allow graft placement. Make the cuts parallel to the dorsal margin of the articular surface and the long axis of the phalangeal shaft. Make the height of the intact articular surfaces equal at both the radial and ulnar margins. Limit thermal osteonecrosis with liberal use of irrigation.
  - The proximal to distal length of the cut usually is only about 5 to 7 mm. Take care to avoid notching the dorsal or distal portion of the cut because this may weaken the shaft.
- Carefully measure the defect in the middle phalanx base to determine the appropriate graft size. Make notes of the dimensions on a drawing created on the back table (**TECH FIG 1D**).
  - ***A*:** Width of the fracture defect. Measure the distance from the radial margin to the ulnar margin of the fracture defect. The graft must be centered on the central ridge of the proximal phalanx. Prepare the fracture site so that radial and ulnar extent of the fracture defect are equal.

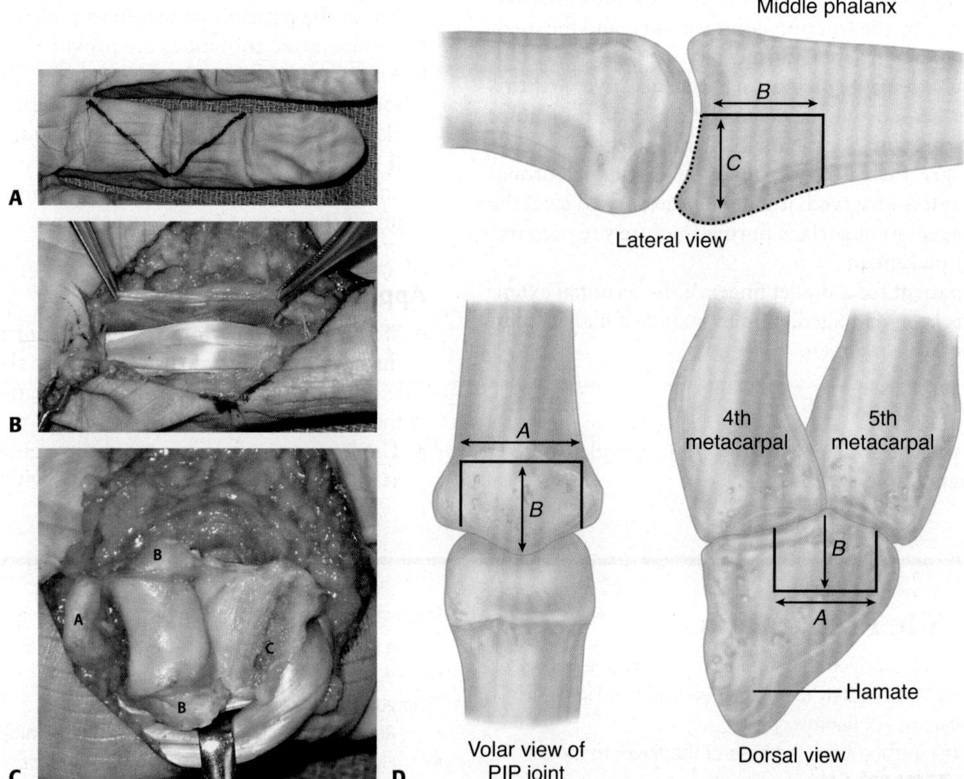

TECH FIG 1 • **A.** A Brunner incision, as depicted in this cadaver dissection, provides excellent visualization of the neurovascular structures, the flexor tendons, and the fracture site. **B.** Creating a flexor tendon sheath flap. Elevate a flap of the flexor tendon sheath from the distal end of the A2 pulley to the proximal edge of the A4 pulley. Preserve the flap so that it may be used to cover the palmar plate and the graft during closure. **C.** Shotgun the joint and prepare the fracture site. The PIP joint has been hyperextended 180 degrees to expose the fracture site. Note the palmar plate (*A*), the collateral ligaments (*B*), and the fracture defect (*C*). The fracture defect must be prepared so that it is of equal height and thickness on the radial and ulnar sides of the middle phalanx. **D.** Measuring graft dimensions. Measure the fracture defect to determine the medial to lateral width (*A*), proximal to distal depth (*B*), and anterior to posterior height (*C*) of the needed graft. Transfer these measurements to the dorsal surface of the hamate.

- ***B***: The proximal to distal size of the defect. To avoid creating an uneven joint surface that causes angulation in the coronal plane, the proximal to distal defect size should be equal on the radial and ulnar margins or the middle phalanx.
- ***C***: Height of articular surface at the central ridge. Measure the distance from the dorsal aspect of the fracture defect to what would be the most palmar extent of the middle phalanx palmar lip. It will be necessary to estimate this based on a lateral view of the proximal phalanx and from the preoperative radiographs (percentage of joint involvement).
- Return the joint to neutral and place a moist sponge on the finger incision while the graft is harvested.

Harvesting the Hamate Graft

- Identify the distal articular margin of the hamate with fluoroscopy and mark the skin with a transverse line.
- Make a transverse 2-cm incision just proximal to the articular line.
- Bluntly dissect to mobilize the subcutaneous nerves, vessels, and extensor tendons.
- Longitudinally incise the hamate–CMC joint capsule, and then subperiosteally elevate the flaps to provide adequate visualization of the articular surfaces and the dorsum of the hamate (**TECH FIG 2A**).
- The apex of the distal articular surface between the fourth and fifth metacarpal articular surfaces will become the new central ridge of the middle phalangeal base once the graft is transferred.
- A 12-mm segment is trimmed from the flexible plastic ruler that accompanies the marking pen. A fine-tipped marker is preferred because it will not bleed as much on the bone. Less soft tissue on the dorsum of the hamate also helps prevent the ink from bleeding.
- Using a fine-tip marker and ruler, mark the dimensions of the graft on the hamate. To ensure stability of the CMC joints, leave at

least 2 mm of the radial edge of the fourth metacarpal–hamate articulation and 2 mm of the ulnar edge of the fifth metacarpal–hamate surface.

- Harvest a graft that is of adequate height to fill the middle phalanx defect, but do not fracture the dorsal cortex of the hamate.
- Use an oscillating saw to make the cuts in the hamate very carefully. Alternatively, define the graft dimensions with a series of holes made with a K-wire, and then make the cuts with an osteotome (**TECH FIG 2B**).
  - To ensure that the graft is not too small, make the osteotomies on the outside of the measured lines.
  - Protect the articular surfaces at the base of the fourth and fifth metacarpals with a Freer elevator.
  - Estimate the depth of the cuts by marking the saw blade or osteotome and measuring how deeply it penetrates the hamate.
- Create a notch in the hamate cortex proximal to the most proximal cut using a rongeur or by making an angled cut from proximal to distal with the saw. The notch is necessary to allow the final coronal cut to be made with a curved osteotome (**TECH FIG 2C**).
- Using extreme care, make the final cut in the hamate and complete the graft harvest.
  - Gently advance an angled osteotome from proximal to distal, aiming to complete the cut through the distal hamate articular surface at the predetermined depth.
  - Protect the metacarpal articular surfaces with an elevator.
  - Take slightly more bone than needed. It is easier to trim excess than to deal with a graft that is too small.
- Keep the graft protected in a moist saline sponge during wound closure.
- After the wound is irrigated, securely close the capsule over the fourth and fifth CMC joints with a 4-0 braided, nonabsorbable suture. Close the skin in layers.

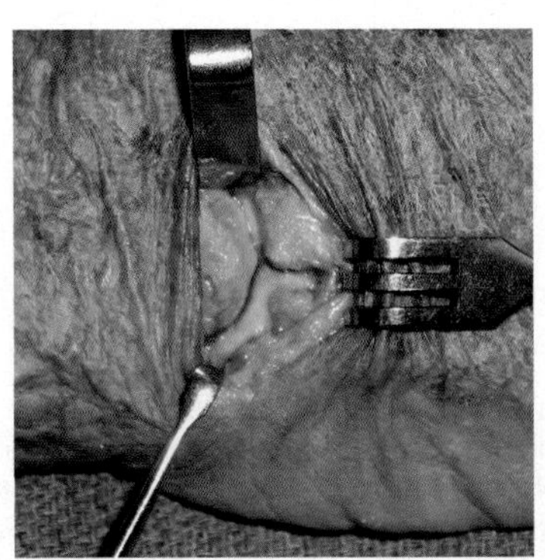
A

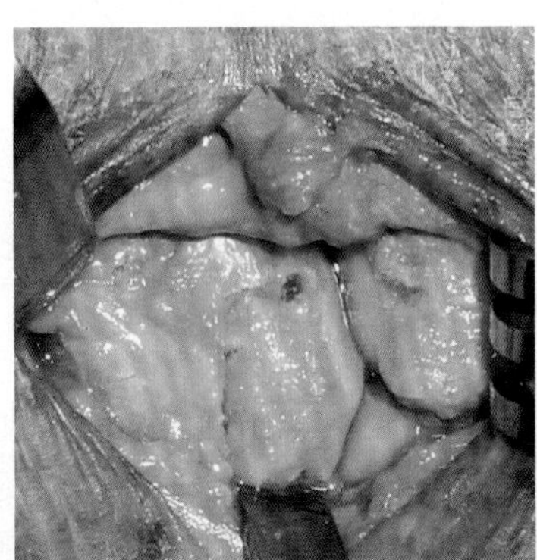
B

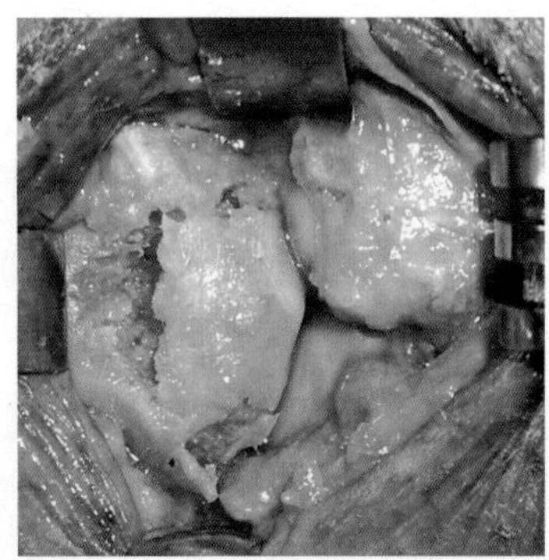
C

TECH FIG 2 • **A.** Exposure of the fourth and fifth metacarpal–hamate joints. Through a transverse skin incision and longitudinal capsular incision, as demonstrated in this cadaver dissection, expose the distal hamate articular surface and mark the graft dimensions. **B.** Use an oscillating saw or, as depicted in this cadaver dissection, K-wire holes and an osteotome to make the cortical cuts in the dorsal surface of the hamate. **C.** Making the final hamate cut. A curved osteotome is used to make the final coronal cut that separates the graft from the hamate. It is necessary to make a back cut in the proximal hamate cortex to allow the osteotome to approach the cut at the proper angle. (**A–C:** Wrist is to the left and fingers are to the right.)

Graft Fixation

- Shotgun the PIP joint open to expose the fracture site.
- Carefully trim the graft with a rongeur or oscillating saw so that it fits precisely into the prepared defect at the middle phalanx base.
- It is very important to tailor the graft so that it restores the cup-shaped contour of the middle phalanx base. Joint stability will be restored only by restoring a concave middle phalanx articular surface that includes a stout palmar lip (**TECH FIG 3A–C**).
- A common error is to set the graft at an angle that creates a dorsal–proximal to palmar–distal slope. This carpentry error fails to restore joint stability and encourages the dorsal migration of the middle phalanx on the proximal phalangeal head (**TECH FIG 3D,E**).
- Temporarily fix the graft with a centrally placed 0.028-inch K-wire.
- Lag 1.0- or 1.3-mm screws on either side of the provisional K-wire.
- If the graft is large enough, augment the fixation with a third screw placed into the hole that remains once the K-wire is removed (**TECH FIG 3F**).
- Relocate the middle phalanx on the proximal phalanx, and assess the joint for stability and alignment.
  - The joint should remain in position throughout a full ROM. Dorsal subluxation suggests that the graft has been set too flat, failing to restore a concave articular surface.
  - The joint should exhibit neutral alignment. Varus or valgus angulation suggests that the graft has not been set perpendicular to the long axis of the middle phalanx.
- Assess screw length and graft placement with fluoroscopy. The hamate articular cartilage is thicker than the middle phalanx cartilage. This discrepancy creates the illusion that the hamate has not been set flush with the middle phalanx, but a lack of step-off already has been confirmed by direct inspection of the joint surface (**TECH FIG 3G**).
- Often, the distal edge of the graft protrudes beyond the volar cortex of the middle phalanx fracture defect. Shave the graft edge to smooth the transition from graft to middle phalanx.

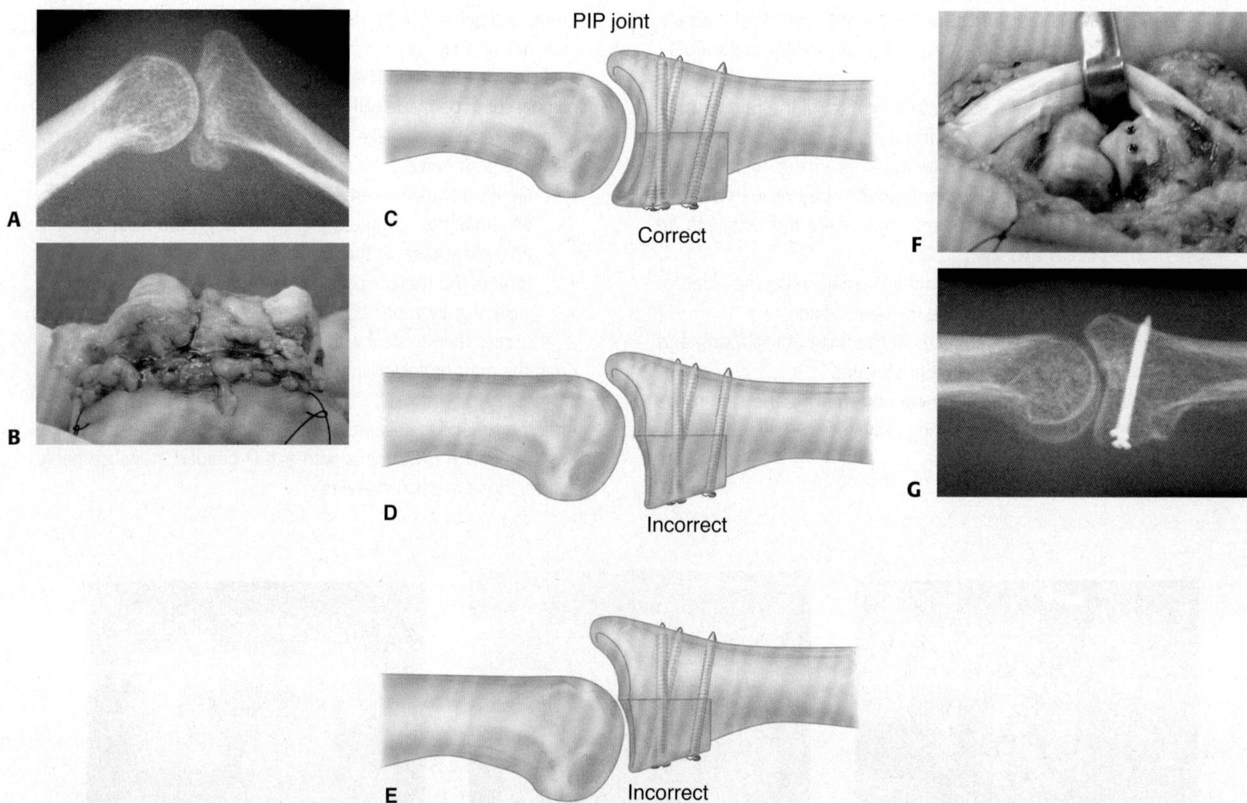

TECH FIG 3 • A. This lateral preoperative radiograph demonstrates a chronic, unstable PIP fracture-dislocation in a 19-year-old woman. Joint flexion occurs as the middle phalanx hinges at the palmar fracture margin and the proximal phalanx falls into the fracture defect. **B.** The graft has been inset to recreate a middle phalanx articular surface that is concave and matches the curvature of the proximal phalanx head. **C.** The graft must be contoured and set into the middle phalanx in a manner that restores the cup-shaped geometry of the middle phalanx base. Failure to restore a concave joint surface creates a flat surface (**D**) that encourages dorsal subluxation of the middle phalanx (**E**). **F.** Relocation of the joint. The joint has been relocated and stability confirmed by taking the joint through a full ROM and ensuring that subluxation does not occur. Note how nicely the hamate graft recreates the palmar lip of the middle phalanx. **G.** Lateral radiograph of the graft. The lateral radiograph gives the false appearance that a step-off exists between the graft and the remaining middle phalangeal articular cartilage.

Closure

- Repair the palmar plate and palmar margin of the middle phalanx. It may be necessary to secure the sutures through small drill holes.
- Repair the collateral ligaments to the stumps that were left on the middle phalanx during the approach.
- Interpose the flexor tendon sheath flap under the flexor tendons and over the PIP joint.
- Obtain hemostasis after the tourniquet is deflated.
- Close the skin.
- Apply a bulky dressing and splint holding the PIP joint in slight flexion.

PEARLS AND PITFALLS

Recurrent dorsal subluxation	■ This is most commonly caused by failure to inset the graft in a position that restores the cup-shaped middle phalanx base. ■ Failure to repair the palmar plate also may contribute to recurrent dorsal subluxation.
Angulation in the coronal plane	■ The graft must be positioned perpendicular to the long axis of the middle phalanx. After provisional graft fixation, clinically assess the finger for varus or valgus angulation and adjust the graft to achieve neutral alignment.

POSTOPERATIVE CARE

- The goal of hemi-hamate arthroplasty is to operatively restore osseous PIP stability. Assuming that this goal has been attained and confirmed with lateral radiographs in extension that demonstrate concentric reduction, ROM is begun within the first week.
- Apply a postoperative dressing that controls edema and supports the PIP joint in a slightly flexed posture.
- Within the first week, begin active PIP flexion within an extension block splint that prevents extension past 20 degrees. The therapists may choose to fabricate a hand-based dorsal extension block splint if swelling is excessive, but a figure-8 splint is preferable.
- Encourage full active and passive motion at the metacarpophalangeal (MP) and DIP. If a concomitant mallet injury is being treated, splint the DIP joint in full extension, but do not inhibit motion at the other joints.
- If the radiographs at 3 weeks show concentric joint reduction and solid graft fixation, begin gentle active-assisted ROM.
- At 6 weeks postoperatively, again confirm solid graft fixation and concentric joint reduction radiographically, discontinue figure-8 splinting, and then begin passive ROM into flexion and correction of an excessive PIP flexion contracture with dynamic extension splinting.

OUTCOMES

- Our initially reported results of 13 hemi-hamate arthroplasties followed for an average of 16 months were encouraging.[18] Pain relief was consistently good, PIP ROM averaged 85 degrees (range 65 to 100 degrees), all grafts incorporated, and no degenerative change were noted.
- We have subsequently reported on the long-term outcome of hemi-hamate arthroplasty.[2]
  - At an average of 4.5-year follow-up (range from 1 to 7 years), 22 patients who had undergone hemi-hamate arthroplasty were evaluated. Fourteen patients were treated within 6 weeks of injury (acute) and 8 patients at an average of 30 weeks (chronic).
  - Motion
    - PIP ROM averaged 70 degrees (range 0 to 100 degrees).
    - Average PIP flexion contracture was 19 degrees (range 0 to 80 degrees).
    - The ROM of the DIP joint averaged 54 degrees (range 0 to 85 degrees).
  - Grip strength measured 95% of contralateral uninjured hand.
  - Functional outcome was good with a mean Visual Analog Scale (VAS) functional score of 1.9 and mean Disability of the Arm, Shoulder, and Hand (DASH) score of 5.
  - The results of acute (<6 weeks) and chronic (mean of 30 weeks) reconstructions were compared. Chronic reconstructions were more likely to exhibit decreased grip strength, more residual pain, and a higher DASH score.
  - Radiographs
    - Forty-three percent of patients (six joints) showed signs of joint space narrowing; however, these radiographic findings did not correlate with poorer patient outcomes.
    - No grafts showed signs of osteonecrosis.
  - Five patients from the original study[18] were reexamined in this long-term follow-up. PIP arcs of motion and VAS-rated pain scores were stable with increases in DIP arcs of motion.
- Afendras et al[1] followed eight patients for a minimum of 4 years after hemi-hamate osteochondral graft.
  - PIP ROM of 67 degrees (range 45 to 95 degrees), grip strength equal to 91% of the uninjured side, and a VAS pain rating of 10 out of 100
  - Radiographs showed grade II arthritic changes in two patients and grade IV arthritic changes in two patients, but only one of these patients was symptomatic.
- The long-term reported outcomes of hemi-hamate arthroplasty continue to be encouraging; however, evidence of some joint space narrowing warrants continued study.

COMPLICATIONS

- The complication rate for this procedure is low.
  - There are no reported cases of infections.
  - Dorsal subluxation postoperatively has been reported. An incompetent palmar plate or inappropriately contouring the graft to restore the cup-shaped geometry of the middle phalanx base are two proposed etiologies.
- Reported cases of revision surgery for complications associated with this procedure are sparse. These include flexor tenolysis for postoperative stiffness, removal of hardware for prominent dorsal screw tips, and revision to silastic interpositional arthroplasty.
- Donor site morbidity is rare.

REFERENCES

1. Afendras G, Abramo A, Mrkonjic A, et al. Hemi-hamate osteochondral transplantation in proximal interphalangeal dorsal fracture dislocations: a minimum 4 year follow-up in eight patients. J Hand Surg Eur Vol 2010;35:627–631.
2. Calfee RP, Kiefhaber TR, Sommerkamp MD, et al. Hemi-hamate arthroplasty provides functional reconstruction of acute and chronic proximal interphalangeal fracture-dislocations. J Hand Surg Am 2009;34: 1232–1241.
3. Eaton RG, Malerich MM. Volar plate arthroplasty for the proximal interphalangeal joint: a ten year review. J Hand Surg Am 1980;5: 260–268.
4. Freeland AE, Benoist LA. Open reduction and internal fixation method for fractures at the proximal interphalangeal joint. Hand Clin 1994;10:239–250.
5. Hamilton SC, Stern PJ, Fassler PR, et al. Mini-screw fixation for the treatment of proximal interphalangeal joint dorsal fracture-dislocations. J Hand Surg Am 2006;8:1349–1354.
6. Hastings H, Capo J, Steinberg B, et al. Hemicondylar hamate replacement arthroplasty for proximal interphalangeal joint fracture-dislocations. Abstract. Presented at the 54th Annual Meeting of The American Society for Surgery of the Hand, September 3–5, 1999, Boston, MA.
7. Hastings H II, Carroll C IV. Treatment of closed articular fractures of the metacarpophalangeal and proximal interphalangeal joints. Hand Clin 1988;4:503–527.
8. Hastings H II, Hamlet WP. Critical assessment of PIP joint stability after palmar lip fractures dislocations. Abstract. Presented at the 56th Annual Meeting of The American Society for Surgery of the Hand, October 3–6, 2001, Baltimore, MD.
9. Inanami H, Ninomiya S, Okutsu I, et al. Dynamic external finger fixator for fracture-dislocation of the proximal interphalangeal joint. J Hand Surg Am 1993;18:160–164.
10. Jupiter JB, Sheppard JE. Tendon wire fixation of avulsion fractures in the hand. Clin Orthop Relat Res 1987;(214):113–120.
11. Kiefhaber TR, Stern PJ. Fracture-dislocations of the proximal interphalangeal joint. J Hand Surg Am 1998;23:368–380.
12. Krakauer JD, Stern PJ. Hinged device for fracture involving the proximal interphalangeal joint. Clin Orthop Relat Res 1996;(327):29–37.

13. McElfresh EC, Dobyns JH, O'Brien ET. Management of fracture-dislocations of the proximal interphalangeal joints by extension-block splinting. J Bone Joint Surg Am 1972;54:1705–1711.
14. Morgan JP, Gordon DA, Klug MS, et al. Dynamic digital traction for unstable comminuted intra-articular fracture-dislocations of the proximal interphalangeal joint. J Hand Surg Am 1995;20:565–573.
15. Schenck RR. Dynamic traction and early passive movement for fractures of the proximal interphalangeal joint. J Hand Surg Am 1986;11:850–858.
16. Viegas SF. Extension block pinning for proximal interphalangeal joint fracture-dislocations: preliminary report of a new technique. J Hand Surg Am 1992;17:896–901.
17. Williams RM, Hastings H II, Kiefhaber TR. PIP fracture-dislocations treatment technique: use of a hemi-hamate resurfacing arthroplasty. Tech Hand Up Extrem Surg 2002;6:185–192.
18. Williams RM, Kiefhaber TR, Sommerkamp TG, et al. Treatment of unstable dorsal proximal interphalangeal fracture/dislocations using a hemi-hamate autograft. J Hand Surg Am 2003;28:856–865.

Operative Treatment of Distal Interphalangeal Joint Fracture-Dislocations

56

CHAPTER

Leo T. Kroonen and Eric P. Hofmeister

DEFINITION

- Injuries about the distal interphalangeal joint (DIP) consist of avulsion injuries of the terminal extensor tendon or the flexor digitorum profundus (FDP) tendon, isolated dislocations of the DIP joint, and complex tuft fractures.
- A "bony" mallet finger (ie, mallet fracture) is an intra-articular bony avulsion at the insertion site of the terminal extensor tendon on the dorsal base of the distal phalanx that results in inability to actively extend the DIP joint.
- A "non-bony" mallet finger is an injury to the extensor mechanism at or near the insertion onto the distal phalanx that typically results in inability to actively extend the DIP joint.
- "Jersey finger" is an avulsion of the FDP tendon, with or without its bony attachment, from the volar base of the distal phalanx. It typically results in inability to actively flex the DIP joint.
- Isolated dislocations of the DIP joint are rare injuries in which the distal phalanx is dislocated either dorsal or volar relative to the middle phalanx.
- An intra-articular or tuft fracture can have a component of a mallet or FDP avulsion, and should be treated accordingly, while also taking into consideration the additional instability associated with the fracture.

ANATOMY

- The DIP joint is stabilized by the radial and ulnar collateral ligaments, the volar plate, and the firm insertions of the FDP and terminal tendons of the extensor mechanism.
- The extensor mechanism terminates with the confluence of the lateral bands into a single terminal tendon, which inserts on the dorsal base of the distal phalanx. The terminal tendon is a strong, flat, thin segment that averages 10.1 mm in length and 5.6 mm in width.[15]
- The terminal tendon insertion, on average, is 1.4 mm proximal to the germinal matrix of the fingernail.[15]
- The volar surface of the terminal tendon usually is adherent to the dorsal capsule of the DIP joint.[15]
- The FDP tendon inserts on the volar surface of the base of the distal phalanx. It is surrounded by the flexor tendon sheath. The A4, A5, and C3 pulleys secure the FDP tendon around the level of the DIP joint.
- The vinculum longus profundus and vinculum brevis profundus are thin mesenteries providing vascular supply to the distal portion of the FDP tendon. They also provide a weak attachment of the FDP tendon to the flexor tendon sheath.[8]

The views expressed in this chapter are those of the authors and do not reflect the official policy or position of the Department of the Navy, Department of Defense, or the United States Government.

PATHOGENESIS

- Mallet finger injuries are the result of a disruption to the extensor mechanism at or near the insertion to the base of the distal phalanx. Such disruptions can occur as a result of a laceration or a sudden flexion force to an extended DIP joint. The disruption of the extensor mechanism allows unopposed pull of the FDP tendon, leaving the DIP joint in a flexed posture and sometimes volar subluxation of the joint.
- Jersey finger injuries occur as a result of disruption to the FDP, from either a laceration or a sudden extension force applied to a flexed DIP joint during an eccentric contraction. The disruption of the FDP tendon leaves the pull of the extensor mechanism unopposed, resulting in a flaccid and often extended posture of the DIP joint.
- Dislocations of the DIP joint are rare due to the inherent stability provided by the collateral ligaments, the volar plate, and the flexor and extensor tendon insertions. However, when a dislocation does occur, the distal end of the middle phalanx usually "buttonholes" through these structures, making reduction more difficult.
- Complex intra-articular distal phalanx fractures and tuft fractures can occur as a result of crushing injuries or axial loading injuries. Careful attention should be given to these injuries to determine whether or not they demonstrate accompanying characteristics of a mallet injury or FDP avulsion. Characteristics such as a transverse shaft fracture impart further instability to the injury pattern and should be treated with stabilization first in order to have a firm foundation on which to base further fixation.

NATURAL HISTORY

- Mallet finger injuries can occur in any digit but most commonly are seen in the three most ulnar digits.
  - Left untreated, a mallet finger injury can progress to a secondary "swan neck" deformity.
    - With the disruption of the extensor mechanism at the DIP joint, the pull of the lateral bands adds to the extension force of the central slip at the PIP joint, thereby creating an imbalance in forces at the PIP joint and a hyperextension deformity at that joint.[17]
  - Despite treatment, residual deformity, usually in the form of a dorsal prominence, can be seen in up to 80% of cases.[17] Additionally, lack of terminal extension or a mild flexion contraction may persist.
- Approximately, 75% of cases of FDP avulsions involve the ring finger. Some authors theorize that this is because the ring finger protrudes the farthest distally when the hand is held in a flexed position; however, no literature has proven this theory.

- Leddy[6] proposed the classification system that is still widely used today for FDP avulsion injuries, based on the level of retraction of the tendon. Other authors since have made additions to this injury.
  - Type I FDP avulsions retract into the palm, thereby disrupting the vincular system and leading to poor blood supply. Surgery should be performed within 7 to 10 days.
  - Type II injuries retract to the level of the PIP joint or distal A2 pulley. An associated small bony fleck often is seen on the lateral radiograph. Because the proximal blood supply is preserved through the long vincula, these injuries can be successfully treated as late as 6 weeks from the time of injury.
  - Type III injuries usually are associated with a bony avulsion and as a result do not retract proximal to the A4 pulley. These injuries are treated as bony injuries with open reduction and internal fixation and can be treated late if required.
  - Type IV injuries are bony avulsion injuries in which the tendon also has separated from the avulsed bony fragment. Time to treatment depends on the level of tendon retraction.[16]
  - Type V injuries are bony FDP avulsion injuries coupled with a distal phalanx fracture.
  - Type Va subtype is with an associated extra-articular fracture.
  - Type Vb subtype is with an associated intra-articular fracture.[1,14]

PATIENT HISTORY AND PHYSICAL FINDINGS

- As with all hand injuries, patients should be questioned about their hand dominance and occupational requirements to aid the surgeon in better understanding individual needs and goals.
- The following examinations should be performed to determine possible injuries:
  - FDP function
    - Inability to flex at the DIP joint implies disruption of the FDP tendon.
    - Limited, weak, or painful flexion may indicate a partial injury or a complete disruption with intact vinculae or pseudotendon.
  - DIP joint extensor mechanism function
    - Inability to extend at the DIP joint implies disruption of the terminal extensor tendon. Weak extension implies a partial or less severe injury. Loss of passive extension indicates a possible fracture or dislocation.
- Axial injuries to an extended DIP joint often are the culprit in mallet finger injuries.
  - The history often reveals an axial blow to the fingertip, such as when an incoming ball strikes an extended fingertip.
  - The patient will be unable to actively extend at the DIP joint.
- Jersey finger injuries often are the result of a sudden extension force on a flexed DIP joint, such as when grabbing for another player's shirt while playing football.
  - Patients will be unable to actively flex through the DIP joint.
  - Active PIP flexion will be present but may be moderately diminished due to pain or stiffness.
- Most dislocations of the DIP joint are the result of sporting injuries.[12,13] In addition to a deformity, there will be lack of active and passive motion of the joint.
- The tenodesis effect can also be used to test the continuity of the terminal flexor or extensor tendons.
  - Passively flexing the wrist should result in extension of the DIP joint by tensioning the extensor tendons at the level of the wrist. If a flexed position is maintained at the DIP joint despite full wrist extension, then an extensor tendon injury should be suspected.
  - Passively extending the wrist should cause flexion of the DIP joint. If the injured finger does not flex with the neighboring digits, FDP injury should be suspected.

IMAGING AND OTHER DIAGNOSTIC STUDIES

- Plain radiographs of the affected hand (posteroanterior [PA], lateral, and oblique) and dedicated views of the affected finger (PA, lateral, and oblique) should be obtained and usually are sufficient for making the diagnosis in association with a thorough clinical examination.
  - Mallet finger injuries can be associated with a bony avulsion. Any joint subluxation should be noted, and the size of the avulsed fragment should be estimated (**FIG 1**).
  - In FDP avulsion injuries, the location of the retracted flexor tendon often can be appreciated by finding a bony fragment on the lateral radiograph of the affected digit (**FIG 2A,B**).
- Ultrasound sometimes can be helpful in determining continuity of the flexor tendon or identifying the location of the retracted proximal flexor tendon stump.[3,7,14]
- Magnetic resonance imaging (MRI) can be useful in determining flexor tendon continuity and level of tendon retraction (**FIG 2C**).

DIFFERENTIAL DIAGNOSIS

- Osteoarthritis
- Inflammatory arthropathy (such as gout, rheumatoid arthritis [RA], etc.)
- FDP rupture
- FDP laceration

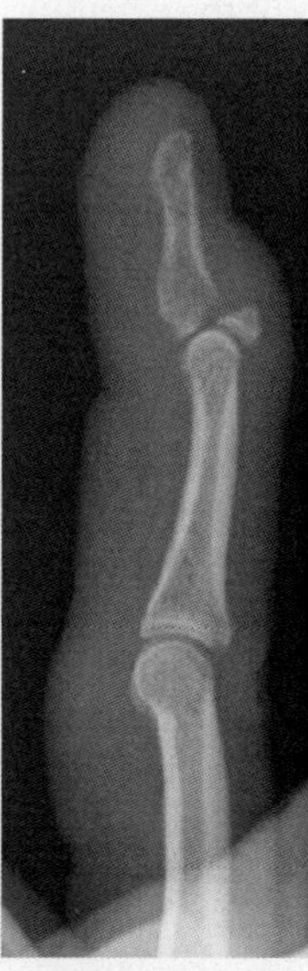

FIG 1 • Lateral radiographs usually are the most helpful in identifying a mallet fracture. Note that in this image, the avulsed fragment includes more than 50% of the articular surface. There is no significant volar subluxation in this case.

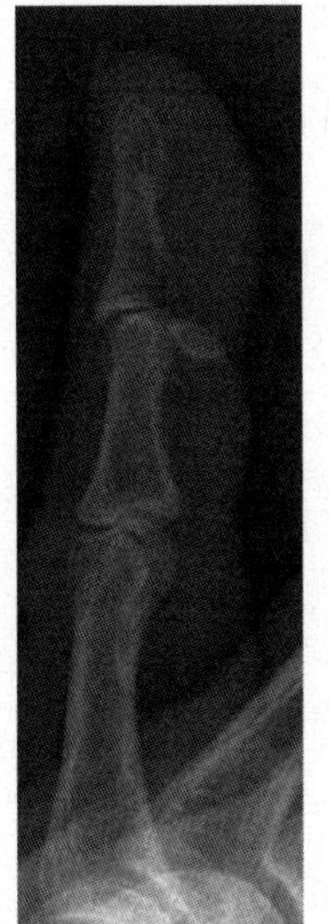
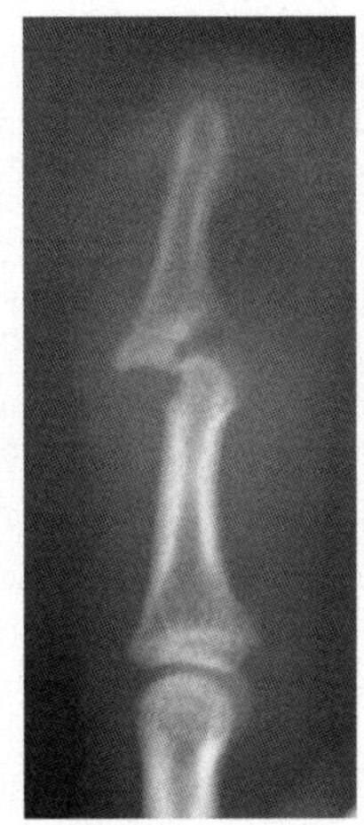
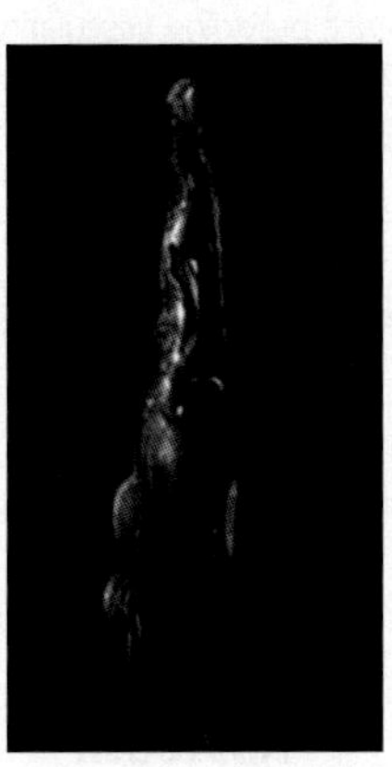

FIG 2 • **A.** FDP avulsion in which a bony fragment has been caught up at the A4 pulley. **B.** Lateral radiograph of a finger demonstrates chronic dorsal dislocation of the DIP joint with associated arthrosis. **C.** Sagittal cut MRI shows the FDP tendon retracted back to the level of the PIP joint.

- Terminal extensor tendon rupture (mallet finger)
- Mallet fracture

NONOPERATIVE MANAGEMENT

- For tendinous mallet fingers and mallet fractures involving less than one-third of the articular surface and without joint subluxation, a variety of splints are available.
  - We prefer immobilizing the DIP joint with a prefabricated polyethylene extension splint.
  - For hygiene assistance, the patient is given two splints that can be alternated to assist in keeping the skin dry. They should be carefully instructed to always keep the digit in full extension when changing splints. This can be accomplished by keeping the entire digit flat against a countertop while sliding the splints on and off.
  - Casting of the DIP joint also has been described.
  - Full-time splinting in extension is recommended for 6 weeks, followed by 6 weeks of part-time splinting. During this second 6 weeks, patients are advised to wear the splint for any heavy activity and at night.
  - Gentle DIP joint flexion is initiated at 6 weeks, not exceeding 20 degrees in the first 2 weeks. Motion is then gradually increasing to full flexion over the course of 6 weeks. If any loss of extension is experienced during this time, the patient is instructed to return immediately to full-time splinting and to follow-up for reevaluation.
- Nonoperative treatment of acute FDP lacerations or ruptures at the DIP joint is not recommended unless the patient is unwilling or unable to comply with postoperative splinting or rehabilitation.
- In subacute and chronic FDP lacerations or avulsions, the functional necessity of DIP joint motion should be carefully considered, and nonoperative treatment should be considered.
  - Literature directing treatment in cases of delayed diagnosis is scarce.
  - If the patient does not have any functional limitations as a result of the injury, we prefer to defer surgical management.
  - If the patient is troubled by a tender mass in the palm but the hand is functional, excision of the distal tendon stump is recommended.
  - Instability and weakness of pinch can become problematic. In such cases, tenodesis[3] or arthrodesis is recommended.
  - Only if the function of the DIP is *crucial* to the performance of daily activities do we recommend a staged reconstruction of the flexor tendon.
- Closed reduction of isolated DIP joint dislocations can be attempted under a digital block.
  - For dorsal dislocations, the FDP tendon or the volar plate can be interposed, blocking the reduction as the head of the middle phalanx buttonholes through the interval between the FDP tendon and the collateral ligament.[13]
    - For dorsal dislocations, gentle traction and extension through the DIP joint can assist in reducing the interposed volar plate.
- In volar dislocations, the head of the middle phalanx can buttonhole through the interval between the terminal extensor tendon and the collateral ligament.[12]
  - For volar dislocations, gentle traction can be used while guiding the condyle of the middle phalanx back through the interval between the terminal extensor tendon and the collateral ligament.
- In the case of a dislocation, a gentle reduction maneuver should be attempted, keeping in mind the structures that are likely to be interposed in the joint. Care should be taken to avoid excessive traction, which may tighten the tendon and ligament, preventing reduction.

SURGICAL MANAGEMENT

- Surgical treatment of mallet fractures is reserved for those fractures associated with joint subluxation.
- Operative treatment is recommended for all acute flexor tendon avulsions at the DIP joint and selected subacute or chronic cases.
  - The level of retraction of the tendon on the flexor side determines the urgency with which the injury needs to be addressed (Table 1). We recommend treating these injuries as soon as possible to optimize recovery and function.
- For isolated dislocations of the DIP joint, surgical management is indicated in those cases where closed reduction is unsuccessful. Generally, no surgical stabilization is required

Table 1 Classification of Flexor Digitorum Profundus Avulsion Injuries

Type	Level of Tendon Retraction	Vascularity	Approximate Time to Surgery
I	Palm	Vinculae are disrupted, leading to dysvascularity of tendon.	7–10 days
II	Distal A2 pulley or PIP joint	Vinculae remain intact, providing vascularity and preventing further retraction.	Up to 6 weeks
III	A4 pulley	Bony attachment prevents retraction beyond the A4 pulley.	6 weeks +
IV	The tendon is avulsed from a bony avulsion fracture and can retract to any level.	Determined by the level of tendon retraction	Determined by the level of tendon retraction
V	Bony FDP avulsions associated with a distal phalanx fracture.	Determined by the level of tendon retraction	Determined by the level of tendon retraction
a	Associated extra-articular fracture		
b	Associated intra-articular fracture		

FDP, flexor digitorum profundus.

unless the injury is chronic in nature or closed reduction cannot be maintained.

Preoperative Planning

- All images should be reviewed.
- For isolated dislocations, a review of the relevant anatomy, including the volar plate, flexor and extensor tendons, and collateral ligaments, is essential to understand which structures might be interposed in the DIP joint.
- For FDP avulsions, an understanding of the flexor tendon sheath, pulley system, and the flexor tendon anatomy should be well understood.

Positioning

- The patient is placed supine on the operating room table with the affected arm outstretched on an arm board. When treating a flexor tendon injury, a flexible aluminum hand holder can be useful for positioning the hand during the exploration.
- For most DIP joint dislocations, tuft fractures and mallet fingers, a digital tourniquet can be used; however, a well-padded tourniquet placed high on the arm is necessary for flexor tendon avulsions, as a more distal tourniquet may prevent complete tendon excursion making reduction more difficult.

Approach

- Mallet fingers
  - We prefer to treat mallet fingers with percutaneous techniques.
    - Percutaneous treatment is more likely to succeed if the injury is treated within the first 3 to 5 days after the injury, although we have successfully treated cases at as late as 6 weeks.
  - If open treatment is to be attempted, a variety of incisions can be used, including straight longitudinal, lazy S-type, H-type, and Bruner incisions. Meticulous soft tissue handling is vital to minimize trauma and necrosis to the skin. Great care must be taken to avoid injury to the germinal matrix proximal to the nail fold.
- Jersey fingers
  - A volar Bruner incision is used and is extended proximal enough to identify or retrieve the proximal tendon stump.
  - In type I injuries, an oblique limb or two limbs of a Bruner incision over the A1 pulley region often can be used to retrieve the retracted tendon.
  - Care is taken to preserve the A2 and A4 pulleys.
- For open reduction of isolated DIP dislocations, the approach is dictated by the direction of the dislocation.
  - Dorsal dislocations are approached volarly, and volar dislocations are approached dorsally.

TECHNIQUES

Treatment of Mallet Fingers

Extension Block Pinning of Mallet Fractures

- The DIP joint is flexed initially, pulling the avulsed fragment volarly.
- A dorsal block pin is inserted obliquely from distal to proximal under fluoroscopy. A 0.045-inch K-wire usually is ideal, although a 0.035-inch K-wire is sometimes preferred if the digit is small.
  - The pin should enter at the dorsal edge of the articular surface of the middle phalanx, and bicortical purchase should be obtained (**TECH FIG 1A,B**). The dorsal blocking pin should *not* engage the fracture fragment, as this may result in comminution of the bone.
  - Anteroposterior and lateral views on fluoroscopy should be obtained to ensure appropriate positioning (**TECH FIG 1C**).
- The distal phalanx is then extended, reducing and compressing the fracture.
- A second K-wire is inserted in a retrograde manner from the distal tip of the distal phalanx to the level of the DIP joint (**TECH FIG 1D**).
- While holding the digit extended with the fracture and DIP joint reduced, the second smooth K-wire is advanced retrograde across the DIP joint into the middle phalanx (**TECH FIG 1E,F**). It is not necessary to have the DIP joint in full extension.
- The K-wires are cut, and protective plastic caps are placed over the exposed ends.
- The finger is then placed in a protective dressing.

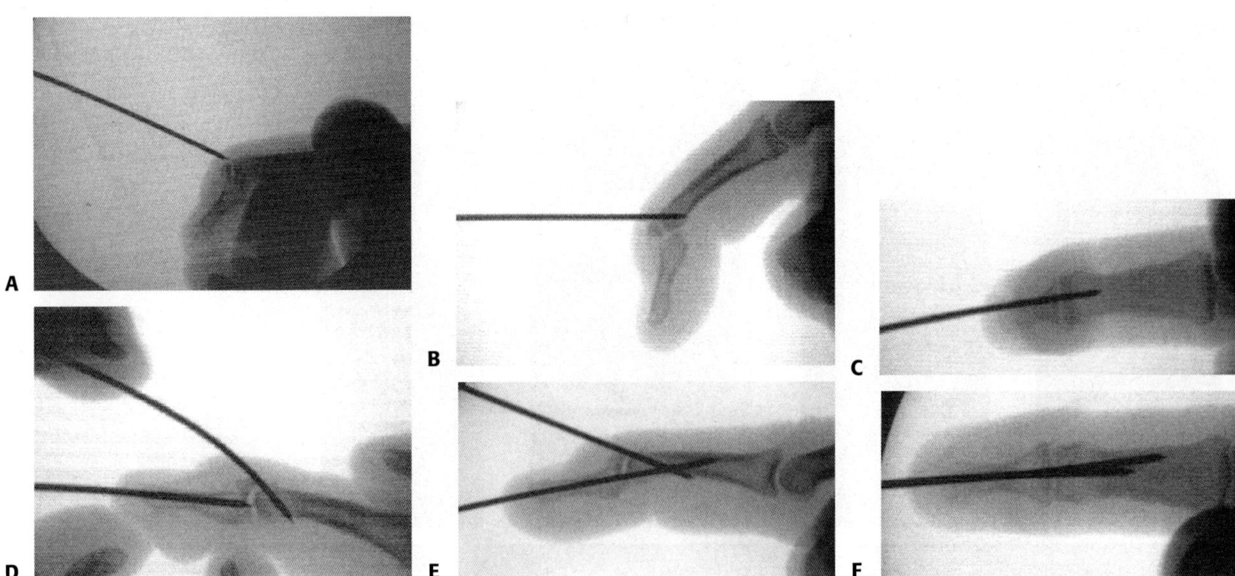

TECH FIG 1 • **A.** With the DIP joint flexed, a K-wire is inserted at the dorsal edge of the articular surface of the middle phalanx. **B.** Bicortical purchase is obtained. **C.** PA fluoroscopic image confirms good bony purchase in both the dorsal and volar phalanx. **D.** With the DIP joint extended, a retrograde K-wire is introduced through the tip of the distal phalanx. **E.** Once reduction is confirmed, this retrograde pin is advanced into the middle phalanx. **F.** A final PA image confirms good placement of pins.

Pinning of Non-Bony Mallet Fingers

- For patients whose compliance is in doubt, or to assist with occupational requirements, a single 0.045-, 0.054-, or 0.062-inch K-wire can be inserted in a retrograde manner through an extended DIP joint.
- The pin can be left either protruding through the skin and covered with a pin cap or just under the skin.
- The patient is counseled on not tapping or hitting the distal tip of the digit against anything hard, as this may force the pin deeper into the distal tuft, making removal much more difficult.

Pull-through Button Technique for Flexor Digitorum Profundus Avulsions

- The fingers are held in an extended position using an aluminum hand.
- The volar surface of the injured finger is exposed through a Bruner incision, and the edges of the avulsed tendon are identified (**TECH FIG 2A**).
- The proximal segment of the tendon is retrieved, pulled out to length, and secured using a small-gauge needle directed transversely across the tendon (**TECH FIG 2B**).
- Using a 2-0 monofilament nonabsorbable suture (or other permanent suture appropriate for tendon repair), the proximal segment of the avulsed tendon is captured using a Krackow or Bunnell suture technique (**TECH FIG 2C**).
- The proximal segment of tendon is then threaded through the flexor pulley system.
- The volar base of the distal phalanx is prepared with a rongeur to expose the bleeding bone.
- Two straight Keith needles are introduced into the volar wound and, using a wire driver, driven from the volar base of the distal phalanx, through the nail bed, and exiting through the center of the fingernail on the dorsal side (**TECH FIG 2D,E**).
- A small square of sterile felt and a plastic sterile button are placed over the exposed tips of the Keith needles (**TECH FIG 2F**).
- The two free ends of suture are threaded through the eyelets of the Keith needles, and the needles are advanced through the nail bed, felt, and button.
- The distal end of the avulsed tendon is pulled into its prepared footprint at the volar base of the distal phalanx, and the suture is then carefully tied over the button (**TECH FIG 2G,H**).
  - Additional fixation is obtained by securing the tendon to tendon remnants at the insertion site.
- As an alternative to tying over the nail and a button, the Keith needles may be advanced through the proximal portion of the distal phalanx, avoiding the germinal matrix. A 3-mm transverse incision is then made over the exiting Keith needles, and the suture is tied down on bone.
- The wound is closed in standard fashion, and the hand is secured in a dorsal extension blocking splint (**TECH FIG 2I**).

Suture Anchor Technique for Flexor Digitorum Profundus Avulsions

- The approach, identification, and suture of the avulsed profundus tendon are the same as in the pull-through button technique.
- One or ideally two small suture anchors are introduced into the volar base of the distal phalanx in a trajectory from proximal volar to distal dorsal or in a distal volar to proximal dorsal direction.[9] Special care is required to ensure the dorsal cortex is not violated. This placement ensures maximum bony purchase in the thickest portion of the distal phalanx and ensures maximum pullout strength.
- Fluoroscopic imaging can be used to ensure proper anchor placement and document that the suture anchors have not penetrated the dorsal cortex or the joint.
- A modified Kessler pattern of suturing can then be used to secure the FDP tendon in place at the base of the distal phalanx.
- The wound is closed and a dorsal extension block splint applied.

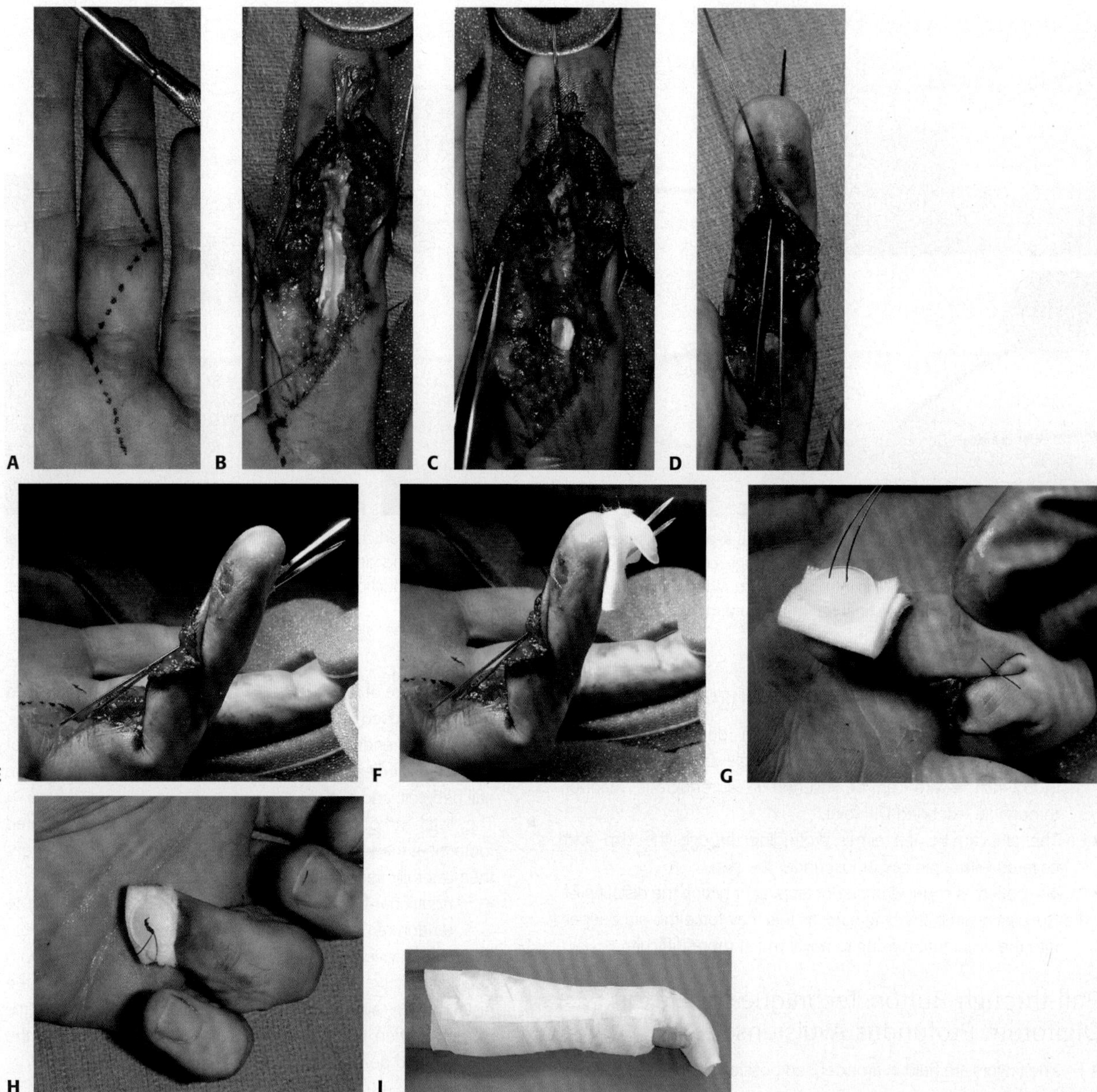

TECH FIG 2 • **A.** A volar Bruner incision is planned. **B.** The avulsed tendon is identified and held in the wound with a small-gauge needle. **C.** The avulsed tendon is captured with a Krackow technique. **D.** Keith needles are advanced through the volar wound to exit in the center of the fingernail. **E.** A side view shows the Keith needles exiting through the fingernail. **F.** Sterile felt and a plastic button are threaded over the needles. **G.** The finger is flexed down, and the sutures are pulled through. **H.** The suture is securely tied over the button. **I.** The patient is immobilized initially in an extension block splint.

Treatment Technique for Flexor Digitorum Profundus Disruption with Bony Avulsion

- If the avulsed fragment is small, the bony fragment can be excised and the tendon repaired as previously described.
- If the avulsed fragment is large enough, open reduction and internal fixation using small screws, intraosseous wiring, or even a small plate is recommended (**TECH FIG 3A–C**).[5,10]
- If there is an associated fracture with the bony FDP avulsion, further fixation may be required and often includes pinning the DIP joint (**TECH FIG 4A–C**). In addition to providing further support, this often eases the difficulties of reducing the FDP fragment.
- It is recommended that the fragment have a diameter at least 2½ times the diameter of the screw to avoid comminution of the bony fragment.[9]
- If comminution of the avulsed fragment precludes fixation, then the bony fragment can be removed from the tendon and placed in the defect as simple bone graft. The remaining tendon can then be secured using a pull-through technique as described earlier.
- Intraoperative radiographs are imperative to confirm reduction.

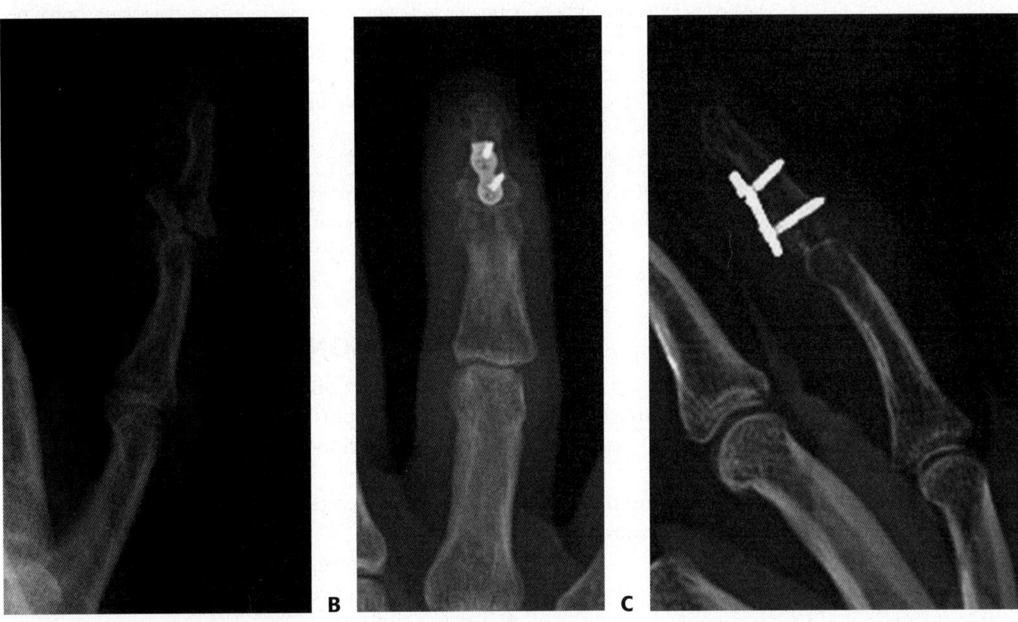

TECH FIG 3 • **A.** When a large bony fragment is present, plate fixation can control the fragment more precisely than a pull-through technique.[5] A large bony fracture is seen in this type 3 avulsion. **B,C.** Postoperative images of successful plate fixation of the large fragment.

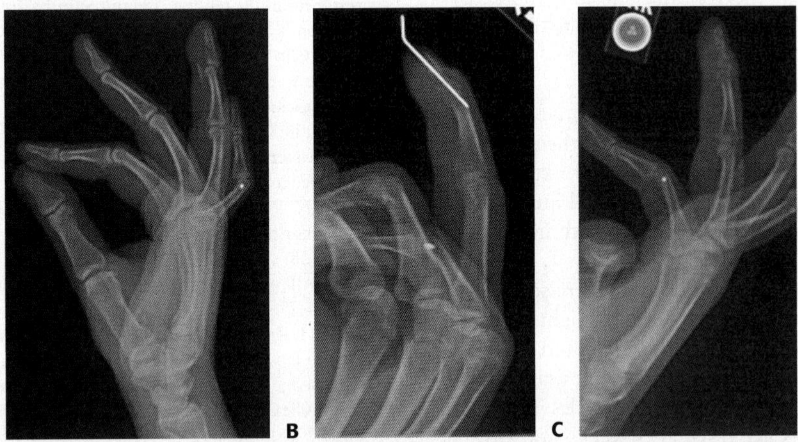

TECH FIG 4 • **A.** In this injury type 5A avulsion, the large FDP bony avulsion was coupled with a transverse shaft fracture. **B.** A single K-wire was placed across the shaft fracture and the DIP joint to provide a stable foundation for FDP repair. The first attempt at plate fixation resulted in comminution of the bony fragment, so the bony fragments were excised and packed in the defect at the volar surface of the distal phalanx. The tendon was then repaired using a pull-through technique. **C.** Final imaging demonstrates complete healing of the bony avulsion and the transverse shaft fracture at 8 weeks.

PEARLS AND PITFALLS

Prevent proximal pin migration in non-bony mallet fingers	■ For cases in which the pin is buried, we prefer to make a small 90-degree bend in the distal end of the wire to prevent proximal migration of the pin into the phalanges.
Tendon retrieval in FDP avulsions	■ It is helpful to use a "milking" technique from proximal to distal in the forearm and palm, with the wrist in a flexed position, to deliver the proximal end of the tendon. Doing so can often decrease the length of the incision that is required for the repair.
Skin irritation with the use of button	■ It is recommended to place a small piece of felt between the patient's nail and the button to decrease irritation (see **TECH FIG 2F,G**).

PIP flexion contracture	▪ Delayed treatment of a type I FDP avulsion can result in a PIP flexion contracture. If nearly full passive joint extension is not obtainable following tendon reinsertion, the repair should be abandoned.
Extension block pinning	▪ Full DIP extension is not required to achieve reduction of the fracture. ▪ Avoid multiple attempts at K-wire placement. ▪ Avoid forced extension of the DIP joint, which may result in fracture at the entrance site of the dorsal block K-wire. ▪ Early treatment is often easier and more effective.
Improper length of screw	▪ Too short will lead to difficulty maintaining the reduction ▪ Too long will cause irritation to the extensor, pain, and possible germinal matrix/nail damage

POSTOPERATIVE CARE

- Mallet fractures (extension block pinning technique)
  - The patient is allowed nearly full activity immediately postoperatively including PIP joint and MCP joint motion.
  - An antibiotic ointment may be applied to the pin sites twice daily, but avoid constant moisture and resultant maceration to the skin.
  - The patient should be counseled thoroughly on keeping pin sites clean.
  - The patient is seen for follow-up around postoperative day 10 and as needed for 4 weeks.
  - Pins are removed in the office setting when there is no tenderness to palpation at the fracture site and there is evidence of bridging trabeculae at the fracture site (usually about 4 to 5 weeks).
- FDP avulsions/lacerations
  - The patient is evaluated 3 to 5 days postoperatively, and if a strong repair has been accomplished and the patient is deemed compliant, a forearm-based dorsal extension block splint is fitted, and the patient is enrolled into a directed hand therapy rehabilitation protocol with immediate edema control.
  - In the compliant patient, place-and-hold exercises, initially in the splint and then with the wrist in slight extension, are started between postoperative days 5 and 7.
  - Further progression is based on the protocol described by Cannon and Strickland,[2] and typically includes tendon glides and wrist tenodesis activities at 5 weeks and progressive strengthening at 7 to 8 weeks.

OUTCOMES

- For extension block pinning of mallet fractures, one study by the primary author reported average time to bony union of 35 days.
  - At an average follow-up time of 74 weeks, range of motion averaged 4 to 78 degrees.[4]
- Most patients with FDP avulsions treated acutely are able to work between 8 and 18 weeks after the surgery, with some studies suggesting that an earlier return to work is seen with a suture anchor repair.
  - An 8- to 10-degree flexion contracture and a similar lack of terminal flexion at the DIP joint often are encountered.[11]
- For isolated dislocations of the DIP joint, case studies suggest that active range of motion at the DIP joint from 0 to 65 degrees is regained by 4 to 12 months postreduction.[12,13]

COMPLICATIONS

- Pin tract infection
- Migration of pins
- Loss of reduction
- Nail deformity
- Dorsal skin necrosis
- Joint stiffness
- Loss of grip strength
- Tendon adherence
- Tendon rupture

REFERENCES

1. Al-Qattan MM. Type 5 avulsion of the insertion of the flexor digitorum profundus tendon. J Hand Surg Br 2001;26(5):427–431.
2. Cannon NM, Strickland JW. Therapy following flexor tendon surgery. Hand Clin 1985;1(1):147–165.
3. Hofmeister EP, Craven CE Jr. Zone I rupture of the flexor digitorum profundus tendon caused by blunt trauma: a case report. J Hand Surg Am 2008;33(2):247–249.
4. Hofmeister EP, Mazurek MT, Shin AY, et al. Extension block pinning for large mallet fractures. J Hand Surg Am 2003;28(3):453–459.
5. Kang N, Pratt A, Burr N. Miniplate fixation for avulsion injuries of the flexor digitorum profundus insertion. J Hand Surg Br 2003;28(4):363–368.
6. Leddy JP. Avulsions of the flexor digitorum profundus. Hand Clin 1985;1:77–83.
7. Lee DH, Robbin ML, Galliott R, et al. Ultrasound evaluation of flexor tendon lacerations. J Hand Surg Am 2000;25(2):236–241.
8. Leversedge FJ, Ditsios K, Goldfarb CA, et al. Vascular anatomy of the human flexor digitorum profundus tendon insertion. J Hand Surg Am 2002;27(5):806–812.
9. Lubahn JD, Hood JM. Fractures of the distal interphalangeal joint. Clin Orthop Relat Res 1996;(327):12–20.
10. Markenson DB, Mughal M, Subramanian P, et al. The simple wire interosseous fixation technique (SWIFT) for reattachment of FDP avulsions with a large bony fragment. Tech Hand Up Extrem Surg 2012;16(4):220–224.
11. McCallister WV, Ambrose HC, Katolik LI, et al. Comparison of pull-out button versus suture anchor for zone I flexor tendon repair. J Hand Surg Am 2006;31(2):246–251.
12. Morisawa Y, Ikegami H, Izumida R. Irreducible palmar dislocation of the distal interphalangeal joint. J Hand Surg 2006;31:296–297.
13. Pohl AL. Irreducible dislocation of a distal interphalangeal joint. J Plast Reconstr Aesthet Surg 1976;29:227–229.
14. Rizis D, Mahoney J. A rare presentation of flexor digitorum profundus type V avulsion injury with associated intra-articular fracture: a case report. Can J Plast Surg 2011;19:62–63.
15. Schweitzer TP, Rayan GM. The terminal tendon of the digital extensor mechanism: part I, anatomic study. J Hand Surg Am 2004;29:898–902.
16. Smith JH Jr. Avulsion of a profundus tendon with simultaneous intraarticular fracture of the distal phalanx—case report. J Hand Surg Am 1981;6:600–601.
17. Wehbé MA, Schneider LH. Mallet fractures. J Bone Joint Surg 1984;66:658–669.

Corrective Osteotomy for Metacarpal and Phalangeal Malunion

Nilesh M. Chaudhari, Mohamed Khalid, and Thomas R. Hunt III

DEFINITION

- *Malunion* results when a fracture fragment heals in incorrect anatomic alignment.

ANATOMY

- Metacarpals and phalanges are tubular structures with a smooth dorsal surface covered by the extensor tendon and its expansions.
- Metacarpals are triangular in cross-section. The medial and lateral surfaces meet at the volar ridge, providing attachment to the interossei. These attachments together with the intermetacarpal ligaments proximally and distally help splint fractured bones, making functionally significant malunions of the ring and small metacarpals less common.
- Phalanges are bean-shaped in cross-section. The volar aspects of the proximal and middle phalanges are in intimate relation to the flexor digitorum profundus (FDP) and flexor digitorum superficialis (FDS) tendons, particularly in the region of the annular pulleys (**FIG 1**).
  - As a result, the tendons are vulnerable to damage from drills and screws used in a dorsovolar direction. This problem is especially significant in the region of the annular pulleys, where the tendons are strapped against the volar cortex, rendering them vulnerable to damage.

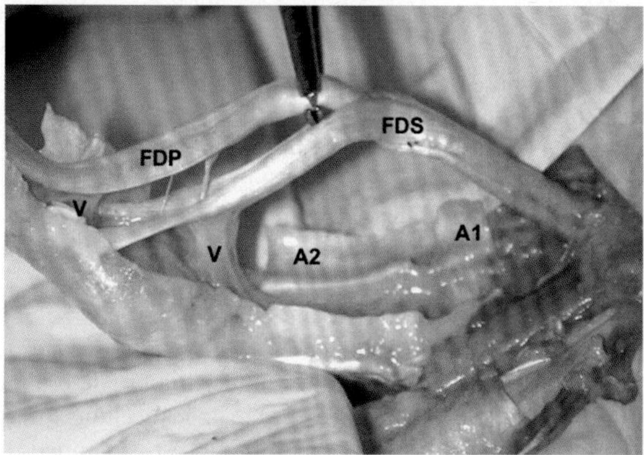

FIG 1 • Structures on the volar aspect of the metacarpals and phalanges. The flexor digitorum profundus (*FDP*) and flexor digitorum superficialis (*FDS*) tendons are intimately associated with the volar aspect of the phalanges and, to a lesser extent, the metacarpals. This dissected specimen also depicts the vinculae (*V*) and the A1 and A2 annular pulleys. (From http://www.turntillburn.ch.)

PATHOGENESIS

- Malunions most often occur secondary to lack of treatment or inadequate nonoperative care.[9]
  - Malunion following internal fixation is uncommon, but when present usually results from inadequate stability or poor patient compliance.
- Extra-articular malunions (EAM) often are multiplanar, but usually there is one major component to the deformity that causes the functional deficit.[8]
- The more proximal the malunion, the greater the deformity.
  - Just 1 degree of rotation at the fracture site may translate to 5 degrees at the fingertip.[6]
  - Five degrees of fracture malrotation can cause 1.5 cm of digital overlap when the fingers are flexed.[2]
- Soft tissue pathology such as neurovascular deficits, trophic changes, joint contractures, and tendon adhesions can coexist.
  - Results of corrective osteotomy are significantly poorer in the presence of such complicating factors.[1]

NATURAL HISTORY

- Significant EAM can cause crossing or scissoring of fingers, pain due to distortion of joints, disturbance of muscle/tendon balance, and reduction of grip strength.[1]
- EAMs associated with shortening can lead to an extension lag proportional to the degree of shortening. The effect is more pronounced in proximal phalanges compared to metacarpals.[13]
- Intra-articular malunion (IAM) with a significant step (0.5 mm) or gap (1 mm) may cause joint surface incongruity, synovitis, capsular loosening or stiffness, and, ultimately, painful posttraumatic arthrosis.[1,4]

PATIENT HISTORY AND PHYSICAL FINDINGS

- The value of a good history and physical examination cannot be overemphasized. The decision as to whether surgical treatment is to be offered depends almost entirely on a history suggestive of a significant functional impairment or pain.
- Injury specifics
  - The original injury and method(s) of treatment
  - Location
    - Phalanx versus metacarpal
    - Extra-articular versus intra-articular versus combined deformities
  - History of complicating factors, for example, infection and chronic mediated pain syndrome

- Duration of malunion, particularly relevant in deciding surgical strategy (reducing the fracture vs. osteotomy)
- Associated injuries such as soft tissue defects and neurovascular injuries
- Specific patient characteristics
  - Skeletal maturity
  - Hand dominance
  - Degree of deformity, swelling, stiffness, weakness of grip, and pain
  - Occupation and avocational pursuits as well as patient expectations and goals
  - Ability to cooperate with postoperative therapy regimen

IMAGING AND OTHER DIAGNOSTIC STUDIES

- Good-quality radiographs taken in three precise planes (anteroposterior, lateral, and oblique) are sufficient for simple EAMs.
  - Radiographs of the opposite hand are helpful in preoperative planning for complex EAMs.
- IAMs and combined malunions may require computed tomography (CT) scans with three-dimensional reconstruction.

DIFFERENTIAL DIAGNOSIS

- Fibrous nonunion
- Nonunion with soft tissue contracture
- Sequelae of epiphyseal injury or growth arrest
- Erosive arthritis

NONOPERATIVE MANAGEMENT

- Hand therapy is directed toward maximizing the range of motion (ROM) of the digits, promoting optimal tendon excursion, and improving the grip strength.
- In less dramatic deformities, physical therapy is the first-line treatment. Many patients will gain enough functional improvement that they decide to "live with" the deformity.
- Initiation of therapy allows the opportunity to assess the patient's personality with respect to compliance and realistic expectations.

SURGICAL MANAGEMENT

Timing of Correction

- Treatment of nascent malunions results in improved outcomes.
- IAMs must be corrected as soon as possible if there is a significant articular step and no overwhelming technical difficulties are anticipated.[1]
- In the case of an EAM, after 6 to 8 weeks from the injury, a "wait and watch" policy before osteotomy is advisable to see whether the malunion causes significant functional or cosmetic problems.

Location of Correction

- At or near the apex of the deformity for angular and complex EAMs
- In the proximal metaphysis of the malunited bone for rotational EAMs. With improved osteotomy techniques and fixation implants, a proximal metacarpal osteotomy is no longer recommended for treatment of a P1 rotational malunion.[1]

Type of Osteotomy

- For most angular EAMs, a closing wedge osteotomy is preferable, especially in the setting of intrinsic tightness. This approach is most commonly used for dorsal apex metacarpal malunions.
- An opening wedge osteotomy is best for angular EAMs in the setting of an extension lag and pseudoclaw deformity, which are more commonly seen in apex volar phalangeal malunions.
- An incomplete osteotomy may be used for either of these cases.
- For rotational and combined rotational/angular EAM correction, a complete osteotomy is required.[6] Metacarpal neck EAM from a previous boxer's fracture without significant shortening may be corrected with a pivot osteotomy.[12]
- Condylar advancement osteotomy[11] is suitable for IAM correction in many cases.
- Step cut osteotomy[3,5,7] provides correction for rotational deformity providing large surface area of bone healing and allows early mobilization.

Severity of Deformity

- Malunion does not always mandate a corrective osteotomy. Patients possess a significant capacity to adapt to minor deformities. For instance, slight overlap of adjacent digits due to rotational malunion may be unsettling and unsightly, but it is consistent with good hand function.[8] Similarly, a proximal diaphyseal malunion of the small finger metacarpal can contribute to tendon imbalance and flexion contracture of the proximal interphalangeal (PIP) joint, but the hand may function effectively.[10]
- Multifragment IAMs and those with established posttraumatic arthrosis are best treated by arthrodesis or arthroplasty rather than repositioning osteotomy.

Preoperative Planning

- In addition to precise evaluation of the bony deformity, careful assessment of the soft tissue envelope, gliding capacity of the flexor and extensor tendons, joint mobility, and neurovascular status is critical.
  - Plan for adjunct procedures (eg, tenolysis, capsulotomy) that may be required.
  - Determine the optimal location for placement of internal fixation.
  - Decide on opening or closing wedge osteotomy. In the presence of an extension lag, an opening wedge is preferred, whereas in the presence of intrinsic tightness, a closing wedge is preferred.
  - Provide for soft tissue coverage as needed.
- Preoperative templates are created for bony correction.
  - The proximal and distal fragments are each outlined then superimposed over an outline of the contralateral uninjured bone.
  - The type and location of the osteotomy, the size of the bone graft needed (in the case of an opening wedge osteotomy), as well as the method of fixation are determined.
  - In the rare cases requiring large corticocancellous interposition grafts, iliac crest bone graft harvest is planned.

Positioning

- The patient is positioned supine with the shoulder abducted to 90 degrees, elbow extended, and the extremity on an arm table.
- Place a proximal arm, nonsterile tourniquet.
- If required, prep for ipsilateral iliac crest graft harvest.

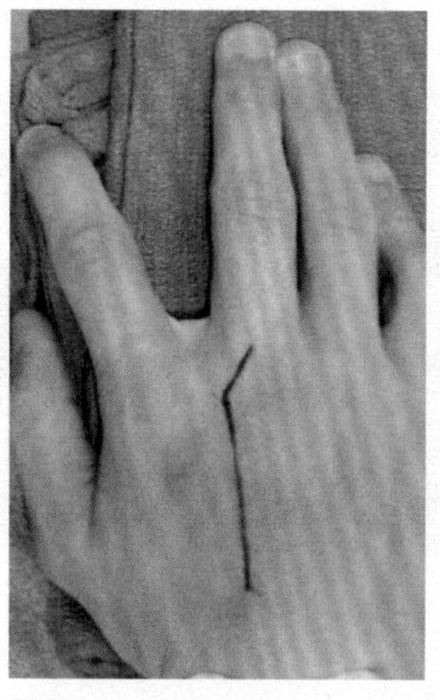
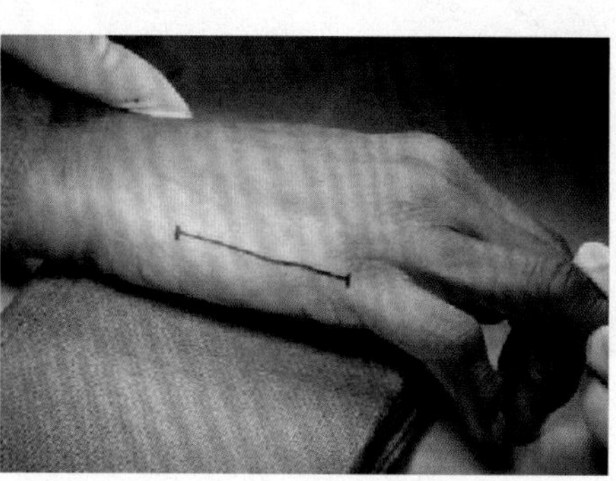
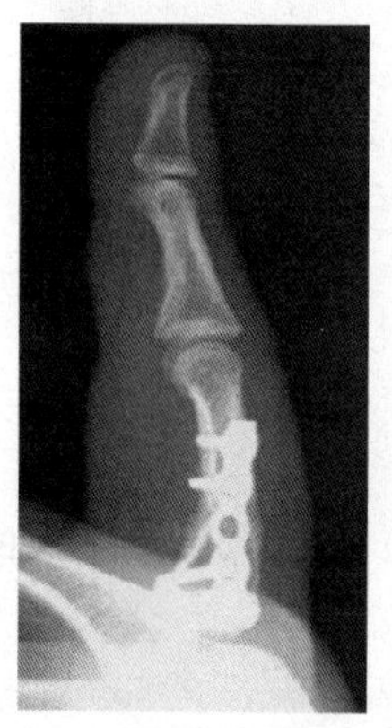
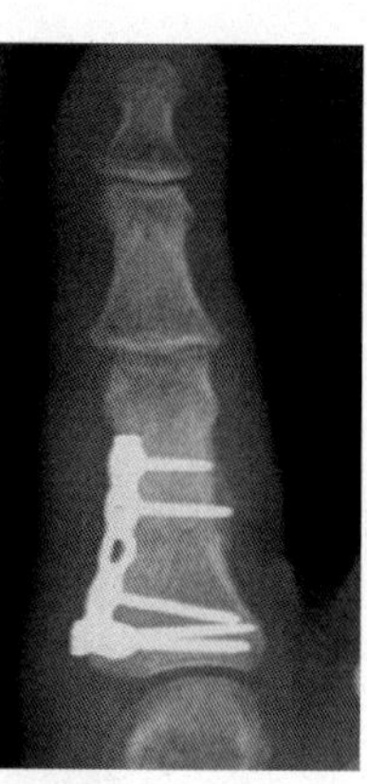

FIG 2 • **A.** Skin incision used for a dorsal approach to a third metacarpal malunion. The longitudinal limb of the skin incision runs between the metacarpals, and depending on whether the malunion is proximal or distal, the appropriate end is curved. **B.** Skin incision at the junction of the glabrous skin for an osteotomy of the fifth metacarpal. A similar midaxial incision is employed for phalangeal malunion correction. **C,D.** Coronal plane correction of a proximal phalangeal malunion. The plate has been placed laterally to avoid interfering with the extensor mechanism as well to avoid damage to the flexor tendons while drilling and inserting screws.

- Perform an examination under anesthesia to determine joint ROM and stability.

Approach

- A dorsal approach through a dorsal skin incision in the intermetacarpal space is used for the second through fourth metacarpals (**FIG 2A**).
- A midaxial approach through a midaxial skin incision at the junction of the wrinkled dorsal and smooth volar skin is used for the fifth metacarpal and the proximal and middle phalanges (**FIG 2B**).
  - Coronal plane correction is best accomplished with a lateral buttress plate placed over the bone graft (**FIG 2C,D**).
  - Dorsal plates should be avoided in the phalanges due to extensor tendon adhesions and resulting loss of motion.

Method of Fixation

- Kirschner wire (K-wire): allows adequate fixation for basal extra-articular osteotomy
- Interfragmentary lag screw: ideal fixation for step cut and condylar advancement osteotomies and allows early mobilization
- Plate fixation: provides rigid fixation that allows early mobilization. Locking plates allow unicortical screw fixation that minimize the potential of tendon penetration on the far side of the bone.

TECHNIQUES

Incomplete Osteotomy for Angular Correction

Metacarpal Closing Wedge Osteotomy

- Make a dorsal incision in the interval between either the index–long or ring–small metacarpals, depending on the bone to be treated (see **FIG 2A**).
  - An incision at the junction of the glabrous skin often is appropriate for small metacarpal malunion correction (see **FIG 2B**).
- Retract the extensor tendon to expose the metacarpal (**TECH FIG 1A**).
- Make a dorsolateral incision through the metacarpal's periosteum and carefully free this layer from the dorsum of the metacarpal with a no. 15 blade (**TECH FIG 1B**).
  - At completion of the operation, this periosteal and muscle layer will be closed, serving to protect the extensor tendons from the underlying internal fixation.
- Subperiosteally expose the circumference of the bone at the planned osteotomy site.
- Pass two small Hohmann retractors, one radially and one ulnarly, to protect the tendons and neurovascular structures.
  - Take care not to put undue tension on these structures.
- Precisely identify the apex of the deformity by determining the intersection between the true anatomic axis of both the proximal and distal fragments.
  - Place a 0.35-mm K-wire parallel to the proximal fragment, and under radiographic guidance, mark the anatomic axis using diathermy or a marking pen.
  - Mark the distal fragment in a similar manner.
- Design the osteotomy around the intersection of these two marks (**TECH FIG 1C**).
  - Plan the cuts perpendicular to the long axis of each fragment.
  - The size of the bone wedge to be removed is determined based on preoperative templates and intraoperative measurements.
- Center and apply a six- or seven-hole 2.0- to 2.7-mm compression plate to the dorsum of one fragment using two screws.
  - Moderately tighten the screws.

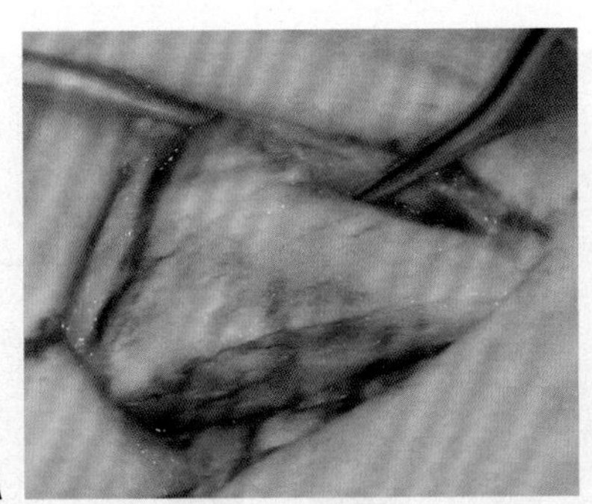
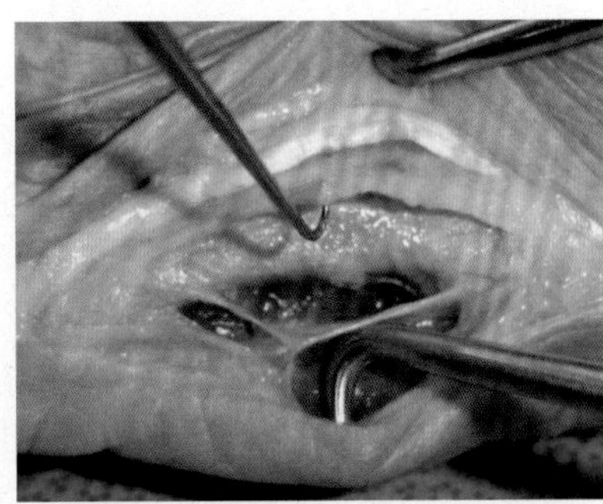
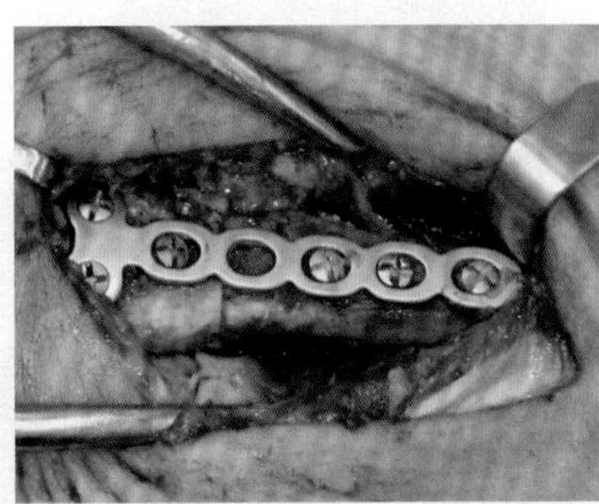
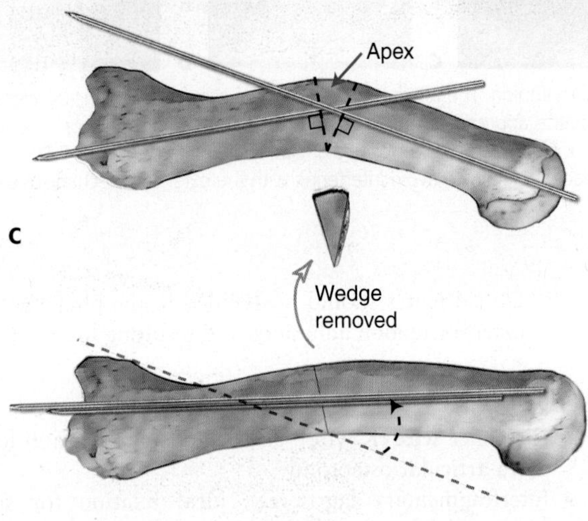

TECH FIG 1 • A. Extensor tendons have been retracted to expose the dorsal surface of the metacarpal sagittal plane malunion. **B.** The deep subtendinous layer of the metacarpal is demonstrated. Note that the periosteum is still intact. This layer is repaired covering the implant to prevent tendon adhesions. **C,D.** Method using K-wires to determine the apex of the deformity. After removing a wedge, the size of which is determined by preoperative templating (**C**), deformity correction is confirmed when the K-wire markings are observed to be parallel (**D**). **E.** Dorsally applied T plate with three screws distal and three screws proximal to the osteotomy.

  - Plan for six cortices of fixation proximal and distal to the osteotomy if possible.
  - Juxta-articular osteotomies are best stabilized using condylar plates, T plates, or Y plates. Locking plates also may be of value in these cases.
- Remove one screw and rotate the plate away from the osteotomy site.
- Create an incomplete osteotomy, starting on the dorsal convex surface and using a water-cooled sagittal saw or sharp osteotome.
  - Complete the distal bone cut before making the proximal bone cut.
  - An elastic pillar of bone is left intact volarly on the concave side to act as a hinge.
  - In some cases, complete correction and osteotomy reduction can be obtained only if the volar cortex is cut and only the volar periosteum is left intact as the hinge.
- Correction is adequate when the true anatomic axes of the proximal and distal fragments are parallel (**TECH FIG 1D**).
  - The dorsal plate often will serve as a guide to reduction when it sits flat on the dorsum of both fragments.
- Reapply the plate, tightening the two screws. Reduce the osteotomy, and secure the other fragment by applying the other side of the plate in compression (**TECH FIG 1E**).
- Insert the remaining screws and assess reduction clinically and radiographically.
- Close the periosteal and muscle layer between the plate and the extensor tendons with absorbable suture and close the skin in the usual manner.
- Place a forearm-based splint with the wrist mildly extended and the metacarpophalangeal (MP) joints immobilized in 60 to 70 degrees of flexion. The PIP joints are left free.

Phalangeal Opening Wedge Osteotomy

- Make a midaxial skin incision (**TECH FIG 2A**).
- Protect against injury to the dorsal sensory nerve branch (**TECH FIG 2B**).
- Incise the lateral band as required (**TECH FIG 2C**), and expose the circumference of the bone subperiosteally at the site of the planned osteotomy.
- Use a "no touch" technique with the extensors and insert small Hohmann retractors to visualize the bone and the deformity.
- Apply K-wires to precisely locate the site of the deformity and serve as a guide for correction in the manner detailed earlier (**TECH FIG 2D,E**).
- Make an incomplete osteotomy on the concave side at the apex of the deformity perpendicular to the distal fragment.
  - Contouring of the bone graft is simplified if the osteotomy is made perpendicular to the distal fragment. This leaves only the proximal portion of the graft irregular.
- Provisionally stabilize the fragments with a longitudinal K-wire and assess clinically and radiographically.

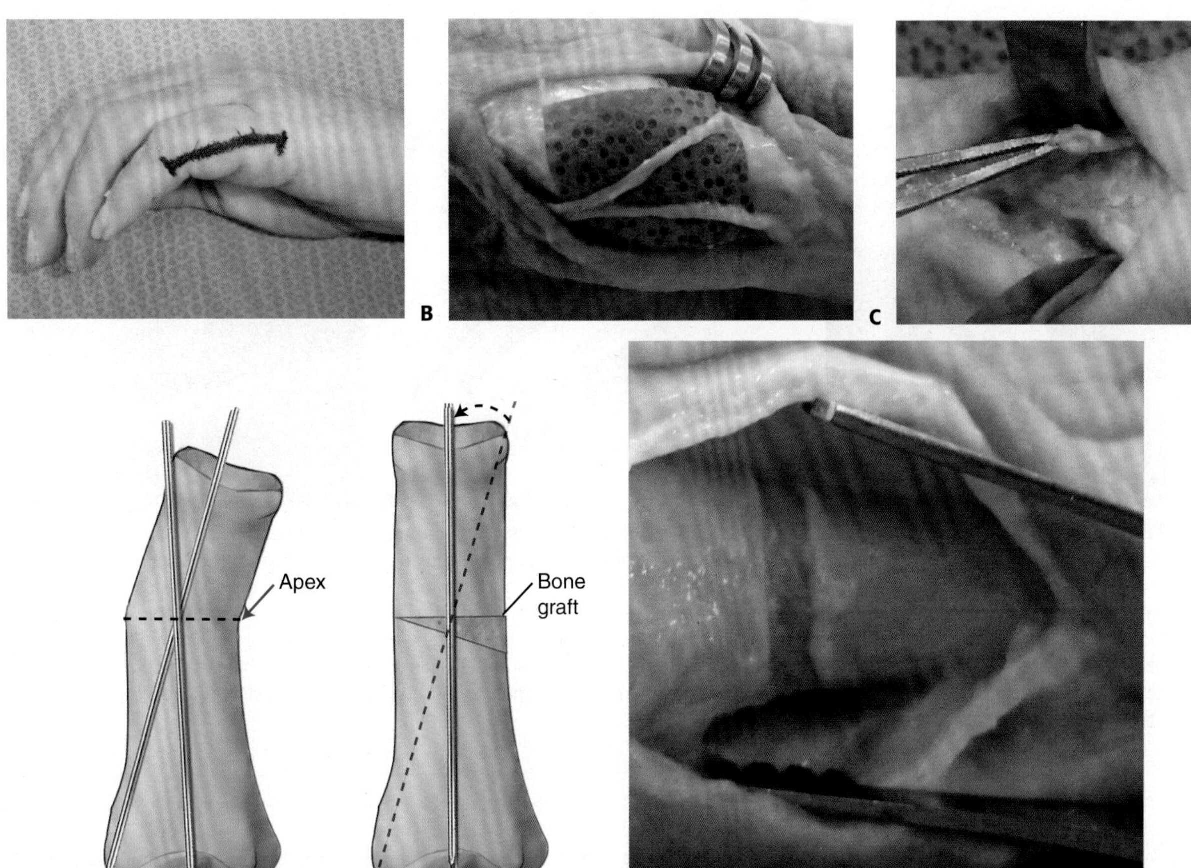

TECH FIG 2 • **A.** Lateral incision for proximal phalangeal osteotomy. **B.** Dorsal cutaneous nerve. **C.** Lateral approach to the proximal phalanx. The sagittal band has been cut and elevated to expose the proximal phalanx. **D.** Method of determining the apex of the deformity for an opening wedge osteotomy. **E.** With the deformity adequately corrected, the wire markings are parallel or overlapping. **F.** The corticocancellous graft has been inserted into the defect correcting the deformity.

- Harvest either a corticocancellous wedge of bone or cancellous bone from the dorsal distal radius just proximal and ulnar to Lister's tubercle.
  - The size of the graft is determined by preoperative templating and intraoperative measurement.
- Contour the graft using a water-cooled sagittal saw.
- Insert the graft to correct the deformity and apply a lateral six-or seven-hole 1.5- to 2.0-mm compression plate (**TECH FIG 2F**).
  - Plan for six cortices of fixation proximal and distal to the osteotomy, if possible.
  - Juxta-articular osteotomies are best stabilized using condylar plates, T plates, or Y plates. Locking plates also may be of value.
- If possible, close the thin periosteal layer between the plate and the extensor tendons with absorbable suture and close the skin in the usual manner.
- Do not repair the lateral band. Check the correction clinically and compare with the preoperative pictures.
- Place a forearm-based splint with the wrist mildly extended and the MP joints immobilized in 60 to 70 degrees of flexion. The interphalangeal joints are immobilized in full extension.

Complete Osteotomy for Rotational and Combined Rotational/Angular Malunions

- Perform a dorsal approach for malunions of the second through fourth metacarpals and a lateral approach for the fifth metacarpal and phalangeal malunions, as detailed earlier.
- Identify and mark the true anatomic axis of the proximal and distal fragments using 0.35-mm K-wires under radiographic guidance in the manner already reviewed. Define the apex of the angular deformity (see **TECH FIGS 1C** and **2D,E**).
- Insert one K-wire proximal and one distal to the malunion, perpendicular to the long axis and in a true dorsovolar direction. This defines the rotational deformity.
- In the manner detailed previously, perform the osteotomy (opening vs. closing) needed to correct the angular portion of the malunion using a water-cooled sagittal saw or a sharp osteotome.
  - Insert a longitudinal K-wire to temporarily stabilize the fragments.
  - Early correction of the angular malunion aids in plate contouring and placement.

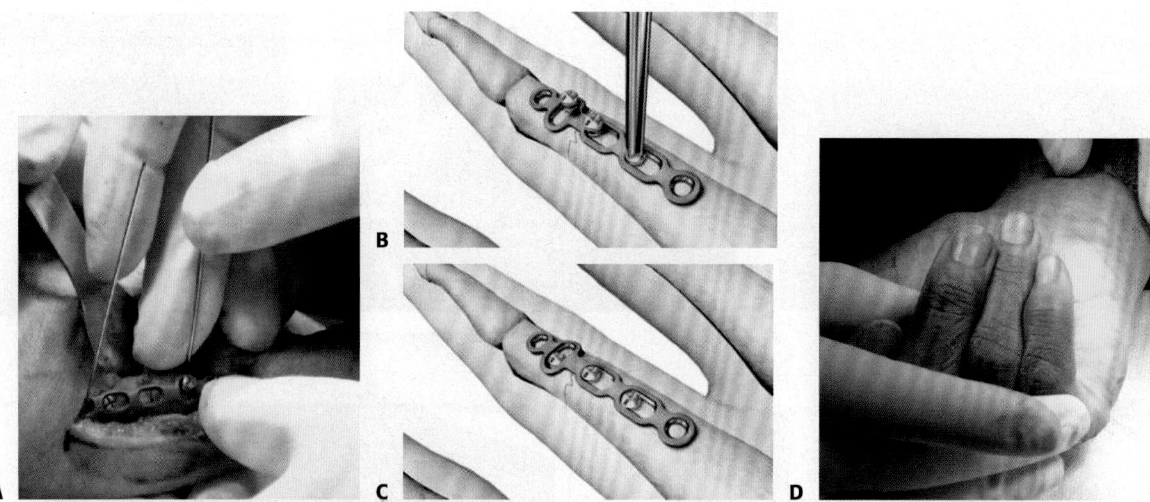

TECH FIG 3 • A. K-wires previously were inserted in the dorsovolar plane, perpendicular to the dorsal surface of the proximal and distal fragments. The position of these K-wires defines the degree of rotational malunion. After correction of the sagittal plane deformity, the K-wires are manipulated into a parallel position to achieve rotational correction. **B,C.** Use of the rotation plates (in this case, VariAx Hand Locking Plate Module [Stryker]). The screw in the perpendicular gliding hole is positioned (but not tightened) ulnar or radial, depending on the direction of the rotational correction desired. The osteotomy is compressed, and the screws in the parallel oblong holes are tightened first. The rotational correction is then obtained, and the gliding hole screw is tightened to obtain controlled correction. **D.** View after correction of a combined rotational and angular malunion of the fifth metacarpal. (**B,C:** Courtesy of Stryker Osteosynthesis.)

- Select a suitable plate (1.5 to 2 mm for P1 and 2.0 to 2.7 mm for metacarpals), contour it to the lateral bony surface of the proximal fragment, align it to the anatomic axis, and insert screws through the plate fixing it to that fragment.
- Harvest, contour, and insert bone graft if required.
- Remove the longitudinal K-wire and correct the rotational portion of the malunion by bringing the dorsovolar K-wires into a parallel position while still maintaining angular correction (**TECH FIG 3A**).
- Secure the distal fragment to the plate in a compression mode.
- Fine-tune the rotational alignment while maintaining the angular correction by using a gliding hole rotation plate (**TECH FIG 3B,C**).
- Check the correction and ROM clinically (**TECH FIG 3D**).
- Close the wound and splint as previously discussed.

Condylar Advancement Osteotomy

- Condylar advancement osteotomy avoids the problem of handling a small condylar malunion (**TECH FIG 4A**), which is difficult to fix securely and is susceptible to osteonecrosis.[12]
- Make a sweeping dorsal, curved skin incision over the involved MP or PIP joint.
  - MP: Incise the sagittal band and then the capsule.
  - PIP: Enter the interval between the lateral band and the central slip and incise the capsule.
  - Protect the origin of the collateral ligament and its accompanying vascularity.
- Carefully dissect the extensor tendon gently off the bone over the region of the proposed osteotomy.
- Evaluate the condition of the joint. If significant arthrosis is present, consider a salvage procedure rather than a repositioning osteotomy.
- Resect a wedge of bone between the condyles with a water-cooled sagittal saw (**TECH FIG 4B**).
- Make a countercut in the diaphysis and advance the malunited condyle distally to restore articular congruity (**TECH FIG 4C**).
- Stabilize the mobilized fragment using interfragmentary screws (**TECH FIG 4D**).
  - Insert the first screw parallel with the joint to ensure precise joint reduction.

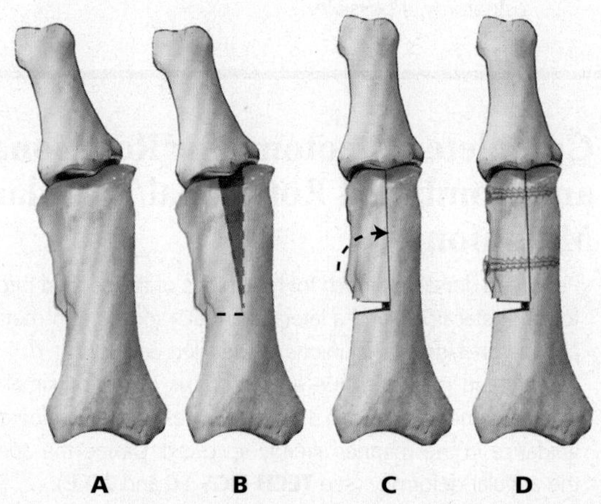

TECH FIG 4 • A–D. Condylar advancement osteotomy for unicondylar malunion.

Step Cut Osteotomy

- It can be used for both metacarpal and phalangeal malunions.
- In the case of a metacarpal EAM, make a dorsal incision in the interval between either index–long or ring–small metacarpals and dorsoulnar for small metacarpal as described earlier.
- Retract the extensor tendons to expose the metacarpal shaft.
- Incise periosteum longitudinally.
- Make hemitransverse cut in the proximal and distal diaphysis 2 to 2.5 cm apart and on opposite sides of shaft as determined by direction of deformity (**TECH FIG 5A**). Place two parallel longitudinal cuts on the dorsal aspect of the shaft connecting the two horizontal cuts. Make sure to leave volar cortex intact. Remove the strip of bone dorsally.
- Close the dorsal gap by using pointed reduction clamp. Crack the volar cortex but leave the periosteum intact.
- Check the digital rotation for correction. Remove another strip of dorsal cortical bone if needed for correction.
- After achieving satisfactory correction, place two parallel 1.5- to 2.0-mm size cortical screws perpendicular to osteotomy site in lag interfragmentary fashion (**TECH FIG 5B**). Check ROM in full flexion and extension.
- Close the periosteum and fascia with absorbable suture and close skin in usual manner.
- Place in forearm-based splint to incorporate the MP joints but allow full ROM of the interphalangeal joints.

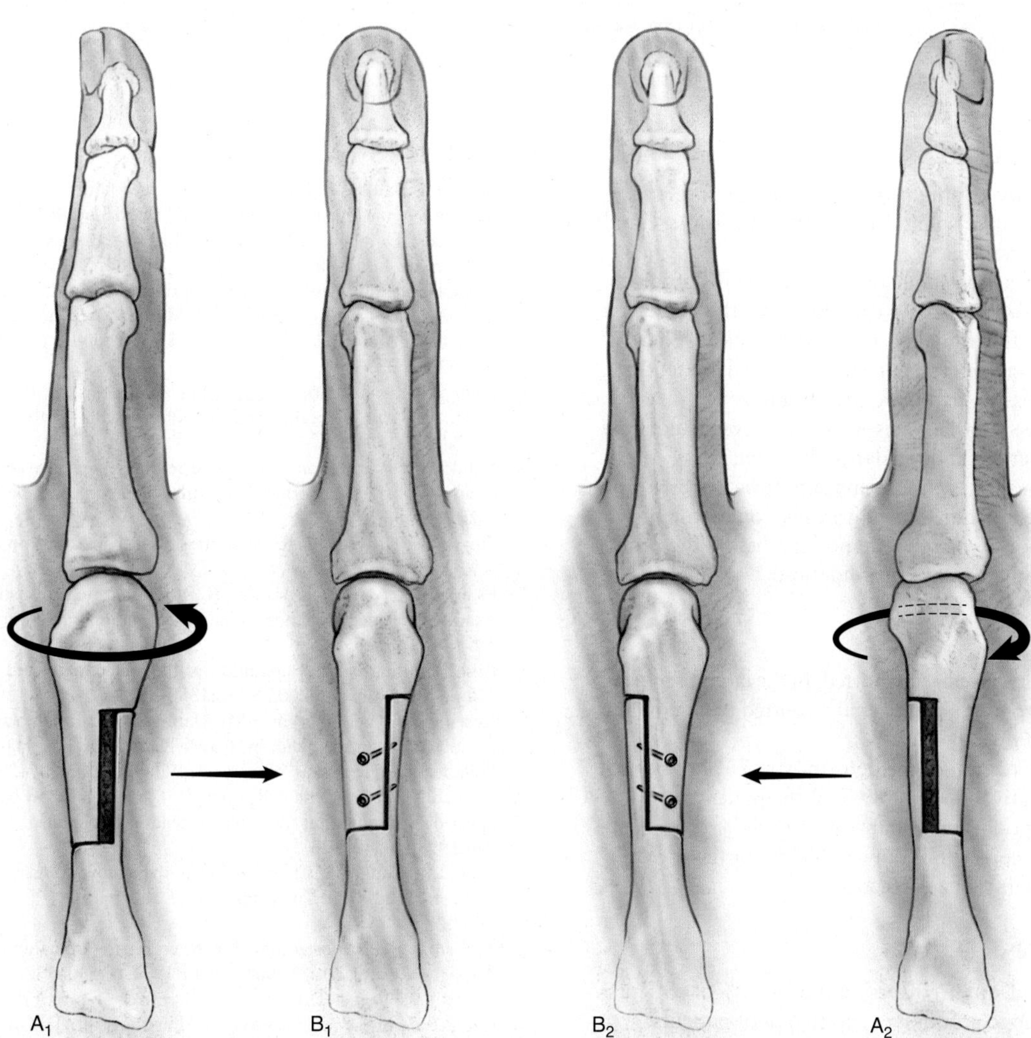

TECH FIG 5 • Step cut osteotomy. **A.** Two horizontal cut are placed in shaft about 2.5 cm apart and a longitudinal wedge cut connecting two horizontal cut is made. Derotation of distal fragment opposite the deformity. **B.** Reduction of the osteotomy and fixation with two interfragmentary screws.

PEARLS AND PITFALLS

Indications	■ Define the goals of treatment with the patient and ensure that they are realistic. ■ In the case of an IAM, consider a salvage procedure rather than a repositioning osteotomy in the face of arthrosis.
Preoperative assessment	■ Understand the "personality" of the malunion as well as the patient. Bony as well as soft tissue aspects of the deformity must be understood.
Operative planning	■ The plane of the deformity and the different components of the deformity, as well as the true extent of the deformity, must be factored in planning the location, orientation, and extent of the osteotomy.
Operative technique	■ Atraumatic bone and soft tissue handling is critical, especially in regard to the extensor mechanism overlying P1. An oscillating power saw with a thin blade and a field of excursion similar to the diameter of the bone is needed. Copious saline irrigation is used to prevent thermal necrosis. ■ Accurate plate and screw placement is essential. A screw offset of 1 mm can cause as much as 10 degrees of rotation.
Implants	■ Stable fixation is needed to allow early ROM. ■ Consider using implants a size larger than used for acute fractures, particularly if extensive soft tissue release has been performed. ■ Newer generation locking plates and screws are valuable when fixation in the metaphysis is required.
Postoperative	■ Institute early postoperative therapy.

POSTOPERATIVE CARE

- If adequate stability is obtained at the time of surgery, remove the postoperative splint 3 to 5 days after surgery and initiate protected motion.
  - Initiate an early active and active-assisted ROM program.
  - When not performing ROM exercises, rest the hand in a volar splint in a functional position (MP joints flexed to 60 to 70 degrees and interphalangeal joints fully extended), apply a compression bandage, and elevate.
- Progress to passive ROM exercises, and use reverse blocking exercises to strengthen and rebalance the extensors.
- If needed, and if healing is progressing appropriately, use static or dynamic splints to address pending joint contractures.
- Encourage functional use of the hand long before the radiographs show complete bony consolidation.

OUTCOMES

- Encouraging results have been reported. In the largest reported series of 59 osteotomies, Büchler et al[1] reported the following:
  - A 100% union rate
  - Satisfactory correction of the deformity in 76% of cases
  - A net gain in active ROM in 89% of the patients
  - Excellent and good functional results in 96% of patients requiring bony corrections only and 64% for those requiring bony and soft tissue correction

COMPLICATIONS

- Incomplete or inadequate correction (up to 24% of patients)
- Iatrogenic damage to soft tissues (up to 4% of patients)
- Residual stiffness

REFERENCES

1. Büchler U, Gupta A, Ruf S. Corrective osteotomy for posttraumatic malunion of the phalanges in the hand. J Hand Surg Br 1996;21:33–42.
2. Freeland AE, Jabaley ME, Hughes JL. Fracture repair: metacarpals and carpals. In: Freeland A, Jabaley M, Hughes J, eds. Stable Fixation of the Hand and Wrist. New York: Springer-Verlag, 1986:35–71.
3. Jawa A, Zucchini M, Lauri G, et al. Modified step-cut osteotomy for metacarpal and phalangeal rotational deformity. J Hand Surg Am 2009;34(2):335–340.
4. Light TR. Salvage of intraarticular malunions of the hand and wrist. The role of realignment osteotomy. Clin Orthop Relat Res 1987;(214):130–135.
5. Manktelow RT, Mahoney JL. Step osteotomy: a precise rotation osteotomy to correct scissoring deformities of the fingers. Plast Reconstr Surg 1981;68:571–576.
6. Opgrande JD, Westphal SA. Fractures of the hand. Orthop Clin North Am 1983;14:779–792.
7. Pichora DR, Meyer R, Masear VR. Rotational step-cut osteotomy for treatment of metacarpal and phalangeal malunion. J Hand Surg Am 1991;16(3):551–555.
8. Ring D. Malunion and nonunion of the metacarpals and phalanges. J Bone Joint Surg Am 2005;87(6):1380–1388.
9. Rosenwasser MP, Quitkin HM. Malunion and other posttraumatic complications in the hand. In: Berger R, Weiss A, eds. Hand Surgery. Philadelphia: Lippincott Williams & Wilkins, 2003:207–230.
10. Strauch RJ, Rosenwasser MP, Lunt JG. Metacarpal shaft fractures: the effect of shortening on the extensor tendon mechanism. J Hand Surg Am 1998;23:519–523.
11. Teoh LC, Yong FC, Chong KC. Condylar advancement osteotomy for correcting condylar malunion of the finger. J Hand Surg Br 2002;27:31–35.
12. Thurston AJ. Pivot osteotomy for the correction of malunion of metacarpal neck fractures. J Hand Surg Br 1992;17:580–582.
13. Vahey JW, Wegner DA, Hastings H. Effect of proximal phalangeal fracture deformity on extensor tendon function. J Hand Surg Am 1998;23:673–681.

Lateral Collateral Ligament Reconstruction of the Elbow

Vikram Sathyendra and Anand M. Murthi

DEFINITION

- Lateral collateral ligament (LCL) injuries most often occur after significant elbow trauma, most commonly after dislocation.
- Attenuation of the LCL can also occur after multiple surgeries to the lateral side of the elbow and after corticosteroid injections.[9] It has recently been reported that even one corticosteroid injection may result in lower complete recovery rates and in recurrence rates after 1 year.[6]
- LCL attenuation has been reported to occur in patients who have residual cubitus varus after malunion of supracondylar humerus fractures.[12]
- Significant injury to the LCL complex can result in posterolateral rotatory instability (PLRI).

ANATOMY

- The LCL is made up of four major components: the lateral ulnar collateral ligament (LUCL), also called the *radial ulnohumeral ligament* (RUHL); the radial collateral ligament (RCL) proper; the annular ligament; and the accessory collateral ligament (**FIG 1**).
- The ligaments originate from a broad band over the lateral epicondyle, deep to the extensor muscle mass, and separate distally into more discrete structures.
- The RUHL is the most important stabilizer against PLRI, and it attaches distally on the supinator crest of the ulna.[11]
- The supinator tubercle resides approximately 15 mm distal to the proximal border of the proximal radioulnar joint (PRUJ).[1]
- The RCL is more anterior and primarily resists varus stress.
- The annular ligament sweeps around the radial head/neck and stabilizes the PRUJ.
- The capsule acts as a static stabilizer, especially at the anterior portion, while the arm is extended.
- The anconeus and extensor muscle groups act as dynamic stabilizers.
- On average, the posterior interosseous nerve crosses the midpoint of the radius 33.4 ± 5.7 mm with the forearm in supination. This distance increases to 52.0 ± 7.8 mm with the forearm in full pronation, thereby increasing the safe zone for exposure of the lateral elbow.[7]

PATHOGENESIS

- Multiple studies have shown that injury to the LCL can lead to PLRI, which is the first stage in elbow instability that can lead to frank elbow dislocation.
- It is controversial whether injury to the RUHL alone can lead to PLRI or whether further injury to the LCL complex is necessary.[10]
- When the forearm is supinated and slightly flexed, a valgus stress with an attenuated LCL causes the ulnohumeral joint to rotate, compresses the radiocapitellar joint, and ultimately causes the radial head to subluxate or dislocate posteriorly from the ulnohumeral joint.

NATURAL HISTORY

- PLRI is not a new condition, but it has only recently been described and studied.
- The prevalence and natural history of this condition are currently not known.

PATIENT HISTORY AND PHYSICAL FINDINGS

- Patients typically report trauma but may have had recurrent lateral epicondylitis or previous surgery.

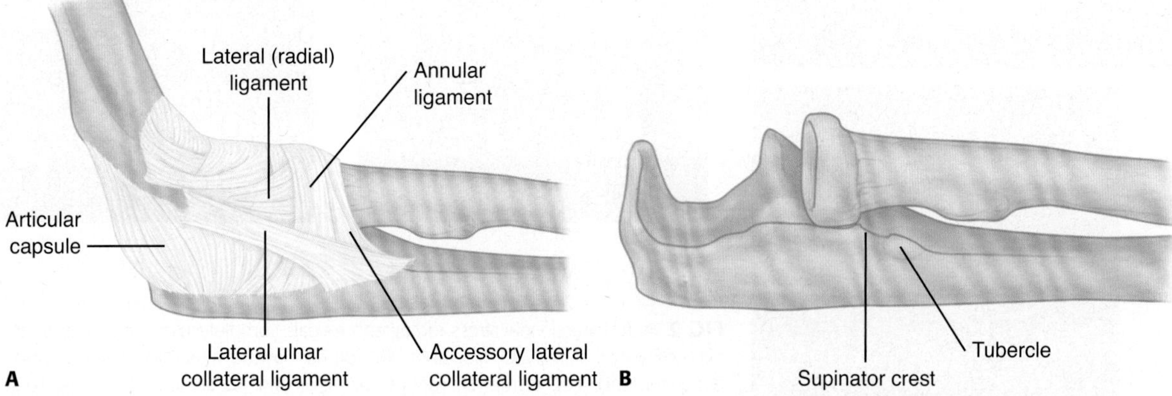

FIG 1 • **A.** The LCL complex is made up of four major components: the LUCL, also called the radial ulnohumeral ligament; the RCL proper; the annular ligament; and the accessory collateral ligament. **B.** Osseous anatomy of the LCL insertion.

- Elderly patients may not have frank dislocation of the elbow, but 75% of patients younger than 20 years report an elbow dislocation.[10]
- Patients typically report mechanical-type symptoms (clicking, popping, and slipping) during elbow supination and extension and rarely report recurrent dislocations. These symptoms may impact activities such as pushing up from a chair with the arms or doing pushups.
- Physical examination can be difficult; provocative tests are described in the following text. It is often necessary to conduct these tests with the patient under anesthesia or with the aid of fluoroscopy.
  - Inspection for effusion: With acute injuries, lateral gutter soft spot effusion is likely to be present, but in more chronic situations, it may be absent.
  - Range of motion (ROM): Locking of the elbow can represent loose bodies; stiffness may indicate intrinsic capsular contracture.
  - Supine lateral pivot shift test: When the elbow is slightly flexed, the radial head can be palpated to subluxate or frankly dislocate, and as the elbow flexes past 40 degrees, it relocates, often with a palpable clunk.[11] This test is often difficult to perform on an awake patient because apprehension is felt and the patient does not allow the test to continue.
  - Prone pivot shift test: Radial head or ulnohumeral subluxation constitutes a positive test, same as the supine lateral pivot shift test. Examination under anesthesia may be required.
  - Push-up test: Reproduction of the patient's symptoms of apprehension during supination and not pronation constitutes a positive test. Inability to complete the push-up also constitutes a positive test.
  - Chair push-up: Elicited pain constitutes a positive test.
  - Table top relocation test: Elicited pain or apprehension as the elbow reaches 40 degrees constitutes a positive test.
  - Elbow drawer test: Ulnohumeral subluxation constitutes a positive test.
- A thorough examination of the elbow should also be completed to rule out other injuries.
  - Valgus instability with the forearm in pronation and 30 degrees of flexion suggests medial collateral ligament (MCL) injury.
  - Lateral epicondylitis or radial tunnel syndrome can present with tenderness over the proximal extensor mass and with resisted extension of the wrist (Thompson test) and long finger.
  - Loose bodies may present with crepitus or locking of the elbow during ROM.

IMAGING AND OTHER DIAGNOSTIC STUDIES

- Standard anteroposterior (AP) and lateral view radiographs often indicate normal findings but may reveal small lateral epicondyle avulsion fractures and radiocapitellar wear.
- Stress AP and lateral view radiographs may reveal widening of the ulnohumeral joint and posterior subluxation of the radial head (**FIG 2A**).
- Magnetic resonance imaging (MRI), especially with intra-articular contrast enhancement, may reveal injuries to the LCL complex. The proximal extensor mass requires attention (**FIG 2B**). Chronic PLRI may lead to evidence of a posterolateral osteochondral defect coined the Osborne-Cotterill lesion (**FIG 2C,D**).[8]

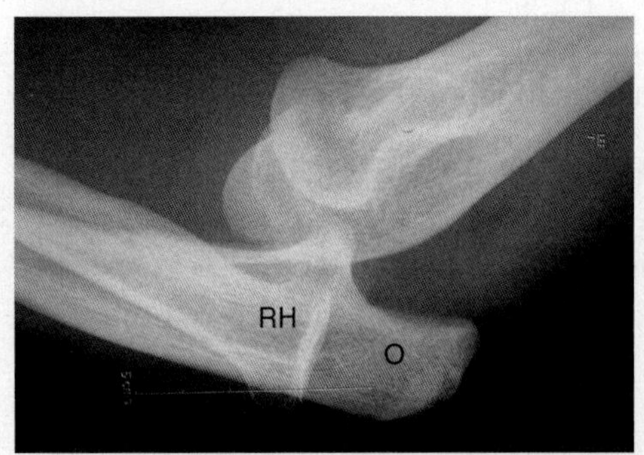

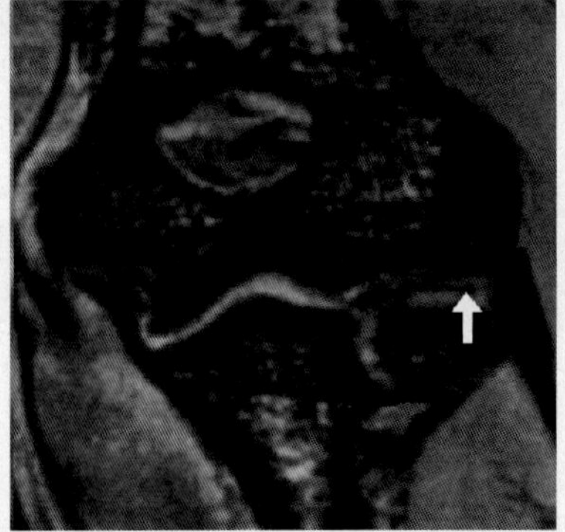

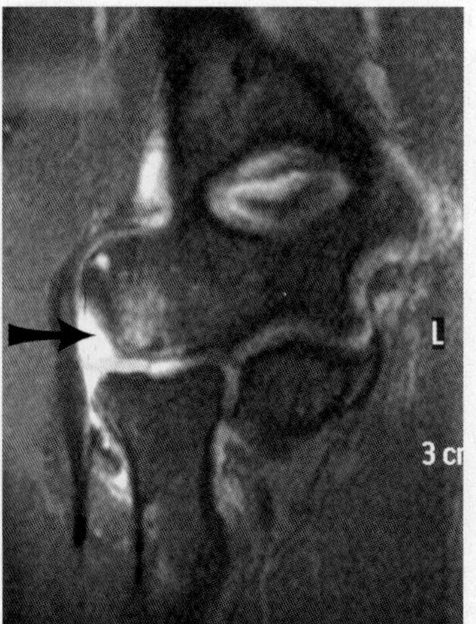

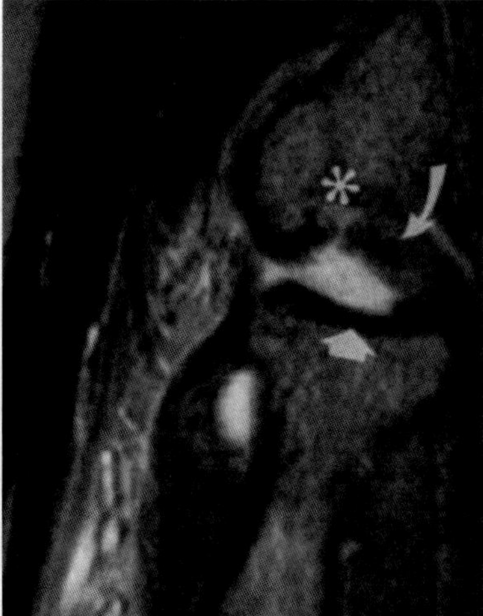

FIG 2 • **A.** Lateral view stress radiograph reveals complete ulnohumeral and radial head (*RH*) rotatory instability. *O*, olecranon. **B.** Coronal oblique view MRI of elbow (with contrast enhancement). LCL disruption can be seen (*arrow*). **C.** Sagittal MRI showing Osborne-Cotterill lesion (*asterisk* and *white arrows*). **D.** Coronal MRI showing Osborne-Cotterill lesion (*white arrow*).

- Diagnostic arthroscopy of the elbow can be performed, although we do not recommend routine diagnostic arthroscopy for this injury.
  - The drive-through sign occurs when the scope can easily be "driven through" the lateral gutter into the ulnohumeral joint from the posterolateral portal.
  - The pivot shift test also can be performed during arthroscopy, and the radial head will subluxate posteriorly.

DIFFERENTIAL DIAGNOSIS

- Lateral epicondylitis
- Extensor tendon tear
- Loose bodies
- Elbow fracture-dislocation
- MCL injury
- Radial head dislocation

NONOPERATIVE MANAGEMENT

- If the injury is diagnosed early, immobilization in a hinged elbow brace in pronation for 4 to 6 weeks may prevent chronic instability.[5]
- Removable neoprene sleeves may offer support.
- A trial of elbow extensor strengthening with progressive ROM can be performed.

SURGICAL MANAGEMENT

Indications

- Recurrent symptomatic PLRI despite nonoperative treatment

Preoperative Planning

- All imaging studies should be reviewed, and informed consent obtained.
- An examination of the elbow should be performed with the patient under anesthesia, especially the pivot shift test.
- If there is any doubt regarding the diagnosis, a pivot shift test should be performed under fluoroscopy.

Positioning

- The patient is placed supine on the operating room table.
- The arm can be placed on an arm board or across the patient's chest with a sterile tourniquet applied to the upper arm and the entire arm draped free (**FIG 3**).
- During the approach, the forearm should be pronated to protect the posterior interosseous nerve.

Approach

- The main approach is the Kocher interval between the anconeus and extensor carpi ulnaris muscles. Care must be taken to gently elevate the anconeus off the underlying LCL complex.
- This can be accomplished through a lateral skin incision or through a utilitarian posterior incision.
  - A posterior incision should be considered if a medial approach will also be needed to repair concomitant ligamentous or bony injury.

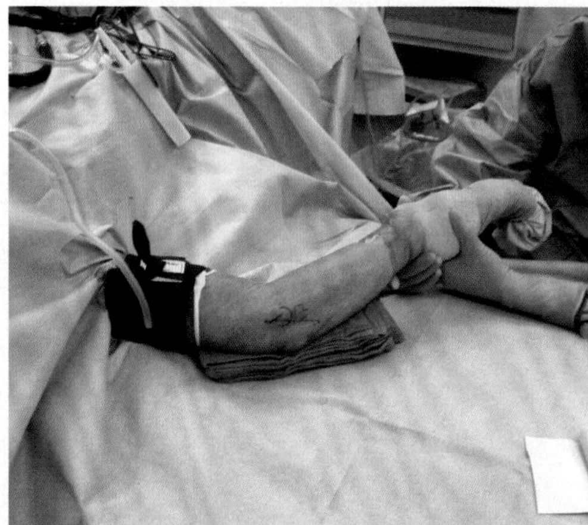

FIG 3 • The patient is placed supine on the operating room table. The arm is placed on an arm board with a sterile tourniquet applied to the upper arm and the entire arm draped free. During the approach, the forearm should be pronated to protect the posterior interosseous nerve.

TECHNIQUES

Figure-8 Yoke Technique

Surgical Approach

- A 10-cm incision is made over the Kocher interval.
  - The interval between the anconeus and the extensor carpi ulnaris is developed, and the remainder of the LCL complex is identified along with the supinator crest and the lateral epicondyle.
- The lateral epicondyle and 2 cm of the supracondylar ridge are exposed.

Tunnel Placement

- Two drill holes for the graft insertion site are made in the ulna.
  - One is drilled near the tubercle of the supinator crest (palpate in supination and varus stress), the other is 1.25 cm proximal to that, near the insertion of the annular ligament (**TECH FIG 1A**).
- A suture is passed through the two holes and tied to itself. The suture is then held up against the lateral epicondyle as the elbow is ranged in flexion and extension to determine its isometric point.
  - The isometric ligament insertion occurs at the point where the suture does *not* move.
  - The isometric point is usually more anteroinferior than expected (**TECH FIG 1B,C**).
- A Y-shaped tunnel is made with the base exiting at the isometric point.
  - The hole is widened to accept a three-ply graft. (Ipsilateral palmaris longus is usually harvested; if not present, gracilis or allograft is used.) A 16-cm graft is usually sufficient.

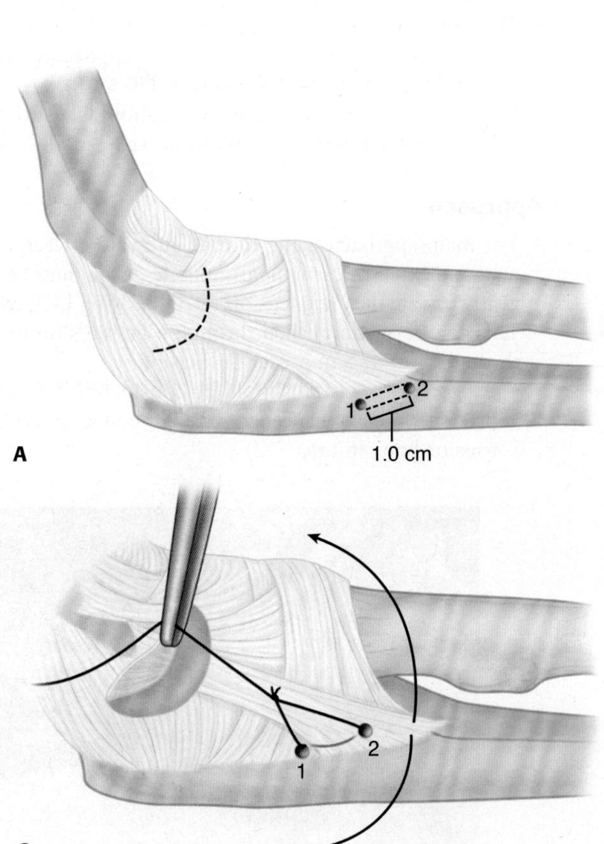

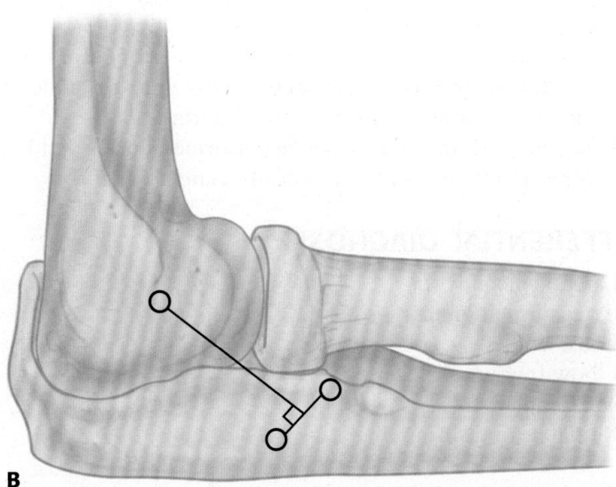

TECH FIG 1 • A. Two drill holes for the graft insertion site are made in the ulna. One is drilled near the tubercle of the supinator crest (palpate while varus and supination applied); the other is drilled 1.25 cm proximal, near the insertion of the annular ligament. *1*, proximal hole near insertion of annular ligament; *2*, tubercle of supinator crest. **B.** The ulnar holes should lie perpendicular to the intended direction of the LUCL. **C.** A suture is passed through the two holes and tied to itself. The suture is then held up with a hemostat against the lateral epicondyle as the elbow is ranged in flexion and extension to determine its isometric point. No movement occurs if the suture is at the isometric point.

Graft Passage and Tensioning and Wound Closure

- The graft is passed through the ulnar tunnel with enough length to just reach the isometric point.
  - The end is then sutured to the long end of the graft (the Yoke stitch).
  - The long end is then passed through the isometric point and exits the superior humeral tunnel (**TECH FIG 2A**).
- The long end is wrapped around the supracondylar ridge and passed through the distal tunnel, exiting back through the isometric point and into the ulnar tunnel.
  - The graft is then tensioned in 40 degrees of flexion, full pronation, and axial tension.
  - If the graft is not long enough to reach the ulnar tunnel, it can be sutured back to itself (**TECH FIG 2B**).
- The reconstruction can be reinforced by weaving a no. 2 FiberWire suture (Arthrex, Inc., Naples, FL) from distal to proximal through the course of the figure 8, thus sewing the graft to itself.
- Plicate the anterior and posterior capsule as needed.
- The extensor origin is repaired to the lateral epicondyle, and the extensor carpi ulnaris fascia is reapproximated to the anconeus muscle with absorbable sutures.

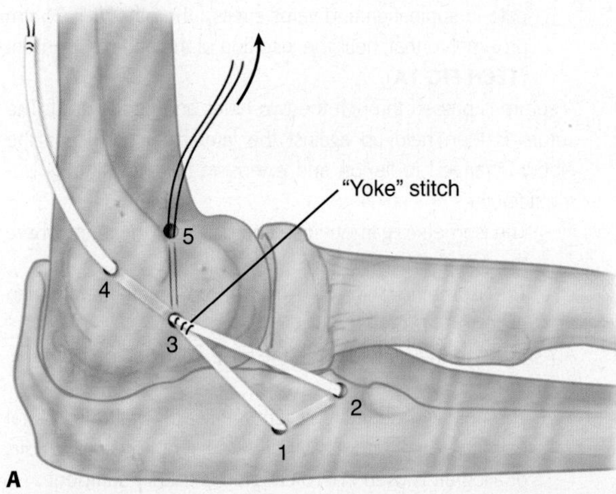

TECH FIG 2 • A. A Y-shaped tunnel is made with the base exiting at the isometric point (*3*). The hole is widened to accept a three-ply graft. The tendon graft is passed through the ulnar tunnel (*1→2*) with enough length to just reach the isometric point. The end is then sutured to the long end of the graft (the Yoke stitch). The long end is then passed through the isometric point and exits the superior humeral tunnel (*3→4*). *(continued)*

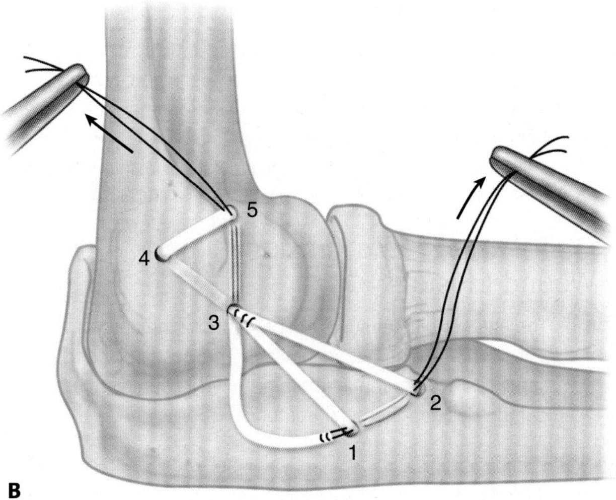

TECH FIG 2 • *(continued)* **B.** The long end is then passed through the distal tunnel, exiting back through the isometric point (*5→3*) and into the ulnar tunnel (*3→1→2*). The graft is then tensioned in 40 degrees of flexion, full pronation, and axial tension. If the graft is not long enough to reach the ulnar tunnel, it can be sutured back to itself.

Split Anconeus Fascia Transfer

- We have developed a reproducible technique for LCL reconstruction that has proven biomechanical strength and reproducibility.
- Advantages include using only local autograft tissue and the minimal creation of bone tunnels.[3,4]

Surgical Approach

- A 6- to 8-cm skin incision is made over the Kocher interval, exposing the underlying Kocher interval between the extensor carpi ulnaris and anconeus (**TECH FIG 3A,B**).
- The interval between the anconeus and extensor carpi ulnaris muscles is developed, taking care to preserve the remainder of the underlying LCL complex.
  - The annular ligament, lateral epicondyle, and 2 cm of supracondylar ridge are isolated (**TECH FIG 3C**).

Graft Preparation

- The anconeus and distal triceps fascia are isolated in continuity. A 1.0-cm wide × 8.0-cm long band of fascia is mobilized off the underlying muscle, leaving the ulnar insertion intact (**TECH FIG 4A,B**).

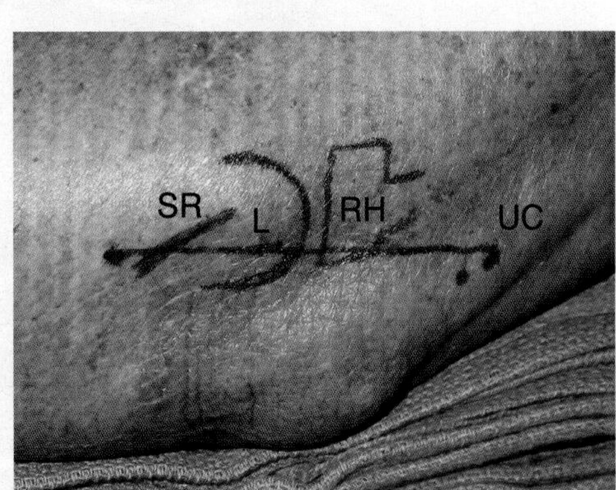

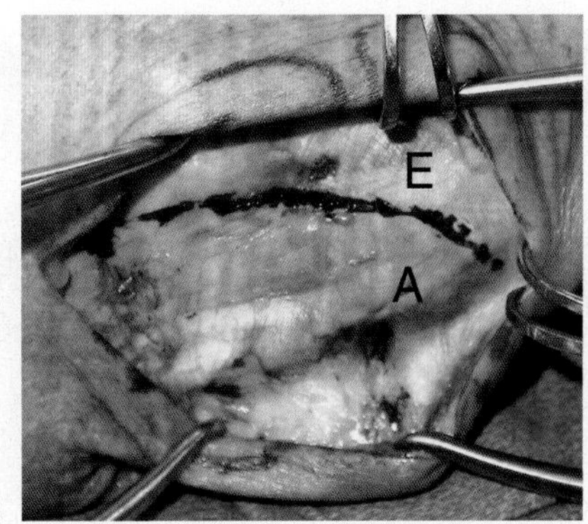

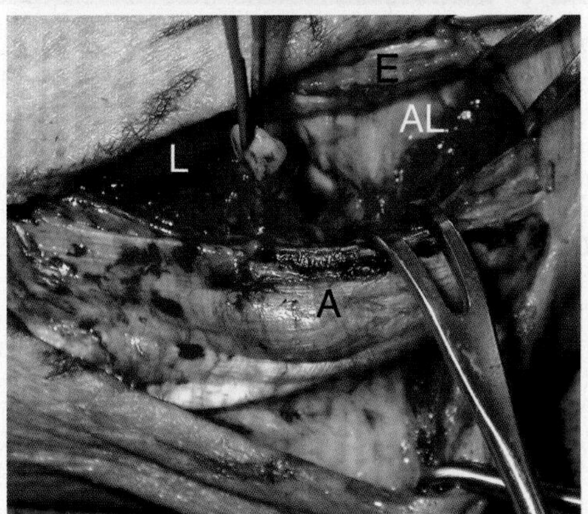

TECH FIG 3 • **A.** A 6- to 8-cm skin incision is made over the Kocher interval. *SR*, supracondylar ridge; *L*, lateral epicondyle; *RH*, radial head; *UC*, ulnar crest. **B.** The underlying Kocher interval between the extensor carpi ulnaris (*E*) and anconeus (*A*) is exposed. **C.** The interval between the anconeus (*A*) and the extensor carpi ulnaris (*E*) is developed, taking care to preserve the remainder of the underlying LCL complex (held in forceps). The annular ligament (*AL*), lateral epicondyle (*L*), and 2 cm of the supracondylar ridge are isolated.

- The band is then divided longitudinally into two bands of equal width (**TECH FIG 4C**).
- The anterior band is passed through an incision just distal to the annular ligament, whereas the posterior band is passed under the anconeus muscle (**TECH FIG 4D**).
- The isometric point of the lateral epicondyle is then located by holding the two bands against the epicondyle while ranging the elbow (**TECH FIG 4E**).
- The final lengths of the fascial bands are estimated by holding the bands along their respective paths. The bands are then trimmed appropriately to prevent them from "bottoming out" prematurely in the humeral docking tunnel.
- Separate Krackow sutures are placed in each band with no. 0 FiberWire suture.

Tunnel Preparation

- A 5-mm round burr is used to create a 1.5-cm long (depth) docking tunnel into the humerus at the isometric point. A 1-mm side-cutting burr is then used to make anterior and posterior bone bridge holes. The holes are separated by 1.5 cm. Individual suture lassos are placed from proximal to distal into the docking tunnel from the separate humeral tunnels (**TECH FIG 5**).

Graft Passage and Tensioning and Wound Closure

- The anterior band sutures are brought out the anterior humeral exit hole by using suture passers. The posterior band passes superficial to the annular ligament and its sutures are brought out the posterior humeral exit tunnel.

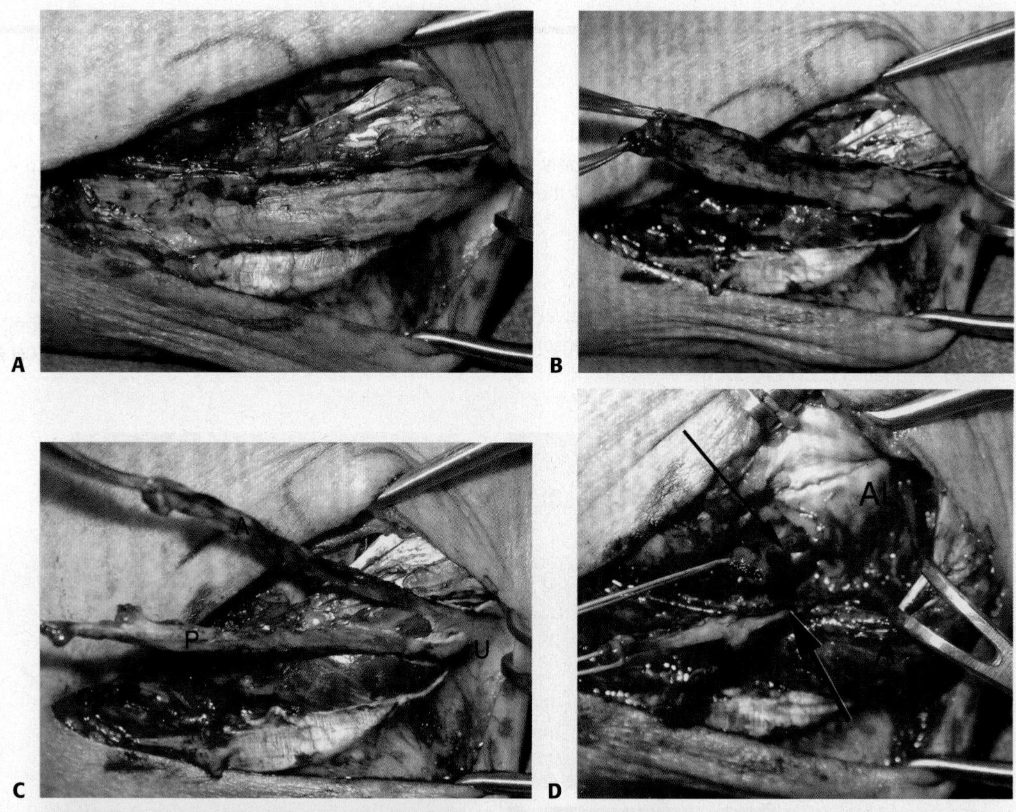

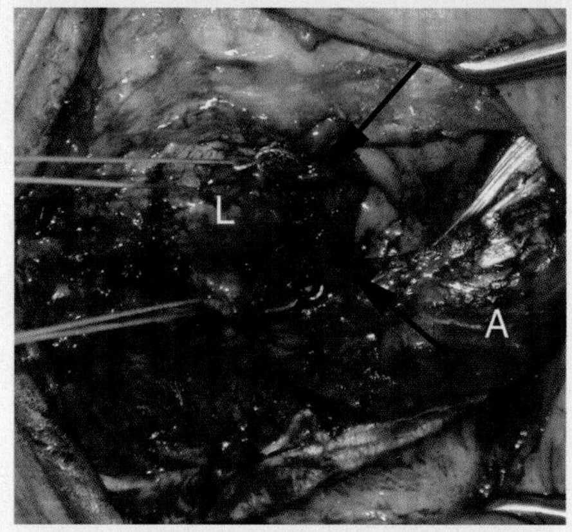

TECH FIG 4 • **A.** The anconeus and distal triceps fascia are isolated in continuity. **B.** A 1.0-cm wide × 8.0-cm long band of fascia is mobilized off the underlying muscle, leaving the ulnar insertion. **C.** The split anconeus fascia band is then divided longitudinally into two bands of equal width. *A*, anterior band; *P*, posterior band; *U*, ulnar insertion point. **D.** The anterior band (*thin arrow*) is passed through an incision just distal to the annular ligament (*AL*), whereas the posterior band (*thick arrow*) is passed under the anconeus muscle (*A*). **E.** The isometric point of the lateral epicondyle (*L*) is then located by holding the two bands against the epicondyle while ranging the elbow. The point of minimal tension loss in either band while ranging the elbow is the optimal isometric point. *Arrows*, anterior and posterior split anconeus fascia bands.

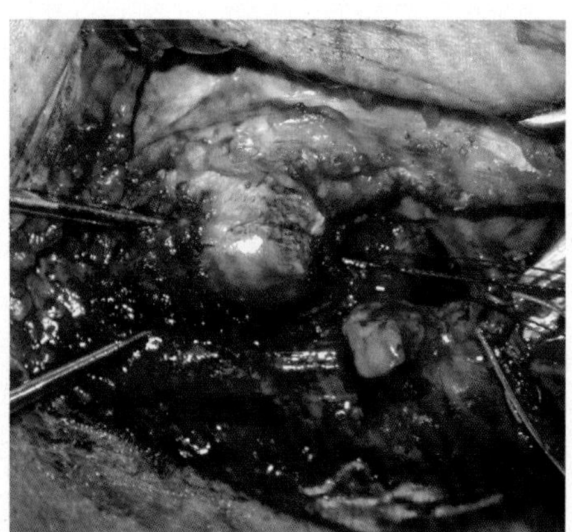

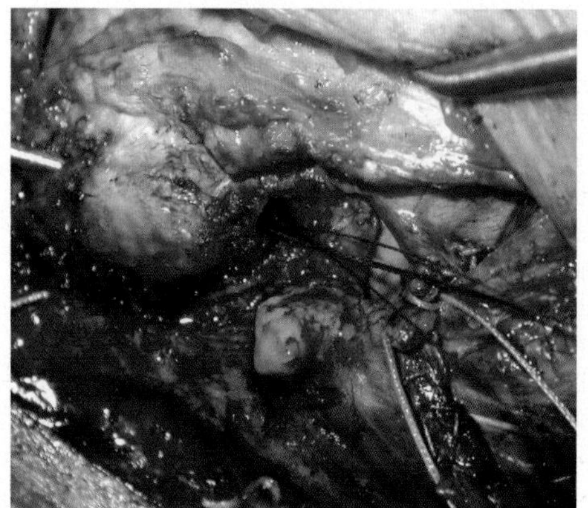

TECH FIG 5 • **A.** Suture lassos passed through exit holes out to the distal docking tunnel. **B.** Suture lasso wires exiting docking tunnel.

- The ends of the fascial bands are docked into the humeral tunnel, and the grafts are tensioned with the elbow in 40 degrees of flexion, in full pronation, and with a valgus stress.
- The sutures are then tied over the bony bridge on the supracondylar ridge (**TECH FIG 6A**).
- The grafts can be augmented with any remaining LCL complex.
- The extensor origin is then repaired to the lateral epicondyle, and the extensor carpi ulnaris fascia is reapproximated to the anconeus muscle with absorbable sutures.
- The skin is closed with a running subcuticular suture (**TECH FIG 6B**).

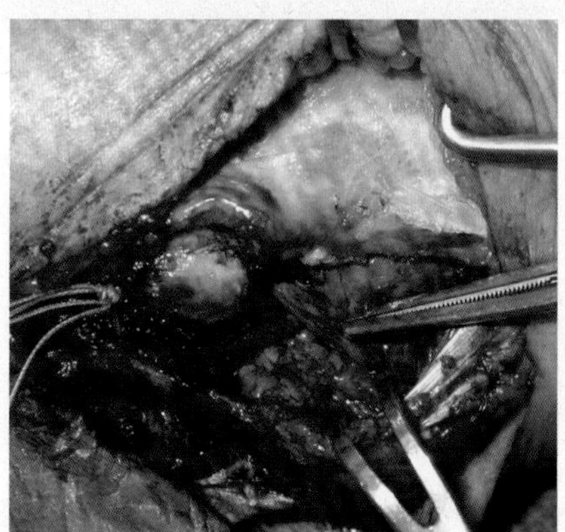

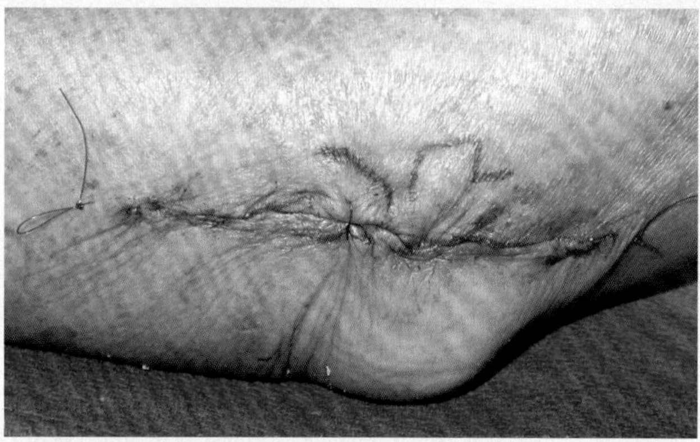

TECH FIG 6 • **A.** The ends of the fascial bands are docked into the humeral tunnel, and the grafts are tensioned with the elbow in 40 degrees of flexion, full pronation, and valgus stress. Sutures are then tied over the bony bridge on the supracondylar ridge (clamp on posterior band). **B.** The incision is closed with subcuticular suture.

Docking Technique

- As previously discussed, the Kocher approach is used for the docking technique.
- Preparation of the ulnar drill holes is described in the section on the figure-8 Yoke Technique elsewhere in this chapter.
- A 5-mm round burr is used to create a 1.5-cm long (depth) docking tunnel into the humerus at the isometric point. A 1-mm side-cutting burr is then used to make anterior and posterior bone bridge holes. The holes are separated by 1.5 cm. Individual suture lassos are placed from proximal to distal into the docking tunnel from the separate humeral tunnels (see **TECH FIG 5**).
- After passage of the graft through the ulnar tunnels, the final lengths of the two graft strands are estimated by holding the strands against the docking tunnel with the arm in the "reduced" position of 40 degrees of flexion, full pronation, and axial tension.
- The strands are then trimmed appropriately to prevent the strands from bottoming out prematurely in the humeral docking tunnel.
    - Separate Krackow sutures are placed in each graft strand with no. 0 FiberWire suture for 1 cm.
- The anterior graft strand sutures are brought out to the anterior humeral exit hole by using suture passers. The posterior graft strand sutures are brought out to the posterior humeral exit tunnel.
- The ends of the humeral graft portion are docked into the humeral tunnel, and the grafts are tensioned with the elbow in 40 degrees of flexion, in full pronation, and with a valgus stress.
- The sutures are then tied over the bony bridge on the supracondylar ridge.
- Standard incision closure is performed.

Direct Repair

- As previously discussed, the Kocher approach is used for direct repair.
- If the LCL complex is intact but traumatically avulsed from its ulnar or humeral attachments (or both), it can be directly repaired to its correct anatomic location with suture anchors or bone tunnels. This most commonly occurs in the setting of acute, traumatic injuries.
- A running locked no. 2 FiberWire suture is placed into the detached LCL complex and repaired back to its origin on the lateral epicondyle through the anterior and posterior drill holes (**TECH FIG 7**).
- A careful repair of the extensor origin and the interval between the anconeus and the extensor carpi ulnaris is performed.

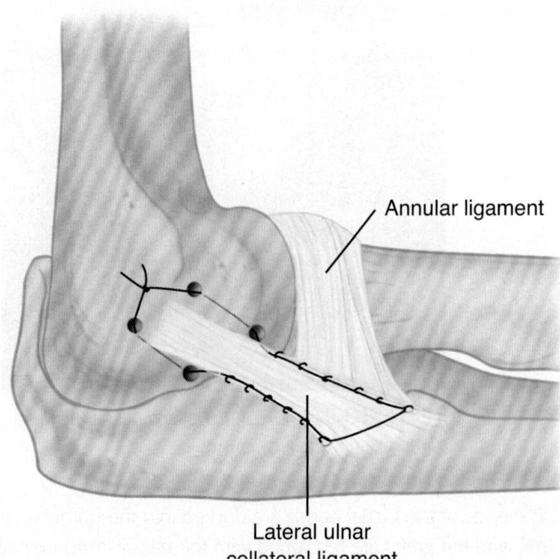

TECH FIG 7 • Primary LUCL repair. Running locked suture placed through detached LUCL. A relaxing incision can be made at its attachment to the base of the annular ligament. Repair through drill holes in the lateral epicondyle.

PEARLS AND PITFALLS

Indications	▪ Iatrogenic causes (eg, "tennis elbow" surgery) very common. ▪ Careful history and physical examination to exclude other pathologic conditions ▪ History of numerous lateral elbow corticosteroid injections
Split anconeus fascia technique: exposure	▪ Isolate Kocher interval; fatty stripe within interval. ▪ Anconeus fibers oblique to extensor carpi ulnaris ▪ Identify LCL disruption. ▪ Isolate annular ligament; protect posterior interosseous nerve.
Splint anconeus fascia preparation	▪ Be careful to harvest long enough fascial band (proximal to humeral bone tunnels). ▪ Be careful not to detach from ulnar insertion. ▪ Isolate LCL complex isometric point of origin. ▪ Harvest fascial band in line with old LUCL.
Figure-8 yoke technique	▪ Carefully isolate isometric point on lateral epicondyle, usually more anterior and inferior; err on inferior placement. ▪ Make ulnar tunnel perpendicular to direction of LUCL. ▪ Chamfer bone tunnels to prevent graft impingement and breakage.
Bone tunnel preparation	▪ Maintain sufficient bony bridge between tunnels. ▪ Smooth edges to prevent graft irritation.
Arm position for final graft tensioning	▪ Forty degrees of elbow flexion ▪ Full pronation ▪ Axial load, valgus stress

POSTOPERATIVE CARE

- Stage I (0 to 3 weeks)
  - Elbow immobilization in posterior splint or brace at 40 degrees of flexion
  - Wrist and hand isometrics as tolerated
  - Shoulder active and passive ROM
- Stage II (3 to 6 weeks)
  - Hinged elbow brace or orthoplast splint, with limits set by surgeon
  - Begin flexor–pronator isometrics
  - Continue with wrist and hand strengthening
  - Continue shoulder as described earlier
  - Active-assisted ROM: 20 to 120 degrees of flexion; keep forearm pronated at all times
- Stage III (6 to 12 weeks)
  - Discontinue immobilization
  - Passive ROM and active-assisted ROM to full motion, including supination
  - Begin unrestricted strengthening of flexor–pronators and extensors
- Stage IV (3 to 6 months)
  - Avoid varus stress to elbow and ballistic movement in terminal elbow ranges

- Begin shoulder strengthening with light resistance (emphasis on cuff)
- Start total body conditioning
- Terminal elbow stretching in flexion and extension
- Resistive elbow exercises as tolerated

OUTCOMES

- Nestor et al[10] have shown successful functional outcomes in patients using the figure-8 reconstruction technique with reproducible results.
- Our early experience with the split anconeus fascia reconstruction technique has shown excellent results, with no failures to date in 22 patients at an average follow-up of 2 years. All elbows have achieved stability without loss of motion.

COMPLICATIONS

- Recurrent elbow instability in up to 8%[2]
- Elbow stiffness
- Infection
- Graft harvest site morbidity (if remote autograft is used for reconstruction)
- Humerus stress fracture through bone tunnels
- Ulnar stress fracture through bone tunnels
- Bone bridge compromise

REFERENCES

1. Anakwenze OA, Khanna K, Levine WN, et al. Characterization of the supinator tubercle for lateral ulnar collateral ligament reconstruction. Orthop J Sports Med 2014;2(4).
2. Anakwenze OA, Kwon D, O'Donnell E, et al. Surgical treatment of posterolateral rotatory instability of the elbow. Arthroscopy 2014;30(7):866–871.
3. Chebli CA, Murthi AM. Lateral collateral ligament complex: anatomic and biomechanical testing. Presented at the 73rd Annual Meeting and Scientific Program of the American Academy of Orthopaedic Surgeons, Chicago, March 2006.
4. Chebli CM, Murthi AM. Split anconeus fascia transfer for reconstruction of the elbow lateral collateral ligament complex: anatomic and biomechanical testing. Presented at the 22nd Open Meeting of the American Shoulder and Elbow Surgeons, Chicago, March 2006.
5. Cohen MS, Hastings H II. Acute elbow dislocation: evaluation and management. J Am Acad Orthop Surg 1998;6:15–23.
6. Coombes BK, Bisset L, Brooks P, et al. Effect of corticosteroid injection, physiotherapy, or both on clinical outcomes in patients with unilateral lateral epicondylalgia: a randomized controlled trial. JAMA 2013;309(5):461–469.
7. Diliberti T, Botte MJ, Abrams RA. Anatomical considerations regarding the posterior interosseous nerve during posterolateral approaches to the proximal part of the radius. J Bone Joint Surg 2000;82(6):809–813.
8. Jeon IH, Micic ID, Yamamoto N, et al. Osborne-cotterill lesion: an osseous defect of the capitellum associated with instability of the elbow. AJR Am Roentgenol 2008;191(3):727–729.
9. Kalainov DM, Cohen MS. Posterolateral rotatory instability of the elbow in association with lateral epicondylitis: a report of three cases. J Bone Joint Surg Am 2005;87(5):1120–1125.
10. Nestor BJ, O'Driscoll SW, Morrey BF. Ligamentous reconstruction for posterolateral rotatory instability of the elbow. J Bone Joint Surg Am 1992;74(8):1235–1241.
11. O'Driscoll SW, Bell DF, Morrey BF. Posterolateral rotatory instability of the elbow. J Bone Joint Surg Am 1991;73(3):440–446.
12. O'Driscoll SW, Spinner RJ, McKee MD, et al. Tardy posterolateral rotatory instability of the elbow due to cubitus varus. J Bone Joint Surg Am 2001;83-A(9):1358–1369.

CHAPTER 59
Ulnar Collateral Ligament Reconstruction of the Elbow

Sameer Nagda and Michael Ciccotti

DEFINITION

- The ulnar collateral ligament (UCL) is a primary stabilizer of the medial side of the elbow. A tear in this ligament can cause pain and disability, primarily in an overhead athlete. When reconstruction is performed, the anterior band of the ligament is reconstructed.

ANATOMY

- The UCL originates from the inferior aspect of the medial epicondyle and inserts onto the sublime tubercle of the ulna.
- There is an anterior band, a posterior band, and a transverse band (**FIG 1**).
- The anterior band provides the primary resistance to valgus stresses between 20 and 120 degrees and is further divided into anterior and posterior bundles that tighten in a reciprocal fashion as the elbow is flexed and extended.

PATHOGENESIS

- Injury to the UCL occurs with a valgus force applied to the elbow. This can occur from trauma such as a fall on an outstretched hand. Injury is most commonly seen in the overhead athlete who applies a significant and repetitive valgus force to the elbow during sports.
- Injury is most common in baseball, javelin, and volleyball but can be seen in numerous other sports such as football, wrestling, and tennis.

NATURAL HISTORY

- Injury to the UCL can occur in one instance with immediate onset of pain or can be progressive over a period of time.
- Patients who do not repeatedly expose the injured ligament to continued stress have a high rate of success with nonsurgical treatment if gross elbow instability is not present.
- Athletes participating in sports that place a valgus stress on the elbow and who wish to continue to participate will usually require surgical reconstruction to resume participation.

PATIENT HISTORY AND PHYSICAL FINDINGS

- Patients will complain of pain on the medial side of the elbow. There may be associated complaints of numbness and/or tingling if there is concurrent irritation to the ulnar nerve.
- Patients may describe feeling a pop in the elbow with one incident of a valgus force, such as a baseball pitch or javelin throw. Conversely, there may be a history of several days or weeks of progressive, worsening medial elbow discomfort, tightness, or trouble with activity involving valgus force to the elbow.
- Patients with isolated UCL injury will rarely complain of instability. Unless concurrent flexor–pronator mass (FPM) or ulnar nerve injury is present, patients will rarely complain of weakness.
- In addition to a thorough basic elbow examination as described previously, provocative tests to diagnose UCL tears

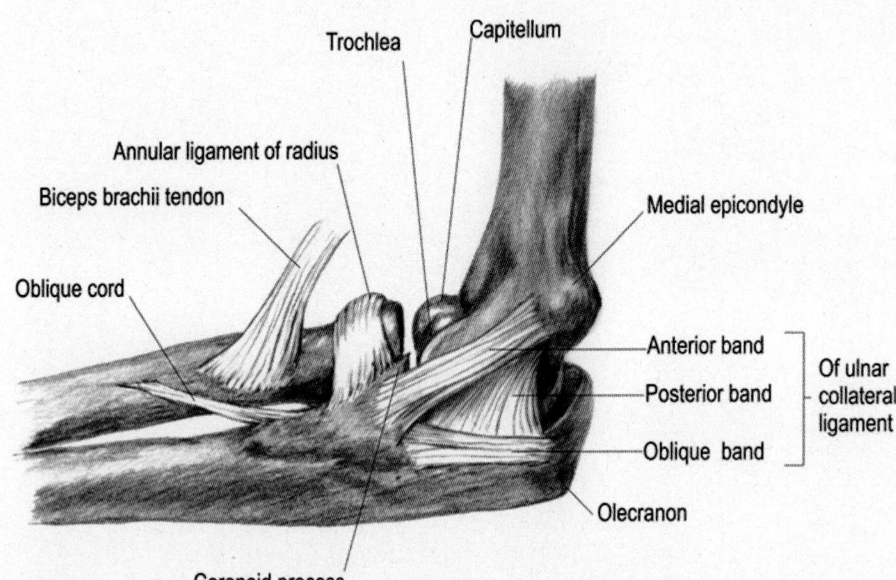

FIG 1 • Anatomy of the medial aspect of the elbow. (Reprinted with permission from Leversedge FJ, Goldfarb CA, Boyer MI. Pocketbook Manual of Hand and Upper Extremity Anatomy: Primus Manus. Philadelphia: Lippincott Williams & Wilkins, 2010.)

include the moving valgus stress test and the milking test. Pain along the UCL elicited with these tests is indicative of a UCL tear.

- The milking test is performed by pulling or "milking" the thumb of the involved elbow while placing a valgus force on the elbow. The involved shoulder is held in an abducted and externally rotated position while the test is performed.
- The moving valgus stress test is performed in a similar position, but the involved elbow is moved from 30 to 120 degrees while valgus stress is applied to the elbow.
- Direct valgus stress testing may also cause pain. However, the examiner will rarely appreciate laxity with this test. This test should be performed in approximately 30 to 60 degrees of elbow flexion.
- Palpation of the posteromedial olecranon may elicit pain in chronic situations of valgus extension overload.
- Chronic microlaxity may also result in lateral-sided compression, causing overload of the radiocapitellar joint. Palpation of this area should be performed for pain or crepitans.

IMAGING AND OTHER DIAGNOSTIC STUDIES

- Initial plain radiographs are helpful especially in younger individuals. These may reveal bony avulsion of the ligament, growth plate fracture, posteromedial olecranon osteophytes, or osteochondritis dissecans (OCD) of the capitellum. Plain radiographs in more mature throwing athletes often show calcifications and or osteophytes. Stress radiographs may be helpful in cases of significant instability.
- The imaging of choice is an elbow magnetic resonance imaging (MRI) with or without intra-articular contrast.
- The T-sign is a finding often seen on an MRI and is suggestive of injury to the UCL (**FIG 2**). In cases where an MRI cannot be attained, a computed tomography (CT) arthrogram can be used to diagnose injury to the UCL.
- Stress ultrasound has more recently been proposed to compliment MRI/magnetic resonance angiography (MRA) particularly in athletes with a clinically subtle injury, partial injury on MRI/MRA, failed nonoperative treatment, or recurrent injury after previous UCL reconstruction[2] (**FIG 3**).

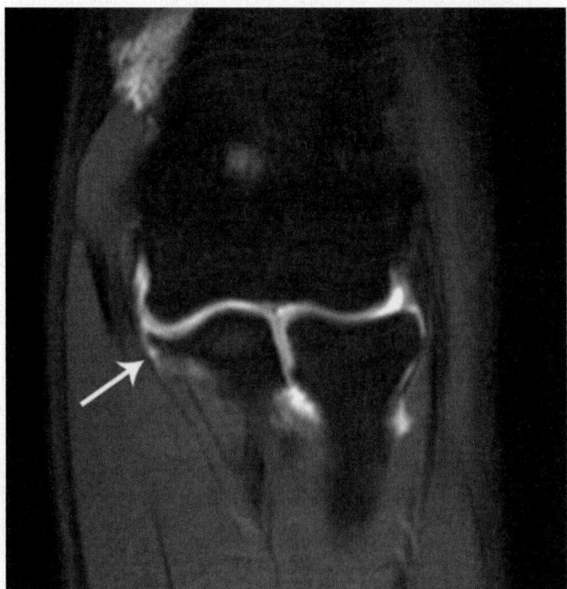

FIG 2 • MRI of the elbow showing the T-sign (*arrow*).

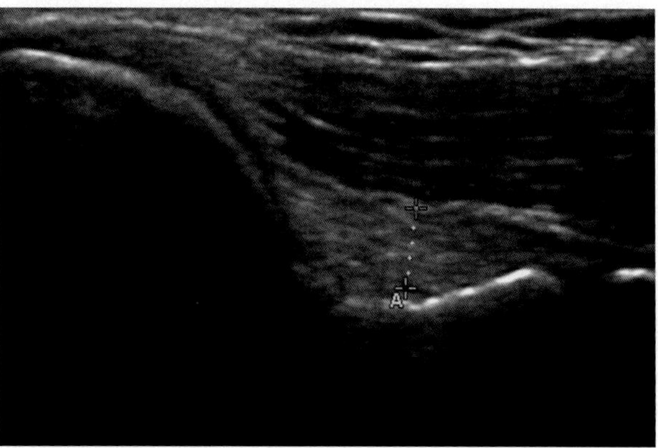

FIG 3 • Ultrasound of the UCL.

DIFFERENTIAL DIAGNOSIS

- FPM injury/medial epicondylitis
- Medial epicondyle fracture
- Ulnar neuritis
- Ulnar stress fracture

NONOPERATIVE MANAGEMENT

- Nonoperative treatment consists of rest, oral nonsteroidal anti-inflammatory drugs (NSAIDs), and rehabilitation focused on shoulder and scapular strengthening along with evaluation of the specific mechanics involved in each athlete's sport.
- Athletes who are not involved in overhead sports may return when symptoms allow and may participate with a hinged elbow brace.
- Athletes involved in overhead sports often require a 3- to 6-week period of rest, during which time a coordinated rehabilitation program including leg, core, and shoulder strengthening and flexibility is carried out. Once preinjury range of motion (ROM) and strength are restored without pain, then a progressive throwing program is initiated. This program includes tossing at increasing distance up to ~180 to 200 feet; pitchers then begin a mound program throwing fastballs first with increasing effort, followed by off-speed pitches. This thorough nonoperative program may require 8 to 12 weeks before return to sport.
- Certain overhead-throwing athletes have high success with nonoperative measures. Dodson et al[6] noted that professional football players, specifically quarterbacks, have a high rate of return with nonoperative treatment.
- Podesta and associates[12] reported an 88% return to competition for athletes with partial tears of the UCL treated with platelet-rich plasma (PRP) in short-term follow-up.

SURGICAL MANAGEMENT

- Surgical management is considered for all athletes who fail nonoperative treatment.
- Surgical management consists of reconstruction of the anterior band of the UCL. Most commonly, a palmaris longus autograft is used if available. Alternatives include contralateral hamstring, plantaris, or medial strip of Achilles

tendon autograft. Allograft reconstruction has also been described recently with good results.[14]

Preoperative Planning

- Preoperative planning should include evaluating if the patient has an available palmaris longus tendon. If not, alternative graft options should be discussed with the patient. The palmaris longus tendon has been identified in 85% of the population.
- Patients with ulnar nerve symptoms should be evaluated for possible ulnar nerve decompression or transposition performed at the time of UCL reconstruction. A subluxing ulnar nerve should also be identified and considered for surgical treatment.
- Concurrent intra-articular pathology such as loose bodies can be managed with arthroscopy at the time of reconstruction.
- Patients with acute injuries should be evaluated for return of full elbow motion prior to undergoing surgery.

Positioning

- The patient is placed in the supine position with a hand table. If elbow arthroscopy is to be performed, the patient should be positioned for this in the desired position first and then switched to the supine position.
- Either a sterile or nonsterile tourniquet can be used.
- If a hamstring, plantaris, or medial Achilles strip autograft is to be taken, the contralateral leg should also be draped out and a nonsterile tourniquet should be used.

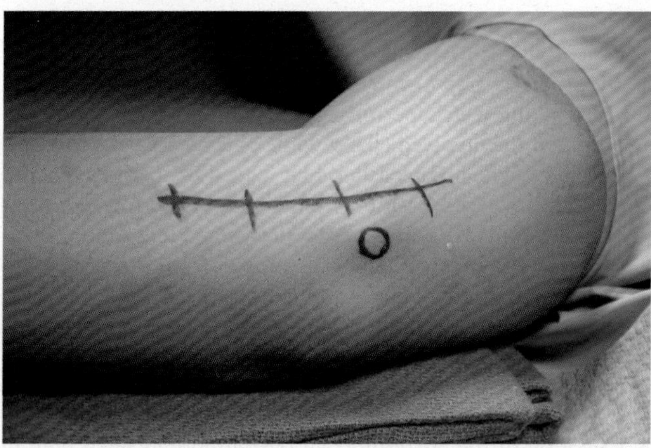

FIG 4 • Incision centered over the medial epicondyle.

Approach

- The approach consists of a standard medial incision centered over the medial epicondyle (**FIG 4**). The initial surgery described by Jobe et al[11] consisted of a takedown of the FPM and ulnar nerve transposition.
- More recent modifications describe an FPM split and ulnar nerve transposition only if indicated.[15]
- Commonly used techniques include the Jobe figure-of-eight technique and the docking technique. Biomechanical evaluation of both techniques has revealed valgus stability comparable to the native ligament.[3]

TECHNIQUES

Figure-of-Eight Reconstruction—Jobe Technique

- An extensile medial incision is used centered over the medial epicondyle.
- Care should be taken to identify and protect the branches of the medial antebrachial cutaneous nerves (**TECH FIG 1A**).
- The medial epicondyle, ulnar nerve, and the fascia overlying the FPM should be identified. The sublime tubercle can often be palpated 2 to 3 cm distal to the medial epicondyle.
- The raphe between the middle and posterior thirds of the FPM should be identified and split from the medial epicondyle distally in line with the fibers, past the sublime tubercle (**TECH FIG 1B**).
- Blunt dissection using a periosteal elevator will bring the ligament into visualization (**TECH FIG 1C**).
- Once the ligament is identified from the inferior border of the medial epicondyle to the sublime tubercle, it should be incised in line with its fibers. This will expose the joint. An assessment of ligament integrity can be performed at this point by applying valgus stress and noting any joint gapping (**TECH FIG 1D**).
- The origin of the ligament at the inferior aspect of the epicondyle as well as the anterior and medial aspect of the epicondyle are exposed for drilling of the tunnels.
- The anterior and posterior aspects of the sublime tubercle are exposed using sharp dissection (**TECH FIG 1E**). Enough area must be exposed to allow for a sufficient bone bridge between the tunnels to prevent fracture. Ideally, one should have at least 8 to 10 mm between the ulnar tunnels.
- Once the exposure has been performed and ligament laxity has been confirmed, the holes may be drilled or the graft can be obtained.
- Using a 3.5-mm drill bit, the ulnar tunnels are drilled anterior and posterior to the sublime tubercle at ~5 to 7 mm from the articular margin and with a 10-mm bone bridge. These tunnels should converge at a point within the ulna below the sublime tubercle (**TECH FIG 1F**). Fracture of the bone bridge between the tunnels is a pitfall that should be avoided.
- Once the tunnels are drilled, a curette should be used to assure connection of beneath the sublime tubercle. Inadequate preparation of this tunnel will result in difficulty with graft passage.
- A curved suture passer should be used to pass a suture through this tunnel. This will be used for graft passage. The loop should be passed from posterior to anterior. This can also be used to identify the isometric point of the humeral tunnel (**TECH FIG 1G**).
- The humeral tunnel is drilled using a 4.5-mm drill bit in a retrograde direction starting at the origin of the ligament midway between the base and tip of the epicondyle (**TECH FIG 1H**). This tunnel is drilled to a depth of approximately 10 to 15 mm. Care should be taken not to fracture the epicondyle or to drill out the back wall into the cubital tunnel.
- The FPM is then split at the junction of the anterior and middle thirds, exposing the superior surface of the medial epicondyle. Two smaller tunnels are then drilled with a 3.5-mm drill bit in an anterograde direction starting on the anterior and medial aspects of the epicondyle converging onto the larger, 4.5-mm tunnel (**TECH FIG 1I**).

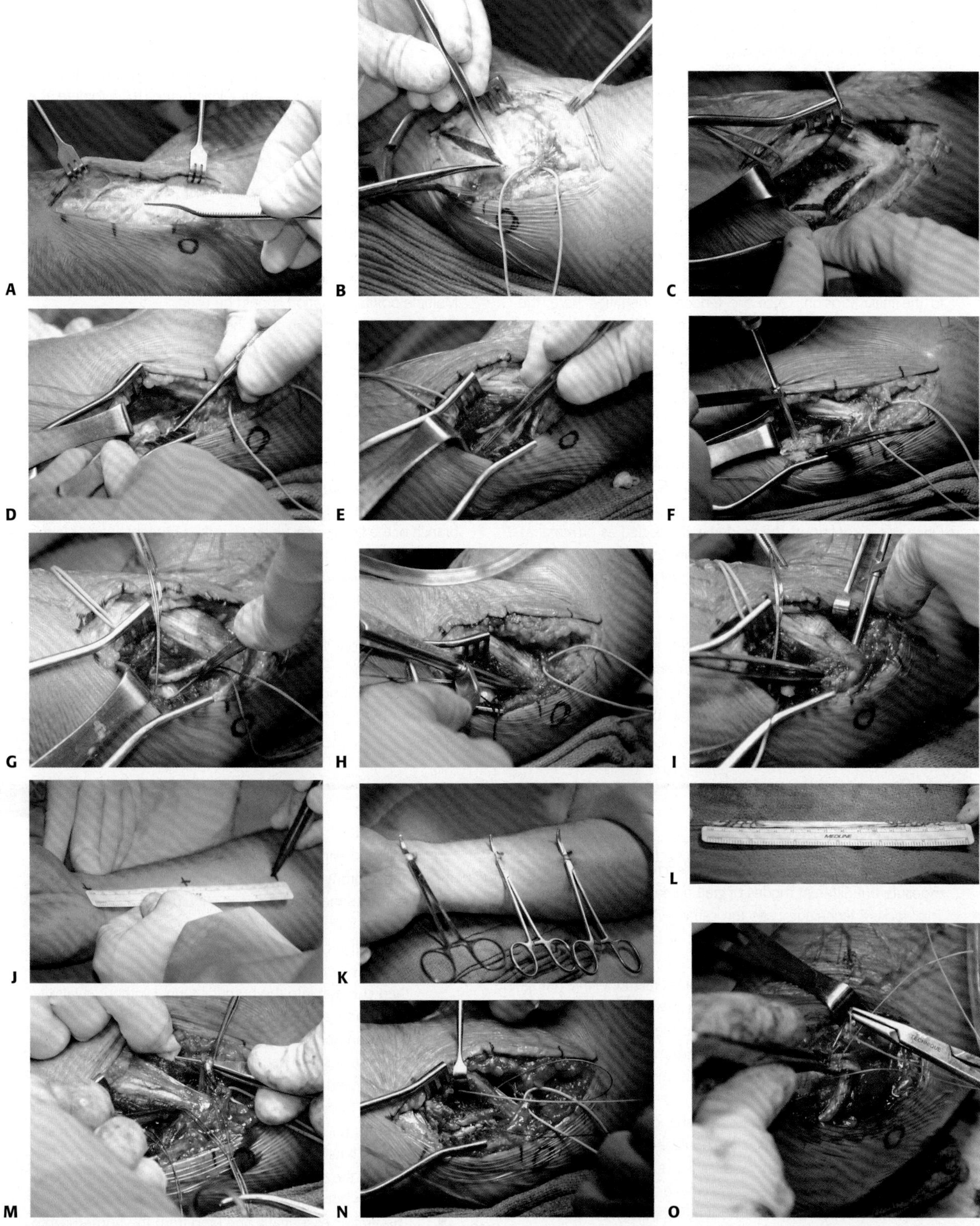

TECH FIG 1 • **A.** (*Left, right*) Jobe technique and docking technique for UCL reconstruction. **B.** Incision with identification of the medial antebrachial cutaneous nerve. **C.** Split in the FPM. **D.** Blunt dissection exposing the UCL. **E.** Exposure of the sublime tubercle for drilling. **F.** Drilling of the ulnar tunnels. The drill is prepared for the anterior tunnel and the forceps is in the posterior tunnel. **G.** Suture in the ulnar tunnels and pointing toward the humeral starting point. **H.** Drilling of the 4.5-mm humeral tunnel. **I.** Split of the FPM exposes the superior surface of the medial epicondyle for drilling. **J.** Measuring for the palmaris longus harvest. **K.** Harvesting of the palmaris longus graft. **L.** Prepared graft. **M.** Graft has been passed and is ready to be secured. **N.** Suturing of the graft to itself and to the native ligament. **O.** Ulnar nerve transposition with fascial sling.

- A curette should be used to assure connection of these tunnels. Vicryl sutures should be passed in opposite directions such that a looped end is present at the origin of the ligament on the humerus and one looped end is located at the opening of the anterior tunnel.
- At this point, three sutures should be in the tunnels for passage of the graft.
- The palmaris longus graft is harvested using three transverse incisions approximately 1 cm in length starting distally at the wrist crease. Once the tendon is identified distally just beneath the skin, a hemostat is placed under the tendon and used to pull the tendon distally. This will allow for easy visualization of the subcutaneous position of the tendon.
- A second incision is made approximately 6 to 8 cm proximal to the initial incision. Once the tendon is identified here, the process is repeated and a hemostat is placed under the tendon to allow for traction to be applied. The third incision is placed approximately 15 cm from the wrist crease at the muscle tendon junction of the palmaris (**TECH FIG 1J**).
- Once all three incisions are created and the tendon is identified, the tendon can be cut distally and pulled out through each incision sequentially until the tendon is entirely located external to the most proximal incision (**TECH FIG 1K**). The entire tendon length should be at least 15 cm.
- Once this is confirmed, the tendon is transected as proximal as possible. Any muscle fibers should be removed.
- The tendon ends should be tagged using a no. 2 suture to aid in passage of the graft. Care should be taken not to make the end too bulbous (**TECH FIG 1L**).
- The graft is then passed in a retrograde fashion through the 4.5-mm distal humeral tunnel and out through the 3.5-mm superomedial humeral tunnel. The graft is then passed through the adjacent 3.5-mm anterior humeral tunnel and back out through the 4.5-mm distal humeral tunnel to create the proximal loop of the figure-of-eight.
- The posterior limb of the graft that is exiting the humerus should be brought over the top and into the anterior ulnar tunnel. This will then exit out the posterior ulnar tunnel to complete the figure-of-eight (**TECH FIG 1M**).
- Both limbs are then pulled to tension the graft. The elbow should be placed in approximately 45 to 60 degrees of flexion. An assistant should maintain a varus force on the elbow for the rest of the procedure.
- Prior to suturing the graft, the palmaris longus graft incisions should be closed.
- The graft is then tied to itself using a nonabsorbable suture. Multiple points of fixation should be used.
- The native ligament can then be closed over the top of the reconstruction to add more collagen tissue to the reconstruction (**TECH FIG 1N**).
- The ulnar nerve is usually not visualized during the procedure. If a transposition is performed, the nerve can be identified and dissected out at the onset of the procedure.
- The most common transposition performed in this setting is an anterior subcutaneous transposition, which avoids takedown of the FPM. The nerve is freed proximally and distally to the motor branch of the flexor carpi ulnaris. It is then brought anterior to the epicondyle and secured there loosely in a subcutaneous pocket or fascial sling with absorbable sutures (**TECH FIG 1O**).
- Closure of the FPM fascial splits can be performed using absorbable suture.
- The subcutaneous layer and the skin are closed using absorbable suture and a static splint is applied with the elbow at 90 degrees of flexion, the forearm in neutral rotation including the wrist.

Docking Technique

- Several other techniques have been described that use the same exposure but different modes of graft passage and fixation.
- The docking technique uses the same ulnar tunnel but only one proximal humeral tunnel for the graft. It is a common technique used.
- After drilling the ulnar and the central humeral tunnel in a retrograde fashion, two smaller holes are drilled in an anterograde fashion from the superior and anterior aspect of the medial epicondyle through the anterior FPM split. These tunnels are made with a 2.0-mm drill bit sufficient for passage of sutures. This bridge should be at least 8 to 10 mm in size.
- The two smaller proximal holes will also converge on the central humeral tunnel. Sutures or wire should be passed through each smaller tunnel in an anterograde fashion exiting the distal humeral tunnel. These should be kept separate so as to avoid crossing the sutures. The looped end of both sutures should come out the distal end of the tunnel.
- The graft is prepared in a slightly different fashion than the figure-of-eight technique. A nonabsorbable no. 2 suture is placed in a Krackow pattern on one end. The other end can be tagged with a temporary stitch.
- The graft is first passed through the ulna (**TECH FIG 2A**). The end with the nonabsorbable suture is passed first and is brought into the humeral tunnel so as to sit flush in the tunnel. The sutures should exit out one of the smaller drill holes in the humerus.
- The graft should be tensioned and then the other limb of the graft is sized for the appropriate length. The graft is then cut to fit into the humeral tunnel without any laxity. This tunnel should be 10 to 15 mm in length.
- A second nonabsorbable 2.0 suture is then placed using a Krackow stitch pattern along approximately 1 cm of the exposed end of the graft. The ends of this suture are passed through the humeral tunnel and out the other 2.0-mm drill hole docking the graft into the humerus. It is then tensioned, and the sutures coming out through each of the smaller humeral drill holes are tied together over the bone bridge.
- The graft is essentially one loop from the humerus into the ulna and back (**TECH FIG 2B**). After the graft is tied, the two limbs can also be sutured together to provide additional tension. All this should be done with a varus force applied to the elbow.
- The closure is as previously described.

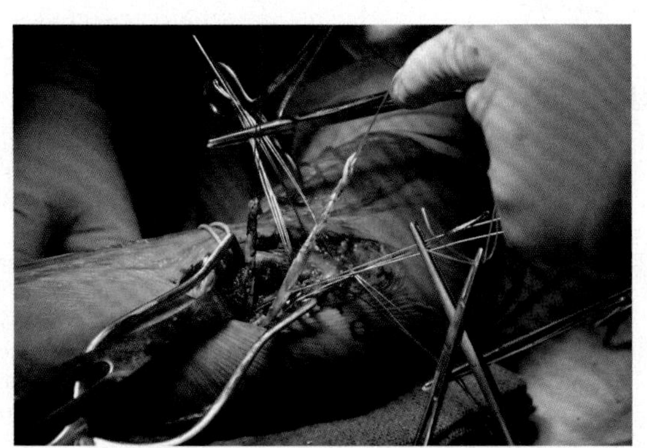

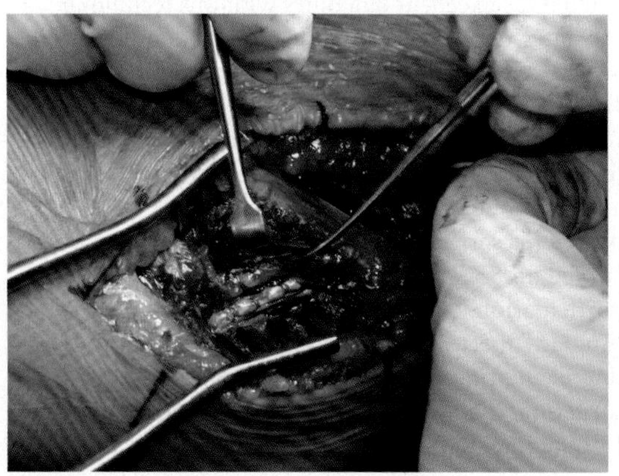

TECH FIG 2 • **A.** Graft passed through the ulnar tunnel. **B.** Graft in place for docking technique.

Other Techniques

- Other techniques have been described using interference screws or suture implants. One such technique, the DANE technique, uses an interference screw on the ulna and the docking technique on the humerus. This technique has also resulted in good outcomes.[5]

PEARLS AND PITFALLS

Difficulty in passing the graft	▪ The tunnels should be meticulously cleaned of any fragments or ridges of bone that may prevent passage. In addition, the end of the graft should not be too large and suture should be used judiciously on each end to prevent enlarging the graft. Mineral oil can be applied to the graft to aid in passage.
Fracture of the bone bridge between the tunnels	▪ A backup option should be available during surgery. Care should be taken to avoid this, but if it occurs, interference screw or EndoButton fixation can be successful in salvaging the reconstruction.
Hamstring autograft is used.	▪ Unlike the palmaris longus graft, the hamstring is much thicker and should be thinned sufficiently to facilitate passage.
Neurologic awareness	▪ Care should be taken to identify the medial antebrachial cutaneous nerve during exposure and protect it throughout the surgery and during closure to prevent a neuroma in continuity. ▪ One should also remain vigilant of the close proximity to the ulnar nerve during drilling of the posterior ulnar tunnel to prevent postoperative neurologic symptoms.

POSTOPERATIVE CARE

- The patient is placed in a posterior splint at the time of surgery for 7 to 10 days.
- After that, the patient is placed in a hinged elbow brace with progressive advancement of elbow flexion and extension weekly until full ROM is achieved at 4 to 6 weeks.
- Gentle strengthening is initiated between weeks 6 and 12. Special attention is directed toward optimizing leg, core, and shoulder strength and flexibility.
- Swinging a bat, golf club, or racquet may begin at 3 months after surgery. A throwing program is begun at 4 months. Progressive tossing proceeds from ~30 feet to ~180 to 200 feet. Pitchers begin to throw from the mound at 6 to 8 months.
- Full recovery in overhead athletes that place a repetitive valgus load on the elbow will take 12 to 18 months.
- Other athletes can return to full activity by 8 to 12 months.

OUTCOMES

- Most outcome studies after reconstruction have been performed in baseball players.
- The original article by Jobe et al[11] showed a 63% return to participation. A second article published by Conway et al [4] showed a 68% return to previous level of competition with reconstruction.
- More recent articles have evaluated the modified Jobe technique, which incorporates a muscle-splitting approach and

ulnar nerve transposition only if needed. Thompson and associates[15] reported 93% excellent outcomes with this technique.

- Cain and associates[1] reviewed 743 athletes with a minimum 2-year follow-up and found that 83% return to the same or higher level of competition.
- Rohrbough and associates[13] and Dodson et al[7] evaluated outcomes of the docking technique and reported 90% to 92% return to the same or higher level of play.
- Savoie[14] reported his series of UCL reconstructions using allograft and noted an 83% return to the same or higher level of athletic participation.
- Vitale and Ahmad[16] performed a systematic review of published studies evaluating outcomes of patients following UCL reconstruction. They found that 83% of patients had an excellent outcome with an overall 10% complication rate.
- Factors related to better outcomes included use of the muscle-splitting approach in lieu of the FPM takedown. Also, series in which patients only had an ulnar nerve transposition if needed resulted in better outcomes.[16]
- Research done on professional baseball pitchers reveals a rate of return of 82% to 83%[8,9] and no significant loss of pitching velocity.[10]
- Athletes not participating in repetitive overhead activity with large valgus force have a high rate of return to the prior level of competition with nonsurgical management.
- Concurrent injury to the FPM, ulnar nerve, or intra-articular structures can decrease the chances of returning to the preinjury level of competition.

COMPLICATIONS

- Elbow stiffness is a complication that can occur with any elbow surgery. Progressive advancement of elbow ROM in the first 4 weeks postoperatively should be initiated. In cases where ROM is lacking, an NSAID can be beneficial in decreasing inflammation and can aid in achieving full ROM. In more difficult cases, dynamic splinting can be used.
- Injury to the ulnar nerve can occur during surgery. When retracting around the sublime tubercle, care should be taken to avoid excessive pressure on the nerve. If the nerve is already irritated preoperatively, this may increase the possibility of postoperative nerve symptoms.
- Injury to the medial antebrachial cutaneous nerve can occur. Neuroma in continuity can give medial elbow pain that may cause persistent symptoms in the overhead athlete.
- Undiagnosed intra-articular pathology can cause persistent symptoms. Preoperative MRI or diagnostic elbow arthroscopy will minimize this possibility.
- Cain and associates[1] reported a complication rate of 20% in their series. Only 4% of these were considered major complications.

REFERENCES

1. Cain EL Jr, Andrews JR, Dugas JR, et al. Outcome of ulnar collateral ligament reconstruction of the elbow in 1281 athletes: results in 743 athletes with minimum 2-year follow-up. Am J Sports Med 2010;38:2426–2434.
2. Ciccotti MG, Atanda A Jr, Nazarian LN, et al. Stress sonography of the ulnar collateral ligament of the elbow in professional baseball pitchers: a 10-year study. Am J Sports Med 2014;42(3):544–551.
3. Ciccotti MG, Siegler S, Kuri JA II, et al. Comparison of the biomechanical profile of the intact ulnar collateral ligament with the modified Jobe and the Docking reconstructed elbow: an in vitro study. Am J Sports Med 2009;37:974–981.
4. Conway JE, Jobe FW, Glousman RE, et al. Medial instability of the elbow in throwing athletes. Treatment by repair or reconstruction of the ulnar collateral ligament. J Bone Joint Surg Am 1992;74:67–83.
5. Dines JS, ElAttrache NS, Conway JE, et al. Clinical outcomes of the DANE TJ technique to treat ulnar collateral ligament insufficiency of the elbow. Am J Sports Med 2007;35:2039–2044.
6. Dodson CC, Slenker N, Cohen SB, et al. Ulnar collateral ligament injuries of the elbow in professional football quarterbacks. J Shoulder Elbow Surg 2010;19:1276–1280.
7. Dodson CC, Thomas A, Dines JS, et al. Medial ulnar collateral ligament reconstruction of the elbow in throwing athletes. Am J Sports Med 2006;34:1926–1932.
8. Erickson BJ, Gupta AK, Harris JD, et al. Rate of return to pitching and performance after Tommy John Surgery in Major League Baseball pitchers. Am J Sports Med 2014;42(3):536–543.
9. Gibson BW, Webner D, Huffman GR, et al. Ulnar collateral ligament reconstruction in major league baseball pitchers. Am J Sports Med 2007;35:575–581.
10. Jiang JJ, Leland JM. Analysis of pitching velocity in major league baseball players before and after ulnar collateral ligament reconstruction. Am J Sports Med 2014;42(4):880–885.
11. Jobe FW, Stark H, Lombardo SJ. Reconstruction of the ulnar collateral ligament in athletes. J Bone Joint Surg Am 1986;68:1158–1163.
12. Podesta L, Crow SA, Volkmer D, et al. Treatment of partial ulnar collateral ligament tears in the elbow with platelet-rich-plasma. Am J Sports Med 2013;41:1689–1694.
13. Rohrbough JT, Altchek DW, Hyman J, et al. Medial collateral ligament reconstruction of the elbow using the docking technique. Am J Sports Med 2002;30:541–548.
14. Savoie FH III, Morgan C, Yaste J, et al. Medial ulnar collateral ligament reconstruction using hamstring allograft in overhead throwing athletes. J Bone Joint Surg Am 2013;95:1062–1066.
15. Thompson WH, Jobe FW, Yocum LA, et al. Ulnar collateral ligament reconstruction in athletes: muscle-splitting approach without transposition of the ulnar nerve. J Shoulder Elbow Surg 2001;10:152–157.
16. Vitale MA, Ahmad CS. The outcome of elbow ulnar collateral ligament reconstruction in overhead athletes: a systematic review. Am J Sports Med 2008;36:1193–1205.

Reconstruction for Interosseous Ligament Disruption

60 CHAPTER

Check C. Kam, Christopher M. Jones, and E. Anne Ouellette

DEFINITION

- An Essex-Lopresti injury or longitudinal radioulnar dissociation (LRUD) occurs when a violent compressive load to the wrist results in a triad of injuries: distal radioulnar joint (DRUJ) disruption, interosseous ligament complex (IOLC) tear, and radial head fracture.

ANATOMY

- The radial head is the primary axial stabilizer of the radius, preventing proximal radial migration during axial wrist loads by its abutment with the capitellum.[20]
- The most important secondary stabilizer of the forearm longitudinal axis is the IOLC, which is responsible for 71% of the longitudinal stiffness of the forearm after radial head resection.[10]
- The triangular fibrocartilage complex is another secondary stabilizer and contributes 8% to forearm longitudinal stiffness.[10]
- The IOLC is composed of five segments with the central band being the stoutest, most important, and consistently present. The mean width of the central band is 9.7 mm. It is 1 to 2 mm thick and 40 mm long[17] (**FIG 1**).
- The central band fibers run, on average, 24 degrees to the long axis of the ulna, originating about 9 cm from the ulnar head (or 34% of the length) and inserting onto the radial interosseous ridge about 14 cm from radial styloid (or 57% of the radial length).[3]

PATHOGENESIS

- At the wrist, the radius transmits 80% of the axial load and the ulna 20%.[18]
- As force travels proximally along the forearm, it is redistributed by the IOLC; so at the elbow, the radiocapitellar joint bears 57% of the load, whereas the ulnohumeral articulation bears 43%.[2,7]
- In cases of LRUD, inserting a radial head prosthesis may restore axial stability but will not address load distribution at the elbow if the IOLC does not heal. The radiocapitellar joint may be subject to supraphysiologic loads without the IOLC to redistribute forces, leading to pain and early degenerative changes.
- Healing of the IOLC cannot be assured even if LRUD is diagnosed early and treated appropriately.[6] This may be due to the substantial herniation of the muscle bellies through the interosseous membrane which would interfere with coaptation of the torn ligament ends.[1,15] Additionally, the ligament has intrinsic properties that makes healing difficult.[16] Reports of immediate shortening of the radius after late removal of a radial head implant[24] and accelerated radiocapitellar wear due to an incompetent IOLC have been reported.[13] Radial head arthroplasty alone for the treatment of chronic LRUD is inadequate and this treatment has been shown to fail in 63% of patients within 3 years.[8]

NATURAL HISTORY

- The incidence of LRUD is likely underdiagnosed and recent literature suggests it may result in 3% of radial head fractures.[9,12,27,28]
- Axial forearm instability, in the absence of a competent radial head, results in progressive proximal radius migration with ulnocarpal abutment and DRUJ dislocation.
- Even with an appropriately repaired or replaced radial head, LRUD can lead to accelerated radiocapitellar wear due to altered forearm mechanics.
- Delayed treatment is associated with unsuccessful results in 80% of patients.[27]

PATIENT HISTORY AND PHYSICAL FINDINGS

- A high index of clinical suspicion is essential to make the diagnosis of LRUD as it is often missed at initial presentation.[13]
- Patients present with a history of a high-energy axial loading of the forearm, that is, fall from height onto outstretched arms.
- Initially, the primary complaint may be isolated to the elbow and the radiographically obvious radial head fracture. Forearm and wrist pain might also be present.
- In the acute setting, all patients with a radial head fracture should be examined for DRUJ laxity and tenderness, forearm swelling, and tenderness along the interosseous space. Positive examination findings indicate the need for further imaging workup.

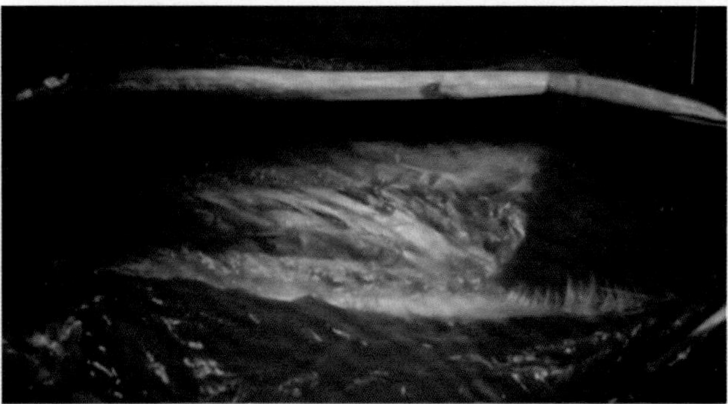

FIG 1 • IOLC and central band.

- Frequently, patients present subacutely with ulnocarpal abutment after a radial head excision or shortened fracture malunion. Recurrent radius shortening can occur after a wrist joint leveling procedure if the underlying LRUD is not addressed.
- In one series, ulnar-sided wrist pain started on average of 9 months following radial head excision.[1]
- Intraoperatively, following radial head excision, the radial pull test can help diagnose IOLC disruption. If the ulnar variance increases greater than or equal to 3 mm with 20 pounds of proximal radius traction, the IOLC is likely disrupted. An intact IOLC will have less than 1 mm increase in ulnar variance and will have an elastic rebound following release.[23]

IMAGING AND OTHER DIAGNOSTIC STUDIES

- In addition to standard radiographs of the affected elbow and forearm, bilateral neutral forearm wrist posteroanterior (PA) views are used to compare ulnar variance.
- Magnetic resonance imaging (MRI) and ultrasound have been shown to be similarly effective in diagnosing IOLC injury in cadaver arms with over 90% sensitivity and specificity.[5] However, the accuracy of these studies for clinical use has been questioned.[24]
- Bilateral comparison of maximum forearm interosseous space might help to confirm the diagnosis. In a cadaver LRUD model, we found the maximum interosseous space measured radiographically increased 70% from 13.9 to 23.4 mm after IOLC disruption. The measurements were made with the forearm in full supination and the results were statistically significant (unpublished data) (**FIG 2**).

DIFFERENTIAL DIAGNOSIS

- Isolated radial head fracture
- Partial IOLC disruption

NONOPERATIVE MANAGEMENT

- Patients with a Mason type 1 radial head fracture can be immobilized in a Muenster cast in a position where the DRUJ is reduced (usually maximum supination). At least 8 weeks of immobilization is required. However, the IOLC may not heal with structural integrity.

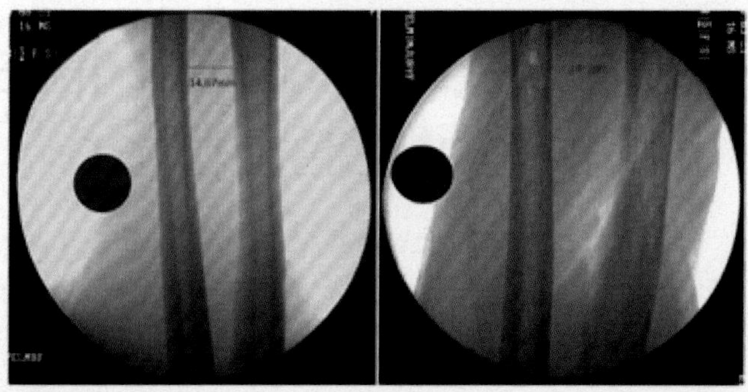

FIG 2 • Comparison of maximum interosseous space in a cadaver arm before and after IOLC disruption.

SURGICAL MANAGEMENT

- Surgical management will depend on whether the injury is acute or chronic. In acute situations, repairing or replacing the radial head and stabilizing the DRUJ either by splinting in supination or pinning the DRUJ can lead to a satisfactory outcome.[27]
- Chronic conditions require addressing the deficient radial head, ulnocarpal abutment, and incompetent IOLC. Radial head arthroplasty (if possible), ulnar shortening osteotomy, and central band reconstruction are usually required.
- IOLC reconstruction has been described using pronator teres rerouting,[4] autograft and allograft tendon, suture and suture-button constructs, and bone–patellar tendon–bone graft.[11,14,15,19,21,22,26]

Preoperative Planning

- Radiographically estimate the amount of ulnar shortening required to level the wrist joint.

Positioning

- Supine with radiolucent hand table
- General anesthesia or regional block is used.
- A nonsterile tourniquet is used on the upper arm.

TECHNIQUES

■ Radial Head Arthroplasty

- An extensor digitorum communis (EDC) splitting approach to the radial head is used.
- Distract the radius to open the radiocapitellar space and assess feasibility of a radial head arthroplasty.
  - In the setting of chronic radial capitellar abutment after radial head excision, it might be impossible to insert a radial head. Ilizarov techniques have been used in the past to gradually regain radius length prior to allograft radial head replacement in two stages in chronic LRUD.[25]
  - Marcotte and Osterman[15] did not perform radial head arthroplasties in their series of 16 patients with chronic LRUD with good results.
- Excise the malunited radial head or make necessary radial neck cuts to insert an implant.
- Place the appropriately sized radial head implant. Do not overstuff the joint, as this will increase radiocapitellar impingement, decreased motion, and increase elbow pain.

Ulnar Shortening Osteotomy

- A 10-cm incision is made over the distal third of the ulna in the interval between extensor carpi ulnaris (ECU) and flexor carpi ulnaris (FCU).
- Distally, the dorsal ulnar sensory nerve is identified and protected.
- The ulna is exposed subperiosteally.
- Considering the amount of radial lengthening, if any, achieved after radial head arthroplasty, the appropriately sized ulnar osteotomy is performed followed by compression plating.
    - Keep in mind, tightening the IOLC reconstruction will likely result in 2 to 4 mm of further ulnar shortening.
- The goal is to achieve 1 to 2 mm ulnar negative variance postoperatively.

Central Band Interosseous Ligament Complex Reconstruction

- Of the many procedures discussed for IOLC reconstruction, bone–tendon–bone has been the most extensively described and clinically evaluated.[1] We believe the suture-button reconstruction is easier to perform and better restores the forearm mechanics by placing the repair at the anatomic axis of forearm rotation. Combining this with allo- or autograft tendon weave could provide lasting stability. Both procedures are described in the following text.

Bone–Patellar Tendon–Bone Central Band Reconstruction

- The previous ulnar incision is used.
- A Kelly clamp is used to create a path under the extensor musculature, about 24 degrees to the axis of the ulna and exiting around the pronator teres insertion.
- Blunt dissection is used to develop the plane under the extensor compartment and over the IOLC, being mindful of the posterior interosseous nerve (PIN).
- An incision is made proximally over the radial shaft, and the interval between the brachioradialis and ECRL is developed. The pronator teres insertion is identified (**TECH FIG 1**).
- With a small burr, obliquely oriented troughs approximately 15 mm wide × 5 mm deep are made in the distal ulna and proximal radius, corresponding to the anatomic origin and insertion of the central band (at 34% of the ulnar length and at 57% of the radial length).
    - The origin and insertion points might need to be adjusted to fit the given patellar tendon length.
- Bone–patellar tendon–bone allograft blocks are trimmed to fit snugly in the troughs after being passed under the extensor musculature.
- The forearm is placed in semisupination. Holding distal traction on the radius with a bone clamp, the bone blocks are individually secured with the graft held taut using 3.5-mm bicortical screws (see **TECH FIG 1**).
- Wounds are closed in layer fashion.

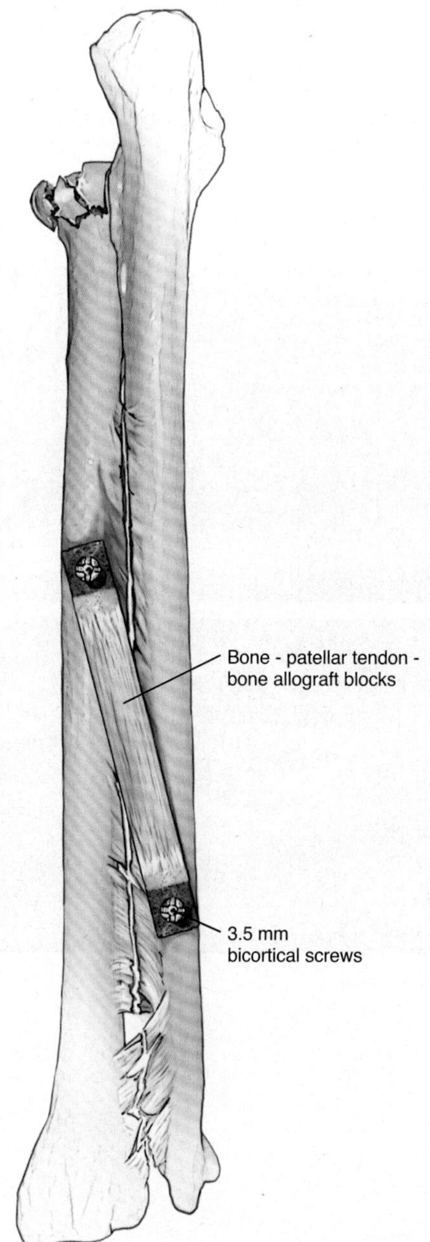

TECH FIG 1 • Drawing depicting the final bone–patellar tendon–bone reconstruction of the central band.

Suture-Button Construct with Allograft Tendon (Alternative Method)

- An Arthrex Mini-Tightrope (or Graftrope) is used for the reconstruction.
- The previous ulnar incision is used. As described earlier, a plane is created under the extensor musculature. The pronator teres insertion is exposed through a separate incision (**TECH FIG 2A**).
- A guidewire for the Tightrope is drilled through the radial shaft at the pronator insertion, aiming about 24 degrees to the ulnar axis (**TECH FIG 2B**).
- Under direct visualization from the ulnar incision, the guidewire is advanced under the extensors and into the ulnar shaft.
  - Keep in mind, the trajectory of the wire is highly dependent of the rotation of the forearm. The forearm should be gently rotated so that the wire can be advanced into the central axis of ulnar shaft.
  - If this proves too challenging, a separate guidewire can be placed through the ulna, from the ulnar incision, in the estimated trajectory.
- Fluoroscopy is used to ensure the guidewire is in the proper anatomic path.
- The guidewire path is overdrilled with the appropriate cannulated drill separately from the radial and ulnar sides (**TECH FIG 2C**).
  - With the Graftrope, a 6-mm drill is required, necessitating that the guidewire be in the central axis of the bone, to prevent off-center drilling. Due to the size of the drill holes, the Graftrope might be inappropriate for small stature patients.
- The suture-button construct (with allograft tendon for the Graftrope) is assembled on the back table and advanced through the radial to ulnar tunnels using the included lasso and pull-through suture (**TECH FIG 2D**).
- The button is flipped on the outer ulnar cortex and tensioned appropriately. It is secured with the forearm in neutral rotation (**TECH FIG 2E**).
- Full passive forearm rotation is assured as well as appropriate ulnar variance.
- Wounds are closed in layered fashion, and an above-elbow splint is applied.
- Final construct should be as depicted in **TECH FIG 2F**.

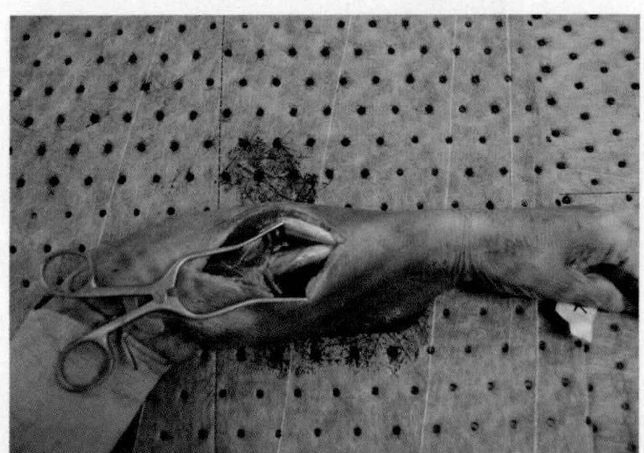
A

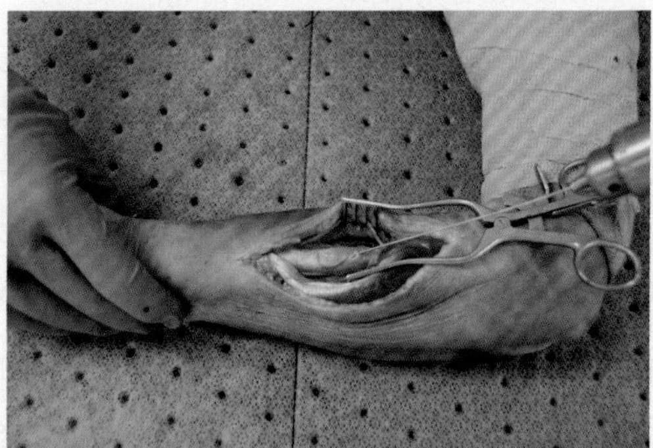
B

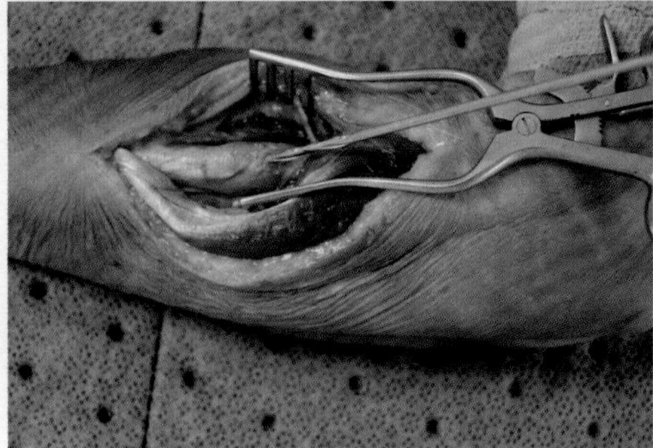
C

TECH FIG 2 • A. Proximal radial exposure is made between the brachioradialis and the wrist extensors. The superficial radial nerve is deep to the brachioradialis. **B.** Trajectory for radial tunnel placement at the pronator teres insertional site. **C.** The guidewire for the radial tunnel is overdrilled with the cannulated drill. *(continued)*

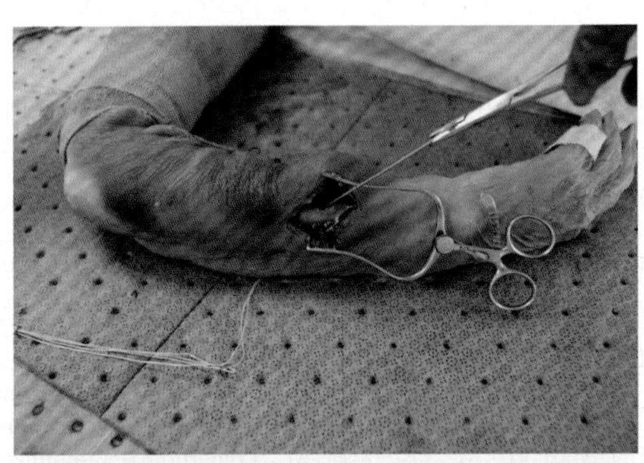

D

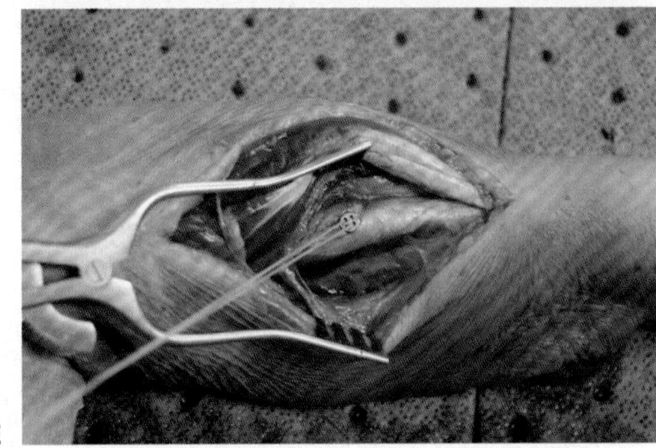

E

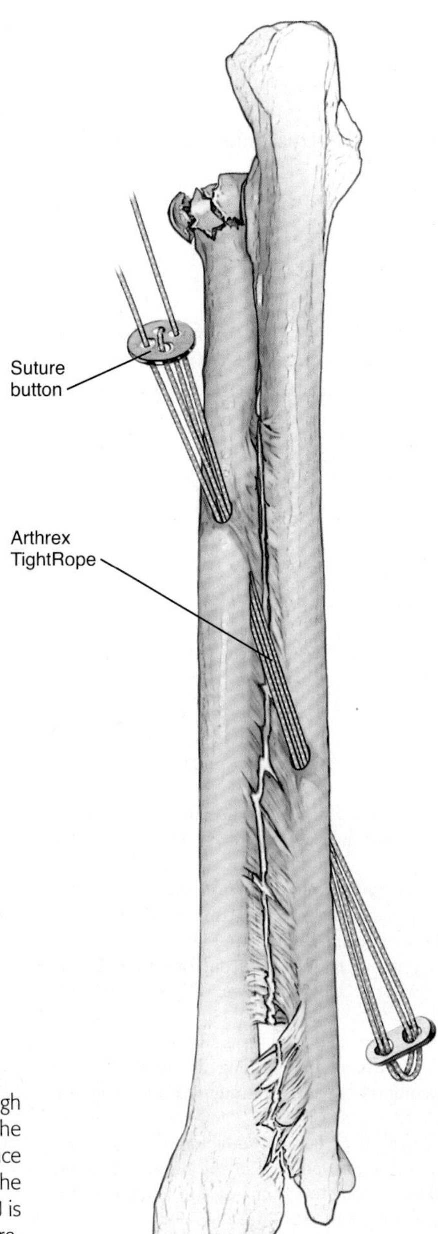

F

TECH FIG 2 • *(continued)* **D.** The lasso and pull-through suture is passed through the predrilled ulnar tunnel until the suture button engages the outer cortex of the ulna. **E.** Once the button is engaged securely on the far ulnar cortex, the sutures are then tensioned on the radial side until the DRUJ is reduced and then tied. **F.** Drawing depicting the final suture-button construct used to reconstruct the central band.

PEARLS AND PITFALLS

Bone–patellar tendon–bone reconstruction	▪ Use allograft tissue to avoid knee pain. ▪ Place ulnar shortening osteotomy plate volarly so the bone trough can sit on the dorsal ulnar cortex.
Suture-button reconstruction or Graftrope reconstruction	▪ Avoid unicortical or eccentric bone tunnels with drilling. ▪ Use a hemostat to clamp sutures to check final tension and DRUJ under fluoroscopy before tying down.
Radial head implant for stability	▪ Ulnar variance is used to assure proper length of the radial head implant. Unlike simple radial head arthroplasty where the IOLC is intact, proper radial head implant length cannot be judged by tension of the reduction or widening of the lateral ulnohumeral joint.

POSTOPERATIVE CARE

- Long-arm splint with forearm and wrist in neutral position until suture removal at 2 weeks
- Munster splint applied at 2 weeks and elbow active range of motion (AROM) initiated
- Four to 6 weeks: Muenster splint discontinued and AROM of wrist and forearm initiated
- Strengthening starts at 3 months postoperative and return to sports at 6 months postoperative.

OUTCOMES

- At 78 months, Osterman showed 15 of 16 patients had improved wrist pain. Grip strength in this cohort improved from 59% to 86% compared with the unaffected limb, and there was maintenance of the ulnar variance at −1.5 mm.[15]

COMPLICATIONS

- Ulnar nonunion
- Extensor tendon adhesions
- Progression of radiocapitellar arthritis
- Radial head prosthesis loosening

REFERENCES

1. Adams JE, Culp RW, Osterman AL. Interosseous membrane reconstruction for the Essex-Lopresti injury. J Hand Surg Am 2010;35(1):129–136.
2. Birkbeck DP, Failla JM, Hoshaw SJ, et al. The interosseous membrane affects load distribution in the forearm. J Hand Surg Am 1997;22(6):975–980.
3. Chandler JW, Stabile KJ, Pfaeffle HJ, et al. Anatomic parameters for planning of interosseous ligament reconstructionusing computer-assisted techniques. J Hand Surg Am 2003;28(1):111–116.
4. Chloros GD, Wiesler ER, Stabile KJ, et al. Reconstruction of Essex-Lopresti injury of the forearm: technical note. J Hand Surg Am 2008;33(1):124–130.
5. Fester EW, Murray PM, Sanders TG, et al. The efficacy of magnetic resonance imaging and ultrasound in detecting disruptions of the forearm interosseous membrane: a cadaver study. J Hand Surg Am 2002;27:418–424.
6. Gong HS, Chung MS, Oh JH, et al. Failure of the interosseous membrane to heal with immobilization, pinning of the distal radioulnar joint, and bipolar radial head replacement in a case of Essex-Lopresti injury: case report. J Hand Surg Am 2010;35(6):976–980.
7. Halls AA, Travill A. Transmission of pressures across the elbow joint. Anat Rec 1960;150:243–247.
8. Heijink A, Morrey BF, van Riet RP, et al. Delayed treatment of elbow pain and dysfunction following Essex-Lopresti injury with metallic radial head replacement: a case series. J Shoulder Elbow Surg 2010;19(6):929–936.
9. Helmerhorst GT, Ring D. Subtle Essex-Lopresti lesions: report of 2 cases. J Hand Surg Am 2009;34(3):436–438.
10. Hotchkiss RN, An KN, Sowa DT, et al. An anatomic and mechanical study of the interosseous membrane of the forearm: pathomechanics and proximal migration of the radius. J Hand Surg Am 1989;14(2 pt 1):256–261.
11. Jones CM, Kam CC, Ouellette EA, et al. Comparison of 2 forearm reconstructions for longitudinal radioulnar dissociation: a cadaver study. J Hand Surg Am 2012;37(4):741–747.
12. Jungbluth P, Frangen TM, Arens S, et al. The undiagnosed Essex-Lopresti injury. J Bone Joint Surg Br 2006;88(12):1629–1633.
13. Jungbluth P, Frangen TM, Muhr G, et al. A primarily overlooked and incorrectly treated Essex-Lopresti injury: what can this lead to? Arch Orthop Trauma Surg 2008;128:89–95.
14. Kam CC, Jones CM, Fennema JL, et al. Suture-button construct for interosseous ligament reconstruction in longitudinal radioulnar dissociations: a biomechanical study. J Hand Surg Am 2010;35(10):1626–1632.
15. Marcotte AL, Osterman AL. Longitudinal radioulnar dissociation: identification and treatment of acute and chronic injuries. Hand Clin 2007;23(2):195–208, vi.
16. McGinley JC, Kozin SH. Interosseous membrane anatomy and functional mechanics. Clin Orthop Relat Res 2001;(383):108–122.
17. Noda K, Goto A, Murase T, et al. Interosseous membrane of the forearm: an anatomical study of ligament attachment locations. J Hand Surg Am 2009;34(3):415–422.
18. Palmer AK, Werner FW. Biomechanics of the distal radioulnar joint. Clin Orthop Relat Res 1984;(187):26–35.
19. Pfaeffle HJ, Stabile KJ, Li ZM, et al. Reconstruction of the interosseous ligament restores normal forearm compressive load transfer in cadavers. J Hand Surg Am 2005;30(2):319–325.
20. Rabinowitz RS, Light TR, Havey RM, et al. The role of the interosseous membrane and triangular fibrocartilage complex in forearm stability. J Hand Surg Am 1994;19(3):385–393.
21. Sellman DC, Seitz WH Jr, Postak PD, et al. Reconstructive strategies for radioulnar dissociation: a biomechanical study. J Orthop Trauma 1995;9(6):516–522.
22. Skahen JR III, Palmer AK, Werner FW, et al. Reconstruction of the interosseous membrane of the forearm in cadavers. J Hand Surg Am 1997;22:986–994.
23. Smith AM, Urbanosky LR, Castle JA, et al. Radius pull test: predictor of longitudinal forearm instability. J Bone Joint Surg Am 2002; 84-A(11):1970–1976.
24. Stevenson JD, Radesh L, Pickard S, et al. Falsely reassuring magnetic resonance imaging appearance of the forearm interosseous membrane following an Essex-Lopresti injury: does it ever completely heal? Should Elb 2010;2:287–290.
25. Szabo RM, Hotchkiss RN, Slater RR Jr. The use of frozen-allograft radial head replacement for treatment of established symptomatic proximal translation of the radius: preliminary experience in five cases. J Hand Surg 1997;22(2):269–278.
26. Tejwani SG, Markolf KL, Benhaim P. Graft reconstruction of the interosseous membrane in conjunction with metallic radial head replacement: a cadaveric study. J Hand Surg Am 2005;30(2): 335–342.
27. Trousdale RT, Amadio PC, Cooney WP, et al. Radio-ulnar dissociation. A review of twenty cases. J Bone Joint Surg Am 1992;74(10): 1486–1497.
28. Van Riet RP, Morrey BF, O'Driscoll SW, et al. Associated injuries complicating radial head fractures: a demographic study. Clin Orthop Relat Res 2005;441:351–355.

Radiocarpal Fracture-Dislocations

Chris J. Williamson and Asif M. Ilyas

61 CHAPTER

DEFINITION

- The radiocarpal joint's stability is provided by the carpal articulation at the scaphoid and lunate fossae as well as the soft tissue restraints of the capsule and extrinsic radiocarpal ligaments.
- Radiocarpal dislocations occur through a traumatic separation of the proximal carpal row from the articular surface of the distal radius.
- Radiocarpal dislocations can occur in either a volar or dorsal direction, with the most common direction being dorsal.
- Radiocarpal dislocations can occur with only soft tissue disruption or, more commonly, in association with marginal rim fractures of the distal radius or ulnar styloid.
- Radiocarpal dislocations are often confused with distal radius fractures of the marginal rim or volar/dorsal shear fractures (ie, "Barton" fractures) (**FIG 1**).
  - Radiocarpal dislocations represent a shear or avulsion injury of the wrist that may or may not be associated with an avulsion fracture of the distal radius or ulna (**FIG 1A**).
  - Barton fractures of the distal radius represent compression and/or shear fractures (**FIG 1B**).
- Two classification systems are typically used to describe radiocarpal dislocations.
  - Moneim et al[13] classified radiocarpal dislocations based on the presence or absence of an intercarpal ligament injury.
    - Type 1 dislocations do not have an associated intercarpal injury.
    - Type 2 injuries are associated with a concomitant scapholunate ligament.[13]
  - Dumontier et al[4] classified radiocarpal dislocations based on the presence or absence of an associated avulsion fracture off the radial styloid.
    - Type 1 injuries are considered purely ligamentous with minimal cortical avulsion off the radial styloid.
    - Type 2 injuries are associated with a large radial styloid fracture compromising of at least one-third of the scaphoid fossa.[4]

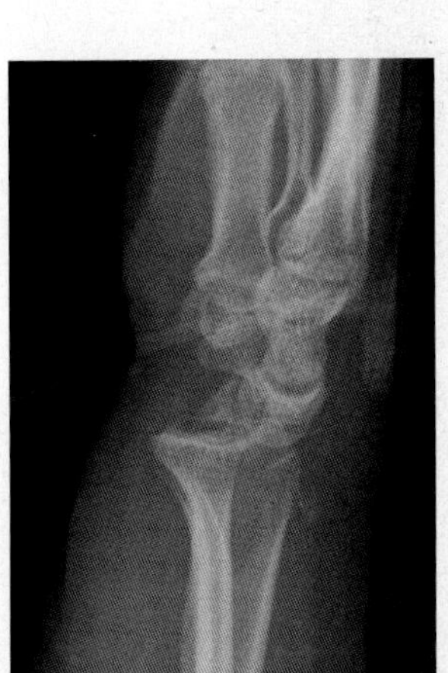
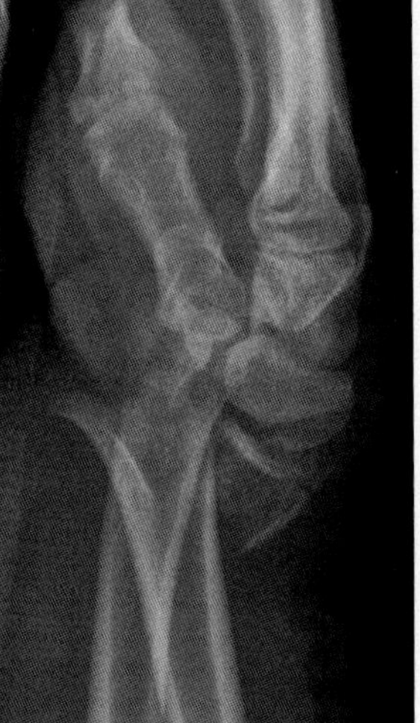

FIG 1 • Radiocarpal dislocations can be confused with shear fractures of the distal radius. **A.** Note the disruption of the carpus from the distal radius in this lateral view of a radiocarpal fracture-dislocation. In contrast, (**B**) note in this lateral view of this distal radius fracture that the relationship between the carpus and distal radial articular surface is maintained.

ANATOMY

- The average arc of motion in a normal wrist ranges from 68 degrees of flexion to 50 degrees of extension.[10]
- Radiocarpal joint stability is provided by both the osseous joint articulation between the scaphoid and lunate bones and their corresponding fossae of the distal radius, along with the extrinsic radiocarpal ligaments and the wrist capsule (**FIG 2**).
- Among the various volar radiocarpal ligaments, the primary ligaments important to radiocarpal stability are the short radiolunate and the radioscaphocapitate ligaments.
  - The short radiolunate ligament originates from the stout margin of the lunate facet of the volar distal radius and serves as the primary restraint against volar translation of the carpus.
  - The stout radioscaphocapitate ligament originates from the radial styloid and resists ulnar translation of the carpus.
- The ulnocarpal ligaments, including the ulnolunate and the ulnotriquetral ligaments, take their origin from the ulnar styloid. Along with the triangular fibrocartilage complex (TFCC), they assist in providing radiocarpal and ulnocarpal joint stability.
- The dorsal radiocarpal ligaments are highly variable[12] and also assist in imparting stability to the radiocarpal joint, although to a much lesser extent than the volar radiocarpal ligaments.

PATHOGENESIS

- Radiocarpal dislocations can occur in either a volar or dorsal direction, with dorsal being far more common (~85%).[4]
- The injury requires pronation and hyperextension of the wrist with a shear force across the joint. With increasing amounts of supination, the risk of a perilunate dislocation rather than a radiocarpal dislocation increases.[11]
- Disruption of the radiocarpal ligaments, the most critical of which are the radioscaphocapitate and the short radiolunate, is necessary to dislocate the radiocarpal joint.
- A pure dislocation without a bony injury is less common. More often, a fracture of the radial styloid, volar marginal rim, or ulnar styloid is identified representing an avulsion of the origin of the radioscaphocapitate, short radiolunate, or ulnocarpal ligaments, respectively.

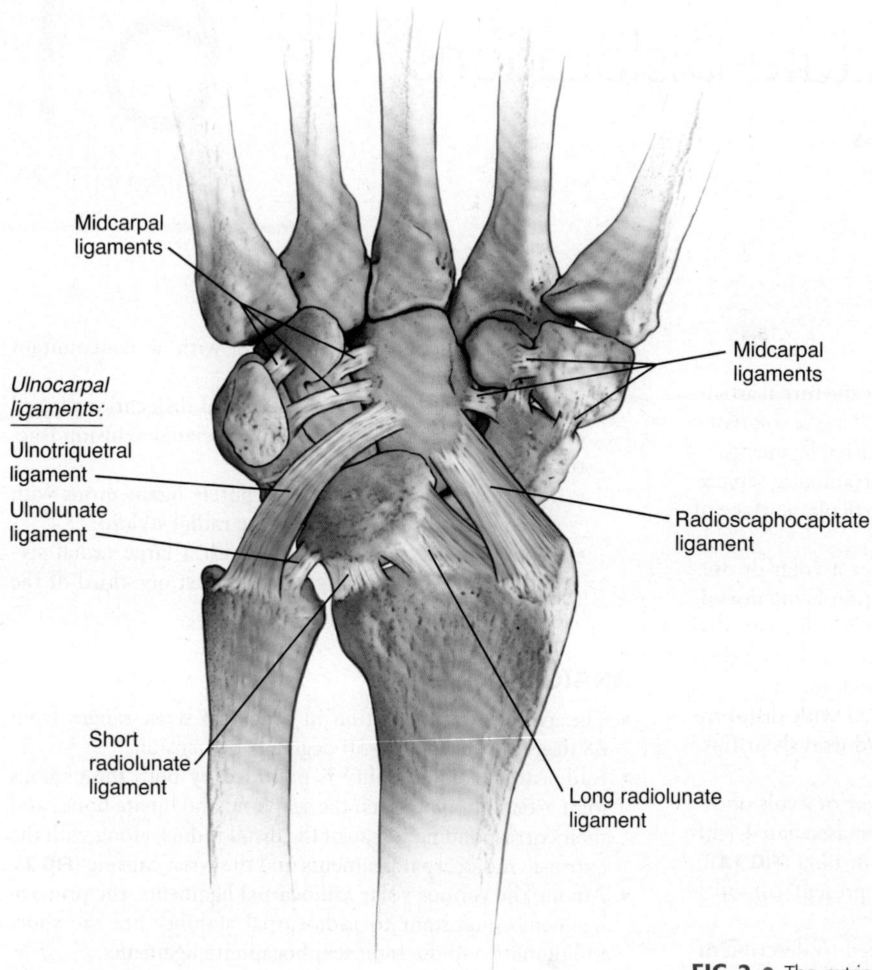

FIG 2 • The extrinsic volar radiocarpal ligaments of the wrist include radioscaphocapitate (RSC), long radiolunate (LRL), short radiolunate (SRL), ulnolunate (UL), ulnotriquetral (UT) ligaments.

NATURAL HISTORY

- Radiocarpal dislocations are high-energy injuries most often seen in males aged 20 to 40 years.[4,9]
- Mechanisms of injury are typically falls from a height, industrial injuries, and motor vehicle accidents.
- The incidence of radiocarpal dislocations has been published to be as low as 0.2%[5] of all hand and wrist dislocations.[5] More recent studies have found incidence of radiocarpal dislocations to be as high as 2.7% of all distal radius fractures and wrist dislocations.[9]
- Due to the high-energy nature of these injuries, there is a high association of associated injuries including neurologic injuries, vascular injuries, and open wounds.[1,4,13]
- Residual radiocarpal instability and posttraumatic wrist degeneration is common, particularly with purely ligamentous injuries (Dumontier type 1).[4]

PATIENT HISTORY AND PHYSICAL FINDINGS

- Radiocarpal dislocations typically present with a very swollen and painful wrist, with likely deformity (**FIG 3**).
- Physical examination should include a thorough neurologic, vascular, and tendon examination.
  - Neurologic deficits, particularly of the median nerve, are common with displaced radiocarpal dislocations.

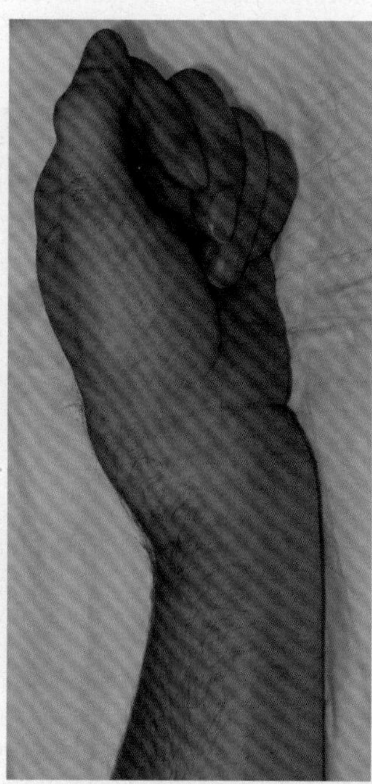

FIG 3 • Typical deformity following a dorsally displaced radiocarpal dislocation.

- Vascular embarrassment to the hand may occur with prolonged displacement and swelling.
- Incarceration of the dorsal extensor tendons can occur pre- and postreduction.
- Close inspection of the skin should also be performed, as open wounds can also be present possibly signifying an open arthrotomy of the wrist or an associated open fracture.[16]
- A full secondary survey is mandatory, as these injuries are typically high-energy and may be associated with concomitant fractures of other limbs and visceral injuries,[14] which have been reported to occur in 58% and 37% of cases, respectively.[4]

IMAGING AND OTHER DIAGNOSTIC STUDIES

- Evaluation should begin with plain radiographs including a posteroanterior and lateral views of the wrist (**FIG 4**). Additional oblique views can help in assessment.
  - On the lateral view, the radiograph should be scrutinized for the alignment of the arcs of Gilula, representing the relationship between the midcarpal and radiocarpal joints. Disruption between the lunate and the distal radius signifies a radiocarpal disruption, whereas disruption between the capitate and lunate may represent a perilunate injury (**FIG 5**).
  - On the posteroanterior view, the radiograph should be scrutinized for associated avulsion fractures of the distal radius or ulna, ulnar translation of the carpus relative to the distal radius, and intercarpal diastasis.
- Computed tomography (CT) may be helpful in identifying marginal rim fractures and to further evaluate intra-articular fracture patterns (**FIG 6**).
- Magnetic resonance imaging (MRI) is useful in evaluating the soft tissue stabilizers of the radiocarpal joint. In addition, MRI can provide better evaluation of associated injuries such as to the intercarpal ligaments and TFCC.

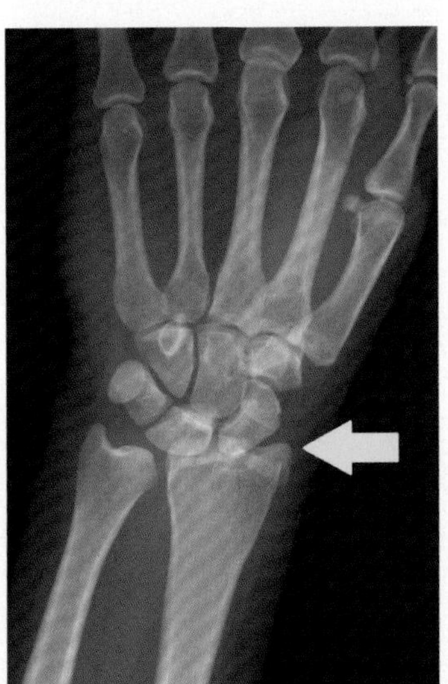

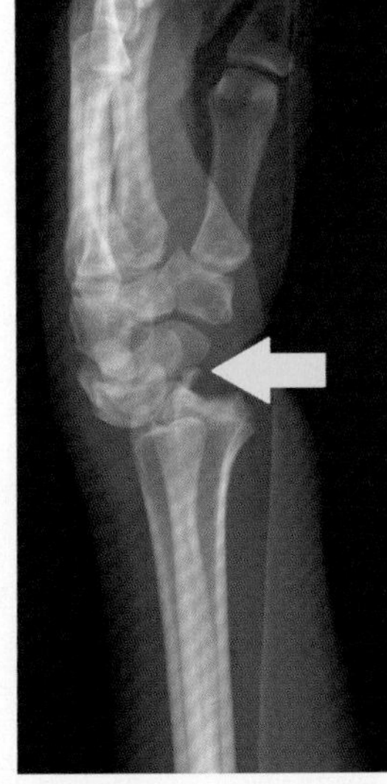

FIG 4 • Anteroposterior and lateral views of a radiocarpal dislocation. **A.** On the anteroposterior view, note the *yellow arrow* is pointing to the avulsed fracture of the radial styloid. **B.** On the lateral view, the *yellow arrow* is pointing to a volar radiocarpal ligament avulsion fracture following disruption of the proximal carpal row relative to the distal radius.

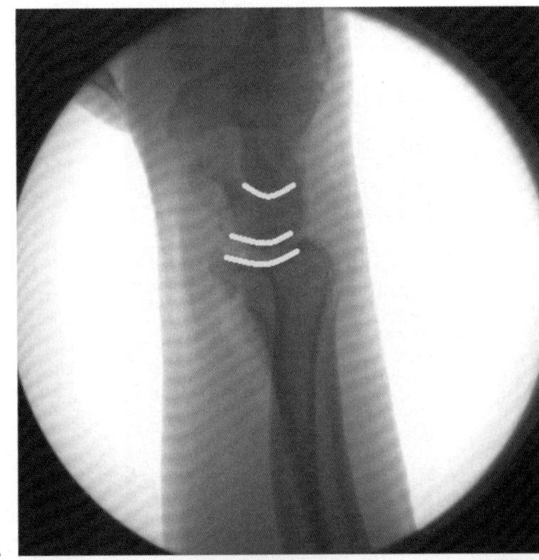

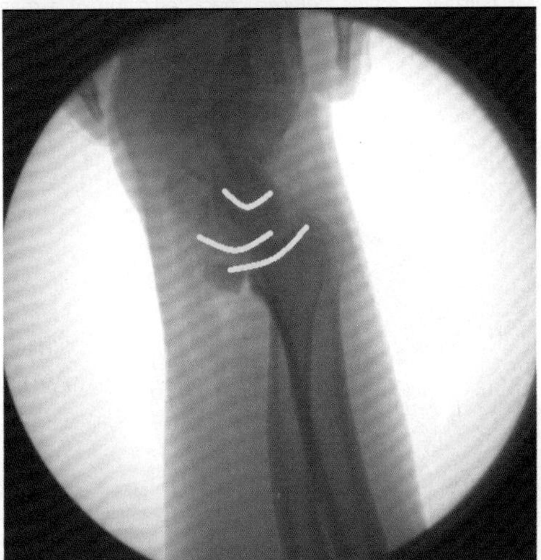

FIG 5 • The arcs of Gilula represent the "cup-shaped" (*yellow lines*) alignment of the capitates, lunate, and distal radial articular surfaces on the lateral view. **A.** When the wrist is reduced, the "cups" stack up symmetrically. **B.** When the radiocarpal joint is subluxed or dislocated, as is the case with this radiocarpal dislocation with an associated volar marginal rim fracture, the cups will not be aligned.

DIFFERENTIAL DIAGNOSIS

- Colles fracture
- Smith fracture
- Barton fracture
- Perilunate dislocation

NONOPERATIVE MANAGEMENT

- Surgical repair is indicated for all displaced radiocarpal dislocations. Uniformly poor outcomes have been shown with nonoperative management and minimal repair techniques due to the high risk of persistent radiocarpal instability and resulting posttraumatic degeneration.[2]

SURGICAL MANAGEMENT

- Successful management of radiocarpal dislocations is dependent on achieving concentric joint reduction and ligament or fracture repair to restore stability.

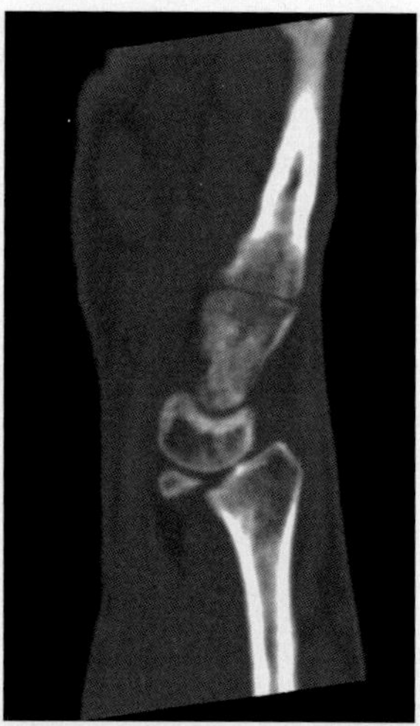
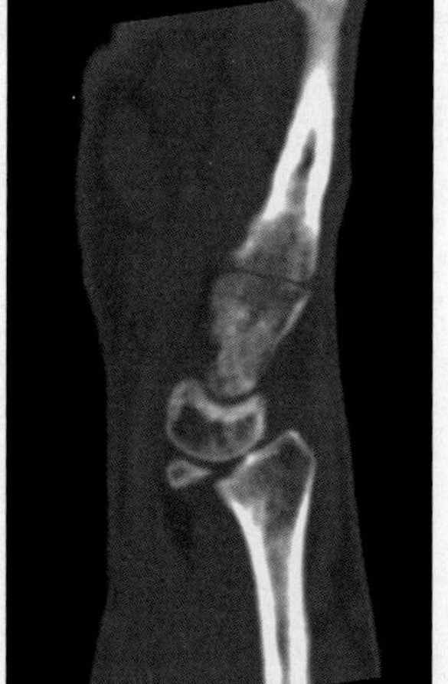

FIG 6 • CT image provide detailed characterization of a marginal rim fracture and subluxated radiocarpal joint.

- Although we recommend routine operative treatment for all cases of radiocarpal dislocations due to their inherent instability, the following are absolute indications for surgery:
  - Open injuries
  - Injuries with neurovascular compromise
  - Irreducible dislocations
- Timing of surgery depends on the ability to achieve a provisional closed radiocarpal reduction, soft tissue status, and neurovascular function.
- Successful management of radiocarpal dislocations requires adherence to three treatment principles:
  - Concentric, stable reduction of the radiocarpal joint
  - Repair of intercarpal ligament injuries, if present
  - Repair of extrinsic ligament avulsion injuries
- Preoperative planning should take into account the presence of any intercarpal ligament injuries and the extent of involvement of the three columns of the wrist including the radial, intermediate, and ulnar columns (**FIG 7**). Surgical intervention should then follow a stepwise approach:
  - Provisional reduction of the radiocarpal joint
  - Decompression of the median nerve, if paresthesias are present

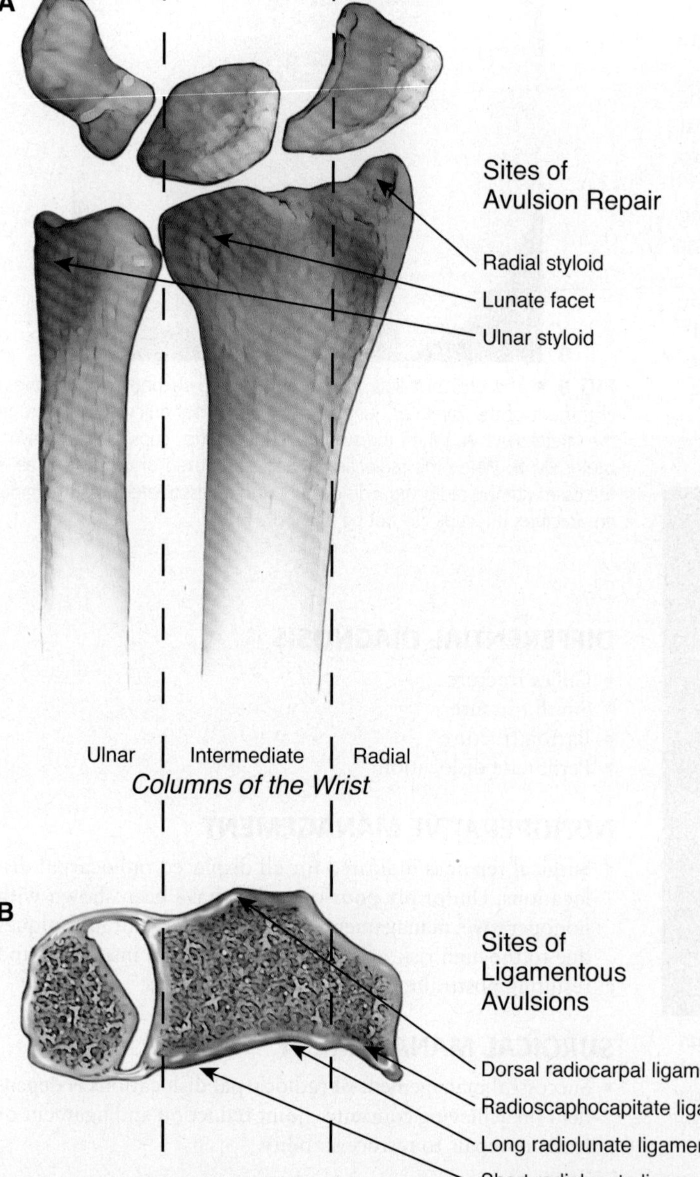

FIG 7 • **A,B.** The three columns of the wrist including the radial, intermediate, and ulnar columns. Each column consists of respective bone, joint, and ligaments.

- Joint exposure and débridement
- Repair of intercarpal ligament injury, if present
- Repair or fracture fixation of extrinsic ligamentous avulsion injuries
- Confirmation of reduction and stability of the three columns of the wrist

- When approaching step 5, repair or fracture fixation of extrinsic ligamentous injuries, the three columns of the wrist should be approached in a stepwise order and associated fractures and ligamentous injuries repaired to restore radiocarpal stability (**FIG 8**).
  - Radial column
    - Radial styloid fracture
    - Radioscaphocapitate ligament injury
  - Intermediate column
    - Lunate facet fracture
    - Short radiolunate ligament injury
  - Ulnar column
    - Ulnar styloid fracture
    - Ulnocarpal ligament injury

Preoperative Planning

- As these are typically young individuals with a high-energy injuries, patients should be counseled regarding the long-term risk of developing posttraumatic arthritis. Those with intercarpal ligament injuries are at higher risk.
- Standard and traction radiographs may be useful in evaluating for radiocarpal alignment, associated fractures, and intercarpal ligament injuries.
- Consider advanced imaging in the form of CT scanning for better fracture characterization or MRI scanning for better intercarpal and extrinsic ligament injury visualization.
- Necessary equipment to have available include suture anchors, Kirschner wires, small fragment or modular hand set, distal radius plating system, external fixator set, tension band materials, arthroscopy equipment, and bone graft/substitutes.
- Arthroscopy can assist in evaluating the extent of ligament and cartilage injury.
  - Use arthroscopy with caution, as excessive extravasation of fluid may occur due to the underlying capsular injury.
- Surgical repair may require use of several approaches to the wrist, including volar extensile and radial and dorsal approaches (**FIG 9**).

Positioning

- Axillary or interscalene block anesthesia is helpful for muscle relaxation as well as postoperative pain control. General anesthesia is recommended over monitored anesthesia care (MAC).
- The patient is positioned supine on the operating table with the operative extremity extended on a radiolucent hand table. This allows for adequate pronation/supination in order to access both the dorsal and volar surfaces of the wrist.
- Tourniquet hemostasis and loupe magnification should be used to maximize visualization.
- Ready access to an image intensifier intraoperatively is necessary.

Approach

- Volar approach[7]
  - The volar approach will be indicated to facilitate joint reduction, joint débridement, and fracture or ligament repairs. This approach will also facilitate median and ulnar nerve decompression, if necessary.
  - Landmarks are identified on the volar surface of the hand and wrist, including Kaplan cardinal line, the hook of hamate, the thenar crease, the transverse wrist crease, and the flexor carpi radialis and palmaris longus tendons.

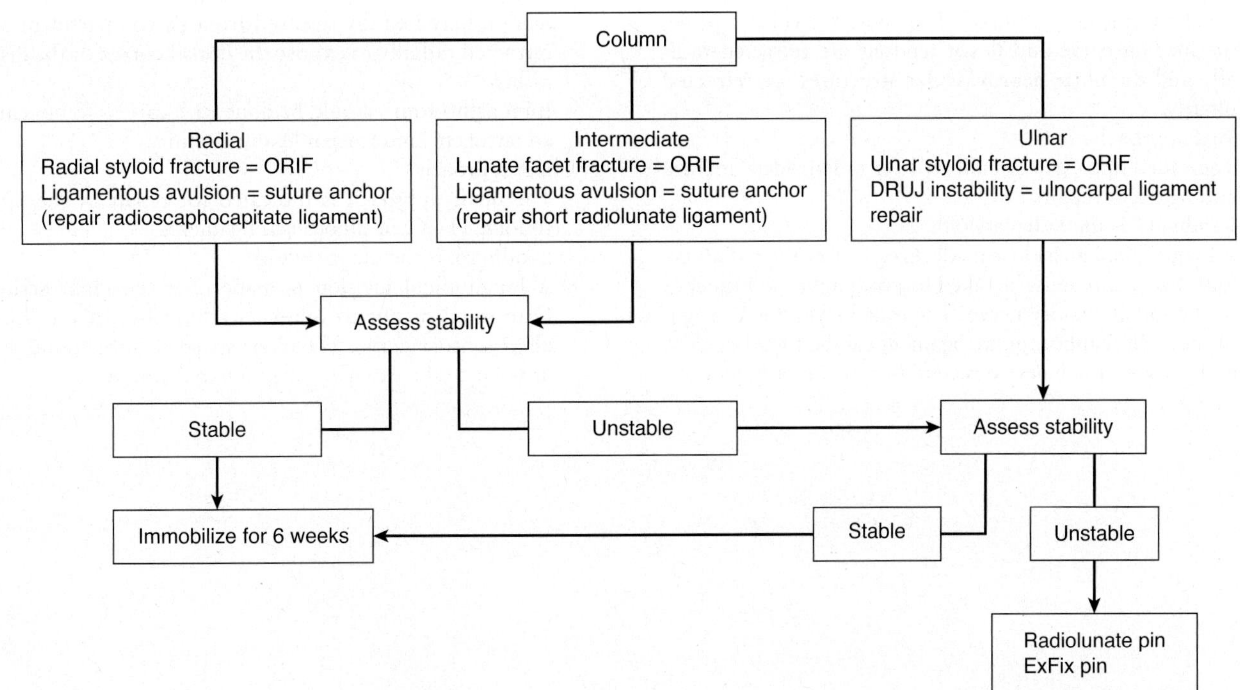

FIG 8 • Algorithm for repair of the columns of the wrist.

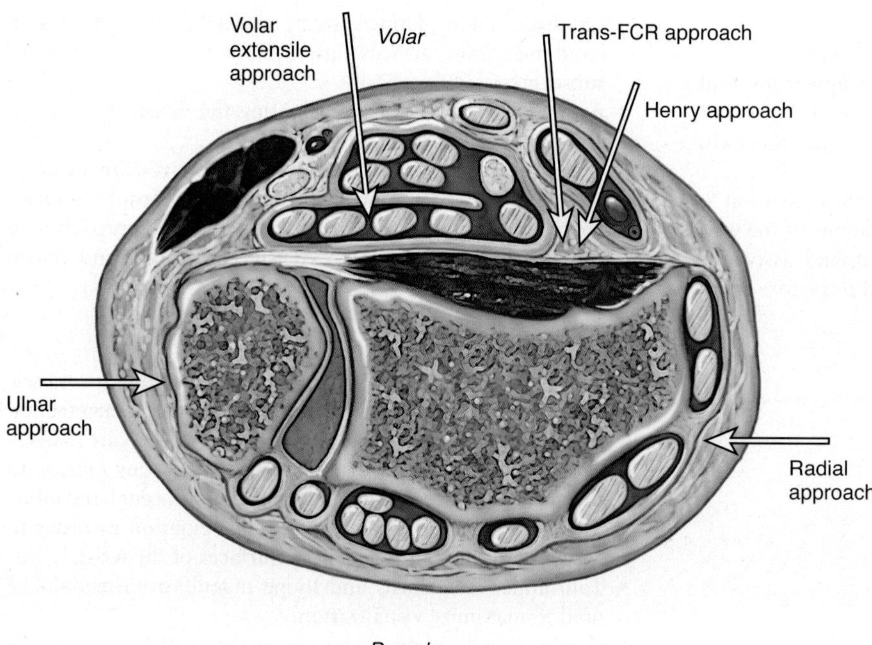

FIG 9 • Multiple approaches to the wrist are possible including ulnar, between the extensor and flexor carpi ulnaris tendons; radial, between the extensor pollicis brevis and extensor carpi radialis longus tendons; the distal extent of the approach of Henry, between the flexor carpi radialis (FCR) tendon and radial artery; the trans-FCR approach; and the volar extensile approach, that is developed between the palmaris longus and flexor carpi ulnaris tendons. In the extensile approach, the median nerve and finger flexor tendons are taken radially and the ulnar neurovascular structures are taken ulnarly.

- The standard volar approach can be performed through the floor of the flexor carpi radialis tendon or through the distal extent of Henry approach between the radial artery and the brachioradialis tendon (see **FIG 9**). Elevation of the distal extent of the pronator quadratus may be necessary to maximize exposure of the avulsed radiocarpal ligaments or fractures.
- An extensile volar approach to the wrist may be used beginning ulnar to the thenar eminence and extending proximally ulnar to the contents of the carpal tunnel (see **FIG 9**). This allows for access and decompression to both Guyon canal and the carpal tunnel. To expose the volar capsule, the median nerve and flexor tendons are retracted radially and the ulnar neurovascular structures are retracted ulnarly.

- Radial approach[7]
  - The radial approach is indicated for radial-sided fracture and ligament repairs.
  - Landmark is the radial styloid.
  - A longitudinal incision is made directly over the radial styloid. Great care must be taken to avoid injury to branches of the radial sensory nerve. The radial styloid and origin of the radioscaphocapitate ligament can be found deep to and between the first and second dorsal compartments.
- Dorsal approach[7]
  - The dorsal approach is indicated for intercarpal ligament injury repair and to facilitate joint reduction and débridement.
  - Landmarks include the radial and ulnar styloids and Lister tubercle.
  - A longitudinal incision is made just ulnar to Lister tubercle, crossing the dorsal wrist crease. The extensor retinaculum is identified and the capsule is exposed between the third and fourth compartments. The extensor pollicis longus tendon in the third compartment is left in place unless more exposure is necessary, and then the tendon may be fully released from its compartment and retracted radially to expose the dorsal cortex of the distal radius.
  - Joint arthrotomy should be done with care as to not cause an iatrogenic intercarpal ligament injury.
- Ulnar approach[7]
  - The ulnar approach is indicated for repair of the ulnar styloid, TFCC, or ulnocarpal ligaments.
  - Landmark is the ulnar styloid.
  - A longitudinal incision is made over the ulnar styloid. Care is taken not to injure any branches of the dorsal ulnar sensory nerve. The ulnar styloid can be found deep or volar to the extensor carpi ulnaris tendon.

Volar Exposure for Decompression of the Median Nerve, Identification of the Disrupted Radiocarpal Ligaments or Avulsion Fractures, and Provisional Joint Reduction and Débridement

- If decompression of the median nerve is deemed necessary, an extensile volar approach to the wrist may be used that will facilitate both complete decompression of the median nerve as well as access to the radial and intermediate columns of the wrist. Alternatively, a standard volar approach can be used (**TECH FIG 1**).
- Following exposure of the volar wrist, soft tissue avulsion and/or marginal rim fractures will be encountered at the radiocarpal joint level. Their elevation will allow direct visualization of the joint and identification of impaction injury and/or articular defects.
- The joint should be provisionally reduced and thoroughly irrigated and débrided of any loose bone or cartilage fragments.
  - Displaced and incarcerated intra-articular fragments can potentially block concentric reduction.
- Stay sutures are placed in the ends of the disrupted radiocarpal ligaments and wrist capsule but not initially sewn down. Once the intercarpal ligament injuries have been addressed, the capsular avulsion will be repaired.

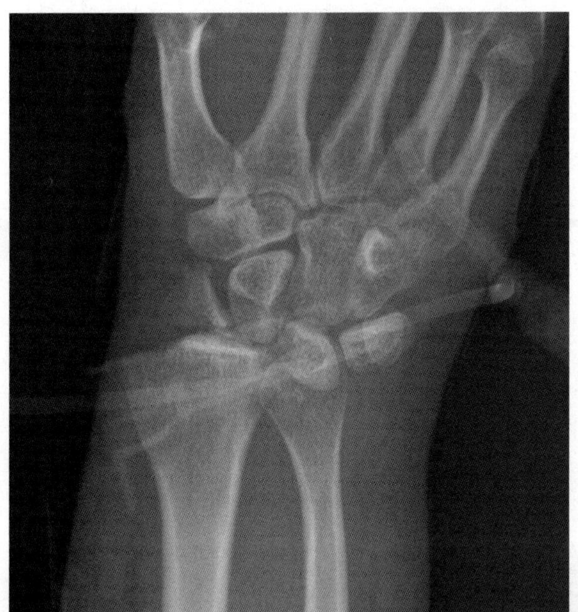
A

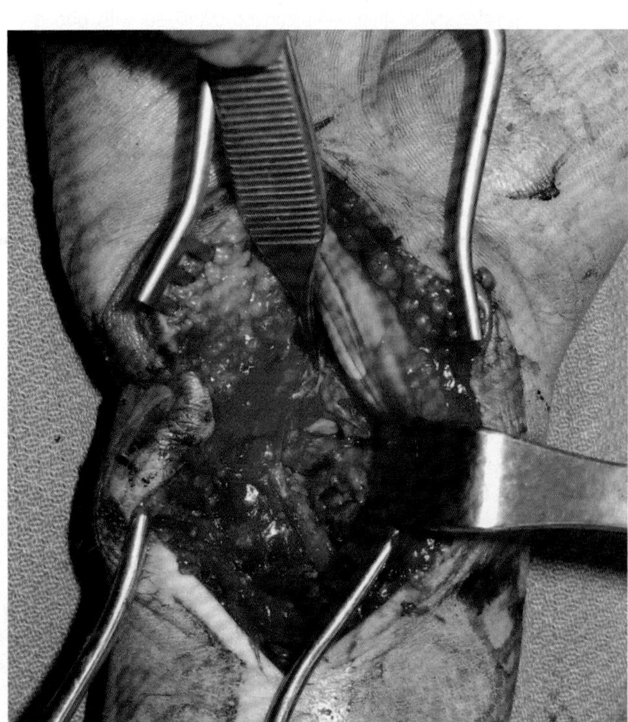
B

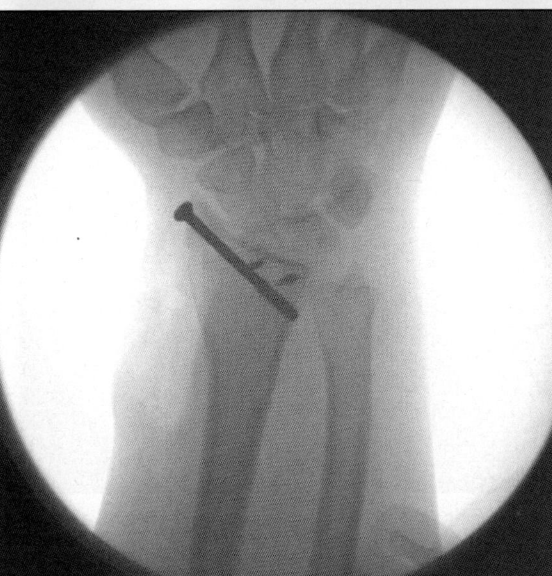
C

TECH FIG 1 • **A.** Radiocarpal dislocation, displaced dorsally with a radial styloid avulsion fracture. **B.** Exposure through a volar extensile approach demonstrating the avulsed radiocarpal ligaments. **C.** Repair consisted of radial styloid internal fixation to stabilize the radial column and suture anchor repair of the intermediate column's avulsed volar radiocarpal ligaments.

Dorsal Exposure and Intercarpal Ligament Stabilization

- If intercarpal ligament injuries are present requiring repair, they should be approached through a separate dorsal incision and repaired definitively prior to returning volar.
- In addition, the dorsal approach to the wrist can facilitate joint exposure, débridement, and reduction.
- If necessary, the dorsal approach can also allow for repair of the avulsed dorsal capsule. Stay sutures can be placed in the avulsed capsule and repaired to the dorsal cortex of the distal radius with suture anchors. Alternatively, if large dorsal marginal rim avulsion fractures are present, they can similarly be repaired with any internal fixation of choice.

Radial Column

- Fractures of the radial styloid are common and require diligent anatomic reduction and stable fixation.
  - Smaller styloid fragments can be stabilized with one or two Kirschner wires.
  - Screw fixation is preferable when the fragments are of appropriate size.
  - Larger radial styloid fragments may be amenable to radial plate fixation.
  - Volar plating can also be used to repair a radial styloid fracture. However, volar plate fixation of the styloid may be tenuous, as it is at a mechanical disadvantage to counter the shear stress that a radiocarpal dislocation will place on the radial styloid fragment. Therefore, caution should be taken when choosing this method of fixation.
- When a radial styloid fracture fragment is not present, avulsion of the radioscaphocapitate ligament must be suspected and repaired to its footprint on the radial styloid with suture anchors.

Central Column

- Fractures of the lunate facet are common and must be precisely repaired if amenable. Fixation options include screws, tension band,[3] or hook plates. Alternatively, a volar plate may be applied to serve as a buttress but must be used with care and placed adequately distal to fully buttress and reduce the lunate facet fracture (**TECH FIG 2**).
- Lunate facet fracture reduction may be facilitated with provisional pinning of the radiolunate articulation. The pin, however, should be removed at the end of the procedure.
- In cases of small lunate facet avulsion fractures or exclusively soft tissue avulsion of the volar wrist capsule, repair of the capsule and short radiolunate with suture anchors placed in the volar distal radius should be performed to recreate the volar capsular buttress.

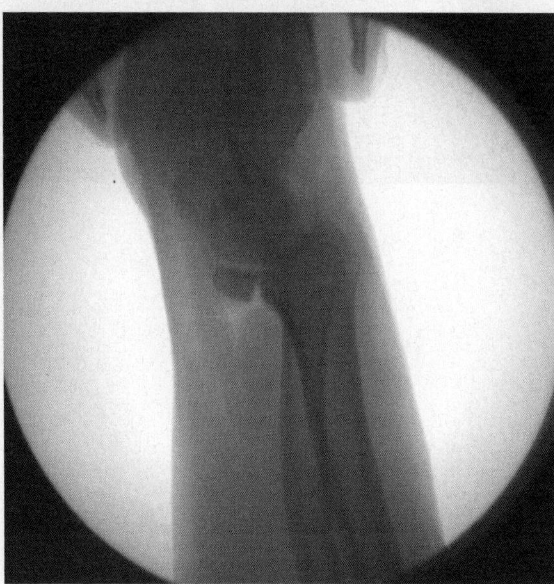

A

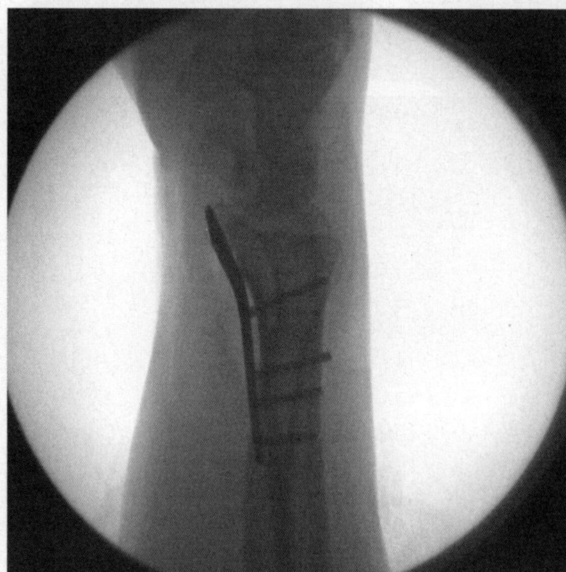

B

TECH FIG 2 • **A,B.** Buttress plate fixation of a radiocarpal dislocation with an associated volar rim marginal rim fracture.

Ulnar Column

- Indicators of potential ulnar column instability include an associated large ulnar styloid base fracture, distal radioulnar joint instability on examination, or MRI findings consistent with peripheral tear of the TFCC and/or injury to the ulnolunate or ulnotriquetral ligaments.
- We recommend routine repair of large ulnar styloid fragments using either a screw or tension band construct.
- If the ulnar column remains unstable after styloid fixation, repair of the ulnocarpal ligaments should be considered.

Evaluation of Wrist Stability

- Upon repair of the columns of the wrist and intercarpal ligament injuries, the operative wrist should be gently taken through a full range of motion under fluoroscopy. Any residual wrist instability should be addressed to avoid poor long-term outcomes.
- If additional stabilization is deemed necessary, consider temporary use of an external fixator or an internal bridge plate.

PEARLS AND PITFALLS

Diagnosis	▪ These are high-energy injuries with other extremity fractures or head and visceral organ injuries. ▪ In the setting of a prolonged unreduced dorsal radiocarpal dislocation, the risk of median neuropathy and acute carpal tunnel syndrome increases.
Imaging	▪ These injuries can be missed on radiographs when not associated with a fracture or confused with a distal radius fracture if the radiographic alignment of the radiocarpal joint is not scrutinized. ▪ CT scan may be helpful in assessing marginal rim and articular fractures. ▪ MRI scan may be helpful in assessing concomitant intercarpal ligament and TFCC injuries.
Surgical management	▪ Use a stepwise approach: ▪ Provisional reduction of the radiocarpal joint ▪ Decompression of the median nerve, if paresthesias are present ▪ Joint exposure and débridement ▪ Repair of intercarpal ligament injury, if present ▪ Repair or fracture fixation of extrinsic ligamentous avulsion injuries of all three columns of the wrist ▪ Confirmation of reduction and stability of the three columns of the wrist

POSTOPERATIVE CARE

- Unlike with standard distal radius fractures, where postoperative motion is often initiated early, secure immobilization for a minimum of 6 weeks following radiocarpal dislocation repair is recommended to allow sufficient soft tissue healing.
- Once satisfied with maintenance of concentric radiocarpal joint reduction, protected range of motion can be initiated after 6 weeks under the supervision of a therapist.
- It is highly recommended to inform the patient early that some permanent loss of motion in the flexion–extension arc is to be anticipated.
  - Expect a 30% to 50% loss of total wrist motion.

OUTCOMES

- Limited long-term data exists in the literature specific to radiocarpal dislocations.
- A number of small retrospective series have reported a range of outcomes generally consisting of decreased range of motion and mild pain at short-term follow-up.[4] Range of motion in the flexion–extension arc generally decreases by 30% to 40%.[8] Secondary radiocarpal instability, including late volar and ulnar translation, was seen with inadequate soft tissue or fracture repairs.[4]
- Intercarpal injuries are indicative of poor outcome,[13] as are open injuries and those with neurovascular complications.[16]
- Pure ligamentous injuries demonstrated inferior outcomes relative to fracture-dislocation variants.[4]
- Posttraumatic arthritis was seen in 11% to 25% of cases at final follow-up.[4,6,15] The presence of late arthritic changes was generally attributed to residual radiocarpal instability or the presence of concomitant intercarpal ligament injury.

COMPLICATIONS

- Complications can be separated into preoperative, early postoperative, and late postoperative.
- In the preoperative setting, sources of complication include open wounds, infection, and neurovascular embarrassment including acute carpal tunnel syndrome. These can be minimized with aggressive management of open wounds and early provisional joint reduction.
- In the early postoperative setting, complications can arise from persistent radiocarpal instability or frank dislocation due to inadequate repair and persistent median neuropathy (**FIG 10**).

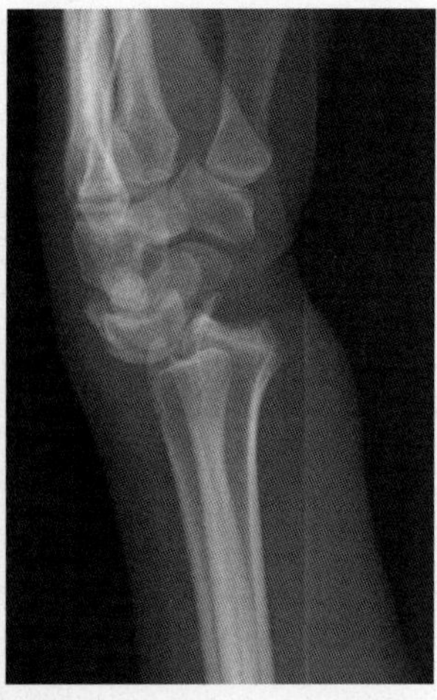
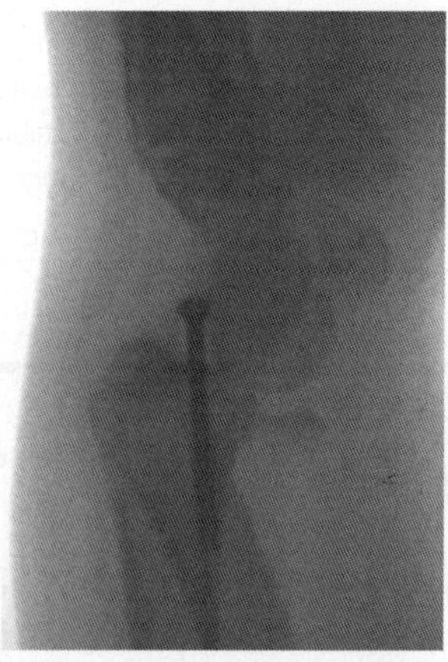

FIG 10 • **A,B.** This is a case of a radiocarpal dislocation treated by repair of the radial column alone with radial styloid fixation but without repair of the intermediate and ulnar columns and resultant failure.

- In the late postoperative setting, complications can include stiffness, decreased range of motion, decreased strength, posttraumatic degeneration, and hardware-related soft tissue irritation.

REFERENCES

1. Bilos ZJ, Pankovich AM, Yelda S. Fracture-dislocation of the radiocarpal joint. J Bone Joint Surg Am 1977;59(2):198–203.
2. Brown D, Mulligan MT, Uhl RL. Volar ligament repair for radiocarpal fracture-dislocation. Orthopedics 2013;36(6):463–468.
3. Chin KR, Jupiter JB. Wire-loop fixation of volar displaced osteochondral fractures of the distal radius. J Hand Surg Am 1999;24:525–533.
4. Dumontier C, Meyer zu Reckendorf G, Sautet A, et al. Radiocarpal dislocations: classification and proposal for treatment. A review of twenty-seven cases. J Bone Joint Surg Am 2001;83-A(2):212–218.
5. Dunn AW. Fractures and dislocations of the carpus. Surg Clin North Am 1972;52(6):1513–1538.
6. Girard J, Cassagnaud X, Maynou C, et al. Radiocarpal dislocation: twelve cases and a review of the literature [in French]. Rev Chir Orthop Reparatrice Appar Mot 2004;90(5):426–433.
7. Ilyas AM. Surgical approaches to the distal radius. Hand 2011;6(1):8–14.
8. Ilyas AM, Mudgal CS. Radiocarpal fracture-dislocations. J Am Acad Orthop Surg 2008;16(11):647–655.
9. Ilyas AM, Williamson C, Mudgal CS. Radiocarpal dislocation: is it a rare injury? J Hand Surg Eur Vol 2011;36(2):164–165.
10. Kaufmann RA, Pfaeffle HJ, Blankenhorn BD, et al. Kinematics of the midcarpal and radiocarpal joint in flexion and extension: an in vitro study. J Hand Surg Am 2006;31(7):1142–1148.
11. Mayfield JK, Johnson RP, Kilcoyne RK. Carpal dislocations: pathomechanics and progressive perilunar instability. J Hand Surg Am 1980;5:226–241.
12. Mizuseki T, Ikuta Y. The dorsal carpal ligaments: their anatomy and function. J Hand Surg Br 1989;14(1):91–98.
13. Moneim MS, Bolger JT, Omer GE. Radiocarpal dislocation—classification and rationale for management. Clin Orthop Relat Res 1985;(192):199–209.
14. Mourikis A, Rebello G, Villafuerte J, et al. Radiocarpal dislocations: review of the literature with case presentations and a proposed treatment algorithm. Orthopedics 2008;31(4):386–392.
15. Mudgal CS, Psenica J, Jupiter JB. Radiocarpal fracture-dislocation. J Hand Surg Br 1999;24(1):92–98.
16. Nyquist SR, Stern PJ. Open radiocarpal fracture-dislocations. J Hand Surg Am 1984;9(5):707–710.

Operative Treatment of Lesser and Greater Arc Injuries

62

CHAPTER

Rick Tosti and Joseph J. Thoder

DEFINITION

- The carpus is a complex, intercalated system of dual rows that allow paired motion within the radial–ulnar and flexion–extension planes. A disruption of the intrinsic ligaments of the carpus or a combination of ligamentous and osseous structures leads to a spectrum of injuries ranging from "wrist sprains" to complex perilunate injuries including lesser and greater arc injuries.[11,12,15]
- Lesser arc injuries are purely capsuloligamentous.
- Greater arc injuries have associated carpal fractures.
- Disruptions of the normal kinematics and stability of the carpal rows lead to a predictable pattern of posttraumatic degenerative changes.

ANATOMY

- The carpus is composed of eight bones arranged in two rows that articulate with the five metacarpals distally and the radius and ulna proximally.
- Complex, three-dimensional motion occurs with wrist movement: radial deviation and wrist dorsiflexion are paired, as are ulnar deviation and wrist volar flexion.
- Motion is passively transmitted through crossing tendons and guided by bony geometry and ligamentous architecture, which also confer stability.
- Volar extrinsic ligaments are oriented in a double V arrangement, with a relative weakness between these V's called the *space of Poirier*.
  - The volar extrinsic ligaments include the inner V ligaments: long radiolunate (LRL), radioscapholunate (RSL), short radiolunate (SRL), and ulnolunate (UL). The outer V consists of the radioscaphocapitate (RSC) and the ulnotriquetrocapitate complex (UTCC) (**FIG 1A**).[18]
- The dorsal extrinsic ligaments provide less structural stability and include the radiotriquetral and dorsal intercarpal (DIC) ligaments (**FIG 1B**).
- The intrinsic ligaments are direct intercarpal connections that provide intrarow stability.
  - In the proximal row, these include the lunotriquetral interosseous ligament (LTIL) and the scapholunate interosseous ligament (SLIL).

PATHOGENESIS

- A high-energy axial load is applied to the thenar eminence causing hyperextension, ulnar deviation, and intercarpal supination. The energy dissipates in a radial to ulnar direction and places the volar structures under tension and the dorsal structures under compression and shear.
- Lesser arc injuries are purely ligamentous and advance through four progressive stages as originally described by Mayfield et al[14] (**FIG 2A**):
  - Stage I: the scapholunate ligament
  - Stage II: the space of Poirier
  - Stage III: the UTCC and lunotriquetral ligament
  - Stage IV: lunate dislocation
- Greater arc injuries proceed in the same direction but involve fractures through the radial styloid, scaphoid, lunate, capitate, triquetrum, and ulna, either solely or in combination (**FIG 2B**).[3,10] The prefix "trans" is given to the fractured carpal bone (eg, trans-scaphoid perilunate fracture-dislocation).
- A perilunate dislocation describes a dorsal dislocation of the capitate and surrounding carpus, but the lunate remains in

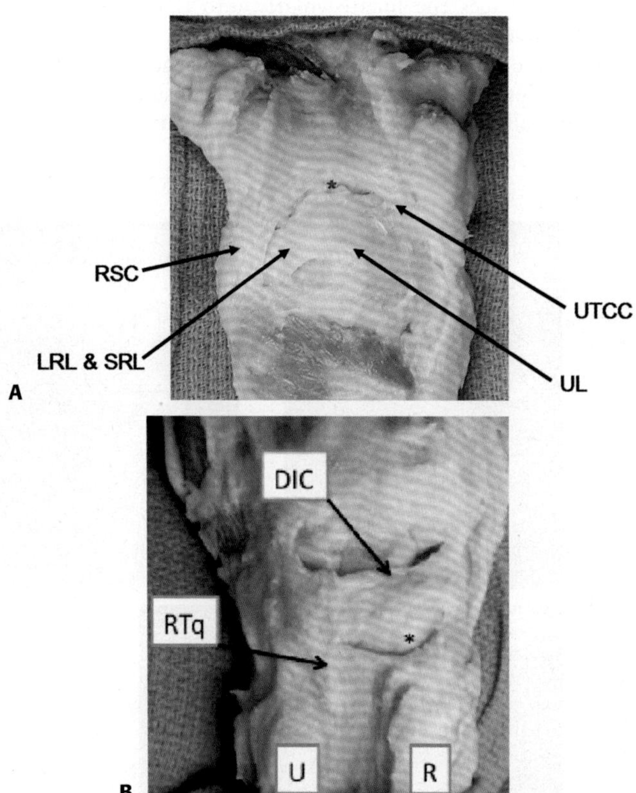

FIG 1 • **A.** Volar extrinsic carpal ligaments. *LRL*, long radiolunate ligament; *SRL*, short radiolunate; *RSC*, radioscaphocapitate ligament; *UL*, ulnolunate ligament; *UTCC*, ulnotriquetrocapitate complex; *asterisk*, space of Poirier. **B.** Dorsal extrinsic carpal ligaments. *RTq*, radiotriquetral ligament; *DIC*, dorsal intercarpal ligament; *asterisk*, scaphoid; *U*, ulna; *R*, radius.

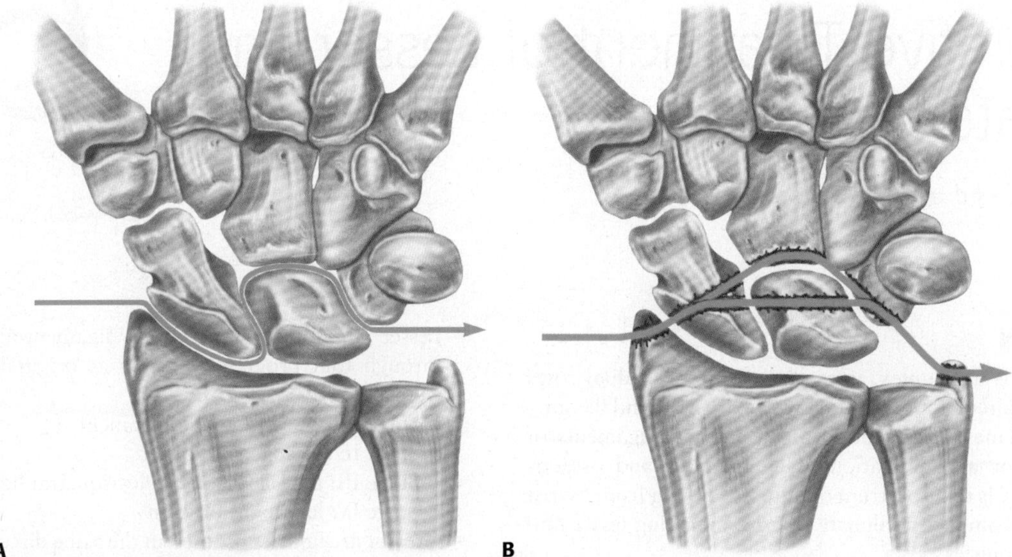

FIG 2 • **A.** Lesser arc injury. Progression of capsuloligamentous injury from radial to ulnar direction. **B.** Greater arc injury. Trans-scaphoid perilunate injury pattern.

the fossa of the distal radius (**FIG 3A,B**). Volar dislocations of the carpus are rare (**FIG 3C**).

- A lunate dislocation describes a more severe progression in which the capitate translocates into the lunate fossa and displaces the lunate volarly into the carpal tunnel (**FIG 3D–F**).
  - As the lunate is ousted through the space of Poirier, a semilunar rent is created in the volar capsule that extends medially and laterally between the V ligaments.

NATURAL HISTORY

- Missed injuries may occur in up to 25% of cases.[8]
- Common sequelae of untreated injuries include pain, weakness, stiffness, acute carpal tunnel syndrome, flexor tendon rupture, early degenerative joint disease, and wrist instability.[11,12,15]
  - Typical instability patterns include scapholunate advanced collapse, scaphoid nonunion advanced collapse, and volar or dorsal intercalated segmental instability.

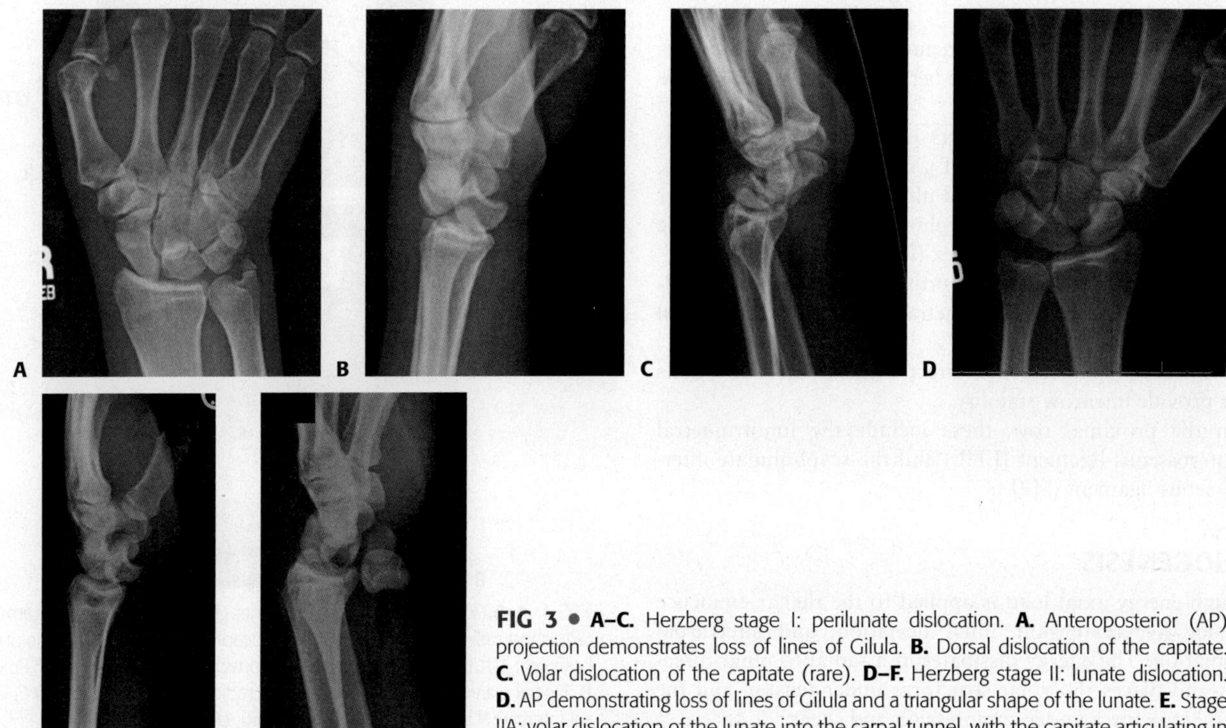

FIG 3 • **A–C.** Herzberg stage I: perilunate dislocation. **A.** Anteroposterior (AP) projection demonstrates loss of lines of Gilula. **B.** Dorsal dislocation of the capitate. **C.** Volar dislocation of the capitate (rare). **D–F.** Herzberg stage II: lunate dislocation. **D.** AP demonstrating loss of lines of Gilula and a triangular shape of the lunate. **E.** Stage IIA: volar dislocation of the lunate into the carpal tunnel, with the capitate articulating in the radial fossa. **F.** Stage IIB: volar dislocation with greater than 90 degrees of rotation.

PATIENT HISTORY AND PHYSICAL FINDINGS

- High-energy injuries (fall from height, motor vehicle collision, or sports injuries) are generally causative.
- Physical examination findings depend on severity of injury and the elapsed time from injury to presentation.
  - Stiffness, tenderness, crepitus, swelling, and resistance to motion are common findings. Deformity is usually minimal.
  - Depending on the severity of injury, the findings can be subtle and easily missed. The examiner must maintain a high index of suspicion.
- A thorough neurologic examination is critical. Acute compression of the median nerve may be present in 16% to 46% of cases and is more frequently associated with lunate dislocations.[15]
- If median nerve symptoms are present, serial examinations are necessary to distinguish between nerve contusion (static findings) and nerve compression (progressive findings).
- Palpation of radial and ulnar styloids or the individual carpal bones in a greater arc injury may reveal tenderness over specific fractures.
- Specific testing of intrinsic and extrinsic ligaments (eg, the Watson test, the lunotriquetral shuck, and the ulnar catch up) may prove difficult and of little value in an acute setting.

IMAGING AND OTHER DIAGNOSTIC STUDIES

- True posteroanterior (PA) and true lateral radiographs should be obtained. The diagnosis is made primarily with these views. Equivocal cases may be compared with identical radiographs of the uninjured wrist.
- The lines of Gilula are disrupted on the PA view.[6]
- If the SLIL is disrupted, widening of the intercarpal joint or a flexed scaphoid (cortical ring sign) may be seen on the PA view, whereas an abnormal scapholunate interosseous angle (normal 30 to 60 degrees) may be seen on the lateral view.
- As the capitate migrates proximally, carpal height may be lost (normal carpal–metacarpal height ratio is >0.5) on the PA view. The concentricity of "the 3 C's," representing the distal radius, lunate, and capitate, is lost on the lateral view.
- As the lunate displaces and rotates volarly, it appears triangular in shape, as opposed to trapezoidal, on the PA view. The "spilled tea cup" sign describes this appearance on the lateral radiograph, which can be quantified by the radiolunate angle (normal <15 degrees).
- Oblique views may help delineate carpal fractures in greater arc injuries. Scaphoid fractures are most common. Capitate, lunate, and triquetral fractures have been described. Fractures of the radial and/or ulnar styloids may also be present.
- Other views such as radial–ulnar deviation, flexion–extension, supinated, and clenched fist views are often difficult to obtain and are of little additional value.
- Computed tomography may be useful for preoperative assessment in greater arc injuries.
- Magnetic resonance imaging (MRI), arthrography, arthroscopy, and bone scan are not indicated in the acute setting after major trauma to the wrist.

DIFFERENTIAL DIAGNOSIS

- Wrist sprain
- Degenerative joint disease
- Isolated intrinsic ligament disruption
- Radiocarpal dislocation
- Midcarpal instability
- Isolated carpal or metacarpal fractures
- Distal radius or ulnar fracture
- Acute carpal tunnel syndrome
- Triangular fibrocartilage complex (TFCC) injury
- Kienböck disease
- Ulnar impaction syndrome

NONOPERATIVE MANAGEMENT

- Closed reduction of perilunate dislocations should be attempted in the emergency room to prevent median nerve compression and cartilage damage. Restoring carpal alignment may also reestablish familiar soft tissue planes at the time of surgery.
  - An intra-articular local anesthetic and in-line traction are helpful for muscle relaxation before reduction. The upper extremity is suspended using finger traps, and weights are hung from the arm with the elbow flexed at 90 degrees for 15 minutes. Conscious sedation is given just prior to manipulation.
  - The surgeon extends the wrist and applies gentle manual traction. The surgeon's thumb stabilizes the lunate volarly and rotates the lunate into extension. The capitate is then translated up and over the lunate by flexing the wrist. A snapping sound may be heard when the capitate reduces over the lunate.[17]
- If closed reduction is successful and median nerve symptoms are nonprogressive, the patient may be immobilized in a sugar-tong splint and return for surgery within a few weeks.
- If closed reduction is unsuccessful or if acute carpal tunnel syndrome is present, then surgery should be scheduled within 24 hours.
- Closed reductions of lunate dislocations are frequently unsuccessful. As traction is applied to the wrist, the volar rent narrows to prevent reduction of the lunate into the wrist joint.
- Herzberg[7] suggested that reductions of lunate dislocations with greater than 90 degrees of volar rotation are more difficult and may cause iatrogenic damage.
- Closed reduction and casting as a definitive treatment has led to poor outcomes including instability, deformity, and early degenerative disease.[1,2]

SURGICAL MANAGEMENT

Preoperative Planning

- Osseous structures should be treated first.
- Carpal bone fractures can be stabilized with Kirschner wires or headless dual-pitch screws. Consider bone graft for comminuted scaphoid fractures.
- Radial styloid fractures can be excised if they are small or stabilized with screws or minifragment plates if they are large.
- Ulnar styloid fractures are stabilized with a tension band construct or a hook plate if distal radioulnar joint instability is present.
- Interosseous ligaments are then repaired or reconstructed.
- SLIL usually avulsed from the scaphoid can be repaired with nonabsorbable sutures or reinserted with suture anchors.
- LTIL repair/reconstruction is controversial.

- Ligament repairs/reconstructions may be reinforced with Kirschner wires or interosseous screws.
- Perform a carpal tunnel release if progressive loss of median nerve function is present.

Positioning

- Supine positioning with a well-padded pneumatic tourniquet on the upper arm
- The use of a radiolucent hand table with fluoroscopic imaging aids in repair and reduction.

Approach

- Surgical approaches to this injury include dorsal approach, volar approach, and combined dorsal and volar approach.
- The dorsal approach uses the universal dorsal wrist incision and the interval between the third and fourth compartments to expose the dorsal capsule and gain access to the joint.
  - The dorsal approach is helpful for open reduction of the dislocation and direct assessment of articular injuries. However, great difficulty may be encountered if attempting to reduce a lunate dislocation through only a dorsal approach.
  - Direct or augmented repair of the scapholunate ligament and open reduction and internal fixation of any concomitant carpal fractures are accomplished through this approach.
- The volar approach is performed through an extended carpal tunnel incision. Retraction of the carpal tunnel contents allows visualization of the volar capsuloligamentous structures and the semilunar rent. Decompression of the carpal tunnel, evacuation of hematoma, and tenosynovectomy of the digital flexor tendons is accomplished.
- Open reduction of a volar lunate dislocation is facilitated by this approach.
  - Repair of the volar capsuloligamentous injuries can also be performed to further stabilize the carpus.
  - An exclusive volar approach does not allow precise repair of the intercarpal ligaments, and bony fixation is difficult.
- The combined dorsal and volar approach combines the advantages of both approaches.

TECHNIQUES

Dorsal Approach

Incision and Dissection

- A universal dorsal skin incision is made under tourniquet control (**TECH FIG 1A**). The extensor retinaculum is exposed, raising medial and lateral skin flaps. Access to the dorsal capsule is gained through the third and fourth extensor compartment interval.
- The extensor pollicis longus (EPL) tendon is dissected distal to the extensor retinaculum and the third compartment is incised. The EPL is transposed radially to prevent injury to the tendon during manipulation and stabilization of the carpus (**TECH FIG 1B**).
- The fourth extensor compartment is incised longitudinally and the tendons are retracted. The dorsal capsule is now visible.
  - One centimeter of the posterior interosseous nerve is excised as part of the procedure (**TECH FIG 1C**).
- A transverse rent extending through the dorsal capsule and radiotriquetral ligament is often found. This rent should be extended in both the radial and ulnar directions to allow visualization of the capitolunate interval.
- A more extensile ligament-sparing incision can also be used to gain considerable access to the carpus.
  - Incise the capsule in a radial direction along the dorsal distal radial lip, leaving a small cuff of tissue attached to the radius for later repair.
  - Incise ulnarly, along the dorsal radiotriquetral ligament and DIC ligament. This generates a radially based capsular flap (**TECH FIG 1D**).
- If the dislocation was not reducible closed, the capitate is prominent and the absence of the lunate is evident.
- The articular injury can now be assessed. Particular attention should be paid to the head of the capitate, as articular shearing occurs as it translocates over the rim of the lunate.

Reduction and Fixation

- Before reduction of the dislocation–subluxation, 0.045- or 0.062-inch Kirschner wire transfixation pins are inserted into the

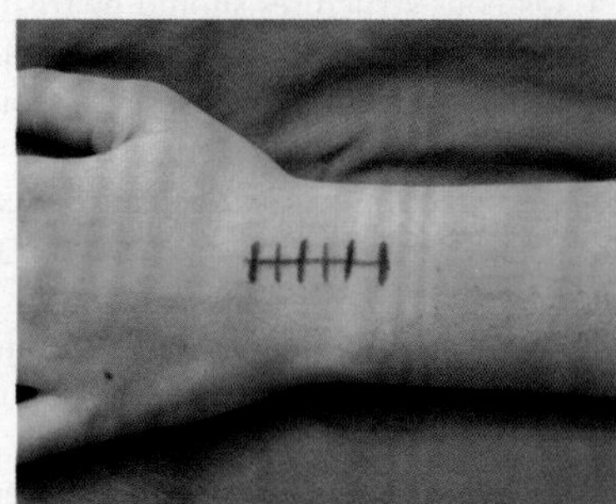

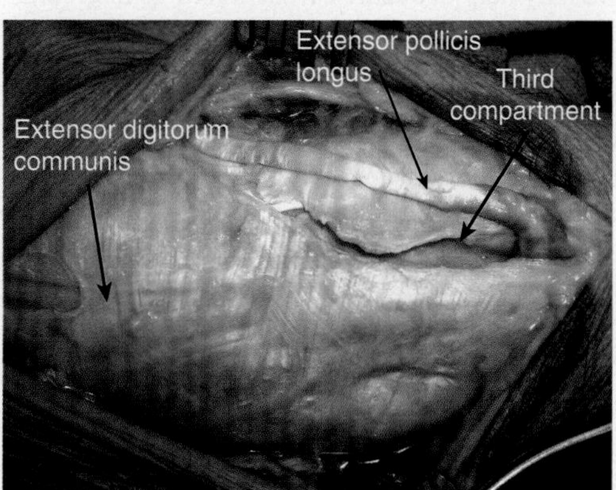

TECH FIG 1 • **A.** Universal dorsal skin incision for the dorsal approach. **B.** The third extensor compartment is incised and the EPL is transposed radially. The extensor digitorum communis (EDC) tendons are visible. (Thumb is at top *left* and wrist is to the *right*.) *(continued)*

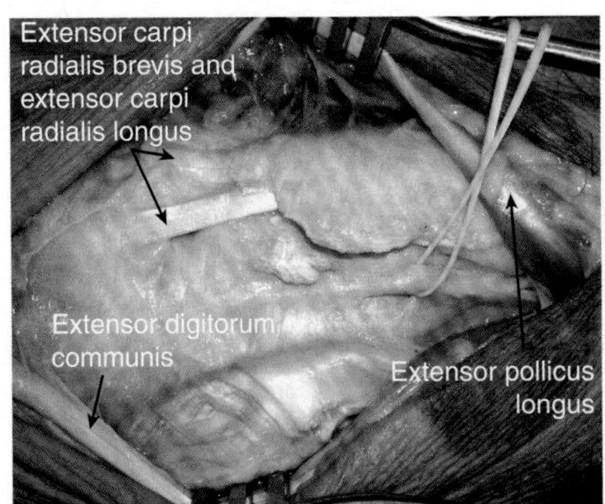

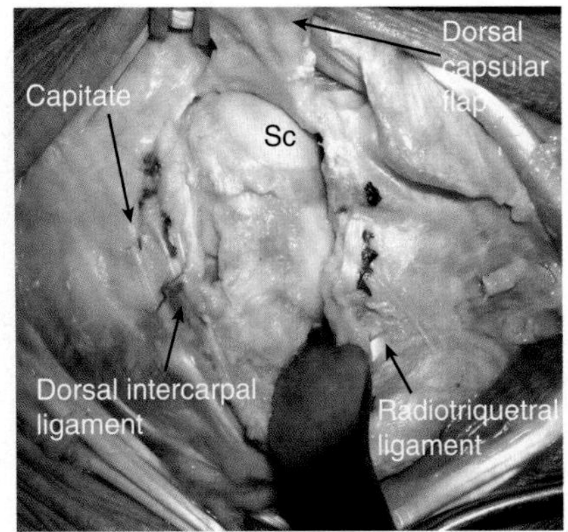

TECH FIG 1 • *(continued)* **C.** The fourth extensor compartment is incised, and the EDC tendons are retracted ulnarly. The sensory branch of the posterior interosseous nerve to the wrist (vessel loop) is sacrificed. **D.** A ligament-sparing capsular incision may be made to visualize the carpus. *Sc*, scaphoid.

triquetrum and scaphoid through the dorsal incision in an in-to-out fashion. These pins are later driven back into the lunate to stabilize the reduction.
  - The starting point for these pins is through the center of the scapholunate and lunotriquetral articulations, respectively (**TECH FIG 2**).
  - Transfixation pins are usually unnecessary in the scaphoid if it is fractured because a screw in the scaphoid will stabilize the radial side of the carpus.
- In combination with manual traction and volar pressure on the lunate, insert a Freer elevator into the capitolunate joint around the proximal pole of the capitate and shoehorn the lunate into place.
- Reduce and stabilize carpal fractures.
- Attention is first directed toward fixation of an associated scaphoid fracture using proximal to distal (antegrade) fixation.
  - The scaphoid is usually fractured at its waist or proximal pole.
  - In a noncomminuted fracture, stabilization is accomplished with a cannulated headless compression screw.
  - If comminution exists, autologous cancellous bone graft is applied before final tightening of the screw.

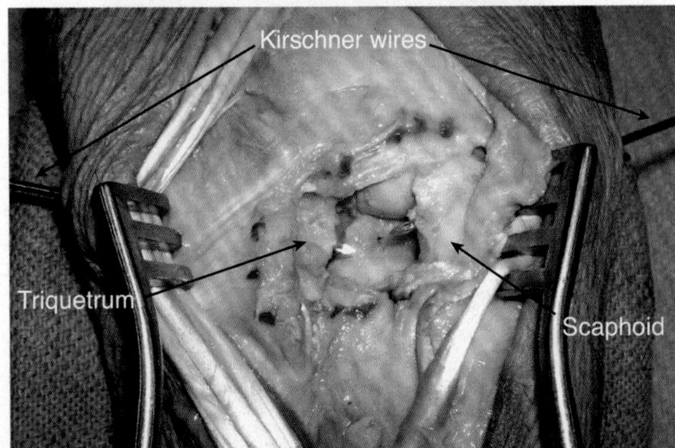

TECH FIG 2 • Transfixation pins are placed through the scaphoid and triquetrum before reduction of the lunate. This facilitates placement of these Kirschner wires and advancement into the lunate after reduction. The entry point is the centroid of the intercarpal joint on the scaphoid and triquetrum. The tips of the Kirschner wires are seen slightly protruding from the scaphoid and triquetrum. The lunate is displaced volarly and is not visible.

Ligament Repair

- Intercarpal ligament injuries may now be repaired.
- In a trans-scaphoid perilunate dislocation, the proximal pole of the scaphoid usually remains attached to the lunate with an intact scapholunate ligament. However, in lesser arc injuries, the scapholunate and the lunotriquetral ligament are disrupted.
- Before ligamentous repair, anatomic carpal realignment is ensured.
  - 0.045-mm Kirschner wires are introduced into the scaphoid, lunate, and triquetrum and used as joysticks to align these bones.
- The previously set Kirschner wires used as transfixation pins are then advanced from the scaphoid and triquetrum into the lunate.
- Transfixation pins are also percutaneously introduced to stabilize the scaphoid and triquetrum to the capitate (**TECH FIG 3A**).
- Intraoperative fluoroscopy aids alignment and placement of Kirschner wires.
  - The scapholunate angle (30 to 60 degrees), capitolunate angle (<15 degrees), and radiolunate angle (<15 degrees) should be reduced and verified. Ulnocarpal translation should also be assessed.
  - The 3 Cs of the distal radius, lunate, and capitate should be concentric (**TECH FIG 3B**).
- Small (about 2 mm) suture anchors with nonabsorbable suture (2-0 to 3-0) are inserted for reattachment of the scapholunate and lunotriquetral ligaments, avoiding the Kirschner wires.
  - Most often, the ligaments avulse from the scaphoid and the triquetrum; therefore, the anchors are placed in those locations.
  - When the intercarpal ligaments are beyond repair, suture anchors are unnecessary, and stability is established via extrinsic capsuloligamentous healing.
- The dorsal capsular injury and extended capsulotomy is closed with nonabsorbable suture.
- The EPL tendon is left transposed in a subcutaneous location (**TECH FIG 3C**).
- The subcutaneous tissue and skin are closed in a standard fashion.

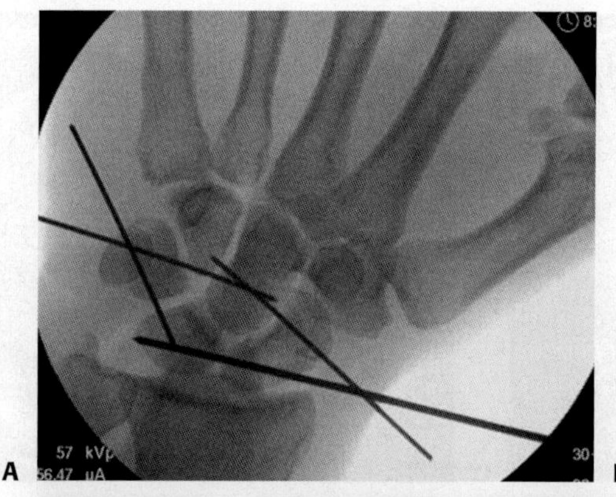

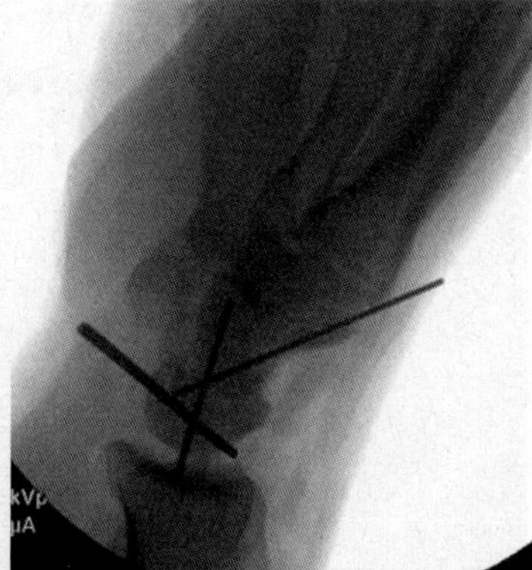

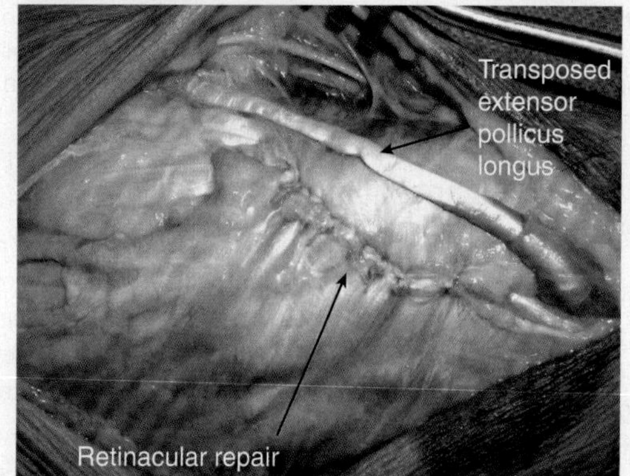

TECH FIG 3 • Transfixation pins are in place protecting the ligament repairs and maintaining anatomic carpal alignment. Suture anchors were not required for repair in this case. The intercarpal ligament injuries were midsubstance. **A.** The PA radiograph shows the reduced trapezoidal shape of the lunate and restoration of the lines of Gilula. **B.** The lateral radiograph shows the reduced scapholunate, radiolunate, and capitolunate angles. The three concentric C's are also visible. **C.** Repair of the extensor retinaculum and transposed EPL.

Combined Dorsal and Volar Approach (Authors' Preferred Method)

Incision and Dissection

- A standard extended carpal tunnel approach is performed under tourniquet control (**TECH FIG 4A**).
  - The median nerve is completely decompressed.
- The contents of the carpal canal are retracted and hematoma is evacuated.
- The volar capsuloligamentous injury, which is represented by an apex distal, semilunar rent, is visualized (**TECH FIG 4B**).
  - This rent courses between the RSC and LRL radially and between the UTCC and UL ligaments ulnarly.
  - In the case of a lunate dislocation, the lunate can be visualized within the carpal canal, having been extruded through the capsular tear.
- Next, the wrist is exposed dorsally as described earlier.
- The degree of injury is assessed.

Reduction, Fixation, and Repair

- Preset transfixation Kirschner wires as previously described.
- Reduce the carpus under direct visualization, with wrist extension and the aid of a Freer elevator to shoehorn the capitate into the lunate fossa.
  - The volar approach facilitates the reduction by allowing direct access to the lunate.

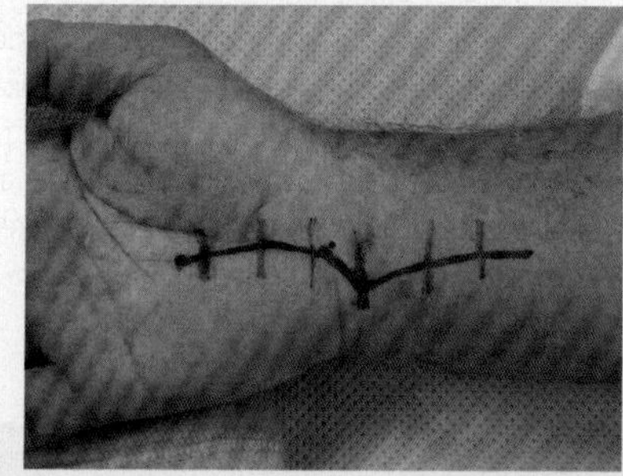

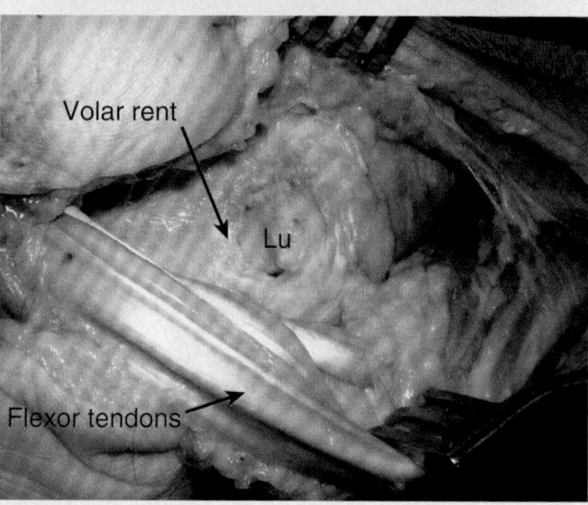

TECH FIG 4 • **A.** Extended carpal tunnel incision used for the volar approach. **B.** A volar, semilunar, apex distal, capsuloligamentous rent is visible at the space of Poirier. The lunate (*Lu*) is seen protruding from the rent.

- Surgical extension of the capsular tear between the RSC and LRL ligaments or between the UTCC and UL ligaments allows greater access to the wrist without further disruption of extrinsic ligaments.
- Through the dorsal incision, reduce, stabilize, and repair any associated carpal fractures and intercarpal ligament injuries in the manner described earlier.
- The volar capsuloligamentous rent is closed with nonabsorbable suture (**TECH FIG 5**).
- The flexor tendons may now be assessed. Often, the tenosynovium surrounding the tendons within the carpal tunnel is thickened. A tenosynovectomy may be performed.
- The EPL should be left transposed dorsally.
- The subcutaneous tissue and skin are closed in a standard fashion.

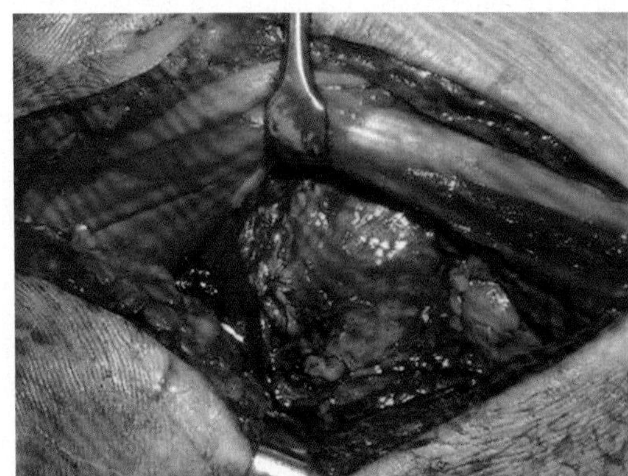

TECH FIG 5 • The volar capsule is closed with nonabsorbable suture.

PEARLS AND PITFALLS

Radiographs	■ This injury is easily missed; therefore, true lateral and PA radiographs are necessary. A high index of suspicion is appropriate in high-energy mechanisms or polytrauma patients.
Timing	■ Delayed repair within a few weeks is acceptable if a stable reduction is achieved and acute carpal syndrome is not present; surgery should otherwise proceed within 24 hours.
Intraoperative reduction	■ The ever-elusive lunate may be stabilized during reduction by placing the thumb through the dorsal incision and the index finger through the volar incision (when a dual-incision approach is used). This facilitates stabilization by transfixion pins in an anatomic position.
Soft tissue repair	■ The bony architecture should be reduced and stabilized in an anatomic position before capsuloligamentous repair. This will ensure proper tension of the soft tissue repair. Overtensioning of the soft tissues by repairing them first may prevent accurate reduction of the carpus.

POSTOPERATIVE CARE

- The immediate postoperative dressing includes a well-padded splint immobilizing the wrist and forearm in a neutral rotational position and 20 degrees of wrist extension.
  - Edema control and prevention of skin maceration can be accomplished with the addition of sterile gauze dressings between the digits and a bulky dressing within the palm.
- Active and passive digital range-of-motion exercises are encouraged immediately to prevent flexor tendon adhesions and digital stiffness.
- Sutures are removed at 10 to 14 days, and full-time cast or splint immobilization is continued for a total of 8 weeks postoperatively.
- Pins may be removed at 8 weeks, and the patient may be converted to a removable splint to promote range of motion of the wrist.
- At 12 weeks, strengthening is permitted with progressive resistance as tolerated.
- Anticipated return to activities is 6 to 12 months.

OUTCOMES

- Delayed treatment, open injuries, chondral damage, instability, and malunions portend a worse prognosis. Prompt recognition and anatomic reduction lead to better results.
- Salvage procedures include proximal row carpectomy, four-corner fusion, or total wrist arthrodesis.
- Sotereanos et al[16] used a dorsal–volar approach in 11 patients with perilunate dislocations and fracture-dislocations. Good to excellent results were achieved in 9 of 11 patients.
- Kremer et al[13] reported on 39 patients with an average of 65.5 months follow-up and noted moderate disability (average Disability of Arm, Shoulder, and Hand [DASH] score of 23) and pain with activity (average visual analog score of 4.8).
- Forli et al[5] reported on 18 patients with a minimum of 10-year follow-up and noted radiographic evidence of arthrosis in 67%; only 1 patient required an arthrodesis.
- Up to 50% loss of flexion–extension motion arc can be anticipated.[4]
- Up to 60% diminished grip strength can be anticipated.[4]
- Progressive arthrosis is common but does not necessarily correlate with outcome.[5,9]

COMPLICATIONS

- Missed diagnosis
- Postoperative pin tract infections
- Median nerve injury
- Transient ischemia of lunate

- Attrition rupture of flexor tendons
- Chondral injury or chondrolysis
- Late carpal instability (scapholunate, lunotriquetral, or midcarpal joints)
- Ulnocarpal translation
- Nonunion or malunion of the scaphoid
- Posttraumatic arthritis

REFERENCES

1. Adkison JW, Chapman MW. Treatment of acute lunate and perilunate dislocations. Clin Orthop Relat Res 1982;(164):199–207.
2. Apergis E, Maris J, Theodoratos G, et al. Perilunate dislocations and fracture dislocations. Closed and early open reduction compared in 28 cases. Acta Orthop Scand Suppl 1997;275:55–59.
3. Bain GI, McLean JM, Turner PC, et al. Translunate fracture with associated perilunate injury: 3 case reports with introduction of the translunate arc concept. J Hand Surg Am 2008;33:1770–1776.
4. Cooney WP, Bussey R, Dobyns JH, et al. Difficult wrist fractures. Perilunate fracture-dislocations of the wrist. Clin Orthop Relat Res 1987;(214):136–147.
5. Forli A, Courvoisier A, Wimsey S, et al. Perilunate dislocations and transscaphoid perilunate fracture-dislocations: a retrospective study with minimum ten-year follow-up. J Hand Surg Am 2010; 35:62–68.
6. Gilula LA, Destouet JM, Weeks PM, et al. Roentgenographic diagnosis of the painful wrist. Clin Orthop Relat Res 1984;(187):52–64.
7. Herzberg G. Perilunate and axial carpal dislocations and fracture-dislocations. J Hand Surg 2008;33:1659–1668.
8. Herzberg G, Comtet JJ, Linscheid RL, et al. Perilunate dislocations and fracture-dislocations: a multicenter study. J Hand Surg Am 1993;18(5):768–779.
9. Herzberg G, Forissier D. Acute dorsal trans-scaphoid perilunate fracture-dislocations: medium-term results. J Hand Surg 2002;27(6):498–502.
10. Johnson RP. The acutely injured wrist and its residuals. Clin Orthop Relat Res 1980;(149):33–44.
11. Jones DB Jr, Kakar S. Perilunate dislocations and fracture dislocations. J Hand Surg Am 2012;37(10):2168–2173.
12. Kozin SH. Perilunate injuries: diagnosis and treatment. J Am Acad Orthop Surg 1998;6(2):114–120.
13. Kremer T, Wendt M, Riedel K, et al. Open reduction for perilunate injuries—clinical outcome and patient satisfaction. J Hand Surg Am 2010;35:1599–1606.
14. Mayfield JK, Johnson RP, Kilcoyne RK. Carpal dislocations: pathomechanics and progressive perilunar instability. J Hand Surg Am 1980;5:226–241.
15. Sawardeker PJ, Kindt KE, Baratz ME. Fracture-dislocations of the carpus: perilunate injury. Orthop Clin North Am 2013;44(1):93–106.
16. Sotereanos DG, Mitsionis GJ, Giannakopoulos PN, et al. Perilunate dislocation and fracture dislocation: a critical analysis of the volar-dorsal approach. J Hand Surg Am 1997;22(1):49–56.
17. Tavernier L. Les deplacements traumatiques du semi-lunaire. Lyon, France; These, 1906:138–139.
18. Walsh JJ, Berger RA, Cooney WP. Current status of scapholunate interosseous ligament injuries. J Am Acad Orthop Surg 2002;10:32–42.

Arthroscopic and Open Triangular Fibrocartilage Complex Repair

63

CHAPTER

A. Lee Osterman and Emily Slate

DEFINITION

- The triangular fibrocartilage complex (TFCC) is a complex anatomic structure located at the ulnar side of the wrist. It has several important biomechanical functions:
  - Extends the gliding surface of the radiocarpal joint
  - Cushions and stabilizes the ulnar carpus
  - Stabilizes the distal radioulnar joint (DRUJ)
- Disorders of the TFCC are responsible for the ulnar-sided wrist symptoms of pain, weakness, and instability that affect the patient's function.
- The diagnosis and treatment of these injuries to the TFCC will restore stability, resulting in pain relief and a generally good prognosis for functional return.

ANATOMY

- The TFCC is a cartilaginous and ligamentous structure interposed between the ulnar carpus and the distal ulna (**FIG 1A**). It arises from the distal aspect of the sigmoid notch of the radius and inserts into the base of the ulnar styloid.[17]
- The TFCC attaches to the ulnar carpus via the ulnocarpal ligament complex (ulnolunate, ulnotriquetral, and ulnar collateral ligament) (**FIG 1B**).
- The radioulnar ligaments stabilize the DRUJ, limiting rotation as well as axial migration.[2]
  - The dorsal and volar radioulnar ligaments are fibrous thickenings within the substance of the TFCC.
  - As a result of this anatomic configuration, they function as a unit rather than as independent ligaments.
- The central, horizontal portion of the TFCC is the thinnest portion, composed of interwoven obliquely oriented sheets of collagen fibers for the resistance of multidirectional stress.
- The vascularity of the TFCC has been carefully studied.[4] The TFCC receives its blood supply from the ulnar artery through its radiocarpal branches and the dorsal and palmar branches of the anterior interosseous artery. These vessels supply the TFCC in a radial fashion (see Bednar et al[4] for a good image of TFCC vascularity).
  - Histologic sections demonstrate that these vessels penetrate only the peripheral 10% to 40% of the TFCC. The central section and radial attachment are avascular.
  - This vascular anatomy supports the concept that peripheral injuries can heal if injured and treated appropriately, whereas tears of the central portion do not heal if sutured and are usually débrided.

Biomechanics

- The TFCC has several important biomechanical functions: it transmits 20% of an axially applied load from the ulnar carpus to the distal ulna, it is the major stabilizer of the DRUJ, and it is a stabilizer of the ulna.[1,6,16,18]
- The amount of the load transferred to the distal ulna varies with ulnar variance. A greater amount is transferred in positive ulnar variance than negative.
  - This results in a corresponding decreased thickness of the central portion of the TFCC in ulnar positive wrists.
- There is a variable load placed on the TFCC with forearm rotation. Supination causes a negative ulnar variance due to the proximal migration of the ulna. This is reversed with pronation as the ulna moves distally, causing it to become ulnar positive.
- The ulnar head also moves within the sigmoid notch in a dorsal direction with pronation and a volar direction with supination.
  - The dorsal and volar radioulnar ligaments, which form the peripheral portion of the TFCC, serve as major stabilizers to translation at the DRUJ during forearm rotation.

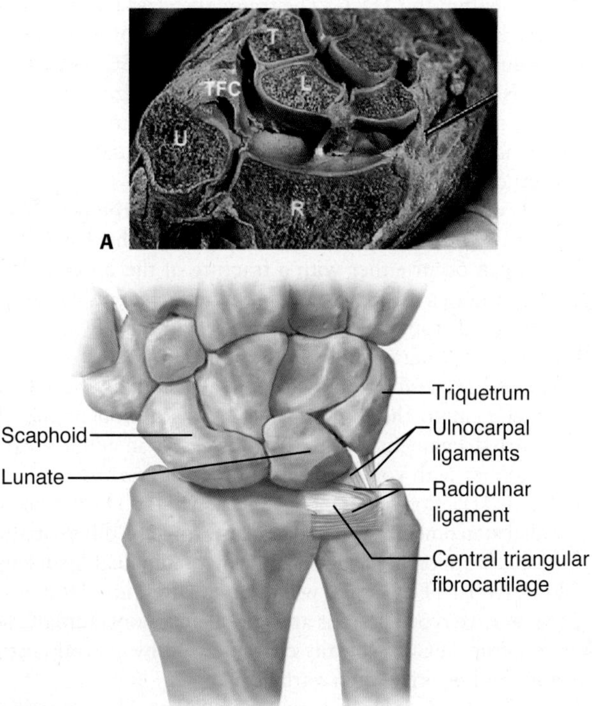

FIG 1 • **A.** Anatomic coronal section demonstrating the triangular fibrocartilage (*TFC*) and its relation to the lunate (*L*), triquetrum (*T*), distal ulna (*U*), and radius (*R*). **B.** TFCC.

PATHOGENESIS

- Traumatic injuries of the TFCC result from either the application of an extension, pronation force to the axially loaded wrist, or a distraction force to the ulnar aspect of the wrist.
  - This will most commonly occur with a fall on the outstretched hand or a resisted torque force.
  - The lesions are more common with ulnar positive and neutral patients and are frequently found in patients with fractures of the distal radius.
- Several authors have examined the incidence of intracarpal soft tissue injuries associated with distal radial fractures.
  - Geissler et al[8] studied 60 patients, finding a TFCC injury in 26 (43%).
  - In Lindau et al's[12] series of 51 patients, 43 had a TFCC injury (84%): 24 had a peripheral tear, 10 had a central perforation, and 9 had a combined central and peripheral tear.
- In a study of 180 wrist joints in 100 cadavers ranging in age from fetuses to 94 years, Mikić[13] found that degeneration of the TFCC begins in the third decade of life.
  - This degeneration increases in frequency and severity as people age.
  - After the fifth decade of life, 100% of TFCCs appear abnormal.
  - However, these age-related TFCC lesions are often asymptomatic.[6]

NATURAL HISTORY

- The classification system described by Palmer[15] is the most useful for describing TFCC injuries, dividing them into traumatic and degenerative.
- Traumatic lesions are classified according to the location of the tear within the TFCC. The traumatic class has been designated by Palmer[15] as class 1, with subclasses of A, B, C, and D assigned to anatomic lesions within the TFCC (**FIG 2A**).
  - A class 1A lesion represents a tear in the horizontal or central portion of the TFCC. The tear is 2 to 3 mm medial to the radial attachment of the cartilage. It is usually oriented from dorsal to volar.
  - A class 1B lesion represents an avulsion of the peripheral aspect of the TFCC from its insertion onto the distal ulna. This can occur either with a fracture of the ulnar styloid or as a pure avulsion from its bony attachment. This type of injury disrupts the stabilizing effect of the TFCC on the DRUJ, resulting in clinical instability.
  - A class 1C lesion represents an avulsion of the TFCC attachment to the ulnar carpus by disruption of the ulnocarpal ligaments. These lesions result in ulnar carpal instability with volar translocation of the carpus.
  - A class 1D lesion represents an avulsion of the TFCC from its radial attachment. Isolated disc tears should be differentiated from disruption of the dorsal and volar radioulnar ligaments. Such global TFCC injury will result in DRUJ instability.
- Degenerative type 2 lesions are age-related, nontraumatic lesions to the TFCC, typically characterized by central perforations and positive ulnar variance.[6,22]
- The natural history of such degenerative lesions, when and if they become symptomatic, is a progressive cascade of degenerative changes, as reflected in Palmer's type 2 classification (**FIG 2B**).
  - The deterioration proceeds from triangular fibrocartilage (TFC) wear through central perforation (type 2C) to lunatotriquetral ligament tear and arthritic changes of the lunate, triquetrum, and distal ulna (type 2D or E).
  - Treatment is based on the stage of involvement.
- Degenerative and traumatic lesions can coexist, and injury can render a degenerative lesion symptomatic.

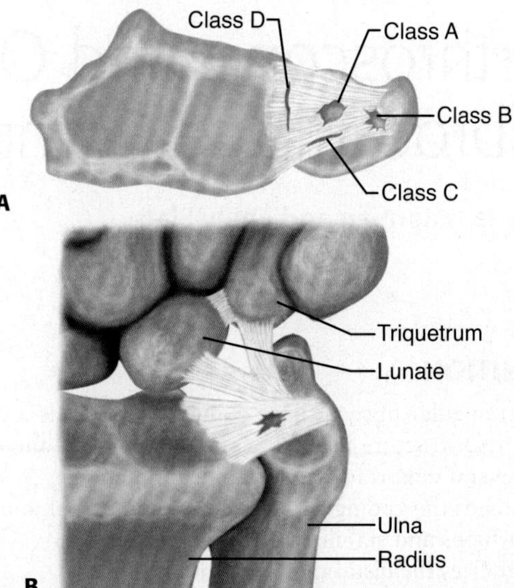

FIG 2 • A. Axial drawing looking at the radius platform and the TFCC. Dorsal is up and volar is down. Palmer classification for acute TFCC injuries. A class 1A lesion involves a tear in the central, horizontal portion of the TFCC. A class 1B lesion is a tear of the TFCC from the distal ulna with or without an ulnar styloid fracture. A class 1C lesion is a tear of the TFCC distal attachment to the lunate and triquetrum through the ulnolunate and ulnotriquetral ligaments. A class 1D lesion is a detachment of the TFCC from its insertion on to the radius at the distal sigmoid notch. **B.** Palmer classification for degenerative TFCC lesions, usually related to positive ulnar variance and ulnocarpal impaction syndrome. The degeneration occurs in a progressive cascade: types 2A and 2B, TFC wear; type 2C, fibrillated central TFC lesion; types 2D and 2E, arthritic chondral changes of the distal ulna and lunate and disruption of the lunatotriquetral ligament. (**A:** Modified From Palmer AK. Triangular fibrocartilage complex lesions: a classification. J Hand Surg Am 1989;14[4]:594–606.)

PATIENT HISTORY AND PHYSICAL FINDINGS

- Symptoms consist of ulnar-sided wrist pain, frequently with clicking, that typically occurs after a fall.
- The initial physical examination reveals swelling over the ulnar aspect of the wrist with inflammation of the tendon of the extensor carpi ulnaris (ECU).
- Point tenderness is present over the TFCC and distal ulna. The more isolated the point of maximal tenderness, the more specific the diagnosis.
  - A fovea sign (point tenderness directly over the ulnar TFC origin) indicates a type 1A or 1B TFC injury or an ulnar extrinsic injury type 1C.
- Ulnar deviation and axial loading of the wrist (TFCC compression test) will elicit a painful response and a click with forearm rotation.
- The DRUJ must be assessed for instability. Instability is best assessed with the forearm in neutral rotation, but it is also checked in full supination and full pronation.
  - The examiner stabilizes the distal radius with one hand and applies a force to the distal ulna, moving it dorsal and

volar, looking for increased motion or subluxation of the distal ulna relative to the radius and comparing it with the opposite uninjured wrist.
  - Significant instability can present as laxity of the distal ulna with a positive "piano key" sign and dorsal prominence of the distal ulna. This may be due to a significant tear or detachment of the dorsal or volar radioulnar ligaments.
- A click produced by ulnar deviation and supination over the ECU sheath at the distal ulna indicates ECU instability with subluxation out of its sixth extensor compartment.
- A visual carpal supination deformity with ulnar prominence that can be passively corrected by a dorsally applied force to the pisiform indicates an ulnar extrinsic ligament tear.
- TFCC injuries do not occur in isolation; they are often a component of a spectrum of injury to the ulnar side of the wrist. The examiner must therefore evaluate all of the commonly injured structures on the ulnar side of the wrist.
  - The lunatotriquetral joint must be assessed for instability due to a lunatotriquetral ligament tear. This would cause tenderness over the lunatotriquetral interval with a positive Shuck test (painful click as the lunate and triquetrum slide abnormally).
  - Point tenderness over the triquetrum may signify a triquetral avulsion fracture.
  - An audible clunk and visual subluxation of the carpus that occur with active ulnar deviation suggest that a midcarpal instability is present.
- Crepitus and pain over the pisotriquetral joint on the shear test may indicate pisotriquetral arthritis.
- The other soft tissue structures around the ulnar wrist should be examined, including the ulnar nerve, the dorsal ulnar sensory nerve branch, and the ulnar artery.
- Grip strength measurements using a Jamar dynamometer, although subjective, are helpful in quantitating patient effort and as a parameter to follow therapeutic progress.

IMAGING AND OTHER DIAGNOSTIC STUDIES

- The diagnostic workup should include plain radiographs and a neutral rotation posteroanterior and lateral view.
  - This will allow assessment for fracture, ligament instability resulting in carpal malalignment, and ulnar variance. It is important to determine ulnar variance because it will influence treatment options (**FIG 3A**).
  - The DRUJ must also be examined radiographically to determine if subluxation, arthritis, or ulnar styloid abnormalities such as an acute or chronic nonunited fracture fragment are present.
- Magnetic resonance imaging (MRI) is useful in the diagnosis of TFCC tears, especially the class 1A and D lesions.[9,11] T2-weighted images in the coronal plane are of the greatest diagnostic value (**FIG 3B**).
  - The TFCC has a homogenous low signal intensity. The synovial fluid of the joint appears as a bright image on T2 and will outline tears in the TFCC.
  - A gadolinium arthrogram enhances the visualization of TFCC tears.
- The reported sensitivity and specificity of MRI in diagnosing injuries of the TFCC in the literature is variable.
  - Golimbu et al[9] reported a 95% accuracy of MRI in the detection of TFCC tears. MRI findings were verified arthroscopically.

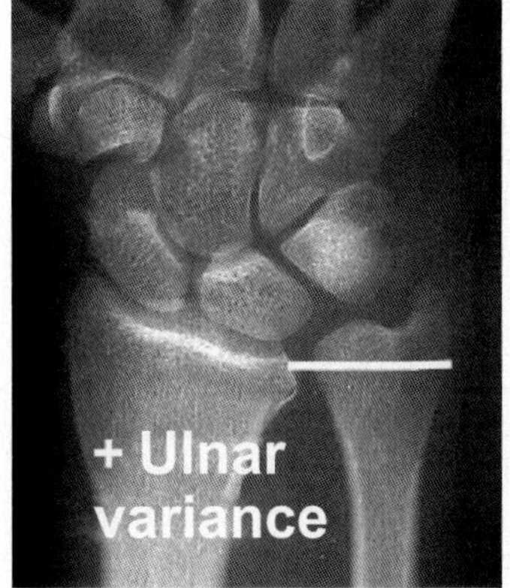

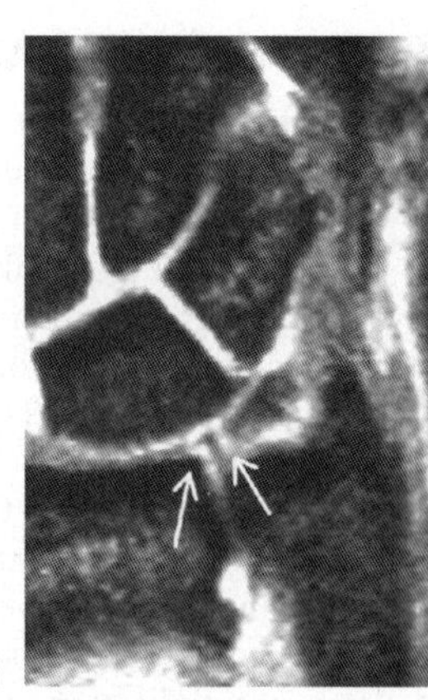

FIG 3 • **A.** Positive ulnar variance is often associated with degenerative TFC tears and ulnocarpal impaction syndrome. The radiograph should be taken in neutral rotation. **B.** Coronal T2 MRI wrist image. High signal of the joint fluid outlines the low signal substance of the TFC complex. Tears will show as high signal within the central region (*arrow at right*) or TFCC periphery. There is a normal clear area (*arrow at left*) at the insertion of the radial TFC into the medial articular cartilage of the radius.

  - Schweitzer et al[19] reported a sensitivity of 72%, a specificity of 95%, and an accuracy of 89%.
  - Arthroscopic findings were correlated with the MRI and clinical examination in a series of patients with TFC injuries reported by Bednar et al.[3] The MRI sensitivity was 44% (the probability of a positive MRI when a TFCC lesion is present) and the specificity was 75% (the probability of a negative MRI when a TFCC lesion is absent). The clinical examination sensitivity was 95%. The MRI correlated with arthroscopic findings in 45% of the wrists studied.
  - Joshy et al[11] reported on a series of patients with a clinical suspicion of a TFCC tear studied by magnetic resonance (MR) arthrography and then wrist arthroscopy. The MR arthrography sensitivity was 74% and its specificity was 80%. They caution that negative results of MR arthrography in patients with clinical suspicion of TFCC tear should be interpreted with caution.
- Wrist arthroscopy has recently become the criterion standard for both diagnosing and treating lesions of the TFCC.[6]
  - When compared to MRI and arthrography, arthroscopy most accurately determines the location of lesions and the size of tears and allows determination of whether a flap is unstable.
  - Wrist arthroscopy can determine the coexistence of other lesions such as tears within the lunotriquetral interosseous ligament, ECU subsheath, or chondral lesions.

DIFFERENTIAL DIAGNOSIS

- ECU subluxation
- Ulnar extrinsic ligament tear
- DRUJ instability
- Triquetral avulsion fracture
- Lunatotriquetral ligament injury
- Pisotriquetral arthritis
- Ulnar artery thrombosis
- Ulnar neuropathy at the canal of Guyon
- Dorsal ulnar sensory neuritis

NONOPERATIVE MANAGEMENT

- The initial treatment of acute TFCC injuries includes immobilization of the wrist and DRUJ.
  - The patient must be examined carefully to look for DRUJ instability or ECU subluxation.
- If the radiographs are negative and instability is not present, then immobilization for 4 to 6 weeks is recommended to allow healing of the TFCC disruption.
- A peripheral tear is expected to heal if the torn edges are held in close contact, due to the good vascularity of the periphery of the TFCC. Many central tears also become asymptomatic with immobilization even though there is no significant vascularity to the central portion.
- After immobilization, a therapy program involving range-of-motion exercises and gradual strengthening is initiated. Forceful grasp or torque is restricted for 8 weeks.
- If there is ongoing synovitis, a well-placed cortisone shot can further help to quiet this inflammation.
- Tears involving the ligamentous portion of the TFCC or those that heal with a flap of cartilage that impinges on the carpus or distal ulna will fail to respond to conservative treatment and will require operative intervention.
  - It is reasonable to wait 3 to 4 months before proceeding to surgical treatment.
- Class 1B lesions without an ulnar styloid fracture and a stable DRUJ can be immobilized for 4 weeks in a cast. If an ulnar styloid fracture is present, closed reduction should be attempted. If adequate reduction is achieved, then cast immobilization is sufficient. If the styloid remains displaced, then open reduction and internal fixation is required.

SURGICAL MANAGEMENT

- Patients who remain symptomatic after adequate immobilization should undergo further workup, including MRI with or without gadolinium.
- The specific treatment for each traumatic type 1 lesion is determined by the type of tear found arthroscopically.
  - Arthroscopic treatment has become increasingly the method of choice for many traumatic lesions.
- The treatment of traumatic radial detachment of the TFCC from the sigmoid notch of the distal radius is controversial. There appears to be no vascularity to this portion of the TFCC, so theoretically, a reattached cartilage would not heal at this repair site. However, clinical experience with open repair of these tears has been positive.[6,20] This may be attributed to vascular ingrowth from the bony radial insertion site that occurs with abrasion of the attachment site, stimulating the formation of new vessels.
  - If the radial tear includes disruption of one or both of the radioulnar ligaments, repair is required to prevent chronic DRUJ instability.
- The algorithm for the treatment of degenerative type 2 tears proceeds from arthroscopy to ulnar shortening osteotomy (see Chaps. 114 and 115).
  - Plain films should identify the ulnar variance, DRUJ alignment, abnormalities of the ulnar styloid, or the presence of arthritic changes. Positive ulnar variance has a strong association with degenerative tears.

Preoperative Planning

- All physical examination findings and radiographic study results must be reviewed.
- Examination under anesthesia is performed, including the tests discussed earlier, before positioning in the arthroscopy tower.

Positioning

- Wrist arthroscopy requires distraction, and the wrist is positioned in the traction tower (**FIG 4**).

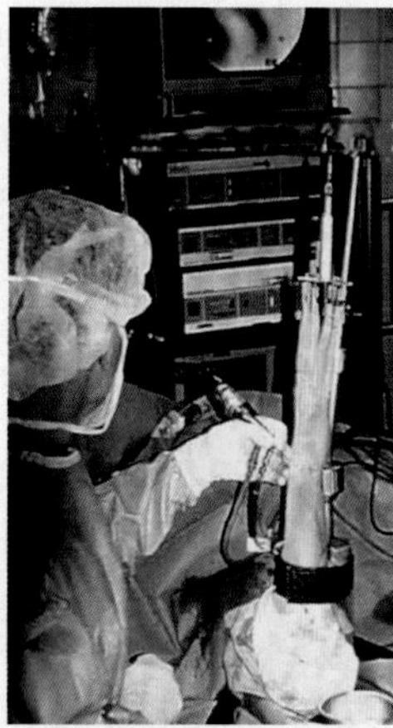

FIG 4 • Positioning for standard wrist arthroscopy. Distraction of the wrist using a wrist traction tower.

TECHNIQUES

■ Wrist Arthroscopy

- Diagnostic wrist arthroscopy of the radiocarpal and midcarpal joints is completed and all pathology is identified.
- Recognize the appearance of a normal TFC (**TECH FIG 1**).
- The type of TFC injury is identified.
  - A trampoline test is positive when the surgeon's probe sinks into the TFCC rather than bouncing off it like a drumstick on a snare drum. Such loss of disc compliance is often seen with a peripheral tear.[10] However, laxity of the TFCC does not necessarily translate into DRUJ instability.
- Loose bodies, if present, are removed.
- Inflamed synovium is removed with a shaver or radiofrequency probe.

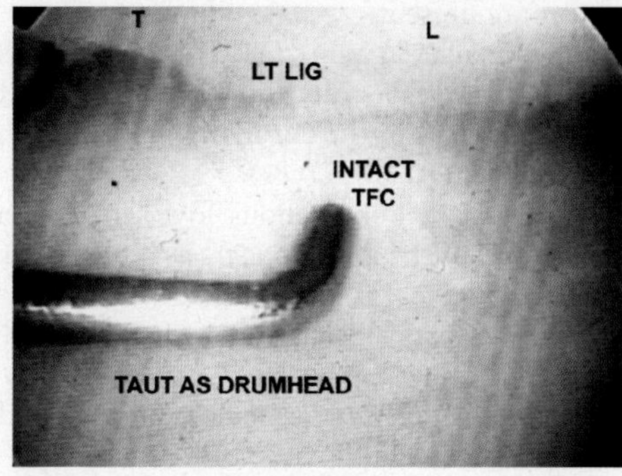

TECH FIG 1 • Normal arthroscopic view of the intact triangular fibrocartilage (*TFC*) with normal "trampoline" tension when probed.

Arthroscopic Repair of Peripheral Triangular Fibrocartilage Tears

- Peripheral TFC tears are well vascularized and amenable to repair using arthroscopic techniques. A two-needle method similar to that employed for the repair of a knee meniscus is described here (**TECH FIG 2A**).
- Visualize the tear through the 3-4 portal.
- Initial arthroscopic evaluation may not reveal a tear of the TFCC periphery, but often synovitis and a thin scar will be seen along the periphery of the TFCC at the location of the tear (**TECH FIG 2B**).
  - A probe placed through the 6R portal will demonstrate loss of the normal trampoline effect of the TFCC, indicating a peripheral tear and loss of mechanical function of the TFCC (**TECH FIG 2C**).
- Débride the edges of the tear and undersurface scarring with a shaver to create mobile edges with fresh areas for healing.
  - Adhesions may be present between the undersurface of the TFCC and the distal ulna. These must be released and the TFC mobilized sufficiently to allow advancement to reattach it and to restore proper tension.
- After débridement, a 1-cm longitudinal incision is made extending the 6R portal.
  - Avoid injury to branches of the dorsal ulnar sensory nerve.
- Open the sixth extensor compartment radially for 1 cm and retract the ECU ulnarly, providing access to its subsheath.
  - The repair includes the subsheath of the ECU compartment, as this is intimately associated with the peripheral TFC.
- Two needles are passed across the tear under arthroscopic vision (**TECH FIG 2D**).
- A wire loop is passed through one needle to retrieve a 2-0 PDS suture, which is passed through the other needle.
  - This allows the placement of a horizontal mattress suture across the tear (authors' preference) (**TECH FIG 2E**).
  - Alternatively, multiple simple vertical sutures placed at the periphery of the TFCC may approximate the torn edges and restore tension to the TFCC. The suture is tied either under the skin over the dorsal wrist capsule (preferred) or out of the skin over a bolster. Usually, two or three sutures are placed.
- Postoperatively, a short-arm splint is applied.
  - We have not found a significant difference between use of a short-arm splint and use of a long-arm or sugar-tong splint in regard to healing and outcome.

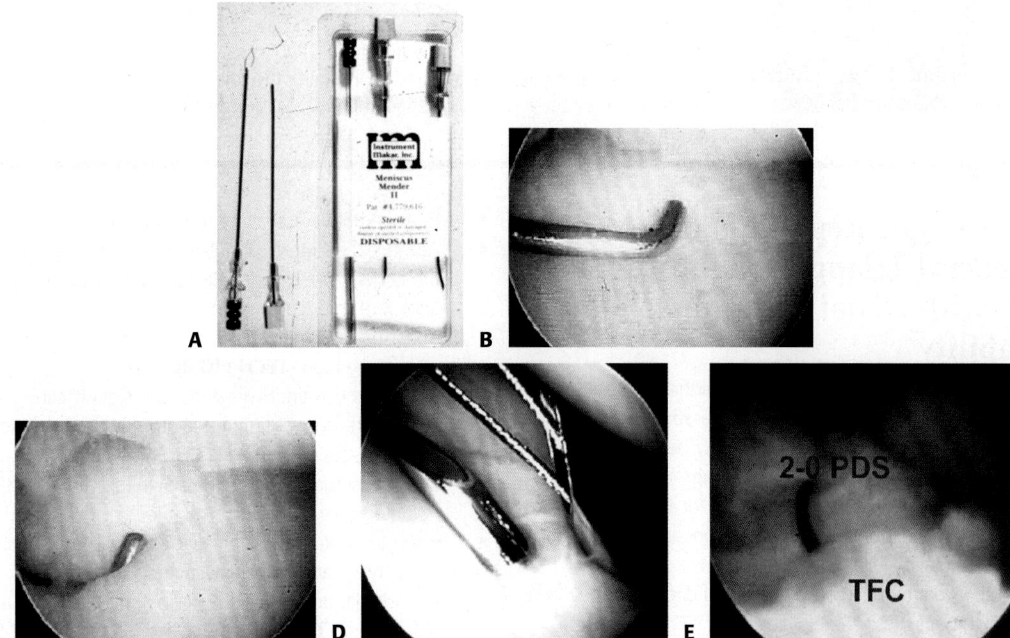

TECH FIG 2 • **A.** Meniscus repair needles with 2-0 PDS suture used for an out-to-in repair. **B,C.** Peripheral TFC tear with loss of compliance such that the probe sinks into the lax surface. Unlike a central tear, fibrous tissue and incomplete healing obscure the actual tear. **D.** Arthroscopic repair of a type 1B peripheral TFC complex tear. Two hollow needles are passed across the tear. A wire loop in one needle is used to pass 2-0 suture across the tear. The suture is tied over the capsule. **E.** The suture approximates the tear and restores tension to the triangular fibrocartilage (*TFC*).

Open Repair of Peripheral Triangular Fibrocartilage Tears without Ulnar Styloid Fracture

- If there is significant DRUJ instability and avulsion of the TFC from the ulna fovea, an open repair is preferred.
- Expose the fifth extensor compartment and retract the extensor digiti quinti minimi tendon.
- Create an L-shaped capsulotomy of the DRUJ and identify the foveal attachment site of the TFC (**TECH FIG 3A**).
- Reattach the TFC with a bone anchor or bone suture (**TECH FIG 3B–D**).
- Postoperative care mirrors that of arthroscopic TFC repair.[11]

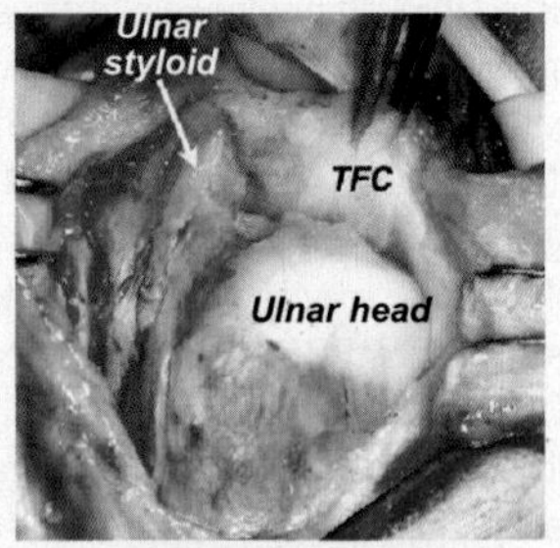

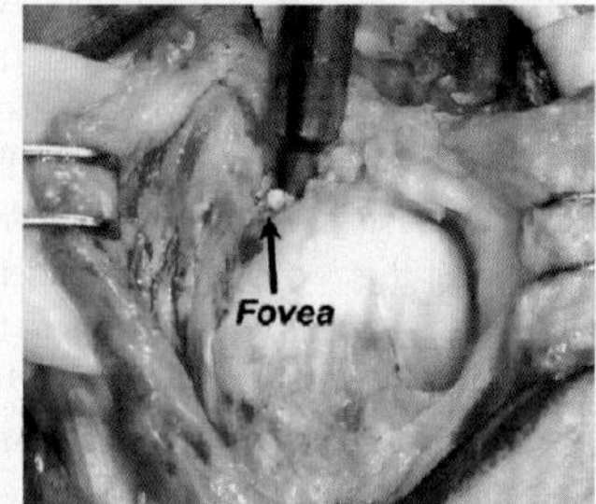

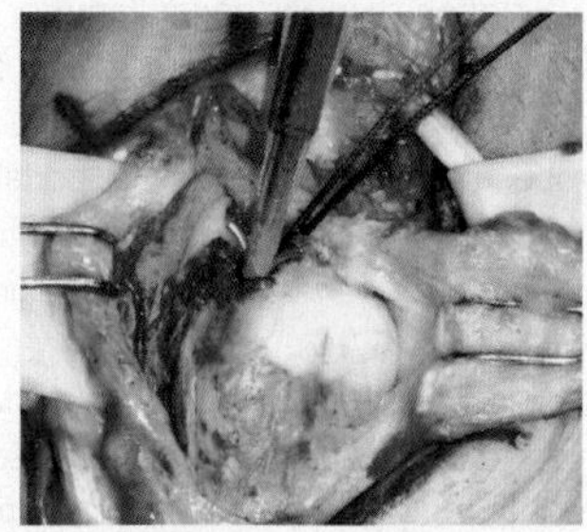

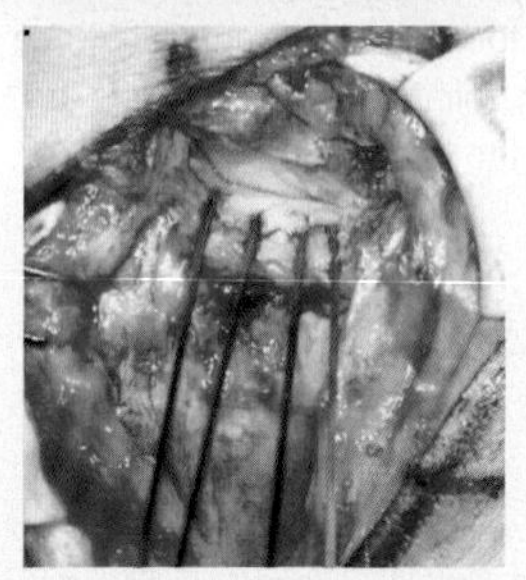

TECH FIG 3 • Open repair of unstable TFC avulsion. **A.** Dorsal exposure through the fifth extensor compartment. A DRUJ capsulotomy has been performed. *TFC*, triangular fibrocartilage. **B.** Defining the foveal insertion site. **C.** Insertion of bone anchor at foveal attachment. **D.** Sutures in place.

Arthroscopic Repair of Foveal Peripheral Triangular Fibrocartilage Tears with Distal Radioulnar Joint Instability

- Geissler[7] has developed a technique of arthroscopic foveal repair valuable in cases of TFCC 1B tears associated with foveal detachment and resulting DRUJ instability. The characteristics of this unique technique include the following:
  - It is entirely arthroscopic with no need for additional incisions.
  - Use of knotless anchors avoids the possibility of superficial nerve irritation from knots.
  - Both layers of the TFCC are repaired directly to their bony attachment sites.
- Perform standard wrist arthroscopy and TFCC débridement as previously described.
- Make an accessory 6R portal under direct visualization. This is done by inserting a needle 1.5 cm distal to and in line with the 6R portal, aimed toward the fovea of the ulna (**TECH FIG 4A,B**).
  - Be aware of extensor digiti quinti and dorsal ulnar sensory nerve.
- Insert the suture lasso through the accessory 6R portal and pass it through the TFCC (**TECH FIG 4C**).
  - View through the 3-4 portal
- Back the suture lasso out of the TFCC without removing it from the joint. Reposition the suture lasso and pass it through the TFCC dorsal or volar to the first pass creating a horizontal mattress stitch (**TECH FIG 4D**).
- Retrieve both sutures into the 6R portal.
- Advance the slotted cannula with obturator into the joint through the accessory 6R portal. Remove the obturator and place a Nitinol wire through the cannula, then retrieve it through the 6R portal using a mini suture hook. Pass the sutures through the nitinol wire loop (**TECH FIG 4E**).
- Retrieve the Nitinol wire from the slotted cannula so that the sutures are now exiting the joint through the slotted cannula in the accessory 6R portal (**TECH FIG 4F**).
- Slide the sutures through the slot in the cannula so that they will not interfere with drilling.
- Insert the obturator and position the assembly just radial to the ulnar styloid at the fovea. Drill the guide wire and check its position with fluoroscopy. Remove the obturator and utilize the cannulated drill (**TECH FIG 4G**).
  - While removing the drill from the joint, secure the cannula so that it remains positioned over the drill hole. The wire may be left in place.
- Thread the sutures through a 2.5 mm mini PushLock anchor (Arthrex, Naples). Advance the anchor through the cannula into the drill hole (**TECH FIG 4H**).
  - Tension the sutures before the tapping the anchor into its final seated position.
  - Once the anchor is fully deployed, the push lock driver is removed by turning the driver counterclockwise, thus disengaging the driver from the anchor.
- Cut the sutures flush inside the joint (**TECH FIG 4I**). Check DRUJ stability.

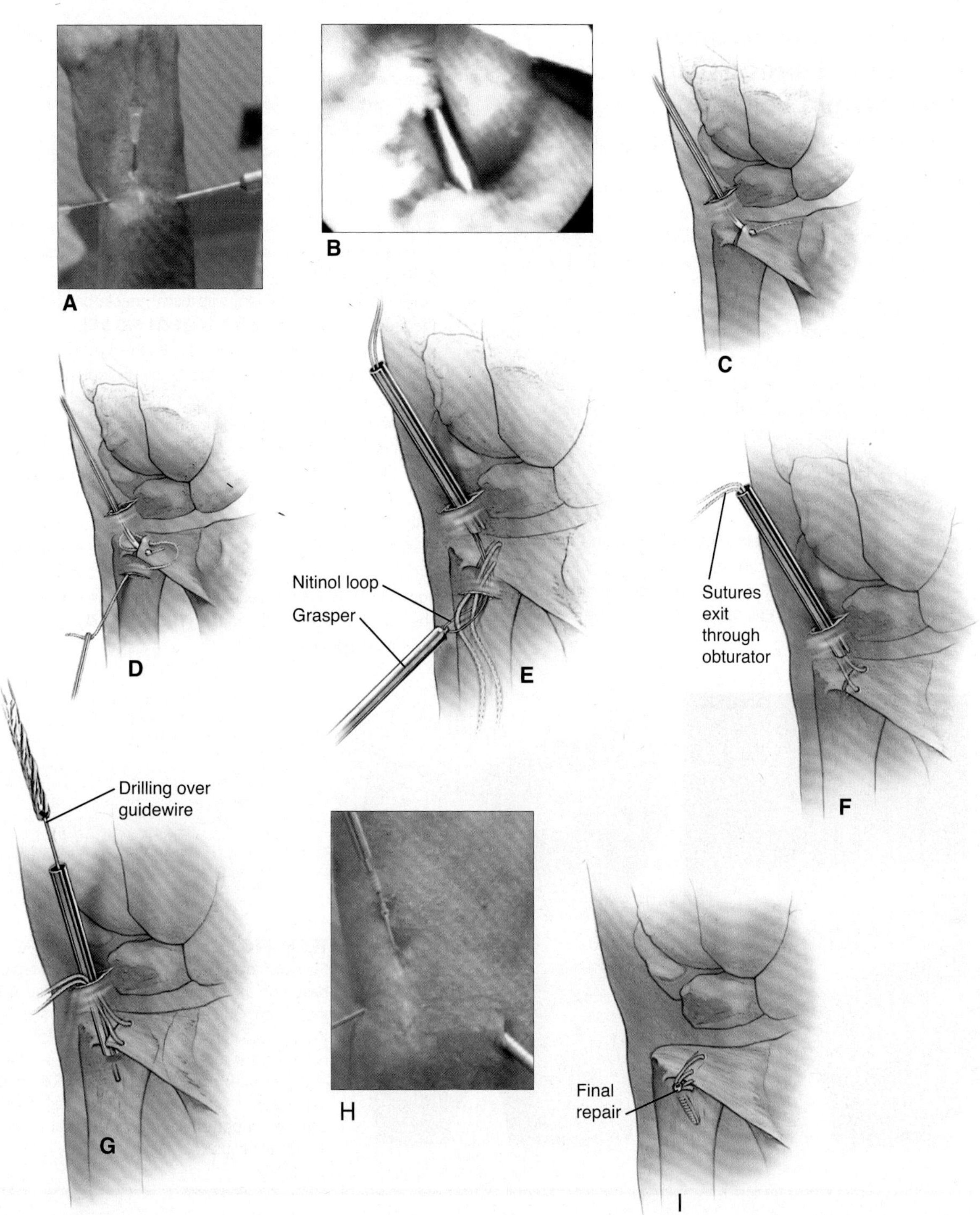

TECH FIG 4 • A. An accessory 6R portal is made under direct visualization 1.5cm distal to and in line with the 6R portal. **B.** A needle is inserted towards the fovea of the ulna as seen in this arthroscopic view. This assures proper portal placement. **C.** The TFCC suture lasso has penetrated the TFCC and the suture is advanced. **D.** A second pass is made through the TFCC using the suture lasso. This creates a horizontal mattress stitch capable of grasping the torn edge of the TFCC. **E.** The nitinol loop is passed into the joint through the slotted cannula from the accessory 6R portal. A grasper is used to retrieve the nitinol loop. It is brought out through the 6R portal and the two suture limbs are advanced through the loop. **F.** The loop, along with the suture ends, is withdrawn through the joint and out the accessory 6R portal. **G.** The cannulated drill is placed over the guide wire and the hole for the anchor is created. **H.** The threaded anchor is inserted through the accessory 6R portal over the guide wire. This may be done through the cannula if preferred. The sutures are tensioned as the anchor is implanted. **I.** A completed knotless repair of the TFCC to the ulna fovea.

TECHNIQUES

Open Repair of Peripheral Triangular Fibrocartilage Tears with Ulnar Styloid Fracture

- Expose the ulnar styloid using an incision just volar and parallel to the ECU tendon.
  - Protect the dorsal ulnar sensory nerve and preserve the ECU sheath.
- Base the method of fixation (longitudinal Kirschner wire, screw, bone anchor, or tension band) on fragment size and surgeon comfort.
- If the ulnar styloid is comminuted and will not allow stable fixation, it can be excised and the TFCC attached to the ulna by a suture placed through drill holes in the ulna proximal to the fracture or using the suture anchor technique described earlier.
- The patient is immobilized in a short-arm splint or cast for 4 weeks before starting rotational motion.

Surgery for Radial-Sided Triangular Fibrocartilage Avulsion Tears

- Assess the tear arthroscopically (**TECH FIG 5A**) and repair it in the manner detailed in the following text if instability is present.
- Place a burr through the 6R portal to roughen the radial attachment of the TFCC (**TECH FIG 5B**).
- Drill two holes using a 0.062-inch Kirschner wire in a retrograde manner, starting at the TFC insertion site. These holes will allow placement of the repair suture.
  - The wires must exit the radius on its radial border, just volar to the first extensor compartment.
- An incision is made over the exiting Kirschner wire to retract and protect the radial sensory nerve and the tendons of the first extensor compartment.
- A cannula is placed in the 6R portal, through which a meniscal repair suture (2-0 PDS suture with a long straight needle at each end) is passed through the torn radial aspect of the TFCC in a horizontal mattress fashion, with each needle passing through the predrilled holes in the radius (**TECH FIG 5C**).
  - The placement of the needles into the predrilled holes can be challenging because the holes are not visible by the scope in the 3-4 portal. Two 18-gauge spinal needles can be placed from the radial side of the radius through the bone until they can be seen in the joint at the attachment site for the TFCC. The needles provide a visible target for the meniscal repair suture needles.
- If the meniscal repair suture with long straight needles is not available, pass 18-gauge needles through the bone tunnels, then directly through the torn radial TFC. A 2-0 PDS suture is passed from one 18-gauge needle to the other using a wire retrieval loop.
- The suture is tied over the radius (**TECH FIG 5D**).
- A short-arm splint is applied.

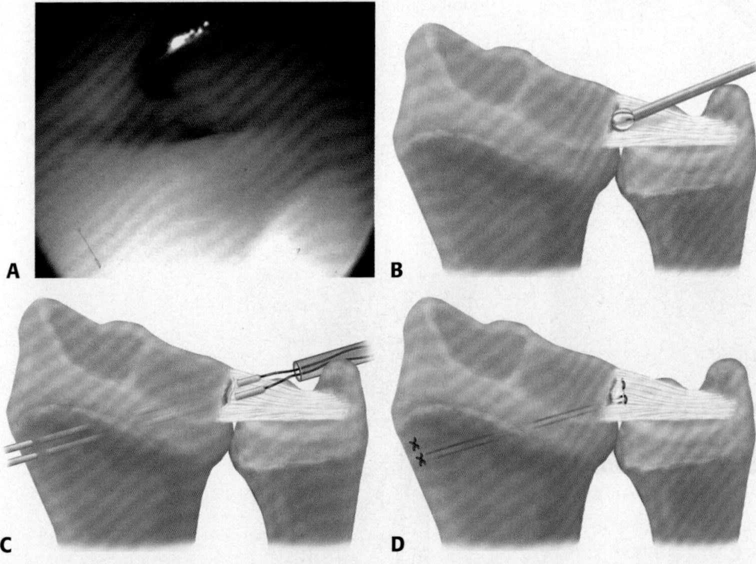

TECH FIG 5 • A. Traumatic radial TFC tear. Such an isolated tear can be débrided or repaired based on the degree of instability. **B.** Radial TFC tear repair. Burring of the attachment site along the sigmoid notch of the radius to bleeding bone is necessary to introduce additional vascularity and promote wound healing. **C,D.** Radial tears are repaired with suture on meniscal needles, tied over a bone bridge on the radial aspect of the distal radius.

PEARLS AND PITFALLS

Indications	▪ Traumatic and degenerative TFC lesions with sufficient symptoms ▪ If the DRUJ is stable, allow 3–4 months of nonoperative treatment.
Preoperative evaluation	▪ Assess ulnar variance. ▪ Physical examination under anesthesia ▪ Complete diagnostic wrist arthroscopy of both radiocarpal and midcarpal joints ▪ A complete history and physical examination of ulnar wrist pain causes

Treatment options related to type of TFC lesion	▪ Class 1A: arthroscopic débridement ▪ Class 1B without fracture: arthroscopic or open repair (DRUJ instability) ▪ Class 1B with ulnar styloid fracture and instability: reattach ulnar styloid ▪ Class 1C: rare 1B repair plus ulnar extrinsic ligament repair ▪ Class 1D: if isolated, débride; if unstable, repair ▪ Degenerative lesions: arthroscopic wafer or ulnar shortening osteotomy
Pitfalls	▪ Excise only unstable central TFC portion. ▪ Protect dorsal sensory nerves and extensor tendons.

POSTOPERATIVE CARE

- After open or arthroscopic TFC repair, a short-arm splint or cast is applied for 4 to 6 weeks.
- Range-of-motion exercises are then progressed, using a removable splint for protection initially.
- Forceful wrist use is restricted for 3 months.

OUTCOMES

- Arthroscopic limited débridement of the central portion of the tear will provide excellent relief of symptoms, with 80% to 85% of patients having a good to excellent result.[14]
  - The biomechanical effect of excision of the central portion of the TFCC has been examined.[1,6] The excision of the central two-thirds of the TFCC with maintenance of the dorsal and volar radioulnar ligaments as well as the ulnocarpal ligaments had no statistical significant effect on forearm axial load transmission. The removal of greater than two-thirds will unload the ulnar column, shifting load to the distal radius and destabilizing the DRUJ.
  - Adams[1] further emphasized that the peripheral 2 mm of the TFCC must be maintained during central débridement in order not to have a biomechanical effect on load transfer.
- The results of arthroscopic repair of class 1B TFCC lesions are equivalent to those reported for open repair. Gratifying outcomes are reached 85% to 90% of the time.[5,6,21]
- The treatment of radial detachment of the TFCC from the sigmoid notch of the distal radius remains controversial.
  - Débridement of an isolated radial tear not associated with joint instability, similar to that for class 1A lesions, yields excellent results.[14]
  - Clinical experience with open repair of radial TFC avulsion tears has also been good.[6,20] Short[20] reported 79% excellent and good results in his series, with return of grip strength to 90%, after arthroscopic repair of radial TFCC tears.

COMPLICATIONS

- Failure to make a complete diagnosis (eg, associated ECU subluxation)
- Failure to appreciate DRUJ instability
- Loss of wrist motion
- Injury to dorsal sensory nerves
- Nonunion of the ulnar styloid or ulnar osteotomy

REFERENCES

1. Adams BD. Partial excision of the triangular fibrocartilage complex articular disk: a biomechanical study. J Hand Surg Am 1993;18(2): 334–340.
2. af Ekenstam FW, Palmer AK, Glisson RR. The load on the radius and ulna in different positions of the wrist and forearm. A cadaver study. Acta Orthop Scand 1984;55:363–365.
3. Bednar JM, Bos M, Giacobetti F. Comparison of the accuracy of clinical exam and MRI in diagnosing TFCC lesions. Presented at the American Society for Surgery of the Hand 52nd Annual Meeting, September 11, 1997, Denver, CO.
4. Bednar MS, Arnoczky SP, Weiland AJ. The microvasculature of the triangular fibrocartilage complex: its clinical significance. J Hand Surg Am 1991;16(6):1101–1105.
5. Corso SJ, Savoie FH, Geissler WB, et al. Arthroscopic repair of peripheral avulsions of the triangular fibrocartilage complex of the wrist: a multicenter study. Arthroscopy 1997;13:78–84.
6. Culp R, Osterman L, Kaufmann R. Wrist arthroscopy: operative procedures. In: Green D, Hotchkiss R, Pederson W, et al, eds. Green's Operative Hand Surgery, vol 1, ed 5. Philadelphia: Elsevier, 2005: 781–803.
7. Geissler WB. Arthroscopic knotless peripheral triangular fibrocartilage repair. J Hand Surg Am 2012;37(2):350–355.
8. Geissler WB, Freeland AE, Savoie FH, et al. Intracarpal soft-tissue lesions associated with an intra-articular fracture of the distal end of the radius. J Bone Joint Surg Am 1996;78(3):357–365.
9. Golimbu CN, Firooznia H, Melone CP Jr, et al. Tears of the triangular fibrocartilage of the wrist: MR imaging. Radiology 1989;173(3): 731–733.
10. Hermansdorfer JD, Kleinman WB. Management of chronic peripheral tears of the triangular fibrocartilage complex. J Hand Surg Am 1991;16(2):340–346.
11. Joshy S, Ghosh S, Lee K, et al. Accuracy of direct magnetic resonance arthrography in the diagnosis of triangular fibrocartilage complex tears of the wrist. Int Orthop 2008;32:251–253.
12. Lindau T, Adlercreutz C, Aspenberg P. Peripheral tears of the triangular fibrocartilage complex cause distal radioulnar joint instability after distal radial fracture. J Hand Surg Am 2000;25(3):464–468.
13. Mikić ZD. Age changes in the triangular fibrocartilage of the wrist joint. J Anat 1978;126:367–384.
14. Osterman AL. Arthroscopic debridement of triangular fibrocartilage complex tears. Arthroscopy 1990;6:120–124.
15. Palmer AK. Triangular fibrocartilage complex lesions: a classification. J Hand Surg Am 1989;14(4):594–606.
16. Palmer AK, Werner FW. Biomechanics of the distal radioulnar joint. Clin Orthop Relat Res 1984;(187):26–34.
17. Palmer AK, Werner FW. The triangular fibrocartilage complex of the wrist—anatomy and function. J Hand Surg Am 1981;6(2):153–162.
18. Schuind F, An KN, Berglund L, et al. The distal radioulnar ligaments: a biomechanical study. J Hand Surg Am 1991;16(6):1106–1114.
19. Schweitzer ME, Brahme SK, Hodler J, et al. Chronic wrist pain: spin-echo and short tau inversion recovery MR imaging and conventional and MR arthrography. Radiology 1992;182:205–211.
20. Short WH. Arthroscopic repair of radial-sided triangular fibrocartilage complex tears. J Am Soc Surg Hand 2001;1:258–266.
21. Trumble TE, Gilbert M, Vedder N. Ulnar shortening combined with arthroscopic repairs in the delayed management of triangular fibrocartilage complex tears. J Hand Surg Am 1997;22(5):807–813.
22. Viegas SF, Ballantyne G. Attritional lesions of the wrist joint. J Hand Surg Am 1987;12(6):1025–1029.

Extra-articular Reconstructive Techniques for the Distal Radioulnar and Ulnocarpal Joints

Christopher J. Dy, E. Anne Ouellette, and Anna-Lena Makowski

DEFINITION

- The diagnostic and therapeutic challenge presented by instability of the ulnocarpal joint reflects the inherent biomechanical and anatomic incongruity of the articulation.
- The triangular fibrocartilage complex (TFCC) provides the majority of anatomic and functional stability of the distal radioulnar and ulnocarpal joints.[1,17]
- As expected, the consequences of TFCC lesions reflect a disruption of its normal function.[3] The Hui-Linscheid procedure and the modified Herbert reconstruction are two approaches to achieve surgical stabilization of the distal radioulnar joint (DRUJ). The Hui-Linscheid reconstruction stabilizes the DRUJ by augmenting function of the ulnocarpal ligament,[7] whereas the modified Herbert reconstruction restores the radioulnar and ulnocarpal functions of the TFCC by ligamentotaxic constraint of the ulnar carpus.[4]

ANATOMY

- The ulnar carpus does not directly articulate with the distal ulna; instead, the ulnar carpus is suspended from the ulnar head by the TFCC.
- The TFCC is a collection of soft tissue structures that stabilizes the radial-ulnar-carpal unit (**FIG 1**). It consists of fibers originating from the subsheath of the extensor carpi ulnaris, the ulnocarpal ligaments, the dorsal and palmar radioulnar ligaments, and the triangular fibrocartilage proper.
- The TFCC provides a continuous gliding surface that spans the distal surfaces of the radius and ulna, allowing carpal movements and acting as a dynamic stabilizer of the forearm during pronation and supination.[13,19] In addition to its radioulnar function, the TFCC stabilizes the ulnar side of the carpus, aids in load transference from the ulnar carpus to the ulna, and cushions ulnocarpal forces.[17]
- The dorsal and volar distal radioulnar ligaments, which are often referred to as the *marginal ligaments*, help to stabilize the radioulnar joint through its extremes of motion.
  - Although controversy exists concerning the exact role of each marginal ligament, several authors have agreed that the ligaments act in concert to stabilize the DRUJ during pronosupination.
- The extensor retinaculum is a thick fibrous band of tissue that holds the extensor tendons against the distal radius and ulna to prevent bowstringing and displacement of the tendons (**FIG 2**). It is continuous with the palmar carpal ligament and shares connecting fibers with the flexor retinaculum just proximal to the pisiform. The extensor retinaculum attaches to the pisiform and triquetrum medially and to the lateral margin of the radius laterally. It is positioned from a proximal-radial to distal-ulnar direction.[16,20]

PATHOGENESIS

- Injuries to the TFCC can occur secondary to trauma, such as a fall on the outstretched hand, or from degenerative changes caused by repetitive loading, especially in patients with rheumatoid arthritis. Palmer has classified TFCC abnormalities by differentiating between traumatic and degenerative pathologies, with further specification within each group.[12]

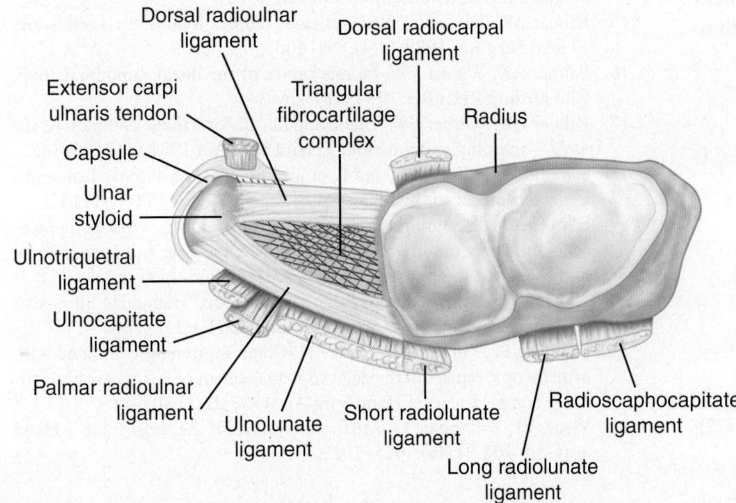

FIG 1 • The soft tissue structures encompassing the TFCC of the wrist stabilizing the radial-ulnar-carpal unit. The triangular fibrocartilage proper originates from the radius medially and attaches to the base of the ulnar styloid. Fibers originating from the subsheath of the extensor carpi ulnaris dorsally cross paths with fibers originating from the ulnocarpal ligaments volarly and blend with the triangular fibrocartilage proper.

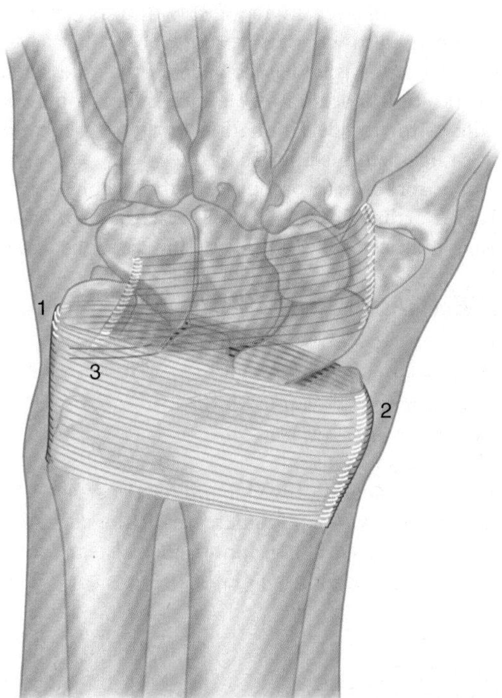

FIG 2 • Extensor retinaculum (*light blue*), flexor retinaculum (*shaded red*), and palmar carpal ligament (*dark blue*). The extensor retinaculum inserts in the pisiform and triquetrum bones (*1*) medially and connects with the lateral margin of the radius laterally (*2*), causing its orientation to be proximal-radial to distal-ulnar. The extensor and flexor retinaculum connects proximal to the pisiform (*3*). The extensor retinaculum is continuous with the palmar carpal ligament, which is superficial to and proximal to the flexor retinaculum.

- Dorsal subluxation of the ulnar head, with or without supination deformity of the radiocarpal complex and ulnocarpal instability, can occur with attenuation or tears of the dorsal radioulnar ligaments.[17,19] The Hui-Linscheid reconstruction repairs these defects through augmentation of ulnocarpal ligament function and an optional imbrication of the attenuated dorsal radioulnar ligament.[5,7]
- Ulnocarpal instability may also result from incompetence of the ulnocarpal ligaments, either secondary to acute trauma or from accumulative attrition.[1,8] The modified Herbert reconstruction addresses ulnocarpal instability by using ligamentotaxis to stabilize both the ulnocarpal and radioulnar aspects of the DRUJ.[4,14]

NATURAL HISTORY

- Ulnocarpal instability is a relatively common finding in the general population. Approximately, two-thirds of asymptomatic volunteers were found to have some form of ulnocarpal instability on physical examination.[11] Medical or surgical intervention is necessary if symptoms are present or are worsening.
- The unstable ulnocarpal joint uses the radiocarpal joint as a pivot. The abnormal rotation in this pathologic state leads to increased pain, weakness, and loss of function during wrist supination. In addition, an ulnar-sided supination deformity may be present.

PATIENT HISTORY AND PHYSICAL FINDINGS

- In both acute and chronic cases, the clinical presentation of the ulnocarpal instability consists of ulnar-sided wrist pain with or without clicking, especially with forearm pronation–supination activities, such as putting topspin on a tennis ball with a forehand shot.
- There may be demonstrable laxity during supination and weakness in passive or active pronation–supination movements. These symptoms may hinder range of motion and function of the wrist.
- On physical examination, patients often localize tenderness to the ulnar carpus on palpation.
  - The examiner should palpate the ulnar styloid.
  - The examiner should palpate between the ulnar styloid and triquetrum.
- Visual inspection of the ulnocarpal area is important, looking for swelling and alignment of the carpal area in relation to the ulna. Swelling may be the result of acute injury. Position of tissues indicates stability or instability.
- In the absence of concomitant pathology, provocative maneuvers such as Watson and Shuck tests are negative.
  - Watson test: Pain and movement of the scaphoid despite blocking its normal capacity to flex in radial deviation is an indication of scapholunate tear or laxity.
  - The Shuck test is performed to evaluate lunotriquetral instabilities.
  - A positive piano key test indicates a complete peripheral tear of the TFCC and/or dorsal radioulnar ligament tear.
  - Midcarpal instability can be ruled out with a negative wrist pivot shift test, as first described by Lichtman et al.[10]
- In patients with ulnocarpal instability, the wrist assumes an ulnar-sided supination deformity similar to that seen in rheumatoid arthritis.
- A key to diagnosing ulnocarpal instability is the supination test, which is a diagnostic maneuver developed by the first author. This examination is performed by stabilizing the affected DRUJ with a firm grasp while stressing the wrist in supination and volar translation.
  - When the wrist is loaded axially and returned through neutral in ulnar deviation, the patient's pain is reproduced. The wrist may also "clunk" back into reduction.
  - The contralateral wrist is also tested for comparison.

IMAGING AND OTHER DIAGNOSTIC STUDIES

- Standard posteroanterior and lateral radiographs have poor diagnostic value for ulnocarpal joint instabilities but can be used to rule out scapholunate interosseous ligament (SLIL) and lunotriquetral interosseous ligament (LTIL) tears. On a pure lateral view, if there is DRUJ instability, the ulna will be dorsally positioned relative to the radius instead of being seen superimposed on the radius.
- Computed tomography is useful for visualizing joint congruity and fractures as well as subluxation or dislocation of the DRUJ.
- Live fluoroscopy during the supination test allows the examiner to evaluate and visualize the presence and amount of ulnocarpal joint instability (**FIG 3**).
  - The changing appearance of the triquetrum, demonstrated by its decreased length while in a position of supination, indicates ulnocarpal instability.

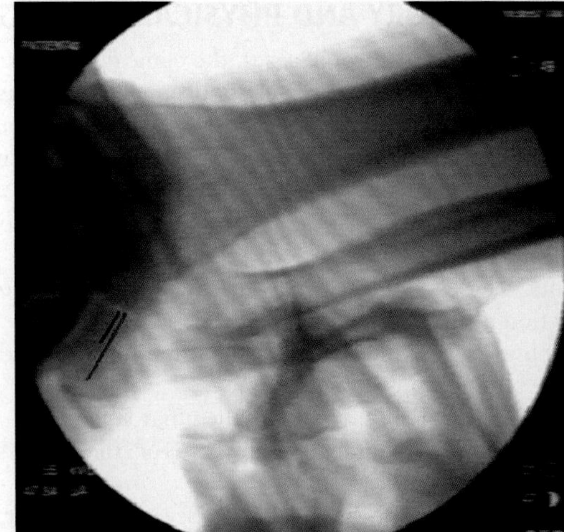

A

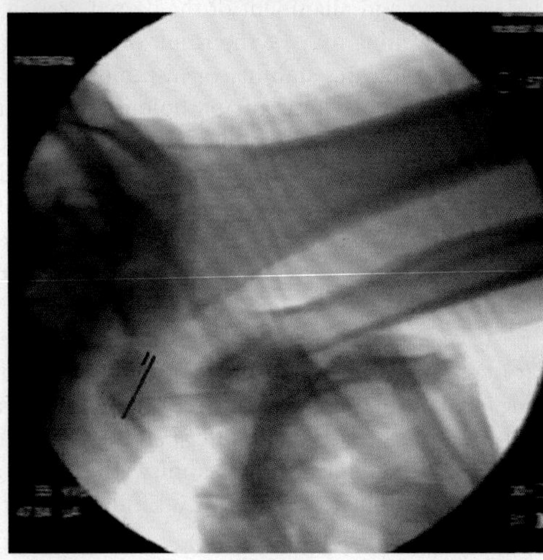

B

FIG 3 • The still photographs shown have been captured from a fluoroscopy video of a wrist with ulnocarpal instability during the supination test. **A.** Top of the examination cycle with the wrist in neutral position. **B.** Bottom of the examination cycle. In both images, the *black line* represents the distance between proximal edges of pisiform and triquetrum. The *red line* indicates the length of the triquetrum. The shorter length of the red and black lines in **B** compared with **A** demonstrates the ulnocarpal instability present during dynamic testing.

  - The pisiform's location in relation to the triquetrum may also indicate the type of ligamentous tear or laxity by either moving together with the triquetrum during the supination test or appearing to be stationary as the triquetrum is moving.[6]
- Triple-injection arthrography of the midcarpal row, radiocarpal joint, and DRUJ can be useful in showing SLIL or LTIL tears, TFCC tears, and ulnar-sided TFCC tears, respectively.
  - The findings must correlate with symptoms for accurate diagnosis.[9,18]
- Standard magnetic resonance (MR) imaging effectively demonstrates the normal anatomy of the TFCC as well as the intrinsic and extrinsic ligaments of the wrist.
  - Abnormalities of these structures can be detected with experience, but the radiographic literature has reported shortcomings of standard MR in diagnosing peripheral TFCC tears.
- MR arthrography, with injection of contrast into the DRUJ, has been shown as an adequate way of diagnosing peripheral TFCC tears, with a sensitivity of 85% and specificity of 76% when compared to wrist arthroscopy.[15]
- Wrist arthroscopy is widely considered the gold standard of diagnostic studies of the wrist joint. Arthroscopic visualization allows for the determination of the size, location, and extent of ligamentous injuries of the wrist.
  - Comparison of arthroscopy to arthrography by Cooney[2] revealed arthroscopy to be the superior method of diagnosing injuries of the TFCC and interosseous ligaments.

DIFFERENTIAL DIAGNOSIS

- Fracture
- DRUJ instability
- Extensor carpi ulnaris subluxation
- TFCC lesions
- Ulnar impaction syndrome
- Degenerative changes of DRUJ and ulnar carpus
- Carpal instability, scapholunate tear (dorsal intercalated segment instability [DISI]), lunotriquetral tear (volar intercalated segment instability [VISI])
- Tendinitis
- Chondromalacia
- Ligament injuries
- Ulnocarpal instability

NONOPERATIVE MANAGEMENT

- Conservative treatment includes the use of a removable soft leather splint that minimizes motion of the wrist, such as those originally designed for use by gymnasts.
  - If the patient wishes to return to athletic activities, he or she should proceed with cautious limitation while wearing a sports splint.
  - Although these splints allow for motion of the wrist and for the use of athletic tools, the patient must understand that he or she must reduce the intensity of activity to a level that the wrist will tolerate.
  - When activity levels are limited or more support is needed, such as while sleeping, a static splint is advised.
- Physical or occupational therapy, including training to increase range of motion and to strengthen the muscles spanning the ulnocarpal joint and DRUJ, may be beneficial.
- Nonsteroidal anti-inflammatories are also recommended before deciding on surgery, with an initial trial of 4 to 6 weeks.

SURGICAL MANAGEMENT

- The main indication for surgery is a painful ulnocarpal joint with diminished grip or pronosupination strength (or both) that does not respond to conservative treatment.
- Individuals with high demand for strong wrist function in weight-bearing supination (eg, golfers, tennis players, certain skilled labor professions) may be considered for surgery even without first receiving conservative treatment.

Preoperative Planning

- The surgeon should review all imaging studies to identify any concomitant pathology of the wrist joint.
- Arthroscopic examination of the wrist is generally undertaken immediately before ulnocarpal reconstruction to address any concomitant lesions or synovitis within the wrist.

- Diagnostic physical examination maneuvers are repeated while the patient is under anesthesia. These maneuvers include the piano key test and ulnocarpal supination test, as described earlier.

Positioning

- Using an arm board, the patient is positioned with the forearm in pronation and the elbow flexed at 45 degrees. The dorsal aspect of the wrist joint is prepared in a sterile manner.

Approach

- Modified Herbert reconstruction
  - Exposure of the dorsal surface of the wrist joint is the only surgical approach needed for the Herbert sling repair.
  - The Herbert sling procedure consists of the development of an ulnar-based flap of the extensor retinaculum, advanced at a 30- to 40-degree angle from distal-ulnar to proximal-radial by securing into the distal radial retinaculum attachments.
- This reduces the radioulnar joint and the carpus to the ulna with a single advancement of the extensor retinaculum (**FIG 4**).
- Hui-Linscheid reconstruction
  - A standard incision on the dorsal surface of the wrist is used to access the ulnocarpal articulation, the ulnar head, and the flexor carpi ulnaris (FCU).
  - A tendon graft is harvested from the FCU and passed through the tunnel in the ulnar head and looped back to its proximal insertion on the pisiform.

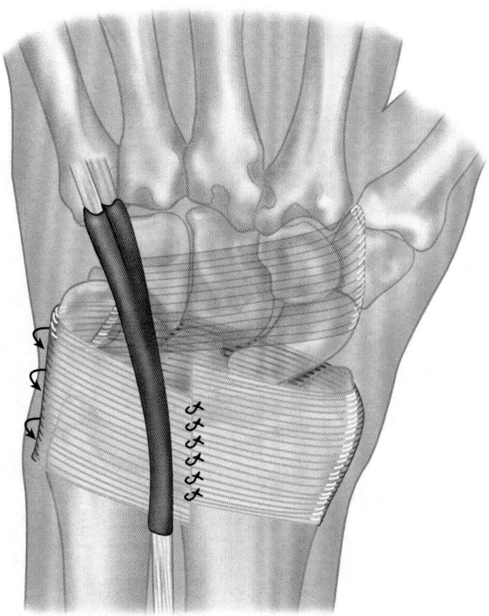

FIG 4 • The EDQ is relocated dorsally of the extensor retinaculum. This procedure uses ligament materials to create an effective sling, providing support to the DRUJ and ulnocarpal joint. The ulnar-based extensor retinaculum flap is advanced in a distal-ulnar to proximal-radial direction. *Arrows* illustrate the direction of the ligamentotaxis.

TECHNIQUES

Modified Herbert Reconstruction

- Create a longitudinal incision over the fifth extensor compartment at the level of the wrist (**TECH FIG 1A**).
- Incise the extensor retinaculum between the fourth and fifth compartments, taking care not to enter the fourth compartment (**TECH FIG 1B**).
- Raise an ulnarly based flap of the distal two-thirds of the retinaculum, and prepare the extensor digiti quinti (EDQ) for transposition dorsal to the retinaculum flap (**TECH FIG 1C**).
- Place the wrist in neutral and apply downward force on the distal ulna to reduce the DRUJ.

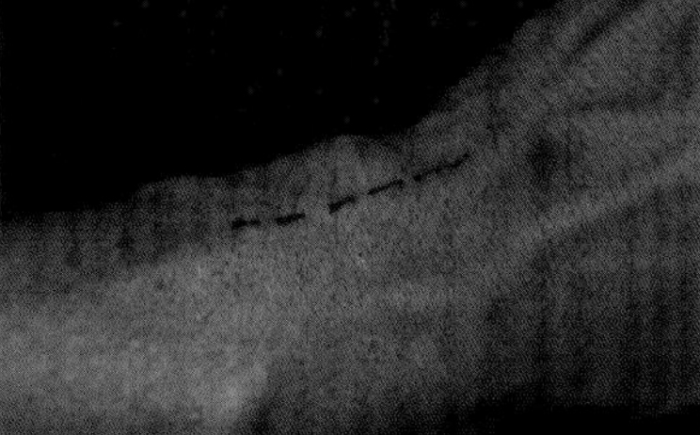

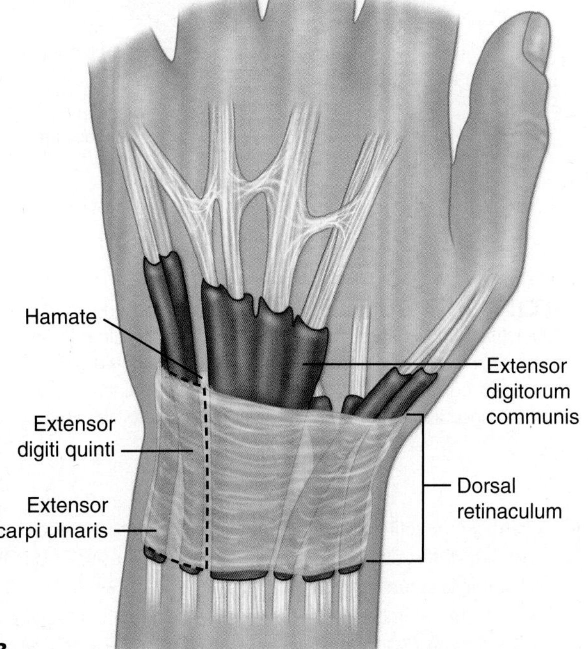

TECH FIG 1 • Modified Herbert reconstruction. **A.** A longitudinal incision over the fifth extensor compartment at the wrist is created. **B.** Plan the transection of the extensor retinaculum along the EDQ. Incise the extensor retinaculum, taking care not to enter the fourth compartment. *(continued)*

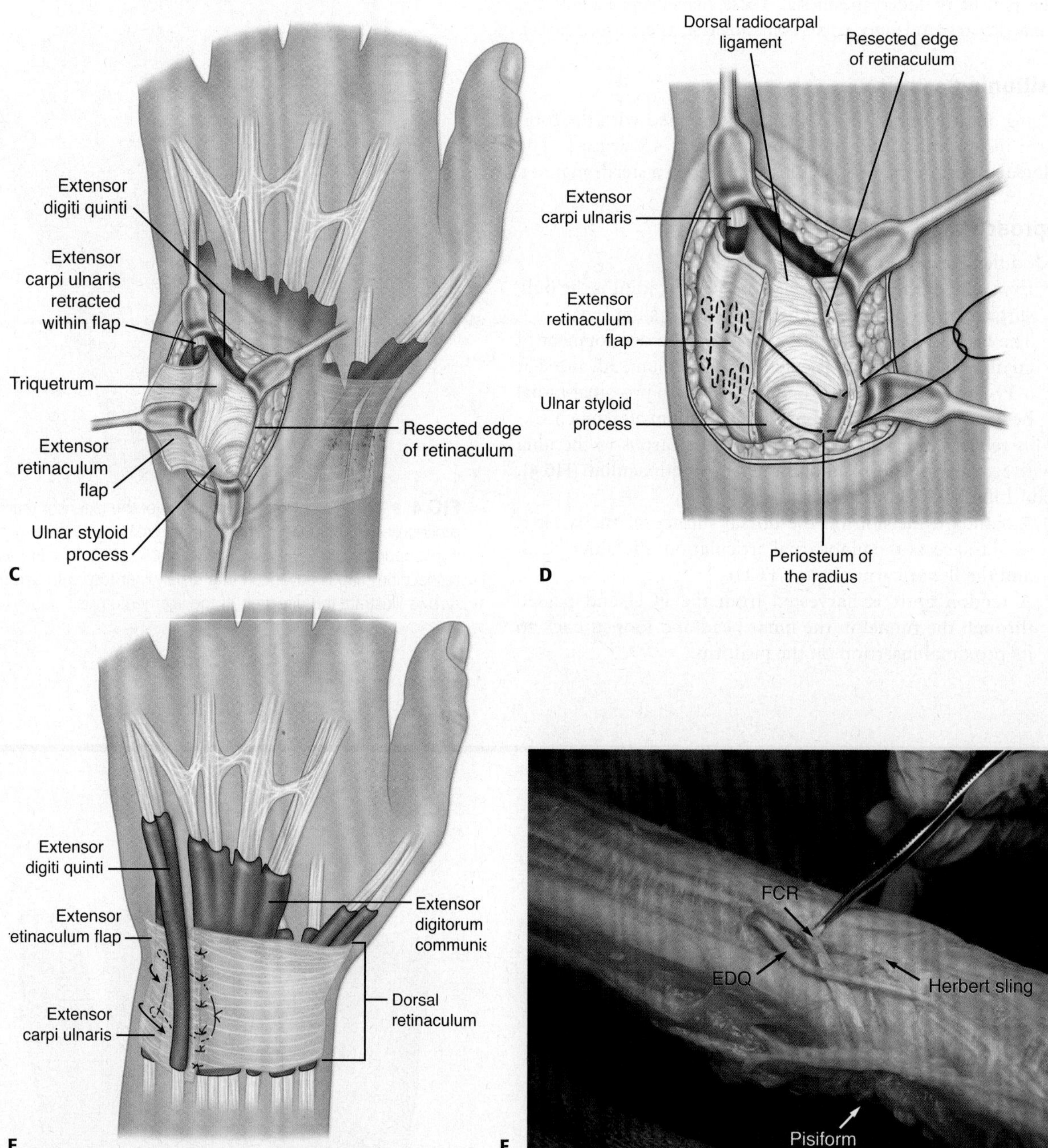

TECH FIG 1 • *(continued)* **C.** Raise an ulnar-based flap. Prepare the EDQ to be transposed dorsal to the extensor retinaculum. **D.** The retinacular flap is sutured to the periosteum of the ulnar border on the distal radius. **E.** Imbricate the extensor retinaculum obliquely in a distal-ulnar to proximal-radial direction. The EDQ should remain dorsally of the imbricated extensor retinaculum flap. **F.** One-half of the FCU is brought from the pisiform proximally along the ulnar border of the ulna along with the extensor retinaculum. It is attached at the same extensor insertion as for the retinacular flap used for the Herbert sling. *FCR*, flexor carpi radialis; *EDQ*, extensor digiti quinti.

- Translate the retinacular flap proximally and suture it to the periosteum of the ulnar border of the distal radius using 2-0 PDS absorbable sutures (**TECH FIG 1D**).
  - Carefully imbricate the extensor retinaculum in an oblique fashion (30 to 40 degrees) from distal-ulnar to proximal-radial (**TECH FIG 1E**).
  - The EDQ is relocated dorsally of the imbricated extensor retinaculum flap.
- A modified Hui-Linscheid procedure can be used to augment the Herbert sling if the ligamentous tissues are poor as seen in rheumatoid arthritis or highly elastic as seen in such syndromes as Ehlers-Danlos.
  - Take one-half of the FCU and bring it from the pisiform proximally along the ulnar border of the wrist. Attach this additional tissue at the same point as is detailed earlier for the retinacular flap (**TECH FIG 1F**).

Hui-Linscheid Reconstruction

Incision and Dissection

- Start the incision at the level of the fifth carpometacarpal joint. Curve the incision over the ulnocarpal joint to reach the far ulnar border and continue to the mid-dorsal forearm for exposure of the dorsal carpal ligament (**TECH FIG 2A**).
- Locate and protect the dorsal sensory branch of the ulnar nerve (**TECH FIG 2B,C**).
- Incise the extensor retinaculum over the sixth extensor compartment, taking care to protect the underlying extensor carpi ulnaris tendon and subsheath.
- Retract the extensor retinaculum medially to expose the capsule over the ulnocarpal joint and the subluxated ulnar head, creating an ulnarly based flap of retinaculum (**TECH FIG 2D**).
- Make a longitudinal incision in the capsule to expose the DRUJ while preserving the dorsal radioulnar ligament (**TECH FIG 2E**).
- Drill a 0.0625-inch Kirschner wire obliquely through the ulnar head beginning near the base of ulnar styloid to the ulnar fovea proximally (**TECH FIG 2F**).
- Placement of the Kirschner wire is confirmed visually, and sequential hand awls are used to create a 4- to 5-mm bone tunnel.

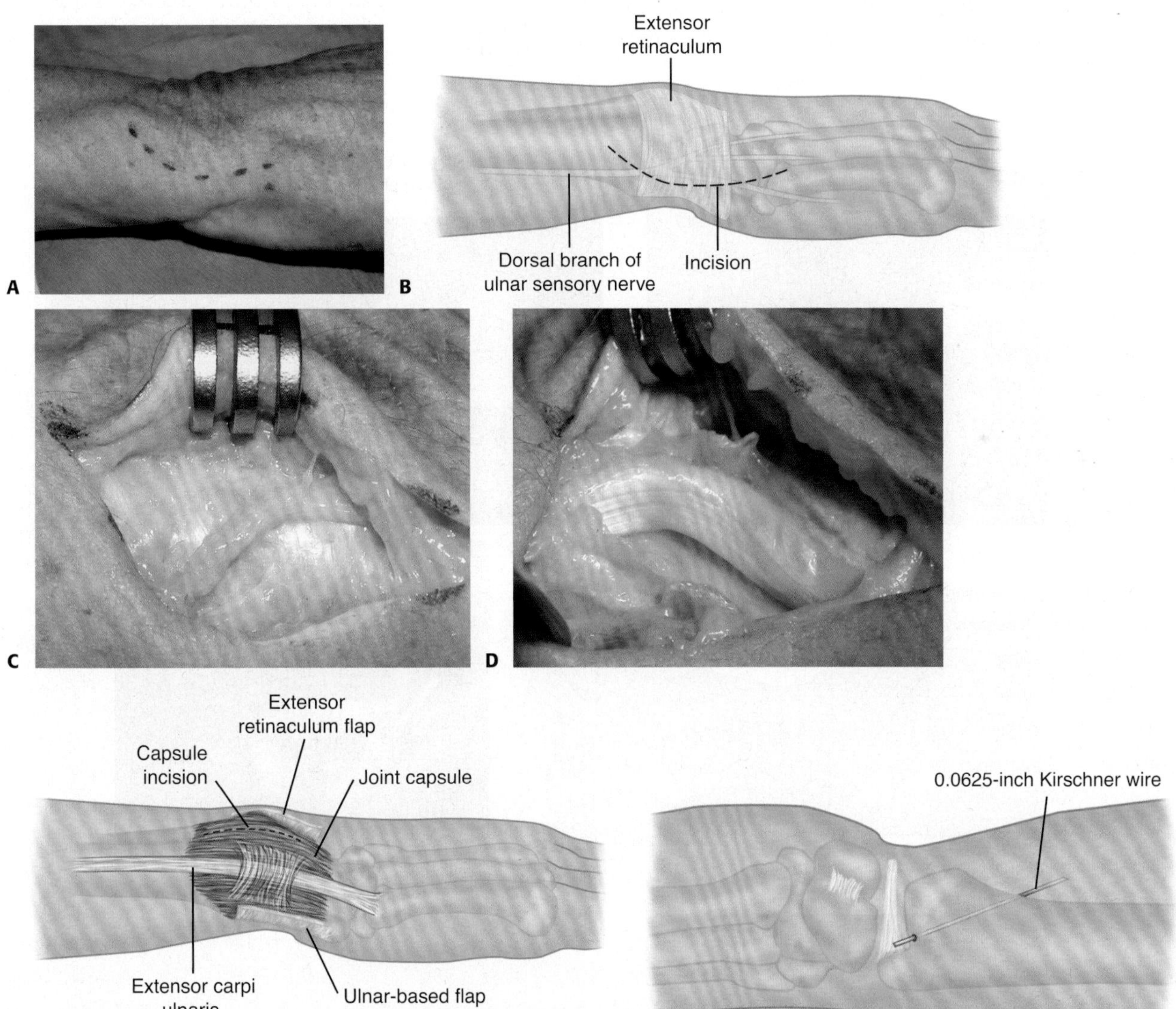

TECH FIG 2 • Hui-Linscheid reconstruction. **A.** Make a slightly curving incision over the ulnocarpal joint to reach the lateral ulnar border and continue it to the mid-dorsal forearm for exposure of the dorsal carpal ligament. **B.** Take care not to injure the dorsal branch of the ulnar sensory branch during the incision and throughout the procedure. **C.** The ulnar nerve is located volar to the incision. The extensor retinaculum is incised at the fifth dorsal compartment. Protect the underlying extensor carpi ulnaris tendon and subsheath. **D.** Retract the extensor retinaculum medially to expose the capsule over the ulnocarpal joint and the subluxated ulnar head, creating an ulnar-based flap. **E.** Incise the capsule to expose the DRUJ while preserving the dorsal radioulnar ligament and taking care not to injure the extensor carpi ulnaris. **F.** Drill a 0.0625-inch Kirschner wire through the ulnar head in a distal to proximal direction. The guidewire should be inserted obliquely starting from the base of ulnar styloid and aiming toward the synovial reflection proximally.

Tendon Graft Harvest

- Locate the FCU in the incision distally and trace it to the musculotendinous junction. This will allow about 10 cm of tendon graft for harvest (**TECH FIG 3A**).
  - If needed, a separate longitudinal incision on the palmar area of the wrist can be used.
  - Alternatively, a free tendon graft from the palmaris longus or other donor area may be used if the FCU tendon is inadequate.
- Split the FCU tendon longitudinally and cut the graft proximally at the musculotendinous junction. Leave the distal portion still attached at its insertion onto the pisiform (**TECH FIG 3B**).
- Perforate the pisotriquetral capsule in a dorsal to volar direction (**TECH FIG 3C**).
- The FCU tendon is passed intracapsularly using a tendon passer or by placing a Kessler suture into the tendon edge and using the suture to pull the tendon through the capsular perforation.
  - Ensure that the graft does not place any tension on the ulnar artery or nerve (**TECH FIG 3D,E**).
- The FCU tendon graft is passed through the TFCC if it is perforated or through an enlargement of the prestyloid recess of the TFCC and through the drill hole in the distal end of the ulna.

Completion of the Reconstruction

- The carpal supination and the ulnar head dorsal subluxation is reduced by pulling the FCU tendon graft taut from its pisiform insertion.
- Hold this reduction by placing the forearm in supination and transfix the distal ulna to the distal radius with two parallel 0.062-inch Kirschner wires.
- Close the DRUJ capsule incision using a 3-0 nonabsorbable suture.

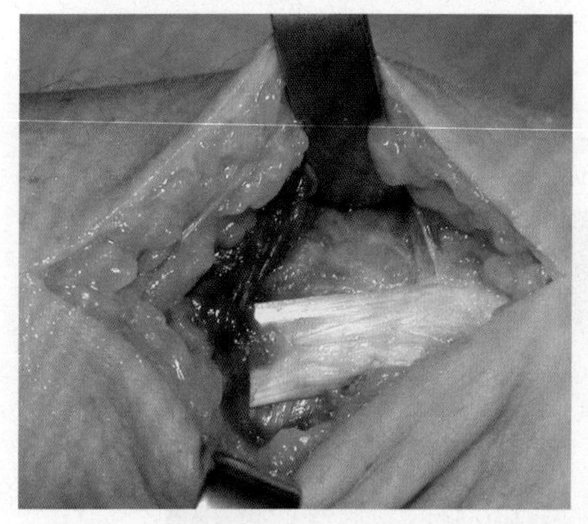

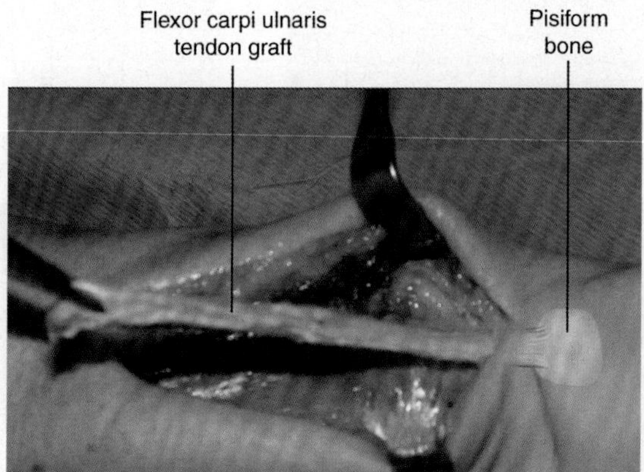

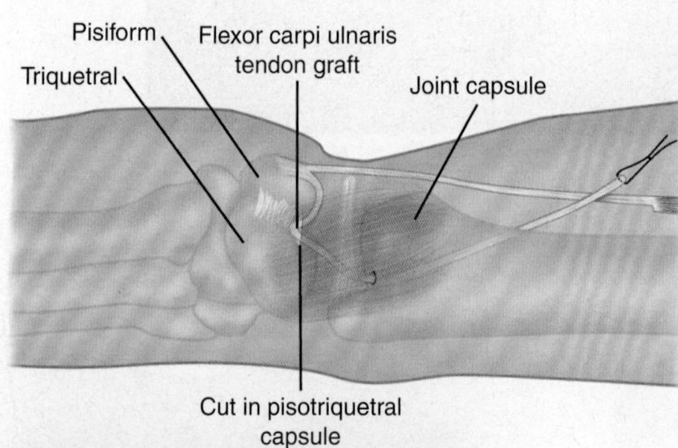

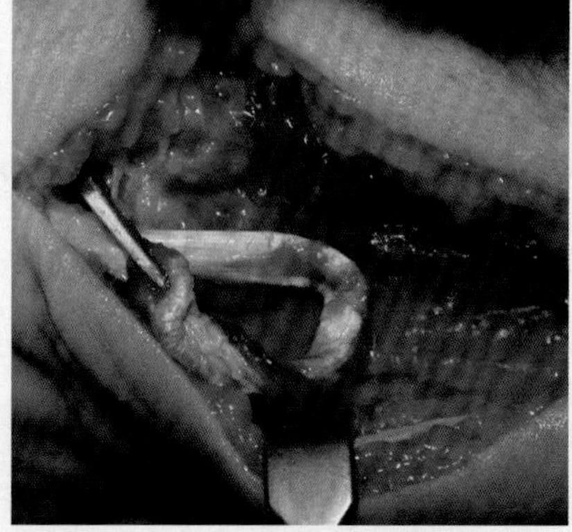

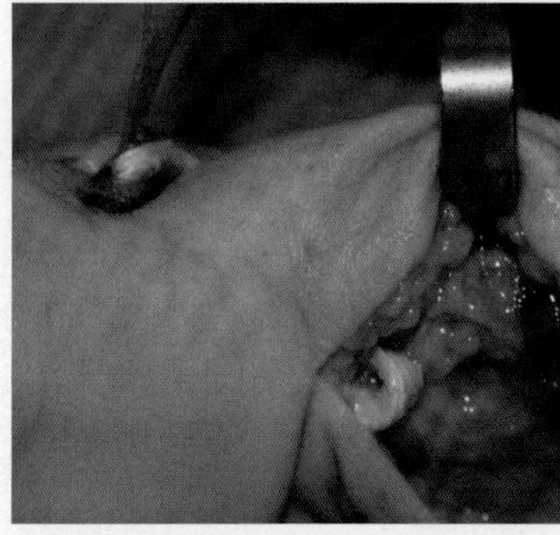

TECH FIG 3 • Hui-Linscheid tendon harvest. **A.** The FCU is located distally and traced into the muscle belly to obtain about 10 cm of tendon graft. **B.** Cut the FCU graft proximally, leaving the distal portion attached distally in its insertion onto the pisiform. **C.** Pass the FCU tendon intracapsularly. **D,E.** Ensure that the graft is not placing any tension on the ulnar artery or nerve.

- The FCU tendon graft is pulled taut through the drill hole and then secured to the periosteum adjacent to the ulna bone tunnel using a 2-0 nonabsorbable suture.
- The FCU graft is doubled back superficially to the radioulnar capsule (**TECH FIG 4A**) and sewn to its pisotriquetral insertion (**TECH FIG 4B**).
- If the dorsal radioulnar ligament is found to be attenuated, imbrication of the ligament is performed.
- The extensor retinaculum is imbricated using a nonabsorbable 3-0 suture.

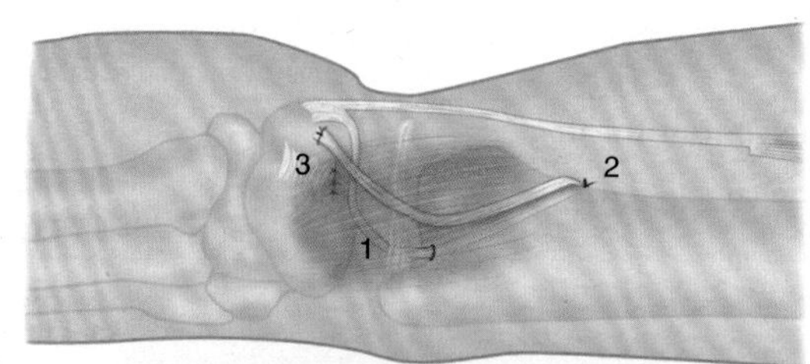

A

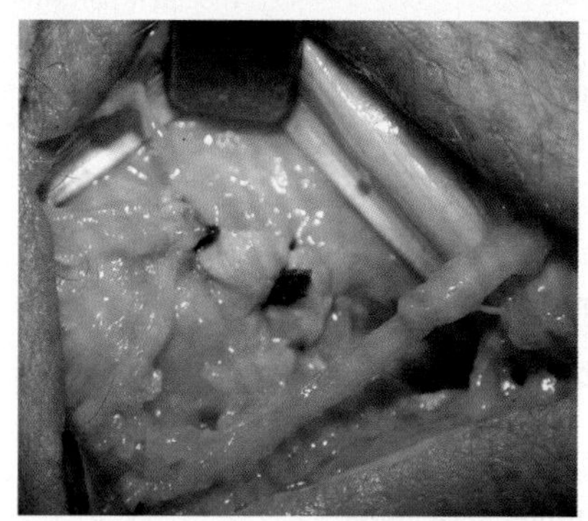

B

TECH FIG 4 • Hui-Linscheid completion. **A.** The FCU tendon graft is passed through the TFCC if it is perforated or through an enlargement of the prestyloid recess of the TFCC (*1*) and through the drill hole in the distal end of the ulna (*2*). The FCU tendon graft is doubled backed superficially to the radioulnar capsule and approached to its proximal insertion in pisiform (*3*). **B.** The FCU graft is pulled through the tunnel in the ulna and is sewn to its pisotriquetral insertion.

PEARLS AND PITFALLS

Modified Herbert reconstruction	
Orientation of the capsulorrhaphy	■ Imbricate the extensor retinaculum in an oblique fashion (distal-ulnar to proximal-radial) to maximize the ulnocarpal ligamentotaxis effect of the repair. This will minimize the risk of postoperative supination deformity. If imbrication occurs at 90 degrees perpendicular to the DRUJ, only the DRUJ will be stabilized, not the ulnocarpal instability.
Augmenting of capsulorrhaphy	■ If the extensor retinaculum is insufficient by itself, a modified Hui-Linscheid reconstruction can be added.
Placement of sutures in extensor retinaculum	■ Avoid injury to surrounding tissues or nerve structures (the dorsal branch of the ulnar nerve and the posterior interosseous nerve, terminal branch) when placing sutures in the extensor retinaculum (**FIG 5**). This will minimize the risk of postoperative wrist pain and dysesthesia.

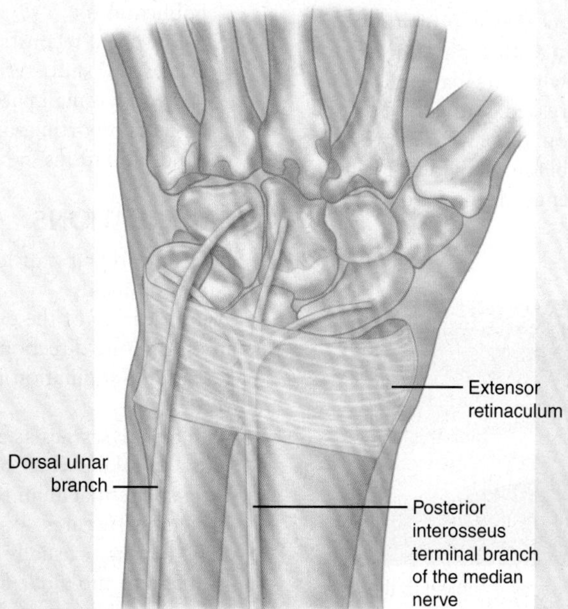

FIG 5 • Note the location of the dorsal branch of the ulnar nerve and the posterior interosseous nerve, terminal branch.

EDQ tendinitis	▪ The tendinitis usually resolves within 6 months.
Postoperative therapy	▪ Advise the patient to avoid aggressive strengthening too soon after surgery, which may lead to loosening of the extensor retinaculum imbrication and failure of the Herbert sling repair.
Hui-Linscheid reconstruction	
Preservation of the nerve	▪ The risk of damaging the dorsal branch of the ulnar nerve can be minimized by being aware of the dorsal ulnar nerve's location during surgical incision, manipulation, and drilling.
Postoperative ulnar fracture	▪ In the postoperative period, the FCU tendon graft may migrate within the ulnar tunnel, which may predispose the distal ulna to fracture. This risk can be minimized by sewing the FCU tendon graft to the ulnar periosteum and local soft tissues around the drill hole, decreasing the chance of the tendon gliding within the tunnel.
Nerve adherence	▪ The ulnar nerve may adhere to surrounding scar tissue at the closing site of soft tissue.

POSTOPERATIVE CARE

Modified Herbert Reconstruction

- Six weeks in a thumb spica Muenster cast with the forearm and wrist both positioned in neutral, followed by 6 weeks in a removable thumb spica splint

Hui-Linscheid Reconstruction

- Long-arm plaster cast for 6 weeks with the forearm and wrist both positioned in neutral. The cast and Kirschner wire are removed after 6 weeks.
- After 6 weeks, an ulnar gutter splint with "boost" padding is applied to the ulnar head dorsally and pisiform palmarly to support the wrist between mobilization exercises (**FIG 6**).

General Suggestions

- Gentle active rotatory motion during temporary splint removal is introduced at 6 weeks postoperatively at the patient's discretion. Passive motion with a physical or occupational therapist is not necessary at this point.
- No heavy lifting or aggressive motion is permitted until 3 months postoperatively.
- Vigorous strengthening exercises to regain pronation are begun 3 months after the operation with a physical or occupational therapist at a pace with which the patient is comfortable, with exercise intensity increased gradually.
- A warm, moist wrap can be used around the wrist to provide additional stretching of the wrist before activities. Ice and nonsteroidal anti-inflammatory agents can be used to provide relief after each session.

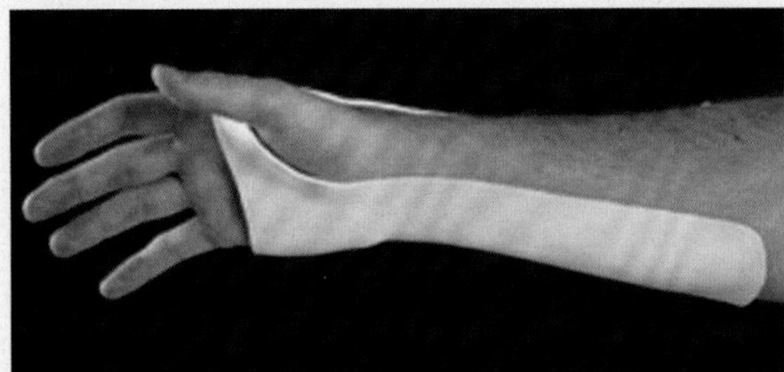

FIG 6 • An ulnar gutter splint with boost padding applied to the ulnar head dorsally and pisiform palmarly can be used in the postoperative period to support the wrist between mobilization exercises.

- Examples of exercises:
  - Pronation and supination: Stretching can be achieved by holding a hammer or frying pan as a weight during the motions.
  - Wrist flexion and extension: Stretching can be achieved using bucket exercises. The patient places his or her arm on a table with the wrist hanging off the edge while holding an empty bucket. The bucket is filled with water until the point of discomfort. The patient holds the bucket for 2 to 3 minutes and repeats the exercise twice daily in flexion and extension.
- If the patient's preoperative activities included sports such as golf and tennis, these activities should be gradually incorporated into the strengthening program.
- A Silastic sheet can be applied to aid scar remodeling. Scar massage may be started after the first 6 weeks.

OUTCOMES

- Modified Herbert reconstruction
  - A recent long-term follow-up study, ranging from 1 month to 13 years, of 39 wrists showed that 85% of the wrists remained stable at the ulnocarpal joint (in preparation for publication).
- Hui-Linscheid reconstruction
  - Successful short-term clinical outcomes have been reported in a small patient series by Hui and Linscheid, with patients reporting satisfactory and excellent outcomes.[7]
  - Mild limitations in pronation may be expected.

COMPLICATIONS

- The sling repair can loosen if aggressive strengthening occurs too quickly.
- If imbrication of the extensor retinaculum is not performed in an oblique direction, the ulnocarpal effect of the sling is lost and a supination deformity of the wrist may occur or recur.
- Pain and dysesthesias at dorsal branch of ulnar nerve: Care must be taken when placing sutures for imbrication of the extensor retinaculum to avoid injury to surrounding tissues or nerve structures.
- EDQ tendinitis usually resolves 6 months after the operation.
- Damage to the ulnar nerve during the surgical procedure is concerning because of its anatomic location. The nerve is immediately exposed after the opening incision and is vulner-

able during drilling of the ulnar tunnel. Dorsal ulnar nerve damage ranging from irritation to neuroma may occur.
  - Additionally, the nerve will be passing directly over an area of soft tissue closure and may be affected by the surrounding scar tissue.
  - A protective covering (such as those used for recurrent nerve entrapments) to protect the dorsal ulnar nerve may minimize damage to the nerve.
- Other potential complications may occur as a result of the Kirschner wire, such as migration, infection, and nerve injury.

REFERENCES

1. Adams BD. Partial excision of the triangular fibrocartilage complex articular disk: a biomechanical study. J Hand Surg Am 1993;18(2):334–340.
2. Cooney WP. Evaluation of wrist pain by arthrogram, arthroscopy, and arthrotomy. J Hand Surg Am 1993;18(5):815–822.
3. Dy CJ, Ouellette EA, Makowski AL, et al. Peripheral triangular fibrocartilage complex tears cause ulnocarpal instability: a biomechanical pilot study. Clin Orthop Relat Res 2012;470:2771–2775.
4. Dy CJ, Ouellette EA, Malik A, et al. Mechanical testing of distal radioulnar instability repair: ligament reconstruction vs. capsulorrhaphy. Proceedings of the Annual Meeting of the American Academy of Orthopaedic Surgeons, San Diego, CA, February 16, 2007.
5. Glowacki KA, Shin AY. Stabilization of the unstable distal ulna: the Linscheid-Hui procedure. Tech Hand Up Extrem Surg 1993;4:229–236.
6. Harrison RJ, Ouellette EA, Latta LL, et al. The biomechanics of diagnosing and treating peripheral TFCC instability. Proceedings of the Annual Meeting of the American Society for Surgery of the Hand, New York, NY, September 9, 2004.
7. Hui FC, Linscheid RL. Ulnotriquetral augmentation tenodesis: a reconstructive procedure for dorsal subluxation of the distal radioulnar joint. J Hand Surg Am 1982;7(3):230–236.
8. Kapindji AI, Martin-Bouyer Y, Verdeille S. Three-dimensional CT study of the carpus under pronation-supination constraints [in French]. Ann Chir Main Memb Super 1991;10:36–47.
9. Levinsohn EM, Rosen ID, Palmer AK. Wrist arthrography: value of the three-compartment injection method. Radiology 1991;179: 231–239.
10. Lichtman DM, Bruckner JD, Culp RW, et al. Palmar midcarpal instability: results of surgical reconstruction. J Hand Surg Am 1993;18(2):307–315.
11. Ouellette EA. Distal radioulnar joint and ulnocarpal instability. Proceedings of the International Wrist Investigators Workshop, American Society for Surgery of the Hand, Washington, DC, September 6, 2006.
12. Palmer AK. Triangular fibrocartilage complex lesions: a classification. J Hand Surg Am 1989;14(4):594–606.
13. Palmer AK, Werner FW. The triangular fibrocartilage complex of the wrist—anatomy and function. J Hand Surg Am 1981;6(2):153–162.
14. Ritt MJ, Stuart PR, Berglund LJ, et al. Rotational stability of the carpus relative to the forearm. J Hand Surg Am 2000;20(2):305–311.
15. Rüegger C, Schmid MR, Pfirrmann CW, et al. Peripheral tear of the triangular fibrocartilage: depiction with MR arthrography of the distal radioulnar joint. AJR Am J Roentgenol 2007;188:187–192.
16. Schmidt HM, Lahl J. Studies on the tendinous compartments of the extensor muscles on the back of the human hand and their tendon sheaths [in German]. Gegenbaurs Morphol Jahrb 1988;134: 155–173.
17. Schuind F, An KN, Berglund L, et al. The distal radioulnar ligaments: a biomechanical study. J Hand Surg Am 1991;16(6):1106–1114.
18. Weiss AP, Akelman E, Lambiase R. Comparison of the findings of triple-injection cinearthrography of the wrist with those of arthroscopy. J Bone Joint Surg Am 1996;78(3):348–356.
19. Wiesner L, Rumehart C, Pham E, et al. Experimentally induced ulno-carpal instability. A study on 13 cadaver wrists. J Hand Surg Br 1996;21(1):24–29.
20. Zancolli EA, Cozzi EP. Atlas of Surgical Anatomy of the Hand. New York: Churchill Livingstone, 1992.

65
CHAPTER

Distal Radioulnar Ligament Reconstruction

Brian D. Adams

DEFINITION

- Distal radioulnar joint (DRUJ) instability may be classified as acute or chronic, unidirectional (volar or dorsal) or bidirectional, and isolated or in association with other injuries.
- There is no consensus regarding the definition of clinically significant instability, although various radiographic criteria have been used. In general, the key physical finding is the presence of increased anteroposterior translation of the DRUJ with passive manipulation when compared with the normal side.
- Although the radius actually rotates around the stable ulna, by convention, DRUJ dislocation or instability is described by the position of the ulnar head relative to the distal radius.

ANATOMY

- The DRUJ consists of the articulation between the ulnar head and the sigmoid notch of the distal radius and the associated supporting soft tissues.
- The DRUJ is not a congruent joint, with the radius of curvature of the sigmoid notch being on average 50% greater than the ulnar head. Although the sigmoid notch is shallow, its dorsal and volar rims are typically augmented by fibrocartilaginous extensions that provide important contributions to joint stability (**FIG 1A**).[12] DRUJ surface contact is maximized between neutral and 30 degrees of supination.[3]
- The soft tissue structures that contribute to DRUJ stability are the pronator quadratus, extensor carpi ulnaris (ECU) and its sheath, interosseous membrane, DRUJ capsule, and several components of the triangular fibrocartilage complex (TFCC). Multiple structures must typically be injured to result in joint instability.[5]
- The palmar and dorsal radioulnar ligaments are the prime components of the TFCC that stabilize the DRUJ.[10] They are thickenings at the combined junctures of the triangular fibrocartilage articular disc, DRUJ capsule, and ulnocarpal capsule.
- As each radioulnar ligament passes ulnarly, it divides in the coronal plane into two limbs. The deep or proximal limbs of the radioulnar ligaments attach at the fovea and the superficial or distal limbs attach to the base and midportion of the ulnar styloid (**FIG 1B**).
- The total pronation–supination arc in a normal individual varies between 150 and 180 degrees. Normal pronation and supination involves a combination of rotation and dorsal palmar translation of the sigmoid notch on the ulnar head.

PATHOGENESIS

- The most common cause of DRUJ injury is a fracture of the distal radius.
- Distal radius angulation greater than 20 to 30 degrees creates DRUJ incongruity, distorts the TFCC, and alters joint kinematics.[1,4] More than 5 to 7 mm of radius shortening results in rupture of at least one of the distal radioulnar ligaments.[1]

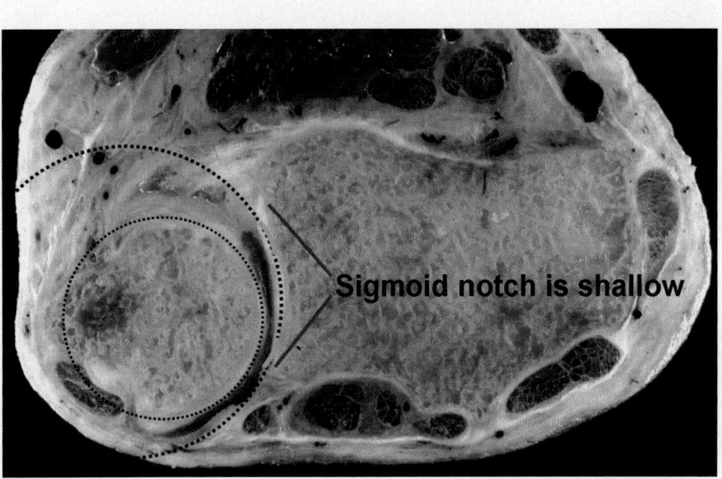

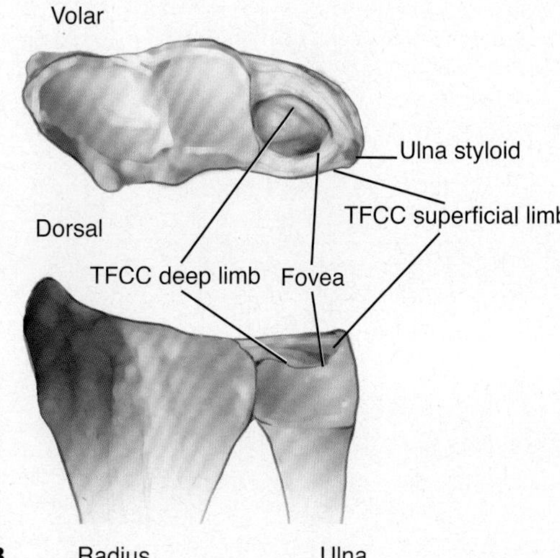

FIG 1 • **A.** DRUJ cross-section. The radius of curvature of the sigmoid notch is much greater than the radius of curvature of the ulnar head. **B.** DRUJ ligaments. (The disc component of the TFCC has been removed to show the deep limbs of the radioulnar ligaments.) The volar and dorsal radioulnar ligaments insert at the fovea and at the base of the ulnar styloid.

- Fractures of the tip of the ulnar styloid are not typically associated with DRUJ instability. Fractures of the base of the ulnar styloid can result in disruption of the radioulnar ligaments, causing DRUJ instability.[8]
- Isolated dorsal DRUJ dislocations (not associated with a fracture) are caused by forceful hyperpronation and wrist extension, such as with a fall on an outstretched hand or the sudden torque of a rotating power tool.
- Isolated volar DRUJ dislocations occur with an injury to the supinated forearm, or forceful torque, or a direct blow to the ulnar aspect of the forearm.

NATURAL HISTORY

- Delayed diagnosis and treatment of acute DRUJ injuries results in worse outcomes.[7]
- Chronic instability rarely improves spontaneously.
- Although there is no proven association between DRUJ instability and the development of symptomatic arthritis, some degeneration should be expected in recurrent dislocations.

PATIENT HISTORY AND PHYSICAL FINDINGS

- Patients may report falling on an outstretched hand or a forced rotation of the wrist followed by ulnar-sided wrist pain and swelling.
- Patients with chronic instability may report a clunk at the wrist during forearm rotation.
- Pain and weakness is exacerbated by activities requiring forceful rotation while gripping, such as turning a screwdriver.
- Increased passive volar–dorsal translation of the ulna relative to the radius is evidence of DRUJ instability.
- When treating an acute distal radius fracture with evidence of DRUJ disruption, the fracture should be reduced and stabilized first, followed by assessment of the DRUJ in comparison with the uninjured wrist.
  - Distal radius fracture management alone usually provides adequate treatment for the DRUJ.
- In the absence of DRUJ arthritis, patients with DRUJ instability typically have full or nearly full wrist range of motion, including flexion, extension, pronation, and supination.
- A thorough patient examination should include the following tests:
  - Passive translation ("piano key" sign). Perform the test and compare results to the unaffected side in pronation, neutral, and supination. A positive test indicates DRUJ instability.[2]
  - Modified press test. Increased depression ("dimple" sign) of ulnar head on the affected side indicates instability.[2] Pain without increased depression may indicate a partial TFCC tear.[6]
  - Passive forearm rotation. A painful clunk indicates joint dislocation and gross DRUJ instability. This should not be confused with more subtle ECU subluxation.

IMAGING AND OTHER DIAGNOSTIC STUDIES

- A zero-rotation posteroanterior view is obtained by abducting the humerus 90 degrees, flexing the elbow 90 degrees, and placing the forearm on a flat surface. Signs of DRUJ instability on this view include the following:
  - Displaced fracture at the base of the ulnar styloid
  - Fleck fracture from the fovea of the ulnar head
  - Widening of the DRUJ
  - Greater than 5 mm of acquired positive ulnar variance compared to the opposite wrist
- A true lateral radiograph is performed with the arm at the patient's side and the elbow flexed 90 degrees. Obtaining a true lateral radiograph is important to avoid inaccurate assessment of DRUJ alignment.
  - Mino et al[9] showed that only 10 degrees of rotation from neutral resulted in an inability to correctly diagnose DRUJ instability on the lateral radiograph.
  - On a true lateral wrist radiograph, the lunate, proximal pole of the scaphoid, and triquetrum should overlap completely and the volar surface of the pisiform should project between the volar surfaces of the capitate and the scaphoid tuberosity.
- Computed tomography (CT) must be performed on both wrists, with axial images obtained with the forearms in identical rotations preferably in neutral and maximum allowed pronation and supination to allow comparison between the normal and symptomatic joints (**FIG 2**).
- Magnetic resonance imaging (MRI) (with or without intra-articular dye) may be used to detect TFCC tears, although the sensitivity and specificity depends on the technique. MRI can be used instead of CT to assess the shape of the sigmoid notch and joint stability if proper settings are used.

DIFFERENTIAL DIAGNOSIS

- ECU tendonitis or subluxation
- Ulnar impaction syndrome
- DRUJ arthritis
- Pisotriquetral arthritis

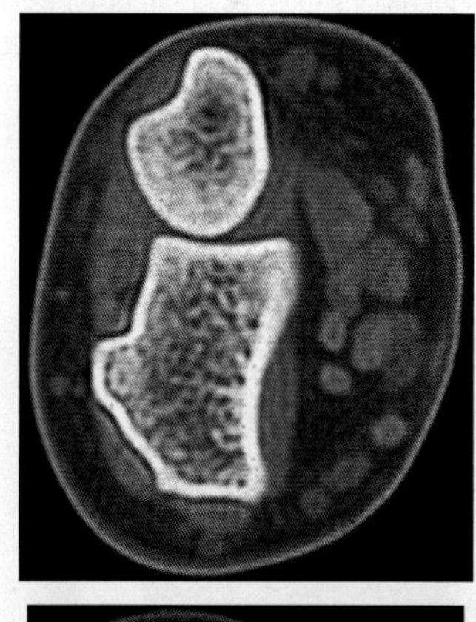

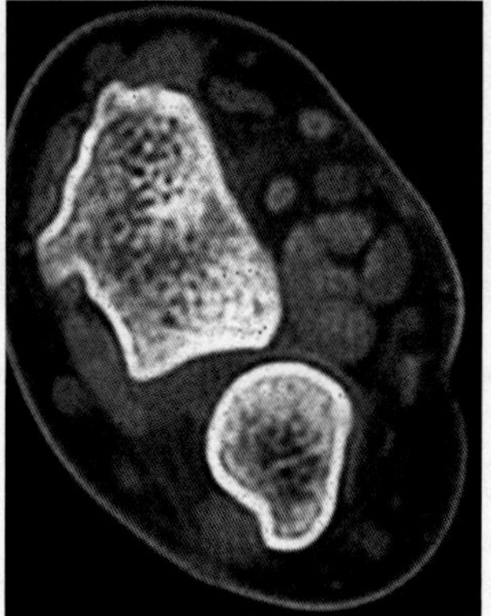

FIG 2 • CT of DRUJ. **A.** Well-reduced asymptomatic DRUJ. **B.** Subluxated DRUJ on the symptomatic side. (**A,B:** Dorsal is left and volar is right.)

- Lunotriquetral ligament tear
- TFCC disc tear

NONOPERATIVE MANAGEMENT

- Patients with mild chronic instability may benefit from a course of nonsteroidal anti-inflammatories, a splint that limits forearm rotation, and a forearm strengthening program.
- Patients with generalized ligamentous laxity and bilateral DRUJ instability have less predictable results following operative reconstruction. In such patients, prolonged conservative management should be used before considering surgery.

SURGICAL MANAGEMENT

- Distal radioulnar ligament reconstruction is indicated for cases of chronic DRUJ instability, where the TFCC is inadequate for primary repair due to chronicity or severity.
- The goal of ligament reconstruction is to restore DRUJ stability and provide a full, painless arc of forearm motion.
- The technique described is designed to restore stability by near-anatomic reconstruction of the dorsal and volar radioulnar ligaments.
- If present, osseous malalignment or sigmoid notch deficiency must be addressed at the time of ligament reconstruction to obtain a good durable result.[12]

Preoperative Planning

- The surgeon should review imaging studies for evidence of osseous deformity or degeneration of the DRUJ articular surfaces. Soft tissue reconstruction in the presence of substantial bony deformity or arthritis will yield poor results.
- Intra-articular radioulnar ligament reconstruction requires a competent sigmoid notch for success. A sigmoid notch that is developmentally flat or that has posttraumatic deficiency of either rim may require a sigmoid notch osteoplasty at the time of ligament reconstruction.
- The surgeon should plan the source of tendon graft. Although the palmaris longus (PL) tendon is typically preferred, it can be too short. Alternative graft sources include the plantaris, extensor digitorum longus, or a strip of the flexor carpi ulnaris tendon.
  - The PL tendon can be identified by having the patient flex the wrist while holding the tips of the thumb and small finger together (see **TECH FIG 1A**).

Positioning

- The patient is positioned supine with the affected limb resting on a hand table. Additional positioning may be necessary to allow access to graft harvest sites.
- A padded tourniquet is placed on the upper arm.

TECHNIQUES

Palmaris Tendon Graft Harvest

- The PL tendon is identified by palpation. It is one of the most superficial structures at the distal wrist crease and lies just ulnar to the flexor carpi radialis tendon (**TECH FIG 1A**).
- A single 1-cm transverse incision is made at the proximal volar wrist crease overlying the PL tendon (**TECH FIG 1B**).
  - A hook is used to pull tension on the tendon to confirm its identity.
- The tendon is transected at the incision site.
- A small tendon stripper is passed distal to proximal along the PL tendon in the forearm to complete the harvest.
- Alternatively, a strip of the flexor carpi ulnaris tendon can be harvested using a tendon stripper through the same volar incision used for graft passage; avoid harvesting too thick of a graft. Additional proximal incisions are usually necessary to complete the harvest.

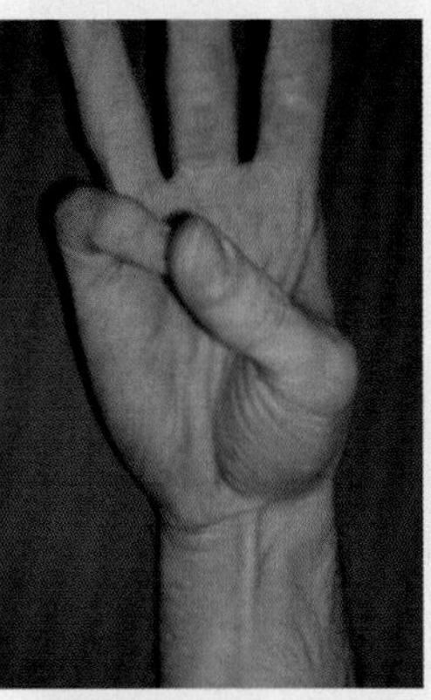
A

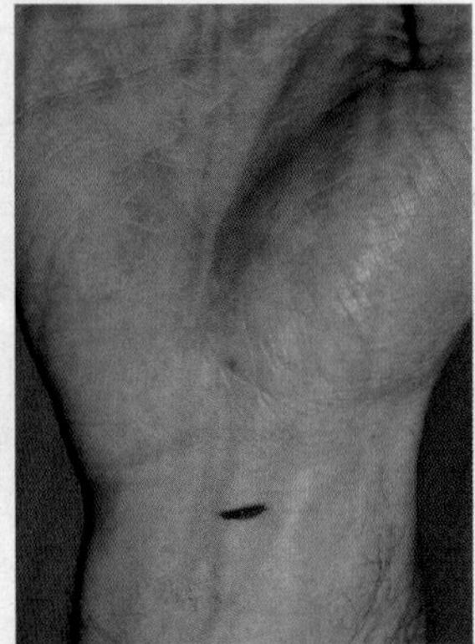
B

TECH FIG 1 • Graft harvest. **A.** The palmaris tendon can be brought into relief by having the patient touch the thumb and small fingers while flexing the wrist slightly. **B.** A small transverse incision is made at the proximal wrist crease.

Dorsal Approach

- A 5-cm skin incision is made between the fifth and sixth extensor compartments overlying the DRUJ (**TECH FIG 2A**).
- The fifth compartment is opened and the extensor digiti minimi is retracted.
- An L-shaped capsulotomy is made in the DRUJ capsule with one limb in the floor of the fifth compartment and the other just proximal and parallel to the TFCC (**TECH FIG 2B**). The ECU tendon sheath marks the ulnar limit of the capsulotomy.
- The ECU tendon sheath is not disrupted during this limited approach.

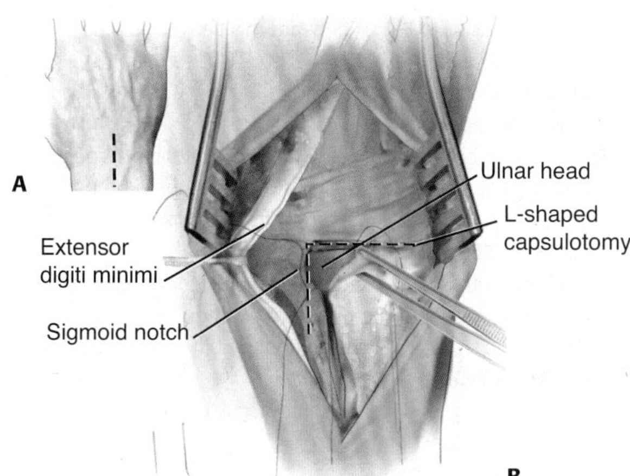

TECH FIG 2 • Dorsal approach to DRUJ. **A.** Dorsal skin incision. **B.** Capsulotomy over the DRUJ.

Bone Tunnel Placement

- Subperiosteal dissection is used to elevate the soft tissue from the dorsal edge of the sigmoid notch for several millimeters.
  - A short cut in the floor of the fourth compartment just proximal and parallel to the distal edge of the radius will help this elevation.
- A distal radius tunnel is planned to be located several millimeters proximal to the lunate fossa and about 5 mm radial to the articular surface of the sigmoid notch (**TECH FIG 3A**).
  - The tunnel should be parallel to the articular surfaces of both the sigmoid notch and lunate fossa.
- A guidewire for a 3.5-mm cannulated drill bit is driven from dorsal to volar through the radius at the site for the tunnel.
- Fluoroscopy is used to confirm guidewire placement, and the tunnel is made with a 3.5-mm cannulated drill bit (**TECH FIG 3B**).
- If a corrective osteotomy of the radius or a sigmoid notch osteoplasty is planned, it is easier to make the bone tunnels before performing the osteotomy, but the tendon graft should not be placed or tensioned until the osteotomy is completed.
- The ulnar flap of the DRUJ capsulotomy is elevated to expose the ulnar head and neck, being careful not to disrupt the ECU tendon sheath.
- The ulnar head tunnel extends from the ulnar fovea to the lateral ulnar neck just volar to the ECU tendon (see **TECH FIG 3A**). Flex the wrist, pronate the forearm, and retract the TFCC remnant to reveal the ulna fovea. Pass a guidewire retrograde from the ulna fovea to exit the lateral ulnar neck just volar to the ECU tendon. Confirm the guidewire position with fluoroscopy.
- If flexing the wrist does not provide adequate exposure, the tunnel is created antegrade from the ulnar neck to the fovea while carefully protecting any TFCC remnant and the ulnar carpus.
  - First, make a hole in the outer cortex on the subcutaneous border of the ulna just volar to the ECU tendon using a standard 3.5-mm drill bit aimed perpendicular to the cortex.
  - The guidewire is inserted through this hole to exit the fovea.
- A 3.5-mm cannulated drill bit is used to create an initial tunnel. (**TECH FIG 3C**).
- Standard drill bits are used to enlarge the bone tunnels as needed to accommodate the previously harvested graft. The ulnar bone tunnel must accommodate both limbs of the tendon graft.

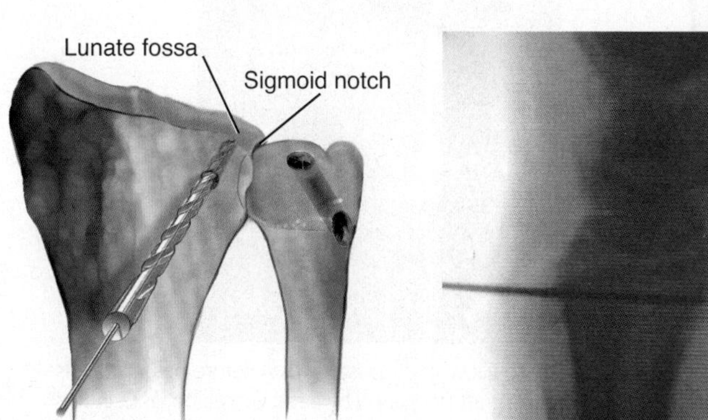

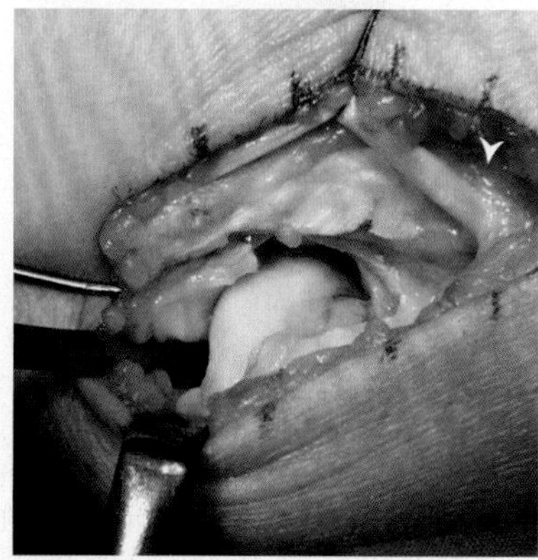

TECH FIG 3 • Tunnel placement. **A.** Bone tunnels are placed to mimic the anatomic attachments of the dorsal and volar radioulnar ligaments. **B.** Fluoroscopy is used to confirm bone tunnel placement. **C.** The probe indicates the location of the fovea on the ulnar head where the drill should exit. The *arrowhead* indicates the ECU tendon being retracted.

Graft Passage

- A second exposure is made to visualize the volar aspect of the radius tunnel.
- A 3-cm longitudinal incision is made extending proximally from the proximal wrist crease (**TECH FIG 4A**).
- Dissection is carried down between the ulnar neurovascular bundle and finger flexor tendons to reach the volar surface of the radius.
- A suture passer is passed through the radius tunnel from dorsal to volar and used to pull one end of the tendon graft back through the distal radius (**TECH FIG 4B**).
- A straight hemostat is passed over the ulnar head and proximal to the TFCC, dorsal to volar, to bluntly pierce the volar DRUJ capsule just distal to the ulnar head. This track should pass adjacent to the ulnar styloid and under the TFCC remnant. The other end of the graft is grasped with the hemostat and pulled back through the capsule.
- At this point, both tendon ends should be visible through the dorsal wound. The suture retriever is used to pass both tendon ends through the ulnar bone tunnel from the fovea to exit at the ulnar neck (**TECH FIG 4C**).
- A right angle grasper is used to guide the tendon ends around the ulnar neck in opposite directions, with one limb of the graft passing deep to the ECU sheath and the other around the volar neck (**TECH FIG 4D**).
- Avoid entrapping any nearby neurovascular structures.

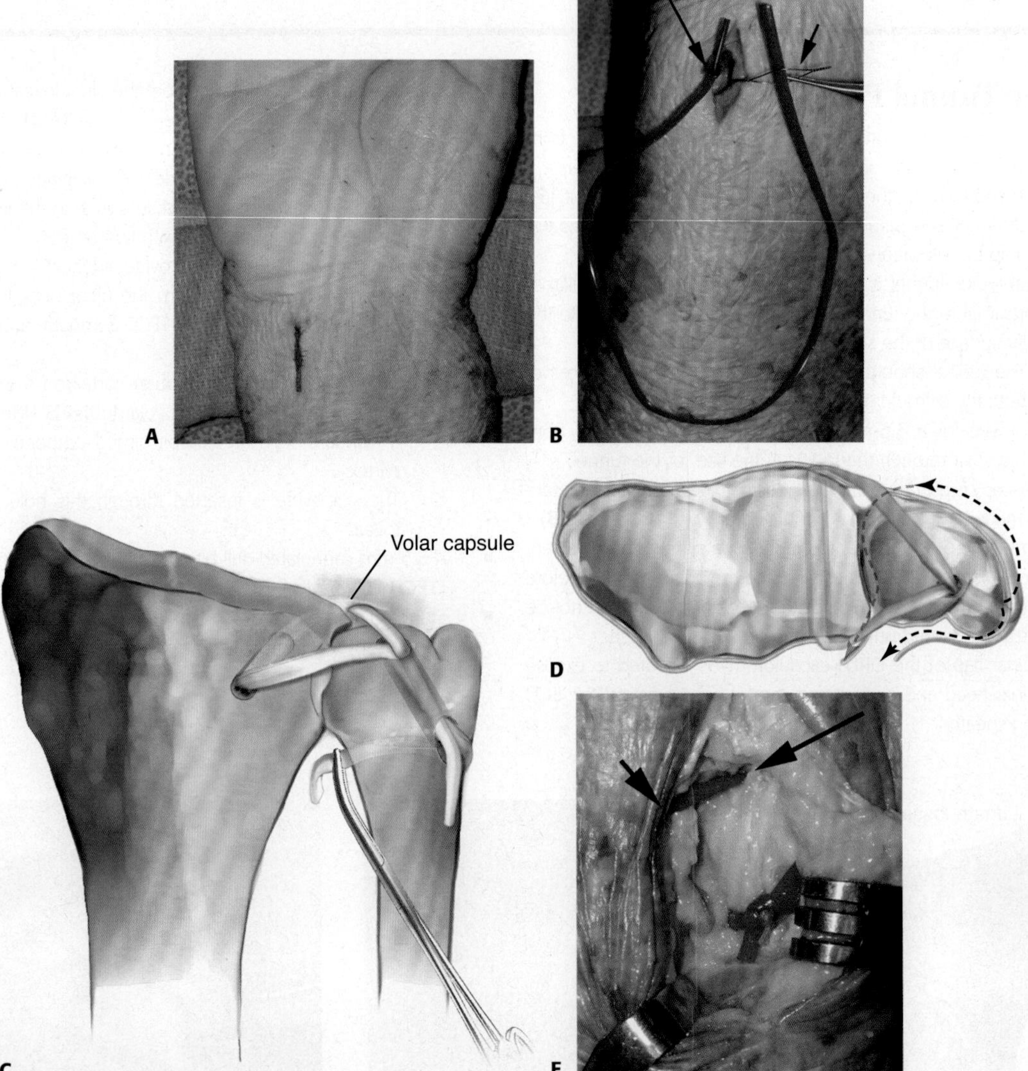

TECH FIG 4 • Graft passage. **A.** A small volar approach is necessary to allow graft passage. **B.** A suture passer travels through the radial bone tunnel (dorsal to volar) to retrieve one limb of the graft (indicated by a red vessel loop). **C.** In this dorsal view, the graft is brought through the volar capsule into the ulnocarpal joint. The two ends are drawn through the ulnar tunnel. **D.** In this axial drawing, the course of the free graft is visualized. The graft provides a near-anatomic reconstruction of the volar and dorsal radioulnar ligaments. **E.** The graft (red vessel loop) exits the radial bone hole (*short arrow*) into the dorsal wound and then enters the ulnar bone hole through the fovea (*long arrow*). The ends of the graft are then wrapped around the ulnar neck.

TECHNIQUES

Graft Tensioning and Fixation

- The forearm is held in slight supination, and the DRUJ is manually compressed.
- The two graft limbs are pulled taut and a half-hitch knot is made against the dorsal aspect of the ulnar neck.
- While maintaining firm tension in the graft, the half-hitch is secured with 3-0 nonabsorbable sutures (**TECH FIG 5**). Additional throws of the graft are made if its length is sufficient.

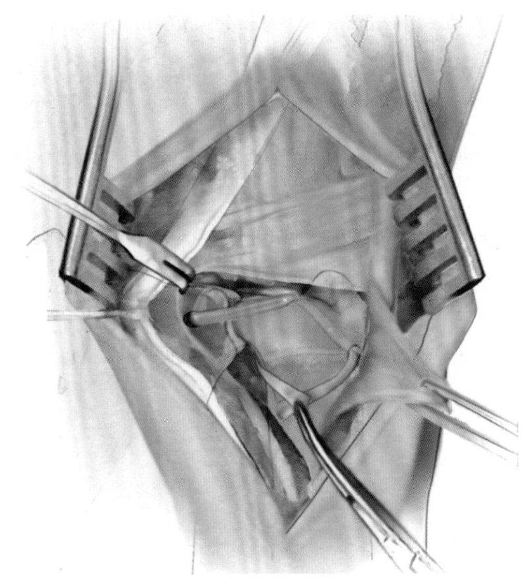

TECH FIG 5 • Graft tensioning. Tension is held on the graft while the knot is secured with a suture.

PEARLS AND PITFALLS

Indications	■ Patients with chronic DRUJ instability in whom the TFCC cannot be repaired ■ Confirm that the patient does not have DRUJ arthritis or a deficient sigmoid notch.
Graft management	■ Harvest the graft early to determine bone tunnel size. ■ Use a suture passer to facilitate graft passage.
Tunnel placement	■ Place the tunnel an adequate distance from the articular surfaces of the DRUJ and lunate fossa to prevent fracturing into the joint. ■ If concurrently performing a corrective osteotomy or sigmoid notch osteoplasty, make the bone tunnels before completing the osteotomy.

POSTOPERATIVE CARE

- The patient is placed in a long-arm splint with the forearm in slight supination. At the first postoperative visit, the patient is transitioned to a long-arm cast for 3 weeks.
- At 4 weeks postoperatively, the patient is placed in a well-molded short-arm cast for an additional 2 weeks.
- At 6 weeks after surgery, the cast is changed to a removable splint, which is worn for an additional 4 weeks.
- The patient should be able to return to most activities by 4 months after surgery, but heavy lifting and impact loading are avoided until 6 months postoperatively.

OUTCOMES

- Patients with a deficient sigmoid notch are more likely to experience recurrent instability if the deficits are not corrected.
- Most patients experience decreased pain and improved strength and stability while maintaining near-normal range of motion. However, full recovery may require 6 to 9 months.
  - The described technique effectively restored stability in 12 of 14 patients while providing about 85% of the strength and range of motion of the contralateral unaffected side.[2] The two failures resulted from deficiencies of the sigmoid notch that were not recognized preoperatively.
- Teoh and Yam[11] reported similar results, with restoration of stability in seven of nine patients using a similar reconstructive method.

COMPLICATIONS

- Joint stiffness
- Recurrent instability
- Persistent pain
- Weakness of grasp
- Infection
- Complex regional pain syndrome

REFERENCES

1. Adams BD. Effects of radial deformity on distal radioulnar joint mechanics. J Hand Surg Am 1993;18(3):492–498.
2. Adams BD, Berger RA. An anatomic reconstruction of the distal radioulnar ligaments for posttraumatic distal radioulnar joint instability. J Hand Surg Am 2002;27(2):243–251.
3. af Ekenstam F. Anatomy of the distal radioulnar joint. Clin Orthop Relat Res 1992;(275):14–18.

4. Kihara H, Palmer AK, Werner FW, et al. The effect of dorsally angulated distal radius fractures on distal radioulnar joint congruency and forearm rotation. J Hand Surg Am 1996;21(1):40–47.
5. Kihara H, Short WH, Werner FW, et al. The stabilizing mechanism of the distal radioulnar joint during pronation and supination. J Hand Surg Am 1995;20(6):930–936.
6. Lester B, Halbrecht J, Levy IM, et al. "Press test" for office diagnosis of triangular fibrocartilage complex tears of the wrist. Ann Plast Surg 1995;35:41–45.
7. Lindau T, Hagberg L, Adlercreutz C, et al. Distal radioulnar instability is an independent worsening factor in distal radial fractures. Clin Orthop Relat Res 2000;(376):229–235.
8. May MM, Lawton JN, Blazar PE. Ulnar styloid fractures associated with distal radius fractures: incidence and implications for distal radioulnar joint instability. J Hand Surg Am 2002;27(6):965–971.
9. Mino DE, Palmer AK, Levinsohn EM. Radiography and computerized tomography in the diagnosis of incongruity of the distal radio-ulnar joint: a prospective study. J Bone Joint Surg Am 1985;67(2):247–252.
10. Stuart PR, Berger RA, Linscheid RL, et al. The dorsopalmar stability of the distal radioulnar joint. J Hand Surg Am 2000;25(4):689–699.
11. Teoh LC, Yam AK. Anatomic reconstruction of the distal radioulnar ligaments: long-term results. J Hand Surg Br 2005;30(2):185–193.
12. Tolat AR, Stanley JK, Trail IA. A cadaveric study of the anatomy and stability of the distal radioulnar joint in the coronal and transverse planes. J Hand Surg Br 1996;21(5):587–594.

Arthroscopic Dorsal Radiocarpal Ligament Repair

66

CHAPTER

David J. Slutsky

DEFINITION

- Tears of the dorsal radiocarpal ligament (DRCL) are more common than previously suspected. They are best seen through a volar radial portal and are amenable to arthroscopic repair.
- DRCL tears appear to be part of a spectrum of radial- and ulnar-sided carpal instability, as evidenced by the frequent association with scapholunate and lunotriquetral ligament injuries as well as triangular fibrocartilage (TFC) tears.
- Isolated DRCL tears can be solely responsible for wrist pain.
- Good results are obtained after arthroscopic repair of isolated DRCL tears. Results of DRCL repairs are less predictable when seen in combination with other types of carpal pathology.[8]
- Recognition of this condition and further research into treatment methods is needed.

ANATOMY

- The DRCL (**FIG 1**) is an extracapsular ligament on the dorsum of the wrist. It originates on the tubercle of Lister and moves obliquely in a distal and ulnar direction to attach to the tubercle of the triquetrum. Its radial fibers attach to the lunate and lunotriquetral interosseous ligament.[2]
- The dorsal intercarpal (DIC) ligament originates from the triquetrum and extends radially to attach onto the lunate, the dorsal groove of the scaphoid, and then the trapezium.

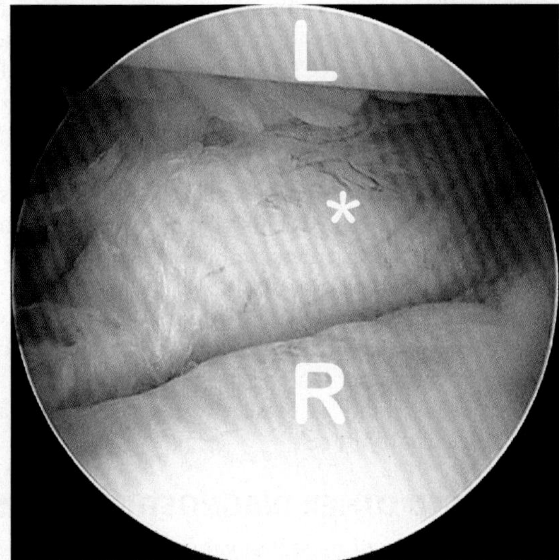

FIG 1 • View of a normal DRCL (*asterisk*) from the volar radial (VR) portal. *L*, lunate; *R*, radius. (Copyright David J. Slutsky MD.)

- The lateral V configuration of the DRCL and the DIC functions as a dorsal radioscaphoid ligament.
  - It can vary its length by changing the angle between the two arms while maintaining its stabilizing effect on the scapholunate joint during wrist flexion and extension.
  - This would require changes in length far greater than any single fixed ligament could accomplish.[9]
- When viewed from a volar radial portal, a DRCL tear can be seen immediately ulnar to the 3-4 portal, just underneath the lunate.
- The DRCL tear can also be seen tangentially from the 6R portal (**FIG 2 A–C**).

PATHOGENESIS

- The wrist has a number of primary and secondary stabilizers.
  - The scapholunate interosseous ligament (SLIL), the lunotriquetral interosseous ligament (LTIL), and the triangular fibrocartilaginous complex (TFCC) are the primary stabilizers.
- The capsular ligaments, including the radioscaphocapitate, radiolunotriquetral, ulnolunate, ulnotriquetral, dorsal radiocarpal, and DIC ligaments, can be thought of as secondary stabilizers.[3]
- A chronic tear of a primary stabilizer may culminate in the attenuation or tearing of the secondary stabilizer.
  - This is seen in patients with a triquetrolunate dissociation of more than 6 months' duration, in whom arthroscopy often reveals fraying of the ulnolunate ligaments and ulnotriquetral ligaments.[12]
- DRCL tears appear to be part of a spectrum of radial- and ulnar-sided carpal instability, as evidenced by the frequent association with SLIL, LTIL, or TFC tears. They have also been associated with midcarpal instability.[4]
- The DRCL tear may occur after or precede these injuries.
- In a recent study, 35 of 64 patients who underwent arthroscopy for the diagnosis and treatment of refractory wrist pain were noted to have associated DRCL tears, for an overall incidence of 55%.[7]
  - Five patients had an isolated DRCL tear.
  - Thirteen patients in this series had SLIL instability, tear, or both; 7 of 13 (54%) also had a DRCL tear. Of this subgroup, 4 patients had Geissler stage 1 or 2 instability and 3 had a Geissler stage 3 or 4 tear.
  - Seven patients had LTIL instability, tear, or both; 2 of 7 (28%) also had a DRCL tear. Of this subgroup, 1 patient had Geissler stage 2 instability and 1 had a Geissler stage 3 or 4 tear.
  - Two patients had a capitohamate ligament tear; one of these patients also had a DRCL tear.

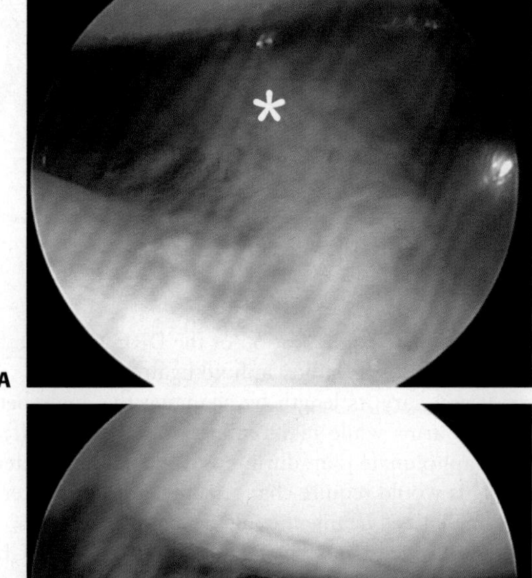
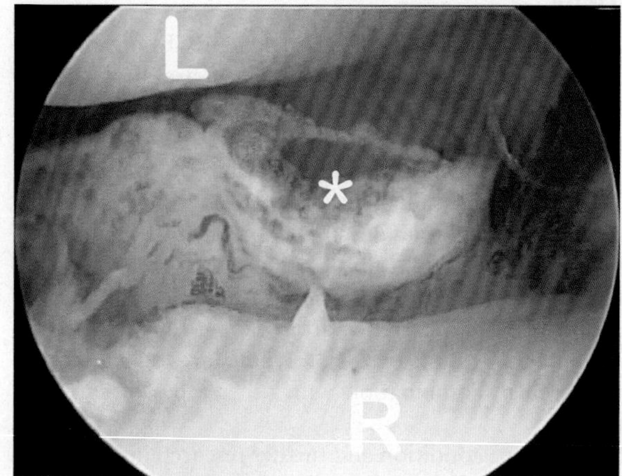

FIG 2 • **A.** View of a DRCL tear (*asterisk*) from the VR portal with dry arthroscopy. **B.** View of a DRCL tear (*asterisk*) from the VR portal with fluid. **C.** View of a DRCL tear (*asterisk*) from the 6R portal with dry arthroscopy. *L*, lunate; *R*, radius. (Copyright David J. Slutsky MD.)

- Seven patients had a solitary TFCC tear; 6 of 7 (86%) were in association with a DRCL tear. One patient had a chronic ulnar styloid nonunion and a DRCL tear. There was TFCC fraying but no tear or detachment.
- Two or more lesions were present in 23 patients; DRCL tears were present in 12 patients (52%). Sixty-two percent of the combined lesions that were associated with a DRCL tear also included a TFCC tear.

NATURAL HISTORY

- The natural history of DRCL tears is not completely certain.[7]
- Unrecognized DRCL tears may be a cause for treatment failures in patients with persistent dorsal wrist pain.
- In nondissociative carpal instability, the pain is believed to be caused by dynamic joint incongruity.[1] Chronic detachment of the ulnar sling on the triquetrum has been implicated as a cause of wrist pain in these cases.[11] It is plausible that impingement of the torn edge of the DRCL against the lunate can have a similar effect.
  - A DRCL repair may relieve this impingement by plicating it to the dorsal capsule with arthroscopic placement of a suture.
- The frequent observation of a DRCL tear in association with the altered kinematics caused by chronic radiocarpal or ulnocarpal instability might be attributed to plastic deformation of the DRCL with cyclical wrist motion that ultimately culminates in a tear.[3]
- An isolated DRCL tear does not necessarily lead to other intracarpal ligament or TFCC tears.[6]

PATIENT HISTORY AND PHYSICAL FINDINGS

- A typical patient with an isolated DRCL tear presents with complaints of intermittent dorsal midline wrist pain that may be sporadic but last 2 or 3 days; the pain is precipitated by repetitive loading or torquing movements of the wrist.
  - When there is an underlying SLIL or LTIL tear or instability or TFCC tear, the pain may be more persistent and localized to the radial or ulnar side of the wrist.
- There are no physical findings that are pathognomonic of a DRCL tear. When there is no other associated wrist pathology, the diagnosis can be made only at the time of arthroscopy.
- Patients with isolated DRCL tears tend not to have localizing carpal tenderness and typically have a normal wrist examination, although some are mildly tender over the tubercle of Lister.[5,8]
- Positive physical findings are usually related to any associated wrist pathology. In patients who have scapholunate instability, scaphoid tenderness and a positive scaphoid shift test are usually present.
- When there is an associated TFC tear, the patient will often have tenderness over the ulnar capsule and may have crepitus and pain with ulnar loading of the pronated wrist.
- If midcarpal instability is present, the patient may have a positive midcarpal shift test.

IMAGING AND OTHER DIAGNOSTIC STUDIES

- Imaging studies are of mostly of value for ruling out associated carpal pathology because they are ineffective at making the diagnosis of an isolated DRCL tear.
- Plain radiographs and arthrograms are normal.

- The magnetic resonance imaging (MRI) is typically normal, although in one patient in the author's series, an MRI was wrongly interpreted as showing a dorsal ganglion due to a high fluid signal intensity over the dorsal capsule (**FIG 3**).

DIFFERENTIAL DIAGNOSIS

- Dynamic scapholunate instability
- Scapholunate ligament tear
- Dorsal wrist syndrome[10]

NONOPERATIVE MANAGEMENT

- Patients should be treated with at least 1 month of wrist splinting, nonsteroidal anti-inflammatories, and activity modification with avoidance of repetitive gripping and lifting.
- Failure to respond is an indication for a radiocarpal cortisone injection followed by 1 additional month of splinting.
- Patients who continue to have wrist pain should then undergo imaging studies to rule out associated intracarpal pathology.

SURGICAL MANAGEMENT

- An arthroscopic repair is especially indicated isolated DRCL tears because the results are quite favorable.
- Repairs may also be considered where the associated interosseous ligament tear or TFCC tear is treated arthroscopically.

Preoperative Planning

- Preoperative investigations should include plain radiographs to rule out a static carpal instability pattern.
- An MRI can be performed to assess the intracarpal ligaments and TFC.

Positioning

- The patient is positioned supine on the operating table with the arm abducted.
- Some method of overhead traction is useful. This may include traction from the overhead lights or a shoulder holder along with 5- to 10-pound sandbags attached to an arm sling. A traction tower such as the Linvatec tower (Conmed Linvatec Corp., Largo, FL) or the ARC wrist traction tower (Arc Surgical LLC, Hillsboro, OR) greatly facilitates instrumentation.

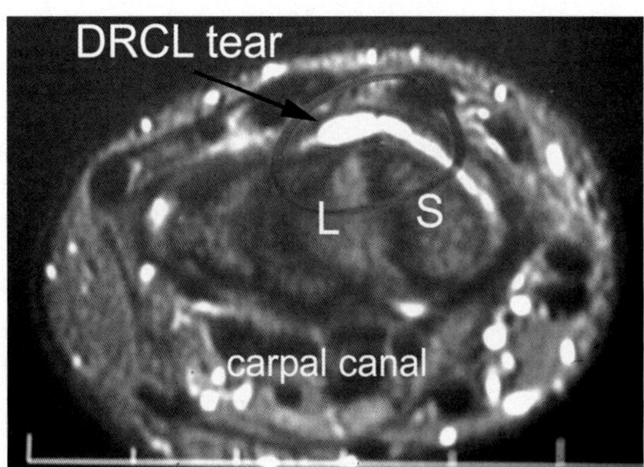

FIG 3 • MRI of an axial view of the carpus at the level of the carpal canal depicting a dorsal radiocarpal ligament (*DRCL*) tear. *S*, scaphoid; *L*, lunate. (Copyright David J. Slutsky MD.)

- A 2.7-mm 30-degree angled arthroscope with a camera attachment is necessary.
  - A fiberoptic light source, video monitor, and printer are also standard equipment.
  - A 3-mm hook probe is needed for palpation of intracarpal structures.
  - A motorized shaver and suction punch forceps are useful for débridement.
- A variety of curved and straight 18-gauge spinal needles are used for passage of an absorbable 2-0 suture for the outside-in repair.
  - A grasper is needed to retrieve the suture ends.

Approach

- An outside-in arthroscopic repair technique of the DRCL ligament is preferred.
- The standard dorsal portals are established, including the 3-4 and 4-5 portals, a midcarpal radial portal, and a midcarpal ulnar portal for an arthroscopic survey.
- Dry arthroscopy without fluid irrigation is often preferred.

TECHNIQUES

Volar Radial Portal

- A 2-cm longitudinal incision is made in the proximal wrist crease, exposing the flexor carpi radialis (FCR) tendon sheath (**TECH FIG 1**).
- The sheath is divided and the FCR tendon retracted ulnarly.
- The radiocarpal joint space is identified with a 22-gauge needle.
- A blunt trocar and a cannula are introduced through the floor of the FCR sheath, which overlies the interligamentous sulcus between the radioscaphocapitate ligament and the long radiolunate ligament.
- A 2.7-mm 30-degree angled arthroscope is inserted through the cannula.

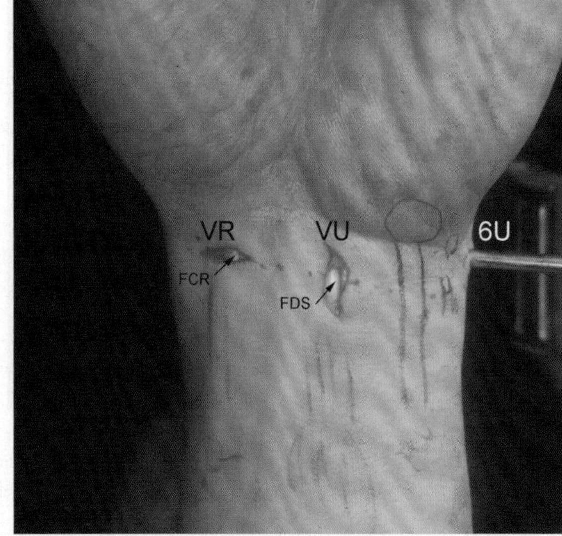

TECH FIG 1 • Demonstration of surface landmarks for the VR portal. *VR*, volar radial; *VU*, volar ulnar; *FCR*, flexor carpi ulnaris; *FDS*, flexor digitorum sublimus. (Copyright David J. Slutsky MD.)

Ligament Repair

- The repair is performed by inserting a curved 21-gauge spinal needle through the 4-5 portal while viewing the DRCL tear through the arthroscope, which is inserted in the volar radial portal (**TECH FIG 2 A–D**).
- A 2-0 absorbable suture is threaded through the spinal needle and retrieved with a grasper through the 3-4 portal.
- A curved hemostat is used to pull either end of the suture underneath the extensor tendons, and the knot is tied either at the 3-4 or 4-5 portal.
- With dorsal traction, the encircling suture pulls the torn DRCL up against the dorsal capsule, preventing it from impinging into the joint.

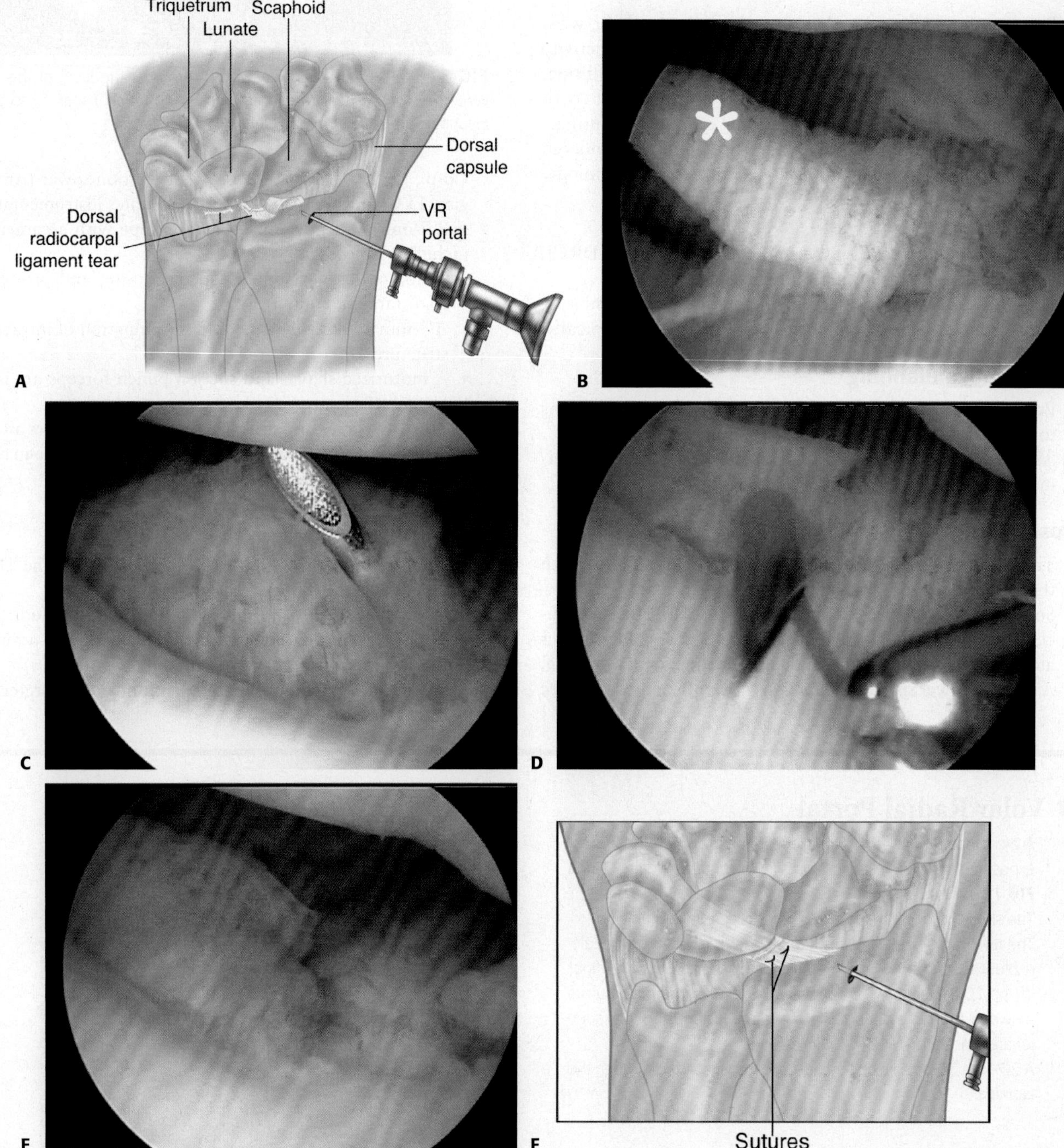

TECH FIG 2 • Outside-in DRCL repair. **A.** Drawing of DRCL tear. **B.** Arthroscopic view of DRCL tear (*asterisk*) from the VR portal. **C.** Insertion of 2-0 PDS suture through a needle in the curved spinal needle through the substance of a DRCL tear. **D.** Retrieval of the suture using a grasper in the 3-4 portal. **E.** Completed repair. **F.** Drawing of completed repair. (Copyright David J. Slutsky MD.)

PEARLS AND PITFALLS

Procedural tips	▪ Use the hook probe in the 3-4 portal to palpate the DRCL. Tears may not be evident until the free edge is pulled into the joint. ▪ Be sure to assess the scapholunate and lunotriquetral intervals from the midcarpal joint to assess any dynamic instability. Consideration may be given to thermal shrinkage of the palmar aspect of the scapholunate ligament when there is an associated dynamic scapholunate instability. ▪ To ensure that the extensor tendons are not entrapped, use a hemostat to thread either end of the suture underneath the extensor compartment. Tie the suture under the skin. ▪ When performing capsular shrinkage, use irrigation to prevent thermal chondral damage.

POSTOPERATIVE CARE

- After an isolated DRCL repair, the patient is placed in a below-elbow splint with the wrist in neutral rotation.
- Finger motion and edema control are instituted immediately. At the first postoperative visit, the sutures are removed and the patient is placed in a below-elbow cast for a total immobilization time of 4 weeks.
- Wrist motion with use of a removable splint for comfort is instituted after cast removal.
- Gradual strengthening exercises are added after 8 weeks.
- Dynamic wrist splinting is instituted at 10 weeks if needed.

OUTCOMES

- The five patients who underwent an isolated DRCL repair graded their pain as none or mild.[7]
  - No patient required pain medication and all had returned to their previous occupation without restriction.
  - The pre- and postoperative wrist motion was unchanged in four of these patients, with less than 15% loss of motion in the fourth patient.
  - Grip strengths were 90% to 130% of the opposite side.
- A dorsal capsulodesis was performed in the seven patients with scapholunate instability.
  - Three of these patients graded their pain level as none or mild, with both returning to full duty.
  - Four patients graded their pain as moderate or severe, with all four changing their occupation.
- Four patients underwent DRCL repair or shrinkage and LTIL pinning.
  - Two patients had no pain and two had chronic, moderate pain.
- Seven patients underwent DRCL repair and TFCC repair or débridement, wafer resection, or both.
  - Two had no pain (with wafer resection), two had occasional mild pain, and three had chronic moderate pain.
- Of the patients with combined injuries who underwent a DRCL repair and treatment for associated tears of the SLIL, LTIL, or TFCC, seven of nine had chronic moderate pain.

COMPLICATIONS

- There were no complications related to the DRCL repair as described.
- Potential complications from use of a volar radial portal would include injury to the radial artery or the palmar cutaneous branch of the median nerve.
- Use of capsular shrinkage is still unproven and cannot as yet be considered a standard of care of the treatment of intercarpal ligament injuries.

REFERENCES

1. Bednar JM, Osterman AL. Carpal instability: evaluation and treatment. J Am Acad Orthop Surg 1993;1:10–17.
2. Mitsuyasu H, Patterson RM, Shah MA, et al. The role of the dorsal intercarpal ligament in dynamic and static scapholunate instability. J Hand Surg Am 2004;29(2):279–288.
3. Short WH, Werner FW, Green JK, et al. Biomechanical evaluation of the ligamentous stabilizers of the scaphoid and lunate, part III. J Hand Surg Am 2007;32(3):297–309.
4. Slutsky D. Arthroscopic repair of dorsoradiocarpal ligament tears. Arthroscopy 2005;21:1486e1–1486e8.
5. Slutsky DJ. Arthroscopic repair of dorsal radiocarpal ligament tears. Arthroscopy 2002;18:E49.
6. Slutsky DJ. The incidence of dorsal radiocarpal ligament tears in patients having diagnostic wrist arthroscopy for wrist pain. J Hand Surg Am 2008;33(3):332–334.
7. Slutsky DJ. The incidence of dorsal radiocarpal ligament tears in the presence of other intercarpal derangements. Arthroscopy 2008;24:526–533.
8. Slutsky DJ. Management of dorsoradiocarpal ligament repairs. J Am Soc Surg Hand 2005;5:167–174.
9. Viegas SF, Yamaguchi S, Boyd NL, et al. The dorsal ligaments of the wrist: anatomy, mechanical properties, and function. J Hand Surg Am 1999;24(3):456–468.
10. Watson HK, Weinzweig J. Physical examination of the wrist. Hand Clin 1997;13:17–34.
11. Watson HK, Weinzweig J. Triquetral impingement ligament tear (tilt). J Hand Surg Br 1999;24(3):321–324.
12. Zachee B, De Smet L, Fabry G. Frayed ulno-triquetral and ulno-lunate ligaments as an arthroscopic sign of longstanding triquetro-lunate ligament rupture. J Hand Surg Br 1994;19(5):570–571.

Arthroscopic Evaluation and Treatment of Scapholunate and Lunotriquetral Ligament Disruptions

Alexander H. Payatakes, Loukia K. Papatheodorou, Alex M. Meyers, and Dean G. Sotereanos

DEFINITION

- Scapholunate interosseous ligament (SLIL) and lunotriquetral interosseous ligament (LTIL) tears are common wrist injuries occurring in isolation or as part of the perilunate injury pattern.
- Interosseous ligament injuries are being diagnosed with an increased frequency as a result of recent advances in imaging and arthroscopy.
- Management of these injuries has proven to be a difficult clinical problem. Surgical treatment has been more reliable in pain relief than in altering the natural history.

ANATOMY

- The scapholunate complex is subject to significant loads, as the scaphoid is the only carpal bone to span from the proximal to the distal carpal row.
- A large amount of potential energy is stored within the proximal carpal row.
  - The proximal carpal row flexes with radial deviation and extends with ulnar deviation.
  - The scaphoid "wants" to flex and the triquetrum "wants" to extend.
  - The lunate (intercalated segment) is tethered between the scaphoid and triquetrum.
- Stability is provided to the scapholunate complex by the intrinsic SLIL as well as extrinsic capsular ligaments, especially the dorsal radiocarpal (DRC), dorsal intercarpal (DIC) ligament, and volar radioscaphocapitate (RSC) and scaphotrapeziotrapezoid (STT) ligaments.
- The SLIL is a C-shaped structure consisting of a stronger dorsal ligamentous portion (2 to 3 mm thick), a volar ligamentous portion (1 mm thick), and a proximal fibrocartilaginous (membranous) portion.[2]
- Isolated injuries to the SLIL appear to be associated with dynamic instability, whereas static instability usually indicates additional injury to the secondary ligamentous stabilizers, including the DIC ligament.[22]
- The lunotriquetral complex is also stabilized by an intrinsic LTIL and extrinsic (volar and dorsal) capsular ligaments.
- The LTIL is C-shaped, analogous to the SLIL, consisting of dorsal and volar ligamentous portions and a membranous proximal portion. In contrast to the SLIL, the volar ligamentous portion of the LTIL is stronger and more significant functionally.[18]
- As with the scapholunate complex, isolated injuries to the LTIL are usually insufficient for the development of static instability. Presence of a static deformity indicates additional injury to extrinsic ligamentous structures (volar ulnotriquetral, ulnolunate, and ulnocapitate ligaments or the DRC and DIC ligaments).[10,27]

PATHOGENESIS

- Mayfield et al[15] postulated that scapholunate disruption is the initial component of the lesser arc perilunate injury pattern, which occurs when force is applied to the thenar area with the wrist in extension, mild pronation, and ulnar deviation. The force results in intercarpal supination.
  - Depending on the amount of kinetic energy involved, the injury may or may not extend to the ulnar side of the wrist.
- SLIL injuries can be sprains, partial tears, or complete tears (with or without injury to the extrinsic ligamentous stabilizers).
  - In a complete SLIL tear with an intact LTIL, the scaphoid flexes and the lunate is pulled by the triquetrum into extension causing a dorsal intercalated segment instability (DISI) pattern.
  - Complete SLIL tears usually fail at the bone–ligament interface off the scaphoid.
- Arthroscopic evaluation has revealed associated SLIL injuries in up to 30% of intra-articular distal radius fractures.[8]
- LTIL disruption may be traumatic or atraumatic in origin.
  - Traumatic LTIL rupture may occur as the final component of a greater or lesser arc perilunate injury pattern.[15]
  - Isolated LTIL tears may result from a fall on an outstretched hand while the wrist is in extension and radial deviation (reverse perilunate injury).[17] The force is applied to the hypothenar region causing intercarpal pronation. In other cases, injury to the LTIL may result from dorsally applied force to the flexed wrist.[32]
  - Atraumatic ruptures of the LTIL may occur secondary to inflammatory arthritis or ulnar impaction syndrome.[24]

NATURAL HISTORY

- Tears of the SLIL or LTIL, with or without extrinsic ligamentous injury, may lead to various degrees of carpal instability (predynamic, dynamic, or static), alteration of normal carpal mechanics and kinematics, and degenerative changes in the radiocarpal and midcarpal joints.
- A complete SLIL tear is associated with the development of a DISI deformity, which may be dynamic or static (if accompanied by injury to the extrinsic ligaments).
  - As a DISI deformity develops, proximal carpal bones shift in position and lose congruency, resulting in abnormal radiocarpal contact loading.

- Abnormal flexion and hypermobility of the scaphoid over time leads to degenerative changes of the radioscaphoid and capitolunate joints and ultimately collapse, termed *scapholunate advanced collapse* (SLAC) wrist degeneration.[29–31]
  - Early degenerative changes have been documented to begin as soon as 3 months after injury.
- A complete LTIL tear is associated with the development of a volar intercalated segment instability (VISI) deformity.
- The natural history of partial tears of the SLIL or LTIL is at present poorly defined.
  - Partial scapholunate and lunotriquetral ligament injuries may cause chronic activity-related wrist pain in the absence of radiologic findings.[30]
- Predynamic or dynamic instability may cause attenuation of extrinsic ligaments with progressive development of further instability and eventual static changes.[36,37]
  - There is evidence that this process typically requires many years.[16]

PATIENT HISTORY AND PHYSICAL FINDINGS

- Dorsoradial or ulnar-sided wrist pain with a history of a fall, sudden loading, or twisting of the wrist should raise suspicion for a SLIL or LTIL tear, respectively. However, it is not uncommon for the patient to deny any significant injury.
- Patients frequently complain of weakness, swelling, and loss of range of motion of the wrist.
- A sensation of instability or "giving way" is often reported, occasionally associated with a painful clunk.
- A detailed physical examination of the wrist may provide significant information for the diagnosis of ligamentous injuries and help to rule out other wrist pathology.
- Examination of the wrist begins with evaluation for any deformity or swelling and determination of wrist range of motion.
- Key tests and maneuvers specifically evaluating the scapholunate and lunotriquetral ligaments are noted in the following text. Comparison with the contralateral uninjured wrist is critical.
  - Grip strength and pain: Diminished grip strength correlates with wrist pathology.
  - The presence of pain at the central aspect of the wrist with attempted grip has also been associated with scapholunate ligament pathology.
  - Deep palpation of scapholunate interval: Point tenderness indicates SLIL injury, scaphoid injury, or ganglion cyst.
  - Watson scaphoid shift test: Pain with or without a clunk or catch sensation is highly suggestive of scapholunate instability.
  - Scaphoid ballottement test: Pain and increased anteroposterior (AP) laxity are highly suggestive of scapholunate instability.
  - Deep palpation of lunotriquetral interval: Point tenderness indicates LTIL injury or triangular fibrocartilage complex (TFCC) pathology.
  - Ulnar wrist loading: A painful snap indicates lunotriquetral instability, midcarpal instability, or TFCC pathology. This maneuver will also be painful if ulnar impaction is present.
  - Lunotriquetral compression test: Pain with this maneuver indicates lunotriquetral or triquetrohamate joint pathology.
  - Lunotriquetral ballottement and shear tests: Pain and increased AP laxity are highly suggestive of lunotriquetral instability.

IMAGING AND OTHER DIAGNOSTIC STUDIES

- Initial imaging of the wrist should always include AP and lateral radiographs, combined with special views depending on the suspected pathology. If scapholunate pathology is suspected, a bilateral pronated grip posteroanterior (Mayo Clinic) view should be obtained. In all cases, comparison with radiographs of the contralateral uninjured wrist is critical.
- Abnormal findings in static scapholunate instability include the following:
  - AP view: increased scapholunate interval (3 mm or more), scaphoid cortical "ring sign," and triangular appearance of lunate
  - Lateral view: flexion of scaphoid and dorsiflexion of lunate, as determined by increased scapholunate angle (more than 60 degrees) and increased lunocapitate angle (over 10 degrees) with dorsal translation of capitate
- Radiographic findings in patients with lunotriquetral tears are often normal. Abnormal findings in static lunotriquetral instability include in following:
  - AP view: Proximal translation of triquetrum or lunotriquetral overlap without gapping and interruption of Gilula arc.
  - Lateral view: flexion of scaphoid and lunate, as determined by normal or decreased scapholunate angle (<45 degrees and increased lunocapitate angle (more than 10 degrees) with volar translation of the capitate
- Provocative views (radial–ulnar deviation, flexion–extension views) or videofluoroscopy may demonstrate asynchronous scapholunate motion (dynamic scapholunate instability) in cases with suspected SLIL injury and normal standard views.[12] Increased, synchronous mobility of the scapholunate complex with diminished motion of the triquetrum indicates an LTIL injury.
- Wrist arthrography has a sensitivity of only 60% compared to arthroscopy and cannot determine the extent of any tear present or its functional significance.[33]
- Magnetic resonance imaging (MRI) (with or without arthrography) has limited value in evaluating interosseous ligament injuries. Reported sensitivity rates for SLIL injuries range from 40% to 65% compared to arthroscopy.[23] MRI is even less reliable in diagnosing LTIL injuries.
- Arthroscopy (radiocarpal, midcarpal with probing) remains the gold standard in evaluation of SLIL and LTIL injuries. This method of evaluation allows a dynamic assessment and determination of the functional significance of the instability.

DIFFERENTIAL DIAGNOSIS

- Differential diagnosis of scapholunate injuries and radial-sided wrist pain[28]
  - Scaphoid fracture or nonunion
  - Scaphotrapezial arthritis
  - Radiocarpal arthritis
  - De Quervain tenosynovitis
  - Dorsal ganglion cyst
  - Dorsal wrist impaction syndrome
  - Perilunate instability
  - Isolated DRC ligament tear
- Differential diagnosis of lunotriquetral injuries and ulnar-sided wrist pain[24]
  - TFCC injury
  - Distal radioulnar joint (DRUJ) instability or arthritis
  - Ulnar impaction syndrome or chondromalacia

- Ulnar styloid impingement syndrome
- Extensor carpi ulnaris (ECU) tendon subluxation
- Pisotriquetral arthritis
- Triquetrohamate instability
- Hamate fracture
- Ulnar neurovascular syndromes

NONOPERATIVE MANAGEMENT

- Scapholunate and lunotriquetral injuries associated with dynamic instability may respond to initial nonoperative treatment for 6 to 12 weeks.
- Conservative management typically includes a combination of the following:
  - Splinting
  - Nonsteroidal anti-inflammatories
  - Intra-articular (radiocarpal) corticosteroid injections
  - Occupational therapy and work restrictions
  - Reeducation of wrist proprioception with flexor carpi radialis (FCR) strengthening

SURGICAL MANAGEMENT

- The selection of surgical treatment for SLIL and LTIL injuries is based on the severity of symptoms, degree of instability (predynamic, dynamic, or static), chronicity (acute, subacute, or chronic), arthroscopic findings (Geissler grade[8]; see **TECH FIG 1**), and reparability of the ligament.
- Dynamic instability (based on positive physical findings with provocative maneuvers, abnormal stress radiographs, or arthroscopic findings) that has failed to respond to nonoperative treatment may be treated arthroscopically.
  - Arthroscopic options include simple débridement, débridement with thermal shrinkage, and débridement (with or without shrinkage) with percutaneous pinning.
- Static instability and severe dynamic instability are typically indications for open surgery, although arthroscopic repair of the SLIL is feasible in select cases.
  - Surgical options include open repair or augmentation (especially of acute or subacute injuries), capsulodesis, tenodesis, or use of the reduction-association scapholunate (RASL) procedure.
- Patients developing carpal collapse with arthritic changes require salvage procedures such as radial styloidectomy, proximal row carpectomy, or limited wrist fusions (eg, STT, scaphocapitate, scaphoidectomy plus four-corner fusion, lunotriquetral fusion).
- The focus of this chapter is arthroscopic management of dynamic scapholunate or lunotriquetral instability. Newer arthroscopic alternatives advocated for management of more advanced pathology are also described.

Arthroscopic Procedures

- Arthroscopic débridement of SLIL and LTIL tears
  - Indications: predynamic or dynamic instability, arthroscopic findings of a partial ligament tear with an unstable tissue flap (Geissler grade II), with or without synovitis[21,34]
  - The ideal patient for this technique is one with mechanical symptoms (pain with clicking) attributable to impingement of unstable tissue flaps and resulting synovitis.
- Arthroscopic débridement and thermal shrinkage of SLIL and LTIL disruptions
  - Indications: predynamic or dynamic instability and arthroscopic finding of a partial ligament tear (Geissler grade I or II).[8,10] The dorsal segment of the SLIL should be intact for this procedure.
  - This technique provides an option for the management of lax, redundant ligaments with no frank tear (Geissler grade I) where simple débridement is not an option.
    - Thermal shrinkage is performed in an attempt to increase stability and improve long-term outcome compared to simple débridement.
  - Radiofrequency probes use a high-frequency alternating current to generate heat. This leads to denaturation (uncoiling) of the collagen triple helix with reduction in overall ligament length.
    - Use of this device is contraindicated in patients with pacemakers or other implantable electronic devices.
- Arthroscopic débridement and percutaneous pinning of SLIL and LTIL disruptions
  - Indications: acute or subacute dynamic instability (Geissler grades II and III)[4,35]
  - This technique aims to induce ligamentous healing and/or the formation of fibrous union (by decortication) between the two involved carpal bones.
- Arthroscopic SLIL repair
  - Indications: Select patients with acute or subacute scapholunate instability (Geissler grades II, III, possibly IV). Dorsal capsuloligamentous repair requires a reparable, midsubstance dorsal SLIL tear with absent or reducible carpal malalignment.[13] Arthroscopic SLIL repair of avulsion-type SLIL tears using bone anchors has also been shown to be technically feasible.[26]
  - This technically demanding technique aims to directly repair the dorsal SLIL (+/− capsulodesis augmentation) without further injury to secondary ligamentous stabilizers.
- Arthroscopic radial styloidectomy
  - Indications: early (stage I) SLAC (ie, radial styloid–scaphoid impingement or arthritis) with focal and reproducible clinical findings of radial styloid pain exacerbated by wrist flexion and radial deviation
  - This procedure may provide significant pain relief until a salvage procedure (proximal row carpectomy, scaphoid excision, four-corner fusion) becomes necessary.
- Arthroscopic RASL procedure and lunotriquetral fusion
  - Indications: static, reducible instability (Geissler grade IV); lunotriquetral arthritis[19,20]
  - Early (stage I) SLAC wrist is not a contraindication.
  - The RASL procedure aims to achieve fibrous union while maintaining limited rotation at the scapholunate joint, thus approximating normal wrist kinematics. On the other hand, osseous fusion is the goal for the lunotriquetral joint.

Preoperative Planning

- A careful review of the patient's history, physical findings, as well as static and stress radiographs may provide the surgeon with a reasonable impression of what will be required.
  - In most cases, however, a decision on the type of procedure to be performed is made intraoperatively based on the arthroscopic findings and associated pathology.
- Consideration must therefore be given to having the following available: arthroscopic resectors, radiofrequency

probes, mini C-arm, drills, Kirschner wires of various widths, and headless compression screws.

Positioning

- The patient is placed in the supine position with the operative extremity on a hand table.
- Any possible donor site for ligament reconstruction or augmentation should also be prepared and draped in a sterile fashion.
- The extremity is placed in a tower distraction device with 10 to 12 pounds (5 to 6 kg) of distraction and 12 to 15 degrees of wrist flexion (**FIG 1**).
- The arthroscope monitor is placed on the opposite side of the hand table from the surgeon.
- If percutaneous pinning or use of other implants is anticipated, a small fluoroscopy unit is placed adjacent to the hand table.

Approach

- Arthroscopic evaluation and management of scapholunate and lunotriquetral injuries can typically be performed through standard dorsal wrist portals (3-4, 4-5, 6R, and midcarpal radial and ulnar).
- The additional use of volar radial (VR) and volar ulnar portals has been advocated for better visualization of the volar portions of the SLIL and LTIL as well as the DRC and DIC ligaments.[1,25]

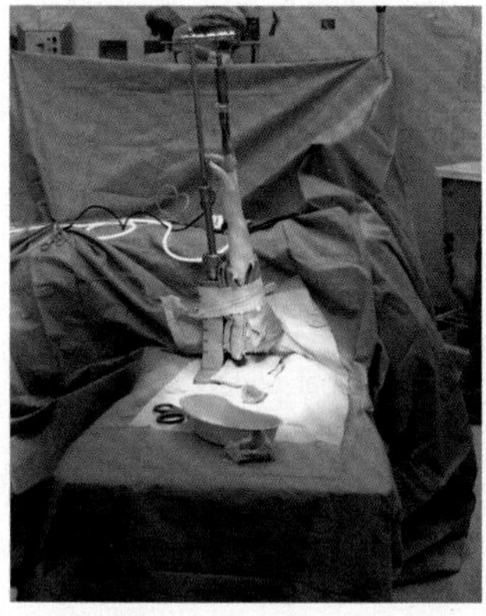
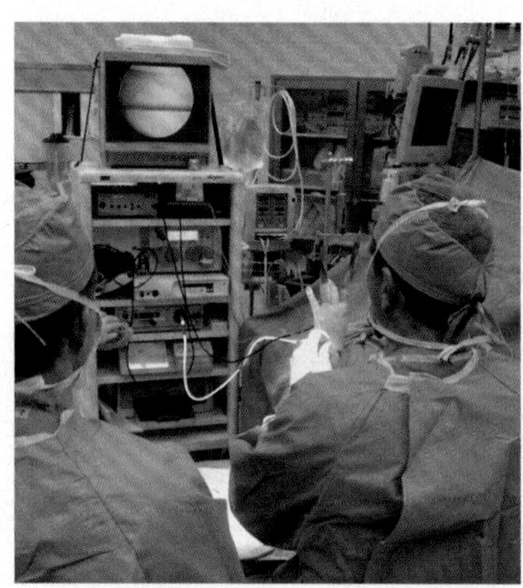

FIG 1 • **A.** Positioning for arthroscopy of the wrist. **B.** The monitor should be visible to the surgeon. If use of fluoroscopy is anticipated, the C-arm is placed adjacent to the hand table.

TECHNIQUES

Arthroscopic Evaluation

- An 18-gauge needle is used to distend the radiocarpal joint with 5 to 8 mL of normal saline.
- A 2.7-mm or smaller, 30-degree arthroscope is preferred for wrist arthroscopy.
- Typical working portals include the 3-4, 4-5, 6R, and midcarpal portals. Outflow is established using an 18-gauge needle through the 6U or 6R portal.
- Portals are established by palpating appropriate anatomic landmarks, making a small incision through the epidermis and dermis using a no. 15 scalpel, followed by blunt dissection using a mosquito clamp. Stab incisions are not used. Either the mosquito clamp or blunt trocars are used to enter the joint.
- The entire radiocarpal joint is evaluated in a systematic manner, usually from radial to ulnar.
- The SLIL is best visualized through the 3-4 portal with a probe insertion through the 4-5 or 6R portal. The 4-5 portal is used for instrumentation.
  - Occasionally, the avulsed portion of the SLIL may make visualization through the 3-4 portal difficult. In this situation, the arthroscope is transferred to the 6R portal and directed radially to facilitate débridement.
- The proximal portion of the SLIL is easily visualized by following the radioscapholunate ligament (ligament of Testut) to its insertion. The volar RSC and long radiolunate ligaments (wider) are visualized radially, whereas the short radiolunate is located ulnar to the ligament of Testut.
- The LTIL is best visualized through the 4-5 or 6R portal, with use of the 3-4 and 6R for instrumentation.
- Both ligaments should be evaluated in their entirety (dorsal, proximal, and volar portions).
  - Placement of the arthroscope in the 6R portal with traction release may allow better visualization of the most distal aspect of the SLIL.
  - If visualization of the volar portions of the SLIL and LTIL is inadequate, an additional VR portal just radial to the FCR sheath may be used.[1]
- In patients with gross scapholunate instability, the arthroscope is finally turned toward the dorsum of the scaphoid and lunate to identify possible avulsion of the DIC or DRC ligament.[22]
- Evaluation of carpal congruence and stability is incomplete without performance of midcarpal arthroscopy.
- The midcarpal portals are placed 1 cm distal to the 3-4 and 4-5 portals.
- The arthroscope is aimed proximally.
  - The scapholunate joint is visualized radially and the lunotriquetral joint ulnarly.
  - Both joints are evaluated for congruity.
  - Stability is assessed with a 1-mm arthroscopic probe.
  - A Watson scaphoid shift test may be performed while visualizing the scapholunate joint.
- The Geissler arthroscopic classification of wrist interosseous ligament tears is shown in **TECH FIG 1**.[8]

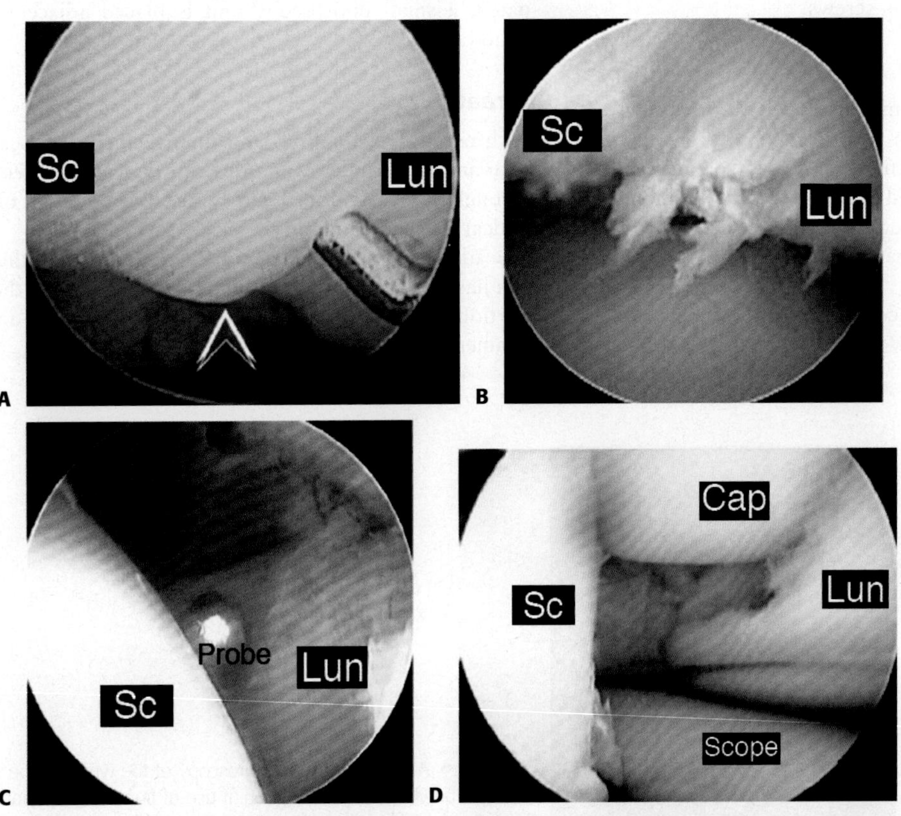

TECH FIG 1 • Geissler arthroscopic classification of interosseous ligament injuries of the wrist.[8] The scapholunate joint is depicted here but the classification is also applicable to the lunotriquetral joint. **A.** Grade I: attenuation of the SLIL as visualized in the radiocarpal joint. No incongruence is noted in the midcarpal joint. **B.** Grade II: partial full-thickness tear with unstable flap but minimal joint incongruity. **C.** Grade III: complete tear of the SLIL with moderate joint incongruity. A 1.5-mm probe can be introduced into the joint (view from midcarpal portal). **D.** Grade IV: complete tear with marked incongruity. The 2.7-mm arthroscope can "drive-through" the joint. *Sc*, scaphoid; *Lun*, lunate; *Cap*, capitate.

Arthroscopic Débridement

- A thorough diagnostic arthroscopy (radiocarpal plus midcarpal) is performed to verify the diagnosis and rule out instability or other associated pathology.
- The inflamed synovium is excised with a 2.5- or 2.7-mm full-radius resector.
- Any unstable tissue flaps are resected with a suction punch or synovial resector.
- Redundant tissue is then resected to a stable rim with the synovial resector or bipolar radiofrequency probe.
- Débridement should generally be limited to the proximal membranous portion of the SLIL or LTIL.
- Unwarranted débridement of the dorsal (SLIL) or volar (LTIL) portions of the ligamentous complex may lead to further instability.
- Carpal stability should be assessed both before and after débridement. This is facilitated by inserting a probe through the 4-5 (or 6R) and midcarpal portals.
- If there is concern regarding stability, consideration should be given to adjunct percutaneous pinning, with or without decortication of the involved joint (see Arthroscopic decortication and percutaneous pinning).

Arthroscopic Débridement and Thermal Shrinkage

- Diagnostic arthroscopy is performed as previously described.
- Geissler grade II tears are débrided with a synovial resector to a stable rim (**TECH FIG 2A**). Thermal shrinkage of the intact portion of the ligament is then performed with a 2.3-mm bipolar radiofrequency probe.
  - Attenuated ligaments (Geissler grade I) are treated with thermal shrinkage alone.
- Thermal shrinkage is performed by applying the radiofrequency probe in a paintbrush fashion (**TECH FIG 2B**). The goal is to evenly distribute the thermal energy throughout the ligament.
  - The 4-5 portal is preferred for this procedure for optimal access to the SLIL.
  - Ligament shrinkage is visually confirmed by a change in its color and consistency (**TECH FIG 2C**).
- Intermittent application of the probe (a few seconds at a time) with adequate cool fluid inflow and outflow prevents ablation of the ligament and overheating of the joint.
  - Radiofrequency probes specially designed for thermal shrinkage have recently become available. They offer additional safety by not reaching ablation temperature.

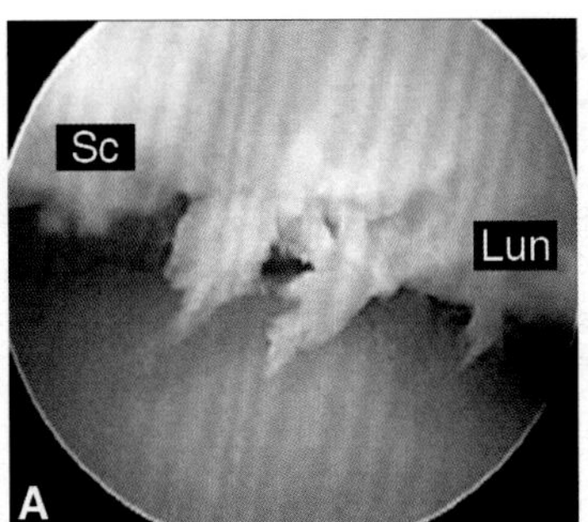

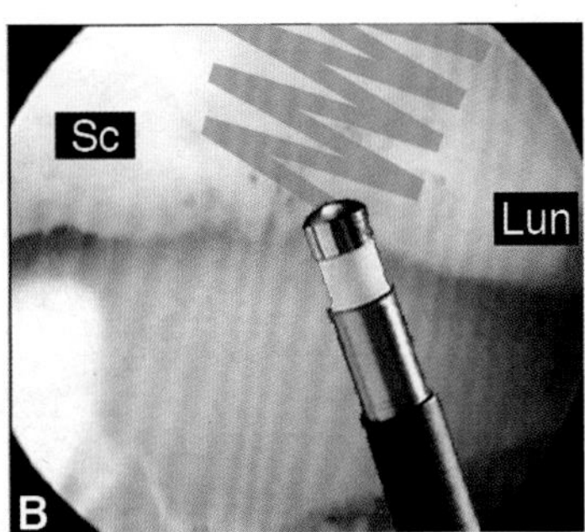

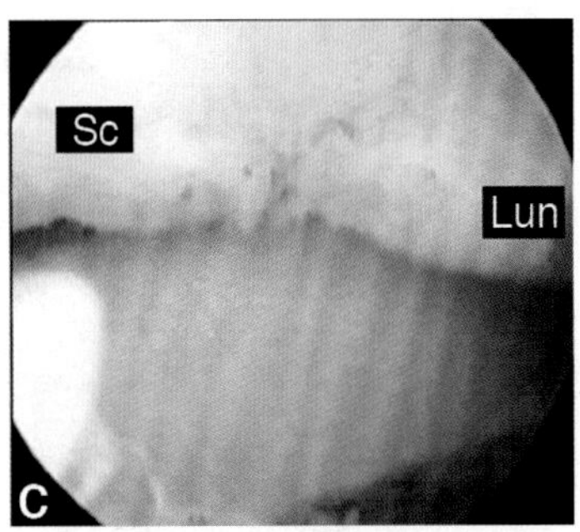

TECH FIG 2 • Débridement and thermal shrinkage. **A.** Geissler grade II SLIL tear as seen through 3-4 portal. **B.** "Paintbrush" technique for thermal shrinkage. The probe is applied intermittently to avoid overheating. **C.** The same ligament after débridement and thermal shrinkage. Note apparent change in color and consistency. *Sc*, scaphoid; *Lun*, lunate.

Arthroscopic Dorsal Capsuloligamentous Scapholunate Interosseous Ligament Repair

- Diagnostic arthroscopy is performed as previously described.
- The scope is placed in the 6R portal to evaluate whether the SLIL tear is suitable for arthroscopic repair (substantial remnants of the dorsal SLIL must be present on both the lunate and scaphoid). Traction release may be necessary to elevate the dorsal capsule off the SLIL for better visualization.[13]
- If necessary, congruity of the joint is improved by external (pressure on the distal pole of scaphoid) or internal maneuvers (percutaneous Kirschner wires used as joysticks).
- A hypodermic needle is inserted into the 3-4 portal, through the dorsal capsule and ulnar (lunate) SLIL remnant, tilted slightly distally so as to end up in the midcarpal joint (**TECH FIG 3A**). The scope is transferred to the ulnar midcarpal (MCU) portal. A 3-0 monofilament absorbable suture is introduced through the needle, then brought out through the radial midcarpal (MCR) portal with a forceps. The process is repeated to pass a second suture through the radial (scaphoid) SLIL remnant and bring it out through the MCR portal (**TECH FIG 3B**).
- The two suture ends exiting the MCR portal are tied together. Traction is applied on the free suture ends protruding through the 3-4 portal, transferring the knot into the midcarpal joint until it abuts the volar surface of the dorsal SLIL (**TECH FIG 3C**).
- A second knot is tied between the two free suture ends and brought to rest on the dorsal capsule through the 3-4 portal (**TECH FIG 3D**).
- The scapholunate joint is stabilized with two Kirschner wires across the scapholunate joint (radial to ulnar) followed by one or two Kirschner wires across the scaphocapitate joint **TECH FIG 3E**.
- The second knot is at this point tied down to complete the capsuloligamentous repair (**TECH FIG 3F**).
- A similar technique has been described for repair of volar SLIL tears.[6]

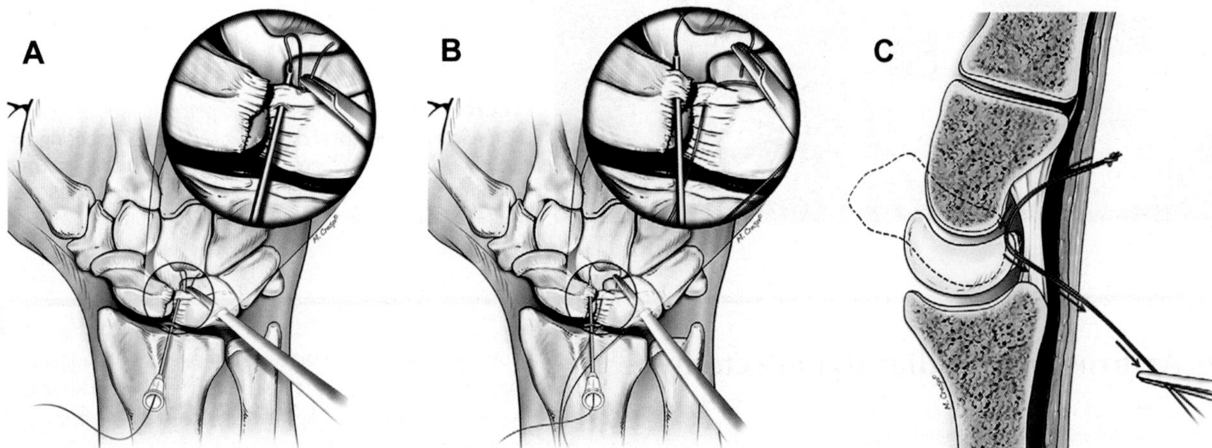

TECH FIG 3 • Dorsal capsuloligamentous SLIL repair (Mathoulin). **A,B.** Sutures are passed through SLIL remnants (via needle through the dorsal 3-4 portal) and retrieved through the MCU portal. **C.** Knot is tied between distal suture ends and pulled into joint against dorsal SLIL by traction on the free proximal dorsal suture ends. *(continued)*

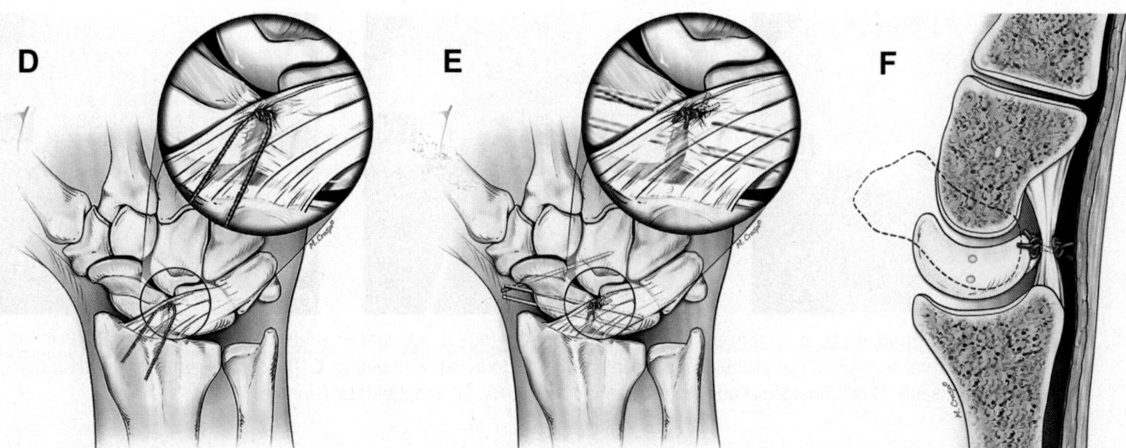

TECH FIG 3 • *(continued)* **D.** Proximal suture ends are tied over the dorsal capsule (through 3-4 portal). **E,F.** Completed capsuloligamentous repair after scapholunate pinning. (Modified from Mathoulin CL, Dauphin N, Wahegaonkar AL. Arthroscopic dorsal capsuloligamentous repair in chronic scapholunate ligament tears. Hand Clin 2011;27[4]:563–572.)

Arthroscopic Decortication and Percutaneous Pinning

- Diagnostic arthroscopy and débridement is performed as previously described.
- If the ligamentous injury is extensive and felt to be irreparable, then all residual tissue of the torn ligament (SLIL or LTIL) is débrided with a 2.5- or 2.7-mm full-radius resector.
- The cartilage of the opposing surfaces of the involved carpal bones is then débrided to bleeding bone with a 2.5- or 2.7-mm aggressive full-radius resector and a 2.9-mm barrel abrader (**TECH FIG 4A**).
- The extremity is then removed from the distraction tower.
- If necessary, congruity of the joint is improved by external (pressure on the distal pole of scaphoid) or internal maneuvers (percutaneous Kirschner wires used as joysticks).
- The joint is stabilized by percutaneously inserting three or four 0.045-inch (1.1 mm) Kirschner wires under fluoroscopic control.
- The scapholunate joint is typically stabilized with two Kirschner wires across the scapholunate joint (radial to ulnar) followed by one or two Kirschner wires across the scaphocapitate joint (**TECH FIG 4B**).
- The lunotriquetral joint is similarly stabilized with two Kirschner wires across the lunotriquetral joint (ulnar to radial) followed by one or two Kirschner wires across the capitotriquetral joint.
- The pins are then cut subcutaneously or bent outside the skin per surgeon preference.

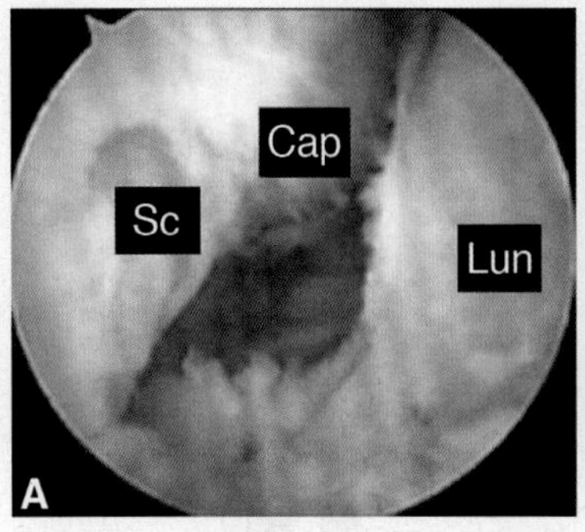

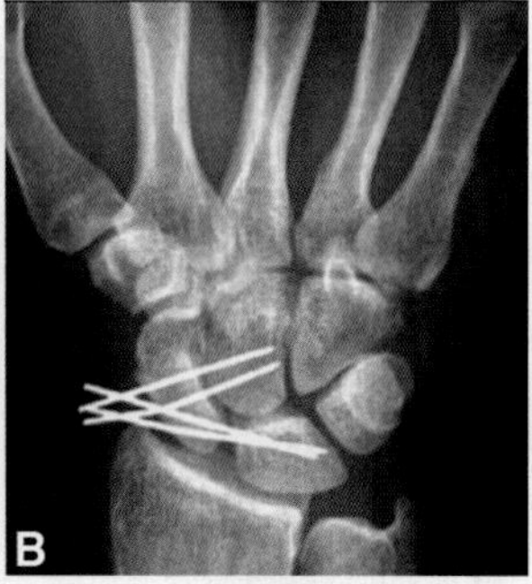

TECH FIG 4 • Decortication and percutaneous pinning. **A.** Remnants of ligament and articular cartilage of opposing surfaces are débrided to bleeding bone. **B.** The joint is stabilized with three or four Kirschner wires placed under fluoroscopic guidance. *Sc*, scaphoid; *Cap*, capitate; *Lun*, lunate.

Arthroscopic Radial Styloidectomy

- Diagnostic arthroscopy is initially performed to delineate the chondral lesions and accurately stage the SLAC wrist.[29]
- The arthroscope is placed in the 3-4 or 4-5 portal.
- Excision of the radial styloid is performed through the 1-2 (or 3-4) portal with a side-cutting 3.5-mm sheathed burr.
- Arthroscopic evaluation of articular cartilage and intraoperative radiographs should be used to determine the extent of resection.
  - The origin of the RSC ligament is visualized and preserved during bone resection.
- Although the tendency is to overestimate the amount of bone resected, excision of more than 4 mm may jeopardize the ligament origin and result in ulnar carpal dislocation.

Arthroscopic Reduction-Association Scapholunate Procedure and Lunotriquetral Fusion

- Diagnostic arthroscopy with evaluation of chondral lesions is performed as described previously.
- The opposing surfaces of the joint to be fused are débrided to bleeding bone with a 2.5- or 2.7-mm aggressive full-radius resector and a 2.9-mm barrel abrader.
  - Complete decortication is verified from both the radiocarpal and midcarpal joints.
  - Failure to perform this step typically results in early failure.
- In the case of the RASL procedure, a side-cutting, 3.5-mm sheathed burr is then used to perform an arthroscopic radial styloidectomy through the 1-2 (or 3-4) portal as described previously.
- Kirschner wires (0.062 inch or 1.6 mm) are then inserted percutaneously from the dorsum into the involved carpal bones (distal scapholunate or lunotriquetral). Positioning of the wires should be slightly eccentric to allow for subsequent placement of the screw centrally. The Kirschner wires are used as joysticks to reduce the joint under fluoroscopic (with or without arthroscopic) control.
  - It is essential to verify adequate reduction of the capitolunate joint on the lateral view.
  - A Kocher clamp may be placed across the Kirschner wires to maintain reduction.
  - An additional 0.045-inch (1.1 mm) Kirschner wire may be inserted through the dorsal rim of the distal radius into the lunate for provisional stabilization of the lunate.
- A 0.035-inch (0.9 mm) guidewire is then placed across the joint (scapholunate or lunotriquetral) under fluoroscopic control.
- In the case of the RASL procedure, the guidewire should be placed through the 1-2 portal, across the scaphoid waist toward the proximal ulnar corner of the lunate, thus approximating the normal axis of rotation of the scapholunate joint (**TECH FIG 5**).

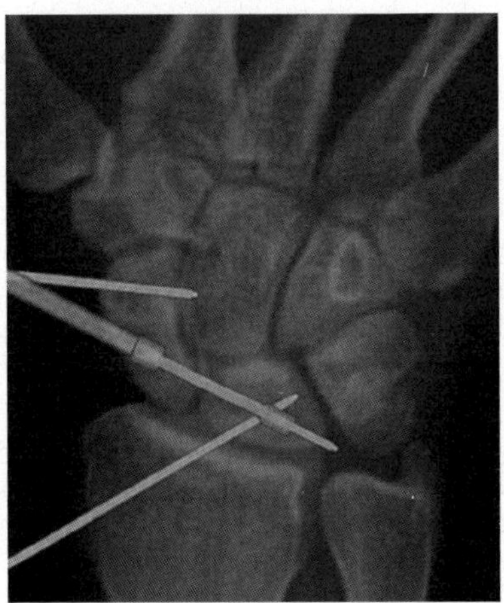

TECH FIG 5 • RASL technique. Scapholunate joint reduction is achieved using two Kirschner wires as joysticks. Optimal positioning of a compression screw is through the scaphoid waist toward the proximal ulnar corner of the lunate and fully countersunk. Note use of screw with smooth shank.

- A cannulated headless compression screw is then placed across the joint. Length measurement should be reduced by about 4 mm to accommodate for joint compression and to ensure that the screw is completely countersunk into bone. Note that, in the case of the RASL procedure, the headless compression screw must have a smooth shank to allow limited rotation through the scapholunate joint.
- After satisfactory reduction and fixation are verified, the wrist capsule incision is repaired.
- In patients with lunotriquetral instability as a result of ulnar impaction syndrome, fusion of the lunotriquetral joint must be combined with an arthroscopic wafer procedure or an ulnar shortening.

PEARLS AND PITFALLS

Diagnosis	■ Meticulous examination and arthroscopy of the entire wrist are necessary to ensure diagnosis and treatment of concomitant pathology.
Indications	■ Arthroscopic débridement with or without thermal shrinkage is not adequate management for static scapholunate or lunotriquetral instability. ■ Arthroscopic repair of the SLIL should be considered in select patients only and requires substantial arthroscopic expertise. Open repair remains the gold standard.
Contraindications	■ Use of radiofrequency probes for débridement or thermal shrinkage is contraindicated in patients with pacemakers or implantable electronic devices.
Surgical technique	■ Wrist arthroscopy for evaluation of SLIL or LTIL tears must include arthroscopy of the midcarpal joint. ■ Carpal stability should be assessed both before and after any débridement of the SLIL or LTIL. ■ Débridement of functionally significant portions of the SLIL (dorsal) or LTIL (volar) should be kept to a minimum to prevent further destabilization. ■ Thermal shrinkage should be performed with specially designed radiofrequency probes. Otherwise, the probe should be applied in a paintbrush fashion for only a few seconds at a time with adequate outflow to avoid reaching ablation temperatures. ■ When performing the RASL procedure, a headless compression screw with a smooth shank must be used to allow for limited rotation through the scapholunate joint. Failure to decorticate the scapholunate joint has resulted in early failure.
Rehabilitation	■ If thermal shrinkage is performed, the wrist should be immobilized for 4 weeks postoperatively and protected for an additional 4 weeks to allow healing of treated tissue. ■ Following scapholunate or lunotriquetral decortication or SLIL capsuloligamentous repair, pins remain in place for 8 weeks.

POSTOPERATIVE CARE

- Patients treated with arthroscopic débridement alone are placed in a cock-up wrist splint postoperatively and instructed to initiate range-of-motion exercises at 48 hours.
- Patients treated with arthroscopic débridement and thermal shrinkage are placed in a full-time short-arm splint postoperatively. Range-of-motion exercises are initiated at 4 weeks, with use of a removable cock-up splint between sessions. Strengthening exercises are initiated at 8 weeks.
- Patients treated with arthroscopic débridement and percutaneous pinning are placed in a short-arm splint; changed to a short-arm cast after suture removal. The cast is maintained until pin removal, which is performed at 8 to 10 weeks for the scapholunate and at 4 to 6 weeks for the lunotriquetral joint. Range-of-motion exercises are then initiated, with progression to strengthening as tolerated.
- Patients treated with an arthroscopic RASL procedure are placed in a long-arm thumb spica cast for 4 weeks, followed by a short-arm spica for another 4 weeks. Range-of-motion exercises are then initiated, with progression to strengthening as tolerated. Patients treated with arthroscopic fusion of the lunotriquetral joint are immobilized until radiographic fusion is obtained.

OUTCOMES

- Ruch and Poehling[21] reported excellent results with arthroscopic débridement alone in 14 patients with partial SLIL or lunotriquetral tears, or both, and predominantly mechanical symptoms. At a minimum follow-up of 2 years, all patients reported complete relief of their mechanical symptoms, whereas pain was significantly reduced and grip strength was restored.
- Weiss et al[34] have treated both partial and complete SLIL and lunotriquetral tears with arthroscopic débridement alone in an attempt to elicit scar formation with some degree of stabilization. Excellent pain relief and increased strength were achieved in 17 of 19 patients with partial tears but only in 17 of 24 patients with complete tears. No radiologic progression was noted at 27 months follow-up.
- Earp et al[7] reported their experience with management of SLIL tears in pediatric and adolescent patients. Long-term improvement was achieved in 24 of 32 patients with arthroscopic débridement of Geissler grade II or III tears.
- Mathoulin and Messina[14] reported their results with arthroscopic débridement and adjunct pinning in 66 patients with acute or subacute SLIL tears. At 36 months, 92% of patients had good or excellent results.
- Darlis et al[5] reported substantial pain relief in 14 of 16 patients with Geissler grade I or II SLIL tears treated with arthroscopic débridement and thermal shrinkage. Wrist motion was maintained, and there was no radiologic evidence of instability at 19 months of follow-up.
- Hirsh et al[9] reported excellent results in 9 of 10 patients with Geissler grade II SLIL tears treated with arthroscopic débridement and thermal shrinkage at 28 months of follow-up.
- Lee et al[11] reported excellent pain relief and improved function in 13 of 16 wrists with Geissler grade I or II SLIL (6 wrists) or LTIL tears (10 wrists) treated with arthroscopic débridement and thermal shrinkage. No progression of carpal instability was noted at 53 months of follow-up.
- Whipple[35] reported his results with arthroscopic decortication and percutaneous pinning in patients with scapholunate instability. Symptom duration of more than 3 months and a side-to-side gap difference of more than 3 mm were associated with poor outcomes. Pain relief was satisfactory in only 53% of patients with both of these factors.
- Darlis et al[4] reported management of chronic (longer than 3 months) dynamic scapholunate instability (Geissler grades III and IV) with arthroscopic decortication and percutaneous pinning in patients who did not wish to undergo open surgery. Results were suboptimal, with significant pain relief and improved grip strength in 6 of 11 patients. At 33 months of follow-up, there was no radiologic evidence of progression to static instability, but 3 patients required additional surgery to address persistent pain.
- Mathoulin et al[13] described arthroscopic dorsal capsuloligamentous repair in 36 patients with scapholunate disruption (Geissler grades II to IV) of varying chronicity. At 11.4 months follow-up, 35 patients reported satisfaction and all patients had returned to work (including 7 professional athletes).
- Clinical experience with the arthroscopic RASL procedure and lunotriquetral fusion is limited. Rosenwasser et al[20] reported excellent results using the open RASL technique in 20 patients with static instability. At 54 months of follow-up, patients had achieved 91% of their normal wrist motion and 87% of contralateral grip strength. The authors noted that the procedure may be performed arthroscopically but felt that experience with the open technique should first be obtained.
- Caloia et al[3] reported their results with arthroscopic RASL in eight patients (nine wrists). At 35 months of follow-up, the procedure was successful in regard to pain relief and grip strength in six patients, but screw removal was necessary in two patients (three screws) due to painful loosening.

COMPLICATIONS

- Injury to branches of superficial radial sensory nerve (especially with use of 1-2 portal) or dorsal branch of ulnar nerve (6R, 6U portals)
- Injury to radial artery (radial volar portal). This portal should be established through the floor of the FCR sheath.
- Persistent pain or instability
- Need for additional surgery (ligament reconstruction, capsulodesis, tenodesis, proximal row carpectomy, partial or complete wrist fusion)

REFERENCES

1. Abe Y, Doi K, Hattori Y, et al. Arthroscopic assessment of the volar region of the scapholunate interosseous ligament through a volar portal. J Hand Surg Am 2003;28(1):69–73.
2. Berger RA. The gross and histologic anatomy of the scapholunate interosseous ligament. J Hand Surg Am 1996;21(2):170–178.
3. Caloia M, Caloia H, Pereira E. Arthroscopic scapholunate joint reduction. Is an effective treatment for irreparable scapholunate ligament tears? Clin Orthop Relat Res 2012;470(4):972–978.
4. Darlis NA, Kaufmann RA, Giannoulis F, et al. Arthroscopic debridement and closed pinning for chronic dynamic scapholunate instability. J Hand Surg Am 2006;31(3):418–424.
5. Darlis NA, Weiser RW, Sotereanos DG. Partial scapholunate ligament injuries treated with arthroscopic debridement and thermal shrinkage. J Hand Surg Am 2005;30(5):908–914.

6. del Piñal F, Studer A, Thams C, et al. An all-inside technique for arthroscopic suturing of the volar scapholunate ligament. J Hand Surg Am 2011;36(12):2044–2046.
7. Earp BE, Waters PM, Wyzykowski RJ. Arthroscopic treatment of partial scapholunate ligament tears in children with chronic wrist pain. J Bone Joint Surg Am 2006;88(11):2448–2455.
8. Geissler WB, Freeland AE. Arthroscopically assisted reduction of intraarticular distal radial fractures. Clin Orthop Relat Res 1996;(327):125–134.
9. Hirsh L, Sodha S, Bozentka D, et al. Arthroscopic electrothermal collagen shrinkage for symptomatic laxity of the scapholunate interosseous ligament. J Hand Surg Br 2005;30(6):643–647.
10. Horii E, Garcia-Elias M, An KN, et al. A kinematic study of lunotriquetral dissociations. J Hand Surg Am 1991;16(2):355–362.
11. Lee JI, Nha KW, Lee GY, et al. Long-term outcomes of arthroscopic debridement and thermal shrinkage for isolated partial intercarpal ligament tears. Orthopedics 2012;35(8):e1204–e1209.
12. Lee SK, Desai H, Silver B, et al. Comparison of radiographic stress views for scapholunate dynamic instability in a cadaver model. J Hand Surg Am 2011;36(7):1149-1157.
13. Mathoulin CL, Dauphin N, Wahegaonkar AL. Arthroscopic dorsal capsuloligamentous repair in chronic scapholunate ligament tears. Hand Clin 2011;27(4):563–572.
14. Mathoulin C, Messina J. Treatment of acute scapholunate ligament tears with simple wiring and arthroscopic assistance [in French]. Chir Main 2010;29(2):72–77.
15. Mayfield JK, Johnson RP, Kilcoyne RK. Carpal dislocations: pathomechanics and progressive perilunar instability. J Hand Surg Am 1980;5(3):226–241.
16. O'Meeghan CJ, Stuart W, Mamo V, et al. The natural history of an untreated isolated scapholunate interosseus ligament injury. J Hand Surg Br 2003;28(4):307–310.
17. Reagan DS, Linscheid RL, Dobyns JH. Lunotriquetral sprains. J Hand Surg Am 1984;9(4):502–514.
18. Ritt MJ, Bishop AT, Berger RA, et al. Lunotriquetral ligament properties: a comparison of three anatomic subregions. J Hand Surg Am 1998;23(3):425–431.
19. Ritt MJ, Maas M, Bos KE. Minnaar type 1 symptomatic lunotriquetral coalition: a report of nine patients. J Hand Surg Am 2001;26(2):261–270.
20. Rosenwasser MP, Miyasajsa KC, Strauch RJ. The RASL procedure: reduction and association of the scaphoid and lunate using the Herbert screw. Tech Hand Up Extrem Surg 1997;1:263–272.
21. Ruch DS, Poehling GG. Arthroscopic management of partial scapholunate and lunotriquetral injuries of the wrist. J Hand Surg Am 1996;21(3):412–417.
22. Ruch DS, Smith BP. Arthroscopic and open management of dynamic scaphoid instability. Orthop Clin North Am 2001;32:233–240.
23. Schädel-Höpfner M, Iwinska-Zelder J, Braus T, et al. MRI versus arthroscopy in the diagnosis of scapholunate ligament injury. J Hand Surg Br 2001;26(1):17–21.
24. Shin AY, Battaglia MJ, Bishop AT. Lunotriquetral instability: diagnosis and treatment. J Am Acad Orthop Surg 2000;8:170–179.
25. Slutsky DJ. The use of a volar ulnar portal in wrist arthroscopy. Arthroscopy 2004;20(2):158–163.
26. Stuffmann ES, McAdams TR, Shah RP, et al. Arthroscopic repair of the scapholunate interosseous ligament. Tech Hand Upper Extrem Surg 2010;14(4):204–208.
27. Trumble TE, Bour CJ, Smith RJ, et al. Kinematics of the ulnar carpus related to the volar intercalated segment instability pattern. J Hand Surg Am 1990;15(3):384–392.
28. Walsh JJ, Berger RA, Cooney WP. Current status of scapholunate interosseous ligament injuries. J Am Acad Orthop Surg 2002;10:32–42.
29. Watson HK, Ballet FL. The SLAC wrist: scapholunate advanced collapse pattern of degenerative arthritis. J Hand Surg Am 1984;9(3):358–365.
30. Watson H, Ottoni L, Pitts EC, et al. Rotary subluxation of the scaphoid: a spectrum of instability. J Hand Surg Br 1993;18(1):62–64.
31. Watson HK, Weinzweig J, Zeppieri J. The natural progression of scaphoid instability. Hand Clin 1997;13:39–49.
32. Weber ER. Wrist mechanics and its association with ligamentous instability. In: Lichtman DM, ed. The Wrist and Its Disorders. Philadelphia: Saunders, 1988:41–52.
33. Weiss AP, Akelman E, Lambiase R. Comparison of the findings of triple-injection cinearthrography of the wrist with those of arthroscopy. J Bone Joint Surg Am 1996;78(3):348–356.
34. Weiss AP, Sachar K, Glowacki KA. Arthroscopic debridement alone for intercarpal ligament tears. J Hand Surg Am 1997;22(2):344–349.
35. Whipple TL. The role of arthroscopy in the treatment of scapholunate instability. Hand Clin 1995;11:37–40.
36. Wolfe SW, Katz LD, Crisco JJ. Radiographic progression to dorsal intercalated segment instability. Orthopedics 1996;19:691–695.
37. Zachee B, De Smet L, Fabry G. Frayed ulno-triquetral and ulno-lunate ligaments as an arthroscopic sign of longstanding triquetro-lunate ligament rupture. J Hand Surg Br 1994;19(5):570–571.

Open Scapholunate Ligament Repair and Augmentation

Loukia K. Papatheodorou, Alexander H. Payatakes, Alex M. Meyers, and Dean G. Sotereanos

DEFINITION

- Scapholunate instability is the most common form of carpal instability.
- Scapholunate interosseous ligament (SLIL) injury can result in a predictable pattern of arthritis over time: scapholunate advanced collapse (SLAC).[14]
- Acute tears (<6 weeks from injury) versus chronic tears (>6 weeks from injury)
  - Acute tears tend to be amenable to primary ligament repair.
  - Chronic tears tend to require ligament reconstruction or stabilization procedures.
- Static or dynamic instability
  - Static instability: Any or all of the five characteristic changes are present on standard plain radiographs (see in the following text).
  - Dynamic instability: Normal plain radiographs; however, with loaded (grip view) plain radiographs, any or all of the five characteristic changes may become present.[12]
- Fixed versus reducible deformity
  - Fixed deformity: The static radiographic changes are not passively correctible.
  - Reducible deformity: The static radiographic changes are passively correctible.
    - This distinction may be determined preoperatively by noting improvement in the static changes on plain radiographs of the wrist in radial deviation compared with anteroposterior (AP) views of the wrist.

ANATOMY, PATHOGENESIS, AND NATURAL HISTORY

- See Chapter 67.

PATIENT HISTORY AND PHYSICAL FINDINGS

- Typical presentation follows a fall onto an outstretched hand with acute onset of wrist pain and mild dorsal wrist swelling.
- Key physical examination findings are reviewed in Chapter 67.

IMAGING AND OTHER DIAGNOSTIC STUDIES

- Plain radiographs may reveal five characteristic findings suggestive of SLIL pathology (**FIG 1**).
  - Scapholunate separation ("Terry Thomas sign"): asymmetric gap between the scaphoid and lunate of more than 3 mm on posteroanterior (PA) radiograph
  - Cortical ring sign: Ring-shaped cortical hyperdensity and scaphoid foreshortening is seen on PA radiograph as the scaphoid moves into increasing flexion.[2]
  - Angular changes in the carpal rows
    - Scapholunate angle: Normal is 30 to 60 degrees (mean 46 degrees); with SLIL injury, more than 60 degrees is suspicious but more than 70 degrees is considered pathognomic.[7]
    - Capitolunate angle: Normal is −15 to 15 degrees (mean 0 degree); with SLIL injury, more than 15 degrees.
    - Radiolunate angle: Normal is −10 to 10 degrees (mean 0 degree); with SLIL injury, more than 10 degrees (lunate tilted dorsally).
  - Triangular lunate: As the lunate moves into extension, it assumes a more triangular appearance on PA radiograph (normally the lunate appears more quadrangular). This corresponds to the dorsal tilt noted on the lateral view.
  - Disruption of Gilula arcs: In the normal wrist, the proximal and distal aspect of the proximal row form gentle concentric arcs. These lines may be disrupted with SLIL tears as the normal relationships between the bones of the proximal row are lost.[5]
- Arthrography: sensitivity 56%, specificity 83%, accuracy 60%[15]
  - False-positive results have been documented with communication of contrast shown in asymptomatic patients.[2]
- Computed tomography (CT) arthrography: sensitivity 86% to 100% (100% sensitive in the detection of dorsal ligament tears), specificity 50% to 79% (79% specific in the detection of dorsal ligament tears), accuracy 78% to 83%[10]
- Magnetic resonance imaging (MRI): sensitivity 25% to 60%, specificity 77% to 100%, accuracy 64% to 78%[11]
  - Specifically, palmar tears of the SLIL were identified with a sensitivity of 60% and specificity of 77% in a cadaveric

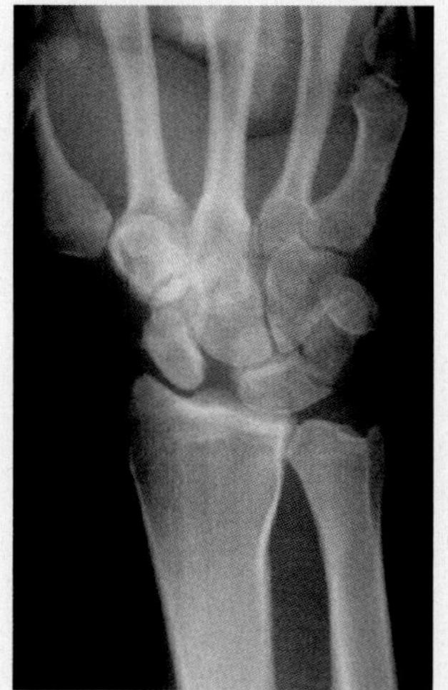

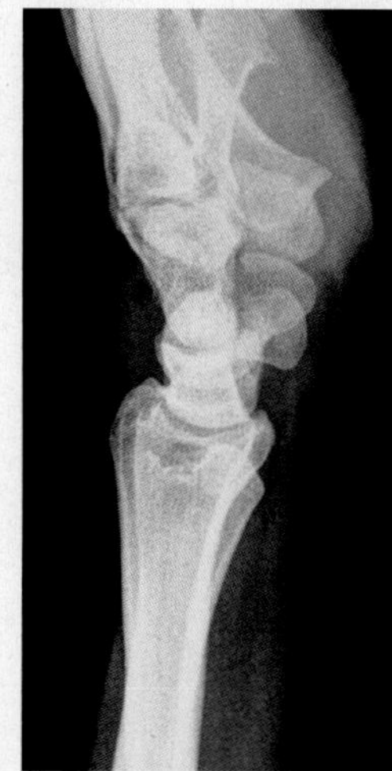

A B

FIG 1 • AP (**A**) and lateral (**B**) plain radiographs of a patient with scapholunate ligament tear.

study. However, the more important stabilizing dorsal portion tears were seen in zero of nine specimens.[10]
- Ultrasound: sensitivity 46%, specificity 100%, accuracy 89%[3]
- A negative result with various imaging studies does not prove an absence of ligamentous injury. Arthroscopy remains the gold standard for the diagnosis of SLIL tears.

DIFFERENTIAL DIAGNOSIS

- Dynamic SLIL instability or partial SLIL tear
- Radiocarpal arthritis
- Scaphoid fracture or nonunion
- Keinböck or Preiser disease

NONOPERATIVE MANAGEMENT

- Nonoperative management is rarely successful in treating dynamic or static acute scapholunate ligament injuries.
  - In one study, 0 of 19 patients with dynamic instability treated with immobilization, nonsteroidal anti-inflammatories, and activity modification had substantial reduction in symptoms even up to 12 weeks into treatment.[16]

SURGICAL MANAGEMENT

- Indications
  - Wrist pain with an acute tear (<6 weeks)
    - These patients may or may not have static radiographic changes.
    - If static radiographic changes are present, plain radiographs in radial deviation may show if the radiographic changes are fixed (and therefore are not amenable to soft tissue repair or reconstruction) or reducible in radial deviation (and therefore are amenable to soft tissue repair or reconstruction).
  - Wrist pain with dynamic instability
  - The authors advocate diagnostic arthroscopy before open treatment.

Preoperative Planning

- General or regional anesthesia
- Equipment
  - Mini suture anchors (1.5 to 2.0 mm)
  - Kirschner wire driver and smooth wires (0.045 and 0.062 inch)
  - Arthroscopic equipment (see Chap. 67)
  - Mini C-arm
- A preoperative examination of both wrists is performed and documented, noting passive range of motion, swelling, and the Watson scaphoid shift test.

Positioning

- The patient is positioned supine with a hand table.
- The bed is rotated 90 degrees so that the hand table extends away from the anesthesia team.
- The arthroscopy tower should be placed adjacent to the feet of the patient and be clearly visible to the surgeon.
- The mini C-arm should be free to move in and out from the opposite corner perpendicular to the patient.
- An upper arm tourniquet should be placed.
- The operative arm is prepared and draped. Slack is left in the arm board portion of the drape to allow the sterile wrist traction tower to slide under the arm above the elbow.
- The operative wrist is suspended in a wrist traction tower with appropriate traction.

Approach

- Arthroscopy is recommended before open repair because of the lack of diagnostic accuracy of available imaging modalities.
  - Wrist arthroscopy remains the gold standard for diagnosis of SLIL pathology and can confirm the diagnosis and degree of instability before making a larger skin incision.
- Geissler staging of SLIL tears[4] is covered in Chapter 67.

TECHNIQUES

Diagnostic Wrist Arthroscopy

- See Chapter 67.
- The 3-4 and midcarpal radial portals are used for viewing.
- The 6U portal is used for outflow (typically an 18-gauge needle with sterile intravenous [IV] tubing).
- The 4-5 and midcarpal ulnar portals are used for introduction of instruments.
- The SLIL is probed in the radiocarpal and midcarpal joints.
  - A 1.5-mm arthroscopic probe passable in the scapholunate interval and rotated 360 degrees is indicative of a grade III Geissler lesion.
  - A "drive-through" sign with a 2.4-mm arthroscope is indicative of a grade IV Geissler lesion.
  - Midcarpal arthroscopy most effectively reveals the degree of instability.

Direct Scapholunate Interosseous Ligament Repair

- Specific indications for direct SLIL repair with or without dorsal capsulodesis
  - Geissler III or IV complete SLIL tear
  - Injury less than 6 weeks old
    - It is rare that a repairable ligament is present more than 3 months after injury.
  - Minimal degenerative changes in the radiocarpal and midcarpal joints
  - Reducible static radiographic changes
  - Adequate SLIL tissue
- A standard longitudinal dorsal incision is made just ulnar to the tubercle of Lister with dissection to the extensor retinaculum.
- Flaps at the level of the extensor retinaculum are raised, exposing the retinacular edges proximally and distally.
  - Superficial radial and ulnar dorsal cutaneous nerve branches will be within these flaps.
- The extensor retinaculum is incised over the third extensor compartment, and the extensor pollicis longus (EPL) tendon is transposed into the radial subcutaneous space.

- The tendons of the second extensor compartment are mobilized radially, whereas the tendons of the fourth extensor compartment are mobilized ulnarly.
- Consideration should be given to performing a formal neurectomy of the posterior interosseous nerve within the radial floor of the fourth extensor compartment.
- The dorsal capsule and dorsal extrinsic ligaments (dorsal radiocarpal [DRC] and dorsal intercarpal [DIC] ligaments) are exposed.
- The dorsal capsule is incised, creating a 1- to 1.5-cm ulnar-based flap (**TECH FIG 1A**).
  - Leaving the capsule attached ulnarly provides a capsular flap available for capsulodesis or augmentation of the repair if desired.
  - This flap of tissue will parallel the DIC and include the capsule and portions of the DIC and DRC.
  - Alternative capsular flap designs may be used per surgeon's preference (see Chap. 69).
- With the scaphoid, SLIL, and lunate exposed, any arthritic changes, the location of the SLIL disruption (typically, it avulses off the scaphoid) (**TECH FIG 1B,C**), and any injury to the DIC ligament are noted.
  - In cases of high energy, the DIC may avulse off its scaphoid and lunate attachment.
- Joystick Kirschner wires (0.062 inch) are placed into the scaphoid and the lunate.
  - These wires are placed parallel to the scapholunate joint about 5 mm from the articular surface.
  - The scaphoid joystick should be angled distal to proximal and the lunate joystick should be angled proximal to distal (**TECH FIG 1D**).
  - The Kirschner wire joysticks are brought together, derotating the scaphoid out of flexion and the lunate out of extension to correct any dorsal intercalated segmental instability (DISI) deformity and reduce the scapholunate joint.

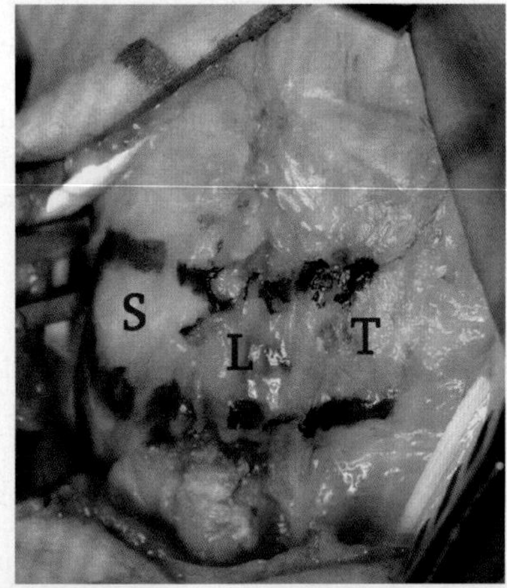

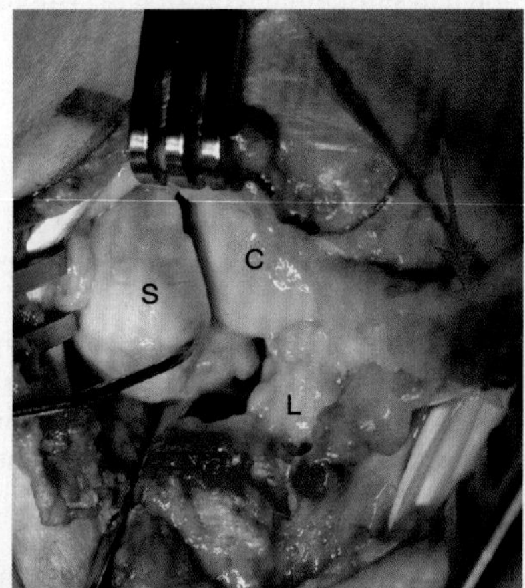

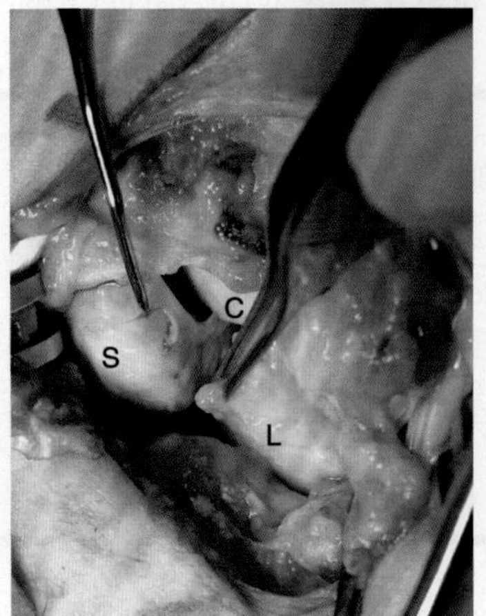

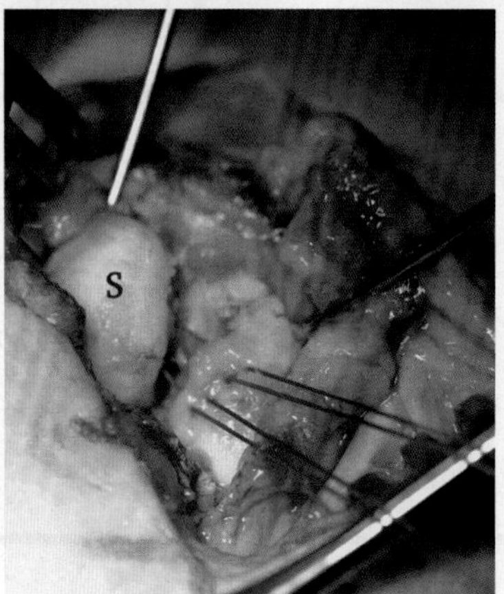

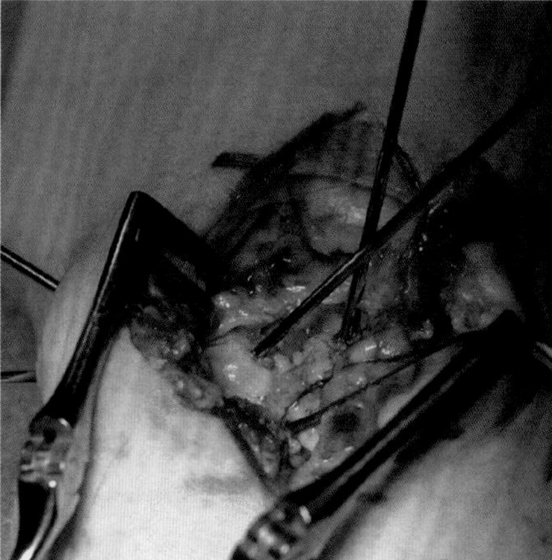

TECH FIG 1 • **A.** Intraoperative photo demonstrating the exposure and location of the dorsal capsular ulnar-based flap. The DIC parallels the more distal transverse limb of the flap. *S*, scaphoid; *L*, lunate; *T*, triquetrum. **B.** Intraoperative photo demonstrating the flexed scaphoid (*S*), the capitate (*C*), and the extended lunate (*L*). A complete disruption of the SLIL is noted. The *arrow* points at the ulnar-based capsular flap. **C.** Intraoperative photo showing the scaphoid on the *left* and the SLIL still attached to the lunate on the *right* (held by forceps). The capitate head is seen distal to the lunate at the *top* of the photo. **D.** Intraoperative photo after suture anchor placement into the scaphoid at the dorsal SLIL footprint on the *left*, then passed through the SLIL shown on the *right*. The joystick Kirschner wires are placed into the scaphoid and the lunate in such a manner that when they are brought together, the DISI deformity will be corrected and the joint reduced. **E.** Intraoperative photo after reduction of the joint and DISI deformity using the joystick Kirschner wires and suture repair of the avulsed SLIL. The Kirschner wires in the scaphoid and in the lunate have been brought together from their divergent positions and are now in the same plane, correcting the DISI deformity. The two Kirschner wires have been placed from radial to ulnar (seen on the *left* of the image), passing through the scapholunate interval and scaphocapitate interval. *(continued)*

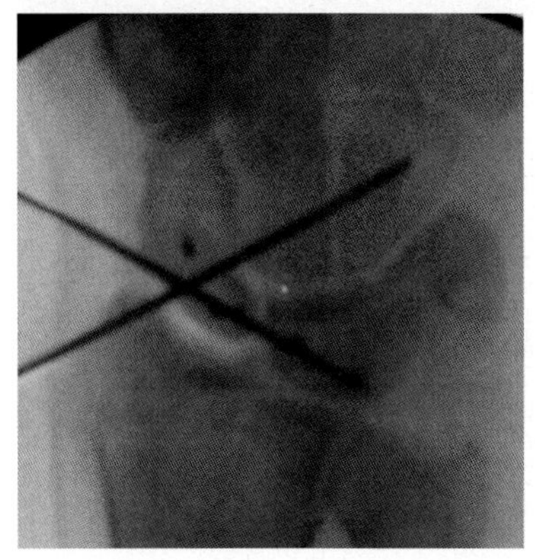

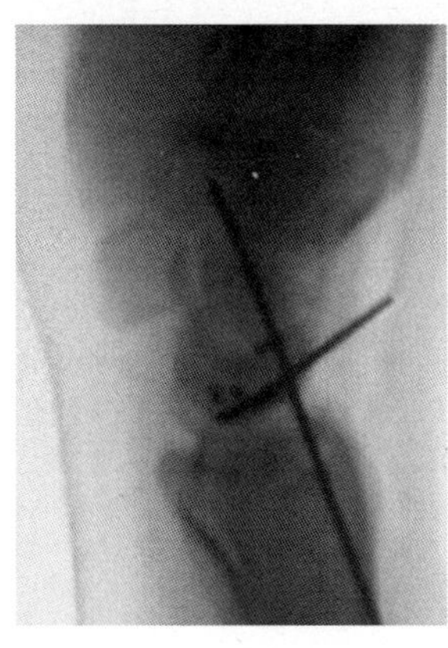

TECH FIG 1 • *(continued)* **F,G.** AP and lateral intraoperative fluoroscopic images demonstrating Kirschner wire placement across the scaphocapitate joint and the reduced scapholunate joint. Suture anchors can be seen in the scaphoid at the dorsal SLIL footprint. This example shows a third, more distal suture anchor at the scaphoid that was used for dorsal capsule augmentation.

- After reduction of the scapholunate joint, the anatomic insertion site for the SLIL is identified.
- The SLIL footprint on the dorsal ulnar portion of the scaphoid is roughened slightly to bleeding bone and one or more mini suture anchors (1.5 to 2.0 mm) are inserted.
- The sutures from the suture anchor are passed through the SLIL stump but are not yet tied (**TECH FIG 1D**).
- With the joint reduced via the joysticks, one or two 0.045-inch smooth Kirschner wires are inserted through the scaphoid into the lunate across the reduced scapholunate joint and one or two 0.045-inch Kirschner wires are inserted through the waist of the scaphoid into the capitate to control rotation (**TECH FIG 1E–G**).
- The SLIL is secured to the prepared site by tying the suture anchor sutures.
- The joystick Kirschner wires are removed and the remainder of the fixation Kirschner wires are cut below the skin.
- Suture anchors are placed at the DIC footprint on the dorsal more distal scaphoid should it be avulsed and need repair or should capsular flap augmentation be desired (see Direct Scapholunate Interosseous Ligament Repair with Dorsal Capsulodesis).
- The capsule is closed with 3-0 absorbable suture.
- The EPL tendon is transposed subcutaneously and the extensor retinaculum is repaired with 3-0 absorbable suture.

Direct Scapholunate Interosseous Ligament Repair with Dorsal Capsulodesis

- Indications
  - Tenuous SLIL repair
  - Chronic scapholunate dissociation (>6 weeks) without arthritis
    - The deformity must be reducible.
- If capsulodesis is required for augmentation, the SLIL repair is performed as described earlier, making the same ulnar-based dorsal capsular incision.
- After the SLIL is repaired, the ulnarly based capsular flap is advanced over the scapholunate interval toward its attachment to the scaphoid waist.
  - The flap will be secured under tension to further stabilize the scapholunate joint.
- One or two mini suture anchors (1.5 or 2.0 mm) are placed into the scaphoid at the determined location and another mini suture anchor dorsal central into the lunate.
- With the capsular flap pulled taut, the sutures from the scaphoid suture anchor(s) are passed through the flap. Then, the sutures from the lunate suture anchor are passed through the central aspect of the flap, selecting suture location to maximize stabilization of the scapholunate joint.
- Once all sutures from the scaphoid and the lunate are placed through the capsular flap, they are then tied down (**TECH FIG 2**).
- Alternative techniques of capsulodesis are described in Chapter 69.

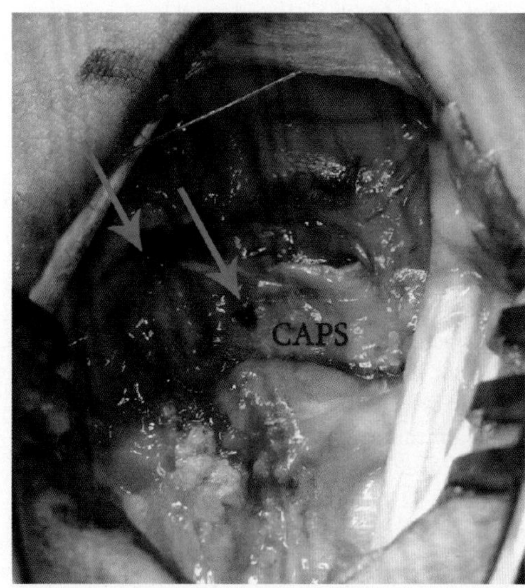

TECH FIG 2 • Repair augmentation with ulnar-based capsular (*CAPS*) flap. Note the suture anchor knots (*arrows*) and the location of the distal suture anchor at the scaphoid at the footprint of the DIC ligament.

PEARLS AND PITFALLS

Fluoroscopy	■ By moving the fluoroscopy unit perpendicular to the patient with the C-arm parallel to the floor and locking all the joints but the most distal fulcrum, the amount of "fighting" with the fluoroscopy unit is minimized. ■ Drape the fluoroscope and keep the C-arm parallel and elevated above the floor (this allows you to keep the fluoroscope sterile and above the hand table).
Buried Kirschner wires	■ Buried Kirschner wires require removal in the operating room but minimize the risk of pin tract infection.
Posterior interosseous nerve neurectomy	■ Neurectomy of the posterior interosseous nerve may be performed during the procedure. The nerve is identified on the radial floor of the fourth extensor compartment and cauterized with its accompanying vessel, then a 1-cm segment is resected distal to this cauterization.
Joystick placement during reduction of the scapholunate joint	■ The scaphoid Kirschner wire is placed distal in the scaphoid, angling proximally. Remember, the scaphoid is flexed and most of the cartilage seen initially is the radiocarpal articular portion of the scaphoid. Similarly, the lunate Kirschner wire is placed proximally, angling in a distal direction to correct its extended position. ■ The joystick Kirschner wires are placed in positions where they will not impede the path of the transarticular scapholunate Kirschner wires.
Kirschner wire placement	■ The fixation Kirschner wires are placed slightly volar to prevent interference with subsequent placement of the suture anchors. A 1-cm longitudinal skin incision with blunt dissection and a guide should be considered to prevent injury to superficial radial nerve branches.
Capsular flap creation	■ When performing dorsal capsulodesis, the flap of capsular tissue is designed to be at least 1 cm wide (providing a strong enough tether for the scaphoid) and to have adequate length to span the scapholunate joint and reach the scaphoid waist.

POSTOPERATIVE CARE

- The wrist is immobilized in a short-arm thumb spica splint immediately after surgery.
- Sutures are removed at 2 weeks and the wrist is placed into a short-arm thumb spica cast for an additional 6 weeks.
  - Radiographs are obtained at 2 and 4 weeks to evaluate reduction and any pin migration.
- Pins are removed at 8 weeks postoperatively and the wrist is placed back into a short-arm thumb spica splint.
  - Gentle active range-of-motion exercises are allowed at 8 weeks, with the splint removed for exercises only.
- Splint immobilization is discontinued at 12 weeks.
- Full activities are allowed at 4 to 6 months.
  - Forced hyperextension (push-ups) and axial loading are especially restricted during the 4- to 6-month postoperative period.

OUTCOMES

- Reported outcomes following early direct SLIL repair have been somewhat variable.
  - Bickert et al[1] reported their results after acute SLIL repair in 12 patients with a mean follow-up of 19 months. Excellent functional results were achieved in 4 patients (33%), good in 4 (33%), satisfactory in 2 (17%), and poor in 2 patients (17%), 1 of whom had developed lunate necrosis. Radiographic evaluation revealed a mean scapholunate angle of 55 ± 8 degrees and a mean scapholunate gap of 3.2 ± 0.8 mm.
  - Rosati et al[9] followed 18 patients after direct SLIL repair for a mean of 32 months. The Mayo Wrist Score at final follow-up was excellent in 13 patients (72%), good in 3 (16%), fair in 1 (6%), and poor in 1 patient (6%). Radiographic assessment demonstrated loss of reduction in only 2 patients (11%).
- Very good results have been demonstrated after SLIL repair augmented with capsulodesis. There is no evidence to support one method of capsulodesis over another when performed as an adjunct procedure to SLIL repair.
  - Lavernia et al[6] reported improvement of range of motion, grip strength, and pain in all patients at a mean of 33 months following combined SLIL repair and capsulodesis. Radiographic evaluation revealed a mean scapholunate angle of 57 ± 18 degrees and a mean scapholunate gap of 1.9 ± 1.8 mm. Degenerative changes developed in 3 of 21 patients, but no correlation between subjective pain scores and radiographic changes was found.
  - Outcomes after SLIL repair and capsulodesis have been shown to correlate with daily job requirements. Pomerance[8] demonstrated that at 5 years, patients with nonstrenuous jobs had less scapholunate gapping (on stress views), higher grip strength, and significantly lower pain scores than those with strenuous jobs. Patients who did not require forceful use of the wrist at work had better wrist range of motion and a rate of higher satisfactory results than patients who require forceful use of the wrist.

COMPLICATIONS

- Pin tract infections (this risk is minimized with buried pins)
- Superficial radial nerve injury
  - The surgeon should create full-thickness skin flaps when dissecting over the extensor retinaculum (thus protecting the superficial radial nerve branches within the flaps).
  - The surgeon should make a small stab incision to bluntly dissect down to bone to minimize risk of nerve injury during pin placement.
- Loss of scapholunate reduction
- Arthritic changes in the radiocarpal and midcarpal joints[13]

REFERENCES

1. Bickert B, Sauerbier M, Germann G. Scapholunate ligament repair using the Mitek bone anchor. J Hand Surg Br 2000;25(2):188–192.
2. Blatt G. Capsulodesis in reconstructive hand surgery. Dorsal capsulodesis for the unstable scaphoid and volar capsulodesis following excision of the distal ulna. Hand Clin 1987;3:81–102.
3. Dao KD, Solomon DJ, Shin AY, et al. The efficacy of ultrasound in the evaluation of dynamic scapholunate ligamentous instability. J Bone Joint Surg Am 2004;86-A(7):1473–1478.
4. Darlis NA, Weiser RW, Sotereanos DG. Partial scapholunate ligament injuries treated with arthroscopic debridement and thermal shrinkage. J Hand Surg Am 2005;30(5):908–914.
5. Geissler WB, Freeland AE, Savoie FH, et al. Intracarpal soft tissue lesions associated with an intra-articular fracture of the distal end of the radius. J Bone Joint Surg Am 1996;78(3):357–365.
6. Lavernia CJ, Cohen MS, Taleisnik J. Treatment of scapholunate dissociation by ligamentous repair and capsulodesis. J Hand Surg Am 1992;17(2):354–359.
7. Linscheid RL, Dobyns JH, Beabout JW, et al. Traumatic instability of the wrist: diagnosis, classification, and pathomechanics. J Bone Joint Surg Am 1972;54(8):1612–1632.
8. Pomerance J. Outcome after repair of the scapholunate interosseous ligament and dorsal capsulodesis for dynamic scapholunate instability due to trauma. J Hand Surg Am 2006;31(8):1380–1386.
9. Rosati M, Parchi P, Cacianti M, et al. Treatment of acute scapholunate ligament injuries with bone anchor. Musculoskelet Surg 2010; 94:25–32.
10. Schmid MR, Schertler T, Pfirrmann CW, et al. Interosseous ligament tears of the wrist: comparison of multi-detector row CT arthrography and MR imaging. Radiology 2005;237:1008–1013.
11. Schweitzer ME, Brahme SK, Hodler J, et al. Chronic wrist pain: spin-echo and short tau inversion recovery MR imaging and conventional MR arthrography. Radiology 1992;182:205–211
12. Taleisnik J. Post-traumatic carpal instability. Clin Orthop Relat Res 1980;(149):73–82.
13. Viegas SF, Patterson RM, Hokanson JA, et al. Wrist anatomy: incidence, distribution, and correlation of anatomic variations, tears, and arthrosis. J Hand Surg Am 1993;18:463–475.
14. Watson HK, Ballet FL. The SLAC wrist: scapholunate advanced collapse pattern of degenerative arthritis. J Hand Surg Am 1984; 9:358–365.
15. Weiss AP, Akelman E, Lambiase R. Comparison of the findings of triple-injection cinearthrography of the wrist with those of arthroscopy. J Bone Joint Surg Am 1996;78(3):348–356.
16. Wintman BI, Gelberman RH, Katz JN. Dynamic scapholunate instability: results of operative treatment with dorsal capsulodesis. J Hand Surg Am 1995;20:971–979.

Capsulodesis for Treatment of Scapholunate Instability

Angel Ferreres, Marc García-Elías, and Andrew Chin

DEFINITION

- Scapholunate dissociation (SLD) is the rupture of the anatomic linkage between the scaphoid and lunate and its subsequent progressive dysfunction, with or without carpal malalignment.
- Classical radiographic signs occur only when there is permanent carpal malalignment. This is preceded by complete scapholunate disruption together with failure of the secondary scaphoid stabilizers, namely the scaphotrapeziotrapezoid (STT) ligament, the scaphocapitate (SC) ligament, and the radioscaphocapitate (RSC) ligament.
- However, in many cases, only partial tears or ligament sprains occur and do not produce positive radiologic signs. These injuries are often seen only arthroscopically.
- Dorsal capsulodesis of the radioscaphoid joint was first described by Blatt.[2] Now it is one of the most commonly used techniques in the treatment of carpal instability. This procedure involves the creation of a dorsal capsular flap.

ANATOMY

- Scapholunate ligaments are divided into three fibrous structures:
  - Dorsal ligament
  - Volar ligament
  - Thin proximal membrane
- Anatomically, the dorsal scapholunate ligament is the thickest and shortest of the fibrous structures, measuring 2 to 3 mm thick and 2 to 5 mm long. Biomechanically, it is the strongest and most resistant to failure under load.[1] The radioscapholunate (Testut) ligament is only a path for vascularization and innervation of the scaphoid and lunate (**FIG 1A**).
- Scaphoid position and relationship with lunate and distal carpal row is maintained by the scapholunate ligaments and by the secondary stabilizers (STT, SC, and RSC ligaments), which prevent excessive scaphoid flexion. These are collectively the secondary stabilizers (**FIG 1B**).
- The flexor carpi radialis (FCR) tendon is closely related to the STT joint and acts as a crucial dynamic stabilizer of the scaphoid, preventing it from rotating into excessive flexion and pronation during grip (**FIG 1C**).

PATHOGENESIS

- Injury to the scapholunate ligaments occurs when the wrist is hyperextended, ulnarly deviated, and supinated during a fall on an outstretched hand. Because of the osseous configuration and disposition of the bones of the proximal carpal row, when the hand hits the floor, the tubercle of the scaphoid is pushed dorsally and extended. The lunate is held in position by the volar radiolunate (RL) ligaments and resists the tendency to extension transmitted by the scaphoid. The impact of the hand on the floor also pushes the pisiform against the triquetrum and because of the configuration of the joint between the triquetrum and the hamate, the former turns into flexion. If forces exceed the ligaments' resistance, they will rupture.
- The sequence of failure of the ligaments is from palmar to dorsal. The first to tear is the volar scapholunate ligament, the weaker of the two scapholunate ligaments, followed by the dorsal scapholunate ligament.[5]
- The participation of the dorsal intercarpal ligament (DICL) in scapholunate instability has been recently supported by the studies of Mitsuyasu et al.[13]

NATURAL HISTORY

- Most SLDs present as the initial stage of a progressive carpal destabilization. The mechanism of injury produces a spectrum of injuries, ranging from mild scapholunate sprains to complete perilunar dislocations, all being different stages of the same progressive perilunar destabilization process as described by Mayfield et al.[11]
- If only the palmar scapholunate ligament and the proximal membrane are disrupted, minor kinematic alterations result in predynamic instability. There is no gross carpal malalignment, but because there is an increased motion between the scaphoid and lunate causing shear stress, these injuries may be sufficient to promote painful synovial inflammation.
- Complete disruption of the scapholunate ligament complex leads to substantial alteration in kinematic and force transmission parameters (demonstrated in cadaver specimens) but not necessarily static carpal malalignment.[13,17] Dynamic instability may be the result. The scaphoid is unconstrained at the proximal end, resulting in increased RL motion and correspondingly decreased radioscaphoid motion. This is accentuated in a loaded wrist.
- When the secondary stabilizers start to attenuate after repeated use of the wrist, carpal malalignment develops, eventually resulting in static instability. Initially, the scaphoid is still reducible, but over time, it becomes permanently flexed and pronated (see Imaging and Other Diagnostic Studies).
- If the alteration in the motion of the scaphoid persists, the cartilage degenerates and arthrosis develops. This pattern of degeneration is known as *scapholunate advanced collapse* (SLAC).
- Once arthrosis is present, surgical techniques directed at replacing or reconstructing the injured ligaments are no longer options.

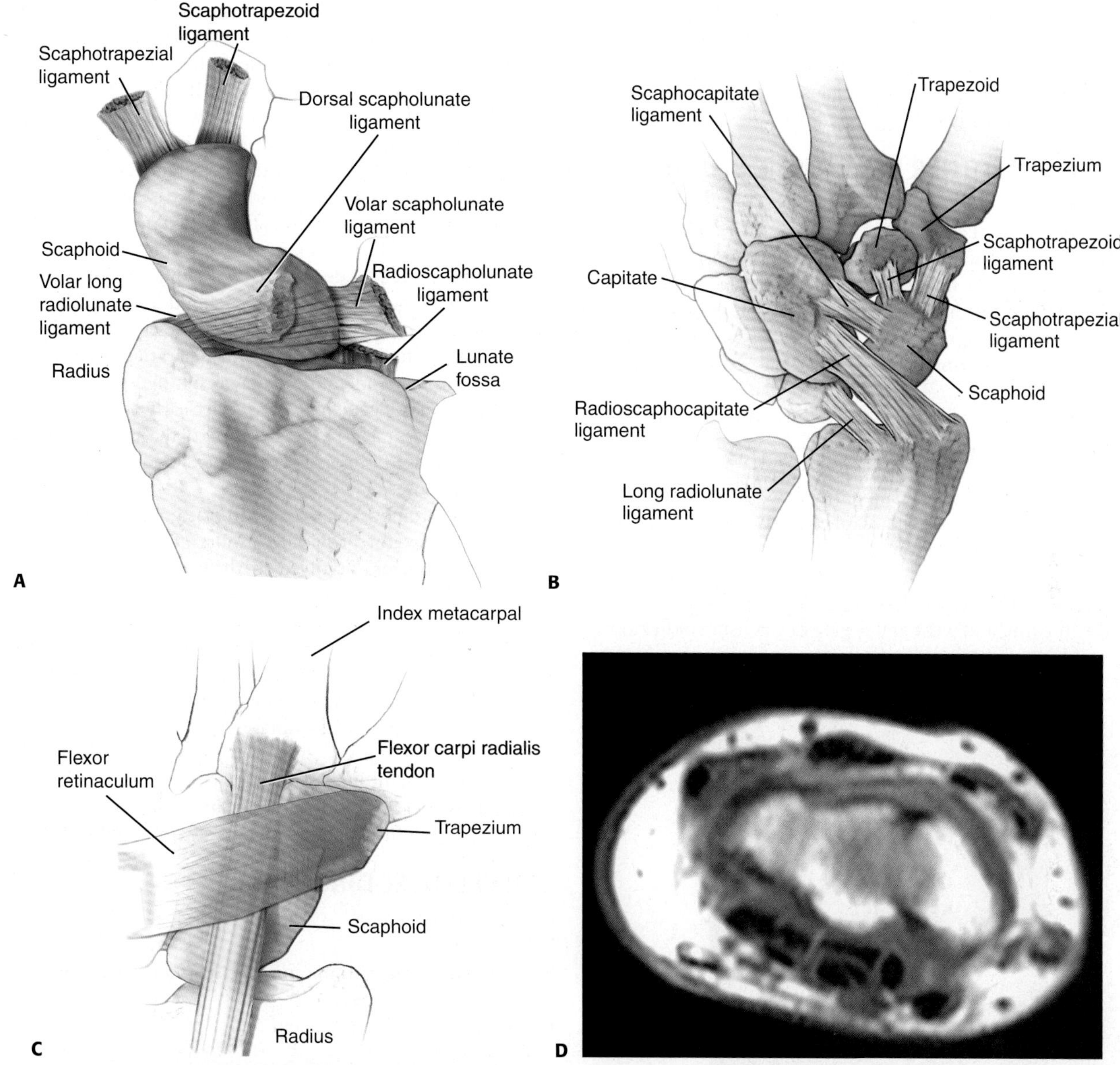

FIG 1 • **A.** The elements that maintain the scaphoid in its normal position. **B.** Volar view of secondary stabilizers. **C.** The dynamic stabilizer of the scaphoid. **D.** MRI vision of the dorsal and volar scapholunate ligaments.

- SLD is a progressive entity. Therefore, reconstruction is advocated as soon as it is diagnosed.

PATIENT HISTORY AND PHYSICAL FINDINGS

- Almost always, patients present after a fall on their outstretched hand. The patient complains of dorsal hand and wrist pain when loading the affected wrist, such as when standing up from a chair.
- Predynamic and dynamic stages of SLD are often missed or overlooked. The injury usually is the result of isolated trauma, which the patient does not clearly remember, or is masked by other more severe or obvious injuries (eg, fractured scaphoid and distal radius). A high index of suspicion is required.
- Weakness of grip strength, occasional swelling over the dorsoradial wrist, point tenderness over the scapholunate interval (more pronounced with gripping), and radial-sided wrist pain after excessive or heavy use are common but subtle physical examination findings.
  - The examiner should palpate the scapholunate interval dorsally (1 cm distal to the tubercle of Lister) with the wrist in 30 to 50 degrees of flexion.
  - On palpation of the anatomic snuffbox and palmar scaphoid tubercle, tenderness may also be present, suggesting ligament involvement, synovitis, or an occult ganglion.
- Provocative tests such as the Watson scaphoid shift test and resisted finger extension test reinforce the possibility of the diagnosis.
- Watson scaphoid shift test: The scaphoid flexes as the wrist goes from ulnar to radial deviation. The examiner's thumb prevents the scaphoid from flexing and if the scapholunate ligament is torn or incompetent, the proximal pole subluxates dorsally out of the scaphoid fossa, causing pain. When the thumb pressure is released, there may be a snap, signifying

spontaneous reduction of the scaphoid back into the scaphoid fossa. This test is not highly specific and may signify synovitis, an occult ganglia, or radioscaphoid impingement.

- Sharp pain on the resisted finger extension test has low specificity but high sensitivity.

IMAGING AND OTHER DIAGNOSTIC STUDIES

- Radiographs
  - Posteroanterior (PA) view
    - Elbow flexed at 90 degrees, neutral pronosupination, and the middle finger aligned with the forearm axis. The palm of the hand is in full contact on the film case.
    - Scapholunate gap greater than 3 mm or wider than the contralateral normal side and a cortical "ring" sign suggest SLD.
    - Decreased space between the radius and the scaphoid signifies cartilage loss and arthrosis.
  - Anteroposterior (AP) view
    - Forearm is in maximal supination.
    - This projection puts the scapholunate interval aligned with the beam of the ray.
  - Lateral view
    - Elbow at 90 degrees of flexion, middle finger aligned with the forearm, and wrist at 0 degree of extension or flexion
    - This projection allows measurement of the scapholunate angle. An angle greater than 60 degrees indicates disruption of the scapholunate ligaments and often corresponds with widening on the PA and AP views.
  - Clenched fist AP view demonstrates a widened scapholunate gap compared to the normal side (**FIG 2A**).
  - Cineradiography reveals abnormal movements between the scaphoid and lunate and an increase in the scapholunate gap as the wrist moves from radial to ulnar deviation.
    - Arthrography is not specific and may be positive in conditions such as degenerative perforations of the scapholunate membrane and osteochondral defects.
- Magnetic resonance imaging (MRI) does not provide much additional information. Minor, degenerative perforation of the scapholunate membrane may result in a positive test.
  - Scapholunate ligaments can be seen clearly only on transverse cuts that pass through the two horns of the lunate (see **FIG 1D**).
  - MRI plays an important role in excluding other differential diagnoses.
- Computed tomography scans do not give additional information except for providing a more accurate measurement of the parameters involved in the diagnosis of static SLD (eg, scapholunate distance and angle; **FIG 2B**).
  - It is useful in looking for other osseous anomalies of the wrist (eg, impacted fracture of the radius, scaphoid fracture).
- Arthroscopy is the gold standard for diagnosing and staging SLD. It allows grading of the instability (Geissler classification) and therefore determination of the degree of injury to the ligament complex.[5]
  - It is also useful in assessing the condition of the cartilage and in locating concomitant carpal injuries that might negatively affect the outcome of a capsulodesis (Table 1).

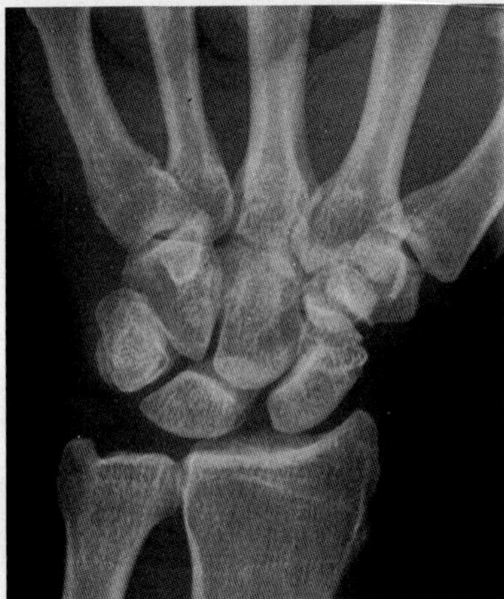

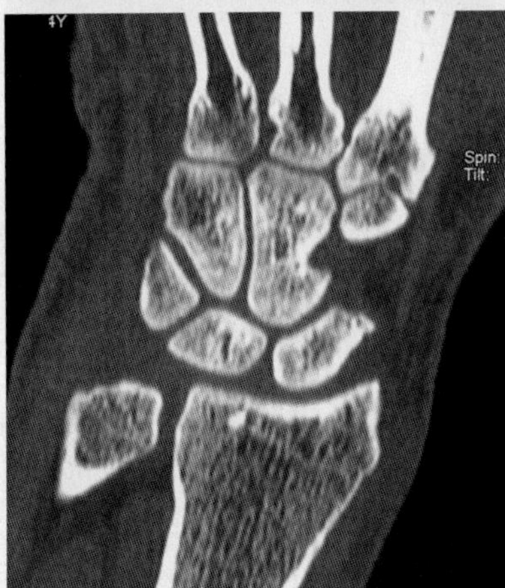

FIG 2 • **A.** Clenched fist PA view with the wrist in supination that shows a significant increase of the scapholunate interval space. **B.** Computed tomography (CT) scan of a patient with pain over the dorsal aspect of his or her left radiocarpal joint, showing a nonwidened space between scaphoid and lunate.

DIFFERENTIAL DIAGNOSIS

- Occult ganglia
- Synovitis
- Scaphoid fracture, nonunion, and avascular necrosis
- Radiocarpal arthrosis
- Radioscaphoid impingement

Table 1 Arthroscopic (Geissler) Grading of Interosseous Ligament Tears

Grade	Description
1	Attenuation or hemorrhage of interosseous ligament as seen from the radiocarpal joint. No incongruency of carpal alignment in midcarpal space.
2	Attenuation or hemorrhage of interosseous ligament as seen from the radiocarpal joint. Incongruency or step-off as seen from midcarpal space. Slight gap (less than the width of 1-mm probe) between the carpal bones.
3	Incongruency or step-off as seen from both radiocarpal and midcarpal spaces. The 1-mm probe is able to pass through the gap between the carpal bones.
4	Incongruency or step-off as seen from both radiocarpal and midcarpal spaces. Gross instability with manipulation noted. A 2.7-mm probe is able to pass through the gap between the carpal bones.

See also Chapter 68.

NONOPERATIVE MANAGEMENT

- Initial conservative management aims at resting the injured limb and decreasing edema. Adequate immobilization with casting or splinting is advocated.
  - This immobilization is frequently therapeutic for patients with predynamic SLD.
  - Elevation of the limb and active finger motion minimize edema.
  - Anti-inflammatory medications can be given for pain relief.
- Physiotherapy may have a role if Geissler grade 1 instability is diagnosed by arthroscopy. As the ligaments have not lost their integrity, a period of short immobilization (2 weeks), followed by proprioception reeducation of the FCR, as dynamic stabilizer of the scaphoid, is suggested.
- Nonoperative treatment is seldom indicated when a significant disruption is diagnosed.

SURGICAL MANAGEMENT

- Capsulodesis is part of the surgical armamentarium for the treatment of SLD. It is indicated for predynamic SLD, resulting from an isolated partial tear of the scapholunate ligament, and for dynamic SLD when the following criteria are fulfilled:
  - Complete disruption of all scapholunate components (palmar and dorsal)
  - Technically repairable dorsal ligament that has good healing potential
  - Intact secondary stabilizers
  - No cartilage degeneration
- Capsulodesis is not indicated when static SLD is present.
- Capsulodesis is used either as an isolated procedure together with Kirschner wire stabilization of the scapholunate joint in predynamic cases or in combination to augment a direct repair of the dorsal scapholunate ligament in dynamic cases.[6]
- Due to its structure and position within the wrist, the scaphoid has an inherent tendency to flex and pronate, especially when the wrist is in flexion and radial deviation. The capsular flap created during dorsal capsulodesis acts as a checkrein to tether the scaphoid, preventing it from going into excessive flexion and pronation.

Preoperative Planning

- All preoperative radiographs and diagnostic studies, especially arthroscopic findings, are reviewed.

Positioning

- The patient is under anesthesia and in the supine position with hips and knees flexed at 30 degrees for low back comfort. The arm is exsanguinated and the tourniquet inflated at 250 mm Hg.
- The arm is on the hand table in pronation, presenting the dorsal aspect of the wrist.

TECHNIQUES

Blatt Capsulodesis

Exposure

- The tubercle of Lister and the radial styloid are identified by palpation.
- An oblique skin incision is made following a line from a point 1 cm distal and ulnar with respect to the tubercle of Lister to a point 1 cm distal to the radial styloid (**TECH FIG 1**).
- Veins are coagulated or ligated.
- Care is taken to identify the branches of the superficial radial nerve and mobilize and retract them with the subcutaneous tissue. This is accomplished taking all the fat with the skin as a flap.

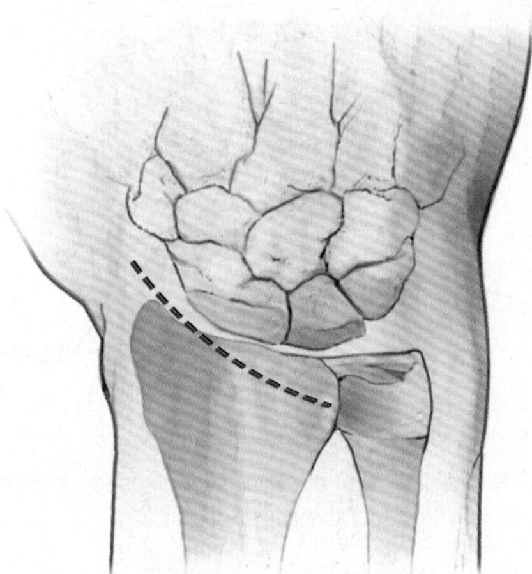

TECH FIG 1 • Incision site.

- Communicating vessels from the superficial layers to the deep arches are divided and coagulated.
- The extensor retinaculum overlying the fourth dorsal extensor compartment is incised. The extensor retinaculum is then raised as two flaps, radially and ulnarly based, to free the extensor tendons from the second to fourth compartments.
- A neurectomy of the posterior interosseous nerve can be performed at this point.
- The extensor digitorum communis (EDC) is retracted ulnarly and the extensor pollicis longus (EPL) and extensor carpi radialis brevis (ECRB) radially to expose the dorsal capsule.

Creation of the Capsular Flap

- A rectangular capsular flap, 25 mm long and 10 mm wide, is created by making a transverse capsular incision just proximal to the vascular dorsal carpal arch and elevating the tissue in a distal to proximal direction, leaving the proximal end still attached to the dorsal rim of the distal radius (**TECH FIG 2A**).
- As the flap is elevated, the scaphoid is exposed (**TECH FIG 2B**).
- At the dorsum of the scaphoid, a trough is created at a point distal to the axis of rotation of the scaphoid (scaphoid neck) (**TECH FIG 2C**).

Reducing the Instability

- If the instability is acute, a primary repair of the scapholunate ligament is performed.
- The space between scaphoid and lunate is reduced, using a 1.1-mm Kirschner wire inserted in the scaphoid as a joystick and then another Kirschner wire is placed in the scaphoid and fixed to the lunate.
  - This step should be performed under radiologic guidance. The scapholunate angle in which these bones are fixed should be 45 ± 5 degrees.

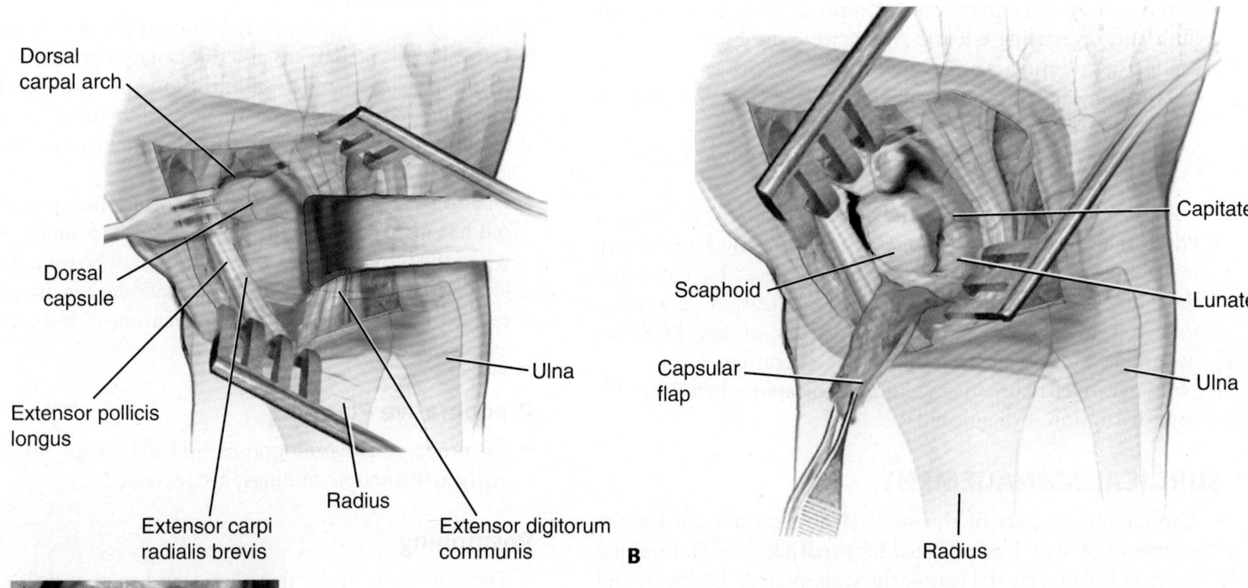

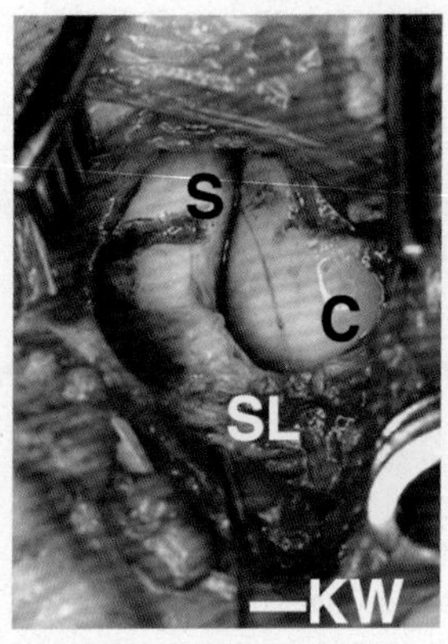

TECH FIG 2 • **A.** The vascular dorsal arch. **B.** Capsular flap is elevated, allowing visualization of the scaphoid, lunate, and head of the capitate. **C.** Intraoperative photo showing the scaphoid (*S*), the capitate (*C*), and the dorsal scapholunate ligament (*SL*). A bone trough has been created in the distal scaphoid for insertion of the capsular flap. *KW*, Kirschner wire in the lunate. (**C:** Courtesy of A. Lluch, Institut Kaplan.)

- When fixing the scaphoid to the lunate, ensure that the lunate is in a neutral position.
- If the capsulodesis is being performed for predynamic instability, the scaphoid is fixed to the lunate in its normal alignment. This is also accomplished by means of a Kirschner wire as described earlier.
- Another Kirschner wire is passed from the scaphoid into the capitate to avoid flexion and pronation (**TECH FIG 3**).

Securing the Capsular Flap and Wound Closure

- The flap is tightly inserted into the notch created on the dorsum of the scaphoid.
- There are two ways of securing the proximally based capsular flap to the scaphoid:
  - The flap is secured through holes created in the notch and transosseous sutures that are tied on the volar surface of the scaphoid tubercle.
  - The flap is secured to the sutures of a bone anchor (authors' preferred method) (**TECH FIG 4**).
- The dorsal capsule is left in situ. The extensor retinaculum is closed with resorbable sutures.
- Layered closure of the wound and skin is performed.

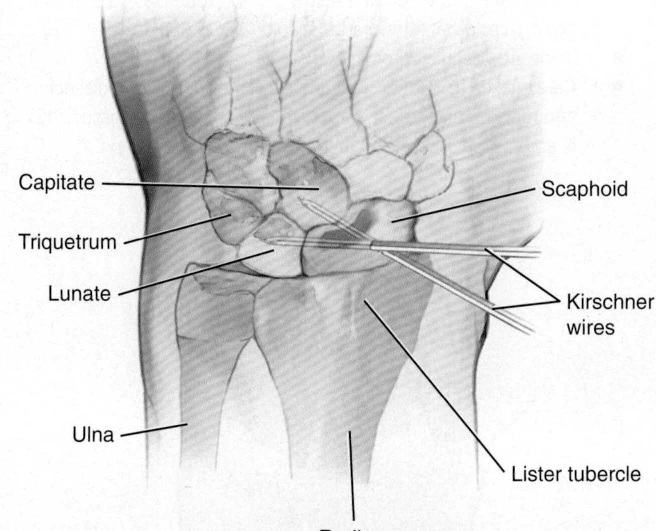

TECH FIG 3 • Orientation of the Kirschner wires recommended to stabilize the joints and protect the capsulodesis.

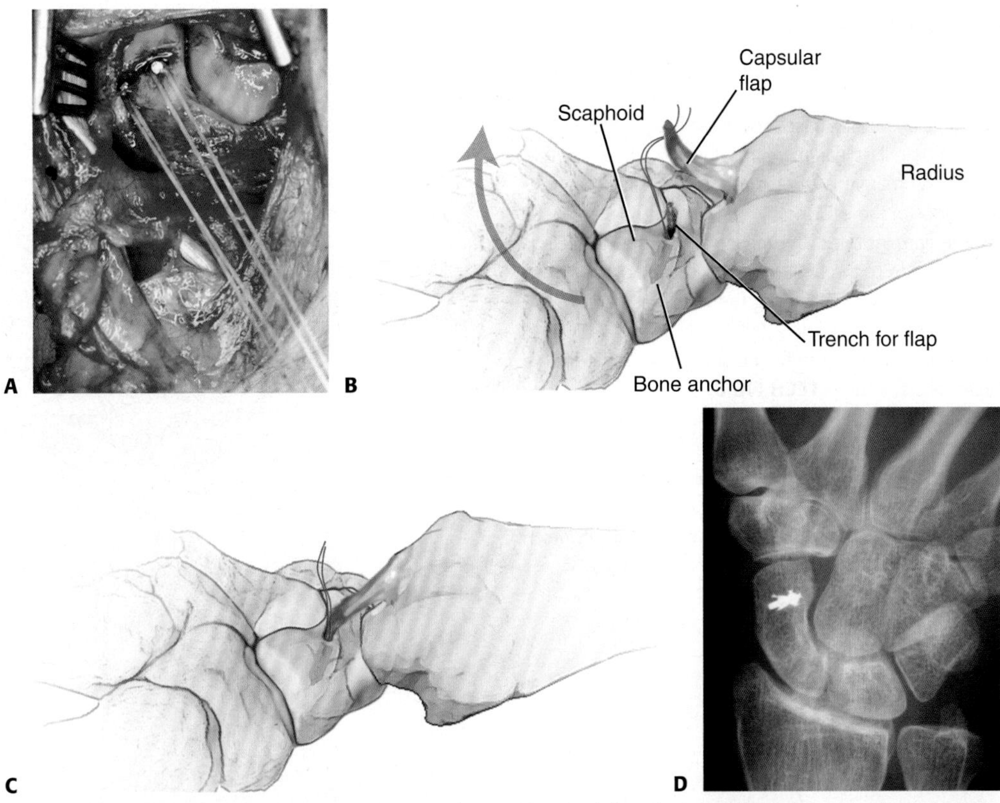

TECH FIG 4 • A. Placement of two bone anchors in the distal dorsal scaphoid. **B.** The proximally based capsular flap is prepared for insertion. **C.** The Blatt capsulodesis is completed. **D.** Radiographic PA view after eventual Kirschner wire removal showing placement of the metallic bone anchors. (**A:** Courtesy of A. Lluch, Institut Kaplan.)

Herbert Technique

- This method is very similar to Blatt's technique, the difference being that the capsular flap is distally based rather than proximally based.
  - There is no clear advantage to this technique over that described by Blatt.
- The same approach is used and the same capsular flap created, except that the tissue is left attached to the distal third of the scaphoid.
- The flap is incised at the radiocarpal joint, tensioned proximally, and anchored to the dorsal radius using a suture anchor. This force extends the distal pole of the scaphoid, reducing the scapholunate joint (**TECH FIG 5**).[7]

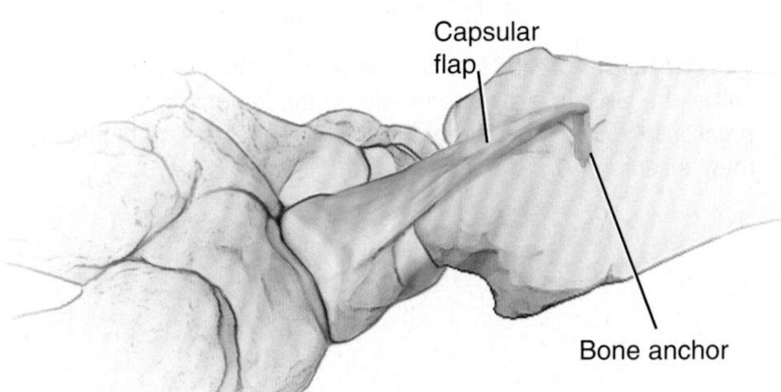

TECH FIG 5 • Drawing depicting the distally based capsulodesis described by Herbert.

Berger Capsulodesis

- Use the same approach and exposure as described for the Blatt capsulodesis.
- Raise a rectangular, radially based, capsular flap to allow exposure of the carpus. Its ulnar margin is the radiotriquetral ligament, its proximal margin is the radius, and its distal margin is the midsubstance of the DICL.
- This elevated flap includes the proximal half of the DICL. Separate this portion of the DICL from the capsular tissue in an ulnar to radial direction, maintaining the radial insertion of the ligament.
- Transfer this strip of ligament to the dorsum of the lunate into a prepared cancellous trough (**TECH FIG 6**).
  - This will create a link between scaphoid and lunate, preventing scaphoid flexion and pronation.
- The ligament is secured by tying to the suture anchor(s) in the lunate.
- This technique represents a variation of a previous version described by Taleisnik and Linscheid[19] and Walsh et al[21] in which the flap was attached to the dorsum of the distal radius.

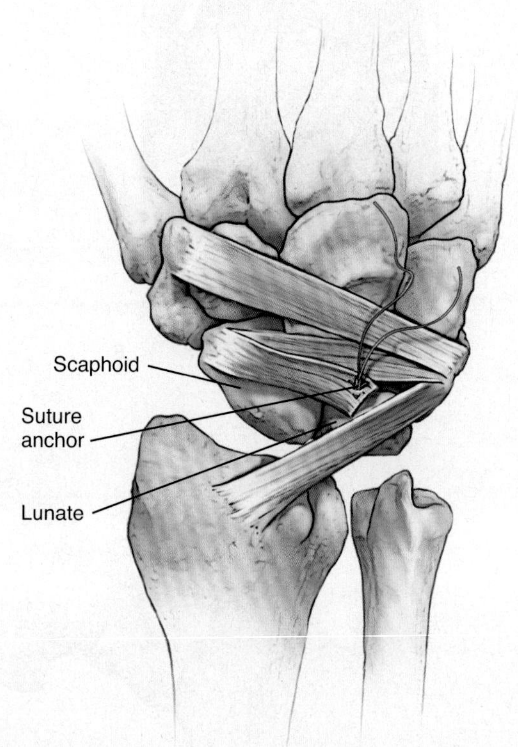

TECH FIG 6 • Berger's technique involves transfer of the proximal half of the DICL to the dorsum of the lunate.

Szabo Technique

- The DICL is used to stabilize the scapholunate interval as described earlier except the ligamentous tissue is ulnarly based and is inserted into the scaphoid rather than the lunate (**TECH FIG 7**).
- Typically, a longitudinal capsular incision is used to expose the carpus.
  - Care is taken to avoid incising the DICL.
- The DICL is defined and its proximal half separated.
- The radial insertion is incised at the level of the trapezium, trapezoid, and distal third of the scaphoid and then transferred to the scaphoid at the level of the scapholunate ligament insertion.
  - The transferred ligament may also be integrated into the scapholunate ligament repair more proximally.
- The transferred ligament is secured using suture anchor(s) into a cancellous trough in the scaphoid.
- Like the Berger capsulodesis, this technique does not specifically limit wrist flexion, as it does not cross the radiocarpal joint.[18]

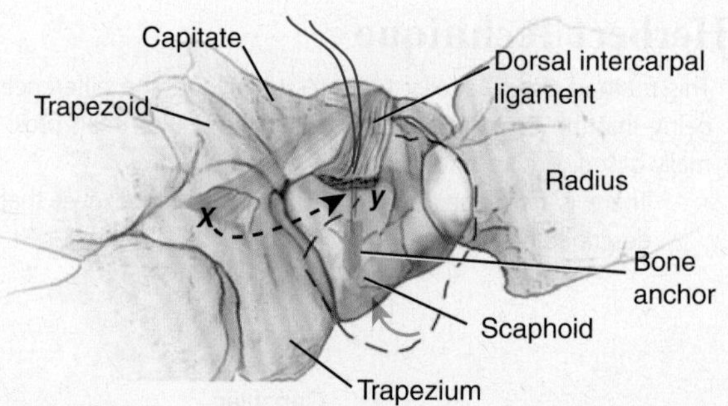

TECH FIG 7 • Szabo's technique involves transfer of the proximal half of the DICL from its attachment on the trapezium, trapezoid and distal scaphoid to the scaphoid at the level of the scapholunate ligament insertion (*y*).

TECHNIQUES

Viegas Technique

- It constitutes a third type of capsulodesis using the DICL. In this case, the proximal part of the whole DICL is displaced proximally but with maintenance of its radial and ulnar attachments on the scaphoid and the triquetrum, respectively.
- After reducing the SLD and stabilizing the bones with Kirschner wires, the elevated proximal part of the DICL is secured to the lunate and scaphoid with two bone anchors (**TECH FIG 8**).
- A third bone anchor may be used if the DSL ligament had been avulsed from the scaphoid or lunate to reinsert it on its original attachement.[19]

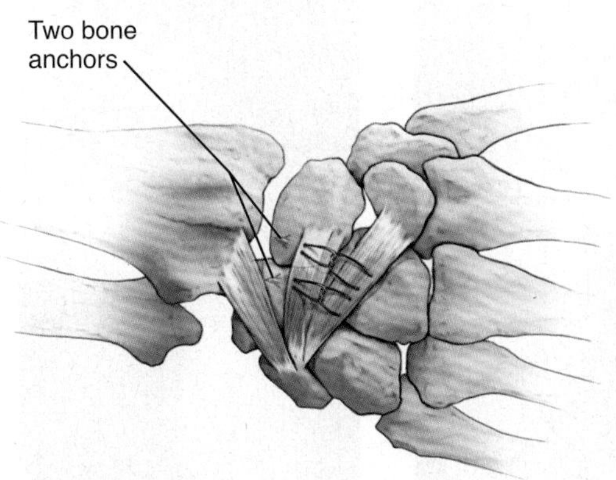

TECH FIG 8 • Viegas technique takes the proximal part of the DICL and fixes it to the lunate and scaphoid through bone anchors.

PEARLS AND PITFALLS

Indication	▪ This procedure should be used only in cases of predynamic and dynamic instability; it is not recommended for static instability.
Approach	▪ Dorsal and oblique from proximal to distal and ulnar to radial
Preparation of the flap	▪ Less than 10 mm wide is not adequate.
Preparation of the scaphoid	▪ Roughen the dorsal aspect of the distal third of the scaphoid. ▪ Use bone anchors; it is the simplest and fastest. ▪ If making holes for attaching the capsule, direct them distally to the tubercle. Then tie the sutures directly on the bone and leave the stitch under the skin.
Reducing instability	▪ If the lunate is not reduced, flexion of the wrist may be limited postoperatively. When securing the scaphoid to the lunate, be sure not to place the scaphoid in more than 70 degrees of extension. This will also limit flexion postoperatively.
Fixing the flap	▪ Tension is adjusted with the wrist in a neutral position.

POSTOPERATIVE CARE

- Blatt recommended wearing a thumb spica cast for 2 months, after which active range-of-motion exercises were begun. The Kirschner wires were left in place for another month before removal, allowing intercarpal motion at 3 months postoperatively. Forceful stress was discouraged for up to 6 months postoperatively.
- We prefer 6 weeks of immobilization in a rigid splint, avoiding extreme motions for one additional month. Kirschner wires can be removed at 8 weeks from the time of surgery.

OUTCOMES

- A number of clinical series have reported good results with these procedures.[2–5,7–9,14–16,18,22–24] The agreement of these series is that tensioning or augmenting the dorsal radioscaphoid capsule offers less surgical morbidity than other alternatives.
- At an average of 2 years of follow-up, these studies noted an absence of symptoms in two-thirds of patients, with 75% grip strength compared to the contralateral side.
- When examined with MRI, these patients demonstrate an increased capsular thickening that prevents rotary subluxation of the scaphoid but with the drawback of limiting wrist flexion by an average of 20 degrees.
- The long-term stabilizing efficacy of this capsule, however, has yet to be determined.
- Poor results have been reported in some series. This may be due to the use of the technique in cases of static instability or even in irreducible forms of SLD.[4,12,14,15,23,24] This procedure is not recommended if the SLD has progressed to the static form because the pathomechanics from the permanent malalignment will increase the risk of a failed procedure. Studies reporting more favorable outcomes are those in which capsulodesis is used mainly for dynamic SLD.[2,8,16,22] Most recent papers report less loss of wrist flexion after the use of techniques based on the DICL.[3,9,10,12,18,20] Long-term results are poor in static instability.[12]

COMPLICATIONS

- Reduction of wrist flexion (**FIG 3**)
- Failure
- Progression of SLD

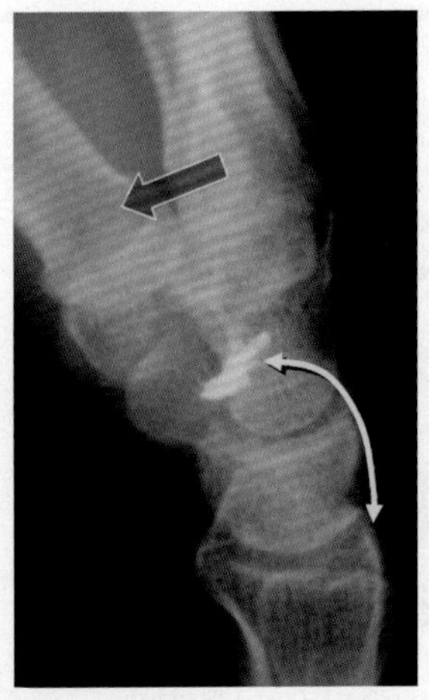

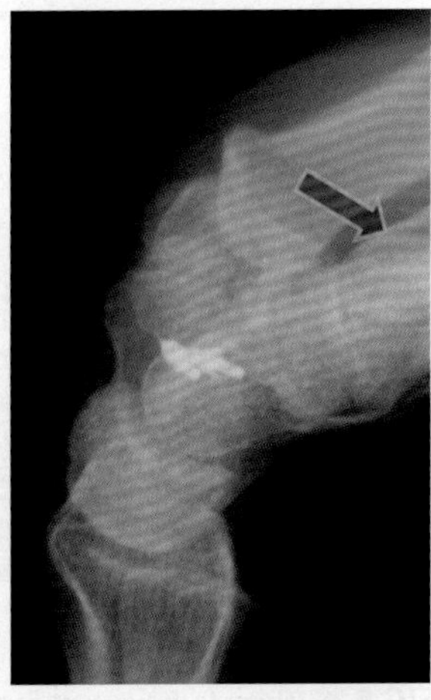

FIG 3 • A. The amount of flexion is reduced because of the dorsal restraint. The *yellow arrow* indicates the origin and insertion of the capsular flap. **B.** Extension is not restricted by the capsulodesis. *Red arrows* indicate the direction of motion.

REFERENCES

1. Berger RA. Ligament anatomy. In: Cooney WP, Linsheid RL, Dobyns JH, eds. The Wrist: Diagnosis and Operative Treatment. St. Louis: Mosby, 1998:73–105.
2. Blatt G. Capsulodesis in reconstructive hand surgery. Dorsal capsulodesis for the unstable scaphoid and volar capsulodesis following excision of the distal ulna. Hand Clin 1987;3:81–102.
3. Camus EJ, Van Overstraeten L. Dorsal scapholunate stabilization using Viegas' capsulodesis: 25 cases with 26 months follow-up. Chir Main 2013;32(6):393–402. doi:10.1016/j.main.2013.09.006.
4. Deshmukh SC, Givissis P, Belloso D, et al. Blatt's capsulodesis for chronic scapholunate dissociation. J Hand Surg Br 1999;24(2):215–220.
5. Garcia-Elias M, Geissler WB. Carpal instability. In: Green DP, Hotchkiss RN, Pederson WC, et al, eds. Green's Operative Hand Surgery, ed 5. Philadelphia: Elsevier, 2005:535–604.
6. Garcia-Elias M, Lluch AL, Stanley JK. Three-ligament tenodesis for treatment of scapholunate dissociation: indications and surgical technique. J Hand Surg Am 2006;31(1):125–134.
7. Herbert TJ, Hargreaves IC, Clarke AM. A new surgical technique for treating rotatory instability of the scaphoid. Hand Surg 1996;1:75–77.
8. Lavernia CJ, Cohen MS, Taleisnik J. Treatment of scapholunate dissociation by ligamentous repair and capsulodesis. J Hand Surg Am 1992;17(2):354–359.
9. Maillot-Roy S, Goubier JN, Dihn A, et al. Scaphotriquetral capsulodesis for scapholunate instability. Chir Main 2011;30:276–281.
10. Mathoulin CL, Dauphin N, Wahegaonkar AK. Arthroscopic dorsal capsuloligamentopus repair in chronic scapholunate ligament tears. Hand Clin 2011;27:563–572.
11. Mayfield JK, Johnson RP, Kilcoyne RK. Carpal dislocations: pathomechanics and progressive perilunar instability. J Hand Surg Am 1980;5(3):226–241.
12. Megerle K, Bertel D, Germann G, et al. Long term results of dorsal intercarpal ligament capsulodesis for the treatment of chronic scapholunate instability. J Bone Joint Surg Br 2012;94:1660–1665.
13. Mitsuyasu H, Patterson RH, Shah MA, et al. The role of the dorsal intercarpal ligament in dynamic and static scapholunate instability. J Hand Surg Am 2004;29(2):279–288.
14. Moran SL, Cooney WP, Berger RA, et al. Capsulodesis for the treatment of chronic scapholunate instability. J Hand Surg Am 2005;30(1):16–23.
15. Moran SL, Ford KS, Wulf CA, et al. Outcomes of dorsal capsulodesis and tenodesis for treatment of scapholunate instability. J Hand Surg Am 2006;31(9):1438–1446.
16. Pomerance J. Outcome after repair of the scapholunate interosseous ligament and dorsal capsulodesis for dynamic scapholunate instability due to trauma. J Hand Surg Am 2006;31(8):1380–1386.
17. Short WH, Werner FW, Green JK, et al. Biomechanical evaluation of ligamentous stabilizers of the scaphoid and lunate. J Hand Surg Am 2002;27(6):991–1002.
18. Slater RR Jr, Szabo RM. Scapholunate dissociation: treatment with the dorsal intercarpal ligament capsulodesis. Tech Hand Up Extrem Surg 1999;3:222–228.
19. Taleisnik J, Linscheid RL. Scapholunate instability. In: Cooney WP, Linsheid RL, Dobyns JH, eds. The Wrist: Diagnosis and Operative Treatment. St. Louis: Mosby, 1998:501–526.
20. Viegas SF, Da Silva MF. Surgical repair of scapholunate dissociation. Tech Hand Up Extrem Surg 2000;4:148–153.
21. Walsh JJ, Berger RA, Cooney WP. Current status of scapholunate interosseous ligament injuries. J Am Acad Orthop Surg 2002;10:32–42.
22. Wintman BI, Gelberman RH, Katz JN. Dynamic scapholunate instability: results of operative treatment with dorsal capsulodesis. J Hand Surg Am 1995;20(6):971–979.
23. Wyrick JD, Youse BD, Kiefhaber TR. Scapholunate ligament repair and capsulodesis for the treatment of static scapholunate dissociation. J Hand Surg Br 1998;23(6):776–780.
24. Zarkadas PC, Gropper PT, White NJ, et al. A survey of the surgical management of acute and chronic scapholunate instability. J Hand Surg Am 2004;29(5):848–857.

70

CHAPTER

Tenodesis for Treatment of Scapholunate Instability

Marc García-Elías and Angel Ferreres

DEFINITION

- Scapholunate dissociation (SLD) is a symptomatic wrist dysfunction that results from partial or total rupture of the scapholunate ligamentous complex, with or without carpal malalignment.[6,7]
- It may appear either as an isolated injury or associated with other local injuries, such as distal radius fractures or displaced scaphoid fractures.
- Usually the result of trauma (hyperextension and ulnar deviation injury to the wrist); SLD may also result from a chronic inflammatory arthropathy (rheumatoid arthritis, chondrocalcinosis).

ANATOMY

- Under load the scaphoid is inherently unstable owing to its oblique alignment relative to the direction of axial forces being transmitted across the wrist.[10] Under load the scaphoid tends to collapse into flexion and pronation. The magnitude of such rotation depends on the following factors:
  - The geometry of the radioscaphoid joint (the deeper the scaphoid fossa, the less unstable tends to be the scaphoid)
  - The stabilizing efficacy of the periscaphoid ligaments (proximal scapholunate interosseous ligament complex, dorsal scaphotriquetral [STq], palmar radioscaphocapitate [RSC], palmar scaphocapitate [SC], and lateral scaphotrapeziotrapezoidal [STT] ligaments)[10]
  - The dynamic action of muscles crossing the wrist.[8] The extensor carpi ulnaris (ECU) has a dorsal position at the level of the ulnar head while inserting at the anteromedial corner of the fifth metacarpal. Because of this obliqueness, when it contracts isometrically, it provokes pronation to the distal row relative to the radius. Other tendons (flexor carpi radialis [FCR], extensor carpi radialis longus [ECRL], abductor pollicis longus [APL]) have opposite obliqueness inducing supination. Intracarpal pronation tends to destabilize the scaphoid by pulling it away from the lunate. Therefore, the more effective the supinators, the more stable the scaphoid will be.
- The scapholunate interosseous ligament complex consists of three structures: the two scapholunate ligaments (palmar and dorsal) and the proximal fibrocartilaginous membrane.
  - The proximal membrane connects the two adjacent convex borders of the two bones from dorsal to palmar, separating the radiocarpal and midcarpal joint spaces (**FIG 1**).
  - The dorsal scapholunate ligament is formed by dense, slightly oblique connective fibers that link the dorsal aspects of the scaphoid and lunate bones.
  - The palmar scapholunate ligament has longer and more obliquely oriented fibers, allowing substantial rotation of the scaphoid relative to the lunate.
  - The dorsal scapholunate ligament has the greatest yield strength (260 Newtons [N] on average), followed by the palmar scapholunate ligament (118 N) and the proximal membrane (63 N).[2]
  - The proximal portion of the membrane often appears perforated in middle-aged and older individuals, which does not cause instability.

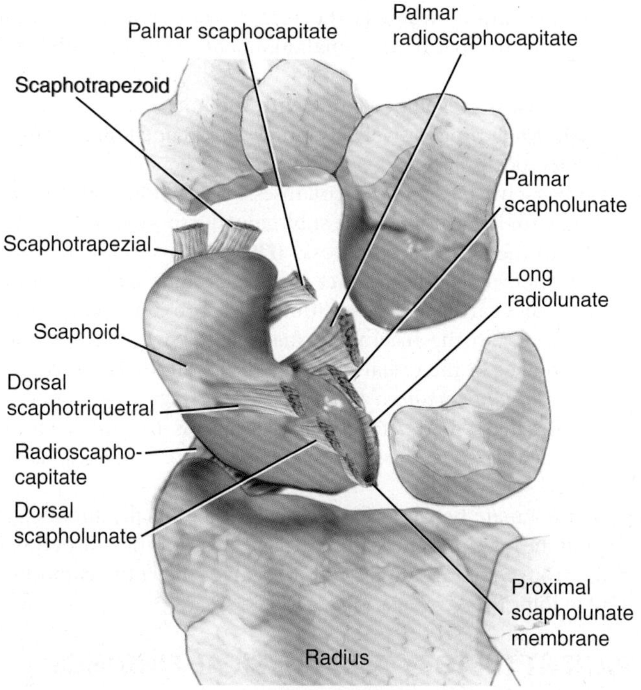

FIG 1 • Schematic representation of the periscaphoid ligaments seen from a dorsoulnar perspective. Both the lunate and the distal row have been drawn away from the scaphoid to better expose the ligaments.

PATHOGENESIS

- When axially loaded, the three proximal bones do not react equally in terms of direction of rotation. The scaphoid tends to rotate into flexion and pronation while the triquetrum is pulled into extension by the dorsally subluxing hamate bone (**FIG 2A**). If both the palmar and dorsal scapholunate and lunotriquetral (LTq) ligaments are intact, such differences in reactive motion generate increasing torques at both scapholunate and LTq levels, resulting in an increasing coaptation of these joints. Such an increased coaptation further contributes to the proximal carpal row stability (**FIG 2B**).
  - If the scapholunate ligaments are completely torn, the scaphoid no longer appears constrained by the rest of the

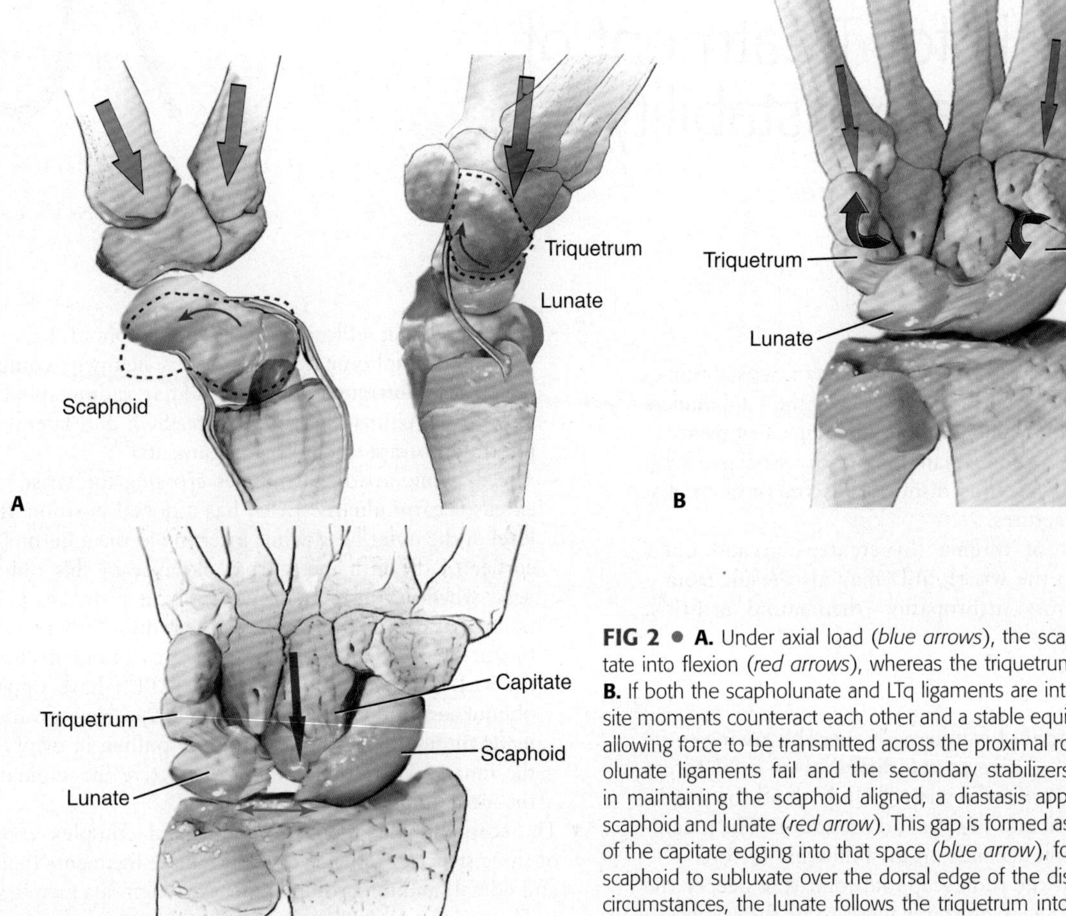

FIG 2 • **A.** Under axial load (*blue arrows*), the scaphoid tends to rotate into flexion (*red arrows*), whereas the triquetrum tends to extend. **B.** If both the scapholunate and LTq ligaments are intact, the two opposite moments counteract each other and a stable equilibrium is reached, allowing force to be transmitted across the proximal row. **C.** If the scapholunate ligaments fail and the secondary stabilizers do not succeed in maintaining the scaphoid aligned, a diastasis appears between the scaphoid and lunate (*red arrow*). This gap is formed as the consequence of the capitate edging into that space (*blue arrow*), forcing the proximal scaphoid to subluxate over the dorsal edge of the distal radius. In such circumstances, the lunate follows the triquetrum into further extension (DISI) and ulnar translation.

proximal row and tends to collapse into an abnormally flexed and pronated posture ("rotatory subluxation of the scaphoid").

- By contrast, the lunate and triquetrum rotate abnormally into extension, a pattern of carpal malalignment known as a *dorsal intercalated segment instability* (DISI) (**FIG 2C**).
- If, in these circumstances, the short radiolunate ligament is also torn or insufficient, the lunate will follow its natural tendency of slide down the ulnarly inclined distal radial surface and will appear translocated ulnarly and palmarly.[4]

NATURAL HISTORY

- Partial scapholunate ligament injury may not be radiologically demonstrable and may not produce symptoms unless the wrist is overloaded and/or there is poor muscle coordination in the stabilization of the carpal bones (predynamic instability).[11]
- If left untreated, a partial scapholunate tear may progress toward a more complete disruption of the three portions of the scapholunate joint, in which case, a symptomatic dysfunction usually appears.
- Radiographically, a gap between the scaphoid and lunate may be seen. This, however, is visible only under certain loading conditions (dynamic instability).
- With time, the secondary stabilizers (STT and SC ligaments) may stretch out and become inefficient. In such circumstances, the scaphoid may collapse into flexion and pronation, whereas the rest of the wrist may progress toward permanent malalignment (static instability) (**FIG 3A,B**).
- The wrist moves abnormally, with the lunate decreasing its range while progressively adopting an extended ulnar translocated position (DISI).
- Conversely, the scaphoid collapses into flexion and pronation, with its proximal pole subluxing dorsoradially over the edge of the radioscaphoid fossa (**FIG 3C**).
- The abnormal joint contact between radius and scaphoid may cause cartilage deterioration of the proximal pole of the scaphoid and the reactive formation of osteophytes at the dorsal edge of the radial styloid. This condition is known as *scapholunate advanced collapse* (SLAC) stage 1.
- If untreated, SLAC stage 1 may progress toward a more extended cartilage loss involving the entire scaphoid fossa (SLAC stage 2).
- As the lunate becomes fixed in DISI, the dorsally subluxing capitate may present with cartilage deterioration progressing from radial to ulnar until it involves the entire capitolunate joint (SLAC stage 3).

PATIENT HISTORY AND PHYSICAL FINDINGS

- Two clinical situations lead to a diagnosis of SLD. One is the patient who presents following violent trauma, such as a fall from a height or a motorcycle accident, who is likely

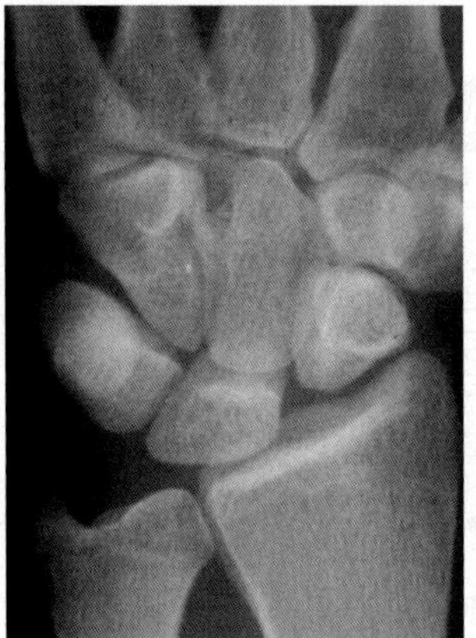

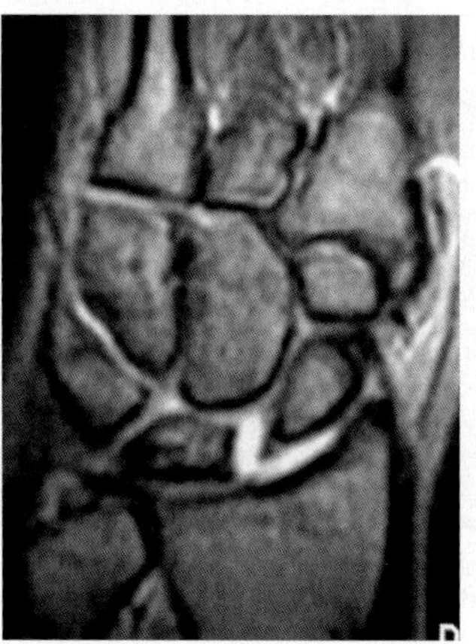

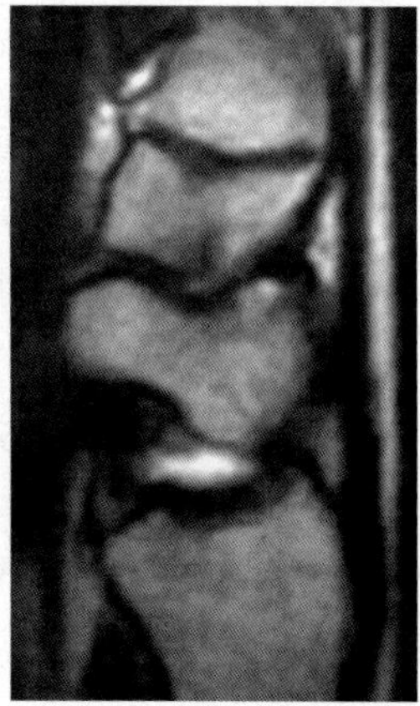

FIG 3 • **A.** Posteroanterior (PA) radiographic view demonstrating a scapholunate gap and a foreshortened scaphoid with the classic ring sign indicating static SLD. **B.** Coronal magnetic resonance imaging (MRI) showing the remnants of the disrupted proximal membrane hanging into the scapholunate gap, which is filled with fluid. **C.** Sagittal MRI showing the abnormal dorsal subluxation of the proximal scaphoid over the edge of the radius.

to have a major carpal derangement. Another is the patient who may not recall specific trauma and yet presents with symptoms.

- In the first case, the diagnosis of a major SLD may be obvious.
- In the second case, identification of the true nature of dysfunction may require a high index of suspicion, careful examination, and appropriate diagnostic tools.
- Not uncommonly, arthroscopy is the only way to fully assess the extent of ligament derangement (see Chap. 68).
- In both dynamic and static SLD, swelling may be moderate. In acute cases, range of motion may be limited by pain, whereas it may be normal in chronic cases.
- Scapholunate point tenderness: If sharp pain is elicited by pressing the scapholunate area—a relatively soft spot located distal to the Lister tubercle—the probability of localized synovitis is high. Not all synovitis represents an injury to the scapholunate joint, however. Occult ganglia may present with a similar type of pain on palpation.
- The resisted finger extension test[11] has low specificity but excellent sensitivity. In the presence of scapholunate injury, sharp pain is elicited at the scapholunate area, representing dorsal subluxation of the scaphoid.
- Scaphoid shift test[11]: If the scapholunate ligaments are completely torn, the proximal pole may sublux dorsally out of the radius in radial deviation, inducing pain on the dorsoradial aspect of the wrist. This test has low specificity: Occult ganglia, hyperlaxity, or radioscaphoid degenerative arthritis may produce similar symptoms.

IMAGING AND OTHER DIAGNOSTIC STUDIES

- Posteroanterior radiographic view of the neutral positioned wrist
- Increased scapholunate joint space compared with the contralateral side (Terry Thomas sign) suggests static SLD.
- A foreshortened appearance of the scaphoid with the scaphoid tuberosity projected in the form of a ring over the distal two-thirds of the scaphoid (ring sign) indicates rotatory subluxation of the scaphoid. The ring sign is not specific for SLD; it may also be present in static LTq dissociations and palmar midcarpal instability.
- Lateral radiographic view
- Increased scapholunate angle compared with the contralateral side. For this to be significant, the wrist needs to be in strict neutral alignment and neutral pronosupination and the angle needs to be greater than 80 degrees.
- Examination of the moving wrist with an image intensifier is always advised. Sometimes, the scapholunate gap only appears in one particular position and/or loading condition; replicating that particular circumstance while scoping the wrist may ensure that the suspected dissociation is, indeed, present.
- Arthroscopy is the gold standard technique in the diagnosis of SLD. It is also useful in describing the degree of injury to the interosseous ligaments.[6]
- Magnetic resonance imaging may provide useful information regarding ligament integrity, bone vascularity, presence of local synovitis, and other soft tissue status.

Staging

- SLD stage 1: partial scapholunate ligament injury, normal wrist alignment, usually diagnosed by arthroscopy, no abnormal scapholunate gap (Table 1)[5]
- SLD stage 2: complete scapholunate ligament injury, reparable; complete disruption of scapholunate ligaments, the dorsal one being still reparable, with good healing potential; normal wrist alignment
- SLD stage 3: complete scapholunate ligament injury, nonreparable, with a normally aligned scaphoid; dorsal scapholunate ligament with poor healing capability; normal carpal alignment
- SLD stage 4: complete scapholunate ligament injury, nonreparable, reducible rotatory subluxation of the scaphoid; complete SLD plus detachment of the dorsal STq ligament off the distal margin of the lunate, plus insufficiency of the distal scaphoid stabilizers (STT and SC ligaments); rotatory subluxation of the scaphoid; radioscaphoid angle greater than 45 degrees. The lunate does not appear ulnarly translated but only in slight DISI.
- SLD stage 5: complete scapholunate and radiolunate ligament injury, nonreparable, reducible rotatory subluxation of the scaphoid plus ulnar translocation of the lunate. The lunate is in substantial DISI and the radiolunate contact surface is reduced.[4]
- SLD stage 6: complete scapholunate and radiolunate ligament injury with irreducible malalignment but normal cartilage; fixed, irreducible long-lasting malalignment, without cartilage degeneration

Table 1 Staging of Scapholunate Dissociation

	I	II	III	IV	V	VI	VII
Partial injury	Yes	No	No	No	No	No	No
Repairable	Yes	Yes	No	No	No	No	No
Normal RS angle	Yes	Yes	Yes	No	No	No	No
Lunate aligned	Yes	Yes	Yes	Yes	No	No	No
Reducible	Yes	Yes	Yes	Yes	Yes	No	No
Normal cartilage	Yes	Yes	Yes	Yes	Yes	Yes	No

Modified from Garcia-Elias M, Lluch A, Stanley JK. Three-ligament tenodesis for the treatment of scapholunate dissociation: indications and surgical technique. J Hand Surg Am 2006;31(1):125–134.

- SLD stage 7: complete scapholunate ligament injury with irreducible malalignment and cartilage degeneration, chronic dysfunctional wrists with cartilage degeneration (SLAC)

NONOPERATIVE MANAGEMENT

- Acute, minimally dysfunctional SLD, stage 1, may respond well to a period of 3 to 5 weeks of wrist immobilization, anti-inflammatory medication, and subsequent physical rehabilitation.
- Proprioception reeducation of the so-called "intracarpal supinator muscles" may be helpful in minimal scapholunate dysfunctions.[8] Particularly useful is to extend and radially deviate the wrist against resistance (ECRL and APL isometric contraction). Optimization of the time response of the FCR muscle to wrist loading may also be useful in preventing progression of scapholunate ligament disruption (**FIG 4**).

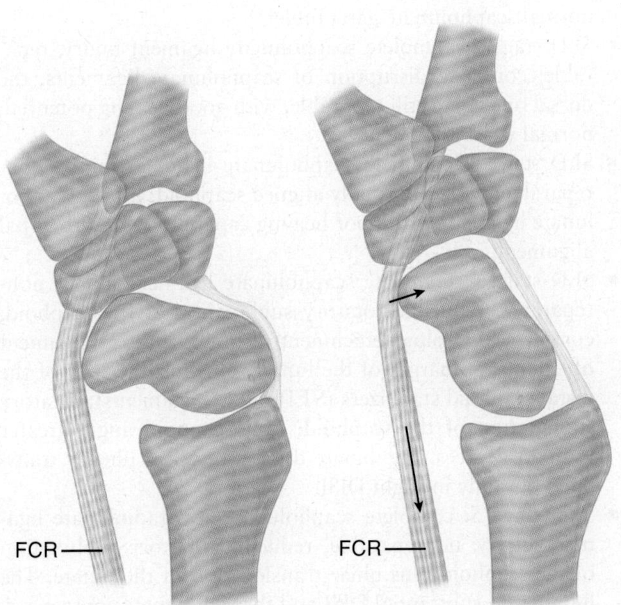

FIG 4 • The FCR tendon is in close relationship to the scaphoid tuberosity. Based on this, the scaphoid flexion tendency that appears when the bone is unstable can be effectively compensated by the dynamic action of the FCR muscle. Indeed, proprioception reeducation of this muscle may be useful in stage 1 SLD.

SURGICAL MANAGEMENT

- Partial ligament injuries may create discomfort from joint irritation by the ligament remnants. Arthroscopic débridement of these fragments may help eliminating symptoms.
- Electrothermal shrinkage of stretched scapholunate ligaments remains controversial. It has shown to be beneficial in selected cases of dynamic instability but there is no evidence of this effect to last long. Careful control of intra-articular fluid temperature is mandatory. Burns are not rare if lasers are carelessly applied.
- Excellent long-term results have been published on the treatment of dynamic SLD stage 3 by transferring the ECRL to the neck of the scaphoid and tenodesing the FCR. It is the so-called "Dyna-desis" procedure described by Seradge et al.[9]
- Tendon reconstruction of the scapholunate linkage is recommended only in SLD stages 3 or 4—that is, when there is a nonreparable complete scapholunate ligament injury causing carpal malalignment.[3,5] For this to be successful, however, it is very important that:
  - The malalignment is easily reducible.
  - The periscaphoid cartilages are completely normal.
  - The radiolunate joint needs to be stable, without ulnar translocation.
- If the radiolunate joint is unstable, tendon reconstruction of only the scapholunate joint is bound to fail. Stability can only be built on a stable bone. To solve a reducible, radiolunate–scapholunate instability (SLD stage 5), the so-called "antipronation spiral tenodesis" is recommended.[4]
- No soft tissue reconstruction can achieve effective carpal stability if the malalignment cannot be reduced with minimal force.
- Intra-articular fibrosis and capsular retraction are the most common causes of irreducibility.
- Heavy manual workers are not good candidates for tendon reconstructions; they may require a more solid form of stabilization, such as a partial fusion.
- Tendon reconstruction cannot solve the loss of protective capsular proprioception, and therefore, tenodeses are likely to deteriorate with time if chronically overstressed.

Preoperative Planning

- A complete set of plain radiographic views and stress views are mandatory.
- Arthroscans (tomograms taken after three-compartment injection of dye) are very useful to assess cartilage status.

- Best quality (ideally 3 Tesla) magnetic resonance imaging may provide useful accessory information regarding bone vascularity, synovitis effects, and soft tissue status.
- Arthroscopy is by far the best tool for preoperative planning.

Positioning

- An axillary block is used. The patient is in the supine position. The arm is exsanguinated.

Approach

- An 8-cm dorsal zigzag, lazy S, or longitudinal incision of the skin and subcutaneous tissue is centered on the tubercle of Lister.
- The dorsal sensory branches of the radial and ulnar nerves are identified and protected.
- The extensor retinaculum is divided along the third compartment and the extensor pollicis longus tendon is retracted radially.
- The retinacular septa between the second and fifth compartments are sectioned and the two retinacular flaps so created are retracted. Most septa contain intraseptal vertical vessels that need to be carefully coagulated (**FIG 5**).

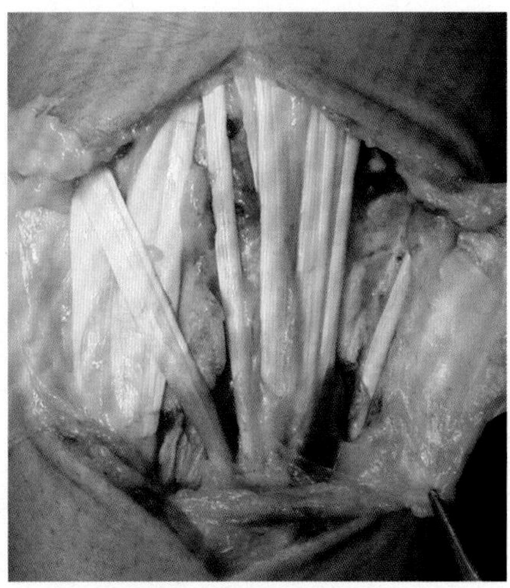

FIG 5 • Dorsal approach to the wrist through a longitudinal incision. The extensor retinaculum has been divided along the third compartment and retracted in the form of two flaps, radial and ulnar. Extensor tendons are uncovered.

Dorsal Ligament-Splitting Capsulotomy (Berger et al)

- The first incision is made along the dorsal rim of the radius to the center of the lunate fossa.
- The second incision is made from the end of the first incision following the fibers of the dorsal radiotriquetral ligament to its distal insertion onto the dorsal ridge of the triquetrum (**TECH FIG 1A**).
- The third incision is made from the STT joint progressing medially along the dorsal intercarpal ligament to its insertion onto the dorsum of the triquetrum.
- By connecting the last two incisions, a radially based capsular flap is created.[1] This flap is carefully elevated by sectioning its connections to the dorsal edge of the three bones of the proximal row (**TECH FIG 1B**).
- It is important to leave enough dorsal radiotriquetral ligament attached to the triquetrum in order to facilitate later tensioning of the tendon reconstruction.
- If the posterior interosseous nerve is normal, a modified capsulotomy may preserve capsular innervation. It consists of a proximally based flap, similar in shape as the one described earlier, except that the first incision along the distal margin of the radius is not done. Instead, a vertical incision connecting the lateral end of the transverse incision to the radial styloid is recommended. When this proximally based capsular flap is elevated, it needs to be detached from the dorsal edge of the proximal row (**TECH FIG 1C**).

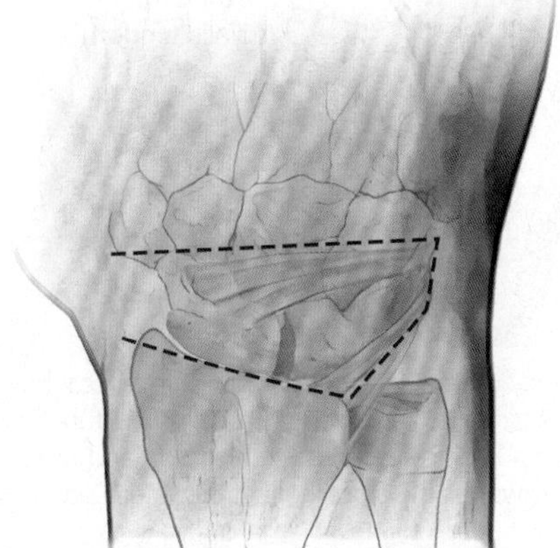

A

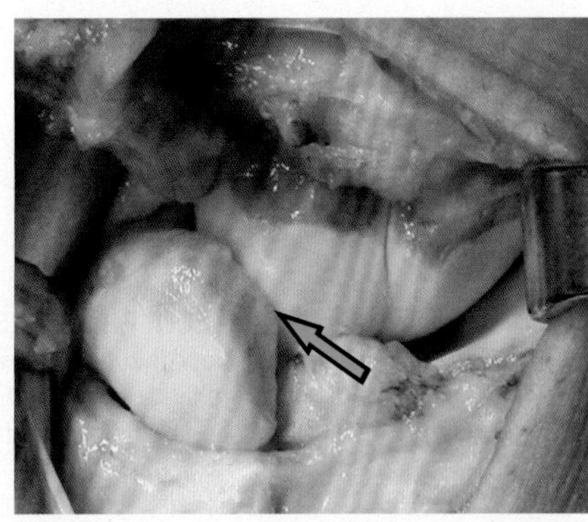

B

TECH FIG 1 • **A.** A radially based capsular flap is created by incising the dorsal capsule along the fibers of both the dorsal radiotriquetral ligament and the dorsal intercarpal ligament. **B.** Once the capsular flap is retracted radially, the scapholunate injury can be inspected (*arrow*) and a final therapeutic decision can be made. *(continued)*

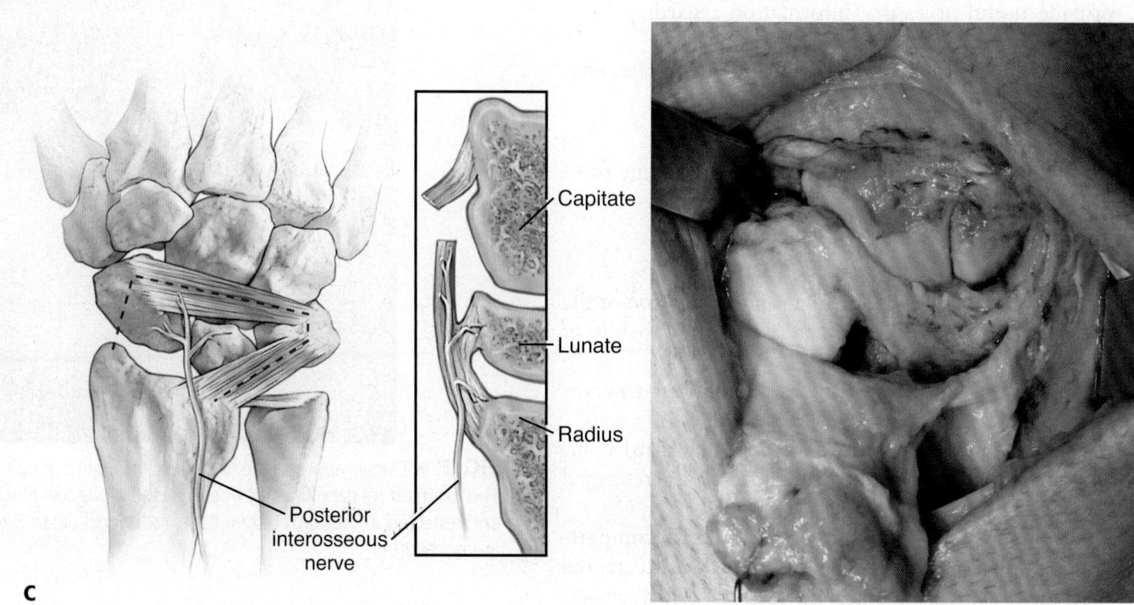

TECH FIG 1 • *(continued)* **C.** A proximally based capsular flap allows good exposure while preserving the integrity of the posterior interosseous nerve (*PIN*). It is a nerve-sparing capsulotomy. *Cap*, capitate; *Lun*, lunate; *Rad*, radius. (Described by Hagert E, Ferreres A, Garcia-Elias M. Nerve-sparing dorsal and volar approaches to the radiocarpal joint. J Hand Surg Am 2010;35(7):1070–1074.)

Palmar Scaphotrapezoid Plus Dorsal Radioscaphoid Tenodesis (Brunelli and Brunelli)

- Beginning at the level of the distal pole of the scaphoid, using small transverse palmar incisions along the course of the FCR, a strip of the FCR tendon is obtained.
  - The strip is incised at the musculotendinous junction and left attached distally.
  - The size of graft harvested depends on the size of the scaphoid and bone tunnel created.
- A 2.7- to 3.2-mm drill hole is started volarly at the distal pole of the scaphoid, entering at the front of the scaphoid tuberosity to emerge dorsally at the level of the scaphoid neck.
- Using a tendon passer or a wire loop, the tendon strip is passed through the bone tunnel.
- While maintaining the proximal pole of the scaphoid reduced on its fossa, two Kirschner wires are passed across the SC joint.
- Fluoroscopic assessment of reduction is important. Slight overreduction (radioscaphoid angle of about 60 degrees) is recommended.
  - Later stretch of the tenodesis is likely, in which case the scaphoid will recover its ideal alignment of 45 degrees.
- While the wrist is maintained in neutral position, the tendon is tightly anchored to the area of the tubercle of Lister using transosseous nonabsorbable sutures or metal suture anchors (**TECH FIG 2**).
- The capsular flap is passed underneath the tenodesis and reattached to its origins by absorbable sutures.
- The extensor retinaculum is repaired, leaving subretinacular drains. The extensor pollicis longus is usually left superficial to the extensor retinaculum.

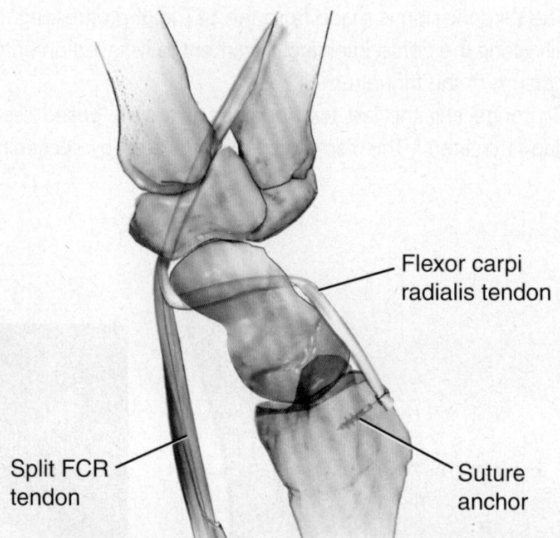

TECH FIG 2 • Schematic representation of the palmar scaphotrapezoid plus dorsal radioscaphoid tenodesis (Brunelli and Brunelli's technique) as seen from a lateral view. Note the location and direction of the bone tunnel as well as the placement of the suture anchor.

Three-Ligament Tenodesis (Modified Brunelli's Tenodesis)

- The transscaphoid tunnel is not transverse across the distal scaphoid (as detailed earlier) but oblique along the longitudinal axis of bone, from dorsal to palmar, entering at the level of the original insertion site of the dorsal scapholunate ligament, aiming at the palmar tuberosity (**TECH FIG 3A**).
  - So as not to damage the medial or lateral articular surfaces of the scaphoid, we recommend using a 2.7- to 3.2-mm cannulated drill over a Kirschner wire preset under fluoroscopy control.
- The FCR tendon strip is passed through the oblique scaphoid tunnel using a wire loop or a tendon passer (**TECH FIG 3B**).
- A transverse trough or channel is then made over the dorsum of the lunate with a rongeur. This trough needs to uncover cancellous bone, the only tissue able to generate proper healing of the tendon into bone (**TECH FIG 3C**).
- To obtain intimate contact between the tendon strip and the lunate cancellous bone, a small anchor suture is placed into the floor of the trough.
- The distal end of the dorsal radiotriquetral ligament is then localized. By its insertion on the bone, a slit is created through which the tendon strip is passed volar to dorsal (**TECH FIG 3D**).
  - The dorsal radiotriquetral ligament is used as a pulley to tension the ligament strip.
- The scaphoid, lunate, and capitate are reduced and stabilized with two 1.5-mm Kirschner wires prior to tensioning the tendon graft. One wire is placed across the scapholunate joint and one across the SC joint.
  - It is critical to ensure reduction of the scaphoid and the lunate, elimination of any DISI deformity, and proper placement of the wires using fluoroscopy.
- Radially directed tension is applied to the tendon graft already placed around and through the dorsal radiotriquetral ligament (**TECH FIG 3E**).
- The tendon graft is secured tightly into the cancellous bone channel created in the lunate (**TECH FIG 3F**).
- The end of the tendon strip is sutured onto itself with nonabsorbable 3-0 sutures (**TECH FIG 3G,H**).
- The capsular flap is brought back, over the tendon reconstruction, to its original position by suturing side by side the split fibers of the two ligaments involved in the capsulotomy. Some sutures are also placed connecting the capsule and the tendon loop to reestablish the normal capsular attachment to the dorsum of the scapholunate joint.
- The extensor retinaculum is finally reconstructed, drains are placed, and the skin is closed.

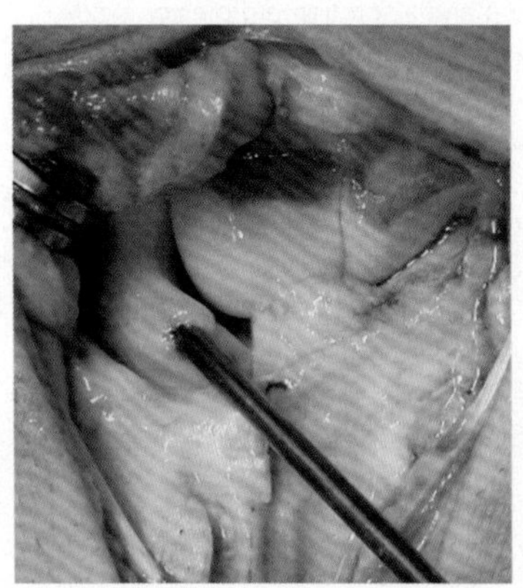

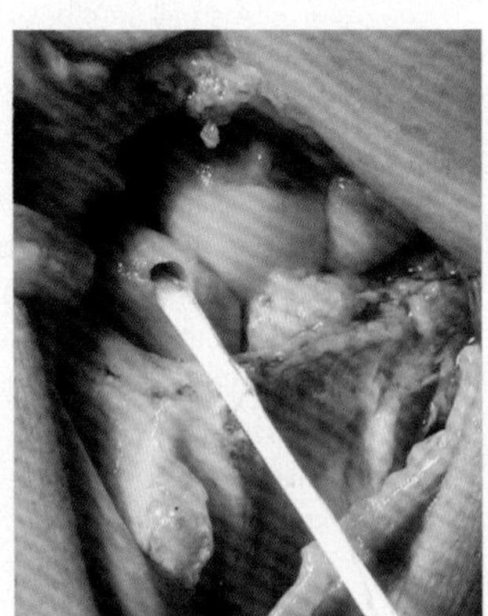

TECH FIG 3 • **A.** A 2.7-mm drill is used to create an oblique tunnel that enters the scaphoid beginning at the site where the dorsal scapholunate ligament originally inserted. The drill exits the scaphoid at the palmar scaphoid tubercle. **B.** With a tendon passer or a wire loop, the strip of FCR tendon is brought through the bone tunnel exiting dorsally. **C.** The strip of FCR tendon has been passed through the scaphoid tunnel. A trough has been carved onto the dorsal cortex of the lunate and a suture anchor inserted at that location. A slit has been developed along the fibers of the dorsal radiotriquetral ligament. **D.** The strip of FCR tendon has been passed through the ligament rent created along the fibers of the dorsal radiotriquetral ligament. **E.** The strip of FCR tendon is tensioned in a radial direction using the dorsal radiotriquetral ligament as a pulley. *(continued)*

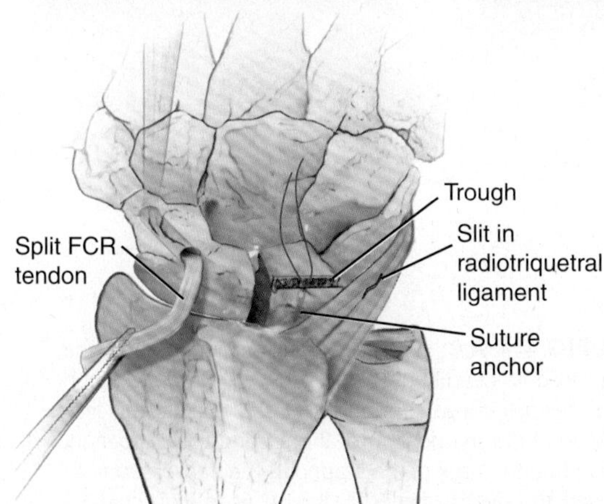

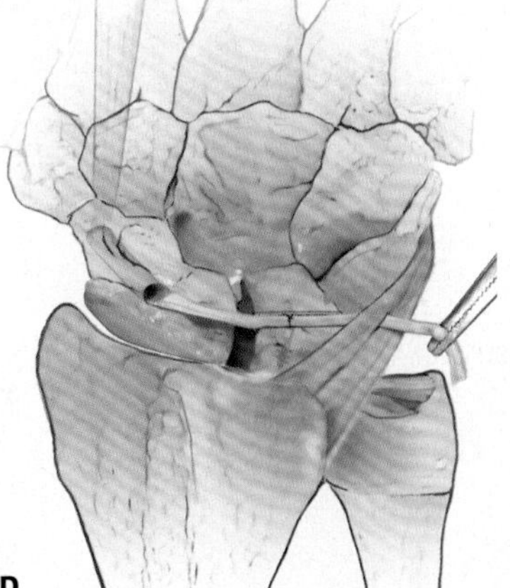

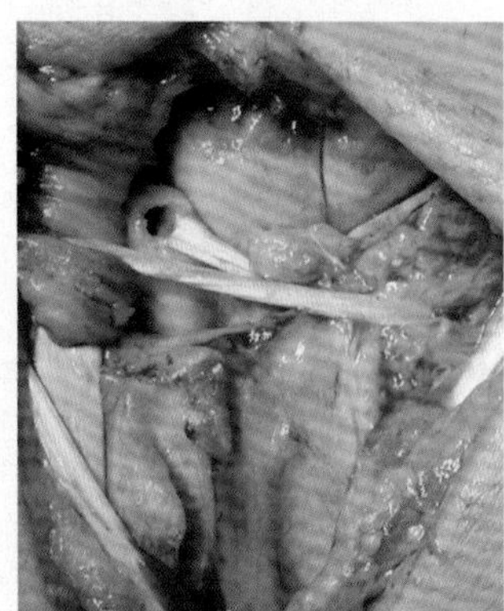

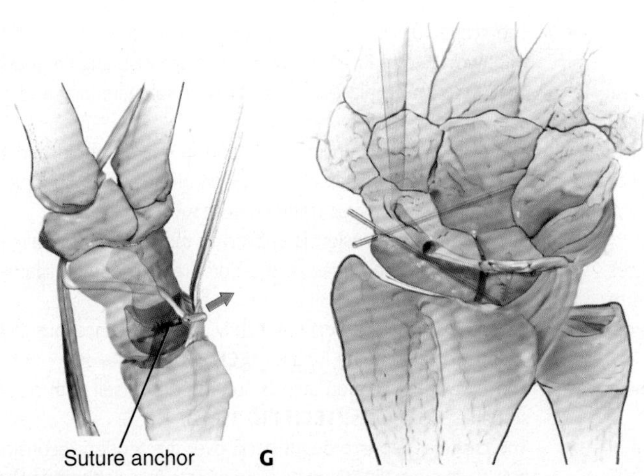

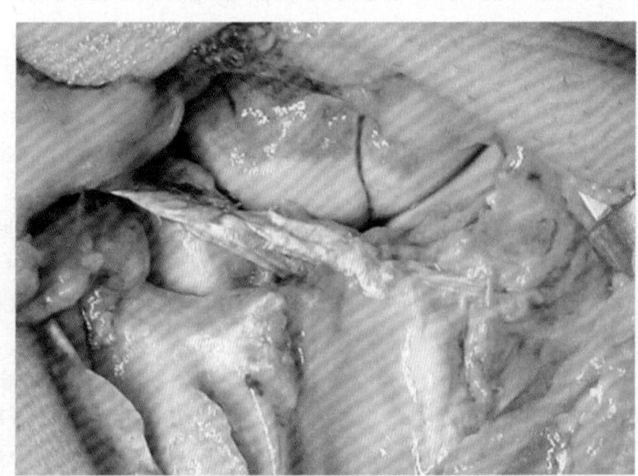

TECH FIG 3 • *(continued)* **F.** Lateral depiction of the tendon graft secured to the dorsal lunate using the suture anchor. **G.** After stabilization of the scaphoid, lunate, and capitate with two Kirschner wires; tensioning of the graft; and suturing of the graft into the lunate trough, the strip of FCR tendon is sutured back to itself. **H.** Final clinical appearance of the tenodesis.

Scaphoid Dyna-desis[9]

- The goal of the so-called Dyna-desis is to reduce and maintain the scaphoid at its normal 45 degrees alignment relative to the radius. This technique does nothing to realign the lunate, should this be in DISI. Therefore, the procedure is only indicated for the dynamic SLD stage 2 or 3.
- It combines two tendons, the ECRL and the FCR. The first is converted into an active scaphoid extensor and the second into a passive tether connecting palmarly the palmar scaphoid tuberosity to the base of the second metacarpal.
- Two incisions are needed: a dorsolateral longitudinal, zigzag, or lazy S incision over the STT joint and a palmar incision at the level of the scaphoid tuberosity.
- Through the first incision, the dorsum of the neck of the scaphoid is decorticated and two dorsopalmar drill holes across the distal scaphoid are made, aiming at the FCR tendon compartment.
- Through the same incision, the ECRL tendon is identified and sectioned at the level of the second carpometacarpal joint.
- Through the palmar incision, the FCR tendon is identified at the medial corner of the scaphoid tuberosity and its sheath is excised for about 3 to 4 mm.
- The scaphoid is then manually reduced by pushing its proximal pole palmarly and its palmar tuberosity dorsally.
- While holding this position, two 1.2-mm Kirschner wires are inserted across the SC, entered distal to the radial styloid.
  - A small snuffbox incision and a soft tissue protector is advised not to injure the dorsal branches of the radial nerve with the wires.
- A nonabsorbable 1-0 suture is then sewn across the FCR tendon, advanced through one of the scaphoid holes, through the end of the transected ECRL, and then back to the volar incision through the second scaphoid drill hole. By tying the two ends of this suture, the ECRL is attached to the neck of the scaphoid and the FCR to the medial corner of the scaphoid tuberosity (**TECH FIG 4**). The first is aimed at extending dynamically the scaphoid; the second will act as a tether preventing scaphoid flexion.

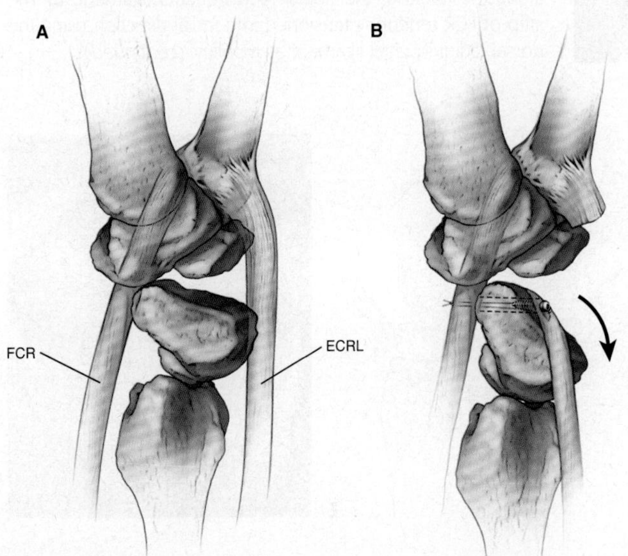

TECH FIG 4 • **A,B.** Schematic representation of the Dynadesis procedure described by Seradge et al.[9] Once the scaphoid has been reduced (*arrow*), the ECRL is detached from its insertion onto the dorsum of the second metacarpal and transferred to the neck of the scaphoid. The transosseous suture used to reattach the ECRL is also used to secure the FCR tendon to the scaphoid in order to create a palmar distal tenodesis effect that prevents scaphoid flexion.

Antipronation Spiral Tenodesis[4]

- This is an extension of a three-ligament tenodesis, except that it does not stop at the dorsum of the LTq joint, but it continues palmarly, across the triquetrum, to reconstruct the palmar radiolunotriquetral ligaments (**TECH FIG 5**).
- In addition to the dorsal longitudinal and the palmar anterolateral incisions described for the three-ligament tenodesis, this intervention requires a standard carpal tunnel incision, extended proximally in a zigzag fashion to uncover the floor of the carpal tunnel.
- The initial steps are the same as for a three-ligament tenodesis. The differences start when the tendon graft has been brought to the dorsum of the triquetrum.
- The tenodesis does not take the dorsal radiotriquetral ligament as an anchor point but is threaded through an anteroposterior tunnel across the triquetrum that has been drilled from palmar to dorsal using the exposure provided through the carpal tunnel incision.
- Once in the carpal tunnel, the tendon is grasped and pulled radially by a curved mosquito that is introduced through the anterolateral incision, under the carpal tunnel contents, following the distal edge of the radius.
  - It is important to protect the radial artery.
- The tendon graft is brought to the volar aspect of the radial styloid and secured by means of either a bone anchor or threaded through another drill hole across the radial styloid, directed at the floor of the second compartment where it can be attached to Lister tubercle with transosseous sutures.
- Capsular, retinacular, and skin closure are identical as for the three-ligament tenodesis, as is the postoperative regimen.

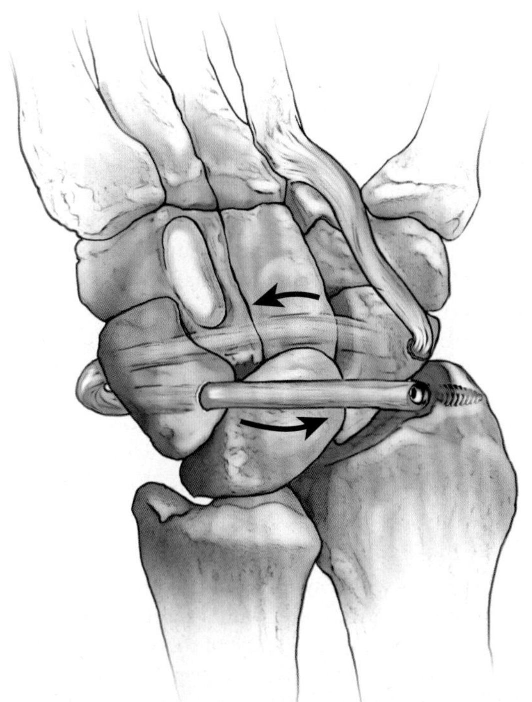

TECH FIG 5 ● A schematic representation of the antipronation spiral tenodesis, seen from the anteromedial corner of the wrist, as described by Chee et al.[4] The use of the FCR tendon graft is similar to that detailed for the three-ligament tenodesis, except that the graft is brought across the dorsal wrist to the triquetrum, then dorsal to volar through a bone tunnel created in the triquetrum, and finally to the radial styloid volarly where it is secured.

PEARLS AND PITFALLS

Indications	■ Never perform a tenodesis if the malalignment is not easily reducible or if there is cartilage wear at the periscaphoid joints. ■ Stability cannot be based on an unstable segment. If the lunate is unstable, a three-ligament tenodesis is likely to fail. In such cases, an antipronation spiral tenodesis is to be chosen.
Scaphoid tunnel placement	■ Drill a Kirschner wire from dorsal to palmar and from proximal to distal, aiming at the tuberosity. After fluoroscopy control, use a cannulated 2.7- or 3.2-mm drill depending on the size of the tendon strip obtained. It is best to have a tighter fit rather than a looser fit in the tunnel so that there is less "slop" in the system and potentially less likelihood of loss of reduction. The bone tunnel size, therefore, depends on the tendon graft thickness and also on the size of the scaphoid.
Pin stabilization	■ One 1.5-mm Kirschner wire enters from the dorsoradial corner of the scaphoid across the scaphoid, aiming at the hook of the hamate. ■ A second Kirschner wire enters from the palmar-radial corner of the scaphoid tuberosity, aiming at the lunate. ■ Avoid Kirschner wires across the anatomic snuffbox (radial artery at risk).
Fixation of the split tendon to the lunate	■ The anchor suture in the lunate is not to be used as anchor point for tendon tensioning but only as a means to maintain the split tendon in full contact to cancellous bone. Tension of the tenodesis relies on the dorsal radiotriquetral ligament.
Tensioning of the tenodesis	■ Avoid excessive reduction of the DISI by applying too much tension to the graft. A "volar intercalated segment instability" may be created, aside from affecting motion, or may even lead to necrosis.

POSTOPERATIVE CARE

- This postoperative regimen can be used, with minimal differences, in the three-wrist stabilizing procedures described earlier. The wrist is immobilized in a well-padded splint including the metacarpophalangeal joint of the thumb for 10 days.
- After stitch removal, the wrist is maintained in a short-arm thumb spica cast for 5 more weeks.
- A protective removable splint is then fabricated. This will allow resting the joint between sessions of supervised physiotherapy. The splint is used for an additional 4 weeks.
- Before wire removal, at 8 weeks, therapy consists of only gentle radiocarpal mobilization. After pin removal, global active mobilization is emphasized. Aggressive passive mobilization is never recommended.
- Intracarpal supinator muscle strengthening exercises are not initiated until 10 weeks after surgery.
- Contact sports are to be avoided for 6 months after surgery.

OUTCOMES

- A review of 38 patients with a symptomatic SLD who had a three-ligament tenodesis procedure, with a mean follow-up of 46 months, showed an average range of motion of about 75% of the contralateral side.[5] Average grip strength was 65%. Pain relief at rest was obtained in 28 patients, with 8 complaining of mild discomfort during strenuous activity and 2 having pain in most activities of daily life. Twenty-nine resumed their normal occupational–vocational activities. There were no signs of scaphoid necrosis. Recurrence of carpal collapse occurred in only two wrists. Nine patients showed mild signs of degenerative osteoarthritis at the tip of the radial styloid, but none had substantial symptoms.
- Seradge et al[9] published the results of the Dyna-desis in 105 wrists followed an average of 63 months. The average grip strength had increased by 65%. The overall function was excellent in 49%, good in 24%, and fair in 26%. Satisfactory pain relief was obtained in 94% of the patients.
- The antipronation spiral tenodesis has been used in five patients.[4] Reviewed at 17 months, they all had returned to their occupations with a 15% reduction of the global range and a grip strength was also reduced to 70% of the contralateral side. All patient were satisfied with the procedure.

COMPLICATIONS

- Recurrence of the malalignment and subsequent development of degenerative arthritis are common when the technique is used inappropriately, in cases with a poorly reducible SLD (stage 5), or when cartilage deterioration is already present (SLAC).
- When reducibility is in doubt, a more aggressive treatment (partial fusion or proximal row carpectomy) is recommended.

REFERENCES

1. Berger RA, Bishop AT, Bettinger PC. New dorsal capsulotomy for the surgical exposure of the wrist. Ann Plast Surg 1995;35:54–59.
2. Berger RA, Imaeda T, Berglund L, et al. Constraint and material properties of the subregions of the scapholunate interosseous ligament. J Hand Surg Am 1999;24(5):953–962.
3. Brunelli GA, Brunelli GR. A new technique to correct carpal instability with scaphoid rotary subluxation: a preliminary report. J Hand Surg Am 1995;20(suppl 3, pt 2):S82–S85.
4. Chee KG, Chin AY, Chew EM, et al. Antipronation spiral tenodesis—a surgical technique for the treatment of perilunate instability. J Hand Surg Am 2012;37(12):2611–2618.
5. Garcia-Elias M, Lluch A, Stanley JK. Three-ligament tenodesis for the treatment of scapholunate dissociation: indications and surgical technique. J Hand Surg Am 2006;31(1):125–134.
6. Kitay A, Wolfe SW. Scapholunate instability: current concepts in diagnosis and management. J Hand Surg Am 2012;37(10):2175–2196.
7. Linscheid RL, Dobyns JH, Beabout JW, et al. Traumatic instability of the wrist. Diagnosis, classification, and pathomechanics. J Bone Joint Surg Am 1972;54(8):1612–1632.
8. Salva-Coll G, Garcia-Elias M, Leon-Lopez MT, et al. Effects of forearm muscles on carpal stability. J Hand Surg Eur Vol 2011;36(7):553–559.
9. Seradge H, Baer C, Dalsimer D, et al. Treatment of dynamic scaphoid instability. J Trauma 2004;56:1253–1260.
10. Short WH, Werner FW, Green JK, et al. Biomechanical evaluation of ligamentous stabilizers of the scaphoid and lunate. J Hand Surg Am 2002;27(6):991–1002.
11. Watson HK, Ashmead D IV, Makhlouf MV. Examination of the scaphoid. J Hand Surg Am 1988;13(5):657–660.

Reduction and Association of the Scaphoid and the Lunate for Scapholunate Instability

CHAPTER 71

Joseph M. Lombardi, James A. Wilkerson, and Melvin P. Rosenwasser

DEFINITION

- Scapholunate instability occurs as a result of injury to the scapholunate interosseous ligament (SLIL) and represents the most common type of carpal instability.
- Instability can be categorized based on physical and radiographic findings.
  - Static instability: abnormal alignment of the scaphoid and lunate evident on routine radiographs
  - Dynamic instability: abnormal alignment of the scaphoid and lunate present only on stress radiographs
  - Predynamic instability: no radiographic abnormalities present but history and physical findings consistent with a SLIL injury
- Reduction and association of the scaphoid and the lunate (the RASL procedure) is used to correct static scapholunate instability.

ANATOMY

- The stability of the scapholunate joint depends on extrinsic capsular ligaments and the robust SLIL.
- The SLIL can be divided into three components: dorsal, palmar, and proximal. Of these, the dorsal component is the thickest and contributes the most to scapholunate stability.[2]
- Normally, the interval between the scaphoid and the lunate measures less than 3 mm, but this can vary between patients. The interval should be compared to the contralateral wrist (**FIG 1A**).
- The normal angle between the scaphoid and the lunate measures 46 degrees with the wrist in neutral position (**FIG 1B**).[6]
- With wrist flexion and extension, there is 25 degrees of obligatory rotation between the scaphoid and the lunate. With radial and ulnar deviation, there is 10 degrees of rotary motion.[9]

PATHOGENESIS

- SLIL injury typically occurs after a fall onto an extended wrist. The combination of axial load, wrist extension, intercarpal supination, and ulnar deviation leads to supraphysiologic loads across the SLIL.
- Injury can also occur in association with other injuries, such as the constellation seen in perilunate dislocations and distal radius fractures.

NATURAL HISTORY

- The motion of the scaphoid and that of the lunate are linked, such that both bones flex with wrist flexion and radial deviation and extend with wrist extension and ulnar deviation.[4] After complete disruption of the SLIL, the synchronous movement between the scaphoid and lunate is lost and the scaphoid flexes while the lunate extends.
  - Increased scaphoid flexion leads to point stress at the radial styloid–scaphoid articulation. This is the first stage of scapholunate advanced collapse (SLAC) and osteoarthritis.
  - Dorsal intercalated segment instability (DISI) occurs because of unlinked lunate extension, leading to scapholunate diastasis, carpal descent, and altered kinematics (**FIG 2**). This results in pain, weakness, and progressive osteoarthritis.
- This predictable, progressive arthritis has been coined SLAC.[12]
  - Arthritic changes first arise between the radial styloid and the scaphoid (stage 1), followed by progressive changes at the proximal scaphoid fossa (stage 2). Next, the midcarpal joint is affected (stage 3), in particular the capitolunate joint, and ultimately pancarpal arthritis results (stage 4).

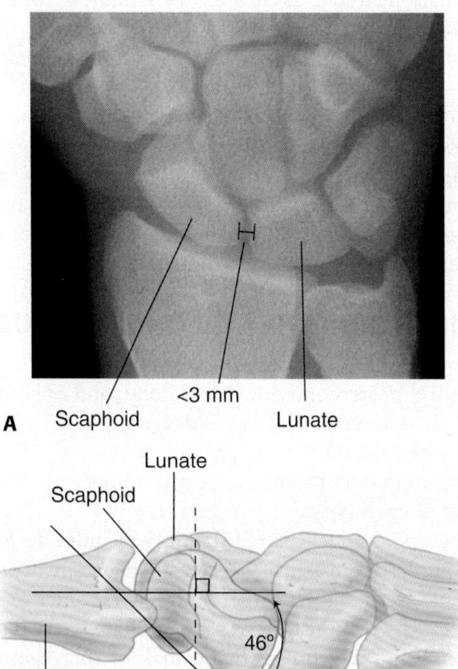

FIG 1 • **A.** The scapholunate interval normally measures less than 3 mm. **B.** The scapholunate angle normally measures 46 degrees with the wrist in neutral position.

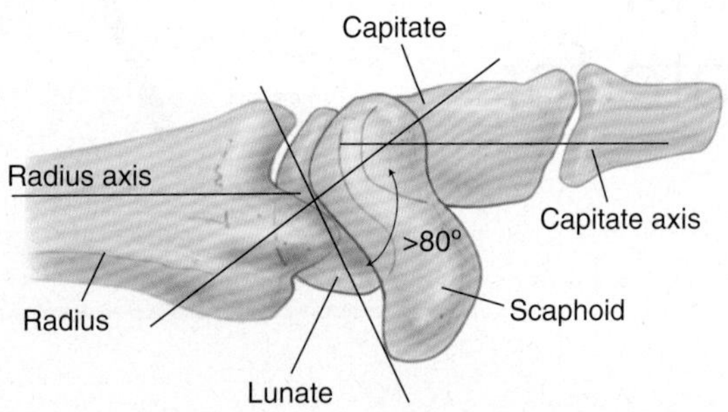

FIG 2 • DISI occurs as a result of lunate extension. Consequently, the capitate and distal carpal row migrate proximally and translate dorsally.

PATIENT HISTORY AND PHYSICAL FINDINGS

- History should include details of prior wrist trauma, especially in regard to mechanism and timing.
  - Patient reporting of injury dating is unreliable and most injuries have acute on chronic etiologies. The number of months should not dictate the treatment options. What is important is the integrity of the ligament for repair and this should be assessed at surgery.
  - After acute trauma, there is usually a reparable scapholunate ligament, whereas in the setting of subacute or chronic injury, the ligament may be attenuated or resorbed. The presence of adequate ligament tissue for repair should dictate surgical strategy.
  - Instability may be the result of cumulative trauma, and the patient may report several minor wrist sprains that culminate in chronic wrist pain.
- Physical examination should include the following:
  - Palpation of the wrist: dorsal tenderness over the scapholunate ligament associated with fullness corresponding to dorsal capsular synovitis
  - Range of motion: Pain with range of motion may indicate instability, synovitis, and chondral wear.
  - Provocative maneuvers such as Watson scaphoid shift test: dorsal wrist pain with reduction clunk consistent with SLIL instability
- Imaging of the contralateral asymptomatic wrist may mimic radiographic findings of scapholunate diastasis or DISI and can represent a hyperlaxity syndrome.

IMAGING AND OTHER DIAGNOSTIC STUDIES

- Plain radiographs and stress views should be performed first.
  - Neutral posteroanterior (PA), lateral, and oblique views
  - PA views in ulnar and radial deviation
  - Clenched fist PA view in pronation
- Contralateral wrist films are helpful to uncover bilateral instability/hyperlaxity.
- Radiographic evidence of SLIL injury includes the following:
  - Scapholunate diastasis greater than 3 mm. Comparison should be made with the contralateral side, as ligamentous laxity demonstrates a scapholunate interval of greater than 3 mm which may be normal for that ligamentously lax individual (**FIG 3A**).[5]
  - Scaphoid cortical ring sign, which occurs when the scaphoid is in a flexed posture and the distal tubercle aligns with the proximal scaphoid (see **FIG 3A**)
  - Scapholunate angle greater than 60 degrees (**FIG 3B**)[8]

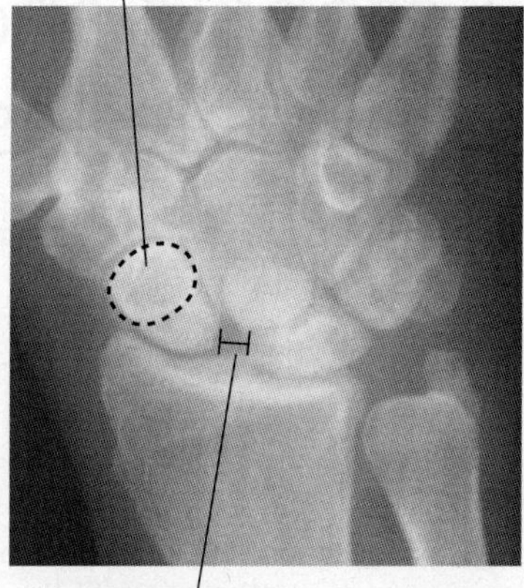

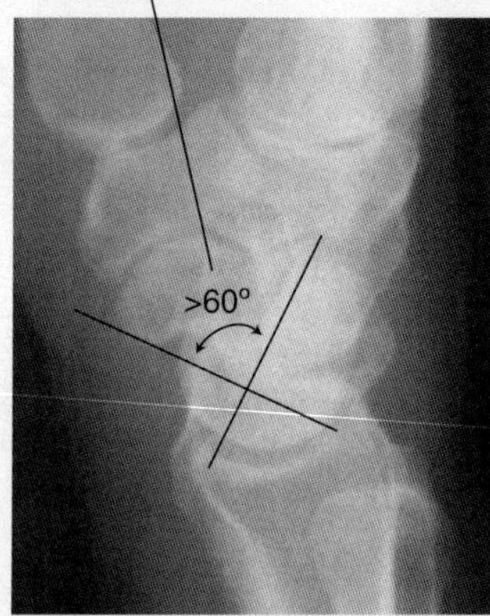

FIG 3 • **A.** A widened scapholunate interval (>3 mm) and a scaphoid cortical ring sign are seen on an AP view of the wrist. **B.** An obtuse scapholunate angle (>60 degrees) is appreciated on a lateral view of the wrist.

  - DISI deformity pattern with capitate dorsal translation and decreased carpal height measurements
- The resolution of ligament anatomy by magnetic resonance imaging (MRI) is affected by the strength of the magnet and the use of dedicated wrist coils.
  - Sensitivity ranges from 63% to 92%.
  - Specificity ranges from 86% to 100%, depending on the degree of injury and the type of MRI used.[10,11]

DIFFERENTIAL DIAGNOSIS

- Scaphoid fracture
- Capitolunate arthritis
- Scaphotrapeziotrapezoidal (STT) arthritis
- Midcarpal instability
- Dorsal carpal ganglion
- Dorsal impaction syndrome

NONOPERATIVE MANAGEMENT

- Normal clinical alignment with persistent wrist pain with or without a Watson scaphoid shift sign is managed with resting splints and nonsteroidal medications until symptoms resolve.
- Occasionally, intra-articular steroid injections are helpful if the dorsal synovitis is severe.

SURGICAL MANAGEMENT

Contraindications to Reduction and Association of the Scaphoid and Lunate

- A repairable SLIL
  - A primary ligament repair is preferable if a ligament of adequate substance is present.
  - This is most likely seen in acute injuries (<3 weeks) but may be possible in chronic injuries. At surgery, repair is done if possible and can be augmented with a trans-scapholunate screw as desired.
- Presence of significant capitolunate or pancarpal arthritis
  - If significant midcarpal or radioscaphoid arthritis is present, other procedures, such as a proximal row carpectomy or a limited carpal fusion, are preferred.
- Focal arthritis between the scaphoid and radial styloid is not a contraindication because a radial styloidectomy is routinely performed during the RASL procedure.

Positioning

- The procedure is performed with the patient supine and the arm on a standard hand table.
- The operating table should be rotated 90 degrees to facilitate the use of the image intensifier during the procedure.

Approach

- The RASL procedure can be performed either arthroscopically or via an open dorsal approach.
- The arthroscopic RASL should be attempted only after obtaining experience with the open technique or by a master arthroscopist.
- We prefer the open technique to facilitate débridement and anatomic reduction.
- The open technique is performed using a dorsal intercarpal ligament–sparing approach.

TECHNIQUES

Dorsal Ligament–Sparing Capsulotomy

- Make a longitudinal incision on the dorsal wrist, staying just ulnar to the tubercle of Lister (**TECH FIG 1A**).
- Bluntly dissect the soft tissue down to the level of the extensor retinaculum, taking care to preserve dorsal veins and cutaneous nerve branches wherever possible.
- Incise obliquely the extensor retinaculum parallel to the course of the extensor pollicis longus (EPL) tendon (**TECH FIG 1B**).
  - This will open the third and fourth extensor compartments.
  - The EPL is retracted radially and the fourth compartment tendons are retracted ulnarly.
- Make an oblique incision through the dorsal wrist capsule parallel and proximal to the dorsal intercarpal ligament (**TECH FIG 1C**).
- The dorsal radiocarpal (DRC) ligament should be identified and preserved.

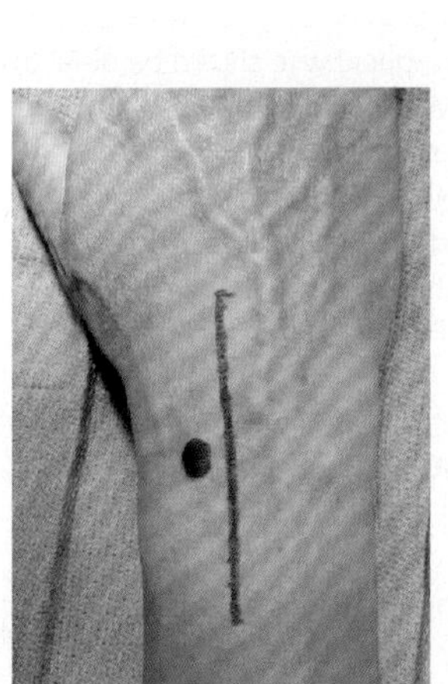

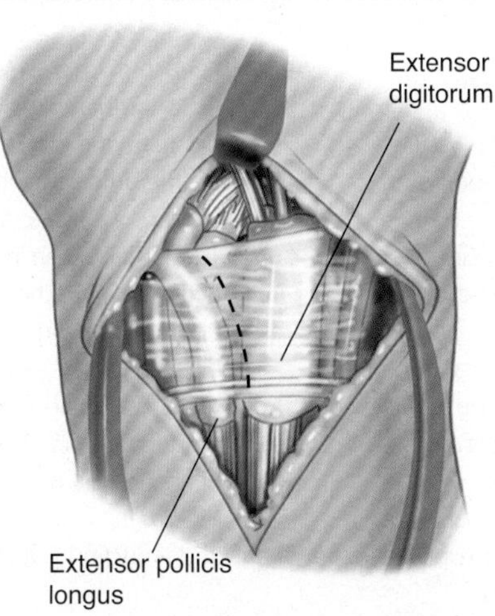

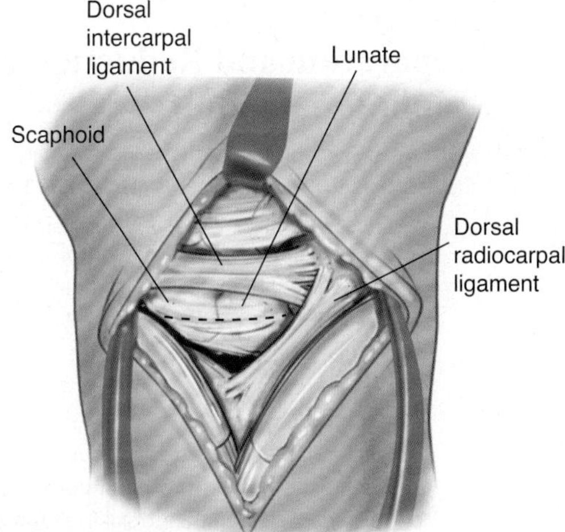

TECH FIG 1 • **A.** A dorsal midline incision is made just ulnar to the tubercle of Lister. **B.** An oblique incision is made through the extensor retinaculum parallel to the EPL tendon. The EPL is retracted radially and the fourth compartment tendons are retracted ulnarly. **C.** An oblique incision is made through the dorsal wrist capsule parallel and proximal to the dorsal intercarpal ligament. The DRC ligament should also be identified and preserved.

Styloidectomy

- Once the capsulotomy is performed, identify the scapholunate interval and the SLIL and inspect the radiocarpal and intercarpal joints.
  - If significant arthrosis is present in areas other than the radial styloid–scaphoid articulation, a salvage procedure is indicated.
- Perform a second incision in the midaxial line over the first dorsal compartment (**TECH FIG 2A**).
  - The dorsal branch of the radial artery and the major branch of the superficial radial nerve should be seen, protected, and isolated with a vessel loops.
- Release the first compartment retinaculum and retract the tendons dorsally.
- Incise the capsule longitudinally through the wrist capsule, thereby exposing the radial styloid (**TECH FIG 2B**).
- Elevate the periosteum overlying the radial styloid, and use an osteotome to perform a radial styloidectomy.
  - Remove just enough of the radial styloid so that radial deviation of the wrist does not cause impingement of the scaphoid and radius.
  - This is done with two cuts of the osteotome so that the origin of the volar radioscaphocapitate ligament can be seen and preserved.

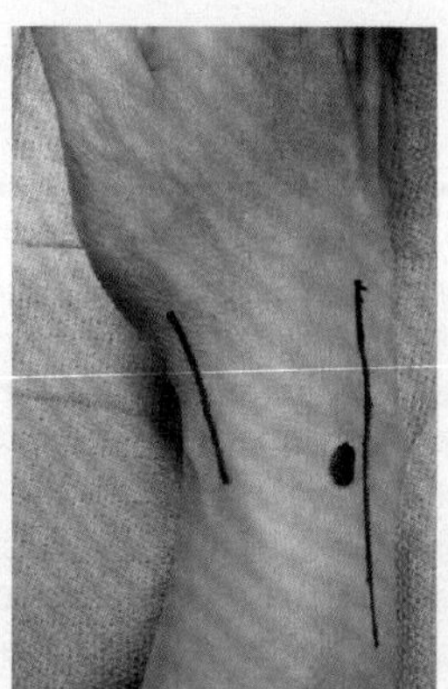

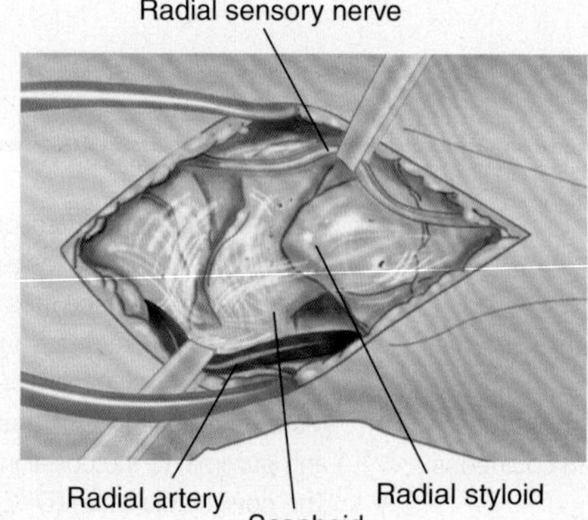

TECH FIG 2 • **A.** A longitudinal incision is made over the first dorsal extensor compartment. **B.** The first compartment is released and a longitudinal incision is made down to the radial styloid.

Preparation and Reduction of the Scapholunate Joint

- Place a 0.062-inch Kirschner wire in the lunate and another in the scaphoid to serve as joysticks (**TECH FIG 3A**).
  - To bring the lunate out of extension, place the Kirschner wire in the most proximal portion of the exposed dorsal surface, angled from proximal to distal.
  - A second Kirschner wire may need to be placed and the step repeated if full counterclockwise rotation of the lunate does not bring it into neutral alignment. The first wire is then removed.
  - Similarly, to bring the scaphoid out of flexion, place the Kirschner wire in the most distal portion of the exposed dorsal surface, angled from distal to proximal.
  - Keep in mind the eventual path of the screw when placing the Kirschner wires. The scaphoid wire should be distal to this path and the lunate wire should be proximal.
- Remove the articular cartilage at the interface of the scapholunate joint using a side-cutting burr (**TECH FIG 3B**).
  - The joysticks can be used to separate the two bones to better visualize the articular surfaces.
  - Remove the cartilage until cancellous bone and punctate bleeding are visualized.
- Reduce the scaphoid and lunate by flexing the lunate and extending the scaphoid (**TECH FIG 3C**).
  - A Kocher clamp is used to hold the reduction (**TECH FIG 3D**).
- Verify the reduction with an image intensifier (**TECH FIG 3E**).

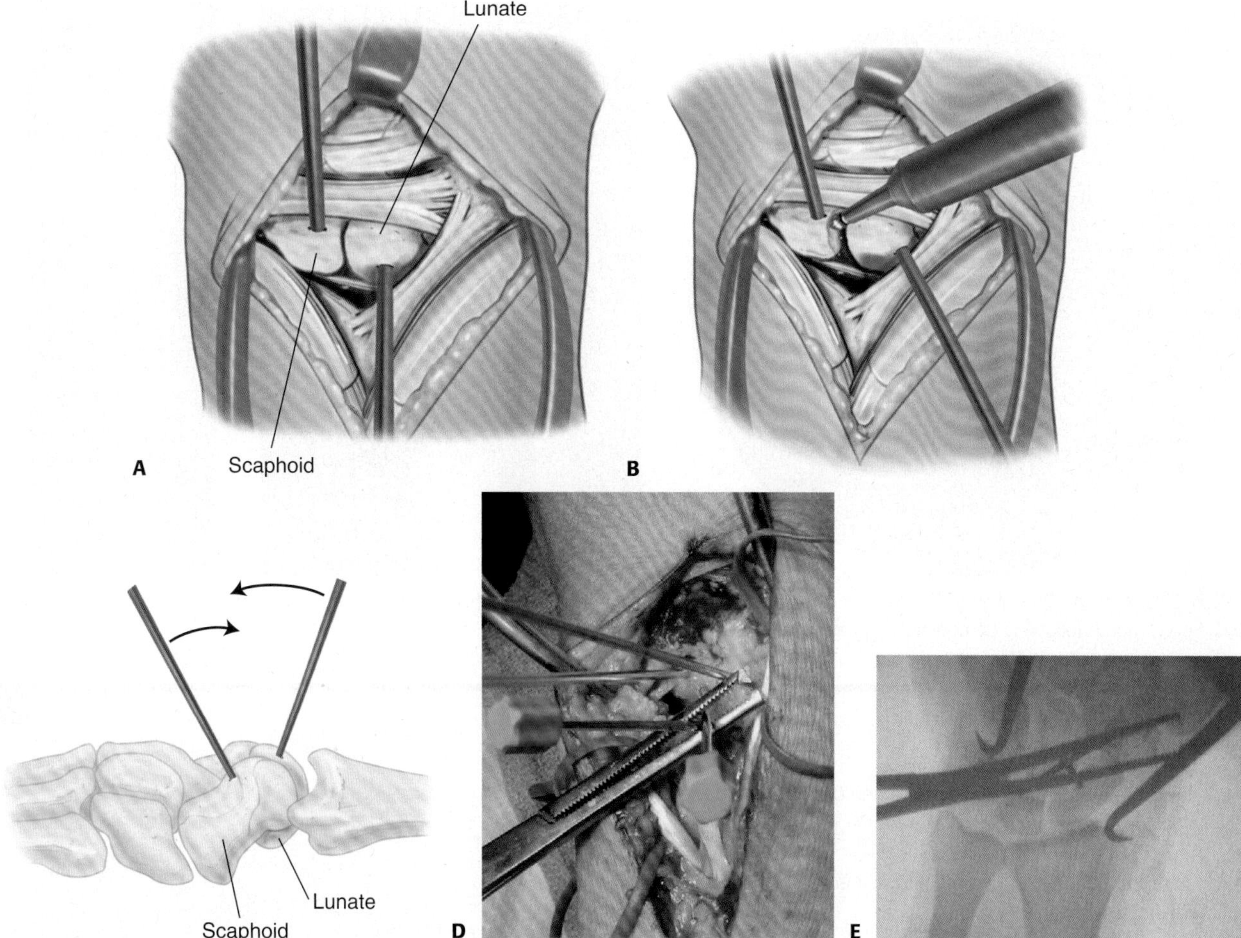

TECH FIG 3 • **A.** 0.062-inch Kirschner wires are placed in the lunate and scaphoid to serve as joysticks. **B.** A side-cutting burr is used to remove the cartilage within the scapholunate joint. **C.** The joysticks are used to extend the scaphoid and to flex the lunate. **D.** A Kocher clamp is used to hold the reduction. **E.** The reduction is verified with an image intensifier.

Headless Bone Screw Placement

- A cannulated headless screw with a smooth central shank is used to secure the reduction, aiming for the center axis of rotation of the lunate.
- Start the guidewire through the radial midaxial incision into the waist of the scaphoid.
- Direct the wire from midlateral on the scaphoid to the medial corner of the reduced lunate on the anteroposterior (AP) view (should be at approximately 20 degrees to match the radial inclination of the distal radius) (**TECH FIG 4A**).
  - Kirschner wire joysticks may need to be repositioned to facilitate screw passage.
- Do not violate the lunotriquetral interosseous ligament.
- Once the guidewire position is confirmed on AP and lateral views, overdrill the wire with a cannulated drill by hand to prevent binding and possible breakage of the 1-mm wire.
- Measure the screw length with cannulated guide or a second guidewire, then subtract 2 to 4 mm for your final screw length so that threads will be completely buried.
- Insert the screw into the scaphoid so that it is below the chondral surface.
- Correct screw placement should be confirmed by fluoroscopy (**TECH FIG 4B,C**).
- Remove the Kocher clamp and the joystick wires.
- Check the stability of the scapholunate reduction while ranging the wrist. It is normal for differential rotation to exist between the scaphoid and lunate.

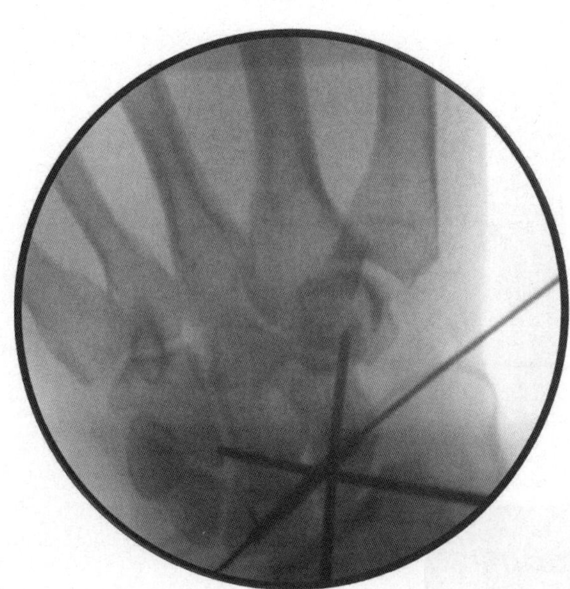

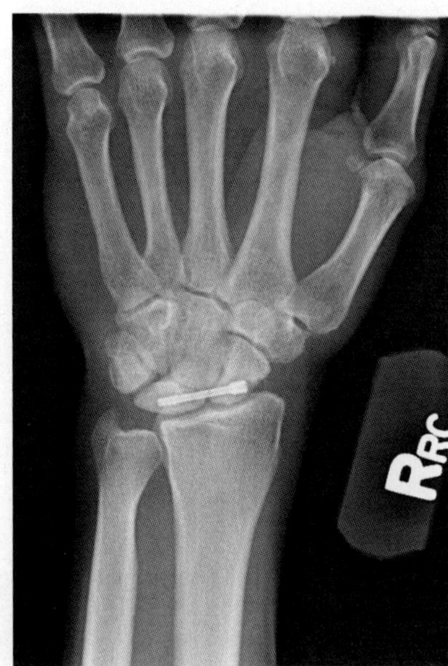

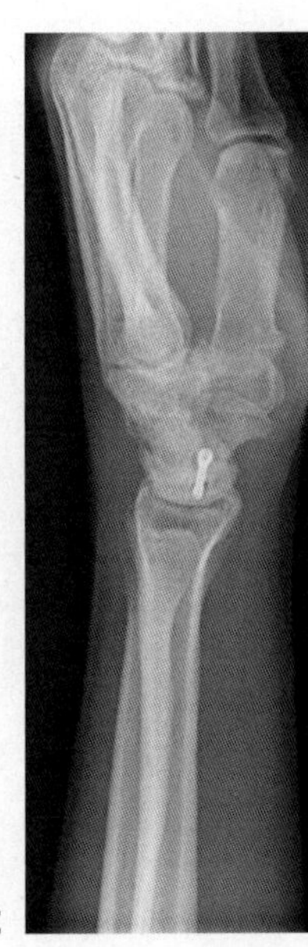

TECH FIG 4 • **A.** The insertion angle of the headless bone screw should be roughly parallel to the radial inclination of 20 degrees. **B,C.** Seven-month follow-up demonstrating proper screw positioning.

Wound Closure

- Release the tourniquet and achieve hemostasis using Bovie or bipolar electrocautery.
- The dorsal capsular incision is left open.
- Close the skin using 5-0 nylon suture and apply a sterile bulky dressing and volar wrist splint.

PEARLS AND PITFALLS

Indications	▪ Good imaging and possible arthroscopy are essential to ensure no capitolunate arthritis exists before a RASL procedure is performed.
Dorsal and radial approaches	▪ Identify superficial radial sensory nerve branches and prevent excessive traction via self-retaining retractors. ▪ Identify the dorsal radial artery just distal to the screw insertion site before screw placement.
Radial styloidectomy	▪ Sequential radial styloid osteotomies are performed: one to visualize the scaphoid facet and one to preserve the volar radioscaphocapitate ligament. ▪ Remove just enough to prevent radioscaphoid impingement.
Kirschner wire joystick placement	▪ Do not place the Kirschner wires in the centers of the scaphoid and lunate. ▪ Aim for the proximal ulnar corner of the lunate and the distal radial corner of the scaphoid to avoid interfering with the eventual path of the screw.
Bone preparation	▪ Burr down the chondral surfaces at the scaphoid and lunate interface to expose cancellous vascular bone. ▪ Do not remove articular cartilage of the superior and inferior surfaces of the scaphoid or lunate so that good contact will continue postreduction and realignment.
Screw placement	▪ A central smooth shank screw is essential. The RASL will not work with a fully threaded screw because it will block scapholunate rotation. ▪ The guidewire must be in ideal position, central to slightly volar on the sagittal image, and directed toward the medial corner of the lunate on the coronal image. ▪ If screw is placed dorsal to the midsagittal line, the off-axis motion will result in failure.
Follow-up	▪ It is expected that the threads at the lunate end of the screw will show lucency over time secondary to resorption as motion is regained. This will not result in scapholunate diastasis because of soft tissue healing at the scapholunate junction.

POSTOPERATIVE CARE

- The wrist splint and sutures are removed at 10 to 14 days.
- The wrist is placed into a custom removable thermoplast splint, and supervised, gentle active range of motion is initiated.
- Occupational therapy for mobility and activities of daily living (ADLs) for 3 months
- Progressive activity at 3 to 6 months
- Unrestricted activity at 6 months

OUTCOMES

- Lipton et al[7] reported on a series of 21 patients and currently a longer term follow-up of 31 patients is submitted for publication.[13]
  - The average time to follow-up was 6.2 years. Patients had a mean Disability of the Arm, Shoulder, and Hand (DASH) of 16.6 and Visual Analog Score (VAS) of 0.58 resting and 1.65 with activity. Patients scored an average of 48.7 for the physical component of the SF-36 and a 53.8 for the mental component.
  - Twenty-three patients were available for physical examination. The average flexion/extension arc of motion was 108 degrees compared to a contralateral arc of 136 degrees ($P = .01$). Average radial and ulnar deviation were 19 and 26 degrees, respectively, representing no statistically significant difference versus the contralateral side ($P = .24$). Additionally, there was no significant difference in grip strength versus the contralateral side.
  - There were no major intraoperative or perioperative complications in this cohort. Of the 32 patients, 4 went on to have further surgery of which 3 were considered treatment failures. The fourth had removal of hardware due to pain but had an otherwise successful outcome with DASH of 18.3.
  - The average preoperative scapholunate angle was 77 degrees versus 55 degrees postoperatively ($P < .0001$). The average scapholunate gap decreased from 4.5 mm preoperatively to 2.1 mm postoperatively ($P < .01$).
- Caloia et al[3] reported a case series of arthroscopic RASL procedures done in eight patients (nine wrists). The average follow-up was 34.6 months. Patients' VAS scored improved from 5.4 to 1.5 following surgery and had a postoperative grip strength that averaged 78% of the contralateral side. The average wrist range of motion was reduced by 20% with a scapholunate angle reduction from 70.5 to 59.3 degrees.
- Aviles et al[1] reported good outcomes for an arthroscopic approach to the RASL for the treatment of static instability in seven patients between the ages of 28 and 77 years old. Six of the seven patients reported good pain relief at an average follow-up of 19 months. The patient who experienced failure had advanced radiocarpal and midcarpal osteoarthritis. The entire cohort experienced reduction in total arc of wrist motion by 17.6%. The average scapholunate diastasis was reduced from 4.2 to 1.75 mm and the average scapholunate angle was reduced from 81.6 to 61.8 degrees.
- Zubairy et al[14] attempted a scapholunate fusion in 13 patients with chronic scapholunate instability. They noted absolute fusion in 4 of the patients and 10 patients altogether reported subjective improvement in symptoms. Two of the patients went on to receive total wrist fusions. The group concluded that although a firm fibrous union is all that is achieved in most patients, it is often sufficient to alleviate pain.

POTENTIAL COMPLICATIONS

- Residual instability
- Screw migration
- Superficial radial sensory nerve injury

REFERENCES

1. Aviles AJ, Lee SK, Hausman MR. Arthroscopic reduction-association of the scapholunate. Arthroscopy 2007;23:105. e101–e105.
2. Berger RA, Imeada T, Berglund L, et al. Constraint and material properties of the subregions of the scapholunate interosseous ligament. J Hand Surg Am 1999;24(5):953–962.
3. Caloia M, Caloia H, Pereira E. Arthroscopic scapholunate joint reduction. Is an effective treatment for irreparable scapholunate ligament tears? Clin Orthop Relat Res 2012;470:972–978.
4. Garcia-Elias M, Geissler WB. In: Green DP, Hotchkiss RN, Pederson WC, et al, eds. Green's Operative Hand Surgery, ed 5. Philadelphia: Elsevier/Churchill Livingstone, 2005.
5. Linscheid RL. Scapholunate ligamentous instabilities (dissociations, subdislocations, dislocations). Ann Chir Main 1984;3:323–330.
6. Linscheid RL, Dobyns JH, Beabout JW, et al. Traumatic instability of the wrist: diagnosis, classification, and pathomechanics. J Bone Joint Surg Am 1972;54(8):1612–1632.
7. Lipton CB, Ugwonali OF, Sarwahi V, et al. Reduction and association of the scaphoid and lunate for scapholunate ligament injuries (RASL). Atlas Hand Clin 2003;8:249–260.
8. Rosenwasser MP, Miyasajsa KC, Strauch RJ. The RASL procedure: reduction and association of the scaphoid and lunate using the Herbert screw. Tech Hand Up Extrem Surg 1997;1:263–272.
9. Ruby LK, Cooney WP III, An KN, et al. Relative motion of selected carpal bones: a kinematic analysis of the normal wrist. J Hand Surg Am 1988;13(1):1–10.
10. Schädel-Höpfner M, Iwinska-Zelder J, Braus T, et al. MRI versus arthroscopy in the diagnosis of scapholunate ligament injury. J Hand Surg Br 2001;26:17–21.
11. Schmitt R, Christopoulos G, Meier R, et al. Direct MR arthrography of the wrist in comparison with arthroscopy: a prospective study on 125 patients [in German]. Rofo 2003;175:911–919.
12. Watson HK, Weinzweig J, Zeppieri J. The natural progression of scaphoid instability. Hand Clin 1997;13:39–49.
13. White NJ, Raskolnikov D, Crow SA, et al. Reduction and association of the scaphoid and lunate (RASL): long-term follow-up of a reconstruction technique for chronic scapholunate dissociation [abstract]. Am Soc Surg Hand 2012;94-B:51.
14. Zubairy AI, Jones WA. Scapholunate fusion in chronic symptomatic scapholunate instability. J Hand Surg Br 2003;28(4):311–314.

Lunotriquetral Ligament Repair and Augmentation

Eric R. Wagner and Alexander Y. Shin

DEFINITION

- Isolated injury of the lunotriquetral (LT) interosseous ligament complex is less common and less well understood compared with the other proximal row ligament injury, scapholunate (SL) dissociation.
- LT ligament disruption can occur in isolation or in combination with other wrist pathology, such as a perilunate fracture or dislocation or a distal radius fracture.
- It may result from acute trauma and chronic degenerative or inflammatory processes.
- LT ligament injuries occur in a spectrum of severity ranging from partial tears with dynamic dysfunction (most common) to complete dissociation with static collapse.
  - Dynamic LT instability occurs when the ligament complex is intact but incompetent or attenuated, such as in the case of chronic or inflammatory degradation. Instability can occur in the absence of ligament dissociation (complete disruption).
  - LT dissociation occurs when the LT ligament is completely ruptured (both dorsal and volar portions).
  - Static carpal collapse results when a complete disruption of the LT ligament is combined with an injury to the dorsal radiotriquetral ligament (and other secondary restraints). This results in volar flexion of the lunate in continuity with the scaphoid, termed *volar intercalated segment instability* (VISI). It is important to note that static VISI carpal collapse cannot be reproduced by simply sectioning the dorsal and palmar subregions of the LT ligament but also requires a loss of the radiotriquetral ligament (**FIG 1**).

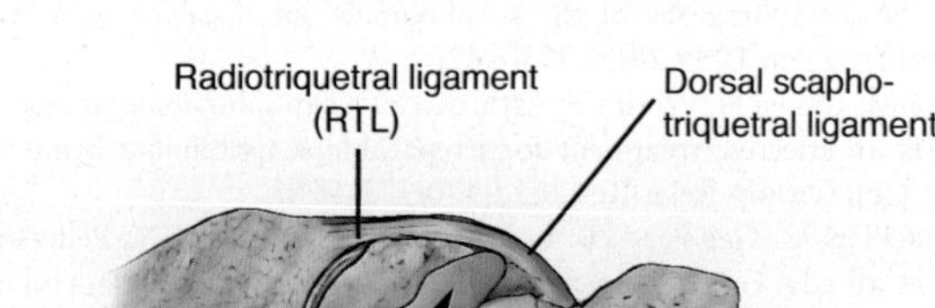

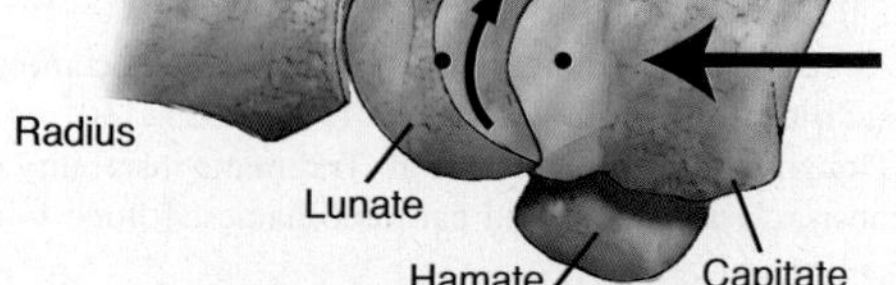

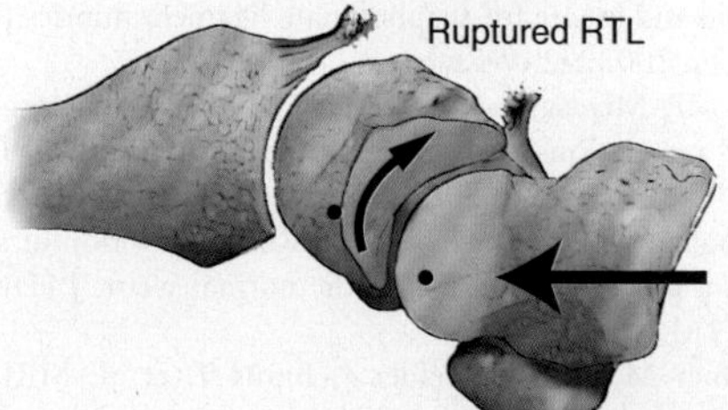

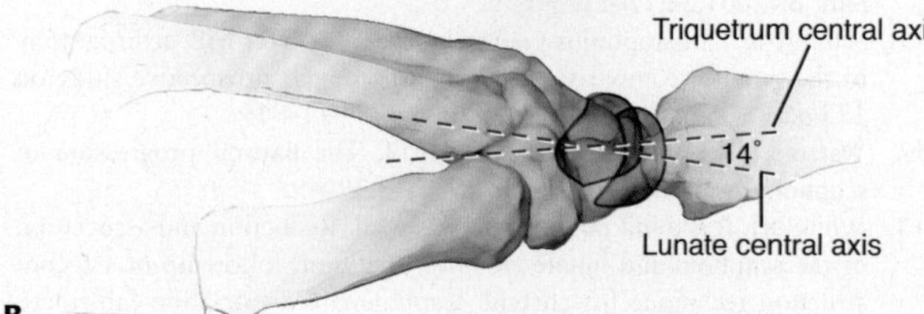

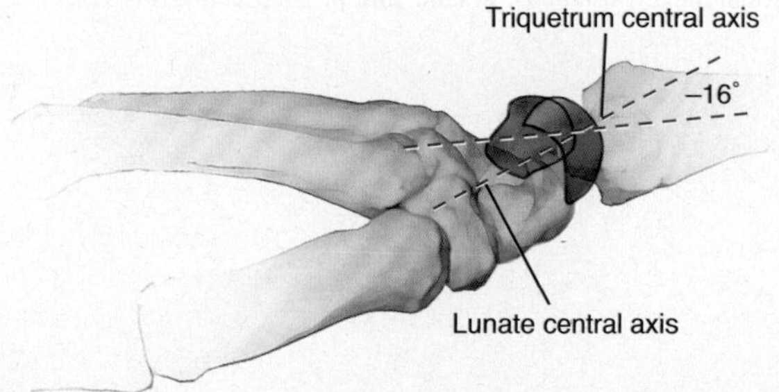

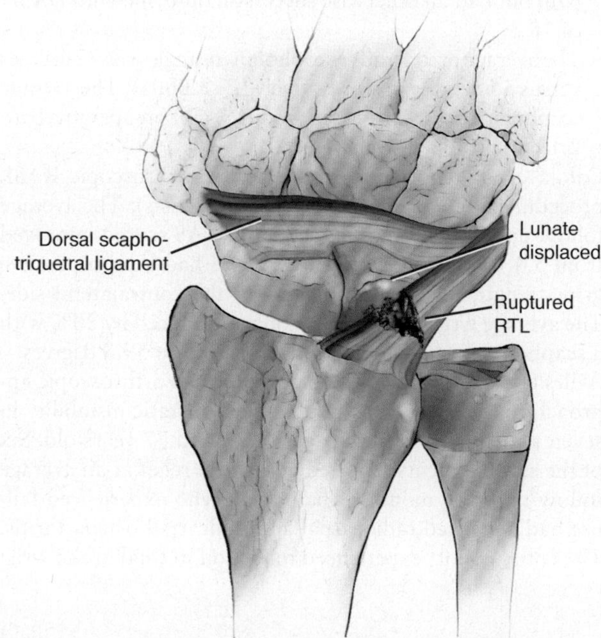

FIG 1 • **A.** Intact dorsal ligaments and normal carpal alignment. Loss of integrity of these secondary restraint structures, the volar-flexed position of the lunate, and the resulting VISI carpal collapse. **B.** Normal anatomic alignment of the carpus as viewed from a lateral radiograph. The LT angle is +14 degrees. **C.** VISI carpal collapse visible on lateral radiograph. The lunate is volar-flexed and the LT angle is −16 degrees. **D.** Rupture of the LT interosseous ligament and the dorsal secondary restraint.

ANATOMY AND KINEMATICS

- Like the SL ligament, the LT interosseous ligament is C-shaped, spanning the dorsal, proximal, and palmar edges of the joint surfaces.
- The palmar portion of the LT ligament is the thickest and most biomechanically important region of the entire complex, interweaving with the ulnocapitate ligament.[18]
  - In contrast, the dorsal component of the SL ligament has been shown to be the strongest.[3]
- The dorsal LT ligament is important as a rotational constraint, whereas the palmar portion is the strongest and transmits the extension moment of the triquetrum as it engages the hamate.
- The proximal region is composed of fibrocartilage, with little rotational or translational strength.
- In the uninjured state, the lunate is "balanced" between the torques of the scaphoid and triquetrum. The scaphoid has a tendency to palmar flex, whereas the triquetrum has a tendency to extend. Through the LT and SL ligaments, these two forces are offset and the proximal carpal row is balanced around the lunate.

PATHOGENESIS

- The exact mechanism of traumatic LT ligament injuries is not fully understood. Many mechanisms may play a role.
- LT ligament injuries can occur in Mayfield III and IV perilunate injuries (**FIG 2A**).
- An isolated traumatic LT ligament injury may occur in a reverse perilunate injury (**FIG 2B**).[17]
- Acute LT Injuries may result from a fall on a pronated wrist combined with either radial deviation or volar flexion.[21]
- In the absence of trauma, degenerative LT instability can result from inflammatory arthritis or ulnocarpal impingement.[15]
- Positive ulnar variance may lead to LT ligament degeneration by wear mechanisms or altered intercarpal kinematics (ulnar impaction syndrome).[16]

NATURAL HISTORY

- The natural history of acute LT injuries has not been fully elucidated, but they may lead to degenerative joint changes.

PATIENT HISTORY AND PHYSICAL FINDINGS

- LT ligament injuries present as vague ulnar-sided wrist pain either acutely after trauma or as chronic wrist pain.[21]
- The examination should encompass the entire wrist, focused on the ulnar side (Table 1).

Table 1 Perilunate and Reverse Perilunate Injury

Stage	Ligament or Bony Injury
Perilunate injury	
1	SL ligament and long radiolunate disruption or scaphoid fracture
2	Volar capitolunate capsule tear in the space of Poirier
3	LT ligament dissociation
4	Dorsal radiolunate capsule tear and lunate subluxation
Reverse perilunate injury	
1	Ulnolunate and ulnotriquetral
2	LT
3	Midcarpal joint and SL

- Dorsal LT joint tenderness should be elicited in LT joint injuries.[9,17]
- Ulnar deviation with pronation and axial compression may elicit dynamic instability with a painful snap "catch up" clunk.
- A palpable wrist click is occasionally significant, particularly if painful and occurring with radioulnar deviation.
- Provocative tests that demonstrate LT laxity, crepitus, and pain are helpful to accurately localize the site of pathology. Three useful tests to perform include the following:
  - Ballottement[17]: The test is positive if increased anteroposterior (AP) laxity and pain occur.
  - Compression: Pain with this maneuver may indicate pathology of the LT or triquetral hamate joints.[2]
  - Shear test[7]: positive with pain, crepitance, and abnormal mobility of the LT joint
- Other common findings on physical examination include limited range of motion and diminished grip strength.[9]
- Comparison of findings with the contralateral wrist is essential.

IMAGING AND OTHER DIAGNOSTIC STUDIES

- Plain radiographs are often normal in LT ligament injuries because the most common presentation is dynamic dysfunction that manifests only with loading or certain positions of the wrist.
  - Dissociation of the LT ligament can lead to disruption of Gilula arcs I and II, demonstrating proximal translation of the triquetrum, with or without LT overlap (**FIG 3A,B**).

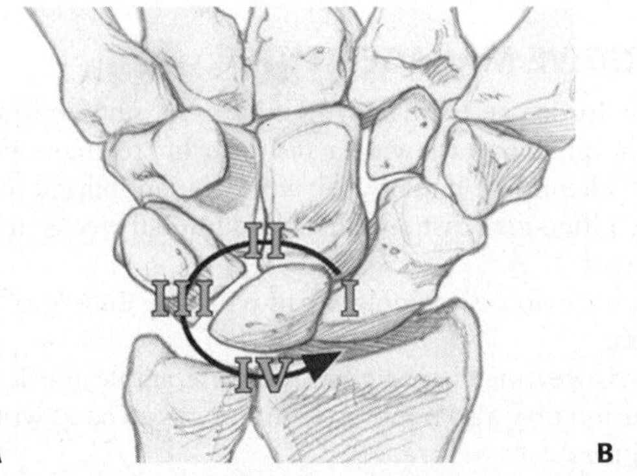

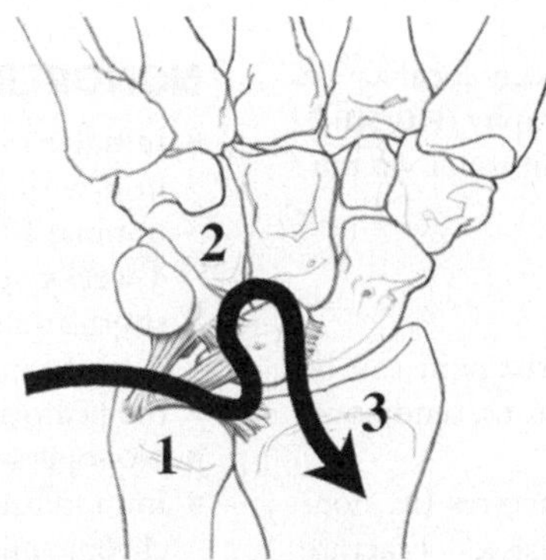

FIG 2 • **A.** Perilunate dislocation. *I–IV* represent the stages of Progressive Perilunar instability as described by Mayfield et al.[10] **B.** Reverse perilunate injury. *1–3* represent the stages of reverse perilunar instability described by Murray et al.[12] (Copyright © Mayo Clinic.)

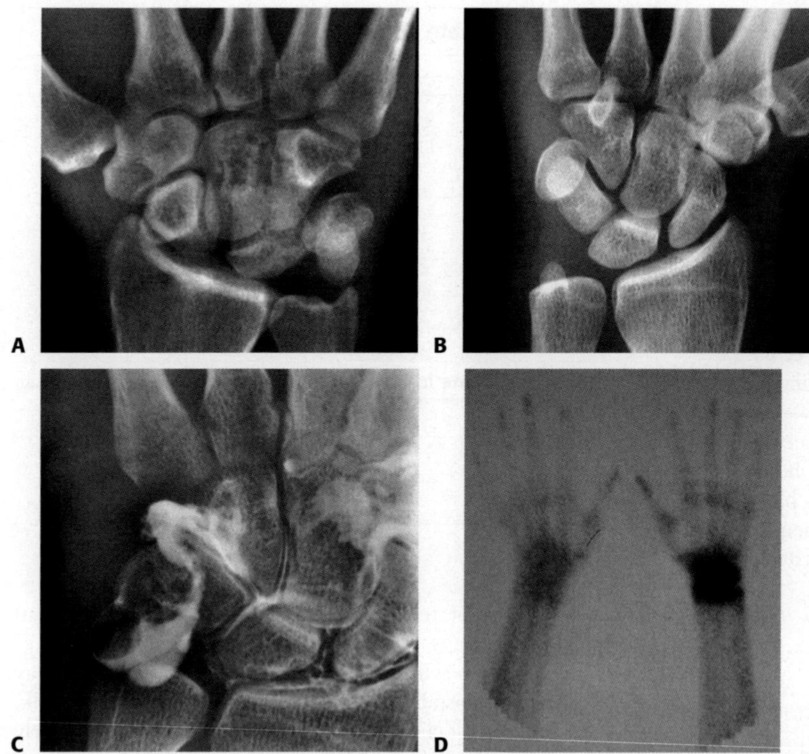

FIG 3 • AP projections of patients with LT ligament dissociation. **A.** The proximal row appears abnormal because both the lunate and scaphoid are volar-flexed. **B.** Disruption of the arcs of Gilula. **C.** Wrist arthrography showing contrast dye pooling, indicative of a LT ligament injury. **D.** Bone scan of a patient with LT ligament injury demonstrates increased radiotracer uptake centered at the LT joint.

- In contrast to SL tears, usually no LT gap occurs.
- A static VISI deformity indicates not only LT ligament injury but also damage to the dorsal radiotriquetral ligament.
- Additional helpful views include radial and unlar deviation view as well as the clenched-fist AP view. In these views, LT dissociation will manifest as a decrease in triquetral motion combined with an increase in the movement of the lunate, scaphoid, and distal row.[2]

- Injection of local anesthetic into the midcarpal space can be useful to localize the cause of the patient's pain.
  - Addition of corticosteroid to the injection may provide temporary relief by decreasing local inflammation and may serve as a positive prognostic sign for surgical treatment.
- Arthrographic dye leakage through the LT interspace can indicate ligamentous injury (**FIG 3C**). However, correlation with the physical examination is necessary because age-dependent degenerative changes and asymptomatic LT instability have been reported.
- Real-time videofluoroscopy can illustrate a "clunk" with ulnar deviation, as the triquetrum "catches up" when the wrist is moved into maximal ulnar deviation.
- Technetium 99m diphosphate bone scan can localize an acute injury but is less specific than arthrography (**FIG 3D**).[6]
- Magnetic resonance imaging is improving but is not yet reliable for imaging of LT ligament injuries.

DIFFERENTIAL DIAGNOSIS

- The differential diagnosis of ulnar-sided wrist pain can be divided into six categories: osseous, ligamentous, tendinous, vascular, neurologic, and tumors.
- Osseous injuries include the sequelae of fractures (ie, nonunion or malunion) and degenerative processes. Fracture nonunions can affect the hamate, pisiform, triquetrum, base of the fifth metacarpal, ulnar styloid process, and distal part of the ulna or radius.
- Degenerative processes involving the pisotriquetral joint, midcarpal (triquetrohamate) articulation, fifth carpometacarpal joint, or distal radioulnar joint. Ulnar impaction or abutment into the radius or carpus can contribute to these processes.
- Ligamentous injuries include any of the ulnar-sided intrinsic (LT or capitohamate) or extrinsic (ulnolunate, triquetrocapitate, or triquetrohamate) ligaments as well as the triangular fibrocartilage complex (TFCC).
- Tendinopathy of the extensor carpi ulnaris (ECU) or flexor carpi ulnaris
- Vascular lesions include ulnar artery thrombosis or hemangiomas.
- Neurologic processes such as entrapment of the ulnar nerve in Guyon canal, neuritis of the dorsal sensory branch of the ulnar nerve, and complex regional pain syndromes
- Although relatively rare, tumors include osteoid osteomas, chondroblastomas, and aneurysmal bone cysts.

NONOPERATIVE MANAGEMENT

- Initial care for most LT ligament injuries is immobilization with a splint or cast with a pisiform lift to maintain optimal LT alignment. Initially, the wrist is immobilized for 4 weeks in a long-arm cast and then 4 additional weeks in a short-arm cast.
- A pisiform lift involves molding a pad palmarly underneath the pisiform.
- Nonoperative treatment is indicated for acute, stable injuries.
- Immobilization may also improve symptoms associated with chronic injuries.

- Midcarpal injections with local anesthetic and corticosteroid often provide significant relief for a prolonged time.
- A trial of nonoperative treatment does not seem to jeopardize the outcome of subsequent surgical intervention.
- Physical therapy targeting ECU strength and proprioception may help to stabilize the deforming forces in a LT tear.[8]

SURGICAL MANAGEMENT

- Operative management is indicated in acute or chronic injuries unresponsive to conservative treatment.
- The goal of surgery is to return rotational stability of the proximal carpal row and restore the natural alignment of the lunocapitate axis.
- Functional reconstruction of the LT ligament can be accomplished with direct ligament repair, ligament reconstruction with a strip of ECU tendon graft, or arthrodesis.
- The choice of intervention should be discussed with the patient. Our preference, based on outcomes studies performed at our institution, is tendon repair or reconstruction.[22]
  - Arthrodesis is avoided whenever possible secondary to higher complication rates and lower patient satisfaction.
  - If significant degenerative changes have occurred in the LT, radiocarpal, or midcarpal joints, partial or total carpal arthrodesis or proximal row carpectomy may be indicated.
  - Static VISI deformity is also best treated with partial intercarpal arthrodesis or radiolunate arthrodesis.
- Significant ulnar positive wrists may be treated with ulnar shortening osteotomy alone or in combination with LT treatments.

Preoperative Planning

- The senior author's preference is to perform diagnostic arthroscopy on patients with LT ligament injuries to evaluate the articular surface and assess other intercarpal pathology.
  - The Geissler classification system grades LT tears and associated instability arthroscopically based on inserting a probe or the camera through the midcarpal portal.[5]
  - Anterior interosseous and posterior interosseous nerve neurectomies can be performed at this time as well.
  - The findings of the arthroscopy are discussed with the patient at a second meeting, and a reconstructive or salvage procedure can then be performed 6 weeks later.
  - Alternatively, a definitive surgical procedure can be performed at a single surgical setting following a thorough preoperative discussion with the patient.
- When an LT dorsal ligament repair is planned, preparations should also be made to proceed with ligament reconstruction if the quality of the LT ligament (especially volarly) is poor.

Positioning

- The patient is positioned supine on a standard operating room table with the affected arm on a hand table.
- A long-acting axillary regional anesthetic block placed preoperatively is helpful with postoperative pain control.
- A nonsterile tourniquet is applied above the surgical drapes.
- Preoperative intravenous antibiotics are routinely administered before beginning the procedure.
- The hand and arm are prepared and draped in standard fashion.
- An examination under anesthesia is always performed initially to evaluate for catch up intercarpal clunks as well as radioulnar clunks.

TECHNIQUES

Diagnostic Arthroscopy and Débridement

Portal Placement and Arthroscopy

- A dorsal 3-4 radiocarpal portal is made just distal to Lister tubercle between extensor digitorum communis (EDC) and extensor pollicis longus (EPL) tendons.
- A dorsal 4-5 radiocarpal portal is made in line with the ring finger metacarpal between the EDC and extensor digiti minimi (EDM) tendons, just proximal to the 3-4 portal.
- Dorsal midcarpal portals are established about 1 cm distal and in line with the radiocarpal portals.
  - Radial midcarpal portal is made on the radial aspect of the third metacarpal.
  - Ulnar midcarpal portal is made in line with the fourth metacarpal.
- Diagnostic arthroscopy is carried out using the 3-4 radiocarpal as the viewing portal with the 4-5 radiocarpal for the probes and shavers.
- LT ligament débridement involves shaving any frayed ligament edges, along with removal of any loose bodies in the joint.
  - It is important to perform the débridement using the radiocarpal and midcarpal portals.

Direct Lunotriquetral Ligament Repair

Incision and Dissection

- A longitudinal incision is made centered over the carpus in line with the third metacarpal ray (**TECH FIG 1**).
  - Alternatively, a curvilinear incision can be used.
- The dorsal sensory branch of the ulnar nerve is identified and protected.
- The extensor retinaculum is divided over the EPL from distal to proximal, releasing it from the third compartment (**TECH FIG 2**).
- Ulnar-based flaps of extensor retinaculum are developed by dividing the septa separating the third through the fifth extensor compartments (**TECH FIG 3**).

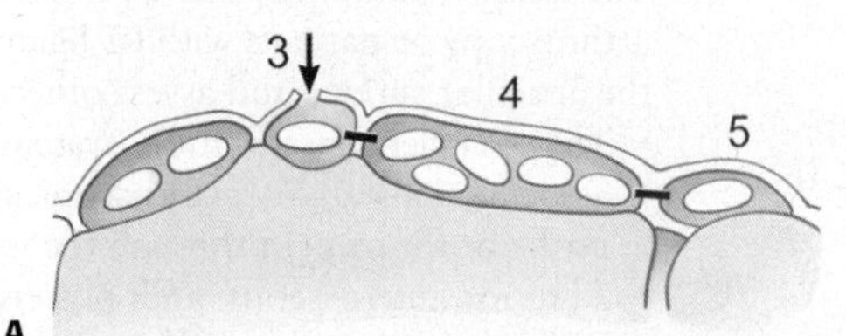

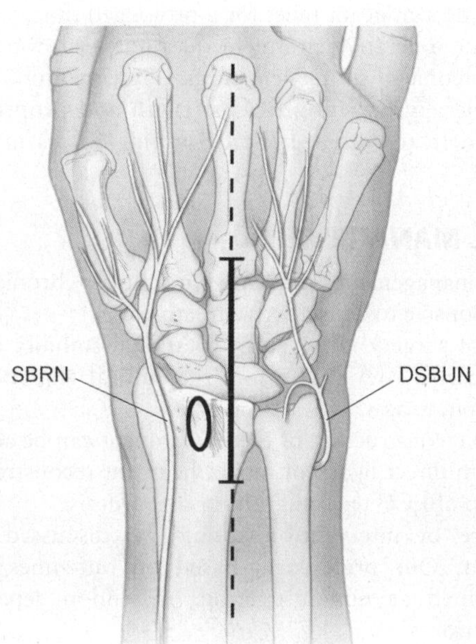

TECH FIG 1 • **A.** Axial image of dorsal wrist compartments with *arrow* indicating location for skin incision over third compartment. **B.** Skin incision centered over third dorsal compartment with superficial branch of the radial nerve (*SBRN*) and dorsal sensory branch of the ulnar nerve (*DSBUN*). *Oval* indicates tubercle of Lister. (Copyright © Mayo Clinic.)

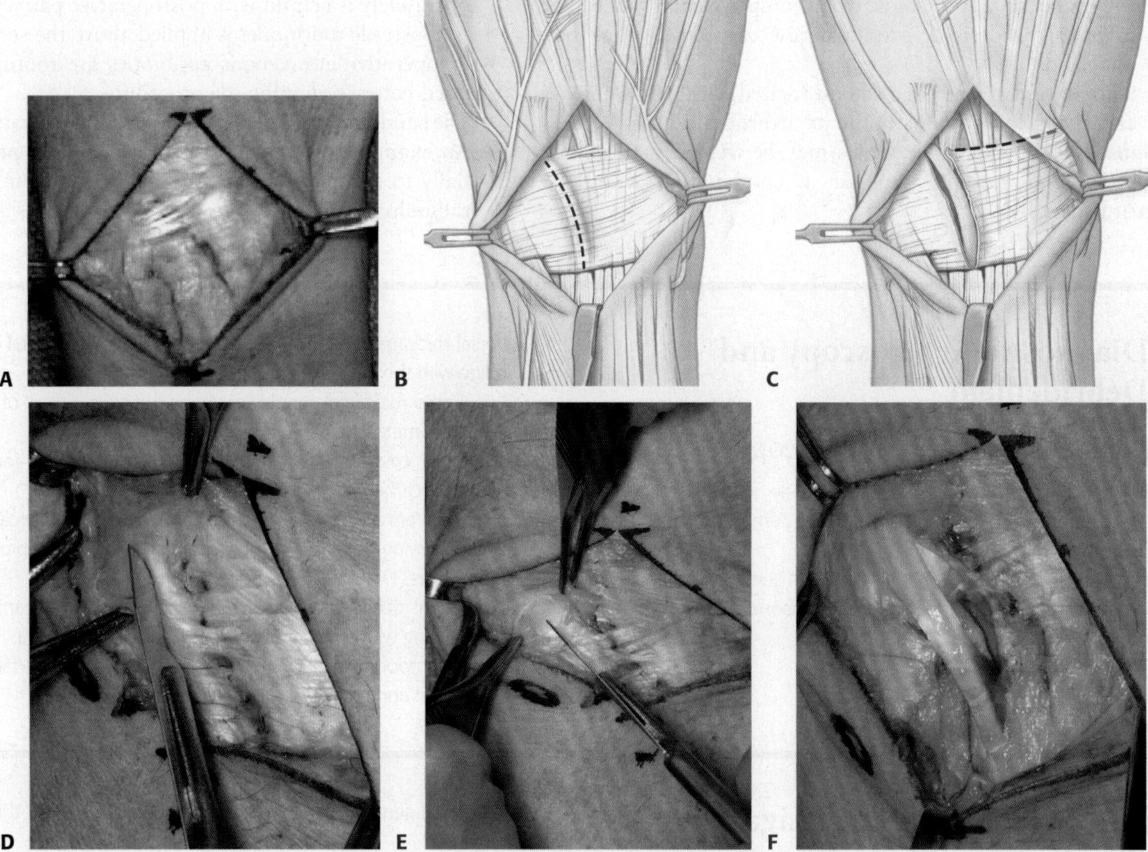

TECH FIG 2 • **A.** Superficial dissection with extensor retinaculum visible. **B.** *Dotted line* indicates incision of third compartment to release the EPL tendon. **C.** EPL released from third compartment. The *dotted line* represent the division of the extensor retinaculum over the third compartment and transversely over the distal portion of the extensor retinaculum. **D.** Incision of extensor retinaculum over EPL. **E.** Incision of extensor retinaculum over EPL. EPL tendon is visible distally. **F.** EPL released from third compartment. (**B,C:** Copyright © Mayo Clinic.)

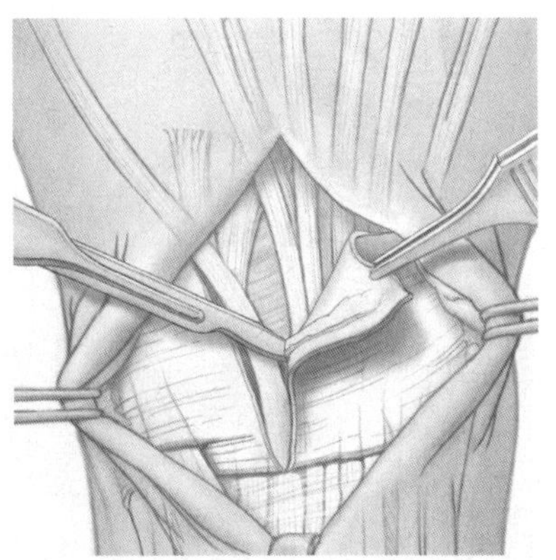
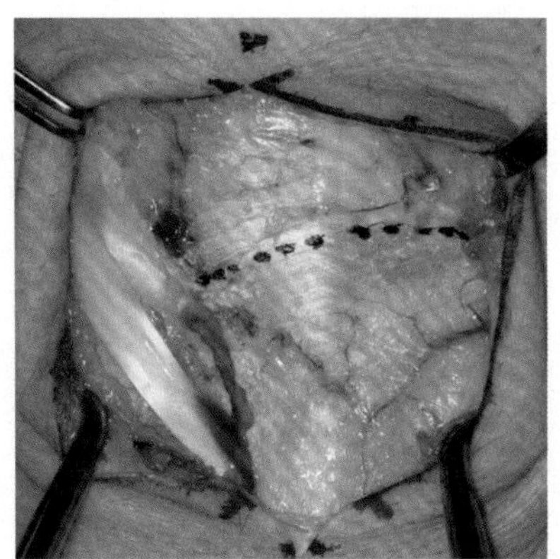
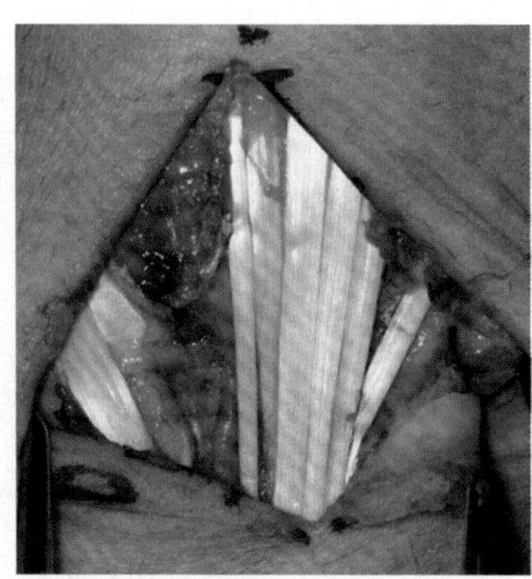

TECH FIG 3 • **A.** Dissection of septa to create ulnar-based flap of extensor retinaculum. **B.** Preparing to reflect extensor retinaculum. **C.** Retinaculum has been reflected ulnarly, and extensor tendons are released. (**A:** Copyright © Mayo Clinic.)

- If not done previously, a posterior interosseous neurectomy is performed to partially denervate the dorsal wrist capsule (**TECH FIG 4**).
- The dorsal radiocarpal and intercarpal ligaments are identified and a ligament-splitting capsulotomy made as described by Berger and Bishop[4] (**TECH FIG 5A–D**).
- When elevating the capsule, it is important not to dissect too deep over the region of the LT area. The dorsal LT ligament is intimately related to the radiotriquetral ligament and can be injured if attention is not paid during the capsulotomy.
- The midcarpal and radiocarpal joint surfaces are exposed and examined for arthritic changes (**TECH FIG 5E**).
- The SL and LT ligaments are thoroughly examined.
  - The dorsal aspect of the LT ligament is inspected to determine if it is suitable for repair. The articular surfaces of the radiocarpal and midcarpal joints are also inspected.
  - The volar portion of the LT joint is examined, and the integrity of the volar LT ligament is indirectly inspected. If it is completely incompetent, then a direct repair of the dorsal LT ligament is contraindicated and one should proceed to a ligament reconstruction as described later in this chapter.
  - Intra-articular step-off of the LT articulation is also assessed as well as the presence of a separate lunate facet with the hamate (type II lunate).

Reattaching the Ligament

- The LT ligament is reattached to the site of avulsion, usually the triquetrum.
- Two techniques for reattachment of the ligament exist: the use of drill holes or suture anchors. Multiple horizontal drill holes or suture anchors are placed in the dorsal, nonarticular surface of the triquetrum (**TECH FIG 6A**).
- Numerous strands of nonabsorbable suture (size 2-0) are used to repair the avulsed ligament (**TECH FIG 6B**).
- Before tensioning and tying the sutures, the diastasis of the LT joint must be reduced and the articular incongruity at the midcarpal joint reduced. The reduction is secured by two 0.045-inch smooth Kirschner wires (K-wires) (**TECH FIG 6C–E**).
  - The K-wires can be used to assist with reduction of the LT joint as well as to maintain anatomic alignment postreduction.
- The sutures are then tensioned and tied but not cut short.

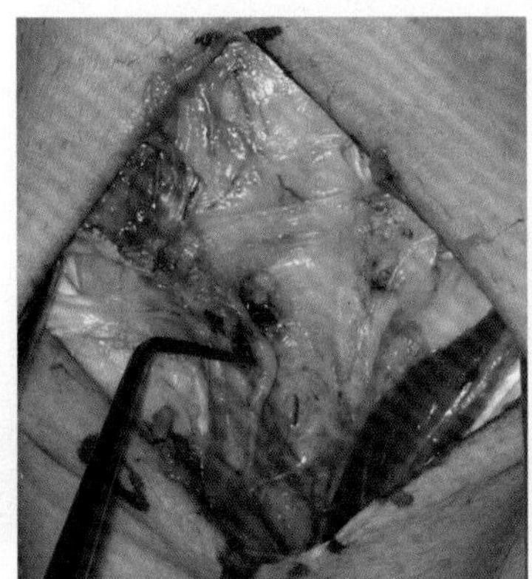
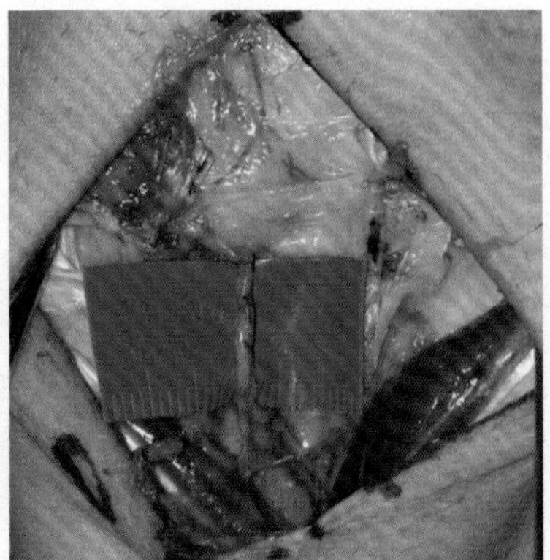
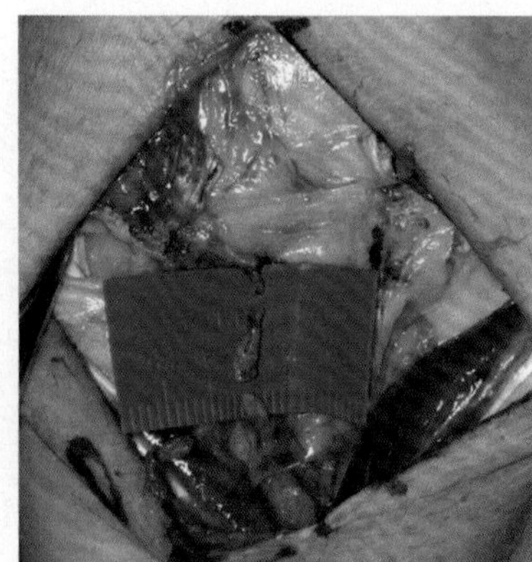

TECH FIG 4 • **A.** Posterior interosseous nerve (PIN) visible overlying wrist capsule. **B.** PIN identified and isolated. **C.** Segment resected from PIN.

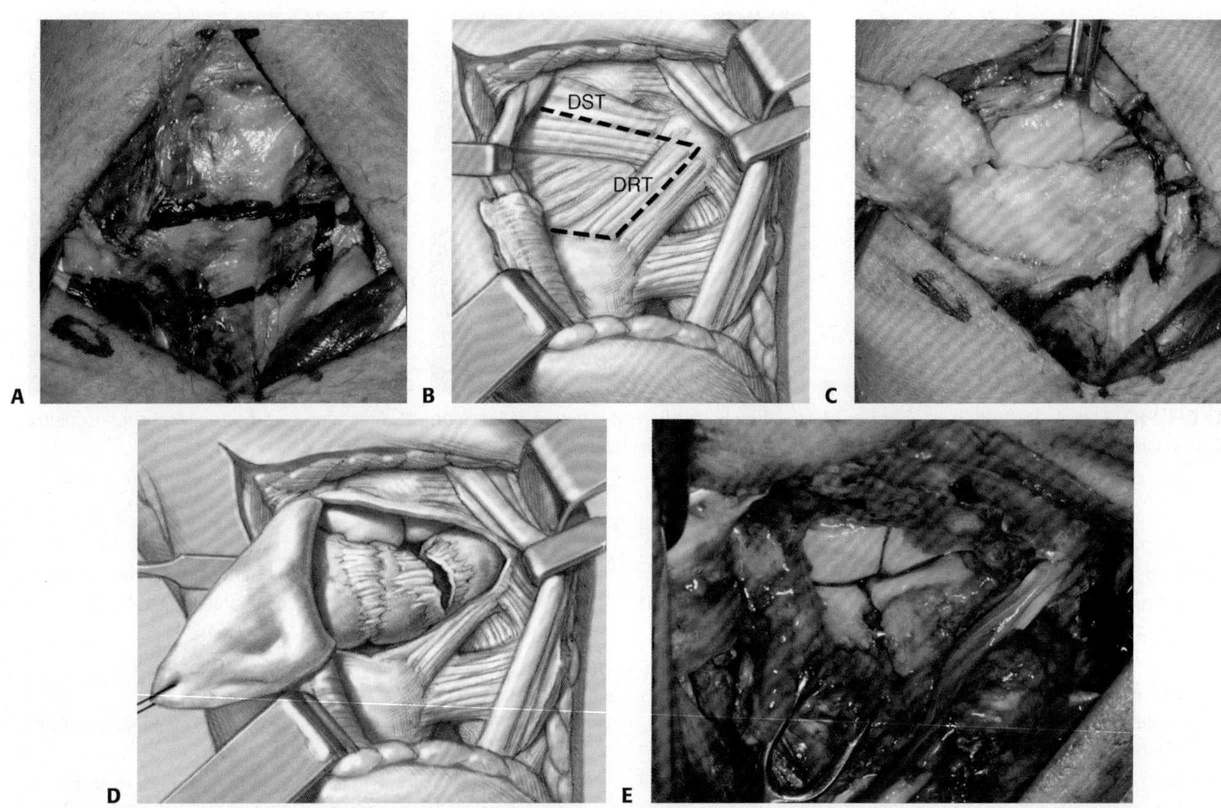

TECH FIG 5 • **A.** Dorsal ligament-splitting capsulotomy planned. **B.** Dorsal ligament-splitting capsulotomy showing location of the dorsal radiotriquetral (*DRT*) and dorsal scaphotriquetral (*DST*) ligaments. **C.** Dorsal capsule reflected radially. **D.** Dorsal capsule reflected radially showing LT ligament disruption. **E.** Dorsal capsulotomy performed. The dorsal LT ligament is visibly torn. (**B,D:** Copyright © Mayo Clinic.)

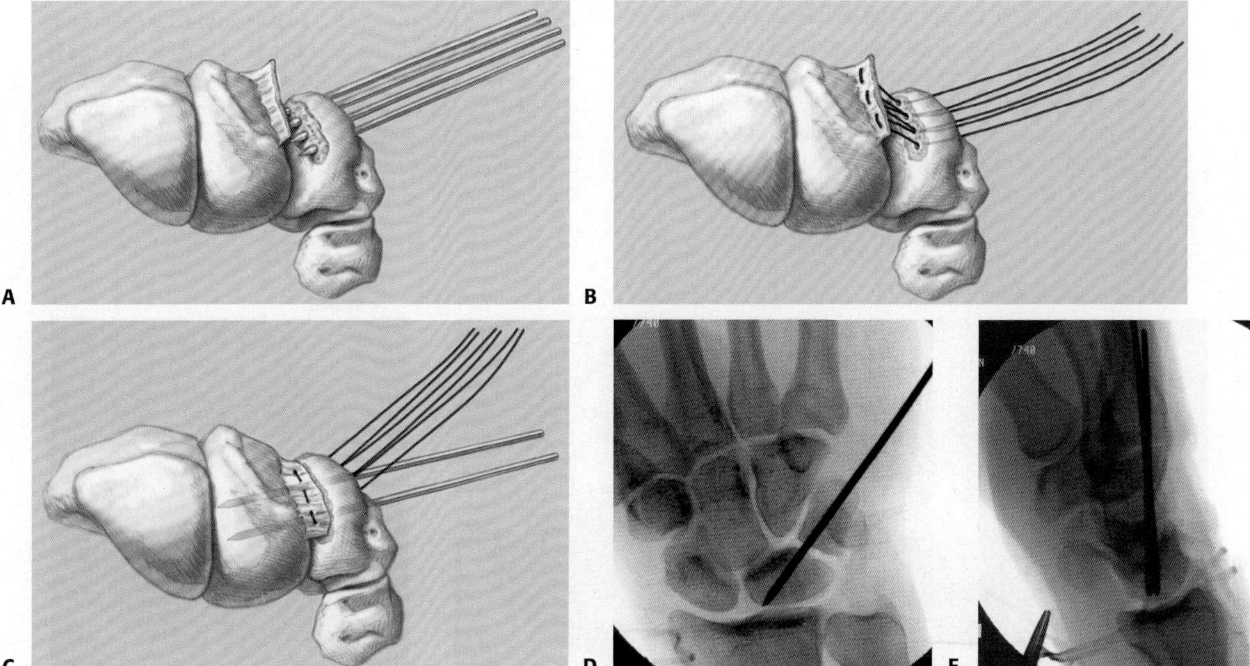

TECH FIG 6 • **A.** Drill holes in the dorsal, nonarticular surface of the triquetrum. **B.** Nonabsorbable sutures passed through drill hole and dorsal LT ligament. **C.** LT joint reduced and stabilized with K-wires. Sutures ready to be tied. **D,E.** Postreduction AP (**D**) and lateral (**E**) fluoroscopy showing LT joint reduction and position of K-wires. *(continued)*

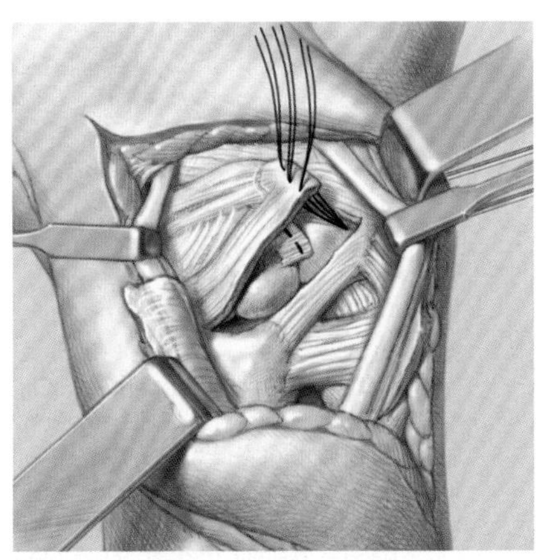

TECH FIG 6 • *(continued)* **F.** Dorsal capsulotomy repaired with heavy, nonabsorbable sutures. (**A–C,F:** Copyright © Mayo Clinic.)

- Dorsal capsulodesis can be then performed to augment the LT ligament.
  - Capsulodesis recreates or augments the dorsal LT ligament using the radiotriquetral ligament.
  - Capsulodesis is performed by placing additional suture anchors into the dorsal aspects of the lunate and triquetrum. Using these anchors to attach a portion of the radiotriquetral ligament to the lunate and triquetrum, it acts to augments the dorsal LT ligament.
- The ligament-splitting capsulotomy is repaired with nonabsorbable sutures (**TECH FIG 6F**).
- The extensor retinaculum is repaired with the EPL dorsally transposed.
- The skin is closed in the standard fashion.
- A long-arm, bulky splint is applied.

Lunotriquetral Ligament Reconstruction with Distally Based Extensor Carpi Ulnaris Strip

Harvesting the Graft

- To avoid disrupting the ECU subsheath,[20] a 2-cm transverse incision is made through the skin and the ECU sheath 6 cm proximal to the ulnar styloid. The ECU tendon is identified (**TECH FIG 7A**).
- A small right angle clamp or 90-degree retractor is used to isolate and elevate the ECU tendon (**TECH FIG 7B**).
- A 4-mm incision is made on the radial side of the ECU tendon to create a strip of tendon graft. A piece of 28-gauge wire is tied to the free end of the tendon graft (**TECH FIG 7C**).
- The ECU sheath is opened at the level of the carpometacarpal joint. The wire is looped and passed from proximal to distal through the sheath into the distal incision. The wire and tendon are gently pulled distally, creating a distally based tendon graft (**TECH FIG 7D**).
- The graft is passed deep to the extensor retinaculum.
- The 28-gauge wire is left tied to the end of the graft and a moist sponge is wrapped around the graft while the bone tunnels are prepared.

Bone Tunnel Creation and Graft Passage

- 0.045-inch K-wires are advanced through the lunate and the triquetrum.
  - The correct starting points for these K-wires are the dorsal ulnar aspect of the triquetrum and the dorsal radial edge of the lunate.
  - The holes should converge at the volar margin of the LT joint and must *not* be intra-articular (**TECH FIG 8A**).
- If a reducible VISI deformity exists, it is important to place the K-wires while the deformity is held reduced. Joysticks in the scaphoid and triquetrum are useful to maintain the reduction while the lunate and triquetral wires are placed (**TECH FIG 8B**).
- The position of the wires is checked with fluoroscopy to confirm the ability to safely enlarge the drill holes without fracture.

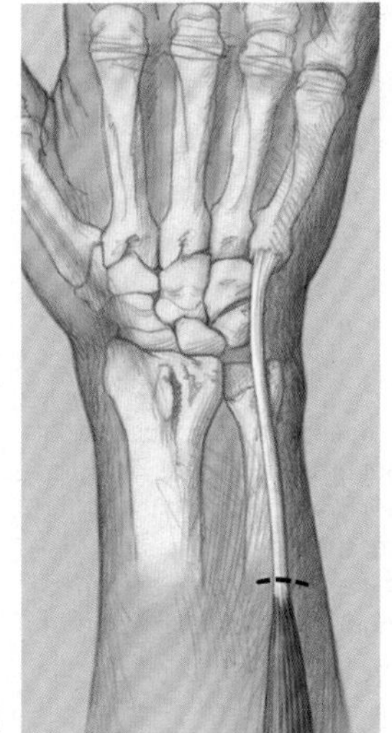

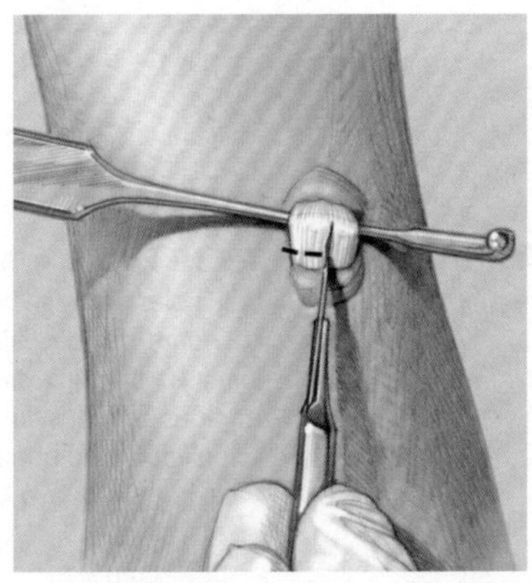

TECH FIG 7 • **A.** Location of 2-cm transverse skin incision located 6 cm proximal to ulnar styloid overlying ECU tendon. **B.** Isolation of the radial 4 mm of ECU tendon to create tendon strip for reconstruction. *Dotted line* shows tendon to be transected. *(continued)*

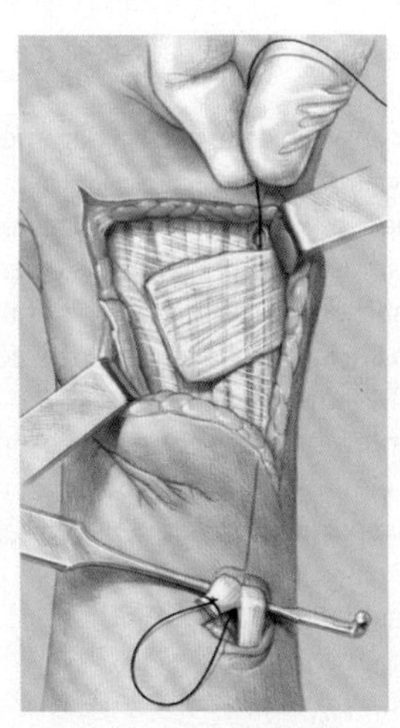

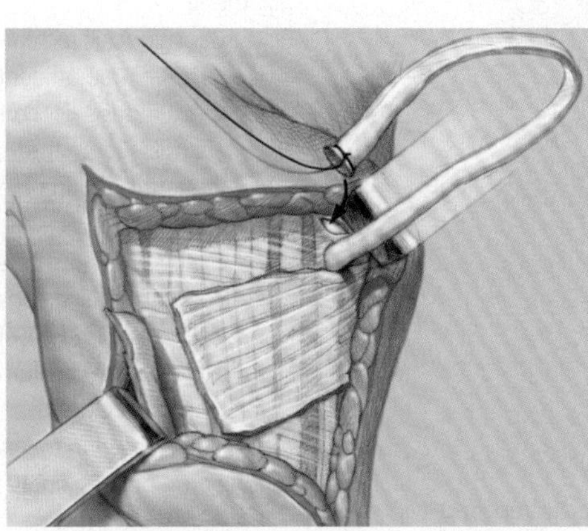

TECH FIG 7 • *(continued)* **C.** A 28-gauge wire tied around ECU tendon strip and passed through ECU tendon sheath. The wire and tendon strip pass deep to the extensor retinaculum. **D.** ECU tendon strip has been passed distally through ECU tendon sheath. (Copyright © Mayo Clinic.)

- The tunnels are created using a series of sharp awls or drill bits, gradually increasing the diameter until a 4- to 5-mm tunnel is created in both the lunate and triquetrum (**TECH FIG 8C**).
  - Alternatively, a cannulated drill system can be used.
- The wire previously secured to the end of the graft is looped and passed through the triquetral tunnel toward the lunate (**TECH FIG 9A–C**).
- An arthroscopic hook or probe is useful to hook the wire loop and pull it through the lunate bone tunnel (**TECH FIG 9D,E**).
- The wire is used to pass the tendon graft through the tunnels (**TECH FIG 10A**).
- While maintaining tension on the tendon graft, the articular surfaces of the lunate and triquetrum are reduced and two 0.045-inch K-wires are passed percutaneously across the LT joint.
- Reduction, pin position, and length are checked with fluoroscopy.
- The tendon graft is then woven through itself on the dorsum of the lunate and triquetrum and firmly secured with nonabsorbable suture (**TECH FIG 10B,C**).
- Excess tendon is trimmed, and the wound is irrigated with normal saline solution.
- The wound is closed as previously described in the ligament repair section.

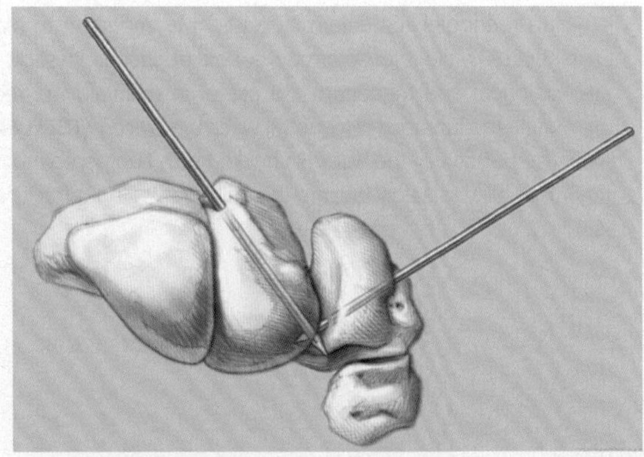

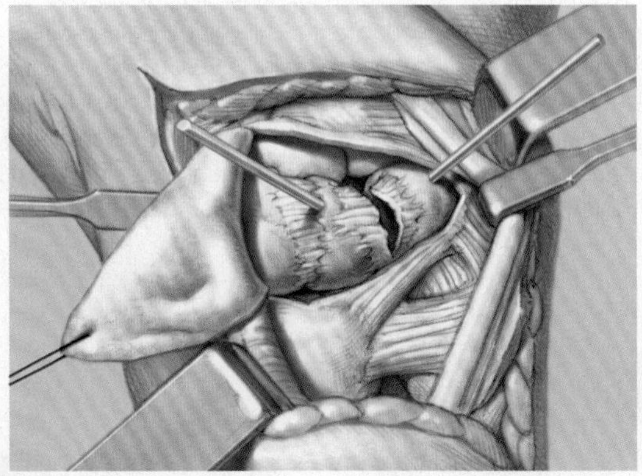

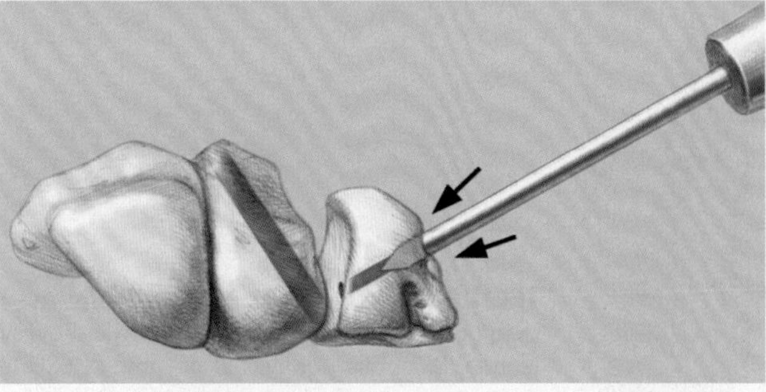

TECH FIG 8 • **A.** K-wires showing position of drill holes through triquetrum and lunate. The tips converge on the palmar, nonarticular surface of the joint. **B.** Dorsal exposure showing LT ligament disruption and position of K-wires for bone tunnels. **C.** Enlarging the bone tunnels to a diameter of 5 mm. (Copyright © Mayo Clinic.)

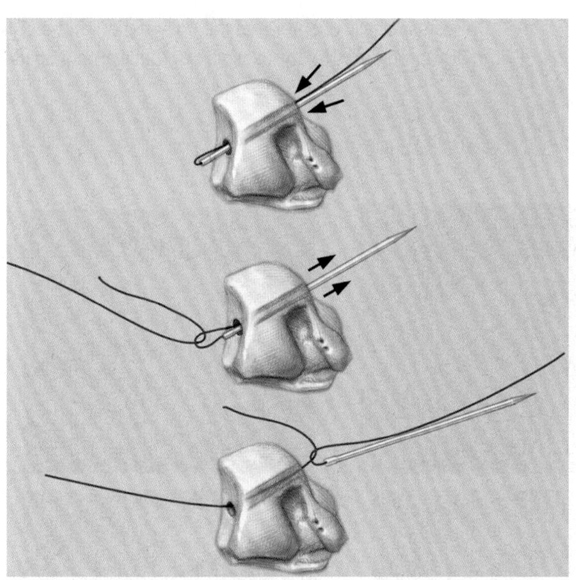
A–C

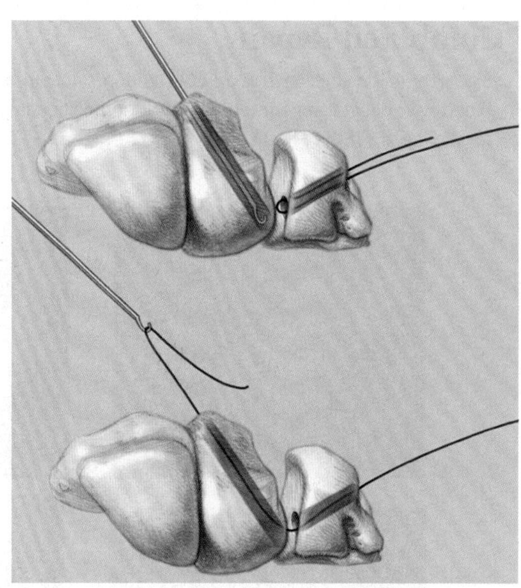
D,E

TECH FIG 9 • A–C. Straight Keith needle used to shuttle wire or heavy suture to assist in passing the ECU tendon strip through bone tunnels—first through the triquetrum and then through the lunate. In the illustration, the drill hole is placed in the articular surface. This is in error, and should be on the volar radial portion of the triquetrum. **D,E.** Arthroscopic hook used to pass wire or heavy suture through bone tunnels. (Copyright © Mayo Clinic.)

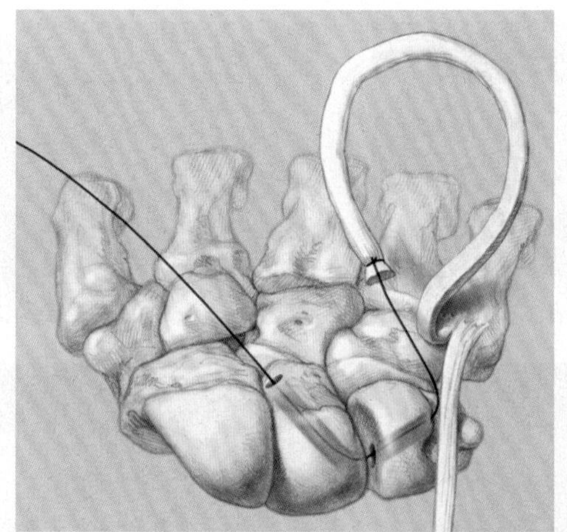
A

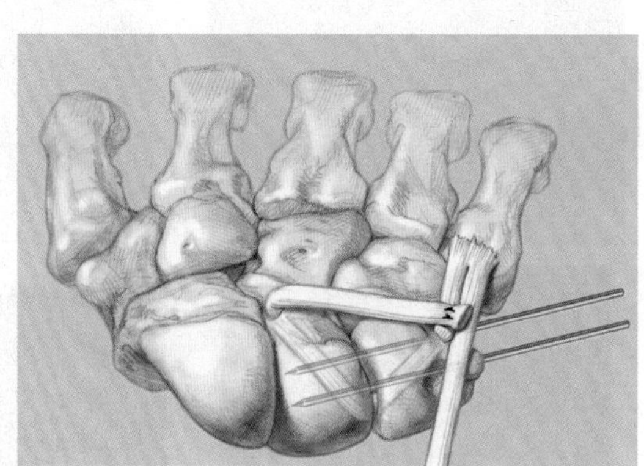
B

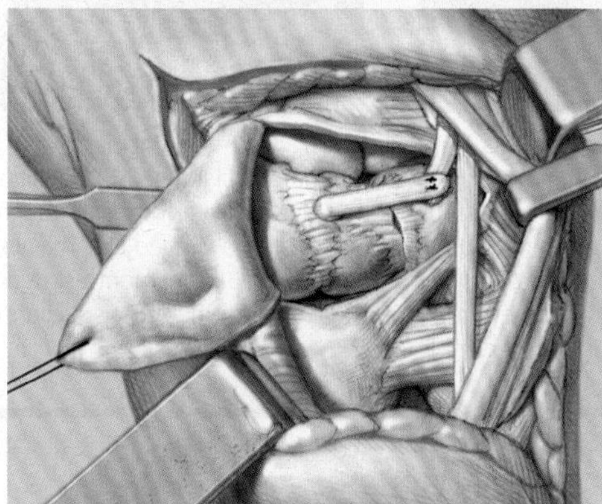
C

TECH FIG 10 • A. Passing ECU tendon strip through bone tunnels. **B.** ECU tendon has been passed through bone tunnels, tensioned, and sutured into itself. K-wires placed percutaneously to maintain LT joint reduction. **C.** Dorsal view of ligament reconstruction with ECU tendon strip. Ready for capsular repair. (Copyright © Mayo Clinic.)

Combined Repair

- Ligament reconstruction with an ECU tendon strip can be combined with direct ligament repair to provide additional strength for the repair (**TECH FIG 11**).
- This is especially useful when the volar region of the LT ligament is disrupted and the dorsal aspect of the ligament is attenuated.

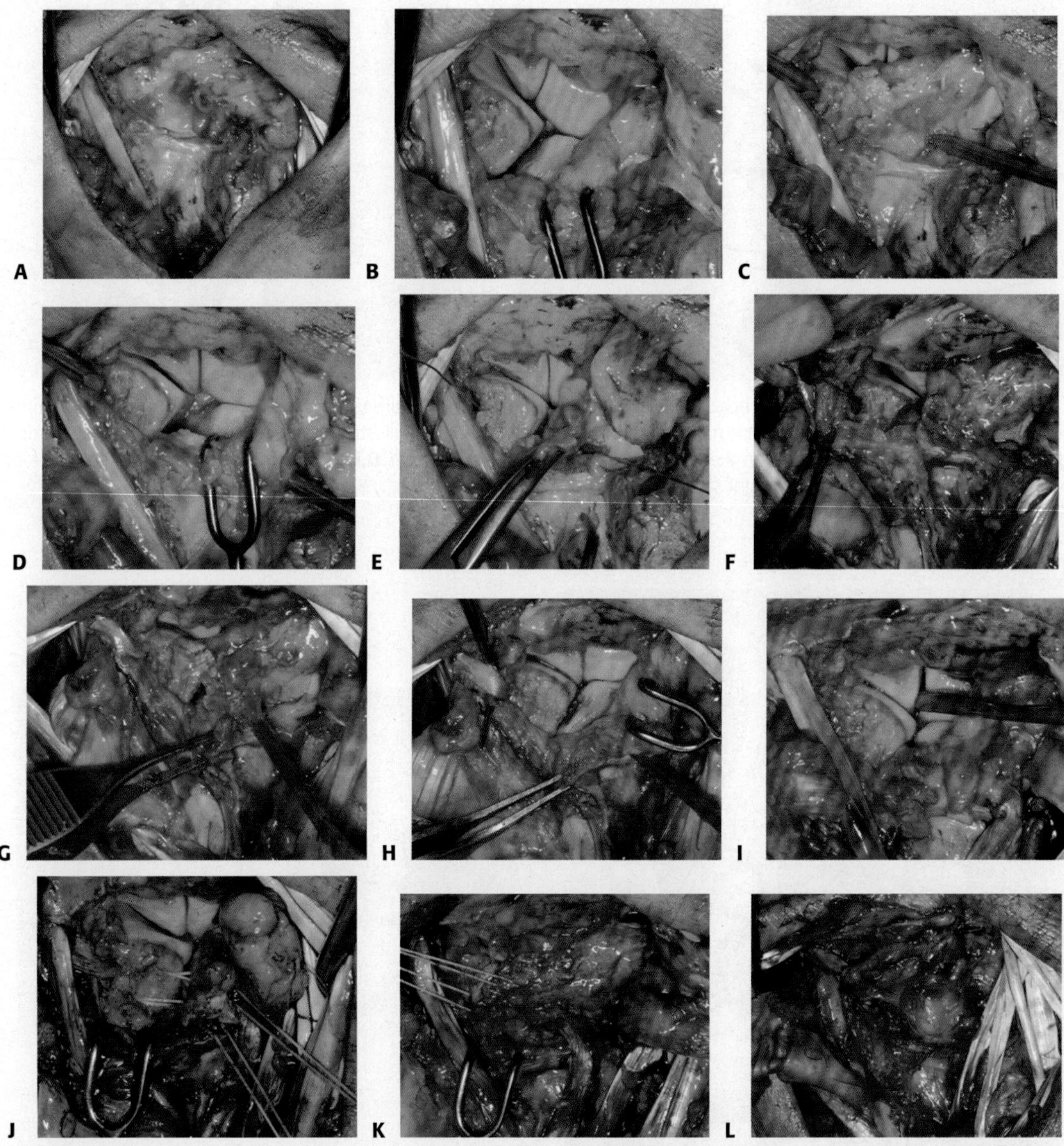

TECH FIG 11 • **A.** Dorsal exposure before capsulotomy (fingers are to the bottom and the thumb is to the left). **B.** LT joint diastasis with dorsal LT ligament disruption. The ligament remains attached to the dorsal lunate. **C,D.** Positioning K-wires for drill holes. **E.** A 28-gauge wire passes through bone tunnels. **F,G.** The tendon graft is first advanced through the triquetrum and then through the lunate. **H.** The tendon graft is tensioned. **I.** Reduction should be verified and maintained with LT K-wires before final ligament tensioning and suture placement. **J.** Direct repair of dorsal LT ligament using suture form anchors placed into the triquetrum. **K.** Tensioning direct LT ligament repair. **L.** Final view of the reconstruction after capsulotomy repair. Heavy, nonabsorbable sutures secure the capsular repair.

PEARLS AND PITFALLS

Direct repair	■ Position the drill holes in the triquetrum so that a strong bridge of bone remains to support the sutures and knots. Holes placed too close to the edge of the bone will allow the suture to pull through when tensioned. ■ Pass the sutures through sufficient substance of the LT ligament so that the suture does not tear or pull out of the ligament. ■ The use of heavy, nonabsorbable suture is important for an adequate capsular repair. ■ It is important to visualize and ensure the adequacy of the reduction before placing the K-wires across the LT joint. ■ The senior author prefers to cut the K-wire below the level of the skin. Other authors advocate percutaneous placement for easy removal.
Ligament reconstruction with distally based ECU strip	■ Positioning the ECU tendon strip through the drill holes can be difficult. Stainless steel wire or heavy monofilament suture can be passed first and used to shuttle the strip of tendon in the correct position. ■ Tensioning the tendon and suturing it into itself can be challenging. A surgical clamp such as a Kocher or Allis can be attached to the proximal free edge of the tendon strip and used as a handle to apply traction to the tendon strip as it is being secured. ■ Tension the tendon strip while the LT joint is reduced. ■ It is important to visualize and ensure the adequacy of the reduction before placing the K-wires across the LT joint. ■ Adequate duration of postoperative immobilization is important to ensure a successful outcome.

POSTOPERATIVE CARE

- Edema control and range-of-motion exercises of the digits are initiated immediately postoperatively.
- Seven to 10 days after the procedure, the surgical splint is removed, sutures are removed, and a long-arm cast is applied for 6 weeks. A short-arm cast is then applied for an additional 4 to 6 weeks for a total period of immobilization of 10 to 12 weeks.
- The K-wires are removed 10 to 12 weeks after surgery, and wrist range-of-motion exercises are commenced.

OUTCOMES

- A high-quality tendon repair is vital for a successful outcome of the LT tenodesis.
- Several studies have shown that direct LT ligament repair results in a successful clinical result.[4,16,17,20]
  - Dorsal capsulodesis has been shown to augment LT repair with successful clinical outcomes in patient's chronic LT instability.[1,14]
- Reagan et al[17] reported that six of seven cases of direct LT ligament repairs were successful, whereas all four patients who underwent arthrodesis did not experience symptom resolution. Cast immobilization successfully treated six of seven acute injuries but only one of four chronic LT tears.
- Favero et al[4] reported patient satisfaction of 90% with only one failure in 21 cases.
- In high-demand patients such as laborers and athletes, rerupture or attenuation can occur and lead to late failure.[22] Reconstruction with a strip of ECU tendon should be considered in this patient subgroup.
- Weiss et al[23] demonstrated that arthroscopic débridement followed by 2 weeks of immobilizaiton led to clinical improvements in 78% of wrists. In contrast, Westkaemper et al[24] reported poor outcomes in four of five patients with a similar treatment protocol.
- A review of clinical outcomes comparing LT ligament repair, ligament reconstruction, and LT joint arthrodesis at our institution showed that patients treated with ligament reconstruction have the lowest reoperation rate.[22]
  - Rerupture after trauma and late attenuation appear to be common modes of long-term failure of direct repair.
- Review of the clinical outcomes at our institution showed that reconstruction with a strip of ECU tendon as described can be an effective treatment.[3]
- Mirza et al[11] reported reduced clinical symptoms in the majority of 53 consecutive patients with an isolated posttraumatic LT tear treated with an ulnar shortening osteotomy.

COMPLICATIONS

- LT arthrodesis have relatively high rates of nonunion, ulnocarpal impingement, and other complications with variable rates of pain relief and clinical improvement.[13,17,19,22]

REFERENCES

1. Antti-Poika I, Hyrkäs J, Virkki LM, et al. Correction of chronic lunotriquetral instability using extensor retinacular split: a retrospective study of 26 patients. Acta Orthop Belg 2007;73:451–457.
2. Beckenbaugh RD. Accurate evaluation and management of the painful wrist following injury. An approach to carpal instability. Orthop Clin North Am 1984;15:289–306.
3. Berger RA. The gross and histologic anatomy of the scapholunate interosseous ligament. J Hand Surg Am 1996;21:170–178.
4. Berger RA, Bishop AT, Bettinger PC. New dorsal capsulotomy for the surgical exposure of the wrist. Ann Plast Surg 1995;35(1):54–59.
5. Geissler WB, Freeland AE, Savoie FH, et al. Intracarpal soft-tissue lesions associated with an intra-articular fracture of the distal end of the radius. J Bone Joint Surg Am 1996;78:357–365.
6. Gilula LA, Weeks PM. Post-traumatic ligamentous instabilities of the wrist. Radiology 1978;129:641–651.
7. Kleinman WB. Diagnostic exams for ligamentous injuries. Am Soc Surg Hand, Correspondence Club Newsletter 1985:51.

8. León-Lopez MM, Salvà-Coll G, Garcia-Elias M, et al. Role of the extensor carpi ulnaris in the stabilization of the lunotriquetral joint. An experimental study. J Hand Ther 2013;26:312–317; quiz 317.
9. Linscheid RL, Dobyns JH. Athletic injuries of the wrist. Clin Orthop Relat Res 1985;(198):141–151.
10. Mayfield JK, Johnson RP, Kilcoyne RK. Carpal dislocations: pathomechanics and progressive perilunar instability. J Hand Surg Am 1980;5(3):226–241.
11. Mirza A, Mirza JB, Shin AY, et al. Isolated lunotriquetral ligament tears treated with ulnar shortening osteotomy. J Hand Surg Am 2013;38:1492–1497.
12. Murray PM, Palmer CG, Shin AY. The mechanism of ulnar-sided perilunate instability of the wrist: a cadaveric study and 6 clinical cases. J Hand Surg Am 2012;37(4):721–728. doi:10.1016/j.jhsa.2012.01.015.
13. Nelson DL, Manske PR, Pruitt DL, et al. Lunotriquetral arthrodesis. J Hand Surg Am 1993;18:1113–1120.
14. Omokawa S, Fujitani R, Inada Y. Dorsal radiocarpal ligament capsulodesis for chronic dynamic lunotriquetral instability. J Hand Surg Am 2009;34:237–243.
15. Palmer AK. Triangular fibrocartilage complex lesions: a classification. J Hand Surg Am 1989;14:594–606.
16. Palmer AK, Werner FW. Biomechanics of the distal radioulnar joint. Clin Orthop Relat Res 1984;(187):26–35.
17. Reagan DS, Linscheid RL, Dobyns JH. Lunotriquetral sprains. J Hand Surg Am 1984;9:502–514.
18. Ritt MJ, Bishop AT, Berger RA, et al. Lunotriquetral ligament properties: a comparison of three anatomic subregions. J Hand Surg Am 1998;23:425–431.
19. Sennwald GR, Fischer M, Mondi P. Lunotriquetral arthrodesis. A controversial procedure. J Hand Surg Br 1995;20:755–760.
20. Shin AY, Bishop AT. Treatment options for lunotriquetral dissociation. Tech Hand Up Extrem Surg 1998;2:2–17.
21. Shin AY, Deitch MA, Sachar K, et al. Ulnar-sided wrist pain: diagnosis and treatment. Instr Course Lect 2005;54:115–128.
22. Shin AY, Weinstein LP, Berger RA, et al. Treatment of isolated injuries of the lunotriquetral ligament. A comparison of arthrodesis, ligament reconstruction and ligament repair. J Bone Joint Surg Br 2001;83:1023–1028.
23. Weiss AP, Sachar K, Glowacki KA. Arthroscopic debridement alone for intercarpal ligament tears. J Hand Surg Am 1997;22:344–349.
24. Westkaemper JG, Mitsionis G, Giannakopoulos PN, et al. Wrist arthroscopy for the treatment of ligament and triangular fibrocartilage complex injuries. Arthroscopy 1998;14:479–483.

Open and Arthroscopic Treatment of Lateral Epicondylitis

73 CHAPTER

Abhishek Julka and Peter J. Evans

DEFINITION

- Lateral epicondylitis involves tendinosis at the origin of the common wrist extensors.
- It is commonly referred to as *tennis elbow* and is likely more correctly termed *lateral elbow tendinopathy*.[15]

ANATOMY

- The common extensor origin is located on the lateral epicondyle.
- The common extensor origin includes the extensor carpi radialis brevis (ECRB), extensor digitorum communis (EDC), extensor digiti minimi, and extensor carpi ulnaris.
- The ECRB is the primary muscle–tendon unit affected, followed by the EDC with the tendons becoming confluent at their origin.[13]

PATHOGENESIS

- Epicondylitis results from repetitive microtrauma, followed by an incomplete reparative response, resulting in chronic tendinosis.[13]
- Functionally, this condition can more correctly be described as "gripper's elbow," as synergistic wrist extension increases finger flexion strength. Patients afflicted with lateral epicondylar tendinopathy commonly engage in repetitive forceful gripping activities as they lift, pull, twist, and push objects.
- Recently, concurrent radiocapitellar cartilage lesions have been noted in a high prevalence on arthroscopic examination.[14]

NATURAL HISTORY

- Lateral epicondylitis is a self-limiting condition that resolves in over 80% of patients over the course of 1 year.[4]
- Most patients receiving active treatment (ie, anti-inflammatory medication, orthotics, ultrasound, physical or occupational therapy, injections) improve with nonoperative treatment.
- Typically, fewer than 10% of patients require surgical intervention.

PATIENT HISTORY AND PHYSICAL FINDINGS

- Acute phase: Lateral elbow pain or ache occurs with activities that typically resolves with rest, ice, or anti-inflammatory medication.
- Intermediate phase: Lateral elbow pain or ache occurs with activity and at rest and may not resolve without prolonged activity restriction.
- Chronic phase: Pain or ache occurs with sleep and is unresponsive to rest, medication, and injections.[13]
- Examination methods include the following:
  - Palpation of the lateral epicondyle for tenderness, a universal finding in lateral epicondylitis
  - Pain either at the epicondyle or radiating distally along the ECRB is a positive finding in any of these circumstances:
    - *Passive stretch test:* With the elbow in full extension, the wrist is flexed, and the forearm is pronated.
    - *Mill test:* With the elbow flexed, the forearm slightly pronated, and the wrist slightly dorsiflexed, the patient actively supinates against the examiner, who resists this rotation.
    - *Thompson test:* With the elbow extended, the wrist in slight dorsiflexion, and making a fist, the patient dorsiflexes against the examiner, who resists this motion.

IMAGING AND OTHER DIAGNOSTIC STUDIES

- Plain radiographs may show calcifications at the extensor origin.
- Magnetic resonance imaging (MRI)
  - Increased intratendon signal is reliably demonstrated on T2-weighted sequences.
  - Most also show increased intratendon signal or tendon thickening on T1-weighted sequences.
  - A small percentage of patients may show increased T2 signal in the lateral epicondyle or anconeus edema.[9]
  - Periosteal reaction is *not* commonly seen on MRI.[9]
  - Lateral collateral ligament tears often are over interpreted on MRI reports, but this possibility must be ruled out by an accurate history and pre- and intraoperative examinations.

DIFFERENTIAL DIAGNOSIS

- Synovial plica
- Lateral collateral ligament tear
- Radial tunnel syndrome
- Loose bodies
- Degenerative joint disease (typically early radiocapitellar joint)
- Avascular necrosis of the capitellum

NONOPERATIVE MANAGEMENT

- Appropriate initial treatment includes avoidance of painful activities and symptomatic relief with ice and nonsteroidal anti-inflammatory drugs (NSAIDs).
- Daytime strapping is biomechanically and clinically effective.
- Nighttime wrist bracing to prevent palmar wrist flexion and prolonged tension on the extensor tendons
- Physical or occupational therapy to supervise and instruct on stretching and strengthening protocol for patients not otherwise inclined to perform these exercises

- Corticosteroid injection have repeatedly not outperformed placebo injections in the literature and have even shown inferior results. They may be used sparingly once other nonoperative measures are exhausted.[2,3,5]
- Platelet-rich plasma injections showed some promising early results[1,11] but have not held up to more critical scrutiny.[8]

SURGICAL MANAGEMENT

- A minority of patients fail nonoperative management.
- Careful patient selection is critical to ensure an excellent outcome following surgical management.
- No prospective randomized studies have yet been done to examine the advantages of open versus arthroscopic techniques for the treatment of lateral epicondylitis. However, the authors choose arthroscopic treatment if there are any signs of a plica or synovial irritation (end point pain) as it allows for direct examination and treatment of these additional pathologies.
- Two relatively new methods of percutaneous tenotomy are available and undergoing evaluation: Tenex Microtenotomy (Tenex Health Inc., Lake Forest, CA) and Topaz MicroDebrider (ArthroCare, Austin, TX). Both are percutaneous methods that allow for a minimally invasive approach to replicate outcomes of open and arthroscopic methods.
- The Topaz MicroDebrider provides a preset amount of energy to débride and stimulate neovascularization as its mechanism of action, whereas the Tenex Microtenotomy has a proposed advantage of removal of pathologic tissue as well via a phacoemulsification mechanism of action.
- Studies examining results from percutaneous tenotomy have been optimistic in the short term,[7,10] but comparative studies of percutaneous methods have yet to be published.

Preoperative Planning

- Be prepared to address concurrent extensor tendon rupture.
- Be prepared to address lateral collateral ligament rupture.

Positioning

- The patient is placed in the supine position.
- The arm is internally rotated at the shoulder, and padding is placed under the elbow, and the ulnar nerve is protected.
- The arm should rest in a position that allows ready access to the lateral aspect of the elbow without requiring constant holding by an assistant.
- The elbow should be examined after the administration of anesthesia to ensure stability, and the result is documented in the operative note.
- The goal of surgery is to débride the degenerative tissue at the extensor origin and create an environment conducive to proper healing of the tendon.

TECHNIQUES

Open Lateral Epicondylar Fasciectomy and Partial Ostectomy

- A 3- to 5-cm incision through skin only is made beginning at the proximal edge of the center of the lateral epicondyle and extending distally through the mid-radiocapitellar joint plane along the axis of the forearm (**TECH FIG 1A**).
- Blunt dissection with scissors is carried out through the subcutaneous tissues to expose the EDC aponeurosis and the ECRL.
- The more anterior and reddish ECRL and the more tendinous EDC originating on the epicondyle are identified (**TECH FIG 1B**).
  - The interval between the ECRL and the EDC aponeurosis is then split in line with the mid-radiocapitellar joint plane. Distally, a fat stripe along the aponeurosis typically is seen along this dissection plane.
  - A small posterior EDC flap is created for later closure, and the ECRL is elevated anteriorly revealing the underlying ECRB origin. The origin may be obliterated by degenerative tissue.
- The abnormal tendon tissue to be excised can be identified by its grayish, unorganized mucoid appearance and should be sharply excised. Care is taken to dissect the ECRB off the underlying capsule.
  - Abnormal tissue typically will scrape away with a no. 15 blade but normal tendon will not (Nirschl scratch test). Sometimes, the ECRB tissue cannot be dissected free from the underlying capsule or it has already ruptured from its origin, and the underlying joint becomes exposed (**TECH FIG 1C**). This will not affect outcome.

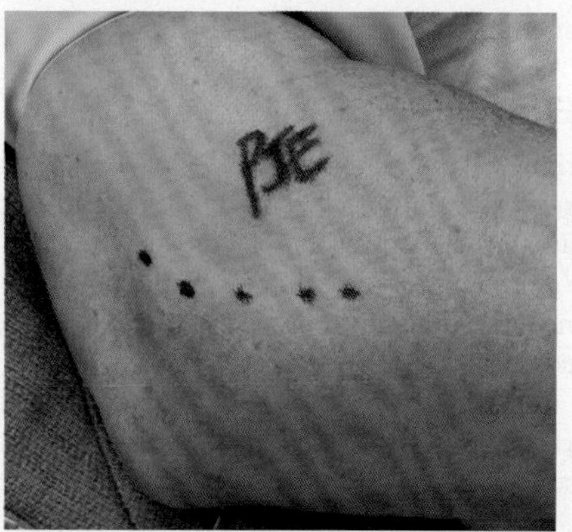

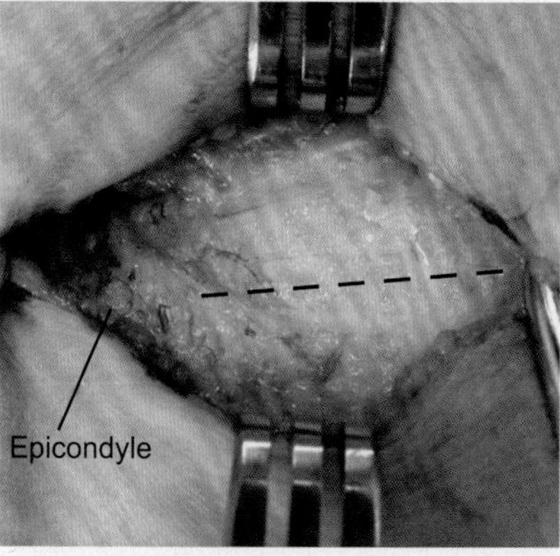

TECH FIG 1 • **A.** Surgical approach uses a 3-cm incision over the lateral epicondyle and can be extended in line with the forearm axis to avoid injury to the lateral collateral ligament. **B.** The interval between the tendinous EDC aponeurosis and the darker muscle of the ECRL is entered, and the ECRL is elevated off the underlying ECRB. (The patient's hand is to the right.) *(continued)*

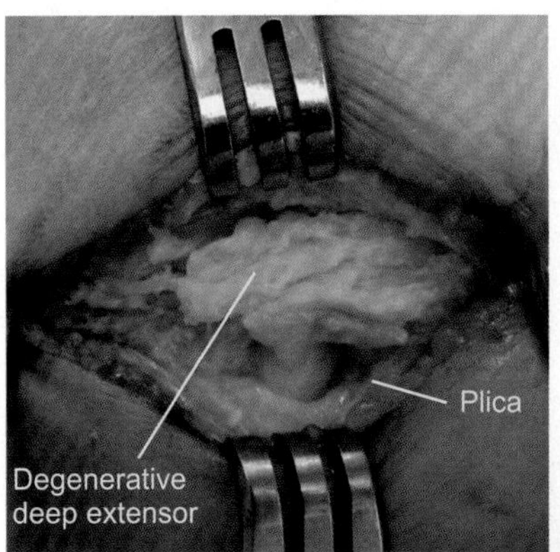

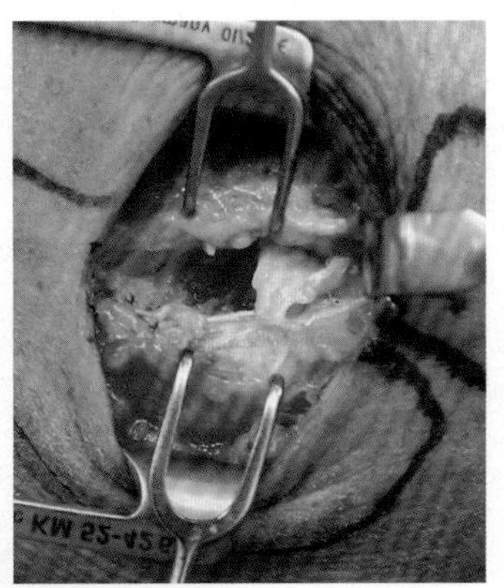

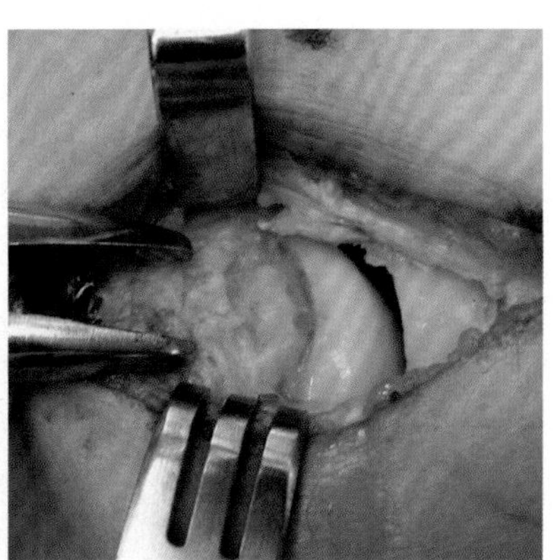

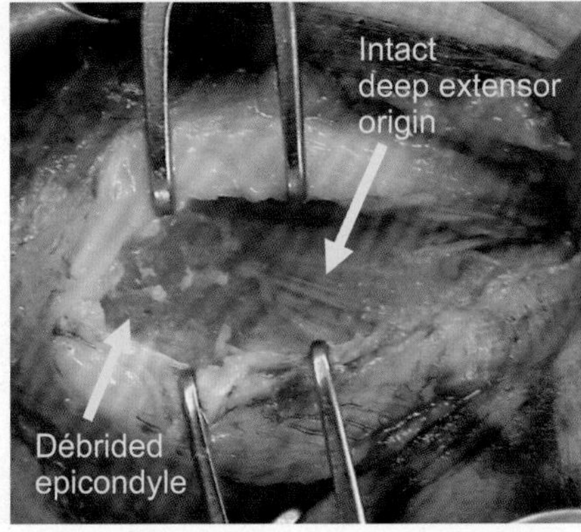

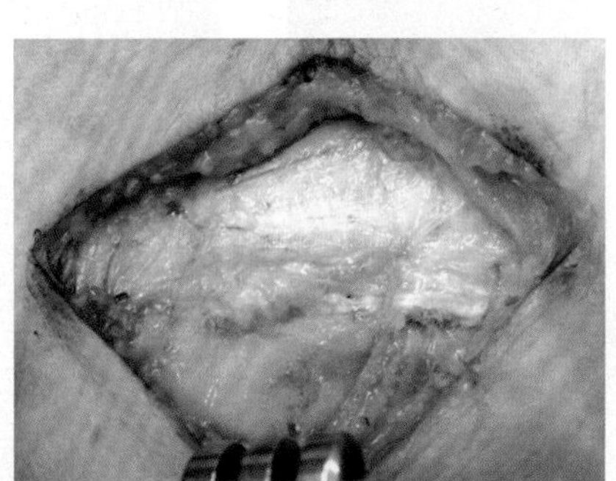

TECH FIG 1 • *(continued)* **C.** The degenerative ECRB is sharply excised. At times, as in this example, it is not possible to separate the ECRB and capsule, and a portion of the capsule also is excised. Neighboring tendon of the EDC is scraped with a no. 15 blade to remove loose degenerative tissue. **D.** In this example, it was possible to excise the degenerative portion of the ECRB without the underlying capsule. **E.** The anterior portion of the lateral epicondyle is scratched clean of degenerative tissue with a no. 15 blade or rongeur but not decorticated. **F.** Some intact, normal ECRB fibers are left if they are present. **G.** Closure is done with an inverted stitch, size 0 Vicryl suture on a tapered needle in a running fashion.

  - If exposed, the joint should be inspected for degenerative change, which, if present, typically is found beneath a plica. The plica should be removed (**TECH FIG 1D**).
- The pathologic tissue is débrided to margins showing an organized, tendinous appearance. Complete resection of the ECRB origin is not necessary if healthy viable portions remain (**TECH FIG 1E**).
  - The proximal stump of the ECRB should not be repaired because it has ample attachments and will not retract significantly.
  - The area of excision usually is 1 to 2 cm long and 5 to 10 mm wide.
  - The undersurface of the EDC often is affected, and degenerative tissue should be similarly removed.
- A rongeur or knife blade is used to roughen the anterior portion of the lateral epicondyle to a bleeding surface without removing cortical bone.
- Drilling of the epicondyle is not done, as it has been shown to confer no benefit and results in increased discomfort and stiffness for the patient.[6]
  - In some cases, patients have a significantly prominent epicondylar tip. This can be removed, especially if patients are focused on this finding and they are very thin, but the early recovery period will be more painful (**TECH FIG 1F**).
- The defect in the tendon is closed with a single running or multiple inverted, simple absorbable suture, using 0 or 1-0 suture material with a tapered needle. If a capsular rent occurs, there is no need to make a separate capsular closure, but the proximal tendon repair should be watertight to avoid a postoperative ganglion (**TECH FIG 1G**).
- The subdermal layer is closed with buried, interrupted absorbable sutures, followed by a subcuticular skin closure and Steri-Strips.

Arthroscopic Lateral Epicondylar Fasciectomy and Partial Ostectomy

- The patient is positioned according to surgeon's preference for elbow arthroscopy.
  - We prefer the lateral decubitus position with the aid of the Tenet Spider Arm Holder (Smith & Nephew, Andover, MA).
  - If prone or lateral, it is advantageous to keep the elbow well above the plane of the chest wall to optimize anterior superomedial portal camera positioning.
- The elbow is filled with 30 to 50 mL of irrigating solution until distended. An anterior superomedial portal is established.
  - A small longitudinal portal incision is made about 2 cm proximal to the medial epicondyle and just anterior to the

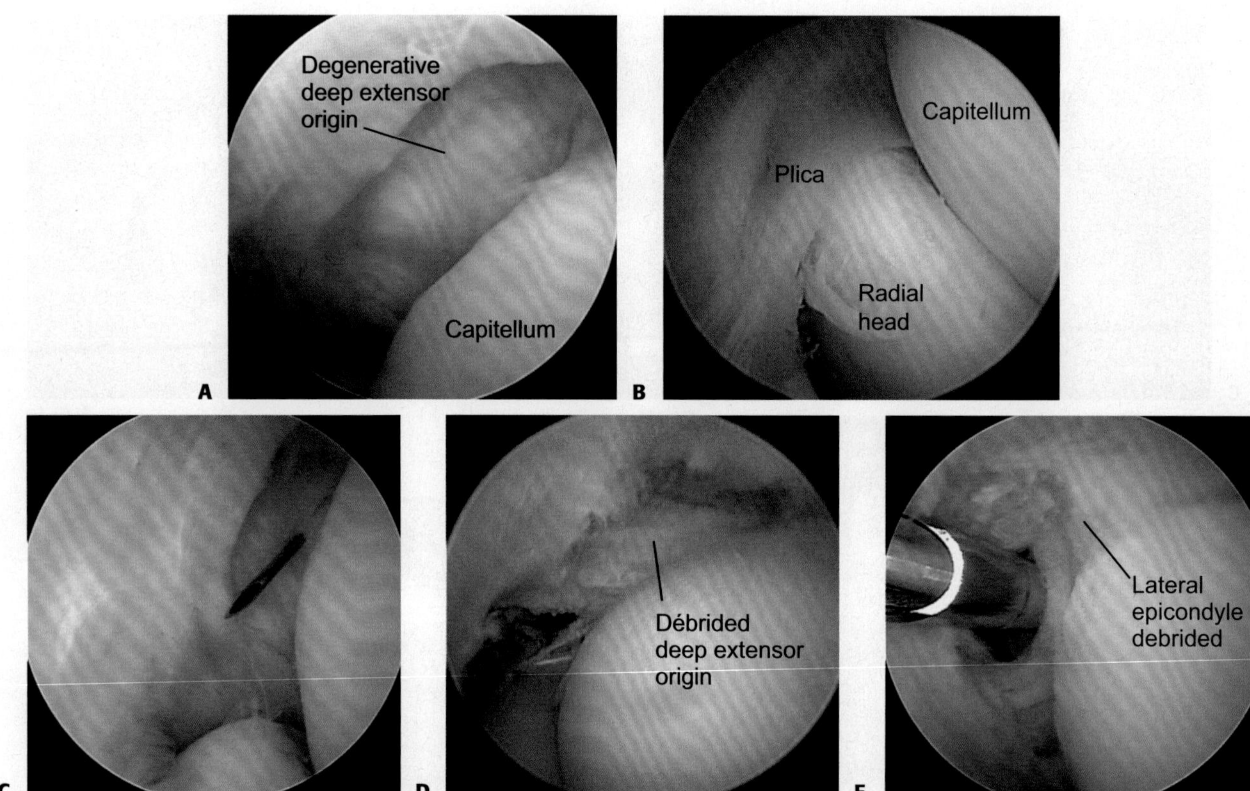

TECH FIG 2 • A. Arthroscopic view showing a capsular invagination lining a ruptured ECRB tendon. **B.** A radiocapitellar plica that is pathologic, causing degenerative changes on the radial head outer rim. **C.** A lateral portal is established at the anterior rim of the radial head at or just proximal to the radiocapitellar joint, often directly through the primary pathology. **D.** A shaver is used to excise abnormal capsule and ECRB tendon, leaving intact, shiny ECRL tendon. **E.** The shaver or burr (in reverse) can be used to clear degenerative ECRB tendon of the anterior portion of the lateral epicondyle from the capitellum back to the portal.

medial intermuscular septum. A curved hemostat is used to spread underlying tissues and feel the medial intermuscular septum and then is slid along its anterior surface to the lateral, then anterior humerus.
  - This is repeated with the scope trocar, which is then passed distally along the anterior humerus toward the radiocapitellar joint, piercing the capsule and entering the joint.
- Documentation of intra-articular (eg, loose bodies, plica [**TECH FIG 2A**], osteochondritis dissecans, arthritis) and lateral capsular or tendon pathology (**TECH FIG 2B**) is made, and they are treated appropriately.
- A 25-gauge needle is placed from outside-in to choose an optimal radiocapitellar portal at the upper rim of the radial head at or just proximal to the radial head (**TECH FIG 2C**).
- A shaver is used to débride the abnormal capsule lining the EDC origin. Abnormal ECRB is débrided until normal superficial tendon fibers are identified and protected. If ruptured, all degenerative portions of the ECRB are excised. Normal, shining ECRL fibers can be seen superficially as well as the dark muscular appearance (**TECH FIG 2D**).
- Débridement should not proceed posteriorly to the mid-radiocapitellar plane to avoid injury to the lateral collateral ligament.
- A bone-cutting shaver or a less aggressive burr used in reverse will roughen, but not decorticate, the anterior aspect of the lateral epicondyle from the capitellum back to the portal entry site (**TECH FIG 2E**).
  - A hooked electrocautery probe is useful to divide a plica to facilitate its resection.
- Lateral and posterior portals are closed with 3-0 Prolene sutures, and the medial portal is left open for rapid resolution of fluid distention and pain relief.

Percutaneous Tenotomy: Tenex

- The console is used to set the desired amount of cutting power and intensity of aspiration.
- Ultrasound is used to identify the area of pathologic tissue, which appears as a hypoechoic focus.
- A stab incision is made distal to the ultrasound probe and the extensor tendon origin.
- The microdebrider tip is introduced retrograde into the pathologic tissue under ultrasound guidance.
- The device is activated until all ultrasound evidence of previously hypoechoic tissue is removed.
- Once satisfied with the treatment, the wound is irrigated with normal saline.
- The incision is closed with a single stitch or adhesive dressing.

TECHNIQUES

Radiofrequency Microtenotomy: Topaz

- A 1-inch incision is made overlying the extensor tendon origin at the lateral epicondyle.
- Blunt dissection is carried out to visualize the extensor tendon origin
- The Topaz MicroDebrider device is then assembled.
- The saline rate of flow is adjusted till it reaches 2 to 3 drops per second.
  - The device is placed perpendicular to the tendon surface with gentle pressure and activated for 0.5 seconds.
  - Multiple applications are spaced 0.5 mm apart with altering depth to create a three-dimensional pattern within the pathologic extensor origin (**TECH FIG 3**).
- Once we are satisfied with the treatment, the wound is irrigated with normal saline.
- The incision is closed identical to closure for the open technique.

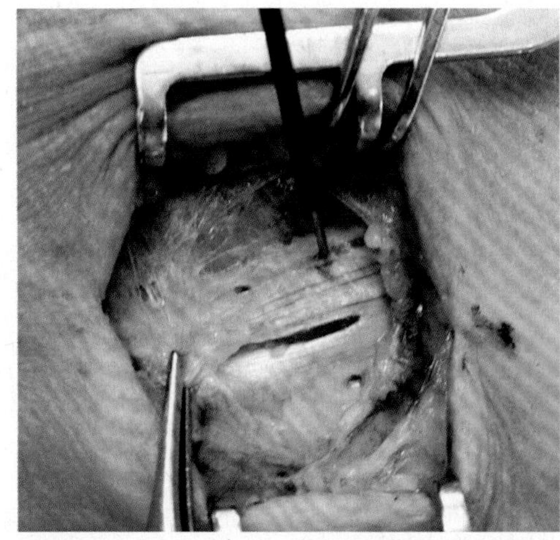

TECH FIG 3 • Demonstration of multiple perforations in the common extensor origin created with Topaz MicroDebrider.

PEARLS AND PITFALLS

Indications	▪ A minimum of 3–6 months of symptoms and failed nonoperative management
Coexisting conditions	▪ Extensor tendon origin rupture may require débridement and repair. ▪ Medial epicondylitis occurs in 30% of cases.
Failure to fully excise devitalized tendon	▪ This will result in a poor result or recurrence; the rehabilitation protocol can be delayed in cases that require more significant débridement.
Injury to the lateral collateral ligament	▪ The ligament is posterior to the mid-radiocapitellar joint, and dissection in this area should be avoided.
Extensor tendon rupture	▪ Rupture of the ECRB is of no consequence and should not be repaired. ▪ Rupture of the EDC mandates repair and can be achieved by advancing the ECRL posteriorly and the extensor carpi ulnaris anteriorly to close the gap. If this cannot be repaired, the anconeus muscle can be rotated to cover the defect.

POSTOPERATIVE CARE

- Postoperatively, the patient is placed in a soft dressing and a removable cock-up wrist brace.
- The elbow is not immobilized, and gentle range of motion is allowed immediately.
- The dressing is removed in 2 to 5 days. The patient may perform activities of daily living as tolerated with the wrist brace, removing the wrist brace several times daily for range of motion exercises.
- Exertion is avoided.
- A strengthening program is initiated at 6 weeks.
- All restrictions are removed at 3 months, but impact activities are not allowed until 4 to 6 months postoperatively. Pain-free full activity may require 6 to 12 months.

OUTCOMES

- Over 85% to 90% of all patients will have return to full activities with no pain. The remaining 10% to 15% have significant pain relief and strength improvement but do not return to normal preinjury levels. These outcomes hold true for both short follow-up and more than 10 years of follow-up.[12,13,16] Future prospective randomized trials will elucidate whether the reported more rapid recovery of the arthroscopic treatment is realized.
- Good short-term outcomes have been described for percutaneous procedures mentioned earlier.
- It is uncommon (<5% of cases) for a patient to have absolutely no improvement in pain after surgery, even if the subjective outcome is unsatisfactory. Such a result should prompt consideration of incorrect diagnosis or the possibility of secondary gain issues.

COMPLICATIONS

- Hematoma
- Infection
- Lateral collateral ligament injury
- Weakness in grip strength

REFERENCES

1. Ahmad Z, Brooks R, Kang S-N, et al. The effect of platelet-rich plasma on clinical outcomes in lateral epicondylitis. Arthroscopy 2013;29(11):1851–1862.
2. Altay TT, Günal II, Oztürk HH. Local injection treatment for lateral epicondylitis. Clin Orthop Relat Res 2002;(398):127–130.

3. Coombes BK, Bisset L, Brooks P, Khan A, Vicenzino B. Effect of corticosteroid injection, physiotherapy, or both on clinical outcomes in patients with unilateral lateral epicondylalgia: a randomized controlled trial. JAMA 2013;309(5):461–469
4. Greenbaum B, Itamura J, Vangsness CT, et al. Extensor carpi radialis brevis: an anatomical analysis of its origin. J Bone Joint Surg Br 1999;81(5):926–929.
5. Hay EM, Paterson SM, Lewis M, et al. Pragmatic randomised controlled trial of local corticosteroid injection and naproxen for treatment of lateral epicondylitis of elbow in primary care. BMJ 1999;319: 964–968.
6. Khashaba A. Nirschl tennis elbow release with or without drilling. Br J Sports Med 2001;35(3):200–201.
7. Koh JSB, Mohan PC, Howe TS, et al. Fasciotomy and surgical tenotomy for recalcitrant lateral elbow tendinopathy: early clinical experience with a novel device for minimally invasive percutaneous microresection. Am J Sports Med 2013;41(3):636–644.
8. Krogh TP, Fredberg U, Stengaard-Pedersen K, et al. Treatment of lateral epicondylitis with platelet-rich plasma, glucocorticoid, or saline: a randomized, double-blind, placebo-controlled trial. Am J Sports Med 2013;41(3):625–635.
9. Martin CE, Schweitzer ME. MR imaging of epicondylitis. Skeletal Radiol 1998;27:133–138.
10. Meknas K, Odden-Miland A, Mercer JB, et al. Radiofrequency microtenotomy: a promising method for treatment of recalcitrant lateral epicondylitis. Am J Sports Med 2008;36(10):1960–1965.
11. Mishra AK, Skrepnik NV, Edwards SG, et al. Efficacy of platelet-rich plasma for chronic tennis elbow: a double-blind, prospective, multicenter, randomized controlled trial of 230 patients. Am J Sports Med 2014;42(2):463–471.
12. Nirschl RP, Davis LD. Mini-open surgery for lateral epicondylitis. In: Yamaguchi K, King GJW, McKee M, et al, eds. Advanced Reconstruction—Elbow. Rosemont, IL: American Academy of Orthopaedic Surgeons, 2007:129–135.
13. Nirschl RP, Pettrone FA. Tennis elbow. The surgical treatment of lateral epicondylitis. J Bone Joint Surg Am 1979;61A:832–841.
14. Sasaki K, Onda K, Ohki G, et al. Radiocapitellar cartilage injuries associated with tennis elbow syndrome. J Hand Surg Am 2012;37(4): 748–754
15. Stasinopoulos D, Johnson MI. "Lateral elbow tendinopathy" is the most appropriate diagnostic term for the condition commonly referred-to as lateral epicondylitis. Med Hypotheses 2006;67: 1400–1402.
16. Verhaar J, Walenkamp G, Kester A, et al. Lateral extensor release for tennis elbow: a prospective long-term follow-up study. J Bone Joint Surg Am 1993;75(7):1034–1043.

Open Treatment of Medial Epicondylitis

74 CHAPTER

Peter J. Evans and Sebastian C. Peers

DEFINITION

- Medial epicondylitis involves tendinosis at the origin of the flexor–pronator mass.
- It is commonly referred to as *golfer's elbow*, although there is a stronger association with racquet sports and manual labor.[4]

ANATOMY

- The common flexor–pronator origin is primarily on the anterior aspect of the medial epicondyle.
- The common flexor–pronator origin includes the humeral head of the pronator teres (PT), the flexor carpi radialis (FCR), the flexor carpi ulnaris (FCU), and a small portion of the flexor digitorum superficialis (FDS).
- The palmaris longus also shares the origin, although this is not likely to be clinically relevant.

PATHOGENESIS

- Epicondylitis results from repetitive microtrauma followed by an incomplete reparative response that results in tendinosis, a pathologic state in which the degenerative tendon cannot heal itself effectively.
- Epicondylitis can be seen with medial collateral ligament instability whereby myotendinous overload occurs in an attempt to dynamically stabilize the ulnohumeral joint. In this scenario, ulnar neuropathy often is part of a trio of pathology.
- The most common tendon insertions affected are the PT and FCR; however, any tendon insertion of the common flexor–pronator origin can be involved.

NATURAL HISTORY

- Most patients improve with conservative treatment.
- However, a greater percentage of patients with medial epicondylitis go on to surgical treatment when compared to patients with lateral epicondylitis.[3]

PATIENT HISTORY AND PHYSICAL FINDINGS

- Patients commonly complain of forearm pain rather than elbow pain. At times, the inflammation is significant enough to cause irritation of the ulnar nerve as it enters the FCU, causing ulnar nerve symptoms (eg, local irritability and distal numbness and tingling).
- Onset usually is insidious, but the patient may recall an inciting event.
- Medial epicondylitis can be present simultaneously with lateral epicondylitis.
- Examination methods include the following:
  - Palpation of the medial epicondyle for tenderness, a universal finding in medial epicondylitis
- Resisted pronation is highly sensitive for medial epicondylitis.[1]
- A decreased range of motion (ROM) suggests intra-articular pathology such as arthritis.
- If resisted wrist flexion reproduced symptoms, it supports a diagnosis of medial epicondylitis.
- Tap the ulnar nerve in the cubital tunnel and along its path into the FCU. Presence of a tingling sensation locally prompts further nerve investigation.
- Flex patient's elbow maximally, then compress the ulnar nerve just proximal to the cubital tunnel. Presence of hand numbness or tingling prompts further nerve investigation.

IMAGING AND OTHER DIAGNOSTIC STUDIES

- Plain radiographs may show calcifications at the flexor–pronator origin.
- Magnetic resonance imaging (MRI) will reliably demonstrate increased intratendon signal on T2-weighted sequences. Most will also show increased intratendon signal and/or tendon thickening on T1-weighted sequences.
  - A small percentage of patients may show increased T2 signal in the medial epicondyle or anconeus edema.[2]
  - Periosteal reaction is *not* commonly seen on MRI.[2]
- Electrophysiologic testing (electromyography and nerve conduction studies) are warranted if patients have ulnar nerve symptoms; but with mild ulnar neuropathy, these tests have a very low sensitivity.

DIFFERENTIAL DIAGNOSIS

- Pronator syndrome
- Medial collateral ligament injury
- Ulnar neuropathy
- Arthritis
- Cervical radiculopathy
- Malingering

NONOPERATIVE MANAGEMENT

- Appropriate initial treatment includes avoidance of painful activities and symptomatic relief with nonsteroidal anti-inflammatory drugs and ice.
- Daytime wrist bracing for exertional activities
- Physical or occupational therapy to supervise and instruct on stretching and strengthening protocol for patients not otherwise inclined to comply with those instructions
- Although corticosteroid injection at the medial epicondyle has been shown to provide temporary symptomatic relief, it does not affect the natural history.[5] Repeat injections should be avoided as they can lead to tendon weakening and rupture.
  - Ulnar nerve injury has been reported with injection, so careful attention should be paid to the location of the nerve and whether or not it is subluxed.

SURGICAL MANAGEMENT

- A minority of patients fail nonoperative management.
- Careful patient selection will ensure an excellent outcome with surgical management.

Preoperative Planning

- Be prepared to address concurrent ulnar nerve pathology. If necessary, ulnar nerve decompression should be performed in situ, using subcutaneous or submuscular transposition.
  - In thin patients, and especially those who have lifestyles in which the inner elbow is struck frequently, we prefer submuscular transposition with flexor–pronator lengthening, which definitively treats epicondylitis as well.
- Be prepared to address flexor–pronator tears or avulsion. These typically will present more abruptly, with acute or chronic pain, ecchymosis, and swelling.
  - It will be necessary to débride the ruptured degenerative tissue (**FIG 1**) and repair it by retensioning it close to the origin and closing the gap with healthier medial and lateral portions of the flexor–pronator origin down to the medial epicondyle (as shown in **TECH FIG 2D**).

Positioning

- The patient is placed in the supine position.
- The arm is externally rotated at the shoulder and padding is placed under the elbow.
- The arm should rest in a position allowing ready access to the medial aspect of the elbow without requiring constant holding by an assistant.

Approach

- The elbow should be examined after the administration of anesthesia to ensure stability, and the result documented in the operative note.
- The goal of surgery is to débride the degenerative tissue at the flexor–pronator origin and create an environment conducive to proper healing of the tendon.

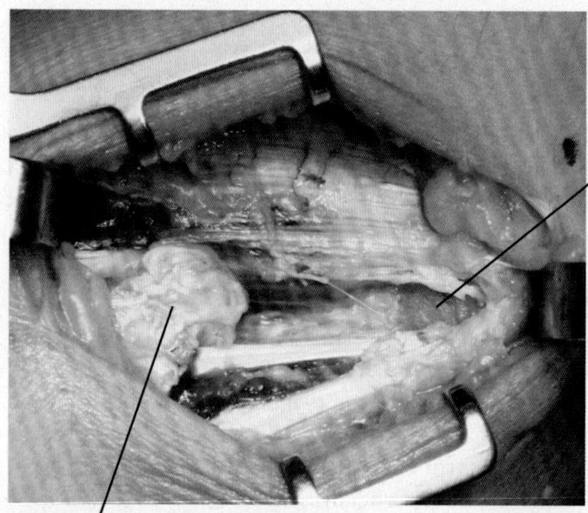

FIG 1 • The common flexors can be seen ruptured and retracted distal to the medial epicondyle.

TECHNIQUES

Medial Epicondylar Fasciectomy and Partial Ostectomy

Incision and Dissection

- A 3- to 5-cm incision through the skin only is made beginning just proximal to and in the center of the medial epicondyle and extending distally along the axis of the forearm (**TECH FIG 1A**).
- Blunt dissection with scissors is carried through the subcutaneous tissues, taking care to preserve medial antebrachial cutaneous nerve branches, which commonly cross the field (**TECH FIG 1B**).
- The subcutaneous tissues are gently swept away, exposing the fascia of the flexor–pronator mass.
- The ulnar nerve is palpated, and the elbow is put through a ROM to check for ulnar nerve subluxation. The result is documented in the operative note.

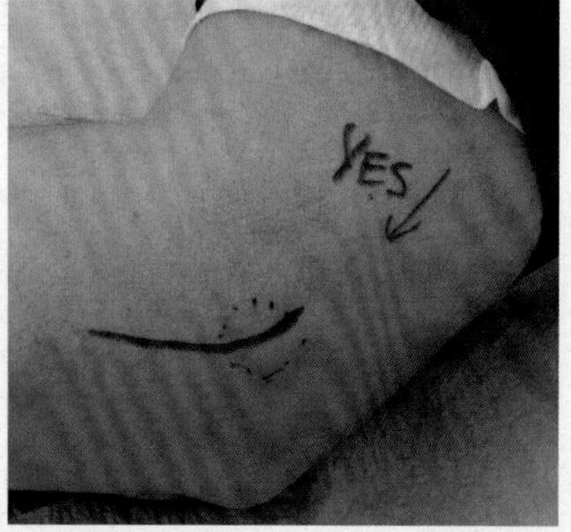

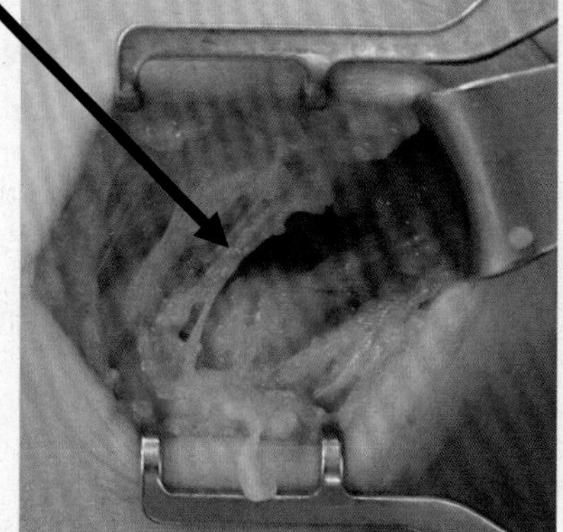

TECH FIG 1 • **A.** A 3- to 5-cm incision is started just proximal to the medial epicondyle. **B.** The medial antebrachial cutaneous nerve is identified and protected. *(continued)*

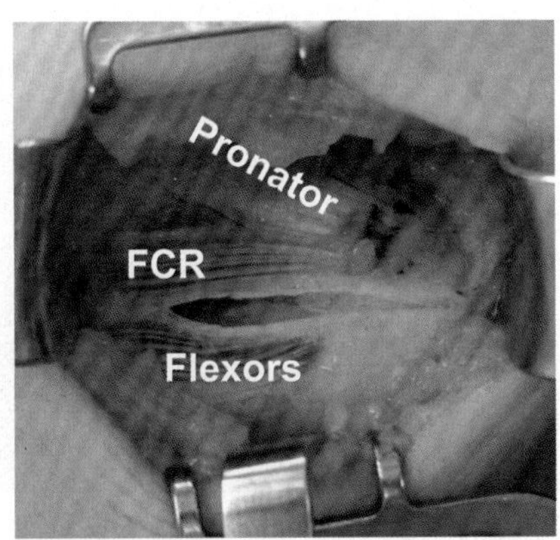

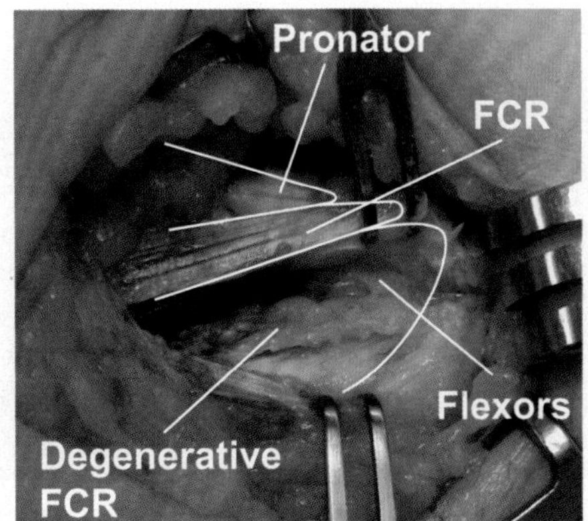

TECH FIG 1 • *(continued)* **C.** The interval between the FCR and common flexors is used and split in line with the fibers. **D.** The FCR is elevated, and the deeper degenerative tendon is identified.

- Most commonly, the fascia overlying the interval between the PT and FCR is then incised in line with the fibers to expose the tendon origin. Observe the orientation of the fibers of the overlying fascia to identify the correct interval. The fibers of PT can be seen coursing toward the radius while the rest of the flexor–pronator tendons are oriented more longitudinally.
- The exact interval can be altered depending on clinical and intraoperative examination. In the figure shown, the interval between FCR and the common flexors was chosen to better access the diseased tissue (**TECH FIG 1C**).
- The selected interval is then developed, exposing the abnormal, deeper tendon tissue (**TECH FIG 1D**).

Fasciectomy and Partial Ostectomy

- The abnormal tissue is excised. It can be identified by its grayish, unorganized mucoid appearance. Abnormal tissue will scrape away with a no. 15 blade, but normal tendon will remain attached (ie, Nirschl scratch test).
- The pathologic tissue is débrided to margins showing an organized, tendinous appearance.
- The area of excision usually is 1 to 1.5 cm long and 3 to 5 mm wide (**TECH FIG 2A**).
- A rongeur is used to roughen the anterior portion of the medial epicondyle to a bleeding surface without removing cortical bone (**TECH FIG 2B,C**).
- The defect in the tendon is closed with a running absorbable suture, using 0 or 1-0 suture material with a tapered needle (**TECH FIG 2D**).
- The subdermal layer is closed with buried, interrupted absorbable sutures, followed by a subcuticular skin closure and Steri-Strips (**TECH FIG 2E**).

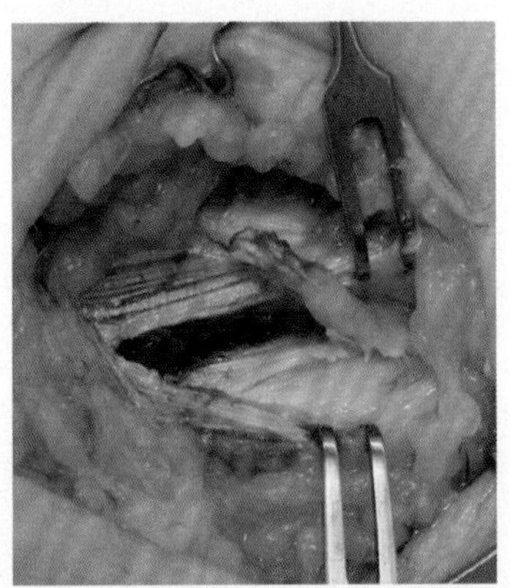

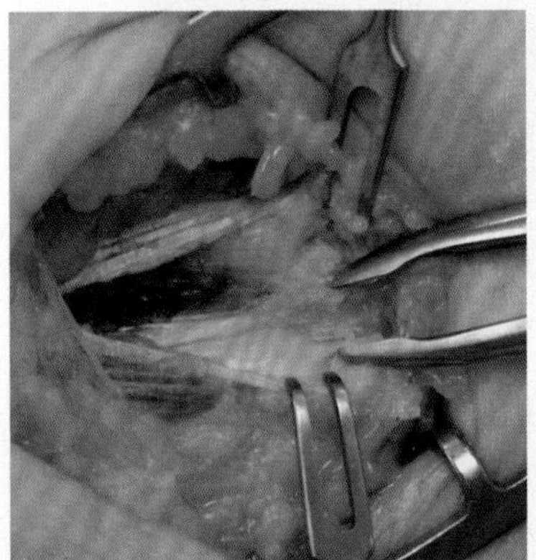

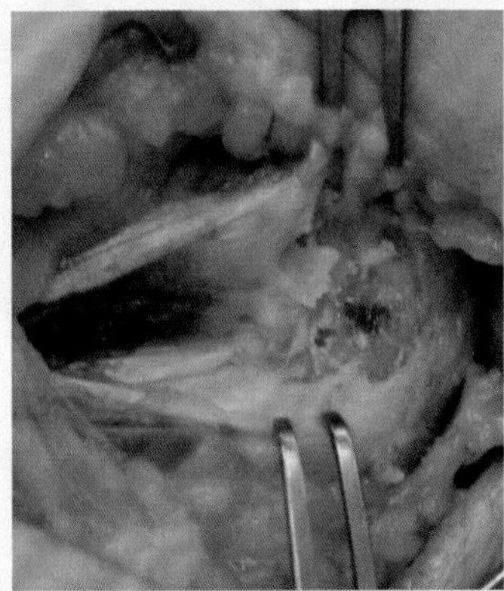

TECH FIG 2 • **A.** Degenerative tissue is excised. The remaining healthy tendon is stable and cannot be scraped away with a no. 15 blade. **B.** The anterior portion of the medial epicondyle is scraped or rongeured to remove any remaining degenerative tendon. **C.** The bony cortex is not violated, however. *(continued)*

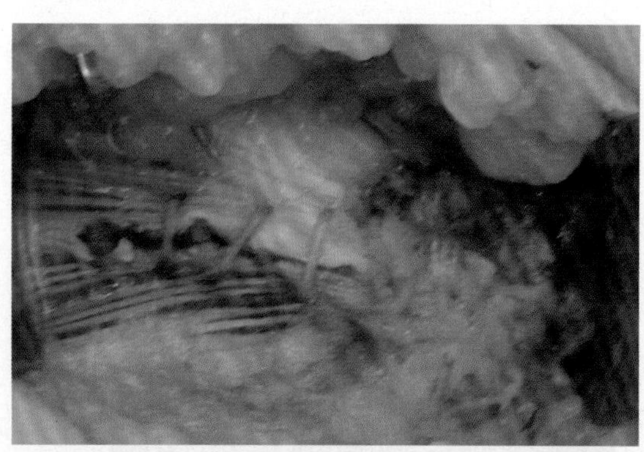

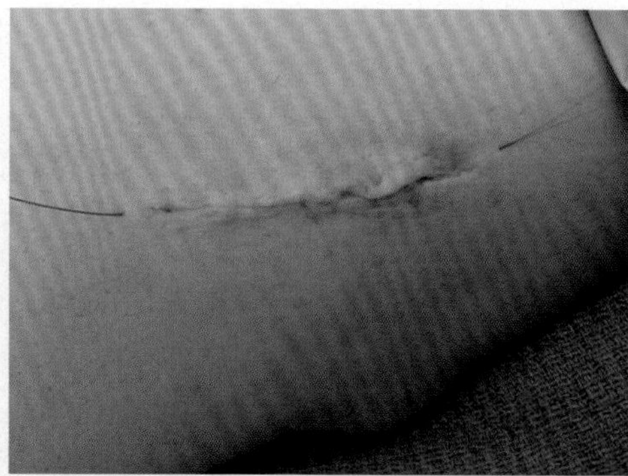

TECH FIG 2 • *(continued)* **D.** The muscle interval is closed with a running size 0 Vicryl suture and tied with inverted knots. **E.** Skin closure is done with a running 3-0 Prolene suture.

Minimally Invasive Radiofrequency Débridement

- In selected cases, a minimally invasive approach using the ArthroCare TOPAZ MicroDebrider (ArthroCare Sports Medicine, Sunnyvale, CA) may be used.
- This procedure is indicated for areas of tendinosis within the common flexor–pronator tendon origin.
- Contraindications include acute trauma, partial or complete tendon tear, neurogenic disease, and bone and joint abnormality.

Incision and Dissection

- A 1.5-cm incision through the skin only is made over the area of tenderness. The incision usually begins at the medial epicondyle and extends distally along the axis of the forearm.
- The origin of the flexor–pronator mass is exposed and the location of the ulnar nerve is verified as described in the previous section.

Radiofrequency Débridement

- Place the tip of the device on the tendon perpendicular to the surface (**TECH FIG 3**).
- Using light pressure, perforate the tendon in the area of tendinosis to the desired depth.
- Repeat this process with multiple perforations in a grid-like pattern (separating the perforations by approximately 5 mm) until the affected area has been covered.
- Irrigate the wound and close the subdermal layer with buried, interrupted absorbable sutures followed by a subcuticular skin closure and Steri-Strips.

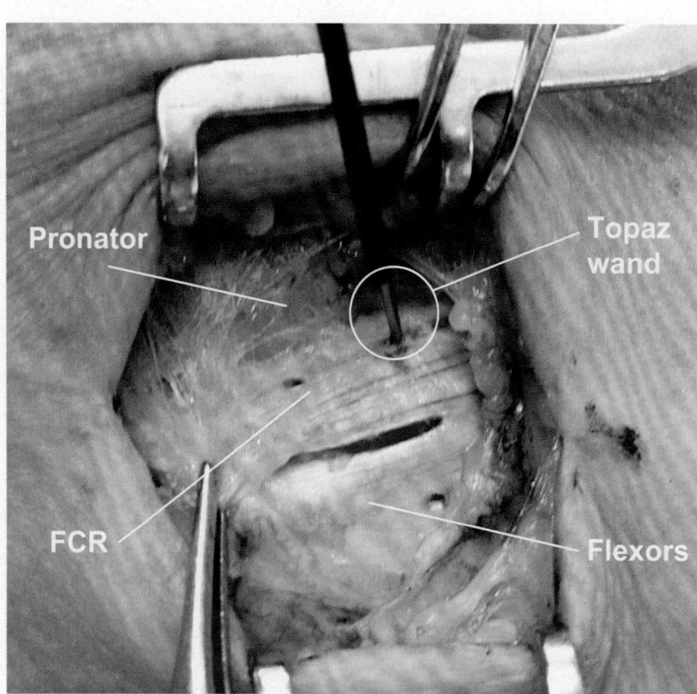

TECH FIG 3 • The tip of the ArthroCare TOPAZ MicroDebrider is placed perpendicular to the surface of the area of tendinosis. In this figure, the FCR is the area being treated.

PEARLS AND PITFALLS

Indications	▪ A minimum of 3–6 months of symptoms and failed nonoperative management
Coexisting conditions	▪ Ulnar nerve irritation, neuropathy, and subluxation may require decompression and anterior transposition. ▪ Flexor tendon origin rupture may require débridement and repair.
Failure to fully excise devitalized tendon	▪ This will result in a poor result or recurrence; the rehabilitation protocol can be delayed in cases that require more significant débridement.
Injury to the medial collateral ligament	▪ The ligament is deep to the tendon and lies on the anterior capsule, more posterior than the area of tendinosis, and can be distinguished from the rougher tendon origin.

POSTOPERATIVE CARE

- Postoperatively, the patient is placed in a soft dressing and a removable cock-up wrist brace.
- The elbow is not immobilized, and gentle ROM is allowed immediately.
- The dressing is removed in 3 to 5 days. The patient may perform activities of daily living as tolerated with the wrist brace, removing the wrist brace several times daily for ROM.
- Exertion is avoided.
- A strengthening program is initiated in 6 weeks with a counterforce brace.
- All restrictions are removed at 3 months, but impact activities are not allowed until 4 to 6 months postoperatively. Return of full, pain-free activity can take 6 to 24 months.

OUTCOMES

- Over 85% of all patients will have return to full activities with no pain or only mild, occasional pain. Among high-level athletes, 75% to 85% will return to their previous level. In patients with mild or no ulnar nerve symptoms, the success rate is greater than 95%.[1,6]
- In patients with more than moderate ulnar nerve symptoms, there is a trend toward less favorable and less predictable outcomes, although a satisfactory result still is possible.
- It is uncommon for a patient to have absolutely no improvement in pain after surgery, even if the subjective outcome is unsatisfactory. Such a result should prompt consideration of incorrect diagnosis or the possibility of secondary gain issues.

COMPLICATIONS

- Medial antebrachial cutaneous nerve injury
- Grip weakness
- Weakness with wrist flexion or pronation
- Hematoma
- Infection
- Ulnar nerve injury
- Medial collateral ligament injury

REFERENCES

1. Gabel GT, Morrey BF. Operative treatment of medial epicondylitis. Influence of concomitant ulnar neuropathy at the elbow. J Bone Joint Surg Am 1995;77(7):1065–1069.
2. Martin CE, Schweitzer ME. MR imaging of epicondylitis. Skeletal Radiol 1998;27:133–138.
3. O'Dwyer KJ, Howie CR. Medial epicondylitis of the elbow. Int Orthop 1995;19:69–71.
4. Ollivierre CO, Nirschl RP, Pettrone FA. Resection and repair for medial tennis elbow: a prospective analysis. Am J Sports Med 1995;23:214–221.
5. Stahl S, Kaufman T. The efficacy of an injection of steroids for medial epicondylitis: a prospective study of sixty elbows. J Bone Joint Surg Am 1997;79:1648–1652.
6. Vangsness CT Jr, Jobe FW. Surgical treatment of medial epicondylitis: results in 35 elbows. J Bone Joint Surg Br 1991;73:409–411.

CHAPTER

Distal Biceps Tendon Disruptions: Acute and Delayed Reconstruction and One- and Two-Incision Techniques

Matt Noyes and Edwin E. Spencer, Jr.

ANATOMY

- Mean length of the distal biceps insertion is 22 to 24 mm and the mean width is 15 to 19 mm on the proximal radius.
- The biceps tendon inserts like a ribbon on the ulnar aspect of radial tuberosity.
- Left tendon spirals clockwise, right tendon counterclockwise.[12]
- A relatively avascular zone exists just proximal to the tendon insertion site.
- The lacertus fibrosus typically originates from the distal short head of biceps tendon.[1]

NATURAL HISTORY

- Complete ruptures
  - Distal biceps tendon ruptures are most common in the dominant extremity of men in the fourth and sixth decade.
  - Injury typically results from an eccentric muscle contraction. This often occurs when an extension force is applied to the supinated arm in 90 degrees of flexion.
  - The initial pain subsides quickly, but there is usually a noticeable deformity in the anterior brachium as the biceps muscle contracts and retracts. The degree of the retraction can be mitigated by the lacertus fibrosus which may remain intact.
  - The patients usually reports loss of flexion and supination strength. This is especially noted in patients that require repetitive supination such as mechanics and plumbers. Pain is usually not a predominant complaint, although some patients will experience fatigue-type pain and cramping in the retracted muscle belly.
  - Studies have revealed a 30% reduction in flexion strength and a 40% loss of supination strength.[3,15]
- Partial ruptures
  - Partial distal biceps tendon injuries are usually more painful than complete tears. Patients usually present with pain in the antecubital fossa especially with resisted flexion and supination. There is an absence of clinical deformity.
  - These can progress to complete tears.
  - Women typically present with partial tears of the distal biceps, usually at a more advanced age (mean age of 63 years).[7]
  - A distinct palpable cystic mass can be found occasionally in women.[7]
  - Partial tears are typically from chronic degeneration without acute trauma.
  - Predisposing factors: anabolic steroids, smoking, cubital bursitis, and bony irregularities on bicipital ridge[17]

PHYSICAL FINDINGS

- In acute cases of a complete distal biceps tendon rupture, there is usually a significant amount of ecchymosis in the antecubital fossa and distal brachium.
- The distal biceps tendon is easily palpated in the antecubital fossa and lack thereof is confirmed by comparing the involved side to the uninvolved side. Local edema can make the diagnosis a little more difficult; however, the "hook test" has been found to be a very reliable diagnostic tool. To perform the test, the patient actively supinates the forearm while the examiner attempts to "hook" the distal biceps tendon lateral side to medial.[16]
  - The hook test has been found to have 100% sensitivity and specificity.[16]
- The degree of proximal retraction of the tendon can be mitigated by the lacertus fibrosus.
- A magnetic resonance imaging (MRI) is usually not necessary to make the diagnosis. However, the only caveat is that if the examiner feels that the distal biceps tendon is intact, then the injury might be more proximal at the myotendinous junction or only a partial tear at its insertion. It is important to make the distinction between the common complete avulsion from the radial tuberosity and an injury at the myotendinous junction, as the more proximal injuries are best treated nonoperatively.[19]
- Partial tears occur at the radial tuberosity and are usually not associated with ecchymosis and demonstrate no proximal retraction. Partial tears present late with pain during resisted flexion and supination. The distal biceps tendon is palpable and frequently tender. An MRI can aid in the diagnosis of partial tendon ruptures.

DIFFERENTIAL DIAGNOSIS

- Cubital bursitis
- Elbow dislocation
- Radial head fracture
- Entrapment of lateral antebrachial cutaneous nerve

NONOPERATIVE MANAGEMENT

- Nonoperative management of complete distal biceps tendon ruptures entails the use anti-inflammatories and physical therapy to reduce pain and swelling. Patients are allowed to use the extremity as tolerated. Strengthening should focus on elbow flexion and supination.
- It should be discussed that complete distal biceps tendon ruptures are not usually associated with residual pain but rather

loss of flexion (30%) and supination (40%) strength.[3,15] If that is compatible with the patient's job and lifestyle, then nonoperative management is acceptable.

- Partial biceps tendon ruptures and ruptures at the myotendinous junction are treated in a similar manner. The patient should proceed to strengthening when full painless range of motion (ROM) is obtained. Operative intervention is considered when nonoperative management fails for partial ruptures. Usually, a minimum 3 to 4 months of observation is appropriate. Patients should be counseled that pain rather than weakness is more of a predominant complaint with these injuries.

SURGICAL MANAGEMENT

Complete and Partial Ruptures

- The EndoButton (Smith & Nephew, Andover, MA) method of fixation has been shown to have highest ultimate tensile load.[14,22] Clinical studies with the EndoButton have also demonstrated good results with few complications.[2,6]
- Other methods are suture anchor and interference screw fixation.

Chronic Disruptions

- The definition of "chronic" is vague. Some authors have stated that greater than 8 weeks is chronic and that a graft is needed in these situations. However, the authors have been able to primarily repair distal biceps tendon ruptures out to 3 months. In these situations, the elbow might not extend beyond 60 degrees on the table, but within 3 months after the repair, the patient's ROM is full. The biceps brachii like the pectoralis major has a significant ability to stretch back out over time.
- The surgeon should discuss with the patient that a more chronic rupture might require a graft and discuss the type of graft to be used. Semitendinosus (either autograft or allograft),[23] Achilles tendon allograft[18] (with the bone plug inserted into the radial tuberosity or just soft tissue repair), flexor carpi radialis (FCR) autograft,[13] and fascia lata[9] have been described.
- Any of the techniques of radial tuberosity fixation described in the acute section can be used. We use the EndoButton for the chronic reconstructions.

Positioning

- The patient is placed in supine position on an arm board with a sterile tourniquet on the upper arm.

Approach

Two Incision

- Originally described by Boyd and Anderson,[4] a small incision was made in antecubital fossa to identify tendon. A second longitudinal incision is made 1 cm radial to the subcutaneous border of the ulna in the proximal forearm at the level of the biceps tuberosity.
- Pronation of the forearm when making the second incision protects the posterior interosseous nerve, which is often not visualized.
- Kelly et al[10] modified the approach by using a dorsal approach that split the extensor carpi ulnaris and avoids dissection of supinator to potentially avoid synostosis.
- May be associated with a higher rate of heterotopic ossification than the single-incision approach

Single Incision

- Initially described as extended S-shaped Henry approach centered over antecubital fossa and has been associated with higher rate of neurologic complications than the two-incision technique.
- Must maintain supination throughout case to keep posterior interosseous nerve out of surgical field.
- Advent of newer fixation methods has facilitated a safer approach through a limited antecubital fossa incision.
- Interval between brachioradialis and pronator teres is developed.
- Must protect lateral antebrachial cutaneous and posterior interosseous nerves by limiting aggressive retraction laterally.
- May ligate recurrent branch of radial artery to minimize hematoma formation

TECHNIQUES

EndoButton

- A longitudinal 4- to 5-cm anterior incision starting at the antecubital fossa and extending distally along the ulnar border of the brachioradialis is used. The lateral antebrachial cutaneous nerve and superficial radial nerve are identified and should be protected.
- The distal biceps tendon is retrieved into the wound. This can be accomplished by flexing the elbow and using a retractor to elevate the tissue of the distal brachium anteriorly for exposure. The tendon can be adherent to the adjacent tissues or the lacertus fibrosus. This may require a limited tenolysis to mobilize the tendon stump. Care must be taken to protect and isolate the lateral antebrachial cutaneous nerve and the brachial artery.
- On occasion, the biceps tendon is not able to be retrieved through the anterior incision. In that case, an incision can be made medially along the distal aspect of the brachium. The tendon is isolated and prepared and then passed into the distal wound.
- Once the tendon is isolated, a no. 2 nonabsorbable suture is woven into the distal biceps tendon using a locking Krackow technique or other locking suture technique. The locking sutures should extend 4 to 5 cm above the stump. The goal is to create a locking stitch proximally and allow about 1 cm of the distal biceps tendon to be unlocked.
- The two sutures extending from the tendon stump are then passed through the two central holes of the EndoButton. The sutures are then tied leaving no space between the end of the tendon and the EndoButton. Alternatively, one suture from the tendon can be passed through one of the central holes of the EndoButton and then back through the other central hole, and the knot is then tied, thus placing the knot in between the EndoButton and the tendon stump (**TECH FIG 1A**). Passing sutures (kite strings) are placed in the other two holes of the EndoButton (**TECH FIG 1B**).

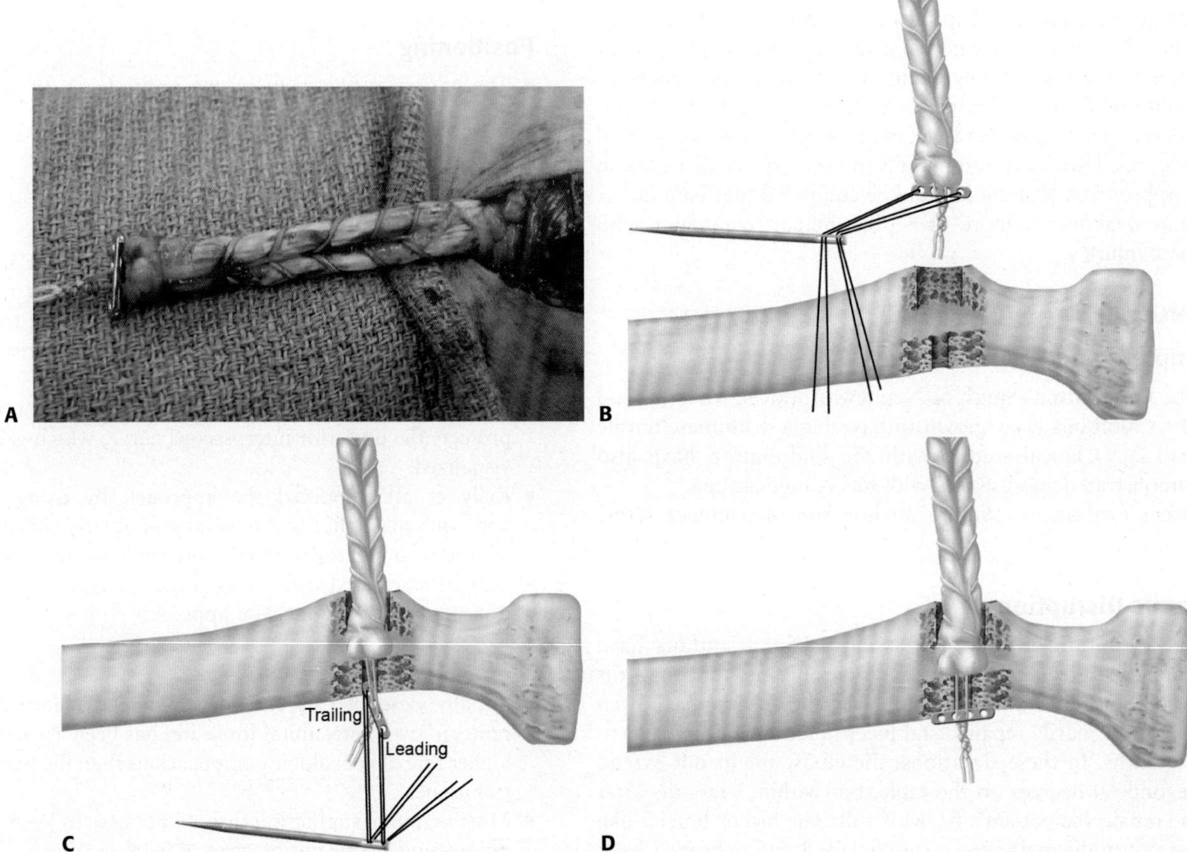

TECH FIG 1 • **A.** EndoButton attached to the distal end of the biceps tendon. **B.** Passing sutures are placed through the two outer holes of the EndoButton and then passed through a Keith needle for passage through the proximal radius. **C.** The tendon is pulled into the proximal radial hole as the EndoButton is advanced through the distal hole. **D.** The EndoButton is flipped to secure it on the other side of the radial cortex.

- The radial tuberosity is exposed, and a burr is used to create an oval cortical window approximately the same dimension as the distal tendon stump. This is performed while an assistant holds the forearm in full supination. Two small Bennett retractors can be placed on either side of the radial tuberosity. Then, the EndoButton drill is used to create a hole in the far cortex to pass the button.
- Keith needles or a Beath needle are used to pass the passing sutures (kite strings) through the bicortical hole and are retrieved as they pass through the skin on the dorsal side of the forearm.
- One of the passing sutures is independently pulled, thereby drawing the tendon into the radial tuberosity. Continued tension on this kite string draws the EndoButton in its vertical orientation through the hole in the far cortex of the radius. Once the EndoButton is on the far side of the radius, the other suture is pulled to flip the EndoButton and lock it in its horizontal orientation on the far side of the radius. The authors use fluoroscopy to confirm placement of the button. The passing sutures are then pulled completely out after anatomic tendon placement is visually confirmed (**TECH FIG 1C,D**).

Tension Slide Technique

- The rationale for development of this technique was to maintain strength of a suspensory cortical button fixation while reducing gap formation at repair site.
- Biomechanical studies have proven that tension slide technique (TST) maintains the strength of standard cortical button repair but significantly reduces gap formation and motion at repair site.[21]
- Standard single-incision approach is used for this technique, similar to an EndoButton.
- A 3.2-mm drill is used to create a bicortical hole in the radial tuberosity for passing the button. An 8.0-mm cannulated reamer is used to ream the anterior cortex and intramedullary canal to allow for flush seating of tendon. Do not ream bicortically.
- The button is placed bicortically on the far cortex of radius and flipped. As suture limbs are tensioned, the tendon is "walked" into the reamed hole.
- A 7- × 10-mm interference screw is then inserted on the radial aspect of the hole, pushing the tendon ulnar to mimic the natural anatomy and potentially increase supination strength.
- The advantages of TST include the ability to tension the repair from the anterior incision, minimal displacement of tendon after fixation, and no need to predetermine length of suture between tendon and button.[20]

Suture Anchor or Interference Screw Fixation

- The same anterior approach is used, and the tendon is retrieved in a similar manner with both the suture anchor and interference screw fixation. However, the radial tuberosity is prepared differently.
- In the case of interference screw fixation, a hole is drilled in the radial tuberosity. The diameter of the hole depends on the system (and the size of the screw) that is being used.
- In the case of suture anchor fixation, the radial tuberosity is lightly decorticated and suture anchors of choice are placed. Some authors have reported using two suture anchors, and most use some kind of a sliding knot to advance the tendon onto the bone.[8]
  - The disadvantage of this technique is that the tendon is repaired to the surface of the proximal radius instead of into the medullary canal.

Two-Incision Technique

- Anterior incision is made transverse in the antecubital flexion crease and used to locate the distal tendon stump. A second longitudinal incision is made 1 cm radial to the subcutaneous border of the ulna in the proximal forearm at the level of the biceps tuberosity.
- Dissection is initially made in the ECU muscle and then through the supinator muscle. Great care is taken to avoid subperiosteal dissection on the ulna.
- The forearm is placed in maximal pronation, and an oval cavity is created in the biceps tuberosity with a burr. Three drill holes are then placed anterior to this cavity by slightly supinating the arm.
- Two no. 2 FiberWire suture is then placed in the distal tendon in a Krackow technique.
- The sutures are then passed from anterior to the posterior incision with long hemostat and retrieved. It is critical to pass the sutures in the interosseous space.
- The sutures are then passed through the drill holes and tied over bone with the forearm in supination after drawing the tendon stump into the proximal radius.

Chronic Distal Biceps Tendon Reconstructions

- More exposure of the biceps tendon and the myotendinous junction is required for the chronic reconstructions. This can be accomplished by creating a second incision at the medical aspect of the distal brachium. One could connect the two anterior incisions but you risk creating a skin pterygium which could limit extension.
- A more meticulous dissection is required to protect the lateral antebrachial cutaneous and musculocutaneous nerves. Invariably, there will be significant scarring and adhesions especially between the biceps tendon and lacertus fibrosus. Some of the lacertus can be used in the reconstruction.
- The authors have used semitendinosus autograft which is harvested in a fashion similar to that used for ACL reconstructions. The tendon is doubled up, and the two free ends are woven into the remaining distal biceps tendon and the myotendinous junction (**TECH FIG 2A**).
- A Bunnell tendon passer is very effective at passing the tendon ends.
- The length of the graft is chosen so that the reconstruction is tight at 60 degrees of elbow flexion. This can be accomplished by fixing it distally first and then performing the weave or vice versa.
- A nonabsorbable suture is passed through the graft/tendon construct and this is secured to the radial tuberosity (**TECH FIG 2B**).

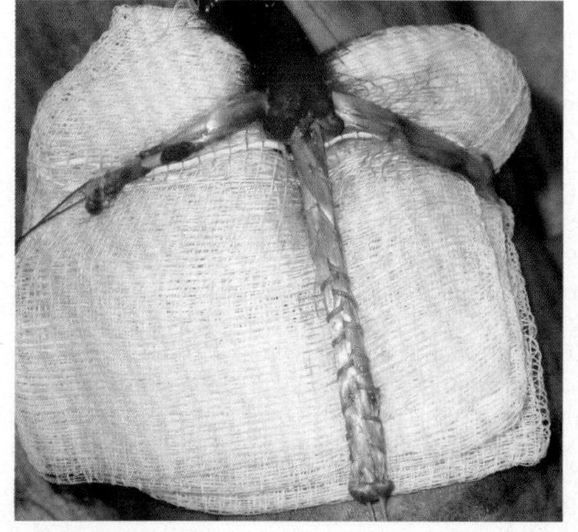

A

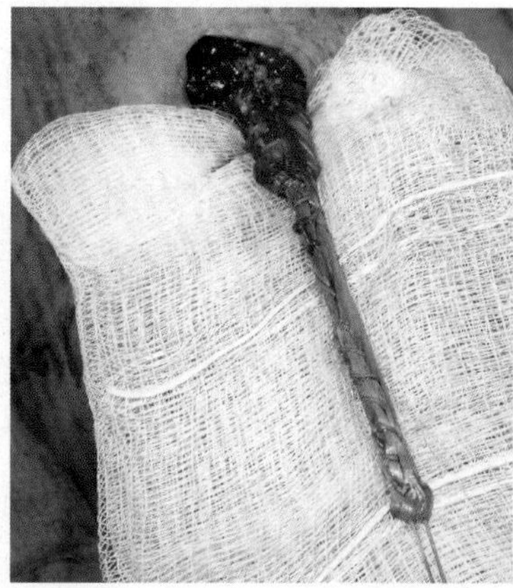

B

TECH FIG 2 • A. Hamstring tendon is doubled up and folded on itself, and the free ends are passed into the distal end of the biceps tendon stump to add length. The free ends of the tendon graft exit laterally. **B.** A nonabsorbable suture is placed through the distal end of the graft and used to attach it to the radial tuberosity.

PEARLS AND PITFALLS

One-incision technique	■ Avoid excessive retraction on the radial side. ■ Prepare the biceps tendon prior to the radial tuberosity. ■ Maintain maximum supination to protect posterior interosseous nerve. ■ If using TST, place interference screw radial to direct tendon toward ulnar aspect of tuberosity for anatomic repair.
Two-incision technique	■ Avoid any subperiosteal dissection or exposure of the ulna. ■ Avoid bone tunnel fracture by providing enough space between drill holes. ■ Maintain maximum pronation to protect posterior interosseous nerve.

POSTOPERATIVE CARE

- If an EndoButton or other radiopaque fixation device is used, radiographs are obtained at the time of surgery and at the first postoperative visit to ensure that the fixation is in good position.
- For the EndoButton repair, the authors remove the splint at 2 weeks and allow active and passive ROM, but no lifting greater than a cup of coffee for 4 weeks. Strengthening is then started but rarely is formal physical therapy necessary.
- Other authors have reported good results with early ROM therapy.[2]
- Others use a more conservative approach and limit full extension until 6 to 8 weeks after surgery. Typical protocol for this therapy approach includes using a hinged elbow brace and increasing extension 10 degree per week until full extension achieved.

OUTCOMES

- Patient-weighted outcome measures such as the (Disability of the Arm, Shoulder, and Hand) DASH and the Mayo Elbow Performance Score (MEPS) have been used in many studies and have demonstrated excellent results with primary repair.[2,8]
- Objective data including strength testing have also demonstrated good results with anatomic repair especially with regard to restoring supination strength.[11]
- Chronic repairs/reconstructions have also performed well, although the results are not as good as those following acute repair and there is a higher complication rate.[23]

COMPLICATIONS

- Reruptures are rare in most series, irrespective of the method of fixation.
- Certain fixation methods have been associated with a higher occurrence of certain complications.
  - Classic two-incision technique—heterotopic ossification, radioulnar synostosis, stiffness, and posterior interosseous nerve palsy. Bone tunnel fractures are also unique to the two-incision technique. Heterotopic ossification and radioulnar synostosis rates have been decreased by avoiding the ulnar periosteum.[5,10]
  - Single-incision technique—lateral antebrachial cutaneous (most common) and posterior interosseous nerve palsies, rerupture, stiffness, anterior elbow pain, radioulnar synostosis, and complex regional pain syndrome (CRPS).

REFERENCES

1. Athwal GS, Steinmann SP, Rispoli DM. The distal biceps tendon: footprint and relevant clinical anatomy. J Hand Surg Am 2007;32(8): 1225–1229.
2. Bain GI, Prem H, Heptinstall RJ, et al. Repair of distal biceps tendon rupture: a new technique using the Endobutton. J Shoulder Elbow Surg 2000;9(2):120–126.
3. Baker BE, Bierwagen D. Rupture of the distal tendon of the biceps brachii. Operative versus non-operative treatment. J Bone Joint Surg Am 1985;67(3):414–417.
4. Boyd HB, Anderson DL. A method for reinsertion of the distal biceps brachii tendon. J Bone Joint Surg Am 1961;43(7):1041–1043.
5. Failla JM, Amadio PC, Morrey BF, et al. Proximal radioulnar synostosis after repair of distal biceps brachii rupture by the two-incision technique. Report of four cases. Clin Orthop Relat Res 1990;(253):133–136.
6. Greenberg JA, Fernandez JJ, Wang T, et al. EndoButton-assisted repair of distal biceps tendon ruptures. J Shoulder Elbow Surg 2003;12(5):484–490.
7. Jockel CR, Mulieri PJ, Belsky MR, et al. Distal biceps tendon tears in women. J Shoulder Elbow Surg 2010;19(5):645–650.
8. John CK, Field LD, Weiss KS, et al. Single-incision repair of acute distal biceps ruptures by use of suture anchors. J Shoulder Elbow Surg 2007;16(1):78–83.
9. Kaplan FT, Rokito AS, Birdzell MG, et al. Reconstruction of chronic distal biceps tendon rupture with use of fascia lata combined with a ligament augmentation device: a report of 3 cases. J Shoulder Elbow Surg 2002;11(6):633–636.
10. Kelly EW, Morrey BF, O'Driscoll SW. Complications of repair of the distal biceps tendon with the modified two-incision technique. J Bone Joint Surg Am 2000;82-A(11):1575–1581.
11. Klonz A, Loitz D, Wöhler P, et al. Rupture of the distal biceps brachii tendon: isokinetic power analysis and complications after anatomic reinsertion compared with fixation to the brachialis muscle. J Shoulder Elbow Surg 2003;12(6):607–611.
12. Kulshreshtha R, Singh R, Sinha J, et al. Anatomy of the distal biceps brachii tendon and its clinical relevance. Clin Orthop Relat Res 2007;456:117–120.
13. Levy HJ, Mashoof AA, Morgan D. Repair of chronic ruptures of the distal biceps tendon using flexor carpi radialis tendon graft. Am J Sports Med 2000;28(4):538–540.
14. Mazzocca AD, Burton KJ, Romeo AA, et al. Biomechanical evaluation of 4 techniques of distal biceps brachii tendon repair. Am J Sports Med 2007;35(2):252–258.
15. Morrey BF, Askew LJ, An KN, et al. Rupture of the distal tendon of the biceps brachii. A biomechanical study. J Bone Joint Surg Am 1985;67(3):418–421.
16. O'Driscoll SW, Goncalves LB, Dietz P. The hook test for distal biceps tendon avulsion. Am J Sports Med 2007;35(11):1865–1869.
17. Safran MR, Graham SM. Distal biceps tendon ruptures: incidence, demographics, and the effect of smoking. Clin Orthop Relat Res 2002;(404):275–283.
18. Sanchez-Sotelo J, Morrey BF, Adams RA, et al. Reconstruction of chronic ruptures of the distal biceps tendon with use of an achilles tendon allograft. J Bone Joint Surg Am 2002;84-A(6):999–1005.

19. Schamblin ML, Safran MR. Injury of the distal biceps at the musculotendinous junction. J Shoulder Elbow Surg 2007;16(2):208–212.
20. Sethi P, Cunningham J, Miller S, et al. Anatomic repair of the distal biceps tendon using tension slide technique. Tech Shoulder Elbow Surg 2008;9:182–187.
21. Sethi P, Obopilwe E, Rincon L, et al. Biomechanical evaluation of distal biceps reconstruction with cortical button and interference screw fixation. J Shoulder Elbow Surg 2010;19(1):53–57.
22. Spang JT, Weinhold PS, Karas SG. A biomechanical comparison of EndoButton versus suture anchor repair of distal biceps tendon injuries. J Shoulder Elbow Surg 2006;15(4):509–514.
23. Wiley WB, Noble JS, Dulaney TD, et al. Late reconstruction of chronic distal biceps tendon ruptures with a semitendinosus autograft technique. J Shoulder Elbow Surg 2006;15(4):440–444.

76 CHAPTER

Triceps Tendon Ruptures

Andrea Celli

DEFINITION

- Elbow extension against gravity or resistance may be difficult or impossible when the distal triceps tendon is ruptured or avulsed from the olecranon insertion.
- Complete ruptures of all three heads tendon insertion (long, lateral, and medial heads) generally require surgical treatment.
- Partial lesions are functionally well tolerated in patients with low functional demand.

ANATOMY

Origin

- The triceps brachii (**FIG 1**) has three heads:
  - The long head arises from the infraglenoid tubercle of the scapula.
  - The lateral head has a linear attachment from the upper margin of the radial grove of the humerus.
  - The medial head originates below the lateral margin of the radial groove that contains the radial nerve. Its insertion covers the entire rear surface of the lower part of the humerus.

Insertion

- In the distal third of the posterior aspect of the arm, the lateral head joins with the long head to form the superficial tendinous part of the insertion on the posterior surface of the olecranon. The medial head (deep part of the triceps) inserts through muscular and tendinous fibers directly onto the olecranon.
- The superficial tendon forms two components as it approaches its insertion area (**FIG 2**):
  - A lateral part that is more expansive and relatively thin and in continuity with anconeus muscle and fascia

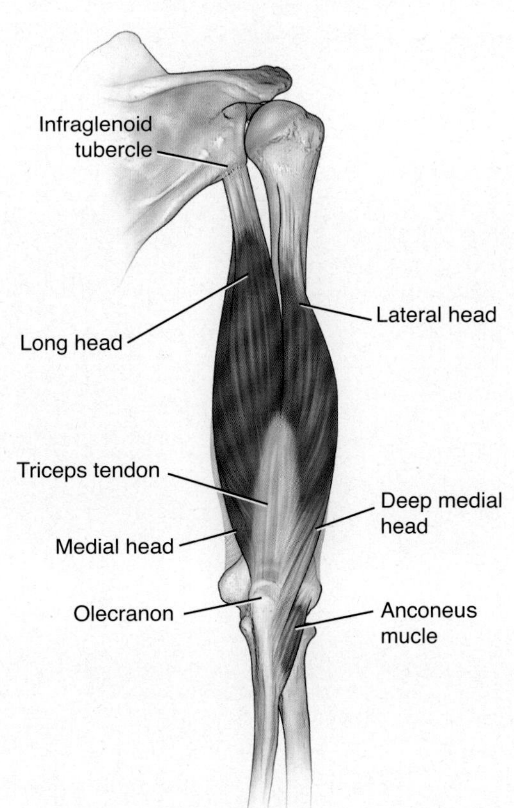

FIG 1 • Triceps brachii anatomy.

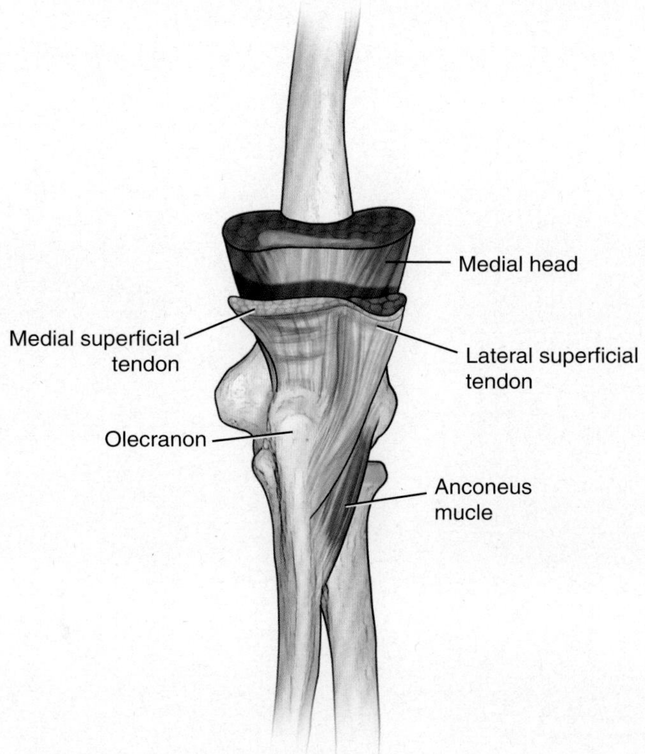

FIG 2 • The distal triceps tendon insertion (superficial and deep components): The lateral aspect of the tendon is more expansive, relatively thin, and in continuity with anconeus muscle and fascia. The medial part is thicker than the lateral aspect and forms the proper triceps tendon. It inserts directly onto olecranon.

- A medial part of the tendon that is thicker than the lateral aspect and forms the proper triceps tendon and inserts directly onto olecranon
- In some cases, a well-defined interval is located between the lateral triceps expansion and medial triceps tendon just proximal to the olecranon. This interval is located along the crest of the ulna and is well known as *triceps decussation*.
- The deep tendon is covered by a thin layer of muscle fibers both medially and laterally.
- The deep medial head of the triceps shows a broad and flat tendon centrally and laterally, whereas medially is a narrow thickened tendon.[22]
- Medially, the superficial and deep tendons are confluent and form the proper triceps tendon that insert into the medial olecranon footprint.
- Magnetic resonance imaging (MRI) often demonstrates a bipartite insertion between the deep and superficial tendon of the triceps into the olecranon[7] (**FIG 3**).
- However, all three heads of the triceps contribute to the formation of the triceps olecranon dome-shaped footprint[1] (**FIG 4**).

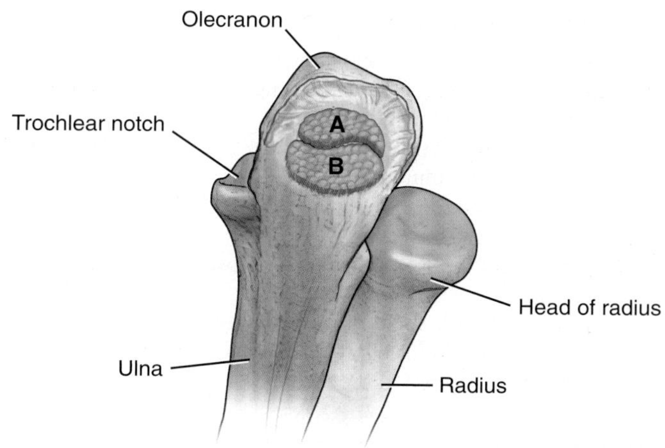

FIG 4 • The mean width (*A*) of the medial head footprint is about 16 mm and the mean thickness is 4 mm. The mean width of the common superficial tendon footprint is 19 mm and the mean thickness is 8 mm (*B*).

Olecranon Footprint

- The mean medial to lateral width of the insertion area is about 20 mm and the mean proximal to distal length[22] is about 13 mm.
- The mean distance from the olecranon tip to the most proximal aspect of the medial head insertion[4,22] is between 14.8 and 16 mm.
- The mean width (medial to lateral distance) of the medial head footprint is 16 mm and the mean thickness is 4 mm.

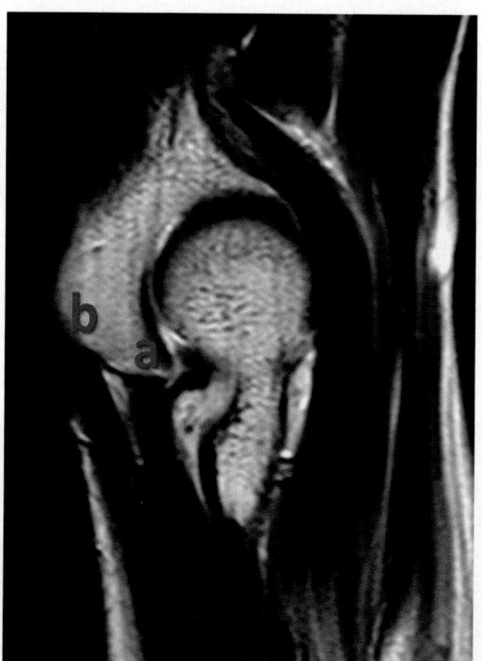

FIG 3 • The MRI demonstrating a bipartite insertion between the deep (*a*) and superficial (*b*) components of the triceps tendon into the olecranon.

- The mean width of the common superficial tendon footprint is 19 mm and the mean thickness[4] is 8 mm.
- Understanding the anatomy of the triceps tendon is the key to good outcomes following posttraumatic triceps repair or triceps reinsertion after deep surgical exposure.

PATHOGENESIS

- Triceps tendon injuries are probably one of the rarest tendon injuries in the body. There is a male predominance (3:1, male to female) with a wide range of age in which it can occur.[56]
- Triceps tendon ruptures can be simply classified into one of four groups:
  - Traumatic lesion (most common)
  - Spontaneous rupture
  - Overuse injury
  - Following total elbow arthroplasty

Traumatic Lesions

- Triceps tendon ruptures most commonly occur acutely when a patient falls on an outstretched hand with the elbow in some flexion and a forced load is applied to the contracting triceps. Traumatic tears can occur at several different anatomic regions, but they are most commonly observed at the insertion of the tendon such as an olecranon avulsion. More rarely, they can occur at the musculotendinous junction or within the muscle belly.[3,5,39]
- The traumatic distal tendon lesions can be partial or total[5,23] and are often isolated. Associated lesions of the radial head,[30,31] the medial collateral ligament (MCL),[24,32,49] and the capitellum[57] have been described.
- Partial traumatic tendo-osseous avulsions with one small fragment of bone visible proximal to the olecranon (flake sign) often occur associated with the radial head fractures[31] or simultaneous radial head and MCL-associated injuries.[57]
- The combination of a triceps avulsion, radial head fractures, and MCL rupture were reported by Yoon et al[57] as triad injury.

Spontaneous Ruptures

- Triceps injury can occur spontaneously due to attrition conditions if the tendon integrity is compromised. Loss of integrity can be caused by the following:
  - Rheumatoid arthritis
  - Chronic renal failure
  - Endocrine disorders
  - Metabolic bone diseases
  - Steroid use (local or systemic corticosteroids or anabolic steroids)[18]
- Tenosynovial pathologic tissue proliferation in the tendon combined with low local blood supply and mechanical attrition results in rupture of the tendon.

Overuse Injuries

- The cumulative submaximal loading of the tissue is referred to as *overuse injuries*, and complete rupture often occurs through abnormal tendon with intrinsic pathologic disorders.[19]
- A classification of progressive Achilles tendon disorders[46] can be useful to understand the structural manifestations of triceps tendon overuse injury.
  - Peritendinitis
  - Tendinosis with or without peritendinitis
  - Partial rupture
  - Total rupture
- Triceps tendinosis during sporting activities is not infrequent. In cases of chronic tendon pain, the pathologic lesion is typical of a degenerative process with areas of marked degeneration and lack of local vascular supply.[2] These characteristic changes, especially if associated with a repetitive use of local corticosteroids, predispose to triceps tendon rupture, possibly by decreasing the tendon tensile strength.
- Surgical treatment is recommended in chronic tendinosis when clinical and MRI assessments detect partial rupture of the tendon.

Following Total Elbow Arthroplasty

- Failure of triceps reattachment can be seen following surgical treatment in which a triceps takedown is performed.
- When the total elbow arthroplasty is performed, the surgical triceps takedown or slide is usually well tolerated, but some patients have an unsuccessful postsurgical attenuation or ruptures of the triceps reattachment.
  - At the Mayo Clinic, this complication occurred in 16 elbows following 887 total elbow arthroplasties, about 2% of the procedures.[10]
- Predisposing factors are inflammatory arthropathies with poor tissue quality.
- The triceps weakening is a frequent and a well-recognized problem following the total elbow arthroplasty.
- The causes of the triceps weakness or rupture following arthroplasty may be related to the following:
  - Changes of the triceps moment arm which is a function of location of the axis of the prosthetic joint.[14] The offset of the triceps tendon decreases (reducing the strength of the muscle) when the prosthesis design is not anatomic. Insufficient reinsertion related to poor quality of tendon tissue or tendon devascularization during the approach.
  - Aggressive rehabilitation program during the postoperative period with active exercises that can attenuate or detach the triceps reinsertion

PATIENT HISTORY AND PHYSICAL FINDINGS

- In patients with suspected rupture of triceps tendon, the physician should gather a precise history including:
  - Age, dominant arm
  - Presence of preexisting pain from overuse injuries[44]
  - Repetitive use of local corticosteroids or systemic anabolic steroids[12]
  - Previous elbow surgery
- The patient most commonly describes a sudden pain in the posterior aspect of the elbow after a history of direct blow or fall on outstretched hand.[16,17,29,38] The usual mechanism of injury is a forceful sudden flexion of extended elbow.[48–50]
- Laceration and open injuries with or without elbow fracture-dislocation can also cause distal triceps rupture.[27]
- In general, the triceps lesions is characterized by the following:
  - Tenderness and a palpable defect in the tendon that can be seen proximal to the olecranon
    - Swelling, ecchymosis, and body habitus can obscure the tendon defect in the acute stage. Once swelling subsides, most patients demonstrate a palpable gap in the tendon.
  - Active extension is typically diminished or absent, depending on whether or not there is a complete or partial tear.[9,40]
- A partial rupture of the medial head is frequently undiagnosed. The diagnosis can be difficult, but care should be taken when evaluating radiographs to assess for the presence of the flake sign.
- The clinical findings of the triceps insufficiency following total elbow arthroplasty are as follows[10,11]:
  - A change in the posterior contour of the elbow with visual and palpable prominence of the implant
  - The presence of olecranon bursitis
  - Atrophy of the triceps muscle
  - Proximal retraction or lateral subluxation of the extensor mechanism
- The most universal physical finding with a triceps rupture is the inability to extend the arm against gravity (**FIG 5**).
- A tear can be seen and palpated in the tendon during attempts at resisted extension (**FIG 6A,B**).
- Discerning between partial or complete ruptures can be a diagnostic challenge. The test to evaluate the triceps function against gravity and resistance is performed by the physician

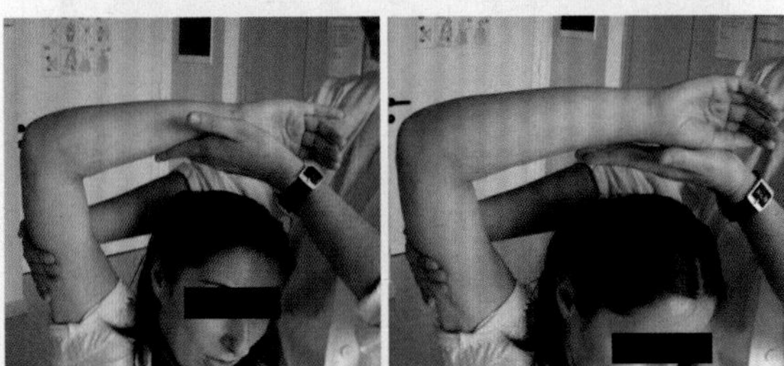

FIG 5 • The triceps extension tests can be performed observing the ability of the patient to extend the elbow over his or her head, against gravity.

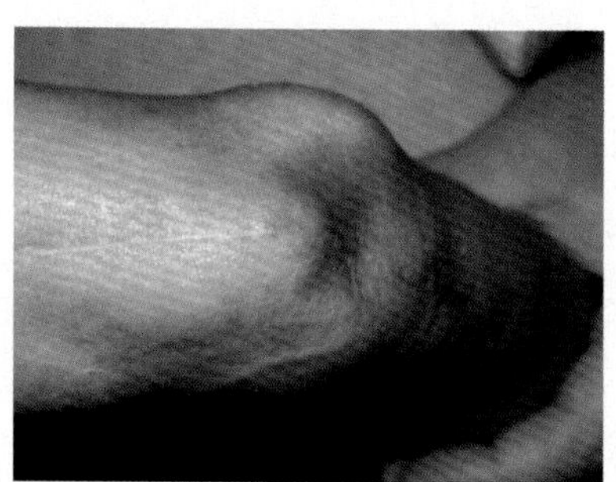

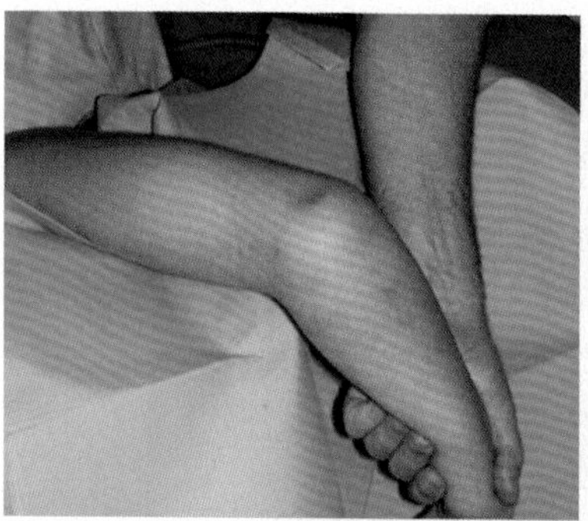

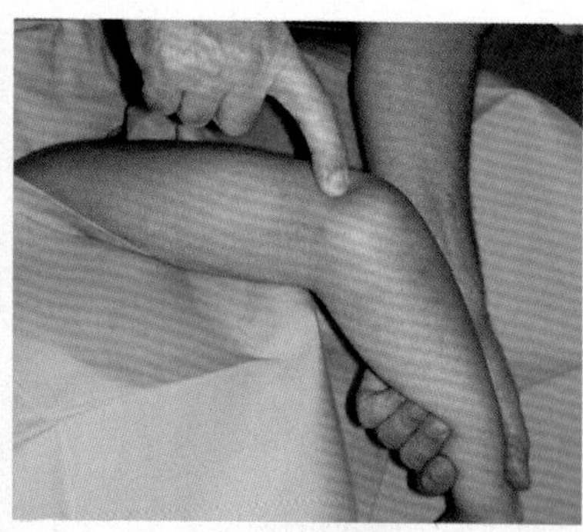

FIG 6 • A. The clinical findings of the triceps insufficiency are a change in the posterior contour of the elbow with visual and palpable prominence of bone. **B.** A tear can often be palpated in the triceps tendon.

with the patient in the prone position with the elbow flexed to 90 degrees, the upper arm supported on the table, and the forearm hanging free (**FIG 7**).

- A partial tendon lesion is manifested by weakness and ability to actively extend the elbow against the gravity but not against resistance. This finding is likely secondary to an intact lateral expansion or a compensating anconeus muscle.

- A total tendon tear is manifested by loss of extension strength against gravity, and active elbow extension is impossible. Viegas[51] described a provocative test similar to the Thompson test that can be employed in diagnosing triceps tendon rupture. With the patient in the prone position and the forearm hanging over the side of the table, the physician squeezes the triceps muscle belly. Slight elbow extension is indicative of a partial tear, whereas no motion signals a complete rupture (**FIG 8**).
- We have defined a test for triceps rupture called the *fall down triceps test*. This test assesses the inability of the patient to keep the forearm in maximum extension against gravity. The patient stands up with the shoulder at 90 degrees of abduction and internal rotation, the examiner stays behind and keeps the forearm in full passive extension. If the forearm falls when the examiner releases it, there is a triceps tendon rupture (**FIG 9**).

IMAGING AND OTHER DIAGNOSTIC STUDIES

- Imaging studies can help to identify the level of lesion (olecranon insertion, myotendinous junction, or intramuscular), discriminate partial from complete tear, and estimate the amount of the tendon retraction and to exclude associated osseous injuries.[16,29,52]
- Lateral x-rays can demonstrate the flake sign. The bony fragment is usually small and easy to ignore, but its presence is pathognomonic of distal triceps avulsion (**FIG 10**). X-rays are also useful for the diagnosis of associated injuries such as radial head and capitellum fractures.
- Ultrasonography may be used, but it provides limited anatomic details. It is useful immediately after an injury,[20] when the diagnosis is in doubt.
- MRI is the best technique for assessment of the tendon lesions[13,55] because it allows for distinguishing partial versus complete lesions, the degree of tendon retraction, and any muscle atrophy as well as the location of the tear[25] (**FIG 11**).

DIFFERENTIAL DIAGNOSIS

- Neurologic weakness from radial nerve problems (compression or lesion)[21]
- C7 isolated nerve root lesions
- Olecranon fracture

FIG 7 • Elbow extension can be evaluated with the patient in the prone position with the elbow flexed to 90 degrees, the upper arm supported on the table, and the forearm hanging free.

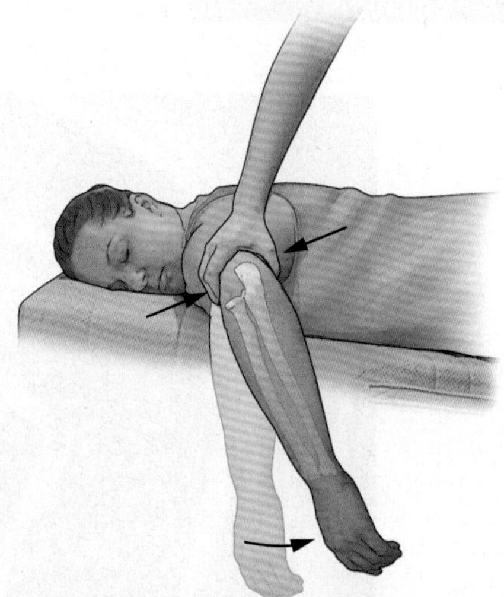

FIG 8 • Viegas' test. With the patient in the prone position and letting the forearm relaxed hang over the table, the physician squeezes the triceps muscle belly.

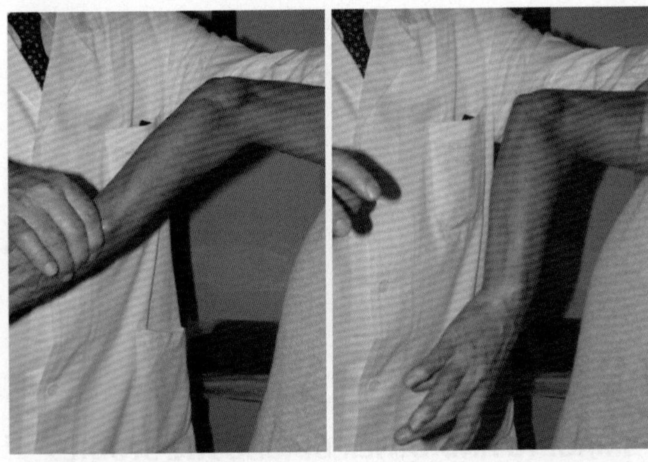

FIG 9 • Fall down triceps test. The forearm falls down when the examiner leaves forearm in maximum extension. If a complete rupture is present, the elbow drops down to 90 degrees of flexion; for partial ruptures, the forearm drops down only partially.

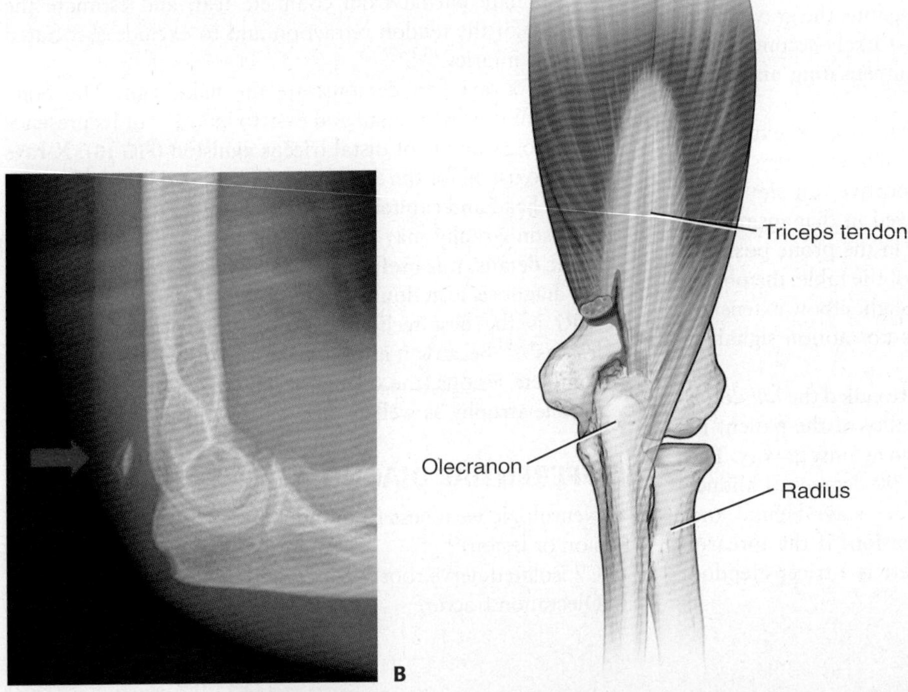

FIG 10 • **A,B.** Lateral x-rays of the elbow are useful in confirming the diagnosis if a small extra-articular avulsion fracture (*arrow*) of the olecranon (flake sign) is present.

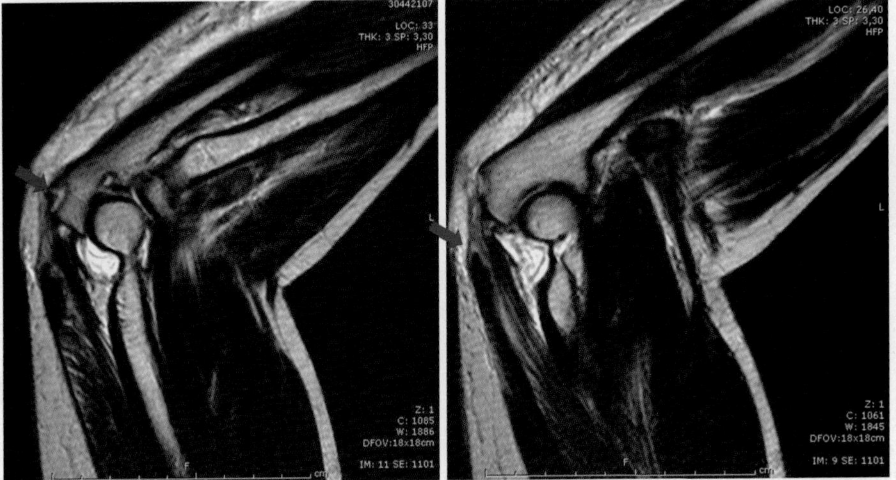

FIG 11 • Sagittal MRI scans demonstrating (**A**) partial and (**B**) complete rupture of the triceps tendon (*arrows*).

NONOPERATIVE MANAGEMENT

- Conservative management plays a role in partial triceps injuries when there is no significant loss of the extension power against gravity.
  - Patient age and lifestyle are important factors in deciding to treat these injuries nonoperatively. This group can include injuries to the nondominant arm injury, sedentary lifestyles, and the elderly patients who are at a higher risk for complications with surgical management.
- Nonoperative treatment ranges from no specific treatment to elbow immobilization for 4 weeks in an extension splint.[37]
- The surgeon must be careful when selecting nonoperative treatment in healthy active patients, as it may lead to permanent loss or weakness of power extension.

SURGICAL MANAGEMENT

- Several surgical techniques and different approaches offer variable options for the surgical management of acute complete or chronic tears.
- The choice depends on the tissue quality, the amount of the muscle retraction, and the chronicity of the lesion. The quality of the olecranon also has to be considered, particularly following total elbow arthroplasty.
- For a successful direct repair, the repair has to be performed between 90 and 70 degrees of elbow extension, without tension at the tendon–bone reinsertion. Direct repair under tension increases the risk of secondary rupture and loss of elbow flexion.
- The surgical options are as follows:
  - Direct repair to the olecranon
  - Augmentation with autograft or allograft
  - Anconeus rotation flap
  - Achilles tendon allograft with or without calcaneus bone

Preoperative Planning

- With the patient under anesthesia, the elbow is assessed for concomitant elbow instability. Varus–valgus stability is evaluated, and the pivot shift test is used to exclude rotational instability.
- Passive range of motion in pronosupination and flexion–extension should also be assessed.

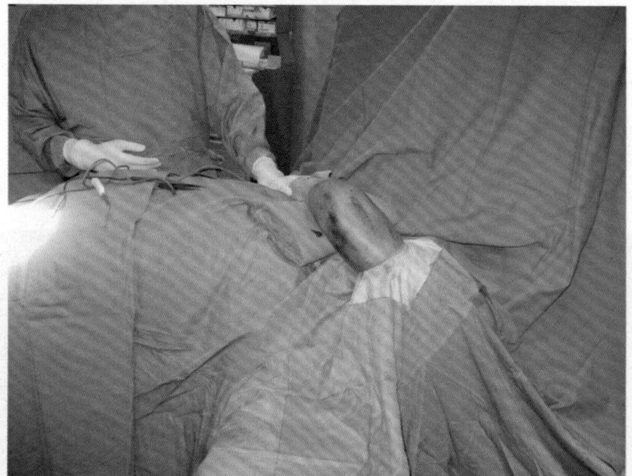

FIG 12 • The patient is placed in supine position with the body rotated 30 to 40 degrees toward the contralateral side, with the arm and elbow folded over the chest.

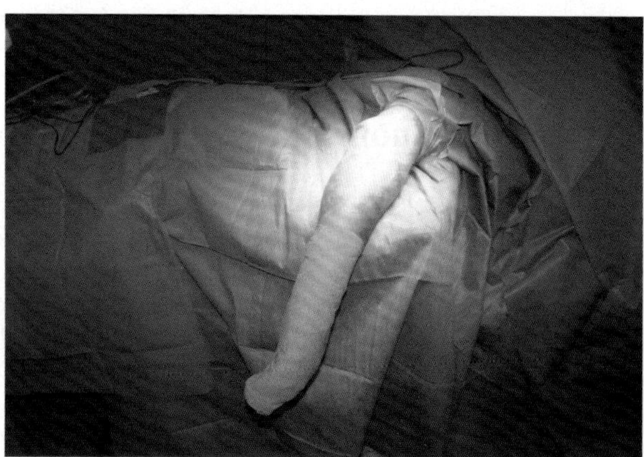

FIG 13 • Alternatively, the patient is placed in the lateral position and with the affected arm over a bolster and the elbow flexed.

Positioning

- The patient is placed supine with the body rotated 30 to 40 degrees toward the contralateral side with the arm and elbow folded over the chest (**FIG 12**).
- Alternatively, the patient can be placed in the lateral position and with the affected arm over a bolster, the elbow flexed, and the forearm free (**FIG 13**).
- A tourniquet is not always necessary because the tendon is relatively superficial and the tourniquet may limit the anatomic reinsertion of the tendon to its attachment on the proximal ulna.
- For cases with significant tendon retraction that require an extensive release of the muscle, it is useful to use a sterile tourniquet for the surgical exposure to help identify the ulnar or the radial nerves. The tourniquet is released during tendon reinsertion to facilitate mobilization of the triceps muscle.

Approach

- A posterior skin incision is made just lateral to the midline (**FIG 14**).
- Skin and subcutaneous flaps are elevated off the triceps, olecranon, and ulna. The proximal insertions of the anconeus and flexor carpi ulnaris are identified.
- Olecranon bursitis is removed, if it is present.
- The ulnar nerve is isolated and protected.

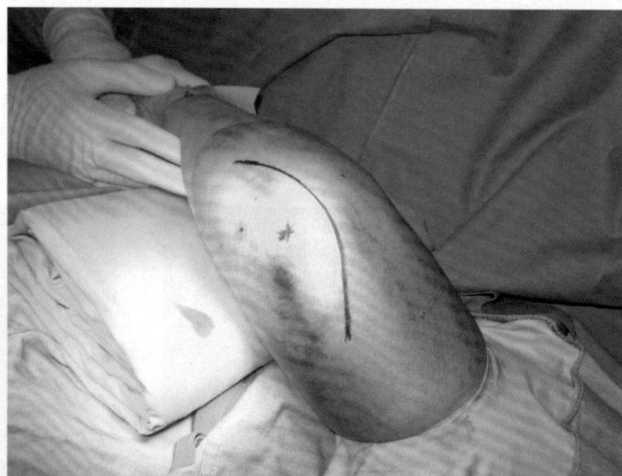

FIG 14 • Posterior straight skin incision is made just lateral to the midline.

Direct Reattachment to the Olecranon

Partial Lesion Reattachment

- The triceps tendon usually retracts no more than 3 to 5 cm. The preserved lateral continuity to anconeus triceps and aponeurotic fascia avoids significant proximal migration of the tendon.
- The proximal stump of the tendon lesion is identified and débrided back to normal tendon that is directly reinserted into the olecranon (**TECH FIG 1A,B**).
- For partial lesions without a bony fragment, the tendon is reinserted directly into the olecranon bone (**TECH FIG 2A–C**).
- In a chronic case with bony fragments attached to the tendon, the bone is débrided and the tendon is reinserted into the olecranon bone with sutures.

Complete Lesion Reattachment

- The tendon and muscle belly are mobilized, and a heavy, nonabsorbable suture is passed through the tendon using a Bunnell- or Krackow-type running locking stitch (**TECH FIG 3A–D**).
- Before reattaching the tendon to the olecranon footprint, the bone is decorticated with a burr.
- Two transverse holes are drilled (2.5-mm drill hole), starting at the triceps insertion and exiting on the dorsal side of the olecranon.
- The sutures are passed through the drill holes using a suture pass.
- Maintaining the elbow at 90 degrees of flexion, the tendon is advanced to the olecranon and tied with the knot placed on the radial side of the ulnar crest avoiding skin postoperative irritation (**TECH FIG 4**).

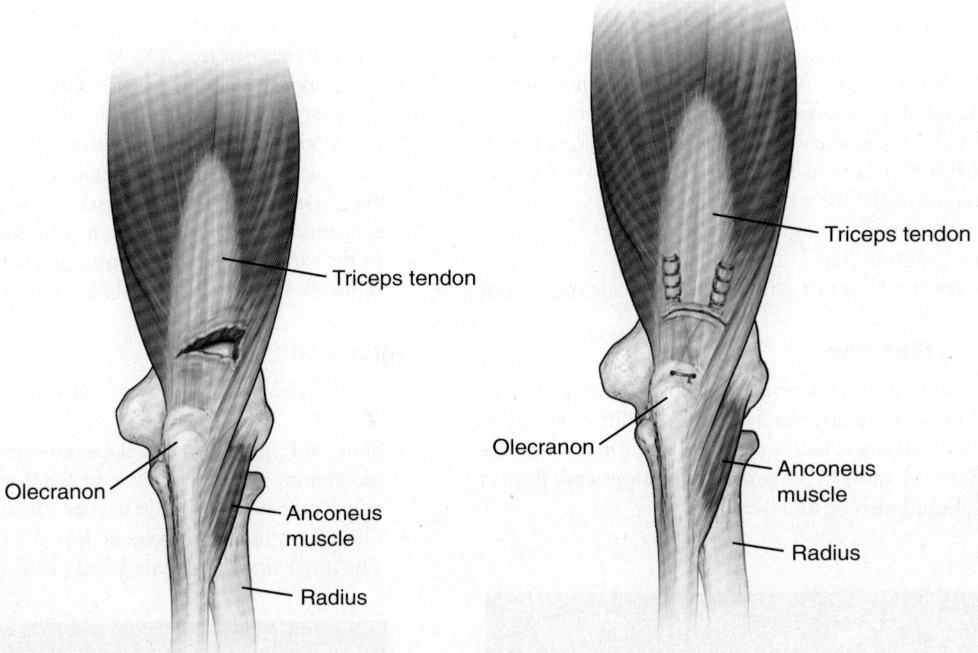

TECH FIG 1 • **A,B.** The proximal stump of a partial or complete lesion is identified and débrided back to normal tendon which is directly reinserted into the olecranon.

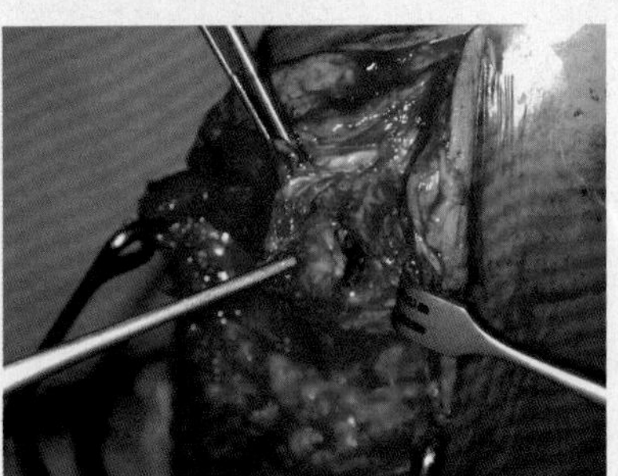

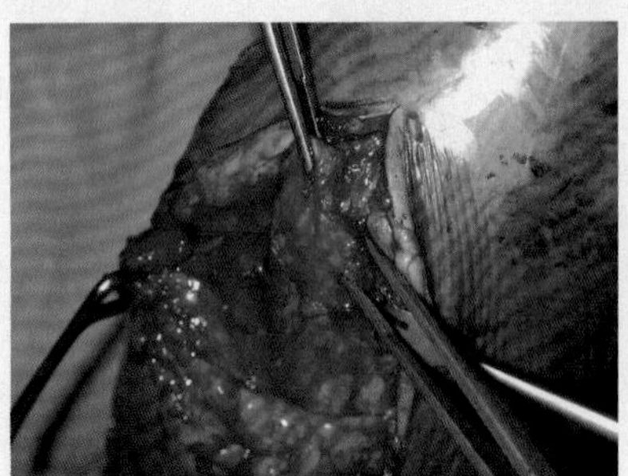

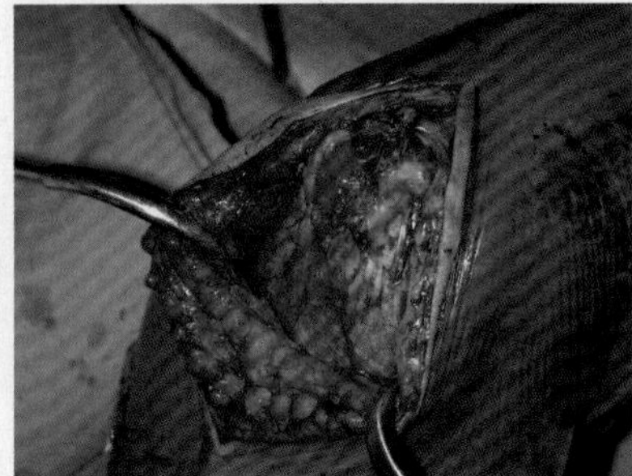

TECH FIG 2 • **A–C.** A partial lesion without a bony fragment is reinserted directly into the olecranon.

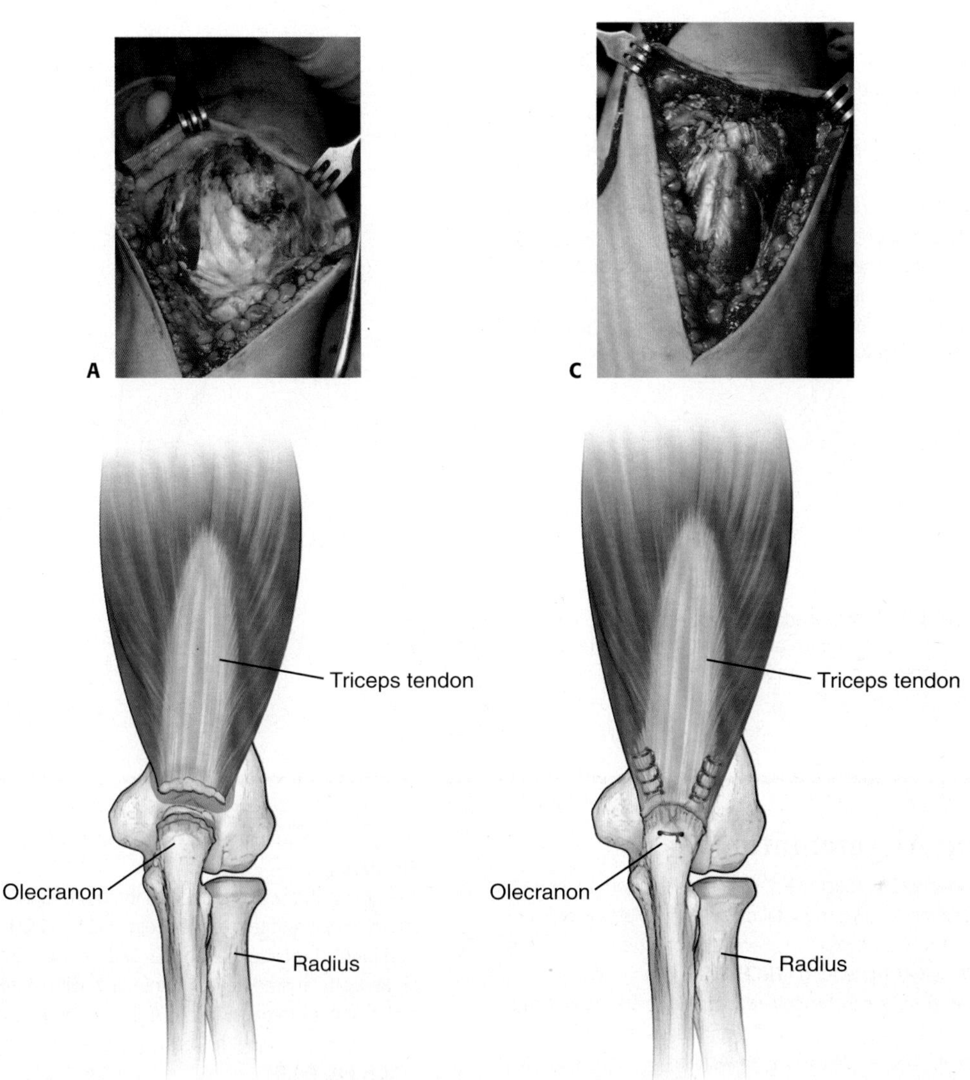

TECH FIG 3 • A–D. The tendon and muscle belly are mobilized, and a running locking stitch with a heavy nonabsorbable suture is placed through the tendon. The sutures are then passed through bone tunnels in the proximal ulna.

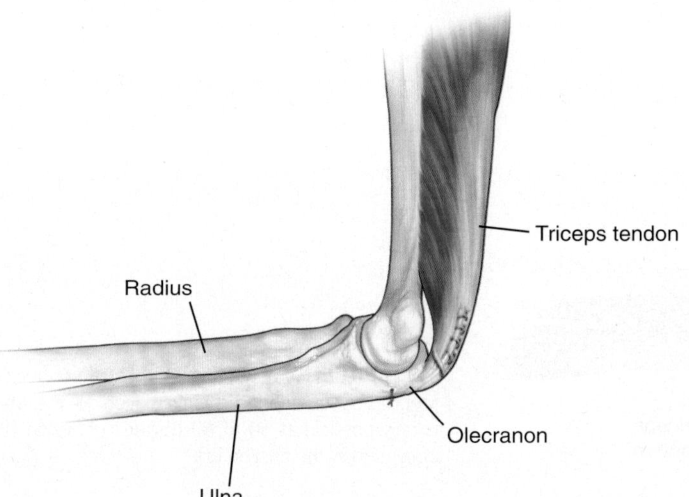

TECH FIG 4 • Direct reattachment to the olecranon is possible when the tendon can be reinserted with the elbow in 90 degrees of elbow flexion.

- An additional fixation can be obtained by using proximal suture anchors (double-row repair) to improve the fixation of the anatomic footprint of the tendon (**TECH FIG 5**).
- The medial and lateral skin flaps are mobilized, and sutures are placed between the fascia and the subcutaneous tissue of the two flaps to reduce the risk of a potential dead space.
- Elbow motion is checked in particular for limitation in flexion due to overtensioning of the repair.
- A posterior subcutaneous drain is placed for the first 24 hours.
- Skin and subcutaneous tissue are closed.
- After surgery, the patient's arm is immobilized in a posterior splint, with the elbow flexed about 30 to 40 degrees.

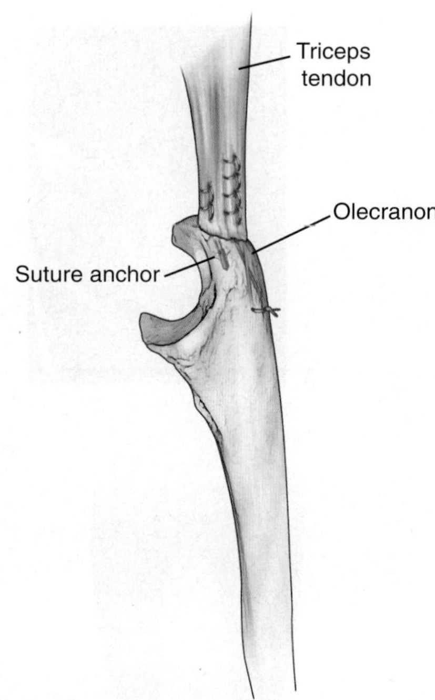

TECH FIG 5 • An additional fixation can be obtained by using a proximal row of suture anchors to improve the fixation of the anatomic footprint of the tendon.

Tendon Augmentation

- When the direct reattachment of triceps tendon to bone in chronic lesions or following total elbow arthroplasty is only possible at 50 to 60 degrees of elbow flexion, then tendon augmentation is recommended (**TECH FIG 6**).
- Small size defects can be covered using the palmaris longus, plantaris tendon autograft, flexor carpi radialis, or semitendinosus allograft. For larger defect, an Achilles tendon allograft is useful.
- The olecranon bone footprint and the tendon defect margins are prepared similar to the direct repair.
- The palmaris longus, the plantaris, flexor carpi radialis, or semitendinosus tendons transfer are harvested and woven through the stump of the ruptured tendon and sutured to the triceps tendon using running locking, nonabsorbable sutures (**TECH FIG 7A,B**).
- The graft is then passed through the bone tunnels into the olecranon similar to direct tendon reinsertion (**TECH FIG 8**).
- Combined procedures can be performed using an autograft or allograft augmentation reinforced with a rotational proximal sleeve of forearm fascia. A flap of fascia is detached from the forearm, leaving its base attached to the olecranon[8,12] (**TECH FIG 9A,B**).
- The tendon graft is secured to the bone in moderate tension at about 90 degrees of elbow flexion, and the forearm fascia is turned up to cover the autograft and the triceps tendon (**TECH FIG 10A–D**).

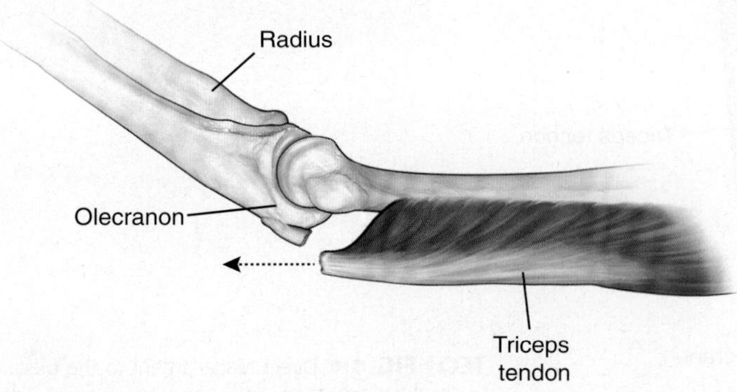

TECH FIG 6 • The tendon augmentation is recommended when tendon approximation to the bone is only possible at 50 to 60 degrees of flexion (the *arrow* shows the traction line).

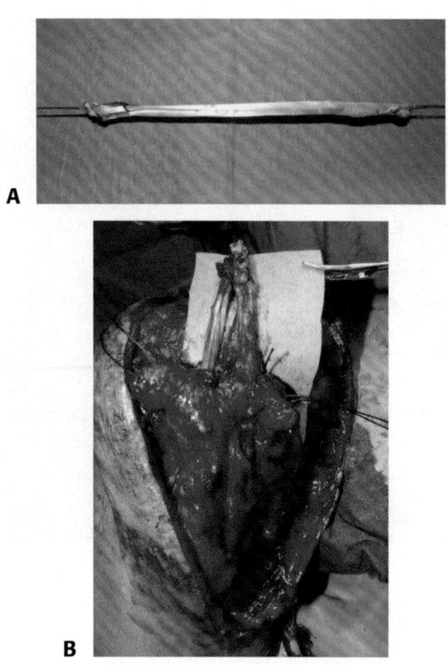

TECH FIG 7 • **A,B.** The tendon graft is harvested, woven through the stump of the ruptured tendon, and sutured to the triceps tendon.

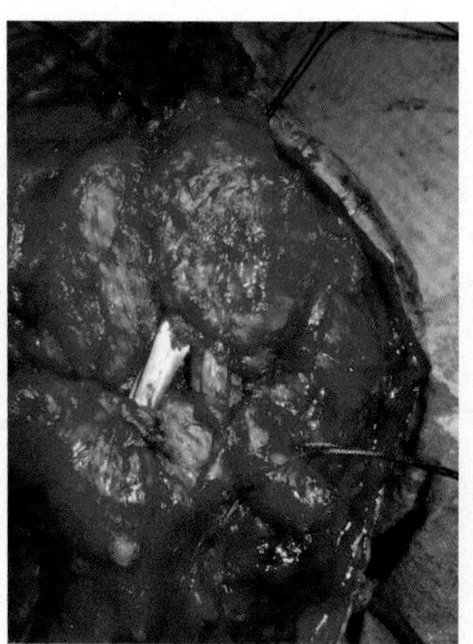

TECH FIG 8 • The graft is then passed through the bone tunnels into the olecranon similar to direct tendon reinsertion.

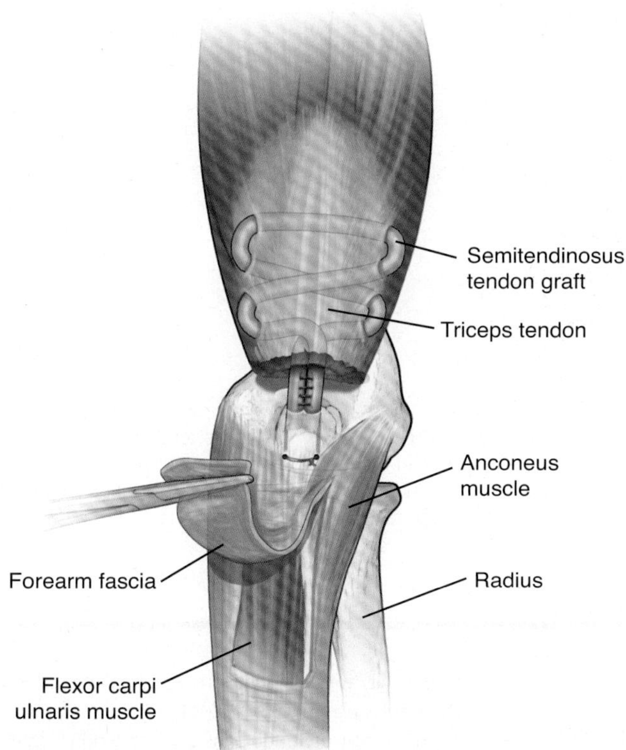

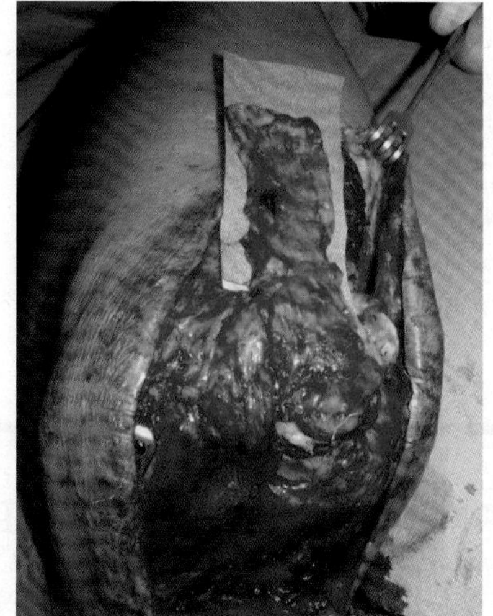

TECH FIG 9 • **A,B.** Combined procedure using tendon autograft and a flap of fascia detached from the forearm leaving its base attached to the olecranon.

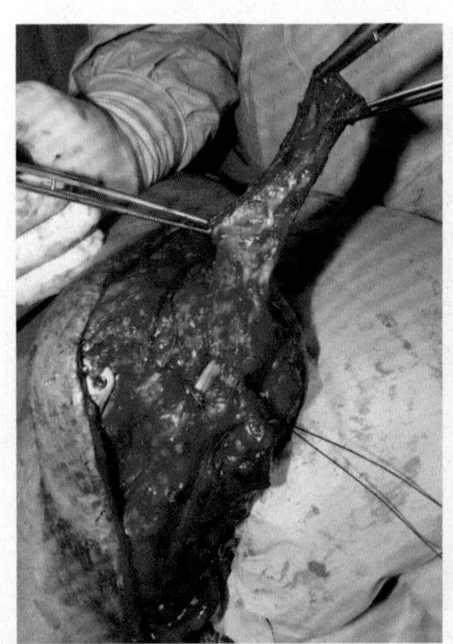
A

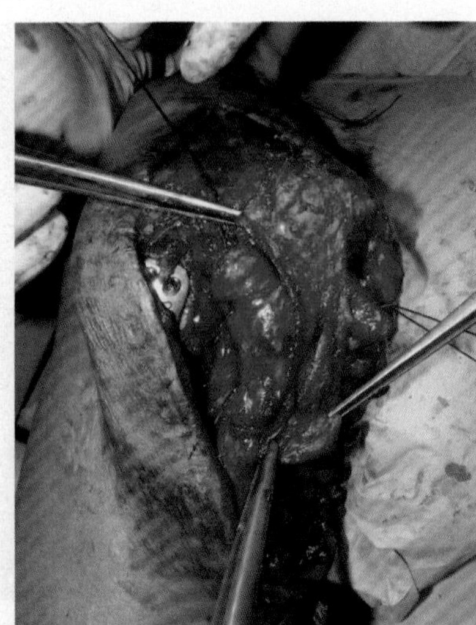
B

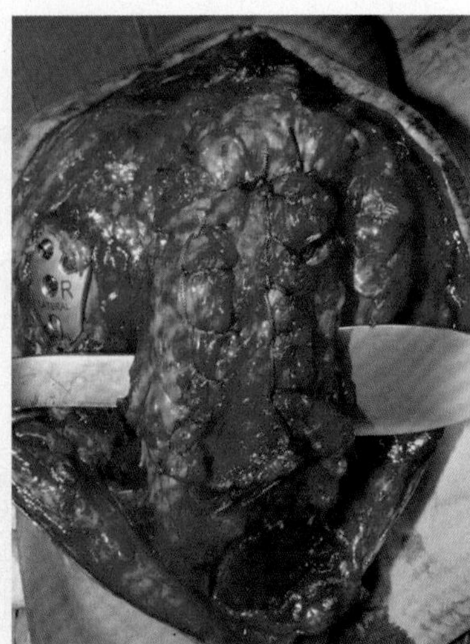
C

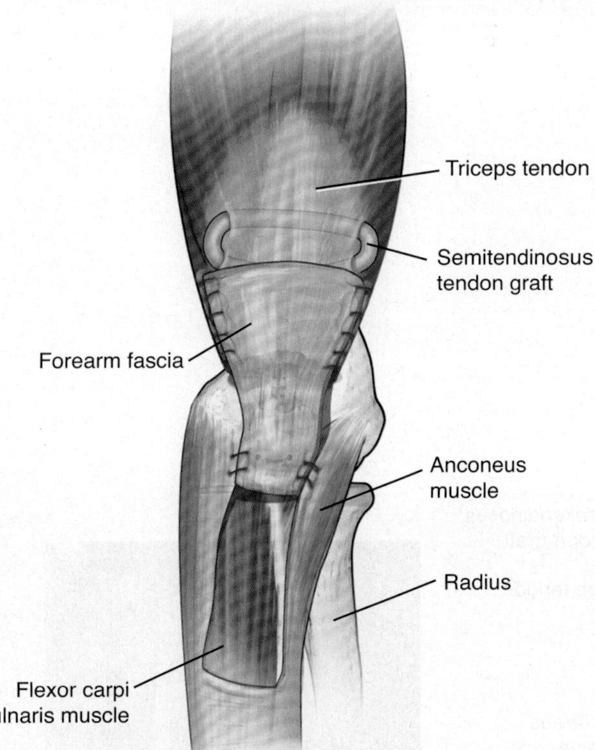

D

TECH FIG 10 • A–D. The tendon graft is secured to the bone in moderate tension at about 90 degrees of elbow flexion, and the forearm fascia covers the tendon autograft and the triceps tendon.

The Anconeus Rotational Flap

- The anconeus rotational flap described by Morrey,[35–37] is a useful procedure when direct reattachment is impossible due to degenerative and fragile triceps tendon. It is indicated when the triceps defect is small, and the lateral triceps fascia and anconeus are preserved as well as for lateral triceps dislocation in continuity with the anconeus as complication following total elbow arthroplasty (**TECH FIG 11**).
- The olecranon bone footprint and the tendon defect margins are prepared similar to the direct repair.
- The Kocher interval between the anconeus and extensor carpi ulnaris is exposed. Care is taken to preserve its superficial fascial connection to the lateral triceps (**TECH FIG 12**).

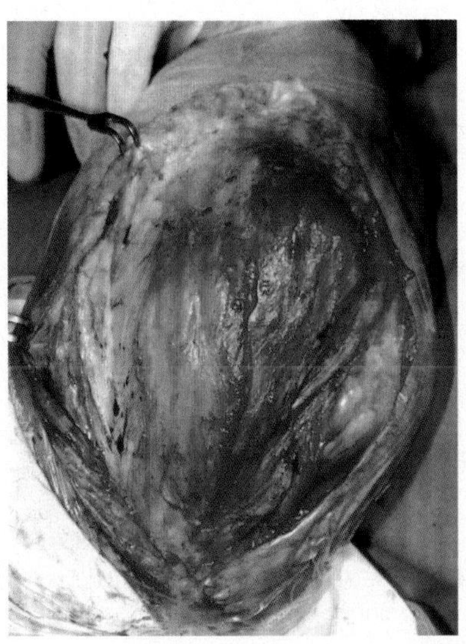

TECH FIG 11 • Lateral triceps dislocation in continuity with the anconeus muscle as a complication following total elbow arthroplasty.

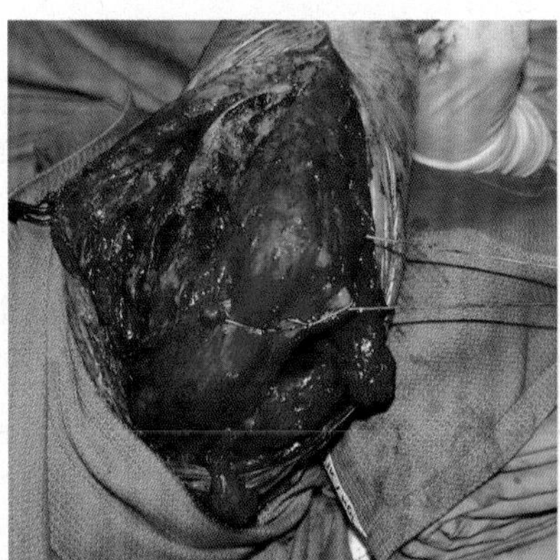

TECH FIG 12 • The Kocher interval between the anconeus and extensor carpi ulnaris is exposed. Care is taken to preserve its superficial fascial connection to the lateral triceps.

- The anconeus is mobilized off the ulna and the humerus without detaching the distal insertion, and the entire muscle and the lateral triceps are transferred medially to close the tendon defect.
- The anconeus flap is mobilized and then oriented over the tip of the olecranon and sutured on it through drill holes (**TECH FIG 13A,B**).
- The anconeus is stabilized to the olecranon, and the medial fascia of the anconeus is sutured to the tendinous portion of the triceps ruptured stump.

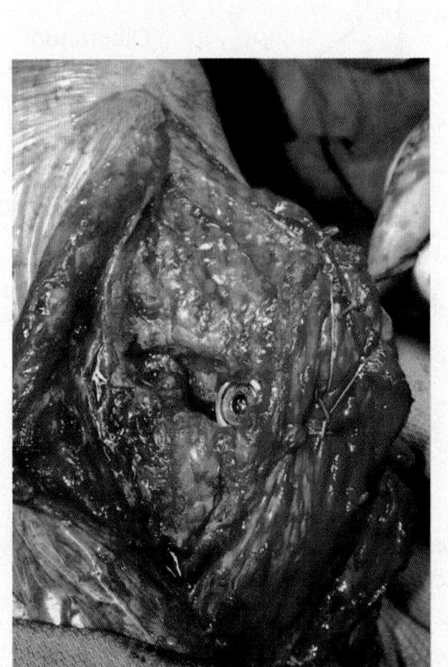

A

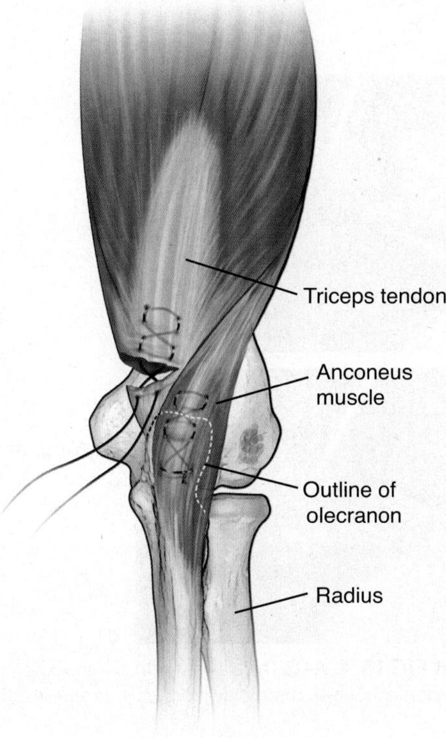

B

TECH FIG 13 • **A,B.** The anconeus flap is mobilized and then oriented over the tip of the olecranon and sutured on it through drill holes.

Achilles Tendon Allograft

- When a chronic rupture has a significant muscle retraction and there is tendon tissue deficiency, the Achilles allograft reconstruction is indicated (**TECH FIG 14**).
- The Achilles tendon allograft with a small piece of calcaneus can be used to reconstruct the continuity of the triceps tendon and also as an osseous graft to olecranon if it is deficient.[35–37]
- The standard posterior approach is used, and tendon and olecranon preparation are identical for primary repair.
- The triceps muscle and tendon are elevated from the posterior humerus, removing any scarring tissue deep in the muscle belly as well as in the subcutaneous tissue.
- Care must be taken with this maneuver because the radial nerve is vulnerable to injury in the spiral groove between the middle and distal thirds of the humerus.
- Two reconstructive techniques may be used:
  - Attach the allograft tendon directly to the olecranon through drill holes. The distal Achilles tendon is secured to the proximal ulna using drill holes as described for the direct repair.
  - Fix the calcaneal portion of the allograft to the remaining olecranon with a screw or a tension band wire. The allograft with calcaneal bone provides an ideal reconstructive unit, especially if the olecranon is deficient as is common in triceps insufficiency following total elbow arthroplasty[10,11] (**TECH FIG 15A–C**).
- With either technique, locking nonabsorbable sutures are placed through the distal stump of the triceps tendon and tied to the allograft (**TECH FIG 16**).

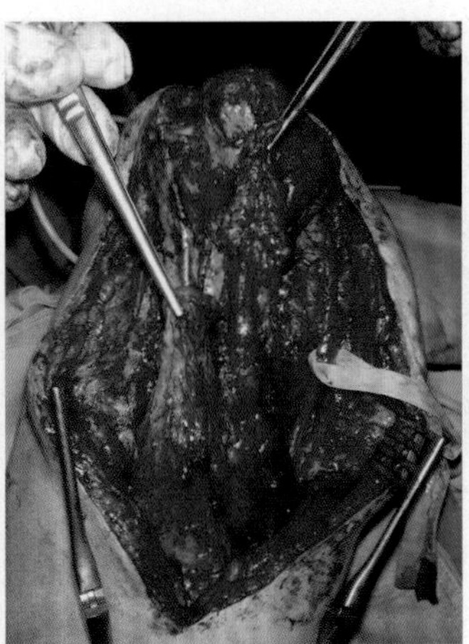

TECH FIG 14 ● Achilles allograft reconstruction is indicated in cases of chronic rupture with significant muscle retraction and tendon tissue deficiency.

- The proximal expansion of the allograft is used to wrap the remaining triceps contractile muscle as well as the remaining tendon and secured with heavy nonabsorbable sutures (**TECH FIG 17A–D**).
- The procedure is performed in at about 90 degrees of elbow flexion.
- Motion is delayed with the osteotendinous allograft technique to allow adequate bone graft revascularization.

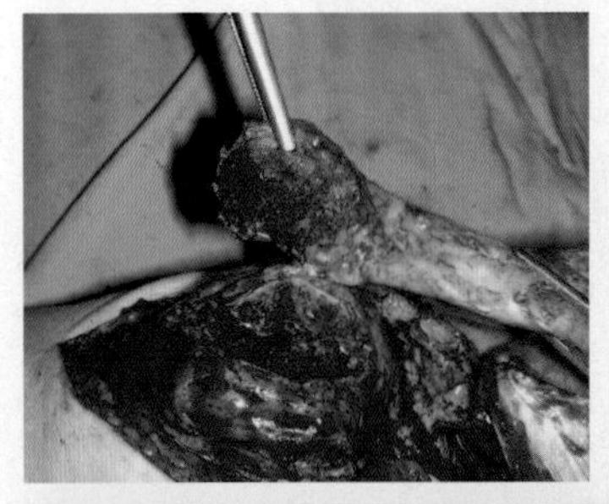

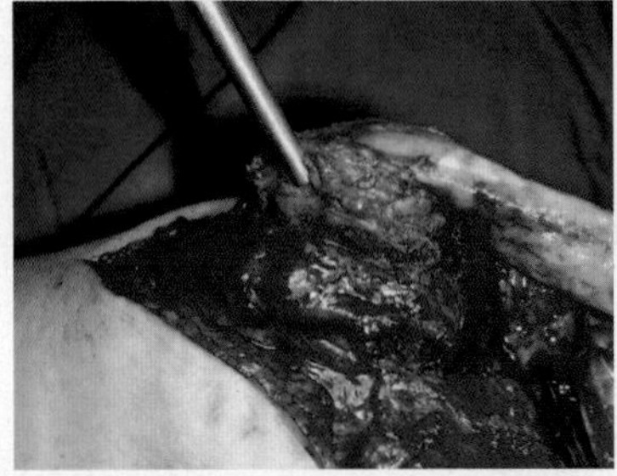

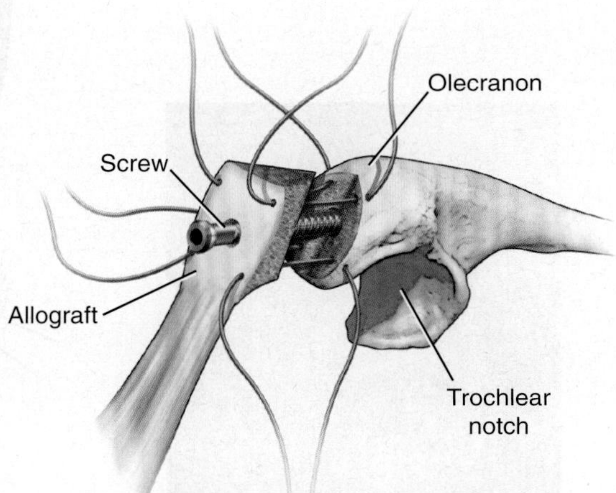

TECH FIG 15 ● **A–C.** The allograft with calcaneal bone provides an ideal reconstructive unit especially with the olecranon deficiency, commonly it occurs in triceps insufficiency following total elbow arthroplasty.

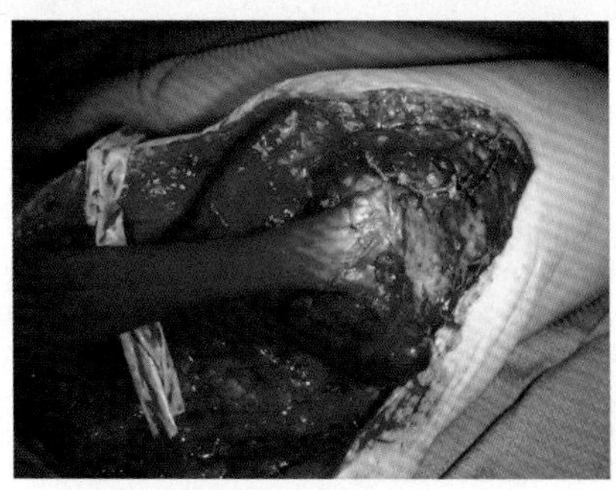

TECH FIG 16 • The distal stump of the triceps tendon is tied to the allograft.

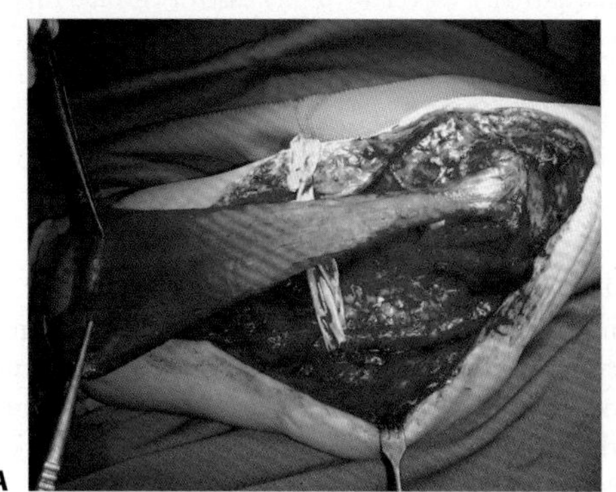

A

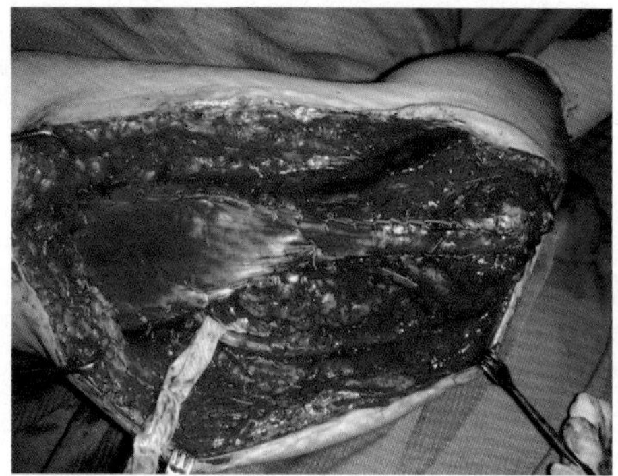

B

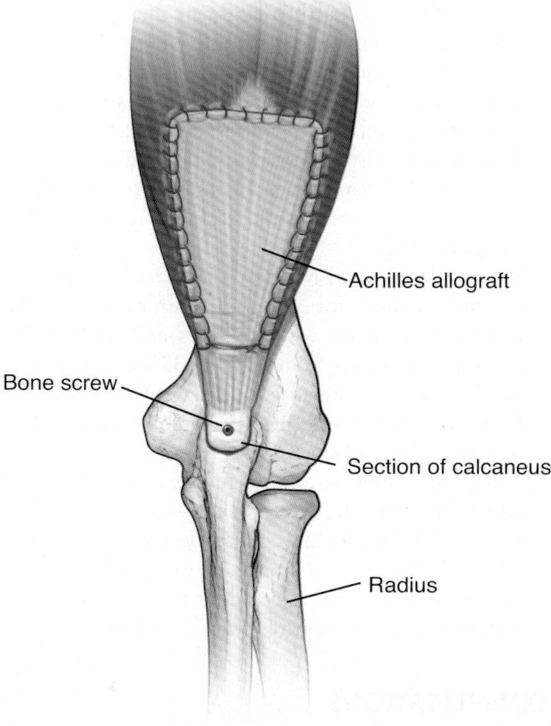

C

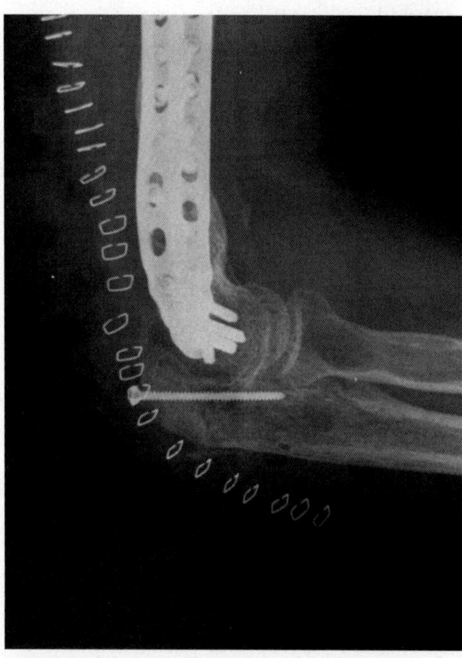

D

TECH FIG 17 • **A–D.** The proximal expansion of the allograft is used to wrap the remaining triceps muscle as well as the remaining tendon using nonabsorbable sutures.

PEARLS AND PITFALLS

Acute versus chronic lesions	▪ Acute ▪ In acute lesions, swelling and body habitus may not allow the examiner to palpate the tendon rupture. It is palpable when the swelling subsides. ▪ Chronic ▪ In the chronic lesions, the olecranon bursa is often associated with the torn tendon. ▪ The anconeus rotational flap is a useful procedure to reinforce the tendon reinsertion when the triceps defect is small and the lateral triceps fascia and anconeus are preserved. Surgeons must ensure that the fascia release laterally is complete and that the muscle and fascia transfer laterally and not slip back with flexion of the elbow. The anconeus has to be well incorporated in the torn triceps while the elbow is extended. ▪ With Achilles tendon allograft reconstruction, the surgeon has to consider: ▪ Excess bulk of allograft tendon might compromise wound closure. ▪ Appropriate length of the transfer to avoid insufficiency or retraction of the extensor mechanism ▪ Long postsurgical time for allograft healing
Imaging studies	▪ MRI is useful for identifying the level of the lesion, discriminating partial from complete tear, and defining the amount of the tendon retraction and muscular atrophy, especially in the case of chronic ruptures. The x-ray and computed tomography (CT) excluded associated osseous injuries.
Management	▪ Be careful to advise nonoperative treatment for partial rupture in healthy active patients.

POSTOPERATIVE CARE

- The postoperative protocol consists of immobilization in 30 to 40 degrees of elbow flexion for 2 weeks (it will be increasing in chronic lesion if augmentation is used to recovered the extensor mechanism).
- Following the first period, a dynamic brace is used for an additional 4 weeks.
- Passive range of motion is permitted after primary repair, and active range of motion begins at 6 weeks following surgical repair. Complete return to previous activities is expected after 3 months from surgery. In cases of tendon augmentation or Achilles allograft, postoperative immobilization is used for 4 weeks and a dynamic brace is used for the following month.

OUTCOMES[6,15,26,41,42,49,54]

- Little information has been described in the literature regarding the outcomes of triceps repairs. All studies reporting triceps repair or reconstruction are small and retrospective. Triceps rupture is the least common of all major tendon injuries.[45,53] It accounts for less than 1% of all tendon ruptures within the upper extremity.[1,34]
- Most investigators described their results as very good to excellent in terms of range of motion, pain relief, and restoration of extensor mechanism function.[5,31,33,47,51]
- The results of immediate or delayed repair are reported to be similar with good results in both series.[37] Outcomes following reconstruction have been shown to be comparable to direct repair,[28,37] although the technique is more challenging and the recovery is slower.[37]
- Good results have been reported with nonoperative management for partial triceps rupture.[3,9] Mair et al[33] reported on 10 professional football players with partial tears, 6 of whom had tears that healed, allowing them to return to competitive football.
- Sierra et al[45] reported the results of treatment of 16 acute triceps tendon ruptures (15 patients) treated from 1976 to 2001.The mean age was 50 years (range, 16 to 71 years). The most common pattern was the triceps avulsion of the insertion from the olecranon (13 elbows). An intratendinous rupture occurred in 2 elbows, and an intramuscular rupture occurred in 1. Eleven elbows underwent surgical repair of the extensor mechanism; the remaining 5 were treated nonoperatively. The surgical repair consisted of advancement of triceps with placement of locking nonabsorbable sutures through tendon and passing through drill holes into the olecranon. Wire was used to augment the repair in one patient who had avulsion of a piece of bone with the tendon. The anconeus muscle was rotated to reinforce the triceps reconstruction in two cases. Three of the 11 surgically treated elbows developed postoperative complications that required reoperation. Postoperatively, patients were followed up for a mean of 1.4 years (range, 7 months to 14 years). Of those elbows treated operatively, strength testing was good and excellent in all.
- Sanchez-Sotelo and Morrey[43] reported the results on seven patients treated for chronic insufficiency of the triceps using the anconeus rotation flaps and the Achilles tendon allograft. At mean follow-up of 33 months (range from 9 to 93 months), one patient underwent a revision surgery for failed anconeus rotation flap 6 months after surgery. The remaining six had slight or no pain with restoration of functional arc of motion and normal or minimal decrease of the power in extension. All of them were satisfied from the results and the final Mayo elbow performance index was 100 points in five and 75 points in one. On the basis of their experience, the authors consider these procedures of choice in case of chronic ruptures with a moderate or large defects.

COMPLICATIONS

- Complications include rerupture, variable loss of extension strength, and transient ulnar nerve palsy.
- Poor tissue quality of the tendon and extensile proximal retraction of the muscle are related to high risk of secondary rerupture, if a direct repair is performed without any augmentation.

REFERENCES

1. Anzel SH, Convey KW, Weiner AD, et al. Disruption of muscles and tendons: an analysis of 1014 cases. Surgery 1959;45:406–414.
2. Apple DV, O'Toole J, Annis C. Professional basketball injuries. Physician Sports Med 1982;10:81–86.
3. Aso K, Torisu T. Muscle belly tear of the triceps. Am J SportsMed 1984;12:485–487.
4. Athwal GS, McGill RJ, Rispoli DM. Isolated avulsion of the medial head of the triceps tendon: an anatomic study arthroscopic repair in 2 cases. Arthroscopy 2009;25(9):983–988.
5. Bach BR Jr, Warren RF, Wickiewicz TL. Triceps rupture. A case report and literature review. Am J Sports Med 1987;15(3):285–289.
6. Bava ED, Barber FA, Lund ER. Clinical outcome after suture anchor repair for complete traumatic rupture of the distal triceps tendon. Arthroscopy 2012;28(8):1058–1063.
7. Belentani C, Pastore D, Wangwinyuvirat M, et al. Triceps brachii tendon: anatomic-MR imaging study in cadavers with histologic correlation. Skeletal Radiol 2009;38:171–175.
8. Bennet BS. Triceps tendon rupture. J Bone Joint Surg Am 1962;44:741–744.
9. Bos CF, Nelissen RG, Bloem JL. Incomplete rupture of the tendon of the triceps brachii. A case report. Int Orthop 1994;18:273–275.
10. Celli A, Arash A, Adams RA, et al. Triceps insufficiency following total elbow arthroplasty. J Bone Joint Surg Am 2005;87(9):1957–1964.
11. Celli A, Morrey BF. Triceps insufficiency following total elbow arthroplasty. In: Morrey BF, Sanchez-Sotelo J, eds. The Elbow and Its Disorders, ed 4. Philadelphia: Saunders Elsevier, 2009:873–879.
12. Clayton ML, Thirupathi RG. Rupture of the triceps tendon with olecranon bursitis. A case report with a new method of repair. Clin Orthop Relat Res 1984;(184):183–185.
13. Gaines ST, Durbin RA, Marsalka DS. The use of magnetic resonance imaging in the diagnosis of triceps tendon ruptures. Contemp Orthop 1990;20:607–611.
14. Guerroudj M, de Longueville JC, Rooze M, et al. Biomechanical properties of triceps brachii tendon after in vitro simulation of different posterior surgical approaches. J Shoulder Elbow Surg 2007;16:849–853.
15. Guitton TG, Doornberg JN, Raaymakers EL, et al. Fractures of the capitellum and trochlea. J Bone Joint Surg Am 2009;91(2):390–397.
16. Herrick RT, Herrick S. Ruptured triceps in powerlifter presenting as cubital tunnel syndrome. A case report. Am J Sports Med 1987;15(5):514–516.
17. Holleb PD, Bach BR Jr. Triceps brachii injuries. Sports Med 1990; 10:273–276.
18. Huxley AF, Niedergerke R. Structural changes in muscle during contraction: interference microscopy of living muscle fibers. Nature 1954;173(4412):971–973.
19. Inhofe PD, Moneim MS. Late presentation of triceps rupture. A case report and review of the literature. Am J Orthop 1996;25(11):790–792.
20. Kaempffe FA, Lerner RM. Ultrasound diagnosis of triceps tendon rupture. A report of 2 cases. Clin Orthop Relat Res 1996;(332):138–142.
21. Kapandji IA. The Physiology of the Joints: Upper Limb. New York: Churchill Livingstone, 1982.
22. Keener JD, Chafik D, Kim HM, et al. Insertional anatomy of the triceps brachii tendon. J Shoulder Elbow Surg 2010;19:399–405.
23. Khiami F, Tavassoli S, De Ridder Bauer L, et al. Distal partial ruptures of triceps brachii tendon in an athlete. Orthop Traumatol Surg Res 2012;98:242–246.
24. Kibuule LK, Fehringer EV. Distal triceps tendon rupture and repair in an otherwise healthy pediatric patient: a case report and review of the literature. J Shoulder Elbow Surg 2007;16(3):e1–e3.
25. Kijowski R, Tuite M, Sanford M. Magnetic resonance imaging of the elbow. Part II: abnormalities of the ligament, tendons, and nerves. Skeletal Radiol 2005;34:1–18.
26. Kim JY, Lee JS, Kim MK. Fractures of the capitellum concomitant with avulsion fractures of the triceps tendon. J Hand Surg Am 2013;38(3):495–497.
27. Lambers K, Ring D. Elbow fracture-dislocation with triceps avulsion: report of 2 cases. J Hand Surg Am 2011;36(4):625–627.
28. Lawrence TM, Evans O, Shahane S. Distal triceps rupture: a case series, anatomical study of the triceps footprint and description of surgical technique. Paper presented at the 21st Annual Meeting of the British Elbow & Shoulder Society, March 25–26, 2010, Oxford, United Kingdom.
29. Lee ML. Rupture of the triceps tendon. Br Med Jr 1960;2:197.
30. Levy M, Fishel RE, Stern GM. Triceps tendon avulsion with or without fracture of the radial head—a rare injury. J Trauma 1978;18(9):677–679.
31. Levy M, Goldberg I, Meir I. Fracture of the head of the radius with a tear or avulsion of the triceps tendon. A new syndrome? J Bone Joint Surg Br 1982;64(1):70–72.
32. Madsen M, Marx RG, Millet PJ, et al. Surgical anatomy of the triceps brachii tendon: anatomical study and clinical correlation. Am J Sports Med 2006;34:1839–1843.
33. Mair SD, Isbell WM, Gill TJ, et al. Triceps tendon ruptures in professional football players. Am J Sports Med 2004;32(2):431–434.
34. McMaster PE. Tendon and muscle ruptures. Clinical and experimental studies on the causes and location of subcutaneous ruptures. J Bone Joint Surg Am 1933;15:705–722.
35. Morrey BF. Open treatment of acute and chronic triceps tendon ruptures. In: Yamaguchi K, ed. Advanced Reconstruction Elbow. Rosemont, IL: American Academy of Orthopaedic Surgeons, 2007:107–113.
36. Morrey BF. Rupture of the triceps tendon. In: Morrey BF, ed. The Elbow and Its Disorder, ed 3. Philadelphia: WB Saunders, 2000:479–548.
37. Morrey BF. Rupture of the triceps tendon. In: Morrey BF, Sanchez-Sotelo J, eds. The Elbow and Its Disorders. Philadelphia: Saunders Elsevier, 2009:536–546.
38. Nirschl RP. Prevention and treatment of elbow and shoulder injuries in the tennis player. Clin Sports Med 1988;7:289–308.
39. O'Driscoll SW. Intramuscular triceps rupture. Can J Surg 1992;35: 203–207.
40. Pina A, Garcia I, Sabater M. Traumatic avulsion of the triceps brachii. J Orthop Trauma 2002;16:273–276.
41. Ring D, Jupiter JB, Gulotta L. Articular fractures of the distal part of the humerus. J Bone Joint Surg Am 2003;85(2):232–238.
42. Ruchelsman DE, Tejwani NC, Kwon YW, et al. Coronal plane partial articular fractures of the distal humerus: current concepts in management. J Am Acad Orthop Surg. 2008;16(12):716–728.
43. Sanchez-Sotelo J, Morrey BF. Surgical techniques for reconstruction of chronic insufficiency of the triceps. Rotation flap using anconeus and tendo achillis allograft. J Bone Joint Surg Br 2002;84(8):1116–1120.
44. Sherman OH, Snyder SJ, Fox JM. Triceps tendon avulsion in a professional body builder. A case report. Am J Sports Med 1984;12(4): 328–329.
45. Sierra RJ, Weiss NG, Shrader MW, et al. Acute triceps ruptures: case report and retrospective chart review. J Shoulder Elbow Surg 2006;15:130–134.
46. Smart GW, Taunton JE, Clement DB. Achilles tendon disorders in runners—a review. Med Sci Sports Exerc 1980;12:231–243.
47. Sollender JL, Rayan GM, Barden GA. Triceps tendon rupture in weight lifters. J Shoulder Elbow Surg 1998;7(2):151–153.
48. Strauch RJ. Biceps and triceps injuries of the elbow. Orthop Clin North Am 1999;30:95–107.
49. Tatebe M, Horii E, Nakamura R. Chronically ruptured triceps tendon with avulsion of the medial collateral ligament: a report of 2 cases. J Shoulder Elbow Surg 2007;16:e5–e7.
50. Van Riet RP, Morrey BF, Ho E, et al. Surgical treatment of distal triceps ruptures. J Bone Joint Surg Am 2003;85-A(10):1961–1967.
51. Viegas SF. Avulsion of the triceps tendon. Orthop Rev 1990;19(6): 533–536.
52. Wagner JR, Cooney WP. Rupture of the triceps muscle at the musculotendinous junction: a case report. J Hand Surg Am 1997;22:341–343.
53. Waugh RL, Hathcock TA, Elliot JL. Ruptures of muscles and tendons with particular reference to rupture or elongation of long tendon, of biceps brachii with report of 50 cases. Surgery 1949;25:370–392.
54. Weistroffer JK, Mills WJ, Shin AY. Recurrent rupture of the triceps tendon repaired with hamstring tendon autograft augmentation: a case report and repair technique. Shoulder Elbow Surg 2003;12:193–196.
55. Wenzke DR. MR imaging of the elbow in the injured athlete. Radiol Clin North Am 2013;51:195–213.
56. Yeh PC, Dodds SD, Smart LR, et al. Distal triceps rupture. J Am Acad Orthop Surg 2010;18(1):31–40.
57. Yoon MY, Koris MJ, Ortiz JA, et al. Triceps avulsion, radial head fracture, and medial collateral ligament rupture about the elbow: a report of 4 cases. J Shoulder Elbow Surg 2012;21:12–17.

CHAPTER 77

Surgical Treatment for Extensor Carpi Ulnaris Subluxation

David H. MacDonald and Thomas R. Hunt III

DEFINITION

- Extensor carpi ulnaris (ECU) subluxation occurs when the separate subsheath of the sixth dorsal compartment is torn or attenuated.
- Incompetence of the ECU subsheath permits subluxation or dislocation of the ECU tendon out of the ulnar groove of the ulna, often with a painful click noted on resisted supination, ulnar deviation, and mild palmar flexion.

ANATOMY

- The dorsal extensor retinaculum of the wrist is composed of two primary layers (**FIG 1**).
  - The supratendinous retinaculum originates 2 to 3 cm proximal to the radiocarpal joint and ends distinctly at the carpometacarpal joints. The most radial attachment on the distal radius forms the radial septum for the first extensor compartment. The supratendinous retinaculum courses medially, surrounding the ulna.[11]
    - The supratendinous retinaculum participates as a block to tendon subluxation for the first through fifth extensor compartments but does not function to prevent subluxation of the ECU.
  - The infratendinous retinaculum runs from the radiocarpal to the carpometacarpal joints. It is found deep to the fourth and fifth extensor compartments on the radius. The ECU lies in its own separate fibro-osseous subsheath, which represents a duplication of the infratendinous retinaculum.
    - The ECU sheath is separated from the supratendinous retinaculum by loose areolar tissue.
- The fibro-osseous subsheath of the sixth dorsal compartment overlies 1.5 to 2.0 cm of the distal ulna and arcs from the radial to ulnar wall of the ECU osseous groove. It ensheathes the ECU and maintains the tendon tightly in the groove (**FIG 2**).
  - The ECU subsheath contributes to the dorsal portion of the triangular fibrocartilage complex (TFCC).

PATHOGENESIS

- The mechanism of a traumatic injury most commonly involves active ECU contraction combined with forced supination, palmar flexion, and ulnar deviation.
  - Injuries resulting from trauma can range from simple attenuation to complete rupture of the ECU fibro-osseous sheath.
- Traumatic ECU subluxation is commonly reported in association with racket sports, baseball, and golf.

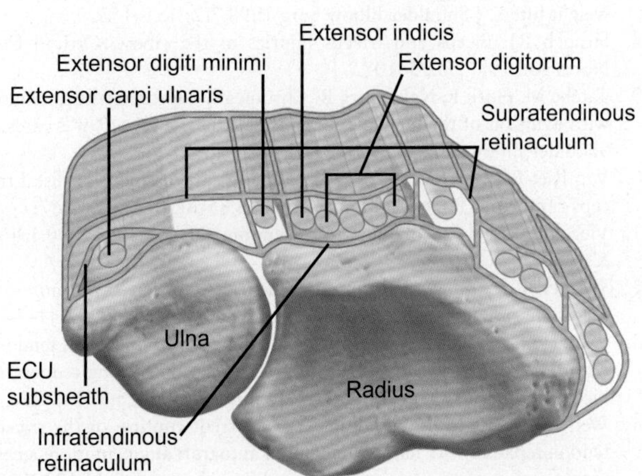

FIG 1 • Axial representation of dorsal extensor compartments. The ECU tendon has a separate compartment along the dorsum of the ulna. The supratendinous retinaculum courses ulnarward over the sixth compartment and does not communicate with the separate ECU fibro-osseous subsheath in any significant way.

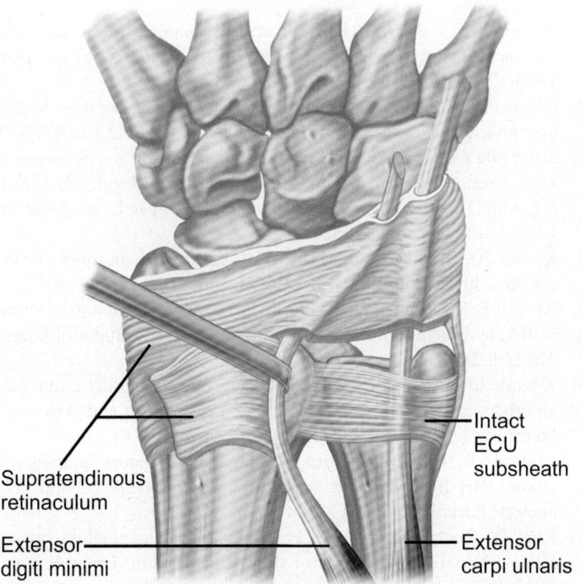

FIG 2 • Dorsal anatomic view of the sixth dorsal component. This representation shows the relation between the deep ECU subsheath and the superficial supratendinous extensor retinaculum.

NATURAL HISTORY

- Chronic subluxation of the ECU tendon over the ulnar prominence of the groove in the distal ulna can lead to painful snapping of the tendon with supination and pronation. This can progress to ECU tendinopathy and partial tendon tears.
- An injury to the ECU sheath resulting in volar dislocation of the ECU tendon can result in distal radioulnar joint (DRUJ) instability. This joint laxity may cause pain and dysfunction, eventually leading to degenerative changes.
- Dislocation of the ECU tendon removes a dynamic stabilizer of the DRUJ.
  - The subsheath of the sixth extensor compartment represents a component of the dorsal peripheral TFCC. Disruption can result in static instability of the DRUJ.
- Some patients may experience relatively minor ECU subluxation and related symptoms that do not progress and often improve with minimal intervention.

PATIENT HISTORY AND PHYSICAL FINDINGS

- Patients may present following an acute injury or, more commonly, in the subacute phase, complaining of persistent ulnar wrist pain aggravated by activities requiring pronation and supination. They may relate the sensation of a "click."
- A complete physical examination of the patient's ulnar-sided wrist complaints should be conducted to elucidate associated pathology and rule out confounding conditions in the differential diagnosis.
  - Palpation and inspection of sixth dorsal compartment and ECU tendon helps to localize the area of discomfort and focus the physical examination. Most patients with acute sheath ruptures and tendinopathies will be tender to palpation at the level of the distal ulna and groove. Tenderness at the joint line may indicate an associated TFCC tear.
  - In range-of-motion testing, an inflamed ECU tendon usually will be most painful with full passive radial wrist flexion, although motion most often is full except in the acute setting.
  - If the tendon dislocates with passive supination, palmar flexion, and ulnar deviation, the ECU is grossly unstable. If the addition of ECU contraction is required for frank dislocation, some inherent stability remains. Pain with subluxation is the critical finding when contemplating surgical treatment.
  - In resisted finger abduction, pain over the wrist and ECU tendon signifies an inflammatory ECU condition, possibly due to subluxation or overuse.

IMAGING AND OTHER DIAGNOSTIC STUDIES

- Routine anteroposterior (AP), lateral, and oblique radiographs in neutral rotation are important.
- Pronated grip views and other specialized plain radiographs of the wrist can provide information on other pathologies that contribute to ulnar-sided wrist pain (see Differential Diagnosis).
- Magnetic resonance imaging (MRI) is the most sensitive and specific imaging modality to detect ECU subluxation (**FIG 3A**).
  - The sensitivity increases in studies with both wrists positioned in pronation, neutral, and supination. This allows side-by-side comparison with the asymptomatic wrist and adequately shows the position of the ECU relative to the ulnar osseous groove in all three positions.
    - The actual subsheath tear may or may not be visualized.
    - Often, inflammation and partial interstitial tendon disruption are visualized.
- An MRI arthrogram of the wrist may depict a subsheath tear and, therefore, an injury to the peripheral TFCC.
  - Contrast may extravasate into the sixth extensor compartment (**FIG 3B**).
  - The study will also provide additional information concerning the remainder of the TFCC and the integrity of the intercarpal ligaments.
- Ultrasound allows dynamic assessment of ECU stability and can be useful in quantifying the degree of ECU tendon subluxation.[7,9]

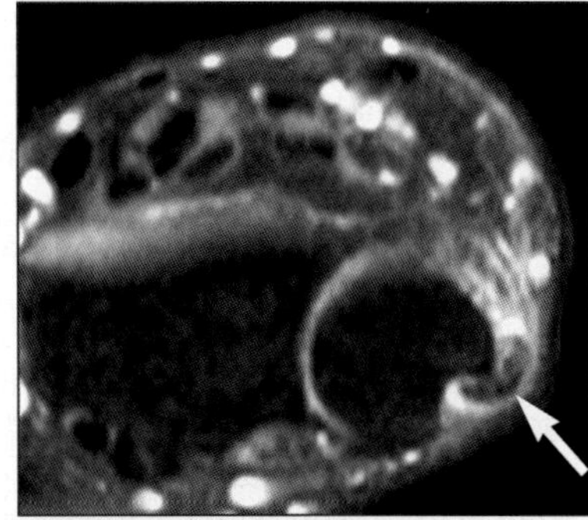

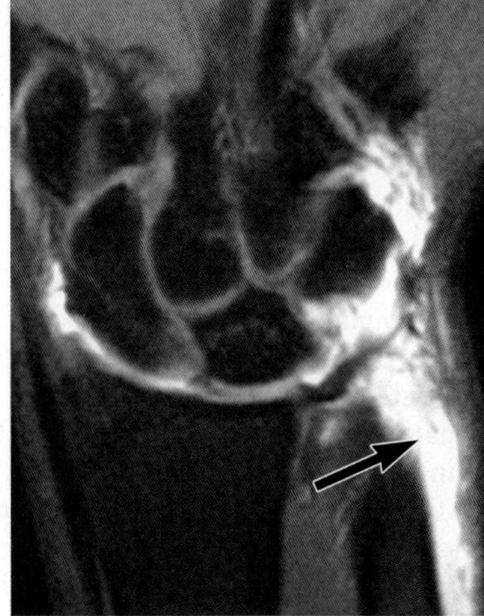

FIG 3 • **A.** This MRI scan shows a "perched" ECU tendon, out of the dorsal ulnar groove. Notice the increased signal in the tendon substance. **B.** The coronal MRI arthrogram projection illustrates leakage of the opaque dye into the ECU fibro-osseous subsheath.

DIFFERENTIAL DIAGNOSIS

- ECU tenosynovitis
  - Fullness and pain with palpation of the sixth dorsal compartment
  - The patient often can reproduce a painful snap or click with supination and ulnar deviation, even in the absence of ECU subluxation.
- TFCC injury
  - Tenderness with direct palpation of the TFCC
  - Pain with axial loading and rotation of the ulnar-deviated wrist (TFCC compression test)

- Instability of the DRUJ with manual manipulation when compared to the contralateral wrist
- Lunotriquetral ligament injury
  - Tenderness to palpation over the dorsal lunotriquetral articulation
  - The patient may also describe pain and crepitance with ulnar deviation of the wrist.
  - Provocative maneuvers for lunotriquetral ligament injuries (ie, ballottement test, ulnar snuff box test) have sufficient sensitivity but poor specificity.
- Ulnocarpal impaction syndrome
  - More common in patients with ulnar positive variance
  - Usually a dynamic phenomenon occurring during forceful activity or pronated gripping
  - The physical examination findings will be similar to those of TFCC injury, with pain on forced ulnar deviation of the wrist (TFCC stress test) that increases with rotation through the loaded ulnocarpal articulation.
  - Tenderness will be elicited along the ulnar border of the triquetrum and the distal ulna.
- Ulnar styloid nonunion
  - Uncommon; occurs more commonly with widely displaced styloid fractures at the time of injury
  - The intimate relationship with the ulnar TFCC attachment means that symptomatic nonunion can be associated with TFCC dysfunction and DRUJ instability.
- DRUJ arthrosis
  - Patients present with complaints of pain, swelling, and stiffness. The pain is exacerbated by forearm rotation, particularly when performed with manual compression of the DRUJ.

NONOPERATIVE MANAGEMENT

- In the acute setting (<3 weeks since injury), immobilize the patient in an above-elbow cast. The wrist should be in neutral to slight pronation, neutral to slight radial deviation, and neutral to slight extension.
  - The cast is removed about 4 to 5 weeks later, and therapy is initiated. A sugar-tong splint is fabricated with the forearm in slight pronation, and a progressive active and active-assisted ROM protocol is initiated.
  - Three weeks later, a forearm-based splint is provided and the patient slowly progresses back to activities.
  - Unprotected, full activity is allowed 3 to 4 months after the initiation of treatment.
- The literature does not agree on the efficacy of nonoperative treatment. Rowland[8] produced a compelling case report of surgical treatment in acute, traumatic ECU subluxation.
  - In this case, the intraoperative findings showed the edges of the ruptured subsheath to be separated by a minimum of 7 mm, regardless of the position of the wrist.
  - These findings suggest that nonoperative treatment could routinely lead to clinical ECU subluxation and persistent symptoms.

SURGICAL MANAGEMENT

- Surgical reconstruction of the ECU subsheath should be considered in patients with clinically significant symptoms related to painful subluxation of the ECU tendon, especially if the injury is more than 3 weeks old. Treatment must be individualized based on the needs and expectations of the patient.
- The guiding principles for surgical repair depend on the essential osteofibrous sheath lesion present at the time of surgery.
- Inoue and Tamura[5,6] classified three distinct patterns of injury (Table 1).
  - Treatment of types A and B lesions
    - In the acute setting, suture repair is sometimes possible and may be augmented using suture anchors.
    - When the fibro-osseous sheath is ruptured and deemed irreparable, reconstruction is accomplished using a retinacular sling or free retinacular graft (see Techniques box).
    - Because of its simplicity and the ability to place a gliding surface between the bone and tendon, the sling is preferred.
  - Treatment of type C lesions
    - Separation of the fibro-osseous sheath from bone necessitates repositioning of the tissue at the ulnar margin of the groove (see False Pouch Reconstruction and Imbrication for Type C Lesions).
    - Stretching and attenuation of the sheath without separation from bone may be effectively treated by suture imbrication, depending on the quality of the tissue.
- Although this chapter describes reconstruction of traumatic ECU subluxation, reconstruction also may be considered in the patient with inflammatory arthropathy and secondary volar dislocation of the ECU tendon. The opportunity to stabilize the ulnar wrist and DRUJ while forestalling progression of deformity may lead the patient and surgeon toward surgical care even in the absence of pain.

Preoperative Planning

- All preoperative information obtained from the history, the physical examination, and imaging studies should be thoroughly reviewed and synthesized into the operative plan. For example, a patient with joint line tenderness and an MRI indicating a TFCC injury might benefit from wrist arthroscopy before any open procedure is done.
  - Dorsal synovitis or tenosynovitis requiring débridement
  - The existence of a shallow ulnar osseous groove and the need to deepen the groove surgically for added stability
  - The paucity of soft tissue for reconstruction and the need for another graft choice for subsheath reconstruction. Graft options include the palmaris and flexor carpi ulnaris tendons.

Positioning

- The patient is positioned supine on the operating table with the injured extremity extended on an arm board in the usual manner.
- Initially, the procedure is performed with the arm extended and pronated. If the wrist must be placed in a neutral or supinated position, the elbow is flexed.

Approach

- A precise incision is chosen to allow for the predetermined method of reconstruction.
- Make a Brunner zigzag incision over the sixth extensor compartment.
  - The incision begins 1 to 2 cm distal to the ulnocarpal joint and is carried proximally 5 cm.

Table 1 Classification of Extensor Carpi Ulnaris Subsheath Lesion with Recommended Surgical Treatment

Lesion Type	Illustration	Description of Pathology	Recommended Surgical Treatment
A		The fibro-osseous sheath is disrupted from the ulnar wall. The tendon may lie beneath the disrupted sheath.	If injury is fairly acute and if adequate tissue is present, a direct repair may be attempted. If nonreconstructible, a sheath reconstruction with retinacular free graft or retinacular sling is employed.
B		The fibro-osseous sheath is disrupted from the radial wall. The tendon may rest on top of the sheath and prevent healing.	A sheath reconstruction with retinacular free graft or retinacular sling is suggested.
C		The fibro-osseous sheath is stripped from the periosteum but remains in continuity, forming a false pouch.	Imbrication of false pouch is reinforced with suture anchors or drill holes.

- Identify and protect the dorsal cutaneous branch of the ulnar nerve in the distal incision.
- Incise the extensor retinaculum on its far ulnar border and carefully separate it from the underlying sixth extensor compartment fibro-osseous sheath (see **FIG 2**).
  - Conservation of and planned incision in the extensor retinaculum is critical to allow for its use as a sling to stabilize the ECU tendon (see Retinacular Sling Reconstruction for Types A and B Lesions)
- Following exposure, inspect the separate fibro-osseous sheath of the ECU and note the position of the tendon through pronosupination.
- Perform a tenosynovectomy as indicated.

Retinacular Sling Reconstruction for Types A and B Lesions

- Retinacular sling reconstruction[2] is performed when the sheath is ruptured and not repairable.
- At the level of the ulnar groove, create a rectangular flap of tissue, 2 to 3 cm wide, based on the septum separating the fifth and sixth extensor compartments (**TECH FIG 1A**).
- Pass this radially based sling in an ulnar direction, volar to the ECU tendon, then fold it back radially over the tendon and secure it to the ulnar portion of the fifth compartment (**TECH FIG 1B**).
  - This places the superficial surface of the retinaculum in contact with the ECU tendon.
- Avoid constricting the ECU tendon by ensuring that the sling is wide and loose, which still prevents subluxation of the tendon.
- The portion of the extensor retinaculum not used for the sling is repaired anatomically.

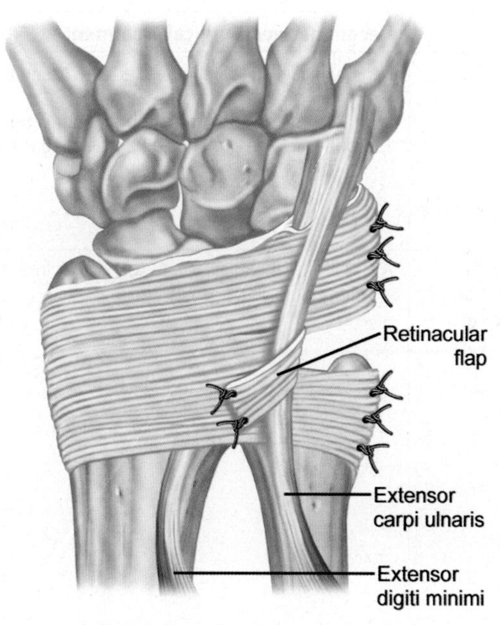

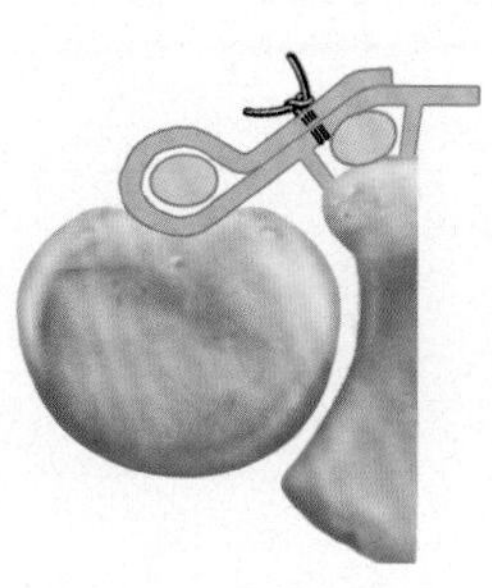

TECH FIG 1 • Retinacular sling reconstruction of types A and B lesions. **A.** Creation of a radially based extensor retinaculum sling. **B.** The retinacular flap is brought deep to the ECU tendon, then looped back over the tendon and sewn to the extensor retinaculum overlying the ulnar compartment. This places the superficial surface of the retinaculum in contact with the ECU tendon when the reconstruction is completed.

Alternate Retinacular Sling Reconstruction for Types A and B Lesions

- An alternate retinacular sling reconstruction[10] requires the development of an ulnarly based, rectangular flap, 2 to 3 cm wide, of supratendinous retinacular tissue, beginning at Lister tubercle or over the second extensor compartment if more length is required (**TECH FIG 2A**).
  - The flap is based on the ulnar septum of the fifth extensor compartment.
- Pass the tissue ulnarly, deep to the ECU tendon, then back over the tendon to create the sling.
  - This places the deep surface of the retinaculum in contact with the ECU tendon.
- Insert suture anchors on the radial and ulnar margins of the ulnar groove and use this suture to stabilize the flap (**TECH FIG 2B**).
  - Avoid constricting the ECU tendon, as discussed previously.

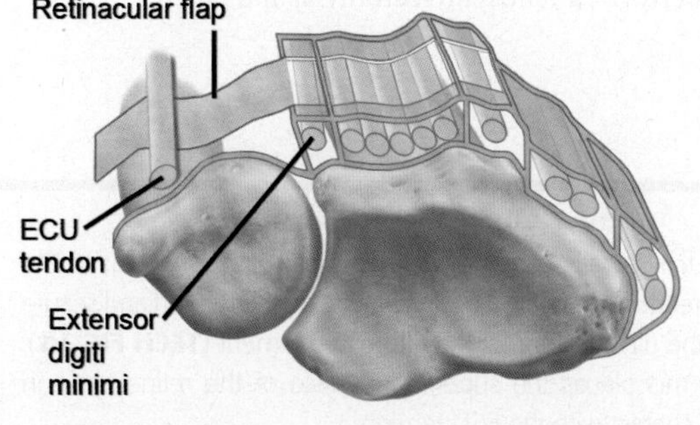

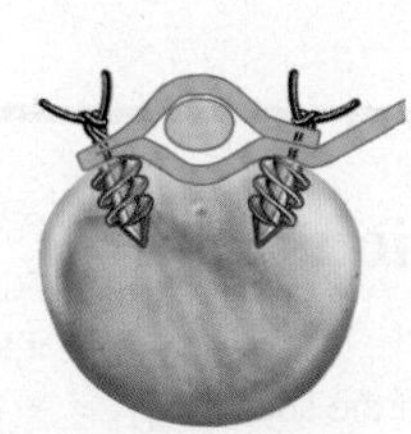

TECH FIG 2 • Alternate retinacular sling reconstruction of types A and B lesions. **A.** The ulnarly based extensor retinaculum flap is harvested, then swung ulnarward, deep to the ECU tendon. **B.** The tissue is then brought back over the tendon and secured to itself and the ulna, using bone anchors. The remaining retinaculum is repaired in an anatomic fashion. This places the deep surface of the retinacular flap in contact with the ECU tendon when the reconstruction is complete.

Retinacular Graft Augmentation for Types A and B Lesions

- Retinacular graft augmentation[4] is performed when the sheath is ruptured and not repairable.
- Harvest a 2- × 2-cm square graft from the distal supratendinous retinaculum (**TECH FIG 3A**).
- Secure this graft to the periosteum on the ulnar and radial borders of the ulnar osseous groove to maintain the ECU tendon within the groove.
- Roughen the bone surface to encourage attachment, and place suture anchors at the anatomic attachment sites along the radial and ulnar borders of the ulnar osseous groove.
- Secure the harvested graft to the margins of the ulnar groove, allowing bony contact between the graft and the ulna (**TECH FIG 3B**).
  - Place the deep surface of the graft against the tendon.
  - This provides secure fixation and does not rely on questionable soft tissue for early fixation.

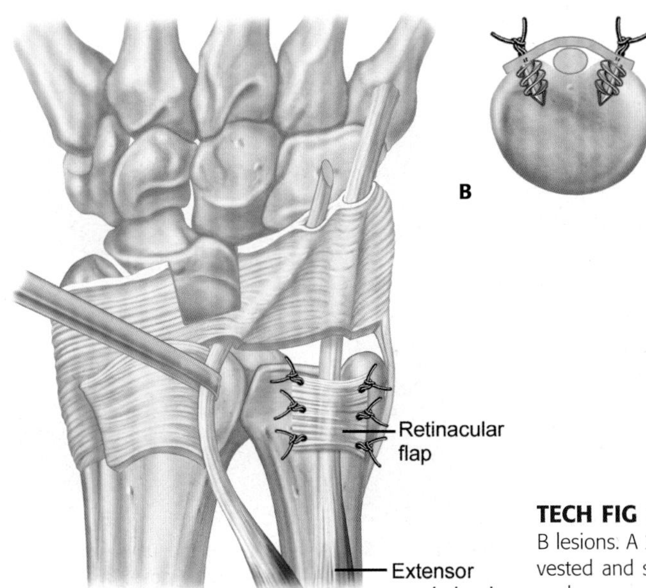

TECH FIG 3 • Free retinacular flap reconstruction of types A and B lesions. A 2- × 2-cm portion of distal extensor retinaculum is harvested and secured to the ulnar osseous groove using small bone anchors.

False Pouch Reconstruction and Imbrication for Type C Lesions

- False pouch reconstruction and imbrication[6] is done when the fibro-osseous sheath of the ECU tendon is attenuated and stretched but intact. The tendon subluxates out of the ulnar groove during forearm rotation (**TECH FIG 4A,B**).
- Incise the sheath on its ulnar margin (**TECH FIG 4C**)
- Alternately, one can attempt subperiosteal dissection of entire sheath off the ulna.[7]
- If the sheath has separated from the deep periosteum, roughen the medial surface of the ulna deep to the false pouch (**TECH FIG 4D**).
- Insert suture anchors at the site of the true ulnar attachment of the sheath (**TECH FIG 4E**).
- Use suture from the bone anchors to capture and repair the fibro-osseous sheath, securing it to the prepared bone bed and forming a barrier to ECU subluxation (**TECH FIG 4F**).
  - The effect is to imbricate the attenuated sheath and obliterate the false pouch.
- Place additional permanent sutures to complete the repair (**TECH FIG 4G**).

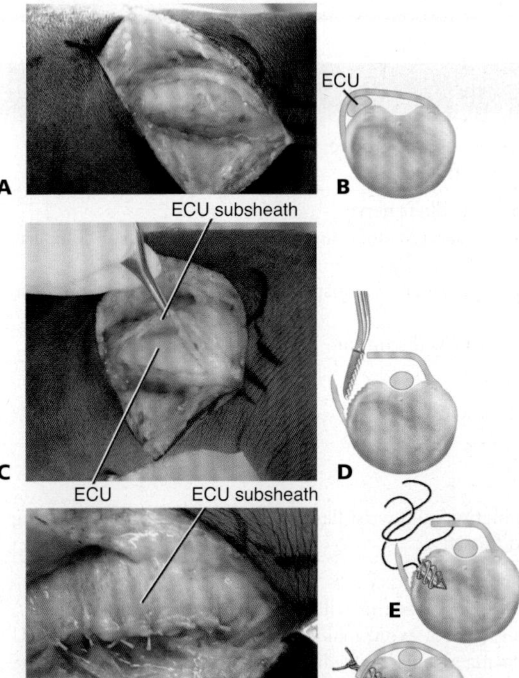

TECH FIG 4 • Type C lesion. **A.** The supratendinous retinaculum has been incised, revealing the ECU subsheath. The subsheath is inflamed, stretched, and attenuated, allowing tendon subluxation. **B.** Diagrammatic representation of a type C lesion in which the sheath has pulled away from the bone. **C.** An incision is made in the attenuated subsheath, allowing visualization of the tendon. Despite MRI findings that indicate potential intrasubstance injury (see **FIG 3A**), the tendon itself appears normal. **D.** The bone underlying the ulnar subsheath flap is roughened with a rasp. **E,F.** Mini bone anchors are used to secure the tissue to the ulnar border of the groove and imbricate the subsheath. **G.** Additional permanent sutures complete the repair.

TECHNIQUES

Deepening of the Ulnar Osseous Groove

- Deepening of the ulnar osseous groove is an optional technique that may be used to address all lesion types.
- This technique is added to the reconstruction when preoperative studies or intraoperative findings suggest that a shallow ulnar osseous groove contributes significantly to subluxation of the ECU tendon (**TECH FIG 5A**).
- Retract the ECU tendon out of its groove.
- Carefully elevate the periosteum and a thin layer of bone along the ulnar 2 to 3 cm of the ulnar osseous groove using a sharp, curved osteotome (**TECH FIG 5B**).
  - The radial border is used as a hinge to expose the underlying cancellous bone.
  - Precise elevation of the osteoperiosteal flap ensures adequate coverage of the raw bony surfaces.
- Remove cancellous bone using a small curette or burr (**TECH FIG 5C**), no deeper than 2 to 3 mm.
- The cortical bone flap is then returned to its position and tamped down using a small bone tamp (**TECH FIG 5D**). The periosteum is repaired (**TECH FIG 5E**).
- Treat any remaining exposed bony surface with bone wax.

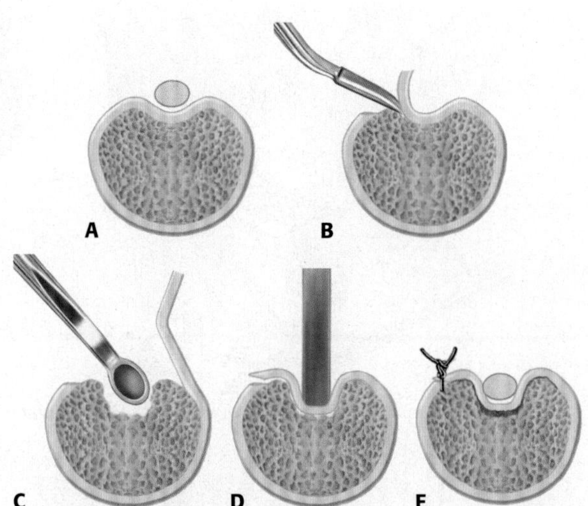

TECH FIG 5 • Deepening of the ulnar osseous groove. **A.** ECU tendon in a shallow ulnar groove. **B.** A sharp curved osteotome is used to create an osteoperiosteal "trapdoor" with a hinge of periosteum radially. **C.** A curette is used to remove cancellous bone. **D.** A bone tamp is used to close the trapdoor gently and deepen the osseous groove. **E.** The periosteum is then secured using 4-0 suture if feasible.

Closure and Splinting

- Perform passive motion testing to ensure that the ECU tendon is stable in its groove following reconstruction or repair.
- Close the extensor retinaculum in a side-to-side fashion using absorbable suture.
- Deflate the tourniquet and obtain hemostasis.
- Following routine skin closure and dressing placement, place a sugar-tong splint with the forearm mildly pronated and the wrist in mild extension and radial deviation.

PEARLS AND PITFALLS

Indications	▪ Symptomatic subluxation of the ECU tendon at the ulnar osseous groove ▪ Acute injuries often are effectively treated with immobilization.
Approach	▪ Protect against injury to the dorsal cutaneous branch of the ulnar nerve ▪ Incise the supratendinous retinaculum along its ulnar border, remembering that the sixth extensor compartment is a separate, deeper structure. ▪ Carefully inspect the ECU subsheath for rupture or attenuation, and adjust the reconstruction based on those findings. ▪ Evaluate the ECU subsheath looking for a concomitant TFCC disruption.
Inspecting the ulnar osseous groove	▪ Consider deepening the ulnar groove to augment stability.
Subsheath repair versus reconstruction	▪ Repair the subsheath if the tissues appear substantial. ▪ Reconstruct the sheath if in doubt. ▪ Perform passive motion testing in the extremes of supination mild wrist flexion and ulnar deviation following the procedure to ensure that the problem has been addressed.
Pitfalls	▪ Avoid injury to the dorsal cutaneous branch of the ulnar nerve. ▪ Do not repair the supratendinous retinaculum to the ulna because this will limit forearm rotation. ▪ If creation of an ulnar extensor retinaculum sling is required, avoid making it overly tight, inhibiting ECU tendon gliding. This can be easily accomplished by placing a pediatric feeding tube beside the ECU during the sling construction.
Return to activity	▪ Full activity is not considered until 3 to 4 months following surgery.

POSTOPERATIVE CARE

- The sutures are removed 2 weeks after surgery, and an above-elbow cast is applied with the forearm and wrist positioned in the manner described.
- This cast is removed 2 weeks later, and therapy is initiated with use of a fabricated sugar-tong splint and progressive range of motion as described in Nonoperative Management.

OUTCOMES

- No large conclusive studies on which to base outcomes have yet been published.
- A few case reports and smaller series have reported good results following surgical treatment for ECU subluxation.[1–4,6–8,10] Our experience mirrors these reports.

COMPLICATIONS

- The uncommon nature of ECU subluxation, the uniformly acceptable surgical outcomes, and the lack of large surgical case series result in a sparse list of postoperative complications. Trends with which to define "routine" postsurgical complications are simply not present.
- Complications that have been reported in the literature include the following:
  - Complex regional pain syndrome[1]
  - Decreased wrist motion
  - Decreased grip strength

REFERENCES

1. Allende C, Le Viet D. Extensor carpi ulnaris problems at the wrist—classification, surgical treatment and results. J Hand Surg Br 2005;30(3):265–272.
2. Burkhart SS, Wood MB, Linscheid RL. Posttraumatic recurrent subluxation of the extensor carpi ulnaris tendon. J Hand Surg Am 1982;7(1):1–3.
3. Chun S, Palmer AK. Chronic ulnar wrist pain secondary to partial rupture of the extensor carpi ulnaris tendon. J Hand Surg Am 1987;12:1032–1035.
4. Eckhardt WA, Palmer AK. Recurrent dislocation of extensor carpi ulnaris tendon. J Hand Surg Am 1981;6:629–631.
5. Inoue G, Tamura Y. Recurrent dislocation of the extensor carpi ulnaris tendon. Br J Sports Med 1998;32:172–177.
6. Inoue G, Tamura Y. Surgical treatment for recurrent dislocation of the extensor carpi ulnaris tendon. J Hand Surg Br 2001;26:556–559.
7. MacLennan AJ, Nemechek NM, Waitayawinyu T, et al. Diagnosis and anatomic reconstruction of extensor carpi ulnaris subluxation. J Hand Surg Am 2008;33(1):59–64.
8. Rowland SA. Acute traumatic subluxation of the extensor carpi ulnaris tendon at the wrist. J Hand Surg Am 1986;11:809–811.
9. Pratt R, Hoy GA, Bass Franzcr C. Extensor carpi ulnaris subluxation or dislocation? Ultrasound measurement of tendon excursion and normal values. Hand Surg 2004;9:137–143.
10. Spinner M, Kaplan E. Extensor carpi ulnaris. Its relationship to the stability of the distal radio-ulnar joint. Clin Orthop Relat Res 1970;68:124–129.
11. Taleisnik J, Gelberman RH, Miller BW, et al. The extensor retinaculum of the wrist. J Hand Surg Am 1984;9:495–501.

Repair of Acute Digital Flexor Tendon Disruptions

Christopher H. Allan and Matthew Iorio

DEFINITION

- Flexor tendon injuries can occur in any of the five described zones within the finger, hand, wrist, or forearm. All such injuries require surgical repair to restore active finger flexion.
- The most challenging injuries to manage are those in zone II, where two flexor tendons occupy a narrow fibro-osseous sheath. Successful repair requires meticulous technique and a careful postoperative therapy regimen balancing the risks of adhesion formation versus rupture.

ANATOMY

- The flexor tendons form two layers in the forearm (zone V; **FIG 1A**), with the thumb's flexor pollicis longus (FPL) and the fingers' flexor digitorum profundus (FDP) muscles deep to the flexor digitorum superficialis (FDS) muscle. At the wrist, the FPL and FDP tendons remain deep, with the index and small FDS tendons above, and the middle and ring FDS tendons most superficial.
- The median nerve runs down the forearm beneath the fascia of the FDS on its undersurface, becoming superficial within the carpal tunnel just proximal to the volar wrist crease (zone IV), with the flexor tendons closely packed together.
- Exiting the carpal tunnel, the flexor tendons cross the palm (zone III) toward the individual digits. Here, the lumbrical muscles take origin from the radial side of the finger FDP tendons and continue deep to the deep transverse intermetacarpal ligaments.
- The two tendons of each nonthumb digit (the thumb has just the FPL) enter the fibro-osseous sheath (zone II) at the level of the metacarpophalangeal (MP) joint. The two FDS slips then rotate laterally and dorsally, with the medial FDS slips forming the decussation termed the *chiasm of Camper*, through which the FDP passes from deep to superficial (**FIG 1B**).
- The two lateral slips of the FDS then insert along the proximal aspect of the volar surface of the base of the middle phalanx, and the FDP proceeds distally to insert along the volar surface of the base of the distal phalanx.
- The flexor sheath extends from the level of the MP joint to the distal interphalangeal (DIP) joint. Multiple condensations of discrete fibers are found along its course and are named as either *annular* or *cruciate pulleys*, reflecting the orientation of the fibers forming the pulley (**FIG 1C**).
- The thicker annular (A1 through A5, from proximal to distal) pulleys hold the tendons close to bone, whereas the more slender cruciate (C1 through C3) pulleys collapse with digit flexion, allowing the sheath to shorten without buckling. Zone II is that part of the sheath where both FDS and FDP tendons are present and zone I is distal to the FDS insertion.
- Tendon nutrition within the sheath is provided indirectly via synovial fluid and directly via vascular inflow through mesenteric folds called *vincula*, with one vinculum longus

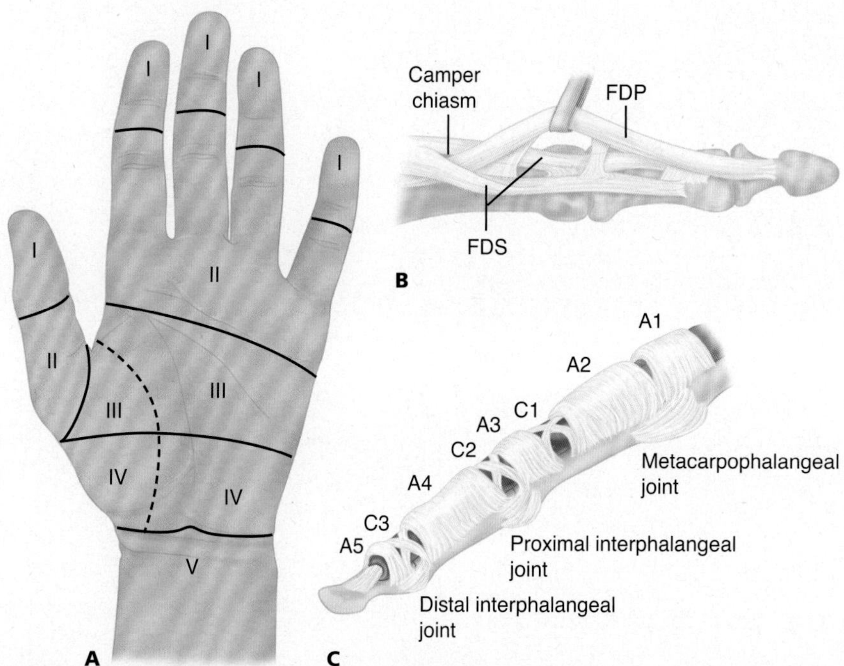

FIG 1 • **A.** Flexor tendon zones (*I* to *V*). **B.** Flexor tendon anatomy in zone II. **C.** Flexor sheath pulley anatomy and distribution in zones I and II.

and one vinculum brevis to each flexor tendon. Following lacerating injury, these vincula help to further limit the proximal retraction of the flexor tendons in the fingers. This mechanism is absent in the thumb, as the FPL lacks a defined vincula, and therefore, proximal counter incisions are frequently required to retrieve the tendon following complete transection.

PATHOGENESIS

- Most acute flexor tendon injuries are the result of open trauma, with sharp transection of the tendon. In such cases, other structures are often injured as well. In particular, examination should include assessment of sensibility and capillary refill to identify injury to the digital nerves and vessels that would affect preoperative planning.
- A less common injury mechanism is closed avulsion of the FDP from its distal attachment to bone. The term *jersey finger* is sometimes used for this injury, as it is often the result of an athlete's fingers forcibly flexing to grab an opponent's jersey, followed by sudden and forceful extension of the DIP joint against resistance as the opponent pulls away. This avulsion injury is addressed elsewhere.

NATURAL HISTORY

- Flexor tendon injuries require surgical repair to restore active digit flexion. Early repair is crucial, with several studies pointing to better results when repairs are performed within the first 7 days after injury.[3,7]
- Outcomes aside, as a practical matter, it is easiest to repair the tendon before proximal tendon retraction occurs, requiring additional incisions. Late repair with tendon retraction and muscle shortening can also result in tension at the repair site, leading to gapping of the repair (which increases the failure rate) or influencing the surgeon to splint the wrist or digits in excessive flexion, leading to joint contractures.

PATIENT HISTORY AND PHYSICAL FINDINGS

- Methods for examining the hand or upper extremity with an acute flexor tendon injury
  - Isolate FDP: While maintaining the injured digit's proximal interphalangeal joint extended, the examiner asks the patient to actively flex the DIP joint (**FIG 2A**).
  - Isolate FDS: While maintaining all uninjured digits in full extension, the examiner asks the patient to actively flex the injured digit's proximal interphalangeal joint (**FIG 2B**).
- Uncooperative or unresponsive patient
  - Tenodesis effect: The examiner extends the wrist; flexion is observed at the interphalangeal joints if the flexor tendons are intact.
  - Forearm compression: Pressure applied to flexor tendon muscle bellies results in interphalangeal joint flexion if flexor tendons are intact.
  - The examiner inspects for normal flexion cascade (**FIG 2C**).
- Examination of the digit to rule out associated digital nerve injury is required.

PHYSICAL FINDINGS

- Laceration
- Affected digit held in unopposed extension
- Inability to actively flex interphalangeal joints (if both tendons are cut), isolated DIP joint (if FDP only is cut), or isolated proximal interphalangeal joint (if FDS only is cut)

IMAGING AND OTHER DIAGNOSTIC STUDIES

- The sudden loss of active flexion after a laceration overlying the flexor sheath almost always represents a tendon injury. Radiographs should be obtained to rule out associated fractures that would require treatment at the time of tendon repair. Lacerations due to glass, metal fragments, and so forth should be imaged to localize any residual foreign bodies for removal.
- In the setting of a closed injury with the sudden loss of active flexion, one must consider the possibility of a tendon avulsion from its insertion. Radiographs may demonstrate an avulsed fleck of bone. In the more common cases of an FDP avulsion, this bone fragment may remain in the region of the distal phalanx or may be pulled proximally into the flexor sheath. If no bony fragment is seen on a plain radiograph and the diagnosis is still in doubt, ultrasound may help.

DIFFERENTIAL DIAGNOSIS

- Pain after injury may cause a patient (especially a child) to hold a digit or hand immobile, mimicking tendon injury.

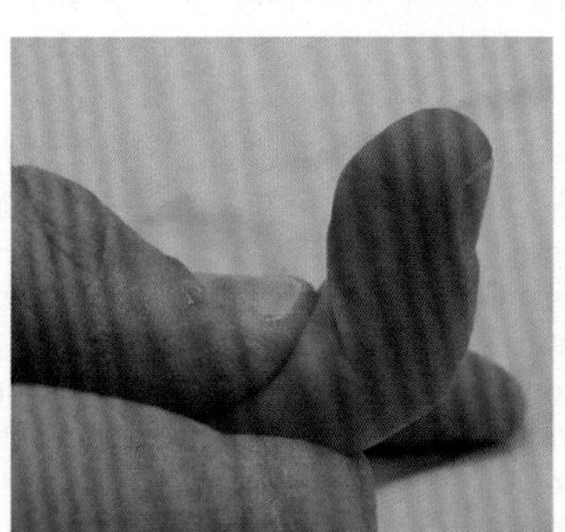
A

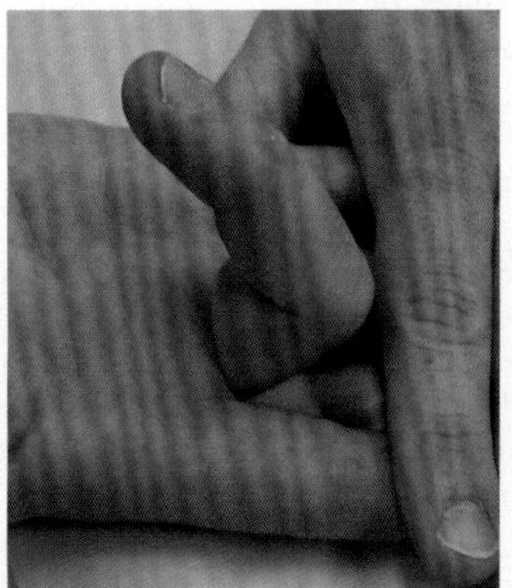
B

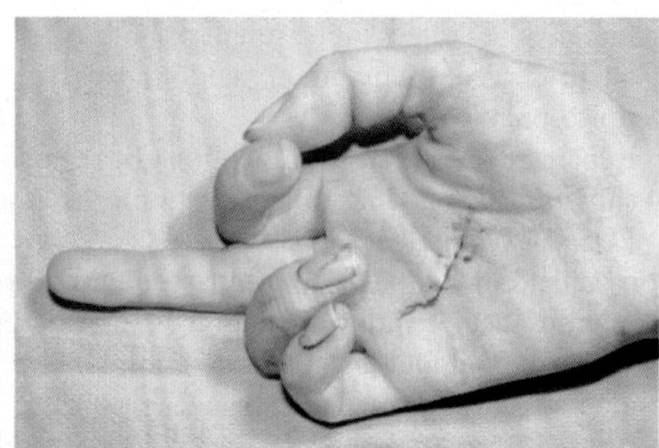
C

FIG 2 • **A.** Isolation of DIP flexion to test FDP. **B.** Isolation of proximal interphalangeal flexion to test FDS integrity. **C.** Loss of normal flexion cascade after tendon laceration in palm.

- Testing for the tenodesis effect (digits passively flex with wrist extension) or compressing the flexor musculature in the forearm to assess for digit flexion should help with diagnosis in these situations.

NONOPERATIVE MANAGEMENT

- There is no nonoperative means of restoring active flexion to a digit whose flexors have been cut, as the tendon ends retract and do not heal to one another.
- If a flexor tendon laceration is encountered within the first 4 weeks after injury, it is probably worthwhile attempting primary repair. After that time, discussion should be held with the patient regarding other options.
- For late presentation of an isolated FDP laceration in zone I, it may be practical to do nothing, as full proximal interphalangeal motion should still be present. If the DIP joint is or becomes unstable, a DIP joint fusion or tenodesis of the distal FDP stump can be performed. One large series reported successful primary tendon grafting for isolated FDP lacerations even in zone II, but this is not widely performed.
- For late presentation of zone II injuries involving both tendons, staged tendon reconstruction (see Chap. 79) may be an option.

SURGICAL MANAGEMENT

- The goal of flexor tendon surgery is a repair that will allow early motion, will not fail due to gap formation or suture pullout, and will not develop adhesions limiting final range of motion.
- Several variables under control of the surgeon contribute to repair strength:
  - Number of strands (most important determinant; a four-strand repair with an epitenon suture added has been shown in laboratory studies to withstand limited early active motion)[6,11]
  - Suture size (3-0 or 4-0 is sufficient; larger suture increases resistance to gliding)
  - Configuration of repair (cruciate repair requires only one knot, buries the knot within the repair site, and allows for equal distribution of force across all four strands)[5]
  - Use of locking stitches (adds resistance to suture pullout)
  - Addition of an epitenon suture (increases repair strength and decreases gap formation and gliding resistance)[6]
  - Presence of a gap (>3 mm at any point will likely result in rupture)
  - Bunching of repair (due to taking too large a "bite" of tendon end; increases gliding resistance and therefore risk of rupture)
  - Integrity of pulleys (at least half of both A2 and A4 should be preserved to maintain tendon excursion and allow tip-to-palm contact)
  - Repair of one versus both tendons (if repair of both FDS slips impedes gliding, one slip should be resected or the FDS not repaired at all)
- It is well accepted that core suture strength is directly related to the number of suture strands crossing the repair site between proximal and distal tendon ends; all else being equal, using more strands means a stronger repair.[11]
  - This concept must be balanced against other factors: Too many sutures crossing the repair site limits the available surface area for exposed tendon ends to heal; more sutures and knots increase the gliding resistance of the tendon; and the more sutures placed, the longer the surgical time, which is associated with risks such as infection and anesthesia-related issues.
  - Strickland[6] showed that a four-strand zone II repair with an epitenon suture is strong enough to tolerate an immediate light active range-of-motion protocol, which allows for early gliding of the repair and decreases the risk of adhesion formation.
- Suture size contributes to repair strength, but one study showed 3-0 and 4-0 suture to resist repair rupture equally well and 2-0 suture to increase gliding resistance significantly.[1]
- Adding at least one locking stitch (making an additional pass to capture more tendon fibers) has been shown to increase repair strength and minimize gap formation.
- Multiple studies suggest that when both tendons are cut in zone II, repair of the FDP and only one slip of FDS rather than both slips results in decreased gliding resistance and improved range of motion.[9,10,13]
  - My present compromise remains a four-strand cruciate repair using 3-0 nonabsorbable suture, with a 6-0 Prolene running epitenon suture, with repair of one slip of FDS and resection of the other slip when both tendons are lacerated in zone II.

Preoperative Planning

- As noted previously, it is usually preferable to perform tendon repair early (if other circumstances allow).[3,7] The upper limit of time past which proximal tendon stump retraction is likely to cause technical difficulty is variable. Although 3 to 4 weeks is a commonly cited limit for primary tendon repair, in rare cases, the vincula may prevent retraction and allow repair even later.
- Patients presenting late should be fully counseled regarding other options, including the potential for intraoperative changes in plan.

Positioning

- Flexor tendon surgery, like most hand surgery, is generally performed with the affected extremity on a hand table, with the shoulder abducted 90 degrees and the elbow extended. The forearm is supinated, exposing the volar surface of the digits.
- A positioning device such as a lead hand can be helpful in stabilizing digits for surgery (once tendon ends have been delivered into the wound) and keeping other digits out of the way.

Approach

- Incisions should be planned so as to incorporate the laceration into the exposure.
  - Bruner (zigzag) or midlateral approaches both work well; they can be combined if needed.
  - Midlateral incisions extending proximally on one side of the digit and distally on the other can give large flaps and excellent exposure.
- The chief concern is not to cross a flexion crease at a right angle because the resultant scar will tend to contract and limit extension.

Primary Repair in Zone II

Retrieval of Tendon Ends

- A Bruner (zigzag) or midlateral incision is made (**TECH FIG 1A**). Consideration should be given to the existing laceration and the use of a combination of midlateral and Bruner-type incisions to avoid small, injured skin flaps and a wound healing complication.
- Often, some manipulation is needed to bring the tendon ends into the wound; for the proximal tendon end, wrist flexion and "milking" of the forearm may succeed. The distal stump is best exposed by extending the incision so that the repair can be performed without holding the digit flexed.
- Initial exposure should include both digital neurovascular bundles, whether or not they were injured along with the tendon or tendons.
  - If digital nerve or artery repair is needed, this should be done after the tendon repair so that the more delicate microsuture used is not disrupted with manipulation of the digit. Exposure of these bundles even when uninjured allows much more freedom for manipulating the cut tendon ends.
- Once the neurovascular bundles are exposed and protected, the sheath should be cleared of overlying soft tissues and inspected.

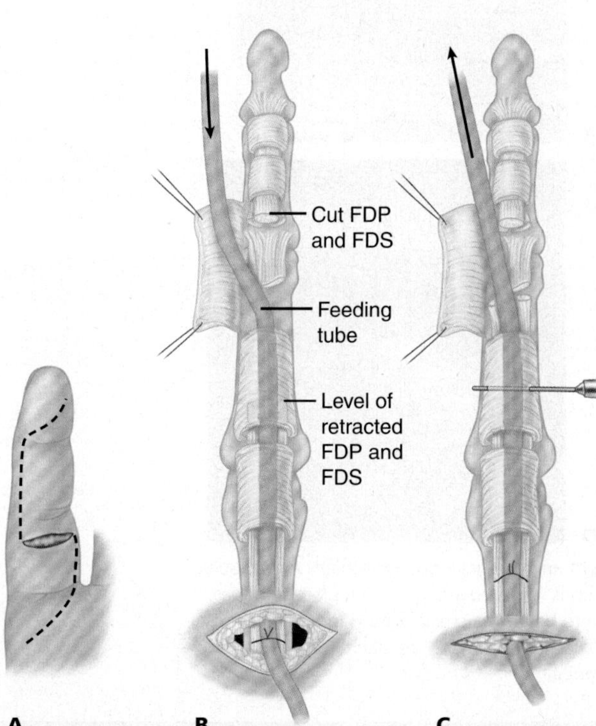

TECH FIG 1 • Exposure (**A**), retrieval (**B**), and temporary transverse pinning through sheath of cut tendon ends (**C**) to allow tension-free repair.

The sheath laceration can be extended with a side cut to form an L-shaped flap, always preserving as much as possible of the A2 and A4 pulleys. Creating such flaps can facilitate retrieving the tendon ends.

- Because most flexor tendon injuries occur with the digit in flexion, the skin laceration is generally more proximal than the tendon laceration. This means that exposure of the distal stump often requires considerable distal extension of the incision, frequently past the level of the DIP joint and obliquely across the pulp of the distal phalanx.
- The proximal tendon end may be held in place near the laceration by its vincula, but it will often have retracted well proximally.
  - It is reasonable to make several attempts to retrieve the proximal tendon end through the sheath with an appropriately small instrument (curved tendon passer, small hemostat, etc.), keeping in mind that the less damage to the tendon end and sheath, the easier the repair and the less scarring that will result. Flexing the wrist and milking the forearm will sometimes encourage a proximally migrated tendon to protrude into the wound.
  - If these measures fail, a short transverse incision along the distal palmar crease can be made, as if exposing the A1 pulley for a trigger finger release, and the tendon exposed at this level.
- A pediatric feeding tube can be threaded from one wound to the other and sutured to the tendon in the proximal wound (**TECH FIG 1B**).
- The tube and flexor tendon can then be retrieved into the distal wound and the tube and suture cut free.
- Following retrieval of the FDP tendon, it should be carefully brought back through the FDS decussation to prevent bunching or a mechanical block to finger flexion.
- Once the proximal end is in the planned repair site, the tendon can be pinned with a 25-gauge needle to prevent retraction back into the sheath (**TECH FIG 1C**).
- Often, the distal location of the distal stump requires that the proximal tendon end be threaded past the original laceration site to a more distal "window" made in the sheath for tendon repair. This, coupled with flexion of the DIP joint, should allow for apposition of the tendon ends and repair under minimal tension.

Tendon Repair

- Four-strand cruciate repair is effected using 3-0 nonabsorbable suture, with a 6-0 Prolene running locking epitenon suture, and repair of one slip of FDS (**TECH FIG 2**).

Epitenon-First Repair

- For very oblique lacerations, it may be easier to perform an epitenon-first repair, coapting the cut tendon ends smoothly, and then performing the core stitch beginning through a slit on the outside of the tendon, burying the knot in this same slit (**TECH FIG 3**).
- The repair is otherwise the same as a four-strand cruciate repair.

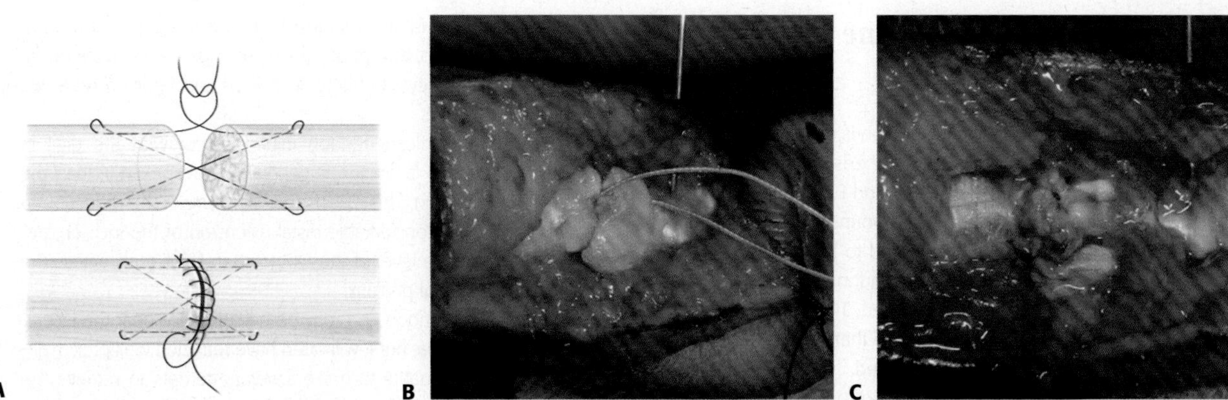

TECH FIG 2 • A. Four-strand cruciate repair with epitenon stitch. **B,C.** The hand is to the right and the fingertips to the left. **B.** Distal zone II FDP laceration with tendon ends pinned in place and core stitch being placed. **C.** Completed repair with epitenon stitch.

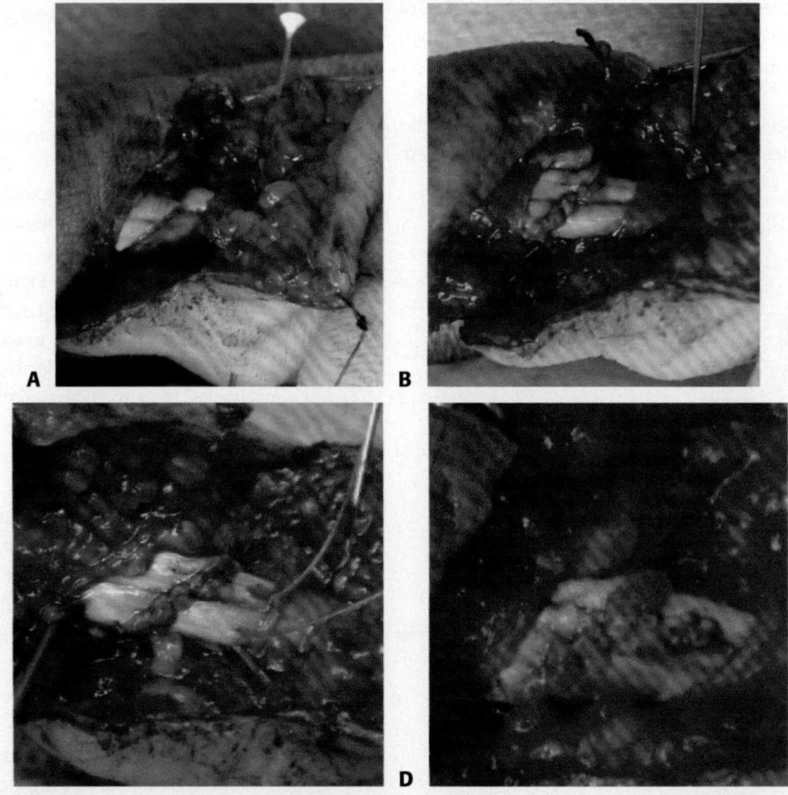

TECH FIG 3 • A–D. The hand is to the right and the fingertips to the left. **A.** Oblique laceration of flexor tendons in zone II; tendon ends retrieved and pinned in place for repair. **B.** Epitenon repair performed first. **C.** Core suture begun via small incision in tendon proximal to repair; otherwise, similar to standard cruciate repair. **D.** Core stitch completed and knot buried in small incision used for starting point.

PEARLS AND PITFALLS

- Early repair is easiest and gives best results.
- Midlateral incisions give wide exposure.
- Hold tendon ends in place with 25-gauge needles to allow tension-free repair.
- A four-strand locking cruciate repair using 3-0 nonabsorbable suture combined with a 6-0 absorbable running epitenon stitch will allow protected early active motion and has been shown to maximize the outcome.
- Limiting repair of FDS to one slip minimizes overcrowding in zone II and allows better tendon gliding.
- For partial lacerations, no repair is necessary unless greater than 60% of the cross-sectional area of the tendon has been divided. Any flap of tendon should be trimmed to prevent later triggering.[2,4,12]

POSTOPERATIVE CARE

- If a primary repair has been performed as described earlier, an immediate light active "place and hold" therapy regimen can usually begin safely as long as the patient is reliable.

OUTCOMES

- A recent meta-analysis of multiple studies over the past 15 years found a rupture rate of 4% to 10% and good to excellent results in about three quarters of patients.[8] Present-day techniques should allow for continued improvement in these results.
- Injury mechanism is a predictor of outcome and is beyond the surgeon's control. An uncomplicated, isolated sharp flexor tendon laceration that is treated acutely represents the best possible scenario for a highly functional digit. Additional injury to bone, tendon, or nerve negatively affects outcome.

COMPLICATIONS

- The two extremes of undesirable outcomes are tendon rupture and tendon adhesions. Ruptures are rare, but adhesions and resultant limited motion are common.
- If rupture is strongly suspected acutely, a repeat repair should be performed, although the patient and surgeon should be prepared for the need to proceed intraoperatively with other reconstructive options.
- The management of tendon adhesions is discussed in Chapter 79.

REFERENCES

1. Alavanja G, Dailey E, Mass DP. Repair of zone II flexor digitorum profundus lacerations using varying suture sizes: a comparative biomechanical study. J Hand Surg Am 2005;30(3):448–454.
2. Erhard L, Zobitz ME, Zhao C, et al. Treatment of partial lacerations in flexor tendons by trimming. A biomechanical in vitro study. J Bone Joint Surg Am 2002;84-A(6):1006–1012.
3. Gorriz GJ, Cooke J. Assessment of the influence of the timing of repair on flexor tendon injuries in chickens. Br J Plast Surg 1976;29:82–84.
4. Hariharan JS, Diao E, Soejima O, et al. Partial lacerations of human digital flexor tendons: a biomechanical analysis. J Hand Surg Am 1997;22(6):1011–1015.
5. McLarney E, Hoffman H, Wolfe SW. Biomechanical analysis of the cruciate four-strand flexor tendon repair. J Hand Surg Am 1999;24(2):295–301.
6. Strickland JW. Flexor tendon injuries: I. Foundations of treatment. J Am Acad Orthop Surg 1995;3:44–54.
7. Tang J, Shi D, Gu Y. Flexor tendon repair: timing of surgery and sheath management [in Chinese]. Zhonghua Wai Ke Za Zhi 1995;33:532–535.
8. Tang JB. Clinical outcomes associated with flexor tendon repair. Hand Clin 2005;21:199–210.
9. Tang JB. Flexor tendon repair in zone 2C. J Hand Surg Br 1994;19(1):72–75.
10. Tang JB, Xie RG, Cao Y, et al. A2 pulley incision or one slip of the superficialis improves flexor tendon repairs. Clin Orthop Relat Res 2007;456:121–127.
11. Thurman RT, Trumble TE, Hanel DP, et al. Two-, four-, and six-strand zone II flexor tendon repairs: an in situ biomechanical comparison using a cadaver model. J Hand Surg Am 1998;23(2):261–265.
12. Wray RC Jr, Weeks PM. Treatment of partial tendon lacerations. Hand 1980;12:163–166.
13. Zhao C, Amadio PC, Zobitz ME, et al. Resection of the flexor digitorum superficialis reduces gliding resistance after zone II flexor digitorum profundus repair in vitro. J Hand Surg Am 2002;27(2):316–321.

Tenolysis following Injury and Repair of Digital Flexor Tendons

David Netscher and Kate Kuhlman-Wood

DEFINITION

- Before the late 1960s, tendon repair within the flexor sheath was so wrought with complications (mainly stiffness and adhesions) that primary repair was never undertaken, leading to the term *no man's land*, until the work of Harold Kleinert dispelled these misgivings.[28]
- Originally, tendon adhesions were felt to be a necessary part of flexor tendon healing within the flexor tendon sheath.[42]
- However, it was subsequently understood that intrasynovial intrinsic tendon healing was adequate to support tendon repair.[35,37]
  - Nonetheless, gapping of the repair site of 3 mm or more is sufficient to cause restrictive tendon adhesions.[18,44,48]
  - Improved tendon suture techniques with strength sufficient to enable early motion in postoperative therapy combined with early active postoperative range of motion aim to reduce tendon adhesions.[19,22]
  - In spite of these innovations, tendon adhesions still may occur following digital flexor tendon repair with a reported incidence of about 10%, and so these repairs in zone II still remain a challenge.
- Tendon adhesions may occur between both the flexor digitorum profundus (FDP) and flexor digitorum superficialis (FDS) as well as between the tendons and the flexor tendon sheath. This results in limited tendon excursion within the sheath and consequently reduced and dysfunctional digital range of motion.
- Tenolysis is the surgical release of tendon adhesions to restore tendon gliding and digital motion. This is only undertaken when
  - The patient is motivated and cooperative and will undertake the directed postoperative hand therapy.
  - A minimum of 3 to 6 months has elapsed since initial tendon repair—risk of devascularizing rupture of the tendon is much higher if tenolysis is performed before that time.
  - Maximum maturation of the healing scars has occurred so that the wound after the initial tendon repair is soft and supple.
  - Maximum passive mobility of interphalangeal joints has been reached. It makes no sense to perform flexor tenolysis in the face of a stiff and swollen finger.
  - The patient has plateaued in hand therapy with no further functional advances being made.
  - There is a substantial difference between active and passive digital range of motion, with the former being considerably less. Furthermore, outcome of tenolysis correlates significantly with total passive range of motion before tenolysis.[64]
  - The skin condition is adequate. Even if scar maturation has fully occurred but there are skin scar contractures due to soft tissue deficiency or linear scarring, this problem must be treated first by Z-plasty or local flap or skin graft before embarking on flexor tenolysis.
  - Overall condition of the digit—for example, a painful dysesthetic finger will be no more functional if improved range of motion is achieved.
- When embarking on flexor tenolysis, both patient and physician should have a clear understanding that intraoperatively, depending on the quality of the repair site and the extensiveness of the scarring, one may need to make a decision for tendon grafting and even two-stage tendon repair with pulley reconstruction.
- Proper patient selection is crucial to outcome of tenolysis. Interphalangeal joint fusion and even digit amputation may potentially be a better decision for the patient based on time away from work, older patient age, extent of external scarring, and joint stiffness.

ANATOMY

- Tenolysis needs to take into consideration the pulley system of the flexor tendon sheath. Thus, access to the tendon must be carefully planned, avoiding destruction especially of A2 and A4 pulleys.[11]
- Digital tenolysis is made even more complex by the changing interrelationships between the bifurcating FDS and its return to the midline dorsal to the FDP in the Camper chiasm.

PATHOGENESIS

- The repair response to tendon injury is similar to elsewhere in the body.
- Adhesions occur as a response to the healing process, and in zone II, the opportunity for restricting adhesions is much greater, occurring between two gliding tendons in a confining fibro-osseous tunnel.
- Both the tendon(s) and tendon sheath are injured and thus the body repair response occurs at both locations, resulting in scarring between the tendons as well as of the tendons to the tendon sheath.
- There is initially an inflammatory phase of tendon healing (48 to 72 hours), followed by the fibroblastic (collagen) phase (5 days to 6 weeks) and remodeling that lasts up to 6 months (similar to other body tissue types). The initial cellular response is largely phagocytic, followed by collagen deposition. When extrinsic healing predominates, adhesions between tendon and surrounding tissues are likely, whereas healing that is predominantly intrinsic cellular activity results in fewer adhesions.

- Factors that may influence formation of excursion-restricting tendon adhesions include the extent of the initial trauma to tendon and tendon sheath,[43] tendon ischemia (including loss of vincular blood supply),[40] tendon immobilization, and gapping at the repair site.
- Early passive and especially active therapy protocols apply stress across the repaired tendon and lead to increased repair site tensile strength, fewer adhesions, and better excursion.[19,22] Thus, primary tendon repair now has as its goal a strong, gap-resistant suture technique, followed by early postoperative motion protocol.
- Although motion-restricting scar-forming adhesions are no longer felt to be an inevitability following zone II flexor tendon repair, it is unrealistic to expect a tendon to heal without any adhesions at all. Exclusive intrinsic tendon healing can only occur with in vitro experimental situations. Loose adhesions may then possibly be disrupted by postoperative therapy protocols.
- The role of distant cytokines has been evaluated in the pathogenesis of scar tissue and adhesions,[31,57] most prominent of which has been transforming growth factor beta (TGF-β), although its exact role is still under research, and also fibronectin. The importance of understanding this cytokine activity lies in the potential to modify its activity in adhesion formation, and experiments have been performed on physical factors, such as shear stress,[16] neutralizing antibodies,[65] and chemical modulations (such as 5-fluorouracil).[39]

NATURAL HISTORY

- Once mature tendon adhesions have developed, the only effective treatment is tenolysis because the adhesions will not resolve.
- Progressive stretch (serial casting and dynamic external fixation with Digit Widget, [Hand Biomechanics Lab, Sacramento, CA]) may resolve joint contractures but will have no effect on tendon excursion.
- Untreated, the patient remains with reduced active range of motion to the finger. The patient may learn adaptive measures by catching the affected finger between the adjacent digits into a clenched fist.
- Symptomatic tendon adhesions may result in substantial morbidity through diminished range of motion and reduced hand strength. They may lead to secondary joint contractures.
- Tenolysis is by far the most common secondary procedure after digit replantation.[60] Even with more current forms of tendon repair and postoperative therapy, it is estimated that 10% of repaired digital flexor tendons require surgical tenolysis.[54] Proximal to zone II, the need for flexor tenolysis is less common.

PATIENT HISTORY AND PHYSICAL FINDINGS

- The hallmark of the diagnosis of flexor tendon adhesions is that active finger flexion is substantially less than passive flexion.
- The aims of the examination are fourfold:
  - Assess that scars are fully mature and that joints are maximally supple before embarking on tenolysis.
  - Assess the quality of volar scars and soft tissue. Preliminary scar releases may potentially be required, or even provision of added quality soft tissue through flaps or skin grafts may be necessary.
  - Determine if tenolysis should be undertaken at all. This may be relatively contraindicated or even deemed unnecessary or delayed until conditions are more favorable—in patients of older age or age younger than 11 years,[54] patients with mild functional deficits, patients with low-demand functional needs, uncooperative and noncompliant patient, very severe scarring or dysesthetic finger (in which case a "salvage" procedure such as arthrodesis or even amputation may be better options), duration since the original tendon repair (generally considered to be at least 3 months since primary repair and 6 months since tendon graft before performing tenolysis out of concern for devascularizing the tendon and sustaining tendon rupture),[15,62] and vascularity of the digit (either due to direct prior traumatizing vascular injury or due to systemic effects such as in a smoker or diabetic or patient with preexisting peripheral vascular or collagen vascular disease).
  - Making the correct diagnosis and excluding other differential diagnoses. This involves not only excluding but also considering other potential associated conditions that may limit active finger flexion and also potentially result in joint flexion contracture.
- Thus, specifically, the clinical assessment of the digit involves the establishment of a definitive diagnosis of flexor tendon adhesion (and exclusion of other causes) as well as determination of the severity of these adhesions. The examination therefore involves the following:
  - Have the patient actively flex the affected digits. Measure the angle of flexion of the metacarpophalangeal (MP), distal interphalangeal (DIP), and proximal interphalangeal (PIP) joints as well as determination of the total arc of active motion (summation of all three joints). Next, passively flex the finger.
  - Evaluate the seesaw defect.[30] This results when a contracted element spans two joints:
    - If, for example, the extrinsic flexor tendons are adherent proximal to the level of the MP joint, passive flexion of that joint will result in correction of an apparent PIP flexion contracture that results from tethering of the flexor tendons. Failure to correct the PIP contracture would mean that the contracture is inherent to the PIP joint itself (**FIG 1**).
    - In contrast, if the extrinsic extensor tendon is adherent to the metacarpal, the limitation of extensor tendon excursion distal to that joint will prevent simultaneous flexion of the MP and PIP joints (**FIG 2**). This is the test of extrinsic extensor tightness.[32,33] Additionally, passive flexion in this case will also be limited.
    - The Bunnell test for intrinsic tightness results from a seesaw phenomenon in which the band occurs across two joints but is an extensor at one joint and a flexor at the next adjacent joint.[12] If this system is foreshortened, extension of the MP joint, actively or passively, will restrain flexion of the PIP joint (**FIG 3**). If flexion of the PIP joint is greater when the MP joint is flexed than when it is extended, intrinsic tightness is present.
    - A similar volar to dorsal seesaw effect may occur at the DIP joint secondary to the action of the oblique retinacular ligament and lateral bands, resulting in an

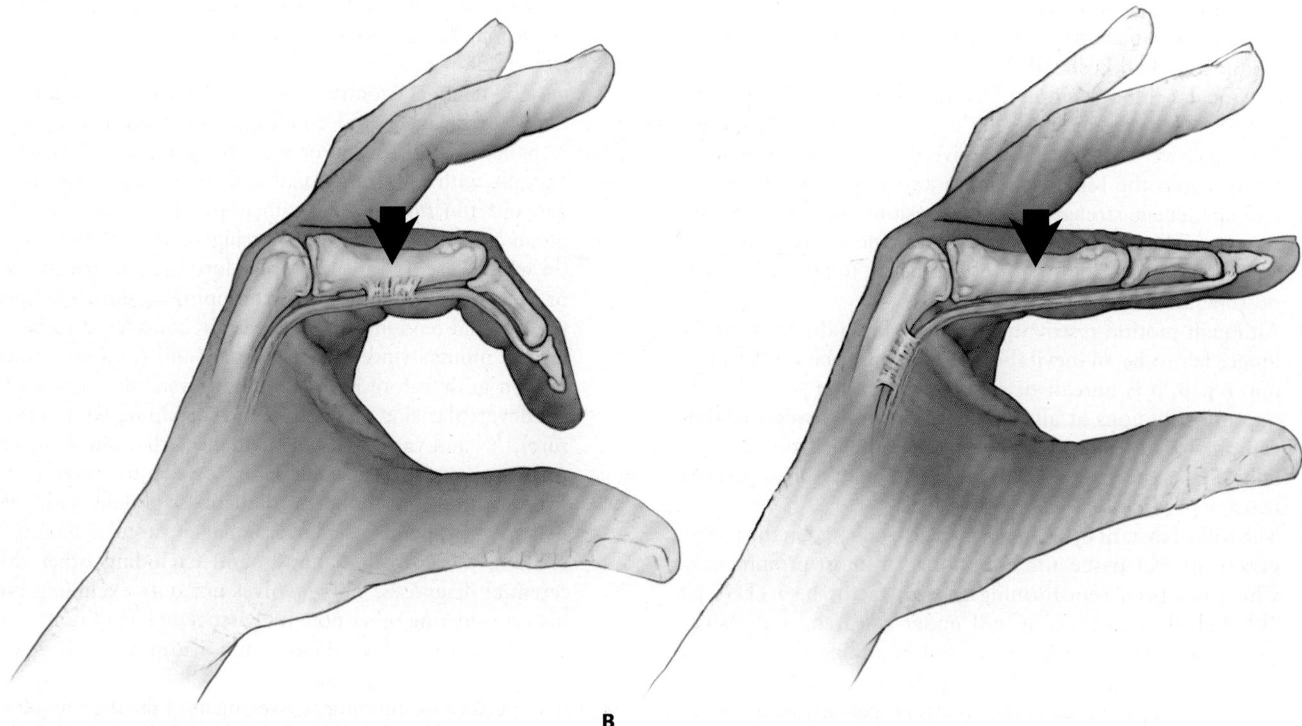

FIG 1 • Seesaw effect. Adjust the joints proximal to the joint that has the contracture. If there are extrinsic flexor tendon adhesions at the proximal phalanx, MP joint positioning in flexion will have no effect on the PIP joint contracture (**A**). If the flexor tendon adhesions are proximal to the MP joint, positioning of the joint in flexion will improve the apparent flexion contracture at the PIP joint (**B**).

extension contracture at that joint (ie, difficulty flexing that joint). In this boutonniere test (sometimes also called the *Landsmeer test*), because the oblique retinacular ligament is foreshortened, when the PIP joint is extended, passive DIP joint flexion is difficult[34] (**FIG 4**).

- Distinguish between tendon rupture and tendon adhesions. Immediately following flexor tendon repair, this distinction may be difficult because the finger is still swollen, painful, and stiff. However, later, this distinction is seldom difficult, as there is, at least, some active finger flexion with generation of stabilizing tension in the more distal joints. If active range of motion is, however, very poor, it may either be due to dense tendon adhesions or an intact but attenuated repair or even tendon ends connected through scar tissue. Special imaging will help in these circumstances.
- Finally, assess for flexor tendon bowstringing. Palpate for the tensing flexor tendon immediately under the skin with resisted finger flexion (**FIG 5**). If there is bowstringing, linear tendon excursion is "wasted" and not available for finger flexion as the tendon is displaced forward from the joint (**FIG 6**).[6] Scar will also form dorsal to the tendon sheath in the concavity of the affected joint and add to the intrinsic joint contracture. In the presence of volar soft tissue scarring from prior injury and tendon repair, potential tendon bowstringing may be difficult to assess and may require special imaging if it is suspected.

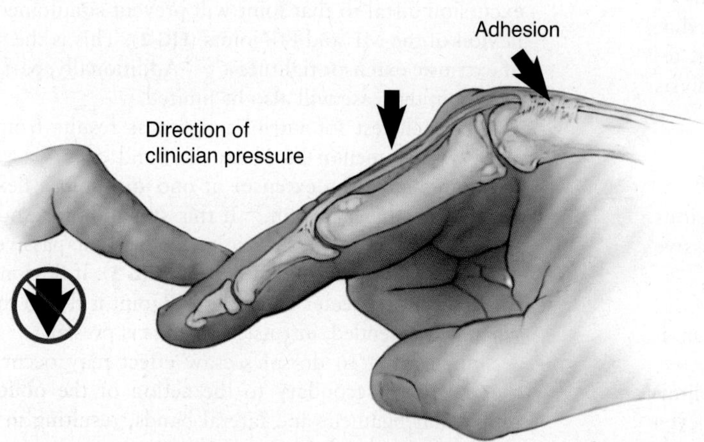

FIG 2 • Extrinsic extensor tendon adhesion. Extrinsic extensor tendon adhesions proximal to the MP joint will prevent simultaneous MP and PIP joint flexion. Both passive and active digital flexion will be restricted.

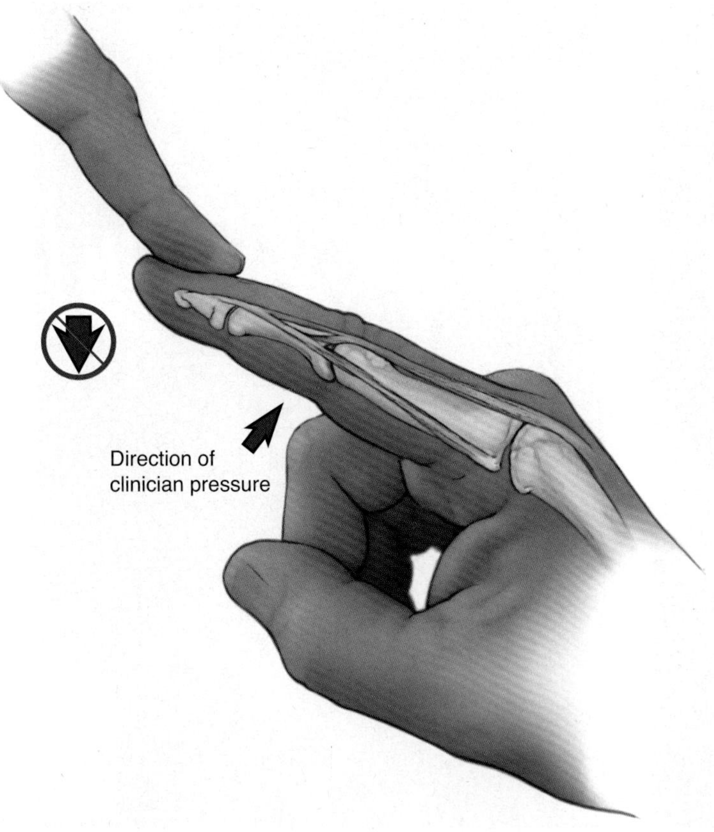

FIG 3 • Intrinsic extensor mechanism tightness. With intrinsic extensor tightness, passive MP joint extension restricts PIP joint flexion (Bunnell test).

IMAGING AND OTHER DIAGNOSTIC STUDIES

- Standard radiographs of the hand are necessary to evaluate for bone or articular pathology. A true lateral image of contracted joints is important to assess the congruity of the articular surfaces.
- Computed tomography (CT) scans may occasionally be selected to assess bone and articular pathology.
- Magnetic resonance imaging (MRI) or ultrasound may sometimes be necessary to assess potential attenuation or disruption of a prior tendon repair.[53] They may also be helpful in evaluating for the potential presence of flexor tendon bowstringing (**FIG 7**).

DIFFERENTIAL DIAGNOSIS

- Following flexor tendon injury, either through sharp laceration or crushing injury, or even from previous replantation (where both flexors and extensors were repaired), active finger flexion may be reduced secondary to the following:
  - Rupture of the original tendon repair
  - Quadriga phenomenon (but adjacent uninjured fingers are also affected), if excessive advancement of tendons have been performed at the original repair site
  - Intrinsic tightness (if associated with severe crushing injury of the hand)

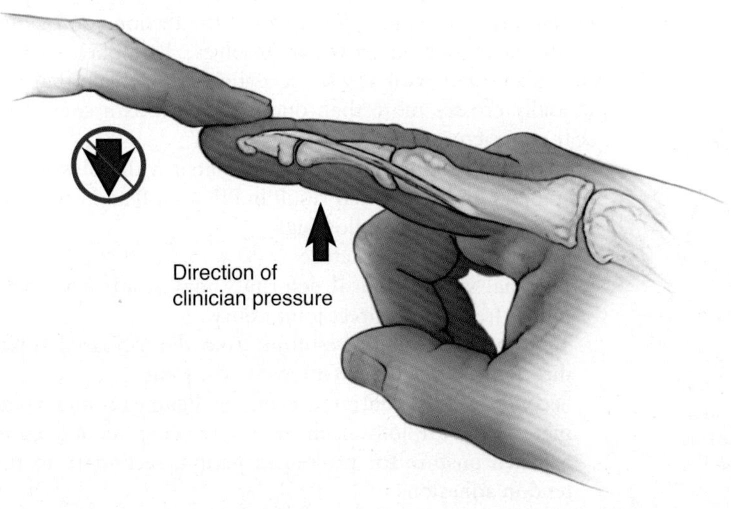

FIG 4 • Landsmeer test. When the oblique retinacular ligament is foreshortened, extension of the PIP joint results in more difficult passive DIP joint flexion.

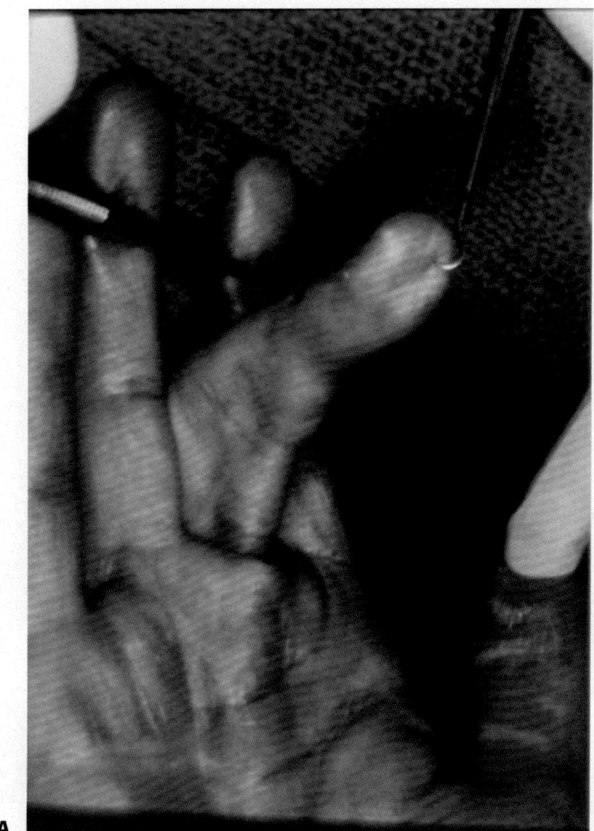

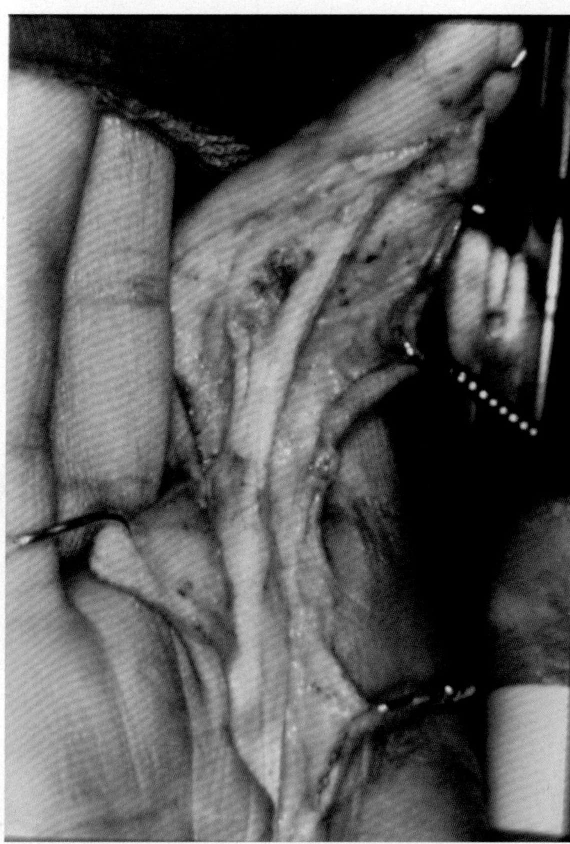

FIG 5 • A,B. Bowstringing. Tensing of the flexor tendon immediately under the skin indicates bowstringing.

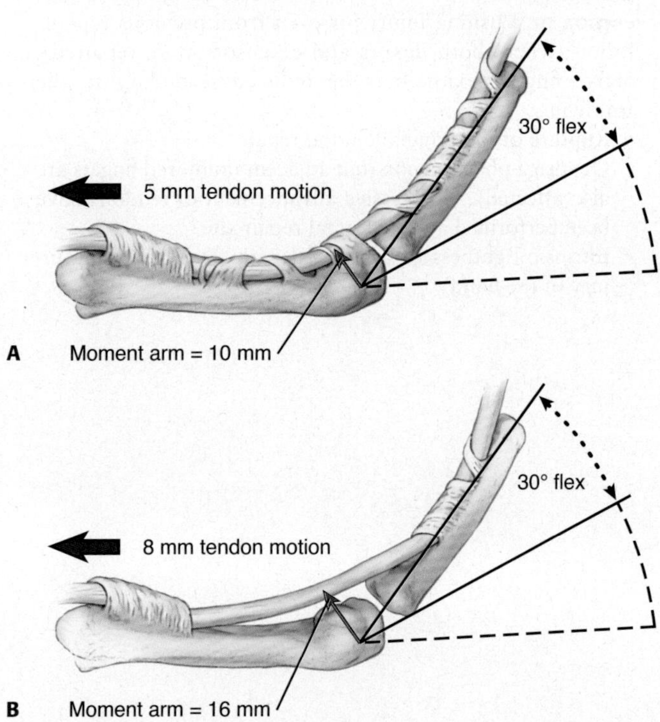

FIG 6 • Bowstringing. Drawing **A** represents normal anatomy and Drawing **B** depicts bowstringing. Without the pulleys to keep the tendon close to the bone, the moment arm away from the bone increases as seen in B (*red arrow*). This means that more tendon excursion is needed to generate the same amount of active finger flexion.

  - Lumbrical plus phenomenon (generally applies more to tendon grafting where the graft is relatively too long and slack)
  - Associated extensor tendon injuries where not only is active flexion limited but there is also restriction of passive flexion
- Flexor tendon adhesions, if sufficiently tight, may cause a deforming flexion force on the next most distal joint, resulting in a flexion contracture. This distinction may be partly resolved by eliciting "the seesaw effect" and flexing the preceding more proximal joint to see if the flexion contracture at the next joint improves or resolves. This phenomenon may also occur with any other associated problem that potentially crosses more than one joint, such as a soft tissue scar contracture.
- Specifically, conditions initially associated with a flexor tendon injury and repair that result in PIP joint flexion contracture may include the following:
  - Soft tissue scar contracture
  - External visible clinical deformity may result from malunited fracture or direct joint injury.
  - Tendon bowstringing resulting from the increased volar-directed vector by the tendons on the joint
  - Secondary scar contracture of the ligaments and volar plate of the PIP joint itself by simply being maintained in a flexed posture for prolonged period, secondary to the tendon adhesions

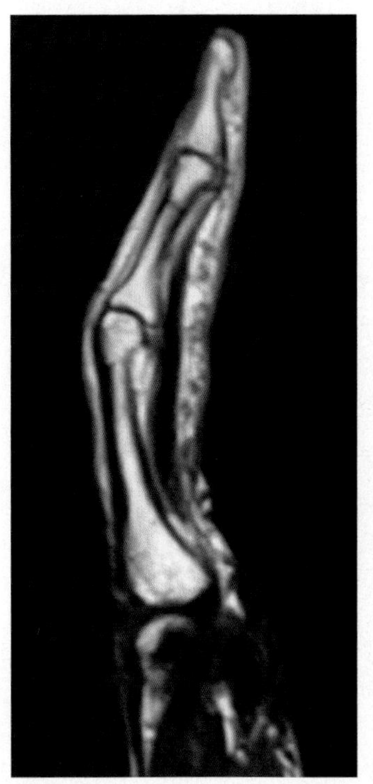

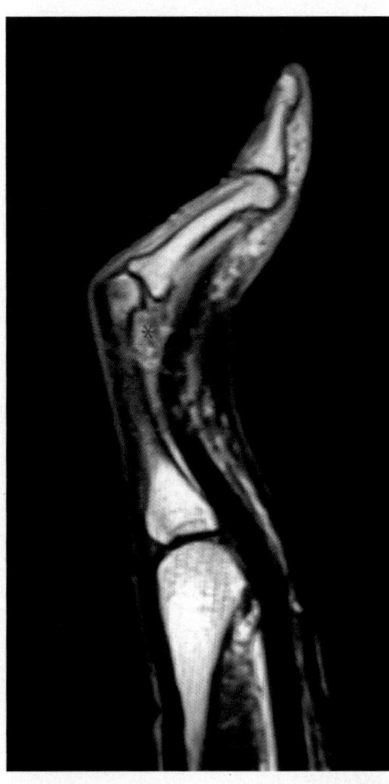

FIG 7 • MRI. **A.** Normal position of flexor tendon on MRI. **B.** Flexed PIP joint and volar displaced flexor tendons (bowstringing). Also, note scar formation dorsal to the flexor tendon in the concavity of the PIP joint (*red asterisk*).

NONOPERATIVE MANAGEMENT

- The goals of nonoperative management are threefold:
  - Improving pliability of soft tissue scars and joint suppleness
  - Resolution of joint contractures by passive stretches
  - Improvement of tendon gliding by active range of motion
- Once all these goals have been maximized, there is no further improvement, and if the patient still requires enhanced finger range of motion and function, then surgical tenolysis is entertained as the next option.
- If at all possible, before embarking on tenolysis, joints should be free of contracture. Many types of static splints are available to overcome PIP flexion contractures. Serial finger casting is another possible modality. A variety of wire-foam splints enable continued PIP joint active flexion but maintain extension stretch of the joint itself (**FIG 8**).
- Initial splinting displaces tissue fluid, which is the rapid gain phase of splinting. Once tissue edema has been displaced, then the external splint forces collagen remodeling. Prolonged splinting over weeks is necessary to achieve the desired effect on collagen.[8]
- Other hand therapy measures such as edema reduction (by extremity elevation and compression gloves), moist heat, and ultrasound may enhance the beneficial changes accomplished by splinting.[4]
- Linear tendon excursion and tendon gliding are encouraged by active finger flexion. This helps break up the loose tendon adhesions. Differential tendon gliding between FDP and FDS is encouraged by respective joint blocking at the PIP and MP levels. Ultrasound, by inducing deep heat, may help the collagen deforming changes induced by progressive stretching.[4] Functional electrical stimulation may enhance active myostatic contractions to encourage tendon pull-through and excursion.

SURGICAL MANAGEMENT

- Tenolysis requires intact tendon and pulleys. This may be determined only at the time of tenolysis surgery. Thus, the patient should be prepared and willing to undergo tendon grafting and even two-stage tendon reconstruction depending on intraoperative findings.

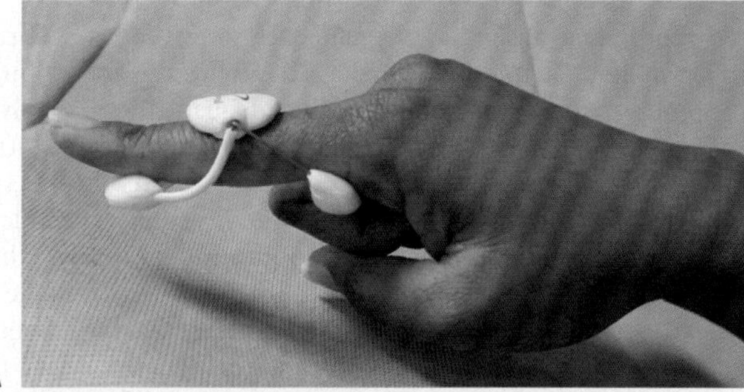

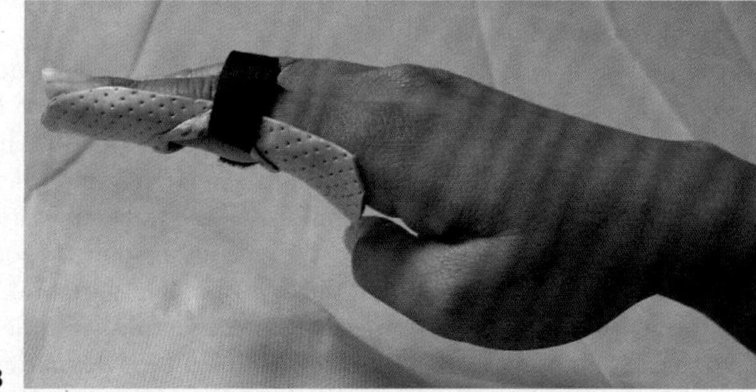

FIG 8 • Dynamic and static finger splints. **A.** Three-point LMB. **B.** PIP drop out. (Courtesy of Kimberly Goldie-Staines, OTR, CHT.)

- Timing of tenolysis is debated but is generally accepted to be at least 3 months following primary repair (with 4 to 8 weeks of no further measurable improvements with active therapy)[51] and 6 months after prior tendon grafting.[15]
- Prerequisites to tenolysis require that all fractures be healed, that wounds are soft and pliable, and that joints are passively supple.
- Concomitant surgical procedures together with tenolysis should generally be avoided out of concern for compromising the result, but on occasion, simultaneous concomitant procedures may be entertained:
  - Volar plate and joint releases at the PIP and DIP joints are frequently necessary for associated joint flexion contractures and may be performed[51] but may also potentially result in inferior outcomes.[55] This will depend partly on the severity of the joint contracture. A contracture of minor functional impairment (<30 degrees) may best be left untreated. A more severe contracture may more optimally be treated on its own merits first with joint release and then performance of tenolysis at a later stage procedure.
  - Simultaneous pulley reconstruction should generally be avoided, although there are reports of successful combined procedures with tenolysis.[17]
  - Because optimum results following tenolysis require immediate postoperative active digital range of motion, procedures that will require immobilization should generally be avoided as simultaneous procedures—these include complex flaps and skin grafts, osteotomies, tendon lengthening or shortening, and tendon repair.[17,58]
- Anesthesia choices are varied:
  - General or regional brachial plexus block anesthesia may be selected where there is a possibility of questionable patient cooperation or where the procedure may be judged too long to tolerate local anesthesia alone. In this situation, a separate counterincision must be made in the forearm to test flexion at the end of the tenolysis procedure by traction on the relevant flexor tendons (**FIGS 9** and **10**).[10,17]
  - Local anesthesia supplemented by intravenous sedation was popularized by Schneider[46] and has the attraction of intraoperative assessment of the adequacy of the tenolysis by having the patient actively flexing the fingers during surgery. The patient can also see the results during surgery, providing additional patient motivation to be able to achieve the same range of motion postoperatively. Ulnar nerve wrist block may have a potential disadvantage of also blocking the motor branch and removing intrinsic muscle power and so diminishing the patient's active finger flexion capability. Thus, whenever possible, perform a sensory nerve block only
  - Lalonde[21,29] has popularized the technique of "wide awake" anesthesia in which tumescent infiltration of lidocaine with epinephrine is performed (see **Video**). This provides both local anesthesia and a relatively bloodless operative field. We prefer initial use of the tourniquet and some intravenous sedation to provide an absolute bloodless field, which is helpful in the exposure and initial takedown of adhesions. This needs to be accomplished in less than 30 minutes because it may be difficult for the patient to tolerate the tourniquet for longer and longer duration would also lead to muscle paralysis. The tourniquet is then released for patient involvement in active finger flexion and further takedown of remaining adhesions. On occasion, the forceful finger flexion of the patient (in the absence of pain) will actually break some of these adhesions, as well.

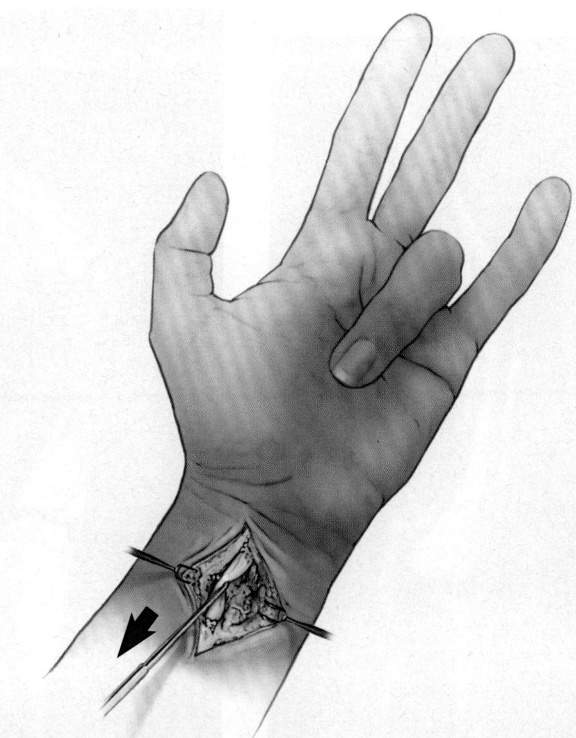

FIG 9 • Proximal traction on the flexor tendon in the distal forearm will result in flexion of the digit, indicating completeness of the finger tenolysis.

- Tourniquet. A totally bloodless field is helpful in the detail that is necessary to accomplish tenolysis within the narrow confines of the flexor tendon sheath. The patient may better tolerate a forearm tourniquet. There is a disadvantage of compressing the forearm flexor muscles, which reduces their active range of motion and ability to flex. Also, the pressure of the tourniquet may cause flexor tightness of the fingers. If a nonsterile forearm tourniquet is used, then it has to be draped out of the operative field, thus reducing the amount of room in the sterile field. The authors thus prefer use of an upper arm tourniquet but strictly limiting the duration of tourniquet use.

Preoperative Planning

- Preoperative discussion with the anesthesiologist is necessary, especially if the patient is to be "awake" for the procedure. A balance is required between patient comfort and patient cooperation intraoperatively. This requires a coordinated effort between surgeon and anesthesiologist for a potentially taxing surgical procedure.
- Ensure availability of necessary instrumentation for accomplishing tenolysis.
- Surgical supplies, to include silicone tendon spacers of different sizes, may be necessary if recourse has to be made intraoperatively to staged tendon reconstruction.

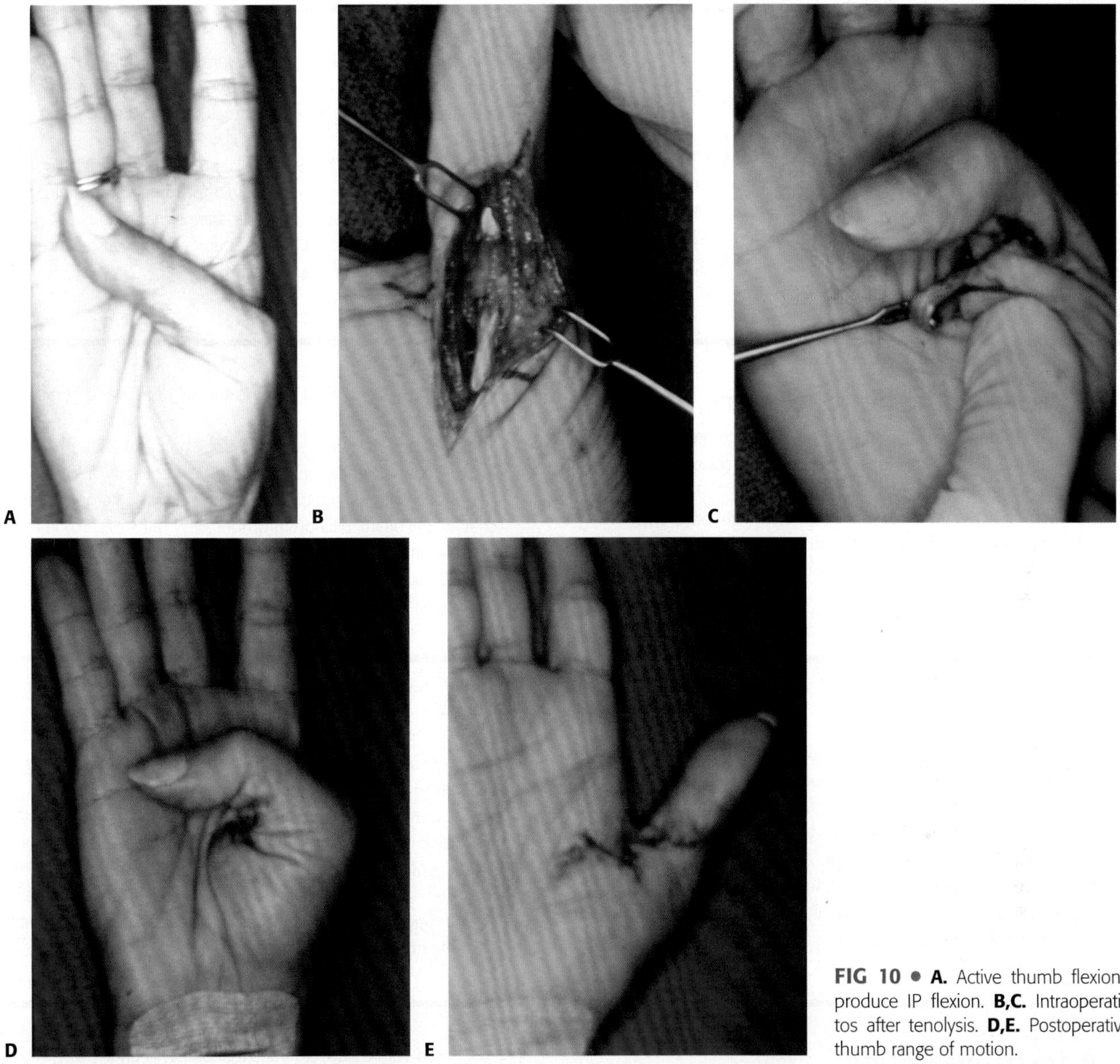

FIG 10 • **A.** Active thumb flexion fails to produce IP flexion. **B,C.** Intraoperative photos after tenolysis. **D,E.** Postoperative active thumb range of motion.

- Assess the patient preoperatively for presence of palmaris longus tendon. If tendon grafting becomes necessary, one should have backup plans for graft sources, which may include palmaris longus, the residual FDS, or even a toe extensor.
- Preoperative consent should not only include the tenolysis but also the potential for tendon reconstruction.

Positioning

- The patient is positioned supine with the upper extremity on a hand table. An aluminum foam hand splint (Instrument Specialists, Inc., Boerne, TX) is useful to stabilize the digits (**FIG 11**).

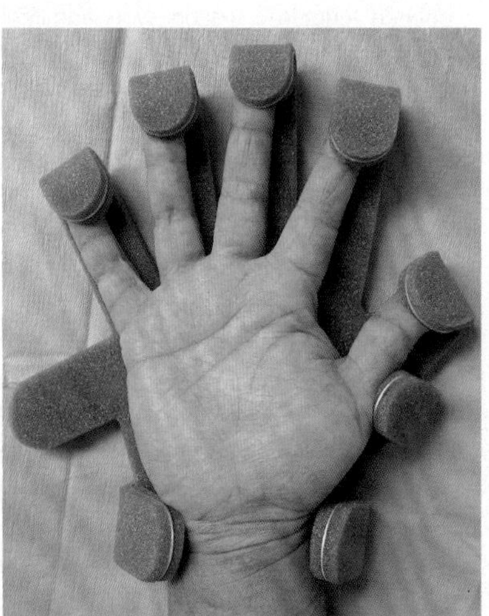

FIG 11 • Aluminum foam hand splint (Instrument Specialists).

Approach

- This is often predetermined by the original surgical incisions for the tendon repair.
- Wide exposure is necessary to reveal the full extent of the flexor tendon sheath. Dissect down the sides of the scarred flexor tendon sheath. In this way, the digital neurovascular bundles (often themselves encased in dense scar tissue) are teased out laterally individually. It may be unnecessarily dangerous to dissect out the neurovascular bundles individually.
- The exposure should extend beyond the distal and proximal limits of the scar for the original tendon repair. In that way, one identifies first the nonadherent structures and then dissects into the scar tissue.
- Wide exposure can be accomplished by a Bruner zigzag incision[7] or by a midlateral incision with proximal and distal zigzag extensions. The advantage of the latter is that it does not place incisional scars directly over the tendon and may also cause less wound tension during hand therapy.

Preserve the Pulley System

- It is critical to preserve A2 and A4 pulleys to prevent bowstringing and thereby the potential loss of capability to achieve full finger flexion down into the palm.[11]
- Mark out the A2 and A4 pulleys (which may be disguised in scar) with an indelible pen. Transverse incisions between these pulleys enable access for instrumentation down the flexor sheath.
- Windows can be created distal to the A4, at A3, and at A1 pulleys if necessary.
- Partial A2 and A4 pulley resection may be permissible.[38]
- Pulley widening may, on occasion, be necessary and can be performed by pediatric urethral dilators, cardiac coronary artery dilators, or Fogarty balloon thrombectomy catheters. Some have even recommended that this pulley widening always be done at the culmination of the tenolysis procedure to allow for smoother postoperative tendon gliding.[52]

Adhesiolysis

- Identify flexor tendons in the palm, starting in the unaffected region, initially raising the adherent FDP and FDS tendons as one. Lyse adhesions around these tendons.
- Retraction on the tendons will withdraw them from within the pulley system, enabling some adhesiolysis to be done under direct vision with scalpel or tenotomy scissors. Handle the tendons as atraumatically as possible by retraction with a blunt instrument or Penrose drain.
- If possible, then separate out the FDS and FDP tendons.
  - FDS may need to be sacrificed (either the entire tendon or a slip of the tendon) in the face of extreme scarring in order to achieve smooth gliding under the pulleys.[46,66]
  - It may be preferable to leave FDS and FDP adherent in the case of severe adhesions and in order to prevent weakening of the individual tendons, allowing them to act as one.
  - Débride the tendon of extraneous residual suture material or frayed edges so that these do not hang up on the leading edges of the pulleys.

Instrumentation

- When performed under direct vision, a no. 15 scalpel and pointed tenotomy scissors work admirably, depending on the density of the adhesions.
- Dissection within the scarred pulley system may require special instrumentation:
  - A 69 Beaver blade can be modified by bending it at 45 degrees to the flat surface.[36] This gives a comfortable angle for circumferential tendon dissection.
  - Knee arthroscopic blades are small and long enough to fit within the tendon sheath.[47]
  - A braided suture of 2-0 gauge or a dental wire may be used as a snare-saw to release adhesions between the dorsal aspect of the tendons and the phalanx and also between the two tendons.[1,2,13] Steady traction or a back-and-forth motion may separate the adhesions. Alternative methods of suture loop retrieval have been devised, such as a blunt elevator with a hole at its distal tip.
  - A Freer elevator may serve well as a "blind" dissector within the pulley system but is sometimes too large. A Cottle elevator (often retrieved from a rhinoplasty set) has a cobra head with a semicutting surface at one end. The working end of the Cottle elevators comes in different sizes, and this is an excellent instrument for working within the flexor tendon sheath (**TECH FIG 1**).

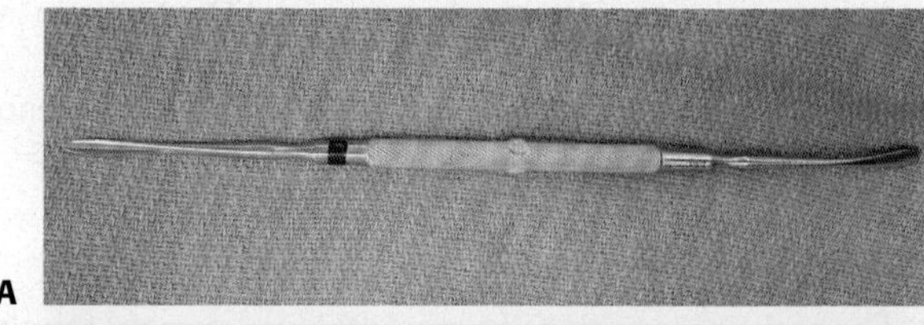

A

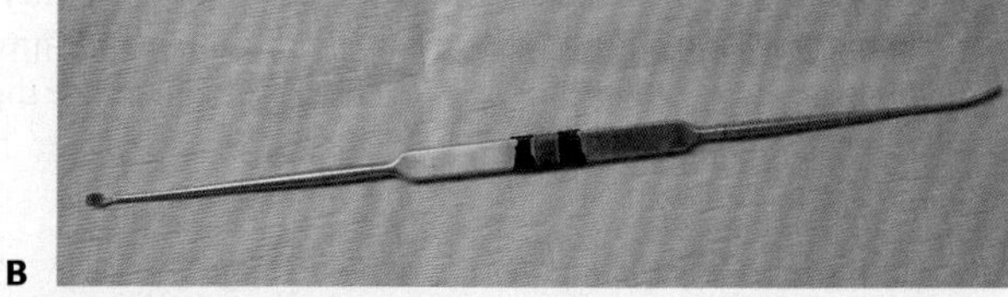

B

TECH FIG 1 • Elevators have working ends that are suitable for passing down the flexor tendon sheath. **A.** Freer. **B.** Cottle.

TECHNIQUES

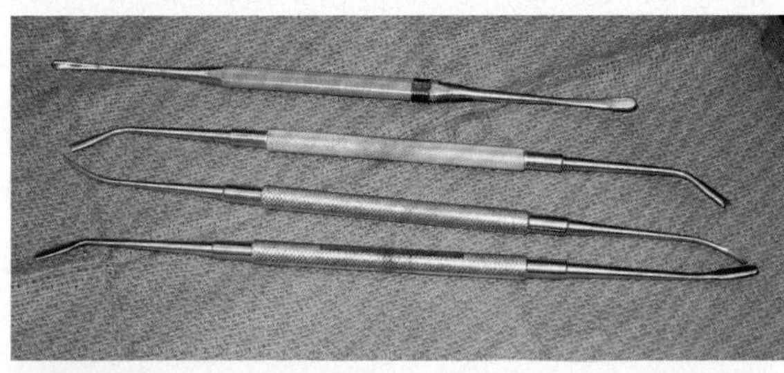

A

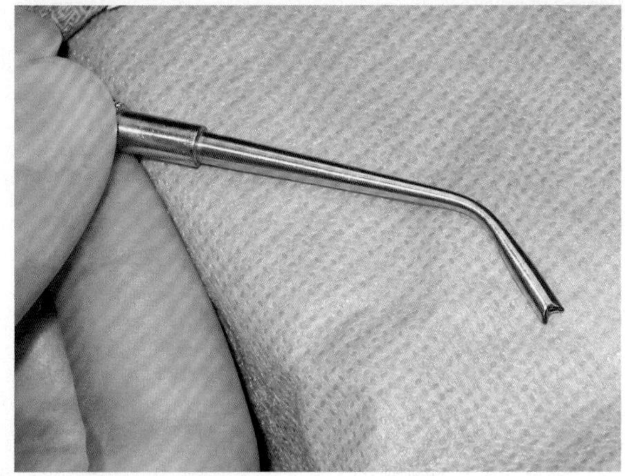

B

TECH FIG 2 • Tenolysis knives designed by Meals have semisharp blades and natural curvature that facilitate working within the digital flexor sheath. **A.** Overview. **B.** Close-up.

- There is a set of instruments specifically designed by Meals for flexor tenolysis within the flexor tendon sheath (George Tiemann & Co., Hauppauge, NY) (**TECH FIG 2**).[1] The necks of these tenolysis knives follow the natural curvature of the finger and they have semisharp blades that conform to the circumference of the tendon sheath with either a convex or concave edge (**TECH FIG 3**).

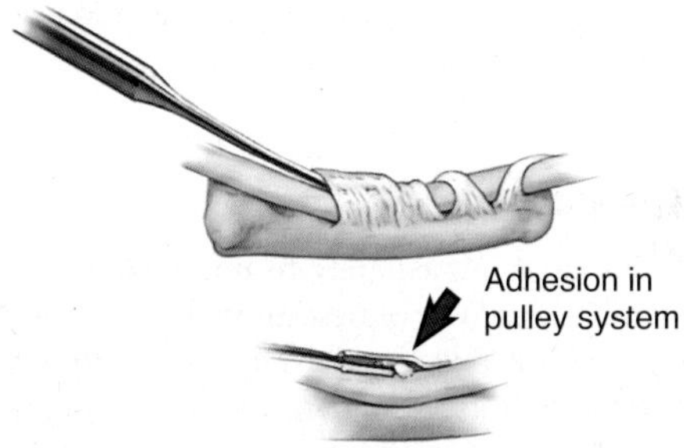

TECH FIG 3 • Diagram showing release of tendon adhesions within the flexor sheath using a Meals tenolysis knife.

Evaluation of Adequacy for Release

- Several techniques are available to assess the functional adequacy of the tenolysis and effective longitudinal tendon excursion:
  - If the patient is awake, active digital flexion reveals adequate finger motion.
  - Traction on the tendon at the distal and proximal ends of each intact pulley will reveal adequacy of segmental tendon releases within each part of the tunnel when "troubleshooting" to determine where adhesions may persist. Also check for adhesions deep to the distal insertion of the FDP, which may limit adequate active DIP flexion.
  - If the patient is not awake, then make a counterincision proximal to the release (in the palm or distal forearm) and apply traction with, for example, a blunt hook on each of the FDS and FDP tendons separately.[17] This traction should flex the finger down into the palm.

Closure

- If the tourniquet has not yet been released, it should be deflated before wound closure to ensure proper hemostasis. Postoperative hematoma and finger swelling will adversely affect postoperative recovery and function.
- Skin closure is accomplished with monofilament sutures that are strong enough to minimize the risk of wound disruption by early postoperative finger motion.
- Dressings should be absorbent but not confining to allow immediate range of finger motion.

PEARLS AND PITFALLS

Indications	■ Appropriate patient selection is as much a key to success as the procedure itself. An uncooperative patient and a patient who is too young or too frail and elderly to understand or adhere to the postoperative therapy may be unsuitable.
Intraoperative evaluation	■ Assess adequacy of tenolysis either by the flexion traction test in the forearm or have patient actively flex the fingers. ■ If there is a tendon gap filled with scar at the repair site, or more than half of the tendon width is missing, aborting tenolysis and grafting may be a better solution. ■ If critical pulleys are destroyed, consider pulley reconstruction and two-stage tendon repair.
Surgical technique	■ Start from the unscarred region and work into scarred areas. ■ Wide exposure of the flexor tendon sheath is necessary. ■ Initially, both flexor tendons are raised in a block. When possible, FDS and FDP should then be separated from each other. ■ Specially designed instruments may facilitate tenolysis within the confines of the pulley system. ■ If there is doubt about tendon integrity at the end of the procedure and if there is sufficient room, one can place a rod adjacent to the tendon. Then, if during the postoperative therapy the tendon were to rupture, only the second-stage graft pull-through would be necessary.[51]

POSTOPERATIVE CARE

- Hand therapy is initiated immediately to minimize the risk of repeat tendon adhesions. The tumescent wide awake local anesthesia technique gives a lasting sensory nerve block for many hours, enabling pain-free range of motion during this time period. A word of caution, however, for potential tendon rupture if the tendon is at all attenuated because gripping can be particularly forceful during this time in the absence of painful sensory feedback.
- This active range of motion is a crucial component of flexor tenolysis to retain the motion achieved during the operation.[13,14,52,59]
- Oral analgesics are generally sufficient to alleviate pain in the postoperative period, although some have recommended local sensory nerve block and installation of bupivacaine through intraoperatively placed catheters[27,52] to ensure freedom from pain and maintenance of the postoperative therapy protocol.
- If there are concerns about the tendon integrity, then a more cautious attitude may be indicated, perhaps even recourse to a protected mobilization protocol akin to primary flexor tendon repair, such as the "place and hold technique" or even a Kleinert rubber band brace.[49] These exercises attempt to maintain maximal tendon excursion but to minimize the tensile forces across a potentially weak tendon (**FIG 12**).
- Intraoperative findings should be discussed with the hand therapist and the specific protocol should be tailored accordingly.[9,50]
- Whatever protocol is initiated, exercises must be done on a routine by the patient and adhering to the prescribed frequency and number of repetitions.
- Blocking and strengthening exercises are added later, usually only after 4 to 6 weeks when they are considered to no longer endanger tendon integrity. Light resistance exercises are begun at 6 weeks, progressively adding more resistance after 8 weeks.[56]
- Protective splints may be prescribed if one is concerned about tendon or pulley integrity. A protective wrist and finger splint to keep the wrist slightly flexed and the MP joints flexed (as in primary tendon repair) may be initially recommended, with the patient coming out of the splint

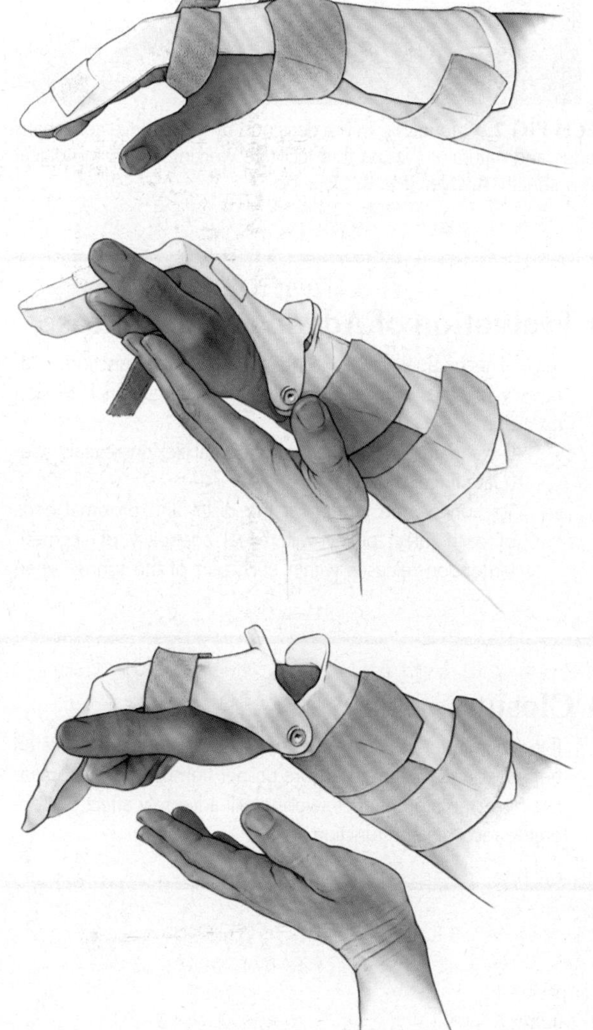

FIG 12 • Protective postoperative therapy may follow a modified Strickland protocol. The patient remains in a fixed brace at all times, except when performing place and hold exercises.

periodically to perform the exercises.[17] A fabricated external finger pulley ring may be used during active digital motion if pulleys are felt to be tenuous.[56]

- Static progressive or dynamic splints may be added if joint stiffness and contracture start to develop.
- Edema and swelling management are important, both by arm elevation and use of compressive gloves or compression taping from distal to proximal. Postoperative edema is an expected sequel of tenolysis and will hinder tendon gliding and joint movement.
- Continuous passive motion (CPM) is of questionable value because maximal tendon excursion requires active motion. However, it is of value for the uncooperative patient or if passive joint range of motion is limited. There have been reports of tendon rupture because of the force required to achieve passive range of motion.[50]

OUTCOMES

- One of the problems with outcomes is that various investigators use different measures for range of motion. The outcomes for tenolysis must take into account the preoperative and postoperative differences, the residual difference between passive and active range of motion, and the potential arc of motion lost through joint flexion contracture. Three of the more commonly used measures of total digital range of motion are as follows:
  - Total active motion (TAM). This takes into account the starting point of the motion that may be due to the flexion contracture. The formula used is TAM = (active flexion of MP + PIP + DIP) − (extension deficit of MP + PIP + DIP).
  - Potential active motion (PAM) takes into account the possible limits in passive range of motion (total passive motion or TPM): PAM = TAM / TPM.
  - In the Strickland formula, a comparison is drawn between the passive and active range of motion achieved with the procedure expressed as a percentage of the preoperative ranges: $[100 - (TPM_{pre} - TAM_{post} / TPM_{pre} - TAM_{pre})] \times 100$. Excellent is reported in 75% to 100%; good as 50% to 74%; fair, 25% to 49%; and poor, less than 24%.
- Strickland[50] reported that 64% of tenolysed digits after zone II injury had at least 50% improvement in active range of motion, 20% with no improvement, and 8% had tendon rupture.
- Jupiter and coauthors[24] used the Strickland formula for evaluation of 37 replanted digits following flexor tenolysis and reported good to excellent results in 24. Factors found to have a negative impact on results were injury classification (crush or avulsion), number of amputated digits, the need for capsulotomy, and inferior results for the thumb.
- Goloborod'ko[20] reported on 20 fingers evaluated between 6 and 12 months after surgery and in whom motion was started immediately after tenolysis. There were excellent results in 18, fair in 1, and poor in 1, with 3 sustaining tendon ruptures.
- Foucher and colleagues[17] reported on 78 digits (9 were thumbs) and excluded replantations. Active motion improved from 135 to 205 degrees in 84% of fingers. Four digits had no improvement and 9 were worse. There were two tendon ruptures. Thumbs achieved less success than fingers.
- There are few reports that deal exclusively with tenolysis in children. One such report concluded that substantial improvement in active flexion can be expected only in children older than 11 years of age.[3] They felt that without patient cooperation for hand therapy in a young child, inferior outcomes would otherwise result.

COMPLICATIONS

- The most common complication is failure to improve active range of motion. Range of motion may less commonly be actually worsened.
- Wound complications may occur, including flap necrosis, dehiscence, and infection. These wounds may be more prone to complications because of previous scarring and trauma and decreased skin vascularity with less pliable skin flaps. If these complications occur, they may further compromise the final range of motion achieved.
- Tendon rupture is relatively uncommon but may be a disastrous complication.
- Reflex sympathetic dystrophy is infrequently reported but again can lead to worse final functional outcome.
- Complications may potentially lead to staged tendon grafting, arthrodesis, or even amputation.

PREVENTION OF RECURRENCE

- A variety of options that inhibit scarring and adhesions may at first seem attractive, but they have met with mixed outcomes. These are divided into two groups:
  - Chemical agents: Some have advocated bathing the operative bed with a steroid solution, citing improved outcomes but acknowledging tendon and wound healing liabilities.[23,26,63]
  - Interpositional devices: Biologic and artificial membranes have been used as mechanical barriers to separate the tendon from adjacent tissues. These have included cellophane,[61] silicone sheeting,[25] amniotic membrane,[41] and hyaluronic acid derivatives.[41] We do not use these barrier devices. They may function as a foreign body and may hinder revascularization and have met with mixed results.[5] One study significantly improved results for tenolysis in a randomly controlled study that evaluated a hyaluronan-based gel that was used intraoperatively.[45]

REFERENCES

1. Azari KK, Meals RA. Flexor tenolysis. Hand Clin 2005;21:211–217.
2. Bain GI, Allen BD, Berger AC. Flexor tenolysis using a free suture. Tech Hand Up Extrem Surg 2003;7:61–62.
3. Birnie RH, Idler RS. Flexor tenolysis in children. J Hand Surg Am 1995;20:254–257.
4. Bissell JH. Clinical perspectives: therapeutic modalities in hand surgery. J Hand Surg 1999;24:435–448.
5. Bora FW Jr, Lane JM, Prockop DJ. Inhibitors of collagen biosynthesis as a means of controlling scar formation and tendon injury. J Bone Joint Surg Am 1972;54:1501–1508.
6. Brand PW, Hollister A. Clinical Mechanics of the Hand, ed 2. St. Louis: Mosby, 1993:70–78.
7. Bruner JM. The zig-zag volar-digital incision for flexor tendon surgery. Plast Reconstr Surg 1967;40:571–574.
8. Buckwalter JA. The effects of early motion on healing of musculoskeletal tissues. Hand Clin 1996;12:13–24.
9. Cannon NM, Strickland JW. Therapy following flexor tendon surgery. Hand Clin 1985;1:147–165.

10. Curtis RM. Stiff finger joints. In: Grabb WC, Smith JW, eds. Plastic Surgery, ed 3. Boston: Little, Brown, 1979:598–603.
11. Doyle JR. Anatomy of the flexor tendon sheath and pulley system: a current review. J Hand Surg Am 1989;14:349–351.
12. Eaton RG. The extensor mechanism of the fingers. Bull Hosp Joint Dis 1969;30:39–47.
13. Eggli S, Dietsche A, Eggli S, et al. Tenolysis after combined digital injuries in zone II. Ann Plast Surg 2005;55:266–271.
14. Feldscher SB, Schneider LH. Flexor tenolysis. Hand Surg 2002;7(1):61–74.
15. Fetrow KO. Tenolysis in the hand and wrist. A clinical evaluation of two hundred and twenty flexor and extensor tenolyses. J Bone Joint Surg Am 1967;49:667–685.
16. Fong KD, Trindade MC, Wang Z, et al. Microarray analysis of mechanical shear effects on flexor tendon cells. Plast Reconstr Surg 2005;116:1393–1404.
17. Foucher G, Lenoble E, Ben Youssef K, et al. A post-operative regime after digital flexor tenolysis. A series of 72 patients. J Hand Surg Br 1993;18:35–40.
18. Gelberman RH, Manske PR. Factors influencing flexor tendon adhesions. Hand Clin 1985;1:35–42.
19. Gelberman RH, Woo SLY. The physiological basis for application of controlled stress in the rehabilitation of flexor tendon injuries. J Hand Ther 1989;2:66–70.
20. Goloborod'ko SA. Postoperative management of flexor tenolysis. J Hand Ther 1999;12:330–332.
21. Higgins A, Lalonde DH, Bell M, et al. Avoiding flexor tendon repair rupture with intraoperative total active movement examination. Plast Reconstr Surg 2010;126:941–945.
22. Hitchcock TF, Light TR, Bunch WH, et al. The effect of immediate constrained digital motion on the strength of flexor tendon repairs in chickens. J Hand Surg Am 1987;12:590–595.
23. James J. The use of cortisone in tenolysis. J Bone Joint Surg 1959; 41:209–210.
24. Jupiter JB, Pess GM, Bour CJ. Results of flexor tendon tenolysis after replantation in the hand. J Hand Surg Am 1989;14:35–44.
25. Karakurum G, Buyukbebeci O, Kalender M, et al. Seprafilm interposition for preventing adhesion formation after tenolysis. An experimental study on the chicken flexor tendons. J Surg Res 2003;113:195–200.
26. Ketchum LD, Martin NL, Kappel DA. Experimental evaluation of factors affecting the strength of tendon repairs. Plast Reconstr Surg 1977;59:708–719.
27. Kirchoff R, Jensen PV, Nielsen NS, et al. Repeated digital nerve block for pain control after tenolysis. Scand J Plast Reconstr Surg Hand Surg 2000;34:257–258.
28. Kleinert HE, Kutz JE, Ashbell TS, et al. Primary repair of lacerated flexor tendons in "no man's land." J Bone Joint Surg Am 1967;49:577.
29. Lalonde DH. Wide-awake flexor tendon repair. Plast Reconstr Surg 2009;123:623–625.
30. Laseter GF. Management of the stiff hand: a practical approach. Orthop Clin North Am 1983;14:749–765.
31. Lilly SI, Messer TM. Complications after treatment of flexor tendon injuries. J Am Acad Orthop Surg 2006;14:387–396.
32. Littler JW. The finger extensor mechanism. Surg Clin North Am 1967;47:415–432.
33. Littler JW. Principles of reconstructive surgery of the hand. In: Converse JM, ed. Reconstructive Plastic Surgery. Philadelphia: WB Saunders, 1964:1612–1632.
34. Littler JW, Eaton RG. Redistribution of forces in correction of boutonniere deformity. J Bone Joint Surg Am 1967;49:1267–1274.
35. Lundborg G, Rank F. Experimental studies on cellular mechanisms involved in healing of animal and human flexor tendon in synovial environment. Hand 1980;12:3–11.
36. McDonough JJ, Stern PJ. Modified 69 blade for tenolysis. J Hand Surg Am 1983;8:610–611.
37. Menon J, Frykman G, Swann OJ. Role of synovial fluid cells in the healing of flexor tendons. Clin Orthop Relat Res 1985;199:300–305.
38. Mitsionis G, Fischer KJ, Bastidas JA, et al. Feasibility of partial A2 and A4 pulley excision: residual pulley strength. J Hand Surg Br 2000;25:90–94.
39. Moran SL, Ryan CK, Orlando GS, et al. Effects of 5-fluorouracil on flexor tendon repair. J Hand Surg Am 2000;25:242–251.
40. Pennington DG. The influence of tendon sheath integrity and vascular blood supply on adhesion formation following tendon repair in hens. Br J Plast Surg 1979;32:302–306.
41. Pinkerton M. Amnioplastin for adherent digital flexor tendons. Lancet 1942;239:70–72.
42. Potenza AD. Critical evaluation of flexor tendon healing and adhesion formation without artificial tendon sheaths: an experimental study. J Bone Joint Surg Am 1963;45:1217–1233.
43. Potenza AD. Prevention of adhesion to healing digital flexor tendons. JAMA 1964;187:187–191.
44. Pruitt DI, Tanaka H, Aoki M, et al. Cyclic stress testing after in vivo healing of canine flexor tendon lacerations. J Hand Surg Am 1996;21:974–977.
45. Riccio M, Battiston B, Pajardi G, et al. Efficiency of Hyaloglide in the prevention of the recurrence of adhesions after tenolysis of flexor tendons in zone II: a randomized, controlled, multicentre clinical trial. J Hand Surg Eur Vol 2010;35(2):130–138.
46. Schneider LH. Tenolysis and capsulectomy after hand fractures. Clin Orthop Relat Res 1996;(327):72–78.
47. Schreiber DR. Arthroscopic blades in flexor tenolysis of the hand. J Hand Surg Am 1986;11:144–145.
48. Seradge H. Elongation of the repair configuration following flexor tendon repair. J Hand Surg Am 1983;8:182–185.
49. Strickland JW. Development of flexor tendon surgery: twenty-five years of progress. J Hand Surg Am 2000;25:214–235.
50. Strickland JW. Flexor tendon injuries. Part 5. Flexor tenolysis, rehabilitation and results. Orthop Rev 1987;16:137–153.
51. Strickland JW. Flexor tendon surgery. Part 2: free tendon grafts and tenolysis. J Hand Surg Br 1989;14:368–382.
52. Strickland JW. Flexor tenolysis. Hand Clin 1985;1:121–132.
53. Sugun TS. Validity of ultrasonography in surgically treated zone 2 flexor tendon injuries. Acta Orthop Traumatol Turc 2010;44(6): 452–457.
54. Tang JB. Clinical outcomes associated with flexor tendon repair. Hand Clin 2005;21:199–210.
55. Taras JS, Kaufmann RA. Flexor tendon reconstruction. In: Green DP, Hotchkiss RN, Pederson WC, et al, eds. Green's Operative Hand Surgery, ed 5. Philadelphia: Elsevier Churchill Livingstone, 2005: 241–276.
56. Trumble TE, Sailer SM. Flexor tendon injuries. In: Trumble TE, ed. Principles of Hand Surgery and Therapy. Philadelphia: WB Saunders, 2000:231–262.
57. Tsubone T, Moran SL, Amadio PC, et al. Expression of growth factors in canine flexor tendon after maceration in vivo. Ann Plast Surg 2004;53:393–397.
58. Verdan C. Tenolysis. In: Verdan C, ed. Tendon Surgery of the Hand. Edinburgh: Churchill Livingstone, 1979:137–142.
59. Vucekovich K, Gallardo G, Fiala K. Rehabilitation after flexor tendon repair, reconstruction, and tenolysis. Hand Clin 2005;21(2):257–265.
60. Wang H. Secondary surgery after digit replantation: its incidence and sequence. Microsurgery 2002;22:57–61.
61. Wheeldon C. The use of cellophane as a permanent tendon sheath. J Bone Joint Surg Am 1939;21:393–396.
62. Wray RC Jr, Moucharafieh B, Weeks PM. Experimental study of the optimal time for tenolysis. Plast Reconstr Surg 1978;61:184–189.
63. Wrenn RN, Goldner JL, Markee JL. An experimental study of the effect of cortisone on the healing process and tensile strength of tendons. J Bone Joint Surg Am 1954;36-A(3):588–601.
64. Yamazaki H, Kato H, Uchiyama S, et al. Results of tenolysis for flexor tendon adhesion after phalangeal fracture. J Hand Surg Eur Vol 2008;33(5):557–560.
65. Zhang AY, Pham H, Ho F, et al. Inhibition of TGF-beta-induced collagen production in rabbit flexor tendons. J Hand Surg Am 2004;29:230–255.
66. Zhau C, Amadio PC, Zobitz ME, et al. Resection of the flexor digitorum superficialis reduces gliding resistance after zone II flexor digitorum profundus repair in vitro. J Hand Surg Am 2002;27:316–321.

Staged Digital Flexor Tendon Reconstruction

CHAPTER 80

Sebastian C. Peers and Kevin J. Malone

DEFINITION

- Staged flexor tendon reconstruction is required in the settings of delayed diagnosis of a flexor digitorum profundus (FDP) and flexor digitorum superficialis (FDS) disruption or failed previous attempt at primary repair within zone II of the digital tendon sheath.
- During the first stage of the reconstruction process, a silicone rod is placed within the flexor tendon sheath. The role of this implant is to help reestablish a frictionless inner lining of the sheath that will accommodate the placement of a tendon graft in the second stage.

ANATOMY

- Flexor tendons can be divided into five zones (**FIG 1A**).
- Bunnell originally described the region between the A1 pulley and the FDS insertion, zone II, as "no man's land" because the initial results after attempted primary tendon repair were so poor he felt that no one should attempt this procedure.
- In the limited confines of zone II, the two flexor tendons function together and rely on the digital sheath and its frictionless synovial interface for gliding and proper function.
- Another complicating anatomic characteristic of zone II is the chiasm of Camper. Here, FDP passes through the slips of FDS, creating another potential region for adhesions (**FIG 1B**).

PATHOGENESIS

- Zone II has the highest probability of developing adhesions and the poorest prognosis after repair.
- Violation of the sheath, the lining, or the blood supply to the tendons by trauma or infection may lead to dense scar and adhesion formation and can compromise the results after either a primary repair or an attempt at single-stage reconstruction with a tendon graft.[1]

NATURAL HISTORY

- Flexor tendon injuries that are not reconstructed can progress to a stiff and sometimes painful digit.
- If both tendons are not functional, no active proximal interphalangeal (PIP) or distal interphalangeal (DIP) motion will be possible, but if only the FDP tendon is disrupted, active PIP flexion will be present.
- If a digit with incompetent flexor tendons is subjected to repeated extension stress, as in pinch, the volar supporting structures will become lax over time, leading to hyperextension and an unstable joint.

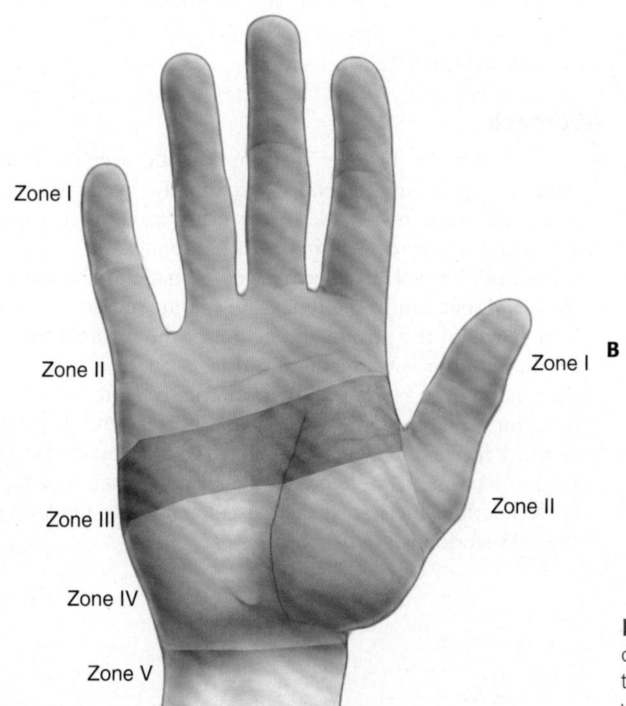

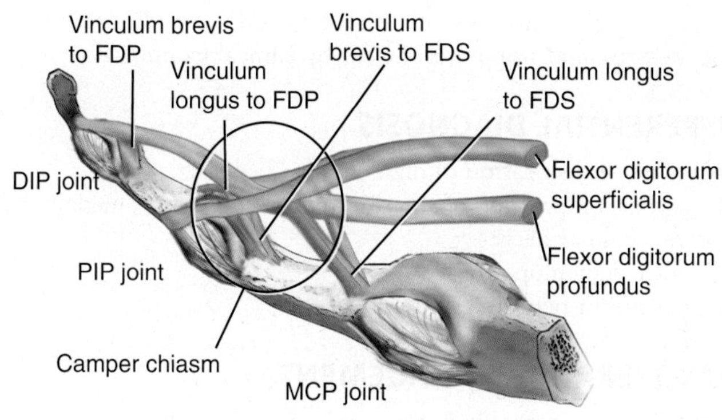

FIG 1 • **A.** The five flexor tendon zones of injury. **B.** The decussation of the flexor digitorum sublimus produces the chiasm of Camper. Both the flexor digitorum sublimus and FDP receive their blood supply via the vinculum longus and brevis.

PATIENT HISTORY AND PHYSICAL FINDINGS

- The examiner should elicit information about the initial injury, such as when it occurred and if there were associated injuries (fractures, laceration of digital nerves or vessels).
- The examiner should determine when the patient first noticed a decrease in the function of the digit (if flexor tendon repair has already been attempted).
- Staged flexor tendon reconstruction is contraindicated in the setting of an active infection, and for that reason, an infection history must be sought.
  - If an infection is identified, it should be treated aggressively with antibiotics and débridement to minimize the destruction of the flexor tendon sheath from the inflammatory process.
- Tests for tendon function include the following:
  - Finger cascade: Loss of the normal cascade suggests disruption or loss of function of the flexor tendons.
  - FDP examination: Loss of active DIP flexion suggests disruption or loss of FDP function.
  - FDS examination: Loss of active PIP flexion suggests disruption or loss of FDS function.
  - Tenodesis effect: Loss of the tenodesis effect suggests disruption of the flexor tendons.
- It is also important to assess the vascular supply and the digital sensation to determine if there is a concomitant injury to the digital neurovascular structures.
- Both active and passive range of motion must be recorded for the metacarpophalangeal (MP), PIP, and DIP joints.
  - If contractures are present, as evidenced by decreased passive joint motion, intensive therapy should be initiated before proceeding with staged flexor tendon reconstruction.

IMAGING AND OTHER DIAGNOSTIC STUDIES

- Radiographs should be obtained to rule out fractures or other associated injuries to the hand and digits.
- Ultrasound or magnetic resonance imaging (MRI) can be used to help localize the site of tendon rupture and position of the proximal stump if not clear by clinical examination.

DIFFERENTIAL DIAGNOSIS

- Fracture or dislocation of digits
- Proximal compression of anterior interosseous nerve, median nerve, or ulnar nerve
- Cervical radiculopathy
- Upper motor neuron lesion

NONOPERATIVE MANAGEMENT

- There is no acceptable nonoperative management for combined FDS and FDP tendon lacerations. Alternatives to staged flexor tendon reconstruction include arthrodesis and amputation.
- Isolated chronic disruption of the FDP tendon with an intact FDS tendon is best treated nonoperatively. Attempts at reconstruction of the FDP tendon risk function of the FDS tendon.
- Buddy taping or trapping of the injured finger by an adjacent figure during finger flexion may allow concealment of the functional deficit between stage 1 and stage 2 or in the patient who is not a candidate for staged tendon reconstruction.

SURGICAL MANAGEMENT

- Indications for two-stage flexor tendon reconstruction include the following:
  - Loss of FDP and FDS
  - Protective sensation
  - Nearly full passive range of motion
  - Good-quality skin in the region of zone II
  - A cooperative patient willing to participate fully in rehabilitation
- The patient will need to have access to a good hand therapist before and after each of the stages of this complex reconstructive process.

Preoperative Planning

- For the second stage of the procedure, a tendon must be harvested to use for the reconstruction. Often, a palmaris longus graft is used. If the patient does not have a palmaris longus, then a long toe extensor or plantaris tendon can be used. In this situation, the lower extremity must also be prepared out into the surgical field.
- As an alternative to a traditional free tendon graft, the proximal end of the lacerated FDS may be used as graft. Paneva-Holevich[7] first described this technique in 1965. It has since been refined and is described as the modified Paneva-Holevich technique[6] in this chapter. If this technique is selected, the proximal tendon stumps of FDS and FDP are sutured together in the shape of a "loop" during the first stage.

Positioning

- For both stages of the procedure, the patient is placed supine on the operating table with the arm abducted on a hand table. A nonsterile tourniquet is placed around the upper arm for hemostasis.

Approach

- Stage 1: A volar Brunner incision is made over the flexor tendon sheath and extended proximally into the palm. A second incision is made in the distal forearm to ensure placement of the rod within the carpal tunnel.
- Stage 2: A limited Brunner incision is made at the level of the distal junction of the repair. A separate incision is made at the level of the proximal junction of the repair. This can be the same incision in the distal forearm as in stage 1 if the tendon graft is long enough. Alternatively, the proximal junction will be in the palm with shorter tendon grafts. A third incision or set of incisions will be made for the tendon harvest. If the modified Paneva-Holevich technique is used, a third incision at the musculotendinous junction of the FDS tendon is used.

Stage 1

- A volar Brunner incision is made over the course of the flexor tendons.
- The flexor tendon sheath is incised, taking care to preserve the A2 and A4 pulleys. L-shaped flaps can be made within the flexor sheath to aid in access to the flexor tendons and protect the A2 and A4 pulleys (**TECH FIG 1A**).
- The scarred tendon is excised, leaving a portion of the distal stump of the FDP intact at its insertion.
  - This is useful in securing the tendon rod in stage 1 and the tendon graft in stage 2.
- If a digital nerve laceration is identified, it should be repaired at this stage.
- Release any adhesions within the sheath.
- Release any flexion contractures of the joints by releasing the volar plate and accessory collateral ligaments.
  - Be sure to preserve the proper collateral ligaments.
- If the A2 or A4 pulleys are absent or have been excised with the scar release, they need to be reconstructed. A tendon graft can be used to reconstruct the pulleys (**TECH FIG 1B**).
  - The tendon should be passed between the proximal phalanx and the extensor tendon for A2 reconstruction.
  - For A4 reconstruction, the tendon can be passed dorsal to the extensor tendon.
- A silicone Hunter rod is inserted into the sheath. Distally, it is secured to the remnant of the FDP tendon with nonabsorbing suture.
  - If there is not enough of the tendon remnant, it can be secured to surrounding tissue at the base of the distal phalanx.
  - Some Hunter rods can be secured using a screw placed in the distal phalanx.
- Proximally, the silicone rod is passed through the carpal tunnel and allowed to glide free with the flexor tendons in the distal forearm (**TECH FIG 1C**).
- All skin incisions are closed with 4-0 nylon after ensuring hemostasis.
- The patient is then placed into a dorsal blocking splint holding the fingers into an intrinsic plus posture.
- Rehabilitation is started early after surgery, often within 1 week, to ensure that the patient regains full passive range of motion. The scar tissue must be soft and supple before the patient is scheduled for the second stage of tendon reconstruction. On average, this takes 3 months.

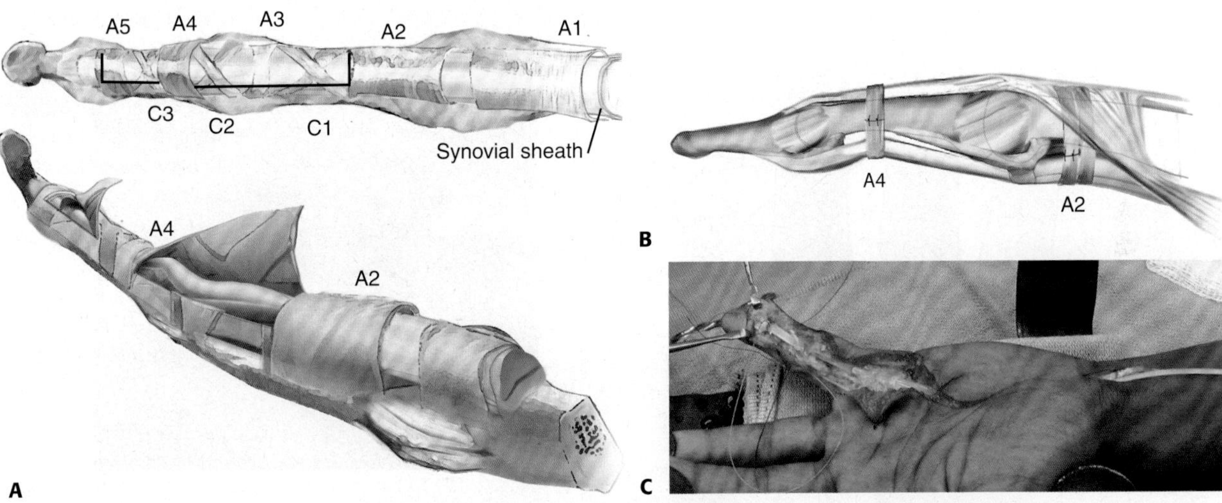

TECH FIG 1 • **A.** Creating an L-shaped flap can aid in accessing the underlying flexor sheath contents while preserving the important A2 and A4 pulleys. **B.** Tendon weaves for reconstruction of A2 and A4 pulleys. **C.** A passive silicone implant running under A2 and A4 pulleys is secured distally to the FDP stump and extends proximally to the distal forearm.

Stage 2

Incisions and Graft Harvest

- A limited Brunner incision is made distally at the level of the DIP joint so that the distal FDP stump can be located within the sheath. The sutures securing the silicone rod to the profundus stump are released.
  - Do not extend the incision or dissection into zone II, as this will compromise the reestablished tendon sheath that has been created by the body's reaction to the silicone rod.
- A second incision is made in the distal forearm so that the proximal portion of the silicone rod can be localized.
- A third set of incisions is then made for tendon graft harvest. This is typically from the palmaris longus, long toe extensor, or plantaris tendon (**TECH FIG 2**).
  - Plantaris often makes the best donor if a long segment of tendon is needed.

Graft Placement

- The tendon graft is then sutured to the proximal end of the silicone rod. The silicone rod is then retrieved from the distal wound, pulling the tendon graft into the tendon sheath (**TECH FIG 3A**).

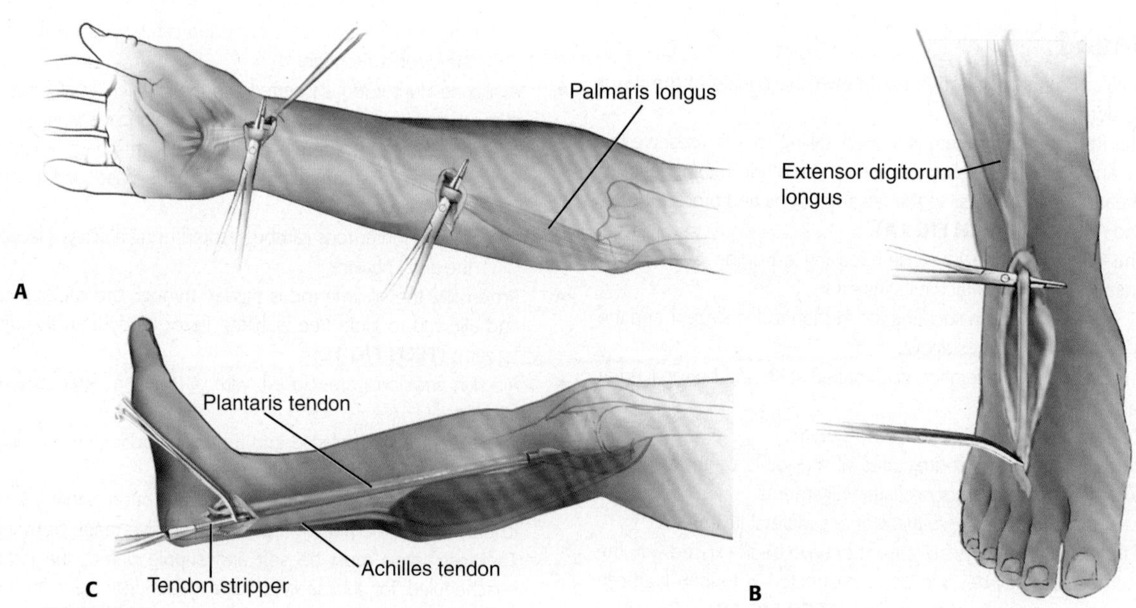

TECH FIG 2 • **A.** Technique for harvesting palmaris longus tendon graft. **B.** Technique for harvesting long toe extensor tendon graft. **C.** Technique for harvesting plantaris tendon graft.

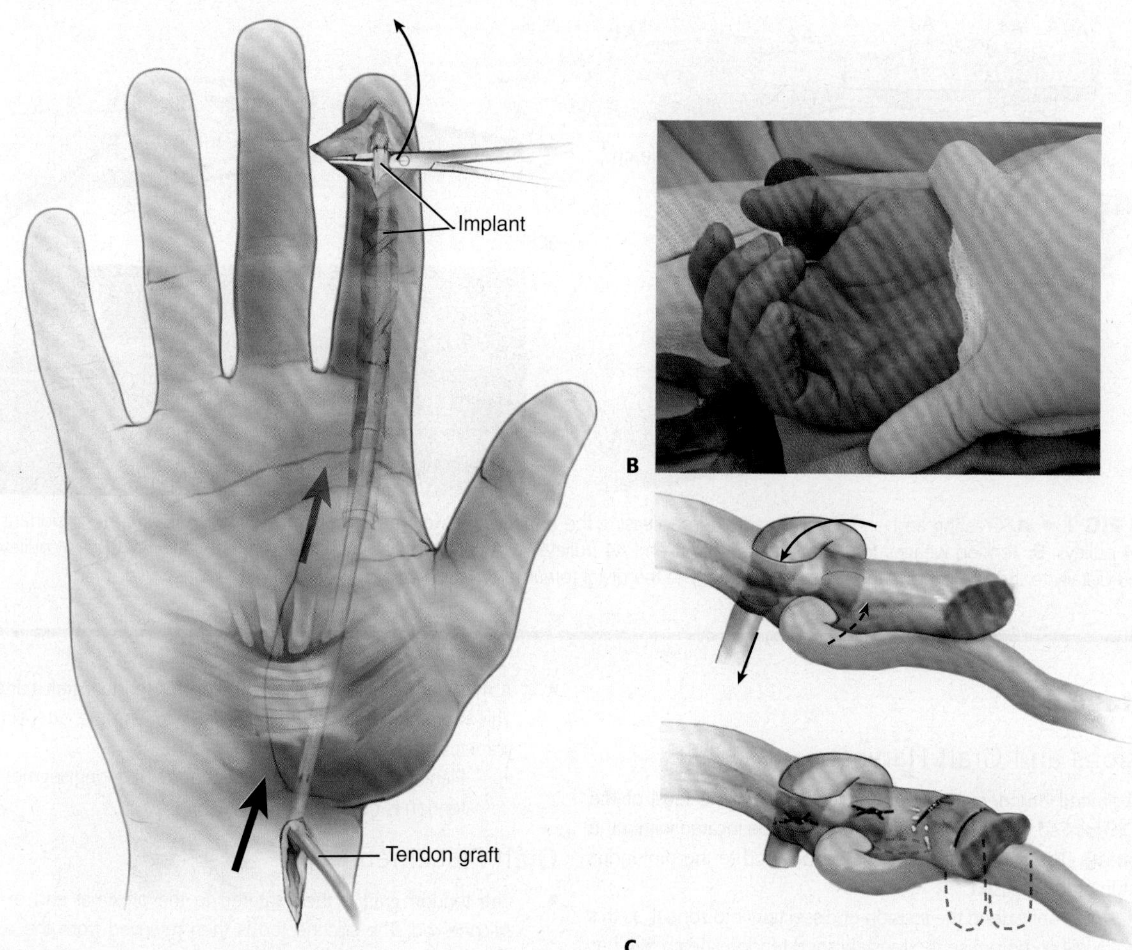

TECH FIG 3 • **A.** Technique for using the silicone rod to draw the tendon graft into the flexor tendon sheath and out through the distal incision. **B.** Recreation of the normal finger cascade. **C.** A Pulvertaft weave is used for the proximal junction between the tendon graft and the FDP or FDS in the forearm.

- The distal end of the tendon graft is secured to the distal phalanx with bone anchors. The anchors should be inserted in the footprint of the FDP stump and angled slightly proximally. The proximal angle will ensure that the anchor stays within the bone rather than penetrating the dorsal cortex. It is important to ensure that the anchor does not penetrate the DIP.
  - Alternatively, the tendon graft can be secured to the distal phalanx with a pullout suture tied over the nail, as in a zone I flexor tendon repair. This has been associated with deformities to the nail after suture removal and has no proven biomechanical advantage over suture anchors.
  - Additional fixation can be provided by using the remaining FDP stump and securing this to the tendon graft with a nonabsorbable suture in figure-8 fashion.
- The distal incision is closed at this point. It will become difficult to gain access to this incision after graft tension is set.
- Tendon graft tension is set from the proximal wound. The correct amount of tension is determined with the wrist in a neutral posture and is set by evaluating digital flexion cascade (**TECH FIG 3B**).
  - It may be wise to exaggerate the cascade slightly so that as the graft relaxes and lengthens, the normal flexion cascade is created.
  - If the cascade is significantly exaggerated, however, a quadriga effect will result.
- The proximal end of the tendon graft is then woven into the proximal recipient tendon stump with a Pulvertaft weave (**TECH FIG 3C**).
  - The recipient stump proximally can be either the FDS or the FDP to the injured finger. If the initial injury is more than a few months old, the muscle belly of the injured FDP or FDS may be atrophic or scarred proximally in the forearm, which would limit postoperative results. In this setting, the recipient tendon can be a side-to-side anastomosis to the neighboring FDP, which will provide the appropriate excursion.
- All skin incisions are closed after ensuring hemostasis. The patient is then placed into a dorsal blocking splint with the wrist slightly flexed and the MP and interphalangeal (IP) joints flexed.
- Rehabilitation is started within a few days (see Postoperative Care).

Tenolysis

- This is often necessary after stage 2 of tendon reconstruction. Tenolysis is indicated when passive range of motion is greater than active range of motion. This surgery should not be performed until 3 to 6 months after stage 2.
- The tendon must be exposed within zone II of the tendon sheath and tenolysis performed within the flexor sheath, taking care to preserve the A2 and A4 pulleys. If residual resistance is noted after tenolysis in the finger, an additional incision may be made at the level of the proximal junction to address any adhesions at that level.
- Immediate hand therapy must be initiated postoperatively and can be easier on the patient if a wrist block is performed with a long-acting local anesthetic to preserve motor function while producing an effective sensory block.

Alternative to Stage 1

- The silicone rod that we use is considered "passive" and has no attachment to the proximal flexor motor.
- An "active" alternative exists in which the rod can be secured to the tendon proximally and function as a graft. This can eliminate the need for stage 2 (**TECH FIG 4**).
- These implants have been associated with a higher rate of complication in the limited number of studies that have examined them.

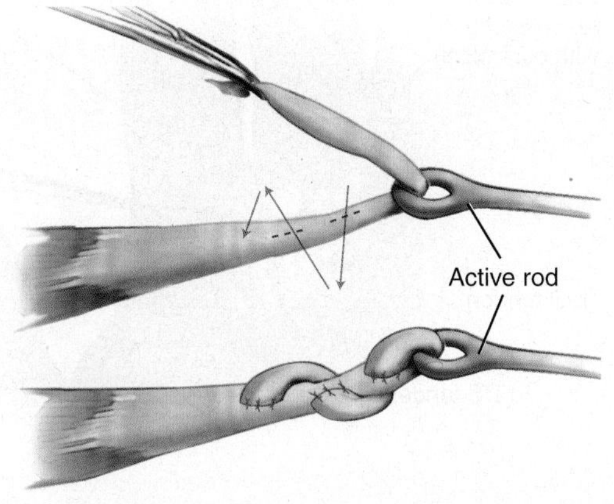

TECH FIG 4 • In an active tendon rod, the motor tendon is looped through the ring in the proximal rod, woven through itself, and fixed with nonabsorbable suture so that active motion can be performed.

Modified Paneva-Holevich Technique

- This technique uses the proximal end of the lacerated FDS tendon as graft. It also allows the proximal tenorrhaphy to heal prior to the second stage of the reconstruction.
- The first stage begins in a similar fashion to the traditional first stage reconstruction.
  - A volar Brunner incision is made, the tendons distal to the laceration are débrided, any necessary contracture releases are performed, the pulleys are addressed, and the rods are placed as previously described.

- It is important to note that hunter rod selection can be tailored to the size of the FDS tendon. When between two sizes, select the larger size hunter rod.
- A loop between FDS and FDP is created at the level of the lumbrical origin. Creating the loop at the lumbrical origin ensures that there will be no impingement with the A1 pulley once motion is allowed after the second stage. A fresh blade is used to cut the FDP and FDS tendons at this level. The freshly cut ends of FDS and FDP are sutured together in an end-to-end fashion using core sutures. The result is a loop of tendon (**TECH FIG 5**).
- The tourniquet is released, hemostasis is obtained, and the wound is closed in standard fashion as previously described.
- A postoperative dorsal blocking splint is applied and postoperative rehabilitation is initiated as in the traditional first stage.
- A minimum interval of 3 months is allowed before the second stage. The tenorrhaphy between FDS and FDP heals during this time.
- The second stage begins by opening the volar incision in the palm and identifying the healed loop tenorrhaphy and the proximal end of the hunter rod.
- The FDS tendon is released from its muscle belly proximally. This is done through a small incision in the forearm at the musculotendinous junction. Care is taken to identify the correct FDS tendon by pulling traction proximally and observing the loop distally.
- The proximal FDS tendon is delivered into the palmar wound by pulling traction on the tendon loop.
- The distal end of the FDS tendon graft is sutured to the proximal end of the hunter rod. The incision over the native FDP insertion is opened, and the distal end of the hunter rod is identified. The hunter rod is used to deliver the graft into the distal most incision.
- The native FDP footprint is identified, and any soft tissue is removed.
- Tension on the graft is evaluated. Tension can be estimating by temporarily fixing the graft to the FDP insertion to the surrounding skin and soft tissue using a small hypodermic needle. Stance of the digit and tenodesis effect is evaluated and tension can be adjusted as necessary. Overtensioning is preferable to undertensioning; however, significant overtensioning will result in quadriga.
- Once proper tension is established, the tendon is marked at the insertion and excess tendon is removed using a fresh blade.
- The FDP footprint is prepared and the tendon is secured to the native FDP insertion using bone anchors or a pullout suture as previously described in the traditional second stage.
- Wound closure and application of a dorsal blocking splint are performed in the same way as in a traditional second stage procedure.
- Postoperative rehabilitation is identical to traditional second stage rehabilitation. Theoretically, because the proximal tenorrhaphy is already healed, more aggressive therapy could be considered.
- Advantages of this technique include FDS is a synovial tendon graft, FDS is a better size-matched graft, it is easier to size match hunter rod size, it is easy to find the tendon loop after stage two, there is decreased risk of failure after stage two because the proximal tendon-to-tendon junction is already healed, more aggressive postoperative therapy may be used, and this procedure is easily converted to a traditional two-stage reconstruction.
- The disadvantage of this technique is that it is more difficult to judge and adjust tension of the repair at the distal tendon-to-bone junction. The traditional reconstruction easily allows tension to be adjusted as it is done through the proximal Pulvertaft weave.

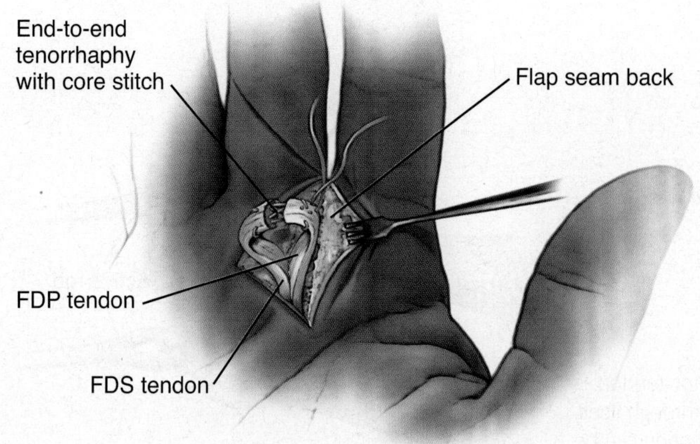

TECH FIG 5 • FDS and FDP are identified through a Brunner incision. They are divided at the level of the lumbrical origin on FDP. They are sutured together in an end-to-end fashion using a core suture.

PEARLS AND PITFALLS

Pulley preservation	■ Both the A2 and A4 pulleys must be maintained or reconstructed at stage 1 to prevent bowstringing and maximize the amount of active flexion (**FIG 2**; see **TECH FIG 1B**).

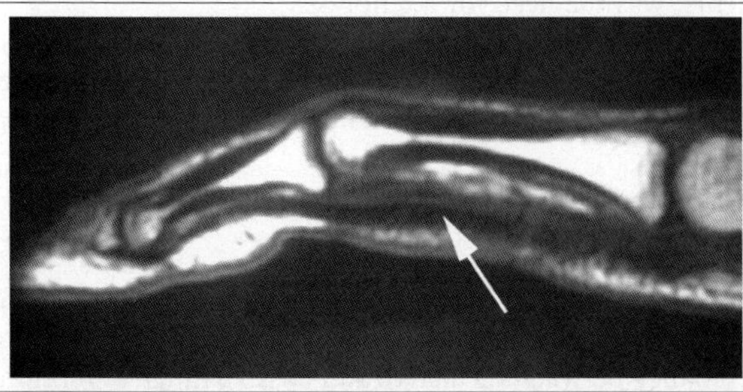

FIG 2 ● Sagittal MRI showing bowstringing of a flexor tendon (*arrow*) over the proximal phalanx due to an incompetent A2 pulley.

Full passive range of motion	■ Full passive range of motion should be achieved before stage 1 and again before stage 2. Less than maximum passive range of motion preoperatively will markedly worsen the functional result after stage 2.
Finger cascade	■ Establishing the correct cascade with the appropriate amount of tension on the tendon graft in stage 2 is important. The graft will likely relax and lengthen as the patient goes through rehabilitation. A slight exaggeration of the cascade at the time of surgery may ultimately produce the normal cascade as the tendon graft lengthens. Gross exaggeration of the cascade, however, will produce a quadriga effect. The uninjured digits will be less than fully flexed when the injured digit has reached full flexion in the palm (**FIG 3**).
Hand therapy	■ A good therapist and a motivated patient are critical for a good outcome for this surgery.

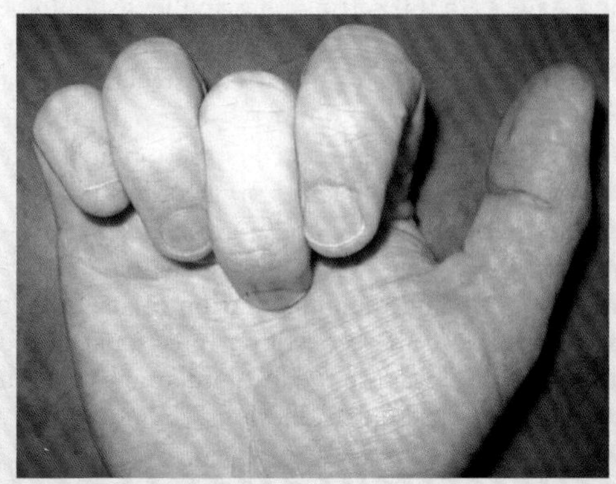

FIG 3 ● Clinical photograph of the quadriga effect. The long finger, in which the FDP has been repaired with too much tension, is maximally flexed into the palm and the adjacent fingers cannot be actively flexed further.

POSTOPERATIVE CARE

- The pre- and postoperative hand therapy is perhaps the most important component of this reconstruction procedure.
  - Patients must be motivated and compliant.
  - Therapists must be knowledgeable.
- Before stage 1 and stage 2, the patient must have nearly full passive range of motion and a soft tissue envelope that will accommodate the subsequent stages of the process.
- Stage 1 postoperative therapy is initiated within 48 hours and continues until the patient is ready for stage 2.
  - If pulley reconstruction was performed, the therapist can make ring splints for the patient to wear to protect the pulleys.
- In general, the patient needs to be monitored for signs of infection. Edema should be controlled with elevation and compressive dressings as needed.
- A custom splint is used when not exercising. This splint should hold the injured fingers in an intrinsic-plus posture, with the MP joints in 70 degrees of flexion and the IP joints held in full extension. The wrist is held at neutral.
- Passive range of motion of all involved digits is initiated, with emphasis on obtaining full composite flexion and full PIP extension.
- Active range-of-motion exercises are also used to establish full active extension of all digits and full flexion of the uninvolved digits. Buddy taping can be employed to facilitate motion of the operated digit.
- The protocol for postoperative therapy after stage 2 is as follows:
  - Zero to 3 weeks postoperatively
    - Precautions: no active finger flexion, no passive finger extension
    - The patient is splinted with a dorsal extension block splint holding the involved digits in an intrinsic-plus posture and the wrist at neutral. The splint should be worn at all times.
    - Therapist-directed exercises begin with passive flexion and active extension in the splint. The PIP and DIP joints are secured to the splint in extension between exercise sessions.
    - Wound care and edema control are also incorporated, and the patient must be observed for signs of infection.

- Three to 6 weeks postoperatively
  - Precautions: monitor closely for PIP flexion contractures, no passive finger extension, no splint removal
  - Active range of motion is initiated with "place and hold" exercises and progressed to full active range-of-motion exercises by 4 weeks after surgery while still in the splint.
  - Once the surgical wounds have healed, soft tissue massage should be incorporated to soften the volar tissues.
- Six to 9 weeks postoperatively
  - Precautions: no resisted active motion, light functional activities only
  - Reliable patients can be weaned from the dorsal blocking splint.
  - The active flexion and extension exercises should be continued. Blocking exercises are initiated for PIP and DIP flexion to facilitate tendon glide and pull-through. Combined finger extension exercises are slowly initiated with the wrist in slight flexion. If the patient is a heavy scar former, this begins at 6 weeks; if average, at 7 weeks; if light, at 8 weeks.
- Nine to 12 weeks postoperatively
  - Precautions: no lifting or uncontrolled use
  - Splinting should be modified to correct any residual joint contractures and increase soft tissue excursion.
  - The patient can be allowed to begin progressive strengthening and should continue active range-of-motion and tendon-gliding exercises as well as scar management as needed.
- Twelve to 14 weeks postoperatively
  - Precautions: no heavy lifting
  - Splinting is continued as needed to address contractures.
  - Active range-of-motion and strengthening activities are continued. Resistance is gradually increased up to about 30 pounds by week 14.
- Fourteen to 16 weeks postoperatively
  - The patient progresses to full resistive strengthening exercises and activities.
  - A work hardening program is initiated if needed to prepare for return to work.
  - If the patient is less reliable, the previously mentioned protocol is followed except that dorsal blocking splinting is continued for up to 9 weeks and active motion is delayed until at least 4 weeks.

OUTCOMES

- Because there are few alternatives to this staged process of reconstruction, there are limited articles comparing this treatment to another. Most of the investigations in the literature are retrospective reviews documenting overall postoperative motion and outcome ratings based on objective and subjective rating systems.
- The larger studies have shown good and excellent results in the 70% to 80% range, depending on the grading system used.[3–5]
- Final total active motion is about 70% of the contralateral uninjured digit.
- Typically, a significant discrepancy exists between ultimate total passive motion and total active motion. A flexion contracture of about 20 degrees at the DIP joint is common.[3]
- The most common reported complication, seen in 30% of patients, was the need for a tenolysis.[2–5,8]
- Other common complications that resulted in the need for further surgery included infection, tendon rupture, pulley rupture with bowstringing, and incorrect tendon tensioning.[2–5,8]

COMPLICATIONS

- The most common complication is the development of adhesions that limit active motion. This can be assessed by a discrepancy between the active and passive range of motion. If there are significant discrepancies after at least 3 months of therapy after stage 2, then a tenolysis is recommended. This is followed immediately by a rigorous course of therapy to regain active motion. By 3 months, the tendon graft and junction sites should be strong enough to allow for unrestricted active motion.
- Bowstringing is common if the A2 and A4 pulleys are compromised by initial trauma or released with the scar and adhesions during stage 1. In this setting, these pulleys should be reconstructed during stage 1. If they are found to be incompetent during the stage 2, then pulley reconstruction must be performed and the tendon graft must be delayed until the patient has healed from the pulley reconstruction and once again demonstrated nearly full passive range of motion.
- Infection should be monitored closely, given the previous history of a penetrating wound that caused the tendon laceration in the first place and the implantation of a synthetic material during stage 1 of the procedure. Infections should be managed aggressively because the local inflammation can produce further contractures and adhesions.

REFERENCES

1. Amadio PC, Hunter JM, Jaeger SH, et al. The effect of vincular injury on the results of flexor tendon surgery in zone 2. J Hand Surg Am 1985;10(5):626–632.
2. Beris AE, Darlis NA, Korompilias AV, et al. Two-stage flexor tendon reconstruction in zone II using a silicone rod and a pedicled intrasynovial graft. J Hand Surg Am 2003;28(4):652–660.
3. Frakking TG, Depuydt KP, Kon M, et al. Retrospective outcome analysis of staged flexor tendon reconstruction. J Hand Surg Br 2000;25(2):168–174.
4. Hunter JM. Staged flexor tendon reconstruction. J Hand Surg Am 1983;8(5 pt 2):789–793.
5. Hunter JM, Singer DI, Jaeger SH, et al. Active tendon implants in flexor tendon reconstruction. J Hand Surg Am 1988;13(6):849–859.
6. O'Shea K, Wolfe SW. Two-stage reconstruction with the modified Paneva-Holevich technique. Hand Clin 2013;29:223–233.
7. Paneva-Holevich E. Two-stage plasty in flexor tendon injuries of the fingers within the digital synovial sheath. Acta Chir Plast 1965;7:112–124.
8. Trumble TE, Sailer SM. Flexor tendon injuries. In: Trumble TE, ed. Principles of Hand Surgery and Therapy. Philadelphia: WB Saunders, 2000:231–262.

Repair following Traumatic Extensor Tendon Disruption in the Hand, Wrist, and Forearm

81

CHAPTER

David B. Shapiro, Mark A. Krahe, and Nathan A. Monaco

DEFINITION

- Traumatic disruptions of the extensor mechanism represent a broad spectrum of injuries, frequently occurring because of the tendons' superficial location, and frequently associated with concomitant injury to bone, skin, and joint.[17]
- Repair can be technically demanding. The extensor tendons are thin, have limited excursion, and are intolerant of shortening, especially in the digits.
- Reconstruction of subacute and chronic extensor tendon injuries are more challenging and less effective than early repair, underscoring the importance of appropriate treatment in the acute setting.

ANATOMY

- Extensor tendon zones of injury (Verdan) (**FIG 1A**)[14]
  - The extensor mechanism is divided into eight zones in the fingers and five in the thumb, numbered from distal to proximal.
  - Even-numbered zones are over bones and odd-numbered ones are over joints.
- Extrinsic extensors (**FIG 1B**)
  - Digital and wrist extensor muscles originate from the lateral epicondyle and condyle, with musculotendinous junctions 3 to 4 cm proximal to the wrist joint. The extensor indicis proprius (EIP), extensor pollicis longus (EPL),

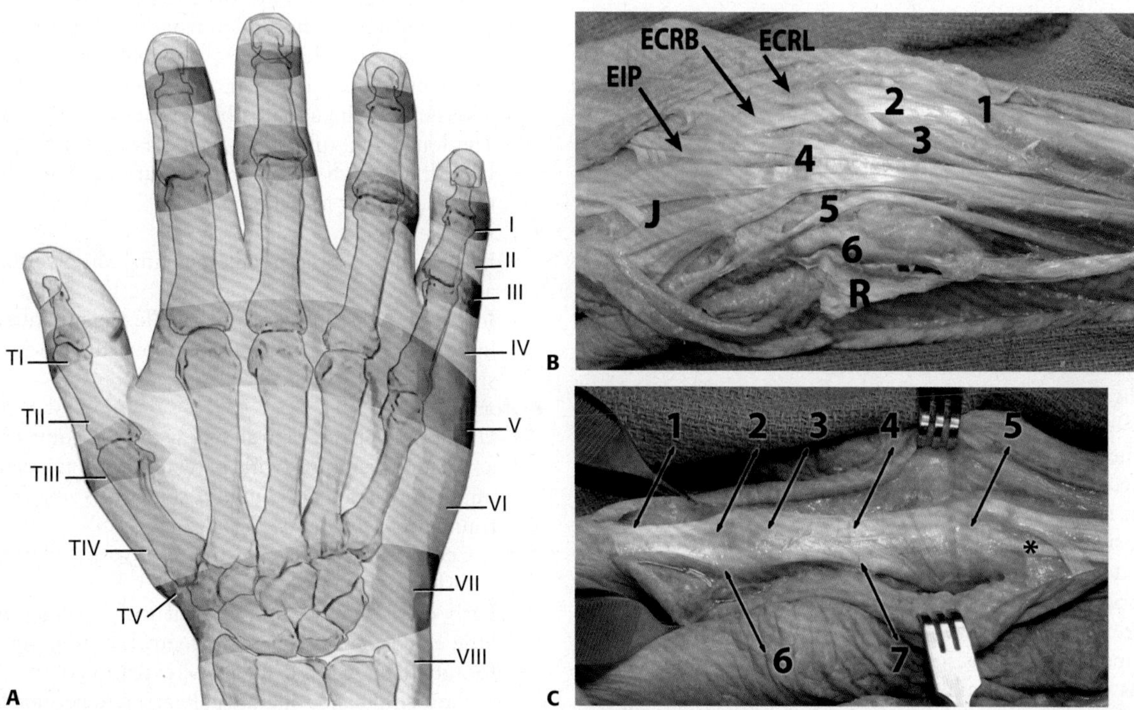

FIG 1 • **A.** Extensor tendon zones of injury. **B,C.** The digits are to the *left* and the wrist is to the *right*. **B.** The *top* of the figure is radial and the *bottom* is ulnar. Wrist and hand extensor tendon anatomy, with numbers (1 to 6) to identify the extensor tendon compartments. *R* is the reflected extensor retinaculum and *J* is a junctura tendinum. Note the combined EDC tendon to the ring and small fingers. In the fourth compartment, the EIP tendon is deep to the EDC tendons and has more distal muscle fibers. In the hand, it is just deep and ulnar to the index EDC tendon. See Table 1 for more details. **C.** The digital extensor mechanism. *1*) Terminal tendon. *2*) Triangular ligament. *3*) PIP joint. *4*) Central slip tendon. *5*) Sagittal band. *6*) Lateral band, which will become the terminal tendon distally. *7*) Conjoined lateral band, with fibers to the base of middle phalanx and to the lateral band. This patient has an unusual proprius tendon to the long finger (*asterisk*), passing ulnar to the EDC tendon and beneath the junctura.

Table 1 Extrinsic Extensor Tendons

Compartment	Muscle	Abbreviation	Comment
1	Abductor pollicis longus Extensor pollicis brevis	APL EPB	Compartment is more palmar than others.
2	Extensor carpi radialis longus Extensor carpi radialis brevis	ECRL ECRB	Two wrist extensors
3	Extensor pollicis longus	EPL	Third compartment tendon goes to the thumb.
4	Extensor digitorum communis Extensor indicis proprius	EDC EIP	Four EDC tendons and "fore"finger tendon
5	Extensor digiti quinti or extensor digiti minimi	EDQ or EDM	Fifth finger independent extensor tendon
6	Extensor carpi ulnaris	ECU	Most ulnar extensor tendon

abductor pollicis longus (APL), and extensor pollicis brevis (EPB) all originate more distally from the ulna, the radius, or both and have more distal extension of muscle fibers.

- The four extensor digitorum communis (EDC) tendons originate from a common muscle belly and have progressively limited independence moving from the index to small fingers.
- The fascia over the extensor tendons thickens at the wrist to form the extensor retinaculum, with vertical septa separating the six extensor compartments (see **FIG 1B**; Table 1).
- Juncturae tendinum provide interconnections between the EDC tendons just proximal to the metacarpophalangeal (MCP) joints.
- The EIP and extensor digiti minimi are ulnar and deep to the EDC in the hand and at the MCP joint. The EIP passes beneath the junctura tendinum between the index and long common extensors.
- At the level of the wrist, the EIP is deep to the other extensors, with a more distally extending muscle belly, making it easy to identify.
- There can be considerable variability of the extensor tendons on the dorsum of the hand, with less than 50% of people having a separate EDC tendon to the small finger.[21] Duplicated and interconnected tendons are common.[12]
- The sagittal band holds the extensor tendon centered over the metacarpal head at the MCP joint and, through its connection to the volar plate, extends the joint.

- Intrinsic extensors (**FIG 1C**)
  - Intrinsic extensors originate in the hand and include the four dorsal interossei, three palmar interossei, and four lumbricals. The thenar and hypothenar muscles also contribute to interphalangeal extension and MCP flexion.
  - The intrinsic tendons join to form the conjoined lateral bands volar to the axis of the MCP joint and continue dorsal to the axis of the proximal interphalangeal (PIP) and distal interphalangeal (DIP) joints.[21] This allows them to simultaneously flex the MCP joint and extend the PIP and DIP joints.
  - The palmar interossei insert on the lateral bands and sometimes to the proximal phalangeal bases—ulnar at the index finger and radial at the ring and small fingers.[12]
  - The dorsal interossei also attach to the lateral bands and proximal phalangeal bases—radial on the index finger, ulnar on the ring finger, and to both sides on the long finger.[12]
  - The lumbrical muscles originate on the radial side of the deep flexor tendons and insert into the radial conjoined lateral bands, serving as powerful MCP flexors.
  - Small finger abduction is via the abductor digiti minimi.

PATHOGENESIS

- Zone I
  - Disruption of the extensor tendon over the DIP joint will result in a terminal extensor lag after an open or closed injury (**FIG 2**).
  - Sudden forced flexion of the extended DIP joint can lead to an avulsion of the tendon from its insertion on the distal phalanx (mallet finger), possibly with an associated distal phalanx fracture. Large bony fragments may be associated with palmar subluxation of the DIP joint.
  - The long, ring, and small fingers are most frequently involved, although closed mallet injuries can also be seen in the index finger and thumb.[2]
- Zone II
  - Laceration over the middle phalanx can give the clinical appearance of a zone I injury.
  - Injury to the periosteum and middle phalanx often lead to increased swelling, extensor tendon adherence, and DIP stiffness.
- Zone III
  - Disruption of the central slip at the PIP joint may occur as a closed rupture (with or without an associated bone injury) or as an open injury, sometimes associated with traumatic arthrotomy.
    - Central slip avulsions are seen with volar PIP joint dislocations.
  - Early closed injuries may present with swelling, pain, and little extension loss but can progress to a boutonnière deformity (flexion of PIP and hyperextension of the DIP joint) as the lateral bands migrate palmarly and become flexors of

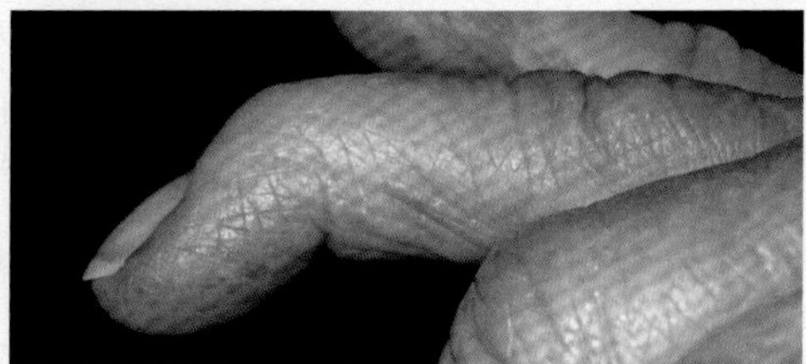

FIG 2 • Mallet finger (zone I extensor tendon injury).

the PIP joint in the weeks after injury.[21] Close follow-up and PIP extension splinting is warranted for suspicious injuries.

- Zone IV
  - Injuries occur over the proximal phalanx and typically involve only a portion of the extensor mechanism but may involve the entire central slip.
    - Some portion of the extensor mechanism usually remains intact, making examination more difficult. With a complete central slip laceration, PIP extension may be maintained (through the lateral bands) initially, although a boutonnière deformity may develop later.
  - A complete central slip injury will often be associated with pain or weakness with resisted PIP extension (especially from an initially flexed position). As discussed earlier, close follow-up is warranted for suspicious injuries.
- Zone V
  - Tendon injury occurs over the MCP joint.
  - There may be an open laceration of the extrinsic extensor, often related to a "fight bite," or a closed injury to the sagittal band with extensor tendon subluxation.
    - Closed sagittal band injuries often result in ulnar subluxation of the extensor tendon.
  - Lacerations at this level should be assumed to extend into the MCP joint.
- Zone VI
  - Disruption of extensor tendon is over the dorsum of the hand.
  - Single tendon and partial tendon lacerations may be difficult to identify due to maintenance of some digital extension through an intact junctura tendinum and EDC tendon from an adjacent digit (see **FIG 3**).
- Zone VII
  - Lacerations occur over the wrist and through the extensor retinaculum.
  - Chronic disruptions can be seen in this zone following traumatic distal radius fractures or from prominent hardware after volar or dorsal fixation.
- Zone VIII
  - Pathology is located in the forearm at the musculotendinous junction or muscle belly.
  - It may be difficult to detect concurrent posterior interosseous nerve injury in the presence of proximal extensor muscle lacerations.
- Thumb
  - The terminal extensor tendon is thicker than in other digits—mallet injury is rare.
  - Tendon lacerations at, and distal to, the MCP joint are not associated with retraction of tendon ends, and primary repair is straightforward. Lacerations proximal to the MCP joint are associated with EPL retraction (often to the wrist) and require more timely repair.

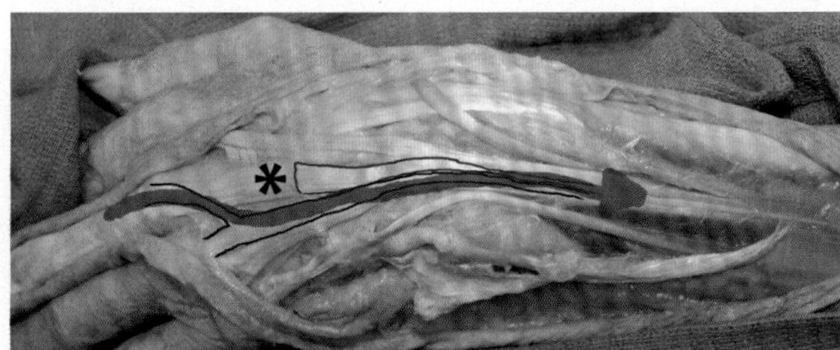

FIG 3 • EDC laceration to the long finger at the *asterisk*. The long finger can still be extended by action of the ring extensor and junctura tendinum. This may be associated with long-term weakness, pain, or extensor lag.

NATURAL HISTORY

- Untreated complete tendon lacerations at and distal to zone V will lead to persistent (and sometimes progressively worsening) digital deformity, often with continued pain and development of a flexion contracture.
  - Untreated terminal tendon injuries may lead to a swan-neck deformity due to proximal retraction of the digital extensor mechanism and increased extension force at the PIP joint.
  - Delayed treatment of central slip injuries may lead to boutonnière deformity and PIP flexion contracture as the lateral bands migrate palmarly, flexing the PIP joint and hyperextending the DIP joint.
- Untreated tendon lacerations proximal to zone V will heal in lengthened fashion with pseudotendon formation. There may be a persistent extensor lag, weakness, or pain. Gradual loss of muscle length and elasticity (sometimes within as little as a week or two) can make delayed primary repair more difficult.
- EPL tendon lacerations proximal to the MCP joint may be difficult to primarily repair as little as 2 weeks after the injury, requiring tendon grafting or EIP transfer.
- Partial tendon lacerations involving less than 50% of the tendon width, longitudinal lacerations, and single lateral band lacerations will generally function well without repair.

PATIENT HISTORY AND PHYSICAL FINDINGS

- Assessment and documentation of skin and soft tissue injury is important to aid in planning for débridement and extension of the skin incision for exposure and in determining the need for soft tissue coverage.
- A complete neurologic and tendon examination is critical to rule out concurrent or remote injury that will alter treatment or outcome.
  - The EIP and EDQ are examined by testing independent index and small finger MCP joint extension.
  - The extrinsic extensor tendons are examined with the wrist in neutral, testing MCP extension against resistance. (Isolated PIP extension can be performed by the intrinsic muscles via intact lateral bands even in the presence of complete extrinsic extensor tendon lacerations.)
  - Examination of the digits may identify extensor lag, weakness, or pain with resistance to extension at the PIP or DIP joints.
  - The resting posture of the hand and absence of a tenodesis effect (MCP extension with passive wrist flexion) can also suggest an extensor tendon injury.
  - The Elson test can be used to diagnose a central slip injury.[6] With loss of the central slip, lateral bands can migrate proximally to allow DIP extension with PIP flexion. Patients demonstrate a rigid DIP with attempted PIP extension from a flexed position with this test.
- Active and passive range of motion and strength are assessed. Active motion loss helps determine tendon deficits, whereas loss of passive motion may be pain-related or represent remote injury or arthritis. Lacerations proximal to the juncturae tendinum may have nearly full motion but with weakness on strength testing and a small extensor lag (**FIG 3**).

IMAGING AND OTHER DIAGNOSTIC STUDIES

- Plain radiographs are necessary to evaluate for any fractures, foreign bodies, preexisting injury, or arthritis that may alter treatment or affect the final result.
- Ultrasound or magnetic resonance imaging (MRI) is occasionally useful for suspected radiolucent foreign bodies. Although both studies can be used to more fully evaluate tendon injuries, treatment decisions are usually based on history and physical examination. Ultrasound may offer some value in diagnosis of lacerations of the central slip.[24]

DIFFERENTIAL DIAGNOSIS

- Radial or posterior interosseous nerve injury
- Extensor tendon subluxation at the MCP joint
- Chronic PIP flexion contracture and "pseudoboutonnière" deformity (no DIP hyperextension)
- Physiologic swan-neck deformity or DIP joint osteoarthritis with apparent mallet deformity
- Underlying joint deformity and arthrosis

NONOPERATIVE MANAGEMENT

- Disruption of the terminal extensor tendon (mallet finger)
  - Treatment consists of full-time static DIP splinting for 6 to 8 weeks, followed by an additional 6 weeks of protective splinting at night and during high-risk activities.
  - Patients must be counseled as to the importance of maintaining full DIP extension, even during splint changes.
  - A dorsal splint (**FIG 4A**) can allow the patient nearly full use and sensibility of the digit, although palmar or thermoplastic splints can be used in some cases (provided that full DIP extension can be ensured). A good fit without excessive DIP hyperextension (which can cause skin injury) is critical.
  - The PIP is generally left free and motion encouraged. For patients with moderate PIP hyperextension, the PIP may be flexed 30 degrees and incorporated in the splint for the first 3 weeks of treatment. A thermoplastic "figure-of-eight" extension block splint for the PIP joint may be used with a DIP static splint.

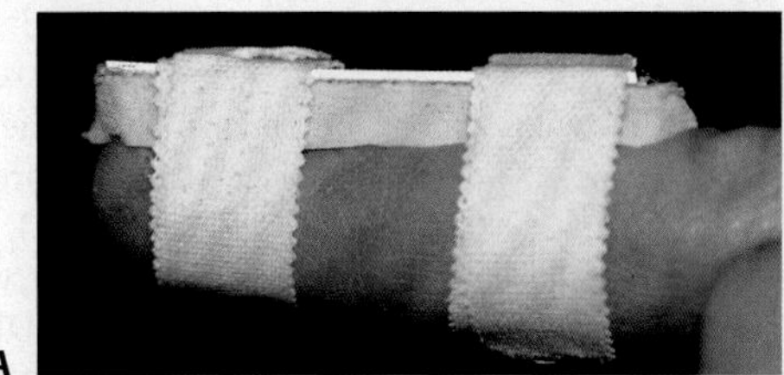

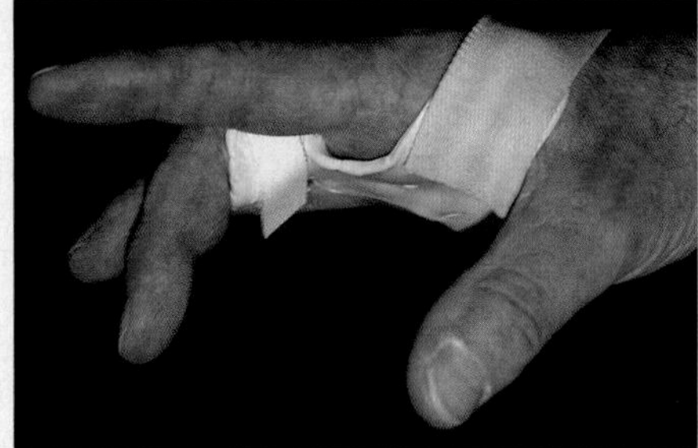

FIG 4 • **A.** Example of mallet finger splint. Any type of DIP joint splint will work as long as the DIP is extended to neutral and the splint is worn full time. **B.** Example of hand-based splint to support MCP joint.

  - Treatment can be initiated as late as 4 months after the original injury and still lead to a good result, although a couple more weeks of full-time splinting may be necessary.[8]
  - Controversy exists regarding the role of conservative management of mallet fractures with subluxation of the DIP joint. Many of these (especially in younger patients) should be treated surgically.[9,23]
  - Final results: About 80% of patients should regain full flexion with less than a 10-degree extensor lag. Patients with a greater extension lag after 6 weeks may benefit from 2 or 3 more weeks of full-time splinting. Swelling and tenderness around the DIP joint can persist for months.
- Central slip avulsion
  - This is treated with full-time static PIP splinting in extension, with active and passive DIP flexion encouraged, for 6 weeks, followed by 6 weeks of night splinting.
  - Intermittent use of dynamic or static progressive extension splint is warranted for PIP flexion contracture in patients who present later.
- Closed sagittal band rupture
  - The patient is placed in a below-elbow cast with the MCP joints supported in full extension (to allow no more than 10 to 20 degrees of flexion) for 6 weeks. Be sure the tendon does not sublux with PIP flexion.
  - Compliant patients can be switched to a hand-based splint after 3 weeks of casting with the MCP joint supported in 30 degrees of flexion and the PIP joints left free (**FIG 4B**).
  - Surgical treatment is indicated for closed ruptures presenting more than 2 weeks after injury or those that do not respond to conservative treatment.
- Partial extensor tendon lacerations
  - Conservative treatment is indicated if the laceration is known to involve less than 50% of the tendon width and in longitudinal tendon lacerations.
  - If the degree of injury is unknown, conservative treatment should be considered in patients with full active extension, minimal or no pain with resisted extension, and good extension strength. Surgical exploration and repair is indicated if there is an extensor lag, weakness, or pain with resisted extension.
    - Partial digital extensor tendon lacerations are treated, with splinting for 2 to 3 weeks, followed by a monitored gradual exercise program to ensure that an extensor lag does not develop.
    - Partial hand and forearm extensor tendon injuries are treated similarly. A splint or cast is used for 3 weeks with mild wrist extension and 30 degrees of MCP flexion. The PIP joints are left free.

SURGICAL MANAGEMENT

Preoperative Planning

- A careful examination is performed to determine the structures that are injured or will need repair (eg, open joint injuries, fractures, flexor tendon or nerve injuries) and to inform the patient of the extent of the procedure, anticipated rehabilitation, need for occupational and nonoccupational restrictions, and expected outcome.
- If the wound is infected at the time of presentation, irrigation and débridement should be followed by a course of antibiotics. Delayed primary tendon repair can be carried out

7 to 14 days later (sooner for EPL lacerations proximal to the MCP joint and EDC lacerations proximal to the junctura).

- The surgeon should anticipate the need for tendon graft or transfer for subacute injuries or those with tendon loss.
- Local anesthesia and a digital tourniquet can be used for injuries distal to the PIP joint. The need for an upper arm tourniquet for more proximal injuries may necessitate a general or regional anesthetic, unless the anticipated surgical time is less than 30 minutes. Regional anesthesia can offer extended postoperative pain relief and muscle relaxation during the initial recovery period.
- "Wide awake local anesthesia with no tourniquet (WALANT)" using 1% lidocaine with 1:100,000 epinephrine is an acceptable alternative.[15]

Positioning

- Standard positioning is used with the hand on a hand table and the surgeon at the head.
- Skin preparation and draping is done above the elbow to allow dressing and splint application before removal of drapes.
- A carefully padded tourniquet is applied, set to 100 mm Hg above systolic blood pressure (sometimes more for obese patients and less for children or those with small arms).

Approach

- Wound exploration and débridement are performed in a bloodless field, with appropriate light and magnification. Injuries over a joint usually require joint exploration and irrigation.
- The skin laceration can be extended to improve exposure, allow retrieval of retracted tendons, provide access to place sutures, and to decrease skin tension during retraction. Long, narrow skin flaps are avoided. Longitudinal incisions on the dorsum of the hand and fingers can cross over joints (unlike on the digital flexor surface).
- Bipolar electrocautery is used as needed, with care taken not to injure dorsal cutaneous nerves. If there is any doubt regarding hemostasis, the tourniquet is deflated before closure. Drains are seldom needed.
- Only the skin in the fingers, hand, and distal forearm is closed, with limited subcutaneous sutures more proximally if needed.

TECHNIQUES

Suture Techniques

- Suture technique is determined by the thickness and shape of the tendon and the nature and character of the laceration (**TECH FIG 1**).
  - Thin tendons (eg, in digits) can be repaired with a horizontal cross-stitch suture (Silfverskiöld), simple running, figure-8, or horizontal mattress suture using 4-0 or 5-0 braided or monofilament nonabsorbable material.
    - Buried knots may be helpful in patients with thinner skin.
  - Thicker tendons can support a two- or four-strand grasping repair with a 2-0, 3-0, or 4-0 nonabsorbable braided suture (eg, Ethibond, Ticron, or FiberWire), optionally reinforced with a 5-0 or 6-0 monofilament epitendinous suture placed in a simple running or cross-stitch fashion.
- In general, repair strength is related to number of suture strands crossing the repair site, the thickness of the suture, and the locking style of the stitch.

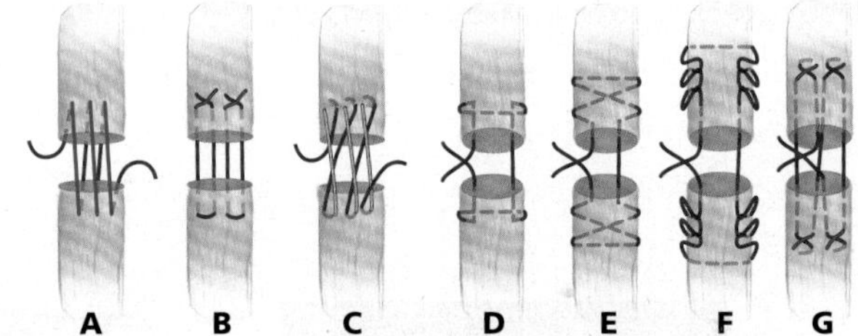

TECH FIG 1 • Some suture techniques for extensor tendon repair. The strongest repairs are the Silfverskiöld cross-stitch for flat tendons and the four-strand cruciate suture for tendons able to accept a core suture. **A.** Running suture. **B.** Horizontal mattress. **C.** Silfverskiöld cross-stitch (which can also be used as a circumferential epitendinous tidying suture over a core suture). **D.** Modified Kessler. **E.** Modified Bunnell. **F.** Krackow. **G.** Four-strand cruciate suture.

Repair in the Fingers

Zone I (Distal Interphalangeal Joint)

Soft Tissue Mallet Treatment

- In patients with closed tendon disruptions who cannot tolerate a splint for occupational reasons, percutaneous pinning across the DIP joint with a 0.045-inch Kirschner wire exposed at the tip or buried under the skin may be indicated. Pin removal is performed 6 weeks later, followed by motion exercises and 6 weeks of splinting at night and during vigorous activity.
- Lacerations in zone I are treated with primary surgical repair.
  - A figure-8 or running cross-stitch with a 5-0 nonabsorbable suture can be placed in the tendon, taking care to avoid shortening the tendon. This is supported with a 0.045-inch Kirschner wire across the DIP joint for 6 weeks. The DIP should be in neutral extension, without hyperextension.
  - An easier and often better alternative is use of a "tenodermodesis" stitch of 4-0 nylon through both the tendon and skin (**TECH FIG 2**).[5,11] This can be especially useful in cases treated in the emergency room, or in children, where the small tendon is difficult to accurately repair.
    - Full-time extension splinting (as in a closed mallet finger) or a 0.045-inch Kirschner wire across the extended DIP joint is required.
    - The suture can be removed in 2 to 3 weeks, but the splinting should continue for a total of 6 weeks full time and another 6 weeks at night.

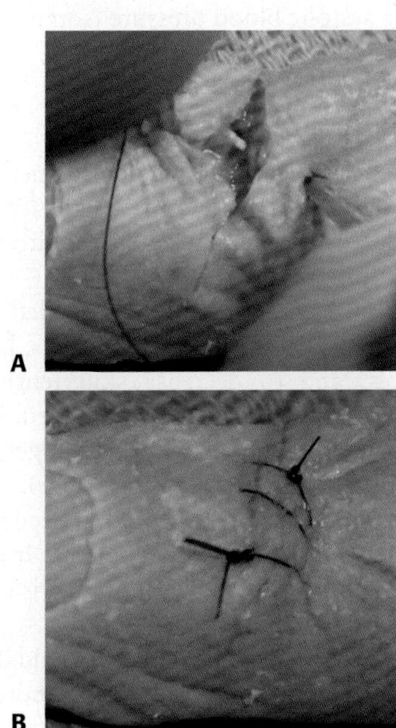

TECH FIG 2 • A,B. Tenodermodesis can be a useful way of suturing terminal tendon lacerations, especially in the emergency department or office. The suture (passing from left to right in **A**) goes through the skin and tendon proximally and distally.

Bony Mallet Treatment

- It remains controversial whether mallet fractures with greater than 50% of the distal phalanx involved or with DIP joint subluxation should be treated surgically or by splinting alone. Surgery is more likely warranted in younger patients and those with subluxation of the DIP joint.[9,23] If conservative management is being considered, be sure to obtain a good lateral radiograph with the digit in the DIP splint, as DIP extension to neutral may show subluxation that was not apparent when the joint was flexed. A large fragment without subluxation can be treated conservatively.
- A large bone fragment is present, with subluxation of the DIP joint (**TECH FIG 3A,B**).
- Place a 0.045-inch Kirschner wire down the shaft of the distal phalanx, almost to the DIP joint.
- Maximally flex the DIP and place a 0.035-inch Kirschner wire at the anticipated location of the reduced dorsal fragment of the distal phalanx. The skin entry point is relatively distal to enable pin movement in the next step. Hold the pin against the middle phalanx (**TECH FIG 3C**).
- Angle the wire distally, pushing the fragment distally and buttressing it. Advance the wire into the middle phalanx (**TECH FIG 3D,E**).

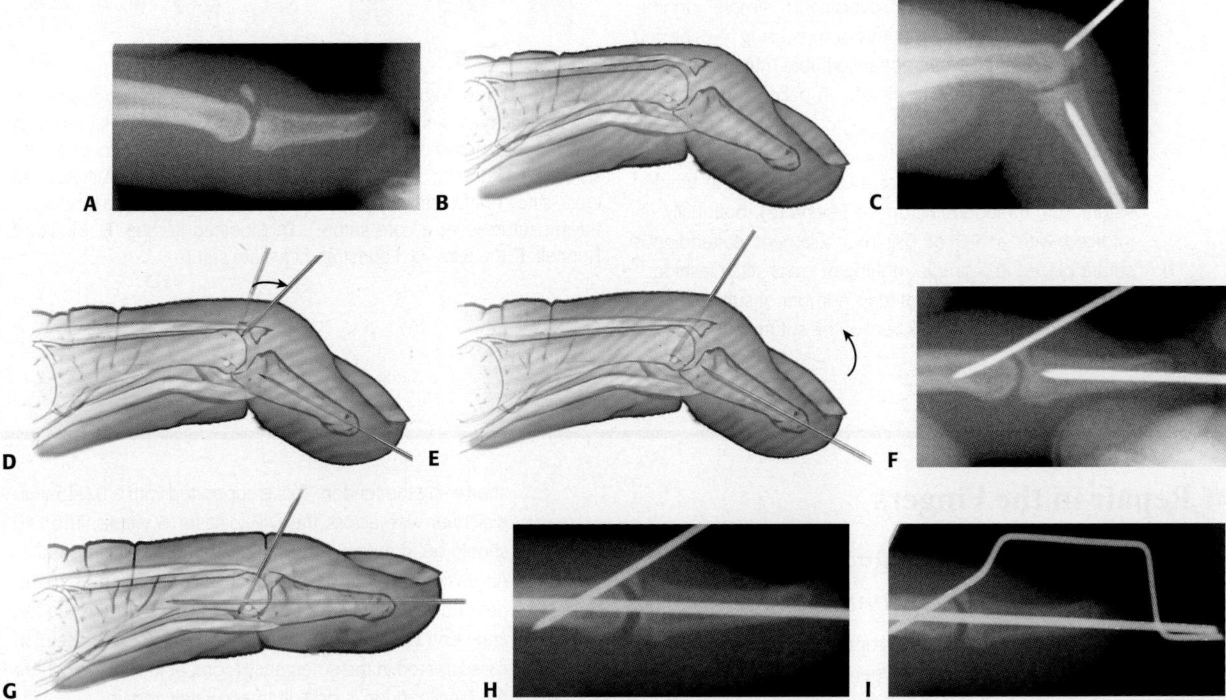

TECH FIG 3 • Technique for pinning a mallet fracture. **A,B.** Large bone fragment is present, frequently with subluxation of the DIP joint. **C.** A pin is placed in the distal phalanx. Maximally flex the DIP and place a 0.035-inch Kirschner wire where you would anticipate the dorsal edge of the distal phalanx to be. The skin entry point is relatively distal to enable pin movement in the next step. **D,E.** Angle the wire distally, pushing the fragment and buttressing it. Advance the wire into the middle phalanx. **F,G.** Extend and reduce the distal phalanx, bringing it up to the fragment and stabilizing it by advancing the 0.045-inch Kirschner wire across the DIP joint. If a significant articular step-off persists after a couple tries, leave the longitudinal wire and allow the fragment to heal where it lies. **H.** Dorsal pins buttress the fragment and the longitudinal pin reduces the flexion and subluxation. **I.** Pins bent to fit in a single pin cap.

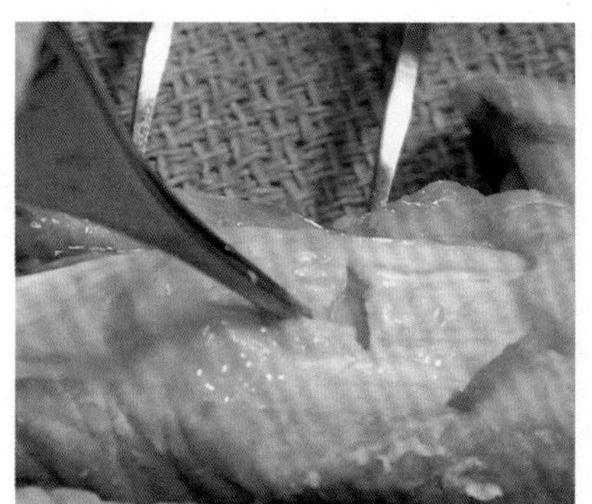

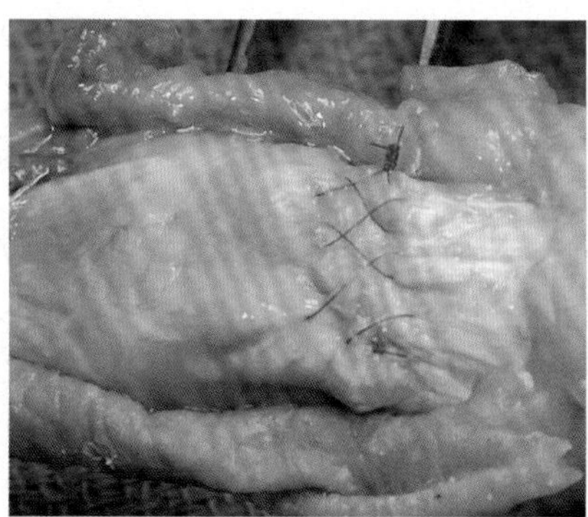

TECH FIG 4 • **A,B.** Simulated central slip laceration on a cadaver specimen. Note how difficult it would be for a laceration to cut all the way around the extensor mechanism. This example has been repaired with a running, cross-stitch suture (Silfverskiöld).

- Extend and reduce the distal phalanx, bringing it up to the fragment. Drive the 0.045-inch wire across the DIP joint. Maintain full extension and correction of any subluxation (**TECH FIG 3F–H**).
- Bend the pins so they can be included in a single pin cap to prevent rotation or movement of the proximal pin (**TECH FIG 3I**).
- If an articular step-off persists after a couple of attempts, remove the dorsal wire but leave the longitudinal wire in place supporting the joint in neutral extension and correcting the subluxation. This may leave a dorsal prominence but will correct the subluxation.
- Pins can be removed in about 6 weeks with institution of a protected motion program and 4 to 6 weeks of additional night splinting.

Zone II (Over Middle Phalanx)

- Perform primary tendon repair with a running 4-0 or 5-0 cross-stitch suture.
- The DIP joint can be splinted or pinned extended for 4 to 6 weeks, followed by splinting for vigorous activity and at night for 6 weeks.

Zone III (Over Proximal Interphalangeal Joint)

- Use a running 4-0 or 5-0 suture to repair the central slip in the manner detailed earlier (**TECH FIG 4**).
- Repair the lateral band or bands with single 4-0 or 5-0 monofilament suture in a figure-8 fashion.
- Pinning the PIP joint in extension for 4 to 6 weeks will protect the repair and enable DIP flexion exercises.

Reconstruction in Cases with Tendon Loss

- Consider V-Y advancement of the central tendon or a "turndown" of the central slip proximal to the laceration to cover the defect.[22]
- Extend the skin incision proximally, almost to the MCP joint.
- Incise a V in the central slip, with the apex just distal to the MCP joint, and the distal end the width of the tendon, taking care not to damage the overlying epitenon (**TECH FIG 5A**, *red line*).
- Advance the tendon distally. Disrupt the loose alveolar tissue between the tendon and periosteum as little as possible.
- Close the V into a Y with a 4-0 or 5-0 suture, and repair the distal end of the advanced central slip as described earlier (**TECH FIG 5B**).
- An alternative method involves creating a rectangular flap of central slip proximally and turning it up to attach distally (**TECH FIGS 5A,C,D**).[22]
- Suture anchors or small holes drilled in the middle phalanx are occasionally needed to secure the tendon to the dorsal base of the middle phalanx, especially if the dorsal margin of the base of the phalanx is lost.
- Techniques using free grafts or passage of a slip of the FDS through the base of the middle phalanx have also been described.[1]

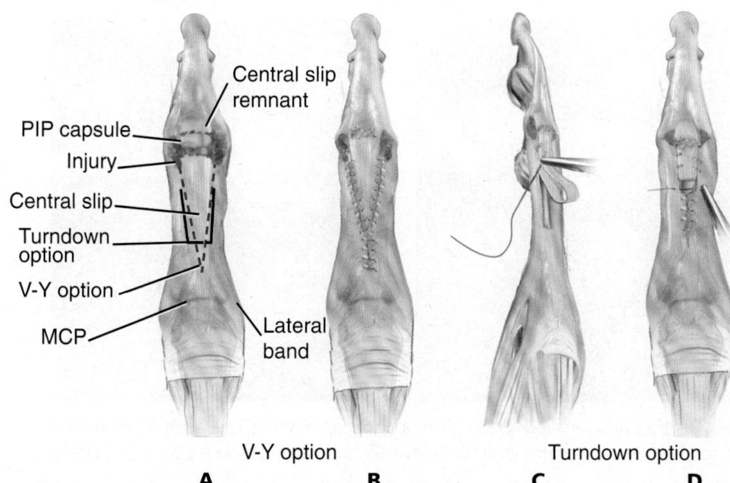

TECH FIG 5 • **A.** Central slip loss (eg, abrasions, grinders) can lead to significant stiffness. **B.** V-Y advancement of the central tendon. **C,D.** Turndown of a portion of the central slip.

Postoperative Management

- Postoperative rehabilitation for children, less compliant adults, and cases with a tenuous repair involves static splinting or pinning of the PIP joint in full extension for 4 weeks, followed by a protected motion program.
- For compliant adults, an early motion protocol can be initiated.[7]
  - Zero to 30 degrees of active PIP flexion and extension is allowed starting a few days after surgery, using a palmar flexion block splint with a free wrist and MCP joint.
  - Ten to 20 repetitions are performed each hour, with a static PIP splint in full extension when not exercising.
  - DIP flexion exercises are performed in the static PIP extension splint.
  - If no extensor lag develops, PIP motion can be increased to 40 degrees after 2 weeks, 50 degrees after 3 weeks, and 70 degrees after 4 weeks. The splinting is discontinued at 6 weeks.
- Results are often less than perfect, especially in cases with tendon loss, where some loss of motion should be expected.

Zone IV (Over Proximal Phalanx)

- The tendon at this level may be thicker and support a grasping or locking core stitch with a 4-0 braided nonabsorbable suture, reinforced with a running 5-0 monofilament suture.
- If the tendon is too thin, repair as in zone III.
- Postoperative management is as in zone III. Intraoperative examination of the repair should be done as the MCP joint is taken through a full range of motion. If gapping or undue tension is noted, MCP splinting in 30 degrees of flexion may be required for a few weeks.

Repair in the Hand, Wrist, and Forearm

Zone V (Over the Metacarpophalangeal Joint)

- The tendon is much thicker at this level and can sometimes support a 3-0 or 4-0 braided nonabsorbable core suture with a running simple or cross-stitch suture over the repair, incorporating any laceration of the sagittal band.
- An abnormal resting cascade of the digits suggest a tendon laceration (**TECH FIG 6A**).
- Lacerations over the MCP joint often extend into the joint. The skin laceration is extended and débrided and the wound explored. Large capsular rents (*arrow* in **TECH FIG 6B**) can be repaired with a simple running 5-0 absorbable monofilament suture. Small capsular lacerations are left open.
- The tendon end is retrieved, and a 3-0 nonabsorbable core suture is placed. The first loops of the cruciate stitch are shown (**TECH FIG 6C**).
- The distal locking stitch is placed on one side of the tendon but not pulled tight until the tendon ends are accurately approximated. The limbs of the "X"—the area where the suture crosses—are individually tightened (**TECH FIG 6D**).
- The core suture is completed and will not slide (**TECH FIG 6E**).
- The repair is reinforced with a 5-0 nonabsorbable monofilament suture. This can be circumferential proximal to zone V but only over the dorsal surface of the tendon distally (**TECH FIG 6F**).
- The resting cascade of the digits shows the repaired finger to be slightly "tighter" than normal immediately after the repair (**TECH FIG 6G**).
- A forearm-based splint is applied with 30 degrees of wrist extension, less than 30 degrees of MCP flexion, and fully extended PIP and DIP joints (**TECH FIG 6H**).
- After 8 to 10 days, this splint is converted to a short-arm cast supporting the MCP joints in extension (including all fingers for index lacerations and the ulnar three for other lacerations) but leaving the PIP joints free for another 3 weeks before institution of a therapy program.
- Alternatively, an early protected motion program can be initiated.[4,10]

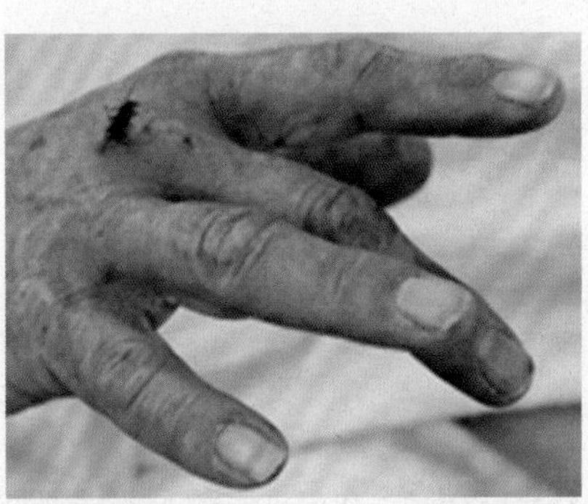
A

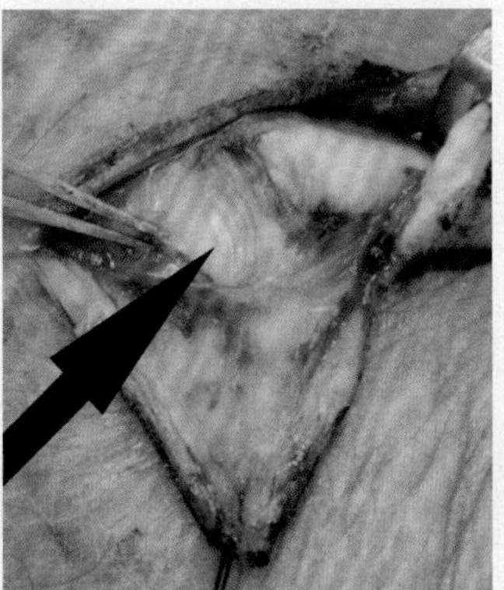
B

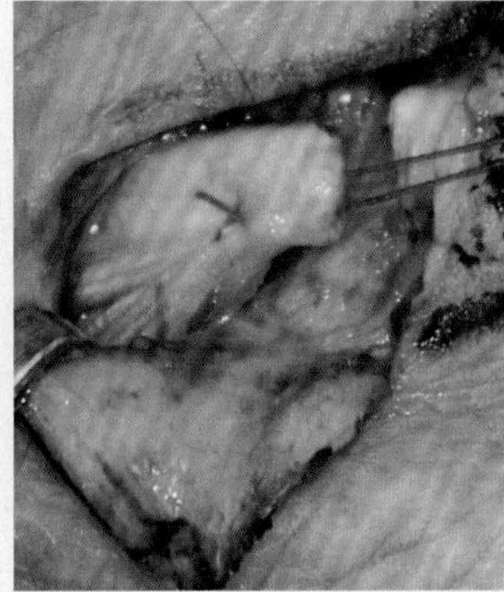
C

TECH FIG 6 • Zone V repair. **A.** There is a preoperative laceration around the MCP joint and loss of long finger extension. **B.** The *arrow* points to a rent in the MCP joint capsule, seen only with flexion of the joint. **C.** The first loops of the cruciate stitch are placed. *(continued)*

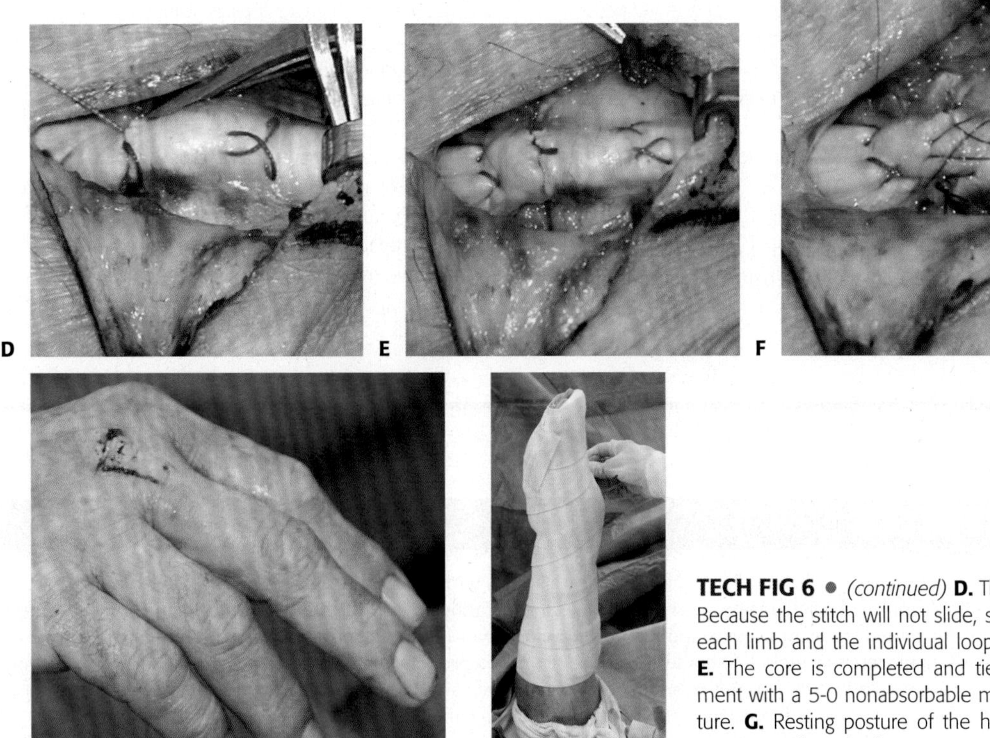

TECH FIG 6 • *(continued)* **D.** The gap is closed. Because the stitch will not slide, slack is taken off each limb and the individual loops are tightened. **E.** The core is completed and tied. **F.** Reinforcement with a 5-0 nonabsorbable monofilament suture. **G.** Resting posture of the hand after repair. **H.** Forearm-based splint.

Repair of Distal "Compromised" Zone V Lacerations

- In this clinical situation, a standard end-to-end repair may be tenuous or may not be possible secondary to contracted or lost tendon substance. A tendon interposition graft may be required.
- Partially incise the distal tendon and extensor apparatus over the MCP joint transversely, approximately 5 mm distal to the cut edge.
- Weave the tendon graft in a volar to dorsal direction through this transverse incision in the distal stump.
- Sew the graft to the distal stump and back to itself using nonabsorbable material (**TECH FIG 7**).
- Use a Pulvertaft weave to secure the other end of the tendon graft to the proximal stump.

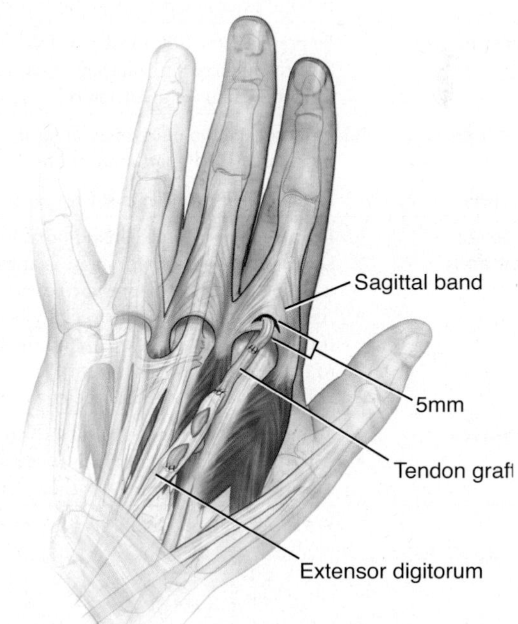

TECH FIG 7 • Tendon graft is woven volar to dorsal through the transverse incision in the distal tendon stump. A Pulvertaft weave is used to secure the graft to the proximal tendon stump.

Zone VI (Metacarpal Level)

- The tendon is thicker and repair is similar but technically easier than in zone V.
- Tendons lacerated proximal to the junctura may retract. If several tendons are cut, be careful to align them correctly.
- Use a 3-0 or 4-0 braided nonabsorbable suture, reinforced with a circumferential running simple or cross-stitch 5-0 or 6-0 monofilament suture.
- Rehabilitation is as for zone V.

Zone VII (Wrist and Extensor Retinaculum)

- Suture repair and postoperative management are as in zone VI.
- The extensor retinaculum is incised for repair and retrieval of the proximal tendon stump.

- Retinacular closure is performed with a 4-0 absorbable suture to prevent tendon bowstringing. A portion of the retinaculum may need to be excised to allow the repair site to glide smoothly.
- The EPL can be repaired outside of the retinaculum and left in the subcutaneous tissue.
- Postoperative management is the same as for zone V injuries.

Zone VIII

- Make a generous incision to determine the resting orientation of the tendons before débridement and repair. It may be helpful to tag proximal tendon ends with labels to define them before further dissection changes their position.
- WALANT may be valuable here to make sure correct proximal and distal connections are made.
- In the distal forearm, conventional repair with grasping sutures is possible. EDC tendons can be repaired as a group if necessary, making sure the resting digital cascade is maintained.
- Proximally, repair can be much more difficult. 3-0 interrupted absorbable sutures can be used in fibrous septa within muscle along with repair of epimysium.
- Postoperative management is as for zones V to VII.

PEARLS AND PITFALLS

Tetanus prophylaxis[20]	▪ Tetanus toxoid "booster" should be given to patients with at least three previous doses but last dose more than 5 years ago for tetanus-prone wounds (>1-cm laceration; crush; burn, high-energy injury; or with infection, devitalized tissue, or gross contamination) or more than 10 years ago for wounds not prone to tetanus. ▪ Tetanus immune globulin should be given for tetanus-prone wounds in patients with unknown or incomplete vaccination history. It is not clear, however, that "tetanus-prone wounds" are more likely to cause tetanus. ▪ The greatest protection against tetanus is a completed childhood vaccination series. ▪ A tetanus booster at the time of injury does not change the likelihood of developing tetanus.
Lacerations proximal to juncturae tendinum	▪ Extensor lag may be more subtle, sometimes noted only with lack of active MCP hyperextension, pain with resisted range of motion, or lack of palpable EDC tendon on dorsum of hand. ▪ Full PIP extension may be possible through the lateral bands even in the presence of a complete tendon laceration.
Subacute lacerations	▪ Be prepared for EIP transfer or free tendon graft for delayed treatment of EPL lacerations. ▪ Side-to-side repair to adjacent extensor tendons or use of a free tendon graft is occasionally needed for treatment of chronic injuries involving other tendons.
Clenched fist injuries	▪ Extensor tendon injury may be well proximal to the skin injury. ▪ Associated MCP joint injuries are common.
Shortened repair	▪ Digital extensor mechanism is very sensitive to shortening, with resulting loss of flexion.
Forearm extensor tendon lacerations	▪ Before exploring a proximal injury, locate and label individual tendon ends (based on location). ▪ Detailed exploration (for incision and drainage, foreign body removal, etc.) may distort tendon position, making it impossible to determine correct proximal motor to attach to each distal tendon end. ▪ Associated nerve injury (especially the posterior interosseous nerve) can make diagnosis and treatment difficult. ▪ If the laceration is proximal and the EPL does not function, then the likelihood of nerve injury is greater (due to the EPL's more distal origin). ▪ Lack of tenodesis effect suggests extensor tendon injury.
Suture techniques	▪ To most easily do the Silfverskiöld cross-stitch, start on the side of the tendon closest to the surgeon. ▪ After the first knot is tied, advance away across the tendon, keeping the needle pointed back at the surgeon for the horizontal component of the stitch.
Anesthesia[15]	▪ WALANT can be useful for many of these injuries.

POSTOPERATIVE CARE

- Postoperative care is detailed under the surgical technique for each individual location.

OUTCOMES

- Good or excellent results can be anticipated in most patients, with worse outcomes seen in the digits and with concomitant soft tissue or bone injury. Loss of digital flexion is a greater problem than small losses of extension.[3,18]
- Stronger suture techniques and early dynamic postoperative protocols may result in better functional outcomes earlier,[19] although few controlled studies show improvement in long-term results when compared to static splinting programs, which are easier, more predictable, and less expensive.[13,16] Early motion programs may be most beneficial in zone III and proximal.

COMPLICATIONS

- Infection
- Rupture of repaired tendons
- Stiffness
  - Primary joint stiffness after immobilization
  - Adherence of repaired tendon to surrounding skin, bone
- Extensor lag

REFERENCES

1. Ahmad F, Pickford M. Reconstruction of the extensor central slip using a distally based flexor digitorum superficialis slip. J Hand Surg Am 2009;34(5):930–932.
2. Bendre AA, Hartigan BJ, Kalainov DM. Mallet finger. J Am Acad Orthop Surg 2005;13:336–344.
3. Carl HD, Forst R, Schaller P. Results of primary extensor tendon repair in relation to the zone of injury and pre-operative outcome estimation. Arch Orthop Trauma Surg 2007;127:115–119.
4. Crosby CA, Wehbé MA. Early protected motion after extensor tendon repair. J Hand Surg Am 1999;24(5):1061–1070.
5. Doyle JR. Extensor tendons: acute injuries. In: Green DP, Hotchkiss RN, Pederson WC, eds. Green's Operative Hand Surgery, ed 4. New York: Churchill Livingstone, 1999:1950–1987.
6. Elson RA. Rupture of the central slip of the extensor hood of the finger. A test for early diagnosis. J Bone Joint Surg Br 1986;68(2):229–231.
7. Evans RB. Early active short arc motion for the repaired central slip. J Hand Surg Am 1994;19(6):991–997.
8. Garberman SF, Diao E, Peimer CA. Mallet finger: results of early versus delayed closed treatment. J Hand Surg Am 1994;19(5):850–852.
9. Hofmeister EP, Mazurek MT, Shin AY, et al. Extension block pinning for large mallet fractures. J Hand Surg Am 2003;28(3):453–459.
10. Howell JW, Merritt WH, Robinson SJ. Immediate controlled active motion following zone 4-7 extensor tendon repair. J Hand Ther 2005;18(2):182–190.
11. Iselin F, Levame J, Godoy J. A simplified technique for treating mallet fingers: tenodermodesis. J Hand Surg Am 1977;2(2):118–121.
12. Kaplan EB, Hunter JM. Extrinsic muscles of the fingers. In: Spinner M, ed. Kaplan's Functional and Surgical Anatomy of the Hand, ed 3. Philadelphia: JB Lippincott Company, 1984:93–112.
13. Khandwala AR, Webb J, Harris SB, et al. A comparison of dynamic extension splinting and controlled active mobilization of complete divisions of extensor tendons in zones 5 and 6. J Hand Surg Br 2000;25(2):140–146.
14. Kleinert HE, Verdan C. Report of the Committee on Tendon Injuries (International Federation of Societies for Surgery of the Hand). J Hand Surg Am 1983;8(5 pt 2):794–798.
15. Lalonde D. Reconstruction of the hand with wide awake surgery. Clin Plast Surg 2011;38:761–769.
16. Mowlavi A, Burns M, Brown RE. Dynamic versus static splinting of simple zone V and zone VI extensor tendon repairs: a prospective, randomized, controlled study. Plast Reconstr Surg 2005;115:482–487.
17. Newport ML. Extensor tendon injuries in the hand. J Am Acad Orthop Surg 1997;5:59–66.
18. Newport ML, Blair WF, Steyers CM Jr. Long-term results of extensor tendon repair. J Hand Surg Am 1990;15(6):961–966.
19. Newport ML, Williams CD. Biomechanical characteristics of extensor tendon suture techniques. J Hand Surg Am 1992;17(6):1117–1123.
20. Rhee P, Nunley MK, Demetriades D, et al. Tetanus and trauma: a review and recommendations. J Trauma 2005;58:1082–1088.
21. Rockwell WB, Butler PN, Byrne BA. Extensor tendon: anatomy, injury, and reconstruction. Plast Reconstr Surg 2000;106:1592–1603.
22. Snow JW. A method for reconstruction of the central slip of the extensor tendon of a finger. Plast Reconstr Surg 1976;57:455–459.
23. Wehbé MA, Schneider LH. Mallet fractures. J Bone Joint Surg Am 1984;66(5):658–669.
24. Westerheide E, Failla JM, van Holsbeeck M, et al. Ultrasound visualization of central slip injuries of the finger extensor mechanism. J Hand Surg Am 2003;28(6):1009–1013.

Tendon Transfer and Grafting for Traumatic Extensor Tendon Disruption

John S. Taras and Jason C. Saillant

DEFINITION

- Traumatic injury to the extensor tendons of the hand and forearm results in the disruption of tendon substance, causing a loss of active wrist or digital extension.
- Primary repair of the extensor tendon usually can be performed within 7 days after appropriate irrigation and débridement of wounds and stabilization of any fractures.[5]
- Late reconstruction of extensor tendon injuries presents an operative challenge and often requires the use of tendon transfer and grafting techniques.

ANATOMY

- The extensor mechanism of the hand and wrist is a complex system involving balanced interplay between extrinsic and intrinsic components (**FIG 1**).
- The extrinsic extensor tendons are divided into superficial and deep groups in the forearm:
  - Superficial: extensor carpi radialis longus (ECRL) and extensor carpi radialis brevis (ECRB), extensor digitorum communis (EDC), extensor digiti minimi (EDM), extensor carpi ulnaris (ECU), and anconeus

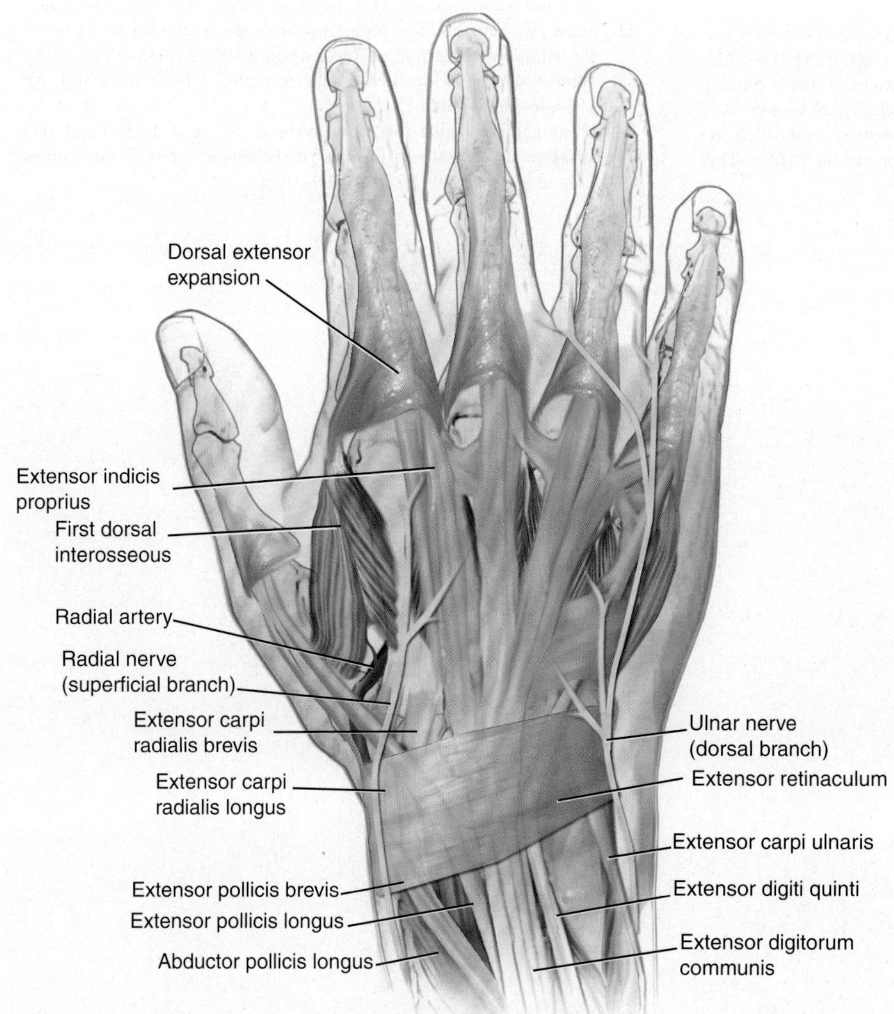

FIG 1 • Tendons on the dorsum of the hand, extensor retinaculum.

- Deep: abductor pollicis longus (APL), extensor pollicis brevis (EPB) and extensor pollicis longus (EPL), extensor indicis proprius (EIP), and supinator
- Wrist extension is provided by the ECRB, ECRL, and ECU.
- Finger and thumb extension is provided by the APL, EPB, EPL, EDC, EIP, and EDM.
- The radial nerve innervates all extensor muscles of the hand, except the intrinsics, which are innervated by the median and ulnar nerves. The radial nerve's deep motor branch becomes the posterior interosseous nerve (PIN).
- There are six fibro-osseous dorsal compartments at the level of the wrist covered by the extensor retinaculum. The contents of each compartment are as follows:
  - I: APL, EPB
  - II: ECRL, ECRB
  - III: EPL
  - IV: EDC, EIP
  - V: EDM
  - VI: ECU
- The intrinsic system of the hand consists of the seven interosseous muscles (three palmar and four dorsal) and four lumbrical muscles.
  - The intrinsic muscles pass volar to the axis of the metacarpophalangeal (MP) joints and dorsal to the interphalangeal (IP) joints; thus, the intrinsic system will flex the MP joints and extend the IP joints.
- On the dorsum of the hand, proximal to the MP joint, there are three fibrous bands of the juncturae tendinum that connect the extensor digitorum tendons of the index, long, ring, and small fingers. There is a high degree of variability in this anatomy.[7]
  - This interconnection is what allows grouped extension of the fingers.
  - The EIP and EDM are ulnar and deep to their respective EDC tendons and function as independent extensors of the index and small fingers.
- Over the MP joints, tendons are held in a central position by the sagittal bands, which envelop the MP joint and attach to the volar plate.
- The dorsal extensor apparatus is formed distal to the MP joint from contributions of both extrinsic and intrinsic tendons.
  - Proximal to the proximal interphalangeal (PIP) joint, the EDC tendon trifurcates.
- The central slip, the continuation of the extrinsic extensor tendon, is joined by medial bands from the interossei and lumbricals. It then inserts into the dorsal base of the middle phalanx.
  - The lateral bands are formed from the intrinsic muscles on either side of the finger and send fibers to the middle phalanx as well as contributions to the central slip.
  - The lateral bands combine dorsally over the middle phalanx to form the terminal extensor tendon, which inserts on the dorsal base of the distal phalanx.
  - The transverse and oblique retinacular ligaments stabilize the tendons of the dorsal apparatus.
- Traumatic injuries to the extensor tendons can be described in terms of nine anatomic zones (Table 1).[3]
- Traumatic injuries to the extensor tendon of the thumb have a separate numbering system and are divided into five anatomic zones (Table 2).
  - Even-numbered zones overlie bones and odd-numbered zones overlie joints.

Table 1 Extensor Tendon Zones of Fingers

Zone	Location
I	Distal interphalangeal
II	Middle phalanx
III	PIP
IV	Proximal phalanx
V	MP
VI	Metacarpal
VII	Wrist
VIII	Distal forearm
IX	Proximal forearm

- Vascular supply[5]
  - Forearm: nutrition via small arterial branches from the surrounding fascia
  - Wrist: derived from mesotenon; nutrition via diffusion
  - Hand: derived from paratenon; nutrition via perfusion

PATHOGENESIS

- Extensor tendons are susceptible to traumatic injury because of their relatively superficial location and thin tendon substance.
- Acute repair within 7 days is recommended, but direct repair of acute injuries is occasionally impractical in cases with extensive soft tissue damage or segmental tendon loss.
  - In these cases, skeletal stabilization is obtained first (**FIG 2**), followed by soft tissue coverage, and finally late reconstruction of the disrupted extensor mechanism.
- Also, late presentation of traumatic disruptions of an extensor tendon makes direct repair difficult because of tendon retraction and subsequent extrinsic tightness.
- Traumatic injury to the extensor tendons can also occur after upper extremity fractures.
  - Acute rupture of the EPL tendon has been associated with displaced distal radius fractures.
  - Delayed EPL rupture has been associated with minimally displaced distal radius fractures. These attritional ruptures are generally attributed to compromise the tendon's vascular supply by soft tissue damage and hemorrhage after fracture with an intact third extensor compartment.[4]
- Delayed extensor tendon ruptures of the EPL, EDC, and EIP have been reported as a complication after volar and dorsal plate fixation of distal radius fractures.[2]

Table 2 Extensor Tendon Zones of Thumb

Zone	Location
T-I	IP
T-II	Proximal phalanx
T-III	MP
T-IV	First metacarpal
T-V	Wrist

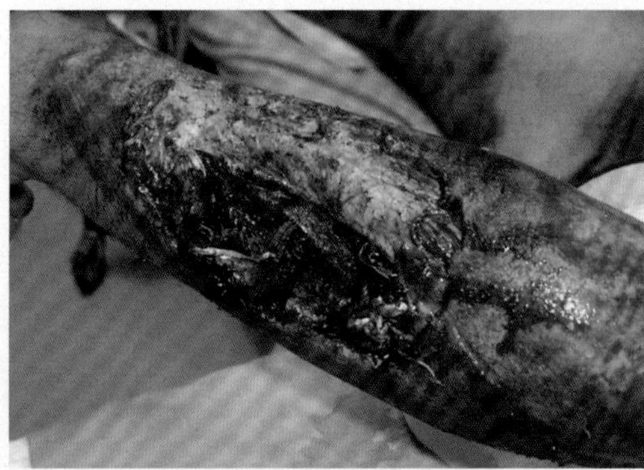

FIG 2 • Preoperative picture of a patient with severe soft tissue loss, including extensor muscle, after a motorcycle accident, which required extensor tendon reconstruction.

- Attritional ruptures will also render the tendon incompatible with primary repair necessitating the need for tendon transfer or grafting procedures.

NATURAL HISTORY

- Without treatment, complete extensor tendon disruptions will result in a persistent loss of active extension or incomplete extension of the wrist or digits (or loss of active abduction and extension of the thumb, depending on which tendon or tendons are involved).
- A late tendon imbalance resulting from pull of the flexor tendons against a disrupted or weakened extensor mechanism with or without fixed joint contracture may develop if reconstruction is not performed.

PATIENT HISTORY AND PHYSICAL FINDINGS

- The patient most commonly has a history of penetrating or blunt trauma to the dorsal forearm or hand with resultant loss of active extension of the wrist, fingers, or thumb (**FIG 3**). Loss of soft tissue may be associated with the original injury.
- In cases of attritional rupture of the EPL tendon, the patient may have a recent or remote history of a distal radius fracture, usually only minimally displaced.
- Physical examination methods include the following:
  - MP extension. Incomplete MP extension indicates extensor tendon disruption in zones proximal to the MP. If the other fingers are not kept flexed, the patient may be able to fully extend the affected finger in the presence of a completely lacerated tendon.
  - EPL test. An EPL rupture manifests as a loss of extension of the thumb IP and MP joints.

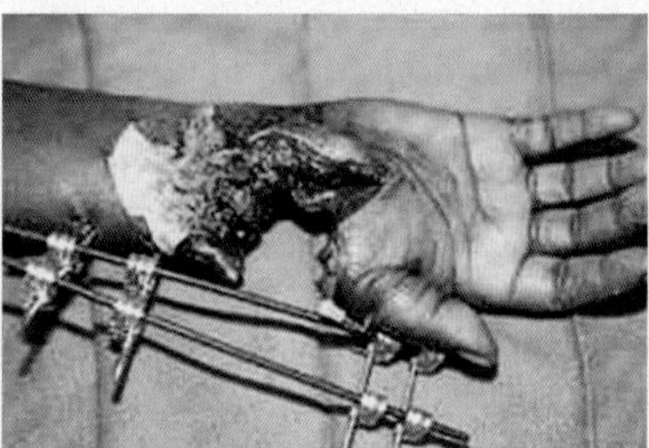

FIG 3 • Segmental loss of extensor and flexor tendons from a shotgun blast.

  - Tenodesis test. A loss of extensor tendon continuity will result in loss of the tenodesis effect. Wrist flexion will have no effect on finger extension.
  - Careful evaluation should be given to lacerations proximal to the juncturae tendinum. Digital extension may be maintained through the juncturae tendinum and an adjacent EDC tendon.[6]
- A complete evaluation of the elbow, forearm, wrist, or hand begins with a thorough inspection of all open wounds and an assessment of the extent of soft tissue compromise.
  - Local or regional anesthesia can assist with patient comfort during the examination.
- A comprehensive neurovascular examination must be performed before using any anesthetic. Special attention is directed to the status of the radial nerve, specifically the PIN.
  - Compromise in PIN function may result from compression neuropathy, direct injury, or underlying elbow pathology.
- If there is a suspicion of joint violation, then injection of sterile saline with or without methylene blue into the joint can verify whether the joint capsule has been disrupted.

IMAGING AND OTHER DIAGNOSTIC STUDIES

- Anteroposterior (AP), lateral, and oblique plain radiographs of the affected area (elbow, forearm, wrist, or hand) are obtained to rule out the presence of a foreign body, underlying fracture, or bony deformity or pathology.
- In cases of late presentation of suspected extensor tendon rupture, magnetic resonance imaging (MRI) is occasionally useful to confirm the diagnosis and identify the location of the retracted tendon ends.

DIFFERENTIAL DIAGNOSIS

- Radial nerve or PIN palsy
- Flexor tendon injury
- Intrinsic tightness
- Tendon adhesions
- Tendon subluxation (MP joint level)
- Joint contracture, subluxation, or deformity
- Soft tissue contracture

NONOPERATIVE MANAGEMENT

- Conservative treatment of injuries proximal to the metacarpals usually is not possible because of tendon retraction and muscle contracture and will result in persistent loss of extension of the wrist or digits.[4]
- Chronic extensor mechanism disorders distal to the metacarpals without fixed deformity will respond to splinting and intensive therapy. Such conservative management may result in an acceptable functional outcome for select patients.

SURGICAL MANAGEMENT

- Most extensor tendon lacerations are amenable to direct primary repair if treated relatively early.
- Indications for reconstruction of extensor tendon injuries include loss of extension of the wrist, fingers, or thumb resulting in a functional deficit.
- When delay or loss of tendon substance precludes a direct repair, tendon grafting or transfer may restore function successfully.

Preoperative Planning

- The patient must be provided with a realistic assessment of the potential gains from surgery as well as details of the treatment plan.
- Any fixed joint contractures should be identified and treated with therapy and splinting before extensor tendon reconstruction to optimize outcomes.
- In cases of severe soft tissue loss, coverage must be obtained before proceeding with extensor system reconstruction.
  - This may include free or island muscle, fascial, or skin flaps in addition to full- or split-thickness skin grafts.

Positioning

- The patient is positioned supine with a hand table attached to the operative side.
- A tourniquet is usually used to operate in a bloodless field.

Approach

- The approach depends on the tendon transfer or grafting technique required and is detailed in the Techniques section.

TECHNIQUES

End and Side Weave Junctures

- Tendon transfer or graft junctures are often best secured using an end weave technique (**TECH FIG 1**).
- The Pulvertaft method is a common weave used.
  - A pointed tendon-grasping and -passing instrument is invaluable and allows one tendon to be brought through the substance of the other tendon with minimal trauma.
  - The tendon weave is performed at right angles. For example, the first entry is horizontal, the next vertical, and then the third horizontal. At least three weaves are needed.

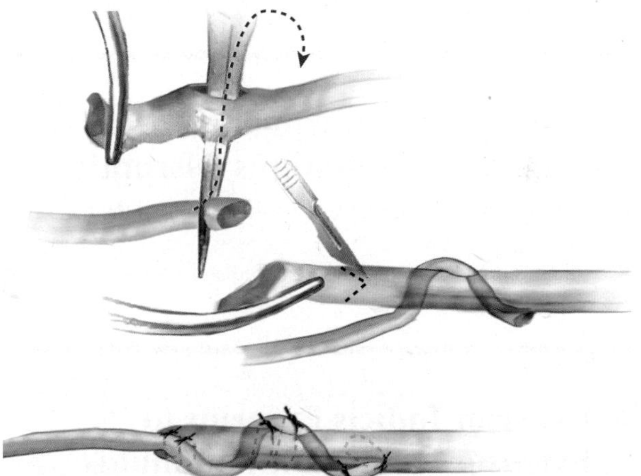

TECH FIG 1 • End weave technique. The smaller tendon is passed through and sutured.

Extensor Indicis Proprius to Extensor Pollicis Longus Transfer

- The distal EIP tendon is identified through a 1-cm incision over the index finger MP joint. The EIP is ulnar to the EDC II.
- A second incision is made just distal to the extensor retinaculum at roughly the radiocarpal joint level, and the EIP tendon is identified in the radial aspect of the fourth extensor compartment.
  - The EIP is readily identified by its distal muscle belly.
- The EIP tendon is separated from the EDC II and transected through the incision over the MP joint.
- The tendon is then brought through to the proximal incision.
- A third incision is centered over the scaphotrapeziotrapeziodal joint and the distal stump of the disrupted EPL tendon is identified (**TECH FIG 2A**).
- A subcutaneous tunnel is created to connect the incision at the wrist and the incision near the base of the thumb.
- The EIP tendon is passed through the tunnel and attached to the distal stump of EPL using an end weave technique (**TECH FIG 2B**).
- Tension should be set so that when the wrist is extended, the thumb IP joint flexes, allowing the tip of the thumb to touch the tip of the index finger. The thumb IP joint should fully extend when the wrist is flexed (**TECH FIG 2C**).
- The thumb is immobilized, with the wrist extended about 20 degrees and the thumb IP joint at 0 degrees for 4 weeks.

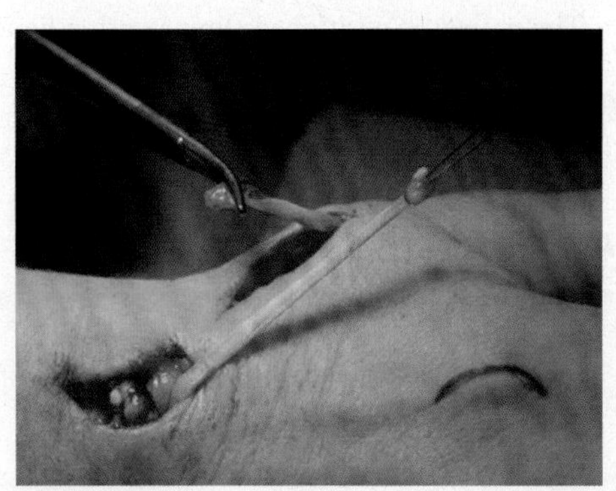
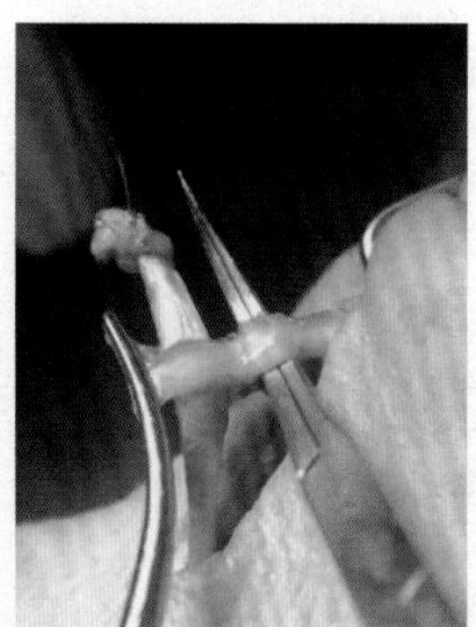
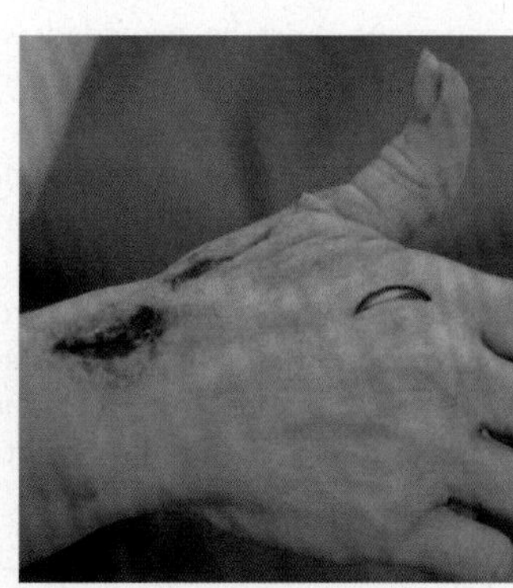

TECH FIG 2 • EIP to EPL transfer. **A.** After the EIP tendon is identified, it is brought through the proximal incision. The distal stump of the EPL tendon is identified as well. **B.** The EIP tendon is passed through and is woven into the EPL tendon. **C.** After proper tensioning, the thumb should extend as the wrist flexes.

End-to-Side Suturing for Extensor Digitorum Communis Disruptions

- A longitudinal incision is made on the dorsum of the hand over the appropriate area.
- The disrupted tendon end is identified and isolated.
- An end-to-side repair is performed to the adjacent intact tendon.
- Tension must be set so that the fingers are in extension when the wrist is flexed and the MP joints are flexed 20 to 30 degrees when the wrist is extended about 20 degrees. The normal flexion cascade must be reestablished.

Extensor Indicis Proprius to Extensor Digitorum Communis (Fourth/Fifth) Transfer

- The EIP tendon is isolated and freed in a manner similar to that described for the EIP to EPL transfer.
- An incision is made dorsally on the hand, over the disrupted extensor tendons of the ring and small fingers.
- The EIP is mobilized and inserted into the distal stump of the disrupted tendon of the small finger.
  - If disrupted, the extensor digiti quinti (EDQ) is sewn side to side to the transfer.
- The distal stump of the ring finger is attached to the adjacent intact common extensor tendon of the long finger. If the EDC to the long finger is also ruptured, it is sewn to the intact EDC to the index, whereas the EDC to the ring is sewn to the EIP transfer (**TECH FIG 3**).

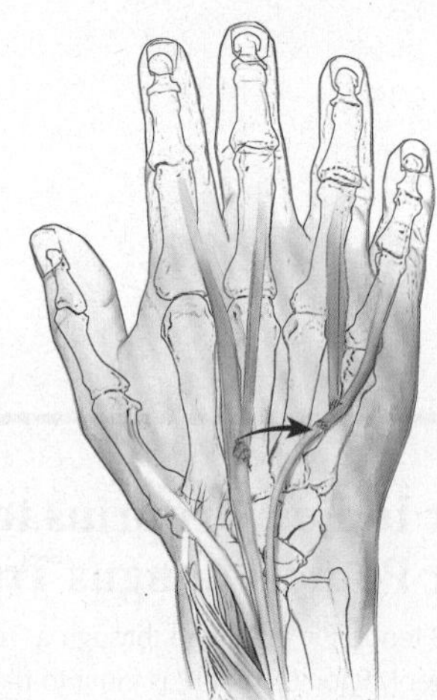

TECH FIG 3 • EIP to EDC IV/V tendon transfer.

Flexor Carpi Ulnaris to Extensor Digitorum Communis Transfer

- A longitudinal incision is made over the flexor carpi ulnaris (FCU) in the distal forearm.
- The FCU tendon is transected just proximal to the pisiform and is freed up proximally.
- A second oblique incision is made 5 cm below the medial epicondyle in the proximal forearm.
- The FCU fascial attachments are incised to free up the entire muscle belly.
- A third incision begins on the dorsoulnar midforearm and angles distally toward the tubercle of Lister to expose the disrupted EDC tendons.
- A tendon passer or Kelly clamp is passed subcutaneously around the ulnar border of the forearm to pull the FCU tendon into the dorsal wound.
- Muscle may be excised from the FCU to reduce bulk.
- The FCU tendon is woven through the EDC tendons at a 45-degree angle just proximal to the dorsal retinaculum.
- The FCU is secured under maximum tension, with the wrist and MP joints in neutral.

Flexor Carpi Radialis to Extensor Digitorum Communis Transfer

- A longitudinal incision is made over the flexor carpi radialis (FCR) in the distal forearm.
- The FCR tendon is identified and transected near its insertion.
- The tendon is freed up proximally to allow additional excursion.
- A second longitudinal incision is made on the dorsal forearm, extending from the midforearm to just distal to the dorsal retinaculum.
- The FCR is then passed subcutaneously around the radial border of forearm and delivered into the dorsal wound.
- The FCR tendon is then inserted into the EDC tendons and positioned superficial to the retinaculum.
- The transfer is secured with the FCR under maximum tension and wrist and MP joints in neutral (**TECH FIG 4**).

Pronator Teres to Extensor Carpi Radialis Brevis Transfer

- An incision is made over the volar radial aspect of the midforearm.
- The pronator teres (PT) tendon is identified and followed to its insertion into the radius.
- A strip of periosteum is kept intact when freeing up the insertion to ensure sufficient length of the transferred tendon.
- The PT muscle is freed up proximally to improve excursion.
- The PT muscle and tendon is then passed subcutaneously around the radial border of the forearm.
- The tendon is inserted into the ECRB just distal to the musculotendinous junction through a second incision if needed (**TECH FIG 5**).
- The transfer is secured with PT in maximum tension and the wrist in 45 degrees of extension.

Flexor Digitorum Superficialis Transfer for Multiple Extensor Disruption

- A transverse incision is made in the distal palm to expose the long and ring superficialis tendons.
- The flexor digitorum superficialis (FDS) tendons to III and IV in the distal palm are divided proximal to the chiasma.
- A longitudinal incision is made on the volar radial midforearm and the interosseous membrane is exposed.
- The two tendons are then delivered into the proximal wound.
- Two openings are excised from the interosseous membrane, large enough to pass the muscle bellies through to minimize adhesions.
- A J-shaped incision is made on the dorsum of the distal forearm, and the tendons are passed through the interosseous membrane.
- The FDS III is routed radially, and the FDS IV is routed ulnarly to the profundus muscle mass.
- The FDS III is interwoven into the tendons of the EIP and EDC II and III (**TECH FIG 6**).
- The FDS IV is interwoven into EDC IV and V.
- Tension is set with the FDS under maximum tension, the wrist in 20 degrees of extension, and the fingers and thumb held in a fist.

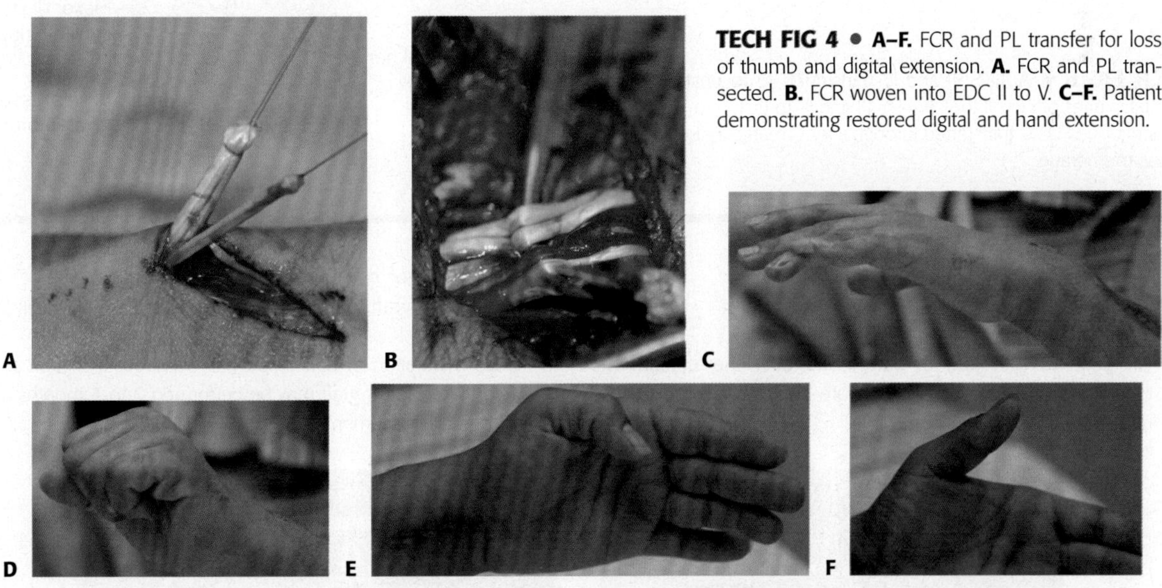

TECH FIG 4 • A–F. FCR and PL transfer for loss of thumb and digital extension. **A.** FCR and PL transected. **B.** FCR woven into EDC II to V. **C–F.** Patient demonstrating restored digital and hand extension.

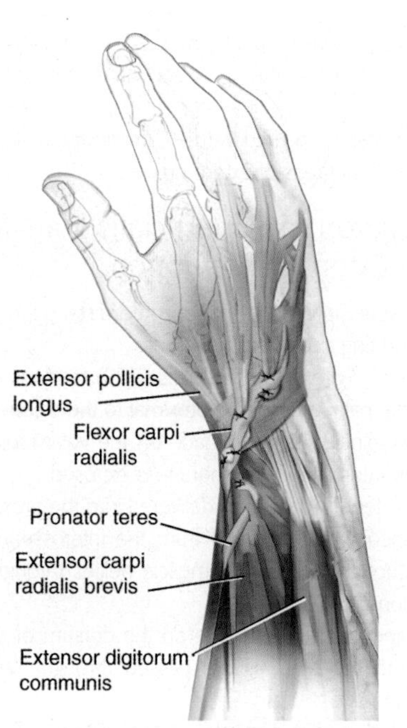

TECH FIG 5 • FCR to EDC and PT to ECRB tendon transfer.

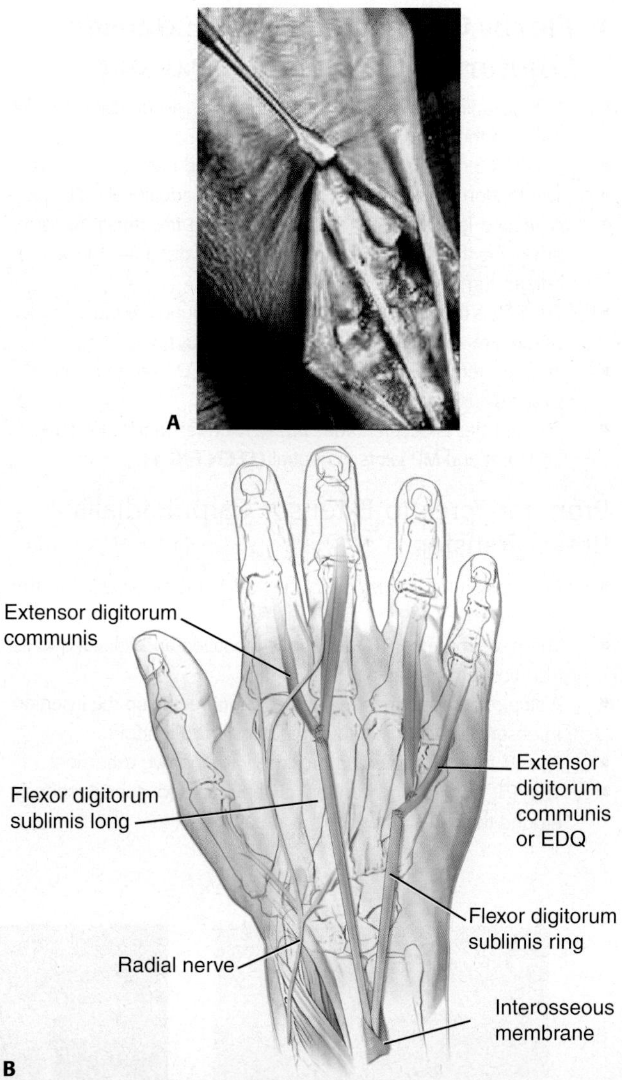

TECH FIG 6 • **A.** FDS III and IV transferred to reconstruct segmental injuries of EDC II to V. **B.** FDS III and IV to EDC II to V tendon transfers. The FDS is transferred through a rent created in the interosseous membrane.

Staged Reconstruction with Silicone Rods

- In patients with loss of soft tissue over the dorsum of the hand and forearm, appropriate soft tissue coverage is obtained first.
- At the time of coverage, the proposed path of the tendon transfer or graft is preserved with the use of a silicone tendon rod.
- Once maturation of soft tissue has occurred, the appropriate tendon transfer or graft may be performed 2 to 3 months after silicone rod placement (**TECH FIG 7**).

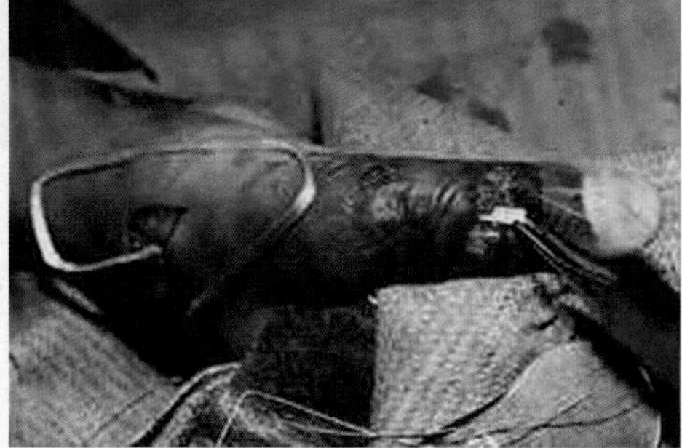

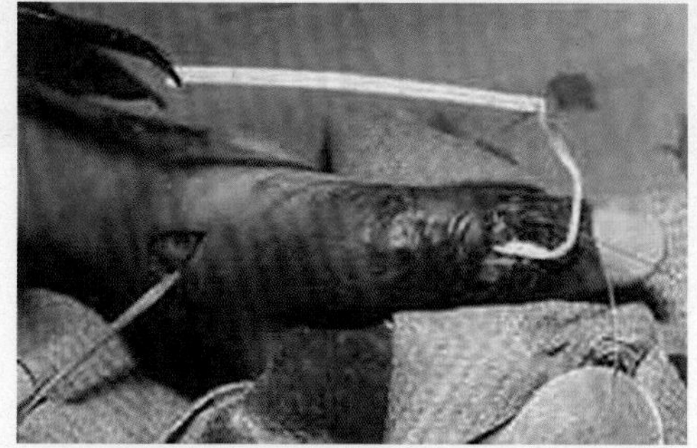

TECH FIG 7 • **A.** Silastic spacer (tendon rod) used to create adhesion-free bed. **B.** Silastic spacer replaced by tendon graft after soft tissue healing and remodeling.

TECHNIQUES

Free Interposition Tendon Graft

- In patients with either segmental tendon loss, muscle contracture, or atritional rupture, consideration may be given to performing an interpositional tendon graft.
- Prerequisite soft tissue coverage is necessary before either local autograft (ie, PL, EDM) or allograft is chosen.
- The tendon stump is freshed sharply, and the distance needed to bridge the gap is carefully measured and taken from the graft.
- The donor tendon caliber is also modified to approximate the recipient.
- A Bunnell crisscross suture is placed in the proximal motor end of the tendon with 3-0 polyester (**TECH FIG 8**).
- The graft is threaded on straight needles, and the distal juncture is completed by another crisscross suture in the distal portion.
- The appropriate resting posture of the finger is obtained. Proper tension is crucial.

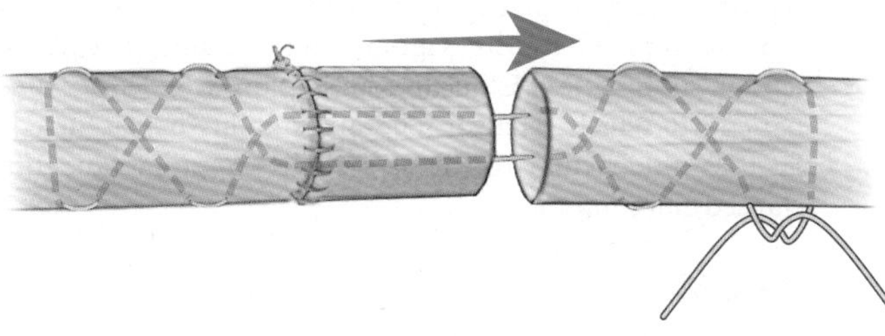

TECH FIG 8 • Interposition graft suture technique. By using short segments of available graft material, a gap can be closed in the late repair.

PEARLS AND PITFALLS

Preoperative issues	▪ In patients with severe soft tissue compromise, skeletal stabilization is obtained first, followed by soft tissue coverage. Reconstruction of the extensor mechanism is addressed later. ▪ Joint contractures should be addressed prior to extensor tendon reconstruction.
Selection of transfer	▪ The type of transfer performed depends on the tendon to be reconstructed and on surgeon preference. We generally prefer using the FCR for EDC reconstruction.

POSTOPERATIVE CARE

- Initial splinting should immobilize the wrist in about 30 degrees of extension, the MP joints in about 15 degrees of flexion, and the IP joints in full extension.
- If transferred tendons originate proximal to the elbow, the elbow should be immobilized in 90 degrees of flexion with appropriate forearm rotation.
- The thumb IP and MP joints should be immobilized in full extension.
- After 4 weeks, active range of motion is started under the supervision of a certified hand therapist and with a protective splint. Active-assisted and passive range of motion follows 2 weeks later.

OUTCOMES

- Staged extensor tendon reconstruction using a silicone implant followed by tendon grafting for restoration of PIP joint extension was reported to have good results in six fingers with severe dorsal soft tissue injuries, improving hand function in all cases.[1]
- Interpositional grafting technique using local autograft has been reported to have no difference in clinical outcome when compared with EIP to EPL transfer techniques.[5]

COMPLICATIONS

- Extrinsic tightness
- Intrinsic tightness
- Rupture
- Donor deficits
- Joint stiffness

REFERENCES

1. Adams BD. Staged extensor tendon reconstruction in the finger. J Hand Surg Am 1997;22:833–837.
2. Al-Rachid M, Theivendran K, Craigen MA. Delayed ruptures of the extensor tendon secondary to the use of volar locking compression played for distal radius fractures. J Bone Joint Surg Br 2006;88(12):1610–1612.
3. Baratz ME, Schmidt CC, Hughes TB. Extensor tendon injuries. In: Green DP, Hotchkiss RN, Pederson WC, eds. Green's Operative Hand Surgery, ed 5. Philadelphia: Elsevier Churchill Livingstone, 2005:187–217.
4. Burton RI, Melchior JA. Extensor tendons—late reconstruction. In: Green DP, Hotchkiss RN, Pederson WC, eds. Green's Operative Hand Surgery, ed 4. New York: Churchill Livingstone, 1999:1988–2021.
5. Chung US, Kim JH, Seo WS, et al. Tendon transfer or tendon graft for ruptured finger extensor tendons in rheumatoid hands. J Hand Surg Eur Vol 2010;35(4):279–282.
6. Newport ML. Extensor tendon injuries in the hand. J Am Acad Orthop Surg 1997;5:59–66.
7. von Schroeder HP, Botte MJ. The functional significance of the long extensors and juncturae tendinum in finger extension. J Hand Surg Am 1993;18(4):614–617.

Extensor Tendon Centralization following Traumatic Subluxation at the Metacarpophalangeal Joint

Byung J. Lee, Ross J. Richer, and Craig S. Phillips

DEFINITION

- Instability of the extensor digitorum tendons at the metacarpophalangeal (MCP) joint has been subdivided into two categories: subluxation and dislocation.
  - Subluxation of the extensor digitorum tendons at the MCP joint is defined as lateral displacement of the tendon with its border reaching beyond the midline but remaining in contact with the condyle during full MCP joint flexion.
  - Dislocation describes the condition in which the extensor tendon is located in the groove between the metacarpal heads.[14]
- Instability of the extensor digitorum tendons at the MCP joint usually occurs in patients with underlying inflammatory conditions (ie, rheumatoid arthritis).
- Traumatic injury to the sagittal bands, particularly the radial sagittal band, can cause instability of the extensor tendon. Although ulnar-sided injuries have been reported, the overwhelming majority of injuries occur to the radial sagittal band.
- Instability of the extensor tendon is relatively rare in nonrheumatoid patients.
- The sagittal bands are sometimes referred to as the *shroud* ligament because of the way they cover, or wrap, the MCP joint.
- Sagittal band injuries are classified as type I, II, or III, depending on the degree of extensor tendon instability.[14]
- Traumatic extensor tendon subluxation at the MCP joint level is classified as type II injury; dislocation is type III. These injuries have been given the eponym "boxer's knuckle."[6]
- Not all injuries to the sagittal bands result in extensor tendon subluxation. Clinical examination will identify those patients in which extensor tendon instability has occurred.
- Factors influencing treatment include symptoms and time elapsed since injury.

ANATOMY

- The digital extensor mechanism at the level of the MCP joint consists of the extensor tendon, sagittal bands, and volar plate. The sagittal bands are part of a complex extensor retinacular system that includes the triangular ligament between the lateral bands, the transverse retinacular ligament, and the oblique retinacular ligament at the proximal interphalangeal (PIP) joint level (**FIG 1A**).
- The sagittal bands are dynamic structures that envelop the extensor tendons, centering them over the MCP joint during flexion, preventing bowstringing during hyperextension, and controlling tendon excursion. The sagittal bands insert onto the volar plate overlying the MCP joint (**FIG 1B**).[15]
- The sagittal bands are the primary stabilizers of the extensor digitorum tendons at the MCP joints, and their integrity is essential for normal extensor tendon function.[12,15,17,20]

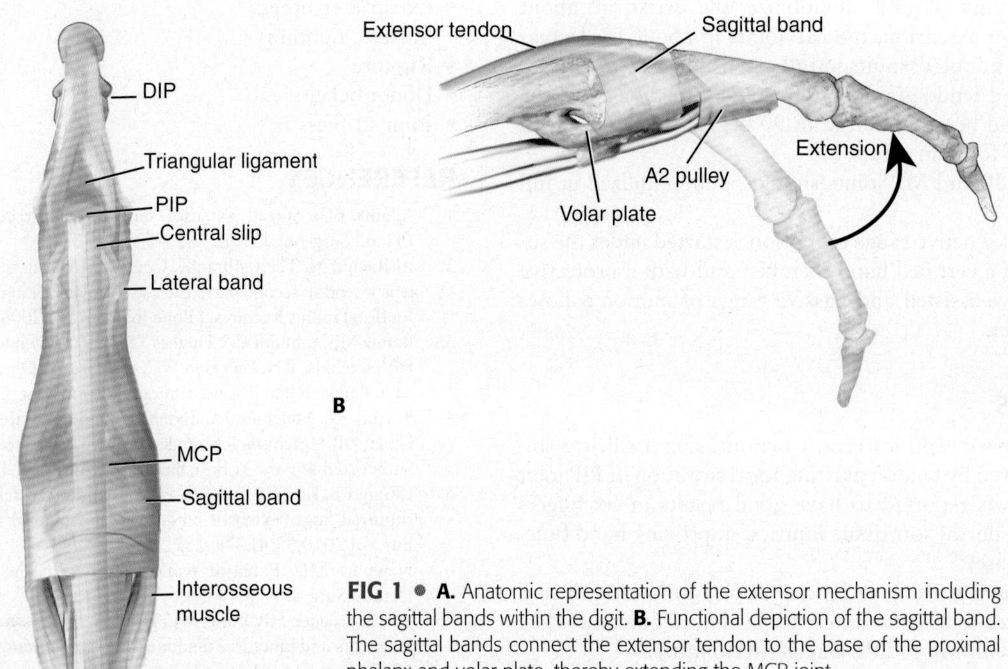

FIG 1 • **A.** Anatomic representation of the extensor mechanism including the sagittal bands within the digit. **B.** Functional depiction of the sagittal band. The sagittal bands connect the extensor tendon to the base of the proximal phalanx and volar plate, thereby extending the MCP joint.

- When the MCP joint is maintained in neutral extension, the sagittal bands are oriented perpendicular to the tendon.
- The sagittal bands are anatomically and physiologically distinct from the deeper collateral ligaments.
- The radial sagittal band is often thinner and longer than its ulnar counterpart.
- The greatest tension on the sagittal bands occurs with wrist and MCP flexion and radioulnar deviation.
- The lumbrical muscles function to flex the MCP joint and extend the interphalangeal (IP) joint through the lateral bands. They originate on the flexor digitorum profundus (FDP) tendon and traverse on the radial aspect of the digit inserting into the extensor expansion.
- The intermetacarpal ligaments are stout ligaments that originate and insert on adjacent metacarpal necks. These ligaments pass dorsal to the lumbrical tendons and volar to the interosseous tendons.

PATHOGENESIS

- The mechanism of sagittal band injury commonly involves a direct blow to a flexed MCP joint.
- Injury may result indirectly from forced flexion or directly from shear forces across the sagittal band.
- Other described mechanisms include forceful deviation of the digit against resistance, usually with the MCP joint extended.
- In open injuries, the sagittal band is usually lacerated.
  - Sometimes, laceration of the junctura tendinum can also lead to extensor tendon subluxation.
- Extensor tendon subluxation typically occurs with at least 50% disruption of the proximal sagittal band.[20] The extensor tendon no longer remains centralized over the MCP joint through flexion but rather subluxates ulnarly.
- It has been suggested that frequency of injury among the digits is related to the cross-sectional diameter of the sagittal band, the extent of distal attachment, and the length of the sagittal band.[7,14,15] The long finger is most commonly injured.
- It has been suggested that traumatic subluxation occurs when there is tearing of both the superficial and deep layers of the sagittal band enveloping the extensor tendon.[8]
- When underlying inflammatory conditions are present, the sagittal bands become attenuated and atrophic, allowing for atraumatic subluxation of the extensor tendons into the troughs (usually ulnar) between metacarpal heads.

NATURAL HISTORY

- Symptoms from acute injuries typically resolve within 3 weeks with appropriate treatment. However, pain can persist for up to 9 months before fully dissipating.[6]
- When sagittal band injuries associated with discomfort, swelling, and subluxation are neglected, patients will experience ongoing symptoms that may worsen over time. The extensor tendon may become fixed in the valley between the metacarpal heads, leading to loss of MCP extension and deviation of the digit. These patients will require surgical treatment for resolution of their symptoms.[7,14,16]

PATIENT HISTORY AND PHYSICAL FINDINGS

- This chapter deals with traumatic subluxation. Treatment protocols for inflammatory subluxation differ and are beyond the scope of this chapter.
- A critical aspect of treatment involves understanding the circumstances surrounding the injury. This information will help identify those at risk for infection in open injuries (eg, clean laceration, fight bite) or the possibility of underlying systemic disease contributing to closed injuries caused by low-energy trauma.
- Shortly after injury, soft tissue swelling may obscure the alignment of the tendon over the MCP joint.
- Initially after traumatic injury to the sagittal bands with subsequent extensor tendon instability, symptoms and signs include the following:
  - Localized pain
  - Swelling over the involved MCP joint
  - Limited motion (**FIG 2A**)
  - Limited or deviated MCP joint extension or both (**FIG 2B**)
  - Weak MCP extension
  - A potentially painful snapping of the tendon over the MCP joint with active flexion (**FIG 2C**)
  - Ulnar deviation deformity and difficulty adducting (or abducting in the case of the index) the affected finger
- Chronic cases of tendon instability often exhibit pain during MCP joint flexion, such as during grip, along with localized tenderness and swelling over the injured sagittal band.[16]
- MCP extension can be actively maintained when the joint is passively placed into extension; however, difficulty is usually encountered when attempts are made to extend the MCP joint from flexion or when flexing the MCP joint from full extension.

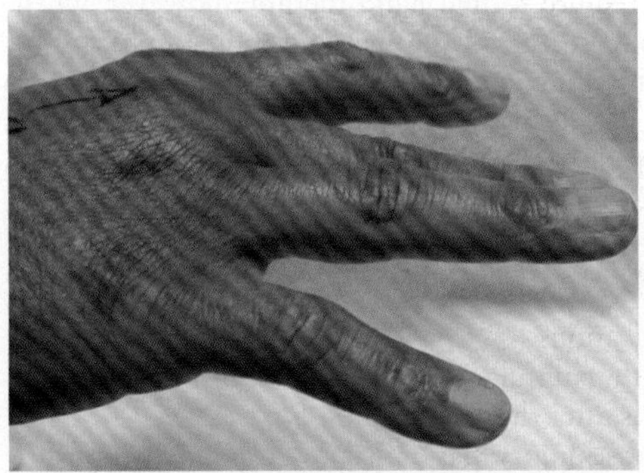
A

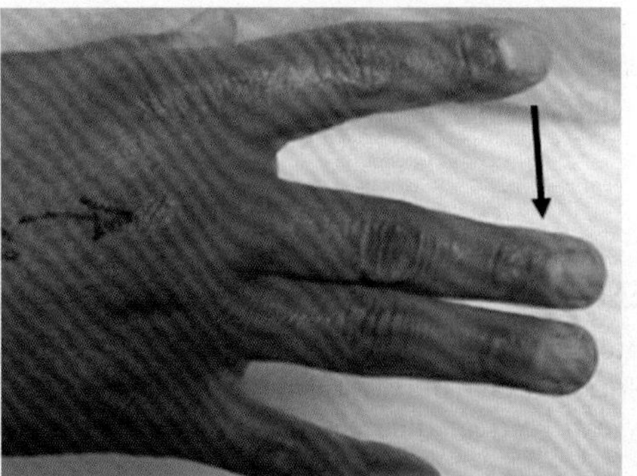
B

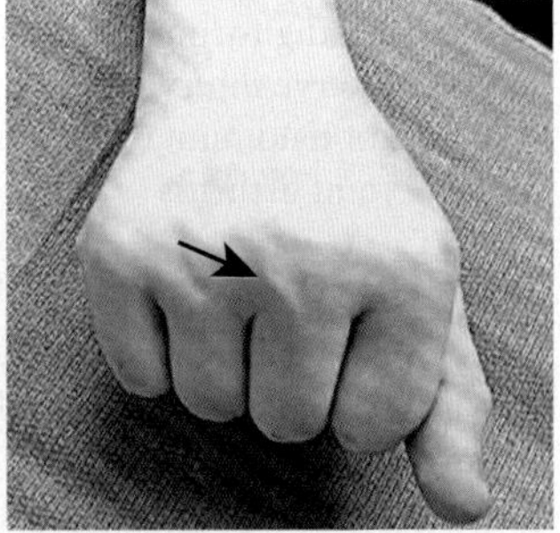
C

FIG 2 • **A.** Lack of complete active digital extension at the MCP joint associated with a sagittal band disruption. **B.** Ulnar deviation of the long finger associated with a radial sagittal band disruption. **C.** Dislocation of the long finger extensor tendon into the ulnar trough of the fourth web space (*arrow*). (**A,B:** Courtesy of Brian Hartigan.)

- Methods for examining extensor tendon instability over the MCP joint include the following:
  - Assess sagittal bands throughout MCP range of motion.
  - Assess swelling, open injuries, and so forth. Determine location of pathology.
  - Palpate over the MCP joints and in the groove between the metacarpal heads.
    - Sagittal band injuries will exhibit pain with superficial palpation. In contrast, pain associated with collateral ligament injury is usually deeper, within the groove between the metacarpal heads.
- Perform tendon and ligament instability examination.
- Ask the patient to flex the MCP joint and wrist. This position places the maximum amount of ulnar force on the extensor tendon at the MCP joint. This will help to determine the amount of instability.
- Pain provocation test: With the distal and proximal IP joints extended and the MCP joint flexed, ask the patient to try to extend the MCP joint against resistance.

IMAGING AND OTHER DIAGNOSTIC STUDIES

- A standard radiographic series, including posteroanterior, lateral, and oblique views of the MCP joint.
  - These views will exclude any mechanical or bony pathology limiting extension of or predisposing the sagittal band to dislocate.
- A Brewerton view (anteroposterior [AP] view with dorsal surface of the fingers touching the cassette and the MCP joints flexed 45 degrees) or stress views may be needed to rule out collateral ligament avulsion injury.
- Magnetic resonance imaging (MRI) has been used with success to identify patients with sagittal band injuries, especially when the physical examination is obscured by swelling and patient discomfort.[13] MRI with the injured MCP joint flexed facilitates the diagnosis.
  - Acute injuries demonstrate morphologic and signal intensity abnormalities within and around the sagittal bands on axial T1- and T2-weighted images, together with poor definition, focal discontinuity, and focal thickening.[4]
- Dynamic ultrasound has been reported as a useful modality for diagnosis of extensor tendon subluxation when swelling obscures the physical examination.[11]

DIFFERENTIAL DIAGNOSIS

- MCP joint collateral ligament injury
- Trigger finger
- Ulnar nerve palsy
- Congenital sagittal band deficiency
- Extensor digitorum communis tendon rupture
- Radial nerve injury
- Junctura tendinum disruption
- MCP joint arthritis

NONOPERATIVE MANAGEMENT

- In our experience, most symptomatic patients presenting within 3 weeks of injury with acute sagittal band disruptions and extensor tendon instability can be treated successfully nonoperatively with a splint.[14]
  - Success in the literature varies, however. Studies have shown that 44% to 100% of patients treated conservatively will be asymptomatic at an average of 13.5 months.[1–3,7,14]

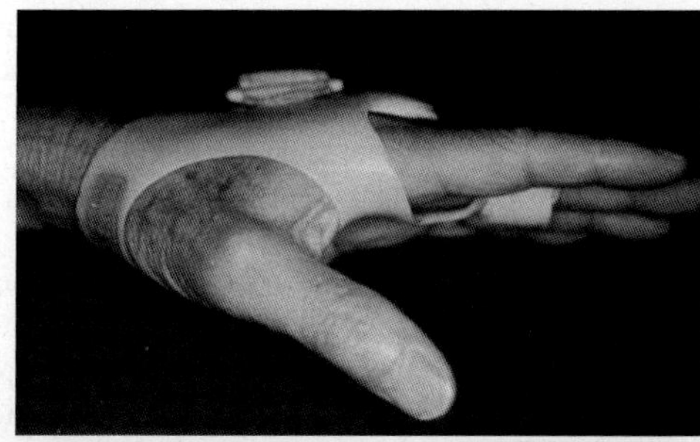

A

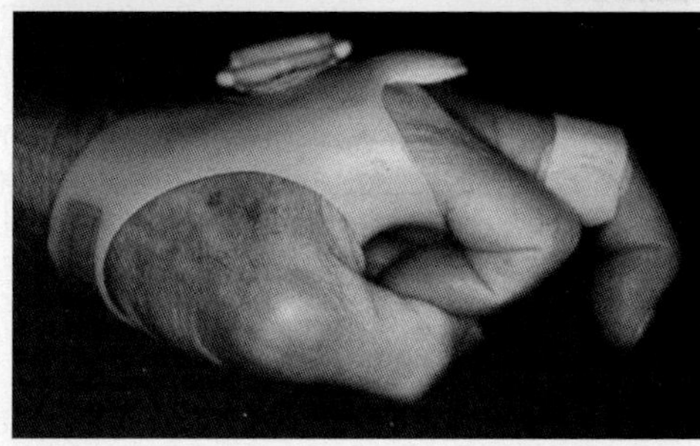

B

FIG 3 • **A,B.** Typical splint used for the conservative treatment of sagittal band disruption. The IP joints are free and no more than 30 degrees of MCP joint flexion is allowed.

  - Certainly, except in special circumstances such as the professional athlete, conservative therapy should initially be attempted.
- Although several different protocols and splints have been described, most share one common objective: maintaining the MCP joint in neutral (full extension) for a period of weeks. In all situations, motion of the IP joint should be accommodated and encouraged.
  - A hand-based, custom orthoplast splint holding the involved digit in 0 to 20 degrees of MCP joint flexion (**FIG 3**) is worn for 4 to 6 weeks, depending on the patient's progress at the 2- and 4-week follow-up visits.
  - After 6 weeks of MCP immobilization in extension, the splint is weaned except for sporting endeavors and other heavy activities, in which case the splint is used for another 2 weeks. Buddy taping can provide long-term support as may be indicated.
  - Active range-of-motion activities are initiated and slowly progressed to gentle passive flexion of the involved MCP joint.
  - Thereafter, unrestricted use of the hand is promoted. It is unusual to require formal hand therapy; however, when excessive joint stiffness is present and radiographs fail to document any bony pathology, a short course of therapy focusing on flexion along with modality use can be helpful.
  - If the injury clearly is not responding to immobilization, surgery is recommended.

SURGICAL MANAGEMENT

- Operative indications
  - Patients with painful extensor tendon instability more than 3 weeks after the injury
  - Patients whose injury has failed to respond to nonsurgical management and have persistent, painful tendon instability beyond 6 weeks of conservative care
  - Professional athletes[6] and other high-demand individuals

- When possible, direct repair of the sagittal band should be performed.
  - Although we believe that this is usually not possible more than 8 weeks after injury, Hame and Melone[6] reported on 11 direct repairs at an average of 3.3 months out from time of injury. No patient had prior splinting. All patients were asymptomatic with full recovery of range of motion and return to professional sports at an average of 5 months.
  - Carroll et al[2] reported on five patients who underwent reconstruction after failed conservative management. All patients regained full, asymptomatic range of motion.
- If tissue deficiency or scarring exists, reconstruction as opposed to primary repair will be required.

Preoperative Planning

- With open injuries, the surgeon should determine if the cause was related to a bite. In this situation, MCP joint contamination is likely and surgical irrigation and débridement as well as antibiotic treatment is warranted. When severe contamination is present, delayed sagittal band repair is indicated.
  - Concomitant MCP joint capsular injury is possible. Once surgically exposed, methylene blue injection into the joint, out of the zone of injury, can help to reveal any rents in the MCP joint capsule. These defects should be débrided with subsequent irrigation of the joint. Afterward, no capsular repair is necessary.[6]
- The surgeon should be prepared to perform either a sagittal band repair or a reconstruction.
- Local anesthesia with sedation is preferred, but regional or general anesthesia is acceptable.

Positioning

- The patient is placed supine on the operating table with the affected hand outstretched onto a hand table.
- A tourniquet is applied to the arm and inflated to the appropriate pressure before starting the procedure.

TECHNIQUES

Exposure

- A curvilinear incision is placed dorsally over the ulnar aspect of the affected MCP joint.
  - This is used for primary sagittal band repair.
- A longitudinal incision is centered dorsally over the affected MCP joint.
  - This is used for reconstructive cases requiring greater exposure.
- Sensory branches of the radial or ulnar nerves, or both, are identified and protected.
- The extensor tendon is exposed, the tear identified, and scar tissue débrided.
- The MCP capsule, which is deep to the extensor tendon, is usually left undisturbed; however, when MCP joint pathology needs to be addressed, the capsule may be incised.

Primary Repair

- The sagittal band disruption is identified and the extensor tendon centralized (**TECH FIG 1A,B**).
- Excess tissue is excised from the area between the torn sagittal band and the common extensor tendon.
- The sagittal fibers are then repaired using 4-0 or 5-0 nonabsorbable suture (Ethibond). The knots are buried where possible.
  - The repair is performed with the joint in 60 to 70 degrees of flexion to avoid tension on the repair and stiffness of the joint.
- The joint is flexed and extended to ensure midline stability (**TECH FIG 1C–E**).
- The wound is closed with interrupted 4-0 nylon sutures.

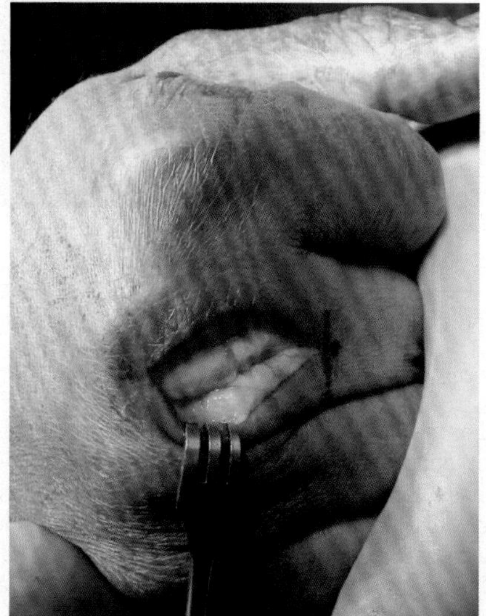
A

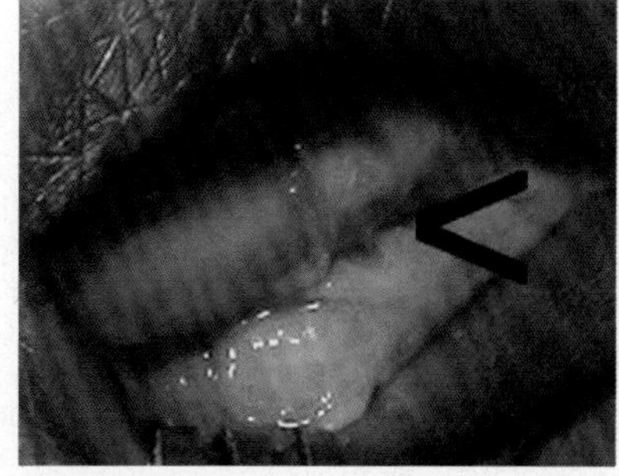
B

TECH FIG 1 • **A.** Traumatic extensor tendon dislocation (ulnar) over the MCP joint with the MCP joint extended. **B.** Extensor tendon subluxation over the MCP joint (*arrowhead*) with the joint flexed. *(continued)*

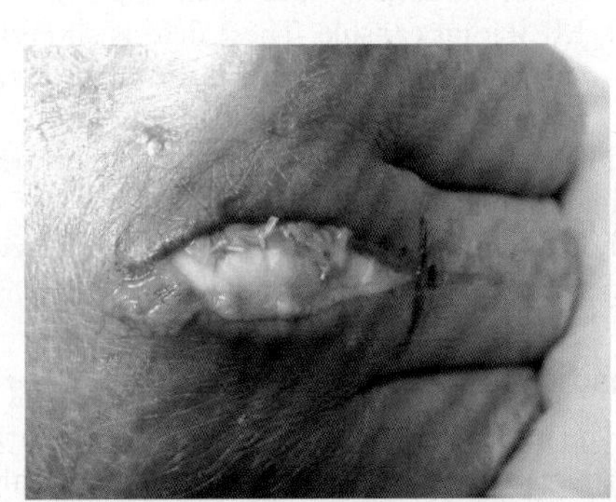

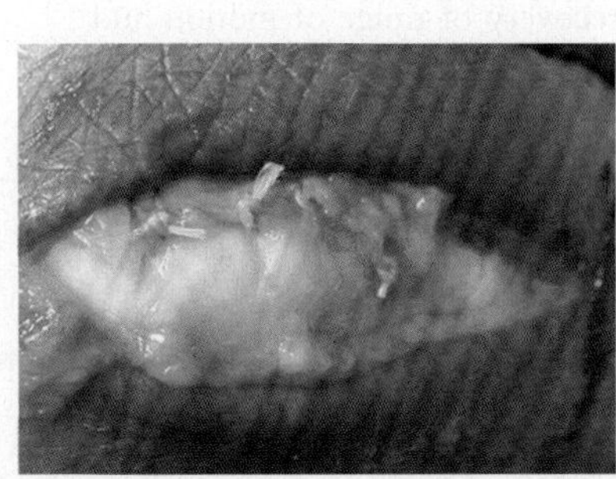

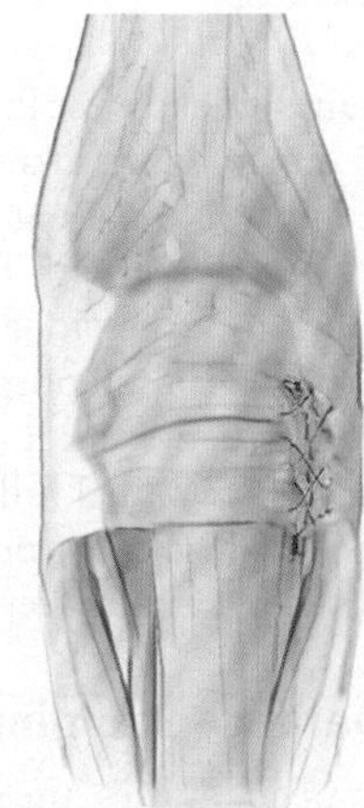

TECH FIG 1 • *(continued)* **C.** Primary repair of the sagittal band with the MCP joint extended. **D.** Primary sagittal band repair with the MCP joint flexed. The extensor tendon remains centralized dorsally with flexion. **E.** Primary repair of the deficient sagittal band. (**A–D:** Courtesy of Brian Hartigan.)

Reconstruction with Extensor Tendon Slip (Carroll/Kilgore) (Authors' Preferred Technique)

- Release of the ulnar sagittal band may be necessary to mobilize the scarred tendon dorsally and radially (**TECH FIG 2A,B**).
- A distally based radial (or ulnar) slip of extensor tendon (about one-third) is fashioned and routed deep to the intact extensor tendon (**TECH FIG 2C**).
- The distally based tendon graft is rerouted deep to the extensor tendon.
- In a distal to proximal direction, the tendon graft is then looped around the radial collateral ligament (if subluxed ulnarly) (**TECH FIG 2D**).
- Once proper tension is determined, the slip is then sutured back to the main tendon with interrupted, nonabsorbable suture or woven through the tendon in a Pulvertaft fashion (**TECH FIG 2E,F**).
  - As with all reconstruction techniques, tension is determined by taking the joint through a full range of motion and documenting stability dorsally.
- The wound is closed with interrupted 4-0 nylon sutures.[2,10]

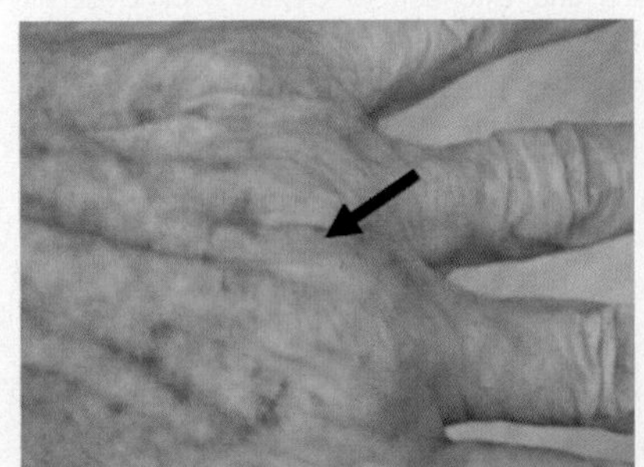

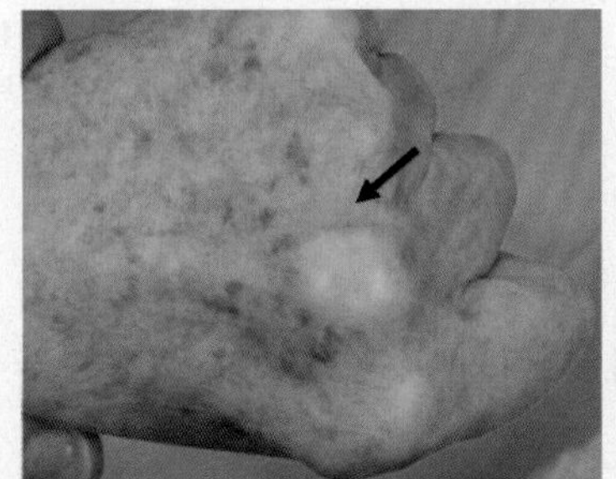

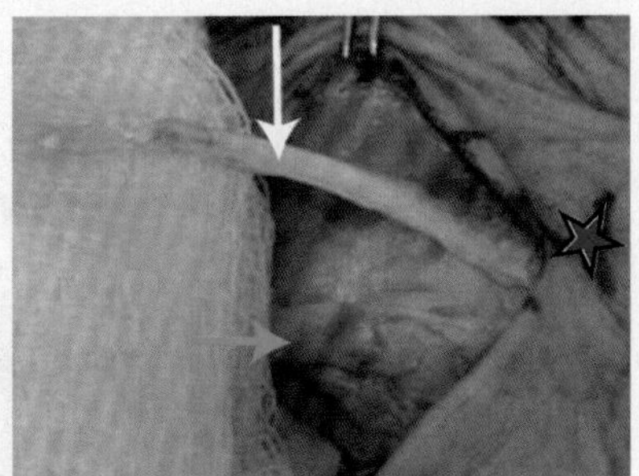

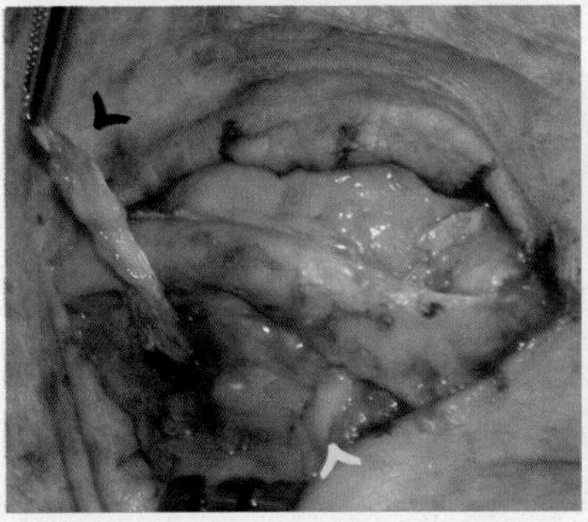

TECH FIG 2 • **A.** Long finger extended at the MCP joint, still with evidence of extensor dislocating into the ulnar trough. **B.** Extensor tendon dislocating when the MCP joint is flexed (*arrow*). **C.** A distally based slip of the extensor tendon is fashioned (*white arrow*). The ulnarly subluxed extensor tendon is indicated with a *blue arrow*. The *red asterisk* indicates the distal aspect of the digit. **D.** The distally based slip of extensor tendon (*black arrowhead*) has been rerouted volar to the radial collateral ligament (RCL; *yellow arrowhead*) from a distal to proximal direction. *(continued)*

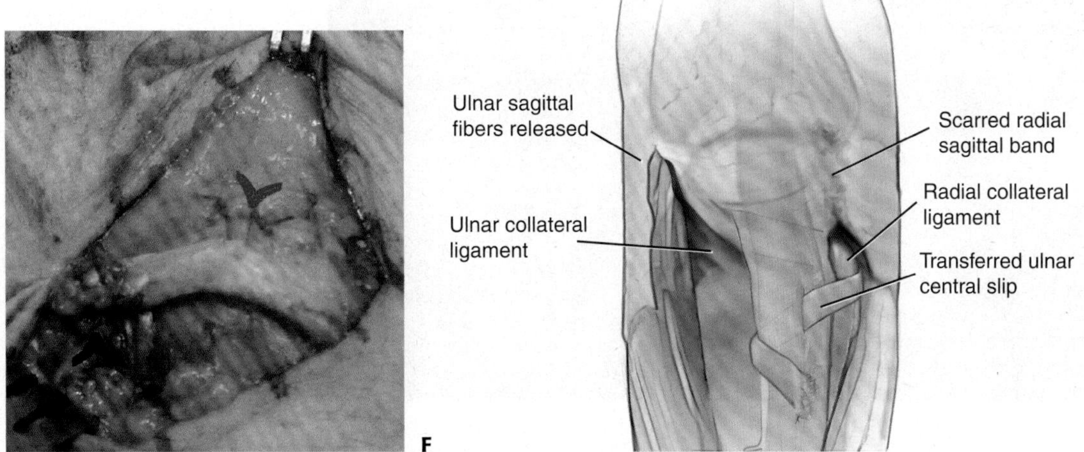

TECH FIG 2 • *(continued)* **E.** The distally based slip of extensor tendon has been secured to the extensor tendon proximal to the MCP joint (*black arrowhead*). The remaining ulnar sagittal band was repaired to prevent radial subluxation of the extensor tendon (*red arrowhead*). **F.** Reconstruction of the sagittal band using a distally based radial slip of extensor tendon wrapped around the RCL and reattached to the extensor tendon (with a weave).

Dynamic Lumbrical Muscle Transfer (Segalman)

- The lumbrical muscle is identified on the radial side of the joint and mobilized (**TECH FIG 3A,B**).
- Begin proximally by separating the lumbrical muscle from the more dorsal interossei.
- Once the lumbrical muscle is separated, continue distally to identify its tendinous insertion.
- The lumbrical tendon is harvested just proximal to its insertion into the lateral band (**TECH FIG 3C**).
- With the extensor tendon reduced, an isometric point in the extensor tendon must be identified. This is achieved by gently ranging the finger or asking the patient to flex. Once it is identified, a small longitudinal slit is made and the lumbrical tendon is passed through from volar to dorsal (**TECH FIG 3D**).
- Tension is set appropriately while gently ranging the finger to confirm the absence of subluxation. The tendon is sutured back to itself using interrupted, nonabsorbable suture.
- The wound is closed with interrupted 4-0 nylon sutures.[18]

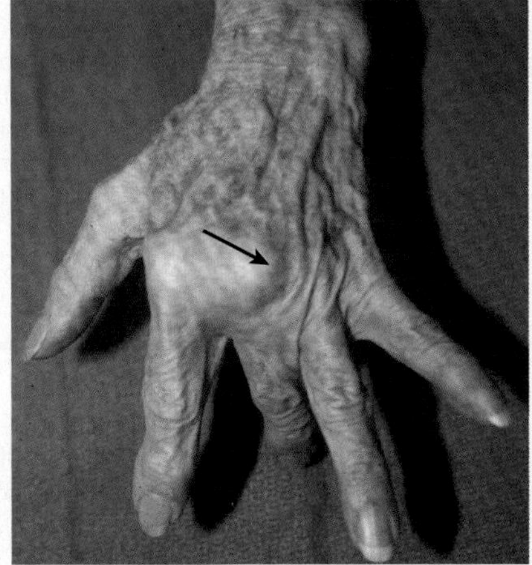

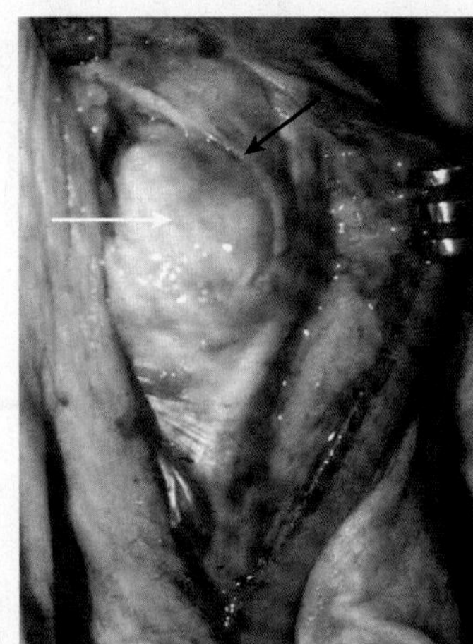

TECH FIG 3 • Technique using the lumbrical muscle for dynamic extensor tendon stabilization. **A.** Ulnar dislocation of the extensor tendon over the long finger MCP joint (*arrow*). **B.** Surgical exposure identifying the extensor dislocation (*black arrow*) with a large chronic defect in the radial sagittal band (*white arrow*). *(continued)*

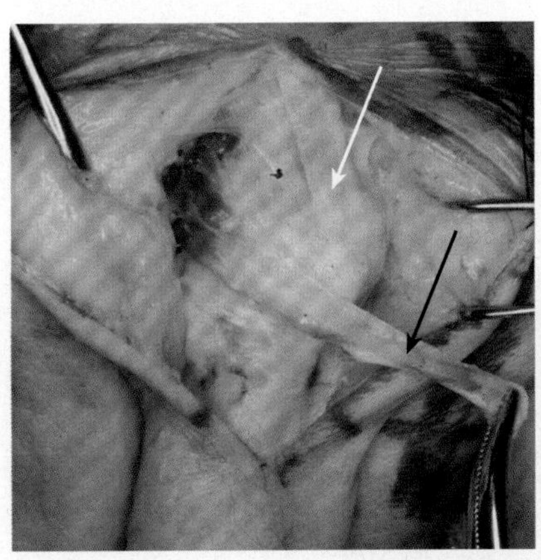

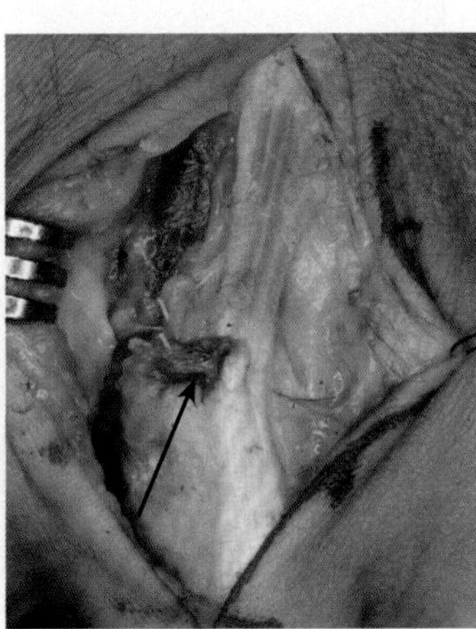

TECH FIG 3 • *(continued)* **C.** The lumbrical muscle–tendon unit is isolated and mobilized for transfer (*black arrow*). The extensor tendon is indicated by the *white arrow*. **D.** The lumbrical tendon is woven into the extensor tendon (*arrow*), now stabilizing the extensor tendon during MCP motion. (Courtesy of Keith Segalman, MD.)

Sagittal Band Reconstruction to the Deep Transverse Intermetacarpal Ligament (Watson)

- A 4-cm, distally based slip of extensor tendon consisting of no more than one-third the tendon width is harvested starting proximal to the MCP joint on the affected side (**TECH FIG 4A**).
- This segment of tendon is then passed through a small slit in the remaining tendon at the level of the deep transverse change to intermetacarpal ligament to prevent further propagation of the tendon split.
- The segment is then passed around or through the deep transverse intermetacarpal ligament using a curved clamp (**TECH FIG 4B**).
- The free end of the tendon graft is then woven through and sutured to the remaining extensor tendon once it has been centralized and properly tensioned using nonabsorbable suture (**TECH FIG 4C**).
- Wounds are closed with interrupted 4-0 nylon sutures.

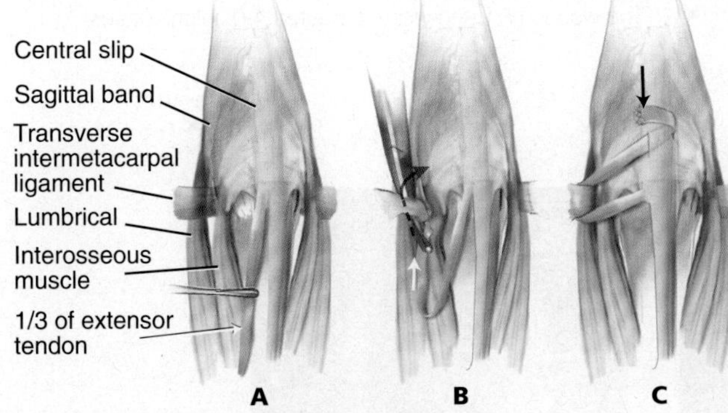

TECH FIG 4 • **A.** A distally based slip of extensor tendon constituting no more than one-third the width of the tendon is harvested. **B.** The slip of extensor tendon is rerouted from proximal to distal, around the deep intermetacarpal ligament. **C.** The tendon slip is then attached to the extensor tendon (usually radially) through a weave distal to the MCP joint.

Centralization Using Junctura Tendinum

- A longitudinal incision is centered dorsally over the affected MCP joint.
- The extensor tendon is identified and held in a centralized position.
- The MCP joint is flexed to reveal the more proximal, ulnar-sided junctura tendinum to the adjacent tendon.
- The junctura tendinum is released from its ulnar-sided insertion into the adjacent tendon.
- It is then brought over to the radial side of the affected finger, still in continuity with the tendon, and sutured to the palmar portion of the remaining sagittal band after correct tension has been set to centralize the tendon.
- In one variation of this technique, the junctura tendiunm is released in continuity with an ulnar slip of the extensor tendon. This slip is passed through the tendon at the isometric point and sutured to the radial deep transverse metacarpal ligament. The remaining slip is then folded back and sutured to itself and the radial extensor hood in an interrupted fashion.[5]
- Wounds are closed with interrupted 4-0 nylon sutures.

Sagittal Band Reconstruction Using Bone Tunnels (Kang)

- A dorsal transverse skin incision is made over the affected MCP joint.
- Three to 4 cm of palmaris longus tendon is harvested through two small incisions in the wrist and volar distal forearm.
- A bone tunnel is created from the dorsal midline of the metacarpal neck to the radial aspect of the head–neck junction using a 1.6-mm drill bit.
- The graft is passed through the bone tunnel creating a radially based pulley over the central extensor tendon.
- Proper tension is determined by taking the digit through a full range of motion and then the pulley is tied down with buried nonabsorbable sutures.
- The wound is closed with 4-0 nylon sutures.[9]

PEARLS AND PITFALLS

Range of motion	▪ Preoperatively, ensure that there is good passive range of motion of the MCP joint. ▪ Avoid overtensioning and malpositioning of the repair or reconstruction. A reconstruction too proximal will limit extension. A reconstruction too distal will lead to recurrent subluxation.
Anesthesia	▪ Local anesthesia will enable the patient to actively flex the MCP joint during the procedure, allowing the surgeon to intraoperatively assess centralization after the repair or reconstruction.
MCP joint capsule	▪ Identify and débride rents in the MCP joint capsule. Repair is unnecessary.[5] Also, be aware of any injury to the junctura tendinum; this should be repaired.
MCP flexion	▪ Range the MCP joint once the tendon is exposed, both before and after repair or reconstruction. The repair or reconstruction should be performed with the MCP joint in 60–70 degrees of flexion.
Additional releases	▪ Sometimes, the sagittal band, as well as the junctura tendinum, on the uninjured side will require release to centralize the tendon.

POSTOPERATIVE CARE

- Wounds are sterilely dressed immediately after the procedure and a splint is applied.
  - A volar and dorsal splint is used with the wrist slightly extended, the MCP joints at 0 to 30 degrees flexion, and the IP joints extended.
- On postoperative day 5, the patient is seen in the office. Sutures are removed and a short-arm cast is applied with the wrist slightly extended, the MCP joints at 0 to 30 degrees of extension, and the IP joints free.
  - Sometimes, in the compliant elderly patient, we favor a hand-based splint fabricated to include the MCP joints in 30 degrees of flexion and the IP joints free.
- Several postoperative protocols have been described for nondynamic reconstructions.
  - Inoue and Tamura[7] placed the involved finger in a plaster cast for 3 weeks with the MCP joint in neutral or slightly flexed, allowing active IP joint motion.
  - Carroll et al[2] splinted the MCP joint neutral for 6 weeks. At 2 weeks after surgery, they began PIP joint range of motion, and at 6 weeks active range of motion, the MCP was initiated.
  - Watson et al[19] used a splint and Kirschner wire to immobilize the MCP joint at 15 to 20 degrees of flexion for 3 weeks.
  - Hame and Melone[6] used cast immobilization of the MCP joint in 60 to 70 degrees of flexion for 6 weeks, with active flexion, but not extension, allowed.
- For dynamic transfers, the patient is immobilized for 4 weeks in a short-arm cast with the wrist in slight hyperextension, MCP joints in extension, and the PIP joints free. Active motion is begun 4 weeks after surgery and strengthening at 6 weeks. Therapy is then continued for 6 to 8 weeks.

OUTCOMES

- Rayan et al[15] treated three type II injuries nonoperatively with 3 weeks of splinting the MCP joint at 0 degree of extension, followed by 2 to 3 weeks of protected range of motion out of the splint three times a day, with a final 4 weeks of buddy splinting. They reported full range of MCP joint motion and no tenderness or pain with resisted digital abduction in all three patients. However, one patient did experience residual painless subluxation.
- Carroll et al[2] treated nine subluxed extensor tendons. Four were treated nonoperatively with 6 weeks of splinting the MCP joint in 0 degree of extension, followed by range-of-motion therapy. Five were treated operatively using a slip of extensor tendon looped around the collateral ligament. After splinting and therapy, all patients were pain-free with full extension and active flexion to 90 degrees or more.

There were no recurrences of symptoms in either group and no complications in the surgical group.

- Watson et al[19] described 16 patients treated operatively with a slip of extensor tendon looped through the deep transverse metacarpal ligament. They reported an average MCP joint flexion of 90 degrees postoperatively, with no subluxation of the tendon. All patients were pain-free. There were no complications and no need for further surgery.
- Hame and Melone[6] reported on eight professional athletes who underwent immediate repair of sagittal band injuries with subluxation of the extensor tendon. There were 11 injured fingers in total. Seven of the 11 had capsular injuries; they were all débrided but not repaired. Each athlete demonstrated full range of motion postoperatively and all returned to professional sport at 5 months on average. No additional intervention was necessary and there were no complications.

COMPLICATIONS

- Complications are rare. Most series in the literature do not report any complications.
- With nonoperative therapy, possible complications include joint stiffness, skin irritation from splinting, and failure of treatment.
- With operative therapy, possible complications include infection, joint stiffness, injury to neurovascular structures, and failure of treatment with recurrent subluxation or dislocation either in a radial or ulnar direction.

REFERENCES

1. Araki S, Ohtani T, Tanaka T. Acute dislocation of the extensor digitorum communis tendon at the metacarpophalangeal joint. J Bone Joint Surg Am 1987;69(4):616–619.
2. Carroll C IV, Moore JR, Weiland AJ. Posttraumatic ulnar subluxation of the extensor tendons: a reconstructive technique. J Hand Surg Am 1987;12(2):227–231.
3. Catalano LW III, Gupta S, Ragland R III, et al. Closed treatment of nonrheumatoid extensor tendon dislocations at the metacarpophalangeal joint. J Hand Surg Am 2006;31(2):242–245.
4. Drape JL, Dubert T, Silbermann P, et al. Acute trauma of the extensor hood of the metacarpophalangeal joint: MR imaging evaluation. Radiology 1994;192:469–476.
5. ElMaraghy AW, Pennings A. Metacarpophalangeal joint extensor tendon reconstruction: a reconstructive stabilization technique. J Hand Surg Am 2013;38(3):578–582.
6. Hame SL, Melone CP Jr. Boxer's knuckle in the professional athlete. Am J Sports Med 2000;28:879–882.
7. Inoue G, Tamura Y. Dislocation of the extensor tendons over the metacarpophalangeal joints. J Hand Surg Am 1996;21(3):464–469.
8. Ishizuki M. Traumatic and spontaneous dislocation of extensor tendon of the long finger. J Hand Surg Am 1990;15(6):967–972.
9. Kang L, Carlson MG. Extensor tendon centralization at the metacarpophalangeal joint: surgical technique. J Hand Surg Am 2010;35(7):1194–1197.
10. Kilgore ES, Graham WP, Newmeyer WL, et al. Correction of ulnar subluxation of the extensor communis. Hand 1975;7:272–274.
11. Lopez-Ben R, Lee DH, Nicolodi DJ. Boxer knuckle (injury of the extensor hood with extensor tendon subluxation): diagnosis with dynamic US—report of three cases. Radiology 2003;228:642–646.
12. Milford LW Jr. Retaining Ligaments of the Digit of the Hand: Gross and Microscopic Anatomic Study. Philadelphia: WB Saunders, 1968.
13. Pfirrmann CW, Theumann NH, Botte MJ, et al. MRI imaging of the metacarpophalangeal joints of the fingers: part II. Detection of simulated injuries in cadavers. Radiology 2002;222:447–452.
14. Rayan GM, Murray D. Classification and treatment of closed sagittal band injuries. J Hand Surg Am 1994;19(4):590–594.
15. Rayan GM, Murray D, Chung KW, et al. The extensor retinacular system at the metacarpophalangeal joint: an anatomical and histological study. J Hand Surg Br 1997;22(5):585–590.
16. Saldana MJ, McGuire RA. Chronic painful subluxation of the metacarpophalangeal joint extensor tendons. J Hand Surg Am 1986;11(3):420–423.
17. Schweitzer TP, Rayan GM. The terminal tendon of the digital extensor mechanism: part I, anatomic study. J Hand Surg Am 2004;29(5):898–902.
18. Segalman KA. Dynamic lumbrical muscle transfer for correction of posttraumatic extensor tendon subluxation. Tech Hand Up Extrem Surg 2006;10:107–113.
19. Watson HK, Weinzweig J, Guidera PM. Sagittal band reconstruction. J Hand Surg Am 1997;22(3):452–456.
20. Young CM, Rayan GM. The sagittal band: anatomic and biomechanical study. J Hand Surg Am 2000;25(6):1107–1113.

Flexor and Extensor Tenosynovectomy

84

CHAPTER

Kyle P. Kokko, John T. Capo, Sanjiv Naidu, and Jay T. Bridgeman

DEFINITION

- Synovium lines the joint spaces and tendon sheaths and secretes a lubricant (hyaluronan and synovial fluid constituents from type B synoviocytes) needed for tendon gliding and reduces friction in synovial joint motion.
- Tendons may be both extra- and intrasynovial.
- Flexor tendons in the carpal tunnel have the added feature of subsynovial connective tissue, which can become inflamed.
- Tenosynovitis is defined as the inflammation of tendon sheaths in extrasynovial tendons and the inflammation of the synovial lining in intrasynovial tendons.[4]

ANATOMY

- The extensor tendons lie under the dorsal retinaculum in six separate extensor (or dorsal) compartments. They are numbered in succession from one to six, beginning radially and ending ulnarly. The portions of the extensor tendons that lie under the dorsal retinaculum are lined with synovial sheaths (**FIG 1A**).
- The extensor tendons that occupy the first dorsal compartment are the abductor pollicis longus (APL) and the extensor pollicis brevis (EPB). They originate as "outcropper" muscles from the distal third of the forearm and cross over the second dorsal compartment tendons—the extensor carpi radialis longus (ECRL) and the extensor carpi radialis brevis (ECRB)—distally at the level of the wrist approximately 4 cm proximal to the radial styloid.
- The extensor pollicis longus (EPL) in the third extensor compartment makes an acute angle at the Lister tubercle at the level of the wrist and crosses superficial to the second dorsal compartment.
- The fourth extensor compartment tendons—the extensor digitorum communis (EDC) and the extensor indicis proprius (EIP)—lie under a broad retinaculum. The posterior interosseous nerve (PIN) lies in the floor of the fourth extensor compartment deep to the EDC and EIP tendons on the radial aspect of the compartment.
- The extensor digitorum quinti (EDQ) in the fifth extensor compartment often is the only tendon to motor the small finger metacarpophalangeal (MCP) joint in the act of extension.
- The extensor carpi ulnaris (ECU) tendon in the sixth dorsal compartment lies in a fibro-osseous tunnel and is intimately held in the ulnar groove by a subsheath that is critical for distal radioulnar joint stability and is a component of the triangular fibrocartilage complex (TFCC).
- The wrist flexor tendons—the flexor carpi radialis (FCR), the palmaris longus (PL), and the flexor carpi ulnaris (FCU)—are extrasynovial tendons.
- The FCR passes through a tight fibro-osseous tunnel in the trapezium before inserting on the base of the second metacarpal (**FIG 1B,C**). Whereas the FCU, attaches first on the pisiform bone that functions as a sesamoid bone and then has distal attachments to the base of the fifth metacarpal.

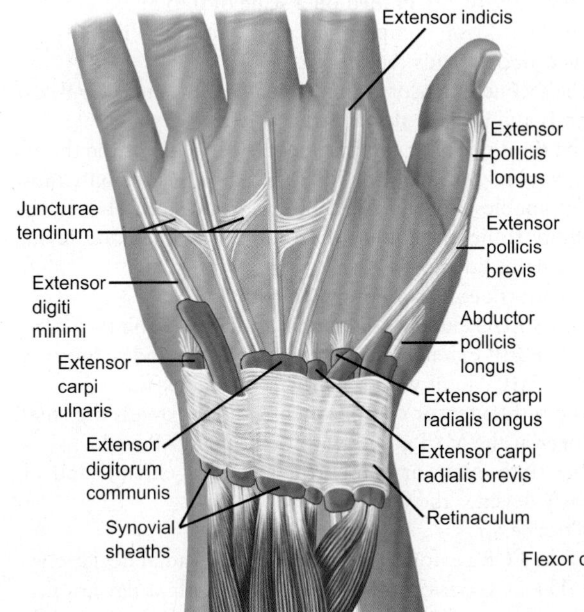

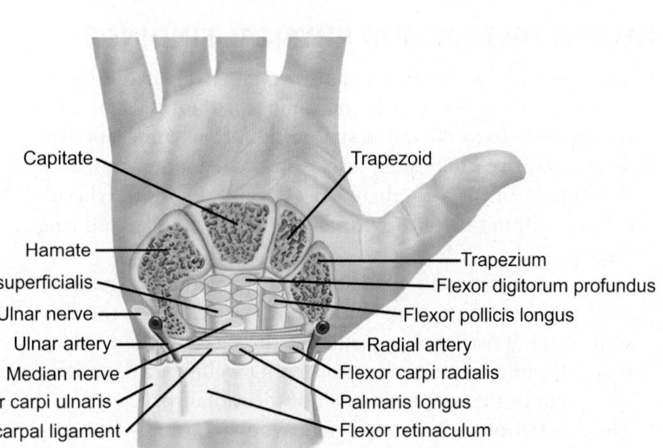

FIG 1 • **A.** Extensor compartments of the hand. **B.** Flexor tendons. *(continued)*

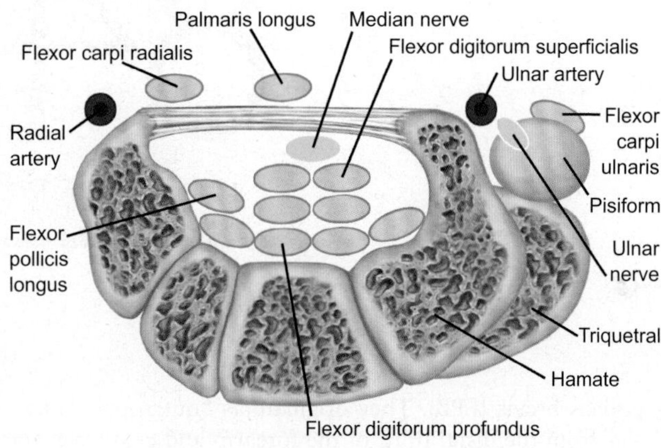

FIG 1 • *(continued)* **C.** Carpal tunnel.

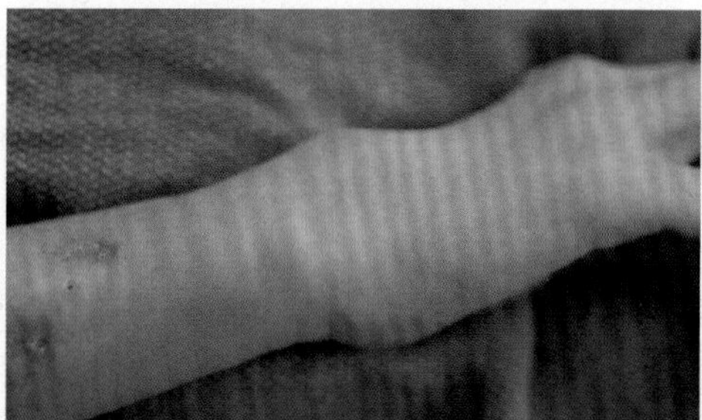

FIG 2 • Dorsal swelling secondary to extensor tenosynovitis.

- The digital flexor tendons lie under the transverse carpal ligament in the carpal tunnel. Unlike digital extensor tendons, flexor tendons are almost entirely intrasynovial.
- The flexor tendons in the digits lie in a fibro-osseous canal formed by the annular and cruciate ligaments.[3]

PATHOGENESIS

- Rheumatoid arthritis is a disease of synovial tissue that can lead to inflammatory tensosynovitis. However, proliferative extensor tenosynovitis has been described in the absence of rheumatoid arthritis.[2]
  - Flexor and extensor tenosynovitis is commonly a sequelae of rheumatoid arthritis.
  - Rheumatoid arthritis causes formation of hypertrophic synovium in the joint spaces, thereby destabilizing joints. The hypertrophic synovium invades the tendon sheaths and synovial lining of all tendons.[4]

NATURAL HISTORY

- Inflammatory tenosynovitis usually is painless and can be the first sign of rheumatoid arthritis.
- The dorsal and volar wrist, as well as the volar digits, are most commonly affected.
- The synovial tissue proliferates in the tendon sheath and eventually may invade the tendon.
- The end result can be weakening and rupture of the tendon.[4]

PATIENT HISTORY AND PHYSICAL FINDINGS

- Tenosynovitis of the first extensor compartment (de Quervain tenosynovitis) reveals thickening of the EPB and APL tendon sheaths at the radial styloid. This thickening can produce a positive Finkelstein test: pain elicited along course of the APL and EPB with ulnar wrist deviation with the thumb cupped within the loose grasp of the index, middle, and ring fingers.
- Second compartment extensor tenosynovitis (intersection syndrome) often presents with painless swelling of the dorsum of the wrist 4 cm proximal to the radial styloid. There is focal tenderness to palpation with swelling and positive Tinel sign of the sensory branch of the radial nerve.
- Third extensor compartment tenosynovitis usually presents with rupture of the EPL tendon. This results in inability to raise the thumb (thumb retropulsion) when the hand is placed flat on a table.
- Chronic fourth extensor compartment tenosynovitis often presents with focal swelling in extensor zone 7 along with multiple tendon ruptures (**FIG 2**).
- Fifth extensor compartment tenosynovitis usually is accompanied by dorsal distal ulna instability and tendon rupture.
- Sixth extensor compartment tenosynovitis is manifested as ECU instability in addition to significant intrasynovial inflammation at the level of the ulnar styloid.
- Pain at the wrist indicates that the radiocarpal or radioulnar joint is affected.
- Flexor tenosynovitis at the wrist can cause median nerve compression in the carpal tunnel as well as decreased active and passive range of motion of the fingers.
- Flexor tenosynovitis of the digits can cause triggering.[3]
- The flexor tendon that most commonly ruptures due to rheumatoid arthritis is the flexor pollicis longus (FPL) (Mannerfelt syndrome) and results in loss of thumb interphalangeal joint flexion.
- The following examinations, all of which may detect weakness or rupture, are graded on a scale of 0 to 5:
  - The first dorsal compartment (APL and EPB) radially abducts and extends the thumb.
  - The second extensor compartment (ECRL and ECRB) extends and radially deviates the wrist.
  - The third extensor compartment (EPL) extends the thumb in combination with the EPB and APL. It is the only muscle capable of producing thumb retropulsion. That is, the ability to lift the thumb off a table with the hand laying flat, palm side down.
  - The fourth extensor compartment
    - The EDC extends the fingers at the MCP joints.
    - The EIP extends and hyperextends the index finger at the MCP joint with the other fingers flexed.
  - The fifth extensor compartment (EDQ) extends the small finger at the MCP joints with other fingers flexed.
  - The sixth extensor compartment (ECU) extends and ulnarly deviates the wrist.
  - Wrist flexors
    - The FCR performs wrist flexion and radial deviation.
    - The FCU performs wrist flexion and ulnar deviation.
  - The flexor digitorum superficialis (FDS) flexes the proximal interphalangeal joint of the fingers independently from one another. This is best tested with all of the FPD (distal interphalangeal [DIP] joints) tendons blocked.

- The flexor digitorum profundus (FDP) tendons flex the DIP joint and share a common muscle belly. The small and ring fingers are innervated by the ulnar nerve, whereas the middle and index fingers are innervated by the median nerve.
- The FPL flexes the thumb interphalangeal joint against resistance.

IMAGING AND OTHER DIAGNOSTIC STUDIES

- Magnetic resonance imaging (MRI) may be useful to evaluate low-grade tenosynovitis and mechanical dysfunction of the fibro-osseous digital pulley system.
- In general, flexor or extensor tenosynovitis is a clinical diagnosis made on physical findings.

DIFFERENTIAL DIAGNOSIS

- Extensor tendon weakness
  - Rupture of sagittal bands
  - PIN palsy
  - Intrinsic muscle tightness or contracture
  - Extensor tendon rupture
- Flexor tendon weakness
  - Flexor tendon rupture
  - Nerve palsy (median nerve, anterior interosseous nerve, ulnar nerve)

NONOPERATIVE MANAGEMENT

- Medical control of rheumatoid arthritis
- Splinting
- Cortisone injections are only *very* rarely indicated due to the risk of tendon rupture.

SURGICAL MANAGEMENT

- Extensor tenosynovectomy is indicated if no improvement is observed after 4 to 6 months of adequate medical treatment, pain recalcitrant to medical treatment, or if tendon ruptures are detected.[4,5]
- Flexor tenosynovectomy is relatively indicated if active digit motion becomes worse than passive motion.[4]

Preoperative Planning

- Consider withholding rheumatoid medications (eg, methotrexate, etanercept, Imuran) 1 week before and 1 week after surgery.[4]

Positioning

- The patient is positioned supine with an arm board or hand table.
- A tourniquet is recommended and placed on the upper arm.

Approach

- For an extensor tenosynovectomy, a dorsal midline approach to the wrist is used (**FIG 3A**).
- For a flexor tenosynovectomy, an extended carpal tunnel approach is used (**FIG 3B**).
- A digital tenosynovectomy is done using a Brunner style approach to the digits (**FIG 3C**).

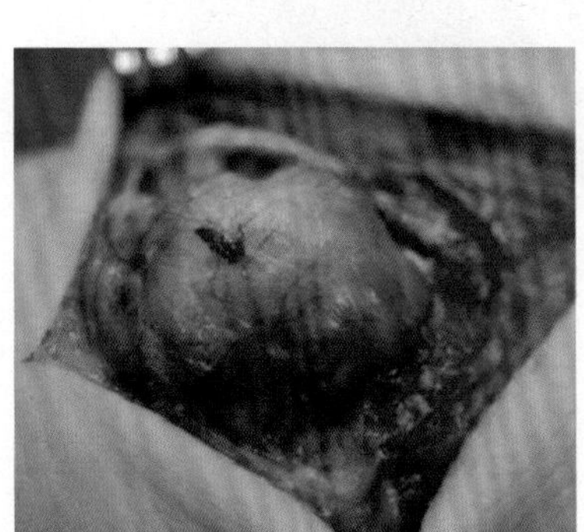

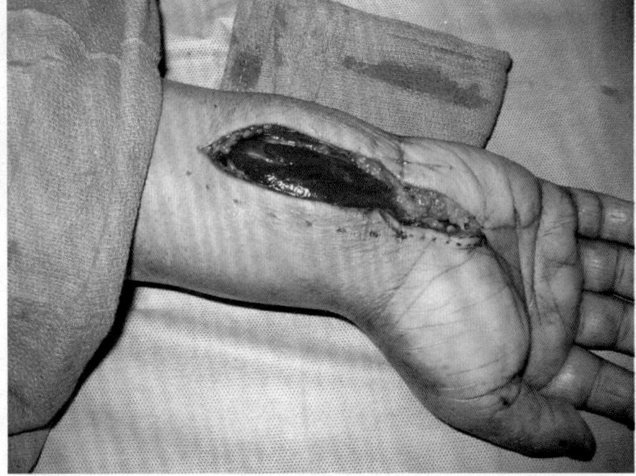

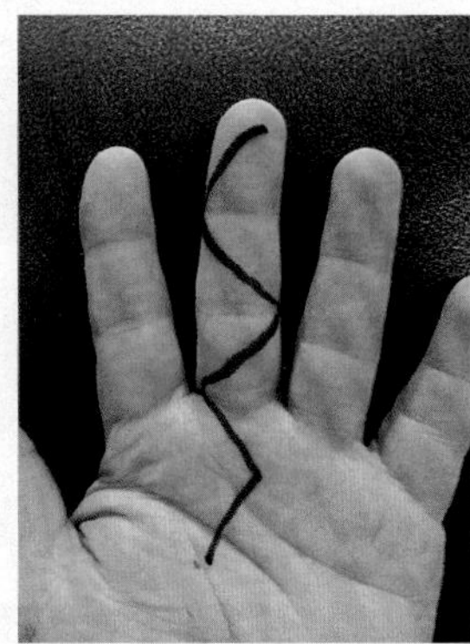

FIG 3 • **A.** Dorsal extensor tenosynovitis. **B.** Volar flexor tenosynovitis. **C.** Zigzag (Brunner) approach to digital flexor tendons.

Extensor Tenosynovectomy

- A straight longitudinal incision is made.
- Full-thickness skin flaps are created, exposing the extensor retinaculum (**TECH FIG 1A**).
- A straight longitudinal incision is made of the extensor retinaculum over the third compartment.
- Transverse incisions are made over the proximal and distal borders of the retinaculum, creating a radially based flap.
- Divide the vertical septum, opening each extensor compartment.
- Excise hypetrophic synovium from each tendon sheath with a combination of blunt and sharp dissection (**TECH FIG 1B**).
- Frayed tendons are repaired with fine interrupted sutures.
- Tendons at risk for rupture should be sutured to adjacent tendons.
- If synovitis of the wrist is encountered, wrist synovectomy is performed and, if possible, the capsule is closed.
- The distal ulna should be resected (Darrach procedure) if it is prominent dorsally or if significant distal radioulnar joint arthrosis is noted. Alternatively, a dorsal osteoplasty of the distal ulna can be done by removing dorsal osteophytes if the distal radioulnar joint is stable and nonarthritic.
- A portion of the retinaculum is passed deep to the extensor tendons and sutured (**TECH FIG 1C,D**), whereas the remaining portion of the retinaculum is sutured over the extensor tendons to prevent bowstringing.[3]

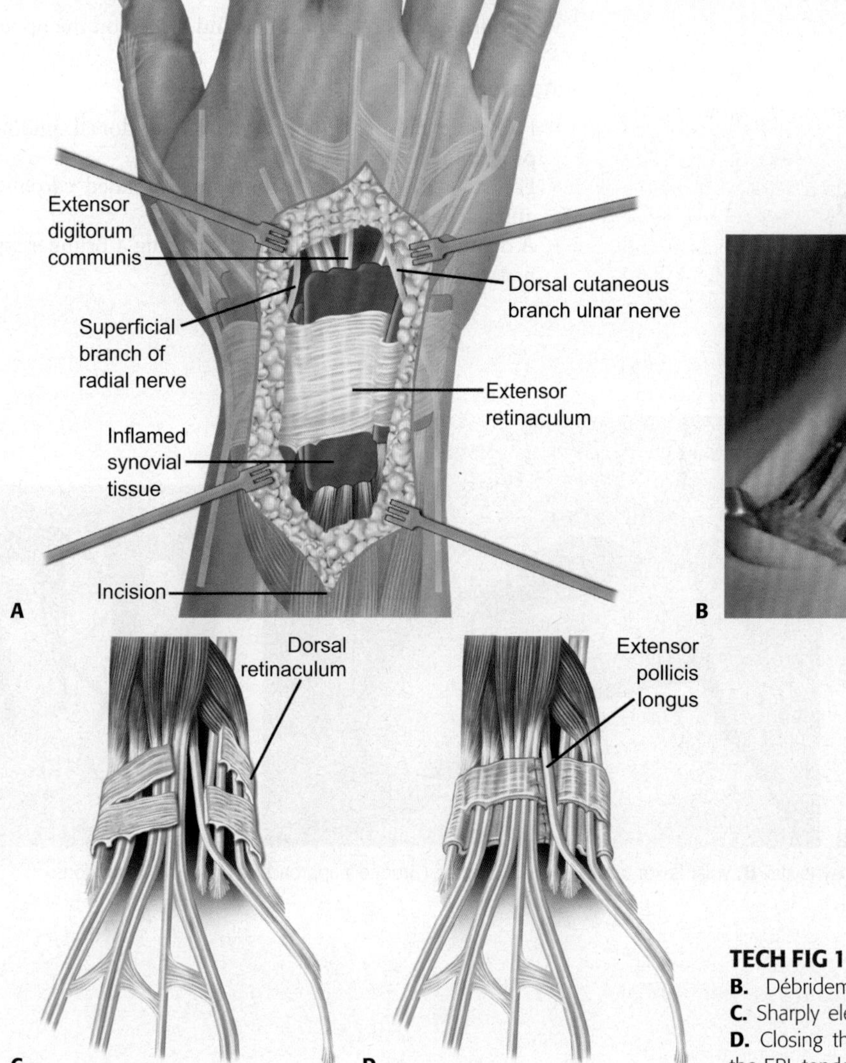

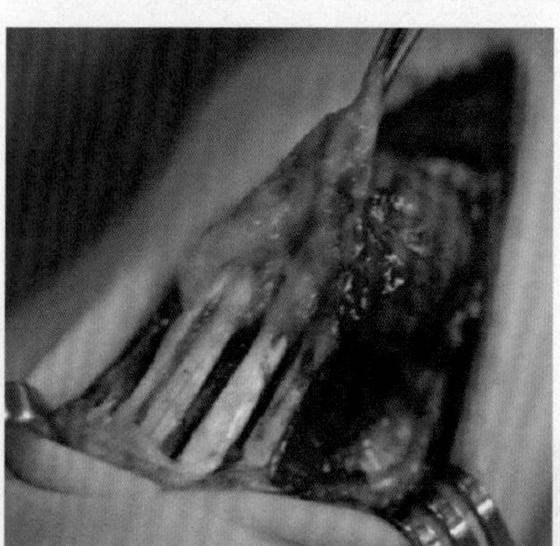

TECH FIG 1 • **A.** Dorsal midline approach. **B.** Débridement of dorsal tenosynovitis. **C.** Sharply elevating the dorsal retinaculum. **D.** Closing the dorsal retinaculum deep to the EPL tendon.

Flexor Tenosynovectomy

- Use a standard carpal tunnel approach with a midpalm incision parallel to the thenar crease in line with central axis of the ring finger.
- Extend the incision proximally and ulnarly in a zigzag fashion across the wrist crease and then for an additional 5 cm proximally.
- Protect the palmar cutaneous branch of the median nerve at the wrist flexion crease.
- Divide the volar antebrachial fascia and protect the median nerve in the forearm.
- Divide the palmar fascia and transverse carpal ligament longitudinally.
- Excise hypertrophic synovium surrounding the flexor tendons (**TECH FIG 2**).
  - A complete synovectomy is not required when the excess synovium involves more than half of the tendon diameter. Synovectomy in this case would lead to loss in function.
- Inspect the floor of the carpal tunnel. Any bony spicules (commonly originating from the scaphoid) are removed with a rongeur.
- Check flexor tendons for decreased excursion, indicating digit tenosynovitis.[3]

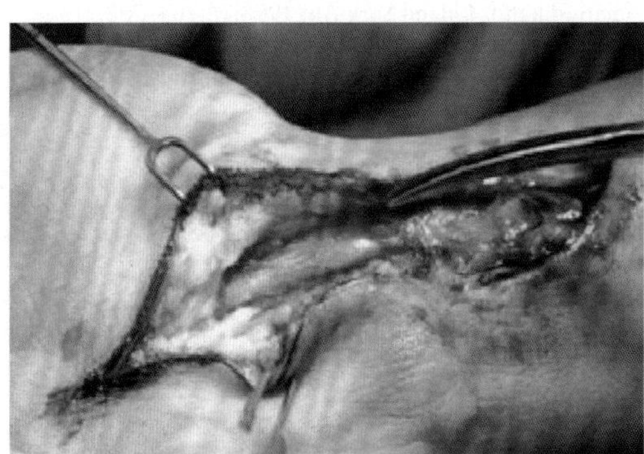

TECH FIG 2 • Extended carpal tunnel approach to flexor tendons.

Digital Flexor Tenosynovectomy

- Use a volar zigzag (Brunner type) incision to explore the flexor tendons in the digit extending the incision proximally and distally for more exposure as necessary.
- Excise all hypertrophic synovium (**TECH FIG 3**).
- Carefully preserve the second and fourth annular pulleys to prevent bowstringing.
- Excise nodules in the tendon and close defects with fine suture.
- Check tendon excursion for smooth gliding.
- Passive flexion of the finger should equal the flexion obtained when pulling on the tendon (simulating active flexion).
- If passive and active flexion are not equal, additional synovectomy is required.[3]

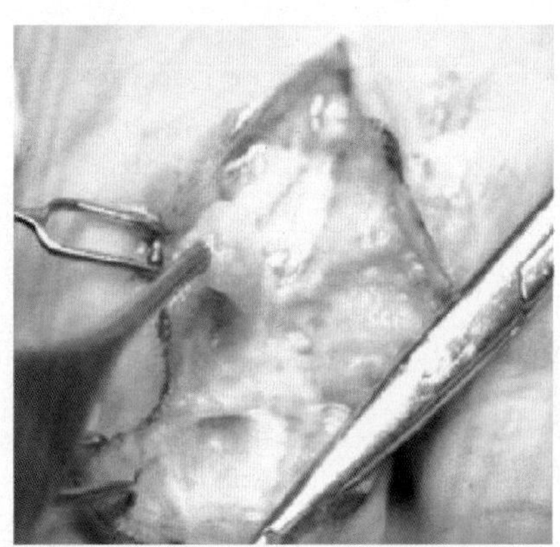

TECH FIG 3 • Débridement of digit flexor tenosynovitis.

PEARLS AND PITFALLS

Indications	■ Failed adequate medical management for 4–6 months or recalcitrant pain
Extensor tenosynovectomy	■ Débride radiocarpal synovitis if present. ■ Resect or contour the distal ulna if prominent or dislocated. ■ Be cautious of ulnar translation of the carpus if a Darrach procedure is performed. If present, a radiolunate fusion is also required.
Flexor tenosynovectomy	■ Débride bony spicules on the carpal tunnel floor (ie, scaphoid).
Digital flexor tenosynovectomy	■ Preserve annular pulleys to prevent bowstringing. ■ Passive flexion of the finger should be the same as the flexion observed when the surgeon pulls on the tendon.

POSTOPERATIVE CARE

- Splint the wrist in neutral position.
- Early (within 48 hours) active and passive digit range-of-motion exercise is key to maintaining motion.[1]

OUTCOMES

- Long-term studies show less than 10% tendon rupture and recurrent tenosynovitis at 5 years.

COMPLICATIONS

- Wound dehiscence
- Tendon adhesions
- Tendon rupture[1]

REFERENCES

1. Brown FE, Brown ML. Long-term results after tenosynovectomy to treat the rheumatoid hand. J Hand Surg Am 1998;13:704–708.
2. Cooper HJ, Shevchuck MM, Li X, et al. Proliferative extensor tenosynovitis of the wrist in the absence of rheumatoid arthritis. J Hand Surg Am 2009;34:1827–1831.
3. Feldon P, Terrano A, Nalebuff E, et al. Rheumatoid arthritis and other connective tissue disease. In: Green DP, Hotchkiss R, Pederson WC, eds. Green's Operative Hand Surgery, ed 5. New York: Churchill Livingstone, 2005:2060–2068.
4. Millender LH, Nalebuff EA, Albin R, et al. Dorsal tenosynovectomy and tendon transfer in the rheumatoid hand. J Bone Joint Surg Am 1974;56(3):601–610.
5. Thirupathi RG, Ferlic DC, Clayton ML. Dorsal wrist synovectomy in rheumatoid arthritis—a long-term study. J Hand Surg Am 1983;8:848–856.

Tendon Transfers Used for Treatment of Rheumatoid Disorders

85 CHAPTER

Raymond J. Metz, Jr., Rey N. Ramirez, and John D. Lubahn

DEFINITION

- Rheumatoid arthritis is a progressive disease that, if uncontrolled, leads to joint destruction, secondary to progressive synovitis, ligament instability, joint dislocation or subluxation, and attrition of adjacent tendons either by bony erosion or direct tenosynovial infiltration.
- When tendon rupture occurs on the dorsum of the hand or wrist, patients cannot extend their fingers and have difficulty grasping objects.
- The most common tendon ruptures on the dorsum of the hand begin on the ulnar side and usually are a result of subluxation of the distal radioulnar joint (DRUJ), the so-called Vaughan-Jackson or caput ulnae syndrome.[13]
- On the volar side of the wrist, the most common tendons to rupture are the flexor pollicis longus and the adjacent flexor digitorum profundus (FDP) tendon to the index finger or possibly the long finger. This is referred to as *Mannerfelt syndrome*.[9]

ANATOMY

- The extensor tendons of the hand and forearm pass beneath the extensor retinaculum at the wrist. The retinaculum is divided into six separate compartments lined by tenosynovium, which can become involved in the pathology of rheumatoid arthritis.
  - The first compartment contains the tendons of the abductor pollicis longus and the extensor pollicis brevis. The former tendon often contains multiple slips, which can contribute to limited space in its respective compartment and secondary de Quervain tenosynovitis.
  - The second compartment consists of the extensor carpi radialis longus (ECRL) and extensor carpi radialis brevis (ECRB), the former tendon inserting at the base of the index metacarpal and the latter at the base of the long finger.
  - The third compartment contains only the tendon of the extensor pollicis longus (EPL), which passes around the tubercle of Lister at a fairly sharp angle. Although frequently involved in tendon ruptures in rheumatoid arthritis, the EPL may also present as an isolated tendon rupture after nondisplaced fractures of the distal radius.
  - The fourth compartment contains the extensor indicis proprius (EIP) and the extensor digitorum communis (EDC), sending tendons from the common extensor muscle in the forearm to each of the fingers. The EIP is a separate muscle tendon unit located within the fourth compartment. It can be differentiated by its distal muscle belly.
  - The fifth extensor compartment contains the extensor digiti quinti (EDQ), often consisting of two slips and passing almost directly over the DRUJ.
  - The sixth compartment contains only the extensor carpi ulnaris (ECU).
- On the palmar side of the wrist, the flexor pollicis longus is located most radially and passes over the radiocarpal joint adjacent to the trapeziometacarpal joint of the thumb. The flexor pollicis, along with the median nerve and the profundus and sublimis tendons to each digit, passes beneath the deep transverse carpal ligament and represents the contents of the carpal canal.
  - Tenosynovial proliferation can exist within the carpal tunnel, arising from the undersurface of the ligament but more commonly proliferating along the tendons themselves.

PATHOGENESIS

- Tendon rupture on the dorsum of the wrist is usually the result of instability in the DRUJ, leading to secondary subluxation and bony erosion through the capsule of the joint and then the tendon.
  - The tendon initially affected is the EDQ. As the carpus supinates and subluxates volarly, causing the distal ulna to be more dorsal, tendons typically rupture sequentially in an ulnar to radial direction.
  - The tendons may also be compromised by direct infiltration from the tenosynovium.
  - Although the ulnar tendons are involved most commonly, it is possible for all of the tendons crossing the dorsum of the wrist to rupture, making reconstruction more difficult.
- On the volar side of the wrist, the flexor pollicis longus may become compromised through erosion by osteophytes and rough bony surfaces at the level of the trapeziometacarpal joint of the thumb or the scaphotrapezial articulation. The adjacent profundus tendon to the index and, occasionally, the long finger can rupture as well.
- Tendons of the flexor surface of the wrist and forearm are also subject to rupture via direct tenosynovial infiltration, but this is less common.
  - In addition to tendon attrition and eventual rupture, tenosynovitis in the carpal tunnel may cause median nerve compression that leads to weakness of the median nerve innervated intrinsics. These include the opponens pollicis and abductor pollicis brevis (APB), the flexor pollicis brevis (usually only the deep head), and the radial two lumbricals. Weakness of these muscles is uncommon but should be checked in all patients with carpal tunnel syndrome (CTS).

NATURAL HISTORY

- Before the advent of treatment for rheumatoid arthritis, the natural history was one of relentless progression. The disease would occasionally "burn itself out," however, with the radiocarpal joint subluxating in a volar and radial direction, leading to instability and loss of function.

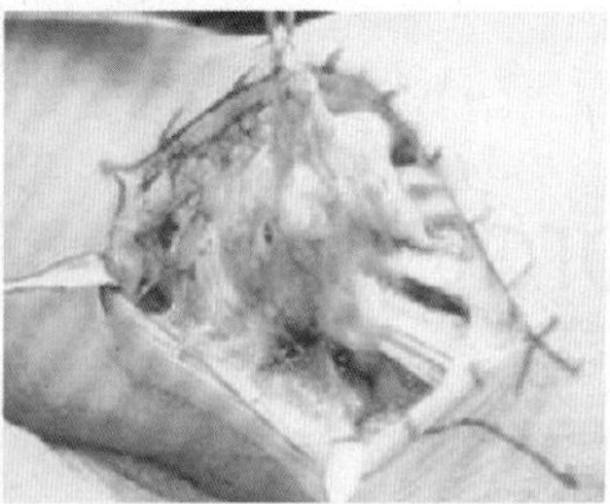

FIG 1 • Exposure of the extensor tendons of the wrist shows proliferative tenosynovitis originating from the tenosynovial lining of the extensor retinaculum. If left unchecked, such proliferative tenosynovitis can contribute to extensor tendon rupture at the level of the wrist.

- Also, before the development and routine use of antitumor necrosis factor drugs, patients were occasionally refractory to nonsteroidal medication, corticosteroids, and stronger anti-inflammatory drugs such as methotrexate. When these drug combinations failed, proliferative tenosynovitis occasionally occurred on the dorsum of the wrist, secondary to a "pannus" of diseased, thickened synovium growing directly into the tendons causing collagen destruction and rupture (**FIG 1**).
- The worst-case scenario is secondary rupture of all of the finger extensors, with subluxation of the ECU volar to the axis of wrist motion such that it becomes more of a wrist flexor and ulnar deviator than a wrist extensor. The radial wrist extensors may also rupture; however, in part as a result of the more robust nature of the tendons themselves, they tend to remain intact even with progressive disease.
- The French impressionist painter Pierre Auguste Renoir was said to have had such severe rheumatoid arthritis that in his later years, he would tape a brush to his hand to paint.

PATIENT HISTORY AND PHYSICAL FINDINGS

- Patients often note a spontaneous loss of finger motion, but there may be minimal swelling and discomfort. Patients occasionally report a snap or twinge of discomfort as the tendon ruptures.
- With an extensor tendon rupture, patients cannot actively extend the metacarpophalangeal (MCP) joints of the involved digit.
  - In the case of isolated rupture of the EDQ, an intact EDC to the small finger may make it difficult to confirm the diagnosis.
  - The proximal and distal interphalangeal joints of the finger may be extended through the intrinsics even when the extensors are ruptured.
  - Wrist flexion should result in MCP joint extension through tenodesis if the extensor tendons are intact. When the finger extensors are ruptured, this tenodesis effect is absent (**FIG 2A,B**).
  - The patient should also be examined for subluxation of the extensor tendons, which may mimic tendon rupture. In this case, the tendon will subluxate ulnarly to lie between the MCP joints. Patients with subluxation rather than rupture should be able to maintain extended position if the MCP joints are passively extended.
- On the volar side of the wrist, the examiner should check closely for the possibility of associated tenosynovial proliferation proximal and deep to the transverse carpal ligament.
  - Active digital motion may cause palpable crepitus at this level.
- Such proliferation may result in coexisting CTS. The examiner should question the patient regarding symptoms of CTS and should assess for signs of CTS.
  - Examination findings suggestive of CTS include decreased sensation or paresthesias in the thumb, index, middle, and radial ring finger; thenar pain; Phalen compression test; and APB weakness.

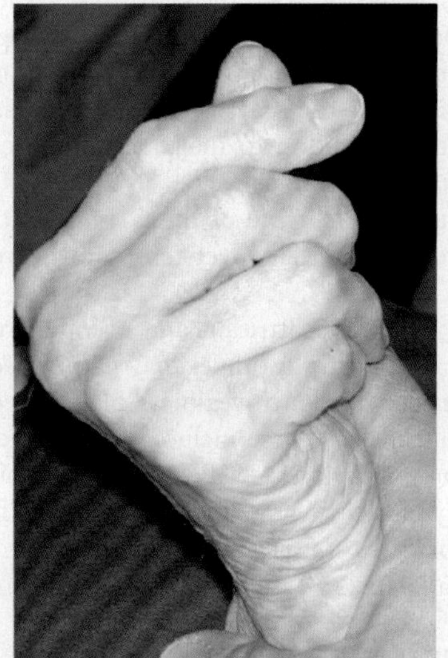
A

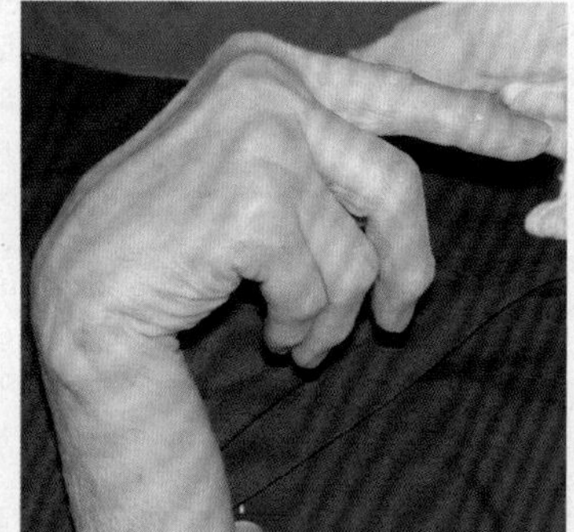
B

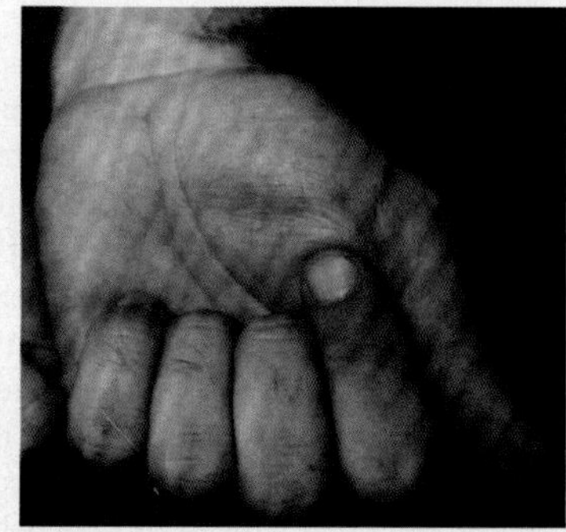
C

FIG 2 • **A.** Passive wrist extension results in passive finger flexion with intact finger flexors. **B.** Passive wrist flexion should result in passive finger extension when the finger extensor tendons are intact. In this situation, however, those tendons are not intact and passive wrist flexion results in the long, ring, and small extensor fingers remaining in a flexed position. **C.** In a patient with Mannerfelt syndrome, attempted active flexion of the thumb and fingers results in absent flexion of the interphalangeal joint of the thumb and, in this situation, the distal interphalangeal joint of the index finger. Clinically, this is similar to anterior interosseous nerve syndrome and must be distinguished clinically and often by electromyography.

- The patient should also be examined carefully for active flexion at the distal interphalangeal joints of the index and long fingers as well as the interphalangeal joint of the thumb.
  - Absence of flexion should alert the surgeon to the possibility of rupture of the flexor pollicis longus and the FDP to the index and occasionally the long finger.
  - These tendons are particularly vulnerable when subluxation and spur formation are present at the trapeziometacarpal or scaphotrapezial joints as well as the volar radiocarpal joint.
  - Tendon rupture at this level is referred to as Mannerfelt syndrome (**FIG 2C**) and needs to be differentiated from anterior interosseous nerve palsy.
    - Direct pressure on the flexor pollicis longus muscle in the forearm should lead to passive flexion in the interphalangeal joint of the thumb if the tendon is intact.
    - The tenodesis test also is effective for the flexor pollicis longus and profundus and sublimis tendons to the fingers; however, in patients with progressive rheumatoid arthritis, the radiocarpal joint and the interphalangeal joints may become arthritic, making passive motion of the wrist and fingers somewhat more difficult and therefore the test more unreliable.

IMAGING AND OTHER DIAGNOSTIC STUDIES

- Anteroposterior (AP) and lateral radiographs of the hand and wrist should be obtained to look for subtle changes of the DRUJ, such as subluxation or a small osteophyte (**FIG 3**), which may be consistent with the physical findings of tendon rupture (**FIG 4**).
- Similar attention should be paid to the volar surface of the radiocarpal joint and the trapeziometacarpal joint of the thumb as well as the scaphotrapezial and trapezoidal joints.
- Radiographs should be examined for arthrosis and deformity, which may mimic tendon rupture by causing motion loss.
- Radiographs of the cervical spine may reveal subluxation, possibly causing nerve compression and secondary sensory loss or weakness.
- Computed tomography (CT) and magnetic resonance imaging (MRI) are not routinely needed.

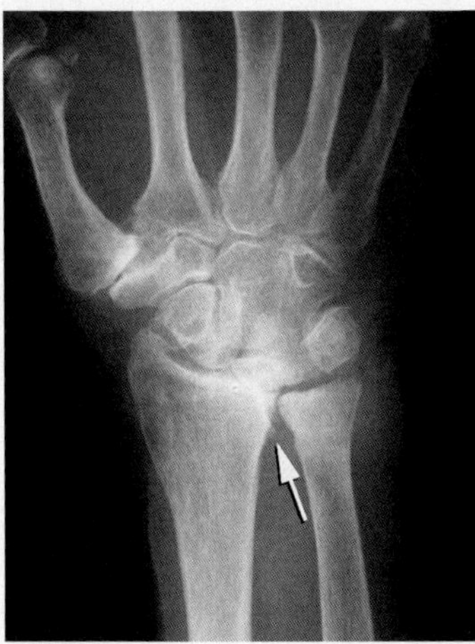

FIG 3 • AP radiograph of the wrist of the patient in **FIG 4** shows osteophyte formation in the DRUJ (*arrow*). (From Lubahn JD, Wolfe TL. Surgical treatment and rehabilitation and tendon ruptures in the rheumatoid hand. In: Mackin EJ, Callahan AD, Skirven TM, et al, eds. Rehabilitation of the Hand and Upper Extremity, ed 5. St. Louis: Mosby, 2002:1598–1607.)

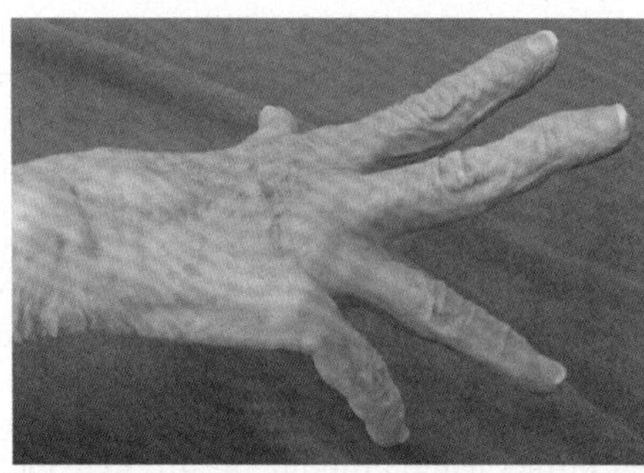

FIG 4 • The clinical consequences of a spur in the DRUJ: rupture of the EDQ and EDC to the ring and small fingers. When the patient attempts to actively extend the fingers, the ring and small fingers remain flexed. (From Lubahn JD, Wolfe TL. Surgical treatment and rehabilitation and tendon ruptures in the rheumatoid hand. In: Mackin EJ, Callahan AD, Skirven TM, et al, eds. Rehabilitation of the Hand and Upper Extremity, ed 5. St. Louis: Mosby, 2002:1598–1607.)

- Electromyography and nerve conduction studies may be helpful in the evaluation of the patient with potential tendon ruptures, particularly if tenodesis testing is normal in the face of a loss of active finger extension or flexion.
  - Compression of both the anterior interosseous and posterior interosseous nerves can occur in rheumatoid arthritis, usually secondary to ganglion cyst formation at the level of the elbow joint.

DIFFERENTIAL DIAGNOSIS

- In the case of tendon ruptures on the dorsum of the hand and wrist, the differential diagnosis is primarily that of posterior interosseous nerve compression or posterior interosseous nerve syndrome.
  - Compression of the posterior interosseous branch of the radial nerve, or the radial nerve itself more proximally, needs to be considered as the cause of the patient's inability to extend the fingers. Careful physical examination of the proximal forearm and elbow is therefore important to include a large cyst, lipoma, radiocapitellar effusion, or other elbow abnormality that may be causing compression of the radial nerve more proximally and leading to muscle paralysis. Electrophysiologic testing may also prove helpful.
- With respect to Mannerfelt syndrome, absence of flexion at the interphalangeal joint of the thumb and the distal interphalangeal joints in the index and long fingers should be differentiated from the anterior interosseous nerve syndrome, which when present in rheumatoid arthritis is usually due to a large ganglion originating on the volar surface of the elbow.

NONOPERATIVE MANAGEMENT

- Nonoperative management probably is more feasible with respect to Mannerfelt syndrome than with the Vaughn-Jackson or caput ulnae syndrome. Although the functional deficit is generally greater with loss of finger extensors than loss of active flexion of the interphalangeal joint of the thumb and distal interphalangeal joints of the index and long fingers, some patients may still function remarkably well.
- Supportive measures in patients who for one reason or another are not deemed suitable surgical candidates may be provided by a certified hand therapist or occupational therapist able to assist the patient with his or her activities of daily living.

- With median nerve entrapment and compression from the proliferative tenosynovitis at the level of the radiocarpal joint, disability becomes more progressive and nonsurgical treatment more difficult. There may be a role for corticosteroid injection at the level of the radiocarpal joint, and certainly, referral to a rheumatologist is crucial for the control and management of the disease before any surgical intervention.
- In the case of wrist or finger extensor tendon rupture, nonsurgical treatment may be beneficial in terms of resting the radiocarpal joint and interphalangeal joints of the fingers to prevent further tendon rupture by attrition. Splinting the wrist or hand may prove beneficial for pain control and to prevent further damage to the joints and soft tissues.
- Nonoperative management of thenar atrophy may be justified if there is an ulnar innervated deep muscle head of the flexor pollicis brevis to serve as a strong palmar flexor of the thumb. Lack of opposition may be of minimal functional significance, especially in the nondominant hand. If there is lack of sensation, the benefits of opposition transfer will be even smaller. Careful patient selection is critical.

SURGICAL MANAGEMENT

Basic Principles of Tendon Transfer

- A large variety of donor options exist. Considerations for donor selection include (1) expendability, (2) synergistic function between original and new function, (3) independent function, (4) good voluntary control, (5) straight line of pull or requirement of minimal (no more than one) pulleys, (6) avoidance of scarred or skin grafted areas, (7) sufficient muscle excursion, and (8) sufficient muscle power. Transferred muscles can be expected to lose one grade of strength.[6]
- Use of a Pulvertaft weave rather than end-to-end repair will greatly decrease the risk of rupture.
- Restore full range of motion prior to tendon transfer. Transfers will not be able to move stiff joints.
- Avoid surgery in patients with open wounds or uncontrolled disease.
- Insensate areas are less likely to benefit from transfer.
- If diagnosed early, an interposition graft may be used to reconstruct the ruptured tendon.[7] The palmaris tendon, a strip of the flexor carpi radialis (FCR), and a slip of the EDQ are suitable choices.
  - Outcomes are similar between tendon transfer and tendon reconstruction with graft. Results correlate inversely with number of fingers involved or chronicity of injury.[5]

Extensor Tendon Rupture

- A variety of tendon transfers are available for reconstruction of single and multiple extensor tendon ruptures.
- It is important for the surgeon to locate the site of tendon rupture and identify as well as treat the cause.
  - Usually, rupture is secondary to the distal ulna subluxating dorsally through the attenuated fibers of the DRUJ. When subluxation occurs at this level, it erodes through the floor of the fourth and fifth extensor compartments.
  - Tendon reconstruction is therefore not complete unless it involves removal of the dorsal osteophyte by a modified Darrach procedure and coverage of the distal ulna with a flap of extensor retinaculum.
  - When the distal ulna is unstable, the pronator quadratus may be brought dorsal to stabilize the bone. The ECU or flexor carpi ulnaris (FCU) combined with ECU[2] may also be considered.
- Small finger extension loss
  - Single tendon rupture of the EDQ may go unnoticed, particularly if there is a strong EDC to the small finger. Often, however, EDC contribution to the small finger is hypoplastic or absent and all that is present is a junctura tendinae from the small finger to the adjacent ring finger. Isolated loss of function in the EDQ is manifest by weakness or lack of extension of the small finger.
  - The distal stump of the ruptured tendon is sewn end to side to the intact ring finger EDC tendon. The risk of this transfer, however, is excessive abduction of the small finger when the distal tendon is short (**FIG 5A**). In general,

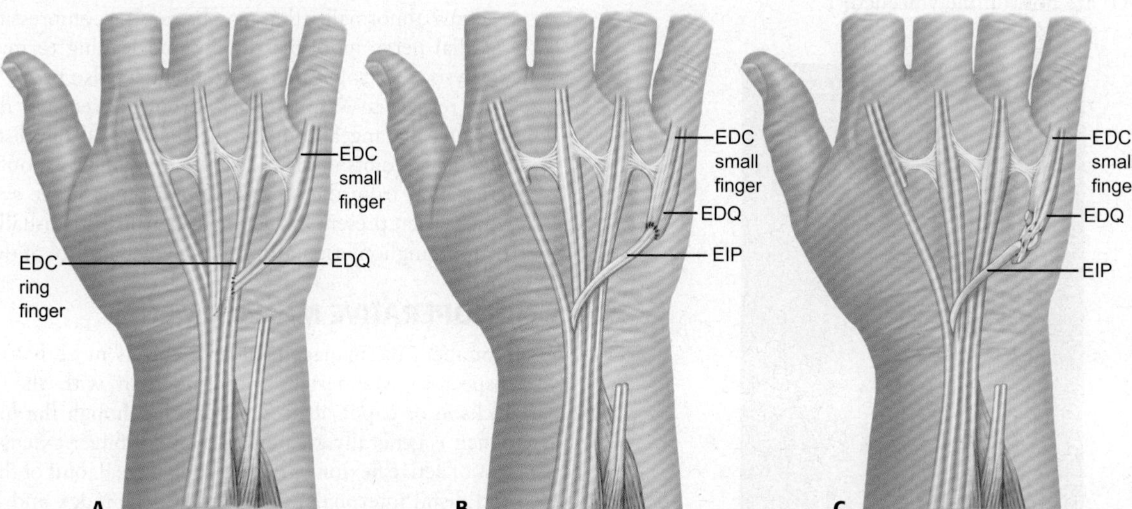

FIG 5 • A. When extensor tendon rupture leads to loss of extension in only one digit, such as the small finger, end-to-side transfer of the distal ruptured tendon to the more proximal adjacent EDC tendon of the ring finger can be performed. **B.** If the ruptured end is distal to the midmetacarpal region, this transfer may lead to abduction of the small finger metacarpal, and under these circumstances, tendon transfer of the EIP to the distal stump of the EDQ is undertaken (depicted here as an end-to-end transfer). **C.** EIP to EDQ, depicted here as a Pulvertaft weave between the distal tendon and the proximal transferred EIP.

the transfer should be performed to the tendon of the adjacent EDC of the ring finger with the weave as far proximal as the distal stump of the EDQ will allow.
- Alternatively, an EIP transfer may be performed (**FIG 5B,C**).
- Ring and small fingers extension loss
  - In addition to the EDC tendons to the ring and small fingers, the EDQ usually will have ruptured.
  - The EIP is transferred to the EDQ.
  - The distal ring finger EDC tendon is transferred end to side to the adjacent intact long finger EDC tendon (**FIG 6**). Alternately, the distal stumps of the EDC ring and small and EDQ may each be woven to the EIP.
  - Another alternative is transferring the FCR to EDC of ring and small with EDQ. This allows maintenance of powerful independent index finger extension. This can be helpful with a concomitant partial or total wrist fusion (**FIG 7A–F**).
- Long and ring fingers extension loss (**FIG 8A**)
  - Although two fingers are seemingly involved, the EDC tendon to the small finger is usually ruptured as well. The EDQ remains intact.
  - If the index finger EDC tendon is intact, EIP transfer to the long and ring finger EDC tendons is performed (**FIG 8B**).

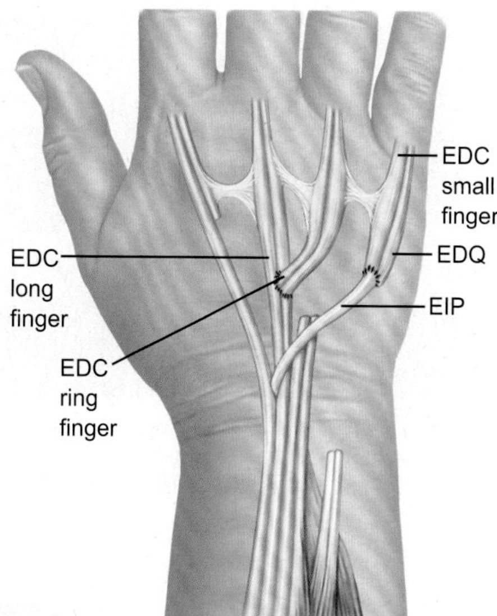

FIG 6 • In cases of double rupture in the ring and small fingers, transfer of the EIP to the distal EDQ, with end-to-side transfer of the distal EDC of the ring finger to the adjacent EDC to the long finger, is a standard transfer.

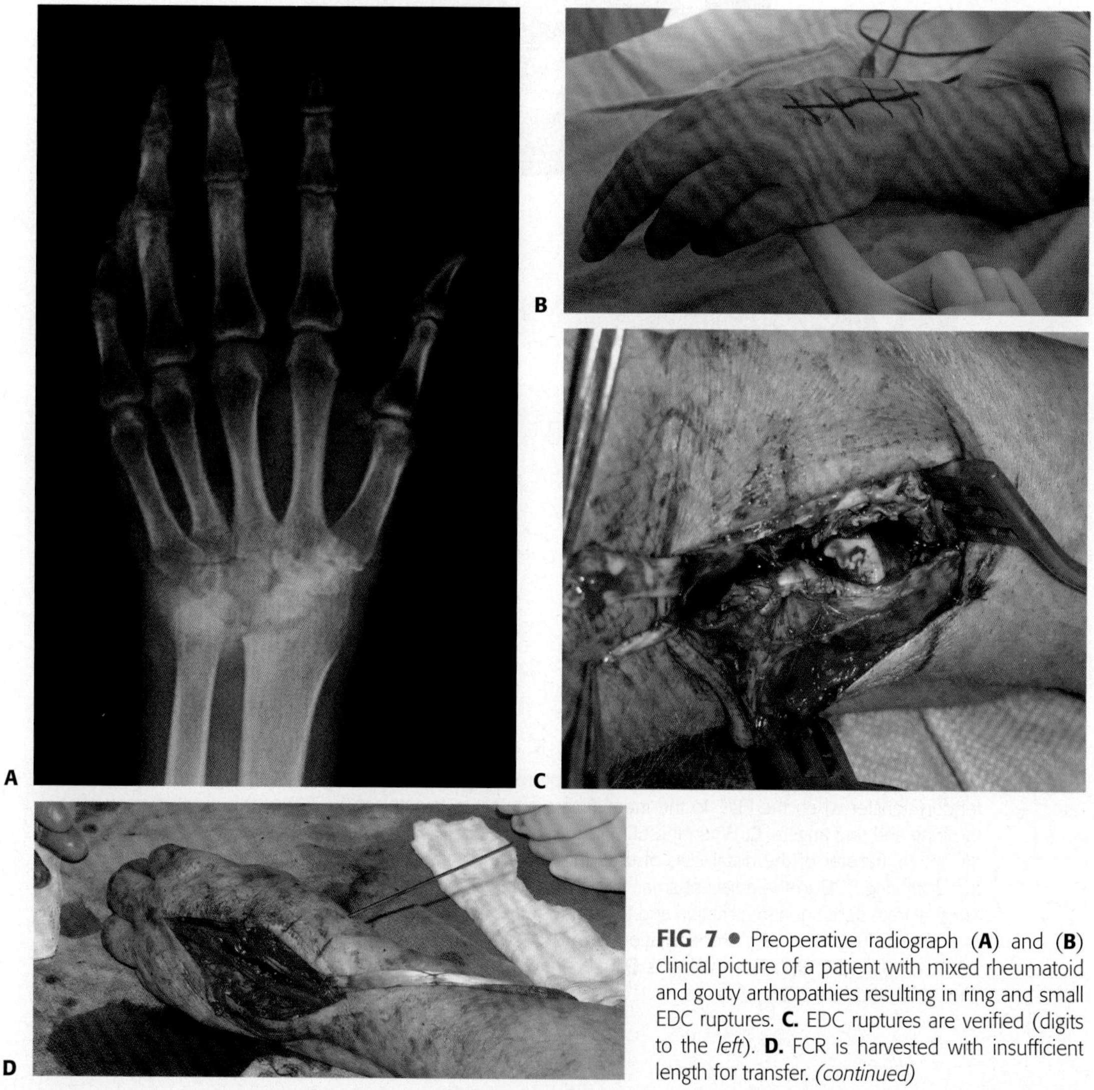

FIG 7 • Preoperative radiograph (**A**) and (**B**) clinical picture of a patient with mixed rheumatoid and gouty arthropathies resulting in ring and small EDC ruptures. **C.** EDC ruptures are verified (digits to the *left*). **D.** FCR is harvested with insufficient length for transfer. *(continued)*

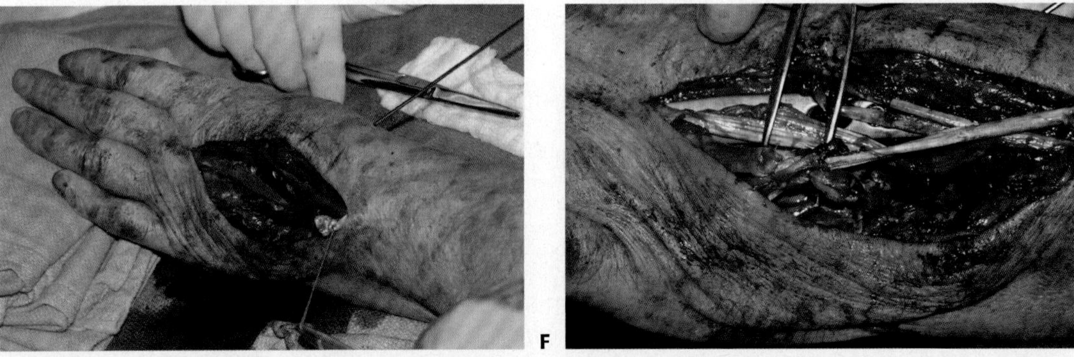

FIG 7 • *(continued)* **E.** A suture is first placed at the distal most portion of the FCR before splitting the tendon proximally and flipping of one slip of FCR distally to extend the tendon transfer. **F.** The transfer is completed with lengthened the FCR to EDQ, EDC ring and EDC small (digits to the *left*).

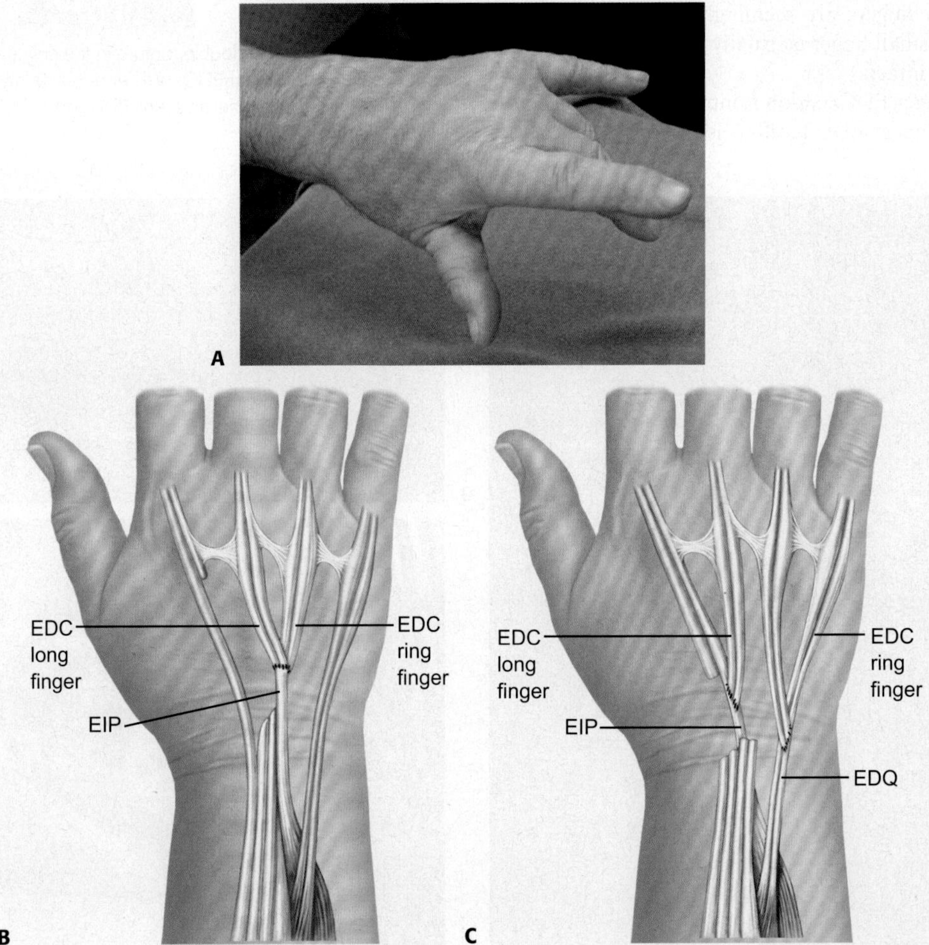

FIG 8 • **A.** Clinical appearance of a hand with rupture of the EDC to the long and ring fingers. **B.** Optional tendon transfer when the EDC to the index finger is intact is transfer of the EIP to the distal stumps of the long and ring fingers. **C.** When the EDC to the index finger has been ruptured and EIP transfer is not an option, transfer of the distal EDC of the long finger to the adjacent EIP of the index and transfer of the distal ring EDC to the adjacent small finger extensor, is shown here. (**A:** From Lubahn JD, Wolfe TL. Surgical treatment and rehabilitation and tendon ruptures in the rheumatoid hand. In: Mackin EJ, Callahan AD, Skirven TM, et al, eds. Rehabilitation of the Hand and Upper Extremity, ed 5. St. Louis: Mosby, 2002:1598–1607; **B,C:** From Williams DP, Lubahn JD. Reconstruction of extensor tendons. Atlas Hand Clin 2005;10:209–222.)

- If the EDC tendon to the index finger has ruptured, end-to-side transfer of the distal tendon of the long finger EDC to the adjacent intact EIP and transfer of the distal tendon of the ring finger EDC to the adjacent intact EDQ may be considered (**FIG 8C**).
- Long, ring, and small fingers extension loss
  - If the EIP and EDC tendons to the index finger are intact, the EIP can be transferred to the distal stumps of the ring and small fingers EDC tendons using end-to-end or end-to-side techniques, depending on the length of the distal stumps.
  - The EDC to the long finger is transferred end to side to the adjacent intact index EDC tendon (**FIG 9**).
  - If only the EIP is intact and all remaining tendons on the dorsum of the wrist have ruptured, transfer of the flexor digitorum sublimis (FDS) of the ring finger around the radial or ulnar border of the forearm is the next logical choice.
  - In patients with partial or complete wrist fusion, or in patients with limited wrist motion, transfer of the ECRL may be considered. Although not "in phase" with the finger extension, the line of pull matches reasonably well.
- Index, long, ring, and small fingers extension loss
  - The two most common transfers are the FDS around the radial and ulnar sides of the forearm or through the interosseous membrane (**FIG 10A,B**).
  - Transfer of one of the radial wrist extensors is a suitable alternative (**FIG 10C**).
- Loss of thumb extension
  - EPL rupture is common and often results in minimal loss of function.
  - Late or chronic ruptures require transfer of the EIP to the distal end of the EPL. The proximal muscle will usually begin to atrophy and become nonfunctional by 6 months after the injury.

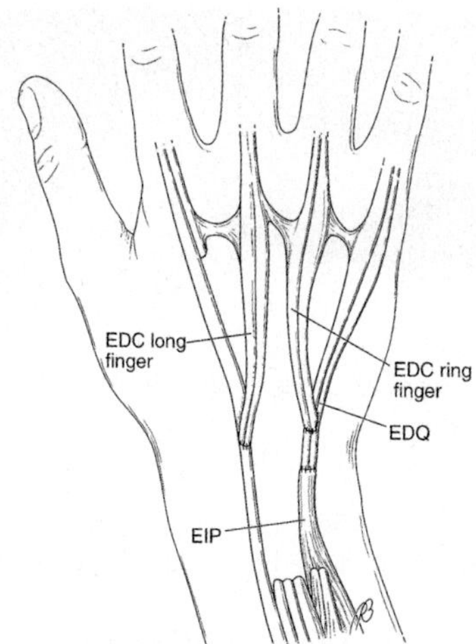

FIG 9 • Rupture of the common extensors to the long, ring, and small fingers with extensor digiti quinti (EDQ) rupture can be treated, as shown here, with transfer of the extensor indicis proprius (EIP) to the distal stumps of the ring and small fingers with distal end-to-side transfer from the extensor digitorum communis (EDC) to the long finger to the adjacent index EDC.

  - If the EIP is not available, transfer of the FDS from the long or ring finger can be considered. The FDS can be routed through the interosseous membrane or around the radial side of the forearm as described for transfer to restore finger extension.[14]
  - A recent transfer that has been described is a partial ECRL turnover tendon. It may be useful when the EIP is not available, as it allows reconstruction of even very distal ruptures without need for graft.[4]

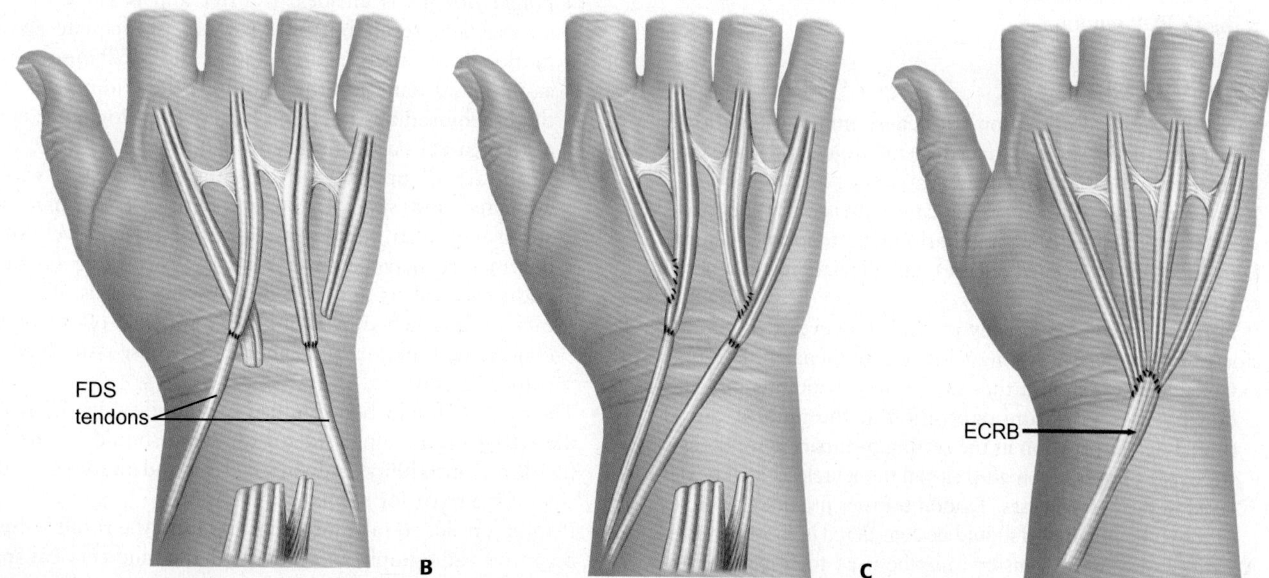

FIG 10 • **A.** Rupture of all four finger extensors may be treated alternatively with transfer of the flexor digitorum superficialis (FDS) to the long and ring fingers, harvested in the distal palm and transferred around the radius and ulna, with the two forearm bones serving as pulleys for the transferred tendon. **B.** Alternatively, both FDS tendons may be transferred around the radial side of the forearm and sutured to the distal stumps of the EDC tendons. **C.** With rupture of all common extensor tendons to the fingers as well as the EIP and the EDQ, extension may be restored through transfer of one of the radial wrist extensors. This is ideal when a partial wrist fusion is being planned, as shown.

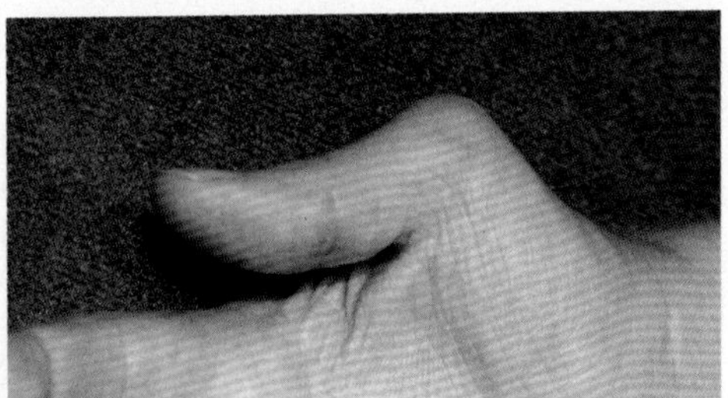

FIG 11 • Extensor pollicis brevis rupture. Boutonnière deformity of the thumb (Nalebuff type I).

- Chronic synovitis at the thumb MCP joint may lead to attritional rupture of the dorsal capsule and the extensor pollicis brevis.
  - This boutonnière deformity of the thumb is a type I as described by Nalebuff[10] and Nalebuff and Millender[11] (**FIG 11**).
  - The deformity usually progresses after extensor pollicis brevis rupture. The EPL shifts ulnarly, the collateral ligaments weaken, and the thumb metacarpal becomes abducted radially. The interphalangeal joint hyperextends as a reciprocal response to the MCP joint flexion.
  - Transfer of the EPL to the extensor pollicis brevis insertion in the base of the proximal phalanx and the dorsal capsule of the MCP joint of the thumb is performed. Local anesthesia is typically adequate.

Flexor Tendon Rupture

- Tendon transfer for the treatment of flexor tendon disruption in the rheumatoid patient is much less common than for extensor tendon rupture.
- Mannerfelt syndrome should be treated by transfer of the brachioradialis tendon to the flexor pollicis longus.
  - Associated disruption of a FDP tendon is usually treated by transferring the distal stump end to side to the adjacent digit's FDP tendon.

Lack of Opposition

- Lack of opposition function may cause minimal functional deficit in patients with advanced rheumatoid arthritis. Many patients may be managed conservatively.
- If chronic CTS is the underlying cause, division of the transverse carpal ligament in combination with tenosynovectomy (as in open carpal tunnel release) will alleviate median nerve compression.
- If intrinsic wasting is already present, however, decompression of the median nerve may not restore thenar function.
  - Consideration should thus be given to simultaneous tendon transfer to restore opposition at the time of carpal tunnel decompression in the setting of intrinsic weakness
  - Recovery of opposition after carpal tunnel release will be delayed in the best of cases. Tendon transfer provides rapid return of function and so should be considered in most patients.
- A variety of tendon transfers may be used to restore opposition. These include the palmaris longus,[3] EIP, FDS, and abductor digiti minimi.[8]
  - If performed at the same time as carpal tunnel release, the palmaris longus transfer is preferred, as it is done through the same incision and has minimal extra morbidity.
  - Otherwise, transfer of the extensor indicis is reliable, has minimal morbidity, and has the most reliable pulley (ulnar border of the wrist).
  - FDS transfer is also very reliable. It has two main drawbacks. Sacrifice of a FDS tendon may decrease grip strength. Donor site morbidity including swan-neck deformity or flexion contracture of the proximal interphalangeal joint may occur. Women tend to be more at risk for the former and men the latter. Donor site morbidity may be minimized by not removing the tendon portion distal to the A1 pulley.
- A variety of insertion sites may be used. Typically, the tendon is sutured to the APB tendon using a Pulvertaft weave. Suture anchors or a bone tunnel may also be used.
  - Additional insertions have been described including the proximal phalanx, the extensor mechanism, or dorsal capsule. A portion of the tendon may also be used to reconstruct the collateral ligament. This allows the tendon transfer to restore additional functions including thumb MCP extension or stability. In these cases, a dual insertion is generally performed, with the tendon being attached to the APB tendon as well as a second location. This second insertion may weaken tendon transfer function and is generally unnecessary unless there is additional deficit of the thumb (eg, extensor pollicis brevis dysfunction or collateral ligament insufficiency).

Preoperative Planning

- All patients with rheumatoid arthritis require a thorough general physical examination as well as careful evaluation of their cervical spine, including posteroanterior and lateral radiographs, often with flexion and extension views to evaluate cervical spine instability.
- Limited joint mobility is a contraindication to tendon transfer.
  - Directed therapy may be used to improve contracture.
  - For example, brachioradialis tendon transfer to the flexor pollicis longus is an ideal transfer and is likely to yield an excellent result but only if there is adequate passive motion at the interphalangeal joint and MCP joint as well as the basal joint and the thumb. If these joints are stiff, the brachioradialis might be better saved for other needs as the patient's arthritis progresses.
  - With lack of opposition, the thumb metacarpal will be adducted and supinated. Contracture of the first web space may also be present. Intraoperatively, web space contracture may be treated by release of the fascia of adductor pollicis and first dorsal interosseous. The skin may be lengthened by skin graft, flap, or Z-plasty. Severe contractures may require metacarpal base osteotomy or trapeziectomy.
- The carpus should be examined for stability. In particular, the DRUJ on the ulnar side of the wrist should be checked for dorsal instability and subluxation and the volar radial side of the wrist for palmar subluxation.
- Planning needs to take into consideration the results of preoperative radiographs of the wrist, hand, and cervical spine as well as electromyographic tests.
  - If the findings on electromyography are negative and the surgeon is certain that tendon rupture is responsible for the lack of active finger motion, plans should be made to transfer expendable existing tendons to those that

have ruptured. In the case of multiple extensor tendon ruptures to the fingers, the ECRL and the FDS from the long and ring fingers are two of the most common donor tendons.
  - If radiographs reveal significant joint destruction and instability, appropriate arthrodesis or arthroplasty should be considered rather than tendon transfer.
- Instruments designed for tendon weaves are extremely valuable.
  - Sharp tendon passers facilitate a Pulvertaft weave. When sharp, pointed tendon passers are not available, a no. 11 blade can be passed through the tendon followed by a hemostat to grasp the knife and guide the hemostat through the tendon. The hemostat then grasps the transferred tendon, weaving it through the recipient tendon.
  - 3-0 and 4-0 braided nonabsorbable sutures on appropriate needles are recommended for tendon repairs.

Positioning

- Most tendon transfers are done with the patient in the supine position on the operating table.
- The contralateral arm or lower extremity may be sterilely draped in the event that a tendon graft is needed.
- Anesthesia may be either general or an axillary block, depending on the patient's preference and the stability of the cervical spine.
  - Although isolated carpal tunnel release may be performed under local anesthesia, carpal tunnel release combined with palmaris longus opponensplasty requires block or general anesthesia.

TECHNIQUES

Extensor Indicis Proprius Tendon Transfer

- Isolate the EIP through a 1-cm longitudinal or curvilinear incision on the dorsoulnar aspect of the index MCP joint.
  - The EIP is usually the ulnar tendon of the two located dorsal to the MCP joint of the index finger.
- Make a second 2- to 3-cm incision over the mid-dorsal wrist (unless a dorsal wrist incision has already been made for another procedure).
- Incise the retinaculum overlying the fourth extensor compartment and locate the EIP tendon ulnar and deep to the EDC tendons.
  - The EIP is identified by its muscle belly, which is the most distal in the fourth extensor compartment.
- Once the identity of the EIP is confirmed proximally and distally, suture the index EIP and EDC tendons together as far distal as possible using 4-0 nonabsorbable braided suture. This will allow the EDC to index finger to pull on the EIP distal remnant.
  - Invert or bury the knot to void prominence under thin rheumatoid skin.
- Incise the EIP just proximal to the stitch, and then free any tendinous interconnections over the dorsum of the hand.
  - Some authors advocate to take a segment of extensor hood with the EIP tendon. This should only be done if the additional length is needed for the transfer. If performed, repair the extensor hood using small nonabsorbable suture to prevent EDC subluxation.
- Use a blunt instrument or Penrose drain to pull the EIP tendon into the wrist wound.
- Transfer the EIP to the exposed recipient tendon using a Pulvertaft weave.
  - A single weave, although usually sufficient for smaller tendons, should be supplemented with an additional one or two weaves if possible. This will significantly strengthen the repair site.
  - If insufficient distal tendon is present for a weave, either an end-to-end repair or a weave in which the transferred tendon is brought through a transverse incision in the distal recipient stump from volar to dorsal is an effective option. As many as three distal tendons may be sewn to the proximal EIP using single weaves. Usually, the EDQ would be most proximal followed by the EDC ring and long.
- Skin incisions are closed and a splint is applied for 3 to 4 weeks after which time therapy is begun under the supervision of a hand therapist.

Flexor Carpi Radialis Tendon Transfer for Finger Extension

- Works best when combined with partial or total wrist fusion
- Primary skin incision for wrist fusion is made over the fourth dorsal compartment. The wrist fusion is performed before tendon transfer as to have a fixed tension for the transfer.
- The FCR may be harvested with a single longitudinal incision on the volar wrist, taken with a portion of the palmar aponeurosis, or, alternatively, it may be harvested through a series of incisions volarly. It is important to free the proximal muscle from its fascial attachments.
- The FCR is then passed subcutaneously around the radius and delivered into the primary skin incision.
- The FCR may then be woven into the EDC of ring and small with EDQ.
- If the FCR transfer is of insufficient length to reach the EDC stumps, the FCR may be split proximally and a portion flipped distally. It is helpful to place a stitch in the distal aspect of the transfer as to not strip the tendon completely.
- Similar to other tendon transfers, the tension must be set at the time of transfer. The FCR is sewn into the extensors with the fingers in full extension.
- The skin incisions are then closed and the hand is splinted with the fingers fully extended.

Flexor Digitorum Superficialis Tendon Transfer for Finger Extension

- In the case of rupture of all of the extensor tendons on the dorsum of the wrist and when wrist motion is still intact, tendon transfer of the FDS, as suggested by Boyes,[1] is a reliable method to restore finger extension.
  - The FDS and FDP to each of the donor fingers must be intact.
  - Preexisting swan-neck deformity in a donor digit may worsen after harvest of the FDS tendon.
  - Long and ring FDS tendons are used most often.
- Make a transverse incision in the distal palm and divide the FDS tendon proximal to the bifurcation between the A1 and A2 pulleys. This leaves the chiasm of Camper intact to provide proximal interphalangeal stability and helps prevent development of a swan-neck deformity (**TECH FIG 1**).
  - Splinting the proximal interphalangeal joint in flexion postoperatively will also help to minimize the risk of developing a swan-neck deformity.
- Isolate the FDS tendon proximally through a Henry-type incision in the distal forearm and atraumatically deliver it into that incision.
- Pass the tendon deep to the median nerve, the FDP, the FCR, the flexor pollicis longus, and the radial artery and the nerve at the wrist with a blunt tendon passer, hemostat, or Kelly clamp.
  - The transferred tendon sits on the radius using the bone as a pulley to enhance the effectiveness of the transfer.
- If the FDS to the ring finger is too short to pass around the radial side of the wrist, an alternative route is beneath the FDP, FCU, and ulnar artery and nerve around the ulnar side of the forearm using the ulna as the pulley.
  - In general, the radial path is preferred to minimize ulnar deviation of the digits.
- Alternatively, the FDS tendon is passed volar to dorsal through an incision in the interosseous membrane just proximal to the DRUJ.
  - The membrane functions as the pulley.
- Weave the smaller distal tendon stumps through the larger transferred FDS tendon in the manner described by Pulvertaft.[12]
  - Adjust tension such that with slight wrist flexion, the fingers are maintained in full extension.
- Immobilize the hand and wrist with the wrist in 40 degrees of extension and the fingers flexed until tension is noted at the suture line (**TECH FIG 2**).
  - Ideally, this should be close to the "safe position" with slight MCP joint flexion and relative interphalangeal joint extension.

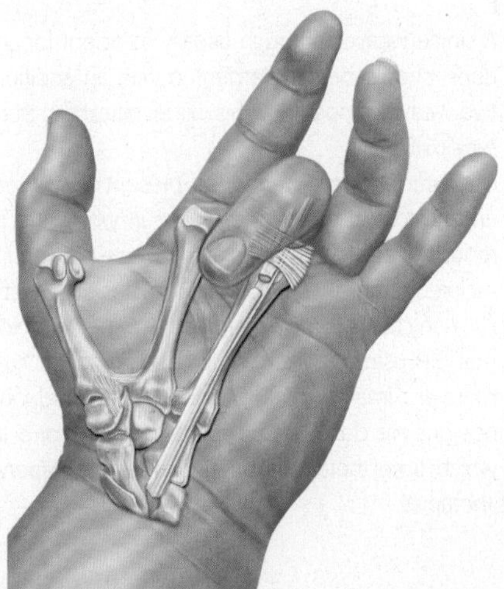

TECH FIG 1 • Transfer of the FDS to the long and ring fingers. The distal incision in the palm is used to isolate the sublimis tendon as far distal as possible by flexing the finger so that the chiasm of Camper is visible in the wound. The tendon is divided just proximal to the chiasm, leaving enough distal tendon to contribute to the stability of the proximal interphalangeal joint in extension and thereby avoiding a secondary instability of that joint and possible swan-neck deformity.

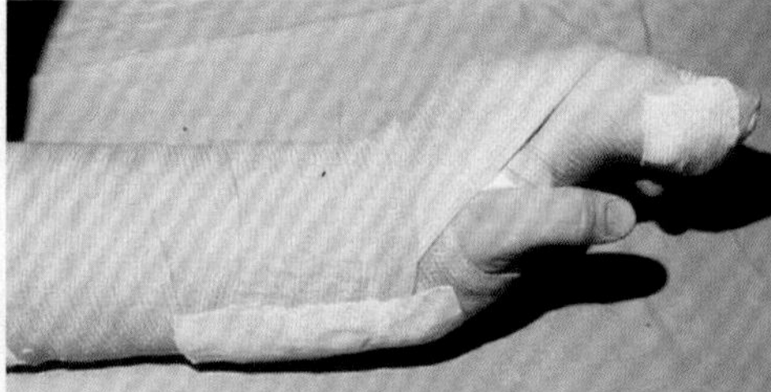

TECH FIG 2 • The ideal splint for transfer to the extensor tendons of the finger immobilizes the wrist in the so-called safe position. With wrist extension, tension at the site of transfer is usually minimal. Finger flexion at the MCP joint is ideal to prevent scarring of the collateral ligaments and secondary loss of finger flexion. The amount of flexion possible is judged in the operating room by passive flexion of the finger until a minimum amount of tension is seen at the repair site. (From Williams DP, Lubahn JD. Reconstruction of extensor tendons. Atlas Hand Clin 2005;10:209–222.)

Extensor Carpi Radialis Longus or Brevis Transfer

- When all of the finger extensors have ruptured, wrist motion is severely limited (ie, after a partial or complete wrist fusion), and the radiocarpal joint is stable, the wrist extensors become potential muscles for use as transfers.
  - The ECRL and the ECRB are located in the second dorsal compartment of the wrist adjacent to the fourth compartment and are separated only by the tubercle of Lister and the EPL.
- Expose the ECRL or ECRB using a straight dorsal incision or a limited transverse incision over the base of the index and long metacarpals at their respective insertion sites.
- Divide the tendon selected for transfer, usually the ECRL, at its insertion and transfer it ulnarly to the recipient tendon stump.

Brachioradialis Tendon Transfer (Reconstruction of Mannerfelt Syndrome)

- Expose the forearm muscles and the brachioradialis tendon insertion on the distal radial aspect of the radius through a Henry-type incision. The brachioradialis is detached from its insertion and carefully released proximally to increase its excursion.
- Confirm the tendon rupture by direct exposure of the slightly more distal and radial tendon of the flexor pollicis longus.
- Mobilize the distal tendon stump and perform a tenolysis to remove adhesions.
- Weave the distal flexor pollicis longus through the brachioradialis in a Pulvertaft fashion. Sharp tendon passers facilitate this technique (**TECH FIG 3**).
- Adjust tension such that with wrist flexion, the MCP and interphalangeal joints of the thumb extend fully and with wrist extension, they flex 30 to 40 degrees.
- Secure the weaves with 3-0 or 4-0 braided nonabsorbable sutures.
- If the index or long FDP tendons also are ruptured, isolate the distal tendon stumps and repair them end to side.

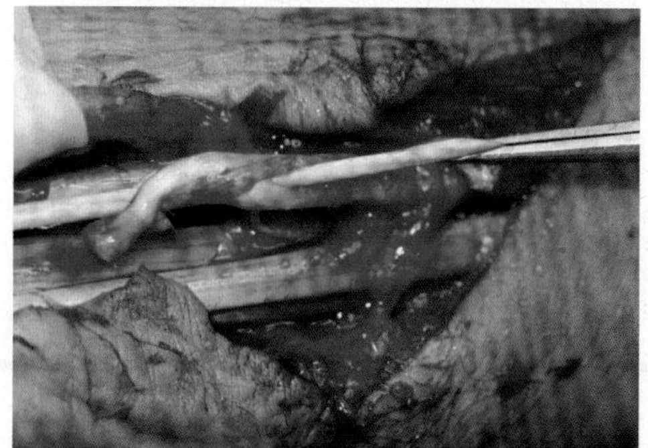
A

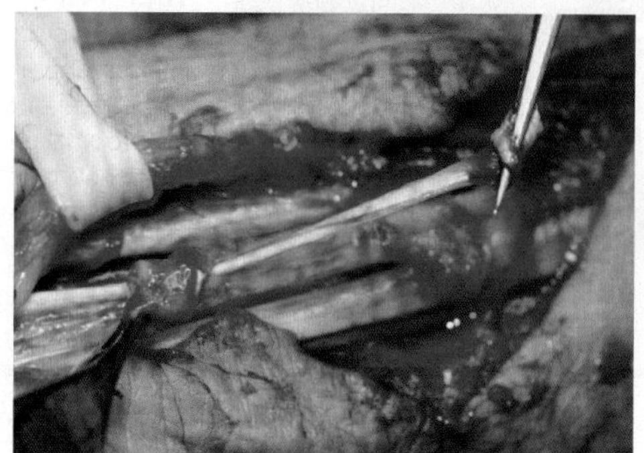
B

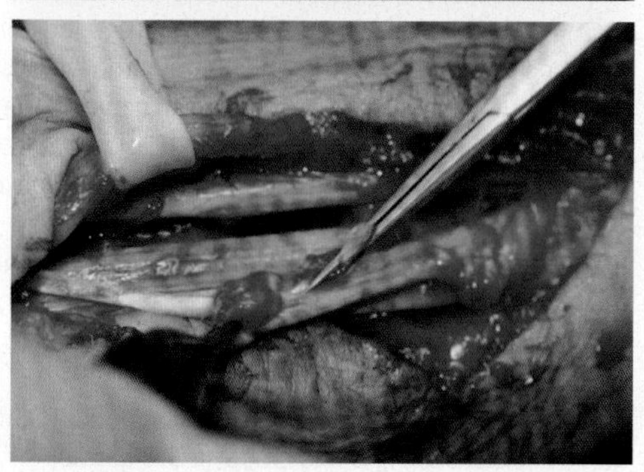
C

TECH FIG 3 • A,B. Pulvertaft weave shown sequentially as a sharp tendon passer is used to puncture the tendon through and through and then grasp the tendon being transferred and weave it through the recipient tendon. **C.** The transfer is secured at each weave with one or two nonabsorbable braided nylon sutures. (From Lubahn JD, Wolfe TL. Surgical treatment and rehabilitation and tendon ruptures in the rheumatoid hand. In: Mackin EJ, Callahan AD, Skirven TM, et al, eds. Rehabilitation of the Hand and Upper Extremity, ed 5. St. Louis: Mosby, 2002:1598–1607.)

Extensor Pollicis Longus Tendon Transfer (Reconstruction of Thumb Boutonnière Deformity)

- Make a longitudinal incision to expose and identify the EPL tendon at its insertion onto the base of the distal phalanx.
- Incise the tendon at that level and mobilize it proximally (**TECH FIG 4A**).
  - Carefully protect the intrinsic tendon, which will now be the sole extensor for the thumb interphalangeal joint.
- Expose the dorsal base of the proximal phalanx and weave the EPL tendon through the dorsal capsule, securing it using a 3-0 or 4-0 nonabsorbable braided suture (**TECH FIG 4B**).
  - Alternatively, secure the EPL tendon in place using drill holes or a suture anchor in the proximal phalanx (**TECH FIG 4C,D**).
- The thumb is splinted or casted for 4 weeks, and a protective splint is worn for strenuous activities for 6 to 8 weeks.

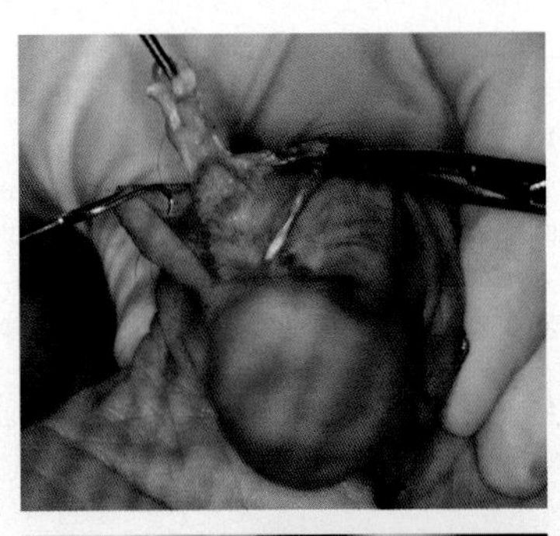
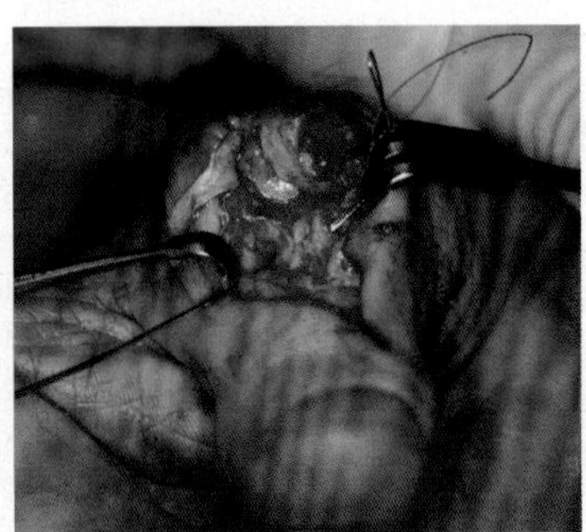
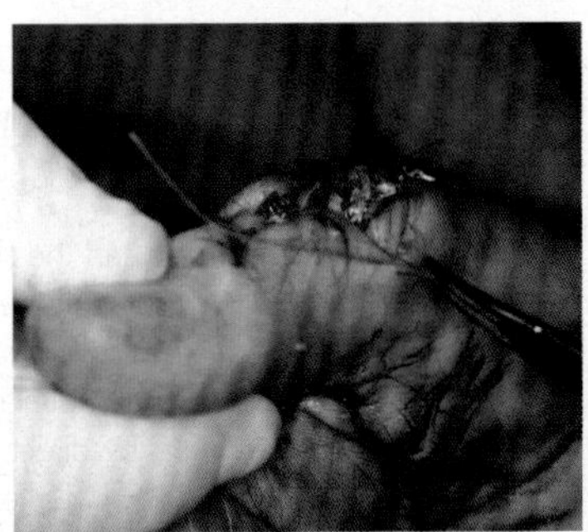
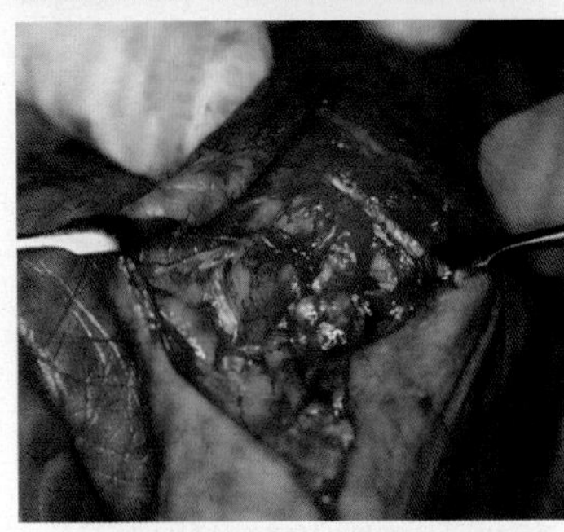

TECH FIG 4 • Extensor pollicis brevis rupture. **A,B.** Tendon transfer of the EPL proximally to the site of insertion of the extensor pollicis brevis, allowing the hyperextended interphalangeal joint to drop into a more flexed position and allowing active extension at the level of the MCP joint. **C,D.** EPL is anchored through drill holes to the base of the proximal phalanx. (From Lubahn JD, Wolfe TL. Surgical treatment and rehabilitation and tendon ruptures in the rheumatoid hand. In: Mackin EJ, Callahan AD, Skirven TM, et al, eds. Rehabilitation of the Hand and Upper Extremity, ed 5. St. Louis: Mosby, 2002:1598–1607.)

Flexor Digitorum Superficialis Opposition Transfer (TECH FIG 5A–F)

- The FDS tendon is harvested as described earlier (see Flexor Digitorum Superficialis Tendon Transfer for Finger Extension).
- The forearm incision is made on the ulnar aspect of the wrist to expose the FCU. The incision is curved proximally to allow access to the finger flexors.
- The donor tendon is isolated and brought into the forearm.
- A pulley is made using the FCU. The FCU is split longitudinally without detaching it from the pisiform. One limb is then divided to create a distally based slip. The cut end is passed back through the intact tendon near the pisiform to create a loop closed by a tendon weave. The weave is sutured with small nonabsorbable suture.
- The FDS tendon is passed through the FCU loop.
- A subcutaneous tunnel is made between the pulley and a small incision on the radial side of the thumb MCP joint. The tunnel should be superficial to the median nerve. The tendon is passed through this tunnel.
  - The transverse carpal ligament or Guyon canal may also be used as a pulley.
- The tendon is sutured to the APB tendon using a Pulvertaft weave.
  - The tendon is tensioned with the thumb in opposition and the wrist in neutral.
  - Because of the large excursion of the FDS tendon, precise tensioning is less crucial in this transfer.
- A thumb spica cast is worn for 4 weeks and then transitioned to a removable splint.

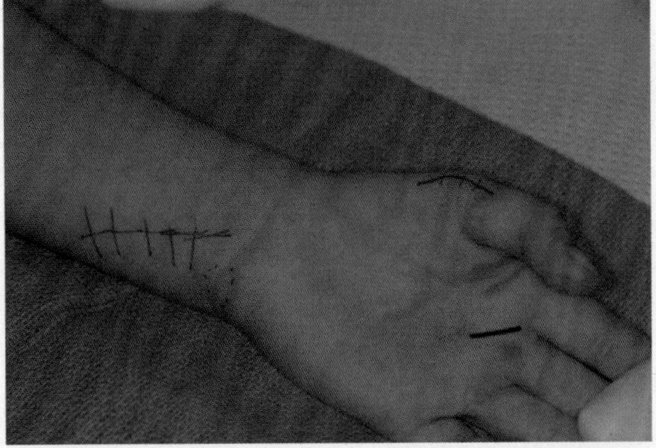
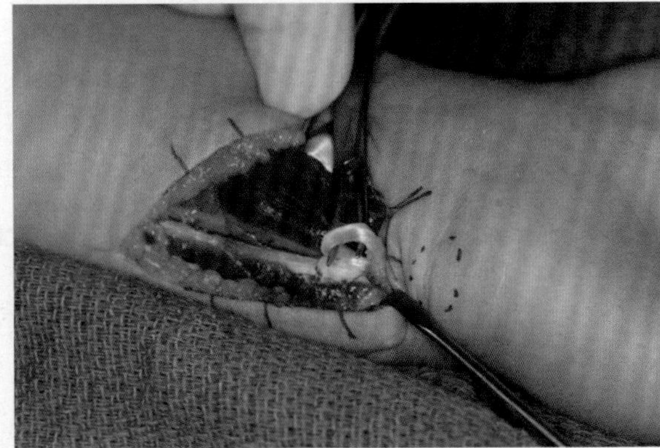

TECH FIG 5 • Flexor digitorum superficialis transfer. **A.** The skin markings are at the distal palmar crease (middle finger was used in this patient only because the ring finger FDS had been previously used), radial thumb, and ulnar forearm. **B.** Through the forearm incision, a portion of FCU is used to create a pulley. *(continued)*

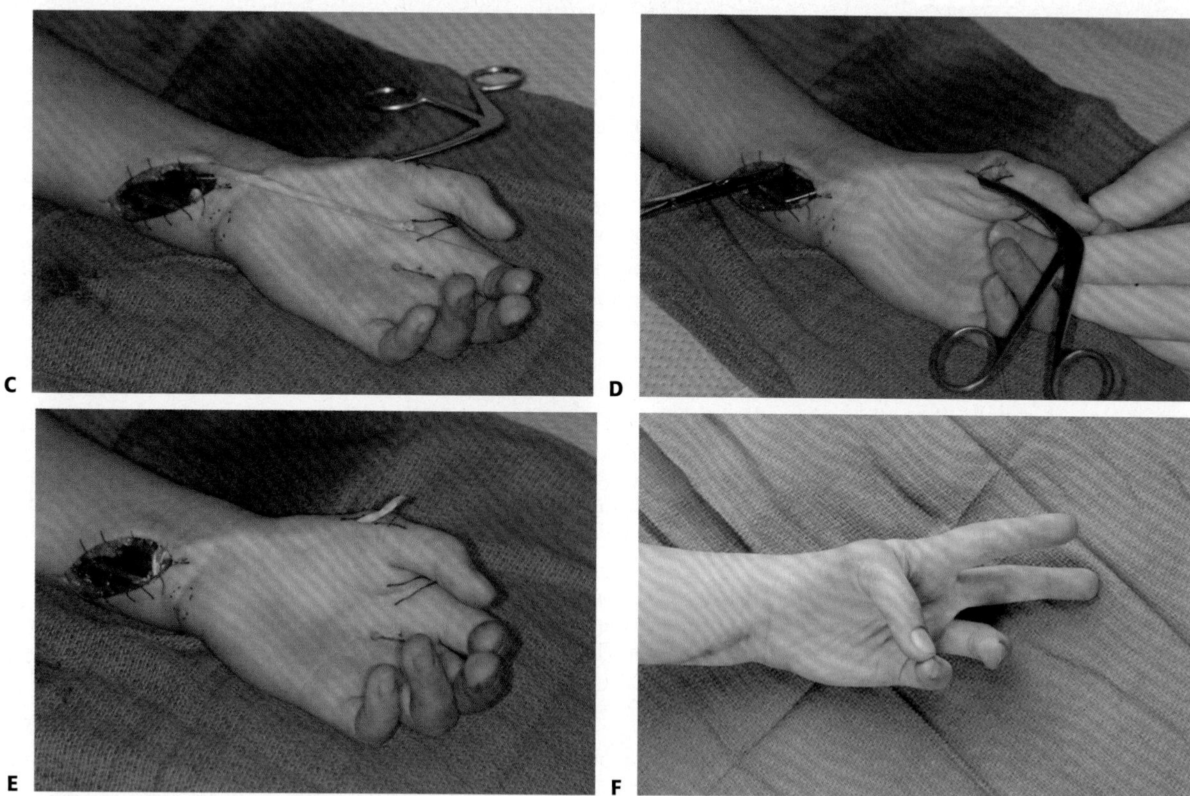

TECH FIG 5 • *(continued)* **C,D.** After dividing the superficialis tendon in the distal palm and drawing it into forearm, a tunnel is made from the thumb to forearm. **E.** The tendon graft is then passed through the FCU loop and the subcutaneous tunnel to its point of attachment at the thumb. **F.** Excellent opposition was restored in this patient.

Palmaris Longus Opposition Transfer

- Preoperatively, confirm presence of the palmaris longus by physical examination. Because the tendon is not long enough to reach the thumb, it is augmented by including a strip of the palmar fascia.
- A longitudinal incision is made from the proximal palmar crease to the forearm. The palmar cutaneous branch of the median nerve arises radial to the palmaris longus tendon and should be identified and protected. After division of the skin, a 1-cm band of the palmar fascia is removed in continuity with the palmaris longus tendon. This additional tissue provides the length required for the palmaris longus to reach the thumb. This will also accomplish the carpal tunnel release. The tendon is then freed from the forearm to palm.
- A second incision is made on the radial aspect of the thumb MCP joint. A subcutaneous tunnel is made between this and the forearm incision.
- The tendon with attached fascia is passed from the forearm to second incision. It is inserted into the APB tendon with a weave.
  - The transfer is tensioned with the thumb in full opposition, MCP joint in full extension, and wrist in neutral.
  - A thumb spica cast is worn for 4 weeks and then transitioned to a removable splint.

Extensor Indicis Proprius Transfer for Lack of Opposition

- The EIP tendon is obtained as in the section Extensor Indicis Proprius Tendon Transfer and passed around the ulnar side of the distal dorsal forearm.
- A second incision is made along the radial aspect of thumb MCP joint.
- A subcutaneous tunnel is around the ulnar border of the wrist from the dorsal forearm incision to this second incision. Care should be taken to not entrap or damage the ulnar neurovascular bundle. This can be done by staying superficial to the FCU. This task is made easier by making an additional small incision proximal to the pisiform. The tendon is first passed into this incision, then a second time across the palm.
- The EIP is passed around the ulnar side of the wrist through the tunnel and inserted into the APB tendon with a weave.
  - The transfer is tensioned with the thumb in full opposition and the wrist in slight flexion.
- A thumb spica cast is worn for 4 weeks and then transitioned to a removable splint.

PEARLS AND PITFALLS

EIP harvest	■ Obtain the EIP transfer by tracing the ulnar most inserting tendon in the MCP joint region of the index finger proximally at the level of the wrist. In a certain percentage of patients, the ulnar most tendon is in fact the EDC rather than the EIP. The EIP, however, is always the deeper, more volar tendon at the level of the wrist. Tracing this independent muscle tendon unit from the wrist to the index finger MCP joint will help assure the surgeon that the correct tendon is being released for transfer. ■ Distal repair of the dorsal apparatus at the site of EIP harvest is somewhat controversial. Although some experts recommend repair, others feel confident that the defect can be left with no risk of extensor lag. The surgeon needs to be aware of the potential risk of extensor lag, and we recommend attention to the defect by suture repair.
EDQ transfers	■ Sufficient length of the distal segment of the EDQ should be available to allow tendon transfer to the adjacent EDC without abducting the small finger. If this transfer is tight, the side-to-side transfer of EDQ to the EDC of the ring finger should be abandoned and tendon transfer to the EIP or another suitable donor pursued.
Unstable DRUJ	■ At the time of tendon transfer, inspect the DRUJ to be certain that any osteophytes have been débrided and a localized flap rotated to cover the exposed bone created. If the DRUJ is deemed unstable, transfer of the pronator quadratus dorsally may be used to stabilize the distal ulna.
Suturing	■ When suturing tendon grafts at the site of tendon weave (ie, where a graft or transfer is passed through another tendon), one or two sutures should be sufficient. Take care that the needle does not pass through the tendon near the thread from another suture. If this occurs, the suture is weakened or possibly cut in two by the needle and the graft or transfer is predisposed to rupture. Cutting needles should never be used, as they place both the suture and the tendon at risk.
Tendon transfer	■ Ensure adequate size of tunnel for passage of tendon. ■ When passing tendons from one compartment to another, make sure to pull in line with the tendon instead of up and out of the wound, as this may avulse the tendon. This may be accomplished by "winding" the tendon using an Allis retractor placed into the wound. ■ Avoid passing tendon through scarred areas. ■ Avoid surgery in the setting of open wounds. ■ Full range of motion should be obtained *prior* to transfer.

POSTOPERATIVE CARE

- Postoperative care for each of these tendon transfers is similar.
- In the case of tendon transfer to restore loss of finger extensors, the hand and wrist are immobilized with the wrist extended about 40 degrees. More may be desirable in certain instances, but too much extension could damage already fragile joints.
  - The MCP joints are brought into flexion until tension is noted at the suture line. Forty degrees or more is ideal to maintain the desired length of the collateral ligaments and prevent MCP joint extension contractures.
  - Immobilization is continued for 3.5 to 4 weeks, and gentle active motion is begun, maintaining the hand in a splint for protection.
  - At 6 weeks, some resistive exercises may be added to the program. By 12 weeks, the patient should be able to resume normal activities.
- In the case of flexor tendon rupture, the hand and wrist are immobilized with the wrist in 60 degrees of flexion, the MCP joints in 40 degrees of flexion, and the interphalangeal joints allowed to extend until tension is noted at the suture line. Immobilization is continued for 6 weeks, at which time a gentle active range-of-motion program is begun without resistance.
  - At 12 weeks, resistive exercises are added and the patient is permitted to gradually resume normal activity.
- In the case of opposition transfer, the thumb is immobilized in full opposition and the wrist in neutral to slight flexion. A thumb spica cast is worn for 4 weeks and then transitioned to a removable splint.

OUTCOMES

- Outcomes in tendon transfer surgery in rheumatoid arthritis are highly dependent on the patient's medical condition and ability to cooperate with the postoperative splinting and rehabilitation program. Most patients who are supervised by a therapist achieve a better result than those who try to make it on their own.
  - With good medical management of rheumatoid arthritis, when the disease is well controlled, and in cooperative patients who are motivated to improve, good results should be expected.
- Tendon transfer should always be delayed in patients with active disease, as results will be poor.
- The only surgical procedure to be performed in poorly controlled patients is synovectomy and with the caveat that success hinges on eventual good medical control of the disease.
- Outcomes correlate inversely with the number of ruptured tendons and chronicity of injury.[5]

COMPLICATIONS

- Infection
- Skin or surgical wound breakdown
- Attenuation of the transferred tendon
- Rerupture of the tendons
- Loss of motion due to improper tensioning of the transferred tendon
- Joint stiffness

REFERENCES

1. Boyes JH. Bunnell's Surgery of the Hand, ed 5. Philadelphia: JB Lippincott, 1970.
2. Breen TF. Jupiter JB. Extensor carpi ulnaris and flexor carpi ulnaris tenodesis of the unstable distal ulna. J Hand Surg Am 2012;14:612–617.
3. Camitz H. Surgical treatment of paralysis of opponens muscle of thumbs. Acta Chir Scand 1929;65:77–81.
4. Chetta MD, Ono S, Chung KC. Partial extensor carpi radialis longus turn-over tendon transfer for reconstruction of the extensor pollicis longus tendon in the rheumatoid hand: case report. J Hand Surg Am 2012;37:1217–1220.
5. Chung US, Kim JH, Seo WS, et al. Tendon transfer or tendon graft for ruptured finger extensor tendons in rheumatoid hands. J Hand Surg Eur Vol 2010;35:279–282.
6. Davis TR. Median and ulnar nerve palsy. In: Wolfe SW, Hotchkiss RN, Pederson WC, et al, eds. Green's Operative Hand Surgery, vol 2, ed 6. Philadelphia: Elsevier, 2011:1093–1137.
7. Hamlin C, Littler JW. Restoration of the extensor pollicis longus tendon by an intercalated graft. J Bone Joint Surg Am 1977;59(3):412–414.
8. Littler JW, Cooley SG. Opposition of the thumb and its restoration by abductor digiti quinti transfer. J Bone Joint Surg Am 1963;45:1389–1396.
9. Mannerfelt L, Norman O. Attrition ruptures of flexor tendons in rheumatoid arthritis caused by bony spurs in the carpal tunnel: a clinical and radiological study. J Bone Joint Surg Br 1969;51(2):270–277.
10. Nalebuff EA. Diagnosis, classification and management of rheumatoid thumb deformities. Bull Hosp Joint Dis 1968;29:119–137.
11. Nalebuff EA, Millender LH. Surgical treatment of the boutonniere deformity in rheumatoid arthritis. Orthop Clin North Am 1975;6:753–763.
12. Pulvertaft RG. Tendon grafts for flexor tendon injuries in the fingers and thumb: a study of technique and results. J Bone Joint Surg 1956;38B:175–194.
13. Vaughan-Jackson OJ. Rupture of extensor tendons by attrition at the inferior radio-ulnar joint: report of two cases. J Bone Joint Surg Br 1948;30B(3):528–530.
14. Williamson SC, Feldon P. Extensor tendon ruptures in rheumatoid arthritis. Hand Clin 1995;11:449–459.

A1 Pulley Release for Trigger Finger with and without Flexor Digitorum Superficialis Ulnar Slip Excision

David H. MacDonald and Alexander M. Marcus

DEFINITION

- Trigger finger is an entrapment of the digital flexor tendon(s) by the flexor tendon sheath.
- Trigger finger progressively causes inflammation, pain, catching, locking, and reduced range of motion (ROM).

ANATOMY

- The flexor digitorum profundus and superficialis (flexor pollicis longus in the thumb) pass under (dorsal to) the flexor sheath, which consists of annular and cruciate pulleys.
- The A1 pulley, which is volar to the metacarpophalangeal (MCP) joint, is the most proximal pulley (except for a thickening known as the *palmar aponeurotic pulley*[7]) and is almost always the primary site of entrapment (**FIG 1**).

PATHOGENESIS

- High angular loads at the A1 pulley and often other causes of local inflammation result in a flexor tendon sheath whose inner diameter is too narrow to accommodate the flexor tendon(s).
- This size mismatch causes hypertrophy (thickening) of the A1 pulley and tendinous swelling.
- These changes exacerbate the size discrepancy, setting up a cycle in which entrapment causes hypertrophy and hypertrophy causes entrapment.

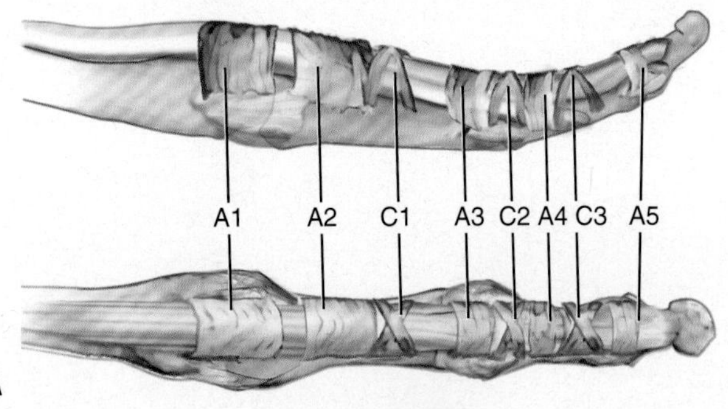

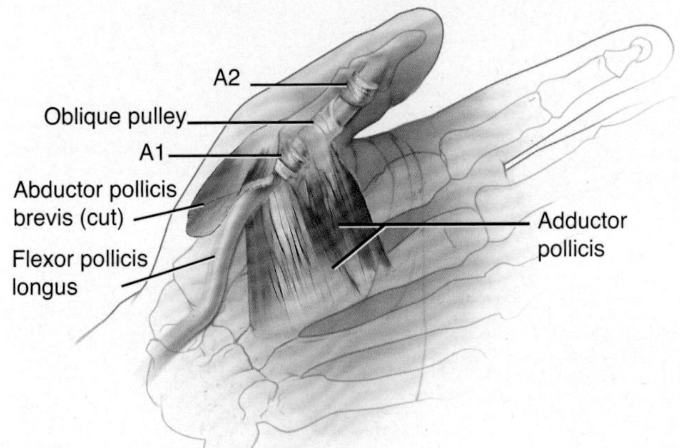

FIG 1 • To understand trigger finger and its release, an appreciation of the flexor tendon pulley system of the finger (**A**) and thumb (**B**) is required.

NATURAL HISTORY

- Trigger digits may develop spontaneously or may occur after swelling, from either trauma or a period of heavy use.
- Trigger digits may:
  - Resolve spontaneously (especially in mild cases)
  - Persist with the same level of symptoms
  - Advance to passively correctable locking
  - Become indefinitely locked in either flexion or extension

PATIENT HISTORY AND PHYSICAL FINDINGS

- The history may include any of the following:
  - Pain in the distal palm, often radiating proximally along the path of the flexor tendon(s)
  - Pain occurring with use and difficulty grasping objects or flexing the digit
  - Clicking or locking with digital flexion and extension, which is often perceived by the patient to be at the proximal interphalangeal (PIP) joint
  - The finger being stuck in flexion, often in the morning, requiring the other hand to straighten it
  - Being unable to flex or extend the digit fully or at all (**FIG 2**)
- The history should elicit the following information:
  - Whether the patient has had a trigger finger before, in either the currently involved or any other digit

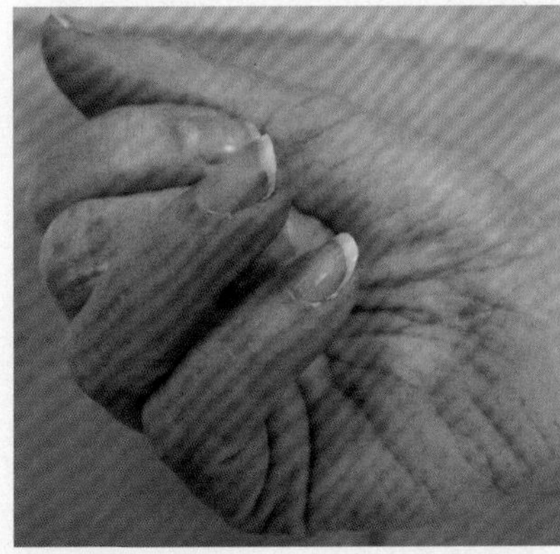

FIG 2 • Reduced flexion caused by ring finger triggering.

    - Previous treatments for trigger finger and the extent and duration of the result
    - Whether the condition began after a particular incident or period of increased hand use
- The patient's medical history should be evaluated for conditions that may cause trigger fingers and alter treatment as well as commonly associated conditions, including the following:
    - Diabetes
    - Rheumatoid arthritis and other inflammatory arthropathies
    - Amyloidosis, most commonly secondary to renal disease requiring dialysis
    - Lysosomal storage diseases
    - Carpal tunnel syndrome (often seen in patients with trigger finger but not causally related)
- The history and physical examination should exclude other conditions that cause overlapping symptoms, including the following:
    - Nerve compression
    - Muscle weakness
    - Tendon interruption from laceration (partial or complete) or rupture
    - Pulley rupture and bowstringing
    - Joint or soft tissue contracture or swelling or both
    - Extensor tendon laceration or subluxation, especially at the MCP joint
    - Joint dislocation
    - MCP joint collateral ligament injury
- The physical examination should include the following:
    - ROM test, which is the most objective measure of severity. If the patient has absolutely no active motion at the PIP (or thumb interphalangeal [IP]), consider tendon interruption.
    - Palpation of the palm. If the A1 pulley is not tender, strongly consider other diagnoses. Examine for other causes of the patient's symptoms, including Dupuytren contracture, tendon sheath ganglion, PIP joint injury, and A3 pulley triggering.
    - Examination of the extensor apparatus. Rule out extensor mechanism abnormalities and stress test the collateral ligaments of the MCP joint (radially and ulnarly) to rule out conditions that may cause overlapping signs or symptoms, including a popping sensation with ROM.
    - Examination of the collateral ligaments at the MCP joint. Stress the collateral ligaments radially and ulnarly.
    - Perform a neurovascular examination. Carpal tunnel syndrome often is associated with trigger finger. Muscle weakness may cause similar findings. Any neurovascular deficit should be documented before treatment.

IMAGING AND OTHER DIAGNOSTIC STUDIES

- Radiographs can exclude some unusual causes of trigger finger symptoms and can assess for arthritis but are not required to make the diagnosis of trigger finger.
- Ultrasound/dynamic ultrasound has been increasingly useful in confirmation of diagnosis and in guiding corticosteroid therapy for trigger finger.[9]
- If other pathology is suspected, magnetic resonance imaging (MRI) can be useful.
- Nerve conduction studies can evaluate for anterior interosseous nerve (AIN) compression, which may mimic a trigger thumb or concomitant carpal tunnel syndrome.

DIFFERENTIAL DIAGNOSIS

- Extensor tendon subluxation at the MCP joint
- Joint contracture or injury, including MCP locking due to collateral ligaments and a swollen PIP joint
- Soft tissue swelling or contracture, including Dupuytren contracture
- Partial tendon laceration
- Triggering at the A3 pulley (rare)
- Muscle weakness, including flexor pollicis longus weakness secondary to AIN palsy
- Masses (especially tendon sheath ganglions), which may cause A1 pulley tenderness

NONOPERATIVE MANAGEMENT

- Observation and splinting
- Mild, early cases often resolve spontaneously or do not bother the patient significantly.
- Use of a night extension splint may help minimize morning locking.
- Unless the PIP joint remains locked, in either flexion or extension, for several weeks, delayed treatment usually does not significantly change either the options available or their results.
- Injection
    - Long-term relief in most affected digits with one to three injections[2]
    - Results in diabetic patients are not as good,[1,4] but it still is worth trying. The patient should be warned that there glucose level may temporarily go up.
- Injection technique (**FIG 3**)
- One milliliter of 2% plain (no epinephrine) lidocaine and 1 mL of a soluble corticosteroid solution (eg, betamethasone or dexamethasone) in a single syringe with a 25-gauge needle is given.
- The A1 pulley area is prepped with an antiseptic solution such as alcohol or Betadine.
- A topical spray may be used to reduce discomfort.
- One to 2 mL is injected in the sheath or subcutaneously around the A1 pulley.[13] Avoid injecting into the tendon itself; if increased resistance is encountered, this may be the cause.
- Ultrasound guidance may provide increased accuracy and avoid possible complications especially in the thumb.[9]

SURGICAL MANAGEMENT

- Indications for surgical treatment include the following:
    - Symptoms that persist despite conservative management
    - Inability to flex or extend the finger even passively: This is an indication for earlier release to prevent secondary joint contracture.
- Open A1 pulley release is indicated for any routine trigger finger.
- Percutaneous trigger finger release:
    - Requires an actively triggering digit so the patient can flex to confirm needle placement and pulley release
    - Is used primarily for the middle and ring fingers. Use in the other digits may place digital nerves in jeopardy.[15]
- In patients with very extensive synovitis, such as that seen in rheumatoid arthritis, lysosomal storage diseases, or amyloidosis associated with end-stage renal disease, releasing the A1 pulley percutaneously or through a routine, small

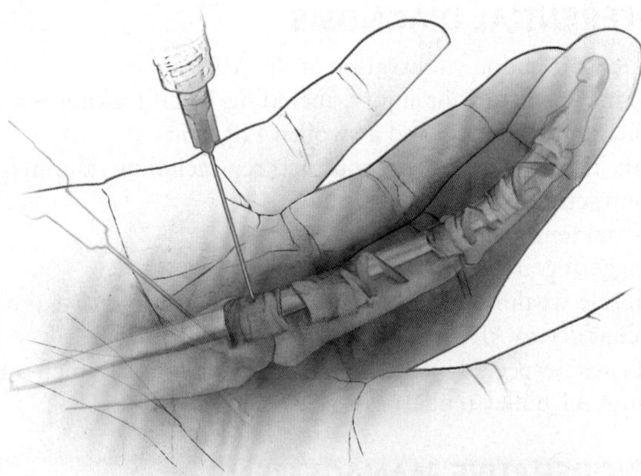

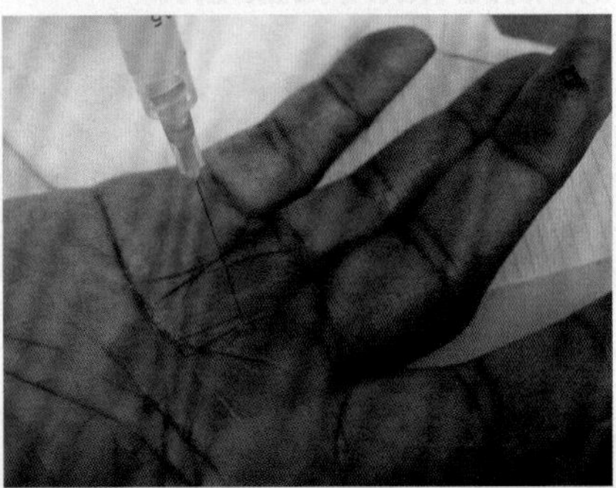

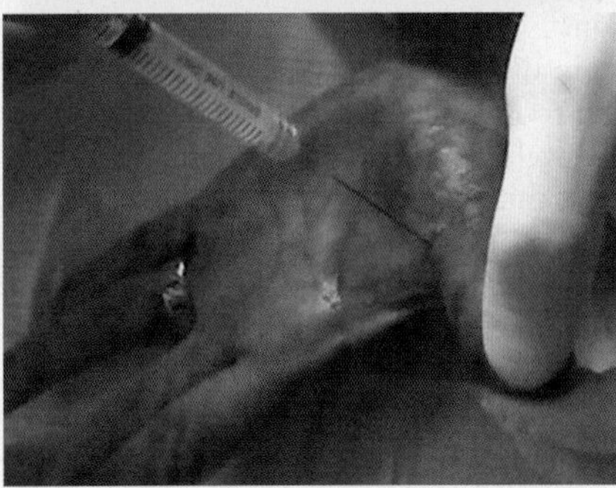

FIG 3 • Technique for trigger digit injection.

incision is often not sufficient. A more extensive tenosynovectomy and sometimes ulnar slip of the flexor digitorum superficialis resection (USSR) is often required.

Preoperative Planning

- Clinical notes and any studies obtained preoperatively should be reviewed.
- If procedures beyond an A1 pulley release are considered likely to be necessary (eg, possible resection of the ulnar slip of the flexor digitorum superficialis [FDS]), they should be discussed with the patient preoperatively.

Positioning

- The patient is supine.
- The extremity is positioned so that the palm is facing up on a hand table.
- For index, middle, ring, and small digits, a hand holder (eg, a "lead hand") may be helpful.
- For the thumb, it is more useful for the surgeon and assistant to position the hand and thumb throughout the procedure or to use a specialized thumb holder.
- Place a padded tourniquet and inflate it just before making the incision.

Approach

- Anesthesia is obtained by injecting 2% plain (no epinephrine) lidocaine subcutaneously around the incision and in the tendon sheath.
  - Sedation will mitigate the discomfort associated with the injection and the tourniquet. If sedation is used, the patient should be allowed to wake up in time to demonstrate complete active digital flexion and extension without locking, documenting successful pulley release.
- A standard volar approach to the A1 pulley is made with either an oblique Bruner-type, transverse, or longitudinal incision.
- For resection of the ulnar slip of the sublimis, a Bruner-type or midaxial longitudinal incision is used over the distal portion of the proximal phalanx.

TECHNIQUES

Open A1 Pulley Release

Incision and Exposure

- A 1-cm incision is placed over the A1 pulley.
  - Longitudinal (**TECH FIG 1A**)
  - If a transverse incision is used, it is placed in a palmar skin crease (**TECH FIG 1B**):
    - Distal palmar crease for small and ring fingers
    - Proximal palmar crease for index finger
    - An incision between creases may be required for middle finger release.
  - Oblique or Bruner-type
- Avoid crossing palmar skin creases at a right angle with any incision type.
- Incise only the skin and dermis with a no. 15 blade.
- Bluntly spread subcutaneous tissue to avoid injury to the digital nerves.

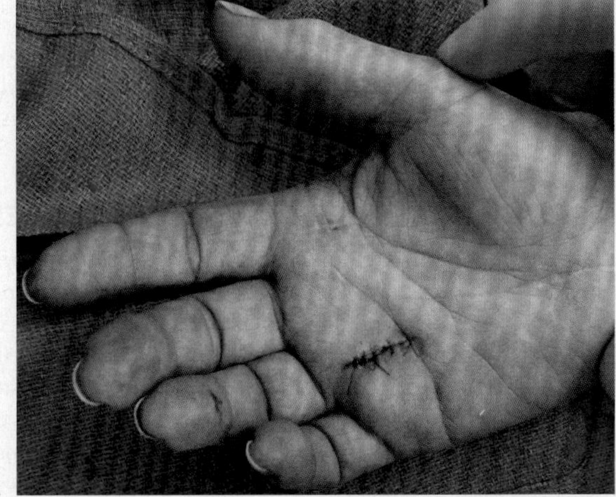

A

TECH FIG 1 • **A.** A longitudinal incision for ring finger A1 release. Index finger demonstrates a well-healed longitudinal incision without any contracture. *(continued)*

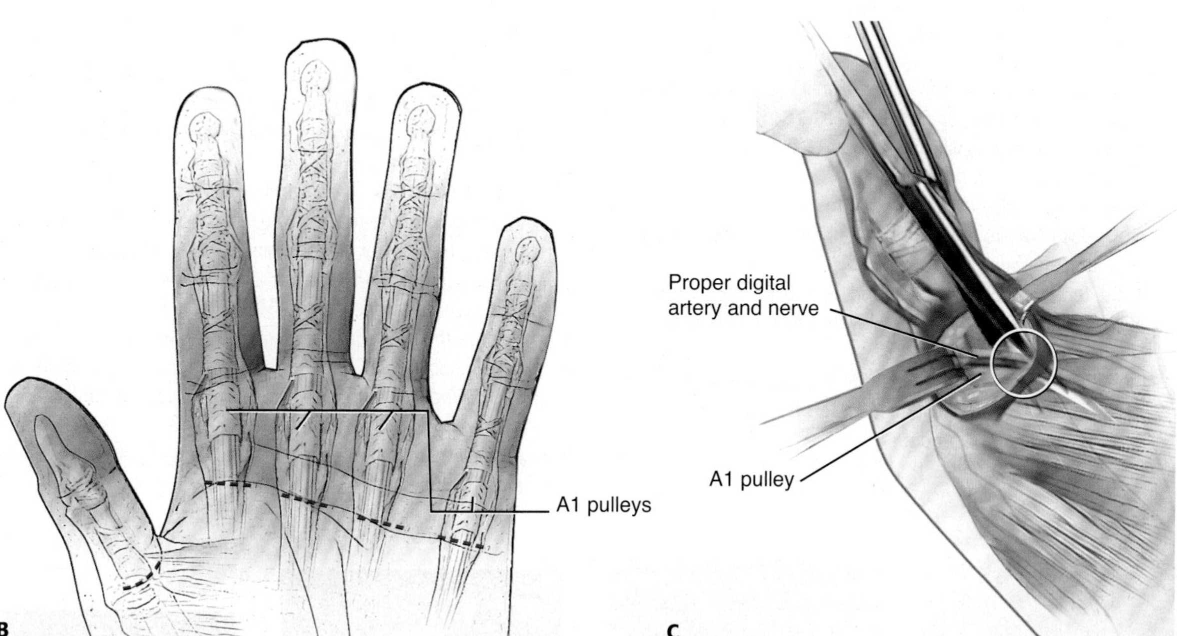

TECH FIG 1 • *(continued)* **B.** Position of transverse incisions for trigger finger release in relation to the palmar skin creases and the A1 pulley. **C.** The digital neurovascular structures are right next to the A1 pulley and must be protected. The *circle* demonstrates the proximity of the digital nerves and arteries. Because the radial digital nerve of the thumb may cross at the level of the A1 pulley, it is particularly vulnerable.

- The digital neurovascular structures adjacent to the A1 pulley must be retracted and protected.
  - Extensive dissection and exposure of these structures are not required.
  - The radial digital nerve of the thumb is at the greatest risk because it typically crosses the surgical field[16] (**TECH FIG 1C**).

Performing the Release

- Clear off the A1 pulley with sponge dissection.
- The A1 pulley is not incised until it is clearly visualized (**TECH FIG 2A**).
  - Use of small right angle retractors helps provide needed visualization.

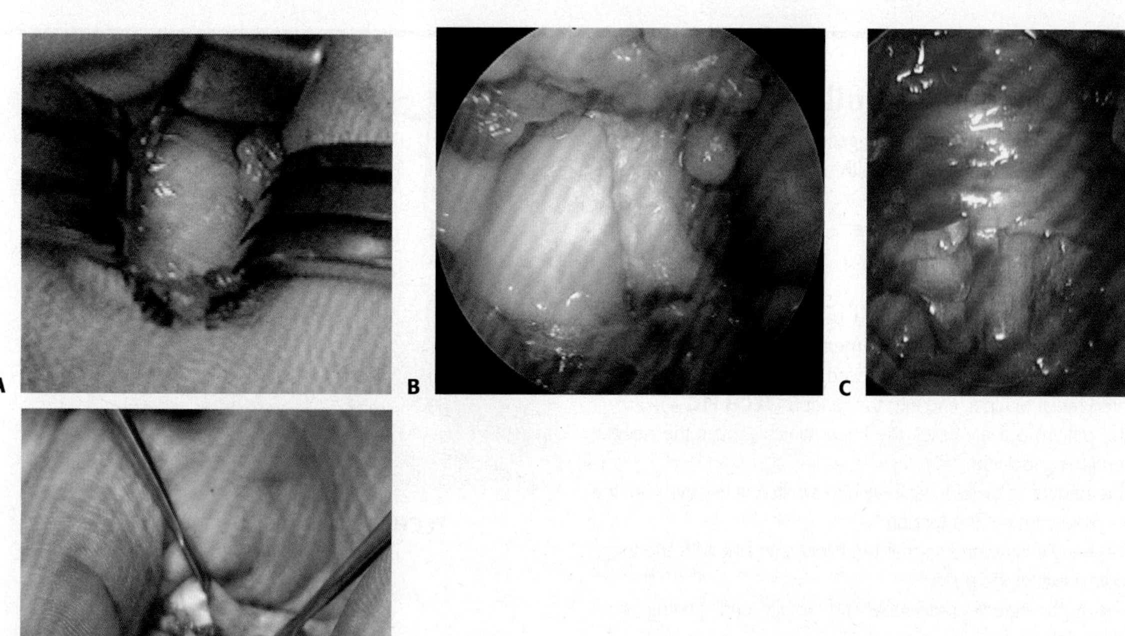

TECH FIG 2 • **A.** The digital neurovascular structures are retracted, and the A1 pulley has been cleared of all overlying soft tissue. **B.** The A1 pulley has been completely released. **C.** The palmar pulley remaining after A1 release. **D.** The flexor tendons are bluntly separated and pulled out of the wound, which then flexes the digit. (**A–D:** Top is proximal.)

- Begin the A1 pulley incision with a knife, taking care not to cut deep into the tendon.
- Complete the release with scissors until the pulley leaflets can be spread completely apart (**TECH FIG 2B**).
- Avoid cutting any significant portion of the A2 pulley (or the oblique pulley in the thumb).
  - The A2 pulley is separated from the A1 pulley either by a space (where there is no sheath) or a section of very thin sheath tissue.[11]
- If the tendons appear constricted by the palmar aponeurotic pulley[7] proximal to the A1 pulley, it should also be released (**TECH FIG 2C**).
- Bluntly separate the tendons (in the fingers) and pull the tendon(s) out of the wound (**TECH FIG 2D**). Minimize any direct handling of the tendons.

Completion

- A limited tenosynovectomy may be performed if required (**TECH FIG 3A**). Any unusual resected tissue or mass is sent to the pathology department for analysis (**TECH FIG 3B**).
- Confirm that the patient can actively flex and extend the finger (**TECH FIG 3C,D**). If the active ROM is not full or significantly improved or if the tendons are not passing under the remaining pulleys, recheck for any portions of the A1 pulley or palmar aponeurotic pulley and consider USSR as well as etiologies other than standard trigger finger.[6,8,10,12]
- Release the tourniquet, and irrigate the wound.
- Obtain hemostasis, usually with manual compression. Reinspect the wound, check for any arterial bleeding, and confirm the finger has brisk capillary refill.
- Close the skin with interrupted sutures and place a mildly compressive dressing.

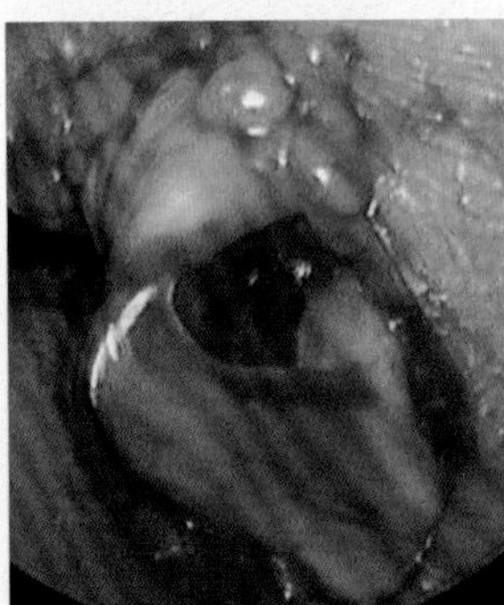

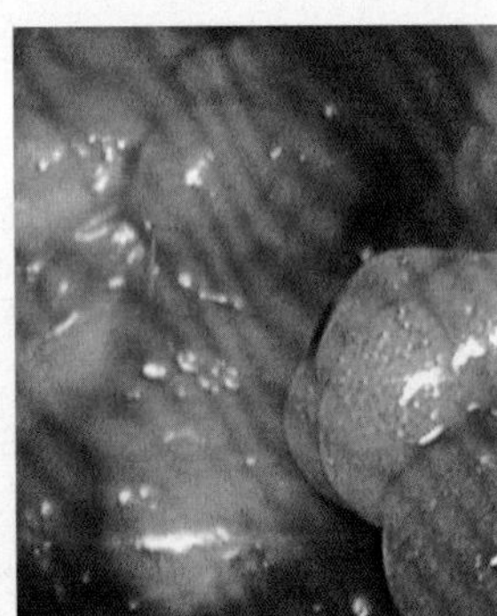

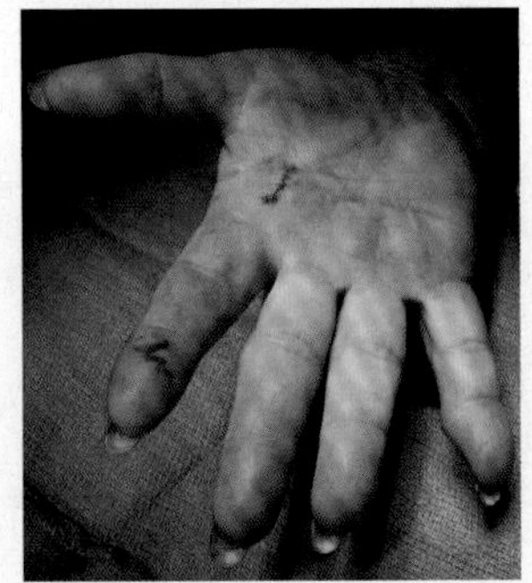

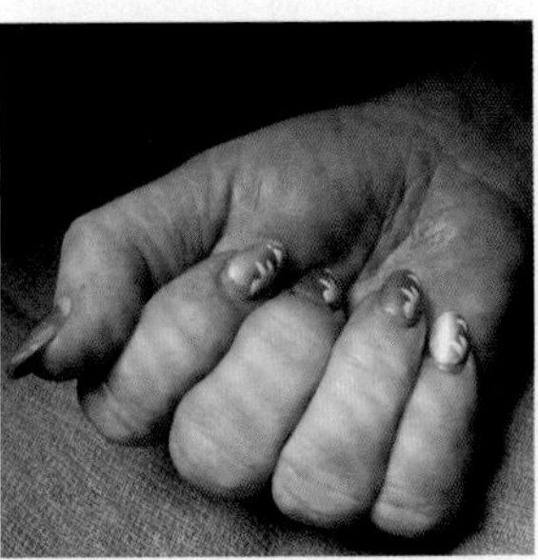

TECH FIG 3 • **A.** Tenosynovium between the tendons can be gently removed. **B.** A tendon sheath mass. Pathologic analysis confirmed it was a tendon sheath ganglion. **C,D.** Full active extension and flexion after release.

Percutaneous A1 Pulley Release

- The patient must have active triggering.
- The procedure is performed with a sterile prep in either the office or operating room.
- Hyperextend the MCP joints over a towel to help displace the neurovascular structures dorsally.
- Palpate the A1 pulley.
- Inject the local anesthetic (with or without corticosteroid) as described for nonoperative treatment.
- An 18- or 19-gauge needle is placed through the A1 pulley, centered radial to ulnar, and into the tendon (**TECH FIG 4**).
- The patient actively flexes the finger which moves the needle, confirming location.
- The needle is pulled back slightly so that it remains in the A1 pulley but not the tendon.
- The needle is rotated so that the bevel is in line with the longitudinal axis of the pulley.
- Sweep the needle proximally and distally until grating is no longer felt.
- The patient should be able to actively flex and extend the finger without triggering, confirming release.

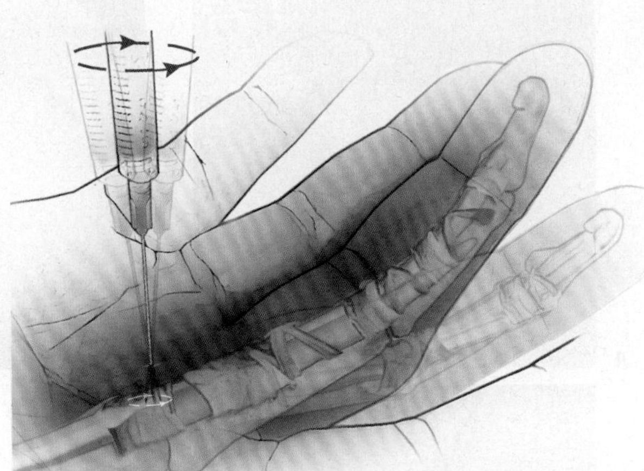

TECH FIG 4 • Percutaneous A1 release.

Open A1 Pulley Release with Flexor Digitorum Superficialis Ulnar Slip Excision

- The initial steps are performed in the same manner as described for an open A1 pulley release.
- A Bruner-type or ulnar midaxial incision can be used.
- Bruner-type incision (**TECH FIG 5**)
  - A zigzag skin incision is made with the points over the finger flexion creases.
  - The skin *only* is opened with a no. 15 blade, and blunt dissection is used to separate the neurovascular bundles as a unit. Formal dissection of the nerve and artery, or separating them from each other, is not required.
  - Care should be taken to stay more centrally as the incision proceeds distally (over the PIP and distal interphalangeal joints) because the neurovascular bundles can become less radial and ulnar on the digit.
- Ulnar midaxial incision (less invasive alternative)
  - A 1- to 1.5-cm incision is made beginning at the PIP flexion crease and proceeding proximally.
  - The dissection plane proceeds dorsal to the digital neurovascular bundle, isolating the ulnar aspect of the flexor sheath.
- Inspect the tendon distal to the A2 pulley, confirming that there is no catching under the A3 pulley[10] and that an enlarged, bulbous flexor digitorum profundus is not catching under the distal end of the A2 pulley.[12] In either of these cases, USSR may or may not relieve the problem.
- Ulnar slip excision is then performed in either distal to proximal fashion[8] or with a proximal to distal technique.[6]
- In extremely severe cases of recalcitrant trigger finger, both FDS slips can be removed.[5] Although there is historical evidence to suggest the increased possibility of developing a swan-neck deformity, there is no consensus. It should probably be avoided in the rheumatoid population.

Distal to Proximal Ulnar Slip Excision

- Just distal to the A2 pulley, incise the tendon sheath, creating a radially based flap. This flap may be repaired later with 6-0 Prolene if desired.
- With the PIP joint maximally flexed, isolate and cut the ulnar slip of the FDS distally, taking care to preserve the vinculum brevis.
- Pull the tendon into the proximal wound and cut it as far proximal as can be reached safely.
- Confirm that the tendons now pass smoothly under the pulley system through a complete ROM.
- Release the tourniquet. Irrigate the wounds.
- Obtain hemostasis, usually with manual compression. Reinspect the wound, check for any arterial bleeding, and confirm the finger has brisk capillary refill.
- Close the skin with interrupted sutures and place a mildly compressive dressing.

Proximal to Distal Ulnar Slip Excision

- Examine the part of the tendon meant to glide under the A1 and A2 pulleys for enlargement, degeneration, longitudinal splitting, or loss of its smooth surface (**TECH FIG 6A**).
- Fully flex the finger, identify the ulnar and radial slips of the FDS distally, and split them longitudinally in a proximal direction (**TECH FIG 6B**).
- With the finger and wrist flexed, cut the ulnar slip of the FDS as far proximal as possible. Pull the ulnar slip distally, carefully separating it through the chiasm, and, with the PIP joint flexed, cut it distally at the edge of the A3 pulley. The tendon slip is then removed from either direction; a loop of 3-0 wire can be used to separate adhesions if necessary (**TECH FIG 6C**).
- Release the tourniquet. Irrigate the wound.
- Obtain hemostasis, usually with manual compression. Reinspect the wound, check for any arterial bleeding, and confirm the finger has brisk capillary refill.
- Close the skin with interrupted sutures and place a mildly compressive dressing.

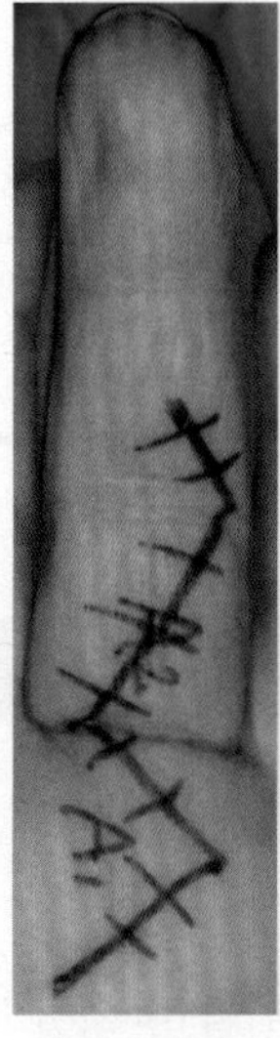

TECH FIG 5 • A Bruner-type incision. (Courtesy of Dominique Le Viet.)

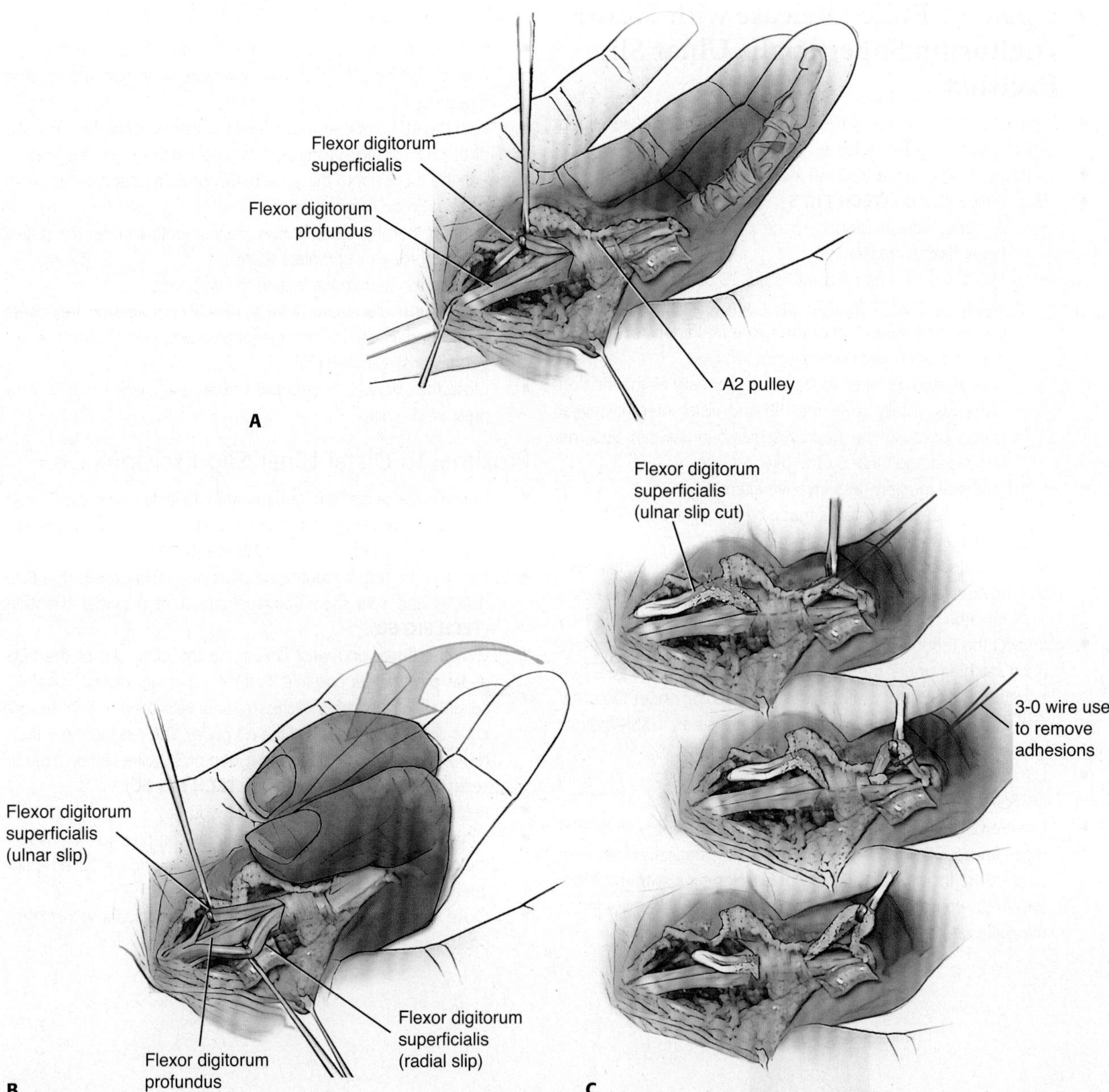

TECH FIG 6 • Open A1 pulley release with FDS ulnar slip excision. **A.** Enlargement of tendon proximal to A2 pulley (after A1 release). **B.** Separating the FDS tendon slips. **C.** Use of a wire loop to separate tendon adhesions after cutting the FDS tendon proximally. (**A,B:** Modified from Le Viet D, Tsionos I, Boulouednine M, et al. Trigger finger treatment by ulnar superficialis slip resection [U.S.S.R.]. J Hand Surg Br 2004:29[4]:368–373.)

PEARLS AND PITFALLS

Satisfactory release	▪ Confirm that the tendon glides freely after release. ▪ If there was no joint contracture preoperatively, the patient should have significantly improved active (or passive, if the patient is under general anesthesia) ROM. ▪ If not, assess the cause and correct.
Avoid injury to A2 pulley.	▪ Release of more than 25% of the A2 pulley may cause bowstringing, reducing flexion ROM, and require pulley reconstruction.

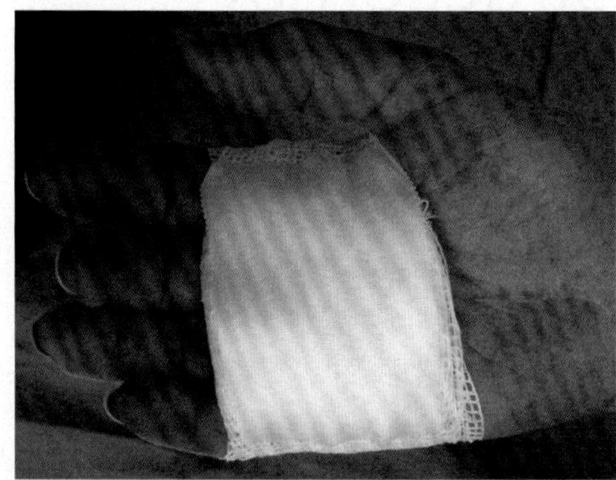

FIG 4 • A soft dressing is applied with all the digits free.

POSTOPERATIVE CARE

- A soft dressing is applied with all of the digits free (**FIG 4**). Active ROM as tolerated is encouraged. Minimize dressing bulk to avoid inhibiting motion.
- Formal therapy is required only if the patient has difficulty regaining ROM.
- Patients whose digits were locked preoperatively are more likely to need therapy. This may be started within the first week.
- Scar massage is encouraged after the wound is sealed.

OUTCOMES

- Surgical release of trigger digits has a high success rate with a low complication and recurrence rate.[3,14]

COMPLICATIONS

- Injury to digital nerve or artery
- Bowstringing
- Wound infection or dehiscence resulting in a flexor sheath infection
- Postoperative stiffness
- Incomplete release
- Recurrence
- Incisional tenderness

REFERENCES

1. Baumgarten KM, Gerlach D, Boyer MI. Corticosteroid injection in diabetic patients with trigger finger. A prospective, randomized, controlled double-blinded study. J Bone Joint Surg Am 2007;89(12):2604–2611.
2. Benson LS, Ptaszek AJ. Injection versus surgery in the treatment of trigger finger. J Hand Surg Am 1997;22:138–144.
3. Gilberts EC, Wereldsma JC. Long-term results of percutaneous and open surgery for trigger fingers and thumbs. Int Surg 2002;87:48–52.
4. Griggs SM, Weiss AC, Lane LB, et al. Treatment of trigger finger in patients with diabetes mellitus. J Hand Surg Am 1995;20:787–789.
5. Husain SN, Clarke SE, Buterbaugh GA, et al. Recalcitrant trigger finger managed with flexor digitorum superficialis resection. Am J Orthop 2011;40(12):620–624.
6. Le Viet D, Tsionos I, Boulouednine M, et al. Trigger finger treatment by ulnar superficialis slip resection (U.S.S.R.). J Hand Surg Br 2004; 29:368–373.
7. Manske PR, Lesker PA. Palmar aponeurosis pulley. J Hand Surg Am 1983;8:259–263.
8. Marcus AM, Culver JE Jr, Hunt TR III. Treating trigger finger in diabetics using excision of the ulnar slip of the flexor digitorum superficialis with or without A1 pulley release. Hand 2007;2: 227–231.
9. Mardani Kivi M, Lahiji FA, Jandaghi AB, et al. Efficacy of sonographically guided intra-flexoral sheath corticosteroid injection in the treatment of trigger thumb. Acta Orthop Traumatol Turc 2012;46(5):346–352.
10. Rayan GM. Distal stenosing tenosynovitis. J Hand Surg Am 1990; 15:973–975.
11. Ryzewicz M, Wolf JM. Trigger digits: principles, management, and complications. J Hand Surg Am 2006;31:135–146.
12. Seradge H, Kleinert HE. Reduction flexor tenoplasty. J Hand Surg Am 1981;6:543–544.
13. Taras JS, Raphael JS, Pan WT, et al. Corticosteroid injections for trigger digits: is intrasheath injection necessary? J Hand Surg Am 1998;23:717–722.
14. Turowski GA, Zdankiewicz PD, Thomson JG. The results of surgical treatment of trigger finger. J Hand Surg Am 1997;22:145–149.
15. Wilhelmi BJ, Mowlavi A, Neumeister MW, et al. Safe treatment of trigger finger with longitudinal and transverse landmarks: an anatomic study of the border finger for percutaneous release. Plast Reconstr Surg 2003;112:993–999.
16. Wolfe SW. Tenosynovitis. In: Green DP, Hotchkiss RN, Pederson WC, et al, eds. Green's Operative Hand Surgery, ed 5. Philadelphia: Elsevier, 2005:2137–2158.

87 CHAPTER

Operative Reconstruction of Boutonnière and Swan-Neck Deformities

Jun Y. Matsui, Samantha L. Piper, and Martin I. Boyer

DEFINITION

- Rheumatoid arthritis is a poorly understood systemic disease affecting the synovium of joints and tendon sheaths. The synovial tissue in rheumatoid arthritis is characterized by a proliferation of synovial lining cells, angiogenesis, and relative lymphocytosis.[15]
  - A combination of cartilage degeneration, synovial expansion, periarticular erosion, and ligamentous laxity creates an imbalance within the extrinsic and intrinsic tendon systems of the digit, causing progressive deformity.
- A boutonnière ("buttonhole") deformity involves attenuation or disruption of the central slip and attenuation of the triangular ligament. It results in a characteristic deformity with flexion at the proximal interphalangeal (PIP) joint and hyperextension (as well as an inability to flex actively) at the distal interphalangeal (DIP) joint.
- A swan-neck deformity is characterized by hyperextension of the PIP joint and flexion of the DIP joint.
  - In the posttraumatic setting, it results from laxity of the PIP joint volar plate and an inability of the terminal tendon to extend the DIP joint (chronic mallet finger deformity).

Classification

- Rheumatoid thumb deformity[25,34]
  - Type I—boutonnière deformity: metacarpophalangeal (MCP) joint flexion and interphalangeal joint hyperextension. The carpometacarpal (CMC) joint is not primarily involved.
  - Type II—rare: a combination of types I and III involving MCP joint flexion and interphalangeal joint hyperextension and associated CMC joint subluxation or dislocation
  - Type III—swan-neck deformity: MCP joint hyperextension, interphalangeal joint flexion, and thumb metacarpal adduction, resulting from progressive CMC joint pathology
  - Type IV: gamekeeper's deformity. Attenuation of the ulnar collateral ligament of the thumb MCP joint results in radial deviation of the MCP joint and secondary metacarpal adduction deformity or contracture.
  - Type V: results from attenuation of the MCP volar plate with progressive MCP joint hyperextension and secondary interphalangeal joint flexion. There is no metacarpal adduction deformity.
- Boutonnière deformity
  - Stage I—mild: PIP joint synovitis and a mild, fully correctable extension lag
  - Stage II—moderate: flexion deformity of the PIP joint, either flexible or fixed
  - Stage III—severe: PIP joint articular destruction
- Swan-neck deformity
  - Type I: PIP joint is fully mobile.
  - Type II: Active and passive motions of the PIP joint are limited, with the MCP joint held in extension due to intrinsic tightness.
  - Type III: decreased PIP joint motion in all positions of MCP joint flexion and extension
  - Type IV: fixed PIP joint hyperextension with advanced destruction of the PIP joint articular surfaces

ANATOMY

Bone and Joint

- The MCP joint is a condyloid joint with average range of motion from 15 degrees hyperextension to 90 degrees flexion.
  - A cam effect for collateral ligaments is due to the shape of the metacarpal head; collateral ligaments are taut with MCP joint flexion and lax with MCP joint extension.
- The PIP joint (**FIG 1A**) is a hinge joint with greater inherent osseous stability than the MCP joint due to the configuration of the two condyles of the head of the proximal phalanx, which articulates with the median ridge at the base of the middle phalanx.
  - The collateral ligaments are taut throughout the joint arc of motion.
  - The volar plate resists PIP joint hyperextension; it originates on the proximal phalanx and inserts into the base of the middle phalanx.
- The DIP joint is stabilized by the collateral ligaments, the terminal extensor tendon insertion, the flexor digitorum profundus (FDP) insertion, and the volar plate.

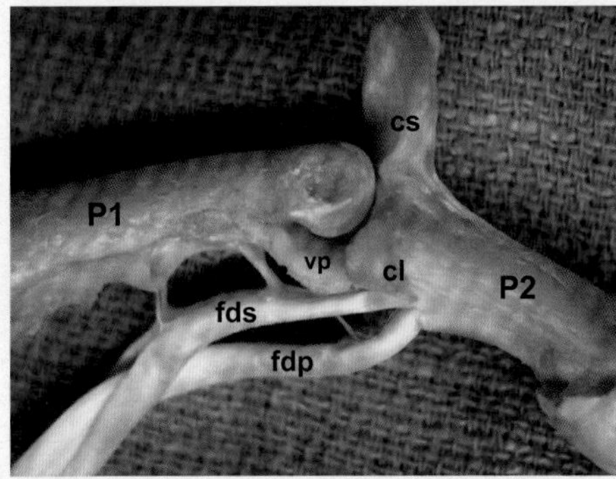

FIG 1 • **A.** PIP joint relationships. The flexor tendons (flexor digitorum superficialis [*FDS*] and flexor digitorum profundus [*FDP*]) have been removed from the proximal digital flexor sheath at the A2 pulley. The FDP and FDS tendon orientation is demonstrated before they reenter the flexor sheath at the A4 pulley. The PIP joint collateral ligament (*cl*) and the insertion of the central slip (*cs*) at the dorsal base of the middle phalanx have been reflected distally to highlight the volar plate (*vp*) and its proximity within the flexor sheath. *P1*, proximal phalanx; *P2*, middle phalanx. *(continued)*

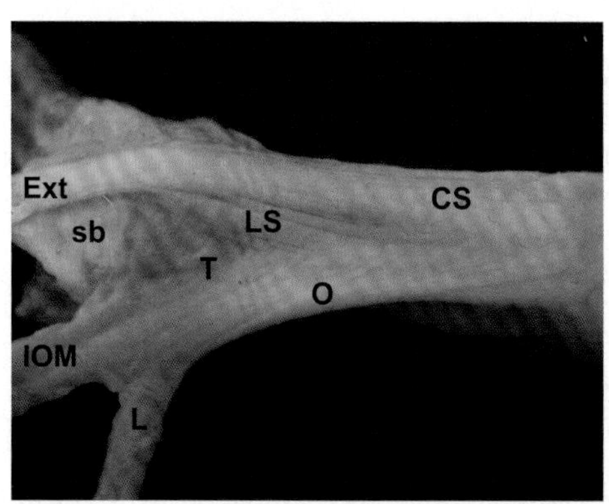

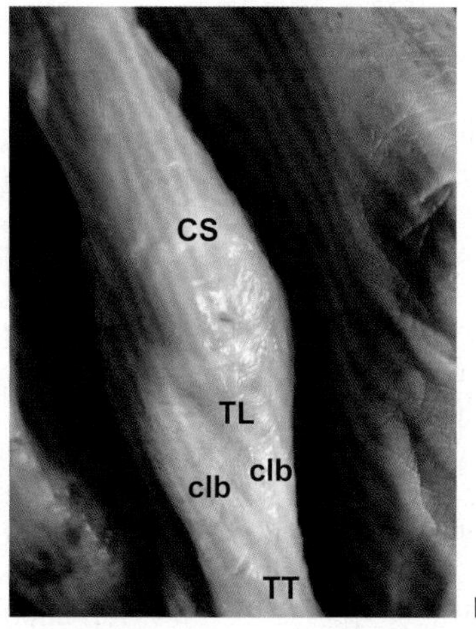

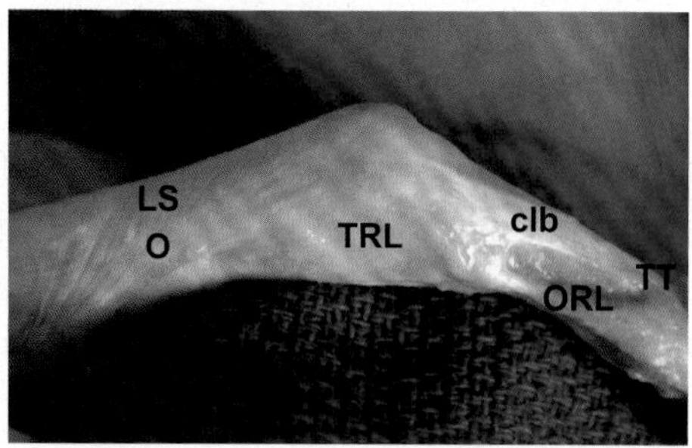

FIG 1 • *(continued)* **B.** The dorsal digital extensor apparatus is derived from contributions of the extrinsic extensor tendons and the intrinsic musculature of the hand. The extrinsic extensor tendon (*Ext*) is identified at the level of the distal hand and splits into two lateral slips (*LS*) and the central tendon slip (*CS*). At the dorsal MCP joint, the extensor tendon is stabilized by the vertically orientated fibers of the sagittal band (*sb*), which originate from the radial and ulnar sides of the volar plate of the MCP joint and the volar base of the proximal phalanx. The MCP joint is extended via a sling-like mechanism of the sagittal band, as there is no direct fiber insertion from the extrinsic extensor tendon at the proximal phalanx. The deep head of the interosseous muscle (*IOM*) courses superficial to the sagittal band (*sb*) at the level of the MCP joint and runs parallel and distal to the sagittal band over the proximal phalanx to form the transverse fibers (*T*) of the extensor apparatus. The lumbrical muscle (*L*) on the radial aspect of the digit forms the oblique fibers (*O*) of the extensor apparatus, which join with the lateral slip of the extrinsic extensor tendon to form the conjoined lateral band. **C.** The extrinsic extensor tendon divides into a central slip (*CS*) and two lateral slips. The central slip inserts at the dorsal base of the middle phalanx to extend the PIP joint, and the two lateral slips receive contributory fibers from the lumbricals via oblique fibers of the extensor hood to form the conjoined lateral bands (*clb*). These conjoined lateral bands coalesce to form the terminal tendon (*TT*), which inserts at the dorsal base of the distal phalanx to extend the DIP joint. The triangular ligament (*TL*) stabilizes the conjoined lateral bands from volar subluxation. **D.** Lateral view of the digit demonstrating the coalescing fibers of the lateral slip (*LS*) and oblique fibers (*O*) of the extensor apparatus, which combine to form the conjoined lateral band (*clb*). The two conjoined lateral bands combine to form the terminal tendon (*TT*), which inserts into the dorsal base of the distal phalanx. The transverse retinacular ligament (*TRL*) prevents dorsal subluxation of the lateral bands. The oblique retinacular ligament (*ORL*) passively links the PIP and DIP joints as it travels from volar to dorsal from the fibro-osseous gutter (middle third of the proximal phalanx and A2 pulley) to the proximal aspect of the distal phalanx through the extensor tendon. (Photographs © Copyright of Fraser J. Leversedge, Charles A. Goldfarb, and Martin Boyer.)

Dorsal Restraining Structures of the Digit

- The sagittal bands originate on both sides of the MCP joint, from the volar plate and the base of the proximal phalanx, and insert into the lateral margins of the extensor tendon over the dorsal MCP joint (**FIG 1 B–D**).
  - They stabilize the extrinsic extensor tendon over the MCP joint to prevent lateral subluxation.
  - They contribute indirectly to MCP joint extension and prevent extensor bowstringing.
- The triangular ligament stabilizes the two conjoined lateral bands over the dorsal aspect of the middle phalanx and prevents volar subluxation of the conjoined lateral bands.
- The transverse retinacular ligament is composed of fibers oriented in a volar–dorsal direction at the level of the PIP joint. It prevents dorsal subluxation of the conjoined lateral bands.
- The oblique retinacular ligament is a static restraining ligament, linking the PIP and DIP joints. It runs from the fibro-osseous gutter at the A2 flexor pulley and the middle third of the proximal phalanx to insert into the terminal extensor tendon and couples PIP joint and DIP joint extension.

Flexor Tendon: Digit

- At the level of the A1 pulley, the flexor digitorum superficialis (FDS) tendon flattens and bifurcates to allow the more dorsal FDP tendon to pass distally within the flexor sheath to insert at the volar base of the distal phalanx.
- The FDS tendon slips rotate laterally and dorsally around the FDP and then divide again into medial and lateral slips. The medial slips rejoin dorsal to the FDP tendon and insert into the distal aspect of the proximal phalanx. The lateral slips continue distally to insert into the base of the middle phalanx.

Extensor Tendon: Digit

- At the base of the proximal phalanx, the extrinsic extensor tendon trifurcates with the central portion inserting into the dorsal base of the middle phalanx as the central slip.
- The lateral slips are joined by the oblique fibers of the lumbrical tendons to form the conjoined lateral band. The conjoined lateral bands converge over the middle phalanx to form the terminal tendon, which inserts at the dorsal base of the distal phalanx, where it functions to extend the DIP joint.
- The interosseous muscles contribute to the dorsal extensor apparatus through their deep muscle belly, which travels superficial to the sagittal band as the lateral tendon, becoming the transverse fibers of the extensor hood (MCP joint flexion).

PATHOGENESIS

Posttraumatic Boutonnière Deformity

- Disruption of the central slip and triangular ligament is the inciting pathology in the development of the boutonnière deformity.
- Injury patterns can be grouped into two broad categories, closed and open.
  - Closed injuries: Forceful hyperflexion of the PIP joint may result in a detachment of the central slip from its insertion. An associated avulsion fracture involving the insertion of the central slip may be identified from the dorsal base of the middle phalanx.
    - Volar dislocations of the PIP joint or digital crush injuries may disrupt the central slip.
  - Open injuries: Dorsal laceration or deep abrasions over the PIP joint may disrupt the integrity of the central slip.
- Disruption of the central slip and attenuation of the triangular ligament allows for the migration of the lateral bands volar to the PIP joint axis of rotation. This results in flexion at the PIP joint and extension at the DIP joint through the action of the displaced lateral bands.
  - The displaced lateral band becomes a flexor of the PIP joint and an extensor of the DIP joint.

Posttraumatic Swan-Neck Deformity

- Unrecognized volar plate injury at the PIP joint may result in volar plate insufficiency. Although this injury usually leads to scarring volar to the PIP joint and the subsequent development of a PIP fixed flexion deformity without coexistent DIP hyperextension deformity (a so-called "pseudoboutonnière deformity"), this leaves the action of the central slip unchecked by the volar plate, resulting in a progressive PIP joint hyperextension deformity.
  - Recurrent dorsal dislocation of the PIP joint is an example of an injury pattern that may result in volar plate incompetence.
- Avulsion of the terminal tendon from its insertion at the base of the dorsal distal phalanx (a soft tissue mallet finger) results in an imbalance in the extensor mechanism. Extension forces are concentrated at the central slip and by the lateral bands dorsal to the axis of rotation of the PIP joint, producing a progressive hyperextension deformity of the PIP joint.
  - Patients predisposed to volar plate laxity (such as from generalized ligamentous laxity, inflammatory conditions, and collagen vascular disorders) are more susceptible to the development of deformity.
- An extension-type malunion of the middle phalanx or peritendinous adhesions secondary to previous digital fracture injury may contribute to the development of a swan-neck deformity, although an extensor lag at the PIP joint from dorsal adhesions may also lead to an inability to actively extend the finger at the PIP joint (not a boutonnière deformity because there is no DIP hyperextension deformity and not a pseudoboutonnière deformity because the PIP flexion deformity is passively correctible).
- Hyperextension of the PIP joint and attenuation of the transverse retinacular ligament permits dorsal migration of the lateral bands relative to the PIP joint axis of rotation. The displaced lateral bands act to extend the PIP joint and to flex the DIP joint.

Rheumatoid Boutonnière Deformity

Fingers

- Boutonnière (buttonhole) deformity results from pathologic synovitis of the PIP joint that causes progressive attenuation of the central slip, transverse retinacular ligaments, and triangular ligament. The PIP joint essentially buttonholes through the extensor mechanism.[31] Characteristic flexion of the PIP joint and hyperextension deformities of the MCP and DIP joint prevail due to the extensor imbalance[22] (**FIG 2A**).
- Subluxation of the lateral bands, volar to the axis of PIP joint rotation, occurs due to the loss of these restraints. The lateral bands become flexors of the PIP joint rather than extensors.
  - It is important to differentiate this pathologic involvement of the extensor mechanism from a flexion contracture of the PIP joint.
- Due to persisting PIP joint flexion, the volar plate, collateral ligaments, and oblique retinacular ligaments become increasingly contracted, resulting in a stiff and subsequently fixed boutonnière deformity.

Thumb

- Type I boutonnière deformity is the most common rheumatoid deformity of the thumb.[30,38] It is characterized by MCP joint flexion and interphalangeal joint hyperextension (**FIG 2B**).
- The pathologic changes affecting the thumb typically involve synovitis of the MCP joint with resulting attenuation of the extensor mechanism (dorsal joint capsule, extensor pollicis brevis tendon insertion, extensor hood). This relative

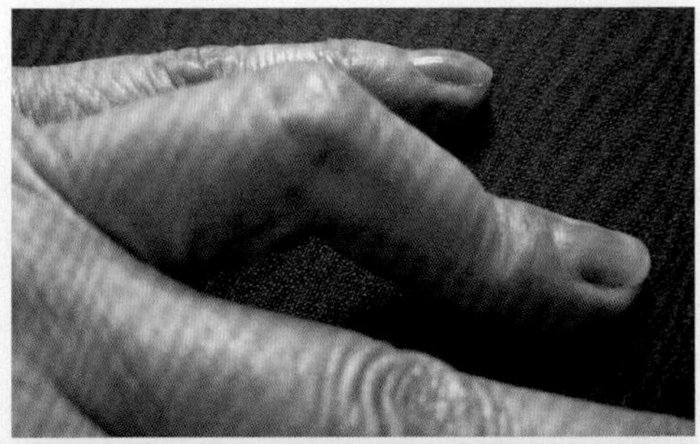

A

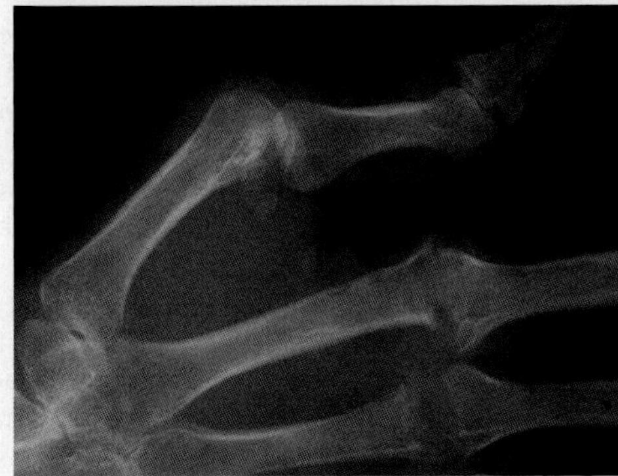

B

FIG 2 • **A.** Boutonnière deformity of the finger. Note the flexion posture of the PIP joint and hyperextension of the DIP joint. **B.** Lateral radiograph of the thumb demonstrating a boutonnière deformity. (Photographs © Copyright of Fraser J. Leversedge, Charles A. Goldfarb, and Martin Boyer.)

extensor imbalance results in MCP joint flexion and possible joint subluxation.

- Attenuation of the sagittal band permits ulnar and volar subluxation of the extensor pollicis longus (EPL) tendon, which accentuates MCP joint flexion and interphalangeal joint hyperextension as it translates volar to the axis of MCP joint rotation.

- The destructive influence of prolific MCP joint synovitis can cause progressive articular erosion and altered joint surface mechanics, resulting in progressive joint instability and deformity.
- As the MCP joint flexion posturing increases in severity, compensatory radial abduction deviation of the thumb metacarpal ensues.
- Rupture of the EPL tendon at the wrist can result in a similar "extrinsic-minus" deformity of the thumb.[21,27]
- Boutonnière deformity can result, also, from a hyperextension deformity of the thumb interphalangeal joint secondary to joint synovitis with attenuation of the volar plate or to rupture of the flexor pollicis longus tendon.[20]
  - Generally, these primary interphalangeal joint etiologies present with less dramatic MCP joint flexion deformity.[34]

Rheumatoid Swan-Neck Deformity

Fingers

- Swan-neck deformity may result from pathologic rheumatoid synovitis of the MCP, PIP, or DIP joints and is characterized by PIP joint hyperextension and MCP and DIP flexion deformities.
  - Progressive attenuation of the volar plate, collateral ligaments, and insertion of the FDS tendon results in the development of a PIP hyperextension deformity.
  - Attenuation of the transverse retinacular ligaments may occur from synovitis, thereby resulting in a loss of the normal restraints to dorsal translocation of the lateral bands. As the lateral bands subluxate dorsal to the axis of PIP joint rotation, they become a constant hyperextension force on the PIP joint.
- The DIP joint may be the primary cause of swan-neck deformity where synovitis results in the attenuation and possible rupture of the terminal extensor tendon. This leads to a concentration of the extensor forces at the PIP joint and a resultant hyperextension deformity.
- Pathologic alterations in MCP joint mechanics may initiate the development of a swan-neck deformity. Progressive flexion deformity and ulnar drift of the digit results in an imbalance of the extensor mechanism whereby the lateral bands are drawn dorsally, concentrating an extension–hyperextension force at the PIP joint. Flexion deformity at the MCP joint may be secondary to several causes (**FIG 3A,B**):
  - Chronic synovitis and associated attenuation of the sagittal bands
  - Articular destruction with associated joint deformity and volar joint subluxation
  - The influence of intrinsic tightness or contracture
- Persisting PIP hyperextension results in contracture of the extensor apparatus, particularly the triangular ligament as well as the skin. These progressive changes result in a stiff and subsequently fixed PIP joint hyperextension contracture.
- Digital flexor tenosynovitis may contribute to poor initiation of digital flexion and an increased extension imbalance at the PIP joint.
- Chronic synovitis of the PIP joint, combined with altered joint mechanics, may result in progressive articular destruction that leads to greater joint deformity, a progressively

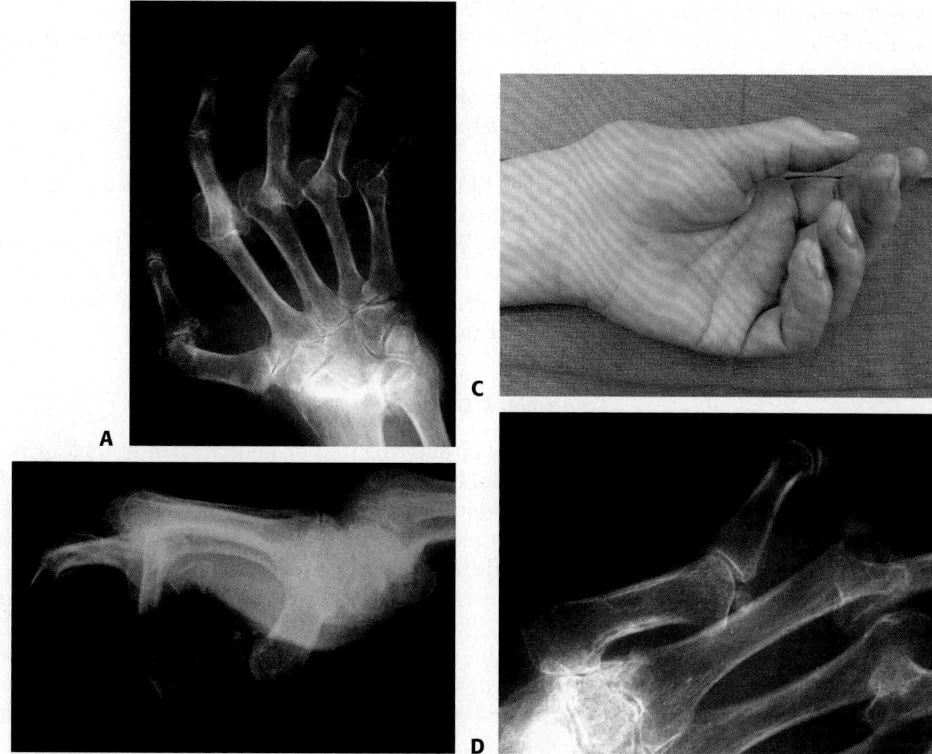

FIG 3 • **A,B.** Anteroposterior (AP) and lateral radiographs demonstrating the volar dislocation and ulnar drift of the MCP joints of the fingers. **C.** Swan-neck deformity of the thumb. **D.** Lateral radiograph of the thumb demonstrating a swan-neck deformity involving CMC joint subluxation, metacarpal adduction contracture, hyperextension of the MCP joint, and thumb interphalangeal joint flexion. (Photographs © Copyright of Fraser J. Leversedge, Charles A. Goldfarb, and Martin Boyer.)

fixed contracture, and, potentially, painful dysfunction of the digit.

Thumb

- Type III rheumatoid thumb deformity is the second most common thumb deformity after boutonnière deformity.[27,30]
- The deformity occurs as the result of CMC joint synovitis and associated alterations in thumb mechanics.
  - Progressive dorsal and radial subluxation of the thumb CMC joint occurs with the deleterious effects of chronic synovitis, including capsular attenuation and articular erosions.
- The force vectors associated with pinch and grasp activities accentuate the CMC deformity and accentuate a progressive thumb metacarpal adduction contracture due to a loss of thumb abduction.
- As the adduction contracture worsens, hyperextension of the MCP joint (permitted by volar plate laxity) and interphalangeal joint flexion becomes a functional compensation (**FIG 3C,D**).

NATURAL HISTORY

Traumatic Injury

- Early diagnosis is critical for achieving satisfactory outcomes. Reconstructive options become limited as the deformity becomes rigid.

Boutonnière Deformity

- Deformity may not be evident immediately after injury but may develop over 2 to 3 weeks.
- The pathologic finger posture develops through five stages[9]:
  - Disruption of the central slip results in resting flexion of the PIP joint and weak extension of the middle phalanx via the lateral bands.
  - Attenuation of the triangular ligament and contracture of the transverse retinacular ligaments results in the volar migration of the lateral bands. Active PIP joint extension is absent.
  - Extension forces are transmitted through the lateral bands, causing hyperextension at the DIP joint.
  - Progressive contracture of the PIP joint volar plate and the oblique retinacular ligament results in fixed flexion contracture at the PIP joint.
  - Progressive articular degeneration occurs after prolonged and untreated pathology.

Swan-Neck Deformity

- The deformity may be subclassified into four groups that describe the natural history[26]:
  - Presence of full passive range of motion at the PIP joint
  - Prolonged hyperextension of the PIP joint results in intrinsic tightness. The PIP joint exhibits full range of motion when the MCP joint is flexed. However, with the MCP joint extended, PIP flexion becomes limited.
  - As the transverse retinacular ligament attenuates and the triangular ligament contracts, the subluxated lateral bands become fixed dorsal to the PIP joint axis of rotation. Hyperextension of the PIP joint becomes fixed regardless of MCP joint position.
  - Progressive PIP joint articular degeneration occurs with chronic, fixed deformity.

Rheumatoid Deformity

- The rate of progressive rheumatoid arthritis-related upper extremity deformity appears to be slowing due to improved medical management of this systemic disease process.
- The incidence of uncorrectable boutonnière and swan-neck deformities during the first 2 years after the onset of systemic disease is about 16% and 8%, respectively.[9]
- The prevalence of finger deformities in patients with established rheumatoid arthritis is about 36% for boutonnière and 14% for swan-neck deformities.[9]
- The wrist, MCP, and PIP joints are the most commonly affected joints of the upper extremity, and pathologic proliferation of the flexor and extensor tenosynovium may influence digital function and deformity.

PATIENT HISTORY AND PHYSICAL FINDINGS

Posttraumatic Injury

Boutonnière Deformity

- A history of blunt trauma to the digit with swelling and tenderness over the PIP joint should arouse suspicion as to the condition. Often, patients report "jamming" or spraining the digit. History of a dorsal digital laceration is similarly concerning.
- Deformity may not develop until 10 to 21 days after the injury, making early diagnosis challenging and diligent follow-up imperative. Laceration, ecchymosis, or tenderness over the dorsum of the PIP joint may be diagnostic when a PIP joint extension lag is present.
- If the examination is limited due to pain, a digital block should be considered to facilitate a comfortable examination.
- The following physical findings are supportive in confirming an early diagnosis:
  - A 15- to 20-degree PIP joint extension lag with the wrist and MCP joint fully flexed[5]
  - Weak extension of the middle phalanx against resistance[2]
  - Elson test: Effort to extend the PIP joint accompanied by rigidity of the DIP joint suggests that the central slip is ruptured and forces are being transferred by the lateral bands.
    - The Elson test is most reliable in diagnosing early boutonnière deformities.[32]
- Boyes test: When the central slip is disrupted, passive extension of the PIP joint causes tension across the lateral bands, resulting in loss of active flexion at the DIP joint. When flexion at the PIP joint is restored, motion at the DIP joint returns.

Swan-Neck Deformity

- A history of unrecognized or undertreated trauma or multiple dorsal PIP joint dislocations is common. A patient who presents with a long-standing "mallet" deformity should arouse suspicion, particularly if there is associated hypermobility in the PIP joint of unaffected digits.
- Physical examination begins with inspection of the involved digit.
  - Typically, the PIP joint is hyperextended and the DIP joint is flexed. MCP joint flexion may be present also.
- Active and passive range of motion of the PIP joint should be assessed.

- In the presence of a flexible deformity, a Bunnell test for intrinsic tightness should be performed.
  - This test assists the examiner in determining the relative contribution of intrinsic tightness to the deformity.
  - Increased resistance to passive PIP flexion with the MCP joint in extension compared with flexion indicates a relative shortening of the intrinsic muscle–tendon units.

Rheumatoid Deformity

- Diagnostic criteria for rheumatoid arthritis are based on the American College of Rheumatology's 1988 recommendations.[2]
- Current medications and medical comorbidities may influence decision making for treatment and the timing for surgical intervention.
- The evaluation of digital deformities associated with rheumatoid arthritis requires careful global assessment, including neurologic assessment (cervical spine, peripheral compressive neuropathy); appreciation for shoulder, elbow, and wrist involvement; and the awareness of lower extremity deformities that will need reconstructive surgery for which the use of ambulatory aids might be necessary.
- As progressive deformity of the wrist occurs, its pathologic influence on digital function and deformity should be recognized.
  - The carpus typically collapses into supination, with concomitant volar translation and ulnar translocation.[4]
  - Relative dorsal prominence of the distal ulna may involve a loss of distal radioulnar joint (DRUJ) congruity and may be associated with ruptures of the extensor carpi ulnaris tendon and extensor tendons to the small and ring fingers (caput ulnae syndrome). Inspection of the extrinsic digital extensors, including the EPL,[21] should be done, particularly in the presence of active synovitis of the radiocarpal joint and DRUJ (**FIG 4**).
- The MCP joint should be assessed for active synovitis and for characteristic volar subluxation and ulnar drift.
- Just as pathologic changes to both the wrist and MCP joints may influence the development of swan-neck and boutonnière deformities of the digits, these changes may adversely affect the outcomes of digital reconstruction if they are not addressed.
- Evaluation of the digits should be performed individually with inspection of the resting posture of each digit, assessment of the active and passive motion of each digital joint, and inspection for joint synovitis or tenosynovitis. Skin integrity is assessed for attenuation and for its contribution to joint contracture.
- Flexor tenosynovitis may be identified by a palpable fullness in the distal volar forearm or along the digital flexor sheath. Swelling, palpable crepitus along the digital flexor sheath, and a discrepancy between active and passive digital motion are hallmarks of flexor tenosynovitis of the digit.
  - Flexor tendon rupture may be present, often secondary to attenuation at the volar carpus,[20] and should be addressed in the presence of a loss of active digital joint flexion.
- Extensor tenosynovitis at the wrist may be determined by palpable tenosynovial hypertrophy, or fullness, and crepitus along the dorsal extensor compartments, proximal and distal to the extensor retinaculum.
  - Tendon ruptures may be identified by a lack of active digital extension despite active muscular contraction, by palpable tendon deficit, and by a lack of digital extension through tenodesis with passive wrist flexion.
  - The adhesion of a ruptured tendon to the surrounding tissues and the influence of the junctura tendinea may limit the accuracy of these evaluations.
- As described earlier, the Bunnell intrinsic tightness test should be performed for all fingers of patients with rheumatoid arthritis, particularly for patients with swan-neck deformity of the digits. This test assists the examiner in determining the relative contribution of intrinsic tightness to the development of the deformity.
- Tightness of the oblique retinacular ligament, often appreciated in digits with early boutonnière deformity, is evaluated by assessing the relative degree of resistance to passive DIP joint flexion with the PIP joint held by the examiner in maximum extension.

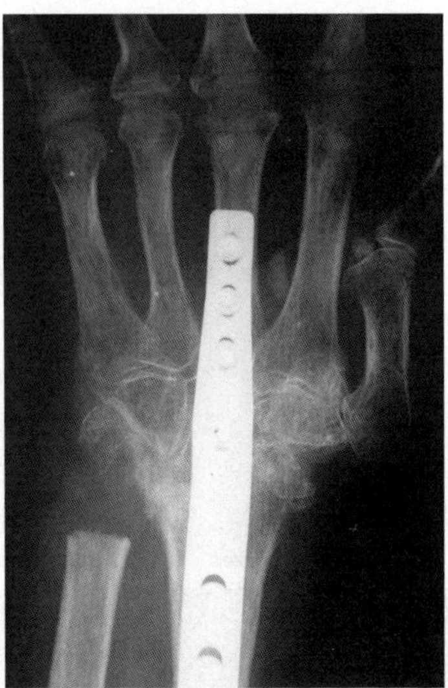

FIG 4 • Preoperative assessment of the digits should include evaluation of the wrist and MCP joints due to their influence on digital function. Wrist stabilization with total wrist arthrodesis and concomitant distal ulnar resection may include soft tissue reconstruction such as tendon repair or tenodesis; such reconstruction should occur before digital reconstructions due to its influence on the outcomes of swan-neck or boutonnière reconstructions. Reconstruction of the MCP joints should occur before or simultaneously with digital swan-neck or boutonnière reconstructions. (Photographs © Copyright of Fraser J. Leversedge, Charles A. Goldfarb, and Martin Boyer.)

IMAGING AND OTHER DIAGNOSTIC STUDIES

- Plain radiographs (four views) are the mainstay of hand and wrist evaluation in the patient with either a traumatic or rheumatoid cause for deformity.
  - Staging of arthritis-related joint pathology and identification of joint subluxation or dislocation, important for diagnostic and management considerations, is performed using plain radiographs (**FIG 5A**).
- Avulsion fractures from the dorsal base of the middle phalanx, volar subluxation of the PIP joint, or both suggest a central slip injury (**FIG 5B**).
- In the presence of a fixed PIP joint flexion deformity, concomitant avulsion fracture of the volar plate suggests pseudoboutonnière pathology.

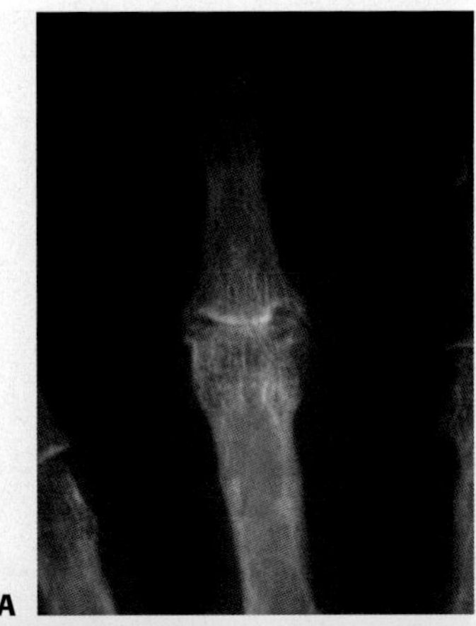

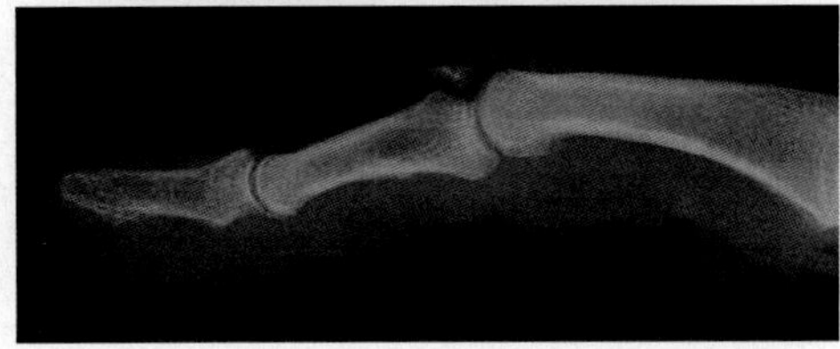

FIG 5 • **A.** Radiographic appearance of periarticular (PIP joint) soft tissue swelling and synovitis and moderate articular erosions involving the PIP joint. **B.** Lateral radiograph of the finger demonstrating a central slip avulsion injury involving an avulsion fracture from the dorsal base of the middle phalanx. There is no volar subluxation of the PIP joint in this example. (Photographs © Copyright of Fraser J. Leversedge, Charles A. Goldfarb, and Martin Boyer.)

- Fluoroscopic imaging or stress views may be helpful in differentiating collateral ligament injury from disruption of the central slip.
- Avulsion fractures from the dorsal base of the distal phalanx suggest terminal tendon injury.
- The presence of volar plate avulsion fractures in the setting of PIP joint hyperextension suggests volar plate incompetence.
- Magnetic resonance imaging (MRI) may be useful in assessing for soft tissue pathology such as tenosynovitis and tendon rupture, especially in rheumatoid patients.

DIFFERENTIAL DIAGNOSIS

Posttraumatic Injury

- Pseudoboutonnière deformity
- Collateral ligament injury
- Mallet finger
- Volar plate avulsion fracture

Rheumatoid Deformity

- Osteoarthritis
- Psoriatic arthritis
  - Similar deformities as seen in rheumatoid arthritis, but skin lesions are common and DIP joint "pencil-in-cup" deformities may be present
- Connective tissue disorders (scleroderma, systemic lupus erythematosus)
  - Systemic lupus erythematosus primarily affects soft tissue structures (ligamentous laxity, tendon subluxation) rather than joint destruction. Radiographs typically demonstrate joint deformities with well-preserved joint spaces. The thumb may be the first digit affected; lateral subluxation of the interphalangeal joint and flexion deformity of the MCP joint (secondary to extensor tendon subluxation) are common.
  - Patients with scleroderma often develop PIP joint flexion contractures and compensatory hyperextension posturing of the MCP joints.
- Crystal-induced arthropathy (gout, calcium pyrophosphate deposition disease)
- Hemochromatosis
- Remitting symmetric seronegative synovitis

NONOPERATIVE MANAGEMENT

Posttraumatic Injury

Boutonnière Deformity

- Nonoperative management is indicated if correction of the deformity restores the anatomic length relationship between the central slip and the lateral bands. It is most appropriate in those with closed injuries who present within 8 to 12 weeks of injury. It may be attempted in those with central slip avulsion fractures or volar dislocation if satisfactory reduction and PIP joint stability can be obtained.
- For patients with full passive extension of the PIP joint, PIP joint extension splinting is the treatment of choice.
  - A transarticular Kirschner wire maintaining the PIP joint in full extension is an alternative or adjunct to external splinting.
- For patients with a PIP joint flexion contracture without secondary joint degenerative changes, progressive static or dynamic extension splinting should be pursued.
  - Full passive extension of the PIP joint should be sought before surgical intervention is considered.
- Active and passive DIP joint range of motion should be emphasized while the PIP joint is being treated. Restoration of active DIP joint flexion while the PIP joint is extended suggests successful treatment. Restoration of full active extension at the PIP joint is the goal.
- For most injuries, PIP joint extension splinting should be maintained for 6 to 8 weeks at all times, transitioning to protective buddy straps for daily activity and nighttime extension splinting for an additional 4 to 6 weeks.

Swan-Neck Deformity

- Once the deformity has developed, nonoperative treatment is rarely effective.
- Some patients with flexible deformities are capable of initiating PIP joint flexion with little impairment. They may complain of "snapping" or "cogwheeling" as the lateral bands relocate volarly during PIP joint flexion. These patients may benefit from a digital splint, such as a figure-8 ring splint, to prevent continued PIP joint hyperextension and to maintain the lateral bands in their anatomic position (**FIG 6**).

Rheumatoid Deformity

Boutonnière Deformity

- Nonoperative management of an early boutonnière deformity includes low-profile PIP joint extension splinting.
- Oral anti-inflammatory medications, intra-articular corticosteroid injection of the PIP joint, or both are used to minimize joint synovitis.

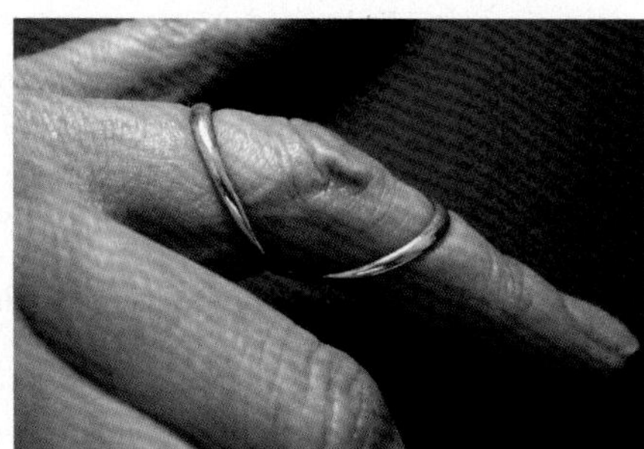

FIG 6 • A figure-8 ring splint (Silver Ring Splint Co., Charlottesville, VA) used to prevent PIP joint hyperextension in a mild, flexible swan-neck deformity. (Photographs © Copyright of Fraser J. Leversedge, Charles A. Goldfarb, and Martin Boyer.)

Type I Swan-Neck Deformity

- The goals of treatment for the flexible swan-neck deformity are prevention of PIP joint hyperextension and improvement in PIP joint flexion.
- In the presence of minimal PIP joint synovitis, use of digital splints, such as a figure-8 ring splint, is advocated to prevent PIP joint hyperextension (see **FIG 6**).

SURGICAL MANAGEMENT

Posttraumatic Injury

Boutonnière Deformity

- Surgical intervention is indicated for patients who fail to respond to at least 3 months of extension splinting, patients with open injuries, and patients with fixed deformity with associated degenerative joint changes.
- Surgical decision making should be tempered by the observations of Burton and Melchior[5]:
  - Boutonnière reconstructions are most successful on supple joints. If necessary, joint contracture release can be performed as a first stage. If the release is followed by an intensive exercise and splinting program, the second stage may be avoided.
  - An arthritic joint usually precludes soft tissue reconstruction. The surgeon should consider either a PIP joint fusion or arthroplasty with extensor reconstruction.
  - Boutonnière deformities rarely compromise PIP joint flexion and grip strength. The surgeon should not trade extension at the PIP joint for a stiff finger and a weak hand.

Swan-Neck Deformity

- Surgery is indicated for patients with a flexible deformity who cannot actively initiate PIP joint flexion and in those with fixed deformities.
- Patients with flexible deformities benefit from volar mobilization of the lateral bands and tenodesis to prevent PIP joint hyperextension.
- Patients with fixed deformities have difficulty grasping objects. Often, functional contact is limited to the volar surface of the hyperextended PIP joint.
  - If the articular surfaces are well preserved, PIP joint release with concomitant procedures to restore flexion may be beneficial.
  - If the articular surfaces are damaged, PIP arthrodesis is a practical option.

Chronic Mallet Finger (with or without Swan-Neck Deformity)

- Described by Fowler,[13] tenotomy of the central slip of the extensor tendon at the level of the PIP joint is a simple and effective treatment option for flexible chronic mallet finger deformities, which can progress to hyperextension at the PIP joint and swan-neck deformity.
  - This procedure allows the extensor mechanism to glide proximally, transmitting the force of the extensor mechanism through the lateral bands to the terminal tendon, improving DIP joint extension, and decreasing PIP joint hyperextension.
- Surgery is indicated for patients whose mallet finger injuries are no longer amenable to extension splinting and have functional limitations due to DIP joint extensor lag.
- If the articular surfaces are damaged, DIP arthrodesis is an option.

Rheumatoid Deformity

- Principles of surgical correction of rheumatoid deformities in the hand should be guided by the relief of pain and the improvement of function.[29]

Boutonnière Finger Deformity

- Stage I—mild
  - For progressive boutonnière deformity associated with persistent PIP joint synovitis unresponsive to oral medication and intra-articular corticosteroid injection, PIP joint synovectomy may be considered. Concomitant central slip reconstruction and lateral band repositioning may be indicated due to soft tissue attenuation over the dorsal PIP joint.
  - Functional limitation due to DIP joint hyperextension may be treated by sectioning the terminal extensor tendon over the dorsal middle phalanx.
- Stage II—moderate
  - For patients with moderate boutonnière deformity and preservation of the articular cartilage of the PIP joint, central slip reconstruction and terminal extensor tendon release may be indicated.[12,44]
- Stage III—severe
  - If articular destruction is evident or if a severe fixed flexion contracture of the PIP joint is present, even without articular changes, then arthrodesis of the PIP joint is a reliable option for reducing pain and for improving function.
  - Implant arthroplasty of the PIP joint and concomitant terminal extensor tendon release is a less reliable option, particularly when there is attenuation of the dorsal extensor apparatus.

Swan-Neck Finger Deformity

- Type I
  - The primary cause of the flexible swan-neck deformity must be determined before proceeding with surgical intervention. Although PIP synovitis and a resulting weakness of the volar PIP joint restraining structures are the most common findings, DIP joint synovitis may be a source of progressive deformity secondary to the transfer of extension forces to the PIP joint.

- The potential influence of MCP joint pathology must be assessed. Extensor tendon subluxation at the level of the MCP joint or flexion contracture of the MCP joint should be addressed before, or concurrently with, surgical correction of the swan-neck deformity.
- In a primary rheumatoid mallet finger where full PIP joint flexibility is preserved, DIP joint arthrodesis is a reasonable option. Postoperatively, the PIP joint is not immobilized, although the DIP joint is protected in a mallet finger splint.
- Frequently, patients with a flexible swan-neck deformity cannot initiate active PIP joint flexion from a resting, hyperextension position. Soft tissue reconstructive procedures that provide a checkrein to prevent PIP joint hyperextension may be considered, including volar skin dermodesis, oblique retinacular ligament reconstruction, lateral band tenodesis,[14,45] and PIP joint flexor tenodesis.[10]

- Type II
  - In type II swan-neck deformities, active and passive PIP joint motion is limited, with the MCP joint held in extension secondary to intrinsic tightness. MCP joint arthritis may be present. Therefore, MCP joint implant arthroplasty, intrinsic release, or both should be considered in planning for this swan-neck reconstruction.
  - Intrinsic release is accomplished via a dorsal approach to the MCP joint with exposure of the lateral band and extensor hood. A 1-cm segment of lateral band with attached sagittal band fibers is excised as described by Nalebuff.[26,28] Release of the ulnar intrinsic tendon, with or without tendon transfer, may reduce the deforming force on the digit and reduce ulnar drift at the MCP joint.
  - If intrinsic release or MCP joint arthroplasty is performed, concomitant flexor tenodesis of the PIP joint may be required.
- Type III
  - Type III swan-neck deformity is characterized by decreased active and passive PIP joint flexion irrespective of MCP joint positioning. The lateral bands are adherent dorsal to the PIP joint axis of rotation and a PIP joint soft tissue contracture is often present. Reconstruction involves lateral band release and volar translocation, combined with dorsal PIP joint capsulectomy, collateral ligament release, and extensor tenolysis.[4,17,35]
- Type IV
  - There is a fixed hyperextension deformity of the PIP joint as well as destructive changes to the articular cartilage of the PIP joint.
  - Soft tissue procedures will not reliably relieve pain nor restore joint motion or function, and definitive treatment is limited to arthrodesis or implant arthroplasty.[4]

Rheumatoid Thumb

- Type I: boutonnière deformity
  - Mild: passively correctable MCP and interphalangeal joints
    - Soft tissue reconstruction is indicated, as this may improve function despite a high incidence of deformity recurrence.[39]
    - Synovectomy of the MCP joint combined with EPL tendon rerouting will increase the extensor moment at the MCP joint through EPL attachment to the dorsal MCP joint capsule.[25]
  - Moderate: fixed MCP joint deformity
    - The condition of the adjacent CMC and interphalangeal joints must be considered to determine whether to proceed with MCP arthrodesis or arthroplasty. Often, treatment at this stage of disease reduces the progression of thumb deformity.
    - If the extent of interphalangeal joint involvement warrants intervention, treatment of the interphalangeal joint is limited to arthrodesis. Therefore, preservation of motion at the MCP joint may be optimal through MCP implant arthroplasty, although function after MCP and interphalangeal arthrodeses is generally good.
    - Arthroplasty of the thumb MCP joint involves resection of the involved joint surfaces and prosthetic placement, most commonly with a flexible silicone implant. Extensor reconstruction, including EPL rerouting, is considered to augment extensor forces acting at the MCP joint. Postoperatively, the thumb MCP joint is splinted in extension for 4 to 6 weeks, allowing for controlled CMC and interphalangeal joint exercises. Good functional results with minimal progression of CMC or interphalangeal joint arthritis have been reported.[11]
    - Arthrodesis of the MCP joint is accomplished by one of several methods, including tension band wire fixation, crossing Kirschner wires, a headless compression screw, or plate and screw fixation. The joint is typically placed in 15 degrees of flexion and the arthrodesis site may be augmented with bone graft as needed to maximize bone surface contact area. The arthrodesis site is protected in a splint until radiographic union is confirmed. Early interphalangeal joint range of motion is encouraged to minimize extensor adhesions and stiffness.
  - Severe: fixed deformities of MCP and interphalangeal joints
    - In this advanced stage, the treatment rationale is similar to that for moderate deformity, except that interphalangeal joint contracture or joint deterioration requires intervention. Rarely, interphalangeal joint capsular release may be indicated to improve motion, in the absence of articular deterioration. For cases involving interphalangeal joint instability or progressive arthritis, interphalangeal arthrodesis is indicated.
  - CMC joint involvement
    - As rheumatoid arthritis has the potential to involve greater numbers of joints, motion-sparing procedures of the CMC joint are preferred compared to arthrodesis.
    - Although total trapezial implant arthroplasty is relatively contraindicated in the rheumatoid patient due to the higher risk for implant failure or dislocation, resection or hemiresection arthroplasty with ligament reconstruction and soft tissue interposition arthroplasty should be considered.[34]
- Type III: swan-neck deformity
  - Mild: isolated CMC joint involvement
    - In the absence of symptomatic relief from conservative treatment, CMC hemitrapeziectomy or trapeziectomy and ligament reconstruction with soft tissue interposition arthroplasty is indicated.
  - Moderate: CMC joint pathology with mild MCP joint involvement (flexible deformity)
    - For CMC joint pathology with progressive MCP joint hyperextension deformity, CMC hemitrapeziectomy or

trapeziectomy and ligament reconstruction with soft tissue interposition arthroplasty and simultaneous MCP joint volar plate capsulodesis, sesamoidesis, or volar tenodesis are considered. Temporary transarticular pin stabilization of the MCP joint in 20 degrees of flexion for 3 to 4 weeks postoperatively permits early motion of the interphalangeal joint.

- Severe: CMC joint dislocation with metacarpal adduction contracture and fixed MCP joint hyperextension deformity
  - Treatment for this advanced stage requires:
    - CMC joint reconstruction with resection arthroplasty and ligament reconstruction or tendon interposition arthroplasty
    - Correction of the metacarpal adduction contracture
    - MCP arthrodesis
  - Often, adduction contracture of the thumb metacarpal may be adequately treated with resection of the thumb metacarpal base and release of the restraining ligaments of the CMC joint during resection arthroplasty. If the adduction contracture persists, then fasciotomy of the first dorsal interosseous and adductor muscles may be completed.[34] Web space reconstruction with Z-plasties is rarely indicated.

Preoperative Planning

- The surgeon must plan ahead. Extended procedures associated with multiple digital reconstructions or the combined treatment of multiple joints should warrant careful and efficient use of tourniquet time.
- Regional anesthesia (axillary block, intravenous [IV] regional) may be preferred for the reconstruction of digital deformities. This form of anesthesia may provide a greater duration of postoperative pain control and may minimize the systemic effects of general anesthesia.
  - Avoidance of general anesthesia may minimize the potential risks of cervical spine positioning in patients with cervical instability secondary to rheumatoid arthritis.
- Procedures that may require the use of bone grafting should involve preoperative discussion with the patient to explain the potential need for bone grafting and to identify potential sources for the graft (ie, iliac crest, olecranon, distal radius, allograft or synthetic bone substitutes).

Posttraumatic Injury

- A detailed history and physical examination should be performed.
- Active and passive PIP joint range of motion should be assessed. Chronic, rigid deformities may require staged procedures with surgical release of the PIP joint before subsequent reconstructive procedures.
- Radiographs should be reviewed for fractures, joint subluxation or dislocation, and degenerative joint changes.
- Adjacent joint injuries and preexisting degenerative changes should be considered during surgical planning.

Rheumatoid Deformity

- Before surgical reconstruction of rheumatoid swan-neck or boutonnière deformities of the digits, a global assessment is completed to characterize the systemic involvement of rheumatoid disease.
  - Coordination of medical clearance and perioperative care may be pertinent for patients with medical comorbidities and for patients taking perioperative medications such as corticosteroids.
  - Preoperative cervical spine evaluation may be indicated to confirm stability of the spine for safe anesthesia administration.
- Timing of rheumatoid swan-neck or boutonnière reconstruction should account for other musculoskeletal pathology as reviewed earlier. Postoperative protocols and anticipated prognosis for recovery should be reviewed carefully with patients to minimize potential conflicts with other medical or surgical management.

Positioning

- Surgical reconstruction of the hand is performed typically in a supine position, with the upper limb placed on a well-padded hand table.
- A brachial tourniquet is used.
- Preoperative shoulder and elbow assessment will minimize potential difficulties with surgical positioning, particularly for patients with severe limitations to joint mobility or joint instability.

Approach

- Careful soft tissue handling is observed to minimize the risk of wound or soft tissue complications. Full-thickness skin flaps are raised during operative exposure.

Dorsal Approach

- A longitudinal midline or curvilinear incision from the proximal phalanx to the DIP joint provides excellent visualization of the extensor mechanism.
- Sharp dissection through the subcutaneous tissue and careful elevation of full-thickness flaps are performed to expose the central slip and lateral bands.
- Exposure of volar structures is limited with this approach but can be enhanced by extending the incision proximally and distally.
- Volarly, the Cleland ligament is divided, taking care to protect the neurovascular bundle, which is volar to the plane of dissection. The underlying PIP joint collateral ligament, PIP joint volar plate, and flexor sheath are exposed.
- A small window can be made in the membranous flexor sheath between the A2 and A4 pulleys to improve exposure of the volar plate.

Volar Approach

- Access to volar structures may be necessary to release the PIP joint. This can be accomplished via a midlateral or a Brunner incision centered at the PIP joint.
- Dissection is carried down to the flexor sheath, elevating full-thickness flaps and preserving the digital neurovascular bundles.
- Between the A2 and A4 pulleys, the membranous portion of the flexor sheath can be elevated to expose the flexor tendons and the underlying volar plate of the PIP joint.
- Arthrodesis and arthroplasty techniques are detailed in separate chapters.

■ Boutonnière Reconstruction

Primary Central Slip Repair

- Primary repair is accomplished through a dorsal approach.
- After isolating the central slip, assess the redundant tissue with the PIP joint held in full extension.
  - Excise a chevron-shaped segment of redundant fibrous tissue, permitting repair of the free tendon edges with 4-0 braided suture using a multistrand, grasping or locking repair method.
- V-Y advancement may be necessary to facilitate repair.
- In the case of an avulsion fracture, identify and carefully elevate the fragment, preserving the attachment of the central slip.
  - For smaller fragments inappropriate for Kirschner wire or screw fixation, the fragment may be excised and the central slip repaired directly into the dorsal base of the middle phalanx using a pullout suture or suture anchor method.
  - If the fracture fragment is larger, reduce the fragment anatomically and stabilize it using appropriate fixation such as small screws or two small Kirschner wires.
- The lateral bands must be restored to their anatomic location, dorsal to the axis of rotation of the PIP joint. Mobilize them by excising the triangular ligament and incising both transverse retinacular ligaments as necessary.
  - Approximate the lateral bands distal and dorsal to the PIP joint and suture them together using 4-0 nonabsorbable, braided suture.
- The repair is protected and the PIP joint is held fully extended, usually using a transarticular Kirschner wire, for 6 weeks.

Central Slip Reconstruction Using Local Tissue

- Central slip reconstruction using local tissue may be considered for patients with a flexible deformity and insufficient central slip for direct primary repair. Several methods have been described using a dorsal approach to the extensor apparatus.

Snow's Technique

- Identify the proximal stump of central slip and dissect it free of the surrounding tissues.[33]
- Elevate a distally based flap of extensor tendon sharply, preserving sufficient length to span the tendinous defect.
- Turn the flap down on itself and suture it to any distal tissue as well as the lateral bands using 4-0 braided, nonabsorbable suture.
- After repair, passive PIP joint flexion of no less than 60 degrees must be possible without excessive tension across the repair site.

Aiache's Technique

- Isolate the radial and ulnar lateral bands and divide them longitudinally from the trifurcation of the extrinsic tendon to the triangular ligament.[1]
- Mobilize the dorsal half of each lateral band dorsally and suture them together using 5-0 nonabsorbable, braided suture.
- Lateral band relocation is recommended when the lateral bands are fixed volar to the PIP joint axis of rotation.

Littler and Eaton's Technique

- Carefully isolate the radial and ulnar lateral bands.[19]
- Incise the lateral bands over the middle phalanx. Preserve at least one oblique retinacular ligament; otherwise, DIP joint extension will be compromised.
- Mobilize the incised lateral bands dorsally and suture them into the insertion of the central slip.
- If excessive attenuation of the central slip precludes suture stabilization, this repair method is contraindicated.

Matev's Technique

- After isolating the lateral bands from the surrounding soft tissue, incise the ulnar lateral band at the level of the DIP joint and incise the radial lateral band at the midpoint of the middle phalanx.[23]
- Suture the proximal stump of the ulnar lateral band to the distal stump of the radial lateral band over the dorsal digit, thereby lengthening the terminal slip (**TECH FIG 1**).
- Weave the proximal stump of the radial lateral band into the remnants of the central slip and suture it to the base of the middle phalanx to restore PIP joint extension.
- Postoperatively, the PIP joint is held in full extension for 6 weeks. A temporary transarticular Kirschner wire may be placed to protect the repair.

Central Slip Reconstruction Using Tendon Graft

- When a flexible deformity is present but there is insufficient local tissue for use in central slip reconstruction, a tendon graft reconstruction may be considered.
- Expose the extensor mechanism via a dorsal, curvilinear incision. Identify the proximal stump of the central slip and isolate it from the surrounding tissues.
- Harvest an autologous tendon graft, preferably the ipsilateral palmaris longus tendon (if present).
- Create a transverse bone tunnel through the dorsal base of the middle phalanx.

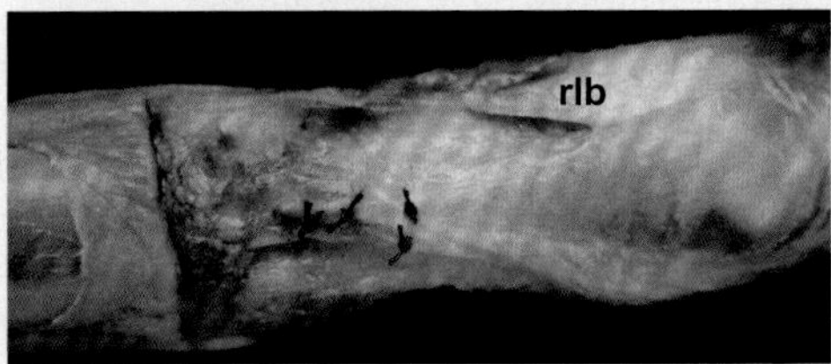

TECH FIG 1 • Boutonnière reconstruction using Matev's technique of lengthening the terminal tendon and reconstructing the central slip using the lateral bands. The ulnar lateral band is incised slightly proximal to the DIP joint and the radial lateral band is incised more proximally, at the level of the midaspect of the middle phalanx. The proximal stump of the ulnar lateral band is then sutured into the distal stump of the radial lateral band as shown here. The free proximal stump of the radial lateral band (*rlb*) is then repaired into the dorsal base of the middle phalanx. (Photographs © Copyright of Fraser J. Leversedge, Charles A. Goldfarb, and Martin Boyer.)

- Pass the palmaris longus tendon through the bone tunnel and weave the two limbs into the lateral bands with the digit held in neutral (**TECH FIG 2**).
- The repair is protected for 6 weeks by maintaining PIP joint extension with a transarticular Kirschner wire.

Extensor Tenotomy

- Hyperextension deformity of the DIP joint may be addressed with extensor tenotomy.[24]
- Tenotomy is indicated in the presence of mild, flexible deformities and for patients who have failed prior surgery directed at the PIP joint.
- Extensor tenotomy may be considered as an adjunct to PIP joint arthrodesis performed for chronic boutonnière deformity with associated PIP joint arthritis.
- Make a dorsal incision over the distal two-thirds of the middle phalanx.
- Identify the terminal tendon and elevate it proximally over a distance of 1.5 cm from the underlying phalanx and DIP joint.
- Incise the terminal tendon distal to the triangular ligament.
- Preserve the radial oblique retinacular ligament so that DIP joint extension is not compromised.
- Passively extend the PIP joint and passively flex the DIP joint to separate the incised tendon ends.

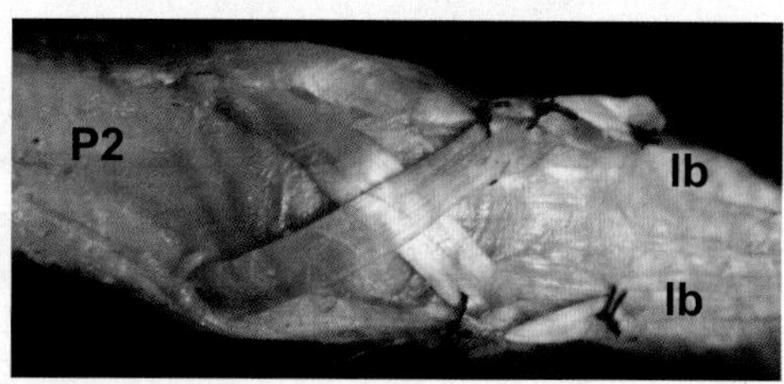

TECH FIG 2 • Boutonnière reconstruction using a tendon graft. The tendon graft is passed through a transverse osseous tunnel in the dorsal base of the middle phalanx (*P2*) and the limbs of the graft are woven into the lateral bands (*lb*). (Photographs © Copyright of Fraser J. Leversedge, Charles A. Goldfarb, and Martin Boyer.)

Swan-Neck Reconstruction

Oblique Retinacular Ligament Reconstruction Using a Free Tendon Graft

- Reconstruction of the oblique retinacular ligament is indicated when a flexible swan-neck deformity develops secondary to an untreated mallet finger. This procedure is suited for patients with a well-preserved DIP joint.[18,40]
- Make an incision from the ulnar margin of the MCP joint flexion crease and continue it volarly and distally along the radial midaxial line before curving it dorsally to end over the DIP joint.
- Isolate the radial neurovascular bundle from the surrounding tissue. Proximally, identify the A2 pulley. Distally, identify the terminal slip.
- Harvest the ipsilateral palmaris longus tendon using a tendon stripper through a 1-cm transverse incision proximal to the wrist crease.
  - Alternatively, make a second transverse incision proximally, overlying the musculotendinous junction. Confirm the inserting muscular fibers at the musculotendinous junction before tendon harvest. If the palmaris longus is not present, obtain another suitable autologous tendon graft.
- The DIP joint is held in full extension and the PIP joint is held in 25 degrees of flexion with transarticular Kirschner wires.
- Suture the tendon graft to the terminal slip using nonabsorbable, braided suture.
- Pass the graft deep to the radial neurovascular bundle and bring it to the volar surface of the digit. Suture it to the distal edge of the A2 pulley after tensioning the graft appropriately (**TECH FIG 3**).

Proximal Interphalangeal Joint Flexor Tenodesis

- Creation of a checkrein to PIP joint hyperextension can be accomplished by PIP joint flexor tenodesis or by lateral band tenodesis (described in the following text).
- Via a Brunner or midaxial incision, elevate full-thickness skin flaps to expose the digital flexor sheath, protecting the digital neurovascular bundles.
- Raise as a flap the membranous portion of the flexor sheath, from the distal aspect of the A2 pulley to the proximal edge of the A4 pulley, to expose the underlying flexor tendons.
- Identify one slip of the FDS tendon and divide it proximally at the level of the decussation, leaving its insertion into the base of the middle phalanx intact (**TECH FIG 4A,B**).

A

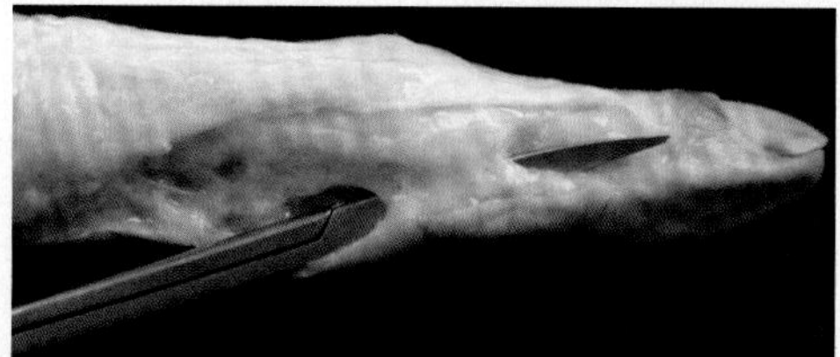

B

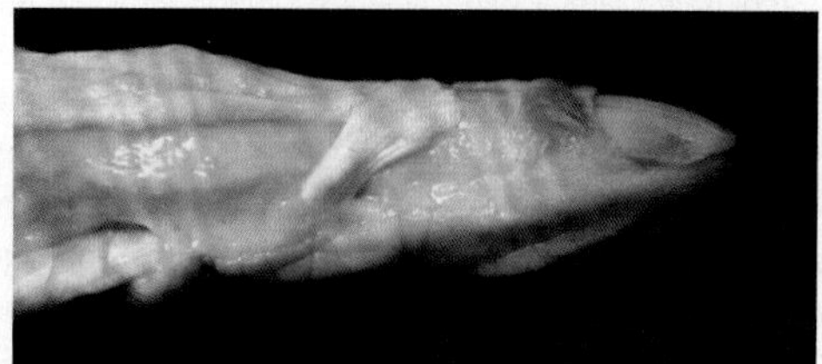

TECH FIG 3 • **A.** Oblique retinacular ligament reconstruction. The scissors illustrate the anatomic plane of dissection for the passage of a tendon graft for reconstruction. The plane extends from the A2 pulley volarly to the dorsal surface of the terminal extensor tendon. **B.** The palmaris tendon graft has been inserted, coursing from volar to the Cleland ligament to be secured to the dorsal aspect of the terminal extensor tendon insertion. The neurovascular bundle is carefully protected. (Photographs © Copyright of Fraser J. Leversedge, Charles A. Goldfarb, and Martin Boyer.)

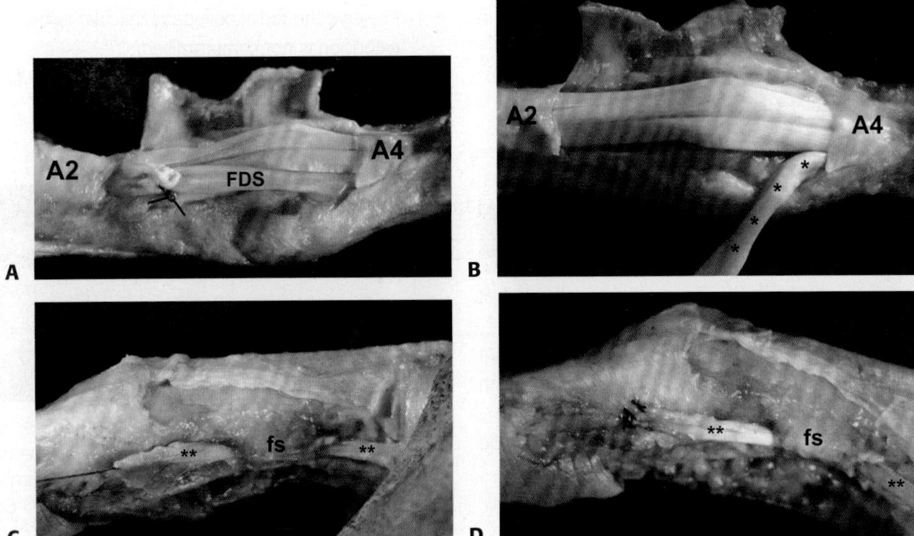

TECH FIG 4 • **A.** PIP joint flexor tenodesis with exposure of the flexor tendons between the A2 pulley and the A4 pulley. One slip of the flexor digitorum superficialis (*FDS*) tendon is divided at the level of the decussation, leaving its insertion intact. **B.** The harvested FDS tendon (*asterisks*) is brought through an opening created in the distal aspect of the A2 pulley to be repaired to itself with the PIP joint held in 20 degrees of flexion. **C,D.** Lateral band tenodesis to provide a checkrein to PIP joint hyperextension. The lateral band (*asterisks*) has been detached distally (**C**) and has been rerouted within the flexor sheath (*fs*) before repair distally (**D**). (Photographs © Copyright of Fraser J. Leversedge, Charles A. Goldfarb, and Martin Boyer.)

- Pass the divided tendon end from dorsal to volar through a transverse incision in the A2 pulley, about 3 mm from the pulley's distal margin, and suture it back onto itself with the PIP joint held in about 20 degrees of flexion (**TECH FIG 4C,D**).
- Postoperative immobilization with a dorsal block splint maintains the joint in more than 20 degrees of flexion for 6 weeks. Flexion exercises for the PIP and DIP joints are started at 3 weeks postoperatively.

Lateral Band Tenodesis

- The lateral band is rerouted so that it lies volar to the PIP joint axis of rotation and forms a restraint to PIP hyperextension.[42,45]
- Approach the extensor apparatus via a dorsal curvilinear incision. Expose the Cleland ligament and divide it to access the flexor sheath with preservation of the digital neurovascular bundles.
- Leaving its proximal and distal attachments intact, dissect the dorsally subluxated lateral band free from the central slip and from its distal attachment to the triangular ligament overlying the base of the middle phalanx. Translocate the lateral band volar to the PIP joint axis of rotation, assisted by flexion of the PIP joint.
- At the level of the PIP joint, elevate a dorsally based flap of the flexor sheath 0.5 to 1 cm wide and place the mobilized lateral band volar to the flap. Repair the flap to its anatomic position, restraining the lateral band as an effective pulley.
- Alternatively, the lateral band may be detached from its insertion into the terminal tendon slip and rerouted within a roughly 0.5- to 1-cm segment of the flexor sheath at the A2 pulley before repairing it to the terminal tendon distally (see **TECH FIG 4A,B**).
  - Confirm unimpeded gliding of the lateral band beneath the flexor sheath by gentle proximal and distal traction on the translocated lateral band.[45]
- Postoperatively, a dorsal block splint maintains the joint in more than 30 degrees of flexion. Digital flexion exercises are encouraged early in the postoperative period. Full active PIP joint extension is not allowed for 6 weeks.

Type III Swan-Neck Reconstruction

- Reconstruction of a type III swan-neck deformity must address the fixed translocation of the lateral bands dorsal to the PIP joint rotation axis and the associated PIP joint soft tissue contracture.
- Management of these pathologic changes includes lateral band release from the central tendon and from the triangular ligament; translocation of the lateral bands to a position volar to the PIP joint rotation axis; dorsal PIP joint contracture release, with dorsal capsulectomy and collateral ligament release; extensor tenolysis of the digit; and possible limited flexor tenolysis, as indicated, for flexor tenosynovitis.
- Via a dorsal curvilinear incision, raise full-thickness skin flaps to expose the underlying extensor apparatus.
- Release the lateral bands along their dorsal attachment to the central tendon, from the proximal phalanx to their confluence over the dorsal aspect of the middle phalanx.

- Complete a dorsal PIP joint capsulectomy and gradually release the radial and ulnar collateral ligaments, from dorsal to volar, until the PIP joint can be passively flexed to 90 degrees.
- Because the mobile lateral bands will passively translate volar to the PIP joint axis of rotation with passive joint flexion, the lateral bands do not require stabilization.
- After soft tissue releases, the PIP joint is stabilized in 20 degrees of flexion with a temporary transarticular Kirschner wire. The digital reconstructions are protected in a forearm-based splint, removed to permit MCP and DIP joint motion. The wire is removed 2 to 3 weeks postoperatively.

Chronic Mallet Finger Deformity

Central Slip Tenotomy

- A straight or curvilinear dorsal incision is made, centered over the PIP joint, and full-thickness flaps are elevated to expose the extensor mechanism.
- The central slip is carefully separated from the lateral bands, preserving the triangular ligament to prevent volar subluxation of the lateral bands. The central slip is then detached from its insertion on the dorsal aspect of the middle phalanx and allowed to slide proximally.
  - Immediate postoperative range of motion is permitted.

PEARLS AND PITFALLS

Patient selection	■ The PIP joint should be assessed for flexibility. ■ Reconstructive options are limited in the presence of PIP joint degenerative changes. Arthrodesis may be the only practical solution. ■ Assess for intrinsic tightness in all patients with digital deformity. ■ In rheumatoid patients, carefully evaluate the wrist and MCP joint before surgical reconstruction of the interphalangeal joints. ■ Tendon ruptures may not be clinically apparent in rheumatoid patients with severe deformity.
Boutonnière deformity	■ The deformity develops from injury to the central slip. ■ Delayed development of the deformity may occur after injury to the central slip. ■ Early diagnosis is important. The Elson test is useful in confirming early diagnosis. ■ Extension splinting is an effective treatment in those who present within 2 to 3 months from the time of injury. A transarticular Kirschner wire holding the PIP joint in extension may serve as an effective internal splint. ■ It is important to differentiate boutonnière deformity from PIP joint contracture (pseudoboutonnière deformity).
Swan-neck reconstruction	■ In rheumatoid patients, a swan-neck deformity can arise from any of the MCP, PIP, or DIP joints. It is critical to identify which type of deformity is present in order to guide treatment.
Thumb CMC reconstruction	■ Implant interposition arthroplasty may have an increased failure rate due to poor soft tissue restraints and an increased risk of implant dislocation.
PIP joint implant arthroplasty	■ Avoid implant arthroplasty in patients with a severe PIP joint flexion contracture (>45–50 degrees). ■ Consider arthrodesis for the index PIP joint due to lateral stresses on the joint with pinch. ■ A volar approach, in the absence of extensor tendon attenuation, may preserve the extensor mechanism and minimize perioperative adhesions and stiffness. ■ Care should be observed with implant broaching to reduce the risk of implant instability or iatrogenic fracture.

OUTCOMES

Traumatic Deformity Reconstruction

- Surgery for established boutonnière and swan-neck deformities is technically challenging.
- A variety of surgical options exist; there is little consensus regarding a preferred technique.
- There are relatively few studies evaluating the long-term results after surgery for posttraumatic boutonnière and swan-neck deformities. Direct comparisons may be difficult due to the variations in clinical stage at the time of presentation.

Boutonnière Deformity

- Towfigh and Gruber[43] reported on the results of surgical treatment of 114 flexible posttraumatic boutonnière deformities. The central slip was repaired directly, with local tissue, or reconstructed with a tendon graft. Follow-up averaged 40 months. Seventy-eight patients report good or excellent results. Satisfactory results were observed in 22 patients and poor results in 14 patients.
- Meadows et al[24] reported on the results of extensor tenotomy performed on 14 fingers with posttraumatic boutonnière

deformity. The average preoperative PIP joint flexion contracture was 36 degrees. All the digits had DIP joint extension contractures with an average arc of motion from 6.5 degrees of hyperextension to 4.2 degrees of flexion. Postoperatively, DIP flexion improved to 44 degrees. Ten of the digits had an extension lag averaging 13 degrees. Seven digits had improved extension at the PIP joint by an average of 27 degrees.

Swan-Neck Deformity

- Tonkin et al[42] reported outcomes of lateral band tenodesis for swan-neck deformity. Thirty digits with swan-neck deformity of various causes were included. Preoperative PIP joint deformity averaged 16 degrees of hyperextension; this was improved to 11 degrees of flexion postoperatively.
- Reconstruction of the oblique retinacular ligament was first described by Thompson et al.[40] They reported improvement in PIP joint hyperextension and DIP joint flexion with this technique. Kleinman and Peterson[18] described similar results with reliable correction of DIP joint flexion and secondary PIP joint hyperextension.

Chronic Mallet Finger Deformity

- Two biomechanical studies have evaluated Fowler's central slip tenotomy for chronic mallet deformity. Chao et al[7] produced a mallet deformity in 15 cadaver fingers, performed central slip tenotomy, and recorded DIP extensor lags before and after tenotomy. They produced an average extensor lag of 45 degrees from terminal tendon lengthening; after central slip tenotomy, this was corrected on average 36 degrees for an average residual postoperative extensor lag of 9 degrees.
- Hiwatari et al[16] evaluated 16 cadaver fingers in order to quantify the extent of release required to minimize DIP extensor lag and minimize boutonnière deformity. They produced a similar DIP extensor lag of 44 degrees, corrected to an average postoperative lag of 6 degrees with detaching the central slip and lateral bands over two-thirds of the middle phalangeal length, without producing a boutonnière deformity. Four fingers had some extensor lag at the PIP joint, all less than 15 degrees and all with one-half or less phalangeal length release.
- In one series of 23 patients treated with central slip tenotomy[3] on average 42 months after the injury, mean preoperative extensor lag at the DIP was 44 degrees and mean postoperative extensor lag was 7 degrees. Two patients had temporary extensor lags at the PIP joint that responded to splinting.
- Advantages of the procedure include that it is technically straightforward, can be performed under local anesthesia, corrects a swan-neck deformity, and does not require postoperative immobilization, although there is the possibility of iatrogenic extensor lag at the PIP joint and some surgeons prefer not to operate on an uninjured part of the finger and rely on the indirect effect on the injured part.

Rheumatoid Deformity Reconstruction

- There is a relative lack of clinical outcomes studies evaluating the long-term results of surgical management for swan-neck and boutonnière deformities in patients with rheumatoid arthritis.
- Kiefhaber and Strickland[17] reported on the results of surgical treatment for type III swan-neck and stage II boutonnière deformities. In 92 patients undergoing lateral band release, extensor tenolysis, and PIP joint dorsal capsulectomy for type III swan-neck deformity, the authors reported an initial increase of 55 degrees flexion at the PIP joint; however, of 15 fingers assessed at 3 and 12 months postoperatively, there was a 17-degree loss of the early postoperative motion gains. Despite this deterioration of postoperative results, the arc of PIP motion shifted toward flexion, improving functional grasp.
  - In 19 patients undergoing central slip reconstruction for stage II boutonnière deformity, the authors found unpredictable results and reported that the deterioration of postoperative correction was greater with time. Four of 19 patients were able to extend the PIP joint beyond 20 degrees of flexion and 11 of 19 patients had a PIP joint extension deficit of greater than 45 degrees.
- Tonkin et al[41,42] published two separate studies assessing the outcomes of treatment for swan-neck deformities with lateral band translocation and with synovectomy and lateral band release and translocation. Although these studies are limited in their conclusions because of the varying stages of disease and their small patient populations, the trend toward positioning the arc of motion into flexion was observed, similar to the study results of Kiefhaber and Strickland.[17]
- Several long-term clinical outcomes studies of PIP and MCP joint implant arthroplasties have demonstrated poor correction of preoperative swan-neck or boutonnière deformities and in general have reported poorer results with respect to pain relief and range-of-motion recovery as compared to arthroplasties done for conditions of osteoarthritis or post-traumatic arthritis.[6,36,37]
- A review of surgical treatment of varying stages of thumb boutonnière deformity by Terrono et al[39] concluded that MCP joint synovectomy and EPL rerouting for early, correctable boutonnière deformity had a high rate of deformity recurrence (64%). The authors recommend MCP joint arthrodesis for cases of moderate severity with isolated joint involvement, but in severe cases, MCP joint arthroplasty and interphalangeal arthrodesis is considered.

COMPLICATIONS

- Perioperative complications in the treatment of post-traumatic boutonnière and swan-neck deformities can be avoided by careful patient selection, appropriate intervention, and adherence to proper surgical technique.
  - Thorough perioperative patient counseling and education is imperative to avoid unrealistic patient expectations and unanticipated outcomes.
- A successful operative result and the avoidance of perioperative complications in the treatment of a boutonnière or swan-neck deformity in the rheumatoid hand is largely dependent on a thorough preoperative evaluation, correct staging of the pathologic condition, and appropriate timing of operative intervention. Although the goals of reducing pain and improving function are primary, patient education is critical for avoiding unrealistic expectations and unanticipated results.

REFERENCES

1. Aiache A, Barsky AJ, Weiner DL. Prevention of boutonniere deformity. Plast Reconst Surg 1970;46:164–167.
2. Arnett FC, Edworthy SM, Bloch DA, et al. The American Rheumatism Association 1987 revised criteria for classification of rheumatoid arthritis. Arthritis Rheum 1988;31:315–324.

3. Asghar M, Helm RH. Central slip tenotomy for chronic mallet finger. Surgeon 2013;11(5):264–266.
4. Boyer MI, Gelberman RH. Operative correction of swan-neck and boutonniere deformities in the rheumatoid hand. J Am Acad Orthop Surg 1999;7:92–100.
5. Burton RI, Melchior JA. Extensor tendons: late reconstruction. In: Green DP, Hotchkiss RN, Pederson WC, eds. Green's Operative Hand Surgery, ed 4. New York: Churchill Livingstone, 1999:215–221.
6. Carducci T. Potential boutonniere deformity: its recognition and treatment. Orthop Rev 1981;10:121–123.
7. Chao JD, Sarwahi V, Da Silva YS, et al. Central slip tenotomy for the treatment of chronic mallet finger: an anatomic study. J Hand Surg Am 2004;29(2):216–219.
8. Cook SD, Beckenbaugh RD, Redondo J, et al. Long-term follow-up of pyrolytic carbon metacarpophalangeal implants. J Bone Joint Surg Am 1999;81(5):635–648.
9. Coons MS, Green SM. Boutonniere deformity. Hand Clin 1995;11:387–402.
10. Curtis R. Sublimis tenodesis. In: Edmonson AS, Crenshaw AH, eds. Campbell's Operative Orthopaedics, ed 6. St. Louis: CV Mosby, 1980:319.
11. Figgie MP, Inglis AE, Sobel M, et al. Metacarpal phalangeal joint arthroplasty of the rheumatoid thumb. J Hand Surg Am 1990;15(2): 210–216.
12. Flatt AE. The Care of the Arthritic Hand. St. Louis: Quality Medical Publishing, 1995.
13. Fowler SB. Extensor apparatus of the digits. J Bone Joint Surg Br 1949;31-B:477.
14. Gainor BJ, Hummel GL. Correction of rheumatoid swan-neck deformity by lateral band mobilization. J Hand Surg Am 1985;10(3): 370–377.
15. Harris ED Jr. Rheumatoid arthritis: pathophysiology and implications for therapy. N Engl J Med 1990;18:1277–1289.
16. Hiwatari R, Kuniyoshi K, Aoki M, et al. Fractional Fowler tenotomy for chronic mallet finger: a cadaveric biomechanical study. J Hand Surg Am 2012;37(11):2263–2268.
17. Kiefhaber TR, Strickland JW. Soft tissue reconstruction for rheumatoid swan-neck and boutonniere deformities: long-term results. J Hand Surg Am 1993;18(6):984–989.
18. Kleinman WB, Peterson DP. Oblique retinacular ligament reconstruction for chronic mallet finger deformity. J Hand Surg Am 1984;9(3):399–404.
19. Littler JW, Eaton RG. Redistribution of forces in correction of boutonniere deformity. J Bone Joint Surg Am 1967;49(7):1267–1274.
20. Mannerfelt LG, Norman O. Attrition ruptures of flexor tendons in rheumatoid arthritis caused by bony spurs in the carpal tunnel. A clinical and radiological study. J Bone Joint Surg Br 1969;51(2): 270–277.
21. Mannerfelt LG, Oetker R, Ostlund B, et al. Rupture of the extensor pollicis longus tendon after Colles fracture and by rheumatoid arthritis. J Hand Surg Br 1990;15(1):49–50.
22. Massengill JB. The boutonniere deformity. Hand Clin 1992;8:787–801.
23. Matev I. Transposition of the lateral slips of the aponeurosis in treatment of long-standing "boutonniere deformity" of the fingers. Br J Plast Surg 1964;17:281–286.
24. Meadows SE, Schneider LH, Sherwyn JH. Treatment of the chronic boutonniere deformity by extensor tenotomy. Hand Clin 1995;11:441–447.
25. Nalebuff EA. Diagnosis, classification and management of rheumatoid thumb deformities. Bull Hosp Joint Dis 1968;29:119–137.
26. Nalebuff EA. The rheumatoid swan-neck deformity. Hand Clin 1989;5:203–214.
27. Nalebuff EA. The rheumatoid thumb. Clin Rheum Dis 1984;10: 589–607.
28. Nalebuff EA, Millender LH. Surgical treatment of the boutonniere deformity in rheumatoid arthritis. Orthop Clin North Am 1975;6:753–763.
29. O'Brien ET. Surgical principles and planning for the rheumatoid hand and wrist. Clin Plast Surg 1996;23:407–420.
30. Ratliff AH. Deformities of the thumb in rheumatoid arthritis. Hand 1971;3:138–143.
31. Rizio L, Belsky MR. Finger deformities in rheumatoid arthritis. Hand Clin 1996;12:531–540.
32. Rubin J, Bozentha DJ, Bora FW. Diagnosis of closed central-slip injuries. A cadaveric analysis of non-invasive tests. J Hand Surg Br 1996;21(5):614–616.
33. Snow JW. Use of a retrograde tendon flap in repairing a severed extensor at the PIP joint area. Plast Reconstr Surg 1973;51:555–558.
34. Stein AB, Terrono AL. The rheumatoid thumb. Hand Clin 1996;12:541–550.
35. Strickland JW, Boyer M. Swan neck deformity. In: Strickland JW, ed. The Hand: Master Techniques in Orthopaedic Surgery series. Philadelphia: Lippincott-Raven, 1998:459–470.
36. Swanson AB, Maupin BK, Gajjar NV, et al. Flexible implant arthroplasty in the proximal interphalangeal joint in the hand. J Hand Surg Am 1985;10(6 pt 1):796–805.
37. Takigawa S, Meletiou S, Sauerbier M, et al. Long-term assessment of Swanson implant arthroplasty in the proximal interphalangeal joint of the hand. J Hand Surg Am 2004;29(5):785–795.
38. Terrono A, Millender L. Surgical treatment of the boutonniere rheumatoid thumb deformity. Hand Clin 1989;5:239–248.
39. Terrono A, Millender L, Nalebuff E. Boutonniere rheumatoid thumb deformity. J Hand Surg Am 1990;15(6):999–1003.
40. Thompson JS, Littler JW, Upton J. The spiral oblique retinacular ligament (SORL). J Hand Surg Am 1978;3(5):482–487.
41. Tonkin MA, Gianoutsos MP, Ryan D, et al. Synovectomy, joint release and lateral band translocation for stiff swan neck deformity. Hand Surg 1996;1:69–74.
42. Tonkin MA, Hughes J, Smith KL. Lateral band translocation for swan-neck deformity. J Hand Surg Am 1992;17(2):260–267.
43. Towfigh H, Gruber P. Surgical treatment of the boutonniere deformity. Oper Orthop Traumatol 2005;17:66–78.
44. Urbaniak JR, Hayes MG. Chronic boutonniere deformity—an anatomic reconstruction. J Hand Surg Am 1981;6(4):379–383.
45. Zancolli E. Structural and Dynamic Bases of Hand Surgery, ed 2. Philadelphia: JB Lippincott, 1979.

Nerve Injury and Compression

Primary Repair and Nerve Grafting following Complete Nerve Transection in the Hand, Wrist, and Forearm

Matthew E. Hiro and Randy R. Bindra

DEFINITION

- *Complete transection* of a peripheral nerve is defined as interruption of all of the axons within the nerve.
- *Primary nerve repair* is the tension-free reapproximation of severed nerve ends performed within a week of injury.
- *Delayed primary repair* is performed up to 3 weeks from injury when local soft tissue injuries do not permit primary wound closure.
- The healing of an injured peripheral nerve is different from the healing of other tissue types.
- Injury is followed by an immediate degeneration, followed by incomplete recovery.
- Irreversible changes in the motor and sensory end organs make timing of repair critical to achieve useful recovery.

ANATOMY

- The anatomy of the peripheral nerve can be simplified by examining its component parts (**FIG 1**).
- *Axon.* The basic unit of a nerve is composed of a cell body, dendrites, and longer axons.
  - All axons are surrounded by Schwann cells, which produce the myelin sheath surrounding the axon.
  - Interruptions in the myelin sheath are referred to as *nodes of Ranvier*. Impulse propagation is faster in myelinated axons using a process called *saltatory conduction*, as the depolarization potential "jumps" between nodes.
  - Myelinated fibers are between 2 and 22 μm in diameter. The larger the fiber, the faster the conduction speeds.
  - Axonal transport of cytoskeletal elements and neuronal factors is oxygen-dependent. Antegrade transport along the axon occurs at roughly 1 to 4 mm per day. The transport is the rate-limiting step in nerve regeneration.
- *Endoneurium.* Delicate connective tissue that supports and surrounds each axonal fiber and associated Schwann cells
  - Consists of longitudinally arranged collagen fibrils and intrinsic blood vessels
- *Perineurium.* The connective tissue that surrounds groups of axons, creating bundles referred to as *fascicles*. The fascicle is the smallest visible unit of the nerve at surgery.
  - The fascicle is several layers thick and acts as a protective membrane and a barrier to diffusion.
- *Epineurium.* Surrounds groups of fascicles to form the superstructure of a peripheral nerve
  - Forms a sheath about the entire nerve and also supports the fascicular structure by passing between all the fascicles
  - Forms 60% to 85% of the cross-sectional area of a peripheral nerve
  - Composed on longitudinally oriented collagen fibers, fibroblasts, and intrinsic vessels
- *Paraneurium or mesoneurium.* Loose areolar tissue surrounding the epineurium
  - Limited to the outer surface of the nerve
  - Location for the extrinsic vascular supply of the nerve
  - Makes up the gliding apparatus of a peripheral nerve
- Fascicles have a definite topographic arrangement within a peripheral nerve.
  - Fascicular segregation into motor and sensory components is important when aligning a sectioned nerve before primary repair or nerve grafting.
  - This concept of functional segregation allows for use of part of a donor healthy nerve for nerve transfer with minimal functional deficit.

FIG 1 • Schematic of ultrastructure of the nerve. The smallest nerve unit visible to the naked eye is the nerve fascicle.

PATHOGENESIS

- Injuries involving peripheral nerves can be simply classified as tidy or untidy.
- *Tidy wounds* involve sharp transections with minimal to no tissue loss:
  - Sharp lacerations from glass or knife wounds
  - Most iatrogenic nerve injuries
- *Untidy wounds* involve crushing or avulsion of tissues in the area:
  - Bony injury may be present.
  - Surrounding soft tissue may have been lost or rendered nonviable and is expected to heal with significant scarring. This corresponds to the *zone of injury*.

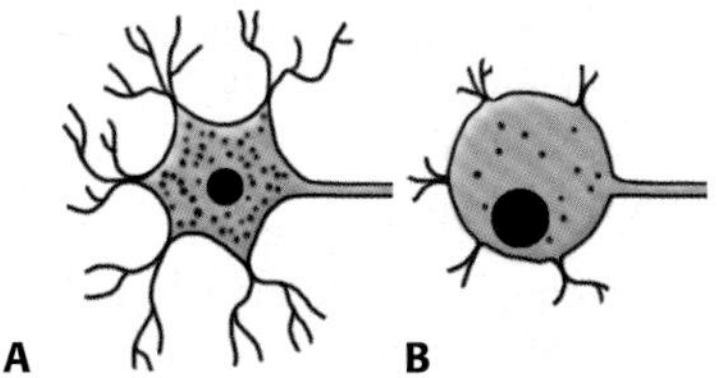

FIG 2 • Comparison of a normal neuron cell body (**A**) with that of a nerve after transection (**B**). Note cellular swelling, dissolution of Nissl granules in the cytoplasm, and retraction of the dendritic processes.

NATURAL HISTORY

- Complete transection of a nerve results in retraction of the nerve ends. The nerve will not heal without surgical intervention to approximate the nerve ends.
- Wallerian degeneration occurs in the nerve segment distal to the level of transection.
  - The axon distal to the injury degenerates and does not directly contribute to repair. The axonal and myelin debris are cleared by macrophages. Schwann cells proliferate, releasing nerve growth factors or neurotrophic factors. The distal stump does produce a complex protein, neurotropic factor, that attracts regenerating axons from the proximal stump.
  - The cell body swells, Nissl granules in the cytoplasm diminish, and its dendritic processes retract. Several cells rupture and die, especially with more proximal nerve injuries (**FIG 2**).
- Regenerating axons sprout from the surviving axons and migrate toward the empty tubules in the degenerate distal stump at a rate of 1 to 3 mm per day.
  - Proliferating Schwann cells myelinate the newly regenerated axons.
  - In an unrepaired nerve, the random proliferation of axons from the proximal stump forms a tender mass of disorganized axons and fibrosis termed a *neuroma*.

PATIENT HISTORY AND PHYSICAL FINDINGS

- History of trauma
  - Penetrating, ballistic, burn, stretch, blunt, fracture, or previous surgery
  - Timing of onset of symptoms: at initial presentation; after procedure, for example, manipulation and casting or internal fixation of a fracture
  - Depth and location of the injury
  - Severity of bleeding-associated blood vessel injury
- Patient reports
  - Paresthesias (pins and needles) or absent sensation (numbness) in fingers
  - Weakness
  - Paralysis due to nerve or associated tendon injury
  - Pain: neurogenic type; can be constant and severe
  - Rarely, a sensation of warmth or anhydrosis
- Physical examination
  - Note the distribution of sensory loss. The area of sensory loss varies with the nerve that is injured (**FIG 3**).
  - Examine the skin for trophic changes or dry skin. Dry, warm skin implies sympathetic interruption.
  - Perform thumb abduction test to check for paralysis of the abductor pollicis brevis from median nerve injury.

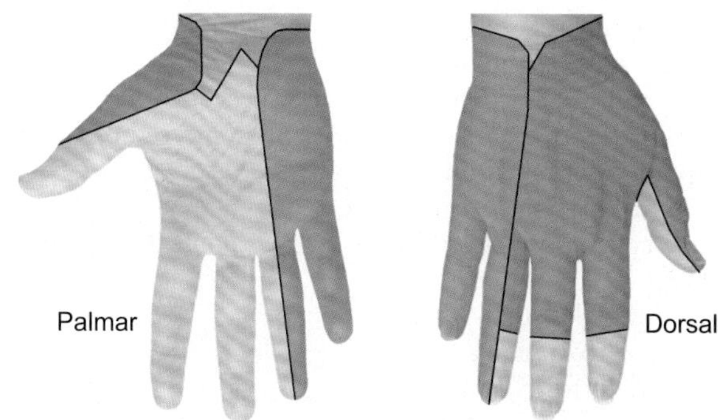

FIG 3 • Distribution of sensory loss with nerve injury. *Yellow*, median nerve; *blue*, ulnar nerve; *pink*, radial nerve.

  - Perform the Froment sign test. The test is positive if paper is held by flexing the thumb interphalangeal (IP) joint, indicating recruitment of the flexor pollicis longus, which implies paralysis of the adductor pollicis from ulnar nerve injury.
  - The thumb IP hyperextension test may indicate paralysis of the extensor pollicis longus due to posterior interosseous palsy.
  - Perform the Tinel sign test. The test is positive if the patient notes a tingling sensation in the sensory distribution of the nerve. Serial progression of Tinel sign distally is useful to monitor axon progression after repair.
- When performing physical examinations, it is helpful to use motor function grading according to the Medical Research Council system. This grading allows for qualitative measurement of function and allows the clinician to chart recovery objectively:
  - M0: no contraction
  - M1: palpable contraction with only a flicker of motion
  - M2: movement of the part with gravity eliminated
  - M3: muscle contraction against gravity
  - M4: ability to contract against moderate resistance
  - M5: normal function
- Quantitative measurements using grip and pinch strength dynamometers and comparing results to the contralateral normal side may also be useful.
- Sensory grading is also useful in evaluation. Sensory function is evaluated within the anatomic distribution of the nerve in question. Sensation is quantified using two complementary tests—(1) Semmes-Weinstein monofilaments, which measure innervation threshold, and (2) two-point discrimination, which measures innervation density. Vibratory, pain, and temperature sensation should also be evaluated. Semmes-Weinstein filaments demonstrate subtle and early sensory loss and are more useful in evaluation of compressive neuropathy. Two-point discrimination measurements help gauge the severity of nerve injury, with two-point discrimination of less than 12 mm indicating neurapraxic injury and readings greater than 15 mm suggesting complete disruption. Used together, the various sensory tests allow for qualitative measurement of function and allow for the clinician to objectively chart recovery:
  - S0: lack of sensation
  - S1: recovery of deep cutaneous pain sensibility within the autonomous area of the nerve

- S2: return of some degree of superficial cutaneous pain and tactile sensibility
- S3: return of function (S2) without evidence of hypersensibility
- S3+: return of function (S3) with some return of two-point discrimination
- S4: normal function

- Sensory recovery classification on two-point discrimination alone:
  - Normal: less than 6 mm
  - Fair: 6 to 10 mm
  - Poor: 11 to 15 mm

IMAGING AND OTHER DIAGNOSTIC STUDIES

- Diagnosis in acute injuries is usually based on history and clinical examination alone without need for additional investigations.
- Plain radiographs are of little use in evaluation of the nerves themselves but may be helpful in cases of injury from fracture or projectiles.
- Computed tomography (CT) myelography is useful for evaluation of injuries to the brachial plexus. The formation of a pseudomeningocele is indicative of root avulsion.
- Magnetic resonance imaging (MRI) is useful for evaluation of peripheral injury but is not routinely indicated for peripheral nerve injuries.
  - Short tau inversion recovery (STIR) MRI may show enhancement of the nerve near the site of injury or interruption of the nerve trunk on T1- and T2-weighted images.
  - MRI provides visualization of pseudomeningoceles at the spinal cord levels in root avulsion injuries.
- Electrodiagnostic testing
  - Nerve conduction velocity (NCV) and electromyography (EMG) are useful in evaluation of closed nerve injuries, for example, after fracture or multiple nerve injuries such as brachial plexus injury.
  - If stimulation distal to the suspected injury elicits a motor response about 3 days after injury, then the lesion is likely a conduction block. However, muscle action may be present in the case of complete transection for up to 9 days.
  - Fibrillation potentials on EMG appear after 2 to 3 weeks and indicate muscle denervation and a severe grade nerve injury.
  - Recovery is best evaluated with serial examination of compound muscle action potentials. Early recovery of only a few motor units may indicate reinnervation from adjacent intact nerves and should not be used as an indicator of recovery of the repaired nerve.

DIFFERENTIAL DIAGNOSIS

- Muscle or tendon injury in open lacerations
- Parsonage-Turner syndrome (brachial plexus neuritis)
- Peripheral nerve entrapment
- Partial nerve injury (neuroma in continuity)
- Neurapraxic injury (axonal dysfunction without discontinuity)

NONOPERATIVE MANAGEMENT

- Nonoperative management of a completely transected nerve after an open injury is doomed to failure because cut ends retract and scar tissue forms in the gap.
- Pending recovery of the nerve, splinting of the paralyzed joint maintains functional position and range-of-motion exercises prevent contractures.
- Serial clinical examination and electrodiagnostic testing are helpful to evaluate recovery.

SURGICAL MANAGEMENT

- Nerves that have been completely interrupted require surgical measures to restore continuity.
- All open injuries with neurologic impairment must be explored expeditiously.
- With closed injuries or delayed presentation, consider the overall functional capacity of the injured limb.
- In a largely motor nerve, for example, the radial nerve, tendon transfers may restore function more reliably than nerve repair.

Preoperative Planning

- The cause of the peripheral nerve injury must be identified. The repaired nerve must have a favorable local environment if the repair is to be successful.
- Underlying fractures must be stabilized.
- Adequate soft tissue coverage of the nerve repair must be planned.
- Repair should be delayed when multiple débridements are necessary until the bed for the repaired nerve is optimal and wound can be primarily closed. If delayed repair is considered, the distal and proximal ends should be identified and tagged with a suture in the epineurium.
- Intraoperative nerve stimulation of motor or mixed (motor and sensory) nerves may assist with identification of the proximal and distal nerve stumps within the first 72 hours after injury. During this interval, residual neurotransmitters are present in the distal nerve and stimulation is still possible.
- If segmental loss is suspected, as with a crushing injury, the patient must give informed consent for additional options such as conduit repair or nerve grafting.
- Injuries that present late should be evaluated with electrophysiologic studies to look for signs of recovery.
- If intraoperative nerve stimulation is to be used, muscle relaxants should be avoided at induction of general anesthesia.
- If associated muscle or tendon lacerations are present, muscle relaxation facilitates their repair.
- Regional anesthetics such as supraclavicular block provide excellent muscle relaxation, and a supraclavicular catheter will help in administering postoperative analgesia. However, the motor blockade from the block will prevent the use of intraoperative nerve stimulation.

Positioning

- The patient is positioned supine, with the arm positioned on a hand table.
- Use of a tourniquet facilitates dissection but will interfere with intraoperative nerve stimulation because it results in ischemic conduction blocks after 15 minutes.
- Use of intraoperative magnification (eg, loupes) for the dissection and a surgical microscope during nerve repair is essential.
- Microinstrumentation is needed for nerve handling and repair. Precise atraumatic dissection technique is necessary for optimal results.
- Alcoholic solutions should be avoided for the preparation of open wounds to avoid chemical damage to nerve tissue.

Approach

- The area of injury should be exposed both proximally and distally to allow for visualization of the proximal and distal nerve stumps using extensile approaches.
- After all injured structures have been assessed, repair fractures and tendons first to take tension off the nerve repair.
- Mobilize nerve ends for about 1 to 2 cm at either end, avoiding unnecessary stripping of the mesoneurium over long distances.
- Preserve the common sheath of neurovascular bundles to maintain nerve vascularity and minimize tension on nerve repair.
- Nerve end preparation is critical. Crushing is present even after sharp lacerations.
- Under an operating microscope, the nerve end is stabilized over a sterile wooden spatula and a fresh no. 11 blade is used to progressively cut back 2-mm segments of the nerve end until sprouting fascicles are seen (**TECH FIG 1**).
- The distal and proximal joints are placed in minimal flexion. Excessive flexion is to be avoided because it will result in flexion contractures or tension on healing nerve.
- Additional length can be gained by transposition of the proximal nerve (eg, ulnar nerve at the elbow) or bone shortening (eg, during replantation surgery).
- End-to-end repair should be attempted as long as this can be accomplished with minimal tension on the repair and with minimal mobilization of the nerve.
- If a single epineurial stitch of 8-0 suture fails to maintain nerve approximation, tension is excessive. Additional mobilization or alternative options such as conduit repair or nerve grafting must be considered.

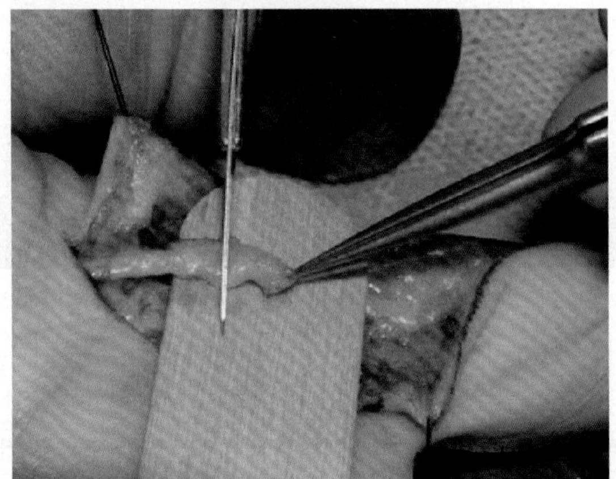

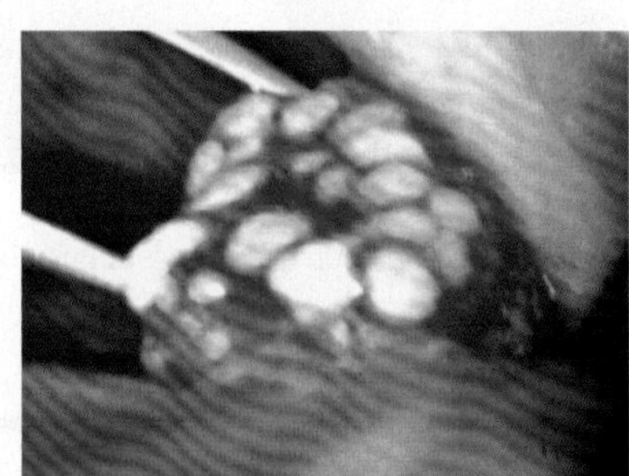

TECH FIG 1 • **A.** Freshening of a lacerated nerve end. The nerve is stretched over a sterile, moistened tongue depressor and cut using a sharp no. 11 scalpel. **B.** Sprouting fascicles must be seen at the cut surface of each nerve end before the repair.

Epineurial Repair

- Epineurial repair, the most common type of nerve repair, consists of alignment and approximation of the nerve ends using sutures placed in the epineurium.
- After clean, pouting bundles of fascicles are exposed, the epineurium is identified circumferentially by resection or pushing back of the mesoneurium.
- Correct alignment of the nerve ends is critical. Line up blood vessels and other external markings in the epineurium and match fascicular bundles in the two ends.
- Suture must be monofilament (eg, nylon) on an atraumatic needle to minimize trauma to the nerve ends. Suture size varies with the size of the nerve. Usually, an 8-0 suture is used in the arm and 9-0 in the fingers. Repair with larger suture dimensions does not add strength to the repair: Sutures fail by pullout of the neural tissue.
- Two simple sutures are placed 180 degrees from one another. Care must be taken to avoid penetrating fascicles with the needle (**TECH FIG 2A**).

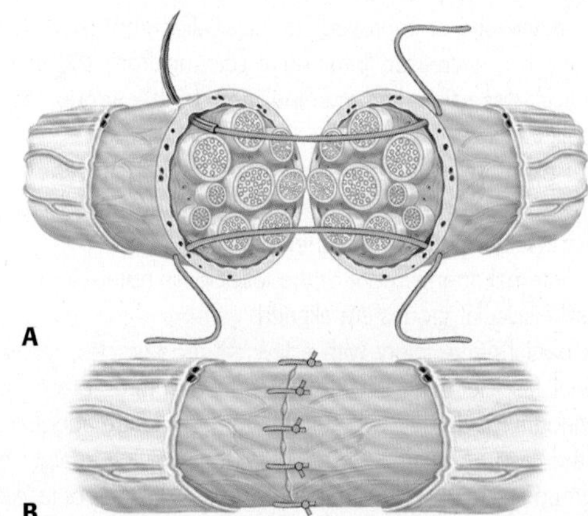

TECH FIG 2 • Steps of epineurial repair. **A.** The nerve ends are aligned, and two sutures are placed 180 degrees from each other. Tension across the repair is tested with two sutures. **B.** Additional sutures are placed in the epineurium.

- One tail of each suture is left long to stabilize the nerve during repair.
- Three or four additional sutures are placed on the anterior face of the repair as necessary to approximate the epineurium and prevent fascicular extrusion (**TECH FIG 2B**).
- By flexing the limb further to relax the nerve, the nerve is turned over, using the suture tails, to expose the posterior wall. Each suture tail can be weighed down with a small vascular clip.
- Posterior wall repair is completed with three or four simple epineurial sutures, as needed.
- The long tails are then cut short, and the nerve is examined carefully to ensure that a complete epineurial seal is achieved (**TECH FIG 3**).

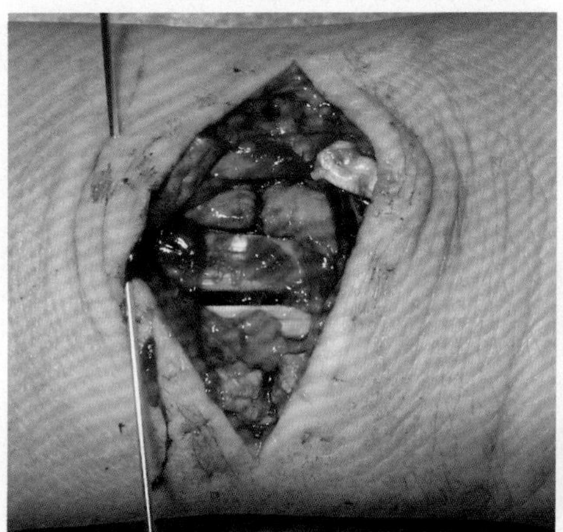

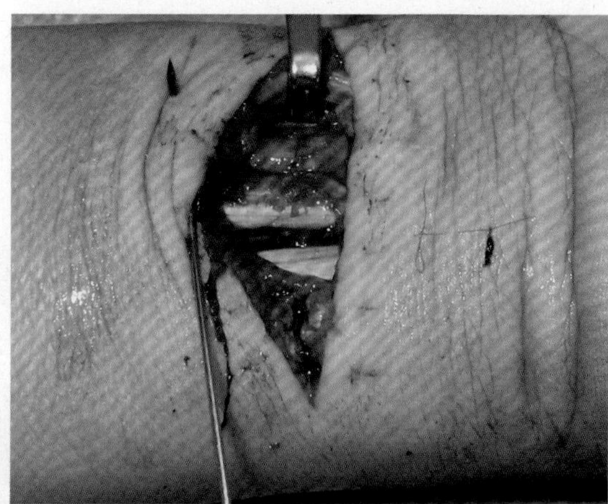

TECH FIG 3 • **A.** A laceration injury of the forearm, just proximal to the wrist. The palmaris longus tendon and the median nerve have been transected. **B.** Epineurial repair using interrupted, circumferential sutures.

Group Fascicular Repair

- Groups of nerve fascicles are approximated by perineurial sutures (**TECH FIG 4**).
- Group fascicular repair is indicated for partial nerve injury involving a few groups of fascicles or in a mixed nerve with distinct motor and sensory components, such as the median nerve proximal to the wrist.
- The advantage of improved fascicular alignment may be counteracted by increased intraneural scarring from the increased surgical dissection and manipulation of the group fascicular repair.
- After exposing clean, pouting bundles of fascicles, the epineurium is resected back for 5 mm to clearly exposed groups of fascicles surrounded by perineurium.
- The internal arrangement of the fascicles is noted, and similarly sized fascicular groups are aligned.
- For partial nerve injury with a few injured fascicles, repair individual fascicles with 10-0 nylon simple sutures placed in the perineurium. Usually, two sutures per fascicle are adequate.
- In the case of a complete nerve injury involving a larger nerve, a group fascicular repair that approximates groups of fascicles is faster and less traumatic.
- When approximating larger groups of fascicles, four to six sutures are placed per group in a circumferential pattern. For additional stability, sutures at the external surface of the fascicular group should be passed through both the epineurium and perineurium. (These sutures are known as *epiperineurial sutures*.)
- After completion of fascicular repair, four additional sutures of 9-0 nylon are placed in the epineurium to take tension off the repair.

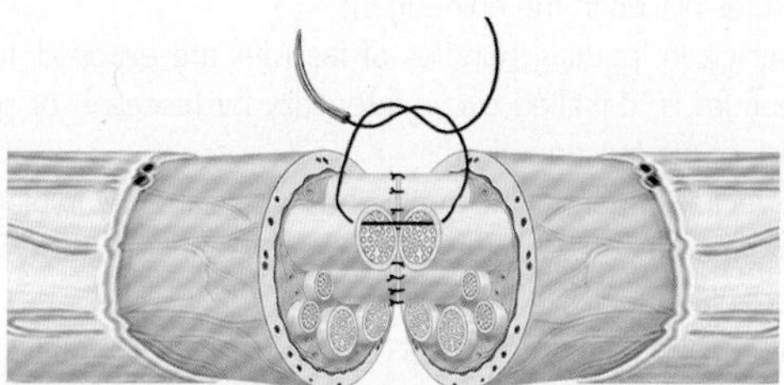

TECH FIG 4 • Technique of group fascicular repair. The epineurium is pulled back, and sutures are placed in the perineurium after fascicular groups have been aligned.

Cable Graft Repair

- Nerve grafting is indicated when end-to-end approximation is not possible, for example, after crushing of the nerve ends, retraction of nerve ends after delay in surgical intervention, or after neuroma resection.
- After the nerve ends are prepared back to pouting bundles of fascicles, the epineurium is identified circumferentially.
- The internal arrangement of the fascicles is noted, and a quick sketch of the fascicular arrangement helps to plan graft alignment (**TECH FIG 5**).
  - An understanding of the normal topography is essential, as the relative position of sensory and motor fascicles changes along the length of the nerve. For example, the deep motor component of the ulnar nerve travels centrally in the proximal forearm, between the dorsal sensory component and the volar sensory component. In the distal forearm and wrist, the deep motor component is positioned dorsally and radially.
- Epineurium is resected to expose the perineurium of the fascicles.
- The gap between the prepared nerve ends is measured.
- When grafting a larger diameter nerve such as the median nerve using a smaller diameter nerve such as the sural nerve, several strands of donor nerve are interposed in the gap as a cable graft.
- The length of nerve graft needed is calculated as follows: graft length = gap + 15% × estimated number of strands
- Donor nerves include the sural (located midway between the lateral border of the tendo Achilles and the lateral malleolus), posterior interosseous (located in the floor of the fourth extensor compartment), and the medial antebrachial cutaneous nerve (located in the anteromedial forearm along branches of the basilic vein).
- The graft must be kept moist from harvest until wound closure.
- Each segment of graft is reversed and attached to a similar-sized group of fascicles at the proximal stump using two sutures of 9-0 nylon, 180 degrees from one another.
- Although the donor nerve allows growth of regenerating axons in either direction, reversing the nerve graft helps to minimize the possibility of regenerating axons growing out along branches of the donor nerve.
- Place the limb in a neutral position; then lay the graft in the defect and align it with a similar fascicular group in the distal stump. The graft is cut and sutured to the distal stump fascicles.
- Follow the same sequence, laying segments of graft across the gap until the gap is filled.
- The repair can be reinforced with fibrin glue placed at the anastomosis and between segments of the graft.

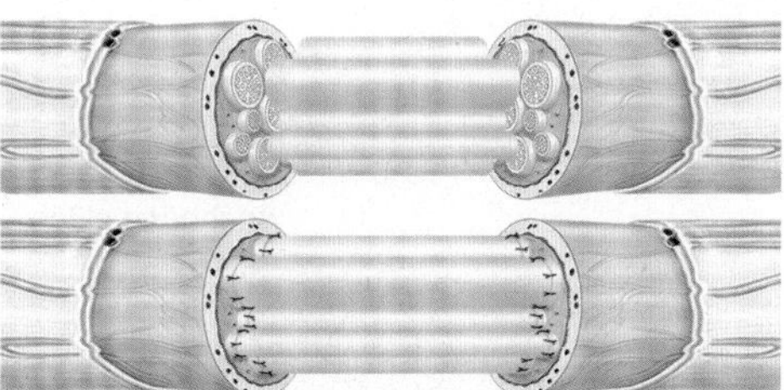

TECH FIG 5 • Nerve grafting using "cables" of nerve graft. After aligning the nerve ends, similar fascicular groups are bridged with segments of nerve graft.

Vascularized Nerve Graft Repair

- Vascularized nerve graft repair may be indicated in cases when the gap is 6 cm or more or in a scarred tissue bed in large proximal nerve reconstruction after brachial plexus injuries.
- The most common vascularized nerve graft donor is the ulnar nerve (following C8 and T1 root avulsion), along with its mesoneurium, containing the superior ulnar collateral vessels.
- For local nerve defects, the ulnar nerve segment is divided, preserving the vascular pedicle. The segment is transposed with its intact pedicle, and epineurial repair is performed.
- If a more remote defect is to be grafted, the vascular pedicle and nerve segment are divided. The nerve is reversed and placed in the defect. Following epineurial repair, microvascular anastomosis is performed between the artery and vein in the vascular leash to a local arterial and venous recipient vessel.
- Other vascularized nerve options include the superficial radial nerve (with radial artery), the vascularized sural nerve (with arterialized lesser saphenous vein), and the vascularized saphenous nerve (with arterialized greater saphenous vein).
- Proposed benefits include faster regeneration due to viable Schwann cells and axons, although no comparative studies have demonstrated a benefit over conventional nerve grafts.

Conduit Repair

- Conduit repair is indicated for clinical use in nerve gaps up to 3 cm.
- Advantages over conventional repair are that it is tension free, less traumatic, permits no axonal escape, and allows spontaneous axonal orientation.
- Two types are in clinical use: reversed autogenous vein or artificial conduits.
  - Artificial conduits may be either manufactured using absorbable materials such as polyglycolic acid and caprolactone or made of collagen engineered from natural xenograft sources such as bovine tendon. Artificial conduits have obvious advantages over a vein conduit in regard to shelf availability, size variation, no additional dissection for harvesting, and resilience and elasticity. Collagen tubes degrade over time with natural processes and without any inflammatory reaction.
  - After nerve end preparation, the nerve diameter is measured. A conduit that is oversized by 1 mm is chosen to avoid constriction of the regenerating nerve.
  - The conduit is rehydrated in saline for 5 minutes.

- The aim of repair is to insert each end of the nerve into the tube for a distance of 5 to 8 mm using a mattress suture followed by a single anchoring suture for stability (**TECH FIG 6**).
- The suture is first passed through the tube from the outside in and about 5 mm from the tube edge. The suture is then passed transversely across the epineurium 3 mm from the edge of the nerve stump and then back through the tube in an inside-to-outside direction.
- Gently ease the nerve into the tube as the knot is tightened.
- Place a simple suture between the epineurium and the edge of the tube at a diametrically opposite point to anchor the tube and prevent rotation.
- Repeat the same steps for the distal stump and fill the tube with saline using a fine cannula (**TECH FIG 7**).

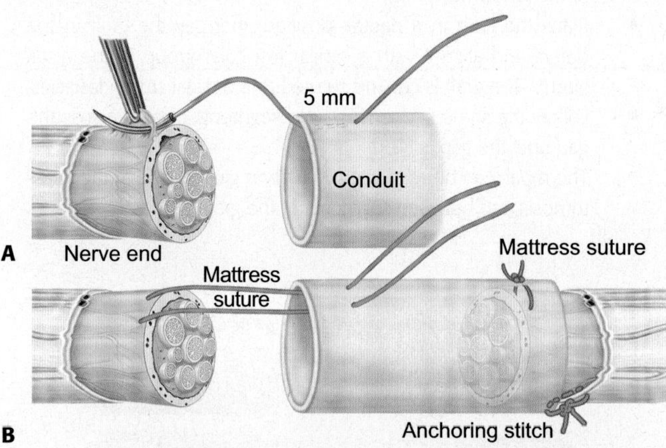

TECH FIG 6 • Technique of conduit repair. **A.** A horizontal mattress suture is placed between the conduit and the epineurium of the nerve. **B.** As the suture is tightened, the nerve is drawn into the conduit. A simple stitch is placed anchoring the epineurium to the tube opposite the location of the mattress suture.

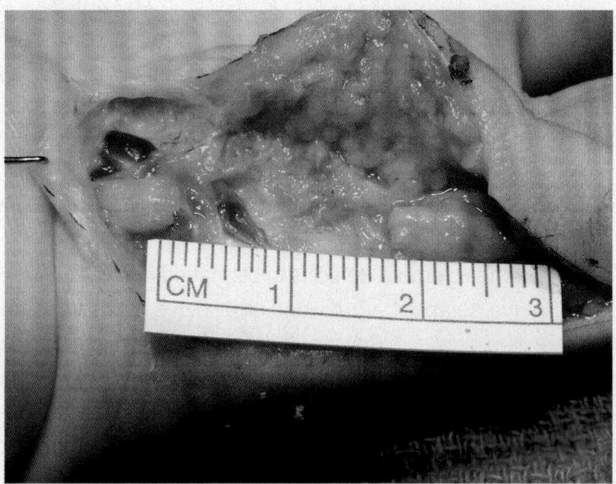

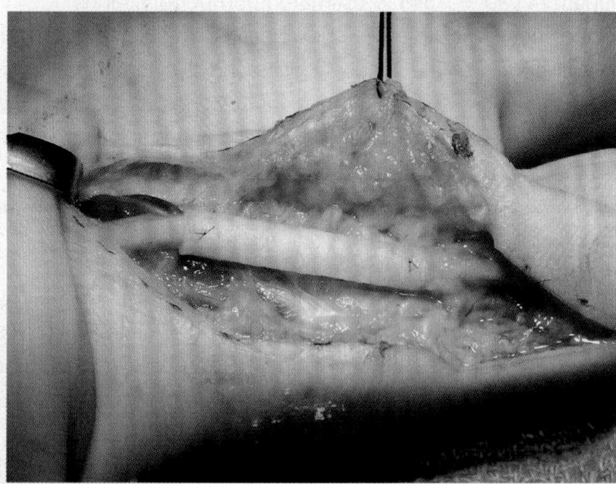

TECH FIG 7 • **A.** Digital nerve injury with a 2-cm gap. The edges have been trimmed back to healthy fascicles. **B.** Nerve repair using a type I collagen conduit to bridge the gap between the nerve ends.

Cadaver Allograft Repair

- Allograft repair is indicated in sensory, motor, and mixed nerve injuries with gaps up to 50 mm.
- Previous allografts required immunosuppression to prevent graft-versus-host disease and rejection. The immunosuppression was only necessary until adequate host Schwann cells migrated across the graft (usually approximately 24 months). Common immunosuppressants (tacrolimus) have been shown to augment neuroregeneration.
- Modern allografts are acellular and must be repopulated with recipient Schwann cells from the proximal nerve stump. Autograft is already populated with autogenous Schwann cells, making autograft a superior graft material. Once the nerve ends are prepared, the nerve diameter at the proximal and distal stumps and the defect length are measured.
- Acellular allograft comes in varying diameters (1 to 5 mm) and various lengths (15 to 70 mm). As with nerve autograft, a graft slightly longer than the measured defect should be chosen to allow a tension-free repair.
- After the appropriately sized graft is chosen, the graft should be thawed using room temperature saline until it is soft and pliable (5 to 10 minutes).
- The allograft should be sutured into position using an epineurial suture technique as described earlier (see **TECH FIG 2A,B**). Cable grafting with allograft can also be used for larger nerves (see **TECH FIG 4**).

Nerve Transfers

- Nerve transfers are indicated in devastating or chronic nerve injuries that are not amenable to primary reconstructive strategies. For example, in the cases of high (proximal) nerve injuries with complete axonal loss and wallerian degeneration, primary reconstructive strategies require the nerve to regenerate from the proximal stump, across the reconstructed gap, and distal to the motor endplates or sensory distribution of the nerve. This regeneration is slow (approximately 1 to 3 mm per day) and may not result in motor endplate reinnervation prior to muscle atrophy.
- With greater understanding of motor and sensory nerve topography, expendable donor nerves have been identified. Multiple donor nerves have been described and catalogued, offering several options for particularly troublesome nerve deficits.
- Keys to nerve transfer surgery include the following:
  - Wide exposure.
  - Precise understanding of the internal topography of the donor and recipient nerves. Transfer often requires intrafascicular dissection of the donor and recipient nerve from the main trunk. Use of a nerve stimulator greatly assists in this technique so be mindful of muscle relaxants and tourniquet palsy during these procedures.
  - Meticulous dissection technique.
    - Use of a microscope and microsurgical instruments is recommended.
    - Iatrogenic injury to the main trunk of the donor nerve may lead to significant morbidity.
  - Tension-free transfer. When designing the transfer, remember "donor distal" and "recipient proximal." The donor nerve should be dissected as distal as possible and the recipient nerve as proximal as possible to allow easy transposition and tension-free repair. If possible, the repair should be lax enough to allow passive range of motion of adjacent joints as well. Often, nerve transposition is required to allow free joint motion without compromising the repair.
  - End-to-end repair. Although end-to-side transfers have been described, end-to-end repair is preferable.

PEARLS AND PITFALLS

Intraoperative precautions	▪ If contemplating intraoperative nerve stimulation, avoid muscle relaxants and tourniquets. ▪ Repair bones and tendons before undertaking fragile nerve repair. ▪ Proceed with nerve repair only if the wound bed is clean and healthy and primary closure is possible. ▪ If delayed repair is planned, place a marking suture in the epineurium to facilitate later identification.
Nerve precautions	▪ Limit handling of nerve and use microsurgical instruments. ▪ Use operating microscope to prepare nerve ends and for fascicular alignment. ▪ Always be prepared to use graft or conduit rather than suture nerve under tension or with joints excessively flexed. ▪ Keep nerves (including grafts) moist. ▪ Repair should be tension free. ▪ Soft tissue coverage is a must.
Instrumentation	▪ Make certain that microinstrumentation is in good repair. ▪ Forceps should be free of spurs and should approximate correctly. ▪ Use 8-0 or 9-0 suture with atraumatic taper-point needles.

POSTOPERATIVE CARE

- Consider use of a local anesthesia infusion pump for postoperative pain control.
- Immobilization is very important to prevent tension across the repair:
  - The elbow should be held at 90 degrees of flexion.
  - Wrist flexion greater than 20 degrees should be avoided.
  - The metacarpophalangeal joints should be held at 70 degrees of flexion.
- Mobilization varies with associated tendon repair. After isolated nerve repair, gentle finger flexion and shoulder range of motion are started soon after surgery to promote nerve gliding and prevent finger stiffness.
- Remove skin sutures after 2 weeks and replace the splint.
- For nerve repairs around the elbow, allow motion in an extension-blocking splint. Full extension is permitted after 6 weeks.
- For repairs in the distal forearm and wrist level, immobilize the wrist at 20 degrees flexion and block metacarpophalangeal hyperextension for 4 weeks. Allow active finger motion within the splint. Bring the wrist to neutral at 4 weeks, and then allow mobilization out of the splint at 6 weeks.
- Nerve regeneration is followed at regular intervals with clinical examination of motor and sensory recovery and Tinel sign.
  - The distal most point at which the Tinel sign is observed is recorded at each visit and its distance from the suture line noted.
  - Expect distal progression of Tinel sign at the rate of about 1 mm per day, with a delay of 1 month after the date of repair.
  - Failure of Tinel progression over serial visits may indicate repair failure: Consider reexploration and grafting.
- Sensory reeducation is initiated early in the postoperative phase with the goal of teaching recognition of new input in a useful manner.

- Three stages to this process are introduced sequentially in the recovery period:
  - *Desensitization:* The patient is presented with graded stimuli to decrease unpleasant sensations.
  - *Early-phase discrimination and localization:* The patient works with static and moving touch, using visual reinforcement.
  - *Late-phase discrimination and tactile gnosis:* The patient works with varying shaped objects.
- Until motor recovery has occurred, regular range-of-motion exercises should continue to prevent joint stiffness or contractures. Strengthening exercises are slowly added after return of voluntary motor function.
- After nerve transfer surgery, the patient must adapt to a new neural pathway from the cerebral cortex. Motor reeducation involves prescribed exercises using voluntary simultaneous contracture of the donor and recipient muscles.

OUTCOMES

- The outcome after nerve repair is generally less favorable than that of repair of other tissues, such as bone or tendon injury.
- It is difficult to predict the outcome because of several variables, including type of nerve (pure sensory vs. mixed), age of patient, and type of injury—clean or crushed, associated soft tissue injuries.
- The single most important factor that correlates with outcome is patient age. The best results are seen in children younger than 10 years of age.
- Pure motor or pure sensory nerves fare better than mixed nerves.
- The outcome also correlates with level of injury. Injuries closer to the end organs fare better because there is less distance for the regenerating axons to cover.
- Peripheral factors that are determined by the injury and cannot be modified by the treating surgeon include axonal cell death, end organ atrophy, and extensive scarring from surrounding crush injury.
- The surgeon can control, to a limited extent, the scarring in and around the nerve repair.
- Central factors that account for poor results include cortical remapping and reorganization, with reduced and disorganized cortical representation of denervated areas.
- Children recover greater function than their adult counterparts with primarily repaired lesions at similar levels due to a combination of better axonal regeneration and cortical plasticity.
- Delayed repairs fare worse than those repaired acutely, with an estimated 1% decrease in performance for every 6 days of delay in the repair.
- The nature of the injury often determines the likelihood of recovery. Massive soft tissue injury or burns involving a peripheral nerve are less likely to regain function than injuries involving sharp or limited transection of a nerve.
- Median nerve outcome after high injuries usually is poor because of hand intrinsic atrophy. After low injuries, useful motor function is regained in 40% to 90% of repairs and useful sensation is restored in 53% to 100% of patients.
- Ulnar nerve injuries show similarly poor results for motor recovery, with functional restoration in 35% of cases and functional sensory recovery in 30% to 68% of cases.
- Because the radial nerve is largely a motor nerve, better results can be expected after acute radial nerve repairs, with functional return in 60% to 75% of patients. Poor results are noted with high injuries, however.
- After repair of digital nerves, about 50% of patients regain static two-point discrimination of less than 10 mm. Younger children demonstrate near-normal sensory recovery due to their cortical adaptability.
- Conduit repair appears superior to primary end-to-side repair in digital nerve reconstruction with gaps less than 4 mm (excellent sensory recovery in 91% vs. 49%) and to standard nerve grafting in digital nerve gaps greater than 8 mm (excellent sensory recovery 42% vs. 0%).
- Lingering symptoms of hypersensitivity and cold intolerance are common with sensory nerve injury in the upper extremity, resolving in most patients after 2 to 3 years. The cause is unclear.
- Complex regional pain syndrome is more likely to be present after untreated nerve injuries. If it does occur, significant joint contractures and atrophic changes can result and the patient generally has a prolonged recovery period and a poor outcome.

COMPLICATIONS

- Causes for failure of repair include the following:
  - Tension on the initial repair
  - An unfavorable local tissue environment with excessive scarring
  - Noncompliance with protective measures or therapy and consequent joint contractures
- Painful neuromas usually form in unrepaired or poorly repaired nerves close to the surface. These usually are treated with desensitization, local padding, and so forth because surgical results are often disappointing.
- Altered sensation is a result of axonal misdirection and cortical misrepresentation and can present as loss of temperature sensation or cold intolerance, hyperesthesia, or neuropathic pain.
- Some amount of altered function is inevitable after all complete nerve injuries in the upper extremity except in young children. It is due to a combination of altered sensation and proprioception along with loss of motor strength.
- Complex regional pain syndrome type II can occur after nerve injury especially in untreated cases or after delayed treatment or failure to control pain. Typical features include dramatic changes in the color and temperature of the skin accompanied by intense burning pain, skin sensitivity, sweating, and swelling. Early recognition is the key with referral to a pain management specialist for stellate blocks along with steroids, antiepileptic drugs, and therapy.

SUGGESTED READINGS

1. al-Ghazal SK, McKiernan M, Khan K, et al. Results of clinical assessment after primary digital nerve repair. J Hand Surg Br 1994;19:255–257.
2. Birch R. Nerve repair. In: Green DP, Hotchkiss RN, Pederson WC, et al, eds. Green's Operative Hand Surgery, ed 5. Philadelphia: Elsevier Churchill Livingstone, 2005:1075–1112.
3. Birch R, Bonney C, Wynn Parry CB. Surgical Disorders of the Peripheral Nerves. Edinburgh: Churchill Livingstone, 1998.
4. Birch R, Raji AR. Repair of median and ulnar nerves. Primary suture is best. J Bone Joint Surg Br 1991;73(1):154–157.
5. Brown JM, Mackinnon SE. Nerve transfers in the forearm and hand. Hand Clin 2008;24:319–340.

6. Chaise F, Friol JP, Gaisne E. Results of emergency repair of wounds of palmar collateral nerves of the fingers [in French]. Rev Chir Orthop Reparatrice Appar Mot 1993;79:393–397.
7. Cho MS, Rinker BD, Weber RV, et al. Functional outcome following nerve repair in the upper extremity using processed nerve allograft. J Hand Surg Am 2012;37(11):2340–2349.
8. Clark WL, Trumble TE, Swiontkowski MF, et al. Nerve tension and blood flow in a rat model of immediate and delayed repairs. J Hand Surg Am 1992;17:677–687.
9. de Medinaceli L, Prayon M, Merle M. Percentage of nerve injuries in which primary repair can be achieved by end-to-end approximation: review of 2,181 nerve lesions. Microsurgery 1993;14: 244–246.
10. Giddins GE, Wade PJ, Amis AA. Primary nerve repair: strength of repair with different gauges of nylon suture material. J Hand Surg Am 1989;14:301–302.
11. Goldberg SH, Jobin CM, Hayes AG, et al. Biomechanics and histology of intact and repaired digital nerves: an in vitro study. J Hand Surg Am 2007;32:474–482.
12. Goldie BS, Coates CJ, Birch R. The long term result of digital nerve repair in no-man's land. J Hand Surg Br 1992;17:75–77.
13. Hudson DA, de Jager LT. The spaghetti wrist. Simultaneous laceration of the median and ulnar nerves with flexor tendons at the wrist. J Hand Surg Br 1993;18:171–173.
14. McAllister RM, Gilbert SE, Calder JS, et al. The epidemiology and management of upper limb peripheral nerve injuries in modern practice. J Hand Surg Br 1996;21:4–13.
15. Parry CB, Salter M. Sensory re-education after median nerve lesions. Hand 1976;8:250–257.
16. Puckett CL, Meyer VH. Results of treatment of extensive volar wrist lacerations: the spaghetti wrist. Plast Reconstr Surg 1985;75:714–721.
17. Shergill G, Bonney G, Munshi P, et al. The radial and posterior interosseous nerves. Results of 260 repairs. J Bone Joint Surg Br 2001;83:646–649.
18. Sullivan DJ. Results of digital neurorrhaphy in adults. J Hand Surg Br 1985;10:41–44.
19. Weber RA, Breidenbach WC, Brown RE, et al. A randomized prospective study of polyglycolic acid conduits for digital nerve reconstruction in humans. Plast Reconstr Surg 2000;106:1036–1045.

Surgical Treatment of Nerve Injuries in Continuity

Matthew E. Hiro and Randy R. Bindra

DEFINITION

- A *nerve injury in continuity* occurs when there is loss of axonal function with preserved structure of the supportive connective tissue.
  - By definition, the epineurium is preserved in a nerve injury in continuity.
- Because varying degrees of axonal interruption may occur, the extent of functional loss in terms of numbness and paralysis is variable.
- The severity of injury varies with degree of preservation of the endoneurium and the perineurium.

ANATOMY

- The cross-sectional anatomy of the peripheral nerve is discussed in detail in Chapter 88.
- Endoneurial tubes form the basic conduit for the Schwann cell–encased axon.

PATHOGENESIS

- Several mechanisms may cause a nerve injury in continuity, but the most common is nerve stretch.
  - When a nerve is subject to blunt injury or stretch, axonal disruption can occur without externally visible injury to the nerve.
  - Stromal elements are more resilient to stretch and remain preserved to a variable extent (**FIG 1**).

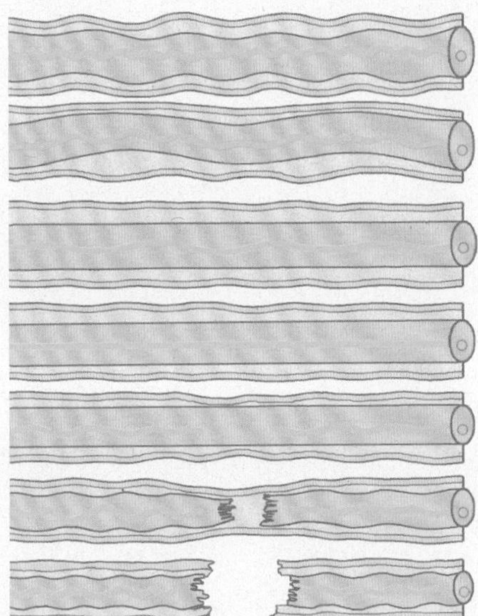

FIG 1 • Pathogenesis of a nerve injury in continuity. The effect of increasing stretch is seen, from normal nerve at the *top* to complete rupture at the *bottom*. Neural elements fail first in response to stretch; epineurium fails last.

  - The type of recovery seen after an injury depends on preservation of the endoneurial tube.
- In the mildest forms of injury, with preserved endoneurial tubes, regenerating axons follow their original path. The destination is reached with good outcome. There is no axonal mismatch, and the recovery is termed *uncomplicated regeneration*.
- When the endoneurial tube is disrupted, axonal regeneration is disorganized. Axons sprout and grow in a different direction and mismatch occurs. This form of repair, termed *complex regeneration*, is associated with a clinically less satisfactory outcome.
- With more severe forms of stretch injury, additional disruption of the perineurium occurs, resulting in a greater fibrotic response and resultant scarring of the nerve.
  - The nerve trunk, which externally appears uninterrupted due to the intact epineurium, demonstrates an injured segment that is enlarged due to intraneural fibrosis surrounding a mass of disorganized axons. This is referred to as a *neuroma in continuity* (**FIG 2**).

NATURAL HISTORY

- Pathoanatomy associated with the injury, pathologic changes resulting from this altered anatomy, and functional recovery are closely related.
- More anatomic disruption results in a stronger pathologic response and worse outcome.
- Sunderland's classification of injury severity is useful to categorize injury and plan treatment.
  - Type I
    - The mildest form of injury involves loss of axonal function without actual structural interruption: *neurapraxia* (**FIG 3A**).
    - Type I injury is seen after mild stretch injuries, tourniquet palsy, and external compression of a nerve, as in radial nerve compression in "Saturday night palsy."
    - Although structurally intact, axons fail to conduct impulses, secondary to malfunction of ion channels along the injured segment.

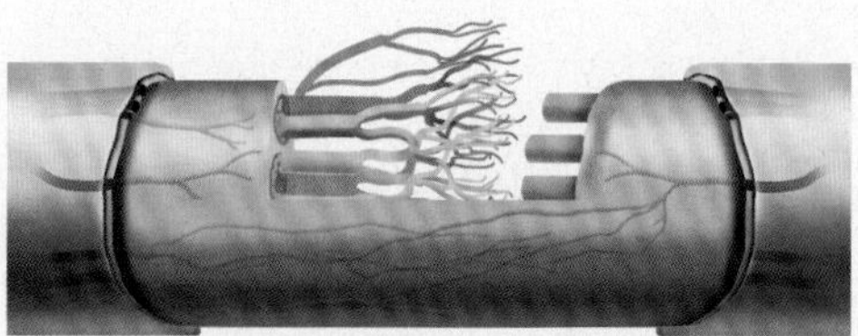

FIG 2 • Neuroma in continuity. The enlarged part of the nerve consists of a mixture of intact and damaged axons surrounded by scar tissue and regenerating axons.

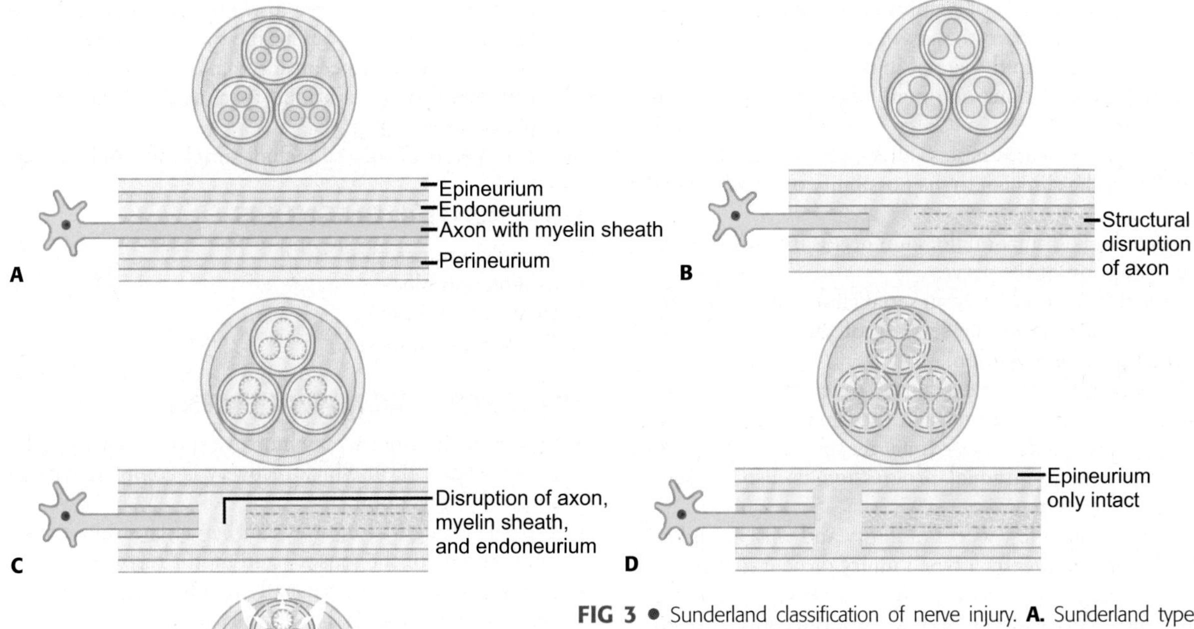

FIG 3 • Sunderland classification of nerve injury. **A.** Sunderland type I, neurapraxia. Nerve injury demonstrating preserved nerve structure with functional loss **B.** Sunderland type II, axonotmesis. Preservation of the endoneurial tube with wallerian degeneration of the distal axon. **C.** Sunderland type III. The fascicular structure is preserved due to intact perineurium. As the endoneurium is disrupted, regenerating axons wander within the fascicle, resulting in a less optimal recovery. **D.** Sunderland type IV. A severe disruption of the nerve. Although the epineurium is intact, loss of fascicular organization makes recovery unlikely without surgical intervention. **E.** Sunderland type V, neurotmesis. Complete structural disruption with loss of continuity.

- No visible change in the microscopic or macroscopic appearance of the nerve is present, and there is no wallerian degeneration of the distal segment.
- Electrophysiologic testing does not reveal a conduction block or denervation potentials.
- Recovery starts within a few weeks and can be expected to be complete.
- Because axons recover conductivity in a variable pattern, clinical recovery follows a random pattern.

- Type II
  - There is structural disruption of the axon, but the endoneurium is preserved (**FIG 3B**).
  - Type II injury is seen after more severe stretch injuries, such as radial nerve palsy resulting from a closed humerus fracture.
  - Wallerian degeneration results and electrophysiologic tests reveal distal conduction block and denervation.
  - As regenerating axons progress distally, proximal muscles are reinnervated first. Clinically, recovery occurs in a proximal to distal direction.
  - Because there is no axonal mismatch, recovery usually is complete but takes longer, usually several months.
- Type III
  - The axon, myelin sheath, and endoneurium are interrupted (**FIG 3C**).
  - Recovery is less predictable because regenerating axons may not follow previous pathways (complicated regeneration).
  - With the perineurium preserved, recovery can take place without surgical intervention but usually is incomplete due to axonal misdirection.
  - Injury to small vessels within the endoneurium leads to an inflammatory response. Fibroblast activation results in a variable degree of interfascicular scarring that may impede nerve regeneration.
- Type IV
  - In more severe stretch injuries, the internal nerve structure is completely disrupted, leaving only an intact epineurium (**FIG 3D**).
  - Retraction of fascicles and scarring within the nerve are present. Even though the nerve is in continuity, no clinically significant recovery can be expected without surgical intervention.
- Type V
  - Complete rupture or laceration of the nerve with retraction of the nerve ends (see Chap. 113) (**FIG 3E**)
- Type VI
  - Mixed injuries with components of types I to V

PATIENT HISTORY AND PHYSICAL FINDINGS

- Stretch injuries that result in nerve injury in continuity usually are proximal. These injuries often take place as the nerve root exits the spinal cord or involve the brachial plexus in the neck or upper arm.
  - At more distal levels, nerve stretch injuries usually are the result of displaced fractures or dislocations.

- There usually is a history of significant trauma, and patients complain of pain and paresthesias with a variable amount of functional loss distal to the site of injury.
  - Incomplete loss of function often indicates an incomplete nerve injury.
  - Severe pain or paresthesias after any closed fracture should alert the clinician to the possibility of an associated nerve injury.
  - Complete loss of function does not necessarily imply complete disruption of the nerve.
- Documented lack of recovery on serial clinical examinations is essential to determine the severity of the injury and the need for surgical intervention.
  - Muscle strength is charted against a timeline at every visit. Progressive muscle recovery in a proximal to distal direction indicates spontaneous axonal regeneration.
  - Tinel sign and its gradual progression is also a useful measure of nerve recovery.
  - Recovery within a few weeks of injury and with a random pattern usually suggests a type I injury or neurapraxia.
- After incomplete injury to a peripheral nerve, function is lost in a predictable order: motor, proprioception, touch, temperature, pain, and sympathetic function.
  - Recovery usually occurs in the reverse order.
- In a closed injury without any obvious fractures, the site of nerve injury is not always obvious.
  - Careful mapping of the motor and sensory deficit will help to distinguish the level of injury.
  - The pattern of sensory loss is a reliable way to determine the level of injury. A more proximal injury usually follows a dermatomal pattern, whereas a distal injury follows the distribution of the nerve.

IMAGING AND OTHER DIAGNOSTIC STUDIES

- Magnetic resonance imaging (MRI) done several weeks after injury may reveal an enlarged nerve segment, suggesting a neuroma in continuity.
- Neurophysiologic studies are useful in evaluating and monitoring an injured nerve when there is no external injury.
  - Conduction blocks usually reverse within 10 to 14 days; therefore, tests should be delayed until this time.
  - Complete loss of muscle action potentials does not necessarily indicate a complete interruption of all axons.
  - Electromyograms (EMGs) will show variable denervation of muscle groups innervated by the nerve in question.
  - Fibrillation potentials on EMG usually appear within 10 to 40 days, indicating complete denervation of a muscle group.
- Electromyographic evidence of reinnervation may precede voluntary muscle contraction by several weeks and may be of use in tracking the progress of nerve regeneration.
  - Return of a muscle action potential requires not only regeneration of the nerve to the level of the end organ but also reestablishment of a physiologic connection between the nerve and the target tissue. Reestablishment of the motor endplate is required before EMG provides evidence of functional return.
- Nerve conduction studies (NCSs) also are useful in the evaluation of a closed nerve injury.
  - In a closed injury, lesions may be localized using NCSs.
  - Continuity of the nerve also may be assessed but should be undertaken at about 10 days after the injury to prevent erroneous results because the axons distal to a complete transection may continue to conduct during this initial period after injury.
  - Parameters evaluated include amplitude and latency.

DIFFERENTIAL DIAGNOSIS

- Complete transection
- Conduction block
- Partial axonal injury
- Compressive injury

NONOPERATIVE MANAGEMENT

- Lesions in continuity may improve spontaneously, especially in types I and II, in which recovery is complete without any surgical intervention.
- Types I through III injuries can be watched closely with serial mapping of the sensory and motor recovery.
- Types IV and V injuries usually require surgical repair of the nerve to restore axonal continuity.
- Preservation of some function distal to the suspected level of the injury within the distribution of the injured nerve suggests a partial injury, and observation is appropriate.
- If there is a complete palsy of a nerve after a closed injury, an initial period of observation may be best until signs of denervation appear in end organs.
  - If signs of reinnervation appear, such as a Tinel sign distal to the level of injury, continued observation is prudent.
  - If no signs of innervation appear, one should strongly consider electrodiagnostic studies to evaluate the continuity of the axonal fibers.
- Physical therapy is very important to maintain mobility during the period of observation.

SURGICAL MANAGEMENT

- If no signs of recovery are present at 2 to 4 months, then surgical exploration may be indicated.
  - Electrodiagnostic testing should be used in this instance to define the level of injury.
  - Longer delays may compromise the efficacy of surgical repair, secondary to end organ degenerative changes.
- Focal injuries are usually observed for shorter periods because the extent of the injured nerve segment usually is smaller.
- Blunt or blast injuries may be observed for up to 6 months, given the often large segments of injured nerve undergoing repair.

Preoperative Planning

- Intraoperative nerve action potentials (NAPs) may provide information about lesions in continuity, including the degree and extent of interruption.
- If NAPs are not recordable across a lesion, then resection and direct repair rather than grafting will likely be required.
  - Resection is performed from the point at which NAPs are lost to the point where they return.

- If NAPs are present, external neurolysis or nerve decompression may be adequate treatment.

Positioning

- The patient is positioned supine, with a hand table.
- If nerve grafts may be required, the opposite leg is prepared to allow access to the sural nerve. Rarely, if bilateral sural nerves are to be harvested, the patient initially is placed prone.
- Use of a tourniquet may result in ischemic conduction blocks, which will render intraoperative nerve stimulation ineffective.
  - It generally is preferable to use a tourniquet for only the first 20 minutes of surgery to facilitate initial dissection.
- The use of an operating microscope and fine soft tissue sets or microinstrumentation is necessary for nerve handling and repair.

Approach

- Surgical exposure should provide adequate access to the section of damaged nerve as well as proximal and distal to this site.
  - Mobilization should be minimized to prevent additional vascular insult to the nerve.
  - Sources of external compression should be identified and alleviated.
  - The bed for repair should be free of scar tissue. Nerve transposition may be required.

External Neurolysis

- External neurolysis is defined as the circumferential freeing of a peripheral nerve from surrounding scar tissue (**TECH FIG 1A**).
- Dissection proceeds from normal nerve (both proximal and distal) to the area of scarring (**TECH FIG 1B**).
- The nerve should be mobilized away from the scar tissue bed to prevent recurrence.
- Use of a xenograft nerve wrap or fat graft may be considered to prevent recurrence of scarring (**TECH FIG 1C**).
- External neurolysis may relieve neuropathic pain associated with compression, but results for sensory and motor recovery are variable.

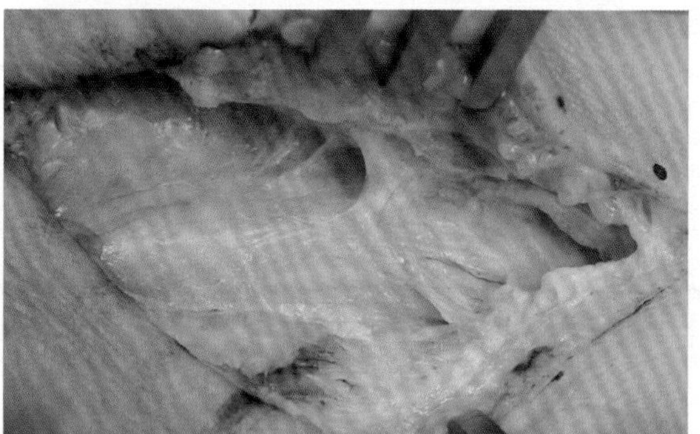
A

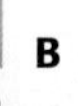

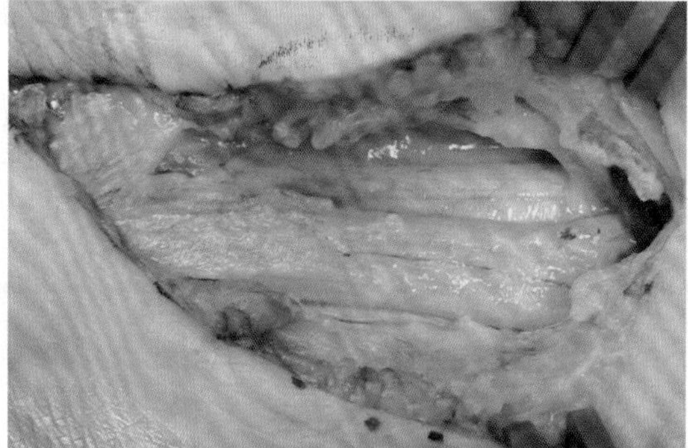
B

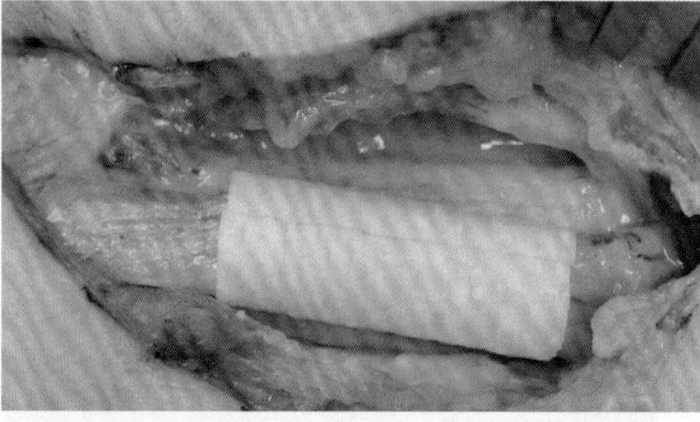
C

TECH FIG 1 • External neurolysis and xenograft nerve wrap. **A.** The median nerve at the wrist developed painful scarring after carpal tunnel release. **B.** External neurolysis has been performed by excision of all scar tissue and thickened epineurium. **C.** A xenograft collagen nerve wrap has been placed around the nerve to minimize scar tissue formation around the nerve.

Internal Neurolysis

- Internal neurolysis is defined as the resection of fibrotic tissue from within the structure of the nerve itself.
- This procedure is indicated for late management of incomplete injuries such as stretch injuries when the nerve has regained partial function that is clinically inadequate.
- Intraoperative recording of NAPs will indicate functioning fascicular groups and help guide the surgeon during this procedure.
- Internal neurolysis is performed along the fascicular segment that has lost NAPs (**TECH FIG 2**).
- This procedure is performed in cases of incomplete functional loss distal to the site of injury.
- Some loss of intact axons can be expected as a result of the dissection, so the patient should be advised that additional loss of function could be possible with this procedure.

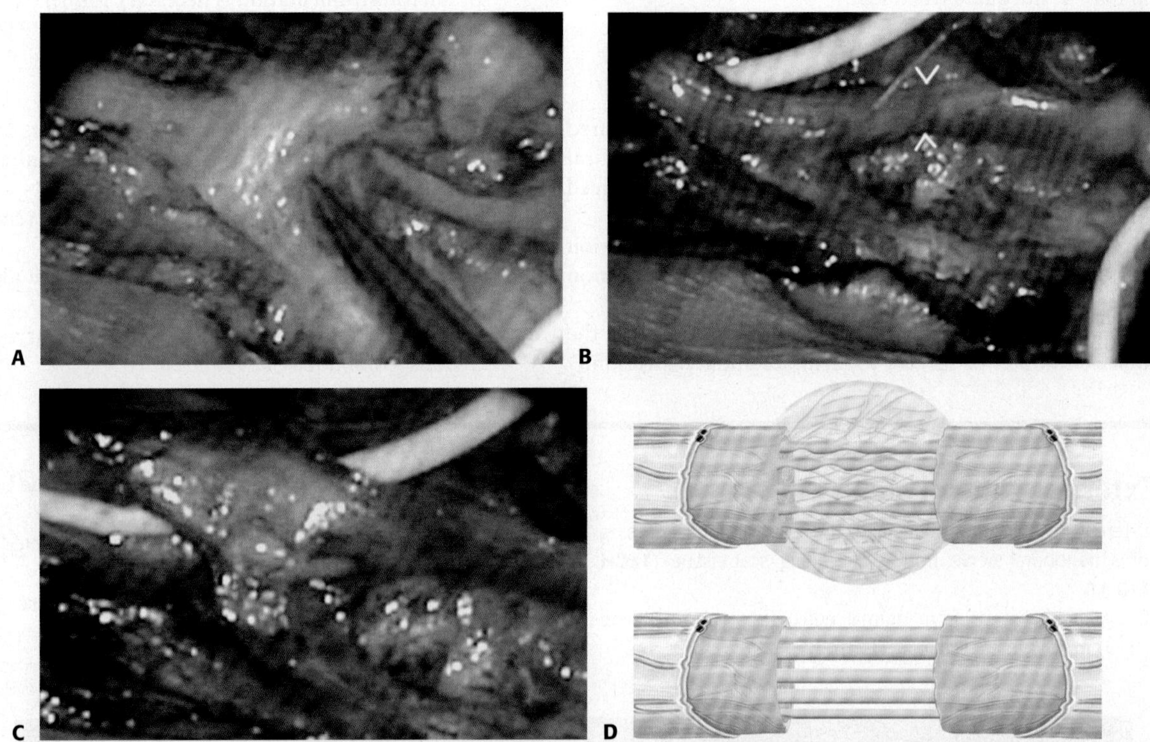

TECH FIG 2 • A–C. Intraoperative microscope images of internal neurolysis of the ulnar nerve at the wrist. **A.** The ulnar nerve is surrounded by dense scar tissue. **B.** After external neurolysis, there is a persistent area of narrowing of the nerve (*arrows*) requiring internal neurolysis. **C.** Appearance after internal neurolysis—the constricting epineurium and scar between fascicles has been excised. **D.** Illustration of a neuroma in continuity treated by internal neurolysis. The segment of scarred epineurium is excised, and all scar tissue between fascicles also is excised.

Split Repair

- *Split repair* is defined as a procedure in which intraoperative NAP recordings are used to guide the resection of individual nonconducting fascicles.
- First, external neurolysis is performed to expose the injured segment of the nerve.
- The epineurium is excised circumferentially to expose the injured fascicles (**TECH FIG 3A**).
- Intraoperative NAP recordings are made to identify the injured fascicular segments (**TECH FIG 3B**).
- Resection of the nonconducting segments is performed using either a blade or sharp microvascular scissors (**TECH FIG 3C**).
- Repair is performed either directly or with autogenous grafting.
  - Cable grafting is the more common technique, using donor nerve from either the sural or antebrachial cutaneous nerve.

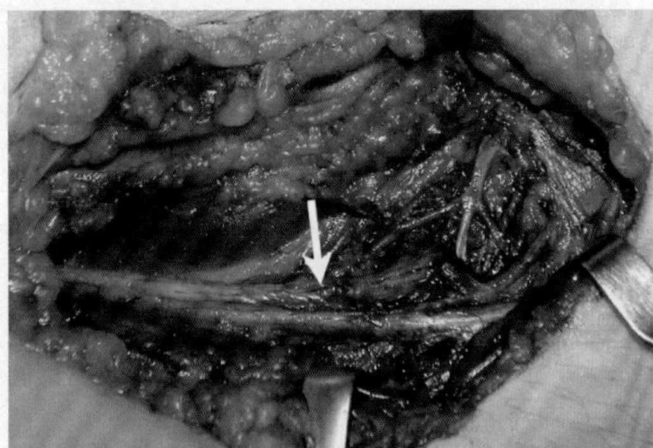

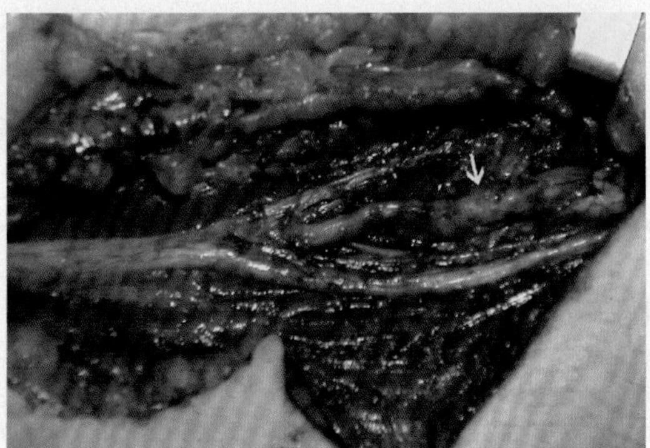

TECH FIG 3 • Exploration and split repair of a partial injury of the posterior interosseous nerve 4 weeks after palsy, following a dog bite at the elbow. **A.** The posterior interosseous nerve demonstrates a neuroma in continuity (*white arrow*). **B.** Internal neurolysis has been performed, isolating intact peripheral fascicles with a central neuroma (*small white arrow*). *(continued)*

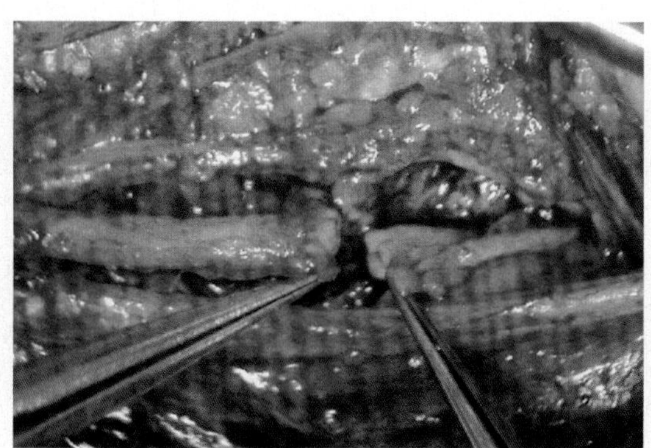

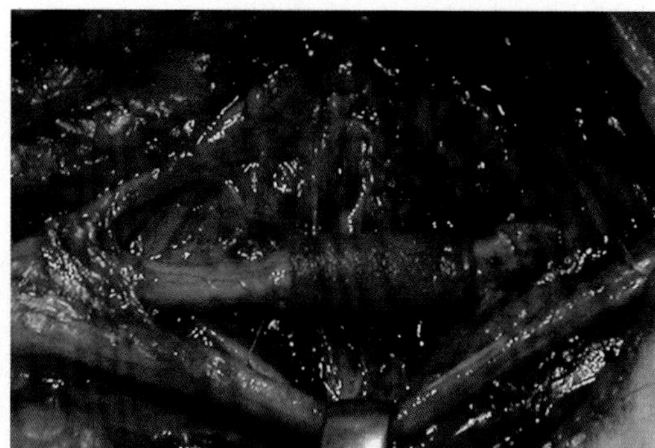

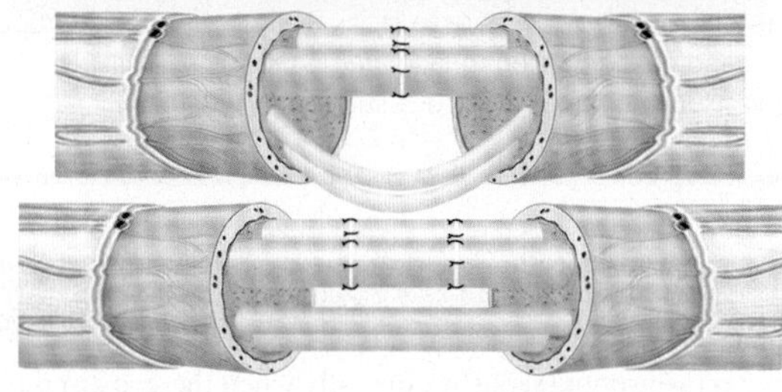

TECH FIG 3 • *(continued)* **C.** A gap remains in the injured fascicular group after neuroma resection. Mobilization of the intact fascicles is limited because of their proximity to the motor branches, making end-to-end repair of the injured fascicles difficult. **D.** Conduit repair of the injured fascicles has been performed. **E,F.** Illustrations of split repair of a partially injured nerve. Nonconducting fascicular segments are excised and either repaired by end-to-end group fascicular repair (**E**) or by interposing nerve grafts (**F**).

- Grouped fascicular repair is then performed (**TECH FIG 3D–F**).
  - The internal arrangement of the fascicles is noted, and a quick sketch of the fascicular arrangement is made to allow alignment of the nerve ends.
  - Nerve grafts will not match the exact fascicular pattern—the aim is to place graft "cables" between groups of fascicles.
  - The gap between nerve ends is measured, and the length of graft needed is calculated.
    - Length = gap + 15% × estimated number of grafts
  - Grafts are attached to a group of fascicles using two sutures of 9-0 or 10-0 nylon, 180 degrees from one another.
  - Each graft is sutured to the proximal and distal stumps before moving on to the next graft, thus allowing for more accurate fascicular matching.
- Check the repair to ensure that no stitches have pulled out. The repair may be reinforced with fibrin glue.
- Handling of the grafts should be minimized.
- Grafts should be kept moist from harvest to repair.

Resection of the Nerve Lesion in Continuity

- If no conduction of NAPs is noted across a lesion after internal neurolysis is performed, then the entire lesion should be resected.
- The proximal and distal portions of the nerve flanking the lesion should be mobilized to prevent undue tension on the repair. During mobilization, longitudinal blood vessels within the epineurium must be preserved.
- The lesion is sharply excised using a fresh, sharp blade against a block (usually a moistened tongue depressor).

Epineurial Repair

- If the extent of the lesion is short, then direct end-to-end epineurial repair without tension often is possible.
- Direct epineurial repair is then performed as described in Chapter 113.

Cable Graft Repair

- Cable graft repair is useful when the extent of the lesion precludes direct repair because of either tension or a large gap (**TECH FIG 4A**).
- Cable graft repair is then performed as described in Chapter 113.
- Sural nerve graft can be harvested through a single longitudinal or multiple transverse incisions (**TECH FIG 4B**).
- The nerve is easily identified by careful spreading dissection in the subcutaneous tissue midway between the lateral malleolus and the tendo Achilles (**TECH FIG 4C**).
- Use of a tendon stripper to harvest the nerve is not recommended.
  - This technique can result in stretch or laceration of the sural nerve.
  - Additionally, the tibial nerve may be inadvertently injured.

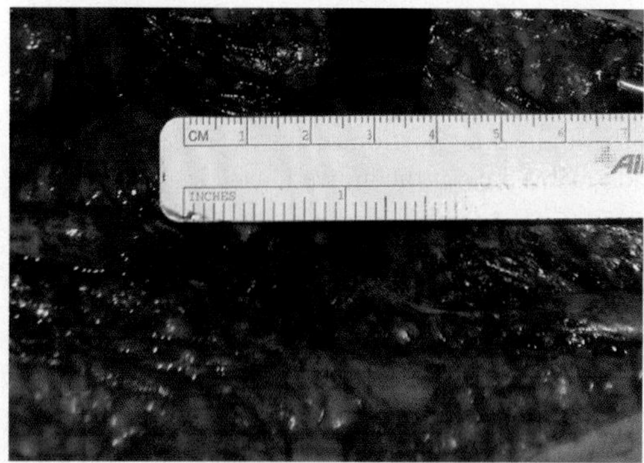

TECH FIG 4 • Cable grafting for reconstruction of a sciatic nerve laceration in the thigh. **A.** The ends of the sciatic nerve lie 6 cm apart. *(continued)*

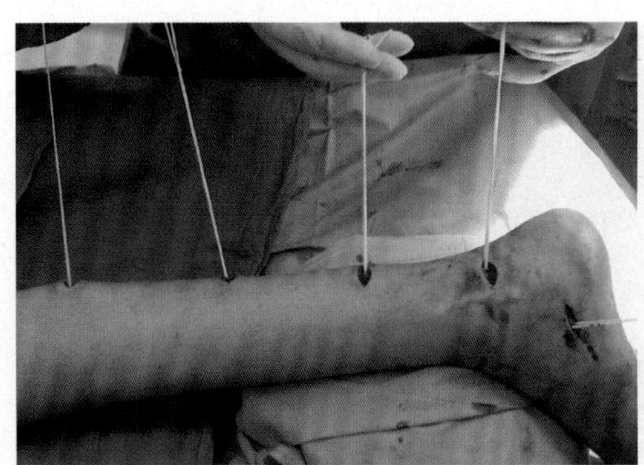
B

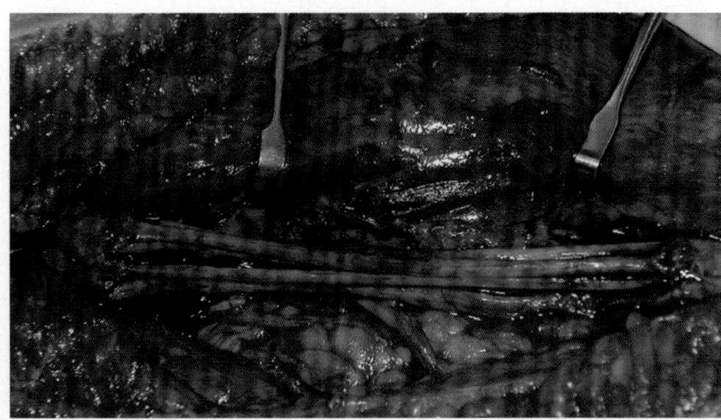
C

TECH FIG 4 • *(continued)* **B.** The ipsilateral sural nerve is harvested by multiple transverse incisions in the leg. Yellow rubber slings have been placed around the nerve at each incision for identification and gentle traction to facilitate dissection. **C.** Multiple segments of the sural nerve have been aligned and inserted in the nerve gap and fixed with group fascicular sutures.

PEARLS AND PITFALLS

Timing of surgical intervention	▪ With lesions in continuity, function may return spontaneously, especially when there is distal functional sparing. Focal injuries can be observed for 2–3 months, whereas lengthy lesions may be observed for up to 5 months.
Is the lesion in continuity?	▪ A combination of clinical and electrodiagnostic testing should be used to evaluate an injury. Serial examinations may provide valuable information about the return of function. Intraoperative measurement of NAPs may provide valuable and objective data of the injured nerve's ability to conduct electrical signals and may guide operative decisions.
Surgical delay	▪ Avoid lengthy periods of observation in the absence of progressive signs of recovery, as irreversible end organ damage may result.

POSTOPERATIVE CARE

- General guidelines for splinting and postoperative care are detailed in Chapter 88.
- Serial examination is important to follow the progress after surgical repair.

OUTCOMES

- Neurolysis
  - If NAPs are recorded through a nerve segment, recovery is thought to be about 90%.
  - NAP recording and subsequent neurolysis without resection have been found to consistently result in better outcomes than direct or graft repair.
- Split repair
  - Outcomes are superior to complete repair when NAPs are recorded through some portion of the nerve.
  - Direct and graft repair of the injured fascicles yield similar results.
- Complete resection with direct repair or graft repair
  - The outcome of direct repairs appears to be superior to those requiring the use of a graft; however, injuries requiring a nerve graft often are more substantial and require regeneration along a greater distance.
  - In general, radial nerve repairs are more successful than median nerve repairs, and both are better than ulnar nerve repairs.
- Children generally have better overall outcomes than adults.
- Internal neurolysis or resection of any lesion in continuity may be related to a decrease in preoperative function as some intact axons may be transected.

COMPLICATIONS

- Infection
- Scarring
- Loss of function
- Increased neuropathic pain
  - Either distal to the lesion or in the form of a painful neuroma
- Failure of recovery of function

SUGGESTED READINGS

1. Birch R, Bonney C, Wynn Parry CB. Surgical Disorders of the Peripheral Nerves. Edinburgh: Churchill Livingstone, 1998.
2. Kline DG. Surgical repair of peripheral nerve injury. Muscle Nerve 1990;13:843–852.
3. Lundborg G, Rosén B, Dahlin L, et al. Tubular versus conventional repair of median and ulnar nerves in the human forearm: early results from a prospective, randomized, clinical study. J Hand Surg Am 1997;22:99–106.
4. Mackinnon SE, Novak CB. Nerve transfers. New options for reconstruction following nerve injury. Hand Clin 1999;15:643–666.
5. Mujadzic M, Ozyurekoglu T, Gupta A, et al. Intraoperative nerve recordings as a useful aid in the management of neuroma-in-continuity. J Reconstruct Microsurg 2005;21:341.
6. Seddon HJ. Nerve grafting. J Bone Joint Surg Br 1963;45(3):447–461.
7. Sunderland S. A classification of peripheral nerve injuries producing loss of function. Brain 1951;74:491–516.

90 CHAPTER

Surgical Treatment of Cubital Tunnel Syndrome

Catherine M. Curtin and Amy L. Ladd

DEFINITION

- Cubital tunnel syndrome is a compression neuropathy of the ulnar nerve that occurs at or around the level of the elbow (*cubis* is Latin for "elbow").
- Cubital tunnel syndrome is the second most common compression neuropathy of the upper limb requiring treatment after carpal tunnel syndrome.

ANATOMY

- The ulnar nerve is the terminal branch of the medial cord of the brachial plexus, with contributions between C8 and T1 nerve roots.
- The ulnar nerve traverses the cubital tunnel, a fibro-osseous tunnel at the elbow. The medial epicondyle, the olecranon, the medial collateral ligament of the elbow (which forms the floor), and the fibrous retinaculum extending from the medial epicondyle to the olecranon make up the anatomic landmarks (**FIG 1**).[13]
- Any of several possible sites of compression of the ulnar nerve around the elbow can result in cubital tunnel syndrome. All of these sites should be considered when selecting the type of surgical decompression.
  - The arcade of Struthers is a controversial site of compression because it is found in only a minority of patients. If present, it is found approximately 8 cm proximal to the medial epicondyle and consists of a fascial band running from the medial head of the triceps to the intermuscular septum.[17]
  - The medial intermuscular septum is a fascial band from the coracobrachialis to the medial humeral epicondyle, especially thick at its attachment to the epicondyle. The ulnar nerve may rest or scissor over the septum as it crosses from the anterior to the posterior compartment, as it approaches the medial epicondyle, or after an anterior transposition if it is not adequately excised.
  - The arcuate ligament of Osborne at the cubital tunnel, which is the fibrous band extending from the medial epicondyle to the olecranon, can cause stenosis of the cubital tunnel and, thus, ulnar nerve compression.
  - Distally, the nerve can be compressed as it passes between the two heads of the flexor carpi ulnaris (FCU), especially if each muscle head from the medial epicondyle and the olecranon converge close to the elbow joint.
  - The presence of an anconeus epitrochlearis (**FIG 2**), an anomalous thin muscle extending from the triceps or olecranon to the medial epicondyle, also can cause ulnar nerve compression.
- The medial antebrachial cutaneous nerve and the medial brachial cutaneous nerve both emanate directly from the medial cord and are thus not ulnar nerve branches, but they importantly may lie in the surgical field. They are usually found deeper than expected, along the fascia of the triceps, brachialis, and FCU.

PATHOGENESIS

- Cubital tunnel syndrome is a compressive neuropathy. Several anatomic factors make the ulnar nerve susceptible to compression at the elbow.
  - The nerve is superficial at the level of the elbow, making it susceptible to minor and major trauma, ranging from mild repetitive contusion to high-energy injury.
  - The bony tunnel and its soft tissue support between the olecranon and medial epicondyle may be shallow, either inherently or traumatically, promoting subluxation, "perching" on the epicondyle, and microtrauma.

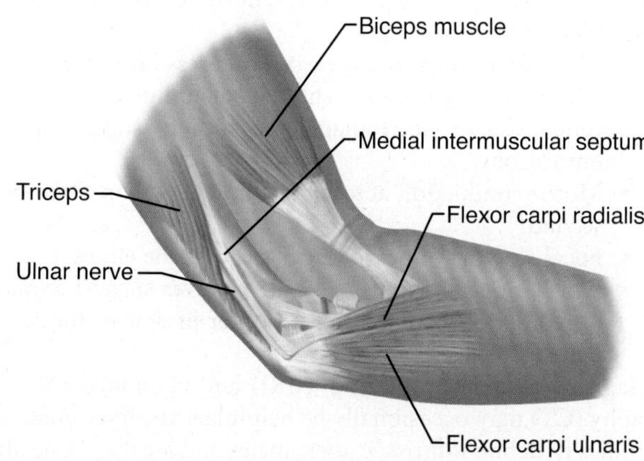

FIG 1 • Anatomy of the cubital tunnel.

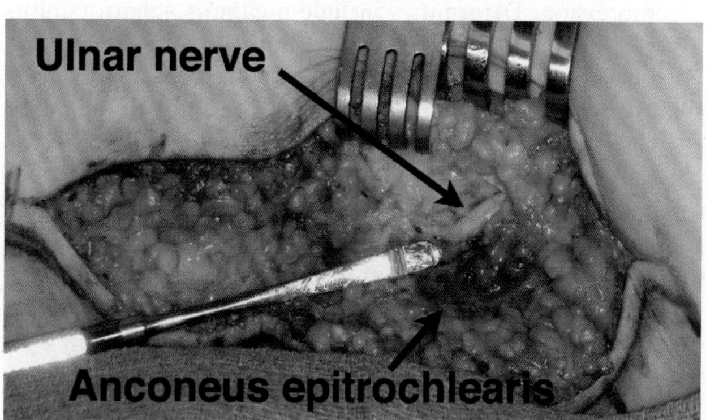

FIG 2 • An anomalous anconeus epitrochlearis encountered overlying the cubital tunnel. Anterior is at *top* and posterior at *bottom*; the forearm is to the *left*.

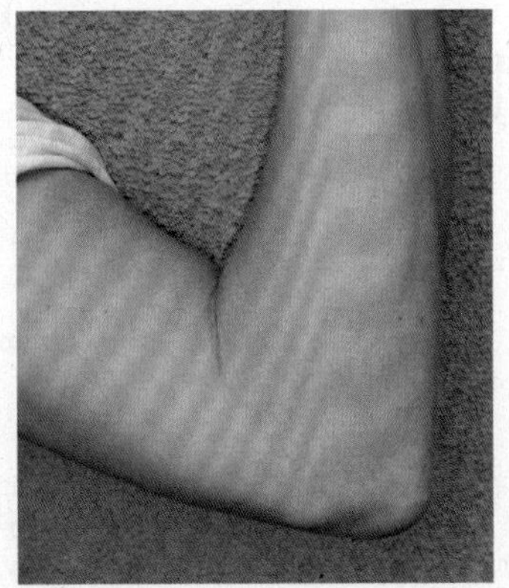

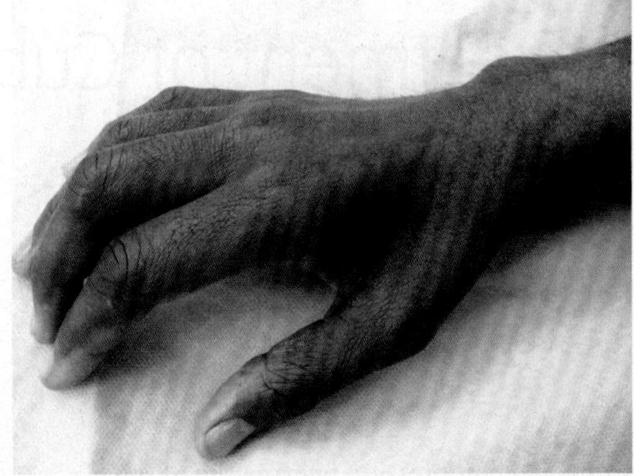

FIG 3 • **A.** "Perched" ulnar nerve. The nerve subluxates anteriorly, sitting on top of the medial epicondyle with the elbow in flexion. **B.** Wasting of first dorsal interosseous nerve. (**A:** Copyright Amy Ladd, MD.)

- Elbow flexion increases pressure on the nerve and decreases the volume of the cubital tunnel, resulting in compression of the nerve.[7]

NATURAL HISTORY

- Without operative intervention, about half of mild cases can resolve with activity modification.[13,14]
- No long-term studies have been done of the natural history for severe disease.

PATIENT HISTORY AND PHYSICAL FINDINGS

- Subjective complaints include numbness in the small and ring fingers, often with accompanying burning pain around the medial epicondyle. Symptoms may be worse at night.
- As the disease progresses, patients may complain of weakness or clumsiness of their hands. More advanced disease will demonstrate wasting of the intrinsics and clawing of the ring and small fingers.
- Systemic diseases such as diabetes, amyloidosis, or alcoholism may cause peripheral neuropathy, which can mimic the symptoms of a compressive neuropathy.
- A smoking history is important not only for impaired vascularity but because it may point to the rare Pancoast tumor, an apical lung tumor, which causes plexus compression, mimicking the symptoms of cubital tunnel syndrome.
- Elbow trauma can create deformity, causing ulnar nerve compression. Deformities include a cubitus valgus, cubitus varus, or malunion. The elbow trauma can be remote and result in tardy ulnar nerve palsy.
- Look for atrophy of the intrinsic muscles of the hand or a clawed posture of the ring and small fingers. Check for masses around the elbow.
- Palpate the elbow and hand to evaluate for tender masses or other anomalous elbow anatomy.
- Put the elbow through its range of motion and assess whether the ulnar nerve subluxates or perches at the medial epicondyle with elbow flexion (**FIG 3A**).[2]
- Visible atrophy of the first dorsal interosseous nerve correlates with significant ulnar nerve compression and can indicate significant motor impairment (**FIG 3B**).
- Perform a sensory examination of the hand, using Semmes-Weinstein monofilaments to obtain threshold measurements. Evaluate sensation on the ulnar dorsum of the hand. If sensation is normal, it suggests the problem may be distal, at the level of Guyon canal.
- Clinical tests that can help with diagnosis include the following:
  - Tinel test. This test may not be specific because many normal individuals will have a positive Tinel response to percussion.
  - Elbow flexion test. This test is sensitive for cubital tunnel syndrome.
  - Scratch collapse test can help localize the site of compression.[3]
  - Crossed finger test. This test demonstrates weakness of dorsal and palmar interossei.
  - Froment sign. A positive Froment sign indicates weakness of the adductor pollicis.
  - Wartenberg sign (in which the small finger assumes an abducted posture with finger extension). This sign is the result of weakness in the palmar interossei, resulting in unopposed ulnar pull of the extensor digiti quinti.

IMAGING AND OTHER DIAGNOSTIC STUDIES

- Radiographs of the elbow define the bony architecture and its alterations: masses, erosions, arthritis, and previous trauma. An axial view is helpful to evaluate the cubital canal (**FIG 4**).
- Normal results on electrodiagnostic studies (eg, nerve conduction and electromyography) do not exclude the diagnosis of cubital tunnel syndrome; the syndrome may be present but not severe.
  - These tests localize the area of compression if the nerve conduction is measured at short segment intervals.
  - Several positive electrodiagnostic findings suggest ulnar compression:
    - Motor conduction across the elbow less than 50 m per second[15]
    - Focal slowing of nerve velocity across the elbow
    - Fibrillation potentials or positive waves suggest axonal degeneration, representing a poorer prognosis for complete recovery.
- Magnetic resonance imaging (MRI) and computed tomography (CT) may occasionally be helpful as ancillary imaging studies to define soft tissue aberrancies and localize bone abnormalities such as osteophytes in the cubital tunnel.

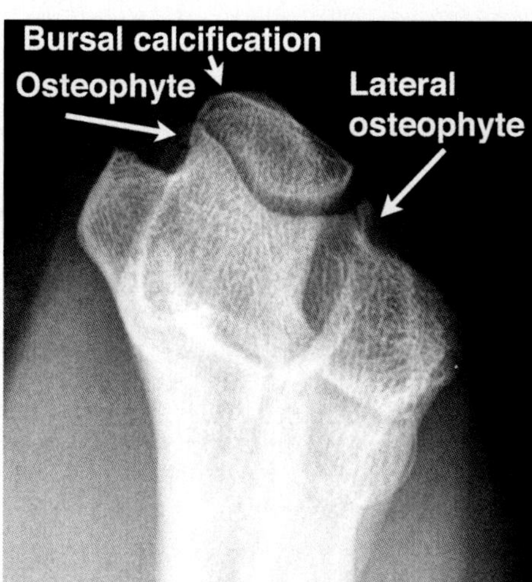

FIG 4 • Axial view of the elbow demonstrates a hooked osteophyte within the cubital tunnel as well as calcification in the bursa and osteophyte. (Copyright Amy Ladd, MD.)

DIFFERENTIAL DIAGNOSIS

- Cervical spine disease affecting C8 and T1
- Compression of the inferior aspect of the brachial plexus from shoulder trauma
- Apical lung tumor (Pancoast tumor)
- Thoracic outlet syndrome
- Entrapment of the ulnar nerve at the wrist (Guyon canal)

NONOPERATIVE MANAGEMENT

- Activity modification
  - Ulnar nerve protection limiting microtrauma to the nerve through elbow padding and limiting direct pressure on the nerve
  - Minimize prolonged elbow flexion, especially at night, through sleep modifications or splints.
- Splinting
  - Splints to prevent elbow flexion; rigid splints are more effective but are less tolerated by patients. If persistent paresthesias exist, a trial of temporary full-time use is recommended. For milder cases, the splint is worn only at night.[4]
  - Nonoperative treatment requires a trial of several months before determining its success.

SURGICAL MANAGEMENT

- Surgical intervention should be considered for patients presenting with motor involvement or permanent sensory changes or for those who have failed nonoperative treatment.

Preoperative Planning

- Review the history and physical examination.
- Review plain radiographs for evidence of old trauma, valgus or varus deformity, or loose bodies.
- Electrodiagnostic testing and examination may correlate with postoperative results.
- A patient with a visible and symptomatic subluxating nerve may be considered for a medial epicondylectomy or transposition.
- Patients with severe disease with muscle wasting are less likely to have complete recovery.[10]

Positioning

- The patient usually is placed in the supine position.
- If a sterile tourniquet is preferred, drape out the forequarter. A standard tourniquet may be used, but position it high in the axilla, with good padding. A proximally placed tourniquet can be challenging to position in the obese arm in either circumstance because the tourniquet tends to gap distally. It is worth the extra time to position it properly because adequate hemostasis and visualized proximal dissection are important aspects of ulnar nerve surgery.
- The patient's shoulder is externally rotated and abducted on an arm table.
- The tourniquet is inflated after exsanguination of the arm.
- Folded towels stabilize and elevate the elbow (**FIG 5**).
- An obese patient with sleep apnea under peripheral nerve block (most commonly supra- or infraclavicular block) may require slight truncal elevation, which may be vexing for the surgeon.

Approach

- The choice of technique depends on the severity of symptoms, the patient's body habitus, the presence of elbow anatomic pathology, and the surgeon's preference.
- The general types of release are in situ release, endoscopic release, in situ release with medial epicondylectomy, and anterior transposition (subcutaneous, intramuscular, and submuscular).
- Table 1 summarizes the surgical options for treating cubital tunnel syndrome.

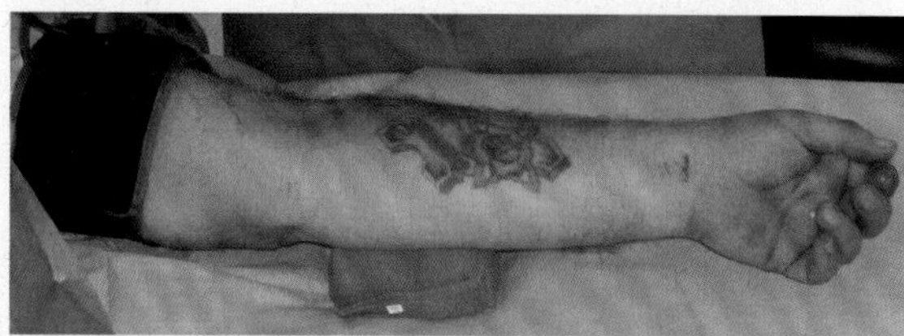

FIG 5 • The arm is draped, the sterile tourniquet is placed proximally, and a bump under the elbow assists visualization. Alternatively, a proximal tourniquet may be placed before the arm is draped.

Table 1 Techniques for Cubital Tunnel Release

Technique	Advantages	Disadvantages	Contraindications	Indications
In situ release	Simplest dissection Does not devascularize the nerve with circumferential dissection Early mobilization	Keeps nerve in same tissue bed Does not address subluxation of the nerve	Subluxating ulnar nerve Abnormal elbow anatomy	Diabetic patient Frail patient Patient with focal compression distal to medial epicondyle
Endoscopic release	Small incision Early mobilization Shortened recovery time	Keeps nerve in same tissue bed Potential iatrogenic nerve compression	Abnormal elbow anatomy Revision surgery	
In situ release with medial condylectomy	Preserves vascular supply to the nerve Early mobilization	Keeps nerve in same tissue bed Risk of destabilizing the medial elbow by damaging the medial collateral ligament of the elbow Tenderness at operative site	Abnormal elbow anatomy Not for throwing athletes	Patients with mild to moderate symptoms
Anterior subcutaneous transfer	Places the nerve in a fresh tissue bed	Nerve is superficial and may be more susceptible to trauma. Greater dissection More prolonged immobilization Possible creation of new point of compression	Very thin patient	Patient with a poor ulnar nerve bed from tumor, osteophyte, heterotopic bone Throwing athlete
Anterior intermuscular transposition	Tension with elbow range of motion is minimized. Nerve is in fresh tissue bed.	Greater dissection Need for longer immobilization	Diabetic patient	Patient with a poor ulnar nerve bed from tumor, osteophyte, heterotopic bone
Anterior submuscular transposition	Tension with elbow range of motion is minimized. Nerve is well padded.	Greater dissection Need for longer immobilization		Thin patient Repeat cubital tunnel release Patients with severe compression

In Situ Release

- Center the longitudinal incision just anterior to the medial epicondyle, making an incision about 6 cm long (**TECH FIG 1A**).
- Dissect through the fat, down to the level of the medial epicondyle.
- Preserve the branches of the medial brachial and antebrachial cutaneous nerves. Although the course is variable, branches can be found from 6 cm proximal to 6 cm distal to the medial epicondyle and often are at the level of the fascia[9] (**TECH FIG 1B,C**).

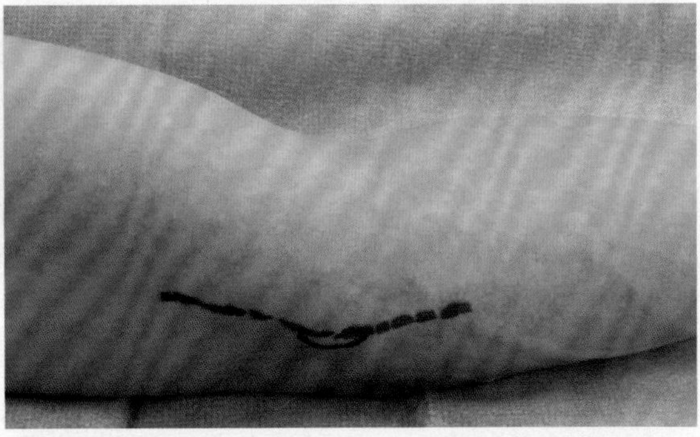
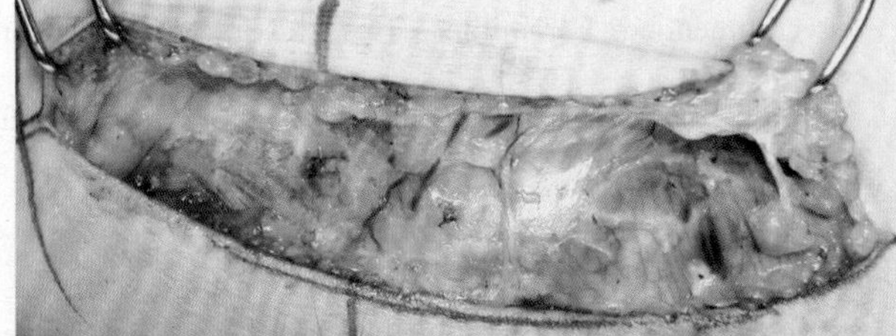
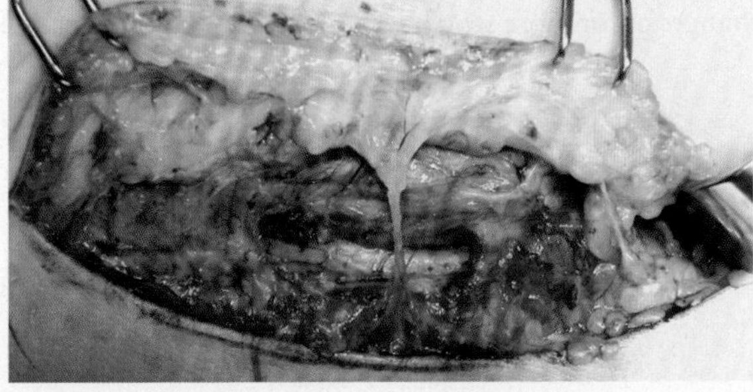

TECH FIG 1 • **A.** The standard incision, centered just anterior or posterior to the medial epicondyle. **B,C.** Preservation of crossing medial brachial and antebrachial nerves. The cutaneous nerves lie deep in the fat, typically on the fascia. Here, two branches are encountered before and after fasciotomies to expose the nerve. (Copyright Amy Ladd, MD.)

- Identify the ulnar nerve and dissect it free proximally until it pierces the medial intermuscular septum. Release any areas of constriction.
- Take the dissection distal to the level of the medial epicondyle and release the band spanning from the medial epicondyle to the olecranon.
- Preserve the branches of the ulnar nerve: the first is the articular sensory branch, followed by the motor branches to the FCU and flexor digitorum profundus (FDP). The FCU branches are found proximally with appearance of the muscle.
- The distal dissection proceeds through the thick arcade of fascia of the flexor pronator aponeurosis. Two layers exist: a superficial layer that covers both heads of the FCU and a deeper one that overlies the nerve as it traverses between the two heads. Continue fascial release into the muscle for several centimeters to ensure that there are no areas of entrapment within the muscle belly, taking care to preserve nerve branches to the muscle.
- Gently palpate to ensure that the entire ulnar nerve is free from compressive bands.
- Range the elbow and check for smooth ulnar nerve excursion. If perching (snapping) over the medial epicondyle occurs, consider medial epicondylectomy. This is often a preclinical determination.
- Close the soft tissues using the surgeon's preferred technique.
- Typically, no drain is placed.
- Place the arm in a bulky supportive dressing or a posterior plaster elbow splint with flexion of about 60 degrees. Remove the splint according to wound care and the surgeon's mobilization preference.

In Situ Endoscopic Release

- Contraindicated in patients with a subluxing ulnar nerve, prior cubital tunnel release, space occupying lesion (osteophyte), elbow contracture
- Equipment: 30-degree arthroscope 4 mm diameter, illuminated speculum, soft tissue dissector (can be dilators or other blunt-tip instrument), long and short scissors
- A 2-cm incision is made over the cubital tunnel (between the medial epicondyle and the retrocondylar groove).
- The ulnar nerve is identified and exposed at the base of the wound.
- A tunnel is dissected above the fascia overlying the nerve, creating a pocket for the scope. Any crossing veins are cauterized.
- Osborne ligament is opened under direct visualization (**TECH FIG 2A**).
- The endoscope and dissector are introduced, and the compressive bands over the nerve are released using the scope for visualization (**TECH FIG 2B**). Care is taken not to cause iatrogenic pressure to the nerve.
- This dissection can release 15 cm of length along the nerve.[18]
- A layered closure and soft dressing are performed.

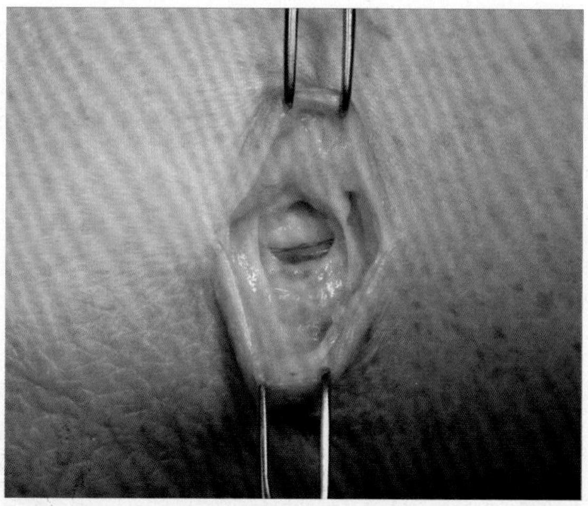
A

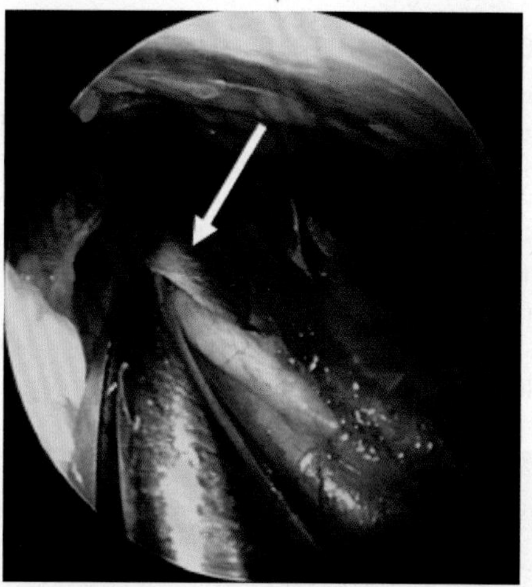
B

TECH FIG 2 • Endoscopic carpal tunnel release **A.** Small incision dissecting down to the ulnar nerve at the cubital tunnel. **B.** View through the scope of release of bands crossing the ulnar nerve (*arrow*). (Courtesy of Dr. Hoffman.)

In Situ Release with Medial Epicondylectomy

- The incision and dissection are the same as the in situ release.
- Excise a strip of the tough fascial intermuscular septum as it attaches to the medial epicondyle to minimize the nerve "scissoring" over the firm edge.
- Once the nerve is free of all areas of entrapment, a longitudinal incision is made slightly anterior to the medial epicondyle with a knife or electrocautery, reflecting the periosteum to reveal the bony prominence of the epicondyle. Carefully protect the ulnar nerve; gentle retraction with a saline-lubricated ¼-inch Penrose drain on a short hemostat is sufficient.
- Expose the medial epicondyle subperiosteally.
- Remove the prominence of the epicondyle, which is most acute in its posterior position, removing 2 to 3 mm of prominence and 6 to 8 mm in length. Use a small, sharp osteotome and smooth with a file while protecting the nerve (**TECH FIG 3A**).

- Place bone wax over the raw bone. This minimizes postoperative hematoma.
- The periosteum is closed with buried sutures, either braided absorbable or nonabsorbable, minimizing contact with the nerve.
- Check that the nerve glides, rather than perches, when the elbow is flexed and extended before closure of the skin (**TECH FIG 3B**).
- Because of potential bony bleeding, a drain can be considered.
- Apply a posterior plaster splint for 10 to 14 days, with protected mobilization thereafter.

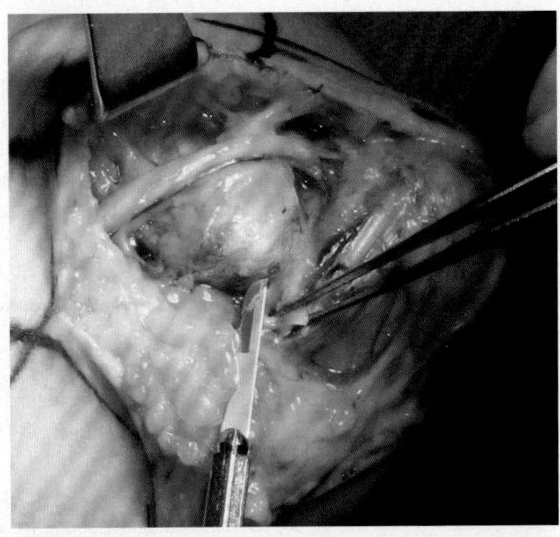

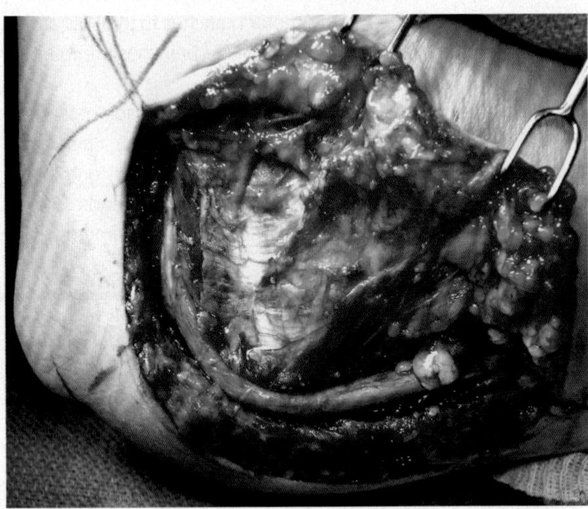

TECH FIG 3 • Medial epicondylectomy. **A.** The medial epicondyle is exposed and the most prominent aspect is removed. We recommend removal of the most prominent and inferior portion, 2 to 3 mm in depth, to avoid disruption of the medial collateral ligament. **B.** Once the epicondylectomy is performed and the fascia closed, the elbow is flexed to visualize smooth movement of the nerve. The nerve no longer perches on the medial epicondyle. (Copyright Amy Ladd, MD.)

Anterior Subcutaneous Transfer

- The incision and dissection are the same as for the in situ release, except that the incision may have to be slightly longer.
- Release the nerve at every potential level of entrapment.
- Circumferentially dissect the nerve to allow it to be moved anterior to the medial epicondyle. Free all posterior attachments to allow for maximal anterior excursion.
- Excise the intermuscular septum from the crossover of the ulnar nerve, anterior to posterior in the proximal dissection, all the way to its tough attachment at the medial epicondyle.
- Preserve the longitudinal vasculature accompanying the nerve to prevent devascularization of the nerve. Use caution around the medial epicondyle and the most fibrous part of the intermuscular septum, where lies an external but vulnerable large venous leash.
- Develop the interval between the skin and the fascia overlying the flexor pronator muscle mass anterior to the medial epicondyle, about 4 cm.
- Transpose the nerve to lie anterior to the medial epicondyle (**TECH FIG 4A**).

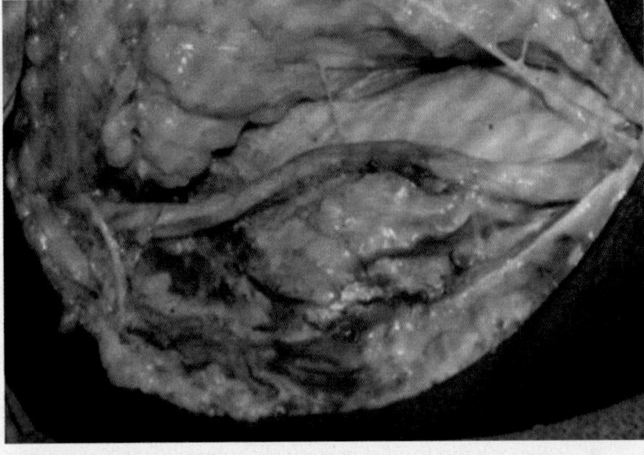

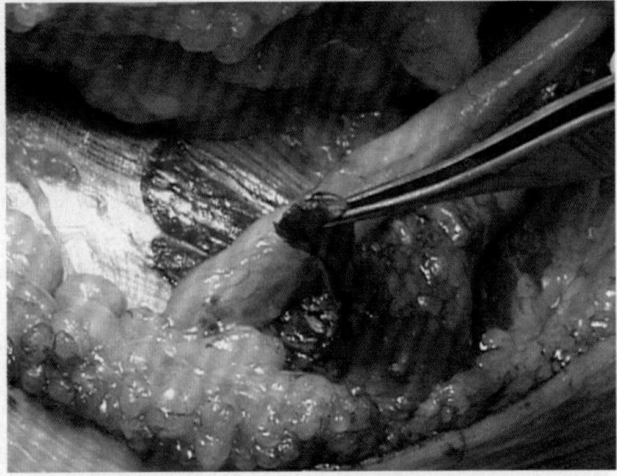

TECH FIG 4 • Anterior subcutaneous transposition. **A.** The subcutaneous flap at the level of the flexor pronator fascia has been developed and the nerve transposed anteriorly. **B.** A 1-cm fascial sling is developed from the flexor pronator mass to provide an inferior restraint for the transposed nerve. (**A:** Courtesy of Thomas R. Hunt, III, MD; **B:** From Black BT, Barron OA, Townsend PF, et al. Stabilized subcutaneous ulnar nerve transposition with immediate range of motion. Long-term follow-up. J Bone Joint Surg Am 2000;82-A(11):1544–1551.)

- The nerve should lie in its new position without any tension or areas of compression. An intraneural dissection to release the motor branches to the FCU may be required proximally.
- To prevent the nerve from subluxating, a 1-cm fasciodermal sling is constructed from the fascia overlying the flexor pronator mass (ie, the FCU, flexor carpi radialis [FCR], and the pronator teres)[5] (**TECH FIG 4B**). This flap is sutured to the skin. This flap prevents the nerve from sliding back to its old position.
- Care must be taken to ensure that this flap does not become a new area of compression.
- No drain is required.
- Apply a posterior plaster splint for 10 to 14 days, with protected mobilization thereafter.

Anterior Intramuscular Transposition

- The nerve is fully released, as described for the subcutaneous transposition.[8]
- The interval between the skin and the fascia is developed anterior to the medial epicondyle to about 4 cm.
- Transpose the nerve so that its rests along the flexor pronator mass (ie, FCU, FCR, and the pronator teres).
- A trough slightly bigger than the nerve is carved out of the muscles along this anterior course (**TECH FIG 5**). Release any fascial bands found within the muscle substance.
  - Flex the elbow and place the nerve in the trough.
  - Suture fascia over the nerve, creating a tunnel.
- Range the elbow to ensure that there is no kinking or tethering of the transposed nerve.
- The arm is immobilized with a pronated forearm in an elbow splint for 2 to 3 weeks at 45 to 60 degrees of flexion with progressive protected mobilization.

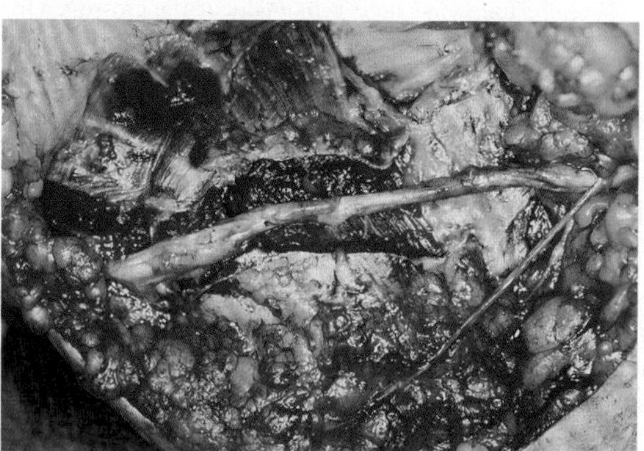

TECH FIG 5 • Intramuscular transposition. The nerve is placed in a tunnel in the muscle, and the fascia is closed. (Courtesy of William Kleinman, Indiana Hand Center.)

Anterior Submuscular Transposition

- The nerve is fully released as described with the preceding procedures, and the skin flap is developed similarly to the intramuscular procedure.
- Divide the flexor pronator mass about 1 cm distal to its insertion on the medial epicondyle, either as a straight incision or in a V-Y fashion (**TECH FIG 6A**).
- Lift the flexor pronator mass distally at the level of the FDS muscle. There is a loose areolar plane between these muscle bellies.
- The median nerve and brachial artery lie in this plane. Transpose the ulnar nerve in the medial position (**TECH FIG 6B**).
  - Take care to avoid injury to the medial collateral ligament complex.
- Flex the elbow and repair the flexor pronator mass with 3-0 Ethibond suture.
- Place a drain.
- The arm is immobilized with a pronated forearm in an elbow splint for 2 to 3 weeks at 45 to 60 degrees of flexion with progressive protected mobilization.

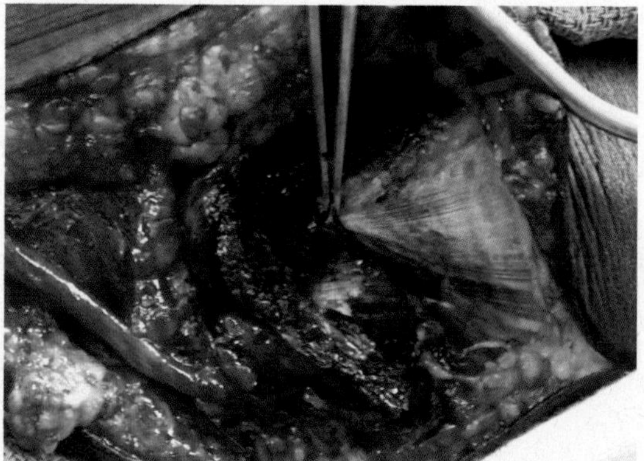

A

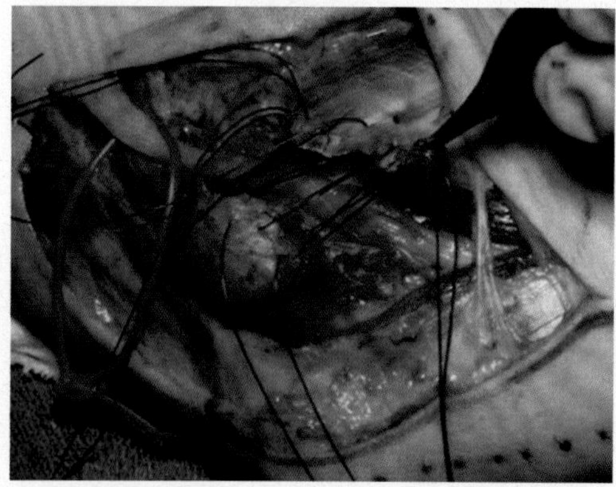

B

TECH FIG 6 • Submuscular transposition. The flexor pronator mass is incised (**A**), and the nerve is passed deep to the flexor pronator muscle mass (**B**). Sutures are in place to repair the muscle origin following use of a simple straight incision. (**A:** Copyright Amy Ladd, MD; **B:** Courtesy of Thomas R. Hunt, III, MD.)

PEARLS AND PITFALLS

Dissection	■ Avoid cutting the medial brachial and antebrachial nerves. Damage to these nerves is the most common cause of pain after cubital tunnel release.[9,16] ■ Make an adequate proximal dissection: Follow the nerve to the crossover of the anterior to posterior compartment, where a thin or thick fascial band is present at the septum, or, rarely, the arcade of Struthers. Make certain the tourniquet is high enough to reach this spot, usually 5–8 cm above the epicondyle. ■ Make an adequate distal dissection: Follow the nerve several centimeters into the muscle bellies to ensure a full release, including the fascia of the FCU encasing its branches.
Transposition	■ Preserve the longitudinal blood supply to the nerve. ■ If transposing the nerve, ensure that a new point of compression is not created. Compression may be created at the following sites: proximally at the crossover from anterior to posterior, the intermuscular septum just proximal to the medial epicondyle, the flexor pronator mass if submuscular or intramuscular transposition is performed, and the entrance to the FCU muscle bellies.

POSTOPERATIVE CARE

- Postoperative care instructions are given individually with the discussion of each technique. In general, the more extensive the dissection, the more protected postoperative splinting and mobilization is required. Strengthening may begin a few weeks after an in situ decompression, for example, and 6 to 8 weeks following a submuscular transposition.

OUTCOMES

- Overall, all procedures have a success rate of about 90% for mild cases. The rate of total relief decreases as severity of disease increases.[11]
- Postoperative outcomes are proportional to disease severity: That is, severe disease is less likely to achieve full recovery.[6]
- Recent studies suggest that outcomes are similar for the different procedure types.[1,6,12]

COMPLICATIONS

- Pain at the elbow
- Decreased sensation around the scar
- Incomplete symptom relief
- Painful neuroma of cutaneous nerves
- Symptomatic subluxating nerve
- Injury to motor branches to the FCU

REFERENCES

1. Bartels RH, Verhagen WI, van der Wilt GJ, et al. Prospective randomized controlled study comparing simple decompression versus anterior subcutaneous transposition for idiopathic neuropathy of the ulnar nerve at the elbow. Part 1. Neurosurgery 2005;56:522–530.
2. Calfee RP, Manske PR, Gelberman RH, et al. Clinical assessment of the ulnar nerve at the elbow: reliability of instability testing and the association of hypermobility with clinical symptoms. J Bone Joint Surg Am 2010;92(17):2801–2808.
3. Cheng CJ, Mackinnon-Patterson B, Beck JL, et al. Scratch collapse test for evaluation of carpal and cubital tunnel syndrome. J Hand Surg Am 2008;33(9):1518–1524. doi:10.1016/j.jhsa.2008.05.022.
4. Dellon AL, Hament W, Gittelshon A. Nonoperative management of cubital tunnel syndrome: an 8-year prospective study. Neurology 1993;43:1673–1677.
5. Eaton RG, Crowe JF, Parkes JC III. Anterior transposition of the u1nar nerve using a noncompressing fasciodermal sling. J Bone Joint Surg Am 1980;62(5):820–825.
6. Gervasio O, Gambardella G, Zaccone C, et al. Simple decompression versus anterior submuscular transposition of the ulnar nerve in severe cubital tunnel syndrome: a prospective randomized study. Neurosurgery 2005;56:108–117.
7. Iba K, Wada T, Aoki M, et al. Intraoperative measurement of pressure adjacent to the ulnar nerve in patients with cubital tunnel syndrome. J Hand Surg Am 2006;31;553–558.
8. Kleinman WB, Bishop AT. Anterior intramuscular transposition of the ulnar nerve. J Hand Surg Am 1989;14:972–979.
9. Lowe JB III, Maggi SP, Mackinnon SE. The position of crossing branches of the medial antebrachial cutaneous nerve during cubital tunnel surgery in humans. Plast Reconstr Surg 2004;114:692–696.
10. Matsuzaki H, Yoshizu T, Maki Y, et al. Long-term clinical and neurologic recovery in the hand after surgery for severe cubital tunnel syndrome. J Hand Surg Am 2004;29;373–378.
11. Mowlavi A, Andrews K, Lille S, et al. The management of cubital tunnel syndrome: a meta-analysis of clinical studies. Plast Reconstr Surg 2000;106:327–334.
12. Nabhan A, Ahlhelm F, Kelm J, et al. Simple decompression or subcutaneous anterior transposition of the ulnar nerve for cubital tunnel syndrome. J Hand Surg Am 2005;30:521–524.
13. O'Driscoll SW, Horii E, Carmichael SW, et al. The cubital tunnel and ulnar neuropathy. J Bone Joint Surg Br 1991;73(4):613–617.
14. Padua L, Aprile I, Caliandro P, et al. Natural history of ulnar entrapment at elbow. Clin Neurophysiol 2002;113:1980–1984.
15. Practice parameter for electrodiagnostic studies in ulnar neuropathy at the elbow: summary statement. American Association of Electrodiagnostic Medicine, American Academy of Neurology, American Academy of Physical Medicine and Rehabilitation. Muscle Nerve 1999;22(3):408–411.
16. Sarris I, Göbel F, Gainer M, et al. Medial brachial and antebrachial cutaneous nerve injuries: effect on outcome in revision cubital tunnel surgery. J Reconstr Microsurg 2002;18:665–670.
17. Siqueira MG, Martins RS. The controversial arcade of Struthers. Surg Neurol 2005;64(suppl 1):S17–S20.
18. Zajonc H, Momeni A. Endoscopic release of the cubital tunnel. Hand Clin 2014;30(1):55–62.

Decompression of the Ulnar Nerve at Guyon Canal

91 CHAPTER

Harris Gellman and Patrick Owens

DEFINITION

- The site of compression must be identified to determine the appropriate treatment for symptoms of ulnar nerve dysfunction. Guyon canal at the wrist is the second most common site of ulnar nerve entrapment.
- Symptoms may be purely motor, purely sensory, or mixed, depending on the site and cause of compression.

ANATOMY

- In the distal half of the forearm, the ulnar nerve is joined on its lateral side by the ulnar artery. Proximal to the wrist, the nerve gives off a large dorsal sensory branch, which supplies sensation to the dorsum of the wrist and the ulnar side of the hand. The ulnar nerve continues into the hand through Guyon canal.
- Guyon canal is a triangular canal at the base of the ulnar side of the palm. It is 4 cm in length, extending from the proximal edge of the palmar carpal ligament to the fibrous edge of the hypothenar muscles.[4] The space functions as a physiologic tunnel with discrete anatomic landmarks (**FIG 1A**).
  - Both the ulnar nerve and artery pass through the canal to enter the hand.
  - The dorsal cutaneous branch of the ulnar nerve usually branches before the nerve enters Guyon canal.
  - It is bordered laterally by the hook of the hamate and the transverse carpal ligament. The medial wall is formed by the pisiform and the attachments of the pisohamate ligament.
- Dividing the tunnel into three zones helps in correlating the clinical symptoms with the specific pathologic cause[4,13] (**FIG 1B**).
  - Zone 1, about 3 cm in length, is the area proximal to the bifurcation of the ulnar nerve into motor and sensory branches. Compression in zone 1 results in combined motor and sensory loss. It is most commonly caused by a fracture of the hook of the hamate or a ganglion cyst.
  - Zones 2 and 3 are located next to each other, from the point where the ulnar nerve divides into a superficial or sensory branch and a deep motor branch to the region just beyond the fibrous arch of the hypothenar muscles.
  - Zone 2 encompasses the motor branch of the nerve, located in the dorsoradial portion of the tunnel. The deep motor branch, along with the deep branch of the ulnar artery, passes between the abductor digiti quinti and the flexor digiti quinti brevis, perforating the opponens digiti quinti. The motor branch then follows the deep volar arch across the palm to innervate the interossei.
    - The nerve supplies the three intrinsic muscles of the small finger, the third and fourth lumbricals, the volar and dorsal interossei, the adductor pollicis, and the deep head of the flexor pollicis brevis.
    - Compression in this area causes pure motor loss to all of the ulnar-innervated muscles in the hand. Ganglions from the pisotriquetral joint and fractures of the hook of the hamate are the most common etiologic factors (**FIG 1C**). Due to the nerve's proximity to the hamate, it is unfortunately easy to damage the nerve while excising the hook of the hamate.
  - Zone 3, located ulnar to zone 2, encompasses the superficial or sensory branch of the bifurcated ulnar nerve. Compression here causes sensory loss to the hypothenar eminence, the small finger, and part of the ring finger but does not usually cause motor deficits. Common causes are aneurysm of the ulnar artery, thrombosis, and synovial inflammation.
    - The superficial branch of the ulnar nerve in Guyon canal supplies the palmaris brevis and the skin of the hypothenar eminence and forms the digital nerves to the small and ulnar side of the ring finger.
- Two specific nerve anomalies can confuse the diagnosis.
  - Martin-Gruber anastomosis in the forearm: Fibers that supply the intrinsic muscles are carried in the median nerve to the middle of the forearm, where they leave the median nerve to join the ulnar nerve. Functioning intrinsic muscles can be observed when the ulnar nerve is injured proximal to this anastomosis.
  - Riche-Cannieu anastomosis: The median and ulnar nerves are connected in the palm. Even with an injury at the wrist, some intrinsic function remains.

PATHOGENESIS

- Causative factors of compression or injury of the ulnar nerve in Guyon canal include repeated blunt trauma from power tools and gripping or hammering with the palm of the hand, which may result in thrombosis or aneurysm of the ulnar artery compressing the nerve (hypothenar hammer syndrome)[2,6,10] (**FIG 2A,B**; Table 1). Direct pressure on the ulnar nerve may occur during activities such as cycling.
- Fractures of the hook of the hamate can impinge on the nerve.
- Idiopathic compression may occur secondary to thickening of the proximal fibrous ligament at the entrance to the canal.
  - Compression also may occur as a result of swelling after distal radius fracture.
- Compression of the ulnar nerve at Guyon canal also has been shown to occur in conjunction with carpal tunnel syndrome. It typically resolves after surgical decompression of the carpal canal.[9,16]
- Other etiologies include tumors such as ganglia or lipomas (**FIG 2C,D**), anomalous muscle bellies,[8,15] or hypertrophy of the palmaris brevis.
  - Ganglia and other soft tissue masses are responsible for 32% to 48% of cases of ulnar tunnel syndrome. Another 16% of cases are due to muscle anomalies.[12]

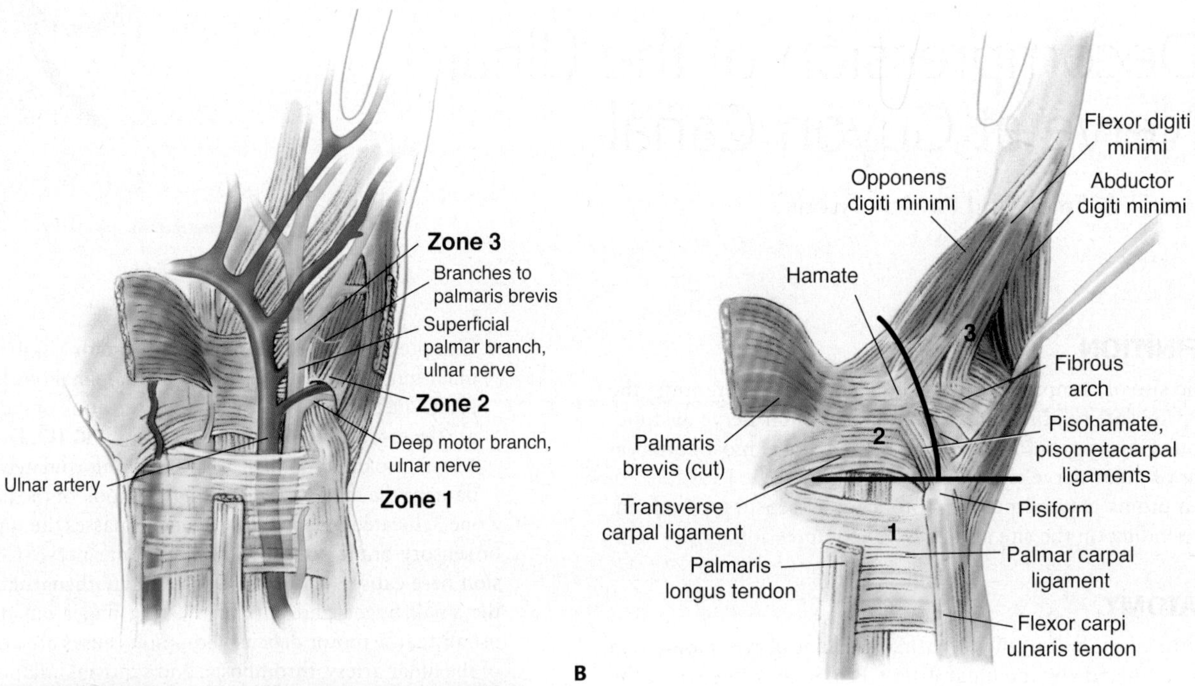

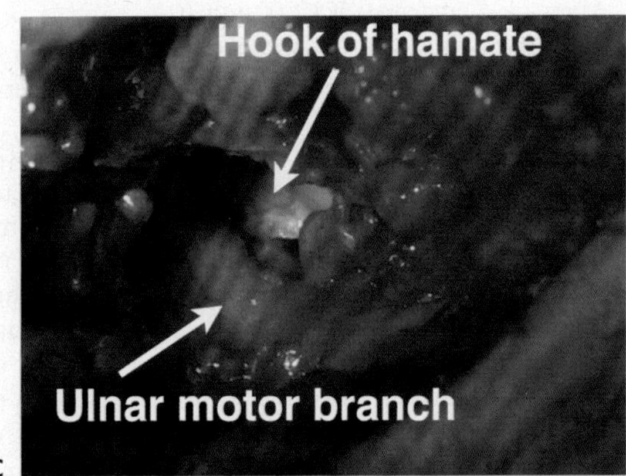

FIG 1 • **A.** Anatomic landmarks of the distal ulnar tunnel (Guyon canal). Zone 1: ulnar nerve in the region proximal to the bifurcation. Zone 2: ulnar nerve motor segment following bifurcation. Zone 3: ulnar nerve sensory segment distal to the bifurcation. **B.** Location of the three zones. Zone *1* is proximal to the bifurcation; zone *2* encompasses the motor branch; zone *3* is the region surrounding the sensory branch. **C.** The proximity of the motor branch of the ulnar nerve to the hook of the hamate as seen during excision of the hook.

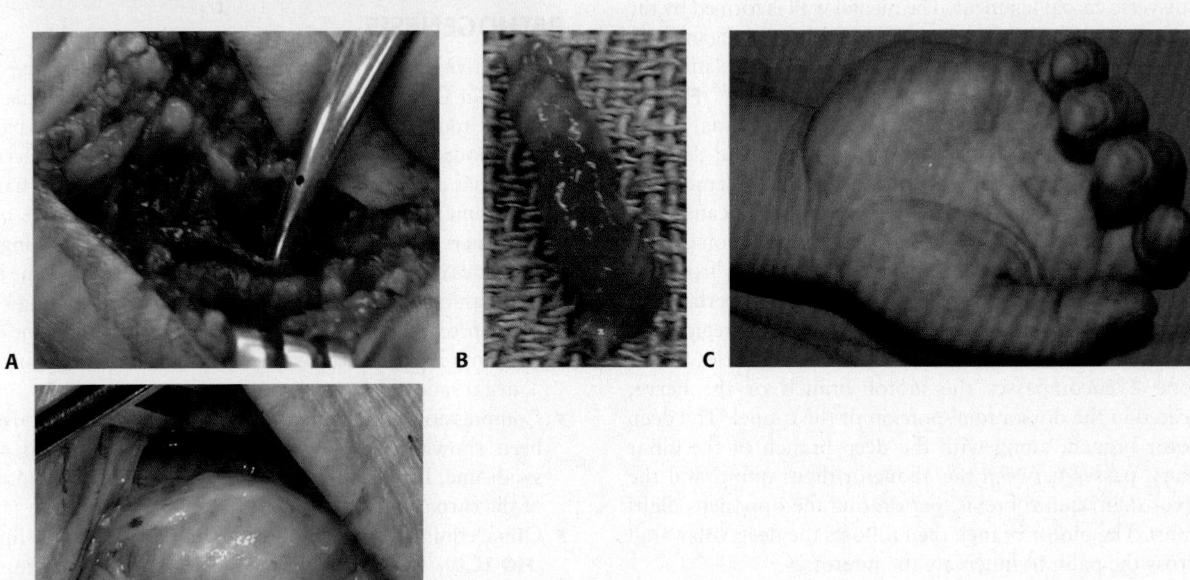

FIG 2 • **A.** Ulnar artery thrombosis. **B.** Resected thrombosed segment. **C.** Hypothenar mass as a cause of compression of the ulnar nerve at the wrist. **D.** Lipoma causing compression of the nerve.

Table 1 Causes of Compression or Injury of the Ulnar Nerve in Guyon Canal

- Ganglia
- Soft tissue masses
- Abnormal muscle bellies
- Hook of hamate fracture
- Distal radial fracture
- Thickening of proximal fibrous hypothenar arch
- Hypertrophic synovium
- Iatrogenic (after opponensplasty)
- Physiology
- Inflammatory conditions
- Tenosynovitis
- Rheumatoid arthritis
- Edema secondary to burns
- Gout
- Coexistent carpal tunnel syndrome
- Vascular conditions
- Ulnar artery thrombosis
- Ulnar artery pseudoaneurysm
- Neuropathic conditions
- Diabetes
- Alcoholism
- Proximal lesion of ulnar nerve (double-crush syndrome)
- Occupation-related
- Vibration exposure
- Repetitive blunt trauma
- Direct pressure on ulnar nerve with wrist extended
- Typing
- Cycling

- Synovitis secondary to rheumatoid arthritis may encroach on the canal and the nerve.
- Metabolic or infectious diseases such as diabetes, thyroid disease, or leprosy may also mimic the symptoms of nerve compression.
- Iatrogenic causes must also be recognized, such as compression by tendon or muscle transfer (Huber opponensplasty).[11]

NATURAL HISTORY

- Untreated compression may result in permanent dysfunction, weakness, and numbness.

PATIENT HISTORY AND PHYSICAL FINDINGS

Clinical History

- Presenting symptoms can vary from mild, transient paresthesias in the ring and small fingers to clawing of these digits and severe intrinsic muscle atrophy.
  - The patient may report severe pain at the elbow or wrist with radiation into the hand or up into the shoulder and neck.
  - Patients may report difficulty or clumsiness when opening jars or turning doorknobs.
  - Early fatigue or weakness may be noticed if work requires repetitive hand motions.
  - Depending on the climate and work conditions, cold intolerance in the ring and small fingers may be present.[5]
- A careful clinical history is imperative, noting the time of occurrence of symptoms. Determine whether symptoms are transient or continuous. Determine whether symptoms are related to work, sleep, or recreation. Elicit duration of symptoms and possible relation to trauma.

Physical Examination

- It is important to determine the level of pathology of the ulnar nerve because compression commonly occurs at four points: the cervical spine, the thoracic outlet, the elbow (cubital tunnel syndrome), or the wrist (Guyon canal).[7,17]
- Begin the clinical examination at the neck and shoulder and move down the affected extremity to the elbow.
  - Pain on neck movement mimicking the patient's symptoms could indicate cervical disc disease.
  - Pain on palpation of the plexus or with shoulder motion could indicate a pathologic condition in the brachial plexus or lung. Results of provocative maneuvers for thoracic outlet syndrome should be assessed.
  - Masses on the medial side of the arm could indicate a soft tissue tumor or hemorrhage compressing the nerve.
  - At the elbow, note any deformity, palpate the nerve, and determine whether abnormal mobility is present.
- The course of the nerve is palpated in the forearm all the way to the wrist.
  - A positive Tinel or Phalen sign often is found at the wrist over the ulnar nerve.
  - Tenderness over the hook of the hamate is particularly important.
- Sensory function is assessed.
  - Semmes-Weinstein monofilament testing may be abnormal but often is normal early in the course of the compression.
  - Two-point discrimination of the ring and small fingers usually becomes abnormal only late in the course of the disease.
- To help differentiate cubital tunnel syndrome from compression of the ulnar nerve at the wrist, assess flexor carpi ulnaris and flexor digitorum profundus strength.
- Intrinsic muscle function is tested by asking the patient to cross the long finger over the index finger (ie, crossed finger test).
- Only two muscles can be tested accurately in the hand—the abductor digiti quinti and the first dorsal interosseous. The tendons or bellies of these muscles can be palpated or visualized.
- Weakness of thumb pinch may be elicited by the Froment sign. Froment sign is ruled positive if the person must flex the thumb interphalangeal joint to maintain grasp.

IMAGING AND OTHER DIAGNOSTIC STUDIES

- Radiographs of the elbow and wrist are mandatory in ulnar nerve compression because entrapment of the ulnar nerve may occur at more than one level.
  - Radiographs of the hand and wrist should include carpal tunnel views as well as standard anteroposterior (AP), lateral, and oblique views. Radiographs of the wrist may reveal fractures of the hook of the hamate, dislocations of the carpal bones, or, less commonly, soft tissue masses and calcifications.
  - Radiographs of the elbow may reveal abnormal anatomy, such as a valgus deformity, bone spurs or bone fragments, a shallow olecranon groove, osteochondromas, or destructive lesions (eg, tumors, infections, abnormal calcifications).
- Radiographs of the neck should be obtained if cervical disc disease is suspected and to rule out cervical ribs.
- Obtain radiographs of the chest if a Pancoast tumor or tuberculosis is suspected.
- Magnetic resonance imaging (MRI) is not usually necessary unless further delineation of soft tissue masses such as lipomas or ganglions[11] or visualization of fractures, aneurysms,

congenital abnormality, or other abnormalities in the nerve is required. MRI also may detect structural abnormalities along the course of the ulnar nerve accounting for compression (eg, fibrous bands).
- Ultrasonography may be used to detect cysts or masses in Guyon canal and to assess ulnar nerve diameter at the elbow.
- Electromyography (EMG) and nerve conduction studies are helpful to confirm the specific area(s) of entrapment as well as document the extent of the pathology.
  - Motor and sensory conduction velocities are more useful in a recent entrapment, whereas conduction velocities and EMG are useful in chronic neuropathies (EMG shows axonal degeneration).
  - Conduction velocity short-segment stimulation (also known as the *inching technique*) can increase the sensitivity of this method and can improve localization by helping the examiner determine exactly where a blockage is occurring.
  - EMG evaluation of motor unit morphology and recruitment patterns ascertains ongoing loss of muscle fibers via detection of abnormal spontaneous activity (eg, fibrillation potentials and fasciculations). It also checks the integrity of the muscle membrane to expand differential diagnosis (eg, myotonia, paramyotonia, periodic paralysis) as manifested by increased insertional activity such as complex repetitive discharges, myokymia, and (para) myotonic discharges.[1]

DIFFERENTIAL DIAGNOSIS

- Cervical disc disease[17]
- Brachial plexus abnormalities, thoracic outlet syndrome, Pancoast tumor
- Elbow abnormalities, epicondylitis
- Infections, tumors, diabetes mellitus, hypothyroidism, rheumatoid diseases, alcoholism
- Wrist fractures
- Ulnar artery aneurysms or thrombosis at the wrist

NONOPERATIVE MANAGEMENT

- Conservative treatment of ulnar nerve compression is most successful when paresthesias are transient. Patient education and insight are important.
- Flexing the wrist at work while typing for long periods and resting the wrist on the handlebars of a bicycle or motorcycle while driving are causes of paresthesia that can be corrected without surgical treatment.
- Avoiding the use of vibrating or power tools, wrist splinting in a neutral position, and correction of ergonomics at work should help alleviate transient palsies.
- Nonsteroidal anti-inflammatory medications also are useful adjuncts to relieve nerve irritation.
- Oral vitamin B_6 supplements may be helpful for mild symptoms. This treatment should be carried out for 6 to 12 weeks, depending on patient response.

SURGICAL MANAGEMENT

- Surgical intervention is indicated if paresthesia increases despite adequate conservative treatment combined with abnormal nerve conduction studies or EMGs and at the first sign of motor changes.
- In a patient who sustains an immediate complete ulnar nerve injury as a result of a fracture of the wrist, the fracture should be reduced as soon as possible.
  - Elimination of any dorsal displacement of the distal radius or ulna should be achieved.
  - If ulnar nerve function does not improve within 24 to 36 hours following satisfactory reduction, the nerve should be explored and decompression carried out.[3,12]

Preoperative Planning

- The diagnosis should be confirmed with EMG and nerve conduction velocity or imaging studies (eg, MRI) before planning surgery.

Positioning

- Patients are operated on in the supine position with the arm extended on an arm board.
- A tourniquet is placed above the elbow and inflated to 250 to 265 mm Hg before the incision is made.

Approach

- Operative treatment is aimed at exploring and decompressing the nerve from the distal forearm into the hand throughout all three zones.

TECHNIQUES

Ulnar Nerve Exploration and Decompression of Guyon Canal

- Palpate and mark the pisiform.
  - The hook of the hamate can be found 1 cm distal and lateral to the pisiform.
- Make a curvilinear incision beginning distally in the interval between the pisiform and the hook of the hamate. Cross the wrist, extending proximal to the distal wrist flexion crease, along the radial border of the flexor carpi ulnaris (**TECH FIG 1A**).
  - The wrist should be crossed in a zigzag fashion to prevent longitudinal contracture of the scar.
- Perform the dissection proximal to distal. Identify the ulnar nerve proximal to the distal wrist flexor retinaculum and follow it distally through Guyon canal by reflecting the flexor carpi ulnaris and the pisohamate ligament.
  - The neurovascular bundle is traced distally to the point at which it enters Guyon canal beneath the palmar carpal ligament.
- Incise the ligament, palmaris brevis muscle, and fibrous tissue, decompressing the nerve along its entire course through the canal.
  - The branches of the ulnar nerve to the hypothenar muscles and palmaris brevis, as well as the deep branch of the nerve, can be identified and protected with this approach.
- The incision should not be carried ulnarly over the hypothenar eminence to avoid injury to the palmar cutaneous branch of the ulnar nerve.

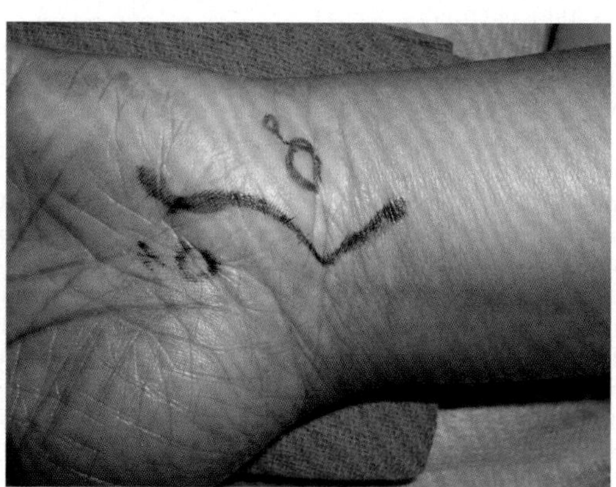

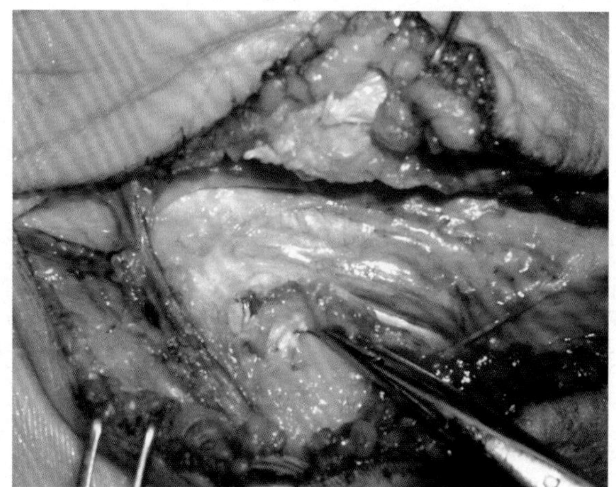

TECH FIG 1 • **A.** The skin incision is marked crossing the wrist at an angle to prevent scar contracture. **B.** The motor branch is followed into the interval between the flexor digiti minimi and abductor digiti minimi muscles.

- The ulnar artery should be examined for areas of thickening or thrombosis, and the ulnar nerve should be examined along its course for intra- or extraneural tumors (eg, schwannoma, neurolemmoma).
- Further exploration of the floor of the canal should be done to identify masses, ganglions, anomalous muscles, fibrous bands, osteophytes, or fracture fragments.
- The motor branch is followed into the interval between the flexor digiti minimi and abductor digiti minimi muscles and through the origin of the opponens digiti minimi (**TECH FIG 1B**).
- After exploration and decompression, release the tourniquet and coagulate all bleeders with a bipolar cautery before the wound is closed.
  - Hematoma in this area could potentially compress the nerve and artery.

PEARLS AND PITFALLS

Pearls	▪ Differentiation between proximal and distal nerve compression: ▪ Weakness of the small finger profundus points to ulnar nerve compression at the elbow. ▪ Involvement of the dorsal sensory branch indicates compression proximal to Guyon canal. ▪ Clawing is seen more commonly in distal (wrist) than proximal (elbow) lesions.
Pitfalls	▪ Inadequate preoperative evaluation, resulting in: ▪ Inaccurate or incomplete diagnosis ▪ Inadequate decompression

POSTOPERATIVE CARE

- Postoperatively, patients are placed into a protective splint for about 2 weeks to prevent excessive wrist flexion and extension.
- Sutures are removed at 10 to 14 days after surgery, at which time gentle active range of motion is started as well as scar care.
- The wrist splint should be continued for 2 to 3 more weeks to prevent scar thickening, which is common in this area.
  - Silicone or Otoform is helpful to prevent hard, firm scars.

OUTCOMES

- Symptoms can be expected to improve in all cases, with fewer than 20% of patients complaining of slight persistent numbness after the surgery.[14]
- The most common cause of failure of surgery is failure in diagnosis, followed by inadequate decompression of all of the branches of the ulnar nerve.

COMPLICATIONS

- Laceration of the ulnar nerve or artery (or both)
- Inadequate decompression
- Injury to the ulnar artery

REFERENCES

1. Agarwal SK, Schneider LB, Ahmad BK. Clinical usefulness of ulnar motor responses recording from first dorsal interosseous. Muscle Nerve 1995;18:1043.
2. Aguiar PH, Bor-Seng-Shu E, Gomes-Pinto F, et al. Surgical management of Guyon's canal syndrome, an ulnar nerve entrapment at the wrist: report of two cases. Arq Neuropsiquiatr 2001;59:106–111.

3. Bartels RH, Grotenhuis JA, Kauer JM. The arcade of Struthers: an anatomical study. Acta Neurochir (Wien) 2003;145:295–300.
4. Beekman R, Schoemaker MC, Van Der Plas JP, et al. Diagnostic value of high-resolution sonography in ulnar neuropathy at the elbow. Neurology 2004;62:767–773.
5. Beekman R, Van Der Plas JP, Uitdehaag BM, et al. Clinical, electrodiagnostic, and sonographic studies in ulnar neuropathy at the elbow. Muscle Nerve 2004;30:202–208.
6. Beekman R, Wokke JH, Schoemaker MC, et al. Ulnar neuropathy at the elbow: follow-up and prognostic factors determining outcome. Neurology 2004;63:1675–1680.
7. Bradshaw DY, Shefner JM. Ulnar neuropathy at the elbow. Neurol Clin 1999;17:447–461.
8. Buzzard EF. Some varieties of toxic and traumatic ulnar neuritis. Lancet 1922;1:317.
9. Campbell WW. Ulnar neuropathy at the elbow. Muscle Nerve 2000;23:450–452.
10. Cooke RA. Hypothenar hammer syndrome: a discrete syndrome to be distinguished from hand–arm vibration syndrome. Occup Med (Lond) 2003;53:320–324.
11. Feindel W, Stratford J. Cubital tunnel compression in tardy ulnar palsy. Can Med Assoc J 1958;78:351–353.
12. Gelberman RH. Ulnar tunnel syndrome. In: Gelberman RH, ed. Operative Nerve Repair and Reconstruction. Philadelphia: JB Lippincott, 1991:1131–1143.
13. Gross MS, Gelberman RH. The anatomy of the distal ulnar tunnel. Clin Orthop Relat Res 1985;(196):238–247.
14. Murata K, Shih JT, Tsai TM. Causes of ulnar tunnel syndrome: a retrospective study of 31 subjects. J Hand Surg Am 2003;28:647–651.
15. Pribyl CR, Moneim MS. Anomalous hand muscle found in Guyon's canal at exploration for ulnar artery thrombosis. A case report. Clin Orthop Relat Res 1994;(306):120–123.
16. Silver MA, Gelberman RH, Gellman H, et al. Carpal tunnel syndrome: associated abnormalities in ulnar nerve function and the effect of carpal tunnel release on these abnormalities. J Hand Surg Am 1985;10:710–713.
17. Szabo RM, Steinberg DR. Nerve entrapment syndromes in the wrist. J Am Acad Orthop Surg 1994;2:115–123.

Tendon Transfers for Ulnar Nerve Palsy

92 CHAPTER

Michael S. Bednar

DEFINITION

- Ulnar nerve palsy refers to loss of sensory and motor function after injury to the ulnar nerve above or below the wrist (high vs. low ulnar nerve palsy).

ANATOMY

- The ulnar nerve is the terminal branch of the medial cord (C8 and T1).
- The ulnar nerve consists of motor and sensory fibers. There are no muscles innervated by the ulnar nerve in the arm. In the forearm, the flexor carpi ulnaris receives its nerve branches after the ulnar nerve passes through the cubital tunnel. The other muscles innervated in the forearm are the flexor digitorum profundus of the ring and small fingers.
- The muscles innervated in the hand (by order of innervation) are the following:
  - Hypothenar muscles
    - Abductor digiti minimi
    - Flexor digiti minimi
    - Opponens digiti minimi
  - Ring and small lumbricals
  - Dorsal and palmar interosseous muscles
  - Adductor pollicis
  - Deep head of flexor pollicis brevis
  - First dorsal interosseous (last muscle innervated by the ulnar nerve)
- The sensory fibers of the ulnar nerve supply the small finger and the ulnar half of ring finger over the entire palmar surface and the dorsal surface distal to the proximal interphalangeal (PIP) joint. The dorsal surface proximal to the PIP joint of the small finger and the ulnar half of the ring finger and ulnar dorsum of the hand are innervated via the dorsal sensory branch of the ulnar nerve, which arises from the ulnar nerve 7 cm proximal to the wrist. The sensory branch crosses from volar to dorsal at the level of the ulnar styloid.

PATHOGENESIS

- Ulnar nerve palsy can arise from a laceration anywhere along its course. Proximal injuries to the medial cord may present with additional sensory loss in the distribution of the medial brachial or antebrachial cutaneous nerves. Nerve compression typically occurs either at the cubital tunnel at the elbow or the canal of Guyon at the wrist.
- A variety of systemic conditions may mimic ulnar neuropathy, including Charcot-Marie-Tooth disease, syringomyelia, and leprosy. In Charcot-Marie-Tooth disease and syringomyelia, there is weakness involving other nerves. In leprosy, there is a profound loss of sensation in the ulnar nerve distribution in addition to the claw deformity of the fingers.

NATURAL HISTORY

- The severity of the nerve palsy depends on the degree of the nerve lesion and the presence of anomalous innervation patterns (Martin-Gruber, Riche-Cannieu) in determining the number of muscles involved and the extent of palsy. Anomalous innervation patterns can confuse the examiner.
- Martin-Gruber anastomosis patterns are divided into four types:
  - Type I (60%): Motor branches from the median nerve are sent to the ulnar nerve to innervate "median" muscles.
  - Type II (35%): Motor branches from the median nerve are sent to the ulnar nerve to innervate "ulnar" muscles.
  - Type III (3%): Motor branches from the ulnar nerve are sent to the median nerve to innervate "ulnar" muscles.
  - Type IV (1%): Motor branches from the ulnar nerve are sent to the median nerve to innervate "median" muscles.
- With prolonged nerve palsy, secondary abnormalities of the hand occur, such as stretching of the central slip of the extensor mechanism at the PIP joint or fixed joint flexion contractures.

PATIENT HISTORY AND PHYSICAL FINDINGS

- An important point is to identify the cause and timing of palsy to determine whether the pathology can be reversed. Treatment is first addressed at improving nerve function by procedures such as decompression of a compressed nerve or acute repair of a lacerated nerve. Recovery can be gauged by progression of symptoms, such as advancing Tinel sign, return of muscle function, and return of sensation. Tendon transfers are indicated when nerve recovery is not expected or possible.
- Loss of sensation in the medial arm or forearm indicates a proximal lesion. Loss of sensation to the dorsal side of the ulnar hand indicates a lesion proximal to the wrist to affect the dorsal sensory branch.
- The following specific tests of motor dysfunction are used to determine the functional loss of the hand:
  - Froment sign: hyperflexion of thumb interphalangeal joint (**FIG 1A**); indicates substitution of flexor pollicis longus (FPL) (median nerve) for adductor pollicis (ulnar nerve)
  - Jeanne sign: reciprocal hyperextension of thumb metacarpophalangeal (MCP) joint (see **FIG 1A**); indicates substitution of FPL for adductor pollicis
  - Wartenberg sign: abduction of small finger at MCP joint; indicates paralyzed palmar intrinsic muscle (ulnar nerve) with abduction from extensor digiti minimi (radial nerve)
  - Duchenne sign: clawing of ring and small fingers, hyperextension of MCP joints, and flexion of PIP joints (**FIG 1B**); indicates paralysis of interosseous and lumbrical muscles of the ring and small fingers (low ulnar nerve), more pronounced in low rather than high ulnar nerve palsy

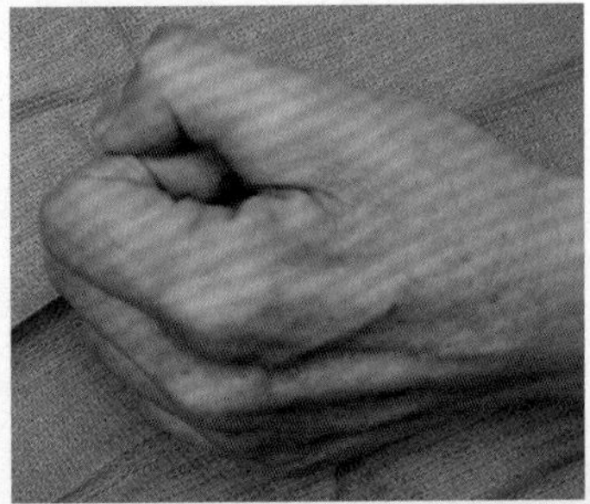
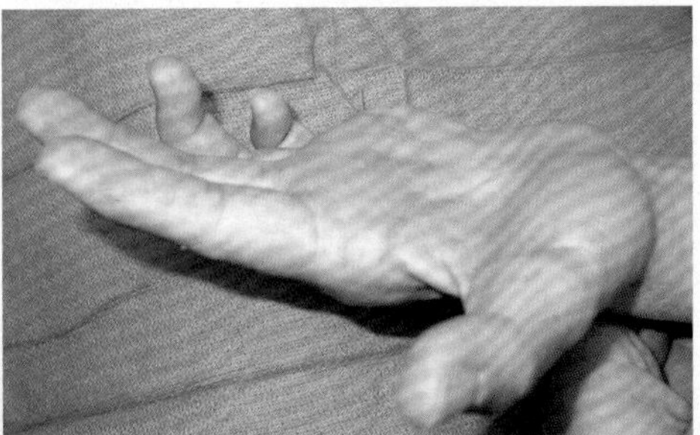
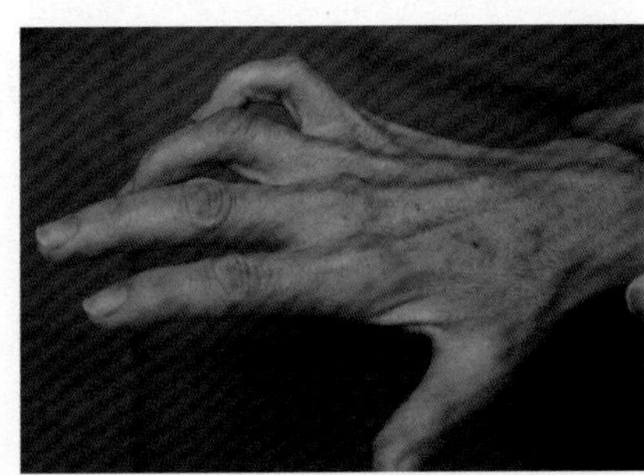
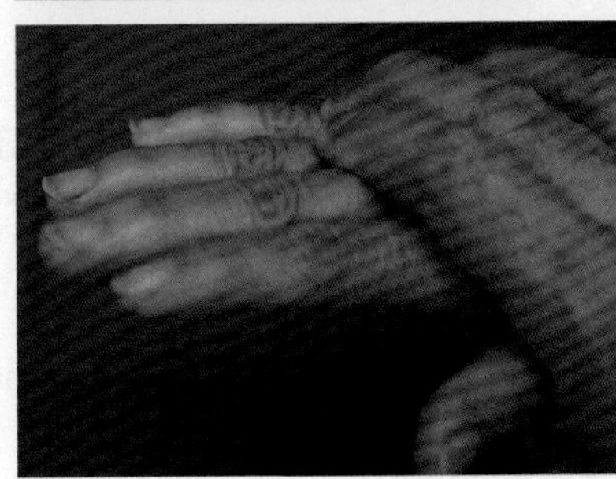

FIG 1 • **A.** With lateral pinch, the thumb interphalangeal joint flexes (Froment sign) and the thumb MCP joint hyperextends (Jeanne sign). **B.** With finger extension, the ring and small fingers hyperextend at the MCP joints and flex at the proximal and distal interphalangeal joints (Duchenne sign). Flattening of the metacarpal arch with loss of the hypothenar muscles produces loss of the small finger to oppose through the carpometacarpal joint (Masse sign). **C.** Clawing of the ring and small fingers when the MCP joints are allowed to extend. This worsens as the patient flexes the wrist to try to aid finger extension (Andre-Thomas sign). **D.** Full extension of ring and small finger PIP joints when MCP hyperextension is blocked indicates a competent central slip (Bouvier maneuver).

secondary to functioning flexor digitorum profundus of ring and small fingers (high ulnar nerve)

- Bouvier maneuver: inability to actively extend PIP joint when MCP joints are hyperextended and ability to actively extend PIP joint when MCP joints are blocked from hyperextension (**FIG 1C,D**). When active PIP joint extension is possible with the MCP joints blocked, this indicates competence of the central slip (positive test). When PIP joints cannot actively extend (negative test), this implies central slip attenuation. In this case, tendon transfers will need to block MCP joint hyperextension and provide PIP joint extension.
- Andre-Thomas sign: clawing of ring and small fingers, hyperextension of MCP joints and flexion of PIP joints, flexion of wrist (**FIG 1C**). An increase in the claw deformity as the patient tries to extend the fingers by flexing the wrist indicates a poor prognosis for tendon transfer surgery.
- Masse sign: flattening of the metacarpal arch (see **FIG 1B**); inability to oppose the small finger carpometacarpal joint
- Pollack sign: inability to flex the distal interphalangeal joint of the ring and small fingers; used to differentiate high from low ulnar nerve palsy

- In assessing for tendon transfers in ulnar nerve palsy, the primary functional concerns are the following:
  - Lack of thumb adduction and lateral pinch
  - Claw deformity of fingers that impairs object acquisition and grip
  - Loss of ring and small finger flexion (high palsy)

IMAGING AND OTHER DIAGNOSTIC STUDIES

- Electromyographic and nerve conduction velocity studies are used to isolate the ulnar nerve pathology and rule out other diagnoses. Serial studies may demonstrate the potential for recovery.

DIFFERENTIAL DIAGNOSIS

- Cervical radiculopathy
- Lower brachial plexopathy
- Charcot-Marie-Tooth disease
- Syringomyelia
- Leprosy

NONOPERATIVE MANAGEMENT

- When the Bouvier test is positive (active PIP joint extension is possible when MCP joint hyperextension is prevented), a dorsal MCP blocking splint for the ring and small fingers is fabricated to preserve the integrity of the PIP joint central slips.
- If a fixed flexion contracture of more than 45 degrees occurs at the PIP joint, a supervised hand therapy program consisting of serial casting is required.
- If the fixed flexion contracture does not respond to therapy, preliminary surgical joint release is necessary before tendon transfers.

SURGICAL MANAGEMENT

- Tendon transfers address the primary functional concerns listed earlier[9]:
  - Lack of thumb adduction and lateral pinch
  - Claw deformity of the fingers that impairs object acquisition and grip
  - Loss of ring and small finger flexion (high palsy)

Considerations

Restoring Thumb Adduction

- The first factor to consider in performing a transfer to restore thumb adduction is what donor muscle to use.
  - The extensor carpi radialis brevis (ECRB)[10] and the flexor digitorum superficialis (FDS)[5] are the most commonly used.
  - The FDS of the ring finger can be used in low ulnar nerve palsy when the flexor digitorum profundus of the ring finger is functioning.[3]
  - In high ulnar nerve palsy, the FDS of the middle finger can be used instead of the FDS of the ring finger.
  - The brachioradialis can be used if the ECRB is required for an intrinsic reconstruction of the fingers.
  - Alternatively, the extensor indicis proprius or abductor pollicis longus can be used.

- The second factor to consider is placement of the pulley.
  - For transfers coming from the dorsum of the hand, the pulley is either the index or middle finger metacarpal. Passing the transfer through the third web space, using the middle metacarpal as the pulley, allows the transferred tendon to lie palmar to the adductor pollicis but dorsal to the flexor tendons and neurovascular bundles.
  - For transfers originating from the palm of the hand (FDS), the vertical septum of the palmar fascia attached to the third metacarpal forms the pulley.
- The third factor is attachment of the transfer to the thumb.
  - The transfer can be inserted directly into the thumb metacarpal, into the adductor pollicis tendon, or into the abductor pollicis brevis tendon.
  - This last technique, favored by Omer,[6] allows the tendon to be sewn to the strong fascia abductor pollicis longus tendon and improves pronation of the thumb to aid in pinch.
- The last factor to address is stability of the MCP and interphalangeal joints.
  - For patients with a persistent Froment sign and mild hyperextension of the MCP joint, the split FPL to extensor pollicis longus tenodesis will stabilize the interphalangeal joint without fusion.
  - When the MCP joint shows substantial instability or arthritic changes, it should be fused.

Correcting Claw Deformity of Fingers

- Procedures to correct MCP hyperextension may be either static or dynamic.
  - A static procedure prevents hyperextension of the MCP joint, improving extension of the fingers. The Bouvier maneuver must be positive. The disadvantage of static procedures, either the MCP volar capsulodesis or tenodesis procedure, is that they tend to stretch with time.
  - A dynamic transfer uses the FDS, extensor carpi radialis longus, ECRB, or flexor carpi radialis as a donor muscle.
  - If the Bouvier maneuver is positive, there is no need to restore PIP joint extension.
  - If the Bouvier maneuver is negative, the procedure must address both MCP joint flexion and PIP joint extension. The insertion site of the tendon transfer determines which joints are affected by the transfer.
- FDS transfers for finger clawing[7]
  - Advantages
    - No need for tendon graft
    - Not passing tendon through interosseous spaces or through carpal tunnel
  - Disadvantages
    - Does not increase grip strength
    - High incidence of swan-neck deformities
    - Cannot use FDS of ring and small fingers in high ulnar nerve palsy
- Wrist motors for transfers for finger clawing[4]
  - Advantage: increases grip strength
  - Disadvantages
    - Requires tendon graft, either palmaris longus, plantaris, fascia lata, or toe extensor
    - Passes tendon through interosseous spaces or through carpal tunnel

Restoring Ring and Small Finger Extrinsic Muscle Function

- In patients with high ulnar nerve palsy, it is important to restore extrinsic flexion power before performing intrinsic transfers.
- Claw deformity of the ring and small fingers will worsen after these transfers.

Preoperative Planning

- Tendon transfers are indicated when no further nerve recovery is anticipated.
- In evaluating a patient for tendon transfer procedures, the examiner assesses the number of functions lost, determines the number of muscles available for transfer, and assesses the strength and excursion of each of the donor and recipient muscles.[2]
- When there are insufficient donor muscles to substitute for all functions that are lost, tenodesis and arthrodesis procedures may partially substitute for the lost function.
- There should be no fixed flexion contractures of the joints affected by the transfers.
- The transferred tendons need to be placed in a smooth, scar-free bed to glide.
- The principle of "one muscle and one function" should apply to each tendon transfer.

Positioning

- The patient is supine with the arm abducted on an arm table.

Approach

- All transfers for thumb adduction must pass distal to the pisiform.
- All transfers for intrinsic reconstruction must pass palmar to the axis of rotation of the MCP joint and dorsal to the axis of the PIP joint.

Transfers to Restore Thumb Adduction

Brachioradialis Extended with Tendon Graft, through Third Web Space, Inserted into Abductor Pollicis Brevis Tendon

- Make an incision between the flexor carpi radialis tendon and the radial artery beginning at the wrist crease and extending to the proximal third of the forearm.
- Dissect free of fascia the brachioradialis tendon and its muscle 7 to 10 cm proximal to the musculotendinous junction.
- Extend the tendon with a palmaris longus graft. Use a three-pass Pulvertaft weave to secure the palmaris longus graft to the brachioradialis tendon (**TECH FIG 1A**).
- Make incisions over the radial thumb MCP joint and in the third web space both palmar and dorsal.
- Sew a tendon graft, using one slip of the abductor pollicis longus tendon, in a three-pass Pulvertaft fashion into the abductor pollicis brevis tendon.
- Pass the tendon palmar to the adductor pollicis but dorsal to the flexor tendons and neurovascular bundles, as identified through the palmar incision over the third web space (**TECH FIG 1B**).

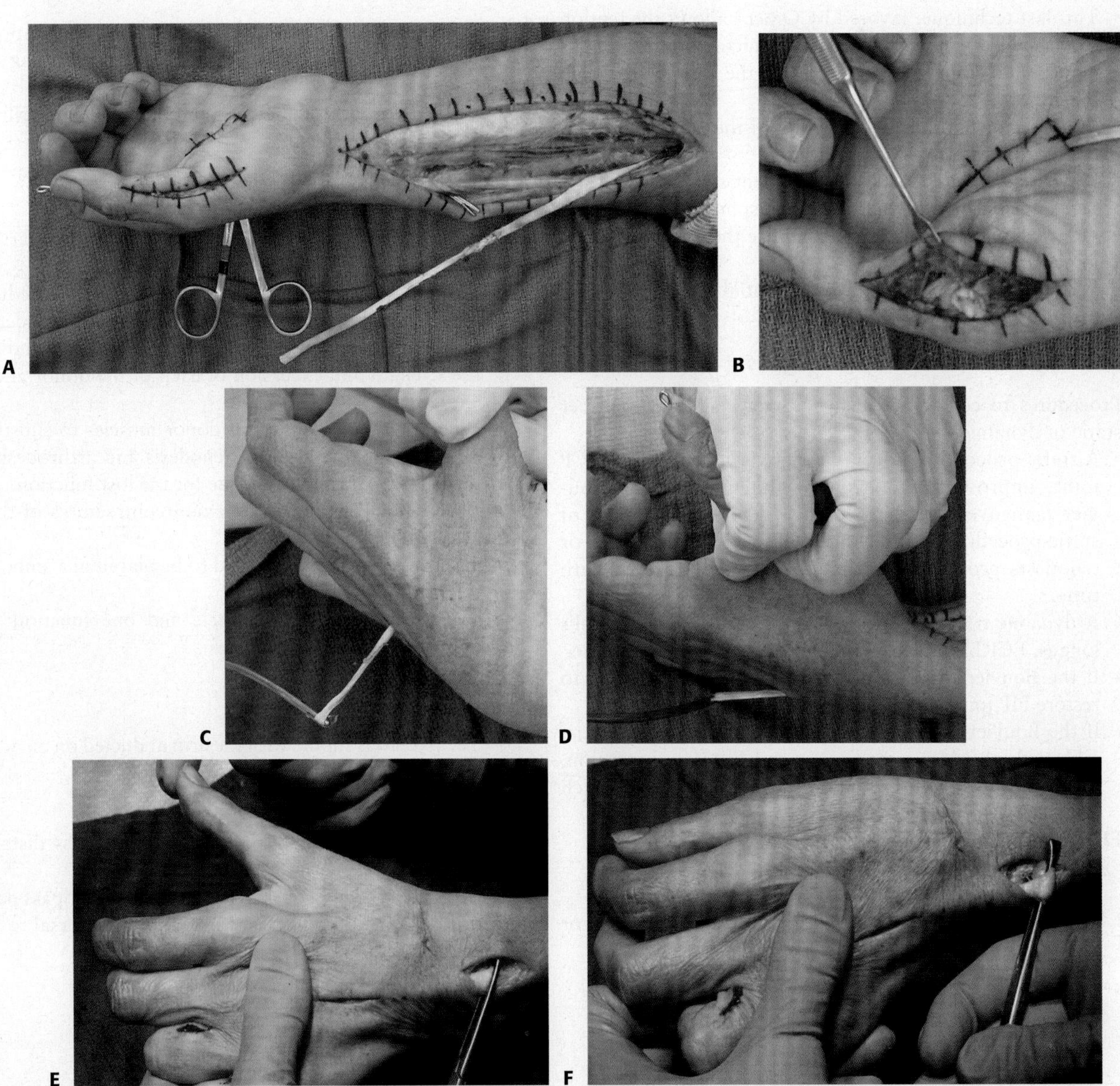

TECH FIG 1 • A. The brachioradialis muscle is freed into the proximal third of the forearm. The tendon is lengthened with a palmaris longus graft via a three-pass Pulvertaft method. **B.** Tendon graft taken from a slip of the abductor pollicis longus is sewn into the insertion of the abductor pollicis brevis tendon. The graft is passed palmar to the adductor pollicis muscle. The tendon is shown through the palmar incision before being passed dorsally through the third web space. **C.** Abductor pollicis longus tendon graft passed dorsally through the third web space. **D.** Brachioradialis with tendon graft passed into the incision over the dorsal hand. **E.** Tensioning of tendon transfer. With the wrist in neutral and no tension on the graft, the thumb should fully extend. **F.** Tensioning of tendon transfer. With the wrist in neutral and moderate tension on the tendon, the thumb strongly adducts to the index finger.

- Use the tendon passer to bring the graft from palmar to dorsal, using the proximal metaphysis of the third metacarpal as the pulley (**TECH FIG 1C**).
- Bring the tendon graft from the brachioradialis to the dorsum of the hand and perform the final Pulvertaft weave (**TECH FIG 1D**).
- Set tension to allow the thumb to rest palmar to the index finger when the wrist is in neutral.
- Take care to weave the tendons proximally enough on the hand such that the weave does not enter the third web space.
- Tension on the graft will pull the thumb into adduction (**TECH FIG 1E,F**).

Split Flexor Pollicis Longus to Extensor Pollicis Longus Tenodesis

- Make an incision along the radial proximal phalanx of the thumb. Identify the FPL and extensor pollicis longus tendons. Take care to preserve the oblique pulley.
- Identify the natural cleft between the radial and ulnar fibers of the FPL and split the tendon (**TECH FIG 2A**).
- Weave the radial half of the FPL tendon into the extensor pollicis longus tendon (**TECH FIG 2B,C**).
- Pin the interphalangeal joint in extension with a 0.045-inch smooth pin.

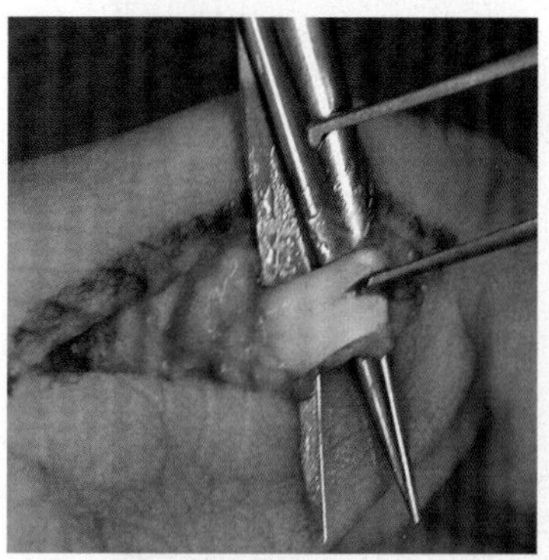
A

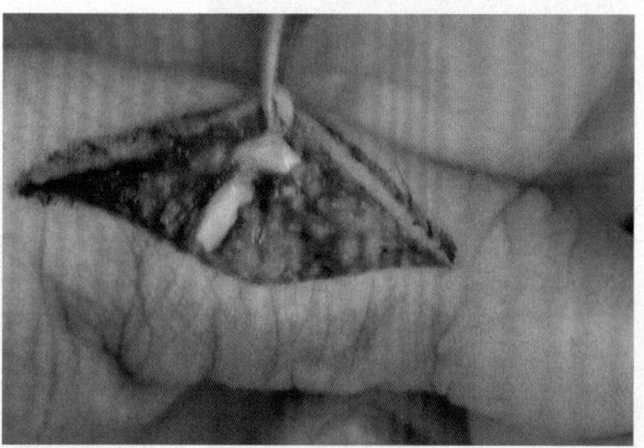
B

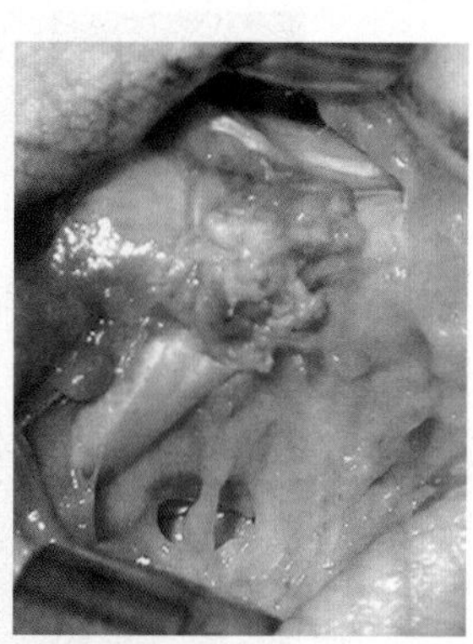
C

TECH FIG 2 • **A.** The FPL tendon is split into radial and ulnar halves at its insertion into the distal phalanx. The radial half is transected at the level of the interphalangeal joint. **B.** The radial half of the FPL tendon is woven into the radial half of the extensor pollicis longus tendon. A pin is placed across the interphalangeal joint in full extension. **C.** FPL split tenodesis sewn into place.

Tendon Transfers for Claw Deformity of Fingers

Zancolli Lasso

- This operation is indicated when there is a positive Bouvier maneuver.
- Make a midpalm Bruner zigzag incision.
- Incise the tendon sheath between the A1 and A2 pulleys. Identify the FDS tendon and transect it just proximal to the bifurcation. Leaving the bifurcation intact will decrease the incidence of PIP hyperextension.
  - Zancolli[11] recommends using the FDS of each finger, but Anderson[1] recommends using the FDS of the middle finger, split into four tails, to control MCP flexion of all four fingers.
- Pull the FDS tendon out of the tendon sheath distal to the A1 pulley, bring it palmar to the A1 pulley, and sew it to itself proximal to the A1 pulley. If insufficient MCP flexion is attained, the tendon exits the pulley sheath in the middle of the A2 pulley to improve the lever arm of the transfer.
- Set tension so the MCP joint is in 40 to 50 degrees of flexion with the wrist in neutral.
- When one FDS tendon is used for all four fingers, transect the FDS middle tendon distal to the A2 pulley through an oblique incision on the finger.
- Make a transverse midpalm incision, retrieve the tendon, and split it into four tails.
- Pass each tail down the lumbrical canal, palmar to the deep transverse metacarpal ligament, and into the flexor sheath proximal to the A1 pulley. Pass the tendon around the pulley and sew the distal end of the tendon back to itself proximal to the A1 pulley, tensioning it while the MCP joint is in 40 to 50 degrees of flexion with the wrist in neutral.
- For either the Zancolli or Anderson technique, the tendon may be sewn to the proximal metaphyseal–diaphyseal junction of the proximal phalanx via suture anchors or pullout drill holes.

Stiles-Bunnell Transfer

- This technique is indicated when the Bouvier maneuver is negative.
- One FDS tendon is used to motor two digits. Make radial midaxial incisions over the proximal phalanges of the digits. Make a midpalmar incision to retrieve the tendon. Cut the FDS ring tendon just proximal to its bifurcation between the A1 and A2 pulleys.
- Split the tendon and pass each half down the lumbrical canal. Pass the tendon passer from distally to proximally, going palmar to the deep transverse intermetacarpal ligament.
- Sew the tendon to the lateral band to restore PIP extension. Set tension with the MCP joint in 40 to 50 degrees of flexion and the PIP joints in full extension with the wrist in neutral. Excessive tension will cause PIP hyperextension.

Dorsal Route Transfer of Extensor Carpi Radialis Brevis

- Make radial midaxial incisions over the proximal phalanges of the digits.
- Pass the tendon passer from distally to proximally, going palmar to the deep transverse intermetacarpal ligament.
- For the ring and small fingers, make an incision in the dorsal fourth web space to retrieve the tendon grafts (**TECH FIG 3A**).
- Sew the distal end of the tendon graft to the proximal metaphyseal–diaphyseal junction of the proximal phalanx via suture anchors or pullout drill holes if the Bouvier maneuver is positive. Tension on the tendon graft will produce MCP flexion (**TECH FIG 3B**).
  - If the Bouvier maneuver is negative, attach the graft to the radial lateral band of the middle, ring, and small fingers and the ulnar lateral band of the index finger.
- Retrieve the ECRB tendon through a dorsal incision. Bring the tendon grafts through the same wound. First, sew the grafts to each other, synchronized to obtain even pull-through the grafts. Then, sew the grafts to the ECRB tendon with the wrist in 30 degrees of extension and the MCP joints in 60 degrees of flexion.

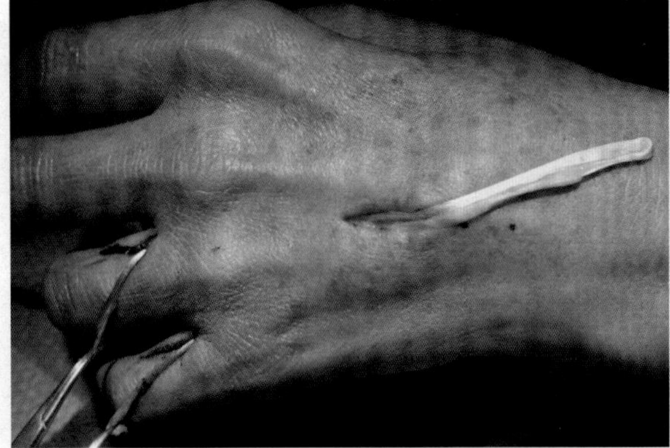

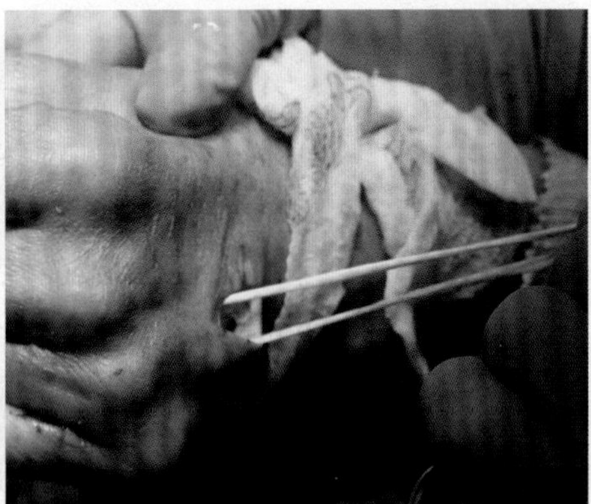

TECH FIG 3 • **A.** Tendon graft is passed from the dorsum of the hand over the fourth web space, palmar to the deep transverse intermetacarpal ligament, and through the lumbrical canals of the ring and small fingers to exit over the radial lateral bands of the fingers. **B.** Tendon grafts have been sewn to the proximal phalanges by suture anchors. Tension on the tendon grafts causes MCP flexion.

Transfer of Flexor Digitorum Profundus Ring and Small to Flexor Digitorum Profundus Middle (High Ulnar Nerve Palsy)

- Make a longitudinal incision over the distal third of the forearm.
- Identify the flexor digitorum profundus tendons.
- After synchronizing the long, ring, and small tendons, place two rows of horizontal sutures between the three tendons.

PEARLS AND PITFALLS

Evaluation	■ Differentiate high from low ulnar nerve palsy. ■ Determine the potential for nerve and muscle recovery. ■ Critically assess the strength of the donor muscles. ■ Determine the integrity of the PIP central slip (Bouvier maneuver). ■ Have the patient prioritize functional impairment.
Adductorplasty	■ Assess both adduction and opposition. ■ Dorsal transfers passed through the third web space allow for strong adduction using a wrist extensor or the brachioradialis muscle. ■ Hyperextension of the MCP joint and hyperflexion of the interphalangeal joint must be addressed with either a capsulodesis and fusion of the MCP joint or a split FPL tenodesis. Both the MCP and interphalangeal joints should not be fused.

Claw finger deformities	■ Determine the integrity of the PIP central slip (Bouvier maneuver). ■ When the Bouvier maneuver shows that the PIP central slip is competent, the tendon transfer should be sewn to the proximal phalanx or the pulleys. If the central slip is not competent, the tendon transfer is sewn into the lateral band. ■ Transfers need to pass palmar to the axis of rotation of the MCP joints.

POSTOPERATIVE CARE

- A knowledgeable hand therapist plays an important role in the postoperative care of tendon transfers for ulnar nerve palsy. Protecting the transfers with well-made splints while mobilizing uninvolved joints requires strict adherence to postoperative protocols.[8]
- For most procedures, the hand is immobilized for 3 weeks, followed by a blocking splint to allow motion within the restraints of the splint for the next 3 weeks.
- Passive exercises are begun at 6 weeks and strengthening at 8 weeks for the adductorplasty and at 10 to 12 weeks for the intrinsic tendon transfers.

OUTCOMES

- After tendon transfers for thumb adduction, pinch strength usually improves from 25% to 50% of normal.
- Tendon transfers to improve intrinsic function maintain good to excellent correction of the claw deformity in 80% to 90% of patients.
- Only the ECRB transfer improves grip strength.

COMPLICATIONS

- More complications occur after intrinsic muscle transfers than adductorplasty because of the delicate balance of the extensor hood mechanism.
- Transfer not strong enough
  - Problems include choice of a muscle with insufficient strength or excursion, use of a soft tissue pulley that stretched, or elongation at the tendon transfer site.
  - Elongation is a particular problem with sewing the transfer into the lateral bands of the extensor hood.
  - Patients with this transfer must be instructed on not hyperextending the MCP joints.
  - Transfers that are not strong enough can be treated with a therapy program to strengthen the muscle but often require surgical revision.
- Transfer too strong
  - Problems include choice of a muscle that is too strong or with too short of an excursion or sewing the transfer in with too much tension.
  - When the transfer is sewn too tightly into the lateral band, it can produce a swan-neck deformity of the digit.
  - Transfers that are too tight can be treated with passive range of motion in therapy, trying to stretch the transfer.

REFERENCES

1. Anderson GA. Ulnar nerve palsy. In: Green DP, Hotchkiss RN, Pederson WC, et al, eds. Green's Operative Hand Surgery, ed 5. Philadelphia: Elsevier, 2005:1161–1196.
2. Brand PW, Beach RB, Thompson DE. Relative tension and potential excursion of muscles in the forearm and hand. J Hand Surg Am 1981;6(3):209–219.
3. Hamlin C, Littler JW. Restoration of power pinch. J Hand Surg Am 1980;5(4):396–401.
4. Hastings H II, Davidson S. Tendon transfers for ulnar nerve palsy. Evaluation of results and practical treatment considerations. Hand Clin 1988;4:167–178.
5. Hastings H II, McCollam SM. Flexor digitorum superficialis lasso tendon transfer in isolated ulnar nerve palsy: a functional evaluation. J Hand Surg Am 1994;19(2):275–280.
6. Omer G. Tendon transfers for combined traumatic nerve palsies of the forearm and hand. J Hand Surg Br 1992;17(6):603–610.
7. Ozkan T, Ozer K, Gülgönen A. Three tendon transfer methods in reconstruction of ulnar nerve palsy. J Hand Surg Am 2003;28(1):35–43.
8. Rath S. Immediate postoperative active mobilization versus immobilization following tendon transfer for claw deformity correction in the hand. J Hand Surg Am 2008;33(2):232–240.
9. Sachar K. Reconstruction for ulnar nerve palsy. In: Berger RA, Weiss APC, eds. Hand Surgery. Philadelphia: Lippincott Williams & Wilkins, 2004:979–990.
10. Smith RJ. Extensor carpi radialis brevis tendon transfer for thumb adduction—a study of power pinch. J Hand Surg Am 1983;8(1):4–15.
11. Zancolli EA. Claw-hand caused by paralysis of the intrinsic muscles: a simple surgical procedure for its correction. J Bone Joint Surg Am 1957;37-A(5):1076–1080.

Decompression of Pronator and Anterior Interosseous Syndromes

E. Bruce Toby, Adam M. Goodyear, and Kyle P. Ritter

DEFINITION

- Pronator and anterior interosseous syndromes are compression neuropathies of the median nerve and its main branch, the anterior interosseous nerve (AIN), at the elbow, and proximal forearm.

ANATOMY

- The median nerve passes in the distal upper arm between the brachialis and the medial intermuscular septum, with the brachial artery sitting lateral to it.
  - A rare supracondylar process may arise from the distal aspect of the humerus, giving origin to a fibrous band extending to the medial epicondyle. This is the ligament of Struthers.
  - If a ligament of Struthers is present, the median nerve passes underneath it.
- At the elbow, the median nerve sits underneath the lacertus fibrosus and then typically passes between the superficial (humeral) head and the deep (ulnar) head of the pronator teres.
  - In 20% of individuals, the deep head is absent or consists of a small fibrous band.
- Motor branches to the palmaris longus, flexor carpi radialis, flexor digitorum superficialis, and flexor digitorum profundus typically branch from the median nerve in an ulnar direction proximal to the pronator teres.
- Under the pronator teres, the AIN branches in a radial direction from the median nerve, and both pass underneath the fibrous arcade of the flexor digitorum superficialis.
- The surgeon should be cognizant of the cutaneous nerves passing over the antecubital and proximal forearm region. Damage to these nerves can result in numbness and paresthesia as well as symptomatic neuromas in the forearm.
- Anomalous muscles and nerve branches may be present, the most common of which is the so-called Martin-Gruber anastomosis.
  - The surgeon should also be aware of more proximal or distal branching of the AIN from the median nerve.
  - The Martin-Gruber anastomosis, which occurs in about 15% of the population, consists of branches from either the median nerve or AIN to the ulnar nerve.

PATHOGENESIS

- Compression of the median nerve in the proximal forearm is rare compared with carpal tunnel syndrome.
- Median nerve compression in the proximal forearm has been labeled as either *pronator syndrome* or *anterior interosseous syndrome.*
- The true incidence of median nerve compression in the proximal forearm is difficult to ascertain, as is the relative contribution of the various potential impinging structures.
- Numerous studies have shown that the most common causes of median nerve compression in the region of the elbow and proximal forearm seem to be fascial bands and muscular anomalies of the pronator teres and the fibrous arcade of the flexor digitorum superficialis.[3,6]
  - Less common sites of nerve compression include the lacertus fibrosus and the ligament of Struthers (in cases with an existing supracondylar process).
  - A large number of additional structures have been identified as potential sources of compression of the median nerve. These include an accessory bicipital aponeurosis[8] and a variety of anomalous muscles, the most frequently cited of which is the accessory head of the flexor pollicis longus muscle, or *Gantzer muscle*.
  - A persistent median artery penetrating the median nerve also has been described.[4]
  - Space-occupying lesions such as lipomas or scarring from trauma can result in nerve compression.
- Anterior interosseous syndrome caused by nerve compression must be differentiated from Parsonage-Turner syndrome or mononeuritis.

NATURAL HISTORY

- Compression of the median nerve in the forearm often is transient due to excessive physical activity or swelling from injury.
- Recovery from Parsonage-Turner syndrome can be prolonged, but the prognosis usually is good without surgical decompression.
- The natural history and prognosis of pronator syndrome is not well understood.

PATIENT HISTORY AND PHYSICAL FINDINGS

- Classically, pronator syndrome presents as paresthesia in the median nerve distribution with minimal or no weakness. The patient also may complain of pain localized to the proximal forearm that is increased with activities. There may be a focal area of increased pain localizing to the specific area of compression.
  - In severe cases, weakness of the anterior interosseous innervated muscles—the flexor pollicis longus, the index and long flexor digitorum profundus, and the pronator quadratus—might be seen as well as select thenar muscles.

- Theoretically, patients may have paresthesia in the distribution of the palmar cutaneous branch of the median nerve, in contrast to carpal tunnel syndrome.
- AIN syndrome presents as diminished motor function of the index (and long) flexor digitorum profundus, flexor pollicis longus, and pronator quadratus without injury or specific known cause.
  - The patient typically complains of spontaneous loss of dexterity and voices specific complaints related to flexion of the thumb interphalangeal (IP) joint and/or index distal interphalangeal (DIP) joint.
  - Decreased sensation is not a common presenting symptom.
    - In cases of space-occupying lesions or scarring from trauma compressing the nerve, one would expect to see sensory symptoms as well as motor abnormalities.
  - Patients suffering from Parsonage-Turner syndrome often will experience a prodromal viral-type illness together with significant pain for several days or weeks before the onset of weakness.
- Physical examinations to perform include the following:
  - *Pronator compression test.* Paresthesia in the median nerve distribution within 30 seconds is considered a positive test. The test is nonspecific and can be seen with carpal tunnel syndrome.
  - *Resisted proximal interphalangeal (PIP) joint flexion of long finger.* Paresthesia in the median nerve distribution and pain in the forearm are considered a positive test. The test is thought to be consistent with compression of the median nerve at the fibrous arcade of the flexor digitorum superficialis.
  - *Resisted pronation test.* Paresthesia in the median nerve distribution and pain are considered a positive test. A positive finding is consistent with compression of the median nerve by the pronator teres.
  - *Elbow flexion test.* Paresthesia and pain are considered a positive test. A positive test is thought to be consistent with lacertus fibrosus compression of the median nerve.

IMAGING AND OTHER DIAGNOSTIC STUDIES

- Electrodiagnostic studies are often not helpful in pronator syndrome. Numerous studies have shown that symptoms and outcome of surgery do not correlate well with electrodiagnostic studies.
- In anterior interosseous syndrome, electrodiagnostic studies will confirm denervation of the anterior interosseous muscles.
- Electrodiagnostic studies are most valuable in the diagnosis of proximal median nerve compression for ruling out carpal tunnel syndrome.
- Ultrasonography and magnetic resonance imaging (MRI) are valuable tests for identifying space-occupying lesions such as lipomas or ganglions.
  - MRI can be a useful investigation to evaluate anterior interosseous syndrome showing edema within the pronator quadratus.[1]
- Plain radiographs of the proximal forearm and elbow may reveal a supracondylar process or anatomic variation.

DIFFERENTIAL DIAGNOSIS

- Carpal tunnel syndrome
- Mononeuritis or Parsonage-Turner syndrome
- Other form of neuritis

NONOPERATIVE MANAGEMENT

- In the acute phase, rest, immobilization, and avoidance of aggravating activities, such as repetitive pronation and heavy gripping, should be recommended.
- Forearm stretching exercises can be tried in chronic cases.
- Modalities such as ultrasound and electrostimulation have been advocated, although there is limited validation of their usefulness.
- Nerve gliding and nerve mobilization remain controversial.
- Spontaneous recovery does appear to occur in the majority of patients with anterior interosseous syndrome, although recovery can take up to 12 months.[7,10]

SURGICAL MANAGEMENT

Approach

- The greatest variation in surgical technique concerns the skin incision.
- For decompression of both pronator and anterior interosseous syndromes, extensile exposures using a modification of Henry approach allows for safe and thorough exposure of the median nerve and decompression of all sites of potential compression.
  - This incision sometimes is associated with unsightly scarring and injuries to the cutaneous nerves.
- Lesser incisions have been described, therefore; these include a lazy S-shape incision in the proximal volar forearm as well as two longitudinal,[2] oblique,[6,11] and transverse[9] incisions.
  - Limited incisions require significant retraction to ensure decompression both proximally and distally.
- Endoscopic decompression has been recently described.[5] Whether the advantages of an endoscopic release outweigh the increased cost and risks remains unknown.
- The surgeon's experience and comfort level may be the determining factors in deciding on the type of incision.

Extensile Approach

- The incision is made on the medial aspect of the distal arm proximal to the elbow flexion crease (**TECH FIG 1A**). It is brought across the elbow flexion crease and extended distally for approximately 10 cm.
- Cutaneous nerve branches, including branches of the lateral brachial and medial antebrachial cutaneous nerves, are identified and atraumatically mobilized.
- The median nerve is identified proximal to the elbow flexion crease and then is traced distally, releasing the lacertus fibrosus (**TECH FIG 1B**).
  - The existence of a ligament of Struthers and supracondylar process can then be ascertained.
- Motor branches of the median nerve to the muscles originating from the medial epicondyle must be protected throughout the operation. These include the palmaris longus, the flexor carpi radialis, and the flexor digitorum superficialis as well as the pronator teres (**TECH FIG 1C**).
- It will be necessary to ligate some vessels, but it will be possible to retract most of them.
- The radial artery lies radial to the nerve and must be protected throughout the procedure.
- The median nerve will be adherent to the pronator teres.
- Retracting the proximal portion of the pronator muscle mass identifies the median nerve and the pronator teres tendon (**TECH FIG 1D**).
- The larger, superficial pronator head is identified.
- It sometimes is possible to retract the entire muscle mass and follow the median nerve into the superficialis arcade. Frequently, however, it is necessary to release the tendinous portion of the pronator teres (**TECH FIG 1E**).
- Considerable variation exists within the pronator teres.
  - The median nerve can either pass between the superficial and deep pronator heads or, less commonly, pass underneath both heads.
  - Up to 20% of the time, the deep head is absent.
  - In the most uncommon variation, the median nerve pierces the humeral head.
- It is critical for all tendinous portions of the pronator teres potentially compressing the nerve to be released in the procedure.
- If scarring of the pronator teres is present as a result of trauma, a Z-lengthening of the pronator teres tendon is advisable.
  - This will improve exposure by allowing the humeral head to be reflected in an ulnar direction, exposing the AIN, the median nerve, and the flexor digitorum superficialis arcade (see **TECH FIG 1E**).

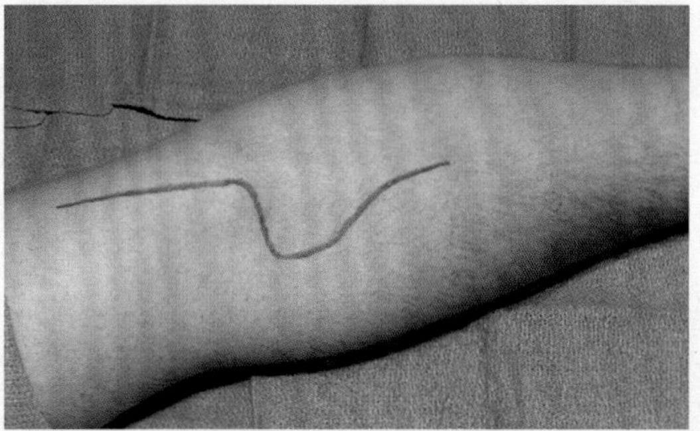

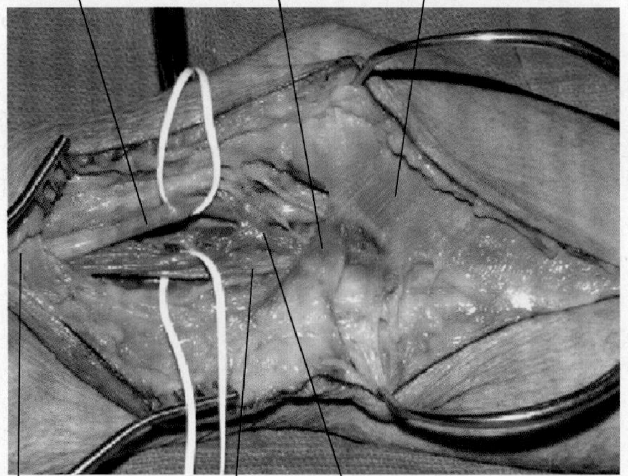

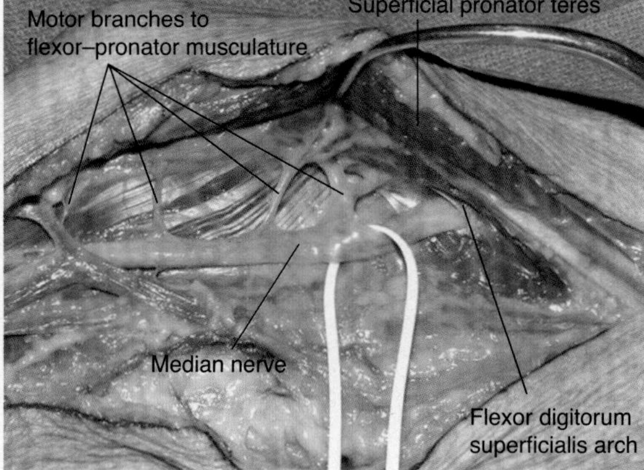

TECH FIG 1 • Extensile exposure. **A.** Skin incision. **B.** Incision with demonstrated lacertus fibrosus. **C.** Retracted but not released superficial pronator teres and intact flexor digitorum superficialis arch. *(continued)*

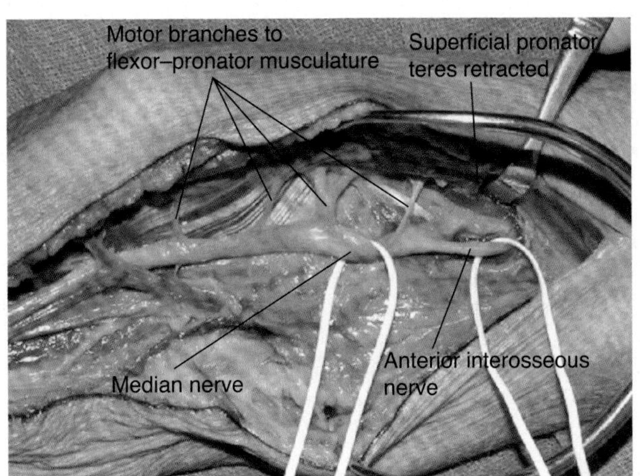

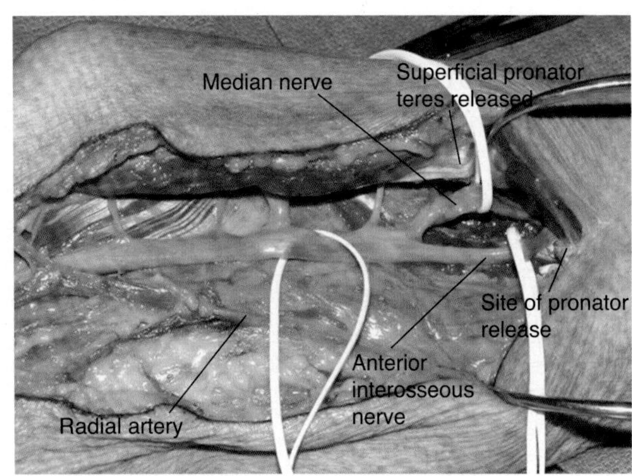

TECH FIG 1 • *(continued)* **D.** Retracted pronator and released superficial arch. **E.** Z-lengthened superficial pronator teres tendon.

- The superficialis arcade can then be released, and the median nerve and AIN are visualized distally by gentle retraction of the muscle fibers.
- AIN branches to the flexor pollicis longus and flexor digitorum profundus must be protected.
- Use of atraumatic technique with careful hemostasis is important to prevent postoperative scarring, with resultant pain and potential weakness.
- If the pronator teres tendon has been released, it should be repaired in a lengthened fashion.
- We prefer to use subcutaneous closure and subcuticular suturing.

Limited Incision

- An oblique or transverse incision can be made in the proximal forearm just distal to the elbow flexion crease (**TECH FIG 2A**).
- Retractors are placed proximally and distally to identify the cutaneous nerve fibers.
- The lacertus fibrosus is released first, and then the median nerve is identified, as previously described.
- Retractors are placed to allow visualization and palpation of the median nerve proximally to permit identification of proximal lesions such as a ligament of Struthers (**TECH FIG 2B**).
- Distally, the pronator teres is identified and the muscle and tendon mobilized.
- If required, the superficial or deep tendons (or both) are released.
- Fascial impinging structures are identified and released as needed.
- The superficialis arcade is identified and released, protecting the median nerve and AIN.

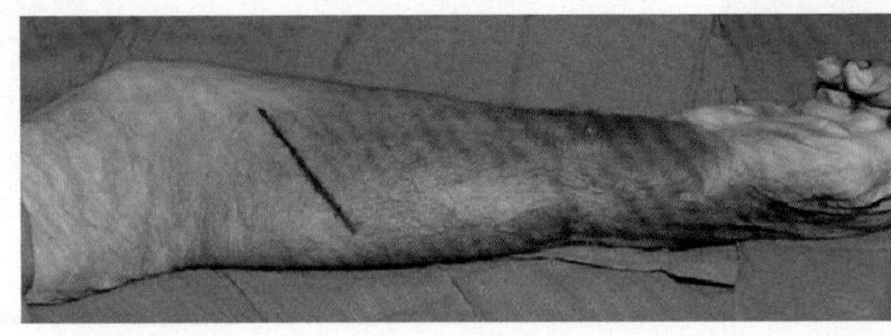

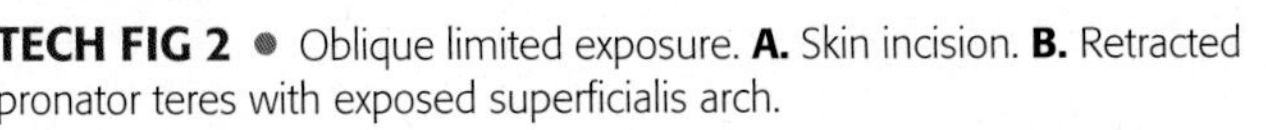

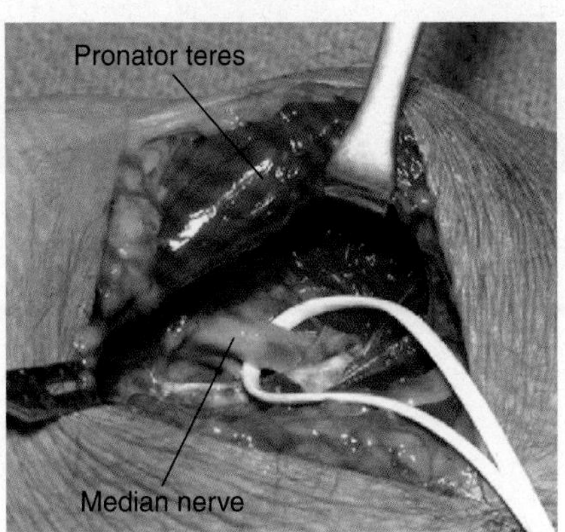

TECH FIG 2 • Oblique limited exposure. **A.** Skin incision. **B.** Retracted pronator teres with exposed superficialis arch.

Endoscopically Assisted Decompression

- A 3-cm incision is made 3 to 4 cm distal to the antecubital crease over the radial border of the flexor mass (**TECH FIG 3A,B**).
- Identification and retraction of the basilic vein is carried out, and the lacertus fibrosus is divided completely under direct visualization.
- The pronator teres is retracted medially, and the biceps and brachioradialis are retracted laterally.
- Blunt dissection then reveals the median nerve which is dissected as distally and proximally as direct vision will allow (**TECH FIG 3C**).
- The endoscope is first inserted proximally, lifting the soft tissues above the median nerve.
- Scissors are then used to release the proximal extension of the bicipital aponeurosis under endoscopic view.
- The endoscope is then directed distally, and the tendinous or fibrous band associated with the pronator teres muscle is identified.
- The fibrous portion of the pronator teres as well as the ulnar and humeral head can be released at this point by a technique combining spreading and cutting.
  - The fibrous arch of the flexor digitorum superficialis is then identified and released using scissors.

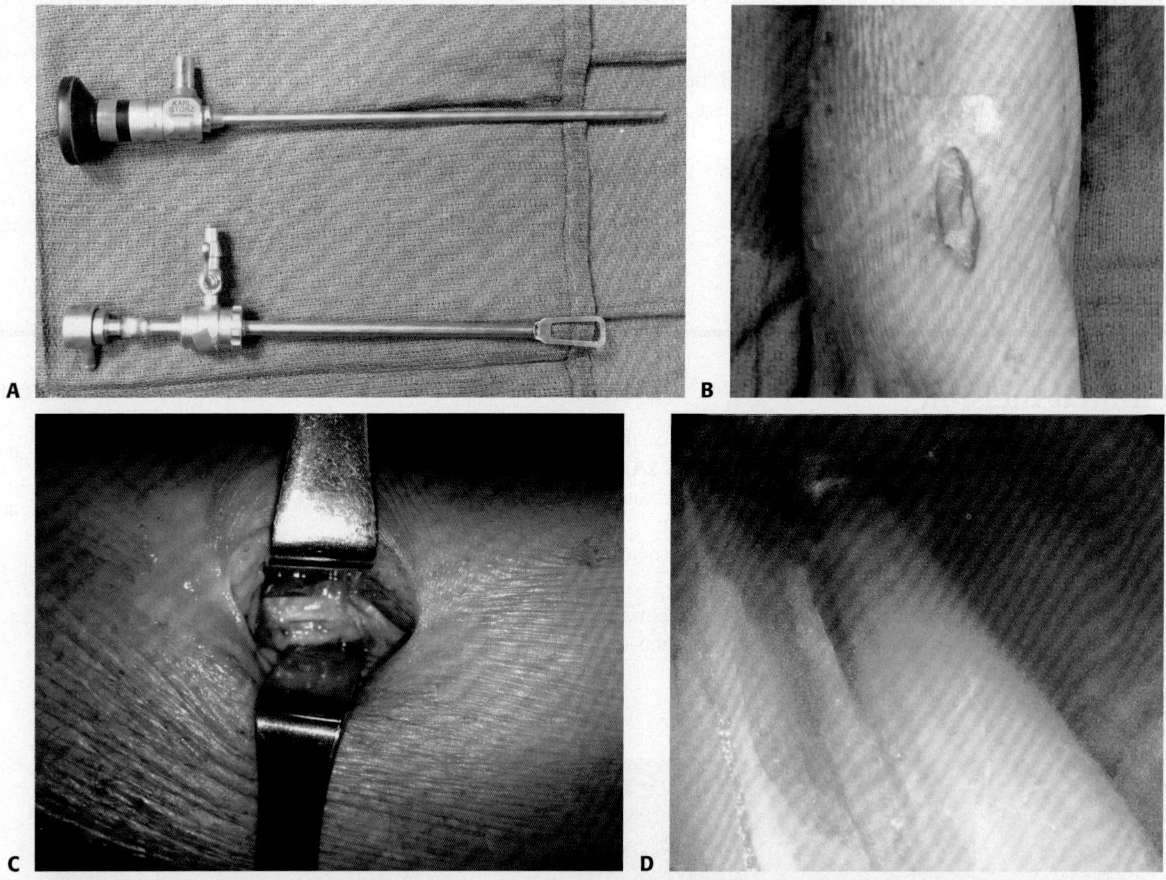

TECH FIG 3 • Endoscopic technique. **A.** Hoffman endoscope sheath (Karl Storz GmbH & Co., Tuttlingen, Germany). **B.** Skin incision. **C.** Median nerve prior to insertion of the endoscope. **D.** Median nerve viewed through the endoscope.

PEARLS AND PITFALLS

Anatomy	■ Tendinous portions of the pronator teres and the fibrous portions of the arcade of the flexor digitorum superficialis are the most common causes of compression. ■ Motor branches that go from the median nerve to the muscles originating from the medial epicondyle branch from the ulnar side of the nerve. ■ The AIN originates from the radial side of the median nerve and under the pronator teres. ■ Considerable variation occurs within the pronator teres. Tendinous portions of the pronator impinging on the median nerve should be released, with preservation of the muscle fibers when possible. ■ The humeral or superficial head of the pronator teres is the largest portion of the muscle. The ulnar head or deep head is far smaller, sometimes absent, and most commonly is deep to the median nerve. Both heads, however, have tendinous insertion sites, which may be sources of impingement. In addition, fascial connections between the heads may be present, impinging on the median nerve.
Surgical technique	■ The fibrous portion of the superficialis arcade can be released with preservation of the muscle. ■ Palpation and visualization proximally and distally can be obtained by appropriate retraction. ■ Extensile exposures result in easier surgery but at the expense of potential unsightly scarring and dysesthesia from cutaneous nerve injury. ■ Judicious release of the pronator teres limits the postoperative morbidity and decreases the recovery time.
Relation to carpal tunnel syndrome	■ Patients often may have both carpal tunnel syndrome and a more proximal compression, resulting in the so-called double crush phenomenon. ■ Some authors have implied that failed carpal tunnel syndrome is due to a misdiagnosis in which the more proximal compression of the median nerve in the forearm was not identified. ■ In cases, however, where electrodiagnostic studies clearly show carpal tunnel syndrome even when proximal forearm symptoms are present, it is wise to merely decompress the carpal canal because the carpal tunnel procedure has a more predictable outcome with less morbidity than proximal forearm median nerve decompression.

POSTOPERATIVE CARE

- Splinting or casting is avoided.
- Early elbow range of motion is encouraged.
- If the pronator tendon has been released, lifting and forearm rotation are restricted for 4 weeks.

OUTCOMES

- Outcome following surgical treatment of proximal forearm median nerve compression has been inconsistent compared to the more uniformly good outcomes associated with carpal tunnel release.
- Many, if not most, patients continue to be at least somewhat symptomatic after surgical decompression.
  - This may reflect persistent compression due to inadequate release or scarring from the surgery itself.
  - It is more likely, however, that it reflects the difficulty in making the diagnosis due to the lack of objective criteria.
- Few studies have evaluated outcome following median nerve decompression in the forearm. Most such studies report results of decompression for pronator syndrome.
- Olehnik et al[6] and Hartz et al[3] both reported results for decompression of pronator syndrome.
  - Olehnik et al[6] showed surgery to be of benefit in 30 of 37 extremities, but 9 of 39 were unchanged and 20 had only partial relief.
  - Hartz et al[3] showed 28 good or excellent results in 36 operations, but a majority of patients still had symptoms.
  - Lee et al[5] showed that 13 patients improved symptomatically as measured by Disability of the Arm, Shoulder, and Hand (DASH) scoring after endoscopically assisted decompression.

COMPLICATIONS

- Persistent symptoms due to incorrect diagnosis
- Damage to cutaneous nerve branches with subsequent dysesthesias
- Damage to or scarring of motor branches of median nerve or interosseous nerve
- Scarring of pronator teres and forearm musculature

REFERENCES

1. Dunn AJ, Salonen DC, Anastakis DJ. MR imaging findings of anterior interosseous nerve lesions. Skeletal Radiol 2007;36:1155–1162.
2. Gainor BJ. Modified exposure for pronator syndrome decompression: a preliminary experience. Orthopedics 1993;1612:1329–1331.
3. Hartz CR, Linscheid RL, Gramse RR, et al. The pronator teres syndrome: compressive neuropathy of the median nerve. J Bone Joint Surg Am 1981;63(6):885–890.
4. Jones NF, Ming NL. Persistent median artery as a cause of pronator syndrome. J Hand Surg Am 1988;13:728–732.
5. Lee AK, Khorsandi M, Nurbhai N, et al. Endoscopically assisted decompression for pronator syndrome. J Hand Surg Am 2012;37(6): 1173–1179.
6. Olehnik WK, Manske PR, Szerzinski J. Median nerve compression in the proximal forearm. J Hand Surg Am 1994;19:121–126.
7. Seki M, Nakamura H, Kono H. Neurolysis is not required for young patients with a spontaneous palsy of the anterior interosseous nerve. J Bone Joint Surg Br 2006;88(12):1606–1609.
8. Spinner RJ, Carmichael SW, Spinner M. Partial median nerve entrapment in the distal arm because of an accessory bicipital aponeurosis. J Hand Surg Am 1991;16:236–244.
9. Tsai TM, Syed SA. A transverse skin incision approach for decompression of pronator teres syndrome. J Hand Surg Br 1994;19:40–42.
10. Ulrich D, Piatkowski A, Pallua N. Anterior interosseous nerve syndrome: retrospective analysis of 14 patients. Arch Orthop Trauma Surg 2011;131:1561–1565.
11. Zancolli ER III, Zancolli EP IV, Perrotto CJ. New mini-invasive decompression for pronator teres syndrome. J Hand Surg Am 2012; 37(8):1706–1710.

Carpal Tunnel Release: Endoscopic, Open, and Revision

Marco Rizzo

DEFINITION

- Carpal tunnel syndrome (CTS) is a compressive neuropathy of the median nerve at the wrist.
- CTS is the most common nerve compression condition in the upper extremity.
- Carpal tunnel release (CTR) is one of the most commonly performed procedures in the United States.
- Early stages of CTS are reversible with treatment.
- Later or more severe stages of CTS may not be (fully) reversible.

ANATOMY

- The carpal tunnel or carpal canal is a space bounded by the carpal bones dorsally, the trapezium and scaphoid radially, the hook of the hamate ulnarly, and the transverse carpal ligament (TCL) palmarly (**FIG 1A**).
- The contents of the carpal canal includes the median nerve and nine digital flexor tendons, along with their accompanying tenosynovium (**FIG 1C**).
- Anatomic anomalies include the following:
  - A persistent median artery
  - Muscle anomalies
  - Median nerve branching anomalies (**FIG 1B**)
- Extraneous masses or structures may be found within the carpal canal, including sarcoid and ganglion cysts.
  - Arthritis or bone spurs from the carpus can diminish the size of the carpal canal and established associations between basal thumb arthritis and CTS exist.[3]

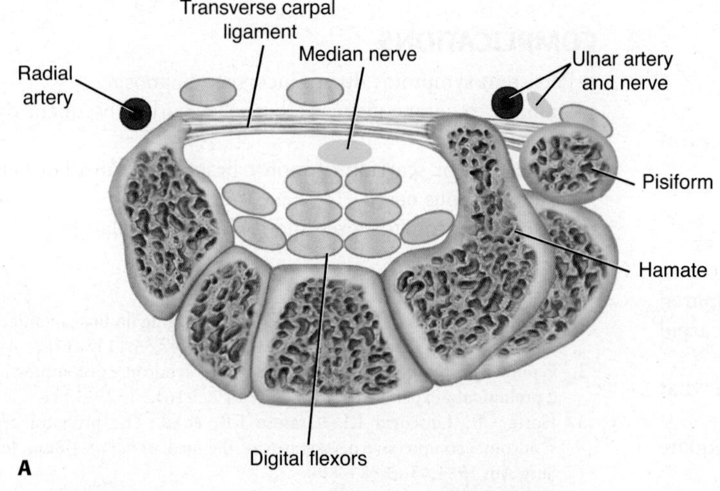

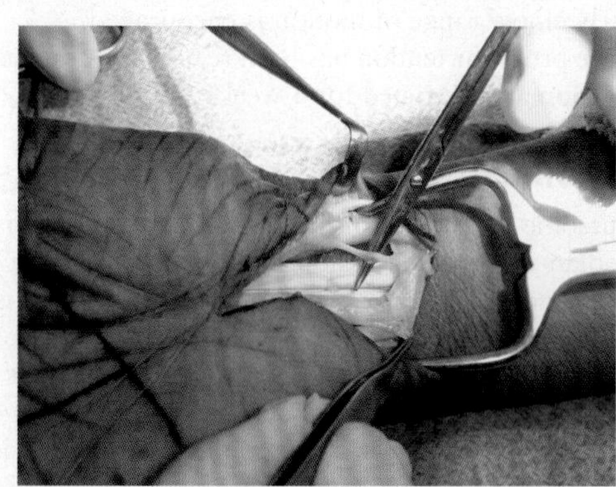

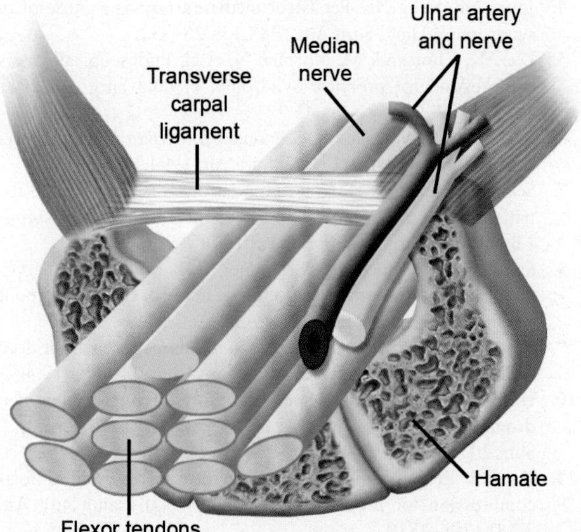

FIG 1 • **A.** Cross-section of the carpal tunnel. **B.** The carpal tunnel has been fully released, and the median nerve motor branch is seen branching from the nerve proximally and penetrating the radial portion of the TCL. **C.** Cross-section of the carpal tunnel with the ulnar artery and nerve superficial to the TCL. *(continued)*

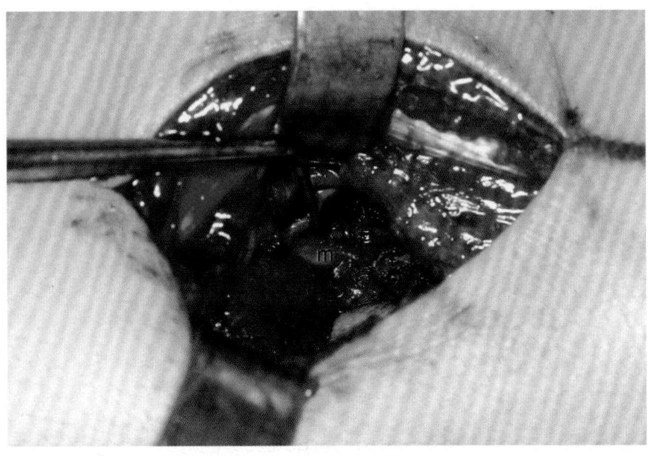

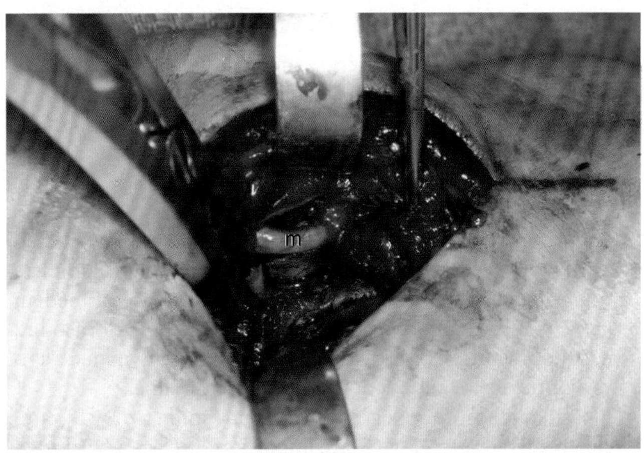

D E

FIG 1 • *(continued)* **D.** Traction on the median nerve secondary to significant displacement of a distal radius and ulna fracture. The nerve was displaced dorsal to the radius and ulna and remained dorsal following reduction. **E.** The nerve is shown after being removed from between the radius and ulna. (**B:** Copyright Thomas R. Hunt III, MD.)

PATHOGENESIS

- Most cases of CTS are idiopathic.[11]
- Some cases are associated with systemic conditions, such as rheumatoid arthritis, diabetes, thyroid disease, chronic renal failure, and sarcoidosis.
- CTS is associated with pregnancy.
- There is an association of CTS with cumulative trauma and repetitive use.[11]
- Increased pressure within the carpal canal is associated with CTS.[2,7,14]
- Peripheral neuropathy and CTS have also been associated with shear forces on the nerve, such as with a traction injury (**FIG 1D,E**).[8]

NATURAL HISTORY

- CTS may have a variable course. It can improve, remain stable, or become more severe.
  - Severity of compression, age, and patient comorbidities help predict natural history.
- Patients with severe CTS have motor and sensory changes and may have muscle weakness and atrophy.[11]
  - Patients with extremely advanced CTS frequently have constant numbness, thenar weakness, and readily visible atrophy.

HISTORY AND PHYSICAL FINDINGS

- Presenting symptoms can be variable: Some patients with mild CTS present with moderate to severe pain, numbness, and paresthesias, whereas other patients have minimal symptoms until their syndrome is severe.
- Symptoms are based in part on severity of disease.
  - Mild disease
    - Intermittent numbness and tingling
    - Provocative symptoms when driving, holding objects, and nocturnal waking
  - Moderate disease
    - Numbness and tingling become constant
    - +/− provocative symptoms
  - Severe disease
    - Dense constant numbness
    - Frequent absence of provocative symptoms
    - Thenar muscle atrophy with weakness and loss of dexterity
- Obtain a full medical history to identify for risk factors for CTS such as hypothyroidism and diabetes.
- The surgeon must understand the patient's occupational and recreational hand activities and any antecedent trauma that might contribute to symptoms.
  - It is helpful to inquire about activity(s) that trigger symptoms.
- Obtain a sense of symptom progression and severity.
  - Questions should be asked about sensory and motor function, pain pattern, and nocturnal waking.
- The physical examination includes evaluation of the neck and shoulder girdle; the supraclavicular, infraclavicular, and axillary area; the humerus and elbow; the forearm; and the wrist and hand.
- It is important to generate a list of findings that may be responsible for the pain or paresthesias *other* than CTS.
- In addition to the standard joint evaluation with range of motion and assessments of stability, it is important to palpate the course of the nerves and elicit the Tinel sign along the course of the paracervical, brachial plexus, median, ulnar, and radial nerves.
  - The Tinel sign is mild, moderate, or severe based on subjective findings of radicular pain in an anatomic distribution. In a patient with peripheral neuropathy, the mechanical external stimulus threshold for nerve depolarization–repolarization is lowered.
  - Phalen sign: Wrist flexion decreases the volume of the carpal canal and raises pressure in patients with CTS. The pattern of paresthesia is important.
  - Carpal tunnel compression test: This is generally considered one of the most sensitive and specific tests for CTS.
  - Two-point discrimination: In peripheral neuropathy, the ability to distinguish one or two points is often diminished.
  - Decreased range of motion, crepitus, and palmar wrist swelling can be indirect indications of tenosynovium in the carpal canal or intra-articular wrist pathology.

IMAGING AND OTHER DIAGNOSTIC STUDIES

- Anteroposterior (AP), lateral, and oblique radiographs are not mandatory in the workup if the wrist examination is completely normal. If there is any possibility of wrist pathology, these studies should be obtained.
- Other imaging studies are generally not indicated in routine cases. However, in patients with recurrent CTS, magnetic resonance imaging (MRI) or ultrasound should be considered as a means to gain further information regarding a complete versus incomplete release of the TCL or evidence of median nerve compression, tenosynovitis, and scarring.[1] Ultrasound has the advantage of providing a real time and dynamic analysis of the nerve and tendons in the carpal tunnel.[10]
- Electrodiagnostics: Nerve conduction studies (NCS) and electromyography (EMG) are important. CTS can be graded based on NCS and EMG findings:
  - CTS mild: increased sensory or motor distal latency; may see decreased amplitude
  - CTS moderate: increased nerve conduction velocity
  - CTS severe: EMG shows signs of chronic denervation with positive fibrillations and sharp waves or unobtainable recordings from the electrodes to median innervated muscles.
  - Although some experts believe the absence of any of the earlier electrodiagnostic findings means that there is no CTS, others believe that false-negatives exist due to sensitivity issues with NCS and EMG.[5]

DIFFERENTIAL DIAGNOSIS

- Cervical radiculitis
- Cervical pathology, joint disease, disc disease, facet disease with foramina stenosis
- Thoracic outlet syndrome
- Brachial plexopathy
- Syringomyelia, motor neuron disease, myelopathy
- "Double crush syndrome"
- Shoulder pain related to instability, intra-articular pathology, subacromial impingement
- Acromioclavicular joint pathology
- Medial epicondylitis
- Lateral epicondylitis
- Cubital tunnel syndrome
- Radial tunnel syndrome
- Pronator syndrome
- Elbow pathology instability or contracture
- Forearm or wrist tenosynovitis
- Wrist tenosynovitis, extensor, flexor, or de Quervain tenosynovitis
- Digital tenosynovitis (trigger finger)
- Guyon canal syndrome
- Hypothenar hammer syndrome
- Wrist or carpal fracture
- Intra-articular wrist pathology

NONOPERATIVE MANAGEMENT

- Mild CTS can often be modulated through conservative means.[6,21]
- Any systemic conditions should be identified and treated.[6,21]
- Activity modification can be attempted, especially if the activity includes highly repetitive loading of the hand, wrist, and upper extremity.

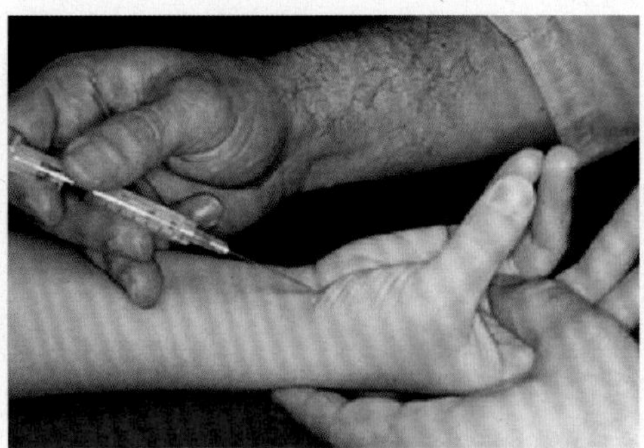

FIG 2 • Cortisone injection.

- Wrist splints can be introduced.
- The physician can recommend or prescribe nonsteroidal anti-inflammatory drugs (NSAIDs).
- Corticosteroid injection into the carpal canal can be considered (**FIG 2**).
  - Temporary relief from such an injection indicates that surgical decompression is likely to be successful.
- Hand therapy can be considered.
- Evidence suggests oral vitamin B_{12} or B_6 treatments can be helpful.[17,18]

SURGICAL MANAGEMENT

- The diagnosis of CTS is confirmed by either the presence of classic clinical symptoms and clinical signs or positive NCS or EMG studies.
  - If the NCS or EMG findings are negative, at least one trial of corticosteroid injection should be considered to evaluate the clinical response. In addition to having a potential therapeutic benefit, it likely has prognostic value for surgery.
- It is important to confirm that a trial of conservative treatment has been undertaken without significant improvement or cure.
- The surgeon should confirm that differential diagnoses have been considered.
- Understanding that the presence of other diagnoses and conditions may affect the overall results of CTS treatment is critical; this needs to be discussed with the patient before, not after, surgery. In fact, one should strongly consider delaying CTS treatment to control or improve other conditions that may be amenable to nonoperative treatment.
- If the earlier conditions are met, CTR will likely provide good to excellent results in more than 90% of cases.[19]
- In the case of recurrent CTS, a key to success is patient selection. Although there are scant data to correlate the preoperative evaluation with results, the patient's clinical course, response to conservative treatment, and interpretation of electrodiagnostic studies and MRI or ultrasound should be carefully considered before revision surgery.

Positioning

- CTR surgery is performed with the arm outstretched on a hand table.
- Pneumatic tourniquet use facilitates accurate identification of critical anatomic structures.
- Loupe magnification is recommended.

- Anesthesia can be by general anesthesia or regional anesthesia such as an axillary block or Bier block.
  - Experienced surgeons can perform CTS safely under wrist block or local infiltration with or without a light anesthetic.

Approach

- The goal of CTR surgery is to decompress the median nerve at the carpal canal by complete division of the TCL to allow the carpal tunnel to expand.
- A volar exposure is used, but incision position and length vary.
- The locations of critical deep structures are defined using superficial landmarks (**FIG 3**). The incision is made along the course of a line drawn down the axis of the fourth ray and another drawn obliquely across the palm in line with the ulnar border of the abducted thumb (Kaplan cardinal line) (see **TECH FIG 1A**).

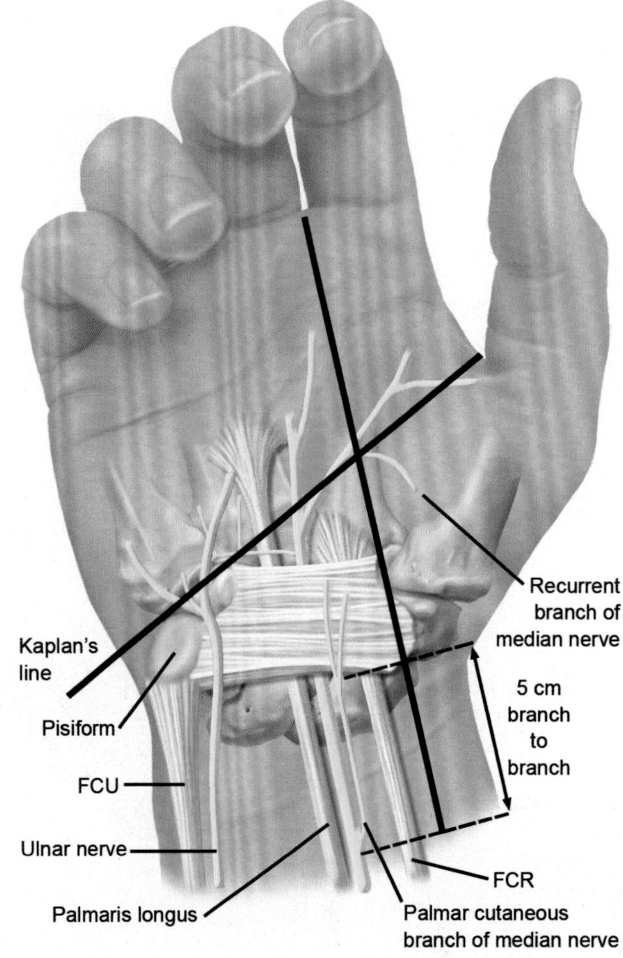

FIG 3 • Surface landmarks are critical when contemplating surgical release of the median nerve. *FCU*, flexor carpi ulnaris; *FCR*, flexor carpi radialis.

Open Carpal Tunnel Release

TECHNIQUES

Exposure

- Mark the skin incision location, beginning at the intersection of the Kaplan cardinal line and a line drawn along the radial border of the fourth ray and ending at the wrist flexion crease (**TECH FIG 1A**).
  - Use of a longitudinal hypothenar crease if available will likely yield a less obvious scar.
  - The incision may be placed anywhere along this mark (**TECH FIG 1B**), depending on the surgeon's preference. I prefer the midpoint of the proximal third of the palm.
  - The incision should be long enough to allow full access to the proximal and distal extents of the TCL in order to ensure full TCL division. This generally can be achieved without having the incision extend proximal to the wrist flexion crease.
- Dissect in line with the incision using a scalpel or scissors, through the subcutaneous fat and the palmar fascia down to the TCL (**TECH FIG 1C**).
  - Frequently, the palmaris brevis muscle is encountered directly superficial to the TCL. It is incised and "feathered" from the ligament for adequate visualization of the TCL.
- Incise the TCL over a small segment, avoiding injury to deep structures (**TECH FIG 1D**).
  - Contents of the carpal canal will have a characteristic appearance due to the tenosynovium.
- Place an instrument such as a mosquito clamp, Saint James, or Carroll elevator into the carpal canal, just deep to the TCL (**TECH FIG 1E**).
  - This defines the undersurface of the TCL, the location of the hamate hook, and the proposed direction for release.
- Visualize the superficial surface of the TCL along its course and place a right angle retractor to protect the critical structures located between the skin and the ligament (**TECH FIG 1F,G**).

Transverse Carpal Ligament Release

- Staying ulnar in the canal but still leaving a 2-mm cuff of TCL attached to the hamate hook, release the TCL under direct vision proximally and distally with a scalpel, scissors, or mini-meniscotome Beaver blade.
  - Keep a radially based TCL leaflet over the median nerve.
- Release the distal forearm fascia proximally (see **TECH FIG 1F**).
  - This tissue may be a secondary compression site, especially in patients with two wrist flexion creases.

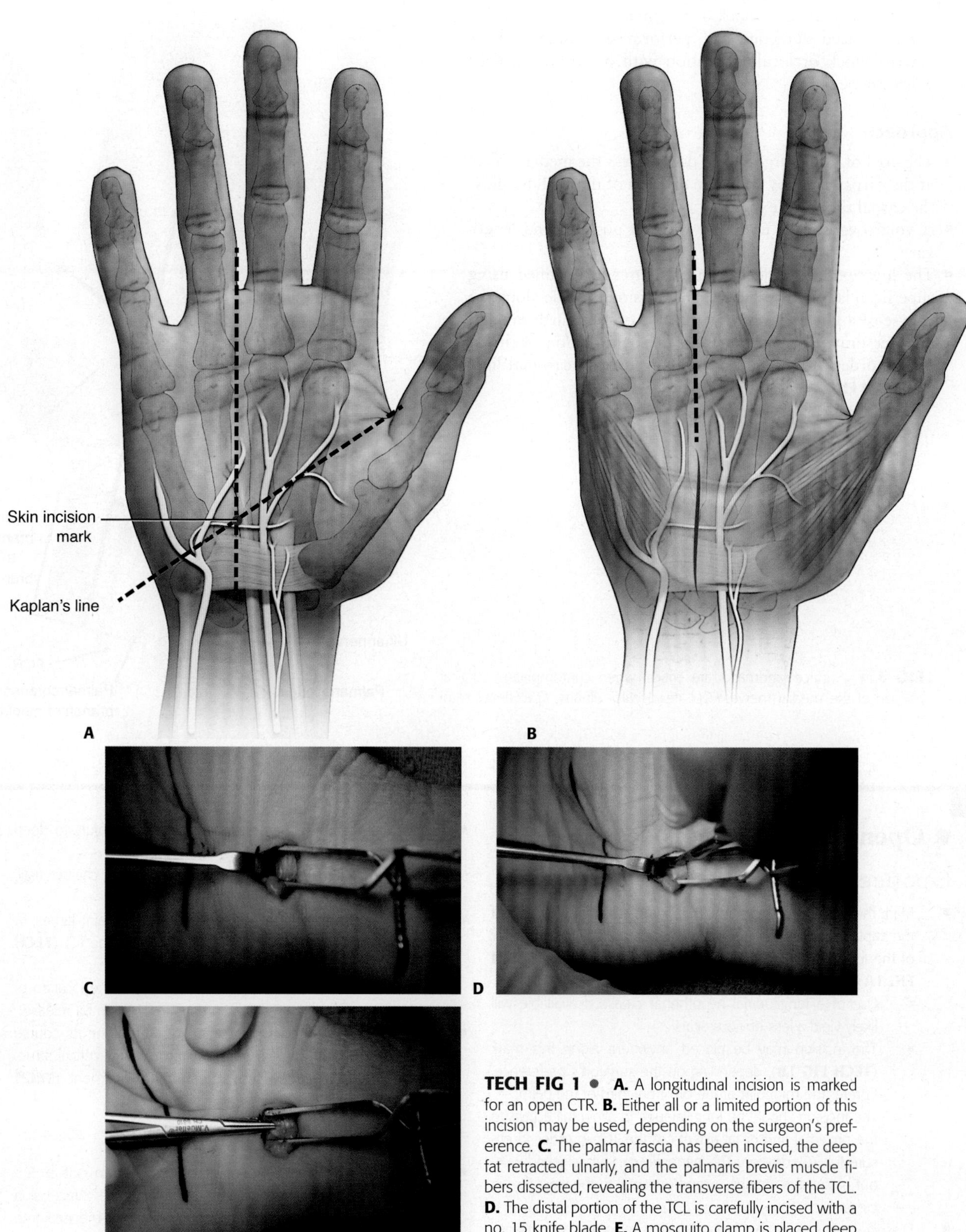

TECH FIG 1 • **A.** A longitudinal incision is marked for an open CTR. **B.** Either all or a limited portion of this incision may be used, depending on the surgeon's preference. **C.** The palmar fascia has been incised, the deep fat retracted ulnarly, and the palmaris brevis muscle fibers dissected, revealing the transverse fibers of the TCL. **D.** The distal portion of the TCL is carefully incised with a no. 15 knife blade. **E.** A mosquito clamp is placed deep to the TCL in a distal to proximal direction. *(continued)*

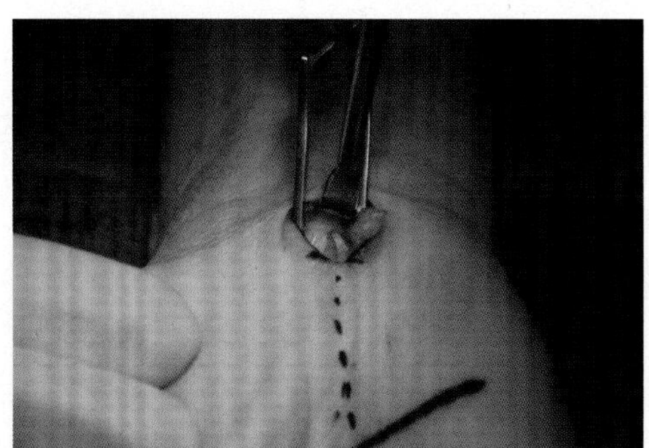

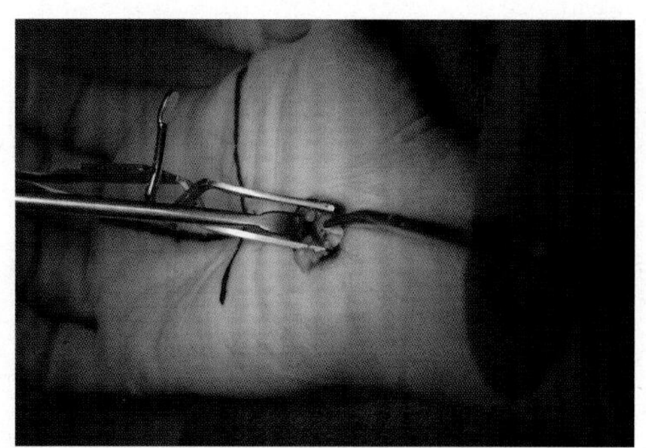

TECH FIG 1 • *(continued)* **F.** A right angle retractor is used to visualize the proximal TCL and the distal forearm fascia. **G.** The same retractor is then used to visualize the distal TCL to allow complete release. (**B–G:** Copyright Thomas R. Hunt, III, MD.)

- Completely divide the TCL and inspect the median nerve and canal contents (see **TECH FIG 1G**).
  - In rare instances, a space-occupying lesion will require removal (ie, "billowing" synovium in a patient with rheumatoid arthritis may require a synovectomy).
  - In primary CTR procedures without systemic disease, there is no role for internal neurolysis or tenosynovectomy (**TECH FIG 2**).[4,9,12]
- The wound is closed and sterile dressings are applied. My preference is interrupted 4-0 Prolene or nylon sutures.
- Use of a splint is based on the surgeon's preference.

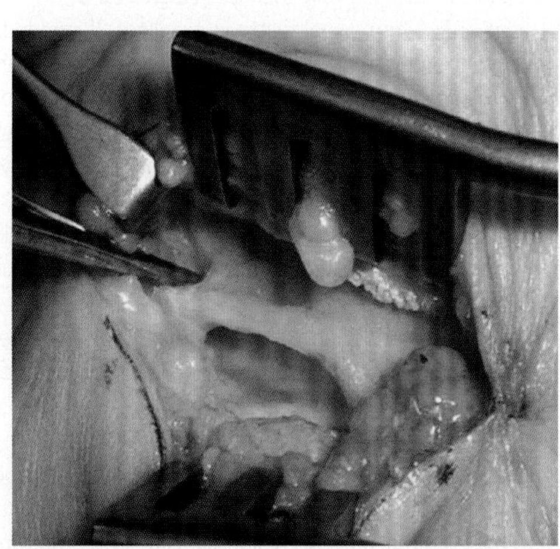

TECH FIG 2 • Open CTR with divided leaflets of the TCL retracted by the retractor jaws. The instrument is on the median nerve which is adherent to the undersurface of the TCL via tenosynovium.

Single-Incision Endoscopic Carpal Tunnel Release (Modified Agee Technique)

Exposure

- Mark out the palmaris longus, the flexor carpi radialis, and the flexor carpi ulnaris.
- Make a transverse 1- to 2-cm incision in a wrist flexion crease centered over or just ulnar to the palmaris longus (**TECH FIG 3A**).
  - If the palmaris longus is not present, incise halfway between the flexor carpi radialis and the flexor carpi ulnaris.
- Expose the palmaris longus and retract it radially with a Ragnell retractor.
- Identify the flexor retinaculum deep to this structure (**TECH FIG 3B**).
- Incise the flexor retinaculum and create a distally based U-shaped flap 1 cm wide. Elevate and retract it with a mosquito clamp.
  - On the undersurface of the retinaculum, adherent tenosynovium is frequently seen.
  - Visible deep to the opening should be the tenosynovium-covered digital flexor tendons and median nerve.
- Pass small and large hamate finders down the carpal canal in an antegrade manner to evaluate the space and the location of the hamate (**TECH FIG 3**).
- Palpate the tip of the instruments as they become subcutaneously distal to the distal edge of the TCL at the Kaplan cardinal line.
  - Make sure these instruments are not palpable subcutaneously in the proximal third of the palm, which would indicate incorrect placement superficial to the TCL and carpal canal and probably within the canal of Guyon.

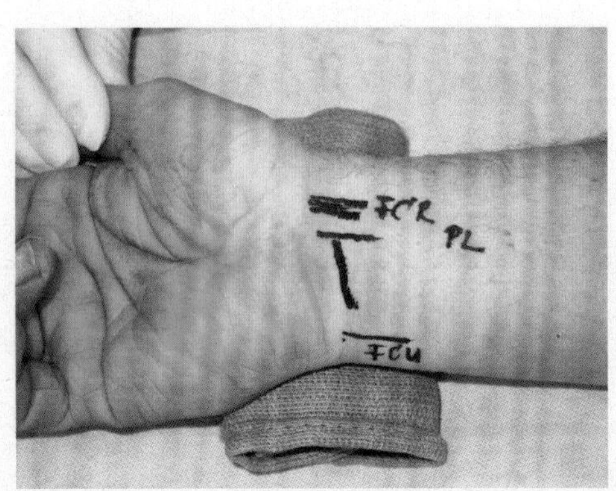

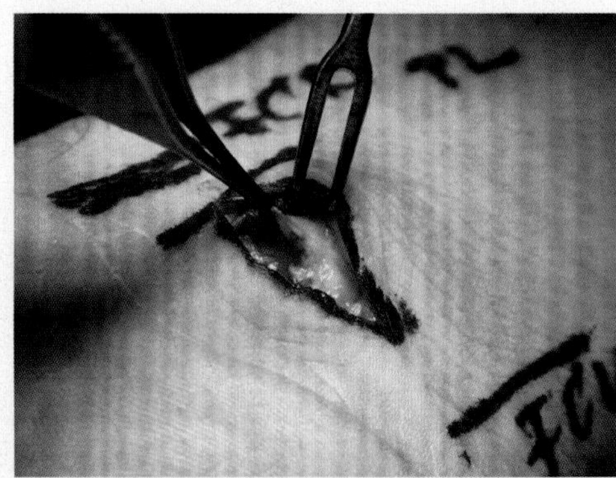

TECH FIG 3 • A. The key landmarks for ECTR are shown here: flexor carpi radialis (*FCR*), palmaris longus (*PL*), flexor carpi ulnaris (*FCU*). The transverse incision is inscribed. **B.** The skin incision has been made and the fascia has also been incised. (Copyright Ekkehard Bonatz, MD.)

- Use the tenosynovial elevator and pass it proximally and distally a dozen times along the axis of the fourth ray to dissect tenosynovium from the undersurface of the TCL.
  - A "washerboard effect" should be felt with this maneuver.

Device Insertion

- Introduce the assembled Agee endoscopic carpal tunnel release (ECTR) device into the carpal canal, with the scope directed palmarly.
  - The undersurface of the TCL with its characteristic transverse striations is visible.
- While viewing the monitor, advance the instrument until the distal edge of the TCL is identified.
  - The distal edge is noted by a transition from the white, transverse fibers of the TCL to the yellow amorphous midpalmar fat, which often contains visible vessels and nerves.
- Using your nondominant hand on the palm, perform a ballottement maneuver to help distinguish the transition between the midpalmar fat and the distal edge of the TCL while viewing the signal from the endoscope within the carpal canal on the monitor.
- In the palm, palpate the tip of the ECTR device as it emerges into the subcutaneous space just distal to the TCL. Drive the device with the other dominant hand (**TECH FIG 4**).
  - The transillumination pattern from the ECTR device light source changes from underneath the TCL to the midpalmar fat.

Transverse Carpal Ligament Release

- Elevate the blade and withdraw the device slowly, cutting the TCL from distal to proximal. Keep the device pressed up against the undersurface of the TCL so no structures come between the blade and the TCL; cut only the TCL (**TECH FIG 5**).
  - Cut only when visualization is excellent. If needed, withdraw the device and redefine the undersurface of the TCL in the manner detailed earlier until visualization is ideal.
- Repeat the earlier step as needed until there is a full release of the TCL, with good separation of radial and ulnar leaflets from proximal to distal.
  - With a full release, it should not be possible to visualize the radial and ulnar leaflets simultaneously with the ECTR device up against the palmar tissues. Also, the ECTR device should be able to be placed within the trough between the radial and ulnar leaflets so neither leaflet is visible, just the fascia overlying the thenar muscles and the subcutaneous space.
- After full TCL release, withdraw the ECTR device.
- Confirm increased volume of the carpal canal by reintroducing the hamate finders down the carpal canal.
- Divide the proximal antebrachial fascia with long tenotomy scissors under direct vision.
  - Adson forceps help to deliver the tissue for cutting.
- The incision is closed and a soft dressing is applied.
- If you cannot safely visualize the structures with the ECTR device, conversion to a two-incision or open CTR method is strongly suggested.

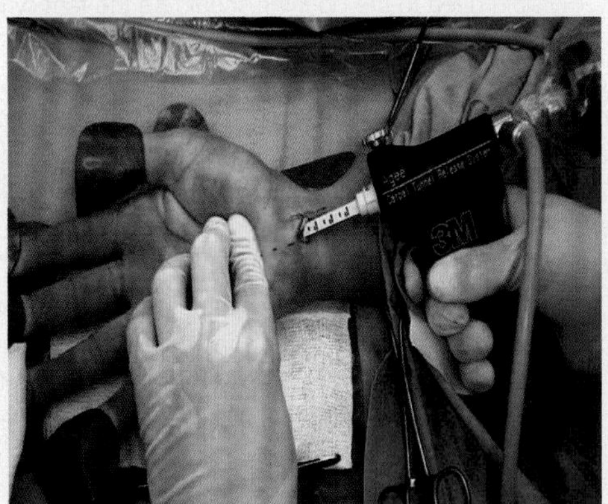

TECH FIG 4 • The surgeon's nondominant index and long digits palpate the tip of the ECTR device as it emerges into the subcutaneous space just distal to the transverse carpal tunnel ligament. The transillumination pattern from the device light source changes from underneath the TCL to the midpalmar fat.

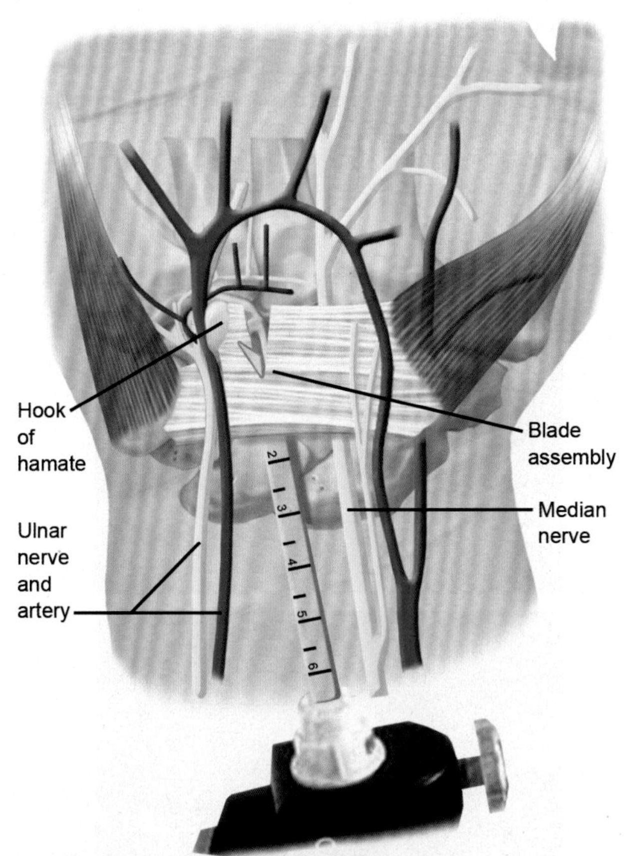

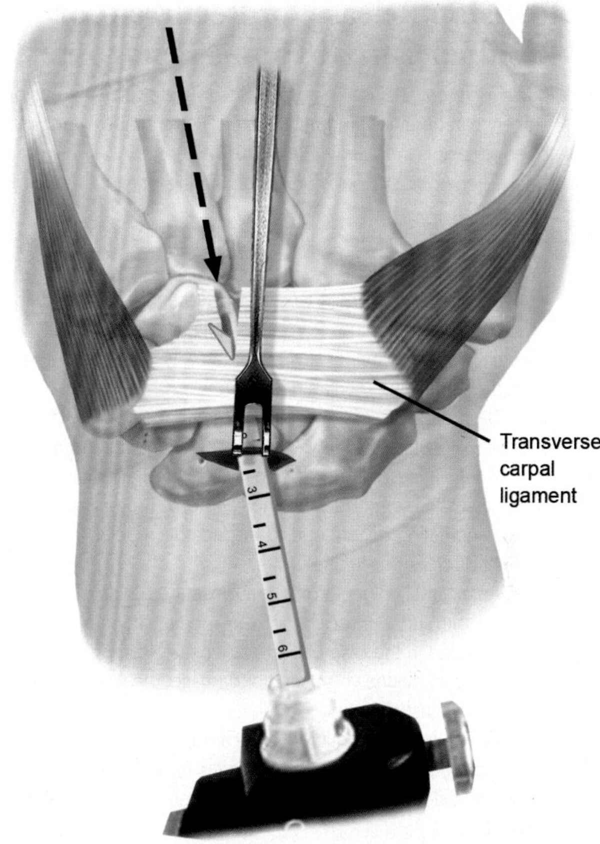

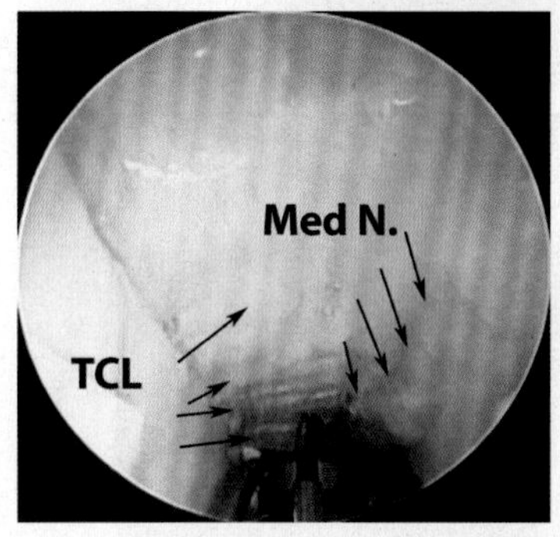

TECH FIG 5 • After careful identification of the distal edge of the TCL (**A**), the ligament is released from distal to proximal (**B**). **C.** This is the start of the transverse carpal ligament (*TCL*) division using the Agee device. The blade is elevated (*center*) and is shown starting to divide the TCL from distal to proximal. The median nerve is just seen radial to the blade. (Copyright Ekkehard Bonatz, MD.)

Two-Incision Endoscopic Carpal Tunnel Release (Chow Technique)

- Make the proximal incision and create the distally based U-shaped flap of antebrachial fascia in the manner described for the single-incision ECTR technique.
- Introduce a clamp, elevator, or trocar under the TCL.
- Advance the instrument until it is palpable in the palm subcutaneously distal to the TCL.
- Make a second small incision to expose the tip of the instrument, usually at the junction of the middle and proximal thirds of the palm.
  - Take care to identify the superficial arch, common digital nerves, and fibers of the distal TCL in the area.
- A variety of techniques (open or scope-assisted) can be used at this point, including slotted trocars for two-incision endoscopic release, or use of a mini-meniscotome blade or scissor or other cutting instrument with a retractor or elevator to protect the median nerve and flexor tendons from the TCL cutting instrument.
- The complete distal TCL division can be ascertained by direct visualization, also taking note that the vessels and nerves have not been injured.
- A pitfall of the two incision techniques, aside from the potential injury to the palmar arterial arch and/or the branches of median or ulnar nerve, is incomplete release of the TCL distally. Therefore, inspection of the operative site with magnifying loupes at the distal incision is important.

Revision Release for Recurrent or Residual Carpal Tunnel Syndrome

- If the recurrent CTS is due to prior incomplete release, revision surgery can be attempted using an ECTR technique; otherwise, open release is indicated (**TECH FIG 6A,B**).
- Use a generous skin incision, incorporating previous incisions as needed.
- Perform the release using a similar technique to that described for primary open CTR.
  - Scarring often requires scalpel dissection, and separation of superficial tissues from the TCL is difficult.
- Carefully separate the TCL (in the area of its previous division) from the underlying median nerve.
  - Dense scarring of the median nerve to the TCL is expected and will place the nerve in jeopardy during this exposure.
- Completely release the TCL and the scarred median nerve, taking great care to protect the median nerve motor branch.
- Use an operating microscope to inspect the median nerve for signs of damage or scarring.
  - An external epineurotomy to expose the bands of Fontana on the surface fascicles of the median nerve is recommended in the case of significant nerve scarring.
- If there is minimal nerve scarring or damage, the wound can be closed in the usual manner.
- If nerve injury is dramatic and rescarring seems likely, cover the damaged nerve with a hypothenar fat pad flap, palmaris brevis muscle flap, vein wrapping, or neural conduit (**TECH FIG 6C**).
- Create a TCL flap through Z-lengthening and tissue rearrangement if flexor tendon prolapse or palmar migration of the median nerve seems likely.

Hypothenar Fat Pad

- When revision CTR reveals median nerve scarring, surgical tactics to improve the environment around the nerve after the neurolysis to reduce rescarring are attractive. Strickland et al[15] has described this technique in several publications. The tissue is readily available and has been shown to be of benefit. In a 1996 article,[15] 62 patients were reviewed. Results were good based on pre- and postoperative patient satisfaction scores, with only three transient minor complications.
- Dissect the fat pad to the level of the ulnar nerve and artery, and advance the radial edge to cover the median nerve.
- Sew this edge to the radial flap of the TCL.

Palmaris Brevis Flap

- Rose et al described this flap in 1991.[13]
- Expose the thin palmaris brevis muscle on the ulnar side of the CTR incision.
- Divide it from its insertion in the subcutaneous space and transpose or rotate it into a position covering the median nerve.

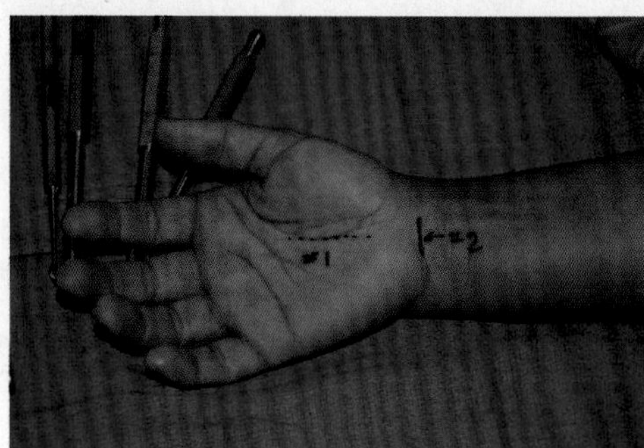

A

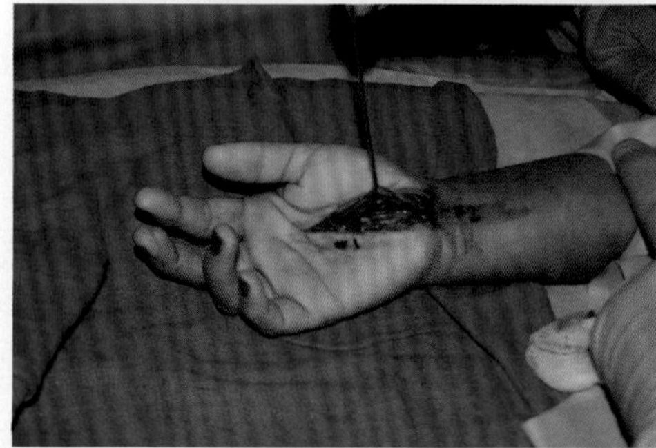
B

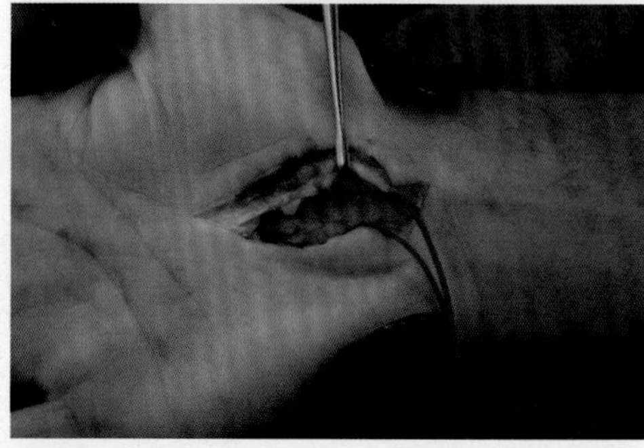
C

TECH FIG 6 • **A,B.** Revision of prior ECTR with open technique. **C.** Revision CTR with NeuraGen tube around scarred branch of median nerve.

PEARLS AND PITFALLS

Poor patient selection	▪ Perform a full history and physical examination and contemplate the entire list of differential diagnoses.
Incomplete release of TCL	▪ Whatever technique is used, make sure it is performed in a technically proficient manner. Confirm complete TCL division, especially distally.
Damage to median nerve	▪ The surgeon must be able to identify the various anatomic structures and distinguish them. The median nerve must be protected during CTR. In techniques where the median nerve is visualized, inspection should be performed after TCL release and before skin closure.

POSTOPERATIVE CARE

- Traditionally, CTR patients were managed in wrist splints for 1 to 3 weeks after surgery. However, multiple studies have shown that faster recovery occurs when the wrist is not splinted postoperatively.
  - Temporary postoperative splints may still be indicated in specific clinical scenarios, such as open revision surgery.
- Hand therapy is helpful in the postoperative period, especially if the patient is having difficulty with full digital active and passive motion.
- Grip and pinch strengths, subjective symptom measures, and functional evaluations are helpful to manage the postoperative course.
- Some patients have prolonged periods of tenderness under the TCL, or pillar pain on the thenar or hypothenar side of the proximal palm, and require extended hand therapy and periods of time to gradually increase hand strength and endurance for hand activities.

OUTCOMES

- There should be greater than 95% good or excellent results.[19] This randomized, double-blinded multicenter study compared open and single portal ECTR and showed statistically significant improvements in the endoscopic group between 6 weeks and 3 months postoperatively in terms of pain and hand strength compared to that of the open group and equivalent good results in both groups at 1 year.
- Stütz et al[16] reported on a retrospective series of 200 patients who underwent a secondary exploration during a 26-month period at a single institution for persistent or recurrent CTS symptoms after CTR. There were 108 cases of incomplete release of the TCL. Twelve patients had evidence of median nerve laceration during the index procedure. Forty-six patients had scarring of the nerve to surrounding tissues. In 13 patients, the cause of their problem could not be determined.
- Varitimidis et al[20] reviewed 22 patients (24 wrists) who underwent revision open CTR after an initial ECTR and who had persistent CTS. Twenty-two patients had incomplete TCL release. One patient had a partial and another a complete median nerve transection. One patient had a Guyon canal release instead of a CTR. Twenty patients returned to work, 15 at the previous level and 5 at lighter duty. The 2 patients with nerve injuries continued to do poorly, 1 patient requiring a vein-wrapping procedure.

COMPLICATIONS

- Incomplete TCL release
- Median nerve scarring or damage (especially the common digital nerve to the third web space and the thenar motor branch)
- Ulnar nerve or artery damage
- Sympathetically mediated pain syndrome
- Damage to palmar arterial arch
- Flexor tendon prolapse

REFERENCES

1. Ablove RH, Peimer CA, Diao E, et al. Morphologic changes following endoscopic and two-portal subcutaneous carpal tunnel release. J Hand Surg Am 1994;19(5):821–826.
2. Diao E, Shao F, Liebenberg E, et al. Carpal tunnel pressure alters median nerve function in a dose-dependent manner: a rabbit model for carpal tunnel syndrome. J Orthop Res 2005;23:218–223.
3. Florack TM, Miller RJ, Pellegrini VD, et al. The prevalence of carpal tunnel syndrome in patients with basal joint arthritis of the thumb. J Hand Surg Am 1992;17(4):624–630.
4. Gelberman RH, Pfeffer GB, Galbraith RT, et al. Results of treatment of severe carpal-tunnel syndrome without internal neurolysis of the median nerve. J Bone Joint Surg Am 1987;69(6):896–903.
5. Grundberg AB. Carpal tunnel decompression in spite of normal electromyography. J Hand Surg Am 1983;8(3):348–349.
6. Kaplan SJ, Glickel SZ, Eaton RG. Predictive factors in the non-surgical treatment of carpal tunnel syndrome. J Hand Surg Am 1990;15:106–108.
7. Lundborg G, Gelberman RH, Minteer-Convery M, et al. Median nerve compression in the carpal tunnel—functional response to experimentally induced controlled pressure. J Hand Surg Am 1982;7(3):252–259.
8. Lundborg G, Rydevik B. Effects of stretching the tibial nerve of the rabbit. A preliminary study of the intraneural circulation and the barrier function of the perineurium. J Bone Joint Surg Br 1973;55(2):390–401.
9. Mackinnon SE, McCabe S, Murray JF, et al. Internal neurolysis fails to improve the results of primary carpal tunnel decompression. J Hand Surg Am 1991;16(2):211–218.
10. Pinilla I, Martín-Hervás C, Sordo G, et al. The usefulness of ultrasound in the diagnosis of carpal tunnel syndrome. J Hand Surg Eur Vol 2008;33:435–439.
11. Rempel DM, Diao E. Entrapment neuropathies: pathophysiology and pathogenesis. J Electromyogr Kinesiol 2004;14:71–75.
12. Rhoades CE, Mowery CA, Gelberman RH. Results of internal neurolysis of the median nerve for severe carpal tunnel syndrome. J Bone Joint Surg Am 1985;67(2):253–256.
13. Rose EH, Norris MS, Kowalski TA, et al. Palmaris brevis turnover flap as an adjunct to internal neurolysis of the chronically scarred median nerve in recurrent carpal tunnel syndrome. J Hand Surg Am 1991;16:191–201.
14. Rydevik B, Lundborg G, Bagge U. Effects of graded compression on intraneural blood flow. An in vivo study on rabbit tibial nerve. J Hand Surg Am 1981;6(1):3–12.
15. Strickland JW, Idler RS, Lourie GM, et al. The hypothenar fat pad flap for management of recalcitrant carpal tunnel syndrome. J Hand Surg Am 1996;21(5):840–848.
16. Stütz N, Gohritz A, van Schoonhoven J, et al. Revision surgery after carpal tunnel release—analysis of the pathology in 200 cases during a 2-year period. J Hand Surg Br 2006;31(1):68–71.
17. Talebi M, Andalib S, Bakhti S, et al. Effect of vitamin b6 on clinical symptoms and electrodiagnostic results of patients with carpal tunnel syndrome. Adv Pharm Bull 2013;3:283–288.
18. Tanaka H. Old or new medicine? Vitamin B12 and peripheral nerve neuropathy [in Japanese]. Brain Nerve 2013;65:1077–1082.
19. Trumble TE, Diao E, Abrams RA, et al. Single-portal endoscopic carpal tunnel release compared with open release: a prospective, randomized trial. J Bone Joint Surg Am 2002;84-A(7):1107–1115.
20. Varitimidis SE, Herndon JH, Sotereanos DG. Failed endoscopic carpal tunnel release. Operative findings and results of open revision surgery. J Hand Surg Br 1999;24(4):465–467.
21. Weiss AP, Sachar K, Gendreau M. Conservative management of carpal tunnel syndrome: a reexamination of steroid injection and splinting. J Hand Surg Am 1994;19(3):410–415.

95 CHAPTER

Tendon Transfers for Median Nerve Palsy

Jeffrey B. Friedrich and Scott H. Kozin

DEFINITION

- The median nerve can be compromised by any number of causes, including trauma, tumor, chronic compression, or synovitis.
- Palsy of the median nerve can result in motor or sensory deficits, or both, within the distribution of this nerve.

ANATOMY

- The median nerve enters the forearm between the two heads of the pronator teres muscle.
- The median nerve travels down the forearm between the flexor digitorum superficialis (FDS) and flexor digitorum profundus (FDP) muscles to enter the carpal tunnel.
- Along its course, the anterior interosseous nerve branches from the median nerve to provide innervation to the flexor pollicis longus, FDP to the index, and the pronator quadratus muscles.
- The median nerve proper provides innervation to the flexor carpi radialis, pronator teres, FDS, palmaris longus (PL), and FDP to the long finger.
- The palmar cutaneous branch arises from the median nerve 5 cm proximal to the wrist joint, crosses the wrist superficial to the transverse carpal ligament, and supplies sensibility to the thenar eminence.
- Just proximal to the wrist, the median nerve becomes superficial and travels within the carpal tunnel.
- The recurrent motor branch originates from the central or radial portion of the median nerve during its passage through the carpal tunnel. The recurrent branch usually passes distal to the transverse carpal ligament to innervate the thenar muscles. The nerve can also pass through the transverse carpal ligament (occurs in 5% to 7% of individuals).[8]
- The thenar muscles are the opponens pollicis, flexor pollicis brevis, and abductor pollicis brevis. The flexor pollicis brevis muscle receives dual innervation from both the recurrent branch (superficial head) and the deep motor branch of the ulnar nerve (deep head).
- The median nerve terminates into multiple sensory branches, which supply sensibility to the thumb, index, long, and ring (radial side) fingers. The sensory branches to the radial side of the index and radial side of the long fingers possess a minor motor component that sends a small branch that innervates the adjacent lumbrical muscle.

PATHOGENESIS

- Most injuries to the median nerve occur at the wrist and affect the thenar muscles. The resultant functional loss is lack of thumb opposition.
- Compression injuries are most common and are usually attributed to prolonged carpal tunnel syndrome.
- Carpal tunnel compression may also be secondary to tumor, adjacent synovitis, or fracture-dislocation.
- Penetrating or perforating injuries may directly damage the median nerve.
- Pediatric causes include lipofibrohamartoma of the median nerve or Charcot-Marie-Tooth disease, a demyelinating process that has a preference for the median and ulnar nerves (**FIG 1**).[6,8]
- High median nerve injuries are rare. Similar causes exist, including trauma and nerve compression.[11]

NATURAL HISTORY

- With a median nerve compression neuropathy (ie, carpal tunnel syndrome), palsy of the median nerve is insidious in onset and manifestation. Over a period of months to years, patients can progress to decreased median nerve function as well as sensory changes in the dermatome of this nerve.
- Acute injuries to the median nerve at the wrist or elbow have a traumatic onset followed by abrupt sensory and/ or motor changes depending on the extent of injury.

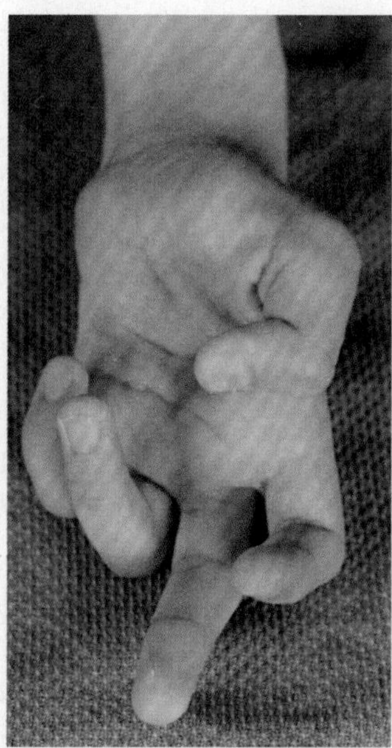

FIG 1 • Left hand of 16-year-old boy with Charcot-Marie-Tooth disorder resulting in median nerve palsy. Note inability to oppose thumb with attempt to touch small fingertip. (Courtesy of Shriners Hospital for Children, Philadelphia.)

PATIENT HISTORY AND PHYSICAL FINDINGS

- Compressive neuropathy of the median nerve
  - Patients report pain, numbness, and tingling in the thumb, index, middle, and sometimes ring finger of the affected hand. They frequently describe problems with fine coordination of the hand, notably pinch. Patients often report pain and numbness that awakens them at night.
  - Physical examination findings include thenar muscle wasting and diminished thumb opposition (defined as the combination of palmar abduction, metacarpophalangeal [MCP] joint flexion, and thumb pronation).
  - Additional signs include the Tinel sign; the Phalen sign; the carpal tunnel compression sign; and increased two-point discrimination in the thumb, index, and long fingers.
  - High median nerve neuropathies have similar findings, in addition to loss of forearm pronation and flexion of the thumb, index, and long fingers.
- Acute median nerve injury
  - There is nearly always a wound on the upper extremity, usually on the volar wrist.
  - Physical findings include diminished sensibility in the thumb, index, and long fingers; increased two-point discrimination in those fingers; a positive Tinel sign; and an inability to touch the thumb tip to the small finger (ie, loss of opposition).
  - Depending on the level of injury, patients may display diminished sensibility of the thenar eminence of the thumb, indicating an injury proximal to the palmar cutaneous branch of the median nerve, or a concomitant injury to the palmar cutaneous branch.
  - Higher median nerve neuropathies have similar findings, in addition to loss of forearm pronation and flexion of the thumb, index, and long fingers.
- Patients with median nerve palsy will not be able to oppose thumb to small finger. There may be some palmar abduction due to function of the abductor pollicis longus or extensor pollicis brevis muscles, but this will be minor. The ulnar-innervated deep head of the flexor pollicis brevis muscle will still function, yielding MCP joint flexion but not true opposition.
- Inability to make an "OK" sign indicates anterior interosseous nerve injury and high median nerve pathology.[11]
- The clinician should ask the patient to try to touch thumb to small finger with the wrist flexed. Due to median nerve palsy, the patient will likely be unable to fully touch the thumb to the small finger.
- The patient is asked to spread his or her fingers apart and hold them against adduction pressure on the small finger to ensure ulnar nerve function. The examiner feels for resistance and palpates the hypothenar eminence at the same time. There should be resistance to adduction force on the small finger, and firmness of the hypothenar eminence should be appreciated.

IMAGING AND OTHER DIAGNOSTIC STUDIES

- Radiographs
  - Plain radiographs are helpful in determining the nature of fractures or dislocations after acute trauma to the upper extremity.
  - Specific carpal tunnel radiographic views may demonstrate osteophytes within the carpal tunnel or a hook of the hamate, but they are not routinely performed.
- Electrodiagnostic studies
  - In the setting of compressive neuropathy of the median nerve, nerve conduction studies typically show increased motor and sensory latencies in the median distribution.
  - In advanced stages of compressive neuropathy, electromyography demonstrates fibrillation potentials in various muscles tested, most commonly the abductor pollicis brevis. These fibrillation potentials indicate denervation of the tested muscle and axonal loss.
  - Advanced high median nerve neuropathy reveals fibrillation potentials in more proximal muscles, such as the flexor carpi radialis and the pronator teres.

DIFFERENTIAL DIAGNOSIS

- Carpal tunnel syndrome
- Anterior interosseous syndrome
- Pronator syndrome
- Wrist synovitis
- Direct injury to the median nerve
- Tumor compression of the median nerve
- Charcot-Marie-Tooth disease
- Brachial plexus injury
- Stroke or other brain injury

NONOPERATIVE MANAGEMENT

- Patients with demonstrable carpal tunnel syndrome can undergo a trial of splinting, wrist corticosteroid injection, or both.
- Work modification is indicated in patients with compressive neuropathy as a result of overuse for both carpal tunnel and pronator syndromes.
- Anti-inflammatory and immunomodulatory medications are indicated in patients with wrist synovitis secondary to inflammatory arthropathy.

SURGICAL MANAGEMENT

- The chief surgical modality for a low or high median nerve palsy that has not responded to surgery or other interventions is tendon transfer.[1,3,8]
- Typically, in a low median nerve palsy, the only function that requires restoration via tendon transfer is thumb opposition, which is a combination of palmar abduction, MCP joint flexion, and thumb pronation.
- In a high median nerve palsy, the additional loss of flexion of the thumb, index, and long fingers requires tendon transfer. In addition, lack of pronation may require tendon transfer.

Preoperative Planning

- The surgeon must ensure that there is good passive range of motion of the joints to be motored by the tendon transfer.
  - In long-standing median nerve palsy, the thumb MCP and carpometacarpal joints can become quite stiff.
  - Physical therapy must be implemented to loosen these joints and increase their passive range of motion.[3] This can usually be accomplished in 3 to 6 weeks.
- A thorough assessment of muscle function and strength is made before selecting a transfer, especially in the setting of combined nerve deficits.
- When performing an opponensplasty, the donor tendon and attachment site are individualized to the particular patient, his or her injury, his or her needs, and the donor muscle–tendon

availability. The vector of transfer is based about the pisiform to provide the most opposition regardless of the donor chosen. As the attachment site onto the thumb moves more dorsal, the amount of pronation and thumb extension is increased.

- Donor options for opponensplasty include the following:
  - FDS[8]
  - Abductor digiti minimi (ADM) (Huber)[4,5]
  - Extensor indicis proprius (EIP)[2]
  - PL (Camitz). The palmaris transfer is associated with more abduction and less opposition compared to other opposition transfers secondary to its inability to transmit force from the pisiform.[3,13]
  - Other less common donors include the extensor pollicis longus, extensor carpi ulnaris, extensor carpi radialis brevis, and extensor digitorum quinti.[4,5]
- Opponensplasty attachment site options include the following[3]:
  - Abductor pollicis brevis tendon. This yields a great deal of thumb abduction and some opposition.
  - Extensor pollicis brevis or longus tendons. This yields thumb abduction, pronation, and MCP joint extension.
  - Single attachment options
    - Riordan's technique involves interweaving the transferred tendon into the abductor pollicis brevis tendon, with continuation onto the extensor pollicis longus tendon distal to the MCP joint.
    - Littler's technique attaches the transferred tendon into the abductor pollicis brevis tendon.
    - Bunnell's method involves passing the tendon through a small drill hole made at the proximal phalanx base from the dorsoulnar to palmar radial direction to provide pronation of the thumb.
  - Dual attachment options
    - These are designed to rotate (pronate) the thumb and either passively stabilize the MCP joint or minimize interphalangeal joint flexion.
    - There is a theoretical benefit in patients with combined median and ulnar nerve deficits who lack all thumb intrinsic function.
    - Some authors question the use of dual insertion techniques because the transfer will only function predominantly on the tighter of the two insertion sites.
    - In Brand's technique, one-half is woven through the abductor pollicis brevis tendon and then passed distal to the MCP joint and attached to the extensor pollicis longus tendon.
    - In the Royle-Thompson method, a slip is passed through a drill hole made in the metacarpal neck, from radial to ulnar, with the metacarpal pulled into as much opposition as possible. This slip is tied to the other half that is initially passed dorsally over the extensor hood at the MCP joint and through a small tunnel in the fascia and periosteum at the base of the proximal phalanx.
- High median nerve palsies require additional restoration of thumb, index, and long finger flexion. On occasion, reestablishment of pronation is required.
- Flexion of the index and long fingers can be accomplished by side-to-side transfers of the FDP tendons of the index and long to the ring and small. The donor tendons are transected proximal to the wrist and woven into the recipient tendons.
- Thumb flexion can be restored by transfer of the brachioradialis to the flexor pollicis longus.
- Loss of pronation can be overcome by rerouting the biceps around the radius, which converts the biceps from a supinator into a pronator.

Positioning

- The patient is positioned supine on the operating table.
- The affected limb is abducted at the shoulder and placed on an attached hand table or arm board.

Approach

- The surgical approach to opponensplasty for median nerve palsy depends on two factors: the donor tendon and the site of attachment.

TECHNIQUES

Low Median Nerve Transfers

Flexor Digitorum Superficialis Transfer (Authors' Preferred Technique)

- Make a palmar transverse skin incision over the first annular pulley of the ring finger.
- Identify the A1 pulley and incise it longitudinally. Isolate the FDS tendon from the FDP tendon.
- Apply traction to the FDS tendon to flex the proximal interphalangeal joint (**TECH FIG 1A**) and divide the FDS tendon transversely just proximal to its bifurcation while protecting the FDP tendon.
- Make a second zigzag incision at the volar ulnar distal forearm in the region of the flexor carpi ulnaris (FCU) tendon insertion.
- Isolate the FCU and the ring finger FDS tendons and protect the ulnar neurovascular bundle.
- Divide the radial half of the FCU tendon transversely about 4 cm proximal to its insertion onto the pisiform.
- Separate the radial half of the tendon longitudinally from the ulnar half, creating a distally based strip of tendon graft.
- Loop the tendon graft distally and pass it through the distal portion of the FCU near the pisiform insertion to create a pulley.

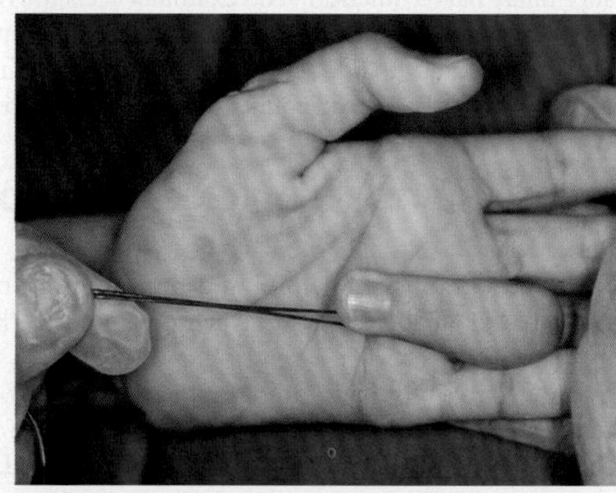

TECH FIG 1 • **A.** Isolation of ring finger FDS to be transferred for thumb opposition. *(continued)*

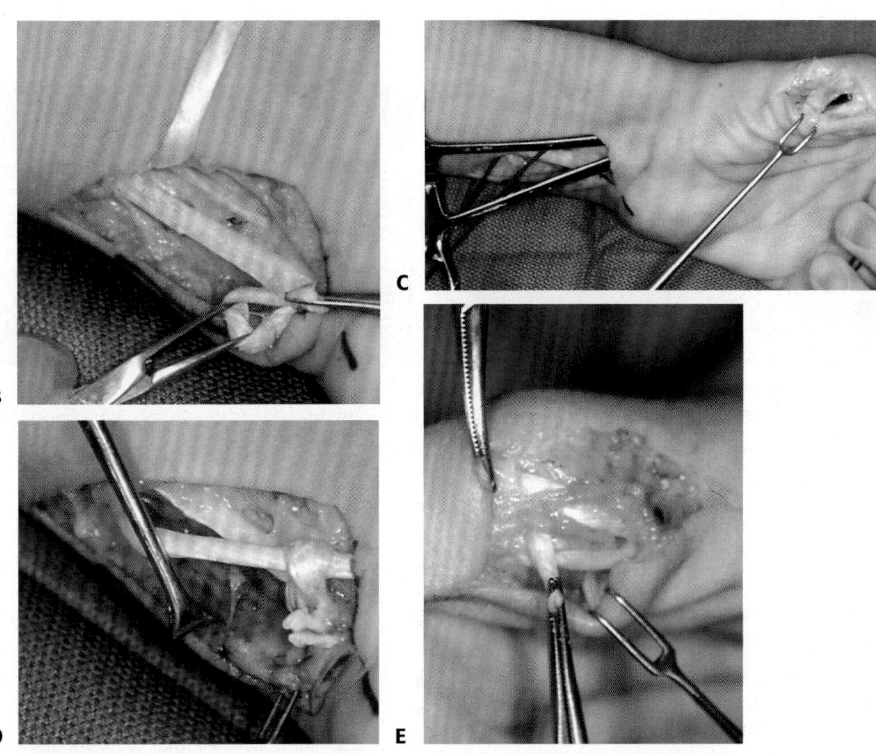

TECH FIG 1 • *(continued)* **B.** Ring finger FDS passed through the FCU loop, which now serves as the pulley for the transferred tendon. **C.** Creation of the subcutaneous tunnel between the ulnar wrist and thumb incisions through which the FDS tendon will be passed. **D.** Ring finger FDS tendon shown passing through both the FCU tendon and the subcutaneous tunnel. **E.** Suture fixation of the FDS tendon to the abductor tendon and extensor hood of the thumb. (Courtesy of Shriners Hospital for Children, Philadelphia.)

- Pull the cut ring finger FDS tendon into the volar ulnar forearm incision and pass it through the constructed pulley (**TECH FIG 1B**).
- Make a third incision on the radial aspect of the thumb MCP joint.
- Create a subcutaneous tunnel between this incision and the wrist incision (**TECH FIG 1C**).
- Pass the ring FDS tendon through this tunnel to the thumb incision (**TECH FIG 1D**).
- Place the thumb into opposition with the small finger.
- Secure the FDS tendon to the thumb with a 3-0 or 4-0 braided polyester suture (**TECH FIG 1E**).
  - The attachment sites usually include the abductor tendon +/− the dorsal capsule and extensor pollicis brevis tendon.

Abductor Digiti Minimi Transfer (Huber)

- Make an oblique or zigzag incision beginning distally on the ulnar border of the small finger proximal phalanx, curving radially along the radial border of the hypothenar eminence.
- Separate the ADM muscle from the flexor digiti minimi. Dissect the ADM distally to its insertion into the proximal phalanx and lateral band.
- Protect the ulnar sensory nerve to the small finger.
- Divide the ADM insertion sites, including a portion of the lateral band to increase its overall length.
- Dissect the muscle proximally to the pisiform (**TECH FIG 2A**).
- Release the origin from the pisiform; identify and protect the neurovascular bundle (on the dorsoradial side).
- Make a longitudinal incision on the radial aspect of the thumb MCP joint.
- Use blunt dissection to create a subcutaneous tunnel in the palm.
- Pass the ADM through the tunnel to the thumb MCP joint (**TECH FIG 2B**).
- Secure the ADM tendon to the thumb using 3-0 or 4-0 braided polyester suture (**TECH FIG 2C**).

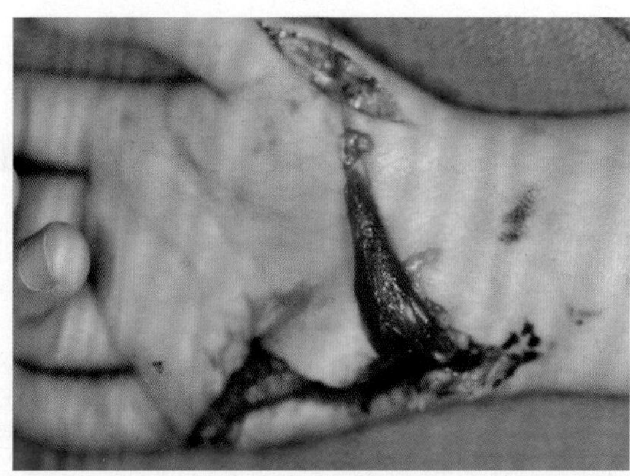

TECH FIG 2 • **A.** Isolated and dissected ADM muscle–tendon unit to be used for transfer for thumb opposition (Huber transfer). *(continued)*

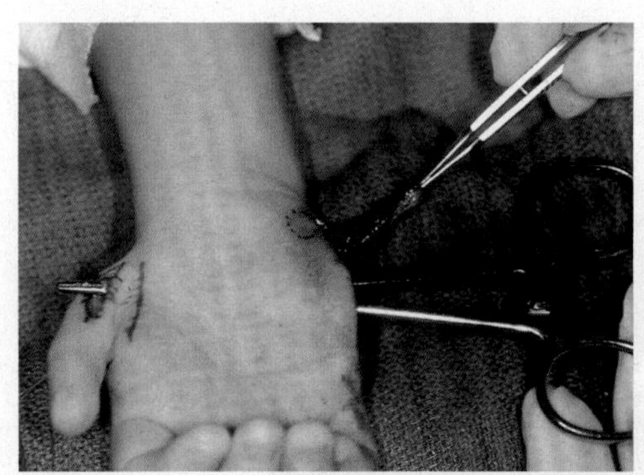
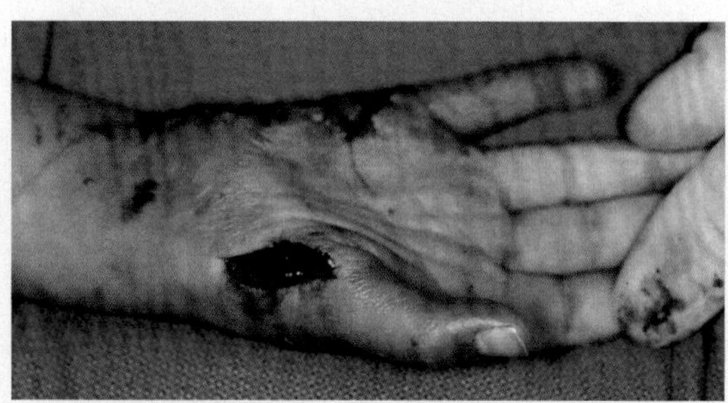

TECH FIG 2 • *(continued)* B. Passage of the ADM muscle–tendon unit through the previously created subcutaneous tunnel to the thumb. **C.** Final position of thumb after suture fixation of the ADM to the thumb. Note opposition and palmar abduction. (Courtesy of Shriners Hospital for Children, Philadelphia.)

Extensor Indicis Proprius Transfer

- Make a longitudinal incision on the dorsum of the index finger MCP joint.
- Locate the EIP tendon deep and ulnar to the extensor digitorum communis tendon to the index finger (**TECH FIG 3A**).
- Identify the EIP tendon along with the extensor hood.
- Divide the EIP tendon on the proximal edge of the extensor hood. The EIP tendon can be elongated by taking a 3- to 4-mm slip of extensor mechanism along the proximal phalanx. Repair the rent in the extensor hood with interrupted 4-0 braided polyester suture.
- Make a longitudinal incision on the dorsoulnar aspect of the wrist, just proximal to the point where the dorsal sensory branch of the ulnar nerve crosses near the ulnar styloid.
- Carry dissection from this incision in a radial direction until the proximal EIP tendon can be identified (just distal to the extensor retinaculum) (**TECH FIG 3B**).
  - The EIP tendon is frequently differentiated from the EDC tendons by its distal muscle belly.
- Divide the distal aspect of the extensor retinaculum over the fourth compartment to mobilize the EIP tendon.
- Bring the EIP tendon out through the ulnar wrist incision (**TECH FIG 3C**).
- Make another small longitudinal incision on the radial edge of the pisiform.
- Make a fourth incision over the thumb MCP joint.
- Create a subcutaneous tunnel from the ulnar wrist incision to the pisiform incision, then on to the thumb MCP joint incision, using blunt dissection.
- Pass the EIP tendon first through the pisiform incision, then on to the thumb incision (**TECH FIG 3D**).
- Suture the EIP tendon to the thumb using a 3-0 or 4-0 braided polyester suture.

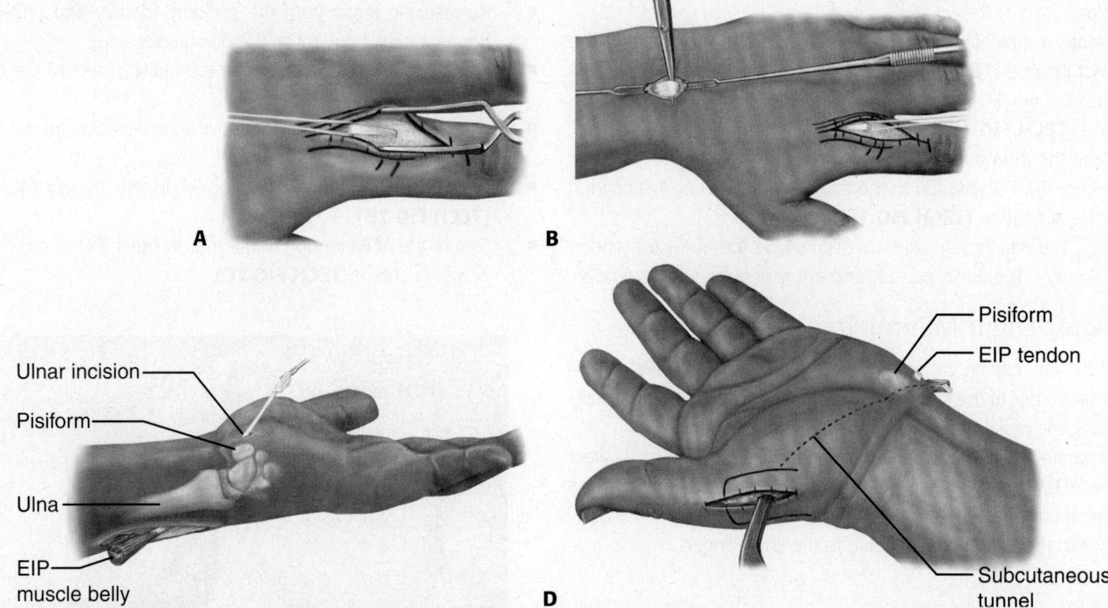

TECH FIG 3 • A. Isolation of EIP tendon ulnar and deep to the extensor digitorum communis tendon to the index finger. **B.** Wrist incision through which the proximal aspect of the EIP is found and isolated. **C.** The EIP tendon is brought out through the previously created ulnar wrist incision. **D.** Passage of EIP tendon through the subcutaneous tunnel between ulnar wrist incision and thumb incision.

Palmaris Longus Transfer (Camitz)

- Confirm the presence of a PL tendon by having the patient attempt to oppose the thumb to the small fingertip with the wrist flexed.
- Make a longitudinal incision beginning at the distal wrist crease and continuing distally to the proximal palmar crease. This incision may be "zigzagged" at the wrist to prevent scar contracture.
- Dissect the PL tendon in a proximal to distal direction.
- Take a small (about 1 cm^2) patch of palmar aponeurosis along with the PL tendon.
- Make an incision over the dorsum of the thumb MCP joint.
- Create the subcutaneous tunnel between the PL tendon and the MCP joint with blunt dissection.
- Pass the PL tendon through the tunnel to the thumb incision.
- Secure the PL tendon to the thumb with 3-0 or 4-0 braided polyester suture.

High Median Nerve Transfers

Brachioradialis Transfer

- Make a long radial incision from the radial styloid to the brachioradialis muscle belly.
- Release the brachioradialis tendon from the radial styloid and mobilize it along the forearm to optimize available excursion (**TECH FIG 4A**).[9]
- Identify the flexor pollicis longus tendon deep to the flexor carpi radialis tendon (**TECH FIG 4B**).
- Weave the harvested brachioradialis tendon into the flexor pollicis longus using a tendon braider and multiple weaves (**TECH FIG 4C**).
- Determine proper tension of the transfer by placing the wrist in flexion and extension and judging tenodesis lateral pinch position and thumb release, respectively (**TECH FIG 4D**).

Biceps Rerouting

- Biceps rerouting is preferred for supple supination deformities of the forearm to correct the forearm position and to apply a pronation moment.
- Surgery is performed under general anesthesia. The upper extremity is prepared and draped in the usual sterile fashion. A sterile circular tourniquet (HemaClear, OHK Medical Devices, Grandville, MI) is applied that exsanguinates during application.
- Design a Z incision with a horizontal limb across the antecubital fossa (**TECH FIG 5A**).
- Identify the lateral antebrachial cutaneous nerve lateral to the biceps tendon and protect it (**TECH FIG 5B**).
- Isolate the biceps tendon and incise the lacertus fibrosus while protecting the underlying median nerve and brachial artery.
- Trace the biceps tendon to its insertion into the radial tuberosity by careful dissection and placement of the elbow in flexion and the forearm into supination (**TECH FIG 5C**).

A

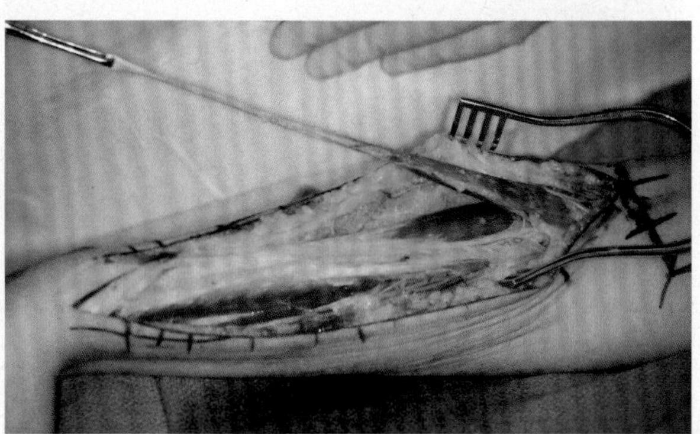

C

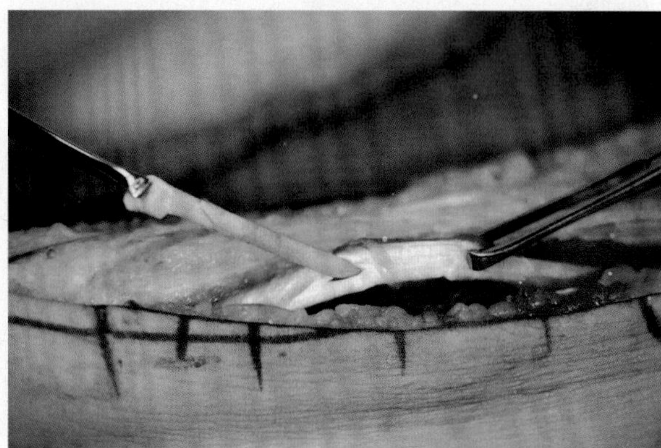

B

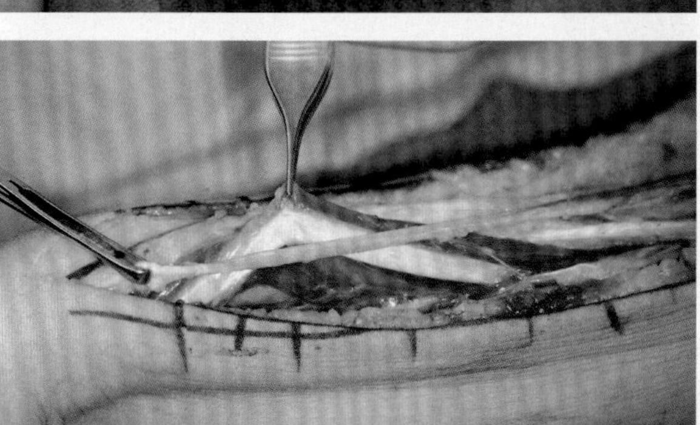

D

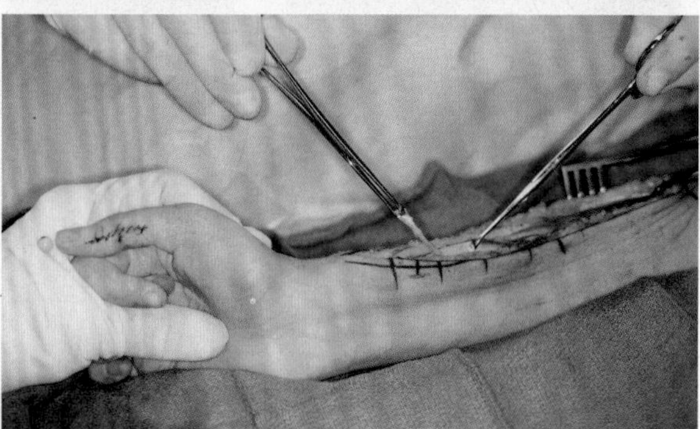

TECH FIG 4 • **A.** Brachioradialis tendon released and mobilized into the proximal one-third of the forearm. **B.** Flexor pollicis longus tendon isolated in volar compartment. **C.** Brachioradialis tendon woven through the flexor pollicis longus tendon. **D.** Tendon transfer tension is adjusted until there is lateral pinch during wrist extension. (Courtesy of Shriners Hospitals for Children, Philadelphia.)

- Plan a Z-plasty of the biceps tendon along its entire length to ensure sufficient tendon length for passage around the radius (**TECH FIG 5D**).
- Leave the distal Z-plasty attached to the insertion site and leave the proximal Z-plasty attached to the muscle belly (**TECH FIG 5E**).
- Reroute the distal attachment around the radius through the interosseous space to create a pronation force. A curved clamp, such as a Deborah cast clamp or Castaneda pediatric clamp (Pilling Surgical, Inc., Research Triangle Park, NC), facilitates tendon passage (**TECH FIG 5F,G**).
- Protect the posterior interosseous nerve during tendon passage.
- Place the elbow in 90 degrees of flexion and the forearm in pronation. Repair the rerouted distal tendon back to the proximal tendon that is still attached to the biceps muscle using a tendon weave augmented by nonabsorbable suture (**TECH FIG 5H**).
- Close the subcutaneous tissue and skin in routine fashion. Apply a long-arm cast with the elbow in 90 degrees of flexion and the forearm in pronation. The cast is worn for 5 weeks.
- After 5 weeks of immobilization, the cast is removed and rehabilitation is started. A posterior long-arm orthosis is fabricated with the elbow in a resting position with the forearm pronated and the wrist in neutral or slightly extended (**TECH FIG 5I**).
- In a gradual fashion, activities of daily living that require pronation are incorporated into the therapeutic regimen (**TECH FIG 5J**).

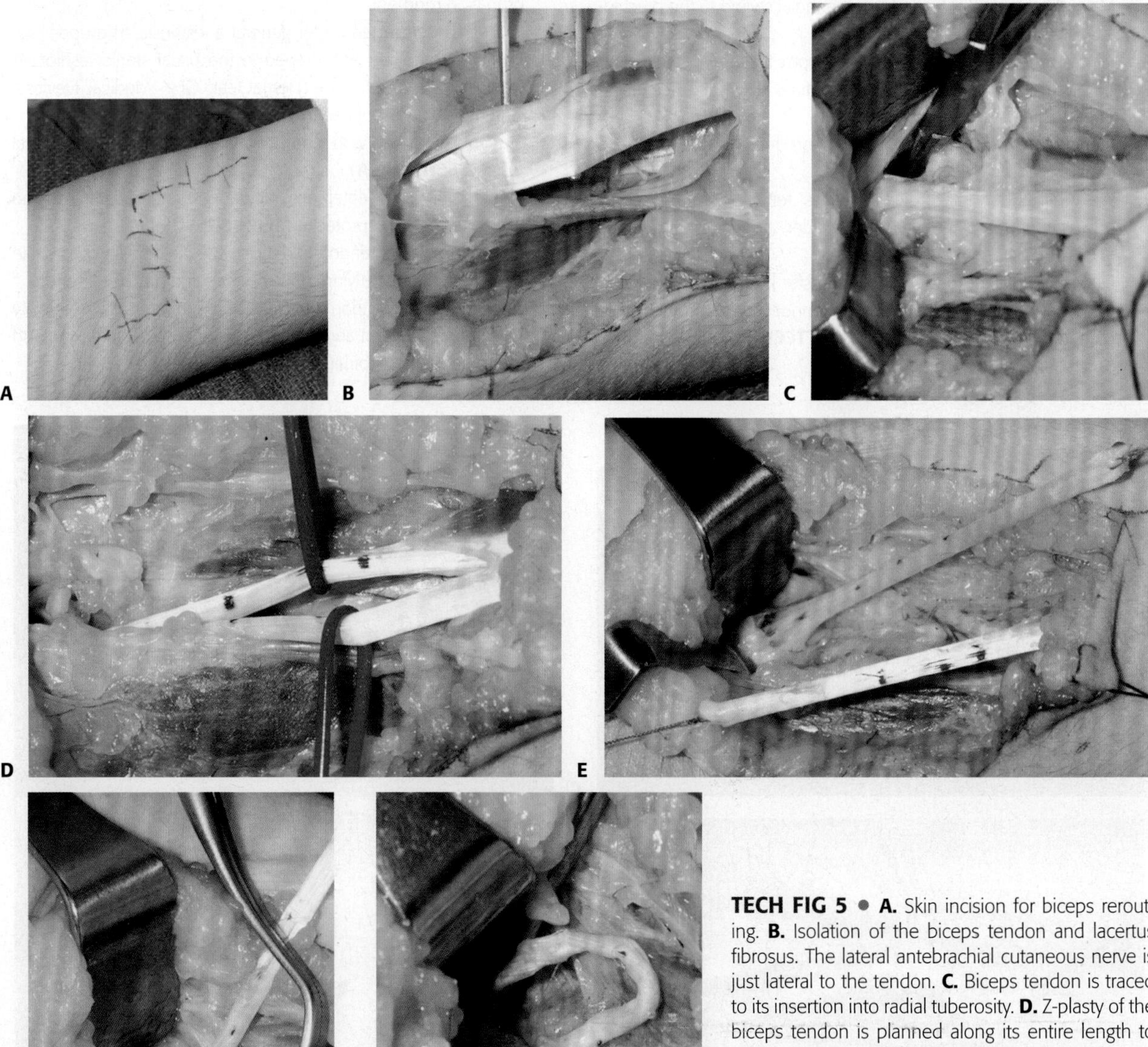

TECH FIG 5 • **A.** Skin incision for biceps rerouting. **B.** Isolation of the biceps tendon and lacertus fibrosus. The lateral antebrachial cutaneous nerve is just lateral to the tendon. **C.** Biceps tendon is traced to its insertion into radial tuberosity. **D.** Z-plasty of the biceps tendon is planned along its entire length to ensure sufficient tendon length for passage around the radius. **E.** Z-plasty of entire biceps tendon. The distal Z-plasty is left attached to the insertion site and the proximal Z-plasty is left attached to the muscle belly. **F.** A curved clamp facilitates tendon rerouting around the radius. **G.** Tendon is passed through interosseous space and around the radius. *(continued)*

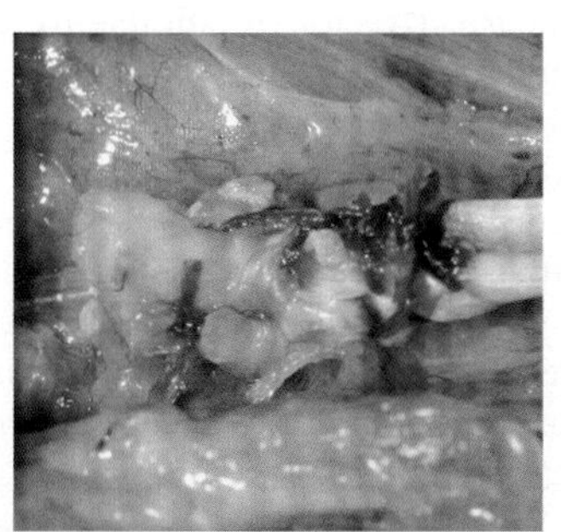

H

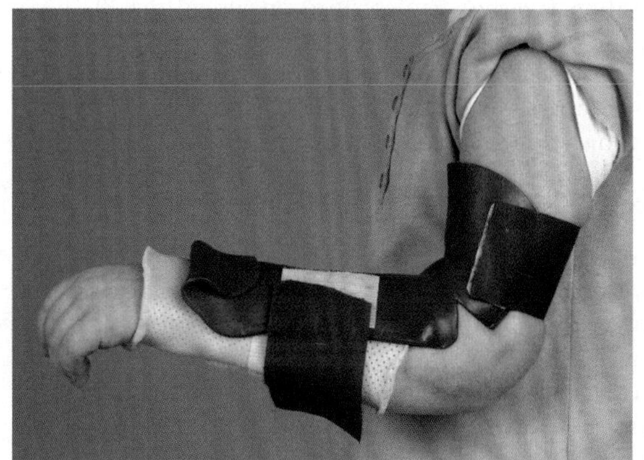

I

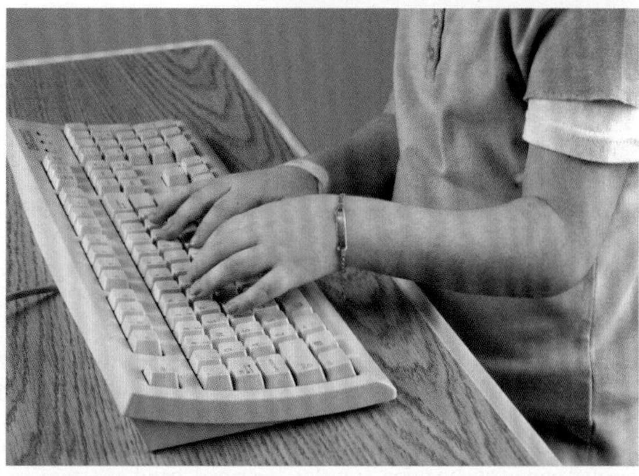

J

TECH FIG 5 • *(continued)* **H.** Distal limb is repaired back to proximal limb using a tendon weave augmented with nonabsorbable suture. **I.** Two-piece supracondylar orthosis is fabricated following cast immobilization. **J.** Activities of daily living that require pronation, such as typing, are incorporated into therapy. The figures are oriented as follows: hand to the left and shoulder to the right. (Courtesy of Shriners Hospital for Children, Philadelphia.)

PEARLS AND PITFALLS

Tendon transfer selection	▪ Patients should be carefully examined prior to surgery to determine donor tendons available for transfer and specific thumb motion(s) needed to regain function for work and daily activities.
Pulley construction	▪ Use the FCU or the pisiform when transferring the FDS ring finger tendon.[3] ▪ Use the pisiform when transferring the EIP tendon. ▪ PL transfer does not require a pulley, but it yield primarily palmar abduction not opposition.
Attachment site	▪ Commonly, the abductor pollicis brevis tendon; however, if additional pronation and extension is necessary, then a more dorsal attachment site is performed.
Subcutaneous tunnel creation	▪ Tunnels should be ample size to allow easy passage of transferred tendons.
Tendon transfer tensioning	▪ After suturing the tendon transfer, the thumb should be in full opposition with the wrist in extension. In flexion, the thumb should relax out of the palm.[8]
Stiff joints before tendon transfer	▪ Affected joints, especially in the thumb, must have good passive range of motion before tendon transfer. Otherwise, transfer risks failure due to inability to motor the joints.

POSTOPERATIVE CARE

- A bulky hand dressing and short-arm plaster splint is placed with the wrist in flexion and the thumb in full opposition.
- Immediate hand therapy commences to maintain motion in the fingers, especially the ring finger after FDS harvest.
- If the ring finger tends to position into flexion, a proximal interphalangeal joint extension splint is fabricated for nighttime wear.
- In contrast, a ring finger that tends to swan-neck secondary to loss of the FDS tendon requires a silver ring splint to prevent deformity until the remaining FDS scars along the volar aspect of the proximal interphalangeal joint.
- After 2 to 3 weeks, the plaster splint is removed and therapy is initiated. Longer periods of immobilization may yield scarring of the FDS tendon within the reconstructed pulley. Earlier mobilization under the auspices of a qualified therapist may be appropriate in the compliant patient.[10]
- An Orthoplast splint is fabricated to maintain mild wrist flexion and thumb opposition. The splint is removed four to six times a day to encourage tendon gliding exercises and retraining of the transferred tendon.

- Similar occupational therapy principles are applied after other opposition transfers as described, including the PL, EIP, ADM, and other transfers.
- Patients are instructed in other modalities, including scar management, muscle–tendon reeducation, and incorporation of the transfer into activities of daily living.

OUTCOMES

- In general, opposition transfers are successful: Most patients regain opposition adequate to perform normal daily activities such as writing, buttoning clothes, and other fine manipulation tasks (**FIG 2**).[12]
- Burkhalter et al[2] reported excellent results in 57 of 65 cases of EIP opponensplasty; excellent results were defined as those with 75% function compared to the opposite normal thumb or those with less than a 20-degree difference between the plane of the opposite thumbnail and the plane of the palm with good power.
- Jacobs and Thompson,[7] using a variety of donor tendons (mainly ring and long finger FDS tendons), pulley designs, and insertion techniques, reported 77 good or excellent, 9 fair, and 17 poor results. Similar results were obtained with ring and long finger FDS tendons.
- In a comparison of FDS versus EIP opponensplasty, Anderson et al[1] compared 50 EIP to 116 FDS ring finger opponensplasty cases. Their analysis demonstrated that the EIP opponensplasty was best in supple hands, whereas the FDS opponensplasty was more suitable in less pliable hands.

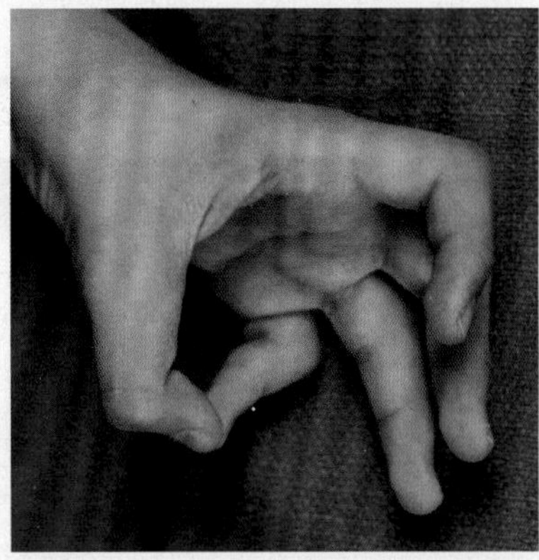

FIG 2 • Postoperative photo of patient from **FIG 1**. This demonstrates good thumb opposition after ring finger FDS transfer for thumb opposition. (Courtesy of Shriners Hospital for Children, Philadelphia.)

COMPLICATIONS

- Suboptimal transfer outcome due to stiff joints
- Selection of suboptimal or weak muscle–tendon unit for transfer
- Incorrect vector of pull due to lack of or poor selection of pulley
- Rupture of transferred tendon
- Tendon adhesions
- Loss of grip strength or independent ring finger function after FDS ring finger transfer
- Difficulty with muscle–tendon reeducation, especially with tendon transfers that are not synergistic. For example, EIP transfer is more difficult to learn compared to FDS tendon transfer.

REFERENCES

1. Anderson GA, Lee V, Sundararaj GD. Opponensplasty by extensor indicis and flexor digitorum superficialis tendon transfer. J Hand Surg Br 1992;17(6):611–614.
2. Burkhalter W, Christensen RC, Brown P. Extensor indicis proprius opponensplasty. J Bone Joint Surg Am 1973;55(4):725–732.
3. Cooney WP. Tendon transfer for median nerve palsy. Hand Clin 1988;4:155–165.
4. Davis T. Median nerve palsy. In: Green D, Hotchkiss R, Pederson W, et al, eds. Green's Operative Hand Surgery, ed 5. Elsevier, 2005:1131–1160.
5. de Roode CP, James MA, McCarroll HR Jr. Abductor digit minimi opponensplasty: technique, modifications, and measurement of opposition. Tech Hand Up Extrem Surg 2010;14(1):51–53.
6. Estilow T, Kozin SH, Glanzman AM, et al. Flexor digitorum superficialis opposition tendon transfer improves hand function in children with Charcot-Marie-Tooth disease: case series. Neuromuscul Disord 2012;22(12):1090–1095.
7. Jacobs B, Thompson TC. Opposition of the thumb and its restoration. J Bone Joint Surg Am 1960;42A:1015–1026.
8. Kozin SH. Tendon transfers for radial and median nerve palsies. J Hand Ther 2005;18:208–215.
9. Kozin SH, Bednar M. In vivo determination of available brachioradialis excursion during tetraplegia reconstruction. J Hand Surg Am 2001;26(3):510–514.
10. Rath S. Immediate active mobilization versus immobilization for opposition tendon transfer in the hand. J Hand Surg Am 2006;31(5): 754–759.
11. Ratner JA, Peljovich A, Kozin SH. Update on tendon transfers for peripheral nerve injuries. J Hand Surg Am 2010;35:1371–1381.
12. Sundararaj GD, Mani K. Surgical reconstruction of the hand with triple nerve palsy. J Bone Joint Surg Br 1984;66(2):260–264.
13. Trumble T. Tendon transfers. In: Trumble T, ed. Principles of Hand Surgery and Therapy, ed 1. Saunders, 2000:343–360.

Radial Nerve Decompression

Mark N. Awantang, Joseph M. Sherrill, and Thomas R. Hunt III

96

CHAPTER

DEFINITION

- Radial tunnel syndrome was first described by Michele and Krueger[7] in 1956 as *radial pronator syndrome*.
- It was described as a compression neuropathy involving primarily the posterior interosseous nerve (PIN), associated with a predominant symptom of pain.

ANATOMY

- The radial nerve pierces the lateral intermuscular septum 10 to 12 cm above the lateral epicondlye. It travels along the lateral border of the brachialis muscle and is covered laterally and anteriorly by the brachioradialis (BR), extensor carpi radialis longus (ECRL), and extensor carpi radialis brevis (ECRB) muscles (see FIG 1B, Chap. 97).
- It divides into the PIN and the superficial radial sensory nerve 3 to 5 cm distal to the lateral epicondyle.
- The PIN then enters the "radial tunnel."
  - The floor of the tunnel begins at the anterior capsule of the radiocapitellar joint and continues as the deep head of the supinator.
  - The roof begins as inconstant fibrous bands between the brachialis and BR and then continues as the medial border of the ECRB. Distally, the roof of the tunnel consists of the superficial or oblique head of the supinator.
  - The radial tunnel ends with the distal edge of the supinator.
- Proximal to the supinator, the nerve often is crossed superficially by branches of the radial recurrent artery known as the *vascular leash of Henry*.

PATHOGENESIS

- Roles and Maudsley[9] described the concept of radial nerve compression in 1972, suggesting that it could result in a wide spectrum of symptoms. Both radial tunnel and posterior interosseous syndrome are thought to be due to compression of the PIN. It is thought that the different clinical presentations may be attributed to a difference in the degree of compression.
  - If the primary complaint is of weakness, the symptom complex is referred to as *posterior interosseous syndrome*.
- The compression may rarely be due to space-occupying lesions such as ganglion, neoplasm, or florid synovitis of the proximal radioulnar, radiocapitellar, or ulnotrochlear joints.
- The sites of compression of the PIN most often cited are the fibrous proximal border of the supinator (arcade of Frohse), the medial border of the ECRB, fibrous bands passing volar to the radial head, and the vascular leash of Henry.
  - The arcade of Frohse and the medial border of the ECRB are thought to be the most common sites of compression.
- Werner et al[13] recorded pressures from 40 to 50 mm Hg exerted on the nerve with passive stretch of the supinator muscle. Pressures exceeding 250 mm Hg have been recorded on the nerve with stimulated tetanic contraction of the supinator muscle. Ischemia of the nerve has been demonstrated at 60 to 80 mm Hg and blockade of axonal transport at 50 mm Hg.
- The documented changes in pressure due to positioning of the forearm in conjunction with the observation that symptoms often are associated with repetitive pronation and supination have led to the theory that the clinical syndrome may be provoked by dynamic and intermittent compression on the radial nerve.
- Although the PIN is considered a motor nerve, it has been well documented that afferent sensory fibers run within the nerve. The muscles innervated by the PIN contain nerve endings corresponding to group IIA fibers and unmyelinated group IV fibers from muscle fibers along its distribution. These fibers are commonly thought to be responsible for the pain from muscle cramps and, therefore, could likely be mediators of pain in radial tunnel syndrome. These small myelinated and unmyelinated fibers are not associated by nerve conduction studies.
- Because of the common association with (or difficulty in distinguishing it from) lateral epicondylitis, some authors have suggested that referred pain from lateral epicondylitis or intra-articular pathology may contribute to radial tunnel syndrome.
  - In 1984, Heyse-Moore[1] suggested that radial tunnel syndrome may be an analog of a musculotendinous lesion of the common extensor tendon, causing lateral epicondylitis in the supinator.

PATIENT HISTORY AND PHYSICAL FINDINGS

- The diagnosis of radial tunnel syndrome is based on clinical findings. Historically, it was described as a cause of treatment-resistant lateral epicondylitis. The two disorders may have similar and overlapping symptoms. The clinician should distinguish when possible between these two diagnoses.
- Symptoms can be variable, but the classic history described by the patient with radial tunnel syndrome is of pain over the lateral forearm musculature distal to the lateral epicondyle (along the course of the radial nerve) that is exacerbated by activity.
  - The pain is often described as a constant "aching" that is aggravated by or prevents activities.
  - Pain is most pronounced with active supination and less severe with activities involving extension of the fingers.
  - Lesser symptoms of weakness of the finger and wrist extensors also may be present, as may dysesthesias over the distal lateral forearm and wrist.
  - Other symptoms include writer's cramp, paresthesias, night cramps, and radiation of pain proximally and distally in the arm and forearm. Some patients complain of a "popping" sensation over the elbow during pronation.

- The most specific finding on physical examination is pain with digital pressure placed on the radial nerve over the mobile wad at the radial neck or over the proximal edge of the supinator approximately 4 cm distal to the lateral epicondyle.
- Two other pathognomonic signs (described by Lister et al[6]) are pain in the lateral forearm with resisted extension of the middle finger and pain with resisted supination.
  - These signs differ from those associated with lateral epicondylitis, which are tenderness over the lateral epicondyle and lateral epicondylar pain elicited by resisted wrist extension with the elbow in extension.
- The most sensitive examination for radial tunnel syndrome involves application of firm constant pressure over the mobile wad onto the radial neck to locate the point of maximum tenderness.
- The middle finger test—extension of the middle finger against resistance with the elbow extended—transmits pressure to the third metacarpal, indirectly tensioning the ECRB and causing increased pressure on the PIN.
- If pain is reproduced at the point of maximal tenderness with supination of the forearm against resistance, the supinator is implicated as the culprit in intermittently increasing pressure on PIN.

IMAGING AND OTHER DIAGNOSTIC STUDIES

- If the patient's clinical examination is suggestive of elbow arthritis or cervical radiculopathy, radiographs of the elbow and a cervical spine series may be helpful in elucidating associated pathology that may contribute to a neuropathy of the radial nerve caused by an anterior osteophyte of the elbow or degenerative disc disease of the cervical spine.
- Magnetic resonance imaging (MRI) can be helpful in identifying possible cervical degenerative disc disease or elbow ganglia.
- Injection of lidocaine into the radial tunnel has been described as a diagnostic tool for radial tunnel syndrome.
  - Because it is difficult to reliably contain the anesthetic within the radial tunnel, the main criticism of this technique is the lack of specificity in differentiating pathology involving the radial nerve from other sources of pain.
- Multiple studies using electromyography (EMG) and nerve conduction velocity have shown no consistent relation between symptoms of radial tunnel syndrome and the findings on these tests.
  - In 1980, Rosén and Werner[10] demonstrated that static motor nerve conduction at rest was not significantly different between symptomatic patients and a nonsymptomatic control group. They did find, however, that active supination of the forearm produced an increase in the conduction time of the PIN across the supinator muscle more often in patients with radial tunnel than in control subjects.
  - Verhaar and Spaans[12] tested patients while holding the forearm in active supination and found that 14 of 16 patients with radial tunnel syndrome had no abnormal latency on nerve conduction studies or abnormality of the EMG.
  - Kupfer et al[3] found that differential latency (ie, different latency measurements recorded in the same nerve in different positions) may be more significant in identifying "pathologic" latency than comparing a measured latency to a standard "normal" latency measurement. Differential latencies were higher in patients with radial tunnel syndrome than in the control group and improved after surgical decompression, correlating with clinical results.

DIFFERENTIAL DIAGNOSIS

- Lateral epicondylitis
- PIN palsy
- Cervical radiculopathy C5–C6
- Neuritis of the lateral antebrachial cutaneous nerve
- Wartenberg syndrome
- Myofascial pain syndrome

NONOPERATIVE MANAGEMENT

- A course of nonoperative treatment should always be attempted.
- Activity modification may be helpful, particularly in patients whose vocation or avocation involves frequent repetitive supination and pronation of the forearm.
- The patient should attempt stretching exercises of the supinator and the ECRB, with pronation of the forearm and wrist flexion with the elbow in extension. Gentle strengthening exercise also may be helpful in improving symptoms.
- An injection of local anesthetic and corticosteroid in the radial tunnel may provide relief in some patients.

SURGICAL MANAGEMENT

- Surgical management should be considered in the patient who has failed nonoperative treatment.
- There is no consensus as to which anatomic structures should be released at the time of surgery. It is agreed, however, that this is typically a clinical decision. Electrodiagnostic studies do not reliably locate the area of pathology.
  - Most authors recommend releasing the PIN as it passes under the superficial head of the supinator by dividing the fibrous arcade of Frohse and the tendinous border of the ECRB, as needed.
  - Lister and others[6] emphasize release of the fibrous bands of the radial tunnel anterior to the radial head.
  - Sponseller and Engber[11] has reported cases where the PIN is compressed by the distal aspect of the supinator muscle.
  - Some surgeons advocate the release of the common extensors as well as structures compressing the PIN to address all potential causes of pain. Ritts et al[8] stated that the pathology of radial tunnel syndrome and that of lateral epicondylitis appear to be interrelated.
  - Little literature has been published supporting release of the superficial sensory branch of the radial nerve. It has been associated with neurapraxia and complex regional pain syndrome.[4]
  - The surgeon should remain mindful of less common causes of pain over the radial tunnel, including radial nerve compression proximal to the supinator.
- When the diagnosis is not clear on physical examination, and the patient has symptoms and examination findings suggestive of lateral epicondylitis, surgical treatment of lateral epicondylitis can be done concomitantly.

Preoperative Planning

- A tourniquet should be placed on the arm to facilitate visualization. If it is thought that more proximal release or exploration of the radial nerve into the arm may be necessary, a sterile tourniquet is used.

Positioning

- The patient is placed in the supine position, with the arm and forearm rotated as needed to facilitate the preferred approach.

Approach

- The most direct dissection path to the radial nerve may be established by palpating the radial nerve through the mobile wad and rolling the PIN under a thumb with enough force to cause an extension flicker of the digits.
- Multiple surgical approaches are possible. Determination of which structures require decompression may influence the approach chosen.
- Anterior approach
  - Advantages: It can easily be extended proximally to decompress the radial nerve in the arm if indicated. This exposure may be of benefit in cases of compression on the nerve by rarer causes such as elbow synovitis or ganglia.
  - Disadvantages: In muscular patients, it can be difficult to retract the BR radially well enough to obtain adequate visualization of the radial tunnel. Distal compression sites often are difficult to release.
- Transbrachioradialis approach
  - Advantage: provides a more direct approach to the radial tunnel, improving exposure
  - Disadvantage: Some surgeons find the intramuscular dissection unappealing, given the relative paucity of definable landmarks.
- Posterior and posterolateral approaches (the authors' favored approaches)
  - Advantage: Dissection between the ECRB and the extensor digitorum communis (EDC), or between the BR and ECRL, allows direct exposure to the entire radial tunnel with relatively less dissection and a bloodless field.
  - Disadvantage: The ECRB–EDC interval is limited in that it does not allow easy extension of the incision to expose the radial nerve more proximally.

TECHNIQUES

Posterior Approach and Nerve Decompression (Extensor Digitorum Communis–Extensor Carpi Radialis Brevis Interval)

Exposure

- The forearm is held in pronation. The radial nerve is palpated just posterior to the mobile wad (**TECH FIG 1A**).
- A 5-cm longitudinal incision is made over the proximal lateral forearm along Thompson cardinal line from Lister tubercle to the lateral epicondyle (**TECH FIG 1B**).
  - The posterior cutaneous nerve of the forearm is identified and protected (**TECH FIG 1C**).
- The interval between the EDC and ECRB is located. The overlying fascia is first incised, beginning distally where the structures are better identified. The incision is extended proximally to the lateral epicondyle.
- The EDC and ECRB muscles are separated bluntly, using finger dissection, or with scissors, as required (**TECH FIG 1D**).
  - Opening of this interval will reveal the superficial fascia of the ECRB to which the fibers of the EDC often are securely attached and from which they must be carefully released.

Releasing the Compression

- The leading edge of the ECRB often is thickened and taut (**TECH FIG 2A**). This potential site of nerve compression is incised.
  - Release of the origin of the ECRB simultaneously treats coexisting lateral epicondylitis.

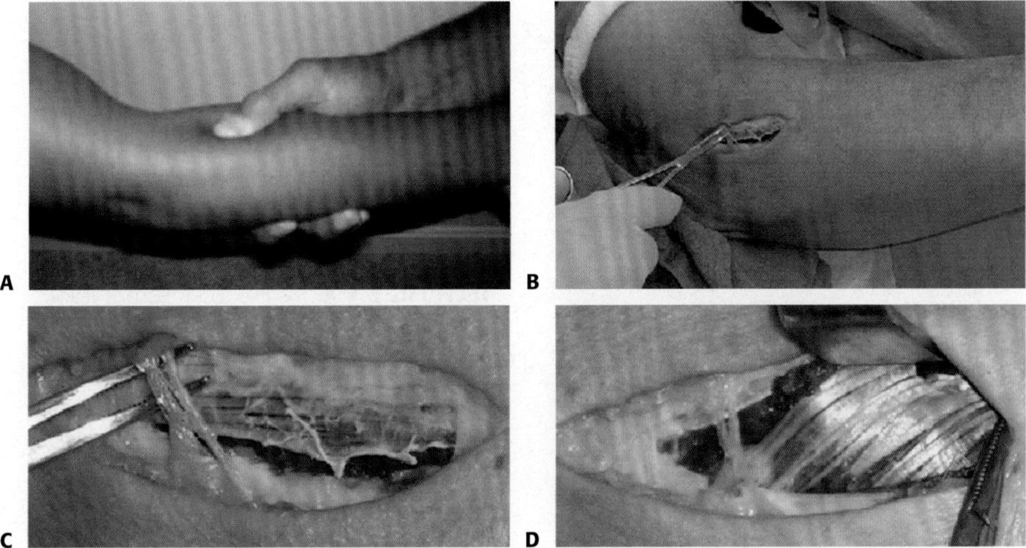

TECH FIG 1 • **A.** The points of maximal tenderness help delineate the course of the nerve and isolate areas of compression. **B.** Standard positioning, use of a sterile tourniquet, and placement of the 5-cm posterior proximal forearm incision. **C.** The posterior cutaneous nerve of the forearm is consistently seen crossing the proximal incision, superficial to the fascia. It must be protected. **D.** The fascia between the EDC and ECRB has been divided, and the supinator is exposed.

- Further blunt dissection in the EDC–ECRB interval reveals fibers of the superficial head of the supinator distally and fat more proximally over the radial neck (**TECH FIG 2B**).
  - The PIN will be found within this fat.
  - Gentle dissection of the nerve is performed through this proximal fat as necessary for complete visualization of the nerve.
- Proximally, the leash of Henry usually is seen running transversely, superficial to the nerve.
  - Typically, the vessels are not large or obviously constricting.
  - If any of the vessels of the leash are substantial enough to appear to cause compression, or if they impede full decompression of the supinator, they are separated and coagulated with bipolar cautery.
- Once the nerve is well visualized proximally, the superficial fascia of the supinator is released in a proximal to distal direction to the most distal border of the supinator.
- A white crescent-shaped band of fibers represents the proximal border of the superficial head of the supinator; this is termed the *arcade of Frohse* (**TECH FIG 2C**).
  - This arcade can be observed to tighten over the PIN as the forearm is pronated.
- These fibers of the superficial head of the supinator are then carefully released. Protect the small motor branches to the ECRB (**TECH FIG 2D**).
  - This release generally results in significant stretching of the remaining underlying supinator muscle fibers and appears to reduce tension over the nerve.
- The nerve is inspected and palpated along its entire course for any other sites of compression.
  - During palpation, special attention is paid to the proximal nerve in the interval between the brachialis and BR.
- A thin fascial layer occasionally is present. This layer is confluent with the fascia of the superficial supinator that extends proximally, causing compression of the nerve. If this is present, it is carefully released.
- Before completion, visualize and palpate the nerve over its entire course to make sure there are no further sites of compression, especially proximally (**TECH FIG 2E**).
- The fascial layer between the ECRB and the EDC is closed with absorbable suture, the skin is closed in the usual manner, and an above-elbow splint is applied with the elbow at 90 degrees and the wrist extended 20 to 30 degrees.

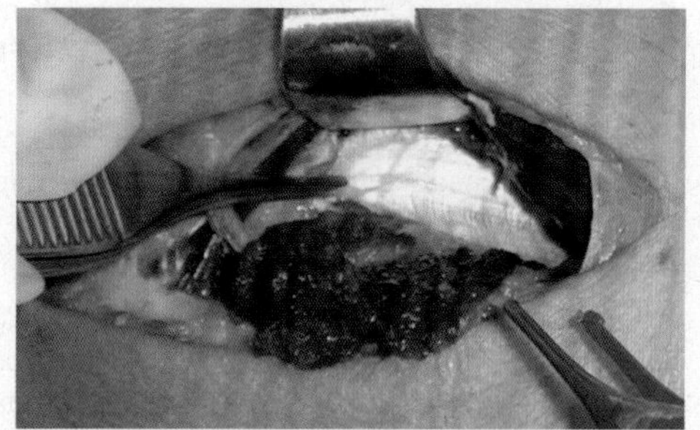
A

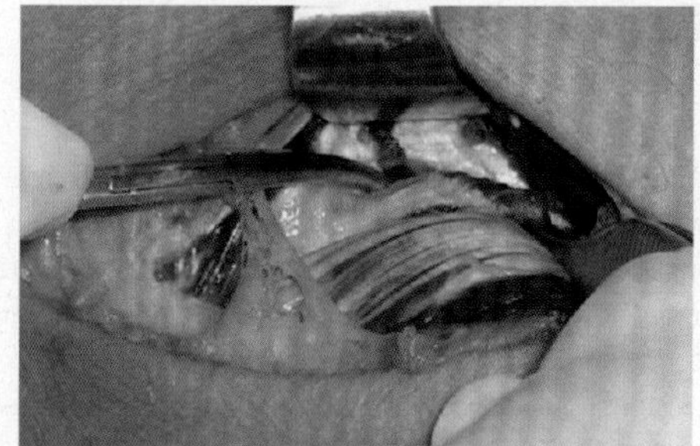
B

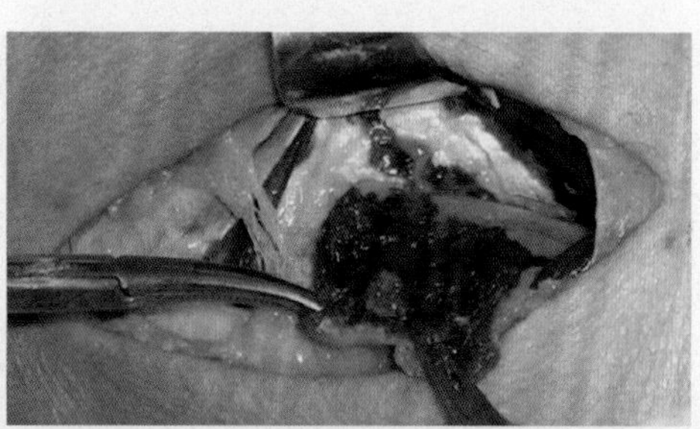
C

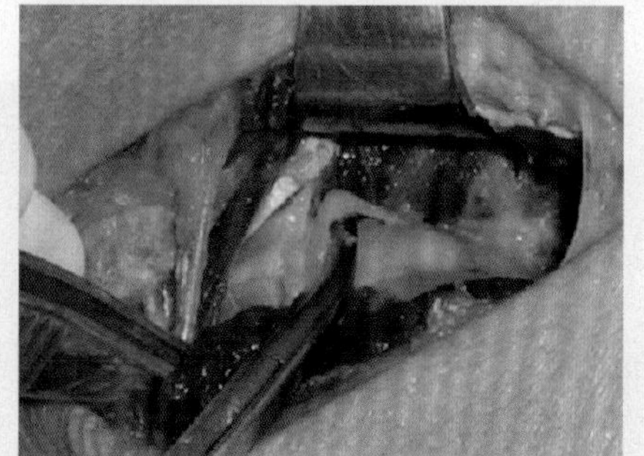
D

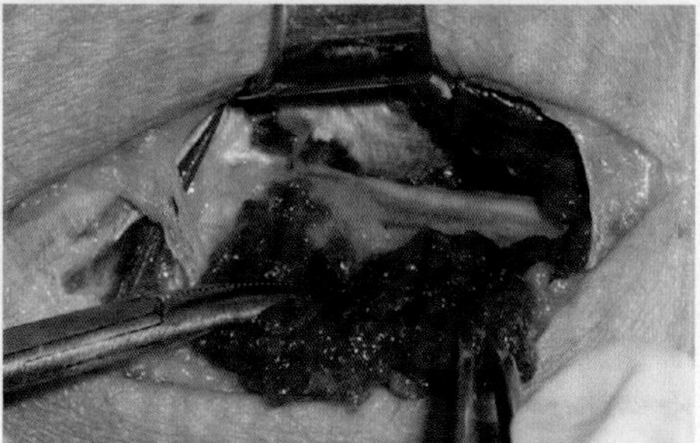
E

TECH FIG 2 • **A.** The thick ECRB fascia is readily visualized once the EDC is separated and retracted posteriorly. Here, the ECRB is fractionally lengthened. **B.** The proximal tendon of the ECRB is visualized and retracted superiorly, revealing the proximal fat (hemostat) covering the PIN and the superficial fascia of the supinator more distally. **C.** The supinator fascia has been incised and the muscle dissected, leaving only the tight arcade of Frohse proximally. **D.** Before release of the arcade, the ECRB motor branches are isolated and protected. **E.** The PIN is now completely released.

Posterolateral Approach and Nerve Decompression (Extensor Carpi Radialis Longus–Brachioradialis Interval)

- A 5- to 7-cm incision is made starting at the lateral epicondyle and heading distally along the posterior border of the BR with protection of the sensory nerve branches.
- The fascial interval between the BR and the ECRL is defined.
  - The BR is a deeper red compared with the ECRL due to its thinner overlying fascia.
- The interval is further developed using blunt finger dissection.
  - Difficulty in dissection usually indicates that the muscular interval is not correct.
- The remainder of the procedure mirrors that detailed for the EDC–ECRB interval.

Brachioradialis Muscle-Splitting Approach and Nerve Decompression

- A 4- to 6-cm longitudinal incision is made over the proximal anterolateral surface of the forearm, starting distal to the elbow flexion crease and 3 cm radial to the biceps tendon and extending over the radial head.
  - A 4-cm transverse incision just distal to the radial head also may be used.
- The deep fascia is divided in the line of the skin incision, and the BR is exposed. Its fibers are parted by blunt dissection.
- Immediately deep to this muscle, the vivid white of the superficial branch of the radial nerve is seen. Inspection at the level of the radial head reveals the fat overlying the PIN.
- The transverse branches of the radial recurrent artery and accompanying veins are divided as they pass between the PIN and radial sensory nerve.
- The radial nerve and its branches are now more fully exposed by dividing adhesions and fibrous bands overlying the nerve as well as the proximal fibrous edge of the ECRB.
- The superficial branch is followed distally anterior to the ECRB.
- The PIN is traced as it disappears beneath the fibrous edge of the superficial proximal border of the supinator, easily distinguished by its prominent oblique striations.
  - This fibrous edge and the muscle are divided longitudinally.
- The nerve is carefully inspected for untreated sites of compression before closure and splinting.

Modified Anterior Approach of Henry and Nerve Decompression

- A 5-cm longitudinal incision is made beginning at the antecubital flexion crease and proceeding distally along the medial border of the BR.
  - More proximal and extensile exposure may be obtained by extending the incision obliquely across the elbow flexion crease in the interval between the brachialis and the BR.
- The deep fascia is incised, and the BR is retracted radially. The proximal radial tunnel can be visualized over the capitellum.
- Any constricting vessels are ligated and divided.
- The superficial sensory branch of the radial nerve and the PIN are identified.
- The PIN is traced distally.
  - Significant retraction of the BR is required for adequate exposure.
  - The medial border of the ECRB is released to aid in exposure and to eliminate a potential site of compression.
- The arcade of Frohse is visualized, and the supinator muscle is divided to its distal border.
- The arm is supinated and pronated to identify constricting structures, and the course of the PIN is carefully inspected.
- Despite closure and splinting, as detailed previously, the scar often is conspicuous.

PEARLS AND PITFALLS

Surgical indications	▪ Attempt a course of nonoperative treatment for at least 3–4 months. ▪ Take care to differentiate radial tunnel syndrome from other pathology using a thorough history and multiple physical examinations.
Surgical approach	▪ Dictated by inciting pathology, coexistent diagnoses, and surgeon comfort.
Decompression	▪ At the time of release, make sure that the PIN is released from the proximal radiocapitellar joint to the distal border of the supinator.

POSTOPERATIVE CARE

- Patients are splinted for 7 to 10 days.
- Gentle active range-of-motion exercises are initiated and progressively advanced. Nerve gliding exercises are emphasized.
- Patients are allowed to resume normal activities in a progressive and graded fashion over the next few weeks.

OUTCOMES

- The efficacy of surgical treatment for radial tunnel syndrome is widely variable.
  - This variability in results may be due to heterogeneous patient populations and varying diagnostic criteria. No randomized controlled trials exist at this time.
- Lister et al,[6] Roles and Maudsley,[9] and Ritts et al[8] all reported high cure rates after release of the PIN.
- Sotereanos et al[11] reported more modest results (11 of 38 good or excellent), although their population did have a high proportion of worker's compensation patients.
- Verhaar and Spaans[12] reported even more modest results (1 of 10 patients had good results; 3 of 10 had fair results). Their diagnostic criterion was limited to tenderness over the radial nerve where it passes under the arcade of Frohse.
- Huisstede et al,[2] in a review of the literature, found a tendency that surgical release of the radial tunnel is effective, with effectiveness ranging from 67% to 92%.
- Lee et al[5] reported good results in 18 of 27 results but found poorer results in patients with concomitant lateral epicondylitis or other compression neuropathies.

COMPLICATIONS

- The incidence of PIN palsy following the procedure is reported to be low.
- Sotereanos et al[11] reported a 31% incidence of paresthesias of the superficial radial nerve.
- Paresthesias of the lateral cutaneous nerve of the arm have also been reported.

REFERENCES

1. Heyse-Moore GH. Resistant tennis elbow. J Hand Surg Br 1984;9(1):64–66.
2. Huisstede B, Midedma H, van Opstal T, et al. Interventions for treating the radial tunnel syndrome: a systematic review of observational studies. J Hand Surg Am 2008;33(1):72–78.
3. Kupfer DM, Bronson J, Lee GW, et al. Differential latency testing: a more sensitive test for radial tunnel syndrome. J Hand Surg Am 1998;23:859–864.
4. Lawrence T, Mobbs P, Fortems Y, et al. Radial tunnel syndrome. A retrospective review of 30 decompressions of the radial nerve. J Hand Surg Br 1995;20:454–459.
5. Lee JT, Azari K, Jones NF. Long term results of radial tunnel release—the effect of co-existing tennis elbow, multiple compression syndromes and workers' compensation. J Plast Reconstr Aesthet Surg 2008;61:1095–1099.
6. Lister GD, Belsole RB, Kleinert HE. The radial tunnel syndrome. J Hand Surg Am 1979;4:52–59.
7. Michele AA, Kreuger FJ. Lateral epicondylitis of the elbow treated by fasciotomy. Surgery 1956;39(2):277–284.
8. Ritts GD, Wood MB, Linscheid RL. Radial tunnel syndrome. A ten-year surgical experience. Clin Orthop Relat Res 1987;(219):201–205.
9. Roles NC, Maudsley RH. Radial tunnel syndrome: resistant tennis elbow as a nerve entrapment. J Bone Joint Surg Br 1972;54:499–508.
10. Rosén I, Werner CO. Neurophysiological investigation of posterior interosseous nerve entrapment causing lateral elbow pain. Electroencephalogr Clin Neurophysiol 1980;50(1):125–133.
11. Sotereanos DG, Varitimidis SE, Giannakopoulos PN, et al. Results of surgical treatment for radial tunnel syndrome. J Hand Surg Am 1999;24:566–570.
12. Verhaar J, Spaans F. Radial tunnel syndrome: an investigation of compression neuropathy as a possible cause. J Bone Joint Surg Am 1991;73:539–544.
13. Werner CO, Haeffner F, Rosén I. Direct recording of local pressure in the radial tunnel during passive stretch and active contraction of the supinator muscle. Arch Orthop Trauma Surg 1980;96(4):299–301.

SUGGESTED READINGS

Eaton CJ, Lister GD. Radial nerve compression. Hand Clin 1992;8:345–357.

Hall HC, MacKinnon SE, Gilbert RW. An approach to the posterior interosseous nerve. Plast Reconstr Surg 1984;74:435–437.

Moss SH, Switzer HE. Radial tunnel syndrome: a spectrum of clinical presentations. J Hand Surg Am 1983;8:414–420.

Sarhadi NS, Korday SN, Bainbridge LC. Radial tunnel syndrome: diagnosis and management. J Hand Surg Br 1998;23:617–619.

Sponseller PD, Engber WD. Double-entrapment radial tunnel syndrome. J Hand Surg Am 1983;8:420–423.

Tendon Transfers for Radial Nerve Palsy

97
CHAPTER

Harry A. Hoyen

DEFINITION

- Radial nerve palsy that is distal to the triceps innervation affects the forearm musculature. A lesion that does not recover results in predictable wrist, finger, and thumb extensor deficits.

ANATOMY

- The brachioradialis (BR) and forearm extensor musculature originate in the lateral humeral epicondyle and the interosseous membrane (IOM) (**FIG 1A**).
  - Each of the extensor muscles has a relatively flat muscle belly before forming a flat, broad tendon.
  - The myotendinous junction for the wrist extensors is in the midforearm, whereas the myotendinous junction of the finger and wrist extensors is in the distal forearm.
- The radial nerve arises from the posterior cord of the infraclavicular brachial plexus (**FIG 1B**). Multiple triceps motor branches are present as the nerve courses in the posterior compartment of the upper arm. The nerve traverses into the anterior compartment through the intramuscular septum. The nerve then lies between the brachialis and BR before it enters the forearm. The BR, extensor carpi radialis longus (ECRL), and extensor carpi radialis brevis (ECRB) are innervated as the nerve divides into the deep radial nerve, the posterior interosseous nerve (PIN), and the superficial radial nerve. The PIN innervates the extrinsic extensors after exiting the supinator musculature.
  - The motor point for each nerve is fairly consistently located just proximal to the myotendinous junction. In most cases, there is one larger motor branch from the radial nerve or PIN to each muscle.
- The sequence of muscle innervation is an important distinction when considering the anatomy of the radial nerve. Whereas some nerves distribute their nerve branches in a tree-like fashion, the radial nerve innervates the extensor musculature in an orderly pattern, from proximal to distal. The proper radial nerve supplies the BR, the ECRL, and occasionally the ECRB.

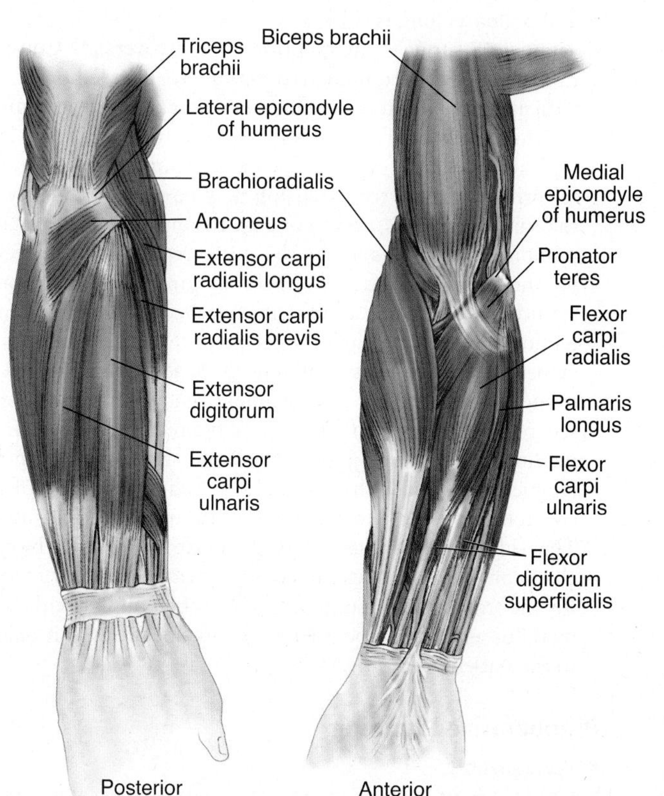

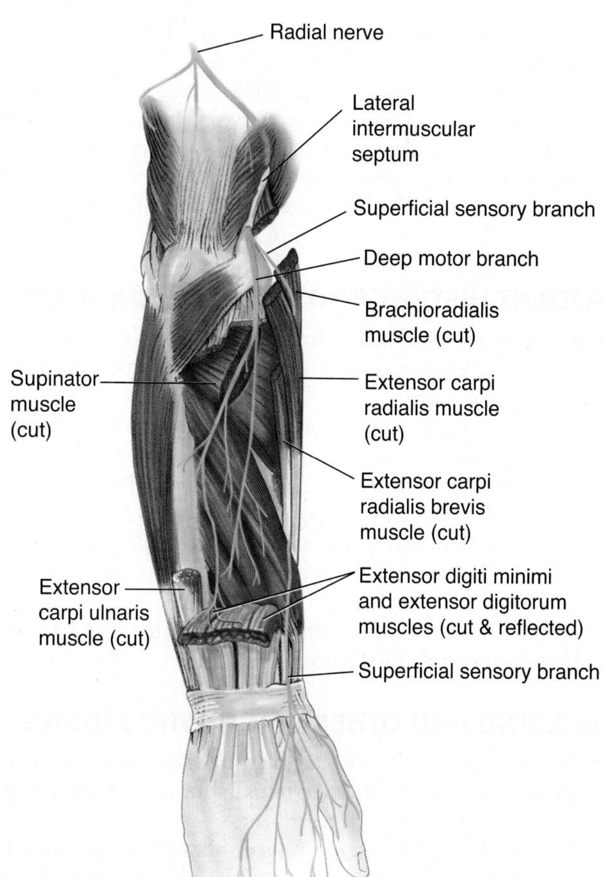

FIG 1 • **A.** Muscles of the forearm. **B.** Course of the radial nerve.

The PIN innervates the ECRB, the extensor digitorum communis (EDC), the extensor carpi ulnaris (ECU), the extensor indicis proprius (EIP), and the extensor pollicis longus (EPL).
- The order of innervation is important in differentiating a radial nerve injury from a mechanical myotendinous injury or muscle disruption after a forearm laceration.
- Understanding the innervation also is helpful while observing and assessing the clinical recovery after radial nerve injury or repair.

PATHOGENESIS

- Most radial nerve deficits result from traumatic injuries. Idiopathic and neoplastic etiologies are less common.
- Radial nerve injury is most commonly associated with mid- to distal shaft humerus fractures.[1,5,25,26,29]

NATURAL HISTORY

- The type of traumatic injury is an important predictor of recovery after humerus trauma.
  - Neurapraxic lesions typically result from low-energy injuries. Recovery can be expected over the course of 3 months. The clinical recovery can be followed by observing the advancing Tinel sign and the previously described reinnervation sequence.
  - Conditions that persist after 3 months can be further evaluated with electrodiagnostic studies. In the clinical setting of a nonadvancing Tinel sign and electromyographic findings of axonal loss, exploration with intraoperative electrophysiologic testing is warranted. Nerve grafting across the injury is indicated in lesions that do not demonstrate improvement after external neurolysis.[19,25,26]
- Exploration of open and penetrating injuries is recommended. The choice of primary repair or nerve grafting depends on the injury zone. Recent evidence warrants exploration of high-energy injuries because these lesions have not demonstrated recovery. It is difficult to determine the injury at the acute setting. Interposition nerve graft is often necessary.[19]

PATIENT HISTORY AND PHYSICAL FINDINGS

- A deficit in radial nerve innervation of the extrinsic wrist and finger extensors results in no active wrist, finger, and thumb extension.
- The clinical presentation of radial nerve and PIN palsies is differentiated by the fact that the BR and ECRL are preserved in PIN palsies. Thus, a patient with a PIN deficit will have some retained composite wrist radial deviation and extension, whereas a radial nerve lesion proximal to the elbow will not have a voluntary wrist extension.
- The BR can be palpated during resisted, neutral position elbow flexion, and the wrist assumes a radial-deviated position during attempted active extension.

IMAGING AND OTHER DIAGNOSTIC STUDIES

- Electrodiagnostic studies (eg, nerve conduction studies and electromyography) are used initially for assessment and for determining subsequent treatment.
  - Axonal loss injuries are evident about 4 weeks after the injury; therefore, the initial study is obtained until at least 4 to 6 weeks after the injury.
  - The electrodiagnostic study also can identify other nerve injuries that were not as evident on the initial evaluation.
  - Recovery can be followed by clinical examination or with supplemental studies. Reinnervation or polyphasic waveforms are seen in the muscles of a regenerating nerve.
  - A final study is obtained before tendon transfer at 12 to 18 months.

DIFFERENTIAL DIAGNOSIS

- Muscle or tendon laceration
- Closed myotendinous rupture
- Cervical spinal disease
- Joint or tendon subluxation (especially if there is lost digital extension)

NONOPERATIVE MANAGEMENT

- Wrist and finger extension splint, especially a wrist extension splint initially after the injury, to counteract the wrist flexion position. Some finger extension can be afforded with the hand intrinsics.
- Active and passive motion exercises to maintain motion and prevent contracture[29] while the nerve is regenerating and in event that transfers may be necessary

SURGICAL MANAGEMENT

- Tendon transfer is the mainstay of treatment. Microvascular repair and nerve graft are discussed in another chapter.
- The goal of treatment is independent wrist, finger, and thumb extension with thumb abduction. Donor muscles include the pronator teres (PT), flexor carpi ulnaris (FCU), flexor carpi radialis (FCR), flexor digitorum superficialis (FDS) 3 and 4, and palmaris longus (PL).
- Timing of surgical intervention is controversial. Conventional surgical recommendations are to proceed after the patient has reached a documented clinical and electromyographic plateau of useful radial nerve regeneration. This typically occurs 1 year after the nerve lesion.[26] Tendon transfer primarily for wrist extension may be performed early, at the same setting as nerve surgery, to improve function and minimize brace reliance as the nerve regenerates. In securing the tendon transfer, two methods can be used. The more traditional method is a Pulvertaft weave in which the donor tendon is passed through the recipient tendon three times at respective right angles. The tension is set with appropriate tension on the donor and recipient tendons. The weave is secured with multiple mattress and figure-8 sutures. Another method involves one pass of the donor tendon through the recipient tendon, with then a side-to-side coaptation of the two tendons over 3 to 5 cm with a running, locking suture. The side-to-side transfer has demonstrated better biomechanical characteristics but require greater recipient tendon for the transfer. The surgeon needs to be familiar with both methods as they can be used in specific locations as it relates to the patient anatomy.[4]

Preoperative Planning

- Prerequisites
- Grade 4+ or 5 median or ulnar nerve–innervated donor musculature

- Maintained passive motion in wrist and finger extension with no contracture
- Controlled systemic disease processes

Positioning

- The patient is positioned supine with arm table support and a tourniquet.

Approach

- Three general exposures are used:
  - Radial incision with volar exposure for FCR and PT and dorsal exposure for the ECRB and ECRL
  - Distal dorsal incision for EDC exposure
  - Individual approaches for harvest of the FCU, FCR, and FDS
- The ideal tendon transfer tension is based on the individual muscle properties. In general, the optimal tension is established at the peak of the length–tension curve for the donor muscle while the wrist and fingers are maintained in the ideal position. Because this donor muscle position is difficult to determine intraoperatively without specialized equipment, this point reasonably corresponds to the midpoint of the passive muscle excursion. The ideal joint position for each transfer is discussed with the individual transfers.

Wrist Extension Restoration through Pronator Teres to Extensor Carpi Radialis Ligament and Extensor Carpi Radialis Brevis[2,9,28]

- Make a longitudinal radial incision over the midshaft of the radius.
  - This allows exposure of the PT and the wrist extensors through a single incision.
- Identify and expose the PT volarly while protecting the radial artery and superficial radial nerve (**TECH FIG 1A**).
- Extend the pronator insertion by harvesting a strip of periosteum distally (**TECH FIG 1B**).
- Release the proximal muscle to improve its excursion (**TECH FIG 1C**).
- Develop the dorsal subcutaneous flap and identify the ECRB and ECRL.
- Deliver the PT dorsally, deep to the BR and superficial radial nerve (**TECH FIG 1D**).
- Perform a Pulvertaft weave into the ECRL and ECRB, and then secure the transfer with 2-0 or 3-0 nonabsorbable braided suture (**TECH FIG 1E,F**).

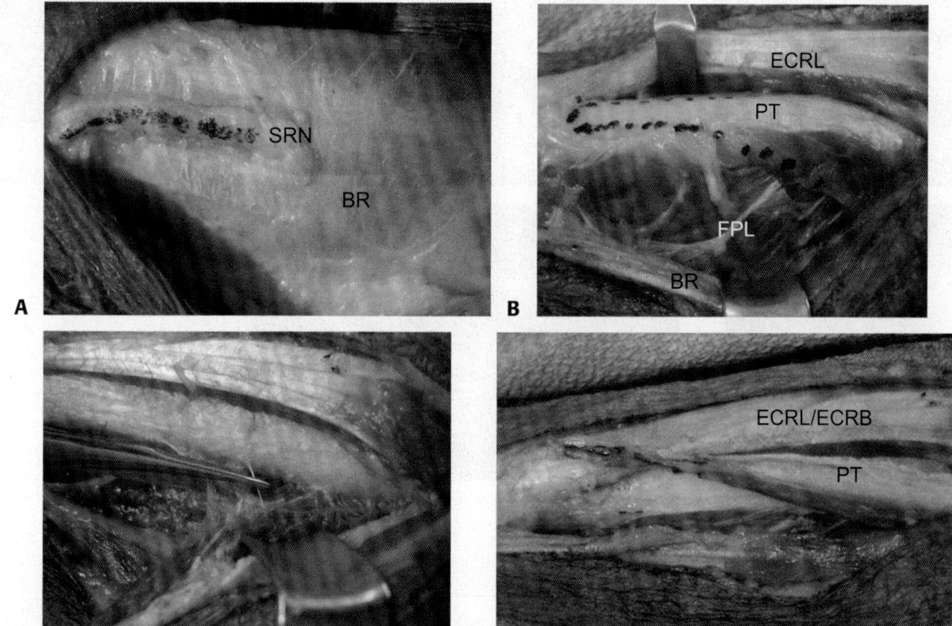

TECH FIG 1 • **A.** The PT is harvested through the volar radial approach. The superficial radial nerve seen here is protected during the exposure between the FCR and BR or between the BR and ECRL. *BR*, brachioradialis; *SRN*, superficial radial nerve. **B.** The PT tendon can be extended by carefully fashioning a distal periosteal sleeve. *ECRL*, extensor carpi radialis longus; *FPL*, flexor pollicis longus. **C.** Muscle excursion can be improved by releasing the PT proximally. **D.** The tendon is transferred deep to the BR. *ECRB*, extensor carpi radialis brevis. *(continued)*

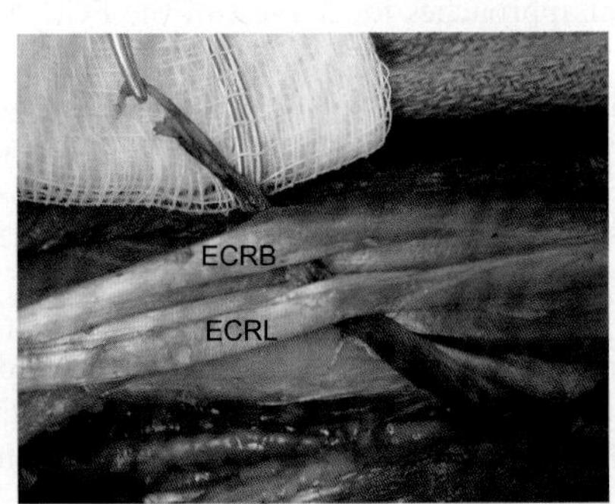

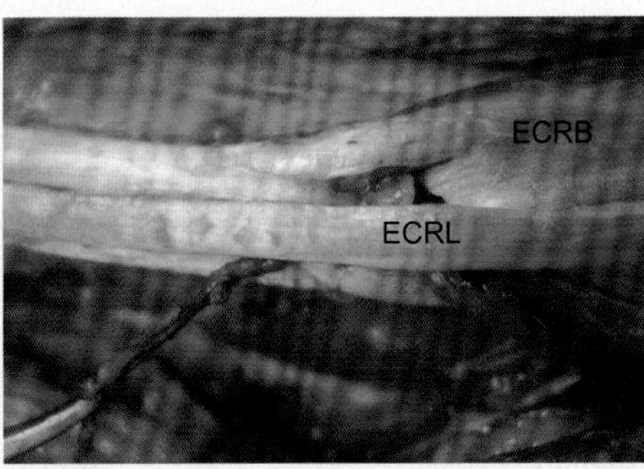

TECH FIG 1 • *(continued)* **E,F.** The PT is then woven through the ECRL and ECRB tendons.

Finger Extension through Flexor Carpi Ulnaris to Extensor Digitorum Communis Transfer[8,17,20,21]

- Make a distal volar longitudinal incision to expose the FCU insertion at the pisiform (**TECH FIG 2A**).
- Extend the exposure proximal to a point 8 cm from the FCU humeral origin and release the FCU periosteal attachments as necessary to improve excursion (**TECH FIG 2B**).
  - Identify the ulnar neurovascular structures.
- Develop a broad subcutaneous dorsal flap to improve the ECU line of pull to the EDC (**TECH FIG 2C**). The ECU may be placed beneath the most superficial subcutaneous fascial layer.
- Trim distal muscle and, if necessary, the tendon to enable passage of tendon into the EDC (**TECH FIG 2D,E**).
- Make a dorsal longitudinal incision 5 to 7 cm long in the retinaculum of the distal forearm.

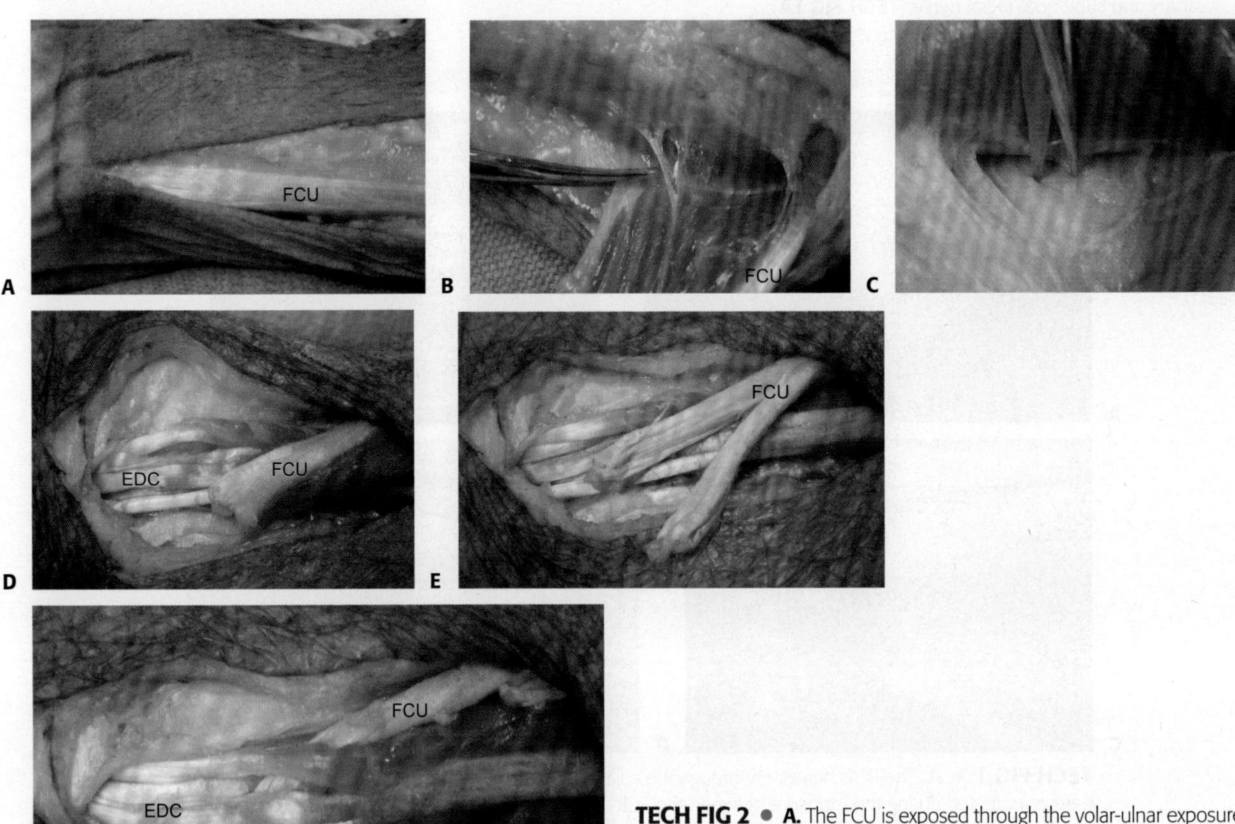

TECH FIG 2 • **A.** The FCU is exposed through the volar-ulnar exposure. **B.** The FCU tendon is mobilized from its ulnar periosteal origin. **C.** Tissues are released to create a broad subcutaneous tunnel to transfer the tendon to the dorsal forearm. **D,E.** The bulky transferred tendon seen here is split and thinned to facilitate the transfer and attachment. *EDC*, extensor digitorum communis. **F.** The tendon is sewn using a Pulvertaft weave.

- Release the proximal extensor retinaculum to permit excursion after transfer.
- Perform a single or double weave into the EDC tendons. Locate the point of insertion into each slip that recreates the normal finger cascade (**TECH FIG 2F**).
- The final transfer tension is set with the metacarpophalangeal (MP) joints in full extension while the wrist is in 30 degrees of extension.
- Secure finger extensor transfers with 3-0 or 4-0 nonabsorbable braided sutures.

Finger Extension through Flexor Carpi Radialis to Extensor Digitorum Communis Transfer[8,10,13]

- Use volar radial exposure to identify the radial artery and the FCR (**TECH FIG 3A**).
- Incise the FCR sheath and transect the tendon while maintaining the wrist in flexion.
- Two different passage techniques may be chosen.
  - In the first, a subcutaneous tunnel to the dorsal incision (similar to the FCU transfer) is developed (**TECH FIG 3B,C**), and the FCR is passed beneath the superficial radial nerve and radial artery to the EDC.
  - In the second, the FDS and median nerve are retracted ulnarly to identify the anterior interosseous artery/nerve bundle and the IOM proximal to the pronator quadratus (**TECH FIG 3D–F**). The FCR tendon is passed volar to dorsal through an enlarged opening in the IOM (**TECH FIG 3G,H**).
    - Be cautious of the anterior interosseous nerve.
    - Do not violate the central band of IOM.
- Tension, weave, and suture into EDC, as with FCU transfer (**TECH FIG 3I,J**).

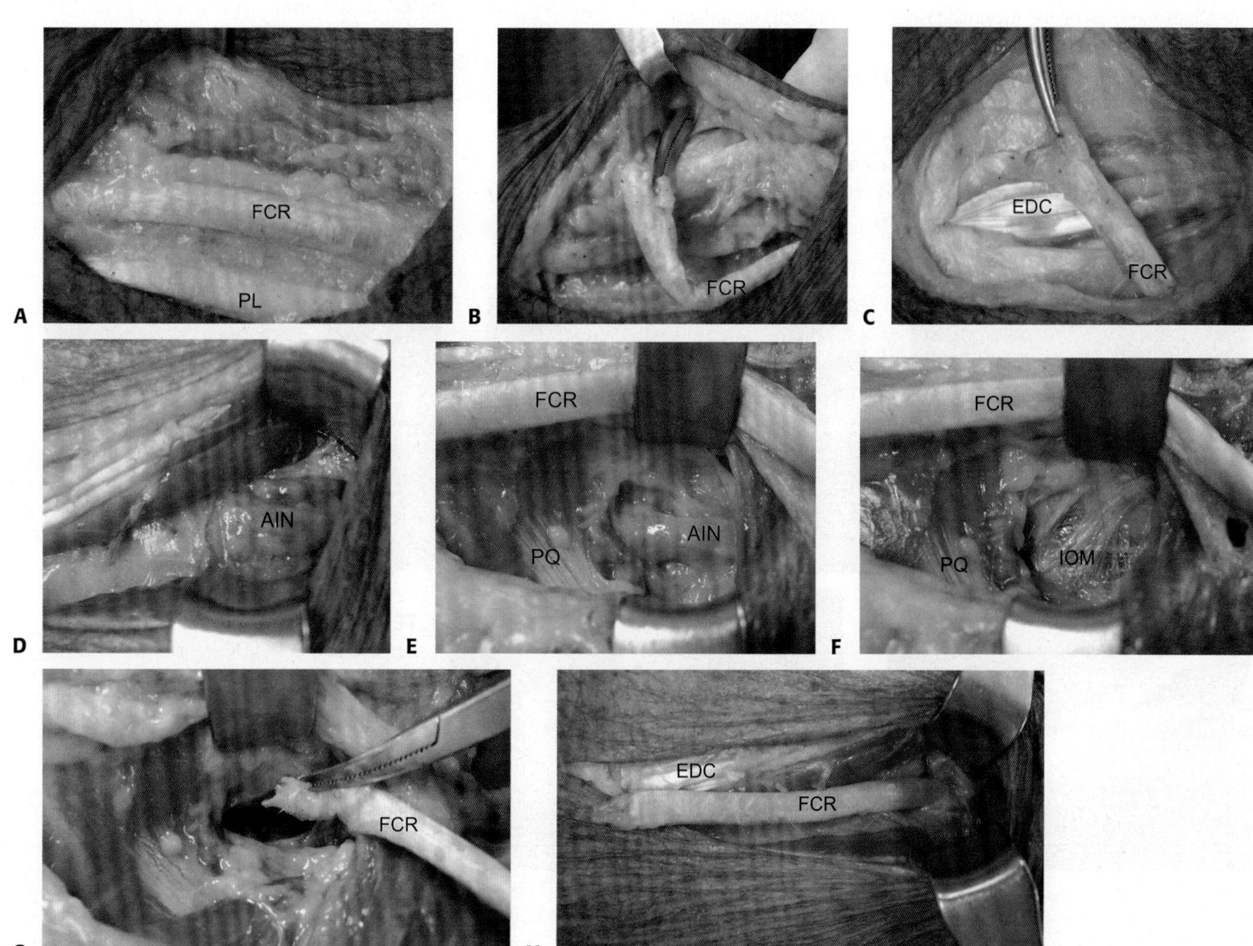

TECH FIG 3 • **A.** The FCR is identified and the tendon mobilized through a volar radial exposure. *PL*, palmaris longus. **B,C.** A radial subcutaneous tunnel is developed, and the FCR tendon is passed deep to the radial sensory nerve, emerging dorsally. Alternatively, the FCR tendon may be passed through the IOM. *EDC*, extensor digitorum communis. **D,E.** The anterior interosseous nerve (*AIN*) is identified and protected. *PQ*, pronator quadratus. **F.** The IOM is exposed just proximal to the pronator. **G,H.** The FCR is transferred through the window in the IOM to the dorsal forearm quadratus. *(continued)*

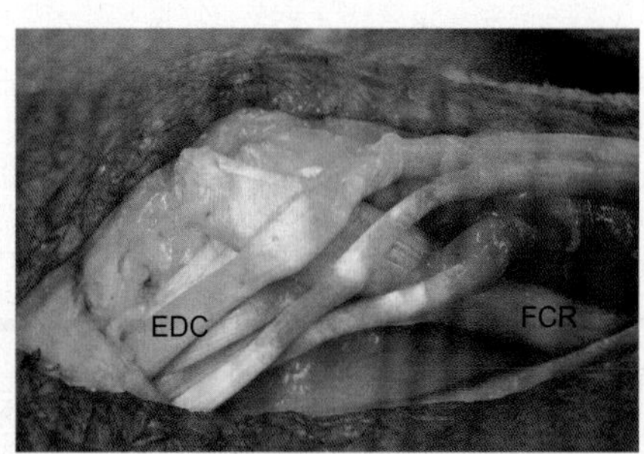

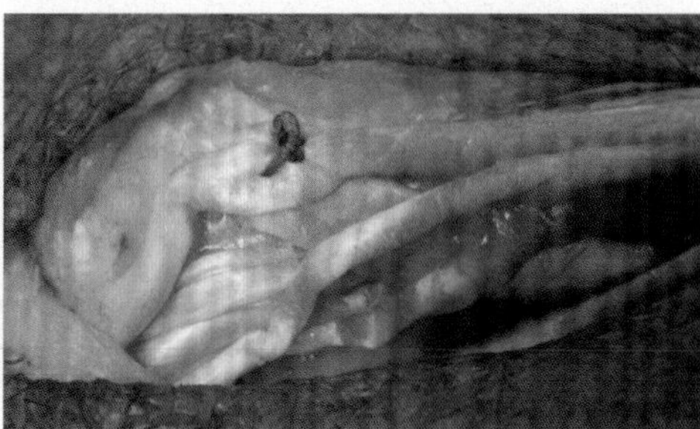

TECH FIG 3 • *(continued)* **I,J.** The transfer is secured with 3-0 nonabsorbable suture.

Thumb Extension through Palmaris Longus to Extensor Pollicis Longus[2,18,22]

- Identify the PL at the wrist crease through the same incision described for exposure of the FCR (**TECH FIG 4A**).
- Dissect and divide the proximal fascial bands to facilitate harvest (**TECH FIG 4B**).
- Develop a subcutaneous tunnel to the dorsal thumb below the cutaneous nerves.
- The EPL may be addressed in either of two ways:
  - Release the EPL from the third compartment to facilitate transfer location. This technique permits the muscle–tendon connection to remain intact if radial nerve recovery is possible (**TECH FIG 4C**).
  - Divide the EPL proximally (only if recovery is not possible) and perform the transfer in a more volar location. The thumb extension vector is improved with the transfer in this location.
- Set the transfer tension at the level of the thumb metacarpal with the wrist in neutral and close to maximum tension on the PL and EPL (**TECH FIG 4D,E**).
- Secure the weave with 3-0 or 4-0 nonabsorbable braided suture.

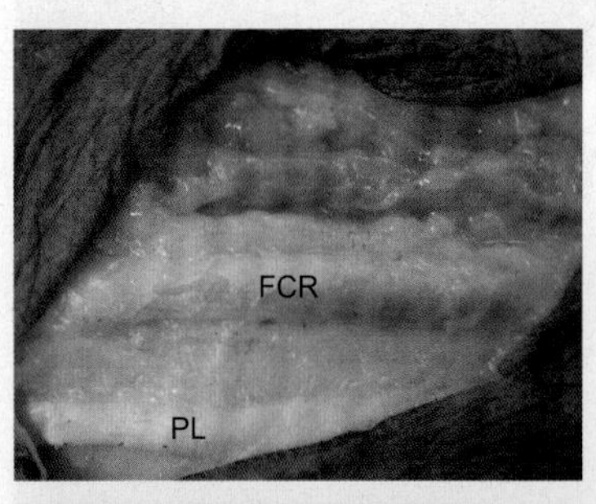

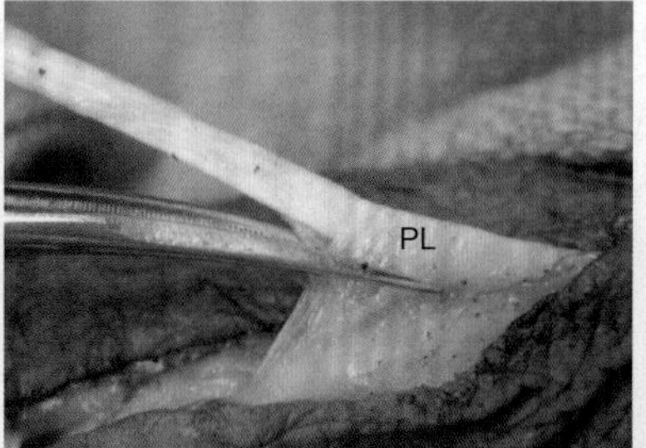

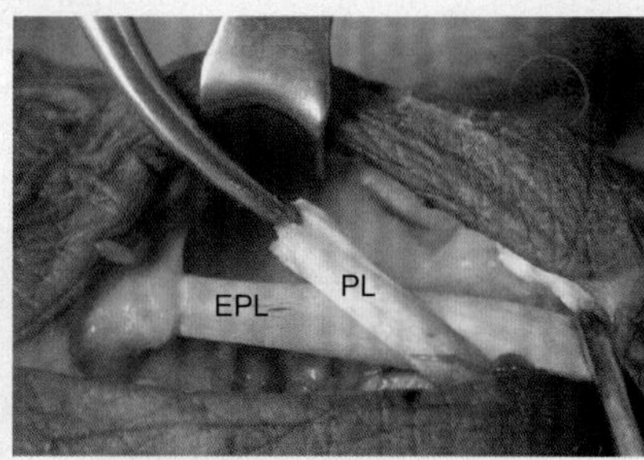

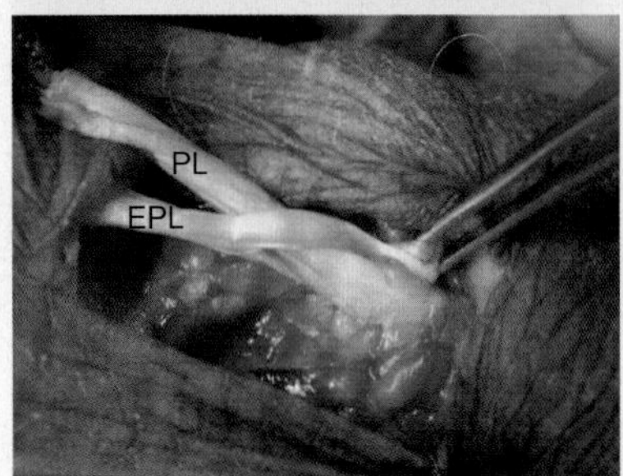

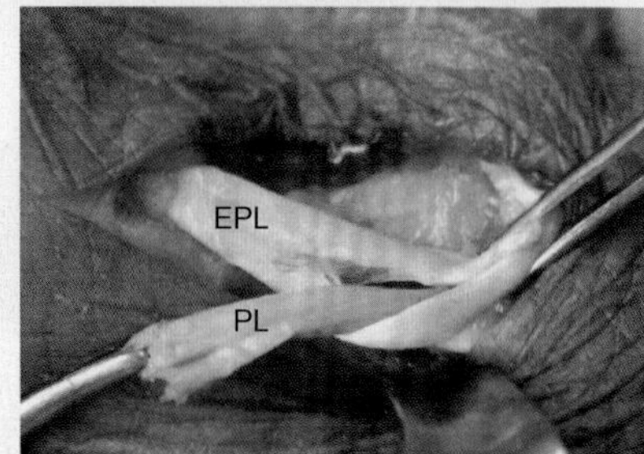

TECH FIG 4 • **A.** This approach was combined with a FCR–EDC transfer with identification of the PL through the same exposure. **B.** Adhesions are released, allowing tendon mobilization. *PL*, palmaris longus. **C.** The EPL is left intact, transposed volarly, and prepared for transfer at the level of the thumb metacarpal. **D,E.** The Pulvertaft weave is initiated and completed once proper tension is set. *EPL*, extensor pollicis longus.

Modification: Finger Extension and Thumb Abduction through Long Finger Flexor Digitorum Superficialis to Extensor Indicis Proprius/Extensor Pollicis Longus; Ring Finger Flexor Digitorum Superficialis to Long, Ring, and Small Extensor Digitorum Communis; and Palmaris Longus to Abductor Pollicis Longus[6,10]

- Perform oblique palmar incisions to harvest the FDS of the long and ring fingers.
  - Include both slips for transfer.
  - Suture the remaining distal tendon to the volar plate or soft tissue to prevent proximal interphalangeal hyperextension.
- Use the volar incision to retrieve the FDS tendons and to harvest the PL.
- Precisely expose the IOM and make preparations for tendon transfer as discussed in the preceding section.
- Perform a dorsal incision and EDC exposure similar to that detailed in the preceding section. Transfer the two FDS tendons dorsally through the IOM.
- The long finger FDS is transferred to the EIP and the EPL. The ring finger FDS is transferred to the long, ring, and small EDC tendons.
- Set tension at the wrist at 30 degrees and at the MP joint at full extension.
- Secure the transfer with 3-0 or 4-0 suture.
- The PL is harvested as detailed for the EPL transfer.
- The radial subcutaneous route also is used to transfer the PL to the abductor pollicis longus (APL), proximal to the retinaculum.
  - The location of this transfer is slightly more proximal to the PL than the EPL transfer due to the length available for the APL.
- Set tension in near-full thumb abduction at wrist 30 degrees; secure with 3-0 or 4-0 suture.

Finger Extension and Thumb Abduction through Flexor Carpi Ulnaris to Extensor Digitorum Communis and Extensor Pollicis Longus and Palmaris Longus to Abductor Pollicis Longus

- Although one donor muscle is not typically transferred to two recipients,[3] an FCU transfer to the EPL and EDC has been described. This may be combined with a wrist extension transfer.
- The technique is similar to that discussed for the FCU to EDC transfer along the ulnar subcutaneous route. The tension is such that the thumb and index metacarpal are parallel.

PEARLS AND PITFALLS

Donor muscle properties	▪ In setting tendon transfer tension, the donor muscle length–tension properties are important to consider. A good clinical approximation of a muscle at the peak of the length–tension curve is to place the muscle near the 50% excursion point. The distal recipient tendon is then pulled proximally until the ideal position of the joints has been achieved.[12]
Pulvertaft weave	▪ In performing a Pulvertaft weave, a curved tendon passer is very helpful. The weaves should be placed at 90 degrees to each other and secured with multiple mattress sutures. The sutures should have small purchase into the donor and recipient tendons to prevent necrosis. At least three weaves should be used.
Goals	▪ With finger extension transfers, it is important to determine the preoperative goals for the FCU/FCR transfers because they do not match the total EDC excursion. Preoperative assessments can determine whether the ideal working range of the transfer should be more in wrist extension or flexion because the force will be less in the opposite position.[12]
Choice of transfer	▪ The choice between the most common extensor transfers—FCR or FCU—is difficult. Usually, the FCU generates greater force and has longer sarcomere excursion and greater fiber length variability. It has better potential excursion than the FCR, but an extensive proximal release is necessary. Because of muscle bulk, the ulnar route is easier to do than the interosseous passage. There may be some loss of ulnar deviation and grip strength as compared to FCR, but it does not appear to have functional implications.[17,23]

POSTOPERATIVE CARE

- Postoperative splint with wrist at 30 to 40 degrees and MP joints in 0 to 10 degrees of hyperextension
- Proximal and distal interphalangeal active and passive motion at 3 to 5 days
- Static immobilization for 3 weeks, then tenodesis motions with activation of wrist extension transfer
- Integration of finger and thumb active extension as wrist motion improves
- The most difficult motion to obtain is independent finger extension with the wrist in the extended position.
- Passive wrist flexion exercises are determined by the recovery of wrist flexion after splint removal. The arc of flexion can be expected to be less than the preoperative level.
- A dynamic splint may be applied so that finger extension may begin at 1 week postoperative. An articulated splint may be used to permit dynamic wrist motion, but the patient must be very adept and have a clear understanding of the therapy regimen.[24,29]

OUTCOMES

- Wrist extension of 40 to 50 degrees (80% M4), wrist flexion 20 to 40 degrees
- Finger extension: at wrist neutral, 0 to 10 degrees flexion; at wrist in 30 degrees of extension, 0 to 30 degrees
- Functional scores: 80% excellent to good[22]; no reported disabilities of the arm, shoulder, or hand

COMPLICATIONS

- If transfer adhesions occur, the therapy can be modified according to postoperative course. Tenolysis should be delayed until at least 9 to 12 months after surgery.
- Transfer attenuation

REFERENCES

1. Amillo S, Barrios RH, Martínez-Peric R, et al. Surgical treatment of the radial nerve lesions associated with fractures of the humerus. J Orthop Trauma 1993;7:211–215.
2. Boyes JH. Selection of a donor muscle for tendon transfer. Bull Hosp Joint Dis 1962;23:1–4.
3. Brand PW. Biomechanics of tendon transfer. Orthop Clin North Am 1974;5:205–230.
4. Brown SH, Hentzen ER, Kwan A, et al. Mechanical strength of the side-to-side versus Pulvertaft weave tendon repair. J Hand Surg Am 2010;35(4):540–545.
5. Burkhalter WE. Early tendon transfer in upper extremity peripheral nerve injury. Clin Orthop Relat Res 1974;(104):68–79.
6. Chuinard RG, Boyes JH, Stark HH, et al. Tendon transfers for radial nerve palsy: use of superficialis tendons for digital extension. J Hand Surg Am 1978;3:560–570.
7. Gousheh J, Arasteh E. Transfer of a single flexor carpi ulnaris tendon for treatment of radial nerve palsy. J Hand Surg Br 2006;31:542–546.
8. Ishida O, Ikuta Y. Analysis of Tsuge's procedure for the treatment of radial nerve paralysis. Hand Surg 2003;8:17–20.
9. Kozin SH, Hines B. Anatomical approach to the pronator teres. Tech Hand Up Extrem Surg 2002;6:152–154.
10. Krishnan KG, Schackert G. An analysis of results after selective tendon transfers through the interosseous membrane to provide selective finger and thumb extension in chronic irreparable radial nerve lesions. J Hand Surg Am 2008;33:223–231.
11. Kruft S, von Heimburg D, Reill P. Treatment of irreversible lesion of the radial nerve by tendon transfer: indication and long-term results of the Merle d'Aubigné procedure. Plast Reconstr Surg 1997;100:610–616.
12. Lieber RL, Pontén E, Burkholder TJ, et al. Sarcomere length changes after flexor carpi ulnaris to extensor digitorum communis tendon transfer. J Hand Surg Am 1996;21:612–618.
13. Lim AY, Lahiri A, Pereira BP, et al. Independent function in a split flexor carpi radialis transfer. J Hand Surg Am 2004;29:28–31.
14. Lowe JB III, Sen SK, Mackinnon SE. Current approach to radial nerve paralysis. Plast Reconstr Surg 2002;110:1099–1113.
15. Omer GE. Tendon transfers for combined traumatic nerve palsies of the forearm and hand. J Hand Surg Br 1992;17:603–610.
16. Omer GE Jr. Tendon transfers in combined nerve lesions. Orthop Clin North Am 1974;5:377–387.
17. Raskin KB, Wilgis EF. Flexor carpi ulnaris transfer for radial nerve palsy: functional testing of long-term results. J Hand Surg Am 1995;20:737–742.
18. Reid RL. Radial nerve palsy. Hand Clin 1988;4:179–185.
19. Ring D, Chin K, Jupiter JB. Radial nerve palsy associated with high-energy humeral shaft fractures. J Hand Surg Am 2004;29:144–147
20. Riordan DC. Radial nerve paralysis. Orthop Clin North Am 1974;5:283–287.
21. Riordan DC. Tendon transfers in hand surgery. J Hand Surg Am 1983;8:748–753.
22. Ropars M, Dréano T, Siret P, et al. Long-term results of tendon transfers in radial and posterior interosseous nerve paralysis. J Hand Surg Br 2006;31:502–506.
23. Skie MC, Parent TE, Mudge KM, et al. Functional deficit after transfer of the pronator teres for acquired radial nerve palsy. J Hand Surg Am 2007;32:526–530.
24. Skoll PJ, Hudson DA, de Jager W, et al. Long-term results of tendon transfers for radial nerve palsy in patients with limited rehabilitation. Ann Plast Surg 2000;45:122–126.
25. Sunderland S. Decision making in clinical management of nerve injury and repair. In: Sunderland S, ed. Nerve Injuries and Their Repair. Edinburgh: Churchill Livingstone, 1991:413–431.
26. Thomsen NO, Dahlin LB. Injury to the radial nerve caused by fracture of the humeral shaft: timing and neurobiological aspects related to treatment and diagnosis. Scand J Plast Reconstr Surg Hand Surg 2007;41:153–157.
27. Tsuge K. Tendon transfer. In: Tsuge K, ed. Comprehensive Atlas of Hand Surgery. Chicago: Year Book Medical Publishers, 1989:485–544.
28. Tubiana R. Problems and solutions in palliative tendon transfer surgery for radial nerve palsy. Tech Hand Up Extrem Surg 2002;6:104–113.
29. Walczyk S, Pieniazek M, Pelczar-Pieniazek M, et al. Appropriateness and effectiveness of physiotherapeutic treatment procedure after tendon transfer in patients with irreversible radial nerve injury. Orthop Traumatol Rehabil 2005;7:187–197.

Arthritis

Synovectomy of the Elbow

Michael J. O'Brien, J. Ollie Edmunds, Jr., and Felix H. Savoie III

DEFINITION

- Elbow synovectomy surgically removes the thickened, inflamed, and painful synovium of the elbow joint.
- Synovectomy is commonly performed for rheumatoid arthritis, hemophiliac synovitis, synovial chondromatosis, and inflammatory arthropathies.
- In the past, synovectomy has been performed through an open arthrotomy, but currently, arthroscopic synovectomy is the treatment of choice.
- Compared with open synovectomy, arthroscopic synovectomy can be performed as an outpatient procedure, allows more rapid recovery, and offers visualization of the entire elbow joint and recognition of concomitant pathology.

ANATOMY

- On the medial side of the elbow, knowledge of the location of the median and ulnar nerves is essential for the safe establishment of medial portals (**FIG 1A**).
- On the lateral side, knowledge of the location of the radial nerve and posterior interosseous nerve (PIN) is essential for the safe establishment of lateral portals (**FIG 1B**).
- Proximal portals are safer than distal portals, as they are further away from the neurovascular structures.
- Posterior portals should never stray medial to midline to avoid iatrogenic damage to the ulnar nerve.
- Proliferation of the synovium and distension of the joint capsule may result in compression neuropathies of the radial or ulnar nerves.

PATHOGENESIS

- Rheumatoid disease is a chronic, systemic autoimmune condition that causes a microvascular disease of the synovium and synovial cell proliferation with perivascular lymphocytosis.[13]
- Synovial tissue hypertrophy is the hallmark of the disease.
- Inflammation of the synovium causes a joint effusion, leading to pain, swelling, and limited range of motion.
- Continued inflammation results in the formation of an erosive, hyperplastic synovium known as a *pannus*. The release of inflammatory cytokines results in continued cartilage damage, periarticular bone erosions, and soft tissue degradation.[14]
- Capsular distension and synovial hypertrophy can lead to gradual ligamentous, cartilaginous, and bony destruction resulting in progressive instability and deformity.
- Recurrent hemarthroses in factor 8 or 9 deficient hemophiliac patients often leads to hemophiliac arthropathy. Hemarthroses lead to blood absorption by the synovium with reactive synovitis which causes the synovium to produce proteolytic enzymes to destroy the blood, articular cartilage, and adjacent bone.

NATURAL HISTORY

- The patient with elbow synovitis will initially present with an elbow effusion, with pain, and restriction of motion. In early stages of inflammatory arthritis, deformity of cartilage and bone are not present. In the case of hemophiliac synovitis, the swollen hypervascular synovium is friable and recurrently bleeds into the elbow joint.

A

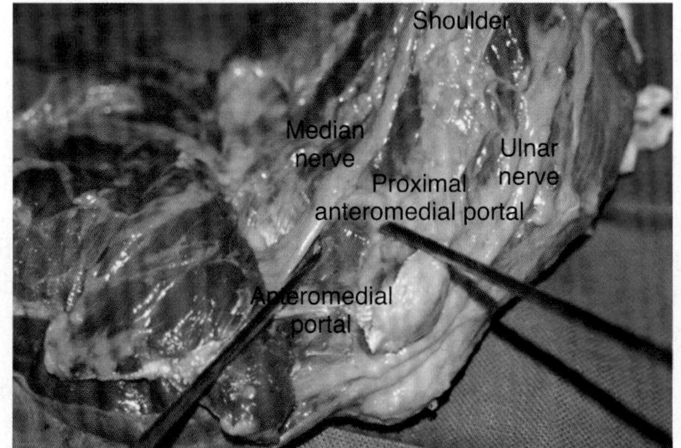

B

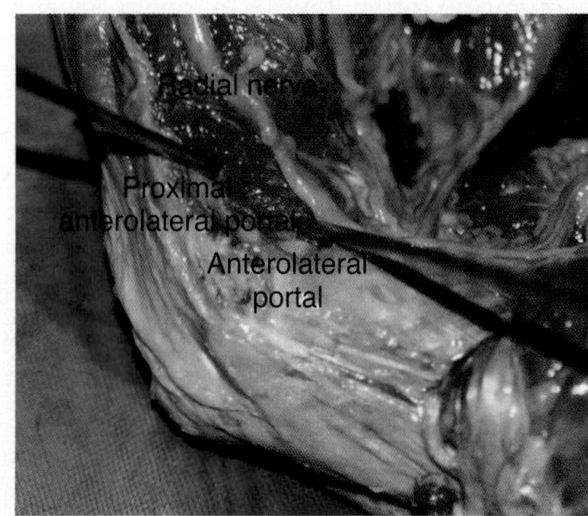

FIG 1 • **A,B.** Cadaveric dissection demonstrating anteromedial and anterolateral portals. The proximal anteromedial portal (**A**) is further from the median nerve than more distal portals. The proximal anterolateral portal (**B**) is further from the radial nerve than more distal portals. (Photographs obtained with permission from Larry D. Field, MD, Mississippi Sports Medicine and Orthopaedic Center, Jackson, MS.)

- In 10% of rheumatoid patients, synovitis will spontaneously resolve.[7]
- In the rheumatoid patient, early medical management may slow natural disease progression.[2] This should be attempted prior to surgical intervention.
- If synovitis persists, secondary changes may occur.
  - A fixed flexion contracture may result from the patient holding the elbow in a flexed position to minimize pain caused by joint motion and capsular distension.
  - The disease may result in atrophy of the brachialis muscle, bringing the median nerve and brachial artery much closer to the synovial lining.
  - Destruction of the annular ligament may cause radial head instability with anterior displacement resulting from the pull of the biceps brachii muscle.
  - Damage to either or both of the medial collateral ligament and lateral collateral ligament (LCL) complexes may result in gross mediolateral elbow instability.
  - Proliferation of the synovium or distension of the joint capsule into the forearm may result in vascular, neural, or muscular dysfunction, particularly compression neuropathies of the ulnar or radial nerves.
- Prolonged synovitis ultimately results in erosion of the articular hyaline cartilage.
- Progressive cartilage degeneration and advancing arthritis is associated with subchondral cyst and marginal osteophyte formation, further weakening the joint capsule and ligamentous supports. Hemophiliac arthropathy of the elbow may create pseudocysts in the adjacent bone.
- The end stage of disease in the elbow is marked by severe loss of joint space, damage to subchondral bone and collapse, and progressive elbow instability. This results in a joint that is painful, weak, and unstable.[7]

PATIENT HISTORY AND PHYSICAL FINDINGS

- Patients will present with a chief complaint of pain and stiffness in the elbow, especially in early stages of synovitis. Stiffness is typically the biggest problem, with loss of terminal flexion and extension. Pain may be present at rest and exacerbated by activities.
- Patients may report swelling and fullness in the elbow with impingement-type symptoms.
- Hemophiliac patients often report recurrent painful bleeding into the joint.
- Physical examination often reveals a boggy swelling posterolaterally, indicative of synovitis or effusion. Effusion and synovial hypertrophy can be palpated in the anconeus triangle and posterolateral gutter.
- Elbow range of motion in flexion, extension, and forearm rotation should be measured with a goniometer. If there is loss of motion, a soft end point suggests a soft tissue cause, such as tense effusion with synovitis or capsular contracture, whereas a firm end point suggests osseous deformity. Limited rotation may be caused by radial head deformity or instability.
- In rheumatoid patients with loss of rotation, examination and imaging of the wrist is important to evaluate for pathology of the distal radioulnar joint, which is commonly involved in these patients.
- Hemophiliac patients most often have an elbow flexion contracture, even if it is painless.
- Ligamentous examination includes varus and valgus stress testing to evaluate the collateral ligaments. The supine lateral pivot shift test and push-off test evaluate for posterolateral rotatory instability (PLRI). The radial head should be palpated during forearm rotation to evaluate for deformity or instability.
- Elbow instability is usually associated with more advanced disease, when joint effusion and synovial hypertrophy have caused ligamentous incompetence. Crepitus may present as degeneration of articular cartilage develops.
  - A routine neurovascular examination is essential. The PIN and ulnar nerve may be compressed by synovitis.

IMAGING AND OTHER DIAGNOSTIC STUDIES

- Plain radiographs include anteroposterior (AP), lateral, and oblique views to evaluate the degree of joint destruction. This aids in predicting the efficacy of synovectomy for pain relief.
- The Mayo classification of rheumatoid elbows[12] grades the severity of disease based on radiographic appearance (**FIG 2A–E**).
  - Grade I is primarily synovitis with no radiographic changes other than periarticular osteopenia or soft tissue swelling (**FIG 2A,B**).
  - Grade II shows narrowing of the joint, but the architecture of the joint is intact (**FIG 2C**).
  - Grade III demonstrates alteration of the subchondral architecture of the joint, such as thinning of the olecranon or resorption of the trochlea or capitellum (**FIG 2D–E**).
  - Grade IV shows gross destruction of the joint.
  - Grade V is ankylosis.
- The Arnold and Hilgartner classification of hemophiliac arthropathy is divided into five stages from mild to severe.[1]
- Computed tomography (CT) is helpful to better define osseous anatomy, such as osteophyte formation, radial head deformity, or loose bodies.
- Magnetic resonance imaging (MRI) can determine the extent of synovitis, intra-articular nonossified loose bodies, and the integrity of the collateral ligament complexes.

DIFFERENTIAL DIAGNOSIS

- Rheumatoid arthritis
- Inflammatory arthropathies (Lupus, psoriatic arthritis)
- Hemophilic arthropathy
- Pigmented villonodular synovitis (PVNS)

NONOPERATIVE MANAGEMENT

- Systemic antirheumatoid agents may help control inflammation in rheumatoid patients.
- Nonsteroidal anti-inflammatory drugs (NSAIDS)
- Infusion of specific clotting factors for factor-deficient hemophilia patients, according to their specific deficiency
- Judicious use of intra-articular corticosteroid injections
- Physical therapy to control swelling and regain range of motion
- Dynamic bracing to improve terminal flexion/extension

SURGICAL MANAGEMENT

- Indications for surgery are persistent, painful synovitis with functional impairment despite a trial of appropriate nonoperative management.

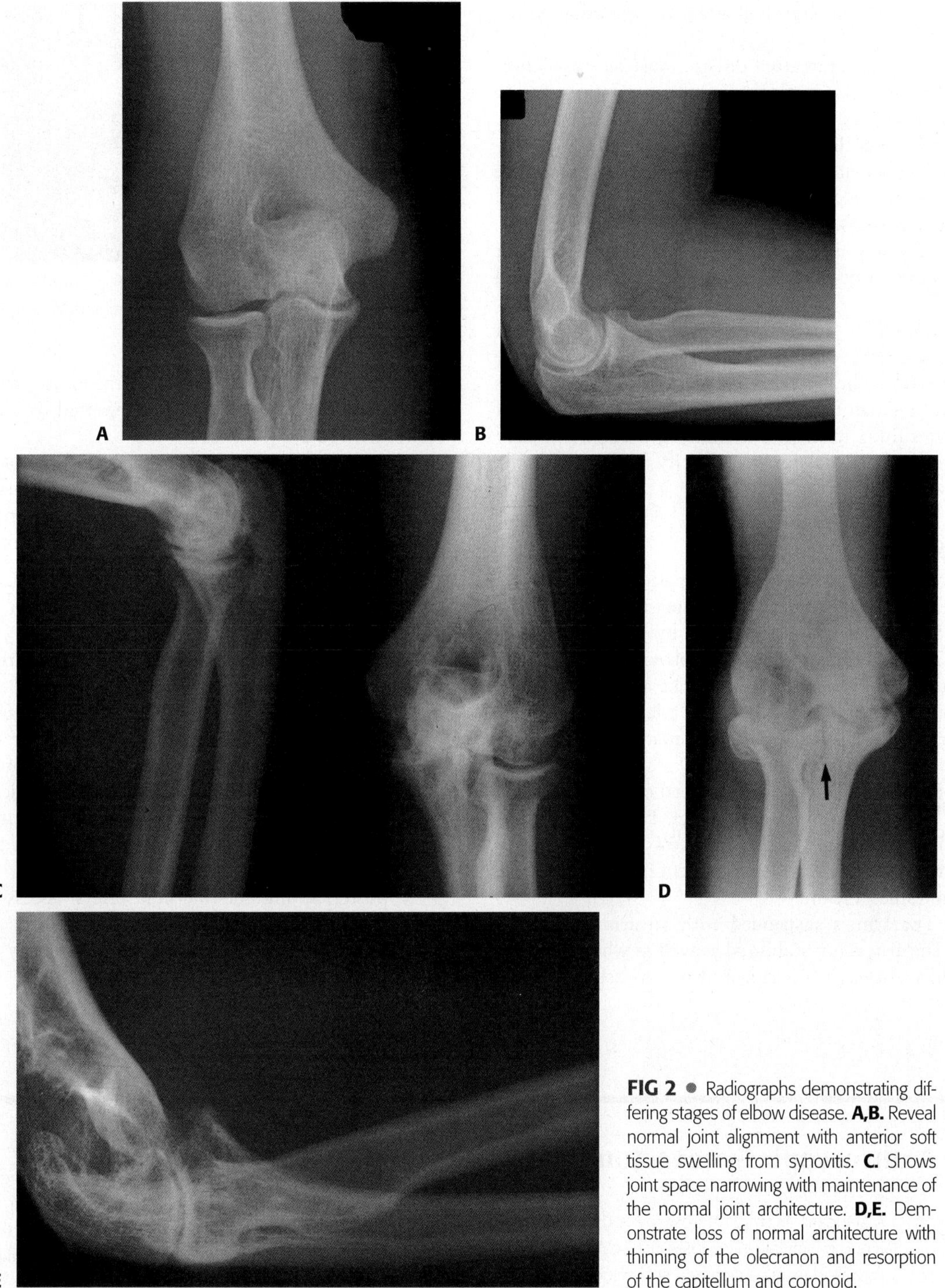

FIG 2 • Radiographs demonstrating differing stages of elbow disease. **A,B.** Reveal normal joint alignment with anterior soft tissue swelling from synovitis. **C.** Shows joint space narrowing with maintenance of the normal joint architecture. **D,E.** Demonstrate loss of normal architecture with thinning of the olecranon and resorption of the capitellum and coronoid.

- Indicated for rheumatoid arthritis (most common), inflammatory arthropathies, hemophilia with recurrent painful elbow hemarthroses, psoriatic arthritis, and acute septic arthritis.
- Contraindications: inadequate medical management for at least 6 months and gross instability of the elbow joint with bony destruction and ligamentous incompetence, as synovectomy alone will not adequately address all of the pathology. Radial head resection is contraindicated in elbows with preexisting instability.
- Contraindications to arthroscopic synovectomy: inadequate expertise of the surgeon, as distorted anatomy with a thin capsule with close proximity of neurovascular structures make iatrogenic injury a concern

Preoperative Planning

- Patients with rheumatoid disease often have multiple joints affected. Typically, the most symptomatic joint will be operated on first. If the elbow and shoulder are equally symptomatic, most surgeons will advocate operating on the elbow first.

- Every patient with rheumatoid disease must receive a thorough evaluation of the cervical spine for instability prior to any purposed surgery.
- Surgery on hemophilia patients must be carefully coordinated with the hematology team to ensure the appropriate delivery of clotting factors in the immediate pre-, intra-, and postoperative periods.
- Patient positioning must be considered if concomitant procedures are to be performed on the elbow, wrist, and shoulder.
- Examination under anesthesia should be performed at the beginning of every case to determine preoperative range of motion, the presence of soft or firm end points to motion, ligamentous stability, and the presence of ulnar nerve subluxation. A subluxating ulnar nerve may necessitate a small incision to identify and protect the ulnar nerve.

Positioning

- For arthroscopic synovectomy, three patient positions are acceptable. Use of a pneumatic tourniquet is standard.
  - Prone: The upper arm is supported by a bolster or arm holder. This stabilizes the arm and provides excellent access to the posterior compartment. The arm can be externally rotated through the shoulder if a lateral approach is necessary. With this position, airway management is more difficult for the anesthesia team.
  - Lateral decubitus: The patient is placed on a beanbag and the arm is supported by an arm holder. This also stabilizes the arm and provides excellent access to the posterior compartment, and airway management is more accessible for the anesthesia team.
  - Supine: The arm is suspended with an arm suspensory device. The arm is not stabilized as well as when using the arm holder. Airway management is not an issue.

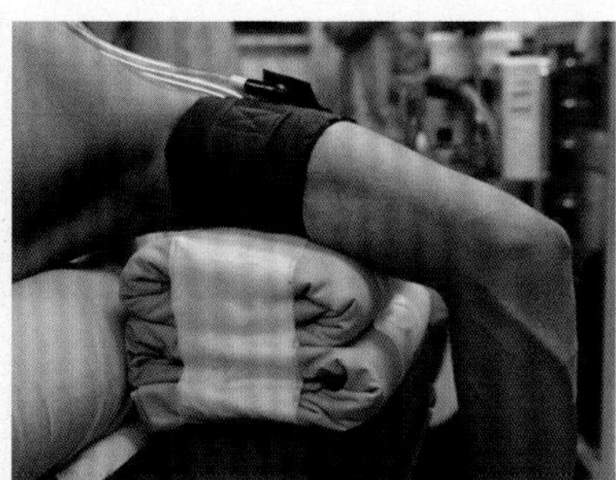

FIG 3 • The prone position for elbow arthroscopy, with the arm supported by a bolster, provides excellent access to the posterior compartment.

- We prefer to perform elbow arthroscopy with the patient prone and the operative arm supported by a bolster or arm holder (**FIG 3**).
- Open synovectomy is typically performed with the patient supine through a lateral approach. A pneumatic tourniquet is used with the arm supported on an arm board. If a posterior midline approach is chosen, the prone or lateral decubitus position may be appropriate.

Approach

- Arthroscopic synovectomy is performed through standard arthroscopic portals.
- Open synovectomy is typically performed through a lateral approach for subtotal synovectomy with or without radial head resection. The extensile Kocher approach provides excellent visualization of the anterior capsule and (with radial head resection) to the synovium of the medial gutter.[10] Access to the olecranon and posterior fossa can be accomplished through this same approach.
- A posterior midline incision offers access to both medial and lateral sides of the elbow. The Bryan-Morrey triceps-reflecting approach is unnecessarily extensive for synovectomy.[3]

TECHNIQUES

Arthroscopic Synovectomy

- *Establish an anteromedial viewing portal.*
  - A standard 4.0-mm arthroscope is used. Gravity inflow or a pump with low inflow pressure (<30 mm Hg) is used to limit fluid extravasation and soft tissue swelling.
  - We prefer to begin the synovectomy in the anterior compartment. The joint is insufflated with 30 mL of saline. A proximal anteromedial portal is established as the viewing portal (**TECH FIG 1A**), by advancing a blunt trocar anterior to the medial intermuscular septum. The initial view is usually poor due to synovial hypertrophy (**TECH FIG 1B**) and capsular tightness resulting in a limited working space.
- *Establish an anterolateral working portal.*
  - A proximal anterolateral working portal is established using a spinal needle and an outside-in technique to localize portal placement. In general, proximal portals are safer than distal portals in the anterior compartment, as they are further away from neurovascular structures.
  - In the presence of significant capsular tightness and a limited working space, a switching stick through the proximal anterolateral portal can be used to elevate the capsule off the anterior humerus proximally. This creates additional working space by increasing capsular volume without disrupting the integrity of the capsule across the front of the joint.
- *Perform anterior compartment synovectomy from lateral portal.*
  - A 4.5-mm full-radius motorized shaver is introduced through the proximal anterolateral portal, and the synovectomy is initiated.
  - Do not begin shaving until the shaver is in full view (**TECH FIG 2A,B**). The joint synovium is removed while preserving the joint capsule, and visualization improves as the synovium is removed.

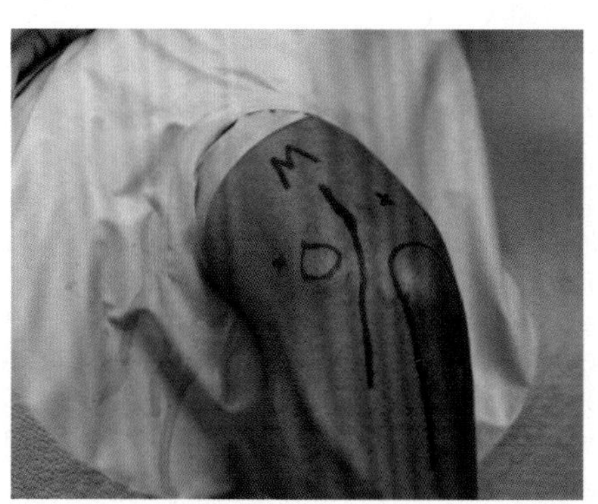

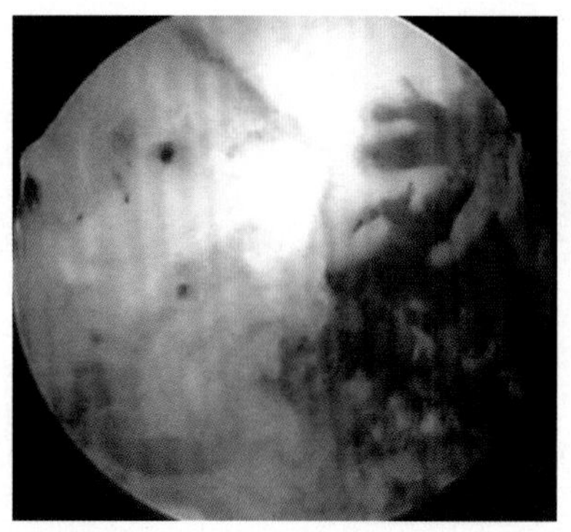

TECH FIG 1 • We typically establish a proximal anteromedial portal as the initial viewing portal (**A**). The initial view may be poor (**B**) due to synovial hypertrophy.

- Use limited suction with the shaver blade facing away from the capsule. Make sure the tip of the shaver is always in the view of the arthroscope. The capsule is often very thin in rheumatoid elbows, and it is best not to disrupt the capsular integrity.
- Judicious use of retractors (either switching sticks or Freer elevators) through more proximal or distal portals can help retract the capsule to improve visualization as well as protect neurovascular structures (**TECH FIG 2C,D**).
- Begin the synovectomy on the lateral side of the elbow to gain visualization of the radial head. Take great caution during synovectomy anterior to the radial head to avoid iatrogenic injury to the PIN.
- Continue the synovectomy across the anterior elbow joint to the medial side of the elbow as far as can be safely visualized.

- *Perform diagnostic arthroscopy, evaluate for osteophytes and radial head deformity.*
  - Once hypertrophic synovium has been removed and visualization has improved, diagnostic arthroscopy can be performed.
  - Evaluate the radial head and radiocapitellar joint for deformity and arthritis (**TECH FIG 3**). Evaluate the annular ligament and LCL complex for laxity. Evaluate the tip of the coronoid and coronoid fossa for osteophytes. Osteophytes and loose bodies may be identified and removed. If severe radiocapitellar arthritis is present, a radial head resection may be indicated and performed arthroscopically.
- *Perform arthroscopic radial head resection if indicated.*
  - When preoperative imaging/examination and arthroscopic evaluation reveal severe radiocapitellar arthritis, radial head resection may be indicated. Radial head resection should be reserved for those patients with a stable elbow and radial head deformity impeding forearm rotation.
  - A motorized burr is introduced through the proximal anterolateral portal, and the anterior half of the radial head can be resected (**TECH FIG 4A**). By pronating and supinating the forearm, the entire anterior half of the

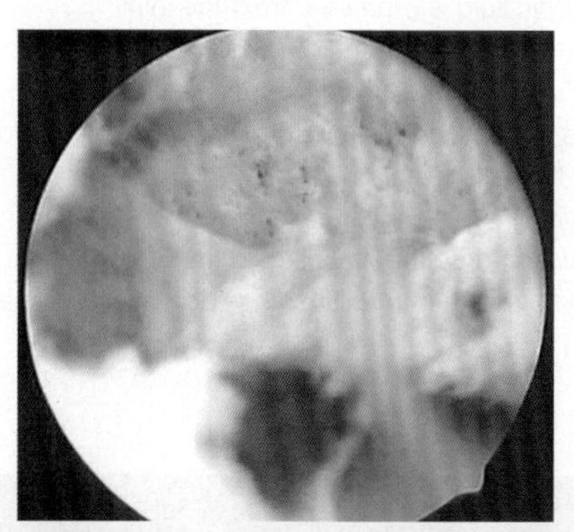

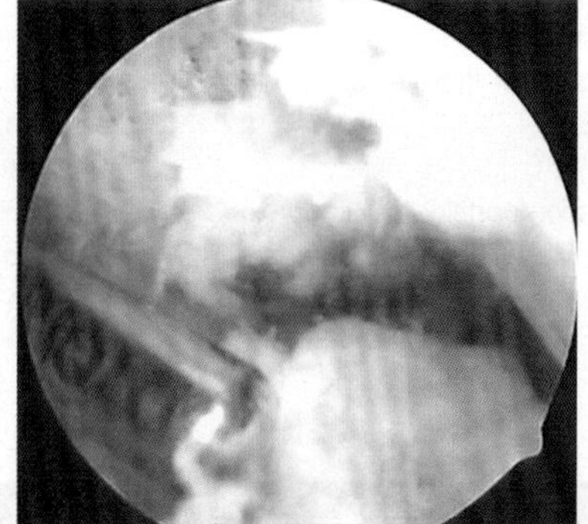

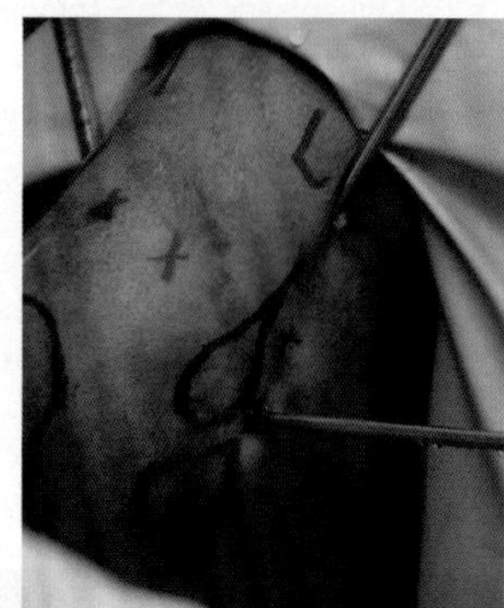

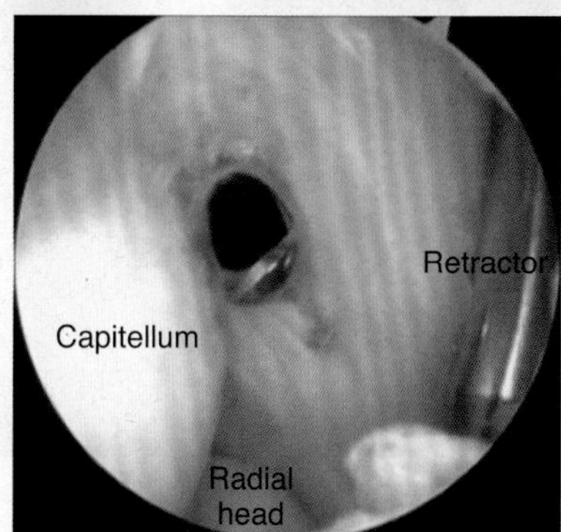

TECH FIG 2 • Initial visualization may be difficult due to capsular tightness and synovial hypertrophy (**A**). Do not begin shaving until the motorized shaver is in full view of the arthroscope (**B**). A switching stick placed through a proximal anterolateral portal (**C**) can be used as an intra-articular retractor (**D**) to elevate the anterior capsule and protect the radial nerve.

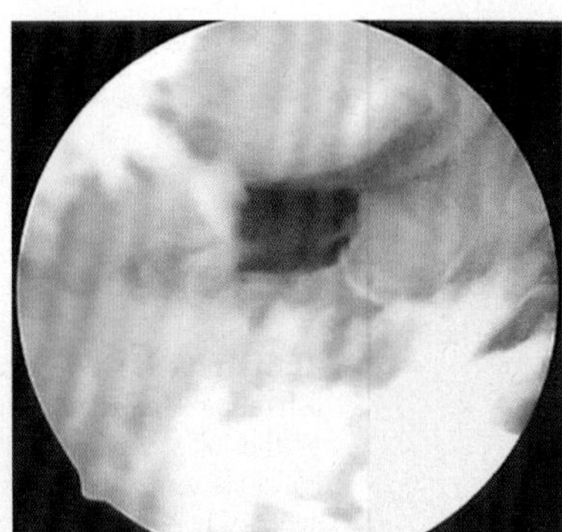

TECH FIG 3 • View of the radiocapitellar joint from a proximal anteromedial viewing portal, demonstrating synovial hypertrophy and severe radiocapitellar arthritis.

  - radial head can be brought into view and resected with the burr.
  - Next, a lateral soft spot portal can be established using a spinal needle, and the burr can be introduced through the posterior aspect of the radiocapitellar joint (**TECH FIG 4B**). The radial head resection can be completed using a cutting block technique level with the anterior resection. The resection should be carried distally to the level of the annular ligament (**TECH FIG 4C**).
- *Perform anterior compartment synovectomy from medial portal.*
  - Use a switching stick to maintain the portals and switch the arthroscope from the medial to the lateral portal. With the shaver in the medial portal, continue the synovectomy from the midaspect of the elbow joint across the front to the medial side of the elbow.
  - Osteophytes in the coronoid fossa or on the tip of the coronoid can be resected with the burr.
  - Use limited suction on the shaver to avoid capsular penetration.
- *Access the posterior compartment.*
  - Make a direct posterior transtendon portal 2 to 3 cm proximal to the tip of the olecranon. Make sure not to stray medial to midline to avoid injury to the ulnar nerve. Advance the blunt trocar through the triceps tendon and into the olecranon fossa.
  - Initial visualization is often poor due to synovial hypertrophy.
  - Establish a posterolateral working portal for the shaver. Place the shaver through the posterolateral portal into the olecranon fossa. Use tactile sensation to feel the tip of the shaver with the tip of the arthroscope, and the shaver should come into view. Begin shaving to clear the olecranon fossa of bursitis and synovitis and create a working space (**TECH FIG 5**). Identify the tip of the olecranon.
- *Remove osteophytes from the tip of the olecranon.*
  - A burr can be introduced through the posterolateral portal, and osteophytes present on the tip of the olecranon can be resected.
- *Perform synovectomy in the posterior compartment.*
  - Advance the arthroscope down the posteromedial gutter. Loose bodies can be identified and removed. Synovectomy can be performed in the posteromedial gutter.
  - Take great care when working in the posteromedial gutter to avoid injury to the ulnar nerve. Do not use suction and keep the shaver blade facing away from the capsule.
  - Next, advance the arthroscope down the posterolateral gutter (**TECH FIG 6**). Loose bodies are often identified in the posterolateral gutter and can be removed.
  - The arthroscope can be advanced down the lateral gutter to view the posterior radiocapitellar joint. An inflamed posterolateral plica will be visualized and can be resected with the shaver through a lateral soft spot portal.
- *Closure of portals with suture.*
  - The arthroscope is removed from the elbow and arthroscopic fluid is expressed from the joint.
  - Portals are sutured with 3-0 nylon using a figure-of-eight portal stitch. Suture closure of portals limits postoperative drainage and decreases risk of postoperative infection and fistula formation.
- *Apply dressing.*
  - A bulky soft dressing is applied to the elbow to limit swelling and facilitate immediate range of motion exercises.

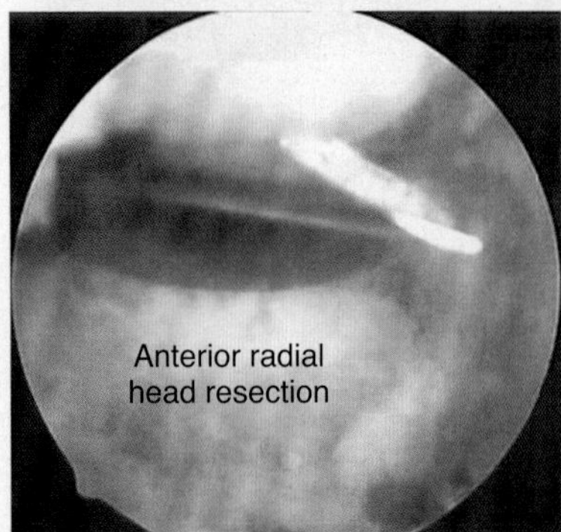

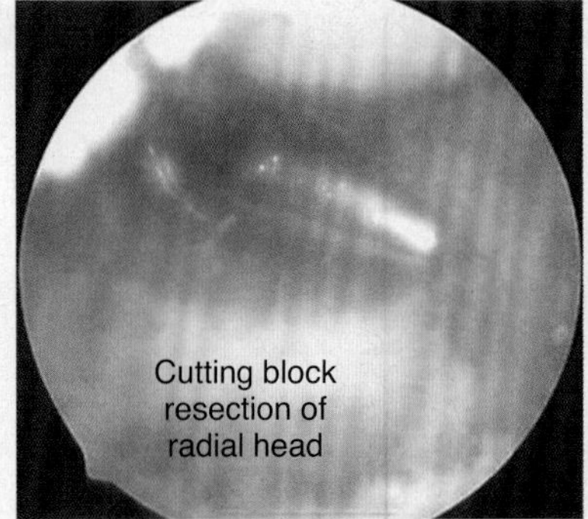

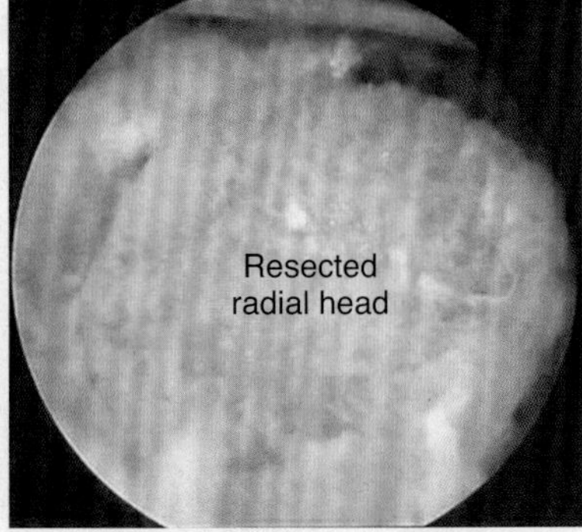

TECH FIG 4 • The anterior half of the radial head can be resected from the anterolateral portal (**A**). A burr is then introduced through the soft spot portal (**B**) to complete the radial head resection (**C**).

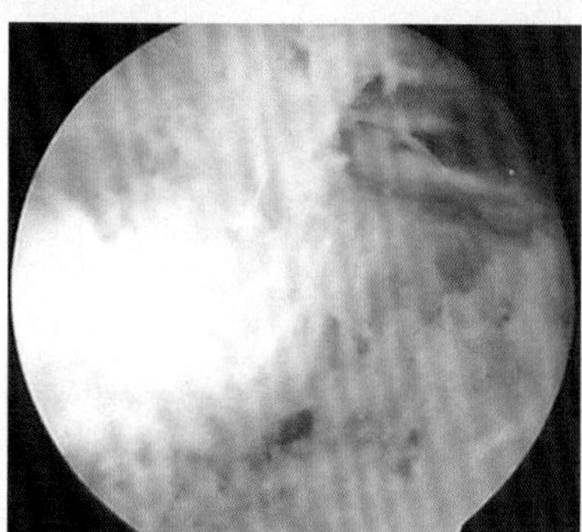

TECH FIG 5 • View of the posterior compartment, with the shaver defining the tip of the olecranon.

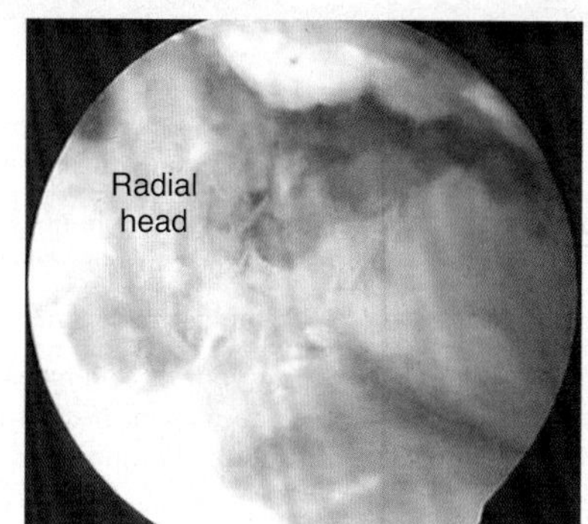

TECH FIG 6 • The posterior radiocapitellar joint can be visualized by advancing the arthroscope down the posterolateral gutter.

Open Synovectomy

- *Lateral approach to the elbow*
  - The arm is elevated and exsanguinated and a pneumatic tourniquet inflated.
  - A 12-cm curvilinear incision is made on the lateral aspect of the elbow centered over the radiocapitellar joint. Dissection is carried sharply with scalpel down to the fascia, and full-thickness skin flaps are raised both anterior and posterior.
  - The extended Kocher approach is typically used.[10] A fatty stripe can be visualized that defines the interval between the anconeus and extensor carpi ulnaris (ECU). The fascia over the fatty stripe is incised, and blunt dissection with an elevator lifts the ECU anteriorly and anconeus posteriorly to expose the joint capsule. Keep the forearm pronated to protect the PIN.
  - Alternatively, the lateral approach to the elbow can be used by developing the interval between the extensor digitorum communis (EDC) and the extensor carpi radialis longus (ECRL) or by splitting the EDC tendon. Through the lateral approach, the PIN is at risk of injury.
  - The capsule and LCL complex should be in view.
- *Make capsulotomy to access the elbow joint.*
  - Incise the capsule anterior to the equator of the radiocapitellar joint in line with the radius.
  - Capsular incision should be made anterior to the lateral ulnar collateral ligament (LUCL) to avoid PLRI. The capsulotomy will go through a portion of the radial collateral ligament (RCL), which can be repaired at the completion of the case.
- *Extend exposure with release of the LCL complex.*
  - With the LCL clearly identified, sharp release of the LCL off of the lateral epicondyle of the humerus allows the elbow joint to "book open" while preserving the integrity of the ligament.
  - This provides excellent exposure to the anterior capsule and anterior compartment.
  - The LCL complex can be repaired at the completion of the case through drill holes in the lateral epicondyle or with use of a double-loaded suture anchor.
- *Incise annular ligament.*
  - The annular ligament can be incised in line with the radius and tagged for later repair.
  - Take great caution in exposure distal to the annular ligament, as the PIN is at risk of injury. If dissection must be carried distal to the annular ligament, the PIN must first be identified and protected.
- *Resect or keep radial head.*
  - At this stage, a radial head resection can be performed if indicated.
  - Place small Hohmann retractors around the radial neck to protect the PIN and resect the radial head with a microsagittal saw.
  - If the radial head is preserved, the anterior capsule can be exposed anterior to the radiocapitellar joint.
- *Perform anterior synovectomy.*
  - Retractors can be placed into the elbow joint so the anterior musculature can be retracted anteriorly. The synovium can be excised with a rongeur, leaving the anterior capsule intact.
  - If using electrocautery, take great care not to damage the articular cartilage.
  - The medial recess cannot be accessed through this exposure.
- *Extend exposure proximally to gain access to posterior compartment.*
  - Proximally, the interval between the triceps and ECRL can be defined. The triceps is retracted posterior and ECRL retracted anterior to gain access to the posterior compartment.
  - A retractor can be placed deep to the triceps to access the posterior compartment.
  - A synovectomy of the posterior compartment and the olecranon fossa can be performed.
- *Expose the ulnar nerve if necessary.*
  - If indicated, the ulnar nerve can be exposed through a medial approach. Once the ulnar nerve is identified and protected, the posteromedial gutter can be exposed to complete the posterior synovectomy.
- *Closure*
  - The LCL complex is repaired back to the lateral epicondyle of the humerus through drill holes or using a double-loaded suture anchor.
  - The capsulotomy is closed with interrupted suture, also repairing the split in the RCL.
  - The interval between the anconeus and ECU is closed with suture.
  - The subcutaneous layer and skin are closed with suture.
- *Apply dressing.*
  - A bulky soft dressing is applied to the elbow to limit swelling and facilitate immediate range-of-motion exercises.

PEARLS AND PITFALLS

Arthroscopic Synovectomy

Avoid excessive soft tissue swelling	■ Keep inflow pressure low (<30 mm Hg if using pump), avoid capsular resection, wrap forearm with elastic dressing during surgery
Create a working space	■ If initial view is limited due to capsular tightness, use a switching stick through the lateral portal to elevate the capsule anteriorly off of the humerus.
Preserve capsular integrity	■ Use a nonaggressive full-radius shaver, keep shaver blades pointed away from capsule, use limited suction
Avoid iatrogenic injury to neurovascular structures	■ Know your three-dimensional anatomy and where nerves are at risk, judicious use of retractors to elevate the capsule and protect neurovascular structures, limited use of suction when working anterior to the radiocapitellar joint and in the medial gutter

Open Synovectomy

Avoid damage to the LCL complex	■ Stay anterior to the equator of the radiocapitellar joint to avoid injury to the radial ulnar humeral ligament (RUHL) and resulting posterolateral instability; taking the entire LCL complex sharply off the lateral epicondyle preserves the integrity of the ligament.
Avoid damage to the PIN	■ Do not carry dissection distal to the annular ligament.
Avoid iatrogenic injury to neurovascular structures	■ Appropriate use of retractors; do not resect the capsule in the anterior compartment; do not attempt synovectomy in the medial gutter through the lateral approach unless the radial head has been removed. Most hemophiliac patients requiring elbow synovectomy will also require radial head resection for the radiocapitellar joint destruction. Bony curettage and osteoplasty may be required for hemophiliac pseudocysts in which the synovium has eroded subchondral bone into the medullary cavity especially between the trochlea and olecranon with telescoping.
Increase exposure	■ Use an extensile approach; flex the elbow to remove tension from the anterior musculature and improve visualization in the anterior compartment; extend the elbow to improve visualization in the posterior compartment

POSTOPERATIVE CARE

- Postoperative management depends on the extent of the surgery.
- Synovectomy alone is an outpatient procedure with initiation of early range of motion.
- Significant osseous resection or capsulectomy may be admitted for 23-hour observation with use of a postoperative drain, continuous passive motion (CPM), and cryocompression device.
- Indomethacin can electively be prescribed for heterotopic ossification prophylaxis.
- Patients are discharged with a continuous brachial plexus block for 72 hours for postoperative analgesia.
- Patients with severe hemophilia requiring factor 8 or 9 infusion during surgery will require infusion postoperative for several days as the hematologists taper the factor replacement dose.
- The bulky soft dressing is removed by the patient 48 to 72 hours postoperative, and range of motion is initiated. The portal sites are dressed with Band-Aids.
- Sutures are removed 7 to 10 days following surgery, and physical therapy is initiated for range of motion, terminal stretching, and edema control. Strengthening is begun at 4 to 6 weeks postoperative.

OUTCOMES

- Elbow synovectomy, with or without radial head resection, is an effective treatment for the rheumatoid elbow and the hemophiliac elbow.
- The best results of elbow synovectomy, either open or arthroscopic, are in younger patients with greater than 90 degrees of flexion/extension, preserved articular cartilage, and mild bony deformities.[12]
- Studies indicate that 70% to 90% of patients have satisfactory outcomes within the first 3 to 5 years, although the results deteriorate with time.[12]
- Arthroscopic synovectomy offers the advantages of being less invasive with less soft tissue injury, which speeds recovery and rehabilitation and limits postoperative pain. The surgeon can visualize all intra-articular pathology and has superior access to the posterior compartment of the elbow.
- In 1997, Lee and Morrey[11] reported on 14 patients who underwent arthroscopic synovectomy, with 93% good and excellent results. These results deteriorated to 57% at 42 months postoperative. Two cases of transient neurapraxia were reported and 4 patients were converted to total elbow arthroplasty.
- Horiuchi et al[6] reported the results of 21 elbows after arthroscopic synovectomy, with good and excellent results for 71% of patients at 2 years. The Mayo Elbow Performance Score improved from 48.3 points preoperatively to 77.5 points postoperatively. The results deteriorated to 43% by 8 years. If elbows with advanced cartilage loss and bony deformity were excluded, the results were 100% and 71% of patients with good and excellent results at 2 and 8 years, respectively. Three patients had transient ulnar nerve paresthesias and two were converted to total elbow arthroplasty.
- In 2006, Tanaka and colleagues[16] reported a prospective comparative study of arthroscopic versus open synovectomy with 23 elbows in each group. At a mean follow-up of

10 years, 48% of those treated arthroscopically and 70% of those treated with open synovectomy had little or no pain. There was no significant difference with respect to pain, range of motion, or level of function. The results of both groups deteriorated with time.

- In 2011, Chalmers and coworkers[4] performed a meta-analysis to compare the effects of arthroscopic versus open synovectomy on pain reduction, recurrence of synovitis, radiographic progression, and need for subsequent total joint arthroplasty. Patients undergoing arthroscopic synovectomy had similar pain reduction, but more frequent recurrences of synovitis and radiographic progression when compared to open synovectomy. The risk of subsequent total elbow arthroplasty was similar between the two groups.
- Kang et al[9] reported on arthroscopic synovectomy in 26 rheumatoid elbows with radiographic changes that were mild to moderate. At a mean follow-up of 34 months, 73% of patients had good to excellent results. Pain decreased from 6.5 to 3.1, the mean flexion arc increased from 98 to 113 degrees, and the Mayo Elbow Performance Score improved from 58.5 to 77.4. Seven patients had radiographic progression of disease and four patients developed recurrent synovitis.
- Limited studies exist in the literature regarding the results of arthroscopic synovectomy for hemophilic arthropathy of the elbow.[5,8,15,17] Studies are limited to very small numbers and often combine results of synovectomy of other joints. Either open or arthroscopic synovectomy dramatically decrease the rate of recurrent hemarthroses.

COMPLICATIONS

- Nerve injury (PIN, median nerve, ulnar nerve)
- Instability with ligamentous injury
- Infection, the risk of postoperative infection is higher in rheumatoid patients taking disease-modifying agents, which should be stopped 7 days prior to surgery
- Heterotopic ossification
- Recurrence of synovitis

REFERENCES

1. Arnold WD, Hilgartner MW. Hemophilic arthropathy. Current concepts of pathogenesis and management. J Bone Joint Surg Am 1977; 59(3):287–305.
2. Breedveld FC. Current and future management approaches for rheumatoid arthritis. Arthritis Res 2002;4(suppl 2):S16–S21.
3. Bryan RS, Morrey BF. Extensive posterior exposure of the elbow joint. A triceps sparing approach. Clin Orthop Relat Res 1982;(166):188–192.
4. Chalmers PN, Sherman SL, Raphael BS, et al. Rheumatoid synovectomy: does the surgical approach matter? Clin Orthop Relat Res 2011;469(7):2062–2071.
5. Dunn AL, Busch MT, Wyly JB, et al. Arthroscopic synovectomy for hemophilic joint disease in a pediatric population. J Pediatr Orthop 2004;24:414–426.
6. Horiuchi K, Momohara S, Tomatsu T, et al. Arthroscopic synovectomy of the elbow in rheumatoid arthritis. J Bone Joint Surg Am 2002;84:342–347.
7. Inglis AE, Figgie MP. Septic and non-traumatic conditions of the elbow: rheumatoid arthritis. In: Morrey BF, ed. The Elbow and Its Disorders, ed 2. Philadelphia: WB Saunders, 1993:751–766.
8. Journeycake JM, Miller KL, Anderson AM, et al. Arthroscopic synovectomy in children and adolescents with hemophilia. J Pediatr Hematol Oncol 2003;9:726–731.
9. Kang HJ, Park MJ, Ahn JH, et al. Arthroscopic synovectomy for the rheumatoid elbow. Arthroscopy 2010;26(9):1195–1202.
10. Kocher T. Textbook of Operative Surgery, ed 3. London: Adam & Charles Black, 1911.
11. Lee BP, Morrey BF. Arthroscopic synovectomy of the elbow for rheumatoid arthritis. J Bone Joint Surg Br 1997;79(5):770–772.
12. Lee BP, Morrey BF. Synovectomy of the elbow. In: Morrey BF, ed. The Elbow and Its Disorders, ed 3. Philadelphia: WB Saunders, 2000:708–717.
13. Morrey BF, Adams RA. Semiconstrained arthroplasty for the treatment of rheumatoid arthritis of the elbow. J Bone Joint Surg Am 1992;74:479–490.
14. Papp SR, Athwal GS, Pichora DR. The rheumatoid wrist. J Am Acad Orthop Surg 2006;14(2):65–77.
15. Tamurian RM, Spencer EE, Wojtys EM. The role of arthroscopic synovectomy in the management of hemarthrosis in hemophilia patients: financial perspectives. Arthroscopy 2002;18:789–794.
16. Tanaka N, Sakahashi H, Hirose K, et al. Arthroscopic and open synovectomy of the elbow in rheumatoid arthritis. J Bone Joint Surg Am 2006;88:521–525.
17. Verma N, Valentino NA, Chawla A. Arthroscopic synovectomy in hemophilia: indications, technique and results. Haemophilia 2007; 13(suppl 3):38–44.

Ulnohumeral (Outerbridge-Kashiwagi) Arthroplasty

Loukia K. Papatheodorou, Alexander H. Payatakes, Filippos S. Giannoulis, and Dean G. Sotereanos

DEFINITION

- Primary osteoarthritis of the elbow is a relatively uncommon but disabling disorder that affects mostly middle-aged men who use the upper extremity in a repetitive fashion. Typically, patients are heavy manual workers or athletes. Osteoarthritis affects the elbow less frequently than other major joints.
- Early stages of arthritis of the elbow may be characterized primarily by pain at the extremes of motion, with some loss of terminal extension and flexion. Some patients present with pain carrying an object with the arm in extension. More advanced stages may present with pain and crepitus throughout the range of motion, stiffness, or locking. Rotation of the forearm may be spared, depending on radiocapitellar involvement.
- Radiographs show osteophyte formation on the coronoid and olecranon but relatively preserved joint space at the early stages. More advanced stages may be associated with significant joint space narrowing.
- Multiple operative techniques have been described for treatment of primary osteoarthritis of the elbow: débridement arthroplasty, interposition arthroplasty, the Outerbridge-Kashiwagi procedure, arthroscopic débridement, and total elbow replacement.
  - Ulnohumeral (Outerbridge-Kashiwagi) arthroplasty was first described in 1978 and became popular a few years later. It is based on a posterior approach to the elbow, removal of any olecranon spur and bony overgrowth of the olecranon fossa, trephination of the fossa to expose the anterior capsule, and excision of the coronoid osteophyte.
  - Recent advancements allow the procedure to be performed with arthroscopic fenestration of the olecranon fossa, débridement, and removal of loose bodies.

ANATOMY

- The elbow joint consists of three separate articulations: the ulnohumeral, the radiocapitellar, and the proximal radioulnar joints.
- The elbow has two main functions: to position the hand in space and to stabilize the upper extremity for motor activities and power.
- The normal range of elbow flexion–extension is 0 to 150 degrees, whereas normal forearm pronation–supination is 80 degrees of each.
- A 100-degree flexion–extension arc of motion (30 to 130 degrees) is required for normal activities of daily living. Functional forearm rotation is quoted as 100 degrees (50 degrees pronation and 50 degrees supination).
- The condyles articulate at the elbow joint, as the trochlea medially and the capitellum laterally. The articular surface is titled about 30 degrees anterior to the axis of the humeral shaft and aligns in approximately 6 degrees of valgus.
- The coronoid fossa and the olecranon fossa, just proximal to the articular surface, accommodate the coronoid process and olecranon process of the ulna in the extremes of flexion and extension, respectively.
- The olecranon and coronoid process coalesce to form the greater sigmoid notch, the main articulating portion of the proximal ulna. It is often not completely covered with articular cartilage centrally.

PATHOGENESIS

- Symptomatic osteoarthritis of the elbow has been found to affect about 2% of the general population and represents only 1% to 2% of all patients diagnosed with degenerative arthritis.
- It has a predilection for males, with a ratio of 4:1 or 5:1. It is most commonly seen in middle-aged and older patients.
- The majority of patients experience symptoms in their dominant extremity.
- The exact etiology of primary degenerative elbow arthritis is still unknown. It is generally attributed to overuse. About 60% of patients report employment or hobbies/sports requiring repetitive use of the limb. The few younger patients who present likely have a predisposing condition such as osteochondritis dissecans.
- There are characteristic pathologic changes that occur within the elbow joint: osteophyte formation on the olecranon, olecranon fossa, coronoid, and coronoid fossa.
- In early stages, the joint space is relatively well preserved. The periarticular bone is typically sclerotic.
- Loose bodies frequently develop within the joint causing clicking or locking of the elbow.
- Capsular fibrosis and contracture of the anterior capsule contribute to loss of extension.

NATURAL HISTORY

- Early stages of primary osteoarthritis of the elbow are characterized by pain at the extremes of motion and some loss of terminal extension and flexion. As the severity of the arthritis progresses, pain and stiffness increase.
- Surgical intervention is indicated when symptoms do not improve with nonoperative management.
- As osteoarthritis is a progressive disease, symptoms may recur over time, typically in the form of impingement pain and flexion contracture.

- Prognostic factors include the etiology of arthritis, the degree of motion loss, mid-arc versus end-range discomfort, the presence of loose bodies, mechanical symptoms, and the presence or absence of cubital tunnel syndrome.

PATIENT HISTORY AND PHYSICAL FINDINGS

- The typical patient with primary degenerative elbow arthritis is a man older than 45 years of age, exposed to repetitive manual labor, and presenting with pain at the end ranges of motion, especially in extension.
- Younger patients may provide a history of sports such as weightlifting, boxing, and other throwing-intensive activities. Arthritic elbows in athletes frequently will include a spectrum of pathologic changes, such as loose bodies and bone spurs.
- Some patients report a history of chronic use of crutches or a wheelchair.
- The chief complaint is pain, especially in terminal extension as a result of mechanical impingement.
- Patients usually hurt while carrying objects with the elbow in full extension.
- The intensity of pain is mild to moderate and only occasionally is described as severe.
- Pain is usually not noted in the midrange of motion until later stages of arthritis.
- Loss of motion is another common presenting symptom.
- Loss of extension is often the result of posterior olecranon and humeral osteophytes and/or anterior capsule contracture.
- Loss of flexion is secondary to osteophytes on the coronoid or its fossa and/or loose bodies.
- Supination–pronation is preserved or is only minimally restricted, owing to limited involvement of the radiocapitellar joint.
- Catching or locking may be present with articular incongruity or when loose bodies are present.
- Crepitus may be present throughout the range of motion.
- Swelling may occur but is not typical.
- Ulnar nerve symptoms may also be present, owing to excessive osteophyte formation. They should actively be sought out because they may influence treatment decisions and even direct the surgical approach.
- Physical examination may reveal a positive Tinel sign and a positive elbow flexion test, with decreased sensation and weakness in the ulnar nerve distribution. Cubital tunnel syndrome may be present in up to 20% of patients.

IMAGING AND OTHER DIAGNOSTIC STUDIES

- Anteroposterior (AP), lateral, and oblique radiographs (**FIG 1**) are diagnostic and illustrate characteristic features of the condition.
- The AP view should be taken with the beam perpendicular to the distal humerus for distal humerus pathology and perpendicular to the radial head for proximal forearm pathology. These views will show ossification and osteophyte formation of the olecranon and coronoid fossae.
- The lateral view should be taken in 90 degrees of flexion with the forearm in neutral rotation. This view will show an anterior osteophyte on the coronoid fossa and process and a posterior osteophyte on the olecranon fossa and process.
- The lateral oblique view provides better visualization of the radiocapitellar joint, medial epicondyle, and radioulnar joint.
- The medial oblique view provides better visualization of the trochlea, olecranon fossa, and coronoid tip.
- A cubital tunnel view may be useful if there is ulnar nerve symptomatology.
- Computed tomography or a lateral tomogram are helpful for preoperative planning to assess the presence and location of loose bodies and subtle osteophyte formation (especially in earlier stages).

DIFFERENTIAL DIAGNOSIS

- Posttraumatic arthritis
- Rheumatoid (inflammatory) arthritis

A 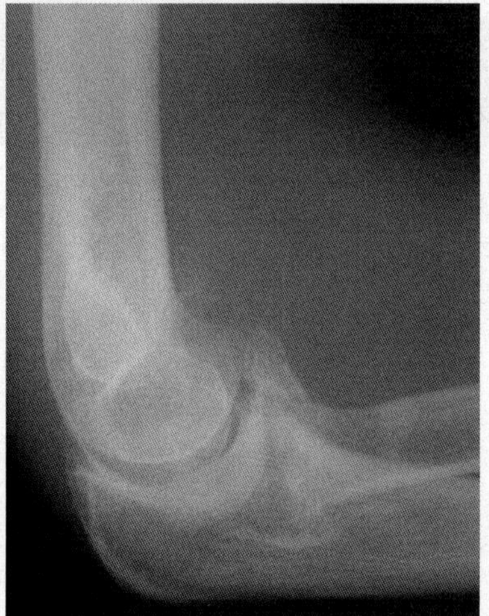
B 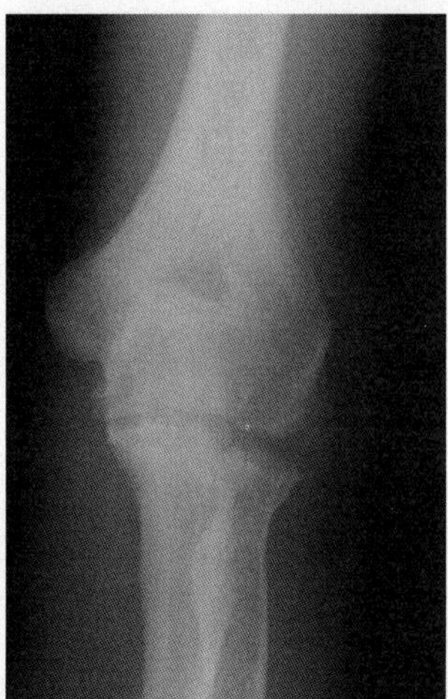
C 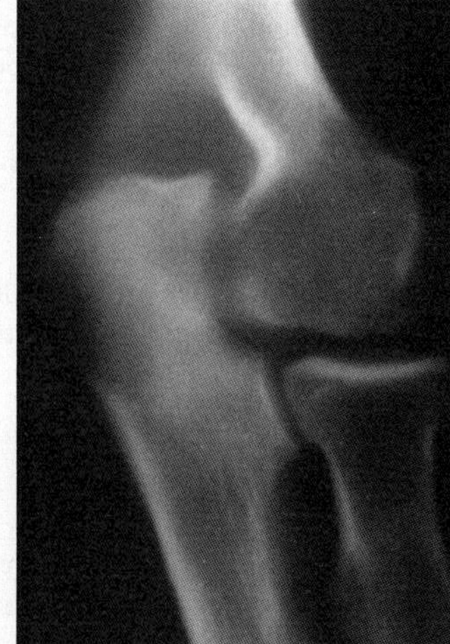

FIG 1 • **A.** Lateral radiograph of a 50-year-old heavy laborer's elbow. The patient had severe pain at the extremes of motion. The radiograph reveals characteristic osteophytes of the olecranon and of the coronoid process. **B.** AP radiograph of the elbow (same patient). This view shows ossification and osteophytes of the olecranon and coronoid fossa. **C.** Lateral oblique radiograph. This view provides better visualization of the radiocapitellar and radioulnar joint. There is an osteophyte at the tip of the olecranon, which causes pain during full extension.

NONOPERATIVE MANAGEMENT

- Nonoperative treatment may be helpful in early stages.
- Patients should limit activities that require heavy elbow use.
- Physical therapy is used to maintain range of motion and strength. Modalities such as heat and cold may be effective.
- Nonsteroidal anti-inflammatory drugs can decrease pain and are of some value. Intra-articular corticosteroid injections may also improve symptoms, but their benefits are usually temporary.
- Avoidance of pressure on the cubital tunnel and avoidance of prolonged elbow flexion are recommended if ulnar nerve symptoms are present.

SURGICAL MANAGEMENT

- Surgical treatment is indicated when symptoms do not improve with appropriate nonoperative management.
- The procedure is indicated in patients with pain in terminal extension or flexion (or both), radiographic evidence of coronoid or olecranon osteophytes (or both), ulnar neuropathy, and functional limitations due to pain or loss of motion.
- The procedure is contraindicated in patients with pain throughout the entire arc of motion, marked limitation of motion with an arc of less than 40 degrees, or severe involvement of the radiocapitellar or proximal radioulnar joints.
- The arthroscopic technique is relatively contraindicated in patients with previous elbow trauma or ulnar nerve transposition because of altered anatomy and potential risk of injury to adjacent neurovascular structures.

Preoperative Planning

- It is very important to carefully review all radiographs (AP, lateral, oblique) before surgery to assess the severity of arthritic changes and evaluate for the presence of loose bodies. Computed tomography may assist in this evaluation. Care should be taken not to overlook any loose bodies, as these may lead to persistent mechanical symptoms postoperatively.
- Specific attention should be paid to the presence of ulnar nerve pathology. If present, this must be addressed at the time of the procedure.

Positioning

- Open or arthroscopic technique
  - The patient is placed in the lateral decubitus position with the elbow flexed at 90 degrees and resting on an armrest.
- Open technique
  - Alternatively, the patient may be placed supine with a sandbag underneath the scapula. The elbow is flexed at 90 degrees and brought across the chest. The patient is rotated about 35 degrees for better access to the posterior aspect of the affected elbow.

APPROACH

- Open technique
  - A posterior approach is used. The incision is longitudinal, starting 6 to 8 cm proximal to the tip of the olecranon and extending 4 cm distal to the olecranon (**FIG 2**).
  - Dissection is carried down to the triceps fascia.
  - The triceps tendon can be split or reflected. In the original description, the triceps muscle is split along the midline, exposing the posterior aspect of the elbow to the lateral and medial supracondylar ridges. Alternatively, the medial margin of the triceps tendon may be reflected from the olecranon.
  - The decision to reflect or to split the tendon is determined based on the size of the distal aspect of the triceps and the need to explore and decompress the ulnar nerve. If the muscle is very bulky, reflection will not provide adequate exposure.

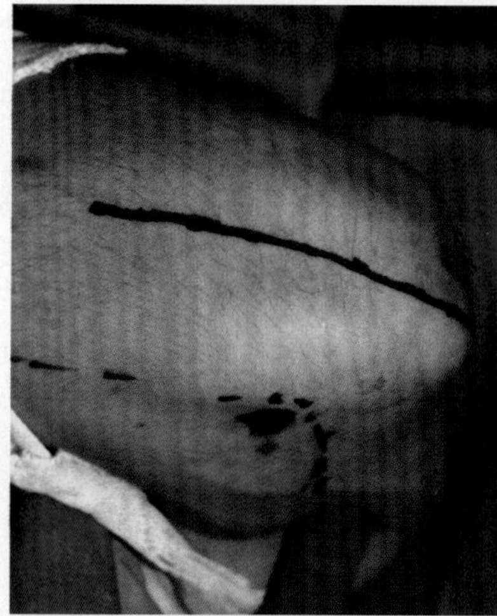

FIG 2 • With the patient in the lateral decubitus position, the elbow is flexed at 90 degrees and is resting on pillows (authors' preferred method). A posterior approach is used via a longitudinal skin incision, which extends distally about 4 cm and proximally 6 to 8 cm from the tip of the olecranon. Note the marked medial epicondyle.

Open Humeral Arthroplasty

Exposure

- After skin incision, the subcutaneous tissue is reflected from the medial aspect of the triceps.
- The ulnar nerve is identified and decompressed at the cubital tunnel if there is evidence of ulnar nerve pathology.
- The triceps muscle–tendon unit is split longitudinally or reflected.
- The triceps is elevated from the posterior aspect of the distal humerus by blunt dissection using a periosteal elevator.
- A capsulotomy is then performed (**TECH FIG 1**).

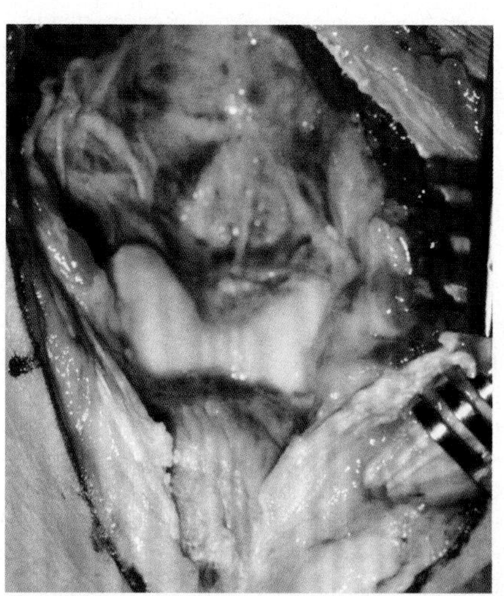

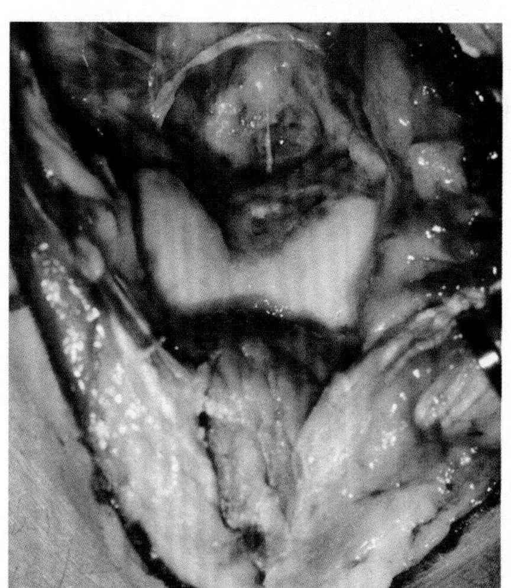

TECH FIG 1 • The triceps muscle has been split to expose the posterior joint. The prominent olecranon osteophyte and the tip of the olecranon process are then removed. The initial cut should be made with an oscillating saw to provide optimal orientation. The osteotomy of the olecranon is completed with an osteotome parallel to each facet of the trochlea.

Osteophyte Removal and Olecranon Resection

- To minimize impingement in extension, the posterior osteophyte and the tip of the olecranon are removed using an oscillating saw. An osteotome is then used to complete the resection. The orientation of the osteotomy should be parallel to each facet of the trochlea.
- A rongeur is used to smooth the edges.
- A hole is drilled in the olecranon fossa to gain access to the anterior elbow compartment and the coronoid process. This requires removal of osteophytes around the olecranon fossa (**TECH FIG 2**).

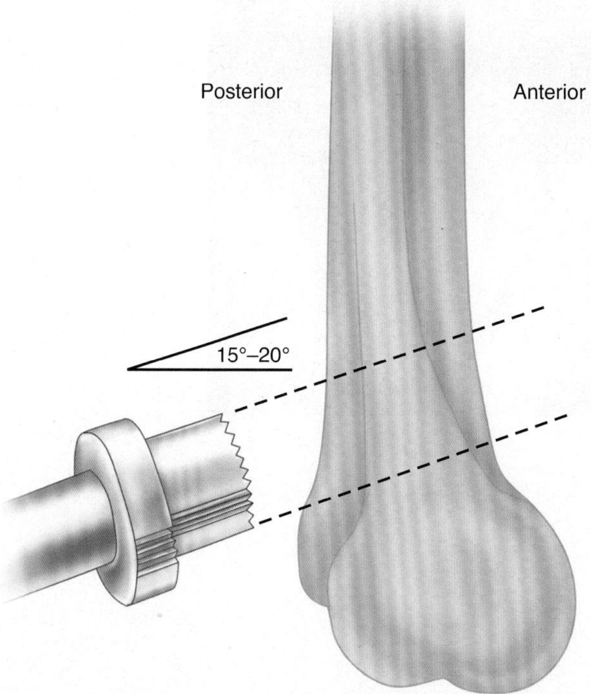

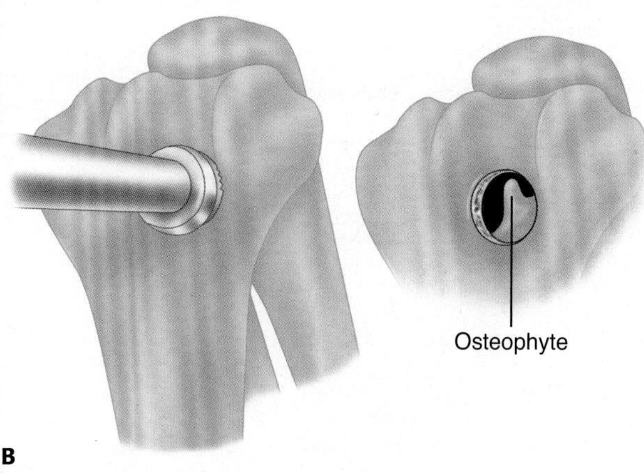

TECH FIG 2 • A neurosurgical dowel is used to make a hole and remove the ossified olecranon fossa. Care should be taken for proper placement of the foraminectomy. The dowel should follow the curvature of the trochlea.

Foraminectomy

- A 1.5-cm neurosurgical dowel is applied to a reaming drill bit, and a drill hole is developed. Proper placement of this foraminectomy is of great importance. The dowel should follow the curvature of the trochlea.
- Once the foraminectomy is complete, a core of bone is removed from the distal humerus. This may include osteophytes from the anterior aspect of the joint (**TECH FIG 3A,B**).
- This hole is used to clean debris and remove loose bodies from the anterior aspect of the elbow (**TECH FIG 3C,D**).
- With maximum elbow flexion, the anterior osteophyte from the coronoid process is removed using a curved osteotome.
- Occasionally, it is necessary to strip the anterior capsule from the anterior humerus using a blunt periosteal elevator to restore extension.
- Care must be taken to ensure that no osteophytes or loose bodies are overlooked.
- Bone wax is used to cover the margins of the foramen, and Gelfoam is inserted into the defect to fill the dead space.
- The wound is meticulously irrigated and closed in standard fashion.
- The elbow is carefully manipulated to maximize the total arc of motion.

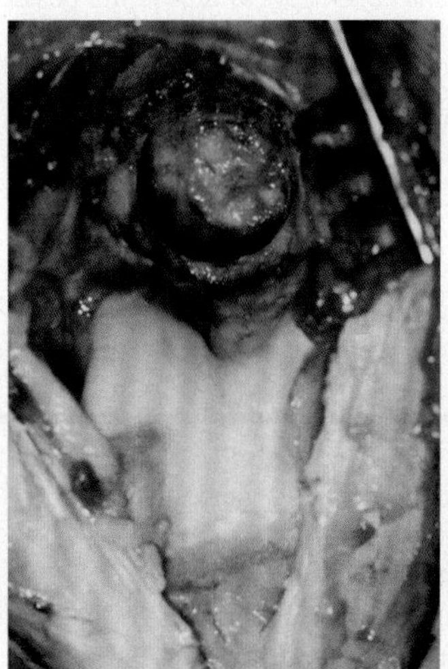

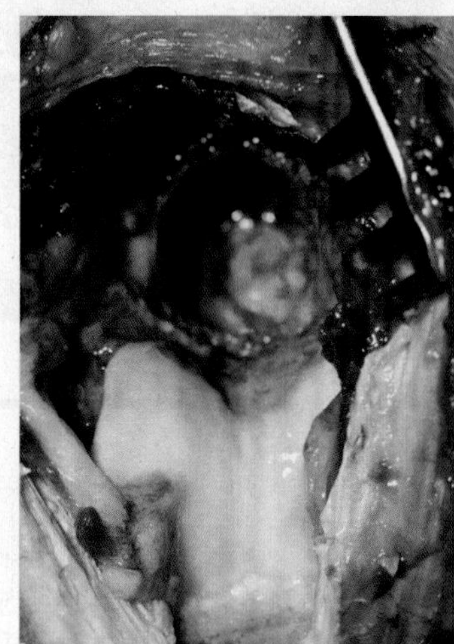

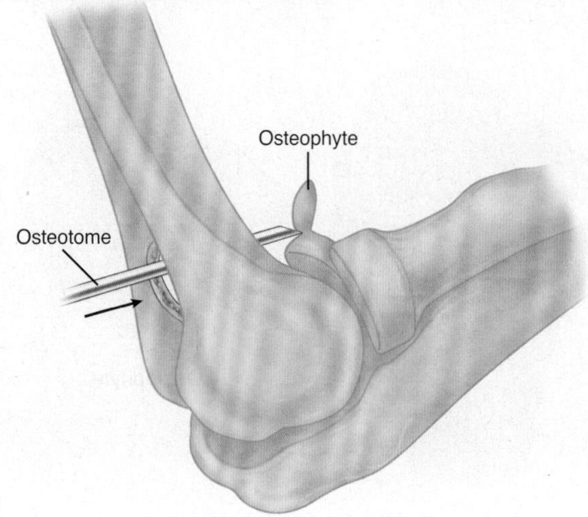

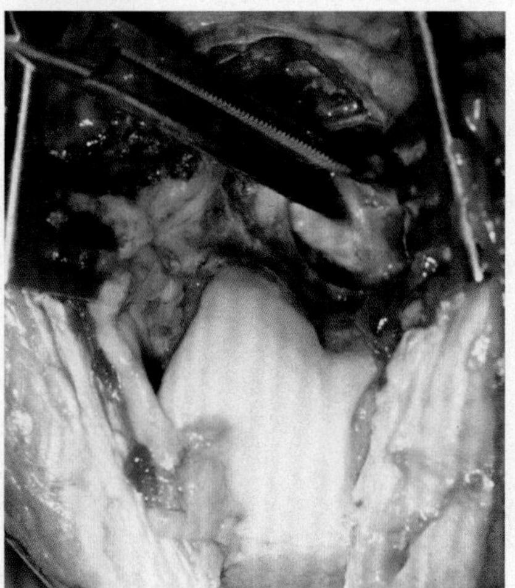

TECH FIG 3 • **A,B.** Once the foraminectomy is completed, the core of bone is removed from the distal humerus. This allows access to the anterior elbow compartment and to the coronoid. At this time, loose bodies of the anterior compartment may be identified and removed. **C.** With maximum elbow flexion, the anterior osteophyte from the coronoid process is removed, using a curved osteotome. **D.** An instrument is then introduced through the foramen, and the osteophyte and a portion of the coronoid are removed.

Arthroscopic Ulnohumeral Arthroplasty

- The elbow joint is insufflated with 15 to 20 mL of normal saline to distend the capsule of the joint.
- An anterolateral portal is established proximally to radiocapitellar joint and anteriorly to the lateral supracondylar ridge of the distal humerus.
- The arthroscope is introduced through the anterolateral portal allowing visualization of any pathologic structures of the anterior compartment of the joint and then an anteromedial portal is established.
- Removal of loose bodies and débridement of the anterior aspect of the elbow can be performed using an arthroscopic grasper and an arthroscopic shaver.
- The posterior aspect of the elbow is then palpated, and a standard posterolateral and posterior central portal are established.
- Débridement of spurs from the olecranon fossa and removal of loose bodies of the posterior aspect of the elbow can be performed through the posterior central portal.
- A 3.2-mm drill is then inserted through the posterior central portal into the center of the olecranon fossa and is angled toward to the center of the coronoid fossa. A drill hole is then developed from posterior to anterior to fenestrate the olecranon fossa.
- Under arthroscopic visualization through the anterolateral portal, the drill hole is enlarged in diameter to at least 1 cm using progressively larger drill bits.
- Once the foraminectomy of the olecranon fossa is complete, removal of the osteophyte from the coronoid process can be performed with maximum elbow flexion using an arthroscopic burr.
- All incisions are closed in standard fashion.

PEARLS AND PITFALLS

Indications	■ Primary osteoarthritis of the elbow presenting with pain at the extremes of motion due to osteophyte formation on the olecranon or coronoid process (or both) and in the olecranon or coronoid fossa (or both)
Contraindications	■ Severe involvement of the radiocapitellar joint ■ Pain throughout the entire arc of motion ■ Previous elbow trauma or ulnar nerve transposition are relative contraindications for arthroscopic technique.
Assessment	■ Careful selection of patients is important. ■ Appropriate imaging studies should be obtained to identify all loose bodies or osteophytes. Computed tomography may be indicated. ■ The surgeon should always evaluate for coexisting ulnar nerve pathology, which should be addressed during surgery.
Operation	■ Proper placement of foraminectomy ■ Meticulous inspection of posterior and anterior aspects of the joint ■ Removal of all loose bodies and osteophytes

POSTOPERATIVE CARE

- A splint is applied with the elbow in relative extension (15 degrees) for 1 week.
- Active range of motion is allowed 7 to 10 days after surgery.
- The patient is reevaluated at 3 weeks, 6 weeks, and 3 months after surgery.
- Continuous passive motion can be initiated on the day of surgery and is discontinued after 3 weeks.
- Sports activities are permitted after 6 weeks to avoid a potential fracture due to the biomechanical weakening of the columns.[5]

OUTCOMES

- A review of the literature shows satisfactory results in over 80% of patients with open or arthroscopic technique.[1,3,4,6,8–20]
- Satisfactory pain relief is achieved in about 90% of patients with both techniques.[1,3,4,6,8–20]
- Extension improves by about 10 to 15 degrees, and flexion improves by about 10 degrees. Overall improvement in the motion arc is about 20 to 25 degrees (**FIG 3**).
- Comparative studies between the open and arthroscopic techniques demonstrated no statistically significant difference in overall effectiveness.[3,4] Higher gain in elbow flexion was achieved with the open procedure likely due to more extensive posterior débridement. Greater pain relief was achieved with the arthroscopic procedure, likely due to decreased scar formation.
- Therefore, arthroscopic technique may be considered in patients with moderate pain and arthritic changes in the anterior compartment of the elbow, whereas open ulnohumeral arthroplasty is preferred when advanced arthritic changes are present in both compartments of the joint.
- There have been no reports of postoperative instability.

COMPLICATIONS

- The complication rate for this procedure is very low, in contrast to most reconstructive procedures of the elbow.[1,3,4,9,10,14–19]
- Symptom recurrence rate is less than 10%.
- Iatrogenic ulnar nerve palsy can occur intraoperatively with the arthroscopic technique as well as with overzealous use of retractors in open technique. Additionally, postoperative ulnar nerve symptomatology has been reported as a result of significant increase of elbow flexion in patients with severe preoperative elbow stiffness.[1,7] We recommend prophylactic release of the ulnar nerve in elbows with less than 100 degrees of preoperative flexion.[21]

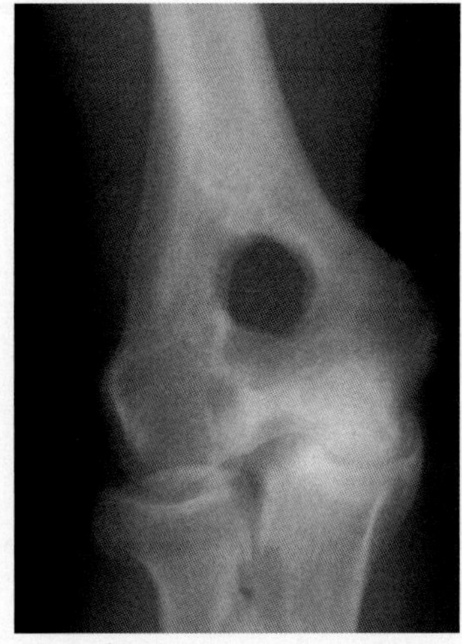

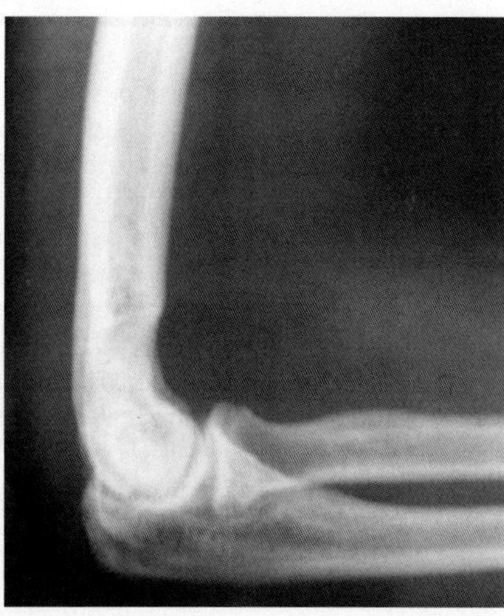

FIG 3 • AP and lateral radiographs after ulnohumeral arthroplasty has been performed. The foraminectomy in the distal humerus can be easily seen. There are no osteophytes of the olecranon and coronoid process and the patient has gained a much better arc of motion without pain.

- Heterotopic ossification with limited elbow motion has been described in one report after open ulnohumeral arthroplasty with a triceps splitting approach.[2] However, development of heterotopic ossification without limitation in motion has also been reported in some cases after arthroscopic technique.[16]
- Improper placement of the foraminectomy may result in a column fracture. Also, a fracture may occur if maximum loading is applied immediately postoperatively due to weakening of the columns of the distal humerus.[5]

REFERENCES

1. Antuna SA, Morrey BF, Adams RA, et al. Ulnohumeral arthroplasty for primary degenerative arthritis of the elbow: long-term outcome and complication. J Bone Joint Surg Am 2002;84-A(12):2168–2173.
2. Chandrasenan J, Dias R, Lunn PG. Heterotopic ossification after the Outerbridge-Kashiwagi procedure in the elbow. J Shoulder Elbow Surg 2008;17:e15–e17.
3. Cohen AP, Redden JF, Stanley D. Treatment of osteoarthritis of the elbow: a comparison of open and arthroscopic debridement. Arthroscopy 2000;16:701–706.
4. Degreef I, De Smet L. The arthroscopic ulnohumeral arthroplasty: from mini-open to arthroscopic surgery. Minim Invasive Surg 2011;(2011):798084.
5. Degreef I, Van Audekercke R, Boogmans T, et al. A biomechanical study on fracture risks in ulnohumeral arthroplasty. Chir Main 2011;30:183–187.
6. Forster MC, Clark DI, Lunn PG. Elbow osteoarthritis: prognostic indicators in ulnohumeral debridement—the Outerbridge-Kashiwagi procedure. J Shoulder Elbow Surg 2001;10:557–560.
7. Jeon IH, Lee SM, Kim PT. Acute ulnar nerve palsy after Outerbridge-Kashiwagi procedure. J Hand Surg Eur Vol 2007;32:596.
8. Kashiwagi D. Outerbridge-Kashiwagi arthroplasty for osteoarthritis of the elbow. In: Kashiwagi D, ed. Elbow Joint: Proceedings of the International Congress, Kobe, Japan. Amsterdam: Elsevier Science Publishers, 1986:177–188.
9. Minami M, Kato S, Kashiwagi D. Outerbridge-Kashiwagi's method for arthroplasty of osteoarthritis of the elbow: 44 elbows followed for 8–16 years. J Orthop Sci 1996;1:11–15.
10. Morrey BF. Primary degenerative arthritis of the elbow. Treatment by ulnohumeral arthroplasty. J Bone Joint Surg Br 1992;74(3):409–413.
11. Morrey BF. Primary degenerative arthritis of the elbow: ulnohumeral arthroplasty. In: Morrey BF, ed. The Elbow and Its Disorders. Philadelphia: WB Saunders, 2000:799–808.
12. Morrey BF. Ulnohumeral arthroplasty. In: Morrey BF, ed. Master Techniques in Orthopaedic Surgery: The Elbow. New York: Raven Press Ltd, 1994:277–289.
13. O'Driscoll SW. Elbow arthritis: treatment options. J Am Acad Orthop Surg 1993;1:106–116.
14. Redden JF, Stanley D. Arthroscopic fenestration of the olecranon fossa in the treatment of osteoarthritis of the elbow. Arthroscopy 1993;9:14–16.
15. Sarris I, Riano FA, Goebel F, et al. Ulnohumeral arthroplasty: results in primary degenerative arthritis of the elbow. Clin Orthop Relat Res 2004;(420):190–193.
16. Savoie FH III, Nunley PD, Field LD. Arthroscopic management of the arthritic elbow: indications, technique, and results. J Shoulder Elbow Surg 1999;8:214–229.
17. Tsuge K, Mizuseki T. Debridement arthroplasty for advanced primary osteoarthritis of the elbow. J Bone Joint Surg Br 1994;76(4):641–646.
18. Tsuge K, Murakami T, Yasunaga Y, et al. Arthroplasty of the elbow. Twenty years' experience of a new approach. J Bone Joint Surg Br 1987;69:116–120.
19. Ugurlu M, Senkoylu A, Ozsoy H, et al. Outcome of ulnohumeral arthroplasty in osteoarthritis of the elbow. Acta Orthop Belg 2009;75:606–610.
20. Vingerhoeds B, Degreef I, De Smet L. Debridement arthroplasty for osteoarthritis of the elbow (Outerbridge-Kashiwagi procedure). Acta Orthop Belg 2004;70:306–310.
21. Williams BG, Sotereanos DG, Baratz ME, et al. The contracted elbow: is ulnar nerve release necessary? J Shoulder Elbow Surg 2012;21:1632–1636.

Total Elbow Arthroplasty for Rheumatoid Arthritis

Bryan J. Loeffler and Patrick M. Connor

DEFINITION

- Rheumatoid arthritis (RA) is a chronic, systemic, inflammatory condition of unknown etiology affecting 1% to 2% of the population.
  - It affects females two to three times as frequently as males, and the incidence increases with age, typically peaking between 35 and 50 years of age.
- Peripheral joints are often affected in a symmetric pattern.
- The elbow is affected in about 20% to 70% of patients with RA, with a wide spectrum of severity.
  - Ninety percent of these patients also have hand and wrist involvement and 80% also have shoulder involvement.
- Juvenile rheumatoid arthritis (JRA) is diagnosed based on the presence of arthritis, synovitis, or both in at least one joint lasting for more than 6 weeks in an individual younger than 16 years old.
- Compared with adult-onset RA, JRA is complicated by severe osseous destruction, deformity, and soft tissue contractures.

PATHOGENESIS

- The cause of RA is unknown.
  - Infectious etiologies have been proposed, but no microorganism has been proven to be causative.
  - Genetic and twin studies have demonstrated that a genetic predisposition clearly exists, and the disease is also associated with autoimmune phenomena.
- In patients with RA, numerous cell types, including B lymphocytes, CD4 T cells, mononuclear phagocytes, neutrophils, fibroblasts, and osteoclasts, have been shown to produce abnormally high levels of various cytokines, chemokines, and other inflammatory mediators.
- The result is inflammatory-mediated proliferation of synovial tissue, leading to soft tissue and finally bony destruction.

NATURAL HISTORY

- Overall, the disease progresses from predominantly soft tissue (synovial) inflammation to articular cartilage damage and ultimately subchondral and periarticular bone destruction.
- Manifestations of RA are initiated by synovitis and synovial hyperplasia resulting in pannus formation. This correlates with a boggy, inflamed elbow that is painful and with limited range of motion.
- Synovial proliferation coupled with joint capsule distention may produce a compressive neuropathy with pain, paresthesias, or weakness in the ulnar or radial nerve distributions, or both.
- Degeneration may progress to ligamentous erosion or disruption, or both. Clinically, the patient experiences progressive instability as ligamentous integrity is compromised.
  - It may affect the annular ligament and produce radial head instability with anterior displacement.
  - Eventually, the medial and lateral collateral ligament complexes may be disrupted, thus causing further instability.
- Prolonged synovitis leads to erosion of the cartilage followed by subchondral cyst formation and marginal joint erosions; the result is end-stage arthritis.
- End-stage disease is marked by severe damage to subchondral bone and gross joint instability. At this stage, patients typically have a painful, weak, and functionally unstable elbow.

PATIENT HISTORY AND PHYSICAL FINDINGS

- Patients typically describe a history of a swollen, tender, and warm elbow with diminished and painful range of motion.
  - This may be accompanied by a report of progressively declining function, constitutional complaints, and often polyarticular involvement.
- In early stages of the disease, the elbow may appear more boggy, with impressive soft tissue swelling and erythema about the elbow.
- As the disease progresses to later stages, soft tissue swelling may become less prominent and the elbow becomes more stiff and painful.

Differences in Examination Findings between Rheumatoid Arthritis and Juvenile Rheumatoid Arthritis

- Elbows affected by JRA occur in younger patients as compared with elbows affected by RA.
- Patients with JRA also have stiffer elbows and therefore typically do not have instability.
- Often, JRA patients have more joints affected by the rheumatoid process, but they also demonstrate a greater tolerance for pain.

IMAGING AND OTHER DIAGNOSTIC STUDIES

- Anteroposterior (AP) and lateral radiographs of the elbow are obtained to assess the degree of rheumatoid involvement and for preoperative planning (**FIG 1**). No further studies are typically required.

Classification

- Although several classification systems have been proposed, the most commonly used is the Mayo Radiographic Classification System (Table 1).[8]
  - It allows monitoring of disease progression and often correlates well with clinical examination findings and patients' functional limitations.
  - The grading system is based on bone quality, joint space, and bony architecture and delineates four grades of progression in order of increasing severity.

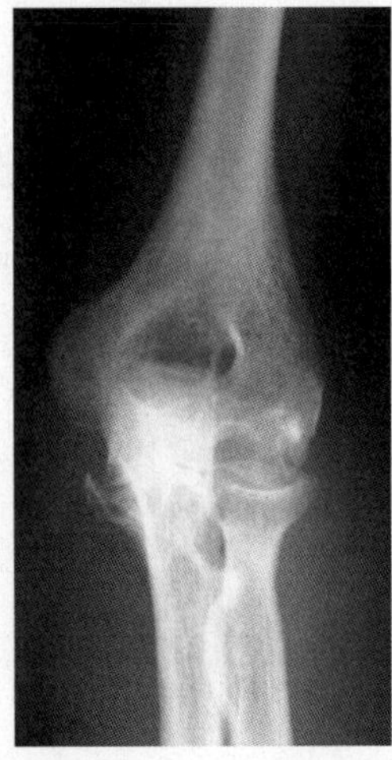
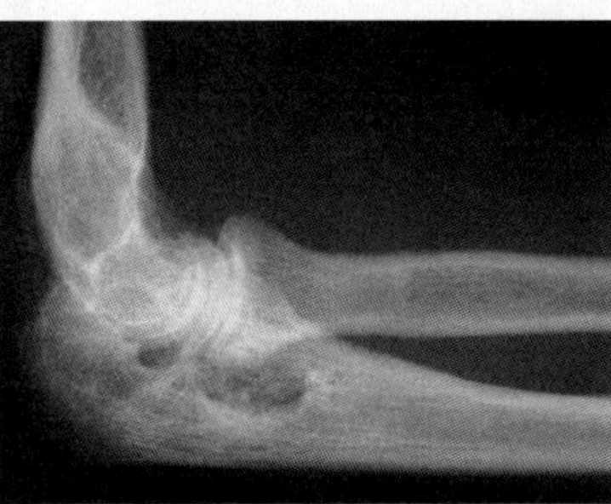

FIG 1 • Preoperative AP and lateral radiographs of a 38-year-old woman with JRA demonstrating advanced changes of osteopenia, joint space narrowing, and changes in subchondral architecture.

DIFFERENTIAL DIAGNOSIS

- Calcium pyrophosphate deposition disease
- Osteoarthritis
- Polymyalgia rheumatica
- Psoriatic arthritis
- Systemic lupus erythematosus
- Fibromyalgia

NONOPERATIVE MANAGEMENT

- Optimal care of the patient with RA requires a team-based approach between the orthopaedic surgeon, rheumatologist, and physical therapists to coordinate the full gamut of nonsurgical and surgical treatment options.

Medical Therapy

- The medical management of RA continues to evolve and is highly effective.
- Medical therapy includes classes of drugs known as *disease-modifying antirheumatic drugs* (DMARDs), *immunomodulators*, *tumor necrosis factor* (TNF) *inhibitors*, as well as other drugs targeting systemic inflammation. These medications may be given alone or as part of combination therapy.
  - DMARDs include medications such as methotrexate, leflunomide, hydroxychloroquine, and sulfasalazine.
  - Immunomodulators such as azathioprine and cyclosporine target the pathologic immune system but may also increase susceptibility to infection.
  - Anti-TNF-alpha agents can reduce pain, morning stiffness, and swollen joints by inhibiting an inflammatory cytokine called *TNF-alpha*. Examples of these drugs include etanercept, infliximab, adalimumab, golimumab, and certolizuman. These medications can also increase the risk of developing severe infection.
  - Other medications which target inflammation include anakinra, abatacept, rituximab, tocilizumab, and tofacitinib.
  - Nonsteroidal anti-inflammatory drugs (NSAIDs) and steroids, such as prednisone, may be prescribed to reduce symptoms of RA as well.
- Judicious use of intra-articular steroid injections also plays a role in symptom management.
- The importance of early referral to a rheumatologist for medical management cannot be overemphasized. Aggressive management of the synovitis can limit or delay the onset and severity of joint involvement. The most reliable and effective responses to antirheumatic medications are observed with therapy initiated in the early stages of the disease.

Physical Therapy

- The goal of physical therapy is to encourage range of motion, functional strength, and maintenance of activities of daily living. This is accomplished by activity modification, rest, ice, and gentle exercise.
- The primary objective of nonoperative management of the rheumatoid elbow is to minimize soft tissue swelling and to optimize range of motion, as preoperative range of motion is often predictive of postoperative total arc of motion after arthroscopic synovectomy as well as total elbow arthroplasty.

SURGICAL MANAGEMENT

- Surgical management of the rheumatoid elbow primarily consists of synovectomy and total elbow arthroplasty.

Surgical Management of the Elbow before Total Elbow Arthroplasty

- For early disease states, excellent clinical results may be achieved with synovectomy performed using open or arthroscopic techniques.
- The goal of synovectomy is to relieve pain and swelling. Although this procedure has not necessarily been shown to alter the natural history of the disease, it reliably produces symptomatic relief for 5 or more years in the majority of cases performed on elbows in the early stages of the disease process.[6]
- The arthroscopic approach is advantageous over the more traditional open approach in that it is less invasive, is associated with less perioperative morbidity, and also allows predictable access to the sacciform recess. When open synovectomy is performed, the radial head must be excised to access and completely débride the diseased synovial tissue that exists in this region.
- Open synovectomy has traditionally been accompanied by radial head excision due to[1] ubiquitous radiocapitellar and proximal radioulnar joint articular destruction and[2] the need to surgically expose the sacciform recess for the requisite complete synovectomy.
  - It has been shown that routine radial head excision may predispose patients with RA to increasing valgus elbow instability due to the loss of the stabilizing effect of the radial head (particularly if the medial collateral ligament is adversely affected by the rheumatoid process).[9]
  - Because the entire synovial proliferation around the radial neck can be accessed arthroscopically, a combined arthroscopic radial head excision is performed only in patients with stable elbows and preoperative elbow symptoms worsened with forearm rotation. Otherwise, a complete arthroscopic synovectomy is performed without excising the radial head.
- In addition, the minimally invasive nature of an arthroscopic approach yields the potential advantages of less pain, faster recovery with earlier range of motion, and a lower rate of infection compared with an open procedure.

Table 1 Mayo Radiographic Classification System

Grade	Radiographic Appearance	Description	Implications
I	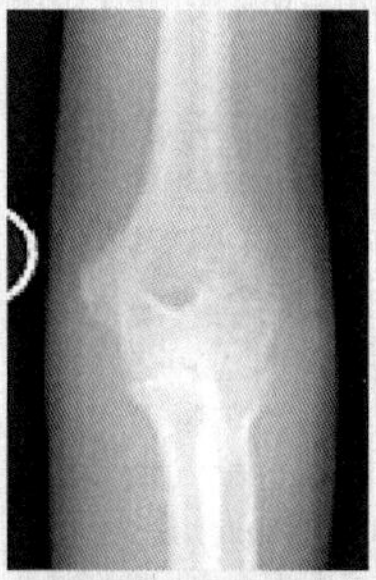	Synovitis in a normal-appearing joint with mild to moderate osteopenia	Often correlates with impressive soft tissue swelling on clinical examination
II	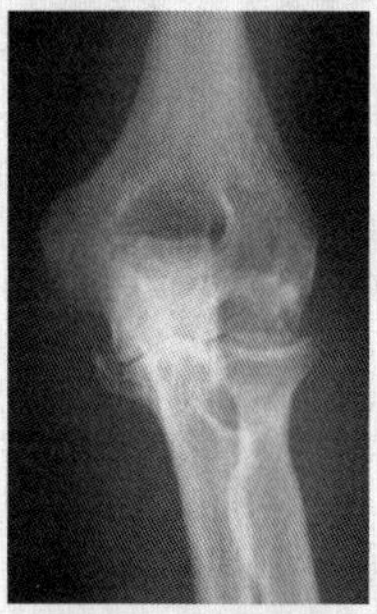	Loss of joint space but maintenance of the subchondral architecture	Varying degrees of soft tissue swelling are present.
III	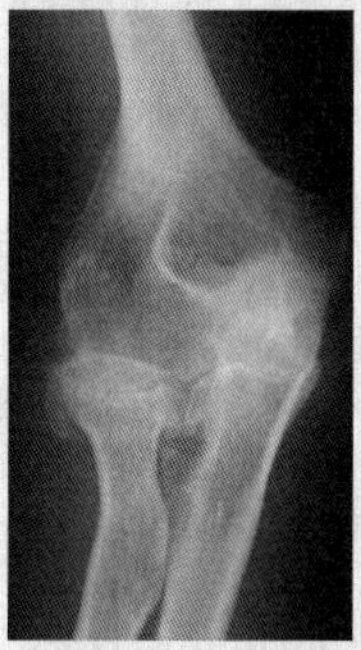	Marked by complete loss of joint space	The synovitis has "burned out" and the elbow is typically more stiff.
IIIA		Bony architecture is maintained	
IIIB		Associated bone loss	
IV	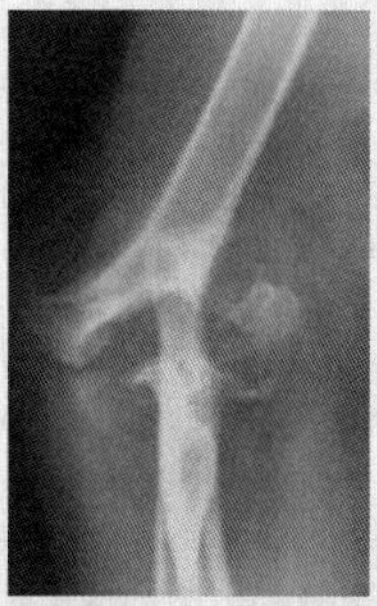	Severe bony destruction	Patients often have severe pain and functional limitations; functional instability may also be present if the joint's bony architecture is destroyed.
V	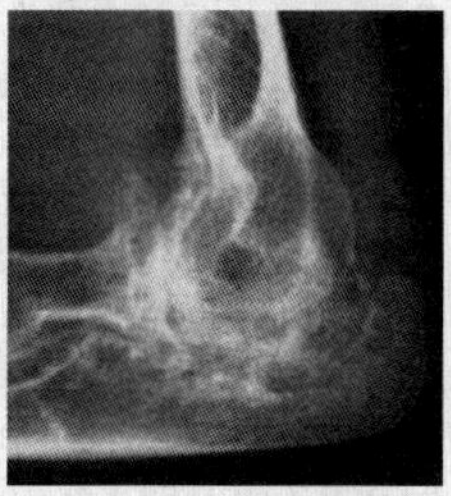	Presence of bony ankylosis of the ulnohumeral joint	Most commonly seen with JRA

Adapted from Morrey BF, Adams RA. Semiconstrained arthroplasty for the treatment of rheumatoid arthritis of the elbow. J Bone Joint Surg Am 1992;74(4):479–490; Connor PM, Morrey BF. Total elbow arthroplasty in patients who have juvenile rheumatoid arthritis. J Bone Joint Surg Am 1998;80(5):678–688.

- An arthroscopic anterior capsular release may be performed at the time of the arthroscopic synovectomy to improve elbow extension. A posterior olecranon plasty may also be performed to reestablish normal concavity of the olecranon fossa.
- Posteromedial capsule release should be avoided to prevent the risk of iatrogenic ulnar nerve injury. If an elbow requires a release of the posterior capsule to regain elbow flexion (typically those with 100 degrees or less of preoperative flexion), then the surgeon should perform an open ulnar nerve decompression and subcutaneous transposition followed by complete posterior capsule release (including the posteromedial band of the medial collateral ligament).

Total Elbow Arthroplasty

- This procedure is indicated for advanced (grade III or IV) RA of the elbow in patients with significant pain and limitations in activities of daily living.
- Absolute contraindications include active infection, upper extremity paralysis, and a patient's refusal or inability to abide by postoperative activity restrictions.
- Relative contraindications include presence of infection at a remote site and a history of infected elbow or elbow prosthesis.

Preoperative Planning

- AP and lateral radiographs of the elbow are reviewed to assess humeral bow and medullary canal diameter as well as angulation and diameter of the ulnar medullary canal.
  - Preoperative radiographic templates may be helpful to assess preoperative radiographic magnification.
- In particular for JRA patients, the canal width may be very small, and therefore the surgeon must ensure that appropriately sized implants as well as intramedullary guidewires and reamers are available.
- If an ipsilateral total shoulder arthroplasty has been performed or is anticipated, a humeral cement restrictor should be used. A 4-inch humeral implant may also be considered; however, shorter, recently introduced humeral components for total shoulder arthroplasty can typically be placed even in the presence of a 6-inch humeral stem. Overlapping cement mantles and/or a short cement gap between the humeral stems of the shoulder and elbow prostheses should be avoided to reduce the risk of subsequent periprosthetic fracture.
- Preoperative limitations in forearm rotation may be due in part to ipsilateral distal radioulnar joint pathology. Thus, radiographs should also be obtained of the ipsilateral shoulder and wrist.

Implant Selection for Total Elbow Arthroplasty

- Implant options have traditionally been classified as linked (semiconstrained) or unlinked.
  - These terms are being used with decreasing frequency, however, as some unlinked implant designs have been developed that have precisely contoured components that create a degree of constraint.
  - Linked, semiconstrained implants inherently have about 7 degrees of varus–valgus and 7 degrees of axial rotation, "play," whereas unconstrained implants typically refer to unlinked, resurfacing components.
  - The stability of unconstrained implants depends on soft tissue and ligamentous integrity. Such tissues may be destroyed by the rheumatoid inflammatory process or surgically released with semiconstrained implants without compromising stability.
- Although no prospective comparisons between linked (semiconstrained) and unlinked implants have yet been performed, studies have generally reported improved survivorship with a semiconstrained design.[7]
  - The semiconstrained design is preferred because it is equally effective in pain relief and in improving range of motion and function while preserving stability without an observed increase in aseptic loosening.[7]
  - The Techniques section describes implantation of a linked, semiconstrained implant.
- Polyethylene bushing wear is a challenging issue which has been implicated as a limiting factor in long-term implant durability following total elbow arthroplasty.[2,5,10] Polyethylene wear has been reported after total elbow arthroplasty with multiple implant designs.[5,10] Osteolysis and loosening from particle-induced bushing wear is an important concern when considering mid- to long-term survivability of the implants, and this is of particular importance for younger patients undergoing total elbow arthroplasty, especially for posttraumatic conditions. Newer bearing designs have recently been created to address the potential issues related to polyethylene wear, including increasing the amount of polyethylene in the bushing as well as designs with conforming polyethylene and metallic-bearing surfaces. The implant described in the Techniques section uses a novel vitamin E highly cross-linked ultra-high-molecular-weight polyethylene bearing to prevent metal-to-metal contact and is designed to have improved polyethylene wear characteristics.
  - Failure of the locking mechanisms used to link ulnar and humeral components in total elbow arthroplasty has been reported for several implant designs.[3,10] The implant described in the Techniques section employs a novel locking mechanism designed to reduce the potential for locking mechanism failure.

Sequence and Timing of Total Elbow Arthroplasty in the Patient with Polyarticular Involvement

- Because RA typically affects multiple joint articulations, the timing of elbow arthroplasty should be considered with regard to the need for arthroplasties of other joints.
- In general, the most disabling articulation should be addressed first. In the case of equivocal involvement in the elbow and a lower extremity joint in which arthroplasty is planned, the surgeon must consider the postoperative effects of surgery and plan accordingly.
- If total elbow arthroplasty is performed first, at least 3 to 6 months should pass before lower extremity reconstruction is performed to allow adequate healing of the elbow. If the lower extremity will be addressed first, total elbow arthroplasty should be delayed until assistive ambulatory devices, which may put strain on the elbow, are no longer required.
  - Patients with total elbow arthroplasty should not bear weight with crutches. A platform walker may be used, provided it does not increase strain on the elbow. This may be achieved by raising the walker's arm rest to an appropriate height such that when the forearm is placed on

the arm rest, the elbow may not be extended beyond 90 degrees of flexion.

Assessment of the Cervical Spine

- Because nearly 90% of patients with RA have cervical spine involvement, approximately 30% of whom have significant subluxation, the cervical spine must be evaluated before any surgery in which intubation is planned.
  - Cervical spine radiographs should be routinely obtained.
  - If patients have neck pain, decreased range of motion, myelopathic symptoms, or radiographic evidence of instability, a magnetic resonance imaging (MRI) study should be ordered with concomitant referral to a spine surgeon to consider addressing the cervical spine pathology before elbow surgery.

Temporary Cessation of Medications before Total Elbow Arthroplasty

- TNF inhibitors affect the immune system and have been found to increase the risk of developing a prosthetic joint infection.
  - In general, anti-TNF agents are typically stopped for a period of time preoperatively based on the half-life of the specific drug and for about 2 weeks after surgery to reduce the risk of perioperative morbidity.
- Methotrexate is generally continued in the perioperative period. Fewer complications, infections, and flares have been reported when methotrexate is continued perioperatively versus discontinuing it.
- Patients on chronic NSAIDs should stop taking those medications approximately 2 weeks before surgery to reduce the risk of increased bleeding.
- For patients on chronic steroids, stress-dose steroids may be required perioperatively.
- Communications with the patient's rheumatologist and the anesthesiologist are imperative to coordinate these efforts.

Positioning

- Intravenous antibiotics are administered 30 to 60 minutes before the incision.
- The patient is placed in a supine position on the operating table with a rolled towel under the ipsilateral scapula. The arm is placed across the chest, and another rolled towel is placed under the elbow to support the arm.
- The entire operative extremity and shoulder girdle is prepared and draped; a sterile tourniquet is placed. An Ioban drape is placed circumferentially over all exposed skin.
- The arm is exsanguinated and the tourniquet inflated.

Approach

- Multiple exposures, including triceps-on approaches, may be used to perform total elbow arthroplasty. The Bryan-Morrey approach (triceps–anconeus "slide") provides excellent exposure and is particularly useful for surgeons with limited experience in triceps-sparing approaches. The Bryan-Morrey approach is described in the following text.

TECHNIQUES

Incision and Exposure

- A straight incision, measuring approximately 15 cm and centered at the elbow joint, is made just lateral to the tip of the olecranon.
- The ulnar nerve is carefully identified and isolated along the medial aspect of the triceps.
- Proximal neurolysis of the nerve is achieved by releasing the arcade of Struthers from the medial head of the triceps. The nerve is then mobilized to beyond its first motor branch distally by dividing Osborne fascia and the fascia between the two heads of the flexor carpi ulnaris (FCU) (**TECH FIG 1A,B**).
- The medial intermuscular septum is excised and a deep pocket of subcutaneous tissue over the flexor pronator group distally and anterior to the triceps proximally is created.
  - The nerve is then anteriorly transposed into this subcutaneous tissue pocket; it must be protected throughout the operation.
- An incision is then made over the medial aspect of the ulna between the anconeus and FCU. The medial triceps and anconeus are subperiosteally elevated off the ulna.
- The medial aspect of the triceps is retracted along with the fibers of the posterior capsule to tension the Sharpey fibers at their ulnar insertion (**TECH FIG 1C,D**).

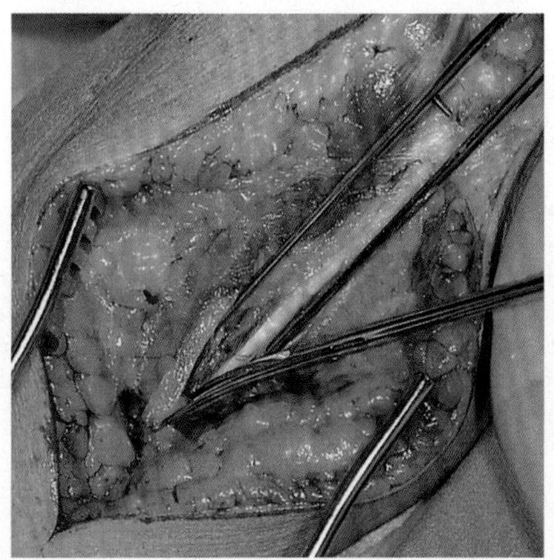
A

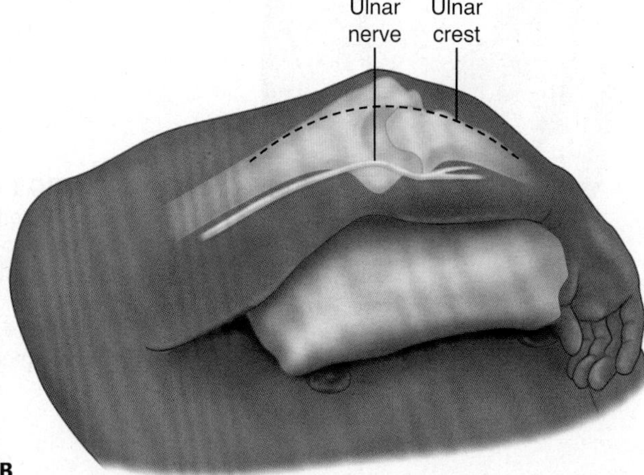

B

TECH FIG 1 • **A,B.** The ulnar nerve is identified along the medial border of the triceps, and a vessel loop is placed. *(continued)*

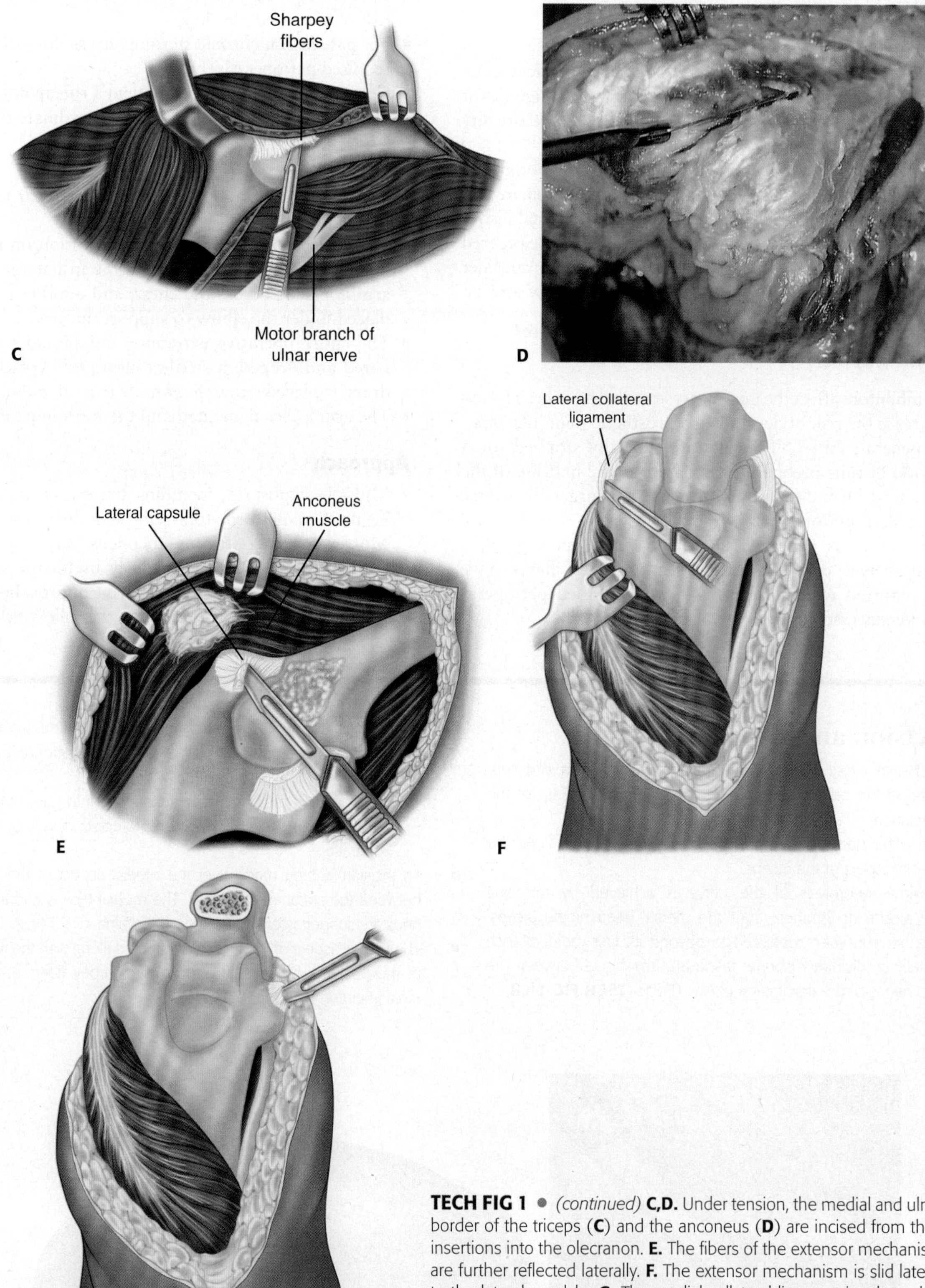

TECH FIG 1 • *(continued)* **C,D.** Under tension, the medial and ulnar border of the triceps (**C**) and the anconeus (**D**) are incised from their insertions into the olecranon. **E.** The fibers of the extensor mechanism are further reflected laterally. **F.** The extensor mechanism is slid lateral to the lateral condyle. **G.** The medial collateral ligament is released to give the elbow maximal motion and to facilitate complete exposure of the ulnohumeral joint.

- These fibers are then sharply dissected, and the triceps in continuity with the anconeus is reflected from medial to lateral (**TECH FIG 1E**).
- The lateral ulnar collateral ligament complex is released from its humeral attachment, thus allowing the extensor mechanism to be completely reflected to the lateral aspect of the humerus (**TECH FIG 1F**).
- If ulnohumeral ankylosis is present, as is sometimes the case in JRA patients, a saw or osteotome may be necessary to reestablish the joint line and to create the osteotomy at the appropriate center of rotation of the ulnohumeral joint.
- The elbow is then progressively flexed, exposing the medial collateral ligament, which is then released subperiosteally from its humeral attachment (**TECH FIG 1G**).
- The tip of the olecranon is removed with a rongeur or oscillating saw, depending on the quality of the bone, and the humerus is then externally rotated and the elbow fully flexed to adequately expose the articulating surfaces of the humerus, ulna, and radial head.
- The anterior capsule is completely released from the anterior aspect of the humerus to accommodate the flange of the humeral component and to allow unencumbered postoperative elbow extension.

Humeral Preparation

- Trochlear resection: The midportion of the trochlea is removed with an oscillating saw if the bone is dense or with a rongeur if the bone is soft, up to the roof of the olecranon fossa.
- The resected bone should be preserved for the anterior distal humeral bone graft needed later in the procedure (**TECH FIG 2A**).
- Humeral canal reaming: The proximal base of the olecranon fossa is entered with a rongeur or burr, and the humeral awl reamer is then used to identify the humeral medullary canal (**TECH FIG 2B,C**). This reamer must be centered and must fit between the remaining portions of the trochlea to ensure that the humeral rasps can be seated in the canal. Additional bone should be resected if needed to accommodate the humeral rasp width.
- Humeral canal rasping: The pilot humeral rasp is used initially (**TECH FIG 2D**) and it is impacted until the solid line on the rasp reaches the axis of flexion (**TECH FIG 2E**). Progressively larger rasps are used to achieve the desired size and fit for the planned implant, and the final rasp is left in place. A humeral alignment rod can be placed through the rasp to help determine the axial alignment (**TECH FIG 2F**).

A
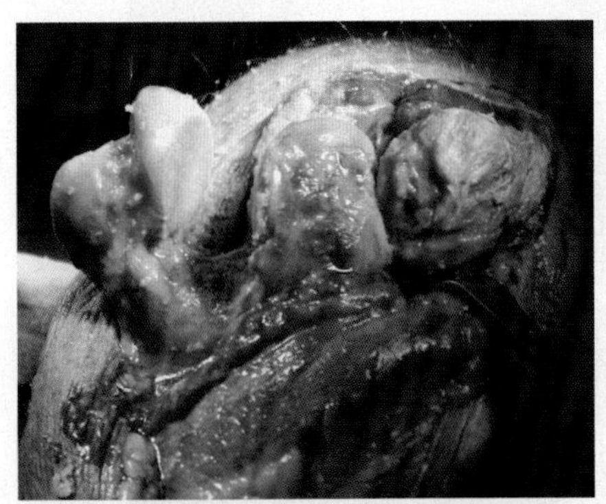

B
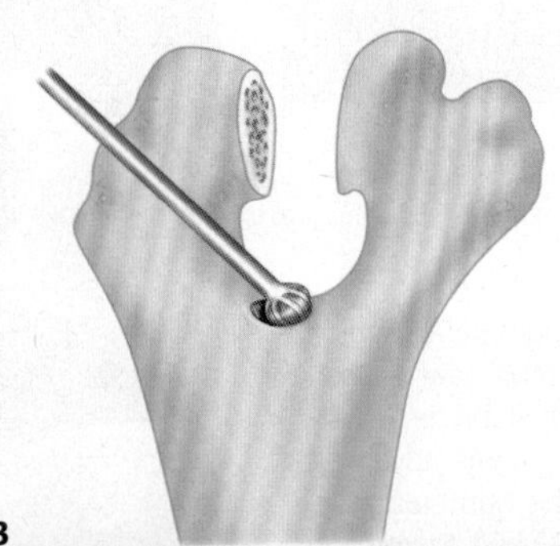

C
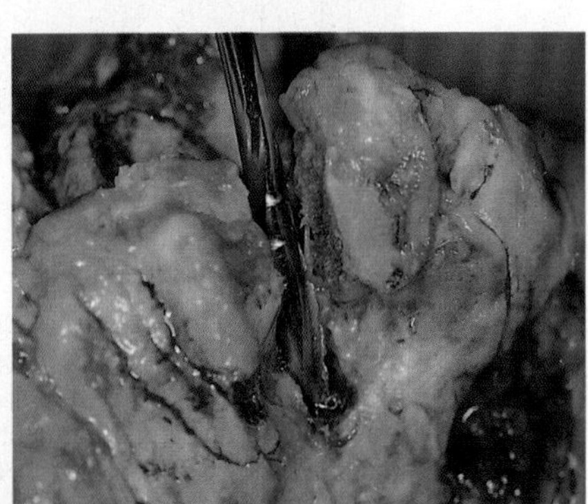

D
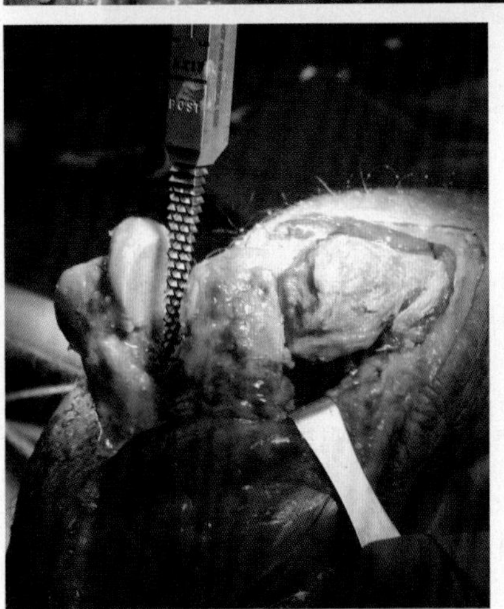

E
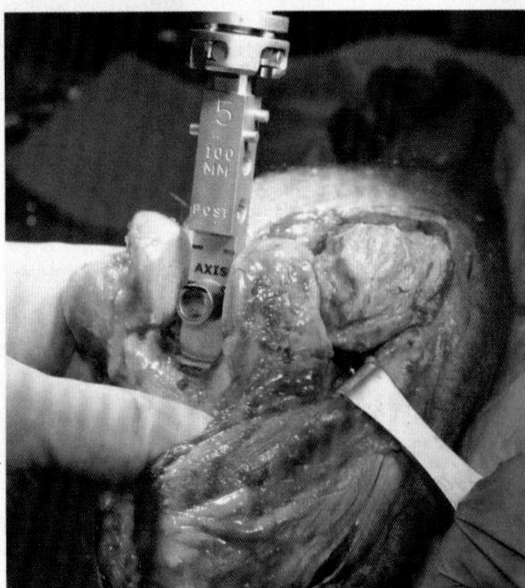

TECH FIG 2 • **A.** Following trochlear resection with an oscillating saw. **B.** A burr is used to enter the roof of the olecranon. **C.** The humeral awl reamer is used to identify the medullary canal. **D.** Progressive humeral canal rasping is performed up to the desired size and fit. **E.** The humeral canal rasp is seated so that the solid line matches the axis of flexion. *(continued)*

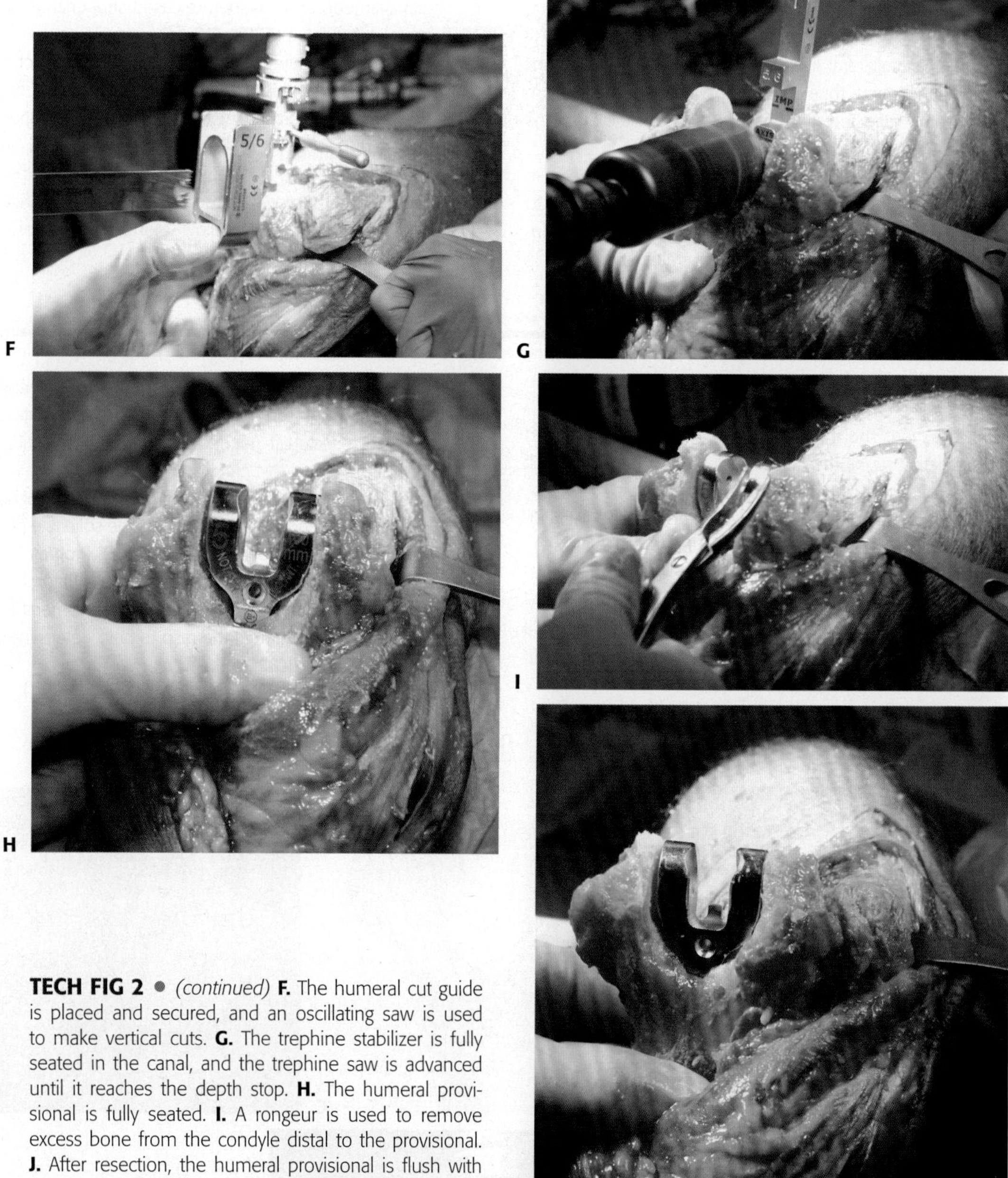

TECH FIG 2 • *(continued)* **F.** The humeral cut guide is placed and secured, and an oscillating saw is used to make vertical cuts. **G.** The trephine stabilizer is fully seated in the canal, and the trephine saw is advanced until it reaches the depth stop. **H.** The humeral provisional is fully seated. **I.** A rongeur is used to remove excess bone from the condyle distal to the provisional. **J.** After resection, the humeral provisional is flush with the distal aspect of the humeral condyles.

- Superficial trephine cut: A size-matched trephine saw based on the final humeral rasp is then used to define the planned humeral cut. A pilot pin is placed into the humeral rasp, and the trephine saw is advanced over this until the depth stop is reached. The posterior aspect of the humerus is scored with the trephine to provide a reference for the final preparation.
- Humeral cut: The humeral cut guide is attached to the humeral rasp, and an oscillating saw is used to excise remaining trochlea with vertical cuts to accommodate placement of the trephine stabilizer (**TECH FIG 2F**).
  - Care must be taken, as this area may be very thin in patients with RA and thus susceptible to fracture.
- The trephine stabilizer is placed into the canal. Full seating may require notching of the coronoid fossa with a burr or rongeur.
  - The trephine's pilot pin is placed into the trephine stabilizer and advanced to its depth stop (**TECH FIG 2G**). The trephine cut is then completed.
  - The size-matched humeral provisional is seated in the canal, and excess bone is removed to make the provisional flush with the distal aspect of the condyles (**TECH FIG 2H**).

Ulnar Preparation

- Ulnar canal exposure: The tip of the olecranon is removed with an oscillating saw. Exercise caution with this step because over-resection weakens the triceps insertion site, whereas underresection causes the intramedullary rasp to be malaligned relative to the axis of the ulna. This may then result in malalignment of the ulnar component and possible dorsal cortex perforation.
- A high-speed burr is angled 45 degrees relative to the axis of the ulnar shaft at the junction of the sigmoid fossa and coronoid to identify the ulnar medullary canal (**TECH FIG 3A,B**).
- The olecranon is notched with a rongeur to allow the reamers and rasps to be placed in line with the ulnar canal.
- Ulnar canal reaming (if necessary): The ulnar awl reamer is centered in the ulna and advanced to open the ulnar canal.
- The ulnar bow should be acknowledged and palpated while inserting the ulnar reamers to avoid ulnar perforation.
- The ulnar canal is progressively reamed with solid flexible reamers until the desired size is reached (**TECH FIG 3C**). Flexible cannulated reamers with a ball-tip guidewire are used to continue reaming as necessary. The ball tip is used to avoid cortical penetration.
- Ulnar canal rasping: The ulnar canal is further prepared with the pilot ulnar rasp. The rasp is fully seated, and the canal is progressively rasped until the desired fit is achieved.
- During advancement of the rasps, it is important to maintain proper rotation of the rasp so that the handle is perpendicular to the flat dorsal aspect of the proximal ulna (**TECH FIG 3D,E**). The final rasp and T handle are left in the canal.
- Sigmoid notch preparation: The ulnar clearance template is placed through the ulnar rasp to ensure adequate clearance around the sigmoid notch to allow articulation (**TECH FIG 3F**). Any osseous impingements encountered when rotating the template are then removed with a burr or rongeur. The template is then moved to the other side of the ulnar rasp, and the process is repeated.
- The tip of the coronoid is removed with a rongeur to eliminate impingement and improve flexion (**TECH FIG 3G**).
- Ulnar provisional: The ulnar provisional is placed into the ulnar canal and lightly impacted if necessary to align the center of the

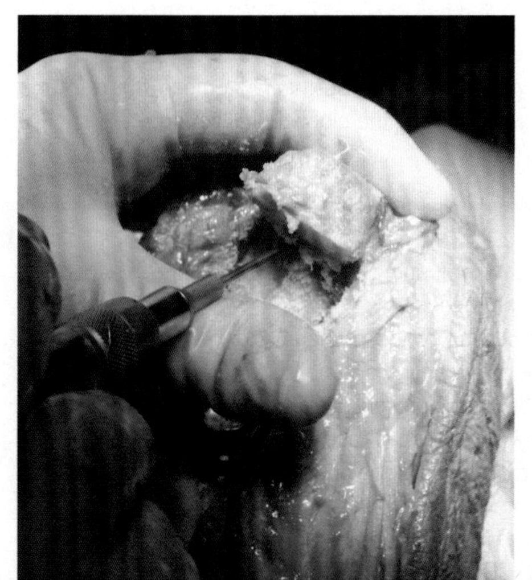
A

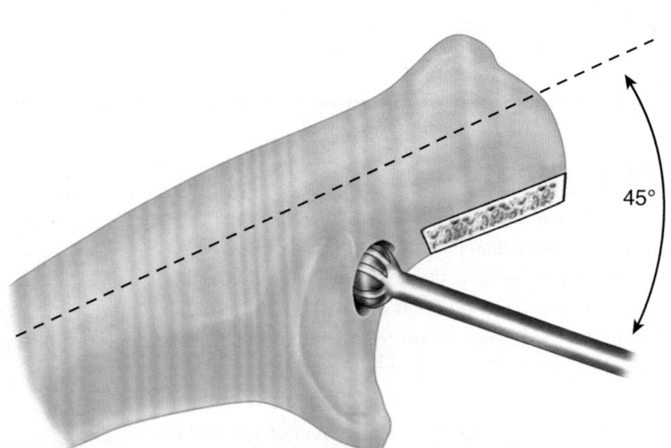

B

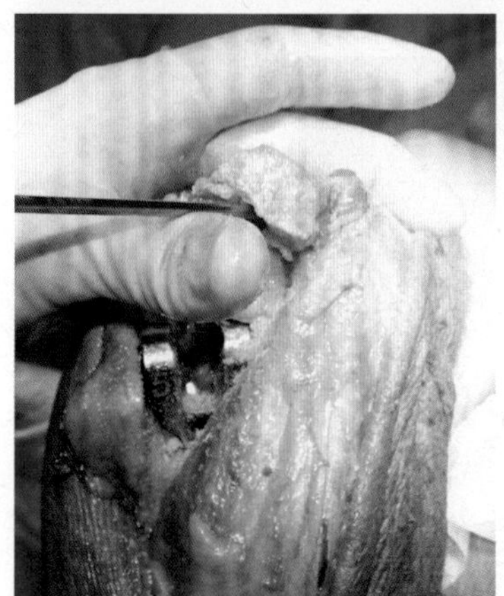
C

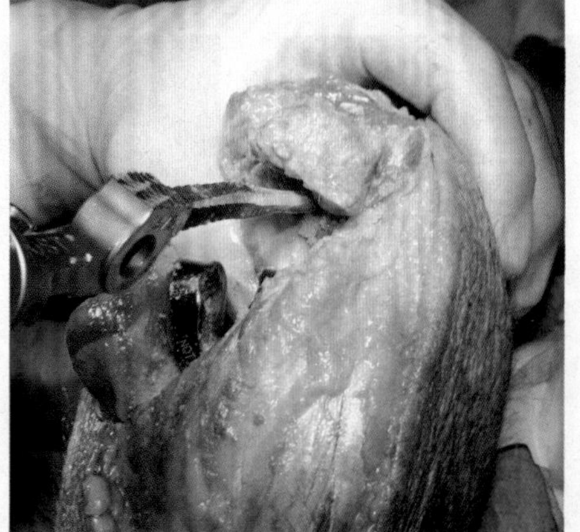
D

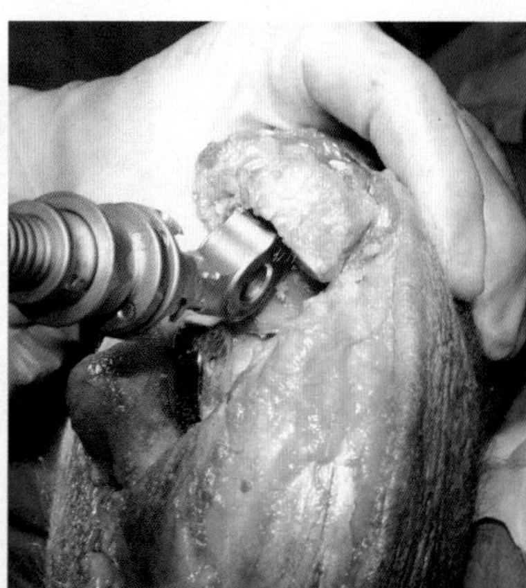
E

TECH FIG 3 • **A,B.** The olecranon tip is resected, and a high-speed burr is used to open the ulnar medullary canal at the base of the coronoid. **C.** The flexible, solid, and cannulated ulnar awl reamers are progressively advanced prior to rasping. The surgeon's hand is placed over the ulnar shaft to guide aiming of the reamers and rasps down the center of the canal. **D,E.** The pilot ulnar rasp is advanced until the center of the rasp matches the center of the sigmoid notch. *(continued)*

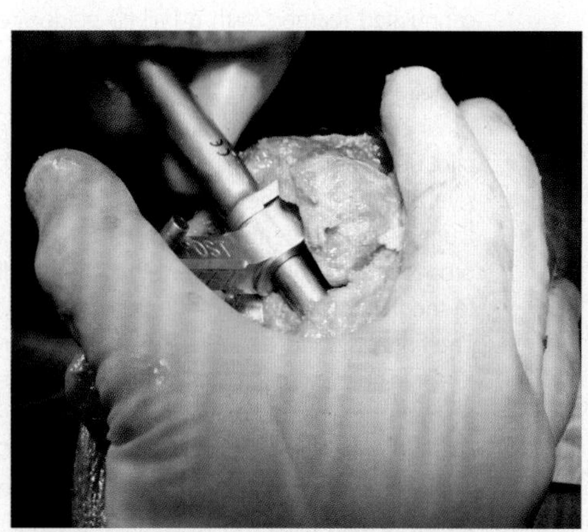

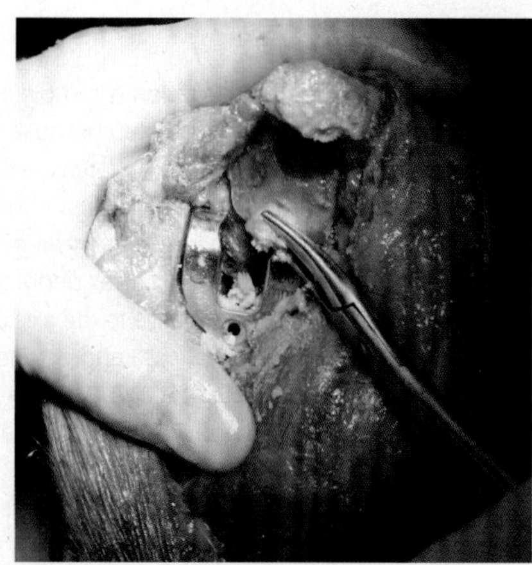

TECH FIG 3 • *(continued)* **F.** The ulnar clearance template is rotated around the sigmoid notch. Any excess bone noted when scoring the surface of the bone is then excised. **G.** The tip of the coronoid is removed to eliminate impingement and improve flexion.

ulnar provisional with the center of the greater sigmoid notch. A humeral-bearing pin may be used to assess rotational and varus/valgus alignment.

- Because proximal radioulnar arthritis is ubiquitous in patients with RA and JRA and the Nexel total elbow arthroplasty does not require proximal radioulnar and radiocapitellar reconstruction, a radial head excision is performed.
- This may be performed by rotating the forearm and using a rongeur to progressively excise the radial head from an axial orientation while holding the elbow in full flexion.

Trial Reduction

- The humeral provisional is then reinserted, the components are coupled, and a trial reduction is performed (**TECH FIG 4A**).
- Range of motion is tested and should be full without limitation in the flexion–extension plane (**TECH FIG 4B**).
- If range of motion is limited owing to inadequate soft tissue release, this should be addressed at this time.
- The components should also be evaluated for bony impingement, which may occur posteriorly (olecranon impingement on the humerus) or anteriorly (coronoid tip on the anterior flange of the humeral component). Any impinging bone should be removed with a rongeur.
- Incomplete seating of the humeral and/or ulnar components may also be a cause for limitations in elbow extension.
- If humeral bowing is present, it may be difficult to fully seat the humeral provisional. In this case, the proximal aspect of the final humeral component may be bowed to match the humeral canal and allow complete seating of the prosthesis.
- After satisfactory trial reduction, the provisional components are removed.

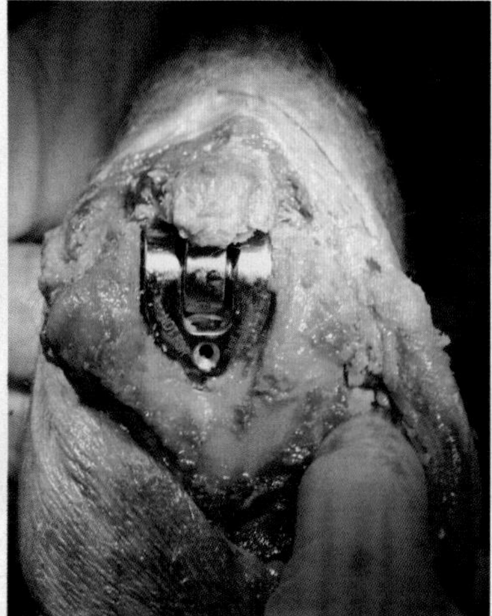

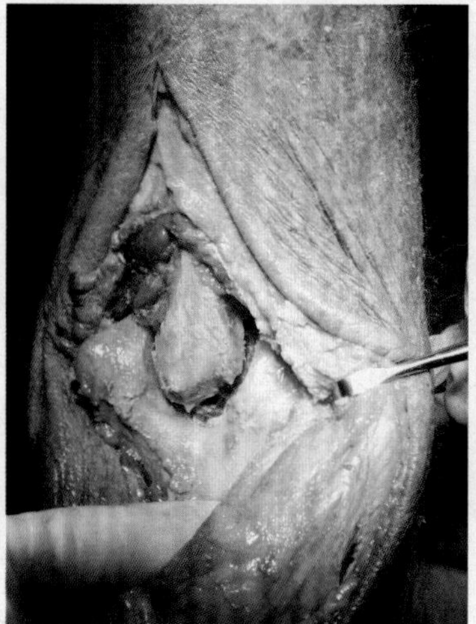

TECH FIG 4 • A,B. A trial reduction of the components is performed and range of motion is assessed to evaluate for bony impingement.

Cementing

- Both medullary canals are then pulse lavaged and dried.
- Based on the trial components used, the length of the cement applicator is measured to equal that of the humeral component.
  - The tip of the applicator is cut at this level to ensure appropriate depth of the cement down the humeral canal (**TECH FIG 5A**).
  - A humeral cement restrictor is placed to the desired depth.
- It is recommended that cementing of the components be performed separately.
  - Cement with antibiotics are mixed and injected with a relatively soft consistency.
- The humeral component is typically cemented first, followed by the ulnar component (**TECH FIG 5B**).
- The ulnar stem inserter is used to protect the ulnar component from being damaged during insertion (**TECH FIG 5C**). The implant must be in line with the flat dorsal surface of the olecranon and it must be fully seated so that the center of the component is in the center of the greater sigmoid notch.
- Care is taken to remove excess cement from around the ulnar component to prevent third-body wear. A plastic curette is used to avoid implant scratching.

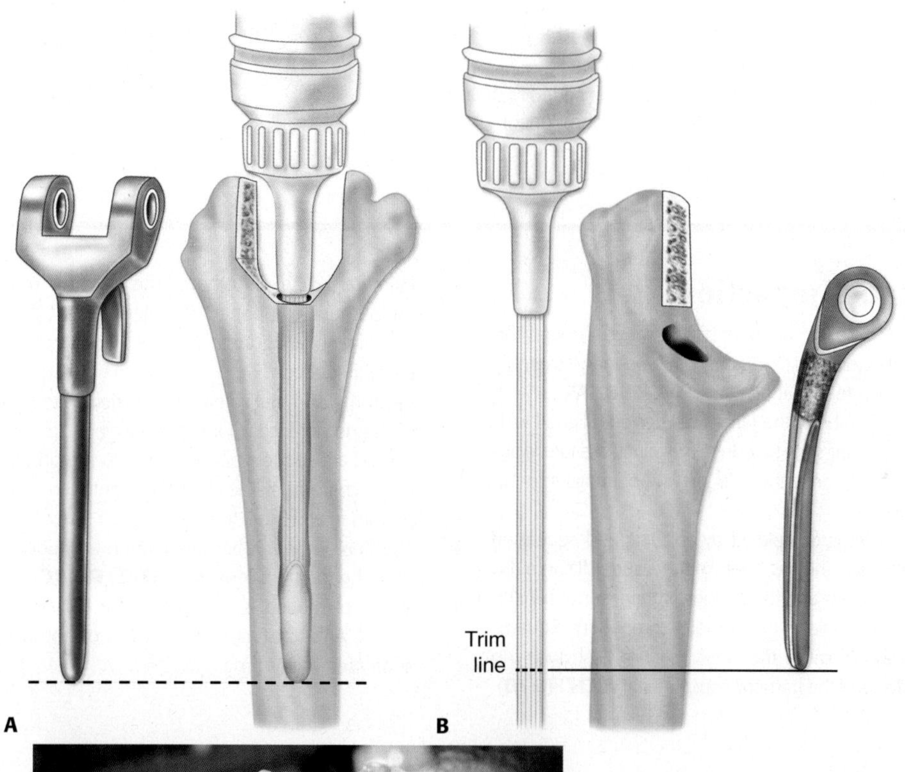

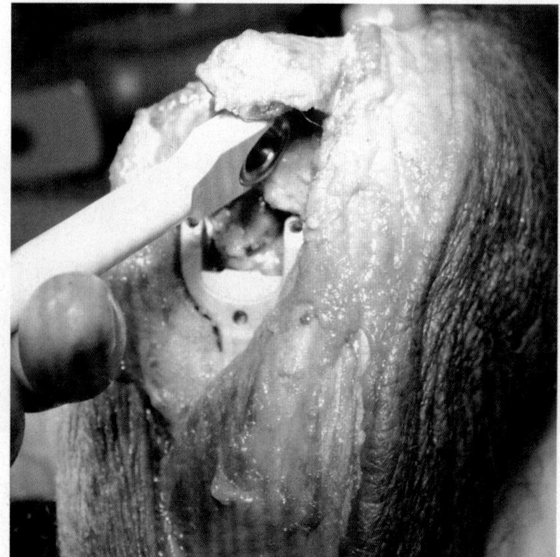

TECH FIG 5 • A,B. Separate cementing of the humeral and ulnar medullary canals is recommended. **C.** The ulnar stem inserter is used to prevent scratching of the ulnar component while fully seating the implant.

Humeral Component and Bone Graft

- A small (about 2 × 2 cm and 2 to 4 mm thick) piece of the removed trochlea is used for the anterior bone graft. Radial head or allograft may be used in revision cases when no bone is resected from the trochlea.
- This bone graft is wedged between the anterior aspect of the humerus and the flange as the humeral component is placed (**TECH FIG 6**).
- This provides the humeral component with rotational stability as well as additional stability in the AP plane.
- Excess cement is removed from the area around the humeral component with a plastic curette.

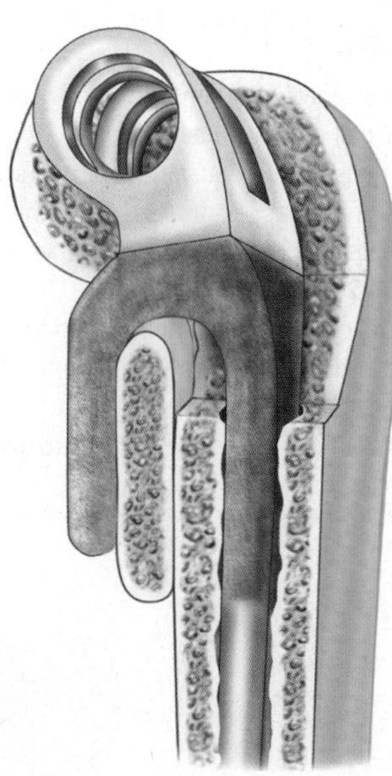

TECH FIG 6 • The humeral component is inserted to the optimal depth that allows proper articulation with the ulnar component.

Assembly and Impaction

- Assembly of ulnar bearing: The axle pin is placed through the eye of the ulnar component, and the ulnar-bearing assembly tool is used to attach the ulnar bearings (**TECH FIG 7A**).
- The axle pin and the tabs of the ulnar bearings are aligned with the humeral component slots to reduce the joint. Pressure is applied to the forearm to drive the axle pin and bearings into the humeral component.
- Reduction of the joint is completed by applying and squeezing the articulation inserter. The top "feet" of the inserter fits into the ulnar-bearing tab pockets and the bottom of the inserter fits into the proximal posterior hole of the humeral component. Squeezing the inserter should make the ulnar bearings flush with the curved distal surfaces of the humeral component (**TECH FIG 7B**).
- Humeral screw placement: The bearings must be flush with the humeral component in order to insert the humeral screws. The ulnar-bearing tamp may be used to press the bearings in place if needed.
- Insert the humeral screws in the medial and lateral screw holes of the humeral component by using the humeral screw holder. Screws are sequentially tightened to the prescribed torque, and each screw should be alternately tightened until it is snug before performing the final torque on either screw.
- The final torque is achieved when an audible "click" is heard from the torque screwdriver (**TECH FIG 7C**).
- Range of motion is checked and a full arc of motion is confirmed. Any soft tissue contractures or bony impingements are addressed at this time.

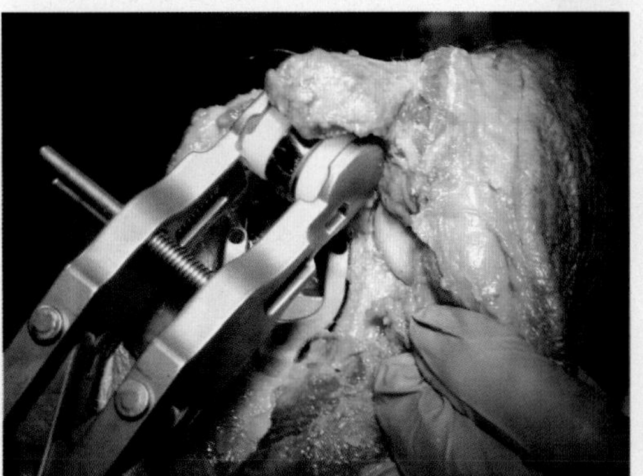

A

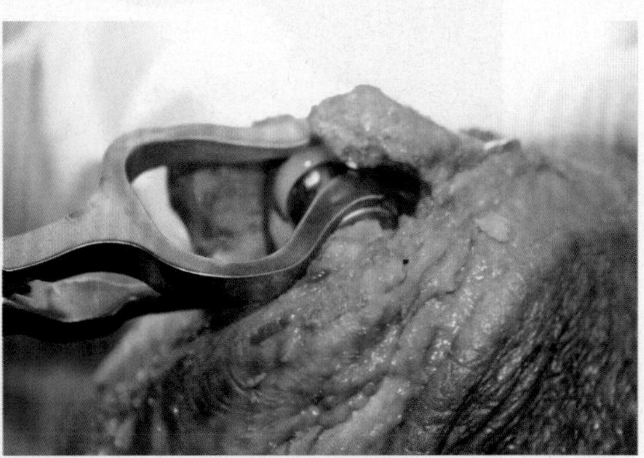

B

TECH FIG 7 • **A.** The ulnar-bearing assembly tool is squeezed until significant resistance is felt to attach the ulnar bearing. There is no audible click. **B.** The articulation inserter is applied and squeezed until resistance is felt and the bearings are seated. There is no audible click with this maneuver. *(continued)*

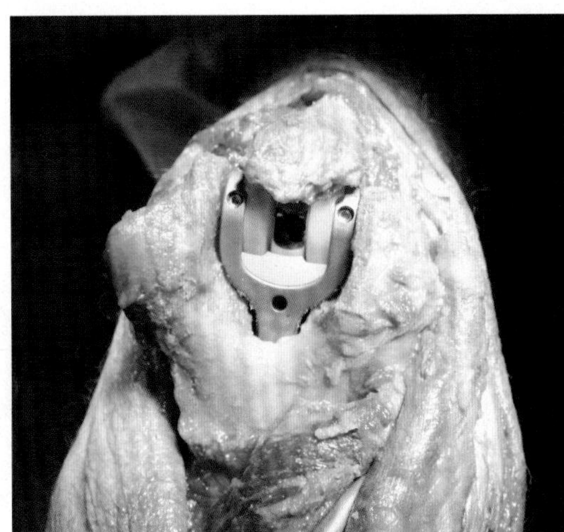

TECH FIG 7 • *(continued)* **C.** Linked components after the humeral screws are tightened.

Triceps Reattachment

- Small cruciate and transverse drill holes are placed through the olecranon at the site of triceps reattachment, and a heavy, nonabsorbable suture (such as no. 5 Ethibond) is placed on a Keith needle and then brought through the distal medial cruciate drill hole and out the proximal lateral hole (**TECH FIG 8A–C**).
- The elbow is flexed to about 60 degrees and the extensor mechanism is reduced over the tip of the olecranon; consider slightly overreducing the extensor mechanism medially to minimize the potential for postoperative lateral subluxation.
- The suture is woven through the triceps tendon in a locking, crisscross pattern such that the suture emerges at the proximal medial hole (**TECH FIG 8D**).
  - The suture is then passed through this hole and out the distal lateral hole such that it is located directly across from the initial suture end.
  - These suture ends are then passed again through the forearm extensor fascia and tied together.
  - Two reinforcing sutures are then passed through the transverse holes and extensor fascia before being tied together.
- Avoid knots directly over the subcutaneous border of the proximal ulna.
- The tourniquet is then deflated, and hemostasis is achieved with bipolar electrocautery.
- The medial soft tissue extensor mechanism is then reapproximated.

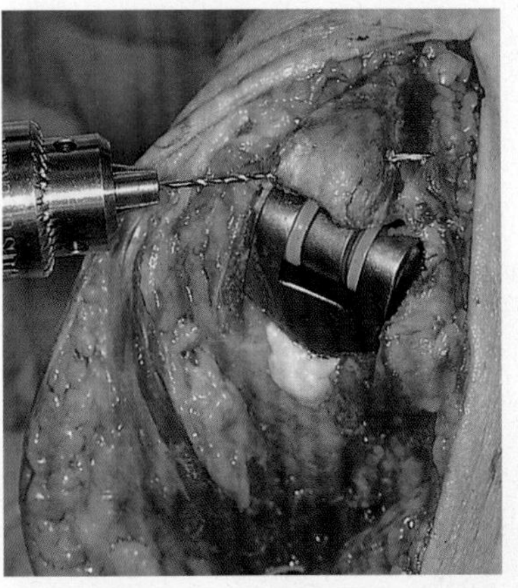

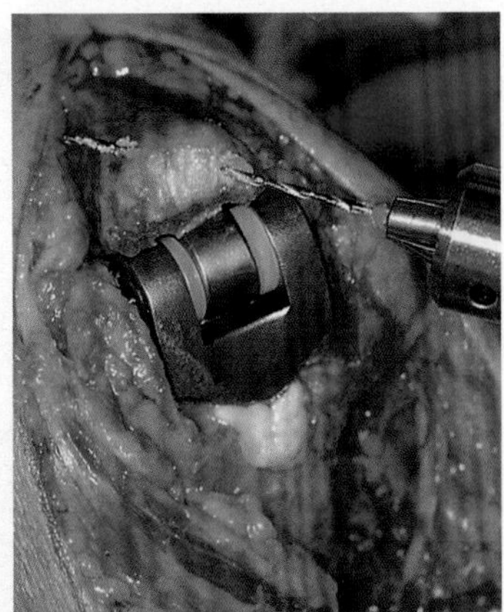

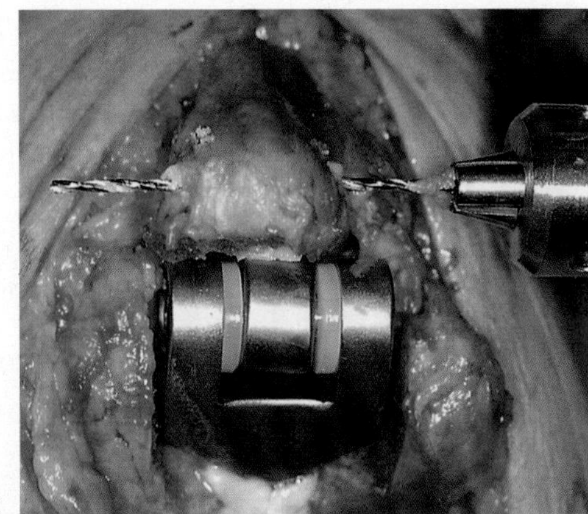

TECH FIG 8 • Cruciate (**A,B**) and transverse (**C**) drill holes are placed in the ulna for triceps reattachment on a Coonrad-Morrey total elbow replacement. The repair for the Nexel total elbow arthroplasty is identical to this repair when the Bryan-Morrey approach is performed. *(continued)*

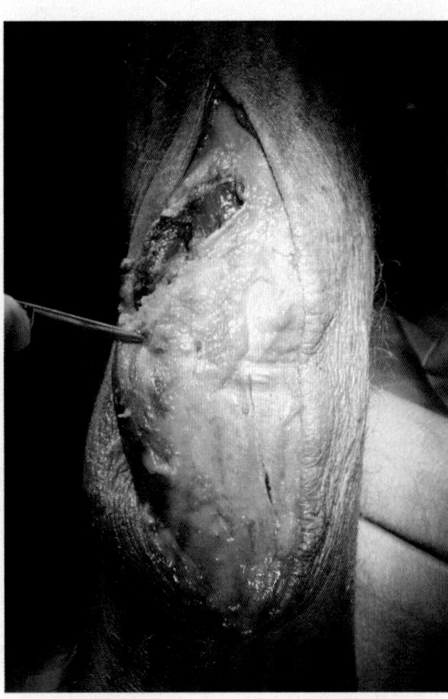

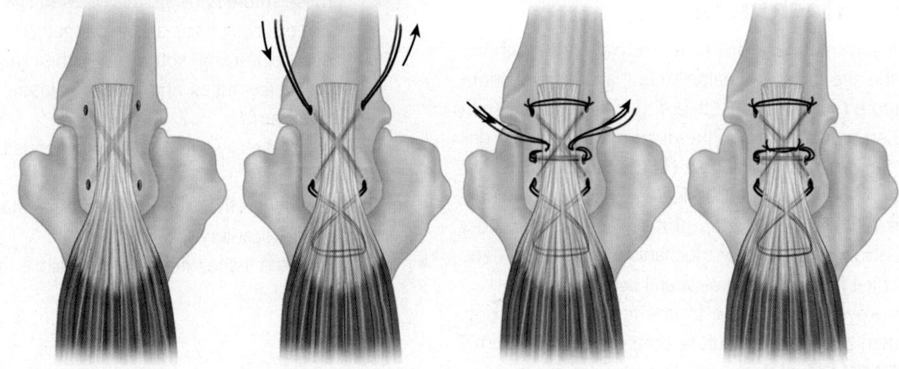

TECH FIG 8 • *(continued)* **D.** Planned triceps repair. **E.** Suture is passed through the proximal ulna and then woven through the triceps tendon before being tied together.

Ulnar Nerve Transposition and Wound Closure

- The protected nerve is in the subcutaneous tissue pocket previously created, and dermal sutures are placed to protect and secure the nerve (**TECH FIG 9**).
- Wounds are closed in layers, and a drain is placed. Staples are used to close the skin.
- An anterior splint is placed with the elbow in full extension, making sure to adequately pad the anterior aspect of the splint both proximally and distally to prevent skin breakdown.

TECH FIG 9 • The ulnar nerve is transposed into the subcutaneous tissue of the medial epicondylar region and secured with sutures in the dermal layer.

PEARLS AND PITFALLS

Approach and exposure	■ Take your time with the Bryan-Morrey approach; maintaining precise subperiosteal elevation of the extensor mechanism will make for a better postoperative extensor mechanism repair. ■ Obtain complete ulnohumeral dissociation before bony preparation. This includes complete releases of the lateral ulnar collateral ligament and medial collateral ligament complexes and a complete anterior capsule release. ■ Consider reflection of common flexors or extensors if severe deformities or arthrofibrosis is present.
Humeral preparation	■ Shorten the humerus by up to 1 cm to augment postoperative range of motion without compromising strength if needed. ■ Use a burr distally to open up the humeral canal if needed rather than forcing with rasps.
Radial and ulnar preparation	■ Excise the radial head and the tip of the coronoid. ■ Always palpate the ulna and consider the ulnar bow before ulnar preparation to avoid perforation.
Cementing	■ Review the cement technique and order mentally before proceeding; use cement that does not rapidly set.
Triceps reattachment	■ Overreduce the triceps–anconeus repair medially.
Postoperative care	■ Use a postoperative extension splint for 24–36 hours. ■ Make all efforts to reduce postoperative swelling.

POSTOPERATIVE CARE

- Postoperatively, the anteriorly placed splint maintains the elbow in full extension for about 24 to 36 hours.
- The elbow is strictly elevated overnight and on postoperative day 1.
- The drain is removed on postoperative day 1 or when output is less than 30 mL in an 8-hour period.
- After splint removal, open-chain active-assisted range of motion is allowed. A formal physical therapy consultation is not usually required.
- The patient is restricted to no pushing and no overhead activities for 3 months to protect the triceps. In addition, no repetitive lifting of objects heavier than 5 pounds and no lifting greater than 10 pounds in a single event is recommented to maximize the survivorship of the implant.

OUTCOMES

- Successful outcomes for total elbow arthroplasty are judged based on relief of pain and improved range of motion, stability, and function.
  - The Mayo Elbow Performance Score assigns numeric values to each of these categories to produce scores for each of these criteria as well as an overall score.[8] Outcomes are often compared using this system.
- Total elbow arthroplasty for RA (**FIG 2**)
  - In the largest study with the longest follow-up in the literature, Gill and Morrey[4] reported 86% good or excellent results with a 13% reoperation rate on 69 patients with RA treated with a semiconstrained total elbow arthroplasty. Forty-four of these patients were followed for more than 10 years.

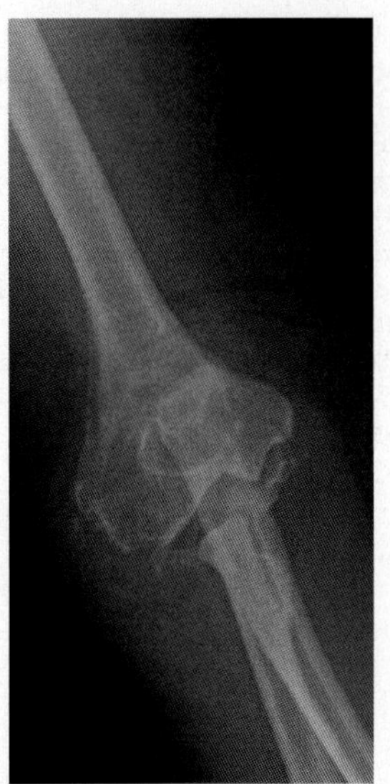

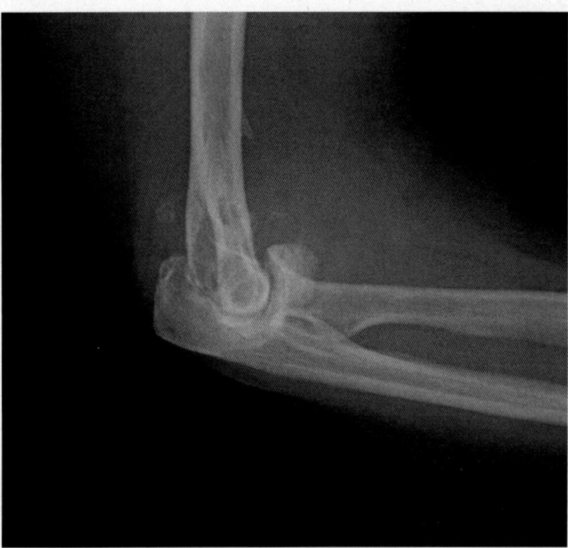

FIG 2 • **A,B.** A 66-year-old female with long-standing RA and Mayo grade IV changes. *(continued)*

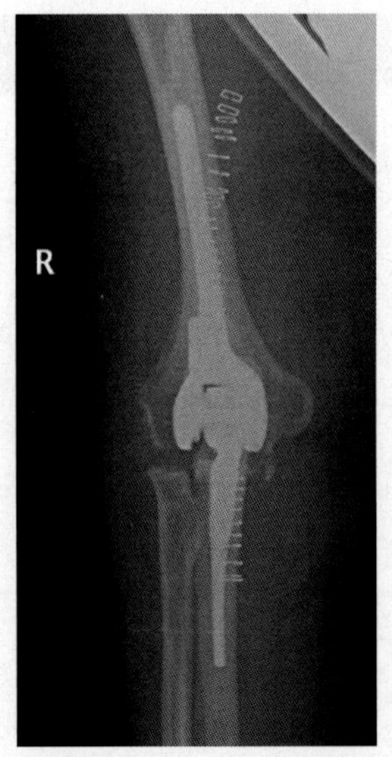

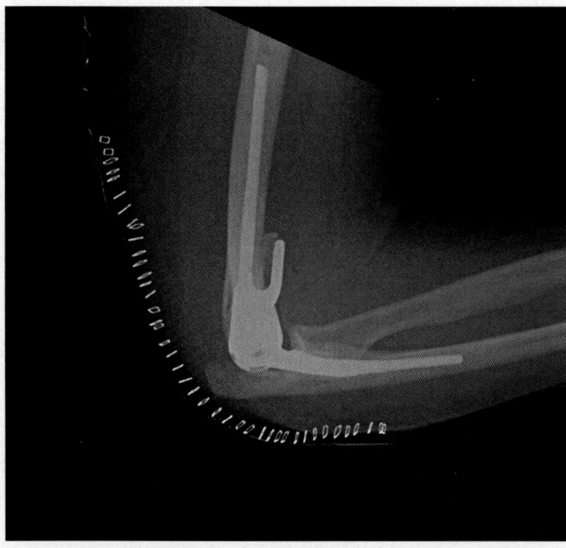

FIG 2 • *(continued)* **C,D.** Postoperative radiographs following Nexel total elbow arthroplasty.

- The prosthetic survival rate was 92.4% at 10 years of follow-up, thus approaching the success of lower extremity arthroplasty.
- Total elbow arthroplasty for JRA
  - Connor and Morrey[1] reported 87% good or excellent results on 19 patients (24 elbows) followed for a mean of 7.4 years.
  - The mean improvement in the Mayo Elbow Performance Score was 59 points, 96% had little or no pain, and there was no evidence of loosening in any prostheses at the latest follow-up.
  - The mean flexion–extension arc of motion improved by only 27 degrees (from 67 to 90 degrees) in this study, which is reflective of the severe soft-tissue contractures associated with JRA.

COMPLICATIONS

- Infection
- Aseptic loosening
- Mechanical failure
  - Short term
  - Long term
- Ulnar nerve injury
- Triceps weakness or avulsion
- Ulnar component fracture
- Ulnar fracture
- Wound healing problems

REFERENCES

1. Connor PM, Morrey BF. Total elbow arthroplasty in patients who have juvenile rheumatoid arthritis. J Bone Joint Surg Am 1998;80(5): 678–688.
2. Day JS, Baxter RM, Ramsey ML, et al. Characterization of wear debris in total elbow arthroplasty. J Shoulder Elbow Surg 2013;22: 924–931.
3. Figgie MP, Su EP, Kahn B, et al. Locking mechanism failure in semiconstrained total elbow arthroplasty. J Shoulder Elbow Surg 2006;15: 88–93.
4. Gill DR, Morrey BF. The Coonrad-Morrey total elbow arthroplasty in patients who have rheumatoid arthritis. A ten- to fifteen-year follow-up study. J Bone Joint Surg Am 1998;80(9):1327–1335.
5. Horiuchi K, Momohara S, Tomatsu T, et al. Arthroscopic synovectomy of the elbow in rheumatoid arthritis. J Bone Joint Surg Am 2002;84-A(3):342–347.
6. Kelly EW, Coghlan J, Bell S. Five- to thirteen-year follow-up of the GSB III total elbow arthroplasty. J Shoulder Elbow Surg 2004;13: 434–440.
7. Little CP, Graham AJ, Karatzas G, et al. Outcomes of total elbow arthroplasty for rheumatoid arthritis: comparative study of three implants. J Bone Joint Surg Am 2005;87(11):2439–2448.
8. Morrey BF, Adams RA. Semiconstrained arthroplasty for the treatment of rheumatoid arthritis of the elbow. J Bone Joint Surg Am 1992;74(4):479–490.
9. Rymaszewski LA, Mackay I, Amis AA, et al. Long-term effects of excision of the radial head in rheumatoid arthritis. J Bone Joint Surg Br 1979;66(1):109–113.
10. Wright TW, Hastings H. Total elbow arthroplasty failure due to overuse, C-ring failure, and/or bushing wear. J Shoulder Elbow Surg 2005;14:65–72.

Total Elbow Arthroplasty for Primary Osteoarthritis

Emilie Cheung and Garet Comer

DEFINITION

- Primary osteoarthritis (OA) of the elbow is a relatively rare condition that has an idiopathic etiology, although it is frequently associated with heavy use of the arm.
- Unlike OA of other large joints, elbow OA is characterized by relatively preserved joint space and articular cartilage but with hypertrophic osteophyte formation and capsular contracture.
- Primary OA at the elbow is characterized by pain and lost motion, strength, and, ultimately, function.

ANATOMY

- The elbow is a modified hinge joint composed of the ulnotrochlear, radiocapitellar, and proximal radioulnar articulations.
- The elbow has two planes of motion: flexion and extension in the sagittal plane and pronosupination in the axial plane.
  - Flexion–extension comes from motion at the ulnotrochlear articulation and has normal range of motion of 0 degree of extension to 145 degrees of flexion.
  - Pronosupination is a result of motion at the radiocapitellar and proximal radioulnar articulation and has a normal range of motion of 80 degrees of pronation and 80 degrees of supination.
- Collateral ligamentous complexes are present on the medial and lateral sides of the elbow that—along with the inherent bony geometry—confer static stabilization to the elbow.
  - Lateral collateral ligamentous complex functions as a lateral stabilizer preventing posterolateral rotatory instability (PLRI) and is described as a Y-shaped confluence of three components.
    - Radial collateral ligament—extends from the lateral epicondyle of the humerus to the annular ligament
    - Lateral ulnar collateral ligament—extends from the lateral epicondyle of the humerus to the crista supinatoris of the ulna
    - Annular ligament—forms a ring around the radial neck, extending from the anterior sigmoid notch of the ulna to the crista supinatoris
  - Medial collateral ligament functions as the most important stabilizer to valgus stress and is composed of three components.
    - Anterior oblique ligament—extends from the medial epicondyle of the humerus to the sublime tubercle of the anteromedial facet of the coronoid
    - Posterior oblique ligament—extends from the medial epicondyle of the humerus and fans out to insert along the sigmoid notch
    - Transverse ligament—this thin band extends transversely from the posterior to anterior margin of the sigmoid notch

PATHOGENESIS

- The cause of primary OA is likely multifactorial with hand dominance, history of heavy use, race, and other factors contributing.[2]

NATURAL HISTORY

- Primary OA is a relatively rare condition that commonly affects the dominant arm of middle-aged males who have a history of heavy use due to sports or heavy equipment use.
- The severity of the presentation is variable and dependent on disease progression.
  - Early OA is characterized by pain at terminal extension and flexion with patients frequently complaining of pain with carrying a heavy object with the elbow extended.
  - Radiographically, early disease is characterized by relatively preserved joint space and impinging osteophytes on the margins of anterior and posterior ulnotrochlear articulation as well as radiocapitellar osteophyte formation.
  - Late-stage OA presents with pain throughout the arc of motion with loss of articular cartilage and joint space narrowing.

PATIENT HISTORY AND PHYSICAL FINDINGS

- Primary OA of the elbow is unique amongst OA of other joints, in that the disease severity and anatomic source of pathology allow for a variety of successful treatment options ranging from simple débridement to arthroplasty.

History

- The classic presentation is a middle-aged male with a history of heavy use who presents with symptoms on his dominant side.
- Symptoms may include pain, loss of motion, mechanical symptoms of catching or locking, or weakness.
- When pain is the primary complaint, it is important to understand the degree of disability and impact on the patient's function; identify the anatomic source of pain whether ulnotrochlear, radiocapitellar, or extra-articular; and identify whether pain occurs at the extremes of flexion and/or extension or throughout the arc of motion.
- Patients with predominantly mechanical symptoms may need only arthroscopic débridement.
- In patients who primarily complain of lost motion, it is important to understand the degree to which this affects the patient and whether the lost motion is in flexion, extension, or both.
- Further history that is necessary to evaluate when considering arthroplasty include prior surgeries, history of trauma, history of infection, and the patient's demand level and posttreatment expectations.

Physical Examination

- The physical examination begins with inspection of the skin for prior surgical scars, other wounds, or evidence of infection.
- Flexion and extension as well as pronosupination range of motion should be assessed.
  - It is essential to document at what point in the arc of motion pain is experienced as well as any catching, locking, or other mechanical symptoms.
  - Rotation through the radiocapitellar joint may not generate significant pain or stiffness despite a degenerative appearance radiographically.
- Neurovascular examination specifically focused on evaluation for ulnar nerve compression at the elbow is essential to document.

IMAGING AND OTHER DIAGNOSTIC STUDIES

- Anteroposterior (AP), lateral, and oblique radiographic views are adequate to make the diagnosis of OA.
  - Characteristic findings on plain films include osteophyte and/or loose body formation emanating from the olecranon and coronoid processes and extending into their fossae (**FIG 1**).
  - The radiocapitellar joint may also be affected and demonstrate osteophytes around the radial head.
- Typically, radiographic changes in the ulnotrochlear joint precede those in the radiocapitellar or proximal radioulnar joints.
- Computed tomography (CT) scan with three-dimensional reconstructions may be performed and is especially helpful for localizing osteophytes not well visualized on plain films.
  - Impinging shelf osteophytes within the olecranon, radial, and coronoid fossae are best appreciated on CT and may be missed on plain films.
  - Similarly, CT is helpful for identifying osteophytes in the medial gutter within close proximity to the ulnar nerve.

DIFFERENTIAL DIAGNOSIS

- Posttraumatic arthritis of the elbow
- Rheumatoid or other inflammatory arthropathy
- Chronic septic arthritis
- Crystalline arthropathy
- Haemophilic arthropathy

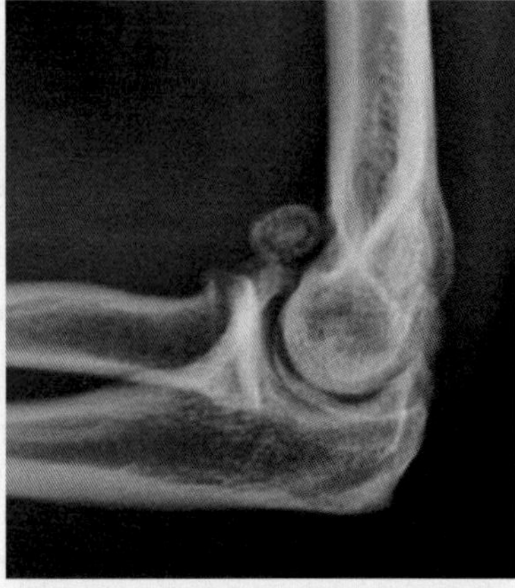

FIG 1 • Lateral x-ray demonstrating osteophyte formation, a loose body, and relatively preserved joint space.

NONOPERATIVE MANAGEMENT

- Nonoperative management is appropriate for the early stages of the disease, when the patient reports mild pain and motion loss of less than 15 degrees.
- Nonoperative treatments include activity modification, nonsteroidal anti-inflammatory drugs, intra-articular corticosteroid injections, and physical therapy.
  - Physical therapy should focus on pain control, anti-inflammatory modalities, and preserving range of motion and strength.
  - Intra-articular injections provide transient relief that is suitable for maintenance therapy.

SURGICAL MANAGEMENT

- Total elbow arthroplasty (TEA) is considered in patients with the following:
  - Disabling elbow OA in patients older than 65 years
    - Mid-arc pain with activity resulting from cartilage loss of the ulnotrochlear joint
  - Willing to comply with low activity levels with their operative extremity
- Prostheses come in several basic designs:
  - Linked prostheses
    - Linked devices have mechanically linked ulnar and humeral components that function as a hinge. Contemporary designs are semiconstrained implants, which about 7 degrees of varus/valgus and rotational laxity at the articulation.
  - Unlinked prostheses
    - Unlinked prostheses have no mechanical connection between the ulnar and humeral components and rely on the ulnar and humeral components' congruence and the capsuloligamentous structures for stability. They have the theoretical benefit of lower bone–cement interface stress leading to less loosening, although clinical data has not yet demonstrated this.
  - Convertible prostheses
    - These implants allow for use in either a linked or unlinked fashion.

Preoperative Planning

- Full-length x-rays of the arm and forearm must be obtained and scrutinized for deformity, prior hardware, or pathologic lesions.
- Preoperative templates are available by many manufacturers and may be used as a guide for intraoperative component selection.
- The condition of the soft tissue must be assessed preoperatively, including prior surgical or traumatic scars. We avoid creating skin bridges of less than 1 cm when there is a prior scar. When any doubt exists about the quality of closure, arrangements should be made preoperatively to have a wound vacuum-assisted closure device available.
- Regional anesthetic infusion through an interscalene catheter is used throughout the perioperative period.

Positioning

- The patient is positioned supine on a standard operating room table.
- A nonsterile tourniquet is applied below the drapes as proximal as possible on the arm.

- The extremity distal to the tourniquet is prepped circumferentially; exposed skin is isolated with the use of an impervious stockinet and an Ioban (3M Health Care, St. Paul, MN) antimicrobial drape.
- The arm is brought over the patient's chest. A padded Mayo stand is brought into the operative field from the patient's contralateral side, and the arm may rest on the Mayo stand during surgery.

Approach

- A roughly 15-cm straight incision with a gentle curve medially around the tip of the olecranon is made and carried down through the subcutaneous tissue to fascia of the forearm and triceps muscle. Wide subcutaneous flaps should be raised over the posterior surface of the elbow and allow for improved exposure and visualization.
- Palpate the ulnar nerve as it lies posterior to the medial epicondyle, dissect it free, and protect it with a vessel loop.
- Mobilize the ulnar nerve from the cubital tunnel, intermuscular septum, and flexor carpi ulnaris aponeurosis to the first motor branch so that it is readily identifiable throughout the case.
- The predominant concern regarding approach to the elbow for TEA is how to manage the triceps. There are three main approaches for dealing with the triceps: triceps-splitting, triceps-reflecting, and triceps-sparing.[1,3]
  - Triceps-splitting (**FIG 2**): Once identified, the triceps tendon is split sharply in its midline from the midpoint of its insertion on the olecranon. Caution should be taken with splitting the triceps proximal to the distal third of the humerus due to the presence of the radial nerve. For further exposure, at the olecranon insertion, the medial and lateral divisions of the triceps are elevated off of the olecranon either subperiosteally or with small wafers of bone. Once the procedure is completed, the triceps is repaired to the olecranon via transosseous sutures if completely elevated. Otherwise, the triceps is repaired side to side with absorbable suture.
  - Triceps-reflecting (**FIG 3**): This approach was described by Bryan and Morrey.[1] The medial border of the triceps is identified and elevated laterally off of the ulna from the intramuscular septum. The antebrachial fascia is incised for about 6 cm distally in line with the medial border of the triceps tendon. The fascia and proximal ulnar periosteum are then elevated from the olecranon, working medially to laterally, maintaining continuity with the triceps. Further subperiosteal dissection is carried out around the lateral surface of the olecranon to elevate the anconeus as well. Once completed, the triceps in continuity with the antebrachial fascia, proximal ulnar periosteum, and anconeus is retracted laterally, exposing the posterior ulnotrochlear and radiocapitellar joints. Once the procedure is completed, the triceps is repaired to the olecranon via transosseous sutures and the sleeve of periosteum and cuff of antebrachial fascia is reapproximated to the intact antebrachial fascia.
  - Triceps-sparing (**FIG 4**): The medial and lateral borders of the triceps are identified and elevated from their intramuscular septa and completely off the posterior surface of the humerus. Laterally, the anconeus is detached from the radial column of the humerus. After release of the collateral ligaments, access to the elbow is gained by delivering the distal humerus through the lateral interval. The proximal ulna is accessed through the medial interval with forearm supination.
- Advocates of the triceps-splitting approach favor this approach for its simplicity. The triceps-reflecting technique has the benefit of even better visualization, although critics argue that both techniques may lead to a potentially higher rate of triceps weakness and risk of postoperative triceps detachment. The triceps-sparing approach is more technically demanding but leaves the triceps intact, reducing associated complications.

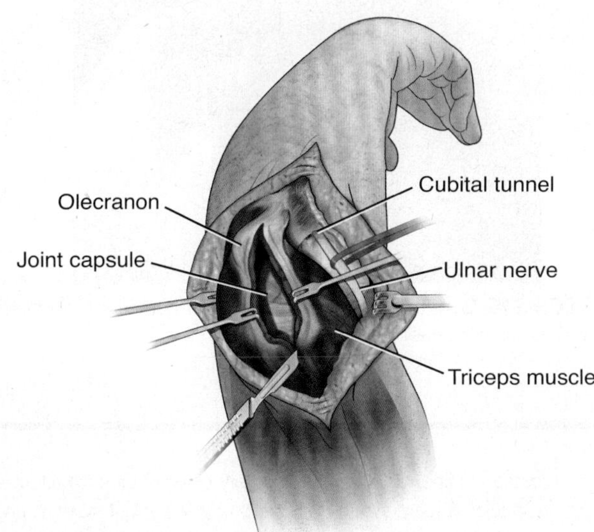

FIG 2 • Triceps-splitting approach: The triceps is split sharply in the midline to the olecranon process where it may be partially detached medially and laterally.

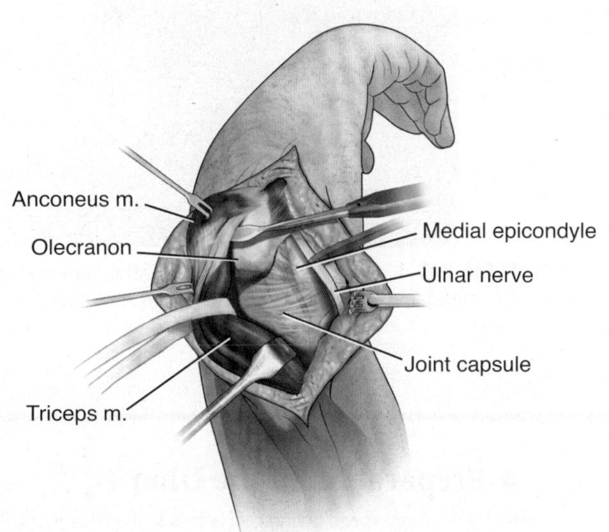

FIG 3 • Triceps-reflecting approach: The triceps in continuity with the antebrachial fascia, proximal ulnar periosteum, and anconeus are elevated and retracted laterally.

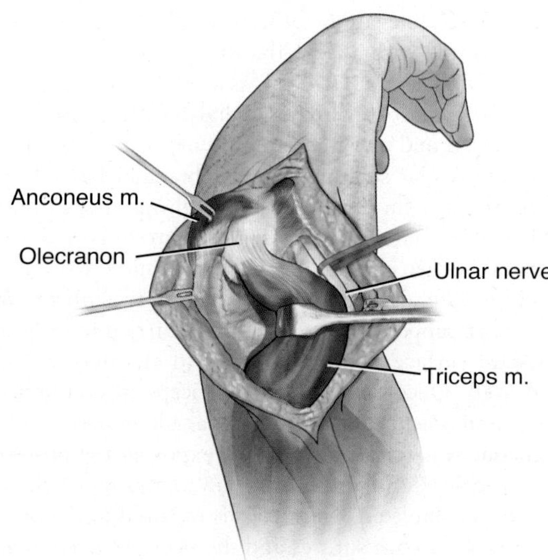

- Regardless of how the triceps is handled, the entire distal humerus must be visualized necessitating the elevation of the collateral ligaments and flexor/pronator and extensor masses from their origins on the medial and lateral epicondyles.
- The elbow may then be dislocated allowing access for bony preparation and prosthesis insertion.

FIG 4 • Triceps-sparing approach: The triceps is elevated from the intermuscular septa and humerus medially and laterally and the anconeus is elevated from the humerus.

TECHNIQUES

Preparation of the Humerus

- With the elbow dislocated and the distal humerus skeletonized, remove a section of bone from the trochlea in line with the midpoint of the olecranon fossa and enough bone should be removed along the proximal extent in order to gain access to the intramedullary canal of the humerus (**TECH FIG 1**).
- Using the humeral medullary canal as a reference point, assemble the distal humeral cutting guide, being careful to ensure neutral rotation in the axial plane. With an oscillating saw, perform the distal humeral cut and save the excised bone for use as bone graft.
- Release the anterior capsule and brachialis along the anterior surface of the humerus proximal to the distal humerus cut. Roughen the anterior surface of the humerus to allow for better incorporation of the bone graft.
- Sequentially rasp the humeral canal to the desired size (**TECH FIG 2**).

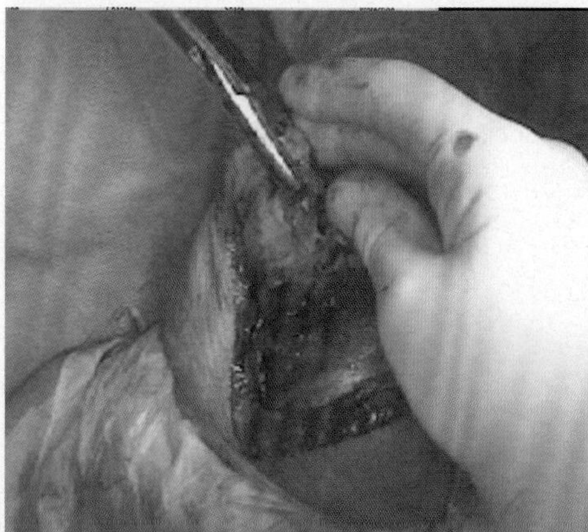

TECH FIG 1 • After skeletonizing, the distal humerus entry into the medullary canal is gained with a rongeur, removing bone from the articular surface in line with the midpoint of the olecranon fossa.

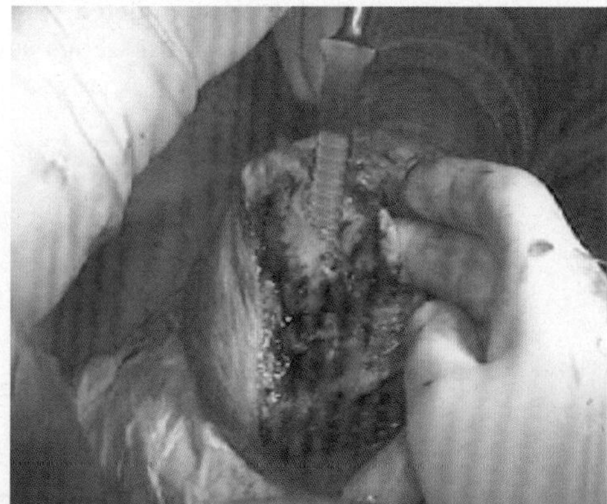

TECH FIG 2 • The medullary canal of the humerus is prepared with rasps of increasing size.

Preparation of the Ulna

- Use a high-speed burr to gain access to the ulnar medullary canal through the chondral surface of the sigmoid notch (**TECH FIG 3**). The proximal inner tip of the olecranon deep to the triceps insertion must be adequately removed such that instruments may be passed in line with the intramedullary canal of the ulna. Flexible cannulated reamers are available on most implant systems and should be used with great care to prevent iatrogenic fracture along the relatively thin ulnar cortex.
- Sequentially rasp the ulnar canal to the desired size (**TECH FIG 4**).

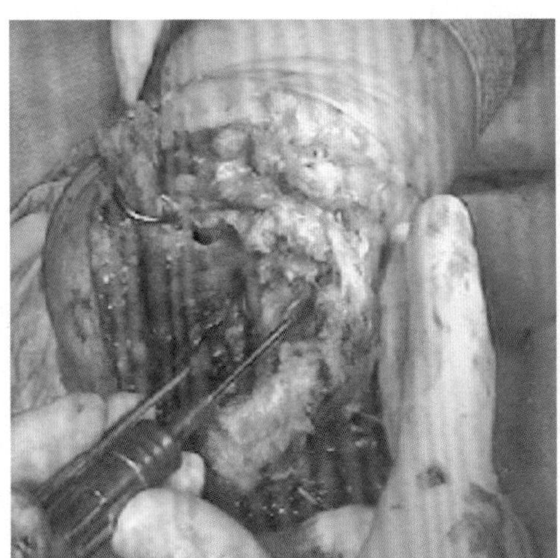

TECH FIG 3 • Entry into the medullary canal of the ulna is gained with a high-speed burr hole through the distal articular surface of the sigmoid notch.

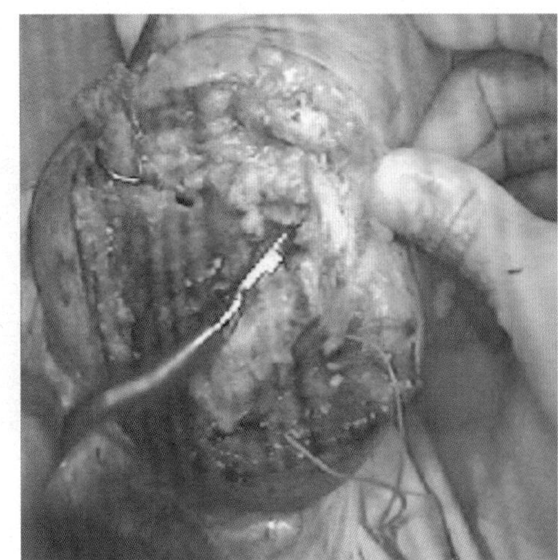

TECH FIG 4 • The medullary canal of the ulna is prepared with rasps of increasing size.

Trial the Components

- The provisional humeral and ulnar components are then inserted.
- The elbow is then reduced, ensuring satisfactory implant placement.
- Range of motion should be assessed. Near full range of motion should be possible with minimal soft tissue tension. Typically, tightness with terminal extension may be addressed by seating either the humeral or ulnar components more deeply. If the radial head has not been resected, ensure that it does not impinge on terminal flexion and forearm rotation. If the radial head causes mechanical impingement, it should be excised. In some implant designs, the radial head may be replaced.
- Examine the reduction for impingement from the radial head, coronoid process, or olecranon process and use a rongeur to resect impinging surfaces.

Component Insertion

- Thoroughly cleanse and dry the humeral and ulnar medullary canals before implant insertion.
- During cementing, use a long-stemmed cement gun to ensure an adequate mantel in the medullary canals (**TECH FIG 5**).
- Fully seat the ulnar implant to the correct depth. Be sure that the rotation of the implant is correct. Typically, the ulnar component will malrotate toward the radius (**TECH FIG 6**).
- A bone graft is placed against the anterior humeral cortex. The humeral component is inserted until the anterior flange engages the bone graft (**TECH FIG 7**).
- If using a linked prosthesis where the components need to be linked prior to seating the implant, engage the linking mechanism prior to fully seating the humeral component (**TECH FIG 8**). Once engaged, fully seat the humeral component.
- Remove excess cement or any impinging bony surfaces.

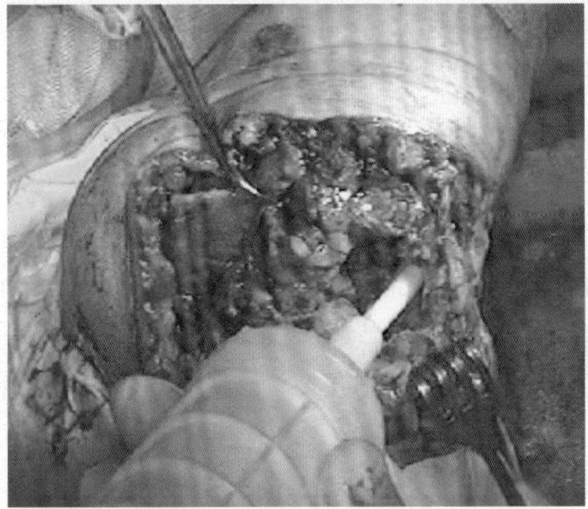

TECH FIG 5 • A long-stemmed cement gun is used to ensure an adequate cement mantle in the ulna and humerus.

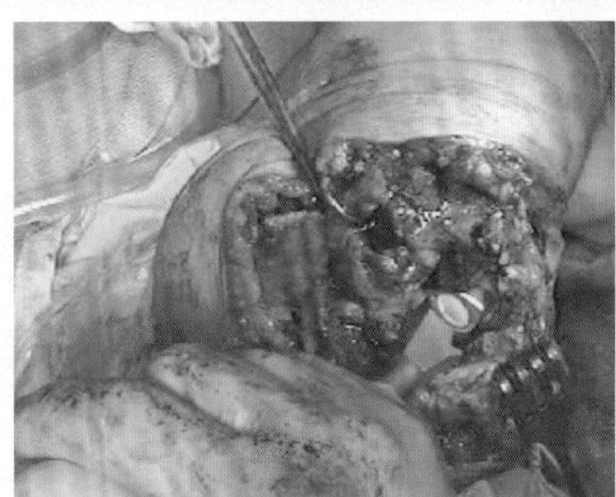

TECH FIG 6 • The ulnar component is seated with gentle mallet blows on its inserter.

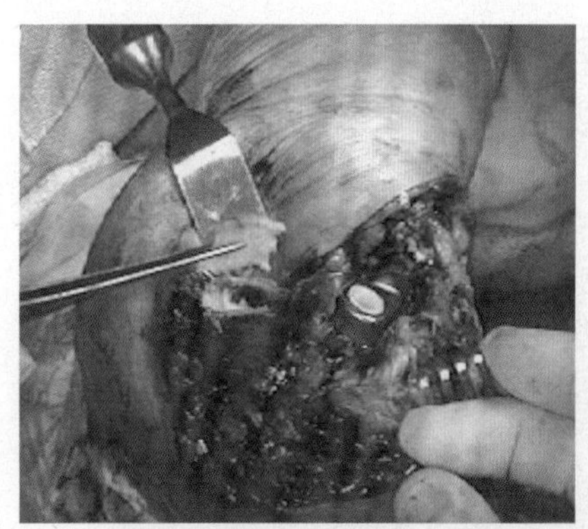

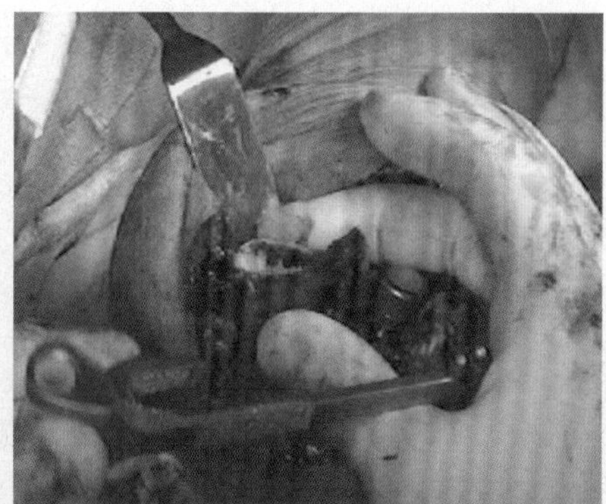

TECH FIG 7 • **A.** A wafer of bone graft from the resected portions of the humerus is contoured to fit along the anterior cortex of the humerus. **B.** The anterior flange of this humeral component seats around the bone graft's position along the anterior cortex.

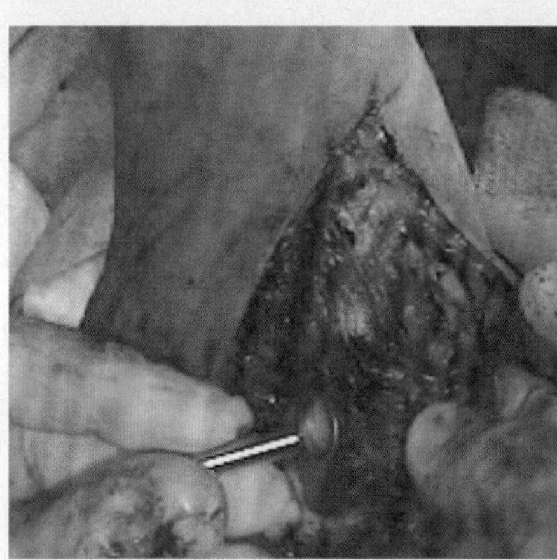

TECH FIG 8 • The ulnar and humeral components are coupled before final seating of the humeral component.

Closure

- Depending on the approach technique, repair the triceps to the olecranon process with nonabsorbable suture.
- We routinely perform an anterior subcutaneous transposition of the ulnar nerve.
- A well-padded anterior splint is placed to maintain the elbow in terminal extension, and instructions are given to elevate the arm as much as possible for the first 1 to 2 weeks. This is thought to minimize skin tension along the incision line, allow for epithelialization to occur, and postoperative edema to subside. The splint should be abundantly padded to prevent pressure necrosis.

PEARLS AND PITFALLS

Wound complications: dehiscence, hematoma formation, drainage, wound infection	■ We emphasize careful and meticulous soft tissue handling. ■ The wound is closed in layers over a drain. ■ The elbow is splinted in a well-padded dressing, in a position of extension to minimize wound tension and allow for epithelialization and edema control.
Infection	■ Antibiotic cement is routinely used.
Ulnar nerve complication	■ Routine transposition of the nerve after it has been carefully isolated and released proximally along the intermuscular septum and distally to the deep fascia of the flexor carpi ulnaris
Aseptic loosening of the prostheses over time	■ Patients should be counseled on permanent activity restrictions.

POSTOPERATIVE CARE

- Sutures are removed 2 weeks following surgery.
- No formal range of motion instructions are imposed following splint removal if the patient had a triceps-sparing approach.
- If the patient had a triceps-reflecting or triceps-splitting approach, then no active extension against resistance is allowed for 8 weeks postoperatively.
- We recommend a lifetime weight-bearing restriction of 5 pounds for the operative extremity.

OUTCOMES

- Results from the Scottish Arthroplasty Project registry identified 1146 primary TEAs of which 108 were performed for primary OA.
  - The 10-year implant survivorship was 85% for TEA for primary OA.[4]
  - Early implant-specific complications rates for all primary TEAs were reported as follows:
    - Infection: 1.9%
    - Dislocation: 0.7%
    - Periprosthetic fracture: 3.1%
- Naqui et al[5] reported on 11 patients with primary OA older than 65 years of age who underwent TEA with the Acclaim (DePuy, Warsaw, IN) convertible prosthesis at an average of 57.6 months.
  - Ten were placed in linked mode and 1 in unlinked.
  - Average arc of motion improved from an average of 70 to 110 degrees, statistically significantly improved American Shoulder and Elbow Surgeons (ASES) scores, and all patients were pain free at rest.
  - There were no cases of loosening, although 4 patients had 1 mm radiolucencies.
  - Complications included 1 patient with an intraoperative periprosthetic fracture and 1 patient with transient ulnar neuritis.

COMPLICATIONS

- Ulnar neuropathy, in the form of paresthesias, is common after this surgery. This condition is usually self-limited and resolves within the first 6 months postoperatively. Careful handling of the ulnar nerve and protecting it from inadvertent stretching or trauma during surgery may minimize these symptoms.
- Infection is one of the most devastating complications after this surgery. The elbow is more prone to infection and wound complications due to its relatively thin soft tissue envelope. Prevention of wound dehiscence and meticulous soft tissue handling are important factors to remember in order to minimize the chance of developing a postoperative infection.
- Aseptic loosening is of greater concern in patients with primary OA than with rheumatoid arthritis given that primary OA patients generally impose higher physical demands on their elbows.
- Strict adherence to postoperative limitations as well as proper implant selection may help limit loosening and early failure. Evolution in implant designs in the future may improve long-term outcomes in this challenging patient population.

REFERENCES

1. Bryan RS, Morrey BF. Extensive posterior exposure of the elbow. A triceps-sparing approach. Clin Orthop Relat Res 1982;166:188–192.
2. Cheung EV, Adams R, Morrey BF. Primary osteoarthritis of the elbow: current treatment options. J Am Acad Orthop Surg 2008;16:77–87.
3. Choo A, Ramsey ML. Total elbow arthroplasty: current options. J Am Acad Orthop Surg 2013;21:427–437.
4. Jenkins PJ, Watts AC, Norwood T, et al. Total elbow replacement: outcome of 1,146 arthroplasties from the Scottish Arthroplasty Project. Acta Orthop 2013;84:119–123.
5. Naqui SZ, Rajpura A, Nuttall D, et al. Early results of the Acclaim total elbow replacement in patients with primary osteoarthritis. J Bone Joint Surg Br 2010;92:668–671.

Surgical Management of Traumatic Conditions of the Elbow: Interposition Arthroplasty

Bernard F. Morrey and Matthew L. Ramsey

DEFINITION AND PATHOGENESIS

- Posttraumatic conditions of the elbow represent a spectrum of disorders involving the elbow as a result of previous trauma. Treatment for posttraumatic conditions is individualized depending on the characteristics of the pathology as well as the functional demands and age of the patient.
  - Posttraumatic arthritis
    - Primary pathology involves posttraumatic degeneration of the articular surface.
    - Secondary pathologies can include contracture, loose bodies, heterotopic bone, and impingement and irritation from retained hardware.
  - Nonunion of the distal humerus
    - May involve all or a part of the articular surface
    - Frequently associated with marked fixed angular and/or rotatory deformity
  - Dysfunctional instability of the elbow
    - Special clinical situation where the fulcrum for stable elbow function is lost
    - Associated with considerable bone loss
    - The forearm may be dissociated from the brachium (**FIG 1**).
  - Chronic instability (dislocation)
    - Chronic ligamentous instability of the elbow can lead to articular degeneration, particularly in the elderly osteopenic patient.
    - Fixed contracture and displacement are characteristic.

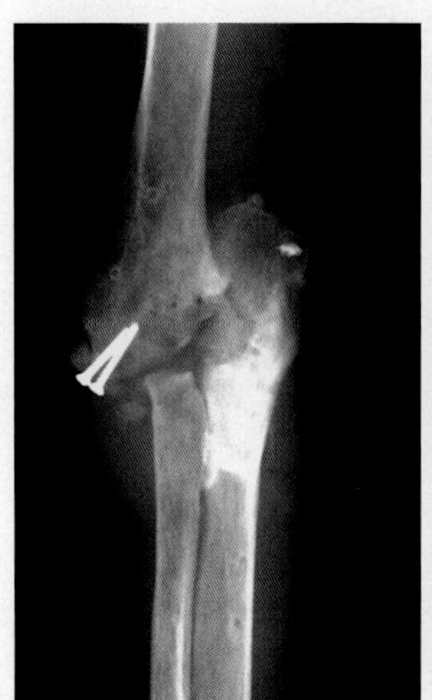
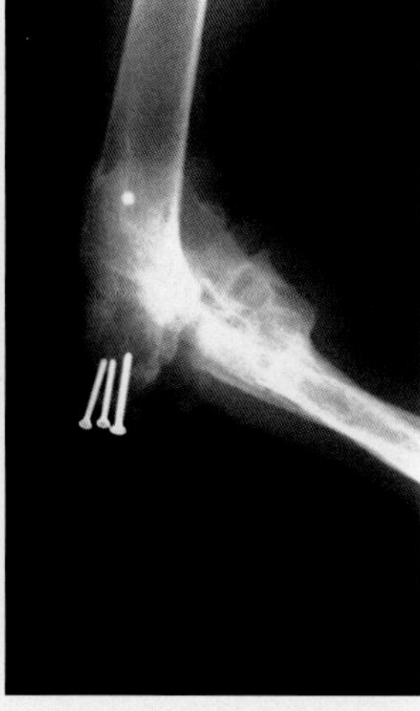

FIG 1 • Radiograph demonstrating dissociation of the forearm from the brachium after four attempts to manage a terrible triad injury. This degree of deformity was not considered amenable to interposition; a total elbow was performed despite the patient's high level of activity.

PATIENT HISTORY AND PHYSICAL FINDINGS

Patient History

- The patient history is directed at gaining information about the initial injury, treatments undertaken, complications of treatment, presenting complaints, and patient expectations.
- Detailed investigation of the patient's symptoms should include questions regarding the degree of pain, presence of instability or stiffness, and mechanical symptoms of catching or locking.
- Presence of radiating pain especially in the ulnar nerve distribution is solicited.
- Special attention is paid to night pain and pain at rest, as these suggest a possibility of sepsis. Note: A history of drainage or any evidence of infection is especially critical to elicit.

Physical Examination

- Physical examination of the elbow should follow a systematic approach.
  - Inspection of the elbow
    - Especially for warmth and redness
    - Presence and location of previous skin incisions or persistent wounds
    - Alignment of the extremity at rest
    - Prominent hardware
  - Range of motion
    - Localization of pain during active and passive motion
    - Active range of motion (AROM) is assessed and compared to the opposite side. The degree of motion, smoothness of motion, and feel of the end point is established.
      - Normal AROM varies but should be symmetric with the opposite unaffected side.
      - Range of motion should be from near full extension (may have hyperextension) to 130 to 140 degrees of flexion.
      - Normal forearm rotation is an arc of 170 degrees, with slightly more supination than pronation.
      - Functional range of motion has been defined as a flexion–extension arc from 30 to 130 degrees and a pronation–supination arc from 50 degrees of pronation to 50 degrees of supination.[10]
    - Passive range of motion (PROM) is then assessed and compared to the active motion arc.
  - Palpation of the elbow
    - Should systematically review all of the bony and soft tissue structures of the elbow

- The ulnar nerve needs to be carefully assessed. If previously surgically manipulated, its location should be identified if possible.
- Examine for the presence of Tinel sign.
- Motor function of the elbow should be assessed. In particular, the flexor (biceps and brachialis) and extensor (triceps) function should be evaluated.

IMAGING AND OTHER DIAGNOSTIC STUDIES

Plain X-rays

- Orthogonal views of the elbow are mandatory.
- A good lateral radiograph can typically be obtained.
- A useful anteroposterior (AP) radiograph can be difficult to obtain, particularly if the patient has a significant flexion contracture.
  - Note: If difficulty is encountered, use fluoroscopic guidance to obtain proper orientation.
- Oblique radiographs can be helpful in obtaining more detail.

Advanced Imaging

- Computed tomography (CT) scan
  - CT scans are particularly helpful in assessing the integrity of the bone and establishing whether the joint space is reasonably preserved.
  - Three-dimensional reconstructions provide a better understanding of complex osseous injuries (**FIG 2**).
- Magnetic resonance imaging (MRI)
  - MRI is rarely needed in the assessment of a posttraumatic joint and is therefore used sparingly.
  - May be helpful to assess suspicious and atypical soft tissue deformity or swelling

DIFFERENTIAL DIAGNOSIS

- Nonunion/malunion of the distal humerus
- Posttraumatic stiffness of the elbow
- Chronic dislocation of the elbow

NONOPERATIVE MANAGEMENT

- The success of nonoperative management depends on specific features of the pathology and the motivation and goals of the patient.
- Activity modification in order to reduce the forces across the elbow

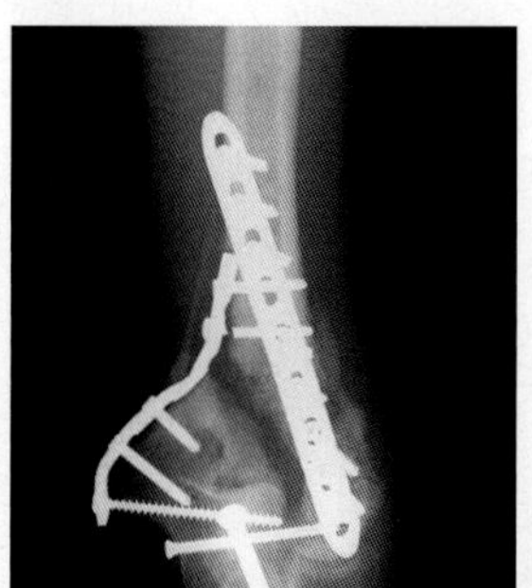
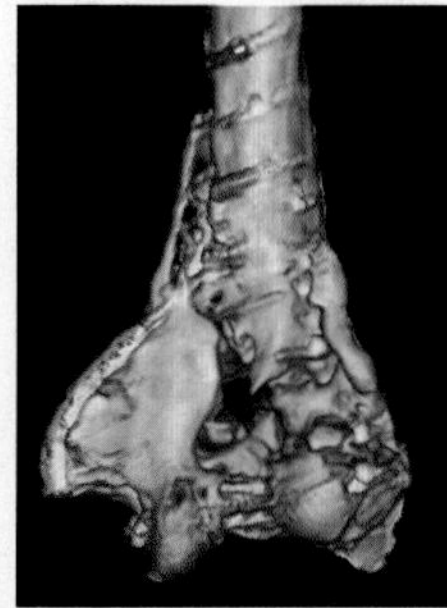

FIG 2 • **A.** Complex injury with unclear joint pathology or state of healing. **B.** The 3-D reconstruction clarifies the extent of the problem.

- Maintain range of motion of the elbow. Aggressive efforts to regain lost motion can inflame and thus aggravate the joint.
- External bracing is occasionally used to support an unstable extremity. However, in general, bracing is poorly tolerated and functionally limiting.

SURGICAL MANAGEMENT

- Surgical management is directed at addressing the underlying cause of disability, taking into consideration the patients age, pathology, physical requirements, and expectations.

Indications

- Age and functional need prompt consideration of this intervention.
- Age is a surrogate for activity.
  - In general, patients younger than age 55 years are always candidates for interposition—all else being equal.
  - Those older than age 70 years with similar pathology are usually better candidates for replacement.
- Patients with pain and/or loss of range of motion who have failed nonoperative management
- Posttraumatic arthritis in patients who are either too young for total elbow arthroplasty (TEA) or who are unwilling to accept the functional restrictions with TEA
- The patients who do best following interposition are those with painful loss of motion when there is no requirement for aggressive, heavy use of the extremity.

Contraindications

- Active or subacute infection (septic arthritis with persistent infection)[8]
- Grossly unstable elbow
- Marked angular deformity (exceeding 15 degrees)
- Inadequate bone stock
- Patients unable or unwilling to follow postoperative instructions
- Inexperience with the technique
- Pain at rest or pain without associated functional loss (relative contraindication)

Preoperative Planning

- Graft options
  - Allograft Achilles tendon[7]: has the advantage of no donor site morbidity
    - The abundance of the tissue allows for variable thickness depending on reconstructive need.
    - Can also be used to reconstruct the collateral ligaments if necessary
  - Autogenous dermis or fascia lata
    - Best used for limited applications (eg capitellum)
  - Allograft dermal tissue
- An articulated (hinged) external fixator must be available.

Patient Positioning

- Supine with the arm across the chest and bump under the ipsilateral shoulder (**FIG 3**)[8]
- Alternatively, the lateral decubitus position with the arm over an arm holder

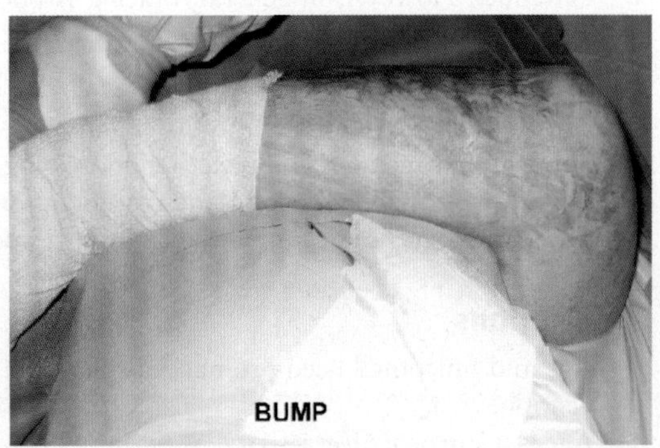

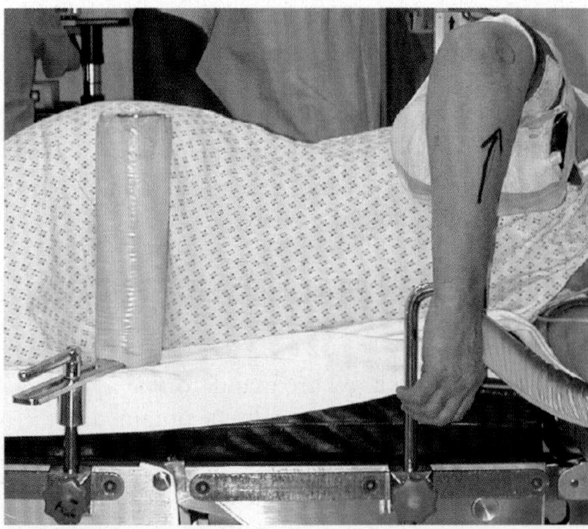

FIG 3 • **A.** Patient is placed in the supine position and the arm is brought across the chest and is supported with a bolster. **B.** Alternative lateral decubitus position with the arm maintained over an arm support.

Interposition Arthroplasty

Surgical Technique[2,7,8]

- Use a posterior skin incision or the posterior most prior incision. Develop medial and lateral subcutaneous flaps. These flaps should be as thick as possible, reflecting from the fascial margin (**TECH FIG 1A,B**).
- Isolate and mobilize the ulnar nerve from the cubital tunnel. Note: We do not routinely transpose an asymptomatic nerve. If stable, it is returned to its anatomic location.
- Deep exposure to the elbow is performed through an extensile Kocher approach (**TECH FIG 1C**).[9]
- The common extensor group is mobilized from the anterior capsule and released proximally with the extensor carpi radialis longus.
- The lateral ulnar collateral ligament is isolated and released from its humeral origin. An anterior and posterior capsular release is performed.
- The triceps can be partially released from the ulna to allow the triceps–anconeus composite to be mobilized. This is sometimes called the *Mayo modification* of the Kocher approach. The lateral aspect of the triceps attachment to the ulna is mobilized and reflected (**TECH FIG 1D**).[11]
- Retracting on the lateral margin of the triceps attachment, flexion of the elbow and supination of the forearm allows the ulna to be rotated off the humerus as it pivots on the intact medial collateral ligament (**TECH FIG 1E**).
- Attempts are made to leave the medial collateral ligament intact as it will improve postoperative stability.
- The cartilage surfaces are inspected.
  - If more than 50% of the articular surface is involved, surgery proceeds to interposition.
- The distal humerus is reshaped to conform to the olecranon. The cartilage is removed from the distal humerus and the bone is smoothed, but aggressive resection of bone is avoided.
- If the distal humerus has architectural changes prompting a varus or valgus joint line, this is corrected.
- The interposition tissue is prepared. The graft of choice is up to the surgeon. However, there is a growing experience with allograft Achilles tendon. In addition to being a robust graft source, it allows for reconstruction of one or both collateral ligaments (**TECH FIG 1F**).

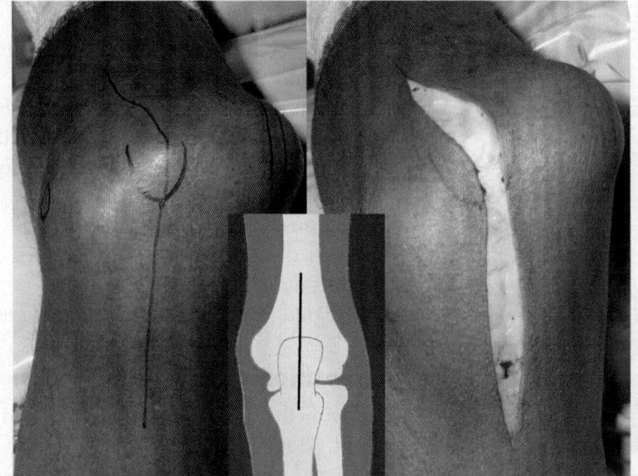

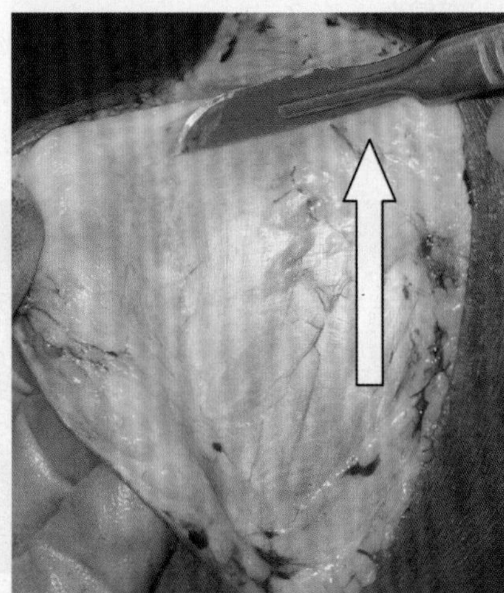

TECH FIG 1 • **A.** Extensile Kocher approach to the lateral elbow. **B.** Subcutaneous flaps are elevated on the fascia allowing identification of Kochers interval and the lateral triceps attachment to the ulna (*arrow*) *(continued)*

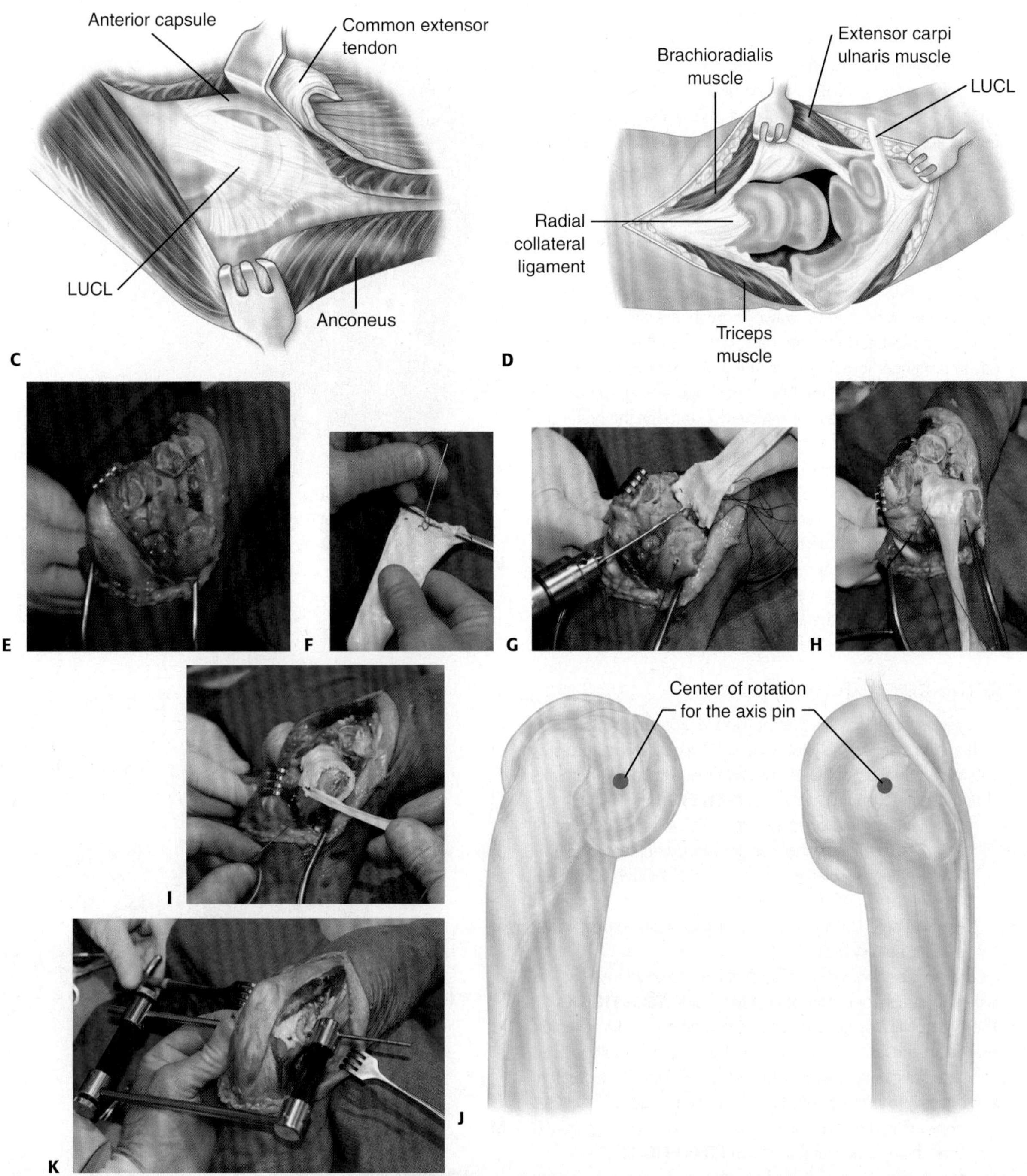

TECH FIG 1 • *(continued)* **C.** The anconeus and triceps are elevated off of the posterolateral capsule whereas the common extensor group is elevated off of the anterior capsule. Exposure can be expanded posteriorly with partial release of the triceps from the lateral aspect of the olecranon. **D.** Deep extensile exposure requires release of the lateral collateral ligament and anterior and posterior capsule. **E.** The released lateral margin of the triceps attachment is retracted. With flexion and supination, the joint is exposed. **F.** The interposition membrane is prepared with mattress sutures placed distally. The Achilles tendon allograft also permits reconstruction of the collateral ligaments if necessary. **G.** Drill holes are placed from posterior to anterior across the supracondylar region to align with the graft as much as possible. **H.** The interposition membrane is secured to the distal humerus. **I.** If necessary the graft can be fashioned to reconstruct the collateral ligaments. **J.** Drawing demonstrating the center of rotation on the lateral and medial side of the elbow. **K.** A stylus is impacted into the axis of rotation using the axis target guide. *(continued)*

- Four nonabsorbable no. 1 sutures are placed in the graft.
  - Note: If the Achilles is used, care is taken to ensure the rough side is applied to the humerus and the smooth side exposed to articulate with the ulna.
- Typically, four drill holes are placed across the supracondylar region from posterior to anterior (**TECH FIG 1G**). These drill holes are placed at the medial aspect of the trochlea, above the trochlear sulcus, at the lateral margin of the trochlea, and at the lateral aspect of the capitellum.
  - Note: Care is taken to align the drill holes with the sutures placed in the graft.
- The interposition tissue is then draped over the distal humerus and secured with sutures drawn through the drill holes from anterior to posterior. They are passed through the graft posteriorly in a manner to tightly apply the graft to the distal humerus and tied (**TECH FIG 1H**). The medial and lateral sutures are first secured, followed by the middle two, through the graft from front to back. If there is collateral ligament insufficiency, the tails of graft (especially when using Achilles tendon) can be fashioned to reconstruct the collateral ligaments (**TECH FIG 1I**).
- The radial head is left intact, especially if medial collateral ligament reconstruction is performed, in order to contribute to the valgus stability of the elbow.
- The lateral collateral ligament is repaired through drill holes at the center of rotation laterally. The ligament is not tied until the external fixator is securely applied.

Hinged Elbow External Fixator

- A hinged external fixator is then applied to protect the interposed graft and to stabilize the joint while soft tissue healing occurs.
- The axis of rotation of the elbow is defined by bony landmarks about the lateral and medial joint (**TECH FIG 1J**).
  - The center of rotation at the lateral elbow is the center point of an arc defined by the articular surface of the capitellum.
  - The center of rotation at the medial elbow is defined by a tightly distributed instantaneous centers of rotation approximated by a point at the anteroinferior aspect of the medial epicondyle.
- An axis pin is established coincident with the center of rotation. This is the foundation for construction of the fixator (**TECH FIG 1K**).
- The type of fixator used dictates the method of pin insertion relative to the axis pin. We prefer the simple laterally placed half-pin configuration, as it has been proven in the laboratory and clinically to provide sufficient stability and rigidity.[4,6]
  - Pins in the proximal humerus are placed no more proximal that the epitrochlear dimension (**TECH FIG 1L**).[5]
- The two 4-mm humeral threaded half-pins are inserted under direct vision and protected with a trocar.
- The humeral side bar is attached with universal couplers.
- The axis pin is removed as the orientation of the fixator is now defined (**TECH FIG 1M**).
- Ulnar pins are introduced with a trocar and placed along the posterolateral aspect of the ulna.
- The joint is reduced and ligament reconstruction, if necessary, is completed.
- With the joint reduced, the fixator is linked to the ulnar pins, and all fitting are secured.
- Two 3 mm of distraction is created with the device.
- If properly placed, near-normal motion is possible (**TECH FIG 1N**).

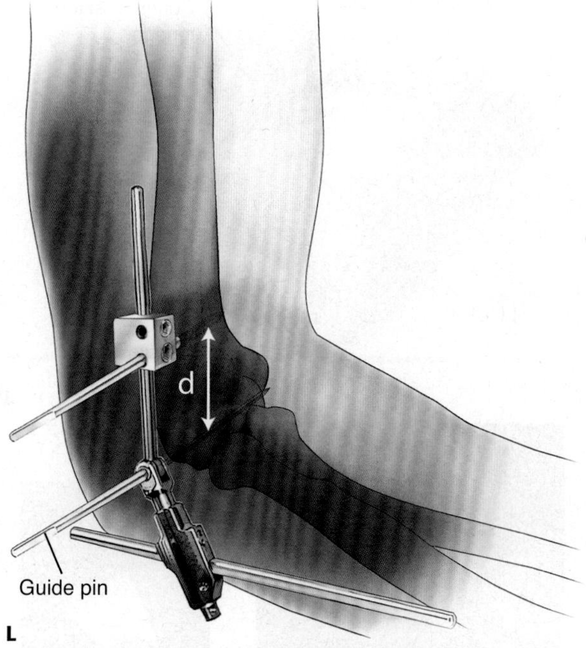

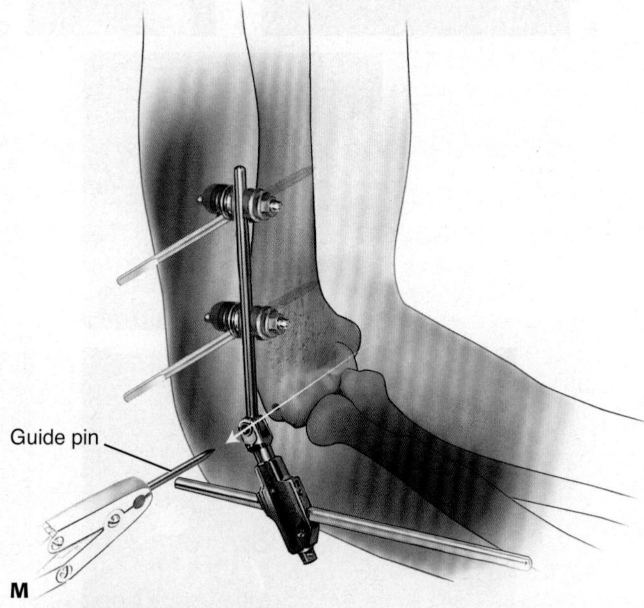

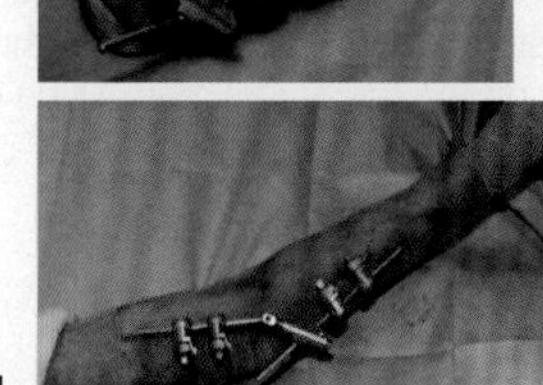

TECH FIG 1 • *(continued)* **L.** The distal humeral pin is placed less than one humeral width dimension proximal to the axis to avoid injury to the radial nerve. **M.** Once the humeral pins are secured, the axis pin is removed. **N.** When properly applied, a markedly functional extension (*top*) and flexion (*bottom*) arc is possible.

PEARLS AND PITFALLS

Indications	■ Interposition arthroplasty is considered in patients with a stable elbow and a limited, painful range of motion. ■ TEA is considered in carefully selected patients where other nonoperative and operative measures have been exhausted.
Goals of treatment	■ Regardless of the treatment undertaken, the goal of treatment is a pain-free, functional arc of motion.
Interposition arthroplasty	■ Predictors of poor outcome ■ Painful, mobile elbow ■ Preoperative instability ■ Fixed deformity ■ Need to reconstruct both the medial collateral ligament and lateral ulnar collateral ligament at the time of interposition ■ Maintain the fixator for 3–4 weeks (do not exceed 6 weeks). ■ Meticulous pin care is required.

POSTOPERATIVE MANAGEMENT

- Range of motion is started as quickly as allowed by the condition of the soft tissues. In general, immediate motion is preferred. However, the prerequisite is a quiet soft tissue envelope. Range of motion may be assisted with a continuous passive motion machine if desired.
- Patients are taught pin care that is performed daily at home.
- Patients are seen at 10 to 14 days postoperatively for staple removal and wound check and every 2 weeks thereafter until pin removal.
- The external fixator is left in place for approximately 3 to 4 weeks and then removed in the operating room (OR) with assessment of elbow stability and motion under anesthesia.
  - Note: At the time of pin removal, access the elbow for stability and smoothness of the flexion arc. We then stretch the arc to regain the flexion and extension arc obtained at the time of surgery.
- Rehabilitation is continued with concentration on obtaining a functional range of motion.

OUTCOMES

- The most predictable results for interposition occur in patients presenting with the following[2,7–9,12]:
  - Stiffness and pain preoperatively
  - Stable elbow
  - One or no ligament reconstruction required at surgery
  - Less than 15 degrees of angular deformity preoperatively
- Poor results noted when
  - Pain, especially pain at rest, is the only presenting complaint
  - Unstable elbow
  - Need to reconstruct both the medial and lateral collateral ligaments at the time of interposition
  - Fixed angular deformity exceeding 15 degrees; rotatory deformity
- Most studies report 70% satisfaction rate among patients with respect to pain relief, and 80% of patients regain a functional range of motion.[9]
  - Cheng and Morrey[2] found 67% of patients treated for rheumatoid arthritis (RA) had satisfactory relief of pain and 75% of patients treated for osteoarthritis (OA) were satisfied at 5-year follow-up. Those with functional arcs of motion did less well than the stiff joint.
  - Larson and Morrey[7] reported 88% of patients would repeat the procedure with a mean surveillance of 8 years.

COMPLICATIONS

- Complications of interposition arthroplasty include the following:
  - Instability
  - Infection
  - Ulnar neuropathy
  - Resorptive bone loss
  - Heterotopic bone formation
- Complications related to the external fixator include the following[3]:
  - Superficial pin tract infections
  - Deep infection (osteomyelitis)
  - Pin breakage
  - Note: Complications with external fixators are statistically correlated to prolonged period of application.[3]
- Complications for the overall procedure have been reported to occur in up to 25% of patients.[7,9]

Revision

- The salvage for a failed interposition arthroplasty is a TEA.[1]
- Interposition arthroplasty should not be undertaken unless the surgeon is comfortable performing a total elbow replacement in the face of failure.

REFERENCES

1. Blaine TA, Adams R, Morrey BF. Total elbow arthroplasty after interposition arthroplasty for elbow arthritis. J Bone Joint Surg Am 2005;87(2):286–292.
2. Cheng SL, Morrey BF. Treatment of the mobile, painful arthritic elbow by distraction interposition arthroplasty. J Bone Joint Surg Br 2000;82(2):233–238.
3. Cheung EV, O'Driscoll SW, Morrey BF. Complications of hinged external fixators of the elbow. J Shoulder Elbow Surg 2008;17(3):447–453.
4. Cobb TK, Morrey BF. Use of distraction arthroplasty in unstable fracture dislocations of the elbow. Clin Orthop Relat Res 1995;(312): 201–210.

5. Kamineni S, Ankem H, Patten DK. Anatomic relationship of the radial nerve to the elbow joint: clinical implications of safe pin placement. Clin Anat 2009;22(6):684–688.
6. Kamineni S, Hirahara H, Neale P, et al. Effectiveness of the lateral unilateral dynamic external fixator after elbow ligament injury. J Bone Joint Surg Am 2007;89(8):1802–1809.
7. Larson AN, Morrey BF. Interposition arthroplasty with an Achilles tendon allograft as a salvage procedure for the elbow. J Bone Joint Surg Am 2008;90(12):2714–2723.
8. Morrey BF. Interposition arthroplasty. In: Morrey BF, Sanchez-Sotelo J, eds. The Elbow and Its Disorders, ed 4. Philadelphia: Saunders Elsevier, 2009:935–948.
9. Morrey BF. Post-traumatic contracture of the elbow. Operative treatment, including distraction arthroplasty. J Bone Joint Surg Am 1990;72(4):601–618.
10. Morrey BF, Askew LJ, Chao EY. A biomechanical study of normal functional elbow motion. J Bone Joint Surg Am 1981;63(6):872–877.
11. Morrey BF, Morrey MC. Exposure of the elbow. In: Morrey BF, Morrey MC, eds. Masters Techniques in Orthopaedic Surgery: Relevant Surgical Exposures. Totowa, NJ: Lippincott Williams & Wilkins, 2008.
12. Nolla J, Ring D, Lozano-Calderon S, et al. Interposition arthroplasty of the elbow with hinged external fixation for post-traumatic arthritis. J Shoulder Elbow Surg 2008;17(3):459–464.

103 CHAPTER

Arthroplasty for Posttraumatic Conditions of the Elbow

Matthew L. Ramsey

DEFINITION

- Posttraumatic conditions of the elbow represent a variety of disorders involving the elbow as a result of previous injury. Included among the posttraumatic conditions are as follows:
  - Posttraumatic arthritis
    - Primary pathology involves posttraumatic degeneration of the articular surface.
    - Secondary pathologies can include contracture, loose bodies, and heterotopic bone.
  - Nonunion of the distal humerus
    - Present with different amounts of bone loss and instability through the nonunion
    - Often results from inadequate internal fixation of distal humerus fractures and typically occurs in the supracondylar region
    - Total elbow arthroplasty (TEA) is considered when reconstruction of the nonunion is deemed impossible or undesirable.
  - Dysfunctional instability of the elbow
    - Special clinical situation where the fulcrum for stable elbow function is lost.[15] The forearm is dissociated from the brachium with the forearm displaced medially and contracted proximally (**FIG 1**). This leads to attenuation of the lateral soft tissues and contracture of the medial soft tissues.
  - Chronic instability (dislocation)
    - Chronic ligamentous instability of the elbow can lead to progressive articular cartilage degeneration and subchondral bone loss, particularly in the elderly, osteopenic patient.
- Treatment for posttraumatic conditions is individualized, depending on the underlying pathology as well as the functional demands and age of the patient.

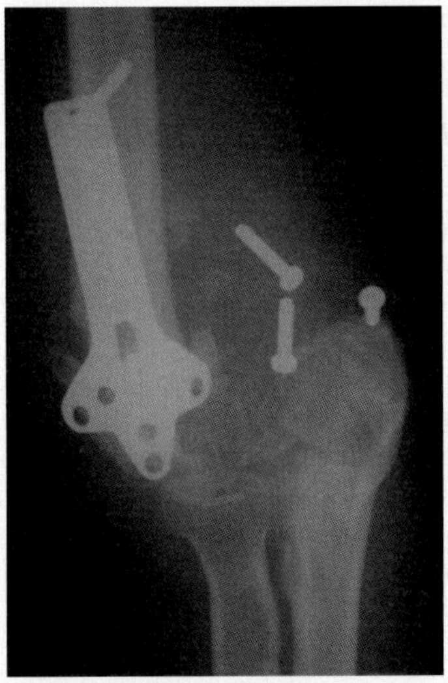

FIG 1 • Radiograph demonstrating dissociation of the forearm from the brachium in a patient with an inadequately treated fracture of the distal humerus with resultant nonunion.

ANATOMY

- The anatomy in posttraumatic conditions can vary widely. The integrity of the bone stock of the distal humerus, proximal ulna, and radial head must be evaluated. In addition, the soft tissue constraints that contribute to stability of the elbow need to be assessed.
  - Posttraumatic arthritis involving only the articular surface maintains the integrity of the regional architecture of the joint. There may be associated soft tissue contracture leading to functional limitation.
  - Nonunion of the distal humerus results in variable deformity. More severe deformity can result in loss of overall alignment of the arm with associated soft tissue contracture.
  - Dysfunctional instability of the elbow typically results from nonunion of the distal humerus, traumatic bone loss, or surgical excision of variable portions of the distal humerus. By definition, the anatomic relationship of the elbow is disrupted, resulting in dynamic or static dissociation of the forearm from the brachium (**FIG 2**).

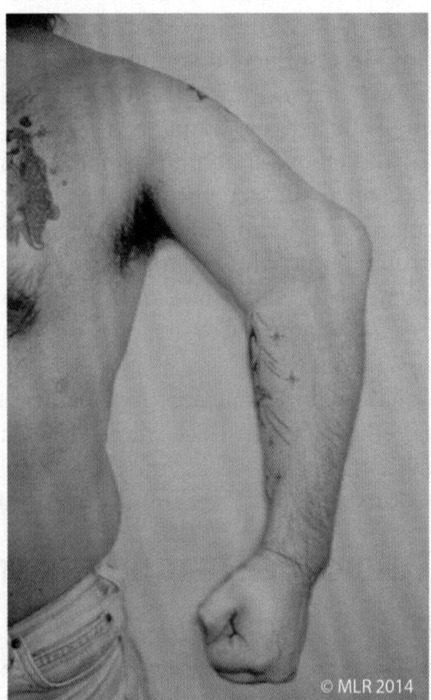

FIG 2 • Photograph of a patient with dysfunctional instability of the elbow. Notice the prominent distal humerus and proximal migration of the forearm medial to the distal humerus.

- Chronic instability of the elbow can result from a persistently unstable elbow following dislocation with or without associated fracture. The articular surface is compromised by the initial injury or persistent instability.

PATHOGENESIS

- The common pathogenesis of all posttraumatic conditions is an injury to the elbow that compromises the integrity of the articular surface with or without nonarticular involvement of the humerus, ulna, or radius.
- The articular surface can be directly injured by trauma or can degenerate over time as a result of a remote traumatic event.
- Periarticular trauma and hemorrhage involving the capsule and musculotendinous tissues about the elbow can lead to intra-articular and periarticular fibrosis leading to intrinsic and extrinsic stiffness of the elbow.

PATIENT HISTORY AND PHYSICAL FINDINGS

Patient History

- The patient history is directed at gaining information about the initial injury, treatments undertaken, complications of treatment, presenting complaints, and patient expectations.
- Detailed investigation of the patient's symptoms should include questions regarding the degree of pain, presence of instability or stiffness, and mechanical symptoms of catching or locking.

Physical Examination

- Inspection of the elbow
  - Presence and location of previous skin incisions or persistent wounds
  - Alignment of the extremity at rest and with attempted motion
  - Prominent hardware
- Range of motion
  - Active range of motion (AROM) is assessed and compared to the opposite side. The degree of motion, smoothness of motion, and feel of the end point is established.
  - Passive range of motion (PROM) is then assessed and compared to the active motion arc.
- Palpation of the elbow should systematically review all of the bony and soft tissue structures of the elbow.
- Neurovascular examination should carefully assess motor and sensory function of the extremity.
  - The ulnar nerve needs to be carefully assessed. If previously surgically manipulated, its location should be identified if possible.
  - A functional requirement for consideration of TEA is functional elbow flexion (biceps and brachialis muscles). Functional extension (triceps muscle) is less critical than active flexion but should be carefully assessed.

IMAGING AND OTHER DIAGNOSTIC STUDIES

Plain X-rays

- Orthogonal views of the elbow are required (**FIG 3**).
  - A good lateral radiograph can usually be obtained except in cases of severe deformity.
  - If there is a significant flexion contracture, it can be difficult to obtain a useful anteroposterior (AP) radiograph. Inability to obtain a proper AP radiograph will typically result in overestimating the amount of joint destruction.
- Oblique radiographs supplement the AP and lateral images.

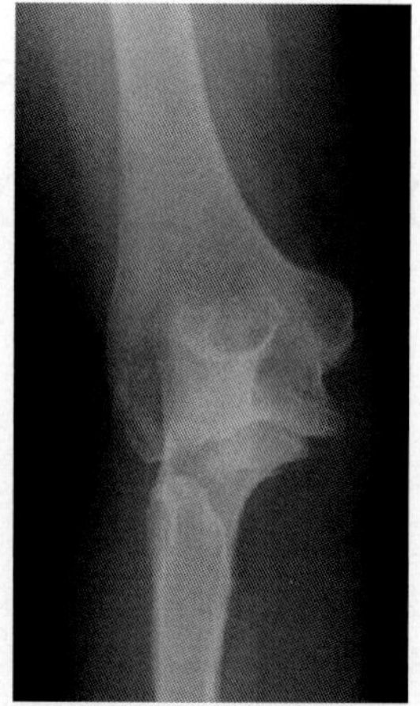

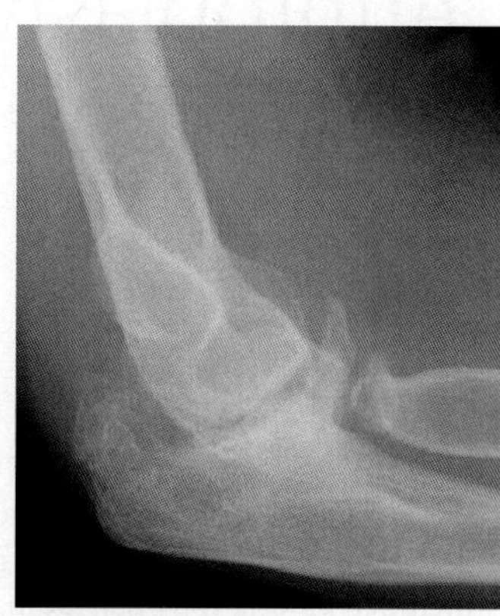

FIG 3 • A,B. AP and lateral radiographs of the elbow in a patient with posttraumatic arthritis of the elbow.

Advanced Imaging

- Computed tomography (CT) scan
  - CT scans are particularly helpful in assessing the structural integrity of the humerus, radius, and ulna.
  - Identifying the presence of periarticular deformity and the integrity of the articulations are facilitated by CT scan.
  - Three-dimensional reconstructions provide a better understanding of any deformity.
- Magnetic resonance imaging (MRI)
  - MRI is rarely needed in the assessment of a posttraumatic joint.

DIFFERENTIAL DIAGNOSIS

- Nonunion/malunion of the distal humerus
- Posttraumatic stiffness of the elbow
- Chronic dislocation of the elbow
- Traumatic bone loss or surgical excision of bone leading to instability

NONOPERATIVE MANAGEMENT

- The success of nonoperative management depends on specific features of the pathology and the motivation and goals of the patient.
- Activity modification attempts to reduce the forces across the elbow.
- Overly aggressive attempts to maintain range of motion of the elbow, although commendable, can cause inflammation that is counterproductive to improved motion.
- External bracing is occasionally used to support an unstable extremity. However, in general, bracing is poorly tolerated and functionally limiting.

SURGICAL MANAGEMENT

- Surgical management is directed at addressing the underlying cause of disability, taking into consideration the patient's age, physical requirements, and expectations.

Total Elbow Replacement

- Patients with posttraumatic conditions of the elbow tend to be younger than other patients undergoing TEA.[4–6,11,14,15,17]
- In this group of patients, TEA should be considered in patients who
  - Have failed appropriate nonoperative management
  - Are not an appropriate candidate for other surgical options
  - Are willing to adopt a more sedentary lifestyle
  - Have no absolute contraindications to the procedure

Preoperative Planning

Implant Selection

- Implants are described in terms of their physical linkage (linked, unlinked, or linkable) and on their constraint (constrained, semiconstrained, minimally constrained).
  - Linkage is determined by whether the components are physically joined.
  - Constraint is a more poorly defined quality of an implant. It depends on the geometry of the implant and its interaction with stabilizing soft tissues about the elbow.[8]
- Linked (semiconstrained) designs
  - Linked implants have the advantage of being universally applicable to all posttraumatic conditions of the elbow.
- Unlinked designs
  - The requirement for the use of unlinked designs in posttraumatic conditions of the elbow is integrity of the collateral ligaments and limited deformity such that normal anatomic relationships can be reestablished.
- Linkable designs
  - Linkable designs have been developed to take advantage of the features of an unlinked implant while capturing the universal applicability of the linked implants. They can be converted from unlinked to linked either at the time of an initial surgery if stability cannot be conferred or remotely if instability becomes an issue postoperatively.

Positioning

- Patients are placed supine on the operating table with a bump under the ipsilateral shoulder. The arm should be freely mobile through the shoulder to allow manipulation of the joint throughout surgery. The arm can then be placed across the body on a bump or externally rotated through the shoulder and flexed at the elbow (**FIG 4**).

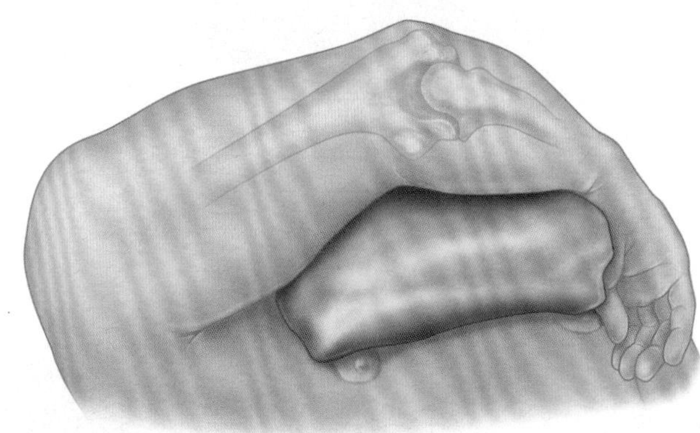

FIG 4 • Patient positioning for TEA with the arm across the body supported on a bolster.

TECHNIQUES

Surgical Approach

- A straight posterior skin incision placed off of the medial aspect of the olecranon is preferred. Previous incisions may modify the location of the incision. Regardless of the incision used, deep access to the medial and lateral aspect of the joint is required.
- The ulnar nerve is identified. If not previously transposed, the nerve is transposed anteriorly. If the nerve was previously transposed, it only needs to be identified but not formally dissected unless the position of the nerve places it at risk during surgery.

Triceps Management

- Triceps-reflecting approaches are preferred over triceps-sparing approaches for posttraumatic conditions. Posttraumatic scarring and deformity can make a triceps-sparing approach difficult unless a nonunited distal humeral segment is to be resected.
- A Bryan-Morrey approach is typically performed[12] (**TECH FIG 1**). The medial aspect of the triceps is developed proximally, whereas the interval between the anconeus and flexor carpi ulnaris (FCU) is developed distal to the olecranon. The triceps is reflected from medially to laterally in continuity with the anconeus. Release of the lateral collateral ligament (LCL) and medial collateral ligament (MCL) completes the exposure and allows separation of the ulna from the humerus.
- The modification of the Bryan-Morrey approach involves release of the triceps insertion onto the ulna through an extra-articular osteotomy of the dorsal tip of the ulna[19] (**TECH FIG 2**). The rationale for this modification relates to the recognized complication of triceps insufficiency that occurs with soft tissue release of the triceps.[1] The osteotomy affords several potential advantages.
  - Bone-to-bone healing of the osteotomy is more reliable than soft tissue healing of the triceps to the ulna.
  - Failure of the osteotomy to heal can be identified radiographically and addressed early.

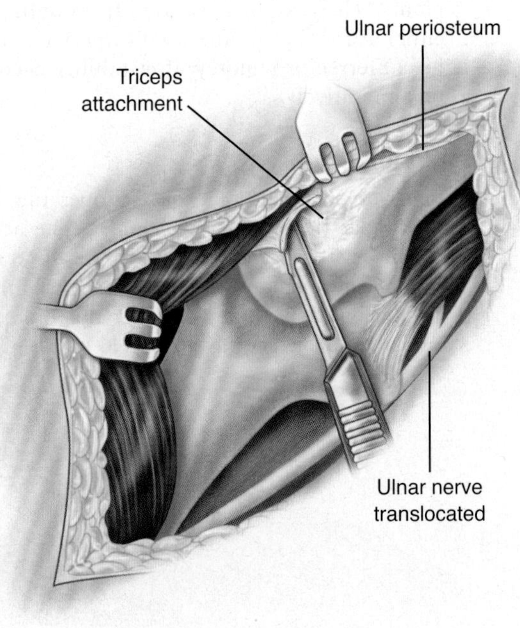

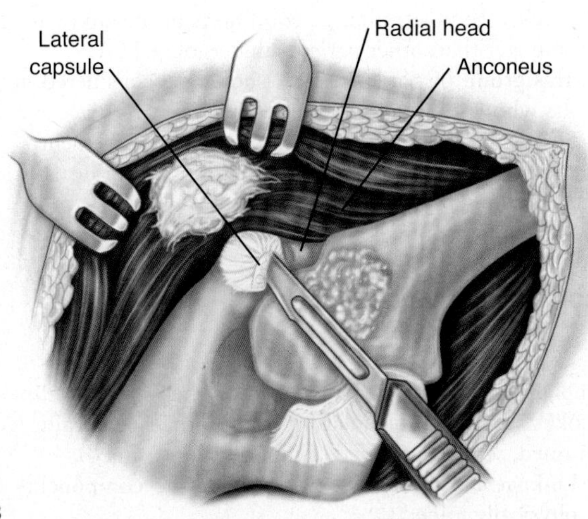

TECH FIG 1 • Bryan-Morrey triceps-reflecting approach. **A.** The triceps insertion is released in continuity with the anconeus from medial to lateral. **B.** Further dissection allows the collateral ligaments to be released.

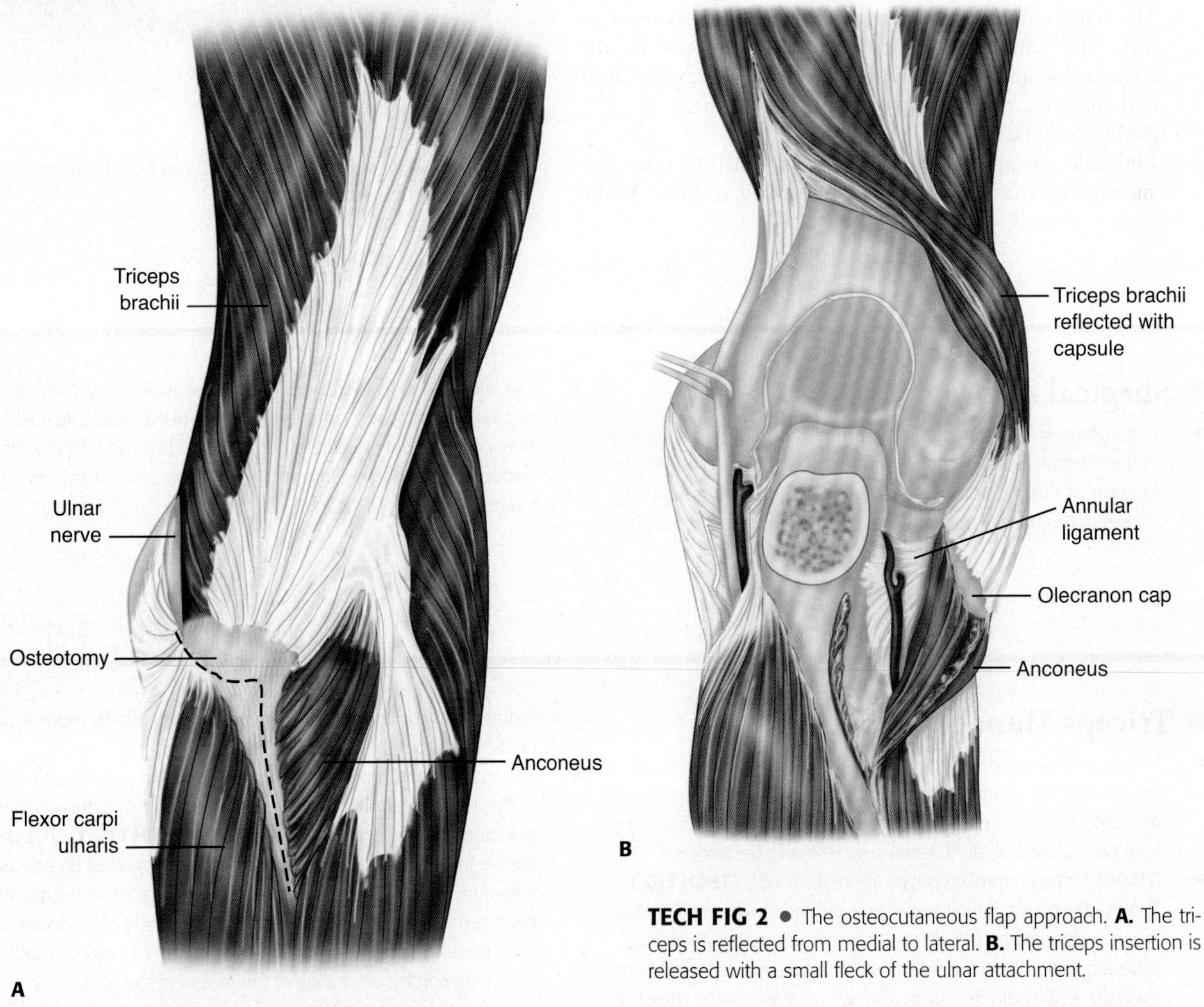

TECH FIG 2 • The osteocutaneous flap approach. **A.** The triceps is reflected from medial to lateral. **B.** The triceps insertion is released with a small fleck of the ulnar attachment.

Deep Dissection

- In either approach, the collateral ligaments and capsule are released (**TECH FIG 3**). This permits the ulna to be separated from the humerus. If ligamentous integrity is necessary (ie, unlinked arthroplasty), then the lateral ulnar collateral ligament (LUCL) and MCL should be tagged with plans at reattachment via bone tunnels in the humerus during closure.
- Contracted muscles (flexor–pronator and common extensor) are released in order to correct deformity that can result in maltracking of the TEA. The scarring about the elbow is sufficiently released to gain unencumbered access to the humerus and ulna for component implantation.

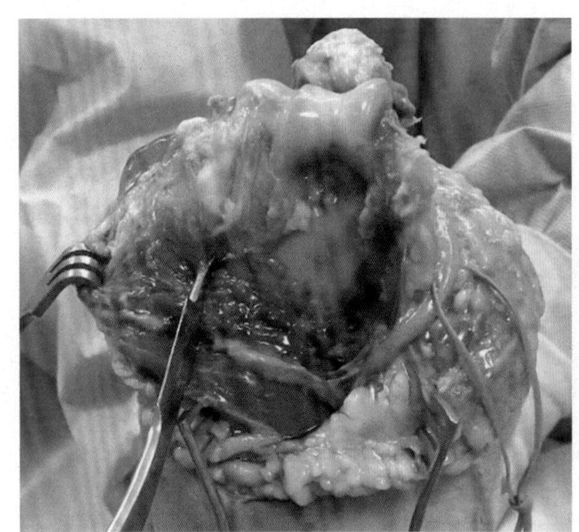

TECH FIG 3 • After the LCL and MCL are released, the shoulder is externally rotated and the elbow is hyperflexed to allow the ulna to be separated from the humerus.

Canal Preparation

Humeral Preparation

- Remove the central portion of the trochlea in line with the intramedullary canal and open the intramedullary canal with a burr (**TECH FIG 4A,B**).
- Insert the humeral awl reamer in order to identify the intramedullary canal and assesses the adequacy of trochlear bone removal.
- Sequentially rasp the humeral canal.
  - Be sure that the depth of insertion aligns the anatomic axis of rotation with the axis line on the humeral rasp (**TECH FIG 5**).
  - Once the final rasp size is identified, leave the rasp in place.
- Insert a trephine saw into the pilot hole in the humeral rasp and score the posterior humeral cortex.
  - There is a depth stop on the trephine saw that will prevent impingement on the humeral rasp.
- Attach the humeral cutting guide to the rasp and secure it with a stabilizing pin. Make vertical cuts in the medial and lateral humerus (**TECH FIG 6**).
- Remove the humeral cutting guide and rasp and inset the trephine stabilizer.
  - The depth of insertion should allow the trephine saw to engage the previous score mark on the posterior score (**TECH FIG 7**). This may require removal of a small amount of bone anteriorly.
- Once all of the cuts are completed, a trial humeral stem is inserted to assess the adequacy of humeral preparation.

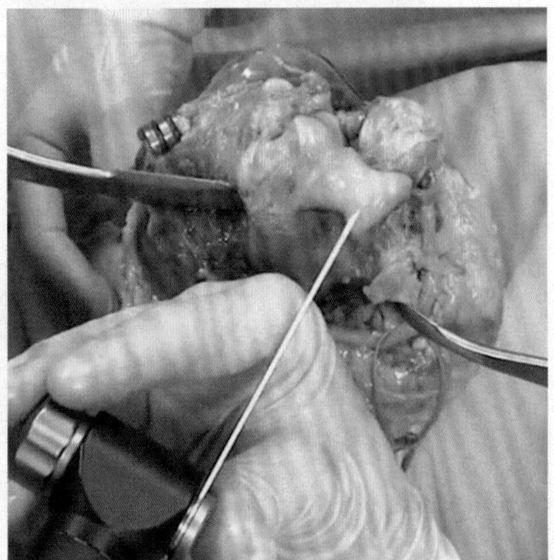

A

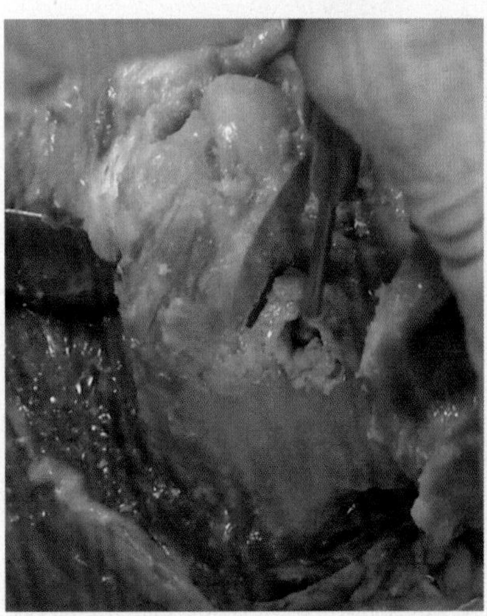

B

TECH FIG 4 • The central portion of the trochlea is removed in line with the intramedullary canal (**A**), and the intramedullary canal is opened with a burr (**B**).

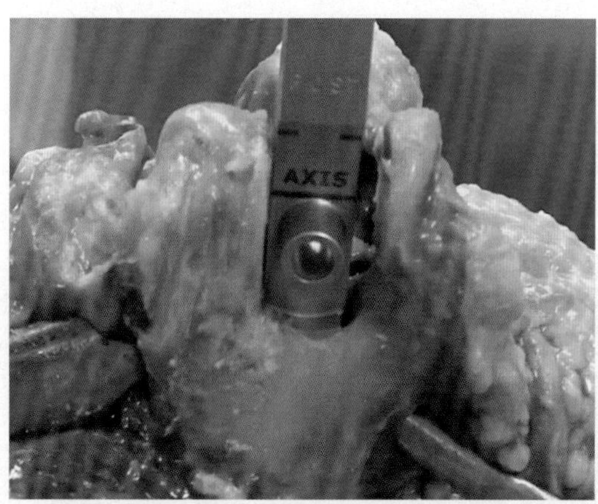

TECH FIG 5 • Humeral rasp is inserted so that the native axis of rotation is coincident with the axis line of the rasp. This guarantees proper depth of insertion of the final humeral component.

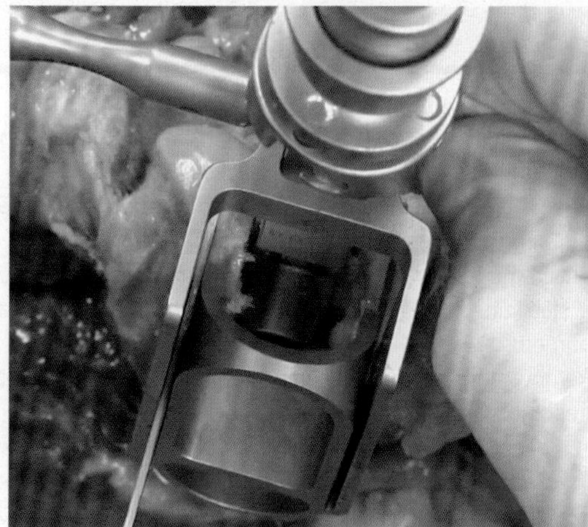

TECH FIG 6 • The vertical cutting guide prepares the medial and lateral aspects of the humeral yoke and connects to the trephine score line.

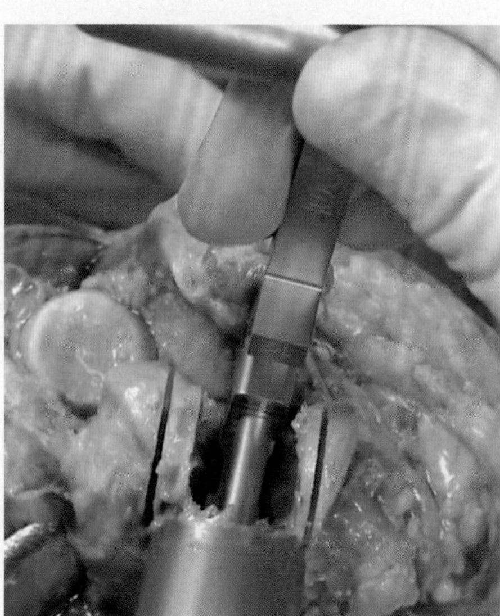

TECH FIG 7 • The trephine stabilizer allows completion of the distal humeral preparation. Proper depth of insertion of this guide may require removal of a small portion of bone from the anterior humerus.

Ulnar Preparation

- The tip of the ulna is removed to the depth of the greater sigmoid notch.
- Prepare the intramedullary canal of the ulna (**TECH FIG 8**).
  - The entrance to the canal is located at the base of the greater sigmoid notch in line with the ulna.
  - Insert a 4.5-mm solid flexible reamer to define the ulnar intramedullary canal. A depth mark on the reamer assists in determining the length of canal preparation.
- A guidewire is inserted into the canal and confirmed fluoroscopically. Sequential reaming with cannulated reamers is performed until the canal is prepared to the desired size.
- Insert the pilot rasp, being sure to maintain the correct orientation of the rasp to the flat surface of the dorsal surface of the olecranon (**TECH FIG 9**).

A

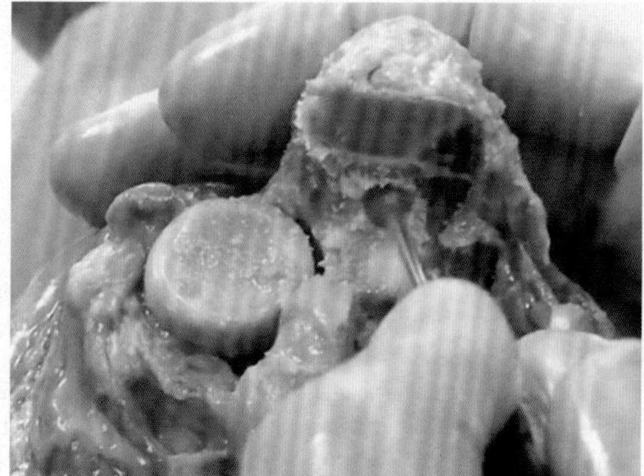

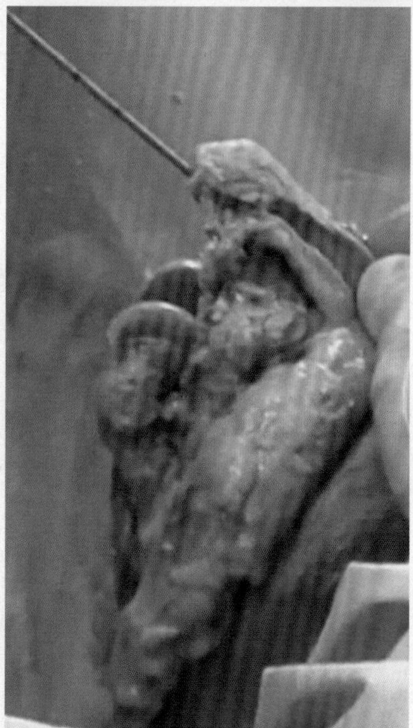

B

TECH FIG 8 • Ulnar canal preparation begins by (**A**) opening the intramedullary canal with a burr then (**B**) defining the intramedullary canal with a 4.5-mm solid flexible reamer.

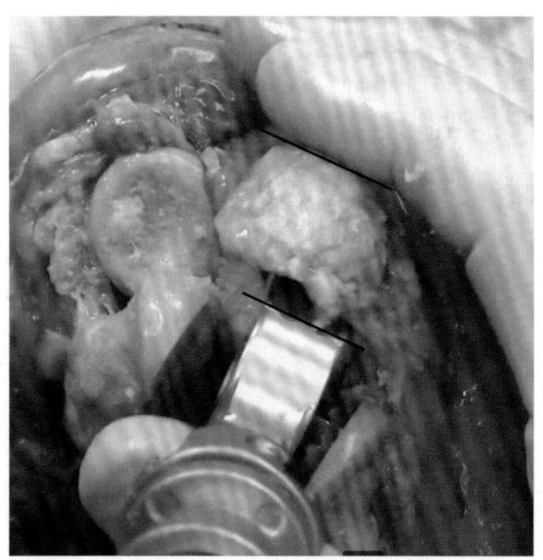

TECH FIG 9 • Proper rotation of the pilot rasp is assured when the back of the rasp is parallel to the flat portion of the dorsal aspect of the olecranon.

- Sequentially rasp the canal to prepare the proximal ulnar canal. The ulnar canal is sequentially rasped until the eye of the final rasp sits centrally within the native greater sigmoid notch (**TECH FIG 10**).
- With the final rasp in place, the ulnar planer is engaged into the medial and lateral aspects of the eye of the rasp to clear bone for the polyethylene ulnar bushing (**TECH FIG 11**).

Trial Reduction

- The appropriate size and length of ulnar trial is inserted to the appropriate depth.
- The ulnar trial is articulated with the humeral trial (**TECH FIG 12**).
- The elbow is taken through a range of motion. If full motion is not achieved, be sure the implant depth of insertion is adequate. Remove any bony impingement and release any contracted tissues to obtain full range of motion.
- Once full range of motion is achieved, disarticulate and remove the humeral and ulnar trials.

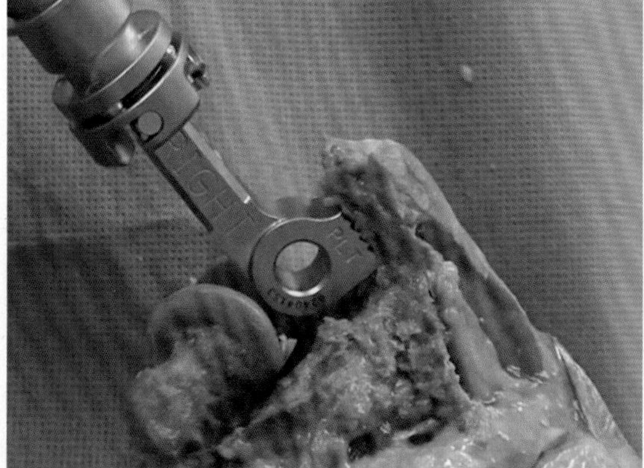

TECH FIG 10 • The final rasp is inserted until the eye sits centrally within the native greater sigmoid notch.

A

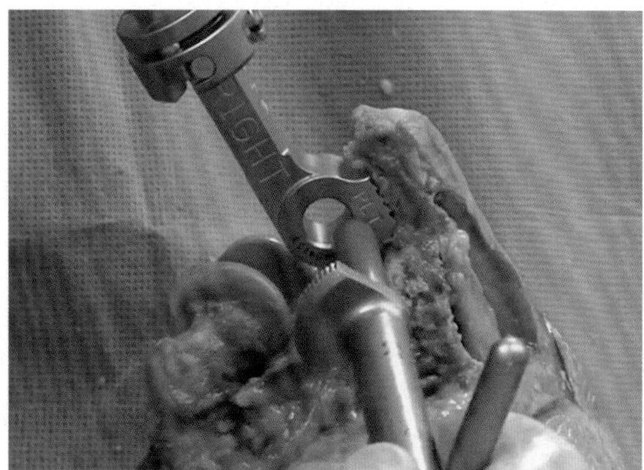

B

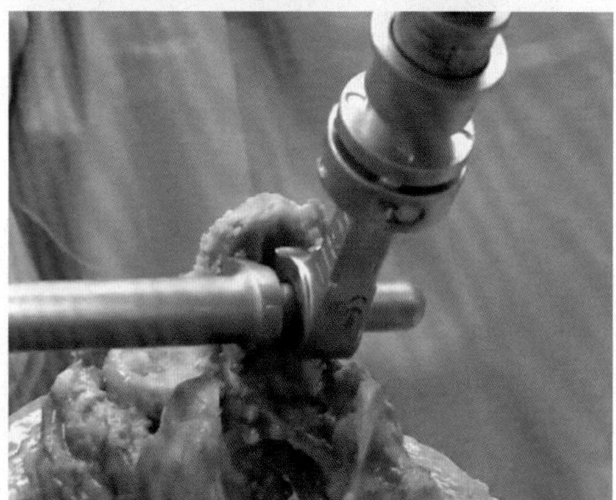

TECH FIG 11 • The medial (**A**) and lateral (**B**) walls of the ulna are prepared with the ulnar rasp which allows proper seating of the ulnar bushings.

Cementing the Implant

- Cement restrictors are placed in the humeral and ulnar canals to limit cement flow and allow pressurization of the cement mantle.
- The humeral and ulnar canals are lavaged and packed with thrombin-soaked sponges to reduce canal bleeding.
- Antibiotic-impregnated cement is injected retrograde into the canals and manually pressurized. A thin nozzle is used with the cement in a relatively liquid state to assist in complete retrograde filling of the canal.

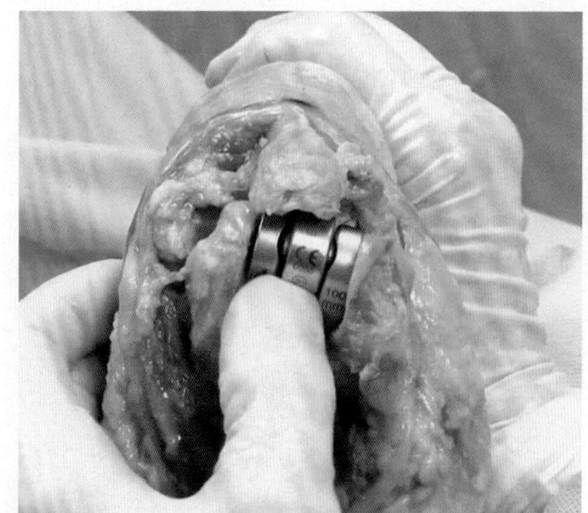

TECH FIG 12 • The humeral and ulnar trial implants are inserted and articulated.

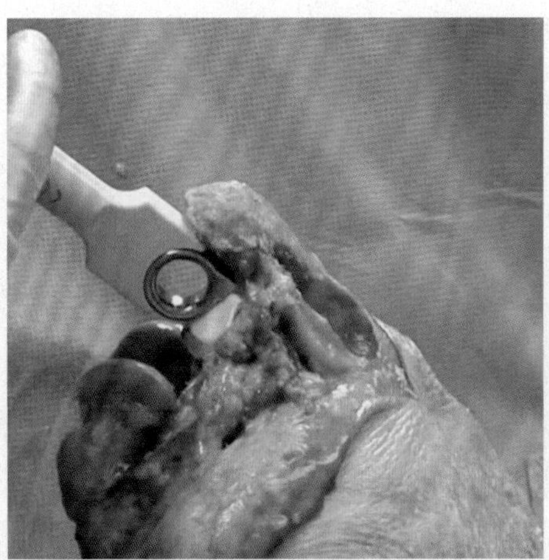

TECH FIG 13 • The ulnar component is inserted so that the ulnar eye sits centered in the greater sigmoid notch.

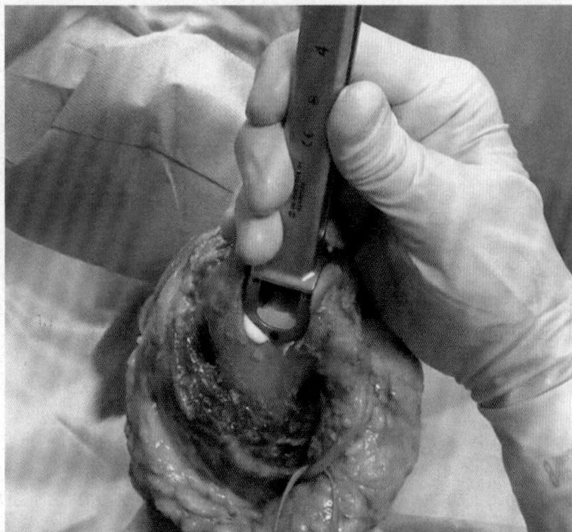

TECH FIG 14 • The humeral component is inserted into the prepared canal. As the component is inserted, a bone graft is placed behind the anterior flange and the anterior humeral cortex.

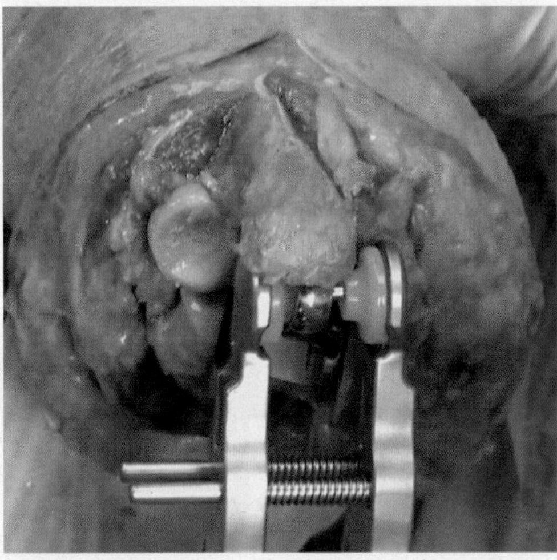

TECH FIG 15 • Once the ulnar component is inserted and the cement has hardened, the ulnar bushings are assembled in situ.

- The ulnar component is inserted to the proper depth and rotation. Any extruded cement is removed and the cement is allowed to fully harden (**TECH FIG 13**).
- The humeral component is inserted with the humeral polyethylene bushing preassembled. During humeral insertion, a bone graft is placed behind the anterior flange (**TECH FIG 14**).
- The ulnar bushings are inserted through the ulnar eye and compressed with the bushing insertion tool (**TECH FIG 15**).
- The components are articulated, and set screws are placed to secure the ulnar bushing to the humeral yoke (**TECH FIG 16**).
- The wound is lavaged to remove any residual bone debris and foreign material.

A

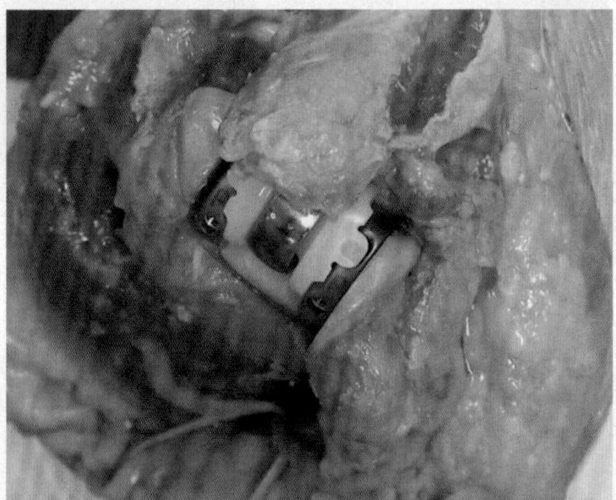

B

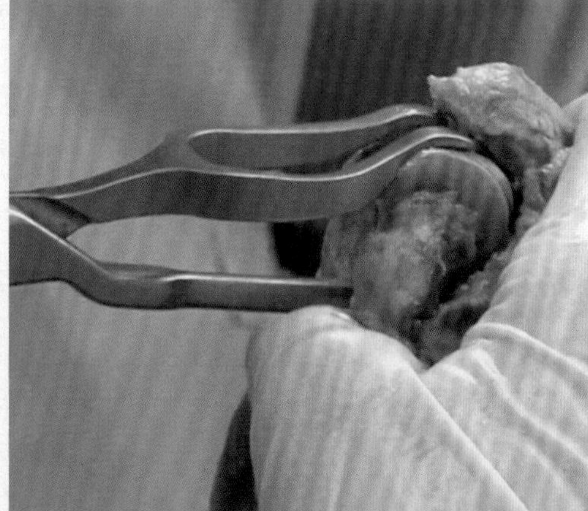

C

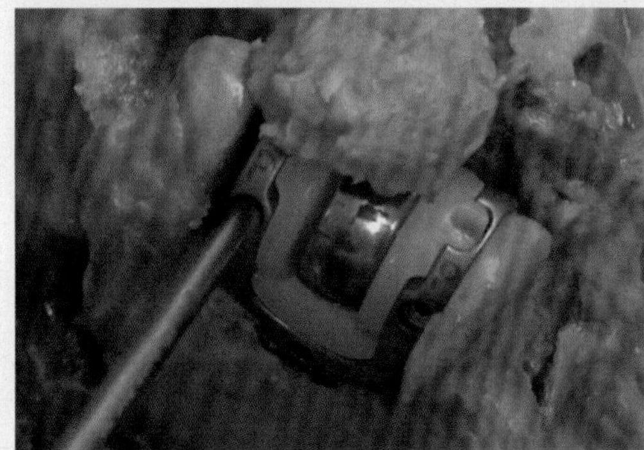

TECH FIG 16 • The ulnar bushings are aligned in the yoke of the humeral component (**A**) and fully seated with the bushing compression tool (**B**). Set screws are inserted and tightened with a torque wrench to secure the articulation (**C**).

Triceps Repair

- Place cruciate and transverse drill holes in the proximal ulna (**TECH FIG 17**).
- Perform cruciate repair of the triceps using a no. 5 nonresorbable suture. Return triceps to a position that is slightly overcorrected medially from its anatomic position.
- Start suture distally on the medial side of the ulna and direct the needle laterally through the drill hole to capture the lateral triceps tendon with a locking stitch. The suture is brought to the midline of the triceps and a second locking stitch is placed slightly more proximal and in the triceps tendon's midline. The third locking stitch aligns with the medial tunnel in the olecranon,

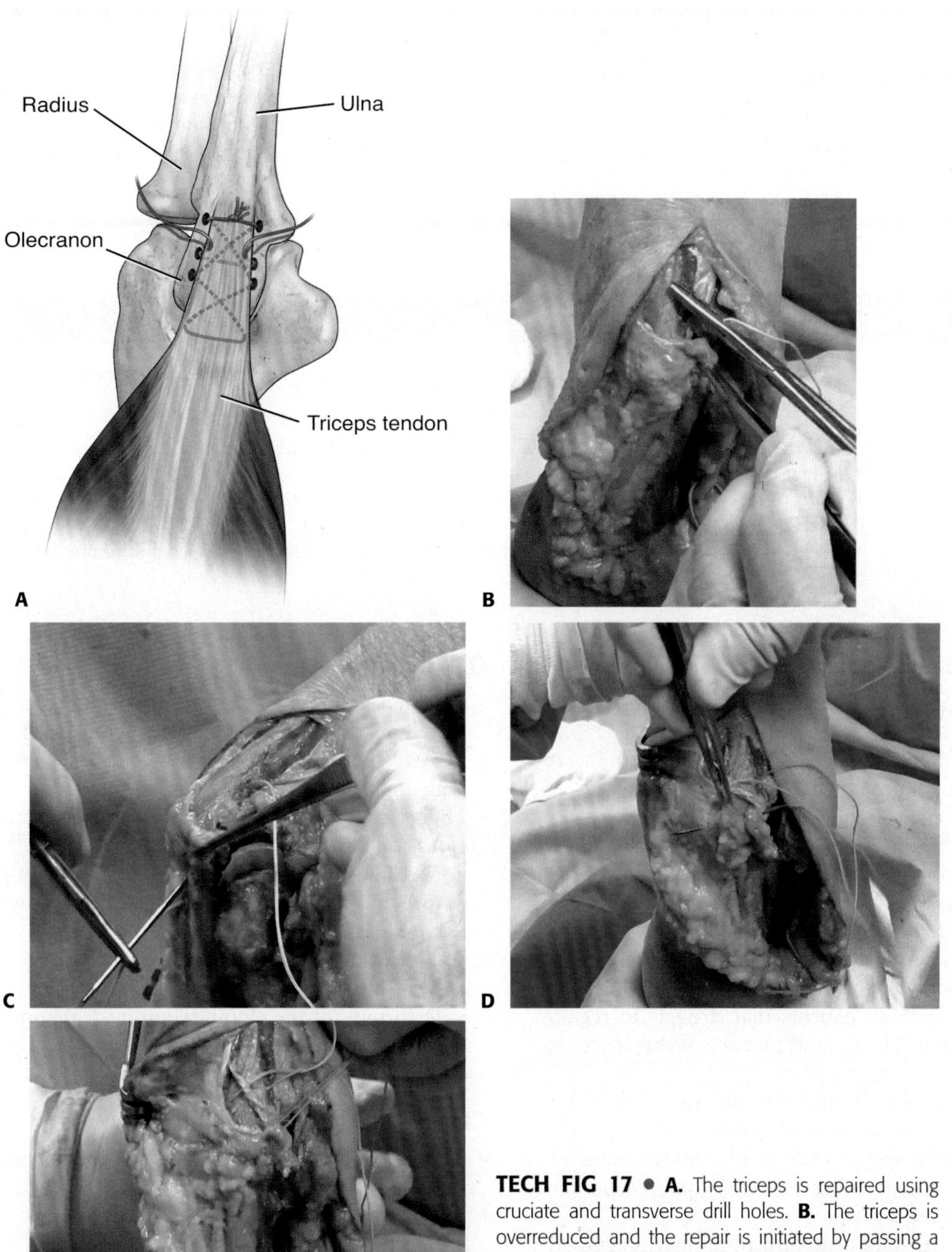

TECH FIG 17 • **A.** The triceps is repaired using cruciate and transverse drill holes. **B.** The triceps is overreduced and the repair is initiated by passing a suture through the distal medial to proximal lateral cruciate drill hole. **C.** A series of locking stitches are placed across the triceps, and the cruciate repair is completed by passing the stitch from proximal medial to distal lateral. **D.** The transverse repair is started by passing the suture from medial to lateral, capturing the triceps. **E.** Sequential locking sutures are placed across the posterior triceps, sealing it to the ulna.

and the suture is drawn through the tunnel emerging on the lateral aspect of the reflected mechanism. It is brought through the sleeve of tissue from lateral to medial.

- The transverse repair starts by passing the suture medial to lateral through the olecranon. After piercing the lateral sleeve of tissue, it is brought to the midportion of the triceps tendon, and a locking stitch is placed slightly proximal to the attachment after which it again pierces the medial aspect of the margin of the triceps.
- The sutures are tied with the elbow in approximately 45 degrees of flexion.
- The FCU fascia and anconeus are then repaired to surrounding tissue.

Wound Closure

- The ulnar nerve is transposed into a subcutaneous pocket and held anteriorly with a fascial sling.
- A subcutaneous drain is place laterally.
- A layered wound closure is performed.
- The arm is immobilized in extension with an anterior splint until the drain is removed on the second postoperative day.

PEARLS AND PITFALLS

Indications	▪ TEA is considered in carefully selected patients where other nonoperative and operative measures have been exhausted.
Goals of treatment	▪ The goal of treatment is a pain-free, functional arc of motion.
TEA	▪ Ulnar nerve transposition in all cases ▪ Triceps-reflecting approach, especially when the joint is very stiff ▪ Release both the MCL and LCL. ▪ Release the flexor–pronator and common extensor, particularly if there is significant preoperative deformity.

POSTOPERATIVE CARE

- The elbow is immobilized in full extension in a well-padded anterior splint.
- The arm is elevated on pillows or suspended from an intravenous (IV) pole to reduce swelling.
- The splint is removed 24 to 48 hours after surgery.
- Gentle AROM is begun in flexion, pronation, and supination. Active extension is avoided for 6 weeks to protect the triceps repair. However, gravity-assisted extension or passive extension is permitted.
- In general, formal physical therapy is rarely required to regain range of motion. However, formal physical therapy may be beneficial in those patients that struggle to regain their range of motion. The general timeline of therapy is as follows:
  - Phase I (0 to 6 weeks): Protect the soft tissue and begin protected active-assistive range of motion.
  - Phase II (6 to 12 weeks): Continue to improve range of motion. Begin strengthening exercises and encourage functional use of the arm.
  - Phase III (12 to 16 weeks): Return to normal functional activities within the restrictions for TEA.
- Postoperative stiffness may be helped with splinting. Static splinting is preferred over dynamic splinting.
- Restrictions
  - Lifetime limitations of the operated extremity include 5-pound repetitive lifting and 10-pound single-event restriction.

OUTCOMES

- Patients undergoing TEA for posttraumatic conditions of the elbow tend to be younger, higher demand.
- TEA for posttraumatic conditions of the elbow is associated with improved clinical outcomes[2–4,9,10,13,15–17]
- Higher complication rate is noted for posttraumatic conditions compared to other indications for TEA.[18]
  - Mechanical complications such as component fracture and increased polyethylene bushing wear are more common.
- Causes of increased complications include the following:
  - Multiple previous surgeries
  - Deformity of the elbow requiring realignment of the extremity through the implant

COMPLICATIONS

- TEA for traumatic conditions is associated with a high complication rate.
- Major complications include the following:
  - Infection[7,20]
    - Current reports indicate an infection rate of 2% to 5% for primary TEA.
    - Higher infection rates are noted with posttraumatic arthritis and a history of prior surgery.
  - Loosening
  - Triceps insufficiency
    - Underrecognized problem

- Neurologic injury
  - Incidence of transient ulnar neuropathy is as high as 26% and permanent nerve injury is up to 10%.
- Wound complications
  - Associated with prior surgery
  - Avoid wound complications by the following:
    - Manage wound by immobilizing in extension postoperatively.
    - Use of a subcutaneous drain to avoid hematoma formation
  - A significant postoperative hematoma should be evacuated.
- Periprosthetic fracture
  - Can occur intraoperatively or postoperatively
  - Incidence ranges from 1% to 23%.

REFERENCES

1. Celli A, Arash A, Adams RA, et al. Triceps insufficiency following total elbow arthroplasty. J Bone Joint Surg Am 2005;87(9):1957–1964.
2. Cil A, Veillette CJ, Sanchez-Sotelo J, et al. Linked elbow replacement: a salvage procedure for distal humeral nonunion. J Bone Joint Surg Am 2008;90(9):1939–1950.
3. Espiga X, Antuna SA, Ferreres A. Linked total elbow arthroplasty as treatment of distal humerus nonunions in patients older than 70 years. Acta Orthop Belg 2011;77(3):304–310.
4. Figgie HE III, Inglis AE, Ranawat CS, et al. Results of total elbow arthroplasty as a salvage procedure for failed elbow reconstructive operations. Clin Orthop Relat Res 1987;(219):185–193.
5. Figgie MP, Inglis AE, Mow CS, et al. Salvage of non-union of supracondylar fracture of the humerus by total elbow arthroplasty. J Bone Joint Surg Am 1989;71(7):1058–1065.
6. Inglis AE, Inglis AE Jr, Figgie MM, et al. Total elbow arthroplasty for flail and unstable elbows. J Shoulder Elbow Surg 1997;6(1):29–36.
7. Jeon IH, Morrey BF, Anakwenze OA, et al. Incidence and implications of early postoperative wound complications after total elbow arthroplasty. J Shoulder Elbow Surg 2011;20(6):857–865.
8. Kamineni S, O'Driscoll SW, Urban M, et al. Intrinsic constraint of unlinked total elbow replacements—the ulnotrochlear joint. J Bone Joint Surg Am 2005;87(9):2019–2027.
9. Kodde IF, van Riet RP, Eygendaal D. Semiconstrained total elbow arthroplasty for posttraumatic arthritis or deformities of the elbow: a prospective study. J Hand Surg Am 2013;38(7):1377–1382.
10. LaPorte DM, Murphy MS, Moore JR. Distal humerus nonunion after failed internal fixation: reconstruction with total elbow arthroplasty. Am J Orthop 2008;37(10):531–534.
11. Moro JK, King GJ. Total elbow arthroplasty in the treatment of posttraumatic conditions of the elbow. Clin Orthop Relat Res 2000;(370):102–114.
12. Morrey BF. Surgical exposures of the elbow. In: Morrey BF, Sanchez-Sotelo J, eds. The Elbow and Its Disorders, ed 4. Philadelphia: Saunders Elsevier, 2009:115–142.
13. Morrey BF, Adams RA, Bryan RS. Total replacement for post-traumatic arthritis of the elbow. J Bone Joint Surg Br 1991;73(4):607–612.
14. Morrey BF, Schneeberger AG. Total elbow arthroplasty for posttraumatic arthrosis. Instr Course Lect 2009;58:495–504.
15. Ramsey ML, Adams RA, Morrey BF. Instability of the elbow treated with semiconstrained total elbow arthroplasty. J Bone Joint Surg Am 1999;81(1):38–47.
16. Sanchez-Sotelo J, Morrey BF. Linked elbow replacement: a salvage procedure for distal humeral nonunion. Surgical technique. J Bone Joint Surg Am 2009;91(suppl 2):200–212.
17. Schneeberger AG, Adams R, Morrey BF. Semiconstrained total elbow replacement for the treatment of post-traumatic osteoarthrosis. J Bone Joint Surg Am 1997;79(8):1211–1222.
18. Throckmorton T, Zarkadas P, Sanchez-Sotelo J, et al. Failure patterns after linked semiconstrained total elbow arthroplasty for posttraumatic arthritis. J Bone Joint Surg Am 2010;92(6):1432–1441.
19. Wolfe SW, Ranawat CS. The osteo-anconeus flap. An approach for total elbow arthroplasty. J Bone Joint Surg Am 1990;72(5):684–688.
20. Yamaguchi K, Adams RA, Morrey BF. Infection after total elbow arthroplasty. J Bone Joint Surg Am 1998;80(4):481–491.

CHAPTER 104

Elbow Arthrodesis

Mark A. Mighell, Robert U. Hartzler, and Thomas J. Kovack

BACKGROUND

- Elbow arthrodesis (EA) is rarely performed in orthopaedic surgery and indicated only as a salvage procedure.
- Historically, EA was performed for tuberculous septic elbow arthritis, with about 50% successful rate of primary fusion.[8,19]
- With modern techniques, especially compression plating, primary fusion rates have improved somewhat from 50% to 86%,[9,10,16] with final fusion rates including reoperation ranging from 83% to 100%.[6,9,16]
- Reoperation for nonunion, infection, wound healing complications, and hardware prominence is common (average 1.4 to 1.6 reoperations per patient).[9,16]
- EA results in greater functional disability than arthrodesis of the ankle, hip, or knee joints.
- Loss of motion in the elbow is disabling and can only be partially compensated by trunk, shoulder, forearm, and wrist motion.[4,12]

PATIENT HISTORY AND PHYSICAL FINDINGS

- Skin and soft tissue defects are evaluated.
- The quality and quantity of bone available for fusion are assessed.
- The surgeon should anticipate the need for bone graft or soft tissue coverage preoperatively.
- If soft tissue coverage is necessary, a plastic surgery consultation is recommended.
- Shoulder, forearm, wrist, and spinal column motion is evaluated.
- Neurologic and motor deficits are documented.
- Blood flow to the hand is determined.

IMAGING AND OTHER DIAGNOSTIC STUDIES

- Standard orthogonal radiographs of the elbow are obtained.
- Computed tomography (CT) scans of the elbow are obtained for more detailed bony anatomy.
- If infection is suspected:
  - Blood work is obtained for complete blood count, sedimentation rate, and C-reactive protein.
  - The joint is aspirated or an indium scan is performed.

SURGICAL MANAGEMENT

- The elbow is one of the most difficult joints to fuse because of the long lever arm and strong bending forces across the fusion site.
  - Average time to fusion is usually around 6 months.[3,10]
  - Reoperation to achieve fusion is common.[9,16]
- EA should be considered a salvage procedure when no other satisfactory surgical option exists. The patient should be counseled regarding the high rate of complications.

Indications

- Septic arthritis, postseptic arthrosis, or chronic osteomyelitis
- Complex traumatic or war injuries with unreconstructable bone and soft tissue defects
- Elbow degenerative joint disease in patients who are too young or active for total elbow arthroplasty (eg, laborer)
- Painful, severe instability
- Failed internal fixation for nonunions or pseudarthrosis
- Failed elbow arthroplasty (rare)[2]

Contraindications

- Massive bone loss preventing successful arthrodesis
- Massive soft tissue loss not amenable to flap reconstruction
- Compromised function of the ipsilateral hand, wrist, shoulder, or spinal column

Preoperative Planning

- The intended fusion position is of paramount importance, as no optimal position for arthrodesis exists.
  - No fusion position will allow all activities to be performed.[4,11,12,18]
  - Historically, a fusion position of 90 degrees has been used,[15] although fusion angles from 45 to 110 degrees have been recommended.[12]
- The position of fusion should be dictated by the needs of the patient.
  - Factors for choosing the best position include gender, occupation, hand dominance, functional requirements, associated joint involvement, and unilateral versus bilateral arthrodesis.
  - If possible, preoperatively, the elbow is immobilized in various angles to determine the patient's preferred fusion angle.
- Suggested fusion angles for patient and surgeon consideration:
  - Male, dominant arm: 90 degrees[2,11]
  - Females seem to prefer the cosmetic appearance of lower fusion angles (45 to 70 degrees).
  - Angles greater than 90 to 100 degrees (ie, 110 degrees) allow for better hand-to-mouth function and facial hygiene.[4,9,18] Conversely, cosmesis may be poor at a higher fusion angles.
  - Fifty to 70 degrees is better for extrapersonal needs.[18]
  - Bilateral EA: dominant arm at 110 degrees, nondominant arm at 65 degrees[9,15]
- The need for vascularized bone or flap coverage may significantly affect preoperative planning:
  - Healing by secondary intention has been described with acceptable results, even in the setting of exposed hardware.[15]
  - Consider staging flap coverage and the use of external fixation.[3]
  - Vascularized fibular autograft for bone loss[17] and pedicled rib–latissimus dorsi flap[13] for combined bone and soft tissue defects have been described.

- Assess bone loss and the need for bone graft or alternative fusion methods:
  - For cases with no or minimal bone loss, consider demineralized bone matrix, cancellous allograft, or autograft.
  - For large bone defects, autograft cancellous bone is preferable.
  - Radiohumeral arthrodesis in the setting of inadequate ulnar bone has been described.[14]
- Compression with lag screws plus plating or external fixation has improved the rate of primary fusion compared with historical techniques and should be part of the surgical tactic.
- The addition of a 3.5-mm locked plate placed medially as a strut to enhance the rigidity of the construct has been described.[5]
- Most authors recommend routine excision of the radial head, especially in the setting of infection.[1,3,5,10] Alternatively, if the radiocapitellar and proximal radioulnar joints are relatively preserved, it is acceptable to maintain the radial head if it does not interfere with the arthrodesis.[9,16]
- Some loss of forearm rotation should be anticipated.[9,10,15]

Special Instruments

- Large fragment locking set (4.5-mm locked narrow plate)
- A 3.5-mm locked plate may be substituted in smaller patients.
- External fixator of surgeon's preference, if applicable
- Sterile goniometer
- Plate press
- High-speed burr
- Power drill
- Osteotomes
- Oscillating saw
- Kirschner wire set

Patient Positioning

- A tourniquet is placed as high on the arm as possible. A sterile tourniquet is required to increase the zone of sterility.
- The patient is placed in the lateral decubitus position with the operative arm resting on a padded arm rest.
- Adequate intraoperative fluoroscopic imaging should be ensured.

Anesthesia

- Antibiotics are given 30 minutes before the incision.
- General anesthesia is used for intraoperative pain control and allows paralysis if necessary.
- A supraclavicular block can be used for intraoperative and postoperative pain management.

TECHNIQUES

Surgical Approach

- Mark existing surgical scars and use prior incisions if possible.
- The preferred incision is a direct posterior approach to the elbow.
- If flap coverage is present, a plastic surgeon may be required for exposure to preserve the vascular pedicle to the flap.
  - With flaps with vascular pedicles, the location of the vessel can be located intraoperatively with a Doppler.
- Create full-thickness flaps right down to the bone.
- Limit subcutaneous dissection.
  - Split the triceps tendon longitudinally.
  - Carry the triceps split distally in the interval between the flexor carpi ulnaris (FCU) and the anconeus.
- Identify the ulnar nerve and make sure it remains protected.
  - Identify neurovascular structures in known areas before following structures through areas of heavy scar tissue.

Arthrodesis

Osteotomy and Reduction

- Expose the dorsal surface of the distal humerus and proximal ulna.
- Use osteotomes to "fish scale" the exposed bone.
- Open the medullary canal of the humerus and ulna.
- Perform a step cut osteotomy of the proximal ulna and distal humerus to increase the surface area for fusion (**TECH FIG 1A**).
- Contour the bone so that it can be reduced at the appropriate angle chosen for arthrodesis.
  - It is often necessary to excise the radial head to allow for adequate reduction of the humerus and ulna.
- Reduce the distal humerus to the proximal ulna.
  - Confirm the fusion angle with a sterile goniometer (**TECH FIG 1B**).
  - Provisionally, hold the reduction at the desired angle with 1.6-mm Kirschner wires.

Screw and Plate Fixation

- Drill from distal to proximal for lag screw insertion (**TECH FIG 2A**).
  - Use two or three lag screws (4.5 mm) whenever possible.
- Apply the 4.5-mm locking plate posteriorly, prebent at the chosen angle of arthrodesis (**TECH FIG 2B**).
  - A long plate should be selected with a minimum of 10 to 14 holes.
  - A plate press is easier to use than bending irons.
- The plate functions as a neutralization device.
  - All compression is achieved with the lag technique employed for screw placement.
- The plate is pulled down to the bone and secured with cortical screws before adding locked screws.
- Use at least one locked screw proximal and distal to the fusion site to increase the torsional strength of the construct (**TECH FIG 2C**).

Completion

- Check the position and fixation of the construct intraoperatively with fluoroscopy.
- The final construct should demonstrate compression across the fusion site.
  - The plate should conform securely to the bone at the desired angle of fusion (**TECH FIG 3A**).
- Irrigate and close the wound.
  - We recommend the use of one or two deep flat drains.
- Final radiographs should be taken intraoperatively (**TECH FIG 3B,C**).

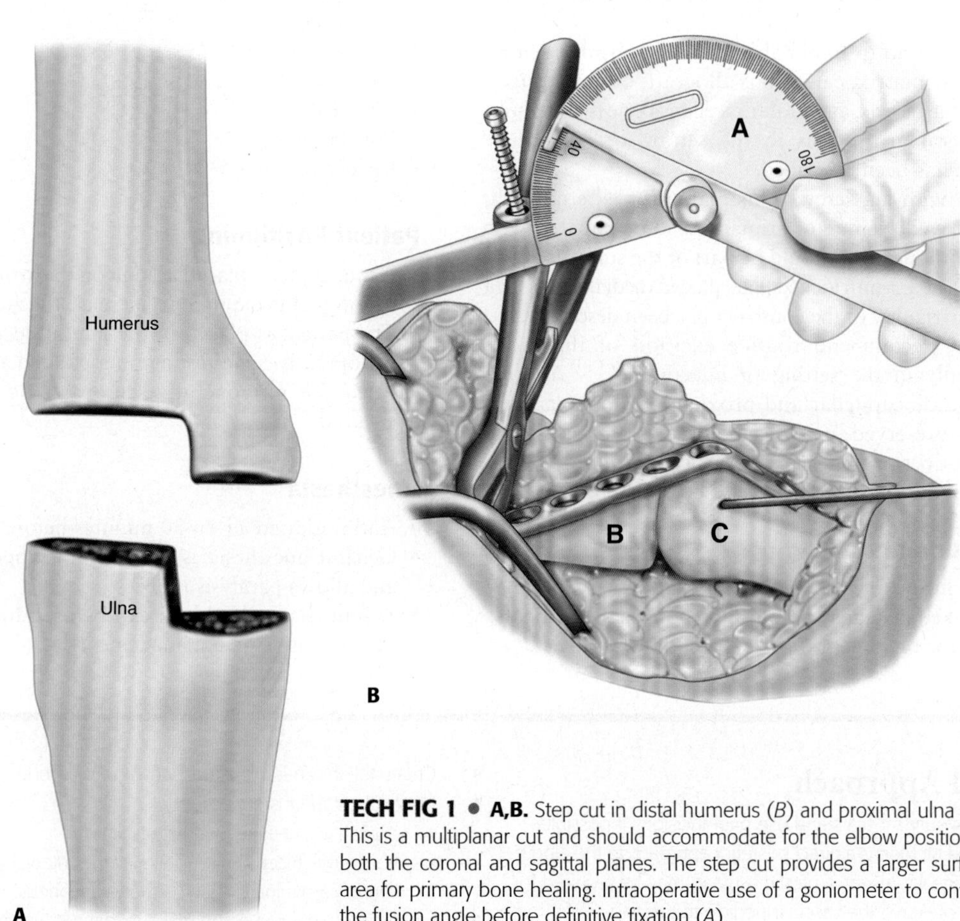

TECH FIG 1 • A,B. Step cut in distal humerus (*B*) and proximal ulna (*C*). This is a multiplanar cut and should accommodate for the elbow position in both the coronal and sagittal planes. The step cut provides a larger surface area for primary bone healing. Intraoperative use of a goniometer to confirm the fusion angle before definitive fixation (*A*).

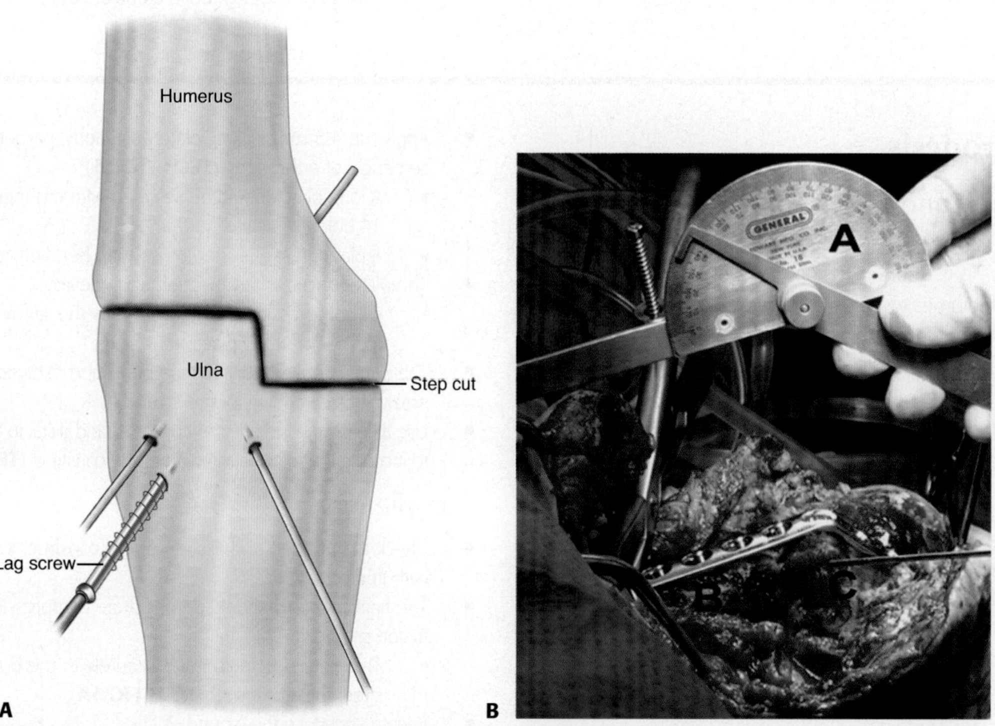

TECH FIG 2 • A. Placement of lag screw. **B.** Provisional fixation is obtained with Kirschner wires and the fusion position is measured with a goniometer (*A*). Screws are placed from distal (*C*) to proximal (*B*) in a crossed configuration. Two or three lag screws are placed before plate application. Plate placement after the fusion angle has been confirmed. *(continued)*

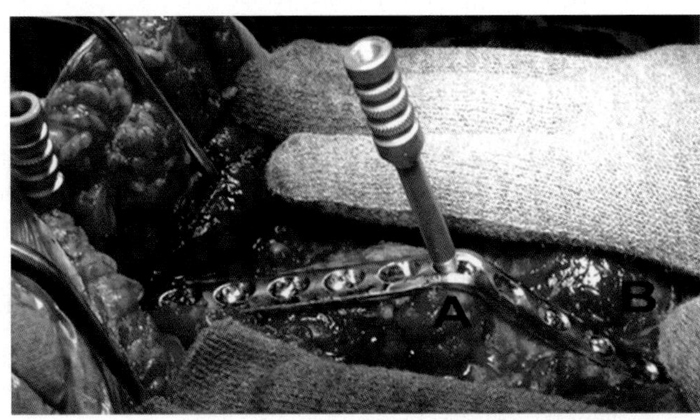

C

TECH FIG 2 • (continued) C. A guide for locking the screw through the plate and across the step cut osteotomy. Compression must be achieved before locking screws are placed. *A*, distal humerus; *B*, proximal ulna.

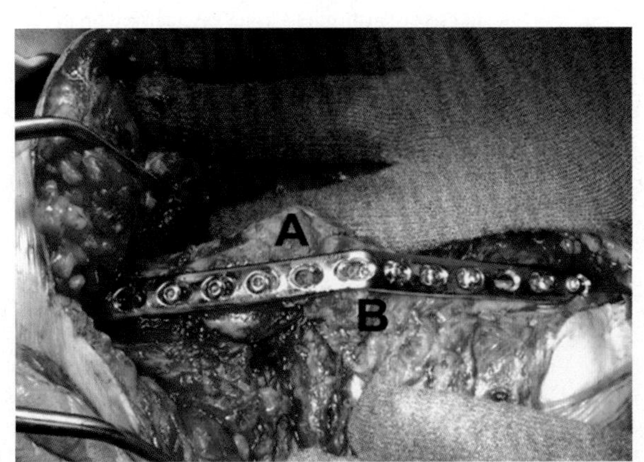

A

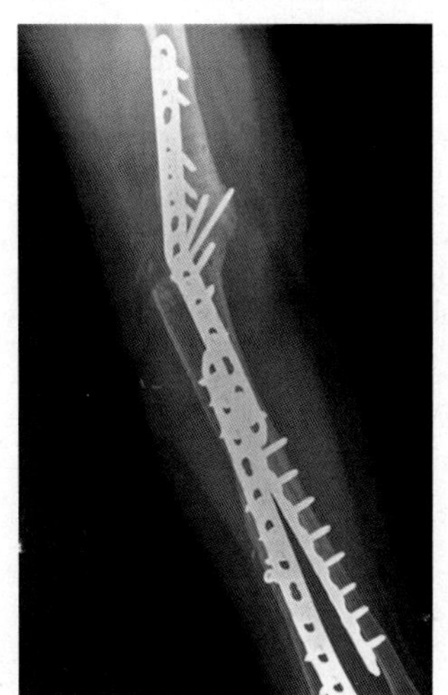

B

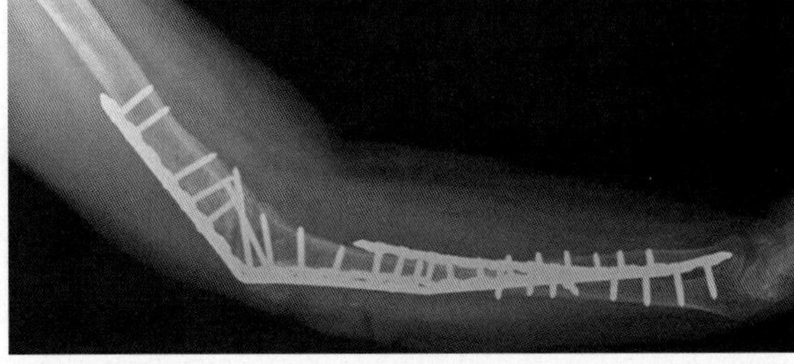

C

TECH FIG 3 • A. Completed EA using step cut osteotomy and 3.5-mm locking plate and lag screw technique. *A*, distal humerus; *B*, proximal ulna. **B,C.** Anteroposterior (AP) and lateral postoperative radiographs of left elbow fusion using step cut osteotomy and locked plating technique.

PEARLS AND PITFALLS

- Step cut bone to increase the surface area for healing.
- Place lag screws in both vertical and horizontal planes to increase compression.
- Maintain full-thickness dorsal tissue, including the periosteum.
- Use lag technique to compress the bone ends.
- Never identify neurovascular structures in areas of extensive surgical scarring. Work from known to unknown surgical fields.
- Open the medullary canal to facilitate blood flow.
- Select a plate of sufficient length to span the fusion site. Longer plates are desirable.
- Place locking screws only after reduction and compression of the bone ends and the plate is compressed to bone with conventional screws.
- Keep patients in a cast until fusion occurs, typically a minimum of 4–6 months.

POSTOPERATIVE CARE

- Drains are removed before hospital discharge.
- Intravenous antibiotics are continued for 48 hours or longer, depending on intraoperative cultures.
- Sutures or staples are removed at 2 weeks.
- The arm is placed in a long-arm cast at the 2-week visit.
- Cast or splint immobilization is continued until there is radiographic evidence of union, typically 4 to 6 months at minimum.[3,7,10]

COMPLICATIONS

- Postoperative fracture after bony union has been achieved is not uncommon[8,9] but may be successfully treated with immobilization in the majority of cases.

REFERENCES

1. Arafiles RP. A new technique of fusion for tuberculous arthritis of the elbow. J Bone Joint Surg Am 1981;63(9):1396–1400.
2. Beckenbaugh R. Arthrodesis. In: Morrey BF, ed. The Elbow and Its Disorders, ed 3. Philadelphia: WB Saunders, 2000:731–737.
3. Bilic R, Kolundzic R, Bicanic G, et al. Elbow arthrodesis after war injuries. Mil Med 2005;170(2):164–166.
4. de Groot JH, Angulo SM, Meskers CG, et al. Reduced elbow mobility affects the flexion or extension domain in activities of daily living. Clin Biomech 2011;26(7):713–717.
5. Galley IJ, Bain GI, Stanley JC, et al. Arthrodesis of the elbow with two locking compression plates. Tech Shoulder Elbow Surg 2007;8(3): 141–145. doi:110.1097/BTE.1090b1013e31812dfb31885.
6. Hahn MP, Ostermann PA, Richter D, et al. Elbow arthrodesis and its alternative [in German]. Orthopade 1996;25(2):112–120.
7. Irvine GB, Gregg PJ. A method of elbow arthrodesis: brief report. J Bone Joint Surg Br 1989;71(1):145–146.
8. Koch M, Lipscomb PR. Arthrodesis of the elbow. Clin Orthop Relat Res 1967;50:151–157.
9. Koller H, Kolb K, Assuncao A, et al. The fate of elbow arthrodesis: indications, techniques, and outcome in fourteen patients. J Shoulder Elbow Surg 2008;17(2):293–306.
10. McAuliffe JA, Burkhalter WE, Ouellette EA, et al. Compression plate arthrodesis of the elbow. J Bone Joint Surg Br 1992;74(2):300–304.
11. Nagy SM III, Szabo RM, Sharkey NA. Unilateral elbow arthrodesis: the preferred position. J South Orthop Assoc 1999;8(2):80–85.
12. O'Neill OR, Morrey BF, Tanaka S, et al. Compensatory motion in the upper extremity after elbow arthrodesis. Clin Orthop Relat Res 1992;(281):89–96.
13. Ozer K, Toker S, Morgan S. The use of a combined rib-latissimus dorsi flap for elbow arthrodesis and soft-tissue coverage. J Shoulder Elbow Surg 2011;20(1):e9–e13.
14. Presnal BP, Chillag KJ. Radiohumeral arthrodesis for salvage of failed total elbow arthroplasty. J Arthroplasty 1995;10(5):699–701.
15. Rashkoff E, Burkhalter WE. Arthrodesis of the salvage elbow. Orthopedics 1986;9(5):733–738.
16. Reichel LM, Wiater BP, Friedrich J, et al. Arthrodesis of the elbow. Hand Clin 2011;27(2):179–186, vi.
17. Ring D, Jupiter JB, Toh S. Transarticular bony defects after trauma and sepsis: arthrodesis using vascularized fibular transfer. Plast Reconstr Surg 1999;104(2):426–434.
18. Tang C, Roidis N, Itamura J, et al. The effect of simulated elbow arthrodesis on the ability to perform activities of daily living. J Hand Surg Am 2001;26(6):1146–1150.
19. Van Gordner GW, Chen CM. The central-graft operation for fusion of tuberculous knees, ankles, and elbows. J Bone Joint Surg Am 1959;41-A:1029–1046.

Wrist Denervation

Carlos Heras-Palou

DEFINITION

- Arthrosis of the wrist often presents with functional movement but with substantial disability due to pain. The purpose of wrist denervation is to decrease pain by surgically dividing the nerves that transmit the afferent pain signal from the wrist.

ANATOMY

- The posterior interosseous nerve (PIN) is considered to be the most important nerve innervating the wrist joint.
- Other nerves involved are branches from the anterior interosseous nerve (AIN), the radial nerve, the dorsal branch of the ulnar nerve, the palmar branch of the median nerve, and recurrent intermetacarpal nerve branches.[1]

PATHOGENESIS

- Common causative conditions include scaphoid nonunion advanced collapse, scapholunate advanced collapse, degeneration secondary to crystalline arthropathy, inflammatory arthritis, and trauma.

NATURAL HISTORY

- The natural history of wrist arthrosis is slow progression, but the correlation between radiologic staging and symptoms is sometimes poor.

PATIENT HISTORY AND PHYSICAL FINDINGS

- Patients with wrist arthrosis present with wrist pain, weakness of the grip, swelling, and stiffness.
- Often, there is a sensation of grating during wrist movement and occasionally clicking or clunking.
- Some patients report a history of wrist injury years previously but many do not recall any wrist trauma.
- It is important to inquire about neurologic symptoms to identify any associated compressive neuropathy at the carpal tunnel, the canal of Guyon, or both.
- Examination of the wrist usually reveals dorsoradial swelling, loss of movement, weak grip strength secondary to pain, and crepitation.

Local Anesthetic Blocks

- Although controversial in the literature, selective injection of a local anesthetic can be used to predict the results of wrist denervation.
- Local anesthetic is injected about 1 cm ulnar and 3 cm proximal to the tubercle of Lister, delivering 1 mL Marcaine 0.5% around the PIN (**FIG 1A**). The needle is pushed forward through the interosseous membrane to deliver 1 mL of local anesthetic adjacent to the AIN.
- One milliliter Marcaine is then injected under the branches of the radial nerve (**FIG 1B**), under the dorsal cutaneous branch of the ulnar nerve (**FIG 1C**), under the palmar branch

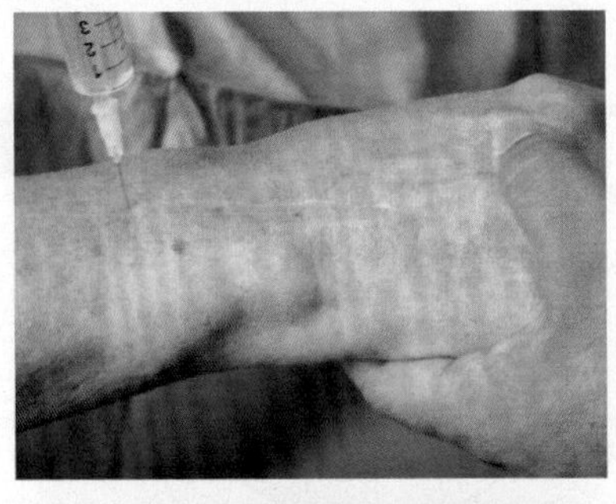
A

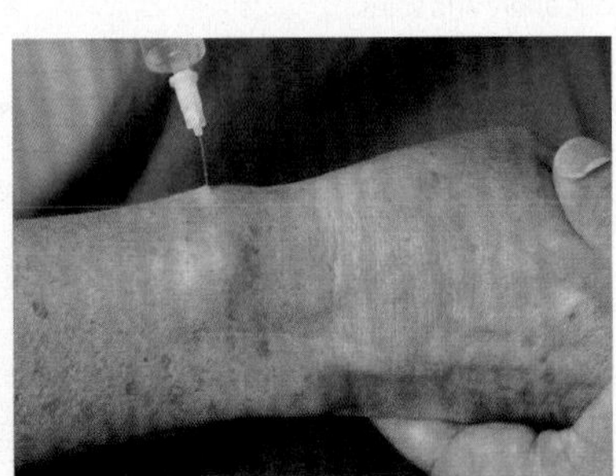
B

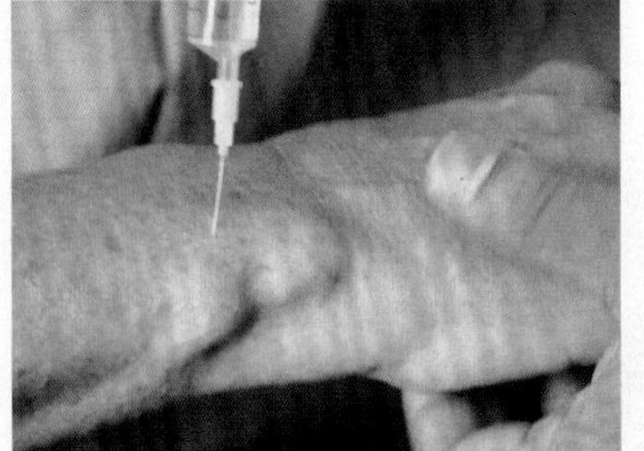
C

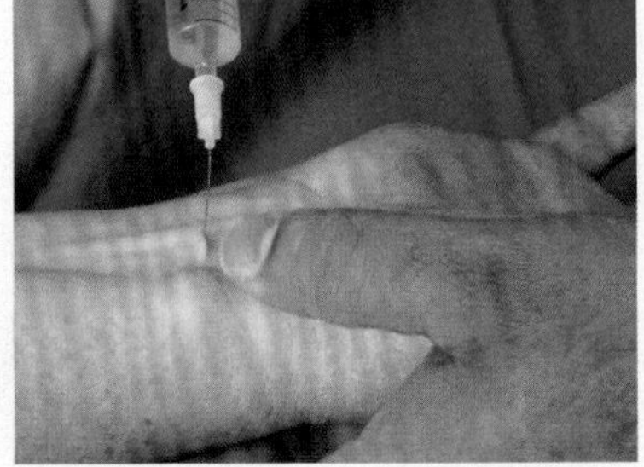
D

FIG 1 • One milliliter of 0.5% bupivacaine is injected to block the PIN and AIN (**A**), the branches of the radial nerve (**B**), the branches of the dorsal cutaneous ulnar nerve (**C**), the palmar branch of the median nerve (**D**), and the branches of the intermetacarpal nerve. (Reprinted from Hunt T, Herlas-Palou C. Wrist denervation. In: Chung K, ed. Operative Techniques: Hand and Wrist Surgery. Philadelphia: Elsevier, 2008:209–230.)

of the median nerve (**FIG 1D**), and finally between the base of the second and third metacarpals to block the recurrent intermetacarpal branches.

- The wrist is examined before the injections and again 20 minutes afterward. Baltimore Therapeutic Equipment is used where available.
  - A decrease in pain rating by 90% and an increase in work output of more than 200% indicate a significant improvement.
  - Patients with these results are considered good candidates for surgical denervation.

IMAGING AND OTHER DIAGNOSTIC STUDIES

- Posteroanterior and lateral radiographs of the wrist confirm the degenerative changes in the wrist joint.
- If there is any doubt about the degree of degeneration, an advanced imaging study (eg, magnetic resonance imaging [MRI]) or wrist arthroscopy can provide more precise information, but these are seldom required.

DIFFERENTIAL DIAGNOSIS

- Wrist denervation is a good option for patients with wrist pain secondary to degeneration. It is important to rule out other causes of pain, such as infection.
- Patients with frank wrist instability and patients with active inflammatory arthritis are unlikely to benefit from wrist denervation.

NONOPERATIVE MANAGEMENT

- For patients with wrist degeneration, conservative management, including anti-inflammatory drugs and splints, should be tried before considering surgery.

SURGICAL MANAGEMENT

- Wrist denervation is indicated in a patient with considerable pain due to wrist degeneration, recalcitrant to conservative measures.
- Alternatives to wrist denervation include open or arthroscopic wrist débridement, radial styloidectomy, partial carpal arthrodesis, proximal row carpectomy, and wrist arthrodesis. Some of these procedures can be combined with a denervation.

Positioning

- The patient is positioned supine with the affected arm on a hand table, under regional block, with a high arm tourniquet, and the procedure is carried out under loupe magnification.

Approach

- Standard denervation of the wrist is carried out through four incisions: dorsal, dorsal–ulnar, volar–radial, and dorsal, over the base of the metacarpals.
- A partial denervation is carried out through one dorsal incision.

TECHNIQUES

Partial Denervation of the Wrist

- Partial denervation involves excision of the PIN with or without excision of the AIN just proximal to the radiocarpal joint.
- Make a 2-cm transverse dorsal incision 3 to 5 cm proximal to the wrist.
- Incise the fourth extensor compartment in a longitudinal direction and retract the extensor tendons ulnarward.
- Isolate the PIN on the radial floor of the fourth extensor compartment.
  - The PIN travels with the posterior interosseous artery and veins.
- Excise a 1-cm segment of nerve.[2,3]
- Retract the fourth compartment extensor tendons radially and make a small window in the interosseous membrane.
- Excise a segment of AIN just deep to the interosseous membrane.
- Close the extensor retinaculum with absorbable suture and close the skin in a routine manner.
- Apply a soft dressing with or without a temporary splint.

Full Denervation of the Wrist

- A full wrist denervation involves four separate incisions (**TECH FIG 1**).

Incision 1

- Make the same transverse incision described for a partial denervation 3 to 5 cm proximal to the wrist on the dorsal forearm.
  - If a more distal incision is used, some articular branches from the PIN may not be completely eliminated.
- Excise the PIN (**TECH FIG 2A**) and branches of the AIN (**TECH FIG 2B**) as discussed earlier.

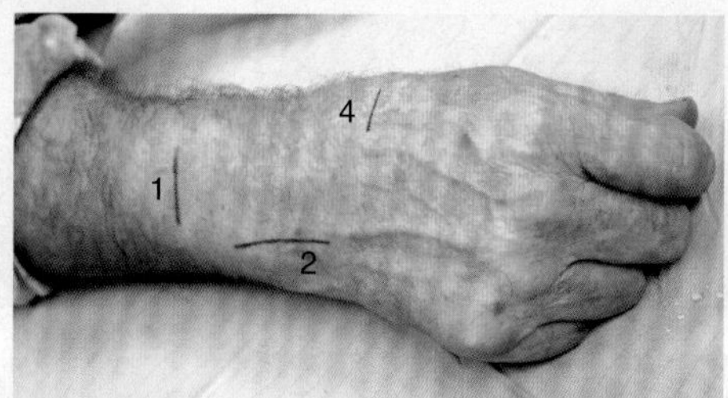

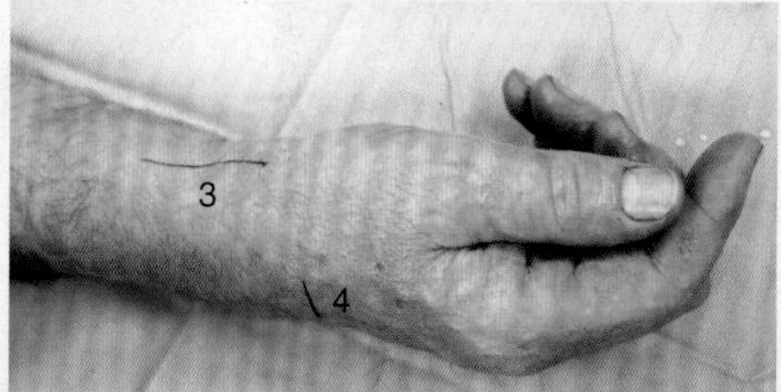

TECH FIG 1 • **A,B.** The four incisions (*1* to *4*) for a complete wrist denervation are marked on the skin. (Reprinted from Hunt T, Herlas-Palou C. Wrist denervation. In: Chung K, ed. Operative Techniques: Hand and Wrist Surgery. Philadelphia: Elsevier, 2008:209–230.)

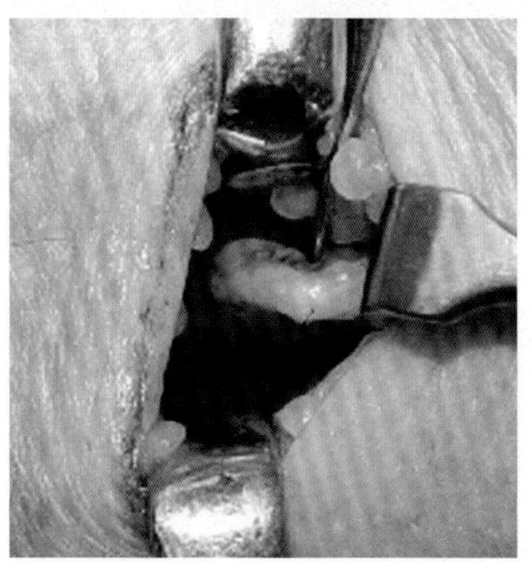
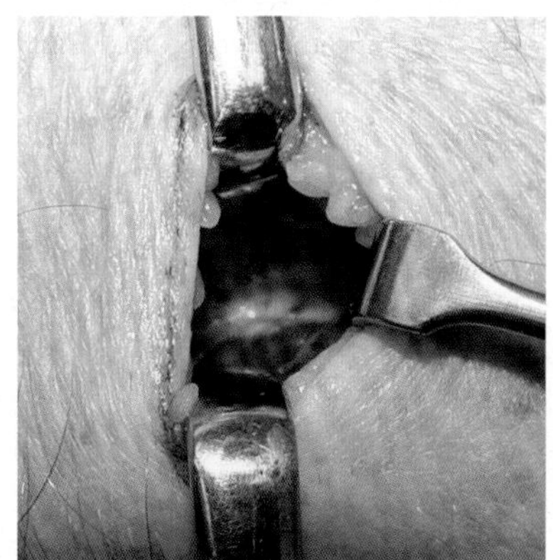

TECH FIG 2 • A. The PIN is isolated on the radial floor of the fourth extensor compartment. **B.** A longitudinal incision in the interosseous membrane reveals the AIN. (Reprinted from Hunt T, Herlas-Palou C. Wrist denervation. In: Chung K, ed. Operative Techniques: Hand and Wrist Surgery. Philadelphia: Elsevier, 2008:209–230.)

Incision 2

- Make a 2- to 3-cm dorsal–ulnar incision over the wrist at the level of the ulnar head.
- Dissect to the level of the extensor retinaculum.
- In the subcutaneous flap, isolate the dorsal branch of the ulnar nerve along with its small articular branches to the wrist joint (**TECH FIG 3**).
- Divide these small branches close to the point where they enter the extensor retinaculum.

Incision 3

- Make a 2- to 3-cm volar–radial incision centered over the radial artery at the level of the wrist and distal forearm.
- Resect a portion of perivascular tissue from around the radial artery.
- Eliminate sympathetic branches to the wrist by using finger dissection to develop planes deep to the vessel, deep to the palmar cutaneous branch of the median nerve, and deep to the radial sensory nerve.

Incision 4

- Make a 2-cm transverse incision over the dorsal base of the second and third metacarpals.
- Dissect through the fascia to expose and resect the recurrent intermetacarpal branches (**TECH FIG 4**).
- Close in standard fashion.
- Apply a soft dressing with or without a temporary splint.

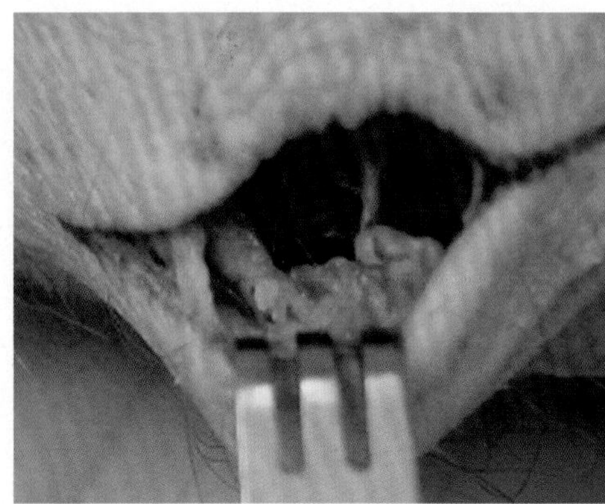

TECH FIG 3 • Through a dorsal–ulnar incision, a subcutaneous flap is raised containing the dorsal cutaneous branch of the ulnar nerve and its small branches, seen here heading toward the retinaculum. (Reprinted from Hunt T, Herlas-Palou C. Wrist denervation. In: Chung K, ed. Operative Techniques: Hand and Wrist Surgery. Philadelphia: Elsevier, 2008:209–230.)

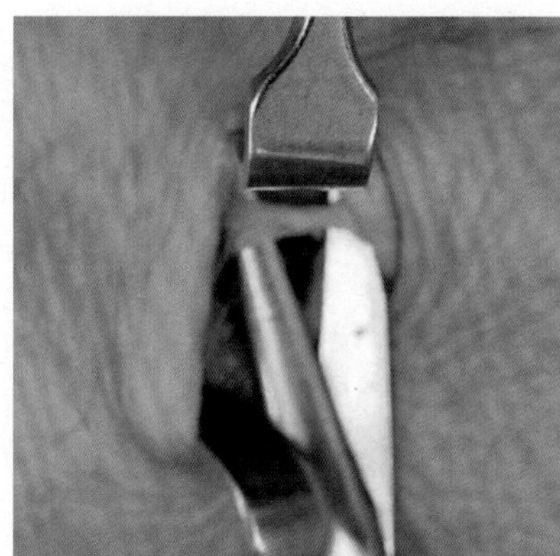

TECH FIG 4 • The recurrent intermetacarpal branch is exposed and resected between the bases of the second and third metacarpals. (Reprinted from Hunt T, Herlas-Palou C. Wrist denervation. In: Chung K, ed. Operative Techniques: Hand and Wrist Surgery. Philadelphia: Elsevier, 2008:209–230.)

PEARLS AND PITFALLS

Indications	■ Patients with wrist degeneration and substantial pain but some useful wrist movement ■ Avoid denervation in patients with frank wrist instability or active inflammatory arthritis. ■ Use local anesthetic blocks to help in patient selection.
Options	■ Partial denervation ■ Full denervation ■ Denervation combined with other procedures
Alternatives to denervation	■ Arthroscopic or open wrist débridement ■ Radial styloidectomy ■ Partial carpal arthrodesis ■ Proximal row carpectomy ■ Wrist arthrodesis

POSTOPERATIVE CARE

- Early range of motion is initiated but little formal therapy is required.
- A removable splint may be provided for comfort initially.
- Patients usually return to work 2 to 4 weeks after surgery.

OUTCOMES

- Wrist denervation is successful in providing pain relief in the long term in two-thirds of patients.
- A partial wrist denervation seems to provide good results initially, but there is often deterioration after 12 months.

COMPLICATIONS

- Although there is a theoretical risk of causing a neuropathic Charcot joint, to our knowledge, this has never been reported. This proves that a complete denervation of the wrist joint is never achieved.
- Neuroma formation has been reported in 2% of patients.

REFERENCES

1. Buck-Gramcko D. Denervation of the wrist joint. J Hand Surg Am 1977;2(1):54–61.
2. Ferreres A, Suso S, Foucher G, et al. Wrist denervation. Surgical considerations. J Hand Surg Br 1995;20(6):769–772.
3. Weinstein LP, Berger RA. Analgesic benefit, functional outcome, and patient satisfaction after partial wrist denervation. J Hand Surg Am 2002;27(5):833–839.

106 CHAPTER

Open and Arthroscopic Radial Styloidectomy

Bruce A. Monaghan

DEFINITION

- Arthritis between the radial styloid and the distal aspect of the scaphoid can lead to pain, weakness of grip, and limitation of motion. This arthritis can occur in the early stages of a variety of pathologic states of the radiocarpal joint.
- Radial styloidectomy is a technique that involves resection of the distalmost aspect of the articular surface of the distal radius.
- A radial styloidectomy can be performed as a distinct procedure via an open incision or by arthroscopic means. It is more commonly undertaken as an adjunct procedure with reconstructive or salvage procedures for scaphoid nonunions, carpal instabilities, Kienböck disease, or posttraumatic arthritis of the radiocarpal joint.[10,22]

ANATOMY

- The radial styloid is the distalmost projection on the lateral aspect of the terminal end of the radius (**FIG 1A,B**).
  - When viewed from the lateral aspect, the styloid has a gentle slope volarly, placing it below the midcoronal longitudinal axis of the radius.
  - The intra-articular component of the radial styloid encompasses part of the scaphoid facet.
  - The extra-articular aspect of the styloid serves as the origin of several dorsal, palmar, and radial extrinsic ligaments that are vital to normal carpal kinematics (**FIG 1C**).
- The palmar radiocarpal ligaments serve as a constraint to radiocarpal pronation, ulnar translation, and distal pole scaphoid stabilization. Global disruption of this complex has been implicated in perilunate dislocation. The palmar radiocarpal ligaments are composed of the following structures:
  - The radial collateral ligament (RCL) is a thin structure that originates from the tip of the radial styloid and inserts into the waist and distal aspect of the scaphoid. The integrity of the ligament is always sacrificed with a radial styloidectomy, but no untoward effects have been reported.[3,4]
  - The radioscaphocapitate (RSC) ligament originates from the palmar cortex of the distal radius coursing distally and ulnarly, attaching to the waist and proximal cortex of the distal pole of the scaphoid and the body of the capitate.[3,4]
  - The long radiolunate (LRL) ligament originates from the palmar cortical margin of the distal radius immediately adjacent and medial to the RSC ligament. It is separated from the RSC by a distinct sulcus that serves an arthroscopic landmark.[3,4]
- The dorsal radiocarpal (DRC) ligament originates broadly from the dorsal rim of the distal radius around the tubercle of Lister, coursing ulnarly, distally, and obliquely to insert on the dorsal tubercle of the triquetrum.
  - The radialmost fibers of this ligament also insert on the dorsal lunate.

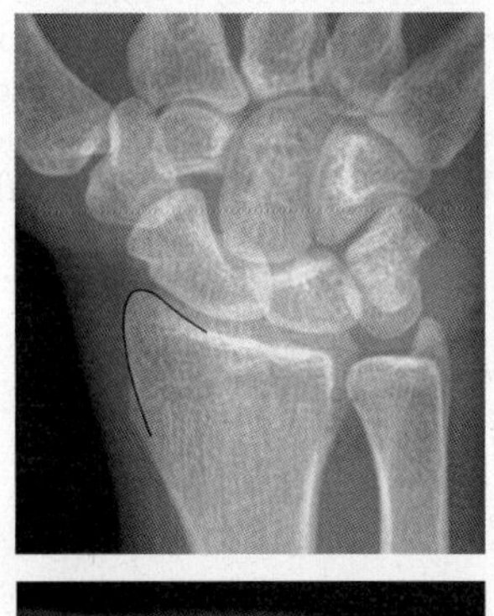

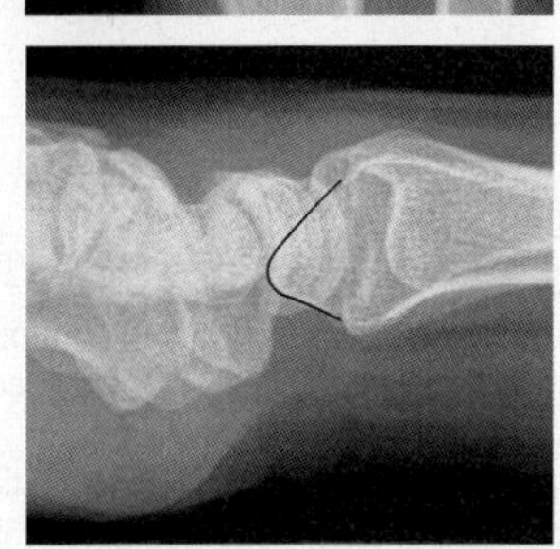

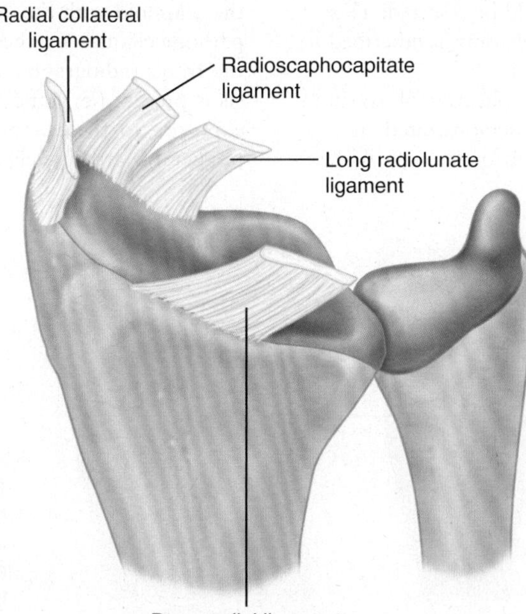

FIG 1 • **A,B.** The radial styloid outlined on a standard posteroanterior (PA) and lateral wrist radiograph. **C.** Palmar and dorsal extrinsic ligaments of the radiocarpal joint. Note the broad origin of the dorsoradial ligament. The RCL originates from the tip of the styloid. The RSC and LRL ligaments are separated by a well-defined sulcus readily seen arthroscopically.

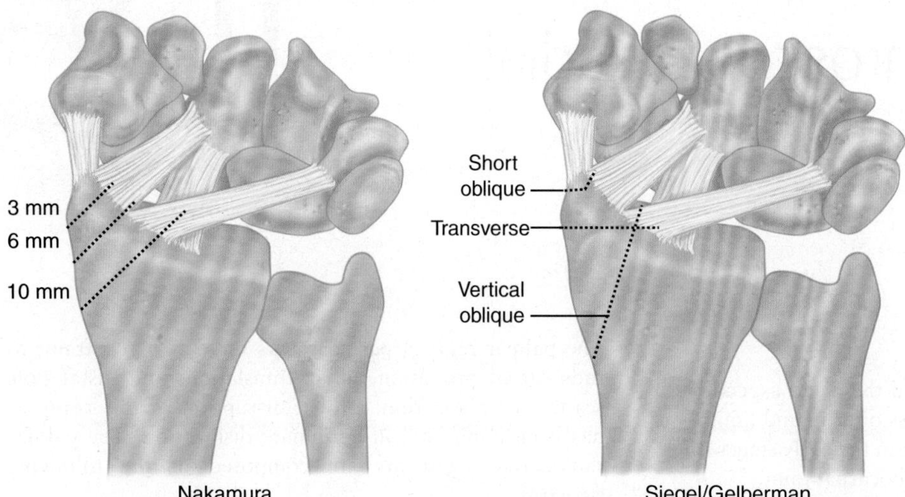

FIG 2 • Styloidectomies as described by Nakamura[12] and Siegel and Gelberman.[16]

- The DRC ligament, in concert with the dorsal intercarpal ligament, has a crucial role in maintaining normal carpal kinematics and carpal stability and preventing ulnar translation of the carpus.[19,20]
- Siegel and Gelberman[16] examined the effect of three different styloidectomy configurations on palmar radiocarpal ligament integrity in a cadaver model (**FIG 2**).
  - The most conservative osteotomy (short oblique) removed only 9% of the RSC and none of the LRL ligaments.
  - A vertical oblique osteotomy sacrificed 92% of the RSC and 21% of the LRL ligaments.
  - A transverse styloidectomy was the most aggressive and resulted in loss of 95% of the RSC and 42% loss of the LRL ligaments.
- Nakamura et al[12] examined the effect of radial styloidectomy on carpal alignment and ulnar translation in cadaveric limbs. They demonstrated that as a larger segment of the radial styloid was resected (see **FIG 2**), a greater tendency toward ulnar translation, as manifested by decreased stiffness, was observed. No frank ulnar translation with axial loading was observed.
  - Based on their analysis, they recommended that no more than 3 to 4 mm of radial styloid should be resected. This correlated with a short oblique styloidectomy as described by Siegel and Gelberman.[16]
- Although ulnar translation is a stated complication of overly vigorous styloidectomy, Viegas et al[19] demonstrated in a cadaver model that ulnar translation can occur only with resection of the DRC, RSC, LRL, and short radiolunate (SRL) ligaments.

PATHOGENESIS AND NATURAL HISTORY

Scapholunate Instability

- Watson and Ballet[21] reviewed radiographs of individuals with scapholunate dissociation to establish the sequential progression of arthritis in the scapholunate advanced collapse (SLAC) wrist (**FIG 3**).
  - SLAC I: Degenerative changes are confined to the radial styloid area.
  - SLAC II: Changes are characterized by joint space narrowing involving the entire radioscaphoid articulation.
  - SLAC III: Changes involve additional arthritis between the capitate and lunate.
- Several authors have examined the mechanics of scapholunate dissociation in cadaver models and have demonstrated that scapholunate instability leads to a shift in the contact pressures from the proximal pole of scaphoid articulation with the radial articular surface toward the distal pole of the scaphoid with the dorsal lip of the radial styloid.[7,8] The pathomechanics of these changes can occur even before the frank radiographic appearance of scapholunate diastasis is present (ie, static scapholunate instability). Prolonged exposure to these abnormal contact stresses leads to the predictable arthritic changes described earlier.

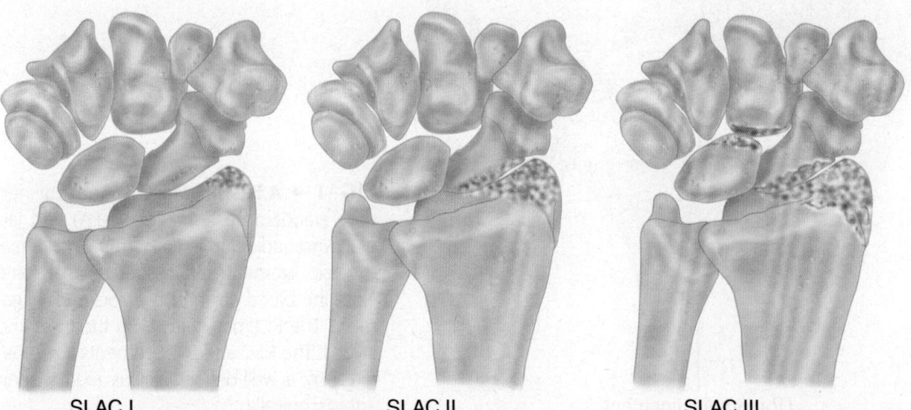

FIG 3 • Stages of arthritis with SLAC. SLAC I: degenerative changes are confined to the radial styloid. SLAC II: joint space narrowing of the entire radioscaphoid articulation. SLAC III: chondral changes in the radioscaphoid and capitolunate joint.

- Scaphoid nonunion
  - With an unstable scaphoid fracture, the proximal pole of the scaphoid remains firmly fixed to and extends with the lunate through an intact scapholunate interosseous ligament. The distal pole adopts a flexed posture, which can then impinge on the radial styloid, leading to abnormal contact stresses and arthritic changes.
  - The natural history of scaphoid nonunion has not been established by rigorous prospective analysis. Nonetheless, most surgeons believe that unstable scaphoid fractures result in abnormal carpal kinematics with a dorsal intercalated segment instability (DISI) deformity and subsequent arthritis (scaphoid nonunion advanced collapse [SNAC] wrist).
  - Vender et al[18] examined the radiographs of 64 patients with symptomatic scaphoid nonunions and showed a high frequency of degenerative changes that occurred in a predictable sequence similar to the findings of SLAC wrist. Initial degenerative changes were seen between the radial styloid and the distal fragment of the scaphoid nonunion. Changes then progressed to include the midcarpal joint with sparing of the proximal pole scaphoid and radiolunate articulation.[18] Inoue and Sakuma[9] reviewed 102 patients with scaphoid nonunions clinically and radiographically; they found that arthritis initially developed at the scaphoid–radial styloid articulation and subsequently the midcarpal joint. All patients had radiographic arthritis within 10 years of injury. They also demonstrated that although radiographic progression did not correlate with wrist pain, it did correlate with a decrease in grip strength and range of motion.
- Impingement after triscaphe (scaphoid-trapezoid-trapezium) fusion
  - Rogers and Watson[14] reviewed 93 patients after triscaphe fusion and found a 33% incidence of painful impingement between the fusion mass and the radial styloid that resolved after limited radial styloidectomy. They hypothesized that the fixed scaphoid could no longer be accommodated in the fossa and impacted on the radial styloid.
- Proximal row carpectomy
  - Although not all surgeons routinely perform a radial styloidectomy in the setting of a proximal row carpectomy, a recent cadaveric study demonstrated that radial deviation after proximal row carpectomy was limited by impingement of the trapezoid on the radial styloid.[6]

PATIENT HISTORY AND PHYSICAL FINDINGS

- Patients with clinically significant radial styloid arthritis or impingement frequently complain of pain along the dorsoradial aspect of the wrist that is exacerbated by extension of the wrist or gripping activities. They may also note focal swelling or a decrease in the range of motion.
- A complete physical examination of the radiocarpal, the midcarpal, and the first carpometacarpal joints is necessary to assess for associated conditions and to rule out alternative diagnoses.
- Styloid impingement typically causes radial-sided wrist pain that is exacerbated by radial deviation, extension, and axial loading of the wrist.
- Physical findings of styloid impingement are centered around the anatomic snuffbox (**FIG 4**).
  - The anatomic snuffbox is triangular, with its radial border formed by the extensor pollicis brevis tendon, its ulnar border by the extensor pollicis longus tendon, and its proximal border by the dorsal rim of the distal radius at the level of the styloid. The waist of the scaphoid and a small segment of the trapezium are palpable in the floor of the snuffbox, more readily with ulnar deviation.
  - Focal tenderness and synovitis along the proximal edge of the snuffbox made worse by forced radial deviation and extension may be indicative of styloid impingement.
- More diffuse tenderness, synovitis, and global limitations of motion may be indicative of a more advanced stage of posttraumatic arthritis or an inflammatory process (ie, rheumatoid arthritis, gout, pseudogout), which would preclude the success of an isolated radial styloidectomy.

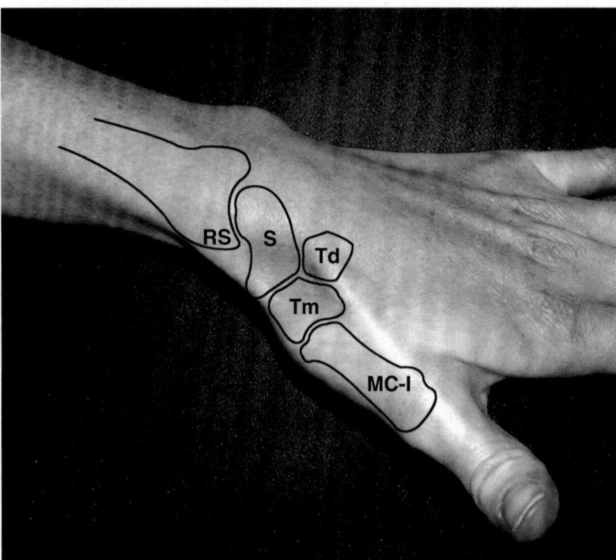

FIG 4 • Meticulous and systematic physical examination of this region can rule out diagnoses other than radial styloid impingement. *RS*, radial styloid; *S*, scaphoid; *Tm*, trapezium; *Td*, trapezoid; *MC-I*, thumb metacarpal.

IMAGING AND OTHER DIAGNOSTIC STUDIES

- Plain radiographs of the wrist
  - To diagnose and stage SNAC and SLAC (**FIG 5**)
  - To rule out scaphoid fracture or other acute injury

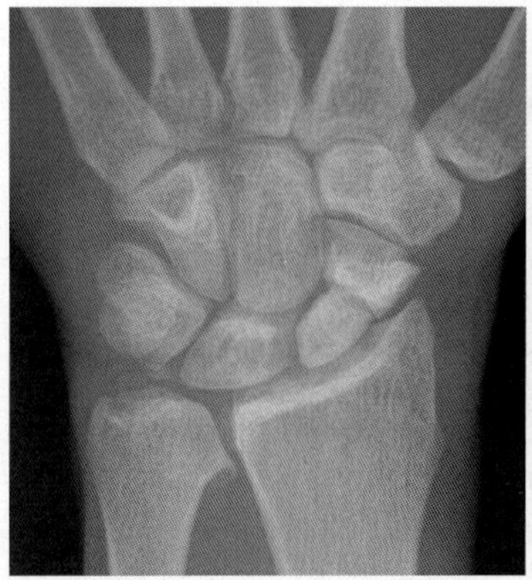
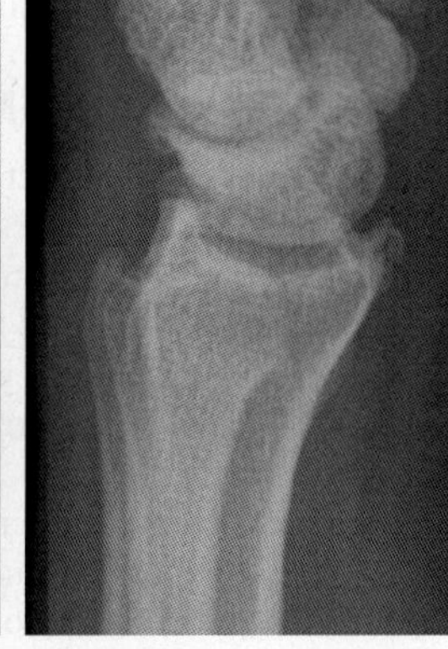
FIG 5 • Impingement of the flexed distal pole of the scaphoid nonunion against the radial styloid leading to arthritic changes.

- Stress radiographs (clenched fist and radial–ulnar deviation posteroanterior) of the wrist can yield information concerning dynamic impingement between the scaphoid and the radial styloid.

DIFFERENTIAL DIAGNOSIS

- De Quervain stenosing tenosynovitis: Tenderness usually extends along the extra-articular component of the radial styloid, proximally and radially over the first dorsal compartment. A positive Finkelstein test is highly suggestive of this disorder.
- Scaphoid-trapezoid-trapezium arthritis: focal tenderness in the distal ulnar aspect of the snuffbox under the extensor pollicis long tendon along the axis of the second metacarpal
- Thumb carpometacarpal instability or arthritis: tenderness distal to the anatomic snuffbox that is worsened by loading of the thumb ray (carpometacarpal grind test)
- Scaphoid fracture: After an acute injury, advanced imaging (bone scan or magnetic resonance imaging [MRI]) may be required to rule out an acute scaphoid fracture.
- Preiser disease
- Inflammatory arthritis (ie, rheumatoid arthritis, gout, pseudogout)
- Radial sensory neuritis or neuroma
- Tenosynovitis of the extensor carpi radialis longus and brevis
- Not uncommonly, styloid impingement coexists with other diagnoses, especially basilar thumb arthritis and de Quervain stenosing tenosynovitis.

NONOPERATIVE MANAGEMENT

- Individuals with chronic SLAC or SNAC wrist arthritis frequently present with acute pain after a recent injury. After obtaining an accurate medical history of prior injury and radiographic assessment, the chronicity of the problem is usually evident.
  - In this situation, a course of conservative treatment with activity modification, nonsteroidal anti-inflammatory drugs, rest in a forearm-based thumb spica splint, and selective corticosteroid injection in the radial styloid area is appropriate.
  - If the arthritic changes are truly isolated to the area of articulation between the scaphoid and the styloid, the surgeon may elect earlier operative intervention with the theoretical goal of slowing or preventing progressive symptomatic arthrosis and the need for a more extensive reconstructive procedure.

SURGICAL MANAGEMENT

- Isolated radial styloidectomy is a limited procedure to treat the early stage of progressive posttraumatic arthritis.
  - It cannot be expected to prevent its pathologic progression.
- It can also be employed as a temporizing solution in a low-demand individual or in a patient unfit or unwilling to undertake a more extensive procedure and postoperative rehabilitative course.
  - In that instance, patient expectations with respect to motion and pain relief must be assiduously managed.
- Arthroscopic radial styloidectomy has the theoretical advantages of being minimally invasive and allowing more precise control of the level of bony resection to minimize injury to the palmar radiocarpal ligaments. In addition, arthroscopic evaluation of the radiocarpal and midcarpal joints can allow for diagnosis and treatment of concomitant intra-articular pathology.[22]

Preoperative Planning

- Precise radiographic assessment and patient selection are critical in ensuring a good outcome. The surgeon must review all radiographic studies and the severity, characteristics, and nature of the patient's symptoms and physical findings.
- In some cases, final staging of the severity of articular degeneration can be made only by direct visualization with diagnostic wrist arthroscopy (**FIG 6**). In situations where there is incompetency of the RSC ligament (eg, rheumatoid arthritis, gout, pseudogout) radial styloidectomy may be contraindicated in that it might cause ulnar translocation of the carpus. An isolated radial styloidectomy or a more extensive reconstructive procedure can be done at the time of arthroscopy or at a later time, after the implications of the arthroscopic findings are discussed with the patient.

Positioning

- The patient is positioned supine on a stretcher with an attached hand table and the arm centered on the hand table with the shoulder abducted 90 degrees. A mini-fluoroscopy unit is draped in a sterile fashion and placed in a plane perpendicular to the hand table.
- For arthroscopic procedures, the arm is stabilized to the hand table with a strap that allows countertraction.
  - The shoulder is abducted 90 degrees, the elbow is flexed 90 degrees, and finger traps are placed on the index and middle fingers.
  - The forearm is suspended in a standard wrist traction tower with 8 to 12 pounds of traction employed.
  - A mini-fluoroscopy unit is draped in a sterile fashion and placed in a plane parallel to and above the hand table.

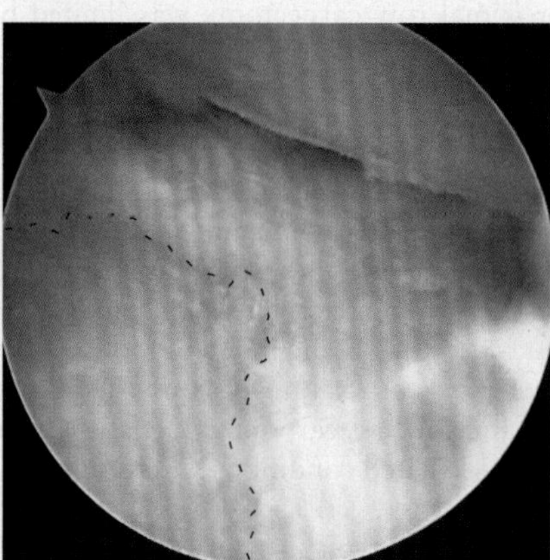

FIG 6 • Arthroscopic findings of full-thickness cartilage loss in the entire scaphoid facet (*dashed line*) and proximal pole of the scaphoid as viewed from the dorsal 3-4 portal. These degenerative changes were not readily apparent on plain radiographs. An isolated radial styloidectomy cannot be expected to confer pain relief in this instance.

- Alternatively, the hand can be suspended via finger traps using a nonsterile overhead traction boom (ie, an arthroscopic shoulder holder); with this method, the wrist traction tower will not be an impediment to intraoperative fluoroscopic assessment (**FIG 7**).

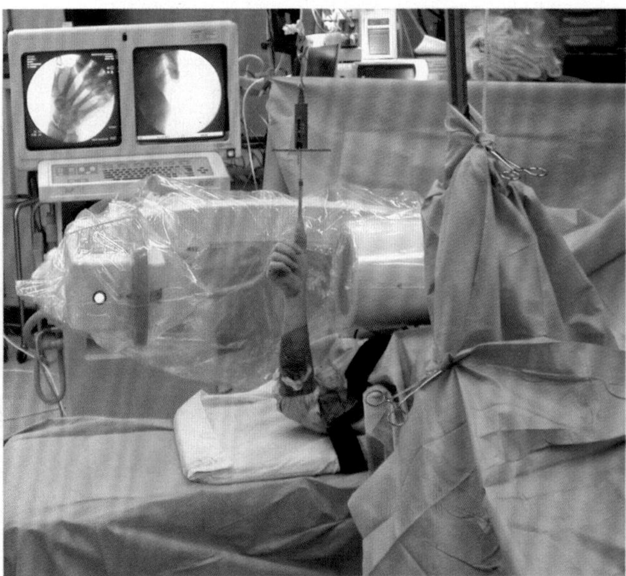

FIG 7 • An alternative arthroscopic setup can be useful. A nonsterile overhead traction boom (an arthroscopic shoulder holder) is used from the contralateral side of the operating room table to suspend the limb via finger traps with countertraction provided by a strap on the arm. With this method, the fluoroscopic images of the wrist can be obtained without being obscured by the arthroscopic wrist tower.

Approach

- A radial styloidectomy can be performed in conjunction with other reconstructive procedures such as proximal row carpectomy, intercarpal fusion, or bone grafting for a scaphoid nonunion.
  - In these instances, the primary procedure usually requires wide exposure through a standard dorsal approach to the wrist.
- An isolated styloidectomy can be performed through a limited radial incision.
- An arthroscopic styloidectomy can be performed through standard arthroscopic portals.

TECHNIQUES

Open Radial Styloidectomy

- Palpate the distalmost aspect of the radial styloid on the volar radial aspect of the wrist. Make an incision from that point for 2 or 3 cm proximally and obliquely between the first and second extensor compartments (**TECH FIG 1A**).
  - Alternatively, a transverse incision may provide a more cosmetically pleasing scar but also may limit exposure.
- At this level, there will be arborization of the terminal branches of the radial sensory and lateral antebrachial cutaneous nerves in the subcutaneous tissue.[2] Use blunt dissection and gentle retraction to expose the first and second compartments.
  - Distal placement of the incision may place the dorsal branch of the radial artery at risk and should be recognized.
- Incise the extensor retinaculum in the 1-2 interval and expose the radial styloid by subperiosteal dissection. Alternatively, the radius can be approached through the floor of the first compartment (**TECH FIG 1B**).
- Expose the radial styloid by sharp dissection (**TECH FIG 1C**).
- Using a sharp osteotome, remove the distal 3 to 4 mm of radial styloid. The plane of the cut should be perpendicular to the articular surface (**TECH FIG 1D**).
  - Fluoroscopic imaging of the level of resection can be useful at this point in the procedure.
- A narrow malleable retractor can be placed in the radiocarpal joint to prevent damage to the scaphoid as the styloid is being resected (**TECH FIG 1E**).
- After styloidectomy, fluoroscopic examination with the wrist in radial and ulnar deviation to assess for impingement confirms adequacy of the resection level (**TECH FIG 1F,G**).
- Loosely reapproximate the periosteum with resorbable suture, allow the extensor compartments to fall back into their anatomic position, and suture the skin. A bulky dressing and volar splint holding the wrist is applied.

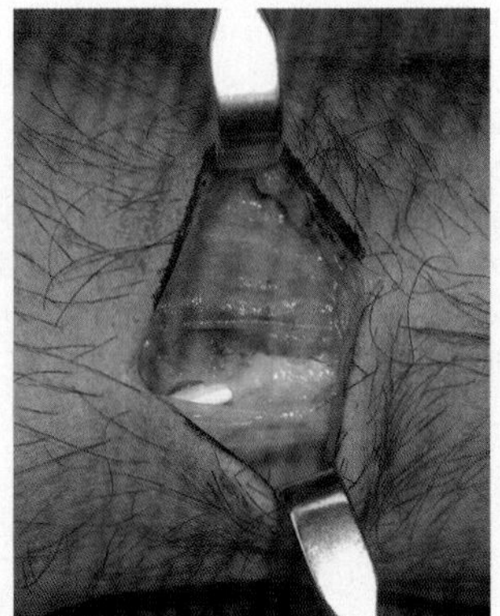

A

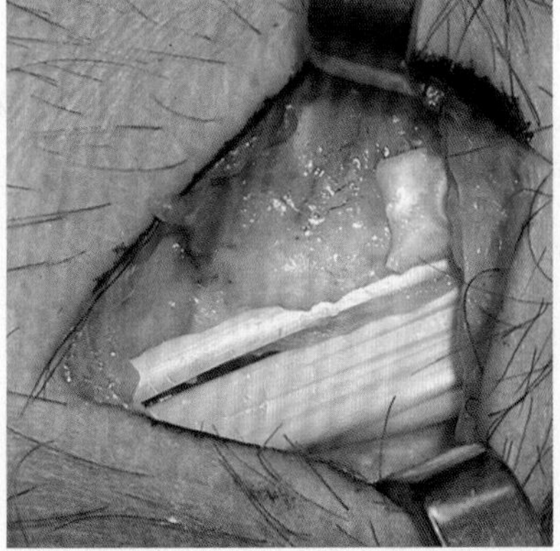

B

TECH FIG 1 • Open radial styloidectomy. **A.** A 2- to 3-cm oblique skin incision is made between the first and second extensor compartments. Note the branches of the radial sensory and lateral antebrachial cutaneous nerves. **B.** The first dorsal compartment is then opened. *(continued)*

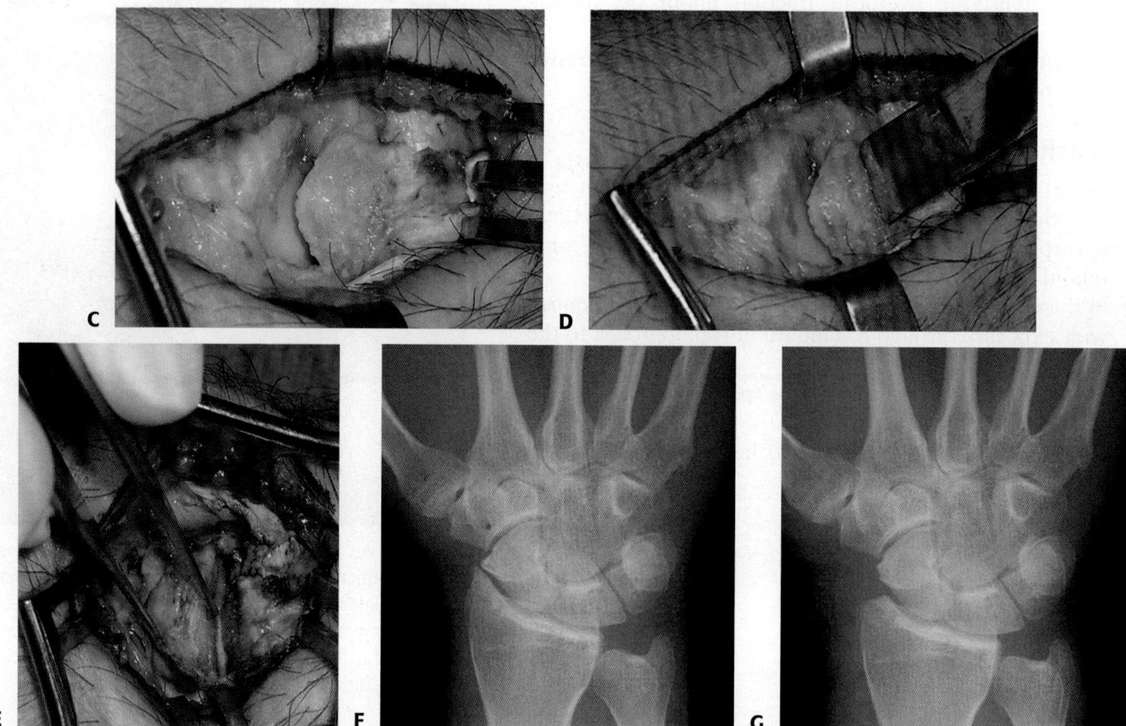

TECH FIG 1 • *(continued)* **C.** The radial styloid is extraperiosteally exposed by sharp dissection. **D.** An osteotome is used to resect the distal 3 to 4 mm of radial styloid. The osteotome should be angled perpendicular to the joint surface. **E.** The resected radial styloid is removed. **F,G.** Preoperative and postoperative PA radiographs of the wrist with early SNAC undergoing open radial styloidectomy. (Courtesy of Dr. John J. Fernandez.)

Arthroscopic Styloidectomy

- After patient positioning as previously described, insufflate the joint with 5 to 10 mL of sterile saline and establish the 3-4 portal. Outflow is achieved by placing an 18-gauge needle in the 6U interval. Perform a complete arthroscopic evaluation of the radiocarpal joint.
- Establish the radial and ulnar midcarpal portals and perform an arthroscopic evaluation to confirm capitolunate joint preservation.
- Place a localization needle into the styloscaphoid joint space, in the interval between the first and second compartments to localize and establish the 1-2 arthroscopic portal. Angling the needle about 24 degrees proximal to mirror the radial inclination will avoid damage to the scaphoid articular surface.
  - Confirm the adequacy of the position of this working portal by arthroscopic evaluation from the 3-4 interval. The volar radial portal can also be used interchangeably with the 3-4 portal for viewing and instrumentation to assure complete access to the radial styloid.[17]
  - Develop the portal by sharp dissection through skin only and blunt dissection in the subcutaneous tissues to the capsule to prevent damage to the radial sensory nerve, the lateral antebrachial cutaneous nerve, and the radial artery. This is best accomplished by a starting point within 4 mm of the palpable tip of the radial styloid.[17]
  - The full-radius resector is first placed in the 1-2 portal to débride the soft tissue radial, dorsal, and volar to the styloid so that the anticipated bone resection can be more easily defined (**TECH FIG 2A**). Resect the radial styloid with a 2.9-mm full-radius resector, an arthroscopic covered burr, or both. This is initiated at the radial margin of the RSC ligament and carried radially. The diameter of the burr can be used as a gauge for the amount of bone being resected. The degenerative cartilage changes of the radial styloid facet can also serve as a useful guide to the ulnar most margin of resection that is required.
- Intraoperative fluoroscopy is critical in the assessment of the resection level (**TECH FIG 2B**).
- After completing the styloidectomy, the wrist is brought out of traction and arthroscopic and fluoroscopic assessment is used to confirm that no further carpal impingement exists. Remove the arthroscopic instruments and suture the portals. Apply a sterile bulky dressing and volar splint to the wrist and forearm.

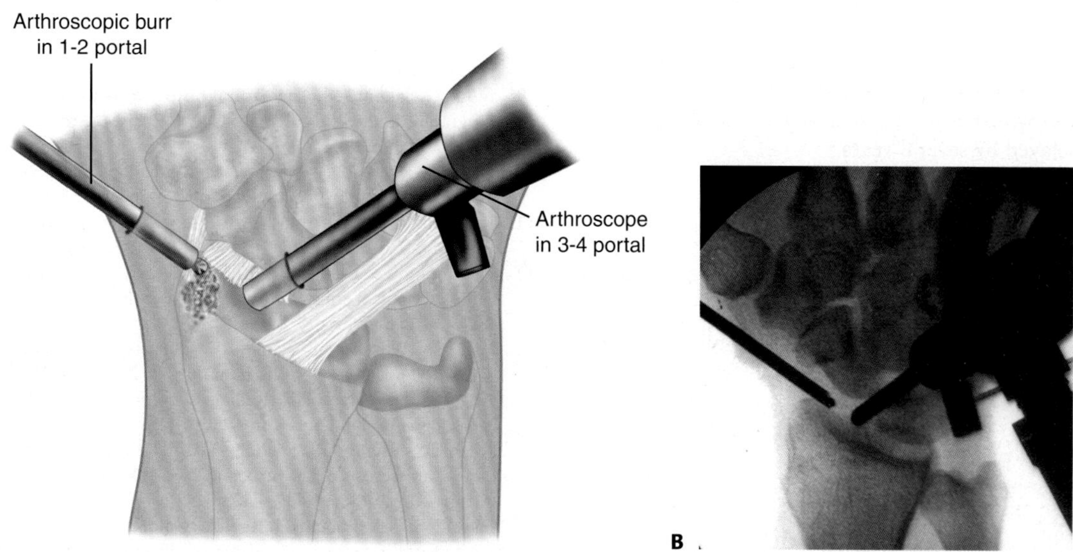

TECH FIG 2 • Arthroscopic radial styloidectomy. **A.** The arthroscopic burr is in the 1-2 portal and the arthroscope is in the 3-4 portal. **B.** Fluoroscopic image obtained during arthroscopic radial styloidectomy for scapholunate instability and secondary degeneration. Note the disruption of the line of Gilula in the proximal carpal row.

PEARLS AND PITFALLS

Indications	■ A complete history and physical examination emphasizing clinical staging is essential. The final decision to proceed with styloidectomy may require staging arthroscopy.
Insufficient or excessive styloid resection	■ Arthroscopic visualization of the RSC ligament to prevent significant injury and to assure its competency ■ Using the diameter of the burr as a gauge for the amount of bone resected ■ Intraoperative fluoroscopic evaluation
Poor arthroscopic visualization	■ Convert from arthroscopic to open procedure.

POSTOPERATIVE CARE

- If the radial styloidectomy is performed concomitantly with another reconstructive procedure (PRC, four-corner arthrodesis, scaphoid bone grafting and fixation), the rehabilitation is dictated by the requirements of that additional procedure.
- After either open or arthroscopic radial styloidectomy, the postoperative dressing and sutures are removed in 7 to 10 days. Early active, active-assisted, and passive motion is initiated under the guidance of a hand therapist. Usually, a removable splint is used initially for patient comfort. As the patient's symptoms permit, graded strengthening and unrestricted activities are allowed.

OUTCOMES

- Barnard and Stubbins[1] first described a radial styloidectomy as part of an operative treatment strategy for scaphoid nonunion in 14 patients in 1948. They thought that the styloidectomy removed impingement, enhanced exposure of the scaphoid, and provided material for bone grafting from the same operative field. Since that time, there have been no series of outcomes in the indexed English literature for outcomes after isolated open radial styloidectomy. Several reports of radial styloidectomy performed with open reduction and internal fixation of scaphoid nonunion or with triscaphe fusion have demonstrated good pain relief but no significant improvement in range of motion.[14,21]
- Ruch et al[15] were the first to describe the use of an arthroscopic radial styloidectomy in the treatment of avascular necrosis of the proximal pole following scaphoid nonunion. Page et al[13] presented their experience with the arthroscopic technique in 22 patients to the European Federation of National Associations of Orthopaedics and Traumatology in 2003. In short-term follow-up, they reported 75% good and satisfactory results. Levadoux and Cognet[11] reviewed their results in 12 patients with SLAC I and SLAC II arthritic changes with average follow-up of 39 months. They showed an 18% increase in grip strength and high patient satisfaction; 80 % of their patients experienced complete relief of their wrist pain. Birman et al[5] performed arthroscopic radial styloidectomy combined with arthroscopic débridement and selective anterior and posterior interosseous neurectomies in advanced SLAC wrist (II and III) in an effort to delay or avoid salvage procedures in eight wrists. At an average of 28 months post procedure, they had maintained good motion and had a 71% satisfaction rate. The authors, however, did caution that this is best thought of as an intermediate procedure to relieve pain and preserve motion.

- Radial styloidectomy is most often performed as a limited procedure to address posttraumatic arthritis of the wrist early in its pathogenesis. Although it can provide long-lasting symptomatic relief, it cannot be expected to halt the progression of the arthritis. A successful radial styloidectomy could be one in which a more extensive reconstructive procedure was delayed by several years.

COMPLICATIONS

- Incomplete resection leading to persistent pain
- Excessive resection leading to extrinsic ligament incompetence and wrist instability with ulnar translocation
- Nerve injury to the terminal branches of the radial sensory nerve or lateral antebrachial cutaneous nerve
- Arthrofibrosis
- Infection
- Complex regional pain syndrome

REFERENCES

1. Barnard L, Stubbins SG. Styloidectomy of the radius in the surgical treatment of nonunion of the carpal navicular: a preliminary report. J Bone Joint Surg Am 1948;30(1):98–102.
2. Beldner S, Zlotolow DA, Melone CP Jr, et al. Anatomy of the lateral antebrachial cutaneous and superficial radial nerve in the forearm: a cadaver and clinical study. J Hand Surg Am 2005;30(6):1226–1230.
3. Berger RA. The ligaments of the wrist. A current overview of anatomy with considerations of their potential functions. Hand Clin 1997;13:63–82.
4. Berger RA, Landsmeer JM. The palmar radiocarpal ligaments: a study of adult and fetal human wrist joints. J Hand Surg Am 1990;15(6):847–854.
5. Birman MV, Danoff JR, Rosenwasser MP. Arthroscopic wrist debridement and radial styloidectomy for late stage scapholunate advanced collapse wrist. Presented at the Arthroscopy Association of North America annual meeting, Orlando, FL, May 2012.
6. Blankenhorn BD, Pfaeffle HJ, Tang P, et al. Carpal kinematics after proximal row carpectomy. J Hand Surg Am 2007;32(1):37–46.
7. Blevens AD, Light TR, Jablonsky WS, et al. Radiocarpal articular contact characteristics with scaphoid instability. J Hand Surg Am 1989;14(5):781–790.
8. Burgess RC. The effect of rotatory subluxation of the scaphoid on radio-scaphoid contact. J Hand Surg Am 1987;12(5 pt 1):771–774.
9. Inoue G, Sakuma M. The natural history of scaphoid non-union. Radiographical and clinical analysis in 102 cases. Arch Orthop Trauma Surg 1996;115:1–4.
10. Kalainov DM, Cohen MS, Sweet S. Radial styloidectomy. In: Geissler WB, ed. Wrist Arthroscopy. New York: Springer-Verlag, 2005:134–138.
11. Levadoux M, Cognet JM. Arthroscopic styloidectomy [in French]. Chir Main 2006;25(suppl 1):S197–S201.
12. Nakamura T, Cooney WP III, Lui WH, et al. Radial styloidectomy: a biomechanical study on the stability of the wrist. J Hand Surg Am 2001;26(1):85–93.
13. Page RS, Waseem M, Stanley JK. Clinical outcome of arthroscopic radial styloidectomy. J Bone Joint Surg Br 2004;86B:280.
14. Rogers WD, Watson HK. Radial styloid impingement after triscaphe arthrodesis. J Hand Surg Am 1989;14(2 pt 1):297–301.
15. Ruch DS, Chang DS, Poehling GG. The arthroscopic treatment of avascular necrosis of the proximal pole following scaphoid nonunion. Arthroscopy 1998;14:747–752.
16. Siegel DB, Gelberman RH. Radial styloidectomy: an anatomical study with special reference to radiocarpal intracapsular ligamentous morphology. J Hand Surg Am 1991;16(1):40–44.
17. Slutsky DJ. Wrist arthroscopy. In: Wolfe SW, Pederson WC, Hotchkiss RN, et al, eds. Green's Operative Hand Surgery. Philadelphia: Elsevier, 2011:709–741.
18. Vender MI, Watson HK, Wiener BD, et al. Degenerative change in symptomatic scaphoid nonunion. J Hand Surg Am 1987;12(4):514–519.
19. Viegas SF, Patterson RM, Ward K. Extrinsic wrist ligaments in the pathomechanics of ulnar translation instability. J Hand Surg Am 1995;20(2):312–318.
20. Viegas SF, Yamaguchi S, Boyd NL, et al. The dorsal ligaments of the wrist: anatomy, mechanical properties, and function. J Hand Surg Am 1999;24(3):456–468.
21. Watson HK, Ballet FL. The SLAC wrist: scapholunate advanced collapse pattern of degenerative arthritis. J Hand Surg Am 1984;9(3):358–365.
22. Yao J, Osterman AL. Arthroscopic techniques for wrist arthritis (radial styloidectomy and proximal pole hamate excision). Hand Clin 2005;21:519–526.

Proximal Row Carpectomy

Kathryn A. Heim, Alex M. Meyers, Thomas B. Hughes, and Mark E. Baratz

DEFINITION

- Proximal row carpectomy (PRC) involves removal of the proximal carpal row (scaphoid, lunate, and triquetrum).
- PRC has been described as a treatment option for a number of pathologic conditions:
  - Scaphoid nonunion advanced collapse (SNAC) wrist
  - Scapholunate advanced collapse (SLAC) wrist
  - Kienböck disease
  - Chronic or missed perilunate dislocation
  - Scaphoid osteonecrosis or Preiser disease
  - Wrist deformity or contracture

ANATOMY

- The proximal row of the wrist consists of three bones: scaphoid, lunate, and triquetrum.
- The proximal row moves as a single unit through intercarpal ligamentous attachments and bony congruity.
  - The proximal row flexes with radial deviation and extends with ulnar deviation.
- The capitate, in the distal row, articulates with the lunate.
  - The proximal capitate articular surface is relatively, although not completely, congruous with the lunate facet of the radius.

PATHOGENESIS

- A number of pathologic conditions lead to wrist degeneration requiring PRC. Patients with progressive pain and limited motion can gain relief following this procedure.
  - SNAC and SLAC
    - Stage I: degenerative changes along the radial half of the radioscaphoid articulation. In SNAC wrists, the degenerative changes are typically limited to the articulation between the distal scaphoid fragment and the radius.
    - Stage II: degenerative changes involving the entire radioscaphoid articulation (**FIG 1**). In SNAC wrists, the articulation between the proximal scaphoid fragment and the radius is preserved, and instead, stage II degeneration occurs in the scaphocapitate joint.
    - Stage III: degenerative changes at the capitolunate joint. The radiolunate joint is spared.
  - Kienböck disease
    - Stage I: normal plain radiographs with wrist pain and positive magnetic resonance imaging (MRI) finding
    - Stage II: sclerosis without collapse of the lunate
    - Stage IIIa: lunate collapse without instability
    - Stage IIIb: where there is lunate collapse with carpal instability (dorsal intercalated segmental instability [DISI]: flexion of the scaphoid with extension of the lunate)
    - Stage IV: fixed carpal instability with pancarpal degenerative changes
  - Missed perilunate dislocation
  - Scaphoid osteonecrosis (Preiser disease)
- Congenital or spastic wrist and hand flexion contractures severe enough that a PRC allows deformity correction that tendon lengthening procedures alone would be unable to correct.

PATIENT HISTORY AND PHYSICAL FINDINGS

- Determine the cause of the wrist degeneration.
- Mechanical wrist pain is aggravated by use and relieved by rest. The history must support this for the proposed treatment to be successful.
- The history defines the patient's symptoms, level of severity, and progression over time as well as any previous attempts at treatment.
- Limited and painful wrist motion with diminished grip strength tends to be a common denominator regardless of the initial source of pathology.
  - Normal range of motion: wrist extension, 70 degrees; wrist flexion, 75 degrees; radial deviation, 20 degrees; ulnar deviation, 35 degrees. This varies considerably.
  - Normal grip strength: Mean grip for males is 103 to 104 for the dominant extremity and 92 to 99 for the nondominant extremity. Mean grip for females is 62 to 63 for the

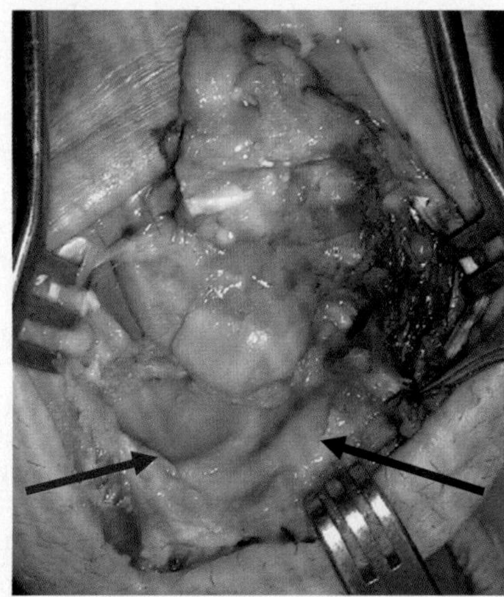

FIG 1 • Intraoperative photograph showing wear at the dorsal half of the scaphoid fossa seen with SLAC wrist, as indicated by the *black arrow*. Cartilage integrity is preserved in the lunate fossa, as indicated by the *red arrow*.

dominant extremity and 53 to 55 for the nondominant extremity.[6]
- Radioscaphoid joint line tenderness on palpation implies radioscaphoid arthritis.
- Swelling over the dorsal and dorsoradial aspects of the wrist can be associated with radiocarpal and intercarpal arthritis. Most often, dorsoradial wrist swelling will be visible and palpable in cases of SLAC and SNAC.

IMAGING AND OTHER DIAGNOSTIC STUDIES

- Plain radiographs assist with making the underlying diagnosis (eg, SNAC wrist, SLAC wrist, Kienböck disease).
  - Evaluate the articular facets and surfaces, specifically the head of the capitate and lunate facet of the radius.
  - Look for other sources of limited wrist motion, diminished grip strength, and pain (eg, thumb carpometacarpal arthritis, scapholunate instability without degenerative changes, fracture).
- MRI has limited use with the exception of suspected Kienböck disease or Preiser disease.

DIFFERENTIAL DIAGNOSIS

- Triangular fibrocartilage complex or distal radioulnar joint pathology
- Extensor carpi ulnaris, flexor carpi ulnaris, flexor carpi radialis tendinitis
- De Quervain tenosynovitis
- Thumb carpometacarpal arthritis
- Scapholunate or lunotriquetral instability without degenerative changes

SURGICAL MANAGEMENT

- The integrity of the articular cartilage on the head of the capitate and the lunate facet of the radius are critical. The ultimate assessment is made intraoperatively.
- Indications
  - SLAC and SNAC wrist degeneration: stage I, II, or III (only if the degenerative changes at proximal capitate are limited to thinning or minor fissuring)
  - Kienböck disease (stage IIIb)
  - Chronic or missed perilunate dislocations
  - Scaphoid osteonecrosis (Preiser disease)
  - Wrist deformity or contracture
- Contraindications
  - Active inflammatory arthritis (rheumatoid arthritis). PRC may be used for inflammatory arthritis patients with "burnout" disease (those without active synovitis).
  - Advanced degenerative changes at the proximal articular surface of the capitate or lunate facet of the radius
  - Ulnar carpal translation or subluxation of the radiocarpal joint
- Relative contraindications
  - Heavy laborers
  - Young (younger than 35 years) active patients[8]

Preoperative Planning

- Review the plain radiographs of the wrist. Scrutinize the location of degenerative changes.
- Obtain consent for alternative procedures from the patient (ie, if you find excessive degenerative changes on the capitate head, you might proceed with an intercarpal arthrodesis).
- Regional anesthesia, general anesthesia, or a combination of the two (for postoperative analgesia) is suitable.

Positioning

- The patient is supine with the arm on a radiolucent arm board.
- A nonsterile tourniquet preset at 250 mm Hg is on the upper arm.
- The shoulder, elbow, and hand are positioned such that the hand rests in pronation at the center of the arm board.

TECHNIQUES

Incision and Exposure

- Make a dorsal longitudinal skin incision over the fourth dorsal compartment or a transverse incision across the dorsal wrist crease just distal to the tubercle of Lister.
  - The longitudinal incision is more extensile and versatile.
  - The transverse incision tends to be more cosmetic.
- Expose the extensor retinaculum.
  - Maintain full-thickness flaps when elevating soft tissues off the extensor retinaculum to minimize the risk of damage to the radial and ulnar sensory nerves (**TECH FIG 1A**).
- Incise the extensor retinaculum in line with extensor pollicis longus (EPL) and transpose the EPL radially, dorsal to the retinaculum.
- Incise the radial septum of the fourth dorsal compartment and expose the wrist capsule by retracting the fourth compartment extensor tendons ulnarly and the EPL and radial wrist extensor tendons radially.
- Look for the distal extent of the posterior interosseous nerve (PIN) in the proximal portion of the incision on the radial floor of the fourth compartment. Perform a PIN neurectomy after coagulating the accompanying vessels.
- Create a distally based "inverted U-shaped" capsular flap by first incising the wrist capsule transversely over the radiocarpal joint (from radial to ulnar) and then, at the margins, extending the incision distally (**TECH FIG 1B**).
  - Making a U-shaped capsular hood provides flexibility should one elect to add a dorsal capsular interposition arthroplasty in the setting of mild midcarpal arthrosis.
  - The dorsal branch of the radial artery is radial to the second compartment, so take care at the radial aspect of the capsulotomy.
- Inspect the articular cartilage on the proximal capitate and lunate facet of the radius for any degenerative changes.
  - If the cartilage is in good condition, proceed with PRC; if not, consider alternative procedures (**TECH FIG 1C**).

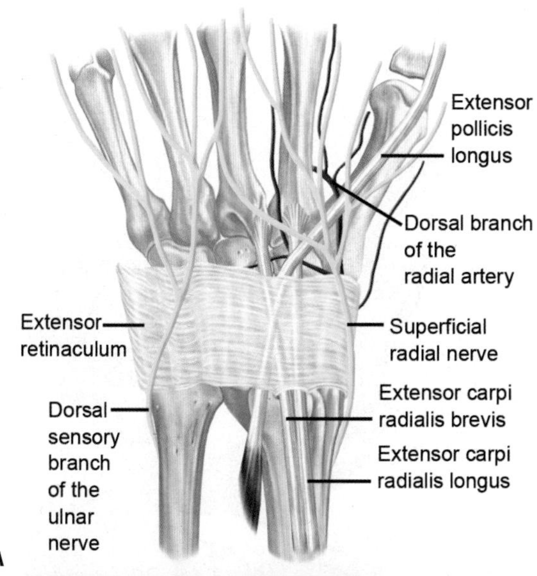

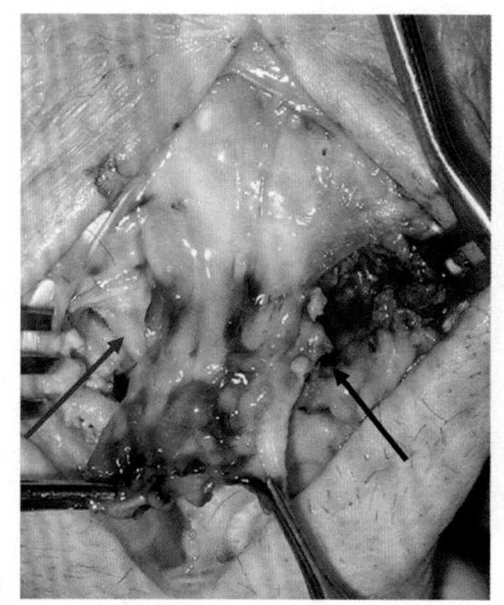

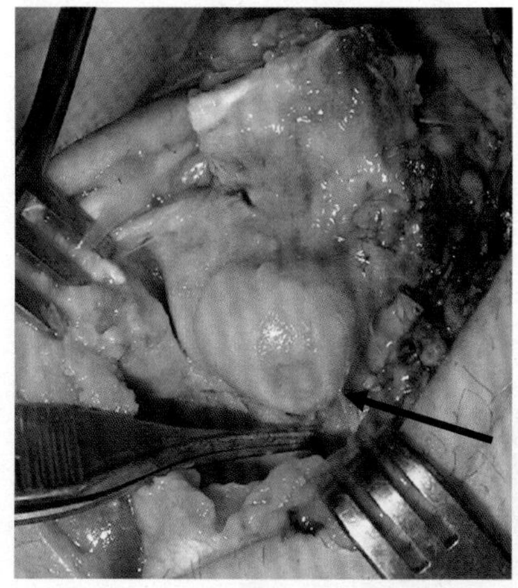

TECH FIG 1 • **A.** Superficial branches of the radial nerve and the dorsal cutaneous branch of the ulnar nerve. The dorsal branch of the radial artery is in danger deeper in the dissection as the wrist joint capsule is incised. **B.** Intraoperative photograph showing the distally based U-shaped dorsal capsular flap. This flap is centered over the capitate. The radial margin is just adjacent to the ulnar border of the extensor carpi radialis brevis tendon. The proximal margin is taken directly off the dorsal lip of the radius. (*Red arrow* points to distal articular surface of the hamate; the triquetrum has not yet been removed. *Black arrow* points to the dorsal lip of scaphoid fossa.) The ulnar margin is just radial to the extensor digiti minimi. **C.** Wear on the ulnar aspect of the head of the capitate is visualized in this case. (*Arrow* points to a cartilage defect on the capitate head.) Arthrosis affecting the non–weight-bearing portion of the capitate does not preclude the use of a PRC, but one may want to include a capsular interposition. This is usually employed in older, lower demand individuals.

Carpectomy

- Divide the scapholunate ligament, if it is intact.
- Split the scaphoid at its waist with a straight osteotome to facilitate scaphoid excision.
- Note that the radioscaphocapitate ligament crosses obliquely at the waist of the scaphoid.
- Orient the osteotome parallel with its fibers. If the osteotome should accidentally plunge beyond the scaphoid, the fibers will be split rather than divided (**TECH FIG 2A,B**).
  - The distal pole of the scaphoid is particularly difficult to remove (especially with SNAC wrist deformities).
- Avoid iatrogenic injury to the cartilaginous surfaces of the capitate head and lunate facet of the radius.
- Consider using a threaded Kirschner wire (0.062 inch) or a large threaded Steinmann pin (5/32 inch) as a joystick to control the bone to be removed (**TECH FIG 2C**). Try to create tension between the proximal carpal bones during dissection (a combination of no. 15 blade; Beaver blade; periosteal, Freer, or Carroll elevator; and small straight or curved curettes is valuable; **TECH FIG 2D**).
- If possible, remove the carpal bones whole rather than piecemeal (**TECH FIG 2E**).

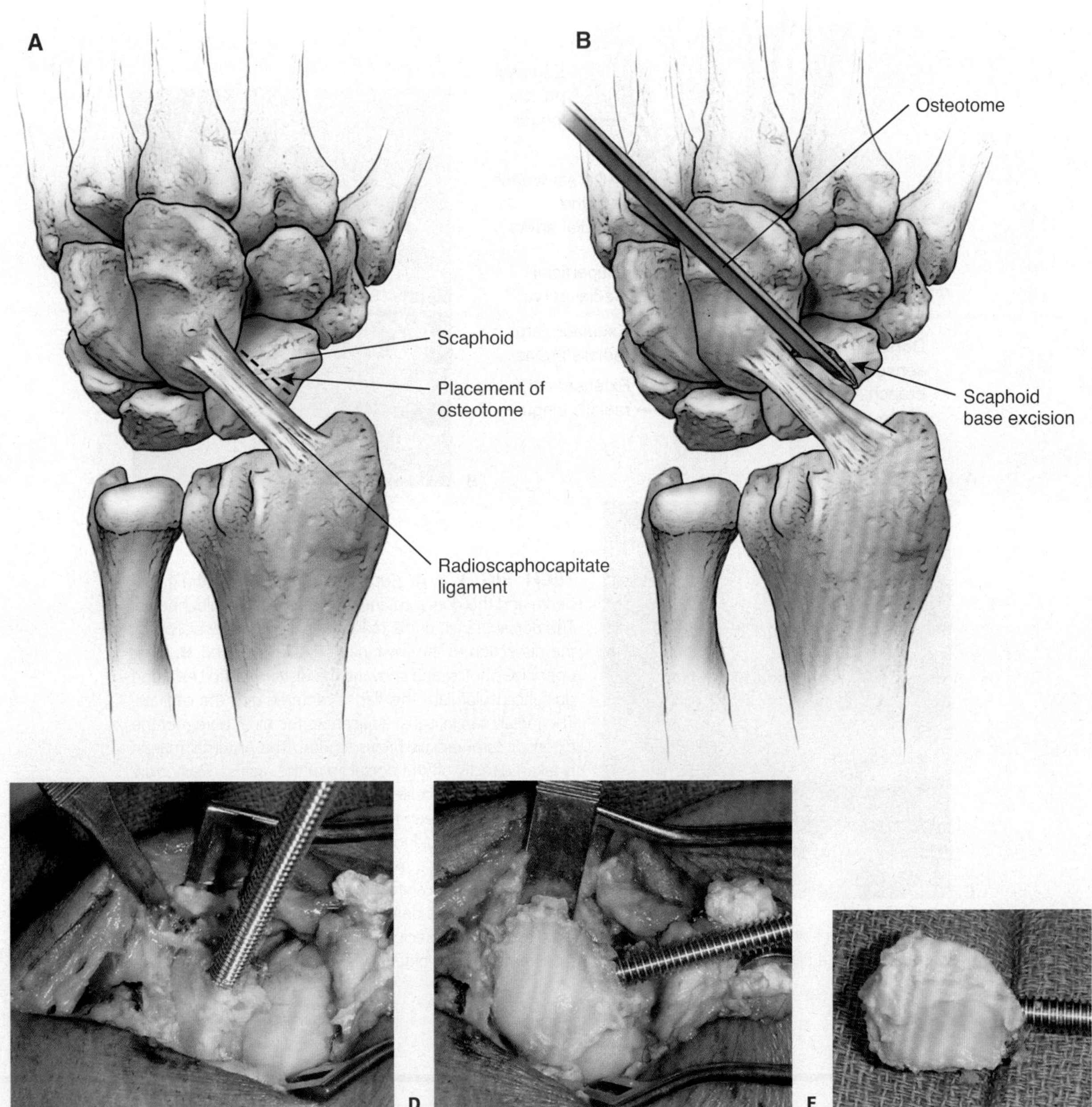

TECH FIG 2 • **A,B.** The appropriate location for the scaphoid osteotomy. **C.** A large threaded pin inserted into the lunate is used to facilitate resection. **D.** An elevator placed in the lunotriquetral joint and then levered against the triquetrum helps strip the volar capsule off the lunate. **E.** Resected lunate.

Assessment of Reduction and Impingement

- Once the proximal row is removed, ensure that the capitate sits in the lunate facet without translating ulnarly.
- If the lunate translates easily, check to see if the radioscapho-capitate ligament is intact.
- Check for impingement between the trapezium and radial styloid with extreme radial deviation.
  - The trapezium is volar to the styloid, making impingement less common than once thought.
  - If radial-sided impingement is a concern, proceed with a radial styloidectomy.

Radial Styloidectomy

- See Chapter 106.
- Elevate the tendons of the second and then the first extensor compartments off the radial styloid through the same dorsal incision.
  - Take care to avoid injuring the dorsal branch of the radial artery just radial to the second dorsal compartment.
- The styloidectomy can be performed from proximal radial to distal ulnar with a straight osteotome (remove no more than 5 to 7 mm) (**TECH FIG 3**).

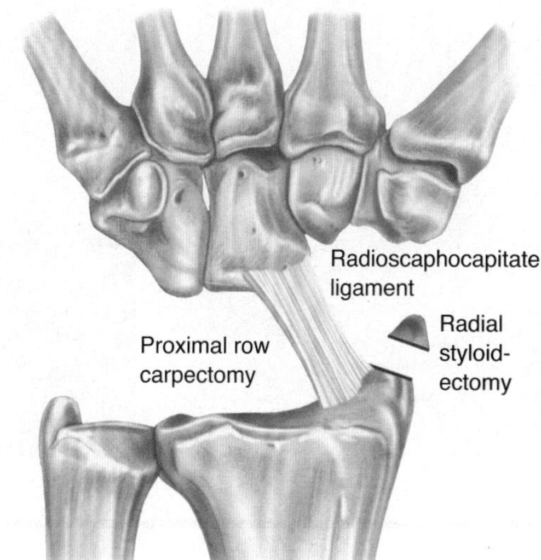

TECH FIG 3 ● The amount of radial styloid that is removed and the direction of the osteotomy. The origin of the radioscaphocapitate ligament is carefully preserved.

Wound Closure

- Close the capsule with nonabsorbable 2-0 suture.
- Plain radiographs or fluoroscopic images should be obtained in anteroposterior (AP) and lateral planes to ensure that the capitate is seated in the lunate fossae.
  - Although uncommon, radiocarpal subluxation is possible with a PRC.
  - Maintenance of the volar ligaments (especially the radioscaphocapitate, which is most at risk during removal of the scaphoid) minimizes any risk of radiocarpal instability after PRC.
- Close the retinaculum with nonabsorbable 3-0 suture, leaving the EPL superficial to the retinaculum.
- Close the skin with a 3-0 running subcuticular monofilament, absorbable stitch reinforced with Steri-Strips.
- Cover the incision with nonadherent gauze.
- Fashion a volar splint over a bulky dressing.
  - Keep the fingers and the thumb free proximal to the metacarpophalangeal joints.
  - Hold the wrist at neutral or slight extension (10 degrees).

Proximal Row Carpectomy with Interposition Arthroplasty

- If mild to moderate chondral changes are noted on the capitate head, a PRC may still be possible with the addition of an interpositional arthroplasty between the capitate head and lunate fossae.
- Use the previously created distally based inverted U-shaped capsular flap as the interpositional material.
- Place three simple stitches (2-0 polydioxanone [PDS]) connecting the dorsal capsular flap to the palmar capsule.
- Place and tag all stitches into the dorsal capsule (passing from deep to superficial) and into the palmar capsule (passing from proximal to distal) before tying them down to the palmar capsule (**TECH FIG 4A**).
- Loosely reapproximate the lateral margins of the dorsal flap to the residual dorsal capsule after interposing the dorsal capsule (**TECH FIG 4B**).
- Postoperative management is not altered.

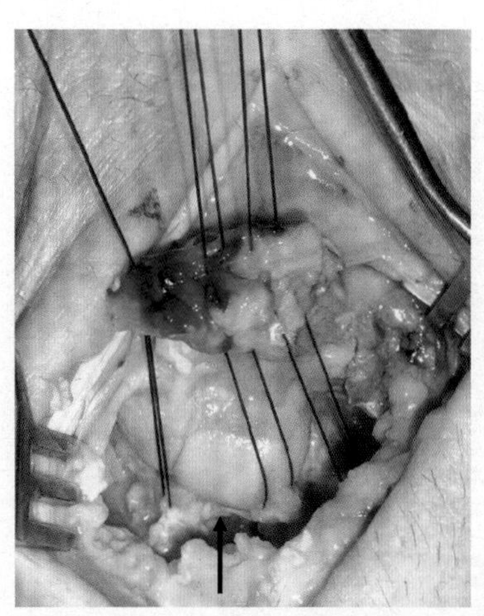

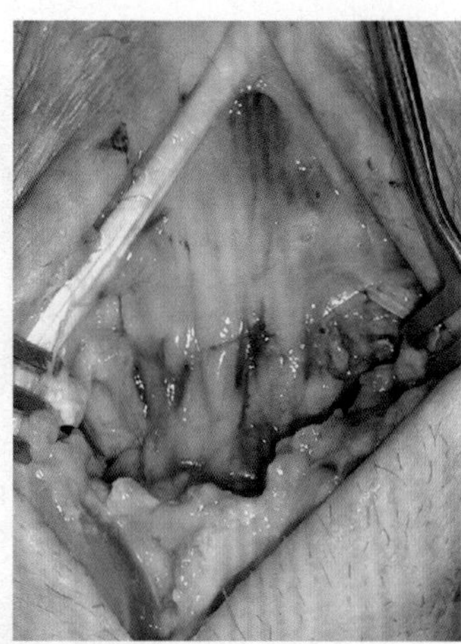

TECH FIG 4 • A. Sutures are passed in a mattress fashion through dorsal capsule, volar capsule, and then dorsal capsule to interpose the dorsal capsular flap between the capitate and lunate fossa. (*Arrow* points to the head of the capitate.) **B.** The dorsal capsule interposed between the capitate (shown *above*) and the radius (shown *below*) after the PDS sutures have been tied down.

PEARLS AND PITFALLS

Intraoperative pearls	▪ Threaded Kirschner wires (0.062 inch) or large threaded Steinmann pins (5/32 inch) in the scaphoid, lunate, or triquetrum can serve as a joystick or fulcrum to assist in removing the carpal bones.
Excessive styloidectomy	▪ Removing more than 5–7 mm of the radial styloid has been associated with compromise of the radioscaphocapitate ligament, with resultant ulnar carpal translation and radiocarpal instability.
Reflex sympathetic dystrophy	▪ Thought to be minimized by accelerated rehabilitation (immediate finger motion) and by avoiding tight postoperative dressings.
Damage to the radial sensory and dorsal ulnar sensory branches	▪ Dissect directly down to the extensor retinaculum and elevate subcutaneous fat in full-thickness flaps off the extensor retinaculum to minimize the risk of nerve injury.

POSTOPERATIVE CARE

- PRC tends to be an outpatient procedure; an overnight stay may be necessary for postoperative pain or nausea.
- A short splint is applied in the operating room with the wrist in neutral and the fingers and thumb free at the metacarpophalangeal joints.
- Passive thumb and finger motion is encouraged immediately postoperatively, along with elevation and ice for the first 48 hours.
- At the first postoperative follow-up visit (in 10 to 14 days), the splint is removed, plain wrist AP and lateral radiographs are obtained to ensure the capitate is located in the radial lunate facet, and sutures are removed.
- At 2 weeks postoperatively, gentle active wrist extension and flexion and radioulnar deviation are added and a removable cock-up wrist splint or custom Orthoplast wrist splint is worn between exercises.
- Scar massage can begin once the incision is healed.
- Edema control may be necessary with compressive dressings.
- The removable splint can be discontinued as the patient feels comfortable (typically in 3 to 4 weeks).
- Therapy is initiated if the patient struggles to regain finger motion by 10 to 14 days. Therapy for wrist motion is initiated, if necessary, at 6 to 8 weeks.
- At 3 months, full activities are permitted.

OUTCOMES

- A broad range in grip strength outcome has been reported postoperatively.
  - A 60% to 100% grip strength of the contralateral wrist (and a 20% to 30% increase in postoperative grip vs. preoperative grip) can be expected.[1,4,8]
  - A decrease in postoperative wrist motion can be expected, as well as a decrease in flexion–extension by 20%, a decrease in radioulnar deviation by 10%,[4] and a 72- to 76-degree arc of motion in flexion and extension.[3,7,8]
- Satisfactory pain relief can be expected in 80% to 100% of patients.[4,5]

- A Brazilian prospective randomized control trial comparing four-corner fusion to PRC showed similar functional results, decreased pain in both groups, and no statistically significant differences in range of motion or grip strength.[2]
- Return to work for manual laborers after PRC has been unpredictable, varying from 20% in one series[4] to 85% in another.[5]
- A study with a minimum of 20-year follow-up showed 65% survival of the PRC, with failure (conversion to arthrodesis) at an average of 11 years postoperatively.[9]
- Age younger than 35 years has been shown to be predictive of early failure with PRC.

COMPLICATIONS

- Use of pins has been associated with pin site infections and rapid degenerative changes when placed through the radiocapitate articulation (because of this, pins are not routinely recommended as they once were).
- Reflex sympathetic dystrophy
- Excessive styloidectomy and compromise of the radioscaphocapitate ligament
  - Compromise of the radioscaphocapitate ligament can lead to ulnar carpal subluxation.
  - Conversely, failure to check intraoperatively for radial-sided impingement may lead to radial-sided wrist pain postoperatively.
- Damage to sensory nerves (radial sensory and dorsal ulnar branches)
- Progressive arthritis

REFERENCES

1. Begley BW, Engber WD. Proximal row carpectomy in advanced Kienböck's disease. J Hand Surg Am 1994;19(6):1016–1018.
2. Bisneto EN, Freitas MC, Paula EJ, et al. Comparison between proximal row carpectomy and four-corner fusion for treating osteoarthrosis following carpal trauma: a prospective randomized study. Clinics 2011;66:51–55.
3. Calandruccio JH. Proximal row carpectomy. J Am Soc Surg Hand 2001;1:112–122.
4. Culp RW, McGuigan FX, Turner MA, et al. Proximal row carpectomy: a multicenter study. J Hand Surg Am 1993;18:19–25.
5. Imbriglia JE, Broudy AS, Hagberg WC, et al. Proximal row carpectomy: clinical evaluation. J Hand Surg Am 1990;15:426–430.
6. Mathiowetz V, Kashman N, Volland G, et al. Grip and pinch strength: normative data for adults. Arch Phys Med Rehabil 1985;66:69–74.
7. Richou J, Chuinard C, Moineau G, et al. Proximal row carpectomy: long-term results. Chir Main 2010;29:10–15.
8. Stern PJ, Agabegi SS, Kiefhaber TR, et al. Proximal row carpectomy. J Bone Joint Surg Am 2005;87(suppl 1, pt 2):166–174.
9. Wall LB, Didonna ML, Kiefhaber TR, et al. Proximal row carpectomy: minimum 20-year follow-up. J Hand Surg Am 2013;38:1498–1504.

108 CHAPTER

Limited Wrist Arthrodesis

Michael N. Nakashian, Andrew W. Cross, and Mark E. Baratz

DEFINITION

- Limited wrist arthrodeses are salvage procedures for posttraumatic and degenerative conditions of the wrist as well as symptomatic instabilities.
- The goal is to reduce pain by selected fusion of the affected joints, thereby sparing motion, and improving the function of the remaining joints.

ANATOMY

- The carpus consists of four bones in the proximal row (scaphoid, lunate, triquetrum, pisiform) and four bones in the distal row (trapezium, trapezoid, capitate, hamate).
- The scaphoid and lunate bones are intimately joined by the scapholunate ligament both dorsally and volarly. This ligament is critical to the kinematics of the wrist.
- Many other named ligaments hold the carpal bones stable as the wrist moves through its five planes of motion (flexion, extension, radial and ulnar deviation, and circumduction).
- Most reconstructive wrist procedures require a dorsal approach to the wrist. The wrist and finger extensor tendons are separated into six compartments by the dorsal extensor retinaculum. The most common interval for exposure of the wrist is the third and fourth interval between the extensor pollicis longus (EPL) and extensor digitorum communis and extensor indices proprius tendons.

PATHOGENESIS

- Distraction forces across the joint as well as twisting motions while the wrist joint is being loaded can both result in a ligament injury.
- Failure of the scapholunate interosseous ligament, either by trauma or inflammatory arthritis, allows the scaphoid to flex and the lunate to extend, leading to dorsal intercalated segment instability (DISI).[20,35] When this occurs, abnormal loading of the carpal bones results. This eventually leads to degenerative arthritis, particularly at the radioscaphoid joint due to the abnormal distribution of force across this elliptical joint.[7] This has been termed *scapholunate advanced collapse* (SLAC).
  - Scaphoid nonunion advanced collapse (SNAC), perilunate dislocations, calcium pyrophosphate dihydrate deposition, and rheumatoid arthritis can also lead to this pattern of arthritis.
- Other ligament injuries, Kienböck disease, and localized arthritis can lead to wrist pain, instability, and deformity.

NATURAL HISTORY

- Much of our knowledge of the natural history of scaphoid nonunion was reported by Mack et al.[23] We have learned that most ununited fractures of the scaphoid and SLAC wrists develop progressive osteoarthritis in a predictable pattern.
- Cyst formation and bony resorption are the hallmarks of arthritis and are usually seen 5 to 10 years after injury.
- Arthritis of the radioscaphoid joint can appear within a year after scaphoid nonunion. At that point, most patients become symptomatic.[13,33]

PATIENT HISTORY AND PHYSICAL FINDINGS

- Typically, the patient describes a traumatic injury to the wrist. The absence of trauma should not exclude traumatic causes.
- Painful wrist motion and a limited arc of motion are common findings.
- Methods for examining the wrist include the following:
  - Finger extension test.[32] The wrist is passively flexed while the examiner resists active finger extension. A positive test yields pain and may represent periscaphoid inflammatory changes, radiocarpal or midcarpal instability, or Kienböck disease. A negative test essentially excludes dorsal wrist syndrome, Kienböck disease, midcarpal instability, and SLAC as the cause of pain.
  - Anatomic snuffbox palpation.[32] The examiner palpates the anatomic snuffbox with the index finger while moving the wrist from radial to ulnar deviation.[30] A positive test yields severe pain at the articular–nonarticular junction of the scaphoid. Periscaphoid synovitis, scaphoid instability, and radial styloid arthrosis from SLAC are possible causes.
  - Triscaphe (scaphotrapeziotrapezoid [STT]) joint palpation.[32] The examiner palpates the second metacarpal proximally until it falls into a recess, the triscaphe joint. Pain with palpation indicates pathology of the distal scaphoid or the triscaphe joint.

IMAGING AND OTHER DIAGNOSTIC STUDIES

- Plain radiographs, including anteroposterior (AP), lateral, oblique, and scaphoid views, should be obtained.
- The stage of wrist arthritis, as seen on plain radiographs, helps to determine the treatment options. Watson and Ballet[31] classified the radiographic findings into stages I to III.
  - Stage IV, not originally described, demonstrates arthritis in most all joints of the wrist. Fortunately, the radiolunate joint is rarely involved and serves as the basis for several treatment options.
  - Arthritis involving the radiolunate joint is usually seen only in patients with inflammatory wrist arthritis.

DIFFERENTIAL DIAGNOSIS

- SNAC
- SLAC
- Arthritis after perilunate dislocation
- Gout

- Pseudogout
- Rheumatoid arthritis
- Infectious arthritis
- Kienböck disease

NONOPERATIVE MANAGEMENT

- Nonoperative measures include rest, anti-inflammatory medications, splinting, occasional casting for flare-ups of arthritis, and cortisone injections.

SURGICAL MANAGEMENT

- Indications
  - Four-corner (capitate–hamate–lunate–triquetral [CHLT]) arthrodesis
    - Stage II or III SLAC wrist arthritis
    - Chronic symptomatic volar intercalated segmental instability (VISI) deformity or midcarpal instability
  - STT arthrodesis
    - Chronic static or dynamic scapholunate instability
    - STT arthritis
    - Kienböck disease
    - Radiocarpal instability
  - Lunotriquetral arthrodesis
    - Lunotriquetral ligament tears
    - Posttraumatic instability
  - Scapholunate arthrodesis
    - Posttraumatic instability
    - Scapholunate instability
    - DISI deformity
  - Scaphocapitate arthrodesis
    - Scaphoid nonunion
    - Chronic DISI deformity with rotatory scaphoid instability
    - Kienböck disease
    - Lunate nonunion
  - Radiolunate arthrodesis
    - Rheumatoid arthritis primarily involving the radiolunate joint
    - Ulnar translocation of the carpus (relative indication)
  - Capitolunate arthrodesis
    - Scaphoid nonunion
    - SLAC wrist arthritis

Preoperative Planning

- The patient's history and pertinent physical examination findings are reviewed.
- Any prior surgical scars are noted.
- All radiographs are reviewed, noting any associated pathology that might need to be simultaneously addressed to yield the best outcome.
- Postoperative pain control should be discussed with the patient and the anesthesia team, and a local or axillary block should be considered for prolonged pain relief after surgery.

Positioning

- The patient is placed in the supine position on the operating table with the arm draped to the side on a radiolucent arm board.
- A tourniquet is used to control bleeding during the procedure.

Approach

- The wrist is approached through a dorsal longitudinal incision between the third and fourth extensor compartments.
  - Alternatively, the fourth and fifth extensor compartment interval may be used to better visualize the CHLT articulations.
- The EPL tendon sheath is opened and it is released both proximally and distally. The tendon is allowed to be transposed out of its compartment in a radial direction.
  - Although the EPL tendon is typically exposed and subsequently transposed, a more limited incision beginning just distal to the tubercle of Lister and proceeding distally may avoid significant exposure of the EPL tendon altogether.
- All joints are exposed fully and a precise decortication is performed down to bleeding bone.
- In almost every case, bone graft is harvested from the distal radius and used to augment the fusion.
  - Iliac crest graft may be substituted but is associated with higher donor site morbidity.

TECHNIQUES

Four-Corner (Capitate-Hamate-Lunate-Triquetral) Arthrodesis Using Kirschner Wire Fixation

- Make a standard dorsal longitudinal incision between the third and fourth extensor compartments using the tubercle of Lister as a landmark (**TECH FIG 1A**).
- Incise the retinaculum over the third extensor compartment.
- Incise the radial septum of the fourth extensor compartment and retract the tendons ulnarly.
- Perform a ligament-splitting dorsal approach to the carpus as described by Berger et al.[4]
  - This capsular incision allows access to the carpus while preserving the dorsal intercarpal ligament and dorsal radiotriquetral ligament (see Chap. 70).
- Inspect the radiolunate joint for articular cartilage wear (**TECH FIG 1B**).
- Identify and excise the scaphoid either piecemeal with a rongeur or sharply using a scalpel (**TECH FIG 1C**).
  - Kirschner wires and tenaculum clamps facilitate the visualization and excision of the distal volar scaphoid.
  - Take care to protect the volar radioscaphocapitate ligament.
- Once the scaphoid is excised, decorticate the opposing joint surfaces of the lunate, triquetrum, capitate, and hamate (**TECH FIG 1D**).
  - Longitudinal traction with fingertraps helps to distract these joints, making decortication easier.
  - Thorough removal of the volar-third cartilage from the lunate and capitate facilitates correction of the preexisting DISI deformity but shortens the intercarpal bone distances. This may restrict final wrist range of motion.
- Once these joint surfaces are denuded, harvest distal radius bone graft and place it into the fusion bed.
- Use a 0.062 Kirschner wire to joystick the lunate into a more flexed position, and apply dorsal pressure to volarly translate the

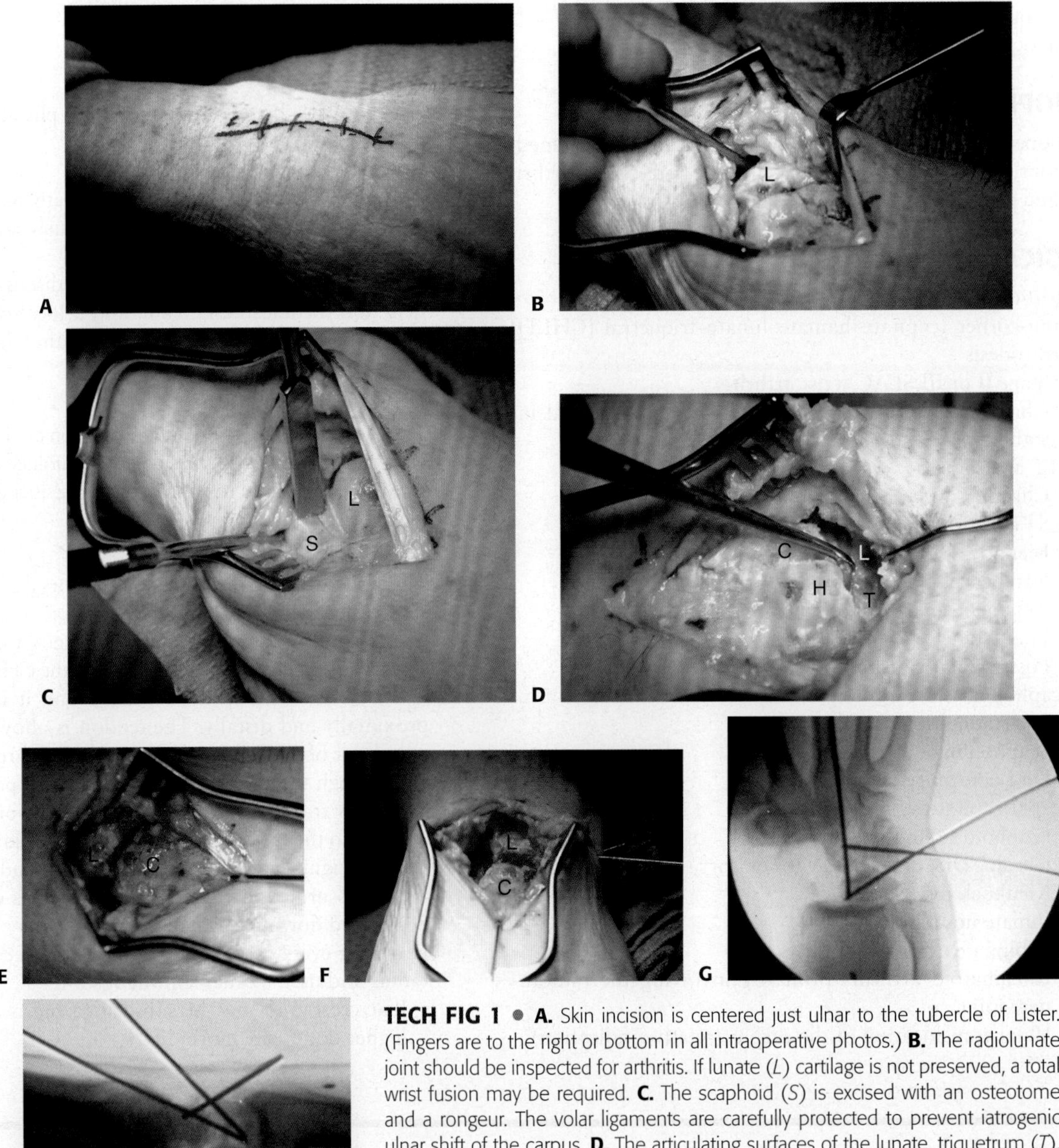

TECH FIG 1 ● **A.** Skin incision is centered just ulnar to the tubercle of Lister. (Fingers are to the right or bottom in all intraoperative photos.) **B.** The radiolunate joint should be inspected for arthritis. If lunate (*L*) cartilage is not preserved, a total wrist fusion may be required. **C.** The scaphoid (*S*) is excised with an osteotome and a rongeur. The volar ligaments are carefully protected to prevent iatrogenic ulnar shift of the carpus. **D.** The articulating surfaces of the lunate, triquetrum (*T*), capitate (*C*), and hamate (*H*) are decorticated. **E.** The capitate is secured to the lunate (*L*) with a retrograde 0.062 Kirschner wire. **F.** Remaining joints are secured with Kirschner wires in a triangular pattern. **G,H.** AP and lateral radiographs showing Kirschner wires properly positioned.

capitate on the lunate. Place one or two 0.062 Kirschner wires across this joint (**TECH FIG 1E**).

- Verify correction of the DISI deformity using fluoroscopy.
- Pin the lunotriquetral joint and the capitohamate joint with two 0.062 Kirschner wires (**TECH FIG 1F**).
  - Intraoperative fluoroscopic images should reveal a stable triangular construct of Kirschner wires traversing the four bones (**TECH FIG 1G,H**).
- The Kirschner wires may be cut under the skin or left external, depending on the surgeon's preference.
- After irrigation, close the capsule with absorbable suture and repair the extensor retinaculum, leaving the EPL tendon transposed subcutaneously.
- Close the skin in a routine manner.
- Apply a large bulky dressing including a dorsal and volar forearm-based splint.
- The previously described technique is taken from published data.[2]

Four-Corner Arthrodesis Using a Circular Plate

- The approach, scaphoid excision, and joint preparation are analogous to those described earlier.
- Place a 0.062 Kirschner wire through the distal radius articular surface. Use a separate 0.062 Kirschner wire as a joystick to hold the lunate reduced in neutral alignment while advancing the Kirschner wire across the radiolunate joint in a dorsal to volar direction.
  - Obtain fluoroscopic images to verify correction of the dorsally tilted lunate.
- After volarly translating the capitate (as described earlier) and fully correcting the DISI deformity, secure the triquetrum to the hamate and the lunate to the capitate with two additional Kirschner wires.
  - Place these Kirschner wires as volar as possible to avoid interference during rasping and plate placement.
- Center the power rasp over the four bones in the AP and lateral planes and bury the rasp down to subchondral bone.
  - Ideal rasp placement does not always coincide with the central point between the four bones.
- Pack bone graft, obtained preferably from the distal radius or iliac crest, between the four prepared bones.
- Center the plate over the four bones in the AP and lateral planes and place the circular plate into the bony crater created by the rasp.
- Rotate the plate to maximize screw purchase into each of the four bones. Two screws should be planned for each of the four carpal bones.
  - All screws must be placed in a unicortical fashion.
- Place the first screw through the plate into the lunate. Do not tighten this screw completely or it will cause the circular plate to tilt up and compromise screw fixation in the remaining bones.
- Place a second screw into the hole opposite the first screw. This sets the plate position.
- Check a lateral fluoroscopic image to ensure the plate is well seated and there is no impingement with wrist extension.
- Fill in the remainder of the holes with screws.
  - Placing the screws opposite one another and tightening them sequentially helps prevent malpositioning of the plate.
- Obtain final images to check screw length and position, carpal reduction, and construct stability (**TECH FIG 2**).
- Close the wound as described earlier. Apply the dressing and splint.
- The previously described technique is taken from published data.[9,15,34]

A 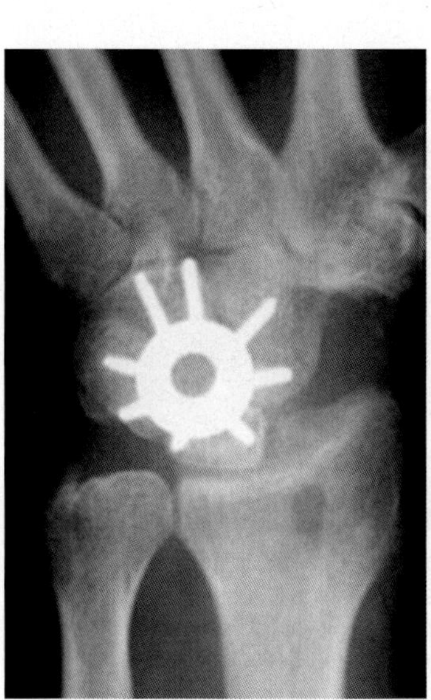

B 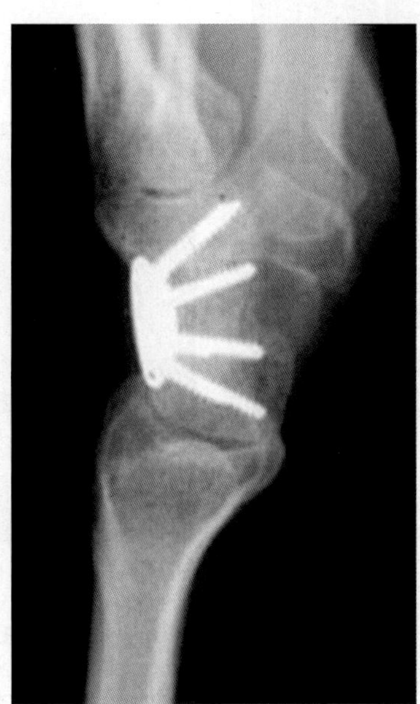

TECH FIG 2 • A,B. AP and lateral radiographs showing a circular plate fusion construct. On the lateral view, the plate is nicely seated to prevent dorsal impingement.

Four-Corner Arthrodesis Using Headless Compression Screws

- Perform exposure, excision, and decortication as above the Kirschner wire fixation technique
- Capitolunate screw is placed antegrade through the proximal ulnar corner of the lunate
  - Place 0.045 wire into radial aspect of capitate neck and advance into the head.
- Correct DISI, then drive guidewire retrograde into the lunate.
- Flex the wrist and place the guidewire of a headless screw (2.5 to 3.0 in diameter) into the proximal ulnar corner of the lunate. Advance into the capitate.
- Measure the pin length and then advance the wire.
- Drill over the wire and place a screw that is countersunk 3 to 4 mm beneath the articular surface.
- Place two pins percutaneously from the ulnar aspect with the drill set on oscillate: one across the lunotriquetral joint and the second across the triquetrohamate joint.
- Apply cancellous bone graft.
- Perform irrigation, closure, and apply splint as previously described.
- The pins are removed at 4 weeks.
- The previously described technique is taken from published data.[24]

Scaphotrapeziotrapezoid Fusion

- Make a transverse or dorsoradial incision centered over the STT joint.
- Protect the superficial radial nerve branches, and coagulate the small perforators from the dorsal branch of the radial artery (**TECH FIG 3A**).
- Make a longitudinal capsulotomy over the STT joint, and reflect the capsule to expose the bone surfaces (**TECH FIG 3B**).
- Verify scaphoid alignment with fluoroscopy. The ideal scapholunate angle is 41 to 60 degrees.
  - Failure to correct this malalignment could lead to persistent pain.
  - Overcorrection of an increased scapholunate angle may limit postoperative motion.
- Remove only the dorsal 70% of the articular cartilage from the three bones.
  - Preserving the volar 30% maintains the intercarpal bone distances but still ensures successful fusion.
- Perform a radial styloidectomy.
  - Resect no more than 3 or 4 mm of the styloid to avoid iatrogenic injury to the origin of the radioscaphocapitate and long radiolunate ligaments.
- Fixation may be accomplished with Kirschner wires or a circular plate.
- Place two 0.045 Kirschner wires anterograde into the trapezium and trapezoid (**TECH FIG 3C**). Add a third 0.045 Kirschner wire in an ulnar to radial direction from the trapezoid toward the trapezium.
  - The aforementioned wires are preset in place and should be advanced across the joints after bone graft placement.
- Alternatively, excision of the lunate has been advocated in cases of advanced collapse.
- Done arthroscopically, this is performed through the midcarpal portal prior to opening the joint. A burr is used to divide the lunate. Pieces are removed with a pituitary forceps.
- Done open, the transverse incision is extended ulnarly to the dorsum of the lunate.
- Harvest cancellous bone graft from the distal radius and pack it into the interstices of the STT joints.
- Reduce the joints and advance the preset Kirschner wires.
- The Kirschner wires can be cut and buried under the skin or left out of the skin to facilitate removal.
- Perform a routine closure and apply a well-padded forearm-based thumb spica splint.
- The previously described technique is taken from published data.[3,6,19]

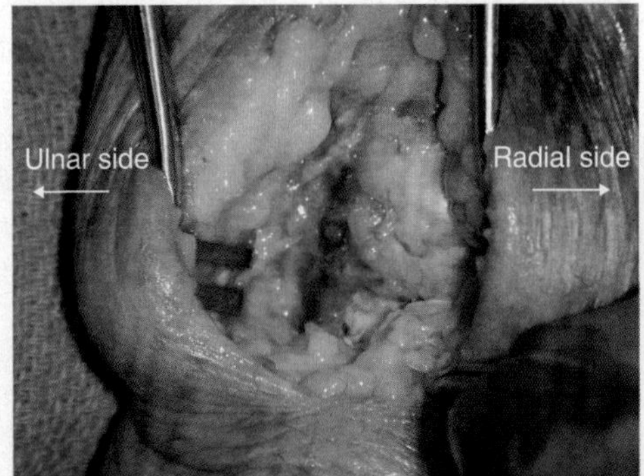

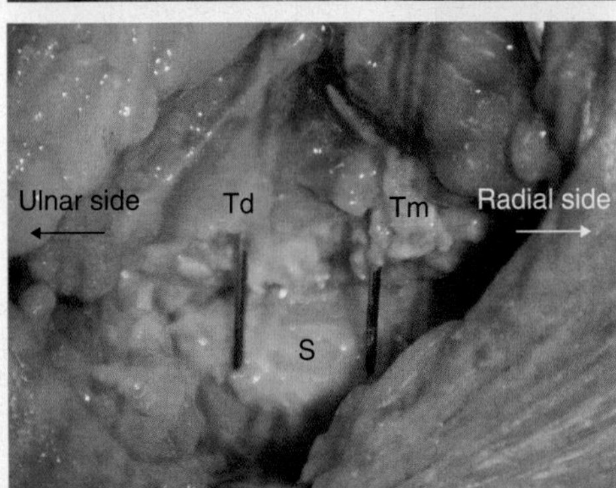

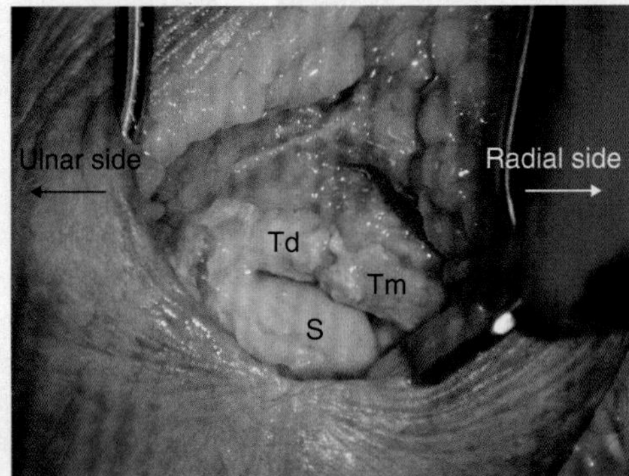

TECH FIG 3 • **A.** Location of the dorsal branch of the radial artery as it crosses the STT joints. (Fingers are at top in all images.) **B.** Exposed STT joints. *Td*, trapezoid; *Tm*, trapezium; *S*, scaphoid. **C.** Kirschner wire position in the trapezium and trapezoid bones before advancement into the scaphoid bone. A separate pin traversing the trapeziotrapezoidal joint is added for stability.

Lunotriquetral Fusion

- Make a transverse incision over the dorsal and ulnar aspect of the radiocarpal joint.
- Retract the extensor tendons and incise the capsule transversely to expose the lunotriquetral joint.
- Remove any remaining lunotriquetral ligament with a small rongeur.
- Decorticate the lunotriquetral articulation, leaving the volar 25% of the joint surface intact to maintain intercarpal distances (**TECH FIG 4A**).
- Harvest distal radius bone graft and pack it into the void created.
- Place two cannulated screw guidewires through the triquetrum, and after reducing the joint, advance the pins across the lunotriquetral joint into the lunate.
  - Verify pin position using fluoroscopy.
- Advance two partially threaded cannulated screws over the guide pins across the lunotriquetral joint (**TECH FIG 4B**).
  - Make sure the thread length on the screw is short enough to allow compression across the lunotriquetral joint.
  - Alternatively, headless screws, staples, or Kirschner wires may be used for fixation.
- Perform routine wound closure and apply a wrist splint.
- The previously described technique is taken from published data.[26]

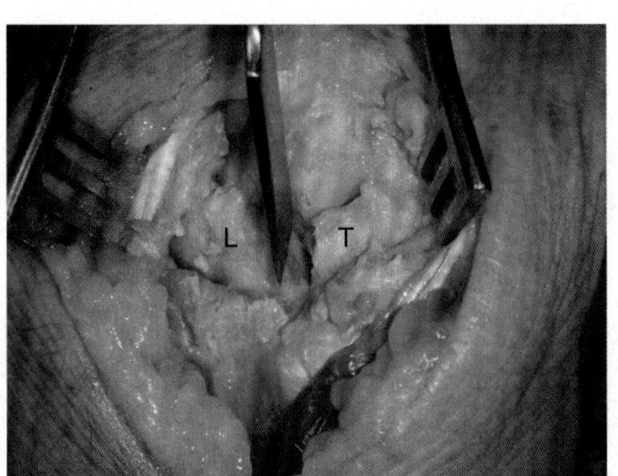

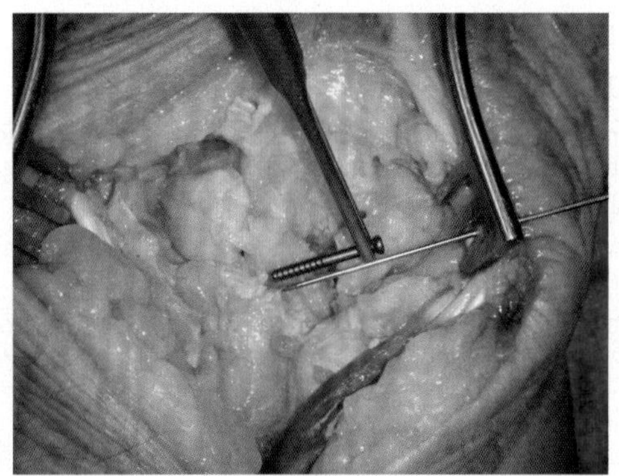

TECH FIG 4 • **A.** Lunotriquetral joint during decortication. (Fingers are at top in all images.) **B.** Lunotriquetral joint fusion construct with a partially threaded cannulated screw and a derotation pin.

Scapholunate Fusion

- Use a standard dorsal incision ulnar to the tubercle of Lister and perform a longitudinal capsular incision.
- Place two dorsal joystick Kirschner wires, one into the palmarflexed scaphoid distally, directed proximally and ulnarly, and a second into the dorsiflexed lunate proximally, directed distally.
    - When these two wires are brought together, the joint is reduced.
- Decorticate the bone surfaces and obtain bone graft from the distal radius.
- Reduce the scaphoid and lunate with the Kirschner wires and hold them in place with a Kocher clamp.
- Verify scapholunate reduction via fluoroscopy before proceeding.
- Stabilize the scapholunate joint with headless cannulated screws, multiple 0.045 to 0.062 Kirschner wires, or staples.
- Perform routine closure and apply a standard dressing and thumb spica splint.
- The previously described technique is taken from published data.[26]

Scaphocapitate Fusion

- Use the third and fourth extensor compartment approach followed by a longitudinal capsulotomy directly over the scaphocapitate interval between the second and fourth compartments.
- Denude the articulating scaphoid and capitate surfaces of articular cartilage down to bleeding cancellous bone.
- For cannulated screw fixation, make a V-shaped incision on the radial aspect of the wrist superficial to the radial styloid. A styloidectomy performed through this incision creates a superior view of the lateral aspect of the scaphoid. Preset two guidewires in the scaphoid, aimed toward the capitate (radial to ulnar).
    - A radial styloidectomy is an option to facilitate accurate positioning of the Kirschner wires.
    - Compression screws (our preference), Kirschner wires, or staples may be used for fixation.
- Harvest distal radius cancellous bone graft and place it between the two prepared bones.
- Reduce the articulation, advance the guidewires, and verify pin placement with fluoroscopy.
    - Obtain a scapholunate angle of about 45 degrees.
- Advance the threaded compression screws across the scaphocapitate joint (**TECH FIG 5**).
- Perform a routine closure and apply the dressing and splint as earlier.
- The previously described technique is taken from published data.[1,3,4]

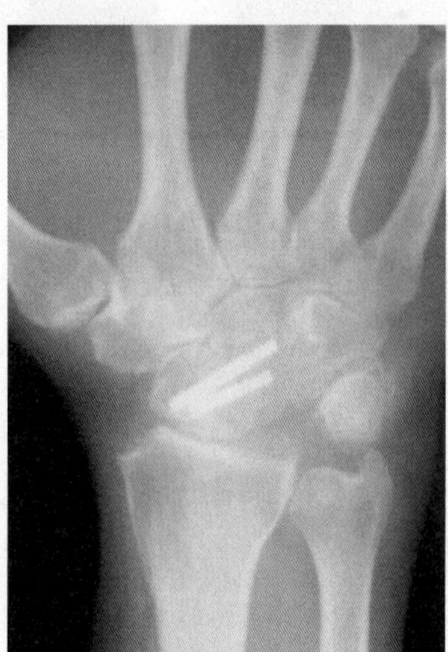

TECH FIG 5 • Scaphocapitate fusion construct using two headless, cannulated compression screws. Note the addition of a radial styloidectomy. (Fingers are at top.)

Radiocarpal (Radiolunate) Arthrodesis

- Use the third and fourth extensor compartment approach followed by a ligament-sparing incision to the wrist capsule as described earlier (**TECH FIG 6**).
- Remove the dorsal lip of the radius over the lunate to facilitate visualization.
- Maintaining general bony contours, decorticate the lunate facet of the radius and the proximal lunate articular surface using curettes, rongeurs, and curved osteotomes.
- Under fluoroscopy, correct any preoperative VISI or DISI deformity.
  - A Kirschner wire inserted into the dorsal lunate may be used as a joystick to effect correction.
- Stabilize the lunate in the reduced position with provisional Kirschner wires from the radius into the lunate.
- Harvest bone graft from the distal radius or iliac crest and pack the graft tightly into the palmar radiolunate joint.
- Secure the lunate to the radius with Kirschner wires, headless screws, staples, or small blade plates.
- Pack the remaining bone graft into the dorsal radiolunate joint.
- Perform a routine closure and apply a splint.
- The previously described technique is taken from published data.[14,27]

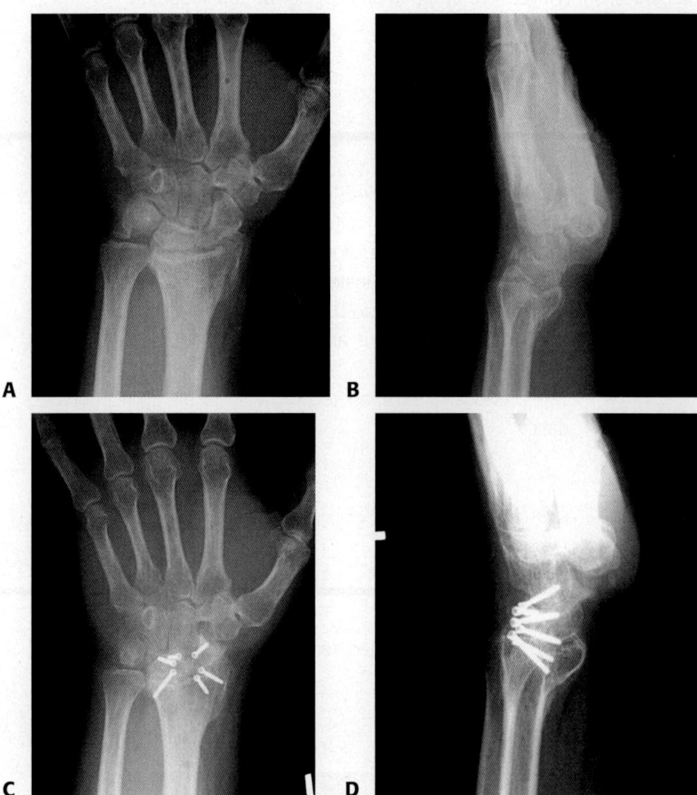

TECH FIG 6 • **A,B.** Preoperative AP and lateral radiographs. **C,D.** Postoperative AP and lateral radiographs following radiocarpal arthrodesis.

Capitolunate Arthrodesis

- Make a dorsal incision from base of second metacarpal to Lister tubercle.
  - Use the third and fourth extensor interval as described earlier.
- Perform an inverted "T" capsulotomy to visualize the scapholunate and capitolunate joints.
- Perform a limited styloidectomy (~3mm) and excise the proximal pole of scaphoid.
  - Stabilize distal scaphoid to capitate with a Kirschner wire.
  - Alternatively, the entire scaphoid can be excised.
- Denude the capitolunate articulation.
- Harvest bone graft from distal radius or iliac crest and pack it into this prepared joint.
  - Tricortical iliac crest graft allows maintenance of carpal height.
- Assure capitolunate alignment with a Kirschner wire as described earlier for CHLT fusion.
- Place a guidewire followed by headless screw into proximal ulnar corner of lunate as described earlier for CHLT fusion.
- Take wrist through a range of motion to be certain a mechanical block is not present.
- Perform a standard closure and apply a splint.
- The previously described technique is taken from published data.[12,15]

PEARLS AND PITFALLS

Pearls

CHLT Kirschner wire arthrodesis/ headless screw arthrodesis	■ For excellent visualization of the wrist capsule, incise the distal most aspect of the extensor retinaculum between the third and fourth compartments to the level of the tubercle of Lister.[2] ■ Protect the volar radioscaphocapitate ligament when excising the scaphoid to prevent iatrogenic ulnar translation of the carpus.[2] ■ Preserve the dorsal intercarpal and radiotriquetral ligament during the capsulotomy.[2]
CHLT circular plate	■ Place the screws opposite one another in the circular plate and tighten them sequentially to help prevent plate malpositioning.[14]
CHLT circular plate and STT arthrodesis	■ The bones here are extremely hard, and a high-speed burr may be needed for adequate decortication.[2]
Lunotriquetral arthrodesis	■ Leave the volar 25% of the articular surface intact during decortication to maintain proper intercarpal distances.
Scapholunate arthrodesis	■ Use Kirschner wires as joysticks and clamp the Kirschner wires together with a Kocher clamp to maintain the reduction during fixation.
Scaphocapitate arthrodesis	■ Correct intercarpal alignment is between 45 and 60 degrees.
Radiolunate fusion	■ Maintaining the normal joint space distance between the radius and lunate is desired to preserve as much wrist motion as possible at the surrounding joints.
Capitolunate arthrodesis	■ When using iliac crest graft, fix the graft in place with a 1.1-mm Kirschner wire, then check flexion–extension, and change graft height if restricted.[15]

Pitfalls

CHLT Kirschner wire arthrodesis/ headless screw technique	■ Expect less predictable pain relief and poorer recovery of motion in elderly individuals and in patients with severe wrist stiffness.[2] ■ One common mistake is not completely correcting the DISI deformity of the wrist before fusion.[2] This will limit wrist motion postoperatively.
CHLT circular plate	■ Dorsal placement of the Kirschner wires will interfere with bone rasping and plate application.[14] ■ Optimal rasp placement does not always coincide with the central point between the four bones. ■ A plate that is not adequately seated will result in dorsal impingement of the plate against the distal radius.[14]
STT arthrodesis	■ Headless screws may cause midcarpal compression and alter joint kinematics. ■ Overcorrection of an increased scapholunate angle may decrease motion postoperatively.
STT arthrodesis and scaphocapitate arthrodesis	■ The radial sensory and lateral antebrachial cutaneous nerves may be injured during exposure and Kirschner wire placement.
Scapholunate arthrodesis	■ There is an extremely high nonunion rate with this procedure, likely due to the high degree of motion between these bones and the relatively small area of contact between them.
Radiolunate arthrodesis	■ Inadvertent bone graft placement in the adjacent joints may be a cause of persistent wrist pain. A small osteotome can be used to block the passage of bone graft into the adjacent joints. ■ Avoid Kirschner wire penetration into the carpal tunnel.
Capitolunate arthrodesis	■ Avoid overcompression, as this could fracture iliac crest graft and lead to carpal height reduction.[15]

POSTOPERATIVE CARE

- The sutures are removed from the wound in 10 to 14 days and a short-arm cast is applied.
- Immobilization is typically 8 to 12 weeks, but this period may be shortened if stable fixation is obtained with screws.
- Plain radiographs are taken at the first postoperative visit and at all subsequent visits until signs of consolidation at the fusion site are noted.
- At this time, the pins are removed and a functional brace is applied to support the wrist but still allow controlled range of motion of the wrist during supervised therapy.
- Strengthening begins about 12 to 16 weeks after surgery.

OUTCOMES

- Nonunion rates range from 4% to 63%, depending on the joints being fused and the stresses placed across the joints before fusion.[5,11,18,26]
- For limited wrist fusions, a loss of grip strength on the order of 25% can be expected.[5,11,18,26]
- About 50% of patients will have some chronic wrist pain.[5,11,18,26]
- For stage I and II SLAC arthritis, four-corner arthrodesis yields clinical results comparable to those of proximal row carpectomy (**FIG 1**).[10,28,35]

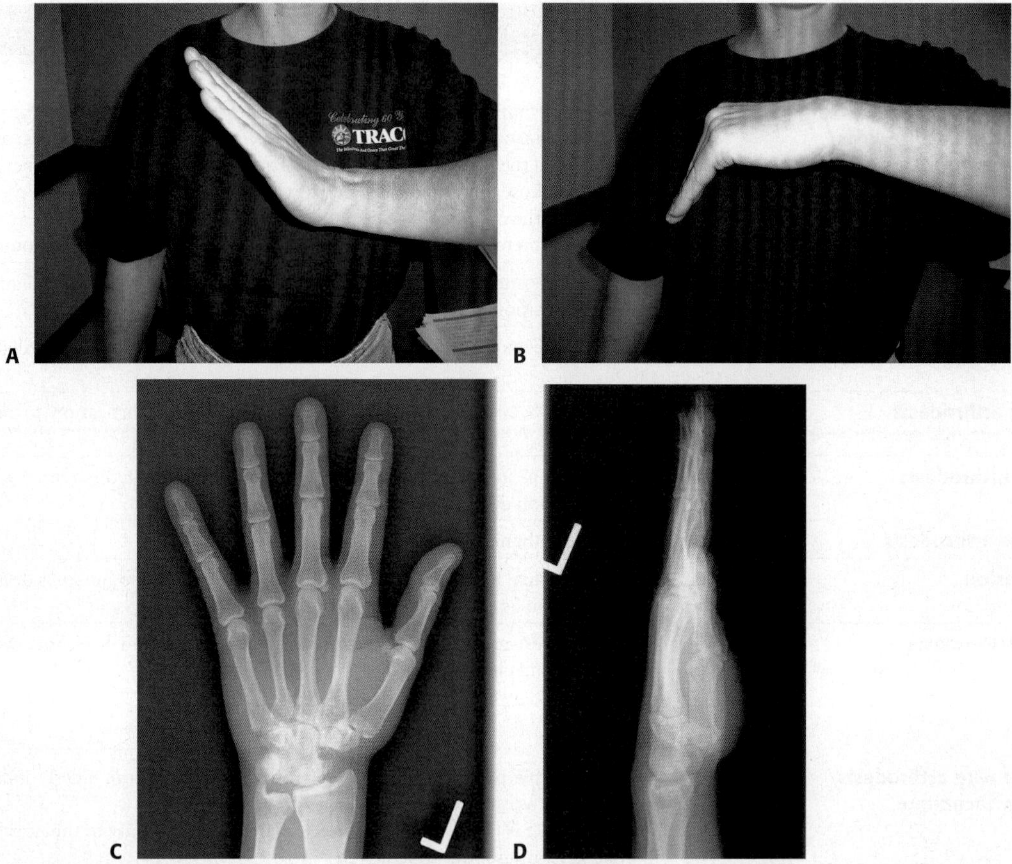

FIG 1 • Nine-year follow-up of four-corner fusion. **A,B.** Maximal active wrist extension and flexion. **C,D.** AP and lateral radiographs.

- Stage III SLAC arthritis can be managed with either a four-corner fusion or a proximal row carpectomy with dorsal capsular interposition.[28]
- In patients 35 years of age or younger at the time of proximal row carpectomy, subjective and objective function may decline over time, and they may eventually require a wrist fusion.[28]
- Circular plate fixation for CHLT fusion is a newer trend. Weiss et al[34] reported a union rate approaching 100% and high patient satisfaction.[14] However, several subsequent studies have documented higher nonunion rates, higher hardware failure rates, higher pain scores, and an overall lower rate of patient satisfaction compared to other traditional methods of fixation.[8,16,25,29]
- Recently, use of a locked radiolucent polyetheretherketone (PEEK) circular plate has shown union in 92% of patients, 66% ROM and 70% grip strength compared to contralateral, and good functional outcomes.[21]
- Biomechanical analysis of four-corner fusion with Kirschner wires versus dorsal circular plate versus locking dorsal circular plate showed that dorsal locked plates were significantly more stable.[17]
- At an average of 67-month follow-up, patients with lunate excision and STT fusion for lunate collapse due to Kienböck disease maintained motion and pain relief, although the scaphoid had a tendency to shift toward the lunate fossa, suggesting a risk of progression to radioscaphoid arthritis if the lunate is excised.[19]
- Scaphocapitate arthrodesis for chronic scapholunate instability in manual laborers has shown an 87 degrees arc in flexion/extension and 41 degrees arc in radioulnar deviation, with 60% of normal grip strength and maintained pain reduction with 90% return to work rate at 10-year follow-up. Incidence of radiocarpal arthritis was 30%.[22]
- In a small series, capitolunate arthrodesis with tricortical iliac crest bone graft, proximal pole scaphoid excision, distal pole scaphocapitate fusion, and radial styloidectomy lead to 100% union rate and 70% Mayo wrist score at 4-year follow-up.[15]
- Capitolunate arthrodesis has shown a decrease of 25 degrees from preoperative and loss of 6-kg strength, allowing a pain-free and functional wrist in 8 of 11 patients reviewed at 10-year follow-up.[12]
- Four-corner fusion with headless screw technique resulted in 94% union with average flexion–extension arc of 71 degrees, maintained carpal height, and 80% grip strength.[24]

COMPLICATIONS

- Pin tract infections
- Osteomyelitis
- Avascular necrosis of the lunate
- Radiolunate arthritis
- Reflex sympathetic dystrophy
- Tendon ruptures
- Persistent wrist pain
- Nonunion

- Fracture through fusion
- Neurapraxia
- Hardware failure
- Neuroma
- Pseudarthrosis

REFERENCES

1. Baratz ME, Rosenwasser MP, Adams BD, et al. Scaphocapitate fusion with lunate excision. In: Baratz ME, Rosenwasser MP, Adams BD, et al, eds. Wrist Surgery: Tricks of the Trade. New York: Thieme, 2006:167–169.
2. Baratz ME, Rosenwasser MP, Adams BD, et al. Scaphoid excision with capitolunate triquetohamate arthrodesis. In: Baratz ME, Rosenwasser MP, Adams BD, et al, eds. Wrist Surgery: Tricks of the Trade. New York: Thieme, 2006:133–134.
3. Baratz ME, Rosenwasser MP, Adams BD, et al. Scaphotrapeziotrapezoid joint fusion. In: Baratz ME, Rosenwasser MP, Adams BD, et al, eds. Wrist Surgery: Tricks of the Trade. New York: Thieme, 2006:138–140.
4. Berger RA, Bishop AT, Bettinger PC. New dorsal capsulotomy for the surgical exposure of the wrist. Ann Plast Surg 1995;35:54–59.
5. Brown RE, Erdmann D. Complications of 50 consecutive limited wrist fusions by a single surgeon. Ann Plast Surg 1995;35:46–53.
6. Burge PD. Scaphotrapeziotrapezoid and scaphocapitate fusions. In: Berger RA, Weiss AP, eds. Hand Surgery. Philadelphia: Lippincott Williams & Wilkins, 2004:1299–1308.
7. Burgess RC. The effect of a simulated scaphoid malunion on wrist motion. J Hand Surg Am 1987;12(5 pt 1):774–776.
8. Chung KC, Watt AJ, Kotsis SV. A prospective outcomes study of four-corner wrist arthrodesis using a circular limited wrist fusion plate for stage II scapholunate advanced collapse wrist deformity. Plast Reconstr Surg 2006;118:433–442.
9. Cohen MS. Four-corner fusions. In: Berger RA, Weiss AP, eds. Hand Surgery. Philadelphia: Lippincott Williams & Wilkins, 2004: 1309–1318.
10. Cohen MS, Kozin SH. Degenerative arthritis of the wrist: proximal row carpectomy versus scaphoid excision and four-corner arthrodesis. J Hand Surg Am 2001;26(1):94–104.
11. Dacho A, Grudel J, Holle G, et al. Long-term results of midcarpal arthrodesis in the treatment of scaphoid nonunion advanced collapse (SNAC-wrist) and scapholunate advanced collapse (SLAC-wrist). Ann Plast Surg 2006;56:139–144.
12. Delclaux S, Rongières M, Aprédoaei C, et al. Capitolunate arthrodesis: 12 patients followed-up an average of 10 years [in French]. Chir Main 2013;32(5):310–316.
13. Düppe H, Johnell O, Lundborg G, et al. Long-term results of fracture of the scaphoid. A follow-up study of more than thirty years. J Bone Joint Surg Am 1994;76(2):249–252.
14. Enna M, Hoepfner P, Weiss AP. Scaphoid excision with four-corner fusion. Hand Clin 2005;21:531–538.
15. Giannikas D, Karageorgos A, Karabasi A, et al. Capitolunate arthrodesis maintaining carpal height for the treatment of SNAC wrist. J Hand Surg Eur Vol 2010;35:198–201.
16. Kendall CB, Brown TR, Millon SJ, et al. Results of four-corner arthrodesis using dorsal circular plate fixation. J Hand Surg Am 2005; 30(5):903–907.
17. Kraisarin J, Dennison DG, Berglund LJ, et al. Biomechanical comparison of three fixation techniques used for four-corner arthrodesis. J Hand Surg Eur Vol 2011;36:560–567.
18. Larsen CF, Jacoby RA, McCabe SJ. Nonunion rates of limited carpal arthrodesis: a meta-analysis of the literature. J Hand Surg Am 1997;22(1):66–73.
19. Lee JS, Park MJ, Kang HJ. Scaphotrapeziotrapezoid arthrodesis and lunate excision for advanced Kienböck disease. J Hand Surg Am 2012;37(11):2226–2232.
20. Linscheid RL, Dobyns JH, Beaubout JW, et al. Traumatic instability of the wrist. Diagnosis, classification, and pathomechanics. J Bone Joint Surg Am 1972;54(8):1612–1632.
21. Luegmair M, Houvet P. Effectiveness of four-corner arthrodesis with use of a locked dorsal circular plate. Clin Orthop Relat Res 2012; 470:2764–2770.
22. Luegmair M, Saffar P. Scaphocapitate arthrodesis for treatment of scapholunate instability in manual workers. J Hand Surg Am 2013; 38(5):878–886.
23. Mack GR, Bosse MJ, Gelberman RH, et al. The natural history of scaphoid non-union. J Bone Joint Surg Am 1984;66(4):504–509.
24. Ozyurekoglu T, Turker T. Results of a method of 4-corner arthrodesis using headless compression screws. J Hand Surg Am 2012;37(3):486–492.
25. Shindle MK, Burton KJ, Weiland AJ, et al. Complications of circular plate fixation for four-corner arthrodesis. J Hand Surg Eur Vol 2007; 32(1):50–53.
26. Siegel JM, Ruby LK. A critical look at intercarpal arthrodesis: review of the literature. J Hand Surg Am 1996;21(4):717–723.
27. Taliesnik J. Radiolunate arthrodesis. In: Blair WF, ed. Techniques in Hand Surgery. Baltimore: Williams & Wilkins, 1996:879–886.
28. Tomaino MM, Miller RJ, Cole I, et al. Scapholunate advanced collapse wrist: proximal row carpectomy or limited wrist arthrodesis with scaphoid excision? J Hand Surg Am 1994;19(1):134–142.
29. Vance MC, Hernandez JD, DiDonna ML, et al. Complications and outcome of four-corner arthrodesis: circular plate fixation versus traditional techniques. J Hand Surg Am 2005;30(6):1122–1127.
30. Watson HK, Ashmeade D IV, Makhlouf MV. Examination of the scaphoid. J Hand Surg Am 1988;13(5):657–660.
31. Watson HK, Ballet FL. The SLAC wrist: scapholunate advanced collapse pattern of degenerative arthritis. J Hand Surg Am 1984;9(3): 358–365.
32. Watson HK, Weinzweig J. Intercarpal arthrodesis. In: Green DP, Hotchkiss RN, Pederson WC, eds. Green's Operative Hand Surgery, ed 4. New York: Churchill Livingstone, 1999:108–130.
33. Watson HK, Weinzweig J, Zeppieri J. The natural progression of scaphoid instability. Hand Clin 1997;13:17–34.
34. Weiss AP. Principles of limited wrist arthrodesis. In: Berger RA, Weiss AP, eds. Hand Surgery. Philadelphia: Lippincott Williams & Wilkins, 2004:1289–1298.
35. Wyrick JD. Proximal row carpectomy and intercarpal arthrodesis for the management of wrist arthritis. J Am Acad Orthop Surg 2003; 11:277–281.

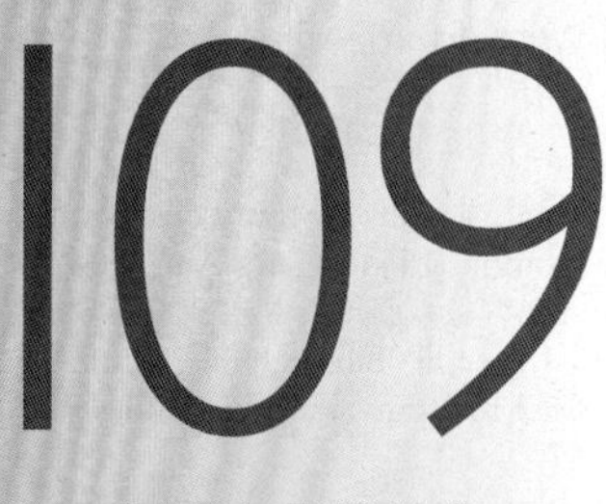

Complete Wrist Arthrodesis

John C. Elfar and Andrew D. Markiewitz

DEFINITION

- Wrist arthritis occurs when the codependent joints of the wrist lose the ability to rotate normally around one another, thereby impairing wrist kinematics.
- Wrist arthritis can originate from many causes including osteoarthritis, degenerative arthritis, and inflammatory arthritis.
- Although sacrificing motion at the wrist, arthrodesis has been shown to reliably relieve pain.

ANATOMY

- The wrist is perhaps the most complex set of joints in the body.
- The eight bones of the wrist work together to provide motion in multiple planes, governed by the complex array of soft tissue ligaments that unite them.
  - Single ligament disruptions can cause degenerative change in nonadjacent bones and at times unlikely sites.
  - Untreated fractures can lead to malunions or nonunions that can disrupt the delicate balance of the wrist.
- In broad terms, the wrist is divided into two distinct rows of bones.
  - The distal row, including the trapezium, trapezoid, capitate, and hamate, is united to the hand and shows little gross motion relative to the metacarpals.
  - As such, the most significant articulations in the wrist occur in the proximal row bones, which are the scaphoid, lunate, and triquetrum. These proximal row bones allow the wrist to flex, extend, deviate both radially and ulnarly, and pronosupinate.

PATHOGENESIS

- Because of the many possible routes to the eventual destruction of the wrist joint, it is difficult to describe a single chain of events that leads to end-stage arthritis, most suitably treated by complete wrist fusion.

NATURAL HISTORY

- Causes of wrist degeneration and the often-predictable pattern and pace of wear are detailed in other chapters.

PATIENT HISTORY AND PHYSICAL FINDINGS

- Patients describe pain and stiffness as their major reasons for presentation. Pain limits their function and their strength.
  - Most patients are less concerned with motion loss if their dominant extremity is not involved. Wrist flexion and extension is typically more involved than supination and pronation.
  - If their dominant wrist is involved, patients prefer to preserve some motion even if faced with low-grade persistent pain after treatment. In this clinical setting, complete wrist fusions are less often performed as the index operation.
- Physical examination findings may include deformity, tenderness, soft tissue swelling, loss of motion, instability, and pain with motion. Pinch and grip strength are reduced compared with age-matched peers and the uninvolved contralateral extremity.

IMAGING AND OTHER DIAGNOSTIC STUDIES

- Wrist arthritis is best studied with standard posteroanterior and lateral radiographs of the wrist.
  - These images often reveal the cause of the degeneration together with its pattern and progression.
  - Special attention is paid to the alignment of the wrist and the bone stock available for fusion and fixation.
- Computed tomography helps plan limited fusions or salvage procedures when arthritis may have spared areas of the midcarpal or proximal carpal rows.

DIFFERENTIAL DIAGNOSIS

- Limited wrist arthritis
- Extrinsic joint contracture (including calcific tendinitis)
- Inflammatory arthritis and synovitis (ie, rheumatoid, gout, or pseudogout)
- Infection
- Posttraumatic changes
- Connective tissue diseases

NONOPERATIVE MANAGEMENT

- In most every case, the first form of treatment for wrist arthritis is nonoperative:
  - Nonsteroidal anti-inflammatory medications (NSAIDs)
  - Disease-modifying medications (if the cause of the degenerative process can be identified and is appropriate)
  - Splinting
    - A custom-made thumb spica splint allows interphalangeal motion of the thumb but limits painful wrist motion.
    - A padded glove (similar to weight lifting or cycling glove) helps decrease the load across the wrist and the motion necessary for a satisfactory grip.
  - Narcotics should be avoided as addiction, dependency, and diversion may occur.

- Local steroid injections placed in the wrist
  - These should be placed with a sterile technique and can be repeated as needed if the joint is destroyed and limited salvage options are available.

SURGICAL MANAGEMENT

- Alternative motion-sparing procedures, including partial wrist fusions and proximal row carpectomy, should be considered before performing a complete wrist fusion, especially in patients who have at least 60 degrees of wrist flexion–extension and have isolated articular degeneration.
- Wrist arthroplasty remains in its infancy and is associated with high revision rates and frequent implant design changes.
  - Wrist arthrodesis after arthroplasty is more difficult due to bone stock loss.
- Wrist arthrodesis is the final treatment method for end-stage wrist degeneration due to multiple causes or as a salvage procedure in patients who have failed the more limited procedures mentioned earlier.
  - Arthrodesis can be obtained reliably and provides a stable wrist in a high-demand patient.[1,2,13,15]
  - In patients who have undergone lower extremity joint replacements and therefore require support for ambulation, fusion of the wrist is generally regarded as a reliable procedure.
- The two most popular methods used to fuse a wrist are plate osteosynthesis and rod osteosynthesis.[2,8,15] A new locked intramedullary rod has been proposed to limit dorsal plate prominence.[10]
- The chief considerations when choosing between these two options are the desired position of fusion, the quality of the bone and available soft tissue coverage, and the possibility of future infection.
  - The strongest grip is achieved when the wrist is fused in 20 to 30 degrees of extension. Advocates of fusion in this position favor the use of a plate and screw construct that is fabricated to reproduce this position.[2,4,16] Straight wrist fusion plates are also available, and all these devices include screws and plates that match the size of the radius and the metacarpal.
  - A neutral wrist position obtained with rod osteosynthesis may be more favorable for activities of daily living, including perineal care.[2,3,5,13]
  - Plate and screw constructs rely on solid screw purchase and stable soft tissue coverage. If good-quality bone and viable soft tissues are not present, as might be the case in a patient with severe rheumatoid disease, intramedullary rod fixation may be a more effective means of fixation.
  - In patients taking aggressive disease-remitting medications, the possibility of late infection should be considered. These patients may benefit from metal removal, which is often more easily accomplished after rod osteosynthesis.

Preoperative Planning

- Patients should be assessed for comorbidities including first carpometacarpal joint arthritis and carpal tunnel syndrome (CTS). CTS untreated at the time of fusion may worsen acutely and lead to emergency management.
- Although the use of aspirin may be continued, clopidogrel (Plavix) should be discontinued to avoid bleeding and flap complications. Warfarin (Coumadin) may be continued if the international normalized ratio (INR) is kept low in the 2 to 2.5 range. The continued use of disease-modifying medicines may be continued at the surgeon's discretion.[12]
- Radiographs should be reviewed before performing a wrist arthrodesis. Specific attention should be paid to the amount of available bone stock and the bony alignment. Special plates may need to be ordered if prior surgeries have been performed on the radius.
- Intraoperative evaluation will require a fluoroscopic device. Appropriate alignment, reduction, screw length, and implant length should be confirmed before closure.

Positioning

- Patients are placed supine with the operative hand extended on a hand table extension.
- A tourniquet is applied to the proximal arm over padding.
- Before anesthesia is induced, the patient's comfortable shoulder position should be assessed. The arm board should not place the shoulder above this position. This test is especially important in rheumatoid patients with limited joint mobility.

Approach

- Both arthrodesis procedures are performed through a standard dorsal approach to the wrist.[11,14–16] A longitudinal midline dorsal incision ulnar to the tubercle of Lister is used.
- The extensor pollicis longus tendon is released from its sheath and retracted radially.[11,14]
- The fourth extensor compartment is subperiosteally elevated from the dorsum of the distal radius and retracted ulnarly.
  - The posterior interosseous nerve can be dissected free and excised for pain relief.
- The dorsal capsule is incised in line with the skin incision and elevated off the carpus.[14]
- This exposure allows for performance of concomitant procedures such as a distal ulna excision and dorsal tenosynovectomy.

Plate and Screw Osteosynthesis

- In addition to the approach described earlier, the proximal portion of the third metacarpal is exposed subperiosteally.
- Expose the radioscaphoid, radiolunate, scaphocapitate, capitolunate, and third carpometacarpal joints (**TECH FIG 1A**); clean them of any remaining cartilage and soft tissue; and then fully denude them to below the subchondral bone.
  - Maintain the general bony geometry to allow the prepared carpal bones to interdigitate effectively.
  - A combination of a no. 15 blade, small curettes, and rongeurs is usually adequate for preparing the joint surfaces. Use of a water-cooled power burr and repeated penetration of the articular surfaces with a 0.045-inch smooth Kirschner wire are sometimes helpful.
  - The triquetrolunate, triquetrohamate, scaphotrapeziotrapezoid, and capitohamate joints may be left undisturbed if not arthritic.
  - If one expects to remove the plate at a second surgery, the second and third carpometacarpal joints can be left intact. This limits the fusion mass to the radiocarpal and midcarpal joints, preserving motion at the carpometacarpal level.
- Obtain autologous bone graft from the distal radius in two forms, a corticocancellous graft and cancellous bone chips. In osteoporotic patients, bone graft substitute may be used.
  - Take care to avoid disrupting the radial cortex of the distal radius (and thereby destabilizing the bone) and removing the cortex on which the plate will eventually sit.
  - Outline the graft using a wire driver and a 0.045-inch Kirschner wire, and then harvest it with a sharp osteotome and mallet.
- After removing this graft, harvest cancellous bone from the site and tightly pack it between the prepared bony surfaces.
  - In cases of severe deformity, the carpus may be held in general alignment with temporary Kirschner wires.
  - With severe bone loss, the pelvis should be used as the site for bone graft. A corticocancellous graft of appropriate length and width may be harvested to fill the void.

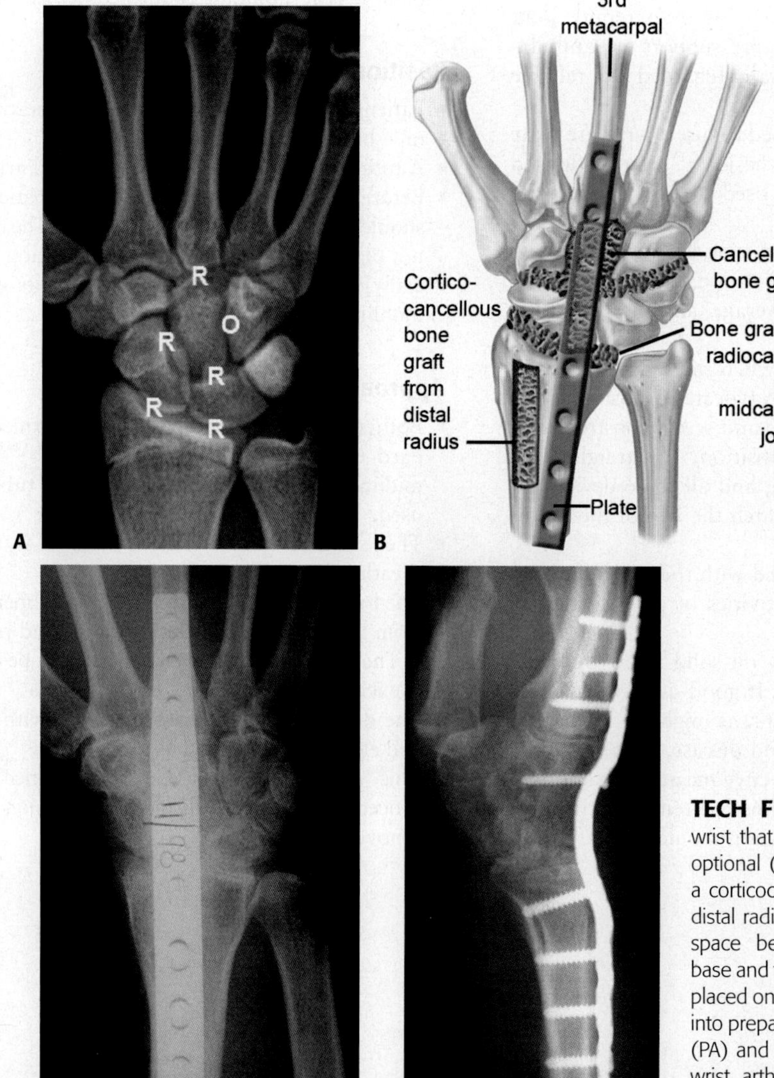

TECH FIG 1 • A. Joints within the wrist that are decorticated and grafted: optional (*O*) or required (*R*). **B.** Use of a corticocancellous bone graft from the distal radius. The graft is keyed into the space between the third metacarpal base and the radius platform. The plate is placed on top. Cancellous graft is packed into prepared joints. **C,D.** Posteroanterior (PA) and lateral radiographs following a wrist arthrodesis using a dorsal plate. (**C,D:** Courtesy of P.J. Stern, MD.)

- Key the corticocancellous graft into the space between the third metacarpal base and the radius platform.
  - This graft will be located directly under the plate (**TECH FIG 1B**).
- Choose the desired wrist fusion plate and secure it distally to the third metacarpal with appropriately sized screws.
  - Plate options include a long bend, a short bend, and a straight plate (Synthes, West Chester, PA).
  - In selected instances, the second metacarpal may be used rather than the third metacarpal. This position may be preferred by the patient for their specific positioning needs.
- With the carpus aligned and the prepared joints reduced and grafted, apply the plate to the distal radius in a compression mode using appropriately sized screws. Complete the fixation with additional screws (**TECH FIG 1C,D**).
- Any remaining bone graft is added in and around the prepared joints.
- Close the capsule with absorbable suture. If needed, the extensor retinaculum may be split, with one portion repaired deep to the extensor tendons to allow coverage of prominent portions of the plate. The other portion is repaired superficial to the tendons to resist "bowstringing." Transpose the extensor pollicis longus tendon dorsally into the subcutaneous space radial to Lister tubercle. Close the skin in the usual manner.
  - Strongly consider using a drain especially in anticoagulated patients.
- A sterile dressing and below-elbow volar splint are applied.

Fusion with Steinmann Rods

- Fusion with Steinmann rods is performed using a technique similar to that described earlier, typically in patients with advanced inflammatory arthritis.
  - Because bone loss and deformity are substantive, precise joint preparation and reduction is not possible and the goal is generation of a fusion mass.
  - Typically, cancellous autograft taken from the distal radius is used between the prepared bony surfaces.
- Fixation may be accomplished using an intramedullary rod inserted through the head of the third metacarpal (**TECH FIG 2A–D**).
  - As an alternative, two rods can be inserted between the second and third and third and fourth metacarpals (**TECH FIG 2E,F**). These are usually smaller pins that produce an interference fit in the radius shaft.
- Placing an intramedullary rod through the third metacarpal head necessitates an incision in the dorsal web space and in the sagittal band.
  - Metacarpophalangeal joint replacement may eventually be required.
- Choose the largest pin that will fit within the metacarpal and advance it retrograde through the reduced carpus and into the radius.
  - A second smaller derotation pin can be placed through the radial styloid into the carpus and metacarpals to prevent rotation.
  - Alternatively, a figure-8 wire can be placed around the third metacarpal and through the radius to compress the construct.
- If the metacarpophalangeal joints have already been replaced, two Steinmann pins through the second and third web spaces may be effective.
- Closure is similar to that described earlier.

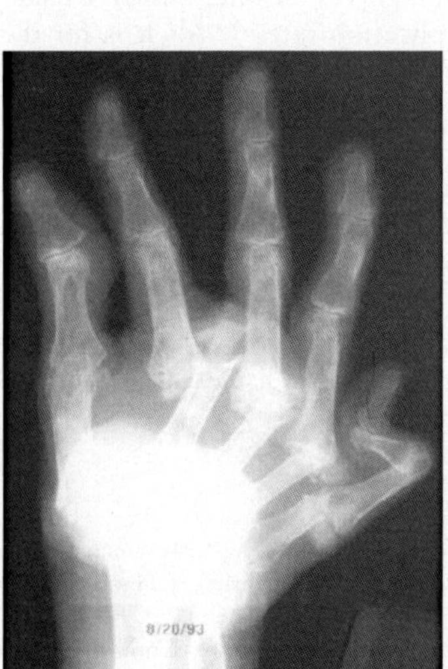

A

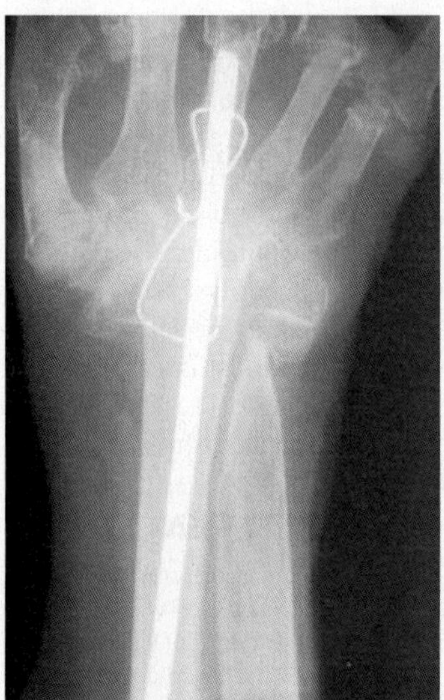
B

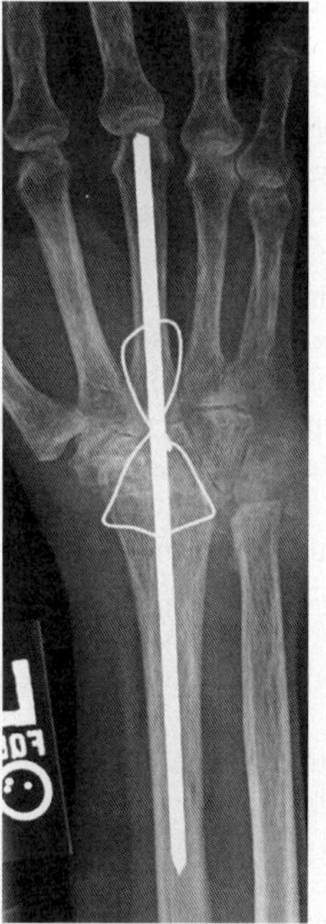
C

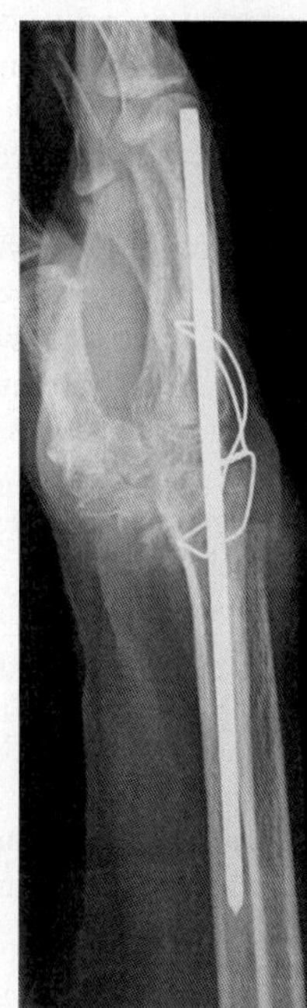
D

TECH FIG 2 • **A,B.** Complex wrist collapse secondary to rheumatoid arthritis treated with an intramedullary rod and wiring. Ulnar impaction symptoms developing at the distal radioulnar joint. **C,D.** Less severe wrist disease in a different patient was treated with a Darrach resection and wrist arthrodesis. *(continued)*

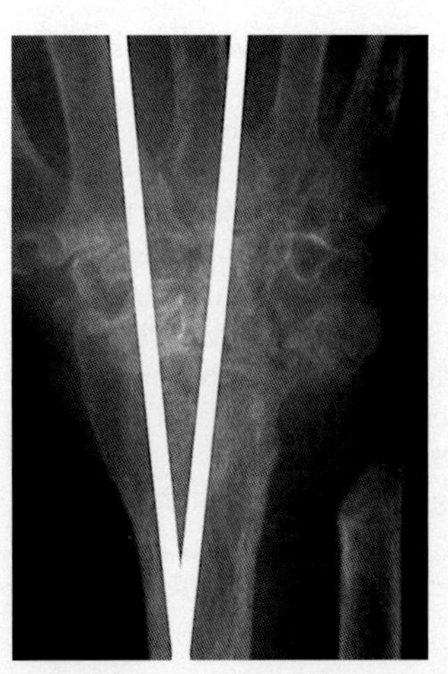

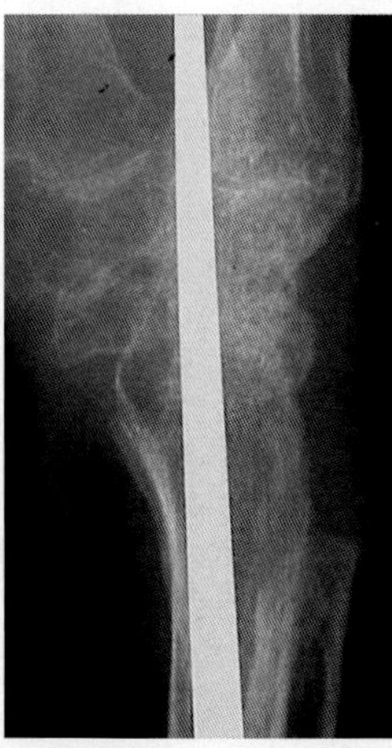

TECH FIG 2 • *(continued)* **E,F.** PA and lateral radiographs after wrist arthrodesis in a different patient with rheumatoid arthritis was undertaken using two Steinmann pins inserted through the second and third and third and fourth intermetacarpal spaces. (**A–D:** Courtesy of P.J. Stern, MD; **E,F:** Copyright Thomas R. Hunt III, MD.)

PEARLS AND PITFALLS

- The third metacarpal should be aligned with the radius. This alignment is essential when applying a plate.
- Patients prefer to be in slight wrist extension without significant radial or ulnar deviation; significant deviation into flexion or radial deviation leads to problems and weakness. Patients already stiff at neutral may prefer a neutral position.
- Bilateral fusions may not be preferred but rarely affect function.[2]
- If the proximal row has displaced, proximal row carpectomy and fusion has been shown to be successful.[4]
- If the ulnar head appears arthritic or prominent, it will need to be addressed using a Darrach procedure, hemiresection techniques, or head replacement. If not addressed, it may be a source of pain postoperatively.
- If a locked plate design is used due to osteoporosis, one should place the first metacarpal and radius screws as nonlocking screws to pull the plate to the bones.

POSTOPERATIVE CARE

- Patients are placed into a removable brace 2 weeks after surgery and started on active finger flexion–extension exercises as well as pronation and supination.
- Osteoporotic patients may benefit from the short-term use of a thumb spica cast before being advanced into a splint.
- Patients with an extensor lag due to dorsal swelling are started on a program of dynamic extension with an outrigger splint until full active extension is regained.
- Strengthening is initiated when motion is recovered and the radiographs demonstrate union. Union usually takes 6 to 8 weeks but is prolonged in smokers. Comorbidities may also affect healing rates. Bone stimulation devices (ultrasound) may be of benefit to accelerate healing especially in at-risk patient populations.
- If patient compliance is an issue, a cast may be used for the first 4 weeks to protect the plate construct.
- A cast is recommended for 4 to 6 weeks when using Steinmann rods until the patient's wrist is nontender on examination indicating healing.
- Therapy may also need to be modified depending on any additional procedures performed.

COMPLICATIONS

- Infection
- Nonunion, delayed union, and malunion
- Dorsal wrist tenderness
- Tendon adhesions and ruptures
- Neuromas and complex regional pain syndromes
- Pin migration
- Wound breakdown

OUTCOMES

- Wrist arthrodesis boasts a high fusion rate, a high satisfaction rate, and a low complication rate.[1,5,7–9,15] It is for this reason that fusion of the wrist is selected in patients who can tolerate fewer trips to the operating room for secondary procedures.
- Although more satisfying than rod stabilization in rheumatoid patients (74% vs. 37%), plate fixation may require tenolysis or plate removal after arthrodesis.[1,13] Satisfaction may be affected by the patient's underlying disease.
- Houshian and Schrøder[6] found that plate removal was common (15%) due to the complications listed earlier but was successful in relieving symptoms.

REFERENCES

1. Barbier O, Saels P, Rombouts JJ, et al. Long-term functional results of wrist arthrodesis in rheumatoid arthritis. J Hand Surg Br 1999;24(1):27–31.
2. Calundruccio JH. Osteoarthritis of the wrist. In: Trumble TE, ed. Hand Surgery Update 3. Rosemont, IL: American Academy of Orthopaedic Surgeons, 2003:528–529.
3. Clendenin MP, Green DP. Arthrodesis of the wrist: complications and their management. J Hand Surg Am 1981;6:253–257.

4. Hartigan BJ, Nagle DJ, Foley MJ. Wrist arthrodesis with excision of the proximal carpal bones using the AO/ASIF wrist fusion plate and local bone graft. J Hand Surg Br 2001;26(3):247–251.
5. Hayden RJ, Jebson PJ. Wrist arthrodesis. Hand Clin 2005;21:631–640.
6. Houshian S, Schrøder HA. Wrist arthrodesis with the AO titanium wrist fusion plate: a consecutive series of 42 cases. J Hand Surg Br 2001;26(4):355–359.
7. Jebson PJ, Adams BD. Wrist arthrodesis: review of current techniques. J Am Acad Orthop Surg 2001;9:53–60.
8. Krimmer H. Radiocarpal and total wrist arthrodesis. In: Berger RA, Weiss AP, eds. Hand Surgery. Philadelphia: Lippincott Williams & Wilkins, 2004:1319–1337.
9. Mack GR, Bosse MJ, Gelberman RH, et al. The natural history of scaphoid non-union. J Bone Joint Surg Am 1984;66(4):504–509.
10. Orbay JL, Feliciano E, Orbay C. Locked intramedullary total wrist arthrodesis. J Wrist Surg 2012;1(2):179–184.
11. Ruby LK, Stinson J, Belsky MR. The natural history of scaphoid non-union. A review of fifty-three cases. J Bone Joint Surg Am 1985;67(3): 428–432.
12. Thorsness RJ, Hammert WC. Perioperative management of rheumatoid medications. J Hand Surg Am 2012;37(9):1928–1931.
13. Toma CD, Machacek P, Bitzan P, et al. Fusion of the wrist in rheumatoid arthritis: a clinical and functional evaluation of two surgical techniques. J Bone Joint Surg Br 2007;89(12):1620–1626.
14. Weil C, Ruby LK. The dorsal approach to the wrist revisited. J Hand Surg Am 1986;11(6):911–912.
15. Weiss AC, Wiedeman G Jr, Quenzer D, et al. Upper extremity function after wrist arthrodesis. J Hand Surg Am 1995;20(5): 813–817.
16. Weiss AP, Hastings H II. Wrist arthrodesis for traumatic conditions: a study of plate and local graft application. J Hand Surg Am 1995;20(1):50–56.

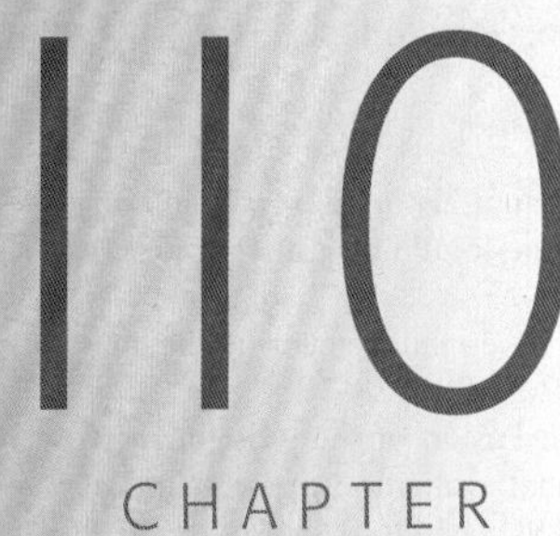

Wrist Implant Arthroplasty

Thomas Ebinger and Brian D. Adams

DEFINITION

- The wrist is a common site for end-stage joint degeneration, particularly in patients with rheumatoid disease. Osteoarthritis and posttraumatic arthritis following distal radius fractures, scaphoid nonunion advanced collapse (SNAC), and scapholunate advanced collapse (SLAC) are other common causes for advanced arthritis.
- The gold standard of treatment for severe wrist arthritis has historically been complete wrist arthrodesis. Although arthrodesis provides good pain relief and durability, it is associated with substantial functional loss, especially if both wrists have arthritis.[1,9,13]
- Total wrist arthroplasty is a motion-preserving alternative to arthrodesis that provides excellent pain relief. Sufficient motion and strength is retained for activities of daily living.
- Preservation of wrist joint motion is of particular importance for patients who are debilitated by arthritis affecting multiple joints and those with specific joint motion requirements.[9]
- Similar to arthroplasty in other joints, early wrist arthroplasty implants had poor long-term survivorship.[2,3,7]
- Wrist arthroplasty has continually improved since the introduction of articulated implants more than 40 years ago. Advancements in design include distal component fixation being primarily within the carpus and not the metacarpal; intercarpal fusion to provide broad, solid support for the component; screw augmentation for carpal component fixation; minimal bone resection; preservation of the wrist capsule; cementless fixation; a broad semiconstrained ellipsoid articulation; and an option to preserve the distal radioulnar joint (DRUJ).
- Through improved materials, designs, and fixation techniques, total wrist arthroplasty has emerged as a viable option for selected patients with end-stage wrist arthritis.
- Regardless of the desire for arthroplasty, patients must commit to a lifetime of restricted activities to obtain a durable outcome.
- There are currently three total wrist implant systems in the United States: Re-Motion (Small Bone Innovations, Inc., Morrisville, PA), Maestro (Biomet, Warsaw, IN), and most recently Freedom (Integra LifeSciences, Plainsboro, NJ) (**FIG 1**). The Freedom wrist system evolved from its predecessor, the Universal 2 (Integra LifeSciences).
  - The Re-Motion wrist offers a mobile bearing attached to the carpal component that theoretically improves motion and load transfer, thus reducing stresses known to contribute to loosening.
  - The Maestro allows complete resection of the proximal carpal row and has a polyethylene surface proximally. The system is also approved for hemiarthroplasty using the distal component alone.
  - The Freedom wrist is the newest design, with a more anatomic articulation that provides physiologic wrist motion, improved bone fixation, and precise instrumentation.

ANATOMY

- The wrist joint consists of the distal radial articular surface, distal ulna, triangular fibrocartilage complex (TFCC), eight carpal bones arranged in two rows (proximal and distal), and five metacarpal bases.
- There are four major wrist articulations: radiocarpal (and ulnocarpal), midcarpal, carpometacarpal (CMC), and distal radioulnar joints.

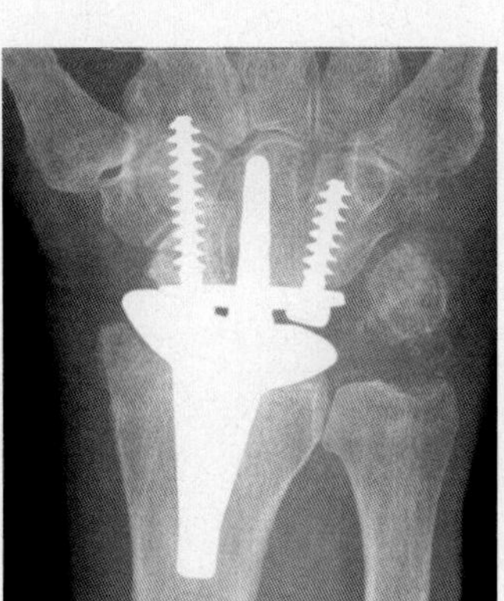
A

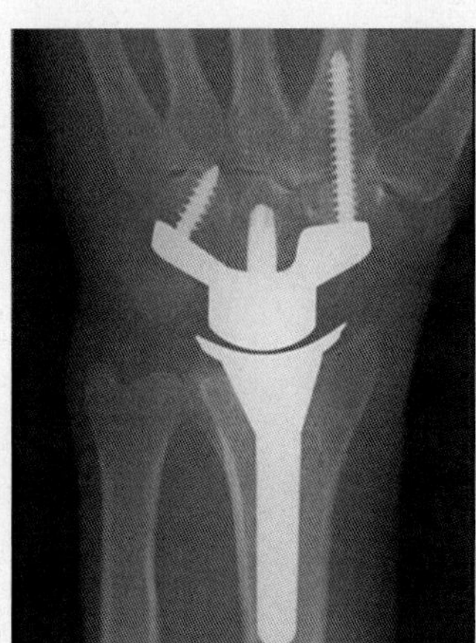
B

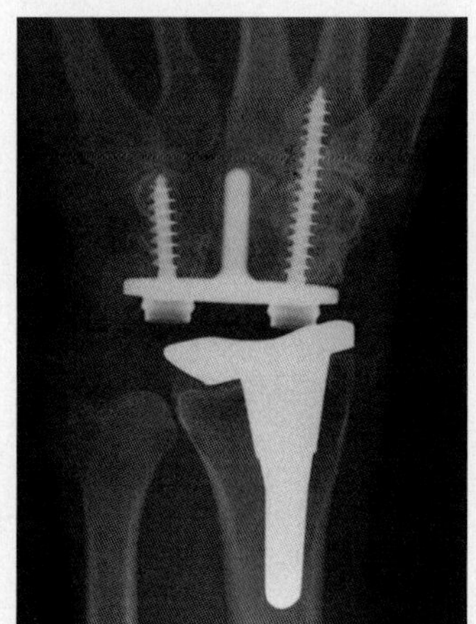
C

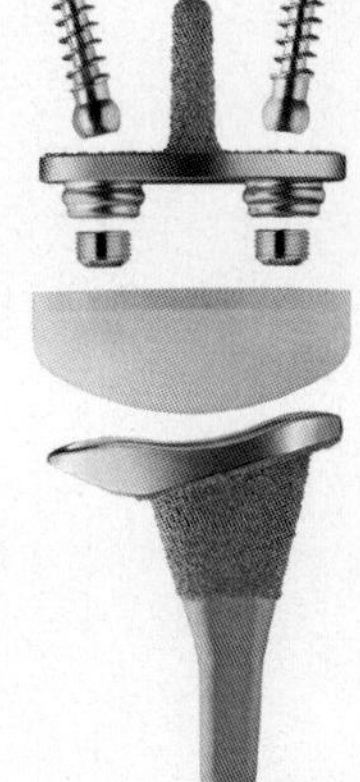
D

FIG 1 • **A–D.** Total wrist arthroplasty implants (from *left* to *right*): Re-Motion (Small Bone Innovations), Maestro (Biomet), Universal 2 (Integra LifeSciences), and Freedom (Integra LifeSciences).

- In addition to the wrist capsule, multiple interosseous, intrinsic and extrinsic ligaments provide joint stability, with intrinsic ligaments referring to those between carpal bones and located primarily within the joint and extrinsic ligaments located within the joint capsule.
- Normal radiographic parameters of the distal articular surface of the radius include 11 degrees of volar tilt, 22 degrees of radial inclination, and 11 mm of radial height.
- Ulnar variance refers to the length of ulna relative to the radius, with positive variance indicating the ulna is longer. Approximately 70% of the population is ulnar neutral.
- The sigmoid notch of the distal radius provides the radial articulation for the DRUJ. The DRUJ is stabilized by dorsal and volar radioulnar ligaments. Current implant systems are designed to preserve both the joint surfaces and ligaments of the DRUJ.
- The center of wrist motion is located near the center of the head of the capitate.

PATHOGENESIS

- Severe wrist arthritis is commonly caused by rheumatoid arthritis.
  - Early rheumatoid arthritis begins with minor joint erosions at synovial reflections such as the scaphoid waist and fovea of the ulnar head.
  - Progression of rheumatoid arthritis results in radial deviation and ulnar translocation of the carpus (**FIG 2A**), followed by carpal supination and volar subluxation (**FIG 2B**).
  - DRUJ deformity is very common in rheumatoid arthritis, resulting in dorsal subluxation of the ulna, often referred to as *caput ulna*.
  - Progression of rheumatoid disease may cause substantial ligament damage and bone erosion resulting in wrist deformity and decreased function.
- Posttraumatic arthritis may develop years after an intra-articular distal radius fracture or fracture-dislocation of the carpus. In regard to implant arthroplasty, a malunion of the radius presents additional surgical challenges, but with proper planning and technique, a successful outcome is possible.
- SNAC and SLAC wrist conditions are the most common causes of nonrheumatoid wrist arthritis, often with predictable degenerative patterns but only modest deformity.

NATURAL HISTORY

- End-stage wrist arthritis, no matter the cause, is a painful condition resulting in progressive stiffness and diminished function.
- In addition to pain and functional loss, deformity may be a cosmetic concern for patients.
- Inflammatory arthritis may cause severe deformity and bone loss, precluding wrist implant arthroplasty.

PATIENT HISTORY AND PHYSICAL FINDINGS

- The history should confirm the presence of substantial pain that indicates the need for wrist arthroplasty.
- Age, activity desires, hand dominance, presence of contralateral wrist arthritis, use of walking aids, and occupation are important factors in the preoperative assessment.
- In rheumatoid patients, disease activity should be optimally controlled medically prior to surgical treatment because highly active disease reduces the durability of an arthroplasty.[12]
- Lower limb surgery, such as total hip or knee arthroplasty, should be done prior to wrist replacement surgery to avoid weight bearing through the wrist implant during rehabilitation.
- The ideal candidate for total wrist arthroplasty is an elderly patient with a low-demand lifestyle who desires pain relief

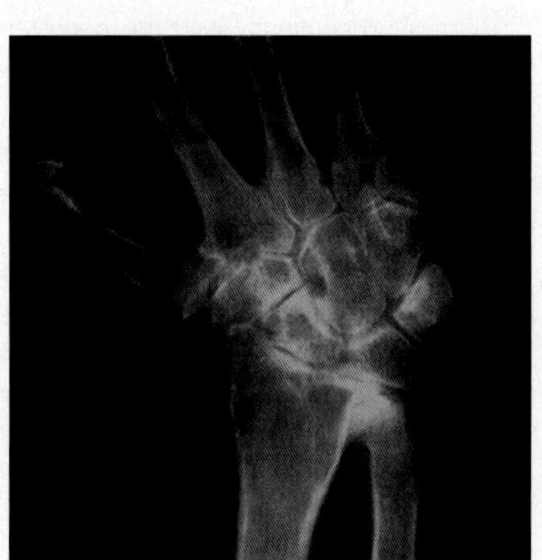
A

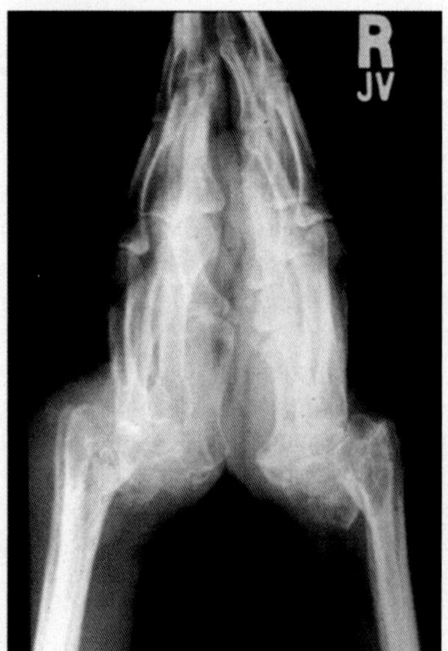

B

FIG 2 • **A.** PA radiograph of a rheumatoid wrist showing ulnocarpal translocation and radial deviation deformity. **B.** Lateral view of a rheumatoid wrist showing severe arthritis with volar subluxation of the carpus.

and can accept modest motion and strength and be willing to avoid stressful use.

- Younger patients may qualify for wrist arthroplasty if activities can be modified, particularly when the nondominant wrist is involved.

IMAGING AND OTHER DIAGNOSTIC STUDIES

- Standard posteroanterior (PA), lateral, and oblique views of the wrist are adequate to assess the extent of disease, alignment, and bone stock.
- In patients with rheumatoid arthritis, cervical spine radiographs are indicated to assess for instability.

DIFFERENTIAL DIAGNOSIS

- Rheumatoid arthritis
- Posttraumatic arthritis
- Osteoarthritis, including SLAC and SNAC wrists
- Avascular necrosis (eg, Kienböck disease)
- Other inflammatory arthritis (eg, psoriatic)

NONOPERATIVE MANAGEMENT

- Conservative treatment for severe wrist arthritis includes activity modification, bracing, nonsteroidal anti-inflammatory medications, and corticosteroid injections.
- Failure of pain relief by conservative treatment or progression of deformity are indications for surgical treatment.

SURGICAL MANAGEMENT

- Relative contraindications include poor bone stock, lack of wrist motor control, and wrist instability due to severely damaged tendons or ligaments,
- Active infection locally or systemically is an absolute contraindication to total wrist arthroplasty.
- Inflammatory arthritis should be well controlled medically prior to proceeding with surgical treatment.

Preoperative Planning

- If severe bone loss or erosive disease is suspected but not confirmed by preoperative imaging, then the surgical permit should include other options such as arthrodesis. Proper instruments and devices should be available.
- The proper implant size is estimated using PA and lateral wrist x-rays; however, final sizing is determined intraoperatively.
- The DRUJ is assessed preoperatively for arthritis and instability.
  - A partial or complete resection of the distal ulna is planned when needed.
  - If the DRUJ is unaffected, then the DRUJ is not exposed.

Positioning

- The patient is positioned supine with the affected limb resting on a hand table.
- A padded tourniquet is placed on the upper arm.
- Prophylactic antibiotics are administered intravenously.

TECHNIQUES

Freedom Total Wrist Prosthesis

- Although the technique for the Freedom wrist arthroplasty is described here, the principles apply to other wrist arthroplasty systems.
- Preoperative prophylactic antibiotics are recommended.
- The procedure can be completed under general or regional anesthesia.
- A strip of transparent adhesive film is applied across the dorsum of the hand, wrist, and distal forearm to protect the skin from damage during instrumentation.
- The surgical exposure described here preserves the DRUJ.
- Although this system is approved for cement fixation, it is typically implanted using a cementless technique.

Dorsal Approach

- A dorsal longitudinal incision is made over the wrist in line with the third metacarpal, extending proximally from its midshaft to approximately 8 cm proximal to the wrist joint.
  - The skin and subcutaneous tissue are elevated from the extensor retinaculum, with care to protect the superficial radial nerve and dorsal cutaneous branch of the ulnar nerve.
  - The extensor digitorum quinti component is opened, and the entire retinaculum is elevated radially to the septum between the first and second extensor compartments.
  - An extensor tenosynovectomy is performed if needed, and the tendons are retracted.
- The dorsal wrist capsule is raised as a broad distally based rectangular flap to the level of the midcapitate. The capsule is raised in continuity with the periosteum over the distal 1 cm of the radius to create a longer flap for closure (**TECH FIG 1**).
  - The radial side of the flap is made in the floor of the second extensor compartment and the ulnar side extends from the radius to the triquetrum, avoiding the TFCC and DRUJ.
  - The first extensor compartment is elevated subperiosteally from the distal 1 cm of the radial styloid and the remaining dorsal wrist capsule is elevated ulnarly from the triquetrum.
  - The wrist is fully flexed, and a synovectomy is performed as needed.

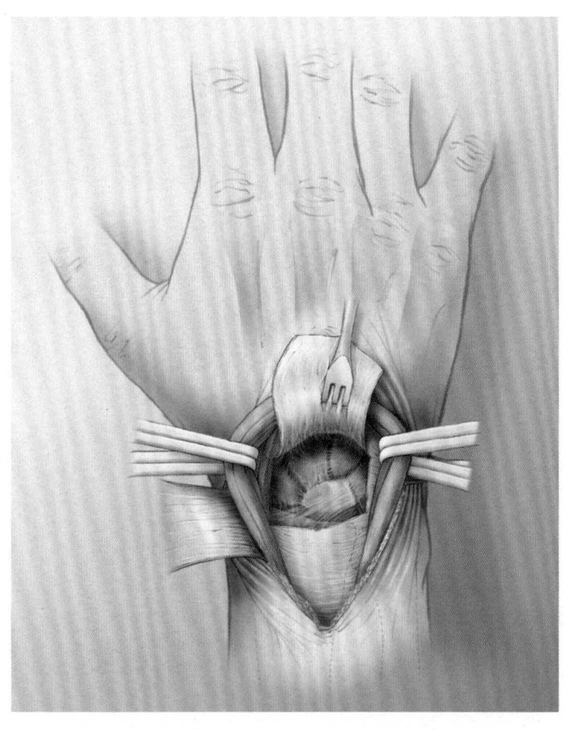

TECH FIG 1 ● To expose the joint, the extensor retinaculum is elevated as a radially based flap and the joint capsule is raised as a distally based flap.

Preparation of the Carpus

- Carpus preparation is facilitated by first temporarily pinning the scaphoid and triquetrum to the capitate and hamate in positions that create maximum joint contact, but do not impede the carpal osteotomy or screw placements.
- The lunate is excised by sharp dissection and rongeur.
- Carpal resection passes approximately through the proximal 1.5 mm of the hamate and capitate head, the scaphoid waist, and the midtriquetrum.
- Implant size is determined by the distance between the proximal pole of the hamate and the center of the capitate head, as measured by the carpal sizer. Implant size options are 1, 2, and 3.
- The modular drill guide is applied with the barrel pressed against the center of the capitate head and the saddle on the third metacarpal shaft (**TECH FIG 2A**).
- A guidewire is inserted through the capitate head and into the third metacarpal.
  - Fluoroscopy is used to ensure the wire is directed down the center of the capitate.
- Place the 3.5-mm cannulated drill bit over the guidewire and drill to the appropriate depth marked on the bit.

A

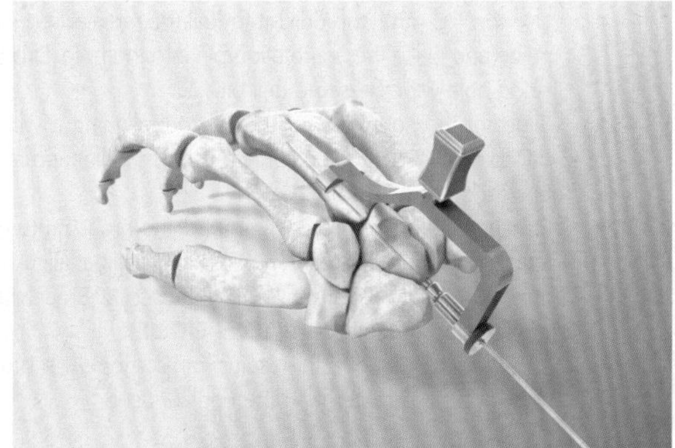

B

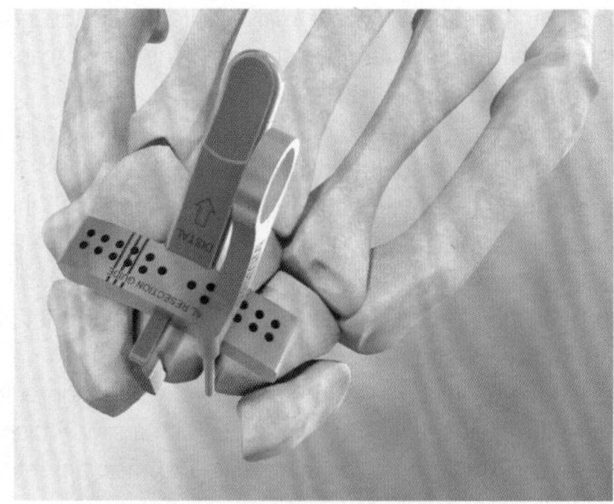

TECH FIG 2 ● **A.** The lunate is excised to expose the capitate. The modular drill guide is applied with the barrel pressed against the center of the capitate head and the saddle on the third metacarpal. A guidewire is inserted through the center of the capitate into the third metacarpal. **B.** Insert the carpal guide bar into the capitate and mount the resection guide with the hamate feeler just touching the proximal pole of the hamate. *(continued)*

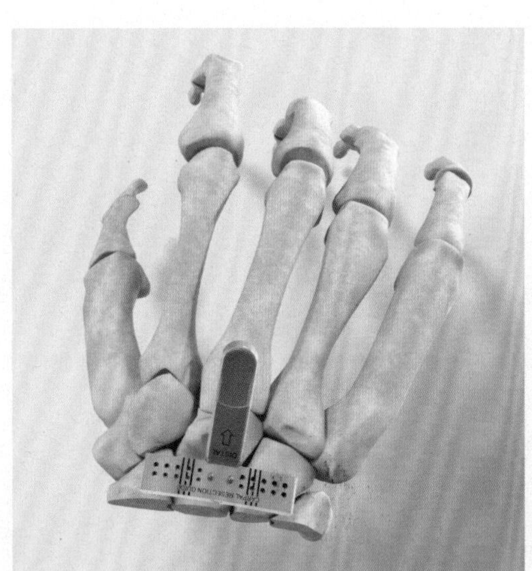

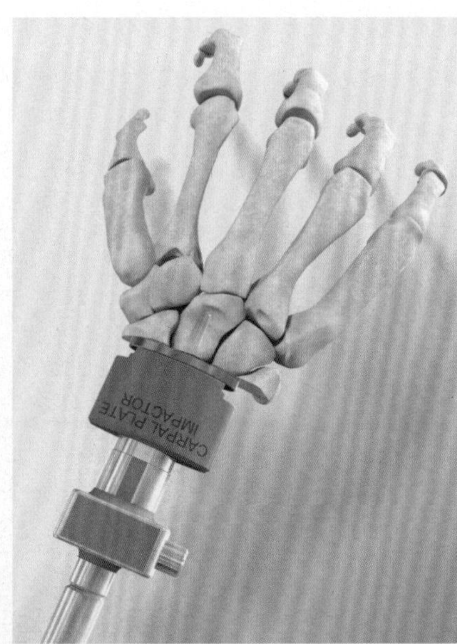

C D

TECH FIG 2 • *(continued)* **C.** Secure the resection guide to the carpus and ensure the osteotomy will pass through the proximal pole of the hamate, a small portion of the capitate head, and approximately half of the scaphoid and triquetrum (avoid excessive carpal resection). **D.** Impact the carpal plate trial into the capitate and confirm that it seats properly at the osteotomy site.

- Insert carpal guide bar into the capitate and mount the carpal resection guide with hamate feeler. Slide the carpal resection guide distally until the hamate feeler contacts the proximal pole of the hamate (**TECH FIG 2B**).
- Pin the resection guide to the capitate using the two innermost holes. Remove the hamate feeler and carpal guide bar.
- Recheck the position of the cutting guide to resect 1.5 mm of the proximal hamate. Complete the carpal cut with an oscillating saw. Save resected bone for later grafting (**TECH FIG 2C**).
- Select an appropriately sized carpal reamer and ream by hand until its flange abuts capitate.
- Impact the trial carpal plate into the capitate while aligning its dorsal edge with the dorsal contour of the carpus (**TECH FIG 2D**).

Preparation of Radius

- Align the radius template with the dorsal and radial edges of the radius. Using the notch on the template, mark the site for guidewire insertion into the canal of the radius.
- Apply the modular drill guide with its saddle on top of the dorsal radius and the barrel at the marked site. Insert the guidewire and confirm its central position within the radius canal using fluoroscopy (**TECH FIG 3A**).
- Use a 3.5-mm cannulated drill over the guidewire and drill to the last laser mark line on the drill bit.
- Insert the radius intramedullary (IM) guide rod until the radius feeler abuts the articular surface. Apply the appropriately sized radius resection guide and adjust its position to resect the dorsal surface of the radius (**TECH FIG 3B**). Insert Kirschner wires to fix the guide to the radius.
- Attach the radius score guide to the radius resection guide and score the radius 1 to 2 mm in depth with a saw, which marks the ulnar extent of the radius resection to maintain integrity of the DRUJ (**TECH FIG 3C**).
- Resect the distal radius with an oscillating saw blade. Remove volar osteophytes and any remaining bony prominences using a rongeur (**TECH FIG 3D**).
- Reinsert the radius IM guide rod and place the radius drill guide over it and against the distal radius in proper rotational alignment.
- Use the 4.0-mm stop drill bit to drill the radial-sided hole in the guide and place the antirotation pin into the hole. Drill the ulnar-sided hole with the same drill bit.
- Slide the box punch over the IM rod, aligning it with the two drilled holes. Seat the box punch using a mallet and remove the enclosed bone (**TECH FIG 3E**).
- Starting with a size 1 broach, impact the broach into the radius canal hole in proper rotational and longitudinal alignment. Confirm appropriate alignment with fluoroscopy. Broach up to size of the selected radius trial (**TECH FIG 3F**).
  - If using cement, the radius canal should be broached to one size greater than the implant used.

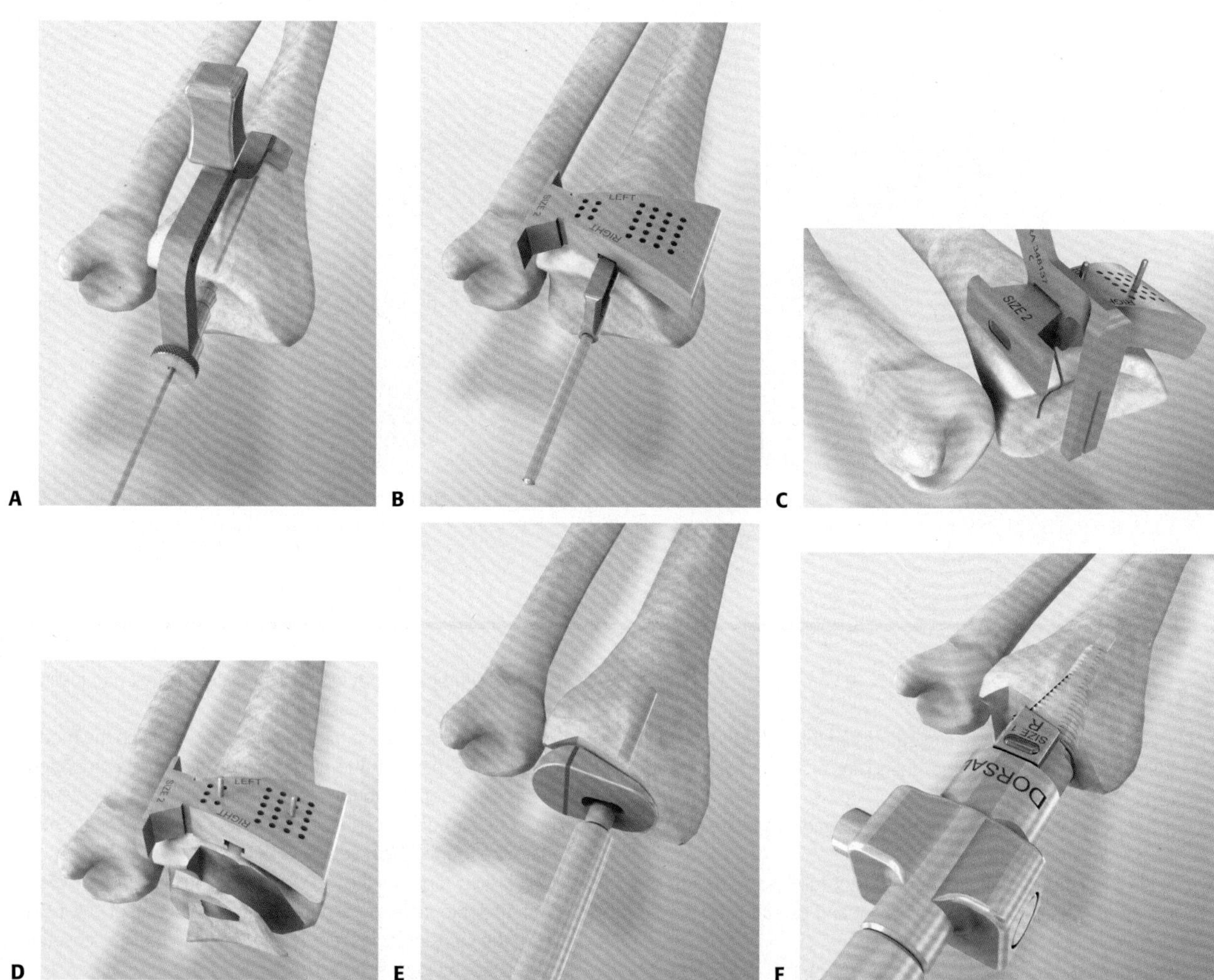

TECH FIG 3 • **A.** Using the modular drill guide, a guidewire is inserted through the articular surface of the radius and down the center of the radius canal (confirm correct position with fluoroscopy). Drill the hole for the guide rod using the cannulated drill bit. **B.** Apply the radius resection guide in a position that will resect only the articular surface of the distal radius (a laser mark on the guide arm corresponds to the level where the barrel is pressed against the articular surface). **C.** Use the radius score guide to make an initial vertical cut, which will mark the ulnar extent of the horizontal cut to protect the DRUJ. **D.** Complete the distal radius articular surface resection. **E.** After reinserting the guide rod, use the radius drill guide followed by the box punch to remove the remaining hard subchondral bone of the distal radius. **F.** Perform sequential broaching to the appropriate size.

Trial Reduction

- Impact the radius trial into place (**TECH FIG 4A**).
- Apply the standard carpal poly trial to the carpal plate trial and reduce the joint (**TECH FIG 4B**).
- Assess motion and stability, with the goal of 35-degrees extension and 35-degrees flexion.
- If the volar capsule is too tight in limiting extension, then additional resection of the radius can be performed.
- If volar instability is present, the volar capsule should be inspected. If the capsule is detached, it is repaired to the volar rim of the radius. If the capsule is intact, then a larger carpal poly trial may be used to improve stability.

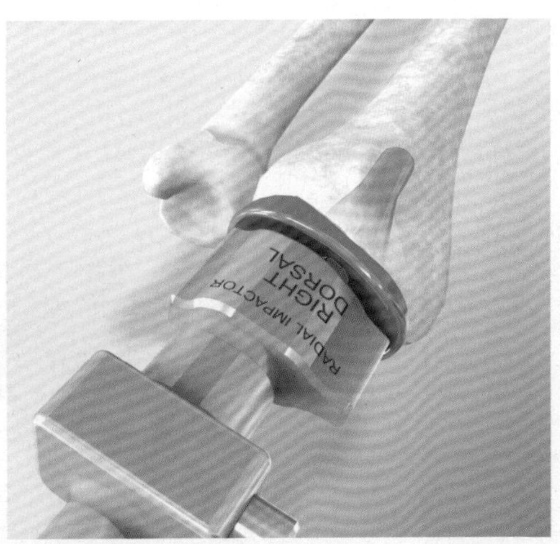

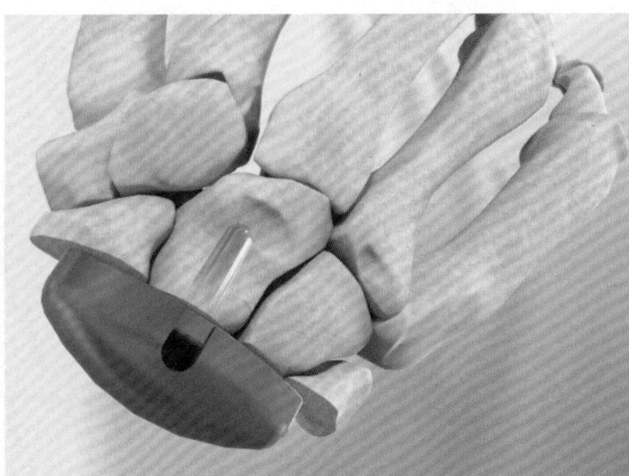

TECH FIG 4 • A. Insert the radius trial component into the prepared radius. **B.** Insert the carpal component and apply the trial poly bearing.

Implantation

- Three horizontal 3-0 polyester sutures are placed through small bone holes made along the dorsal rim of the radius for later capsule closure.
- If being cemented, inject cement into the radius and the capitate prior to implant insertion.
- Insert the radius component and seat it fully using the impactor. Insert the carpal plate component and use the carpal plate impactor to fully seat.
- Position the modular drill guide barrel in the radial hole of the carpal component and its saddle on the second metacarpal shaft. Insert a guidewire into base of second metacarpal. Confirm the position with fluoroscopy and measure the depth.
- Drill to the proper depth with a cannulated drill bit and insert a 4.5-mm screw of the measured depth.
- Using a similar technique for the ulnar screw, position the modular drill guide barrel in the ulnar hole of the carpal component and its saddle on the fourth metacarpal shaft. Insert a guidewire, measure, and drill. Insert a screw of proper length. Do not penetrate the fourth CMC joint (**TECH FIG 5A**).
- Apply locking caps over the two carpal screw heads (**TECH FIG 5B**).
- Confirm appropriate carpal poly thickness using carpal poly trials.
- Apply the carpal poly implant and impact it into place, ensuring there is no impinging soft tissue.
- Reduce the joint and make a final assessment of the balance and stability (**TECH FIG 5C**).

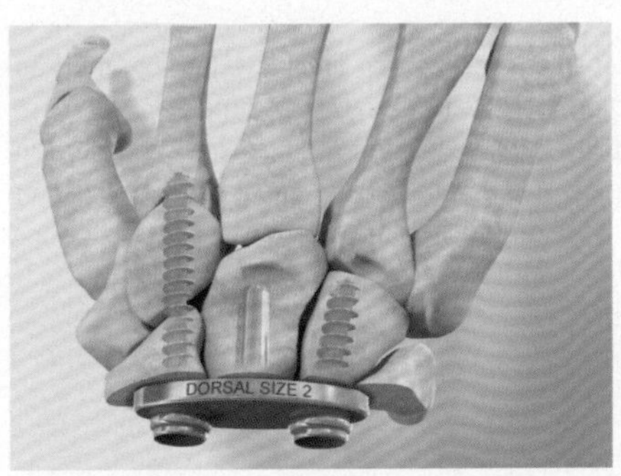

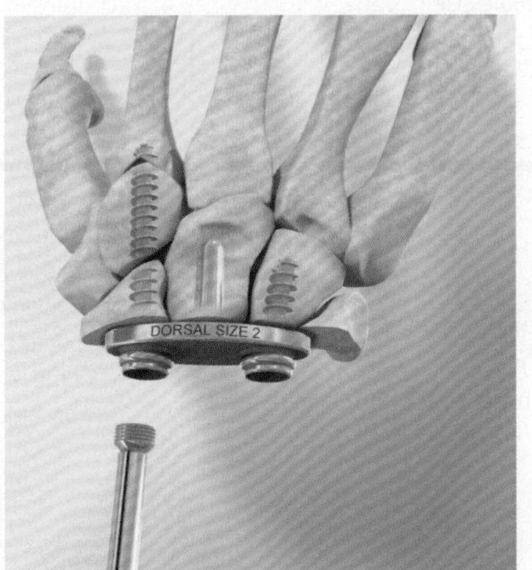

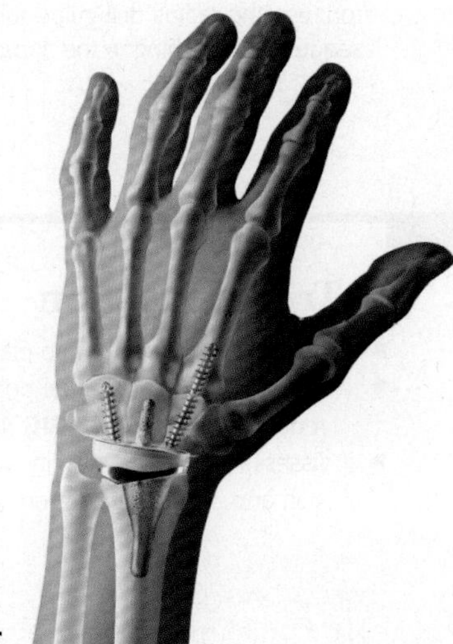

TECH FIG 5 • A. Impact the carpal component and insert the fixation screws, beginning with the radial screw using the modular drill guide, guidewire, and cannulated drill for preparation. **B.** Apply the locking caps over radial and ulnar carpal screws. **C.** Impact the radial component, apply the appropriate poly bearing, reduce the joint, and assess range of motion and joint stability.

TECHNIQUES

Bone Graft and Closure

- Perform an intercarpal fusion by carefully resecting portions of the joint surfaces and then inserting cancellous bone chips from the previously resected bone into the prepared fusion sites.
- Reattach the dorsal capsule to the dorsal rim of the radius using the previously placed sutures. The medial and lateral edges of the capsule are also closed.
- If the capsule is insufficient for closure with the wrist flexed 30 degrees, it is supplemented with a portion of the extensor retinaculum.
- A suction drain is placed, skin is closed, and a bulky dressing with a below-elbow plaster splint is applied.

PEARLS AND PITFALLS

Indications	▪ Wrist degeneration resulting from all causes of arthritis serves as an indication for this surgery; however, patients should be of appropriate age and have fewer activity demands. ▪ Severe loss of bone stock and active and aggressive inflammatory arthritis are contraindications.
Surgical technique	▪ Adequate exposure is mandatory to achieve accurate component implantation. ▪ Intercarpal arthrodesis is a key factor in obtaining long-term fixation of the implants.
DRUJ management	▪ Preservation of the DRUJ including the TFCC improves stability of the wrist and overall functional outcome. ▪ When treatment is needed, expose the DRUJ through the same skin incision but through a separate capsulotomy.

POSTOPERATIVE CARE

- Strict elevation and early active digital range of motion are encouraged.
- At 2 weeks postoperatively, the sutures are removed. Implant reduction is confirmed by x-ray and gentle wrist exercises are begun, including active flexion, extension, radial and ulnar deviation, and pronation and supination. A removable splint is applied.
- The splint is weaned at 4 weeks postoperatively, and strengthening is added to the rehabilitation.
- The patient is advised against impact loading of the wrist and repetitive forceful use of the hand.

OUTCOMES

- Long-term outcomes of modern generation implants have been reported with the first generation Universal implant by Ward et al.[12]
  - Carpal component loosening was found to be the most common reason for revision surgery.
  - Survival of stable implants was found to be 75% at 5 years and 60% at 7 years.
  - Early failures in this series of patients all had highly active inflammatory arthritis and severe wrist laxity, demonstrating the importance of medical control of rheumatoid arthritis.
- Cooney et al[2] performed a retrospective review comparing the 16 Biaxial resurfacing implants to a series of 30 anatomic implants (Re-Motion and Universal 2). At an average of 6 years follow-up, they found that 50% of the Biaxial implants had failed, whereas 1 out of 30 of the new generation implants had failed indicating significant improvements in implant design.
- The Universal 2 implant has been reported in several midterm follow-up series with positive results.
  - Ferreres et al,[4] Morapudi et al,[8] and van Winterswijk[11] reported three separate series with follow-up between 3 and 5 years.
  - All studies demonstrated high levels of patient satisfaction and improved postoperative standardized outcome scores (Disability of the Arm, Shoulder, and Hand [DASH] and Patient-Rated Wrist Evaluation [PRWE]).
  - There was only 1 revision in the combined total of 57 wrists in these series. Average arc of motion ranged from 52 to 68 degrees; average motion was improved postoperatively in each study.

- The Maestro prosthesis has shown promising results in short follow-up.
  - Nydick et al[10] retrospectively reviewed 23 total wrist arthroplasties at mean 28-month follow-up and found pain scores improved from 8.0 to 2.2. A 30% complication rate was reported in this series. There was only one failure due to infection.
- Results of the Re-Motion prosthesis reported by Herzberg[5] showed good to excellent outcomes in 16 of 20 wrists at an average 32-month follow-up.
  - These results were part of a larger multicenter web-based database which included 215 wrists. At average follow-up of 4 years, they reported a 96% survival rate in patients with rheumatoid arthritis and a 92% survival in nonrheumatoid arthritis patients. Average postoperative motion was 60.5 degrees, and there were significant improvements in postoperative pain scores.[6]
- The Freedom total wrist has yet to be reported in clinical follow-up; however, it has been designed based on the successful concepts of the Universal 2 implant. Improvements in design aim to decrease rates of loosening and increase range of motion.

COMPLICATIONS

- Superficial or deep infection
- Stiffness or contracture
- Joint imbalance or instability
- Implant loosening

REFERENCES

1. Adey L, Ring D, Jupiter JB. Health status after total wrist arthrodesis for posttraumatic arthritis. J Hand Surg Am 2005;30(5):932–936.
2. Cooney W, Manuel J, Froelich J, et al. Total wrist replacement: a retrospective comparative study. J Wrist Surg 2012;1(2):165–172.
3. Dennis DA, Ferlic DC, Clayton ML. Volz total wrist arthroplasty in rheumatoid arthritis: a long-term review. J Hand Surg Am 1986;11(4):483–490.
4. Ferreres A, Lluch A, Del Valle M. Universal total wrist arthroplasty: midterm follow-up study. J Hand Surg Am 2011;36(6):967–973.
5. Herzberg G. Prospective study of a new total wrist arthroplasty: short term results. Chir Main 2011;30(1):20–25.
6. Herzberg G, Boeckstyns M, Sorensen AI, et al. "Remotion" total wrist arthroplasty: preliminary results of a prospective international multicenter study of 215 cases. J Wrist Surg 2012;1(1):17–22.
7. Kistler U, Weiss AP, Simmen BR, et al. Long-term results of silicone wrist arthroplasty in patients with rheumatoid arthritis. J Hand Surg Am 2005;30(6):1282–1287.
8. Morapudi SP, Marlow WJ, Withers D, et al. Total wrist arthroplasty using the universal 2 prosthesis. J Orthop Surg 2012;20(3):365–368.
9. Murphy DM, Khoury JG, Imbriglia JE, et al. Comparison of arthroplasty and arthrodesis for the rheumatoid wrist. J Hand Surg Am 2003;28(4):570–576.
10. Nydick JA, Greenberg SM, Stone JD, et al. Clinical outcomes of total wrist arthroplasty. J Hand Surg Am 2012;37(8):1580–1584.
11. van Winterswijk PJ, Bakx PA. Promising clinical results of the universal total wrist prosthesis in rheumatoid arthritis. Open Orthop J 2010;4:67–70.
12. Ward CM, Kuhl T, Adams BD. Five to ten-year outcomes of the universal total wrist arthroplasty in patients with rheumatoid arthritis. J Bone Joint Surg Am 2011;93(10):914–919.
13. Weiss AC, Wiedeman G Jr, Quenzer D, et al. Upper extremity function after wrist arthrodesis. J Hand Surg Am 1995;20(5):813–817.

Resection Arthroplasty of the Distal Radioulnar Joint

Jeffrey A. Greenberg

DEFINITION

- The distal ulna resection attributed to Dr. William Darrach was described by Severinus in 1644, Rognetta in 1834, and Dupuytren in 1839.[13] Malgaine in 1855 and Moore in 1880 also described distal ulna resections.[9] Dr. William Darrach described the distal ulna resection that bears his name in 1912 and 1913 for the treatment of a posttraumatic volar distal radioulnar joint (DRUJ) dislocation. This operation continues to have a place for the treatment of a variety of afflictions of the DRUJ.
- In an effort to preserve some of the critical stabilizing soft tissue elements of the distal ulna, alternative treatments to complete ablation of the distal ulna have been developed.
  - Bowers[2] published his results of the hemiresection interposition technique (HIT). This procedure differs from the Darrach in that the weight-bearing seat and pole are resected, preserving the styloid and soft tissue elements of the triangular fibrocartilage (TFC).
  - Watson and Gabuzda[24] and Watson et al[25] advocated the matched resection procedure.
  - The essential element is matching the profile of the resected distal ulna to the medial side of the radius.

ANATOMY

- The DRUJ is formed by the articulation between the sigmoid notch and the head of the ulna (**FIG 1A,B**). The sigmoid notch is the articular cartilage surface on the medial aspect of the distal radius. This concave surface matches the corresponding convex surface or "seat" of the distal ulna. The arc of curvature of the sigmoid notch ranges between 47 and 80 degrees, with an average radius of 12 to 18 mm.
- The articulation is constrained loosely, allowing both forearm rotation through a 150-degree arc and proximal and distal migration as well as dorsal and palmar translation of the ulna relative to the radius during forearm rotation. The articular cartilage-covered "cap" of the distal ulna can be divided into two functional regions. The seat of the ulna is the concave portion that articulates with the sigmoid notch. The arc of curvature ranges between 90 and 135 degrees, with an average radius of 8 to 13 mm. This region is covered by articular cartilage around 270 degrees of its surface. This is the region that supports the compressive loads of the distal radius during most activities of daily living and can be considered the fulcrum for load support.
- The pole is the distal portion of the ulna that lies deep to the cartilaginous TFC. This region supports the centrum of the TFC as compressive loads pass from the ulnar carpus to the bony elements of the forearm. The medial distal portion of the ulna projects as the ulnar styloid. The base of the styloid contains the critical attachment of the deep layer of the TFC, the ligamentum subcruentum (**FIG 1C**).
  - Distal to this, and in a more peripheral location, is the attachment of the superficial layer of the TFC. The dorsal and volar portions of the TFC are thickened, forming the limbi of the TFC, the volar and dorsal radioulnar ligaments. These ligaments play critical roles in stabilizing the DRUJ.

PATHOGENESIS

- Conditions that cause DRUJ degenerative change or altered DRUJ mechanics can lead to pain and DRUJ dysfunction. Most commonly, distal ulna resection is performed in

A 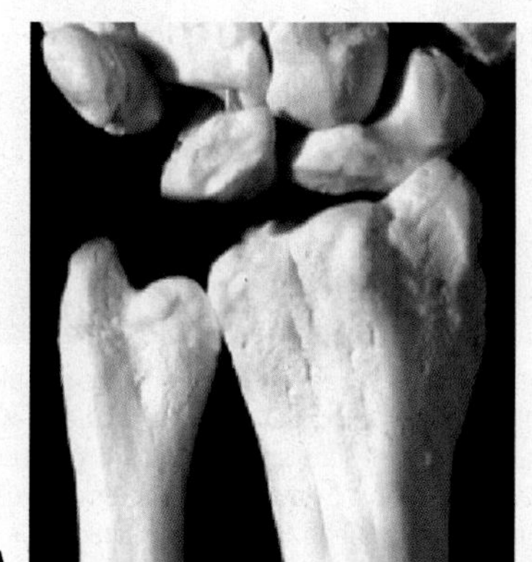

B 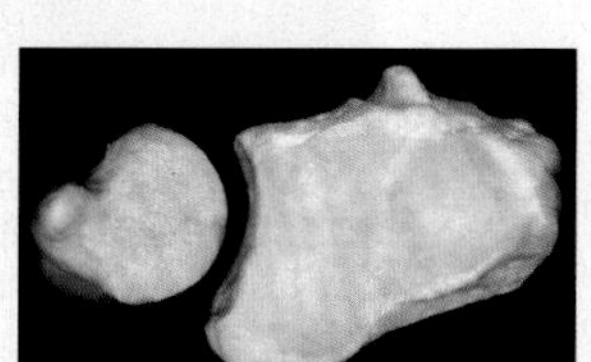

C 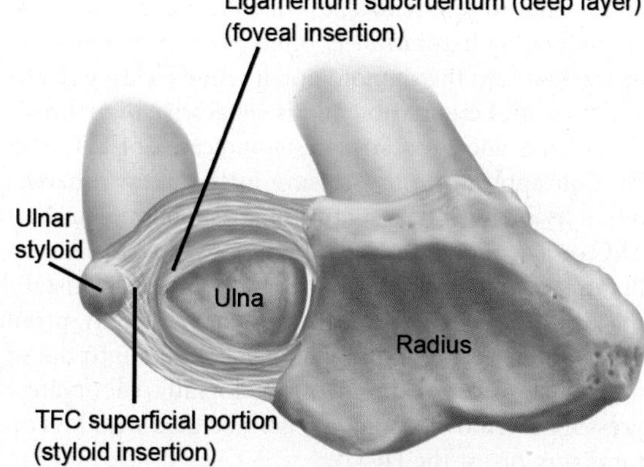

FIG 1 • Diagrammatic representations of the bony anatomy (**A**) and relationship of the radius and ulna at the DRUJ (**B**). **C.** Soft tissue elements of the DRUJ, including the deep (ligamentum subcruentum) and superficial peripheral attachments of the TFC.

patients with inflammatory arthropathy, usually rheumatoid arthritis. Frequently, treatment of the DRUJ is performed in conjunction with other bone or soft tissue reconstructions.

- DRUJ instability secondary to trauma or attritional changes of the supporting soft tissue elements can lead to degenerative change of this articulation.
- Malunions of the distal radius can negatively affect the sigmoid notch by alterations in angulation or length and can disrupt DRUJ kinematics.
- A less common cause of DRUJ arthritis is primary osteoarthritis, which may also lead to osteophytes and loose bodies.
- Developmental conditions, such as Madelung deformity, can alter DRUJ joint mechanics. Painful forearm rotation and degenerative changes as well as ulnar impaction can develop.

PATIENT HISTORY AND PHYSICAL FINDINGS

- Patients with DRUJ problems present with pain and limited forearm rotation.
  - In isolated DRUJ arthrosis, the patients usually localize their pain at the DRUJ articulation.
  - In patients with concomitant associated pathology of the soft tissue elements and DRUJ stabilizers, the ulnar-sided pain is more diffuse.
- Pain occurs with activities that require forearm rotation, such as turning doorknobs, turning keys in locks, starting a car, and opening jars. Lifting activities with the arm away from the body are difficult because the DRUJ is loaded in this position.
- Limited forearm motion may be secondary to an arthritic DRUJ; however, other conditions (eg, capsular contracture) must be considered.
- Prominence and deformity of the distal ulna is common in patients with inflammatory changes and in patients with distal radius fracture malunions.
- Inspection is usually unremarkable in patients with isolated DRUJ osteoarthritis. In contrast, DRUJ deformity and prominence is common in patients with rheumatoid arthritis.[19] Fullness due to synovial proliferation may be visible and secondary attritional changes of surrounding soft tissue elements, such as extensor tendon rupture, can lead to abnormal hand posture.
- Radius malunions with shortening and angulation produce visible prominence of the distal ulna (**FIG 2**).
- Tenderness with pressure on the dorsal aspect of the DRUJ is frequently elicited. In patients with associated impaction or TFC pathology, tenderness may be more diffuse. Palpable crepitance with rotation is often present. Compressing the distal ulna into the sigmoid notch while rotating the forearm elicits painful crepitation and is suggestive of arthrosis.
- Pain on the ulnocarpal stress test is indicative of TFC pathology.
- Pain on application of pressure in the interval between the ulnar styloid and flexor carpi ulnaris tendon is indicative of TFC or capsuloligamentous pathology (foveal sign).[22]
- Piano key maneuver: Visible dorsal winging or instability of the distal ulna is noted. If the ulna is dorsally prominent, the examiner can manually reduce the ulna into the sigmoid notch. The ulna spontaneously dorsally subluxates when pressure is removed. Winging is associated with loss of structural support of the DRUJ.
- Grip strength is frequently limited secondary to painful compressive loading of the DRUJ.

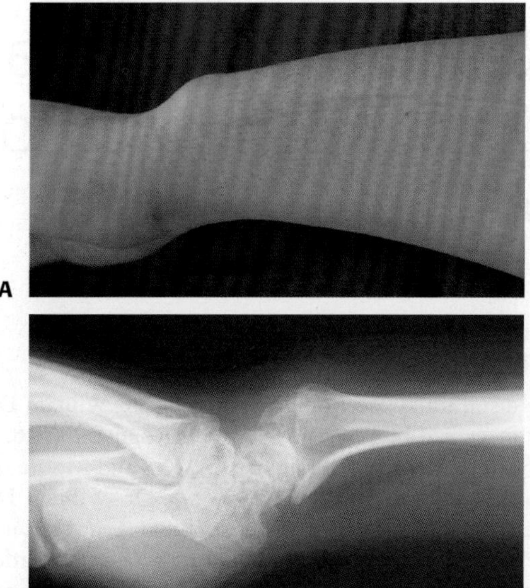

FIG 2 • Loss of the soft tissue support with or without associated degenerative change or malunion of the radius with resultant sigmoid notch incongruity leads to dorsal prominence and winging of the ulna relative to the radius. **A.** Dorsal prominence of the ulna relative to the radius is seen in a patient with a radius malunion. **B.** Radiograph of a wrist of a patient with rheumatoid arthritis shows the volar translation and secondary changes in the carpus that are associated with dorsal ulna prominence.

IMAGING AND OTHER DIAGNOSTIC STUDIES

- Plain radiographs are usually sufficient to supplement physical examination findings. It is essential to obtain a neutral forearm rotation posteroanterior (PA) and lateral views (**FIG 3A**) to accurately assess ulnar variance, styloid morphology, inclination of the sigmoid notch, and position of the ulnar styloid. These factors are important in selecting the appropriate surgical management for disorders of the distal ulna.

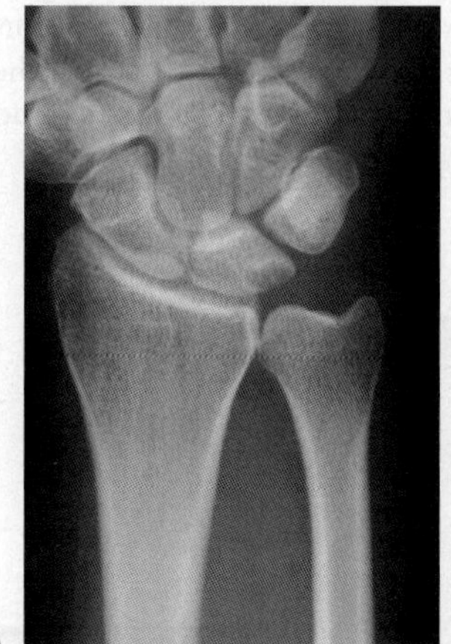

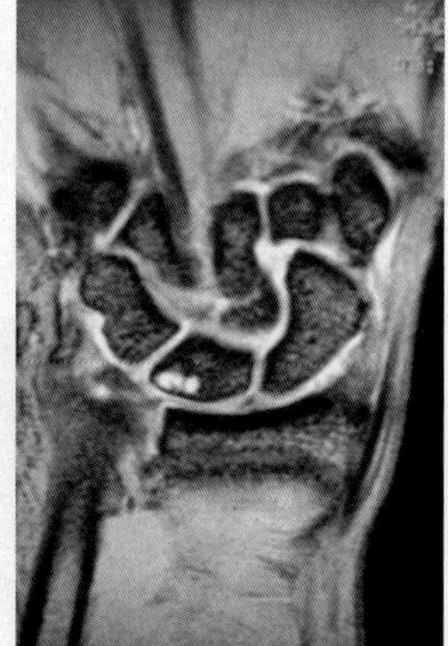

FIG 3 • **A.** The zero rotation view is taken with the patient's shoulder abducted at 90 degrees, the elbow flexed 90 degrees, and the wrist pronated in the PA position. The ulnar styloid is seen in full profile in this view. This view is the standard radiographic view used to determine ulnar variance. **B.** Although not part of the routine imaging evaluation for the TFC, MRI can confirm the diagnosis for related conditions. This MRI in a patient with an ulnar positive wrist shows a discrete intense lesion at the ulnar base of the lunate consistent with ulnar impaction.

- Thin-section computed tomography (CT) scanning can provide useful additional information about DRUJ articular surfaces and subluxation.
- Magnetic resonance imaging (MRI) evaluation is rarely necessary to diagnose arthritic disorders of the DRUJ but can be useful when detailed information about the radioulnar ligaments or surrounding bony ligaments of the TFC is necessary (**FIG 3B**).

DIFFERENTIAL DIAGNOSIS

- DRUJ arthritis
  - Inflammatory
  - Osteoarthritis
  - Traumatic
  - Iatrogenic (eg, altered joint mechanics after ulnar shortening)
- DRUJ instability
- TFC tears
- Ulnar impaction
- Lunotriquetral ligament tears or instability
- Extensor carpi ulnaris tendinitis
- Extensor carpi ulnaris instability
- Pisotriquetral disorders
- Nerve entrapment (canal of Guyon)
- Nerve injury (eg, neuromas of dorsal ulnar sensory nerve)
- Madelung deformity with DRUJ dysfunction

NONOPERATIVE MANAGEMENT

- Patients with mild symptoms and minimal functional impairment may be managed with oral anti-inflammatories, intra-articular injections, or splinting.
- Splinting must include the elbow to eliminate forearm rotation.

SURGICAL MANAGEMENT

- Maintaining the distal ulna has gained recent popularity as resection can be associated with considerable postoperative complications and functional disability. Meticulous attention to preoperative, intraoperative, and postoperative detail is essential for a successful result.

Adjunctive Procedures

- After complete or partial resection of the distal ulna, convergence between the radius and ulna can develop.[14] Loss of the weight-bearing fulcrum of the ulna seat can yield convergence with grip or loaded lifting with the arm extended and the forearm in neutral rotation (**FIG 4**).
- Adjunctive procedures incorporate some type of tendon transfer or interpositional material to stabilize the resected ulnar stump (**FIG 5**). The pronator quadratus, extensor carpi ulnaris, and flexor carpi ulnaris tendons have been used alone and in combination.
- In addition to tendon transfer, some authors have recommended suturing the ulnar capsule to the dorsal ulnar stump to help stabilize the remaining ulna.[21] Kleinman and Greenberg[11] advocated use of a dynamic pronator quadratus interosseous transfer in conjunction with an extensor carpi ulnaris distal tenodesis for failed distal ulna resections. More recently, allograft soft tissue interposition has been advocated[12] as well as distal ulna implant arthroplasty.[27]
- Most adjunctive procedures have been described for treatment of a failed symptomatic Darrach procedure; however, they can be incorporated during the initial surgery.

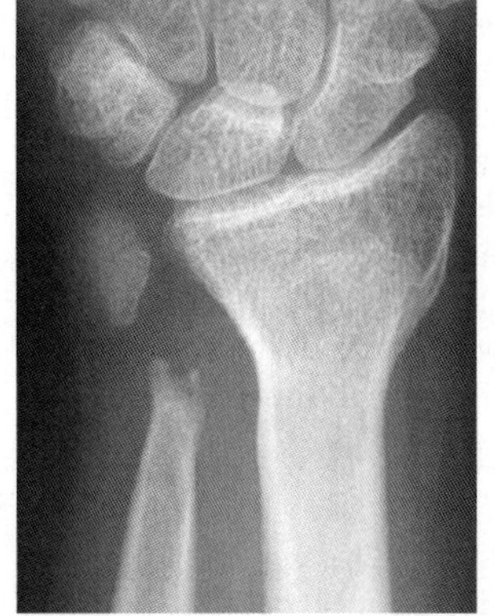
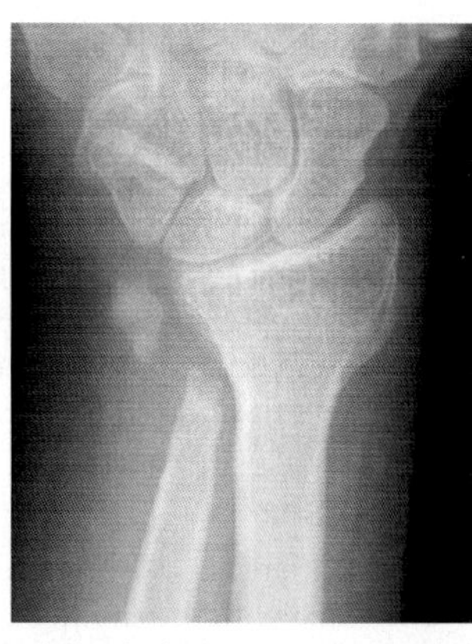

FIG 4 ● Impingement of the resected distal ulna against the medial wall of the radius is common after distal ulna resection. It can be demonstrated radiographically even in patients who may be asymptomatic after distal ulna resection. Convergence is demonstrated with a weighted PA radiograph. **A.** Radiograph of a patient who has undergone Darrach resection shows a wide separation between the ulna and radius without external load. **B.** Significant convergence is noted on a weighted, loaded view.

Symptomatic convergence tends to develop in a relatively younger, higher demand patient. If distal ulna resection is necessary in this patient population, use of an adjunctive procedure is recommended.

Preoperative Planning

- The ideal candidate for a Darrach resection is a patient with a relatively low-demand upper extremity that does not require the load-bearing DRUJ.
- Coexisting pathology is frequently present in patients with distal ulna dysfunction, especially in patients with inflammatory arthropathy.[19] Assessing for associated tenosynovitis and tendon ruptures is necessary.
  - The status of the radiocarpal joint is critical. Patients with loss of radial-sided carpal support due to tenosynovitis often have ulnar translation. In advanced cases, the carpus may abut the distal ulna and isolated Darrach resection without carpal stabilization is contraindicated to avoid exacerbating ulnar translation.

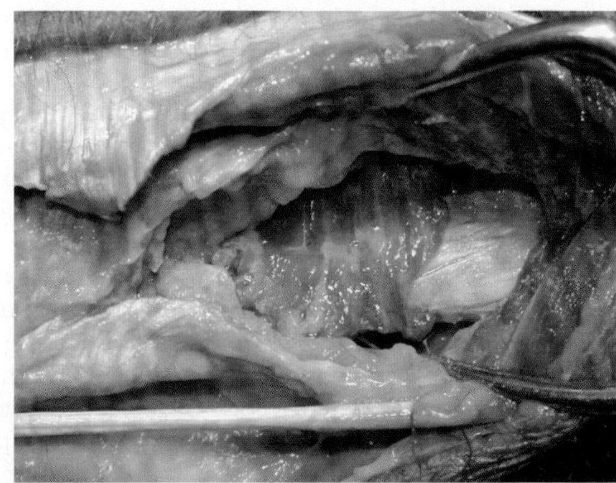

FIG 5 ● After resection of the distal ulna, the pronator quadratus muscle has been transferred dorsally through the interosseous space, providing a dynamic interpositional material to help mitigate impingement and dorsal translation of the ulna relative to the radius.

- If a limited resection of the distal ulna is considered, one must evaluate the length of the ulna, ulnar variance, and position of the styloid. If stylocarpal abutment exists, it will persist after limited resection. Therefore, consideration needs to be given to a joint leveling procedure or styloid recession in conjunction with limited resection.
  - Alternatively, a complete distal ulna resection that addresses the ulna head as well as the styloid or a Sauvé-Kapandji DRUJ arthrodesis may be considered.

Positioning

- The patient is positioned supine. The operative arm is extended with the shoulder abducted at 90 degrees. The arm is supported on a standard table used for upper extremity surgery.
- A tourniquet is used.
- The motion of the elbow and shoulder should be noted before surgery. Limited passive motion can create awkward arm positioning.

Approach

- The incision used for distal ulna resection is based on whether the resection is performed alone or in conjunction with other procedures (**FIG 6**).
- The recommended approach for distal ulna resections is dorsal, deep to the fifth extensor compartment.

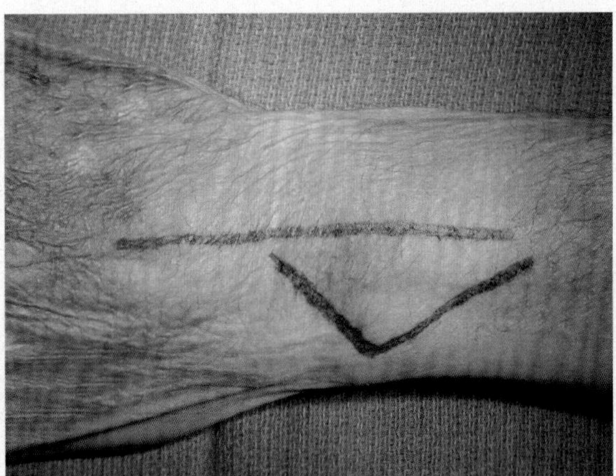

FIG 6 • Options for incisions when approaching the DRUJ and TFC. The longitudinal incision is frequently used in patients undergoing complex reconstructions involving the DRUJ and radiocarpal or midcarpal joint. This incision is also recommended in patients requiring extensor tendon reconstruction in conjunction with treatment of the DRUJ. The chevron incision, with its distal limb paralleling the dorsal sensory branch of the ulnar nerve, is recommended for isolated arthroplasty of the DRUJ.

- A medial approach between the extensor carpi ulnaris and flexor carpi ulnaris tendons is not recommended. This approach has greater potential for disrupting the linea jugata, with resultant potential extensor carpi ulnaris destabilization.

TECHNIQUES

Complete Distal Ulna Resection: The Darrach Procedure

Incision and Dissection

- Frequently, Darrach resection is performed in conjunction with other procedures, especially in patients with inflammatory arthropathies. In this situation, the surgical incision is usually dorsal midline longitudinal, which enables all aspects of the wrist reconstruction (wrist fusion, arthroplasty, tenosynovectomy, tendon transfer, etc.) to be completed via a single approach.
- If the Darrach procedure is to be performed independently, a single oblique or chevron dorsal approach is made (see **FIG 6**) overlying the fifth dorsal compartment.
- During the dissection to the retinacular layer, take care to avoid injury to the transverse retinacular branch and dorsal sensory branch of the ulnar nerve that pass from the medial forearm to the dorsal hand between the ulnar styloid and pisiform (**TECH FIG 1A**).
  - Keep the oblique incision or distal limb of the chevron approach parallel to this nerve to minimize this complication.
- Frequently, dorsal capsular reinforcement is necessary after distal ulna resection. This is especially true in patients with inflammatory arthropathies and multiple extensor tendon ruptures.
  - When performed in conjunction with other procedures, raise opposing extensor retinacular flaps so that one of the flaps can be used to reinforce the dorsal capsule and create a stabilizing extensor carpi ulnaris sling during closure (**TECH FIG 1B,C**).
  - When performed as an isolated procedure, raise a retinacular flap from the margin of the fourth dorsal compartment (**TECH FIG 1D**).

Capsulotomy and Osteotomy

- Perform a longitudinal capsulotomy deep to the fifth dorsal compartment (**TECH FIG 2A**). This capsular approach starts proximal to the dorsal radioulnar ligament and proceeds in a proximal direction.
  - Extend the capsular release parallel and just proximal to the dorsal radioulnar ligament to facilitate exposure. Take

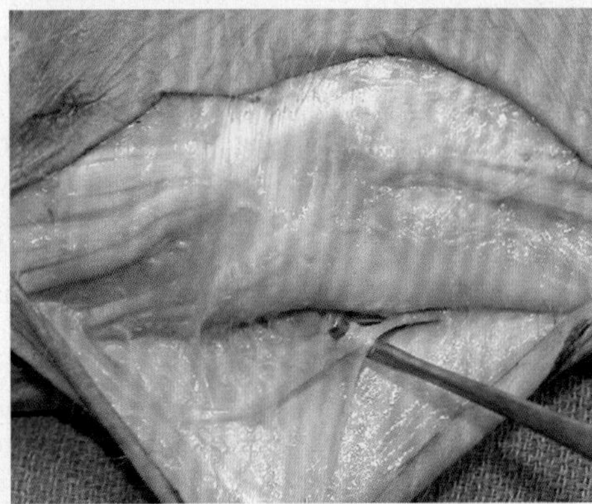

TECH FIG 1 • **A.** The dorsal sensory branch of the ulnar nerve, held in the retractor, passes from volar to dorsal just distal to the head of the ulna. It is vulnerable in all approaches to the DRUJ and TFC and should be protected. *(continued)*

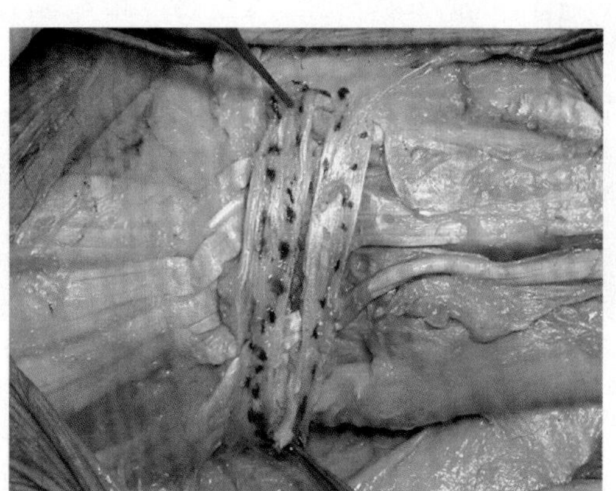

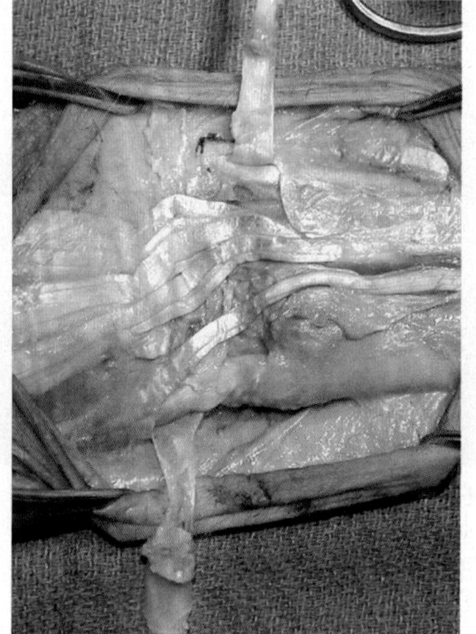

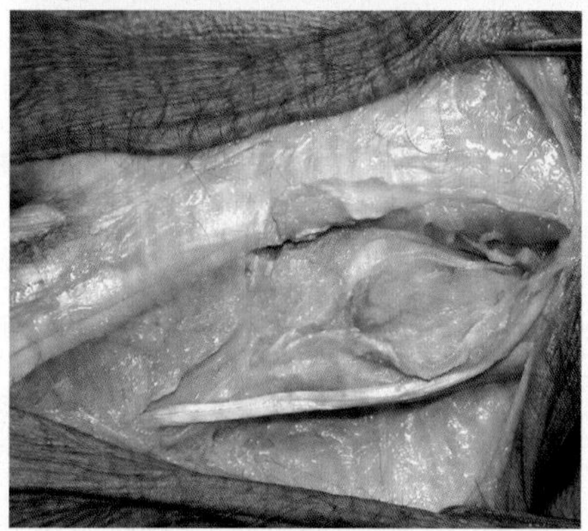

TECH FIG 1 • *(continued)* **B,C.** Opposing retinacular flaps are raised to provide wide exposure and access to all extensor compartments. This approach is frequently necessary in patients with concomitant extensor tendon dysfunction. One of the flaps can then be used to reinforce the capsule deep to the extensors at the termination of the procedure. **D.** The fifth compartment is opened, exposing the EDQP tendon. An ulnarly based retinacular flap is raised, preserving the wall of the fourth dorsal compartment for later repair. All figures in the technique section are oriented as follows: fingers to the left and elbow to the right.

care during the deep periosteal dissection to elevate and maintain as thick a periosteal sleeve as possible.

- Osteotomize the distal ulna using a power oscillating saw just proximal to the sigmoid notch (**TECH FIG 2B**). Enough ulna is sacrificed to completely decompress the DRUJ. Keep resection to 2 cm or less.
- Intraoperative fluoroscopic guidance is frequently helpful to assist with the location of the osteotomy.
- Once the distal pole and seat are resected, there is no advantage to preserving the ulnar styloid, and the entire styloid should be removed with the distal ulna.

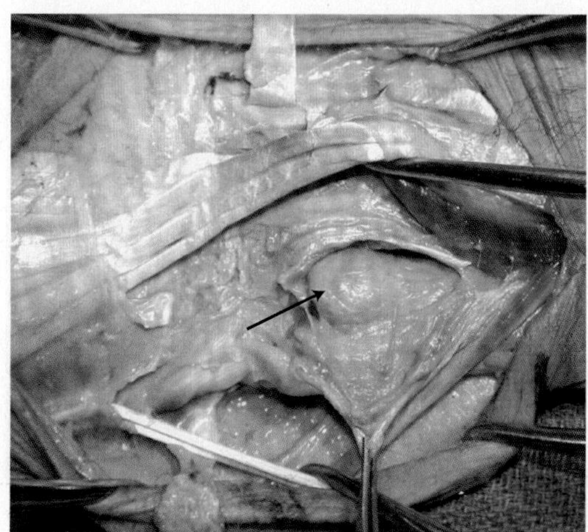

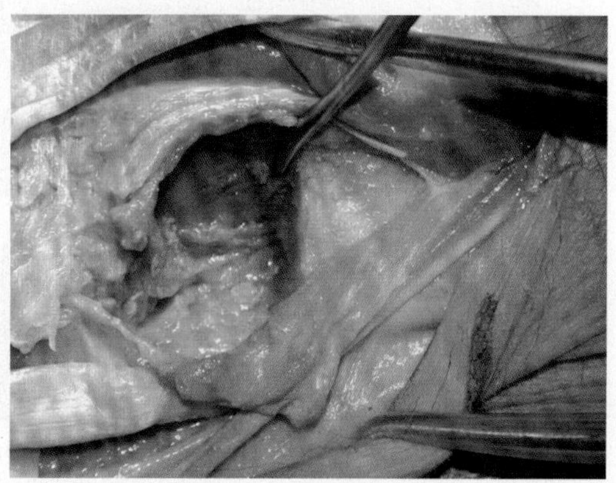

TECH FIG 2 • **A.** A longitudinal capsulotomy exposes the distal ulna (*arrow*) and allows access to the distal metaphysis, depending on the reconstruction being performed. **B.** The distal ulna has been osteotomized just proximal to the sigmoid notch. The resection should be less than 2 cm and should clear all abnormal bony elements that may affect rotation from within the sigmoid notch.

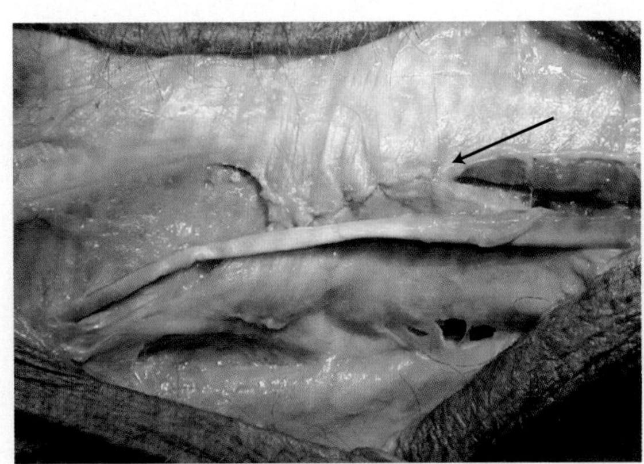

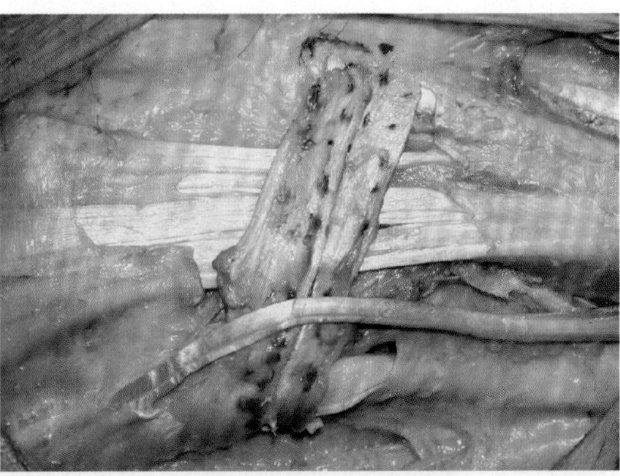

TECH FIG 3 • **A.** Closure is performed (*arrow*), leaving the EDQP superficial to the retinaculum. **B.** In another example, both retinacular flaps have been closed deep to the EDQP but superficial to the other extensors. If capsular reinforcement is necessary, the distal flap can be closed deep to the extensors. The ulnar portion of the proximal radially based flap is used to reinforce the sixth dorsal compartment.

Wound Closure

- Meticulous attention to closure is imperative.
- Perform a secure multilayered closure. Perform separate closure of the periosteal and capsular layers with nonabsorbable sutures.
- Suture the retinacular flaps for capsular reinforcement.
  - Transpose the extensor digiti quinti proprius (EDQP) tendon dorsal to the extensor retinaculum. This does not create any functional disability (**TECH FIG 3**).
- Routine skin closure follows.

Distal Ulna Hemiresection Interposition Technique

- The surgical approach for the HIT procedure as developed by Bowers is identical to the Darrach resection. The difference lies in the treatment of the bone and soft tissue interposition after bone resection.
- Instead of resecting the distal ulna at the proximal margin of the sigmoid notch, the osteotomy removes the seat and pole of the ulnar head (**TECH FIG 4A,B**). The entire shaft and the styloid are left intact.
- After resection, the forearm is rotated through a full arc. This ensures that prominent osteophytes or bone that may interfere with forearm rotation have been removed.
- The resected shaft should be round in cross-section and should taper distally. The resection is lateral to the insertion of the deep portion of the TFC, so the integrity of both the deep and superficial components of the TFC is maintained. If the TFC is incompetent or cannot be made functionally competent by reconstruction, then there are no advantages over the Darrach complete distal ulna resection.

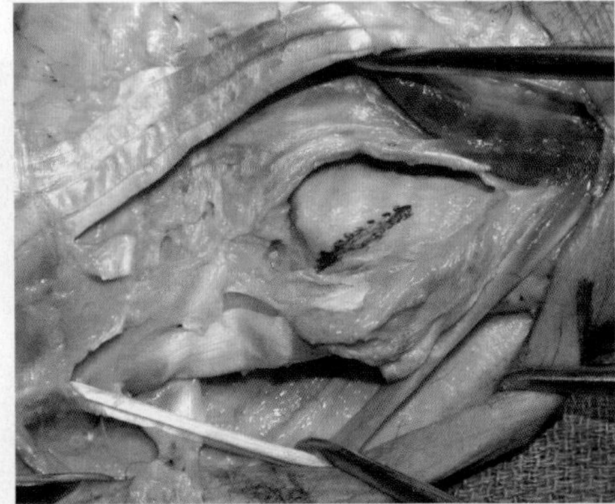

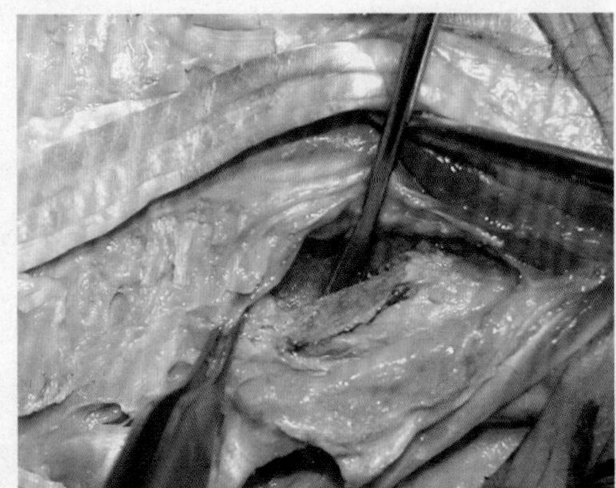

TECH FIG 4 • **A.** The level of osteotomy for the HIT procedure is marked before osteotomy. **B.** This osteotomy eliminates the entire ulnar head but leaves the attachments of the TFC intact. *(continued)*

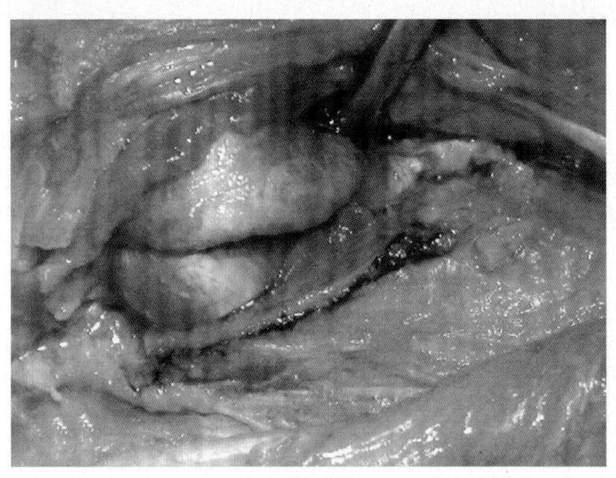

TECH FIG 4 • (continued) C. After osteotomy and removal of the ulnar head, the space is filled with a free tendon graft that provides bulky tissue and mitigates impingement of the resected ulna against the medial wall of the distal radius.

- Convergence of the radius and ulna develops after ulnar head resection. To mitigate this, the ulnarly based capsular flap raised during the approach is interposed between the radius and resected ulna. Interposition bulk may be increased by using a free tendon graft (**TECH FIG 4C**).

Modification

- In an effort to avoid an interpositional tendon graft, Adams[1] advocates a modification of the HIT procedure.
- In this technique, an ulnar-based retinacular flap is raised from the radial margin of the extensor carpi ulnaris sheath.
- Only 3 to 7 mm of bone is resected, and the ulna is tapered distally in a dowel shape. The fovea is not violated, thereby preserving all TFC attachments.
- The retinacular flap is then interposed and sutured to the volar DRUJ capsule. As in other procedures, attention is paid to avoid stylocarpal impingement.

Matched Distal Ulna Resection

- In this modification, developed by Watson, the distal ulna is resected in a long, sloping convex curve that matches the opposing concave radius (**TECH FIG 5**).
- The surgical approach is identical to the approaches listed for prior procedures. Although Watson advocated a transverse incision just proximal to the DRUJ, I prefer a more utilitarian longitudinal or chevron incision as previously described.
- The entire 270-degree arc of the ulna is addressed. Similar to the HIT procedure, great care is taken after bone resection to ensure full, unimpeded forearm rotation. Any osteophytes or prominent bone that may interfere with rotation must be removed.
- This technique differs from the HIT procedure because the ulna is reshaped over a longer distance and no interposition material is used. Although this technique is advocated to preserve the ulnar sling, by necessity, the resection sacrifices both the deep and superficial insertions of the TFC. Any resultant stability of the residual stump of the ulna is generated only by soft tissue scarring.

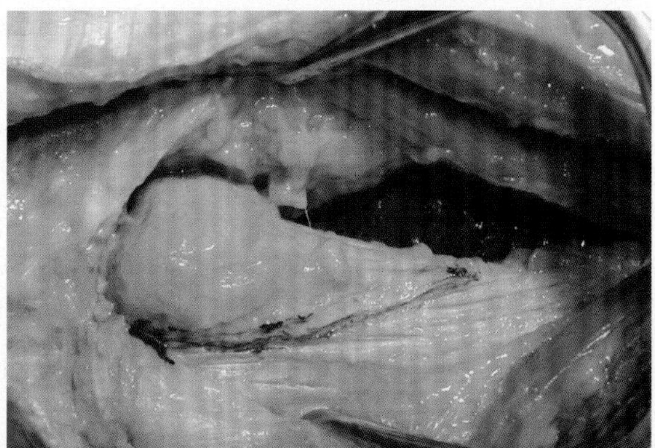

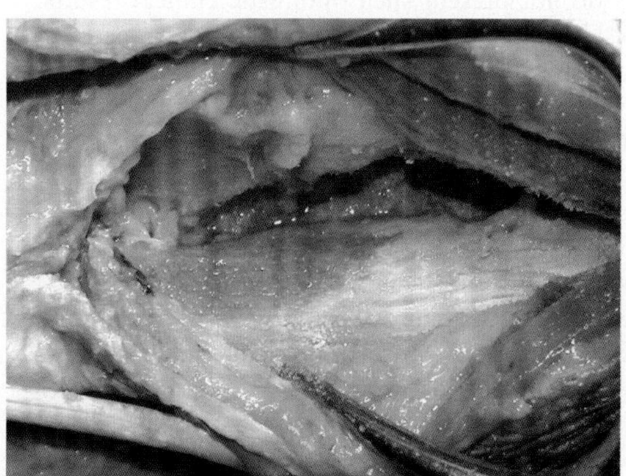

TECH FIG 5 • The matched resection osteotomy is more proximal than the Bowers osteotomy (**A**) and is resected in a long, sloping curve matching the opposite concave surface of the radius through a complete 270-degree arc (**B**).

PEARLS AND PITFALLS

Indications	■ Consider distal ulna resection as a final salvage procedure. Consider alternative procedures that will preserve the load-bearing fulcrum of the DRUJ. Distal ulna resections are tolerated in a relatively older, lower demand patient.
Associated conditions	■ Diagnose and treat associated bone and soft tissue pathology. Consider the effects of distal resection on the radiocarpal joint.
Approach	■ Meticulous attention to soft tissue handling and avoiding injury to cutaneous nerves is essential. Raise retinacular and capsular flaps carefully so they can be used for stabilization or interposition if necessary. Avoid destabilizing the extensor carpi ulnaris. If the extensor carpi ulnaris sheath is violated and stability needs to be restored, reconstruct the sheath using retinacular flaps.
Bone resection	■ Decompress the entire length of the sigmoid notch when performing a Darrach resection. Avoid removing the insertions of the TFC during the HIT procedure. Ensure that full forearm rotation is possible after bone resection. Similarly, after partial distal ulna resection, eliminate any remaining osteophytes or bony prominences to ensure full range of motion. Assess for postresection stylocarpal impingement and correct length if impingement is present.
Convergence and instability	■ Consider additional procedures that may stabilize or prevent symptomatic convergence and impingement, especially in the younger, more active, higher demand patient.
Aftercare	■ Maintain neutral forearm rotation with a long-arm or Munster-type splint for the first 3 postoperative weeks. Allow gentle forearm rotation until 6 weeks postoperatively. Full activity is allowed at 3 months postoperatively.

POSTOPERATIVE CARE

- Postoperatively, the extremity is maintained in a long-arm bulky dressing with the elbow at 90 degrees and the forearm supinated for 3 weeks. At 3 weeks postoperatively, long-arm splintage between exercises and at night begins and persists until 6 to 8 weeks postoperatively. Strengthening without splint immobilization can begin at that time.

OUTCOMES

- In general, distal ulna resections are associated with relief of pain and restoration of function. Elderly patients with lower demands on the upper extremities tend to have more favorable results than younger, active, higher demand patients.
- Good results regarding relief of pain and recovery of function can be expected in 60% to 95% of patients with rheumatoid arthritis.[4] Early clinical reports on the Darrach resection demonstrated marked improvement in pain and range of motion in greater than 80% of patients; however, other series do not present such optimistic clinical results. Two reviews describe improved functional results in patients undergoing distal ulna resections; however, caution is advised regarding patient selection and potential postoperative complications.[18,30]
- Leslie et al[13] in 1990 and Melone and Taras[15] in 1991 demonstrated 85% and 86% favorable results, respectively. Fraser et al's[6] 1999 study supported the use of the Darrach resection in patients with rheumatoid arthritis, finding 85% good to excellent results in 23 patients with rheumatoid arthritis versus only 36% satisfactory results in 27 patients with posttraumatic arthritis.
  - Despite significant attrition within their patient cohort, Grawe et al[9] demonstrated satisfactory functional, subjective, and objective long-term (13-year average follow-up) results in a group of patients that had Darrach resections in conjunction with wrist trauma. Interestingly, half of the patients demonstrated dynamic radioulnar convergence.
  - Yoneda and Watanabe[28] used the Darrach distal ulna resection as primary treatment for a comminuted distal ulna fracture in conjunction with distal radius fractures. This study evaluated 23 patients older than 70 years old. They concluded that a primary Darrach resection in this clinical situation was an effective treatment alternative. Reduction of pain and improvement in forearm rotation after trauma was also demonstrated by De Witte et al,[5] even though some patients in this cohort still had pain after the procedure.
- George et al[7] demonstrated satisfactory results in 21 patients treated with Darrach resections compared to a group who underwent Sauvé-Kapandji resection. They concluded that results were comparable and unpredictable. Despite reported complications, authors have advocated the use of the Darrach resection for patients with rheumatoid arthritis, emphasizing attention to correct technique as a critical factor in the procedure's success.[10,16]
- Compiled results using the HIT procedure for a variety of afflictions indicate that 76% of patients are pain-free and 24% report mild pain.[3,8,17,29]
- Minami et al[16] demonstrated better clinical outcomes using the HIT or Sauvé-Kapandji procedure than the Darrach procedure in 61 patients with osteoarthritis. This study supports the use of the Darrach procedure for the lower demand, elderly patient. Van Schoonhoven and Lanz[23] advocate use of partial resection of the ulnar head in cases of instability or radial malunion associated with arthrosis. These authors feel that maintaining the remaining contact of the TFC adds a biomechanical advantage to prevent secondary problems after resection.
- Two publications on the matched resection report good to excellent results in 24 of 32 patients with posttraumatic or mechanical disorders of the DRUJ[24] and no or mild pain in 44 patients, most with rheumatoid arthritis.[25] Weinzweig and Watson[26] report excellent results in their entire series of 97 wrists over 21 years. Pain was improved in 14 of 15 patients with rheumatoid arthritis in Srikanth et al's[20] clinical study.

COMPLICATIONS

- Persistent pain
- Distal ulnar stump instability (coronal, sagittal)
- Radioulnar impingement
- Loss of forearm rotation
- Ulnar translation due to loss of ulnar support in rheumatoid arthritis
- Extensor tendon rupture
- Soft tissue irritation
- Cutaneous nerve injury
- Stylocarpal impingement
- Complex regional pain syndrome
- Extensor carpi ulnaris tendinitis or instability

REFERENCES

1. Adams BD. Distal radioulnar joint instability. In: Green DP, Hotchkiss RN, Pederson WC, et al, eds. Green's Operative Hand Surgery, ed 5. Philadelphia: Churchill Livingstone, 2005:605–644.
2. Bowers WH. Distal radioulnar joint arthroplasty: the hemiresection-interposition technique. J Hand Surg Am 1985;10(2):169–178.
3. Bowers WH, Zelouf DS. Treatment of chronic disorders of the distal radioulnar joint. In: Lichtman DM, Alexander AH, eds. The Wrist and Its Disorders, ed 2. Philadelphia: WB Saunders, 1997:429–441.
4. De Smet L. The distal radioulnar joint in rheumatoid arthritis. Acta Orthop Belg 2006;72:381–386.
5. De Witte PB, Wijffels M, Jupiter JB, et al. The Darrach procedure for post-traumatic reconstruction. Acta Orthop Belg 2009;75: 316–322.
6. Fraser KE, Diao E, Peimer CA, et al. Comparative results of resection of the distal ulna in rheumatoid arthritis and post-traumatic conditions. J Hand Surg Br 1999;24(6):667–670.
7. George MS, Kiefhaber TR, Stern PJ. The Sauvé-Kapandji procedure and the Darrach procedure for distal radioulnar joint dysfunction after Colles' fracture. J Hand Surg Br 2004;29(6):608–613.
8. Glowacki KA. Hemiresection arthroplasty of the distal radioulnar joint. Hand Clin 2005;21:591–601.
9. Grawe B, Heincelman C, Stern P. Functional results of the Darrach Procedure: a long-term outcome study. J Hand Surg Am 2012;37(12): 2475–2480.
10. Greenberg JA. Resection of the distal ulna: the Darrach procedure. Hand Clin 2000;5:19–30.
11. Greenberg JA, Kleinman WB. Salvage of the failed Darrach procedure. In: Gelberman RH, ed. Master Techniques in Orthopaedic Surgery: The Wrist, ed 2. Philadelphia: Lippincott Williams & Wilkins, 2002:331–337.
12. Greenberg JA, Sotereanos D. Achilles allograft interposition for failed Darrach distal ulna resections. Tech Hand Upper Extrem Surg 2008;12:121–125.
13. Leslie BM, Carlson G, Ruby LK. Results of extensor carpi ulnaris tenodesis in the rheumatoid wrist undergoing a distal ulnar excision. J Hand Surg Am 1990;15(4):547–551.
14. McKee MD, Richards RR. Dynamic radio-ulnar convergence after the Darrach procedure. J Bone Joint Surg Br 1996;78(3):413–418.
15. Melone CP Jr, Taras JS. Distal ulna resection, extensor carpi ulnaris tenodesis, and dorsal synovectomy for the rheumatoid wrist. Hand Clin 1991;7:335–343.
16. Minami A, Iwasaki N, Ishikawsa J, et al. Treatments of osteoarthritis of the distal radioulnar joint: long-term results of three procedures. Hand Surg 2005;10:243–248.
17. Minami A, Kaneda K, Itoga H. Hemiresection-interposition arthroplasty of the distal radioulnar joint associated with repair of triangular fibrocartilage complex lesions. J Hand Surg Am 1991;16(6):1120–1125.
18. Murray PM. Current concepts in the treatment of rheumatoid arthritis of the distal radioulnar joint. Hand Clin 2011;27:49–55.
19. Papp SR, Athwal GS, Pichora DR. The rheumatoid wrist. J Am Acad Orthop Surg 2006;14:65–77.
20. Srikanth KN, Shahane SA, Stilwell JH. Modified matched ulnar resection for arthrosis of distal radioulnar joint in rheumatoid arthritis. Hand Surg 2006;11:15–19.
21. Syed AA, Lam WL, Agarwal M, et al. Stabilization of the ulna stump after Darrach's procedure at the wrist. Int Orthop 2003;27:235–239.
22. Tay SC, Tomita K, Berger RA. The "ulna fovea sign" for defining ulna wrist pain: an analysis of sensitivity and specificity. J Hand Surg Am 2007;32(4):438–444.
23. Van Schoonhoven J, Lanz U. Salvage operations and their differential indications for the distal radioulnar joint [in German]. Orthopade 2004;33:704–714.
24. Watson HK, Gabuzda GM. Matched distal ulna resection for post-traumatic disorders of the distal radioulnar joint. J Hand Surg Am 1992;17(4):724–730.
25. Watson HK, Ryu JY, Burgess RC. Matched distal ulnar resection. J Hand Surg Am 1986;11(6):812–817.
26. Weinzweig J, Watson HK. Matched ulnar resection arthroplasty. In: Gelberman RH, ed. Master Techniques in Orthopaedic Surgery: The Wrist, ed 2. Philadelphia: Lippincott Williams & Wilkins, 2002: 355–361.
27. Willis AA, Berger RA, Cooney WP III. Arthroplasty of the distal radioulnar joint using a new ulnar head endoprosthesis: preliminary report. J Hand Surg Am 2007;32(2):177–189.
28. Yoneda H, Watanabe K. Primary excision of the ulnar head for fractures of the distal ulna associated with fractures of the distal radius in severe osteoporotic patients. J Hand Surg Eur Vol 2014;39(3):293–299.
29. Zelouf DS, Bowers WH, Osterman AL. Distal radioulnar joint reconstruction: hemiresection-interposition technique and Sauvé-Kapandji. In: Katzman B, Feldon P, eds. Rheumatoid Arthritis of the Wrist (Atlas of the Hand Clinics). Philadelphia: WB Saunders, 2005:319–325.
30. Zimmerman RM, Kim JM, Jupiter JB. Arthritis of the distal radioulnar joint: from Darrach to total joint arthroplasty. J Am Acad Orthop Surg 2012;20:623–632.

Sauvé-Kapandji Procedure for Distal Radioulnar Joint Arthritis

Robert M. Szabo

DEFINITION

- Disorders of the distal radioulnar joint (DRUJ) are a significant source of wrist pain that is typically caused by one or a combination of conditions: instability, impingement, impaction, and inflammatory arthritis.
- The etiology of impingement or impaction symptoms referable to this joint includes displaced fractures or malunions of the distal radius, which cause pain during forearm pronation–supination, and tears of the foveal attachment of the triangular fibrocartilage (TFC) complex, which result in DRUJ instability, mechanical symptoms, and pain.
- Both Madelung deformity[23] and rheumatoid arthritis (RA) can display secondary incongruity of the DRUJ, causing pain and loss of forearm rotation. Radial head fracture treated by resection and subsequent shortening of the radius (Essex-Lopresti lesion) also can result in painful incongruity or instability of the DRUJ.
- Management of DRUJ pain, incongruity, or instability alone is challenging, but the Sauvé-Kapandji procedure is one solution that treats all three disorders.[11,17,19,20]

ANATOMY

- The DRUJ is a distal articulation in the biarticulate rotational arrangement of the forearm that allows 1 degree of motion: pronation and supination. The sigmoid notch of the radius is concave, with a 15-mm radius of curvature.
  - The ulnar head is semicylindrical, with a radius of curvature of 10 mm, and has an articulate convexity of 220 degrees. It is surrounded by the ulnolunate and ulnotriquetral ligaments, which originate from the palmar radioulnar ligament near the ulnar styloid.
  - The TFC is a fibrocartilaginous disc originating at the junction of the lunate fossa and the sigmoid notch inserting at the base of the ulnar styloid. Its central portion is cartilaginous and avascular and is designed for weight bearing.
  - The peripheral margins, the dorsal and palmar radioulnar ligaments, are thick lamellar cartilage designed for tensile loading. They are well vascularized from the palmar and dorsal branches of the anterior interosseous artery and from the ulnar artery.
  - The ulnar styloid acts as a strut on the end of the ulna to stabilize the ulnar soft tissues of the wrist. The sheath of the extensor carpi ulnaris (ECU), the ulnocarpal ligaments, and the TFC attach at the base of the ulnar styloid to the fovea and together are known as the triangular fibrocartilage complex (TFCC).
- The radius of curvature of the head of the ulna does not equal that of the sigmoid notch. In the extremes of pronation–supination, less than 10% of the ulnar head may be in contact with the notch. In pronation, the ulnar head translates 2.8 mm dorsally from a neutral position and in supination, the ulnar head translates 5.4 mm volarly from a neutral position.
  - The stability of the DRUJ comes from the joint surface morphology, the joint capsule, the dorsal and palmar radioulnar ligaments, the interosseous membrane (particularly the distal oblique bundle), and the musculotendinous units that cross the joint, primarily the ECU and pronator quadratus. The pronator quadratus actively stabilizes the joint by coapting the ulnar head in the sigmoid notch in pronation and passively by viscoelastic forces in supination. The ECU is retained over the dorsal distal ulna by a separate fibro-osseous tunnel deep to and separate from the extensor retinaculum, allowing unrestricted rotation of the radius and ulna.[18]

PATHOGENESIS

- Traumatic injury to the wrist can lead to derangement of the DRUJ, which can result in instability and eventually painful degenerative changes.
- Distal radial malunions with dorsal or volar subluxations or dislocations of the DRUJ produce secondary rupture, elongation, or functional shortening of the distal radioulnar ligaments. Shortening of the radius due to malunion can result in ulnar impaction against the lunate and incongruity of the DRUJ.
- Arthritis of the DRUJ is a common complication of Colles fractures, particularly when fractures involve the sigmoid notch.
- Congenital disorders such as Madelung disease as well as traumatic epiphyseal closures of the distal radius can produce marked positive ulnar variance with dorsal dislocation of the DRUJ.
- In the rheumatoid wrist, progression of distal radioulnar synovitis typically results in the "caput ulnae syndrome" as described by Backdahl,[1] which consists of the following:
  - Wrist weakness with pain on pronation and supination
  - Dorsal prominence of the ulnar head
  - Limitation of pronation and supination
  - Swelling of the distal radioulnar area
  - Secondary tendon changes with possible extensor tendon rupture and ECU subluxation[1]
  - If allowed to progress without intervention, the carpus will eventually fall in a more ulnarward and palmarward direction, with strength, mobility, and function all suffering.[21]

- A chronically unstable DRUJ without degenerative changes can be treated with various soft tissue reconstructions, depending on the abnormalities and underlying pathology.
  - As a group, many of these reconstructions fail to restore stability; even if stability is restored, limitation of forearm motion persists.

NATURAL HISTORY

- The natural history of DRUJ derangement is painful limitation of forearm rotation, often with additional functional deficits.
  - When positive ulnar variance exceeds a few millimeters, additional limitations of wrist flexion–extension as well as radial–ulnar deviation movements can occur.

PATIENT HISTORY AND PHYSICAL FINDINGS

- Clinical evaluation begins with a detailed and accurate history.
  - A history of fracture involving the forearm or wrist is clearly important. Patients may recall a specific injury involving damaging forces of torque with axial load applied to the involved wrist and forearm. In the absence of trauma, congenital conditions may also be considered.
  - The patient's occupation or hobbies may give insight into the mechanism of injury as well as the most important functional deficits currently experienced by the patient.
  - A complete medical history is important, including questions about inflammatory arthritis or osteoarthritis.
- DRUJ pathology most often causes ulnar-sided wrist pain, diminished grip strength, limited forearm pronation and supination, and limited wrist ulnar deviation.
  - Pain is exacerbated with activity and increases with resisted rotation of the forearm.
  - With large ulnar length discrepancy (positive ulnar variance), limited flexion–extension also can be seen.
- During the physical examination, the clinician should determine whether loss of forearm rotation is solely due to DRUJ pathology or if there is a concurrent problem at the proximal radioulnar joint or interosseous membrane. Other sources of wrist pain and dysfunction must be ruled out.
  - The clinician should check for instability or chronic dislocation of the joint, comparing the injured with the uninjured wrist.
  - The patient's normal and affected wrist and forearm ranges of motion, both active and passive, should be measured. A rigid end point with loss of motion suggests bony pathology such as fracture malunion, whereas a soft end point with limited motion suggests soft tissue contractures.
  - The clinician should carefully palpate, ballote, and compress around the DRUJ and compare the findings to the opposite side. Grip strength measurements should be checked bilaterally. The presence of isolated pain on palpation of the fovea should lead the examiner to consider other etiologies such as a TFCC tear or split ulnotriquetral ligament tear.
  - When evaluating patients with RA, the clinician should try to distinguish the pain and instability of the DRUJ from radiocarpal and midcarpal joint symptoms by careful palpation, ballottement, and compression of areas around the DRUJ, comparing the degree of symptoms elicited by forearm rotation versus wrist flexion–extension.
- Examinations to perform include the following:
  - Piano key test. The test, which isolates DRUJ disorders, is positive if it causes pain and/or crepitus.
  - Selective anesthetic injections. The test is positive when precise, selective injection of anesthetic into the area eliminates pain and improves function. Injections help to confirm pathologic changes and can be used to distinguish intra-articular from extra-articular lesions.
  - Ulnocarpal compression test. A positive test reproduces the ulnar-sided wrist pain and grinding by translating force across the TFC. It also isolates pathologic changes in the TFC.
  - Lunotriquetral (Regan) shuck test. Pain, sometimes with increased joint mobility and grinding, represents a positive test. This test detects and assesses abnormalities or pathologic conditions associated with the lunotriquetral joint.

IMAGING AND OTHER DIAGNOSTIC STUDIES

- Standard neutral rotation posteroanterior (PA), lateral, and ulnar variance radiographs of the wrist should be obtained and compared with the normal side. The clinician should look for evidence of fractures, arthritic changes, bone lesions, and distal ulna position relative to the radius.
- Forearm and elbow radiographs are obtained if there is a history of an elbow injury (especially a radial head fracture) or forearm injury.
- If ulnocarpal abutment is suspected, a PA radiograph is obtained with the forearm in pronation and the fist clenched. This will increase ulnar variance and potentially reveal ulna impaction.
- Computed tomography (CT) is best to evaluate subluxation and articular congruity of the DRUJ.[4,18] To assess the distal radioulnar articular surfaces, simultaneous views are obtained of both extremities with the forearms in neutral rotation, full supination, and full pronation.
- Magnetic resonance imaging (MRI) with single-injection gadolinium arthrography is a good way to evaluate TFC lesions as well as the integrity of the scapholunate and lunotriquetral interosseous ligaments.

DIFFERENTIAL DIAGNOSIS

- ECU tendinitis or subluxation
- Flexor carpi ulnaris (FCU) tendinitis
- Pisotriquetral arthritis
- Lunotriquetral ligament tear
- TFCC tear
- Acute DRUJ dislocation
- Split ulnotriquetral ligament tear

NONOPERATIVE MANAGEMENT

- A trial of nonoperative management is helpful for some patients with DRUJ disorders.
- Minor strains of the DRUJ capsule or sprains of other ulnar-sided wrist ligaments may respond to rest, ice after activity, wrist splints, and oral anti-inflammatory medications.
- Easily reducible dislocations of the DRUJ can be treated by immobilization in a rigid splint or cast for 6 weeks.

- Inflammation of the ulnar-sided wrist tendons often accompanies DRUJ problems.
  - Tendinitis should be treated first with stretching exercises, other physical therapy modalities, and sometimes a steroid injection before addressing the DRUJ surgically.

SURGICAL MANAGEMENT

- The Sauvé-Kapandji procedure is especially useful for patients with RA. Despite advanced radiographic findings of radiocarpal or midcarpal arthritis, complaints of wrist pain can be relieved in many RA patients by addressing the DRUJ pathology with a Sauvé-Kapandji procedure.
  - Commonly, resection of the distal end of the ulna, the Darrach procedure, is recommended for patients with RA and ulnar-sided wrist pain. However, the inflammatory changes and deforming forces acting on the hand and wrist in RA tend to cause palmar and ulnar translocation of the wrist and secondary radioulnar impingement resulting in decreased mobility, strength, and function. Removal of the distal ulna exacerbates and accelerates the problem.
  - With the Sauvé-Kapandji procedure, the retained distal ulna provides bony support for the ulnar corner of the wrist to help stabilize against the palmar–ulnar slide of the carpus (**FIG 1**). In addition, the important attachments of the ulnocarpal complex are preserved.[21]
- The Sauvé-Kapandji procedure is also beneficial in the treatment of DRUJ disorders resulting from trauma.[2]
  - In cases of wrist trauma with ulnar-sided ligamentous injury and incompetence, retaining the ulnar head, as is performed with a Sauvé-Kapandji reconstruction, maintains the ulnocarpal buttress and the TFC to allow a more physiologic transmission of load from the hand to the forearm.
  - The osteotomy made in the ulna in the Sauvé-Kapandji procedure allows as much shortening as is needed to match the level of the radius while retaining supination and pronation.
- Other surgical options include hemiresection and interposition arthroplasty, matched resection of the distal part of the ulna, Darrach resection, and more recently prosthetic replacements of either constrained or unconstrained design.[2]

Preoperative Planning

- The clinician should review preoperative radiographs carefully for marked positive ulnar variance to assess whether fixation of the ulna head can be performed before the osteotomy or if the osteotomy and excision of ulna segment should be done first to restore proper length and head position into the sigmoid fossa.

Positioning

- The patient is positioned supine with the upper extremity on a hand table.
- A pneumatic tourniquet is placed on the arm.
- An intraoperative fluoroscope is draped sterile and made available throughout the procedure.

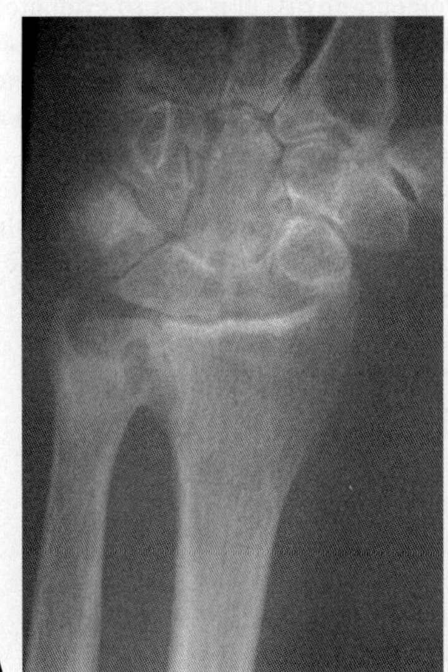
A

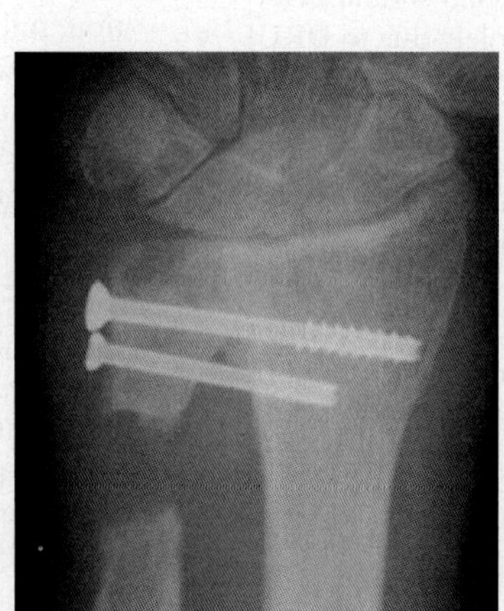
B

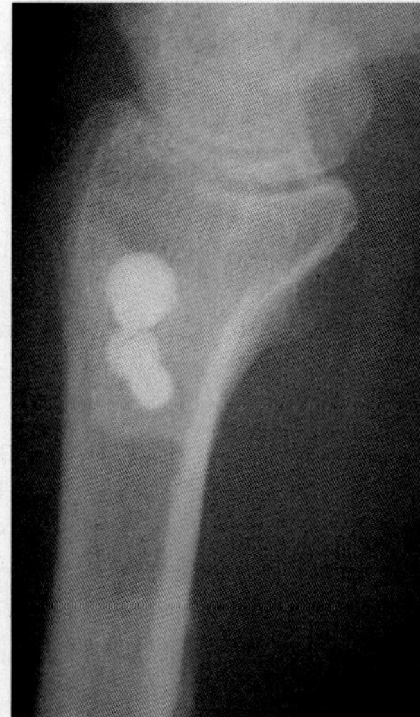
C

FIG 1 • Radiographs from a patient with RA before (**A**) and after (**B,C**) a Sauvé-Kapandji procedure.

Author's Preferred Technique for the Sauvé-Kapandji Procedure

Incision and Dissection

- Make a straight longitudinal incision, 6 to 8 cm long, along the ulnar border of the distal forearm.
  - An alternative incision may be used if additional procedures are planned at the same sitting. For example, in patients with RA, often the Sauvé-Kapandji procedure needs to be combined with another soft tissue procedure such as a dorsal wrist synovectomy, tenosynovectomy, or tendon transfer to treat extensor tendon ruptures that result from the caput ulnae syndrome. If that is the case, start the incision more dorsally to facilitate exposure for the additional procedure, and then extend it proximally and obliquely to expose the distal ulna.
- Identify the dorsal cutaneous branch of the ulnar nerve and protect it throughout the case (**TECH FIG 1**).
- Expose the distal 4 to 6 cm of the ulna extraperiosteally through the interval between the ECU and FCU.

Osteotomy of the Ulnar Diaphysis

- Select the appropriate level for an osteotomy of the ulnar diaphysis (**TECH FIG 2A**).
- Cut the bone just proximal to the flare of the ulnar head; this will leave enough of the distal ulna to accommodate two fixation screws.
- Confirm with fluoroscopy that the proposed osteotomy site is appropriate.
- Make a second cut proximal and parallel to the first (**TECH FIG 2B**) and remove a 10- to 14-mm segment of ulna (**TECH FIG 2C**). Resect the periosteum in the region of the gap and irrigate thoroughly to remove bone debris.
  - If there is a positive ulnar variance, remove a correspondingly longer segment of the ulna so that when the ulnar head is recessed to neutral ulnar variance, the resulting gap will be adequate.
- Save the removed bone for subsequent grafting into the DRUJ arthrodesis site (**TECH FIG 2D**).

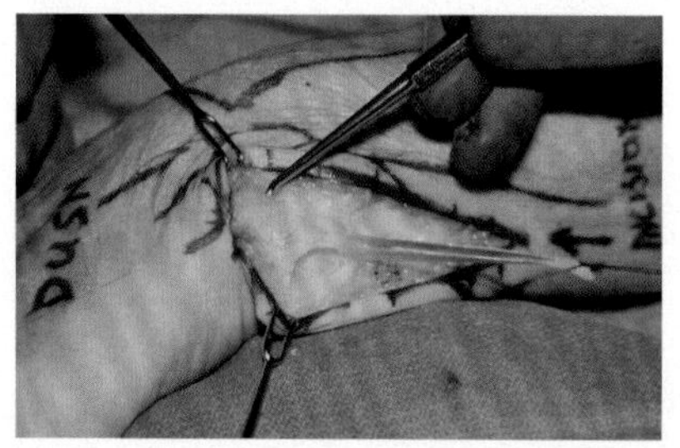

TECH FIG 1 ● Identification and mobilization of the dorsal sensory ulnar nerve, which is tagged with a rubber dam. Notice a dorsal branch under the probe.

Distal Radioulnar Joint Exposure and Preparation

- Incise the retinaculum over the fifth dorsal compartment and retract the extensor digiti minimi radially. Expose the DRUJ with a dorsoulnar capsulotomy just radial to the ECU tendon.
- Denude both the ulnar head and sigmoid fossa of the radius of all remaining cartilage to create flush surfaces of cancellous bone on each side of the arthrodesis site and pack the harvested cancellous bone from the removed ulna segment (**TECH FIG 3**).
  - In patients with severe bone loss, after decortication of the corresponding articular surfaces of the DRUJ, sculpt the resected segment of the ulna to fit into the space between the ulnar head and sigmoid notch as a corticocancellous bone graft.

Fixation

- Cannulated 3.0- to 4.0-mm self-tapping screws are preferable to Kirschner wires (K-wires) for fixation of the arthrodesis site.
  - K-wires can irritate cutaneous nerves when buried or can cause wound problems when placed percutaneously.
  - There is usually no need to remove hardware when screws are used, and rehabilitation can begin sooner because of secure fixation.

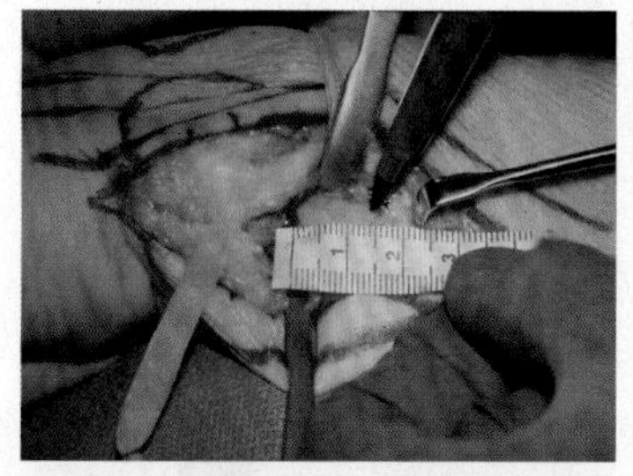
A

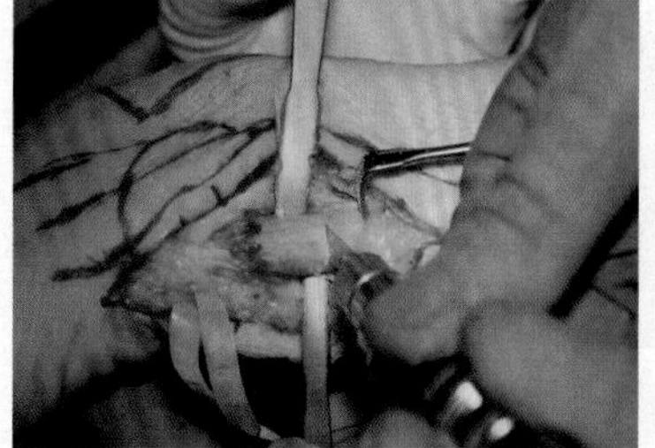
B

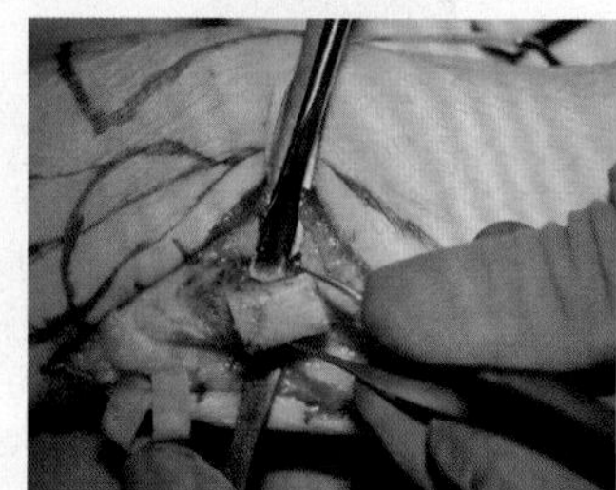
C

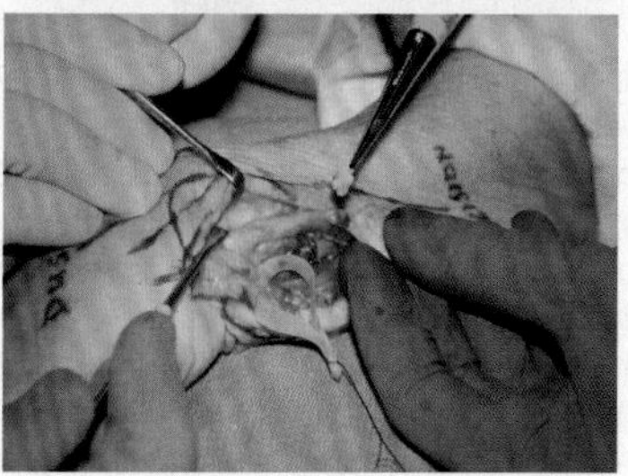
D

TECH FIG 2 ● **A.** Measure the osteotomy resection. As shown here, take into consideration the amount of shortening needed to obtain neutral ulnar variance. **B.** Make the proximal and distal osteotomies using a microsaw. **C.** Removal of the resected ulna. Preserve the pronator quadratus, which is left behind for later use. **D.** Harvest the cancellous bone from the resected ulna.

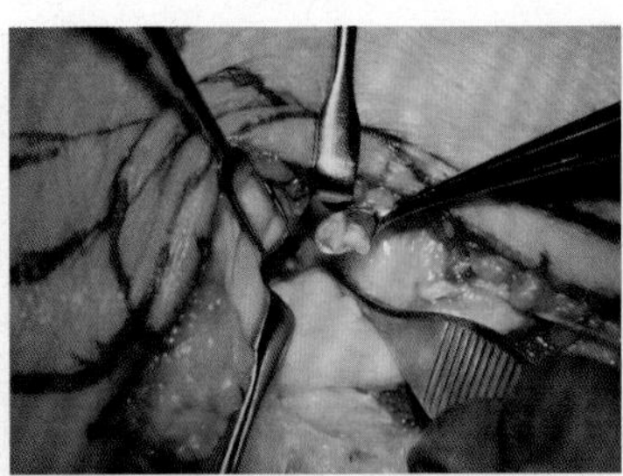

TECH FIG 3 • Curette the sigmoid notch of any remaining cartilage and then pack in the bone graft from the resected ulna.

   - Cannulated screws over guidewires allow accurate screw placement and facilitate the alignment of the cortices of the distal ulna and radius.
- Establish ulnar neutral variance by moving the ulnar head proximally or distally to bring its distal surface parallel with the distal radius surface; confirm correct placement fluoroscopically.
   - Do this while holding the forearm in neutral rotation with the patient's elbow resting on the operating table while supporting the forearm perpendicular to the table in neutral rotation.
   - Temporarily fix the ulnar head to the sigmoid notch of the distal part of the radius with a single K-wire and ensure proper position with fluoroscopy.
- While maintaining neutral forearm rotation, drill two guidewires across the DRUJ to stabilize the ulnar head in proper position.
   - Place one wire a few millimeters proximal to the subchondral bone of the distal ulna and position the second wire proximal enough to allow for seating of both screw heads without impingement (**TECH FIG 4A**).
   - Confirm correct placement of the guidewires with fluoroscopy.
- Advance the distal wire into the far (radial) cortex of the radius and measure for screw length.
   - The proximal screw provides rotational control and needs only tricortical fixation. It can be 5 mm shorter than the distal screw.

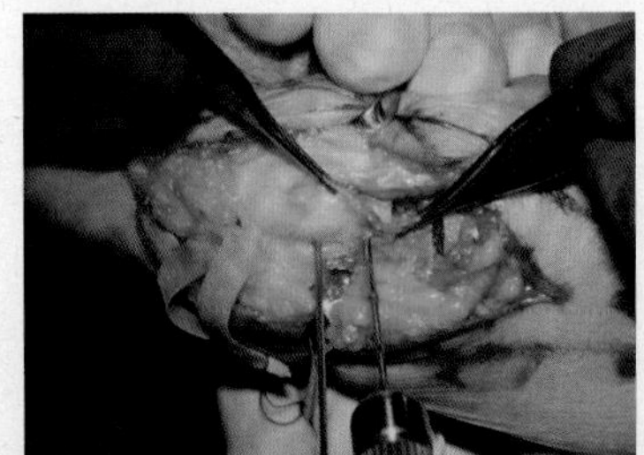

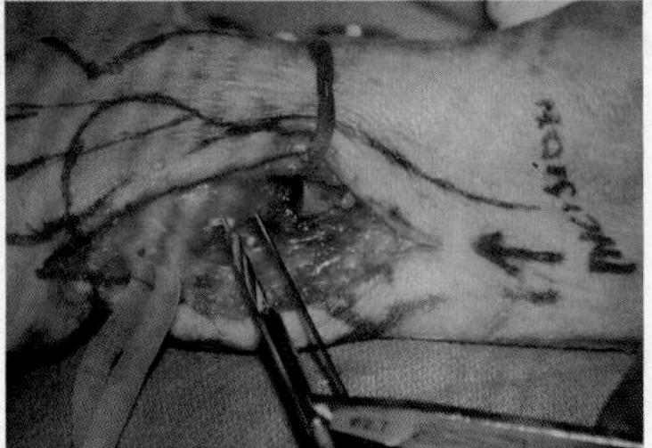

TECH FIG 4 • **A.** Placement of the two K-wires to stabilize the ulnar head. **B.** Drill over the K-wires, measure, and put in the screws.

- After the screw lengths are measured, advance the wires through the skin to the radial side of the forearm with a mallet and grasp them with a clamp to avoid having the wire come out during drilling and screw placement.
   - With a mallet, the chances of injuring a branch of the radial sensory nerve branch are less than those with a power driver.
- Drill over the guidewires with a cannulated drill bit (**TECH FIG 4B**).
- Pack additional cancellous bone harvested from the excised ulnar segment into the DRUJ space.
- Insert the selected screws over the guidewires while manually compressing the ulnar head against the radius.
- Tighten the distal screw first to avoid compressing the radial and ulnar shafts together and levering the ulnar head out of position.
- Do not use lag screw technique on the proximal screw, and avoid tilting the head of the ulna; it must remain parallel to the long axis of the ulnar shaft.

Extensor Carpi Ulnaris Stabilization of the Proximal Ulnar Stump

- After fixation of the DRUJ, drill a 3.5-mm hole from the dorsoulnar aspect of the ulnar shaft proximal stump into its intramedullary cavity.
- Split the ECU tendon in the central sulcus and release the radial half at the ulnocarpal level.
- Reflect this half of the ECU proximally, leaving it attached at the musculotendinous junction.
- Pass this proximally based strip, approximately 6 to 8 cm long, into the medullary canal through the drill hole and retrieve it at the distal stump of the ulna, pulling it distally under moderate tension, and then suture it back onto itself in an interlacing fashion (**TECH FIG 5**).

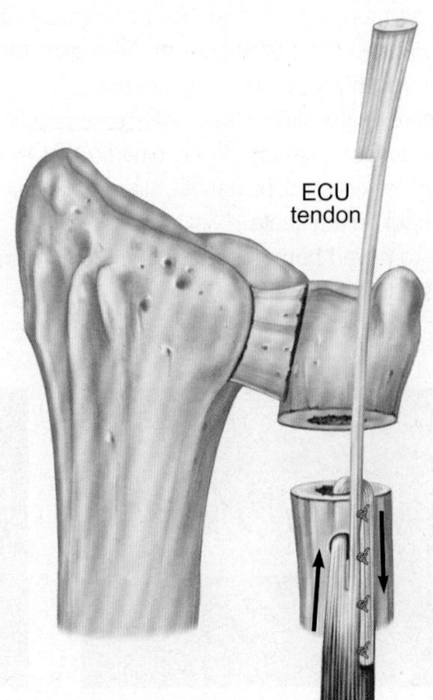

TECH FIG 5 • Modification of the Sauvé-Kapandji procedure with ECU tenodesis as described by Minami et al.[14,15] After the Sauvé-Kapandji procedure, a 3.5-mm hole was drilled from the dorsoulnar aspect of the ulnar shaft into the intramedullary cavity. The ECU tendon was then split in the central sulcus and the radial half released at the ulnocarpal level. It was then reflected proximally, leaving it attached at the musculotendinous junction. This proximally based strip was then passed into the medullary canal through the drill hole, retrieved at the distal stump of the ulna, and then sutured back on itself in an interlacing fashion.

Flexor Carpi Ulnaris Stabilization of the Proximal Ulnar Stump

- Over a distance of 8 to 10 cm through the volar aspect of the incision, isolate a distally based slip of FCU tendon (measuring about half the width of the tendon) attached to the pisiform.
- Drill a 4- to 4.5-mm hole on the volar cortex, 1 cm proximal to the end of the osteotomized surface of the proximal ulnar segment.
  - This is facilitated by inserting the drill bit obliquely through the medullary cavity in a dorsal to volar direction.
- Pass the slip of FCU tendon deep to the FCU muscle through the distal end of the ulnar stump and loop it back on itself, securing it with nonabsorbable suture (**TECH FIG 6**).
- Suture the tendon under moderate tension, keeping the forearm in neutral rotation and the wrist in neutral flexion–extension and neutral radioulnar deviation.
- Pull the pronator quadratus muscle into the gap in the ulna and suture it to the volar aspect of the tendon sheath of the ECU.

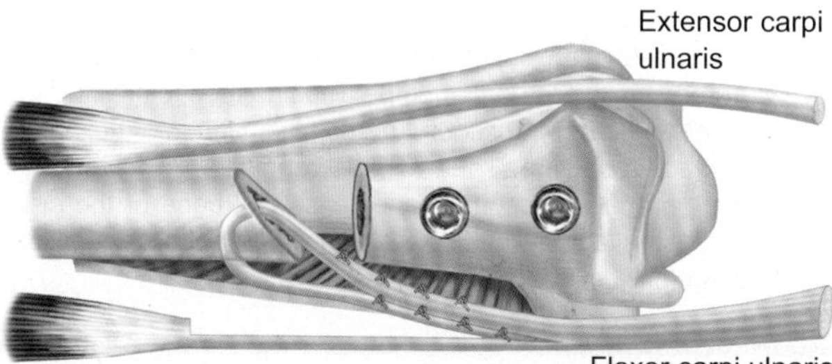

TECH FIG 6 ● Modification of the Sauvé-Kapandji procedure with FCU tenodesis as described by Lamey and Fernandez.[12] Lateral aspect of the wrist, showing stabilization of the proximal ulnar segment with use of a distally based slip of the FCU tendon.

- Reattach the sixth dorsal compartment within the groove on the ulnar head and close the wound.

Wound Closure

- Make sure that there is a gap of 10 to 12 mm between the proximal and distal ulnar segments.
- Suture the fascia of the underlying pronator quadratus into the gap to prevent reossification across the pseudarthrosis site and stabilize the stump of the ulnar shaft (**TECH FIG 7A**).
- Repair the joint capsule and retinacular compartments (**TECH FIG 7B**) and close the skin in routine fashion.

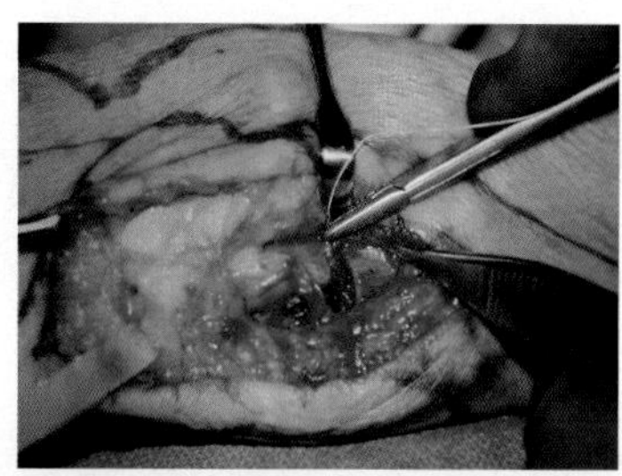

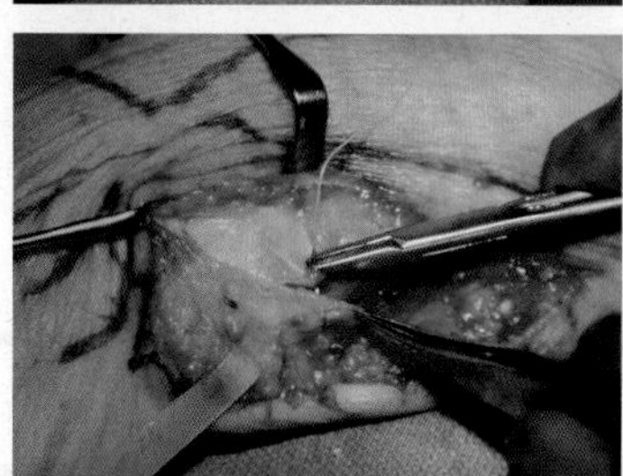

TECH FIG 7 ● **A.** Suturing the pronator quadratus into the gap. **B.** Closure of the retinaculum.

Technique for Cases Characterized by Poor Bone Quality (Fujita Technique)

- Make a 7-cm longitudinal skin incision on the dorsal aspect of the wrist centered on the ulnar head (**TECH FIG 8A**).
- Open the fourth dorsal compartment. Divide the septum between the fourth and fifth compartments and reflect the retinaculum ulnarly to preserve a single common retinacular flap.
- Retract the extensor digitorum communis and extensor digiti minimi tendons radially and perform a neurectomy of the terminal branch of the posterior interosseous nerve.
- Incise the capsule of the DRUJ and dissect the distal part of the ulna subperiosteally.
- Perform an oblique osteotomy with an oscillating saw 30 mm proximal to the distal end of the ulna and excise the ulnar head (**TECH FIG 8B**).
- Perform a synovectomy of the DRUJ and remove the periosteum of the resected portion of the ulna.
- Interpose the pronator quadratus muscle at the osteotomy site.
- Drill a hole 10 mm in diameter at the sigmoid notch of the radius while viewing the distal articular surface of the radius through the TFC, which is usually ruptured. Do not penetrate the subchondral bone (**TECH FIG 8C**).
- Remove all soft tissue from the resected portion of the ulna and then rotate it 90 degrees and insert the cut end of the ulnar graft into the hole in the radius, creating a shelf 12 to 15 mm long.
- Impact the ulnar graft into the subchondral and cancellous bone of the distal part of the radius without penetrating the radial cortex and fix it in the drill hole with a cancellous bone screw (**TECH FIG 8D**). Do not overtighten the screw.
- Cover the graft with the joint capsule contiguous with a periosteal flap.
- Mobilize and relocate the ECU tendon by dissecting the septum between the fifth and sixth compartments.
- If subluxation of the ECU tendon is evident during rotation of the forearm, reflect the distal portion of the periosteal flap ulnarly beneath the ECU tendon to act as a sling and suture it to the adjacent soft tissue to restrain the ECU in a dorsal and radial position over the graft.
- Close in the fashion previously outlined.

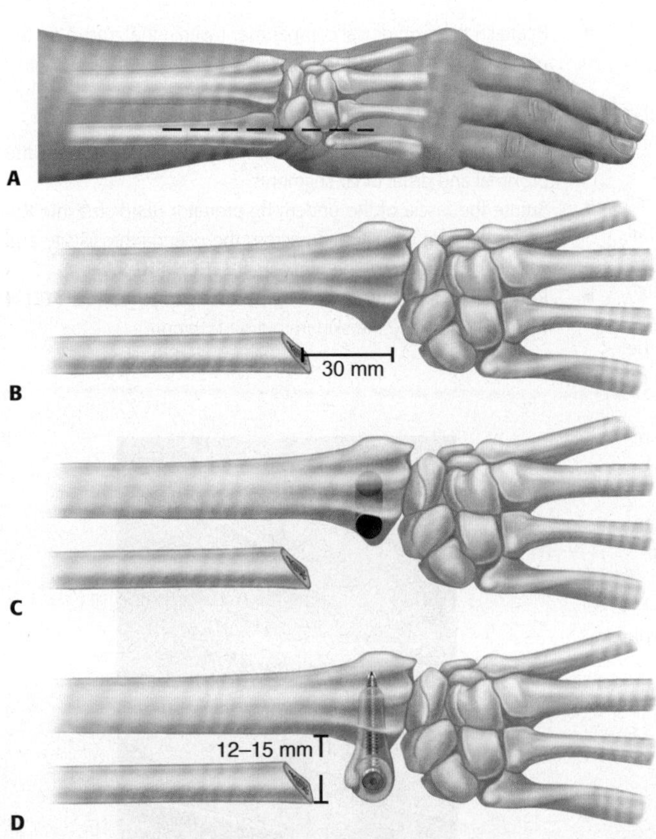

TECH FIG 8 • Modification of the Sauvé-Kapandji procedure with the distal ulna used as a bone peg as described by Fujita et al.[8,9] **A.** Make a 7-cm longitudinal skin incision on the dorsal aspect of the wrist centered on the ulna head. **B.** Perform an oblique osteotomy with an oscillating saw 30 mm proximal to the distal end of the ulna and excise the ulna head. **C.** Drill a hole 10 mm in diameter at the sigmoid notch of the radius while viewing the distal articular surface of the radius through the TFC, which is usually ruptured. Do not penetrate the subchondral bone. **D.** Remove all soft tissue from the resected portion of the ulna and then rotate it 90 degrees and insert the cut end of the ulnar graft into the hole in the radius, creating a shelf 12 to 15 mm long. Impact the ulnar graft into the subchondral and cancellous bone of the distal part of the radius without penetrating the radial cortex and fix it in the drill hole with a cancellous bone screw.

PEARLS AND PITFALLS

Indications	■ Ulnocarpal pain should be distinguished from DRUJ pain. This procedure should not be done for a pain-free, stable DRUJ. ■ If the DRUJ is unstable and arthritic, use of either the FCU or ECU tenodesis of the proximal ulnar stump should be strongly considered. ■ In patients with RA, DRUJ symptoms should be distinguished clinically, not radiographically, from radiocarpal symptoms. Many patients can be treated with the Sauvé-Kapandji procedure successfully despite radiocarpal changes on radiographs.
Technical details	■ The dorsal sensory branch of the ulnar nerve should be identified and protected to avoid neuromas and stretch injuries. ■ Osteotomy of the ulna should be performed as distal as possible. To avoid stump instability, no more than 1 cm of ulna should be excised.

POSTOPERATIVE CARE

- Rehabilitation after the Sauvé-Kapandji procedure follows guidelines published by Skirven.[16]
  - Postoperatively, a bulky dressing with plaster splints extending above the elbow, maintaining the forearm in neutral position, is applied for 7 to 10 days.
  - Sutures are then removed and the patient is given a removable, lightweight splint to support the wrist.
  - Hand therapy is initiated with an emphasis on gentle active wrist, digit, and forearm rotation exercises.
  - Except for exercise sessions and bathing, the splint is worn at all times.
  - In the postoperative period, the goal is to allow adequate healing by supporting and protecting the arthrodesis site from stress, followed by gradual restoration of functional mobility without sacrificing the stability of the ulnar shaft or the arthrodesis.
- The arthrodesis is protected from loading forces for 4 to 6 weeks.
  - When the arthrodesis appears healed radiographically, usually 8 weeks postoperatively, light strengthening exercises are initiated. Heavy lifting and forearm torque are avoided until 3 months postoperatively.
- For conservative management of postoperative instability of the ulnar shaft, Skirven[16] has recommended a small, cuff-style splint to support the pseudarthrosis site and help stabilize the ulnar shaft.
  - The splint, which is made of thermoplastic material, extends from the distal radius ulnarly to a few centimeters proximal to the pseudarthrosis site.

- An adjustable strap allows the patient to set the tension on the splint to provide comfort and the level of stability required for specific activities.

OUTCOMES

- There is a broad international experience with this operation on many patients.
- Zimmermann in Austria retrospectively reported on 43 patients' clinical results and Disability of the Arm, Shoulder, and Hand (DASH) questionnaires 8 years (range 5 to 12 years) after a Sauvé-Kapandji operation.[24] Forearm rotation improved in all patients. Ulnar wrist pain was diminished in 97% of the patients, and 9% had mild pain at the proximal ulnar stump. Grip strength compared to the contralateral side improved from a preoperative mean of 38% to a postoperative mean of 55%. The mean DASH score was 28 points (range 0 to 53 points). In all cases, the arthrodesis fused within 8 weeks.
- In Australia, Millroy reported on 81 procedures in 71 patients and found that "almost all patients were pain-free during normal activity, although 7 experienced discomfort with overuse."[13]
- In Belgium, De Smet conducted a prospective survey on 84 patients treated for posttraumatic arthritis of the DRUJ with the procedure.[7] According to the Mayo wrist score, there were 20 excellent, 34 good, 18 fair, and 12 poor results, with an overall satisfaction rate of 74%.
- In Denmark, Jacobsen found that 15 of 17 employed patients returned to work.[10]
- In England, Carter found that 86% of his patients would have the operation again.[3]
- In Germany, Daecke looked at the functional outcomes of 56 patients with the DASH and Mayo wrist scores as well as clinical results.[6] Although only 50% of patients were free of symptoms during heavy labor, 95% had excellent results. The postoperative DASH score was 24.2 ± 22.5 and the Mayo wrist score was 76.1 ± 17.6.
- In Switzerland, Lamey reported on 18 patients who underwent the Sauvé-Kapandji procedure with the FCU tenodesis of the ulnar stump.[12] There were 6 excellent, 7 good, 4 fair, and 1 poor Mayo wrist scores. Eight of the patients who had performed heavy manual labor before the injury were able to return to work full-time without restrictions.
- Many other studies report similar outcomes, confirming the use and broad appeal of this operation.

COMPLICATIONS

- The main source of complications from the Sauvé-Kapandji procedure is the distal stump of the ulna.
- Pain, ulnar impingement syndrome, and a feeling of instability of the ulnar shaft have been reported, but these symptoms are usually transient and resolve by 3 months postoperatively.
- Significant instability of the ulnar shaft is more commonly reported after the Darrach procedure, but it can also occur if too much bone is resected during the described procedure.[5]
  - To prevent instability, the surgeon should carefully stabilize the ulnar stump with pronator quadratus fascia advancement, should place the osteotomies as far distally as possible, and should not resect too much bone.
  - The surgeon should also avoid excessive stripping of the interosseous membrane. A soft tissue tube should surround the pseudarthrosis site to connect and stabilize the proximal and distal ulnar segments.
  - Despite these precautions, painful instability of the distal ulnar stump can occur. In this scenario, the stump can be stabilized by using a strip of the ECU or FCU tendon based on its distal attachment.
- Another complication from the Sauvé-Kapandji procedure is ossification of the pseudarthrosis site.[5]
  - The pronator quadratus should be interposed in the ulnar gap after the osteotomy is complete and the ulnar segment should be removed extraperiosteally to minimize the occurrence of this complication.
  - If ossification does occur, the bone may be resected when mature. The patient should then immediately begin forearm rotation exercises.
- Injury of the dorsal cutaneous branch of the ulnar nerve is a potential problem and can be avoided with careful dissection.
- Wada and Ishii reported closed rupture of a finger extensor tendon after the Sauvé-Kapandji procedure. They postulated that this was due to the ulnar shaft stump's being left distal to the edge of the extensor retinaculum, causing attritional rupture of the tendon trapped between the bone edge and the retinaculum.[22]
  - This could be avoided by contouring the ulnar shaft edge to a smooth edge and covering the stump with the interposed pronator quadratus.
- Painful neuromas of the dorsal sensory branch of the ulna nerve have also been reported.
  - Lamey and Fernandez[12] noted that this may be more common when harvesting a distally based slip of the FCU from one incision. They recommend this be done from a second incision.[12]
- Some patients may develop hardware pain from palpable screw heads. These screws can be removed.

REFERENCES

1. Backdahl M. The caput ulnae syndrome in rheumatoid arthritis: a study of the morphology, abnormal anatomy and clinical picture. Acta Rheum Scand Suppl 1963;5:1–75.
2. Bowers WH. Distal radioulnar joint arthroplasty: current concepts. Clin Orthop Relat Res 1992;(275):104–109.
3. Carter PB, Stuart PR. The Sauvé-Kapandji procedure for post-traumatic disorders of the distal radio-ulnar joint. J Bone Joint Surg Br 2000; 82(7):1013–1018.
4. Cone RO, Szabo R, Resnick D, et al. Computed tomography of the normal radioulnar joints. Invest Radiol 1983;18:541–545.
5. Daecke W, Martini AK, Schneider S, et al. Amount of ulnar resection is a predictive factor for ulnar instability problems after the Sauvé-Kapandji procedure: a retrospective study of 44 patients followed for 1–13 years. Acta Orthop 2006;77:290–297.
6. Daecke W, Martini AK, Streich NA. Kapandji-Sauvé procedure for chronic disorders of the distal radioulnar joint with special regard to the long-term results [in German]. Handchir Mikrochir Plast Chir 2003;35:164–169.
7. De Smet LA, Van Ransbeeck H. The Sauvé-Kapandji procedure for posttraumatic wrist disorders: further experience. Acta Orthop Belg 2000;66:251–254.
8. Fujita S, Masada K, Takeuchi E, et al. Modified Sauvé-Kapandji procedure for disorders of the distal radioulnar joint in patients with rheumatoid arthritis. J Bone Joint Surg Am 2005;87(1):134–139.

9. Fujita S, Masada K, Takeuchi E, et al. Modified Sauvé-Kapandji procedure for disorders of the distal radioulnar joint in patients with rheumatoid arthritis. Surgical technique. J Bone Joint Surg Am 2006;88(suppl 1, pt 1):24–28.
10. Jacobsen TW, Leicht P. The Sauvé-Kapandji procedure for post-traumatic disorders of the distal radioulnar joint. Acta Orthop Belg 2004;70:226–230.
11. Kapandji IA. The Kapandji-Sauvé operation. Its techniques and indications in nonrheumatoid diseases. Ann Chir Main 1986;5:181–193.
12. Lamey DM, Fernandez DL. Results of the modified Sauvé-Kapandji procedure in the treatment of chronic posttraumatic derangement of the distal radioulnar joint. J Bone Joint Surg Am 1998;80(12):1758–1769.
13. Millroy P, Coleman S, Ivers R. The Sauvé-Kapandji operation. Technique and results. J Hand Surg Br 1992;17(4):411–414.
14. Minami A, Kato H, Iwasaki N. Modification of the Sauvé-Kapandji procedure with extensor carpi ulnaris tenodesis. J Hand Surg Am 2000;25(6):1080–1084.
15. Minami A, Suzuki K, Suenaga N, et al. The Sauvé-Kapandji procedure for osteoarthritis of the distal radioulnar joint. J Hand Surg Am 1995;20(4):602–608.
16. Skirven T. Rehabilitation following surgery for the distal radioulnar joint. Tech Hand Up Extrem Surg 1997;1:219–225.
17. Slater RR Jr, Szabo RM. The Sauvé-Kapandji procedure. Tech Hand Up Extrem Surg 1998;2:148–157.
18. Szabo RM. Distal radioulnar joint instability. J Bone Joint Surg Am 2006;88(4):884–894.
19. Szabo RM, Anderson KA, Chen JL. Functional outcome of en bloc excision and osteoarticular allograft replacement with the Sauvé-Kapandji procedure for Campanacci grade 3 giant-cell tumor of the distal radius. J Hand Surg Am 2006;31(8):1340–1348.
20. Taleisnik J. The Sauvé-Kapandji procedure. Clin Orthop Relat Res 1992;(275):110–123.
21. Vincent KA, Szabo RM, Agee JM. The Sauvé-Kapandji procedure for reconstruction of the rheumatoid distal radioulnar joint. J Hand Surg Am 1993;18(6):978–983.
22. Wada T, Ogino T, Ishii S. Closed rupture of a finger extensor following the Sauvé-Kapandji procedure: a case report. J Hand Surg Am 1997;22(4):705–707.
23. White GM, Weiland AJ. Madelung's deformity: treatment by osteotomy of the radius and Lauenstein procedure. J Hand Surg Am 1987;12(2):202–204.
24. Zimmermann R, Gschwentner M, Arora R, et al. Treatment of distal radioulnar joint disorders with a modified Sauvé-Kapandji procedure: long-term outcome with special attention to the DASH Questionnaire. Arch Orthop Trauma Surg 2003;123:293–298.

Ulnar Head Implant Arthroplasty

Sam Fuller and Randy R. Bindra

DEFINITION

- As with any synovial joint, the distal radioulnar joint (DRUJ) can degenerate due to osteoarthritis, inflammatory arthritis, chronic instability, infection, and trauma.[4]
- Standard treatments such as partial ("matched resection") or complete (Darrach procedure) distal ulnar resection have the potential to destabilize the forearm axis and cause painful forearm rotation.
  - The normal compressive muscle forces acting between the radius and ulna help stabilize the DRUJ.[1]
  - When the distal ulna has been resected and the forearm is rotated under such a compressive load, a palpable grinding between the ulnar stump and the radius may develop; this is referred to as *ulnar impingement*.[6] This may progress from minor irritation to painful erosion of the radius. These patients present with pain on stress loading of the upper extremity, weakness in grip strength, decreased forearm rotation, and difficulty with lifting.[2]
- Ulnar head implant arthroplasty is designed to maintain the DRUJ, thereby avoiding ulnar impingement. An adequate soft tissue envelope repaired over the implant provides stability.
  - The first prosthesis used was a silicone cap designed to provide a soft end to the ulnar stump. These prostheses understandably failed under loading.
  - Newer designs aim to restore the ulnar head using a metallic prosthesis to articulate with the sigmoid notch.

ANATOMY

- See Chapters 26, 63, 64, 65, 111, 112, and 115.

PATHOGENESIS

- See Chapters 111 and 112.

NATURAL HISTORY

- See Chapters 111 and 112.

PATIENT HISTORY AND PHYSICAL FINDINGS

- Patients who have had an ulnar head resection complain of painful forearm rotation, often associated with instability of the forearm axis, decreased strength, and joint grinding.
- In addition to recording the range and fluidity of DRUJ motion, the examiner must determine the stability of the joint and the contribution of ulnar impingement to the patient's pain.
- Radioulnar compression creates radioulnar impingement by external passive compression.
  - The examiner should encircle the patient's distal forearm with his or her hands and apply firm compression.
  - A positive sign is reproduction of the patient's pain.
- Active radioulnar impingement is reproduced by active muscle contraction, specifically the brachialis.
  - The patient has pain lifting a load of 2 pounds with the forearm in neutral position.
- Ulnar stump instability results from compromised soft tissue stabilizers of the distal stump, which tends to fall away from the radius as the forearm is rotated.
  - The patient is asked to actively rotate the forearm. Dorsal and palmar subluxation of the ulnar stump is visible.

IMAGING AND OTHER DIAGNOSTIC STUDIES

- Standard posteroanterior, lateral, and oblique radiographs of the wrist
  - These x-rays demonstrate scalloping of the ulnar cortex of the radial metaphysis and some corresponding pencilling of the distal ulnar stump.
- Posteroanterior stress-loaded radiographs
  - May demonstrate impingement between the radius and ulna
  - The patient stands with the involved forearm facing the x-ray tube. The wrist is stress-loaded by asking the patient to hold a 2.2-kg lead cylinder with the shoulder adducted, the elbow flexed to 90 degrees, and the forearm in the position of neutral rotation.
  - The forearm rests on the x-ray cassette and the radiograph is then taken with the beam aligned in the coronal plane, creating a posteroanterior view of the neutral forearm.
  - Radiographs are obtained before and after stress-loading.
- Computed tomography (CT) scanning
  - In patients with osteoarthritis of the DRUJ, axial scans are essential for evaluation of the extent of degenerative changes in the ulnar head and the need for total or partial replacement.
  - CT scanning is also essential for evaluation of the sigmoid notch for osteophytes and erosion in patients with painful ulnar head replacement.
  - CT scanning with forearm in pronation and supination is also useful in detecting radioulnar instability if clinical examination is equivocal.

DIFFERENTIAL DIAGNOSIS

- In addition to radioulnar impingement, a patient who has pain at the DRUJ after resection of the ulnar head may have pain due to the following conditions:
  - Ulnar neuropathy
  - Painful surgical scar due to sensory nerve injury or scarring
  - Radiocarpal or midcarpal arthritis

NONOPERATIVE MANAGEMENT

- Activity modification to minimize forearm rotatory movements will diminish pain.

- A Russe splint is partially helpful for patients with instability of the distal ulnar stump but is of no help in preventing radioulnar impingement pain.

SURGICAL MANAGEMENT

- The most common indication for distal ulnar implant arthroplasty is to relieve impingement symptoms in patients who have undergone previous ulnar head resection.
- Other less common indications include the following:
  - Treatment of patients with primary degenerative arthritis of the DRUJ who have failed to respond to splinting and steroid injections
  - Reconstruction of the ulna after excision of a tumor involving the ulnar head
  - After unreconstructable fractures of the ulnar head as either a primary or delayed procedure
  - Relative indication: patients with well-controlled inflammatory arthritis but well-preserved bone stock
- The amount of the DRUJ that is replaced may vary for any given case.
  - Partial ulnar head replacement
  - Unconstrained replacement of the entire distal ulna with or without sigmoid notch resurfacing
  - Constrained total DRUJ replacement, including the sigmoid fossa of the distal radius
- Partial ulnar head replacement preserves the styloid process and the attachment of the triangular fibrocartilage.
  - This procedure is indicated when the disease process, typically arthritis, is limited to the distal ulnar articular surface.
  - Contraindications include active infection, inadequate soft tissue coverage or poor bone stock, instability of the distal ulna, excessive ulnar positive variance, and degeneration at the sigmoid notch.
  - Two types of implants are available: a one-piece stemmed metal prosthesis and a two-piece prosthesis with a titanium stem and an articulating pyrolytic carbon disc that replaces the head (**FIG 1**).[5]
  - Long-term results of partial ulnar head replacement are not known. The articulating two-piece prosthesis has the theoretical advantage of less radius erosion from articulation with the pyrocarbon head.
- Unconstrained complete ulnar head replacement is indicated for reconstruction of ulnar impingement after resection or replacement of an arthritic DRUJ associated with instability of the distal ulna. With mild instability, repair of the soft tissue envelope is adequate to restore stability. In cases with more obvious instability, an additional soft tissue procedure is indicated along with ulnar head replacement.
  - Ulnar head prostheses are generally spherical and made of metal or ceramic. An eccentric-shaped metallic head has been designed to more closely approximate the shape of the normal head. However, biomechanical studies have demonstrated normal tracking patterns of the distal ulna around the radius, closely simulating the normal joint, even with the use of spherical heads.[8]
  - Ulnar head prostheses may articulate with a metal-backed polyethylene resurfacing of the sigmoid notch in an unconstrained manner (**FIG 2**).
  - An adequate soft tissue envelope is essential to prevent subluxation of a complete ulnar head replacement. The triangular fibrocartilage complex (TFCC) is no longer attached to the distal ulna, making the prosthesis prone to dislocation. Thus, an essential part of the surgical technique is reconstructing the capsuloligamentous envelope surrounding the ulnar prosthesis.
  - Other contraindications include previous open fracture, infection in or around the joint, skeletal immaturity, and known sensitivity to the implant materials.
- In cases of marked instability, with lack of an adequate soft tissue stabilizing envelope and ablation of the DRUJ

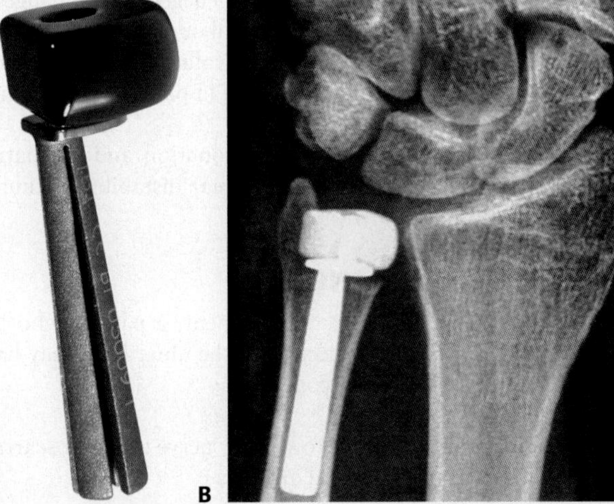

FIG 1 • The Eclypse partial ulnar head replacement (Tornier Surgical Implants, Tornier, Inc., Rodborough Road, FR) consists of an expandable titanium stem with a mobile pyrocarbon spacer (**A**). When implanted, the prosthesis preserves the ulnar styloid and attachment of the TFCC (**B**).

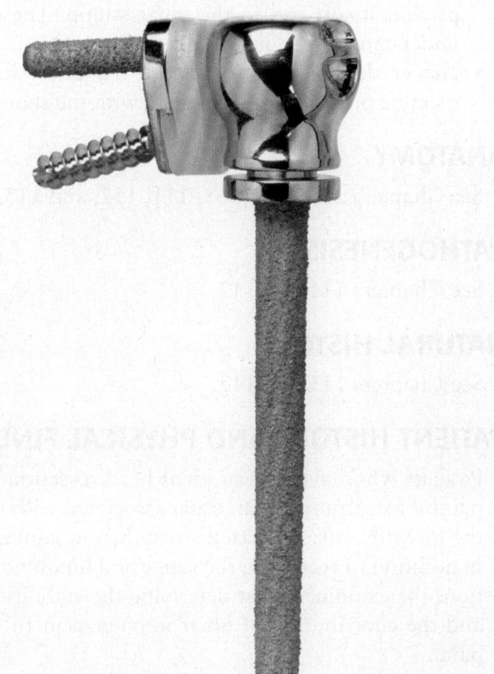

FIG 2 • The Stability total ulnar head arthroplasty system (Small Bone Innovations, Inc., Morrisville, PA) consists of a metal ulnar head component that articulates with a metal-backed polyethylene sigmoid notch. The ulnar head component can be used individually as a hemiarthroplasty.

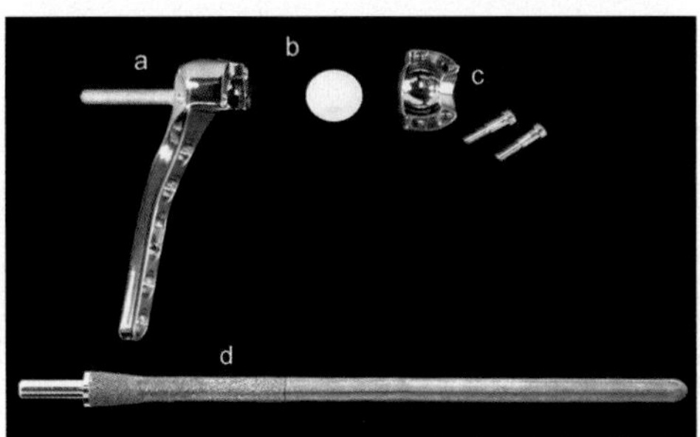

FIG 3 • The Aptis system (Aptis Medical, Louisville, KY) replaces the entire DRUJ with a constrained articulation. The components include (*a*) radial plate with socket, (*b*) polyethylene ball, (*c*) hemisocket with screws, and (*d*) ulnar stem with peg.

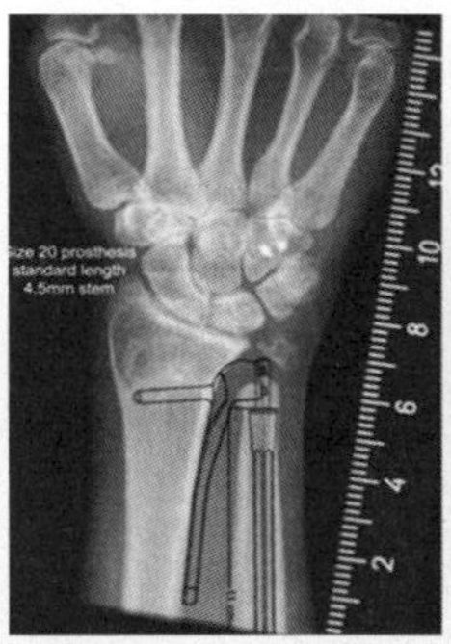

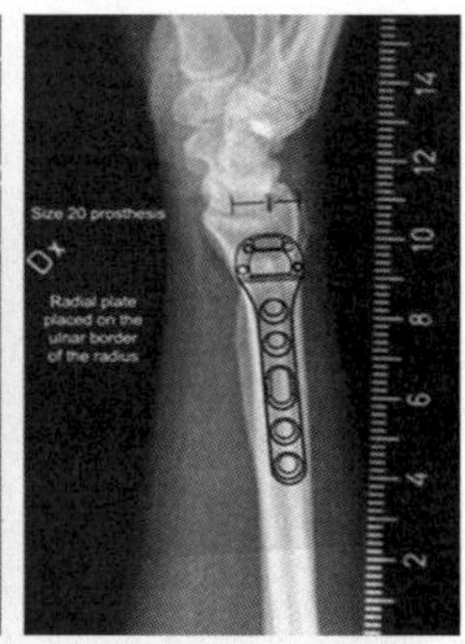

FIG 4 • Preoperative templating for the Aptis system is done in the frontal and lateral planes to determine the appropriate size of implants to be used at surgery.

after trauma or tumor resection, a constrained total DRUJ replacement should be used (**FIG 3**).

- The radial component consists of a plate with a polyethylene-lined metal sphere affixed to the interosseous surface of the radius.
- The ulnar stem has a protruding peg that is captured and rotates within the polyethylene liner. The stem has limited freedom of proximodistal and limited dorsopalmar motion, simulating normal DRUJ mechanics.

Preoperative Planning

- Preoperative radiographs of both sides are used for templating (**FIG 4**).
  - Normal anatomy and ulnar variance are reproduced to the extent possible.
  - The appropriate implant size is chosen.

Positioning

- Standard positioning and tourniquet application are used.

Approach

- An incision is made along the ulnar border of the shaft of the distal ulna in line with the ulnar styloid. The interval between the flexor carpi ulnaris (FCU) and extensor carpi ulnaris (ECU) tendons is developed for access to the ulna.
- A dorsal approach is an alternative and is indicated for partial head replacement. Access to the articular portion of the ulnar head is gained through the floor of the fifth extensor compartment.

Partial Ulnar Head Replacement Arthroplasty

- Evaluate preoperative radiographs (**TECH FIG 1A**).
- Make a longitudinal skin incision over the DRUJ between the fifth and sixth extensor compartments (**TECH FIG 1B**).
- Divide the extensor retinaculum of the fifth compartment (**TECH FIG 1C**).
- Retract the extensor digiti minimi tendon.
- Create an ulnarly based combined retinaculum and DRUJ rectangular capsular flap, with care to make the distal limb of the capsulotomy just proximal to the dorsal radioulnar ligament.
- Leave the ECU subsheath and ECU tendon in place.
- Dorsally subluxate the ulnar head from sigmoid notch using a small Hohmann retractor placed under the head.

A 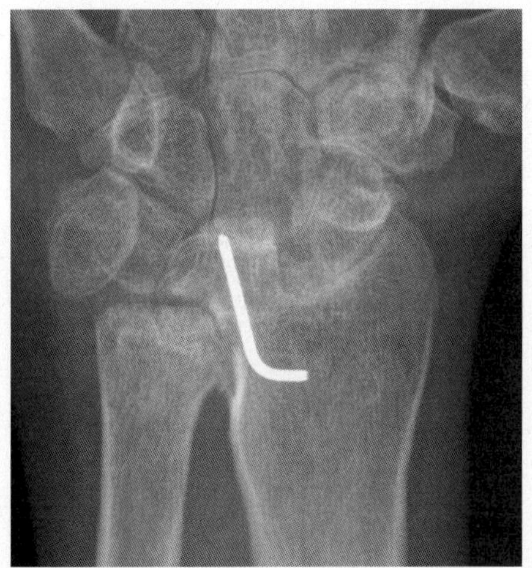

B 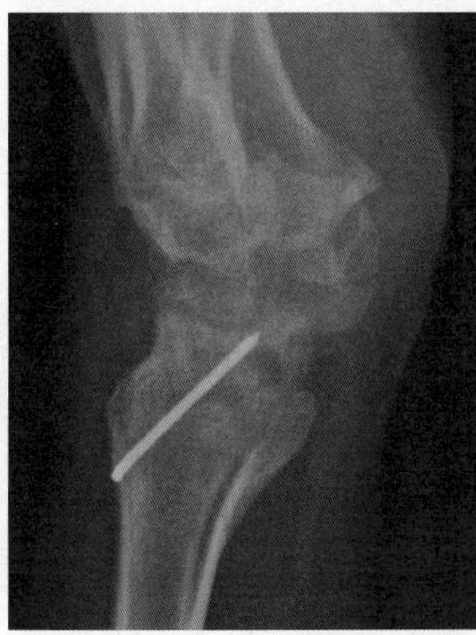

TECH FIG 1 • A,B. Preoperative radiographs of a patient with rheumatoid arthritis and previous radiolunate fusion who treat with First Choice partial ulnar head arthroplasty (Integra LifeSciences, Plainsboro, NJ). *(continued)*

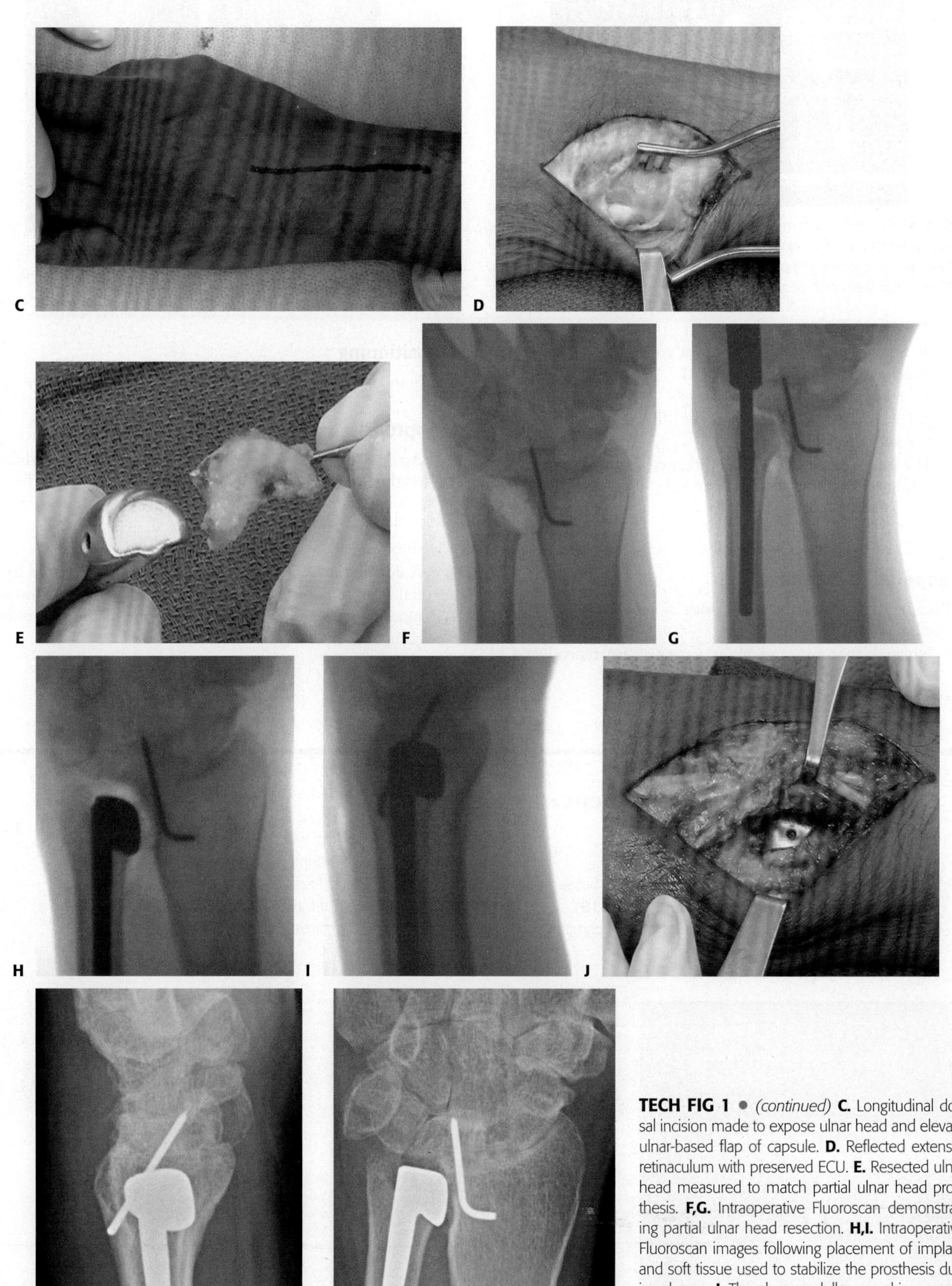

TECH FIG 1 • *(continued)* **C.** Longitudinal dorsal incision made to expose ulnar head and elevate ulnar-based flap of capsule. **D.** Reflected extensor retinaculum with preserved ECU. **E.** Resected ulnar head measured to match partial ulnar head prosthesis. **F,G.** Intraoperative Fluoroscan demonstrating partial ulnar head resection. **H,I.** Intraoperative Fluoroscan images following placement of implant and soft tissue used to stabilize the prosthesis during closure. **J.** The ulnar medullary canal is reamed. **K,L.** Postoperative radiographs of partial ulnar head prosthesis.

- Resect the articular portion of the ulnar head using a customized jig specific to the implant system to be used (**TECH FIG 1D,E**).
- Ream the ulnar medullary canal and place a trial prosthesis of the appropriate size (**TECH FIG 1F**). Obtain intraoperative radiographs to confirm correct sizing of head and ulnar variance.
- Ascertain range of motion and stability and insert a definitive prosthesis. Repair the capsular flap and retinaculum together and imbricate it only if necessary for stability (**TECH FIG 1G**).
- Confirm stability with postoperative radiographs (**TECH FIG 1H**).

Ulnar Head Hemiarthroplasty (without Sigmoid Notch Resurfacing)

- Make a longitudinal skin incision on the ulnar border of the distal forearm (**TECH FIG 2A**).
- Incise the extensor retinaculum along the medial border of the distal ulna between the ECU and FCU.
  - Identify and protect the dorsal cutaneous branch of the ulnar nerve as it crosses from volar to dorsal across the most distal part of the incision.
- Elevate the ECU tendon subsheath subperiosteally off the distal ulna along with the TFCC and ulnar collateral ligament distally.
- Determine the resection level of the distal ulna using a template and mark it with a pen or osteotome (**TECH FIG 2B**).
  - The aim is to create ulnar neutral variance after the implant is in place.
  - When the distal ulna has been previously excised, use the distal end of the sigmoid fossa of the distal radius as a landmark to determine the ulnar osteotomy level.
- With soft tissue retractors in place, use an oscillating saw to osteotomize the distal ulna (**TECH FIG 2C**).
  - Take care to ensure that the cut is perpendicular to the long axis of the ulna.
- Remove and size the ulnar head.
  - To allow for easy identification for soft tissue repair, place a tagging suture into the TFCC attachment in the fovea before releasing it from the ulna.
- Inspect the sigmoid notch of the distal radius for incongruity. Remove osteophytes.
- Define the intramedullary canal of the distal ulna using an awl or sharp broach. Gently enlarge the canal to the appropriate stem size using broaches of increasing diameter (**TECH FIG 2D**).
- Gently impact the appropriate trial stem into the shaft of the distal ulna (**TECH FIG 2E**). The collar should seat firmly against the resected surface of the distal ulna.
  - In cases with previous excessive ulnar resection, a prosthesis with an extended collar may be indicated.
  - To ascertain the need for an extended collar, place a trial spacer on the neck of the trial stem before placing the trial head.

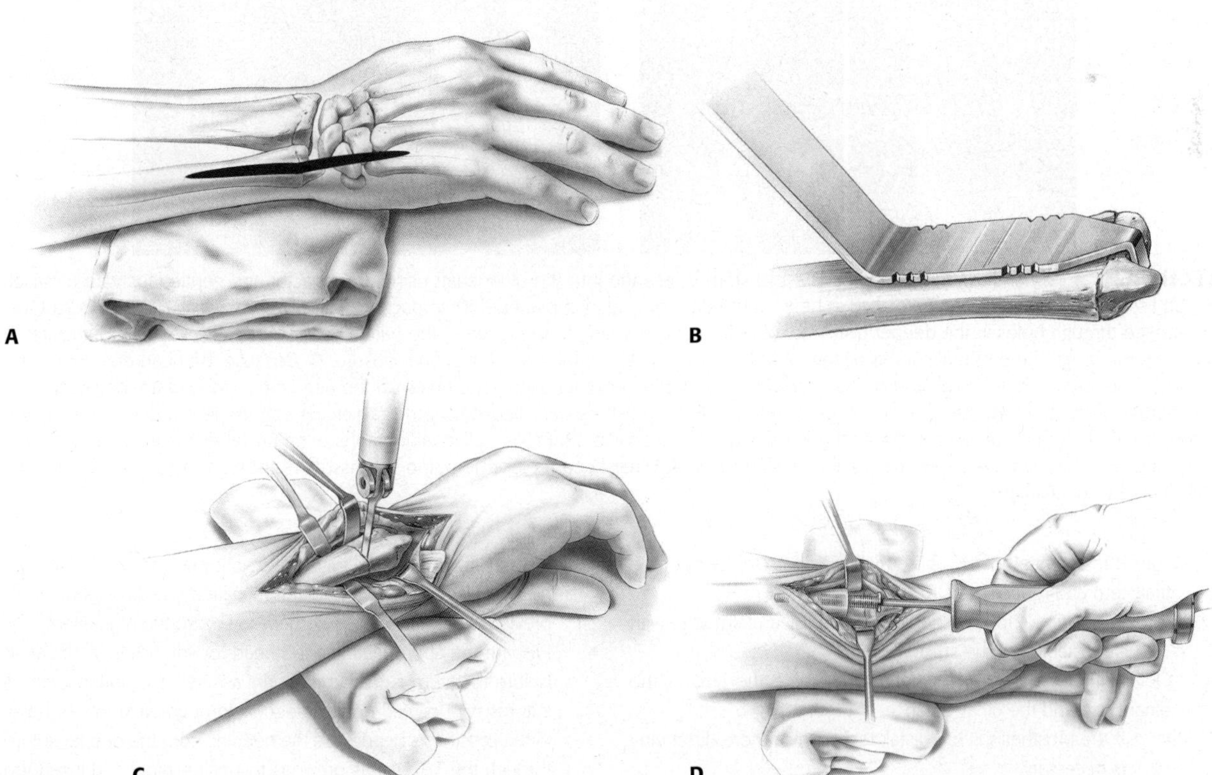

TECH FIG 2 • **A.** A longitudinal incision is made between the FCU and ECU tendons on the ulnar border of the distal forearm and wrist. **B.** The cutting guide helps determine the level of resection of the ulnar head. The distal notches are for use with the three head sizes and standard stem, and the proximal notches are for use with a collared stem in cases of previous resection or resorption of the distal ulna. **C.** An oscillating saw is used to resect the ulnar head at the determined level. **D.** The ulnar medullary cavity is reamed using broaches. *(continued)*

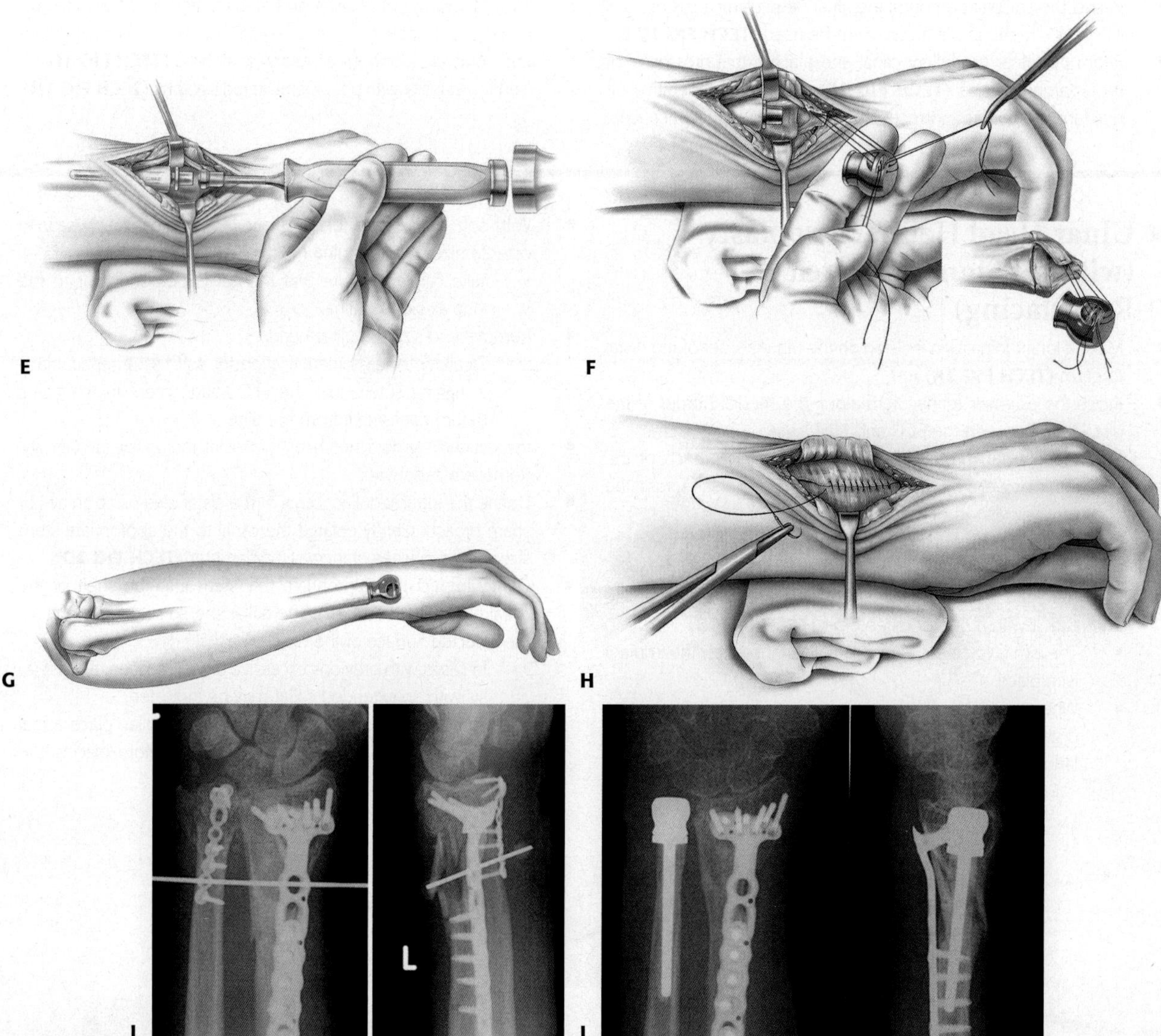

TECH FIG 2 • *(continued)* **E.** The appropriate trial stem is inserted into the ulnar shaft using an impactor and gentle taps with a mallet. **F.** Soft tissue–stabilizing sutures are placed in holes in the definitive head implant before impaction onto the stem (*inset*). The TFCC sutures are passed through holes in the deeper distal row of holes corresponding to the fovea of the native head. Sutures from the ECU subsheath are passed through the proximal superficial row of holes. The sutures are left untied until final closure. **G.** Because the head does not freely rotate on the stem, it is essential to align the head before impaction onto the stem. The holes on the head are lined up with the subcutaneous border of the ulna. **H.** After the pull-through sutures of the prosthesis are tied down, the remaining soft tissue envelope deep to the extensor retinaculum is approximated with the forearm in neutral position. **I.** Preoperative radiographs of an unstable and incongruous ulnar head after comminuted fracture of the distal radius and ulna. **J.** Ulnar head replacement and soft tissue imbrication restored congruity and stability to the articulation.

- Place the trial head of the appropriate size onto the neck of the trial stem and reduce the DRUJ.
  - Supination and pronation should be full and smooth, with no instability at the articulation.
- Obtain intraoperative radiographs to evaluate the size of the ulnar head and the ulnar variance.
  - If the prosthesis is too distal, resection of more distal ulna is necessary.
- Remove the trial implant by gently applying anteriorly directed pressure on the distal ulna to dislodge the ulnar head from the sigmoid notch.
- If a firm fit is obtained with the trial, a press-fit technique may be used with the final implant. In patients with osteopenia or previous wrist fusion, use cement to secure the ulnar stem.
- Prepare the appropriately sized head for soft tissue stabilization before the stem is fully impacted. Pass two 3-0 nonabsorbable sutures with curved double needles through each row of holes in the prosthesis head. Pass the needles from the deeper suture through the TFCC at its previous foveal insertion, and insert the needles from the superficial suture into the ECU subsheath. Leave the sutures untied (**TECH FIG 2F**).
- Insert and impact the final stem (with or without cement) using the stem impactor.

- Align the head of the prosthesis such that the two rows of suture holes are along the subcutaneous border of the ulna (**TECH FIG 2G**). Then place it onto the tapered neck of the stem and gently impact it.
- Advance the soft tissues ulnarly over the head of the prosthesis as it is reduced into the sigmoid notch. With the forearm in midrotation, tie down the sutures placed in the head, closing the ECU subsheath over the top of the prosthesis.
- Imbricate the remaining soft tissue envelope over the distal ulna while approximating the FCU–ECU interface (**TECH FIG 2H**).
- Check the stability of the prosthesis in supination and pronation.
- Close the extensor retinaculum over the capsule.
- Obtain final radiographs (**TECH FIG 2I,J**).
- Obtain hemostasis after the tourniquet is deflated.
- Obtain repeat radiographs at the first postoperative follow-up to confirm stability of prosthesis within the sigmoid notch (**TECH FIG 3A–C**).

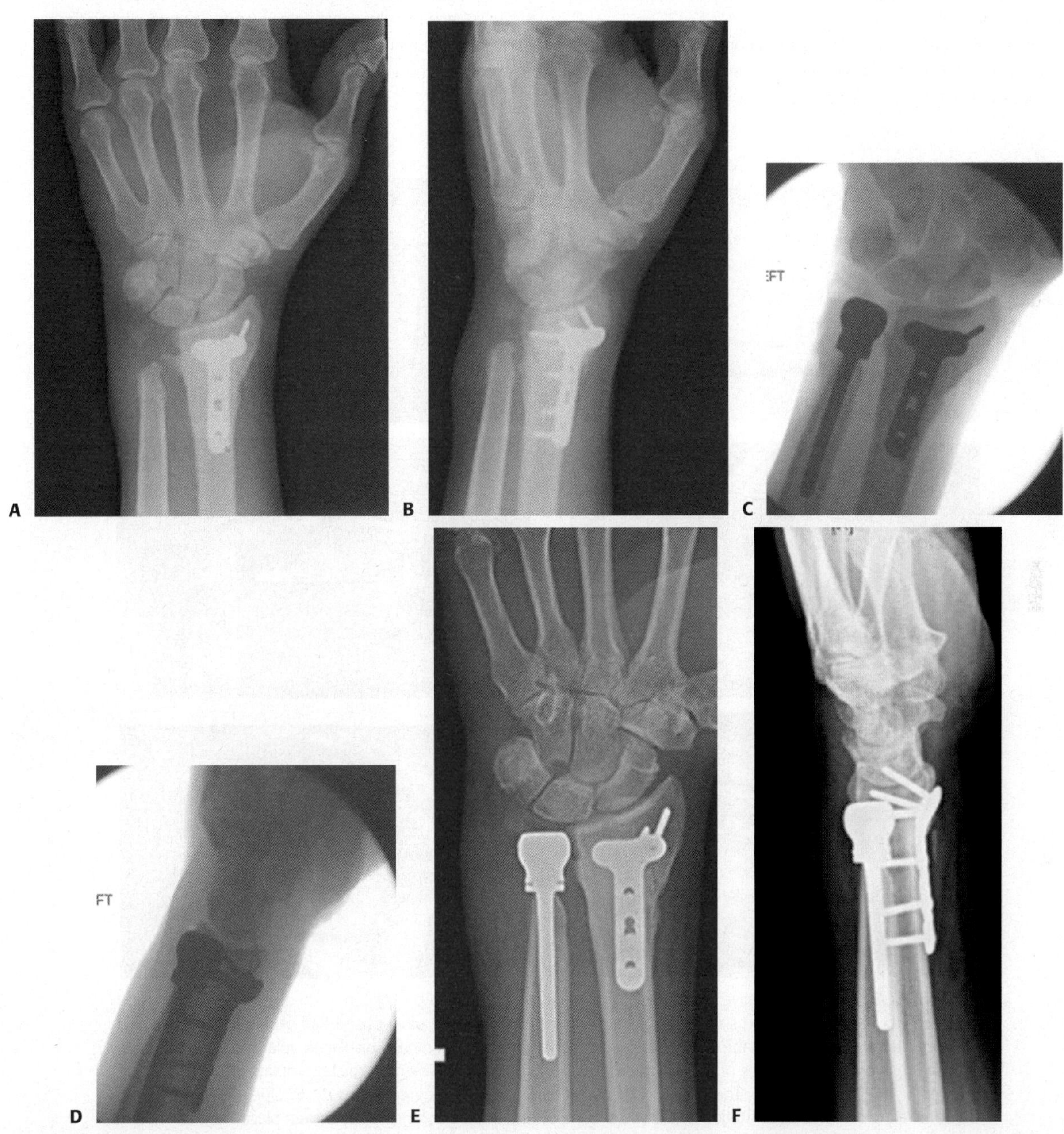

TECH FIG 3 • **A,B.** Preoperative posteroanterior (PA) and oblique radiographs demonstrating previous Darrach procedure and distal radius plate for a distal radius fracture treated 1.5 years prior to presentation. **C,D.** Intraoperative Fluoroscan images status post ulnar head prosthesis insertion. **E,F.** Six-week postoperative radiographs of ulnar head prosthesis demonstrating stability of implant.

Constrained Distal Radioulnar Joint Arthroplasty

- Make an 8-cm longitudinal incision in the shape of a hockey stick along the ulnar border of the distal forearm between the fifth and sixth dorsal extensor compartments (**TECH FIG 4A**).
- Create a rectangular ulnarly based fascia flap (**TECH FIG 4B**). Use the flap to create a barrier between the prosthesis and the ECU at closure.
  - The width of the flap should cover the head of the implant and may include the most proximal part of the extensor retinaculum.
- Expose the distal ulna through the floor of the fifth extensor compartment and mobilize the tendons of the extensor digiti minimi proximally for a distance of 8 cm.
- Divide the sensory branch of the posterior interosseous nerve to avoid avulsion of the nerve from the thumb extensors when placing an elevator between the extensor mass and the radius.
- Incise the ECU sheath to its insertion at the base of the fifth metacarpal.
  - This is to avoid pressure against the distal end of the implant.
- Excise the remaining head of the ulna at a level just proximal to the cartilage or where the DRUJ would have been.
- Leave the radial attachment of the TFCC undisturbed to provide a barrier between the prosthesis and the carpal bones.
- Displace the ulnar shaft in a volar direction to expose the radius and sigmoid notch (**TECH FIG 4C**).
- Elevate the interosseous membrane along the distal 8 cm of the radius.

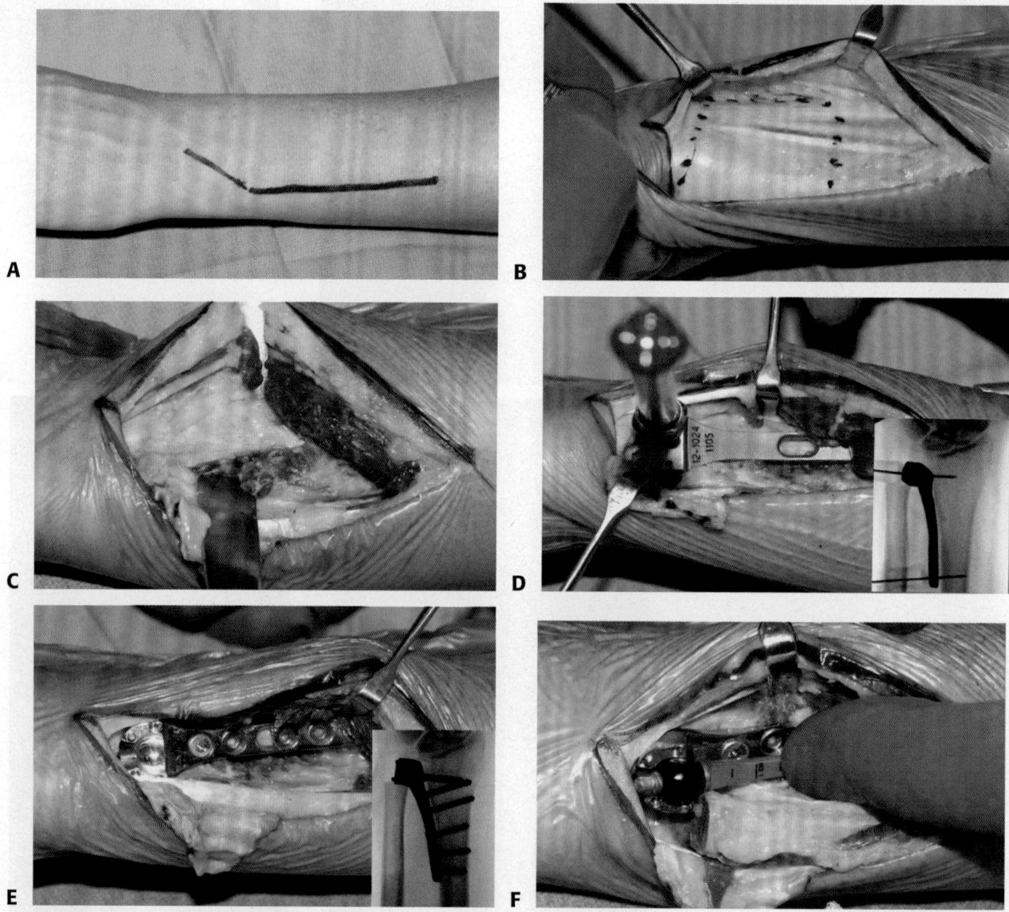

TECH FIG 4 ● **A.** Intraoperative photograph of implantation with the Aptis system. The dorsoulnar skin incision is placed between the fifth and sixth extensor compartments. **B.** A large ulnar-based flap of retinaculum is raised for later interposition between the ECU tendon and the implant. **C.** The ulna is displaced volarly with retractors to expose the interosseous surface of the radius and the sigmoid notch. **D.** The radial plate template is positioned and temporarily fixed to the radius. The plate's position is checked with radiographs (*inset*). **E.** Operative photograph demonstrating completion of fixation of the radial component. Radiographs confirm correct placement of implant and screw length (*inset*). **F.** A sizer with an attached ball is used to determine the level of ulnar resection. This ensures that the ulnar implant with seated polyethylene ball will be level with the radial socket. *(continued)*

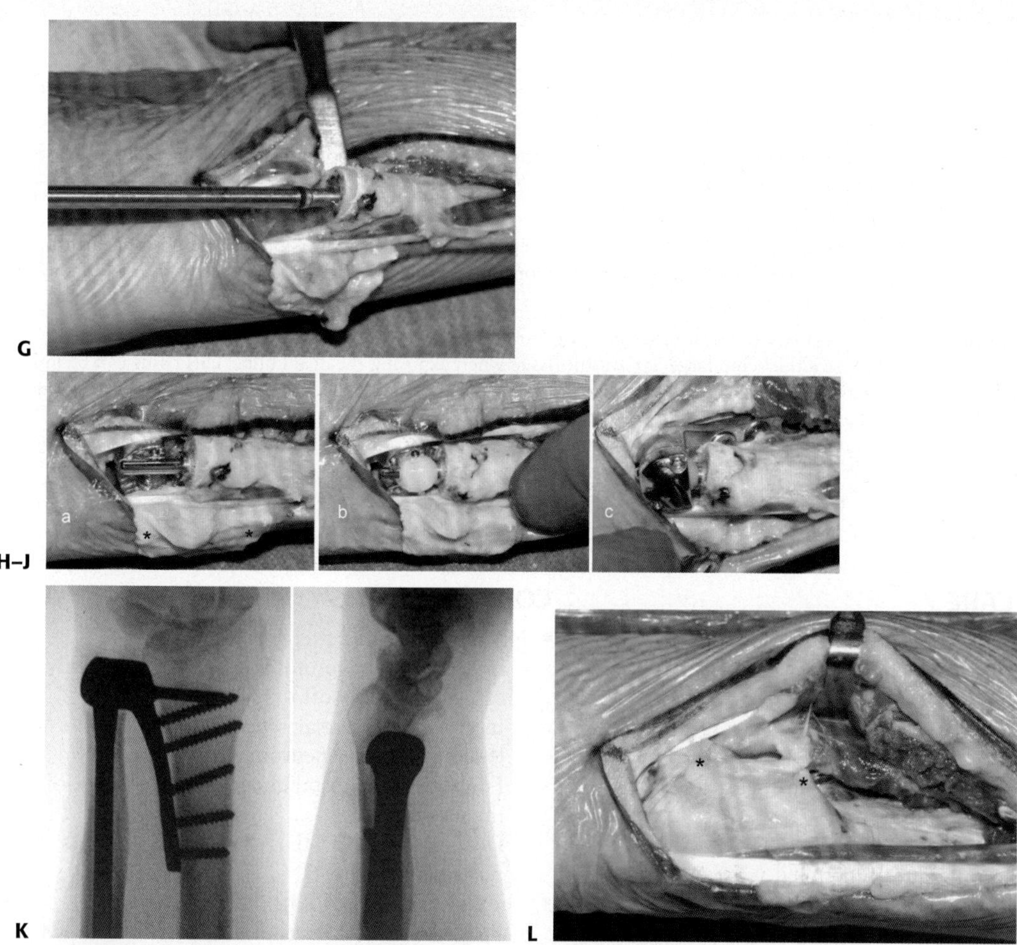

TECH FIG 4 • *(continued)* **G.** Medullary broaches are used to enlarge the medullary canal of the distal ulna. **H–J.** Steps for final assembly of the system. After the ulnar stem is inserted, the polyethylene ball is placed over the peg. The ball is then aligned with the radial socket and the cap is placed over it and secured with two screws. **K.** Final radiographs demonstrate correct placement of the implant. **L.** The previously raised retinacular flap (marked by *asterisks*) is then placed over the prosthesis and beneath the ECU tendon.

- Place the radial trial plate over the interosseous crest of the radius with the volar border aligned with the volar surface of the radius (**TECH FIG 4D**).
  - The plate should lie at least 3 mm proximal to the distal end of the sigmoid notch of the radius to avoid impaction with the carpus.
- Use a burr to contour the distal radius as necessary to accommodate the plate. Position the plate and hold it temporarily with Kirschner wires passed through the plate.
- Use intraoperative imaging to check the position of the plate.
- After drilling the hole for the radial peg, remove the trial and gently impact the final radial component in place. Insert fixation screws into the radius to secure the implant and take radiographs (**TECH FIG 4E**). Remove the Kirschner wires.
- With the forearm fully pronated, seat a sizer with attached ball into the hemisocket of the radius and align it with the ulna (**TECH FIG 4F**). Determine the level of ulnar resection.
- After resecting the distal ulna, insert a 1.6-mm guidewire into the medullary canal and use a cannulated drill to ream the canal.
- Insert a medullary broach of the appropriate size into the canal to bevel the distal ulna and plane its distal end (**TECH FIG 4G**).
- Irrigate the medullary canal and insert the stem of the ulnar component (**TECH FIG 4H**). Place the ultra-high-molecular-weight polyethylene ball over the distal peg and position the ulnar component within the hemisocket of the radial component (**TECH FIG 4I**).
- Position the cover of the socket over the ball and secure it with two small screws (**TECH FIG 4J**).
- Obtain radiographs to confirm satisfactory positioning of the prosthesis (**TECH FIG 4K**).
- Position the fascia and retinacular flap between the prosthesis and the ECU tendon and suture them to the radius before doing a layered closure (**TECH FIG 4L**).

PEARLS AND PITFALLS

Scar sensitivity or tenderness	▪ Identify and protect the sensory branch of the ulnar nerve.
Intraoperative fracture of the distal ulna	▪ Broach the distal ulna with caution. In hard cortical bone, use a drill to enlarge the cavity before impacting a broach in the ulna.
Incorrect ulnar variance	▪ Before making the ulnar osteotomy, identify the correct level of the DRUJ using radiographs or along the distal edge of the sigmoid notch.
Loosening of prosthesis	▪ Rule out metal allergy, infection. ▪ Revision options include (1) explanting prosthesis, (2) conversion to interposition arthroplasty with Achilles tendon allograft, (3) conversion to total linked distal DRUJ arthroplasty, or (4) conversion to a one-bone forearm.
Instability of the prosthesis	▪ Correct soft tissue insufficiency prior to prosthesis implantation. ▪ Raise a thick and large flap of soft tissue when exposing the distal ulna. This tissue can be imbricated to stabilize the prosthesis if needed. Alternatively, a distally based strip of the FCU can be wound around the prosthesis to provide volar stability. ▪ Stability of the implant may not be to demonstrate intraoperatively until the soft tissue envelope is closed over the prosthesis.

POSTOPERATIVE CARE

- The forearm is immobilized in neutral rotation and held in a supportive long-arm or Muenster-type splint or cast for 3 weeks.
- Active range of motion of the wrist and forearm is initiated at 3 weeks.
  - A removable splint is required between therapy sessions for 3 weeks.
- Therapy is advanced as tolerated after 6 weeks, with strengthening starting only after functional wrist and forearm motion has been obtained.
- For a patient with rheumatoid arthritis, poor-quality soft tissue coverage, or mild instability intraoperatively, immobilization in supination for up to 6 weeks must be considered.
- Postoperative radiographs should be obtained at 6 weeks, 6 months, and then yearly.

OUTCOMES

- Outcomes vary with the indication and type of prosthesis used.[3]
- The pain of radioulnar impingement is relieved in patients with previous excision arthroplasty and stability is restored.[9]
- The range of motion of the forearm after prosthetic replacement remains largely unchanged, as it depends on previous scarring.
- Grip strength recovered depends on the underlying problem, but in patients with severe pain and weakness preoperatively, final grip averages about 60% of the opposite side.
- Long-term results are limited and variable.
- One study reported 6-year survival of implant as 83%.[7]
- Implant failure was associated with a history of previous surgery, use of an extended collar, lucency greater than 2 mm around the implant stem, and pedestal formation at the tip of the implant.[7]
- Continued pain relief and no deterioration or revision requirements were seen in other small, longer term follow-up studies.[10,11]

COMPLICATIONS

- Immediate- or short-term complications
  - Infection and wound breakdown, especially in revision cases with poor soft tissue cover
  - Injury to the dorsal sensory branch of the ulnar nerve, leading to tender neuroma
  - Fracture of the distal ulna during reaming or impaction of the prosthesis
  - Dislocation of the prosthesis from the DRUJ postoperatively
- Long-term complications
  - Progressive degeneration of the sigmoid notch
  - Implant loosening
  - Tenosynovitis of the ECU tendon
  - Erosion of the radius sigmoid notch with pain
  - Ectopic bone formation around the distal ulna
  - Stress shielding and resorption of distal ulna
  - Prosthetic fracture

ACKNOWLEDGMENTS

The authors thank Small Bone Innovations for permission to use their illustrations for demonstration of operative technique, Dr. Luis Scheker for the images of the Aptis system and Dr. Marc Garcia-Elias for the images of the Eclypse prosthesis.

REFERENCES

1. Berger RA. Implant arthroplasty for treatment of ulnar head resection-related instability. Hand Clin 2013;29:103–111.
2. Berger RA, Cooney WP III. Use of an ulnar head endoprosthesis for treatment of an unstable distal ulnar resection: review of mechanics, indications, and surgical technique. Hand Clin 2005;21:603–620.
3. Bizimungu R, Dodds S. Objective outcomes following semi-constrained total distal radioulnar joint arthroplasty. J Wrist Surg 2013;2:319–323.
4. Conaway DA, Kuhl TL, Adams BD. Comparison of the native ulnar head and a partial ulnar head resurfacing implant. J Hand Surg Am 2009;34(6):1056–1062.

5. Garcia-Elias M. Eclypse: partial ulnar head replacement for isolated DRUJ arthrosis. Tech Hand Upper Extrem Surg 2007;11:121–128.
6. Gordon KD, Roth SE, Dunning CE, et al. An anthropometric study of the distal ulna: Implications for implant design. J Hand Surg Am 2002;27(1):57–60.
7. Kakar S, Swann P, Perry KI, et al. Functional and radiographic outcomes following distal ulna implant arthroplasty. J Hand Surg Am 2012;37:1364–1371.
8. Scheker LR, Babb BA, Killion PE. Distal ulnar prosthetic replacement. Orthop Clin North Am 2001;32:365–376.
9. Van Schoonhoven J, Fernandez DL, Bowers WH, et al. Salvage of failed resection arthroplasties of the distal radioulnar joint using a new ulnar head prosthesis. J Hand Surg Am 2000;25(3):438–446.
10. Van Schoonhoven J, Muhldorfer-Fodor M, Fernandez DL, et al. Salvage of failed resection arthroplasties of the distal radioulnar joint using an ulnar head prosthesis: long-term results. J Hand Surg Am 2012;37:1372–1380.
11. Yen SN, Dion GR, Bowers WH. Ulnar head implant arthroplasty: an intermediate term review of 1 surgeon's experience. Tech Hand Up Extrem Surg 2009;13:160–164.

Arthroscopically Assisted Triangular Fibrocartilage Complex Débridement and Ulnar Shortening

Brandon P. Donnelly and Randall W. Culp

DEFINITION

- The triangular fibrocartilage complex (TFCC) is a homogenous anatomic structure located on the ulnar aspect of the wrist that is responsible for distal radioulnar joint (DRUJ) stability and transfers load across the wrist from the ulnar carpus to the distal ulna.[21]
- Injury to the TFCC and subsequent synovitis is associated with ulnar-sided wrist pain, weakness of grip, and painful clicking about the DRUJ often resulting in patient disability.
- Ulnocarpal abutment or ulnar impaction syndrome is characterized by ulnar-sided wrist pain associated with a TFCC tear and accompanying variable chondromalacia of the ulnar head, lunate, and triquetrum surfaces. The degenerative process typically occurs in ulnar positive or neutral variance from chronic compressive overloading of the ulnocarpal joint.
- Arthroscopic TFCC débridement is indicated for centrally based lesions and may be combined with ulnar shortening in light of concomitant ulnocarpal abutment.

ANATOMY

- The TFCC is a confluence of cartilaginous and ligamentous structures that span and support the DRUJ and ulnocarpal articulations. It arises from the distal aspect of the radial sigmoid notch and inserts into the base of the ulnar styloid and fovea (**FIG 1**).
  - The ulnocarpal complex, consisting of the ulnolunate ligament, ulnotriquetral ligament, and extensor carpi ulnaris (ECU) subsheath, spans the ulnocarpal joint.
  - The superficial limbs of the dorsal and palmar radioulnar ligaments insert onto the base of the ulnar styloid, whereas the deep limbs insert into the fovea.[11]
  - The central articular disc is a thin fibrocartilage structure, spanning from the distal rim of the sigmoid notch and blends with the radioulnar ligaments.

PATHOGENESIS

- Acute, Palmer I, TFCC injuries typically result from an axial load in ulnar deviation, combined with forearm rotation. Biomechanically, the TFCC becomes compressed and stretched between the ulna and lunate producing a tear.
  - These injuries typically occur in falls on a pronated outstretched hand or activities that require forceful ulnar deviation of the wrist (eg, golf and racquet sports).
- Intra-articular distal radius fractures show a high incidence of concomitant tears of the triangular fibrocartilage, 50% to 84%.[6,13] However, many of these tears are minimally symptomatic and do not require surgical intervention.[16]
- Chronic degenerative tears of the TFCC are associated with ulnar positive variance and ulnar carpal impaction (**FIG 2**).
  - Ulnar positive variance occurs with any condition that causes a relative greater ulnar than radial length at the wrist. These include distal radius malunion, Essex-Lopresti lesion, developmental positive ulnar variance, and premature radial physeal closure.

FIG 1 • TFCC anatomy.

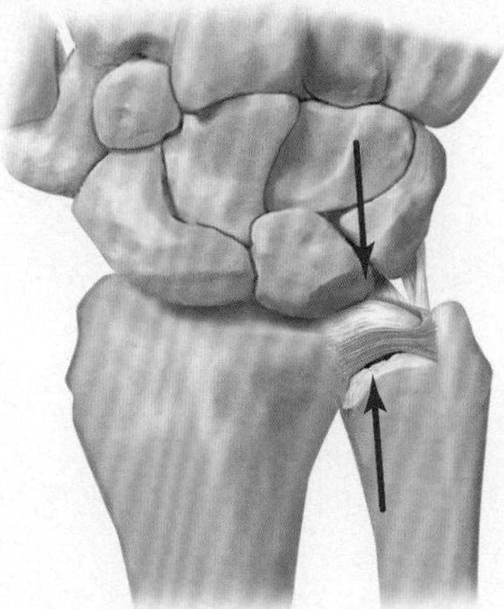

FIG 2 • Ulnar abutment. The TFCC is compressed between the proximal ulnar lunate and the distal ulnar head.

- Degenerative tears result from chronic load to the ulnar side of the wrist. In an ulnar neutral wrist, the ulnar carpus absorbs 18% of axial load. This increases to 42% when ulnar variance is increased 2.5 mm and decreases to 4.3% when ulnar variance is decreased 2.5 mm.[20]

NATURAL HISTORY

- The natural history of Palmer type I TFCC tears is not well understood. Many type IA lesions without instability respond to nonoperative management.[22] In a long-term follow-up, Mrkonjic et al[16] showed that distal radius fracture associated TFCC tears with a stable DRUJ showed some increased laxity and decreased grip strength but did not require routine surgical treatment.
  - Surgical débridement for failed conservatively treated type IA lesions showed excellent success.[18] However, high failure rates were noticed when TFCC débridement alone was performed in the ulnar positive wrist.[15]
  - Types I B, C, and D tears may result in clinical instability of the DRUJ and require surgical intervention to restore stability.
- Degenerative tears (type II) are nontraumatic with a natural history that shows TFCC attrition in more than half of patients older than 50 years of age.[3] Also, after the fifth decade, 100% of TFCCs evaluated showed an abnormal appearance but usually asymptomatic.[4]
  - Symptomatic degenerative tears typically have progressive degenerative changes that involve the ulnocarpal joint surfaces, which may or may not strictly follow the progressive cascade in accordance with Palmer's classification: TFCC wear (IIA), ulnar or lunate chondromalacia (IIB), central TFCC perforation (IIC), lunotriquetral ligament tear (IID), and arthritic changes of the lunate and triquetrum (IIE).
- It is possible to have components of a type I traumatic tear in a wrist with a preexisting degenerative TFCC, in which an acute flap causes mechanical symptoms. In this case, arthroscopic débridement alone may not improve symptoms and ulnocarpal decompression is warranted.

PATIENT HISTORY AND PHYSICAL EXAMINATION

- Patients often report ulnar-sided wrist pain occurring after a fall. They may also complain of clicking, catching, weakness, localized swelling, and a sense of instability.
- Physical examination reveals swelling over the ulnar wrist, with focal tenderness over the TFCC and distal ulna.
  - Fovea sign—direct pressure applied to the fovea region that reproduces their pain had 95.2% sensitivity and 86.5% specificity for TFCC foveal disruption and/or ulnotriquetral ligament injury.[24]
  - Ulnocarpal palpation—pain at the ulnocarpal joint suggests synovitis or TFCC pathology.
  - TFCC stress test—ulnar deviation and axial loading of wrist reproduces a painful click with forearm rotation.
  - Ulnocarpal stress test—pain reproduced during pronation and supination of the forearm with the wrist in ulnar deviation
  - Pisiform boost test—increased pain of passive and active ulnar deviation with dorsally directed pressure applied over the palmar aspect of the pisiform, resulting in a lifting of the carpus
- The DRUJ must be assessed for instability with shuck or "piano key" test. The distal radius is held in one hand and the other hand stresses the distal ulna volarly and dorsally in neutral rotation, pronation, and supination. This must be compared to the contralateral side.
  - Instability suggests disruption of the radioulnar ligaments.

IMAGING AND OTHER DIAGNOSTIC STUDIES

- The radiographic evaluation of a patient with ulnar abutment should include a standard wrist series, a Palmer 90 × 90 neutral rotation view[19] and a fully pronated grip stress view.[25]
  - The Palmer 90 × 90 view places the forearm in neutral rotation while the elbow is flexed to 90 degrees and the shoulder is abducted to 90 degrees. The static ulnar variance is calculated from this view (**FIG 3**).
  - The fully pronated grip stress view has the shoulder adducted to the patient's side and slightly externally rotated, the forearm is pronated, and the patient is asked to make a fist of maximum intensity. An increase ulnar variance indicates dynamic variance.
  - Ulnar impaction is suspected in a patient with an ulnar-zero or ulnar-plus variance. Subchondral cystic and sclerotic joint changes in the lunate indicate probable ulnar impaction (**FIG 4**).
- Magnetic resonance imaging (MRI) evaluation of the triangular fibrocartilage can aid in diagnosis especially in central tears. Magnetic resonance (MR) arthrogram has been shown to be more sensitive than standard MR imaging but can have higher false positives.[12,23]
  - On T2 imaging, an intact TFCC has a homogenous low signal.
  - An MRI should be considered for ulnar impaction syndrome in the absence of clear radiographic findings. Characteristic early findings include bone hyperemia in the lunate, triquetrum, and ulnar head, which has low signal intensity on T1-weighted images and high signal intensity on T2-weighted images (**FIG 5A,B**).[9]
  - Computed tomography (CT) arthrography has been shown to have high sensitivity and specificity in diagnosing central TFCC tears and can be used when MRI is contraindicated.[12,17,23]

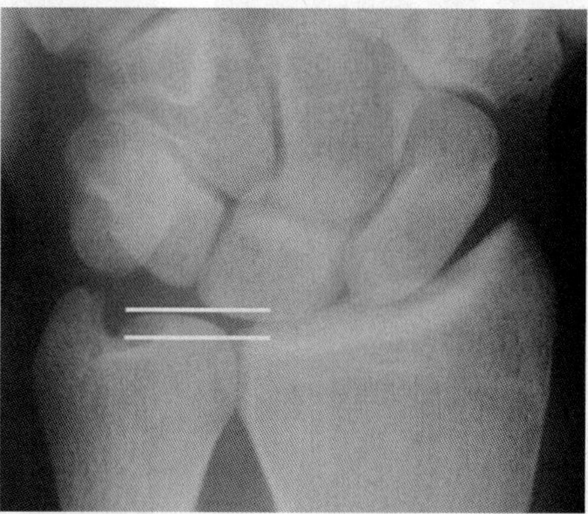

FIG 3 • Ulnar-plus variance is shown on a 90 × 90 neutral rotation view.

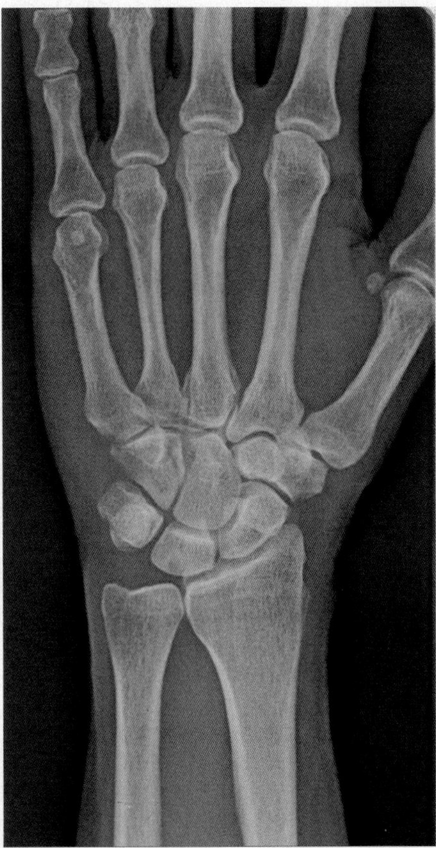

FIG 4 • PA radiograph of a wrist with ulnar abutment showing positive ulnar variance and cystic changes within the lunate.

DIFFERENTIAL DIAGNOSIS

- TFCC tear
- Ulnocarpal impaction
- Ulnocarpal synovitis
- Ulnar extrinsic ligament tear
- Lunotriquetral joint instability
- DRUJ instability
- DRUJ arthritis
- Ulnar styloid nonunion
- Pisotriquetral arthritis
- Kienböck disease

NONOPERATIVE TREATMENT

- Nonoperative management is indicated for the initial treatment of TFCC tears in the absence of DRUJ instability.
  - Immobilization of the wrist and forearm with a sugar-tong or long-arm splint for 4 weeks, combined with a course of nonsteroidal anti-inflammatories
  - Intra-articular steroid injection can be helpful in patients who present acutely.
  - Activity modifications are used to avoid movements that exacerbate the pain.
- Postimmobilization therapy includes gradual range of motion and strengthening, but avoid torque or forceful grasp for 8 weeks.
- Three to 4 months of nonoperative treatment is a reasonable plan prior to surgical intervention.

SURGICAL MANAGEMENT

- Surgical treatment is indicated in the symptomatic patient after failure of nonoperative management.
  - Wrist arthroscopy is performed to evaluate the TFCC, ulnocarpal articular surfaces, and intercarpal ligaments.
- Type IA tears have been shown to respond well to arthroscopic débridement in the absence of ulnar positive variance. Types I B to D tears are often treated with repair and discussed elsewhere in this text.
- Treatment of degenerative fibrocartilage complex tears begins with arthroscopic TFCC débridement and includes ulnar shortening in the ulnar positive or neutral patient (IIA to IIC). Additional lunotriquetral ligament débridement and possible pinning along with diaphyseal ulnar shortening osteotomy are indicated for IID and IIE TFCC tears.
  - Mechanical débridement of the triangular fibrocartilage with a 2.5- or 2.7-mm shaver has been successful,

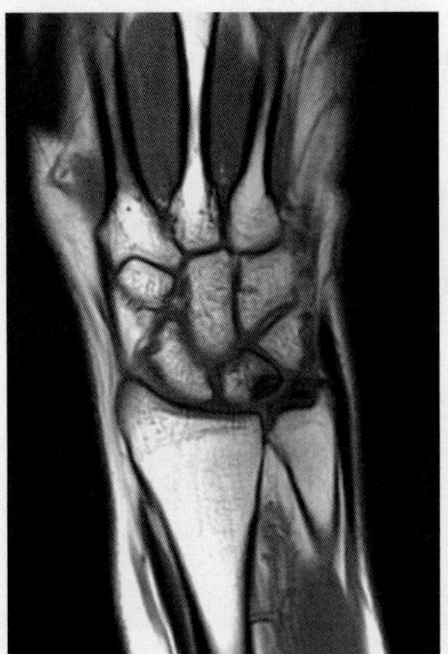

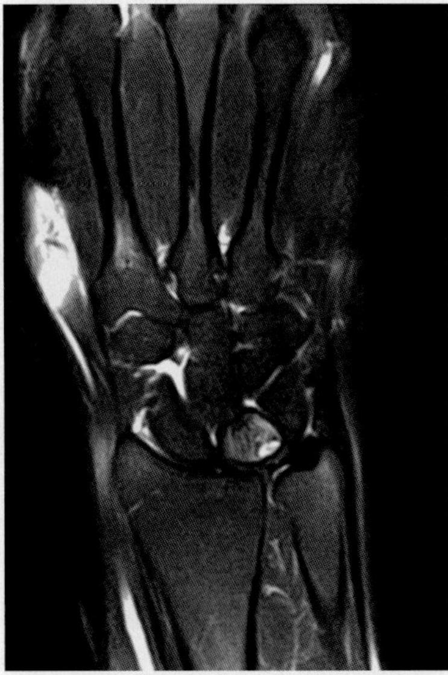

FIG 5 • **A.** T1-weighted MRI of a wrist with ulnar abutment demonstrating low signal intensity at the proximal lunate. **B.** T2-weighted MRI of a wrist showing increased signal intensity within the proximal lunate and TFCC demonstrating ulnar abutment.

although it can be challenging, particularly in regard to the débridement of the ulnar and dorsal aspects of the triangular fibrocartilage tear.
  - Radiofrequency ablation probes have become increasingly popular for TFCC débridement and are useful for removal of torn fragments of fibrocartilage.[5]
- Arthroscopic ulnar shortening by burr excision of the ulnar dome is indicated in patients with a TFCC tear who have ulnar impaction with less than 4 mm ulnar-plus variance that do not respond to nonoperative treatment.
  - The goal of the surgery is to create an ulnar neutral to minus variance of 2 mm.

Preoperative Planning

- Preoperative radiographic evaluation is paramount to determine ulnar variance and evidence of ulnar impaction.
  - The patient must be informed that an arthroscopically assisted ulnar shortening may not be possible should there be laxity of the ulnocarpal ligaments, a peripheral TFCC tear, or lunotriquetral laxity.
  - The amount of shortening should be calculated preoperatively, with no more than 4 mm resection possible for arthroscopic shortening.
  - The surgeon should verify that the operating room is equipped with a mini C-arm to confirm intraoperatively the amount of ulna resected.

Positioning

- The patient is placed supine, using the hand table, with the arm in a position accessible to fluoroscopic imaging.
- A well-padded pneumatic tourniquet is placed on the proximal arm.
- The involved extremity is prepared and draped in the usual fashion.
- The wrist is distracted (10 to 12 pounds) using a commercially available wrist traction device.

TECHNIQUES

Triangular Fibrocartilage Complex Débridement

Portals and Arthroscopic Examination

- The standard dorsal 3-4, 4-5, 6R, and midcarpal radial portals are used. Incision is made just through skin. A hemostat is used for blunt dissection and penetration through capsule into the joint to reduce the risk of nerve or tendon injury.
- A diagnostic arthroscopic examination of the radiocarpal, ulnocarpal, and midcarpal joints is performed to assess the intrinsic and extrinsic ligaments, the articular surfaces, and synovium for potential pathology and causes of symptoms that could affect the treatment plan.
- Perform a synovectomy to ensure clear visualization of the joint.
- The TFCC is evaluated for injury. All joint surfaces are assessed for evidence of ulnar impaction including the lunotriquetral ligaments (**TECH FIG 1A,B**).
  - The TFCC is probed to assess the integrity of its peripheral attachments.

Triangular Fibrocartilage Complex Débridement

- With the scope in the 3-4 portal, a working 6R portal is used to débride the radial, palmar, and a portion of the dorsal aspect of the TFCC tear (**TECH FIG 2**).
  - Alternating working portals between 6R and 4-5 may provide easier access to the tear.
  - Placing scope in 6R or 4-5 allows visualization and débridement of ulnar aspect of TFCC with instrumentation in the 3-4 portal.

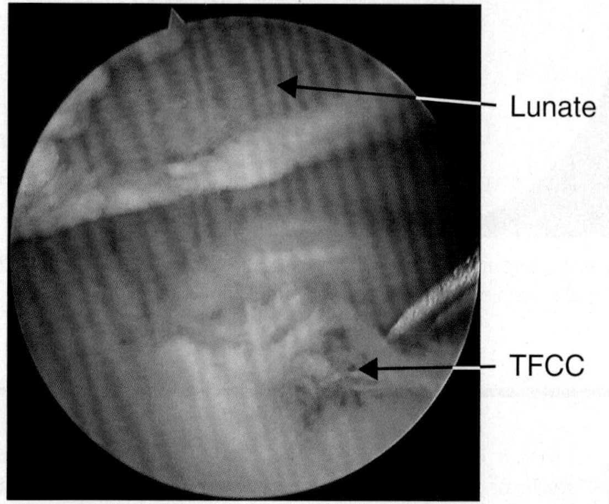

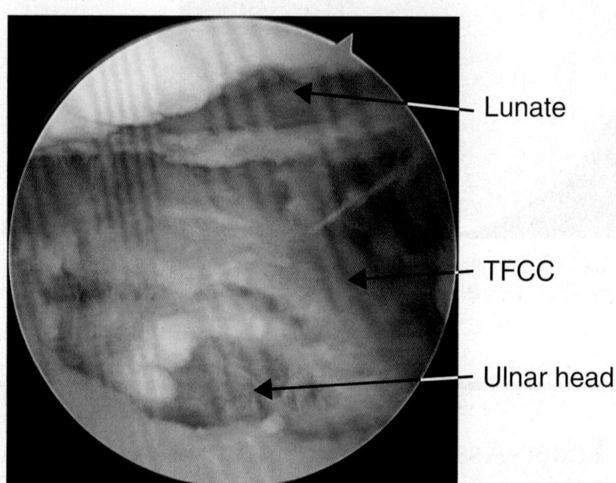

TECH FIG 1 • **A.** Arthroscopic evaluation of ulnar carpal impaction from 3-4 portal with lunate chondromalacia and degenerative TFCC tear. **B.** Arthroscopic ulnar impaction with degenerative TFCC tear and exposed ulnar head with chondromalacia.

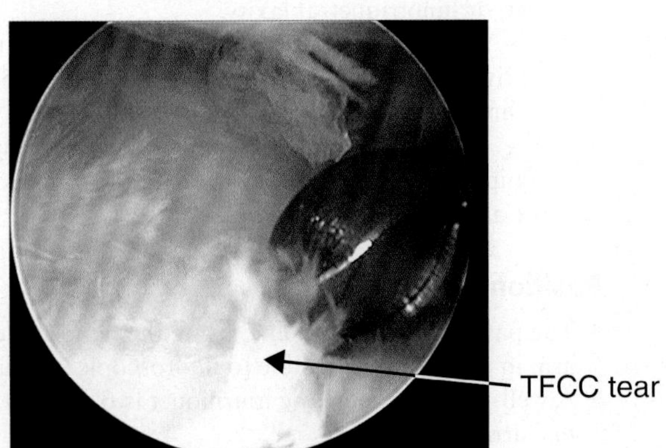

TECH FIG 2 • Mechanical débridement of the TFCC. The arthroscope is in the 3-4 portal looking ulnar while the suction punch enters through the 6R portal to débride the TFCC.

- Use small joint punches (straight and angled), graspers, or an 18-gauge needle to débride the TFCC. The suction punch is particularly useful.
- Take care not to injure the underlying ulnar head and overhanging lunate and triquetrum.
- Keep three points in mind while débriding the ulnar aspect of the TFCC:
  - Avoid injuring the attachment of the triangular fibrocartilage at its insertion on the base of the ulnar styloid.
  - Avoid injuring the dorsal or palmar radioulnar ligaments. If the ulnar attachment of the TFCC is transected, or if the dorsal and palmar radioulnar ligaments are injured, DRUJ instability could result.
  - Avoid scuffing the articular surfaces while passing the cutting and grasping instruments from the 3-4 portal across the radiocarpal joint into the ulnocarpal joint.
- After the TFCC has been mechanically débrided, the edges are smoothed using a shaver or radiofrequency ablator. If done appropriately, ablation of the tissue is also thought to cause shrinkage, which could tighten the peripheral edge of the TFCC and prevent unstable flaps.[14]
  - A 2.0- or 2.9-mm shaver can be used to smoothen the TFCC rim (**TECH FIG 3A**).
- The end point of TFCC débridement is reached when the ulnar head is visible through the TFCC and a stable, smooth TFCC rim remains (**TECH FIG 3B**).
  - Typically, a central defect measuring approximately 1 cm in diameter is created and up to 80% of substance can be resected without creating iatrogenic instability.[1]
- After confirming that ulnar recession is not necessary, the wrist is removed from traction and a TFCC stress test is performed (ulnarly deviate, axially load, and repeatedly supinate and pronate the wrist).
  - The presence of popping or clicking is a sign that further débridement might be needed or that some other pathology is present.
  - One source of such postdébridement popping is thickened synovium in the DRUJ just proximal to the TFCC.
- Wounds are closed with 4-0 nylon in simple or mattress fashion and a well-padded short-arm volar splint is applied.

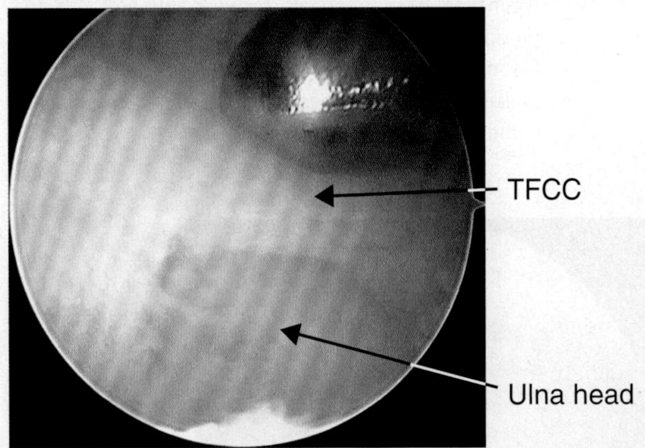

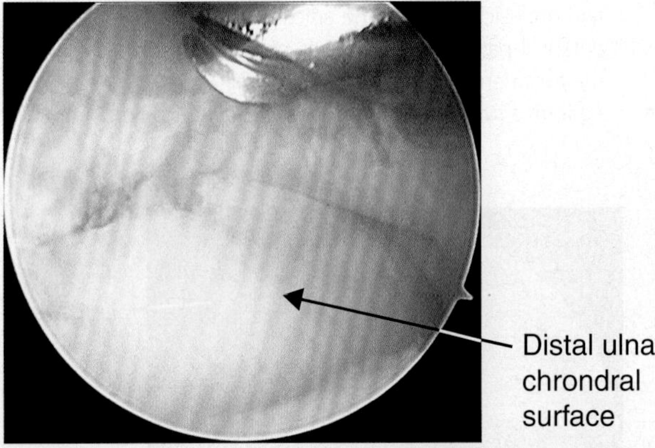

TECH FIG 3 • **A.** The arthroscope is in the 3-4 portal and the shaver is passed through the 6R portal to smooth the edges of the débrided central TFCC tear. **B.** The débridement of the TFCC is complete. The ulnar head is visible and ready for shortening if indicated.

Laser-Assisted Triangular Fibrocartilage Complex Débridement

- The technique of laser-assisted TFCC débridement is similar to that of mechanical débridement, with the exception that the arthroscope can be left in the 3-4 portal, whereas the laser probe is kept in the 4-5 portal.
- The laser is set to 1.4 to 1.6 joules at a frequency of 15 pulses per second. With the help of a side-firing 70-degree laser tip, the triangular fibrocartilage can be rapidly and precisely débrided.
  - The 70-degree laser tip permits ablation of not only the radial and palmar portions of the TFCC tear but also the ulnar and dorsal components.
  - There is no need to bring the laser probe in through the 3-4 portal.

- During the débridement, take care not to injure the ulnar head by firing the laser tangentially to the head of the ulna or passing the probe beneath the triangular fibrocartilage and firing distally (**TECH FIG 4**).
  - This latter technique presents minimal danger to the lunate or triquetrum, as the fluid used to expand the joint acts as a heat sink and absorbs the laser energy as it emerges from beneath the triangular fibrocartilage.

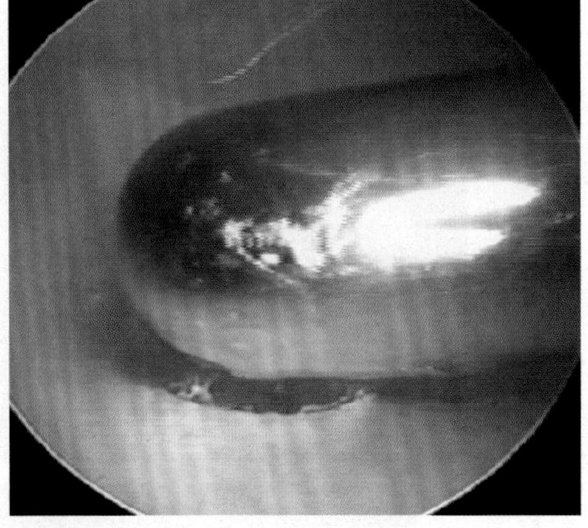

TECH FIG 4 ● Laser-assisted débridement of a TFCC tear. The laser probe is placed 1 mm from the TFCC.

Arthroscopic Ulnar Shortening

- The objective is to create a smooth and level distal ulna with neutral to 2 mm negative variance.
  - Small irregularities, however, tend to flatten out with the passage of time.
- After TFCC débridement, arthroscopic ulnar shortening is accomplished by placing the scope in the 3-4 portal and introducing the instruments through the 4-5 portal.
  - Occasionally, the 6R portal can be used, as can the DRUJ portal.
- The small joint arthroscopic burr abrader (2.9 mm) is placed in the 4-5 portal (**TECH FIG 5**).
  - Alternating the burr between portals enables access to the entire ulnar head.
- The distal ulnar cartilage is then removed through the defect in the central TFCC.
- A 3 to 4 mm of distal ulna is then removed with the burr; however, sufficient ulnar head must remain for proper joint loading to avoid arthritis from excessive contact stress.
- During burring, the forearm is fully supinated and pronated by the assistant to ensure circumferential débridement of distal ulna.
- The burr should be removed intermittently from the wrist and irrigated to cleanse the ulnocarpal joint of bone fragments.
- Frequent fluoroscopic imaging is used to confirm the level of resection.
- Avoid burring at the ulna fovea to prevent injury to deep TFCC attachment.
- After completing the resection, there should be neutral to 2 mm negative ulnar variance.
- The wrist is removed from the traction tower and examined with ulnar deviation, axial load, and supination and pronation to ensure no crepitance or clicking is felt which require further ulnar leveling or TFCC débridement.
- The holmium:YAG laser can be used for ulnar resection. It is introduced through the 4-5 portal and the cartilage and subchondral bone of the ulnar seat of the distal ulna are rapidly vaporized, using similar technique as burring (**TECH FIG 6A,B**). The laser is set to 1.4 to 1.6 joules at a frequency of 15 pulses per second.
  - The laser becomes less efficient once the trabeculae of the distal ulna are visible (**TECH FIG 6C**). At that point, the 2.9-mm arthroscopic burr is brought in to finish the shortening.
  - Frequent fluoroscopic monitoring is again used to ensure appropriate resection.
  - Saline inflow must be adequate to prevent thermal injury.
- Wounds are closed with 4-0 nylon in simple or mattress fashion, and a well-padded short-arm volar splint is applied.

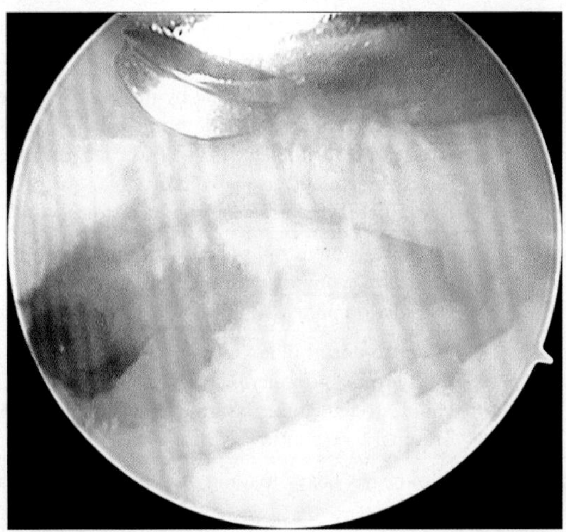

TECH FIG 5 ● Arthroscopic 2.9-mm burr in the 4-5 portal débriding articular cartilage and subchondral bone of ulnar head.

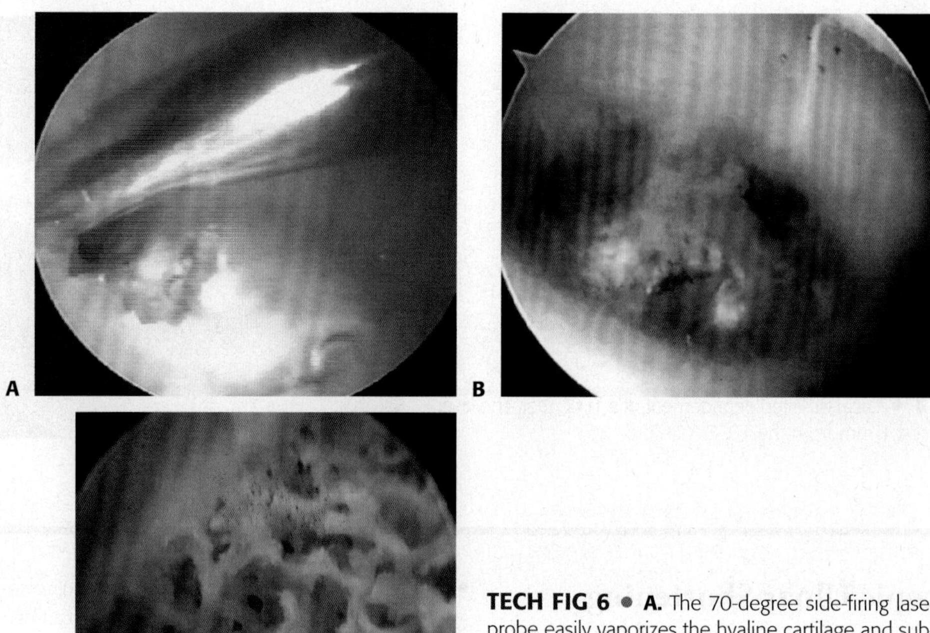

TECH FIG 6 • **A.** The 70-degree side-firing laser probe easily vaporizes the hyaline cartilage and subchondral bone of the ulnar head. **B.** The laser has cleared the ulnar head of its cartilage and subchondral plate. **C.** The spacing of the bony trabeculae of the ulnar head decreases the laser's efficiency. The final leveling of the ulnar head is achieved with the small joint burr.

PEARLS AND PITFALLS

TFCC débridement

Indication	■ Symptomatic Palmer types IA and IIA tears without evidence of static or dynamic ulnar impaction that failed nonoperative management
Pearls	■ All portals should be made by incising only the skin (avoid plunging blade beneath skin). Once the skin is cut, a small hemostat should be used to bluntly dissect through the subcutaneous tissue and penetrate the wrist joint capsule. ■ Excise only unstable central TFCC, leaving the periphery intact (at least 2 mm). ■ Assess lunate and triquetrum articular surfaces and ulnar head for evidence of chondromalacia. ■ Reevaluate wrist after débridement for absence of preoperative TFCC click.
Technical points	■ Scope viewing in 3-4 portal with a 6R working portal (but can adjust for needed visualization) ■ Cauterize synovitis with thermal probe. ■ Use suction punch and 2.0–3.0-mm shaver to remove unstable TFCC flap.
Pitfalls	■ Injury to dorsal ulnar sensory nerve ■ Injury to the peripheral attachments of the TFCC and the dorsal and palmar radioulnar ligaments ■ Failure to recognize unstable DRUJ with repairable TFCC tear ■ Traumatic central tear with positive ulnar variance may need ulnar shortening.
Rehabilitation	■ Avoid early heavy loading of the wrist for at least 4 weeks.

Arthroscopic ulnar shortening

Indications	▪ Symptomatic TFCC tear with ulnar carpal impaction (Palmer types IIA to IIC)
Pearls	▪ Preoperative neutral posteroanterior (PA) and pronated grip x-rays to determine ulnar variance ▪ Resect only 3–4 mm of bone. ▪ Midcarpal arthroscopy is used to evaluate lunotriquetral joint stability.
Technical points	▪ Pronate and supinate the wrist during distal ulnar resection to ensure complete resection. ▪ Preserve peripheral attachment of TFCC and radioulnar ligaments. ▪ Avoid resection into the ulnar fovea. ▪ Use 2.9-mm burr for ulnar head resection (can use burr size as guide for resection). ▪ Intermittent fluoroscopic evaluation to assess resection
Pitfalls	▪ Injury to dorsal ulnar sensory nerve ▪ Destabilization of the DRUJ with detachment of TFCC or radioulnar ligaments ▪ Excessive head resection that disrupts loading across sigmoid notch ▪ Failure to recognize lunotriquetral ligament perforation (IID and IIE) which require débridement and/or pinning with ulnar shortening osteotomy to tighten ulnocarpal ligaments

POSTOPERATIVE CARE

Triangular Fibrocartilage Complex Débridement

- Postoperative care includes immediate immobilization in volar short-arm splint with digital range of motion.
  - Active wrist and forearm range of motion is begun at 2 weeks.
- Strengthening exercises are initiated at 6 weeks; avoid repetitive rotation or wrist loading.
  - Premature return to activities can lead to ulnocarpal synovitis and associated pain.
- Return to normal activities and lifting can resume at 3 months.

Arthroscopic Ulnar Shortening

- Similar protocol is used for patients undergoing ulnar shortening with brief immobilization followed by early active range of motion.

OUTCOMES

- The results of arthroscopic débridement of type IA TFCC tears have a very good prognosis, revealing 80% to 85% good to excellent results.[8,15]
- However, multiple studies have shown that simple TFCC débridement alone, in the setting of ulnar positive variance and in particular ulnar impaction, has inferior outcomes.[2,7,10]

A

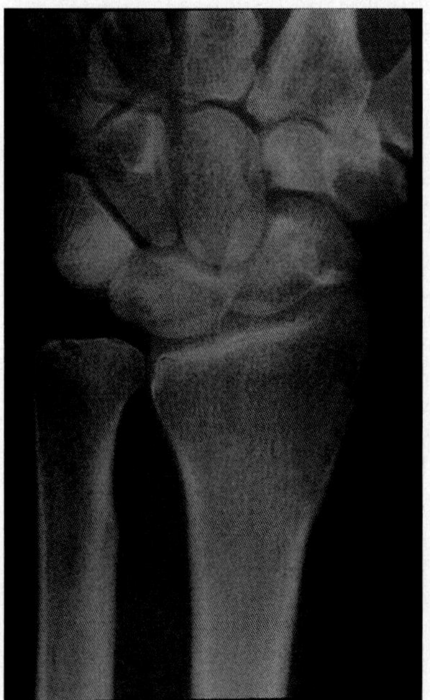

B

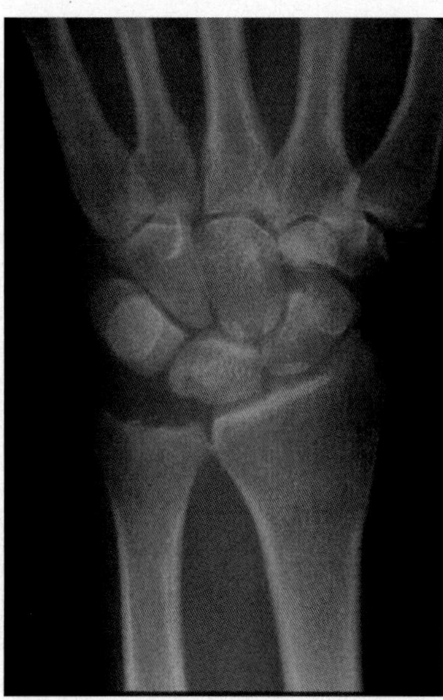

FIG 6 • **A.** Preoperative radiograph showing ulnar abutment. **B.** Postoperative radiograph after arthroscopically assisted ulnar shortening.

- Arthroscopic TFCC débridement, when combined with an arthroscopically assisted ulnar shortening, has been shown to provide excellent and good results in over 80% of patients.[18,26,27]
- This technique offers comparable results with ulnar shortening osteotomy, without the risk of hardware irritation or ulnar nonunion (**FIG 6A,B**).[2]

COMPLICATIONS

- TFCC débridement
  - Injury to the dorsal branch of the ulnar nerve
  - Instability secondary to excessive débridement of the TFCC (dorsal and palmar radioulnar ligaments, attachment in the ulnar fovea)
  - Continued symptoms due to unrecognized ulnar impaction
- Arthroscopic ulnar shortening
  - Continued symptoms due to inadequate or uneven resection
  - Disruption of the DRUJ from excessive resection
  - Detachment of the TFCC from the ulnar fovea
  - Loss of forearm rotation

REFERENCES

1. Adams BD, Holley KA. Strains in the articular disk of the triangular fibrocartilage complex: a biomechanical study. J Hand Surg Am 1993; 18(5):919–925. doi:10.1016/0363-5023(93)90066-C.
2. Bernstein MA, Nagle DJ, Martinez A, et al. A comparison of combined arthroscopic triangular fibrocartilage complex debridement and arthroscopic wafer distal ulna resection versus arthroscopic triangular fibrocartilage complex debridement and ulnar shortening osteotomy for ulnocarpal abutment syndrome. Arthroscopy 2004;20(4):392–401. doi:10.1016/j.arthro.2004.01.013.
3. Brown JA, Janzen DL, Adler BD, et al. Arthrography of the contralateral, asymptomatic wrist in patients with unilateral wrist pain. Can Assoc Radiol J 1994;45(4):292–296.
4. Culp RW, Osterman AL, Kaufmann RA. Wrist arthroscopy. In: Green DP, Hotchkiss RN, Pederson WC, et al, eds. Green's Operative Hand Surgery, ed 5. Philadelphia: Elsevier, 2005:781–803.
5. Darlis NA, Weiser RW, Sotereanos DG. Arthroscopic triangular fibrocartilage complex debridement using radiofrequency probes. J Hand Surg Br 2005;30(6):638–642. doi:10.1016/j.jhsb.2005.06.016.
6. Geissler WB, Freeland AE, Savoie FH, et al. Intracarpal soft-tissue lesions associated with an intra-articular fracture of the distal end of the radius. J Bone Joint Surg Am 1996;78(3):357–365.
7. Hulsizer D, Weiss AP, Akelman E. Ulna-shortening osteotomy after failed arthroscopic debridement of the triangular fibrocartilage complex. J Hand Surg Am 1997;22(4):694–698. doi:10.1016/S0363-5023(97)80130-X.
8. Husby T, Haugstvedt JR. Long-term results after arthroscopic resection of lesions of the triangular fibrocartilage complex. Scand J Plast Reconstr Hand Surg 2001;35(1):79–83.
9. Imaeda T, Nakamura R, Shionoya K, et al. Ulnar impaction syndrome: MR imaging findings. Radiology 1996;201(2):495–500. doi:10.1148/radiology.201.2.8888248.
10. Kim BS, Song HS. A comparison of ulnar shortening osteotomy alone versus combined arthroscopic triangular fibrocartilage complex debridement and ulnar shortening osteotomy for ulnar impaction syndrome. Clin Orthop Surg 2011;3(3):184–190. doi:10.4055/cios.2011.3.3.184.
11. Kleinman WB. Stability of the distal radioulna joint: biomechanics, pathophysiology, physical diagnosis, and restoration of function what we have learned in 25 years. J Hand Surg Am 2007;32(7):1086–1106. doi:10.1016/j.jhsa.2007.06.014.
12. Lee RK, Ng AW, Tong CS, et al. Intrinsic ligament and triangular fibrocartilage complex tears of the wrist: comparison of MDCT arthrography, conventional 3-T MRI, and MR arthrography. Skeletal Radiol 2013;42(9):1277–1285. doi:10.1007/s00256-013-1666-8.
13. Lindau T, Adlercreutz C, Aspenberg P. Peripheral tears of the triangular fibrocartilage complex cause distal radioulnar joint instability after distal radial fractures. J Hand Surg Am 2000;25(3):464–468. doi:10.1053/jhsu.2000.6467.
14. Medvecky MJ, Ong BC, Rokito AS, et al. Thermal capsular shrinkage: basic science and clinical applications. Arthroscopy 2001;17(6): 624–635.
15. Minami A, Ishikawa J, Suenaga N, et al. Clinical results of treatment of triangular fibrocartilage complex tears by arthroscopic debridement. J Hand Surg Am 1996;21(3):406–411.
16. Mrkonjic A, Geijer M, Lindau T, et al. The natural course of traumatic triangular fibrocartilage complex tears in distal radial fractures: a 13-15 year follow-up of arthroscopically diagnosed but untreated injuries. J Hand Surg Am 2012;37(8):1555–1560. doi:10.1016/j.jhsa.2012.05.032.
17. Omlor G, Jung M, Grieser T, et al. Depiction of the triangular fibrocartilage in patients with ulnar-sided wrist pain: comparison of direct multi-slice CT arthrography and direct MR arthrography. Eur Radiol 2009;19(1):147–151. doi:10.1007/s00330-008-1118-3.
18. Osterman AL. Arthroscopic debridement of triangular fibrocartilage complex tears. Arthroscopy 1990;6(2):120–124.
19. Palmer AK, Glisson RR, Werner FW. Ulnar variance determination. J Hand Surg Am 1982;7(4):376–379.
20. Palmer AK, Werner FW. Biomechanics of the distal radioulnar joint. Clin Orthop Relat Res 1984;(187):26–35.
21. Palmer AK, Werner FW. The triangular fibrocartilage complex of the wrist—anatomy and function. J Hand Surg Am 1981;6(2):153–162. doi:10.1016/S0363-5023(81)80170-0.
22. Park MJ, Jagadish A, Yao J. The rate of triangular fibrocartilage injuries requiring surgical intervention. Orthopedics 2010;33(11):806. doi:10.3928/01477447-20100924-03.
23. Smith TO, Drew B, Toms AP, et al. Diagnostic accuracy of magnetic resonance imaging and magnetic resonance arthrography for triangular fibrocartilaginous complex injury: a systematic review and meta-analysis. J Bone Joint Surg Am 2012;94(9):824–832. doi:10.2106/JBJS.J.01775.
24. Tay SC, Tomita K, Berger RA. The "ulnar fovea sign" for defining ulnar wrist pain: an analysis of sensitivity and specificity. J Hand Surg Am 2007;32(4):438–444. doi:10.1016/j.jhsa.2007.01.022.
25. Tomaino MM. The importance of the pronated grip x-ray view in evaluating ulnar variance. J Hand Surg Am 2000;25(2):352–357. doi:10.1053/jhsu.2000.jhsu25a0352.
26. Tomaino MM, Weiser RW. Combined arthroscopic TFCC debridement and wafer resection of the distal ulna in wrists with triangular fibrocartilage complex tears and positive ulnar variance. J Hand Surg Am 2001;26(6):1047–1052. doi:10.1053/jhsu.2001.28757.
27. Wnorowski DC, Palmer AK, Werner FW, et al. Anatomic and biomechanical analysis of the arthroscopic wafer procedure. Arthroscopy 1992;8(2):204–212.

Ulnar Shortening Osteotomy

Lance G. Warhold and Nelson L. Jenkins

DEFINITION

- Ulnar impaction syndrome (ulnocarpal abutment) results from a chronic compressive overloading of the ulnocarpal articulation secondary to static or dynamic ulnar positive variance.
- Ulnar variance defines the relationship of the length of the ulna to that of the radius.
- Ulnar positive variance can be the result of a congenital anomaly; traumatic radial shortening from a distal radius, Essex-Lopresti, or Galeazzi fracture; injury to the distal radius physis; or a variant of normal anatomy.
- An ulnar shortening osteotomy is designed to decompress the ulnocarpal joint while simultaneously tightening the ulnocarpal and radioulnar marginal ligaments of the triangular fibrocartilage complex (TFCC).[16]
  - Ulnar shortening osteotomy has been shown to be an effective alternative to TFCC repair in in the management of Palmer type IB tears.[20]
  - Ulnar shortening osteotomy has been shown to be effective in reducing symptoms of isolated posttraumatic lunotriquetral ligament tears regardless of preoperative ulnar variance.[13]

ANATOMY

- The distal radius has three articular surfaces: the scaphoid fossa, the lunate fossa, and the sigmoid notch.
- The radius articulates with and rotates around the ulnar head via the sigmoid notch. The sigmoid notch has well-defined dorsal, palmar, and distal margins, whereas the proximal margin is indistinct.
- The distal radioulnar joint (DRUJ) and ulnocarpal relationships are maintained by numerous ligamentous structures (**FIG 1A**).
- The interosseous membrane is a complex structure with a thickened central portion. It almost completely spans the radius and ulna, acting as a hinge for forearm rotation.
- The diaphysis of the distal half of the ulna is supplied by small segmental branches from the anterior and posterior interosseous arteries. These enter the ulna in 1- to 3-cm intervals from the direction of the interosseous membrane and must be protected during the surgical approach.[26]

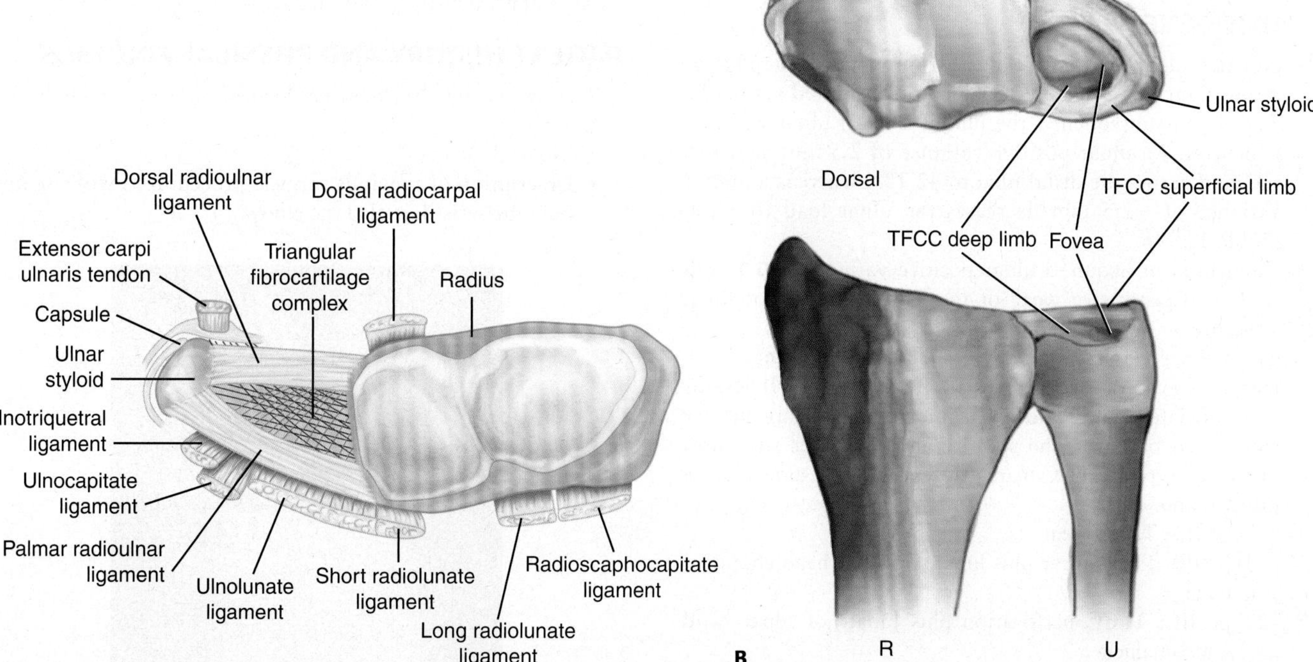

FIG 1 • **A.** The soft tissue structures encompassing the TFCC of the wrist stabilizing the radioulnocarpal unit. The TFCC proper originates from the radius medially and attaches to the base of the ulnar styloid. Fibers originating from the subsheath of the ECU dorsally cross path with fibers originating from the ulnocarpal ligaments volarly and blend with the TFCC proper. **B.** DRUJ ligaments. (The disc component of the TFCC has been removed to show the deep limbs of the radioulnar ligaments.) The volar and dorsal radioulnar ligaments are the major soft tissue stabilizers of the DRUJ and insert onto the base of the ulnar styloid. *R*, radius; *U*, ulna.

- The dorsal capsule of the DRUJ contains two ligaments: the proximal metaphyseal arcuate ligament and the distal radioulnar ligament. The palmar capsule is composed of a single radioulnar ligament.[1]
- The TFCC spans the ulnocarpal joint and connects the distal radius to the distal ulna (**FIG 1B**). The TFCC functions to cover the distal ulna, to partially dampen and transmit a portion of the axial load of the wrist through the ulna, to stabilize the DRUJ, and to provide support for the ulnar side of the carpus.
- The TFCC contains a central avascular articular disc composed of types I and II collagen. It is of variable thickness (average, 2 mm) and chiefly functions in load transmission between the ulnar head and ulnar carpus.
  - The articular disc is connected to the peripheral palmar and dorsal radioulnar (marginal) ligaments, which originate on the medial border of the distal radius and insert into the base of the ulnar styloid at the fovea. These ligaments are composed of linear type I collagen and are stabilizers of the DRUJ.
  - The ulnolunate and ulnotriquetral ligaments originate from the ulnar fovea and pass palmar to the palmar radioulnar ligament. They traverse the palmar surface of the TFCC to insert on their respective carpal bones. These ulnocarpal ligaments stabilize the ulnar side of the carpus relative to the ulna and resist carpal supination.
- The periphery of the TFCC is supplied by dorsal and palmar branches of the anterior interosseous artery and the ulnar artery. Because of this vascular distribution, injuries to the periphery of the TFCC are capable of healing and are often amenable to repair. Injuries to the central avascular portion of the articular disc do not heal in a predictable manner and are often treated with débridement.

PATHOGENESIS

- Normal ulnar variance ranges from neutral to plus or minus 2 mm. The average axial load transmitted across the TFCC and subsequently the ulna is 20% if ulnar variance is neutral. An ulnar positive variance of 2.5 mm increases the load across the distal ulna to 42.7%, whereas an ulnar variance of −2.5 mm decreases the ulnar load to 3.1% (Table 1).[19]
- Congenital or acquired ulnar positive variance (**FIG 2**) can lead to degenerative wear of the TFCC and surrounding structures.
- The Palmer classification divides TFCC lesions into traumatic (type I) or degenerative (type II).[18] Type II lesions are associated with ulnocarpal impaction and are further subdivided based on the severity and the other structures involved. Type II TFCC tears are generally not amenable to direct repair.
  - Type IIA: TFCC wear
  - Type IIB: TFCC wear plus lunate or ulnar head chondromalacia
  - Type IIC: TFCC perforation plus lunate or ulnar head chondromalacia
  - Type IID: TFCC perforation plus lunate or ulnar head chondromalacia plus lunotriquetral ligament perforation
  - Type IIE: TFCC perforation plus lunate or ulnar head chondromalacia plus lunotriquetral ligament perforation plus ulnocarpal arthritis

Table 1 Percentage of Force Transmitted through the Ulna (Nine Arms)

Ulnar Length (mm)	Amount Removed of the Articular Disc of the Triangular Fibrocartilage Complex			
	None	1/3	2/3[a]	All[a]
Neutral	17.6%	16.1%	13.4%	8.0%
−2.5	3.1%	2.7%	2.4%	2.3%
+2.5	42.7%	41.9%	36.1%	26.3%

[a]Removal of two-thirds or more of the horizontal portion of the triangular fibrocartilage complex statistically decreased the percentage of force through the nine ulnas tested. (Adapted from Palmer AK, Werner FW. The triangular fibrocartilage complex of the wrist—anatomy and function. J Hand Surg Am 1981;6[2]:153–162.)

NATURAL HISTORY

- Defining the natural history of ulnocarpal impaction syndrome is at best challenging.
- The Palmer classification provides an accurate anatomic description of the degenerative changes seen in the ulnocarpal structures, but it does not dictate treatment, suggest prognosis, or indicate timing of progression.
- Deterioration of the ulnocarpal structures is very common regardless of ulnar variance. Numerous cadaveric studies have found TFCC perforations and chondromalacia of the ulnar head, lunate, and triquetrum in up to 70% of "normal specimens."[12,19]
- Ulnar positive variance and persistent heavy demand across the ulnocarpal joint can hasten the development of the disease.
- An individual's ability to unload the ulnar side of the wrist with conservative measures and change of lifestyle may slow or even prevent progression.

PATIENT HISTORY AND PHYSICAL FINDINGS

- The patient history must be detailed and must include the following:
  - Medical history
  - Description of previous surgical procedures involving not only the wrist but also the elbow

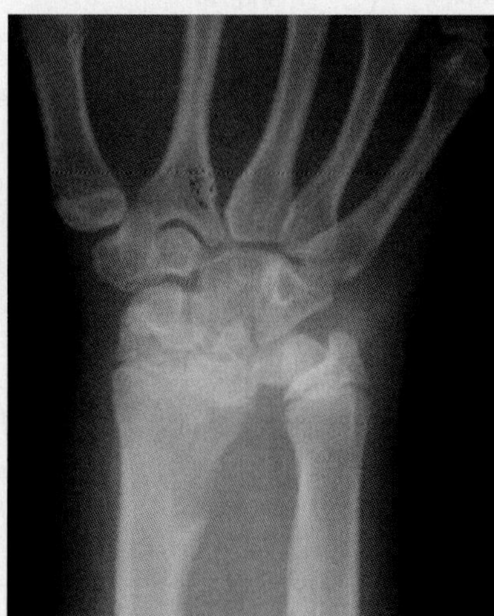

FIG 2 • Radiograph of Madelung deformity showing congenital ulnar positive variance.

- Analysis of whether the pain was caused by an acute injury or brought on by repetitive motion activities
  - A distal radius or radial head fracture can lead to ulnocarpal impaction, as can a chronic distal radius physeal injury (ie, the gymnast's wrist).
- Characterization of the pain
  - Description of the location, duration, and radiation of the pain as well as any associated swelling, burning or tingling sensations, or sounds (clicks, etc.)
  - Aggravating and alleviating factors
- The physical examination should always begin with inspection.
  - The wrist and elbow should be examined for surgical scars.
  - Prominence of the ulna either palmarly or dorsally may indicate instability of the DRUJ. A palmar sag and a supination posture of the wrist may indicate the capsuloligamentous instability that occurs in rheumatoid arthritis.
  - Swelling, bruising, perforations of the skin, or obvious dislocations may indicate trauma.
  - Intrinsic atrophy and clawing may indicate ulnar nerve pathology.
  - Splinter hemorrhages beneath the nails and decreased turgor in the volar digital pads suggest vascular insufficiency.
- Single-finger palpation should proceed in a systematic fashion by isolating anatomic structures. The examination should be performed with the patient's elbow resting on a table, the hand pointing toward the ceiling, and the forearm in a neutral position.
  - Tenderness over any anatomic structure suggests a specific clinical diagnosis.
- Active and passive range-of-motion (ROM) maneuvers may illicit pain, suggesting pathology. Limitations of ROM may be the result of swelling or obstruction (blocking). The examiner should listen for sounds of pathology throughout ROM.
- Specific provocative tests should be performed in an attempt to further define the injured structure(s).
  - Piano key test: A positive result is characterized by painful laxity in the affected wrist compared with the contralateral wrist, suggesting DRUJ synovitis.
  - Ulnar compression test: A positive test is exacerbation of pain, which suggests arthritis or instability; dorsal or palmar subluxation may be noted.
  - Lunotriquetral ballottement test: Used to elicit laxity associated with pain and crepitus in the presence of lunotriquetral instability
  - Reagan shuck test: Positive if pain and clicking at the lunotriquetral joint is present, suggesting lunotriquetral ligament perforation or disruption

IMAGING AND OTHER DIAGNOSTIC STUDIES

- Plain radiographic views should include neutral rotation posteroanterior and lateral projections of both wrists. These are obtained with the patient seated and the elbow flexed at 90 degrees and the shoulder abducted at 90 degrees.
  - The contralateral wrist films may be used as a template for reconstruction.
  - Radiographic assessment of ulnar variance has used a neutral rotation radiographic view of the wrist that provides an image of the radioulnar length with the wrist unloaded. Such views may underestimate variance in wrists in which power grip and pronation result in significant proximal migration of the radius. Tomaino[25] found that ulnar variance increased an average of 2.5 mm using the pronated grip view and ranged from an increase of 1 to 4 mm (**FIG 3A**).
- Other plain views may be obtained based on clinical suspicion.
  - The carpal tunnel (**FIG 3B**) view visualizes the hook of the hamate and the pisotriquetral joint.
  - An oblique view in 30 degrees of pronation (**FIG 3C**) allows evaluation of the dorsoulnar wrist.
  - The reverse oblique view (30 degrees of supination) (**FIG 3D**) allows evaluation of the palmar ulnar wrist with a profile of the pisotriquetral joint.
  - An ulnar deviation posteroanterior view (**FIG 3E**) may reveal lunotriquetral instability or evidence of ulnocarpal abutment. If ulnocarpal abutment is suspected, it is often useful to obtain a posteroanterior radiograph with the forearm in pronation and the fist clenched (see **FIG 3A**), which increases ulnar variance.
- Videofluoroscopy is useful for evaluating dynamic ligament instabilities. The wrist should be examined through an entire active and passive ROM as well as with provocative maneuvers in an attempt to demonstrate pathology while reproducing symptoms.
- Arthrography may demonstrate a TFCC defect or interosseous ligament disruption if contrast material injected into one compartment leaks into an adjacent space.
- Magnetic resonance imaging (MRI) can aid in the detection of soft tissue and osseous lesions, including interosseous and extrinsic ligament tears, TFCC defects, tumors, avascular necrosis, and occult fractures (**FIG 3F**).
  - Sensitivity of the MRI increases if it is combined with arthrography. The ability to show marrow changes in the ulnar portion of the lunate and simultaneous central TFCC pathology is very helpful in confirming a diagnosis of ulnocarpal impaction.
- Arthroscopy can confirm a diagnosis suggested by findings from other diagnostic modalities.
  - This is the most sensitive tool for diagnosis of chondral and ligamentous pathology.
  - It has therapeutic applications in the management of ulnar abutment, TFCC defects, interosseous ligament tears, chondral defects, loose bodies, synovitis, and degenerative arthritis.
- Bone scan, ultrasonography, and computed tomography serve a very limited role in the diagnosis of ulnar impaction syndrome.

DIFFERENTIAL DIAGNOSIS

- Extensor carpi ulnaris (ECU) subluxation or tenosynovitis
- DRUJ arthritis (degenerative or inflammatory), incongruity, intra-articular pathology, instability
- Ulnar styloid fracture nonunion
- Isolated TFCC tears
- Lunate and triquetrum lesions: chondromalacia, cyst, interosseous ganglion (lunate/capitate), or intraosseous pathology (enchondroma, osteoid osteoma)
- Kienböck disease

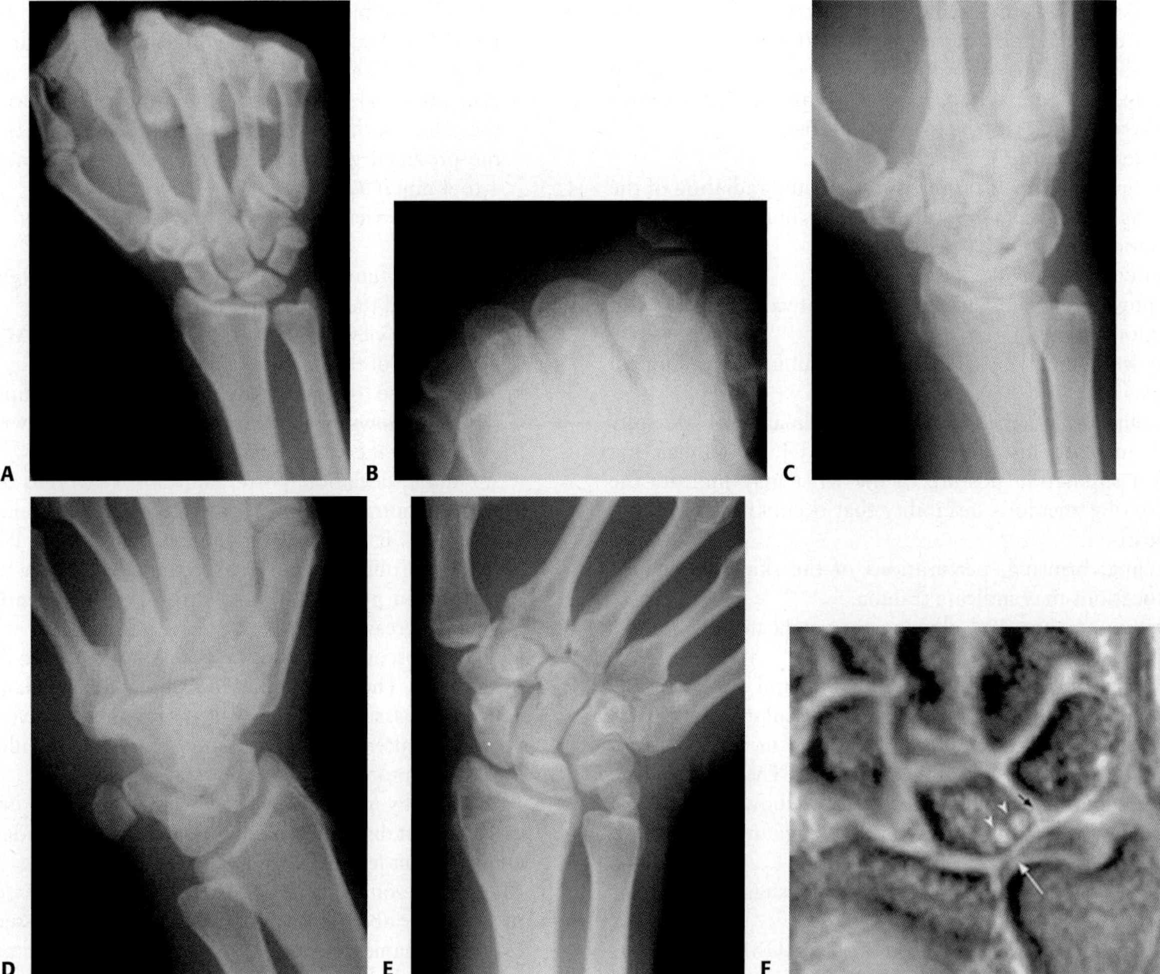

FIG 3 • **A.** Clenched fist view. **B.** Carpal tunnel view. **C.** Oblique view in 30 degrees of pronation. **D.** Oblique view in 30 degrees of supination. **E.** Ulnar deviation view. **F.** Coronal gradient-echo magnetic resonance (MR) image reveals a central triangular fibrocartilage perforation (*white arrow*), subchondral cystic changes in the lunate bone (*arrowheads*), and a lunotriquetral ligament tear (*black arrow*) in a 41-year-old man with ulnar impaction syndrome with positive variance and chronic ulnar-sided wrist pain (Palmer class IID lesion).

- Lunotriquetral instability (trauma or impaction)
- Midcarpal joint arthritis or chondromalacia
- Hamate hook, triquetral, or pisiform fractures
- Flexor carpi ulnaris tendinitis
- Pisotriquetral arthritis
- Guyon canal pathology: ganglion, tunnel syndrome, ulnar artery thrombosis
- Ulnar neuritis

NONOPERATIVE MANAGEMENT

- Rest and avoidance of any aggravating maneuvers are the mainstay of nonoperative management for ulnar impaction syndrome.
  - The success of this treatment lies with the patient's ability to change the way he or she does any number of routine tasks and may involve a change of employment.
- Ice and elevation may help to reduce any swelling associated with overuse or aggravation of a previous injury.
- Nonsteroidal anti-inflammatory medications will also reduce swelling and provide some analgesia.
- Neutral splinting provides support for the wrist and may help to prevent aggravating maneuvers.
- Injection of a steroid and local anesthetic mixture into the wrist may provide some temporary relief of symptoms and decrease swelling.
  - An intra-articular injection may also help differentiate intra- and extra-articular disorders.
- A combination of hand therapy modalities (ie, ultrasound, iontophoresis) and patient education may alleviate some symptoms.

SURGICAL MANAGEMENT

- Surgical treatment of ulnar impaction syndrome is indicated for patients who fail to respond to conservative modalities or those who cannot avoid aggravating maneuvers.
- Patients undergoing ulnar shortening osteotomy must be good surgical candidates, with a high likelihood of healing the osteotomy site.
  - Otherwise, an alternative surgical procedure, such as a wafer resection osteotomy, should be considered.
- Wrist arthroscopy is frequently used to document physical findings consistent with ulnar impaction syndrome before performing a shortening osteotomy, especially in cases of diagnostic uncertainty even after nonoperative management and injections discussed earlier.

Commercial Devices for Ulnar Shortening Osteotomy

- Plates and jigs to assist with ulnar osteotomy are commercially available.[15] These offer features such as low-profile plate design, locking screws, simplicity of use, decreased surgical time, and improved accuracy of the osteotomy cuts.
- The surgeon must consider whether the potential advantages of these systems justify the additional expense.[22]

Preoperative Planning

- Neutral rotation posteroanterior and lateral radiographs of both wrists demonstrate ulnar variance and the morphology of the DRUJ, helping to determine the degree of shortening required to unload the joint and still provide a congruent articulation.
- In principle, a long ulna should be shortened to neutral or 1 mm of negative variance. If there is ulnar neutral variance as a baseline, 2 mm of bone should be removed.[8]
- Care must be taken to prevent excessive shortening of the ulna, as this has the potential to increase pressures across the DRUJ articular surface[12] and can lead to limitation of forearm rotation.
- The absolute amount of possible shortening is limited by the marginal ligaments of an intact TFCC.
  - This is reportedly 15 mm in the setting of posttraumatic ulnar impaction syndrome.[7]
- DRUJ anomalies, congenital disorders, or arthritis should be ruled out.
- DRUJ stability is best assessed with examination under anesthesia.

Positioning

- Preoperative antibiotics with a coverage spectrum for skin flora are given intravenously about 30 minutes before the skin incision.
- The patient is positioned supine on the operating table with the upper extremity on an arm board.
- A single-bladder brachial tourniquet is placed over Webril in the upper brachial region and the arm is prepared and draped to the midbrachial level.
  - Extremity exsanguination is achieved with an elastic bandage wrap from the distal fingertips to midbrachial region, and then the tourniquet is inflated to about 250 mm Hg (the pressure may have to be increased in hypertensive patients).
- Unobstructed access to the elbow during the procedure is crucial to accurately evaluate pronation and supination.
- Intraoperative fluoroscopy helps the surgeon to discern the degree of correction in ulnar variance after the osteotomy.

Approach

- An 8- to 10-cm midaxial incision is made over the distal third of the ulnar diaphysis, ending at, or just proximal to, the distal ulnar metaphysis.
- The interval between the ECU and the flexor carpi ulnaris is developed to expose the ulnar periosteum.
- Although it is unlikely to be encountered, the location of the dorsal sensory branch of the ulnar nerve must be considered and protected.
  - It takes off from the ulnar nerve an average of 6.4 cm proximal to the distal aspect of the head of the ulna and runs along the subcutaneous border of the ulna for about 5 cm proximal to the pisiform.
  - The dorsal sensory branch typically courses along the medial border of the ulnar head with the forearm supinated and runs in a more palmar position with the forearm pronated.[2]
- Circumferential subperiosteal dissection is avoided to prevent injury to the segmental blood supply to the distal ulnar diaphysis, with the exception of a 1-cm zone at the site of the planned osteotomy.[26]

TECHNIQUES

Authors' Preferred Technique for Ulnar Shortening Osteotomy

Exposure

- Make an 8- to 10-cm incision over the subcutaneous border of the ulna as previously described (**TECH FIG 1A**).
- Elevate the ECU muscle–tendon from the distal dorsal aspect of the ulna to allow sufficient room for a six- or seven-hole AO dynamic compression plate (Synthes LC-DCP, Synthes, Paoli, PA) (**TECH FIG 1B**).
  - Take care to avoid disrupting the ECU subsheath distally.

Osteotomy

- Position the limited contact dynamic compression plate (LC-DCP) along the distal dorsoulnar shaft to ensure fit and prebend it into a very slightly concave configuration to ensure compression of the volar cortex with plate application.
  - A 3.5-mm plate is appropriate for most individuals, although a 2.7-mm plate may be used for smaller patients.
- Draw the proposed oblique osteotomy site beneath the third (for a six-hole plate) or fourth (for a seven-hole plate) hole in the plate.
  - The osteotomy is made obliquely in a dorsal to palmar direction so that the osteotomy site can later be secured with an interfragmentary screw applied through the dorsal plate.
  - The oblique osteotomy angle is about 45 to 60 degrees and it is typically 5 to 6 cm proximal to the ulnar styloid (**TECH FIG 2A**).
  - The orientation of the osteotomy (either distal-dorsal to proximal-palmar or vice versa) is designed such that the acute angle (point) of the cut bone is adjacent to the plate on the side of the fragment to be compressed. This technique compresses the bone to the plate, avoiding displacement of the osteotomy.
- Secure the Synthes small distractor–compressor apparatus over the proposed osteotomy site (along the ulnar border) with four 2.5-mm threaded Kirschner wires (**TECH FIG 2B**).
  - Place the pins into the ulna in a region that will later be spanned by the plate to avoid creating unprotected stress risers after removal.

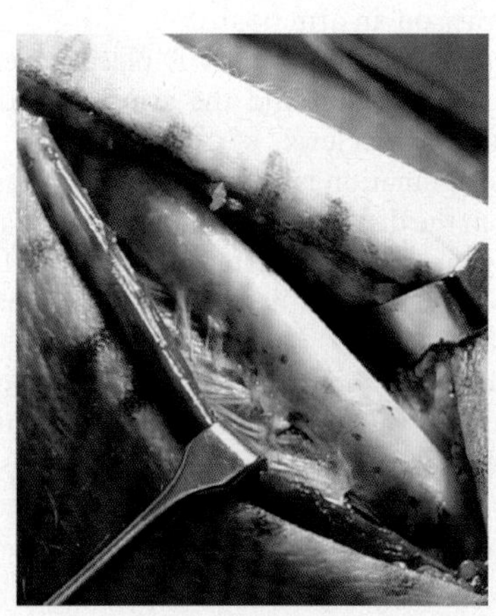

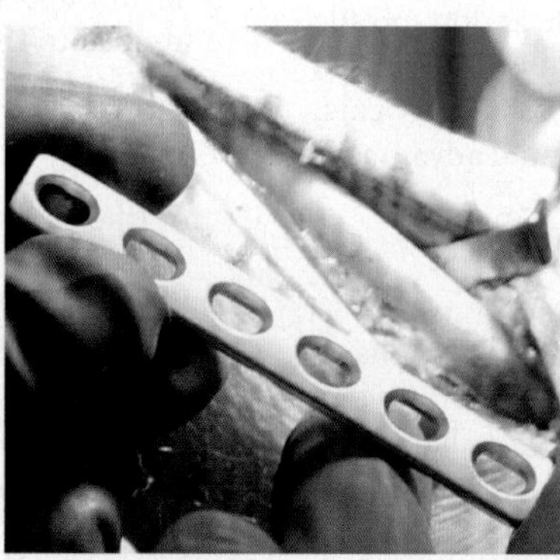

TECH FIG 1 • **A.** An 8- to 10-cm incision over the subcutaneous border of the ulna. **B.** Six-hole AO-type dynamic compression plate (DCP) (Synthes).

- Avoid interfering with the osteotomy when placing the pins by referring to the line drawn at the proposed osteotomy site.
- Place the pins palmar enough to allow the plate to be securely seated over the dorsal surface of the ulna.

Ulnar Osteotomy

- Remove the plate from the operative field and complete the first osteotomy cut using a precise oscillating blade (**TECH FIG 3**).
  - It may be helpful to complete the distal cut first to avoid removing too much distal bone, forcing distal placement of the plate and poor fixation.
  - Take care to continuously irrigate the bone edges while sawing to avoid thermal necrosis of the bone and periosteum.
- The kerf (amount of bone resected by the saw blade itself) must be taken into account when planning the site of the second osteotomy cut to determine accurately the total amount of bone removed.
  - Kerf thickness varies based on the specific blade used and can be obtained from the manufacturer.[7]
- Make the second parallel osteotomy cut proximal to the first, using a freehand technique, and remove the wafer of bone.
- Distract the osteotomy site and inspect it to ensure that there are no bony excrescences or residual uncut bone margins, which could interfere with apposition of the fragments.

Alternative Osteotomy Technique

- Perform a single osteotomy cut using stacked saw blades.[10] This theoretically removes some of the "human element" and provides a more precise cut with improved apposition of the fragments.

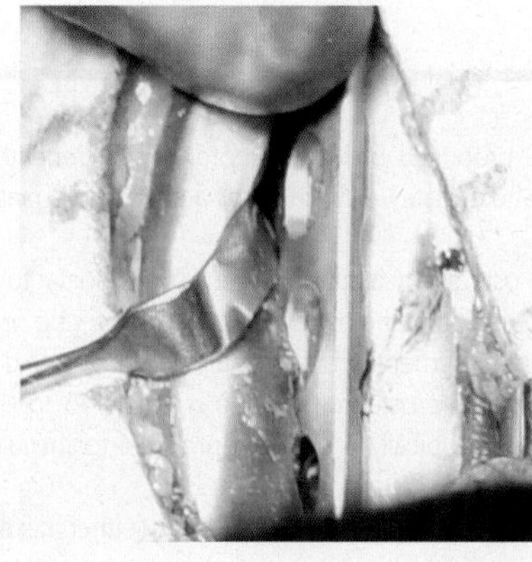

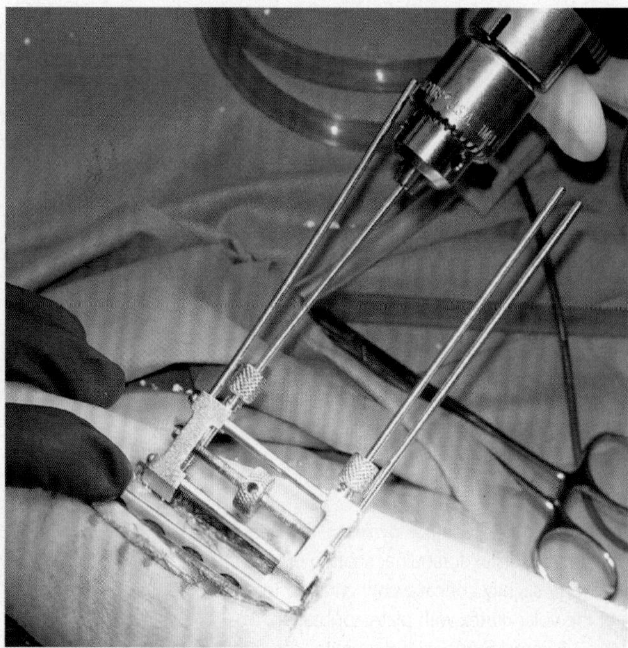

TECH FIG 2 • **A.** Dorsal compression plate in dorsal position. Proposed osteotomy drawn. The oblique osteotomy angle is about 45 to 60 degrees and it is typically 5 to 6 cm proximal to the ulnar styloid. **B.** Synthes small distractor apparatus secured along the ulnarmost border with four 2.5-mm threaded Kirschner wires.

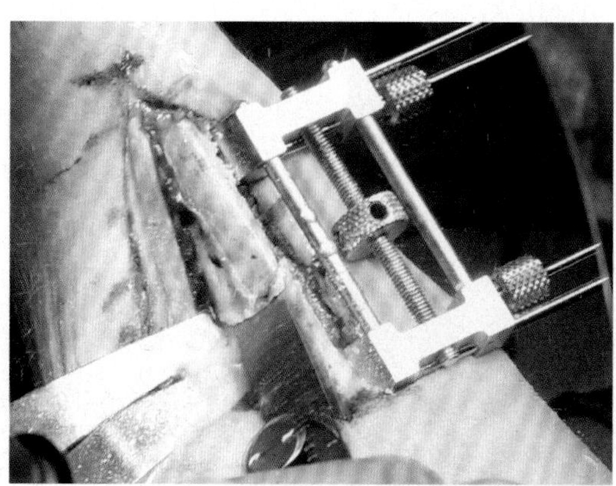

TECH FIG 3 • Oblique osteotomy created.

- Using a single-cut technique, reproducible ulnar shortening with precision within 0.2 mm of the exact desired ulnar variance has been reported.
- A relatively steep angled cut (60 degrees) using stacked blades with a kerf thickness of 4.45 mm can allow for up to 9 mm of shortening with a single cut.
- Cuts may be made at lesser angles and with lesser kerf thicknesses to allow for lesser degrees of shortening.[7]

Reduction and Stabilization

- Dial down the small distractor apparatus to achieve compression at the osteotomy site and bone-to-bone abutment (**TECH FIG 4A**).
  - A reduction clamp is valuable in guiding and then securing the fragments as compression is applied.
- Examine the radioulnar relationship under fluoroscopy to ensure adequate correction of ulnar variance and DRUJ congruence.
  - Additional bone resection followed by repeat reduction and compression can be easily achieved if necessary.
- Again, place the Synthes nonlocking LC-DCP on the dorsum of the ulna, and drill screw holes using a compression or neutral drill guide.
  - With the exception of the interfragmentary lag screw hole, directly over the osteotomy site, all screw holes in the plate are drilled using a 2.5-mm drill followed by a 3.5-mm tap (unless self-tapping screws are used).
- First, secure the plate with static screws to the fragment with the acute angle (point) on the side away from the plate (palmar in this case, using a dorsal plate).
- Reduce and secure the osteotomy, and then place compression screws in the other fragment, the one with the acute angle (point) adjacent to the plate.
  - Place the first compression screw in the second hole away from the osteotomy.
  - Fill the remaining more proximal holes with either compression or static screws.
- As a final step, insert an interfragmentary lag screw through the osteotomy via the hole in the plate directly over the osteotomy (**TECH FIG 4B**).
  - Pass a 3.5-mm drill only through the near cortex, followed by a 2.5-mm drill through the far cortex. Tap this hole and fill it with a 3.5-mm bone screw.
  - Once proximal and distal stabilization has been achieved, it may be necessary to remove the 2.5-mm pins to fill the remaining screw holes.

Completion

- Again, examine the bone under fluoroscopy to ensure good plate-to-bone and osteotomy site apposition and to assess screw lengths. Make a final assessment of the radioulnar relationship using standard posteroanterior and lateral neutral rotation views (**TECH FIG 5**).
- Irrigate the wound with normal saline. Close the deep subcutaneous layer with 3-0 Vicryl and approximate the skin edges with interrupted horizontal mattress 4-0 nylon.
- Apply a palmar, forearm-based plaster wrist splint after the tourniquet is deflated and sterile dressings have been applied.
- The arm is protected in a cast or splint until bony union has occurred.

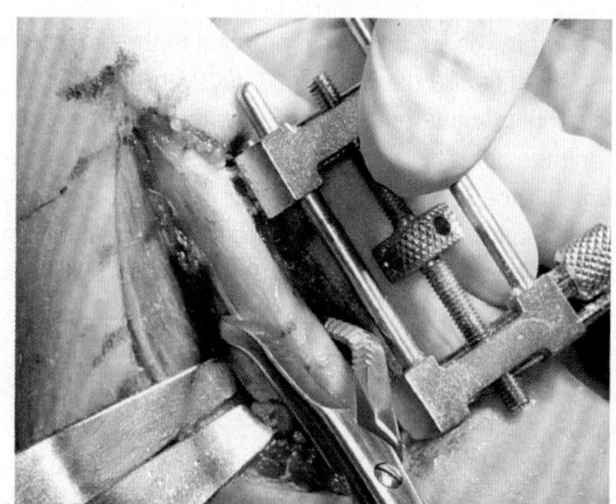

A

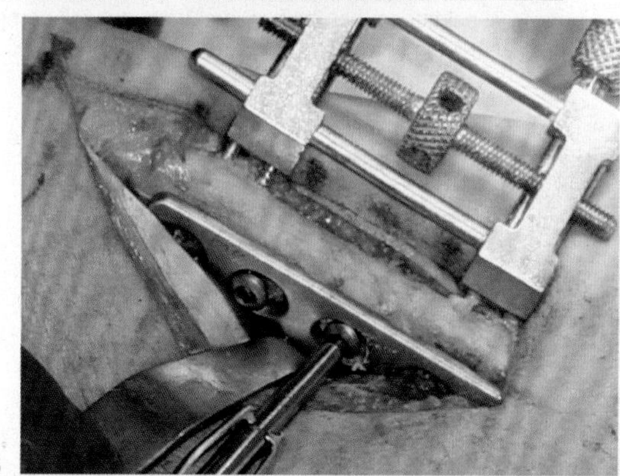

B

TECH FIG 4 • **A.** Osteotomy compression. **B.** An interfragmentary lag screw is placed through the plate.

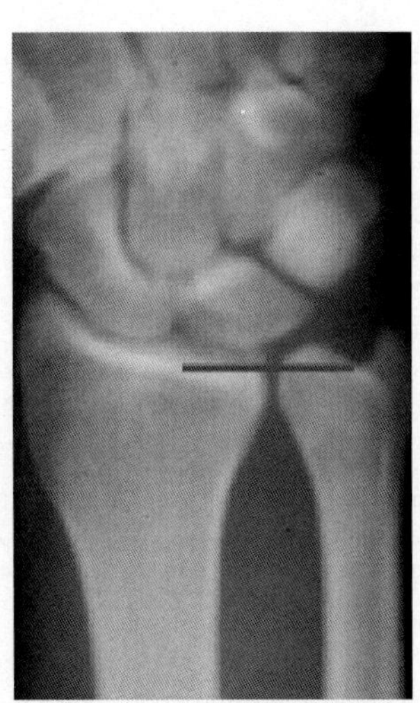

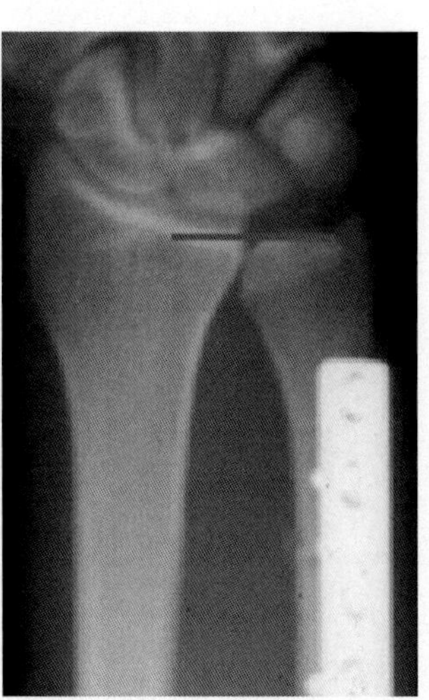

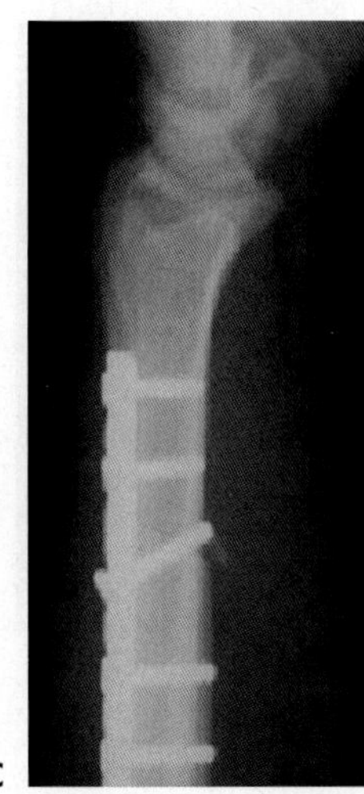

TECH FIG 5 • A. Posteroanterior (PA) wrist radiograph showing ulnar positive variance. **B,C.** PA and lateral radiographs after ulnar shortening osteotomy. The interfragmentary lag screw compresses the osteotomy site.

Ulnar Shortening Osteotomy Using an AO Compression Device

- Expose the ulna in the manner previously described and plan the osteotomy about 5 to 6 cm proximal to the ulnar styloid.
- Place a five- or six-hole 3.5-mm LC-DCP on the flat surface of the distal ulna, centered about the planned osteotomy site, with two or three holes distal, one hole across, and two or three holes proximal to the osteotomy.
  - Although the plate may be placed dorsal or volar, palmar positioning of the plate may be preferable to avoid subcutaneous prominence of the hardware after surgery.
  - Contour the plate in the manner described earlier.
- Fix the plate distally with two or three 3.5-mm cortical screws placed in a static mode.
- For a dorsal plate, draw the planned osteotomy on the bone with a marking pen at an angle of about 45 degrees distal-dorsal to proximal-palmar so that the proximal fragment will compress into the plate (**TECH FIG 6**).

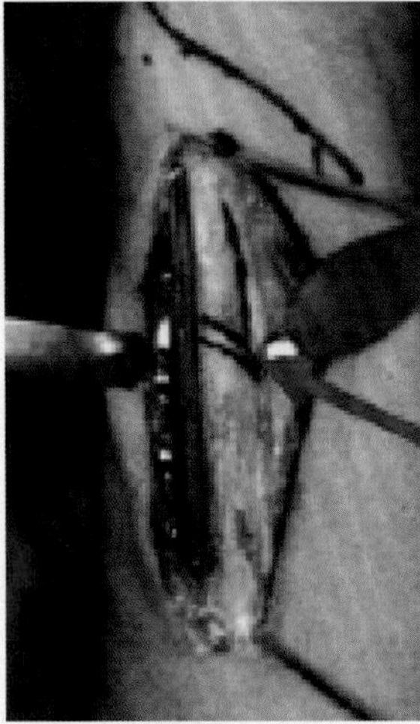

TECH FIG 6 • The proposed site of the osteotomy is marked on the ulna. This will allow for compression of the osteotomy when using a DCP and placement of an interfragmentary lag screw. (Courtesy of Thomas R. Hunt III, MD.)

- Fix the standard AO compression device to the ulna proximally with one unicortical screw and engage the mobile arm in the most proximal plate hole.[5]
  - Place the unicortical screw far enough proximal that adequate compression can be obtained. This distance will vary based on the amount of bone to be removed.
  - Once shortening is complete and the compression device removed, the empty screw hole must not be too close to the proximal margin of the plate in order to avoid a stress riser.
- Remove the compression device and one distal screw and loosen the most distal screw slightly, allowing the plate to be rotated away.
- Using a water-cooled oscillating saw, make the distal cut first using the freehand technique.
  - Interrupt the osteotomy cut after it is two-thirds complete.
  - The saw blade may be left in this initial cut to act as a planar guide for the second parallel and proximal osteotomy cut.
- Place a new blade into the saw and make the proximal cut two-thirds of the way through the bone.
- Complete the initial distal cut, followed by the proximal cut, and remove the perfectly round wafer of bone.
- Replace the previously removed distal screw and tighten both screws.
- Reapply the compression device and compress the osteotomy.
- Place the screw just proximal to the interfragmentary compression hole in a compression mode using the compression guide.
- Place the interfragmentary compression screw by first drilling a gliding hole through the near cortex with a 3.5-mm drill bit.
- Then, using a drill guide ("top hat"), drill the far cortex with a 2.5 mm drill bit. Measure the hole, tap the far cortex with a 3.5-mm tap, and place the interfragmentary compression screw.
- Remove the compression device and fill the remaining proximal screw hole(s) using the static drill guide.
- Irrigate and close the wound and apply a splint as previously described.

Metaphyseal Ulnar Shortening Osteotomy

- Metaphyseal ulnar shortening osteotomy, previously termed by Slade as *osteochondral shortening osteotomy*,[23] has recently increased in popularity due to its potential advantages of improved bone healing and reduced risk for complications.[9] Modifications using an arthroscopy-guided osteotomy[27] and fixation using a distal ulnar hook plate[17] have recently been reported, but it is not clear if the outcomes of these modifications are different when compared to the original technique described by Slade.
- Wrist arthroscopy is performed to both stage and treat any ulnocarpal arthrosis or TFCC tear that may require débridement or repair.
- After arthroscopy, make a longitudinal incision over the fifth dorsal compartment.
  - Take care to identify and protect the dorsal sensory branch of the ulnar nerve.
- Incise the fifth extensor compartment, retract the extensor digiti quinti tendon, and create a capsulotomy through the floor of this fifth compartment.
  - Complete the capsulotomy in an L-shaped fashion by extending the incision transversely just proximal to the dorsal radioulnar ligament of the TFCC, thus preserving its stabilizing function for the DRUJ.
- Based on preoperative determinations, resect a 3- to 5-mm wafer of bone using a microsagittal saw at the level of the proximal margin of the DRUJ.
  - Leave the distal ulnar articular surface and the TFCC foveal attachments intact (**TECH FIG 7A–C**).
- Reduce and compress the osteotomy with a hemostat and a Kirschner wire placed for temporary stabilization.
- Intraoperative fluoroscopy is used to confirm the adequacy of resection and osteotomy reduction.
- More bone can be removed if necessary, up to 5 mm total.
  - Excessive bony resection could lead to DRUJ instability or impingement.
- Thread a cannulated headless compression screw over the previously inserted Kirschner wire while manual compression is maintained (**TECH FIG 7D,E**).
- Remove the Kirschner wire and irrigate the wounds.
- Repair the dorsal capsule with interrupted nonabsorbable sutures.
- Transpose the extensor digiti quinti tendon out of the fifth compartment as the capsule is repaired.
- Close the skin incision with a nonabsorbable monofilament suture, and inject all incisions, as well as the wrist, with a local anesthetic.
- Place the wrist in a bulky dressing with a volar splint.

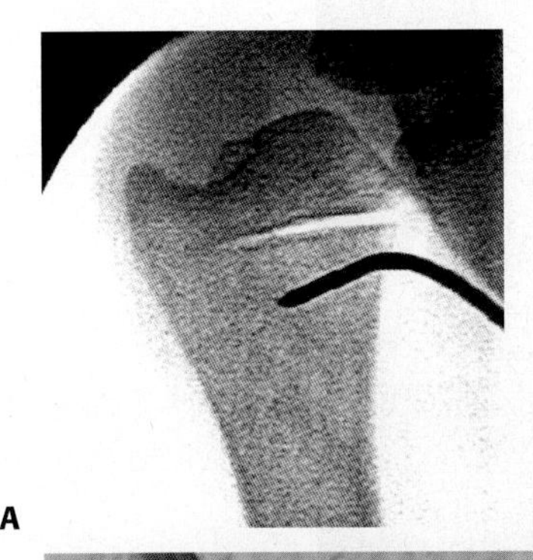
A

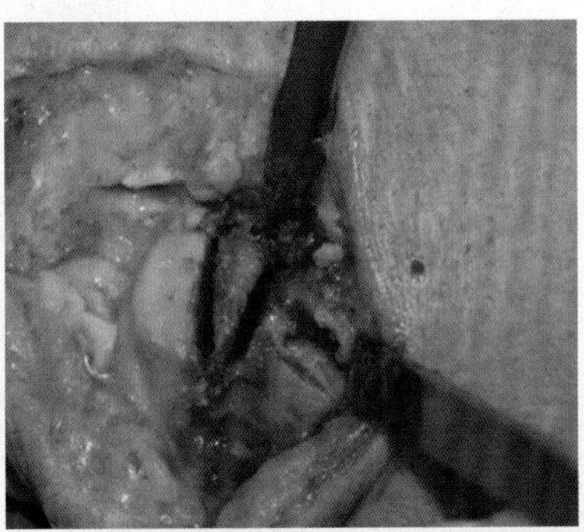
B

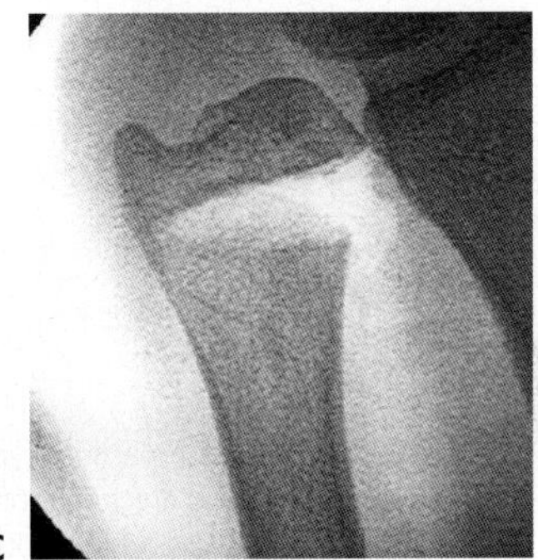
C

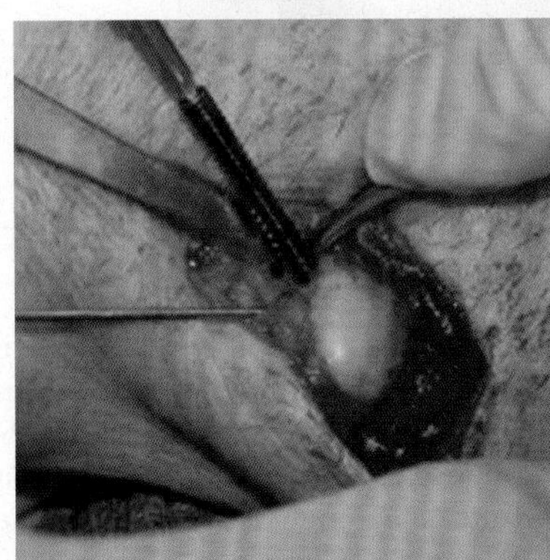
D

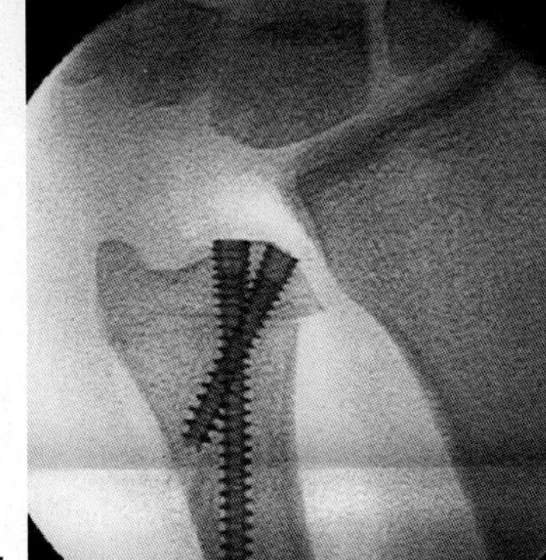
E

TECH FIG 7 • **A.** Fluoroscopic image of distal osteotomy, proximal to the sigmoid notch. **B.** Completion of radial wedge osteotomy. Bone wedge is removed using an osteotome. **C.** Fluoroscopic image of completed radial wedge osteotomy. **D.** Placement of headless compression screw over Kirschner wire. **E.** Radiograph after screw placement showing osteotomy compression. (From Slade JF III, Gillon TJ. Osteochondral shortening osteotomy for the treatment of ulnar impaction syndrome: a new technique. Tech Hand Up Extrem Surg 2007;11:74–82.)

PEARLS AND PITFALLS

- In very osteopenic bone, the surgeon should consider using a longer plate or locking hardware to achieve better bony purchase (**FIG 4**).
- Smokers, malnourished patients, and patients with poorly controlled diabetes or vascular compromise have a higher risk of osteotomy nonunion. The surgeon should consider a procedure that does not require bone healing (Darrach or wafer osteotomy).
- Ulnar shortening osteotomy should be avoided in patients with DRUJ arthritis. The surgeon should consider unloading the ulnocarpal axis with a Sauvé-Kapandji or Darrach procedure.
- The dorsal sensory branch of the ulnar nerve should be protected during the surgical exposure. It runs medial to the ulnar head with the forearm supinated and more palmar with the forearm pronated.[2]
- The surgeon should avoid circumferential exposure of the ulna to avoid injury to the segmental blood supply to the ulnar diaphysis, which typically enters the bone from the region of the interosseous membrane.[26]
- The ECU subsheath should not be disrupted during the surgical approach.
- In smaller patients, the surgeon should consider using a 2.7-mm AO dynamic compression plate.
- The Kirschner wires used in the Synthes distractor apparatus should be inserted far enough away from the osteotomy site such that they will not interfere with the osteotomy cuts. They should be biased palmarly in the ulna if dorsal plating is planned. The four pins should be inserted in the region that will be spanned by the plate to prevent creation of an unprotected stress riser. The surgeon should avoid passing the distal pins through the ulna into the radius, as this will prevent shortening of the ulna.
- Making the distal cut first may help to avoid placing the plate too distally on the ulna.
- The osteotomy site should be continuously irrigated while the bone is being cut to avoid thermal necrosis of the bone and periosteum.
- The surgeon should avoid overshortening the ulna, as this can lead to DRUJ instability, loss of forearm rotation, and increased DRUJ contact pressures.[14] Failure to consider the kerf thickness when planning the osteotomy can lead to excessive shortening.
- After the cuts are made, the surgeon should distract the osteotomy and inspect for bony excrescences or residual uncut bone margins, which can interfere with apposition of the proximal and distal fragments.
- Although the plate may be placed on the dorsal or palmar surface of the ulna, palmar positioning of the plate may be preferable to avoid a subcutaneous prominence of the hardware after surgery in thin or smaller patients.

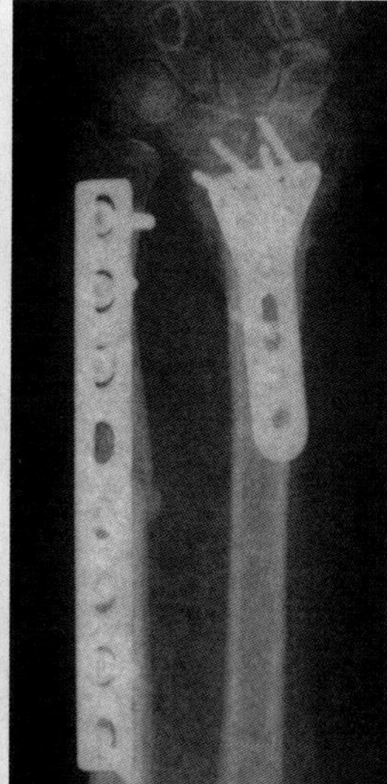

FIG 4 • Ulnar impaction syndrome in a 73-year-old woman after distal radius fracture nonunion and subsequent collapse. She underwent open reduction and internal fixation of the radius fracture as well as ulnar shortening osteotomy to correct the post-traumatic ulnar positive variance. Severe osteopenia prevented stable fixation of the ulnar osteotomy with the standard plate and necessitated a longer eight-hole DCP.

POSTOPERATIVE CARE

- Short-arm below-elbow splint immediately postoperatively
- Ice and elevation to assist with swelling control
- Elbow and finger ROM is encouraged immediately.
- Sutures are removed at 10 to 14 days.
- A removable splint is applied and protected ROM is started at 6 to 8 weeks, depending on the radiographic appearance of healing.
- More aggressive ROM exercises are started with hand therapy after 8 to 10 weeks if necessary.

OUTCOMES

- Chun and Palmer[6] reviewed their series of 30 wrists in 27 patients with an average follow-up of 51 months. Wrists were graded preoperatively and postoperatively according to the Gartland and Werley wrist system. Preoperative wrists graded as poor (28) and fair (2) improved to excellent (24), good (4), fair (1), and poor (1) after ulnar shortening osteotomy. They reported no ulnar nonunions, and complications were rare.
- Loh et al[11] evaluated 23 wrists at a mean follow-up of 33 months. A statistically significant reduction in pain intensity by visual analog scale assessment was seen in 77% of patients. Preoperative versus postoperative change in ROM was not statistically significant, and postoperative wrist function and grip strength also failed to show a statistically significant improvement. Sixty-eight percent of patients complained of local irritation secondary to prominent hardware and 32% eventually had the implant removed.

- We do not think that the use of specialized equipment is necessary to achieve accurate cuts and stable fixation for an ulnar shortening osteotomy.
  - Sunil et al[24] reported no significant differences in duration of surgery, relief of pain, return to work, postoperative complications, time elapsed between surgery and return to work, or osteotomy union in patients undergoing ulnar shortening osteotomy using the Rayhack device versus those undergoing freehand osteotomies.
  - Braun[3] reported a $650 increase in cost with use of the Rayhack device compared to performing the technique freehand.
- Our preferred technique is simple, it does not require specialized equipment (Synthes Small External Fixation and Small Fragment Bone Fixation Systems); it provides for rotational control of the distal segment; it provides compression of the osteotomy site; and it uses only one size of drill bit, tap, and screw except for the single interfragmentary hole at the osteotomy site.

COMPLICATIONS

- Wound infection and osteomyelitis (rare)
- Hardware fracture (rare with 3.5-mm plate)
- Hardware failure with very osteopenic bone
- Delayed union rates in smokers (7.1 months for smokers vs. 4.1 months for nonsmokers)[4]
- Painful, prominent hardware: It is generally not necessary to remove hardware, but 3.5-mm compression plates seem to be removable at 6 to 9 months in symptomatic patients with a low risk for refracture when sequential sets of radiographs confirm healing of the osteotomy site.[21]

REFERENCES

1. Berger RA. The ligaments of the wrist. A current overview of anatomy with considerations of their potential functions. Hand Clin 1997;13:63–82.
2. Botte MJ, Cohen MS, Lavernia CJ, et al. The dorsal branch of the ulnar nerve: an anatomic study. J Hand Surg Am 1990;15(4):603–607.
3. Braun RM. A comparative study of ulnar-shortening osteotomy by the freehand technique versus the Rayhack technique [letter to the editor]. J Hand Surg Am 2006;31(8):1411–1412.
4. Chen F, Osterman AL, Mahony K. Smoking and bony union after ulna-shortening osteotomy. Am J Orthop 2001;30:486–489.
5. Chen NC, Wolfe SW. Ulna shortening osteotomy using a compression device. J Hand Surg Am 2003;28(1):88–93.
6. Chun S, Palmer AK. The ulnar impaction syndrome: follow-up of ulnar shortening osteotomy. J Hand Surg Am 1993;18(1):46–53.
7. Fricker R, Pfeiffer KM, Troeger H. Ulnar shortening osteotomy in posttraumatic ulnar impaction syndrome. Arch Orthop Trauma Surg 1996;115:158–161.
8. Friedman SL, Palmer AK. The ulnar impaction syndrome. Hand Clin 1991;7:295–310.
9. Hammert WC, Williams RB, Greenberg JA. Distal metaphyseal ulnar-shortening osteotomy: surgical technique. J Hand Surg Am 2012;37(5):1071–1077.
10. Labosky DA, Waggy CA. Oblique ulnar shortening osteotomy by a single saw cut. J Hand Surg Am 1996;21(1):48–59.
11. Loh YC, Van Den Abbeele K, Stanley JK, et al. The results of ulnar shortening for ulnar impaction syndrome. J Hand Surg Br 1999;24(3):316–320.
12. Mikić ZD. Age changes in the triangular fibrocartilage of the wrist joint. J Anat 1978;126:367–384.
13. Mirza A, Mirza JB, Shin AY, et al. Isolated lunotriquetral ligament tears treated with ulnar shortening osteotomy. J Hand Surg Am 2013;38(8):1492–1497.
14. Miura T, Firoozbakhsh K, Cheema T, et al. Dynamic effects of joint-leveling procedure on pressure at the distal radioulnar joint. J Hand Surg Am 2005;30(4):711–718.
15. Mizuseki T, Tsuge K, Ikuta Y. Precise ulna-shortening osteotomy with a new device. J Hand Surg Am 2001;26(5):931–939.
16. Nishiwaki M, Nakamura T, Nakao Y, et al. Ulnar shortening effect on distal radioulnar joint stability: a biomechanical study. J Hand Surg Am 2005;30(4):719–726.
17. Nunez FA Jr, Barnwell J, Li Z, et al. Metaphyseal ulnar shortening osteotomy for the treatment of ulnocarpal abutment syndrome using distal ulna hook plate: case series. J Hand Surg Am 2012;37(8):1574–1579.
18. Palmer AK, Werner FW. The triangular fibrocartilage complex of the wrist—anatomy and function. J Hand Surg Am 1981;6(2):153–162.
19. Palmer AK, Werner FW, Glisson RR, et al. Partial excision of the triangular fibrocartilage complex. J Hand Surg Am 1988;13(3):391–394.
20. Papapetropoulos PA, Wartinbee DA, Richard MJ, et al. Management of peripheral triangular fibrocartilage complex tears in the ulnar positive patient: arthroscopic repair versus ulnar shortening osteotomy. J Hand Surg Am 2010;35(10):1607–1613.
21. Pomerance J. Plate removal after ulnar-shortening osteotomy. J Hand Surg Am 2005;30(5):949–953.
22. Rayhack JM. Ulnar shortening. Tech Hand Up Extrem Surg 2003;7:52–60.
23. Slade JF III, Gillon TJ. Osteochondral shortening osteotomy for the treatment of ulnar impaction syndrome: a new technique. Tech Hand Up Extrem Surg 2007;11:74–82.
24. Sunil TM, Wolff TW, Scheker LR, et al. A comparative study of ulnar-shortening osteotomy by the freehand technique versus the Rayhack technique. J Hand Surg Am 2006;31(2):252–257.
25. Tomaino MM. The importance of the pronated grip x-ray view in evaluating ulnar variance. J Hand Surg Am 2000;25(2):352–357.
26. Wright TW, Glowczewskie F. Vascular anatomy of the ulna. J Hand Surg Am 1998;23(5):800–804.
27. Yin HW, Qui YQ, Shen YD, et al. Arthroscopic distal metaphyseal ulnar shortening osteotomy: a different technique. J Hand Surg Am 2013;38(11):2257–2262.

Thumb Metacarpal Extension Osteotomy

Matthew M. Tomaino

DEFINITION

- When ligamentous restraint at the thumb carpometacarpal (CMC) joint is compromised, functional grip and pinch may result in painful synovitis and hypermobility long before the development of cartilage wear and arthritis.
- The so-called Eaton stage 1 disease can be treated with an extension osteotomy at the base of the thumb metacarpal (TM) joint as an alternative to either ligament reconstruction or arthroscopic synovectomy and pinning.[8,9]

ANATOMY

- The TM joint is a biconcave–convex saddle joint with minimal bony constraints, so ligamentous support is extremely important, especially considering the compressive forces transmitted across the joint during functional pinch. Eaton and Littler identified the anterior oblique "beak" ligament, so called for its attachment on the palmar beak of the TM, as the primary stabilizer of the TM joint.
- With the assistance of TM joint arthroscopy, Bettinger et al[1] have further defined the anterior oblique ligament (AOL) into a superficial anterior oblique ligament (sAOL) and deep anterior oblique ligament (dAOL). The dAOL, which is intracapsular, is, in fact, the beak ligament. The dAOL plays an important role in the kinematics of thumb opposition. It acts as a pivot point and becomes tight during pronation, opposition, and palmar abduction. The dAOL limits pronation in flexion and both pronation and supination in extension.
- In their comprehensive assessment of the ligamentous anatomy of the TM joint, Bettinger et al[1] described a total of 16 ligaments that stabilize the trapezium and TM. Seven of these ligaments, including the sAOL, dAOL beak ligament, dorsoradial (DRL), posterior oblique, ulnar collateral, intermetacarpal, and dorsal intermetacarpal, are responsible for directly stabilizing the TM joint.
- The DRL's role in joint stability has been debated, but Bettinger et al[1] showed that the DRL is an important joint stabilizer. The DRL, which covers a large percentage of the posterior aspect of the joint, is a wide, thick ligament that attaches to the trapezium and inserts on the dorsum of the metacarpal base. This ligament tightens with DRL and dorsal translational forces in all positions except full extension. It also tightens in supination and in pronation with joint flexion.

PATHOGENESIS

- Functional incompetence of the basal joint's AOL results in pathologic laxity, abnormal translation of the metacarpal on the trapezium, and generation of excessive shear forces between the joint surfaces, particularly within the palmar portion of the joint during grip and pinch activity. Histologic study has shown that attritional changes in the AOL at its attachment to the palmar lip of the metacarpal precede degeneration of cartilage.[2]

NATURAL HISTORY

- Because the AOL appears to be the primary stabilizer of the TM joint and because its detachment results in dorsal translation of the metacarpal, its reconstruction has been recommended to restore thumb stability not only in cases of end-stage osteoarthritis but also for early-stage disease.
- Pellegrini et al[6] were the first to evaluate the biomechanical efficacy of extension osteotomy. Palmar contact area was unloaded with a concomitant shift in contact more dorsally so long as arthrosis did not extend more dorsal than the midpoint of the trapezium.
- Shrivastava et al[7] studied the effect of a simulated osteotomy on TM joint laxity by flexing the metacarpal base 30 degrees, thus placing the joint in the relationship it would assume if an extension osteotomy was performed.
  - The simulated extension osteotomy reduced laxity in all directions tested: dorsal–volar (40% reduction), radial–ulnar (23% reduction), distraction (15% reduction), and pronation–supination (29% reduction).
  - They hypothesized that the beneficial clinical effects of a TM extension osteotomy may be partially due to tightening of the DRL, which might reduce dorsal translation.

PATIENT HISTORY AND PHYSICAL FINDINGS

- Basal joint arthritis may present with mild symptoms beneath the thenar eminence at the level of the TM joint, particularly during pinch and grip. Ultimately, the greatest functional impairment occurs with advanced disease—limiting breadth of grasp and forceful lateral pinch activities such as brushing teeth, turning a key, opening a jar, or picking up a book.
- Complaints are directed toward the base of the thumb, and pain is frequently associated with a sensation of movement or "slipping" within the joint. An enlarging prominence, or "shoulder sign," inevitably develops at the base as the clinical manifestation of dorsal metacarpal subluxation on the trapezium and metacarpal adduction.
- Early presentation may result in only pain with TM stress and palpation beneath the thenar cone, without deformity, instability, subluxation, or crepitance.
- Methods for examining the thumb CMC joint for hypermobility (stage 1 disease) include the following:
  - Trapeziometacarpal stress test, which may cause pain or a slight shift or subluxation
  - Thenar CMC joint palpation test, which may cause pain

IMAGING AND OTHER DIAGNOSTIC STUDIES

- Radiographic evaluation includes a posteroanterior (PA) 30-degree oblique stress view, lateral view, and a Robert (pronated anteroposterior [AP]) view (**FIG 1**).
- Osteoarthritis may be confined to the TM joint, or it may involve the pantrapezial joint complex. Indeed, the staging system described by Eaton and Littler describes four stages:
  - Stage 1: a normal joint with the exception of possible widening from synovitis
  - Stage 2: joint space narrowing with debris and osteophytes smaller than 2 mm
  - Stage 3: joint space narrowing with debris and osteophytes larger than 2 mm
  - Stage 4: scaphotrapezial joint space involvement in addition to narrowing of the TM joint

DIFFERENTIAL DIAGNOSIS

- CMC arthritis (stages 2 to 4)
- De Quervain tendonitis
- Flexor carpi radialis tendinitis

NONOPERATIVE MANAGEMENT

- Nonoperative treatment includes anti-inflammatory medication, intra-articular steroid injection, hand- or forearm-based thumb spica splint immobilization, and thenar muscle isometric conditioning.
- Although none of these measures may provide permanent or even long-lasting relief from symptoms, they may indeed provide temporary relief. This allows the patient to contemplate surgery, to gain acceptance, and to participate in the surgical decision-making process.

SURGICAL MANAGEMENT

- Until recently, surgical treatment has centered around reconstruction of the palmar beak ligament with a slip of flexor carpi radialis tendon, as described by Eaton and Littler.[3]
- The rationale for TM extension osteotomy involves dorsal load transfer and a shift in force vectors during pinch. Pellegrini et al[6] showed that a 30-degree closing wedge extension osteotomy effectively unloaded the palmar compartment when eburnation involved less than half, and optimally only one-third, of the palmar joint surfaces. Osteotomy in this setting shifted the contact areas to the intact dorsal articular cartilage.
- The most recent biomechanical assessment of metacarpal osteotomy suggested that joint laxity is reduced in lateral pinch because of obligatory metacarpal flexion and resulting increased tightening of the dorsal radial ligament.[7]

Preoperative Planning

- Radiographs should show a normal joint or slight widening from synovitis. A trapeziometacarpal stress test should elicit pain along with palpation of the joint beneath the thenars. Obviously, other causes of discomfort in the region should be excluded.

Positioning

- The extremity is placed on a standard hand table.

Approach

- A dorsal approach is used and subperiosteal exposure of the base of the metacarpal is provided.
- The osteotomy is made 1 cm distal to the base and is 5 mm wide, so the incision should extend 4 cm distal to the base.
  - The base of the wedge is therefore 5 mm wide and is dorsal. Its apex is palmar.

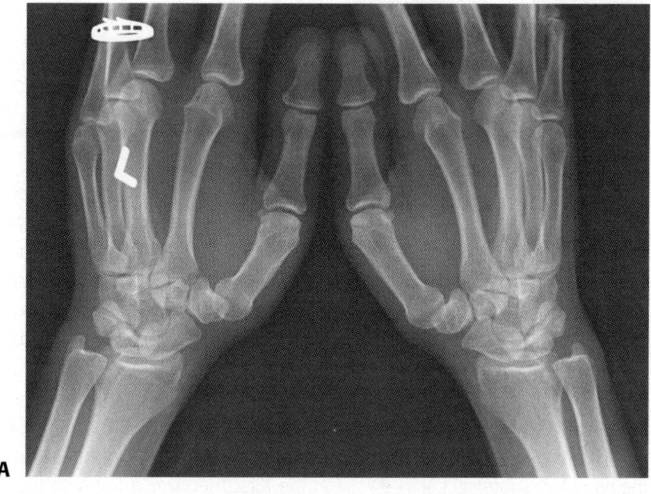

A

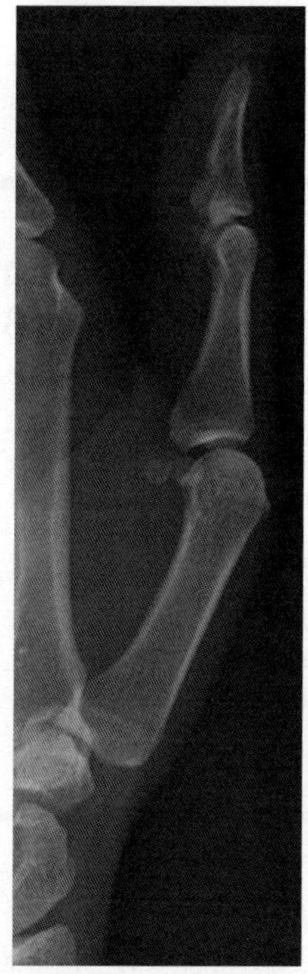

B

FIG 1 • AP (**A**) and lateral (**B**) preoperative thumb radiographs.

Extension Osteotomy with Staple Fixation

- Regional, axillary block anesthesia is performed and a nonsterile tourniquet is placed.
- After exsanguination with an Esmarch bandage and inflation of the tourniquet to 250 mm Hg, make a dorsal incision from the base of the TM distally for about 3 cm.
- In the subcutaneous tissue, identify and protect the sensory branches of the radial and lateral antebrachial cutaneous nerves. Obtain subperiosteal exposure without injuring the extensor pollicis longus, and identify the TM joint with a 25-gauge needle.
  - One centimeter distal to the TM joint, obtain near-circumferential access around the metacarpal in anticipation of the osteotomy.
- Visualize the volar extent of the metacarpal at this location to facilitate accurate resection of a dorsally based 30-degree wedge of bone (**TECH FIG 1A**).
- Use a microsagittal saw to score the metacarpal 1 cm distal to its base transversely, but do not make a complete cut through the volar cortex.
  - Leave a new saw blade in that partial osteotomy site and use a second blade about 5 mm distal to the first cut at an angle of 30 degrees so that the two blades intersect at the volar cortex.
- Remove the wedge of bone, extend the distal metacarpal and compress it against the proximal fragment, and place one 11 × 8 staple (OSStaple, BioMedical Enterprises, Inc., San Antonio, TX).
  - Typically, I maintain the reduced position of the metacarpal while my assistant predrills and then places the staple (**TECH FIG 1B,C**).
- Perform a layered closure of the periosteum and skin and place an overlying thumb spica splint.

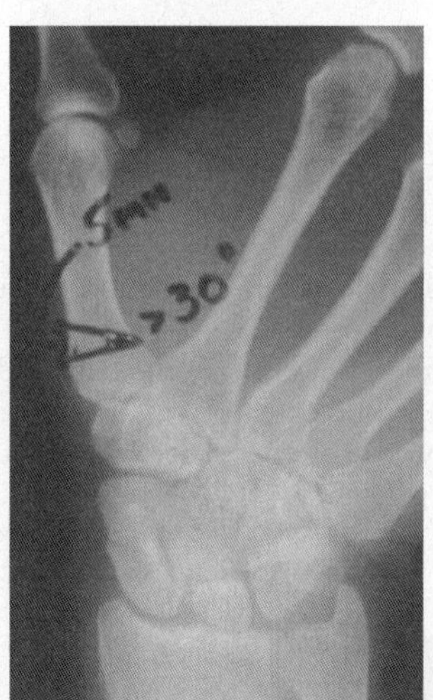

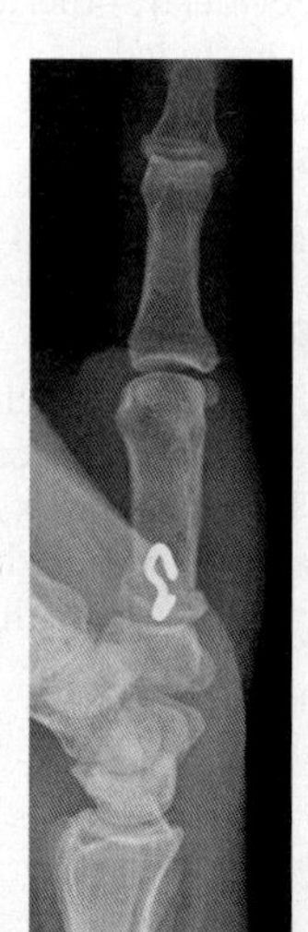

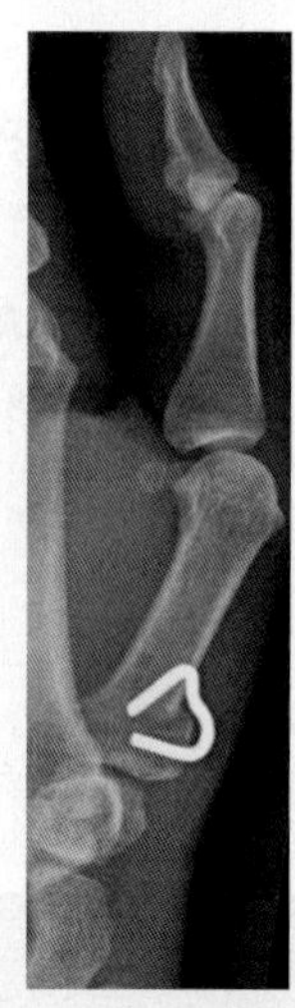

TECH FIG 1 • **A.** Radiograph showing planned osteotomy. **B,C.** AP and lateral postoperative thumb radiographs.

Extension Osteotomy with Kirschner Wire and Tension Band Fixation

- The technique is as described for staple fixation except for the use of Kirschner wires.
- Use a microsagittal saw to score the metacarpal 1 cm distal to its base transversely, but do not make a complete cut through the volar cortex.
  - Leave a new saw blade in that partial osteotomy site and use a second blade about 5 mm distal to the first cut at an angle of 30 degrees so that the two blades intersect at the volar cortex.
- Remove the wedge of bone and use a 0.045-inch Kirschner wire to place a transverse hole on either side of the osteotomy.
  - Pass a 22-gauge wire radial to ulnar and ulnar to radial.
  - Place a 0.045-inch Kirschner wire retrograde through the distal osteotomy site, exiting out the ulnar aspect of the thumb, and compress the osteotomy by extending the distal metacarpal.
  - With an assistant maintaining compression, tighten the wire, cut it, and bend it beneath the thenar musculature. Then advance the Kirschner wire anterograde.
- Cut the Kirschner wire external to the skin to facilitate removal, and repair the periosteal origin of the thenar musculature with absorbable suture.

PEARLS AND PITFALLS

Intra-articular osteotomy	■ Accurately locate the CMC joint with a 25-gauge needle so that the osteotomy is made 1 cm distal to the base.
Accurate execution of a 30-degree osteotomy	■ Make the most proximal cut perpendicular to the metacarpal—with the metacarpal parallel to the table. ■ Make the second cut at an angle of 30 degrees—5 mm distal to the first cut—such that the saw blade intersects the volar cortex at the location of the first blade.

POSTOPERATIVE CARE

- A thumb spica splint is placed for 10 days.
- At that time sutures are removed, and a thumb spica cast with the interphalangeal joint of the thumb left free is placed for an additional 4 weeks.
- About 6 weeks after surgery, a forearm-based thumb spica Orthoplast splint is placed and the patient is instructed to begin gentle TM motion.
- Grip and pinch exercises are started at about 8 weeks after surgery unless union is delayed.

OUTCOMES

- In light of Pellegrini et al's[6] biomechanical data and my own relative dissatisfaction with Eaton ligament reconstruction for stage 1 disease, primarily related to a prolonged recovery period (8 to 10 months) and a stiff TM joint, I prospectively evaluated the efficacy of a 30-degree extension osteotomy in 12 patients (12 thumbs) between 1995 and 1998.[9]
  - TM arthrotomy allowed accurate intra-articular assessment and verified AOL detachment from the metacarpal rim in each case.
  - Follow-up averaged 2.1 years (range 6 to 46 months).
  - All osteotomies healed at an average of 7 weeks. Eleven patients were satisfied with outcome. Grip and pinch strength increased an average of 8.5 and 3 kg, respectively.
- Since that study's publication, I have become even more impressed by the efficacy of the procedure and believe, as Koff et al[4] suggested, that osteotomy decreases laxity and shifts contact area more dorsally. It seems logical that the DRL participates in this effect and this substantiates the contention that the DRL is an important stabilizer.
- In 2008, Parker et al[5] published long-term outcomes following extension osteotomy in eight patients in whom the Eaton stage was I in three patients, II in 3 patients, and III in two patients. Follow-up ranged from 6 to 13 years, and pinch and grip strength increased 129%, 103%, and 108%, respectively. Eaton stage was preserved in five of the eight patients, with excellent functional outcomes in six of eight patients at a mean of 9 years. Although numbers are small, their data suggests that first metacarpal extension osteotomy can be an effective and durable procedure that does not limit future salvage procedures such as trapeziectomy or arthroplasty and supports the use of this treatment in early and moderate Eaton stages.
- Since the publication of the first edition of this text, I continue to use TM extension osteotomy for the painful hypermobile CMC joint Eaton stage I disease. However, rather than using staple fixation, which I advocated earlier, preferentially, over Kirschner wire fixation with a cerclage wire, I now preferentially use the latter technique, which, in my hands, is easier to reliably execute.

COMPLICATIONS

- Nonunion
- Persistent pain necessitating resection arthroplasty with trapezium excision
- Radial sensory nerve injury or dysesthesia

REFERENCES

1. Bettinger PC, Linscheid RL, Berger RA, et al. An anatomic study of the stabilizing ligaments of the trapezium and trapeziometacarpal joint. J Hand Surg Am 1999;24(4):786–798.
2. Doerschuk SH, Hicks DG, Chinchilli VM, et al. Histopathology of the palmar beak ligament in trapeziometacarpal osteoarthritis. J Hand Surg Am 1999;24(3):496–504.
3. Eaton RG, Lane LB, Littler JW, et al. Ligament reconstruction for the painful thumb carpometacarpal joint: a long-term assessment. J Hand Surg Am 1984;9(5):692–699.
4. Koff MF, Shrivastava N, Gardner TR, et al. An in vitro analysis of ligament reconstruction or extension osteotomy on trapeziometacarpal joint stability and contact area. J Hand Surg Am 2006;31(3):429–439.
5. Parker WL, Linscheid RL, Amadio PC. Long-term outcomes of first metacarpal extension osteotomy in the treatment of carpal-metacarpal osteoarthritis. J Hand Surg Am 2008;33(10):1737–1743.
6. Pellegrini VD Jr, Parentis M, Judkins A, et al. Extension metacarpal osteotomy in the treatment of trapeziometacarpal osteoarthritis: a biomechanical study. J Hand Surg Am 1996;21(1):16–23.
7. Shrivastava N, Koff MF, Abbot AE, et al. Simulated extension osteotomy of the thumb metacarpal reduces carpometacarpal joint laxity in lateral pinch. J Hand Surg Am 2003;28(5):733–738.
8. Tomaino MM. Thumb by metacarpal extension osteotomy: rationale and efficacy for Eaton stage I disease. Hand Clin 2006;22:137–141.
9. Tomaino MM. Treatment of Eaton stage I trapeziometacarpal disease with thumb metacarpal extension osteotomy. J Hand Surg Am 2000;25(6):1100–1106.

Thumb Carpometacarpal Arthrodesis

K. J. Hippensteel and Ryan Calfee

DEFINITION

- The trapeziometacarpal joint of the thumb is frequently affected by osteoarthritis, second in frequency only to the distal interphalangeal joint, but often more disabling due to pain and weakness of grip and pinch strength.
- The choice of surgical management for symptomatic thumb carpometacarpal (CMC) joint arthrosis varies according to patient age, medical comorbidities, functional demands, and radiographic staging.
- Arthrodesis of the CMC joint was initially described by Muller[13] in 1949. Despite the popularity of arthroplasty at this joint, arthrodesis can also provide excellent functional outcomes.
- Arthrodesis is ideal for the younger patient with moderate to advanced thumb CMC degeneration (arthritic or posttraumatic) who anticipates higher load pinch and grip requirements.[9]

ANATOMY

- The thumb CMC joint is a biconcave–convex (saddle) joint, permitting motion in three planes: flexion–extension, abduction–adduction, and pronation–supination. These multiplanar motions allow for power grip, power pinch, opposition, and delicate precision pinch.
- Provided minimal osseous constraints, ligamentous structures are largely responsible for stabilizing the thumb CMC joint.
- Sixteen ligaments have been described around the thumb CMC joint.
  - Seven are primary stabilizers of the thumb CMC joint:
    - Superficial anterior oblique ligament (sAOL) and deep anterior oblique ligament (dAOL)
    - Dorsoradial
    - Posterior oblique
    - Ulnar collateral
    - Intermetacarpal
    - Dorsal intermetacarpal
- The remainder stabilize the trapezium, providing a stable foundation for the thumb.[2]

PATHOGENESIS

- The pathogenesis of CMC joint arthrosis is multifactorial, involving biochemical,[16] biomechanical, and genetic influences.
- Osteoarthritis of the thumb CMC joint occurs more commonly in females compared to males.
- Arthritic degeneration begins on the palmar aspect of the thumb metacarpal and trapezium. This may be secondary to compression in this area during pinch.
- The dorsal ligament complex (dorsoradial and posterior oblique ligaments) is the thickest, strongest, and most important ligament stabilizing the thumb CMC joint. It prevents both the thumb metacarpal volar beak from disengaging from the volar recess in the trapezium as well as dorsal subluxation of the metacarpal base during power grip or pinch. Although the anterior (palmar) oblique ligament, or so-called beak ligament, was thought to be the most important stabilizing ligament of the thumb, multiple studies have suggested the dorsal ligament complex is the most critical stabilizer.[3,19,22] The volar beak ligament is completely lax in opposition and taut only in the hitchhiker position.
- Arthritis begins secondary to the compressive, rotational shear forces during power pinch and grip in the volar recess of the trapezium near to the volar beak of the metacarpal. After many years, the volar beak begins to wear down and instability develops during the screw-home-torque rotation seen in opposition.[7] With progression of disease, osteophytes develop and eburnation progresses throughout the entire joint surface.
- Osteoarthrosis can also develop from disruption of the articular cartilage. Any fracture involving the articular surfaces (most commonly the base of the thumb metacarpal) will predispose to, or accelerate the development of, arthrosis. This is the result of direct cartilage injury at the time of the accident or over time secondary to articular incongruity or articular surface irregularity.
  - Anatomic restoration of the joint surface can minimize this progression but not eliminate it completely.

NATURAL HISTORY

- Arthrosis of the thumb CMC joint begins along the palmar aspect of the metacarpal secondary to the compressive rotational shear and dorsal subluxating forces during pinch and grip. These forces can approach 164 kg during power grasp at the CMC joint.[4]
- The entire base of the metacarpal and the distal trapezium experience eburnation of the cartilage, which progresses to develop osteophytes.
- As arthritis progresses, the thumb metacarpal subluxates dorsally and radially. The metacarpal adducts and flexes resulting in compensatory metacarpophalangeal (MCP) joint hyperextension. This hyperextension effectively brings the thumb pulp out of the palm to allow for grasp.
- In fulminant arthritis, the entire surface of the trapezium becomes involved, resulting in degeneration between the proximal trapezium and the distal scaphoid.
- Arthrosis can involve all the trapezial articulations as well as the scaphotrapezoidal joint.[15,21]

PATIENT HISTORY AND PHYSICAL FINDINGS

- Thumb CMC joint arthrosis will often present with pain at the base of the metacarpal.
  - The pain will be exacerbated with activities that load the thumb metacarpal base, such as turning a doorknob, twisting a lid off a jar, or turning a key.
  - Pain at rest may or may not be present.
  - This classic deep-seated pain at the base of the thenar muscles must be distinguished from de Quervain tendonitis, tendonitis of the flexor carpi radialis, radioscaphoid degeneration, and trigger thumb.
- Symptoms do not always correlate with the clinical or radiographic appearance. A patient may have advanced clinical and radiographic disease with minimal symptoms. Conversely, a patient may have significant symptoms with minimal radiographic changes and no clinical deformity.
- Physical examination of the patient with advanced disease reveals deformity.
  - The thumb metacarpal base subluxates in a dorsal direction and the metacarpal becomes fixed in adduction and flexion. This manifests as a metacarpal prominence at the CMC joint with decreased ability to abduct the thumb away from the palm.
  - In an effort to compensate for this limitation, the MCP joint will often hyperextend, creating a zigzag deformity.
  - Asking the patient to place one finger on the point that is most symptomatic helps localize the point of maximal tenderness to the CMC joint or another area.
  - CMC grind test: Reproduction of symptoms while axially loading the thumb and circumducting the thumb metacarpal confirms the CMC joint as a site of disease.
  - Finkelstein maneuver: Maximal tenderness over the radial styloid during ulnar deviation of the hand with a thumb in the fist suggests that de Quervain tendonitis may be a greater source of symptoms.
  - Phalen test: Reproduction of symptoms during wrist flexion indicates carpal tunnel syndrome as a more likely etiology.
  - Carpal tunnel compression test (Durkan test): Reproduction of symptoms with compression over the carpal tunnel indicates carpal tunnel syndrome as a more likely etiology of symptoms.
  - Trigger evaluation: Reproduction of pain, triggering, or locking of the thumb at the interphalangeal joint with activity flexion indicates trigger thumb as an etiology.
  - Allen test: The radial and ulnar arteries are compressed and the hand is exsanguinated. The ulnar artery is released and the circulation of the hand is assessed. The process is repeated, releasing the radial artery while the ulnar artery is occluded. Surgical procedures often involve mobilization of the radial artery in the snuffbox. Damage to this artery will require reconstruction if the ulnar artery cannot compensate.

IMAGING AND OTHER DIAGNOSTIC STUDIES

- Plain radiographs are the imaging modality of choice for evaluation of thumb CMC joint arthrosis (**FIG 1**).
  - These include posteroanterior, pronated anteroposterior (AP) (Robert view), lateral, and Bett views.
- Eaton and Littler[6] have described a radiographic staging system that is commonly used.
  - Stage I: normal-appearing or widened joint space secondary to synovitis

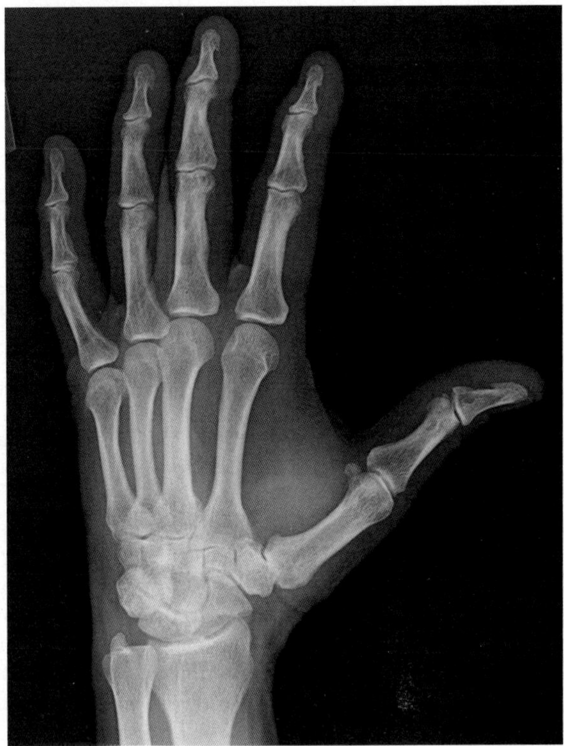

FIG 1 • Posteroanterior (PA) radiograph of wrist showing osteoarthritis of the thumb CMC joint.

  - Stage II: joint space narrowing and osteophyte formation smaller than 2 mm
  - Stage III: joint space narrowing with osteophytes larger than 2 mm
  - Stage IV: stage III appearance with the addition of narrowing or osteophytes in the scaphotrapezial joint
- The scaphotrapezoid joint is not specifically addressed in this system and may be difficult to assess radiographically, but this joint should always be assessed at the time of surgery because it may be a source of continued pain.[21]

DIFFERENTIAL DIAGNOSIS

- Thumb CMC arthrosis
- De Quervain disease
- Trigger thumb or stenosing tenosynovitis
- Flexor carpi radialis tendonitis
- Scaphoid pathology (fracture, nonunion, avascular necrosis)
- Radioscaphoid arthrosis
- Scaphotrapeziotrapezoid (STT) arthrosis
- Carpal tunnel syndrome
- Intramuscular (thenar) processes, such as vascular or tumor etiologies

NONOPERATIVE MANAGEMENT

- Most patients with symptomatic thumb CMC joint arthrosis benefit from a trial of conservative therapy, which may include rest, oral anti-inflammatory medication, intra-articular corticosteroid injection, thenar isometric strengthening exercises, and splinting.[1]
  - Forty percent of patients can have significant and sustained relief of pain with steroid injection and splinting for

3 weeks regardless of radiographic staging. If separated by Eaton's staging, over 80% with stage I can have sustained relief for over 18 months compared to approximately 33% with stage II or III or less than 25% with stage IV.[5]

- Although nonoperative treatment does not eliminate the problem or alter the underlying disease process, it often reduces symptoms and may either negate the need for surgery or at least allow for delay of surgical intervention. During this time, patients are reassured that continued activity is not expected to change the disease course and that despite radiographic progression, the arthritic pain may at times improve over time.

SURGICAL MANAGEMENT

- The indication for surgical intervention for symptomatic thumb basilar joint arthrosis is pain and weakness not sufficiently responsive to conservative treatments.
- There are multiple procedures used to treat symptomatic CMC thumb arthritis, none of which have proven superiority.
- The ideal patients for thumb CMC arthrodesis are younger, active patients who need to maintain power grip and pinch and regularly place high force demand on their thumb. These are typically younger manual laborers with stage II or III disease. However, arthrodesis can provide symptomatic relief in older patients with stage II or III disease.
- The condition of joints around the thumb CMC joint should be considered, as pathology may relatively contraindicate CMC arthrodesis.
  - STT arthritis also contraindicates thumb CMC arthrodesis as the patient would be expected to experience continued symptoms from this joint postoperatively.[9]
  - Thumb MCP hyperextension or arthrosis may require MCP arthrodesis which would markedly limit the thumb if the CMC joint is also fused.[9]

Preoperative Planning

- The patient should be made aware of the decreased mobility, inability to flatten the palm on the table (index MCP joint typically 1 to 2 cm off table when attempting to flatten palm), potential difficulty in placing the hand in tight confined spaces, and possible difficulty placing the hand in a glove.[9]
- Patients also should understand the risks of nonunion, prolonged postoperative casting, potential for hardware complications, and potential for developing degenerative changes at adjacent joints.

Positioning

- The procedure is performed under regional or general anesthesia with the use of a pneumatic tourniquet on either the proximal forearm or upper arm.
- The patient is supine with the arm extended on an arm board.

Approach

- We prefer a dorsal incision be oriented in a longitudinal fashion, along the ulnar aspect of the first dorsal compartment tendons.
- Alternatively, the procedure can be performed through a Wagner-type incision, along the junction of the glabrous and dorsal skin, or through a dorsal incision.

Thumb Carpometacarpal (Trapeziometacarpal) Arthrodesis

Incision and Dissection

- Make a dorsal longitudinal incision along the ulnar aspect of the first dorsal compartment tendons using a knife and then dissect once into subcutaneous tissue with tenotomy scissors (**TECH FIG 1A**).
- Identify and protect sensory branches of the radial nerve and the lateral antebrachial cutaneous nerve in the subcutaneous tissue (**TECH FIG 1B**).
- Identify the interval between the first dorsal compartment tendons and the EPL tendon.
- The first dorsal compartment is released.
- Identify the dorsal branch of the radial artery deep to the abductor pollicis longus and extensor pollicis brevis tendons running in a dorsal and ulnar direction. Carefully mobilize and protect it by retracting it dorsally throughout the remainder of the case (**TECH FIG 1C**). The radial artery courses directly over the STT joint.
- Identify the base of the thumb metacarpal, and complete a longitudinal capsulotomy to expose the base of the metacarpal, the entire trapezium, and the distal aspect of the scaphoid.
- Fluoroscopy is used to confirm the location of the CMC joint if necessary.

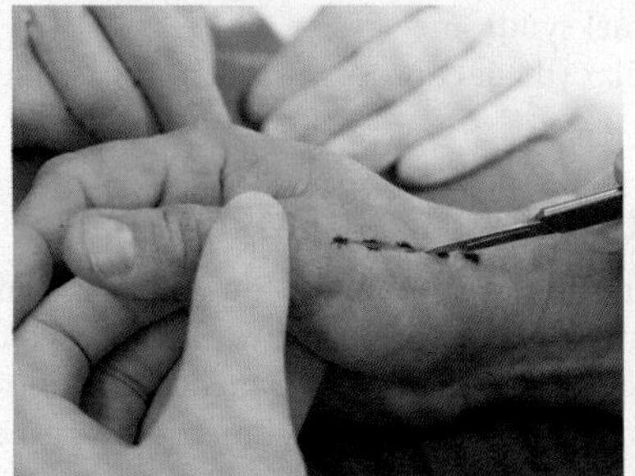
A

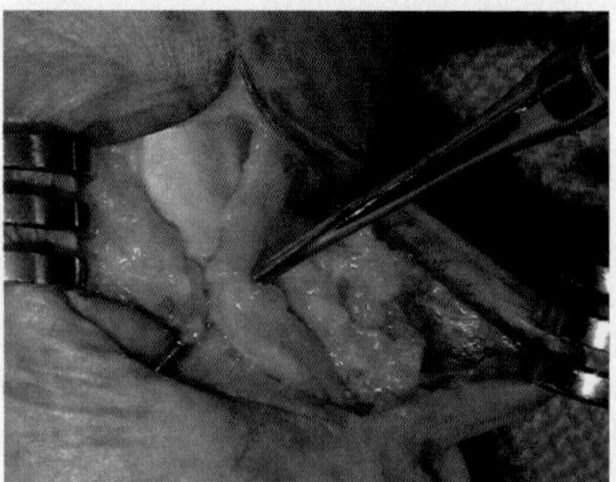
B

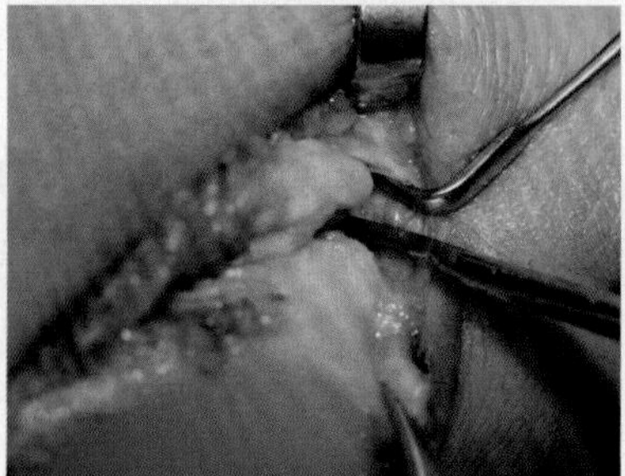
C

TECH FIG 1 • **A.** Dorsal longitudinal incision along the ulnar aspect of the first dorsal compartment. **B.** Surgical incision with identification of the radial sensory nerve. **C.** Dorsal branch of radial artery is mobilized and protected by retracting it dorsally and proximally.

Preparation of the Joint

- Inspect the STT joints.
  - If there is evidence of arthrosis, consideration is given to alternative procedures such as trapeziectomy and possible ligament interposition.
- Inspect the CMC joint (**TECH FIG 2A**).
  - By releasing the surrounding capsular attachments radially and ulnarly, the base of the metacarpal can be flexed to allow better access to the joint.
- Use a rongeur to remove osteophytes (**TECH FIG 2B**), any remaining articular cartilage, and subchondral sclerotic bone to get down to healthy cancellous bone at the base of the thumb metacarpal.
  - Shape the metacarpal base in a convex fashion to match the trapezium (**TECH FIG 2C**).
- Decorticate the distal aspect of the trapezium in a similar fashion (**TECH FIG 2D,E**).
  - Use a water-cooled burr to perform final contouring of the concave surface of the trapezium.
- Per surgeon preference, the articular surfaces can also be prepared as parallel flat surfaces with a water-cooled oscillating saw.

Distal Radius Bone Graft Harvest

- Distal radius autograft is harvested to pack into the arthrodesis site.
- Extend the dorsal incision proximal to Lister tubercle and bluntly spread through the subcutaneous tissues to expose the extensor retinaculum.
- Incise the retinaculum sharply over the radial edge of Lister tubercle to expose the tubercle's surface within the second extensor compartment.

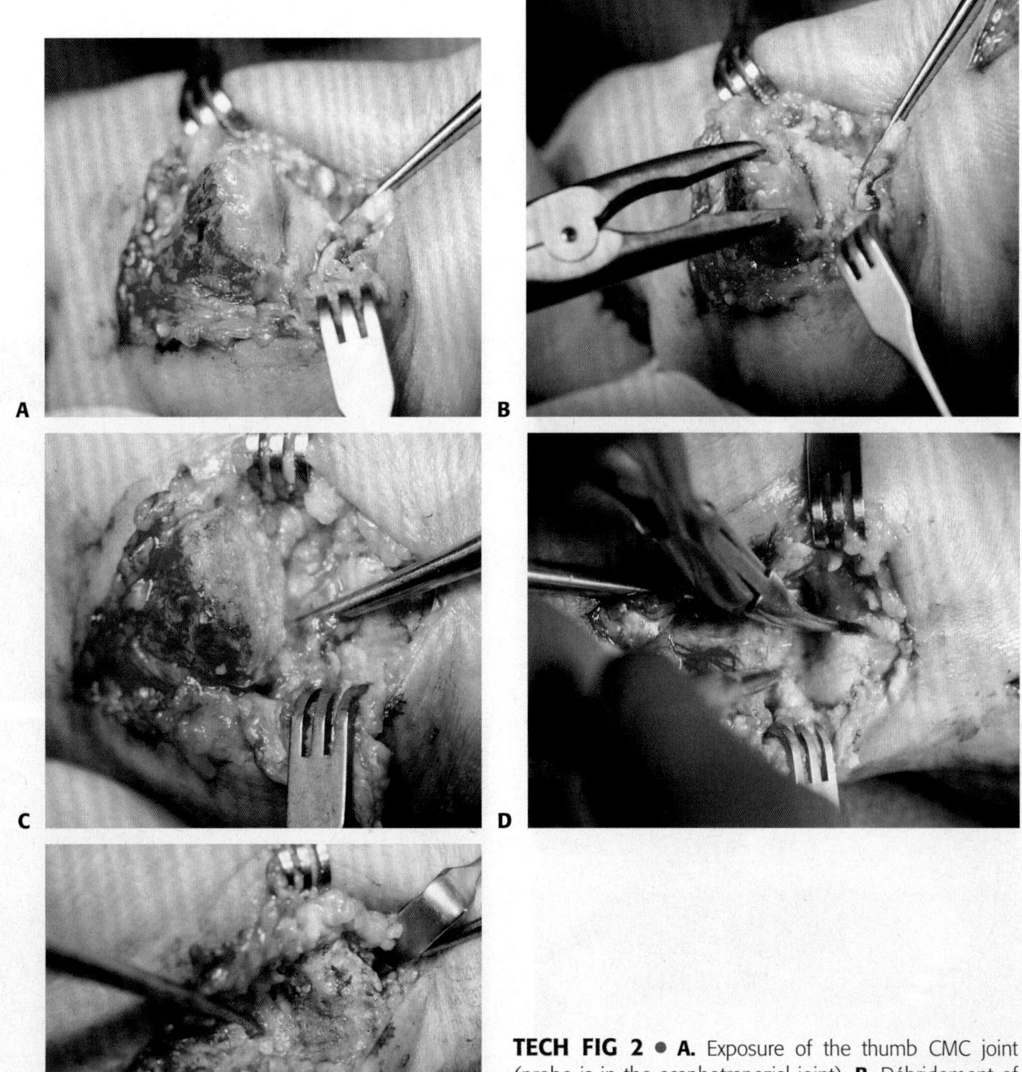

TECH FIG 2 • **A.** Exposure of the thumb CMC joint (probe is in the scaphotrapezial joint). **B.** Débridement of thumb metacarpal with a rongeur. **C.** Thumb metacarpal base fully débrided. **D.** View of the CMC joint while trapezium is being débrided with a rongeur. **E.** Trapezium is fully débrided in preparation for arthrodesis.

- Use a curette as a hand drill (spin with compressive force applied by hand) into the radial border of Lister tubercle. This provides access to the medullary canal through an area of thin cortex. Cancellous bone graft is harvested.

Positioning and Fixation

- The position for arthrodesis should allow the pulp of the thumb to rest against the radial distal aspect of the index middle phalanx when the hand is resting with slight wrist extension.
  - The exact angles to accomplish this position are debated, but in general, there should be about 30 to 45 degrees of palmar abduction and adequate pronation to direct the thumb pulp space toward the index finger.
- Once positioned, provisionally stabilize the CMC joint with a single 0.045 Kirschner wire. This allows for clinical assessment of position and fluoroscopic evaluation.
- A six- to eight-hole plate (two rows of screws) is applied across the CMC joint (**TECH FIG 3A**), and sequentially, two holes in trapezium are drilled and screws placed (**TECH FIG 3B**).
  - Cortical or locking screws can be used based on bony purchase and plate apposition on the trapezium.
  - Care should be taken to ensure that screws in the trapezium do not violate the articular surfaces of the scaphoid, trapezoid, or index metacarpal.
- While maintaining reduction and manual compression of the thumb metacarpal against the trapezium and plate, the remaining four to six holes are drilled and cortical screws placed (**TECH FIG 3C**).
- Distal radius bone graft is then packed into the fusion site (**TECH FIG 3D**).
- At this time, final assessment of clinical alignment and fluoroscopic evaluation (position, bony contact, hardware placement/screw length) are performed (see **FIG 2A,B**).
- Irrigate the wound lightly with saline. Close the capsule with a nonabsorbable suture (3-0 Ethibond), repeat irrigation, and deflate the tourniquet to confirm hemostasis as the radial artery and venae comitantes are within the operative field. Close the skin with 4-0 nylon horizontal mattress sutures.
- If mild thumb MCP joint hyperextension is noted at this juncture, pin the MCP joint in 20 degrees of flexion with a single 0.045 Kirschner wire or consider a volar capsulodesis. In our experience, correction of the fixed flexion and adduction of the thumb metacarpal often improves MCP position with pinch so that operative intervention at the MCP joint is infrequent.
- Apply soft sterile dressings and a well-padded short-arm thumb spica splint.

Fixation Options

- Although we prefer plate fixation, single or multiple smooth Kirschner wires, tension band wiring, cerclage wiring, staples, compression screws, and other types of plate and screw constructs have all been used with documented success.[9]
- Conflicting reports of union rates are reported when comparing Kirschner wires to more rigid fixation devices such as plates and screws.[8,11]

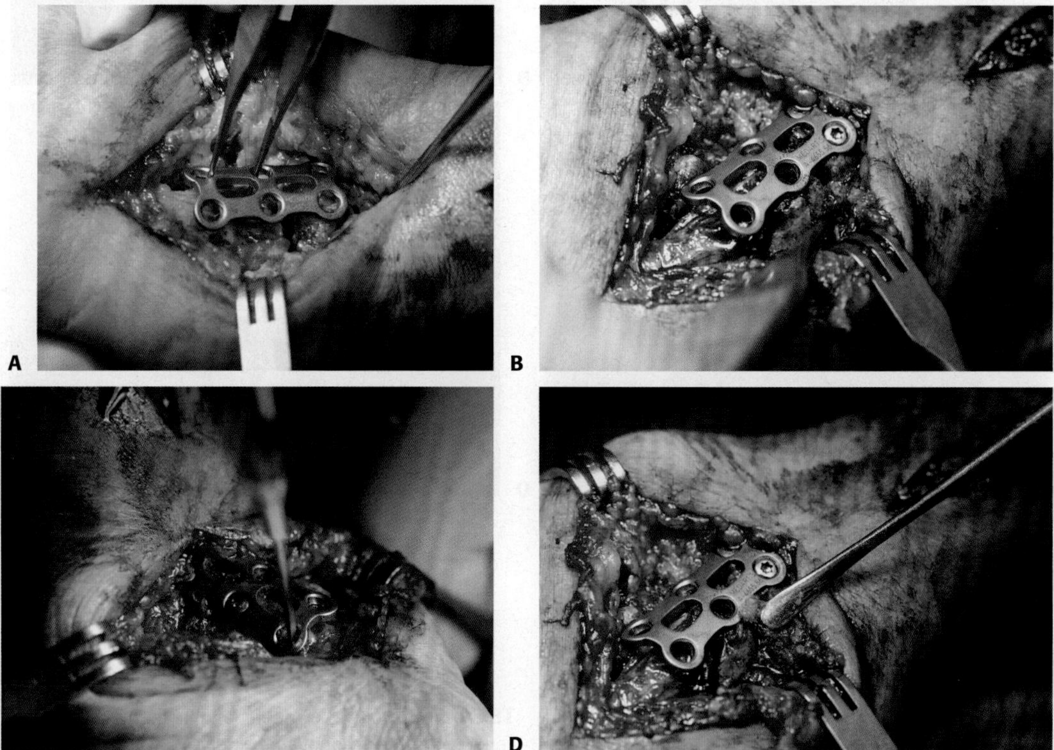

TECH FIG 3 • **A.** A six-hole plate is applied across the CMC joint. **B.** Two screws have been placed through the plate into the trapezium. **C.** Plate being applied onto the thumb CMC. **D.** Distal radius bone graft being packed into the CMC joint.

PEARLS AND PITFALLS

Surgical approach	■ Take care to protect the cutaneous branches of the radial sensory nerve and the lateral antebrachial cutaneous nerve throughout the entire procedure. ■ Protect the radial artery coursing over the STT joint.
Intraoperative joint inspection	■ Carefully inspect the STT joints, as arthritic involvement will preclude success with CMC arthrodesis.
Judicious use of bone graft	■ Make sure there is good apposition of the bony surfaces before closure. Distal radius autograft is ideal to fill any voids.
Radial sensory nerve injury	■ If there is inadvertent injury to the radial sensory nerve and this is recognized, it should be repaired with fine epineurial suture.
Radial artery injury	■ If there is inadvertent injury to the radial artery, it should be temporarily clipped with temporary vascular clamps. After the arthrodesis is completed and the capsule is closed, the tourniquet is deflated. If there is good perfusion to all the digits, the artery can be ligated. If the perfusion is inadequate, microvascular repair must be accomplished.
Nonunion or malunion	■ Inadequate preparation of joint surfaces may lead to nonunion. ■ Improper positioning of thumb metacarpal on the trapezium may lead to malunion.

POSTOPERATIVE CARE

- The patient is seen in the office at 7 to 14 days to check the wound. Sutures are removed and radiographs obtained. If fixation is secure, a well-molded short-arm thumb spica cast is applied and the patient is encouraged to continue active digital motion. The thumb interphalangeal joint can be left free.
- The patient is seen at 4 to 6weeks postoperatively for reassessment with cast removal and repeat x-rays. The patient is placed in a removable Orthoplast thumb spica splint and immobilized for 2 to 4 more weeks. Active and active-assisted thumb motion are initiated.
- Usually, radiographic evidence of fusion will be seen by 6 to 8 weeks after surgery (**FIG 2**). Removable bracing is used until radiographic fusion. Then, the patient is allowed to begin strengthening exercises and gradually progress toward unrestricted activities.
- Final photos of motion from a patient 2 months and 9 days postoperative are shown in **FIG 3A–D**.

OUTCOMES

- The outcomes of trapeziometacarpal arthrodesis are generally good, with predictable pain relief and patient satisfaction.
- Forseth and Stern[8] compared the complication rate with Kirschner wire fixation ($n = 59$) to that with plates (minicondylar blade or T plate, $n = 26$) and screws over an average follow-up of 40 months. They found similar nonunion rates (<10% in their small series), but there were higher rates of secondary procedures and lower patient satisfaction in the plate and screw group.
- Hartigan et al[11] retrospectively reviewed patients who had arthrodesis and compared them to those having trapezial excision and ligament reconstruction with an average follow-up of 69 months.There were no significant differences in pain, function, patient satisfaction, or grip strength. The arthrodesis group had greater lateral pinch and chuck pinch but more difficulty with opposition and the ability to flatten the hand, all of which were statistically significant.

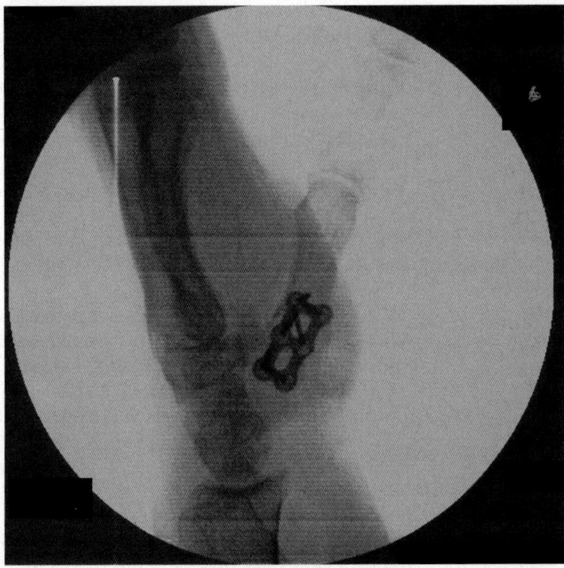

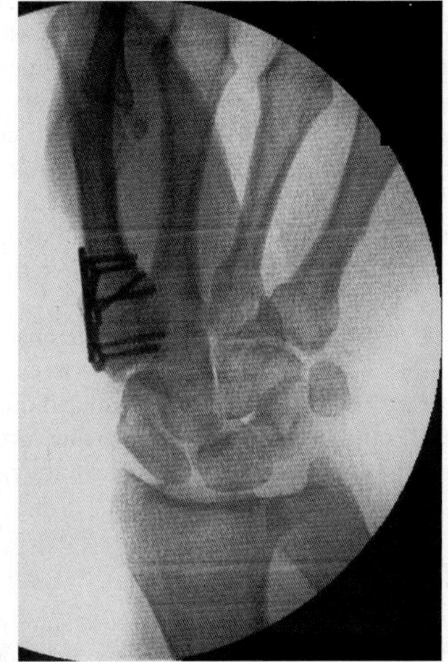

FIG 2 • **A,B.** AP (**A**) and lateral (**B**) fluoroscopic images demonstrating application of plate and screws across thumb CMC joint.

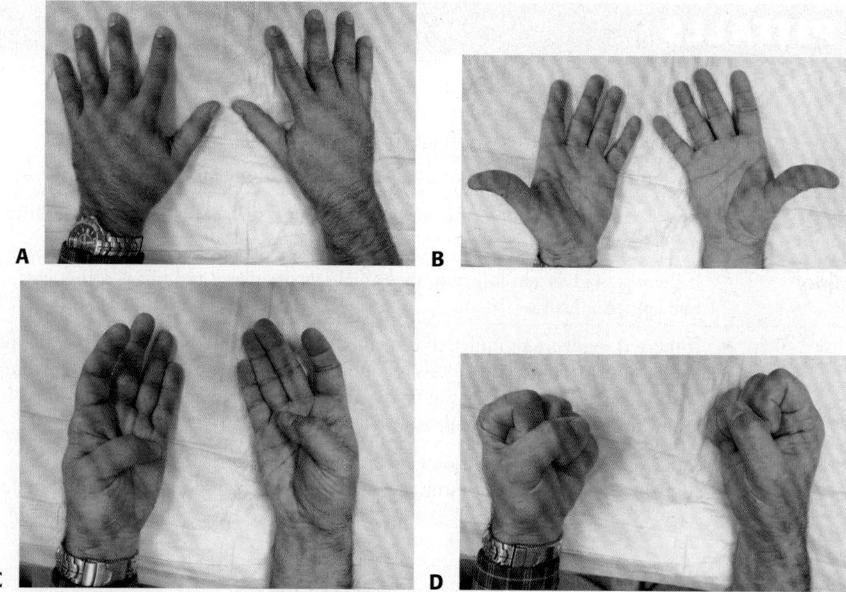

FIG 3 • A–D. Final photos of motion 2 months and 9 days postoperatively after thumb CMC joint arthrodesis with plate and screw fixation. The right side is the operative side. **A.** At rest. **B.** Radial abduction. **C.** Opposition. **D.** Fist.

The arthrodesis group also had a higher complication rate, most of which was attributable to nonunion. There was a 16% nonunion rate using Kirschner wires or tension band, but this rate decreased to 6% after they switched to using a minicondylar plate. Interestingly, all patients with nonunion had improvement in their pain, were able to return to their previous job, and were very satisfied with their outcomes.

- Hartigan et al's[11] data contrasts with Mureau et al[14] who found less subjective improvement with arthrodesis in comparison to arthroplasty and no significant differences in pinch or grip strength. They also found a higher incidence of complications in the arthrodesis group. However, fixation was performed using crossed Kirschner wires with or without iliac crest autograft. In another series, when arthrodesis was performed using a three- to four-hole AO miniplate with cortical screws, no differences in outcomes were found and less complications were found in the arthrodesis group compared to a resection–interposition arthroplasty group.[18]
- Considering the body of available literature, no consensus exists as to the optimal surgical treatment for thumb CMC arthrosis.[10,11,17,18,20] Although complications and reoperations have been found to be more frequent following CMC arthrodesis, this has not been proven to affect the overall outcome.[11,20]
- Two systematic reviews did not show any difference in either subjective or objective outcome measures between all surgical procedures for thumb CMC arthrosis but did comment that high level randomized trials comparing arthrodesis to other surgical procedures are needed to fully assess this question.[12,23]

COMPLICATIONS

- Complications from thumb CMC arthrodesis are generally related to nonunion or hardware problems, including malposition (screws in the trapeziotrapezoid joint), prominence and tendon irritation, and rupture.
- The patient should be made aware of the possible need for secondary procedures to address such complications.

REFERENCES

1. Berggren M, Joost-Davidsson A, Lindstrand J, et al. Reduction in the need for operation after conservative treatment of osteoarthritis of the first carpometacarpal joint: a seven year prospective study. Scand J Plast Reconstr Surg Hand Surg 2001;35:415–417.
2. Bettinger PC, Linscheid RL, Berger RA, et al. An anatomical study of the stabilizing ligaments of the trapezium and trapeziometacarpal joint. J Hand Surg Am 1999;24(4):786–798.
3. Bettinger PC, Smutz WP, Linscheid RL, et al. Material properties of the trapezial and trapeziometacarpal ligaments. J Hand Surg Am 2000;25(6):1085–1095.
4. Cooney WP III, Chao EY. Biomechanical analysis of static forces in the thumb during hand function. J Bone Joint Surg Am 1977;59(1):27–36.
5. Day CS, Gelberman R, Patel AA, et al. Basal joint osteoarthritis of the thumb: a prospective trial of steroid injection and splinting. J Hand Surg Am 2004;29(2):247–251.
6. Eaton RG, Littler JW. Ligament reconstruction for the painful thumb carpometacarpal joint. J Bone Joint Surg Am 1973;55(8):1655–1666.
7. Edmunds JO. Current concepts of the anatomy of the thumb trapeziometacarpal joint. J Hand Surg Am 2011;36(1):170–182.
8. Forseth MJ, Stern PJ. Complications of trapeziometacarpal arthrodesis using plate and screw fixation. J Hand Surg Am 2003;28(2):342–345.
9. Goldfarb CA, Stern PJ. Indications and techniques for thumb carpometacarpal arthrodesis. Tech Hand Up Extrem Surg 2002;6(4): 178–184.
10. Hart R, Janecek M, Siska V, et al. Interposition suspension arthroplasty according to Epping versus arthrodesis for trapeziometacarpal osteoarthritis. Eur Surg 2006;38(6):433–438.
11. Hartigan BJ, Stern PJ, Kiefhaber TR. Thumb carpometacarpal osteoarthritis: arthrodesis compared with ligament reconstruction and tendon interposition. J Bone Joint Surg Am 2001;83-A(10):1470–1478.
12. Martou G, Veltri K, Thoma A. Surgical treatment of osteoarthritis of the carpometacarpal joint of the thumb: a systematic review. Plast Reconstr Surg 2004;114(2):421–432.
13. Muller GM. Arthrodesis of the trapeziometacarpal joint for osteoarthritis. J Bone Joint Surg Br 1949;31B(4):540–542.
14. Mureau MA, Rademaker RP, Verhaar JA, et al. Tendon interposition arthroplasty versus arthrodesis for the treatment of trapeziometacarpal

arthritis: a prospective comparative follow-up study. J Hand Surg Am 2001;26(5):869–876.
15. North ER, Eaton RG. Degenerative arthritis of the trapezium: a comparative roentgenologic and anatomic study. J Hand Surg Am 1983; 8(2):160–166.
16. Pellegrini VD Jr, Smith RL, Ku CW. Pathobiology of articular cartilage in trapeziometacarpal osteoarthritis. I. Regional biochemical analysis. J Hand Surg Am 1994;19(1):70–85.
17. Raven E, Kerkhoffs G, Rutten S, et al. Long term results of surgical intervention for osteoarthritis of the trapeziometacarpal joint. Int Orthop 2007;31(4):547–554.
18. Schröder J, Kerkhoffs GM, Voerman HJ, et al. Surgical treatment of basal joint disease of the thumb: comparison between resection-interposition arthroplasty and trapezio-metacarpal arthrodesis. Arch Orthop Trauma Surg 2002;122(1):35–38.
19. Strauch RJ, Behrman MJ, Rosenwasser MP. Acute dislocation of the carpometacarpal joint of the thumb: an anatomic and cadaver study. J Hand Surg Am 1992;19(1):93–98.
20. Taylor EJ, Desari K, D'Arcy JC, et al. A comparison of fusion, trapeziectomy, and silastic replacement for the treatment of osteoarthritis of the trapeziometacarpal joint. J Hand Surg Br 2005;30(1):45–49.
21. Tomaino MM, Vogt M, Weiser R. Scaphotrapezoid arthritis: prevalence in thumbs undergoing trapezium excision arthroplasty and efficacy of proximal trapezoid excision. J Hand Surg Am 1999;24(6):1220–1224.
22. Van Brenk B, Richards RR, Mackay MB, et al. A biomechanical assessment of ligaments preventing dorsoradial subluxation of the trapeziometacarpal joint. J Hand Surg Am 1998;23(4):607–611.
23. Vermeulen GM, Slijper H, Feitz R, et al. Surgical management of primary thumb carpometacarpal osteoarthritis: a systematic review. J Hand Surg Am 2011;36(1):157–169.

Thumb Carpometacarpal Joint Resection Arthroplasty

Matthew M. Tomaino

DEFINITION

- Osteoarthritis, or more appropriately osteoarthrosis, is a common problem in the hand. The trapeziometacarpal joint is commonly affected, second in frequency only to the distal interphalangeal joint. Trapeziometacarpal joint osteoarthritis, however, can be much more disabling secondary to pain and weakness of grip and pinch strength.
- The surgical management of symptomatic basilar joint arthrosis varies according to the anatomy, radiographic staging, intraoperative confirmation of disease stage, and patient requirements.

ANATOMY

- The thumb carpometacarpal (CMC) joint is a biconcave joint, allowing for motion in three planes: flexion–extension, abduction–adduction, and pronation–supination.
- There are minimal constraints from an osseous standpoint, making the ligamentous structures extremely important in providing stability to the base of the thumb. A total of 16 ligaments have been described around the thumb CMC joint, 7 of which are primary stabilizers of the thumb metacarpal (TM).
- The superficial and deep anterior oblique, dorsoradial, posterior oblique, ulnar collateral, intermetacarpal, and dorsal intermetacarpal ligaments directly stabilize the TM, whereas the remainder serve to stabilize the trapezium, allowing for a stable foundation for the thumb to rest on (**FIG 1**).[1]

PATHOGENESIS

- The pathogenesis of CMC joint arthrosis is multifactorial, involving biochemical and biomechanical influences. The synovial fluid within the joints contains cytokines that invariably play a role in cartilage degradation and decreased ability to withstand the loads generated at the joint during daily activities.[9] Although not clearly delineated, estrogen or estrogen-related compounds probably play some protective role, which may explain the increased incidence of osteoarthritis in postmenopausal women (10 to 15:1).
- The palmar or anterior oblique ligament (AOL), or so-called beak ligament, has been shown to be the most important stabilizing ligament of the thumb. Degeneration or functional incompetence of this ligament leads to laxity, abnormal translation of the metacarpal on the trapezium, increased shear forces, and resultant abnormal wear patterns. This eburnation of the articular cartilage initially occurs along the palmar aspect of the joint.[10] With progression of disease, osteophytes develop and eburnation progresses throughout the entire joint surface.
- Osteoarthrosis can also develop from damage and disruption of the articular cartilage. Any fracture through the metacarpal or trapezium joint surfaces yield arthrosis. Anatomic restoration of the joint surface can minimize this sequela but cannot eliminate the risk entirely. Paradoxically, however, a Bennett fracture may protect the joint from the development of osteoarthritis, assuming subluxation has been treated, by virtue of consequential unloading of the volar aspect of the joint.

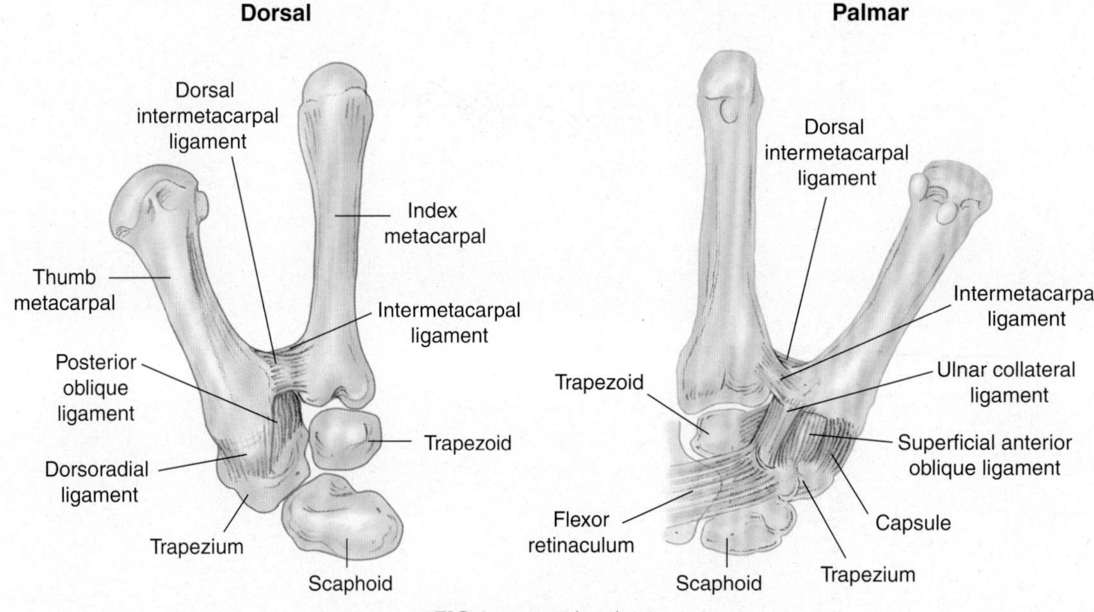

FIG 1 • CMC thumb joint.

NATURAL HISTORY

- Arthrosis of the thumb CMC joint begins along the palmar aspect of the metacarpal secondary to laxity of the AOL. As the process progresses, the entire base of the metacarpal and distal trapezium becomes involved.
- There is initial eburnation of the cartilage, which progresses to osteophyte formation. As the disease continues, the TM assumes an adducted position and the metacarpophalangeal (MCP) joint may compensate by becoming hyperextensile, resulting in varying degrees of MCP joint hyperextension.
- The disease can involve all the trapezial articulations as well as the scaphotrapezoidal joint.[15]

PATIENT HISTORY AND PHYSICAL FINDINGS

- Thumb CMC joint arthrosis often presents with pain at the base of the metacarpal. The pain may or may not be present at rest. It will be exacerbated with activities involving loading the TM base, such as turning a doorknob, twisting a lid off a jar, or turning a key.
- With advanced disease, the thumb subluxes in a dorsal direction and becomes fixed in adduction. This manifests as a prominence at the base of the thumb and decreased ability to abduct the thumb away from the palm. In an effort to compensate for this, the MCP joint will often hyperextend, creating a zigzag deformity.
- Symptoms do not always correlate with the clinical or radiographic appearance, meaning that a patient may have advanced clinical and radiographic disease but be minimally symptomatic. Conversely, a patient may have substantial symptoms with minimal radiographic changes and no clinical deformity at rest.
- Other conditions causing pain at the base of the thumb must be eliminated, such as de Quervain disease, trigger thumb, and carpal tunnel syndrome. Although more than one condition may exist, the physical examination can usually determine the most troubled area.
- Physical examination includes the following:
  - Point tenderness assessment: With the TM adducted, the CMC joint is palpated beneath the thenars. Tenderness confirms the clinical significance of changes seen on radiographs.
  - Reproduction of symptoms on the CMC grind test confirms the CMC joint as a site disease.
  - Key pinch assessment: If dynamic collapse accompanies pinch, MCP joint fusion or capsulodesis is recommended (**FIG 2**).

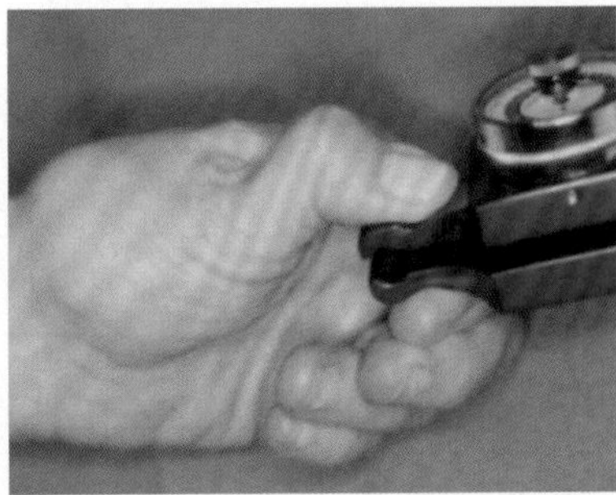

FIG 2 • Dynamic collapse of the thumb on key pinch testing.

IMAGING AND OTHER DIAGNOSTIC STUDIES

- Plain radiographs are the imaging modality of choice for evaluation of thumb CMC joint arthrosis. These include a pronated anteroposterior (AP) (Robert's view), lateral, and a 30-degree posteroanterior stress view (**FIG 3**).
- Eaton and Littler have described a radiographic staging system, which is commonly used, but Tomaino et al[15] have emphasized routine assessment of the scaphotrapezoidal joint, both radiographically and intraoperatively, to rule out scaphotrapezoidal arthritis—what they termed *stage V disease*.
  - Stage I: normal-appearing or widened joint space secondary to synovitis
  - Stage II: joint space narrowing and osteophyte formation smaller than 2 mm
  - Stage III: joint space narrowing with osteophytes larger than 2 mm
  - Stage IV: scaphotrapezial joint space involvement in addition to narrowing of the TM joint

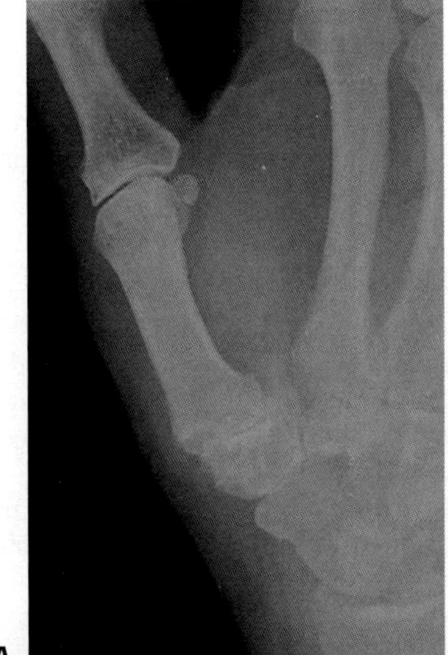

A

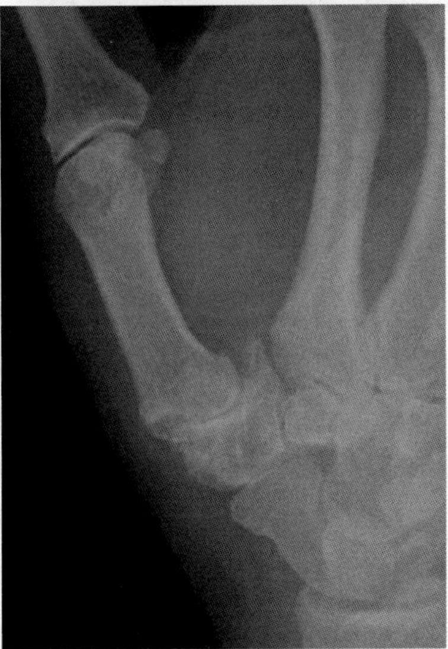

B

FIG 3 • Preoperative posteroanterior (PA) stress and lateral radiographs of the right thumb.

  - Stage V: stage IV appearance with the addition of narrowing or osteophytes in the scaphotrapezoid joint
- The scaphotrapezoid joint is not specifically addressed in this system and may be difficult to assess radiographically, but it should always be assessed clinically during operative intervention because it may be a source of continued pain.

DIFFERENTIAL DIAGNOSIS

- De Quervain disease
- Trigger thumb or stenosing tenosynovitis
- Carpal tunnel syndrome

NONOPERATIVE MANAGEMENT

- Most patients with symptomatic thumb CMC joint arthrosis benefit from a trial of conservative therapy, which may include corticosteroid injection, thenar isometric strengthening exercises, and splinting.
  - Although this will not eliminate the problem or alter the underlying disease process, conservative treatment often reduces symptoms, at least transiently, allowing the patient the opportunity to plan for surgical treatment at the most opportune time.
- Differential injection of steroids can also be helpful to assess how much of a patient's symptoms are coming from the thumb CMC joint versus other areas (carpal tunnel or de Quervain disease).

SURGICAL MANAGEMENT

- The indications for surgical intervention for symptomatic thumb basilar joint arthrosis include pain and weakness.
- There are multiple procedures used to treat symptomatic CMC thumb arthritis, many of which have merit depending on the extent of arthritic involvement.
- Pantrapezial involvement contraindicates the use of arthrodesis or implant arthroplasty, in particular, because of the risk of incomplete pain relief.
- Arthrodesis may be preferable in younger, high-demand patients such as laborers.
- Resection arthroplasty can be performed with ligament reconstruction or without (hematoma distraction arthroplasty).[5,7]
- The flexor carpi radialis (FCR) and abductor pollicis longus (APL) are most commonly used when performing "suspensionplasty."

Preoperative Planning

- Consideration should be given to the age of the patient and the demands placed on the thumb.
- Dynamic collapse of the MCP joint during key pinch necessitates MCP fusion or capsulodesis.
- Intraoperative evaluation of the scaphotrapezotrapezoidal (STT) joint is critical to ensure adequate pain relief after surgery. Thus, hemitrapeziectomy is rarely performed once the decision to proceed with conventional resection arthroplasty is made. If retention of the proximal trapezium is elected because of the absence of STT disease, Artelon resurfacing or joint arthroplasty may be elected.
- Intraoperative assessment of the scaphotrapezoidal joint is recommended, and if changes exist, a 2- to 3-mm resection of the proximal trapezoid is performed.[15] Care is taken not to injure the capitate.
- Suspensionplasty ensures stability of the TM during pinch and grip, resisting the cantilever bending forces that will potentially lead to subluxation and proximal migration compared to trapeziectomy alone.
- Intermediate-term outcome of the hematoma distraction arthroplasty suggests that this procedure may have a role in providing excellent pain relief in well-selected patients for whom grip strength is a less important issue.[5]

Positioning

- The patient is supine, and the involved hand and arm are supported by a hand table.

Approach

- Trapezium excision and ligament reconstruction and suspensionplasty can be performed using the Wagner (volar) approach or a dorsal approach. I prefer the dorsal approach except when performing an Eaton ligament reconstruction, in which case a volar approach is used. I have modified my technique since performing the ligament reconstruction and tendon interposition (LRTI) arthroplasty exclusively during the first 10 years of practice.[12,14]
- Over the past 5 years, I have performed a suspensionplasty using a distally based slip of the APL tendon, which obviates the need for a bony channel. This is a variation of other suspensionplasty techniques.[8,11,16] In addition, I no longer pin the joint or interpose tissue into the space remaining after trapezial resection. The procedure is performed more expeditiously and seems to be associated with equivalent outcomes.[13]

Ligament Reconstruction and Tendon Interposition Arthroplasty Using the Flexor Carpi Radialis Tendon

Incision and Superficial Dissection

- A triradiate is drawn before the tourniquet is inflated to allow palpation of the radial pulse in the vicinity of the anatomic snuffbox; this typically identifies the scaphotrapezial joint.
- When a substantial shoulder sign (prominence associated with dorsal subluxation of the proximal phalanx trapezium) exists, it can be difficult to identify the TM joint. In these cases, palpation of the scaphoid tuberosity is helpful to ensure that the incision is neither too distal nor too proximal.
- The triradiate incision facilitates dissection of the radial artery off the dorsal capsule; when first extensor compartment release is planned, however, a longitudinal incision may be preferred.
- At the outset, the radial sensory nerve must be identified and small branches must not be skeletonized or divided. This may cause postoperative radial sensory neuritis and even transient reflex sympathetic dystrophy.
  - Place blunt retractors beneath the extensor pollicis longus (EPL) in a dorsal and ulnar position and the APL radially and volarly.
  - The radial artery courses within this interval, and deep perforators to the dorsal capsule must be coagulated and divided so the artery can be retracted dorsally and ulnarly.

Capsular Incision and Trapezial Excision

- With gentle traction on the thumb, perform a longitudinal capsulotomy and obtain subperiosteal exposure of the trapezium and the base of the metacarpal (**TECH FIG 1A**). Extend the capsulotomy proximally so the scaphotrapezial joint is identified.
  - Either retractors or tag sutures of 3-0 Vicryl can be used to retract the capsule.
- Before the trapezium is excised, use a microsagittal saw to remove a thin sliver of bone at the base of the metacarpal. This facilitates exposure of the distal extent of the trapezium and, with further traction on the thumb, provides a safer window for sectioning of the trapezium.
- Cut the trapezium into quadrants, beginning with the limb that parallels the expected course of the FCR tendon. Injury to the tendon during this portion of the procedure is unlikely if the saw is not brought completely through the trapezium.
- After making perpendicular cuts in the trapezium, place an osteotome and twist it to break apart its four quadrants. Removal of the trapezium in pieces with a rongeur is facilitated by sharp dissection of the remaining capsule, particularly volarly and around loose bodies. Avoid inordinate ripping and pulling with the rongeurs because damage to the underlying capsule can increase postoperative discomfort, particularly where it abuts the carpal tunnel.
- Remove osteophytic bone between the base of the thumb and index metacarpal so that pain does not accompany key pinch after the procedure. Identify the FCR tendon at the base of the arthroplasty space so it is not injured; remember that the trapezium may encircle the FCR tendon at its volar extent.
- At this portion of the procedure, I routinely have an assistant place traction on the index and long fingers to allow inspection of the scaphotrapezoidal joint. If there is cartilage fraying or eburnation, a motorized burr or rongeur is used to remove 2 to 3 mm of proximal trapezoid so that, with axial compression applied to the index and long finger metacarpals, there is no contact between the remaining trapezoid and scaphoid (**TECH FIG 1B**). I do not interpose soft tissue or FCR tendon into the space. Take care not to remove bone from the capitate.

Creation of the Bony Channel through the Metacarpal Base

- One centimeter distal to the squared-off base of the metacarpal, in the plane of the nail, create a bone tunnel with a motorized 3-mm burr that exits the base of the metacarpal on its volar margin (**TECH FIG 2**).
  - This position is selected rather than central exit point in the metacarpal base because passage of the FCR tendon volarly more closely simulates the original attachment of the beak ligament.
- Enlarge the bony channel with two curettes of increasing size, but do not make it large enough for the entire width of the leading edge of the FCR tendon. Rather, trim the full width of the FCR at its tip to facilitate passage with a Carroll tendon passer. In that light, the bony channel needs to be large enough only for the Carroll tendon passer to be used.

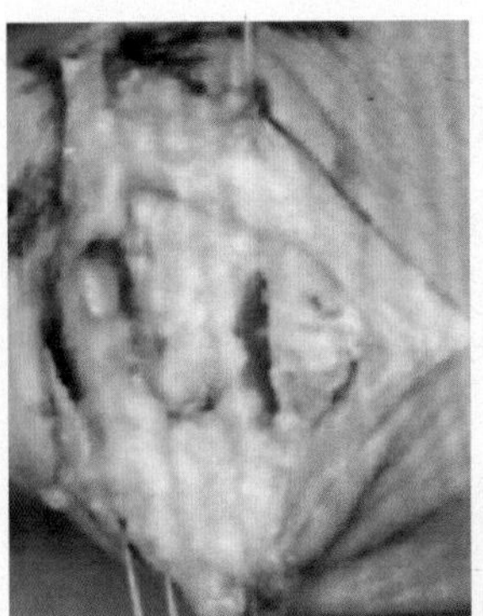

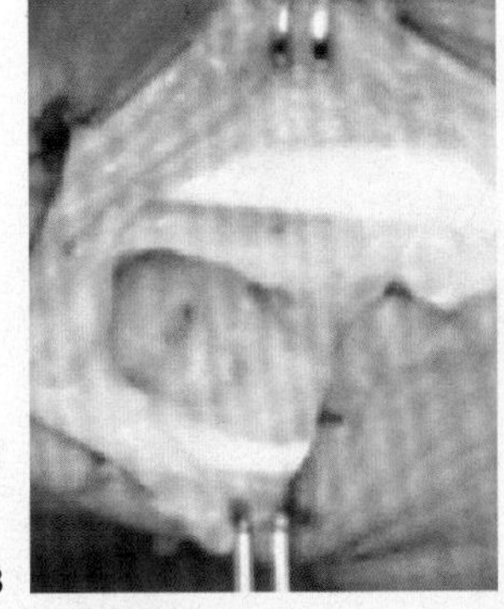

TECH FIG 1 • The base of the metacarpal is resected (**A**), and the trapezium is excised (**B**).

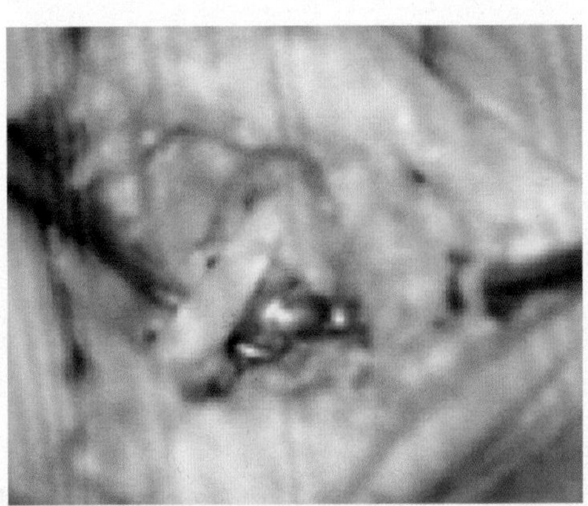

TECH FIG 2 • A tunnel is made at the base of the metacarpal.

Flexor Carpi Radialis Harvest

- Palpate the FCR tendon at wrist level during passive flexion and extension of the wrist, where it is clearly tendinous. More proximally in the forearm, the tendon becomes less discrete. This generally correlates with the proximal one-third to half of the forearm. At that location, make a 1.5-cm transverse incision.
- Open the fascia, maximally flex the wrist, and identify the interval between the FCR tendon and muscle. Lift it into the wound via a curved clamp and divide it. Close this wound with 5-0 nylon sutures.
- Retract the capsular flaps to protect the overlying radial artery dorsally and ulnarly. Place a curved snap beneath the FCR tendon and pull it. This typically delivers the entire tendon into the arthroplasty space.
- Grasp the tendon at its tip and mobilize it to its insertion at the base of the index metacarpal without violating the small blood vessels that perfuse the tendon insertion itself.
  - If adhesions between the FCR and the volar capsule are not released, the vector of the ligament reconstruction is based more proximally and will not closely simulate the original vector of the beak ligament. This, in my opinion, is a potential cause of early subsidence after ligament reconstruction.
- Taper the tendon for about 2 to 3 cm so the diameter of the tip of the tendon will easily fit through the bone tunnel via the Carroll tendon passer.
  - Use a 4-0 Vicryl suture on a small needle to purchase the volar capsule for subsequent stabilization of the tendon interposition.
  - If there are rents in the volar capsule, this same suture can be used to repair them, but I no longer am inordinately preoccupied with repairing small tears in the volar capsule because there is little risk of the tendon interposition extruding into the carpal canal or into the base of the metacarpal.

Stabilization of the Thumb Metacarpal (Optional) and Flexor Carpi Radialis Tendon Tensioning

- Kirschner wire placement, when elected, is one of the more tedious parts of the procedure and must be performed skillfully so that the bony channel is not violated. If the Kirschner wire inadvertently purchases the FCR tendon within the bony channel in the metacarpal, it will impair the ability to pull it tight and properly tension the new ligament.
  - Usually, a 0.045- or 0.054-inch wire is used. It begins obliquely at the dorsoradial aspect of the metacarpal and purchases the ulnar carpus.
- I place the thumb in the "fisted" position as if engaged in key pinch. The TM is suspended at the level of the index metacarpal. Its base should be colinear with the scaphoid articular surface and the thumb tip should rest on the index finger, neither too extended nor flexed at its base.
  - Ideally, this positions the thumb intrinsic muscles optimally on the Blix curve and ensures optimal restoration of pinch strength.
  - Bend the wire external to the skin and cut it.
- A hand probe or the like is used to take the FCR tendon at the base of the metacarpal and pull it proximally (**TECH FIG 3**).
  - When pinning has been performed, it should not prevent free excursion of the FCR through the bone channel. Pull the tendon tightly as it exits the dorsum of the TM and suture it to adjacent periosteum and soft tissue with 3-0 Vicryl suture.
  - If pinning is not performed, at this point, ensure that you have suspended the metacarpal at the level of the index CMC joint.
- The extensor pollicis brevis (EPB) tendon is sutured more radially and divided distally. This completes the EPB tenodesis, rendering it an abductor of the metacarpal as opposed to a potential hyperextender of the MCP joint.
- Place a second suture slightly more proximal to the tenodesis suture so that the ligament reconstruction is stabilized adequately, and perform tissue interposition.

Tissue Interposition (Optional)

- Although Burton's original technique continues to "resurface" the metacarpal base to minimize the chance that interposition material may extrude through the channel, this is unlikely. Studies have suggested that interposition is not a critical element of the procedure if suspension of the metacarpal has been effectively executed.[4] Furthermore, proximal migration, short of causing scaphometacarpal impingement, appears not to affect the functional outcome.[6]

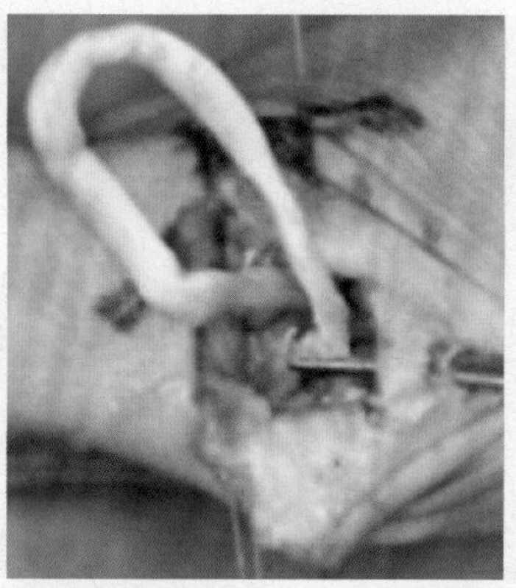

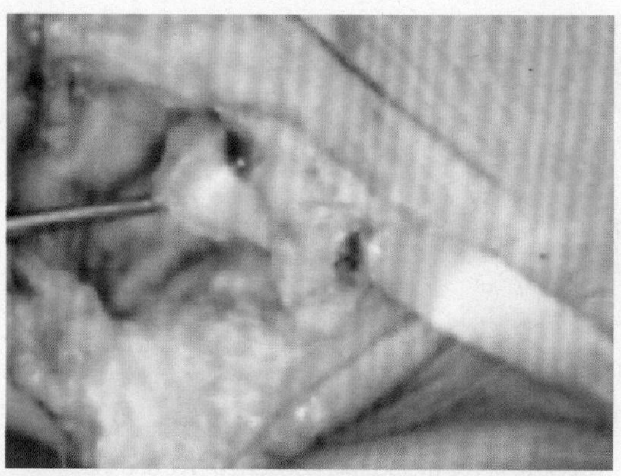

TECH FIG 3 • **A.** The FCR is passed through bony tunnel. **B.** A hand probe indicates FCR suspensionplasty.

- In a higher demand patient, however, residual length of the FCR is available for interposition as follows. The tendon is folded into the volar aspect of the arthroplasty space to ensure that it will sink into its depth. From that point distally, the tendon is folded back and forth about four times on a single Keith needle, like ribbon candy.
- A 4-0 Vicryl suture is used to stabilize each corner of the tendon anchovy, and then a second Keith needle is placed through it, parallel to the first. Apertures in each needle should be volar, the tip of each needle dorsal, and, with the previously placed volar capsular suture, each limb is threaded and the anchovy is slid down and delivered into the arthroplasty space. The two Vicryl limbs are tied, securing the tissue interposition (**TECH FIG 4**).

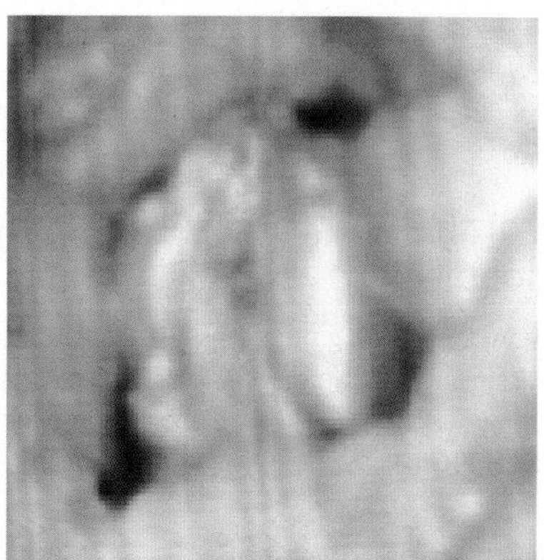

TECH FIG 4 • The tendon anchovy held in place with Vicryl sutures.

Capsular Repair and Wound Closure

- Tightly repair the capsule using 3-0 Vicryl sutures. If redundant capsule is present, a pants-over-vest closure can be performed.
- When closing the capsule, protect radial artery and neighboring radial sensory nerve branches to avoid damage.
- Close the incisions with 4-0 nylon and repeat identification of underlying radial sensory nerve branches to avoid inadvertent injury during skin closure. This may be a cause of dystrophic pain after surgery.
- Place a bulky thumb spica dressing, followed by volar and thumb spica splints.
- The hand is elevated for 3 or 4 days after surgery.

Abductor Pollicis Longus Suspensionplasty

Incision and Deep Dissection

- Make a 6-cm curvilinear incision from two fingerbreadths proximal to the radial styloid process to 1 cm distal to the base of the metacarpal (**TECH FIG 5A**). Expose and retract the radial artery and branches of the radial sensory nerve.
- Release the first extensor compartment retinaculum as would be performed for de Quervain disease, leaving the volar attachment intact.
- At the myotendinous junction of the APL, release the ulnarmost slip of APL and free it to the level of its insertion at the metacarpal base (**TECH FIG 5B**).
- Expose the EPL and APL tendons—in between is the capsule of the TM joint.
- Perform a capsulotomy to expose the trapezium (**TECH FIG 5C**), which is resected after being cut partially into four fragments with a saw and osteotome.
    - The base of the TM is not squared off; not resecting a small sliver from the metacarpal base may help to preserve the intermetacarpal ligament.

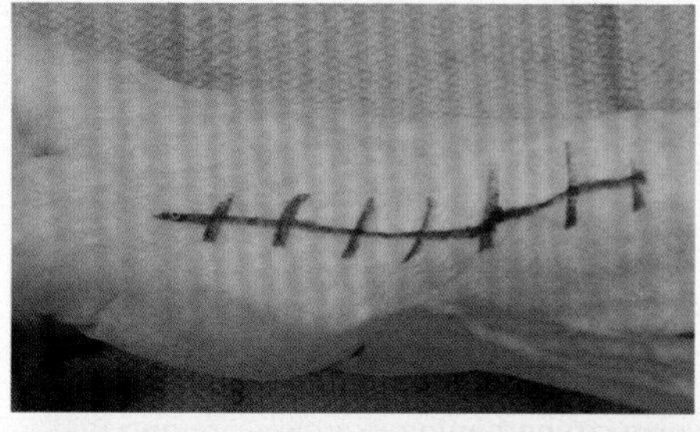

A

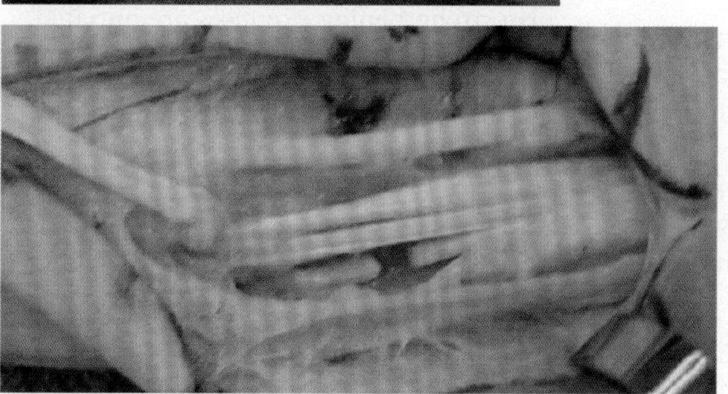

B

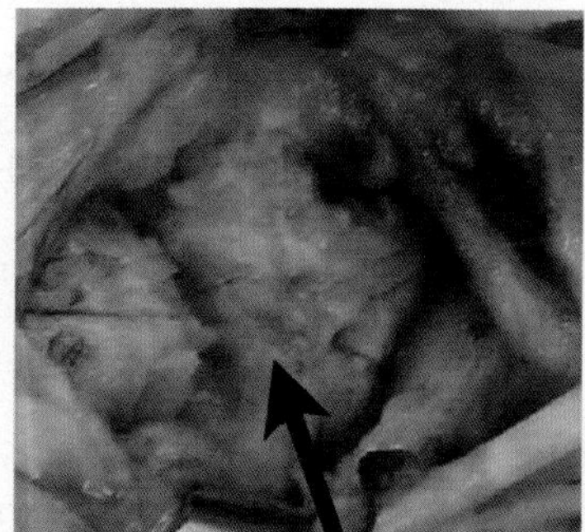

C

TECH FIG 5 • APL suspensionplasty technique. **A.** Skin incision. **B.** Distally based slip of APL. **C.** Trapezium excision (*arrow* identifies the trapezium).

- The FCR tendon is visualized in the base of the arthroplasty space. With traction on the index and long fingers, inspect the scaphotrapezoidal joint; if it is arthritic, resect the proximal trapezoid.

Creation of the Abductor Pollicis Longus Suspensionplasty

- Poke the APL slip through the capsule to within the arthroplasty space. Using a right angle clamp, pass it through a slit in the FCR tendon or around the FCR while grabbing some local capsule as well (**TECH FIG 6**).
- Position the thumb so that it rests on the index finger in the fisted position—distracted so that the metacarpal base is at the level of the index CMC joint. A Kirschner wire is not placed.
- Pull the APL slip taut and place a 3-0 Vicryl suture between the APL slip, at the level of the metacarpal base, and the EPB (radially) and the tissue deep to the EPL (ulnarly).

Capsular Closure and Rehabilitation

- The capsule is closed and a thumb spica splint is placed for 14 days.

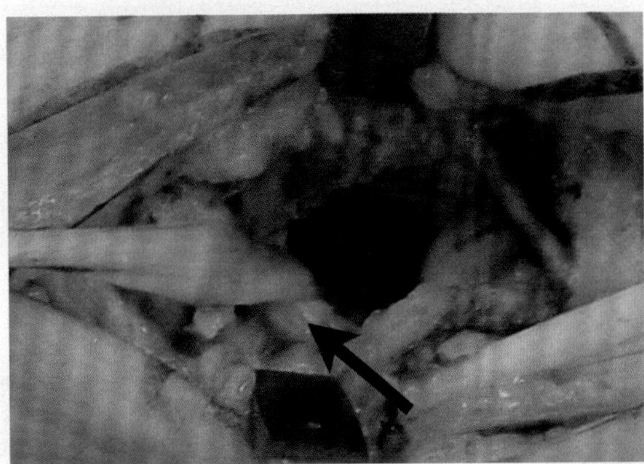

TECH FIG 6 • APL slip is passed through and around FCR (*arrow*).

PEARLS AND PITFALLS

Address MCP joint hyperextensibility	■ Static laxity is no longer viewed as an absolute indication for capsulodesis or fusion. Rather, dynamic collapse during pinch is a relative indication.
Address scaphotrapezoidal disease	■ If proximal trapezoid excision is not performed, pain at this articulation may persist.
Pinning is not essential; tissue interposition is not essential	■ Neither pinning for 4 weeks nor tissue interposition is required. Outcomes appear not to be compromised by modest proximal metacarpal migration. However, these elements of the procedure do have a role if concern about any potential for scaphometacarpal impingement exists.
Ensure stability of the APL suspension	■ The APL should be placed through the FCR or around it and should capture some capsule. This technical point will prevent the APL and TM from sliding proximally along the FCR.
Joint fusion timing	■ When necessary, concomitant MCP joint fusion should be performed after tendon harvest and passage to avoid thumb manipulation after fusion.

POSTOPERATIVE CARE

- First month
  - At 2 weeks, the patient returns for suture removal, wound inspection, and placement of a fiberglass thumb spica cast that allows full motion of the thumb interphalangeal joint, unless MCP joint fusion has been performed.
  - At 4 weeks, the patient returns again, the Kirschner wire is pulled (if one has been placed), and a forearm-based thumb spica Orthoplast splint is fashioned by the hand therapist.
  - Gentle wrist and thumb MCP joint range-of-motion exercises are initiated as well as thenar isometric exercises. The latter are performed with the thumb in the splint.
- Month 2
  - At 6 weeks, if the patient is comfortable, gentle pinch and grip strengthening exercises are initiated.
  - By 8 weeks, flexion–adduction and opposition exercises are begun.
- Month 3
  - By this time, the patient is usually doing well enough that the splint can be discarded.
  - Grip and pinch exercises are typically continued by the patient via a home program.
  - No rigorous attempt is made for the thumb to reach the ring and small finger bases because there is no functional relevance to these activities and they risk stretching the

ligament. In addition, passive range of motion is not a part of the postoperative regimen.

- During months 3 to 6, the patient is encouraged to use the hand and to push the exercises vigorously. Typically, patients return to normal activities, including golf and tennis.

OUTCOMES

Ligament Reconstruction and Tendon Interposition Arthroplasty

- Improvements in grip strength typically exceed improvements in key pinch strength. In 1995, Tomaino et al[14] noted that key pinch strength took at least 6 years to equal preoperative measurements.
- At an average follow-up of 9 years (range 8 to 11), these authors[14] reported on 24 thumbs in 22 patients and found that average grip strength increased 93%, average key pinch strength increased 34%, and tip pinch strength increased 65% compared with preoperative values.
- In contrast to many other studies, stress radiographs showed an average subluxation of the metacarpal base of only 11% and subsidence of only 13%. This compares favorably with the radiographic outcomes after the hematoma distraction arthroplasty.[5,7]
- Even in series in which proximal migration of the metacarpal base averaged greater than 20%, there has been no significant correlation between maintenance of arthroplasty space height and objective or subjective clinical outcome (**FIG 4**).[6]

Abductor Pollicis Longus Suspensionplasty

- My evaluation of outcomes after the APL suspensionplasty found a satisfaction rate and functional return equivalent to the LRTI procedure.[13]
- Evaluation of 23 thumbs in 22 patients at a minimum of 1 year after surgery showed that grip and key pinch strengths were 82% and 77%, respectively, compared to the opposite side. Proximal migration of the metacarpal averaged 50% of the preoperative trapezial height. Experience and the literature show that modest proximal migration does not correlate with outcome.[6] It is interesting to note that a comparative, randomized, and prospective study evaluating outcomes following APL suspensionplasty and the LRTI procedure, in which both subjective and functional parameters were evaluated 8 months following surgery, revealed no significant difference in outcomes.[3] Radiologically, both groups showed an approximate 50% reduction in the height of the trapezial space.
- In summary, APL suspensionplasty is a simple yet effective treatment alternative for basal joint arthritis. The suspensionplasty technique uses our current understanding of the forces involved during pinch and grip[2] as well as the role of normal ligamentous anatomy. APL suspensionplasty appears at least in terms of early outcome to have very similar results to those which have been reported using the LRTI technique.

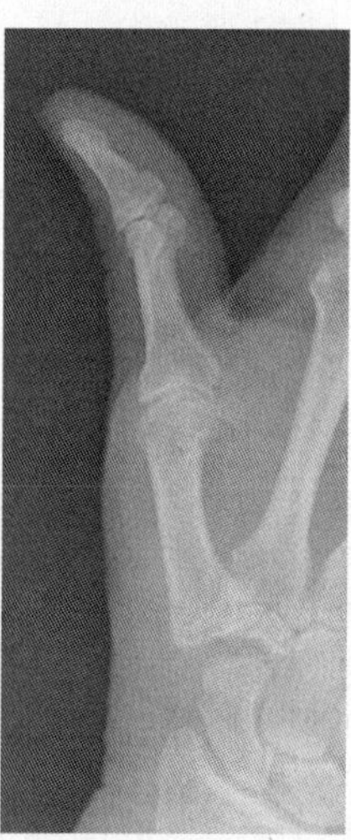

FIG 4 • Postoperative lateral radiograph shows arthroplasty space 1 year after surgery.

COMPLICATIONS

- One cause of unsatisfactory outcome after basal joint arthroplasty is residual pain because of failure to address scaphotrapezial or scaphotrapezoidal disease.[15] Routine complete excision of the trapezium certainly precludes the scaphotrapezial joint pain. Routine intraoperative observation and treatment of the scaphotrapezoidal disease by partial excision of the proximal trapezoid prevents scaphotrapezoidal joint pain.[15]
- Unaddressed instability of the MCP joint can also impair functional outcome after ligament reconstruction. During lateral pinch, MCP joint hyperextension causes reciprocal deformity more proximally, imposing metacarpal adduction and stressing the reconstructed ligament. Accordingly, early identification of hyperextension in excess of 30 degrees during key pinch should prompt stabilization to protect the integrity of the basal joint ligament reconstruction. Even with a sound ligament reconstruction and appropriate stabilization of the MCP joint, it is theoretically possible to develop recurrent laxity at the basal joint due to stretching of the ligament reconstruction.

REFERENCES

1. Bettinger PC, Linscheid RL, Berger RA, et al. An anatomic study of the stabilizing ligaments of the trapezium and trapeziometacarpal joint. J Hand Surg Am 1999;24(4):786–798.
2. Cooney WP III, Chao EY. Biomechanical analysis of static forces in the thumb during hand function. J Bone Joint Surg Am 1977;59(1):27–36.
3. Esenwein P, Hoigne D, Zdravkovic V, et al. Resection, interposition and suspension arthroplasty for treatment of basal joint arthritis of the thumb: a randomized and prospective comparison of techniques using the abductor pollicis longus and the flexor carpi radialis tendon [in German]. Handchir Mikrochir Plast Chir 2011;43(5):289–294.
4. Gerwin M, Griffith A, Weiland AJ, et al. Ligament reconstruction basal joint arthroplasty without tendon interposition. Clin Orthop Relat Res 1997;(342):42–45.
5. Gray KV, Meals RA. Hematoma and distraction arthroplasty for thumb basal joint osteoarthritis: minimum 6.5-year follow-up evaluation. J Hand Surg Am 2007;32(1):23–29.
6. Kriegs-Au G, Petje G, Fojtl E, et al. Ligament reconstruction with or without tendon interposition to treat primary thumb carpometacarpal osteoarthritis. A prospective randomized study. J Bone Joint Surg Am 2004;86-A(2):209–218.
7. Kuhns CA, Emerson ET, Meals RA. Hematoma and distraction arthroplasty for thumb basal joint osteoarthritis: a prospective,

single-surgeon study including outcomes measures. J Hand Surg Am 2003;28(3):381–389.

8. Nylén S, Juhlin LJ, Lugnegard H. Weilby tendon interposition arthroplasty for osteoarthritis of the trapezial joints. J Hand Surg Br 1987;12(1):68–72.
9. Pellegrini VD Jr. Pathomechanics of the thumb trapeziometacarpal joint. Hand Clin 2001;17:175–184.
10. Pellegrini VD Jr, Olcott CW, Hollenberg G. Contact patterns in the trapeziometacarpal joint: the role of the palmar beak ligament. J Hand Surg Am 1993;18(2):238–244.
11. Sigfusson R, Lundborg G. Abductor pollicis longus tendon arthroplasty for treatment of arthrosis in the first carpometacarpal joint. Scand J Plast Reconst Hand Surg 1991;25:73–77.
12. Tomaino MM. Ligament reconstruction tendon interposition arthroplasty for basal joint arthritis. Rationale, current technique, and clinical outcome. Hand Clin 2001;17:207–221.
13. Tomaino MM. Suspensionplasty for basal joint arthritis: why and how. Hand Clin 2006;22:171–175.
14. Tomaino MM, Pellegrini VD Jr, Burton RI. Arthroplasty of the basal joint of the thumb. Long-term follow-up after ligament reconstruction with tendon interposition. J Bone Joint Surg Am 1995;77(3):346–355.
15. Tomaino MM, Vogt M, Weiser R. Scaphotrapezoid arthritis: prevalence in thumbs undergoing trapezium excision arthroplasty and efficacy of proximal trapezoid excision. J Hand Surg Am 1999;24(6):1220–1224.
16. Weilby A. Tendon interposition arthroplasty of the first carpometacarpal joint. J Hand Surg Br 1988;13(4):421–425.

Thumb Carpometacarpal Joint Implant and Resurfacing Arthroplasty

Matthew J. Robon and Matthew M. Tomaino

DEFINITION

- Trapeziometacarpal joint (basal joint) arthritis is a debilitating condition that most commonly affects women in their 50s and 60s.[21,22] The stage of arthritis dictates the treatment for this disorder.[6,7,23]
- Ligament reconstruction and tendon interposition (LRTI) arthroplasty, fusion, and nonbiologic reconstruction of this joint are common techniques to treat this condition.[11,12,24,25]
- This chapter will discuss the role of resurfacing arthroplasty and total joint replacement.

ANATOMY

- The anatomy of the thumb metacarpal (TM) joint is extremely complex and has been well studied.[3,19] The deep anterior oblique ligament (dAOL) ("beak ligament") is the primary stabilizer of the TM joint.[10,11] More recently, 16 ligaments have been described that stabilize the TM joint. Seven of these ligaments, including the superficial anterior oblique ligament (sAOL), dAOL, dorsoradial, posterior oblique, ulnar collateral, intermetacarpal, and dorsal intermetacarpal, directly stabilize the TM joint. The other 9 ligaments indirectly stabilize the TM joint by directly stabilizing the trapezium.[3,18]
- The TM joint is the most complex joint in the hand.[8] It is a biconcave–convex saddle joint with minimal bony constraints. This joint allows flexion–extension, abduction–adduction, and pronation–supination of the thumb ray.[14] For optimal treatment outcomes with joint replacement, normal kinematics—six degrees of freedom—should be restored as closely as possible.

PATHOGENESIS

- Degeneration of the AOL of the TM joint has been linked to the development of osteoarthritis.
- Pathologic laxity, abnormal translation of the metacarpal on the trapezium, and generation of abnormally high shear forces within the TM joint, especially on the palmar aspect of the joint during pinch and grip motions, occur when the AOL becomes incompetent.
- The base of the metacarpal tends to sublux dorsally with AOL detachment, emphasizing the importance of the AOL. In advanced osteoarthritis, adduction and flexion contractures tend to develop, producing further functional impairment and joint overload.

NATURAL HISTORY

- The vast number of described operations to treat osteoarthritis of the TM joint demonstrates the lack of consensus among treating surgeons as to the best way to approach this disorder. This chapter details the role of resurfacing and implant arthroplasty for the treatment of osteoarthritis of the TM joint.
- Various materials, techniques, and prostheses have been used in the past. Hemiarthroplasty and total joint arthroplasty of the TM joint have largely failed, with mediocre long-term results compared with soft tissue arthroplasty.[1,2,7,9,17,23] However, the appeal of a replacement may lie with quicker recovery, more normal kinematics, immediate stability, and the avoidance of metacarpal subsidence.
- Obviously, the perils of prosthetic alternatives revolve around durability, survivability, and complication rate. Joint resurfacing with the Artelon implant (Small Bone Innovations, Inc., Morrisville, PA) was touted to have the most potential, in terms of a biologic resurfacing. This procedure avoids the use of a semiconstrained device—which has been associated with trapezial component loosening and failure, but long-term follow-up has been characterized by a significant complication rate and poor satisfaction.

PATIENT HISTORY AND PHYSICAL FINDINGS

- Arthritis of the TM joint often presents with pain at the base of the thumb during pinch and grip (stressful activities for the TM joint). Women are 10 to 15 times more likely than men to develop this disorder. Asian and Caucasian populations have an increased prevalence as well.
- Common offending activities include brushing teeth, opening a jar, picking up a book, or turning a key. All of these activities involve increasing the breadth of grasp or forceful lateral pinch. Usually, the pain is localized at the base of the thumb on the dorsal or volar radial aspect of the thenar cone. Patients often feel the joint slipping or subluxing radially.
  - A "shoulder sign" is an enlarging prominence (the result of a dorsally subluxing proximal metacarpal on the trapezium and metacarpal adduction) that develops with progressive disease.
- Other causes of pain in the hand should be evaluated (see Differential Diagnosis list) as well. This is important because any concomitant disease, such as a trigger thumb, may hamper the postoperative therapy regimen and negatively affect the patient's final outcome.
- The treating physician should also keep the diagnosis of carpal tunnel syndrome in mind, as it coexists in about 44% of patients with TM joint arthritis. Furthermore, the postoperative swelling from a basal joint arthroplasty may exacerbate even mild cases of carpal tunnel syndrome.
- The Allen test should be performed on every patient who is undergoing surgery for basal joint arthroplasty, as the radial artery will be near or in the operative field and may

need to be mobilized depending on the exact procedure performed. Any injury to the radial artery should be repaired immediately.

- The stability of the metacarpophalangeal (MCP) joint of the thumb is also critical, as this is a source of postoperative stress on the reconstructed beak ligament from either ligament reconstruction or suspensionplasty procedures.
  - MCP joint fusion or volar plate capsulodesis should be performed when the MCP joint hyperextends to greater than 20 degrees.[15]
- Methods for examining the carpometacarpal (CMC) joint of the thumb include the following:
  - CMC grind test: A positive test is suggestive of degenerative disease.
  - CMC instability test: Laxity of the TM joint is common in early stages of degeneration, but as the joint degenerates, it usually becomes stiffer.
  - MCP joint stability test: If the MCP joint is actively hyperextending, this could put undue stress on a reconstructed TM joint and lead to failure. This hyperextendable MCP joint should be stabilized.
  - Metacarpal base compression test: Glickel[13] believed that this is more commonly painful in advanced stages rather than milder stages of TM joint disease.
  - Distraction test: A positive result from this maneuver is thought to be caused by traction on an inflamed TM joint capsule.

IMAGING AND OTHER DIAGNOSTIC STUDIES

- Imaging of the TM joint includes a true anteroposterior (AP) view of the TM joint (called a *Robert view or pronated AP*), lateral, and posteroanterior 30-degree oblique stress view (with thumb tips pressing against each other).
- The most common staging system was originally described by Eaton and Littler[11,12]: stage 1 shows slight widening of the joint, possibly from synovitis; stage 2 demonstrates some joint space narrowing and osteophytes smaller than 2 mm; stage 3, osteophytes larger than 2 mm; and stage 4 disease, scaphotrapezial joint space involvement along with TM joint narrowing.
- The senior author of this chapter has described a "fifth stage" in which the disease process is pantrapezial and there is TM, scaphotrapezial, and scaphotrapezoidal joint degeneration. Scaphotrapezoidal arthritis can be a source of continued pain and this joint should be evaluated intraoperatively in every patient because, unfortunately, preoperative radiographs are only 44% sensitive and 86% specific for diagnosing arthritis at this joint.[26]

DIFFERENTIAL DIAGNOSIS

- Scaphotrapezial arthritis
- Scaphotrapezoidal arthritis
- Thumb sesamoid arthritis
- Carpal tunnel syndrome
- De Quervain tenosynovitis
- Stenosing flexor tenosynovitis (trigger finger)

NONOPERATIVE MANAGEMENT

- Initial management of TM joint arthritis is nonoperative and includes anti-inflammatory medication, thenar cone muscle isometric strengthening exercises, hand- or forearm-based thumb spica splint immobilization, steroid injections, and activity modification.
- These measures may not alleviate any or all of the patient's symptoms, but they may help enough to provide temporary relief, allowing the patient ample time to educate himself or herself and to contemplate the treatment alternatives.
- The time afforded by the nonoperative measures may also allow the patient to schedule the operation at a more convenient time.

SURGICAL MANAGEMENT

- There are several options for surgical treatment of TM joint arthritis. LRTI, suspensionplasty, and CMC joint fusion are discussed in other chapters. This chapter focuses on the role of resurfacing and implant arthroplasty. Resurfacing is an increasingly attractive option in younger, more active patients in whom one might prefer to avoid trapeziectomy to eliminate the risk of metacarpal subsidence with time. Subsidence can result in recurrent pain and weakness.
- The Artelon (Small Bone Innovations) spacer is a bioabsorbable implant (**FIG 1A**) that degrades and is replaced with scar tissue that protects the base of the TM and the distal aspect of the trapezium. This implant is ideal for a younger laborer with TM arthritis in whom grip and pinch strength are of critical importance. The attraction of this alternative is that it is a potentially definitive procedure that does not "burn the bridge" of resection arthroplasty in the future.[20]
- Pyrocarbon resurfacing using the "saddle" implant (Ascension Orthopedics, Austin, TX; **FIG 1B**) is an alternative to Artelon. Its design mimics the articular shape of the metacarpal articular surface, which may more closely restore CMC joint kinematics compared to Artelon implant use. Little information exists in the literature, however, regarding outcomes; in 2009, Mayo Clinic investigators reported on the use of pyrolytic carbon hemiarthroplasty for the treatment of CMC arthritis and 49 patients.[16] This investigation showed that its use was an acceptable option, although a high complication rate was observed in the early cohort, with many cases of subluxation attributed to the creation of a too shallow trapezial cup.
- Total joint arthroplasty, such as with the Avanta CMC implant (**FIG 1C**), is another option. Implant arthroplasty options may require less immobilization, lead to quicker return of functional abilities, obviate metacarpal subsidence, and provide immediate stability.[5] In 2006, the outcomes following 26 procedures in 25 patients were reported.[2] This series intimated that this option was efficacious and feasible for the osteoarthritic thumb. Indeed, a review of implant options published in 2013 acknowledges that a variety of metal total joint prostheses have been developed and that favorable short-term outcomes have been reported.[27] However, the literature is full of articles describing failures of innumerable prosthetic implants for the TM joint, thus appropriate patient selection remains critical.

Preoperative Planning

- Many other hand pathologies can coexist with TM joint arthritis. These other diagnoses should be evaluated before the day of surgery.

- If an Allen test had not been performed previously, it should be performed before the surgery.

Positioning

- The patient is positioned supine on the operating table with the affected hand placed on a hand table extension. A tourniquet is placed above the elbow.
- When using a dorsal approach, we tend to keep the hand in neutral pronation–supination, with an assistant holding the hand stable and at times pulling traction or directly stabilizing the thumb with the nail plate parallel to the floor.

Approach

- There are several different approaches for soft tissue arthroplasties, but for resurfacing or implant arthroplasties, a dorsal approach seems to work the best and to offer the best visualization.

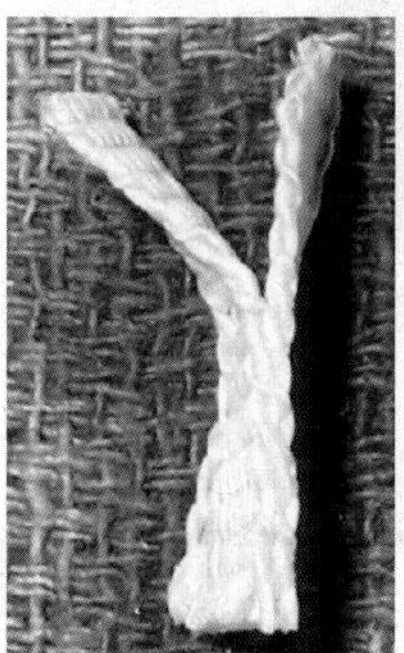
A
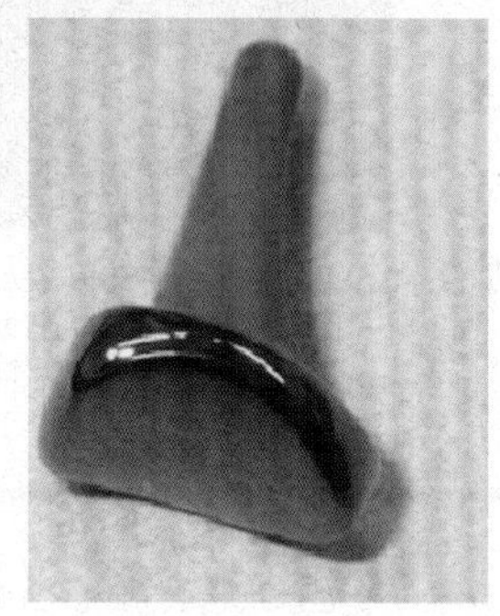
B
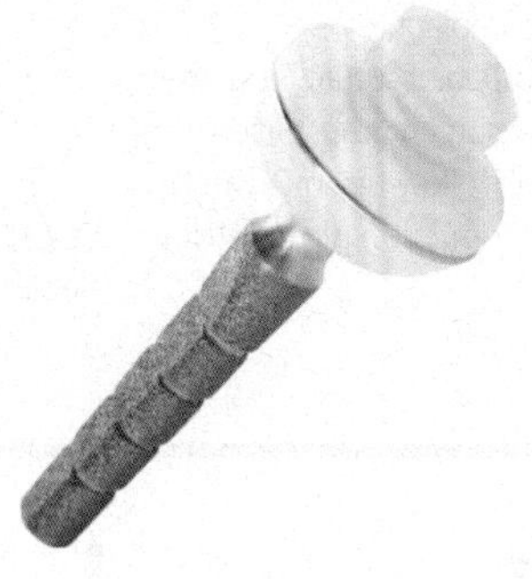
C

FIG 1 • **A.** Artelon implant demonstrating T shape with two dorsal wings. **B.** Pyrocarbon saddle implant. **C.** Avanta CMC implant. (**C:** Courtesy of Small Bone Innovations, Inc., Morrisville, PA.)

Artelon Resurfacing Arthroplasty

Exposure

- A dorsal approach is needed for placement of the Artelon implant between the distal trapezium and the proximal metacarpal of the thumb.
- Make a longitudinal incision centered over the CMC joint. Identify and protect branches of the superficial radial nerve throughout the case, along with the extensor pollicis longus (EPL) and extensor pollicis brevis (EPB).
- After mobilizing and protecting the radial artery, mobilize the EPL and EPB tendons enough to facilitate a longitudinal incision through the capsule. Reflect the capsule enough to completely visualize the joint (**TECH FIG 1**).
- Visualize the scaphotrapezoidal joint; if it is found to have substantial degeneration, this joint surface would need to be addressed as part of the procedure.

Joint Preparation

- Use a high-speed sagittal saw to remove the distal facet of the trapezium. Take care not to injure the flexor carpi radialis (FCR) or flexor pollicis longus (FPL) tendons, which lie on the volar side of the bony cut. Alternatively, a burr can be used to decorticate the trapezial surface while maintaining its native contour.
- Use a high-speed burr to slightly decorticate the dorsum of the proximal metacarpal to stimulate healing but not enough to affect the suture anchor fixation (**TECH FIG 2**).

Implant Placement

- The implant (see **FIG 1A**) comes in two sizes; pick the appropriate size to fill the void from radial to ulnar as well as dorsal to volar between the trapezium and the base of the metacarpal. The larger size may be able to be trimmed down to fit more anatomically.

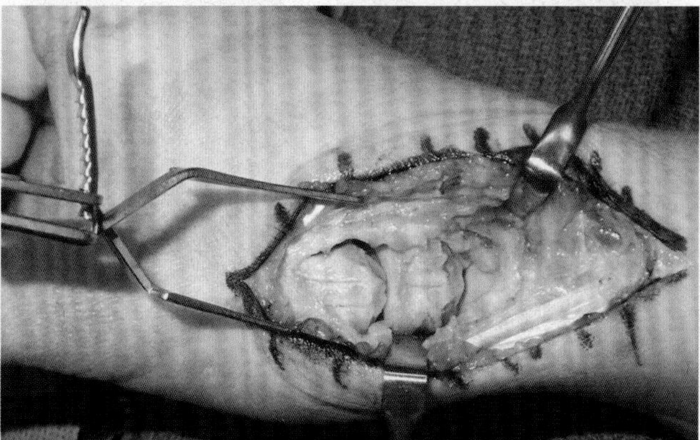

TECH FIG 1 • Dorsal approach to the TM joint after reflecting the joint capsule.

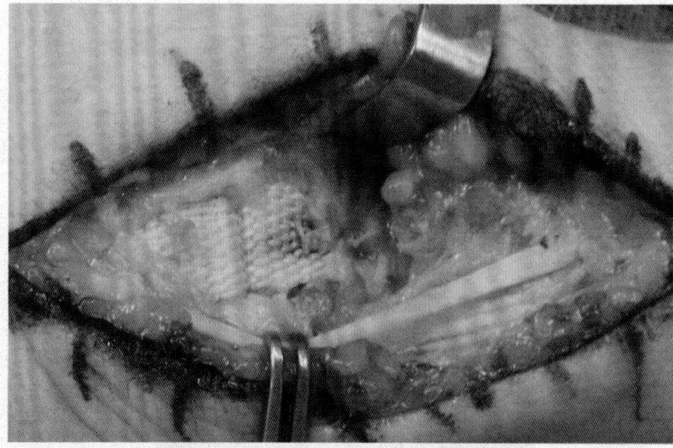

TECH FIG 2 • Appearance of the TM joint after bone cuts on trapezium, burring of proximal TM, and placement of bioabsorbable suture anchors.

- The Artelon implant is shaped similar to a T, with two wings for the dorsum of the trapezium and metacarpal, with the other part to be placed between the fresh bone edges of the trapezium and the base of the metacarpal.
- Bioabsorbable suture anchors (with 2-0 FiberWire or equivalent) are used to hold the dorsal wings down to the bone (**TECH FIG 3**). Although cortical bone screws were recommended to secure the implant early on, experience has shown that screws are a frequent source of complication and may pull through the mesh. Screws should be avoided. Suture anchors are much easier and quicker and provide better fixation of the implant.
- After this, close the capsule with absorbable suture and the skin with 3-0 nylon. At the end of the surgery, the patient is placed into a thumb spica splint and will follow-up in 2 weeks for suture removal and placement into a thumb spica cast for 4 more weeks.

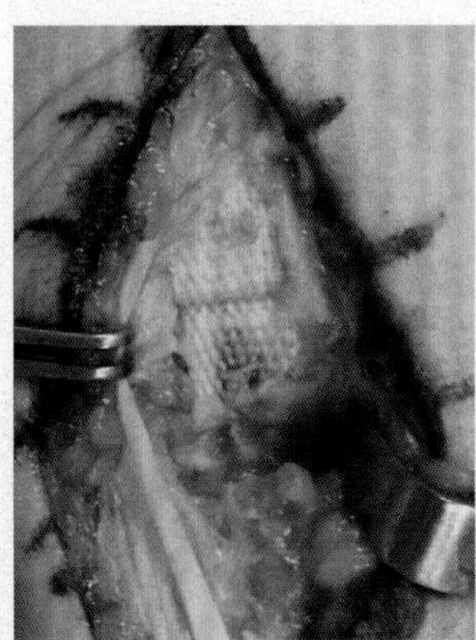

TECH FIG 3 • Appearance of the resurfacing arthroplasty after stabilization of the Artelon implant with suture anchors.

Pyrocarbon Resurfacing Arthroplasty

Exposure

- Make a dorsal longitudinal incision centered over the CMC joint. Identify and protect the branches of the superficial radial nerve throughout the procedure, along with the EPL and EPB.
- After mobilizing and protecting the radial artery, mobilize the EPL and EPB tendons enough to facilitate a longitudinal incision through the capsule. Reflect the capsule enough to completely visualize the joint. Subperiosteal release allows the base of the metacarpal to be dislocated dorsal to the trapezium. Place a Hohmann retractor beneath the palmar surface to maintain exposure.

Joint Preparation

- First, place a sizing guide over the surface as a guide toward what the ultimate size implant is likely to be.
- Resect the base using the cutting guide, which is assembled after an intramedullary rod is inserted. Just the articular surface is removed.

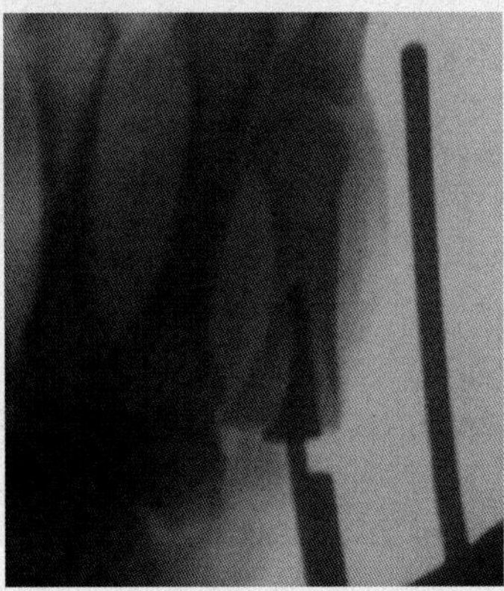

TECH FIG 4 • Extramedullary guide to plan placement of saddle implant.

- Start broaching. Ensure that the broach is started just volar to the central portion of the cut to ensure that the implant is not placed too dorsal (**TECH FIG 4**).

Implant Placement

- Check stability with the final implant in place (**TECH FIG 5A**). Gentle cross-palm pressure before capsular closure should not cause dislocation.
- The implant comes in four sizes. If the trial is not stable, upsizing the implant may be necessary.
- Close the capsule with absorbable suture and the skin with 4-0 nylon.
- At the end of the surgery, the patient is placed into a thumb spica splint and will follow-up in 2 weeks for suture removal and placement into a thumb spica splint for 4 more weeks.
- Radiographs are checked at that time to ensure that the implant is reduced (**TECH FIG 5B**).

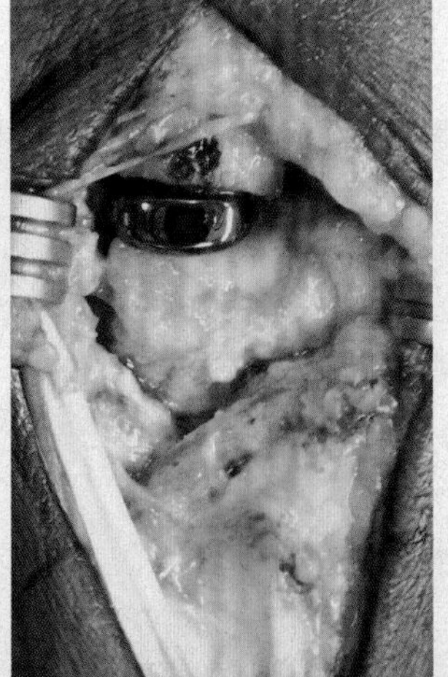

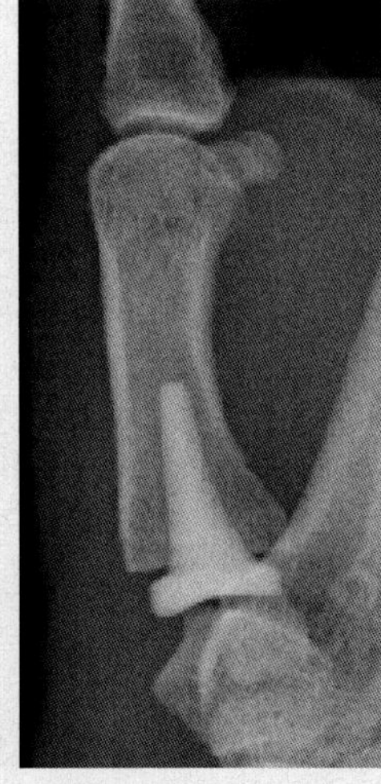

TECH FIG 5 • **A.** Saddle implant in place. **B.** Postoperative lateral radiograph showing implant in place.

Total Joint Replacement

Exposure

- We use a technique and surgical approach similar to that described by Badia and Sambandam[2] for implanting a Braun-Cutter trapeziometacarpal joint prosthesis (or Avanta CMC implant; Small Bone Innovations; see **FIG 1C**) using bone cement.
- Make a 4-cm longitudinal incision over the dorsal aspect of the base of the thumb. Identify and protect branches of the superficial sensory radial nerve. Perform further dissection between the EPL and EPB tendons, isolating and protecting the dorsal branch of the radial artery.
- Open the dorsal capsule of the trapeziometacarpal joint longitudinally. Reflect the periosteum and the dorsal capsule radially and ulnarly as a single flap to be repaired later (**TECH FIG 6**).

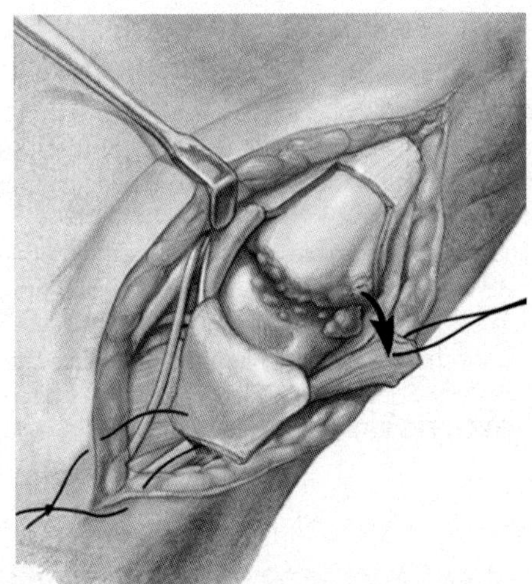

TECH FIG 6 • The first compartment is opened from the volar side and the strands of the abductor pollicis longus (APL) are inspected. A strand of the APL that inserts on the base of the metacarpal in the bone area that will be resected should be freed from its insertion and tagged for later repair. (Courtesy of Small Bone Innovations, Inc., Morrisville, PA.)

Joint Preparation

- Using a sagittal saw, remove about 8 mm of the TM base. This resection is necessary to provide enough exposure to the trapezium (**TECH FIG 7A,B**).
- Release the adductor pollicis if required to allow abduction of the TM away from the palm. At this point, longitudinal traction and flexion are applied to better expose the trapezial surface.
- Use a rongeur to remove the marginal osteophytes and flatten the joint surface of the trapezium.
- With imaging, identify the center of the trapezium with a small burr. Enlarge the center hole to create a deep channel within the trapezium where the polyethylene cup will be cemented (**TECH FIG 7C**).
- For the TM, use a guide to open the intramedullary canal, which is broached with a burr to allow for an ample cement mantle (**TECH FIG 7D**).

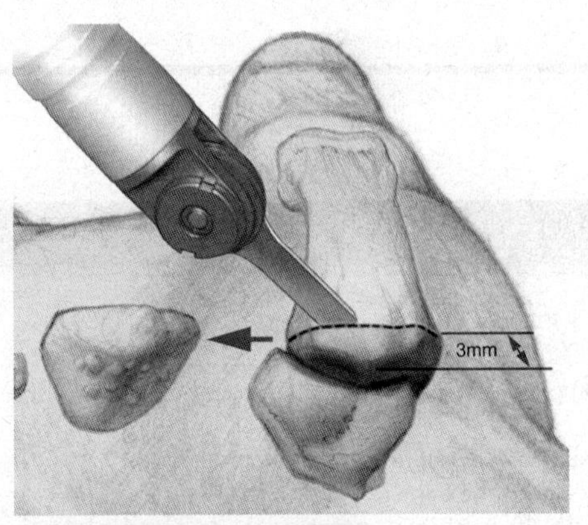

A

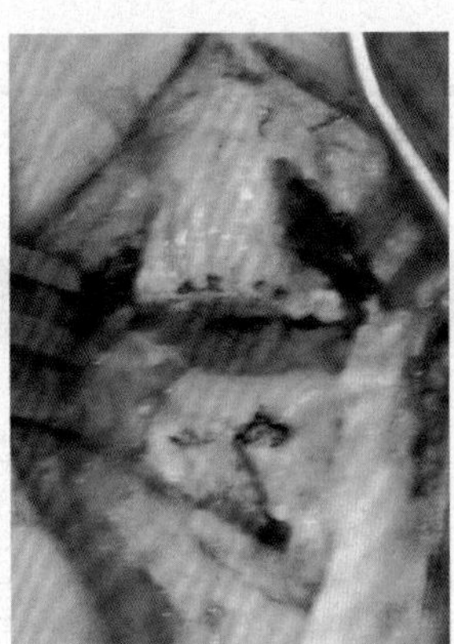

B

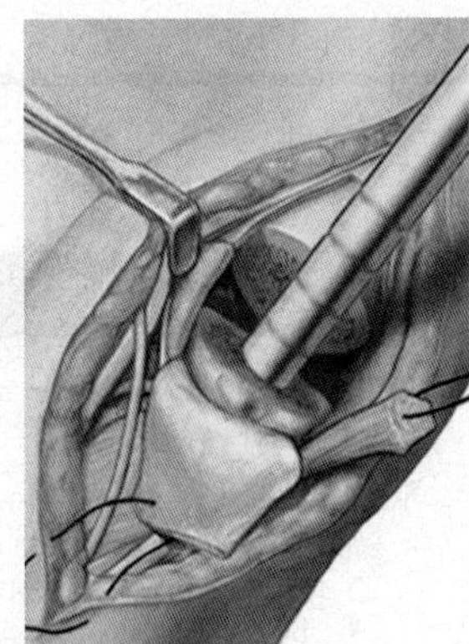

C

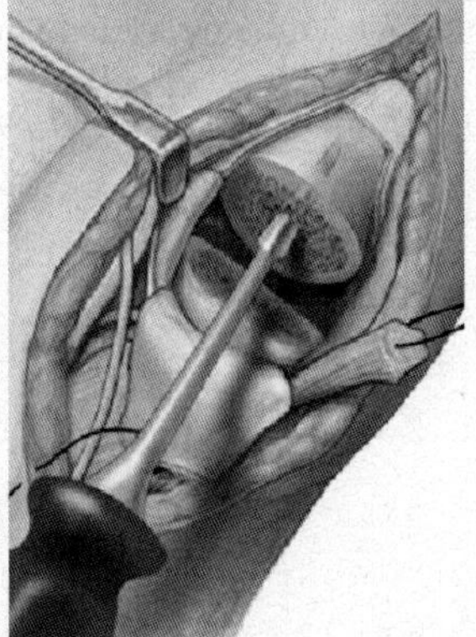

D

TECH FIG 7 • The capsule of the trapeziometacarpal joint is excised (**A**) and the joint is exposed (**B**). **C.** The alignment of the metacarpal component is parallel to the axis of the metacarpal shaft, with slight volar inclination. The trapezial joint surface is evaluated. If the surface is fairly intact, blocking volar, ulnar, and radial osteophytes are removed and the hole is burred for the trapezium component. **D.** The metacarpal canal is reamed and prepared for prosthetic insertion. (**A,C,D:** Courtesy of Small Bone Innovations, Inc., Morrisville, PA.)

Implant Placement

- Place the implant and perform a trial reduction so that motion and fluoroscopic images can be assessed. If there is any bony impingement at the periphery of the residual trapezium, this can be addressed before placing the permanent prosthesis.
- For final placement, first cement the trapezial cup in the trapezium, taking care to impact the cement beneath the subcortical bone.
  - Once the cup has been inserted but before the cement has cured, insert the TM component with bone cement (**TECH FIG 8A**).
  - The two components are linked, but because this stem is collarless, it is important to maintain adequate neck length (to prevent subsidence) until the bone cement has cured. Make sure the stem neck does not impinge on the edge of the trapezium (**TECH FIG 8B**).
  - Assess stability and circumferential motion to ensure there is no impingement on the implant.
- Close the capsule–periosteal flap with absorbable suture.
- After inserting the implant and before closure, use intraoperative fluoroscopy to check proper alignment and placement of the prosthesis (**TECH FIG 8C**).
- Close the skin and subcutaneous tissue with a resorbable suture and place a well-padded short-arm thumb spica splint.

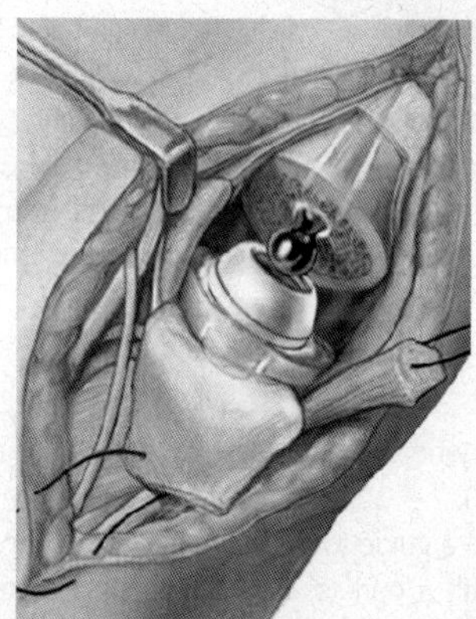
A

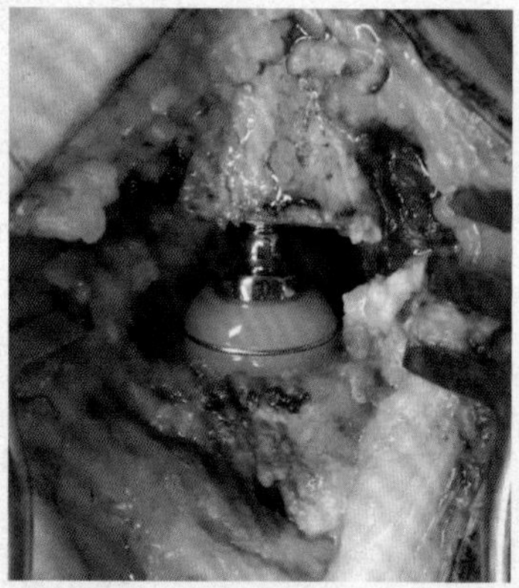
B

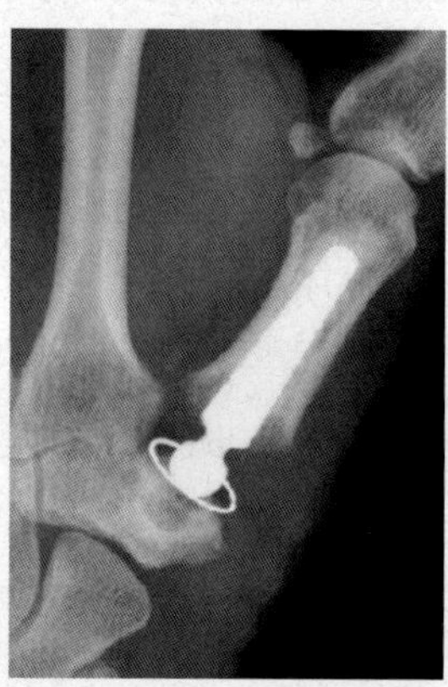
C

TECH FIG 8 • A,B. The components are cemented into place, the trapezium first and the metacarpal second. Compression should be maintained until the bone cement has completely set. **C.** Postoperative lateral radiograph showing implant in place. (**A:** Courtesy of Small Bone Innovations, Inc., Morrisville, PA.)

PEARLS AND PITFALLS

Preoperative	■ Always do an Allen test before surgery. ■ Always evaluate the thumb MCP joint for active instability–hyperextension.
Intraoperative	■ Use extreme caution mobilizing the radial artery. Often, bipolar electrocautery facilitates mobilization, especially of the deep perforators at the volar base of the TM joint. ■ Evaluate the scaphotrapezoidal joint, as preoperative radiographs are not good at predicting disease. ■ Be careful when sawing or drilling not to injure structures deep to the bone. ■ After making the bone cuts on the trapezium and burring the proximal metacarpal, drill and place the suture anchors far enough away from the prepared bone to avoid inadvertent breakout in the fresh cancellous bone surfaces. ■ Once the implant has been secured and the capsule repaired, do not manipulate by the thumb, as this may put undue stress on the soft tissue repair. ■ After the procedure, before contaminating the sterile field, release the tourniquet and observe the reperfusion of the hand to ensure that no unexpected arterial injury occurred.
Postoperative	■ Have a postoperative therapy protocol for patients to follow.

POSTOPERATIVE CARE

- At the end of the surgery, the patient is placed into a thumb spica splint to keep the thumb in opposition. At 2 weeks postoperatively, the sutures are removed and placement into a thumb spica cast continues for 2 more weeks.
- The cast immobilization is discontinued at 6 weeks postoperatively if Artelon resurfacing has been used and at 2 weeks if CMC replacement has been performed. A custom Orthoplast thumb-based spica splint (Johnson & Johnson, New Brunswick, NJ) is worn full time for protection, except during showers and therapy.
- Formal therapy is usually not required after total joint replacement. In the case of resurfacing, therapy will focus on range-of-motion exercises only for postoperative weeks 4 to 6, advancing to thenar isometrics for weeks 6 to 8. At 8 weeks postoperatively, the patient will start grip and pinch strengthening exercises; the splint is also discontinued at this point.

OUTCOMES

- Several long-term studies have shown better than 90% satisfaction and pain relief with soft tissue arthroplasties, but favorable long-term outcome studies in support of the Artelon implant or for total joint arthroplasty are infrequent. In 2013, a retrospective review was published of 38 patients who received an Artelon implant.[4] Twelve of 32 patients (37%) required revision surgery with removal of implant and salvage arthroplasty. Twenty patients with nonrevised Artelon implants were compared with 10 patients who received 13 LRTI procedures; patients with Artelon has significantly less pain improvement compared to those receiving the LRTI procedure. In addition, satisfaction was significantly decreased. As was the conclusion of the arteries of this study,[4] the authors have abandoned the use of Artelon in the treatment of thumb CMC joint osteoarthritis.
- Although the literature supports the use of pyrolytic carbon hemiarthroplasty[16] and total joint arthroplasty[2] in the treatment of thumb CMC joint arthritis, patient selection remains very important because nonimplant options provide favorable outcomes.

COMPLICATIONS

- Superficial branch of the radial nerve injury
- Damage to flexor tendons during saw use
- Radial artery injury
- Dislocation or subsidence of total joint implant
- Subluxation of TM joint
- Continued pain or discomfort
- Failure to recognize other sources of pathology in the hand and wrist

REFERENCES

1. Athwal GS, Chenkin J, King GJ, et al. Early failures with a spheric interposition arthroplasty of the thumb basal joint. J Hand Surg Am 2004;29(6):1080–1084.
2. Badia A, Sambandam SN. Total joint arthroplasty in the treatment of advanced stages of thumb carpometacarpal joint osteoarthritis. J Hand Surg Am 2006;31(10):1605–1614.
3. Bettinger PC, Linscheid RL, Berger RA, et al. An anatomic study of the stabilizing ligaments of the trapezium and trapeziometacarpal joint. J Hand Surg Am 1999;24(4):786–798.
4. Blount AL, Armstrong SD, Yuan F, et al. Porous polyurethaneurea (Artelon) joint spacer compared to trapezium resection and ligament reconstruction. J Hand Surg Am 2013;38(9):1741–1745.
5. Bozentka DJ. Implant arthroplasty of the carpometacarpal joint of the thumb. Hand Clin 2010;26:327–337.
6. Burton RI, Pellegrini VD Jr. Basal joint arthritis of thumb. J Hand Surg Am 1987;12(4):645.
7. Burton RI, Pellegrini VD Jr. Surgical management of basal joint arthritis of the thumb. Part II. Ligament reconstruction with tendon interposition arthroplasty. J Hand Surg Am 1986;11(3):324–332.
8. Cooney WP III, Chao EY. Biomechanical analysis of static forces in the thumb during hand function. J Bone Joint Surg Am 1977;59(1): 27–36.
9. De Smet L, Sioen W, Spaepen D, et al. Total joint arthroplasty for osteoarthritis of the thumb basal joint. Acta Orthop Belg 2004;70: 19–24.
10. Doerschuk SH, Hicks DG, Chinchilli VM, et al. Histopathology of the palmar beak ligament in trapeziometacarpal osteoarthritis. J Hand Surg Am 1999;24(3):496–504.
11. Eaton RG, Littler JW. Ligament reconstruction for the painful thumb carpometacarpal joint. J Bone Joint Surg Am 1973;55(8):1655–1666.
12. Eaton RG, Littler JW. A study of the basal joint of the thumb: treatment of its disabilities by fusion. J Bone Joint Surg Am 1969;51(4):661–668.
13. Glickel SZ. Clinical assessment of the thumb trapeziometacarpal joint. Hand Clin 2001;17:185–195.
14. Haines RW. The mechanism of rotation at the first carpometacarpal joint. J Anat 1944;78:44–46.
15. Lourie GM. The role and implementation of metacarpophalangeal joint fusion and capsulodesis: indications and treatment alternatives. Hand Clin 2001;17:255–260.
16. Martinez de Aragon JS, Moran SL, Rizzo M, et al. Early outcomes of pyrolytic carbon hemiarthroplasty for the treatment of trapezial-metacarpal arthritis. J Hand Surg Am 2009;34:205–212.
17. Naidu SH, Kulkarni N, Saunders M. Titanium basal joint arthroplasty: a finite element analysis and clinical study. J Hand Surg Am 2006;31(5):760–765.
18. Nanno M, Buford WL Jr, Patterson RM, et al. Three-dimensional analysis of the ligamentous attachments of the first carpometacarpal joint. J Hand Surg Am 2006;31(7):1160–1170.
19. Napier JR. The form and function of the carpometacarpal joint of the thumb. J Anat 1955;89:362–369.
20. Nilsson A, Liljensten E, Bergström C, et al. Results from a degradable TMC joint spacer (Artelon) compared with tendon arthroplasty. J Hand Surg Am 2005;30(2):380–389.
21. Pellegrini VD Jr. Osteoarthritis of the trapeziometacarpal joint: the pathophysiology of articular cartilage degeneration. I. Anatomy and pathology of the aging joint. J Hand Surg Am 1991;16(6):967–974.
22. Pellegrini VD Jr. Osteoarthritis of the trapeziometacarpal joint: the pathophysiology of articular cartilage degeneration. II. Articular wear patterns in the osteoarthritic joint. J Hand Surg Am 1991;16(6): 975–982.
23. Pellegrini VD Jr, Burton RI. Surgical management of basal joint arthritis of the thumb. Part I. Long-term results of silicone implant arthroplasty. J Hand Surg Am 1986;11(3):309–324.
24. Tomaino MM. Suspensionplasty for basal joint arthritis: why and how. Hand Clin 2006;22:171–175.
25. Tomaino MM, Pellegrini VD Jr, Burton RI. Arthroplasty of the basal joint of the thumb. Long-term follow-up after ligament reconstruction with tendon interposition. J Bone Joint Surg Am 1995;77(3):346–355.
26. Tomaino MM, Vogt M, Weiser R. Scaphotrapezoid arthritis: prevalence in thumbs undergoing trapezium excision arthroplasty and efficacy of proximal trapezoid excision. J Hand Surg Am 1999;24:1220–1224.
27. Vitale MA, Taylor F, Ross M, et al. Trapezium prosthetic arthroplasty (silicone, Artelon, metal, and pyrocarbon). Hand Clin 2013;29:37–55.

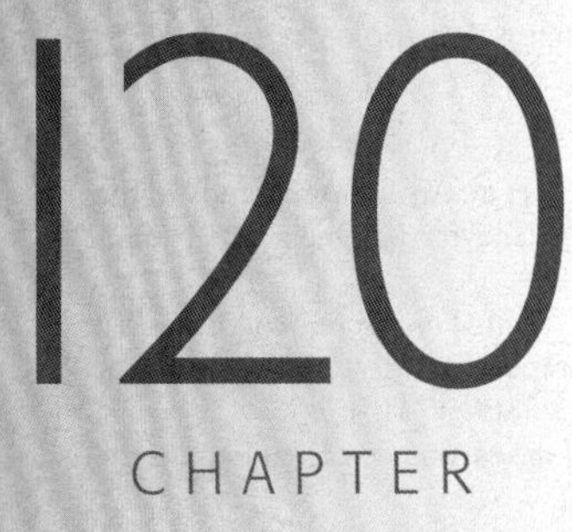

Metacarpophalangeal Joint Synovectomy and Extensor Tendon Centralization in the Inflammatory Arthritis Patient

Andrew L. Terrono, Paul Feldon, and Hervey L. Kimbal III

DEFINITION

- The finger metacarpophalangeal (MCP) joint is commonly and characteristically involved in inflammatory arthritis.
- The MCP joint is often involved early in inflammatory arthritis and usually presents with ulnar extensor tendon subluxation resulting in ulnar deviation of the fingers.
- Occasionally in systemic lupus erythematosus (SLE), radial subluxation of the extensor tendon is seen.

ANATOMY

- The normal MCP joint is a condylar joint that allows flexion and extension as well as radial and ulnar deviation and a combination of these movements. Normally, there is 90 degrees of flexion, although hyperextension can vary.[1,2]
- The stability of the MCP joint is provided by the radial and ulnar collateral ligaments, the accessory collateral ligaments, the volar plate, the dorsal capsule, and the extensor tendon (**FIG 1**).
- The metacarpal head diameter increases in both the transverse and sagittal planes and therefore has a cam effect, making the collateral ligaments tight in flexion and lax in extension. This allows more radial and ulnar deviation of the MCP joint in extension.
- The MCP joint collateral ligaments are asymmetric.
  - The ulnar collateral ligament is more parallel to the long axis of the fingers.
  - The radial collateral ligament is more oblique.
  - This causes supination of the MCP joint with MCP joint flexion.
- The collateral ligament also resists volar-directed forces.
- The volar plate is fibrocartilaginous distally and has a membranous portion proximally. It limits MCP joint extension.
- The transverse intermetacarpal ligament connects the volar plates to each other.
- The accessory collateral ligament connects the collateral ligament and volar plate and keeps the volar plate close to the volar aspect of the MCP joint throughout motion.
- The A1 pulley of the flexor tendon sheath is attached to the volar plate.
- The extensor digitorum tendon is maintained centrally over the MCP joint by the transverse fibers of the sagittal band that attach volarly to the volar plate and the intermetacarpal ligament. This forms a sling mechanism. The ulnar sagittal band is felt to be stronger and denser than the radial sagittal band.

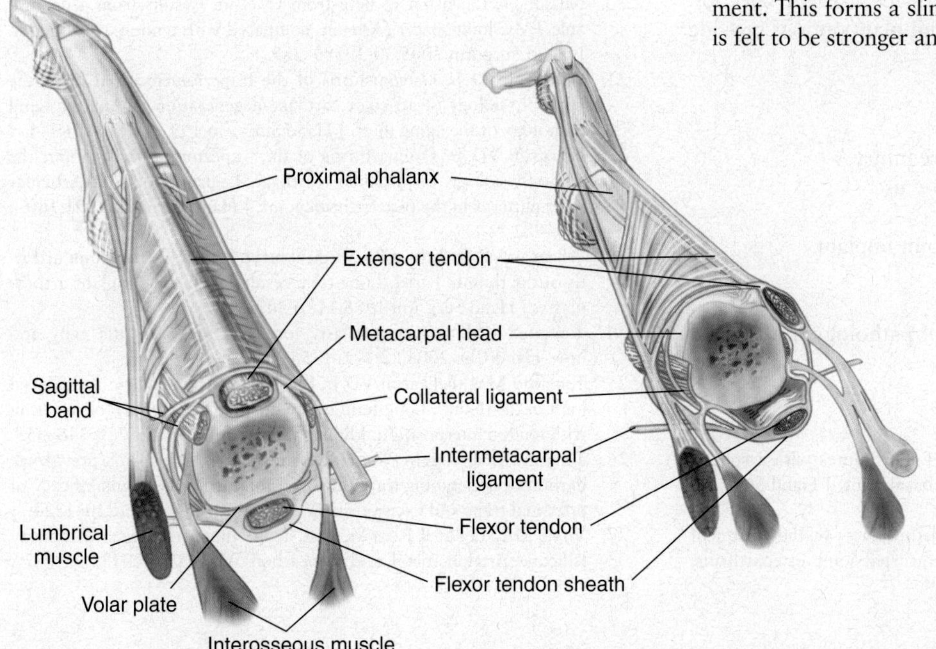

FIG 1 • **A.** Normal anatomy of the MCP joint. **B.** Abnormal anatomy seen in inflammatory arthritis. The extensor tendon is subluxated ulnarly.

- There is usually no direct extensor tendon insertion into the proximal phalanx. The proximal phalanx is extended through the sling mechanism.
- The lumbrical muscle originates from the tendon of the flexor digitorum profundus and is volar to the intermetacarpal ligament. It inserts into the lateral band.
- There are three volar (which adduct) and four dorsal (which abduct) interossei that have tendons that all pass dorsal to the transverse intermetacarpal ligament. They have variable insertions into the proximal phalanx and extensor mechanism.
  - The first dorsal interosseous almost always inserts completely into the radial side of the proximal phalanx of the index finger.

PATHOGENESIS

- The pathology of inflammatory arthritis begins with proliferative synovitis.[1,3]
- Selective changes in static and dynamic stabilizers of the MCP joint occur, resulting in alteration in the equilibrium of the joint. The most common deformity produced is ulnar deviation of the fingers (**FIG 2A**).
  - Which comes first, the changes to the dynamic or static stabilizers, is unclear and may vary.
  - The capsule, radial collateral ligament, and radial sagittal band are stretched by the synovitis and allow the equilibrium to move toward ulnar deviation.
  - The accessory collateral ligament and the membranous portion of the volar plate become lax.
  - The joint capsule becomes thinned and a defect in the dorsal capsule may occur.
  - With increasing ulnar deviation, the ulnar intrinsic muscle tendon unit shortens.
  - The intrinsic muscle contribution to the deformity is unclear. It may be a primary or secondary change. There is a cycle that is set up as the MCP joint ulnarly deviates and the extensor tendon acts as an ulnar deviator and may even act as a flexor of the MCP joint.
  - The laxity of the volar plate and accessory collateral ligament causes the flexor tendons to be further away from the center of rotation of the MCP joint. Therefore, the flexor tendon develops a mechanical advantage and increased flexion force. This results in an increase in the deformity.
- The combination of changes to the capsule, radial collateral ligament, radial sagittal band, accessory collateral ligament, and the membranous portion of the volar plate and the increased mechanical advantage of the flexor tendon is magnified by the normal ulnar and volar slope of the metacarpal condyles and allows ulnar deviation and volar displacement of the proximal phalanx (**FIG 2B**).
- The wrist may be a contributing factor to the development of the MCP joint deformity, and this must be considered in each case before correcting the MCP joint.
  - Radial deviation of the wrist can be a compensatory position to the ulnar deviation of the MCP joints to allow the fingers to line up with the forearm.
  - Ulnar deviation of the digit is more common in patients with radial deviation of the wrist.
- At first, the deformity is correctable passively, but gradually, this mobility is lost and the deformity becomes fixed.

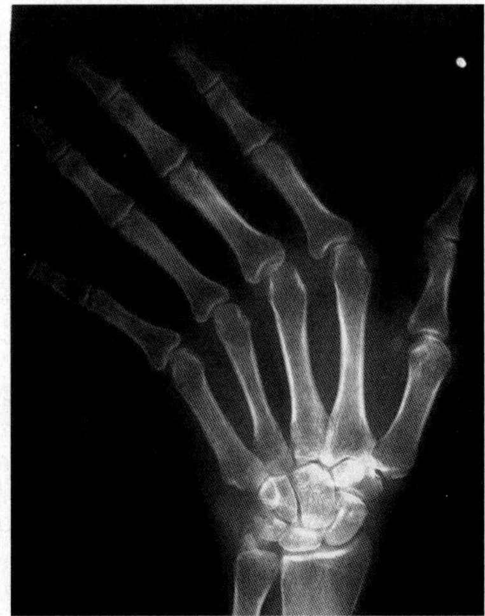

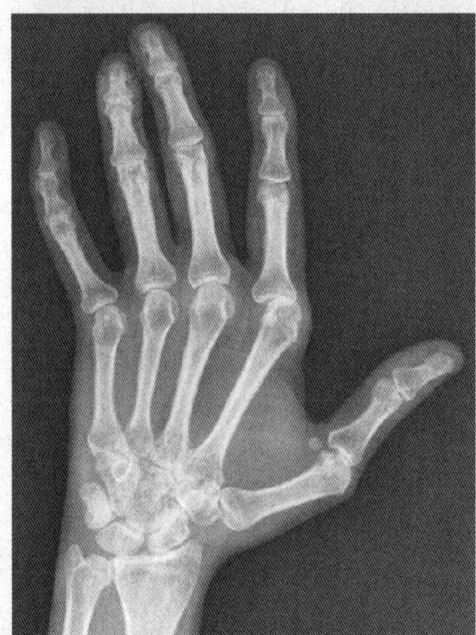

FIG 2 • **A.** Radiograph of a patient with extensor tendon subluxation and ulnar deviation of the MCP joints. The joint spaces are maintained and the joints are not subluxated. **B.** Radiograph of a patient with extensor tendon subluxation and ulnar deviation of the MCP joints with reducible MCP joint subluxation involving the index and middle MCP joints.

- Articular cartilage changes progress from softening of the cartilage to erosion with significant loss of cartilage and bone. This contributes to the deformity.
  - Once there are significant cartilage and bone changes, extensor tendon realignment alone, without joint resurfacing, is not indicated.
- The changes seen in SLE are secondary not to synovitis but rather to alteration in the collagen that results in a change in the equilibrium of the MCP joint and subsequent deformity.
  - The finger deformity in SLE is often ulnar deviation, but radial deviation is not uncommon.
  - In SLE, it is easy to change one deformity to another (ie, ulnar drift into a radial deviation deformity after surgery) because of the global changes to the supporting structures.
  - Despite the MCP deformity becoming fixed, the articular cartilage is usually preserved.

NATURAL HISTORY

- The natural history of the MCP joint changes in inflammatory arthritis is not known and is probably highly variable and influenced by the new disease-modifying medications.

- Mild ulnar deviation of the fingers is normal and increases with MCP joint flexion.
- In inflammatory arthritis, such as rheumatoid arthritis, deformity is initially passively correctable.
- Mild ulnar deviation of the fingers is seen in less than 10% of the patients in the first 5 years of having rheumatoid arthritis.[3]
- Ulnar deviation has been reported in 30% of patients with rheumatoid arthritis, with palmar subluxation in 20%.[3]
- Palmar subluxation almost always occurs with ulnar deviation.[3]

PATIENT HISTORY AND PHYSICAL FINDINGS

- In a patient with inflammatory arthritis who is being considered for MCP joint surgery, the entire upper extremity is evaluated. Involvement of the lower extremities must also be considered, given that the upper extremities may need to assist in ambulation.
  - The need to use the upper extremities for weight bearing can significantly affect the durability of the correction obtained after MCP joint surgery.
  - Ideally, MCP joint surgery is performed when the upper extremity is not needed for such support.
- The wrist is evaluated for the presence of a static deformity at the time of MCP joint surgery. Presence of a static radial deviation deformity will negatively affect the results of MCP joint surgery.
- The skin over the MCP joint is evaluated; it should be in good condition.
- Motion of the MCP joint is assessed. The surgeon should specifically ensure that ulnar deviation and flexion deformities can be easily corrected passively.
- Proximal interphalangeal (PIP) joint motion and alignment must be critically evaluated.
  - If there is a significant boutonnière deformity, this should be corrected before the MCP joint surgery because the PIP flexion will influence the amount of MCP joint flexion obtained postoperatively.
  - If there is a swan-neck deformity, this can be treated at the same time or after the MCP joint. A stiff PIP joint in extension will cause the patient to flex the finger at the MCP joint and can help obtain better flexion postoperatively.
  - Any radial or ulnar deformity at the PIP joint must be corrected before the MCP joint surgery.
- The flexor and extensor tendons must be intact before any MCP joint surgery.

IMAGING AND OTHER DIAGNOSTIC STUDIES

- Radiographs of the hand and wrist are essential before MCP joint surgery to evaluate alignment, congruence, and joint integrity.

DIFFERENTIAL DIAGNOSIS

- The most common cause of inflammatory arthritis that affects the MCP joint is rheumatoid arthritis.
- SLE is more common in black women, and the deformity is secondary to a collagen abnormality causing ligament and tendon imbalance. Articular cartilage loss is a much less common problem in SLE. Soft tissue realignment can be performed even after the condition has been present for a long time.
- Psoriatic arthritis is more common in men and has a characteristic skin rash, although patients may have joint involvement before a clinically obvious skin rash. The patient with psoriatic arthritis often has an asymmetric deformity and more stiffness. The cartilage and bone are also affected.

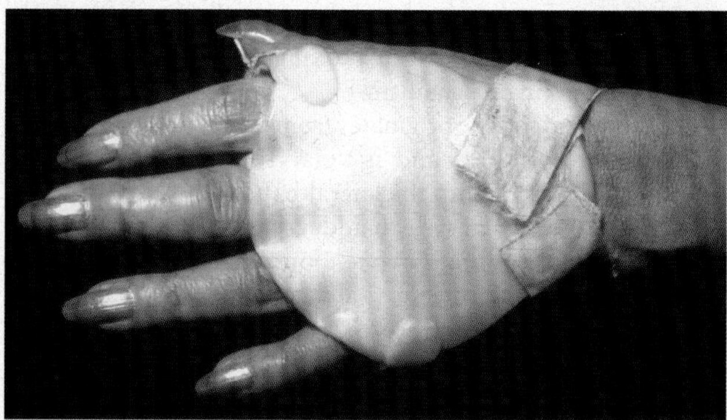

FIG 3 • A splint used to try to prevent progression of the ulnar deviation. Usually, this is not successful and ulnar deviation eventually progresses.

NONOPERATIVE TREATMENT

- A team approach to patients with inflammatory arthritis is important.
- Splinting in a corrected position (**FIG 3**) and joint protection may decrease the forces that contribute to the deformity.
- This may be helpful, but the effect in the long term is unknown, and we have not noticed significant long-term benefit.

SURGICAL MANAGEMENT

- One of the most difficult operations to decide to perform is MCP joint synovectomy and realignment.
  - This is usually best performed early when there is minimal deformity.
  - However, at this time, the patient often has minimal pain and only slight loss of function.
  - With the use of disease-modifying medications, if the anatomy can be restored and the mechanical problems corrected, salvage procedures may be prevented or significantly delayed.
- The ideal patient for surgery is one with increasing deformity and good medical management with control of his or her synovitis.
- The deformity should be passively correctable with good active MCP joint motion.
  - Ideally, the MCP joint is not volarly subluxated because correction and maintenance of correction is more unreliable.
- There should be a well-aligned wrist with good PIP joint function without deformity.
  - If the deformity is passively correctable but cannot be actively corrected, obtaining active ulnar deviation by an extensor carpi ulnaris tendon relocation or transfer should be considered.
- The radiographs should reveal good preservation of the joint space without volar subluxation.
- If all of these criteria are met and the joints are not passively correctable or there is volar subluxation of the MCP joint, surgery can be performed, although the results may not be as reliable.[2]
- A firm diagnosis can help with establishing a prognosis for the maintenance of correction obtained at surgery.
  - The effect of the new disease-modifying medication is not known.

- It is possible that the soft tissue correction obtained at surgery may now last longer and therefore the procedure should be entertained earlier and more often.
- Ideally, earlier surgery will solve the correctable mechanical problem and will end the cycle of deformity.

Positioning

- The procedure is performed using tourniquet control. The hand is supported by a hand table.

Approach

- The procedure usually is performed on all four fingers through a transverse dorsal incision over the MCP joint (**FIG 4**).[2–4]
  - If a single digit is involved, a longitudinal incision should be used.
- If not all of the fingers are going to be corrected, the fingers on the side of the deformity (ie, if there is ulnar deviation deformity, the radial involved digits) must be corrected first to limit recurrent deformity.

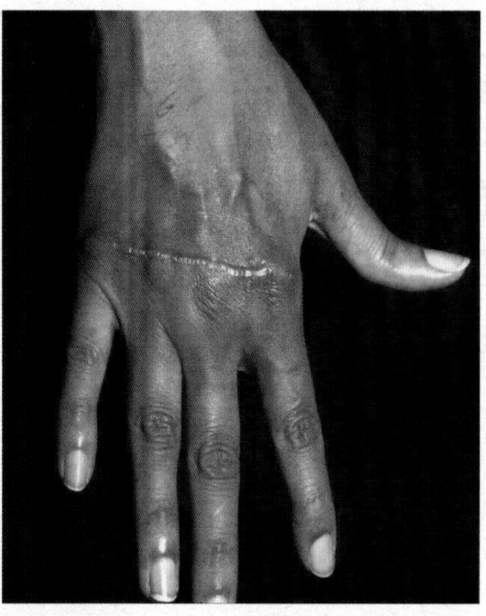

FIG 4 • A transverse incision is used to expose the MCP joints when performing an extensor tendon centralization.

TECHNIQUES

Exposure

- Expose the extensor mechanism at each joint (**TECH FIG 1A**).
- Release the junctura tendinae as needed (**TECH FIG 1B**).
- Develop the interval between the extensor hood and capsule.
- Try to relocate the extensor tendon to the midline.
  - Sometimes, this can be done without releasing the ulnar sagittal band.
- If the extensor tendon can be relocated to the midline, expose the joint by incising the radial sagittal band.
  - The radial sagittal band will be reefed at the end of the procedure.
- If the extensor tendon cannot be relocated to the midline, release the ulnar sagittal band to expose the capsule.
- A central defect in the joint capsule is often present. Open the capsule through this defect using a distally based dorsal capsular flap (**TECH FIG 1C**).

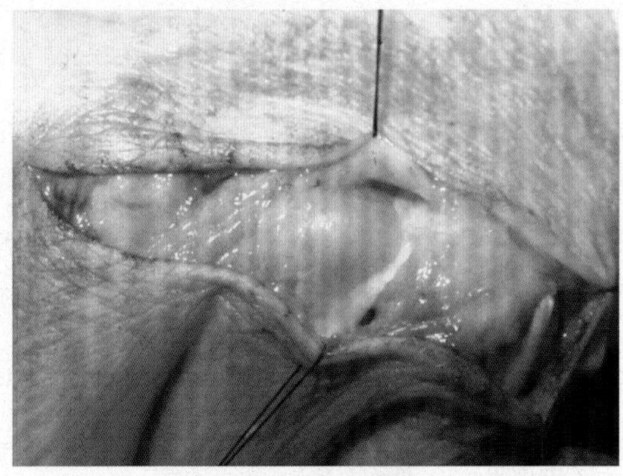

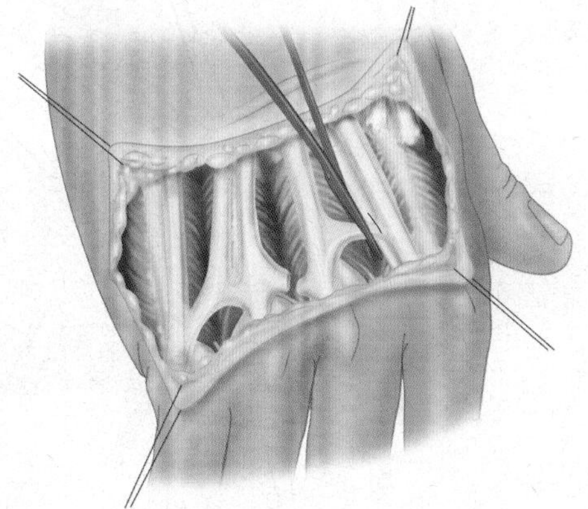

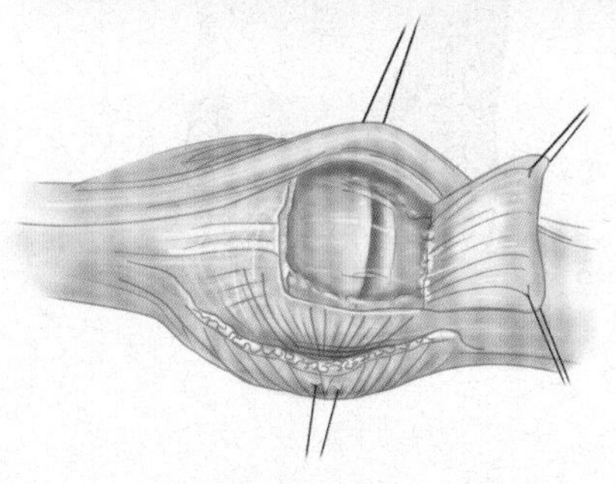

TECH FIG 1 • **A.** The extensor tendons are exposed through a transverse skin incision. The extensor tendons are subluxated ulnarly. **B.** The junctura tendinae are released as needed. **C.** The capsule is opened by creating a distally based dorsal capsular flap.

Synovectomy and Tendon Realignment

- Perform a synovectomy using small rongeurs, curettes, and elevators (**TECH FIG 2A**).
- Evaluate the intrinsics after the extensor tendon is relocated and the joint is in neutral position. Perform an intrinsic tightness test. If positive, intrinsic tightness persists, release the ulnar intrinsic.
  - Incise the sagittal band and expose the intrinsic tendon on the ulnar side of the joint.
    - It is superficial to the collateral ligament and capsule.
  - Pass a curved hemostat beneath the ulnar intrinsic tendon as it inserts into the lateral band (see **FIG 1**) and divide the tendon.
    - A section of the oblique fibers may be excised.
  - If intrinsic tightness continues, release the proximal phalanx insertion by grasping the proximal portion of the tendon with a clamp and sectioning (**TECH FIG 2B**).
  - A step cut lengthening of the ulnar intrinsics may be preferred to complete intrinsic release in patients with SLE to avoid late radial deviation.
- If the joint still cannot be corrected, release the ulnar collateral ligament.
- If the ulnar intrinsic has been released, an intrinsic transfer can be performed, usually attaching it to the radial collateral ligament (**TECH FIG 2C**).
  - The advantage of using the radial collateral ligament as the attachment site is that it does not increase the extensor force at the PIP joint, which could result in a swan-neck deformity.
- If the joint was subluxated volarly preoperatively, pin the MCP joint in extension with a Kirschner wire.
- After the proximal phalanx is reduced, reef or advance the radial collateral ligament as needed (**TECH FIG 2D**).
- Close the capsule in a pants-over-vest manner so that the MCP joint is in extension (**TECH FIG 2E**).
- The extensor tendon is relocated onto the dorsal midline of the joint.
- Strip the periosteum from the dorsum of the proximal phalanx base and tenodese the central tendon to the proximal phalanx using a suture anchor (**TECH FIG 2F,G**).
  - Alternatively, place two drill holes in the proximal phalanx to suture the tendon directly to the bone.
  - A 2-0 PDS suture is used. Nonabsorbable suture may result in prominent knots in this patient population with thin skin.
- Reef the radial sagittal band fibers with a 4-0 absorbable suture to rebalance and support the extensor tendon directly over the joint.
- Repair the junctura tendinae.
- Traction on the central tendon should result in full MCP joint extension.
- Flexion of the MCP joint should not cause extensor tendon subluxation.
- A bulky dressing with fluffs between the fingers is applied, followed by a volar splint supporting the MCP joints in extension and in a slightly overcorrected position.

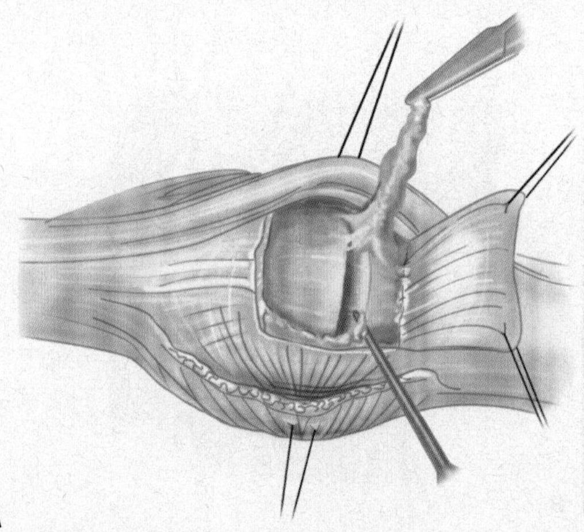

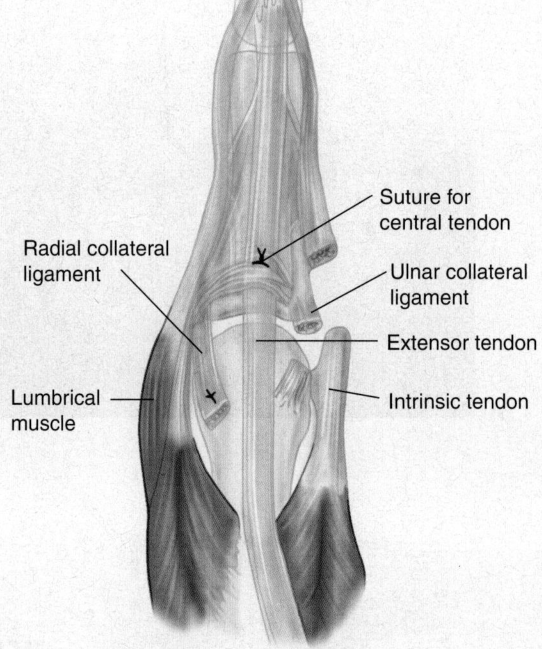

TECH FIG 2 • **A.** An MCP joint synovectomy is performed. **B.** The ulnar intrinsic tendon is sectioned and the ulnar collateral ligament is released. The central tendon is centralized and sutured to the proximal phalanx. *(continued)*

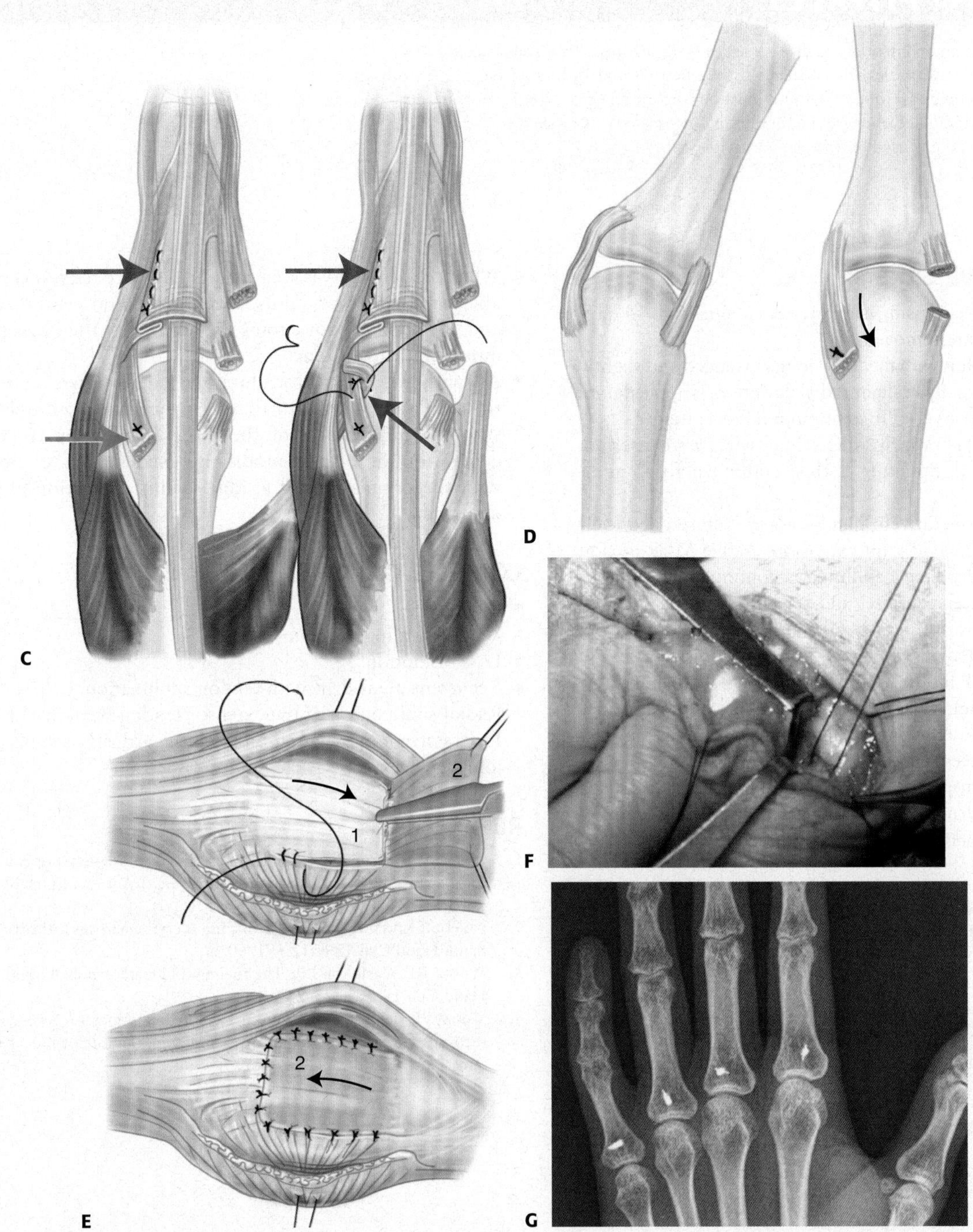

TECH FIG 2 • *(continued)* **C.** The contracted ulnar sagittal fibers are released and the radial sagittal fibers are reefed (*red arrows*) to rebalance and support the extensor tendon in the midline. The radial collateral ligament is advanced (*green arrow*) and the ulnar intrinsic muscle is transferred to the radial collateral ligament (*blue arrow*) of the adjacent digit. **D.** The radial collateral ligament is advanced, as in this case, or reefed. **E.** The capsule is closed in a pants-over-vest manner so that the MCP joint is supported in extension. **F.** The extensor tendon is sutured directly to the dorsal base of the proximal phalanx using absorbable suture. **G.** Postoperative radiograph of a patient showing suture anchors in place after extensor tendon centralization.

PEARLS AND PITFALLS

- Patient selection and control of the disease process are the most important factors.
- Joints with fixed deformities and cartilage loss are best treated with replacement arthroplasty.
- Proximal joint and distal joint correction must be performed before MCP joint surgery.
- Intrinsic transfers do not improve the long-term outcome of this procedure.
- Intrinsic lengthening is used only in patients with SLE.

POSTOPERATIVE CARE

- The postoperative dressing is removed at about 10 to 14 days and the sutures are removed.[2,4]
- An orthoplast splint with the MCP joints extended and slightly overcorrected, usually in slight radial deviation, is applied until 4 weeks postoperatively. PIP joint motion is encouraged.
- At 4 weeks postoperatively, if Kirschner wires were inserted, they are removed. Splinting is then continued for 2 additional weeks.
- At 6 weeks postoperatively, hand therapy is started, concentrating on active MCP joint extension. Active MCP flexion is also started. Protective splinting is continued for another 2 weeks in between exercises and at night.
- To increase the postoperative flexion, the PIP joint is occasionally splinted in extension, concentrating the flexion force at the MCP joint.
- Dynamic splinting can be used to support extension and maintain digital alignment during the early healing stage but is usually not necessary.
- At 8 weeks postoperatively, daytime splinting is decreased and gradual return to functional activities is encouraged.
- Nighttime extension splinting is continued for 3 months.

OUTCOMES

- MCP joint extension and ulnar drift are improved postoperatively.[4]
- MCP flexion is usually slightly less than it was preoperatively.
- Strength is not significantly improved.
- Maintenance of correction is usually good with slight increase in ulnar drift, usually without recurrent subluxation.
- When the deformity is seen early and is still passively correctable with preserved joints, extensor tendon centralization and MCP joint synovectomy (as needed) is often beneficial, improving patient function.
- As with all joint procedures for deformities resulting from inflammatory arthritis, the procedure itself does not stop the progression of the disease. However, the new generation of disease-modifying medications combined with surgery may result in long-lasting correction of joint deformity.

COMPLICATIONS

- Infection
- Wound healing problems
- Loss of motion
- Recurrent ulnar drift with tendon subluxation
- Radial subluxation of the extensor tendon (seen in SLE)
- Progressive joint destruction from the arthritis and need for joint replacement

REFERENCES

1. Abboud JA, Beredjiklian PK, Bozentka DJ. Metacarpophalangeal joint arthroplasty and rheumatoid arthritis. J Am Acad Orthop Surg 2003;11:184–191.
2. Nalebuff EA. Surgery for systemic lupus erythematosus arthritis of the hand. Hand Clin 1996;12:591–602.
3. Wilson RL, Carlblom ER. The rheumatoid metacarpohalangeal joint. Hand Clin 1989;5:223–237.
4. Wood VE, Ichtertz DR, Yahiku H. Soft tissue metacarpophalangeal reconstruction for treatment of rheumatoid hand deformity. J Hand Surg Am 1989;14(2 pt 1):163–174.

Proximal Interphalangeal and Metacarpophalangeal Joint Silicone Implant Arthroplasty

121 CHAPTER

Charles A. Goldfarb

DEFINITION

- Arthritis of the metacarpophalangeal (MCP) or proximal interphalangeal (PIP) joints may cause pain, deformity, and decreased motion. Rheumatoid arthritis (RA), osteoarthritis, and posttraumatic arthritis are common causes.
- Silicone implant arthroplasty may be considered as a surgical option after failure of nonoperative treatment in the patient with pain, functional disability, or both secondary to arthritis at the MCP or PIP joint.
- The primary function of the silicone implant is to serve as a dynamic spacer until the joint is encapsulated; thereafter, the joint can be expected to maintain alignment and provide a satisfactory range of motion.

ANATOMY

Metacarpophalangeal Joint

- The MCP joint is condyloid with motion in three planes: flexion–extension, abduction–adduction, and rotation.
- The head of the metacarpal is wider on its volar aspect, providing greater stability in flexion. The radial condyle is larger as well, contributing to the ulnar deviation posture most commonly seen in RA patients.
- Collateral ligaments arise dorsal to the center of rotation; this, together with the shape of the metacarpal head, contributes to the cam effect that is manifest by collateral ligament laxity in extension and tightness in flexion.
- Hyperextension of the MCP joints is common; however, the volar plate limits excessive motion.

Proximal Interphalangeal Joint

- The PIP joint is a hinge joint with an average arc of motion of 0 to 100 degrees of flexion.
- The bony anatomy is crucial to PIP joint stability in all positions; the base of the middle phalanx is wider volarly, thus helping to prevent dorsal dislocation. The PIP joint is more stable in all positions compared to the MCP joint.
- The proper collateral ligaments originate from the center of rotation of the proximal phalanx head and insert onto the volar base of the middle phalanx; they provide stability in all positions. The accessory collateral ligaments insert onto the volar plate and provide more stability in extension. There is no significant cam effect with the PIP joint.
- The volar plate resists hyperextension and is a key supporting structure of the joint.

PATHOGENESIS

- Arthritis of the MCP or PIP joints may be idiopathic, posttraumatic, or inflammatory (RA).
- Idiopathic osteoarthritis involves the distal interphalangeal joint most commonly, but the PIP joint is also affected; the MCP joint is less commonly involved.
- The PIP joint is the most frequently traumatized finger joint and, thus, has the highest incidence of posttraumatic arthritis. Given the shortcomings of the salvage procedures for PIP joint arthritis, an anatomic joint reduction and aggressive restoration of the normal anatomy after trauma is critical to reduce the risk of arthritis.
- The bony congruity of the PIP joint makes it poorly tolerant of any loss of cartilage; deformity and loss of motion may progress quickly.
- Inflammatory arthritis (RA) most commonly affects the MCP joint but may also involve the PIP joint. In RA, a proliferative synovitis compromises the soft tissue support of the affected joint and may lead to the characteristic deformities at the MCP joint, including volar subluxation (and a flexed posture) and ulnar deviation. The PIP joint is less predictable because attenuation of the volar supporting structures may lead to joint hyperextension, whereas compromise of the central slip insertion will lead to a joint flexion deformity.
- The efficacy of the disease-modifying antirheumatic drugs has dramatically decreased the need for joint arthroplasty in these patients.

NATURAL HISTORY

- The natural history of osteoarthritis or posttraumatic arthritis of the PIP joint is progression with loss of motion, pain, and, in some patients, deformity. The MCP joint is less commonly affected and is also more tolerant of arthritis, given its increased mobility in all planes.
- In the patient with severe RA not controllable by disease-modifying antirheumatic drugs, joint inflammation will lead to progression of the arthritis.
- The functional effect of the arthritis depends on the degree of involvement, the specific joint, and the involvement of the adjacent joints.

PATIENT HISTORY AND PHYSICAL FINDINGS

- It is vital that the surgeon understand how the arthritis specifically affects the function of a particular patient. This depends on many factors, including adjacent joint involvement, specific patient activities, and the degree of pain experienced.

Physical Examination

- Key components in the physical examination are as follows:
  - Palpate along the joint line to confirm the site of pain and presence of synovitis.

- Measure active and passive range of motion of the joint with a goniometer. Joint motion is lost with arthritis. Pain with motion is noted.
- Measure coronal plane deformity (angulation) of the joint with a goniometer. Progressive arthritis leads to joint deformity.
- Stress the joint in a radial–ulnar directions to evaluate the collateral ligaments. The MCP should be tested in flexion; the PIP joint may be tested in any position but is most commonly tested in extension. Attenuation of collateral ligaments may occur in RA or after trauma.
- Assess the integrity of intrinsic and extrinsic tendon function and strength: most commonly abnormal in RA or after prior trauma
  - Assess for tendon shortening or lengthening (eg, after repair of an open injury) and the presence of tendon adhesions, which is most important in posttraumatic conditions.
  - Perform the Elsen test: Integrity of the central slip is important when contemplating PIP joint arthroplasty.
- Evaluate alignment and function of the adjacent joints (including the wrist), as there is an intimate relationship between the joints.
  - In inflammatory conditions, the more proximal joints, most importantly the wrist, are also examined. If wrist deformity is not corrected before surgical correction of distal disease, surgical correction (such as MCP arthroplasty) will have a higher incidence of failure due to the uncorrected deforming forces.
- Assess for intrinsic or extrinsic contractures after hand trauma.
  - Perform the intrinsic tightness (Bunnell) test: If the intrinsics are tight, therapy or surgical intervention may be needed.

IMAGING AND OTHER DIAGNOSTIC STUDIES

- Posteroanterior and lateral plain radiographs provide sufficient diagnostic information. Occasionally, oblique radiographs are helpful (**FIG 1**).
- Magnetic resonance imaging (MRI) and computed tomography (CT) are of limited use in the evaluation of the MCP and PIP joints.

DIFFERENTIAL DIAGNOSIS

- Acute fracture with or without joint subluxation
- Collateral ligament injury
- Joint infection
- Flexor or extensor mechanism injury

NONOPERATIVE MANAGEMENT

- Anti-inflammatory medications
- Steroid injections
- Hand therapy to address contractures, including splinting

SURGICAL MANAGEMENT

- Surgery is considered if nonoperative management fails. Given the limitations of silicone implant arthroplasty as noted in the following text, the decision for surgical intervention should be patient driven.
- The best outcome is expected in patients with joint-based pain and a well-preserved arc of motion and minimal deformity. Patients without pain and presenting with deformity or a lack of motion are not ideal candidates for arthroplasty, especially if the adjacent joints are functioning well. Joint arthroplasty, of any variety, does not reliably increase motion at long-term follow-up.
- In RA, an ulnar drift and volar subluxation of the MCP joints with a flexion posture of the joints may lead to weakness and a loss of the ability to grasp larger objects. These deformities are also unsightly. Surgical intervention in these patients can be expected to improve the appearance and function of the hand.

Preoperative Planning

- All imaging studies are reviewed.
- Involvement of adjacent joints is assessed.

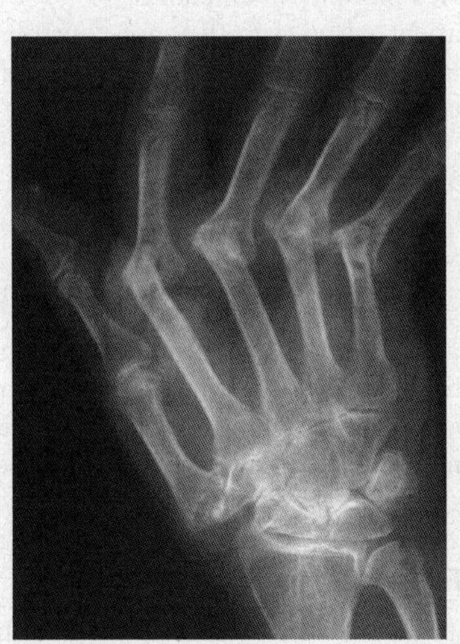
A

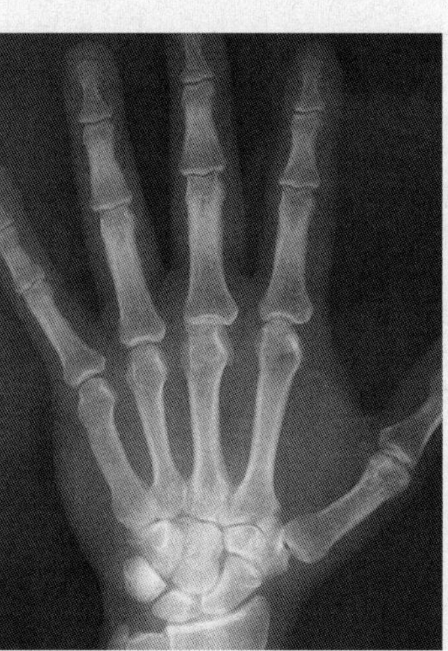
B

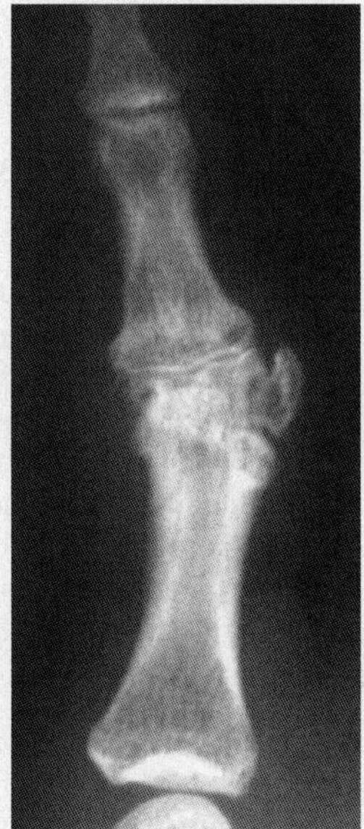
C

FIG 1 • **A.** RA affecting hand, with most notable disease affecting MCP joints. The wrist is also affected. **B.** Isolated osteoarthritis of the MCP joint of the long finger. **C.** Posttraumatic arthritis affecting the small finger PIP joint.

- Multiple MCP or PIP joints can be treated with silicone arthroplasty at the same surgical setting, but we do not typically recommend MCP and PIP joint silicone arthroplasty in the same finger.
  - In patients with symptomatic disease at both the MCP joint and the PIP joint, the MCP is typically treated with silicone implant arthroplasty and the PIP joint is fused.
- An assessment of the ligamentous stability of the MCP and PIP joints is performed under anesthesia.
- MCP and PIP arthroplasty is performed cautiously in the index (or long) finger, as pinch forces may be problematic for joint stability if the collateral ligaments are elongated or compromised with surgery.
- Templating is performed to ensure that appropriate-sized implants are available.

Positioning

- The patient is supine with the extremity on an arm table.
- A nonsterile arm tourniquet is used.
- General or axillary block anesthesia is used.

Approach

- The MCP joint is approached from dorsally with a midline incision.
- The PIP joint may be approached from either the dorsal or volar approach.

Metacarpophalangeal Joint Silicone Arthroplasty

Incision and Dissection

- If a single joint is being addressed (osteoarthritis or posttraumatic arthritis), make a longitudinal incision over the MCP joint. If multiple joints are being addressed, make a transverse incision over the metacarpal necks[2] (**TECH FIG 1A**).
- Protect the superficial veins (most important in RA patients).
- Identify and protect the extensor tendons.
- In RA, the tendons may be translocated in an ulnar direction. If so, divide the sagittal bands on the ulnar side to allow later centralization of the tendons.
  - If the tendons are centralized, the interval between tendons (index and small finger between extensor indicis proprius or extensor digit minimi and extensor digitorum communis) can be used to approach the joint (**TECH FIG 1B**).
- In RA, the ulnar intrinsic tendon is often a deforming force. In fingers with marked ulnar deviation, bring the tendon into the surgical field with a blunt hook and divide it.
- Divide the joint capsule longitudinally for later repair.
- Débride the joint (**TECH FIG 1C**).
- It may be necessary to recess the collateral ligaments off their origin from the metacarpal head. Carefully protect their insertion onto the base of the proximal phalanx.
  - In osteoarthritis or posttraumatic arthritis, the collateral ligaments need not be released if adequate exposure can be obtained.
- If the joint is volarly subluxated, it may exhibit a flexion contracture that must be released.
  - Perform a soft tissue release using a Freer to elevate the volar plate off the volar distal metacarpal; this, together with bony resection, will allow joint reduction.
  - A sufficient release has been accomplished once the proximal phalanx can be mobilized dorsal to the metacarpal head.

Bone Preparation

- Using an oscillating saw, remove the metacarpal head just distal to the collateral ligament origin, staying perpendicular to the axis of the bone in the posteroanterior and lateral planes.
  - The amount of bone removed depends on the degree of deformity and contracture (**TECH FIG 2A**).
  - In severe cases, it is necessary to elevate the collateral ligaments from their origins to resect more metacarpal.

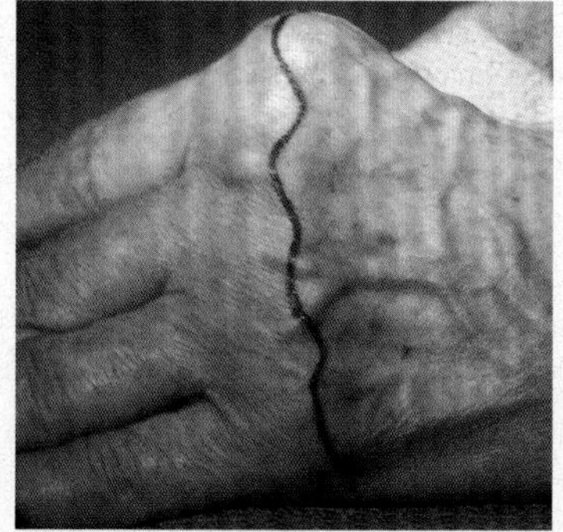
A

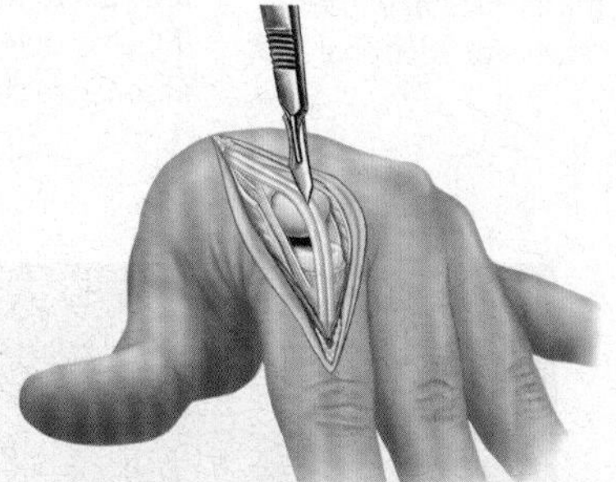
B

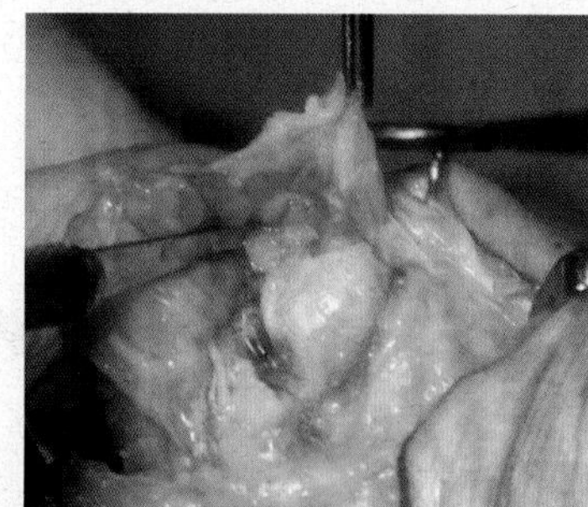
C

TECH FIG 1 • **A.** Transverse dorsal incision for MCP arthroplasty of all four fingers. The incision may be straight or undulating. **B.** The interval between the extensor tendons may be chosen to approach the joint for the index or small fingers. The interval between the extensor digitorum communis and the extensor indicis proprius is illustrated. **C.** The joint is débrided. This can be an extensive process in severe rheumatoid disease.

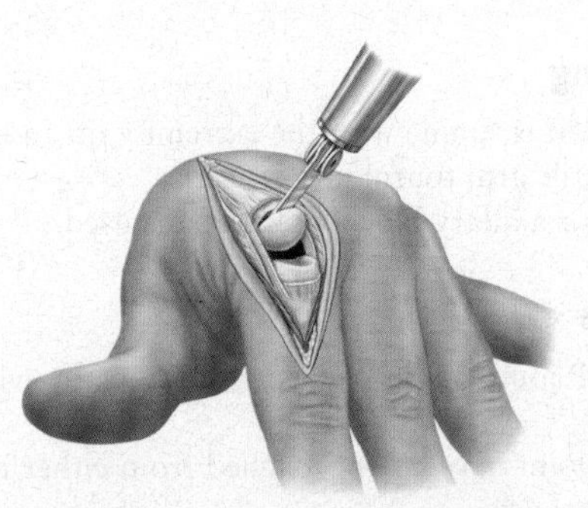

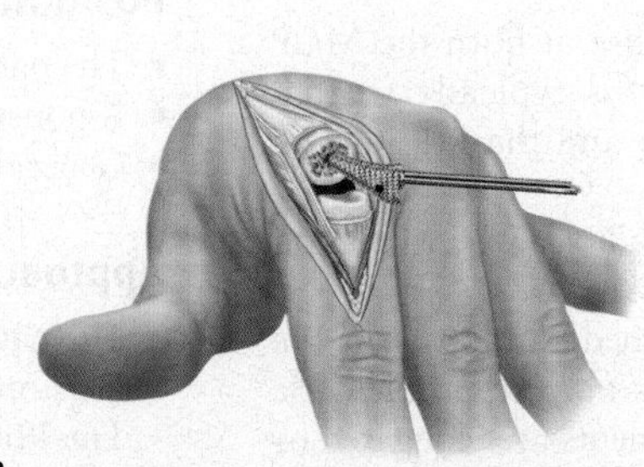

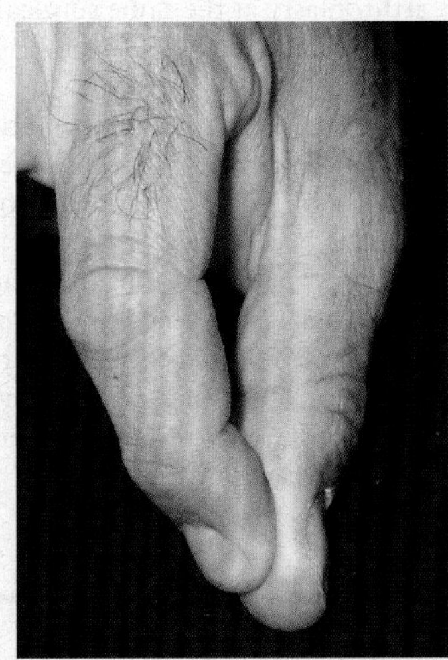

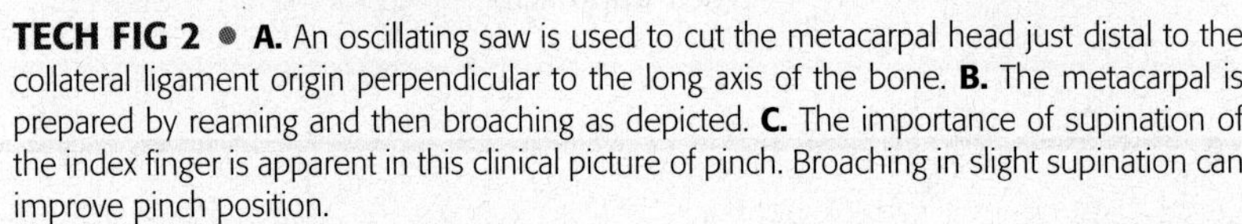

TECH FIG 2 • **A.** An oscillating saw is used to cut the metacarpal head just distal to the collateral ligament origin perpendicular to the long axis of the bone. **B.** The metacarpal is prepared by reaming and then broaching as depicted. **C.** The importance of supination of the index finger is apparent in this clinical picture of pinch. Broaching in slight supination can improve pinch position.

In these cases, radial collateral (and ulnar) ligaments are repaired during closure.

- Prepare the base of the proximal phalanx by removing the articular cartilage using an osteotome or rongeur. Carefully protect the collateral ligament insertions.
- Use an awl to identify the metacarpal medullary canal first.
  - The awl typically enters the canal dorsal to the apparent center of the cut end of the metacarpal given the dorsovolar bone curvature.
- Use hand reamers to prepare the bone.
  - Use progressive broaches, taking care to ensure correct broach alignment and integrity of the cortex (**TECH FIG 2B**).
  - The ring finger metacarpal is frequently narrower and may require more reaming, use of a burr, and potentially a smaller implant.
- Once the metacarpal is prepared, initiate the same procedure for the proximal phalanx.
  - The base of the proximal phalanx can be reamed in slight supination for the index finger to improve pinch (**TECH FIG 2C**).

Implant Placement and Closure

- Place a trial prosthesis, choosing the largest "comfortable" fit that allows full passive joint motion. Ensure proper clinical alignment (**TECH FIG 3A**).
  - If the prosthesis buckles, choose a smaller prosthesis or create more space through soft tissue release or additional bone resection.
  - If the prosthetic stem is too long and is contributing to buckling of the prosthesis, the stem may be trimmed using scissors.
- If the origins of the collateral ligaments were disturbed during the approach, drill holes in the dorsoradial and the dorsoulnar (in the case of osteoarthritis or posttraumatic arthritis) metacarpal and place 2-0 nonabsorbable suture into the collateral ligaments for later repair.
  - The radial collateral ligaments are typically attenuated in RA, especially if the joints have been ulnarly deviated. The ligaments are tightened via imbrication when repaired (**TECH FIG 3B**).
  - A distally based radial slip of the volar plate may be mobilized and integrated into the repair in the case of severely attenuated radial collateral ligaments.
- Place the final implants using a "no touch" technique.
  - To minimize the risk of a reaction between the silicone implant and the sterile gloves, do not directly handle the implants; instead, insert them using forceps.
  - We do not routinely use grommets.
- Insert the proximal stem first; then bend the implant and place the distal stem.
- Once the implant has been placed in a stable position, the collateral ligaments are repaired, imbricated, or reconstructed as required to restore stability (especially against ulnar deviation).
- If the capsule is sufficiently robust, repair it with interrupted 3-0 absorbable suture.

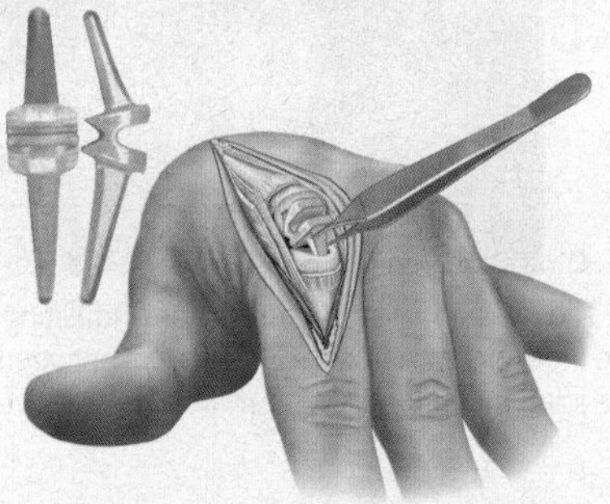

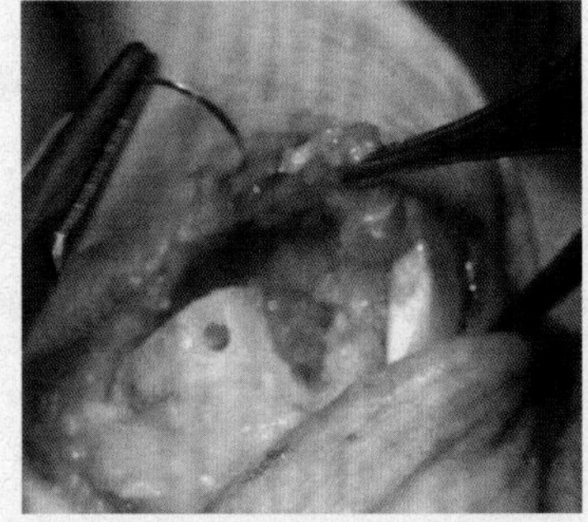

TECH FIG 3 • **A.** A trial implant is placed to test range of motion and implant fit. **B.** After final implant placement, the collateral ligaments are repaired through drill holes placed in the metacarpal. This is most important for the radial collateral ligament in RA.

- Repair the extensor mechanism in a centralized position with nonabsorbable 2-0 suture. Use passive joint range of motion to ensure there is no tendon subluxation after repair.
  - If the radial sagittal band is attenuated, imbricate or incise it and advance it deep to the extensor digitorum communis tendon in a pants-over-vest manner.
  - Additional release of the ulnar sagittal band may also be required to centralize the extensor mechanism.
- Obtain C-arm or standard radiographs to confirm clinical alignment.
- Close the skin with 4-0 nylon suture. Once the wound is closed, deflate the tourniquet.
  - A Penrose drain may be used if excessive bleeding is noted (uncommon). We typically remove the drain the next day.

Proximal Interphalangeal Joint Silicone Arthroplasty

Volar Approach for Proximal Interphalangeal Joint Arthroplasty

Incision and Dissection

- Use a volar, Brunner incision centered at the PIP joint[4,6] (**TECH FIG 4A**).
- Raise full-thickness flaps with careful protection of the neurovascular bundles.
- Divide the C1, A3, and C3 pulleys at their insertion on one side and elevate them to expose the flexor tendons (**TECH FIG 4B,C**).
  - Protect the A2 and A4 pulleys.
- Retract the flexor tendons to either side using a Penrose drain.
- Detach the volar plate proximally and divide the accessory collateral ligaments from their insertion onto the volar plate. Leave the volar plate attached distally (**TECH FIG 4D**).
- Detachment of the collateral ligaments at their insertion is required for optimal exposure and visualization (may be repaired back to volar plate at closure).
- Dislocate the joint in a "shotgun" manner to expose the articular surfaces.

Bone Preparation

- Using an oscillating saw, remove the condyles of the proximal phalanx head, staying perpendicular to the long axis of the bone in both the posteroanterior and lateral planes.
- Carefully prepare the base of the middle phalanx, taking great care not to injure the central slip insertion or proper collateral ligament insertion. Remove remaining cartilage with a rongeur or osteotome. Create a flat surface to accommodate the implant.
- Use awls, hand reamers, and broaches to prepare the medullary canals of the proximal and middle phalanges.
  - The proximal phalanx is typically prepared before the middle phalanx.
  - Use the rectangular shape of the broach base to ensure correct rotation of the final implant.

Implant Placement and Closure

- The trial should allow satisfactory joint range of motion without buckling or displacement.
  - The trial and final implant should remain flush against the cut ends of the bones.
  - The implant can be shortened or additional reaming can be performed as needed for the trial that buckles.

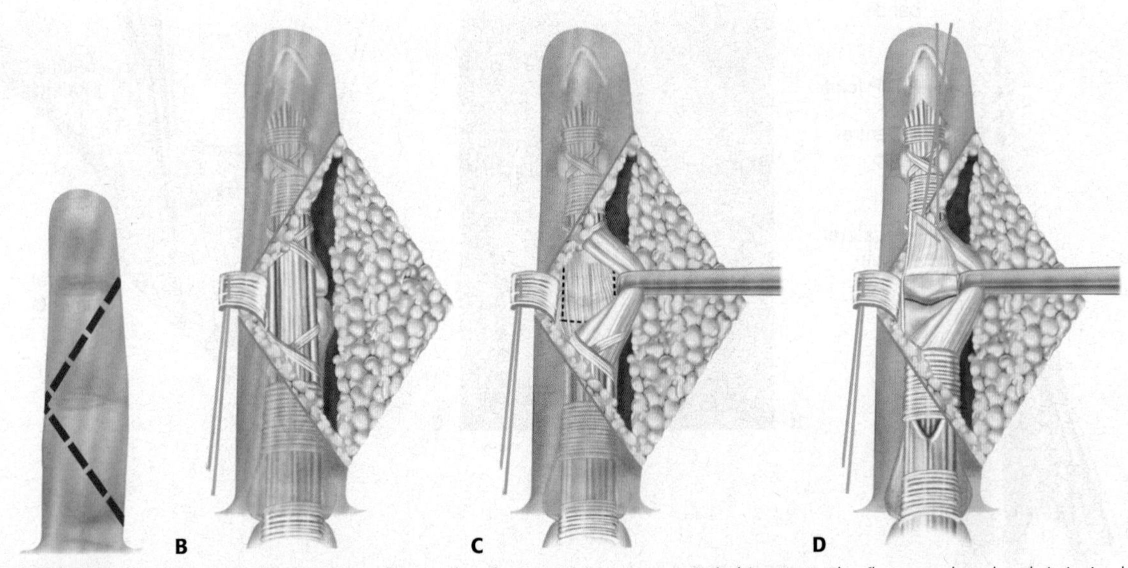

TECH FIG 4 • **A.** A volar skin incision is centered at the PIP joint in a Brunner fashion. **B,C.** The flexor tendon sheath is incised between the A2 and A4 pulleys to allow retraction of the tendons. **D.** The volar plate is released proximally for exposure.

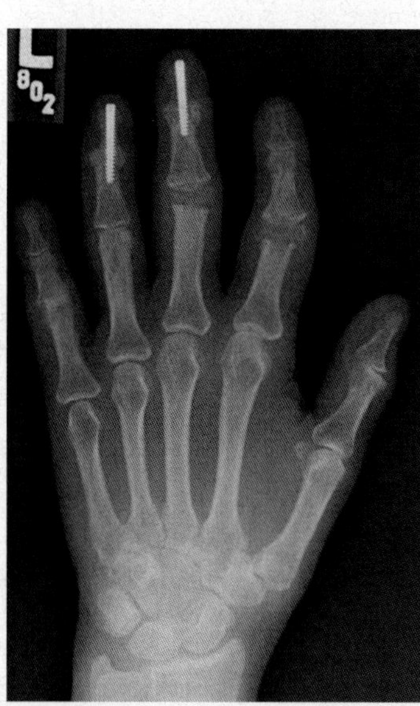

TECH FIG 5 • Postoperative radiograph of patient with diffuse osteoarthritis. Note the silicone implant arthroplasties for the PIP joints of the index and long fingers as well as the fusions of the distal interphalangeal joints of the long and ring fingers. Clinical alignment was excellent.

- Create small drill holes at the radial and ulnar bases of the proximal phalanx before final prosthesis fitting to allow volar plate repair.
- Create dorsal drill holes at the origin of the proper collateral ligaments to be used for repair.
  - The volar plate can be divided longitudinally and used to reconstruct the collateral ligaments if needed.

- Obtain C-arm or standard radiographs to confirm clinical alignment (**TECH FIG 5**).
- The flexor sheath need not be repaired.
- Use 4-0 nylon sutures to close the skin.

Dorsal Approach for Proximal Interphalangeal Joint Arthroplasty

- Make a straight or gently curved longitudinal incision centered over the dorsal PIP joint.
- Raise full-thickness flaps off of the extensor mechanism.
- Split the central slip longitudinally and elevate it radially and ulnarly, taking care not to injure the central slip insertion and create an iatrogenic boutonnière deformity. Other alternatives for improved joint exposure include the following:
  - The longitudinal split of the extensor mechanism may be carried to one or both sides of the central slip insertion for its protection. We prefer the exposure between the lateral and central slips (**TECH FIG 6A**).
  - The Chamay approach may be used. A distally based triangular flap of the extensor mechanism is created; this provides excellent joint exposure and allows adjustment of any preoperative imbalance of the extensor mechanism during later repair (**TECH FIG 6B**).[1]
- Recess the collateral ligaments off their origin on the proximal phalanx head for later repair. Before final implant placement, drill holes adjacent to the collateral ligament origin to allow suture passage for ligament repair (**TECH FIG 6C**).
- The volar plate is protected with the dorsal approach.
- The remaining portion of the procedure is similar to that described as part of the volar approach.

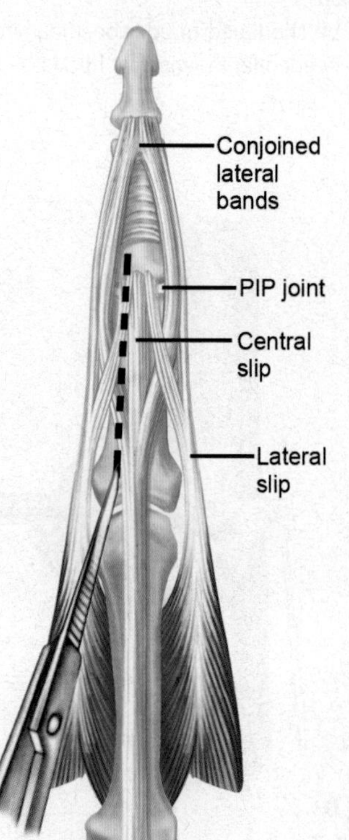

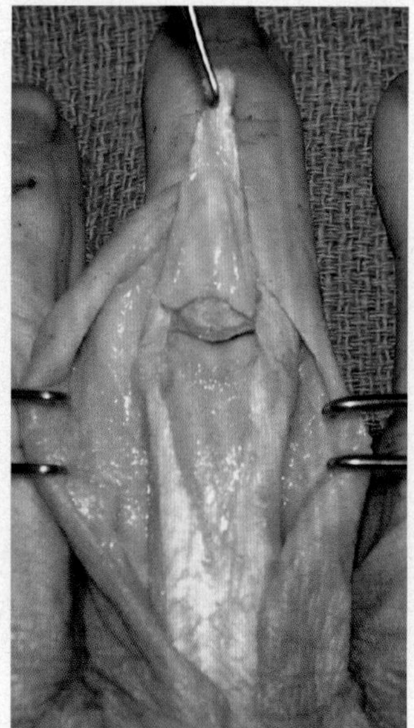

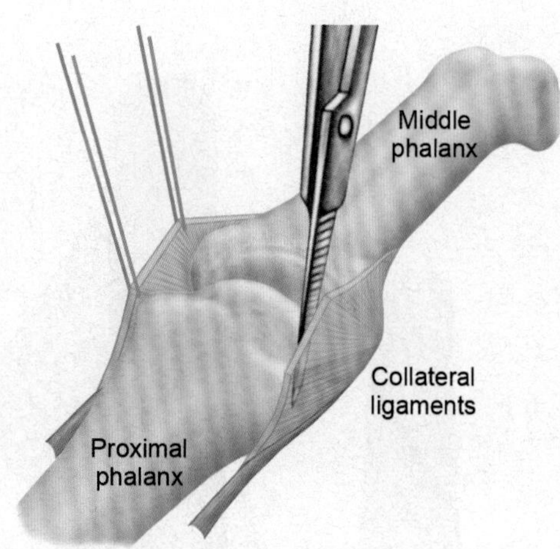

TECH FIG 6 • **A.** Preservation of the central slip is crucial for successful postoperative rehabilitation. **B.** The Chamay approach may be used for PIP joint exposure. **C.** The collateral ligaments may be recessed off the head of the proximal phalanx.

PEARLS AND PITFALLS

Indications	■ Painless loss of motion is not an ideal indication; the operation does not reliably increase motion at long-term assessment. ■ Osteoarthritis and posttraumatic arthritis are more common in the PIP joint than in the MCP joint. ■ MCP arthroplasty has traditionally been performed for RA but has declined in frequency due to better control of disease in RA patients. ■ PIP joint arthroplasty is helpful in maintaining motion in the ring and small fingers (for grip); PIP fusion is more acceptable in the index and long fingers (especially in workers) due to concerns of stability with pinch after arthroplasty. ■ Avoid arthroplasty at both the MCP and PIP joints in one finger.
Technique	■ Broaching is carefully performed to avoid penetration of the cortex or rotation of the implant. ■ Collateral ligament origin and insertion may be compromised with bone preparation; careful repair is performed. ■ The dorsal approach is straightforward but requires careful protection of the central slip insertion. ■ The volar approach minimizes the danger to the central slip and the extensor mechanism. ■ The implant fit is carefully assessed. Buckling of the implant requires bony or soft tissue adjustments to increase space before final implant placement.
Rehabilitation	■ Motion is carefully progressed until joint encapsulation is complete. ■ Rotation or deformity after arthroplasty may be corrected with dynamic splinting.

POSTOPERATIVE CARE

- The patient is placed in a plaster splint after surgery for 3 to 5 days. The MCP and PIP joints are immobilized in extension.
  - Some surgeons advocate 3 to 4 weeks of immobilization after MCP joint implant arthroplasty before the initiation of hand therapy.
- Early joint motion is important for appropriate joint encapsulation.
- An engaged hand therapist is crucial in obtaining a satisfactory surgical outcome.
  - Early therapy emphasizes edema control and patient comfort through splinting.
  - Subsequent therapy focuses on range of motion.
- MCP joint arthroplasty, especially in the rheumatoid patient, requires meticulous postoperative hand therapy.
  - Dynamic extension (daytime) splints, static extension (nighttime) splints, or both are fabricated.
  - The alignment and motion of the fingers are carefully monitored. Adjustments to the splints are commonly required as the encapsulation process and the healing process progress.
  - Active and gentle passive motion are progressively allowed.
- After PIP joint implant arthroplasty through a volar approach, the flexor and extensor mechanism need not be protected. Active and gentle passive motion may be initiated quickly, although the collateral ligament repairs should be protected for at least 6 weeks.
  - Dynamic extension splinting may be used during the first 6 weeks.
- If the central slip was spared during a dorsal PIP joint approach and implant placement, early active motion is initiated with progression to gentle passive motion.
- If the approach for PIP implant arthroplasty required central slip takedown and repair, the extensor mechanism should be carefully protected during the rehabilitation period.

OUTCOMES

- Pain is reliably improved in patients with MCP or PIP joint arthroplasty.[2–7]
- Most patients are improved functionally after silicone MCP arthroplasty. Patients with RA and a marked flexion and ulnar deviation posture of the MCP joints stand to benefit most.[2,3] Although the arc of motion may be improved in the early postoperative period, at long-term follow-up the arc of motion is not dramatically increased; however, the arc is moved to a more extended and a more functional position.[2,3]
- The ulnar drift of the MCP joints most commonly seen in RA is improved (although some recurrence in drift over time may also occur).[2,3]
- MCP arthroplasty for osteoarthritis can be expected to decrease pain and maintain or somewhat improve MCP range of motion and strength. In contrast to RA patients, MCP joint flexion may be increased in patients treated for osteoarthritis.[2,5]
- PIP arthroplasty will place the PIP joint in a more extended and functional posture but should not be expected to increase range of motion at long-term follow-up. Total joint motion depends on the preoperative motion but typically averages about 45 degrees. Pain relief is reliable for most patients no matter the diagnosis.[4,6,7]
- PIP arthroplasty for RA may have a lesser outcome compared for PIP arthroplasty performed for posttraumatic arthritis or osteoarthritis. Patients with a boutonnière or swan-neck deformity are most likely to be unchanged or worse in regard to their deformity.[7]
- PIP silicone implant survivorship decreases from 98% at 2 years to 80% at 10 years to 49% at 16 years (in a mixed population analysis).[7]

COMPLICATIONS

- Infection
- Implant fracture (which may or may not necessitate revision arthroplasty; if the encapsulated joint is stable, a fractured implant may be observed)
- Rotational malalignment
- Joint subluxation

- Silicone synovitis
- In RA patients, recurrent ulnar drift may occur.

REFERENCES

1. Chamay A. A distally based dorsal and triangular tendinous flap for direct access to the proximal interphalangeal joint. Ann Chir Main 1988;7:179–183.
2. Goldfarb CA, Stern PJ. Metacarpophalangeal joint arthroplasty in rheumatoid arthritis: a long- term assessment. J Bone Joint Surg Am 2003;85-A(10):1869–1878.
3. Kirschenbaum D, Schneider LH, Adams DC, et al. Arthroplasty of the metacarpophalangeal joints with use of silicone-rubber implants in patients who have rheumatoid arthritis. Long-term results. J Bone Joint Surg Am 1993;75(1):3–12.
4. Lin HH, Wyrick JD, Stern PJ. Proximal interphalangeal joint silicone replacement arthroplasty: clinical results using an anterior approach. J Hand Surg Am 1995;20(1):123–132.
5. Rettig LA, Luca L, Murphy MS. Silicone implant arthroplasty in patients with idiopathic osteoarthritis of the metacarpophalangeal joint. J Hand Surg Am 2005;30(4):667–672.
6. Schneider LH. Proximal interphalangeal joint arthroplasty: the volar approach. Semin Arthroplasty 1991;2:139–147.
7. Takigawa S, Meletiou S, Sauerbier M, et al. Long-term assessment of Swanson implant arthroplasty in the proximal interphalangeal joint of the hand. J Hand Surg Am 2004;29:785–795.

Proximal Interphalangeal and Metacarpophalangeal Joint Surface Replacement Arthroplasty

122 CHAPTER

Christopher R. Goll and Peter M. Murray

DEFINITION

- Rheumatoid arthritis is a disorder that can affect the hands and can cause systemic symptoms of fatigue, muscle pain, loss of appetite, depression, weight loss, anemia, and immunocompromise. The effect on the hands is a combination of tenosynovitis and inflammation of the metacarpophalangeal (MCP) synovial lining of the joints (synovitis).[14,17]
- Rheumatoid arthritis less frequently involves the proximal interphalangeal (PIP) joints of the hand; more commonly, the PIP joints are affected by degenerative arthritis or psoriatic arthritis. Degenerative arthritis may occur after trauma or infection or may arise as an idiopathic process.[1]

ANATOMY

- Anatomy of the extensor tendon mechanism is shown in **FIG 1**.

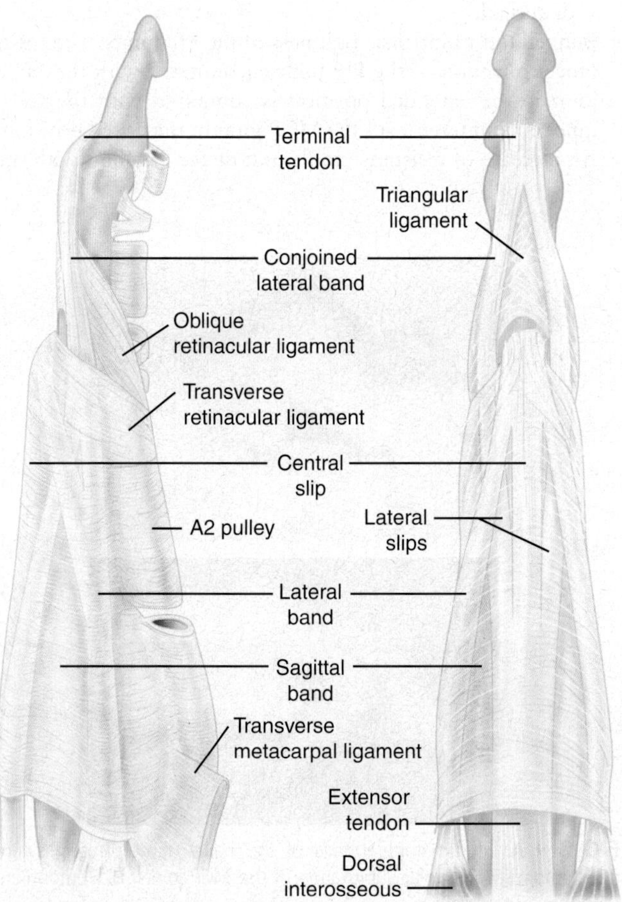

FIG 1 • Anatomy of the extensor mechanism of the finger.

PATHOGENESIS

- Rheumatoid arthritis is a multifactorial entity.
  - The disease is autoimmune mediated and may occur after a bacterial or viral infection.
  - There is a hereditary influence.
  - The B lymphocytes, T lymphocytes, and macrophages lead to proliferation and hypertrophy of synovial cells. The enzymes released by these cells can cause bony erosions, ligamentous laxity, and tendon ruptures.[14]
- MCP joint deformities in rheumatoid patients include concentric joint wear as well as ulnar deviation and volar subluxation or dislocation of the proximal phalanx on the metacarpal head (**FIG 2**).[4,15]
  - These deformities occur after synovial proliferation in the recesses between the collateral ligaments and the metacarpal head, attenuating the collateral ligaments.
  - Radial inclinations of the metacarpals and wrist joint destruction often leads to an ulnar translation of the entire carpus. This translation can cause ulnar and volar extensor tendon subluxation between the metacarpal heads. Ulnar forces generated by the extensor apparatus and volar forces produced by the flexors lead to ulnar drift of the fingers and fixed MCP flexion deformities or volar dislocations of the MCP joints.
- Degenerative arthritis affecting the PIP joints of the hand is a process whereby the articular cartilage develops irreversible wear changes, caused by an incompletely understood mechanism. Subchondral bone stiffens and periarticular new bone formation occurs, which leads to restricted joint motion and pain.[11]
- Less commonly, degenerative arthritis can affect the MCP joints of the hand. This can occur after trauma, infection, and osteonecrosis or may be idiopathic, having a predilection for the index and long MCP joints.[11]

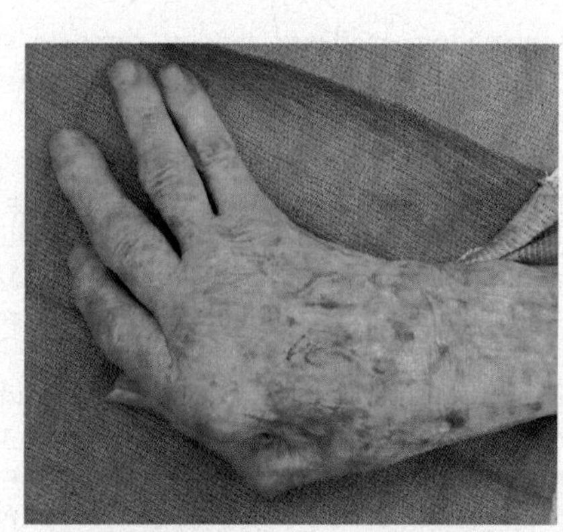

FIG 2 • Ulnar drift of the digits.

NATURAL HISTORY

- Rheumatoid arthritis has a variable prognosis based on the severity of the disease and the structures involved. Mild presentations may go undiagnosed for years, whereas severe presentations may progress to rapid joint destruction in the third or fourth decade of life.
- Three clinical stages of rheumatoid arthritis exist.
  - First, swelling of the synovial lining, which causes pain, warmth, stiffness, redness, and fullness around the joint
  - Second, synoviocyte hypertrophy and proliferation leading to synovial thickening
  - Third, enzymatic release causing bone and cartilage destruction, ligamentous laxity, and tendon ruptures
- Medical management as well as surgical management, including synovectomy, can halt or minimize progression of rheumatoid arthritis.

PATIENT HISTORY AND PHYSICAL FINDINGS

- A thorough patient history and physical examination are important before implant arthroplasty of the fingers.
  - The surgeon should note the patient's occupation, hobbies, and expectations.
  - The history of the patient's condition is helpful in gauging the progression of the disease.
  - The primary indication for surface replacement arthroplasty of the MCP or PIP joints is pain relief. Correction of deformity and improvement in function are secondary considerations. It is important to remember that profound deformity may be painless and functional for some.
- Examination of the entire upper extremity should be performed. Although the order of reconstruction is controversial, deficits of the shoulder, wrist, and elbow should be addressed before addressing hand conditions.
- Particular attention should be paid to elements of radiocarpal instability, including ulnar translation of the carpus as well as distal radioulnar joint instability. In some situations, a wrist arthrodesis or wrist realignment procedure may be necessary before performing MCP arthroplasties.[6]
  - Failure to correct carpal collapse and radial deviation of the metacarpals can result in recurrence of ulnar drift deformity after MCP arthroplasty.
- Careful examination of flexor and extensor tendons of the hand and wrist should be performed. The extensor digiti quinti minimi, extensor pollicis longus, and flexor pollicis longus often rupture in more active forms of rheumatoid arthritis.
  - Extensor tendon or flexor tendon ruptures should be treated before considering implant arthroplasty of the hand.
- Examination of the PIP joint should include range-of-motion assessment of the joint, assessment of volar plate integrity, central slip integrity, and collateral ligament stability.
  - Normal range of motion of the PIP joint is 0 to 110 degrees.
  - Varus and valgus stability should be compared to the contralateral side.
  - Failure of volar plate integrity in rheumatoid arthritis can lead to swan-neck deformity, which is characterized by PIP joint hyperextension, dorsal subluxation of the lateral bands, and flexion of the distal phalangeal joint. The swan-neck deformity is considered a relative contraindication for surface replacement arthroplasty of the PIP joint (**FIG 3A**).
  - A boutonnière deformity is caused by failure of the central slip mechanism. This can occur in rheumatoid arthritis or after trauma (**FIG 3B**). It is characterized by flexion of the PIP joint due to central slip incompetence, volar subluxation of the lateral bands, and hyperextension of the distal interphalangeal (DIP) joint.
- Normal MCP range of motion is between 0 and 90 degrees.
- Instability testing: The individual MCP or PIP joints are tested by the examiner grasping the patient's finger and then applying a valgus and then a varus stress in approximately 30 degrees of flexion. The resultant opening of the joint, or laxity, is compared to the contralateral side. Differences in laxity indicate ligamentous instability. Attempts at hyperextension of the digit at the PIP or the MCP joint can identify volar plate instability and the propensity of the digit to subluxate or dislocate. Surface replacement arthroplasty of either the MCP or the PIP joint is contraindicated in patients with ligamentous instability, as these are semiconstrained devices.
  - Grade 1: no difference in joint line opening compared to the contralateral joint
  - Grade 2: notable opening of the joint line compared to the contralateral joint, but a solid "end point" is reached
  - Grade 3: complete opening of the radial or lateral joint line with valgus or varus stress. This can be demonstrated at either the MCP or the PIP joints. No end point can be discerned.
- Bunnell test of intrinsic tightness of the PIP joints: The resistance to flexion of the PIP joint encountered with the MCP joint in the extended position is compared with the resistance encountered with the MCP joint in the flexed position. An increase of resistance to flexion of the PIP joint with the

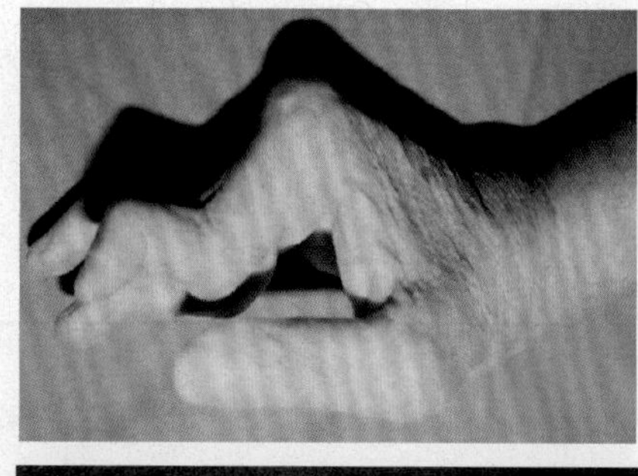

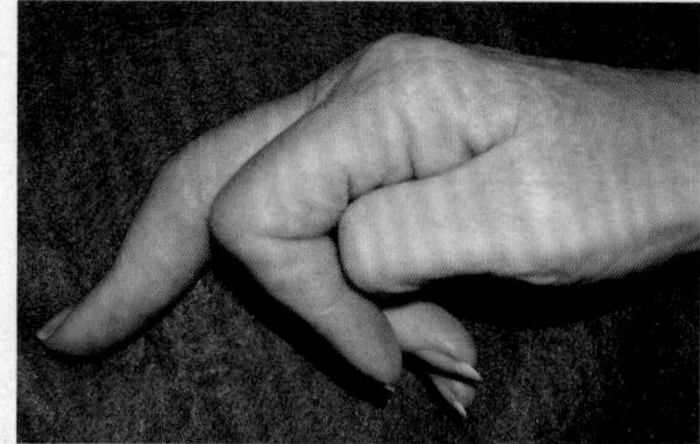

FIG 3 • **A.** Rheumatoid arthritis of the hand demonstrating swan-neck deformity and volar subluxation of the MCP joints. **B.** Boutonnière deformity of the digit.

MCP joint in the extended position indicates intrinsic tightness of that digit.
  - It is important to distinguish intrinsic tightness from extrinsic tightness. Extrinsic tightness is encountered when the long extensors of the digits are adherent to either the surrounding soft tissues or the metacarpals. The result is increased resistance to flexion of the PIP joint with the MCP in flexion. In either instance, the limitation of motion is important to clarify, as it can affect the outcome of implant arthroplasty of the MCP or the PIP joint.

IMAGING AND OTHER DIAGNOSTIC STUDIES

- Posteroanterior, lateral, and oblique views of the hands will adequately image the MCP joints. Brewerton views may add additional information.
- Posteroanterior and lateral views of the digits are preferred to image the PIP joints.

DIFFERENTIAL DIAGNOSIS

- Psoriatic arthritis
- Chronic septic arthritis
- Osteomyelitis
- Gout
- Articular malunions of the MCP and PIP joints
- Scleroderma

NONOPERATIVE MANAGEMENT

- Nonoperative management in rapidly progressing rheumatoid arthritis is largely ineffective.
- In the quiescent forms of rheumatoid arthritis, nighttime wrist and hand splinting in conjunction with medical management may provide pain relief. Various combinations of prednisone, remitting agents (eg, methotrexate, hydroxychloroquine sulfate, sulfasalazine, adalimumab, etanercept, infliximab, minocycline), and nonsteroidal anti-inflammatory agents may prove effective for extended periods in certain cases.
- During periods of active rheumatoid arthritis of the MCP joints, corticosteroid injections into the joint may provide acute pain relief and improve function in the short term.
- The symptoms of MCP and PIP joint degenerative arthritis may come and go, successfully responding to nighttime wrist and hand splinting and nonsteroidal anti-inflammatory agents.
- Corticosteroid injection into the MCP and PIP joints for advanced degenerative arthritis seldom provides long-term benefits.

SURGICAL MANAGEMENT

- The indications for surface replacement or pyrocarbon MCP arthroplasty are similar to those for flexible MCP implants. These include pain in the face of deformity and worsening function.
  - Surface replacement implants are designed to recreate the anatomy of a native joint, potentially resulting in greater stability than with flexible MCP implants.
  - The enhanced stability of these implants is best demonstrated in the index and long fingers, where flexible MCP implants are prone to fracture and failure due to the increased forces born by these joint in pinch.
- Contraindications to surface replacement implant arthroplasty of the MCP joint include infection, lack of adequate bone stock, insufficient radial or ulnar collateral ligament support, lack of adequate soft tissue coverage, and excessively small metacarpal or proximal phalanx medullary canals.
  - These implants rely on intact soft tissue elements. This includes functioning flexors and extensors as well as intact radial and ulnar collateral ligaments.
- Indications for PIP joint surface replacement arthroplasty are pain and diminishing function in the context of advanced radiographic articular degeneration.[1,8]
- Contraindications to PIP joint surface replacement arthroplasty include inadequate bone stock of either the proximal or the middle phalanx, ulnar or radial collateral ligament insufficiency, acute or chronic infection, inadequate soft tissue coverage, insufficient digital flexor function, or disruption of the extensor central slip insertion on the middle phalanx.
  - Relative contraindications include the presence of a static swan-neck or boutonnière deformity.[10]
- The importance of postoperative therapy should be emphasized. To ensure that the implants heal with a stable and a functional range of motion, the patient must wear a combination of static and dynamic splints for several weeks to months after. Patients must also be aware that heavy lifting or gripping must be avoided indefinitely.

Preoperative Planning

- Sizing templates with a 3% parallax enlargement are available for MCP and PIP joint systems and should be used preoperatively to give the surgeon an idea of the size implant required.

Positioning

- The patient is positioned supine, with the arm placed on an arm board for either MCP or PIP joint surface replacement arthroplasty.
- A nonsterile tourniquet is placed proximal to the drapes on the arm and can be accommodated at the forearm or upper level. Some surgeons prefer the use of a simple finger tourniquet.
- The hand is pronated to allow access to the dorsum.

Approach

- For MCP surface replacement arthroplasty, two different incisions can be used.
  - A transverse incision across the dorsum of the hand, centered over the MCP joints, will facilitate access to multiple joints.
  - Alternatively, multiple longitudinal incisions can be used to address all four MCP joints individually.
  - If a single joint is being addressed, a longitudinal incision should be used.
- For PIP joint surface replacement arthroplasty, a midline longitudinal incision is preferred.
  - Alternative approaches include the lateral approach and the volar approach.

Metacarpophalangeal Joint Surface Replacement Arthroplasty

Exposure

- The extensor mechanism is exposed through either a dorsal longitudinal incision or through a transverse incision, depending on surgeon preference.
  - Preserve the dorsal veins.
- Incise the extensor hood just ulnar to the extensor mechanism.
- Retract the extensor hood and extensor mechanism radially.
- In the rheumatoid patient, the extensor tendon ulnarly translates with destruction of the radial sagittal band. If possible, dissect the sagittal bands from the capsule and preserve them so that the extensor tendon can be relocated and the sagittal bands imbricated at the end of the procedure in order to maintain a centralized extensor tendon position.
- Incise the remnants of the MCP joint capsule and use small Hohmann retractors to deliver the head of the metacarpal into the wound.
- After the joint is exposed, perform a synovectomy, carefully preserving the collateral ligaments.
- If the joint is irreducible, it may be necessary to release one or both collateral ligaments from their origins.
  - Tag the ends of the collateral ligaments with 4-0 nonabsorbable suture for later repair to bone at their tuberosity origins.

Joint Preparation and Trial Implant Insertion

- Use a metacarpal sizing template to identify the appropriate amount of metacarpal head to be resected.
- Remove the metacarpal head by first making a vertical saw cut distal to the collateral ligaments. A second cut oriented 45 degrees proximally and volarly removes the remainder of the metacarpal head, retaining the collateral ligament origins.
- Remove the articular surface along with a small portion of the base of the proximal phalanx, preserving the collateral ligaments (**TECH FIG 1A**).
  - Contracture of the ulnar capsule may require detaching the ulnar collateral ligament to achieve alignment of the finger in some circumstances.
- Insert an awl into the dorsal aspect of the intramedullary canal of the metacarpal (**TECH FIG 1B**).
- Perform sequential broaching for the metacarpal until a proper fit has been attained.
  - For the index and long fingers, the broaching is slightly ulnarly displaced. This provides a better moment arm for the radial intrinsic and extrinsic tendons to compensate for ulnar drift.
- Repeat the broaching in a similar fashion for the proximal phalanx.
- A plastic impactor with a concave surface aids insertion of the metacarpal proximal trial component.
  - Avoid forceful impaction in order to avoid fracture.
- A convex impactor aids insertion and seating of the distal component.
- Once the trial components are inserted and the joint is reduced, check component fit and position using an image intensifier. Then assess range of motion, component tracking, and stability.
  - Revisions of bone cuts may be necessary for soft tissue balancing and to ensure adequate range of motion.
- If release of the collateral ligaments was required, drill two holes through the tuberosity at the dorsoradial and dorsoulnar aspect of the remaining metacarpal head for reattachment of the ligaments. Insert sutures for repair of the collateral ligament (4-0 nonabsorbable suture preferred).

Final Implant Insertion

- Irrigate the intramedullary canal with saline and 0.5% neomycin solution, then dry it.
- Inject polymethylmethacrylate (PMMA) in a liquid state into the metacarpal and the proximal phalanx using a size no. 14 plastic Angiocath catheter attached to a 10-mL syringe.
  - Under some circumstances, "finger packing" may be necessary.

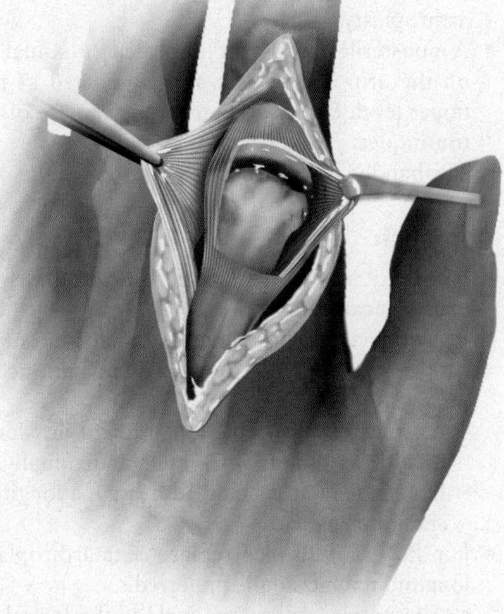

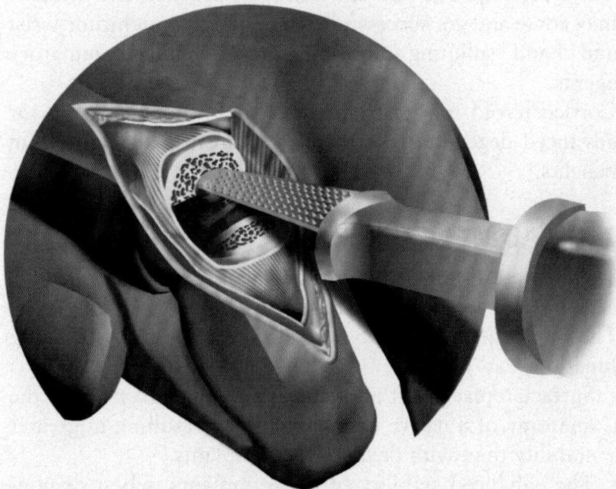

A B

TECH FIG 1 • **A.** Exposure of the MCP joint demonstrating the bone cuts for preparation of MCP surface replacement arthroplasty. **B.** Broaching of the metacarpal preparing for MCP surface replacement arthroplasty. (Courtesy of Small Bone Innovations, Morrisville, PA.)

- Insert the distal component first. Convex and concave plastic impactors are provided to assist in implant insertion (**TECH FIG 2**).
  - Avoid impacting with metallic instruments, which can accelerate prosthetic wear.
- The joint is extended and viewed under the image intensifier before allowing the cement to harden so that last-minute corrections in alignment can be made.
- Cement fixation of one finger at a time is advisable if positioning is difficult.
  - If multiple MCP joints are to be implanted, it may be easier to do the distal components as a group, followed by the proximal components.
- After the cement has cured, check passive range of motion to ensure adequate range without impingement or prosthetic binding.
- For MCP joint arthroplasty using pyrocarbon implants, a press-fit technique is typically used instead of cement.

Closure and Soft Tissue Balancing

- After hardening of the cement, the collateral ligaments are tightened or reattached, depending on the circumstances, with nonabsorbable suture.
  - Ensure proper radial and ulnar stability as well as rotational alignment before securing the sutures.
- Close any remaining capsule with absorbable suture before extensor apparatus closure.
- Centralize the extensor tendon and imbricate the radial sagittal bands in rheumatoid hands using nonabsorbable suture.
  - A pants-over-vest centralization of the sagittal bands may be required in moderate to severe ulnar drift along with intrinsic releases or crossed-intrinsic transfers (**TECH FIG 3**).
  - With the finger held in slight overcorrection, imbricate the radial sagittal band over the extensor tendon.
- The skin is closed in a routine manner and a splint is applied with the MCP joints in slight flexion.

Postoperative Care

- Postoperatively, the MCP joints should be placed in slight flexion and the PIP joints in about 45 degrees of flexion. If there was ulnar deviation before surgery, the fingers should be placed in 10 degrees of radial deviation.
- The dressing is removed 2 to 4 days after surgery and a dynamic splint is applied for daytime exercises. A static rest or nocturnal splint capable of holding the fingers in the corrected position is used for 4 to 6 weeks.

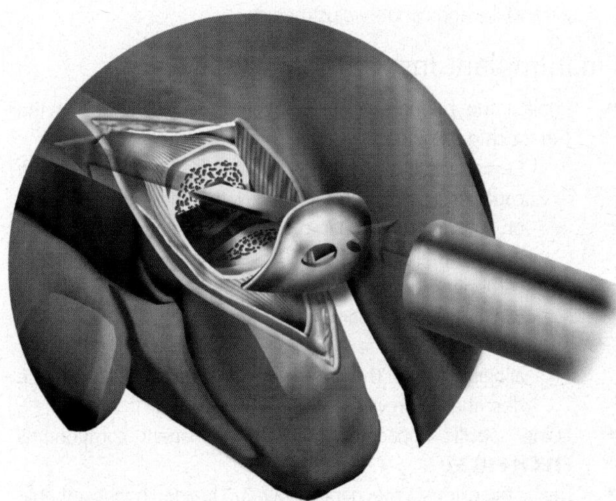

TECH FIG 2 • Insertion of the metacarpal component of the MCP surface replacement arthroplasty. (Courtesy of Small Bone Innovations, Morrisville, PA.)

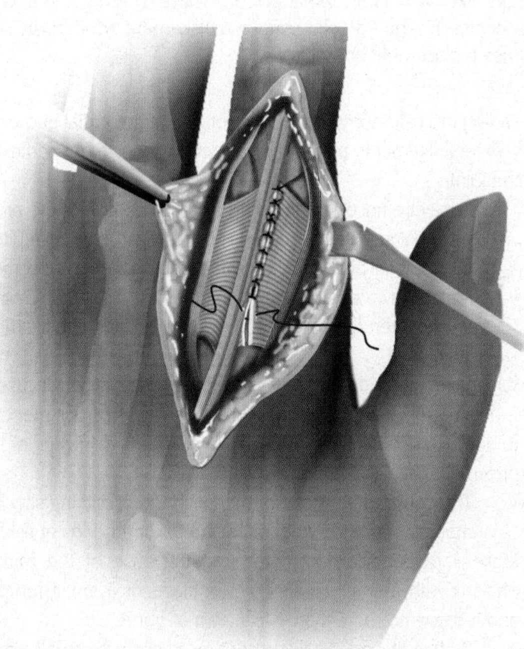

TECH FIG 3 • Radially directed "pants-over-vest" reefing of the extensor mechanism after MCP surface replacement arthroplasty. (Courtesy of Small Bone Innovations, Morrisville, PA.)

Proximal Interphalangeal Joint Surface Replacement Arthroplasty

Exposure

- Through a midline longitudinal incision, reflect the extensor tendon distally by creating a distally based flap, as described by Chamay[2] (**TECH FIG 4A**).
- Identify and incise remnants of the dorsal PIP joint capsule.
- Protect the radial and ulnar collateral ligaments using small Hohmann retractors while bringing the articular surface of the middle phalanx into view.

Joint Preparation and Trial Implant Insertion

- Resect the proximal phalanx head by an osteotomy performed 90 degrees to the long axis of the proximal phalanx, just proximal to the most proximal extent of the articular surface (see **TECH FIG 4A**).

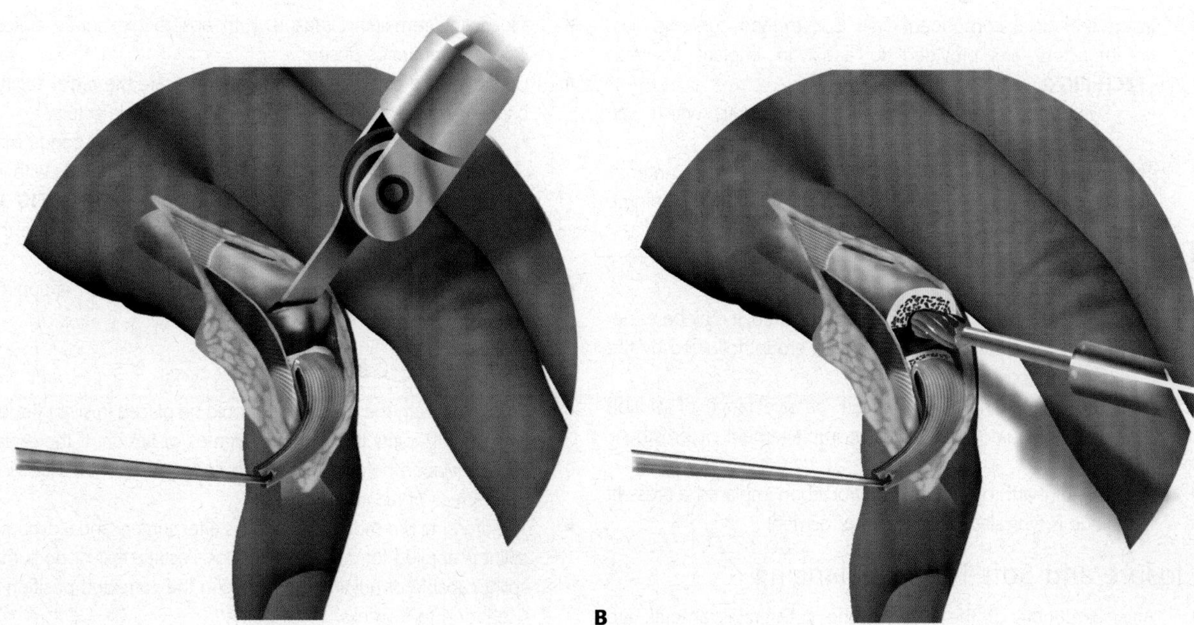

TECH FIG 4 • A. Proximal phalanx exposed using the Chamay approach. An oscillating saw is used to accomplish an osteotomy in preparation for the PIP joint surface replacement arthroplasty placement. **B.** Broaching of the proximal phalanx in preparation for PIP joint surface replacement arthroplasty.

- During the osteotomy, protect the origins of the radial and ulnar collateral ligaments by using small retractors or by hyperflexing the joint.
  - It may be necessary to release a small portion of the proximal phalangeal origin of the collateral ligaments to facilitate the proximal phalangeal osteotomy and prosthesis insertion.
  - Minamikawa et al[10] have shown that the PIP joint remains stable after removal of 50% of the collateral ligament substance.
- While protecting the volar plate with a small retractor, use a 2-mm burr to assist in making a small back cut (or chamfer cut) to accept the posterior aspect of the prosthetic condyles of the proximal phalangeal component.
  - This can also be accomplished with the oscillating saw but that can place the volar plate and flexor tendons at risk.
- Make a perpendicular osteotomy at the base of the middle phalanx with a small oscillating saw blade or a small rongeur and remove no more than 1 to 2 mm of bone.
  - Protect the collateral ligament insertions with small retractors or by hyperflexing the digit.
- Broach the proximal and middle phalanges with specific and sequential instruments.
  - Broach the proximal and middle phalanges to the largest size possible (**TECH FIG 4B**).
  - Undersized components can result in limited motion due to bony impingement during flexion.
- Insert the trial components using proximal and middle phalanx-specific impactors.
  - The components are not modular and are generally not interchanged. Under certain circumstances, such as revision surgery, it is permissible to implant unmatched sizes, but no more than one size up or one size down should be used and this is considered an off-label use of the prosthesis.
- After trial component insertion, examine the digit for implant position, range of motion, and stability as detailed for the MCP joint. Make appropriate adjustments.

Final Implant Insertion and Closure

- Implant the permanent components by "press-fit" using the "no-touch" technique.
  - Cementing is discouraged except perhaps in cases with capacious canals or in patients with substantial bone loss or substantial articular erosion. In these circumstances, the prosthetic stems and flanges are simply coated with cement. Excessive cement packing into the medullary canal is not necessary.
  - Another technique is to pack the canal with morselized allograft bone. This is analogous to the Ling technique described for revision total hip arthroplasty.[5]
- Using specific impactors, seat the permanent components (**TECH FIG 5**).
- Repair the extensor mechanism with 3-0 braided nonabsorbable suture.
- Release the tourniquet before skin closure.
- The patient leaves the operating room with a sterile dressing, splinted in extension.

Postoperative Care

- Initiation of formal postoperative rehabilitation is encouraged by postoperative day 5. A dynamic extension splint permitting active flexion is applied at this time and used for about 6 weeks. A static forearm-based digital extension splint is used at bedtime.
  - During the first 2 weeks after surgery, PIP flexion is limited to 30 degrees.
  - Flexion to 60 degrees is allowed beginning at 4 weeks.
  - By 6 weeks, the extension outrigger splint is discontinued and unrestricted flexion and extension is permitted.

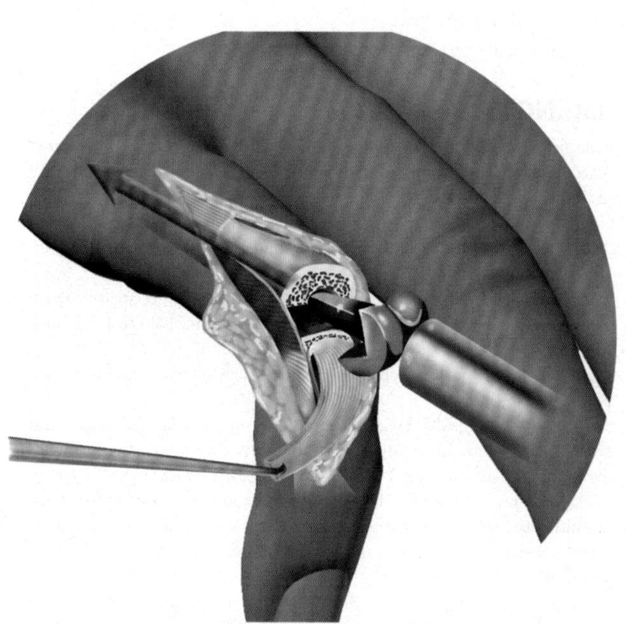

- The static bedtime splint is used for an additional 6 weeks. Heavy lifting or gripping is not permitted.
- The rehabilitation program is enhanced by the close supervision of a hand therapist. The first week of therapy is best carried out with daily supervision.
- Follow-up examinations should include range-of-motion assessment for all the joints of the hand and wrist. Static deformities, grip strength, and pinch strength should also be assessed and recorded.
- Follow-up radiographic examination includes posteroanterior, lateral, and oblique views of the hand. Any residual deformity should also be assessed and recorded.
- For the PIP joint surface replacement arthroplasty, a controlled rehabilitation protocol is needed to prevent central slip failure.

TECH FIG 5 • Insertion of the proximal phalangeal component of the PIP surface replacement arthroplasty. (Courtesy of Small Bone Innovations, Morrisville, PA.)

PEARLS AND PITFALLS

PIP joint surface replacement arthroplasty	■ Take care to preserve the insertion of the central slip. ■ Osteotomy of the proximal phalanx must avoid the origin of the PIP joint collateral ligaments. ■ Remove only a small amount of bone from the middle phalanx. ■ Broach the proximal phalanx to the largest size that can be accommodated. Failure to use appropriate-sized implants may result in subsidence of the implants and posterior cortical impingement of the phalanges.
MCP joint surface replacement arthroplasty	■ Contracture of the ulnar capsule may require detaching the ulnar collateral ligament. ■ Broaching of the index finger should be slightly ulnarly displaced. ■ Centralization of the extensor tendon is generally necessary in rheumatoid hands; it can be achieved by imbricating the radial sagittal bands. ■ Imbrication of the radial sagittal bands should be performed with the digit in radial deviation. ■ "Watertight" closure of the extensor mechanism is necessary to prevent PIP joint flexion lag or contracture.

OUTCOMES

- Initial results after 76 PIP joint surface replacement arthroplasties were published.[9]
  - At a mean follow-up of 4.5 years, 32 joints had good results, 19 fair, and 25 poor.
  - Better results were obtained with arthroplasties performed through a dorsal approach rather than the volar approach.
  - Range of motion at follow-up averaged −14 degrees of extension and 61 degrees of flexion. There was a 12-degree improvement in the flexion–extension arc compared to the preoperative examination.
- A longer term outcome review of 67 metal polyethylene PIP arthroplasties has recently been published from the same institution.[12]
  - With a mean follow up of 8.8 years, the study concluded that this technique yielded joints with minimal pain and ranges of motion similar to preoperative levels.
  - There were 22 complications in 14 patients, resulting in four interphalangeal fusions and two amputations.
- A review of 43 PIP surface replacement arthroplasties in 25 patients was published.[7]
  - Follow-up time averaged 37 months (range, 12 to 72 months).
  - It was notable that 10 of the 11 failed arthroplasties requiring revision were due to loosening associated with lack of cement use.
- A retrospective review of 31 pyrocarbon arthroplasties of the PIP joint performed by a single surgeon in 17 patients with interphalangeal joint osteoarthritis has also been published.[16]
  - At mean follow-up of 55 months, the postoperative range of motion decreased from 57 degrees to 31 degrees.
  - "Complications included implant fracture (one joint), dislocation (five joints), squeaking (eleven), loosening (fifteen), and interphalangeal joint contracture (twenty).

Six joints required a reoperation (an arthrodesis in four joints, a silicone arthroplasty in one, and excision of exostosis in one). Implant migration was severe for seven proximal phalanx implants and three distal phalanx implants, and one implant breached the phalangeal cortex."

- The MCP joint surface replacement arthroplasty (Small Bone Innovations, Morrisville, PA) has been available in Europe for 8 years and is under clinical trial in the United States. No series has been published reporting results of this implant. Although from a theoretical perspective there are advantages to the use of the MCP joint surface replacement arthroplasty, it currently cannot be considered a replacement for the Swanson silastic MCP joint spacer.
- Previous primate studies have shown no evidence of debris or inflammatory reaction after implantation of the pyrolytic carbon MCP joint arthroplasty. Good bone incorporation of the prosthesis was also observed.
- In a 1999 study, a series of 151 pyrolytic carbon MCP prostheses (Ascension Orthopedics, Austin, TX) implanted over an 8-year period, mostly in patients with rheumatoid arthritis, were followed up at an average of 11.7 years.[3]
  - The arc of MCP joint motion improved an average of 13 degrees.
  - The 10-year survivorship was 81.4%.
  - At follow-up, the degree of digital ulnar drift was the same as preoperative.
  - Complications led to 18 implant revisions (12%).

COMPLICATIONS

- PIP
  - Failure of the central slip can occur, resulting in extensor lag or, more commonly, a flexion contracture or boutonnière deformity. An analysis of reoperations following PIP joint arthroplasty found that 76 of 294 PIP joints required reoperation. Extensor mechanisms dysfunction was the most common reason for reoperation which occurred in 51 of the 76 cases.[13]
  - With the volar approach, failure of the volar plate may occur, leading to swan-neck deformity.
  - Tenodesis as well as joint instability and joint subluxation can occur.
  - Postoperative infection or prosthesis loosening is seldom seen.[9]
- MCP
  - Stiffness
  - Loosening
  - Subluxation
  - Proliferative synovitis
  - Squeaking in pyrocarbon implants

REFERENCES

1. Amadio PC, Murray PM, Linscheid RL. PIP arthroplasty. In: Morrey BF, ed. Joint Replacement Arthroplasty, ed 3. New York: Churchill Livingstone, 2003:163–174.
2. Chamay A. A distally based dorsal and triangular tendinous flap for direct access to the proximal interphalangeal joint. Ann Chir Main 1988;7:179–183.
3. Cook SD, Beckenbaugh RD, Redondo J, et al. Long-term follow-up of pyrolytic carbon metacarpophalangeal implants. J Bone Joint Surg Am 1999;81(5):635–648.
4. Flatt AE. Some pathomechanics of ulnar drift. Plast Reconstr Surg 1966;37:295–303.
5. Halliday BR, English HW, Timperley AJ, et al. Femoral impaction grafting with cement in revision total hip replacement. Evolution of the technique and results. J Bone Joint Surg Br 2003;85(6):809–817.
6. Ito J, Koshino T, Okamoto R, et al. Radiologic evaluation of the rheumatoid hand after synovectomy and extensor carpi radialis longus transfer to extensor carpi ulnaris. J Hand Surg Am 2003;28(4): 585–590.
7. Jennings CD, Livingstone DP. Surface replacement arthroplasty of the proximal interphalangeal joint using the PIP-SRA implant: results, complications, and revisions. J Hand Surg Am 2008;33(9):1565. e1–e11.
8. Linscheid RL. Implant arthroplasty of the hand: retrospective and prospective considerations. J Hand Surg Am 2000;25(5):796–816.
9. Linscheid RL, Murray PM, Vidal MA, et al. Development of a surface replacement arthroplasty for proximal interphalangeal joints. J Hand Surg Am 1997;22(2):286–298.
10. Minamikawa Y, Horii E, Amadio PC, et al. Stability and constraint of the proximal interphalangeal joint. J Hand Surg Am 1993;18: 198–204.
11. Murray PM. New-generation implant arthroplasties of the finger joints. J Am Acad Orthop Surg 2003;11:295–301.
12. Murray PM, Linscheid RL, Cooney WP III, et al. Long-term outcomes of proximal interphalangeal joint surface replacement arthroplasty. J Bone Joint Surg Am 2012;94(12):1120–1128.
13. Pritsch T, Rizzo M. Reoperations following proximal interphalangeal joint nonconstrained arthroplasties. J Hand Surg Am 2011;36(9): 1460–1466.
14. Smith RJ, Kaplan EB. Rheumatoid deformities at the metacarpophalangeal joints of the fingers: a correlative study of anatomy and pathology. J Bone Joint Surg Am 1967;49A:31–47.
15. Stack HG, Vaughan-Jackson OJ. The zigzag deformity in the rheumatoid hand. Hand 1971;3:62–67.
16. Sweets TM, Stern PJ. Pyrolytic carbon resurfacing arthroplasty for osteoarthritis of the proximal interphalangeal joint of the finger. J Bone Joint Surg Am 2011;93(15):1417–1425.
17. Wilson RL, Carlblom ER. The rheumatoid metacarpophalangeal joint. Hand Clin 1989;5:223–237.

Distal Interphalangeal, Proximal Interphalangeal, and Metacarpophalangeal Joint Arthrodesis

123 CHAPTER

Charles Cassidy and Jennifer Green

DEFINITION

- Conditions resulting in the need for arthrodesis in the hand include arthritis, unreconstructable soft tissue problems, and certain neurologic conditions.

ANATOMY

- The proximal interphalangeal (PIP) joint and distal interphalangeal (DIP) joint configurations are quite similar.
  - The condylar heads are biconvex but slightly asymmetric, being about twice as wide volarly as dorsally.
  - The reciprocal bases of the distal segment are biconcave, having a central ridge.
- The volar plate extends from the neck of the phalanx to the volar base of the more distal phalanx, preventing joint hyperextension.
- Radial and ulnar collateral ligaments provide additional joint stability. The "true" collateral ligaments have bony attachments at both ends, whereas the accessory collateral ligaments extend from the condylar head to the volar plate.
- The axis of rotation and radius of curvature for a given interphalangeal joint are fairly constant. Consequently, the true collateral ligaments are effectively isometric, whereas the accessory collateral ligaments resist lateral translation when the joint is extended.
- As a result of the ligamentous and bony architecture, the PIP and DIP joints normally function as highly constrained hinge joints.
- The extensor tendon crosses the DIP joint dorsally as the terminal tendon, inserting slightly distal to the dorsal base of the distal phalanx.
  - The germinal matrix of the nail bed is close to the terminal tendon insertion (average of 1.3 mm distal).
- The flexor digitorum profundus (FDP) tendon inserts broadly on the volar aspect of the distal phalanx, extending from the base to the midshaft.
- Over the PIP joint, the extensor apparatus splits into thirds. Contributions from the extensor tendon, the interosseous tendons, and lumbricals form the central slip, which inserts onto the dorsal base of the middle phalanx. The lateral bands travel past the PIP joint along the lateral margins and then combine to form the terminal tendon distally.
- The flexor digitorum superficialis (FDS) tendon splits to insert on the volar lateral margins of the proximal shaft of the middle phalanx.
- Unlike the interphalangeal joints, the metacarpophalangeal (MCP) joints are multiaxial, permitting motion in multiple planes.
- The metacarpal head has a complex, convex shape. Viewed end-on, the metacarpal head is pear-shaped, being wider volarly. In the sagittal plane, the radius of curvature increases progressively from dorsal to volar.
- The metacarpal attachment of the collateral ligaments is dorsal to the axis of rotation. The phalangeal and volar plate attachments are similar to the interphalangeal joint.
- As a consequence of the metacarpal head shape and ligament attachments, the MCP joints are typically more lax in extension and tight in flexion.
- Significant variability exists in the shape of the thumb metacarpal head. Some heads are more square than round, potentially limiting lateral translation and MCP flexion.
- In the thumb, the extensor pollicis brevis (EPB) tendon inserts onto the dorsal base of the proximal phalanx. The size of the EPB tendon is variable.
  - For some patients, the extensor pollicis longus (EPL) tendon assumes the major role in MCP joint extension.
  - In the other digits, no direct extensor attachment exists. MCP joint extension occurs through a sling effect of the sagittal hood fibers lifting the proximal phalanx through the pull of the extensor tendon.
- MCP joint flexion is produced through a combination of direct intrinsic tendon attachments to the volar lateral phalangeal base and indirect actions of the intrinsics on the more distal transverse fibers of the extensor hood.

PATHOGENESIS

- Arthritis is the principal indication for small joint arthrodesis.
- Osteoarthritis (OA) most commonly affects the DIP joints. It is estimated that at least 60% of individuals older than age 60 years have DIP joint arthritis, which may not necessarily be symptomatic.
- In the early stages, the joints may be painful and swollen in spite of normal radiographs. As the arthritis progresses, osteophytes and mucous cysts may develop. Bony prominences (Heberden nodes) and angular deformities in both the coronal and sagittal planes (mallet appearance) may develop. In the final stages, DIP joint motion may be severely restricted.
- OA may also involve the PIP joints and the MCP joints, especially in the index and middle fingers.

- Inflammatory arthritis may also affect the small joints of the hand. About 70% of rheumatoid patients have hand involvement. Synovitis may result in deformity due to attenuation of supporting structures (collateral ligaments, extensor tendons) long before arthritic changes are evident.
    - At the DIP joint, terminal tendon incompetence may result in a secondary swan-neck deformity.
    - At the PIP joint, central slip attenuation results in a boutonnière deformity.
    - At the MCP joint, collateral ligament involvement may contribute to ulnar drift. Persistent synovitis produces cartilage loss.
- Hand involvement in systemic lupus erythematosus (SLE) may mimic rheumatoid arthritis. Supporting structures are affected principally in SLE, which may result in joint subluxation or dislocation with relatively normal-appearing articular cartilage. The capsuloligamentous problems may compromise attempts at joint salvage.
- In contrast, psoriatic arthritis may produce a remarkable degree of bone loss as the arthritis progresses. Pencil-in-cup deformity is a characteristic feature of psoriatic arthritis of the interphalangeal joints. Severe bone resorption is the characteristic feature of arthritis mutilans, most commonly seen in patients with psoriatic arthritis. Arthrodesis is the most reliable method for halting this destructive process.
- Scleroderma typically produces PIP flexion and MCP extension contractures. Impaired vascularity of the digits may result in dorsal PIP ulcer formation and central slip attenuation, compounding the PIP flexion deformity.
- Presentations of crystalline arthropathy in the small joints of the hand may be varied. The process may be indolent, presenting as gouty tophi over the DIP joint, or acute, presenting as an exquisitely painful, swollen, tender joint. Untreated, gout results in a resorptive arthritis.
- Infection is another cause of small joint arthritis.
    - A "fight bite" directly inoculates the MCP joint and, if undertreated, can result in rapid joint destruction.
    - Contiguous spread, for example, from a felon or a wound over the DIP or PIP joint may destroy the adjacent joint.
    - Hematogenous spread is an uncommon cause of septic arthritis in the hand.
- Trauma is another cause of unreconstructable problems in the small joints of the hand.
    - Intra-articular fractures and fracture-dislocations may result in arthritis, particularly in cases of residual joint incongruity. The PIP joint does not tolerate injury well.
    - Severe periarticular soft tissue injuries may cause severe joint stiffness, even if the underlying joint surface is not initially involved. Certain soft tissue injuries, such as central slip disruptions, may confound attempts at reconstruction.
- Central or peripheral nerve injury may produce imbalances in the hand. Arthrodesis can potentially simplify reconstructions in an effort to improve function.

PATIENT HISTORY AND PHYSICAL FINDINGS

- Pain is the most common complaint of patients who are candidates for arthrodesis. Ideally, the location of the pain should correlate with the joint in question.
- In OA, multiple DIP joints may appear abnormal, although they may not necessarily be painful.
- Polyarticular involvement is common in rheumatoid arthritis. A priority list should be elicited from the patient.
- Handedness, occupation, and avocational activities should be documented.
- The functional impact of the problem should be clearly defined.
- When a single joint is involved, a history of trauma should be sought.
- In cases of acute, painful swelling, a history of penetrating injury, gout, or recent infection should be considered.
- The physical examination should include the appearance of joints and overlying skin, active and passive range of motion of the affected joints, stability, grip and pinch strength, and sensibility.
- The status of adjacent joints should be evaluated.
    - For example, chronic DIP OA resulting in a DIP flexion deformity may produce a secondary hyperextension deformity of the PIP (swan neck) that may be more disabling than the primary (DIP) problem.
- Multiple DIP joint bumps (Heberden nodes) are a characteristic feature of OA.
- Mucous cysts are suggestive of underlying DIP OA.
- Onycholysis and eczema are suggestive of psoriatic arthritis.
- Discrepancies between active and passive motion are indicative of an associated tendon problem.
- Stress examination may demonstrate collateral ligament incompetence.

IMAGING AND OTHER DIAGNOSTIC STUDIES

- Plain radiographs (posteroanterior [PA], lateral, oblique) of the affected digit are usually sufficient to make the diagnosis.
- In cases of suspected inflammatory arthritis, a collagen vascular screen is ordered. This blood panel includes a rheumatoid factor, antinuclear antibody (ANA), complete blood count with differential, erythrocyte sedimentation rate (ESR), and C-reactive protein (CRP).
- A uric acid level may be drawn in cases of suspected gout.
- Blood tests are not generally helpful in the setting of an acute finger infection.
- Magnetic resonance imaging (MRI) or ultrasound may rarely be ordered to evaluate tendon pathology if stiffness is associated with tendon abnormality.

DIFFERENTIAL DIAGNOSIS

- OA
- Inflammatory arthritis (rheumatoid, SLE, psoriatic arthritis)
- Crystal arthritis
- Posttraumatic arthritis
- Infection

NONOPERATIVE MANAGEMENT

- The mainstays of nonoperative treatment for unreconstructable small joint problems in the hand include oral medications, splints, and intra-articular corticosteroid injections.
- For OA and posttraumatic arthritis, oral anti-inflammatory agents may reduce pain and stiffness.
    - Glucosamine and chondroitin sulfate appear to be of limited value for hand arthritis.
- Rheumatoid patients can consider modifications in their medication regimen, supervised by a rheumatologist.

- Resting splints may reduce pain and inflammation.
  - At the DIP and PIP joints, a simple padded aluminum splint may suffice.
  - Corrective splints, such as the safety pin static progressive or LMB dynamic splint (DeRoyal), will not be tolerated when the joint is inflamed.
  - For the thumb MCP joint, a hand-based thermoplast splint may lessen discomfort and improve function.
  - Buddy taping to the adjacent digit may be appropriate for some MCP joint problems. Dynamic MCP joint splints are usually reserved for postoperative protection.
- Corticosteroid injections may provide temporary relief of pain and synovitis. The joint may be difficult to access and the joint capacity is quite small.
  - The surgeon should use a 27-gauge needle and inject 0.5 mL of Celestone Soluspan and 0.5 mL of 1% Xylocaine through a dorsal approach.

SURGICAL MANAGEMENT

Arthrodesis versus Arthroplasty

- Arthrodesis is a reliable procedure for managing arthritis and instability of the DIP joint. The functional impairment from loss of motion at the DIP joint is minimal.
- At the PIP joint level, the surgeon and patient must weigh the potential benefits of stability and pain relief against the functional impairment resulting from the loss of PIP joint motion. For the index finger, PIP joint stability is critical for pinch. On the other hand, in the small finger, PIP joint mobility is necessary for grip.
  - As a general rule, for isolated unreconstructable PIP problems, the index finger gets arthrodesis, the middle finger gets arthrodesis or arthroplasty, and the ring and small fingers get arthroplasty.
  - Exceptions to the rule include associated unsalvageable tendon problems and soft tissue coverage issues, in which arthrodesis may be preferred.
- The status of the adjacent joints is an important factor in deciding whether to perform arthrodesis or arthroplasty. In the rheumatoid patient with both MCP and PIP involvement, the temptation is to perform arthroplasties of all involved joints. So-called double-row arthroplasties tend to compromise the results at both the MCP and PIP joints. In such instances, the goal is stability at the PIP joint (arthrodesis) and motion at the MCP joint (arthroplasty).
- Arthrodesis of the thumb MCP joint is a reliable procedure for managing arthritis and unreconstructable ligament problems. Arthrodesis is a far superior procedure to arthroplasty for the thumb. However, before undertaking this, it is important to ensure adequate motion and function of the adjacent joints (interphalangeal, carpometacarpal).
  - The chronic radial collateral ligament tear with static volar ulnar subluxation is a good indication for thumb MCP fusion.
- Arthrodesis of the digital MCP joints is not commonly performed. Indications include multiple failed arthroplasty or inadequate bone stock for arthroplasty, unrelenting infection, refractory instability of the index MCP, and an unreconstructable extensor mechanism.
- Candidates for arthrodesis must understand that all motion in the affected joint will be eliminated and that the principal goals are pain relief and stability.[20]

Arthrodesis Position

- The fusion position varies with the digit and joint involved. Invariably, the decision is a compromise between appearance and function. The ideal posture should replicate the normal digital cascade (**FIG 1**).
- In general, the DIP joints and thumb interphalangeal joint should be fused in 0 to 10 degrees of flexion.[15]
- For the PIP joint, some authors recommend a uniform 40-degree flexion position for all digits,[6] whereas others recommend 40 degrees for the index finger, progressing ulnarward in 5-degree increments to 55 degrees in the small finger.[18]
  - Many prefer a slightly more extended position for the index PIP that will still allow functional tip-to-tip pinch.
- The recommended fusion angle of the MCP joints is a cascade from 25 degrees of flexion in the index digit, progressing ulnarward in 5-degree increments to 40 degrees in the small finger.[15]
- The recommended fusion angle of the MCP joint of the thumb is 10 to 15 degrees of flexion and just resting at the radial border of the index finger mid-distal phalanx.[15]

Fixation Options

- The choice of surgical technique depends on a number of factors, including the affected joint to be fused, the availability and cost of implants, the adequacy of bone stock, and the comfort of the surgeon. The goal is to achieve a solid fusion of the affected joint in a timely manner. Bone preparation is essential.
  - The specific method of fixation may be less important in obtaining union than specific patient factors such as bone quality. Certain constructs, such as the tension band, are more rigid but may be associated with more hardware-related problems.
  - The biomechanical issues must be weighed against potential soft tissue problems when deciding on a form of fixation. Maintenance of motion in the adjacent joints is critical.
- Kirschner wire fixation has been associated with fusion rates of up to 99%.
  - Advantages
    - Simplicity of the technique
    - Ready availability of low-cost implants

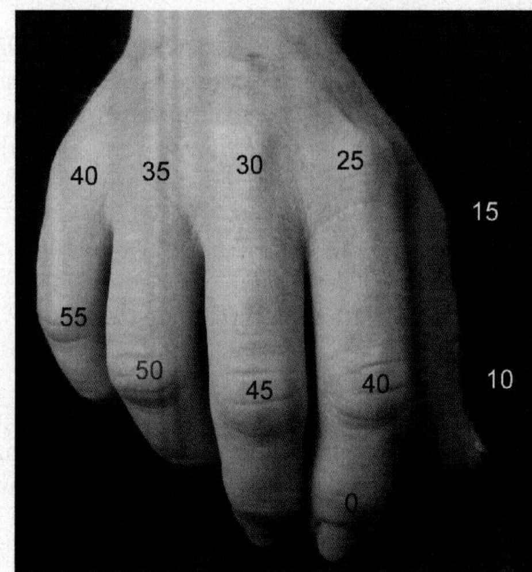

FIG 1 • Recommended positions for digital joint fusion.

- Disadvantages
  - Infection risk, including superficial pin site and deep wound infections, osteomyelitis; pin migration; minimal compression across the fusion site
  - Less rigid fixation,[10] requiring additional external immobilization to enhance stability, possibly leading to stiffness of surrounding joints[9,16]
- Interosseous wiring has been found to be biomechanically stronger than Kirschner wire fixation.[19] It is especially useful for PIP fusion and thumb interphalangeal fusion.
  - Advantages
    - Biomechanically stronger than Kirschner wire fixation[19]
    - Readily available low-cost implants
  - Disadvantages
    - Large amount of soft tissue stripping for appropriate placement of drill holes
    - Higher rate of nonunion, up to 9%[12]
- Tension band fixation is a biomechanically stable method of fixation[17] combining parallel Kirschner wires for rotational control and interosseous wiring for compression. This technique is especially useful for MCP, PIP, and thumb interphalangeal arthrodesis.
  - The tension band construct converts the strong distracting force created by the finger flexors to a compressive force across the arthrodesis interface.
  - This technique is relatively simple, with a high fusion rate and reliable outcomes,[1,17] especially when used for arthrodesis of the MCP and PIP joints.
  - Postoperative immobilization is necessary only in the immediate postoperative period to allow for healing of the incision.[1,9]
  - Advantages
    - Simplicity of the procedure
    - Low rate of infection[17]
    - High fusion rates, reportedly 97% to 100%[1,17]
    - Readily available, low-cost implants
    - Enhanced biomechanical stability and strength of the construct, allowing for early active range of motion.[17] The tension band construct for small joint arthrodesis has been shown to be biomechanically superior compared to crossed Kirschner wire fixation and intraosseous wiring, especially in anteroposterior bending and in axial torsion.[10]
  - Disadvantages
    - Increased soft tissue dissection to place the drill holes, with resultant increased risk of soft tissue and tendon scarring
    - Difficult to remove fully internalized hardware if necessary
- Plate fixation provides biomechanically strong fixation, especially useful for PIP and MCP joint arthrodesis.[4,20]
  - Advantages
    - Excellent fusion rate by 6 weeks, 96% to 100%[17]
    - Ability to correct deformity
    - Useful in cases with segmental bone loss[4]
  - Disadvantages
    - Technically demanding
    - Time-consuming
    - Extensor tendon adhesions, possibly necessitating hardware removal and tenolysis[17]; stiffness in adjacent joints
    - Hardware prominence
- Compression screw fixation is a biomechanically strong fixation technique[21] that is especially useful for arthrodesis of the finger DIP and PIP joints as well as the thumb interphalangeal joint.
- Recent biomechanical studies suggest that an intramedullary linked screw (Extremity Medical, Parsippany, NJ) is stronger than current plate and tension band constructs for PIP arthrodesis. It does, however, sacrifice considerable bone.[5]
- Using a headless screw keeps the fixation hardware low profile and prevents the problems associated with prominent hardware.
- PIP joint fusion uses the same principles but has a slightly different surgical technique.[2]
  - Advantages
    - Fusion rates 85% to 98%[2,3,14]
    - Hardware is buried and low profile.
  - Disadvantages
    - Risk of infection
    - Risk of penetration and fracture of the dorsal cortex,[3] especially with screw fixation of the PIP joint,[21] resulting in poor fixation
    - Risk of nail irregularities from disturbance of germinal matrix[3] in DIP fusion
  - Complications
    - Risk of infection, hardware complications, nail irregularities secondary to penetration of the dorsal cortex of the distal phalanx by the screw, and fractures of the dorsal cortex from screw breakthrough[3]
    - Easily avoided by maintaining adequate space between the dorsal proximal entry site and the arthrodesis site
    - For DIP arthrodesis, the nail-associated complications usually occurred in the small finger because of the large diameter of the screw used relative to the size of the small finger distal phalanx medullary canal.[21] Now that smaller diameter screws are available, this has become less of an issue.[8]

Preoperative Planning

- Radiographs of the affected joint must be reviewed before operative management. Assessment of the bone stock, quality, and size is useful in helping to determine the optimal type of surgical fixation.
- Should a fusion screw be considered, templates may be used to determine the appropriate screw length and diameter.

Positioning

- The patient is placed in the supine position, with the affected limb resting on a hand table. Sterile preparation and draping is performed.
- For arthrodesis of the PIP and DIP joints, local anesthesia with or without sedation is adequate.
  - Two percent mepivacaine provides a rapid rate of onset and lasts about 1 hour.
  - For the PIP joint, a web space block is performed, including the dorsal cutaneous branches.
  - For the DIP joint, the flexor tendon sheath is injected.
  - For the MCP joint, either regional or general anesthesia is necessary.

Distal Interphalangeal Joint Arthrodesis

Exposure

- A digital tourniquet is used.
- Center a dorsal H-shaped incision over the DIP joint (**TECH FIG 1A**).
- Transect the terminal tendon (**TECH FIG 1B**).
- Release the collateral ligaments from the middle phalanx, using a no. 15 blade directed dorsally, parallel to the sides of the phalanx (**TECH FIG 1C**).

Preparation of the Dorsal Interphalangeal Joint

- Hyperflex the DIP joint and remove peripheral osteophytes with a small rongeur.
- Remove the volar condyles of the head of the middle phalanx with the rongeur.
- Identify the periphery of the base of the distal phalanx with a no. 15 blade, protecting the germinal matrix and the neurovascular bundles.
- Remove bone necessary to correct any joint malalignment, but minimize loss of digital length.
- Dechondrify and decorticate the opposing surfaces until healthy-appearing bone is present.
- Contour the head of the middle phalanx into a transversely oriented cylindrical shape (**TECH FIG 2A**), and fashion the base of the distal phalanx into a reciprocal shape.
  - Alternatively, create flat opposing surfaces perpendicular to the shafts.
- On occasion, the base of the distal phalanx is eburnated. Multiple 0.035-inch drill holes may be placed ("pepperpot" technique), which may then be connected with a small rongeur to unveil subchondral bone (**TECH FIG 2B,C**).

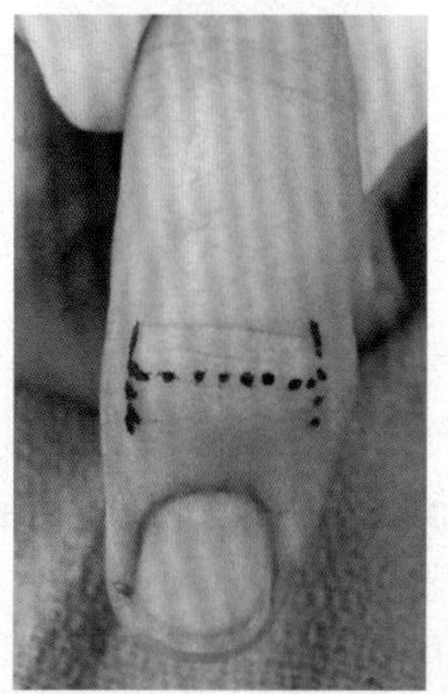
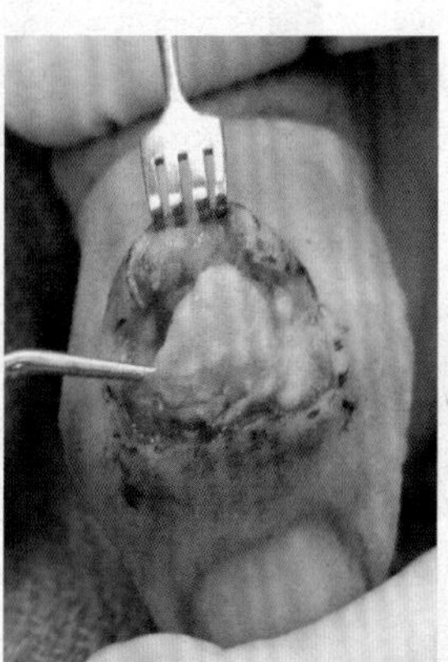
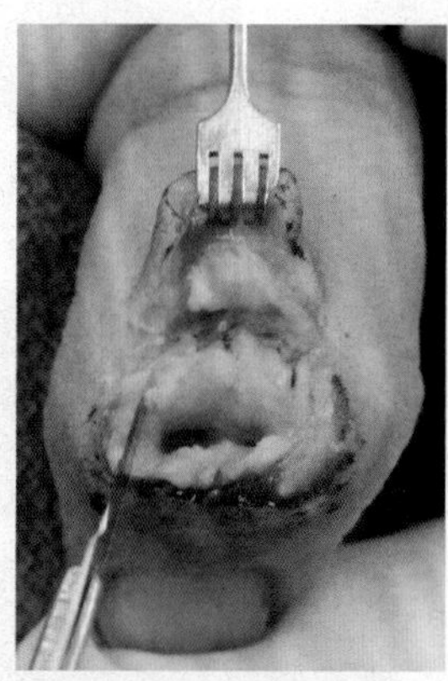

TECH FIG 1 • **A.** Dorsal H-shaped incision, centered over the DIP joint. **B.** The terminal tendon is transected and flaps are elevated. The probe is under a large dorsal loose body. **C.** The collateral ligaments are released from the head of the middle phalanx by orienting a no. 15 blade upward and parallel to the ligament recesses.

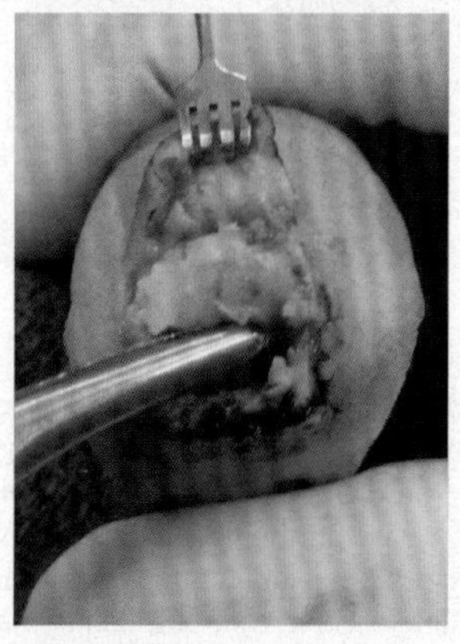
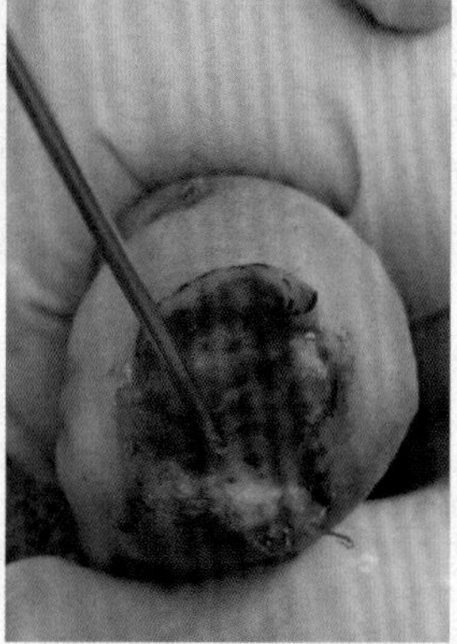
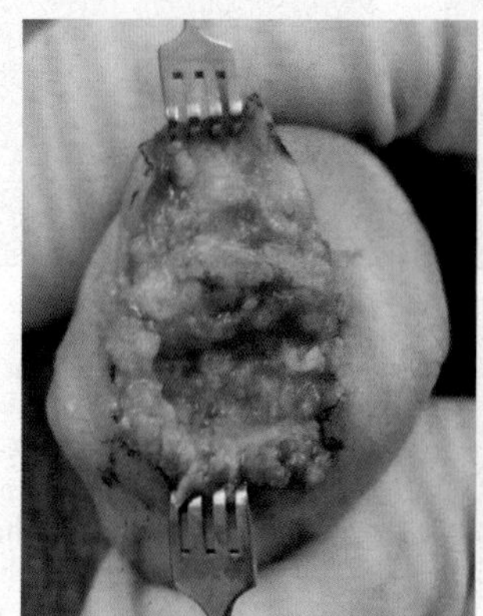

TECH FIG 2 • **A.** The DIP joint is hyperflexed. Peripheral osteophytes and the volar condyles are removed. The remaining articular surface is dechondrified and decorticated with a rongeur, fashioning reciprocal surfaces. **B.** Placing multiple small drill holes facilitates débridement of eburnated bone at the base of the distal phalanx. **C.** Appearance after preparation of the DIP joint.

Reduction and Fixation

- The type of fixation depends on the size of the bone. An Acutrak fusion screw (Acumed, Hillsboro, OR) or similar cannulated, headless, compression screw is preferred when the diameter of the middle and distal phalanges is sufficient to accommodate the screw.
  - If a cannulated screw system is to be used, ensure the appropriate guidewire from the set is used.
- Insert a 0.062-inch Kirschner wire antegrade beginning at the base of the distal phalanx and exiting the tip of the distal phalanx, just volar to the nail plate (**TECH FIG 3A**).
  - If the Kirschner wire penetrates the nail plate, discard it and use another to minimize the likelihood of contamination.
- Drive a smooth 0.062-inch Kirschner wire retrograde into the center of the middle phalanx to create a pilot hole, and then remove it (**TECH FIG 3B**).
- Reduce and compress the joint and then advance the wire retrograde across the DIP joint into the middle phalanx (**TECH FIG 3C**).
- Assess the reduction and Kirschner wire position clinically and fluoroscopically (**TECH FIG 3D**).
- While manually maintaining the joint position, remove the Kirschner wire and replace it with the appropriate drill bit.
  - Proper drill bit size is based on preoperative templating as well as an estimate of the available space based on the lateral fluoroscopic image with the 0.062-inch Kirschner wire in place.

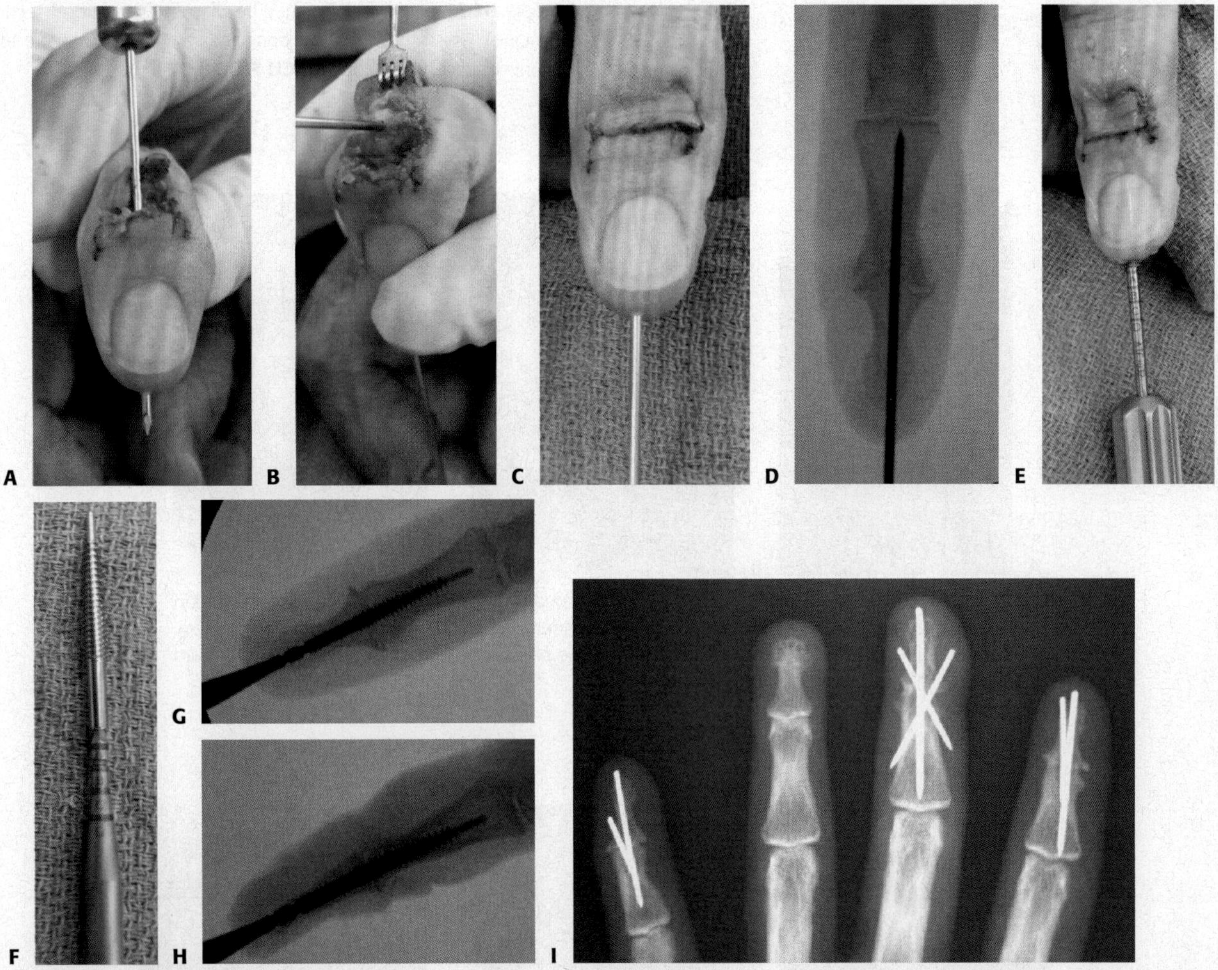

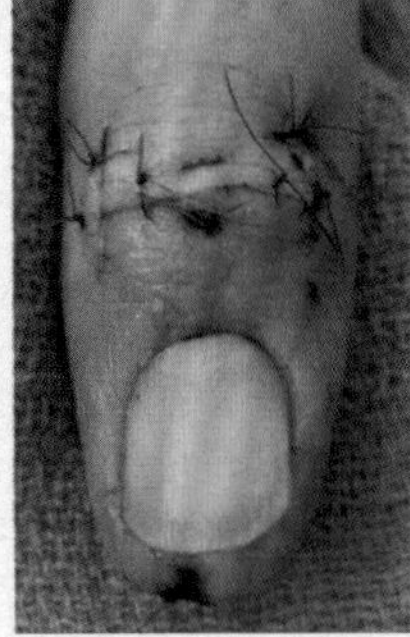

TECH FIG 3 • A. A 0.062-inch Kirschner wire is driven antegrade through the center of the distal phalanx. **B.** A second 0.062-inch Kirschner wire is driven retrograde down the center of the middle phalanx to prepare a path for the screw. **C.** The DIP joint is reduced, and the distal Kirschner wire is driven retrograde into the middle phalanx. **D.** Proper alignment is confirmed fluoroscopically. The diameter of the intramedullary Kirschner wire is used as a reference for determining the screw diameter, based on the lateral radiograph. **E.** The Kirschner wire is removed. While maintaining manual compression across the joint, the appropriate drill bit is advanced by hand retrograde through the Kirschner wire path under fluoroscopic control. External markings on the drill bit serve as a reference for depth. **F.** The appropriate-sized screw is selected and secured to the driver. External markings on the driver correlate with the drill bit. **G,H.** PA and lateral radiographs during screw insertion. **I.** An alternative method of fixation involves the use of two or three Kirschner wires. **J.** Clinical appearance after fixation and closure.

- While maintaining compression across the joint, advance the drill retrograde by hand along the path created by the removed Kirschner wire (**TECH FIG 3E**).
- Determine the proper depth by fluoroscopy, using the external drill bit markings as a reference.
- Remove the drill bit and insert the appropriate-sized fusion screw (**TECH FIG 3F**) while maintaining manual compression across the joint.
  - Final seating of the screw is based on the external reference used for the drill bit.
  - Avoid inadvertent malrotation of the distal segment as the screw is tightened.
- Obtain final fluoroscopic images and evaluate the stability (**TECH FIG 3G,H**).
  - Insert a supplemental 0.035-inch oblique Kirschner wire if necessary for stability.
- If Kirschner wires are used as the sole form of fixation, drive an appropriate diameter pin antegrade into the distal phalanx, reduce the joint, and advance the pin retrograde, preferably into the subchondral plate at the base of the middle phalanx.
  - One or two additional Kirschner wires are inserted obliquely in a retrograde fashion.
  - Final radiographs are obtained, and the pins are cut beneath the skin (**TECH FIG 3I**).

Completion

- Remove the digital tourniquet and achieve hemostasis using bipolar electrocautery.
- Irrigate the wound copiously.
- Approximate the skin with 5-0 nylon interrupted sutures (**TECH FIG 3J**).
  - Repair of the terminal tendon is unnecessary.
- Apply a sterile dressing and dorsal aluminum DIP splint, leaving the PIP joint free.
- Instruct the patient on PIP exercises.

Proximal Interphalangeal Joint Arthrodesis

Exposure

- Make a longitudinal dorsal incision.
  - The surgical approach is similar to the thumb MCP arthrodesis (discussed later).
  - In the multiply operated finger, a preexisting midaxial scar may be used.
- The central slip and capsule are split longitudinally and elevated subperiosteally.
- The collateral ligaments are released from the middle phalanx, using a no. 15 blade directed dorsally, parallel to the sides of the phalanx.

Preparation of the Proximal Interphalangeal Joint

- Hyperflex (shotgun) the PIP joint and prepare the joint in the manner detailed for the DIP joint.
- Correct joint malalignment but minimize loss of digital length.
- As for the DIP joint, contour the head of the proximal phalanx into a transversely oriented cylindrical shape and fashion the base of the distal phalanx into a reciprocal shape.
- Alternatively, use a water-cooled sagittal saw to cut flat surfaces perpendicular to the phalangeal shafts in the coronal plane and with an appropriate degree of flexion in the sagittal plane.
  - The flexion angle is built into the proximal phalanx saw cut. The middle phalanx cut is perpendicular to the axis of the phalanx in the sagittal plane.
  - There is little room for error with the bone cuts. Commitment to the final position of the arthrodesis is made when the bone cuts are made. Any change may result in excessive shortening of the bone.[7]
- On occasion, as with the DIP joint, the base of the middle phalanx is eburnated. Multiple 0.035-inch drill holes may be placed (pepperpot technique), which may then be connected with a small rongeur to unveil subchondral bone.

Kirschner Wire Fixation

- In patients with inflammatory arthritis, the overlying skin is quite thin and may not tolerate prominent hardware. In those instances, crossed 0.035- to 0.045-inch Kirschner wires are used.
- Preset the appropriately sized Kirschner wires into the sides of the middle phalanx.
- Reduce and compress the joint manually, then advance the Kirschner wires in a retrograde manner into the proximal phalanx.
- If the skin is very thin, it may be impossible to cut the Kirschner wires beneath the skin. In those instances, the Kirschner wires are simply bent and left exposed.

Tension Band Fixation

- A tension band technique is used for posttraumatic and OA cases, particularly those involving the index PIP joint (**TECH FIG 4A**).
- Use a 0.035-inch Kirschner wire to make a transverse hole in the middle phalanx, dorsal to the midaxis, about 8 mm distal to the joint.
- Pass a 26-gauge surgical steel wire through the hole.
- With the joint manually reduced, drive parallel 0.035- to 0.045-inch Kirschner wires antegrade across the PIP joint into the subchondral head of the middle phalanx.
  - Begin the Kirschner wires on the dorsoradial and dorsoulnar margins of the proximal phalanx, about 10 mm proximal to the fusion site.
  - The Kirschner wires should remain intramedullary in the middle phalanx.
  - A second option is to displace the prepared joint and advance the Kirschner wires in a retrograde manner from the prepared surface of the proximal phalanx through the dorsoradial and dorsoulnar cortices approximately 1 cm proximal to the distal margin. The joint is then reduced and the Kirschner wires advanced antegrade into the middle phalanx as detailed earlier.

- Loop the 26-gauge wire into a figure-8 configuration around the Kirschner wires proximally and tighten carefully with a needle driver.
  - A gentle distraction force on the needle holder as the device is used to turn the wire and compress the fusion site helps avoid wire breakage.
- Remove the excess knot and impact the knot into bone.
- Withdraw the Kirschner wires slightly, bend them as close to the bone as possible so they can capture the 26-gauge wire, cut the Kirschner wires just distal to the bend, and advance them using the needle holder.
- Obtain final radiographs (**TECH FIG 4B**) and assess stability.
- Remove the tourniquet, achieve hemostasis, and irrigate the wound.
- Reapproximate the extensor tendon using interrupted inverted 4-0 nonabsorbable sutures. Close the skin with 5-0 nylon interrupted sutures.
- Place a sterile dressing and dorsal aluminum splint, leaving the DIP joint free. Instruct the patient on DIP joint exercises.

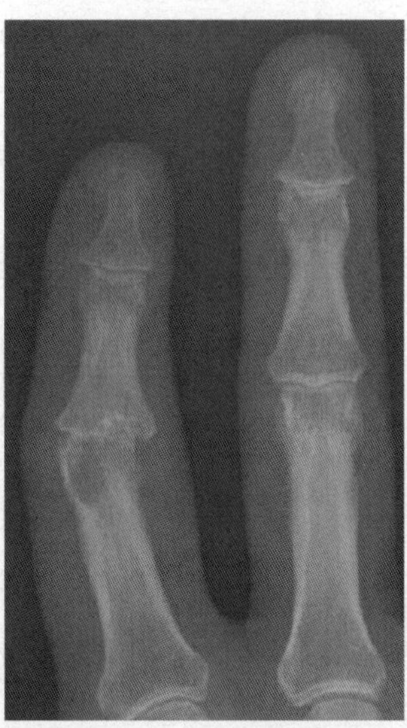

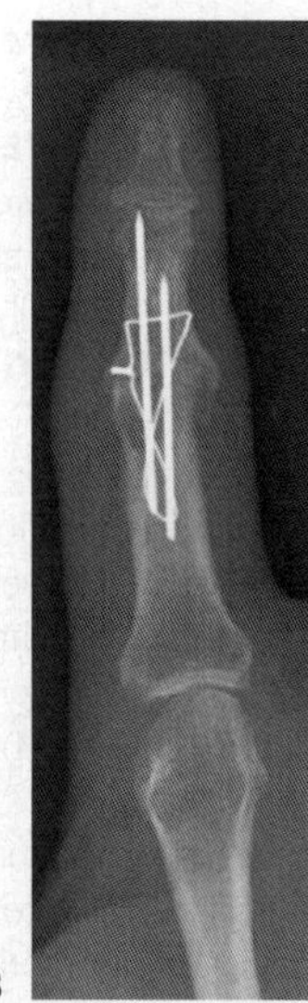

TECH FIG 4 • **A.** Preoperative PA radiograph demonstrating advanced osteoarthritis of the index PIP joint. Note the angular deformity, joint space loss, and large subchondral cyst. **B.** Postoperative PA radiograph demonstrating PIP arthrodesis with tension band fixation.

Thumb Metacarpophalangeal Joint Arthrodesis

Exposure

- Make a longitudinal dorsal incision over the MCP joint (**TECH FIG 5A**).
- Incise the extensor apparatus longitudinally between the EPB and EPL tendons (**TECH FIG 5B**). This will reveal the joint capsule (**TECH FIG 5C**).
- Perform a longitudinal capsulotomy and subperiosteally dissect around the dorsal base of the proximal phalanx (**TECH FIG 5D**).
- Release the collateral ligaments from the metacarpal head (**TECH FIG 5E**) and hyperflex the MCP joint (**TECH FIG 5F**).

Joint Preparation

- Dechondrify the articular surfaces and remove peripheral osteophytes as well as the volar condyles of the metacarpal head with a rongeur (**TECH FIG 6A**).
- Decorticate and prepare the fusion surfaces in a "cup-and-cone" configuration[7,13] using Coughlin reamers (Howmedica, Rutherford, NJ) (**TECH FIG 6B,C**).
  - This method allows for maintenance of thumb length and subtle adjustments in joint position while still maintaining optimal bone contact.
  - The 14 and 16 mm sizes are most often appropriate. Size selection is usually based on the size of the metacarpal head in order to avoid notching.
  - The same dimensions must be used for both metacarpal and phalangeal reaming or the surfaces will be incongruent.
  - Ream the base of the proximal phalanx first to avoid iatrogenic injury to the metacarpal head.
- Place an elevator volar to the base of the proximal phalanx to deliver the phalanx away from the metacarpal head and to protect the flexor pollicis longus.
- Advance a 0.062-inch Kirschner wire antegrade into the proximal phalanx, centered in the coronal plane (**TECH FIG 6D**) and slightly flexed (Kirschner wire tip dorsal) in the sagittal plane (**TECH FIG 6E**).
- Ream the base of the proximal phalanx over the Kirschner wire using the selected phalangeal "cup" reamer until uniform cancellous bone is exposed (**TECH FIG 6F**). Remove the reamer and the pin.
- Prepare the metacarpal head by first advancing a 0.062-inch Kirschner wire retrograde from the center of the head, angled slightly radially (**TECH FIG 6G**) and dorsally (**TECH FIG 6H**).
- Ream the metacarpal head using the matching metacarpal "cone" reamer (**TECH FIG 6I**) until healthy subchondral bone is exposed (**TECH FIG 6J**). Then remove the reamer and the Kirschner wire.

Fixation and Reduction

- Tension band fixation is performed to stabilize the thumb MCP joint fusion in much the same manner as detailed for arthrodesis of the PIP joint.
  - Alternative methods of fixation include Kirschner wires alone, headed or headless, compression screw fixation, and plate and screw fixation.
  - The tension band construct is strong enough to allow for early motion with a hand-based splint.
  - Plate fixation is reserved for cases of bone loss requiring supplemental grafting.
- Use a 0.045-inch smooth Kirschner wire to create a transverse hole in the proximal phalanx, about 1 cm distal to the joint and dorsal to the midline.

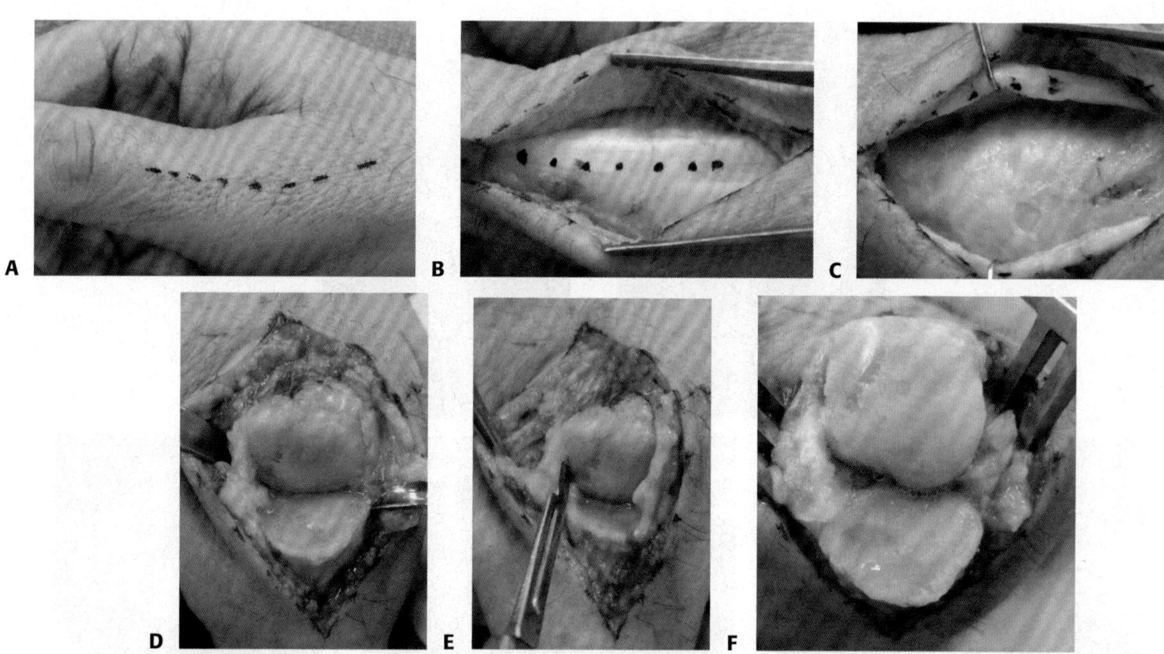

TECH FIG 5 • A. A longitudinal incision is centered over the MCP joint. **B.** The extensor hood is incised between the EPL and EPB tendons (*dotted line*). **C.** The hood has been split, revealing the dorsal joint capsule. **D.** The capsule has been incised longitudinally and reflected subperiosteally from the dorsal base of the proximal phalanx. Note the full-thickness cartilage loss along the ulnar aspect of the metacarpal head and dorsal base of the proximal phalanx secondary to volar ulnar subluxation. **E.** The collateral ligaments are released from the metacarpal head. **F.** The MCP joint is now hyperflexed.

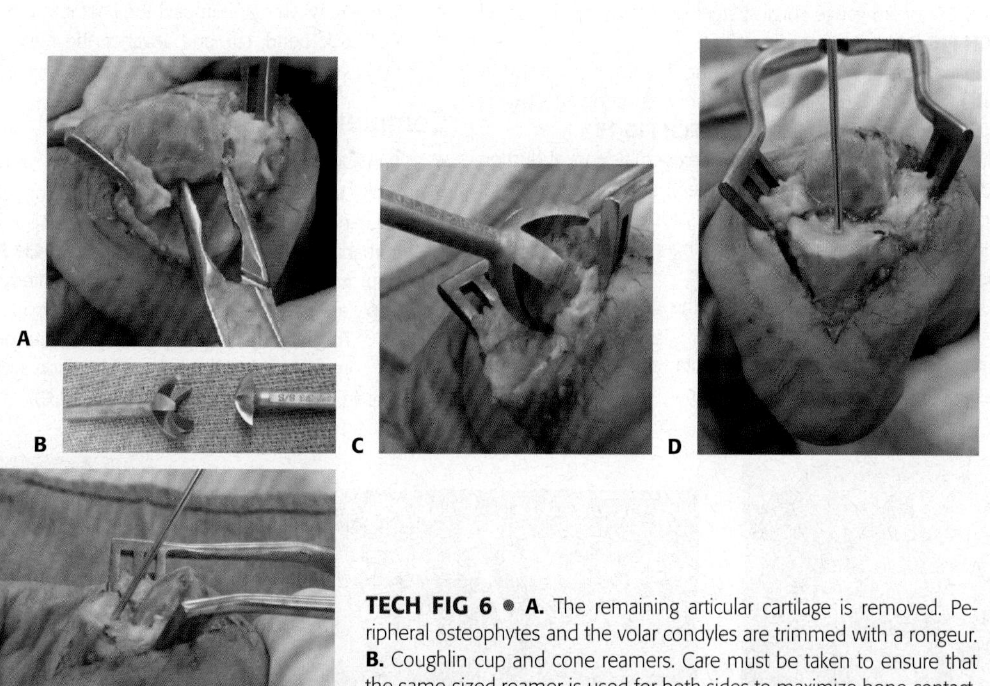

TECH FIG 6 • A. The remaining articular cartilage is removed. Peripheral osteophytes and the volar condyles are trimmed with a rongeur. **B.** Coughlin cup and cone reamers. Care must be taken to ensure that the same-sized reamer is used for both sides to maximize bone contact. **C.** The metacarpal head is used as a reference in determining reamer size. The smallest reamer that will not notch the cortex is selected. **D,E.** A 0.062-inch Kirschner wire is advanced antegrade in the proximal phalanx to be used as a guidewire. The pin is positioned in the center of the bone in the coronal plane (*dot* in the center of the interphalangeal joint) and in slight flexion in the sagittal plane. *(continued)*

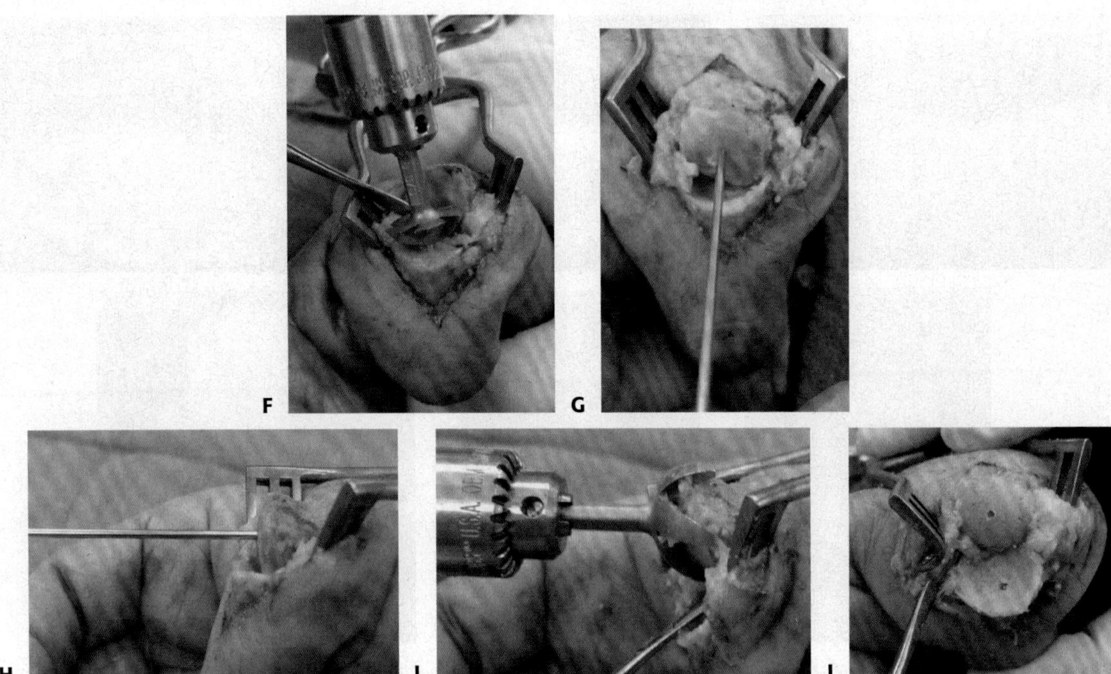

TECH FIG 6 • *(continued)* **F.** The cup reamer is placed over the Kirschner wire under power with frequent irrigation until bleeding subchondral bone is revealed. The asymmetry of the base of the proximal phalanx due to chronic subluxation is corrected. **G,H.** A 0.062-inch Kirschner wire is then inserted retrograde into the metacarpal head. The pin is positioned in slight flexion and slight ulnar deviation. **I.** The matching cone reamer is placed over the Kirschner wire under power with frequent irrigation until bleeding subchondral bone is apparent. **J.** Appearance of the surfaces after joint preparation.

- Pass a 24- or 26-gauge surgical steel wire through the tunnel (**TECH FIG 7A**).
- Anticipating the ultimate position of the thumb fusion, advance parallel 0.054- or 0.062-inch Kirschner wires retrograde, exiting dorsally along the metacarpal shaft (**TECH FIG 7B**).
- Reduce the MCP joint in slight (<25 degrees) flexion, abduction (5 degrees), and pronation (5 degrees), and drive the preset Kirschner wires antegrade. The goal is to have the thumb tip contact the radial border of the index finger just distal to the DIP flexion crease.
  - Take care to avoid perforating the volar cortex into the flexor tendon sheath.
- Loop the wire in a figure-8 configuration around the Kirschner wires and tighten using a needle driver.
- Trim excess wire and impact the knot into the bone.
- Pull back, bend, cut, and advance the Kirschner wires (as detailed earlier) to secure the tension band wire (**TECH FIG 7C**).

Completion

- Remove the tourniquet, achieve hemostasis, and irrigate the wound.
- Close the capsule over the hardware using absorbable 4-0 suture and then close the extensor mechanism using 4-0 nonabsorbable interrupted inverted stitches (**TECH FIG 8A**).
- Approximate the skin using 5-0 nylon interrupted suture, and apply a sterile dressing and radial gutter splint.
  - The interphalangeal joint is left free, and the patient is instructed on interphalangeal motion exercises.
- Obtain final radiographs (**TECH FIG 8B,C**).

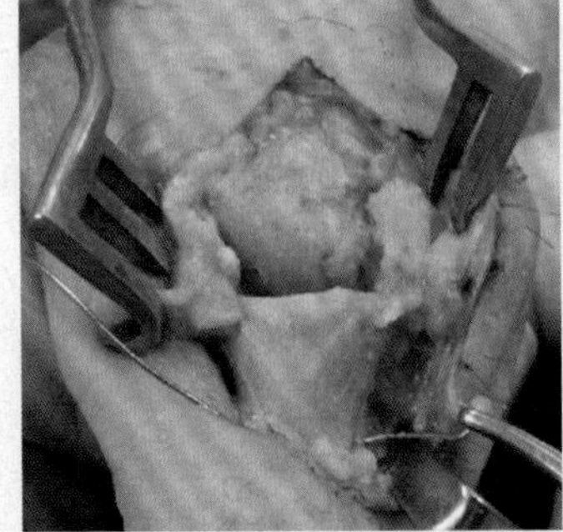

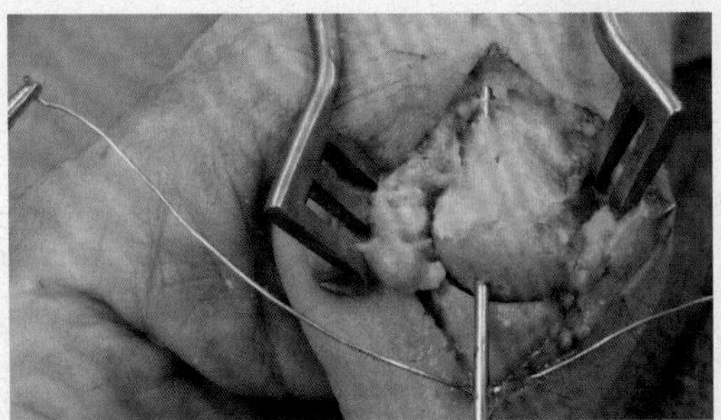

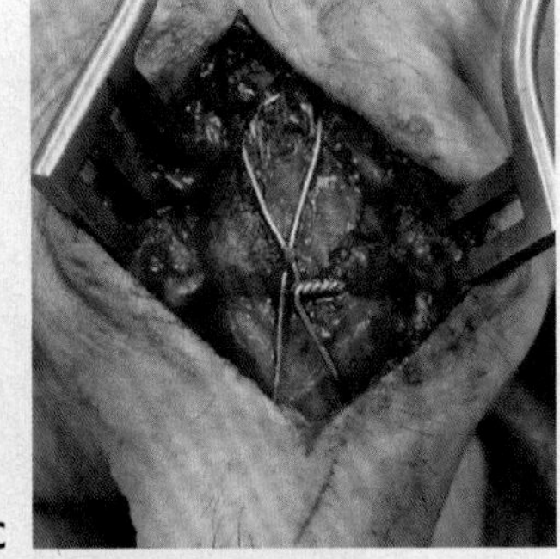

TECH FIG 7 • **A.** A 24-gauge wire is passed through a drill hole in the proximal shaft of the proximal phalanx, dorsal to the midline and parallel to the joint. **B.** A 0.062-inch Kirschner wire is then driven retrograde in the metacarpal head, exiting dorsally, anticipating the ultimate position of the MCP joint. **C.** The 24-gauge wire is looped around the base of the Kirschner wires in figure-8 fashion and tensioned. The Kirschner wires are cut short and the wire knot is tamped against the cortex.

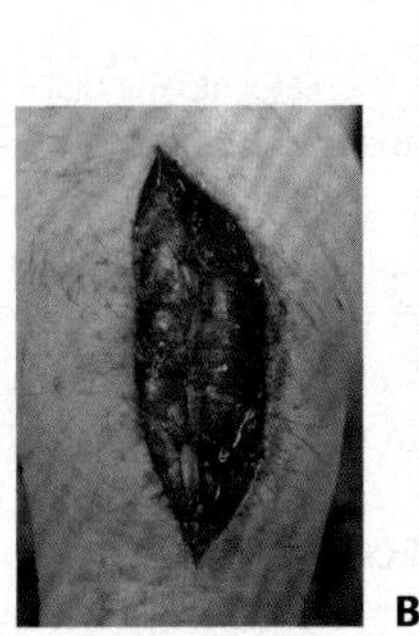
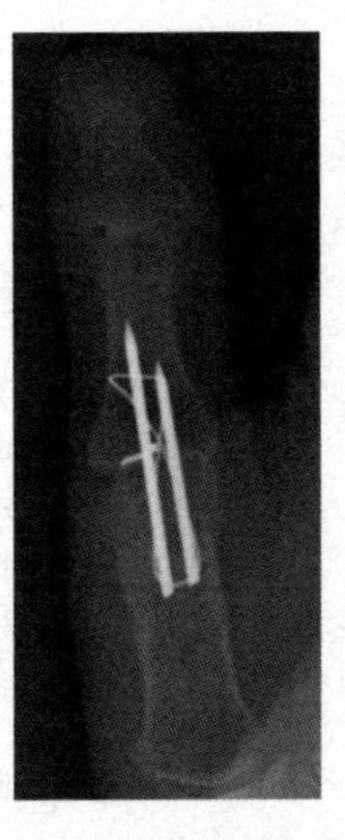
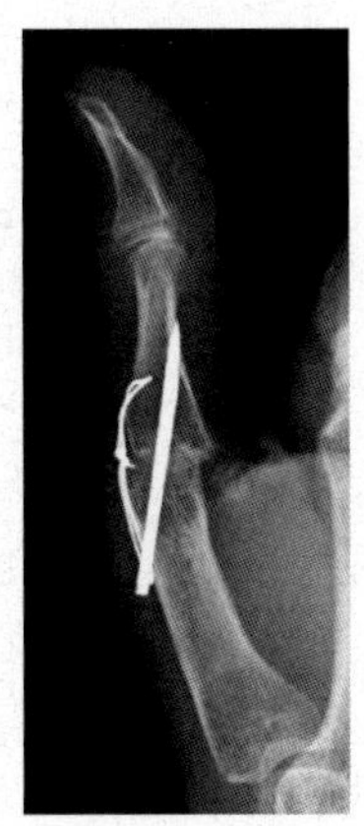

TECH FIG 8 • **A.** The capsule and extensor hood are repaired in layers. **B,C.** Postoperative PA and lateral radiographs demonstrate good joint apposition and alignment.

Index through Small Finger Metacarpophalangeal Joint Arthrodesis

- The approach and bone preparation mirror those described for the thumb.
- Fixation may be achieved with Kirschner wires alone, a tension band construct, screws, or plates (**TECH FIG 9**).
  - Keep in mind the anticipated deforming forces, which may be out of plane with the fixation.
- Immobilization should protect the fused joint from stress while simultaneously permitting motion of the PIP and DIP joints. We prefer to apply a short-arm cast extending out to the PIP joints, allowing PIP and DIP motion.

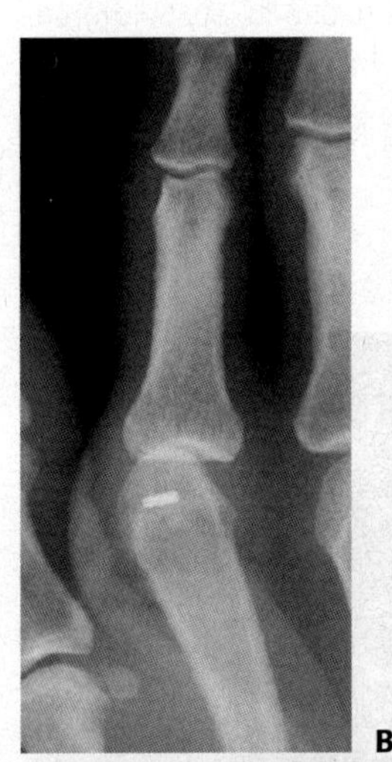
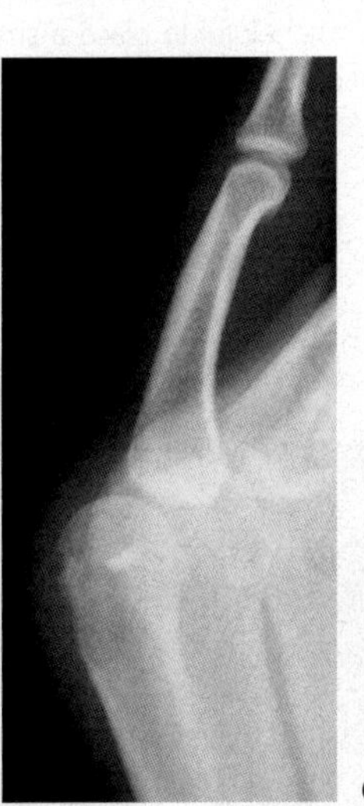
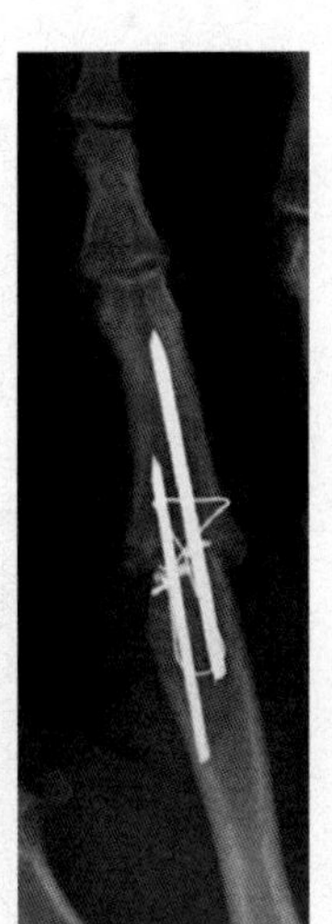
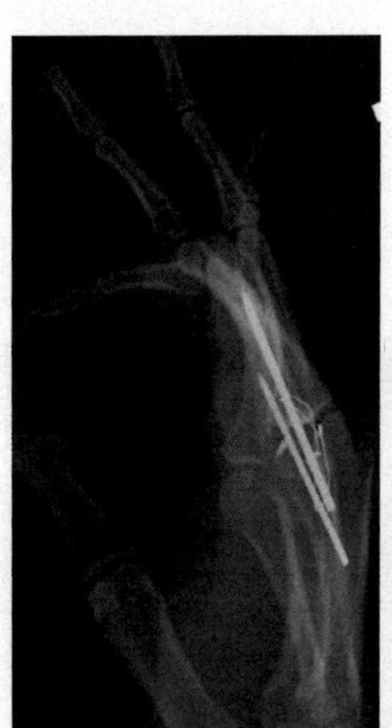
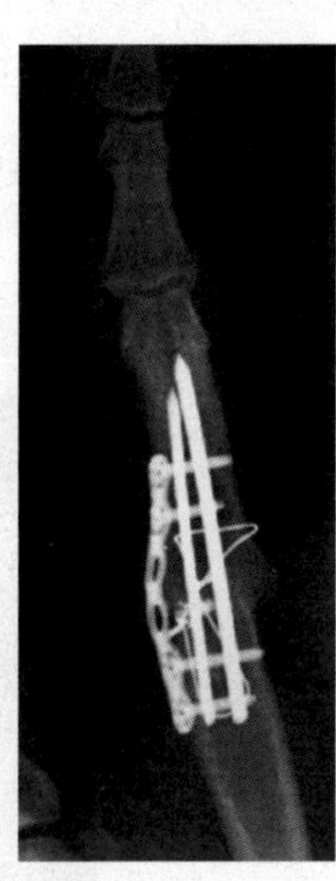
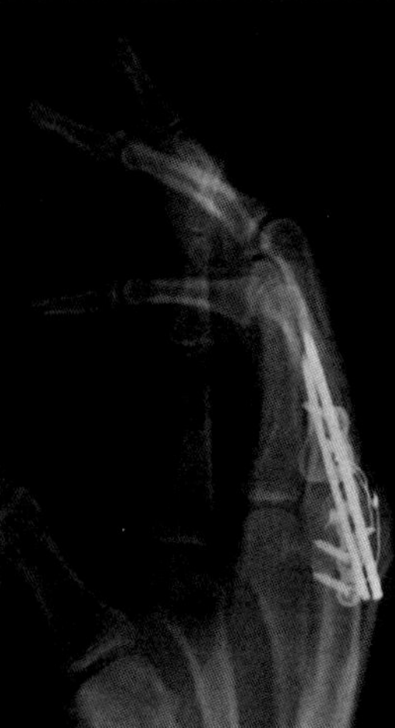
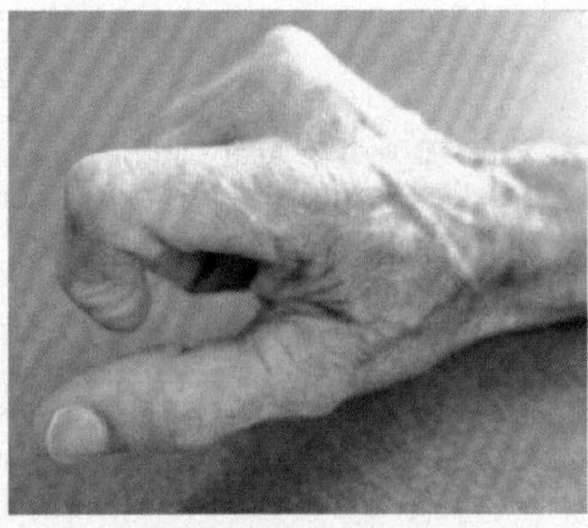

TECH FIG 9 • **A,B.** PA and lateral radiographs showing chronic right index MCP volar ulnar subluxation in patient who had undergone two previous attempts at radial collateral ligament reconstruction. **C,D.** Postoperative PA and lateral radiographs demonstrating loss of fixation after cup-and-cone tension band arthrodesis. **E,F.** PA and lateral radiographs after successful revision of the index MCP arthrodesis. This included redébridement of the bone ends and repeat tension band fixation as well as supplemental fixation using a 2-mm plate to control out-of-plane forces perpendicular to the tension band. **G.** Clinical photograph after index MCP fusion. For this patient, a professional photographer, the MCP joint position was chosen to permit optimal control of the camera shutter.

Additional Fixation Methods

- The surgical approach, bone preparation, and closure are performed as detailed earlier.
- Most frequently, flat bone cuts are used with these fixation techniques.

Interosseous Wiring

- Following bone preparation, drill two parallel holes from dorsal to volar, each 3 to 4 mm away from the arthrodesis site, using a 0.035-inch Kirschner wire.
- Drill two additional holes, this time in the radioulnar plane, again about 3 to 4 mm on either side of the arthrodesis site.
- Thread two 26-gauge surgical steel wires through the drill holes.
  - A 20-gauge hypodermic needle may be used to facilitate wire placement.
- Pass one wire from dorsal to volar through one drill hole and then volar to dorsal in the parallel drill hole, forming a loop.
- Pass the second 26-gauge steel wire through the drill holes in the coronal plane, forming a second loop.
- After the wires are placed, tighten the ends of the wires sequentially and shorten and bend them to decrease their profile.
- This configuration results in two perpendicular loops providing compression and fixation across the arthrodesis interface.

Plate Fixation

- Fill bone defects with intercalary grafts as needed (**TECH FIG 10A,B**).
- Select the largest compression plate that will not be prominent.
  - These range in size from 1.5 to 2.7 mm.
- The plate is precontoured to match the angle of the fusion.
  - A slight increase in concavity is created to allow compression of the volar cortex when the plate is applied (**TECH FIG 10C**).
- Insert a bicortical screw through the plate into the distal fragment.
  - Be certain that this and other screws do not penetrate the volar cortex and impair the function of the flexor tendons.
- Using AO compression technique, place a screw through the plate into the proximal fragment.
  - Drill as proximally and eccentrically as possible within the plate's screw hole so that when the screw is tightened, compression is obtained.
- Place the remaining screws (**TECH FIG 10D**).
  - Four to six cortices on either side of the fusion site provides adequate fixation.[15]

Compression Screw Fixation

- In much the same manner as described for placement of Kirschner wires for tension band fusion of the thumb MCP joint, the guidewire is introduced into the proximal fragment in a retrograde manner, exiting the dorsal cortex at least 5 mm proximal to the arthrodesis site.
  - This protects against inadvertent fracture of the dorsal cortex.
- Manually reduce and compress the prepared joint.
- It may be helpful to place a small (0.028 to 0.035 inch) provisional Kirschner wire away from the anticipated screw site to provide rotational stability.

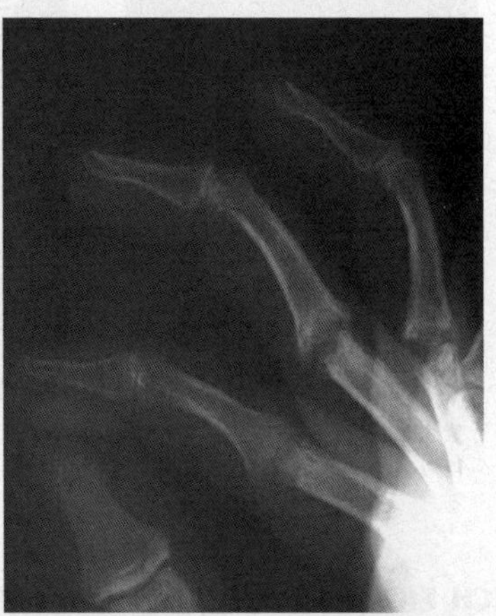
A

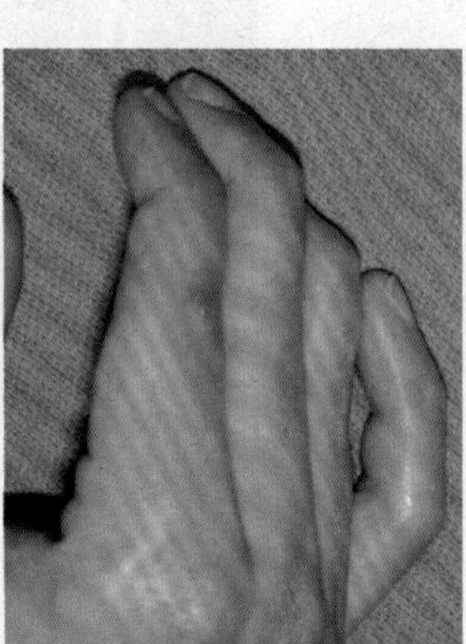
B

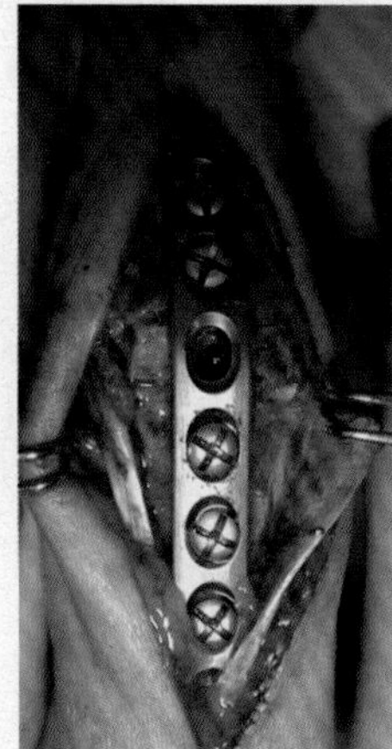
C

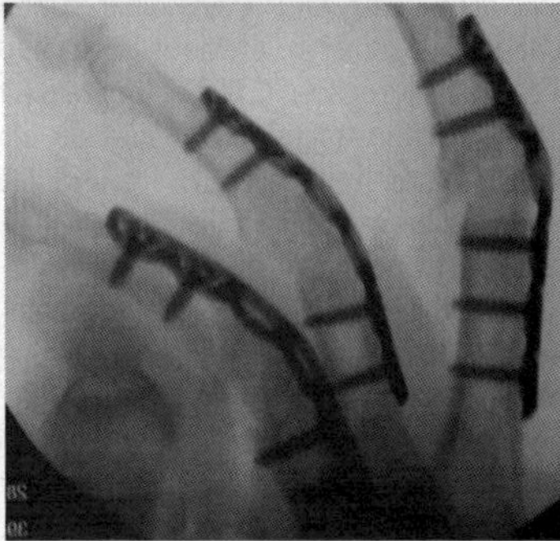
D

TECH FIG 10 • **A,B.** After silicone implant arthroplasty, rigid swan-neck deformities developed. Conversion to arthrodesis in a more functional position was complicated by large bone defects resulting from removal of the implants. **C.** A prebent 2-mm dynamic compression plate is applied to the dorsal surface for the proximal and middle phalanges. **D.** Lateral radiograph depicts placement of intercalary bone graft and compression plate fixation. Screw length is carefully determined to avoid irritation of the flexor tendons. (Copyright Thomas R. Hunt III, MD.)

- Advance the guidewire antegrade from proximal to distal, perpendicular to the fusion interface, and into the medullary canal of the distal segment.
- Advance the wire just beyond the mid-diaphyseal region of the distal fragment.
- Evaluate clinically and fluoroscopically to ensure proper position (**TECH FIG 11**).
- Measure the guidewire and choose the appropriate-length screw to ensure that after compression, the distal screw threads will engage the endosteal cortex and the proximal aspect of the screw will be buried.
  - Drill and place screw. Confirm position with fluoroscopy.
- Remove the derotation Kirschner wire.

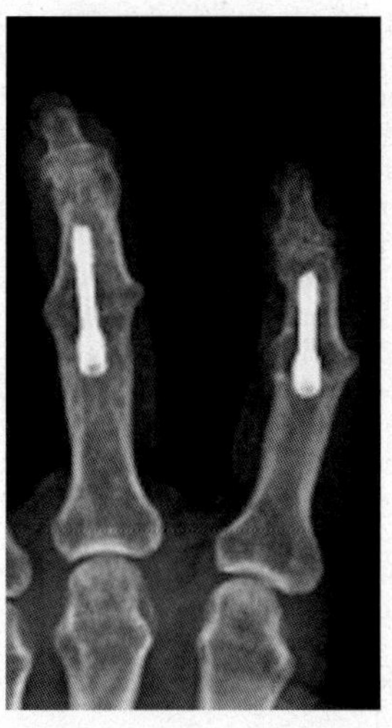

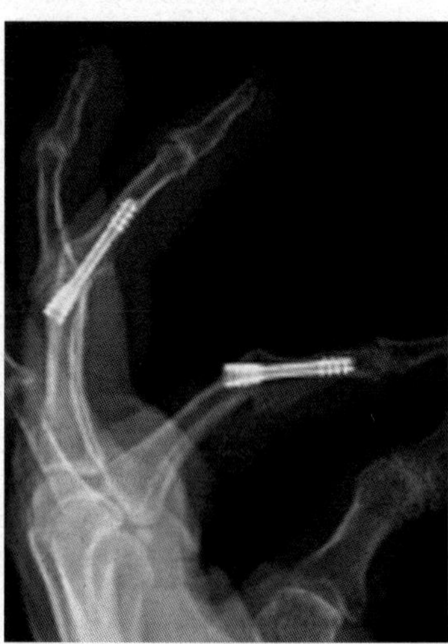

TECH FIG 11 • PA (**A**) and lateral (**B**) radiographs demonstrating arthrodesis of PIP joints with cannulated, headless compression screws. (Copyright Thomas R. Hunt III, MD.)

PEARLS AND PITFALLS

Bone end preparation	▪ If flat bone cuts are to be used, predetermine and create accurate flexion angles for the joint fusion. There is little room for error with this technique. Inaccurate cuts will result in excessive bone shortening. ▪ The cup-and-cone preparation technique is more forgiving, allowing for angular and rotational adjustments while maintaining bone contact. ▪ Ensure that there is no malrotation of fusion interface.
Surgical approach	▪ Preserve joint capsule for later repair to minimize extensor tendon adherence.
Tension band fixation	▪ To minimize hardware problems, position the Kirschner wires within the intramedullary canal and advance them into the subchondral plate.
Compression screw fixation	▪ In the PIP and MCP joints, ensure that the starting point is 5 mm from the bony end of the proximal fragment to prevent fracture of the dorsal cortex.

POSTOPERATIVE CARE

- Postoperative management depends on the involved joint and method of fixation. Early motion of the adjacent joints is critical to minimize stiffness.
- For DIP joint arthrodesis, protection with a simple aluminum splint is sufficient. PIP motion is encouraged. Splinting may be unnecessary if a fusion screw is used. Radiographs are taken at 6 weeks postoperatively. Buried pins may be removed once the fusion is radiographically solid (at least 8 weeks postoperatively).
- For PIP joint arthrodesis, tension band, screw, and plate constructs are usually strong enough to obviate the need for supplemental splinting. Early MCP and DIP motion is encouraged; however, the patient is advised against lateral stress or forceful grip with the affected digit. With simple pin fixation, a supplemental dorsal aluminum or thermoplast PIP splint is used until radiographs demonstrate union.
- For the thumb MCP joint treated with tension band fixation, a protective custom-molded thermoplast hand-based MCP splint is used for about 6 weeks. Early IP joint motion is encouraged.
- In general, arthrodesis of the other MCP joints must be protected with a hand- or forearm-based splint, regardless of the type of fixation. Significant flexion and lateral stresses must be neutralized while simultaneously allowing for PIP and DIP motion. It may be necessary to splint the PIP joint in extension part-time to prevent an extensor lag from developing.

OUTCOMES

- Multiple studies have evaluated the biomechanical advantages of one type of surgical technique versus another in order to establish the most rigid type of fixation that will allow a rapid and complete arthrodesis.
- A comparison between the failure load of a Herbert screw and the failure load of a tension band construct showed no significant difference between the two[2]; the authors concluded that these two methods of fixation have similar biomechanical strength.
- A comparison of multiple fixation techniques showed that arthrodesis by screw fixation had a better fusion rate than Kirschner wires, tension band construct, and plate fixation.[11]
- A comparison of tension band constructs versus Kirschner wire fixation for PIP joint arthrodesis concluded that tension bands provide more rigid fixation.[10]
- Biomechanical testing comparing the Herbert screw and tension band construct for DIP arthrodesis showed that the Herbert screw has significantly higher bending strength as well as more rigidity against axial torsion, although no difference was noted in the bending stiffness between these two methods of fixation.[21]

COMPLICATIONS

- Pin tract infection
- Nonunion
- Malunion
- Vascular insufficiency
- Skin necrosis
- Cold intolerance
- Stiffness of adjacent digits
- Painful hardware

REFERENCES

1. Allende B, Engelem JC. Tension-band arthrodesis in the finger joints. J Hand Surg Am 1980;5(3):269–271.
2. Ayres JR, Goldstrohm GL, Miller GJ, et al. Proximal interphalangeal joint arthrodesis with the Herbert screw. J Hand Surg Am 1988;13(4):600–603.
3. Brutus JP, Palmer AK, Mosher JF, et al. Use of a headless compressive screw for distal interphalangeal joint arthrodesis in digits: clinical outcome and review of complications. J Hand Surg Am 2006;31(1):85–89.
4. Büchler U, Aiken MA. Arthrodesis of the proximal interphalangeal joint by solid bone grafting and plate fixation in extensive injuries to the dorsal aspect of the finger. J Hand Surg Am 1988;13(4):589–594.
5. Capo JT, Melamed E, Shamian B, et al. Biomechanical evaluation of 5 fixation devices for proximal interphalangeal joint arthrodesis. J Hand Surg Am 2014;39(10):1971–1977. doi:10.1016/j.jhsa.2014.07.
6. Carroll RE, Dick HM. Arthrodesis of the wrist for rheumatoid arthritis. J Bone Joint Surg Am 1971;53(7):1365–1369.
7. Carroll RE, Hill NA. Small joint arthrodesis in hand reconstruction. J Bone Joint Surg Am 1969;51(6):1219–1221.
8. Cox C, Earp B, Floyd WE IV, et al. Arthrodesis of the thumb interphalangeal joint and finger distal interphalangeal joints with a headless compression screw. J Hand Surg Am 2014;39(1):24–28.
9. Ijsselstein CB, van Egmond DB, Hovius SE, et al. Results of small-joint arthrodesis: comparison of Kirschner wire fixation with tension band wire technique. J Hand Surg Am 1992;17(5):952–956.
10. Kovach JC, Werner FW, Palmer AK, et al. Biomechanical analysis of internal fixation techniques for proximal interphalangeal joint arthrodesis. J Hand Surg Am 1986;11(4):562–566.
11. Leibovic SJ, Strickland JW. Arthrodesis of the proximal interphalangeal joint of the finger: comparison of the use of the Herbert screw with other fixation methods. J Hand Surg Am 1994;19(2):181–188.
12. Lister G. Intraosseous wiring of the digital skeleton. J Hand Surg Am 1978;3(5):427–435.
13. McGlynn JT, Smith RA, Bogumill GP. Arthrodesis of small joint of the hand: a rapid and effective technique. J Hand Surg Am 1988;13(4):595–599.
14. Moberg E. Arthrodesis of finger joints. Surg Clin North Am 1960;40:465–470.
15. Shin A, Amadio P. Stiff finger joints. In: Green DP, ed. Green's Operative Hand Surgery. Philadelphia: Elsevier, 2006:417–457.
16. Stern PJ, Fulton DB. Distal interphalangeal joint arthrodesis: an analysis of complications. J Hand Surg Am 1992;17(6):1139–1145.
17. Stern PJ, Gates NT, Jones TB. Tension band arthrodesis of small joints in the hand. J Hand Surg Am 1993;18(2):194–197.
18. Tubiana R. Arthrodesis of the fingers. In: Tubiana R, ed. The Hand, vol 2. Philadelphia: WB Saunders, 1985:698–702.
19. Vanik RK, Weber RC, Matloub HS, et al. The comparative strengths of internal fixation techniques. J Hand Surg Am 1984;9(2):216–221.
20. Wright CS, McMurtry RY. AO arthrodesis in the hand. J Hand Surg Am 1983;8(6):932–935.
21. Wyrsch B, Dawson J, Aufranc S, et al. Distal interphalangeal joint arthrodesis comparing tension-band wire and Herbert screw: a biomechanical and dimensional analysis. J Hand Surg 1996;21(3):438–443.

Compartment Syndrome, Vascular Disorders, and Infection

Surgical Decompression of the Forearm, Hand, and Digits for Compartment Syndrome

124 CHAPTER

Marci D. Jones, Rodrigo Santamarina, and Lance G. Warhold

DEFINITION

- Acute compartment syndrome is a condition in which increased tissue pressure compromises the circulation within the enclosed space of fascial compartments. As a result of this elevated interstitial pressure, the blood supply to the soft tissues is impaired. If left untreated, elevated pressures can cause irreversible muscle and nerve damage resulting in fibrosis and contracture.

ANATOMY

- Compartment syndrome is most common in the forearm and hand but can occur in the arm and in the finger.
- The arm is divided into two fascial compartments, the forearm into three compartments, the hand into ten compartments, and the finger into two compartments.
- The two arm compartments are the anterior and posterior, separated by the medial and lateral intermuscular septa (**FIG 1A**).
  - The anterior arm compartment contains the biceps brachii, brachialis, and coracobrachialis.
  - The posterior arm compartment contains the triceps brachii.
- The forearm consists of three compartments: the volar, the dorsal, and the mobile wad of three (**FIG 1B**).
  - The contents of the volar compartment include the flexor muscles and can be subdivided into superficial and deep components. The superficial muscles are the flexor carpi ulnaris, palmaris longus, pronator teres, and flexor carpi radialis. The deep muscles are the flexor digitorum superficialis and profundus, the flexor pollicis longus, and distally the pronator quadratus.
  - The dorsal compartment of the forearm contains the extensor muscles. The superficial extensors include the extensor digitorum communis, extensor digiti minimi, and extensor carpi ulnaris. The deep layer includes the supinator, abductor pollicis longus, extensor pollicis longus, extensor pollicis brevis, and extensor indicis.
  - The mobile wad of three is a distinct muscle compartment that contains the brachioradialis, extensor carpi radialis longus, and extensor carpi radialis brevis.
- The wrist has one significant closed space, the carpal tunnel. Although not a compartment in the strictest sense, increased pressure in this tunnel can be detrimental to the median nerve.
- The hand contains ten distinct compartments (**FIG 1C**).
  - There are seven compartments for the interossei. Each of the four dorsal and three palmar interossei has a separate compartment.
  - The adductor compartment contains the adductor pollicis.
  - The thenar compartment contains the abductor pollicis brevis, the opponens pollicis, and the flexor pollicis brevis.
  - The hypothenar compartment contains the abductor digiti minimi, flexor digiti minimi, and opponens digiti minimi.
- Compartment syndrome can also occur in the finger due to the limited skin compliance from the multiple fascial attachments.

PATHOGENESIS

- The blood flow to a compartment is determined by several factors, including venous pressure, arterial pressure, and local interstitial pressure. Increased pressure within a compartment decreases the blood supply to the soft tissues and can result in tissue ischemia and ultimately necrosis. Increased capillary permeability results from muscle ischemia. This increased permeability leads to intramuscular edema, increases the tissue pressure, decreases blood flow and oxygen transport, and leads to more tissue damage. It is easy to appreciate the vicious cycle that escalates the pathophysiology of the compartment syndrome.
- Many conditions are associated with compartment syndrome. These can be divided into two major categories[3]:
  - Conditions that decrease compartment volume: tight casts or dressings, burn eschar, limb lengthening or application of traction, and increased external pressure on limb from prolonged weight (lying on limb or entrapment under a weight)
  - Conditions that increase compartment contents: bleeding (arterial or venous injury, anticoagulation, trauma), reperfusion injury, edema, infiltrated infusion, snakebite, infection, high-pressure injection

NATURAL HISTORY

- Compartment syndrome results in hypoxic cell damage and ultimately anoxic cell death. Functional changes occur in muscle after 2 to 4 hours of total ischemia. Hypoxia to nerves causes paresthesia and hypoesthesia within 30 minutes of ischemia, but irreversible nerve damage may not occur until 12 hours or more of total ischemia.

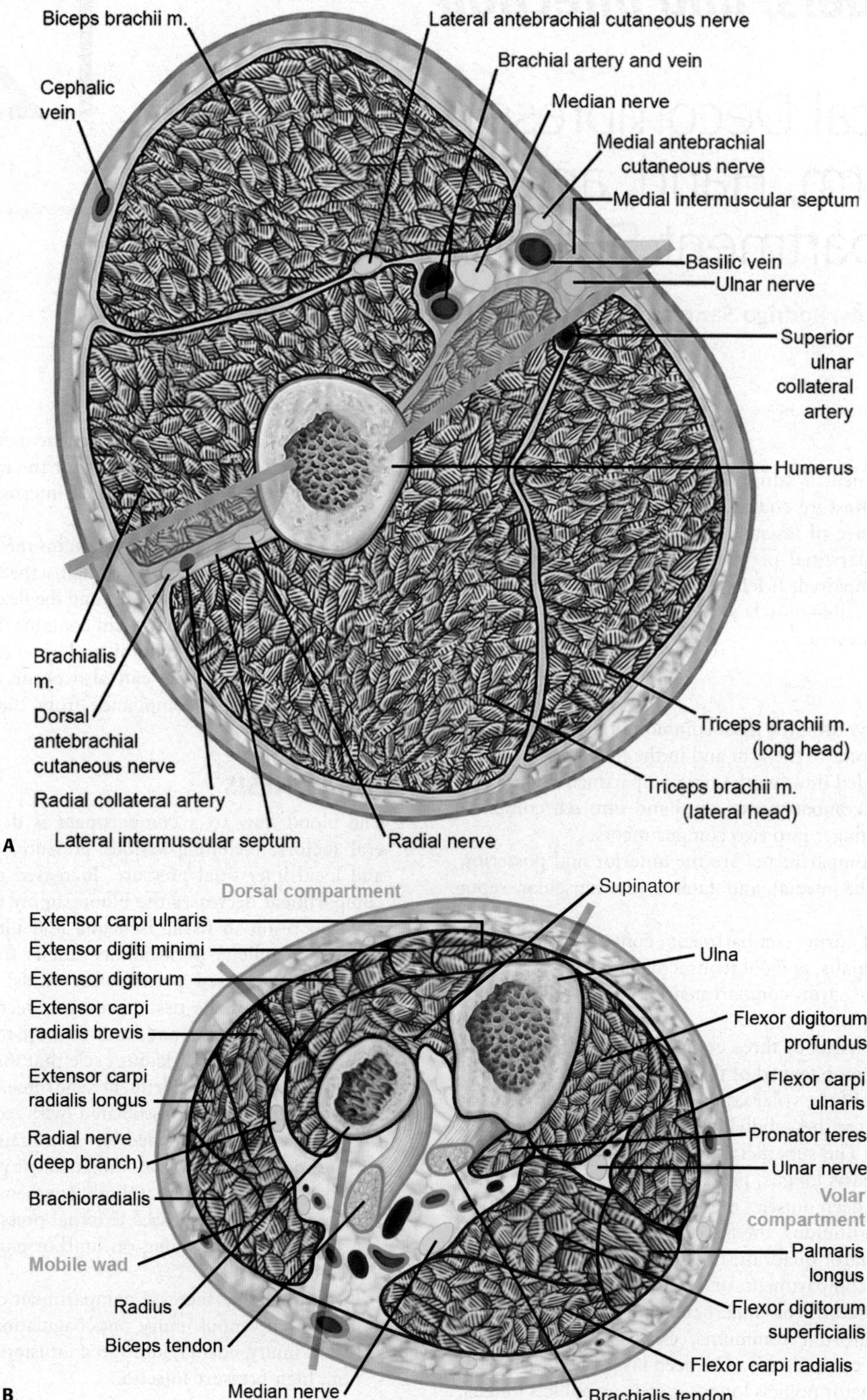

FIG 1 • **A.** Compartments of the arm. **B.** Compartments of the forearm. *(continued)*

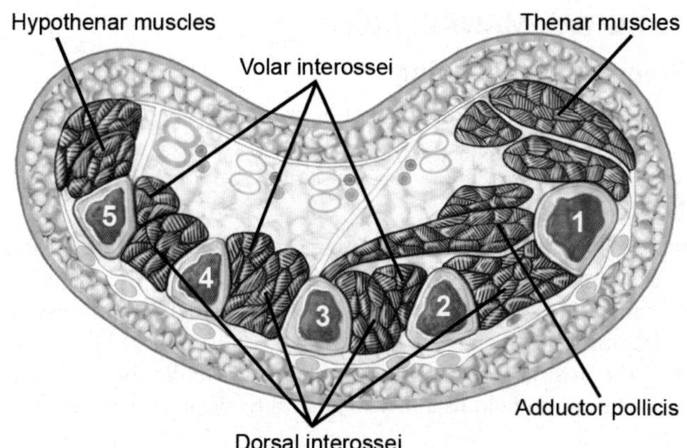

FIG 1 ● *(continued)* **C.** Compartments of the hand.

- An untreated compartment syndrome can result in permanent neural deficit, tissue necrosis, growth arrest, Volkmann contracture, and even wet gangrene.

PATIENT HISTORY AND PHYSICAL FINDINGS

- It is important to elicit a detailed history and evaluate the possible causes of compartment syndrome (discussed earlier).
- Pain out of proportion to physical findings is the most important finding. For patients with this finding, one must have a high clinical suspicion regardless of the presumed severity of the inciting event.
- Most commonly, patients will present with a history of trauma or a crushing injury; however, other causes must not be overlooked.
- Compartment syndrome may involve single or multiple compartments in the extremity.
- Physical examination findings include the following:
  - A tense, swollen, and tender compartment (**FIG 2**)
  - Pain with passive stretch of the muscles within the compartment
  - Paresthesias or sensory disturbances in the nerve distribution of the compressed nerve are intermediate findings. This can be accompanied by motor weakness. Motor paralysis is a later finding.
  - Pallor and pulselessness are late findings.
- The findings of pain out of proportion to physical examination, a tense compartment, and pain with passive stretch are sufficient to warrant intracompartmental pressure measurements. One should not delay definitive diagnosis and treatment until later findings are present.
- In obtunded or sedated patients, a tense, swollen compartment is sufficient to warrant intracompartmental pressure measurements.

IMAGING AND OTHER DIAGNOSTIC STUDIES

- Clinical examination is the cornerstone of the diagnosis, and it is important to have a high degree of suspicion for compartment syndrome.
- Immediate fasciotomy is indicated in patients with unequivocal symptoms and signs of compartment syndrome. Direct measurement of compartment pressures is indicated in all cases when the patient's symptoms and physical

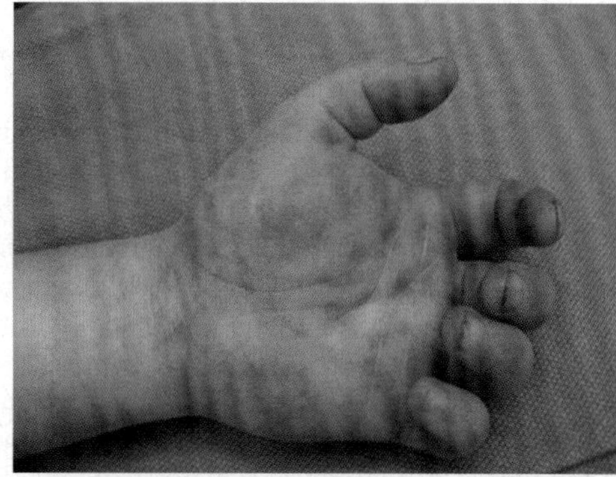

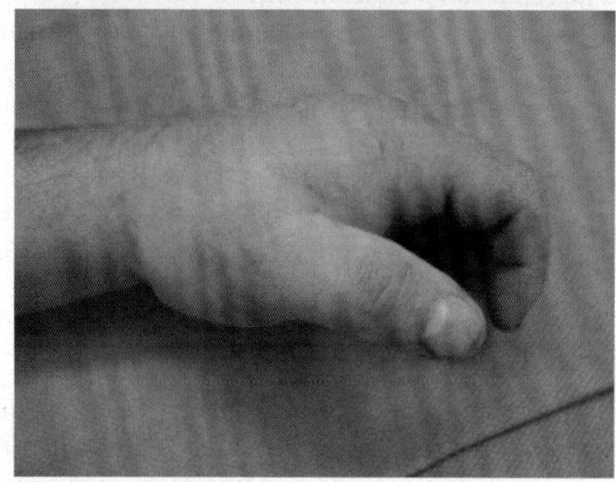

FIG 2 ● Diffuse, tense swelling of the hand. **A.** Palmar view with loss of palmar concavity. **B.** Radial view.

examination signs are indicative of compartment syndrome, and it is especially important in patients who are obtunded or sedated.

- Diagnosis of compartment syndrome of the finger is made clinically and not through the use of pressure measurement.
- Pressure measurement in the arm is made in both anterior and posterior compartments. Anteriorly, the pressure is measured over the biceps muscle and posteriorly over the triceps muscle.
  - The physician must be careful not to injure the radial nerve when measuring the arm compartment pressure. The nerve courses deep to the triceps in the spiral groove of the humerus. Ten centimeters proximal to the lateral epicondyle, it passes through the lateral intermuscular septum to the anterior compartment.
- In the forearm, the pressure is measured over the volar, mobile wad, and dorsal compartments.
  - The median and ulnar nerves are at risk during measurement of the volar compartment. The ulnar nerve courses deep to the flexor carpi ulnaris in the ulnar forearm; the median nerve is between the flexor digitorum superficialis and profundus muscles.
  - When measuring the mobile wad, the superficial branch of the radial nerve is deep to the brachioradialis in the forearm but emerges between the brachioradialis and extensor carpi radialis longus tendons about 8 cm proximal to the radial styloid.
    - The posterior interosseous nerve courses around the radial neck in the proximal radial forearm and should be avoided when measuring the mobile wad and dorsal compartments.

- In the hand, pressure measurements should be made in the affected compartments; measurements are generally made in the area of the planned incisions.
- There is not an absolute increased compartment pressure that warrants fasciotomy. When the pressure approaches 30 to 45 mm Hg, or 30 mm Hg less than the diastolic pressure, with concordant physical examination findings, decompressive fasciotomy should be performed.[4] In the hand, lower pressures (15 to 20 mm Hg) may indicate compartment syndrome.
- Plain radiographs should be performed to evaluate any underlying bony abnormality. Fractures and dislocations should be reduced as anatomically as possible.
- Arterial injury can lead to ischemia and can present similarly. Arteriography is indicated if the history may be significant for arterial injury (fracture, avulsion, or laceration).

DIFFERENTIAL DIAGNOSIS

- Arterial injury
- Nerve injury

NONOPERATIVE MANAGEMENT

- There is no role for nonoperative management of an acute compartment syndrome. In acute cases of compartment syndrome with elevated compartment pressure, prompt decompressive fasciotomies are required to relieve tissue ischemia.
- In patients with early symptoms and signs of compartment syndrome, but without elevated compartment pressures, removal of all compressive dressings and casts and elevation of the affected extremity to the level of the heart is indicated.
  - Frequent close monitoring by physical examination and repeated pressure measurements as necessary are critical.
- In patients presenting late with aseptic muscle necrosis, acute fasciotomy and débridement may not be indicated.

SURGICAL MANAGEMENT

Preoperative Planning

- The surgeon should review radiographs and plan for surgical stabilization as necessary.

Positioning

- The patient is positioned supine on the operating table with the upper extremity on an arm board.
- Tourniquets are not routinely used during decompressive fasciotomy.
- If the arm is affected, the shoulder and axilla are included in the sterile field to allow exposure to the entire extremity.

Approach

- Skin is considered a significant compressive structure, and it is important to create a skin incision of sufficient length to allow complete decompression. Cosmesis is not a concern.
- Incisions are planned to afford complete and rapid decompression of the compartments while maintaining coverage of vital structures and avoiding joint contractures due to scarring.
- The viability of muscles is determined by muscle tone and color, contractility, and bleeding.
  - If the viability is still unclear, the muscle should be left alone and reinspected in 24 to 48 hours.
- The skin is left open, and the wounds are copiously irrigated and covered with wet saline dressings. Occasionally, a wound vacuum dressing can be applied to facilitate care and reduce edema and pain associated with frequent dressing changes.
- Once the wound is considered to be stable and clean, the skin can be closed if under no tension. If tension is present, split-thickness skin grafts are usually applied.

TECHNIQUES

Decompression of the Arm

- Compartment syndrome of the arm is rare. It can be approached from the lateral, posterior, or anteromedial approach.
  - The choice of incision may be based on the need for fracture fixation.[1,2]
- The lateral approach begins at the deltoid insertion and extends to the lateral epicondyle. The fascia overlying the biceps anteriorly and triceps posteriorly is split through the incision (**TECH FIG 1A**).
- The anteromedial approach extends from the medial epicondyle toward the axilla, and the fascia overlying the biceps and triceps is split (**TECH FIG 1B**). This incision can be continued from the forearm skin incisions.
  - The ulnar nerve must be protected in this approach.
- For isolated posterior compartment syndrome, a posterior incision can be made from 8 cm distal to the acromion to the olecranon (**TECH FIG 1C**). The triceps fascia is directly exposed and incised.[5]
  - The radial nerve runs between the long and lateral heads of the triceps and is at risk during muscle débridement.

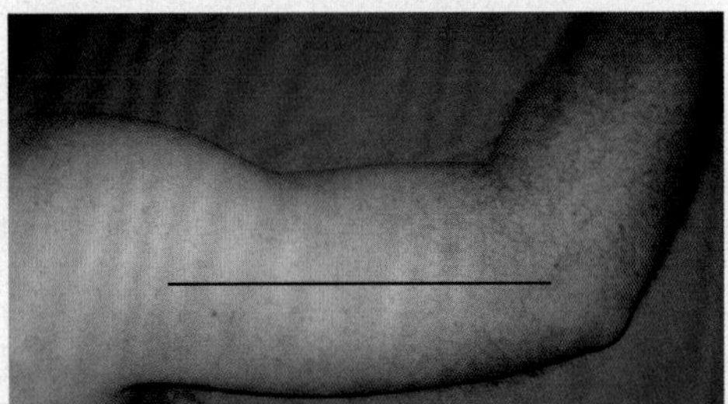

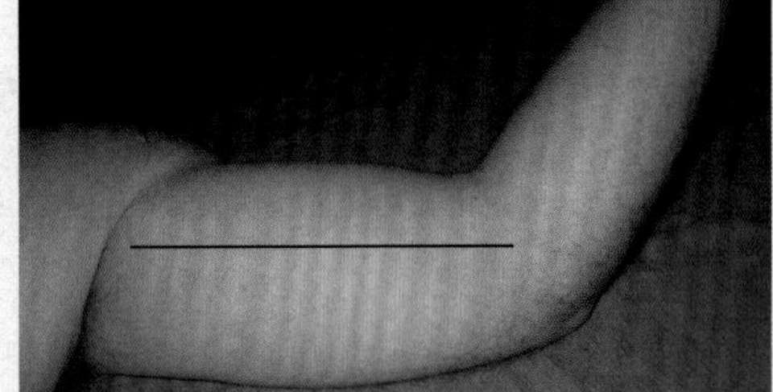

TECH FIG 1 • **A.** Lateral approach to the arm. **B.** Anteromedial approach to the arm. *(continued)*

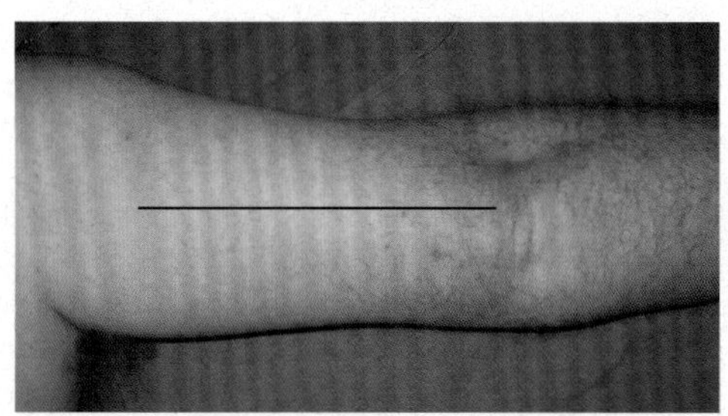

TECH FIG 1 • *(continued)* **C.** Posterior approach to the arm.

Decompression of the Volar Forearm

- Design a curvilinear incision from the carpal tunnel to the antecubital fossa. A complete carpal tunnel release is indicated if symptoms of median nerve compression are present (**TECH FIG 2**).
- Start the incision distally between the thenar and hypothenar eminences in line with the radial border of the ring finger. Release the skin, palmar fascia, and transverse carpal ligament.
- Continue the incision proximally to the distal wrist crease, then curve it ulnarly to the pisiform and extend it proximally along the ulnar side of the distal forearm.
  - This prevents exposure of the flexor tendons and median nerve and protects the palmar cutaneous branch of the median nerve.
- Curve the incision radially in the midforearm and then just anterior to the medial epicondyle at the elbow.
  - Creation of this flap provides coverage of the median nerve.
- At the antecubital fossa, curve the incision slightly anteriorly to meet the incision of the arm, if necessary.
  - This prevents a linear incision at the level of the elbow and provides coverage for the brachial artery.
- Release the fascia covering the superficial and deep compartment of the forearm, as well as the mobile wad, through this incision. Release the lacertus fibrosus at the elbow. Release individual muscle fascia if release of the compartment fascia does not relieve the pressure within each muscle.
- Loosely close the wound over the carpal tunnel; it is generally left open over the forearm.
  - If the swelling is mild, the fascia may be left open and the skin closed or the skin edges may be approximated with a vessel loop-stapling technique.
  - If the wound is left open, it is covered with a sterile nonocclusive dressing. Alternatively, a vacuum-assisted closure (VAC) dressing may be applied.
- An alternative incision uses the Henry approach between the brachioradialis and the flexor carpi radialis, connecting to the carpal tunnel distally and proximally, crossing the antecubital fossa obliquely from radial to ulnar.
  - If this approach is used, take care not to injure the palmar cutaneous branch of the median nerve at the wrist.

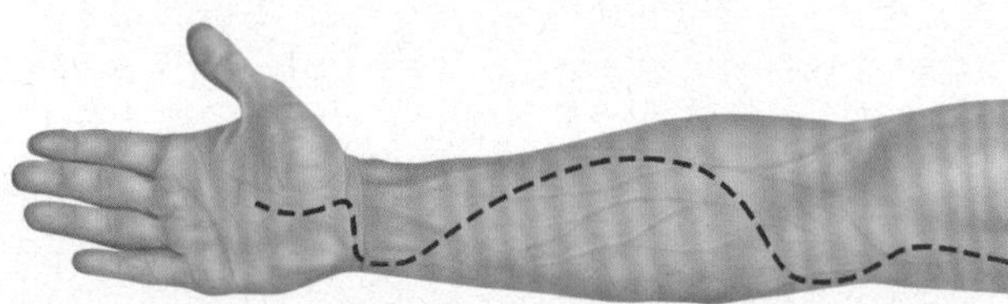

TECH FIG 2 • Incision for decompression of the palmar forearm. Note the incision in the hand used here for release of the thenar compartment.

Decompression of the Dorsal Forearm

- In the forearm, release of the volar compartment and mobile wad may decrease the pressure in the dorsal compartment. Once the palmar fasciotomy has been performed, the dorsal compartment should be reevaluated for the need for fasciotomy.
- Make a longitudinal dorsal incision just ulnar to the tubercle of Lister and extending proximally toward the lateral epicondyle. Release the fascia over the dorsal compartment (**TECH FIG 3**).
- Release individual muscle fascia if necessary.
- If posterior interosseous nerve involvement is suspected, separate the extensor carpi ulnaris and extensor digitorum communis muscles to expose and release the fascia overlying the supinator.
- The wound is managed in a similar way to that described for the volar forearm fasciotomy.

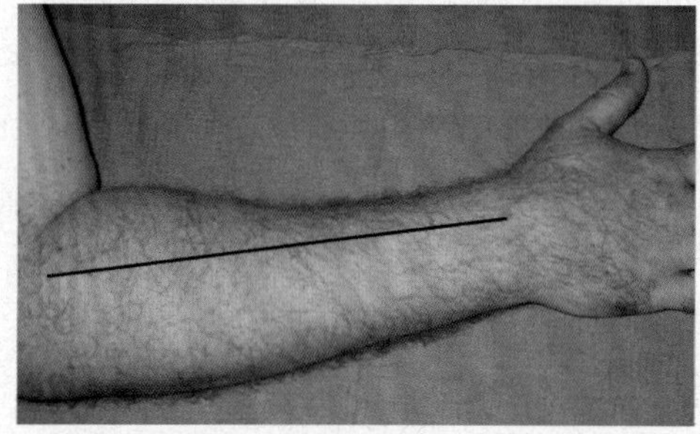

TECH FIG 3 • Incision for approach to the dorsal forearm.

Decompression of the Hand Compartments

- To release the four dorsal and three palmar interosseous compartments and the adductor compartment, make two dorsal longitudinal incisions over the second and fourth metacarpals (**TECH FIG 4A**).
- Take the incisions to the level of the extensor tendons. Avoid the sensory branches of the radial and ulnar nerves, and preserve dorsal veins to minimize postoperative edema.
- Retract the extensor tendons and the dorsal surface of the metacarpal. Release the dorsal compartments on each side of the metacarpal (the first and second dorsal compartments are reached on either side of the second metacarpal, and the third and fourth dorsal compartments are found on either side of the fourth metacarpal). Continue blunt dissection palmarly through the dorsal interosseous to release the three palmar interosseous compartments.
- Release the adductor compartment through the incision over the second metacarpal.
- Release the thenar compartment through a longitudinal incision along the radial border of the thumb metacarpal, and release the hypothenar compartment through an incision along the ulnar border of the fifth metacarpal (**TECH FIG 4B**). Split the underlying fascia longitudinally.
- The wounds are left open (**TECH FIG 4C**) and the hand is placed in a bulky splint in intrinsic-plus position (metacarpophalangeal joints flexed 70 degrees and interphalangeal joints extended).

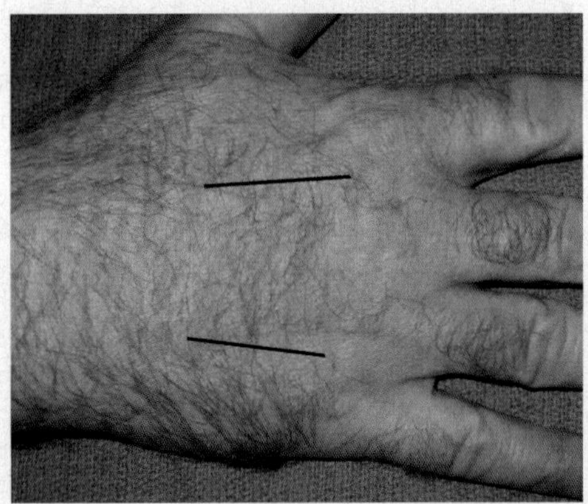
A

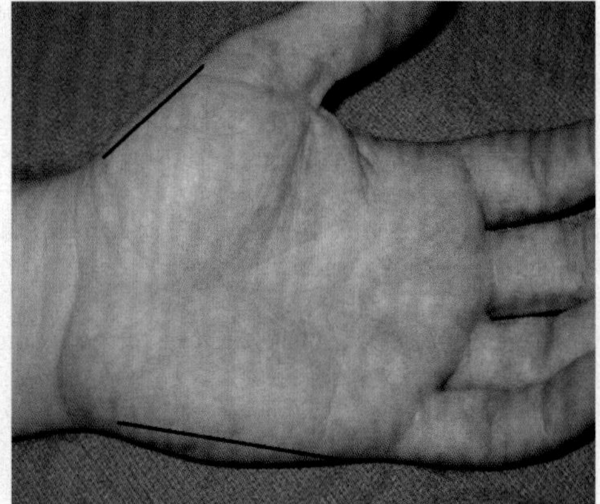
B

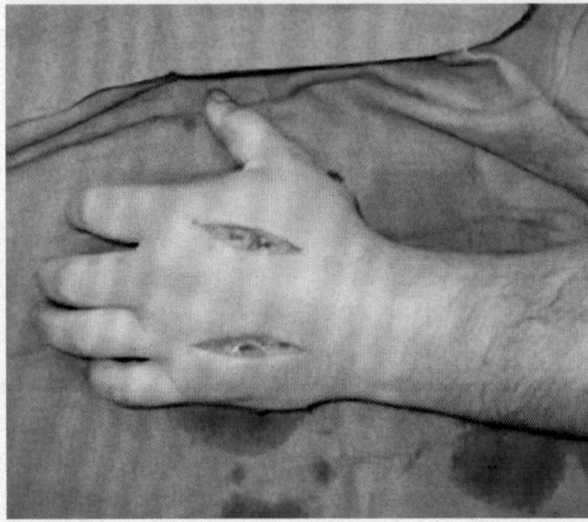
C

TECH FIG 4 • Incisions for the release of the hand compartments. **A.** Dorsal. **B.** Thenar and hypothenar. **C.** Incisions over dorsal, thenar, and hypothenar compartments. These incisions were left open.

Decompression of the Finger

- Make longitudinal midaxial incisions along the finger. These incisions are made by connecting the most dorsal portions of the joint flexion creases (**TECH FIG 5A**). These are more easily seen with the finger in flexion.
- Avoid making a more palmar, midlateral incision to prevent postoperative flexion contracture.
- Carefully divide the transverse retinacular ligament and Cleland ligament to release the neurovascular bundles on both radial and ulnar sides (**TECH FIG 5B**).
- If possible, loosely approximate the skin.

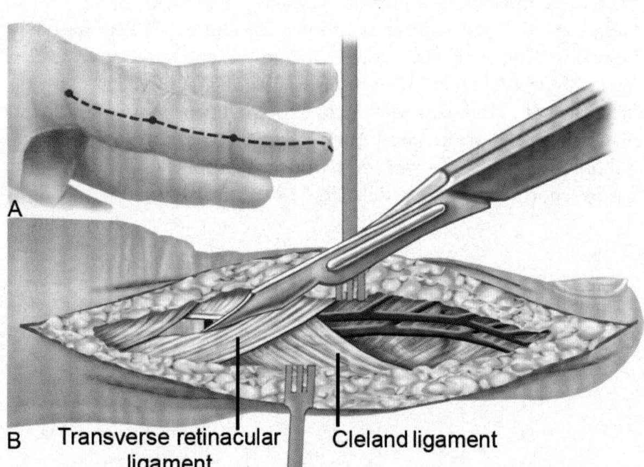

TECH FIG 5 • **A.** Incision for the release of the finger. *Dots* are placed at the apex of each flexion crease and connecting the dots provides the midaxial line. **B.** Division of the transverse retinacular ligament and Cleland ligament.

PEARLS AND PITFALLS

Indications	■ Have a low threshold for measurement of compartment pressures. Perform pressure measurements if clinical examination findings are equivocal.
Surgical management	■ Take care to completely decompress the skin and fascia. ■ Do not injure superficial nerves. ■ Débride any devitalized muscle. ■ Do not close the fascia. ■ Close the skin loosely or leave it open at the initial procedure.
Postoperative management	■ Return to the operating room for a second look if there is muscle of questionable viability. ■ Base closure of the wounds on the skin tension and viability. Choose delayed primary closure, split-thickness skin grafting, or flaps as appropriate.

POSTOPERATIVE CARE

- A second look is planned 48 to 72 hours after the index procedure.
  - Additional débridement of devitalized tissue is performed. Serial débridements are performed until no devitalized tissue remains.
  - Delayed primary closure of the skin (not fascia) may be possible. More frequently, split-thickness skin grafting is performed to cover the wounds (**FIG 3**). If significant soft tissue has been lost with exposed tendon, nerve, or bone, flap coverage is planned.
- Wound coverage should be performed as soon as possible to minimize complications such as infection, desiccation, and amputation.
- The upper extremity should be elevated and splinted in an intrinsic-plus position. Gentle active and active-assisted range of motion of the hand, wrist, and elbow should be initiated as soon as swelling begins to subside, generally within 2 to 3 days after wound closure. Placement of a flap or skin graft may preclude motion at certain joints, but unaffected joints should be ranged.

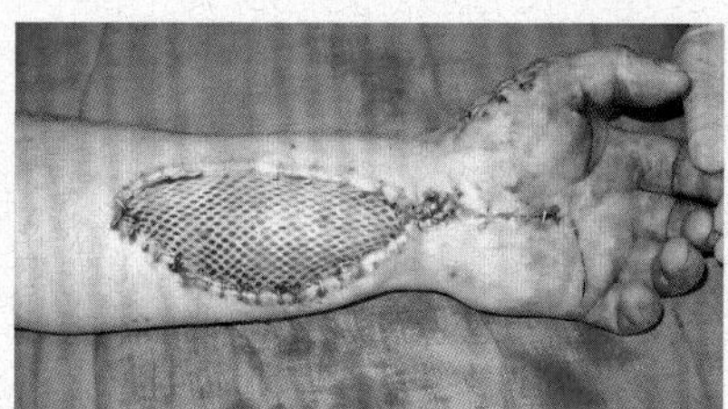

FIG 3 • Wound coverage after second look with delayed primary closure and split-thickness skin grafting.

OUTCOMES

- The outcome after compartment release depends both on the severity of the initial injury and the time elapsed before release.
- Patients with prompt diagnosis and treatment and limited devitalized tissues generally have favorable outcomes.
- Patients with severe initial injuries, delayed treatment, or extensive tissue necrosis have a more guarded prognosis for functional recovery of the upper extremity.

COMPLICATIONS

- Volkmann ischemic contracture is the result of untreated acute compartment syndrome.
- Necrosis and fibrosis of the muscle occur, with a resultant claw hand deformity. This deformity is due to extrinsic flexor and extensor contracture with concomitant intrinsic muscle dysfunction.
- Nerve dysfunction results either from the initial ischemic injury or from subsequent compressive neuropathy due to the dense scarring of the tissues surrounding the nerves.

- The deeper compartments are more severely compromised, with the flexor digitorum profundus alone affected in milder cases, and fibrosis of all muscles in the most severe.

REFERENCES

1. Antebi E, Herscovici D Jr. Acute compartment syndrome of the upper arm: a report of 2 cases. Am J Orthop 2005;34:498–500.
2. Diminick M, Shapiro G, Cornell C. Acute compartment syndrome of the triceps and deltoid. J Orthop Trauma 1999;13:225–227.
3. Gulgonen A. Compartment syndrome. In: Green DP, Pederson WC, Hotchkiss RN, et al, eds. Green's Operative Hand Surgery, ed 5. New York: Elsevier Churchill Livingstone, 2005:1985–2006.
4. Whitesides E, Heckman MW. Acute compartment syndrome: update on diagnosis and treatment. J Am Acad Orthop Surg 1996;4:209–218.
5. Yabuki S, Kikuchi S. Dorsal compartment syndrome of the upper arm: a case report. Clin Orthop Relat Res 1999;(366):107–109.

Surgical Treatment of Injection Injuries in the Hand

125 CHAPTER

Joshua Choo, Rimma Finkel, and Morton Kasdan

DEFINITION

- Injuries caused by high-pressure injection equipment, which can generate pressures of 2000 to 12,000 pound per square inch (psi),[9] are more than sufficient force to break the skin.[15]
- Substances typically injected include grease, paint, paint thinners, diesel fuel, oil, water, and cement. Cases involving molten metal,[3] dry cleaning solvents,[11] and veterinary vaccines[5] have also been documented.
- Hallmark of injury is an innocuous-appearing superficial wound that can greatly underestimate the true extent of injury (**FIG 1**).
- The three most important determinants of morbidity are the (1) type of substance injected, (2) anatomic location of injury, and (3) delay in treatment.
- Treatment of injection injuries is urgent and thorough surgical débridement.
- High-pressure injection injuries occur most frequently in young men, particularly among those who are manual laborers.
- Previously, it was thought that most of these injuries occurred to people who had been on the job for less than 6 months, but more recent studies show that the mean time on the job was 11 years.[12,32]
- Typical scenarios include grasping pressurized tubing in which there is a break in the seal or attempting to unclog the nozzle of a high-pressure injector with the guard removed (**FIG 2**).
- With the increasing use of power contrast injection in computed tomography (CT), contrast extravasation injuries may be classified under injection injuries of the upper extremity. However, the pressures involved are generally much lower (100 psi),[33] the associated injuries are more proximal, and the natural history is generally benign, with surgery rarely being required.

ANATOMY

- Quick facts
  - The nondominant hand (58% to 76%)[8,12] is injured more often than the dominant hand.
  - The index finger, thumb, palm, and small finger are afflicted in descending order.
  - The site of injection is an important determining factor in predicting the zone of deep injury and morbidity.
- Experimental reproductions of high-pressure injections have shown that the anatomic location of entry is an important factor in predicting the distribution of injury:
  - Eccentric sites of injury tend to bypass the palmar tissue and result in dorsal involvement.
  - Injections in the tough glabrous skin overlying and the thicker portions of the fibrous flexor sheaths (annular pulleys) of the finger (midphalanx) tend to be deflected circumferentially in the superficial tissue, as the flexor sheath is less likely to be penetrated.
  - Injection sites in the skin creases, that is, thinner parts of the flexor sheath (cruciate pulleys) overlying the distal or proximal interphalangeal joint, are more likely to result in penetration of the flexor sheath and proximal spread through the tenosynovial space.
  - Injuries that penetrate the tenosynovial space of the index, long, and ring fingers do not spread beyond the distal palmar crease; injuries to these fingers are more likely to be concentrated in the finger itself and cause local inflammation and ischemia.[15,16]
  - In contrast, the tenosynovial sheaths of the thumb and little finger extend into the proximal palm via the radial and

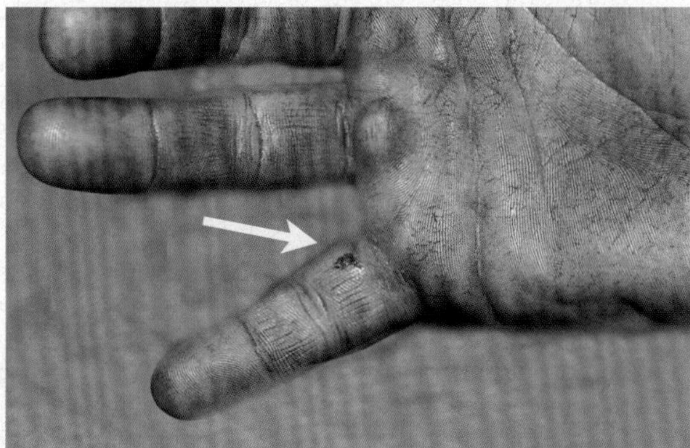

FIG 1 • An innocuous-appearing puncture of the volar radial surface of the right small finger. This may be the only visible point of injury in a high-pressure injection injury.

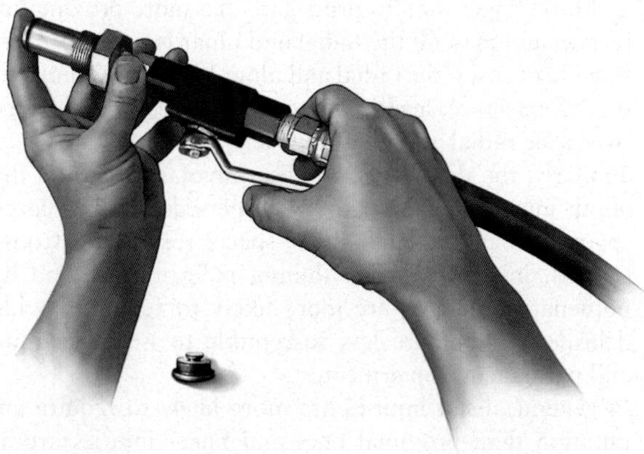

FIG 2 • Injury commonly occurs to the nondominant hand while attempting to clean the nozzle of a high-pressure injector. Note that the nozzle guard has been removed.

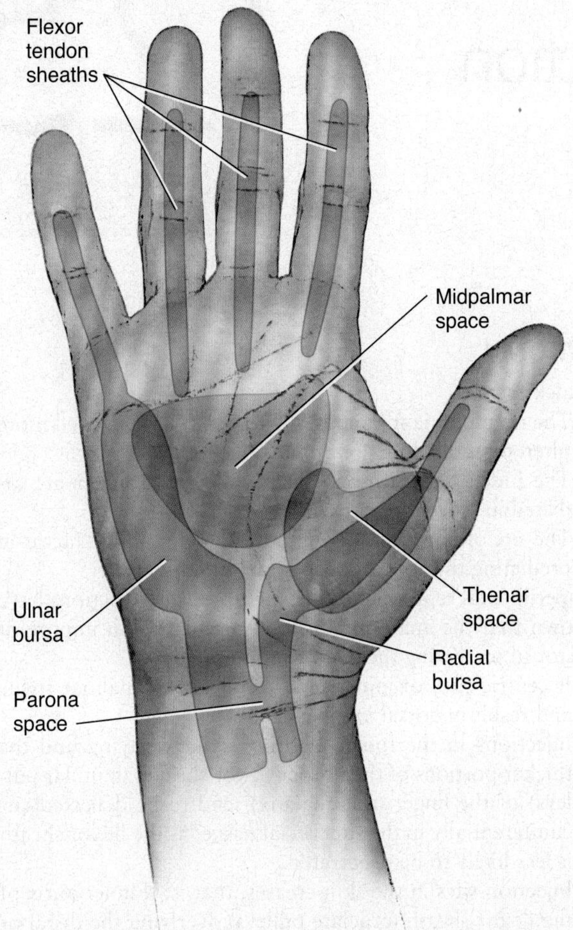

FIG 3 • Synovial spaces (*blue*) and deep myofascial spaces (*green* and *orange*) of the hand. Note the synovial sheaths of the small finger and thumb extend to the ulnar and radial bursae, respectively, whereas the synovial spaces of the index, middle, and ring fingers are confined to the digits. Note also the potential deep spaces of the hand, the midpalmar space (*green*) and the thenar space (*orange*). Not shown is the hypothenar space. In 85% of patients, a communication between the ulnar and radial bursae exists, as shown here.

ulnar bursae and may communicate with the myofascial spaces of the palm (**FIG 3**).[15] Thus, injections in the thumb and little finger tend to propagate in a more proximal direction and may fill the radial and ulnar bursae.
  - In 85% of cases, the radial and ulnar bursae are connected by Parona space, leading to potential spread of injury between the radial and ulnar bursae.[21]
  - Similarly, the palm contains deep myofascial spaces that allow injected material to be dispersed within a larger space (thenar and midpalmar space; see **FIG 3**). Consequently, injections in the thumb, palm, thenar, and hypothenar eminences are more likely to require a wider débridement but are less susceptible to ischemic injury and permanent impairment.
  - In general, distal injuries are more likely to require amputation than proximal ones and finger injuries are associated with higher morbidity and amputation rates than thumb or palm injuries.[14]
- The anatomic studies on which many of these observations were made used pressures of 750 psi. Injections at much higher pressures may be enough to overcome tissue resistance, leading to less predictable patterns of injury.

PATHOGENESIS

- Two key pathogenic mechanisms are responsible for the morbidity of high-pressure injuries: (1) mechanical injury directly resulting from the injected material, which is a function of viscosity, velocity, and volume, and (2) the inflammatory host response, which is a function of the irritant/chemical properties of the injected material.
- The degree of mechanical injury has been shown to be inversely proportional to the viscosity of the material and proportional to the volume of material delivered and the pressure at which it was delivered.[9,13,27] For example, injected material with relatively low viscosity, such as paint thinner,[10] has been shown to result in wider zones of injury and greater morbidity.
- The type of inflammatory response incited by the injected material also has an important effect on degree of injury. Only rare cases of water or air injection have been found to result in amputation. In contrast, organic solvents such as oil paint have been found to have a 10-fold increased incidence of amputation compared to other materials such as hydraulic fluid or grease (58% vs. 6%). The inflammatory response to various materials is clearly different.[14]
- Controversy continues as to which aspect dominates in these injuries; however, they are more likely synergistic, with the inflammatory response compounding the mechanical injury.
- Time elapsed before intervention has a major influence on prognosis (see Natural History, next section). Most agree that surgery should be done within 6 hours after injury to decrease morbidity.[29]

NATURAL HISTORY

- The natural history of high-pressure injuries can be divided into three stages.
  - Acute stage
    - The *acute stage* occurs immediately.
    - The injection causes external compression and spasm of the vessels, leading to compromised blood flow that is manifested by white, mottled tissue; numbness; severe pain; or a combination of these findings.
    - Any initial paresthesias that occur are due to local compression or chemical irritation of the involved nerves.
    - During this stage, the site of injection is key in determining where the material has spread.
    - The volume of material injected also determines the degree of tissue distention and impairment of blood flow.
    - In several studies by Gelberman et al,[9] Schoo et al,[27] and Hayes and Pan,[13] patients with hands that had higher volume injections and longer time to decompression had higher morbidity rates.
  - Intermediate stage
    - During the *intermediate stage*, a foreign body reaction induces granuloma formation and fibrosis.
    - Severity of inflammation that occurs is determined by the volume and type of substance.
    - Injection of paint solvent has a significantly higher morbidity due to its low viscosity, allowing diffusion through the soft tissues. Its corrosive effects cause severe tissue necrosis.[9]

- Grease injections have more chronic inflammatory reactions, leading to prolonged sequelae (foreign body granulomas).[13,28]
- Schoo et al[27] reported that amputation rates associated with various injection injuries were as follows: paint thinner, 80%; paint (soya alkyl base), 58%; automotive grease, 23%; and hydraulic fluid, 14%.

- Late stage
  - Late stage of injury occurs when the granulomas break open, resulting in draining sinuses and cutaneous lesions.[8,27]
  - Chronic sinuses may degenerate into malignancies (squamous epithelioma).[8]
  - Secondary infections may occur in this stage; these may be due to *Staphylococcus aureus*, *Streptococcus epidermidis*, *Pseudomonas* spp., or a variety of polymicrobial flora.[24,26]

PATIENT HISTORY AND PHYSICAL FINDINGS

- Important information includes hand dominance and occupation, sequence of events postinjury, and type of injector and pressure as well as substance injected.
- Comorbidities, including vascular disease, diabetes, and smoking history, are relevant risk factors that influence healing and posttreatment function.[19]
- If possible, a Material Safety Data Sheet (MSDS) for the substance injected should be obtained from the company or online at http://www.msdsonline.com.
- Physical examination should include the following:
  - Determining location of puncture site to determine spread of injected material. It is not uncommon for the site of injury to be small and difficult to find.
  - Observing range of motion when the patient attempts to form a fist
  - Palpation of the digit, hand, and arm to help determine the extent of required débridement

IMAGING AND OTHER DIAGNOSTIC STUDIES

- Radiographs of the hand and forearm are helpful in evaluating the extent of injury.
- Although not all injected substances are radiopaque, air may be present in the compartments of the hand and forearm, which may help in determining how far the substance has traveled.[23,24,31]
- It may be necessary to obtain radiographs of the arm and chest. Extension into the arm, chest wall, and mediastinum from injuries to the hand has been reported.[30]
- Imaging studies also document preexisting pathology.

DIFFERENTIAL DIAGNOSIS

- Snake bite
- Spider bite
- Crush injury
- Suppurative tenosynovitis
- Black thorn tenosynovitis
- *Mycobacterium marina* infection (chronic)

NONOPERATIVE MANAGEMENT

- Most injuries require surgical débridement, and there are only few case reports of nonoperative management for such injuries.
- Cases managed without surgery include air injection into the hand, which leads to subcutaneous emphysema that resolves within hours to days[18] or, occasionally, water injection in an otherwise clean environment may be managed conservatively in some cases.[17]

SURGICAL MANAGEMENT

- Early and aggressive decompression and débridement of all tissues is the cornerstone of treatment. Some authors also include amputation as a major treatment modality.
- The time from injury to surgery is the major determinant of morbidity and prognosis in high-pressure injection injuries.[29]

Preoperative Planning

- Radiographic studies should be reviewed.
  - Attention should be paid to radiopaque areas of the hand and forearm.
  - Air in the soft tissue should be evaluated.
  - Bones should be evaluated for any possible fractures or preexisting lesions.
- Intravenous (IV) lines should be placed in the patient's noninjured extremity, and manipulation of the injured extremity should be limited.

Positioning

- Patient should be placed supine with the arm abducted.
- Arm should not be exsanguinated with an Esmarch bandage to avoid proximal spread of injected material and further trauma to the tissues.
- Regional nerve block can be used, if necessary.
  - If an IV regional (Bier) block is selected, gravity exsanguination is performed without a compression wrap but with 4 minutes of elevation.

Approach

- High-pressure injection injuries must be approached with a view to expose and débride all particulate matter.
- Incisions must follow the general principle of avoiding longitudinal incisions across flexion creases.
- Débridement of the neurovascular bundle, if affected, must be done with extreme caution. Some particulate matter may be left behind in order to preserve vital structures.
- All suspected compartments should be opened and explored.

Bruner Incision

- Hand is prepped and exsanguinated by elevation.
- For longitudinal exposure of the digits, it is important to avoid crossing joint creases in a straight line. This is accomplished by creating diagonal Bruner incisions at joint creases (**TECH FIG 1a**).
- Injectate is removed, avoiding the neurovascular bundles located on the radial and volar ulnar surfaces of the digits.
- Incision is continued into the palm and wrist, if necessary (**TECH FIG 1a,b**). Palmar incisions also are placed in such a manner as to gain access into the thenar or hypothenar compartments in continuity and to avoid postoperative contractures (**TECH FIG 1a,d**).
- If extension is necessary proximal to the wrist crease, the incision should be angled away from midline to avoid injury to the palmar sensory branch of the median nerve (see **TECH FIG 1**).
- Extension onto the forearm may be longitudinal or in an S curve, if compartment decompression is necessary (see **TECH FIG 1**).

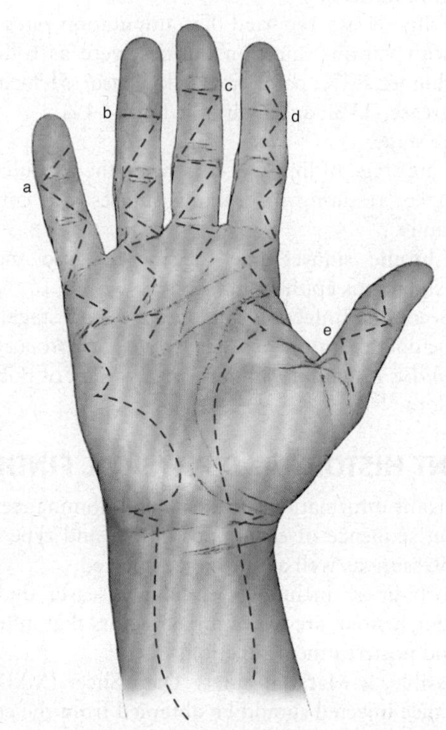

TECH FIG 1 • Various incisions for débridement. All are based on the principle of avoiding longitudinal incisions over flexion creases. (*a*) Bruner incision, extended in continuity with the ulnar bursae and forearm. (*b,c*) Mixed diagonal and transverse incisions. (*d*) Littler incision, extended in continuity with the thenar space and radial bursae. (*e*) Bruner incision of the thumb, which may be extended to the radial bursae and forearm as needed.

Midaxial Incision

- In some cases, longitudinal midaxial incisions are made on the digit, radially and ulnarly.
  - These incisions are made dorsal to the neurovascular bundles (**TECH FIG 2**).
  - Incision across the palm continues as described for Bruner incision.[2]

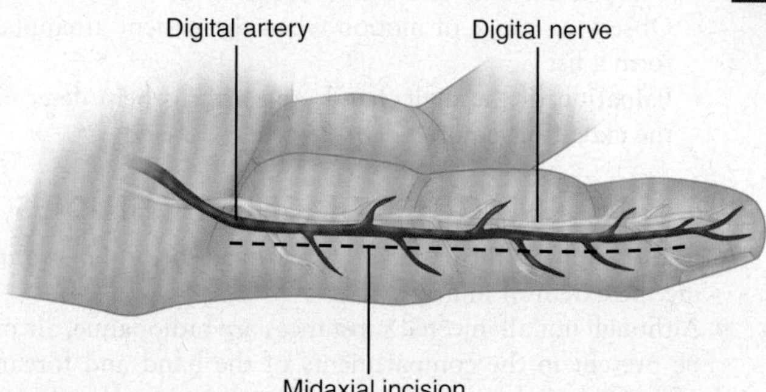

TECH FIG 2 • Midaxial incision of the finger. This sacrifices the dorsal branches of the neurovascular bundle, but the digital nerve and artery are protected.

Other Incisions

- Other diagonal incisions may be used. These are similar to Bruner incision in that they adhere to the principle of avoiding crossing a flexion crease longitudinally. Littler incision (see **FIG 1D**) does not provide as wide as an exposure of the finger but minimizes exposure of the tendon sheath.
- A mixed diagonal–transverse-type incision may also be used in these cases. A transverse incision is made parallel to the flexion crease and the next interphalangeal incision is another oblique Bruner incision (see **TECH FIG 1c**).
- This is continued along the length of the digit onto the palm.
- The authors use a mixed diagonal–transverse incision that is similar to the one described in **TECH FIG 1b**. This technique allows for loose closure of the incision along the creases while allowing drainage along the oblique incisions.

PEARLS AND PITFALLS

- Understand that the underlying pathology will usually be worse than the external wound.
- Managing comorbidities are important in the care of patients with injection injuries.
- Obtain the MSDS to understand the toxic effects of the injected material. This can be obtained from the manufacturer or online at http://www.msdsonline.com.
- Exploration should extend to clearly healthy tissue. Avoid "minimally invasive" treatment.
- Leave the wound open or very loosely closed.

POSTOPERATIVE CARE

- The wound should be left open and packed or very loosely closed. The hand should then be splinted in the "safe" position (**FIG 4AB**).
- Any additional débridement should be performed at 48-hour intervals, as necessary, until the wound can be primarily closed or covered (**FIG 4C**).
  - Less involved injuries often are allowed to heal by secondary intention, especially if critical structures are covered.
  - Occasionally, free tissue transfer may be necessary for coverage.[4,6]
- The use of parenteral corticosteroids to decrease the inflammatory response postoperatively has not been proven, although animal studies have shown a possible benefit in cases where an organic solvent was injected.
  - Although neither animal data nor human clinical findings show such an increase, there is also a concern for increased infection risk.
  - No convincing human studies have been published that show that corticosteroids are effective in limiting tissue loss, and they should be used cautiously.[14]
- Early range-of-motion exercises are important to reduce the risk of stiffness and should be done prior to wound healing.

OUTCOMES

- Outcomes of high-pressure injection injuries are based on the volume, pressure, and kinetic properties of the injected material, resistance of the tissues and other anatomic features of the site of injury, toxicity of the material, and time to surgery.
- Morbidity includes cold intolerance, hypersensitivity, paresthesias, constant pain, infection, oleoma formation (**FIG 5A**), squamous degeneration,[27] and amputation.
- Amputation rates ranging from 14% to 88% have been reported in the literature.[13,22,27]
  - Highest amputation rates are associated with organic solvent injection into the fingers.[14]

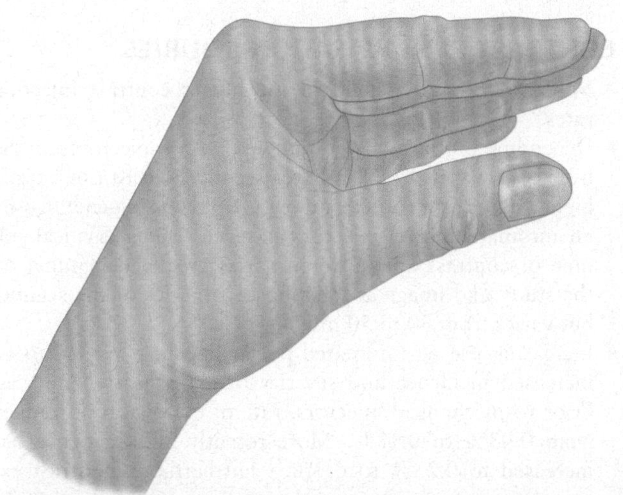
A

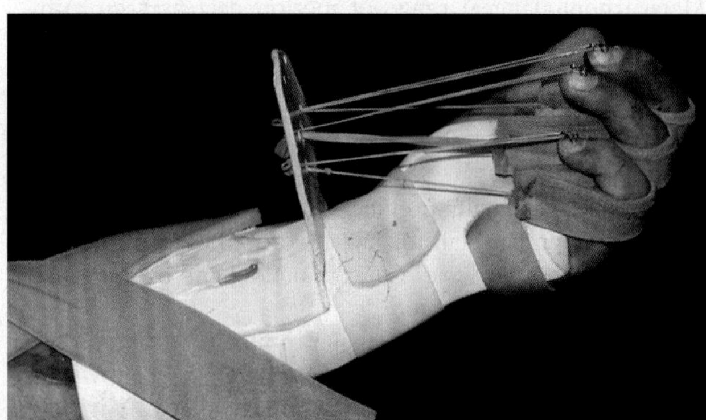
B

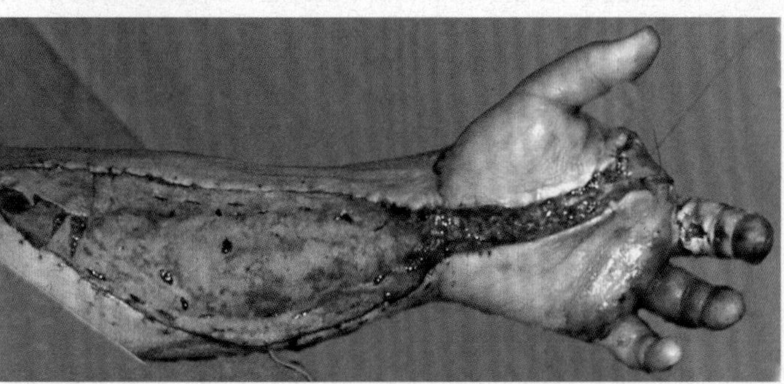
C

FIG 4 • **A.** The safe position for postoperative splinting. The wrist is slightly extended, the metacarpophalangeal joints are fully flexed, and the interphalangeal joints are fully extended. **B.** Dynamic splinting of the hand in flexion to allow for early mobilization. **C.** Primary and split-thickness skin graft closure of a wound after final débridement.

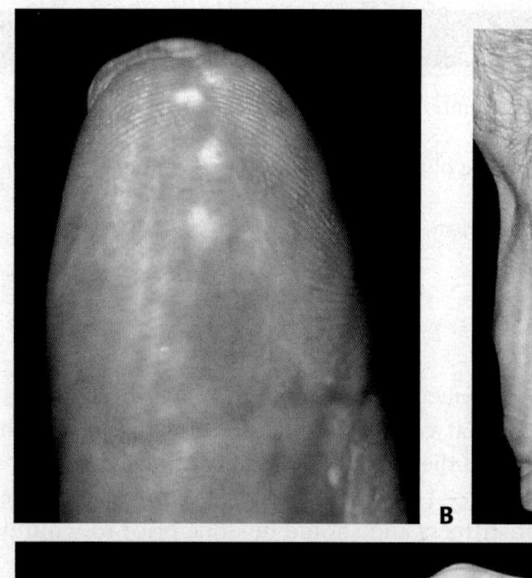

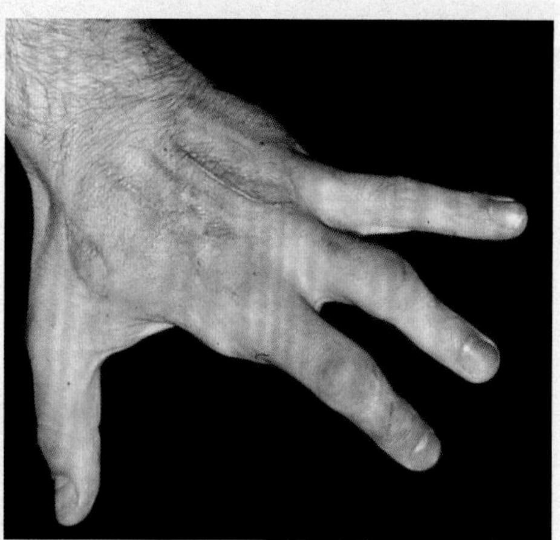

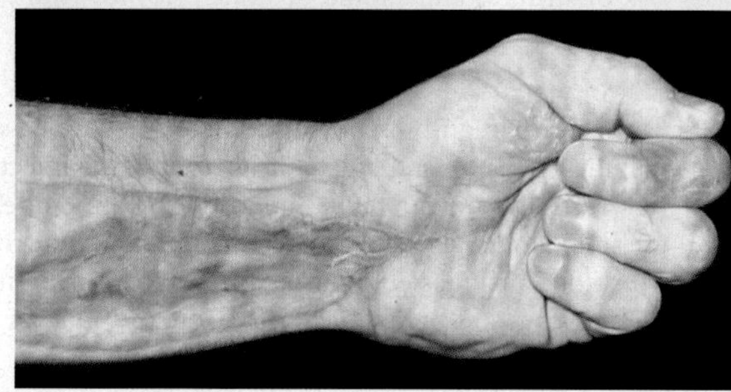

FIG 5 • A. Oleoma formation after débridement and closure of a digital high-pressure injection. The well-healed longitudinal incision on the volar surface of the digit is surrounded by yellow lesions, consistent with oleomas. **B,C.** Well-healed primary closures and split-thickness skin grafts of the volar and dorsal hand and forearm. There is full range of motion of the remaining digits after amputation of the index finger.

- In this subset of patients, time to débridement has a significant impact on amputation rate.
  - Even if surgery occurs within 6 hours of injury, the amputation rate is 40%.
  - If the surgery is delayed for more than 6 hours, the amputation rate increases to 57%.
  - If débridement is delayed to more than 1 week after injury, the amputation rate is 88%.[14]
- Metacarpophalangeal range of motion decreases an average of 8.1%, proximal interphalangeal range of motion decreases 23.9%, and distal interphalangeal range of motion decreases by 29.7%.
  - Maximum grip strength diminishes by 12% and pinch strength decreases by 35%.
  - Two-point discrimination increases by 49%[32] (**FIG 5B,C**).
- The average impairment for injuries caused by spray guns is 15%, by pneumatic hoses is less than 2%, and by hydraulic fluid is 6%.[31]
- If treatment is delayed more than 6 hours after injury, then permanent impairment rate is approximately 17%; however, if treatment is obtained in under 6 hours, that rate is only 4%.[31]
- Loss of work related to these injuries also varies, from 6 to 26 weeks, with about 92% of patients returning to their previous jobs.[13]

COMPLICATIONS

- Infection
- Cold intolerance
- Hypersensitivity
- Oleoma formation
- Malignant degeneration
- Decreased range of motion and function
- Paresthesias
- Diminished two-point discrimination
- Amputation

CONTRAST EXTRAVASATION INJURIES

- Modern CT studies tend to use higher contrast injection rates.[20]
- Depending on the study, automated power injectors can deliver contrast at 4 to 5 mL per second, two to three times higher than for a routine survey CT. Pressures generated by an automated power injector can reach 100 psi. Typical volume of contrast administered varies greatly depending on the study and image acquisition capabilities of the scanner but varies from 30 to 50 mL.[33]
- Increasing use of automated power injectors has led to an increased incidence and severity of extravasation injuries. Prior to mechanical injectors, rate of extravasation ranged from 0.03% to 0.17%. More recently, the incidence has increased to 0.25% to 0.9%.[33] Furthermore, contrast extravasations from automated pressure injectors tend to be higher volume. Accordingly, approximately 60% of contrast extravasations involve volumes greater than 50 mL.[25]
- Pathogenesis of extravasation injuries involve multiple factors, such as (1) volume of contrast extravasation, (2) increased osmolality associated with contrast, and (3) cytotoxic effect of contrast media. The literature shows a general trend toward more severe extravasation injuries with larger volumes of contrast material. The threshold for significant tissue injury from increased osmolality is estimated in the literature to be between 1.025 and 1.420 mOsm/kg water.[1] The higher the osmolality of the contrast, the more fluid is

drawn into the injured tissue, resulting in greater subcutaneous edema. Thirdly, although use of low osmolality nonionic contrast such as iopamidol 300 has decreased the morbidity associated with contrast extravasation,[25] iodinated contrast media is still listed as a vesicant and can cause significant soft tissue injury that manifests as blistering, ulceration, and necrosis.

- The anatomy of the hand and forearm as it relates to the complications of contrast extravasation have not been definitively studied. Similarly, the pathophysiology of compartment syndrome in contrast extravasation has not been clearly established, presumably from the infrequency of this complication. Because the veins used in the extremity for IV access are superficial and proximal, direct infiltration of the muscle compartments or hand involvement is uncommon. It has been the authors' experience that most contrast extravasation injuries involve the subcutaneous tissue and not the muscular compartments. Some authors have suggested that the mechanism of compartment syndrome in contrast extravasation is subcutaneous edema that results in extrinsic compression of the hand or forearm compartments.[7] Usually, patient comorbidities such as collagen vascular disease and peripheral vascular disease are potentiating factors.
- In the workup of the patient with contrast extravasation, it is important to note the type of contrast given, the estimated volume extravasated, and the IV access site. The presence of collagen vascular disease, peripheral vascular disease, diabetes, and other comorbidities must be determined and documented. The presence of swelling of the forearm and hand, blistering, and erythema must be noted on examination. If compartment syndrome is a concern, the importance of a neurovascular examination and compartment pressure measurements cannot be overemphasized.
- The overwhelming majority of cases reported in the literature resolve without surgical intervention; conservative treatment, in the form of elevation, cold compresses, and interval neurovascular examinations during a period of observation for 24 hours is generally all that is required. However, early signs of compartment syndrome should be vigilantly assessed and the appropriate surgical compartment release performed.

REFERENCES

1. Bellin MF, Jakobsen JA, Tomassin I, et al. Contrast medium extravasation injury: guidelines for prevention and management. Eur Radiol 2002;12(11):2807–2812.
2. Bruner JM. The zig-zag volar-digital incision for flexor-tendon surgery. Plast Reconstr Surg 1967;40(6):571–574.
3. Caddick JF, Rickard RF. A molten metal, high-pressure injection injury of the hand. J Hand Surg Br 2004;29(1):87–89.
4. Chan BK, Tham SK, Leung M. Free toe pulp transfer for digital reconstruction after high-pressure injection injury. J Hand Surg Br 1999;24(5):534–538.
5. Couzens G, Burke FD. Veterinary high pressure injection injuries with inoculations for larger animals. J Hand Surg Br 1995;20(4):497–499.
6. del Pinal F, Herrero F, Jado E, et al. Acute thumb ischemia secondary to high-pressure injection injury: salvage by emergency decompression, radical debridement, and free hallux hemipulp transfer. J Trauma 2001;50(3):571–574.
7. Fallscheer P, Kammer E, Roeren T, et al. Injury to the upper extremity caused by extravasation of contrast medium: a true emergency. Scand J Plast Reconstr Surg Hand Surg 2007;41(1):26–32.
8. Fialkov JA, Freiberg A. High pressure injection injuries: an overview. J Emerg Med 1991;9(5):367–371.
9. Gelberman RH, Posch JL, Jurist JM. High-pressure injection injuries of the hand. J Bone Joint Surg Am 1975;57(7):935–937.
10. Gonzalez R, Kasdan ML. High pressure injection injuries of the hand. Clin Occup Environ Med 2006;5(2):407–411, ix.
11. Gutowski KA, Chu J, Choi M, et al. High-pressure hand injection injuries caused by dry cleaning solvents: case reports, review of the literature, and treatment guidelines. Plast Reconstr Surg 2003;111(1):174–177.
12. Hart RG, Smith GD, Haq A. Prevention of high-pressure injection injuries to the hand. Am J Emerg Med 2006;24(1):73–76.
13. Hayes CW, Pan HC. High-pressure injection injuries to the hand. South Med J 1982;75(12):1491–1498, 1516.
14. Hogan CJ, Ruland RT. High-pressure injection injuries to the upper extremity: a review of the literature. J Orthop Trauma 2006;20(7): 503–511.
15. Kaufman HD. The anatomy of experimentally produced high-pressure injection injuries of the hand. Br J Surg 1968;55(5):340–344.
16. Kaufman HD. The clinicopathological correlation of high-pressure injection injuries. Br J Surg 1968;55(3):214–218.
17. Kon M, Sagi A. High-pressure water jet injury of the hand. J Hand Surg Am 1985;10(3):412–414.
18. Lo SJ, Hughes J, Armstrong A. Non-infective subcutaneous emphysema of the hand secondary to a minor webspace injury. J Hand Surg Br 2005;30(5):482–483.
19. Luber KT, Rehm JP, Freeland AE. High-pressure injection injuries of the hand. Orthopedics 2005;28(2):129–132.
20. Macha DB, Nelson RC, Howle LE, et al. Central venous catheter integrity during mechanical power injection of iodinated contrast medium. Radiology 2009;253(3):870–878.
21. Malenfant J, Walters A, Kralovic S, et al. Francesco Parona (1842-1908) and his contributions to our understanding of surgery through anatomy. Clin Anat 2013;26(5):547–550.
22. Neal NC, Burke FD. High-pressure injection injuries. Injury 1991;22(6):467–470.
23. O'Reilly RJ, Blatt G. Accidental high-pressure injection-gun injuries of the hand; the role of the emergency radiologic examination. J Trauma 1975;15(1):24–31.
24. Pinto MR, Turkula-Pinto LD, Cooney WP, et al. High-pressure injection injuries of the hand: review of 25 patients managed by open wound technique. J Hand Surg Am 1993;18(1):125–130.
25. Sbitany H, Koltz PF, Mays C, et al. CT contrast extravasation in the upper extremity: strategies for management. Int J Surg 2010;8(5): 384–386.
26. Schnall SB, Mirzayan R. High-pressure injection injuries to the hand. Hand Clin 1999;15(2):245–248, viii.
27. Schoo MJ, Scott FA, Boswick JA Jr. High-pressure injection injuries of the hand. J Trauma 1980;20(3):229–238.
28. Sirio CA, Smith JS Jr, Graham WP III. High-pressure injection injuries of the hand. A review. Am Surg 1989;55(12):714–718.
29. Stark HH, Ashworth CR, Boyes JH. Paint-gun injuries of the hand. J Bone Joint Surg Am 1967;49(4):637–647.
30. Temple CL, Richards RS, Dawson WB. Pneumomediastinum after injection injury to the hand. Ann Plast Surg 2000;45(1):64–66.
31. Vasilevski D, Noorbergen M, Depierreux M, et al. High-pressure injection injuries to the hand. Am J Emerg Med 2000;18(7):820–824.
32. Wieder A, Lapid O, Plakht Y, et al. Long-term follow-up of high-pressure injection injuries to the hand. Plast Reconstr Surg 2006;117(1):186–189.
33. Wilson BG. Contrast media-induced compartment syndrome. Radiol Technol 2011;83(1):63–77.

126 CHAPTER

Revascularization and Replantation of the Digits

L. Scott Levin

DEFINITION

- *Replantation* is the reattachment of a completely amputated body part.
- *Revascularization* is the restoration of circulation and repair of all injured structures in an incompletely amputated, dysvascular body part. Revascularization always includes repair of blood vessels to reestablish blood flow to the part.
- *Revision amputation* is the procedure performed at the site of amputation to gain soft tissue coverage and to address concomitant injuries to the digit.
- The decision of whether to perform replantation or revascularization and revision amputation of a digit is multifactorial. The relative indications and contraindications for each are discussed later in the chapter.

ANATOMY

- An understanding of the anatomy over the complete length of the digit is essential for successful replantation. The anatomy of the thumb is different from that of the four fingers.
- Palmar and dorsal cutaneous ligaments maintain the position of the neurovascular bundle during range of motion of the digit.
  - Grayson ligament is palmar to the neurovascular bundle, originates from the flexor tendon sheath, and inserts on the skin.
  - Cleland ligament travels dorsal to the neurovascular bundle from the phalanx to the overlying skin.
- A radial and ulnar proper digital artery supplies each digit. Each vessel travels with a respective radial and ulnar proper digital nerve. At the level of the digit, the artery lies dorsal to the nerve.
- The ulnar digital artery is typically larger in the thumb and index fingers. The radial digital artery usually is larger in the small finger.
  - Three major palmar arches arise from the digital arteries. The proximal, middle, and distal arches are consistently located at the level of the C1 pulley, C3 pulley, and just distal to the flexor digitorum profundus (FDP) insertion, respectively.
  - Four palmar and four dorsal branches usually extend from each digital artery.
- Injection studies have demonstrated that the venous system of the digit consists of a series of arcades on the dorsal and palmar surfaces, with connecting oblique and transverse anastomotic veins.[10] The dorsal veins have a larger caliber than the palmar veins, which do not consistently travel with the digital artery and nerve.
- A radial and ulnar proper digital nerve travels with each proper digital artery. The digital nerve is sensory only and typically contains one to three fascicles. It trifurcates at the level of the distal interphalangeal (DIP) joint.
- Each finger has two flexor tendons within the flexor tendon sheath.
  - The FDP tendon inserts at the proximal base of the distal phalanx.
  - The flexor digitorum superficialis (FDS) tendon inserts as two slips into the midportion of the middle phalanx. The FDS tendon splits into two slips, and its relative position to the FDP tendon switches from palmar to dorsal at Camper chiasm. This allows the deeper FDP tendon to continue to its more distal insertion.
- There are a series of five annular and three cruciform pulleys, which are discrete thickenings of the fibro-osseous sheath. The annular pulleys prevent bowstringing of the flexor tendons during flexion, whereas the cruciate pulleys are collapsible, accommodating flexion.
  - The odd-numbered annular pulleys are located over the joints of the finger, and the even-numbered annular pulleys are over the proximal and middle phalanx, respectively.
  - The A2 and A4 pulleys are most important in preventing bowstringing and should be preserved if possible.
- Each lesser digit receives a tendon from the extensor digitorum communis (EDC). The index and small fingers each have a second extensor tendon, the extensor indicis proprius (EIP) and extensor digiti minimi (EDM), respectively. Both of these tendons are ulnar to the EDC tendons.

PATHOGENESIS

- The mechanism of injury has a considerable effect on the potential for replantation.
- Sharp amputations are ideal for replantation because of the narrow zone of injury.
- The degree of tissue injury increases substantially with crush and avulsion mechanisms and may prohibit successful replantation (**FIG 1**).
- Most digit amputations occur as an isolated injury. When amputations occur in the multiply injured patient, consideration of other systemic injuries and adherence to advanced trauma life support (ATLS) protocols may prevent replantation.

NATURAL HISTORY

- Replantation of an amputated digit results in longer hospital stays and more prolonged rehabilitation than revision amputation. Patient satisfaction, however, usually is higher with replantation than with revision amputation or a prosthesis.[8,11,12]
- Functionally, the expected range of motion in a replanted digit is 50% of normal.
- Secondary procedures, such as tenolysis, are common.
- The literature reports rates of reoperation ranging from 3% to 93%. In a series of more than 1000 replants and

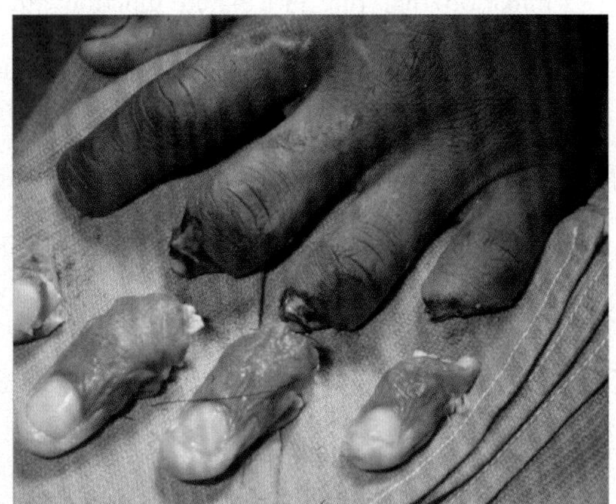

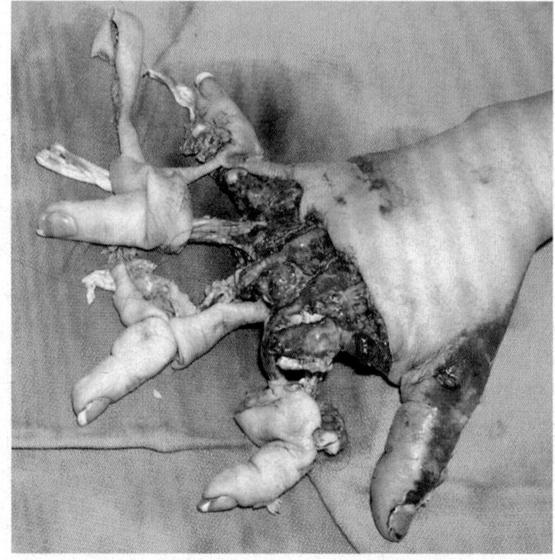

FIG 1 • **A.** This hand sustained sharp amputation of the digits from a table saw. The narrow zone of injury made the digits ideal for replantation. **B.** This hand sustained a crush injury. The resultant wide zone of injury prohibited successful replantation.

revascularizations, 35% of patients required at least one secondary surgery.[18] The incidence is higher for replantations than for revascularizations.

- Expected survival rates of replanted digits are 80% or higher, with even higher survival rates in revascularized digits.

PATIENT HISTORY AND PHYSICAL FINDINGS

- The surgeon must evaluate the patient in the emergency room immediately on arrival. A complete history and physical examination are performed.
- The history should include specific details regarding the mechanism and timing of the injury. Identification of the specific machinery involved often reveals valuable information about potential contamination and the pattern of injury sustained by the amputated part.
- A history of mental instability is relevant because rehabilitation protocols require significant patient compliance to maximize functional outcomes. Furthermore, self-inflicted amputations are unlikely to yield the same functional results after replantation as accidental amputations.
- A history of medical comorbidities should be thoroughly evaluated. Conditions such as diabetes, peripheral vascular disease, hypercoaguability, and tobacco use are not absolute contraindications to replantation but must be considered.
- Similarly, the surgeon must evaluate for medical conditions that prevent the patient from tolerating the blood volume changes associated with major limb replantation. Revision amputation may be the best choice if the patient has a history of previous trauma or arthritis in the amputated part.
- Ischemia time and method of transport should be evaluated for appropriateness. In the digits, a warm ischemia time of less than 6 hours is desired. In more proximal amputations containing muscle, ischemia time is more critical.
  - Cooling the amputated part reduces metabolic acidosis, bacterial growth, and muscle necrosis. Cold ischemia times of up to 12 hours are tolerated for replantation of digits. There are reports of successful replantation of digits with warm ischemia times of 42 hours and cold ischemia times of 96 hours.[2,19]
- Proper transportation of the amputated part is essential. Never place the part directly on ice. The part should be wrapped in a sterile gauze moistened with Ringer lactate or normal saline. The gauze is then placed in a leakproof plastic bag and the bag is placed on ice (**FIG 2**). The temperature should be maintained at approximately 4° C.
  - Alternatively, the part may be immersed in Ringer lactate or normal saline in a plastic bag with the bag then placed on ice.
- The surgeon examines the part and the injured extremity to evaluate suitability for replantation. The number of digits, level of injury, and type of injury are assessed.
- Specifically, the surgeon evaluates the injured parts for the red line sign and the ribbon sign.
  - The *red line sign* refers to a red streak of ecchymosis along the lateral border of the digit, which is the result of hemorrhage from avulsed branches of the digital artery after a traction injury (**FIG 3**).

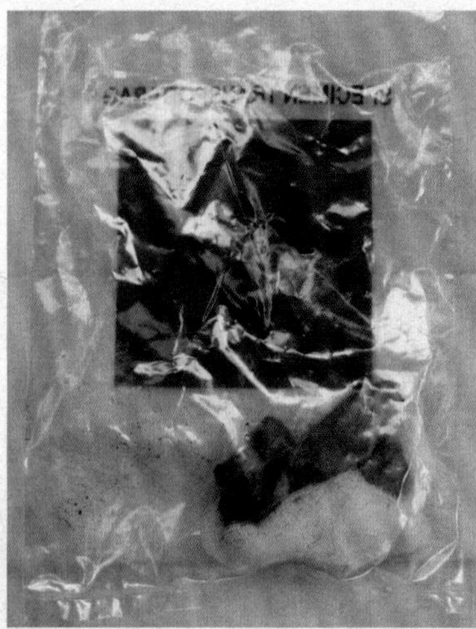

FIG 2 • The amputated part should be wrapped in a sterile gauze moistened with Ringer lactate or normal saline. The gauze is then placed in a leakproof plastic bag, which is placed on ice. The part should never be placed directly on ice.

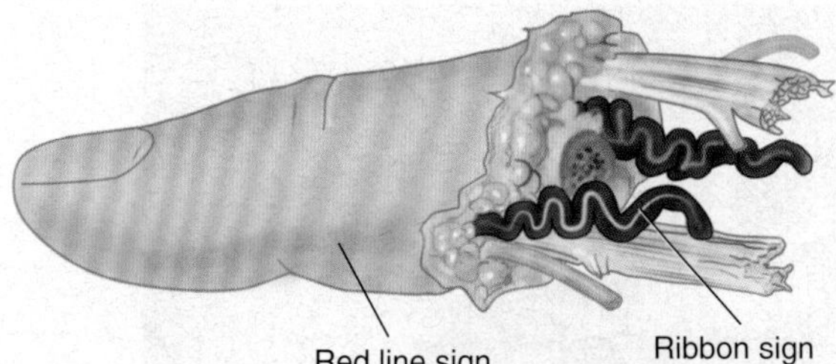

FIG 3 • The red line sign, which represents an avulsion injury, is seen clinically as a red streak of ecchymosis along the lateral border of the digit. This ecchymosis is the result of hemorrhage from avulsed branches of the digital artery after a traction injury. The ribbon sign, which also represents an avulsion injury, refers to the corkscrew appearance of the digital artery resulting from disruption of the vessel wall layers. When these clinical signs are present, the zone of injury must be bypassed with vein grafts if replantation is attempted.

- The *ribbon sign* also represents an avulsion injury (see **FIG 3**). Coiling of the artery at the amputation site results from disruption of the vessel wall layers from traction.[17] If replantation is attempted, vein grafting is often required.

IMAGING AND OTHER DIAGNOSTIC STUDIES

- When the patient arrives in the emergency department, standard radiographs of the amputated parts and the injured limb are obtained (**FIG 4**).
- Laboratory evaluations should include a complete blood count, basic metabolic panel, coagulation panel, drug screen, and blood type and crossmatch. Other preoperative tests are ordered as indicated by the patient's age and comorbidities.

NONOPERATIVE MANAGEMENT

- There is no role for nonoperative management of these injuries.
- Some surgeons advocate performing revision amputations in the emergency department under local anesthesia. It has been our experience that these procedures are best performed in the operating room with appropriate anesthesia, hemostasis, sterile conditions, lighting, and equipment.

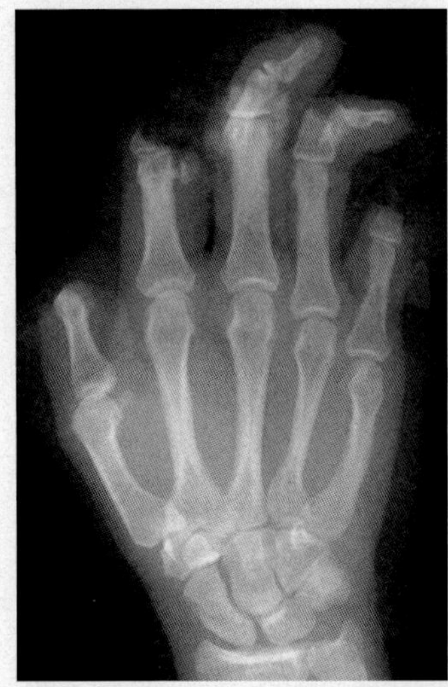
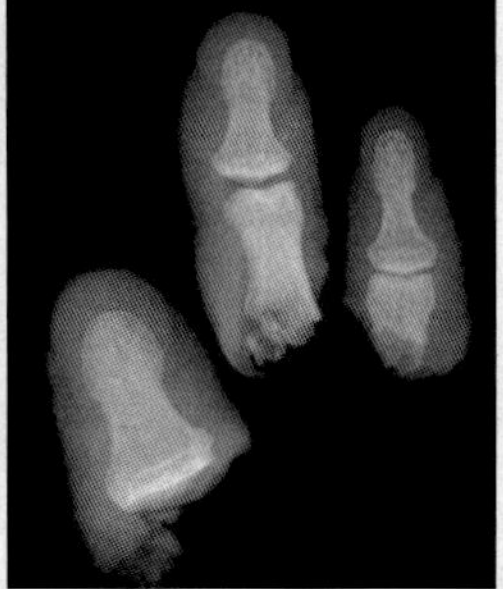

FIG 4 • **A.** Standard posteroanterior (PA) radiograph of the injured hand. **B.** A radiograph of the amputated parts is also obtained by placing the bag containing the parts directly on the x-ray cassette.

SURGICAL MANAGEMENT

- The decision to replant a digit is predicated on the determination that the anticipated function after replantation will be better than that of a revision amputation. This determination is made after careful consideration of the factors influencing the predicted survival of the replanted digit, morbidity to the patient, and functional outcome.
- Specific factors related to the status of the amputated part and the status of the patient include the following:
  - Mechanism of injury (eg, sharp, crush, avulsion)
  - Level of amputation
  - Ischemia time (warm or cold)
  - Health of patient
  - Age of patient
  - Presence of segmental injury
  - Predicted rehabilitation
  - Vocation and hobbies
- Informed consent for replantation versus revision amputation must reference the postoperative care differences.
  - Patients undergoing revision amputation typically are discharged from the hospital much quicker and have much shorter, less intensive rehabilitation protocols.
  - Patients treated by replantation typically require a 5- to 7-day hospital course, avoidance of smoking and caffeine, possible blood transfusions, and prolonged rehabilitation. Furthermore, these patients must be advised about the likelihood of cold intolerance.
- The techniques we use for replantation of amputated digits are described in detail in the following sections. The same techniques and sequence of repair are followed for the revascularization of partially amputated parts.
  - In partial amputations, not all structures will be injured, so it may be that only some structures require repair. For example, if the dorsal skin and its veins remain intact, the procedure does not require venous anastomosis for outflow.
  - Each case should be examined individually, and all structures should be carefully evaluated for injury.

Preoperative Planning

- Broad-spectrum antibiotics and tetanus prophylaxis are administered on presentation in the emergency department.
- The patient, hand, and amputated parts are examined to confirm suitability for possible replantation.
- A urethral catheter should be placed for long procedures.
- Regional anesthesia is preferred to facilitate autonomic blockade, which results in increased peripheral vasodilation. Ideally, an indwelling catheter is placed to allow for continuous postoperative pain relief and sympathetic block. General anesthesia is required for children.
- If an attempt at replantation is determined to be appropriate and desired, the parts are brought to the operating room as soon as possible. Initial preparation of the parts can begin while the anesthesia team evaluates the patient.
- The operating room and patient must be kept warm to prevent peripheral vasoconstriction.
- The sequence of repair is as follows:
  - Débridement and identification of structures
  - Bone shortening and fixation
  - Extensor tendon repair
  - Flexor tendon repair

- Arterial repair
- Nerve repair
- Vein repair
- Skin closure/coverage

Positioning

- The patient is positioned supine on a standard operating room table with a hand table attachment. The table is rotated 90 degrees to allow access for the operating microscope and fluoroscopy.

Approach

- Slightly dorsal midaxial incisions are made on both the radial and ulnar sides of the digits. These incisions allow for rapid identification of both the neurovascular bundles and the dorsal veins. Both the palmar and dorsal flaps can be reflected as needed (**FIG 5**).

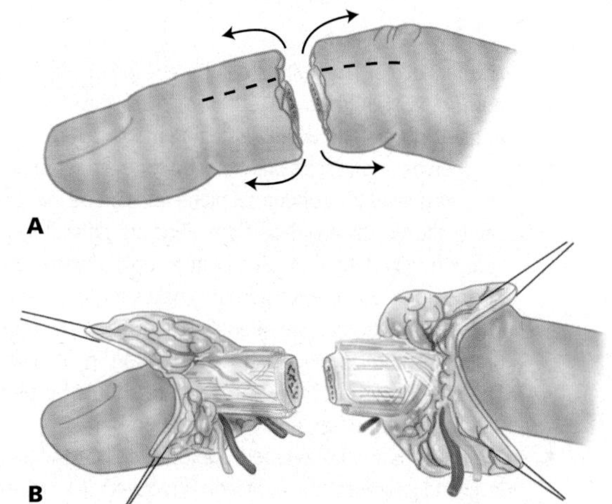

FIG 5 • A,B. Bilateral longitudinal midaxial incisions allow for easy exposure of the neurovascular bundles and dorsal veins.

TECHNIQUES

Preparation of the Amputated Part

- A two-team approach is used. One team prepares the amputated part, whereas the other team prepares the patient.
- The parts should continue to be kept cool until they are reattached. A sterile prep table and a sterile covered ice-filled basin are required for preparation of the parts (**TECH FIG 1**).
  - A sterile metal irrigation basin is filled with ice and covered with a sterile adhesive drape.
  - A moist sterile towel is placed over the drape as a working surface.
  - The basin should be filled such that the ice forms a mound above its rim.
- The parts are brought to the operating room and cleaned on the sterile prep table with Hibiclens and sterile Ringer lactate.
- A nylon suture is passed through the tip of each amputated part and secured to the towel with a small hemostat.
- Under loupe magnification, the contaminated skin edges and subcutaneous tissues are débrided.
- Slightly dorsal midlateral incisions are made on the radial and ulnar sides of the digit. Arteries, nerves, and veins are identified

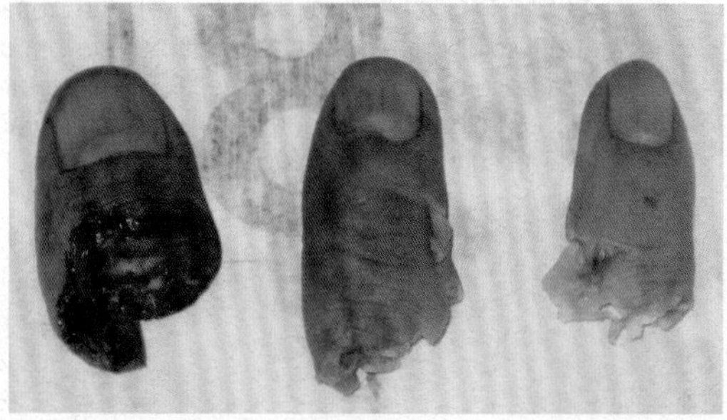

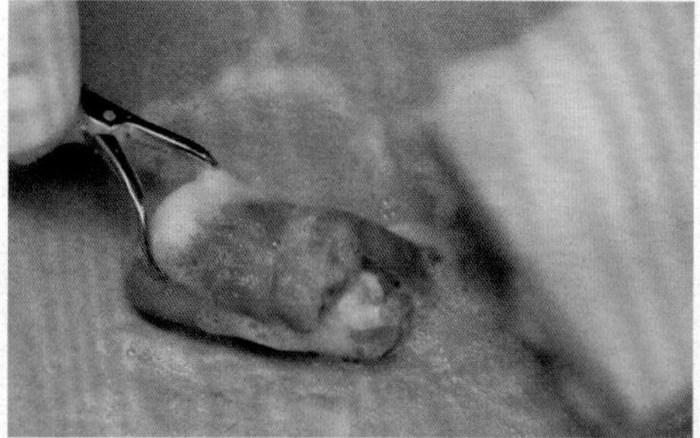

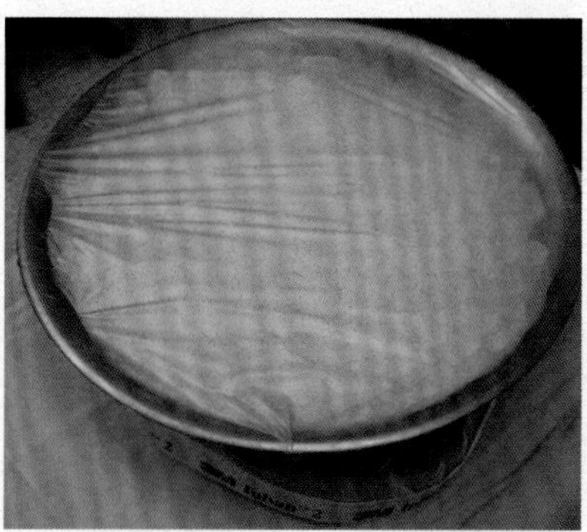

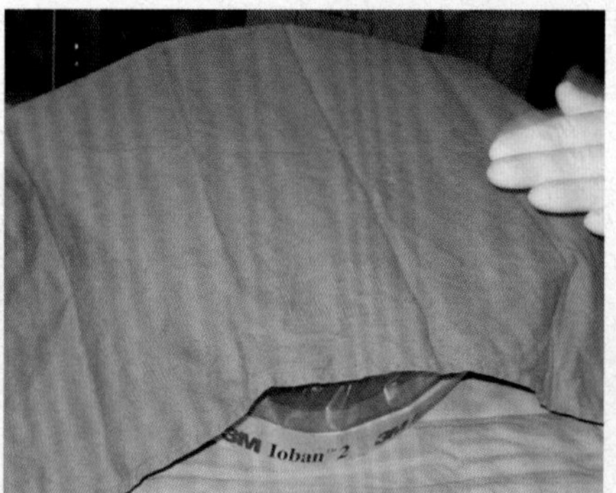

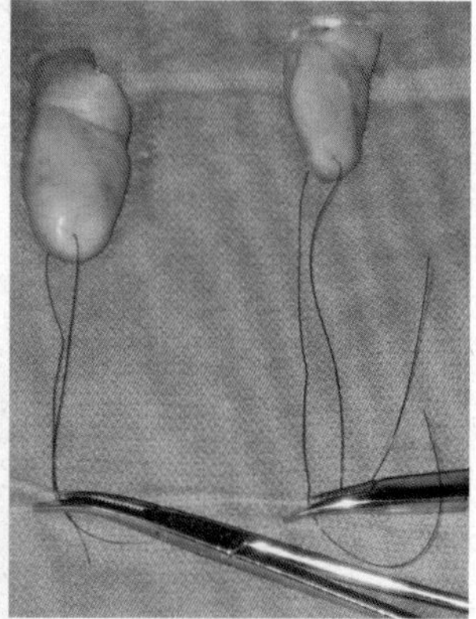

TECH FIG 1 • A,B. The amputated parts are removed from the bag, and a sterile prep is performed on a separate table. **C.** A sterile metal irrigation basin is filled with ice and covered with a sterile adhesive drape. Use as much ice as can be placed without disruption of the sterile environment to maximize contact with the amputated parts. **D.** A sterile surgical towel is then placed over the drape and used as a working surface. **E.** Nylon sutures placed through the amputated parts are secured to the surgical towel. The amputated parts are now ready for débridement and preparation.

and tagged for later with small hemoclips or microsutures. The hemoclips should be placed as close to the vessel and nerve ends as possible to avoid damaging the structures.

- The nerves and vessels are exposed for a length of 1.5 to 2 cm. The veins lie in the subdermal plane and can be identified by elevating the dorsal skin flap. If the veins are difficult to isolate, the surgeon may defer their identification until after the anastomosis of one artery when engorgement makes them more prominent.
- The flexor tendons are identified, and a 4-0 nonabsorbable braided suture is placed in each tendon in a Tajima fashion. The crossing limb of the Tajima suture should be placed 1.0 to 1.2 cm from the free end of the tendon.
- The bone is then shortened appropriately. Consideration of the level and geometry of amputation is required. It is necessary to reference the recipient site to match the orientation of the bone ends.
- In general, 4 to 10 mm of total digit shortening allows for appropriate débridement of nerves and vessels to healthy tissue and subsequent primary repair without tension. Shortening also eases skin coverage of the repair site. The amount of shortening depends partly on the mechanism of injury. Crush injuries typically require more resection than sharp injuries.
- Two 0.045-inch Kirschner wires (K-wires) are placed longitudinally down the long axis of the bone in a retrograde fashion. The K-wires should exit through the tip of the digit just palmar to the nail. The K-wires are advanced until the tips are showing through the bone so that the amputated digit is now ready for immediate attachment.
- The parts should continue to be kept cool under ice packs until they are reattached.

Preparation of the Stump

- The second surgical team initiates preparation of the injured extremity while the amputated parts are being prepared.
- Under tourniquet ischemia and loupe magnification, débridement of the skin and subcutaneous tissues is performed.
- In an identical manner to the amputated parts, the arteries, nerves, and veins are identified, tagged, and exposed through slightly dorsal midlateral incisions. The veins are the most difficult structures to identify on the stump. Once a vein is located, continue the dissection in the same subdermal plane to identify others. If possible, two veins are repaired for each artery.
- Flexor tendons are identified, and a Tajima suture is placed in each (**TECH FIG 2**). If the tendons have retracted proximally, atraumatic retrieval is necessary to avoid inducing spasm or damaging the proximal vessels. If required, a separate proximal incision is made to retrieve the tendons safely.
- After identifying all structures, evaluate the need for grafts. Every attempt should be made to repair all structures primarily. Delayed reconstructions are much more difficult, place the repaired vessels at risk, and subject the patient to additional surgery and rehabilitation.
- Any amputated parts that are not being replanted should not be discarded because these are an excellent source for donor grafts(skin, bone, nerve, vessel).

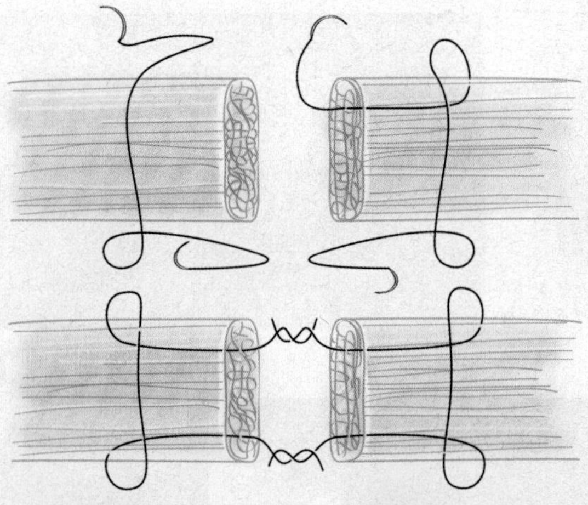

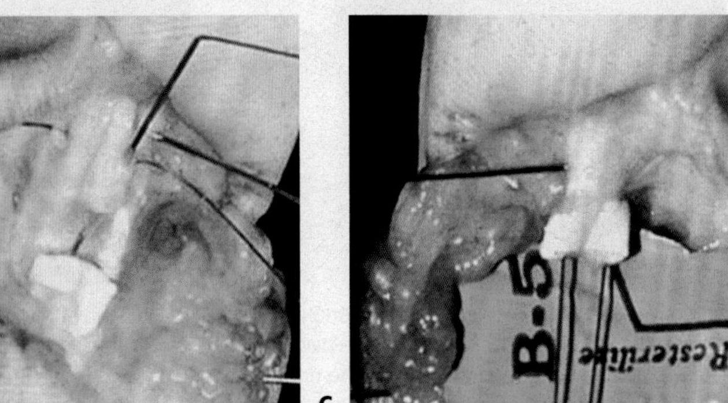

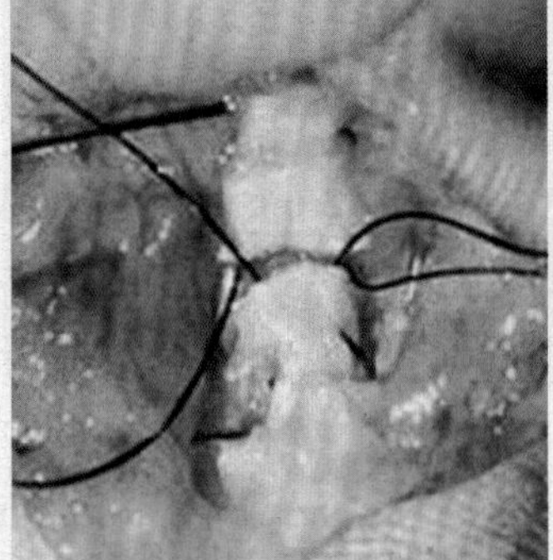

TECH FIG 2 • **A.** A Tajima-type suture repair is used so that the flexor tendons can be opposed and secured at the ideal time. **B,C.** The suture is placed in the proximal and distal ends of the tendon. **D.** The sutures are then tied in the repair site at the appropriate time.

Bone Fixation

- Bone shortening has already been performed at the time of débridement. If shortening was limited by the proximity of joints, the use of vein grafts should be entertained at the time of vessel anastomosis. When shortening the bone in a thumb amputation, the resection should be maximized on the amputated part so that if the replant fails, thumb length is maintained.
- Numerous methods of bone fixation are available, including longitudinal K-wires, crossed K-wires, intraosseous wiring (so-called 90-90 wiring), tension band wiring, intramedullary screw, and plate and screws.
  - Parallel longitudinal K-wires are quick, easy, and have low nonunion and complication rates.[7] When possible, this is our preferred technique (**TECH FIG 3A–D**).
  - Crossed K-wires are also relatively quick and easy to use. The drawback to crossed K-wires is potential risk to the neurovascular bundles, either directly or by tethering (**TECH FIG 3E–H**).
  - Intraosseous wiring takes more time and exposure to perform but allows for early range of motion. Drill holes accepting of a 24-gauge wire are placed in a dorsal to palmar and radial to ulnar orientation at each bone end. Two loops of 24-gauge wire are then passed perpendicular to each other through the analogous drill holes at each bone end and tightened in standard cerclage fashion.
  - The tension band technique is a useful option for arthrodesis because it allows the surgeon to set the desired amount of flexion. Two parallel 0.045-inch K-wires are placed across the fusion site, and a figure-8 loop of 24-gauge wire is used over the dorsum of the finger to complete the construct.
  - The intramedullary screw is most useful in thumb amputations at the metacarpal level. Removal of this hardware is difficult, so its use should be avoided in highly contaminated wounds where the risk of infection is high.
  - Lag screw fixation is appropriate to treat long oblique fractures. However, because most amputations do not result in this fracture pattern, this technique is seldom used in replantation surgery.

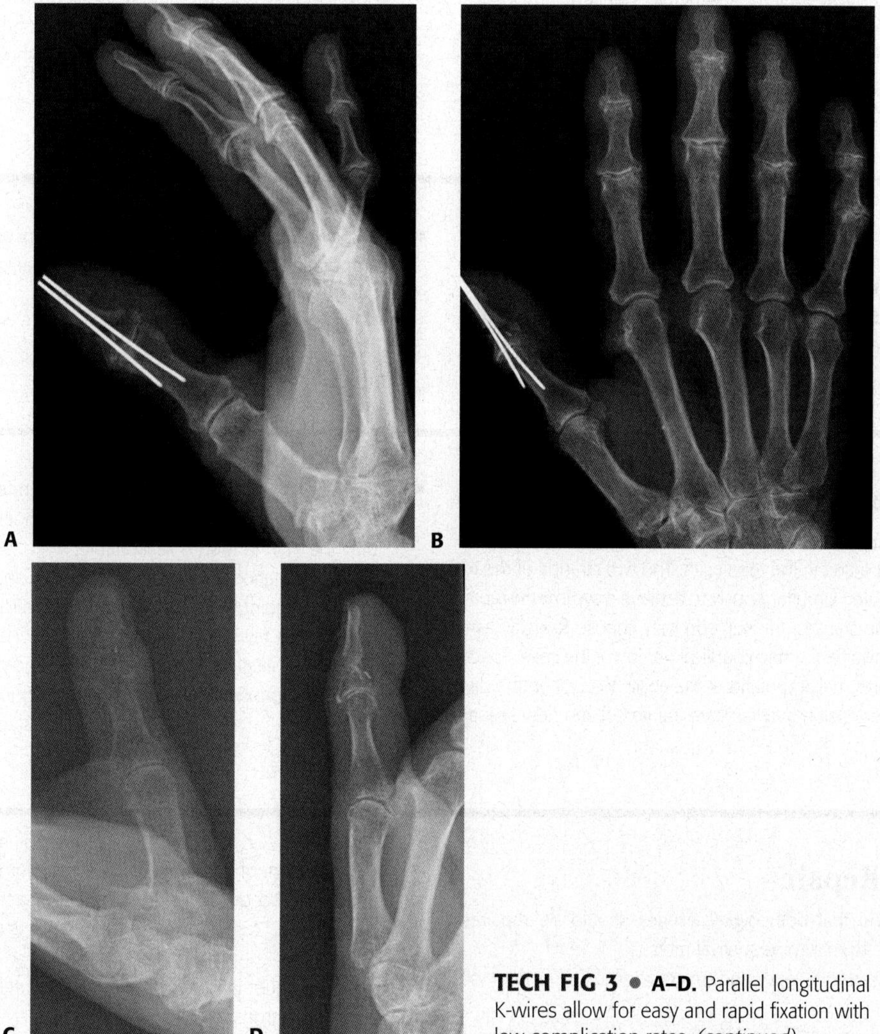

TECH FIG 3 • A–D. Parallel longitudinal K-wires allow for easy and rapid fixation with low complication rates. *(continued)*

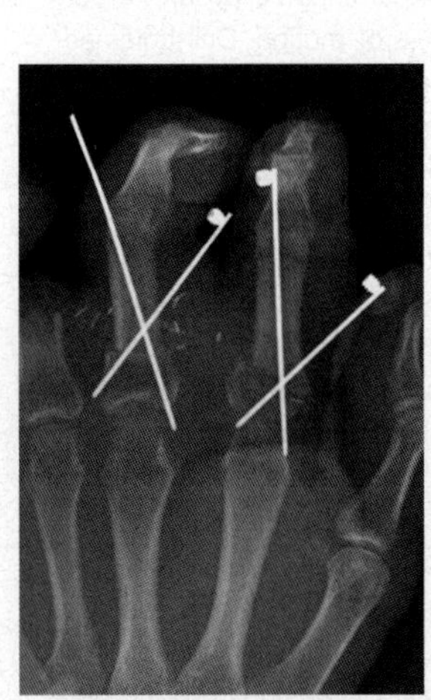
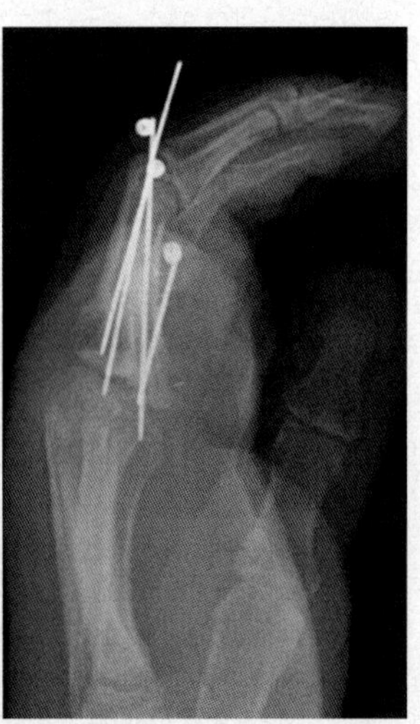
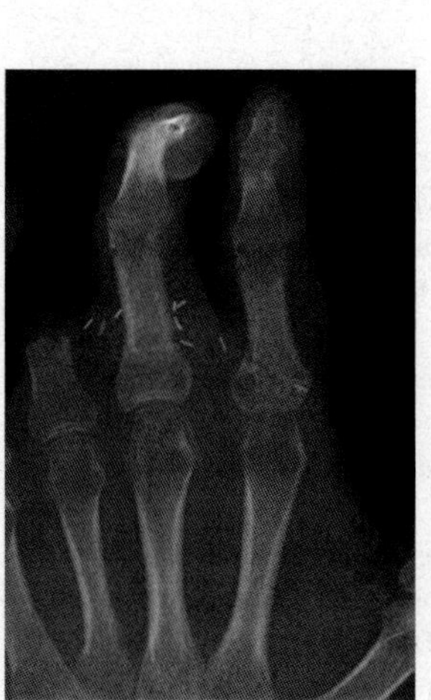
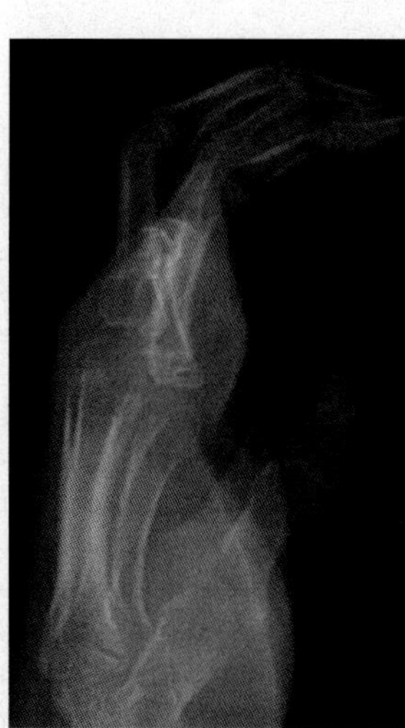

TECH FIG 3 • *(continued)* **E–H.** In more proximal amputations, longitudinal K-wires may not be possible. Crossed K-wires can be used successfully in these injuries.

- Plate-and-screw fixation is generally not required in digit replantation because nonunion is rare. Although it provides rigid fixation, the hardware is bulky, increases tendon adhesions, and requires more time and exposure.
- Regardless of the method of fixation, the surgeon must constantly evaluate alignment and rotation of the digit in both flexion and extension. The flexed fingertips should point toward the distal pole of the scaphoid.

Extensor Tendon Repair

- After bone stabilization, the extensor mechanism is repaired.
- In the digit, the tendon is repaired with two horizontal mattress sutures using a 4-0 nonabsorbable suture.
- It is imperative to repair the entire extensor mechanism. If the amputation is through the proximal phalanx, repair of the lateral bands will optimize functional outcomes.

Flexor Tendon Repair

- Because the Tajima sutures have already been placed, they are now ready to be tied in the repair site. The two strands of the repair should be tied simultaneously to achieve a symmetric repair.
- In certain circumstances, the surgeon may choose to delay tying the sutures until after the microsurgical portion of the case. Specifically, in very proximal amputations, the ability to position the digit in slight hyperextension may facilitate the vessel and nerve repair.
- Both the FDS and FDP are repaired when feasible. If the amputation is in zone 2 and the tendons are not cleanly cut, repair of only the FDP tendon is reasonable.
- If the amputation level is distal to the FDS insertion, but proximal to the DIP joint, we typically do not repair the FDP or extensor tendon. We favor arthrodesis of the DIP joint with K-wires and direct rehabilitation toward early active and passive range of motion of the proximal interphalangeal (PIP) joint.

Arterial Repair

- We have found that both digital arteries should be repaired, when feasible, to maximize survival rates.
- The operating microscope and microsurgical instrument set are used.
- The most important factor affecting survival is achieving a tension-free anastomosis of normal intima to normal intima (**TECH FIG 4A–C**).
- Débridement of damaged arteries is performed under the operating microscope. The surgeon must resect until normal intima is identified. The liberal use of vein grafts is advocated for resulting defects.
- The tourniquet is released to ensure good blood flow from the proximal stumps.
- Sharply trim the proximal stump with angled Potts scissors and dilate the lumen with jeweler's forceps or a lacrimal duct dilator.

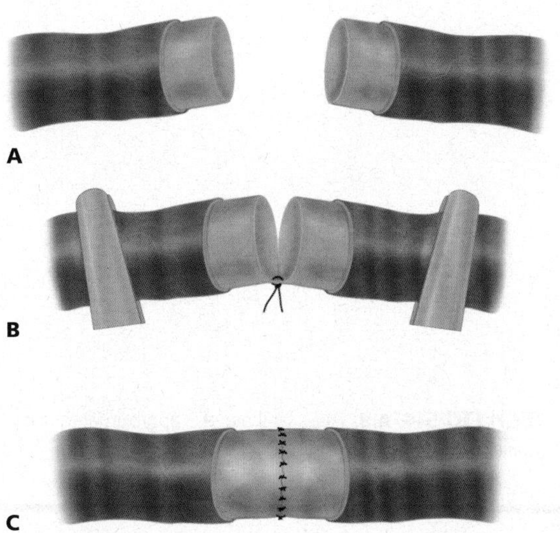

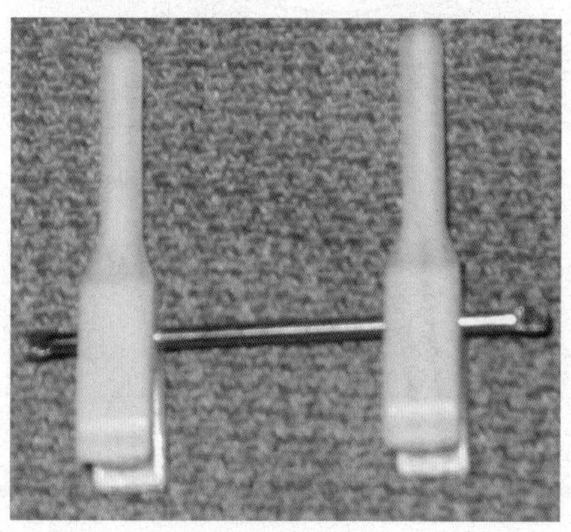

TECH FIG 4 • **A–C.** Arterial repair is performed using the operating microscope. A tension-free anastomosis of normal intima to normal intima is essential for survival of the replanted part. **D.** The vascular approximating clamp should have less than 30 g of closing pressure. Two clamps on a sliding bar allow for tension-free positioning of the vessel ends.

- If adequate blood flow is not obtained, evaluate for all reversible causes of vasospasm, including hypotension, hypovolemia, acidosis, pain, or cold. Double check that the tourniquet was deflated.
- Evaluate the proximal vessel for mechanical constriction.
- Thoroughly irrigate the lumen with warm heparinized Ringer lactate through a 30-gauge blunt-tipped needle on a 10-mL syringe.
- If vasospasm persists, irrigate the proximal vessel with papaverine solution (diluted 1:20 with sterile normal saline).
- After appropriate blood flow is established, the proximal and distal stumps are placed within the vascular approximators. Several types of approximating devices are available. We favor two clamps on a sliding bar. The clamps should have less than 30 g of closing pressure and should be limited to no more than 30 minutes of application time due to the potential for vessel damage (**TECH FIG 4D**).
- Place a microsurgical background deep to the repair site.
- A bolus of 3000 to 5000 U of intravenous heparin is given just before the anastomosis. After the bolus, we typically initiate a heparin drip at 1000 U per hour.
- Repeat inspection of the intima is performed proximally and distally to confirm its integrity. Verify that the anastomosis is tension-free and that no adventitia overhangs the lumen.
- Appropriately sized monofilament nylon sutures (Table 1) are used and initial sutures are placed 180 degrees apart.
- The size of each "bite" should be about one to two times the thickness of the arterial wall.
- Care must be taken to avoid damaging the intima of the vessel.
- One limb each of the initial sutures should be cut long for use in manipulating the vessel without directly handling it.
- Suture the front wall of the artery sequentially between stay sutures.
- Irrigate the lumen after each suture is tied, and inspect the repair site to confirm that the back wall was not captured.
- Flip the approximating clamp to expose the back wall and complete the anastomosis.
- Remove the vessel from the approximating clips and repeat the procedure on the other digital artery.

Table 1 Needle and Suture Sizes

Site of Repair	Suture Size	Needle Size (μm)
Palm	9-0	100
Proximal digit	10-0	75
Distal digit	11-0	50

Nerve Repair

- The proximal and distal nerve ends are examined under the operating microscope.
- The ends are cut sharply with a no. 11 blade against a wooden tongue depressor. The nerve is resected until pouting fascicles are visualized.
- The fascicles are aligned, and an epineurial repair is performed using two or three 9-0 or 10-0 sutures (**TECH FIG 5**).
- If a tension-free repair is not possible, primary nerve grafting is performed. The medial antebrachial cutaneous nerve is the ideal caliber for digital nerves and can be obtained from the ipsilateral extremity. Similarly, any amputated digits that are not candidates for replantation provide an excellent source for grafts.

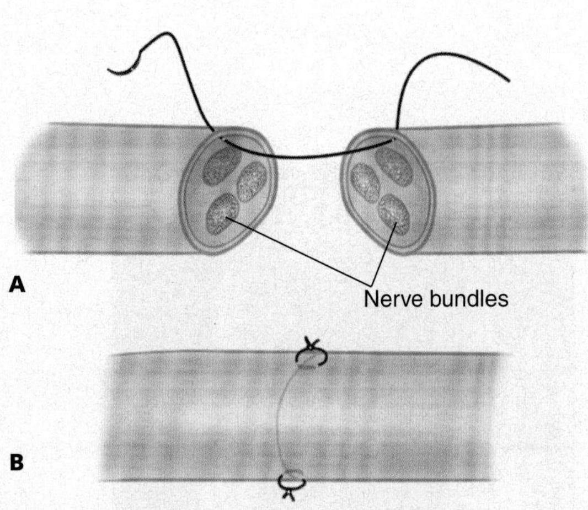

TECH FIG 5 • A,B. The digital nerve is approximated using an epineurial repair consisting of two or three sutures.

Vein Repair

- Ideally, a minimum of two veins are repaired for each artery.[1,7] The largest veins identified should be repaired.
- When performing the anastomosis, each bite should be about two to three times the thickness of the vein wall.
- Constant irrigation with heparinized Ringer lactate helps to "float" the lumen of the vein open.
- Due to the low-pressure flow, the venous anastomosis can be performed with fewer sutures than are required for the arterial anastomosis (**TECH FIG 6**).

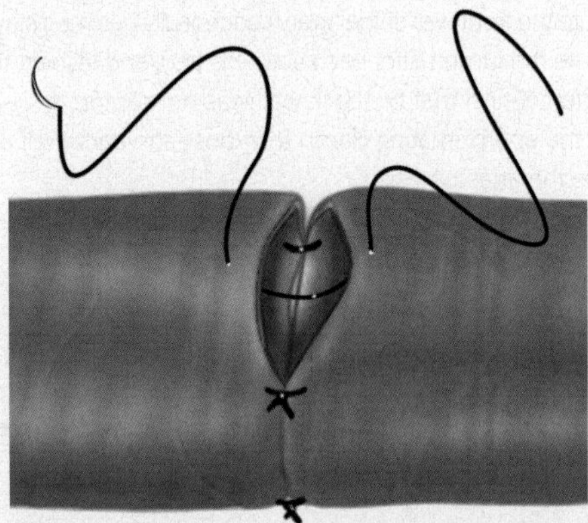

TECH FIG 6 • The venous anastomosis is performed with fewer sutures than the arterial repair due to the low-pressure flow.

- Familiarity with alternatives to venous anastomosis is necessary in the event suitable veins cannot be located.
  - Continuous venous oozing can be encouraged by removal of the nail with subsequent scraping of the matrix. This scraping is performed every 2 hours with a cotton-tipped applicator and is followed by the application of heparin-soaked pledgets.
  - If proximal veins are present but distal veins are not, creation of either an arteriovenous or venocutaneous fistula may facilitate outflow to reduce congestion. This scenario is most common in very distal amputations just proximal to the nail. An arteriovenous fistula may be created possibly if one artery has been successfully repaired and back bleeding is present from the other distal artery. This artery can be anastomosed to the proximal vein. Alternatively, a vein graft can be used to create a temporary shunt from the skin of the pulp to the proximal vein.
  - Medicinal leeches (*Hirudo medicinalis*) can be placed on the engorged part if postoperative venous congestion occurs. They should be changed every few hours and should be used for a minimum of 7 days to allow for the establishment of collateral circulation. Although the leeches may fall off after engorgement, they secrete hirudin, a local anticoagulant that keeps the digit bleeding for 8 to 12 hours. While using leech therapy, the patient should be treated with a third-generation cephalosporin as prophylaxis against *Aeromonas hydrophila* infection, a symbiotic gram-negative rod in the leech gut.

Skin Coverage and Wound Closure

- Before the wound is closed, meticulous hemostasis must be achieved. Even small postoperative hematomas can compress the vascular repairs and result in failure of the replant.
- Interrupted nylon sutures are used to close the wounds, avoiding constriction of underlying structures. The midlateral incisions can be left open without concern for healing difficulties. If the repaired dorsal veins lack local coverage, a split- or full-thickness graft should be applied.
- No part of the postoperative dressing should be circumferential. Small strips of petroleum-impregnated gauze are applied to the incisions. A bulky dressing is constructed with a plaster splint extending above the elbow. The tips of all digits must remain exposed, and a temperature probe is taped to the pulp of the replanted digit for monitoring.
- The limb is elevated in a foam pillow.

PEARLS AND PITFALLS

Amputated parts	■ Take the amputated parts to the operating room to begin débridement and identification of structures as soon as the room is ready.
Heterotopic replantation	■ Prioritize the functional goals for replantation. If multiple digits are amputated, but not all parts are suitable for replantation, put the salvageable digits in the most functional position (eg, replant a finger in the thumb position if the thumb cannot be saved).
Vein grafts	■ If there is concern for intimal damage, resection and the liberal use of vein grafts saves time and frustration. Always reverse the vein graft in case valves are present in the segment. The volar aspect of the wrist contains numerous veins 1–2 mm in diameter.
Spare parts surgery	■ Never discard any amputated parts until the conclusion of the case. Amputated parts that are not suitable for replantation are an ideal source of autologous grafts.
Vascular anastomosis	■ Never perform an anastomosis under tension. Either additional bone shortening or vein grafting should be performed.
Multiple digit replantations	■ The overall duration of surgery is decreased by performing a structure-by-structure repair instead of a digit-by-digit repair (ie, repair the same anatomic structure in all digits before repairing the next structure).[3]

POSTOPERATIVE CARE

- Usually, the hand is elevated, with the level of elevation adjusted for changes in vascular status. If arterial inflow becomes problematic, the hand is lowered. If venous congestion is present, the hand is raised.
- Color, warmth, turgor, and capillary refill are monitored by the surgeon.
- The patient's room should be kept warm, preferably above 22° C (72° F). The temperature probe is monitored by the nursing staff, and the surgeon is notified if the digital temperature is less than 30° C or if the temperature drops 2° C over 1 hour.
- The patient is maintained on bed rest for the first 2 or 3 days, and the room is kept dark with minimal stimulation. Visitors are limited to two at a time.
- The patient is restricted from nicotine and caffeine products.
- The intravenous heparin drip is continued at 1000 U per hour. The rate is adjusted for a goal activated partial thromboplastin time (aPTT) of 1.5 times normal. It is maintained for 5 days, then weaned by 100 U per hour until off.
- Dextran 40 is given as a 50-mL bolus and then maintained at a rate of 20 mL per hour while the patient is in the hospital.
- Enteric-coated aspirin (325 mg daily) and dipyridamole (50 mg three times a day) are initiated and maintained for 6 weeks postoperatively.
- Chlorpromazine (25 mg orally every 8 hours) is useful as both an anxiolytic and a peripheral vasodilator. We generally use it for the duration of the patient's hospital stay.
- Appropriate antibiotics are maintained for 7 days.
- We prefer to leave the operative dressing in place for 7 days to avoid causing vasospasm. Excessive bleeding with formation of a blood cast that would restrict venous outflow should prompt an earlier dressing change.
- Gentle active motion is started on postoperative day 3 within the confines of the splint. Formal hand therapy is initiated after the splint is removed.

OUTCOMES

- A survival rate greater than 80% is expected for replantation surgery.
- Functional outcomes are greatest for replantation of the thumb, proximal hand, and single digit distal to the FDS insertion (**FIG 6A–D**).[5,6,13,16]
- Recovery of sensation is correlated with function. As in other peripheral nerve injuries, age is the most important factor for recovery, with better results in younger patients. The average two-point discrimination in replanted thumbs is 11 mm and in fingers is 8 mm.[4] These values represent the average recovery for sharp amputation. Crush and avulsion mechanisms result in poorer two-point discrimination.
- Range of motion is related to level of amputation. Active PIP joint motion in replantations proximal to the FDS insertion average 35 degrees, whereas replantations distal to the FDS insertion result in 82 degrees of PIP joint motion (**FIG 6E–G**).[7]

COMPLICATIONS

Immediate Complications

- Immediate complications affect the survival of the replanted digit and typically relate to the vascular status.
- Arterial insufficiency may result from unrecognized vessel injury away from the anastomosis, which causes thrombosis or vasospasm.
  - A check for reversible causes is initiated to ensure that the patient is warm, comfortable, hydrated, and calm.
  - Check the dressings to confirm that there is no mechanical constriction.
  - Confirm that the patient's hematocrit is near normal and that all ordered medications are being given appropriately.
  - The hand should be lowered to increase inflow, and an intravenous bolus of heparin (3000 to 5000 U) is given. If the patient has not been anticoagulated or has not achieved therapeutic levels, a regional sympathetic block will aid peripheral vasodilation.

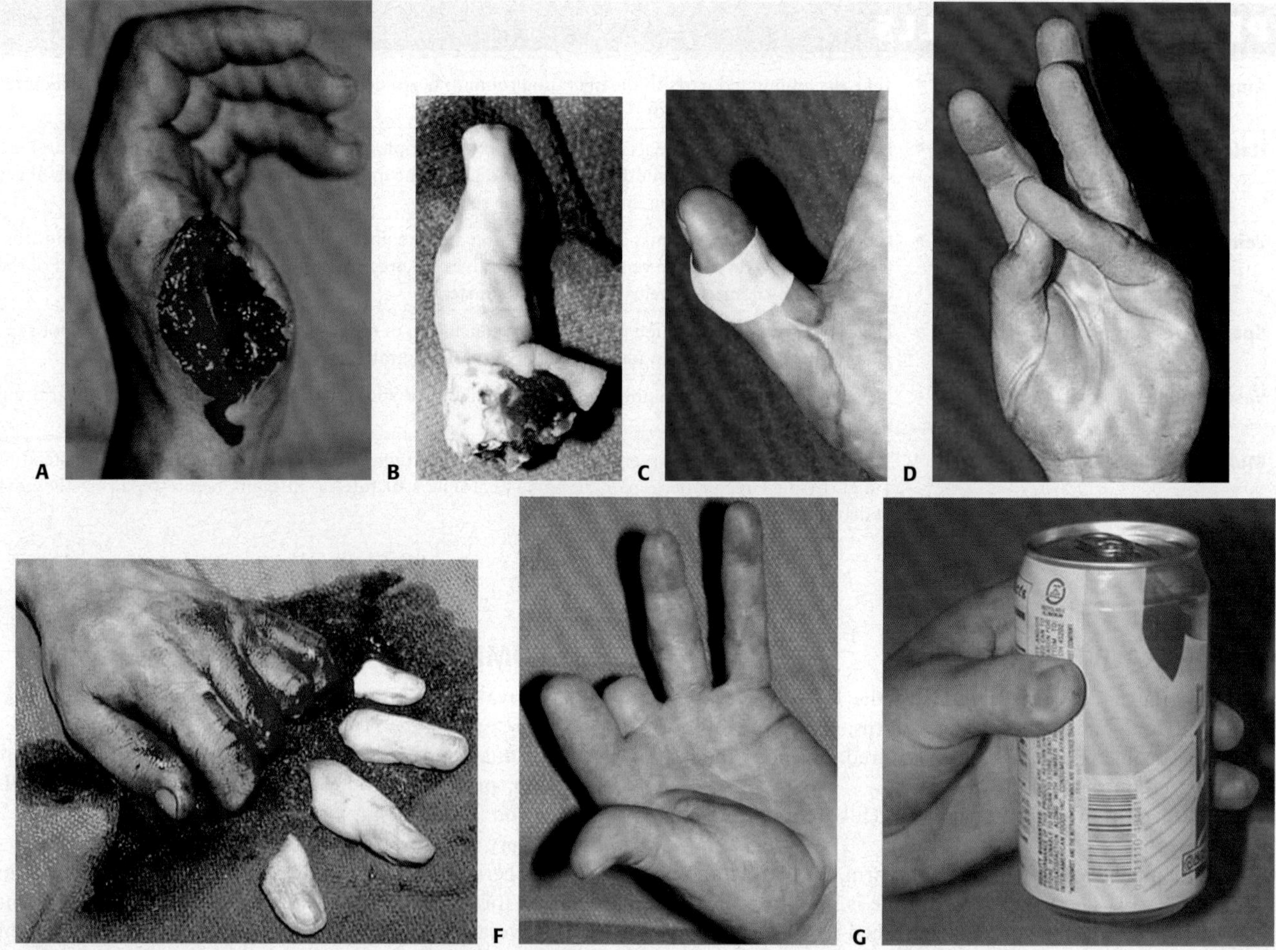

FIG 6 • A–D. This patient sustained an amputated thumb, which was successfully replanted with good cosmetic and functional results. **E–G.** Successful replantation of the ring and small fingers resulted in a functional hand capable of holding common objects.

  - Vigilant reexamination of color, warmth, turgor, and capillary refill is necessary to decide whether exploration in the operating room is indicated. Revisions after 4 to 6 hours of reduced perfusion seldom result in digit salvage.[7]
- If venous engorgement occurs postoperatively, elevate the hand and remove constrictive dressings (including sutures that are too tight).
  - Consideration for return to the operating room is based on intraoperative findings affecting the possibility of revising the venous anastomosis.
  - If this is not possible, leeches or nail removal are used to alleviate venous congestion. These methods typically are used to bridge the first 4 to 6 days until adequate outflow is established.

Long-term Complications

- Long-term complications include pin tract infections, cold intolerance, stiffness, malunion, and nonunion.
- Pin tract infections usually occur more than 4 weeks after surgery. They are easily treated by pin removal and a course of oral antibiotics.
- Cold intolerance is almost universal. (This also is a problem in revision amputations.) Cold intolerance is expected to improve over the first 2 years, but it remains debatable whether it completely resolves.[2,14]
- Digital stiffness is common because both the flexor and extensor tendons are repaired. Tenolysis should be delayed for at least 3 months postreplantation but has demonstrated good results.[9]
- Malunion usually results from malalignment at the time of bone fixation. Intraoperatively, rotational alignment is the most difficult to assess. Malunion is more common in proximal amputations because even slight malalignment at the amputation level is greatly accentuated at the fingertip.
- Nonunion is not common after replantation of the digit. It has been reported in fewer than 10% of digit replantations and rarely requires reoperation.[15,16]

REFERENCES

1. Allen DM, Levin LS. Digital replantation including postoperative care. Tech Hand Up Extrem Surg 2002;6:171–177.
2. Backman C, Nyström A, Backman C, et al. Arterial spasticity and cold intolerance in relation to time after digital replantation. J Hand Surg Br 1993;18:551–555.
3. Camacho FJ, Wood MB. Polydigit replantation. Hand Clin 1992;8:409–412.

4. Glickman LT, MacKinnon SE. Sensory recovery following digital replantation. Microsurgery 1990;11:236–242.
5. Goldner RD, Howson MP, Nunley JA, et al. One hundred eleven thumb amputations: replantation versus revision. Microsurgery 1990;11:243–250.
6. Goldner RD, Stevanovic MV, Nunley JA, et al. Digital replantation at the level of the distal interphalangeal joint and the distal phalanx. J Hand Surg Am 1989;14:214–220.
7. Goldner RD, Urbaniak JR. Replantation. In: Green D, Hotchkiss RN, Pederson WC, et al, eds. Green's Operative Hand Surgery, ed 5. Philadelphia: Elsevier Churchill Livingstone, 2005:1569.
8. Hattori Y, Doi K, Ikeda K, et al. A retrospective study of functional outcomes after successful replantation versus amputation closure for single fingertip amputations. J Hand Surg Am 2006;31:811–818.
9. Jupiter JB, Pess GM, Bour CJ. Results of flexor tendon tenolysis after replantation in the hand. J Hand Surg Am 1989;14:35–44.
10. Lucas GL. The pattern of venous drainage of the digits. J Hand Surg Am 1984;9:448–450.
11. Matsuzaki H, Yoshizu T, Maki Y, et al. Functional and cosmetic results of fingertip replantation: anastomosing only the digital artery. Ann Plast Surg 2004;53:353–359.
12. Ozkan O, Ozgentas HE, Safak T, et al. Unique superiority of microsurgical repair technique with its functional and aesthetic outcomes in ring avulsion injuries. J Plast Reconstr Aesthet Surg 2006;59:451–459.
13. Patradul A, Ngarmukos C, Parkpian V. Major limb replantation: a Thai experience. Ann Acad Med Singapore 1995;24(4 suppl):82–88.
14. Povlsen B, Nylander G, Nylander E. Cold-induced vasospasm after digital replantation does not improve with time: a 12-year prospective study. J Hand Surg Br 1995;20:237–239.
15. Urbaniak JR, Hayes MG, Bright DS. Management of bone in digital replantation: free vascularized and composite bone grafts. Clin Orthop Relat Res 1978;(133):184–194.
16. Urbaniak JR, Roth JH, Nunley JA, et al. The results of replantation after amputation of a single finger. J Bone Joint Surg Am 1985;67(4):611–619.
17. Van Beek AL, Kutz JE, Zook EG. Importance of the ribbon sign, indicating unsuitability of the vessel, in replanting a finger. Plast Reconstr Surg 1978;61:32–35.
18. Waikakul S, Sakkarnkosol S, Vanadurongwan V, et al. Results of 1018 digital replantations in 552 patients. Injury 2000;31:33–40.
19. Wei FC, Chang YL, Chen HC, et al. Three successful digital replantations in a patient after 84, 86 and 94 hours of cold ischemia. Plast Reconstr Surg 1988;82:346–350.

CHAPTER 127 Surgical Treatment of Vasospastic and Vaso-occlusive Diseases of the Hand

Scott L. Hansen and Neil F. Jones

DEFINITION

- Vasospastic and vaso-occlusive diseases of the hands include a wide range of disorders that cause decreased or limited blood flow to the digits, resulting in chronic ulcerations and potentially loss of digits.
- Vasospastic disorders result from constriction of the microvasculature, resulting in decreased blood flow.
  - The most common vasospastic disorder is Raynaud syndrome.
    - Raynaud syndrome may also have an obstructive component.
- Vaso-occlusive disorders produce disruption of blood flow due to a reduction in cross-sectional area of the vessel lumen.

ANATOMY

- The right common carotid artery and right subclavian artery originate from the brachiocephalic trunk, whereas the left subclavian artery branches directly from the aorta.
- The subclavian artery becomes the axillary artery at the distal edge of the first rib and ends at the distal edge of the teres major tendon.
- The brachial artery is a continuation of the axillary artery, beginning at the distal margin of the teres major.
- The hand is supplied by the radial and ulnar arteries, which originate from the brachial artery at the level of the antecubital fossa.
- The radial artery becomes the deep palmar arch; the ulnar artery becomes the superficial palmar arch (**FIG 1**).
- The superficial palmar arch is usually the major arterial inflow to the fingers on the ulnar aspect of the hand, whereas the deep palmar arch supplies blood to the digits on the radial aspect of the hand.
  - The superficial palmar arch lies more distal in the palm than the deep palmar arch.
- In about 80% of patients, the deep and superficial palmar arches are in continuity, a configuration described as a *complete palmar arch*.[4]
- In a very small percentage patients, a persistent median artery also can contribute blood supply to the hand.
- Sympathetic nerves exit the spinal cord along with the ventral roots of the second and third thoracic nerves, passing via the brachial plexus into the forearm and hand.
  - The sympathetic nerve fibers innervate the blood vessel walls, contributing to control of tone of the vascular smooth muscle.

PATHOGENESIS

- Raynaud syndrome, a vasospastic disorder, is characterized by significant structural narrowing of the arterial lumen due to intimal hyperplasia. Vasospasm can occur from increased sympathetic tone in response to temperature, vibratory stimuli, and sometimes emotional stress, causing further ischemia and the clinical manifestation of color changes.
- Vasospasm can also be associated with pheochromocytoma, carcinoid syndrome, and cryoglobulinemia.
- Emboli can shower from a cardiac source (eg, chronic atrial fibrillation) or from microemboli in ulcerated, atherosclerotic plaques, either spontaneously or from iatrogenic cannulation of vessels during vascular procedures.
- Thrombosis may occur spontaneously from atherosclerotic disease or from repetitive blunt trauma to the vessels, as in hypothenar hammer syndrome.
- Low-flow states can occur in sepsis, malignant disease, hypercoagulable states (eg, polycythemia, lupus anticoagulant antibody), and after intra-arterial drug injections.
  - Low-flow states predispose end organs to global thrombosis.
- Focal stenosis and segmental occlusion of vessels may result from intimal proliferation secondary to connective tissue disorders, atherosclerosis, and renal vascular disease.

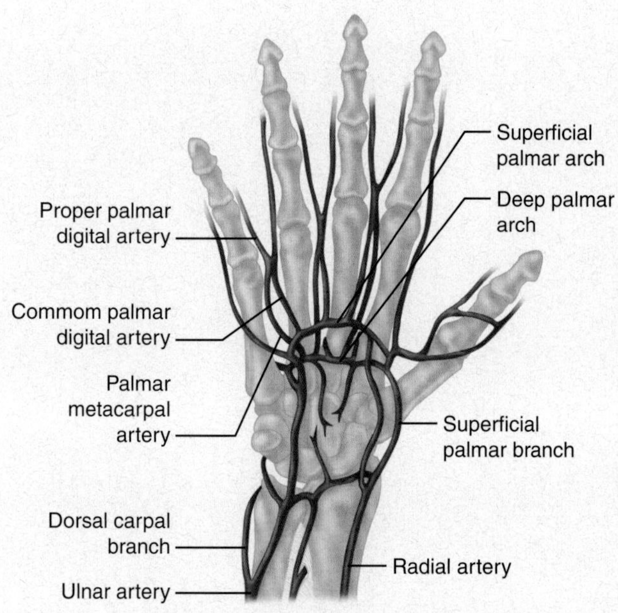

FIG 1 • Vascular anatomy of the hand.

- Vasospastic disorders may result from increased sympathetic tone.
- Vaso-occlusive disorders result in ischemia distal to the site of occlusion.

NATURAL HISTORY

- Clinical manifestations of vasospastic disorders range from episodic digital vasospasm and pain to severe hand and digit ischemia, progressing to gangrene.
- The classic triphasic attack in Raynaud syndrome consists of sudden onset of digital pallor or blanching after cold exposure or emotional stress, followed by a period of cyanosis and then redness with rewarming, resulting in the classic white-blue-red sequence of color changes.[1]
  - The typical Raynaud attack lasts for 15 to 45 minutes.
- Vaso-occlusive disorders follow a more predictable clinical course in that they usually result from fixed lesions that are progressive.
- Cold intolerance and vasomotor color changes in the hand develop, forcing patients to seek treatment.

PATIENT HISTORY AND PHYSICAL FINDINGS

- A complete history and physical examination must be done on each patient, focusing on evidence of connective tissue or cardiovascular disease.
  - Does the patient describe paresthesias, pallor, cold intolerance, pain, and digit ulceration?
- The entire upper extremity is examined for range of motion, skin color and turgor, capillary refill, radial and ulnar pulses, temperature, and presence of ulcerations.
- The distal fingertips and nails of each finger are examined closely.
- The radial and ulnar pulses are palpated and examined by Doppler probe if necessary.
- The palmar arch is assessed with the Doppler probe as well as the radial and ulnar digital arteries to each finger.
- Allen test is performed.
  - After the patient makes a tight fist to exsanguinate the blood form the hand, the radial and ulnar arteries are occluded at the level of the wrist.
  - The arterial flow is then reestablished to the hand by sequentially releasing the radial and ulnar arteries while capillary refill is assessed simultaneously.
  - This test evaluates the patency of arterial inflow to the hand through the radial and ulnar arteries.
  - The same technique can be applied to each digit after compressing or milking the blood in the digit from distal to proximal.
- Any pulsatile masses, chronic skin changes, or superficial vascular lesions are evaluated.

IMAGING AND OTHER DIAGNOSTIC STUDIES

- Posteroanterior (PA), lateral, and oblique radiographs to evaluate bone architecture and the presence of any calcification in the radial and ulnar arteries, palmar arches, or digital arteries
- Doppler examination of the arteries from the wrist to the digits
- Echocardiogram to evaluate potential sources of emboli
- Digital photoplethysmography, which measures digital volume changes over time, can be used to differentiate vasospastic from vaso-occlusive disease.
- Segmental arterial pressure measurements
- Nielsen digital hypothermic challenge test[18]
- Ultrasonography for vascular tumors[10]
- Angiography: remains the gold standard to evaluate blood flow to the hand
- Magnetic resonance (MR) angiography[5]
- Laboratory tests: complete blood cell count (CBC) with platelet count, coagulation studies, markers for collagen vascular diseases

DIFFERENTIAL DIAGNOSIS

- Raynaud disease
- Hypothenar hammer syndrome
- Malignancy
- Trauma
- Buerger disease (thromboangiitis obliterans): an inflammatory occlusive disease of the small and medium-sized vessels of the limbs
- Arteritis: a group of disorders characterized by acute or chronic inflammation in the walls of small, medium, and large arteries. Patients with these conditions often present with concurrent fever, malaise, weight loss, cutaneous lesions, and arthralgias.
- Diabetes
- Peripheral vascular disease, atherosclerosis
- Thoracic outlet syndrome
- Connective tissue disorders (eg, scleroderma, systemic lupus erythematosus, rheumatoid arthritis)
- Illicit drug use
- Vascular tumors
- Pseudoaneurysm
- Iatrogenic injury

NONOPERATIVE MANAGEMENT

- Pharmacologic therapy is the mainstay of treatment of vasospastic disorders of the hand.
- Avoidance of smoking and exposure to cold temperatures may control vasospastic episodes.[9]
- Biofeedback
  - Patients are trained to control certain bodily processes that occur involuntarily.
  - Electrodes are attached to the skin of the patient and physiologic responses monitored.
  - The biofeedback therapist then leads the patient through exercises that bring about desired physical changes.
- Occlusive dressings may be helpful both to protect areas from recurrent trauma and to promote healing of lesions.
- Calcium channel blockers (eg, nifedipine)
- Pentoxifylline decreases blood viscosity and may result in relaxing vascular smooth muscle.
- Prostacyclins[26]
- Nitrates
- Local anesthetic blockade
- Botulinum toxin A[17,25]
- Thrombolytic therapy

SURGICAL MANAGEMENT

- The surgical management of vasospastic and vaso-occlusive diseases should proceed in a systematic fashion.
- Indications for operative management are progressive symptoms (eg, Raynaud syndrome, ulcers, pain, cold intolerance) despite optimal medical management and with angiographically defined occlusion of one or both inflow arteries (ie, radial, ulnar).
- Indications for a digital sympathectomy are progressive symptoms of Raynaud syndrome or ulcerations refractory to medical management with no evidence of major occlusion of the radial or ulnar arteries and with good visualization of three common digital arteries in the palm.
- Cold challenges are very painful for patients with scleroderma and systemic lupus erythematosus and are used on a case-by-case basis.
- The patient should be educated on the outcomes of the various procedures and realize the limitations of each one.
- Newer techniques such as fat grafting may improve symptoms in certain patients.[2]

Preoperative Planning

- The preoperative history and physical examination are reviewed.
- The site of operative intervention is determined primarily by the preoperative imaging studies (eg, angiogram).
- If vascular grafting is indicated, the donor vessels are identified and marked.

Positioning

- The patient is placed in the supine position on the operating room table with the extremity on an appropriately padded hand table.
- An upper arm tourniquet is placed because a bloodless field is essential.
- If a vein graft is anticipated, another extremity (usually a leg) is prepped and a proximal tourniquet is applied.

Approach

- Usually, the surgeon must access proximal arterial inflow vessels when treating either vasospastic or vaso-occlusive disorders of the hand.
- The brachial artery in the upper arm is approached via an incision on the medial aspect of the arm.
- The distal brachial artery and proximal radial and ulnar arteries are approached through a lazy S incision in the antecubital fossa.
  - Care is taken to avoid making a straight line incision across the antecubital fossa.
- The radial and ulnar arteries in the forearm are approached through a longitudinal incision over the specific vessel.
- The palmar arches are accessed via Bruner incisions extending proximally from the proximal phalanges, using natural creases in the palm where possible, or through an inverted J-shaped incision in the palm.
- The digital arteries are approached through Bruner incisions on the palmar aspect of the finger or through midlateral incisions on the digit.

TECHNIQUES

Flatt Digital Sympathectomy

- Flatt digital sympathectomy is used for patients with vasospastic disorders such as Raynaud phenomenon.[6]
- Proximal or cervical sympathectomy has largely fallen out of favor due to the high recurrence rates.
- Peripheral sympathectomy has gained popularity since Pick[21] identified sympathetic nerve fibers innervating the arteries from the wrist to the fingers.
  - Sympathectomy is performed at the level of the digital arteries.
- Make Bruner incisions in the distal palm and expose the digital arteries.
- Disrupt all connections between the digital nerves and digital arteries.
- Strip the adventitia from the digital arteries over a distance of 0.5 to 2.0 cm using the operating microscope (**TECH FIG 1A,B**).
  - Stripping must be performed very carefully to avoid damaging the digital arteries themselves.
- In cases of more widespread vasospasm, when more radical digital sympathectomy is desired, many surgeons recommend to strip the adventitia from the distal radial and ulnar arteries, the superficial palmar arch, and the common digital arteries in the palm[11,12,19] (**TECH FIG 1C,D**).

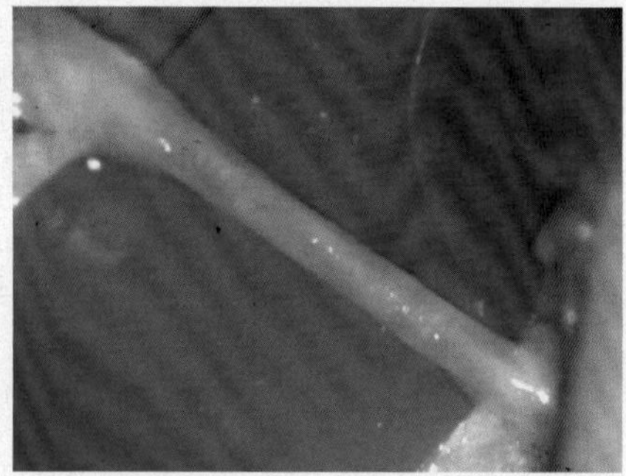
A

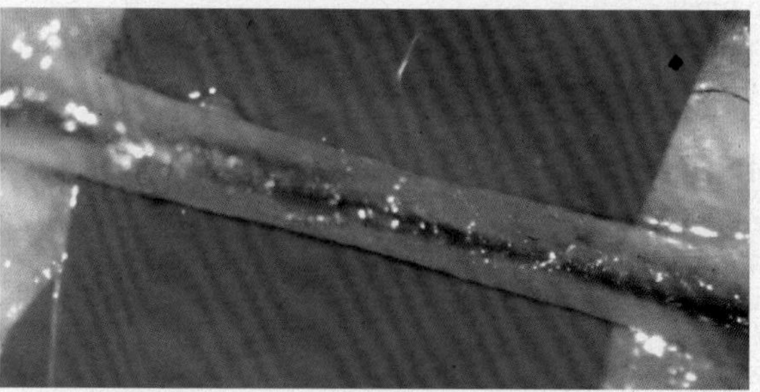
B

TECH FIG 1 • **A,B.** View through the operating microscope before (**A**) and after (**B**) removal of the adventitia from a common digital artery. *(continued)*

C 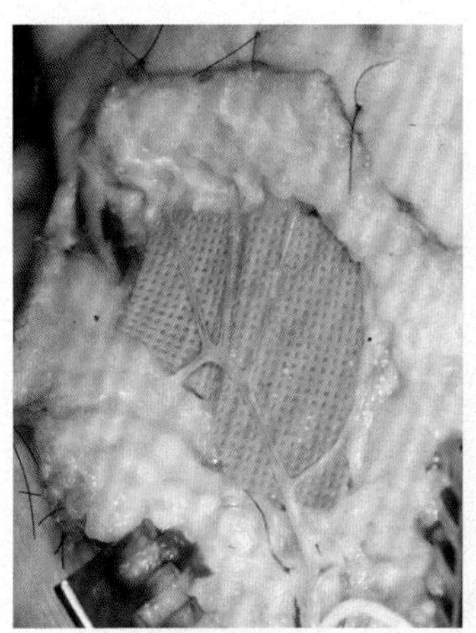

D 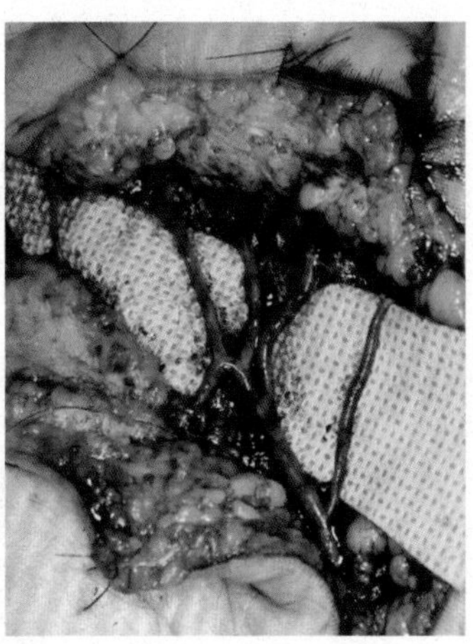

TECH FIG 1 • *(continued)* **C,D.** Radical or extensive digital sympathectomy before (**C**) and after (**D**) stripping the adventitia from the distal ulnar artery, superficial palmar arch, and common digital arteries to the index–middle, middle–ring, and ring–small finger web spaces.

Leriche Sympathectomy

- If adequate collateral flow is present, consider excision of a segment of thrombosed or occluded artery.[15]
- The concept is to reduce the sympathetic discharge from the diseased artery that is producing vasospasm in the more distal vessels.
- Resection is also used to treat a thrombosed or occluded ulnar artery in hypothenar hammer syndrome.

Microsurgical Revascularization

- Reconstruction of a thrombosed or occluded artery is considered if:
  - A discrete segment of artery can be resected and bypassed.
  - Adequate arterial inflow and patent distal arteries with adequate distal "runoff" are present to take advantage of the restored blood flow.
- Resect the arterial segment and measure the defect.
- Reverse vein grafts (eg, cephalic, saphenous) or arterial grafts (eg, deep inferior epigastric artery, lateral circumflex artery, thoracodorsal artery) are harvested in the standard fashion.
- Draw an axial line down the length of the vessel to be harvested while in situ.
  - The line helps prevent inadvertent "twisting" of the graft during the anastomoses.
- Perform standard microsurgical anastomoses using 9-0 or 10-0 nylon sutures and the operating microscope, between the distal radial or ulnar arteries and the deep or superficial palmar arches, respectively, or directly to one or more common digital arteries (**TECH FIG 2**).
- An end-to-side anastomosis of the graft to the inflow artery is preferable to maximize any remaining circulation to the hand, but end-to-end anastomoses are technically easier.
- The distal anastomosis is usually end to end to the superficial or deep palmar arches or end to side to the common digital arteries.
- After the anastomoses are completed, the tourniquet is deflated, and vascular inflow through the other artery is occluded by manual compression for a few minutes to maximize flow across the anastomoses.
- Restoration of arterial flow into the hand is assessed either by using a pencil Doppler probe or by performing an Acland "adventitial strip test" distal to the distal anastomosis.

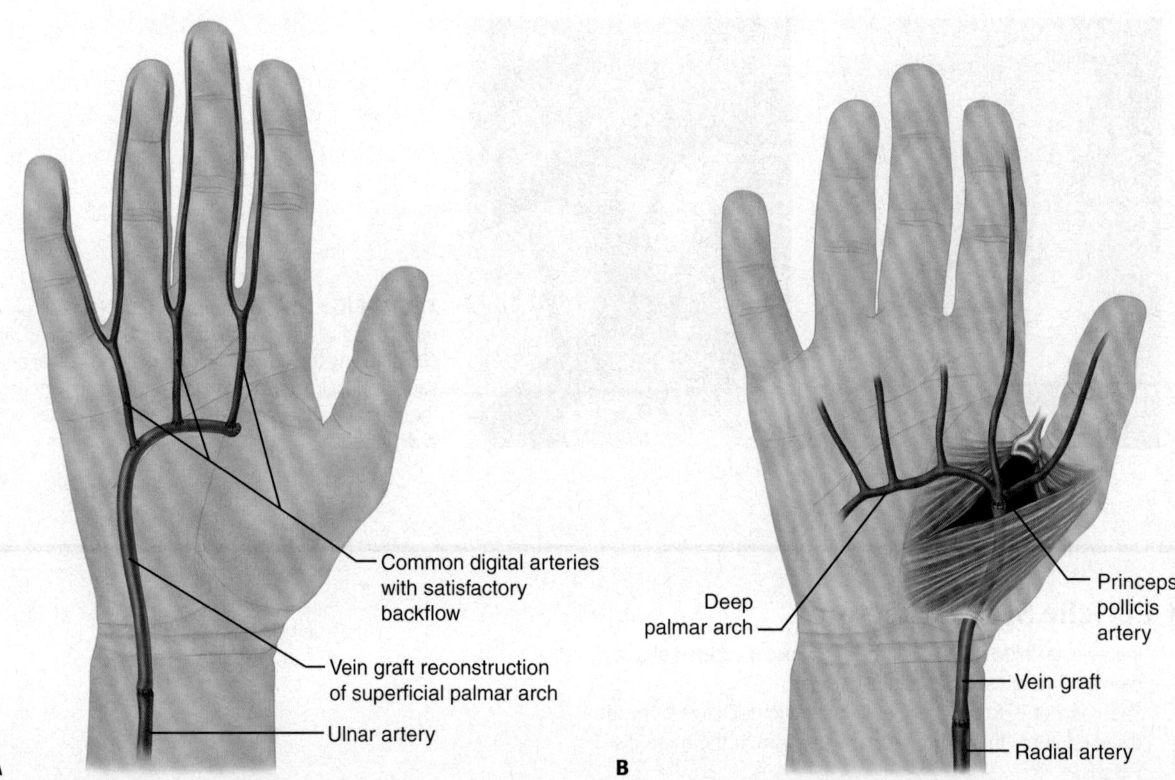

TECH FIG 2 • **A.** Microsurgical revascularization for thrombosis or occlusive disease of the distal ulnar artery and superficial palmar arch, using an interposition vein graft from the ulnar artery to the common digital arteries. **B.** Microvascular revascularization for thrombosis or occlusive disease of the distal radial artery and deep palmar arch, using an interposition vein graft from the radial artery to the princeps pollicis artery.

Embolectomy

- An acute embolus is treated by immediate heparinization to prevent propagation of the embolus more distally into the digits.
- Small Fogarty embolectomy catheters may be used selectively at the arm, elbow, forearm, and wrist levels, but use of embolectomy catheters in the hand and digits is difficult and can itself lead to vascular injury and further thrombosis.
- After identification of the segment involved by embolus, control the affected artery both proximal and distal to the embolus.
- Make a longitudinal arteriotomy proximally to access the vessel lumen.
  - A side branch may be chosen if available.
- Insert the Fogarty catheter into the artery and pass it down the lumen beyond the area of occlusion; then inflate the balloon.
- Gently withdraw the catheter to retrieve any thrombus.
  - Repeat catheterization until the lumen is completely cleared of the embolus, as demonstrated by improved back-bleeding from the distal vessel.
- Suture the arteriotomy and release arterial inflow.
- Assess the restoration of arterial flow into the hand either by using a pencil Doppler probe on the artery more distally or by performing an Acland adventitial strip test distal to the site of embolism.

Arterialization of the Venous System

- Choose a suitable vein on the dorsum of the hand, that is, one that will lie in a straight line following anastomosis to the radial or ulnar artery near the palmar wrist.[20]
- Mobilize the vein and ligate the multiple side branches of the vein with small hemoclips to maximize flow to the fingers.
- Perform valvulotomies in the vein to prevent valvular obstruction.
- Ligate the vein proximally and perform an end-to-side microsurgical anastomosis between the vein and the radial or ulnar artery at the wrist.
- After the anastomosis has been performed, assess arterial flow through the distal vein.
  - Any remaining obstruction due to a valve should be relieved by an open valvulotomy and excision of the valve leaflets, followed by microsurgical closure of the vein.
- Postoperative monitoring is performed using a pencil Doppler probe over the distal arterialized vein to the fingers.

PEARLS AND PITFALLS

Indications	▪ History and physical examination should isolate the probable cause for ischemia. ▪ Preoperative studies should confirm the cause before surgical intervention.
Sympathectomy	▪ Strip the adventitia of the artery over a distance of 0.5–2.0 cm.
Microsurgical reconstruction	▪ A discrete segment of thrombosed or occluded artery are identified to be effective. ▪ Adequate arterial inflow and distal runoff is essential.
Embolectomy propagation of the clot	▪ Identification of an embolus must be treated with heparinization immediately to prevent propagation. ▪ Use of embolectomy catheters in the hand and digits should be done selectively and with caution.
Arterialization of the venous system	▪ Generally used for unreconstructable vascular lesions. ▪ Valvulotomies are performed to prevent vascular obstruction when flow is established. ▪ All venous side branches are ligated to maximize flow distally.

POSTOPERATIVE CARE

- The hand is immobilized in a lightweight splint to protect the operative site, with care taken to avoid any pressure on the underlying anastomoses or vulnerable mobilized arteries.
- The fingertips are assessed for color and capillary refill, temperature using a small temperature probes, or oxygen saturation using a pulse oximeter.
- Microvascular reconstruction with interposition grafts can be monitored using a pencil Doppler probe.
- Relative anticoagulation can be achieved using a continuous infusion of dextran 40 or low-dose aspirin.

OUTCOMES

- Calcium channel blockers are moderately effective in patients with Raynaud phenomenon, with 35% reporting improvement in severity of their symptoms.[23]
- Results of sympathectomy remain variable, although surgeons have reported improvements in pain, ulcer healing, cold intolerance, and quality of life.[8,11,14,22,24]
- Long-term patency rates for vascular bypass grafting secondary to occlusive disease have been reported to range between 53% and 94%.[3,11,13,16]
- Combining sympathectomy with arterial reconstruction may offer improved outcomes versus sympathectomy alone.[7]

COMPLICATIONS

- Bleeding and hematoma
- Infection
- Thrombosis of the interposition graft
- Progression of the underlying systemic disease

REFERENCES

1. Allen E, Brown G. Raynaud's disease: a critical review of minimal requisites for diagnosis. Am J Med Sci 1932;83:187–200.
2. Bank J, Fuller SM, Henry GI, et al. Fat grafting to the hand in patients with Raynaud phenomenon: a novel therapeutic modality. Plast Reconstr Surg 2014;133:1109–1118.
3. Barral X, Favre JP, Gournier JP, et al. Late results of palmar arch bypass in the treatment of digital trophic disorders. Ann Vasc Surg 1992;6:418–424.
4. Coleman SS, Anson BJ. Arterial patterns in the hand based upon a study of 650 specimens. Surg Gynecol Obstet 1961;113:409–424.
5. Dalinka MK, Meyer S, Kricun ME, et al. Magnetic resonance imaging of the wrist. Hand Clin 1991;7:87–98.
6. Flatt AE. Digital artery sympathectomy. J Hand Surg Am 1980;5:550–556.
7. Given KS, Puckett CL, Klienert HE. Ulnar artery thrombosis. Plast Reconstr Surg 1978;61:405–411.
8. Hartzell TL, Makhni EC, Sampson C. Long-term results of periarterial sympathectomy. J Hand Surg 2009;34:1454–1460.
9. Herrick AL. Management of Raynaud's phenomenon and digital ischemia. Curr Rheumatol Rep 2013;15:303.
10. Hutchinson DT. Color duplex imaging. Applications to upper extremity and microvascular surgery. Hand Clin 1993;9:47–51.
11. Jones NF. Acute and chronic ischemia of the hand: pathophysiology, treatment, and prognosis. J Hand Surg Am 1991;16:1074–1083.
12. Jones NF. Ischemia of the hand in systemic disease. The potential role of microsurgical revascularization and digital sympathectomy. Clin Plast Surg 1989;16:547–556.
13. Koman LA, Ruch DS, Aldridge M, et al. Arterial reconstruction in the ischemic hand and wrist: effects on microvascular physiology and health-related quality of life. J Hand Surg Am 1998;23:773–782.
14. Koman LA, Smith BP, Pollack FE Jr, et al. The microcirculatory effect of peripheral sympathectomy. J Hand Surg Am 1999;20:709–717.
15. Leriche R, Fontaine R, Dupertius SM. Arterectomy with follow-up studies on 78 operations. Surg Gynecol Obstet 1937;64:149–155.
16. McCarthy WJ, Flinn WR, Yao JS, et al. Result of bypass grafting for upper limb ischemia. J Vasc Surg 1986;3:741–746.
17. Neumeister MW. Botulinum toxin type A in the treatment of Raynaud's phenomenon. J Hand Surg Am 2010;35:2085–2092.
18. Nielsen SL, Lassen NA. Measurement of digital blood pressure after local cooling. J Appl Physiol Respir Environ Exerc Physiol 1977;43:907–910.
19. O'Brien BM, Kumar PA, Mellow CG, et al. Radical microarteriolysis in the treatment of vasospastic disorders of the hand, especially scleroderma. J Hand Surg Br 1992;17:447–452.
20. Pederson WC, Woodward C, Hermansdorfer J. Arterialization of the venous system for the treatment of end-stage ischemia of the upper extremity. J Reconstr Microsurg 1996;12:414–417.
21. Pick J. The Autonomic Nervous System. Philadelphia: JB Lippincott, 1970.
22. Ruch DS, Koman LA, Smith TL. Chronic vascular disorders of the upper extremity. J Am Soc Surg Hand 2001;1:73–80.
23. Thompson AE, Shea B, Welch V, et al. Calcium channel blockers for Raynaud's phenomenon in systemic sclerosis. Arthritis Rheum 2001;44:1841–1847.
24. Tomaino MM, Goitz RJ, Medsger TA. Surgery for ischemic pain and Raynaud's phenomenon in scleroderma: a description of treatment protocol and evaluation of results. Microsurgery 2001;21:75–79.
25. Van Beek AL, Lim PK, Gear AJ, et al. Management of vasospastic disorders with botulinum toxin A. Plast Reconstr Surg 2007;119:217–226.
26. Wigley FM, Wise RA, Seibold JR, et al. Intravenous iloprost infusion in patients with Raynaud phenomenon secondary to systemic sclerosis. A multicenter, placebo-controlled, double-blind study. Ann Intern Med 1994;120:199–206.

Surgical Treatment of Deep Space Infections of the Hand

Jennifer Etcheson and Jeffrey Yao

DEFINITION

- Deep space infections occur in one of three anatomically defined potential spaces within the hand.
  - Thenar, midpalmar, and hypothenar spaces
  - Interdigital subfacial web space
  - Parona space—a potential forearm space
- Thenar space infections are the most common deep space infections. Midpalmar and hypothenar space infections are much more rare.
- Deep space infections usually result from direct penetrating trauma or spread from an adjacent infection such as a superficial abscess or a flexor tenosynovitis (in the case of thenar and midpalmar space infections).
- The single most common infecting organism is *Staphylococcus aureus*, although most of these infections are mixed. Other common pathogens include streptococci and coliforms.[2]

ANATOMY

- The thenar space (**FIG 1**) is defined by the fascia of the adductor pollicis muscle dorsally and the tendon sheath of the index finger and palmar fascia volarly.
  - The radial border is defined by the insertion of the adductor pollicis tendon and fascia on the thumb proximal phalanx.
  - The ulnar border is the midpalmar (oblique) septum, which extends from the third metacarpal to the palmar fascia.

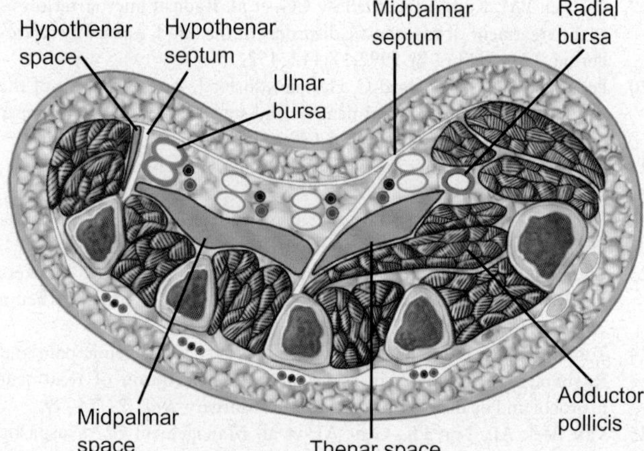

FIG 1 • Cross-sectional anatomy of the hand demonstrating the deep spaces.

- The midpalmar space (see **FIG 1**) is bordered radially by the midpalmar septum and bordered ulnarly by the hypothenar septum, which extends from the fifth metacarpal to the palmar fascia.
  - The dorsal border of the midpalmar space is the fascia of the second and third palmar interosseous muscles, and the volar border is the flexor sheaths of the long, ring, and small fingers and the palmar fascia.
- The hypothenar space (see **FIG 1**) is bordered radially by the hypothenar septum and dorsally by the periosteum of the fifth metacarpal. The fascia of the hypothenar muscles forms the ulnar and palmar borders.
- The interdigital subfacial web spaces are three interdigital spaces at the distal end of the palm containing loose subcutaneous fat. These spaces are located near the metacarpophalangeal joints, just proximal to the deep transverse ligaments.
- Parona space is a deep potential space in the distal forearm superficial to pronator quadratus and deep to the flexor digitorum profundus tendons. It is continuous with the midpalmar space.

PATHOGENESIS

- Thenar space infections may result from penetrating injury or local spread from adjacent flexor tenosynovitis or a subcutaneous abscess.
- If not treated early, the infection may spread to the dorsal side of the hand after destroying the fascia of the adductor pollicis muscles and traveling between the transverse and oblique heads.
- Midpalmar space infections usually result from direct penetrating trauma but may also result from spread of an adjacent flexor tenosynovitis or superficial abscess.
- Hypothenar space infections usually result from direct penetrating trauma but may also result from spread of a superficial abscess.
- Interdigital subfacial web space infections usually result from penetrating injury but may also result from spread of an adjacent lumbrical canal infection or infected palmar blister.[1]
- Parona space infection may result from direct penetrating trauma, in which case the infection may be isolated to Parona space.
  - Infection involving Parona space may also result from contiguous spread from a ruptured radial or ulnar bursae (**FIG 2**). The end result will be involvement of the midpalmar space and a horseshoe abscess (**FIG 3**).

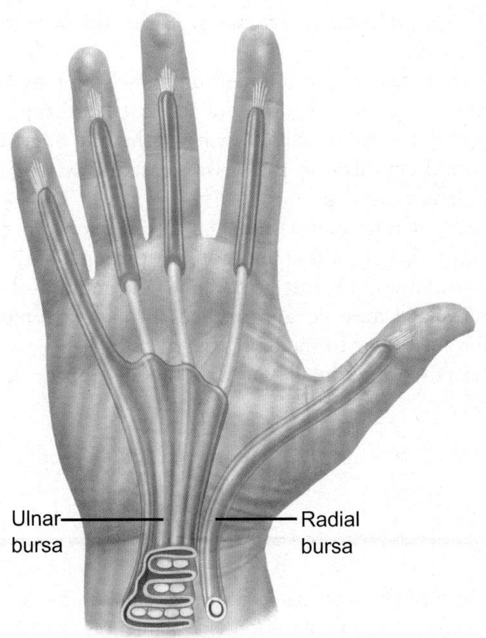

FIG 2 ● Radial and ulnar bursae may communicate in the distal volar forearm (Parona space).

PATIENT HISTORY AND PHYSICAL FINDINGS

- The patient may recall a history of a penetrating injury in the vicinity of the involved deep space.
- In the case of a thenar space infection, the patient will present with swelling and tenderness in the thenar region.
  - The patient will hold the thumb in an abducted position to minimize the pressure for comfort.
  - If the infection has been present for some time, it may have spread dorsally, in which case swelling and tenderness will be found dorsally in the first web space.
- In the case of a midpalmar space infection, there will be tenderness and swelling in the midpalm, although dorsal swelling may be more impressive due to the strength of the palmar aponeurosis.
  - The fingers will be held in a semiflexed posture.

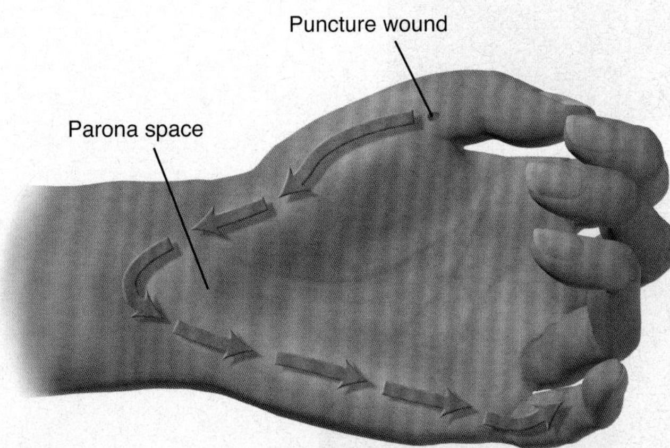

FIG 3 ● Drawing representing the clinical appearance of a horseshoe abscess.

  - This condition is distinguished from flexor tenosynovitis by relative lack of pain with passive motion of the fingers and with direct palpation of the flexor sheath along the digit.
- In the case of interdigital subfacial web space infection, the patient will present with swelling and tenderness in the dorsum of the hand and maximal tenderness on the palmar aspect of the web space.
  - If the infection is severe, the fingers may be abducted on either side of the infected web space.[1]
- Infection of Parona space is characterized by swelling in the distal volar forearm and pain with digital flexion.
  - Infection involving Parona space may also result from contiguous spread from a ruptured radial or ulnar bursae (see **FIG 2**).

IMAGING AND OTHER DIAGNOSTIC STUDIES

- Radiographs should be obtained in all cases to rule out the presence of foreign bodies.
- Radiographs also may reveal underlying osteomyelitis in the setting of more chronic infections.
- Patients suspected to have systemic illness should have an appropriate laboratory workup.

DIFFERENTIAL DIAGNOSIS

- Thenar space infection
- Midpalmar space infection
- Hypothenar space infection
- Flexor tenosynovitis
- Superficial abscess
- Osteomyelitis

NONOPERATIVE MANAGEMENT

- There is no role for nonoperative treatment in the setting of deep space infections.
- Antibiotics should be avoided until adequate cultures can be obtained, unless the patient is systemically ill and there will be a forced delay in operative treatment.

SURGICAL MANAGEMENT

- Drainage of deep space infections should be carried out in the operating room under general anesthesia.
- Gram stain and cultures for aerobes, anaerobes, mycobacteria, and fungi should be obtained intraoperatively just before intravenous [IV] antibiotics are administered.
- Thorough irrigation with 6 to 9 L of normal saline should be performed.
- All nonviable tissue must be débrided sharply.
- Surgical wounds may be closed very loosely over a drain if all necrotic tissue has been thoroughly débrided.
  - If there is any doubt, the wound should be left open to heal by secondary intention using wet-to-dry dressing changes and soaks.
  - In very severe cases, a second irrigation 48 to 72 hours later may be required.

Positioning

- The patient is positioned supine with a standard hand table and nonsterile tourniquet.

Approach

- Drainage of thenar space infections can be performed through a volar incision or a dorsal longitudinal incision (or, sometimes, both).
  - A volar incision involves risk to the recurrent motor branch of the median nerve, the digital nerves to the thumb and index fingers, the princeps pollicis artery, and the proper digital arteries.
  - A volar incision also allows concomitant treatment of a thumb septic flexor tenosynovitis.
  - A dorsal longitudinal incision avoids the painful scar associated with a volar incision.
- Drainage of midpalmar space infections may be performed through a transverse skin incision in, or parallel to, the distal palmar crease over the third and fourth metacarpals.
  - Alternatively, a curved longitudinal incision may be used.
- Hypothenar space infections are approached through an incision in line with the ulnar border of the ring finger extending from 3 cm distal to the wrist crease to just proximal to the midpalmar crease.
- Drainage of interdigital subfacial infections are performed through either a palmar incision, or through both palmar and dorsal incisions, just proximal to the actual web space.
- Parona space may be approached through a longitudinal incision just ulnar to the palmaris longus.
  - Alternatively, a transflexor carpi radialis approach may be used.

TECHNIQUES

Incision and Drainage of Thenar Space Infections

- In the case of a volar approach, make an incision just adjacent and parallel to the thenar crease, beginning 1 cm proximal to the web space and extending 3 to 4 cm proximally (**TECH FIG 1A**).
- After blunt dissection through the palmar fascia, the digital nerves to the thumb and index fingers, the princeps pollicis artery, the proper digital arteries, and the recurrent motor branch of the median nerve are encountered (**TECH FIG 1B,C**).
- The abscess will lie superficial to the adductor pollicis muscle.
- Dissection should then continue dorsally over the distal edge of the adductor muscle to decompress any dorsal extension of the abscess.
- Alternatively, a thenar space infection may be approached dorsally through a longitudinal incision (**TECH FIG 1D**).
- The dorsal incision may be straight or slightly curved and should bisect the space between the first and second metacarpals.
  - Dissection should be carried down to the interval between the first dorsal interosseous muscle and adductor pollicis muscle, where the purulence will be encountered.
- Thoroughly débride all necrotic tissue and irrigate copiously with sterile saline.
- Place a strip of packing strip gauze into the open wound to allow for drainage, and dress the wound appropriately.

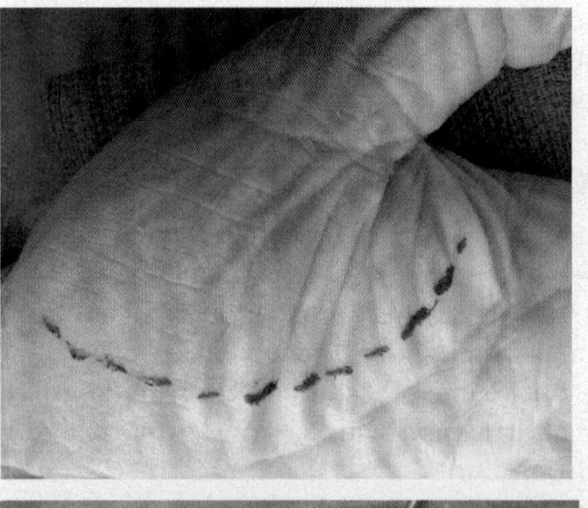
A

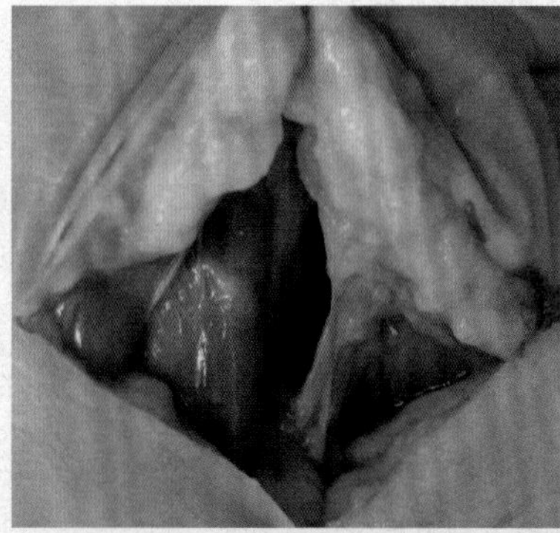
B

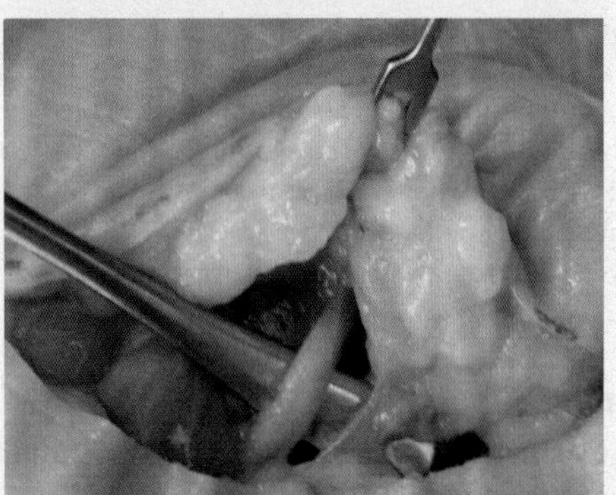
C

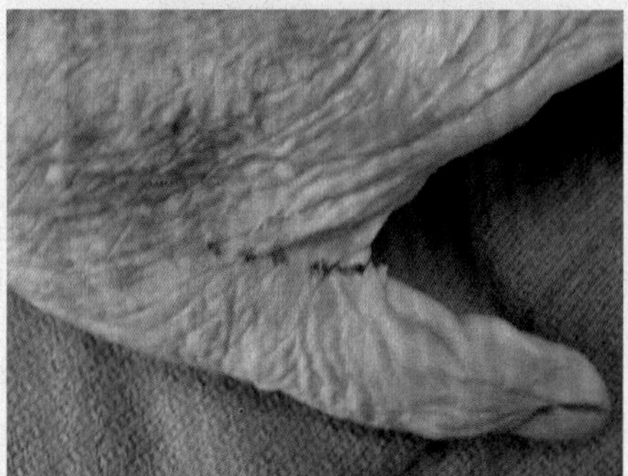
D

TECH FIG 1 • **A.** Thenar incision. **B,C.** Neurovascular bundle. **D.** Alternative dorsal incision for drainage of thenar abscess.

Incision and Drainage of Midpalmar Space Infections

- Make a transverse incision parallel to or in the distal palmar crease over the third and fourth metacarpals (**TECH FIG 2A**).
  - Alternatively, a curved longitudinal incision may be used (**TECH FIG 2B**).
- Bluntly dissect to either side of the flexor tendons to the ring or middle finger, where the abscess will be encountered.
- Protect the neurovascular bundles, which lie on either side of the tendons (**TECH FIG 2C**).
- Thoroughly débride all necrotic tissue and irrigate copiously with sterile saline.
- Place a strip of packing strip gauze into the open wound to allow for drainage, and dress the wound appropriately.

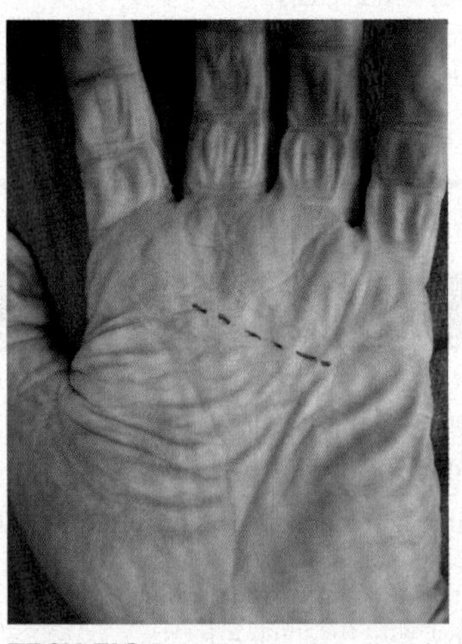
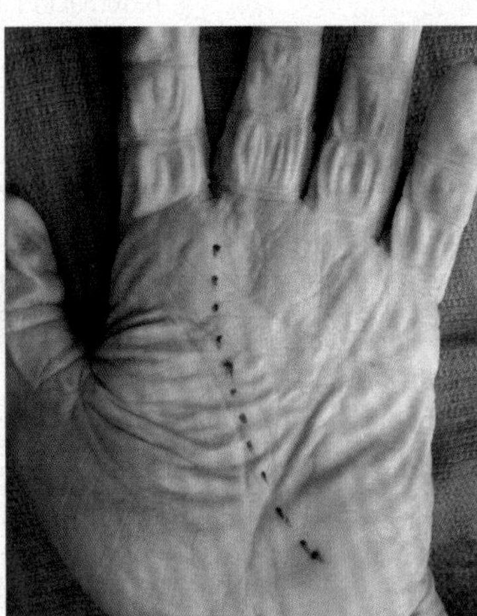
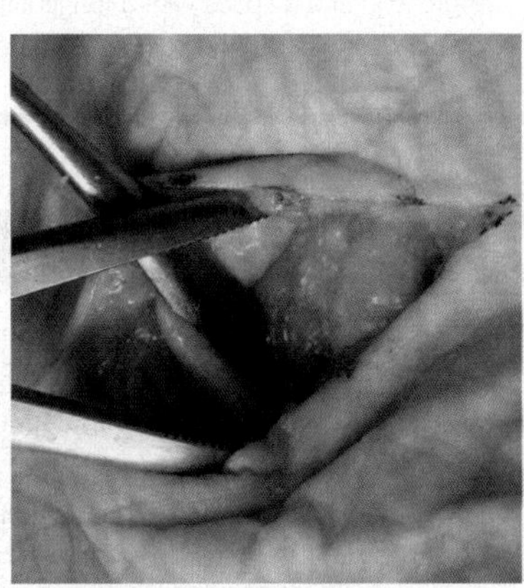

TECH FIG 2 • **A.** Transverse incision for drainage of midpalmar abscess. **B.** Curved longitudinal incision for drainage of midpalmar abscess. **C.** Drainage of midpalmar abscess (neurovascular bundle protected by Freer).

Incision and Drainage of Hypothenar Space Infections

- Make an incision in line with the ulnar border of the ring finger, extending from just proximal to the midpalmar crease to 3 cm distal to the wrist crease (**TECH FIG 3A**).
- Incise the hypothenar fascia in line with the skin incision and the purulence will be encountered (**TECH FIG 3B**).
- Thoroughly débride all necrotic tissue and irrigate copiously with sterile saline.
- Place a strip of packing strip gauze into the open wound to allow for drainage, and dress the wound appropriately.

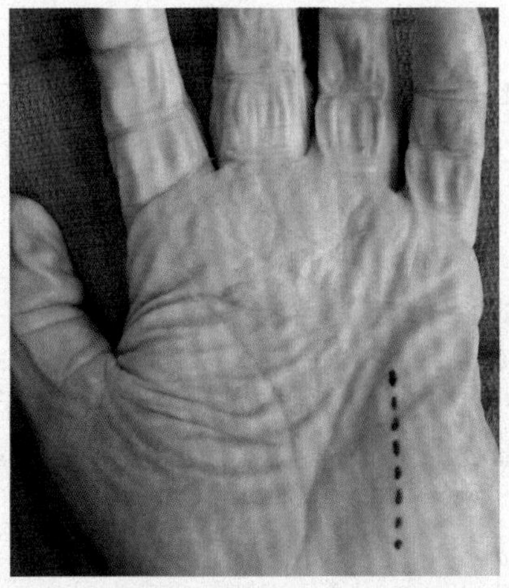
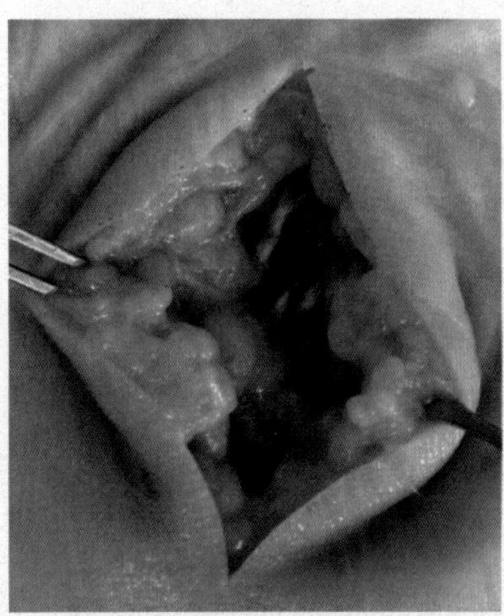

TECH FIG 3 • Incision (**A**) and drainage (**B**) of a hypothenar abscess.

TECHNIQUES

Incision and Drainage of Interdigital Subfacial Web Space

- Approach the interdigital web space with a palmar incision, and excise the palmar fascia lying within the interdigital web space to gain better access for drainage of the infection.[1]
  - Alternatively, both a palmar and dorsal incision may be used.
- Irrigate both the dorsal and palmar extension of the web infection with thoroughly with sterile saline.
- Transverse incisions or extension of incisions into the transverse web should be avoided, as they may cause web contracture.[1]

Incision and Drainage of Parona Space Infections

- Approach Parona space with a longitudinal incision in the distal forearm just ulnar to the palmaris longus.
- If the infection is isolated to Parona space, keep the incision proximal to the wrist flexion crease.
- If the infection is contiguous with a midpalmar space abscess, the incision is carried across the wrist in Brunner fashion.

PEARLS AND PITFALLS

Misdiagnosis	▪ Recognize underlying osteomyelitis in long-standing cases. ▪ Recognize any systemic illness that may hinder resolution of the infection.
Presurgical planning	▪ Always obtain radiographs to evaluate for osteomyelitis or a foreign body.
Technique	▪ When approaching the thenar space, protect the digital nerves to the thumb and index fingers, the princeps pollicis artery, the proper digital arteries, and the recurrent motor branch of the median nerve. ▪ In the midpalmar space, protect the superficial palmar arch and the digital nerves and arteries. ▪ In the hypothenar space, protect the ulnar nerve and its branches, together with the ulnar artery. ▪ Obtain Gram stain and cultures for anaerobes, aerobes, mycobacteria, and fungi. ▪ Administer IV antibiotics intraoperatively once cultures have been obtained. ▪ May close over Penrose drain if débridement is adequate ▪ If there is the possibility of remaining necrotic tissue, the wound should be left open to close by secondary intention.
Postoperative care	▪ Allow open wounds to heal by secondary intention with wet-to-dry dressing changes. ▪ IV oral antibiotics for 7–14 days ▪ Infectious disease consultation, if necessary ▪ Maintain elevation. ▪ Use of a removable splint will rest soft tissues and improve patient comfort. ▪ Perform soaks in warm water three times per day. ▪ Begin early digital range-of-motion exercises. ▪ Be prepared to repeat irrigation and débridement if there is no clinical improvement after 48 hours.

POSTOPERATIVE CARE

- IV antibiotics, initially given intraoperatively, are continued postoperatively.
- The patient may be switched to oral antibiotics once cultures and sensitivities return from the microbiology laboratory and if he or she is responding to IV antibiotic therapy.
- Let open wounds heal by secondary intention using wet-to-dry dressing changes and soaks or whirlpools.
- Remove drains after 24 to 48 hours, depending on the condition of the wound and particulars associated with surgery.
- Begin early range-of-motion exercises during soaks or whirlpool treatments to minimize digital stiffness.
- Treatment of systemic illness is critical.

COMPLICATIONS

- Persistent abscess formation if irrigation and débridement is inadequate or the wound is closed tightly and not allowed to drain
- Systemic spread of the infection if appropriate treatment is delayed

REFERENCES

1. Franko OI, Abrams RA. Hand infections. Orthop Clin North Am 2013;44(4):625–634.
2. Hausman MR, Lisser SP. Hand infections. Orthop Clin North Am 1992;23:171–185.

SUGGESTED READINGS

Burkhalter WE. Deep space infections. Hand Clin 1989;5:553–559.

Leddy JP. Infections of the upper extremity. J Hand Surg Am 1986;11:294–297.

Siegel DB, Gelberman RH. Infections of the hand. Orthop Clin North Am 1988;19:779–789.

Surgical Treatment of Acute and Chronic Paronychia and Felons

129
CHAPTER

Jennifer Etcheson and Jeffrey Yao

DEFINITION

- An *acute paronychia* is an infection of the soft tissue fold around the fingernail.
  - It is the most common soft tissue infection of the hand.
  - The most common infecting organism is *Staphylococcus aureus*, although these infections are commonly mixed infections.
- A *chronic paronychia* is characterized by repeated infection and inflammation of the eponychium.
  - The eponychium becomes thickened and rounded.
  - This problem often occurs in the setting of repeated and prolonged exposure to water.
  - The most commonly isolated organisms are *Candida albicans*, gram-positive cocci, gram-negative rods, and *Mycobacterium* spp.
- *Herpetic whitlow* is caused by an outbreak of herpes simplex virus in the skin of the finger and can be confused with acute paronychia or felon.
  - Herpetic whitlow is common in children and medical personnel who come into contact with oral secretions.
- A *felon* is a tense abscess of the distal pulp of the finger or thumb that involves multiple septal compartments (**FIG 1**).

ANATOMY

- The nail complex consists of the nail bed, nail plate, and perionychium (**FIG 2**).
- The nail plate sits below the proximal nail fold.
- The *perionychium* is the border tissue which surrounds the nail.
- The *eponychium* is the tissue that attaches closely to the nail plate proximally, commonly referred to as the *cuticle*.
- The nail folds consist of skin, which continues underneath the visible edges to form a protective barrier.
- The pulp of each digit consists of multiple compartments separated by fibrous septa.
  - These vertical septa extend from the periosteum of the distal phalanx to the epidermis, lending structural support to the fingertip.

PATHOGENESIS

- Acute paronychia results from the introduction of bacteria into the space between the nail fold and the nail plate, either proximally or laterally.
  - This commonly occurs as a result of a hangnail, nail biting, artificial nails, or an overzealous manicure.
- Chronic paronychia results from colonization and infection by organisms that enter the space between the nail plate and the cuticle, eponychium, and nail fold.
  - Infection may result from repeated exposure to moisture.
  - This chronic infection and inflammation lead to fibrosis of the eponychium, which, in turn, leads to decreased vascularity of the dorsal nail fold.
  - This decreased vascularity predisposes to repeated bacterial insults, resulting in the characteristic clinical exacerbations.
- Felons often result from penetrating trauma or from bacterial inoculation through the exocrine sweat glands contained within the pulp.
  - Cellulitis and local inflammation lead to local ischemia, which, in the setting of the closed spaces defined by septa, leads to increased pressure.
  - Fat necrosis and abscess formation result from the increased pressure, which, in turn, causes a further increase in pressure and, in effect, a compartment syndrome.

NATURAL HISTORY

- If acute paronychia is left untreated, an early infection will turn into an abscess along the nail fold.
  - The abscess may then extend into the pulp space or into the eponychium and then to the opposite side of the nail.
  - Purulence at the base of the nail may cause ischemia of the germinal matrix, which then may lead to temporary or permanent nail growth arrest.
- Herpetic whitlow improves without any intervention in approximately 3 weeks.
  - Many cases of herpetic whitlow are misdiagnosed as acute paronychia or felon.

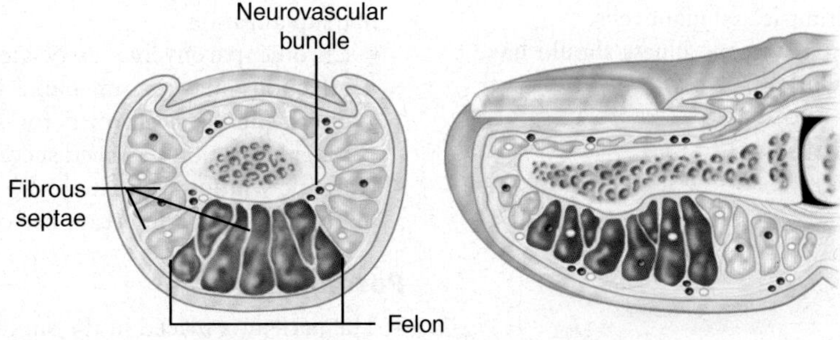

FIG 1 • Felon in coronal and sagittal section.

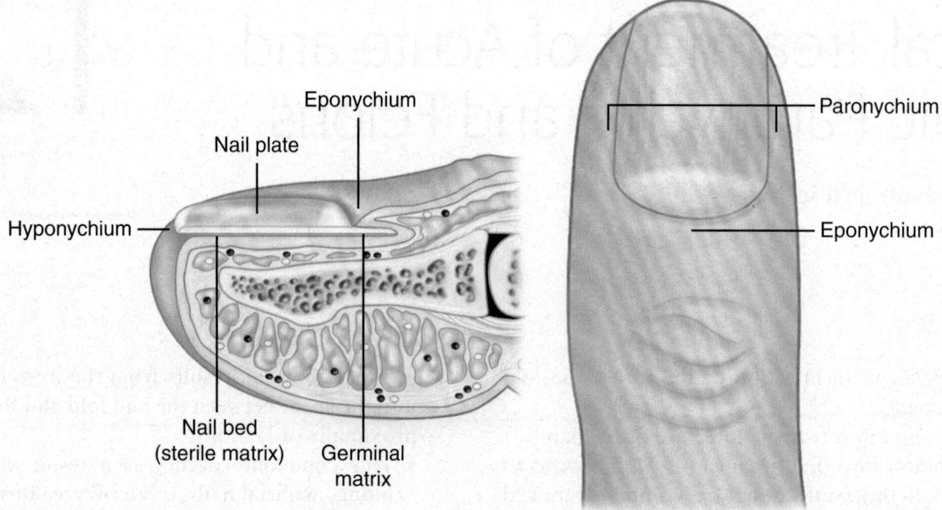

FIG 2 • Anatomy of the nail complex.

- Subsequent incision and drainage may lead to secondary bacterial infection.
- Chronic paronychia are characterized by induration of the eponychium punctuated by episodes of swelling and drainage.
- A felon, if left untreated, may lead to osteomyelitis or septic flexor tenosynovitis.

PATIENT HISTORY AND PHYSICAL FINDINGS

- In acute paronychia, the patient will complain of swelling and pain immediately adjacent to the nail.
  - If an abscess has formed, there may be erythema and purulent drainage.
- In chronic paronychia, the patient will present with a chronically indurated and rounded eponychium characterized by repeated episodes of inflammation and drainage.
- Herpetic whitlow is characterized by pain and swelling followed by the appearance of multiple vesicular lesions.
  - The pain typically is out of proportion to the physical findings, and the fingertip is not tense (in contrast to a felon).
- A patient with a felon will present with severe throbbing pain, swelling, and a tense fingertip pad.
  - A felon will not extend proximal to the distal interphalangeal (DIP) joint flexion crease unless it is associated with septic flexor tenosynovitis.

IMAGING AND OTHER DIAGNOSTIC STUDIES

- Radiographs are indicated to rule out osteomyelitis or if a foreign body is suspected.
- The diagnosis of herpetic whitlow is confirmed by Tzanck smear, which will show multinucleated giant cells.
- Patients suspected of having a systemic illness should have the appropriate laboratory workup.

DIFFERENTIAL DIAGNOSIS

- Acute paronychia
- Chronic paronychia
- Herpetic whitlow
- Felon
- Osteomyelitis
- Septic arthritis of the DIP joint

NONOPERATIVE MANAGEMENT

- Acute paronychia may be treated with warm soaks and oral antibiotics if infection is caught early and if no significant abscess is present.
- Herpetic whitlow is managed by keeping the hands clean to prevent bacterial superinfections; these lesions will resolve on their own.
  - Some recommend treatment with oral acyclovir, but multiple clinical trials have failed to show any definite benefit.
- Nonoperative treatment has no role in the treatment of chronic paronychia unless there is a concomitant fungal infection that may benefit from medical therapy.
- Given the rapid clinical progression of a felon, nonoperative treatment with antibiotics rarely will be successful, except in very early cases.

SURGICAL MANAGEMENT

- If the abscess is superficial, drainage may sometimes be performed without anesthesia.
- If the infection is more extensive or involves both sides of the nail, incision and drainage should be performed under digital nerve block.
  - Use lidocaine or a mixture of lidocaine and bupivacaine without epinephrine.
  - Instillation of the medication at the level of the distal metacarpal from dorsal to volar is the safest and best tolerated technique.
- Chronic paronychia usually are treated with eponychial marsupialization.
  - Chronic paronychia associated with underlying fungal infections may be amenable to more standard surgical treatments as performed for acute paronychia after the fungal infection has been successfully treated medically.
- Herpetic whitlow is treated with incision and drainage *only* if a bacterial superinfection has occurred.

Positioning

- The patient is placed in the supine position with a standard hand table and either digital or forearm tourniquet.

Approach

- The surgical approach is dictated by the location of the infection.
- Infection under the nail plate will require elevation of part of the nail.
- Infection under the eponychial fold will require elevation of the eponychium.
- Infection into the pulp will require incision deep into the pulp space.

Incision and Drainage of an Acute Paronychia

Single Incision

- Use a no. 15 scalpel to incise into the paronychial sulcus, keeping the blade directed away from the nail bed (**TECH FIG 1A**).
- If the abscess extends below the nail plate, then that portion of the nail is freed from the underlying bed, a longitudinal incision is made in the nail, and that section of the nail is removed in an atraumatic manner (**TECH FIG 1B,C**).
  - Alternatively, if the purulence extends into the pulp space, the perionychium may be incised peripheral and parallel to the nail sulcus (**TECH FIG 1D,E**).
- If the abscess extends to the eponychium, the incision may be carried as far proximally as necessary; a portion of nail may then be removed if necessary.
  - Avoid making an incision across the eponychium, as this may result in a late nail fold deformity.

Parallel Incisions

- If the abscess involves the eponychium and is not completely decompressed with a single incision, a parallel incision may be made on the opposite paronychial sulcus. The entire eponychial fold is elevated, and the proximal third of the nail is excised (**TECH FIG 2**).
- This is then irrigated and packed with gauze to prevent premature closure.

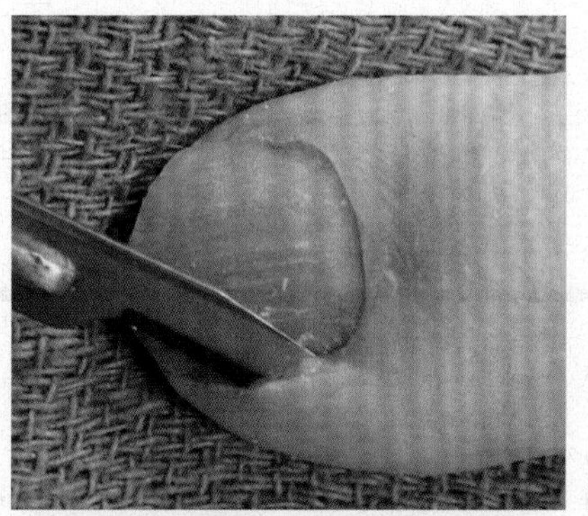

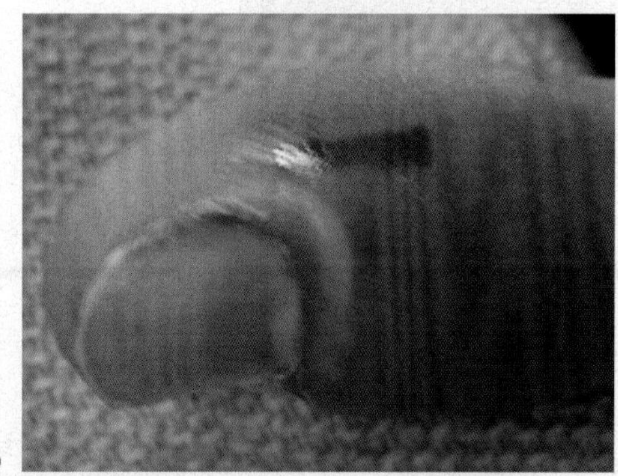

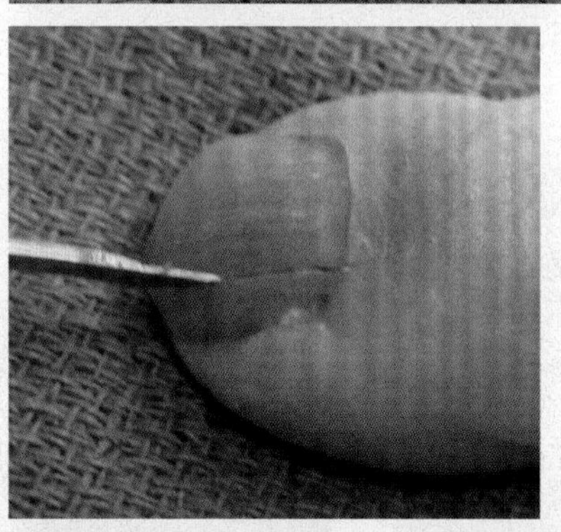

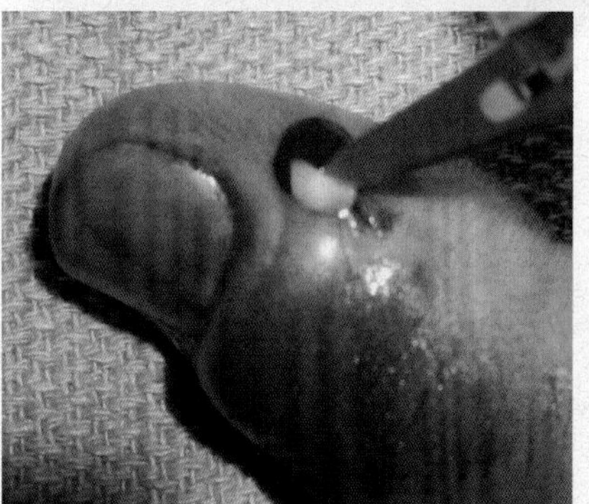

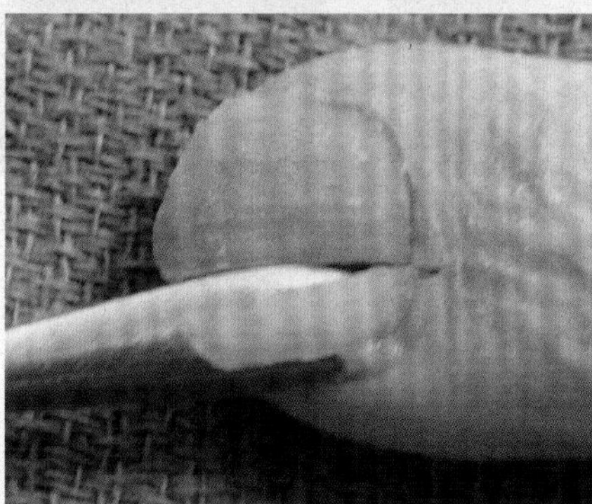

TECH FIG 1 • **A.** Incision to drain the paronychia. **B,C.** Incision and removal of a portion of the nail plate. **D,E.** Alternative incision to drain the paronychia.

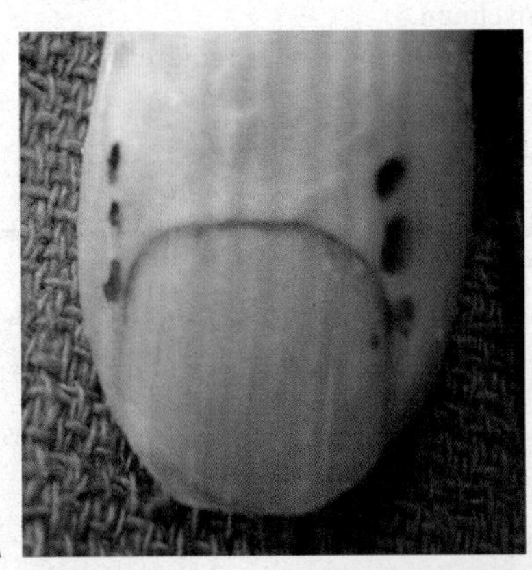

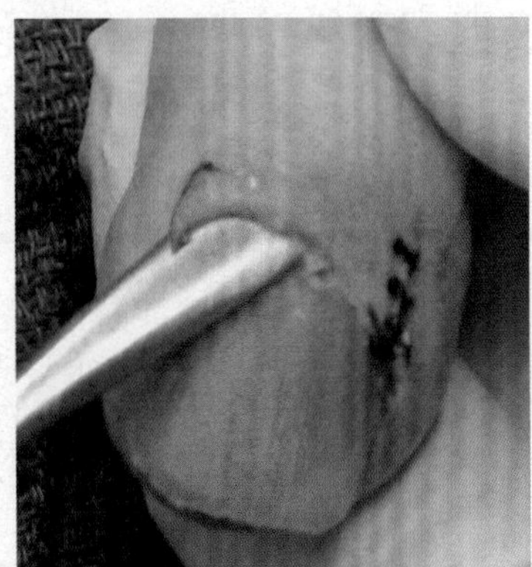

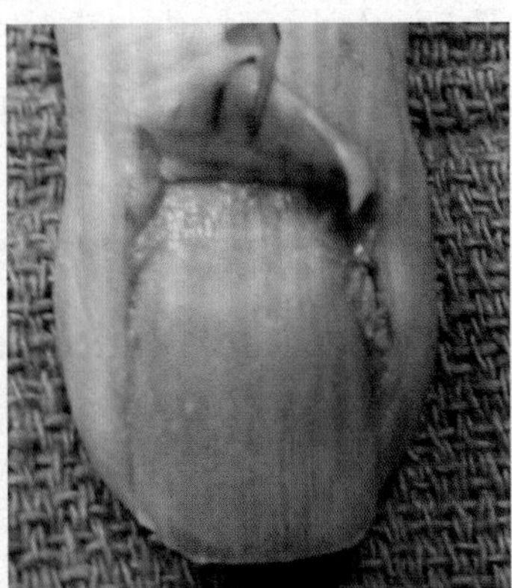

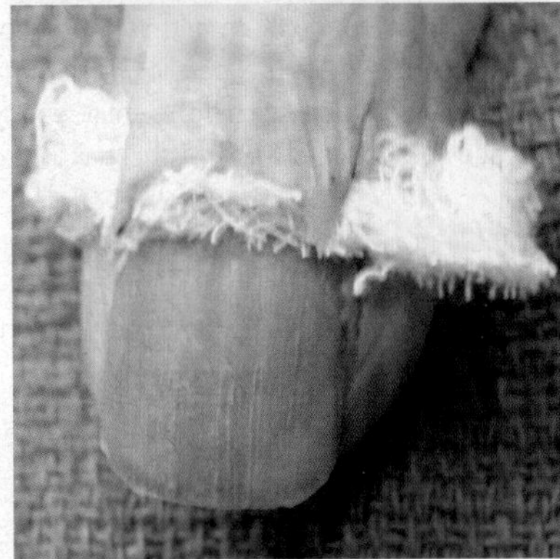

TECH FIG 2 • Incision (**A**) and elevation of the eponychial fold (**B,C**) with removal of the proximal nail to decompress a proximal abscess. **D.** The wound is packed with gauze to prevent premature closure.

Eponychial Marsupialization for a Chronic Paronychia

- Make a crescent-shaped incision 1 to 3 mm proximal to the eponychial fold, extending 3 to 5 mm proximally and extending to the edge of each nail fold (**TECH FIG 3A,B**).
- Excise this tissue, taking care not to damage the underlying germinal matrix (**TECH FIG 3C**).
- Irrigate and dress the wound appropriately.
- Allow the wound to heal by secondary intention.

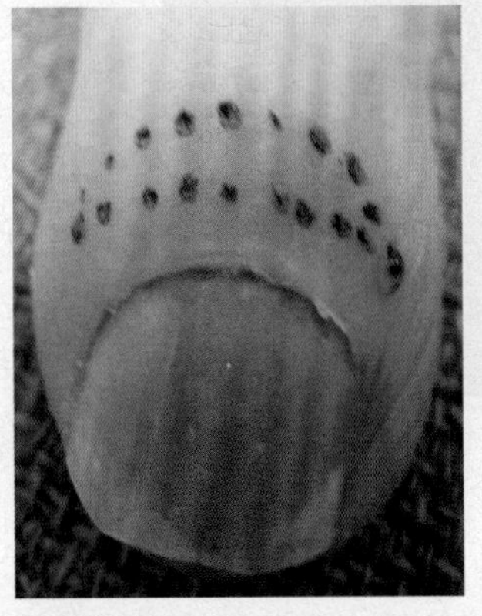

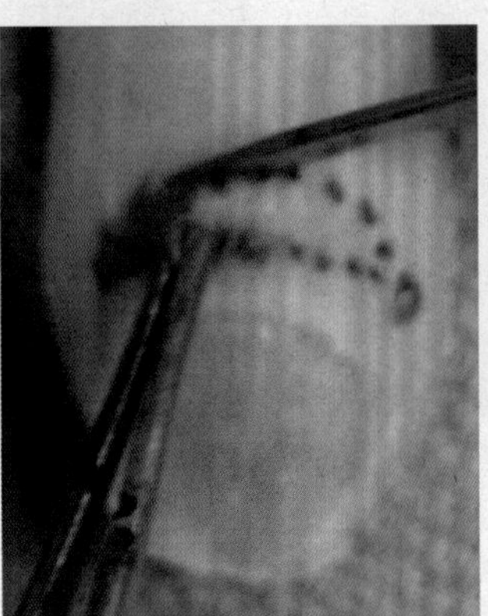

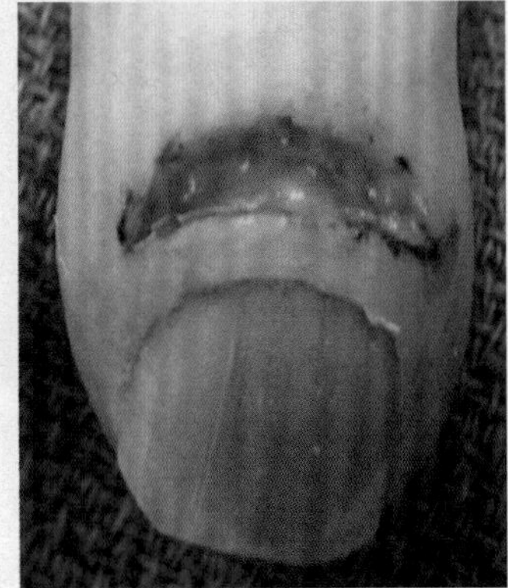

TECH FIG 3 • **A,B.** Incision for marsupialization of chronic paronychia. **C.** Tissue removed with the underlying germinal matrix exposed.

Incision and Drainage of a Felon

- Base the incision over the point of maximal tenderness. Be aware that an incision on the pulp can result in a tender scar.
  - For a volarly oriented abscess, make an incision precisely in the midline distal to the DIP joint flexion crease (**TECH FIG 4A,B**).
  - When the point of maximal tenderness is on the side of the finger pulp, make the incision longitudinally, dorsal to the tactile surface of the finger, not more than 3 mm from the edge of the nail. A more volar incision risks damage to the digital nerve branches (**TECH FIG 4C**).
- Carry the incision deep enough to disrupt all involved septa or spread with a hemostat (**TECH FIG 4D,E**).
  - Avoid proximal probing to avoid the spread of infection to the flexor sheath.
- Irrigate the wound with normal saline.
- Place a strip of gauze into the open wound to allow for drainage, and dress appropriately.

A 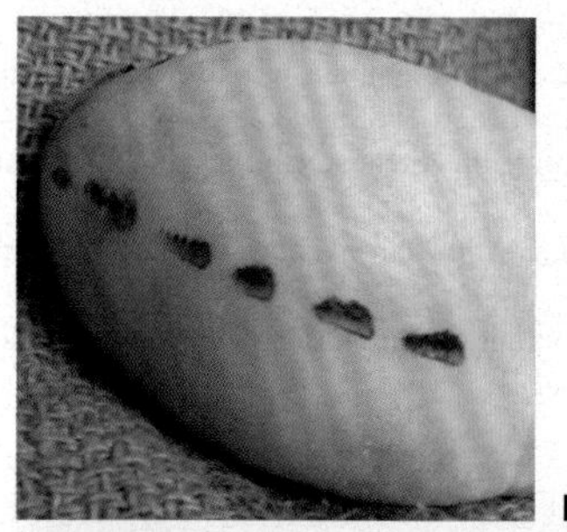
B 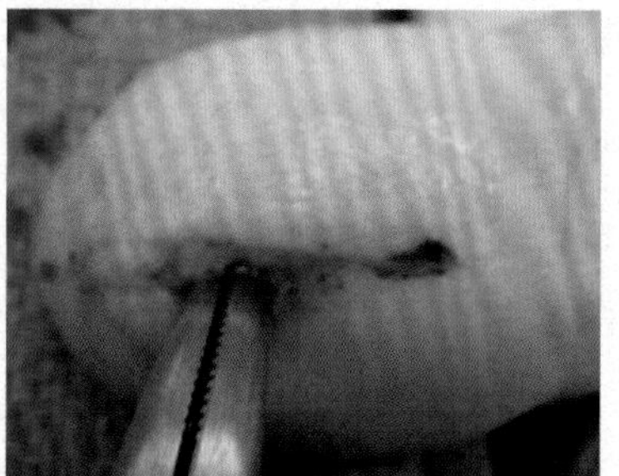
C 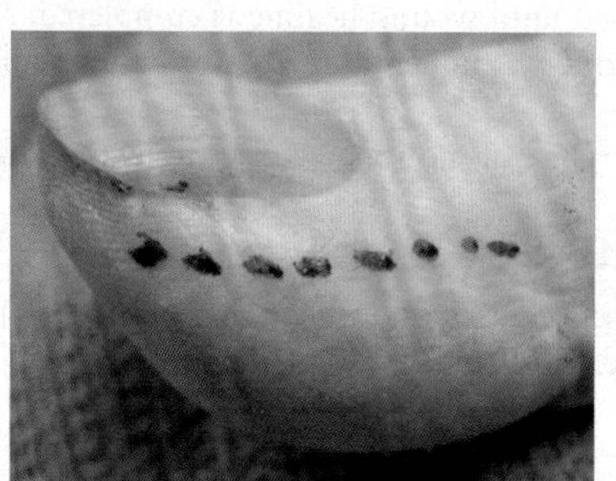
D 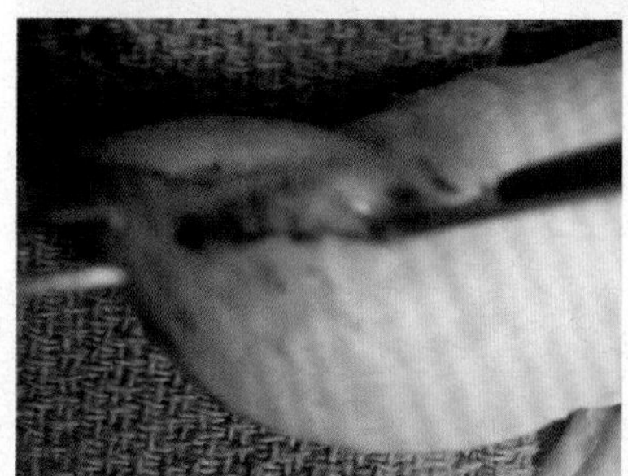
E 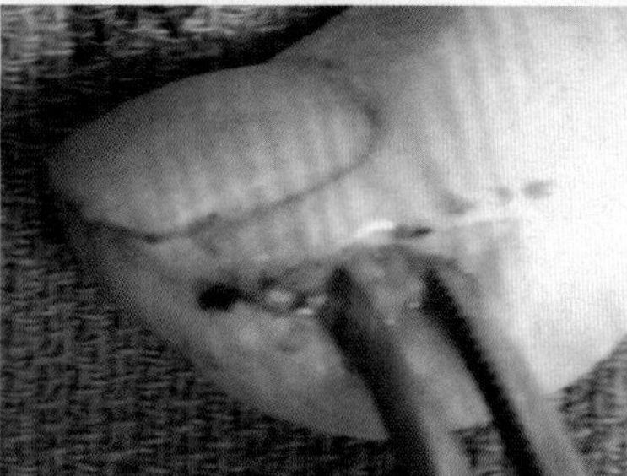

TECH FIG 4 • **A.** Midvolar approach for drainage of a felon. **B.** Spread deeply with a hemostat to disrupt all septa. **C,D.** Lateral incision for drainage of a felon. **E.** Spread deeply with a hemostat to disrupt all septa.

PEARLS AND PITFALLS

Misdiagnosis	▪ Avoid misdiagnosis of herpetic whitlow as an acute paronychia with concomitant overtreatment of this problem resulting in a secondary bacterial infection and no improvement in the herpetic whitlow. ▪ Recognize underlying osteomyelitis in long-standing cases. ▪ Recognize any systemic illness that may hinder resolution of the infection. ▪ Chronic paronychia: Avoid missing a cyst, tumor, or associated fungal infection.
Technique	▪ *Acute paronychia:* Determine whether purulence is present under the nail plate or extending into the pulp. Avoid incising into the sterile matrix by keeping the blade turned away from the nail bed. ▪ *Chronic paronychia:* Excise tissue superficial to the germinal matrix; avoid damaging the germinal matrix. ▪ *Felon:* Base the incision on the location of maximal tenderness. With a lateral incision, avoid damaging the digital nerve branches by remaining within 3 mm of the lateral edge of the nail. With a volar incision, do not cross the DIP joint flexion crease and avoid incising the flexor tendon sheath. Such incisions may lead to septic tenosynovitis.
Postoperative care	▪ *Acute paronychia and felons:* Treat with 10 days of oral antibiotics. Use of a removable splint over the distal digit is valuable early in recovery for patient comfort. Encourage early digital range-of-motion exercises during daily soaks. ▪ *Chronic paronychia:* Failure to modify environmental factors and treat systemic disease may lead to recurrence.

POSTOPERATIVE CARE

- Acute paronychia and felons
  - Oral antibiotics should be started postoperatively.
  - Soaks in a dilute solution of either chlorhexidine or povidone-iodine may be started on postoperative day 2 and continued until wound healing is completed. The packing is removed when the soaks begin.
  - Begin early range-of-motion exercises to avoid stiffness.
- Chronic paronychia
  - Oral antibiotics usually are not necessary.
  - Soaks in a dilute solution of either chlorhexidine or povidone-iodine may be started on postoperative day 2 and continued until wound healing is completed.
  - Correction of environmental factors or systemic illness is critical.
  - Begin early range-of-motion exercises to avoid stiffness.

COMPLICATIONS

- Recurrent infection (systemic spread of the infection)
- Incisional tenderness (pulp)
- Digital nerve injury
  - Decreased sensation
  - Neuroma
- Osteomyelitis
- Nail plate deformity

SUGGESTED READINGS

1. Bednar MS, Lane LB. Eponychial marsupialization and nail removal for surgical treatment of chronic paronychia. J Hand Surg Am 1991;16:314–317.
2. Canales FL, Newmeyer WL III, Kilgore ES Jr. The treatment of felons and paronychias. Hand Clin 1989;5:515–523.
3. Franko OI, Abrams RA. Hand infections. Orthop Clin North Am 2013;44(4):625–634.
4. Gill MJ, Arlette J, Buchan K. Herpes simplex virus infection of the hand. A profile of 79 cases. Am J Med 1988;84:89–93.
5. Hausman MR, Lisser SP. Hand infections. Orthop Clin North Am 1992;23:171–185.
6. Jebson PJ. Infections of the fingertip. Paronychias and felons. Hand Clin 1998;14:547–555.
7. Kesson AM. Use of acyclovir in herpes simplex virus infections. J Paediatr Child Health 1998;34:9–13.

130 CHAPTER

Surgical Treatment of Septic Arthritis in the Hand and Wrist

Asif M. Ilyas

DEFINITION

- *Septic arthritis* is defined as an infection within the closed space of a joint.
- It is usually acute and purulent secondary to a bacterial infection.
- It can cause irreversible damage to articular cartilage and therefore warrants prompt treatment with adequate drainage and an appropriate antibiotic regimen.
- Delay in making the diagnosis and initiating treatment can have serious negative implications to the condition of the joint and health of the patient.[2]

ANATOMY

- The interphalangeal (IP) and metacarpophalangeal (MP) joints of the hand are hinge joints (**FIG 1**).
- The IP joint space is maximized in slight flexion and the MP joint in extension.
- The wrist joint includes the radiocarpal, midcarpal, and radioulnar joints. Septic arthritis may be present in all of these joint spaces, concomitantly or separately, depending on the integrity of the intercarpal ligaments and the triangular fibrocartilage complex (see **FIG 1**).

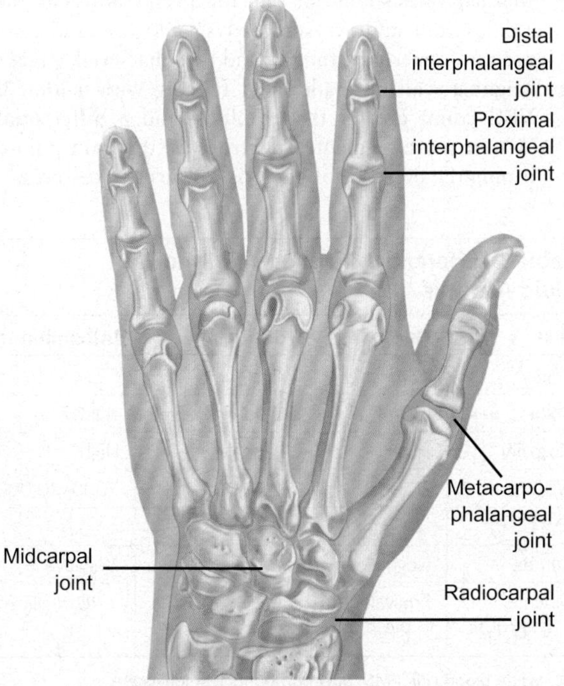

FIG 1 • Anatomy of the IP, MP, and wrist joints.

PATHOGENESIS

- Septic arthritis may affect any joint of the hand or wrist.
- Septic arthritis does not have a gender or race predilection, but it is more common in adults than in children.
- The inoculation of the joint is most likely due to a penetrating injury (ie, lacerations, puncture wounds, and bites). Other causes include hematogenous seeding or contiguous spread.[10]
  - At the distal IP joint, septic arthritis is common from penetrating trauma as well as contiguous infection from a mucous cyst, felon, paronychia, or suppurative flexor tenosynovitis.
  - At the proximal IP joint, contiguous infection is most commonly related to a suppurative flexor tenosynovitis.
  - At the MP joint, septic arthritis is most common after direct inoculation from a clenched fist injury or fight bite.
- Hematogenous spread can result from any concomitant or preceding infection of the body, including oral, upper respiratory, gastrointestinal, and genitourinary infections.
  - The synovium is highly vascular and contains no limiting basement membrane, promoting easy access of blood contents to the synovial space.[3]
- The presence of bacteria within the joint induces a cellular and immunologic response that is detrimental to the joint. Bacteria rapidly replicate, producing toxins. The presence of bacteria stimulates an immunogenic response, resulting in the arrival of leukocytes, which produce proteolytic enzymes. Both the bacterial toxins and leukocytic enzymes destroy the articular cartilage of the joint by degrading proteoglycans and eventually injuring the underlying chondrocytes.
- Multiple risk factors can predispose a patient to septic arthritis[6] (Table 1).
  - Any disorder that results in an immunocompromised state can predispose to septic arthritis.

Table 1 Common Risk Factors Predisposing to Septic Arthritis

Local factors	Systemic disorders
• Penetrating joint trauma	• Rheumatoid arthritis
• Recent joint surgery	• Diabetes mellitus
• Open reduction of intra-articular fractures	• Liver diseases, alcoholism
• Osteoarthritis	• Chronic renal failure, hemodialysis
• Prosthetic joints	• Malignancies
Social factors	• AIDS
• Newborns	• Immunosuppressive medication
• Elderly	• IV drug abusers
• Occupational exposure to animals	
• Low socioeconomic status	

IV, intravenous.

Table 2 Common Microorganisms Causing Septic Arthritis

Gram-positive aerobes
- *Staphylococcus aureus*
- *Streptococcus pyogenes*
- *Streptococcus pneumoniae*

Gram-negative aerobes
- *Haemophilus influenzae*
- *Escherichia coli*
- *P. multocida*
- *N. gonorrhoeae*

Anaerobes
- *Eikenella corrodens*
- *Borrelia burgdorferi*
- Mycobacterial species

Fungus
- Sporotrichosis
- *Cryptococcus*
- Blastomycosis

- Rheumatoid arthritis, in particular, poses a higher risk of infection. This risk is related to a variety of factors including general debilitation, immunosuppressive medication, tumor necrosis factor blockers (eg, infliximab or etanercept), and chronic joint injury.
- In patients with rheumatoid arthritis, a diagnosis of septic arthritis may be delayed because of misinterpretation of a rheumatoid flare. A high index of suspicion must be maintained when evaluating for septic arthritis in patients with rheumatoid arthritis.[9]

- Virtually, any microbial pathogen is capable of causing pyogenic septic arthritis (Table 2).
  - *Staphylococcus aureus* and *Streptococcus* species are the most common offending organisms.
  - Gram-negative, anaerobic, and polymicrobial infections also are possible, especially in intravenous (IV) drug abusers and immunocompromised patients.
  - Specific bacterial pathogens are related to certain circumstances, for example, *Eikenella corrodens* in human bite wounds, *Pasteurella multocida* after domestic animal bites, *Neisseria gonorrhoeae* infections in sexually active young patients, and fungal and mycobacterial infections in immunocompromised patients.

NATURAL HISTORY

- The combination of the growing bacterial load and the ensuing inflammatory response results in a growing effusion that causes synovial ischemia, pressure necrosis of the cartilage, and infiltration of the bacteria into both the subchondral bone and overlying skin.
- Bacterial infiltration out of the joint can result in secondary osteomyelitis, suppurative flexor tenosynovitis, and skin breakdown with spontaneous drainage.

PATIENT HISTORY AND PHYSICAL FINDINGS

- Patients will complain of pain and swelling about the joint.
- Systemic signs of joint infection may include fevers, chills, malaise, and tachycardia.
- The patient should be asked about a history of penetrating trauma; human, animal, or insect bites; recent joint aspirations; recent infections elsewhere; and the presence of an immunocompromising condition.
- On examination, patients will manifest a painful swollen joint, with overlying erythema and warmth.
- The most important physical examination finding is exquisite pain with precise joint motion, different from that typically seen when a noninfectious effusion or overlying cellulitis is present.
  - Use of a regional block for pain relief, often performed by an emergency or primary care physician, will mask the condition and must be discouraged.
  - Attempted active digital motion will result in significant guarding, and passive flexion and extension should induce exquisite pain.
- Physical examination of the wrist often is less dramatic than that of the digits. The joint typically is held in a neutral position.
- Active wrist motion also will induce guarding and pain.
- Passive flexion will also cause the patient to guard secondary to pain.
  - Passive pronation and supination may also help determine involvement of the distal radioulnar joint.

IMAGING AND OTHER DIAGNOSTIC STUDIES

- Laboratory studies should include white blood cell (WBC) count, erythrocyte sedimentation rate (ESR), C-reactive protein (CRP), and blood cultures.
  - The WBC usually is not elevated, but the ESR and CRP levels are consistently elevated (unless the patient is immunocompromised).
- Diagnosis of a septic arthritis is best accomplished by joint aspiration, microscopic analysis, and culture.
  - If an infection is present, increased fluid turbidity will be noted.
  - Joint aspirates should be sent for a cell count with differential, Gram stain, crystal analysis, glucose, and cultures (aerobic, anaerobic, fungal, and mycobacterial) (Table 3).
  - Diagnosis can be made most reliably with a joint fluid WBC count greater than 50,000 (and a differential of 75% or more segmented neutrophils), a Gram stain confirming the presence of bacteria, or positive cultures.[5]

Table 3 Differential Diagnosis of Synovial Fluid Analysis

Test	Normal	Septic	Inflammatory
Clarity	Transparent	Opaque	Straw
Color	Clear	Yellow-green	Yellow
Viscosity	High	Variable	High
WBC count	<200	>50,000	2000–10,000
PMN (%)	<25	>75	>50
Culture	Negative	Often positive	Negative
Glucose (mg/dL)	Equivalent to plasma	−25 < plasma	−40 < plasma

WBC, white blood cell; PMN, polymorphonuclear leukocyte.

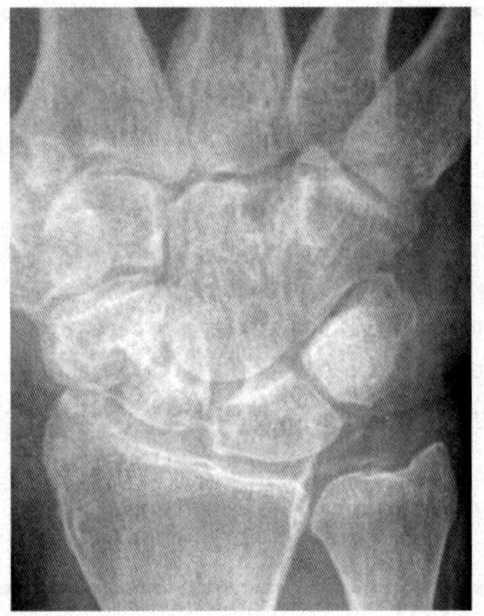
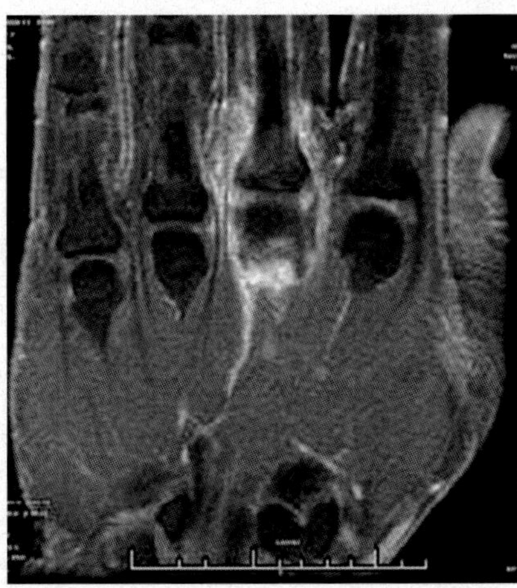

FIG 2 • **A.** Radiograph showing chondrocalcinosis of the triangular fibrocartilage complex from chronic pseudogout. **B.** Coronal T2-weighted MRI of an MP joint with underlying septic arthritis. Note the normal bone signal but the presence of high signal within the joint from the fluid and surrounding soft tissue inflammation.

    - A low WBC count with a high percentage of neutrophils (>90%) may indicate an early septic arthritis.[11]
    - A joint glucose of 40 mg/dL or less compared with the fasting blood glucose level also suggests a septic process.[7]
- Crystal analysis is necessary to rule out the presence of gout or pseudogout because they also can present similarly, including an elevated WBC count in the aspirate.
- The role of imaging studies early in the course of the septic process is limited. Radiographs may reveal joint distention, presence of foreign bodies, osteomyelitis, air in the soft tissues, and chondrocalcinosis (characteristic of both gout and pseudogout) (**FIG 2A**). Later radiographs may reveal joint destruction.
- Magnetic resonance imaging (MRI) is effective in diagnosing early septic arthritis and in differentiating it from osteomyelitis or overlying tenosynovitis (**FIG 2B**).

DIFFERENTIAL DIAGNOSIS

- Rheumatoid arthritis
- Crystalline arthropathies: gout, pseudogout
- Seronegative arthropathies: systemic lupus erythematosus, psoriatic arthritis, Reiter syndrome, ankylosing spondylitis, rheumatic fever
- Lyme disease
- Cellulitis
- Osteomyelitis
- Suppurative flexor tenosynovitis

NONOPERATIVE MANAGEMENT

- Septic arthritis is predominantly a surgical problem warranting operative management.
    - However, if septic arthritis is detected or suspected early enough, antibiotics alone have been suggested in the medical literature to be sufficient in the eradication of the infection.[3]
- In cases where comorbid conditions contraindicate surgery, serial aspiration of the involved joint can be done to decrease the bacterial load, decompress the joint, and allow medical management with antibiotics to treat the infection.
    - However, this technique has been shown to be less effective than open surgical drainage in large joints and, therefore, would be even less reliable in small joints.[4]

SURGICAL MANAGEMENT

- Septic arthritis typically warrants prompt surgical intervention to drain and lavage the joint.
- Open and arthroscopic techniques are available for surgical drainage of the wrist. Arthroscopic intervention is recommended to maximize drainage, visualization, lavage, and débridement while minimizing the surgical morbidity.

Preoperative Planning

- Arrangements for instruments, irrigation fluid, drains, sutures, and assistants should be made in advance of surgery.

Positioning

- Approaches to the hand and wrist can be accomplished with the patient supine and the operative extremity extended on a hand table with the surgeon and assistants seated.
- The hand table should be stable and well-secured and should allow adequate space for both the operative limb and the surgeon's elbow and forearm to minimize surgeon fatigue and enhance stability.
- Tourniquet use is advised to obtain a bloodless field and clear visualization of anatomic structures.
    - The limb usually is exsanguinated via gravity with elevation before inflating the tourniquet to avoid proximal spread of the bacteria with the use of an Esmarch.
- A small joint wrist arthroscopy tower should be used. This will provide appropriate positioning and application of traction during arthroscopy and also facilitate conversion to an open procedure if necessary. Additionally, small joint arthroscopy equipment, including a 30-degree 2.7-mm camera, should be available for use.

Approach

- Multiple approaches to a joint are available. The choice of which approach to use should be based on ease of the approach while still allowing adequate joint exposure for débridement and minimizing contiguous spread of infection.
- All surgical approaches of the hand and wrist warrant a sound understanding of surface anatomy, surgical anatomy, internervous planes, and surgical technique.

Aspiration of Interphalangeal or Metacarpophalangeal Joints

- Prepare the skin with an antiseptic wash, but avoid placing local anesthesia before the aspiration because it may mask the location of the joint space.
- As large a needle as possible should be used, preferably 18 or 20 gauge.
- A syringe no larger than 3 or 5 mL should be used, as larger syringes may cause too great a vacuum upon aspiration and collapse the joint, making them less effective in aspirating the joint.
- The joint space can be identified just radial or ulnar to the extensor mechanism on the dorsal surface.
  - The needle should be inserted in a dorsal to volar direction with a 30- to 45-degree angle toward the midline.
  - A palpable "pop" or sensation of entering the joint should be felt, and the joint should be aspirated.
  - Distraction of the joint can sometimes aid entry.
  - If there is resistance to aspiration, the needle should be redirected while maintaining suction on the syringe.

Surgical Drainage of Interphalangeal or Metacarpophalangeal Joints

- For the MP joint, a dorsal longitudinal incision is made (**TECH FIG 1A**). The extensor mechanism is exposed and also incised longitudinally to expose the capsule.
  - Alternatively, the capsule can be exposed by incising the ulnar sagittal band.
- The joint is exposed by incising the capsule dorsal to the collateral ligaments.
- For the proximal IP joint, a midaxial incision is preferred to avoid injury to the central slip and creation of a septic boutonnière deformity (**TECH FIG 1B**).
  - The neurovascular bundle may be identified and retracted volarly. The dorsal sensory branches are at risk and should be retracted with the dorsal flap.
  - The extensor mechanism, including the lateral bands, is identified and retracted dorsally, thereby exposing the capsule laterally. The accessory collaterals (volar to the proper collaterals) are released to allow entry into the joint.
- The distal IP joint can be approached through a midaxial incision or through a dorsal "H" incision and the terminal tendon retracted laterally, exposing the joint dorsal to the collateral ligaments.
  - Injury to the terminal tendon can result in a mallet finger and possible late swan-neck deformity.
- Obtain cultures and thoroughly irrigate and débride the joint with gravity cystoscopy tubing or a bulb syringe.
  - In-line traction on the digit will help expose the joint space.
- Inspect the joint surfaces for articular damage.
- Leave a small wick in the joint to prevent premature closure of the joint capsule, and reapproximate the extensor mechanism using a monofilament suture. Avoid using deep braided sutures in the face of an infection.
- Loosely close the skin around the wick with one or two 4-0 nylon sutures.
- Place the hand in a volar splint for comfort and emphasize that the patient should keep it elevated.

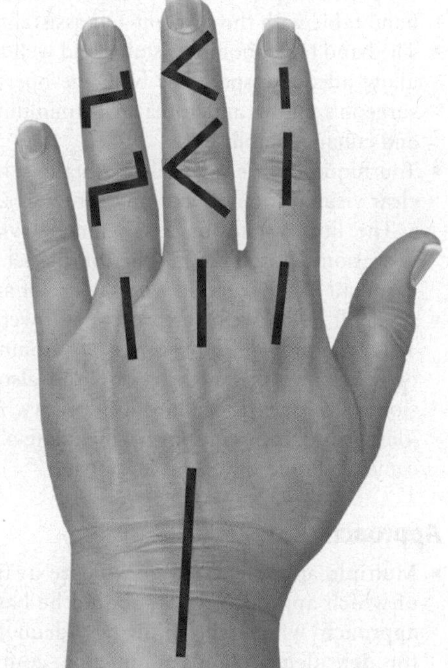

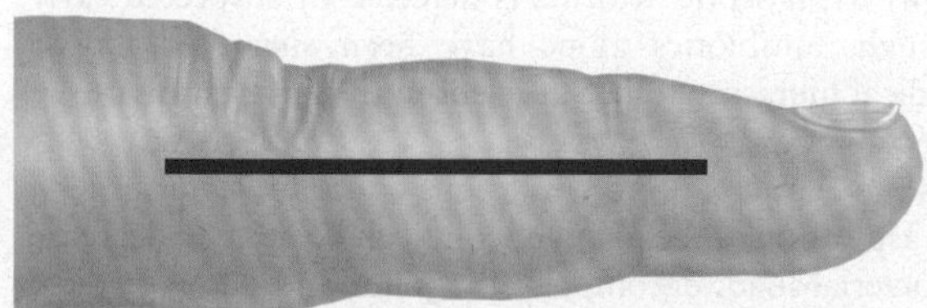

TECH FIG 1 • **A.** Sample incisions for open dorsal drainage of the IP, MP, and radiocarpal joints. **B.** Sample midaxial incision for open drainage of the IP joints.

Aspiration of the Wrist

- Prepare the skin with an antiseptic wash, but avoid placing local anesthesia preaspiration because it may mask the location of the joint space.
- As large a needle as possible should be used, preferably 18 gauge.
- A syringe no larger than 5 or 10 mL should be used, as larger syringes may cause too great a vacuum upon aspiration and collapse the joint, making them less effective in aspirating the joint.
- The joint space can be identified just distal to Lister tubercle on the dorsum of the wrist. The needle should be angled approximately 10 degrees volar to accommodate for the normal volar tilt of the radius.
    - Alternatively, the joint may be easily entered through the dorsal ulnocarpal space, just distal to the triangular fibrocartilage complex.
- A palpable pop or sensation of entering the joint should be felt and the joint should be aspirated. If there is resistance to aspiration, then the needle should be redirected while maintaining suction on the syringe.

Arthroscopic Débridement of the Wrist

- Secure the hand and wrist in a sterile small joint arthroscopy tower. Apply 5 to 10 pounds of traction.
- Identify and mark the dorsal surface anatomy of the wrist. Specifically, palpate the dorsal and distal surface of the radius, ulna, distal radioulnar joint, and Lister tubercle. These landmarks will guide safe establishment of portals and maximize visualization (**TECH FIG 2**).
- The 3-4 portal is the main "viewing" portal and should be established first to visualize the radiocarpal joint. Begin by identifying the soft spot just distal to Lister tubercle. The portal is bordered by the third and fourth dorsal compartments.
    - An 18-gauge needle is directed just distal to Lister tubercle and should be angled about 10 degrees volar to accommodate for the normal volar tilt of the radius.
        - A preliminary joint aspirate should be taken.
        - The joint is then insufflated with 5 to 10 mL of normal saline.
    - Create the portal with a 3-mm longitudinal skin incision using a no. 11 blade directed superiorly. Spread the soft tissue bluntly with a curved hemostat down to the joint, avoiding inadvertent penetration of the capsule.

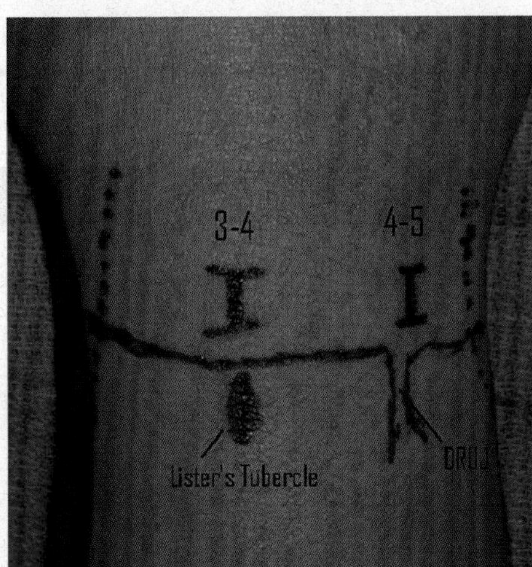

TECH FIG 2 • Dorsal surface anatomy of the wrist. The 3-4 and 4-5 portals are marked. The *dashed lines* represent approximate location of the radial sensory nerve on the radial side and the dorsal ulnar sensory nerve on the ulnar side. *DRUJ*, distal radioular joint.

    - Direct a blunt-tipped cannula and trocar into the joint, again angling about 10 degrees volar just distal to Lister tubercle. Avoid plunging the cannula uncontrolled into the joint because this may cause iatrogenic articular cartilage injury.
    - Replace the trocar with the camera.
- Cultures can be taken through the cannula.
- Systematically explore the radioscaphoid, radiolunate, and ulnocarpal joints for turbid fluid.
    - In addition, evaluate the scapholunate ligament and triangular fibrocartilage complex for tears that may allow the infection to communicate with the midcarpal and distal radioulnar joints, respectively.
- Establish a second "working" portal. Arthroscopic equipment such as the shaver and probe will be used through this portal. A needle is directed into the proposed site under direct arthroscopic visualization before making the skin incision.
    - The 4-5 portal is identified just ulnar to the fourth dorsal compartment and just distal to the distal radioulnar joint (see **TECH FIG 2**).
    - Alternatively, a 6R or 6U portal can be used and can be identified just radial or ulnar, respectively, to the sixth dorsal compartment. Diligent blunt dissection with a curved hemostat must be performed before inserting the blunt cannula and trocar to avoid inadvertent injury to the dorsal ulnar sensory nerve.
- The joint can be both visualized and washed through the camera cannula in the viewing portal and drained through the working portal with a cannula. Drainage can be facilitated by gravity or suction.
- The joint can be further débrided with the aid of a shaver with suction placed through the working cannula.
    - Devitalized tissues and synovial shavings can be taken through the shaver.
- Thorough arthroscopic débridement of the wrist should include visualization and irrigation of the midcarpal joint as well.
    - Palpate a soft spot about 1 cm distal to the 3-4 portal.
    - Place a 25-gauge needle first, and insufflate the joint with 5 mL of normal saline.
    - Direct a blunt cannula and trocar into the midcarpal joint just radial to the base of the capitate.
- After thorough visualization, irrigation, and débridement of the wrist, insert a small Hemovac drain through the working portal cannula.
- Remove the arthroscopic equipment. Close the portals with 4-0 nylon stitches.
- Place the wrist in a volar splint for comfort and encourage limb elevation and active finger motion.

Open Surgical Drainage of the Wrist

- A dorsal longitudinal incision should be placed just ulnar to Lister tubercle (**TECH FIG 3A**). The incision should be approximately 4 cm in length, with about two-thirds distal to the tubercle.
  - Alternatively, a transverse incision may be used. Although more cosmetic, it may not provide adequate exposure.
- Once the extensor retinaculum is exposed with blunt dissection, the distal third is released perpendicular to the fibers and ulnar to the third dorsal compartment.
- The interval between the third and fourth extensor compartments is bluntly dissected and the joint capsule is exposed (**TECH FIG 3B**).
- The joint capsule is incised longitudinally and limited flaps are raised subperiosteally off the dorsal distal radius, like an inverted T (**TECH FIG 3C**).
- Cultures are taken, and synovial tissue should be sent for culture and histology.
- The joint should be thoroughly irrigated with gravity cystoscopy tubing or a bulb syringe.
  - Pulse lavage should be avoided due to its potential to cause additional soft tissue injury.
  - The joint should be ranged during irrigation to maximize the effect of the lavage.
- The joint surfaces are inspected for articular damage.
- Leave a small wick or drain in the joint and loosely close the skin around the wick.
  - Primary closure of the joint risks reaccumulation of the purulence.
  - Typically, two to three loosely placed 4-0 nylon sutures will be sufficient.
- Place the wrist in a volar splint for comfort and encourage limb elevation.

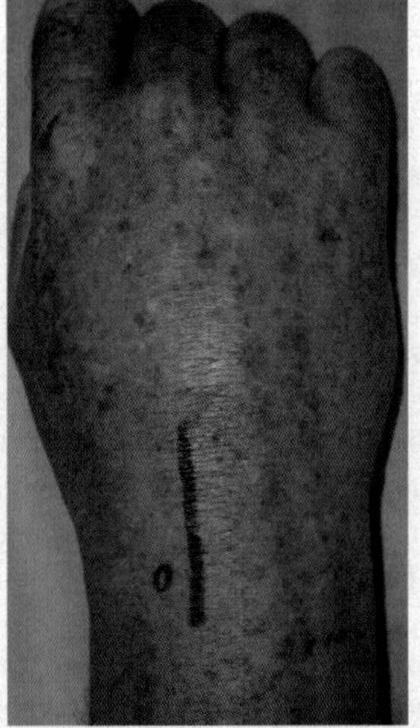
A

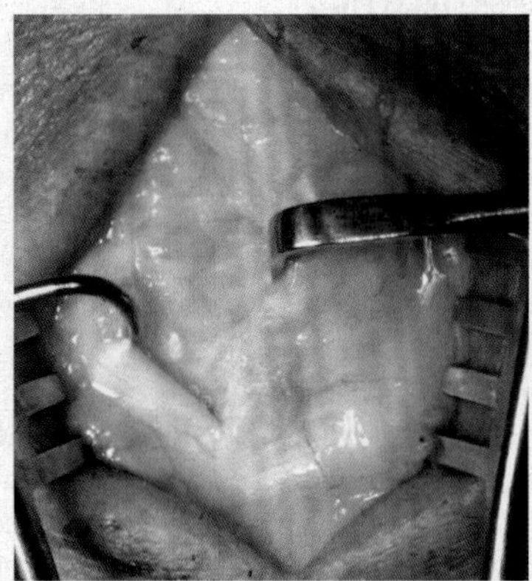
B

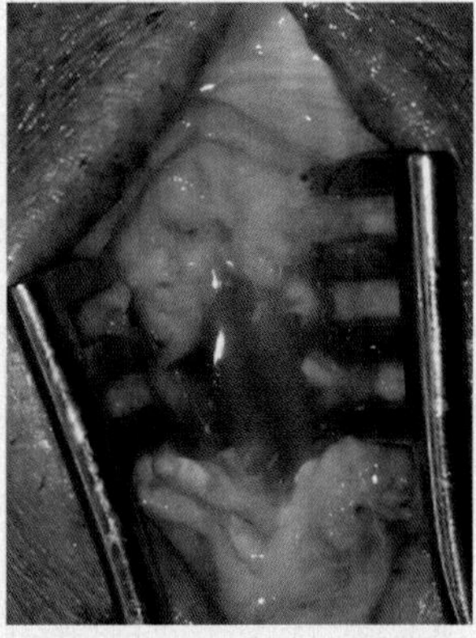
C

TECH FIG 3 • **A.** Incision for open drainage of the wrist. **B.** The distal third of the extensor retinaculum is released and the interval between the third and fourth dorsal compartment developed. **C.** The capsule is arthrotomized with an inverted T.

PEARLS AND PITFALLS

Diagnosis	■ Diagnosis is best accomplished by joint aspiration and analysis.
Antibiotics	■ Obtain cultures before beginning antibiotics. ■ Empiric antibiotics should be tailored to the most likely organism based on mechanism of injury and patient factors.
Aspiration	■ Avoid using larger syringes because the vacuum created can collapse the joint and may be less effective for aspiration.
Arthroscopic drainage	■ Identify the surface landmarks of the joint and avoid inadvertent injury to the dorsal tendons and cutaneous nerve. ■ Be prepared to convert to an open procedure if adequate exposure and débridement are not possible.
Open surgical drainage	■ Be prepared to perform a second open surgical débridement if symptoms do not improve.

POSTOPERATIVE CARE

- Empiric IV antibiotics are initiated immediately after obtaining cultures and then later tailored to the results of laboratory cultures and sensitivities.
- IV antibiotics should be continued for 2 weeks or at least through symptom resolution, followed by oral antibiotics.[8]
- The duration of antibiotics is the subject of some controversy. This should be determined on a case-by-case basis, with consideration of surgical findings, virulence of the offending bacterial pathogen, and the response to treatment.
- Early range of motion (active and active-assisted) in diluted povidone-iodine soaks is initiated three times daily to provide mechanical lavage of the joint and to prevent premature wound closure.
- The wick or drain is removed 1 or 2 days postoperatively.
- As symptoms resolve, the soaks are discontinued to allow the wound to heal and progressive range-of-motion exercises are initiated.
- If symptoms do not improve within 2 days, then a repeat surgical drainage should be considered.

OUTCOMES

- The results of surgical treatment of septic arthritis are not well documented in the literature, and it is difficult to predict the outcome even during the course of treatment.
- Functional outcome is most closely correlated to the duration of symptoms before treatment is initiated.[10]
- Some loss of motion and joint stiffness are expected, even in cases treated with early surgical drainage and rehabilitation.[1,10,12–14]
- Some joint space narrowing usually is seen following treatment, and significant arthrosis and ankylosis may occur in severe cases or when treatment has been delayed.

COMPLICATIONS

- Joint stiffness, arthrosis, osteomyelitis, and secondary tendon adhesions
- Salvage options for postseptic arthritis include arthrodesis, resection arthroplasty, or amputation.
- Implant arthroplasty is controversial and is not generally recommended for a previously infected joint.

REFERENCES

1. Boustred AM, Singer M, Hudson DA, et al. Septic arthritis of the metacarpophalangeal and interphalangeal joints of the hand. Ann Plast Surg 1999;42:623–628.
2. Glass KD. Factors related to the resolution of treated hand infections. J Hand Surg Am 1982;7:388–394.
3. Goldenberg DL, Reed JI. Bacterial arthritis. N Engl J Med 1985; 312:764–771.
4. Leslie BM, Harris JM III, Driscoll D. Septic arthritis of the shoulder in adults. J Bone Joint Surg Am 1989;71:1516–1522.
5. Li SF, Cassidy C, Chang C, et al. Diagnostic utility of laboratory tests in septic arthritis. Emerg Med J 2007;24:75–77.
6. Linscheid RL, Dobyns JH. Common and uncommon infections of the hand. Orthop Clin North Am 1975;6:1063–1104.
7. Moran G, Talan D. Hand infections. Emerg Med Clin North Am 1993;11:601–619.
8. Murray PM. Septic arthritis of the hand and wrist. Hand Clin 1998;14:579–587.
9. O'Dell JR. Anticytokine therapy—a new era in the treatment of rheumatoid arthritis. N Engl J Med 1999;340:310–312.
10. Rashkoff E, Burkhalter W, Mann R. Septic arthritis of the wrist. J Bone Joint Surg Am 1983;65:824–828.
11. Shmerling RH, Delbanco TL, Tosteson AN, et al. Synovial fluid tests. What should be ordered? JAMA 1990;264:1009–1014.
12. Sinha M, Jain S, Woods DA. Septic arthritis of the small joints of the hand. J Hand Surg Br 2006;31:665–672.
13. Willems C. Treatment of purulent arthritis by wide arthrotomy followed by immediate active mobilization. Surg Gynecol Obstet 1919;28:546–554.
14. Wittels N, Donley J, Burkhalter W. A functional treatment method for interphalangeal pyogenic arthritis. J Hand Surg Am 1984;9:894–898.

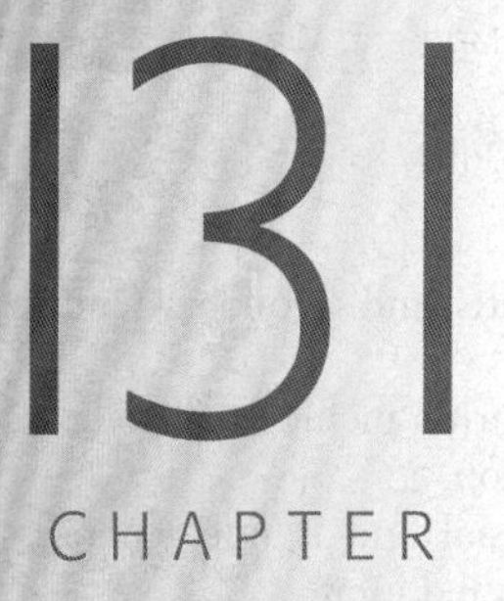

Arthroscopic Treatment of Elbow Loss of Motion

Laith M. Al-Shihabi, Chris Mellano, Robert W. Wysocki, and Anthony A. Romeo

DEFINITION

- Loss of motion is a common sequela of elbow trauma or the natural progression of nontraumatic conditions of the elbow, significantly impairing function of the upper extremity and hindering performance of activities of daily living (ADLs).
  - A functional arc of 100 degrees (30 to 130 degrees) in flexion and extension, along with 100 degrees in pronation and supination (50 degrees each), is required for most ADLs.[19]
  - Neighboring joints offer little compensatory function, making elbow stiffness poorly tolerated.
- Stiffness may be due to intrinsic (intra-articular) or extrinsic (extra-articular) causes (Table 1) or a combination of both.[6,14]
- Posttraumatic stiffness is most common, but osteoarthritis, inflammatory conditions, systemic injuries (head trauma), and neurologic disorders may also cause elbow joint contractures.
- Loss of extension is most common, although loss of flexion is more poorly tolerated due to an inability to reach the face for eating or grooming.[18]
- The key to treatment is identifying and correcting the functional and occupational impairment; decisions should not be based solely on the absolute loss of motion of the elbow.[11]
- Arthroscopic treatment of elbow stiffness is intended to restore motion, function, and relieve pain when present.[23]

Table 1 Classification of Elbow Stiffness Based on Location of Structure in Relation to the Elbow Joint

Type	Location	Description
Intrinsic	Within the elbow joint	Articular incongruity after fracture, degenerative changes and loss of cartilage, intra-articular adhesions, loose bodies, synovitis, infection
Extrinsic	Tissues immediately adjacent	Soft tissue and capsular contracture, muscle fibrosis (brachialis especially), collateral ligament stiffness, to the elbow joint heterotopic ossification, skin contractures
Peripheral	Factors anatomically separate from the elbow	Stroke, neurologic problems, peripheral nerve disorder, head injury, cerebral palsy

From Jupiter JB, O'Driscoll SW, Cohen MS. The assessment and management of the stiff elbow. AAOS Instr Course Lect 2003;52:93–111.

- Arthroscopic treatments may range from capsular release alone to osteocapsular arthroplasty, including the removal of loose bodies, osteophytes, and capsulectomy.[22]

ANATOMY

- The elbow is anatomically predisposed to stiffness by virtue of the close relationship of the capsule to the surrounding ligaments and muscles, along with the presence of three joints within a synovial-lined joint cavity—(a hinge ginglymus) ulnohumeral articulation and rotatory (trochoid) radiocapitellar and radioulnar joints.[11]
- The anterior elbow capsule attaches proximally above the coronoid fossa and distally extends to the coronoid medially and annular ligament laterally. The posterior capsule starts proximally just above the olecranon fossa and inserts at the articular margin of the sigmoid notch and annular ligament (**FIG 1**).
- The anterior capsule is taut in extension and lax in flexion, with strength derived from the cruciate orientation of its fibers.
- The greatest capsular capacity is at 80 degrees flexion.[9,24] The normal capacity of 25 mL can be reduced to as little as 6 mL in a contracted state.[9,24]
- The joint capsule is innervated by branches from all the major nerves crossing the joint along with the musculocutaneous nerve.[16]
- The cubital tunnel, which houses the ulnar nerve at the elbow, becomes compressed in flexion (due to stretching of the retinaculum between the olecranon and medial epicondyle) and loosens in extension.
- Flexion contractures may adversely compress the ulnar nerve, leading to ulnar neuropathy (**FIG 2**).

PATHOGENESIS

- O'Driscoll[23] describes four stages of posttraumatic elbow stiffness:
  - Bleeding: minutes to hours
  - Edema: hours to days. Both bleeding and edema cause swelling within the joint and surrounding tissues, and the capsule become biomechanically less compliant. Early elbow range of motion through an entire range during stages 1 and 2 can help prevent stiffness.
  - Granulation tissue: days to weeks. Splints can be used to regain range of motion.
  - Fibrosis: Maturation of the granulation tissue further decreases compliance. More aggressive splinting is necessary, along with possible surgical management.

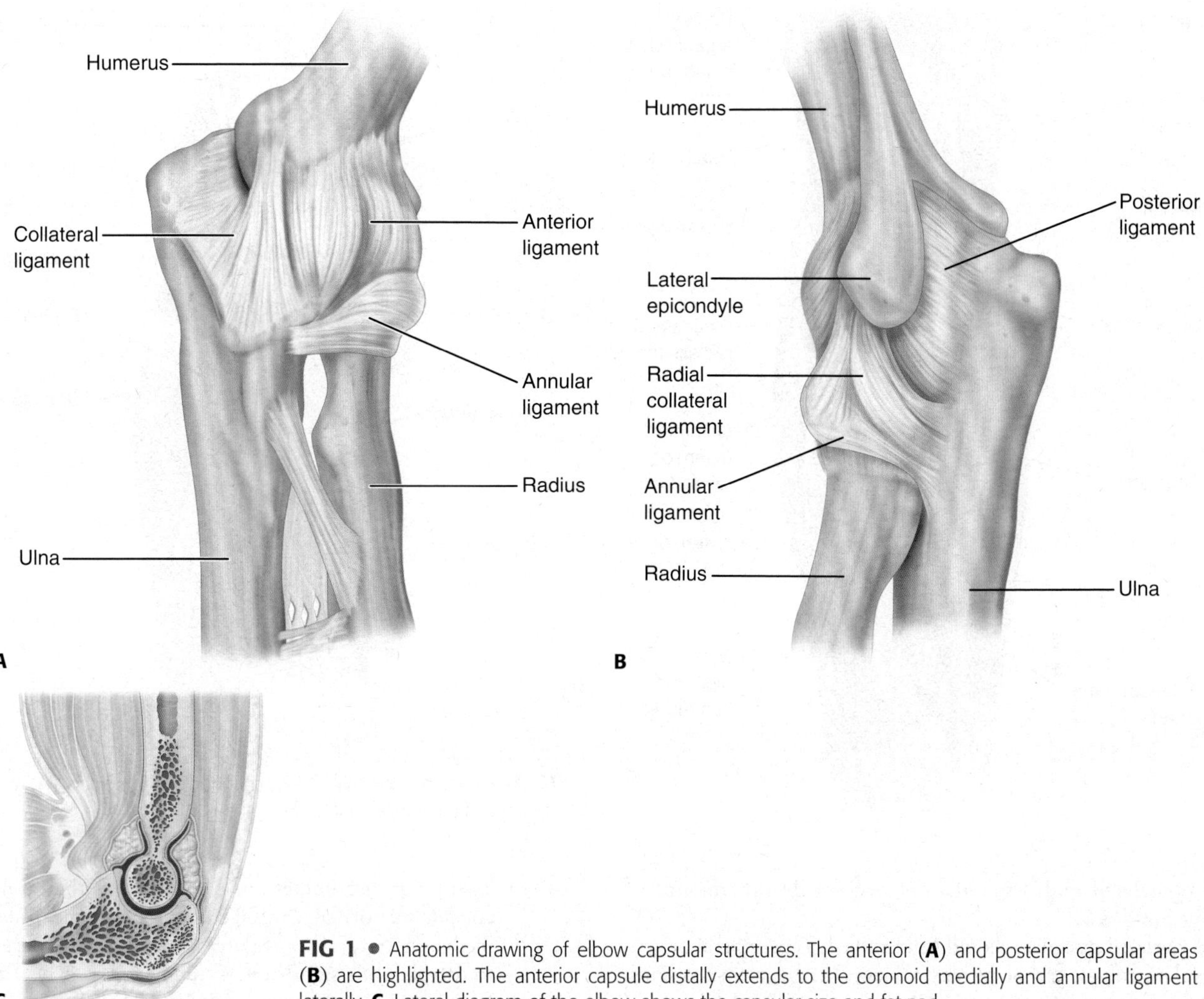

FIG 1 • Anatomic drawing of elbow capsular structures. The anterior (**A**) and posterior capsular areas (**B**) are highlighted. The anterior capsule distally extends to the coronoid medially and annular ligament laterally. **C.** Lateral diagram of the elbow shows the capsular size and fat pad.

- The posttraumatic joint capsule is sensitive to contracture, secondary to an increase in disorganized collagen fiber deposition at the cellular level, resulting in thickening that translates into loss of flexibility and joint volume.[9,16,23]
- The reasons for altered capsular properties are multifactorial and not completely known.
  - Myofibroblasts, cells that enhance collagen production and tissue contraction, increase in number in the posttraumatic anterior capsule.[10]
  - Collagen formation, cross-linking, and hypertrophy increase while water and proteoglycan content decrease in the contracted elbow tissue.[1]
  - Increased matrix metalloproteinase activity and collagen disorganization have also been described in the contracted capsular tissue.[10]
  - Growth factors and other cellular mechanisms may be involved. This is highly variable among individuals.[17]
- Heterotopic ossification may also occur in conjunction with capsular thickening and act as a bony block to motion. Patients most at risk are those with combined head and elbow trauma, burn patients, and those who have undergone surgical approaches to the elbow, all of which are believed to incite a complex inflammatory chain that leads to elbow contracture and heterotopic ossification.[7]

NATURAL HISTORY

- The onset and progression of elbow stiffness is closely related to its inciting causes (see Table 1); most contractures have mixed elements.[14]
  - Posttraumatic contracture is most common and is associated with a failure to regain motion after a direct traumatic injury to the elbow joint rather than progressive elbow motion loss. A posttraumatic contracture will typically remain stable over the long-term unless intra-articular degenerative changes ensue that would worsen motion further.
  - Contractures associated with degenerative or inflammatory arthritis may slowly progress with time due to capsular contraction and impingement on osteophytes or hypertrophic synovium. Such cases will often have episodic flares of swelling and stiffness in combination with steady baseline progression.
- Morrey[17] has also characterized elbow stiffness as static or dynamic based on tissue involvement (Table 2).

PATIENT HISTORY AND PHYSICAL FINDINGS

- It is critical to determine the degree of functional impairment and duration of symptoms for each patient. Management decisions should be based on subjective

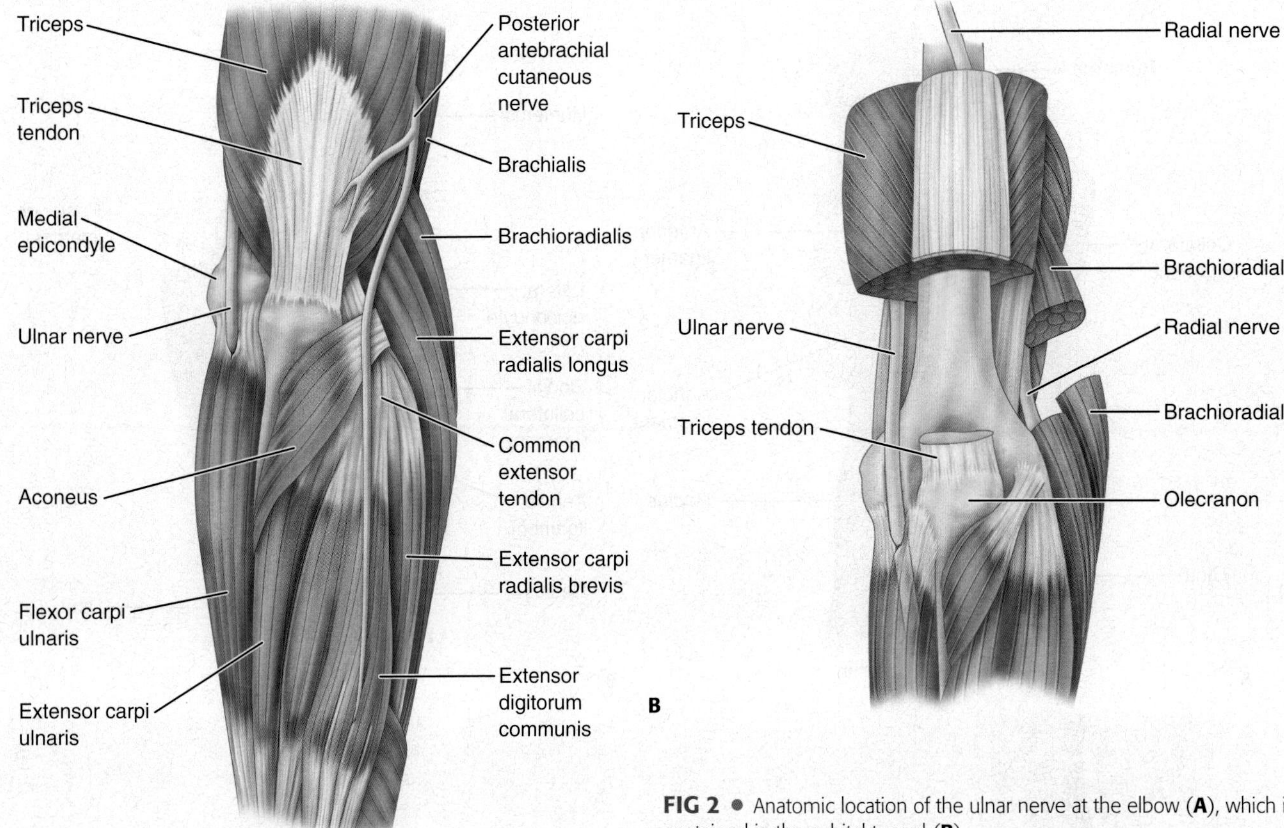

FIG 2 • Anatomic location of the ulnar nerve at the elbow (**A**), which is contained in the cubital tunnel (**B**).

impairment and demands, not necessarily the amount of motion loss.[11]

- Associated disorders should be identified, as peripheral or central neurologic pathology may influence management decisions.
- Hand dominance, the patient's occupation, and the extent of prior therapy should be noted.
- The function of the entire ipsilateral and contralateral upper extremities should be tested.
- Physical examination
  - The cranial nerves and cervical spine should be examined to assess for neurologic pathology.
  - Shoulder motion and strength is assessed.
  - Careful assessment of the ulnar nerve
    - The physical examination is critical, as the patients will often not even recognize the presence of ulnar neuropathy in the setting of their adjacent elbow pathology. The elbow flexion and ulnar nerve compression test is the most sensitive for detection of ulnar nerve entrapment at the elbow.[21]
    - Two-point discrimination: Although less than 6 mm is considered normal, careful comparison to the ipsilateral median nerve and contralateral ulnar nerve is necessary to detect subtle signs of nerve damage.
    - Froment sign and intrinsic hand muscle function: Weakness of the adductor pollicis or interossei may also signify ulnar neuropathy.
    - The cubital tunnel is palpated to assess for tenderness or a positive Tinel sign.
  - Elbow range of motion: Flexion and extension are tested with the shoulder flexed to 90 degrees, whereas pronation and supination are evaluated with the elbow held in flexion at the side of the body.
    - Measure the flat surface of the forearm just proximal to the wrist in comparison to the axis of the humerus. Measurements in supination can be erroneous if tested through the palm because patients can often compensate with significant intercarpal supination.

Table 2 Characterization of Elbow Stiffness by Tissue Involvement

Classification	Relative Occurrence	Location	Description
Static	Most common	Tissues in and around the elbow joint	Capsule, ligaments, heterotopic ossification, articular and cartilaginous components
Dynamic	Less common	Involves muscles around the joint	Poor muscle tone, nerve injuries, and poor excursion of the muscles that cross the elbow joint

From Morrey BF. The stiff elbow with articular involvement. In: Jupiter JB, ed. The Stiff Elbow. Rosemont, IL: American Academy of Orthopaedic Surgeons, 2006:21–30.

- Measurements can also be erroneous in obese patients who cannot fully adduct the arm to the side, as they will appear to have a deficit in supination if the measurement is compared to the trunk axis and not the abducted humerus, which stresses the importance of using the humerus and not the trunk as the reference point.
- Elbow instability: The surgeon should check the ligamentous restraints to varus and valgus stress, as concomitant elbow instability and stiffness may occur after elbow dislocation or subluxation.
  - Ligaments are assessed with varus and valgus stress at 0 and 30 degrees of flexion as allowed by the patient's range of motion.

IMAGING AND OTHER DIAGNOSTIC STUDIES

- Plain radiographs (anteroposterior [AP] and lateral) are usually adequate.
  - The AP provides joint line and subchondral bone visualization.
  - If an elbow is contracted more than 45 degrees, the AP view of the joint line is usually distorted.[17]
- The lateral view may show osteophytes on the olecranon or coronoid processes or within their respective fossae (**FIG 3A,B**).
- Radiographs can be used to follow the maturation process of heterotopic ossification, which usually signifies multiple extrinsic causes of elbow contracture that preclude arthroscopic treatment (**FIG 3C**).
- Computed tomography (CT) is useful to better characterize impinging osteophytes, loose bodies, and intra-articular non- or malunions. These studies are often more for preoperative planning than for diagnostic purposes
- Magnetic resonance imaging (MRI) has a limited role in the management of elbow stiffness but is the favored imaging study for staging and diagnosis of osteochondritis dissecans lesions and ulnar collateral ligament insufficiency, both of which not uncommonly will be accompanied by loss of motion. Fortunately, the age and history in these patients are quite specific, which helps narrow the differential diagnosis.

DIFFERENTIAL DIAGNOSIS

- Elbow fracture-dislocation
- Osteoarthritis/posttraumatic arthritis
- Inflammatory arthropathy
- Osteochondritis dissecans
- Ulnar collateral ligament insufficiency with posteromedial impingement
- Heterotopic ossification
- Closed head injury
- Burns
- Dysplastic radial head (congenital)
- Neuromuscular disease
- Stroke

NONOPERATIVE MANAGEMENT

- Nonoperative management should be considered up to 6 months after contracture onset.[14]
- Response is better if there is a soft "spongy" end point during range of motion[14,23]; bony blocks to motion such as heterotopic ossification or osteophytes are unlikely to respond to stretching protocols.
- The goal is to gain motion gradually without causing additional trauma to the capsule and, subsequently, development of additional capsular contracture (more pain, inflammation, and swelling leads to more contracture).
- Edema control is critical, and therapy should focus on this, not exercises that induce inflammation around the elbow.
- Static-progressive splinting is indicated as a first-line treatment for capsular contracture and should be used three times daily in between therapy sessions.[11,18] Dynamic splints yield results comparable to static progressive but are often less well tolerated as they provide a constant tension over time rather than allowing stress relaxation of soft tissues.[16,20] Care should be taken not to be overly aggressive in stretching as this may incite an inflammatory process leading to further capsular contracture. Regardless of whether static or dynamic splinting is chosen, this type of splinting can be beneficial for up to 1 year in treating posttraumatic elbow stiffness.[16]

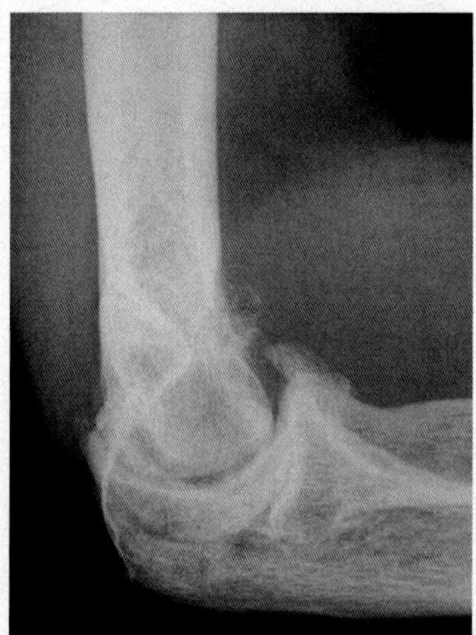
A

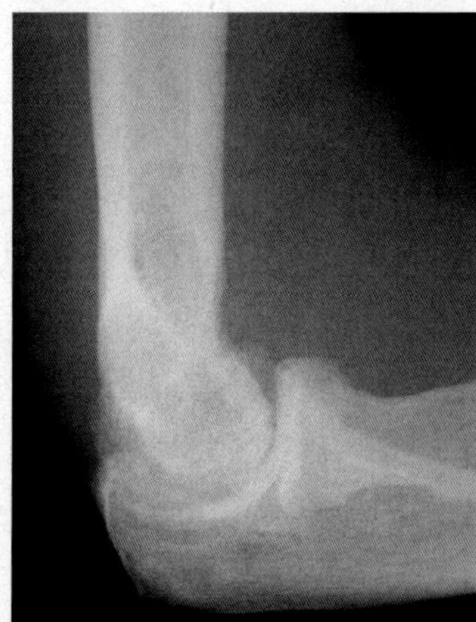
B

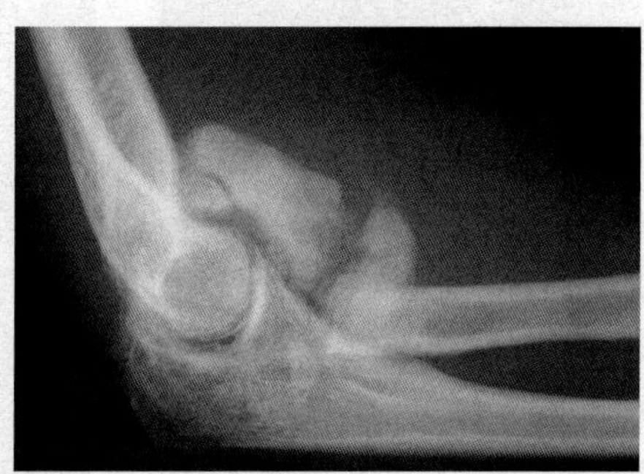
C

FIG 3 • **A.** Preoperative lateral radiograph of an elbow before arthroscopic resection of osteophytes at the olecranon and coronoid, with associated anterior capsular contracture. Heterotopic ossification is absent. **B.** Postoperative radiograph after resection of osteophytes. **C.** Lateral radiograph of an elbow with heterotopic ossification. Arthroscopic resection is not recommended in this type of patient.

- Nonoperative improvements in range of motion vary widely. A systematic review by Müller[20] found an average improvement of 40 degrees with static-progressive splinting, but results of 10 to 50 degrees or more have been reported.[14,17,23]

SURGICAL MANAGEMENT

- The key is to identify the functional disability of the patient—pain, loss of motion, or both—and what would be most beneficial to correct.
- The indications include a loss of function precluding the patient from performing ADLs and occupational or vocational activities.
- Arthroscopic treatment of elbow stiffness should be undertaken only if the offending structures can be treated from an arthroscopic approach. Capsular contractures and intra-articular osteophytes are ideally suited for arthroscopic treatment, whereas articular malunion, heterotopic ossification, or skin and muscle contractures are not amenable to arthroscopic release.
- Appropriate counseling with the patient should cover realistic expectations of range of motion and functional recovery. Will patients be able to get their hand to their mouth, comb their hair, or reach behind their back, or are more extensive demands required?
- There are several contraindications to arthroscopic release:
  - Prior surgery that has altered the neurovascular anatomy, especially of the radial nerve from previous surgery in the area of the radial head
  - Joint deformity that would compromise arthroscopic viewing, such as with severe posttraumatic malunion or inflammatory arthritis
  - Arthroscopy is also less favored for pathology best treated through an open approach such as heterotopic ossification or a fracture malunion that requires osteotomy.[3,26,27]

Preoperative Planning

- An examination under anesthesia helps to distinguish static versus dynamic elbow stiffness and should confirm the preoperative clinical diagnosis.
- A thorough understanding of the pathoanatomy will allow the surgeon to plan the surgical order of events to maximize surgical efficiency and optimize patient safety.
  - In the presence of osteophytes or loose bodies, a CT scan with two-dimensional coronal and sagittal reconstructions as well as three-dimensional surface renderings may be helpful to provide a "road map" for the osteocapsular arthroplasty.
  - If the posterior compartment medial and lateral gutters require extensive work, it may be technically easier to perform this first before significant soft tissue swelling evolves. Visualization of the anterior compartment in the presence of soft tissue swelling can be better accommodated by the use of arthroscopic retractors.
- If the preoperative examination documented ulnar nerve irritation or neuropathy or if the patient has a subluxating ulnar nerve,[3] it should be exposed and an in situ release across the elbow joint be performed.
  - We recommend that the ulnar nerve be released before arthroscopy for ease of soft tissue dissection before fluid distention.
  - In patients with elbow flexion of less than 100 degrees, the nerve should be prophylactically released to prevent compression once flexion is restored postsurgically.[17]
  - Exploration and identification of the nerve prior to arthroscopy is also mandatory for patients who have undergone a prior ulnar nerve transposition. Open release may be preferable for these patients.
  - Following release, the nerve must be protected during placement of the anteromedial portal to prevent iatrogenic injury.

Positioning

- Either the lateral decubitus or prone position can be used, with the operative extremity supported by either an arm cradle or rolled sheets (**FIG 4A,B**).
- A well-padded sterile tourniquet is used to optimize viewing by limiting intra-articular bleeding.
- The remainder of the arthroscopic setup has been described elsewhere.
- The surgeon should clearly mark the course of the ulnar nerve, portal sites, and bony landmarks with surgical marker (**FIG 4C**).

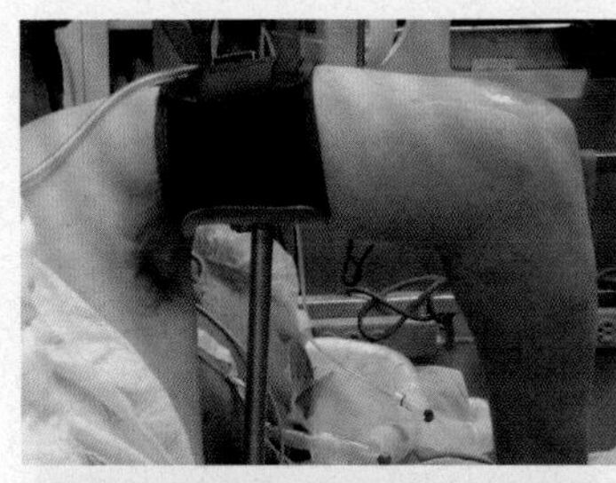

A

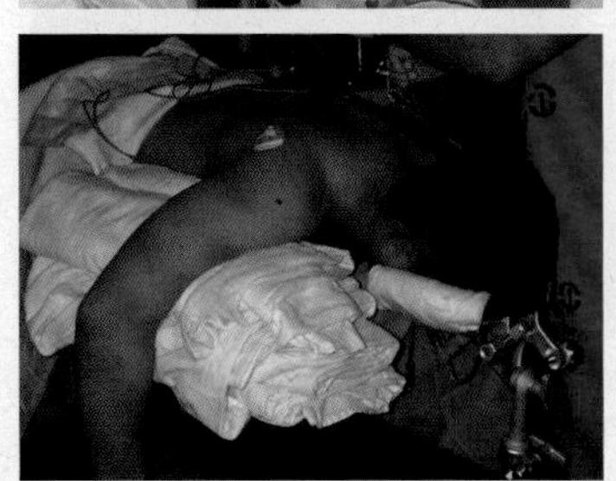

B

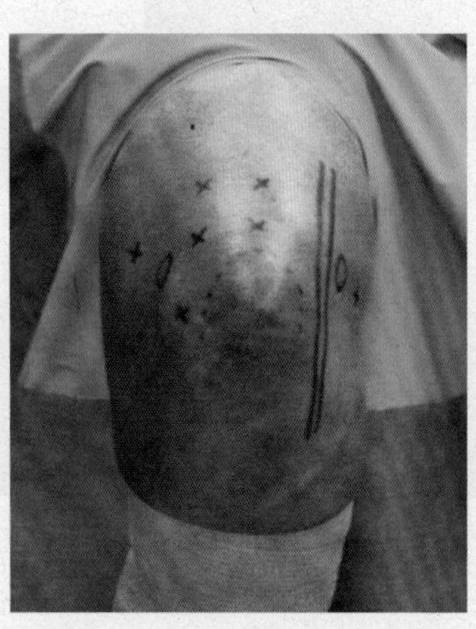

C

FIG 4 • **A,B.** Setup of patient for elbow arthroscopy in lateral (**A**) and prone (**B**) positioning. **C.** Landmarks of the elbow drawn for operative incisions and to identify at-risk structures, including the ulnar nerve, in the prone position.

Approach

- Arthroscopic elbow osteocapsular arthroplasty should proceed in a stepwise fashion.
  - Establish a view—get into the joint and confirm your anatomic orientation.
  - Create a working space—synovectomy and removal of debris
  - Bone removal—retractor is used to hold soft tissue away from burr or shaver blade.
  - Capsulectomy—using a large shaver can optimize fluid outflow and act as a periosteal elevator to strip soft tissue off bone before resection.
- Capsular contraction and loss of volume complicates arthroscopic visualization of the stiff elbow but can be greatly facilitated through the use of arthroscopic retractors placed through proximal medial and proximal lateral portals 1 to 2 cm above the standard medial and lateral portals.[22,23]
- Avoiding nerve injury during the approach and during capsular treatment is critical.
- If required, the ulnar nerve is decompressed and protected prior to arthroscopy in order to avoid soft tissue distortion due to fluid extravasation (**FIG 5**).

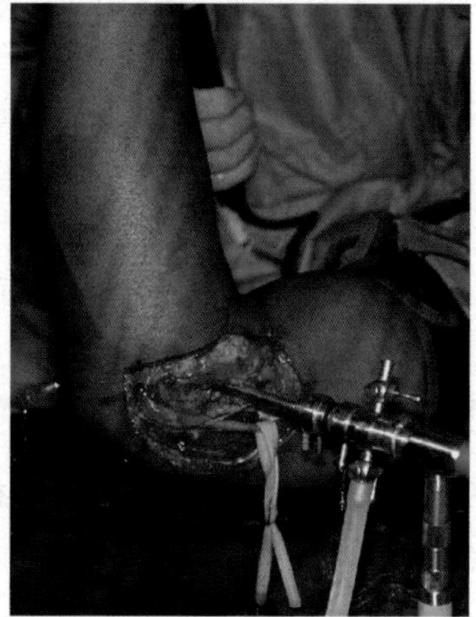

FIG 5 ● If the ulnar nerve is thought to be involved, it may be released before starting the arthroscopy to facilitate dissection without the soft tissue changes that occur after fluid extravasation from the elbow joint. The ulnar nerve is marked with a vessel loop.

TECHNIQUES

Ulnar Nerve Release and Transposition

- Subcutaneous transposition or in situ decompression of the ulnar nerve can be performed; these techniques are described elsewhere within this text.
- The ulnar nerve is exposed before performing the arthroscopic release to allow gentle fluid extravasation from the soft tissue posteromedially.[23]
  - Gentle retraction on the nerve with a Penrose drain can help protect it while performing arthroscopic releases in this area, especially posteromedial osteophytes.

Portal Establishment in the Contracted Elbow

- The joint is distended with saline through the "soft spot" portal (up to 40 mL, as allowed by contracture).
- Portals are established.
  - The proximal anteromedial portal is established first (2 cm proximal to the medial epicondyle and 1 cm anterior to the intermuscular septum). A 4.5-mm, 30-degree scope is used for visualization (**TECH FIG 1A,B**).[2]
  - The proximal anterolateral portal (1.5 to 2 cm proximal to lateral epicondyle) is useful as a retractor portal to improve distention and visualization. The portal is established with either a blunt-tipped Wissinger rod as an inside-out technique or a spinal needle under direct visualization using an outside-in technique. (**TECH FIG 1C**).
- Blunt elevation with the Wissinger rod, a freer elevator, or specially designed retractors will help create a working space by lifting the capsule away from the joint and anterior humerus.

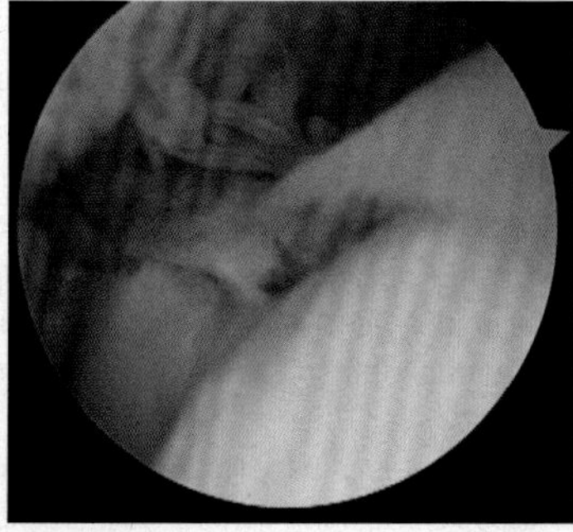

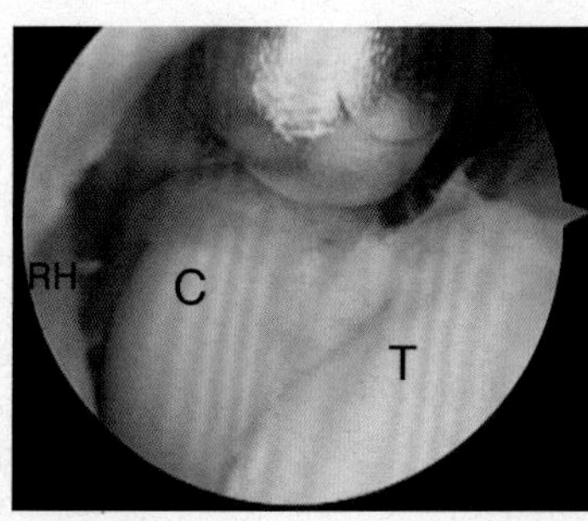

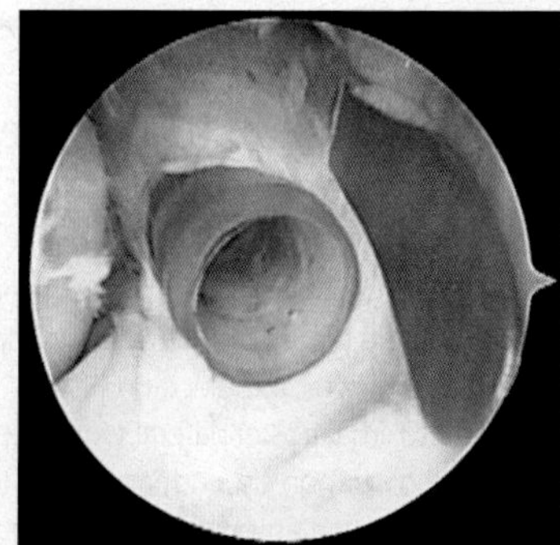

TECH FIG 1 ● **A.** Arthroscopic view of a right elbow joint after first obtaining scope entry into the proximal anteromedial portal, looking laterally. There is synovitis in the joint. **B.** After the synovitis is gently débrided with an arthroscopic shaver, the bony overgrowth of the coronoid and radial fossa is revealed. There is a lack of concavity in the trochlea and capitellum area. **C.** Arthroscopic view of elbow joint viewed from the medial portal, showing the increased visualization of the elbow joint that is obtained with the use of intra-articular retractors. *C*, capitellum; *RH*, radial head; *T*, trochlea.

- Avoid excessive inflow and high-pump pressures (>35 mm Hg), which will lead to increased fluid extravasation and extra-articular soft tissue distention that will impair visualization.
- A 4.5-mm shaver (oscillate function) débrides intra-articular synovitis or loose flaps of articular cartilage.
- A small radiofrequency device can also be used to ablate scar tissue within the joint. Inflow should be increased during the use of thermal energy to prevent cartilage injury.
- Impinging osteophytes of the coronoid tip and coronoid or trochlear fossae can be resected with a burr or shaver, if necessary.
  - Direct the burr away from the capsule to prevent accidental injury to the anterior neurovascular structures.
- The capsule is débrided superficially to define it as a structure and clear any synovitis; however, it is not removed until all intra-articular débridement, both bony and soft tissue, has already been carried out so as to limit fluid extravasation.

Anterior Capsular Release

- Capsulotomy of the anterior capsule is performed with an arthroscopic basket cutter or radiofrequency ablation, from lateral to medial, along the nonarticular distal humerus.
  - The radial nerve rests on the anterior capsule at the level of the radial head. To prevent injury to it, the capsulotomy should be performed as close to the humerus as possible.
  - The posterior interosseous nerve (PIN) is adjacent to the anterolateral capsule at the level of the radial neck.[26]
  - The capsulotomy can be continued to the level of the collateral ligaments on each side, but the ligaments are not incised.
- The brachialis muscle can be visualized and the plane between the capsule and brachialis developed from the lateral working portal (**TECH FIG 2A**).
  - The brachialis protects the median nerve, so the surgeon should avoid penetrating this muscle. The fibers of the brachialis serve as the marker that the capsule has been released to an appropriate depth.
- The arthroscope is then moved to the anterolateral portal and the same steps of capsular release performed to ensure adequate medial release (**TECH FIG 2B**).
- Check passive extension after excision of posterior osteophytes and anterior capsulotomy alone, and if sufficient extension is restored, then complete capsulectomy can be avoided.
- A wide capsulotomy fully from medial to lateral off the humerus is often sufficient for the anterior release without endangering the neurovascular structures that are more at risk with a complete capsulectomy.

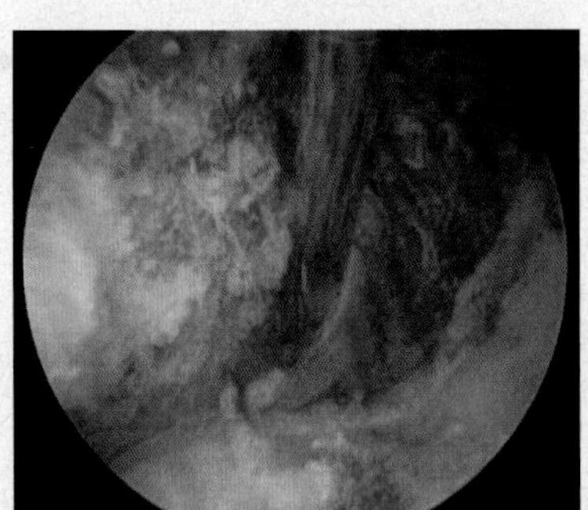
A

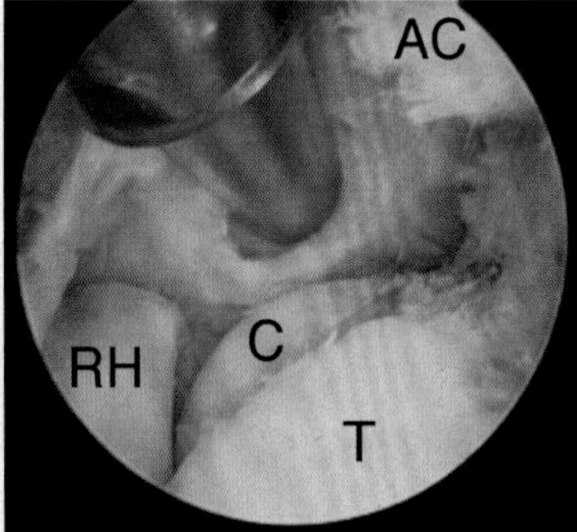

B

TECH FIG 2 • **A.** Arthroscopic view of the elbow joint after capsulectomy and deepening of the coronoid and radial fossae. The dissection is carried down to the fibers of the brachialis muscle but does not violate the brachialis (retracted structure). **B.** View from the lateral portal shows the partially completed release. Bony work and resection are completed before capsulectomy. The concavity of the coronoid and trochlear fossae areas is restored, but anterior capsulectomy is not yet completed. *AC*, anterior capsule; *C*, capitellum; *RH*, radial head; *T*, trochlea.

Posterior Capsular Release

- Portals are established:
  - The posterocentral viewing portal (3 to 4 cm proximal to the olecranon tip, through the triceps) is established first; it must be placed sufficiently proximal to clear the olecranon tip and enter the olecranon fossa.
  - A proximal posterolateral working portal (2 cm proximal to the olecranon tip and lateral to the triceps) is also established using an outside-in technique.
- A shaver is used to débride the posterior fat pad and open the posterior working space, avoiding shaving medial to the midline and certainly in and along the medial gutter until full visualization is obtained.
- The capsule is elevated from the distal humerus using blunt dissection or an elevator.
- Visualization and débridement of the posterior radiocapitellar joint can be facilitated using a midlateral (soft spot) working portal.
  - Viewing through the posterolateral portal, the midlateral portal is made under direct visualization using a spinal needle placed through the soft spot toward the posterior radiocapitellar joint.
  - An arthroscopic shaver is in used in this portal to débride the posterior capsule and arthrofibrosis. Suction is avoided in and along the medial gutter.
- Loose bodies and impinging osteophytes are removed before capsular resection to optimize visualization.

- Osteophytes are resected from the olecranon fossa, posterior capitellum, and olecranon tip using an arthroscopic burr or shaver.
- When necessary, osteophytes involving the medial gutter should be removed with care. Using a burr or serrated shaver may inadvertently draw the ulnar nerve into harm's way. For this reason, it is recommended to use a shaver blade instead.
- Up to 14 mm of the olecranon tip can be resected without injury to the triceps tendon.[12]
- A small open arthrotomy may be required at times for removal of larger loose bodies.

- The posterior capsule is released with a basket cutter or arthroscopic elevator on the medial and lateral sides; care should be taken to avoid capsular release medial to the olecranon fossa to avoid injury to the ulnar nerve.
- The posteromedial capsule (posterior band of the medial collateral ligament) should be resected in the setting of significant flexion loss. Release of this tissue does not risk medial-sided elbow instability.[25]
  - Care should be taken to protect the ulnar nerve, as this tissue represents the floor of the cubital tunnel. If a posteromedial release is planned, a limited open ulnar nerve decompression or full transposition should be performed prior to arthroscopy.
  - Release is performed along the olecranon, rather than the humerus, as this portion of the capsule is furthest from the ulnar nerve.
  - Use of radiofrequency ablation or suction medially should also be avoided to protect the nerve.
- An open arthrotomy through the ulnar nerve incision carries minimal morbidity and can be very useful to access the posteromedial capsule for release and the olecranon tip for excision in cases where the arthroscopic visualization is limited.
- Final inspection from both portals is done to ensure adequate release (**TECH FIG 3**).

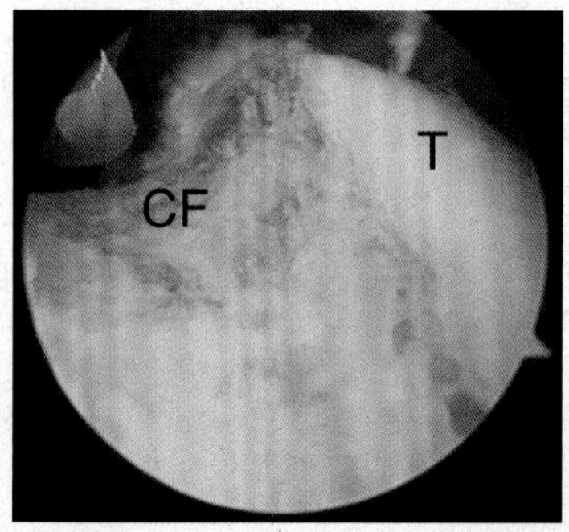

A

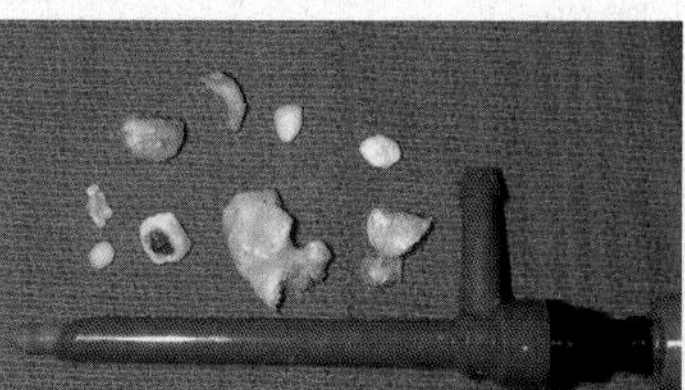

B

TECH FIG 3 • **A.** View from the lateral portal after medial release showing completed capsulectomy and bony débridement in the coronoid fossa area. **B.** Loose bodies are removed during this procedure via a 5-mm smooth cannula. *CF*, coronoid fossa; *T*, trochlea.

Wound Closure and Intraoperative Splinting

- A drain is placed through the proximal anterolateral portal because accumulation of fluid and postoperative bleeding will compromise range of motion.
- Our postoperative dressing is a soft bulky dressing with Webril, Kerlix, and Ace bandages from wrist to shoulder. Material is cut out from the antecubital fossa in order to facilitate flexion (**TECH FIG 4**). Continuous passive motion (CPM) can be initiated on postoperative day 0 at the surgeon's discretion.
  - Alternatively, an anterior plaster slab is placed to keep the elbow near full extension and alternating resting flexion and extension splints are used.
- Indwelling catheters, a long-acting regional block, or cryotherapy may be used to facilitate CPM (from full flexion to extension).

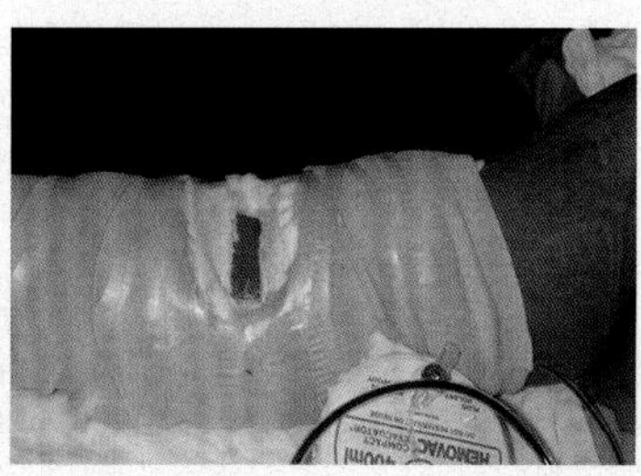

A

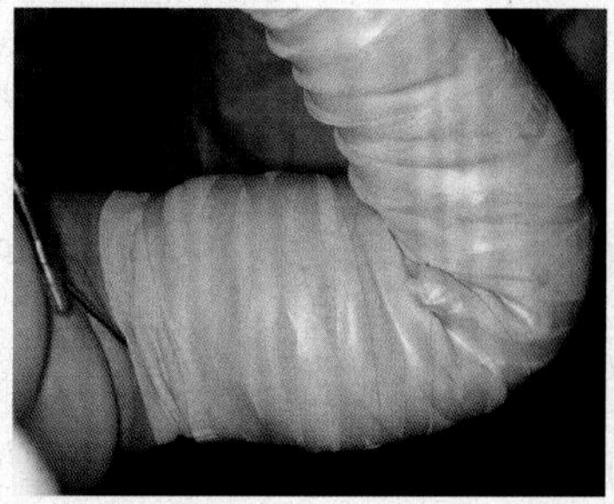

B

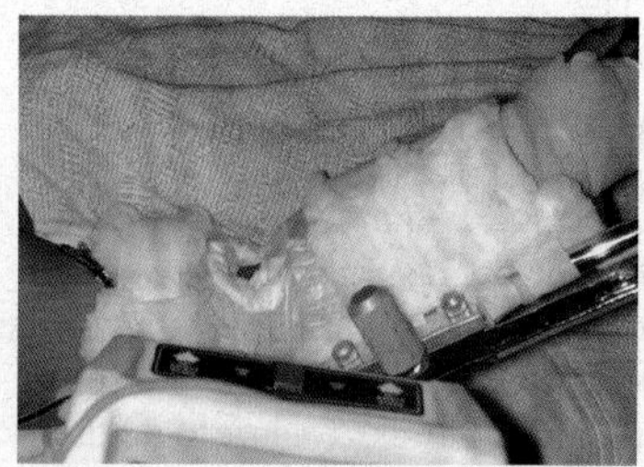

C

TECH FIG 4 • **A.** Postoperative dressing is applied to the patient after capsular release in the operating room with a drain. **B.** Flexion obtained after removing splint material from the antecubital fossa. **C.** Immediate continuous passive motion is instituted.

PEARLS AND PITFALLS

Managing the ulnar nerve	■ Prophylactic release before arthroscopy if flexion contracture is significant or if examination consistent with neuropathy or neuritis.
Optimizing visualization	■ Use arthroscopic retractors to aid visualization in anterior and posterior compartments.
Avoiding neurovascular injury	■ The surgeon should avoid motorized burrs. No suction should be used on the shaver in at-risk areas. Use of arthroscopic retractors is recommended.
Anterior osteocapsular release	■ Using a basket and retractor, develop the plane between capsule and brachialis until the defined fat stripe over the midportion of radiocapitellar joint, which represents the radial nerve. Watch for PIN adjacent to anterolateral capsule distally.
Posterior osteocapsular release	■ Consider performing first if working in medial and lateral gutters. Retract the ulnar nerve and use a shaver blade to avoid iatrogenic nerve injury.

POSTOPERATIVE CARE

- CPM can be continued at home up to 4 weeks and should be used in full range of motion (0 to 145 degrees) with a bolster behind the elbow.[26]
- Daily physiotherapy is instituted immediately postoperatively, with home static- (preferred) or dynamic-progressive splinting.
- The surgeon should consider prophylaxis of heterotopic ossification with indomethacin. Single-dose external beam irradiation is only considered in the most severe cases of heterotopic ossification, in which case, the release is typically performed open.

OUTCOMES

- Patients usually regain about 50% of lost motion.[11,23]
- About 80% of patients obtain a functional arc of motion greater than 100 degrees.[11]
- A systematic review by Kodde et al[15] found a mean gain in arc of motion of 40 degrees (from 84 to 124 degrees) with arthroscopic elbow release, although gains of up to 80 degrees have been reported.[26]
- Ball et al[3] reported high patient satisfaction and recovery of function after surgery, with all patients in the series stating they wound undergo surgery again.
- In high-level athletes undergoing arthroscopic release for loss of terminal extension (<35 degrees), the average loss of flexion improved from 27 degrees to 6 degrees, and 23 of 26 athletes returned to the previous level of performance.[4]
- It is difficult to compare arthroscopic versus open capsular releases as arthroscopic surgery is typically performed for less severe disease, whereas open release is preferred for more complex cases.[15]

COMPLICATIONS

- The overall complication rate for arthroscopic release is low (5% vs. 23% for open surgery).[15]
- Blona et al[5] reported no permanent neurologic injuries in a series of over 500 elbow arthroscopic releases for stiffness. In less experienced hands, a neurologic injury is more likely and the learning curve should be appreciated.
- Persistent stiffness requiring a second surgical release is the most common complication.[15]
- Ulnar nerve
  - Although the overall rate of ulnar nerve injury with elbow arthroscopy is low (1%), the preoperative diagnosis of elbow contracture and performance of a capsulectomy are both risk factors for transient ulnar nerve palsy.[13]
  - In the medial aspect of joint, the surgeon should use retractors to move the capsule medially and avoid resection along the humerus, or identify and protect the ulnar nerve through a small open incision prior to any work in the posteromedial gutter.
- Ulnar neuritis
  - If present preoperatively, or there will be a significant increase in flexion after surgery, the ulnar nerve should be released.
  - Postoperatively, it may be transient; there is a much lower incidence if it is transposed during the initial surgery.
- Radial or PIN
  - The overall rate of radial or PIN nerve palsy with elbow arthroscopy is 1%.[13]
  - Iatrogenic injury can be avoided by refraining from use of suction when working near the capsule anterior to the midline of the radiocapitellar articulation.
  - Retractors of soft tissue are used to improve visualization and distention.
- Median or anterior interosseous nerve
  - Iatrogenic injury is avoided by not penetrating the brachialis muscle.
  - The surgeon should place portals carefully, avoiding moving more anterior than necessary.
- Excessive bony resection leading to iatrogenic fracture or inadvertently aggressive resection of soft tissues surrounding the radial head leading to violation of the collateral ligament and elbow instability
  - When working in the anterolateral joint, avoid débriding further posterior than the equator of the radiocapitellar joint, as this corresponds to the superior margin of the lateral collateral ligament.[8]

REFERENCES

1. Akai M, Shirasaki Y, Tateishi T. Viscoelastic properties of stiff joints: a new approach in analyzing joint contracture. Biomed Mater Eng 1993;3:67–73.
2. An K, Morrey BF. Biomechanics of the elbow. In: Morrey BF, ed. The Elbow and Its Disorders. Philadelphia: WB Saunders, 2000: 43–74.
3. Ball CM, Meunier M, Galatz LM, et al. Arthroscopic treatment of post-traumatic elbow contracture. J Should Elbow Surg 2002;11:624–629.

4. Blonna D, Lee G, O'Driscoll SW. Arthroscopic restoration of terminal elbow extension in high-level athletes. Am J Sports Med 2010;38:2509.
5. Blonna D, Wolf JM, Fitzsimmons J, et al. Prevention of nerve injury during arthroscopic capsulectomy of the elbow utilizing a safety-driven strategy. J Bone and Joint Surg Am 2013;95:1373–1381.
6. Bruno RJ, Lee ML, Strauch FJ, et al. Posttraumatic elbow stiffness: evaluation and management. J Am Acad Orthop Surg 2002;10:106–116.
7. Cohen MS. Heterotopic ossification of the elbow. In: Jupiter JB, ed. The Stiff Elbow. Rosemont, IL: American Academy of Orthopaedic Surgeons, 2006:31–40.
8. Cohen MS, Romeo AA, Hennigan SP, et al. Lateral epicondylitis: anatomic relationships of the extensor tendon origins and implications for arthroscopic treatment. J Should Elbow Surg 2008;17:954–960.
9. Gallay S, Richards R, O'Driscoll SW. Intraarticular capacity and compliance of stiff and normal elbows. Arthroscopy 1993;9:9–13.
10. Hildebrand K, Zhang M, van Snellenberg W, et al. Myofibroblast numbers are elevated in human elbow capsules after trauma. Clin Orthop Relat Res 2004;419:189–197.
11. Jupiter JB, O'Driscoll SW, Cohen MS. The assessment and management of the stiff elbow. AAOS Instr Course Lect 2003;52:93–111.
12. Keener JD, Chafik D, Kim HM, et al. Insertional anatomy of the triceps brachii tendon. J Should Elbow Surg 2010;19:399–405.
13. Kelley ED, Morrey BF, O'Driscoll SW. Complications of elbow arthroscopy. J Bone Joint Surg Am 2001;83:25–34.
14. King GJ, Faber KJ. Posttraumatic elbow stiffness. Orthop Clin North Am 2000;31:129–143.
15. Kodde IF, van Rijn J, van den Bekerom MP, et al. Surgical treatment of post-traumatic elbow stiffness: systemic review. J Should Elbow Surg 2013;22:574–580.
16. Lindenhovius AL, Doornberg JB, Brower KM, et al. A prospective randomized control trial of dynamic versus static progressive elbow splinting for posttraumatic elbow stiffness. J Bone Joint Surg Am 2012;94:694–700.
17. Morrey BF. Anatomy of the elbow joint. In: Morrey BF, ed. The Elbow and Its Disorders. Philadelphia: WB Saunders, 2000:13–42.
18. Morrey BF. The stiff elbow with articular involvement. In: Jupiter JB, ed. The Stiff Elbow. Rosemont, IL: American Academy of Orthopaedic Surgeons, 2006:21–30.
19. Morrey BF, Askey LJ, Chao EY. A biomechanical study of normal functional elbow motion. J Bone Joint Surg Am 1981;63:872–877.
20. Müller AM, Sadoghi P, Lucas R, et al. Effectiveness of bracing in the treatment of nonosseous restriction of elbow mobility: a systematic review. J Should Elbow Surg 2013;22:1146–1152.
21. Novak CB, Lee GW, Mackinnon SE, et al. Provocative testing for cubital tunnel syndrome. J Hand Surg 1994;19:817–820.
22. O'Driscoll SW. Arthroscopic osteocapsular arthroplasty. In: Yamaguchi K, King G, McKee M, et al, eds. Advanced Reconstruction Elbow, 1 ed. Rosemont, IL: American Academy of Orthopaedic Surgeons, 2007:59–68.
23. O'Driscoll SW. Clinical assessment and open and arthroscopic treatment of the stiff elbow. In: Jupiter JB, ed. The Stiff Elbow. Rosemont, IL: American Academy of Orthopaedic Surgeons, 2006:9–19.
24. O'Driscoll SW, Morrey BF, An K. Intra-articular pressure and capacity of the elbow. Arthroscopy 1990;6:100–103.
25. Ruch DS, Shen J, Chioros GD, et al. Release of the medial collateral ligament to improve flexion in post-traumatic elbow stiffness. J Bone Joint Surg Br 2008;90:614–618.
26. Savoie FH III, Field LD. Arthrofibrosis and complications in arthroscopy of the elbow. Clin Sports Med 2001;20(1):123–129.
27. Tucker SA, Savoie FH, O'Brien MJ. Arthroscopic management of the post-traumatic stiff elbow. J Should Elbow Surg 2011;20:S83–S89.

Lateral Columnar Release for Extracapsular Elbow Contracture

Leonid I. Katolik and Mark S. Cohen

DEFINITION

- Extrinsic elbow contracture refers to elbow stiffness secondary to fibrosis, thickening, and, occasionally, ossification of the elbow capsule and periarticular soft tissues.
- In contrast to intrinsic contracture, the articular surface is either uninvolved or minimally involved, without the presence of intra-articular adhesions or articular cartilage destruction.
- Although a distinction is made between extrinsic and intrinsic causes of contracture, these entities often overlap.

ANATOMY

- The elbow is a compound uniaxial synovial joint comprising three highly congruous articulations.
- The ulnohumeral joint is a ginglymus, or hinge, joint. The radiocapitellar and proximal radioulnar joints are gliding joints.
- All three articulations exist within a single capsule and are further stabilized by the proximity of the articular surface and capsule to the intracapsular ligaments and overlying extracapsular musculature.

PATHOGENESIS

- The propensity for elbow stiffness after even trivial elbow trauma is well recognized. After even seemingly trivial injuries, the capsule can undergo structural and biochemical alterations leading to thickening, decreased compliance, and loss of motion.
- Causes of extrinsic elbow contracture include capsular contracture, damage to and fibrosis of the flexor–extensor muscular origins, collateral ligament scarring, heterotopic bone, and skin contracture.
- Prolonged immobilization after trauma may be a separate risk factor for the development of stiffness.

NATURAL HISTORY

- Little consensus exists regarding the natural history of capsular contracture. It is felt that appropriate recognition and treatment of acute elbow injuries, avoidance of prolonged immobilization, and early active range of motion may limit the severity of posttraumatic extrinsic contracture.
- Patients typically do not tolerate elbow stiffness well because adjacent joints do not provide adequate compensatory motion.
  - Morrey[10] showed that the performance of most activities of daily living requires a functional arc of motion from 30 to 130 degrees.
  - Vasen and colleagues[11] have demonstrated that volunteers with uninjured elbows may adapt to a functional arc of motion from 70 to 120 degrees to perform 12 tasks of daily living.
  - Patients typically request treatment for elbow contracture when loss of extension approaches 40 degrees and flexion does not exceed 120 degrees.
  - Patients who do not improve with a concerted effort at nonoperative treatment often require surgical release.
- Stiffness of the elbow typically is incited by soft tissue trauma, hemarthrosis, and the patient's response to pain. Elbow trauma may cause tearing and contusion of the periarticular soft tissues. The patient typically holds the injured elbow in a flexed position to reduce pain. A fibrous tissue response then ensues within the hematoma and damaged muscular tissues. This fibrous tissue may ossify. In addition, overly aggressive therapy may further exacerbate these injuries, potentiating the cycle of pain, swelling, and limitation in motion that leads ultimately to frank contracture.
- Collateral ligament injury may contribute to contracture. Primary fibrosis may develop within the collateral ligaments because of the initial injury. Alternatively, secondary fibrosis may result from immobilization and scar formation.
- Significant injury to the anterior joint capsule and the overlying brachialis muscle may also result in capsular hypertrophy and fibrotic reaction contributing to ankylosis. This is particularly common in association with fracture-dislocations of the elbow.

PATIENT HISTORY AND PHYSICAL FINDINGS

- The cause of contracture should generally be easily elucidated from the history. Particular notation should be made of concomitant injuries, including closed head injury or associated burn injury.
- The duration and possible progression of symptoms should be noted.
- The impact of the contracture on the patient's upper extremity function and any limitations in activities of daily living should be noted.
- Any previous treatment for contracture should be elucidated. This should include the appropriateness, duration, and results of prior physical therapy, splinting, intra-articular injections, and surgeries.
- For patients with prior elbow surgery, the presence and type of any residual internal fixation devices should be noted. In addition, attention should be paid to any remote history of elbow infection.
- Physical examination should include a general physical examination as well as a detailed examination of the involved extremity.
  - Attention must be paid to the examination of the skin and soft tissue envelope about the elbow, with notation made of prior incisions, skin grafts, flaps, or areas of wound breakdown.

- Elbow motion should be measured with a goniometer and active and passive motion should be compared.
- Notation should be made whether motion improves with the forearm in full pronation, which may suggest posterolateral rotatory instability.
- Although rare, symptomatic incompetence of the ulnar collateral ligament may elucidated by examination.
- Strength of the involved limb should be assessed, as a joint without adequate strength is unlikely to maintain motion after release.
- Because many posttraumatic and inflammatory contractures about the elbow are associated with ulnar nerve symptoms, a careful neurologic examination should be performed. A positive Tinel test over the cubital tunnel as well as a positive elbow flexion test should increase the suspicion for concomitant ulnar nerve pathology.

IMAGING AND OTHER DIAGNOSTIC STUDIES

- Anteroposterior (AP) and lateral radiographs are often all that is needed for preoperative planning (**FIG 1**).
- Cross-sectional imaging with computed tomography is helpful in visualizing the articular surfaces, particularly after fracture.
  - We advocate the use of computed tomography for preoperative planning in cases of moderate to severe heterotopic ossification.
- Extracapsular contracture is typically not painful through the remaining arc of motion and is not painful at rest. If pain is a significant component of the patient's symptoms, serologic workup for infection, including a complete blood count, erythrocyte sedimentation rate, and C-reactive protein, is indicated.

DIFFERENTIAL DIAGNOSIS

- Conversion disorder
- Infection
- Inflammatory arthropathy
- Intracapsular contracture

NONOPERATIVE MANAGEMENT

- Alternative measures to improve elbow stiffness include conservative modalities to decrease joint swelling and inflammation and relax or stretch contracted soft tissues. For protracted swelling, edema control sleeves, ice, elevation, active motion (including the forearm, wrist, and hand), and oral agents such as anti-inflammatory medication can be useful.
- A short-term oral prednisone taper can be very effective in difficult cases. In addition, one can consider an intra-articular cortisone injection to decrease inflammation and joint synovitis.
- Rarely, when patients exhibit guarding and involuntary co-contraction, biofeedback may be a helpful adjunct.
- Dynamic splints, which apply a constant tension to the soft tissues, may be helpful.[5]
  - These braces improve range of motion through soft tissue creep. They tend to be more painful to wear and may cause unwanted inflammation.
- Patient-adjusted static braces appear to be more effective. These braces use the principle of passive progressive stretch, allowing for stress relaxation of the soft tissues. They are applied for much shorter periods of time and are better tolerated by patients.

SURGICAL MANAGEMENT

- To improve elbow flexion, one must release any soft tissue structures posteriorly that might be tethering the joint. These include the posterior joint capsule (including the posterior bundle of the ulnar collateral ligament) and the triceps muscle and tendon, which can become adherent to the humerus.[1,6,8,9]
  - Any bony or soft tissue impingement also must be removed anteriorly, including osteophytes off the coronoid process and any bony or soft tissue overgrowth in both the coronoid and radial fossae.
  - There must be a concavity above the humeral trochlea to accept both the coronoid centrally and the radial head laterally for full flexion to occur.
- Similarly, to improve elbow extension, posterior impingement must be removed between the olecranon tip and the olecranon fossa.
  - Anteriorly, any tethering soft tissues must be released, namely the anterior joint capsule and any adhesions between the brachialis and the humerus.[4,7]

Preoperative Planning

- All radiographic studies should be reviewed.
- The presence and type of any retained implants is noted.
- Range-of-motion and pivot shift testing is performed under anesthesia as well as under live fluoroscopy.

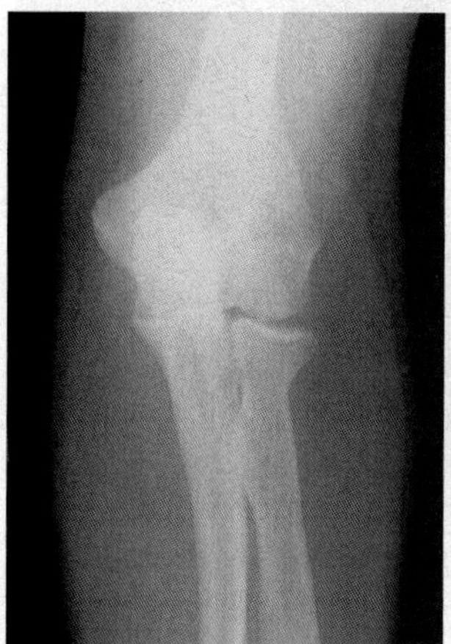

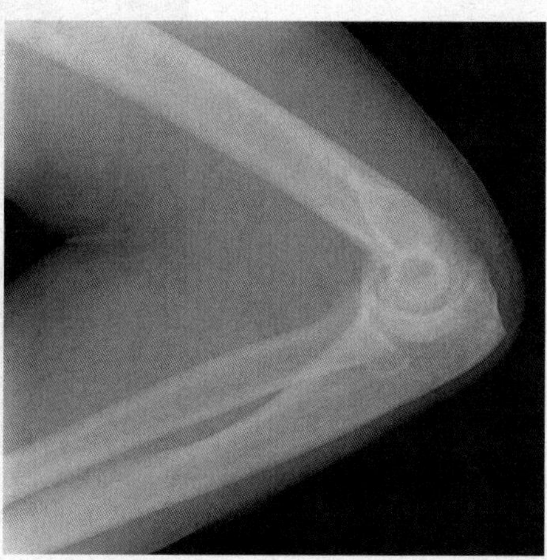

FIG 1 • Routine preoperative AP (**A**) and lateral (**B**) radiographs are obtained in all cases. Contracture may occur after subtle injury. This patient developed stiffness after nonoperative treatment of a nondisplaced radial neck fracture.

Positioning

- Patients are positioned supine with the arm on a hand table.
- The patient's torso is brought to the edge of the operating table to ensure adequate elbow exposure for fluoroscopic imaging.
- A towel bump may be placed under the medial elbow.

Approach

- A direct posterior skin incision or a lateral incision is used.
  - A direct posterior incision has been criticized for an increased propensity toward postoperative seroma formation.
  - It has the advantage of being a utilitarian incision that allows access to the medial and lateral sides simultaneously.
- Advantages to the lateral exposure include its simplicity, less extensor and flexor–pronator disruption, and access to all three joint articulations.
  - The main disadvantage of the lateral exposure is the inability to address the ulnar nerve and posterior bundle of the ulnar collateral ligament when indicated.
- The deep interval for exposure of the anterior capsule lies between the extensor carpi radialis longus (ECRL) proximally and the extensor carpi radialis brevis (ECRB) distally. Posterior access is achieved between the triceps and the humerus.

TECHNIQUES

Surgical Approach

- The procedure can be performed under general anesthesia or under regional anesthesia with a long-acting regional block.
- For the posterior incision, care is taken to avoid placing the line of incision directly over the prominence of the olecranon. Full-thickness fasciocutaneous flaps are elevated laterally to expose the extensor muscle mass.
- For a lateral incision, an extended Kocher approach is used, beginning along the lateral supracondylar ridge of the humerus and passing distally in the interval between the anconeus and the extensor carpi ulnaris (ECU).

Posterior Release

- The Kocher interval between the anconeus and ECU is developed.
- The anconeus is reflected posteriorly in continuity with the triceps. This exposes the posterior and posterolateral joint capsule (**TECH FIG 1A,B**).
- A triceps tenolysis is carried out with an elevator, releasing any adhesions between the muscle and the posterior humerus. The humeroulnar joint is identified posteriorly and the olecranon fossa is cleared of any fibrous tissue or scar that would restrict terminal extension. The tip of the olecranon is removed if there was evidence of overgrowth or impingement (**TECH FIG 1C**).
- The posterior aspect of the radiocapitellar joint is inspected after excision of the elbow capsule just proximal to the conjoined lateral collateral and annular ligament complex through the "soft spot" on the lateral side of the elbow. The proximal edge of this complex lies along the proximal border of the radial head.

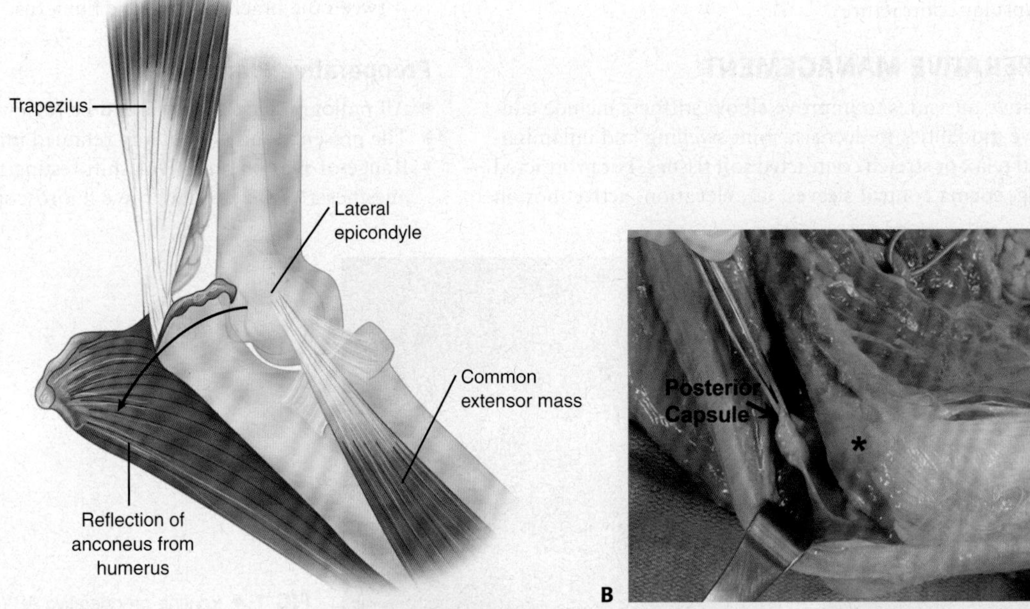

TECH FIG 1 • **A,B.** Exposure of the lateral and posterior ulnohumeral joint. The anconeus and triceps are reflected posteriorly, exposing the posterior capsule, olecranon tip, and olecranon fossa. *Asterisk* indicates the lateral epicondyle. *(continued)*

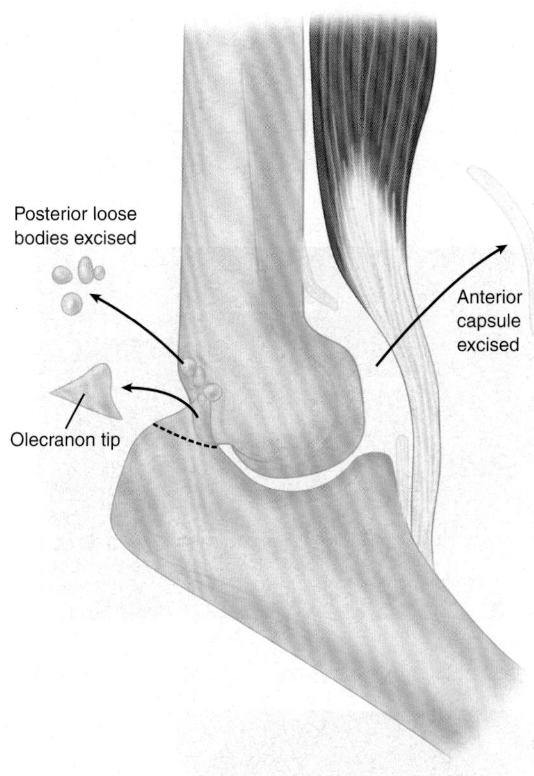

TECH FIG 1 • *(continued)* **C.** Visualization of the posterior compartment permits débridement of the posterior joint, including removing impinging tissue of osteophytes in the olecranon fossa and the tip of the olecranon.

Anterior Release

- Once the posterior release is completed, dissection is carried anteriorly. The anterior interval proximally is between the lateral supracondylar column and the brachioradialis and ECRL. Distally, the interval is between the ECRL and extensor digitorum communis (EDC) (**TECH FIG 2A**).
- The brachialis is then mobilized off the humerus and anterior capsule with an elevator, releasing any adhesions between the muscle and the anterior humerus (**TECH FIG 2B**).
- The brachioradialis and ECRL are released from the lateral supracondylar ridge of the humerus (**TECH FIG 2C**).
- This dissection is continued distally between the ECRL and ECRB, allowing exposure of the anterior capsule with preservation of the lateral collateral ligament and the origins of the ECRB, the EDC and extensor digiti minimi, and the ECU from the lateral epicondyle.
- Dissection is then carried out beneath the elbow capsule between the joint and the brachialis. The capsule is excised as far as the medial side of the joint.

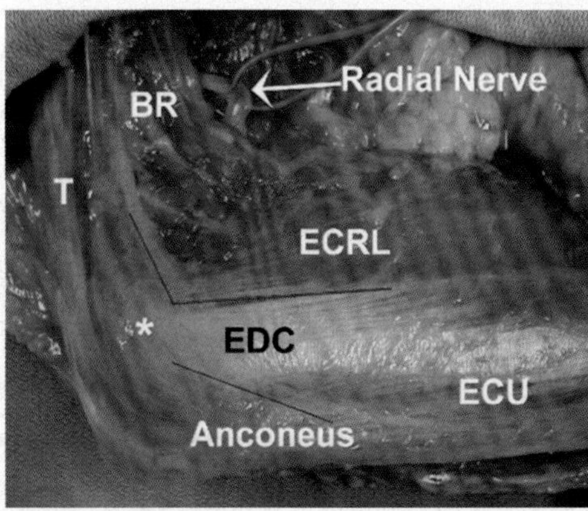

TECH FIG 2 • **A.** The lateral view of a dissected elbow. *Blue lines* mark the fascial intervals for access to the anterior and posterior aspects of the joint, which leaves the extensor carpi ulnaris (*ECU*), extensor digitorum communis (*EDC*), and extensor carpi radialis longus (*ECRL*) origins intact as well as the underlying lateral collateral ligament complex. The anterior elbow capsule is exposed by releasing the ECRL from the lateral supracondylar ridge. Distally, the exposure continues between the ECRL and ECRB. *T*, triceps; *BR*, brachioradialis; *asterisk*, lateral epicondyle. *(continued)*

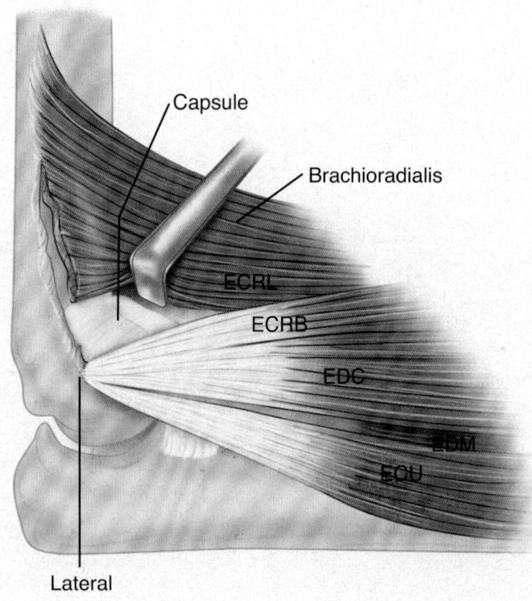

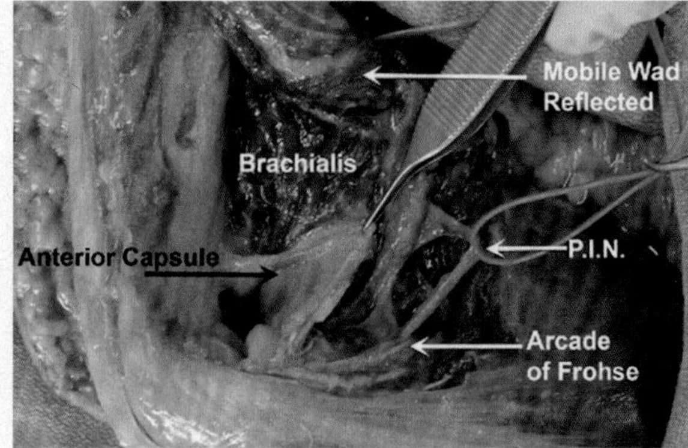

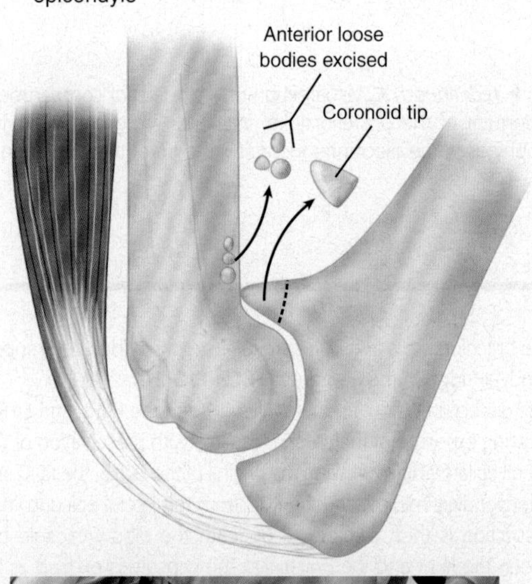

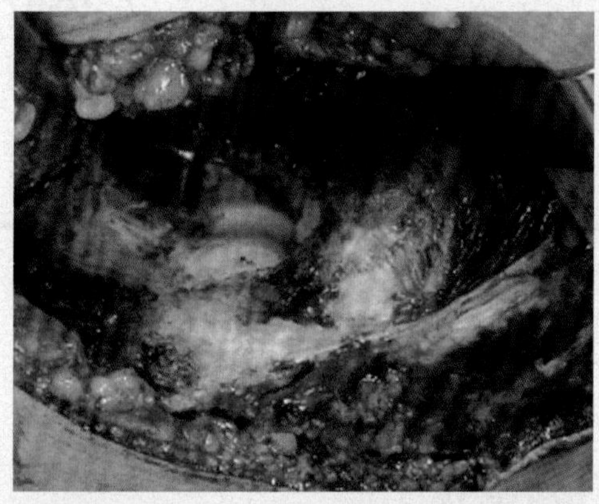

TECH FIG 2 • *(continued)* **B,C.** The anterior exposure for release. The anterior capsule is exposed by detaching the humeral origin of the ECRL proximally and the interval between the ECRL and extensor carpi radialis brevis (*ECRB*) distally. The brachialis is released from the anterior capsule. The capsule should be visualized all the way over to the medial joint with all muscle reflected anteriorly. *EDM*, extensor digiti minimi; *PIN*, posterior interosseous nerve. **D,E.** Anterior compartment débridement removes the tip of the coronoid and clears the coronoid and radial fossae. **F.** Intraoperative extension after contracture release.

- The radial and coronoid fossae are cleared of fibrous tissue and the tip of the coronoid is removed if overgrowth or impingement was noted in flexion. Loose bodies are removed (**TECH FIG 2D,E**).
- After release of the anterior capsule, gentle extension of the elbow with applied pressure usually brings the joint out to nearly full extension.
- In long-standing cases of contracture, the brachialis muscle can be tight, inhibiting full terminal elbow extension. This myostatic contracture can be stretched for several minutes during the procedure and requires attention at subsequent physiotherapy (**TECH FIG 2F**).

PEARLS AND PITFALLS

Indications	■ The importance of prolonged postoperative rehabilitation cannot be stressed enough. A program of active and passive range of motion, weighted elbow stretches with wrist weights, formal therapy, and patient-adjusted elbow bracing is common for 3–6 months after surgery. ■ Postoperative gains may easily be lost in the patient who is not fully committed to rehabilitation or who does not have access to regular supervised therapy.
Ulnar nerve	■ Patients with preoperative signs and symptoms of ulnar nerve irritability should undergo neurolysis and transposition of the ulnar nerve. Although no strict guidelines exist, patients with preoperative flexion less than 100 degrees generally undergo concurrent ulnar nerve release even in the absence of preoperative symptoms. ■ Care should be observed when manipulating the elbow following all soft tissue releases from the lateral approach to regain flexion. Residual limitations in flexion are likely due to contracture of the posterior bundle of the ulnar collateral ligament. Forced manipulation can cause a traction injury to the ulnar nerve.
Median nerve and brachial artery	■ These structures are generally well protected by the brachialis muscle. Their safety is increased if dissection proceeds in the interval between the elbow capsule and the brachialis.
Radial nerve injury	■ The posterior interosseous nerve may be encountered as extracapsular dissection proceeds distal to the radiocapitellar joint. Care must be taken with more distal dissection, and a firm understanding of neural anatomy is mandatory before attempting capsular release. Except in cases of significant anterolateral heterotopic ossification, we do not routinely dissect and isolate the radial nerve from proximal to distal.
Iatrogenic posterolateral rotatory instability	■ Instability may be induced with overly aggressive dissection about the lateral condyle. Care should be taken to stay anterior to the origin of the ECRB.

POSTOPERATIVE CARE

- Although several rehabilitation programs may be effective, we have found continuous passive motion, begun immediately in the recovery room and used continuously until the following morning, to be helpful in maintaining the motion gained at surgery (**FIG 2A**).
- Formal therapy is begun on postoperative day 1.
  - The dressing is removed and edema control modalities (eg, an edema sleeve or Ace wrap, ice) are used to limit swelling.
  - Active and gentle passive elbow motion is combined with intermittent continuous passive motion.
  - To help maintain extension, weighted passive stretches using a 2-pound wrist weight with the arm extended over a bolster are performed several times daily for 10 to 15 minutes as tolerated.
  - Because the collateral ligaments are not released at surgery, no restrictions are typically placed on therapy.[3]
- Static progressive elbow bracing is begun early in the postoperative period. The brace is worn for about 30 minutes, two or three times a day. Flexion and extension are alternated based on the preoperative deficit and the early progress of the elbow (**FIG 2B**).
  - Commercially available braces should be obtained preoperatively, as trying to secure them postoperatively can delay the onset of their use.
- A nonsteroidal anti-inflammatory agent (Indocin) is commonly prescribed as a prophylaxis against heterotopic ossification for several weeks postoperatively. This also helps to limit inflammation of the joint and soft tissues during rehabilitation.

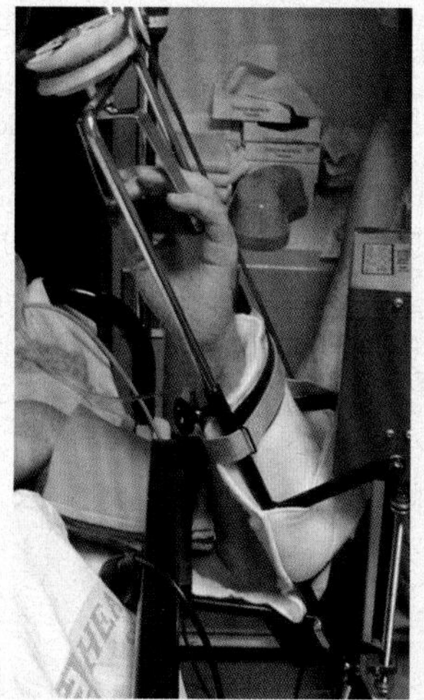
A

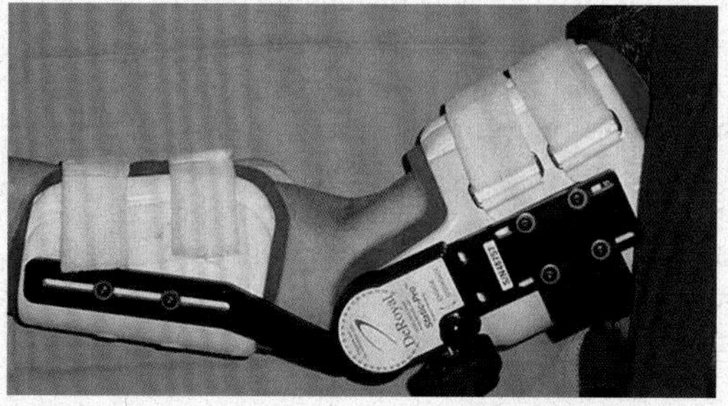
B

FIG 2 • **A.** Elbow continuous passive motion device. **B.** Patient-adjusted static elbow brace.

- Patients are typically discharged home on postoperative day 1. Home therapy is performed daily thereafter, including active and passive exercises, continuous passive motion, weighted stretches, and patient-adjusted bracing.
  - Progress should be closely monitored by a therapist who is familiar with the protocol. The physician must also follow these patients closely.
- Although the bulk of ultimate elbow motion is gained during the first 6 to 8 weeks, patients can continue to make gains in terminal flexion and extension for several months postoperatively. This is especially true for elbow flexion.
- Continuous passive motion is typically discontinued at 3 to 4 weeks, but bracing is continued for several months as required. As long as the patient is able to obtain full elbow flexion and extension once per day (eg, in the brace), a favorable prognosis exists with respect to the ultimate outcome if vigilance is maintained.

OUTCOMES

- In appropriate patients, release of the contracted elbow can be a reliable and satisfying procedure with predictable results.
- We reviewed our results for 22 patents treated for posttraumatic elbow stiffness using a soft tissue release of the elbow through a lateral approach. The average length of follow-up was 29 months.[2]
  - Total elbow motion improved in all subjects. Extension increased from an average of 39 ± 10 degrees preoperatively to 8 ± 6 degrees at follow-up. Elbow flexion increased from 113 ± 18 degrees preoperatively to 137 ± 9 degrees at follow-up. Thus, total ulnohumeral joint motion increased an average of 55 degrees ($P < .001$).
  - Elbow pain, as determined by visual analog scales, decreased in all patients. Elbow function, as determined by standardized scales, also significantly improved.
  - Radiographic analysis revealed no patients with regrowth of excised osteophytes or loose bodies at follow-up.

COMPLICATIONS

- Ulnar nerve
  - The most common complication after elbow release surgery involves the ulnar nerve. This may be related in part to improved elbow flexion after surgery, as ulnar nerve tension increases with flexion. This may precipitate symptoms in a nerve that is already subclinically compromised.
  - Patients with preoperative signs and symptoms of ulnar nerve irritability should undergo neurolysis and transposition of the ulnar nerve.
  - Although no strict guidelines exist, patients with preoperative flexion less than 100 degrees generally undergo concurrent ulnar nerve release even in the absence of preoperative symptoms.
- Median nerve and brachial artery
  - Although generally well protected by the brachialis muscle, these structures are at risk with anterior dissection. Their safety is increased if dissection proceeds in the interval between the elbow capsule and the brachialis.
  - In addition, transient median neuritis is known to occur in our practices after release. This is likely due to stretch of the median nerve with extension of the severely contracted elbow.
- Radial nerve injury
  - The posterior interosseous nerve may be encountered, as extracapsular dissection proceeds distal to the radiocapitellar joint.
  - Except in cases of significant anterolateral heterotopic ossification, the radial nerve does not typically require identification.
- Persistent stiffness
  - The importance of prolonged postoperative rehabilitation cannot be stressed enough. A program of active and passive range of motion, weighted elbow stretches with wrist weights, formal therapy, and patient-adjusted elbow bracing is common for 3 to 6 months after surgery. All of our patients meet preoperatively both with the therapists at our home institutions as well as with their local therapists.

REFERENCES

1. Cohen MS, Hastings H II. Operative release for elbow contracture: the lateral collateral ligament sparing technique. Orthop Clin North Am 1999;30:133–139.
2. Cohen MS, Hastings H II. Post-traumatic contracture of the elbow. Operative release using a lateral collateral sparing approach. J Bone Joint Surg Br 1998;80(5):805–812.
3. Cohen MS, Hastings H II. Rotatory instability of the elbow. The anatomy and role of the lateral stabilizers. J Bone Joint Surg Am 1997;79(2):225–233.
4. Gates HS III, Sullivan FL, Urbaniak JR. Anterior capsulotomy and continuous passive motion in the treatment post-traumatic flexion contracture of the elbow. J Bone Joint Surg Am 1992;74(8): 1229–1234.
5. Green DP, McCoy H. Turnbuckle orthotic correction of elbow flexion contractures after acute injuries. J Bone Joint Surg Am 1979;61(7):1092–1095.
6. Jupiter JB, O'Driscoll SW, Cohen MS. The assessment and management of the stiff elbow. Instr Course Lect 2003;52:93–111.
7. Kasparyan NG, Hotchkiss RN. Dynamic skeletal fixation in the upper extremity. Hand Clin 1997;13:643–663.
8. Mansat P, Morrey BF. The column procedure: a limited lateral approach for extrinsic contracture of the elbow. J Bone Joint Surg Am 1998;80(11):1603–1615.
9. Modabber MR, Jupiter JB. Reconstruction for post-traumatic conditions of the elbow joint. J Bone Joint Surg Am 1995;77(9): 1431–1446.
10. Morrey BF. Post-traumatic contracture of the elbow. Operative treatment, including distraction arthroplasty. J Bone Joint Surg Am 1990;72(4):601–618.
11. Vasen AP, Lacey SH, Keith MW, et al. Functional range of motion of the elbow. J Hand Surg Am 1995;20(2):288–292.

Extrinsic Contracture Release: Medial Over-the-Top Approach

133

CHAPTER

Pierre Mansat, Aymeric André, and Nicolas Bonnevialle

DEFINITION

- Multiple techniques have been described for the release of elbow contractures. The medial approach has the advantages of direct access to both the anterior and posterior aspects of the ulnohumeral joint and direct visualization of the ulnar nerve.
- Medial-based releases were initially proposed by Wilner,[24] whose technique involved medial epicondylectomy and wide dissection.
  - Weiss and Sachar[23] subsequently has described splitting the flexor–pronator mass rather than complete release of the flexor–pronator mass.
  - Mansat et al[12] popularized this approach to deal with extrinsic contracture of the elbow and ulnar nerve involvement.
  - Itoh et al[10] and Wada et al[22] underlined the importance of the posterior oblique band of the medial collateral ligament as a critical structure to identify and release if an extension contracture exists.

ANATOMY

- The medial compartment of the elbow includes the medial side of the ulnohumeral joint, the medial collateral ligament, the flexor–pronator mass, the ulnar nerve, and the medial antebrachial cutaneous nerve (**FIG 1A**).
- The medial ulnohumeral joint is composed of the medial column, the medial epicondyle, the medial side of the proximal aspect of the ulna, and the coronoid process.
- The medial collateral ligament consists of three parts: anterior, posterior, and transverse segments (**FIG 1B**).
  - The anterior bundle is the most discrete component, the posterior portion being a thickening of the posterior capsule, and is well defined only in about 90 degrees of flexion.
  - The transverse component appears to contribute little or nothing to elbow stability.
  - The medial collateral ligament originates from a broad anteroinferior surface of the epicondyle but not from the condylar elements of the trochlea just inferior to the axis of rotation.[18] The ulnar nerve rests on the posterior aspect of the medial epicondyle, but it is not intimately related to the fibers of the anterior bundle of the medial collateral ligament itself.
- The flexor–pronator mass includes the pronator teres, the most proximal of the flexor–pronator group; the flexor carpi radialis, which originates just inferior to the origin of the pronator teres at the anteroinferior aspect of the medial epicondyle; the palmaris longus muscle, which arises from the medial epicondyle and from the septa it shares with the flexor carpi radialis and flexor carpi ulnaris; the flexor carpi ulnaris, which is the most posterior of the common flexor tendons originating from the medial epicondyle and from the medial border of the coronoid and the proximal medial aspect of the ulna; and the flexor digitorum superficialis, which is the deepest from the common flexor tendon but superficial to the flexor digitorum profundus.

IMAGING AND OTHER DIAGNOSTIC STUDIES

- Diagnosis of the contracture is usually made by identifying a characteristic history and performing a physical examination.
- Joint involvement is confirmed by plain radiographs. The anteroposterior (AP) view gives good visualization of the joint line, whereas the lateral view can demonstrate osteophytes on the coronoid and at the tip of the olecranon, even when the joint space is preserved.
- The details of the extent of any boney involvement are best observed on computed tomography.
- Transverse imaging by magnetic resonance imaging (MRI) has little use in our practice.

NONOPERATIVE MANAGEMENT

- Several options have been proposed for the treatment of elbow contracture.
- Nonoperative treatment with mobilization of the elbow through the use of alternating flexion and extension splints[17] or dynamic splints[8] can provide a good result if it is initiated soon after the contracture develops.
- Manipulation with the patient under anesthesia have also been recommended, but loss of motion and ulnar nerve injury have been reported.[6]
- Recently, botulinum toxin has been used to release muscle contracture in order to facilitate elbow rehabilitation and regain motion.[20]
- Nonoperative treatment usually is successful only for extrinsic stiffness that has been present for 6 months or less, and the results can be unpredictable. With failure of nonoperative treatment, surgical release may be indicated. Recently, arthroscopic techniques for capsular release of the elbow have been described; however, open release remains a safe, reproducible option for regaining elbow motion.

SURGICAL MANAGEMENT

Indications

- Contracture release
- Stiff elbow
- Degenerative arthritis with anterior and posteromedial osteophytes
- Ulnar nerve symptoms

Advantages

- Allows exposure, protection, and transposition of the ulnar nerve
- Preserves the anterior band of the medial collateral ligament
- Affords access to the coronoid with intact radial head

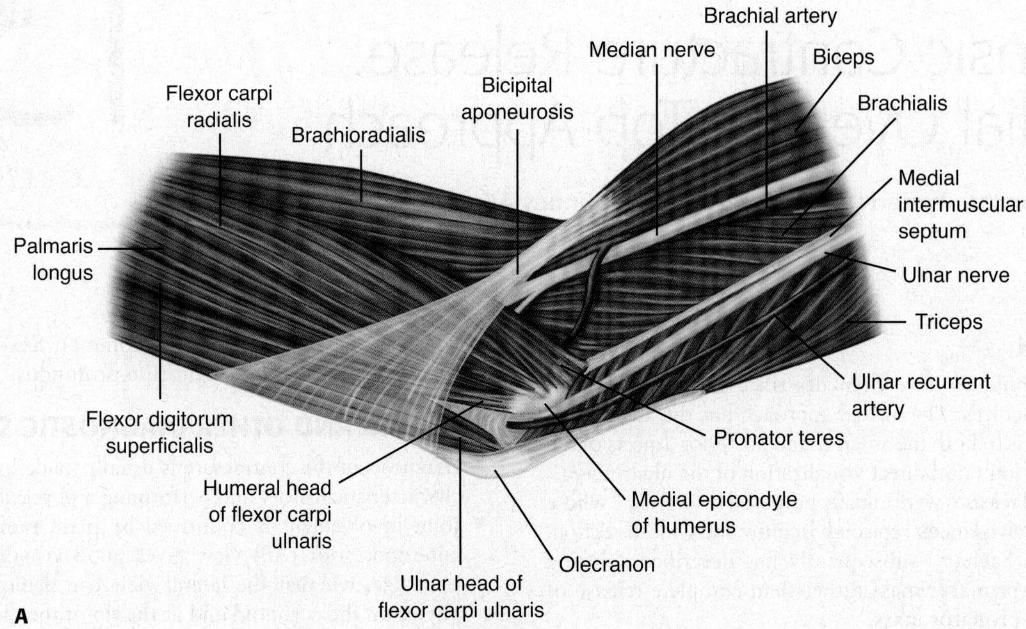

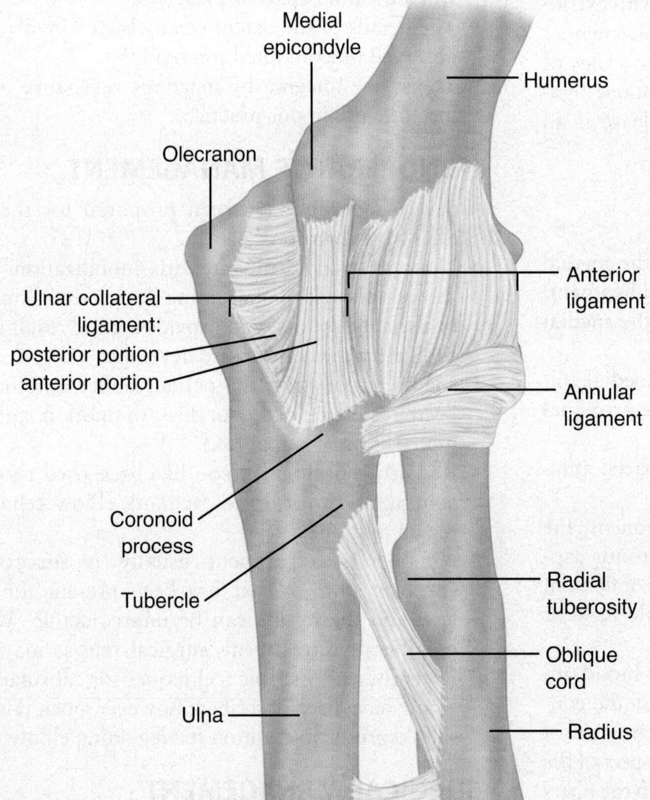

FIG 1 • Superficial (**A**) and deep (**B**) anatomy of the medial side of the elbow.

Disadvantages

- Difficulty in removing heterotopic bone on the lateral side of the joint
- Affords poor access to radial head

Preoperative Planning

- Before surgery, the decision must be made to approach the capsule from the lateral or medial aspect.
- If the ulnar nerve is to be addressed or there is extensive medial or coronoid arthrosis, the medial approach is of value.
- If the radiohumeral joint is involved or if a simple release is all that is required, the lateral "column" procedure is carried out.

Positioning

- The patient is usually positioned supine, supported by an elbow or a hand table.

- Two folded towels should be placed under the scapula.
- A sterile tourniquet is positioned.
- To expose the posterior joint, the patient's shoulder should have fairly free external rotation; otherwise, the arm should be positioned over the chest.

Approach

- The skin incision may be a midline posterior skin incision or a medial one (**FIG 2**).
- The key to this exposure is the identification of the medial supracondylar ridge of the humerus.
- At this level, the surgeon can locate the medial intermuscular septum, the origin of the flexor–pronator muscle mass, and the ulnar nerve.
- This site also serves as the starting point of the anterior and posterior subperiosteal extracapsular dissection of the joint.

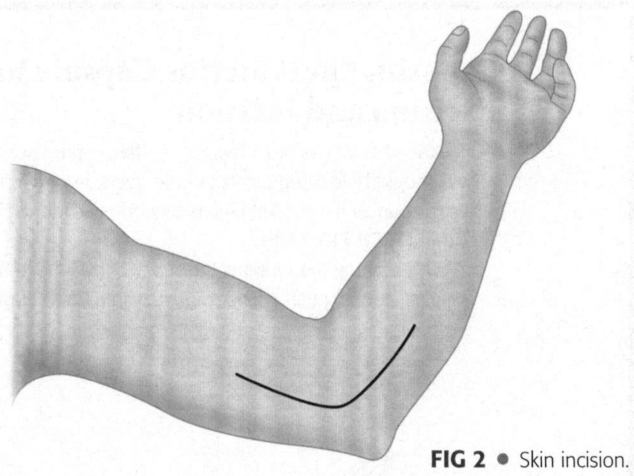

FIG 2 • Skin incision.

Exposing the Ulnar Nerve and the Medial Fascia

- Once the medial intermuscular septum is identified, the medial antebrachial cutaneous nerve is identified, traced distally, and protected.
  - The branching pattern varies, however, so it is occasionally necessary to divide the nerve to gain full exposure and to adequately mobilize the ulnar nerve, especially in revision surgery.
  - If this is necessary, the nerve is divided as proximally as the skin incision will allow, ensuring that the cut end lies in the subcutaneous fat (**TECH FIG 1**).
- If a previous anterior transposition was performed, the ulnar nerve should be fully identified and mobilized before proceeding.
  - The surgeon must be prepared to extend the previous incision proximally as necessary.
  - In this setting, the nerve is often flattened over the medial flexor–pronator muscle mass or it can "subluxate" to a posterior position.
  - This dissection requires patience and may take considerable time. Dissection of the nerve needs to be carried distally far enough to allow the nerve to sit in the anterior position without being kinked distal to the epicondyle.
- The septum is excised from the insertion on the supracondylar ridge to the proximal extent of the wound, usually about 5 to 8 cm.
  - Many of the veins and perforating arteries at the most distal portion of the septum require cauterization.

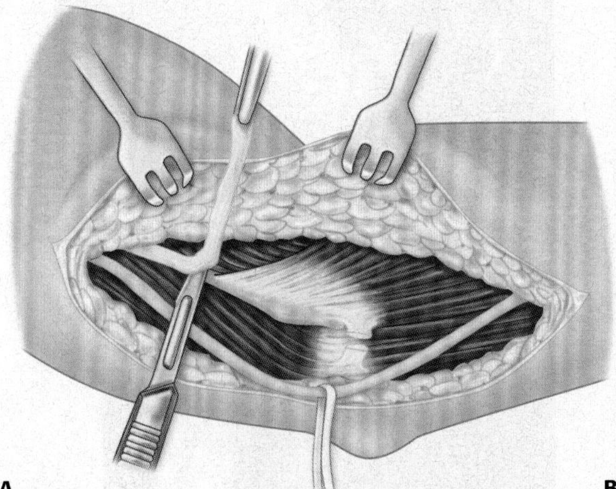

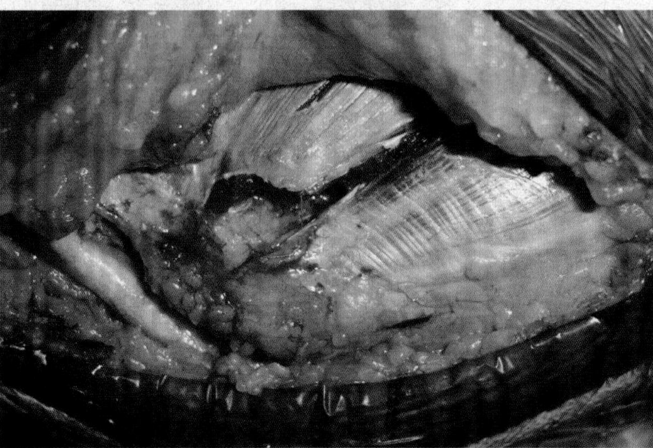

TECH FIG 1 • Exposure of the ulnar nerve and medial fascia.

Exposing the Anterior Capsule for Excision and Incision

- Once the septum has been excised, the flexor–pronator muscle mass should be divided parallel to the fibers, leaving roughly a 1.5-cm span of flexor carpi ulnaris tendon attached to the epicondyle (**TECH FIG 2A,B**).
  - The surgeon then returns the supracondylar ridge and begins elevating the anterior muscle with a Cobb elevator.
- Subperiosteally, the anterior structures of the distal humeral region proximal to the capsule are elevated to allow placement of a wide Bennett retractor. As the elevator moves from medial to lateral, the handle of the elevator is lifted carefully, keeping the blade of the elevator along the surface of the bone.
  - When heterotopic ossification along the lateral distal humerus is profuse, the radial nerve is at risk if it is entrapped in the scar on the surface of the bone.

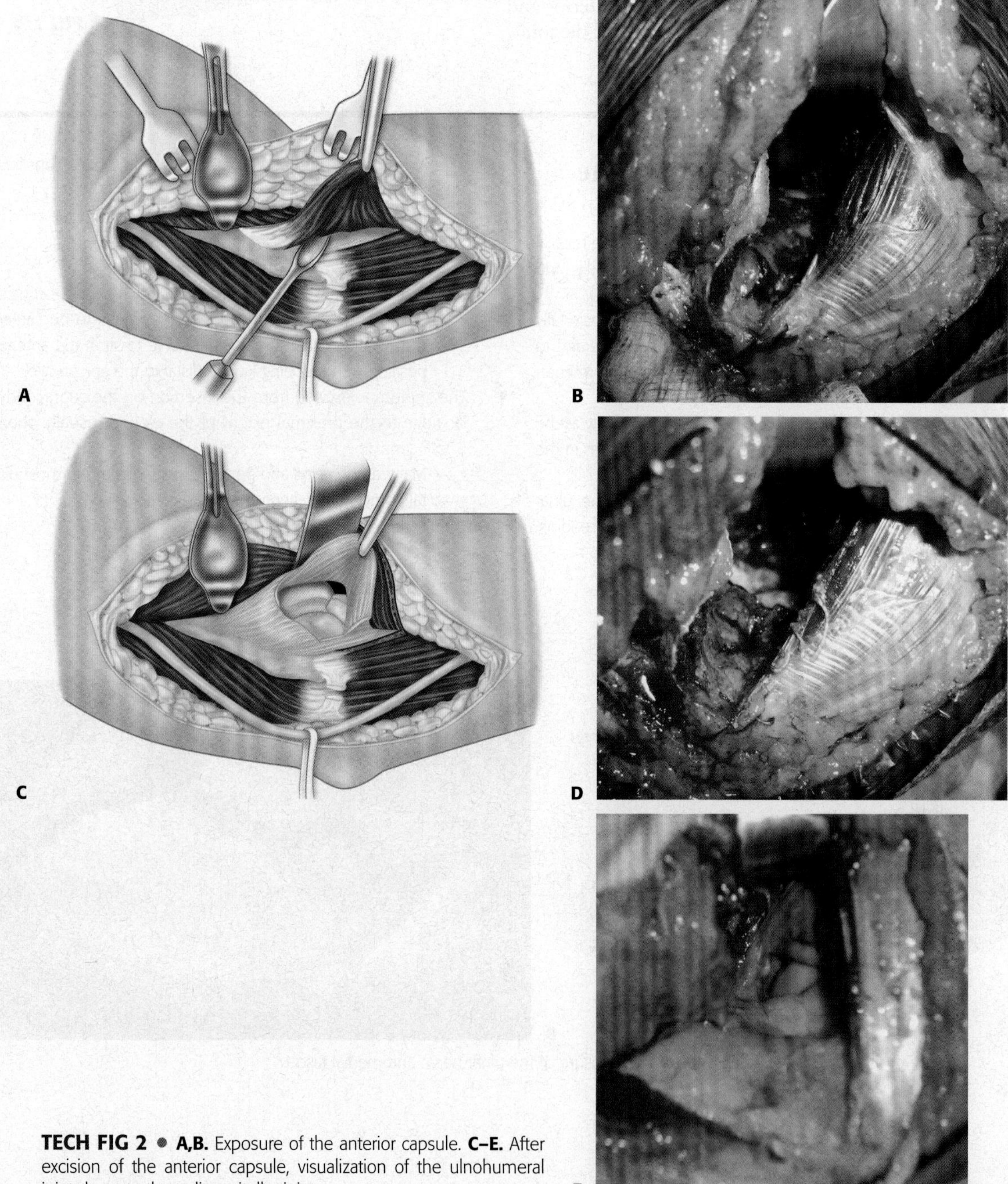

TECH FIG 2 • **A,B.** Exposure of the anterior capsule. **C–E.** After excision of the anterior capsule, visualization of the ulnohumeral joint down to the radiocapitellar joint.

- A separate approach to the lateral side may be required in this situation.
- The median nerve and brachial vein and artery are superficial to the brachialis muscle.
  - A small cuff of tissue of the flexor–pronator origin can be left on the supracondylar ridge as the muscle is elevated. This facilitates reattachment during closing.
  - A proximal, transverse incision in the lacertus fibrosus may also be needed to adequately mobilize this layer of muscle.
- Once the Bennett retractor is in place and the medial portion of the flexor–pronator has been incised, the plane between muscle and capsule should be carefully elevated.
  - As this plane is developed, the brachialis muscle is encountered from the underside. This muscle should be kept anterior and elevated from the capsule and anterior surface of the distal humerus.
  - Finding this plane requires careful attention.
  - The dissection of the capsule from the brachialis muscle proceeds both laterally and distally.
- At this point, it is helpful to feel for the coronoid process by gently flexing and extending the elbow. The first few times that this approach is used, the coronoid seems quite deep and far distal.
  - A deep, narrow retractor is often helpful to allow the operator to see down to the level of the coronoid.
- The extreme anteromedial corner of the exposure deserves special comment.
  - In a contracture release, the anteromedial portion often requires release.
  - To see this area, a small, narrow retractor can be inserted to retract the medial collateral ligament, pulling it medially and posteriorly.
  - This affords visualization of the medial capsule and protection of the anterior medial collateral ligament.
- The anterior capsule should be excised (**TECH FIG 2C–E**) to the extent that is practical and safe.
  - When first performing this procedure, it is helpful first to incise the capsule from the medial to the lateral aspect along the anterior surface of the joint.
  - Once this edge of the capsule is incised, it can be lifted and excised as far distally as is safe. From this vantage, and after capsule excision, the radial head and capitellum can be visualized and freed of scar as needed.
- In cases of primary osteoarthritis of the elbow, removing the large spur from the coronoid is crucial.
  - Using the Cobb elevator, the brachialis muscle can be elevated anteriorly for 2 cm from the coronoid process.
  - With the elevator held in position, protecting the brachialis but anterior to the coronoid, the large osteophyte can be removed with an osteotome.
  - The brachialis insertion is well distal to the tip of the coronoid.

Exposing and Excising the Posterior Capsule and Bone Spurs

- The posterior capsule of the joint is exposed. The supracondylar ridge is again identified (**TECH FIG 3**).
  - Using the Cobb elevator, the triceps is elevated from the posterior distal surface of the humerus.
  - The exposure should extend far enough proximally to permit use of a Bennett retractor.
- The posterior capsule can be separated from the triceps as the elevator sweeps from proximal to distal. The posterior medial joint line should also be identified, as it is often involved by osteophytes or heterotopic bone.
  - In contracture release, the posterior capsule and posterior band of the medial collateral ligament should be excised.
  - The medial joint line up to the anterior band of the medial collateral ligament should also be exposed and the capsule excised. This area is the floor of the cubital tunnel.
- In contracture release and in primary osteoarthritis, the tip of the olecranon usually must be excised to achieve full extension.
  - The posteromedial joint line is easily visualized, but the posterolateral side must also be carefully palptated to ensure clearance.

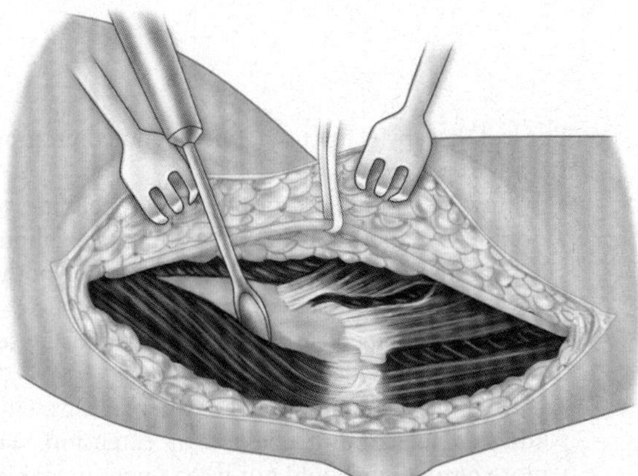
A

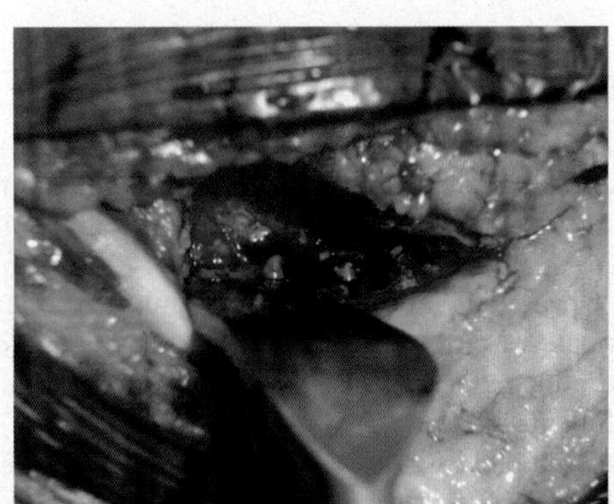
B

TECH FIG 3 • **A,B.** Exposure of the posterior compartment.

TECHNIQUES

Ulnar Nerve Transposition

- The ulnar nerve should be transposed and secured with a fascial sling to prevent posterior subluxation.
  - The sling can be fashioned by elevating two overlapping rectangular flaps of fascia or by using a medially based flap attached to the underlying subcutaneous tissue.
- Once this maneuver is completed, the nerve must not be compressed or kinked.
- The joint should be flexed and extended to ensure that the nerve is free to move.

Closure

- The flexor–pronator mass should be reattached to the supracondylar ridge with nonabsorbable braided 1-0 or 0 suture.
  - If a large enough cuff of tissue was left on the medial epicondyle, no holes need to be drilled in bone.
  - Otherwise, drill holes in the edge of the supracondylar ridge can be made to secure the flexor–pronator mass (**TECH FIG 4**).

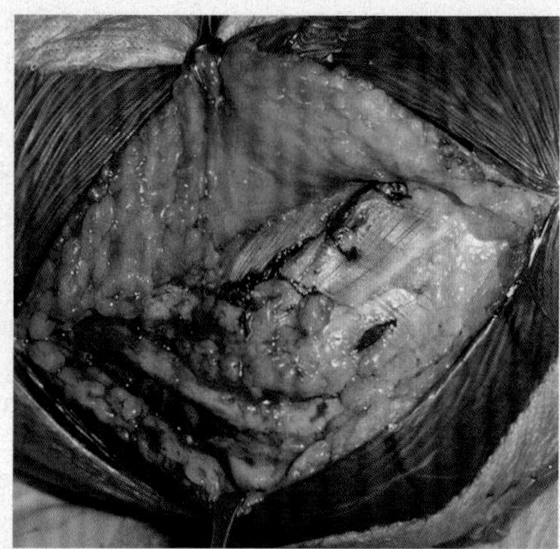

TECH FIG 4 • Closure.

PEARLS AND PITFALLS

Wrong incision	▪ Identification of the medial supracondylar ridge
Injury to the medial antebrachial cutaneous nerve	▪ Identification of the medial antebrachial cutaneous nerve
Injury to the ulnar nerve	▪ Identification, mobilization, and protection of the ulnar nerve
Disinsertion of the flexor–pronator mass from the medial epicondyle	▪ The flexor–pronator muscle mass should be divided parallel to the fibers.
Injury to the anterior vessels and nerves	▪ A Bennett retractor is placed between the anterior muscle and the capsule.
Section of the anterior band of the medial collateral ligament	▪ A small, narrow retractor is inserted to retract the medial collateral ligament, pulling it medially and posteriorly.

POSTOPERATIVE CARE

- If the neurologic examination findings in the recovery room are normal, a brachial plexus block is established and maintained with a continuous pump through a percutaneous catheter.
  - The arm is elevated as much as possible, and mechanical continuous passive motion exercise are begun the day of surgery and adjusted to provide as much motion as pain or the machine itself allows.
  - After 2 days, the plexus block is discontinued, and at day 3, the continuous passive motion machine is stopped.
- Physical therapy is not used, but a detailed program of splint therapy is prescribed.
  - Adjustable splints are prescribed, depending on the motion before and after the procedure. The splints include a hyperextension or a hyperflexion brace or both.
  - A detailed discussion regarding heat, ice, and anti-inflammatory medication, along with a visual schedule for bracing, is provided.
  - During the first 3 months, the patient sleeps with the splint adjusted to maximize flexion or extension, whichever is more needed; it should not be so uncomfortable as to prevent sleeping for at least 6 hours.

- Because the principal objective is to gain motion but to avoid pain, swelling, and inflammation, routine use of an anti-inflammatory medication is prescribed.
- Therapy with splints is continued for about 3 months, during which time the patient is seen at 2- to 4-week intervals, if possible.
- After 4 weeks, an arc of about 80 degrees of motion is obtained, and the amount of time that each splint is worn is gradually decreased.
- Splinting at night is continued for as long as 6 months if flexion contracture tends to recur when the splint is not used.
- Patients are advised that it may take a year to realize full correction.

OUTCOMES

- Recent reports on the results of surgical arthrolysis reveal an absolute gain in the flexion–extension arc between 30 and 60 degrees.[1,3–5,7,9–11,14–16,19,21]
  - A functional arc of motion between 30 and 130 degrees is obtained in more than 50% of cases, and some improvement in motion in more than 90% of the cases has been reported in the literature.[1,3–5,7,9–11,14–16,19,21]
  - In Europe, a combined lateral and medial approach has been used for many years, and gains in flexion arc have averaged between 40 and 72 degrees (in about 400 procedures).[1,3,7,14] Some preferred a posterior extensile approach if medial and lateral exposures are anticipated.
  - The importance of sequential release of tissues has been emphasized, based on an experience with 44 of 46 patients (95%) who were satisfied with such an approach.[13] The preoperative arc improved from 45 to 99 degrees.
    - The authors emphasize the need to release the exostosis and the collateral ligament when contracted, especially noting the need to release the posterior portion of the medial collateral ligament and decompress the ulnar nerve when ulnar nerve symptoms exist preoperatively.[13]
- Using a medial approach, Wada et al[22] obtained improvement of the mean arc of movement of 64 degrees. A functional arc of flexion–extension (30 to 130 degrees) was obtained in 7 of the 14 elbows. None of the patients developed symptoms related to the ulnar nerve. According to those authors, the medial approach has several advantages over both the anterior and lateral approaches:
  - Pathologic changes in the posterior oblique bundle of the medial collateral ligament can be observed and excised under direct vision.
  - Anterior and posterior exposure is possible through one medial incision, through which a complete soft tissue release and excision of part of the olecranon and coronoid process can be undertaken if necessary. Additional lateral exposure is indicated only if the medial approach has proved to be inadequate.
  - In the medial approach, the ulnar nerve is routinely released and protected under direct vision, which decreases the risk of damage.

COMPLICATIONS

- A most important emerging consideration of the proper treatment of elbow stiffness is the vulnerability of the ulnar nerve.
- The most common cause of failure of treatment has been in patients whose preoperative ulnar nerve symptoms were not appreciated or addressed, or patients in whom ulnar nerve symptoms developed postoperatively without adequate treatment. This is attributable to traction neuritis caused by the abrupt increase in elbow flexion or extension during the operation.
- Even in the absence of preoperative neurologic symptoms, the nerve may be compromised subclinically and become symptomatic as elbow motion increases after surgery. Therefore, all patients who have stiff elbows must be evaluated for the presence or absence of ulnar nerve symptoms.
- Antuna et al[2] recommended that elbows with preoperative flexion limited from 90 to 100 degrees in which we expect to improve the motion by 30 or 40 degrees should be treated with inspection and often prophylactic decompression or translocation of the nerve, depending on the appearance of the nerve once the surgical procedure is finished.
  - Furthermore, all patients with preoperative ulnar nerve symptoms, even if they are mild, are treated with mobilization of the nerve.
  - These authors stated that manipulation of the elbow in the early postoperative period must be avoided if the nerve has not been decompressed or translocated.

REFERENCES

1. Allieu Y. Raideurs et arthrolyses du coude. Rev Chir Orthop 1989;75(suppl 1):156–166.
2. Antuna SA, Morrey BF, Adams RA, et al. Ulnohumeral arthroplasty for primary degenerative arthritis of the elbow: long-term outcome and complications. J Bone Joint Surg Am 2002;84-A(12):2168–2173.
3. Chantelot C, Fontaine C, Migaud H, et al. Etude retrospective de 23 arthrolyses du coude pour raideur post-traumatique: facteurs prédictifs du résultat. Rev Chir Orthop 1999;85:823–827.
4. Cikes A, Jolles BM, Farron A. Open elbow arthrolysis for posttraumatic elbow stiffness. J Orthop Trauma 2006;20:405–409.
5. Cohen MS, Hastings H II. Posttraumatic contracture of the elbow. Operative release using a lateral collateral ligament sparing approach. J Bone Joint Surg Br 1998;80(5):805–812.
6. Duke JB, Tessler RH, Dell PC. Manipulation of the stiff elbow with patient under anesthesia. J Hand Surg Am 1991;16:19–24.
7. Esteve P, Valentin P, Deburge A, et al. Raideurs et ankyloses post-traumatiques du coude. Rev Chir Orthop 1971;57(suppl 1):25–86.
8. Gelinas JJ, Faber KJ, Patterson SD, et al. The effectiveness of turnbuckle splinting for elbow contractures. J Bone Joint Surg Br 2000;82:74–78.
9. Husband JB, Hastings H II. The lateral approach for operative release of post-traumatic contracture of the elbow. J Bone Joint Surg Am 1990;72(9):1353–1358.
10. Itoh Y, Saegusa K, Ishiguro T, et al. Operation for the stiff elbow. Int Orthop 1989;13:263–268.
11. Mansat P, Morrey BF. The column procedure: a limited surgical approach for the treatment of stiff elbows. J Bone Joint Surg Am 1998;80(11):1603–1615.
12. Mansat P, Morrey BF, Hotchkiss RN. Extrinsic contracture: the column procedure, lateral and medial capsular releases. In: Morrey BF, ed. The Elbow and Its Disorders, ed 3. Philadelphia: WB Saunders, 2000:447–456.
13. Marti RH, Kerkhoffs GM, Maas M, et al. Progressive surgical release of a posttraumatic stiff elbow: technique and outcome after 2–18 years in 46 patients. Acta Orthop Scand 2002;73:144–150.
14. Merle D'Aubigne R, Kerboul M. Les opérations mobilisatrices des raideurs et ankylose du coude. Rev Chir Orthop 1966;52:427–448.
15. Morrey BF. Post-traumatic contracture of the elbow: operative treatment, including distraction arthroplasty. J Bone Joint Surg Am 1990;72(4):601–618.

16. Morrey BF. The posttraumatic stiff elbow. Clin Orthop Relat Res 2005;431:26–35.
17. Morrey BF. The use of splints for the stiff elbows. Perspect Orthop Surg 1990;1:141–144.
18. O'Driscoll SW, Horii E, Morrey BF. Anatomy of the attachment of the medial ulnar collateral ligament. J Hand Surg Am 1992;17:164.
19. Park MJ, Kim HG, Lee JY. Surgical treatment of post-traumatic stiffness of the elbow. J Bone Joint Surg Br 2004;86(8):1158–1162.
20. Rosenwasser M. Sequelae of fractures of the elbow. Presented at 11th Trauma Course, AIOD, Strasbourg, 2005.
21. Urbaniak JR, Hansen PE, Beissinger SF, et al. Correction of post-traumatic flexion contracture of the elbow by anterior capsulotomy. J Bone Joint Surg Am 1985;67(8):1160–1164.
22. Wada T, Ishii S, Usui M, et al. The medial approach for operative release of post-traumatic contracture of the elbow. J Bone Joint Surg Br 2000;82:68–73.
23. Weiss AP, Sachar K. Soft tissue contractures about the elbow. Hand Clin 1994;10:439–451.
24. Willner P. Anterior capsulectomy for contractures of the elbow. J Int Coll Surg 1948;11:359–362.

Release of Posttraumatic Metacarpophalangeal and Proximal Interphalangeal Joint Contractures

134

CHAPTER

Christopher L. Forthman and Keith A. Segalman

DEFINITION

- Posttraumatic metacarpophalangeal (MCP) joint and proximal interphalangeal (PIP) contractures may develop directly as a result of injury to the joints and adjacent tissues or indirectly as a result of excessive immobilization or poor splinting of the hand.
- The circumstances precipitating the contracture determine the structures most involved:
  - Joint capsule and collateral ligament contracture
  - Flexor tendon adhesions
  - Intrinsic musculature contracture
  - Extensor tendon adhesions
  - Skin and subcutaneous tissue scarring
- The MCP joint generally becomes stiff in the extended position. Flexion contractures are uncommon and, when present, generally do not cause significant disability.
- The PIP joint often becomes contracted in the flexed position, although extension and combined contractures are not uncommon.
- The key to successfully mobilizing a stiff MCP or PIP joint is anticipating the pathologic causes before surgery.

ANATOMY

- MCP joint osteology allows biaxial motion, including circumduction. The articular surface of the metacarpal head is asymmetric, with a relatively flat mediolateral convex arc (abduction–adduction) and a large anteroposterior convex arc (flexion–extension) that extends more volarly (**FIG 1A**).
- The MCP joint is enveloped by a relatively loose capsule inserting onto ridges surrounding the articular cartilage.
- Proper collateral ligaments originate from a dorsolateral tubercle on the metacarpal head and insert on the lateropalmar edge of the phalangeal base (**FIG 1B**).
- The volar plate of the MCP joint is an extension of the phalangeal articular surface. Unlike the volar plate of the PIP joint, the volar plate of the MCP joint is collapsible and there is little tendency to produce checkreins.
  - This is one reason why MCP joint flexion contractures are much less common than those in the PIP joint.
- The flexor and extensor mechanisms surround the MCP joint.
  - Volarly, the flexor sheath lies directly on the palmar plate and is thick, forming the first annular pulley.
  - Dorsally, the extensor tendon gives rise to fibroaponeurotic sagittal bands that wrap around to insert on the palmar plate. The tendons of the lumbricals and interossei join the dorsal expansion of the extensor. A slip of the dorsal interossei inserts on the dorsolateral aspect of the phalangeal base.
- The PIP joint is a simple ginglymus hinge joint stabilized by a boxlike arrangement of structures consisting of the proper and accessory collateral ligaments, the volar plate, and the dorsal capsule (**FIG 1C,D**).
  - The joint is most stable in extension, and stability in flexion is provided by the volar plate, proper and accessory collateral ligaments, and flexor tendons, and less so by the dorsal structures.
  - The collaterals provide radial and ulnar stability. They remain taut throughout the PIP joint range of motion.
  - The accessory collaterals arise from the proximal phalanx and insert into the volar plate. Because there is no insertion of the accessory collateral into the middle phalanx, they will contract when the PIP joint is immobilized in flexion.
  - The volar plate resists PIP hyperextension, and the dorsal capsule is relatively weak.
  - Transverse retinacular ligaments connect the extensor and flexor tendon sheath.

PATHOGENESIS

- The irregular contour of the MCP joint functions as a cam, transforming joint flexion into translation (or elongation) of the collateral ligaments. When flexed, the MCP joint has minimal capsular volume and is maximally constrained. Conversely, extension allows maximal capsular volume and joint laxity.
- Direct trauma to the MCP joint causes joint effusions and hemarthrosis. Hand trauma elsewhere results in edema, which also collects within the MCP joints. In both cases, as the capsule fills with fluid, the MCP joint is hydraulically pushed into a nearly fully extended position.
- With time, the dorsal capsule becomes thick and noncompliant, leading to an extension contracture. The overlying extensor mechanism may become adherent to the capsule. The underlying collateral ligaments shorten and scar laterally to the metacarpal head. The volar recess may fill with adhesions between the volar plate and condyles.
- The extended MCP joint increases flexor tone and relaxes the extensor mechanism, leading to interphalangeal joint flexion, and may *indirectly* result in a fixed flexion contracture of the PIP joint.
  - The combination of extended MCP joints and flexed interphalangeal joints defines the intrinsic-minus hand.
- Injury, infection, excess immobilization, and inappropriate splinting may *directly* result in fixed flexion or extension contracture of the PIP joint.
  - An accumulation of fluid or blood within the capsule leads to stiffness, as does articular damage.

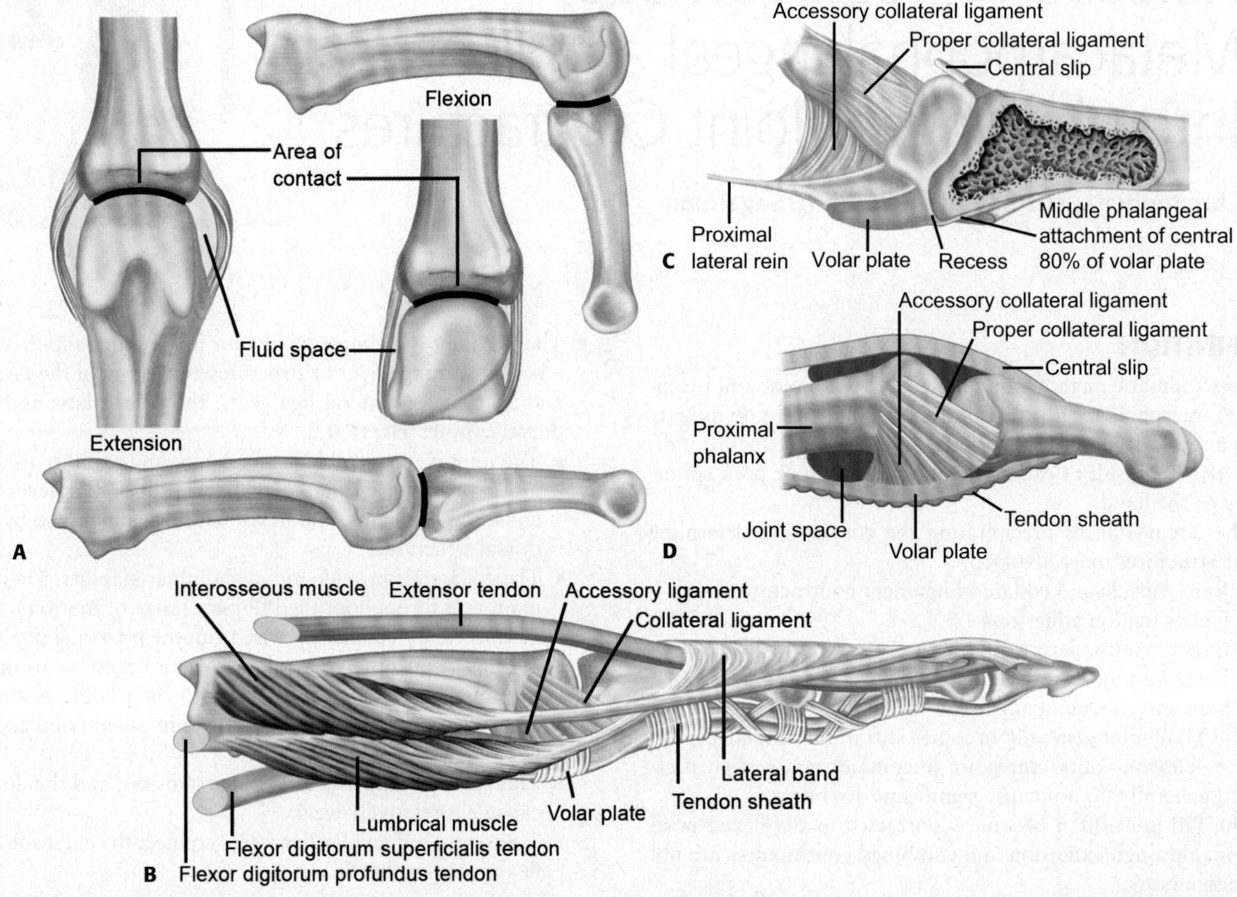

FIG 1 • **A.** The articular surface of the metacarpal head protrudes volarly, making the capsule (and proper collateral ligaments) taut with flexion. **B.** MCP joint anatomy can be considered in two layers: the capsule and collateral ligaments, which lie immediately adjacent to the articular surfaces, and the flexor and extensor mechanisms, which envelop the joint. **C.** Normal anatomy of the PIP joint showing the arrangement of the collateral ligaments and the volar plate. **D.** Normal PIP anatomy showing the arrangement of the proper and accessory collateral ligaments.

- Curtis[3,4] has reported that a contracture of the PIP joint can be due to the following:
  - Contracture of the volar plate or the capsular structures
  - Collateral ligament contracture
  - Scar contracture over the joint
  - Volar skin contracture
  - Flexor sheath contracture
  - Extensor tendon contracture or adhesions
  - Interosseous contracture or adhesions
  - A bony block or exostosis
- Additional causes not pertinent to this chapter include fascia contracture, as in Dupuytren disease.
- Watson et al[11] reported that a flexion contracture of the PIP joint is due to contracture of the checkreins on the proximal surface of the volar plate.

NATURAL HISTORY

- Long-standing scarring and contracture of the MCP or PIP joint capsule almost invariably lead to adhesions to the adjacent flexor sheath and extensor mechanism.
- Residual joint kinetics are often altered with joint motion occurring through incongruous articular motions such as pivoting.
- Cartilage gradually atrophies and softens with disuse. Surface irregularities may develop.

PATIENT HISTORY AND PHYSICAL FINDINGS

- The history should identify the following:
  - The inciting cause of the joint contracture
  - The time of the insult
  - Efforts made to mobilize the digit
- The hand is evaluated for edema and the return of normal skin creases.
  - Ongoing swelling and inflammation (**FIG 2A**) must subside before surgery.
- The dorsal soft tissues are assessed for mobility and compliance.
  - Capsulectomy after burns and crush injuries may fail due to inadequate dorsal coverage.
  - Skin contracture can also be an original inciting cause for digital stiffness.
- The MCP and interphalangeal joints are assessed for differences in active and passive motion. Passive motion is always greater than active; however, a large difference suggests extrinsic tendon adhesions.
- Bunnell intrinsic tightness test: Intrinsic release may be necessary to mobilize a PIP joint with extension contracture.
- Finger threshold sensitivity is checked, along with overall sensitivity to percussion and cold. Vascularity is assessed by checking capillary refill. The painful and insensate stiff finger may be a better candidate for amputation than capsulectomy. Poor vascularity is a relative contraindication to capsulectomy.

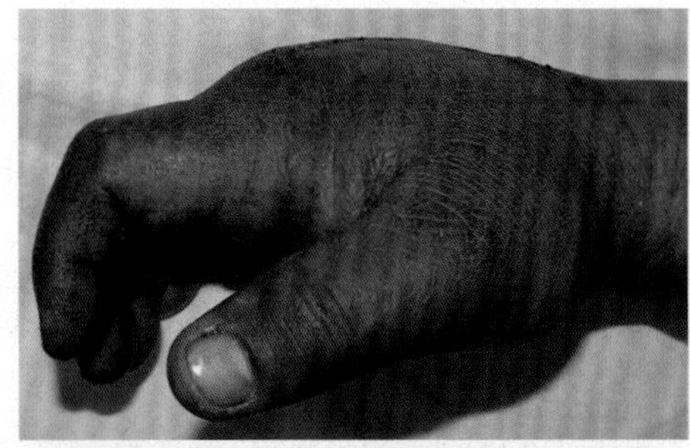

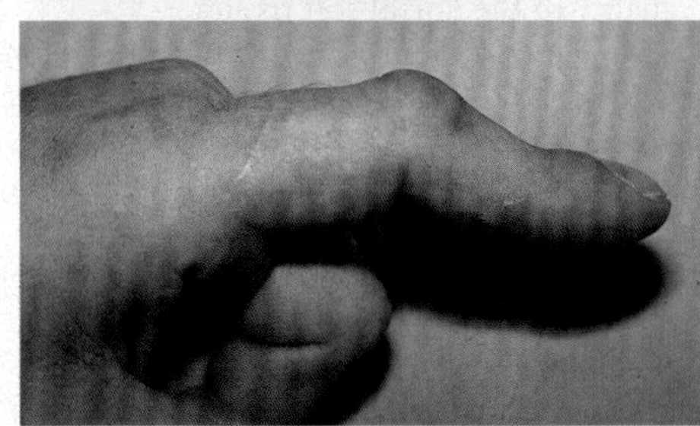

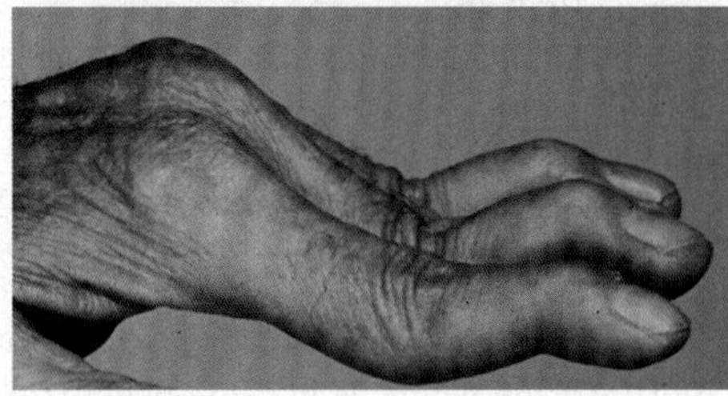

FIG 2 • **A.** Swollen hand. **B.** Boutonnière deformity. **C.** Swan-neck deformity.

- Concomitant PIP flexion and distal interphalangeal hyperextension mark a boutonnière deformity (**FIG 2B**), whereas hyperextension at the PIP joint is a sign of a swan-neck deformity (**FIG 2C**).

IMAGING AND OTHER DIAGNOSTIC STUDIES

- Plain radiographs of the hand are made to evaluate for extrinsic and intrinsic causes of joint stiffness.
  - Extrinsic
    - Metacarpal neck or shaft fracture: Extensor tendon adhesions at the fracture site may restrict MCP joint flexion (passive and active).
    - Metacarpal fracture malunion: Shortening of the metacarpal results in extensor lag (average of 7 degrees for every 2 mm of shortening according to Strauch and colleagues[12]). Apex dorsal metacarpal malunions create a corresponding extensor lag at the adjacent MCP joint.
    - Proximal phalangeal fracture: Flexor and extensor tendon adhesions at the fracture site may limit active PIP (and sometime MCP) joint motion; passive motion may be maintained.
    - Proximal phalangeal fracture malunion: Common apex volar proximal phalanx malunions can cause an apparent limitation of MCP joint flexion.
  - Intrinsic
    - Intra-articular fracture: Articular incongruity may serve as a bony restraint to joint motion.
    - Arthritic changes: Cartilage softening and erosion often result in some degree of radiographically apparent arthritis.
- A "true" lateral radiograph of the involved joint must be closely examined for significant arthritic changes or any subluxation.
- There is little role for computed tomography (CT) scanning or magnetic resonance imaging (MRI) of the digits.

DIFFERENTIAL DIAGNOSIS

- MCP extension contracture from extrinsic extensor muscle spasticity or intrinsic muscle paralysis or denervation
- MCP loss of flexion from proximal phalanx apex volar malunion
- PIP contracture from tendon imbalances, including boutonnière deformity and swan-neck deformity
- Skin contracture
- Dupuytren disease

NONOPERATIVE MANAGEMENT

- Nonoperative efforts to improve joint motion must be tried until motion has plateaued and the soft tissues are absolutely quiescent.
- As a general rule, inflammation and edema will subside and range of motion will improve for a minimum of 3 to 4 months after a traumatic or surgical insult to the hand.
- During this time, a supervised hand therapy program is essential.
  - Most MCP contractures occur in extension. In addition to regular exercises, dynamic flexion splints (daytime) and static extension splints (nighttime) are useful.
  - Most PIP contractures occur in flexion. Treatment begins with application of a nonelastic extension force across the PIP joint for an extended time. This can be done with serial finger casts or commercially available splints such as the Joint Jack (Joint Jack Co., Wethersfield, CT) or wire-foam splints. Once the contracture is corrected, elastic splints such as the Joint Spring or clock-spring splints can be used.
- Prosser[10] presented one of the few studies to follow patients treated conservatively. Using a Capener splint to be worn for 8 to 12 hours per day over an 8-week period, there was an average improvement in the flexion contracture from 39 to 21 degrees.[10] There was no association between time in the splint with final extension or with final stiffness.
- PIP extension contractures are treated conservatively with serial static splints such as a joint-strap system.
- Curtis[3,4] has reported that these joints do not require surgery if the joint can be passively flexed more than 75 degrees.
- The only study in the literature on the results of conservative treatment comes from Weeks et al.[15] In a review of 212 patients with 415 stiff PIP joints, 87% responded favorably to nonoperative treatment. The average improvement in total active motion was 36 degrees.

SURGICAL MANAGEMENT

- A capsulectomy is indicated only for a contracture not associated with articular incongruity or persistent subluxation of the joint.
- A stiff MCP or PIP joint in the face of articular incongruity or subluxation is best treated as an arthritic joint with a salvage type of surgery such as arthroplasty or arthrodesis.
  - Mild to moderate joint wear is not a contraindication to capsulectomy, particularly in younger patients. Focal areas of articular cartilage irregularity and dorsal osteophytes may be débrided at the time of surgery.

- The literature does not give any specifics as to when to recommend surgery. We usually make this decision when a "functional arc of motion" has not been achieved after a minimum of 3 months of therapy.
- There is no absolute functional arc of motion for the MCP joint. In the absence of interphalangeal contractures, we have found that index, middle, ring, and small finger MCP flexion of 30, 35, 40, and 45 degrees, respectively, is generally satisfactory. When the interphalangeal joints have limited flexion, greater degrees of MCP flexion may be useful.
- Similarly, 45 degrees or more of total PIP motion is usually satisfactory. Flexion contractures greater than 45 degrees are poorly tolerated and may benefit from surgical release.
  - Extreme flexion contractures (>60 or 70 degrees) may be best managed with arthrodesis. The results of a capsulectomy are often disappointing.
  - Extension contractures are better tolerated, especially if there is flexion to at least 75 degrees.
- When a patient has exhausted nonoperative management options and joint stiffness exceeds the preceding guidelines, surgery for contracture release is considered.

Preoperative Planning

- The patient is required to demonstrate a commitment to therapy before surgery is undertaken. A preoperative meeting between the patient and the therapist is arranged to plan the first postoperative visit and to fabricate a dynamic flexion splint.
- If possible, surgery is planned under a form of anesthesia that will allow patient cooperation and active motion during the procedure.
  - A wrist block with sedation is optimal; however, a Bier block may be used and reversed with deflation of the tourniquet.
- In severely scarred hands (eg, massive crush injuries and burn patients), the surgeon must anticipate inadequate dorsal soft tissue and extensor tendon excursion. A transverse incision and extensor tenotomy is indicated and coverage of the residual soft tissue defect is planned and discussed with the patient. Kirschner wire fixation of the MCP joints in flexion may be necessary to maintain a flexed joint and protect the dorsal soft tissue reconstruction.

Positioning

- Patients are positioned supine with the affected extremity on a hand table. A brachial tourniquet is applied that allows access to the forearm should a full-thickness skin graft be necessary.

Approach

- The approach for MCP contracture depends on three factors:
  - The number of involved MCP joints
  - The need to operate on the PIP joint
  - The quality of the dorsal soft tissues
- A single MCP joint is approached with a dorsal longitudinal incision. If the PIP joint has an extension contracture, the incision is carried over the PIP in the midline. If the PIP has a flexion contracture, the incision may be extended distally in the midaxial line (**FIG 3A**).
- Multiple MCP joint extension contractures are approached using separate dorsal longitudinal incisions.
  - This is the most extensile method and facilitates management of associated extensor tendon adhesions and PIP contractures (**FIG 3B**).
- Two adjacent MCP joints may also be approached by making a dorsal longitudinal incision centered in the web between affected rays.
  - If necessary, it is safe to extend this incision as a Y onto each digit to complete a tenolysis or operate on the PIP joints.
- Multiple MCP joints may be also approached by making a single transverse incision lying just proximal to the metacarpal heads.
  - This approach is preferred only when the dorsal soft tissues are fibrotic and noncompliant. In this situation, the surgeon should plan for skin graft or flap coverage of the anticipated defect.
- The surgical approach for *isolated* PIP joint contractures varies with the procedure used.
  - A capsulectomy for a flexion contracture is performed through a lateral approach, a checkrein release through a volar approach, and percutaneous release laterally.
  - A dorsal skin incision could be used with a capsulectomy for an extension contracture or when there is a previous dorsal incision or specific hardware to remove.
  - External fixation requires no incision.

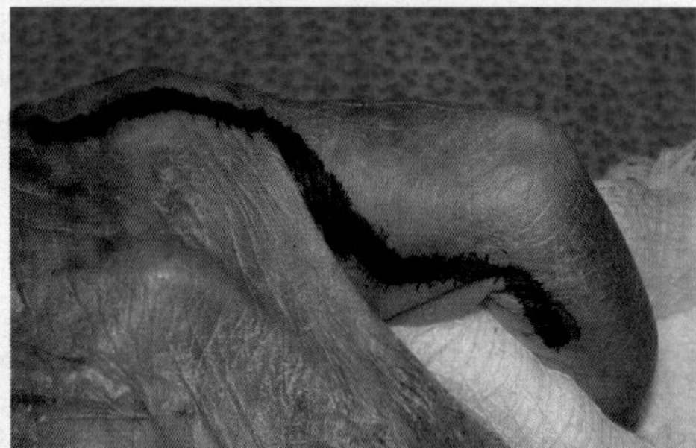

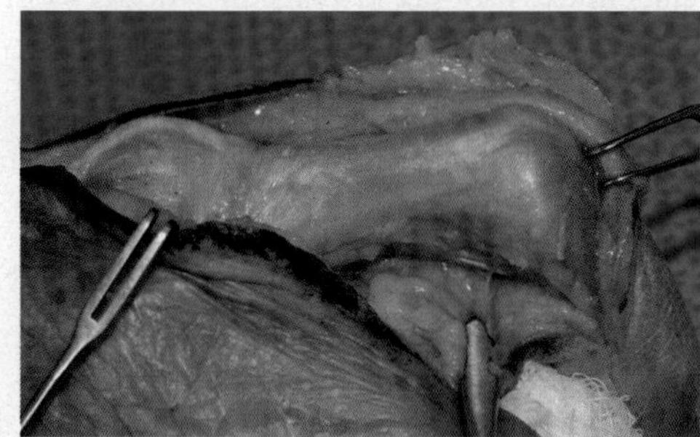

FIG 3 • **A.** A combined MCP extension contracture and PIP flexion contracture of the index finger is approached by extending the dorsal incision distally in the midaxial line. **B.** Excellent exposure of the finger extensor mechanism is coupled with visualization of the volar aspect of the PIP joint.

Metacarpophalangeal Joint Contractures

Dorsal Capsulectomy of the Joint

- Make the skin incision based on the aforementioned considerations (**TECH FIG 1A**).
- Carry dissection down sharply to the extensor mechanism, preserving small dorsal nerves.
  - If the soft tissues about the MCP joint are excessively scarred, identify the extensor mechanism proximally and distally with careful development of soft tissue planes in between.
- Raise full-thickness soft tissue flaps over the length of the extensor mechanism (**TECH FIG 1B**).
- Use a Freer elevator to lyse adhesions beneath the extensor mechanism, especially over the metacarpal proximally (**TECH FIG 1C**).
- As described by Curtis[3,4] and later Tsuge,[13] the extensor tendon is bisected sharply over the MCP joint (**TECH FIG 1D**); the sagittal fibers are preserved. Do not carry the extensor split into the transverse fibers of the extensor hood.
  - In the index or small finger, the split is made between the extensor communis and the extensor proprius tendons.
- Retract each half of the extensor tendon and attached sagittal band to expose the joint capsule.
- At times, it may be painstakingly difficult to develop the interval between the extensor mechanism and capsule, and a combination of both sharp and blunt dissection is necessary.
- The capsule is usually quite thick and generally should be excised rather than released (**TECH FIG 1E**).
- Attempt passive finger flexion; it usually is limited, necessitating release or excision of the collateral ligaments (**TECH FIG 1F**).
  - Start dorsally and release the proper collateral ligaments from the collateral recess and from any adhesions to the metacarpal head. Often, the collateral origin may be gently pried away from the metacarpal head with a Freer elevator.
  - Dense adhesions and excessively thick collateral ligament tissue may need to be incised at the metacarpal origin and removed.

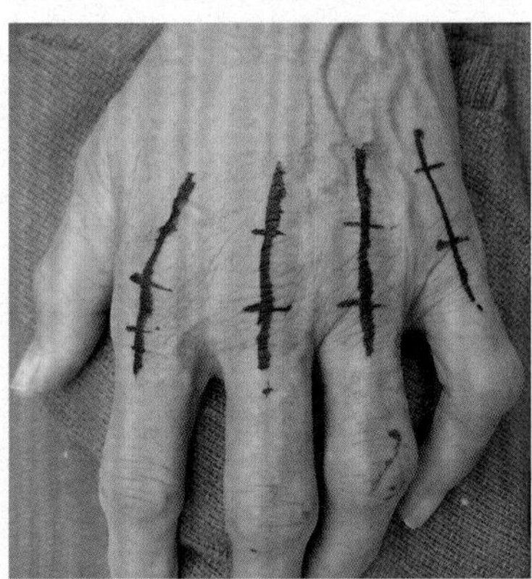

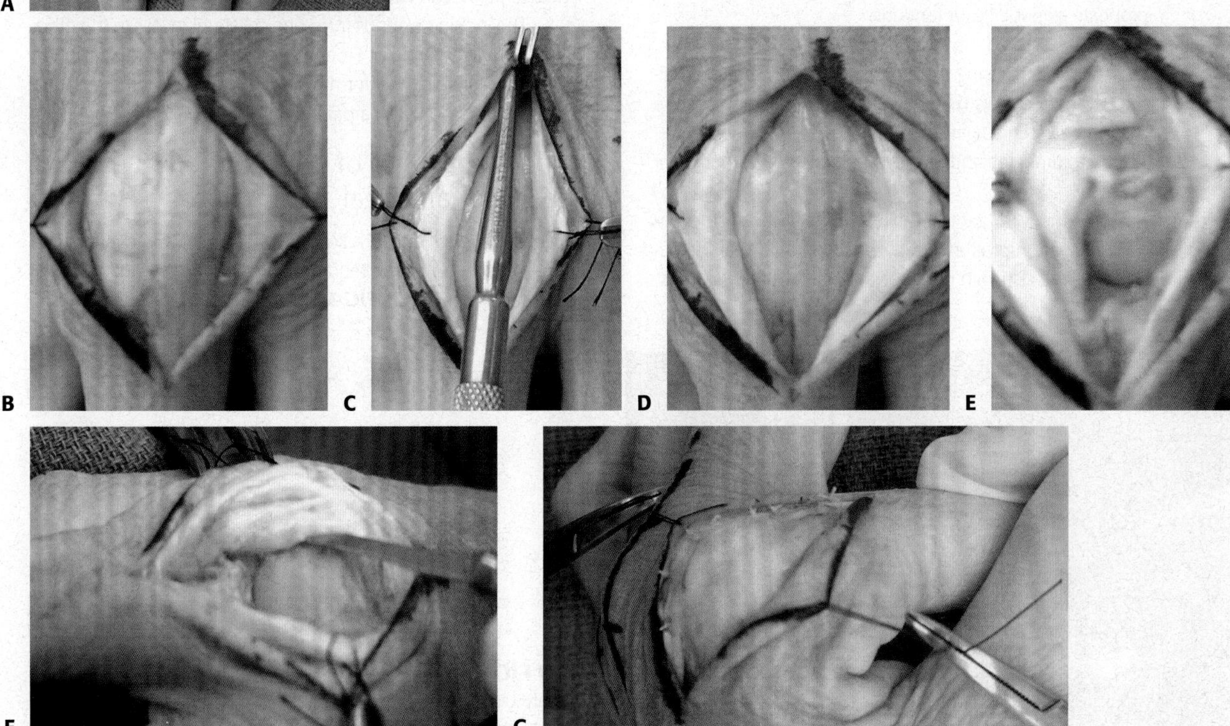

TECH FIG 1 • **A.** Separate dorsal longitudinal incisions are planned for multiple MCP joint extension contractures. **B.** Full-thickness soft tissue flaps are raised at the level of the extensor mechanism. **C.** The extensor mechanism is split longitudinally. **D.** Each side of the extensor tendon is freed of adhesions to the adjacent tissues. **E.** The dorsal capsule is excised. **F.** The proper collateral ligaments are released from the metacarpal head. **G.** MCP flexion is reassessed.

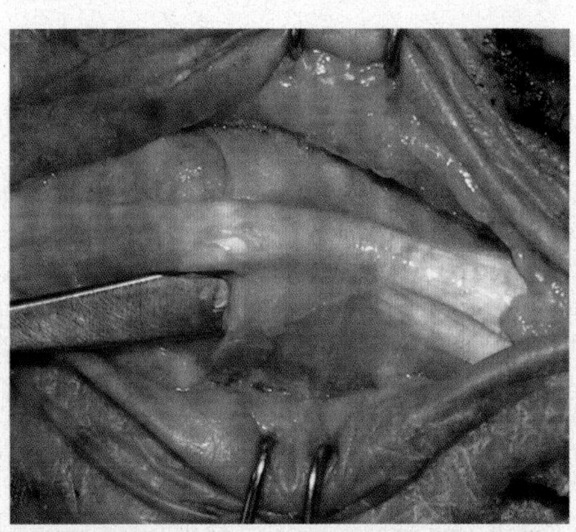

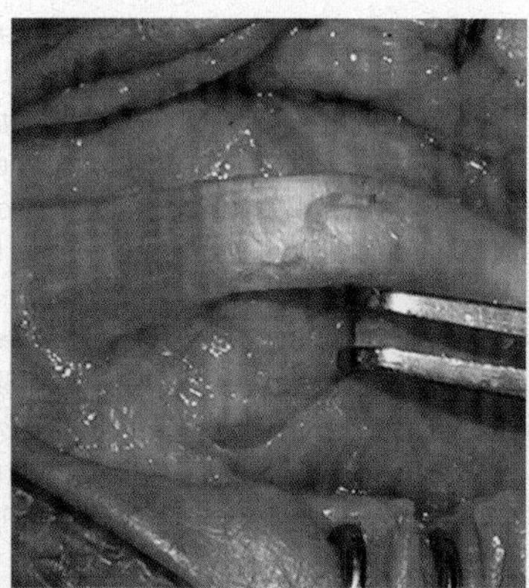

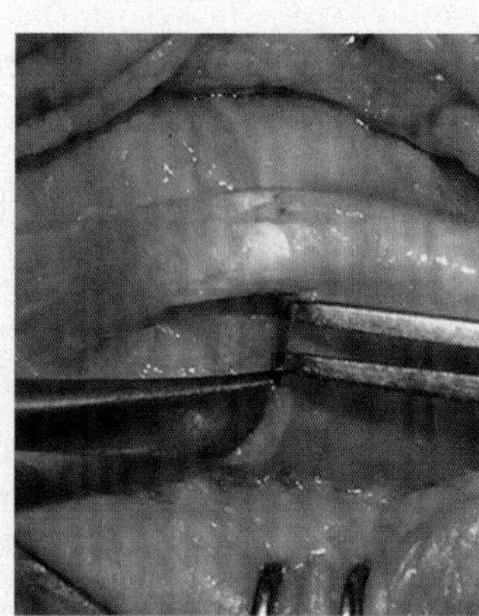

TECH FIG 2 • **A–C.** The wrist is located to the *left* and the finger to the *right* in each figure. **A.** The leading edges of the sagittal fibers are identified and liberated from the underlying dorsal capsule. **B.** Sagittal fibers are retracted distally and the capsule is incised transversely. **C.** A Freer elevator is used to release the proper collateral ligament origins.

- Reassess passive MCP flexion (**TECH FIG 1G**). If flexion remains inadequate or the joint "jumps" or "snaps" when reaching full extension, then the accessory collaterals may need to be released as well.
  - The goal is an incremental collateral ligament release—enough to restore joint motion but not compromise stability, especially on the radial (pinch) side.
- Assess the volar recess and release any adhesions between the volar plate and condyle with a Freer elevator.
  - Failure to release the volar adhesion can result in joint "hinging" with dorsal gapping of the joint during flexion.
- The joint should now have a smooth arc of passive motion without any hinging during flexion or snapping into extension. Ninety degrees of flexion can usually be achieved.
- If the patient is under a wrist or Bier block anesthesia, check active flexion.
  - Alternatively, a short incision may be made on the volar ulnar aspect of the forearm and traction applied to the appropriate extrinsic flexor tendons.
- If active flexion is limited, consider performing a flexor tenolysis.
  - We consider releasing the flexor at the same setting, although the tenolysis may be staged, emphasizing passive motion between surgeries.
- Release the tourniquet and achieve hemostasis with bipolar electrocautery.
- While keeping the MCP joint flexed, close the extensor mechanism with 4-0 interrupted inverted nonabsorbable braided suture and close the skin with nonabsorbable interrupted sutures.
- If bleeding from scar is excessive, then use a small rubber vascular loop or a quarter-inch Penrose drain to stent open the wound to allow drainage for the first 24 hours.
- A dorsal splint is applied to maintain the MCP joints in 70 degrees of flexion.

Limited Dorsal Capsulotomy of the Metacarpophalangeal Joint

- In mild contractures, a dorsal capsulectomy may not be necessary. Bode and Gottlieb[1] have described a limited capsulotomy.
- Expose the extensor mechanism as described earlier (see **TECH FIG 1**).
- Use a Freer elevator to release the extensor mechanism and sagittal bands from the dorsal capsule (**TECH FIG 2A**).
- Retract the dorsal capsule distally.
- Incise the capsule transversely at the distal dorsal aspect of the metacarpal head (**TECH FIG 2B**).
  - The incision extends from one collateral recess to the other.
- Using a Beaver blade or Freer elevator directed to the periphery of the capsulotomy, perform a stepwise release of the collateral ligaments off the metacarpal head (**TECH FIG 2C**).

Extensor Tenotomy of the Metacarpophalangeal Joint

- In long-standing densely scarred multidigit MCP contractures, the extensor communis tendon may need to be tenotomized to achieve flexion (**TECH FIG 3A**).

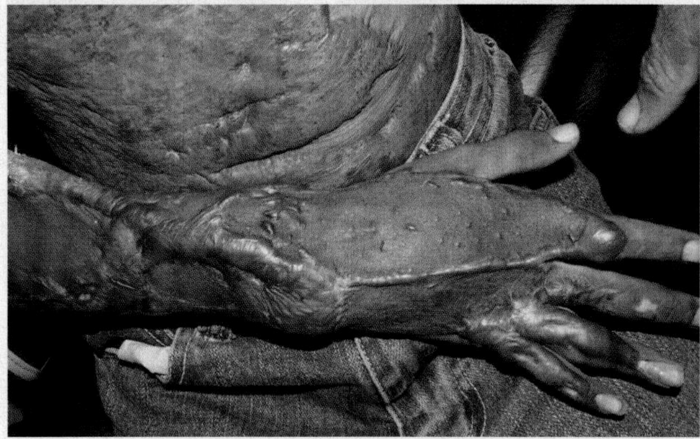

TECH FIG 3 • **A.** Release of MCP extension contractures in the severely burned hand is accomplished through a transverse skin incision and extensor tenotomy. *(continued)*

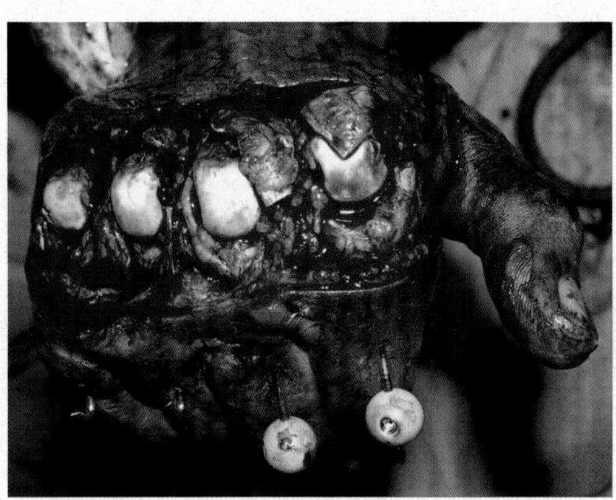

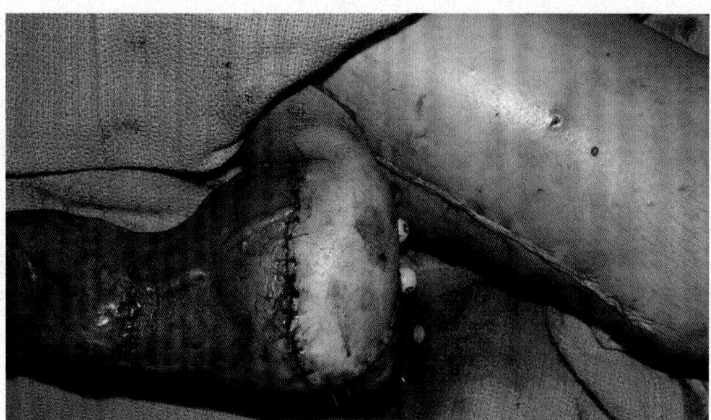

TECH FIG 3 • *(continued)* **B.** The MCP joints are maintained in flexion with Kirschner wires. **C.** The dorsal soft tissue defect is covered with a pedicled tensor fascia lata flap.

- Make a tenotomy at the distal margin of the sagittal bands.
- Capsulectomy and collateral ligament release follow as described earlier.
- At closure, sew the proximal tendon to the sagittal bands; close the extensor hood on itself in the midline dorsally.
- Given the chronicity of these contractures, consider temporary Kirschner wire fixation of the MCP joints in flexion (**TECH FIG 3B**).
  - Kirschner wire fixation is especially useful for protection of skin grafts or flaps when the dorsal soft tissues are deficient (**TECH FIG 3C**).

Proximal Interphalangeal Joint Contracture

Capsulectomy for Proximal Interphalangeal Joint Flexion Contracture

- If there is an adequate skin envelope, the finger is approached through a midaxial incision (**TECH FIG 4A**).
- Make a radial incision centered over the PIP joint; it is usually 4 cm long.
- Retract the neurovascular structures volarly and protect them. Take care to preserve the dorsal branch of the digital nerve, which typically crosses the proximal aspect of the incision.
- Open the flexor sheath just distal to the A2 pulley.
  - Excise a segment of pulley if it is contracted.
- Perform a formal flexor tenolysis as necessary.
  - If a more extensive tenolysis is required, the incision can be extended volarly over the flexor sheath. Take care to avoid injury to the digital nerve and artery that cross the operative field at the level of the web space.

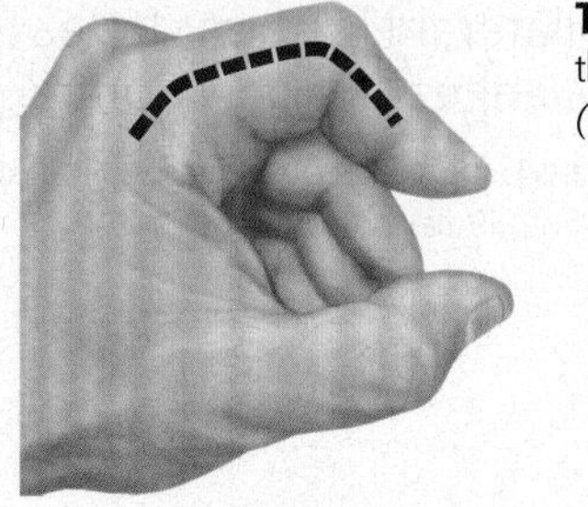

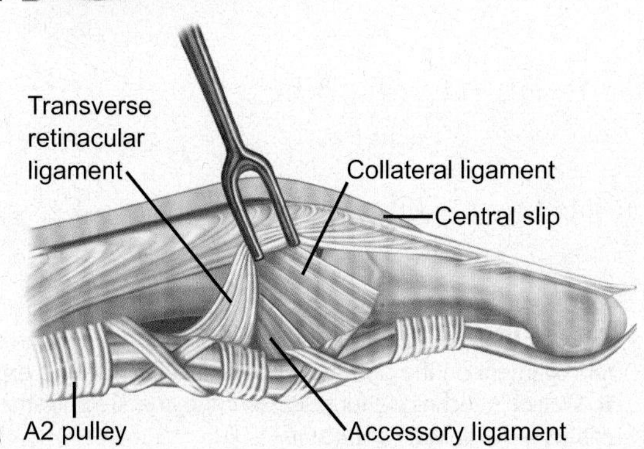

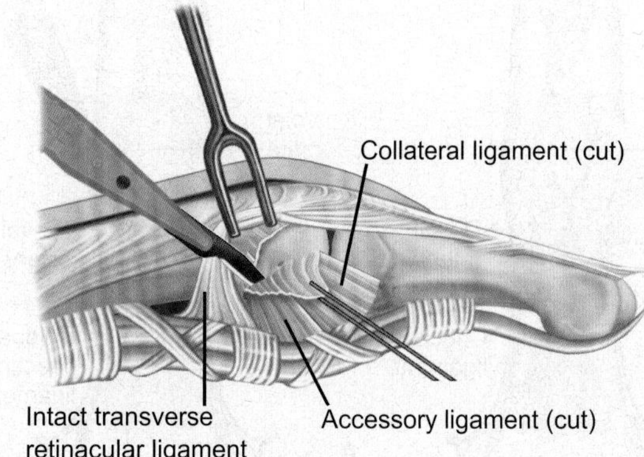

TECH FIG 4 • **A.** Skin incision. **B.** The transverse retinacular ligament is protected and the collateral ligament is exposed for excision. **C.** The collateral ligaments are excised. *(continued)*

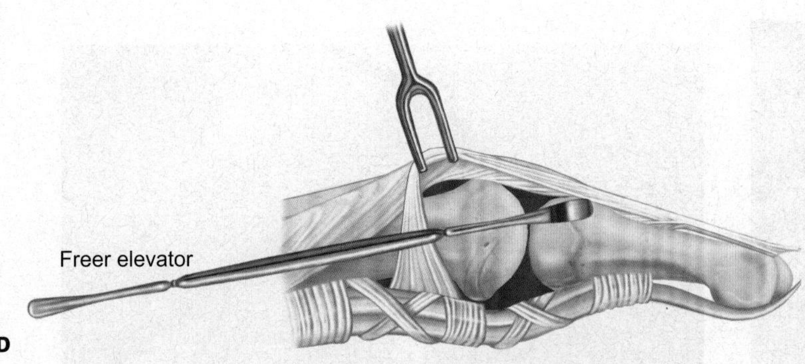

TECH FIG 4 • *(continued)* **D.** Extensor tenolysis is done if required.

- Excise a volar segment of collateral ligament (including the underlying capsule) using a no. 69 Beaver blade while carefully protecting the transverse retinacular fibers (**TECH FIG 4B**). Excise the entire accessory collateral ligament as necessary.
  - Isolate and preserve the transverse retinacular fibers by bluntly dissecting perpendicular to the fibers (**TECH FIG 4C**).
- Do not excise the volar plate (joint capsule), but expand the volar pouch by lifting the volar plate from the phalanges with a Freer elevator. Lengthen the interossei as needed.
- If there is still stiffness after completing the dissection on the radial side of the finger, then make a similar incision on the ulnar side of the digit.
- The ulnar incision is usually only 3 cm long, as the flexor and extensor tendon disorders have already been addressed. If there is concern that extensor tendon adhesions may limit active extension after release of the flexion contracture, then an extensor tenolysis is performed by elevating the dorsal skin. During the extensor tenolysis, protect the central slip insertion (**TECH FIG 4D**).
- A skin graft or local flap may be required if there is inadequate soft tissue coverage after joint mobilization.
  - If there is insufficient volar skin or unstable volar skin, then raise a cross-finger flap from the adjacent finger. When a cross-finger flap is used, make a transverse incision over the volar aspect of the PIP joint and extend it with a radial midaxial incision.
- Curtis[3,4] originally described pinning the joint in extension for 1 week, but most surgeons do not follow this recommendation.
  - Some authors have advocated resecting the superficialis tendon to avoid recurrence. The author's personal experience suggests that this is not helpful. Favre and Kinnen[5] reported their results for release of the superficialis at the time of a trigger release, but there is no data in the literature to support release of the superficialis in routine cases.

Checkrein Ligament Release for Proximal Interphalangeal Flexion Contracture

- According to Watson et al,[14] the volar plate does not flex but rather slides proximally and distally with flexion and extension. PIP joint adhesions causing contracture occur proximal to the volar plate and involve the checkrein ligaments.
  - Excision of the volar plate or division of the collateral ligaments is rarely required to achieve full extension.
- The joint is approached volarly, often with a V-Y incision to address palmar skin contracture.
- Open the theca between the A2 and A4 pulleys and retract the flexor tendons (**TECH FIG 5A**).
- Release the checkrein ligaments, preserving the nutrient vessel (**TECH FIG 5B**).
- If there is still a contracture after release of the checkreins, release the dorsal portion of the collaterals or the oblique retinacular ligament of Landsmeer.
- This technique is helpful if a palmar exposure is required for excision of Dupuytren disease or during flexor tendon reconstruction.

Percutaneous Collateral Ligament Release for Proximal Interphalangeal Flexion Contracture

- Stanley et al[11] described a percutaneous release of the collateral ligaments for persistent PIP flexion contractures.

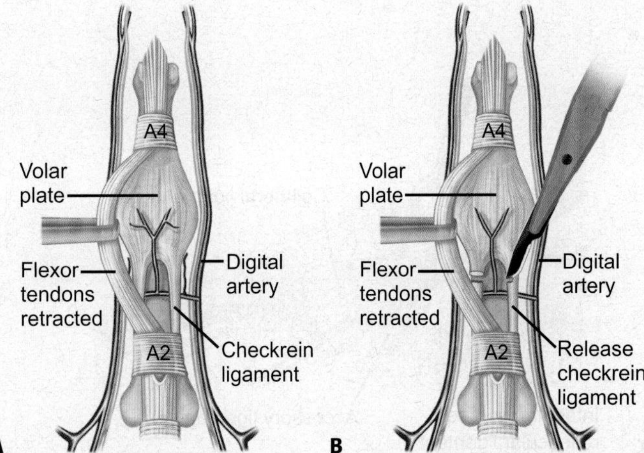

TECH FIG 5 • **A.** The flexor sheath is exposed and the checkrein ligament on the proximal edge of the volar plate is exposed. **B.** Watson's technique for release of the checkrein ligaments to correct a PIP flexion contracture.

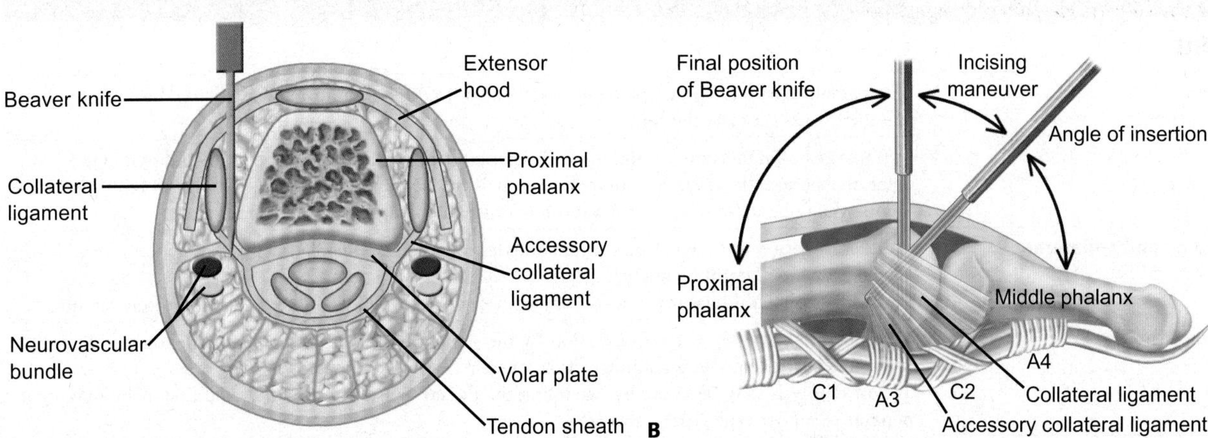

TECH FIG 6 • **A.** Cross-section shows placement of the no. 69 Beaver blade parallel to the proximal phalanx and adjacent to the PIP collateral ligament origin. **B.** Sagittal view demonstrates the technique of "sweeping" the Beaver blade and detaching the collateral ligament from its origin.

- Place a no. 69 Beaver blade percutaneously adjacent to the proximal phalangeal head (**TECH FIG 6A**).
- Disinsert the proper collateral ligaments with a sweeping-type motion (**TECH FIG 6B**).
- Gently manipulate the finger into extension.

Use of an External Fixator for Proximal Interphalangeal Flexion Contracture

- Three types of distractors have been used.
  - Houshian et al[8] used a Pennig mini-external fixator (Orthofix Ltd., Surrey, England) with 2-mm threaded pins.
  - Kasabian et al[9] described the use of a multiplanar distractor used for mandible reconstruction.
  - The use of a Digit Widget (Hand Biomechanics Lab, Inc., Sacramento, CA) has become popular (**TECH FIG 7**).
- An external frame is applied without any soft tissue release.
  - Houshian et al[8] distracts a one-fourth turn (1/4 mm) each day until 5-mm distraction of the joint is achieved.
- The frame is left in place for 4 to 6 weeks. Houshian leaves the frame in place for one week after distraction is stopped.

Capsulectomy for Proximal Interphalangeal Joint Extension Contracture

- Make a dorsal curvilinear incision.
- Preserve the transverse retinacular ligament by blunt dissection and excise the proper collateral ligaments with a no. 69 Beaver blade as described earlier (**TECH FIG 8**).
- Perform a dorsal capsulectomy and an extensor tenolysis. If there is intrinsic tightness, perform a lengthening or release.

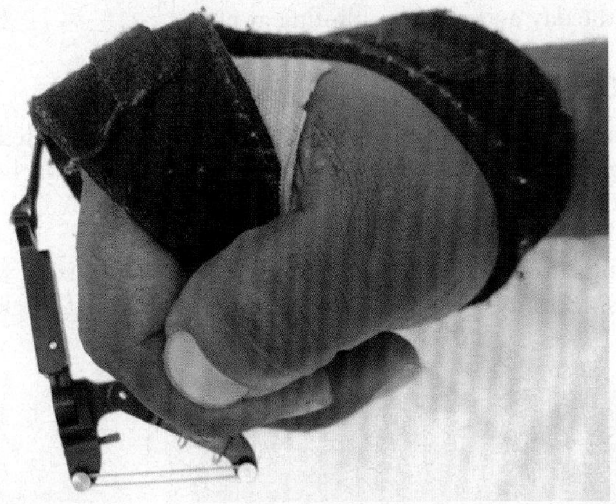

TECH FIG 7 • Application of the Digit Widget for PIP flexion contractures.

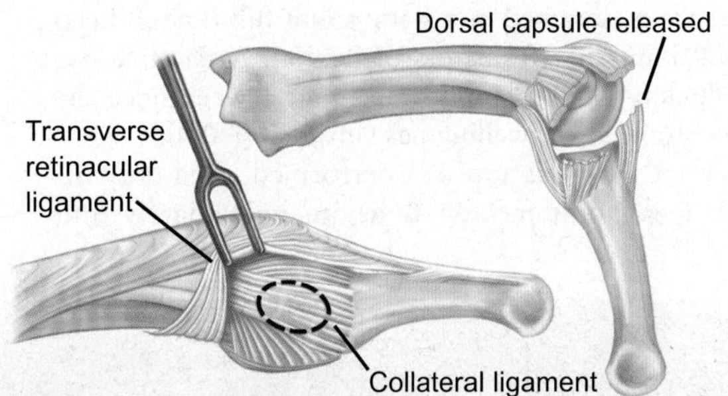

TECH FIG 8 • Through a dorsal incision, the transverse retinacular ligament is protected and the collateral ligament is excised. The dorsal capsule is also released.

PEARLS AND PITFALLS

MCP joint

Indications	▪ The patient must have participated in a well-supervised rehabilitation protocol *and* be committed to another 8–12 weeks of therapy.
Approach	▪ A transverse skin incision is more likely to restrict flexion and more prone to breakdown in the postoperative period; however, a transverse skin incision facilitates soft tissue coverage of multiple MCP joints when operative release of the severely crushed or burned hand is undertaken.
Capsulectomy and collateral release	▪ Adhesions between the volar plate and condyles may be responsible for limited flexion after release of the proper collateral ligaments. ▪ Accessory collateral ligament release may be necessary to achieve full extension without catching.
Associated pathology	▪ Intraoperative attempts at active flexion by the patient will identify associated flexor tendon adhesions in a surprisingly large number of patients. ▪ Flexor tenolysis may be made by extending the dorsal incision in the midaxial line or by making a separate Brunner-type volar approach.

PIP joint

Persistent stiffness	▪ Failure to recognize intrinsic contracture, inadequate skin envelope, and flexor sheath contracture ▪ Unrecognized reflex sympathetic dystrophy
Postoperative instability	▪ Failure to preserve transverse retinacular fibers or excessive release of the soft tissues
Preoperative flexion contracture more than 75 degrees	▪ Consider an arthrodesis rather than soft tissue release.
Best patients for a release	▪ Younger patient, without a crush injury, reflex sympathetic dystrophy, or revascularization ▪ Preoperative flexion contracture of less than 43 degrees

POSTOPERATIVE CARE

- Patients are instructed in strict elevation until the first postoperative visit.
- The wounds are assessed 48 to 72 hours after surgery and, if stable, immediate active-assisted range of motion is begun.
- Wound care and edema control measures are also instituted. A nonadherent gauze should be applied until the wound is watertight. A Coban wrap and gauze finger sleeve limit swelling. Once the wound is healed, compression gloves or elastic finger sleeves further decrease swelling.
- Therapy may quickly advance to include active and passive range of motion as the status of the extensor mechanism allows.
- For MCP extension contractures:
  - Patients are maintained in a static splint full time to keep the MCP joints in 70 degrees of flexion. A daytime dynamic flexion splint is applied at about 1 week once the initial postoperative swelling has subsided (**FIG 4**).
  - If Kirschner wire fixation was performed, then only interphalangeal joint motion is begun immediately and MCP therapy is delayed until wire removal at 7 to 10 days.
  - Patients are reassessed 2 to 3 weeks after surgery. If there is a significant extensor lag (as may follow an extensive extensor tenolysis), a dynamic extension splint can be alternated with the dynamic flexion splint during the day.
  - Nighttime static splinting is continued for a minimum of 6 to 8 weeks.
  - Therapy is usually continued for about 3 months.
- PIP release often benefits from early dynamic splinting during the day and passive splinting at night.

OUTCOMES

- Final motion is often much less than that obtained at surgery but often makes a substantial difference in hand function.
  - Motion plateaus 3 to 6 months after surgery.
- Results are best when the joint can be mobilized with capsulectomy alone. Each additional procedure, such as

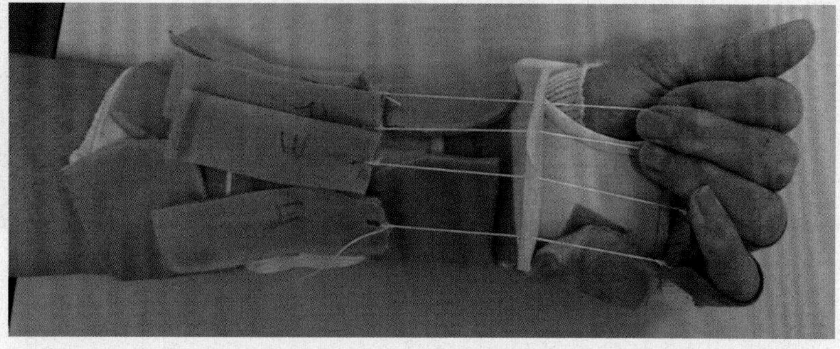

FIG 4 • Dynamic flexion splinting is instituted after surgery for correction of MCP joint extension contracture.

tenolysis, increases postoperative swelling and scar formation, limiting long-term gains.[4]

- In some cases, an improvement in MCP or PIP joint motion of 30 to 45 degrees is a reasonable expectation.[2,16]
- According to Gould and Nicholson,[7] improvement in MCP and PIP motion depends on the cause of the contracture. In a study of 105 MCP capsulectomies and 112 PIP capsulectomies, patients with direct joint trauma (fractures or crush injuries) gained an average of about 20 degrees of active motion, slightly more for the MCP and less for the PIP. Patients with indirect causes of capsular contracture (nerve injury, stroke, or skin burns) did better.[7]
- Ghidella et al[6] reported on the results of 68 PIP capsulectomies. The average overall improvement was a disappointing 7 degrees.[6] The best results occurred in young patients without a history of crush injury, pain syndrome, or revascularization. The average improvement measured 17 degrees in this group compared with 0 degree when there was a "complex diagnosis."
- Houshian et al[8] reported a mean improvement of 67 degrees in 94 patients. Better results were observed in patients younger than 40 years old.[8] Only 12 superficial infections were observed without major complications. There are no reported results using the Digit Widget. Unfortunately, the authors have not been able to reproduce Houshian's results.

COMPLICATIONS

- Wound dehiscence and infection
- Persistent or recurrent contracture
- Extensor rupture
- Ulnar deviation of the finger at the MCP joint
- Postoperative subluxation or dislocation
- Injury to the dorsal branch of the digital nerve

REFERENCES

1. Bode L, Gottlieb M. Dorsal capsulectomy of the metacarpophalangeal joint. In: Blair WF, ed. Techniques in Hand Surgery. Baltimore: Williams & Wilkins, 1996:923–929.
2. Buch VI. Clinical and functional assessment of the hand after metacarpophalangeal capsulotomy. Plast Reconstr Surg 1974;53:452–457.
3. Curtis R. Stiff finger joints. In: Grabb W, Smith J, eds. Plastic Surgery. Boston: Little, Brown, 1979:598–603.
4. Curtis RM. Capsulectomy of the interphalangeal joints of the fingers. J Bone Joint Surg Am 1954;36-A(6):1219–1232.
5. Favre Y, Kinnen L. Resection of the flexor digitorum superficialis for trigger finger with proximal interphalangeal joint positional contracture. J Hand Surg Am 2012;37:2269–2272.
6. Ghidella SD, Segalman KA, Murphey MS. Long-term results of surgical management of proximal interphalangeal joint contracture. J Hand Surg Am 2002;27(5):799–805.
7. Gould JS, Nicholson BG. Capsulectomy of the metacarpophalangeal and proximal interphalangeal joints. J Hand Surg Am 1979;4:482–486.
8. Houshian S, Jing SS, Kazemian GH, et al. Distraction for proximal interphalangeal joint contractures: long-term results. J Hand Surg Am 2013;38:1951–1956.
9. Kasabian A, McCarthy J, Karp N. Use of a multiplanar distracter for the correction of a proximal interphalangeal joint contracture. Ann Plast Surg 1998;40:378–381.
10. Prosser R. Splinting in the management of proximal interphalangeal joint flexion contracture. J Hand Ther 1996;9:378–386.
11. Stanley JK, Jones WA, Lynch MC. Percutaneous accessory collateral ligament release in the treatment of proximal interphalangeal joint flexion contracture. J Hand Surg Br 1986;11:360–363.
12. Strauch RJ, Rosenwasser MP, Lunt JG. Metacarpal shaft fractures: the effect of shortening on the extensor tendon mechanism. J Hand Surg Am 1998;23:519–523.
13. Tsuge K. Contractures. In: Tsuge K, ed. Comprehensive Atlas of Hand Surgery. Chicago: Year Book Medical Publishers, 1989:239–241.
14. Watson HK, Light TR, Johnson TR. Checkrein resection for flexion contracture of the middle joint. J Hand Surg Am 1979;4:67–71.
15. Weeks PM, Wray RC Jr, Kuxhaus M. The results of non-operative management of stiff joints in the hand. Plast Reconstr Surg 1978;61:58–63.
16. Young VL, Wray RC Jr, Weeks PM. The surgical management of stiff joints in the hand. Plast Reconstr Surg 1978;62:835–841.

Needle Aponeurotomy and Collagenase Injection for Treatment of Dupuytren Disease

Frederick N. Meyer

DEFINITION

- Dupuytren disease (DD) is a benign, generally painless, fibroproliferative disorder affecting the palmar fascia that often leads to progressive contractures of the fingers and thumb (**FIG 1**).
- These contractures can be severe having a significant impact on hand function.
- Although most estimates give the incidence of DD as 3% to 6% of Caucasians, some studies have reported rates as high as 42%.[46] This would mean that as many as 13.5 to 27 million people in the United States and Europe could be affected.

ANATOMY

- For a detailed description of normal and pathologic anatomy, please see the excellent description in Dr. Rayan's chapter 143, Surgical Treatment of Dupuytren's Disease.
- A particular concern is the location of the digital nerve when there is a spiral cord. The presence of a spiral nerve can be predicted if the patient has a soft, fatty mass lying between the distal palmar flexion crease and the proximal finger flexion crease. In 44 dissections, if a patient had this mass, there was a spiral nerve 90% of the time.[60]
- The neurovascular bundle usually makes a straight line in the digit. When the pretendinous band, the spiral band, and the lateral digital sheet become involved in DD, they contract and become straight displacing the neurovascular bundle centrally and palmarly (**FIG 2**).[44]

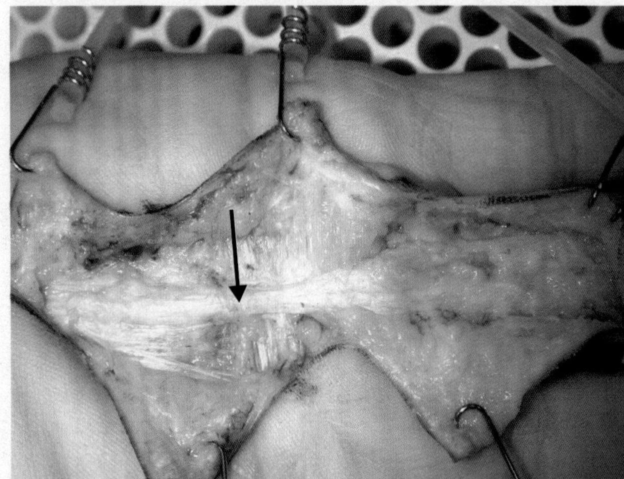

FIG 1 • Surgical dissection showing a pretendinous Dupuytren cord (*arrow*) affecting the palm and finger.

- When the spiral cord contracts, it causes the neurovascular bundle and fibrofatty tissue to become more superficial. This causes redundant skin and fibrofatty tissue to become a soft, pliable mass in the palm that measures approximately 2 cm in diameter.
- The spiral nerve occurs most commonly in the ring and small fingers when there is a proximal interphalangeal (PIP) joint contracture of 30 degrees.[60]

PATHOGENESIS

- DD is believed to be inherited as an autosomal dominant trait with incomplete penetrance. Hu et al[32] was able to identify an autosomal dominant gene for DD on chromosome 16q in a Swedish family.
- The progression of DD is not uniform. Cords can be nodular or nonnodular based on the number of localized cellular nodules in a cord. Nodular cords are hypercellular, the majority of which are alpha smooth muscle actin (α-SMA) positive cells. Nonnodular cords are the most contracted. Cells in nodular cords are responsible for cord contraction. Stress shielding leads to myofibroblast apoptosis that results in cords becoming less cellular.[69]
- Normal palmar fascia is composed largely of type I collagen. DD cords are largely composed of type III collagen.[10]
- DD has been staged histologically[7,58]:
  - *Type I (proliferative stage)*: All lesions show mitotic figures. Mitotic figures are regular in shape and are rare. Cells have round nuclei.
  - *Type II (fibrocellular stage)*: There is high cellularity but no mitotic figures. Cell nuclei are elongated with abundant wavy collagen fibers. Silver stain shows a dense reticulin network in the more cellular areas.
  - *Type III (fibrotic stage)*: There are dense fibrous cords that rarely contain cells with elongated nuclei.
- The highest incidence of recurrence is in patients with the type I histologic group at 54%. By 8 to 9 years postoperatively, the recurrence rate increases to 71%.
- The major source of contraction in DD is the myofibroblast. This cell can generate significant contractile forces and has characteristics of both smooth muscle and fibroblasts.[5,23]
- Prostaglandin $F_{2\alpha}$ stimulates significant contracture of myofibroblasts, whereas prostaglandin E_2 causes relaxation.[5,35]
- DD tissue contains large amounts of transforming growth factor beta (TGF-β_1 and TGF-β_2) that has a significant effect on myofibroblast proliferation.[6]
- TGF-β_1 is a mechanotransduction cytokine that causes increased contractile force of myofibroblasts during the early phase of attachment and contractions as well as an increased contractile response to mechanical stimuli.[9]

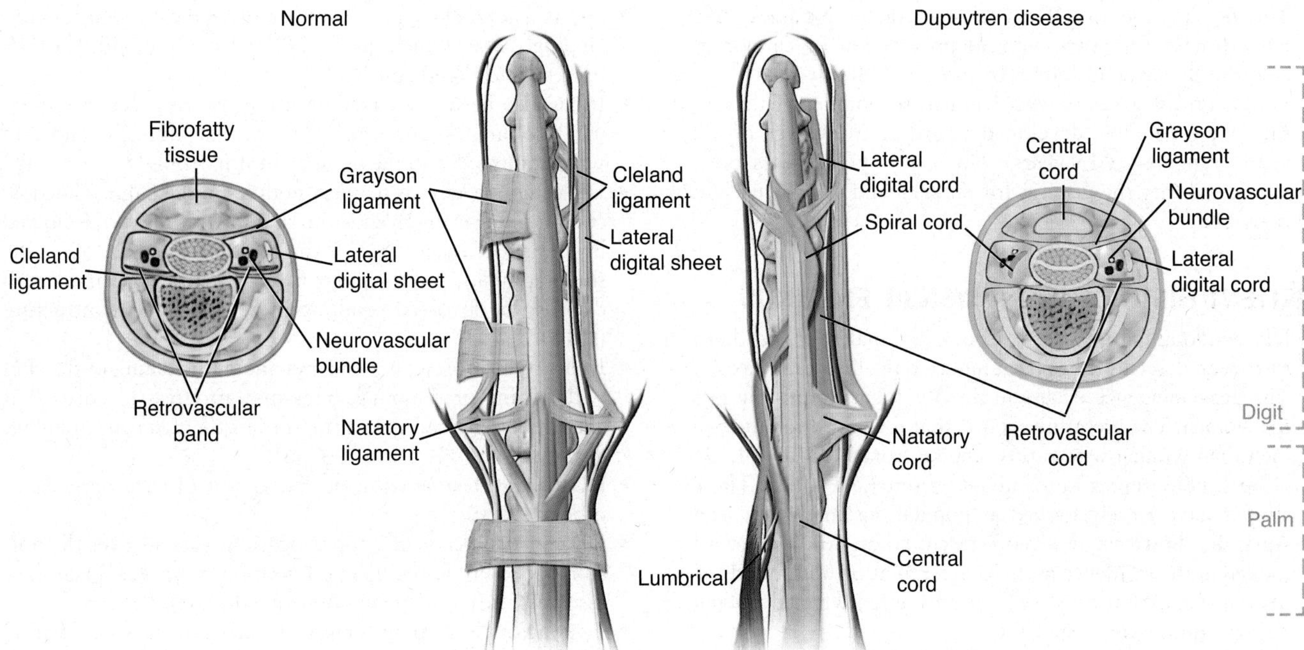

FIG 2 ● The formation of a spiral cord showing displacement of the neurovascular bundle.

- A *Z19* transcription factor gene increases the potency of TGF-β_1.
- Multiple other proteins influence differentiation, growth, and contractility of myofibroblasts. These include platelet-derived growth factor (PDGF), fibroblast growth factor (FGF), epidermal growth factor (EGF), interleukin-1 (IL-1) tenascin and periostin (Tables 1 and 2).[10,49]

NATURAL HISTORY

- DD progresses through three clinical stages[15,42]:
  - *Stage I*: the proliferative or nodular stage. In this stage, patients have a nodule or nodules within the palmar fascia. The nodules are predominantly cellular, composed of peripheral, perivascular spindle-shaped hyperplastic fibroblasts with irregular hyperchromatic nuclei. The nodules tend to be vascular with reactive tissue around the periphery. There is no increase in collagen deposition. The hyperplastic cells disrupt the continuity of the normal palmar fascia.
  - *Stage II*: the involutional or active disease stage. In this stage, there is nodular thickening of the palmar fascia with the beginning of joint contracture. Fibroblasts align themselves along lines of stress. They become more mature and decrease in size and number. The predominate cell type is myofibroblast. There are definite cords composed of well-aligned, mature collagen fibers and few scattered cells.
  - *Stage III*: the residual or advanced disease stage. In this stage, there are diffuse, thick fibrotic cords that become more contracted. The cords are predominantly collagen with few cells that are elongated and compressed by the collagen fibers. Cell types are both fibroblasts and myofibroblasts.

Table 1 Selected Genes and Proteins Upregulated in Dupuytren Disease

- A disintegrin and metalloproteinase domain (ADAM) 12
- Alpha smooth muscle actin (α-SMA)
- β-1 integrin
- Cadherin 11 (CDH11)
- Collagen I, collagen V, collagen VIII
- Contactin 1 (CNTN1)
- Fibronectin
- Heat shock protein 47 (HSP47)
- Laminin
- Leucine-rich repeat (LRR) domain-containing 17
- V-maf musculoaponeurotic fibrosarcoma oncogene homolog B (MafB)
- Periostin, osteoblast specific factor (POSTN)
- Postsynaptic density protein-95 (PSD-95)
- Tenascin C
- Tissue inhibitor of metalloproteinase (TIMP-1)
- Transforming growth factor-β2 (TGF-β2)
- Zonula occludens-1 protein (ZO-1)

From Black EM, Blazar PE. Dupuytren disease: an evolving understanding of an age-old disease. J Am Acad Orthop Surg 2011;19(12):746–757.

Table 2 Selected Genes and Proteins Downregulated in Dupuytren Disease

- Chitinase 3-like protein 2
- Collagen XV
- Cornea-derived transcript 6 (CDT6)
- Cysteine dioxygenase 1 (CDO1)
- Matrix metallopeptidase 27 (MMP27)
- Matrix metalloproteinase-3 (MMP3)
- Superoxide dismutase (SOD)
- Superoxide dismutase 2 (SOD2)

From Black EM, Blazar PE. Dupuytren disease: an evolving understanding of an age-old disease. J Am Acad Orthop Surg 2011;19(12):746–757.

- The progression of DD is unpredictable. Nodules may lay dormant for years without progression or can progress rapidly over a matter of months.[42] Reilly et al[57] reported on 59 patients with Dupuytren nodules. Thirty of the 59 patients had developed a cord at an average of 8.7 years (range 6 to 15 years). However, by 8.7 years only, 5 patients met the criteria for surgery and 7 patients had regressed.[57]

PATIENT HISTORY AND PHYSICAL FINDINGS

- DD predominantly affects Caucasian males of northern European descent. It has been reported in all races, however.
- The peak incidence occurs in the 50s for men and the 60s for women. The literature reports that it is more common in men than women with ratios ranging from 7.5:1 to 5.4:1.[42] Other studies report ratios ranging from 9.5:1 to 3:1. These studies have largely looked at populations in Europe and Australia, however. In a more recent study, Anthony et al[1] looked at the incidence in the U.S. population and found the male-to-female ratio to be 1.7:1 and noted with advancing age, the ratio approached 1:1.
- DD interferes with activities of daily living and work including hair brushing, face washing, holding hands, putting hands in pockets, holding tools, and wearing gloves.
- DD is associated with a number of medical conditions including diabetes mellitus,[3,13] HIV[11] frozen shoulder, a high lipid profile,[29] and epilepsy.[2]
- It has also been associated with lifestyle risk factors including smoking, alcoholism,[12,24,25] manual labor,[41] hand and wrist trauma,[40] and the use of vibratory tools.[64]
- DD usually begins as painless nodules in the palm. The most common finger involved is the ring finger (60.7%), followed by the small finger (51%), the middle finger (22.5%), the thumb (7.0%), and the index finger (5.8%). The thumb web can also be involved resulting in an adduction contracture (**FIG 3A**).[55]
- Early in the disease, patients may note thickening of the skin with pitting or dimpling. This may progress to cords that can ultimately lead to contracture of the metacarpophalangeal (MP) and PIP joints (**FIG 3B**).
- DD usually begins with one finger but often progresses to others (**FIG 3C**).
- DD can also occur in ectopic locations such as over the dorsum of the PIP joints (Garrod nodes), in the feet (Lederhose disease), and in the penis (Peyronie disease).[30]
- Five factors have been identified that indicate a DD diathesis. They include onset younger than age 50 years, bilateral involvement, ectopic lesions, male gender, and a positive family history.[30,33]

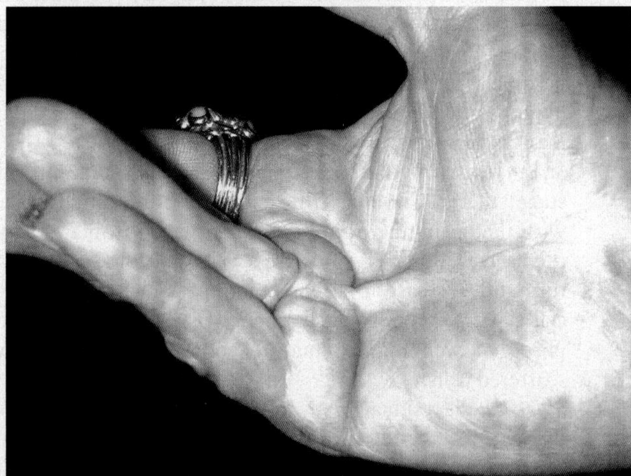
A

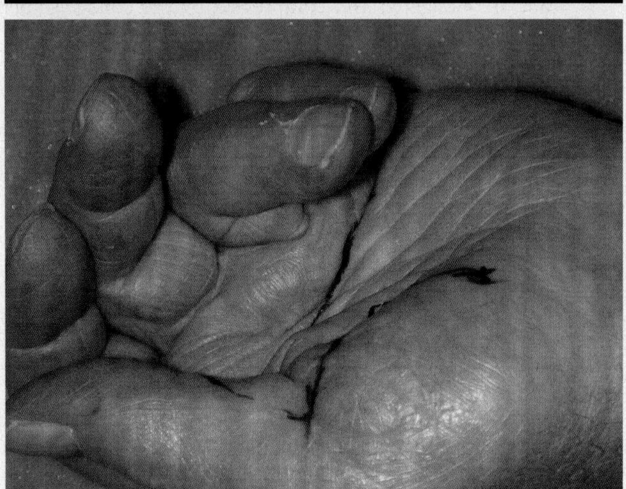
C

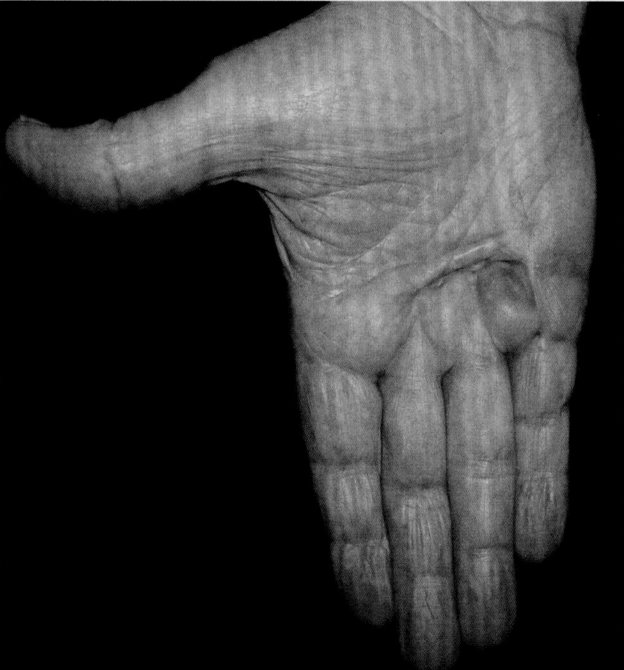
B

FIG 3 • **A.** Dupuytren cord affecting the ring finger. **B.** Pitting and dimpling associated with Dupuytren contracture. **C.** Multiple Dupuytren cords involving all fingers and the thumb.

- Patients with a DD diathesis have a more aggressive disease with higher rates of recurrence.
- The "fasciodesis" maneuver is useful for predicting minimum gain in PIP motion after percutaneous needle fasciotomy (PNF).
  - Flex the MP joint to 90 degrees.
  - Measure the extension gain at the PIP joint.[20]
- Tubiana classified DD based on total passive extension deficit (TPED) of the MP, PIP, and distal interphalangeal (DIP) joints (Table 3).[65]

IMAGING AND OTHER DIAGNOSTIC STUDIES

- In most instances, radiographic imaging is not necessary to adequately evaluate DD. The only time one might consider imaging is if there is a concern for some other pathology such as significant osteoarthritis or neoplasm. If these are suspected, then appropriate imaging studies could be ordered.

DIFFERENTIAL DIAGNOSIS

- The differential diagnosis of DD is well covered in the chapter on Surgical Treatment of Dupuytren's Disease.

NONOPERATIVE MANAGEMENT

- In the past, a number of nonoperative treatments for DD have met with limited success. These include physical therapy, splinting, dimethylsulfoxide injections, topical vitamins A and E, gamma interferon injections, radiation, and the calcium channel blockers such as nifedipine and verapamil.[56]
- In 1971, Hueston[33] performed what he referred to as *enzymatic fasciotomy.* He injected patients with a mixture of trypsin, hyaluronidase, and lidocaine, followed by a forcible extension maneuver. He was able to obtain full extension of all fingers 15 minutes following injection.[33]
- When McCarthy[43] studied the long-term results, however, he found that seven of nine patients had developed recurrence within 2 to 3 years.
- Injection of triamcinolone acetonide directly into the DD nodules resulted in regression in 97% of patients. The average number of injections was 3.2. There was a 50% recurrence rate between 1 and 3 years after the last injection, however.[38]

Table 3 Tubiana Grades of Dupuytren Disease Based on Total Passive Extension Deficit

Grade I	0–45 degrees
Grade II	45–90 degrees
Grade III	90–135 degrees
Grade IV	≥135 degrees

COLLAGENASE *CLOSTRIDIUM HISTOLYTICUM* (XIAFLEX)

- In 2009, Hurst et al[34] reported the results of the multicenter collagenase option for reduction of Dupuytren (CORD) I study. This was a double blind, placebo-controlled study in which they injected Dupuytren cords with 0.58 mg collagenase *Clostridium histolyticum* (CCH) (Xiaflex).[34]
- Xiaflex is a mixture of two synergistic collagenases that tend to rapidly degrade type I and type III collagens.[61]

Indications for Treatment

- A palpable cord with an MP or PIP joint contracture of 20 degrees or more

Contraindications

- Patients who are intolerant of pain are poor candidates.
- The drug is expensive and patients with multiple cords may face months of treatment and a great deal of expense.
- A history of sensitivity to CCH.
- Patients who have been on anticoagulants other than low-dose aspirin within 7 days of CCH injection
- Contractures associated with huge nodules are not good candidates for collagenase.

Preoperative Planning

- Give the patient take-home information describing common side effects and risks.
- Be sure to obtain insurance preauthorization if required.
- Identify the primary cord for treatment.
- Identify secondary and tertiary joints for later treatment.

Injection[28]

- CCH comes as a lyophilized powder containing 0.9 mg of the drug. It is reconstituted with 0.39 mL of sterile diluent for MP joint contractures and 0.31 mL for PIP joint contractures.
- Once reconstituted, the drug should sit for 15 minutes, but if not, refrigerated should be used within 1 hour. Refrigerated CCH may be stored up to 4 hours.
- The dosage for all injections is 0.58 mg.
- The use of local anesthesia prior to injection is not recommended.
- The injection is performed with a 1 mL syringe and a 0.5-inch 27-gauge needle. It is best to use the syringes supplied by the company.
- Gently extend the involved finger to put the cord under tension, displacing it away from the underlying flexor tendon (**TECH FIG 1**).
- Inject a cord where it bowstrings the most and is displaced furthest from the underlying flexor tendon.
- Insert the needle through the skin into the underlying cord. This should feel firm.
- Passively manipulate the PIP or DIP joint to be certain the needle is not in the flexor tendon.
- Inject one-third of the volume. Resistance to injection indicates the needle is in the cord.
- The cord is injected in three different locations. The needle can either be redirected or removed and reintroduced into two other locations 2 to 3 mm away. One-third of the volume is injected in each location (**TECH FIG 2**).

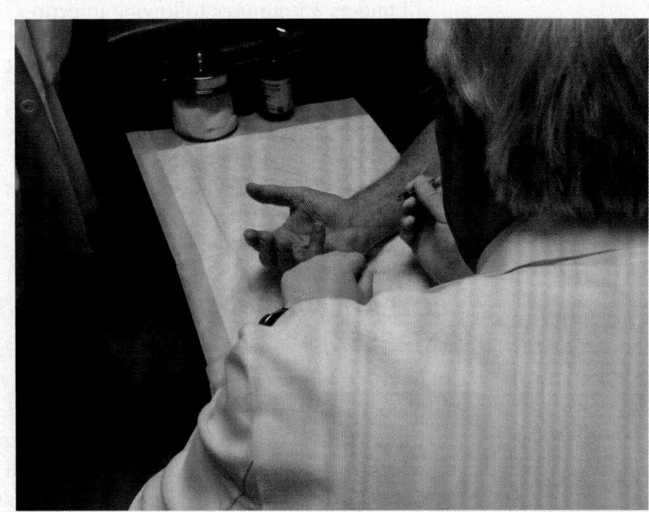

TECH FIG 1 • CCH injection technique.

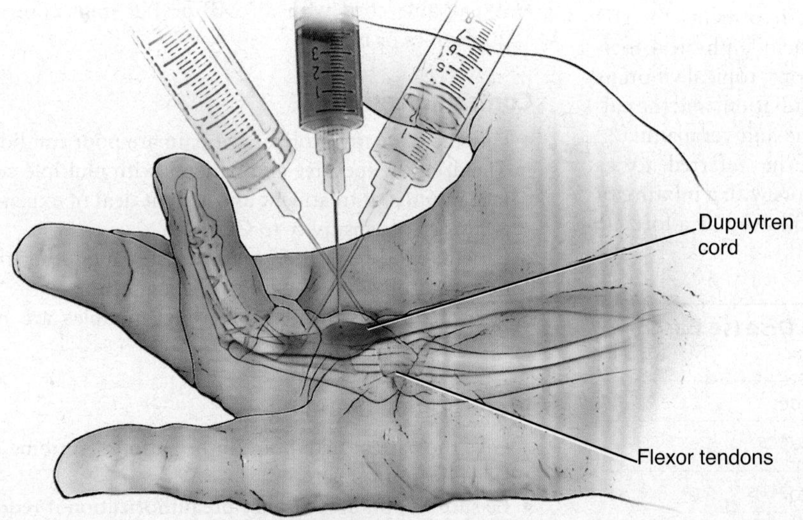

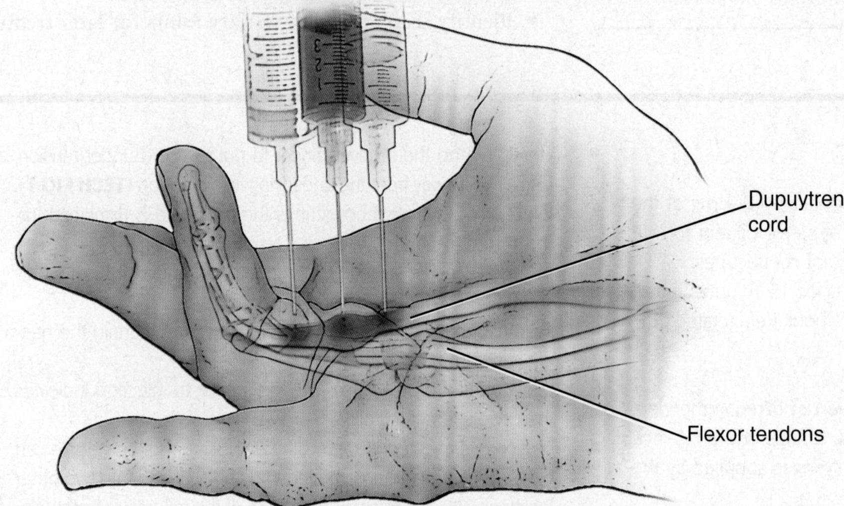

TECH FIG 2 • **A.** Inject by redirecting the needle. **B.** The preferred injection technique is to remove and reinsert the needle.

- MP joint cords are injected with 0.25 mL of CCH.
- PIP joint cords are injected with 0.20 mL of CCH
- Cords causing PIP joint contractures should not be injected more than 4 mm distal to the proximal finger flexion crease (**TECH FIG 3**).
- Insert the needle no more than 2 to 3 mm.
- Currently, the manufacturer recommends injecting only one cord at a time.
- Coleman et al[16] reported on injecting cords affecting two joints in the same hand at one sitting. Although there was an increased incidence of some adverse events, few were serious and the authors concluded it was safe to perform.[16]
- Each cord can be injected up to three times at 30-day intervals.

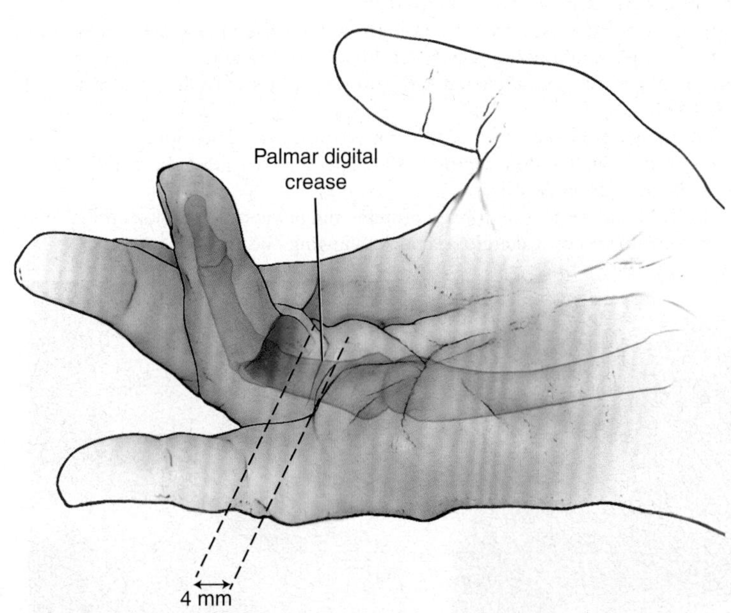

TECH FIG 3 • Do not inject a PIP joint more than 4 mm distal to the proximal finger flexion crease.

Manipulation

- The day following the injection, patients return for manipulation. Manipulation may be safely performed up to 7 days following injection without negatively affecting the results (**TECH FIG 4**).[28,37]
- Prior to manipulation, perform a wrist or digital nerve block with 1% lidocaine.
- The wrist is flexed and moderate passive extension is applied to the involved digit for 10 to 20 seconds.
- If manipulating the PIP joint, the MP joint is flexed.
- Often, a "pop" or tearing noise is heard as the cord breaks.
- Some cords rupture spontaneously.
- Up to three attempts at 5- to 10-minute intervals can be made.
- If unsuccessful after three attempts, the patient should be instructed to return in 30 days for another injection.

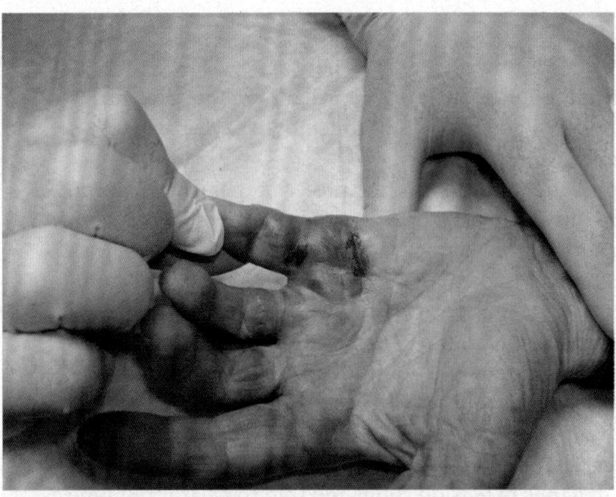

TECH FIG 4 • Manipulation of the finger 2 days following injection with CCH. Note the local reaction at the injection site.

PEARLS AND PITFALLS

- There is significant resistance when injecting into a cord. Sudden loss of resistance may mean the cord has been penetrated. It is safer to remove the needle and inject in another location rather than to try to redirect the needle.
- When injecting, it is best to have the patient or an assistant hold the finger, so two hands can be used to prevent inadvertent advancement of the needle through the cord.
- When injecting a spiral cord, lateral cord, or abductor digiti minimi cord, it is often safer to inject from the side with the needle pointing away from the flexor tendons.
- If there is both a radial and ulnar cord in the same digit, consider splitting the dose and injecting both cords. On occasion, I have used the full vial to do this. This is technically off-label.
- If the patient gets paresthesias during the injection, remove the needle and inject in another location.
- If there is a Y-shaped cord, injecting at the apex of the Y often allows correction of both involved digits.
- Periarticular fibrosis can cause joint contractures that do not respond to collagenase injections. Dynamic splinting following injection may be helpful, but on two occasions, I have had to surgically release the volar plate in order to release the PIP joint contracture.
- Skin tears can be alarming and some authors have reported repairing them with split-thickness skin grafts. However, even dramatic tears heal quickly with simple wound care within 10 days to 3 weeks (**FIG 4A–C**).
- First web contractures can have mixed results because of difficulty applying enough pressure on the cord during manipulation.
- The safety of CCH in patients receiving anticoagulant medications other than low-dose aspirin (150 mg per day) has not been established so it should be used with caution in patients on anticoagulants or with coagulation disorders.
- Although there have been no reports of severe allergic reactions to CCH, it does contain foreign proteins and patients do develop anti-AUX-I and AUX-II antibodies. Therefore, physicians should be prepared to address severe allergic reactions following injections.

A
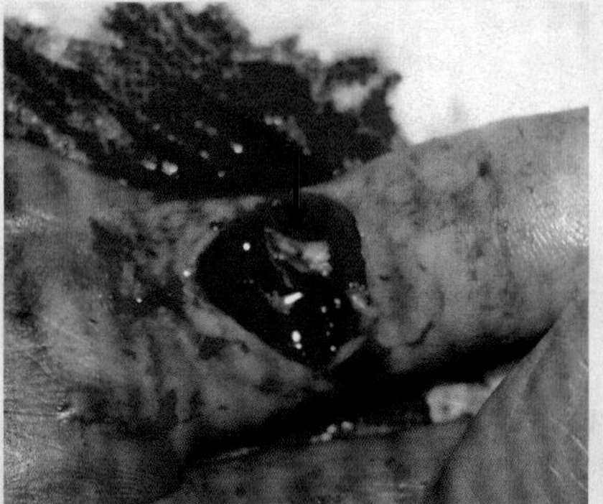
B
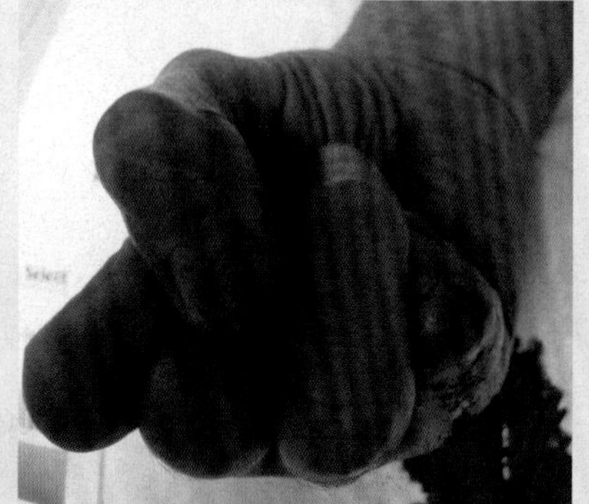
C
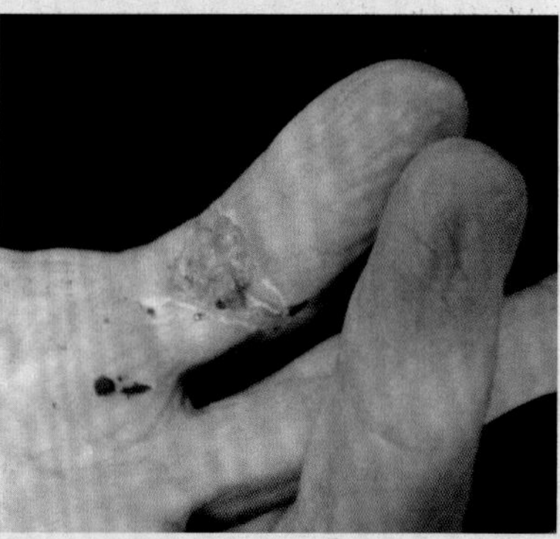

FIG 4 • **A.** There is a large skin tear following the manipulation of a PIP cord. The distal portion of the Dupuytren cord (*arrow*) can be visualized in the wound. **B.** Despite the large tear, the patient still has full ROM. **C.** Two weeks following the tear, it is almost completely healed with simple wound care.

POSTOPERATIVE CARE

- Following the injection of CCH, a light compressive dressing is applied. Patients are told to remove the dressing either that evening or the next day.
- Although some authors do not prescribe pain medication, I prefer to give patients a prescription for a few narcotic pain pills for the first few days.
- Patients are advised to avoid heavy use of their hand until the next day.
- Following manipulation, patients are given a home exercise program and a night splint that holds the fingers in extension. They are told to wear the splint at night for 3 to 4 months.
- For severe PIP joint contractures (≥40 degrees), patients are given a dynamic extension splint and told to wear it full time for 3 to 4 months except for bathing and exercise.
- Patients are advised to avoid heavy use of their hand until pain-free.

OUTCOMES

- In the CORD I study, authors report getting 64% of digits to within 5 degrees of full extension with an average of 1.7 injections given at monthly intervals. Results were better for MP joints (76.7%) than PIP joints (40%) and in mild (MP <50 degrees = 88.9% and PIP <40 degrees = 80.9%) versus severe disease (MP 57.7% and PIP 22.4%) (**FIG 5A–C**).[34]
- Average improvement in range of motion (ROM) for all patients was:
  - From 43.9 to 80.7 degrees (mean improvement 36.7 degrees)
  - MP joint motion improved from 42.6 to 83.7 degrees (mean improvement 40.6 degrees)
  - PIP joint motion improved from 46.6 to 74.9 degrees (mean improvement 29.0 degrees)
- More recent data has shown similar outcomes from an academic and community-based experience with CCH. In this study, patients received an average of 1.08 injections.[53]

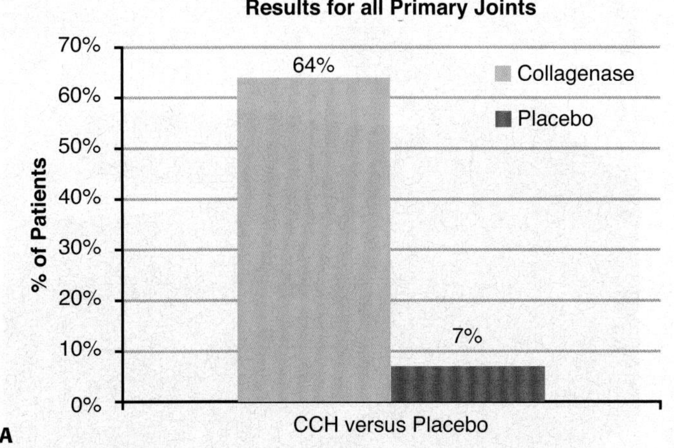

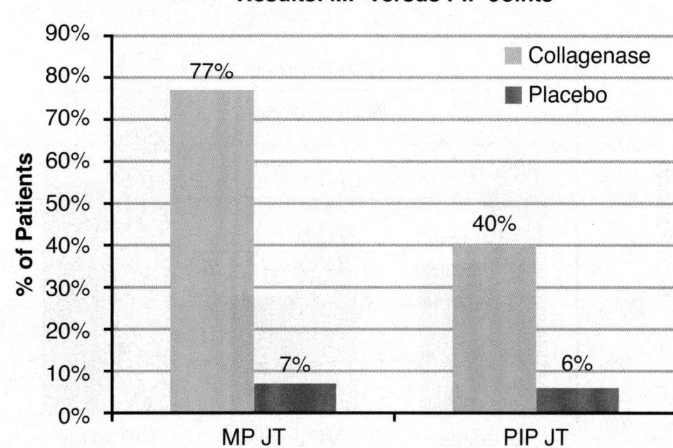

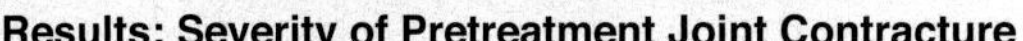

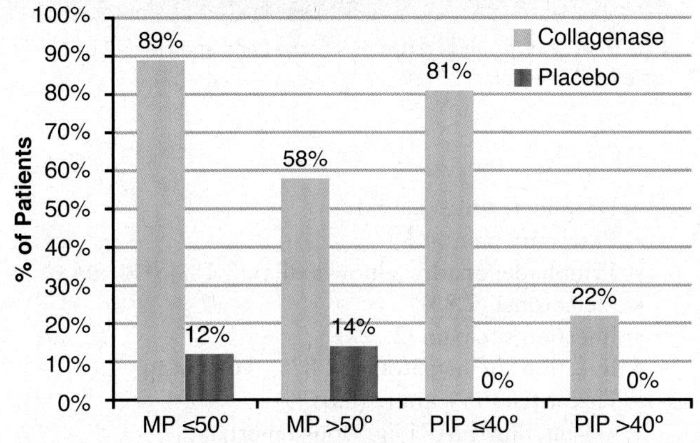

FIG 5 • **A.** CORD I study: overall percentage of results for patients treated with an average of 1.7 injections of CCH. **B.** Percentage of results for patients treated with CCH by joint involved. **C.** Outcomes compared by degree of severity for MP joints (severe = >50 degrees) and for PIP joints (severe = >40 degrees).

- Most patients (≥85.8%) developed antibodies to either type 1 (AUX-I) or type II (AUX-II) CCH or both within 30 days after the first injection. All patients developed antibodies to both AUX-I and AUX-II by the third injection.
- However, there were no meaningful systemic allergic reactions.
- Some patients ultimately require fasciectomy. Unlike surgery following previous limited fasciectomy, there is no significant distortion of anatomy or increased difficulty in dissection in patients previously treated with CCH (**FIG 6**).[26]
- In fingers with both MP and PIP joint contractures, the PIP joint will often correct with treatment of the MP joint cord alone.[27]
- Recurrence rates are difficult to evaluate because there is no agreed definition of what constitutes recurrence. Peimer et al[50] reported on 3-year recurrence rates where he defined recurrence as a contracture of greater than or equal to 20 degrees with a palpable cord or as the need to have further surgical or medical treatment. Of the 1080 CCH treated joints, 35% had recurred. The MP joint had a recurrence rate of 27% and the PIP joint 56%. Only 7% of patients with recurrence received further treatment, however.
- Four-year recurrence data was recently reported. The overall recurrence rate was 42.1%. MP joint recurrence was 34.6% and PIP joint recurrence was 61.6%.[31]
- Some authors have suggested using 30 degrees rather than 20 degrees as the indication of a recurrence.[67,68] If 30 degrees is used, the recurrence rate was 27.9% overall with a 22.2% recurrence at the MP joint and a 43% recurrence at the PIP joint (**FIG 7**).

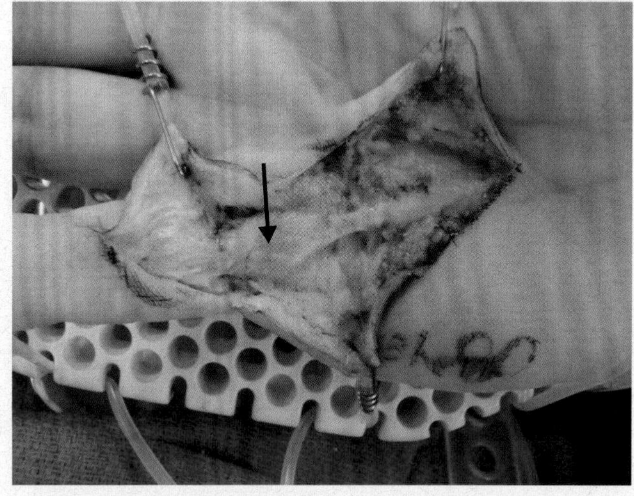

FIG 6 • A patient with a previous CCH injection who ultimately requested surgery. The *arrow* points to the previous site of injection. There is minimal scarring and distortion from the previous treatment.

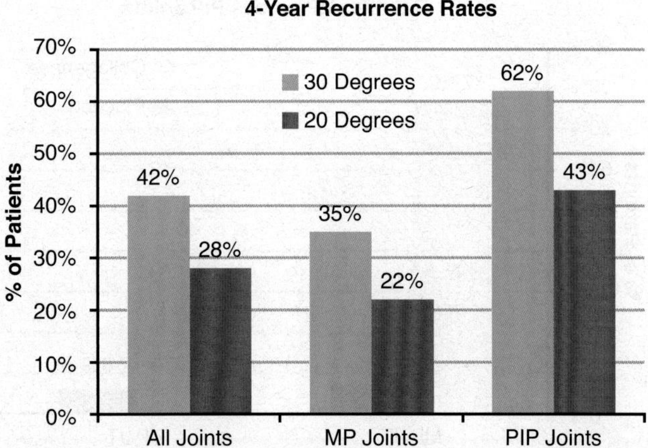

FIG 7 • Four-year recurrence data presented at the 2013 American Society for Surgery of the Hand (ASSH) Annual Meeting by Hotchkiss et al.[31]

- 87.2% of joints successfully treated with CCH did not require further treatment. However, patients treated with fasciectomy had a lower incidence of retreatment.

COMPLICATIONS[4,51,52]

- The most recent data reported 1732 adverse events from 49,078 injections on 846 patients.
- The majority of these adverse events were mild injection site reactions that resolved rapidly. These include the following:
  - Skin tear (13.2%)
  - Ecchymosis (9.7%) (**FIG 8**)
  - Hand and finger edema (9.5%) (**FIG 9**)

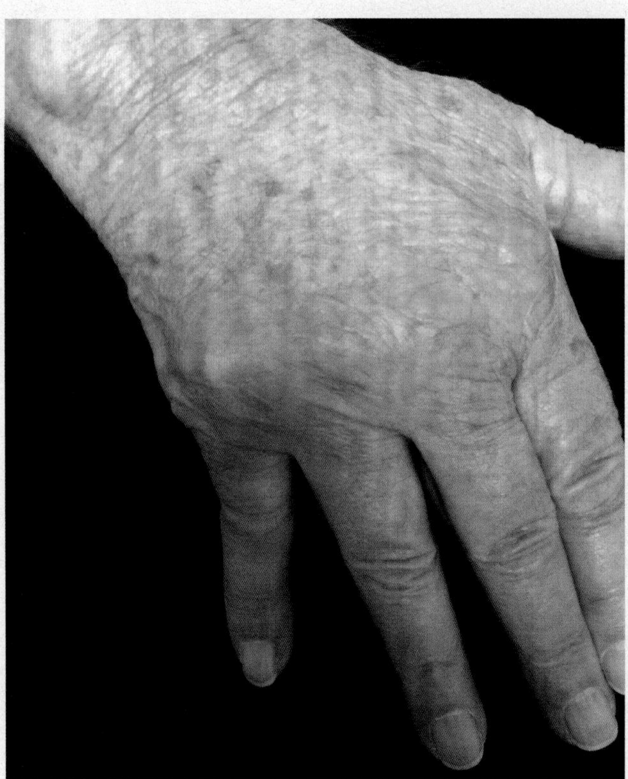

FIG 8 • Ecchymosis of the hand 2 days following a CCH injection.

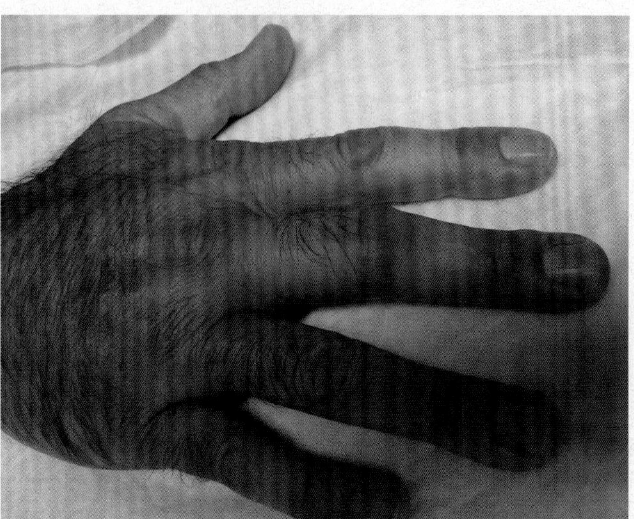

FIG 9 • Swelling and ecchymosis of the hand and finger 2 days following a CCH injection.

  - Drug ineffective (6.1%)
  - Extremity pain (4.6)%
  - Lymphadenopathy (elbow/axilla) (3.1%) (**FIG 10A,B**)
  - Hematoma (2.8%)
  - Injection site pain (2.7%)
  - Injection site hematoma (2.8%) (**FIG 11A,B**)
  - Flexor tendon rupture (0.05%)
    - Ring finger MP joint (four reports)
    - Little finger MP joint (five reports)
    - Little finger PIP joint (eight reports)
  - Complex regional pain syndrome (CRPS) (two reports)
  - A2 pulley injury (one report)
  - Stretch neurapraxia (one report)
  - Flexor pulley injury (one report)
  - Loss of a well-established skin graft (one report)[62]
  - Pruritus or localized rash

SURGICAL MANAGEMENT

- Sir Astley Cooper originally performed percutaneous fasciotomy in 1822 using a bistoury later known as a *Cooper knife*. The procedure came to be known as *Cooper fasciotomy*.[18,36,66]
- In 1979, two French rheumatologists, Lermusiaux and Debeyre,[39] popularized using a 25-gauge needle to perform PNF.

Indications for Treatment[18,20]

- MP joint contracture of 30 degrees or greater
- PIP joint contracture of any degree that results in functional impairment
- A discreet, palpable cord
- An elderly, medically frail patient
- A compliant patient
- Early Tubiana stage I disease with a moderate MP flexion contracture
- PNF can be used to treat recurrent DD.[68]

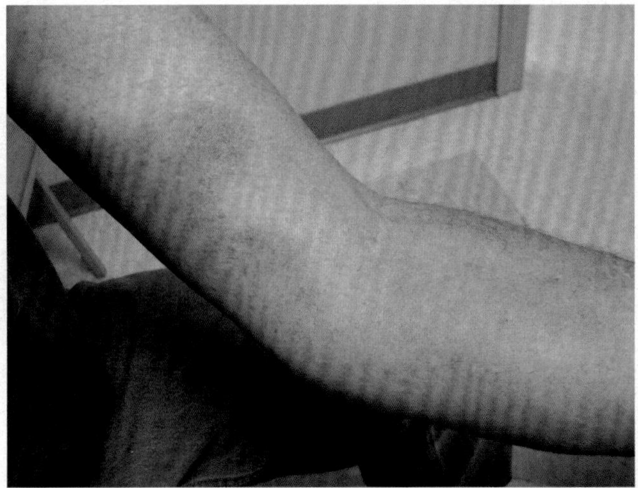

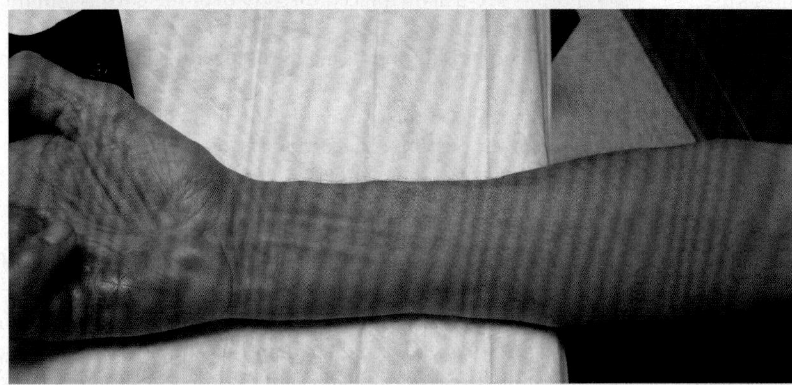

FIG 10 • **A.** Swelling of the arm with epitrochlear lymphadenopathy. **B.** Forearm pain and swelling following an injection of CCH.

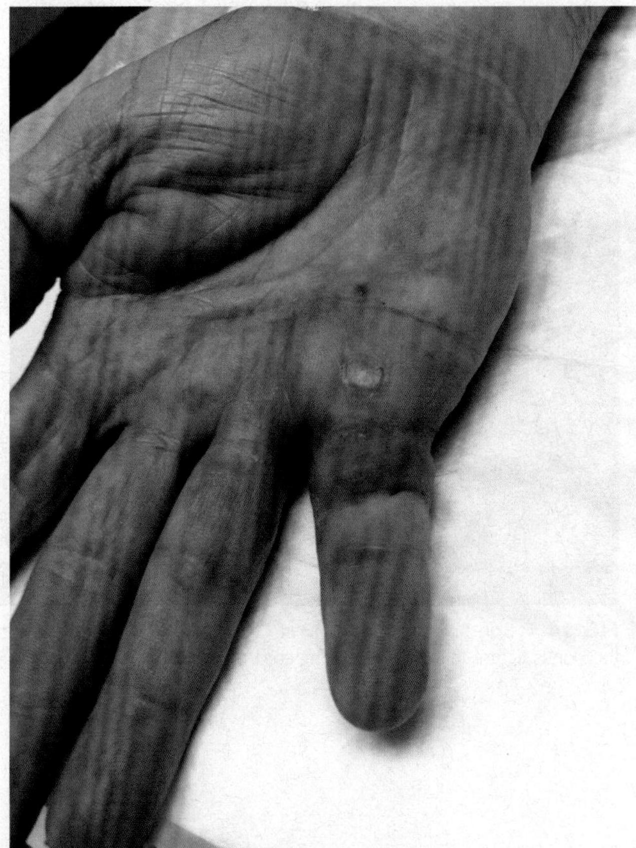

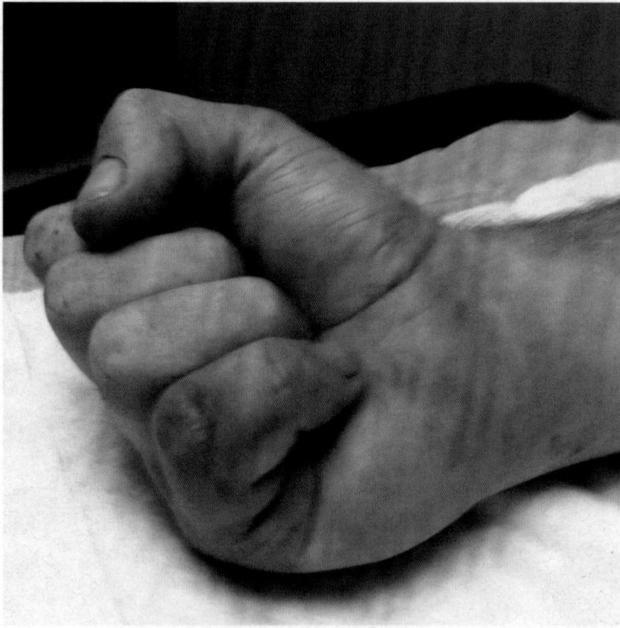

FIG 11 • **A.** Injection site hematoma. These usually resolve rapidly. **B.** Despite the large injection site hematoma, the patient is able to make a complete fist immediately following manipulation.

Contraindications[20]

- Large, bulky ill-defined cord (relative)
- Patients without a distinct, palpable cord[19]
- Recurrent cord after surgery (relative)
- Patients unable to tolerate local procedures
- A cord that allows for full passive finger extension
- Uncooperative or mentally impaired patients
- Nodules without cords
- Long-standing PIP flexion contractures (relative)
- Deep lateral cords
- Contractures resulting from insufficient skin or postsurgical scarring

Preoperative Planning

- Perform a detailed history and physical examination.
- Measure and document the degree of flexion contracture.
- Note the character of the cord or nodules.
- Document preoperative sensation and flexor tendon function.
- Counsel the patient to inform you immediately if they feel electric shocks in the finger.
- Warn the patient of potential complications including skin tears, nerve injury, flexor tendon damage, and recurrence.

Positioning

- The patient is supine with the hand resting on a hand table.
- A 2-inch thick pad of folded towels is placed behind the hand to facilitate MP extension.[19]
- The hand is draped with sterile drapes.

Approach

- The procedure can be performed in either an office setting or an outpatient surgery suite.
- A tourniquet may be used but is usually not necessary.
- The cord is marked on the skin where it is most prominent (**FIG 12**).

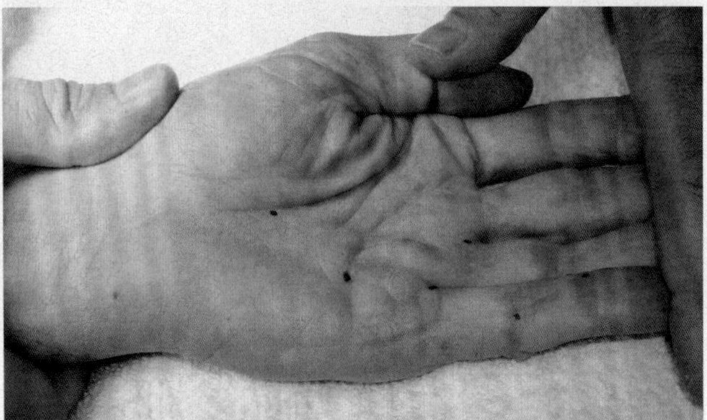

FIG 12 • The skin is marked outlining the cord.

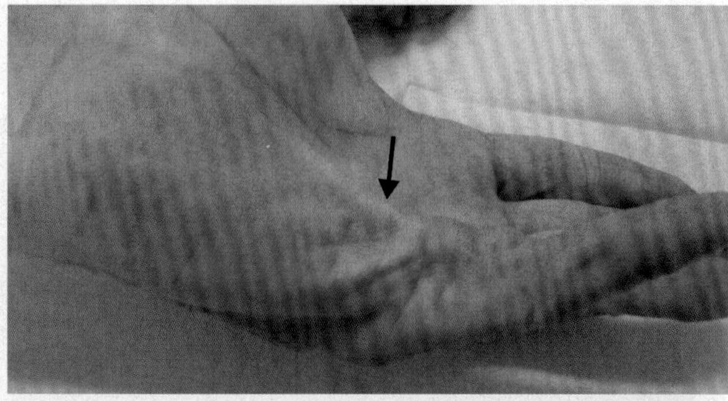

FIG 13 • The figure shows an ideal cord for PNF. The *arrow* points to an ideal position to place a portal.

- Portals are usually placed directly over the cord a minimum of 5 mm apart.
- Dual side-by-side portals maybe used with wide cords (>5 mm in width).
- Plan portals on the convex side of skin creases.
- Whenever possible, place portals in areas where the cord bowstrings maximally (**FIG 13**).
- Avoid nodules and skin creases for portals.
- Beware of skin dimples.
- Doppler examination may help elucidate the location of a suspected spiral cord.
- Look for blanching when tension is applied. No blanching indicates the cord is tighter than the skin and this is a good location for a portal. Once the cord is released, the skin should blanch with tension (**FIG 14**).
- A small amount of 1% plain lidocaine is used to infiltrate the overlying skin (0.1 to 0.2 mL).

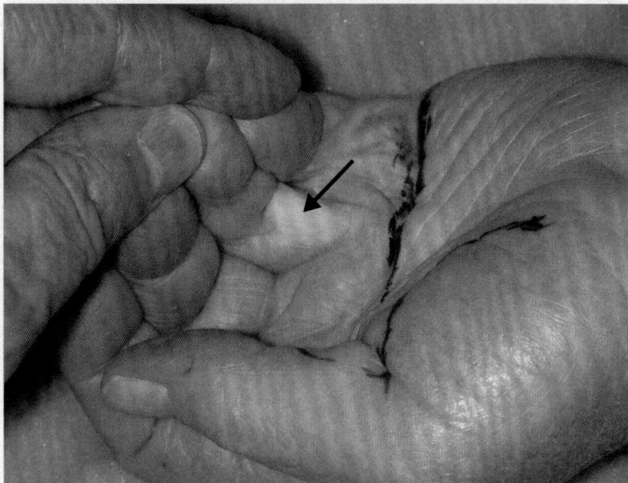

FIG 14 • Skin blanching (*arrow*) with traction on the finger indicates the skin is tighter than the underlying cord.

Collagenase Injection

- Pull the finger into extension, making the cord more palpable and hold it under tension (**TECH FIG 5A**).
- Use a 25-gauge needle to perforate the cord in the area of anesthesia (**TECH FIG 5B**).
- Some authors prefer to use a 19-gauge needle.[20]
- Check fingertip sensation repeatedly during procedure.
- Monitor tendon involvement by asking the patient to flex and extend the DIP and PIP joints during the procedure. The needle should not move with the tendon.
- Begin perforations distally and progress proximally along the cord for approximately 1 cm.
- Initially, use the needle to develop a plane between the skin and the cord.
- Orient the needle to use as a probe to define the width of the cord.
- Perforations should not go completely through the cord.
- Alternately, use the needle in a sawing motion.
- With either technique, there should be a grating feeling. If a grating is not felt, change the needle and move to another portal.
- Following the perforations, the finger is firmly but gently extended while stabilizing the hand. Frequently, a pop is heard as the cord breaks (**TECH FIG 5C**).
- Flex the wrist and ask the patient to actively extend the finger during the manipulation maneuver.
- Extend the finger and palpate for a residual cord.
- Repeat the procedure as necessary until full extension is achieved, the remaining cord is no longer palpable, or further treatment would put the neurovascular bundles at risk.
- A local or wrist block may be helpful if the manipulation is too painful.
- Injecting triamcinolone acetonide (TA) into the portals and nodules following release may be helpful. McMillan and Bidhammer[45] reported significantly improved correction of deformity at 6 months in patients who received TA injection postoperatively.

A
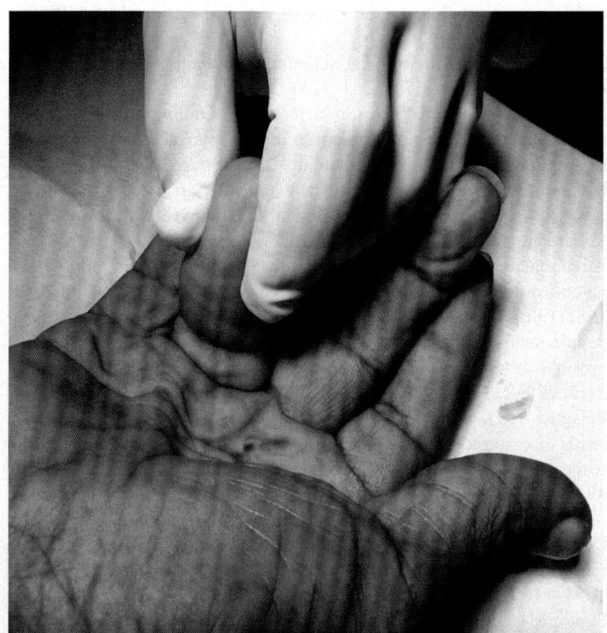

B
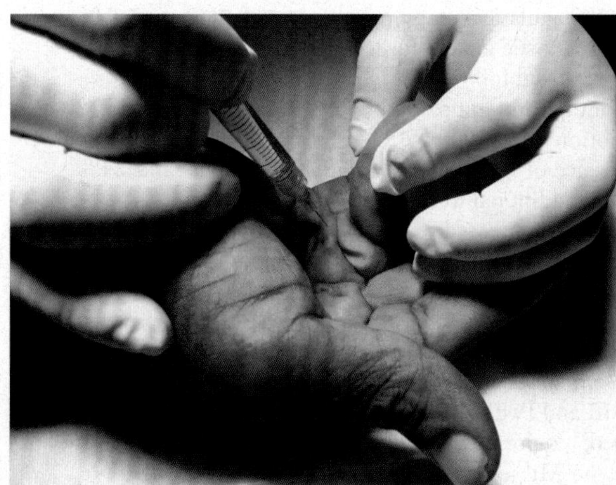

C
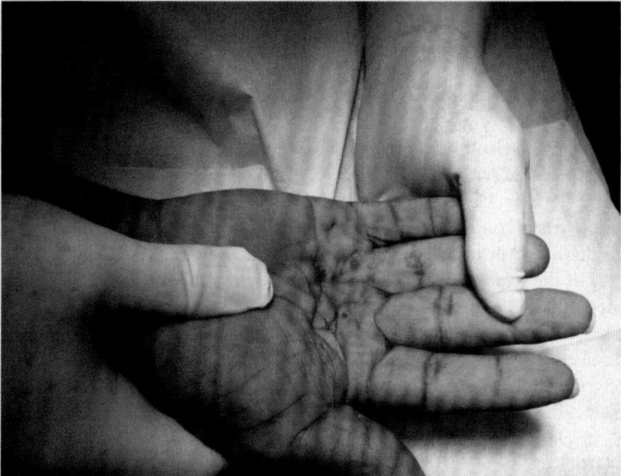

TECH FIG 5 • **A.** A patient with a large Dupuytren cord causing contracture of both the MP and PIP joints. **B.** A 25-gauge needle is used to inject 0.1 to 0.2 mL of 1% lidocaine immediately under the skin. The needle is then used to release the cord as described. **C.** The ring finger is gently manipulated into extension releasing the contracture at both the MP and PIP joints.

PEARLS AND PITFALLS

- A spiral nerve can be predicted with 90% reliability if there is a soft, pulpy mass of skin lying between the distal palmar crease and the proximal finger crease.[60]
- If this soft, pulpy mass is present, perform the fasciotomy proximally at the level of the transverse fibers only.[20]
- Patients will report a strong electrical shock sensation if the nerve is touched.
- If the fingertip becomes numb from the use of local anesthetic, move to a more proximal portal.[19]
- Traction on the skin or nodule is safer than pulling on the fingertips. The flexor tendons should remain relaxed.
- Repeatedly check for nerve or tendon involvement during the procedure.
- Change to a fresh needle and new portal if you no longer feel a grating sensation.

POSTOPERATIVE CARE

- A Band-Aid or light dressing covers the wound for 24 hours.
- Ice and elevate the hand for 48 hours.
- Avoid strenuous gripping for 1 week.
- Skin tears are treated with a light dressing and local wound care until healed.
- Patients are instructed to avoid painful activity.
- Postoperative therapy is rarely necessary.
- A night splint is worn for 1 month.[47]

OUTCOMES

- Patients with diseases such as rheumatoid arthritis, and diabetes, anticoagulant therapy or a history of previous CRPS are bad prognostic factors for treatment.
- Foucher reported follow-up at 3.2 years.[21,22]
  - MP joint motion improved by 79%
  - PIP motion improved by 65%
  - Recurrence of DD occurred in 58% of patients and 24% required additional treatment.
- PNF has been compared to limited fasciectomy (LF).[66]
  - TPED improved 63% in the PNF group and 79% in the LF group.
  - LF recovery took from 21 to 58 days. Most PNF patients are using their hands optimally within 1 week.
  - Poor outcomes are reported in patients with Tubiana stage III and IV DD.
- Pess et al[54] reported initial correction of contractures of 99% at the MP joint and 89% at the PIP joint with PNF. Final follow-up was a minimum of 3 years and the correction was maintained in 72% of the MP joints and 31% of the PIP joints.[54]
- Five-year follow-up recurrence rates have been reported to be 84.9% for PNF compared to 20.9% for LF.[67]
- Comparison of PNF and collagenase demonstrate similar clinical outcomes in the short term.[48]
- Cost analysis comparing LF, PNF, and CCH demonstrate LF is not cost effective. PNF is cost effective if the success rate is high. CCH is cost effective if the cost per injection is significantly less than currently priced in the United States.[8,14,17,59]

COMPLICATIONS

- Vascular injury
- Nerve laceration
- Infection
- Skin tears
- Paresthesias
- CRPS type I
- Increased postoperative pain requiring analgesics
- False aneurysm[63]
- FDP injury (0.05%)[63]

REFERENCES

1. Anthony SG, Lozano-Calderon SA, Simmons BP, et al. Gender ratio of Dupuytren's disease in the modern U.S. population. Hand 2008; 3(2):87–90.
2. Arafa M, Noble J, Royle SG, et al. Dupuytren's and epilepsy revisited. J Hand Surg Br 1992;17(2):221–224.
3. Arkkila PE, Koskinen PJ, Kantola IM, et al. Dupuytren's disease in type I diabetic subjects: investigation of biochemical markers of type III and I collagen. Clin Exp Rheumatol 2000;18(2):215–219.
4. Badalamente MA, Hurst LC. Efficacy and safety of injectable mixed collagenase subtypes in the treatment of Dupuytren's contracture. J Hand Surg Am 2007;32(6):767–774.
5. Badalamente MA, Hurst LC, Sampson SP. Prostaglandins influence myofibroblast contractility in Dupuytren's disease. J Hand Surg Am 1988;13(6):867–871.
6. Badalamente MA, Sampson SP, Hurst LC, et al. The role of transforming growth factor beta in Dupuytren's disease. J Hand Surg Am 1996; 21(2):210–215.
7. Balaguer T, David S, Ihrai T, et al. Histological staging and Dupuytren's disease recurrence or extension after surgical treatment: a retrospective study of 124 patients. J Hand Surg Eur Vol 2009;34(4): 493–496.
8. Baltzer H, Binhammer PA. Cost-effectiveness in the management of Dupuytren's contracture. A Canadian cost-utility analysis of current and future management strategies. Bone Joint J 2013;95-B(8): 1094–1100.
9. Bisson MA, Beckett KS, McGrouther DA, et al. Transforming growth factor-beta1 stimulation enhances Dupuytren's fibroblast contraction in response to uniaxial mechanical load within a 3-dimensional collagen gel. J Hand Surg Am 2009;34(6):1102–1110.
10. Black EM, Blazar PE. Dupuytren disease: an evolving understanding of an age-old disease. J Am Acad Orthop Surg 2011;19(12): 746–757.
11. Bower M, Nelson M, Gazzard BG. Dupuytren's contractures in patients infected with HIV. BMJ 1990;300(6718):164–165.
12. Burge P, Hoy G, Regan P, et al. Smoking, alcohol and the risk of Dupuytren's contracture. J Bone Joint Surg Br 1997;79(2):206–210.
13. Cagliero E, Apruzzese W, Perlmutter GS, et al. Musculoskeletal disorders of the hand and shoulder in patients with diabetes mellitus. Am J Med 2002;112(6):487–490.
14. Chen NC, Shauver MJ, Chung KC. Cost-effectiveness of open partial fasciectomy, needle aponeurotomy, and collagenase injection for dupuytren contracture. J Hand Surg Am 2011;36(11):1826–1834.e1832.
15. Chiu HF, McFarlane RM. Pathogenesis of Dupuytren's contracture: a correlative clinical-pathological study. J Hand Surg Am 1978;3(1): 1–10.
16. Coleman S, Gilpin D, Kaplan FT, et al. Efficacy and safety of concurrent collagenase clostridium histolyticum injections for multiple Dupuytren contractures. J Hand Surg Am 2014;39(1):57–64.

17. De Salas-Cansado M, Cuadros M, Del Cerro M, et al. Budget impact analysis in Spanish patients with Dupuytren's contracture: fasciectomy vs. collagenase Clostridium histolyticum. Chir Main 2013;32(2): 68–73.
18. Diaz R, Curtin C. Needle aponeurotomy for the treatment of Dupuytren's disease. Hand Clin 2014;30(1):33–38.
19. Eaton C. Percutaneous fasciotomy for Dupuytren's contracture. J Hand Surg Am 2011;36(5):910–915.
20. Foucher G, Medina J, Malizos K. Percutaneous needle fasciotomy in dupuytren disease. Tech Hand Up Extrem Surg 2001;5(3):161–164.
21. Foucher G, Medina J, Navarro R. Percutaneous needle aponeurotomy. Complications and results [in French]. Chir Main 2001;20(3): 206–211.
22. Foucher G, Medina J, Navarro R. Percutaneous needle aponeurotomy: complications and results. J Hand Surg Br 2003;28(5):427–431.
23. Gabbiani G, Majino G. Dupuytren's contracture: fibroblast contraction? An ultrastructural study. Am J Pathol 1972;66:131–138.
24. Godtfredsen NS, Lucht H, Prescott E, et al. A prospective study linked both alcohol and tobacco to Dupuytren's disease. J Clin Epidemiol 2004;57(8):858–863.
25. Gudmundsson KG, Arngrimsson R, Jonsson T. Dupuytren's disease, alcohol consumption and alcoholism. Scand J Prim Health Care 2001; 19(3):186–190.
26. Hay DC, Louie DL, Earp BE, et al. Surgical findings in the treatment of Dupuytren's disease after initial treatment with clostridial collagenase (Xiaflex). J Hand Surg Eur Vol 2013;39(5):463–465.
27. Hayton MJ, Bayat A, Chapman DS, et al. Isolated and spontaneous correction of proximal interphalangeal joint contractures in Dupuytren's disease: an exploratory analysis of the efficacy and safety of collagenase collagenase Clostridium histolyticum. Clin Drug Investig 2013;33(12):905–912.
28. Hentz VR. Collagenase injections for treatment of Dupuytren disease. Hand Clin 2014;30(1):25–32.
29. Hindocha S, John S, Stanley JK, et al. The heritability of Dupuytren's disease: familial aggregation and its clinical significance. J Hand Surg Am 2006;31(2):204–210.
30. Hindocha S, Stanley JK, Watson S, et al. Dupuytren's diathesis revisited: evaluation of prognostic indicators for risk of disease recurrence. J Hand Surg Am 2006;31(10):1626–1634.
31. Hotchkiss RN, Peimer CA, Coleman SG, et al. Recurrence of Dupuytren contracture after nonsurgical treatment with collagenase Clostridium histolyticum: summary of 4-year CORDLESS data. Presented at the 68th Annual Meeting of the American Society for Surgery of the Hand, October 3–5, 2010, San Francisco, CA.
32. Hu FZ, Nystrom A, Ahmed A, et al. Mapping of an autosomal dominant gene for Dupuytren's contracture to chromosome 16q in a Swedish family. Clin Genet 2005;68(5):424–429.
33. Hueston JT. Enzymatic fasciotomy. Hand 1971;3(1):38–40.
34. Hurst LC, Badalamente MA, Hentz VR, et al. Injectable collagenase clostridium histolyticum for Dupuytren's contracture. N Engl J Med 2009;361(10):968–979.
35. Hurst LC, Badalamente MA, Makowski J. The pathobiology of Dupuytren's contracture: effects of prostaglandins on myofibroblasts. J Hand Surg Am 1986;11(1):18–23.
36. Hutchison RL, Rayan GM. Astley Cooper: his life and surgical contributions. J Hand Surg Am 2011;36(2):316–320.
37. Kaplan FT, Badalemente M, Hurst L, et al. Delayed manipulation following clostridial collagenase histolyticum injection for Dupuytren contracture. Presented at the 68th Annual Meeting of the American Society for Surgery of the Hand, October 3–5, 2013, San Francisco, CA.
38. Ketchum LD, Donahue TK. The injection of nodules of Dupuytren's disease with triamcinolone acetonide. J Hand Surg Am 2000; 25(6):1157–1162.
39. Lermusiaux J, Debeyre N. Le traitement médical de la maladie de Dupuytren. In: De Seze S, Ryckewaert A, Kahn MF, et al, eds. L' Actualité Rhumatologique. Paris, France: Expansion Scientifique, 1979: 338–343.
40. Logan AJ, Mason G, Dias J, et al. Can rock climbing lead to Dupuytren's disease? Br J Sports Med 2005;39(9):639–644.
41. Lucas G, Brichet A, Roquelaure Y, et al. Dupuytren's disease: personal factors and occupational exposure. Am J Ind Med 2008;51(1):9–15.
42. Luck JV. Dupuytren's contracture; a new concept of the pathogenesis correlated with surgical management. J Bone Joint Surg Am 1959; 41-A(4):635–664.
43. McCarthy DM. The long-term results of enzymic fasciotomy. J Hand Surg Br 1992;17(3):356.
44. McFarlane RM. Patterns of the diseased fascia in the fingers in Dupuytren's contracture. Displacement of the neurovascular bundle. Plast Reconstr Surg 1974;54(1):31–44.
45. McMillan C, Binhammer P. Steroid injection and needle aponeurotomy for Dupuytren contracture: a randomized, controlled study. J Hand Surg Am 2012;37(7):1307–1312.
46. Medjoub K, Jawad A. The use of multiple needle fasciotomy in Dupuytren disease: retrospective observational study of outcome and patient satisfaction. Ann Plast Surg 2014;72(4):417–422.
47. Meinel A. Long-term static overnight extension splinting following percutaneous needle fasciotomy [in German]. Handchir Mikrochir Plast Chir 2011;43(5):286–288.
48. Nydick JA, Olliff BW, Garcia MJ, et al. A comparison of percutaneous needle fasciotomy and collagenase injection for dupuytren disease. J Hand Surg Am 2013;38(12):2377–2380.
49. O'Gorman DB, Vi L, Gan BS. Molecular mechanisms and treatment strategies for Dupuytren's disease. Ther Clin Risk Manag 2010;6: 383–390.
50. Peimer CA, Blazar P, Coleman S, et al. Dupuytren contracture recurrence following treatment with collagenase clostridium histolyticum (CORDLESS study): 3-year data. J Hand Surg Am 2013;38(1): 12–22.
51. Peimer CA, McGoldrick CA, Fiore GJ. Nonsurgical treatment of Dupuytren's contracture: 1-year US post-marketing safety data for collagenase clostridium histolyticum. Hand 2012;7(2):143–146.
52. Peimer CA, McGoldrick CA, Kaufman G. Nonsurgical treatment of dupuytren contracture: 3-year safety results using collagenase *Clostridium histolyticum*. Presented at the 68th Annual Meeting of the American Society for Surgery of the Hand, October 3–5, 2013, San Francisco, CA.
53. Peimer CA, Skodny P, Mackowiak JI. Collagenase clostridium histolyticum for dupuytren contracture: patterns of use and effectiveness in clinical practice. J Hand Surg Am 2013;38(12):2370–2376.
54. Pess GM, Pess RM, Pess RA. Results of needle aponeurotomy for Dupuytren contracture in over 1,000 fingers. J Hand Surg Am 2012; 37(4):651–656.
55. Rayan GM. Clinical presentation and types of Dupuytren's disease. Hand Clin 1999;15(1):87–96, vii.
56. Rayan GM, Parizi M, Tomasek JJ. Pharmacologic regulation of Dupuytren's fibroblast contraction in vitro. J Hand Surg Am 1996; 21(6):1065–1070.
57. Reilly RM, Stern PJ, Goldfarb CA. A retrospective review of the management of Dupuytren's nodules. J Hand Surg Am 2005;30(5): 1014–1018.
58. Rombouts JJ, Noel H, Legrain Y, et al. Prediction of recurrence in the treatment of Dupuytren's disease: evaluation of a histologic classification. J Hand Surg Am 1989;14(4):644–652.
59. Sanjuan Cerveró R, Franco Ferrando N, Poquet Jornet J. Use of resources and costs associated with the treatment of Dupuytren's contracture at an orthopedics and traumatology surgery department in Denia (Spain): collagenase clostridium hystolyticum versus subtotal fasciectomy. BMC Musculoskelet Disord 2013;14:293.
60. Short WH, Watson HK. Prediction of the spiral nerve in Dupuytren's contracture. J Hand Surg Am 1982;7(1):84–86.
61. Starkweather KD, Lattuga S, Hurst LC, et al. Collagenase in the treatment of Dupuytren's disease: an in vitro study. J Hand Surg Am 1996;21(3):490–495.
62. Swanson JW, Watt AJ, Vedder NB. Skin graft loss resulting from collagenase clostridium histolyticum treatment of Dupuytren contracture: case report and review of the literature. J Hand Surg Am 2013;38(3):548–551.
63. Symes T, Stothard J. Two significant complications following percutaneous needle fasciotomy in a patient on anticoagulants. J Hand Surg Br 2006;31(6):606–607.
64. Thomas PR, Clarke D. Vibration white finger and Dupuytren's contracture: are they related? Occup Med 1992;42(3):155–158.

65. Tubiana R. Surgical management. In: Tubiana R, ed. The Hand. Philadelphia: WB Saunders Company, 1999:480.
66. van Rijssen AL, Gerbrandy FS, Ter Linden H, et al. A comparison of the direct outcomes of percutaneous needle fasciotomy and limited fasciectomy for Dupuytren's disease: a 6-week follow-up study. J Hand Surg Am 2006;31(5):717–725.
67. van Rijssen AL, ter Linden H, Werker PM. Five-year results of a randomized clinical trial on treatment in Dupuytren's disease: percutaneous needle fasciotomy versus limited fasciectomy. Plast Reconstr Surg 2012;129(2):469–477.
68. van Rijssen AL, Werker PM. Percutaneous needle fasciotomy for recurrent Dupuytren disease. J Hand Surg Am 2012;37(9): 1820–1823.
69. Verjee LS, Midwood K, Davidson D, et al. Myofibroblast distribution in Dupuytren's cords: correlation with digital contracture. J Hand Surg Am 2009;34(10):1785–1794.

Surgical Treatment of Dupuytren Disease

Ghazi Rayan

136

CHAPTER

DEFINITION

- Dupuytren disease (DD) is a fibroproliferative disorder that affects primarily the palmar fascia of the hand, with occasional secondary involvement of other areas in the hand as well as remote tissues.
- DD has a strong genetic origin that is suggested not only by population studies and family clustering but also by genome-wide association study,[15] which suggest that chromosomes 6, 11, and 16 may contain genes for the disease and that multiple other genes may be involved in its etiology.
- It is a sui generis condition that clinically and pathophysiologically resembles no other known condition.
- Although physiologically DD bears a resemblance to the processes associated with normal wound healing, the difference is the perpetual and progressive proliferation with abnormal collagen deposition and resultant tissue contracture.
- Attempts to classify DD under other headings such as inflammatory and neoplastic disorders have not been born out.

ANATOMY

- The radial; ulnar; and central aponeuroses, palmodigital fascia, and digital fascia are elements of the palmar fascia.[17]
- The radial aponeurosis has four components:
  - Thenar fascia, which is an extension of the central aponeuroses
  - Thumb pretendinous band, which is small and ill defined
  - Distal and the proximal commissural ligaments
- The ulnar aponeurosis has the following components:
  - Hypothenar muscle fascia, which is an extension of the central aponeurosis
  - Pretendinous band to the small finger, which is consistent and substantial
  - Abductor digiti minimi muscle confluence
  - Pisiform ligament complex
- The central aponeurosis is the core of DD activity and has a triangular shape with a proximal apex (**FIG 1A**).
  - Its fibers are oriented longitudinal, transverse, and vertical.
  - The longitudinal fibers fan out as pretendinous bands to the three central digits (index, middle, and ring). Each pretendinous band bifurcates distally and each bifurcation has three layers. The superficial layer inserts into the dermis, the middle layer continues to the digit as the spiral band, and the deep layer passes almost vertically dorsally toward the flexor tendon digital sheath.
  - The transverse fibers make up the natatory ligament (NL) located in the distal palm and the transverse ligament of the palmar aponeurosis (TLPA). The TLPA is proximal and parallel to the NL (**FIG 1B**) and lies deep to the pretendinous bands. Its distal radial extent is the proximal commissural ligament. The TLPA gives origin to the septa of Legueu and Juvara, which protect the neurovascular structures and provide an additional proximal pulley to the flexor tendons.
  - The vertical fibers of the central aponeurosis are the minute but strong vertical bands of Grapow and the septa

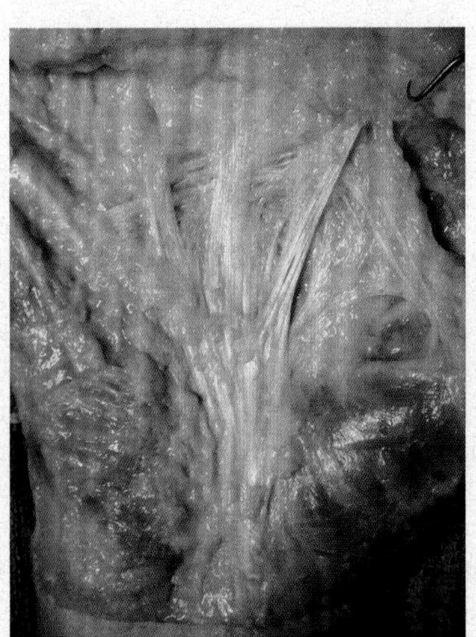

A

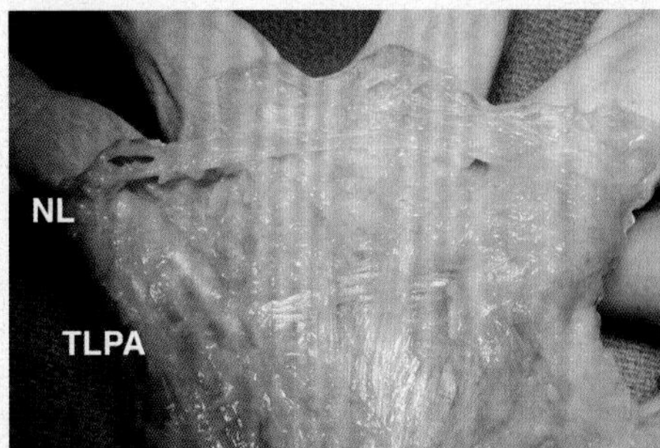

B

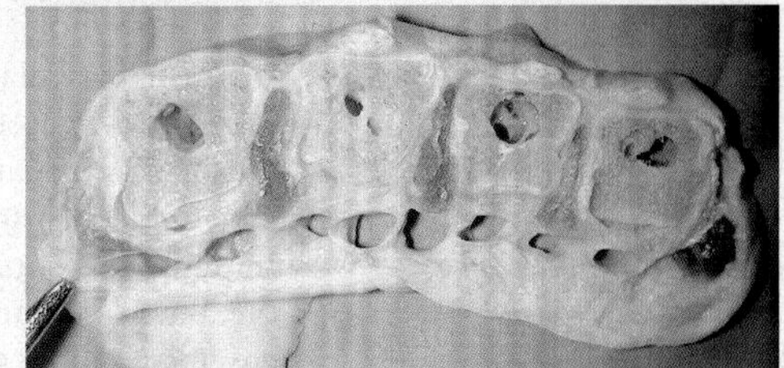

C

FIG 1 • **A.** The central aponeurosis is the core of DD activity and has a triangular shape with a proximal apex. **B.** The transverse fibers make up the natatory ligament (*NL*) located in the distal palm and the transverse ligament of the palmar aponeurosis (*TLPA*). **C.** There are eight septa of Legueu and Juvara that form seven fibro-osseous compartments of two types: four flexor septal canals that contain the flexor tendons and three web space canals that contain common digital nerves and arteries and lumbrical muscles. *(continued)*

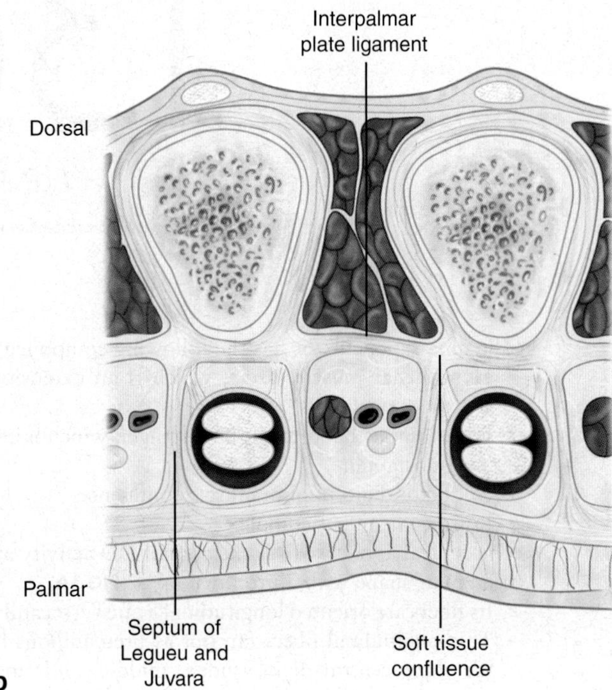

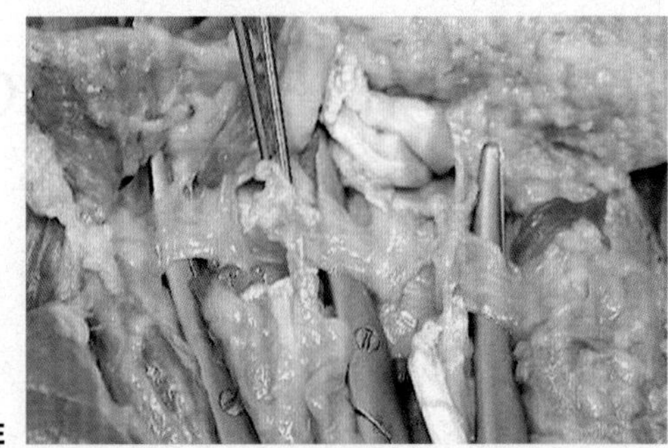

FIG 1 • *(continued)* **D.** IPPL and septum of Legueu and Juvara. **E.** There are three IPPLs: radial (to the *left*), central, and ulnar (to the *right*). These form the floor of the three web space canals.

of Legueu and Juvara (**FIG 1C,D**), which lie deep to the palmar fascia. There are eight of these septa that form seven fibro-osseous compartments[3] of two types: four flexor septal canals that contain the flexor tendons and three web space canals that contain common digital nerves and arteries and lumbrical muscles. These septa insert in a soft tissue confluence that consists of five structures: A1 pulley, palmar plate, sagittal band, interpalmar plate ligament (IPPL; **FIG 1D,E**), and septum of Legueu and Juvara.

- The palmodigital fascia encompasses a number of fascial structures, including the terminal fibers of the pretendinous bands, the spiral bands, the beginning of the lateral digital sheet, and the NL. The middle layer of the bifurcated pretendinous band spirals about 90 degrees and the peripheral fibers run vertically adjacent to the metacarpophalangeal (MCP) joint. They continue distally deep to the neurovascular bundle and NL and emerge distal to this ligament and contribute to the formation of the lateral digital sheet. The proximal fibers of the NL run in a transverse plane, but the distal fibers form a "U" that continues longitudinally along both sides of the digit, forming the lateral digital sheet. The lateral digital sheet therefore has deep and superficial contributions from the spiral band and NL.
- The digital fascia surrounds the neurovascular bundle in the digit and this includes the Grayson ligaments (palmar), the Cleland ligaments (dorsal), the Gosset lateral digital sheet laterally, and possibly fibers from the checkrein ligaments medially and dorsally, which were described previously as the Thomine retrovascular fascia.

PATHOGENESIS

- In DD, normal bands become diseased cords,[13] and Dupuytren nodules and cords are pathognomonic of the disease.[14]
- A nodule usually appears first, followed by the cord.
- The cords form in the palmar, palmodigital, or digital regions and progressively shorten, leading to joint and soft tissue contractures.
- The Grapow vertical bands become microcords, leading to thickening of the skin, which is one of the earliest manifestations of DD.
- Skin pits develop from the diseased first layer of the split pretendinous band.
- The pretendinous cord develops from the pretendinous band and is the most common cord in DD. It leads to MCP joint flexion deformity and often extends distally, contributing to the digital cords. The pretendinous cord may bifurcate distally with each branch extending into a different digit, forming a commissural Y cord (**FIG 2**).
- The vertical cords, or diseased septa of Legueu and Juvara,[2] are short and thick. They are connected to the pretendinous cord and extend deeply in between the neurovascular bundle and flexor tendon fibrous sheath.
- Extensive palmar fascial disease is encountered in severe conditions and affects larger areas of the palm, leading to diffuse thickening of many components of the palmar fascial complex.
- The spiral cord has four components: the pretendinous band, the spiral band, the lateral digital sheet, and the Grayson ligament. It is encountered most often in the small finger, but it may be present in the ring finger.
  - In the palm, this cord is located superficial to the neurovascular bundle. Distal to the MCP joint, it passes deep to the neurovascular bundle, and in the digit, it runs lateral to the neurovascular bundle as it involves the lateral digital sheet and again becomes superficial to the neurovascular bundle as it involves the Grayson ligament.
  - Initially, the cord spirals around the neurovascular bundle, but as it contracts, the cord straightens and the neurovascular bundle spirals around the cord.

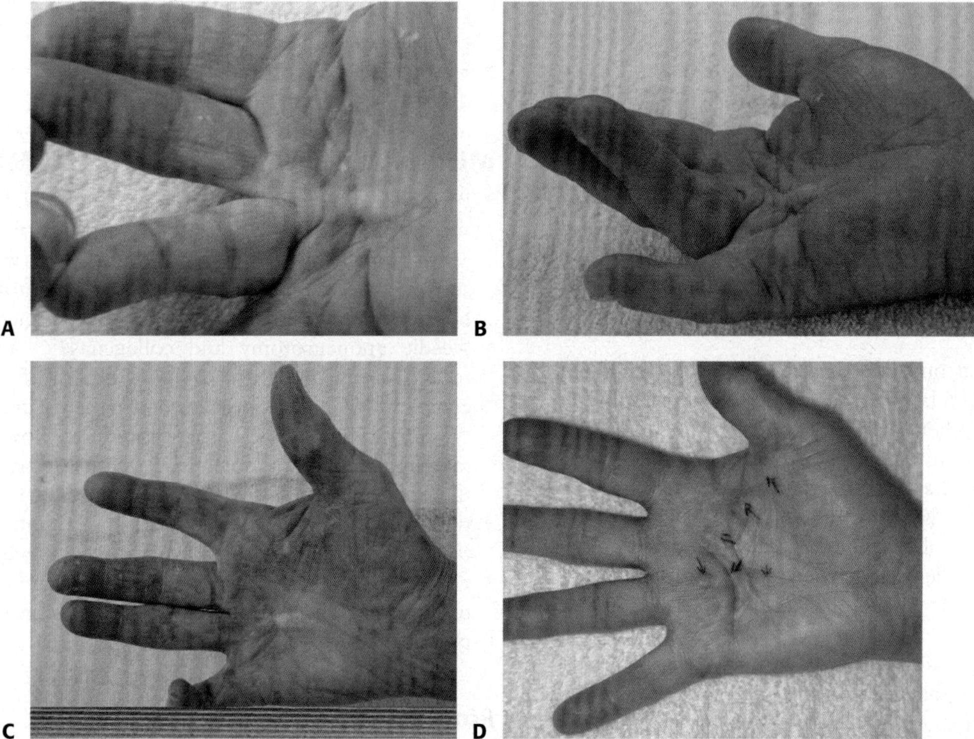

FIG 2 • **A,B.** Pretendinous cord and a nodule in the palm in line with the ring finger causing MCP flexion contracture. **C.** Two pretendinous cords in the palm in line with the small and ring fingers causing MCP and PIP flexion contracture of the small finger. A small proximal commissural cord in the first web space is also present. **D.** Diffuse Dupuytren palmar fascial disease is present with nodular thickening in the entire palm.

  - The distorted anatomy of the neurovascular bundle, which is displaced medially and centrally, and later also proximally, is at risk for injury during surgery.[23]
- The natatory cord develops from the NL, converting the U-shaped web space fibers into a V shape, resulting in contracture of the second to fourth web spaces.
  - This cord extends along the dorsal lateral aspect of the adjacent digits and is best detected by passively abducting the digits and at the same time flexing one digit and extending the other at the MCP joints.
- The most commonly encountered digital cord is the lateral cord, followed by the central and spiral cords. These are responsible for proximal interphalangeal (PIP) joint flexion contractures.
  - The central cord is an extension of the pretendinous cord in the palm.
  - The lateral cord originates from the lateral digital sheet and attaches to the skin or to the flexor tendon sheath near the Grayson ligament. The lateral cord causes a contracture of the PIP joint but can also rarely cause a distal interphalangeal joint contracture.
- The abductor digiti minimi cord, also known as the *isolated digital cord*, takes origin from the abductor digiti minimi tendon but may also arise from adjacent muscle fascia at the base of the proximal phalanx.
  - It courses superficial to the neurovascular bundle and infrequently entraps and displaces the bundle toward the midline.
  - It inserts on the ulnar side of the base of the middle phalanx but may attach on the radial side or have an additional insertion in the base of the distal phalanx, causing a distal interphalangeal joint contracture.
- The distal commissural cord develops from the diseased distal commissural ligament, which is the radial extension of the NL. The proximal commissural cord originates from the proximal commissural ligament, which is the radial extension of the TLPA.
  - Both of these cords cause first web space contracture.
- The thumb pretendinous cord originates from the thumb pretendinous band and causes thumb MCP joint flexion deformity, which is uncommon.

NATURAL HISTORY

- DD has three clinical phases: early, intermediate, and late.[16]
  - Skin changes with loss of normal architecture and skin pitting characterize the early phase.
  - Nodules and cords form during the intermediate phase.
  - Contractures mark the late phase, with the MCP joint most frequently affected, followed by the PIP joint.

PATIENT HISTORY AND PHYSICAL FINDINGS

- The classic DD patient is a Caucasian man with a positive family history. The condition is bilateral and progressive and may extend to the digits, leading to their contracture.
- Palmar involvement usually precedes disease extension into the digits, but the disease may begin and remain in the digits.
  - The ring finger is the most commonly involved digit, followed in order of frequency by the small, middle, and index fingers, and last by the thumb.

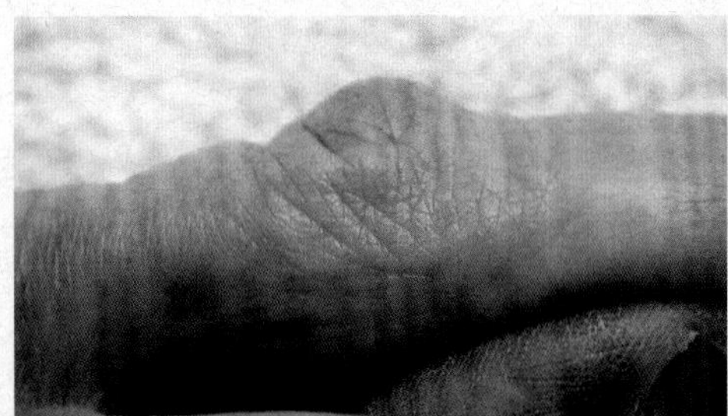

FIG 3 • A Garrod node over the dorsum of the PIP joint.

- DD may affect areas outside the palmar surface of the hand.
  - Ectopic disease can be either regional in the upper extremity or distant in other parts of the body.
  - Garrod nodes are different from knuckle pads, occur on the dorsum of the hand, and are almost always limited to the finger (**FIG 3**). We have shown that DD nodules are pathognomonic of DD, whereas knuckle pads demonstrate similar prevalence in normal and DD populations.[18]
  - Distant ectopic DD affects the plantar fascia and male genitals.
- Patients said to express a Dupuytren diathesis or genetic predisposition typically have faster and more severe development of the condition.
  - Positive family history
  - Young age of onset
  - Ectopic sites of fibromatosis such as the dorsal digital area (Garrod nodes), plantar fascia (Ledderhose disease), and male genitals (Peyronie disease)

DIFFERENTIAL DIAGNOSIS

- Non-DD[19]
  - Occurs in a diverse ethnic group, is unilateral and nonprogressive, usually involves a single digit, and frequently follows trauma or surgery
  - Patients with this disease rarely require surgical treatment. Confusing this with DD will produce contrasting epidemiologic data.
- Epithelioid sarcoma
- Occupational thickening and callus formation that mimic Dupuytren nodules
- Palmar subcutaneous soft tissue lesions, such as localized pigmented villonodular synovitis, palmar ganglions, and inclusion cysts
- Stenosing tenosynovitis without triggering can be associated with thickening and adherence of the skin to the underlying flexor tendon sheath.
- Prominent flexor tendons can be confused with pretendinous cords because of attenuation of annular pulleys, as seen in rheumatoid arthritis.

NONOPERATIVE MANAGEMENT

- No treatment is necessary for non-DD.
- Observation is appropriate for nonprogressive DD with minimal contracture and without compromise of function.
  - Surgical treatment for minor disease or pitting can result in a disease flare and must be avoided.
- Basic science research has shown the potential of certain local agents in the treatment of DD. These include calcium channel blockers, nifedipine, and verapamil,[20] especially for early stages of the disease.
- Steroid injection of nodules has been used to suppress the disease.

MINIMALLY INVASIVE TREATMENT METHODS

- Percutaneous fasciotomy was used initially by the British surgeon Sir Astley Cooper in the early 19th century. The appeal for this procedure has recently reemerged in the pursuit of lower morbidity and fewer complications that may be encountered with conventional open surgical treatment.
- Needle aponeurotomy and collagenase[1,10] injection have recently been used for DD more broadly by treating surgeons and gained appeal among patients because of their "noninvasive" nature. These procedures, however, are mistakenly labeled as nonoperative treatment methods. In fact, these are minimally invasive procedures, which create distinct deep soft tissue wounds with the potential for accidental injury to neurovascular structures or infection.
- For elderly patients with comorbidities, minimally invasive procedures especially percutaneous fasciotomy can be a practical approach for the treatment of DD.

Procedures

Needle Aponeurotomy

- Needle aponeurotomy[6] can be done as an office procedure or outpatient setting.
- Area(s) of percutaneous release in the palm or digit is infiltrated with intradermal anesthetic using 2% lidocaine, avoiding the initiation of digital nerve block. Multiple needle entry portals are made directly over the palpable cord. The combination of puncturing and sweeping motions is made by the tip of a short, 25-gauge needle beneath the skin. Accidental nerve and flexor tendon injuries can be prevented by repeatedly checking fingertip sensibility and active finger motion.
- Passive manipulation of the contracted digit will complete the fasciotomy by elongating or rupturing the diseased cord. This will regain varying amounts of digital extension depending on the severity of cords and contracture.
- Dressings are applied and the hand can be splinted if necessary for 1 week for comfort. During this time, the patient performs active exercises out of the splint three times a day. If a splint is not applied, the patient is allowed to use the hand for light activities but should avoid vigorous gripping for 1 week. If the cord does not rupture, an open procedure is done.
- Complications include failure to rupture the cord, possible neurovascular injury, and disease recurrence, with recurrence being common.
- Needle fasciotomy can be combined with limited partial fasciectomy (**FIG 4A–D**). This combined procedure is especially indicated for cases with a pretendinous cord having extension into the digit, such as a spiral cord in the palm and small finger. In this scenario, needle fasciotomy is done in the palm and a limited incision is made in the digit and the digital cord is excised while protecting the spiral nerve and vessels, which are located superficial. Needle aponeurotomy or collagenase injection in the digit in this case may injure the vulnerable neurovascular structures.

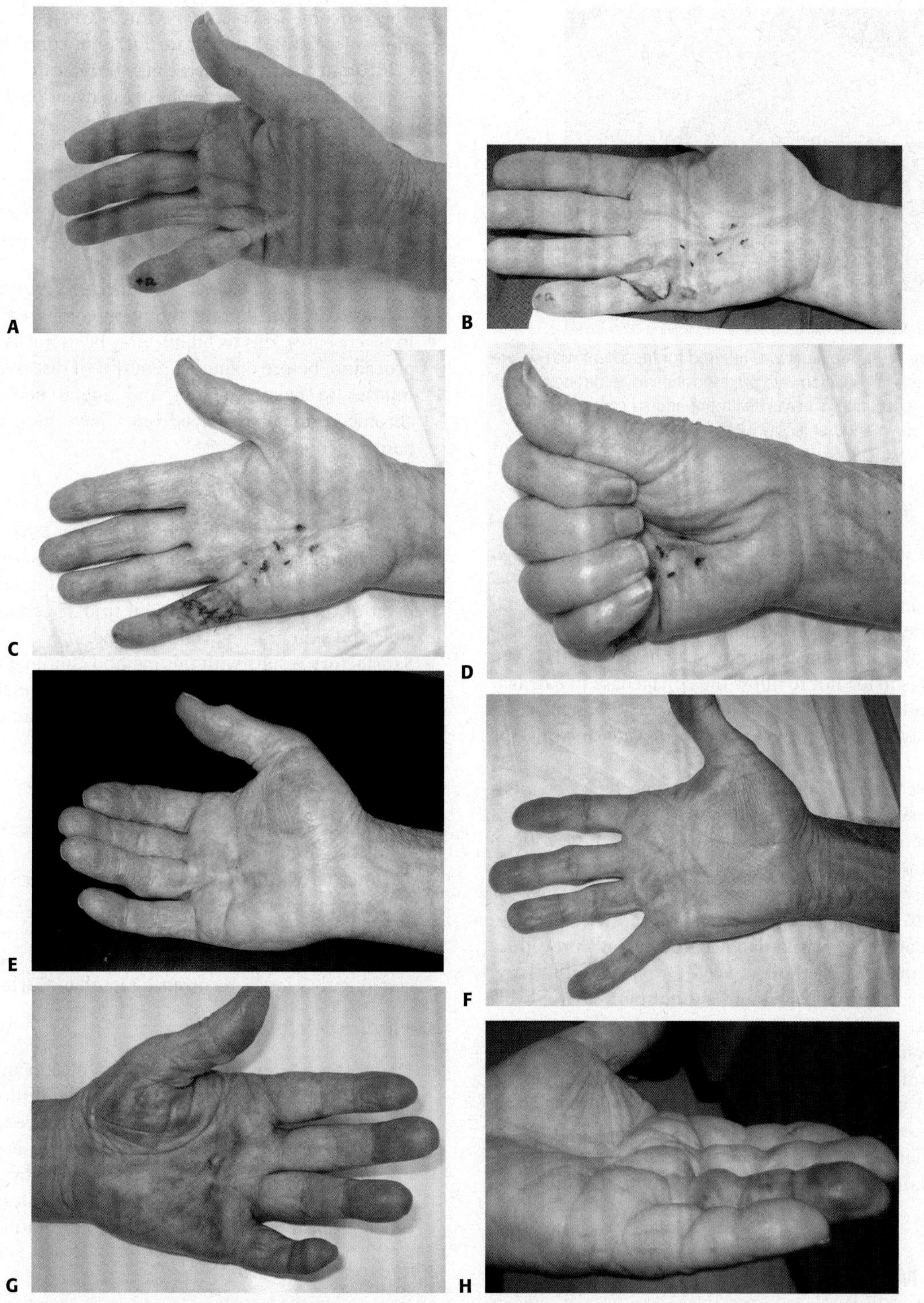

FIG 4 • A. A patient with DD pretendinous digital spiral cord affecting the small finger. **B.** Combined needle fasciotomy in the palm and limited open fasciectomy in the digit were done. **C.** Two weeks postoperatively, the patient had satisfactory correction of the flexion deformity. **D.** He had near full flexion. **E.** A patient with pretendinous cord in the palm along the ring finger with moderate MCP joint contracture, immediately after collagenase injection which is an ideal indication for this treatment. **F.** Six weeks after collagen injection showing satisfactory correction of the deformity. **G.** Second day after collagenase injection of a pretendinous cord showing the ecchymosis in the palm. **H.** Another patient the second day after collagenase injection of a nonspiral digital cord in the ring finger showing the digital ecchymosis. *(continued)*

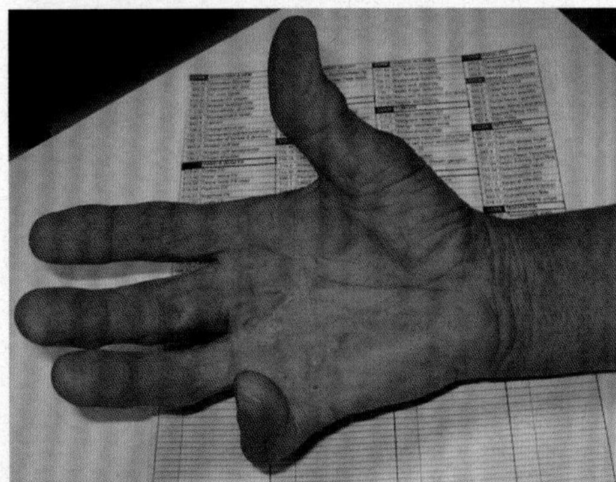

FIG 4 • *(continued)* **I.** A patient was referred for treatment with severe Dupuytren diathesis, a condition with predisposition to recurrence, showing disease recurrence, after surgical treatment and six collagenase injections, all were done in another facility.

Collagenase Injection

- Collagenase injection is a staged office procedure done on two separate consecutive days.
- During the first visit, the diseased pretendinous or digital cord is injected with a 10,000 units (0.58 mg) of collagenase clostridium histolyticum using an insulin syringe (**FIG 4E**). Every effort is made not to allow the collagenase to extravasate subcutaneously or deep to the cord. The patient is instructed to avoid applying pressure to the site or using the hand.
- During the second visit on the following day, finger manipulation is done by passive extension to rupture the cord and achieve extension. The manipulation is often performed with local anesthetic injected into the affected site(s).
- The hand is immobilized in a splint for night use for 4 weeks (**FIG 4F**). If the cord does not rupture, the procedure is repeated 4 weeks later. If the second procedure fails, then an open method is used 2 to 3 months later. Multiple cords in the same hand should be treated at different times.
- Complications include ecchymosis (**FIG 4G,H**), which is common and usually resolves within 3 weeks; failure to rupture the cord; possible infiltration of the collagenase into the flexor tendon, causing tendon rupture[26]; potential neurovascular injury; and disease recurrence, which is common especially among patients with Dupuytren diathesis (**FIG 4I**).

SURGICAL MANAGEMENT

- Surgery remains the most widely used treatment method for symptomatic DD especially in primary cases with severe and multiple digit involvement and in recurrent cases.
  - Outpatient surgery offers substantial savings and should be used in an otherwise healthy patient with moderate hand involvement.
  - Local, regional, or general anesthesia can be used depending on the procedure performed.
- Flexion contractures of the MCP joint of greater than 30 degrees and PIP flexion contractures of 15 degrees interfere with function and, in the presence of a well-developed cord, are indications for surgical treatment.
- The outcome after surgery for MCP joint contracture is more successful than that for PIP joint contracture.
  - PIP joint checkrein release may be indicated if 40 degrees of residual flexion is present after conventional fasciectomy.

Procedures

Percutaneous Fasciotomy

- Percutaneous fasciotomy is indicated for palmar cords in elderly unhealthy patients.
  - This technique carries a higher risk for complications when performed in the thumb as compared to the digits.
- In severe cases, this technique may be useful as a preliminary procedure before definitive removal of diseased tissue.
- Injuries to flexor tendons and digital nerves as well as chronic regional pain syndromes have been reported after percutaneous releases.

Open Palm Fasciectomy

- This method was first used by Dupuytren, who left the transverse palmar incision wound open after fasciectomy.
- Leaving the wound open is indicated for extensive involvement of the palmar fascia and if primary closure is not possible and skin grafting is not desired.
- Satisfactory results with this method continue to be reported in the literature,[8,12,25] including less pain, better motion, and low rates of complication. The primary disadvantage is prolonged postoperative wound healing.

Partial Fasciectomy

- Partial fasciectomy is the excision of the diseased tissue with preservation of normal-appearing fascia.
  - Other terms for this procedure are selective, regional, or limited fasciectomy.
- Partial fasciectomy remains the most widely used technique for treatment of DD among hand surgeons today. It is associated with a lower recurrence rate than fasciotomy.

Dermofasciectomy

- Dermofasciectomy involves excision of skin and diseased tissue simultaneously followed by grafting of the skin defect.[9]
- Dermofasciectomy is considered the procedure of choice by many surgeons for recurrent or aggressive disease with marked adherence of skin to underlying diseased cords. It was reported to have lower recurrence rates compared to other surgical techniques even for recurrent disease.[11]

Extensive Fasciectomy

- Extensive fasciectomy involves a wide, generous fasciectomy of diseased tissue involving most of the palmar fascial complex.
  - This can be combined if necessary with partial fasciectomy in the digits.
  - This technique is indicated when broad involvement of the palmar fascial complex is present.
  - The NL and TLPA may be involved in severe DD and these can be included in the extensive fasciectomy.
  - After extensive fasciectomy, the skin sometimes can be closed primarily. If a defect is present, the wound can be skin grafted or left open.

- Total or radical fasciectomy entails removal of the entire diseased and normal palmar fascia with or without excision of the overlying skin.
  - This highly morbid, radical approach is rarely indicated.

Positioning

- The patient is positioned supine and the hand is placed on a hand table with the shoulder abducted 90 degrees.
- A padded pneumatic tourniquet is placed on the arm as proximally as possible. The upper extremity is exsanguinated and the tourniquet is inflated to 250 mm Hg.

Approach

- The most commonly used incision is the zigzag Brunner incision (**FIG 5A**).
- A midline longitudinal incision that is closed with multiple Z-plasties can be also used (**FIG 5B**).
- Transverse palmar incisions can be used for the open palm method or for removal of extensive palmar fascial complex disease.
- Local rotation flaps sometimes should be used to cover exposed flexor tendons or neurovascular structures, and the remaining secondary defect can be grafted with full-thickness skin.

A 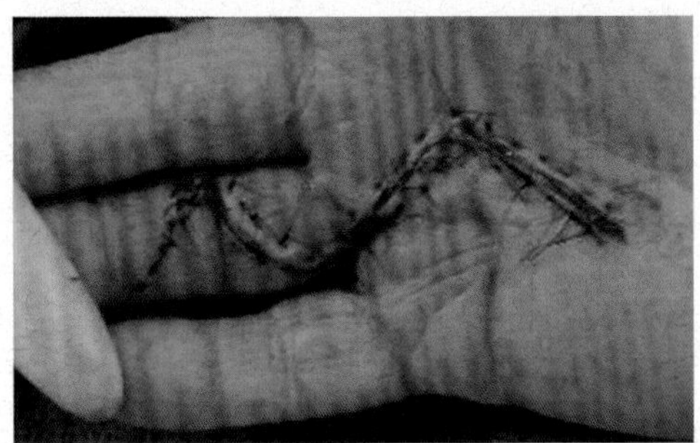

B 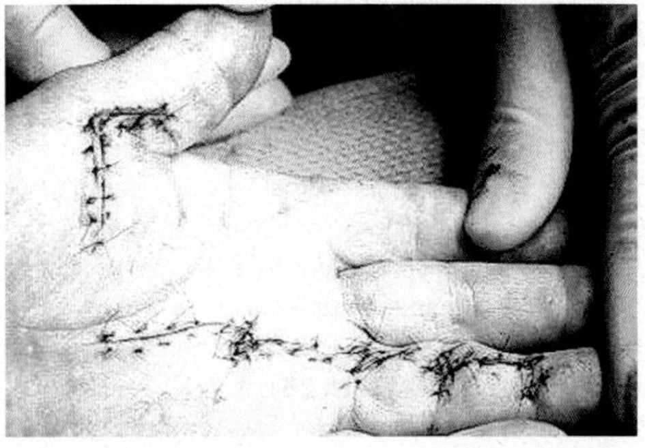

FIG 5 • **A.** Partial fasciectomy through a zigzag Brunner incision. **B.** A longitudinal incision closed with multiple Z-plasties.

Percutaneous Fasciotomy

- Local anesthesia is used.
- A tourniquet is not necessary.
- Select the point of fasciotomy adjacent to the cord.
- Use a no. 11 blade held vertically (**TECH FIG 1**).
- Make a stab wound and turn the blade horizontally to cut the cord while the digit is manually extended.
- A gratifying snap is felt and the finger should extend.

TECH FIG 1 • The no. 11 blade is used to incise the midline cord to improve the PIP joint contracture in this elderly patient.

Open Palm Fasciectomy

- Make a transverse incision in the middle of the palm and extend it if necessary to the digits as a zigzag Brunner incision.
- Undermine the skin flaps and identify the diseased tissue.
- Carry the dissection proximally until a transition between normal and diseased fascia is identified.
  - Isolate the neurovascular structures from the diseased tissue and protect them.
  - Release the diseased tissue proximally; dissection is followed distally and excised.
- The transverse incision is left open to heal by secondary intention but close the extensions of the original incision into the fingers.
- Apply nonadherent gauze to the wound and immobilize the hand in a forearm-based splint with the fingers in extension.

Partial Fasciectomy

- Make a zigzag Brunner incision; it may extend from the proximal palm to the digital pulp in cases of palmar and digital disease. By making the incisions pass through skin pits, the risk of buttonholes is reduced during flap elevation.
- Undermine the skin flaps by careful dissection to separate relatively normal dermis from the diseased tissue. This can be difficult in recurrent cases. Make every effort not to buttonhole the flaps.
- It is better to leave diseased tissue in the dermal flap rather than thinning the flap too much and running the risk of buttonholing the flap.
- Identify the neurovascular structures, dissect them from the diseased cords, retract them, and protect them during the entire procedure (**TECH FIG 2A**).
- Begin the dissection proximally in the palm until a transition between relatively normal and diseased fascia is identified.
- Carry the dissection in a proximal to distal direction.
- Transect the pretendinous cord proximally and follow the cord distally, dividing all connections to adjacent normal fascia.
- If present, include in the excised tissue a vertical cord from the diseased septa of Legueu and Juvara and a natatory cord from the diseased NL (**TECH FIG 2B**).
- Special attention must be given to a spiral cord which originates from spiral band (**TECH FIG 2C**) to prevent injury to the digital nerve and vessel, which are intertwined with and spiraled around the diseased cord.
- If the diseased tissue is confined to the palm in the form of a pretendinous cord, the distal end of the cord can be seen inserted onto the flexor tendon sheath distal to the MCP joint. The cord can be excised at this level.
- If the diseased tissue extends to the digit, follow the digital cord into the finger.
  - Pretendinous cord extension in the digit can be in the form of lateral, central, or spiral cord.
  - The digital cord must be dissected in the finger with great care because of its proximity to the neurovascular bundle.
  - Identify and release the distal insertion of the digital cord.
- Release the tourniquet and coagulate bleeders with a bipolar forceps.
- After adequate hemostasis is achieved, close the wound without a drain.
- If skin shortage is present, particularly in the finger, perform full-thickness skin grafting.
- If the neurovascular bundle or flexor tendons are exposed, a flap may be rotated to cover these structures and skin grafting is done for the secondary defect (**TECH FIG 2D,E**).
- A palmar plaster splint with the digits in the corrected extended position is used for 1 week or less.

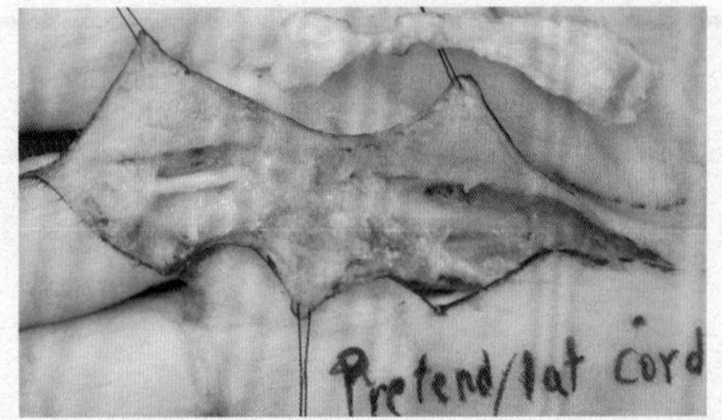

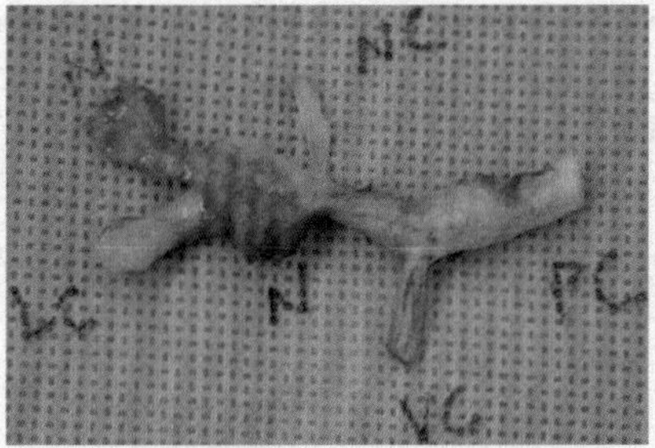

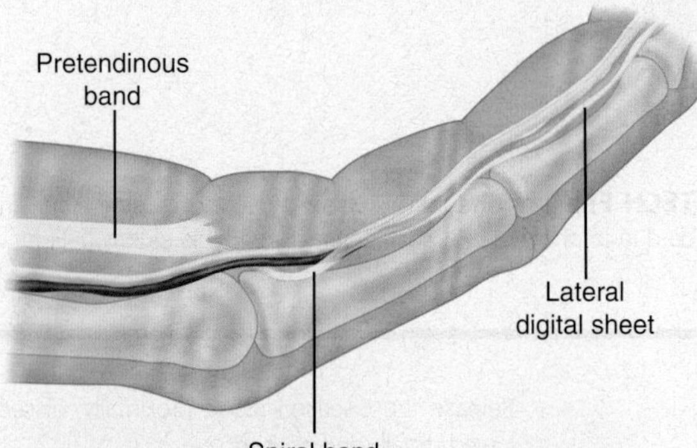

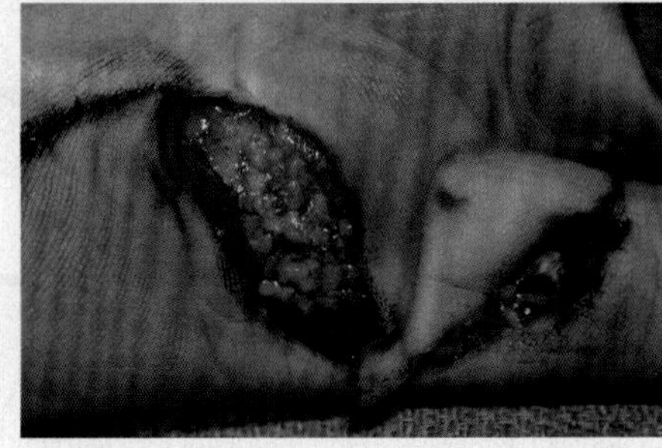

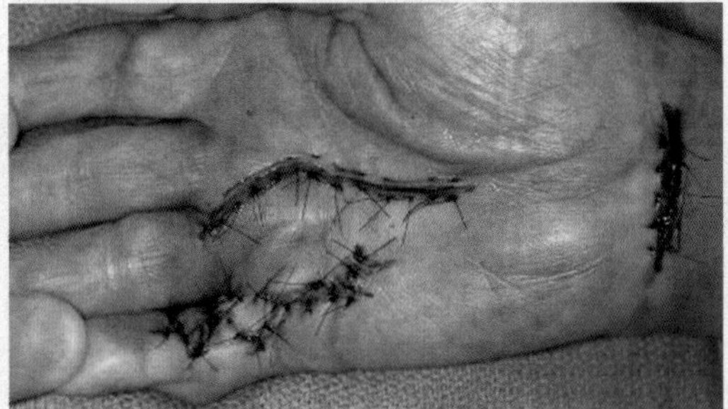

TECH FIG 2 • **A.** The neurovascular structures are dissected and protected during surgery. **B.** An excised specimen showing pretendinous (*PC*), vertical (*VC*), natatory (*NC*), nodule (*N*), and lateral (*LC*) cords. **C.** With a spiral cord, care must be taken to prevent injury to the digital nerve and vessel, which are intertwined with and spiraled around the diseased cord. **D.** A local flap is rotated to cover neurovascular structures. **E.** Skin shortage in the small finger was covered with a full-thickness skin graft from the volar wrist.

Dermofasciectomy

- Plan the incision by mapping the area of diseased tissue and skin with a marker. The remaining exposure is done through a zigzag Brunner incision that extends from the dermofascial island (**TECH FIG 3**).
- Remove the diseased fascia and adherent overlying skin as one component.
- Close the zigzag Brunner incision and cover the skin defect with full-thickness skin graft from the volar wrist.

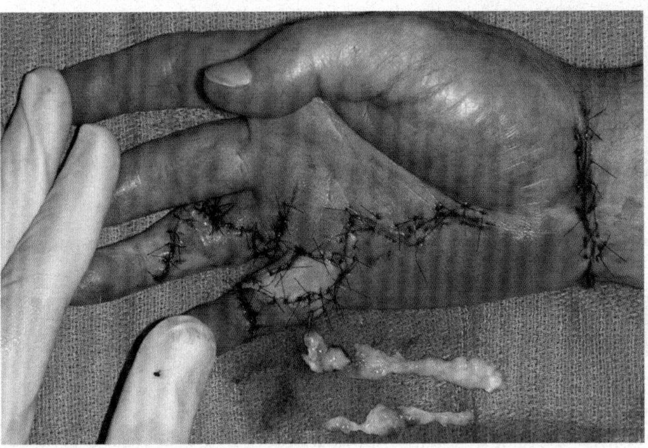

TECH FIG 3 • In a patient with recurrent DD with two pretendinous cords in the palm in line with the small and ring fingers causing severe MCP and PIP flexion contracture of the small finger, dermofasciectomy was done for the small finger and partial fasciectomy through a zigzag Brunner incision was done for the ring finger. Correction of the contractures was achieved. Skin shortage in the small finger was covered with a full-thickness skin graft from the volar wrist.

Extensive Fasciectomy

- Make either a transverse incision in the middle of the palm or a U-shaped incision in the distal palm (**TECH FIG 4A**).
- The incision has two limbs extending proximally on the ulnar and radial aspect of the digits, forming a broad proximally based skin flap. These can be continued if necessary to the digits with zigzag Brunner incisions.
- Undermine the proximal skin flap and distal skin margin by separating the skin from the extensive diseased palmar fascial complex. Retract the flap proximally to expose the deeper structures (**TECH FIG 4B**).
- Carry the dissection proximally and distally to expose the majority of the palmar fascia. A transition between normal and diseased fascia may not be identified. Leave behind any normal-appearing fascial tissue and excise the entire diseased pretendinous cords and adjacent thick nodular structures (**TECH FIG 4C**).
- Keep the neurovascular structures in sight and protected throughout the procedure.
- The TLPA is usually involved, forming a transverse cord that extends from the ulnar to the radial aspect of the palm.
  - This should be removed with the diseased tissue, along with any natatory cords.
  - Divide all the septa of Legueu and Juvara to remove most of the diseased fascial carpet.
  - If these septa are diseased, they will form vertical cords that should be incorporated in the mass of excised tissue.
- Release the tourniquet and achieve adequate hemostasis.
- Close the wound if possible (**TECH FIG 4D**), leaving a Penrose drain; it is removed on the second postoperative day.
- If skin shortage is present, perform full-thickness skin grafting.
- Alternatively, the wound can be left open as in the open palm method.

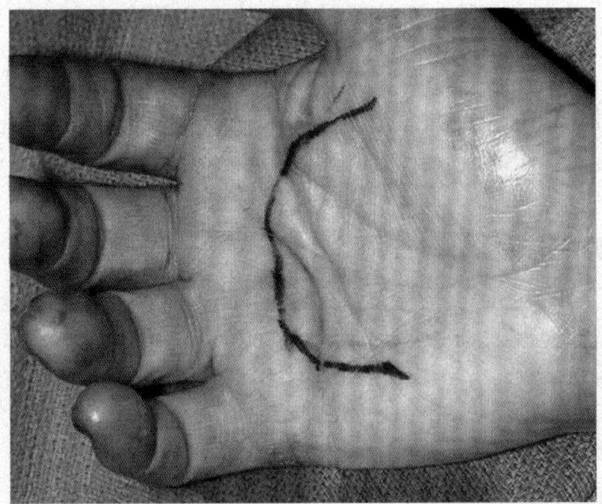

A

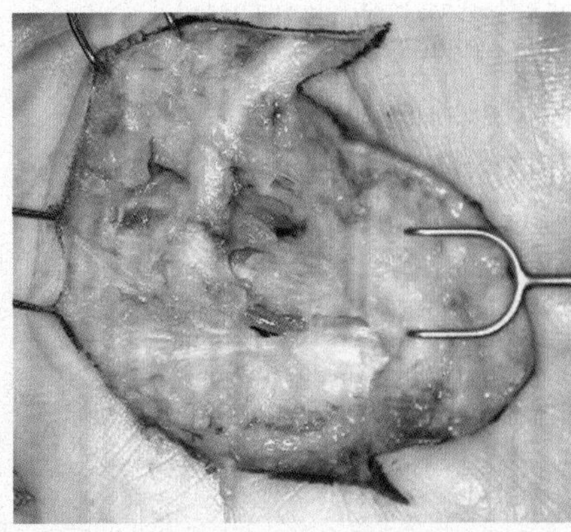

B

TECH FIG 4 • **A.** A U-shaped incision is planned in a patient with diffuse Dupuytren palmar fascial disease with nodular thickening in the entire palm. **B.** The diseased fascia is exposed after reflection of the proximally based skin flap. *(continued)*

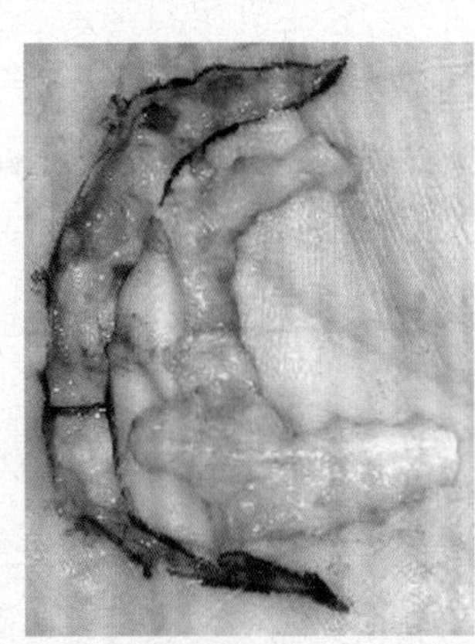

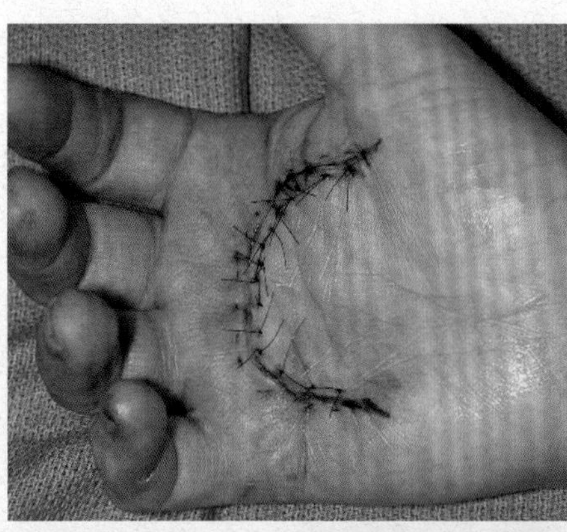

TECH FIG 4 • *(continued)* **C.** The excised specimen includes a pretendinous cord from the ring finger and diseased TLPA. **D.** The surgical wound after skin closure.

PEARLS AND PITFALLS

- Injury to digital nerves is more common in cases with severe MCP and PIP joint contracture and altered nerve anatomy by a spiral cord. Such a complication is especially common in previously operated cases with an exuberant amount of scar tissue. Preventive measures include isolation of the neurovascular bundle by careful dissection, using loupe magnification, and knowledge of pathoanatomy. The dissection is carried out in a proximal to distal direction and is sometimes combined with distal to proximal dissection before removal of the diseased cord. If the nerve is transected, a primary repair should be performed.
- Vascular injury can be in the form of an arterial laceration, arterial spasm, intimal hemorrhage, or vessel rupture from vigorous correction of severe digital joint contracture. Arterial laceration that results in vascular compromise requires immediate repair or interposition vein graft. Arterial spasm and intimal hemorrhage are treated first by repositioning the digit in flexion, then irrigating with warm saline, applying topical lidocaine, even using intravenous heparin, and, if all else fails, vascular reconstruction.
- Separating diseased tissue from adherent skin is difficult, especially in recurrent cases. To reduce the risk of buttonholing the skin, using a no. 15C scalpel and the back of the knife blade as a dissector will allow precise separation of diseased tissue from normal skin. In addition, using an operating room light to transilluminate from the epidermal side of the skin allows visualization of the thickness of the flap and can alert the surgeon when the dissection is too superficial.

POSTOPERATIVE CARE

Open Palm Fasciectomy

- The surgical wound is covered with sterile nonadhesive gauze, which can be changed daily. By 4 weeks, no dressings should be necessary.
- Forty-eight to 72 hours after surgery, the patient begins active range of motion every 2 to 3 hours but maintains nocturnal extension splint immobilization.
- Whirlpool therapy can be used early in the postoperative period if unwarranted or excessive bleeding occurred.
- Wound healing takes place within 6 to 8 weeks, depending on the extent of the incision.

Partial Fasciectomy and Dermofasciectomy

- Range-of-motion exercises are encouraged out of the splint after 1 week. The sutures are removed and splint use is discontinued 2 weeks after surgery in uncomplicated cases.
- Formal hand therapy is used after surgery for extensive disease, especially if residual flexion deformity is present. Range of motion alternating with extension splinting is emphasized.

OUTCOMES

- The recurrence rate varies between 2% and 60%, with an average of 33%. This may be a true recurrence (recurrent disease at the operated site) or disease extension (disease outside the area of prior surgery). Recurrence is more common in patients with PIP joint involvement, disease in the small finger, more than one digit affected, a longer time since surgery, and a secondary fasciectomy.
- Werker et al[24] in a 2012 literature review found that the reported recurrence rates in the literature ranged from 12% to 73% for patients treated with fasciectomy/aponeurectomy and from 33% to 100% for fasciotomy/aponeurotomy.
- Roush and Stern[21] reported that the postoperative total range of motion of recurrent DD was better after fasciectomy and flap converge compared to skin grafting or arthrodesis.
- DD has intrigued basic scientists and clinicians for centuries. Both ancient[7] and current publications[5,22] underscore the interest in and the advances toward understanding the pathophysiology of this disease and improving its treatment.

COMPLICATIONS

- Complications related to patient physiology include postoperative stiffness, chronic regional pain syndromes (CRPS), recurrence, and digital stiffness.[4] The surgeon has little influence in preventing these complications.
- Early postoperative complications
  - Hematoma is prevented by tourniquet deflation and adequate hemostasis before wound closure. Deflating the tourniquet and assessing the skin vascularity before closure to ensure adequate circulation is the best way to prevent skin necrosis.

- Closure under tension should be avoided and consideration should be given to grafting or the open palm method if a primary closure is too tight.
- Skin necrosis develops after excessive thinning of skin flaps and tight skin closure. Small areas of skin necrosis may be allowed to heal by secondary intention, but large areas of necrotic tissue should be excised, and skin graft or flap coverage is done.
- A simultaneous carpal tunnel release with DD surgery, especially in women, is a predisposing factor to CRPS atraumatic technique and gentle handling of nerves and tissues during surgery reduces the risk of this complication.

- Late postoperative complications
  - Inclusion cysts can occur near the scar due to dermal tissue entrapment in the subcutaneous space. This can be prevented by careful attention to skin approximation during wound closure. The risk of hypertrophic scar formation is lessened by careful attention to placement of the skin incisions.

REFERENCES

1. Badalamente M, Hurst L. Enzyme injection as nonsurgical treatment of Dupuytren disease. J Hand Surg Am 2000;25(4):629–636.
2. Bilderback K, Rayan G. Dupuytren's cord involving the septa of Legueu and Juvara: a case report. J Hand Surg Am 2002;27(2):344–346.
3. Bilderback K, Rayan G. The septa of Legueu and Juvara: an anatomic study. J Hand Surg Am 2004;29(3):494–499.
4. Boyer M, Gelberman R. Complications of the operative treatment of Dupuytren's disease. Hand Clin 1999;15:161–166.
5. Brenner P, Rayan G. Dupuytren's Disease: A Concept of Surgical Treatment. Vienna, Austria: Springer, 2002.
6. Eaton C. Percutaneous fasciotomy for Dupuytren's contracture. J Hand Surg Am 2011;36(5):910–915.
7. Elliot D. The early history of Dupuytren's disease. Hand Clin 1999; 15:1–19.
8. Gelberman R, Panagis J, Hergenroeder P, et al. Wound complications in the surgical management of Dupuytren's contracture: a comparison of operative incisions. Hand 1982;14:248–254.
9. Heuston J. The control of recurrent Dupuytren's contracture by skin replacement. Br J Plast Surg 1969;22:152–156.
10. Hurst LC, Badalamente MA, Hentz VR, et al. Injectable collagenase clostridium histolyticum for Dupuytren's contracture. N Engl J Med 2009;361(10):968–979.
11. Ketchum L, Hixson FP. Dermofasciectomy and full-thickness grafts in the treatment of Dupuytren's contracture. J Hand Surg Am 1987;12(5 pt 1):659–664.
12. Lubahn J. Open-palm technique and soft-tissue coverage in Dupuytren's disease. Hand Clin 1999;15:127–136.
13. Luck JV. Dupuytren's contracture; a new concept of the pathogenesis correlated with surgical management. J Bone Joint Surg Am 1959; 41-A(4):635–664.
14. McFarlane RM. Patterns of the diseased fascia in the fingers of Dupuytren's contracture. Displacement of the neurovascular bundle. Plast Reconst Surg 1974;54:31–44.
15. Ojwang JO, Adrianto I, Gray-McGuire C, et al. Genome-wide association scan of Dupuytren's disease. J Hand Surg Am 2010;35(12):2039–2045.
16. Rayan G. Dupuytren disease: anatomy, pathology, presentation, and treatment. J Bone Joint Surg Am 2007;89(1):189–198.
17. Rayan G. Palmar fascial complex anatomy and pathology in Dupuytren's disease. Hand Clin 1999;15:73–86.
18. Rayan G, Ali M, Orozco J. Dorsal pads versus nodules in normal population and Dupuytren's disease patients. J Hand Surg Am 2010;35(10):1571–1579.
19. Rayan G, Moore J. Non-Dupuytren's disease of the palmar fascia. J Hand Surg Br 2005;30(6):551–556.
20. Rayan G, Parizi M, Tomasek J. Pharmacologic regulation of Dupuytren's fibroblast contraction in vitro. J Hand Surg Am 1996;21(6): 1065–1070.
21. Roush T, Stern P. Results following surgery for recurrent Dupuytren's disease. J Hand Surg Am 2000;25(2):291–296.
22. Tubiana R, Leclercq C, Hurst L, et al. Dupuytren's Disease. London: Martin Dunitz, 2000.
23. Ulmas M, Bischoff R, Gelberman R. Predictors of neurovascular displacement in hands with Dupuytren's contracture. J Hand Surg Br 1994;19(5): 664–666.
24. Werker P, Pess G, van Rijssen A, et al. Correction of contracture and recurrence rates of Dupuytren contracture following invasive treatment: the importance of clear definitions. J Hand Surg Am 2012; 37(10):2095–2105.
25. Zachariae L. Operation for Dupuytren's contracture by the method of McCash. Acta Orthop Scand 1970;41:433–438.
26. Zhang AY, Curtin CM, Hentz VR. Flexor tendon rupture after collagenase injection for Dupuytren contracture: case report. J Hand Surg Am 2011;36(8):1323–1325.

CHAPTER 137

Surgical Treatment of Thermal Injuries of the Upper Extremity

Jennifer Waljee, Evan McGlinn, and Kevin C. Chung

DEFINITION

- Thermal injuries of the upper extremity include contact, scald, flame, chemical and electrical burns, and present with both acute and chronic injury that may require surgical intervention.
- Despite aggressive acute care, splinting, and therapy, long-term hand and wrist deformities due to burn injuries are common.
- Following burn injuries, scar contractures are common due to the loss of normal skin pliability, which often require surgical release.

ANATOMY

- Burns yield both a local and systemic response.
- Locally, there are three zones of injury.
  - The zone of coagulation describes the point of maximum damage with irreversible tissue loss.
  - The zone of stasis represents the area of diminished tissue perfusion and is most critical, as it represents the zone of reversible injury with adequate resuscitation and wound care.
  - The zone of hyperemia is most peripheral and typically represents tissue that will recover in the absence of overwhelming infection or hypoperfusion (**FIG 1**).

PATHOGENESIS

- Systemically, burn injuries result in the release of inflammatory mediators that can cause widespread physiologic changes for those injuries that are more than 30% of the total body surface area. For example, cardiovascular collapse can occur from increased capillary permeability and diminished myocardial contractility.
- Inhalational injury can result in bronchospasm and acute respiratory distress syndrome. A catabolic state results from an increase in metabolism greater than three times the basal rate. Finally, patients may be relatively immunocompromised from downregulation of the immune response.

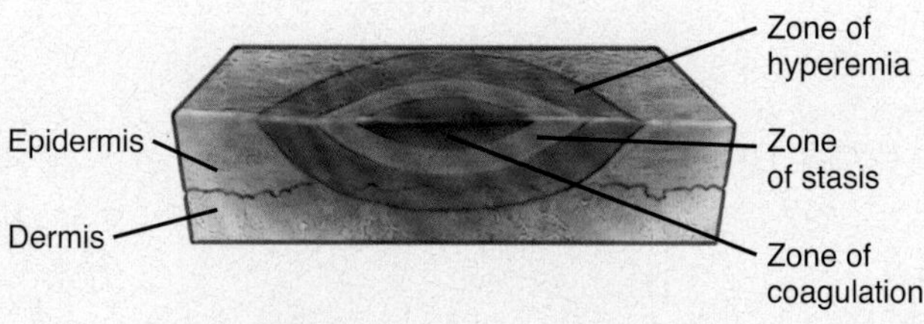

FIG 1 • Burn zones of injury.

- Electrical shock produces a complex pattern of injury in which the severity of injury depends on the intensity of the current and duration of contact.
  - Electric current travels through the body, creating "entry" and "exit" points, damaging any tissue in between these two points.
  - As the electrical current travels, heat is generated along its path, leading to thermal damage. The amount of heat generated (and tissue damage) is proportional to the voltage of the current as well as the resistance of the tissue.
  - Alternating currents can interfere with the cardiac cycle, increasing the risk of arrhythmias.
  - Electrical burns are classified as high voltage (≥1000 V) and low voltage (<1000 V).
  - Electrical injuries often extend far beyond the visible cutaneous burn and involve deeper structures.
  - Tissues with high electrical resistance, such as the skin and bone, generate more heat, causing more damage to both themselves and the surrounding tissues. Therefore, patients with high-voltage electrical burns often sustain extensive deep tissue and muscle injuries that predispose to developing acute compartment syndrome.
- Despite splinting, range-of-motion exercises, compression, and positioning, 80% of patients will have decreased joint motion and up to 10% have difficulties with activities of daily living.
- Increased and disorganized deposition of collagen fibers following burn injuries results in compact, foreshortened scars. The amount and severity of hypertrophic scarring and contracture is directly related to the depth of the burn and the time required for wound healing.

NATURAL HISTORY

- Superficial burn injuries involve only the epidermis.
- Partial-thickness burns involve the entire epidermis and varying levels of the dermis and dermal appendages.
- Full-thickness burns injure all layers of the epidermis and dermis and can extend to deeper structures.
- Superficial burns are painful and involve only the epidermis, which is erythematous and blanches with pressure. These burns will heal with minimal or no scarring and can be managed with local wound care.
- Partial-thickness burn injuries involve the epidermis as well as varying degrees of the dermis. These can be considered as either superficial or deep, depending on the degree of injury to the dermis. Superficial partial-thickness burns are typically sensate, moist, weepy, and painful after sloughing of the epidermis and usually heal within 2 weeks of injury. Deep partial-thickness burns extend into the reticular dermis

and typically heal within 3 to 8 weeks and often require excision and grafting (**FIG 2**).

- Full-thickness burns involve the entire thickness of the skin and are characterized by charred, painless, leathery skin with visible coagulated vessels.

PATIENT HISTORY AND PHYSICAL FINDINGS

Assessment of the Burned Patient

- In addition to routine medical history, it is imperative to obtain the mechanism of burn injury and assess for other concomitant injuries.
  - High-voltage electrical burns, burns that occurred in an enclosed space, or burns from explosions require trauma and critical care to evaluate and treat other potential life-threatening injuries.
- Physical examination should focus on determining the extent of burn injury and vascular status.
- All upper extremities should be assessed for signs of vascular compromise, such as diminished pulses, poor capillary refill, cool skin temperature, and poor turgor.
  - Vascular insufficiency is uncommon with superficial and partial-thickness burns. Patients with crush injuries, full-thickness burns, circumferential injuries, and those in association with lacerations or other trauma may be at risk for vascular insufficiency.

Classification of Burn Injuries

- Superficial burn injuries involve only the epidermis. Partial-thickness burns involve the entire epidermis and varying levels of the dermis and dermal appendages. Full-thickness burns injure all layers of the epidermis and dermis and can extend to deeper structures.
  - Superficial burns are painful and involve only the epidermis and are erythematous that blanch with pressure. These burns will heal with minimal or no scarring and can be managed with local wound care.
- Partial-thickness burn injuries involve the epidermis as well as varying degrees of the dermis. Partial-thickness burns can be considered as either superficial or deep partial thickness, depending on the degree of injury to the dermis.
  - Superficial partial-thickness burns are typically sensate, moist, weepy, and painful after sloughing of the epidermis and usually heal within 2 weeks of injury.
  - Deep partial-thickness burns extend into the reticular dermis and typically heal within 3 to 8 weeks, often requiring excision and grafting.
- Full-thickness burns involve the entire thickness of the skin and are characterized by charred, painless, leathery skin with visible coagulated vessels.

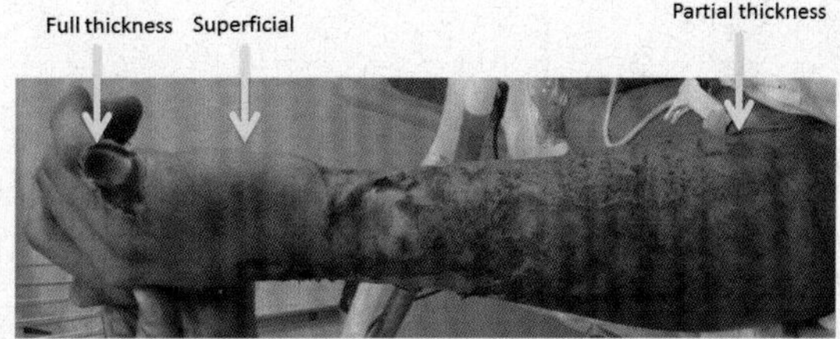

FIG 2 • Upper extremity burn injury demonstrating superficial, partial-thickness, and full-thickness burns.

Compartment Syndrome

- Compartment syndrome may result from burn injuries, especially electrical burn injuries.
- Acute circumferential or near-circumferential full-thickness burns of the extremity may compromise distal perfusion and require escharotomy, in which the unyielding burned tissue is released or excised.
  - The inelastic skin in a circumferential burn acts as a tourniquet, which compromises venous return and capillary perfusion leading to tissue ischemia distal to the burn.
- The differential diagnosis for compartment syndrome includes nerve injuries causing paresthesias and arterial or venous insufficiency from other causes (eg, trauma).
- Compartment pressures can be measured with a commercially available pressure transducer or by creating one using an 18- or 20-gauge needle, a syringe containing saline, a pressure transducer, and a three-way stopcock.
- Treatment for compartment syndrome of the forearm and hand should be initiated based on clinical suspicion. Prompt fasciotomy minimizes functional loss and promotes recovery. Fasciotomy should be performed if compartment pressures are higher than 30 mm Hg for normotensive patients or within 20 mm Hg of the diastolic pressure for hypotensive patients.

IMAGING AND OTHER DIAGNOSTIC STUDIES

- In addition to routine medical history, the mechanism of burn injury and assessment for concomitant injuries is sought. High-voltage electrical burns, burns that occurred in an enclosed space, or burns associated with explosions and inhalation injury require further consultation.
- Plain radiographs are obtained if hand reconstruction for scar contractures is planned to assess for heterotopic ossification or arthritic changes that may require additional treatment, such as capsulotomy and ligamentous releases.

DIFFERENTIAL DIAGNOSIS

- Allergic reactions
- Pressure-induced injury
- Compartment syndrome
- Dermatologic conditions resulting in desquamation or tissue loss (eg, toxic epidermal necrolysis, erythema multiforme)

NONOPERATIVE MANAGEMENT

- Acute superficial or partial-thickness burns over noncritically functioning areas that are expected to heal within 2 to 3 weeks may be managed with dressing changes. Typical options for topical wound care are detailed in Table 1.
  - Topical antibiotic agents (eg, Bacitracin, Silvadene, Sulfamylon, Mepilex Ag, Acticoat) are applied and changed regularly as the burn heals.
  - Empiric systemic antibiotics are not indicated for burn injuries.
  - Burns should be cleaned with soap and water daily and covered with topical antimicrobial agents.
  - For early, immature scarring within 6 months of injury, conservative measures can dramatically improve scar appearance through collagen remodeling.
    - Examples include pressure garments, silicone gel/sheeting, and physical therapy. All have been shown to control hypertrophic scarring with full-time use over several months.

Table 1 Topical Agents and Dressings for Burn Treatment

	Description	Application	Pros	Cons
Acticoat	Silver-coated polyethylene net dressing	Change every 3–7 d	Few dressing changes, painless, large antimicrobial spectrum	Cost
Adaptic	Impregnated mesh	Once daily	Painless, nonadherent, good moisture	No antimicrobial effect, may dry out
Aquacel Ag	Silver rayon mesh dressing	Change every 1–14 d	Painless, large antimicrobial spectrum	Difficult patient maintenance
Bacitracin	Topical agent	1–4 times daily	Painless, inexpensive, uncommon incidence of bacterial resistance	Antibiotic resistance and dermatitis with long-term use
Silvadene (silver sulfadiazine)	Topical agent	1–2 times daily	Painless, cooling effect; fight gram-negative bacteria	Poor deep eschar penetration, daily dressing changes, leukopenia
Mepilex Ag	Silver-impregnated foam dressing	Every few days	Ease of application and excellent patient tolerance	Requires clean, noncontaminated wound bed; not effective for full-thickness injury
Sulfamylon (mafenide acetate)	Topical agent	Daily	Bacteriostatic action	Application may be painful.
Xeroform	Impregnated mesh	Once daily	Nonadherent, bacteriostatic activity	Dessication

SURGICAL MANAGEMENT

Preoperative Planning

- Extent of the burn injury and vascular status is assessed for signs of vascular compromise, such as diminished pulses, poor capillary refill, cool skin temperature, and poor turgor.
- Crush injuries, full-thickness burns, circumferential injuries, and those in association with lacerations are at highest risk for vascular insufficiency.
- The "rule of nines" is useful to estimate the total percentage of body surface area involved (**FIG 3**).
  - Alternatively, the area can be estimated using the patient's palm, which is approximately 1% of the total body surface area.
  - Resuscitation is guided by the total body surface area involved, patient weight, and urine output, with adjustment made for pediatric patients.
- Because burns may continue to evolve over 48 to 72 hours following injury, serial examinations are required to adequately determine burn depth.

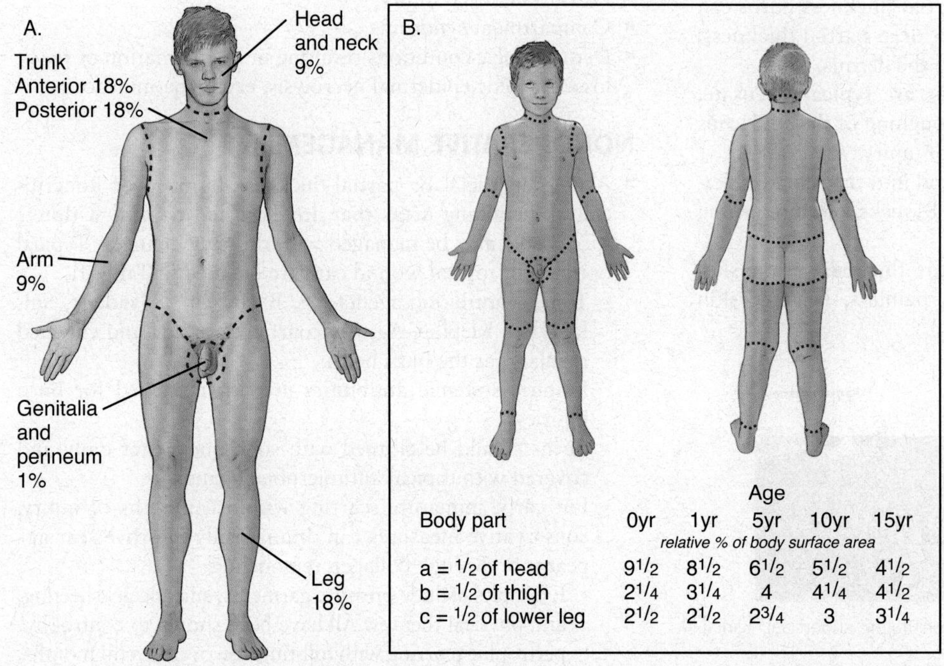

FIG 3 • Lund-Browder diagram to estimate burn wound size.

- Infection, inadequate resuscitation, poor wound care, and malnutrition can result in burns progressing from superficial to deep partial-thickness or full-thickness burn injuries. Close attention to nutrition and resuscitation are imperative.
- In general, burns that are not anticipated to heal within 3 weeks should undergo operative excision and grafting within the first few days of the burn injury.
  - Early tangential excision of the burn is indicated within the first few days of injury and is performed in the operating room under general anesthesia.
- Scar maturation continues for approximately 1 year.
  - True keloid formation is rare; however, hypertrophic burn scars are common and can be managed by the conservative measures listed earlier.

Positioning

- Supine position is used for upper extremity burns, with the arm extended on a hand table and a tourniquet available.
  - Donor sites should be accessible; most commonly the ipsilateral upper thigh.

Approach

- Depending on the size and depth of the burn and the clinical status, burn wounds may undergo débridement and coverage with autologous skin (meshed vs. nonmeshed), cadaveric skin substitutes, or xenograft substitutes (eg, Integra).
- Even without scar resection, surgical release of burn scars often result in large soft tissue defects due to tissue deficiency.
- Thick split- or full-thickness skin grafts can be used to resurface the soft tissue defect, but flap coverage may be necessary if contracture release or scar excision leads to exposure of joint structures, tendons, or neurovascular bundles.
- Burn scar contractures can result in secondary joint contractures and tendon damage requiring release or reconstruction.
- Burn scar contractures in the hand cause a "claw" deformity with flexed wrist and proximal interphalangeal (PIP) joints, extended distal interphalangeal (DIP) and metacarpophalangeal (MCP) joints, and adducted web spaces (**FIG 4A–C**). These contractures should be differentiated from other causes of stiffness, such as intrinsic joint disease or Dupuytren disease.
- Flaps can include local pedicled flaps (eg, radial or ulnar forearm flap), regional pedicled flap (groin flap), or free flap (eg, lateral arm or anterolateral thigh).
- Scar is excised through an incision around the contracted scar and through the subcutaneous fat and underlying structures. Scar is often adherent to underlying fascia, tendons, and joints.
  - Traction is applied to assist in identifying the areolar plane between scar and normal tissue. Scar is lifted in its entirety and tight underlying fibrous bands are broken up with blunt and sharp dissection.
  - After complete excision of scar, affected joints are stretched to evaluate the need for capsulotomy or ligamentous release.

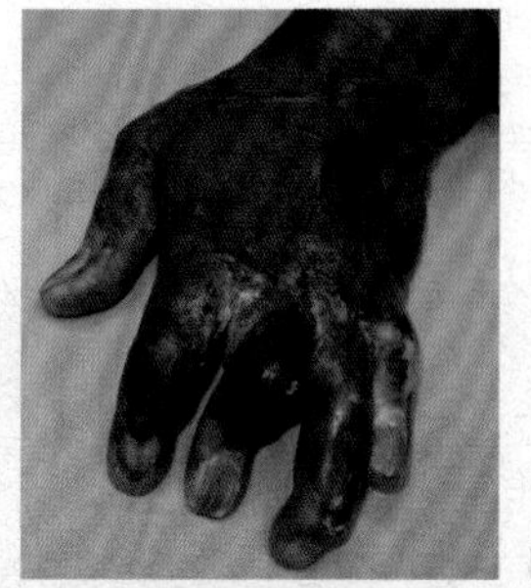
A

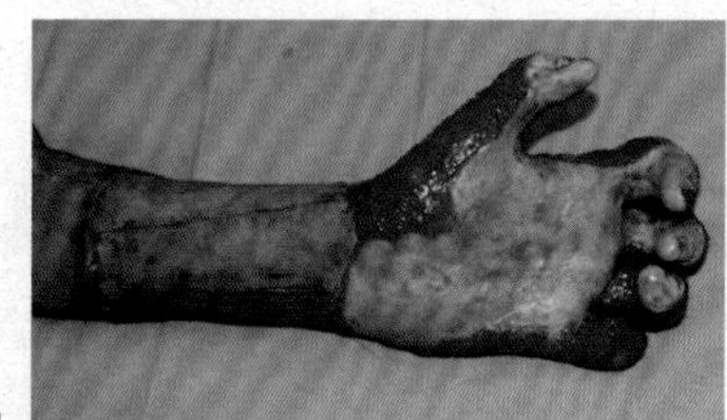
B

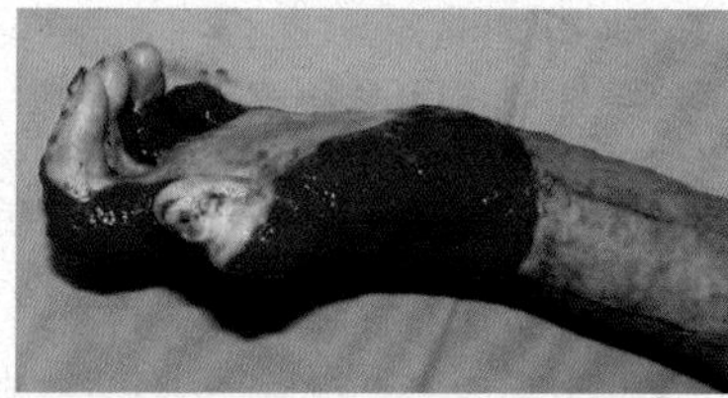
C

FIG 4 • **A–C.** Classic deformities associated with severe hand burn, with flexed PIP joint and extended MCP and DIP joints.

TECHNIQUES

Burn Wound Débridement

- Tangential excision of the burn is performed sharply with specialized blades set to the depth of desired excision (eg, Goulian knives). Alternatively, pressurized knives such as a dermatome or using hydro-débridement instruments such as the Versajet.
- Débridement is completed down through the layers of burn to rid the wound surface of necrotic nonviable debris down to punctate bleeding.
  - Inadequate débridement will lead to graft failure and increase the infection risk.
- If the burn wound is limited to an extremity, débridement may be performed under tourniquet control. The tourniquet is released to confirm adequate débridement prior to coverage.
- Hemostasis is achieved using epinephrine-soaked dressings applied topically and using adjuncts such as thrombin spray. Maintain normotensive and normothermic to prevent intraoperative coagulopathy.
- For clean, adequately débrided burn wounds without exposed vital structures, autologous skin grafting is ideal coverage. Large burn wounds with exposed deep structures or exposed neurovascular bundles are temporarily covered with moist dressing changes and will require local flap, distant flap, or free tissue coverage within 48 to 72 hours.
- Autologous skin can be harvested using either a dermatome or a Goulian blade at approximately 0.012 to 0.018 inch.
  - Thinner skin grafts are preferred for those patients with extensive burn injuries in whom donor sites may need to be used several times.
  - Full-thickness skins grafts are preferred in areas of high function or high aesthetic value but are difficult to obtain in an extensively injured patient.
- Nonmeshed grafts are preferred over the hands and joints to prevent scar contracture (**TECH FIG 1**). Grafts meshed at 1:1.5 to 1:3 provide fluid egress, prevent seroma formation, and provide greater coverage over nonjoint areas, such as the forearm.

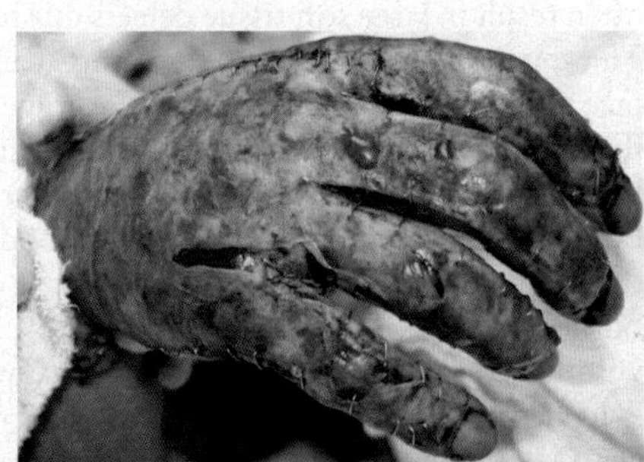

TECH FIG 1 • Split-thickness autograft to dorsal hand burn.

- Grafts are fixed in place with either absorbable sutures (4-0 chromic or Monocryl) or staples. Fibrin glue (eg, Artiss) can be used and diminishes graft loss due to shear.
- For patients with inadequate donor skin, or who are hemodynamically unstable, temporary wound coverage can be achieved with cadaveric skin substitutes or dermal skin substitutes (eg, Integra). Autologous skin grafting can be performed later when donor sites are available and grafting is more favorable.
- Grafted wounds are dressed using antibiotic ointment and antibiotic-impregnated gauze applied with light compression over grafts to reduce shear injury. The hand is splinted in a functional position. Dressings are left in place for approximately 3 to 5 days.
- Donor skin sites are dressed with either occlusive dressings or with antibiotic-impregnated gauze. These wounds typically reepithelize within 1 to 2 weeks and can be reharvested for skin grafts as needed.
- The grafted wounds are inspected in approximately 5 days to assess early graft take, and gentle active and passive range of motion can be initiated. Grafts are then redressed with antibiotic dressings until complete healing (approximately 10 to 14 days).
- For burn wounds that are not amenable to early autologous skin grafting, temporary skin substitutes are available. Cadaveric skin (homograft), porcine xenograft, or dermal skin substitutes (eg, Integra) can affixed to the wound similar to a split-thickness skin autograft. In a healthy wound bed, cadaveric skin will incorporate and provide temporary coverage for 2 to 3 weeks as the wound continues to heal underneath.

Escharotomy

- Escharotomy can be performed at the bedside using electrocautery with the patient under sedation.
- A full-thickness skin incision is made at the length of the full-thickness burn on the radial aspect of the forearm along a line connecting the lateral end of the antecubital flexion crease and radial styloid (**TECH FIG 2**).
  - The incision is deepened until viable tissue is encountered. The incision spans the entire burn, from normal skin to normal skin.
- If the hand and the forearm are still tight after a radial release, a second escharotomy incision is made along a line just volar to the ulna, spanning the entire burn.
- To perform escharotomy of the hand, extend the radial incision onto the hand with the radial incision along the midaxial line of the thenar eminence. The radial sensory nerve will lie along this incision and must be protected.
- The ulnar incision can be carried onto the hypothenar eminence as needed.
- Circumferential finger burns are treated with a digital escharotomy. A midlateral incision down into subcutaneous fat is made along one side of the finger, from the MCP joint to the fingertip.
- Escharotomy wounds are dressed with a moist dressing.

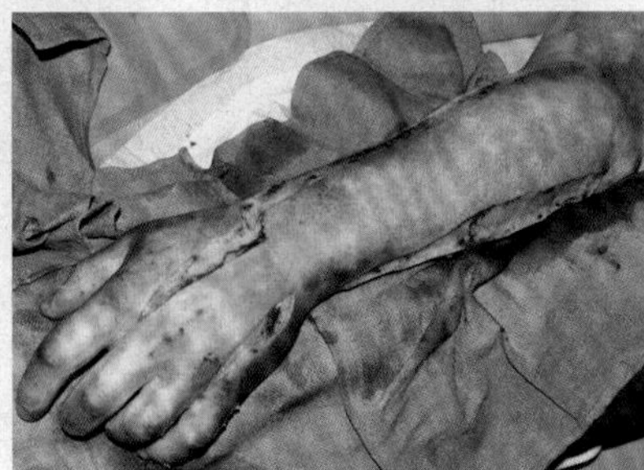

TECH FIG 2 • Escharotomy release.

Fasciotomy of the Hand and Forearm with Carpal Tunnel Release

- Two dorsal incisions, centered over the index and ring metacarpals, are used to release the interosseous muscles and the thumb adductor muscle compartments (**TECH FIG 3A**).
  - Incisions are made ulnar and radial to the index and ring extensors. Dissection is continued until the fascia of the dorsal interosseous muscles is reached. The fascia is opened sharply.
  - Blunt dissection is performed along the ulnar and radial side of the index finger metacarpal to open the first volar interosseous and adductor pollicis muscles.
  - The second volar interosseous muscle is opened with deep blunt dissection along the radial border of the ring finger metacarpal.
  - Through the ring finger metacarpal incision, deep blunt dissection along the radial border of the small finger metacarpal releases the third volar interosseous muscle.
- Thenar muscles are released through an incision on the radial border of the thumb metacarpal between the volar glabrous and dorsal pliable skin. The dissection is volar to the metacarpal to expose the fascia of the thenar muscles, which is sharply opened (**TECH FIG 3B**).
- The hypothenar muscles are released similarly with an incision on the ulnar aspect of the small finger metacarpal (**TECH FIG 3C**).

- The carpal tunnel is released through a standard incision in the palm in line with the ring metacarpal. See **TECH FIG 3B** for the technique.
- We perform fasciotomy of all three forearm compartments to avoid lingering doubts regarding inadequate release.
- For uncomplicated fasciotomy wounds, once adequate débridement has been achieved, moist dressing changes are performed for 7 to 14 days in preparation for primary closure or skin grafting. Large wounds with exposed deep structures or exposed neurovascular structures are temporarily covered with moist dressing changes and will require local flap, distant flap, or free tissue transfer coverage within 48 to 72 hours.
- Negative-pressure dressings can be used for postfasciotomy defects as an alternative to traditional wound care; edema often subsides and allows for primary wound closure. Open defects are covered with a 0.012-inch split-thickness skin graft.

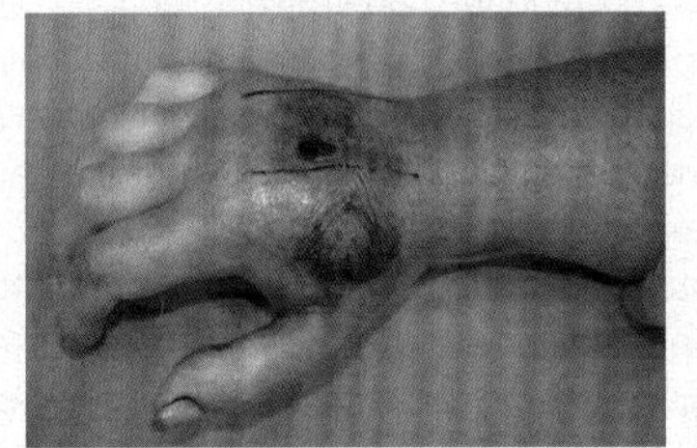
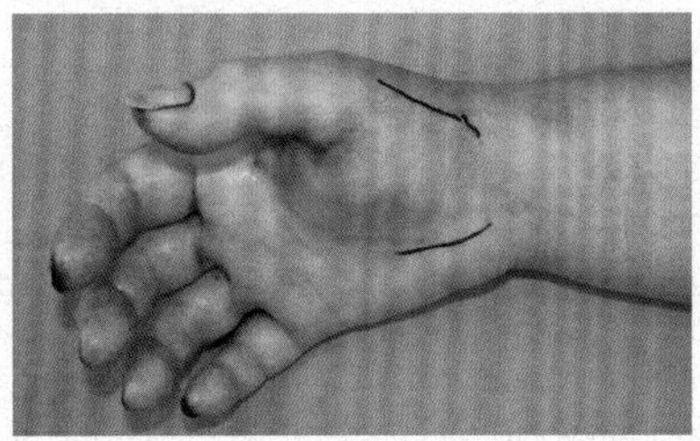
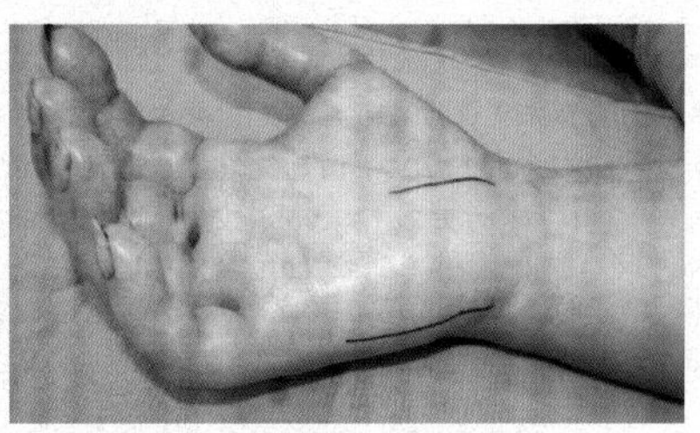

TECH FIG 3 • **A.** Dorsal fasciotomy release. **B.** Thenar muscle release and carpal tunnel release. **C.** Hypothenar release.

Scar Contracture Release with Local Tissue Rearrangement

- Mild linear scar bands can be corrected with scar release and local tissue rearrangement.
- A basic Z-plasty can be used (**TECH FIG 4A**) to interrupt and lengthen a scar.
  - The central limb of the Z is planned along the axis of the scar band, and the angle of the Z-plasty can be varied, with a larger angle providing more release. We prefer 45-degree flaps.
  - The theoretical gain in length is proportional to the angle of the Z-plasty (Table 2).
- One or multiple Z-plasty flaps are used to break up mild to moderate linear contractures (**TECH FIG 4B**).
  - The Z-plasty flaps are elevated just below the dermis, preserving a small cuff of subcutaneous fat on the underside of the flaps.
  - Foreshortened fibrous bands that require release with scissors or a knife often are present in the underlying soft tissue.
  - Care is taken to protect the neurovascular bundle.
  - After release of underlying tissue and extension of the joint, the Z-plasty flaps should fall naturally into a transposed position.
  - The flaps are sutured in place with absorbable sutures.
- Antibiotic ointment is placed on the incision, followed by soft bulky dressings, which remain for 2 days.
- Patients are allowed progressive gentle range of motion. Stretching and scar massage are encouraged to begin 2 to 3 weeks postoperatively.
  - Abduction or extension splints may be used at night to maintain posture.
- Variations on the basic Z-plasty can be performed to accommodate specific areas.
  - For example, a five-flap "jumping man" Z-plasty (combination of two Z-plasty flaps with a V-Y advancement flap) works well to release web space contractures.
  - Compared to a basic Z-plasty, the additional flaps maximize gain in length and the V-Y flap introduces unscarred skin into the reconstruction, providing more pliability and elasticity to the reconstructed web space (**TECH FIG 4C**).

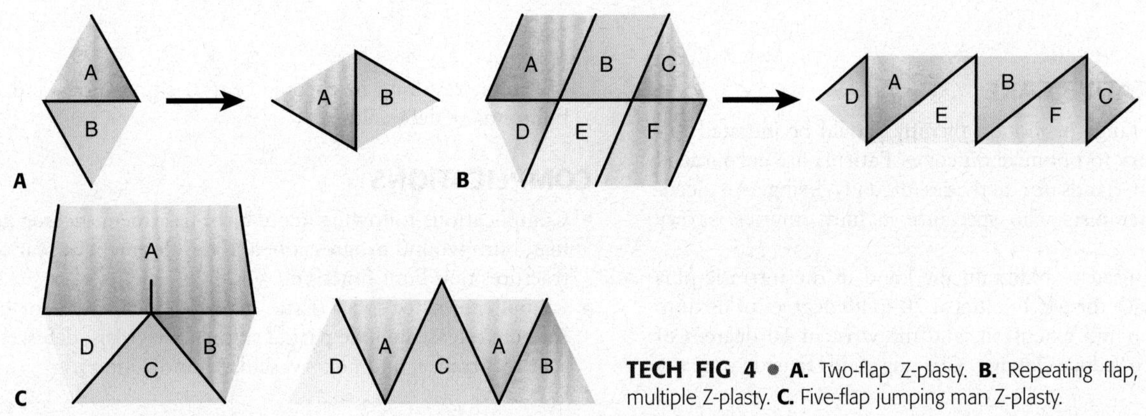

TECH FIG 4 • **A.** Two-flap Z-plasty. **B.** Repeating flap, multiple Z-plasty. **C.** Five-flap jumping man Z-plasty.

Table 2 Z-Plasty Angles for Burn Scar Contracture Release

Z-Plasty Angles (Degrees)	Theoretical Gain in Length
30	25
45	50
60	75
75	100

Laser Therapy for Burn Scars

- In recent years, laser therapy for scar conditions have evolved substantially and can be applied to burn scar injuries to improve scar pliability, symptoms (pain, pruritis), and appearance.
  - Laser therapy stimulates scar remodeling through microscopic thermal injury, which causes an acute inflammatory reaction resulting in metalloproteinase-mediated turnover of extracellular matrix proteins, increased cell proliferation in the dermis and epidermis, recruitment of stem and precursor cells, and sustained production of new dermal matrix proteins including collagen types I and III and elastin.
- Pulsed dye laser treatment at 585 to 595 nm targets hemoglobin and causes selective damage to cutaneous microvessels.
  - It is useful to improve erythematous scars with telangiectasias or inflammatory scars with pruritis and pain.
- Fractional lasers use an array of thin, deep columns of thermal injury by laser microbeam exposures.
  - Treatment can be tailored by modifying the depth of penetration (energy delivered), the width of penetration (duration of the laser delivery), and the density of the area treated.
  - Common ablative fractional lasers include carbon dioxide lasers, erbium:YAG, and thulium.
- Benefits of laser therapy include minimal recovery periods and short, outpatient procedures. However, scars may require multiple treatments to achieve remodeling and complications include pigmentation changes, pain, blistering, bruising, and swelling.

Groin Flap Coverage for Burn Scar Contracture

- An ipsilateral groin flaps can be harvested based on the superficial circumflex iliac artery.
  - A line between the anterior superior iliac spine (ASIS) and pubic tubercle is drawn, identifying the inguinal ligament. A second parallel line is drawn 2 to 3 cm below the midaxis of the flap and corresponds to the course of the superficial circumflex iliac artery.
  - Using a pattern of the defect, a flap is designed inferior to the ASIS to lie along the previously marked midaxis. If necessary, the flap can be extended lateral to the ASIS for additional length.
  - A flap up to 20 × 10 cm can be closed primarily and is sufficient for most hand and wrist defects.
  - The flap is oriented to minimize kinking and twisting of the pedicle after inset.
  - The flap is incised down to the underlying fascia.
    - Inferiorly, the fascia lata and sartorius fascia are identified. The flap is elevated tangentially off the fascia in a lateral to medial fashion until the lateral aspect of the sartorius fascia is encountered.
    - The sartorius fascia is incised at its lateral margin and elevated from the underlying muscle, with care taken to avoid injuring the lateral femoral cutaneous nerve. The dissection concludes at the medial edge of the sartorius.
    - Although the vascular pedicle is not typically identified, it traverses out of the femoral triangle and through the sartorius fascia at the medial edge of the muscle.
  - The proximal portion of the flap is tubularized if possible around the vascular pedicle.
  - The donor defect is closed primarily, including countouring the cutaneous deformity at the lateral aspect; however, a small open area may be left at the base of the flap.
  - The flap is gently thinned along the margins. The defect is brought into the field, and the flap is inset using nonabsorbable sutures. The forearm is secured to the abdominal skin with several large nonabsorbable sutures.
  - Soft bulky dressings are used, followed by an elastic bandage wrapped around the hip to further stabilize the reconstruction.
    - Members of the surgical team must be present at the time of recovery from anesthesia to mitigate the chance of accidental flap avulsion.
- The flap is divided, thinned, and inset in 3 to 4 weeks at an additional operation.

POSTOPERATIVE CARE

- Aggressive range of motion therapy should be initiated following injury to optimize outcome. Patients are encouraged to use their hands for activities of daily living. An occupational therapists who specialize in burn injuries is very helpful.
- Splints are used to maintain the hand in the intrinsic-plus position, with the MCP joints at 70 to 90 degrees of flexion, PIP joints at full extension, and the wrist in 10 degrees of extension to reduce clawing. Clawing yields tension over the PIP joint, resulting in chronic central slip injuries and late boutonnière deformities.

COMPLICATIONS

- Complications following acute burn treatment include graft loss, burn wound progression, and development of scar contractures that limit function.
- Complications of local tissue rearrangement used for contracture release include partial skin flap necrosis, dehiscence, scar recurrence, and neurovascular bundle injury.

SUGGESTED READINGS

1. Dente CJ, Feliciano DV, Rozycki GS, et al. A review of upper extremity fasciotomies in a level I trauma center. Am Surg 2004;70:1088–1093.
2. Esselman PC, Thombs BD, Magyar-Russell G, et al. Burn rehabilitation: state of the science. Am J Phys Med Rehabil 2006;85:383–413.
3. Graham TJ, Stern PJ, True MS. Classification and treatment of post-burn metacarpophalangeal joint extension contractures in children. J Hand Surg Am 1990;15:450–456.
4. Hargens AR, Romine JS, Sipe JC, et al. Peripheral nerve-conduction block by high muscle-compartment pressure. J Bone Joint Surg Am 1979;61(2):192–200.
5. Larson DL, Abston S, Willis B, et al. Contracture and scar formation in the burn patient. Clin Plast Surg 1974;1:653–666.
6. Lee RC, Zhang D, Hannig J. Biophysical injury mechanism in electrical shock trauma. Annu Rev Biomed Eng 2000;2:477–509.

Nail Matrix Repair, Reconstruction, and Ablation

Reuben A. Bueno, Jr. and Elvin G. Zook

DEFINITION

- Injury to the nail usually occurs by traumatic setting. Because of its location at the distal end of the digits, the perionychium is the most frequently injured part of the hand.[9]
  - Restoration of normal nail appearance and function is best achieved by acute repair of the nail matrix.
  - Reconstructive techniques may be used to provide a more normal-appearing nail.
- Excision of benign and malignant tumors involving the nail bed matrix may require techniques of nail bed repair and reconstruction also used for trauma.
- Optimal treatment depends on thorough understanding of the components of the perionychium—skin, sterile matrix, germinal matrix, eponychial fold, and distal phalanx—and their anatomic relationship with each other.

ANATOMY

- The nail serves multiple functions: protecting the fingertip, regulating peripheral circulation, and contributing to sensory feedback of the fingertip.[9,10]
- The perionychium includes the nail plate, nail bed, hyponychium, eponychium and fold, and paronychium (**FIG 1**).
- The proximal portion of the nail matrix (approximately one-fourth of the nail length) is the germinal matrix and the distal three-fourths is the sterile matrix. The germinal matrix produces about 90% of the nail, whereas the sterile matrix produces the remaining 10% of the nail and produces the cells on the undersurface of the nail responsible for nail adherence.
- The hyponychium is the skin distal to the nail bed, the paronychium is the skin on each side of the nail, and the eponychium is the skin over the nail fold.
- The nail bed is adherent to the periosteum of the distal phalanx.

PATHOGENESIS

- The main causes of nail deformity are trauma and tumor.
- The middle finger is the most commonly injured finger because of its length.[13]
- Inadequate treatment in the acute setting often leads to a nail deformity.
- There is an associated distal phalanx fracture in 50% of nail bed injuries. This type of injury should be considered an open fracture and treated as such with irrigation and débridement, reduction of the fracture and fixation if necessary, and repair of the nail bed (**FIG 2**).[1,4]
- Scarring can lead to a split nail deformity.
- Absence of nail matrix can lead to detachment of the nail.
- Lack of support from the distal phalanx leads to the hook nail deformity.
- Benign tumors (glomus tumor, distal interphalangeal joint ganglion) and malignant tumors (squamous cell carcinoma, melanoma) can affect nail appearance.

NATURAL HISTORY

- Repair in the acute injury period provides the best chance for normal appearance of the nail.
- The nail plate grows at about 0.1 mm per day or 2 to 3 mm per month. When the nail plate is removed for nail bed repair, new nail growth is delayed for 3 to 4 weeks.[9]

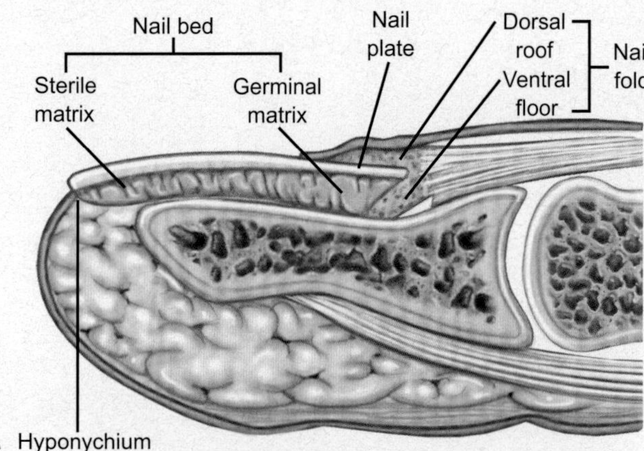

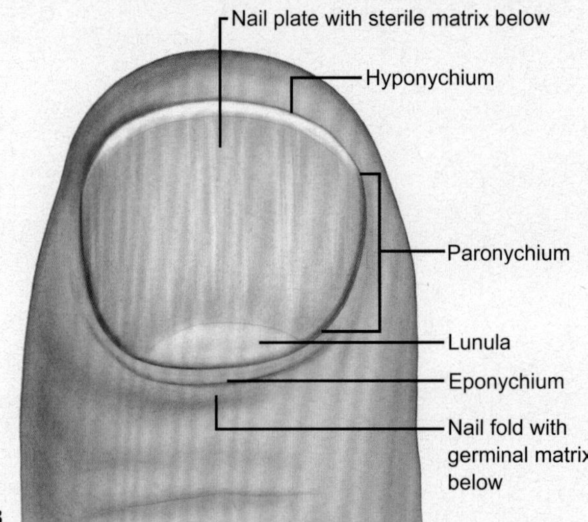

FIG 1 • **A,B.** The perionychium and its associated structures.

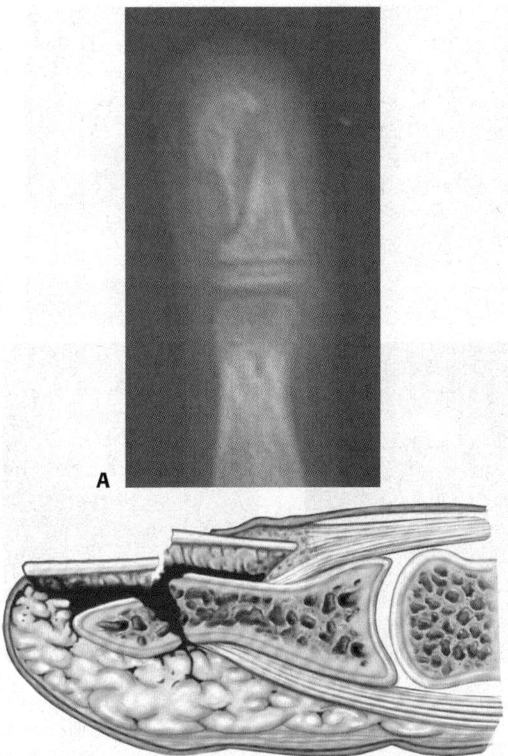

FIG 2 • A. Radiograph showing distal phalanx fracture associated with a nail bed crush injury. B. Nail bed injury with concomitant distal phalanx fracture. With a break in the periosteum, there is communication of the distal phalanx with the outside environment. There is a risk for osteomyelitis if not treated appropriately.

- If placed back on after repair, the old nail will remain adherent for 1 to 3 months and then fall off as a new nail pushes it off.[12]
- After nail repair, it will take about 12 months for the nail to achieve its final appearance. Thickening of the nail proximal to the level of injury is seen for about 50 days (**FIG 3**).[9,12,13]

PATIENT HISTORY AND PHYSICAL FINDINGS

- Traumatic injury to the perionychium is usually caused by a crush injury.[1,4]
- In the acute setting, the status of the entire fingertip must be assessed: quality of the skin, presence of a subungual hematoma, quality of the nail matrix, capillary refill, sensory function, flexion and extension at the distal interphalangeal joint, and presence of a distal phalanx fracture.
- Features of acute nail bed injury
  - Subungual hematoma (**FIG 4A,B**): bleeding beneath the nail from laceration of the nail bed
    - Pain secondary to pressure in the space between the nail plate and the nail bed
    - Treated with evacuation of hematoma by trephination
  - Laceration of nail bed (**FIG 4C,D**)
    - Mechanism of injury usually is crush.
    - Concomitant injury to fingertip skin or distal phalanx fracture may be present.
    - Nail lacerations can be described in one of four ways: simple laceration, stellate laceration, severe crush, and avulsion.
    - Repair of nail bed laceration and Kirschner wire fixation of distal phalanx fracture if unstable
  - Nail bed avulsion (**FIG 4E**)
    - Quality of avulsed nail matrix and size of defect will determine treatment.
    - Treatment options include returning avulsed piece back into the defect or harvesting a split nail graft from the adjacent matrix or from the great toe. (A skin graft will prevent new grooving nail to adhere.)
- Posttraumatic nail deformities
  - Nail nonadherence or split nail (**FIG 4F**)
    - Usually due to injury to the sterile matrix, which produces the cells responsible for adherence
    - Excision of scar and primary closure or nail matrix reconstruction with a split graft from the great toe
  - Hook nail deformity (**FIG 4G**)
    - Due to excessive tension at junction of nail bed and hyponychial skin and loss of support of distal phalanx
    - Revision amputation or reconstruction of nail bed and bone graft to the distal tip of the distal phalanx
  - Nail remnant (**FIG 4H**)
    - Due to presence of residual germinal matrix not completely ablated at the time of initial repair or revision amputation
    - Complete nail matrix ablation or revision amputation
  - Pincer nail deformity (**FIG 4I**): characterized by excessive transverse curvature of the nail and progressive pinching off of the distal fingertip, causing pain and abnormal appearance
    - Partial or complete nail ablation
    - Reconstruction of nail bed with elevation of the lateral nail bed using dermal graft or AlloDerm

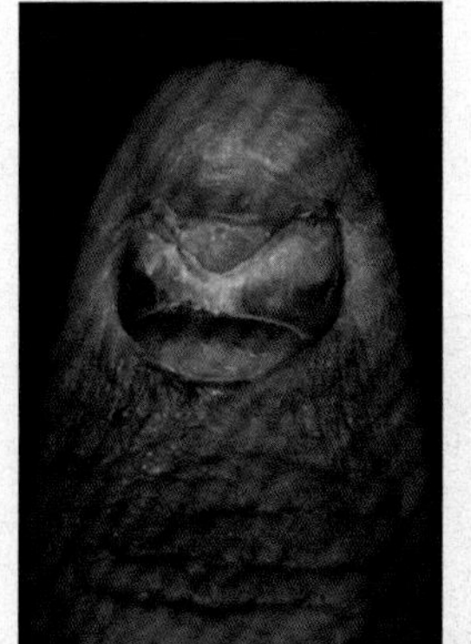

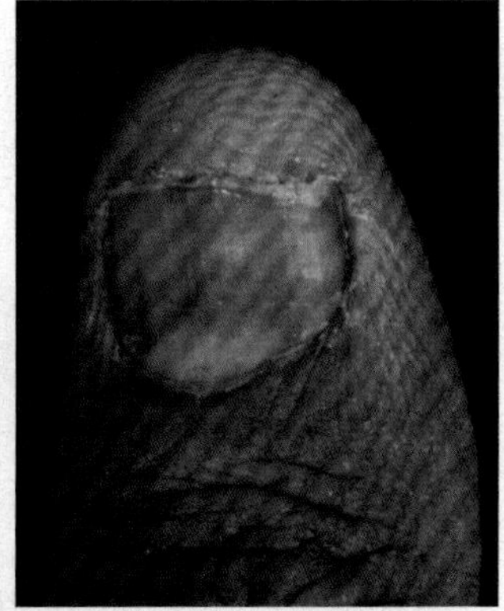

FIG 3 • A. Nail appearance at 3 months after repair. Patients should be aware of the heaped-up appearance as the nail grows distally. B. Nail appearance at 1 year after repair.

IMAGING AND OTHER DIAGNOSTIC STUDIES

- Anteroposterior (AP) and lateral radiographs of the distal phalanx are recommended to rule out a fracture.
  - Depending on the level of injury, the following fractures are seen: distal tuft fracture, comminuted fracture, and a transverse or oblique fracture of the midshaft.
  - Intra-articular fractures at the distal interphalangeal joint are rare with an associated nail bed injury.

DIFFERENTIAL DIAGNOSIS

- Trauma
- Benign tumor
  - Glomus tumor
  - Distal interphalangeal joint ganglion cyst

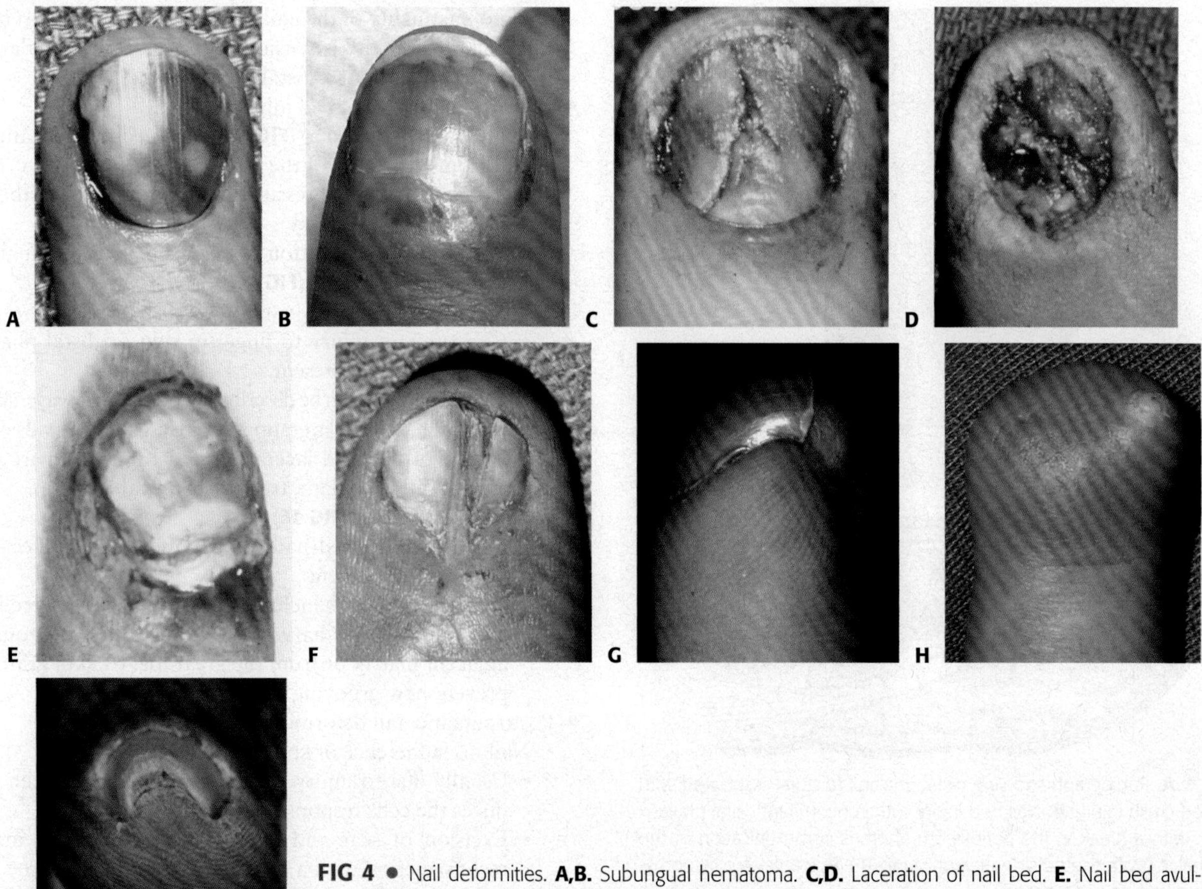

FIG 4 • Nail deformities. **A,B.** Subungual hematoma. **C,D.** Laceration of nail bed. **E.** Nail bed avulsion out of eponychial fold. **F.** Split nail deformity. **G.** Hook nail deformity. **H.** Nail remnant. **I.** Pincer nail deformity.

- Malignant tumor
  - Squamous cell carcinoma
  - Melanoma

NONOPERATIVE MANAGEMENT

- Left untreated, traumatic injury to the nail matrix may result in an abnormal appearance and shape of the nail.

SURGICAL MANAGEMENT

- Repair in the acute period increases the chance of a normal-appearing nail.
- Both surgeon and patient should be aware of the stages of nail growth and characteristic appearance at different points in the healing process as the nail regrows.
- Reconstruction of the nail matrix in a chronic injury should be approached with realistic expectations.
- Reconstruction of the nail matrix after tumor excision will depend on the amount of nail bed excised and the amount remaining.[2,6–8]

Preoperative Planning

- Management of malignant tumors involving the nail bed requires an understanding of the optimal level of amputation (usually to the level of the more proximal joint) and the need for sentinel node biopsy.

Positioning

- To provide a bloodless field, use of a Penrose drain tourniquet at the base of the digit secured with a clamp is recommended (**FIG 5**).
- Use of a portion of a surgical glove as a tourniquet is discouraged because of the risk of leaving the tourniquet at the base of the digit after repair and placement of the dressing. The dressing may then hide the tourniquet, and vascular compromise and subsequent necrosis of the finger is possible in the postoperative period.

Approach

- Sterile preparation and draping is done.
- A digital block with 1% plain lidocaine (maximum dose 7 mg/kg) is administered.

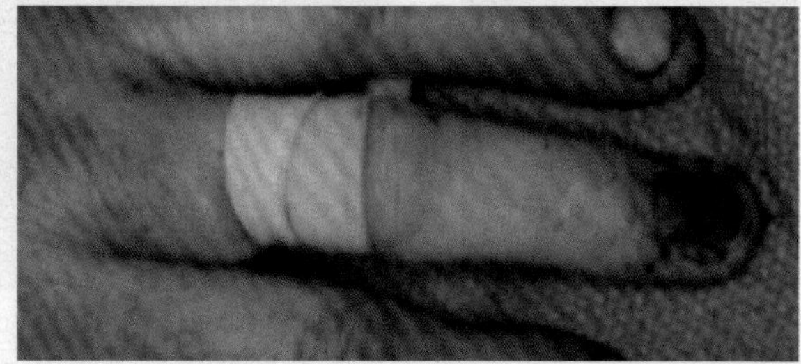

FIG 5 • Use of Penrose drain tourniquet at base of digit.

- Use of surgical loupes (2.5× magnification is sufficient) is recommended for the most accurate repair.
- A Kleinert-Kutz elevator is used to separate the nail plate from the nail matrix.
- The nail plate is cleaned and soaked in povidone-iodine (Betadine) as nail bed repair is done. If the nail plate is not available, a silicone sheet or nonadherent gauze can be used to maintain the eponychial fold after repair.
- Minimal débridement of the nail matrix is performed to preserve as much of the nail bed as possible.
- Incisions perpendicular to the eponychial fold may be necessary for adequate exposure of the germinal matrix (**FIG 6**).

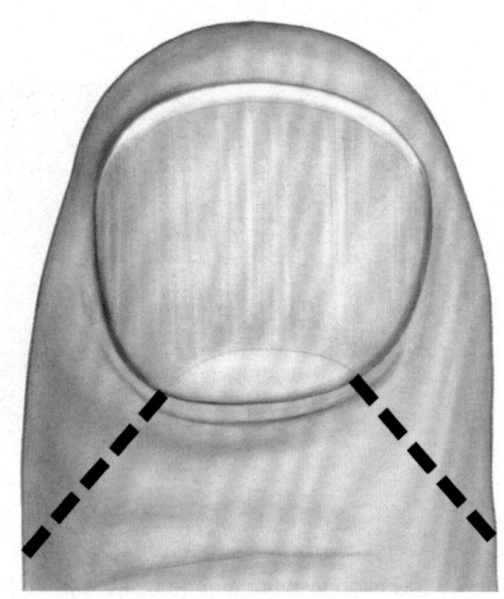

FIG 6 • Incisions made perpendicular to eponychial fold for exposure of the germinal matrix.

TECHNIQUES

Drainage of Subungual Hematoma

- A standard surgical preparation is performed to prevent introducing bacteria into the subungual space.
- Trephination of the nail can be accomplished using a heated paper clip, needle, or handheld battery-powered cautery (**TECH FIG 1**).
- Nail removal and repair is recommended if more than 50% of the nail is lifted up by the underlying hematoma or if the nail edges are not intact.

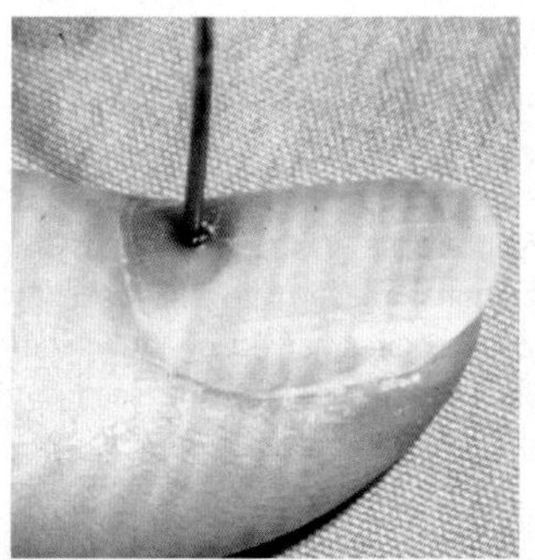

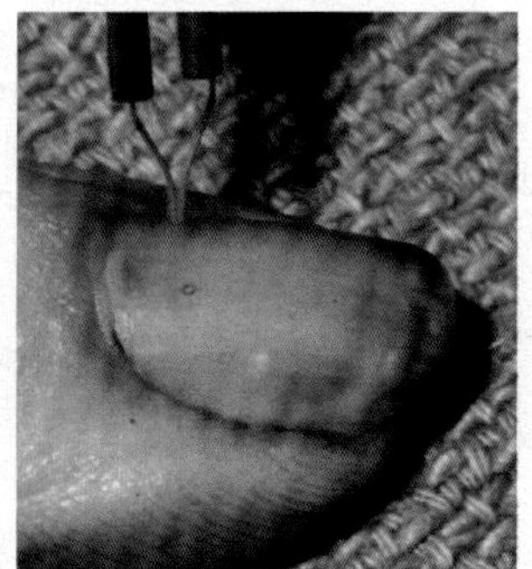

TECH FIG 1 • Trephination of the nail to drain a subungual hematoma using a heated paper clip (**A**) or battery-powered cautery (**B**).

Repair of Nail Bed Laceration

- Use a digital block, standard surgical preparation, and a Penrose drain at the base of the digit to serve as tourniquet.
- Use the Kleinert-Kutz elevator to separate the nail plate from the nail bed for adequate exposure (**TECH FIG 2A**).
- Repair the laceration under loupe magnification using simple sutures of 7-0 chromic (**TECH FIG 2B**).
  - Avoid aggressive débridement of the nail bed.
- Clean the nail plate, soak it in Betadine, and rinse it with normal saline; then place it back into the proximal fold to maintain this space and to serve as a splint for a distal phalanx fracture (**TECH FIG 2C**).

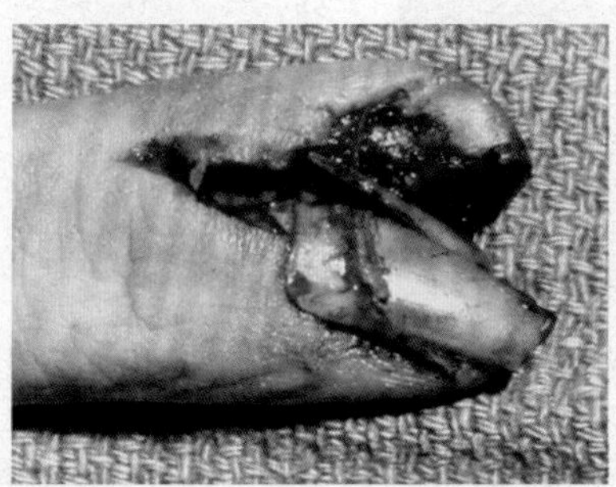

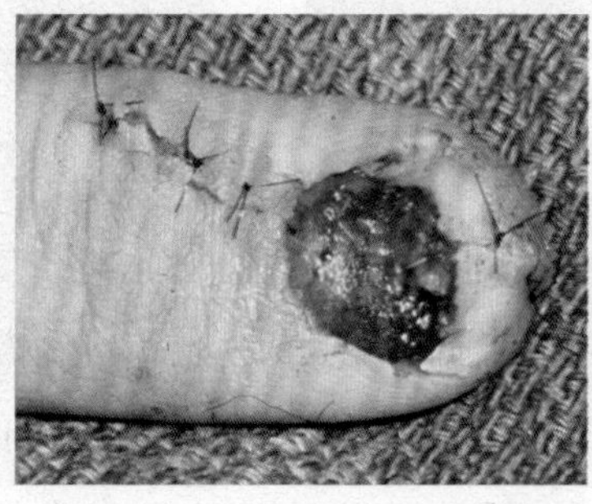

TECH FIG 2 • Repair of nail bed laceration. **A.** Laceration with nail plate present. The nail plate is cleaned and will be used later as a splint to maintain the eponychial fold. **B.** Repair of nail bed and surrounding skin after débridement. *(continued)*

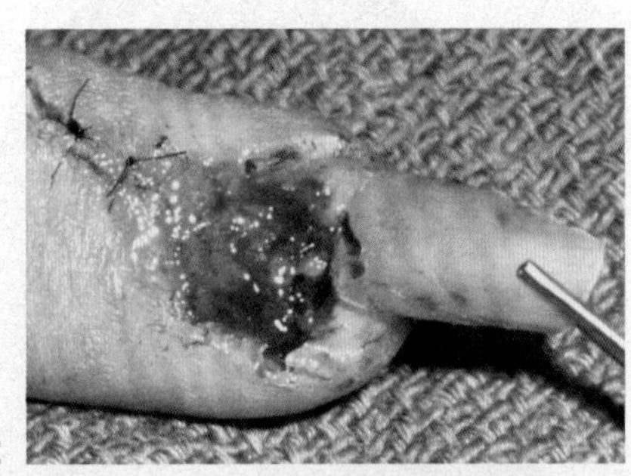

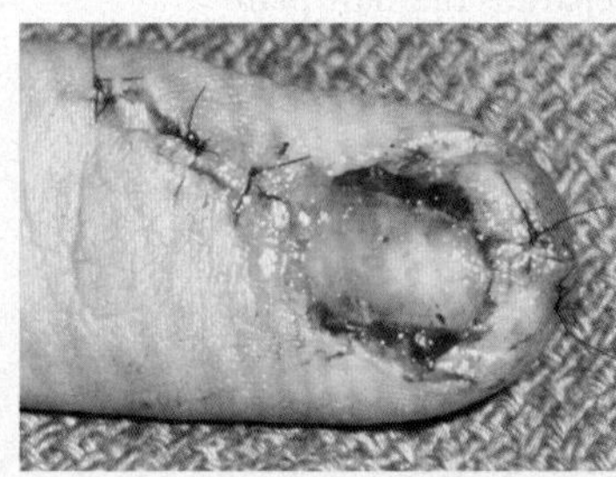

TECH FIG 2 • *(continued)* **C.** Nail plate being placed back into fold. **D.** Completed nail bed laceration repair.

- A figure-of-eight suture of 5-0 nylon or a simple stitch from nail to hyponychium can be used to hold the nail in place if desired (**TECH FIG 2D**).
  - A silicone sheet may be used if the nail plate is not available.
- Repair of a nail bed avulsion and resultant proximal germinal matrix disruption may require incisions perpendicular to the curved portion of the eponychial fold for exposure.

Treatment of Nail Bed Defects

- A defect amenable to reconstruction may be present after excision of scar (causing nonadherence or a split nail deformity) from prior injury to the nail bed (**TECH FIG 3A**).
  - Small areas (<2 mm) can be left to heal by secondary intention but may result in recurrent scarring and nail deformity.
  - Defects larger than 2 mm can be treated with split-thickness nail bed grafts from the adjacent noninjured nail bed, the nail bed from another digit, or the nail bed from a toe (**TECH FIG 3B**).[2,6,9,13]
- Prepare and drape the recipient and donor sites in standard surgical fashion and perform a digital block.
- Exsanguinate the digit and place a Penrose drain tourniquet at its base.
- Expose the nail bed and measure the defect.
- Harvest split-thickness nail bed graft from the sterile matrix of the same donor digit using a no. 15 scalpel blade (**TECH FIG 3C,D**).
  - To reduce the risk of donor site nail deformity, the germinal matrix should not be used as a graft for a defect of the sterile matrix.
  - Graft is carefully harvested by placing the blade parallel to the nail bed and taking it thin enough so that the blade can be seen through the graft.
- Suture the split-thickness nail bed graft in place using 7-0 chromic, as is done in a laceration repair (**TECH FIG 3E**).
- Reconstruction of the germinal matrix with subsequent nail growth on the recipient digit requires harvest of a full-thickness germinal matrix graft from a toe (preferably the second toe) (**TECH FIG 3F**).[11]

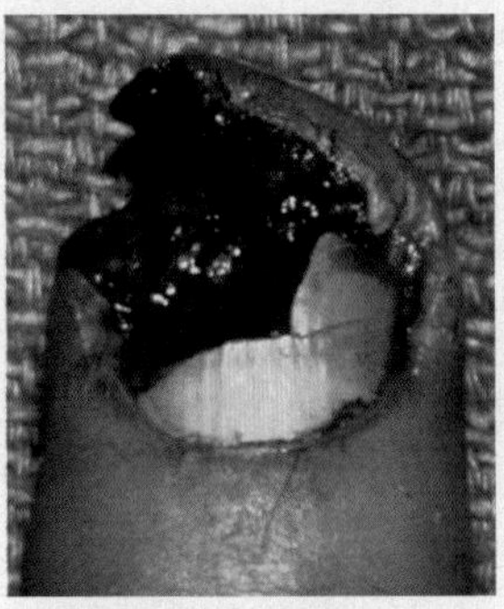

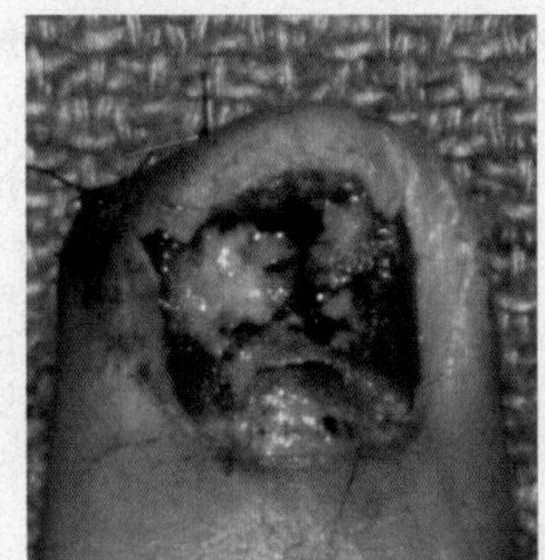

TECH FIG 3 • Treatment of nail bed loss with split nail graft. **A.** Initial presentation of this nail bed crush injury. **B.** Available tissue has been repaired, leaving a significant nail matrix defect. Exposed bone is visualized deep to the defect. **C.** Harvest of split sterile nail matrix graft from toe. **D.** Harvested split sterile nail matrix graft. **E.** Graft inset into defect to cover the exposed bone. **F.** Harvest of germinal matrix from the toe.

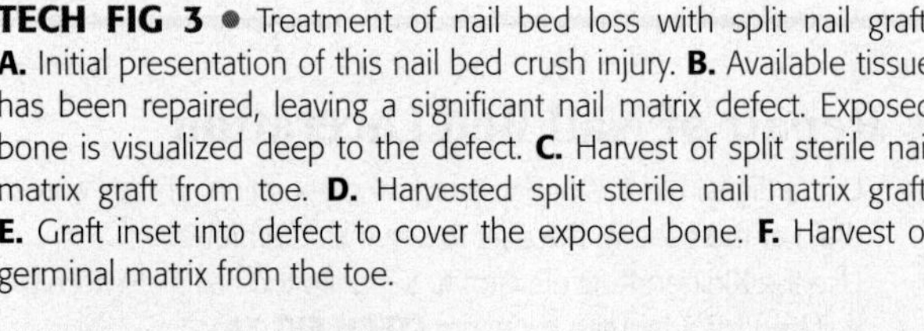

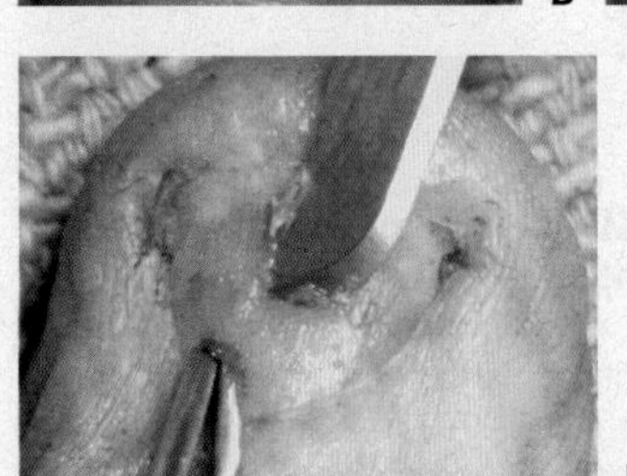

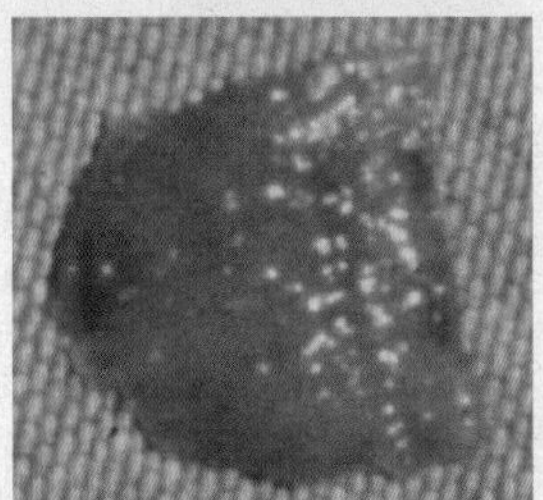

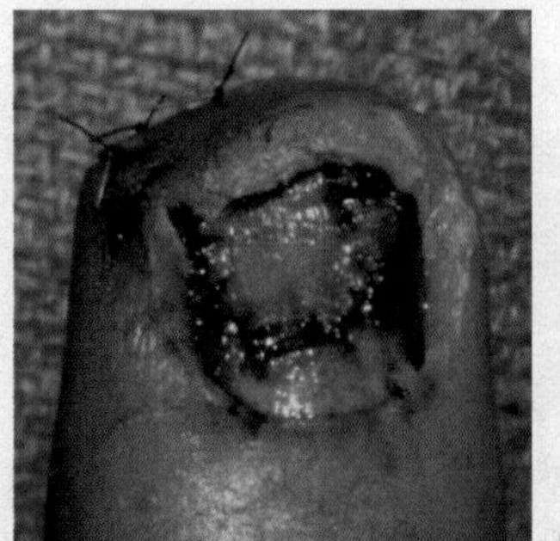

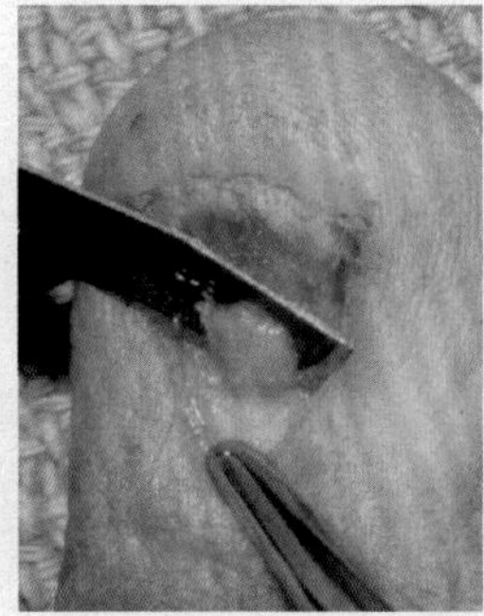

Nail Matrix Ablation

- A nail remnant may grow at the site of a previous nail ablation (**TECH FIG 4A**). It may grow in a dorsal direction, catching on clothes and requiring frequent clipping. This remnant may be a source of persistent pain, irritation, or infection.
  - A cyst may form from a nail remnant after a revision amputation and become a source for a subcutaneous abscess (**TECH FIG 4B**).
  - Complete excision of the residual germinal matrix is the goal of treatment.
  - It is important to tell the patient that a nail will no longer grow at the fingertip.
- Reenter the old incision, preserving skin to allow adequate primary closure.
- Dissect to the proximal portion of the distal phalanx at the expected location of germinal matrix.
  - The distal interphalangeal joint is used as a landmark to guide dissection to the level of the germinal matrix. It may be difficult to distinguish scar from residual germinal matrix after traumatic injury.
- Use a scalpel, curette, or rongeur (or combination) to ablate the residual nail bed germinal matrix (**TECH FIG 4C,D**).
- To preserve length yet fully ablate the nail, a full-thickness skin graft can be used to cover the distal phalanx.
- The distal phalanx is a unique area where a skin graft may survive even after being placed directly on bone without the presence of periosteum.

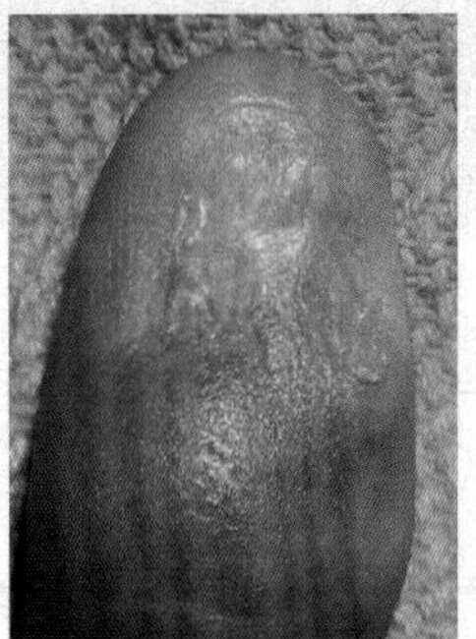
A

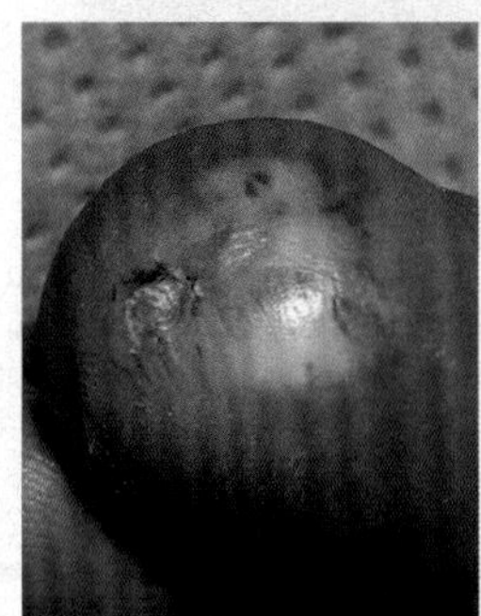
B

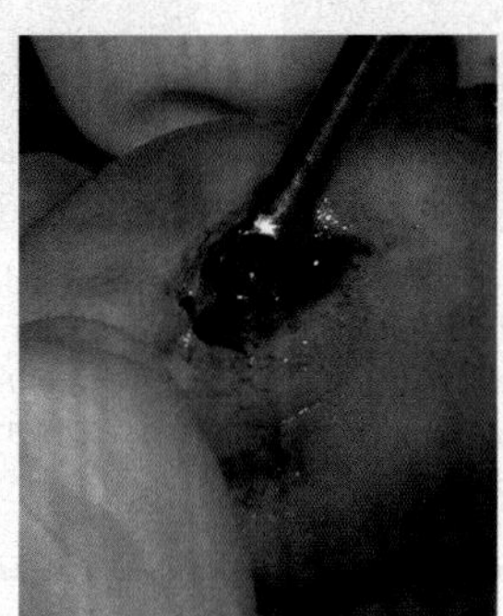
C

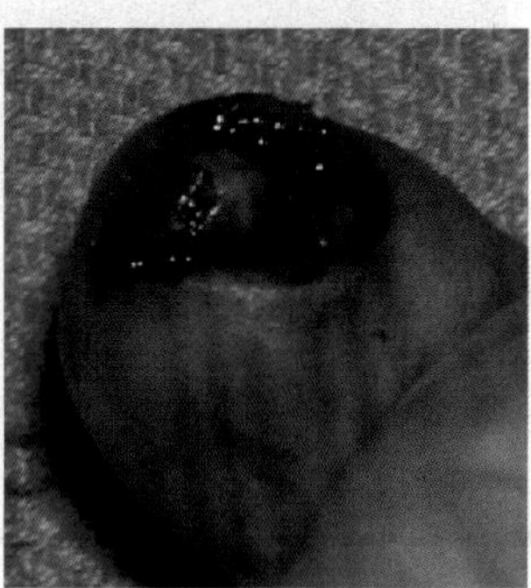
D

TECH FIG 4 • **A.** Right small finger after nail bed avulsion from fingertip trauma treated with nail bed ablation. Full-thickness skin graft was placed directly on the distal phalanx to preserve length and avoid revision amputation. Good take of skin graft was seen, but a nail remnant appeared on the proximal ulnar aspect of the fingertip, causing pain. **B.** Subcutaneous abscess from a nail remnant after revision amputation. **C.** Ablation of symptomatic nail remnant shown in **A**. An elliptical incision was made and all residual germinal matrices were removed with a scalpel. A curette was used to scrape the distal phalanx. **D.** A nail cyst is seen after incision and drainage of the abscess shown in **B**. The nail remnant was found within the cyst. Cyst and nail remnant were removed and symptoms resolved.

Treatment of Hook Nail Deformity

- Hook nail deformity can be caused by overaggressive débridement of the distal phalanx, resulting in lack of support, or by too much tension on a closure of the tip amputation, creating an unnatural, curved appearance of the nail.[5]
  - If the germinal matrix is still present, the nail will continue to grow but will hook downward without adequate bony support.
- Three treatment options exist: doing nothing, reconstruction of the tip to produce a flatter nail with or without bone graft, and revision amputation.
- Additional soft tissue bulk to the volar pad may be required to support the reconstructed nail.
  - A thenar flap may be used for reconstruction of the tip.
- Bone graft can be used for support, but there is a high rate of resorption.
- A favorable cosmetic result is often difficult to achieve.

Treatment of Pincer Nail Deformity

- The goal of treatment is to flatten out the excessive medial curvature of the nail and correct the "pinched-in" appearance of the nail (**TECH FIG 5A**).[3]
- Elevate the lateral margins of the nail bed from the distal phalanx using a Kleinert-Kutz elevator after removing the nail plate. (**TECH FIG 5B**).
  - Avoid injuring the paronychium as the nail bed is elevated.
- Make stab incisions on the ulnar and radial fingertip.
- Through these stab incisions, create subcutaneous tunnels to the radial and ulnar eponychium using the elevator. Make a second set of stab incisions at that proximal location (**TECH FIG 5C**).
- Cut dermal graft or AlloDerm to the appropriate length and place it through each tunnel.
- Pull the graft through the tunnel, distal to proximal, with the aid of a suture. This positions the graft in the desired location (**TECH FIG 5D**).
- Close the stab incisions with 6-0 nylon and replace the nail after it is flattened (**TECH FIG 5E,F**).

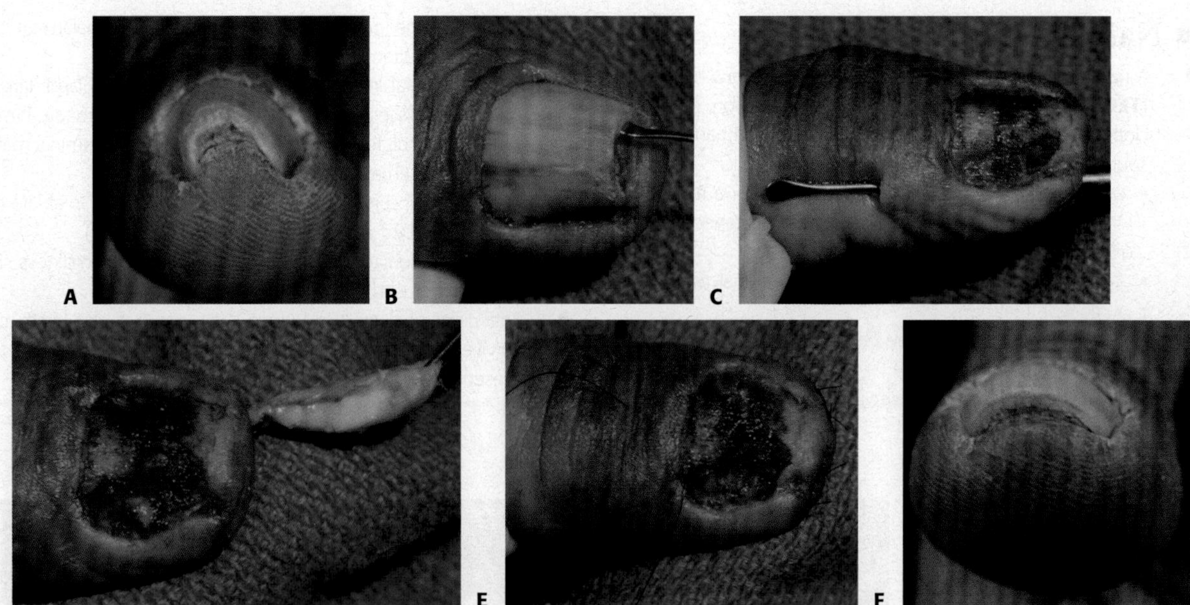

TECH FIG 5 • Treatment of pincer nail deformity. **A.** Pincer nail deformity with characteristic pinched-in appearance. **B.** The lateral borders of the nail are lifted from the distal phalanx in an atraumatic manner with a Kleinert-Kutz elevator. **C.** Creation of subcutaneous tunnels through stab incisions on the radial and ulnar sides. **D.** Placement of AlloDerm or dermal graft in subcutaneous tunnel. The graft is pulled into the tunnels with the aid of a suture in a distal to proximal direction. **E.** The wounds are closed, and the stitch is placed to hold the nail under the proximal nail fold. **F.** Postoperative appearance.

PEARLS AND PITFALLS

Traumatic injury	▪ With prompt treatment of nail bed injury, subacute and chronic problems can be avoided and a more complex reconstruction may be avoided. ▪ Failure to treat a nail bed laceration and concomitant distal phalanx fracture as an open fracture may result in osteomyelitis. ▪ Too much tension at the site of nail bed repair or a lack of support from the distal phalanx may result in a hook nail deformity.
Nail growth	▪ An accurate repair of the nail matrix allows the nail plate to grow out with a smooth appearance and nail shape. ▪ The germinal matrix produces about 90% of the nail. ▪ The sterile matrix contributes cells that are responsible for nail adherence to the underlying nail bed. ▪ The nail grows at 0.1 mm a day. ▪ New nail growth is completed by 6–9 months.
Nail bed reconstruction	▪ The goal of reconstruction is to restore the nail bed after loss due to trauma, scarring, or excision to allow more normal growth. ▪ Reconstruction of the sterile matrix can be accomplished with a split nail bed graft from the adjacent nail bed, an adjacent digit, or a toe. ▪ Reconstruction of the germinal and sterile matrices can be accomplished with a germinal and sterile matrix graft from the second toe but leaves a defect of the donor digit nail.

POSTOPERATIVE CARE

- The postoperative dressing is left on for 5 to 7 days and may need to be soaked in a mixture of hydrogen peroxide and water for removal. The repaired nail is checked for signs of infection, seroma, and hematoma.
- Nonadherent gauze placed to maintain the eponychial fold should be removed. Any suture used to hold the nail or silicone sheet within the fold should also be removed at 5 to 7 days postoperatively.
- Sutures placed in the skin of the hyponychium or paronychium should be removed at 10 to 14 days after repair.
- A fingertip splint that does not include the proximal interphalangeal joint can be used for the first 3 to 5 weeks after injury to protect the nail bed repair and immobilize a distal phalanx fracture if present.
  - Early motion of the proximal interphalangeal joint should be encouraged. The fingertip splint provides protection of the tip and will allow earlier motion of the injured digit.
- Hypersensitivity of the tip may be present for 1 to 3 months after injury, and desensitization exercises may be necessary to promote use of the affected digit.

OUTCOMES

- Although repair in the acute period provides the best chance for a normal-appearing nail (**FIG 7**), scarring at the site of injury may produce a nail deformity and patients should be reminded of this possibility at the time of repair.[11,13,14]
- Results of nail bed repair are adversely affected by avulsion or crush injury of the fingertip, presence of a distal phalanx fracture, three or more sites injured, and the need to use a silicone sheet for replacement of the nail.[1,4,13]
- Late reconstruction of the nail bed is often not as successful as surgeon or patient would desire.[9]
- Management plans must be individualized and realistic expectations must be discussed when treating patients with nail bed injuries.

COMPLICATIONS

- Complications in the acute or subacute setting include soft tissue infection, osteomyelitis of the distal phalanx, nonunion of the distal phalanx fracture, and posttraumatic stiffness and loss of motion at the distal interphalangeal joint.
- Complications or unfavorable outcomes in the chronic setting include scarring in the sterile matrix, leading to a split nail or nonadherent nail; scarring at the eponychial fold, which may interfere with nail plate growth; and persistent nail growth after an unsuccessful attempt at nail ablation.

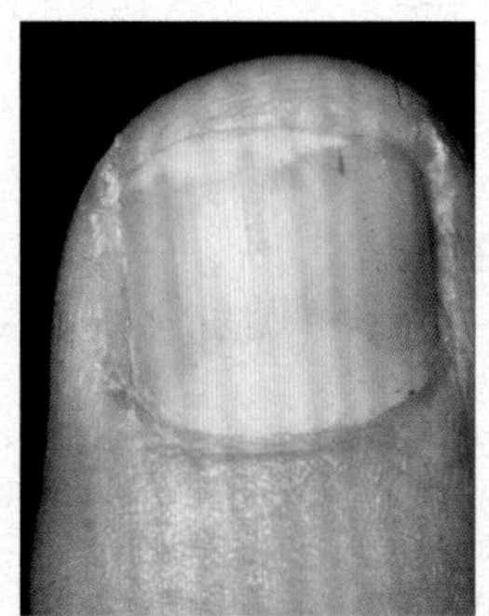

FIG 7 • Appearance of the nail in **TECH FIG 3** 1 year after nail matrix reconstruction with a split graft from the toe.

REFERENCES

1. Brown RE. Acute nail bed injuries. Hand Clin 2002;18:561–575.
2. Brown RE, Zook EG, Russell RC. Reconstruction of fingertips with combination of local flaps and nail bed grafts. J Hand Surg Am 1999; 24(2):345–351.
3. Brown RE, Zook EG, Williams J. Correction of pincer-nail deformities using dermal grafting. Plast Reconstr Surg 2000;105:1658–1661.
4. Guy RJ. The etiologies and mechanisms of the nail bed injuries. Hand Clin 1990;6:9–19.
5. Kumar VP, Satku K. Treatment and prevention of "hook nail" deformity with anatomic correlation. J Hand Surg Am 1993;18(4):617–620.
6. Shepard GH. Nail grafts for reconstruction. Hand Clin 1990;6:79–102.
7. Shepard GH. Perionychial grafts in trauma and reconstruction. Hand Clin 2002;18:595–614.
8. Shepard GH. Treatment of nail bed avulsions with split thickness nail bed grafts. J Hand Surg Am 1983;8:49–54.
9. Van Beek AL, Kassan MA, Adson MH, et al. Management of acute fingernail injuries. Hand Clin 1990;6:23–35.
10. Zook EG. The perionychium: anatomy, physiology, and care of injuries. Clin Plast Surg 1981;8:21–31.
11. Zook EG. Reconstruction of a functional and aesthetic nail. Hand Clin 2002;18:577–594.
12. Zook EG, Brown RE. The perionychium. In: Green DP, ed. Operative Hand Surgery, ed 3. New York: Churchill Livingstone, 1993: 1283–1287.
13. Zook EG, Guy RJ, Russell RC. A study of nail bed injuries: causes, treatment, and prognosis. J Hand Surg Am 1984;9(2):247–252.
14. Zook EG, Van Beek AL, Russell RC, et al. Anatomy and physiology of the perionychium: a review of the literature and anatomic study. J Hand Surg Am 1980;5:528–536.

Soft Tissue Coverage of Fingertip Amputations

Jennifer Etcheson and Jeffrey Yao

DEFINITION

- A fingertip injury or amputation involves trauma to the finger distal to the distal interphalangeal (DIP) crease.
- The fingertip is the most sensitive area of the hand.
- Fingertip injuries are common, accounting for 45% of emergency room hand injuries.

ANATOMY

- **FIG 1** depicts the anatomy of the fingertip.
- Eponychium: the cuticle or the thin membrane over the dorsum of the nail at the nail fold
- Perionychium: the skin at the lateral nail margin
- Hyponychium: the skin below the distal aspect of the nail plate, consisting of a mass of keratin with a high concentration of lymphocytes and polymorphonuclear cells; serves as a barrier to infection
- Nail root: portion of the nail plate proximal to the eponychial fold
- Lunula: the curved white opacity representing the distal, visible portion of the germinal matrix
- Germinal matrix: produces 90% of the nail plate volume
- Sterile matrix: contributes to nail plate adherence
- Nail plate: consists of flattened sheets of anuclear keratinized epithelium
- Nail bed: the floor of the nail plate, comprising proximal germinal matrix and distal sterile matrix
- Distal phalanx: lies deep to the nail bed
- Pulp: composed of fibrous septa

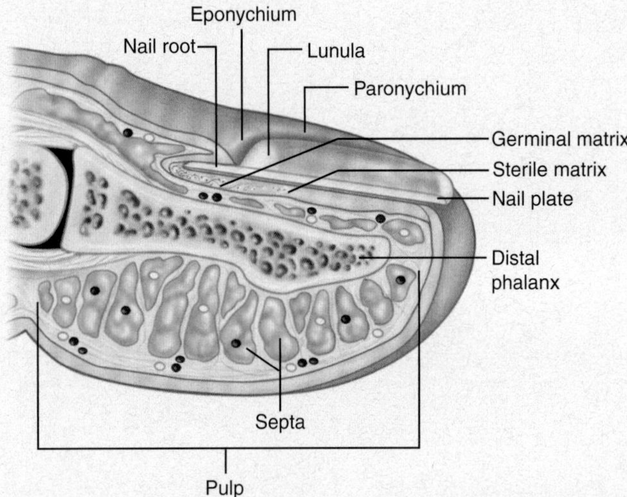

FIG 1 • Cross-section of a fingertip depicting key anatomic structures.

Fingertip Amputation Classification (Tamai)

- Zone I: distal to lunula
- Zone II: DIP joint to lunula

PATHOGENESIS

- Various mechanisms of trauma
  - Avulsion
  - Crush
  - Compression
  - Sharp
  - Dull

NATURAL HISTORY

- Fingertip injuries with no bone exposed will ultimately heal by secondary intention.
- In the setting of wounds less than 1 cm^2, secondary intention healing aided by daily dressing changes actually allows for increased recovery of sensation.
- The use of secondary intention healing for larger injuries involves a prolonged period of dressing changes with associated risk of infection and unfavorable scarring.

PATIENT HISTORY AND PHYSICAL FINDINGS

- Full history and physical examination
  - Mechanism of injury
  - Age
  - Handedness
  - Occupation
  - Level of cooperation and understanding
- Injury assessment
  - Digit or digits involved: thumb versus finger
  - Transverse versus dorsal oblique–volar oblique versus radial–ulnar
  - Damage to nail or nail bed
  - Exposure of bone
  - Static and moving two-point discrimination: There is decreased density of innervation with increased two-point discrimination.
  - Terminal flexion and extension: Injury to tendons will require more significant flap coverage.
  - Vascularity: Prolonged capillary refill is suggestive of arterial injury.

IMAGING AND OTHER DIAGNOSTIC STUDIES

- Plain radiographs in orthogonal planes (posteroanterior, lateral)

NONOPERATIVE MANAGEMENT

- Most fingertip amputations may be treated at the bedside using sterile technique and employing a metacarpal block, finger tourniquet, and loupe magnification.
- There should be a low threshold for operative management.
- If no bone is exposed, options include healing by secondary intention, primary closure, or skin grafting.
- Secondary intention healing aided by daily dressing changes provides the best recovery of sensation and is appropriate for wounds less than 1 cm^2.
- Primary closure is an option only if there is minimal skin loss.
  - Tight closures should be avoided. This can minimize function by causing joint contracture and distal tip tenderness due to poor soft tissue coverage of the bony prominences.
  - Sewing the volar skin tightly to the distal nail may result in a cosmetically displeasing hook nail.
- If a nail bed laceration is suspected, the nail plate should be removed with a Freer elevator, allowing repair of the nail bed with either 6-0 or 7-0 simple interrupted absorbable sutures (chromic gut). Loupe magnification is extremely helpful.
- The eponychial fold should be stented open with either trimmed and carefully cleansed nail or other material (eg, foil from a suture pack) to prevent abnormal growth of the future nail.
- With amputations through the germinal matrix, any remaining unrepairable matrix should be removed to prevent formation of a painful nail remnant.

SURGICAL MANAGEMENT

- The decision to take a patient with a fingertip injury to the operating room depends on the size of the defect, presence of exposed bone, angle of amputation, willingness of the patient to do dressing changes, and surgeon experience.
- The goals are to preserve function and sensation and allow early return to activity.
- In terms of functional outcome, healing by secondary intention provides equal or better results for defects less than 1 cm in diameter.
- Full-thickness grafts are preferable to split-thickness grafts.
  - Split-thickness grafts should be used only on the ulnar side of the index, middle, and ring fingers.
  - Donor site options include the volar wrist skin (should be avoided, as it can mimic a suicide attempt laceration), antecubital skin, medial upper arm skin, and hypothenar skin.
- These donor sites can be closed primarily.
- If salvageable, the original skin from the amputated segment can be defatted and applied as a graft/biologic dressing.
- If bone is exposed, options include bone shortening and primary closure and bone shortening and healing by secondary intention or fingertip flaps.

Preoperative Planning

- Preliminary irrigation and débridement, exploration
- Antibiotics
- Patient comorbidities
  - Is the patient a diabetic? smoker? recreational drug user?
  - Is the tetanus status up-to-date?
- Anesthesia assessment

Positioning

- Supine with standard hand table. An arm, forearm, or digital tourniquet is used. The arm is placed in the center of the hand table for equal access by the surgeon and assistant.

Approach

- Once the decision to perform a flap has been made, the angle of amputation, patient age, and patient gender determines whether an advancement or regional flap is appropriate.

TECHNIQUES

Skin Grafting

- Measure the size of the defect carefully and create a template.
  - This template is used to draw a corresponding defect on the donor site (**TECH FIG 1A**).
- Harvest the full-thickness graft with a no. 15 blade. Take great care to defat the graft down to dermis (**TECH FIG 1B,C**).
- Sew the graft into place and secure it using absorbable suture (**TECH FIG 1D**).
  - At four corners, the suture is left long so that later it may be tied over a bolster.
- Cover the skin graft with Xeroform dressing and mineral oil–soaked sterile cotton balls.
- Tie down the four long sutures over the cotton balls to create a bolster, placing gentle pressure on the graft to minimize shear.
- The finger is padded with gauze and protected with a finger splint, leaving the proximal interphalangeal (PIP) joint free for 5 to 7 days.
- After 5 to 7 days, the splint and dressing should be carefully removed, the graft inspected, and daily Xeroform dressing changes instituted until the graft is fully healed.

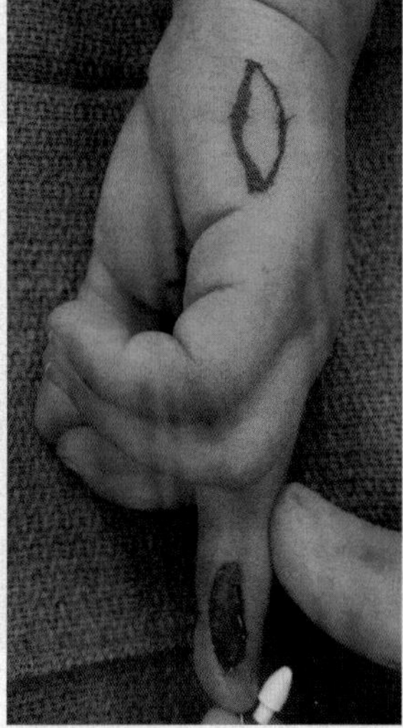

TECH FIG 1 • **A.** Ulnar defect of the long finger with the proposed hypothenar graft drawn out. *(continued)*

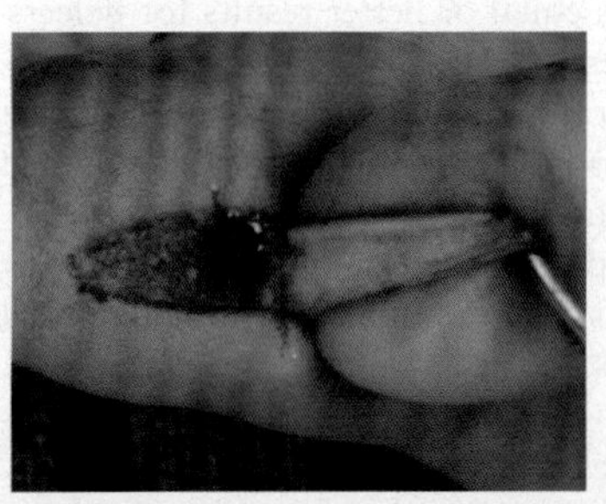

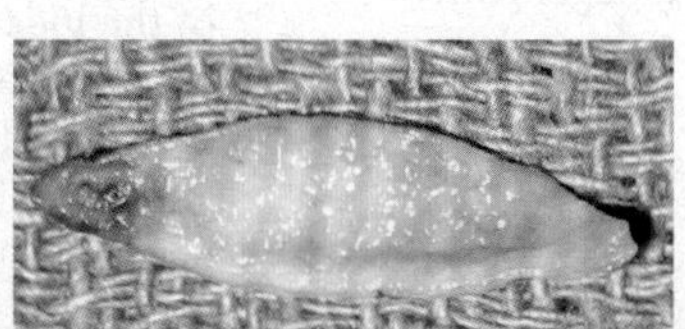

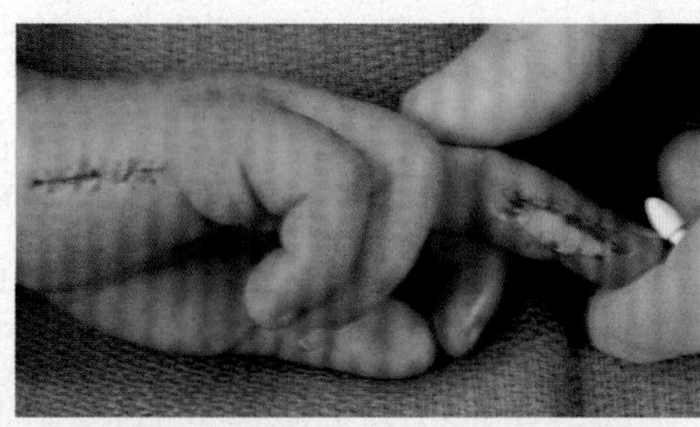

TECH FIG 1 • *(continued)* **B.** The hypothenar full-thickness skin graft is harvested, taking great care to defat the graft; only the dermis and epidermis are harvested. **C.** The hypothenar full-thickness skin graft ex vivo. Note a paucity of fat. **D.** The skin graft is inset using absorbable sutures. Four bolster sutures are then tied over a mineral oil–soaked cotton ball placed on top of the graft (not pictured). A dry dressing is applied. The bolster is left in place for 5 to 7 days.

Moberg Advancement Flap

- Indication: thumb tip amputation less than 1.5 cm; preserves sensation and length (**TECH FIG 2A,B**).
- *Not* indicated for fingertip amputations.
- Make a longitudinal incision just dorsal to the neurovascular bundles, based at the metacarpophalangeal joint flexion crease (**TECH FIG 2C**).
- Elevate a flap elevated from the flexor sheath (**TECH FIG 2D**).
- If the flap is difficult to advance, consider the following (**TECH FIG 2E**):
  - Flexing the interphalangeal joint
  - Extending the lateral incisions toward the palm with excision of skin at base to create an island flap; skin grafting of the secondary defect
- Excise a triangle of skin at the bilateral flap base (ie, triangle of Burow).
- Carefully preserve bridging vessels.
- Close with permanent suture under minimal tension (**TECH FIG 2F**).

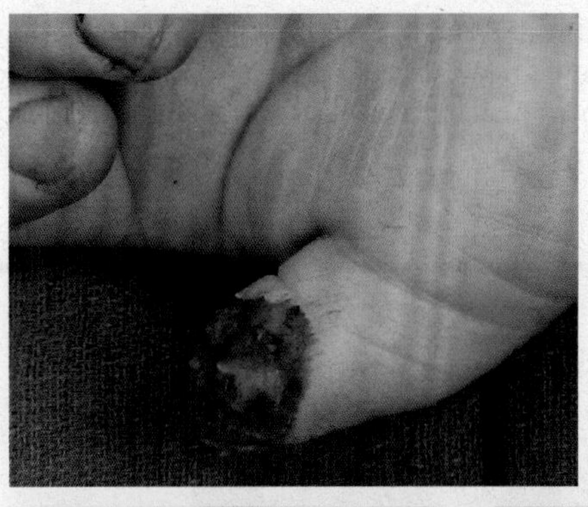

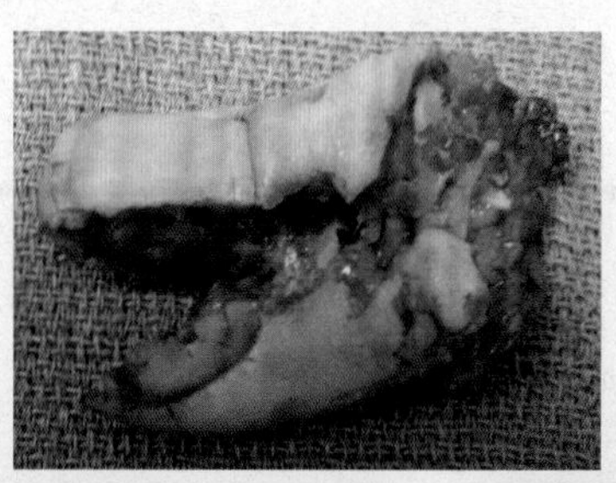

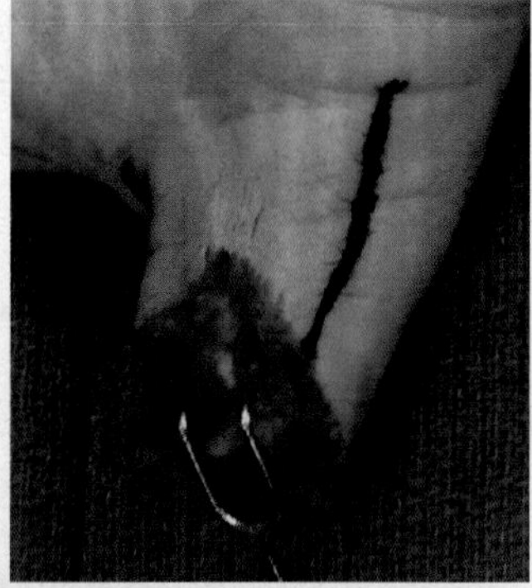

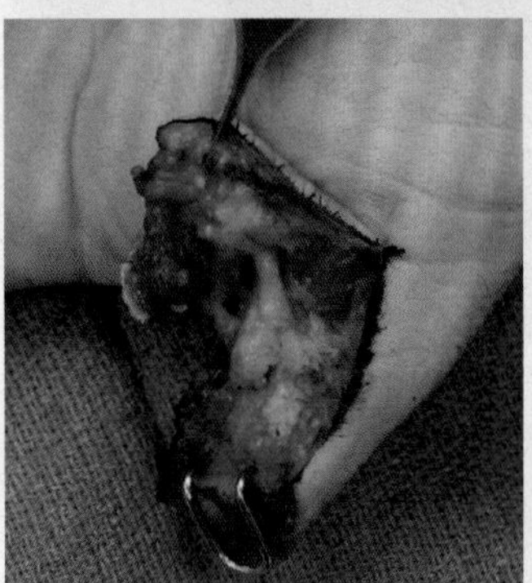

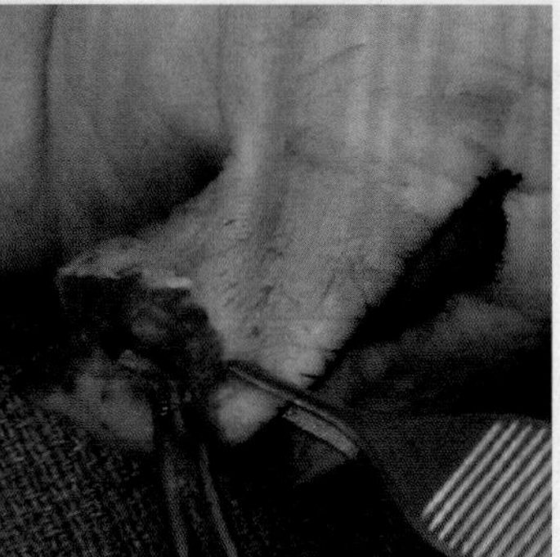

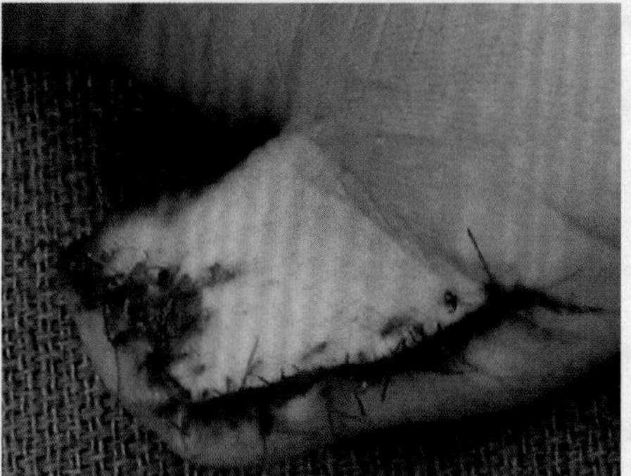

TECH FIG 2 • **A.** Distal thumb defect with exposed proximal phalanx. **B.** Nonreplantable distal phalanx. **C.** Intraoperative photograph indicating planned Moberg flap, with longitudinal incisions just dorsal to neurovascular bundles and based at metacarpophalangeal joint flexion crease. **D.** Moberg flap elevation from flexor sheath. **E.** Advancement of Moberg flap was possible without creation of an island flap or use of a triangle of Burow. **F.** Closure of the defect after advancement of Moberg flap. (Courtesy of James Chang, MD.)

Lateral V-Y Advancement Flaps (Kutler)

- Indication: transverse fingertip amputation with exposed bone
- The apex of the V is located at the lateral distal digital crease (**TECH FIG 3A–D**).
- Adequately mobilize the flap: Only nerves and vessels need to be kept intact.
- Bilateral triangles are advanced and sutured together distal to the nail bed.

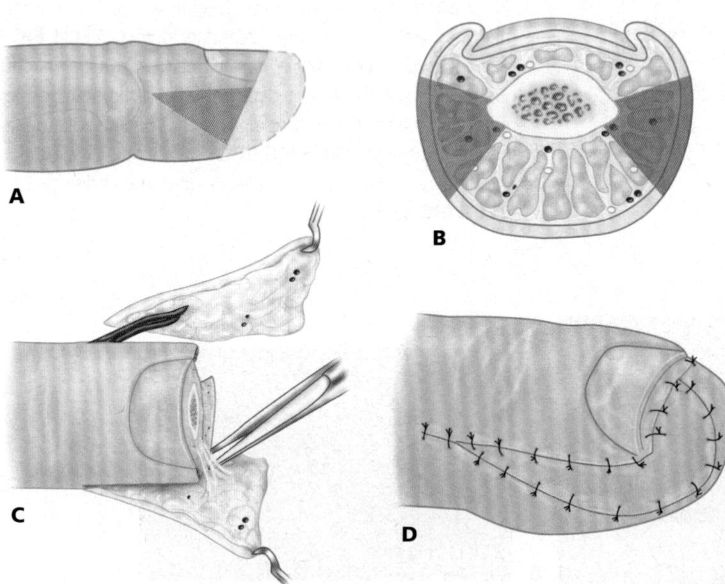

TECH FIG 3 • A. Lateral view of the digit with triangular flaps raised along the midlateral line. **B.** Flaps raised on both the radial and ulnar neurovascular bundles. **C.** Adventitia is released and the flaps are advanced distally to cover the defect. **D.** The flaps are sewn together to cover the defect, and the donor area is closed primarily in a lateral V-Y fashion.

Volar V-Y Advancement Flap (Atasoy-Kleinert)

- Indication: dorsal oblique fingertip amputation (ie, more dorsal than palmar skin loss) with exposed bone
- The apex of the V is at the volar midpoint of the distal digital crease (**TECH FIG 4A–C**).
- The base of the triangle should be as wide as the nail bed.
- Adequately mobilize the flap.

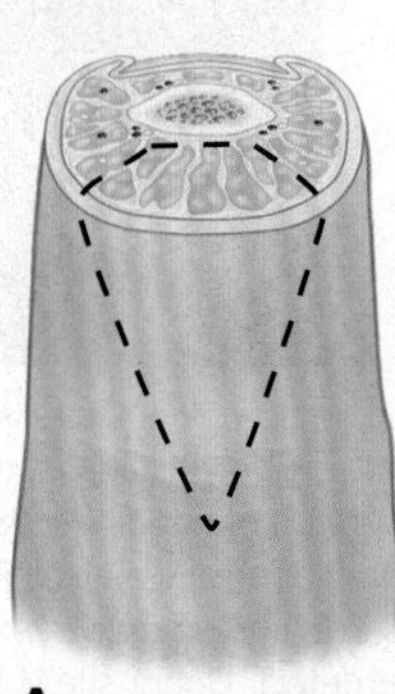

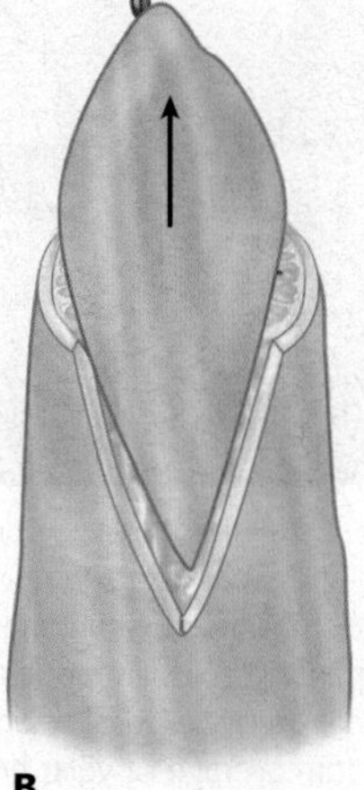

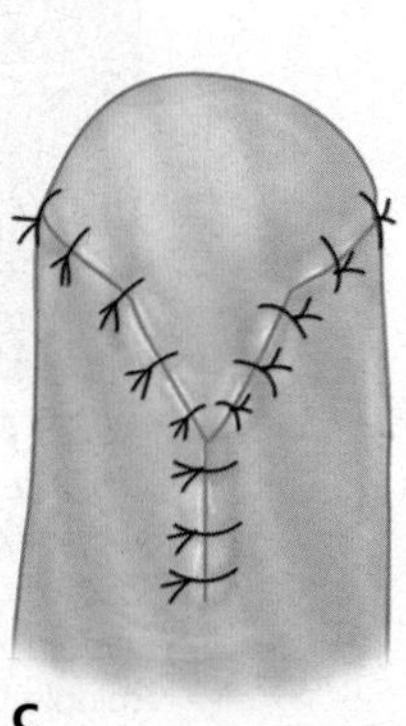

TECH FIG 4 • A. Volar-based V is incised. **B.** The volar flap is advanced distally to cover the distal defect. **C.** The flap is secured distally, and the donor area is closed primarily in a volar V-Y fashion.

Cross-Finger Flap

- Indication: volar fingertip defects up to 1.5 × 2.5 cm with an uninjured adjacent digit present (**TECH FIG 5A–C**)
- The donor area is the dorsal aspect of the middle phalanx skin of the adjacent finger.
  - The middle finger is used for an index fingertip amputation; otherwise, the donor skin is derived from the radial digit.
- Make two transverse midaxial to midaxial incisions on the donor area at roughly the DIP and PIP extension creases. Make one longitudinal midaxial incision on the side of the donor digit away from the injured digit to connect these two transverse incisions.
- Dissection is carried out in the loose areolar plane above the extensor paratenon.
- The paratenon must *not* be violated.
- A dorsal cutaneous nerve may be harvested as well to create an innervated cross-finger flap.
- The graft is mobilized to the midaxial line adjacent to the injured digit (**TECH FIG 5D**).
- Apply a full-thickness skin graft to the secondary defect.
  - The full-thickness graft should be first sewn to the hinge margin of the primary defect.
- The flap and full-thickness graft are then each rotated 180 degrees, allowing the flap to cover the primary defect and the full-thickness graft to cover the secondary defect (**TECH FIG 5E**). If an innervated cross-finger flap is pursued, the dorsal cutaneous nerve from the donor digit (in the flap) is attached to the pulp branch from the proper digital nerve on the volar aspect of the recipient digit (**TECH FIG 5F,G**).
- The flap is divided 2 to 3 weeks after the index procedure (**TECH FIG 5H,I**).

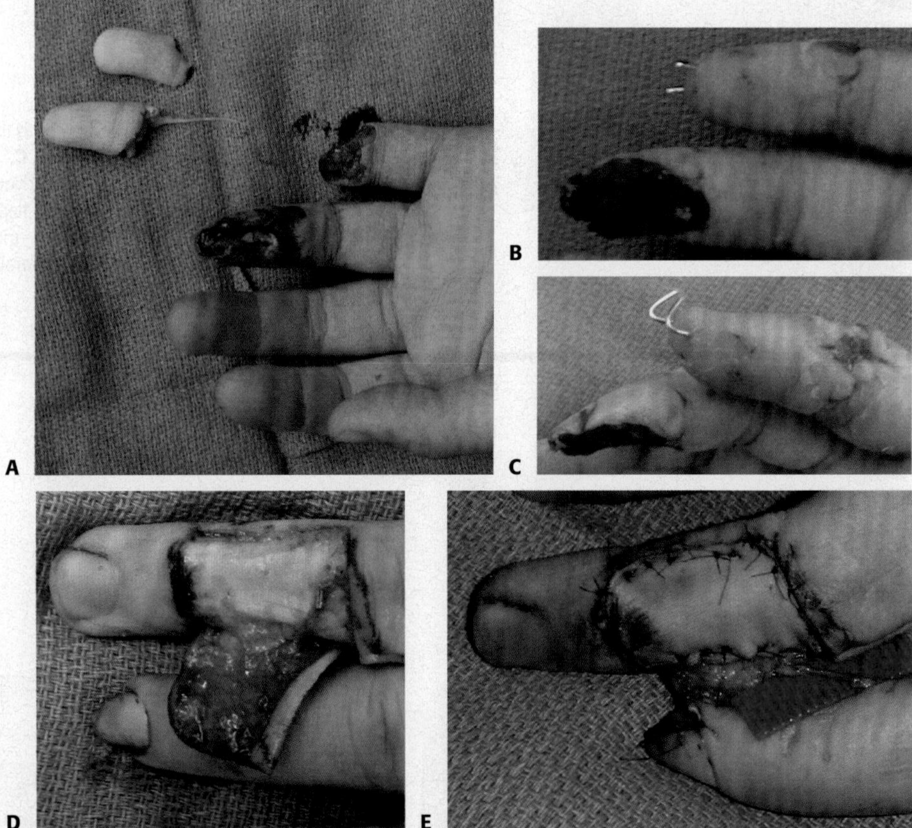

TECH FIG 5 • **A.** Intraoperative photograph depicting ring finger volar fingertip avulsion with exposed flexor tendon and small finger amputation at middle phalanx level. **B,C.** Two weeks after successful replantation of small finger with continued problem of ring finger wound, which had been treated with daily dressing changes. **D.** Intraoperative photograph after elevation of cross-finger flap from dorsal aspect of middle phalanx skin of adjacent finger. **E.** Intraoperative photograph after cross-finger flap from middle finger for coverage of volar ring finger defect. Donor site was covered with a full-thickness skin graft. Blue background indicates preservation of sensory branch. *(continued)*

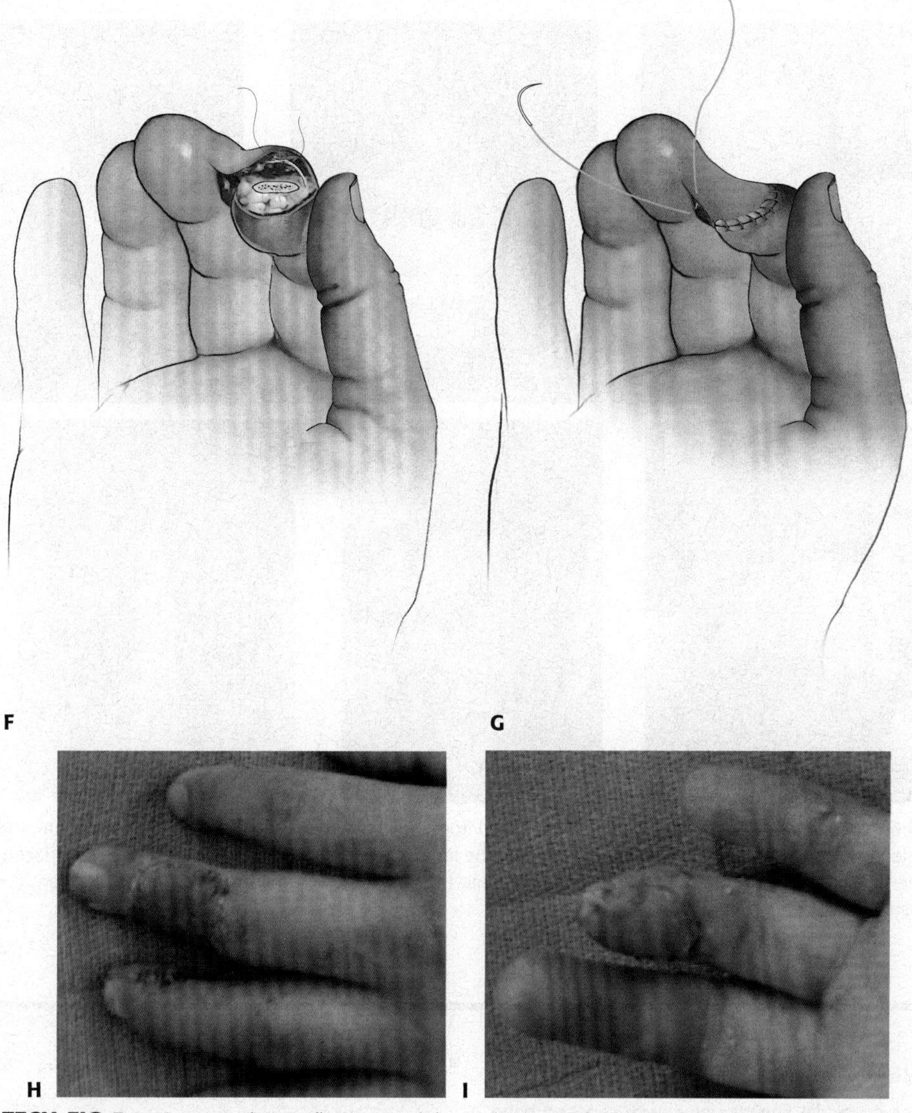

TECH FIG 5 • *(continued)* **F,G.** Illustration of the operative method. **H,I.** Intraoperative photographs after cross-finger flap division at 3 weeks.

Reverse Cross-Finger Flap

- Indication: dorsal fingertip injury
- Raise a deepithelialized full-thickness flap from the dorsal middle phalanx skin (**TECH FIG 6A,B**).
- Elevate the subcutaneous tissues underlying the raised graft (**TECH FIG 6C,D**).
- Cover the primary defect with the elevated deep tissue and then with a full-thickness graft (**TECH FIG 6E**).
- Cover the secondary defect with the previously described native full-thickness flap (**TECH FIG 6F**).
- The subcutaneous flap is divided in 2 to 3 weeks (**TECH FIG 6G**).

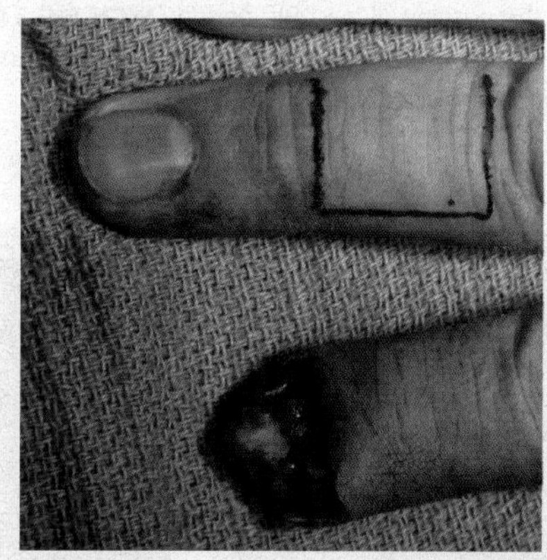

TECH FIG 6 • **A.** Dorsal defect of the right index finger with the flap drawn out on the adjacent long finger. *(continued)*

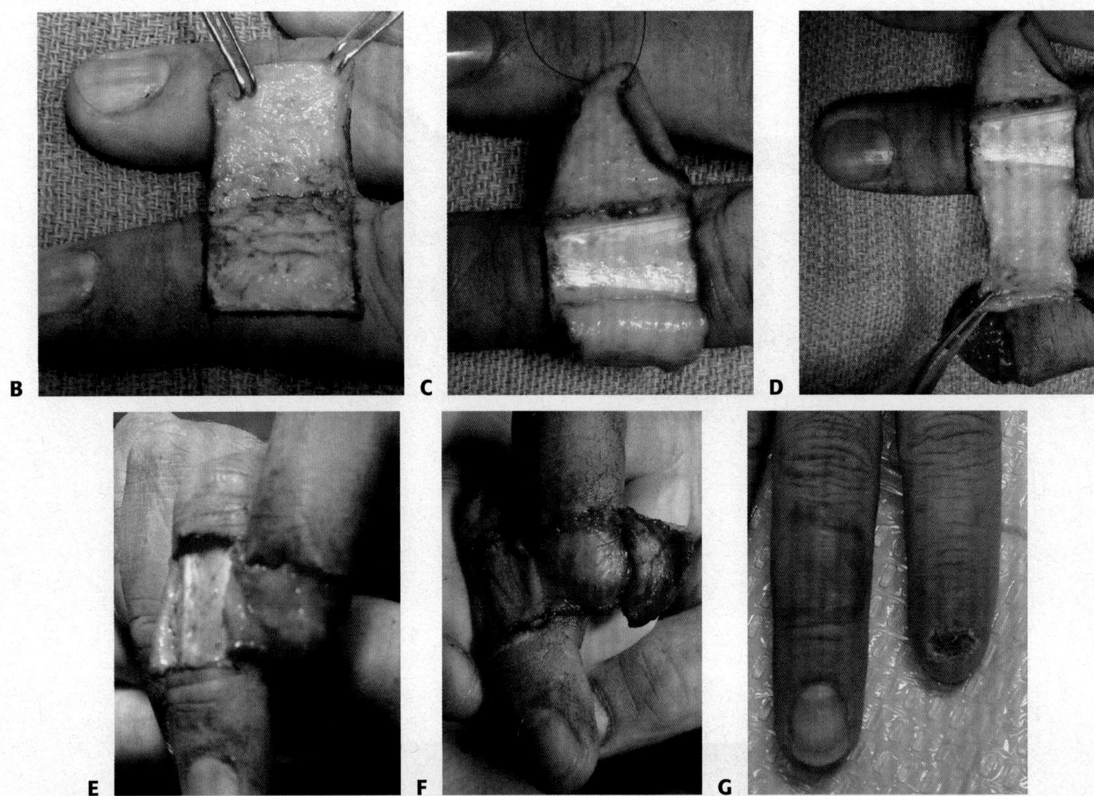

TECH FIG 6 • *(continued)* **B.** Ulnarly based skin flap raised from the long finger. **C,D.** The subcutaneous tissue is elevated off the paratenon of the long finger. **E.** The flap is inset onto the index finger defect. **F.** Split-thickness skin graft placed on the recipient site. The native ulnarly based skin flap is restored onto the long finger. **G.** Three months postoperatively. (Courtesy of Phani Dantuluri, MD.)

Thenar Flap

- Indication: Index or middle fingertip injury with exposed bone and more palmar than dorsal skin loss (defects roughly 1 × 1.5 cm in size) in patients younger than 35 years of age who are less likely to develop PIP joint contractures.
  - Women are better candidates for this flap than men.
- Press the amputated tip against the thenar eminence with the digit in the position of least PIP flexion (**TECH FIG 7A**).
- The position of the H flap is indicated by the bloody imprint from the amputation site (**TECH FIG 7B**).
- The designed H flap should be 50% wider than the defect to fully cover the pulp's semicircular contour.
- Raise the flap at the level of the thenar muscles with as much subcutaneous tissue as possible (**TECH FIG 7C**).
  - Take care to avoid injury to the digital nerves of the thumb.
- The H flaps may either be "tubed" around the defect or one flap may be advanced to fill the defect of the other flap that is sewn to the amputation site (**TECH FIG 7D**).
- The flaps are divided at 3 weeks.
- One or both H flaps can be used to close the donor defect primarily.

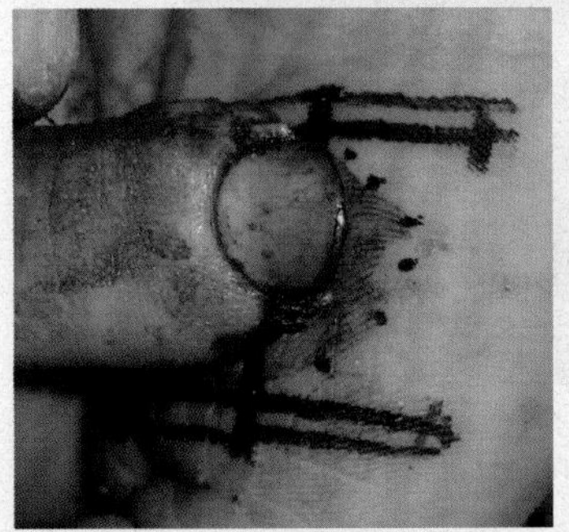

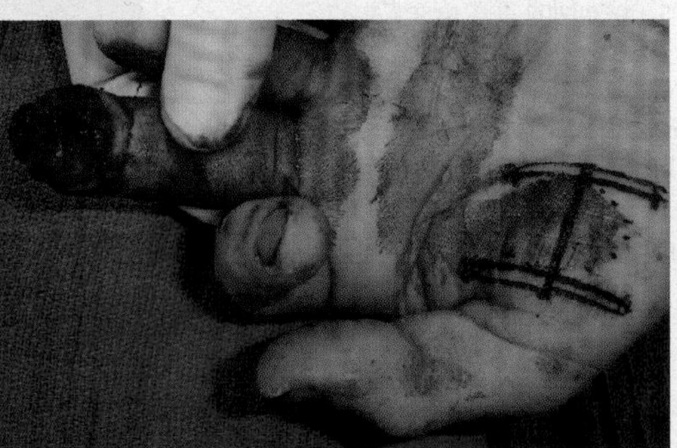

TECH FIG 7 • A. The middle digit is passively flexed to the thenar eminence and the thenar H flap outlined. **B.** The outside *pen lines* reveal that the flap is widened past the bloody impression to accommodate for the contour of the pulp. Note the volar oblique fingertip amputation of the middle digit. *(continued)*

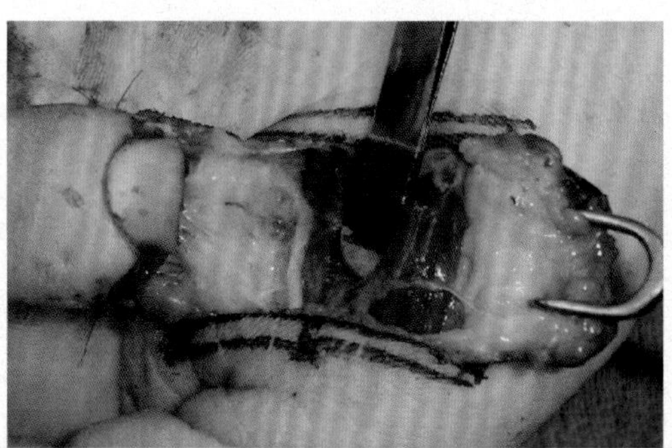

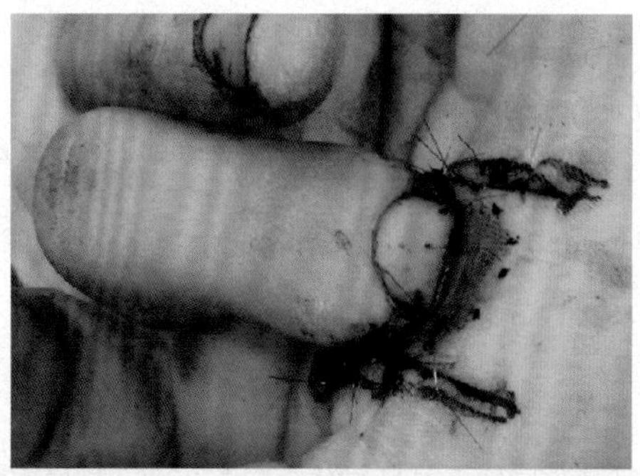

TECH FIG 7 • *(continued)* **C.** Dissection of the flap is performed at the level of the thenar musculature. Note the digital nerve present in the field of dissection. **D.** The flap is sewn in position. (Courtesy of Thomas R. Hunt III, MD.)

Neurovascular Island Pedicle Flap (Littler)

- Indication: volar distal thumb defect as well as volar radial index or volar ulnar small finger defects sufficient to produce a scarred pulp and an anesthetic tip (**TECH FIG 8A,B**)
- Use Doppler to ensure that flow is present in the ulnar digital artery of the ring finger and the radial digital artery of the middle finger.
- Create a template of the defect on the ulnar aspect of the donor digit.
- Apply the pattern to the distal ulnar aspect of the middle finger with small V-shaped indentations at the DIP joint creases.
  - The flap may be continued posteriorly, beyond the midaxial line.
- Make a Bruner incision to the distal flexor retinaculum.
  - Dissection is commenced in the palm to ensure normal anatomy.

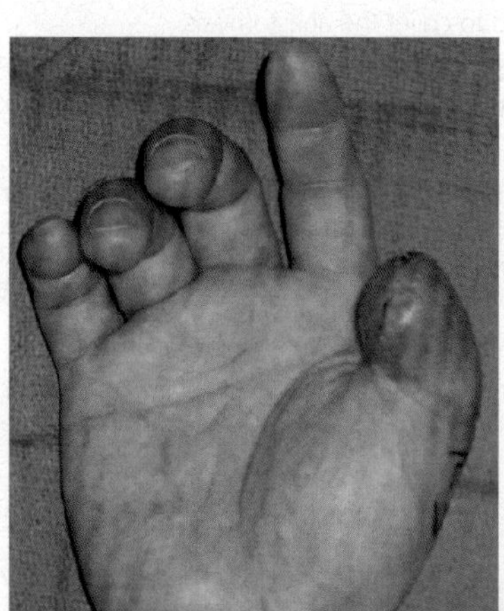

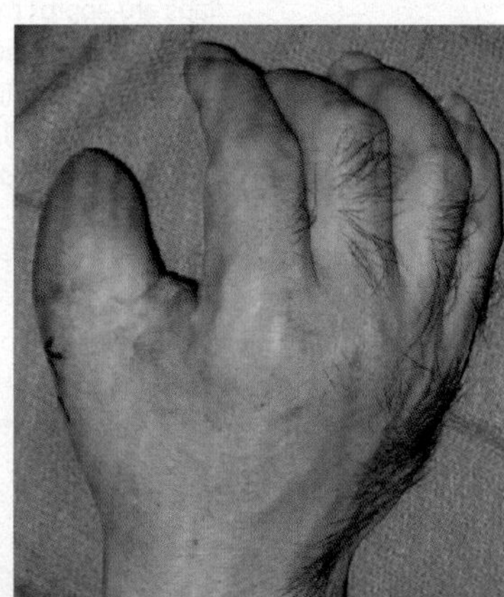

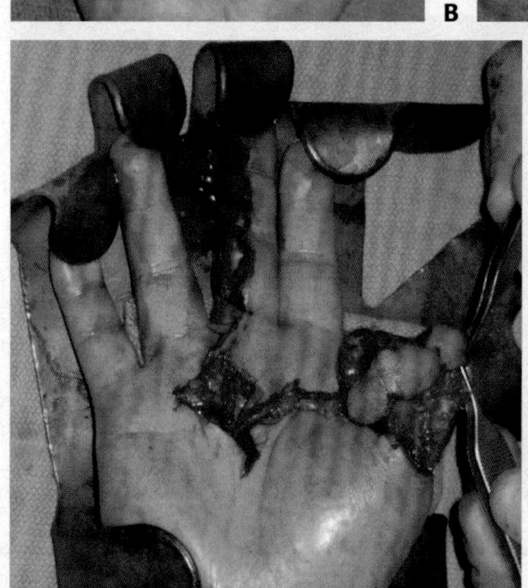

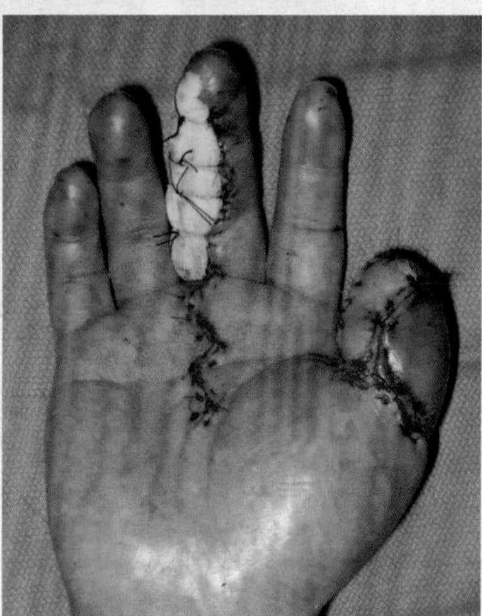

TECH FIG 8 • A,B. Insensate volar distal thumb after coverage of amputation site with free flap. **C.** Intraoperative photograph depicting neurovascular island pedicle flap (Littler) harvested from ulnar aspect of middle finger. **D.** Intraoperative photograph after tunneling of neurovascular island pedicle flap (Littler) to volar distal thumb, closure of wounds, full-thickness skin grafting of donor site, and application of a bolster dressing. (Courtesy of James Chang, MD.)

- Isolate and ligate the radial digital artery to the ring finger.
- Mobilize the vessel to the level of the superficial palmar arch to allow maximum pedicle length (**TECH FIG 8C**).
- Pass the entire pedicle beneath the digital nerve if it causes tension.
- Create a subcutaneous tunnel to the thumb using blunt scissor dissection.
- The tourniquet is released and flap viability assessed.
- The flap is then gently placed into a Penrose drain and secured in place with a 4-0 nylon suture to the tip of the flap skin.
  - The Penrose drain is used to avoid kinking and twisting of the pedicle as the flap is passed through the subcutaneous tunnel to the recipient site.
- The flap is sutured in place under minimal tension and the donor site is closed primarily or with a full-thickness graft (**TECH FIG 8D**).

Distal Tip Replantation

- Indications: amputation of the digit distal to the insertion of the extensor and flexor tendons into the distal phalanx with preserved vein(s) for anastomoses
- If the Tamai zone I amputations are too small to be held by an assistant, the surgeon holds the amputated part (**TECH FIG 9A**).
- Palmar and dorsal oblique full-thickness flaps are raised and sutured back under the microscope for thin flaps to avoid injury to the palmar veins.
- The distal amputated part is stabilized, and osteosynthesis is achieved with a single axial Kirschner wire.
- If in a Tamai zone II amputation, and the DIP joint is destroyed, primary arthrodesis is done with a single axial Kirschner wire for 4 to 6 weeks.
- The nail plate is reinserted into the nail fold in avulsed amputations using horizontal mattress sutures. Do not repair the flexor tendon but instead insert the proximal stump into the volar plate of the DIP joint to maintain better pinch strength.
- Under the microscope, visualize the nerve ends and the stumps of the arteries and veins by gently squeezing the pulp.
  - This can only be done once.
- Subcutaneous fat is removed from the artery and vein once they are identified to make room for the clamps.
- The proximal arterial stump is prepared with a tourniquet.
- Four to five 10-0 nylon sutures are used to repair the large central artery.
  - To aid the visualization and placement of the sutures, heparinized saline is used to irrigate the vessel lumen.
- In zone I, following arterial repair, the clamps are released momentarily to locate the subdermal palmar vein.
- Close the skin from dorsal to palmar, and then anastomose the subcutaneous palmar vein.
- Palmar vein anastomosis is carried out using a 1-V double clamp. If the clamp cannot be applied, the two ends are brought together and the corner sutures are held while the others are put in (**TECH FIG 9B**).
  - A 11-0 suture with 50 μm needle is used.
- Repair the nerve ends with 10-0 nylon suture.
- Artery and vein clamps are removed after the repair, and skin flaps are approximated to cover the anastomosis.
- The limb is kept immobilized in a short-arm cast for 2 weeks. The finger is watched for color change. Bluish coloring with hyperbrisk capillary refill indicates a venous congestion problem and a pale color with poor capillary refill and turgor indicates an arterial inflow problem. Continuous pulse oximetry may be used to monitor the oxygenation of the digit as well.
- The patient is kept on intravenous (IV) antibiotics and continuous infusion of 500 mL Dextran 40 and 5000 units of Heparin for 5 days, followed by 75 mg of aspirin for 3 weeks.

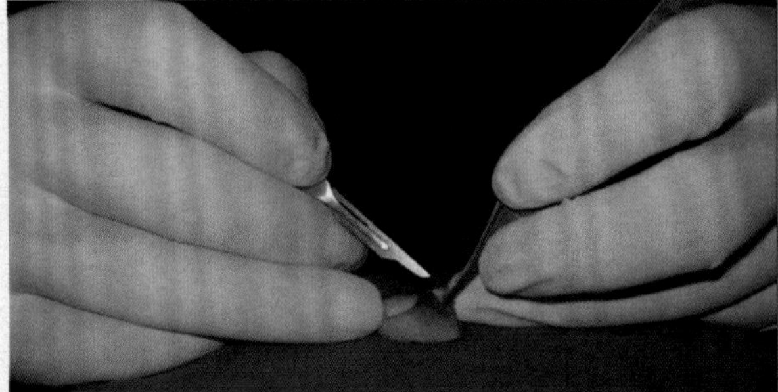
A

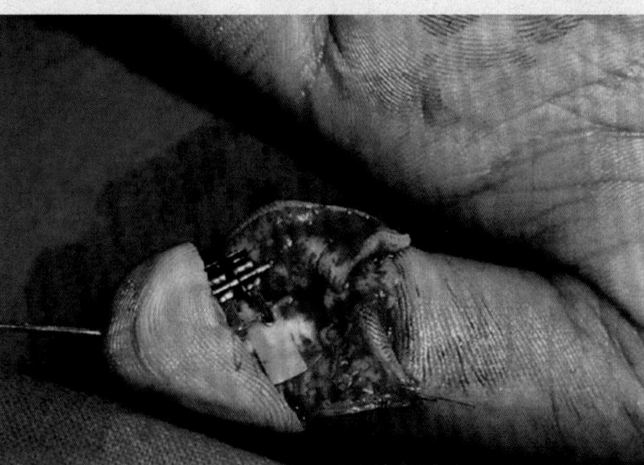
B

TECH FIG 9 • **A.** Positioning the amputated part between the surgeon's ring fingers of both hands. **B.** Palmar vein repair.

PEARLS AND PITFALLS

- Fingertip injuries less than 1 cm^2 can generally be treated with dressing changes with equal or better results than flap closure.
- The bridging vessels should be carefully preserved when performing a Moberg flap to prevent skin necrosis.
- V-Y advancement flaps may lead to scarring and hypersensitivity at the fingertip.
- The radial digital nerve should be carefully preserved and protected when performing a thenar flap.
- Cross-finger flaps (nonglabrous skin) may lead to hair growth on the fingertip and deficiency of pulp.
- Thenar flaps (glabrous skin) allow good sensibility in the flap but may be complicated by development of PIP joint contractures, especially in older male patients.
- Poor sensory outcome in neurovascular island flaps can be minimized by use of the most distal portion of donor skin, preservation of as much subcutaneous skin on the pedicle as possible, and avoidance of tension and kinking in the pedicle.

POSTOPERATIVE CARE

- When possible, the patient should meet the hand therapist preoperatively.
- Active and passive range of motion
- Sensory reeducation
- Scar massage
- Moberg advancement flap: thumb spica splint for 10 days to 2 weeks, followed by range-of-motion exercises
- Lateral V-Y advancement and volar V-Y advancement flaps: finger splintage of only the involved joint for 10 days to 2 weeks, followed by range-of-motion exercises
- Cross-finger flap and reverse cross-finger flap: A nonadherent bolster dressing is applied to the skin graft site and a splint is applied. PIP joints and the DIP joint of the donor finger can be gently ranged 2 weeks after flap inset, taking care to avoid tension on the flap. After flap division at 3 weeks, range-of-motion exercises are directed toward extending the PIP joints. Severe contractures may be treated with static progressive splinting.
- Thenar flap: A splint is applied postoperatively. Gentle range of motion of unaffected digits is started 2 weeks after flap inset, with care taken to avoid tension on the flap. Full range-of-motion exercises are started after flap division at 3 weeks. Severe contractures may be treated with static progressive splinting.
- Neurovascular island flap: The splint is changed 10 days after surgery, when sutures can be removed; gentle active range of motion is started, with full range of motion delayed until 3 weeks after surgery. Sensory reeducation is necessary to help differentiate thumb from middle finger sensation.
- Distal fingertip replantation: The Kirschner wire is removed in 4 weeks and a finger splint is kept on for an additional 2 weeks for lifting and during sleep. Otherwise, therapy for range-of-motion exercises is begun.

OUTCOMES

- Moberg flaps consistently provide return of normal two-point discrimination or within 2 mm of the contralateral digit and may result in a decrease in the hyperextensibility of the interphalangeal joint with no functional impairment.
- V-Y advancement flaps result in return of sensation to within 2.75 mm of the contralateral digit but may also result in paresthesia, hypersensitivity, and cold intolerance (50%).
- Patients who undergo a cross-finger flap have a return of protective sensation (8 mm of two-point discrimination), most predictably in younger patients, but the sensation remains less than the normal pulp.
- Hematoma or seroma significantly impairs the return of sensation.
- Thenar flaps provide superior return of sensation compared to cross-finger flaps but still less than normal.
- Neurovascular island flaps may result in hyperesthesia (23%) and cold intolerance (32%), which can be minimized by proper attention to detail and technique.

COMPLICATIONS

- Moberg flap: interphalangeal joint flexion contracture and skin necrosis
- Lateral V-Y advancement flaps (Kutler): scarring at the fingertip, which may be insensate or painful
- Volar V-Y advancement flap (Atasoy-Kleinert): hook nail or hypersensitivity
- Cross-finger flap: deficiency of fingertip pulp and hair growth on the fingertip
- Thenar flap: PIP joint flexion contracture of recipient finger
- Hematoma
- Seroma
- Infection
- Skin necrosis
- Dysesthesia or altered sensation
- Flexion contractures
- Loss of flap
- Epidermal inclusion cysts
- Nail deformities
- Symptomatic neuromas

SUGGESTED READINGS

1. Atasoy E. Reversed cross-finger subcutaneous flap. J Hand Surg Am 1982;7(5):481–483.
2. Barbato BD, Guelmi K, Romano SJ, et al. Thenar flap rehabilitation: a review of 20 cases. Ann Plast Surg 1996;37:135–139.
3. Blair WF, ed. Techniques in Hand Surgery. Baltimore: Williams & Wilkins, 1996.
4. Baumeister S, Menke H, Wittemann M, et al. Functional outcome after Moberg advancement flaps in the thumb. J Hand Surg Am 2002;27(1):105–114.
5. Fitoussi F, Ghobani A, Jehanno P, et al. Thenar flap for severe fingertip injuries in children. J Hand Surg Br 2004;29(2):108–112.
6. Foucher G, Delaere O, Citron N, et al. Long-term outcome of neurovascular palmar advancement flaps for distal thumb injuries. Br J Plast Surg 1999;52:64–68.

7. Goitz RJ, Westkaemper JG, Tomaino MM, et al. Soft tissue defects of the digits. Coverage considerations. Hand Clin 1997;13:189–205.
8. Green DP, Hotchkiss RN, Pederson WC, eds. Green's Operative Hand Surgery, vol 2, ed 5. Philadelphia: Churchill Livingstone, 1999: 1798–1816.
9. Henderson HP, Reid DA. Long-term follow-up of neurovascular island flaps. Hand 1980;12:113–122.
10. Kappel DA, Burech JG. The cross-finger flap: an established reconstruction procedure. Hand Clin 1985;1:677–683.
11. Koch H, Kielnhofer A, Hubmer M, et al. Donor site morbidity in cross-finger flaps. Br J Plast Surg 2005;58:1131–1135.
12. Lau C, Knutson GH, Brown WA. Thenar and palmar-flap repair in finger-tip amputations. Can J Surg 1969;12:294–301.
13. Lee NH, Pae WS, Roh SG, et al. Innervated cross-finger pulp flap for reconstruction of the fingertip. Arch Plast Surg 2012;39:637–642.
14. Melone CP Jr, Beasley RW, Carstens JH Jr. The thenar flap: an analysis of its use in 150 cases. J Hand Surg Am 1982;7(3):291–297.
15. Nicolai JP, Hentennar G. Sensation in cross-finger flaps. Hand 1981;13:12–16.
16. Nishikawa H, Smith PJ. The recovery of sensation and function after cross-finger flaps for fingertip injury. J Hand Surg Br 1992;17(1): 102–107.
17. Nomura S, Kurakata M, Sekiya S, et al. The modified thenar flap and its usefulness. J Jpn Soc Hand Surg 2000;16:707.
18. Okazaki M, Hasegawa H, Kano M, et al. A different method of fingertip reconstruction with the thenar flap. Plast Reconstr Surg 2005;115:885–888.
19. Shepard GH. The use of lateral V-Y advancement flaps for fingertip reconstruction. J Hand Surg Am 1983;8(3):254–259.
20. Tamai S. Twenty years' experience of limb replantation—review of 293 upper extremity replants. J Hand Surg Am 1982;7:549–556.
21. Trumble TE. Principles of Hand Surgery and Therapy. Philadelphia: WB Saunders, 2000:192–200.

Skin Grafts and Skin Graft Substitutes in the Distal Upper Extremity

140 CHAPTER

James N. Long, Luis O. Vásconez, and Jorge I. de la Torre

DEFINITION

- Upper extremity wounds that are candidates for skin grafting very closely parallel wounds suitable for skin grafting in other areas of the body. Certain wound conditions must be adhered to, and the principles of grafting remain constant, no matter the location of a wound.

Terminology

- *Autograft* refers to skin that is harvested from the same individual to whom it will be applied at a different location.
- *Isograft* refers to skin harvested from an identical twin of the recipient individual. Isograft behaves like autograft.
- *Allograft* refers to skin harvested from an individual of the same species as the recipient individual. Due to histocompatibility mismatch, these grafts eventually separate from the wound, except in immunosuppressed patients, and so provide only temporary coverage.
- *Xenograft* refers to the use of skin grafts from a species different from the recipient individual. Due to histocompatibility mismatch, these eventually separate from the wound, except in the immunosuppressed patient, and so provide only temporary coverage. Xenograft use is associated with an elevated rate of wound bed infection.
- *Split-thickness skin grafts* contain epidermis, along with a varying thickness of dermis that represents less than the full thickness of the dermis.
- *Full-thickness skin grafts* incorporate the full thickness of dermis and epidermis.
- *Donor site* refers to an area from which either a split- or full-thickness skin graft is harvested. Depending on the thickness of the graft, donor site treatment varies, from topical dressings, which typically are used for split-thickness skin graft donor sites, to direct closure, which is the usual method for addressing full-thickness skin donor defects.
- *Skin substitutes* are semisynthetic or purely synthetic constructs designed to act as replacements for lost skin structures. Ideally, they will be incorporated into the host to act as durable long-term replacements for lost tissue. In 1984, Pruitt and Levine[2] described the characteristics of ideal biologic dressings and skin substitutes. Their list of qualities considered to be ideal for skin substitutes still holds true more than 20 years later:
  - Little or no antigenicity
  - Tissue compatibility
  - Lack of toxicity
  - Permeability to water vapor, as would be seen in normal skin
  - Impenetrability to microorganisms
  - Rapid and long-term adherence to the wound bed
  - Capacity for ingrowth of fibrovascular tissue from the wound bed
  - Malleability, which would allow the construct to conform to the wound bed
  - Inherent elasticity that would not impede motion
  - Structural stability against linear and shear forces
  - Smooth surface to hinder bacterial proliferation
  - Good to tensile strength that would allow it resist fragmentation
  - Biodegradability
  - Low cost
  - Ease of storage
  - An indefinite shelf life

Wound Bed

- Before making a decision about using skin grafts or a substitutes, it is important to be familiar with the characteristics of a wound bed that make it suitable for grafting.
  - Graft beds should be properly débrided so that they are free of dead tissue and made as clean as possible to help minimize the risk of graft loss from infection.
  - Beds that are being considered for grafting must have an appropriate substrate from which the graft can derive its blood supply. In the context of upper extremity wounds, the bed specifically should contain no areas of denuded tendon or bone, as these denuded areas will not support inosculation (ie, neovascularization of the graft).
  - A further requirement, once débridement is complete, is the reduction of bacteria in the wound, which usually is effected through the use of a pulse lavage system. Enhanced skin graft survival by means of reducing bacterial counts is supported by studies published by Perry et al[1] in 1989.
- A useful tool in maturing a wound bed for grafting is the vacuum-assisted closure (VAC; KCI, Inc., San Antonio, TX) device. This device provides microdébridement of the wound bed and can help to promote the development of healthy granulation tissue, an ideal substrate for the support of skin graft adherence. Moreover, the VAC device can be used over the top of a skin graft applied to a wound and, through its negative pressure effect, limit fluid collection beneath the graft, also helping to ensure contact between graft and bed through an even distribution of pressure across the interface.
- Elements key to the development of an adequate graft bed are as follows:
  - Débridement of all nonviable tissue

- Minimization of bacterial colonization within the wound bed
- Ensuring that there exists an appropriate substrate for adherence of graft
- Microdébridement and maturation of the graft bed using appropriate dressings, which may include myriad measures ranging from the use of wet-to-moist saline gauze dressings to use of the VAC device.

ANATOMY

- The decision-making process in choosing split- versus full-thickness graft in the distal upper extremity involves both gross and microanatomic considerations.
- The lack of secondary contraction seen in full-thickness skin grafts supports their use on surfaces that overlie or are juxtaposed to joints. This lack of secondary contraction helps minimize the risk of unwanted joint contracture as the grafts mature.
- Over broad flat surfaces, such as the dorsal or volar aspect of the forearm, split-thickness skin grafts perform well.
- Wounds that involve the glabrous surface of the hand ideally are replaced with skin that possesses the same characteristics as the adjacent skin.
  - Harvest of glabrous skin from the sole of the foot or from the contralateral uninjured hand should be considered for such use.
  - In some cases, the wound may be so large that it is not possible to harvest sufficient donor skin while still permitting primary closure of the donor site. When this is the case, the arch within the sole of the foot may yield a full-thickness glabrous skin graft sufficient to cover the area of the original wound; however, the donor site then may require a skin graft itself. The donor site from the arch of the foot can be grafted with nonglabrous, meshed split-thickness graft with minimal morbidity due to its minimal weight-bearing requirement.

Microanatomy

- As suggested earlier, the surgeon must be concerned with the microanatomic conditions of the wound bed.
  - An appropriately vascular substrate is required to ensure proper graft take. Healthy fat, muscle, paratenon, or periosteum must be present within the base of the wound to ensure success.
  - Additional considerations include proper débridement of nonviable tissues from the wound bed as well as the minimization of bacterial contamination.

Donor Sites

- Glabrous skin
  - The sole of foot within the arch, beginning at the junction of glabrous and nonglabrous skin along the medial aspect of the arch
  - The ulnar aspect of the hand, beginning at the junction of the glabrous and the nonglabrous skin along the ulnar aspect of the palm
- Full-thickness skin
- Redundant areas of full-thickness skin available for harvest that maintain ease of primary closure of the donor defect include the lower abdomen, running from the anterior superior iliac spine in a gentle arc around the lower portion of the abdomen to the contralateral anterior superior iliac spine
  - Skin harvested from this area may be hair bearing. Depending on requirements of the recipient site, selection of full-thickness skin graft can range from the relatively hairless portions found laterally to the hirsute areas found centrally.
- Smaller areas of satisfactory full-thickness skin can be harvested from the upper inner arm. This skin, located at the junction of the medial biceps and triceps muscle groups, is thin and usually hairless.
- Split-thickness skin graft
  - Traditionally preferred sites have included the anterior thighs due to the ease of harvest and postoperative care of these areas.
  - Another site that has favorable characteristics in terms of quality of graft donor, as well as healing of donor site, includes the scalp.
  - Harvest of split-thickness skin graft from the scalp requires shaving of the head and the injection of epinephrine-containing wetting solution, for example, Pitkin solution or Klein solution, which is directed via puncture into a subgaleal plane to help minimize blood loss from the harvest.
  - The very rich vascular supply to the scalp makes split-thickness skin grafts from this site quite robust.
  - If the harvest is kept within the hair-bearing portions of the scalp, little to no donor defect can be detected once hair has grown back. Moreover, because of the high density of epidermal appendages in the scalp, reepithelialization of this area is more rapid than at other sites on the body. This rapid reepithelialization helps to minimize the potential for donor deformity (ie, scarring and dyspigmentation).

Harvest

- Skin harvest is greatly facilitated by proper preparation of the chosen site.
- First, a template of the bed to be grafted should be transferred to the donor site to ensure an adequate harvest. This is easily done with gentian violet and a sterile glove wrapper.
- Limiting blood loss from the harvest site is desirable and is easily achieved by preinjecting the hypodermis of the planned harvest area with an epinephrine-containing local anesthetic.
- If a long-acting local anesthetic such as Marcaine with epinephrine is used, the patient will have the additional benefit of prolonged donor site anesthesia postoperatively.
  - As split-thickness donor sites are typically quite painful, use of long-acting local anesthesia is a real benefit and is appreciated by the patient.
- When a large area is planned for harvest, attention must be paid to the appropriate maximum dosage for the local anesthetic selected. Dilute solutions in these cases can provide the benefits sought for these larger surface areas while still respecting the maximum allowed dosages.

PATHOGENESIS

- Wounds in the distal upper extremity requiring coverage arise from a host of different mechanisms. Among the most common are traumatic injuries, which commonly result in avulsive loss of skin. Other causes include burn injury to the upper extremity as well as defects created by tumor removal.

- Any one of these mechanisms may result in a wide range of injuries, from simple skin loss to injuries of deeper structures, including loss of paratenon or periosteum.

NATURAL HISTORY

- Skin graft healing varies from site to site on the body, and each location will vary from person to person.
- Skin in young adults is thick and healthy; however, in about the fourth decade, the skin begins to thin.
- Despite differences in skin thickness at differing anatomic locations, the overall dermal-to-epidermal ratio remains relatively constant: about 95% dermis to 5% epidermis.
- Blood vessels form arborizations into the dermis of the skin through access portals in the dermal papillae.

How Do Grafts Work?

- After application to an appropriately prepared wound bed, both split- and full-thickness grafts undergo a process that has been commonly termed *take*.
- The process involved in adherence of skin graft to wound bed is complex and involves an initial hypermetabolic condition within the graft, supported by plasmatic imbibition. Plasmatic imbibition is the process whereby nutrients and oxygen are drawn into the graft by absorption and capillary action. During this time, the graft remains adherent by a thin and friable film of fibrin between wound bed and graft.
- This early phase of graft support is followed by inosculation and capillary ingrowth. Before inosculation, there is a period during which ischemia and, therefore, hypoxia within the graft, with attendant histologic findings, are present.
- Once capillary ingrowth occurs and makes contact with the vascular network inherently present within the graft, blood flow is reestablished, and the skin graft takes on a pinkish hue. This process likely involves both the use of the inherent network of vessels within the graft and new vascular proliferation.
- Secondary adherence is mediated through fibrovascular ingrowth. The new vascular connections between graft and bed, as well as the new fibrous connections, solidify graft adherence.

Properties of Skin Grafts

- Skin grafts have been used to provide both temporary and permanent coverage, offering the inherent benefit of protection of the host bed from additional trauma while also providing an important barrier to infection.
- Split-thickness grafts tend to adhere to wound beds more easily and under adverse conditions that would not typically support full-thickness graft viability. This characteristic of split-thickness skin grafts provides a considerable advantage in managing difficult wounds; however, certain disadvantages can arise from their use. Once healed, split-thickness skin grafts undergo secondary contraction which, under uncontrolled conditions, can lead to pathologic contracture.
  - *Contracture* refers to a disability in function that arises from secondary contraction.
  - Additional disadvantages arising from the use of split-thickness skin grafts include dyschromia, poor elasticity, and reduced durability when referenced against their full-thickness counterparts.
- Full-thickness skin grafts include the full thickness of the dermis, along with the epidermis. In the initial phases, full-thickness skin grafts tend not to show the hardy "take" often seen with split-thickness skin grafts. To ensure full-thickness graft success, their use should be limited to well-vascularized recipient beds only.
  - Once established, full-thickness grafts offer distinct advantages; specifically, secondary contraction is far less problematic. Their thickness offers more resistance to external trauma and tends to be less likely to experience the dyspigmentation often associated with split-thickness grafts. They have much better inherent elasticity than split-thickness grafts, and for this reason, they are the graft of choice for use over and around joints.

Contraction

- As mentioned earlier, split-thickness skin can undergo a process of secondary contraction that ultimately may lead to pathologic contracture. Immediately on harvest, full- and split-thickness skin grafts behave differently.
  - The phenomenon of *primary contraction* refers to the tendency of a graft to shrink on elevation from the donor site. Substantial primary contraction is more often associated with full-thickness skin grafts than with split-thickness skin grafts. Full-thickness skin grafts contain the entire dermal layer and have more elastin than split-thickness skin grafts.
  - It is clinically important to remember that the immediate- and long-term elasticity of full-thickness skin grafts is much greater that in split grafts. It is this elastic property that makes full-thickness skin grafts an ideal choice for use around joints.
  - Once skin grafts have healed in place, the secondary process of contraction occurs more than in split-thickness grafts.
  - Full-thickness grafts tend to remain about the same size and, for practical purposes, show little to no secondary contraction. Full-thickness skin grafts have the capacity to increase their surface area with limb growth over time, whereas split-thickness grafts tend to decrease in size by a process of contraction or, alternatively, their size remains static.

Reinnervation

- The restoration of sensation in skin grafts is mediated through both peripheral ingrowth and direct growth into the graft from the bed.
- Factors affecting reinnervation of skin grafts include the location and quality of the recipient bed as well as the choice of full- versus split-thickness skin graft.
- Timing of recovery is variable, with some sensory recovery at between 4 and 6 weeks postgrafting. The return of normal sensation occurs between 12 and 24 months.

- The speed with which sensory recovery is realized depends on the accessibility of graft neural sheaths to wound bed nerve fibers. Accessibility of neural sheaths is improved in full-thickness grafts over their split-thickness counterparts, and, therefore, sensory recovery in full-thickness grafts is both more rapid and more complete.

Dyspigmentation

- The harvest of a graft disrupts its normal circulation, causing a loss of melanoblast content. This reduction results in a significant decrease in the number of pigment-producing cells within the graft.
- After graft revascularization, the initial hypoxia is corrected, and the melanocyte population recovers to a normal level.

Skin Substitutes

- The use of skin substitutes for wound coverage in the distal upper extremity typically is considered when the surface area involved is greater than that which could be reasonably covered with a full-thickness skin graft, but for which a split-thickness skin graft is suboptimal, for cosmetic or functional reasons.
- Skin substitutes are available in several classes. These include synthetics, biosynthetics, and biologic classes. The biologic class can be further subdivided into cultured autografts, allografts, and xenografts.
- Of the several skin substitutes on the market, the most clinically relevant are AlloDerm (LifeCell Corp., Branchburg, NJ) and Integra Dermal Regeneration Template (Integra LifeSciences Corp., Plainsboro, NJ). AlloDerm is a deantigenized human cadaveric acellular dermal construct. Integra consists of a bovine collagen dermal matrix sheathed with a silicone top membrane creating a bilaminar structure.

Prognosis

- For beds that have been prepared using proper technique with an appropriate choice of graft type, a high degree of successful take with excellent functional results can be obtained.
- It is important to bear in mind the process whereby the graft becomes mated with the bed to achieve good end results. Improperly prepared beds will not provide the vascularity required to ensure graft take.
- Excessive bacterial colonization of the wound also can lead to graft loss.
- Graft immobilization on the wound bed after placement is key to successful adherence.
  - Additional agents that act to prevent successful adherence include the accumulation of subgraft hematoma or seroma as well as shearing forces acting across the graft–wound interface.
  - Immobilization strategies must be directed toward the prevention of unwanted shear while providing pressure adequate to minimize the accumulation of fluid between graft and bed.
- All efforts should be made to minimize the risk of infection before graft application by means of débridement, lavage, and the use of both topical and systemic antibiotics, as directed by culture results.
- The rigid application of these principles produces high success rates.

PATIENT HISTORY AND PHYSICAL FINDINGS

- When considering a patient for skin grafting, along with the normal complete history and physical examination, special attention should be given to inspection of the wound bed.
- The surgeon should ascertain that all tissues within the prospective graft bed are viable and that bacterial growth within the wound is addressed through both wound débridement and treatment with appropriate antimicrobials. Areas of denuded tendon or bone are not acceptable for graft adherence.
- Other factors that negatively impact graft take are factors known to be responsible for impaired wound healing. The most common of these are cigarette smoking, diabetes mellitus, and malnourished states. It is important to elicit this information before proceeding with the operative plan.

IMAGING AND OTHER DIAGNOSTIC STUDIES

- Wounds with a bacterial content greater than 10^5 colony-forming units (CFUs) have significantly reduced successful graft take. A quantitative culture can be performed to assess this variable before skin grafting.
  - A punch biopsy is used to obtain a portion of vascularized wound bed, and this tissue sample is sent to the laboratory, where it is homogenized and then plated. CFUs on the culture plate are counted and then referenced against the initial sample weight. A concentration of more than 10^5 CFUs per gram of sample tissue is a negative predictor of successful graft adherence.
  - The area of tissue biopsied must be delivered from the viable portions of the tissue bed and not from devitalized tissues, which will show very high colony counts and are not representative of the graftable bed.

DIFFERENTIAL DIAGNOSIS

- Superficial or partial-thickness skin loss
- Full-thickness skin loss
- Full-thickness skin loss concomitant with deep tissue injury
- Loss of paratenon or periosteum
- Wound over or adjacent to joints
- Wound over broad, flat surface that does not overlie a joint

NONOPERATIVE MANAGEMENT

- Superficial abrasions or burns over broad surfaces with maintained viability of the dermal and hypodermal structures can be treated by local wound care without the use of grafting. Areas of skin with abundant epidermal appendages (sebaceous glands, sweat glands, and hair follicles) have inherent source tissue for reepithelialization of these superficial wounds.
  - Conservative management ideally includes a moist wound healing environment that limits bacterial growth and does

not inhibit the process of neoepithelialization, such as the petrolatum-based antimicrobial ointments (eg, Neosporin [Johnson & Johnson, New Brunswick, NJ] and Xeroform gauze [Covidien, Mansfield, MA]).
    - When conservative wound management is being employed, serial observation is advised to ensure that the process of neoepithelialization is underway and is not hindered by the development of local infection or other unforeseen factors.
    - If the process of reepithelialization is complete by the end of 2 weeks after the event of the initial injury, scarring at the site of injury will be minimized.
- Smaller wounds that are deeper and penetrate through dermis into the hypodermis may be treated conservatively as well.
    - Local wound care with serial wet-to-moist changes or by use of the VAC device can help facilitate healing by secondary intention.
- Larger areas of skin loss allowed to heal by secondary intention can result in a substantial delay in wound healing. In addition, functionally limiting contractures can develop as a byproduct of secondary intention healing.
- Larger, superficial dermal wounds such as second-degree burns can be managed nonoperatively by use of synthetic membrane dressings such as Biobrane (Smith & Nephew, Hull, United Kingdom; **FIG 1**) or TransCyte (Smith & Nephew). These dressings are applied immediately after débridement of nonviable skin.
    - This class of dressing is effective for superficial wounds that penetrate only to mid-dermal levels. They depend on retained epidermal appendages (ie, hair follicles, sebaceous and sweat glands) to accomplish the task of reepithelialization.
- Deeper, full dermal thickness areas of wounding require deeper débridements that typically are followed by skin grafting or skin graft substitutes.

SURGICAL MANAGEMENT

Preoperative Planning

- Once appropriate débridement has been performed, and the wound is deemed clean and the wound bed is appropriately vascularized, the surgeon can proceed with skin grafting.
- Before beginning in the operating room, the surgeon should have discussed the proposed donor site with the patient and also should have decided whether a full- or split-thickness graft is most appropriate.

Positioning

- The volar and dorsal aspects of the distal upper extremity can be accessed easily with the patient in a supine position with the arm placed on an arm table.
- Occasionally, patients who have limited range of motion in their joints at the shoulder or elbow must be placed prone to facilitate access to certain areas.
- Decisions about positioning should be made well in advance of initiation of the procedure.

Approach

- Wounds that are being considered for placement of skin graft or skin graft substitutes are, by definition, vascularized wound beds with direct superficial access.
- Logical preoperative planning determines the approach.

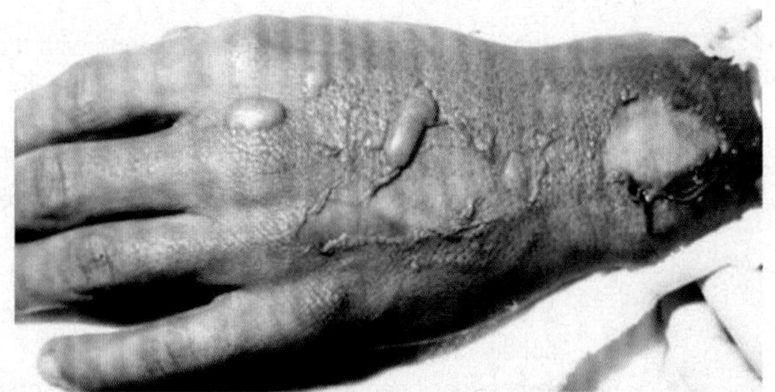
A

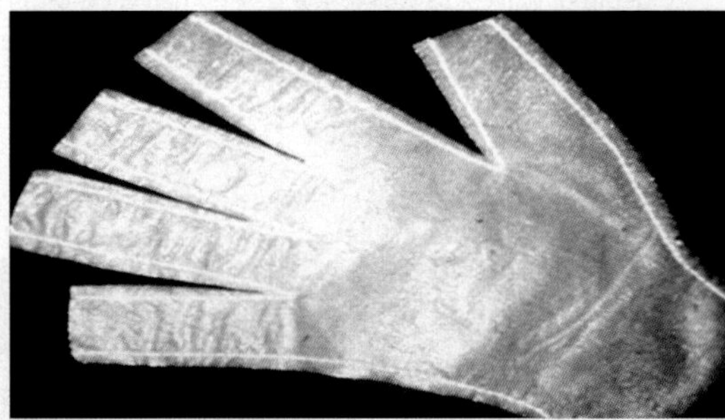
B

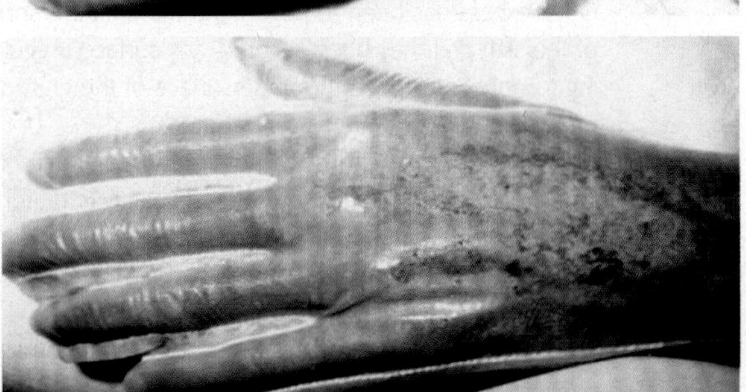
C

FIG 1 • **A.** Superficial second-degree burn to the dorsal hand. **B.** Biobrane glove designed for superficial second-degree hand burns. **C.** Biobrane glove applied.

■ Split-Thickness Skin Graft

Determining Wound Size and Making a Template

- To begin the procedure, a sterile ruler is used to measure the size of the wound to be addressed with skin grafting.
- A simple and effective way to determine the shape of a wound bed is to place a sheet of sterile glove paper within the wound. The mark left on the paper by the wound is a close match of the wound bed. (This technique is not as accurate for wounds with markedly irregular contours.)
- Once the wound has transferred moisture onto the glove paper, the paper can be trimmed with scissors to provide a template of the wound bed. This template then can be transferred to the area of planned skin harvest.
- The shape of the template is marked with a dashed line, using a gentian violet marker, on the skin that is to be harvested.

Harvesting the Graft

- Most modern dermatomes are designed to harvest skin in a quadrangular pattern.
- To ensure that the harvested graft is capable of proper wound coverage, it should be larger than the gentian violet marks on all sides, both to offset shrinkage from primary graft contraction and to compensate for the difficulties in harvesting amorphous shapes with an instrument designed to cut quadrangular patterns.
- The degree of primary contraction is a function of the depth of dermis harvested. For very thin split-thickness grafts, primary contraction is virtually absent.
- Grafts usually are harvested with either nitrogen- or electric-powered dermatomes (**TECH FIG 1**), which can be adjusted for depth of harvest as well as the desired harvest width.
- The usual appropriate depth for harvesting skin to be applied to a wound bed in the distal upper extremity is between 0.012 and 0.014 inch.

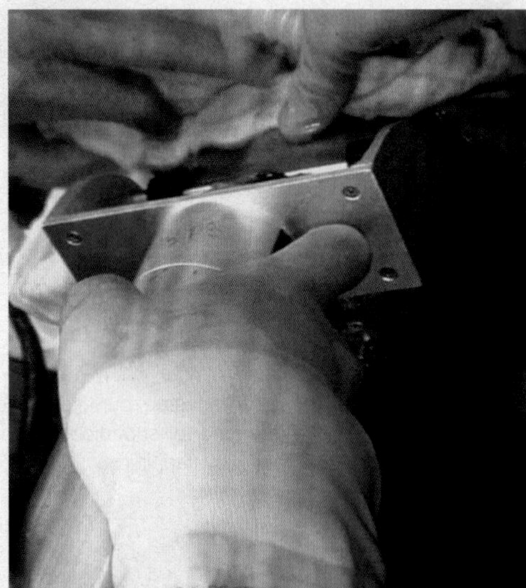

TECH FIG 1 • Technique of split-thickness skin graft harvest.

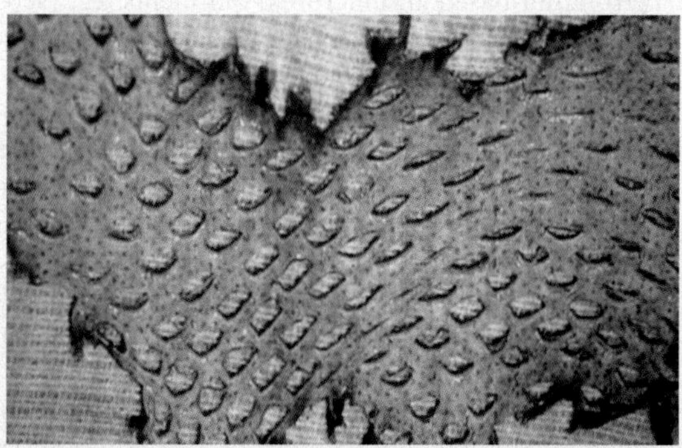

TECH FIG 2 • Meshed graft. Appearance of meshed split-thickness graft, dermis side up.

Unmeshed versus Meshed Grafts

- Once a graft of appropriate size has been harvested, it must be decided whether to use the graft as a sheet graft (unmeshed) versus an expanded graft (meshed) (**TECH FIG 2**).
- Sheet grafts, because of their contiguous nature, have a greater tendency to develop subgraft seromas and hematomas.
  - This complication can lead to graft loss; for this reason, it is worth considering the use of meshed grafts.
- Under ideal circumstances, a meshed graft can be used in its nonexpanded state.
  - To do this, simply mesh the graft using the appropriate device, and after placing it in the wound bed, close the small fenestrations made by meshing.
  - This closure will give a final healed appearance very close to that of a sheet graft but without the complication of accumulated fluid beneath the graft, which can lead to graft loss.

Placing the Graft

- Once the graft has been placed in the wound with the dermis side down, the graft can be secured in place using either staples or sutures around the periphery.
- As this is done, excess peripheral graft may develop. This is the byproduct of the quadrangular shape of the harvest versus the amorphous shape of the typical wound.
  - Excesses are easily trimmed by holding the graft in place and using thin, sharp scissors to skirt just outside the periphery of the wound.
- Once excess has been removed and the entire peripheral edge of the skin graft has been secured, any surface irregularity leading to noncontact with the undersurface of the graft can be addressed by placement of quilting sutures.
  - These sutures are placed through the surface of the graft into the depth of the contour irregularity and then back out of the graft.
  - When tied, the sutures draw the deep surface of the graft into contact with the wound bed.
  - A suitable suture for this purpose is 4-0 chromic.
- A nonadherent interface (eg, Xeroform [Kendall, Mansfield, MA] or Aquaphor [Beiersdorf AG, Hamburg, Germany] gauze) should be placed over the graft to prevent the graft from adhering to the bolster that will further secure the graft in position.
  - If Aquaphor gauze is used and the patient is not allergic to bacitracin ointment, a triple antibiotic ointment doping of

the Aquaphor further inures the graft from injury when the overlying bolster is removed.

- In the upper extremity, lightly applied circumferential dressings work well as bolsters.
- Tie-over bolsters typically are not required, but they can be used if preferred. Reston foam (3M, St. Paul, MN) or saline- and mineral oil–doped cotton batting secured in place with light gauze and an elastic overwrap from the tips of the fingers to a point several centimeters beyond the most proximal aspect of the grafted site is sufficient.
- A sugar-tong splint should then be applied to help prevent the shear stress created between the wound bed and the undersurface of the graft, which occurs as a byproduct of pronation and supination as well as wrist and finger flexion and extension.
- The patient's arm should be elevated to help minimize accumulation of edema at the graft site.

Postoperative Care

- On postoperative day 5, dressings should be removed and the graft examined. Typically, at this time, the graft will have acquired a pink coloration, and although most of the fenestrated areas may not have fully epithelialized, it should be clear that graft take is underway. If this is not the case, the wound should be inspected to determine why the graft is not taking.
- For fenestrated grafts, it is unusual for either hematoma or seroma to be a cause of graft failure. The more common cause for graft failure with fenestrated split-thickness grafts is wound infection.
  - Quantitative cultures obtained preoperatively will help guide the surgeon in appropriate antibiotic treatment for these patients pre-, intra-, and postoperatively.
- Once early graft healing has occurred, wound infection is unlikely, and the application of a hypoallergenic emollient cream helps keep the graft supple and moisturized while at the same time promoting slough of scaling stratum corneum and eschar.

Full-Thickness Skin Graft

Donor Site

- If the area of the wound is over or in proximity to a joint, it may be decided to use a full-thickness graft. Again, a template can be made using sterile glove paper, with this glove paper template then transferred to the area desired for harvest of the full-thickness graft.
- There are limitations on the surface area that can be obtained from full-thickness skin graft donor sites, and, therefore, consideration should be given to the recipient bed surface area when deciding on the type of graft.
- Typical donor sites include the lower abdomen and the inner aspect of the upper arm.

Graft Harvest

- Once the template has been transferred to the skin, harvest can be facilitated by injection of 1% lidocaine with epinephrine into the subcutaneous fat directly beneath the area planned for harvest.
  - Allow approximately 7 minutes for the epinephrine to take effect and help minimize bleeding during harvest.
- A no.15 scalpel blade can be used to accurately incise the periphery of the planned graft harvest, followed by elevation of the full-thickness graft in the plane directly beneath the undersurface of the full thickness of dermis, directly above the subdermal fat and below dermal papillae. The underlying fat should be removed from the underside of the dermis as the graft is being raised to facilitate defatting.
  - In most cases, some fat is still adherent to the underlying dermis after elevation.
    - The full-thickness skin graft can be stretched over the finger and curved scissors used to directly excise fat from the undersurface of the full-thickness graft.
    - The removal of unwanted fat maximizes the surface area of deep dermis in direct contact with the wound bed, which helps to facilitate the inosculation and revascularization process.
- Full-thickness grafts have a greater degree of primary contraction than do split-thickness grafts; therefore, upon immediate harvest, the graft will appear much smaller than it did when in situ. Once sewn in place around the periphery, however, the graft will return to the actual size of the template with little effort.
- This ability to return to the template size, and even extend beyond it, means that when harvesting full-thickness graft, the harvest should not be extended much beyond the periphery of the template, as is done with split-thickness grafts.

Graft Preparation

- To minimize the accumulation of hematoma or seroma beneath the graft, a well-prepared bed is required.
- One measure to help prevent subgraft fluid accumulation is "pie-crusting," a technique in which the surgeon simply makes random perforations through the full thickness of the graft using a no.11 scalpel blade.
  - These perforations provide avenues of egress for accumulated subgraft fluid in much the same way that meshing does for split-thickness grafts.

Graft Placement

- To improve the precision of dermal edge contact of the graft in the wound, suture fixation is preferred over staple fixation. Again, an ideal suture for this purpose is 4-0 chromic.
- The process for dressing this graft is the same as that for a split-thickness graft: the use of either Aquaphor or Xeroform gauze dressings with an overlying bolster of Reston foam or cotton batting secured with gauze and an elastic wrap, followed by appropriate immobilization of the area.
- The VAC can be more challenging to use with unmeshed grafts and so full-thickness skin grafts be pie-crusted. A tie-over bolster can be very effective (**TECH FIG 3**).

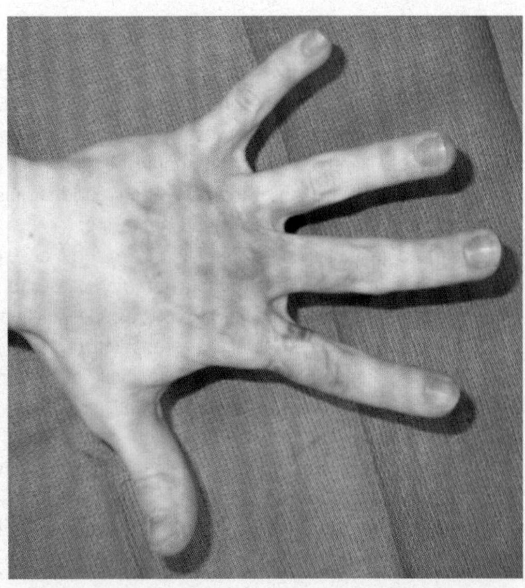

TECH FIG 3 • Full-thickness graft to dorsal hand. Appearance of mature full-thickness skin graft applied over joint.

Skin Substitutes

- The goal with skin substitutes is to place within the wound bed a biosynthetic dermal construct that will offer the advantages of a full-thickness skin graft but without the physical cost of obtaining such a large full-thickness skin graft harvest from the patient.
- The dermal constructs are placed within the wound in much the same manner as a full-thickness graft. They become fibrovascularly integrated into the wound bed as a synthetic neodermis. After maturity, application of a thin split-thickness skin graft (0.008 to 0.010 inch) converts these nonepithelialized constructs to closed wounds.
- The technical application of AlloDerm and Integra is the same as placement of a full-thickness skin graft.
  - AlloDerm and Integra usually are secured in place around the periphery with either 4-0 chromic or staples (**TECH FIG 4A**).
- Once a split-thickness skin graft is applied to a site treated with either AlloDerm or Integra, these split-thickness grafts should be treated in just the same manner as split-thickness skin grafts on any wound bed, observing the postoperative technical requirements of such grafts (**TECH FIG 4B**).

AlloDerm

- When using AlloDerm, bolstering dressings are applied over a petrolatum-doped nonadherent gauze interface and the dermal construct is observed periodically at twice-weekly intervals.
- AlloDerm will demonstrate granulation tissue issuing through the pores of the dermal construct, typically at about 2 to 3 weeks after graft placement.
- Once this has occurred, the AlloDerm is ready for split-thickness skin grafting.

Integra

- On initial placement, Integra appears white, with a transition over the succeeding 2 to 3 weeks to a rosy color, the byproduct of neovascularization. At this point, the silastic layer of the Integra can be separated and the vascularized dermal construct grafted with a thin split-thickness skin graft.
- If desired, Integra can be meshed 1:1 with a specialized mesher designed not to crush the construct (eg, Brennen Medical Skin Graft Mesher, Brennen Medical, LLC, St. Paul, MN).
  - Meshing may help the construct conform to the wound bed and also help limit subgraft fluid accumulations.

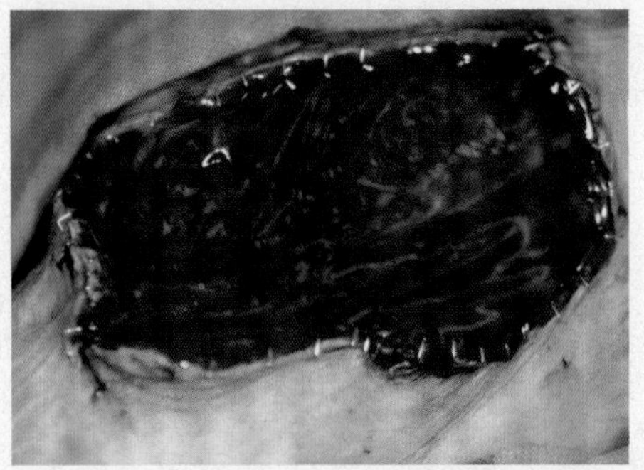

A

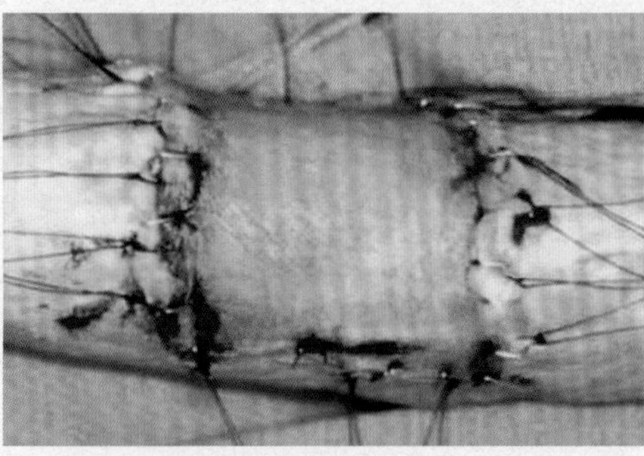

B

TECH FIG 4 • **A.** Appearance of mature Integra applied over open forearm wound. **B.** Very thin split-thickness graft applied and now adherent to mature Integra bed.

- The meshed construct should not be expanded on the wound bed because its purpose is to replace absent dermis. Its expansion thins the Integra construct and diminishes its benefits.
- Fenestrations in Integra are made only for the purpose of creating an avenue for fluid escape. Integra has a silastic membrane that acts as an external barrier.
- Integra's silastic membrane obviates the need for petrolatum-doped dressing and is transparent, which allows direct observation of the process of maturation of the dermal construct beneath.

Biobrane

- Biobrane is appropriate for use only in wounds that have some retained dermis and, because of this distinction, acts as an advanced wound dressing rather than a skin substitute. For wounds with full-thickness loss of skin, Biobrane is not an appropriate choice because epidermal appendages, which are required to act as the source of cells needed for reepithelialization, must be present.
- Biobrane acts as a protective barrier and a scaffold for the healing process. It notably decreases pain; allows for the retention of moisture within the wound, improving the healing environment; acts as a barrier to infection; and promotes more rapid healing.
- Its clinical use is most evident in treatment of burn injuries, but it also may be used to treat split-thickness skin graft donor sites to minimize morbidity in these areas.
- The application of Biobrane includes tangential excision of nonviable tissues or rough débridement with an antibiotic solution–doped lap sponge, followed by drying and then application of the Biobrane to the wound surface.
  - It is secured in place around the periphery using staples.
  - This is followed by application of a nonadherent gauze dressing with placement of an absorbent dressing, such as a sterile absorbent gauze pad held in place with gauze and an elastic wrap.
- The site is immobilized for 24 hours, after which all dressings are removed, leaving Biobrane in place.
  - At this stage, the Biobrane should be adherent to the wound bed.
- Biobrane is observed over time and allowed to separate from the wound without disturbance.
- Small abscesses below the silastic layer, if they develop, can be treated by simple incision and drainage. As edges release, they are trimmed.

PEARLS AND PITFALLS

Primary contraction	▪ Full-thickness grafts tend to shrink immediately on harvest. This primary contraction is easily overcome by application of peripheral sutures to draw the elastic full-thickness graft back out to its original surface area when applied to the wound.
Secondary contraction	▪ Split-thickness grafts tend to shrink over time as a function of harvesting less than the full thickness of dermis. This problem is exacerbated by meshed graft expansion. Secondary contraction can lead to functional contracture, especially when grafts are used over or near joints.
Graft meshing	▪ Meshing of split-thickness graft to provide fenestrations that will allow subgraft fluid accumulations to be expelled. This will help to keep the dermal surface of the graft in apposition to the wound bed, thereby enhancing the opportunity for inosculation and ultimately revascularization to occur.
Wound bed preparation	▪ Preparation requires débridement of nonviable tissue and bacteria. Quantitative culture can assist the surgeon in defining the species and number of bacterial colonies within the wound. More than 10^5 CFUs per gram of harvested tissue increases the likelihood of graft loss secondary to infection.
Enhancing graft adherence	▪ Proper immobilization to prevent shear stress across the wound graft interface cannot be overemphasized.
VAC device	▪ The VAC device may be used as a skin graft bolster over fenestrated grafts. Its negative pressure serves to effectively immobilize graft on the wound bed, as well as draw interstitial fluid from the wound, preventing its accumulation beneath the graft.

POSTOPERATIVE CARE

- On admission to the postanesthesia care unit, the patient's operated extremity should be placed in elevation and kept relatively immobile until time to take down dressings and evaluate the graft.
- Examination of the graft can be done as early as 3 days postoperatively; however, the graft at this point is very sensitive to manipulation.
- If takedown of the dressings is done on postoperative day 5 or 6, allowing time for additional graft maturation, the risk of disturbing the graft is reduced.
- Once maturation of the graft has been noted to be underway, application of a nonadherent dressing such as Xeroform or Aquaphor gauze should be continued, with light overpressure provided by an absorbable gauze dressing held in place by gauze and a light elastic wrap and splinting.
- After the graft has more fully matured, with all interstices fully epithelialized, at between 2 and 3 weeks postoperatively, the graft will require no further application of nonadherent dressings. Instead, light application of a hypoallergenic emollient cream such as Eucerin (Beiersdorf North America Inc., Wilton, CT) is preferred. This helps to keep the graft hydrated while maturation continues without the restrictions of constant compression and splinting.
- An occupational therapist should be consulted to help develop a program of appropriate splinting in tandem with an exercise regimen that will provide the foundation for maximizing the patient's final functional range of motion.

OUTCOMES

- Because of the disparate nature of wounds and the significant variation that exists in patient physiology, it is impossible to provide standardized outcome measures for skin grafting.
- The goal of the general principles defined in this chapter is to assist the surgeon in optimizing outcomes for all cases. Collectively, they will work to help limit complications while maximizing functional outcomes.

COMPLICATIONS

- Wound or graft infection with loss
- Subgraft seroma or hematoma
- Hypertrophic or keloid scarring
- Contractures
- Loss of functional range of motion
- Tendon adherence to graft
- Poor durability
- Hyperpigmentation

REFERENCES

1. Perry AW, Sutkin HS, Gottlieb LJ, et al. Skin graft survival—the bacterial answer. Ann Plast Surg 1989;22:479–483.
2. Pruitt BA Jr, Levine NS. Characteristics and uses of biologic dressings and skin substitutes. Arch Surg 1984;119:312–322.

SUGGESTED READINGS

Birch J, Branemark PI. The vascularization of a free full-thickness skin graft. I. A vital microscopic study. Scand J Plast Reconstr Surg 1969;3:1–10.

Brown D, Garner W, Young VL. Skin grafting: dermal components in inhibition of wound contraction. South Med J 1990;83:789–795.

Burleson R, Eiseman B. Nature of the bond between partial-thickness skin and wound granulations. Surgery 1972;72(2):315–322.

Caldwell RK, Giles WC, Davis PT. Use of foam bolsters for securing facial skin grafts. Ear Nose Throat J 1998;77:490–492.

Conway H, Sedar J. Report of the loss of pigment in full thickness autoplastic skin grafts in the mouse. Plast Reconstr Surg 1956;18:30–36.

Davison PM, Batchelor AG, Lewis-Smith PA. The properties and uses of non-expanded machine-meshed skin grafts. Br J Plast Surg 1986;39:462–468.

Hauben DJ, Baruchin A, Mahler D. On the history of the free skin graft. Ann Plast Surg 1982;9:242–245.

Jeschke MG, Rose C, Angele P, et al. Development of new reconstructive techniques: use of Integra in combination with fibrin glue and negative-pressure therapy for reconstruction of acute and chronic wounds. Plast Reconstr Surg 2004;113:525–530.

Molnar JA, DeFranzo AJ, Hadaegh A, et al. Acceleration of Integra incorporation in complex tissue defects with subatmospheric pressure. Plast Reconstr Surg 2004;113:1339–1346.

Ratner D. Skin grafting. From here to there. Dermatol Clin 1998;16:75–90.

Rehim SA, Singhal M, Chung KC. Dermal skin substitutes for upper limb reconstruction: current status, indications, and contraindications. Hand Clin 2014;30(2):239–252.

Robson MC, Krizek TJ. Predicting skin graft survival. J Trauma 1973;13:213–217.

Rudolph R, Klein L. Healing processes in skin grafts. Surg Gynecol Obstet 1973;136:641–654.

Saltz R, Bowles BJ. Reston. An alternate method of skin graft fixation. Plast Reconstr Surg 1997;99:601–602.

Schneider AM, Morykwas MJ, Argenta LC. A new and reliable method of securing skin grafts to the difficult recipient bed. Plast Reconstr Surg 1998;102:1195–1198.

Smahel J. The healing of skin grafts. Clin Plast Surg 1977;4:409–424.

Smoot EC. A rapid method for splinting skin grafts and securing wound dressings. Plast Reconstr Surg 1997;100:1622.

Waris T, Astrand K, Hämäläinen H, et al. Regeneration of cold, warmth and heat-pain sensibility in human skin grafts. Br J Plast Surg 1989;42:576–580.

Wolter TP, Noah EM, Pallua N. The use of Integra in an upper extremity avulsion injury. Br J Plast Surgeons 2005;58:416–418.

Rotational and Pedicle Flaps for Coverage of Distal Upper Extremity Injuries

141 CHAPTER

L. Scott Levin

DEFINITION

- A *flap* is a composite of tissue (ie, skin, fascia, muscle, bone, or combination) that is moved from its original location to another location in or on the body.[5]
- Several different types of flaps exist, defined by their blood supply.
  - *Random flaps* (eg, Z-plasty, cross-finger flap) depend on preserving enough of the subcutaneous and dermal vascular plexus for flap survival. There are very few "random flaps." Because of the extensive research on cutaneous circulation, the knowledge of vascular perforators, and understanding of angiosomes, this term is rarely used (**FIG 1A**).
  - *Axial flaps* depend on the blood supply from a single consistent (usually named) blood vessel; examples of this include the radial forearm flap and dorsal metacarpal artery flap (**FIG 1B**).

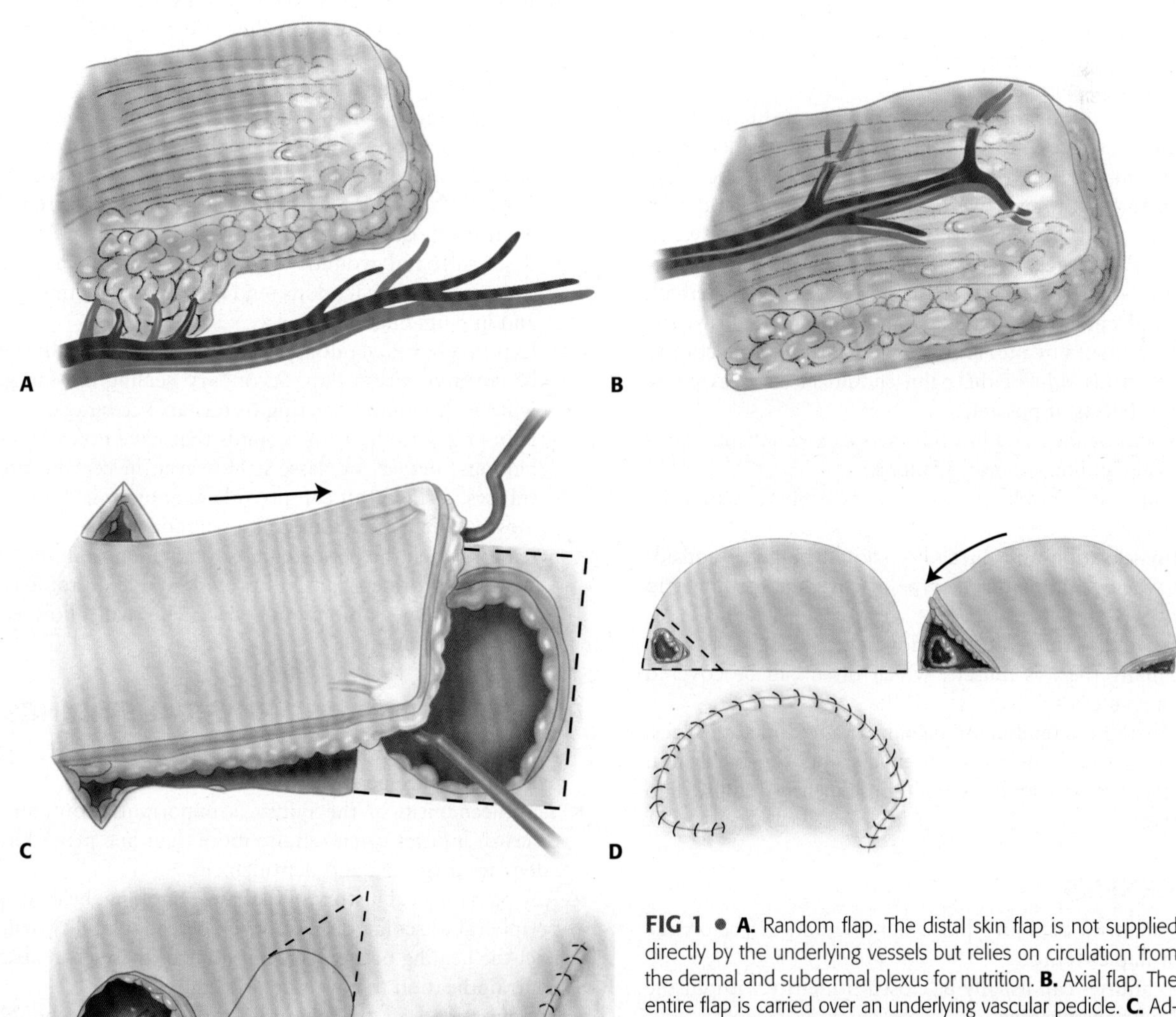

FIG 1 • **A.** Random flap. The distal skin flap is not supplied directly by the underlying vessels but relies on circulation from the dermal and subdermal plexus for nutrition. **B.** Axial flap. The entire flap is carried over an underlying vascular pedicle. **C.** Advancement flap. This is a direct tissue advancement. This figure also shows Burow triangles, which will decrease the dog-ears at the corners. **D.** Rotational flap. The flap rotates into the adjacent defect. The radius of the flap decreases with the rotation. A backcut can be used to extend the arc of coverage. **E.** Transposition flap. This flap is similar to a rotational flap, but the flap is moved across normal tissue to fill the defect.

- *Free flaps* depend on the division and microsurgical anastomosis of the artery and vein to reestablish blood flow to the flap in a different location.
- Flaps also can be defined by how the tissue is moved.
  - *Advancement flaps* are elevated and advanced in a linear direction away from the base of the flap (**FIG 1C**).
  - *Rotational flaps* are elevated adjacent to the defect and re-inset within the same bed[10] (**FIG 1D**).
  - *Transpositional flaps* are elevated and moved across normal tissue to a new defect site (**FIG 1E**).
  - *Island flaps* are elevated on their vascular pedicle and moved to a different location; mobility is limited by the pedicle length.
- Grafts are differentiated from flaps in that there is no native blood supply to the tissue. A skin graft survives initially by osmosis (imbibition) before it obtains vascular ingrowth (inosculation). This process works only for fairly thin tissue grafts.[3,4]

ANATOMY

- A thorough understanding of the anatomy of the area injured and the donor area of the flap is necessary for safe elevation and insetting of these flaps.
- A full description of the anatomy of the forearm and hand is beyond the scope of this chapter, but the key points of the relevant anatomy will be addressed in the separate sections.
- The skin and soft tissue covering the forearm and hand vary by location, and this variation must be accounted for when considering coverage.
- The palm (volar surface) of the hand consists of very thick dermis and epidermis that is structurally anchored to the underlying tissues by numerous vertical fascial connections.
  - The glabrous skin of the palm should be used to cover palmar defects, if possible.
- The dorsum of the hand has thin dermis and subcutaneous fat covering gliding extensor tendons.
  - Coverage here should be as thin as possible to match the lost tissue.
- Fingertip sensation and durability should be given consideration when deciding on the type of coverage for fingertip injury.
- The forearm has thin soft tissue coverage.
  - Proximally there is muscle, which often can be covered with a skin graft.
  - Distally there is tendon on the palmar and dorsal surfaces. Trauma to the soft tissue often disrupts the paratenon and the exposed tendons will subsequently require flap coverage.

PATHOGENESIS

- The mechanism of injury has a considerable effect on the need for flap coverage.
  - Sharp injuries can usually be closed primarily without the need for flap coverage.
  - Abrasive injuries commonly occur as a result of motor vehicle accidents. These usually involve one surface of the hand, and the extent of injury is usually relatively apparent. However, the level of contamination often is high, and extensive débridement of contaminated and devitalized tissue is necessary.
  - Crush injuries can lead to necrosis of skin, tendon, bone, and muscle. The zone of injury often is large and can be underestimated on initial inspection.
- Other systemic injuries may delay treatment of extremity injuries. However, treatment for compartment syndrome and gross contamination must not be delayed any longer than necessary.

NATURAL HISTORY

- The natural history of a wound depends greatly on the type of injury. The degree of original injury is the primary factor contributing to the prognosis for function of the hand.
- A large wound involving the bones, tendons, or joints often has a profound negative effect on future function of the hand.
- Early coverage can decrease total inflammation of the injured area and can limit the detrimental effect of the injury on the return to function.
- Many wounds will heal by second intention without the need for coverage. Secondary healing can lead to acceptable results in some locations but also may lead to very poor results in others. These factors must be taken into account when deciding type of coverage.
  - Small wounds (<1 cm) on the fingertips, without exposed bone or tendon, will likely heal well on their own. This secondary healing often gives the strongest soft tissue coverage with the best sensibility and is the preferred treatment for most wounds of this type.
  - If dorsal hand wounds secondarily heal or "granulate" over tendons, the tendons tend to scar, which limits gliding and impairs finger motion.
  - Exposed bones, tendons, nerves, or vessels usually should be covered with a flap. Secondary healing or skin grafts will result in more scarring or unstable coverage.
  - Skin grafts are best for wounds that have no exposure of tendons, nerves, or vessels. However, in certain circumstances, a skin graft can provide temporary coverage over most viable tissue. Skin grafts will not survive on bone or tendon when the periosteum or paratenon is absent.
  - A well-performed flap will provide stable, durable coverage over any viable wound bed. This will allow earlier therapy and motion.

PATIENT HISTORY AND PHYSICAL FINDINGS

- After a traumatic injury, a complete history and physical examination are performed.
- The mechanism of the injury is important. Contaminated or crush injuries often require more than one procedure for adequate irrigation and débridement.
- Any past medical history of diabetes, smoking, heart disease, peripheral vascular disease, or hypercoagulability will impact the healing of any flap, but none of these is an absolute contraindication to coverage procedures.
- Examination of the wound and extremity should be comprehensive:
  - Assessment of vascular status
  - Imaging for fracture
  - Motor and sensory examination to evaluate for nerve, tendon, or muscle injury
  - Examination for compartment syndrome in severe injuries

IMAGING AND OTHER DIAGNOSTIC STUDIES

- Radiographs of the hand should be obtained to evaluate for bony injury.
- Advanced imaging, such as computed tomography (CT) scan or magnetic resonance imaging (MRI), may be warranted for fracture pattern delineation, but these studies rarely are needed to assess the indications for flap coverage.
- Questionable blood flow or limb perfusion warrants further evaluation, such as angiography.
  - Adequate blood flow to the extremity must be restored before considering flap coverage.

TYPES OF FLAPS

Radial Forearm Flap

- This is a useful flap to cover upper extremity wounds. This flap can be used as a pedicle or free flap and provides excellent thin soft tissue coverage.[9]
- The donor site is the major area of morbidity.
  - The volar forearm donor site is relatively conspicuous.
  - If a skin graft is needed to close the donor site, the donor morbidity is decreased by using nonmeshed split-thickness skin grafts applied carefully.
- The radial artery is divided during isolation of the flap. Therefore, ulnar artery patency is critical. This must be confirmed with an Allen test or with direct Doppler evaluation of the hand with the radial artery occluded with manual pressure.
- The flap can be elevated with a proximal (anterograde) or distal (retrograde or reversed) pedicle.
- The anterograde flap is useful for coverage of the elbow, as either a pedicled flap or a free flap.
- The reverse radial forearm flap can cover the volar and dorsal hand to and can reach the tips of the fingers.
- The reversed radial forearm flap has arterial flow through the ulnar artery and palmar arches and back through the radial artery. The venous return is compromised due to valves in the vein but occurs through interconnections in the vena comitans that bypass the valves.
- Advantages
  - Thin pliable tissue
  - Reliable anatomy
  - Fair color match
  - Can be elevated under tourniquet control
- Disadvantages
  - Possible unsightly donor site
  - Requires patent ulnar artery
  - Reversed flap may appear swollen and slightly congested (but loss of flap is rare)
- Relevant anatomy
  - The brachial artery divides in the proximal forearm to form the radial and ulnar arteries. The ulnar artery is the dominant arterial blood supply to the hand in most people.
  - The radial artery courses distally just deep to the interval between the brachioradialis (BR) and the flexor carpi radialis (FCR) muscles. In the proximal forearm, the superficial branch of the radial nerve is adjacent to the radial artery.
  - The radial artery has paired venae comitantes that are important for venous egress from the flap once it is elevated.

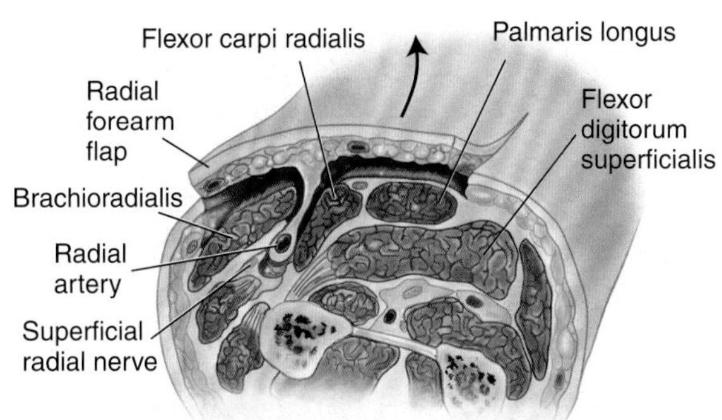

FIG 2 • Cross-section showing the relevant forearm anatomy for a radial forearm flap. The septum lies between the BR and FCR. The skin and subcutaneous tissue and fascia above the volar forearm musculature are elevated as a unit with the radial artery and septum with perforating vessels.

  - There is a loose tissue septum between the FCR and BR. Within this septum, there are perforating branches of the radial artery to the skin that provide blood supply to the overlying skin. These are meticulously preserved to perfuse the flap (**FIG 2**).

Groin Flap

- The groin flap is another commonly used pedicled flap for coverage of larger soft tissue avulsions of the hand.
- This fasciocutaneous flap is based on the superficial circumflex iliac artery (SCIA) and is located on the anterior thigh, just below the inguinal ligament.[8]
- It can be taken as a free flap but more commonly used as a pedicled flap and a two-stage operation.
  - In the first stage, the flap is elevated laterally and inset onto the injured area. It is still attached medially by the pedicle originating from the femoral vessels.
  - In the second stage (2 to 3 weeks later), the pedicle is divided, freeing the arm from its connection to the groin.
- Advantages
  - The flap is thin.
  - It is nearly hairless, which may or may not be an advantage, depending on the recipient site.
  - It is very reliable.
  - Flap elevation is relatively quick.
  - The donor site can be closed primarily with widths up to about 10 cm.
- Disadvantages
  - Mandatory two-stage operation
  - The injured hand is dependent and connected to the patient's groin for 2 to 3 weeks while waiting for vascular ingrowth.
  - Poor color match
  - Postoperative numbness in the lateral femoral cutaneous nerve is common.
- Relevant anatomy
  - The SCIA arises off the femoral artery about 3 cm inferior to the inguinal ligament and deep to the deep fascia of the thigh (**FIG 3**).
  - SCIA travels superolaterally beneath the deep fascia.
  - As the SCIA crosses the sartorius, it supplies branches to the muscle.
  - About 6 cm from the femoral artery, the SCIA travels superficial to Scarpa fascia.

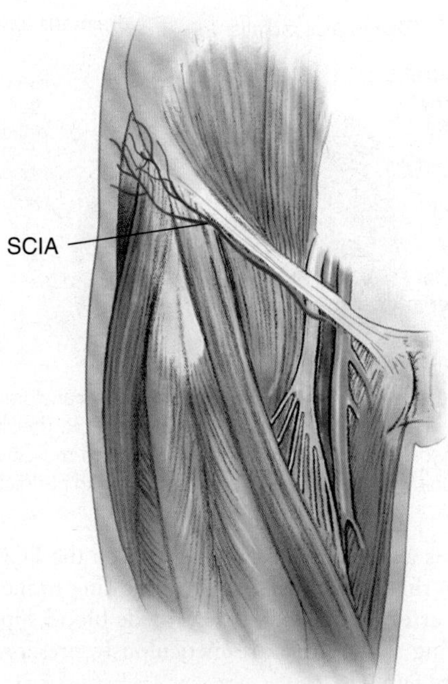

FIG 3 • Relevant groin flap anatomy. The SCIA arises from the femoral artery 3 cm distal to the inguinal ligament. It then travels laterally, anterior to the thigh musculature, parallel and inferior to the inguinal ligament.

Kite Flap

- The kite flap, or first dorsal metacarpal artery flap, is a reliable flap taken from the dorsum of the index finger over the proximal phalanx.
- Its most common use is for reconstruction of palmar thumb defects. Both soft tissue coverage and sensibility can be provided if the dorsal branches of the radial nerve are moved with the flap.[1]
- It also can be used for web space reconstruction or covering smaller defects on the dorsum of the hand or wrist.
- The flap can be 2 × 4 cm in size.
- Relevant anatomy
  - The radial artery travels through the anatomic "snuffbox," then onto the dorsum of the thumb, before diving between the two heads of the first dorsal interosseous muscle. This artery has three main branches:
    - The dorsal carpal arch
    - The princeps pollicis artery to the thumb
    - The first dorsal metacarpal artery
- The first dorsal metacarpal artery extends dorsally out along the surface of the first dorsal interosseous muscle to the dorsum on the index finger (**FIG 4**).
- The venous drainage of the flap is from the dorsal venous system of the finger.
- The radial nerve provides sensation to the dorsum of the radial hand and fingers distally. These small branches can be preserved and included with the flap, if desired.

Posterior Interosseous Flap

- The posterior interosseous flap, a fasciocutaneous flap, is a less commonly used flap taken from the dorsum of the forearm.[11] This flap can be based proximally to cover the elbow or distally to cover the dorsum of the hand or can be harvested as a free flap.

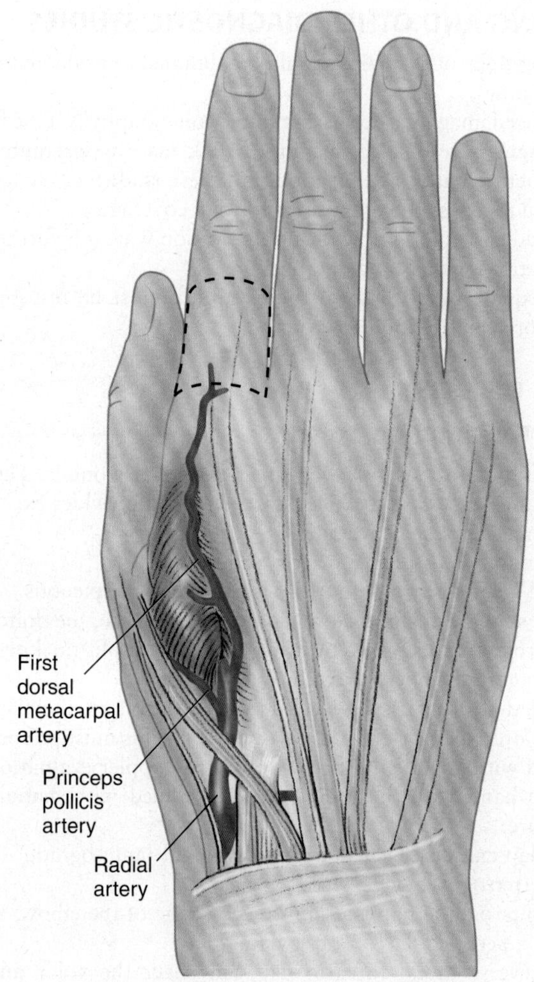

FIG 4 • Anatomy of the dorsal metacarpal artery.

- The reversed flap, if used to cover the hand or wrist, relies on retrograde venous and arterial flow. The valves within the veins are bypassed by interconnections between the paired venae comitantes.
- The donor site on the dorsal forearm is more visible and subsequently less desirable than the radial forearm flap.
- The flap is based on the perforating arteries coming from the posterior interosseous artery.
  - The posterior interosseous artery travels on the posterior side of the interosseous membrane and arises from either a common interosseous artery or the ulnar artery.
- Septocutaneous perforators travel in the septum between the extensor digiti quinti (EDQ) and extensor carpi ulnaris (ECU) to the skin.
- The posterior interosseous artery connects with the anterior interosseous artery near the distal radioulnar joint (DRUJ) and also will get retrograde flow through the dorsal carpal arch. This site is the location of the distal pivot point of the flap.
- Proximally, the posterior interosseous artery enters the posterior compartment of the forearm at the junction of the proximal and middle thirds of the forearm (**FIG 5**).
- Advantages
  - Thin pliable tissue with good match to dorsal hand tissue
  - Preservation of both the ulnar and radial arteries
  - Can be closed primarily if flap width is less than 5 cm

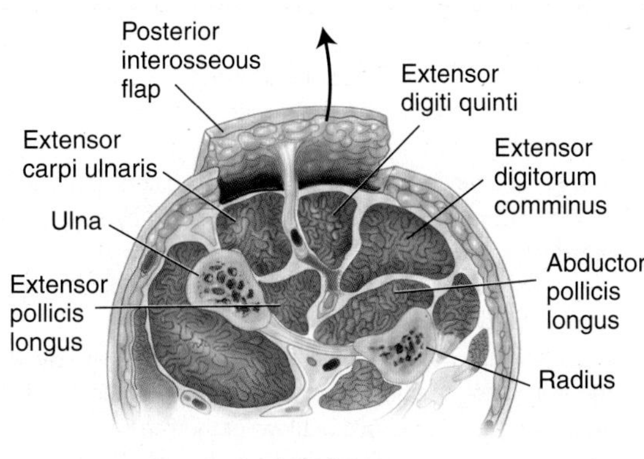

FIG 5 ● The posterior interosseous flap is elevated with the posterior interosseous artery in a retrograde fashion. Perforating vessels are present within a septum that lies between the EDQ and ECU. The skin, subcutaneous tissue, fascia, and septum are all elevated with the artery.

- Disadvantages
  - Technically difficult dissection due to the proximity of the posterior interosseous nerve
  - The anatomy does not always allow safe dissection of the flap, and the surgeon should have a plan for an alternate flap if necessary.
  - Flap repair is contraindicated with wrist trauma due to disruption of the dorsal wrist vascular arcade.

Z-Plasty

- Although Z-plasty is not often used during immediate reconstruction, it is a useful adjunct for secondary reconstruction due to scar contracture.
- This method lengthens or redirects a scar by transposing two triangular flaps to bring normal tissue within a scarred area.
- A prerequisite is good tissue on either side of the area to be lengthened because this tissue is interposed in the place of the original scar.

NONOPERATIVE MANAGEMENT

- As with all reconstructive procedures, if nonoperative management is possible, it should be considered and may be preferred.
- Small wounds often will heal secondarily with good results.
  - Fingertip injuries that do not expose bone or tendon usually heal with good results and with good sensibility. These wounds should be débrided and cleaned, then dressed appropriately and allowed to heal over 2 to 3 weeks.
- Wounds on the distal forearm and hand often have exposure of tendon, bone, nerve, or vessel. Except in rare circumstances, these should all be covered with good tissue.
  - Primary closure is the ideal, but with tissue loss, this may not be possible.
  - Skin grafts provide good coverage for muscle or clean wounds of the hand but often do not offer the best coverage for future function of the hand.
    - A skin graft will heal on bone or tendon if the periosteum or paratenon is intact, but this may create a thin, unstable wound. Skin grafting over tendons is prone to scarring and may decrease tendon excursion.
    - Skin grafts will heal over nerves or vessels but can result in hypersensitivity with nerves or thin coverage over vessels increasing the chance of bleeding.
- In many cases, early flap closure with a good gliding surface (for tendon movement) may be better than delayed healing with increased scar tissue.

SURGICAL MANAGEMENT

- The wound should be débrided back to viable tissue before it is covered.
- If there is gross contamination, the débridement often can be done in several stages to obtain a clean wound.
- The wound depth and size must be taken into consideration.

Preoperative Planning

- If there is tendon or bone involvement of the injury site, the selected reconstruction should consider these factors.
- The affected area should be well perfused when the patient is brought to the operating room for flap coverage.
- Only rarely should flaps be performed on an emergent basis in an unhealthy patient.
- Flap coverage should be performed over a stable skeleton, and devitalized or contaminated tissue should not be covered.

Positioning

- The arm usually is placed on an arm board at a 90-degree angle. The operating table is positioned to allow the surgeon and the assistant to sit on either side of the arm.
- This positioning gives excellent access to the palmar and dorsal forearm, arm, and hand.
- If a skin graft is considered, the ipsilateral groin or thigh is prepped to allow for full- or split-thickness grafting, respectively.
- Small full-thickness grafts can be obtained from the antecubital fossa, the ulnar forearm, or the ulnar side of the palm (for thick glabrous skin).

Approach

- For all procedures, a padded tourniquet is used on the patient's arm and inflated for the duration of the débridement of the wound and for flap elevation.
  - At the end of the flap elevation, the tourniquet is released and bleeding controlled with bipolar electrocautery.
  - Easily visible vessels are divided with clips or ties while the tourniquet is inflated.
- The wound site is always well débrided back to good tissue. Any foreign material is removed, and the wound irrigated with saline. Pulse lavage irrigation is used for heavily contaminated wounds.
- Careful handling of the tissue is imperative. Avoid handling the skin edges with pickups because the corners of flaps are particularly susceptible to trauma. Use retention sutures and skin hooks as much as possible.

TECHNIQUES

Radial Forearm Flap

- A template of the defect is made (**TECH FIG 1A**).[2]
- The position of the radial artery is established using Doppler ultrasound and marked on the forearm (**TECH FIG 1B**).
- The template is placed over the radial artery on the volar forearm and marked in place.
  - If a reversed flap is to be used for hand coverage, it usually is obtained from the proximal forearm.
  - If antegrade flap is to be used, it is obtained from the distal forearm.
  - The proximally based flap can pivot at the bifurcation of the radial and ulnar arteries. The distally based flap will pivot at the level of the radial styloid.
- An incision is made distal to the flap to identify the radial artery.
- Then, starting on the ulnar aspect, the skin and subsequently the forearm fascia are incised.
- The flap is elevated deep to the forearm fascia.
- Care must be taken when approaching the radial artery not to cross and divide the septum between the FCR and BR (see **FIG 2**).
  - The perforating vessels that perfuse the skin paddle lie within this septum.
- Once the radial artery is identified along the course of the flap on the ulnar aspect, the radial aspect of the flap is elevated in a similar fashion.
- The radial artery exposure is facilitated by lateral opposing traction on FCR and BR, which can be provided by a self-retaining retractor.
- The radial artery is then divided proximally (or distally) and the flap elevated (**TECH FIG 1C**).
- It is imperative that the venae comitantes be preserved with the flap during the dissection and elevation of the radial artery. These will provide venous outflow for the flap.
- As the flap is elevated over the tendons of the FCR and palmaris longus, the paratenon must be preserved because this will provide the vascular bed for the skin graft that will cover the donor site.
- Once flap elevation is complete, the flap is inset in the defect and the donor defect covered with a skin graft (**TECH FIG 1D**).

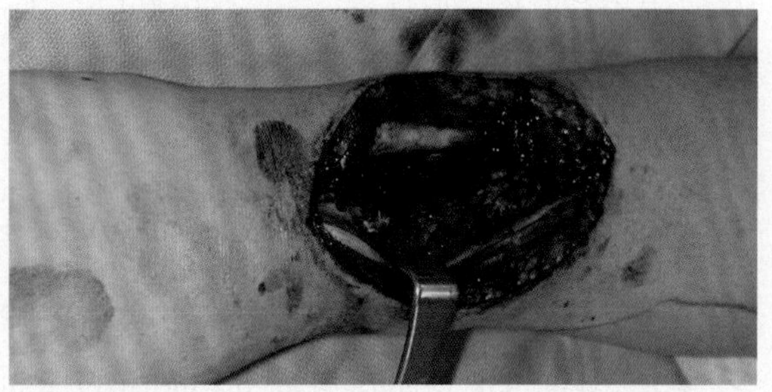
A

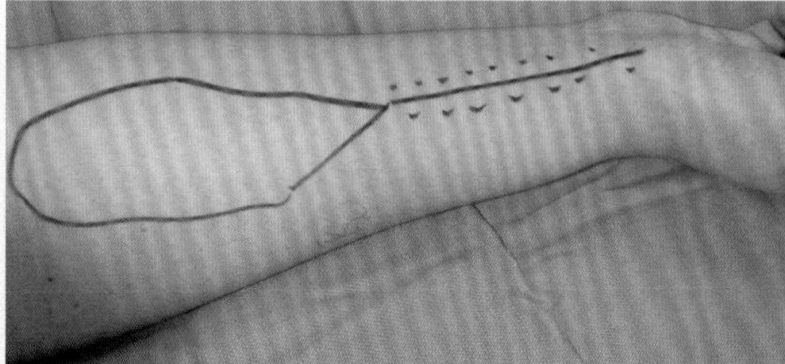
B

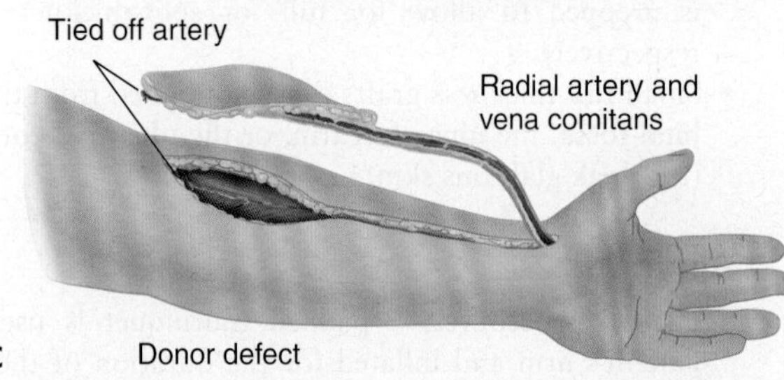

C

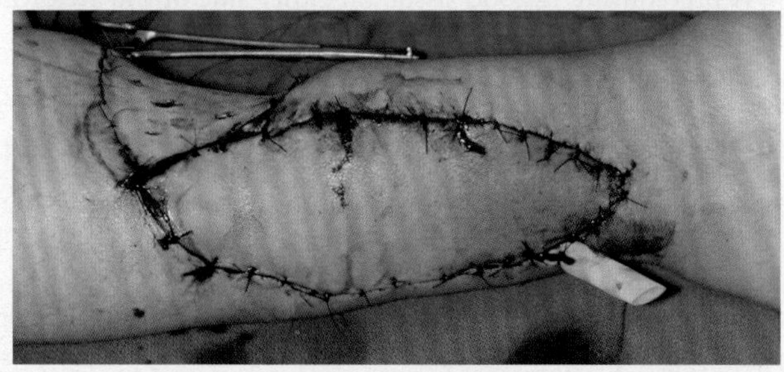
D

TECH FIG 1 • **A.** After resection of a recurrent sarcoma, this patient had a large dorsal defect with exposure of bone and tendon. **B.** The radial forearm flap is planned on the proximal forearm overlying the radial artery. Distal to the flap, the incision is drawn over the radial artery to extend the pedicle length. **C.** The flap is elevated from the proximal forearm, and once freed from its bed, the pedicle dissection is completed to the wrist. **D.** After the flap is elevated, it is inset in the excised wound. The flap defect is covered with a split-thickness skin graft.

Groin Flap

- A template of the defect is made (**TECH FIG 2A**).
- The inguinal ligament is marked from the anterior superior iliac spine to the pubic tubercle (see **FIG 3**).
- The origin of the SCIA is about 3 cm below the inguinal ligament and off the femoral artery.
- A second line is drawn parallel to the first, 3 cm inferior to it, indicating the SCIA.
- The flap can be as large as needed up to the following guidelines—any larger and the donor site may not close primarily. The flap margins are marked as follows[6]:
  - Superior margin: 2 to 3 cm above the inguinal ligament
  - Inferior margin: 7 to 8 cm below the inguinal ligament
  - Lateral margin: 8 to 10 cm lateral to the anterior superior iliac spine
- The flap is then elevated from lateral to medial (**TECH FIG 2B**).

- The skin is incised laterally, and the flap is elevated at the level below the superficial fascia (Scarpa fascia).
- When the lateral border of the sartorius is encountered, the dissection proceeds beneath the deep fascia, just on top of the muscle fascia.
- The penetrating branches to the sartorius are ligated and divided.
- When the medial border of the sartorius is encountered, the dissection stops (for the pedicled flap).
- The donor site is then closed over a drain. Near the origin of the flap, care is taken not to strangulate the flap with the closure.
- The proximal portion of the flap is then tubed if possible; however, there cannot be any tension on the tube.
- The flap is then inset on the hand, usually over a Penrose drain (**TECH FIG 2C**).
- The flap may then be divided 2 to 3 weeks later (**TECH FIG 2D,E**). Perfusion of the flap can be tested before division by temporarily occluding the pedicle with a circumferential Penrose drain and assessing flap perfusion.

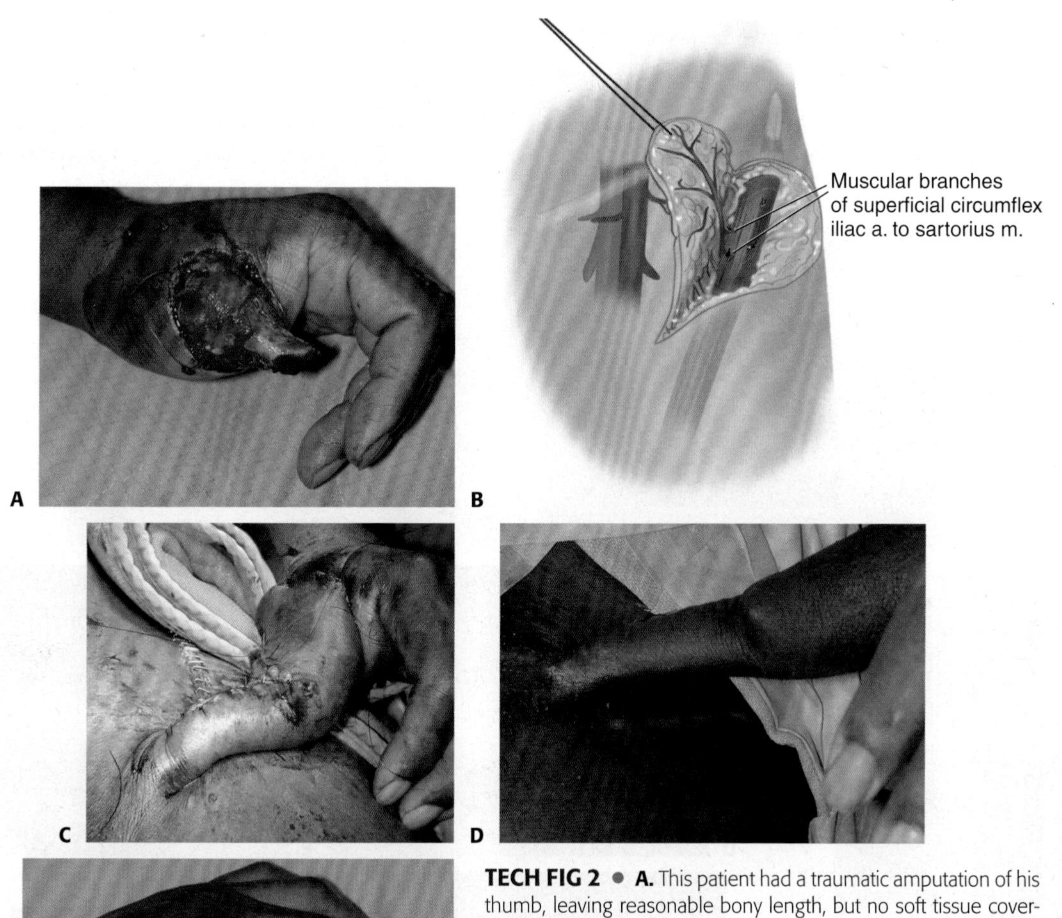

TECH FIG 2 • **A.** This patient had a traumatic amputation of his thumb, leaving reasonable bony length, but no soft tissue coverage. **B.** The groin flap is elevated from lateral to medial. Lateral to the sartorius, the superficial fascia is elevated with the flap. At the lateral border of the sartorius, the deep fascia is elevated and the perforating branches are ligated. Elevation stops at the medial border. **C.** After elevation and inset of the flap, the thumb is well covered. **D.** After 3 weeks, the flap had matured well in place. The pedicle is divided in the operating room. **E.** Three months after pedicle division, the flap is doing well. The preserved length of the thumb allows for a good post for opposition. The bulk of the flap can be reduced operatively over time.

Kite Flap: First Dorsal Metacarpal Artery Flap

- A template of the defect is made (**TECH FIG 3A**).
- The template is transferred to the dorsum of the index finger overlying the proximal phalanx, on the radial aspect.
- The flap is marked, then a proximal incision is marked in a zigzag or curvilinear fashion to extend to the takeoff of the first dorsal metacarpal artery (**TECH FIG 3B**).
- The flap is incised along the sides and distally down to the level of the extensor apparatus. Care is taken to preserve the paratenon of the extensors.
- The first dorsal interosseous artery will be elevated, with the subcutaneous tissue lying above it. The skin above the artery is left in its original location.
- The skin incision is made proximal to the flap. The incision around the proximal border of the flap needs to remain shallow, at the subdermal level as the venous drainage is through the small veins in the subcutaneous tissue.
- The skin proximal to the flap is elevated on the radial and ulnar side of the artery. The skin is elevated off the fat at the subdermal level.
- The pedicle should be elevated, with a total width of about 1 cm. On the ulnar side, the pedicle border is the middle of the metacarpal. On the radial side, the pedicle border is 5 to 10 mm radial to the artery (**TECH FIG 3C**).
- The artery lies on top of the fascia of the first dorsal interosseous muscle. To help preserve the artery and subcutaneous tissue, the muscle fascia is elevated with the pedicle.[1,7,11]
- Once the dissection of the pedicle has reached the radial artery proper, as it dives palmar to the deep palmar arch, the elevation typically ends.
- This should allow enough pedicle length for coverage of many volar thumb defects and some dorsal hand defects (**TECH FIG 3D–G**).

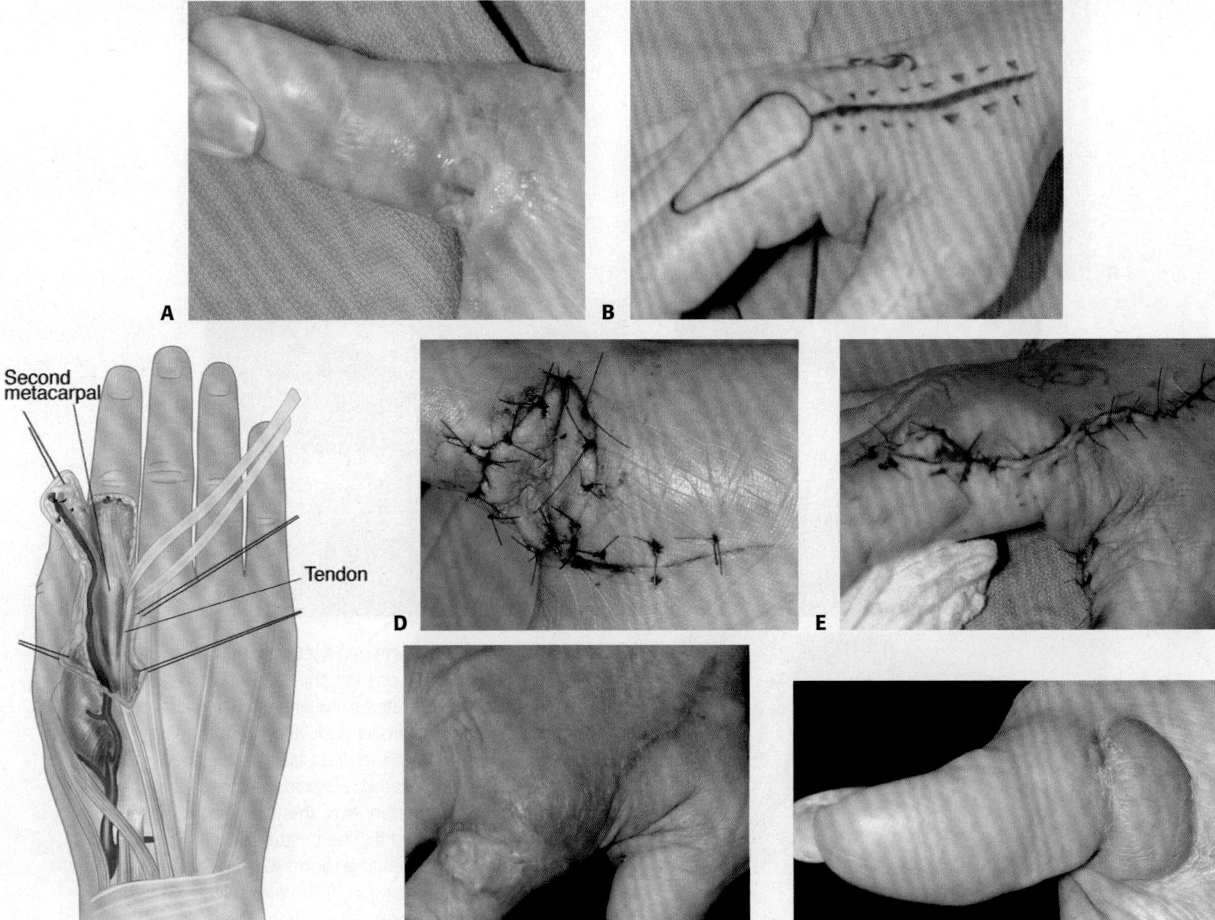

TECH FIG 3 • **A.** This wound of the volar thumb has exposed tendon and will not heal without a vascularized skin flap. **B.** The flap is planned on the dorsoradial aspect of the index finger. The proximal incision is for pedicle dissection. **C.** The first dorsal metacarpal artery flap is a vascularized skin flap from the dorsum of the index finger over the proximal phalanx. The dissection will give a flap that is good for small dorsal defects of the volar thumb. **D.** The flap is inset on the wound. **E.** The defect is closed. A small skin graft is needed to assist in closure. **F.** At 3 weeks postoperatively, the donor defect is healed. **G.** At 6 months postoperatively, the flap is well healed and allows for full tendon excursion.

Posterior Interosseous Flap

- The operation is performed under tourniquet control, but without Esmarch exsanguination, to maintain visibility of the small vessels.
- The wound is débrided and irrigated, and then a template is made (**TECH FIG 4A**).
- A line is drawn from the lateral epicondyle to the DRUJ. The line approximates the position of the posterior interosseous artery (**TECH FIG 4B,C**).
- The template is placed over the line marking the pedicle. It can be placed proximally as close as 6 cm from the lateral epicondyle of the humerus.
- An incision is made along the flap outline proximal to the pivot point. Dissection is carried between the EDQ and ECU to look for the posterior interosseous artery (see **FIG 4**).
- If the artery is found at this location, it is generally consistent with favorable anatomy. If the artery is not satisfactory, the operation is aborted.
- Once the artery has been determined to be acceptable, the radial incision is made. The skin flap is elevated below the level of the muscular fascia. The EDC, extensor indicis proprius, and EDQ muscles are all retracted radially to facilitate exposure of the septum.
- The muscular branches of the posterior interosseous artery are carefully divided, exposing the posterior interosseous artery along the septum.
- Once one good septocutaneous perforator is located, the posterior interosseous artery is divided proximal to this branch. Further dissection to obtain more perforators is discouraged because of the proximity to the posterior interosseous nerve and potential damage to this nerve.
- After locating the major perforator and dividing the posterior interosseous artery proximally, the ulnar incision around the flap is made. This side is also elevated at a subfascial level.
- The flap is then elevated from proximal to distal. This dissection is facilitated with ulnar retraction of the ECU. A generous cuff of surrounding tissue is taken with the posterior interosseous artery to help preserve its vena comitans.
- A superficial vein may be preserved in the elevation for distal reanastomosis to help with venous drainage (**TECH FIG 4D,E**).

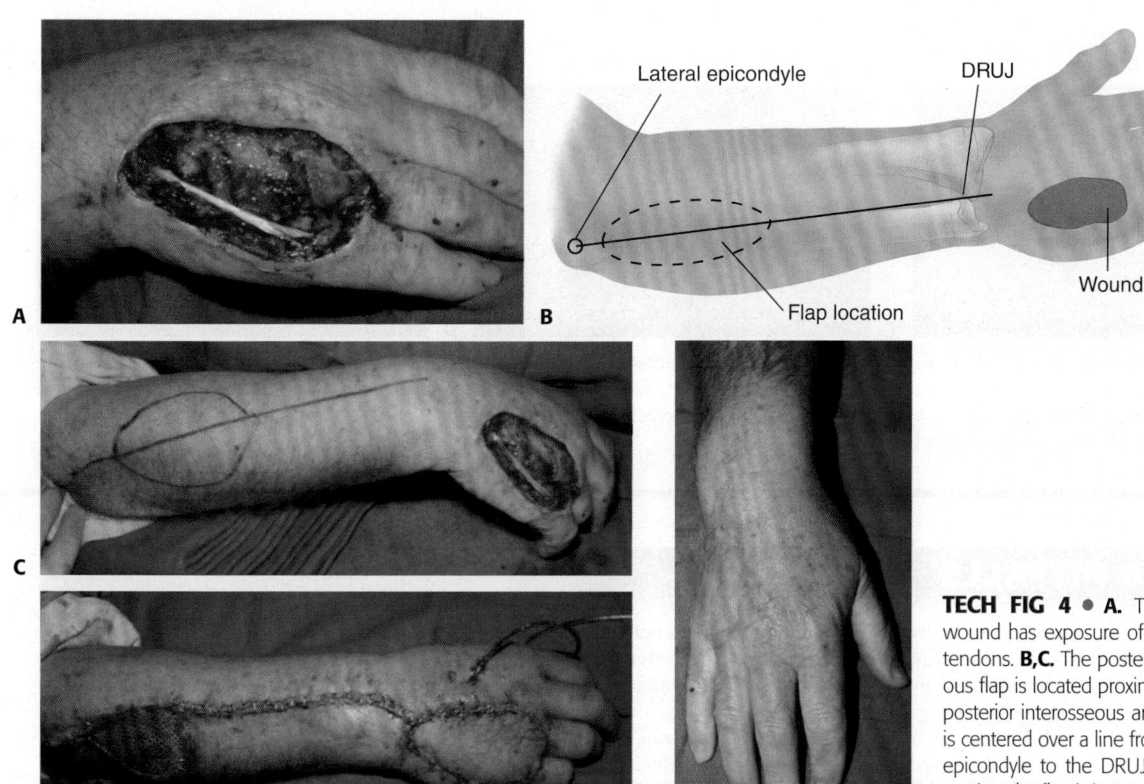

TECH FIG 4 • **A.** This traumatic wound has exposure of the extensor tendons. **B,C.** The posterior interosseous flap is located proximally over the posterior interosseous artery. The flap is centered over a line from the lateral epicondyle to the DRUJ. **D.** After elevation, the flap is inset on the wound. **E.** The wound is well healed.

Z-Plasty

- The angle of the flaps in Z-plasty is most commonly 60 degrees (**TECH FIG 5A**), but it can be varied to give more or less lengthening, depending on the quality of the adjacent tissue. Theoretically, 60-degree flaps will provide a lengthening of 75%.
- The central incision is designed along the tight scar. This scar often is excised during this part of the procedure (**TECH FIG 5B**).
- The two limbs are designed at opposing ends of the scar on opposite sides of the central member. These limbs are placed at about 60 degrees from the central incision (**TECH FIG 5C**).
- The flaps created are then elevated at a subcutaneous level. Then, the two triangular flaps are transposed and sutured into place.
- Once the two flaps are elevated, they often "fall" into the correct position and are easily sutured in place.
- This usually gives an obvious and considerable lengthening immediately after flap transposition and insetting (**TECH FIG 5D**).

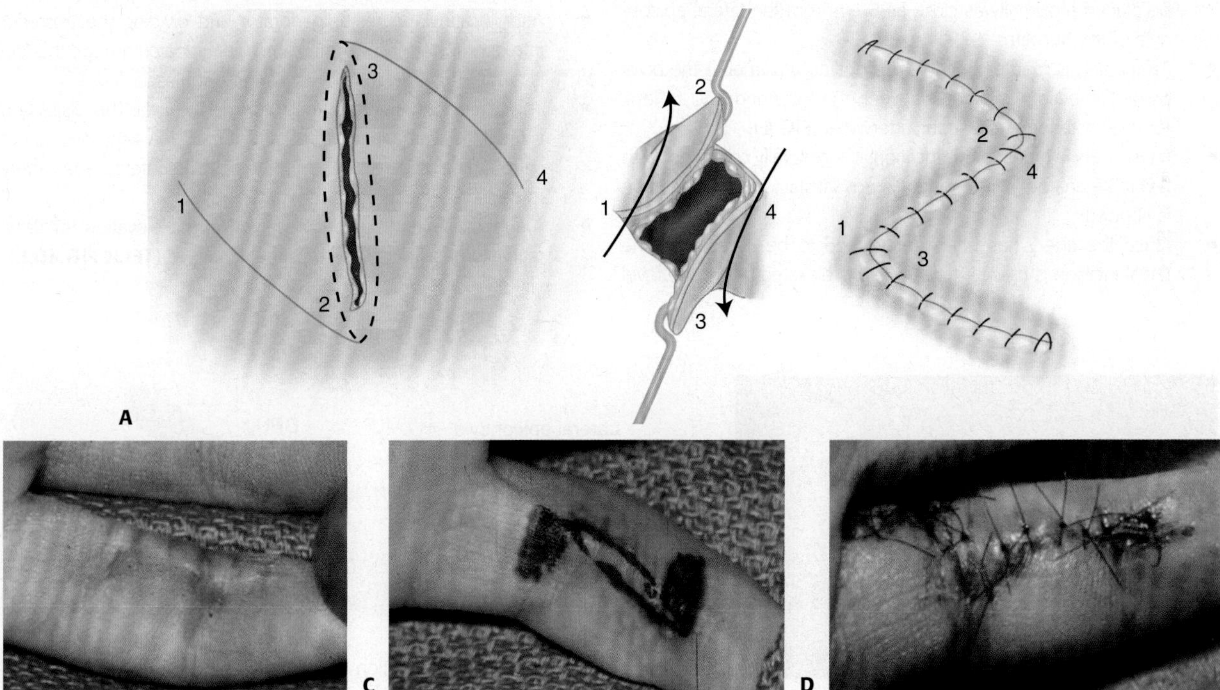

TECH FIG 5 • **A.** With a Z-plasty, two triangular flaps are elevated and transposed to interpose normal tissue into a contracted scar. The angle of the flaps usually is 60 degrees. **B.** This small finger has a contracted scar on the volar radial border. As it crosses both interphalangeal joints, the scar decreases the finger's ability to extend fully. **C.** The Z-plasty is designed. **D.** After the flaps are elevated and transposed, the scar is lengthened, allowing full extension of the finger.

PEARLS AND PITFALLS

Indications	▪ A thorough physical examination must be completed before reconstruction of any defect. ▪ The choice of reconstruction is guided by the reconstructive ladder. Less invasive operations should be considered before more invasive procedures, but, ultimately, the expected outcome of the type of operation will direct the choice. ▪ Before any wound is covered, it must be clean, with no foreign material or dead tissue. Delaying reconstruction a few days until these goals are met is worthwhile.
Flap elevation	▪ Flap elevation must be done with care and precision, with attention to preservation of the feeding blood vessels. The small vessels perfusing the flaps are vital to flap survival. ▪ Frequent use of Doppler ultrasound facilitates vessel identification.
Radial forearm flap	▪ The dissection is safest when the fascia is elevated first from the ulnar side. The septum rises obliquely under the BR. ▪ Preservation of the paired venae comitantes and the septal perforators is critical to survival of the flap. ▪ The reversed flap needs a patent palmar vascular arch.
Groin flap	▪ The patient must be prepared to have the hand connected to the groin and must understand that a second operation is mandatory. ▪ This flap and the radial forearm flap are the workhorse flaps for large soft tissue flaps of the hand.

First dorsal metacarpal artery flap	■ Reliable coverage for volar thumb or small dorsal hand defects ■ Sensation can also be preserved with this flap through branches of the superficial radial nerve. ■ The dissection is somewhat complex due to the small caliber of the vessels.
Posterior interosseous flap	■ This flap is not typically a first choice. ■ It is used when there is not a patent palmar arch (ie, when a radial forearm flap is contraindicated) and when there is a reason not to use a groin flap.

POSTOPERATIVE CARE

- The postoperative care largely depends on the flap that has been used.
- For all of the operations, some of the same principles are followed.
  - Postoperative antibiotics often are indicated because the wounds have been open for some time, have been contaminated, or have associated open fractures. The choice of antibiotic is individualized for each patient.
  - The operative site usually is splinted to allow for healing of the flap without movement. If there is no bony injury, this is usually for 7 to 10 days, but the length of time may vary.
  - The arm should be elevated above the level of the heart as much as possible. This will help decrease both edema within the flap and patient discomfort.
- The radial forearm flap should be monitored in the hospital for 2 or 3 days.
  - When distally based, this flap may be susceptible to venous congestion.
    - Care should be taken during the operation to meticulously preserve the vena comitans.
    - If the cephalic vein has been preserved with the flap, it can be anastomosed to a vein in the field of the flap, but this is rarely necessary with the reversed flap.
    - Care should be taken not to make the splint or dressing too tight.
- If a skin graft is placed during the operation, the bolster dressing is removed at 5 to 7 days and the skin graft is dressed daily with petrolatum-infused gauze or a nonadhering dressing until fully healed.
- Sutures around the flap are removed at 10 to 14 days.
- Early active motion of the fingers is encouraged to promote tendon gliding and lessen edema, unless contraindicated after coverage.
- Hand therapy is initiated in most patients at 1 to 2 weeks following surgery.

COMPLICATIONS

- Short-term complications include those related to flap survival and healing of the wound.
- Long-term complications result from undesirable scarring relating to both the primary injury and the method of closure.
- Complete flap loss due to flap ischemia is uncommon. More often, a small area of the flap margin may not heal to the native skin margin due to inadequate débridement of the skin edges or rough handling of the flap skin.
- As the flaps heal, the function of the hand depends on subsequent scarring, which, if it occurs, leads to poor tendon gliding. Persistent tendon scarring requires later tenolysis. After 3 months, loss of the flap by inadvertent pedicle division is rare, but late flap loss has been reported.
- If scarring from the flap margin creates a contracture across a joint, a Z-plasty may be necessary.
- Overall, the complications related to flap closure are less than complications related to secondary healing. The long-term outcome will be better with flap coverage compared to secondary healing because secondary intention creates an abundance of scar tissue, which can impair function of the hand.

REFERENCES

1. Foucher G, Baun JB. A new island flap transfer from the dorsum of the index to the thumb. Plast Reconstr Surg 1979;63:344–349.
2. Foucher G, van Genechten N, Merle M, et al. A compound radial artery flap in hand surgery: an original modification of the Chinese forearm flap. Br J Plast Surg 1984;37:139–148.
3. Mathes SJ, Nahai F. Introduction: a systematic approach. In: Mathes SJ, Nahai F, eds. Reconstructive Surgery: Principles, Anatomy, and Technique. New York: Churchill Livingstone, 1997:3–15.
4. Pederson WC, Lister GD. Skin flaps. In: Green DP, Hotchkiss RN, Pederson WC, et al, eds. Green's Operative Hand Surgery, ed 5. Philadelphia: Elsevier Churchill Livingstone, 2005:1648–1703.
5. Place MJ, Herber SC, Hardesty RA. Basic techniques and principles in plastic surgery. In: Aston SJ, Beasley RW, Thorne CH, eds. Grabb and Smith's Textbook of Plastic Surgery. Philadelphia: Lippincott Williams & Wilkins, 1997:13–16.
6. Serafin D. The groin flap. In: Serafin D, ed. Atlas of Microsurgical Composite Tissue Transplantation. Philadelphia: WB Saunders, 1996:57–65.
7. Sherif MM. First dorsal metacarpal artery flap in hand reconstruction: I. Anatomical study. J Hand Surg Am 1994;19:26–31.
8. Smith PJ, Foley B, Mcgreggor IA, et al. The anatomic basis of the groin flap. Plast Reconstr Surg 1972;49:41–47.
9. Song R, Gao Y, Song Y, et al. The forearm flap. Clin Plast Surg 1982;9:21–26.
10. Spector JA, Levine JP. Cutaneous defects: flaps, grafts, and expansion. In: McCarthy JG, Galiano RD, Boutros SG, eds. Current Therapy in Plastic Surgery. Philadelphia: WB Saunders, 2006:11–21.
11. Zancoli EA, Angrigiani C. Posterior interosseous island flap. J Hand Surg Br 1988;13:130–135.

The Use of Free Vascularized Fibular Grafts for Reconstruction of Segmental Bone Defects

Arik Zaretski, Ravit Yanko-Arzi, Yehuda Kollender, Eyal Gur, and Jacob Bickels

BACKGROUND

- Wide resection of long bone tumors can create a large intercalary bone defect requiring reconstruction. Such defects were traditionally reconstructed with prosthetic implants, allografts, and allograft prosthetic composites, all of which were associated with considerably high rates of complications and failures.[5]
- Distraction osteogenesis provides biologic reconstruction of only small- to medium-sized intercalary defects. Moreover, it is a prolonged procedure, which requires up to 2 months for an elongation of 1 cm, and complications are frequent, patient compliance is critical, and large soft tissue defects cannot be addressed simultaneously.[8,12] Reported experience regarding safety and efficacy in the oncologic setup is also limited.
- Since the introduction of vascularized autogenous graft for long bone reconstruction after tumor resection in the early 1970s, the use of a free fibular flap has become a viable option for reconstruction of large intercalary bone defects following tumor resection or for the purpose of resection arthrodesis.[3,4,6,9–11,13,15] Its inherent advantage is based on its ability to exploit the biology of normal fracture healing rather than the creeping substitution that is fundamental to the incorporation of a nonvascularized graft.
- The fibula is an optimal vascularized graft source because of its anatomic accessibility and because removing an intercalary segment while preserving the proximal fibula, distal tibial–fibular syndesmosis, and the lateral malleolus would have minimal impact on knee and ankle stability and would not compromise weight-bearing capacity and overall function of the lower extremity. It allows reconstruction of large bone defects because of its independent blood supply, which permits graft incorporation into the host bone even when presence or viability of the surrounding soft tissue are considerably compromised because of previous surgery or radiation therapy.
- Furthermore, a vascularized fibular graft has the capability to hypertrophy over time as a response to continuous pressure load. As a result, vascularized fibula have shown excellent long-term durability.[2,9,16] The fibular head can also be used for joint reconstruction after intercalary resection of bone tumors.[7]
- In summary, a free fibular graft provides a durable true biologic reconstruction with accommodative and regenerative capabilities associated with minimal short- and long-term complications.[16] It requires a combined effort of highly trained and committed teams as well as the patient's compliance throughout a very long, complex, and demanding rehabilitation period.

APPLIED ANATOMY OF THE FIBULAR FLAP

- The fibula is long and narrow and therefore provides a strong cortical strut for reconstruction of long bone defects. It has a square cross-section in its superior part and is triangular in its inferior end. In the adult patient, it can reach a width of 1.5 to 2 cm and a length of 35 cm, 25 to 30 cm of which can be harvested for the purpose of free grafting. Its shape and length can match bone segments of the upper extremity (humerus, radius, and ulna) or fit the medullary canal of bones of the lower extremity (femur, tibia); therefore, it can be used for reconstruction of bone defects at these sites.
- The fibula is circumferentially surrounded by muscle groups on its lateral, anteromedial, and posterior aspects and is also the origin of the four intermuscular septi of the leg. The blood supply and drainage of the fibular shaft are related to the peroneal vessels. The peroneal artery together with the two peroneal venae comitantes follow a course parallel to the fibula and lie between the flexor hallucis longus and tibialis posterior muscles (**FIG 1**). The fibula is dually vascularized through its endosteal and periosteal vessels.
- The endosteal blood supply is based on the nutrient artery, which stems 6 to 14 cm from the peroneal artery bifurcation, enters the middle third of the diaphysis via the nutrient foramen, and then divides into an ascending and a descending branch. The periosteal blood supply is derived from 8 to 9 periosteal branches, mostly in the middle third of the diaphysis. The peroneal artery is also the source of 4 to 6 fascial vessels that pass through the posterior intercrural septum to the skin territory, lateral to the fibula. It provides numerous muscular branches as well; specifically, it supplies multiple small branches to the muscles of the anterior compartment and a few larger branches to the soleus muscle at the deep posterior compartment of the leg.
- The unique morphologic characteristics and blood supply of the fibula allow considerable versatility in the use of the fibular flap for reconstruction of skeletal, soft tissue, and growth plate defects, as required. The fibular flap can be transferred in various configurations and compositions to suit the needs of individual cases:
  - In its straight configuration, it can be used for reconstruction of a relatively narrow bone segment (**FIG 2**). A longitudinal osteotomy that increases the surface area of the flap can serve as an onlay graft to augment the healing process for partial cortical defects. Based on perforating fasciocutaneous branches at the middle and distal thirds of the pedicle, a skin paddle of up to 20 × 10 cm can be transferred simultaneously to facilitate coverage of concomitant large soft tissue defects and to allow the patency

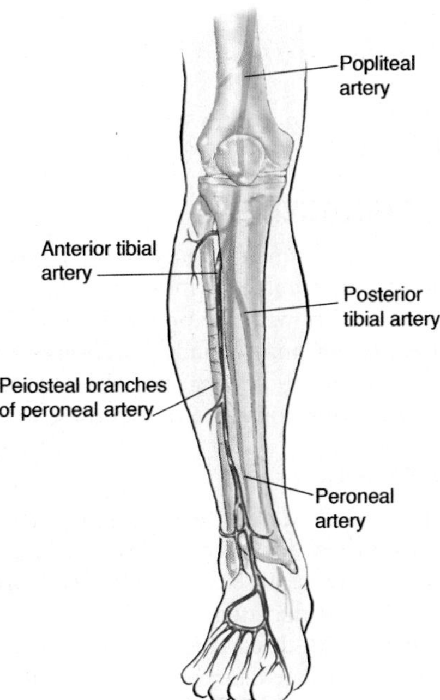

FIG 1 • The blood supply and drainage of the fibula are related to the peroneal artery and two peroneal veins, which follow a course parallel to the fibula. The fibula has a dual blood supply: endosteal and periosteal. The former is based on a nutrient artery that stems 6 to 14 cm from the peroneal bifurcation and the latter is based on multiple periosteal branches along the fibular diaphysis.

of the pedicle anastomosis to be monitored. Part of the soleus or the flexor hallucis longus muscles can also be included with the flap to reconstruct soft tissue defects and cover exposed bone.

- Transverse osteotomies can be made through the mid-diaphysis to produce two or more cortical struts on a single pedicle (double/triple barrel) for reconstruction of a wide bone segment. In these cases when the endosteal vessels are transected, the bone survives on its periosteal system.
- The proximal epiphysis may be included in the flap for joint reconstruction and preservation of longitudinal growth potential (in pediatric patients) after intra-articular resection of bone tumors (**FIG 3**). This flap is based on the anterior tibial vascular flap or the descending geniculate artery and is most commonly used for reconstructions following resections of the proximal humerus and distal radius.

INDICATIONS

- Segmental bone defects larger than 5 cm following resection due to the following:
  - Tumor
  - Radiation-induced bone necrosis
  - Osteomyelitis
- In cases of high-grade sarcomas of bone, the authors generally use spacers for immediate reconstruction following tumor resection rather than performing the definitive reconstruction with vascularized fibula. The latter is carried out 2 years after tumor resection if there had been no tumor recurrence or lung metastases.

CONTRAINDICATIONS

- Systemic/general conditions
  - Cardiovascular, surgical, or hematologic diseases that may affect peripheral blood flow
  - Incompliance with or if patient's physical or psychological states do not allow to withstand a prolonged non–weight bearing and/or rehabilitation
  - Poor general health status

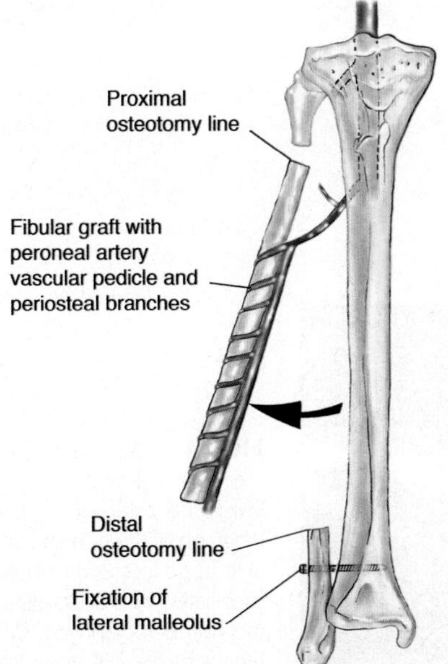

FIG 2 • Diaphyseal fibular graft, used for reconstruction of intercalary bone defects. If a long segment is required and the osteotomy is closed to the lateral malleolus, screw fixation to the tibia is advised to prevent valgus deformity and ankle instability.

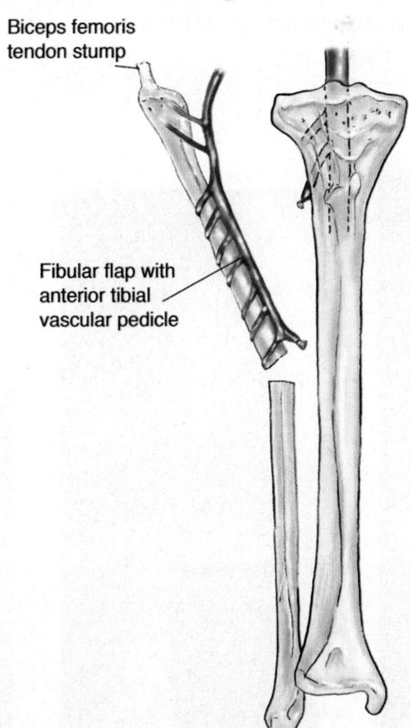

FIG 3 • Proximal fibular graft that includes the proximal fibular epiphysis and based on the anterior tibial vascular pedicle may be used for joint reconstruction and preservation of longitudinal growth in children following intra-articular resection of bone tumors.

- Donor site considerations
  - Fibular deformity following previous injury to the lower extremity
  - Vascular injury or compromise following previous trauma to the leg
  - Vascular anomalies of the leg or plantar arches (eg, single-vessel or peroneal vessel–dominant foot)
- Recipient site considerations
  - Infection around the recipient site
  - Suspected tumor recurrence

IMAGING AND OTHER STAGING STUDIES

- Detailed preoperative evaluation of both the recipient and donor sites is mandatory. Imaging of the recipient site should provide information regarding the dimensions of bone (length and diameter) and soft tissue defects remaining after tumor resection, thus allowing the selection of the appropriate type and size of fibular flap to be used.
- Imaging of the donor site should include the entire leg and is aimed at excluding fibular deformity and at determining maximal flap length.
- The surgeon should verify adequate pulses in both posterior tibial and dorsalis pedis arteries. Evaluation of the deep and superficial plantar vascular arches is done using an equivalent to the palmar Allen test and is confirmed by Doppler ultrasound examination. If those studies are nonconclusive, an angiography or computed tomography angiography (CTA) is performed.

Recipient Site

- Plain radiography (**FIG 4AB**)
- CTA when the vascular anatomy is unclear (**FIG 4C**)
- Magnetic resonance imaging (MRI)

Donor Site

- Plain radiography
- CTA
- Doppler ultrasound (done intraoperatively to detect the skin island perforants)

SURGICAL MANAGEMENT

- To minimize the duration of surgery and if the patient's position on the operating table permits, the fibular flap is harvested simultaneously with the preparation of the recipient site, a procedure that may include resection of the primary bone tumor or removal of a spacer that had been used in a previous surgery for reconstructive purposes.

Intercalary Resection

- As a rule, a vascularized fibula in its straight and simple configuration is sufficient for reconstruction of bone defects of the upper extremity because of the relatively narrow cross-sectional diameter of the latter.
- Reconstruction of such defects of the lower extremity requires graft material of a larger diameter because of the additional mechanical support needed. A double-barrel fibular flap can be used for reconstruction of femoral and tibial defects of up to 13 cm. Longer defects may require the support of an allograft, which provides the initial stability required for bone healing, graft incorporation, and subsequent fibular hypertrophy.
- Furthermore, in cases of failed vascular anastomosis, the combined fibular–allograft construct is still comparable to multiple cortical allogenic struts with a relatively good chance of success, especially if reliable fixation is achieved. The technique of combined reconstruction with an allograft and the vascularized fibula, as described by Capanna and his colleagues,[1,2] provides such stability and is the preferred method of reconstruction used by the authors for long intercalary defects of the lower extremities.

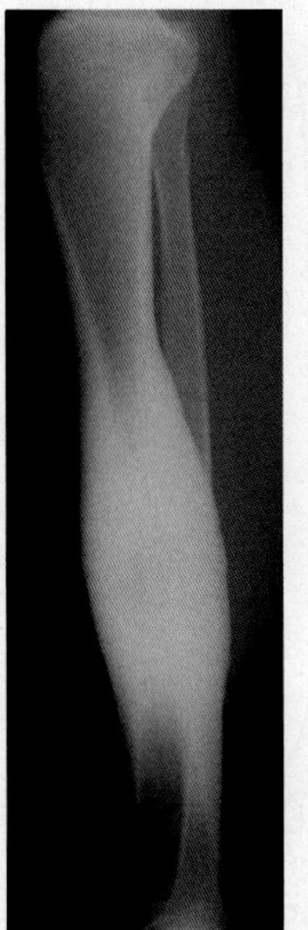
A

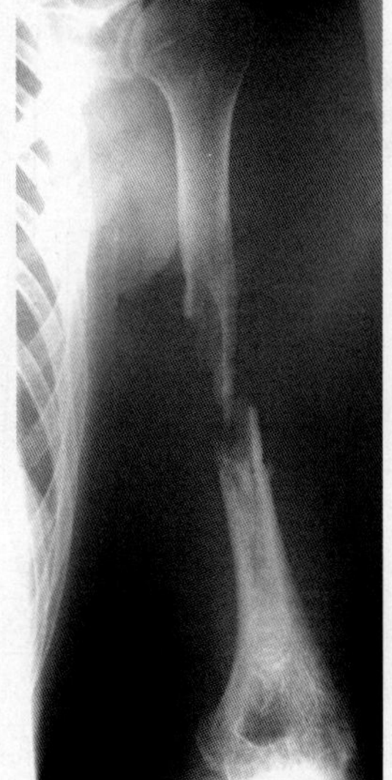
B

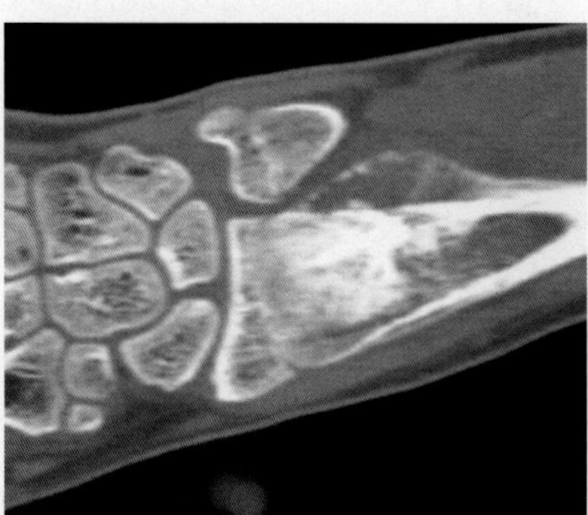
C

FIG 4 • **A.** Plain radiograph of the tibia showing a large diaphyseal low-grade osteosarcoma. **B.** Plain radiograph of the arm showing considerable bone loss and pathologic fracture associated with acute osteomyelitis of the humeral diaphysis. **C.** Coronal CT reconstruction of the distal forearm showing an osteosarcoma of the distal radius.

Position and Incision

- For treating a bone defect of the lower extremity, the patient is placed supine on the operating table with the thighs spread apart. The hip and knee of the donor extremity are flexed (**TECH FIG 1**). The first team, which is responsible for tumor resection, (blue team) is positioned along the medial or lateral side of the recipient extremity.
- If tumor resection is done from the medial side of the extremity, a surgeon can be positioned at that aspect. A second (red) team, responsible for the harvest of the fibular flap from the donor extremity, is positioned along its lateral.

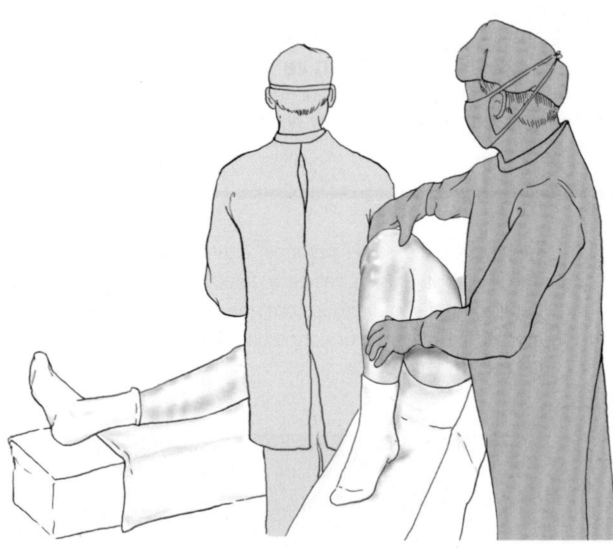

TECH FIG 1 • The patient is placed supine on the operating table with the thighs spread apart with the hip and knee of the donor extremity in flexion. The team responsible for tumor resection (in *blue*) is positioned along the medial or lateral of the recipient extremity, as requires. The team responsible for removal of the fibular graft from the donor extremity (in *red*) is positioned along its lateral aspect of the donor extremity.

Resection of Bone Tumor

- The bone tumor is removed according to the standard techniques, and the length and diameter of the intercalary bone defect are measured (**TECH FIGS 2** to **4**).

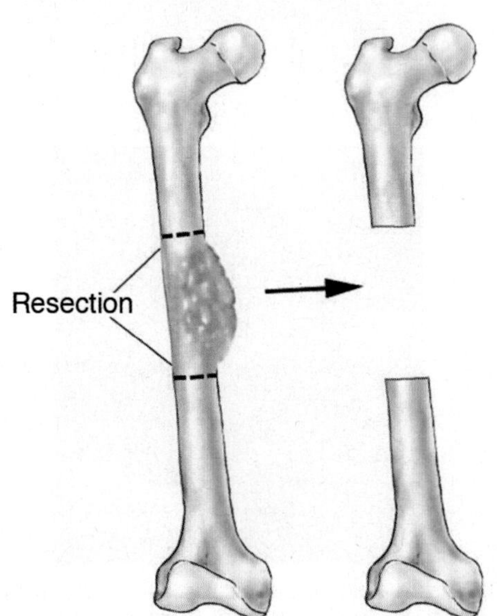

TECH FIG 2 • Diaphyseal tumor is resected with wide margins, leaving a long intercalary bone defect.

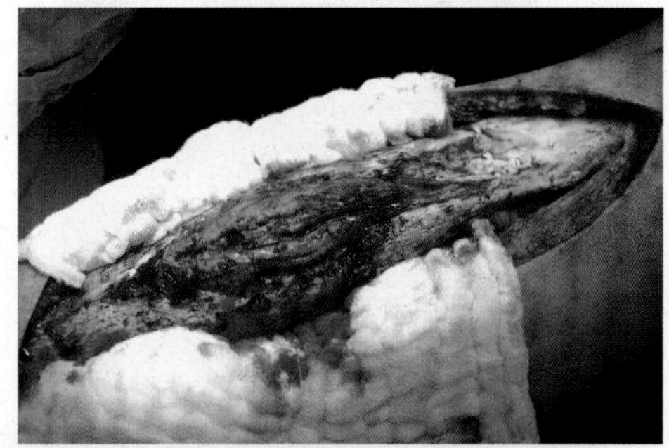

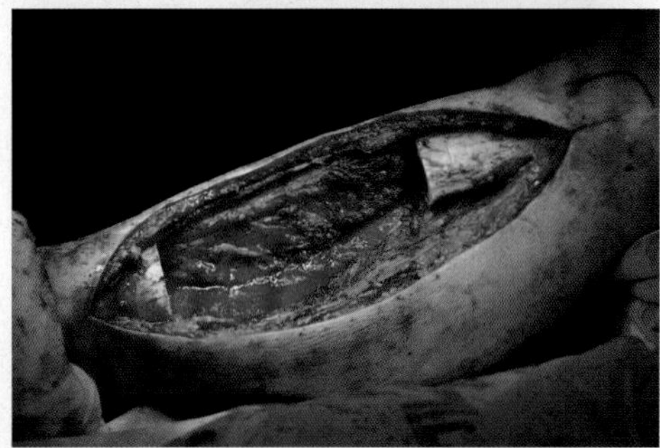

TECH FIG 3 • **A.** Intraoperative photograph of the large diaphyseal low-grade osteosarcoma of the tibia shown in **FIG 4A**. **B.** Large intercalary defect remaining after wide tumor resection.

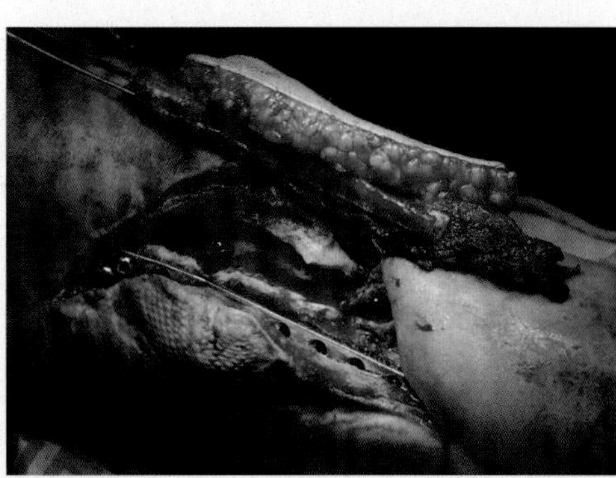

TECH FIG 4 • Following tissue sampling and cultures, administration of intravenous antibiotics, and resolution of acute manifestation of infection, the patient in **FIG 4B** with acute osteomyelitis of the humeral diaphysis underwent resection of the infected bone tissue, leaving a long intercalary bone defect.

Harvest of a Fibular Flap and Allograft

- Using an anterolateral incision at the contralateral leg, an intercalary fibular segment that is 6 cm longer than the bone defect is harvested together with its nutrient vessels and its periosteal cuff (**TECH FIG 5**).
- If a large skin defect is anticipated at the tumor resection site, the fibular flap is harvested with an overlying skin island supplied by the same peroneal artery, which allows tension-free skin closure as well as early detection of flap-compromised viability: Arterial or venous compromise would instantly be expressed by ischemic or congestion changes of the skin island (**TECH FIG 6**).

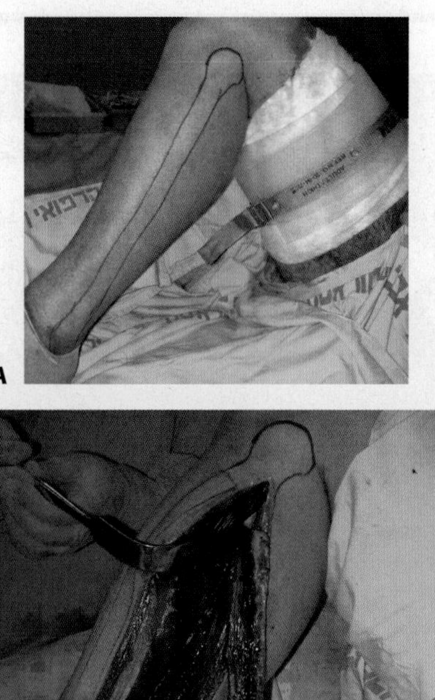

TECH FIG 5 • **A.** An anterolateral leg incision is used for harvesting of the fibular flap. **B.** An intercalary fibular segment, 6 cm longer from the bone defect, with its periosteal cuff is harvested.

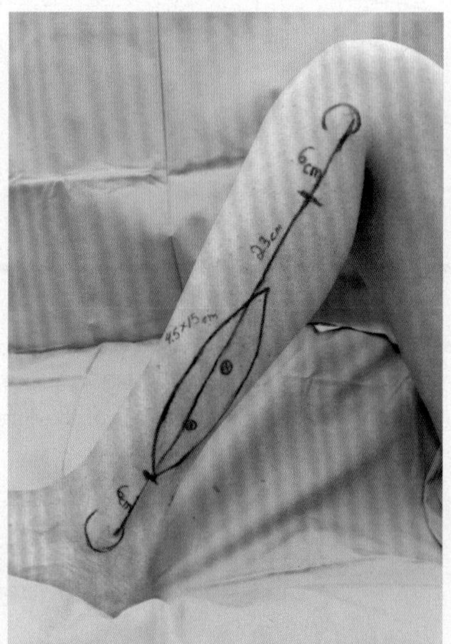

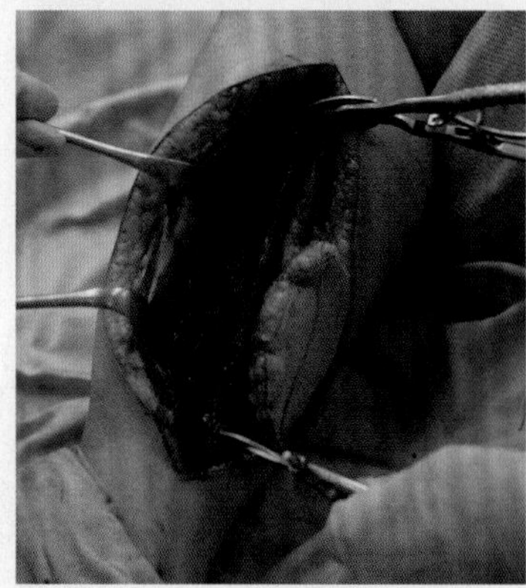

TECH FIG 6 • **A–F.** If a large skin defect is anticipated at the tumor resection site, the fibular graft is removed with an overlying skin island, which is used for coverage of that defect and for monitoring of flap viability. *(continued)*

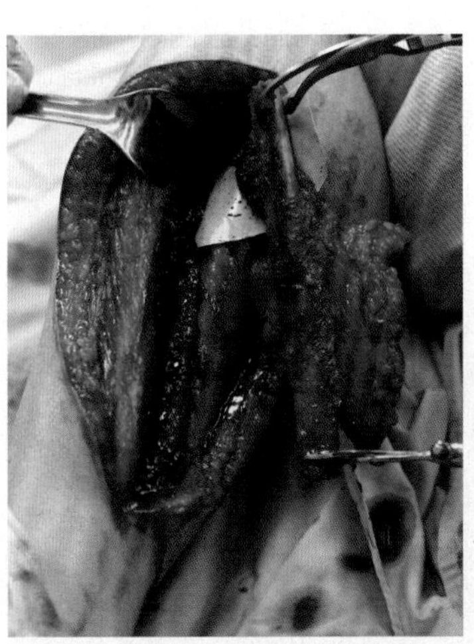
C

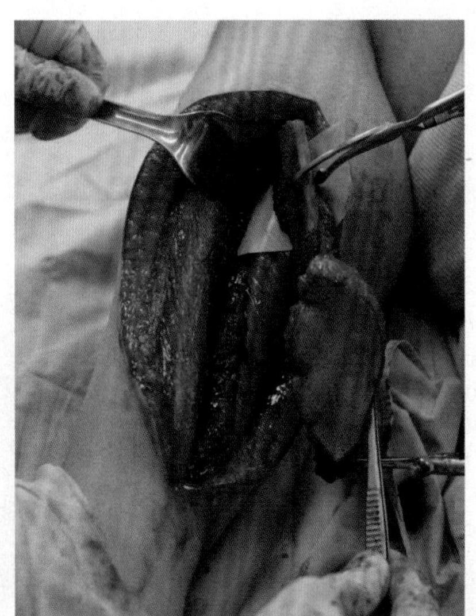
D

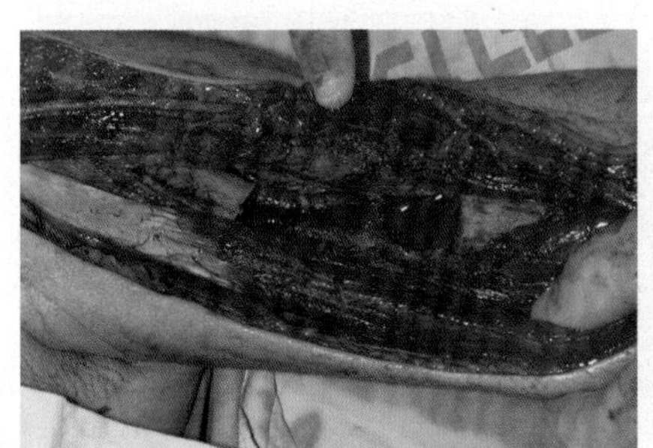
E

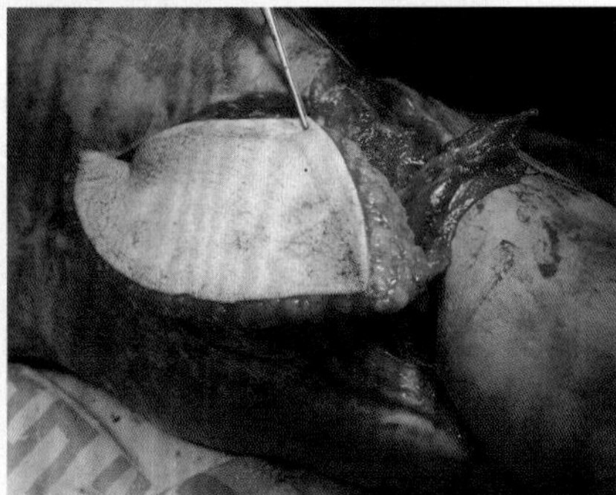
F

TECH FIG 6 • *(continued)*

- The skin island is removed without the underlying fascia; it is preserved to maintain the biologic coverage of the peroneal tendons and allow better skin graft take (**TECH FIG 7**).
- If a long bony segment is required and the osteotomy is close to the lateral malleolus, screw fixation to the tibia is advised to prevent valgus deformity and ankle instability (see **FIG 2**). A skin graft, usually taken from the thigh of the donor extremity, is used to cover the skin defect in that leg.
- The allograft is cut to the same length as the bone defect, and a groove is opened longitudinally by removing as much cortical and cancellous bone as needed to allow insertion of the fibular flap into it.

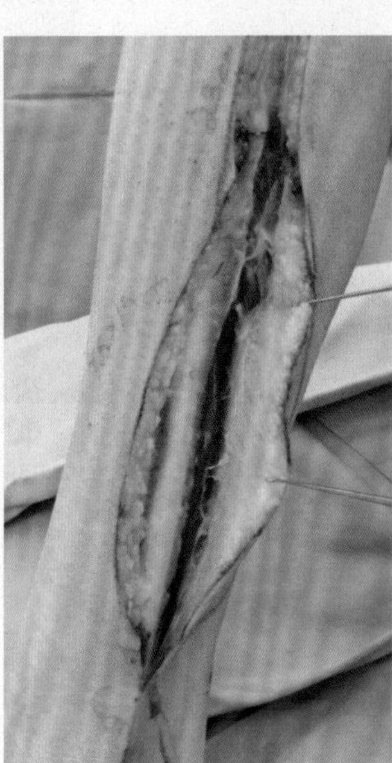

TECH FIG 7 • Skin is harvested and the underlying fascia is left intact over the peroneal tendons.

Reconstruction of the Recipient Site

- The allograft is inserted to fill the bone defect and fixed to its proximal and distal edges with a side plate and screws (**TECH FIG 8**). An intramedullary nail is also used if the diameter of the allograft medullary canal is wide enough to contain both the nail and the fibular graft.
- Using a high-speed burr, a defect is created in the allograft cortex at the appropriate level to allow the passage of the fibular vascular pedicle toward the vascular bundle of the recipient extremity while avoiding traction on the vascular anastomosis.
- The fibular graft is inserted 2 to 3 cm into the medullary canal at both ends and fixed with screws (**TECH FIG 9**). Care is taken to prevent damage to the nutrient vessels of the fibula by those screws. The fibula can be placed in an intramedullary location, inside the allograft or parallel to it. In both options, the fibular osteotomy sites should lie in close approximation to the native long bone resected edges.
- After vascular anastomoses are completed, an autologous bone graft, taken from the fibular flap remnants or the ipsilateral iliac crest, is used to reinforce the interface between the fibula and the recipient bone.

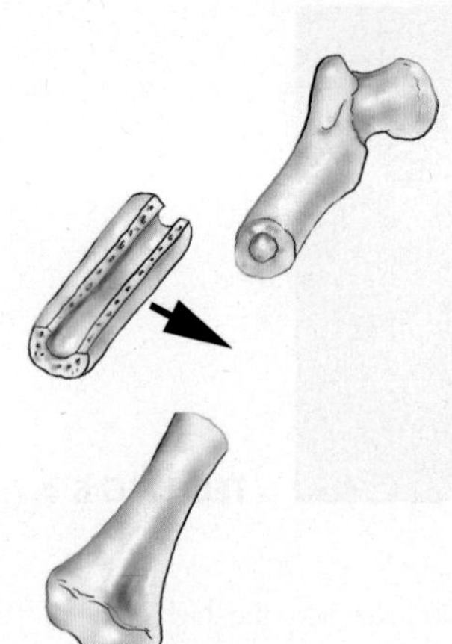

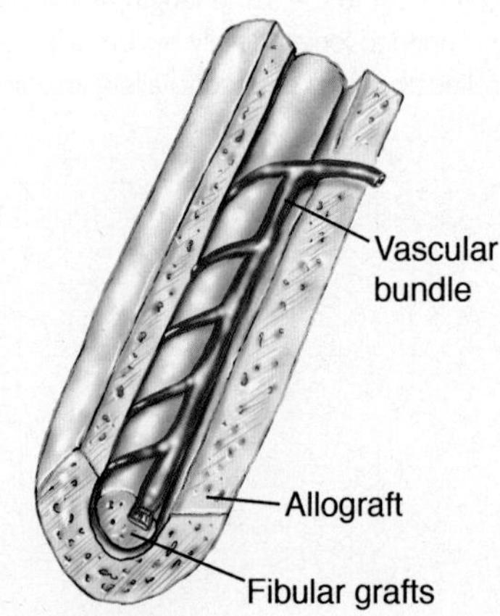

TECH FIG 8 • **A.** The allograft is cut to the same length as the bone defect, and a groove is opened longitudinally by removing as much cortical and cancellous bone as needed to allow insertion of the fibular graft into it. It is then inserted to fill the bone defect and fixed to its proximal and distal edges with a side plate and screws. **B.** A defect is created in the allograft cortex to allow the passage of the fibular vascular pedicle.

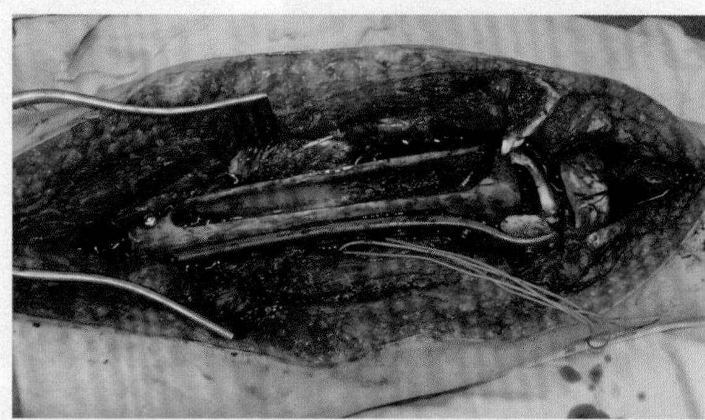

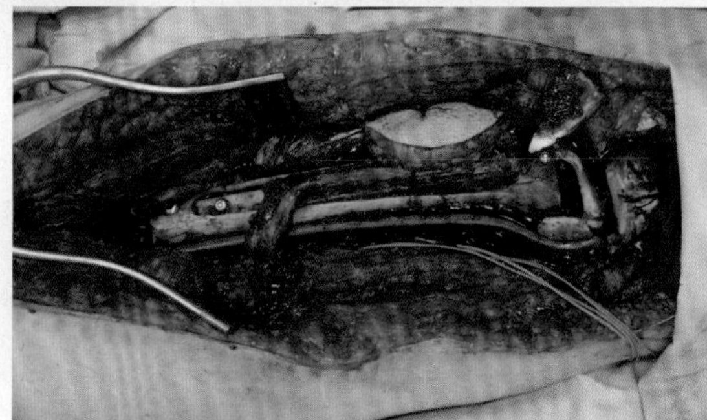

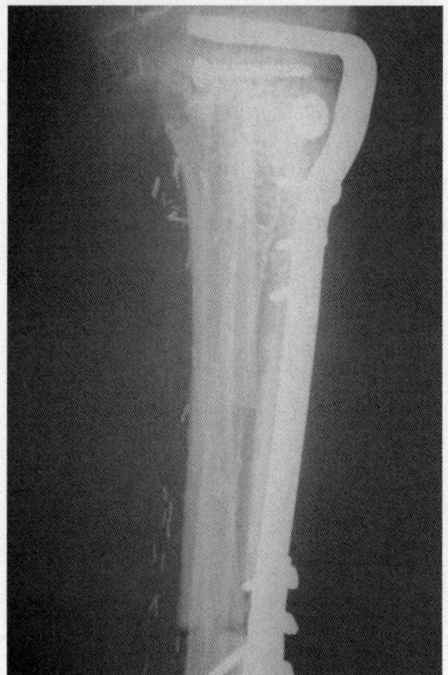

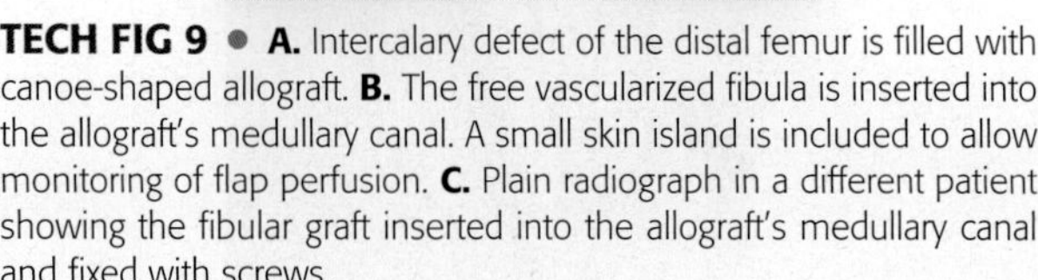

TECH FIG 9 • **A.** Intercalary defect of the distal femur is filled with canoe-shaped allograft. **B.** The free vascularized fibula is inserted into the allograft's medullary canal. A small skin island is included to allow monitoring of flap perfusion. **C.** Plain radiograph in a different patient showing the fibular graft inserted into the allograft's medullary canal and fixed with screws.

Intra-articular Resections

- The proximal fibular epiphysis with variable lengths of the diaphysis and with the anterior tibial vessels as the vascular pedicle or alternatively the inferior geniculate artery is used for reconstruction of defects that include one side of the articular surface.
- Following harvest of the fibular flap, the lateral collateral ligament is secured to the medial tibial metaphysis with a metal staple to preserve lateral knee joint stability (**TECH FIG 10**).
- The proximal aspect of the fibular flap is fixed to the radial or humeral diaphysis with a side plate and screws, and the biceps tendon stump is used for attachment to the opposing articular surface soft tissue envelope (**TECH FIGS 11** and **12**).

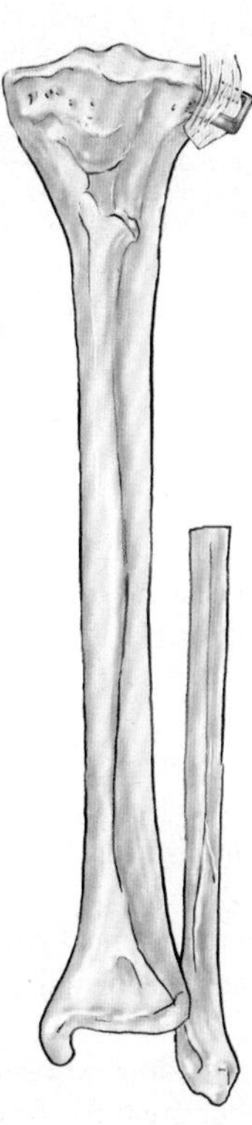

TECH FIG 10 • Following removal of a proximal fibular graft, the stump of the lateral collateral ligament is secured to the lateral tibial metaphysis to restore lateral knee joint stability.

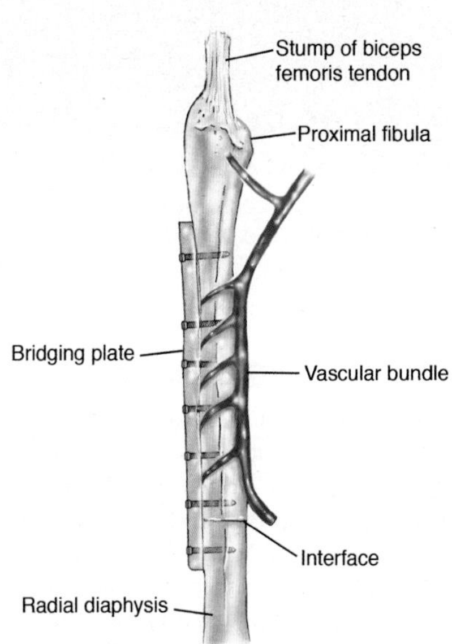

TECH FIG 11 • Reconstruction of proximal fibular graft to the remaining radial diaphysis.

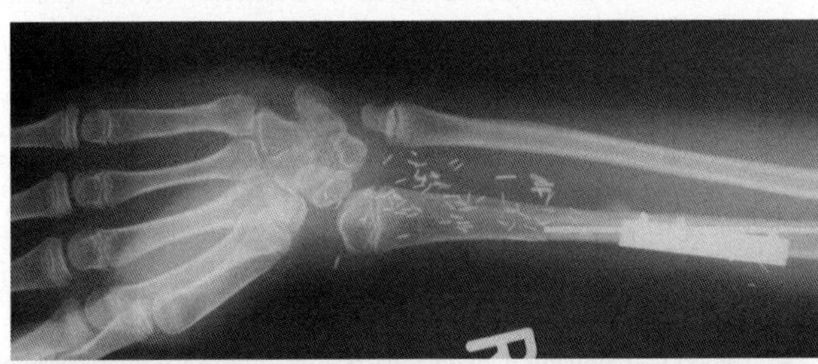

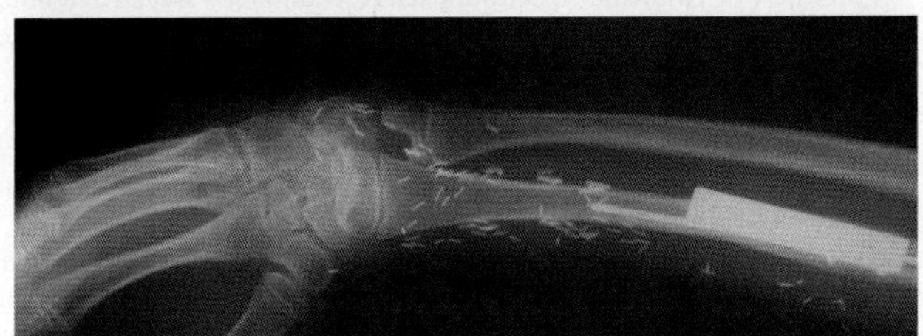

TECH FIG 12 • Anteroposterior (**A**) and lateral (**B**) plain radiographs of the patient in **FIG 4C** with osteosarcoma of the distal radius showing reconstruction of the intercalary bone defect with a proximal fibular graft.

PEARLS AND PITFALLS

Fibular flap monitoring	▪ When a skin island is included in the fibular flap, an external pencil Doppler is used to monitor blood circulation. If the flap is buried, an implantable Cook-Swartz Doppler is used for monitoring. The use of implantable Doppler in surgery also allows detection of impairment of venous outflow during wound closure[14] (**FIG 5**).

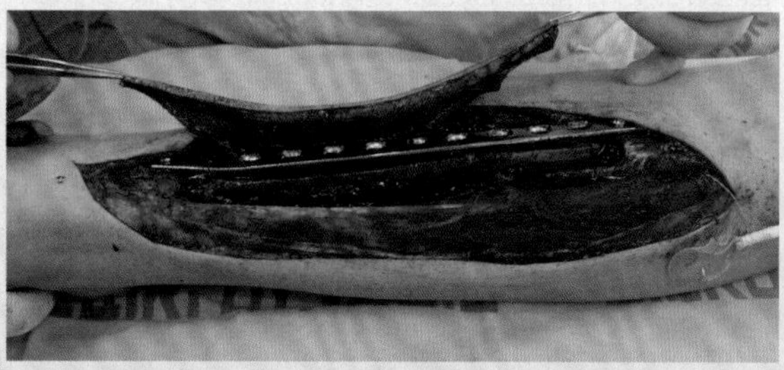

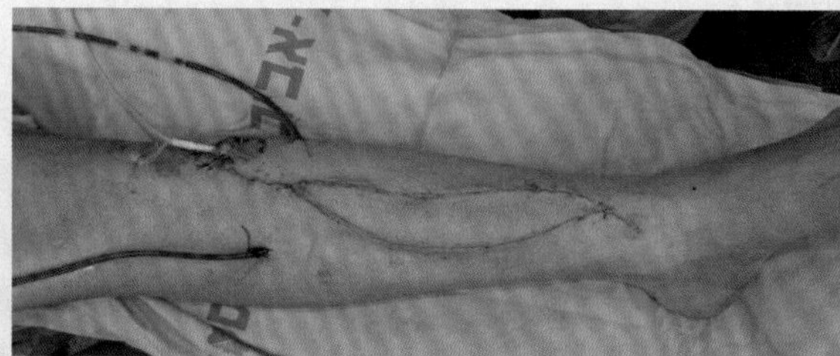

FIG 5 • A. An implantable Cook-Swartz Doppler is used to monitor fibular flap perfusion. **B.** Following wound closure, flap perfusion is monitored by the implantable Doppler and viability of the overlying skin island.

POSTOPERATIVE CARE AND REHABILITATION

- All patients must be treated and monitored postoperatively according to a strict and constant protocol. They are admitted to the department of plastic surgery for the first 5 days after surgery, where they are monitored for vital signs and flap viability and administered a mildly elevated volume of lactated Ringer solution (1.2 times the maintenance) to maintain blood flow through the anastomosis and prevent thrombus formation. This fluid protocol is maintained for a total of 5 days.
- Enoxaparin is given for prevention of deep vein thromboses. Blood samples are drawn twice daily for blood count and electrolytes. Hemoglobin levels are kept between 9 and 10 g/mL to minimize blood viscosity and further decrease the likelihood of anastomotic thrombus.
- Recipient extremities are immobilized for 3 months (an upper extremity by a brace and a lower extremity by a plaster cast) after which gradual passive ranges of motion are practiced.
- Signs of bony union are evaluated radiologically by serial plain radiographs. Bone unions are usually seen after 4 to 5 months in the upper extremity and after 5 to 7 months in the lower extremity. Partial weight bearing is allowed on detection of radiologic evidence of bone union. Gradual physical loads on the limb are recommended until full weight bearing is achieved.

OUTCOMES

- Solid bony unions associated with fibular hypertrophy, full weight bearing, and mechanical load capacities are achieved in the vast majority of patients. Fibular hypertrophy occurs over years and is the result of pressure transport, microfractures, and callus formation.
- Mild to moderate decreases in range of motion are common and of a similar extent to those seen after other types of reconstructive surgeries. The latter is the result of the extent of resection of bone and soft tissues rather than the mode of reconstruction.
- Deep infections are rare, as is hardware failure requiring revision surgery.

COMPLICATIONS

- Recipient site
  - Anastomotic thrombosis and loss of flap viability
  - Partial skin island necrosis
  - Nonunion
  - Infection
  - Hardware failure and breakage
- Donor site
  - Valgus ankle deformity
  - Ankle joint instability
  - Transient or permanent peroneal palsy
  - Transient or permanent peroneal distribution area sensory deficit
  - Skin graft failure and tendon exposure
  - Transient or permanent great toe flexion impairment

REFERENCES

1. Capanna R, Bufalini C, Campanacci M. A new technique for reconstructions of large metadiaphyseal bone defects. Orthop Traumatol 1993;3:159–177.
2. Capanna R, Campanacci DA, Belot N, et al. A new reconstructive technique for intercalary defects of long bones: the association of massive allografts with vascularized fibular autograft. Long-term results and comparison with alternative techniques. Orthop Clin North Am 2007;38:51–60.
3. Chang DW, Weber KL. Use of a vascularized fibula bone flap and intercalary allograft for diaphyseal reconstruction after resection of primary extremity bone sarcomas. Plast Reconstr Surg 2005;116: 1918–1925.
4. Gebert C, Hillmann A, Schwappach A, et al. Free vascularized fibular grafting for reconstruction after tumor resection in the upper extremity. J Surg Oncol 2006;94:114–127.
5. Getty PJ, Peabody TD. Complications and functional outcomes of reconstruction with an osteoarticular allograft after intra-articular resection of the proximal part of the humerus. J Bone Joint Surg 1999;81(8):1138–1146.
6. Innocenti M, Delcroix L, Manfrini M, et al. Vascularized proximal fibular epiphyseal transfer for distal radial reconstruction. J Bone Joint Surg Am 2004;86:1504–1511.
7. Innocenti M, Delcroix L, Manfrini M, et al. Vascularized proximal fibular epiphyseal transfer for distal radial reconstruction. J Bone Joint Surg Am 2005;87:237–246.

8. Kocaoglu M, Eralp L, Rashid H, et al. Reconstruction of segmental bone defects due to chronic osteomyelitis with use of an external fixator and an intramedullary nail. J Bone Joint Surg Am 2006;88:2137–2145.
9. Malizos KN, Zalavras CG, Soucacos PN, et al. Free vascularized fibular grafts for reconstruction of skeletal defects. J Am Acad Orthop Surg 2004;12:360–369.
10. McKee DM. Microvascular bone transplantation. Clin Plast Surg 1978;5:283–292.
11. O'Brien BM, Morrison WA, Ishida H, et al. Free flap transfers with microvascular anastomoses. Br J Plast Surg 1974;27:220–230.
12. Paley D. Problems, obstacles, and complications of limb lengthening by the Ilizarov technique. Clin Orthop Relat Res 1990;250:81–104.
13. Rose PS, Shin AY, Bishop AT, et al. Vascularized free fibula transfer for oncologic reconstruction of the humerus. Clin Orthop Relat Res 2005;438:80–84.
14. Schmulder A, Gur E, Zaretski A. Eight-year experience of the Cook-Swartz Doppler in free-flap operations in microsurgical and reexploration results with regard to a wide spectrum of surgeries. Microsurgery 2011;31(1):1–6.
15. Taylor GI, Miller GD, Ham FJ. The free vascularized bone graft. A clinical extension of microvascular techniques. Plast Reconstr Surg 1975;55:533–544.
16. Zaretski A, Amir A, Meller I, et al. Free fibula long bone reconstruction in orthopedic oncology: a surgical algorithm for reconstructive options. Plast Reconstr Surg 2004;113:1989–2000.

143 CHAPTER

Tumors

Surgical Treatment of Vascular Tumors of the Hand

Joshua Choo, Dean Louis, and Morton Kasdan

DEFINITION

- Vascular tumors are diverse and often have a confusing nomenclature. Part of the confusion resides in the ambiguity of the term *tumor*, which literally means "growth" or "swelling" but usually connotes a proliferative process. Vascular tumors were often named based on clinically descriptive terms (eg, strawberry hemangioma) rather than underlying histopathology. Consequently, the term *vascular tumor* has been applied to both nonproliferative and proliferative lesions.[9] Similarly, the term *hemangioma* has been used to describe various vascular lesions that have different biologic behavior.[14]
- Since 1996, the International Society for the Study of Vascular Anomalies (ISSVA) has adopted a standardized nomenclature to facilitate the classification, diagnosis, and treatment of vascular tumors.[14]
- "Vascular anomalies" is now the widely accepted term for benign congenital vascular lesions that include both vascular tumors and vascular malformations.
  - The majority (90%) of vascular growths of the hand fall within this category (benign congenital lesions).
  - Vascular tumors, or hemangiomas, are true neoplasms characterized by endothelial proliferation. The most common vascular tumor is infantile hemangioma.
  - Vascular malformations are nonproliferative lesions that result from dysmorphogenesis. Examples of vascular malformations include capillary malformations, venous malformations, and congenital arteriovenous fistulas (AVFs). Many of these malformations have been historically mislabeled as hemangiomas (Table 1).
- The remaining 10% of vascular lesions not included in the previously mentioned group include noncongenital vascular tumors, which may be benign (eg, glomus tumor) or malignant (eg, hemangioendothelioma, hemangiosarcomas, glomangiosarcoma, and malignant hemangiopericytoma), and traumatic or iatrogenic lesions, such as AVFs and pseudoaneurysms.
- The incidence of congenital vascular tumors and malformations in the general population is about 2% to 6%.[20]
  - Most are discovered at birth, although some may not be evident until adulthood.
  - About 15% to 26% of vascular anomalies present in the extremities,[24,37] most commonly the hand and forearm.[20]
  - Vascular anomalies are fourth in frequency among upper extremity tumors, after ganglions, giant cell tumors, and inclusion cysts.

Table 1 Historical Terms for Vascular Anomalies

Vascular Anomalies	Tumors 1) Infantile hemangioma (strawberry hemangioma) 2) Lobular capillary hemangioma (pyogenic granuloma) 3) Kaposiform hemangioendothelioma
	Malformations 1) Arteriovenous malformation (arteriovenous hemangioma) 2) Venous malformation (cavernous hemangioma) 3) Capillary malformation (port-wine stain, capillary hemangioma) 4) Lymphatic malformation (lymphangioma)

Vascular anomalies are categorized into tumors and malformations. Note the historical terms in parentheses, which in many cases are misnomers.

ANATOMY

- Arteries in the hand terminate at either a capillary bed or a glomus body. The glomus is a specialized arteriovenous shunt that functions as a neuromyoarterial mechanoreceptor. It lies in the stratum reticularis of the skin, especially in the subungual region and distal pads of the digits. The glomus body acts as a thermoregulator and it regulates peripheral blood flow in the digits and possibly controls peripheral blood pressure. It contains the glomus cells surrounding the Sucquet-Hoyer canals, which are narrow vascular anastomotic channels.

PATHOGENESIS

- Various theories for the pathogenesis of vascular tumors exist. Some implicate endothelial cells originating from disrupted placental tissue that becomes embedded in fetal soft tissue; others link hemangioma formation to abnormal circulating hematopoetic stem cells.[27] Various theories exist as to the pathogenesis of vascular malformations, but broadly speaking, they are thought to occur as a failure of differentiation or involution of common embryonic vascular channels.[24]
- Acquired vascular tumors are usually due to trauma that induces pseudoaneurysms or fistulas.

NATURAL HISTORY

Vascular Tumors

Infantile Hemangiomas

- Also referred to as *strawberry hemangiomas* or *capillary hemangiomas*, infantile hemangiomas are the most common benign vascular tumor in infancy, with a reported incidence of 1% to 4% among Caucasian infants.[37]
- Thirty percent of hemangiomas are visible at birth, but this increases to 70% to 90% before the infant is 4 weeks old.[37]
- Hemangiomas typically are reddish lesions that become raised during the growth phase (**FIG 1**).

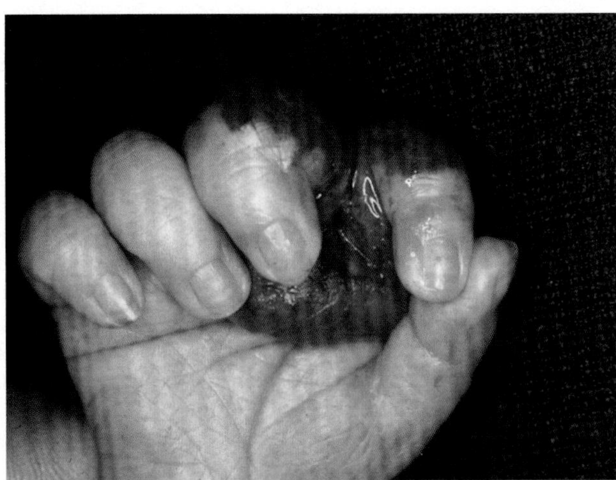

FIG 1 • Infantile hemangioma of the second web space of the right hand. Note the typical red color and raised appearance. During the proliferative phase, these lesions may ulcerate.

- These lesions classically progress through a proliferative phase marked by rapid growth, an involution phase marked by gradual replacement with fibrofatty tissue, and resolution.[34,36] As a general rule, the overall rate of involution among affected individuals occurs at 10% per year; thus, 50% of hemangiomas will involute by the time the child is 5 years old and 70% will involute by the age of 7 years.[37] Exceptions do occur; a subset of infantile hemangiomas (rapidly involuting congenital hemangiomas or RICH) are characterized by a lack of a proliferative phase and complete resolution by 12 to 18 months of age, whereas another subset of hemangiomas (noninvoluting congenital hemangiomas or NICH) do not spontaneously involute.[37] Because these hemangiomas also tend to be fully formed at birth, they are usually categorized separately as congenital hemangiomas to distinguish them from infantile hemangiomas.[27]
- Histologically, hemangiomas are characterized by endothelial proliferation and consist of plump endothelial cells with high turnover rates.[20] They may be further classified by other histologic features and location (superficial, subcutaneous, or intramuscular).[24] Thirty percent of upper extremity hemangiomas will ulcerate, which becomes acute or chronic paronychia, especially in children who suck their fingers.[33] Other complications include bleeding, infection, pain, and permanent skin changes after involution. [37]
- If the hemangioma is associated with thrombocytopenia and consumptive coagulopathy, it is termed *Kasabach-Merritt syndrome*, which is unrelated to the size of the hemangioma and is associated with a 30% to 40% mortality.[13] Multiple treatment modalities exist, including surgical extirpation, ablation, and/or compression, none of which are consistently efficacious.
- Sclerosing hemangiomas contain a perivascular thickening of the lymphatic cells. These lesions have fibrous rather than a hematogenous origin and represent 10% of all hemangiomas.[24]
- Although observation is the rule for infantile hemangiomas, occasionally, complications such as ulceration, slow regression, impairment of function, or psychosocial factors prompt intervention. Common agents include intralesional or oral corticosteroids and vincristine. Propranolol, a nonselective beta-adrenergic agonist, has in recent years been shown to be efficacious and safe in the treatment of hemangiomas. Although no clear protocols for its use in hemangiomas of the upper extremity exist, propranolol is a valuable therapeutic option that has changed the paradigm for hemangioma management and may be considered as an alternative to observation in problematic lesions.[17]

Kaposiform Hemangioendothelioma

- Kaposiform hemangioendotheliomas have been historically included with capillary hemangiomas.[14] Although capillary hemangiomas, or infantile hemangiomas, have been reported to represent about 57% of subcutaneous hemangiomas, the incidence of true kaposiform hemangioendotheliomas is exceedingly small.[19]
- Histologically, these lesions are distinguished from infantile hemangiomas by their characteristic tightly packed "cannonball nests" of endothelial cells within the dermis, sheets of spindle cells, and close resemblance to Kaposi sarcoma.[19]
- Clinically, these lesions do not spontaneously involute and the treatment modality with the most consistent results is vincristine alone or surgical resection.[37]

Lobular Capillary Hemangiomas

- Lobular capillary hemangiomas, or pyogenic granulomas, make up 20% of the vascular tumors of the hand and may be a variant of a capillary hemangioma. They appear as a well-circumscribed lesion.
- They develop rapidly and become pedunculated, friable outgrowths that are easily traumatized and bleed. In children, these lesions are more commonly found on the glabrous portion of the palm and digits as well as in the mouth and around the lips and face. In adults, they are more commonly found on the fingers and toes.
- They may occur spontaneously but more frequently present as an overgrowth of granulation tissue in an area of previous penetrating trauma (**FIG 2**).[7,24,31,36]

Vascular Leiomyomas

- Vascular leiomyomas are very rare tumors of the hand. They arise in the smooth muscle of the tunica media of veins in 50% of cases and are typically well encapsulated, small, round, firm, colorless, and curable (**FIG 3**).[15]

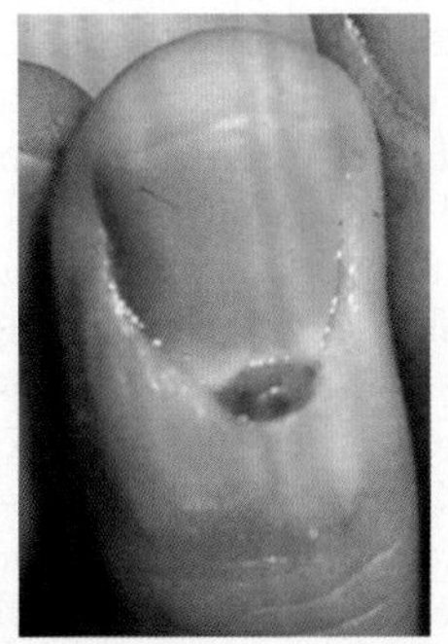

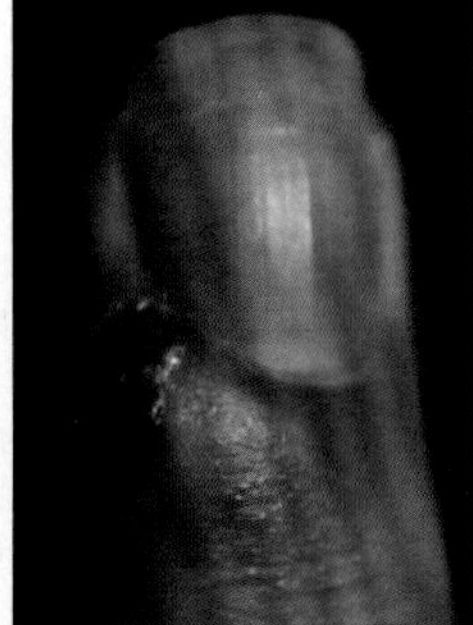

A **B**

FIG 2 • **A.** Pyogenic granuloma of the left ring finger. The patient developed an open lesion of the cuticle that progressively swelled and then blistered over the nail bed. **B.** Pyogenic granuloma of the left index finger. Notice the granular, raised appearance.

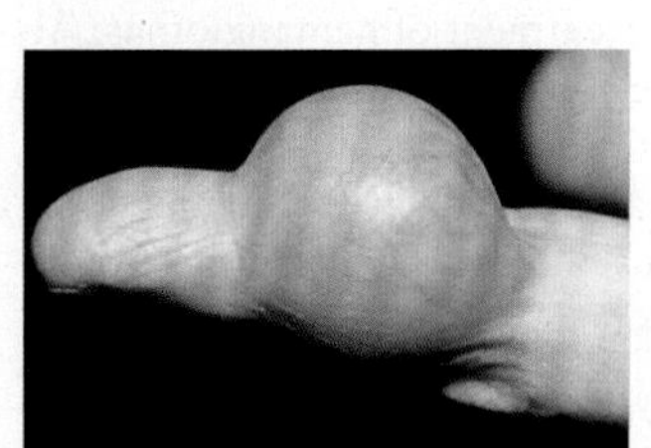

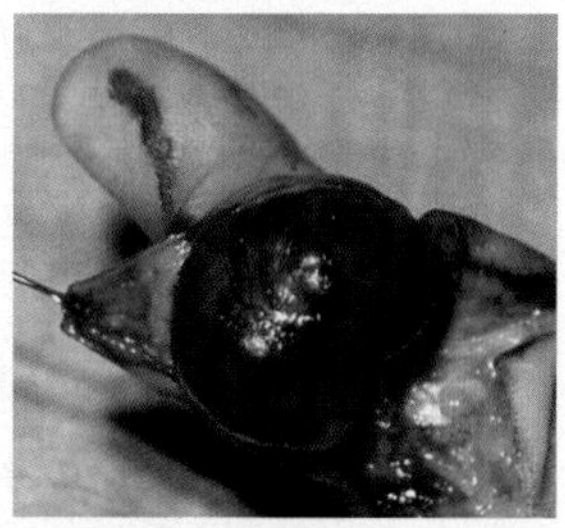

FIG 3 • A. Vascular leiomyoma of the right index finger. The patient presented after a 7-month history of having a trauma at work. She stated that the growth appeared 3 months later and had increased in size since then. **B.** Intraoperative photograph of the above vascular leiomyoma. It is a well-circumscribed lesion that is difficult to differentiate from an aneurysm except on pathology.

Vascular Malformations

- Vascular malformations are uniformly present at birth but may not be visible until childhood, adolescence, or adulthood. Most appear by ages 2 to 5 years.[36] They enlarge proportionately with the child unless they are stimulated by trauma, hormones, infection, or surgery.[4] These lesions have an equal sex distribution. Malformations generally have flat, slowly dividing endothelial cells.
- Vascular malformations present with a mass or skin discoloration depending on the depth of the lesion. They enlarge shortly after birth and grow with the child.[31]
- It is important to differentiate vascular malformations from hemangiomas because vascular malformations do not involute. Growth is due to progressive dilatation of the vessels and recurrence or regrowth after excision is due to alteration in hemodynamics and rerouting of flow through previously quiescent aberrant channels (**FIG 4**).
- Patients with vascular malformations will complain of the mass effect of the lesion, increased size with exercise, or pain due to thrombosis. Elevation of the extremity eases symptoms. These lesions may lead to nerve compression at the forearm and wrist and digital compression may be seen with localized thrombosis.[31,33]
- Vascular malformations consist of venous, capillary, arterial, and lymphatic malformations. Because up to 70% of vascular malformations are mixed, classification is not always straightforward. In the Hamburg classification, vascular malformations of the extremities are classified by the predominant vascular defect and by whether a truncular or extratruncular form, depending on involvement of a major axial vessel.[3]
- Vascular malformations are also classified as either low-flow or high-flow lesions based on their radiographic appearance and clinical characteristics. Before the routine use of magnetic resonance imaging (MRI) and Doppler ultrasound (US), angiography was used to estimate flow rates and shunt volume. Based on these findings, high-flow lesions were distinguished from low-flow lesions by the caliber and rate of opacification of feeding and draining vessels. The use of angiography has been augmented—and increasingly supplanted—by the development of Doppler US, nuclear scanning, and MRI, which have allowed more precise measurement of flow velocities, shunt volumes, and soft tissue anatomy.[18]
  - Low-flow malformations have large channels without intervening parenchyma and often are associated with phleboliths. These lesions are more common than high-flow lesions, representing 90% of vascular malformations. They consist mainly of venous, capillary, and lymphatic malformations.[32]
  - High-flow malformations usually have an arterial component and arteriovenous shunting. Marked enlargement and increased number of arteries, small vessels, and veins are consistent findings.[5]
  - High-flow malformations present early as a painless mass. They have a bimodal occurrence: 40% show up at birth and another 34% after 10 years old.[31] They do not contract with elevation. Later in childhood, they can become painful and lead to distal ischemia or even high-output heart failure if large and untreated. They have been divided into three types:
    - Type A lesions have single or multiple AVFs, aneurysms, or ectasias involving the arterial side. They are localized to a specific anatomic region.[32,36]
    - Type B lesions consist of arteriovenous anomalies with microfistulas or macrofistulas that are localized to a single limb, hand, or digit. They have stable flow characteristics and provoke minimal to no distal symptoms. As with type A lesions, they remain localized to an anatomic region.[32,36]
    - Type C lesions enlarge slowly. They are diffuse, with microfistulas and macrofistulas involving all limb tissues. With increasing size, vascular steal occurs. They can cause distal ischemic pain, tachycardia, and congestive heart failure. Compartment syndrome, compression neuropathies, and ulceration secondary to ischemia or attempted surgical interventions can occur. The result can be unrelenting, progressive pain, eventually leading to amputation.[31,32] These lesions are notoriously difficult to treat.[32]

Venous Malformations

- Historically termed *cavernous hemangiomas* (see Table 1), venous malformations represent the majority of vascular malformations and are also the most common vascular anomaly overall.[31]
- Venous malformations are characterized histologically by thin-walled vessels and abnormally arranged smooth muscle cells that lead to ectatic changes over time, hence the term cavernous hemangioma.
- Clinically, venous malformations present as bluish compressible nodules. Slow commensurate growth, compressibility,

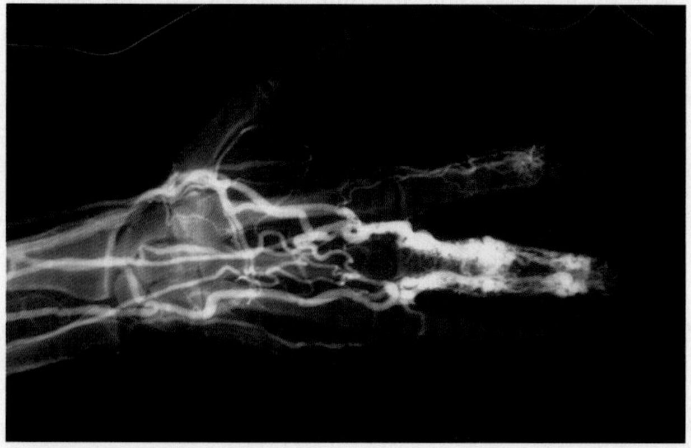

FIG 4 • Vascular malformation of the hand. Note the dilated vasculature. The growth of these lesions is due to progressive ectasia of the vessels and regrowth after excision is due to rerouting of flow through aberrant channels secondary to alterations in hemodynamics.

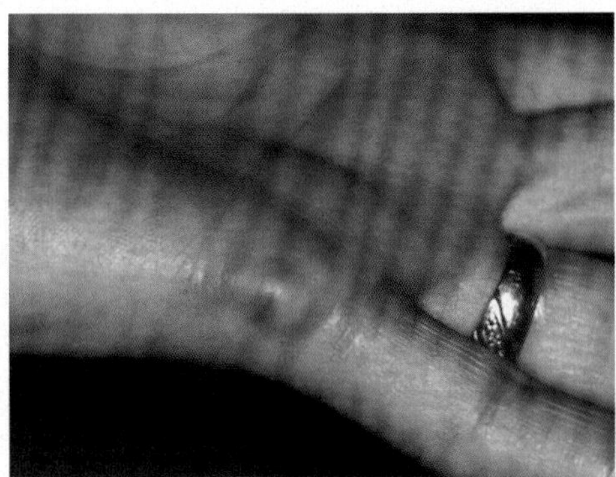

FIG 5 • Venous malformation of the ulnar side of the left hand. Notice the blue color and slightly raised appearance.

and phleboliths are pathognomonic for venous malformations (**FIG 5**).[20]

- They can occur in isolation or with any number of syndromes, including blue rubber bleb nevus syndrome or Klippel-Trenaunay syndrome (see section on Syndromes Related to Vascular Malformations of the Hand and Upper Extremity).[37]
- They may be associated with limb or digit overgrowth.[31]

Capillary Malformations

- Capillary malformations, as known as *port-wine stains* or *nevus flammeus*, are a common congenital vascular malformation.[37] They are dark red to purple and may have other associated vascular lesions. Over time, they become darker and acquire a cobblestone appearance.
- Histologically, these lesions are characterized by a normal number of dilated capillaries and postcapillary venules in the upper dermis.
- The treatment for these lesions is generally nonsurgical and consists of pulsed dye laser. Other modalities include intense pulsed light, photodynamic therapy, and angiogenesis inhibitors such as topical imiquimod and rapamycin.[37]

Arteriovenous Malformations

- Arteriovenous malformations have direct arteriovenous shunts without intervening capillaries and, like venous malformations, may be associated with a number of syndromes, including Parkes-Weber syndrome and Klippel-Trenaunay syndrome. These are more likely to be high flow and be complicated by ulceration and high-output failure as well as amputation (**FIG 6**).
- As with venous malformations, arteriovenous malformations may be associated with limb or digit hypertrophy.[31]

Lymphatic and Mixed Malformations

- Lymphatic malformations enlarge secondary to fluid accumulation, cellulitis, or inadequate drainage of lymphatic channels.[20] They can limit hand motion, and infections are common.[31] They can also cause bone hypertrophy (**FIG 7**).
- Mixed vascular malformations share the characteristics of their combination of vascular malformations.

Syndromes Related to Vascular Malformations of the Hand and Upper Extremity

- Klippel-Trenaunay syndrome is characterized by port-wine stains, combined low-flow vascular malformations (capillary, lymphatic, and venous), and limb enlargement due to hypertrophy of soft tissue and bone.[37] Visceral malformations may occur as well.

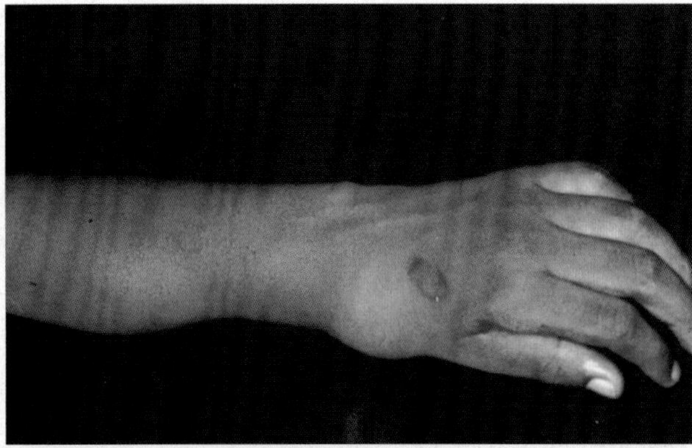

A

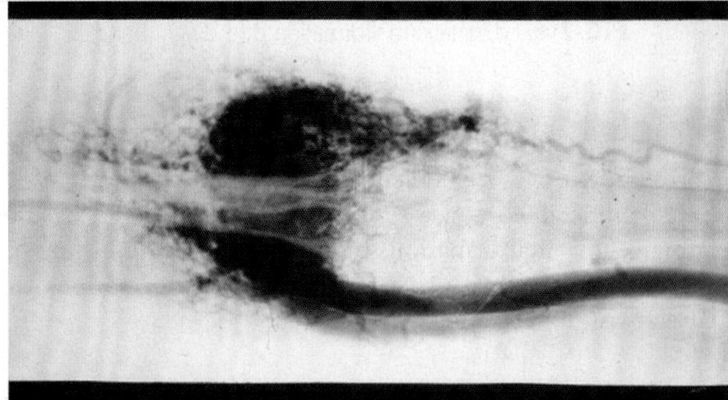

B

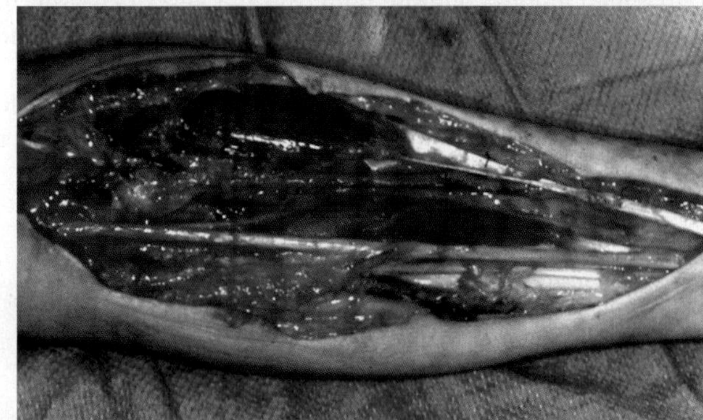

C

FIG 6 • **A.** Arteriovenous malformation involving the entire upper extremity of a teenage boy. **B.** Angiography demonstrating the dense nest of blood vessels at the elbow. Note the enlarged feeding and draining vessels. **C.** Surgical dissection of the forearm. This patient ultimately required an amputation at the shoulder secondary to high-output heart failure.

- Parkes-Weber syndrome, like Klippel-Trenaunay syndrome, is also characterized by combined vascular malformations and skeletal hypertrophy of the affected limb. A distinguishing characteristic is the presence of high-flow lesions and complex multiple AVFs.[18]
- Both of these syndromes may have significant medical sequelae, including congestive heart failure, pulmonary embolism, venous thrombosis, bleeding, and cellulitis.
- Proteus syndrome is a progressive condition characterized by widespread cutaneous and subcutaneous nevi, lipoma, and mixed venous malformations.[18]

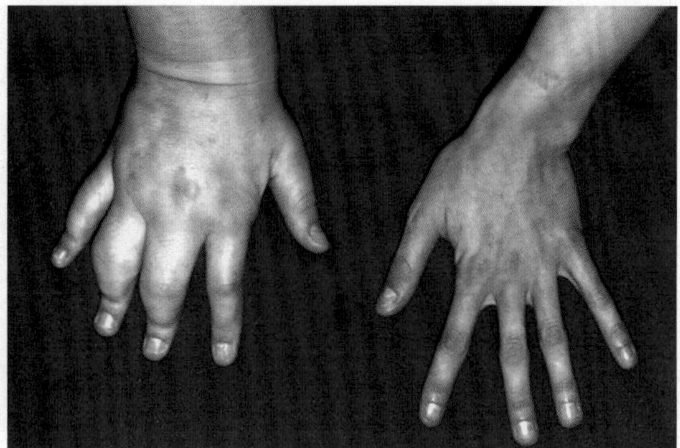

FIG 7 • Lymphatic malformation of the right hand.

- Maffucci syndrome is characterized by multiple endochondromas, exostoses, and venous malformations.[18]
- Blue rubber bleb nevus syndrome is characterized by multiple venous malformations of the skin. A distinguishing feature is the presence of gastrointestinal malformations that are at risk for bleeding.[18]

Acquired Lesions

- Acquired lesions comprise both true and false aneurysms of vessels, glomus tumors, pyogenic granulomas, fistulas, and vascular leiomyomas.
  - True aneurysms contain all three layers of the vessel wall: intima, media, and adventitia. False or pseudoaneurysms do not contain all three layers of the vessel wall.

True Aneurysms

- True aneurysms account for 6% of all tumors of the hand.[24]
- True aneurysms, most notably hypothenar hammer syndrome, usually follow blunt trauma in the area of the vessel. The trauma may be a single event or repeated injury. The vessel dilates in response to injury to the arterial media, leading to fusiform vessel enlargement.
- Aneurysms also occur secondary to disease processes such as arteriosclerosis, metabolic disorders, Kawasaki disease, Buerger disease, hemophilia, osteogenesis imperfecta tarda, granulomatous arteritis, and cystic adventitial disease (**FIG 8**).[20]

Pseudoaneurysms

- Pseudoaneurysms account for most (83%) aneurysms of the hand and generally occur on the palmar surface of the hand.
- They may be secondary to a puncture wound (such as from a knife or pencil) or complete rupture of the vessel wall with continuity maintained by the surrounding soft tissues.[20,24] They typically present with significant soft tissue swelling (**FIG 9**).
- Pseudoaneurysms develop slowly over time and are usually not evident for weeks to months after the injury.
- A bruit may be noted on examination. Like true aneurysms, the most common vessel is in the ulnar artery.

Acquired Arteriovenous Fistulas

- Acquired AVFs occur secondary to trauma or surgical intervention. AVFs consist of a communication between an artery and a vein that shunts away from the higher resistance capillary system.
- Traumatic AVFs occur when there is penetrating injury to an artery and the adjacent vein, leading to a hematoma and

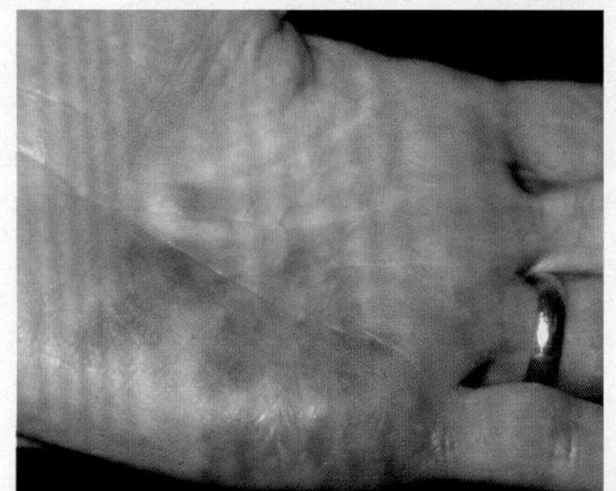

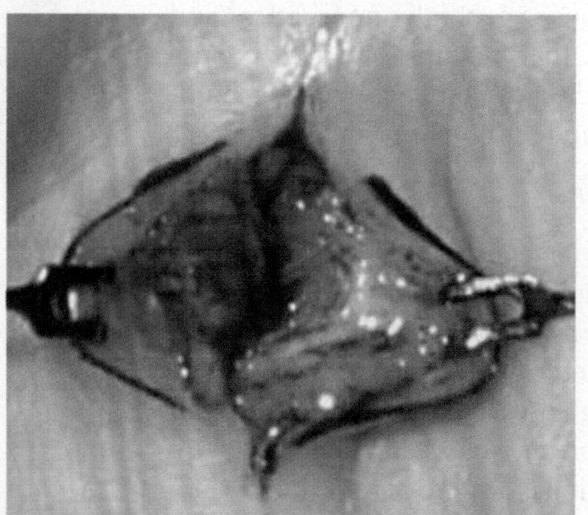

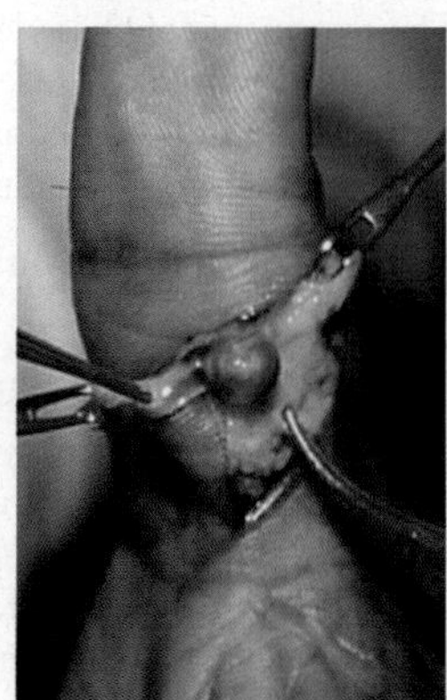

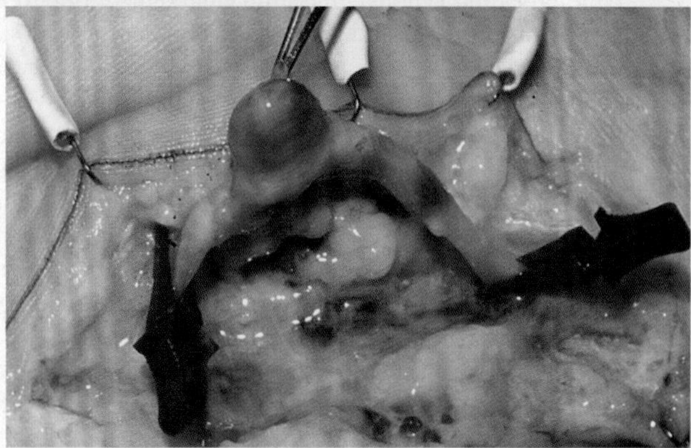

FIG 8 • **A.** Venous aneurysm of the palm. Again, a bluish tinge is noticeable over the lesion. **B.** Intraoperative view of a venous aneurysm. There is dilatation present at the vein. **C.** Ulnar digit artery false aneurysm. The patient sustained a traumatic injury at work and noted an increase in the size of the lesion over the ensuing 6 weeks. **D.** Hypothenar hammer syndrome. The patient was releasing a mechanical latch of a machine by using the heel of his hand, which caused a sharp pain. The patient presented with coolness of the ring fingertip and associated pain.

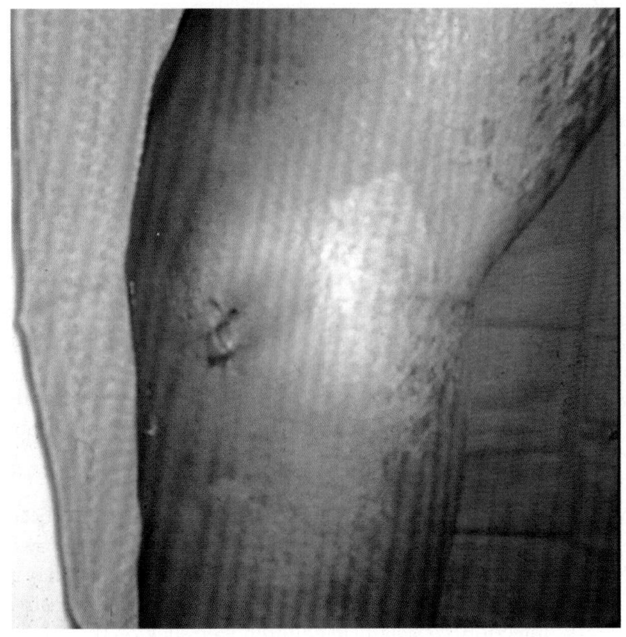

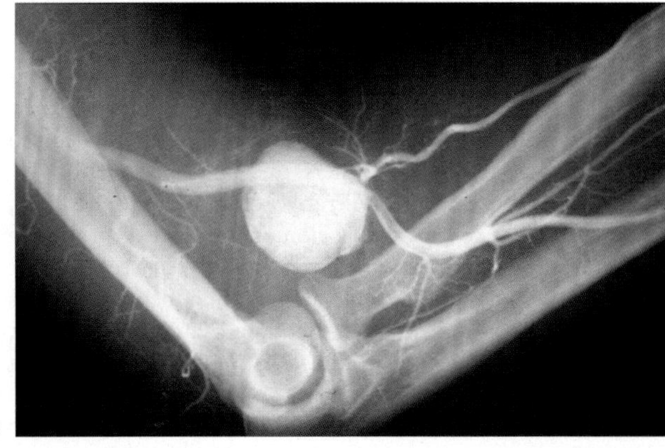

FIG 9 • **A.** Pseudoaneurysm of the radial artery due to injury, associated with significant soft tissue swelling. **B.** Angiogram showing extravasation of blood from the proximal radial artery walled off by surrounding soft tissue.

shunting. This may occur secondary to injury with such objects as small knives or pencils, but it may also be due to venipuncture, arterial cannulation, or catheterization procedures. AVFs secondary to iatrogenic vascular injuries tend to occur slowly, whereas those that occur secondary to other trauma are usually rapid in onset. This may be secondary to the size of the puncture that occurs; iatrogenic injuries tend to be smaller punctures than traumatic ones.[33] Patients with intrinsic coagulation deficiencies are more vulnerable to this complication.

- Surgical AVFs are formed for dialysis access in patients with renal failure and can cause similar symptoms, including vascular steal (ischemia distal to the fistula secondary to shunting of blood), venous arterialization, and hand edema.

Glomus Tumors

- Glomus tumors make up 8% of the vascular tumors of the hand and 1% to 4.5% of all hand tumors.[24,34] They arise in the neuromyoarterial apparatus that was first described by Wood in 1812 and then again by Masson in 1924. These lesions have been found in the stomach, trachea, and retina but are most commonly found in the digits. Glomus tumors are more consistent with a hamartoma than a true tumor.[20] Sixty-five percent of these lesions are found in women 30 to 50 years old.
- Between 26% and 90% of solitary glomus, tumors are located in the subungual region.[20] These lesions tend to be small—normally 5 mm and usually less than 1 cm. They are encapsulated and contain numerous small lumina when found as single tumors. Multiple tumors tend to be nonencapsulated, rarely subungual, with larger shaped vascular spaces.
- Multiple glomus tumors tend to be asymptomatic and present earlier in life, whereas solitary tumors often go undiagnosed or misdiagnosed for years because the lesions are small and not palpable (**FIG 10**).[21]
- The classic triad of pain, tenderness, and cold sensitivity is associated with glomus tumors. Lancinating pain is the most common symptom.[28]

Malignant Tumors

- Malignant vascular tumors account for less than 1% of all vascular hand and forearm tumors.[24] There are several types of malignant vascular tumors: hemangioendothelioma, glomangiosarcoma (malignant glomus tumors), angiosarcoma, Kaposi sarcoma, lymphangiosarcoma, and hemangiopericytoma.
- Hemangioendotheliomas tend to arise adjacent to or within veins. They extend centrifugally from the vessel. They are slow-growing tumors, and tumors that show greater than one mitosis per high-power field on histology are more likely

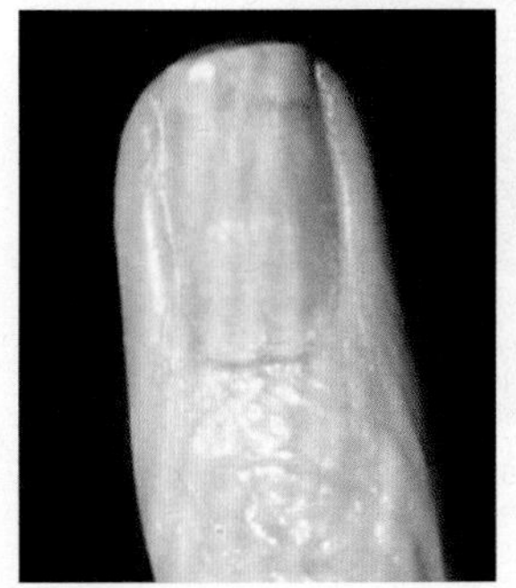

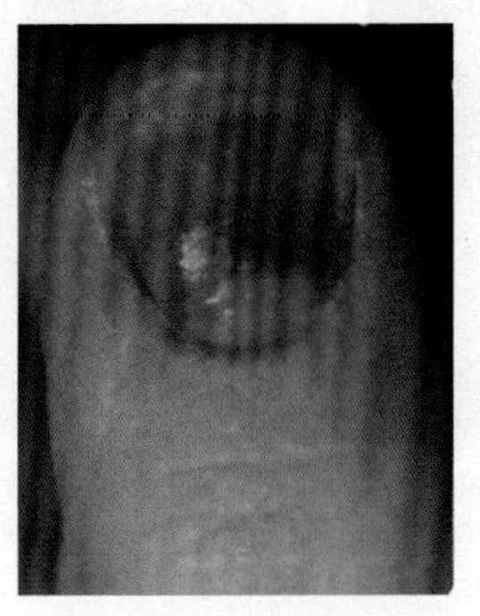

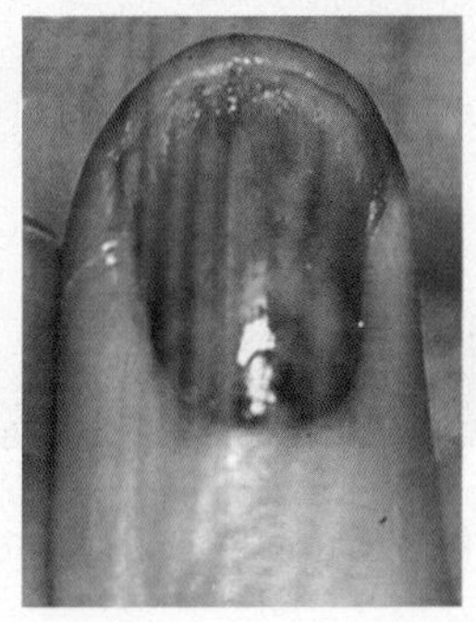

FIG 10 • **A.** Glomus tumor of the left ring finger, subungual region. The patient presented with minimal discoloration and sensitivity to heat and cold. **B.** Glomus tumor of the left thumb. The patient had more significant discoloration of the subungual region consistent with a glomus tumor. **C.** Although the patient had minimal discoloration with the nail plate on, the bluish hue becomes more discernible after the nail is removed.

to metastasize. Metastasis may occur locally to lymph nodes or distantly to the lungs, liver, or bone.[36]

- Glomangiosarcomas are extremely rare and were first described in 1972 by Lumley and Stansfield. They tend to be low-grade tumors that are locally invasive. They occur in adults aged 20 to 89 years. There are three categories of glomangiosarcoma: locally infiltrative glomus tumor (LIGT), which are identical to solitary glomus tumors except for the tendency toward infiltrating growth and recurrence after resection; glomangiosarcoma arising in a benign glomus tumor (GABG); and de novo glomangiosarcoma (GADN), which is a sarcoma with round cells and features of the a benign glomus tumor.[16,25,26]
- Angiosarcomas are rare and aggressive and metastasize early. They may occur after radiation therapy or long-term exposure to polyvinyl chloride. They are sometimes mistaken for hemangioendotheliomas on histology. The prognosis is extremely poor for these tumors; the mean survival after diagnosis is 2.5 years.[20,24,36]
- First described by Kaposi in 1872 in elderly men of Jewish and Mediterranean heritage, Kaposi sarcoma present as small, purple macules. They are a malignant degeneration of the reticuloendothelial system. These lesions tend to start on the hands or lower extremities, progress to the trunk, and coalesce into large papules. In this patient population, the disease has an indolent course and may be treatable with surgery and radiation.
  - Kaposi sarcoma has been closely associated with HIV/AIDS, and in this patient population, the disease is much more aggressive, with a larger number of lesions. In these patients, it is associated with human herpes virus 8.[20,24,36]
- Lymphangiosarcoma is a rare cancer that occurs after long-standing lymphedema, as seen in some postmastectomy patients. These lesions metastasize rapidly.
- Hemangiopericytoma is a diffuse proliferation of capillaries, encased in connective tissue, and surrounded by pericytes. They have no nerve elements and are generally painless. Patients tend to delay treatment secondary to lack of pain. They may present as a nonpigmented bleeding mole; an ulceration with prominent telangiectasia; or a dark blue, hemorrhagic swelling.
  - Histologically, they have sheets of spindle cells surrounding capillaries, regular oval nuclei without anaplasia, indistinct cytoplasmic borders, and a reticulin sheath surrounding each cell on silver stain.[15,35]
  - Pathologists have described three histologic grades based on the previously mentioned criteria: benign, borderline malignant, and malignant. It has an unpredictable behavior and may metastasize years after excision; therefore, long-term (5 to 10 years) follow-up is recommended (**FIG 11**).

PATIENT HISTORY AND PHYSICAL FINDINGS

- A complete history and physical examination of the patient is imperative.
  - It should be determined whether the lesion was present at birth or infancy or appeared later in adolescence or adulthood.
  - The history of rate of growth may help to differentiate between a hemangioma and an arteriovenous malformation in early childhood.
- Hemangiomas
  - Hemangiomas will appear as a reddish lesion that becomes raised. Lesions of the axilla or interdigital region will be chronically macerated. Fingertip hemangiomas may present with findings similar to an acute or chronic paronychial infection, especially in children who suck on their fingers.[32]
- Vascular malformations
  - Low-flow malformations most commonly present as a mass or skin discoloration. If a capillary component is present, there may be a reddish stain of the skin. The presence of a compressive symptoms from the lesion consistent with a mass effect, distention, or pain with exercise would indicate a venous malformation.
    - Ulceration is uncommon in these lesions.
    - If there is a lymphatic component, patients may present with intralesional infections secondary to ruptured vesicles and maceration of large lesions.
    - They may also be found in association with syndromes such as Parkes-Weber, Klippel-Trenaunay, Proteus, and Mafucci (see section on Syndromes Related to Vascular Malformations of the Hand and Upper Extremity).[31,32] When multiple lesions are present, an associated syndrome should be considered.
- High-flow malformations tend to be painless early on but then progress to be warm, painful masses with palpable thrills and bruits as the child grows.
  - Relief of the pain with elevation, increased pain with exercise, and increased warmth in the lesion may help to distinguish these from low-flow lesions.

A
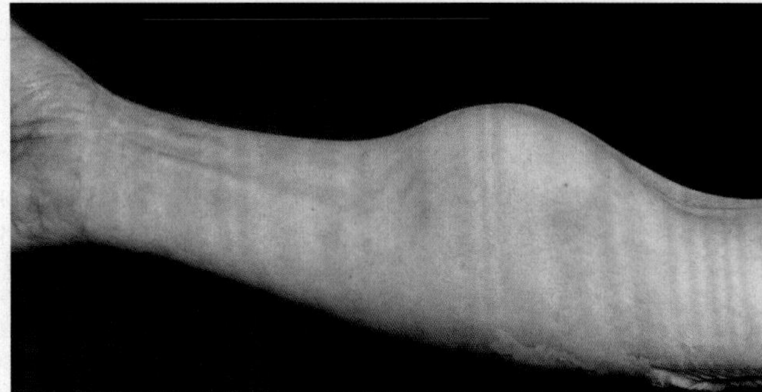
B
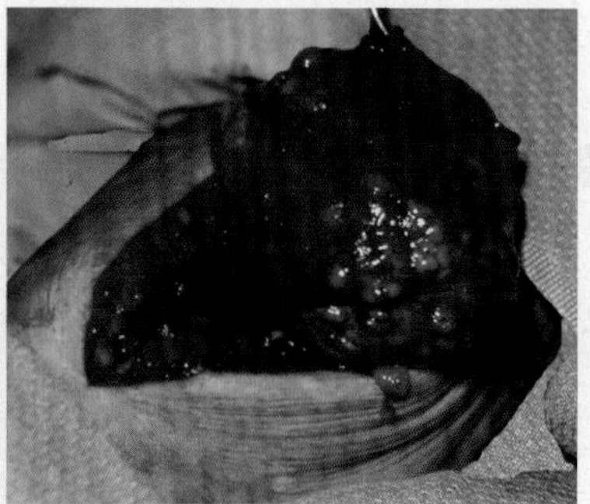

FIG 11 • **A.** Hemangiopericytoma of the right forearm. The patient presented with a large mass of the forearm that had been present for 46 years. **B.** Intraoperative view of hemangiopericytoma. The lesion was 9 × 6.6 × 5 cm and weighed 168 g.

- Presence of symptoms of congestive heart failure, which may occur as sequelae of an untreated high-flow malformation[31]
- Any patient who is suspected of an arteriovenous malformation should be evaluated for other lesions, Nicoladoni sign (decrease in pulse rate with occlusion of the fistula), and any evidence of distal ischemia.[20]
- Aneurysms and pyogenic granulomas
  - A history of trauma in the region, how long the lesion has been present, whether a pulsatile or bleeding mass is present is sought.
- Glomus tumors
  - The classic triad of paroxysmal pain, pinpoint tenderness, and cold intolerance is typical of a glomus tumor.
  - On physical examination, the physician should look for a bluish discoloration (found in 28% of patients) and a pulp nodule or nail deformity (found in 33% of patients).[21]
  - Duration of symptoms can assist in differentiating glomus tumors from other upper extremity tumors because most patients tend to have symptoms for more than 10 years.
  - A patient with multiple glomus tumors tend to be less symptomatic.
- An Allen test should be performed.[1]
- Methods for examining vascular lesions of the hand:
  - Inspect for blue spots, nail ridging, reddish, raised lesions, pulsatile masses, or traumatic injury, which helps to differentiate between malformations, aneurysms, pyogenic granulomas, and glomus tumors.
  - Using a stethoscope placed gently over the lesion, listen for bruits or thrills that are consistent with a fast-flow arteriovenous malformations.
  - If a pulsatile mass is felt, ascertain whether the lesion is compressible and tender.
  - Love pin test: To locate a glomus tumor, use the head of a pin or paper clip pressed gently against the tender area to localize the site of maximum discomfort. In subungual tumors, the pin is placed on the nail plate at various locations to find the tumor.[21]
  - Hildreth test: The digit is exsanguinated by placing a tourniquet at its base or the hand is exsanguinated by elevating it and making a tight fist. The point of tenderness located by the Love pin test is then repeated: If the patient has diminished pain with this maneuver, then the test is considered positive for a glomus tumor.[11]

IMAGING AND OTHER DIAGNOSTIC STUDIES

- Plain radiographs of the digits and hands
  - Phleboliths (in 6%) and bony hypertrophy may be noted.[20,24]
  - There may be evidence of a soft tissue mass or signs of bone erosion or destruction of the cortical surface, which is seen in about 6% of patients with hemangiomas.[24]
- Doppler ultrasonic flow detection is a noninvasive study that does not require the use of contrast.
  - It has been used to confirm high-flow anomalies and to help differentiate between hemangiomas and malformations.[31] Doppler ultrasonography will show these lesions to be monophasic with low-flow velocity averaging 0.22 kHz.[30]
- Computed tomography with contrast enhancement may show bony involvement of the tumor, especially in type A high-flow malformations.[32]
- MRI/magnetic resonance angiography (MRA) can be used to evaluate the site, size, flow rate, and characteristics of the lesion as well as involvement of contiguous structures.[32]
  - It may be used to determine whether a malformation is low flow or high flow and can also distinguish between dense parenchymal lesions and malformations with large vascular channels.[14]
  - It can also be used to evaluate glomus tumors, which have a high signal intensity on T2-weighted spin-echo MRI or after gadolinium injection.[21]
  - MRI has a sensitivity of 90% and a specificity of 50% for glomus tumors, so that it cannot be used as the only diagnostic study for glomus tumors, especially if they are less than 2 to 3 mm in size.[2]
  - Hemangiomas will appear as well-circumscribed mass lesions that enhance with gadolinium and will have a high T1 signal secondary to infiltrative margins and fatty tissue overgrowth as well an extremely high, heterogeneous T2 signal. A serpentine pattern in the mass may also be seen on MRI.[36]
- MRA may be performed at the time of MRI to evaluate lesions in patients who are unable to undergo angiography secondary to renal problems or contrast allergies. It can be used to define the anatomic extent of lesions and their relationship with the surrounding tissue. It can be used to evaluate for both arterial and venous tumors without contrast enhancement.[8]
- Technetium 99m red blood cell perfusion and blood pool scintigraphy will show increased activity on early and late blood pool images with increased perfusion in hemangiomas and may be useful in their diagnosis.[36]
- Angiography is the gold standard evaluation of certain tumors, including vascular malformations. No longer routinely used for diagnosis of a lesion, it is used as an evaluation for operation or embolization.[32] It may show a cluster of anomalous arterial branches with multiple communications with venous trunks draining the site of involvement.[22]
- Closed venous angiography uses contrast injected into the venous system distal to a proximal arterial tourniquet applied on the upper arm. Contrast is injected into the exsanguinated extremity distal to the tumor, and radiographs are taken as the vascular tumor fills to get an accurate assessment of the anatomy.[20] Arterial angiography is performed through a stick into the femoral artery with a catheter that is fed into the involved extremity. Dye is then injected and both the arterial and venous phases of circulation are evaluated. This can be used to evaluate the size of the tumor, locate the feeding vessels, and embolize feeding vessels before operation (**FIG 12**).[20]

DIFFERENTIAL DIAGNOSIS

- Foreign body
- Bacillary angiomatosis
- Pyogenic granuloma
- Glomus tumor
- Hemangioma
- Arteriovenous or lymphatic malformation
- AVFs (traumatic, congenital, iatrogenic)
- Traumatic aneurysm (true or false)
- Mycotic aneurysm (hematogenous or exogenous)
- Arteriosclerotic aneurysm

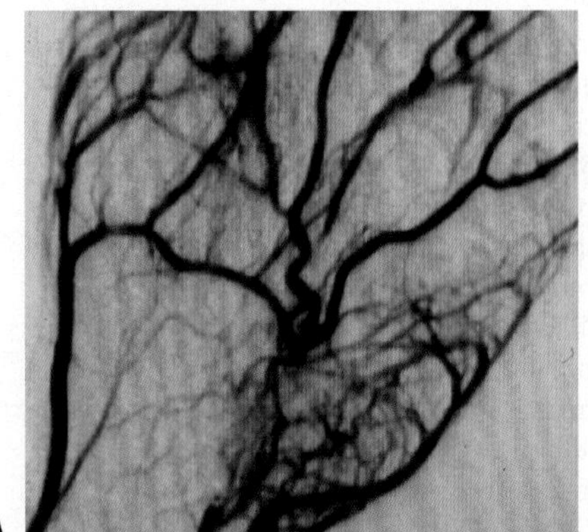

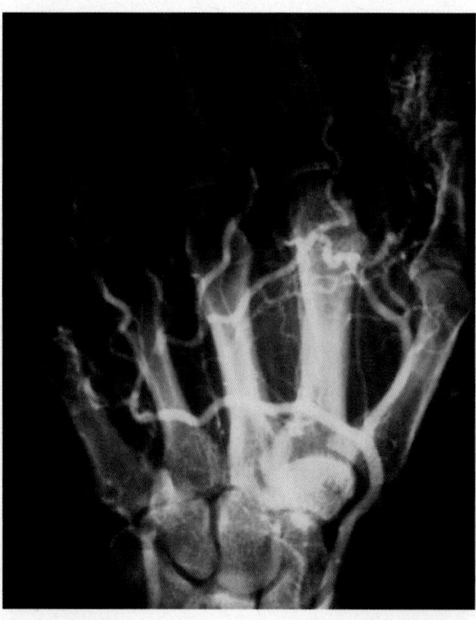

FIG 12 • A. Angiogram of hypothenar hammer syndrome. The ulnar artery flow is absent and collaterals have formed to allow for flow in the palmar arch. This patient was relatively asymptomatic until a trauma to the hand. **B.** Angiogram of a second patient with hypothenar hammer syndrome. In this patient, there are no collaterals present, and he presented with coldness of the ulnar distribution digits.

- Congenital aneurysm
- Metabolic aneurysm (eg, osteogenesis imperfecta, granulomatous arteritis, Buerger disease)
- Vascular leiomyomas
- Glomangiosarcoma
- Angiosarcoma
- Hemangioendothelioma
- Hemangiopericytoma
- Kaposi sarcoma
- Lymphangiosarcoma

NONOPERATIVE MANAGEMENT

- Observation is the mainstay of management for hemangiomas. Up to 90% of these lesions will involute by the age of 9 years.[37]
- Large venous or capillary malformations should be observed for limb growth disturbances and a possible underlying high-flow lesion.
- Limb compression garments can be used to compress massive congenital AVFs that are inoperable, giant venous malformations, lymphatic malformations, or large hemangiomas in the arm and forearm.[24,31] For larger lymphatic lesions, home compression pumps can be used to decrease edema at night.[31]
- Antibiotic prophylaxis is indicated in patients who have recurrent infections in lymphatic malformations. The bacteria most commonly responsible for these infections is penicillin-sensitive beta-hemolytic streptococcus.[31]
- If a patient with venous malformations or capillary–venolymphatic malformation has recurrent intralesional thrombosis, then low-dose aspirin may be added to the compression garments for effective therapy.[31]
- Local wound care and dressings may be required if ulcerations occur in the periungual regions or the central portions of large lesions during the involutional phase.[31]
- Pulsed dye laser or argon laser may be used with some hemangiomas to treat the pigmented lesion without damaging the overlying skin, sweat glands, and hair follicles. Lasers of 585-nm wavelength work well on vascular lesions, such as hemangiomas, which are rich in hemoglobin. The laser heats the hemoglobin, causing coagulation of the vessels in the dermis. Scar formation ensues and replaces the damaged blood vessels.[24]
- Sclerotherapy with 1% sodium tetradecyl sulfate for small superficial lesions or 100% ethanol for large, deep saccular lesions may be used in treating venous malformations.
  - With the larger lesions, there is a possibility of skin ulceration, necrosis, inflammatory changes, and contracture due to the treatment and patients should be warned to watch for these sequelae.[31]
- In arteriovenous malformations interventional radiology may be used for embolization of selectively catheterized vessels with polyvinyl alcohol foam or tissue adhesive. This may be done as a stand-alone treatment or in conjunction with surgery. In small lesions, embolization may completely occlude the malformation and destroy the lesion, eliminating the need for surgical resection. Several embolizations may be necessary.[20] In larger or more complex lesions, embolization is usually followed by surgical resection 24 to 48 hours later.
- Complications of embolization include tissue loss, neurologic deficit, and enlargement of the malformation if the lesion is large and not excised promptly.[12,22]
- Either intralesional or systemic steroids may be useful for the treatment of hemangiomas. A 6-week course may help to treat life-threatening or tissue-threatening lesions. This is also true for interferon alpha-2a or 2b. However, neither of these medications has been shown to have any effects on malformations, and the morbidity (neutropenia, elevation of liver enzymes, and spastic diparesis) of interferon must be considered before its use.[31,36]
- Radiation therapy was used in the past for sclerosis of hemangiomas; however, it leads to atrophic changes in the skin and subcutaneous tissue as well as arrest of skeletal growth.[24]

SURGICAL MANAGEMENT

- Indications for surgery include pain, intralesional thrombi, episodic bleeding or ulceration, recurrent infection, or functional problems related to the size or weight of the extremity. It is important to consider whether the extremity will be functional after the proposed surgical treatment; in many cases, amputation may be a better option.[31]
- Lymphatic malformations have the added difficulties of beta-hemolytic streptococcal septicemia, skin maceration, and vesicular eruptions. This makes the planning of surgical

resection complex. Complications occur in 25% of all procedures. The surgeon should be aware that tumor-free tissues, such as grafts or flaps, may be necessary for coverage.[31]

Preoperative Planning

- Radiographic studies should be reviewed carefully to plan resection of large or complex lesions.
- An Allen test should be performed on the patient to evaluate for the patency of the superficial palmar arch and to see if the patient has an adequate ulnar artery.
  - If the Allen test is abnormal, reconstruction of the radial artery is necessary if it is to be resected.

Positioning

- A proximal arm tourniquet is used, but the arm should not be exsanguinated with an Esmarch bandage to avoid the proximal spread or localized compression of the tumor. Exsanguination with the Esmarch bandage may also obscure the margins of hemangiomas and malformations.
- Injections around the tumor should also be avoided to reduce the risk of local spread and compression of the mass, which could cause incomplete resection.

Approach

- The technique chosen is based on the location of the lesion and the access necessary for excision.

Ligation of Feeding Vessel

- For lesions that are small, with few feeder vessels, direct exploration and ligation of the feeding vessels can lead to involution of the lesion without significant tissue loss.
- If tissue loss occurs, excision of the area and either primary closure, skin grafting, or flap reconstruction can be performed.

Staged Excision

- Staged excision is useful for venous malformations, lymphatic malformations, combined malformations, and types A and B high-flow malformations, especially when large or involving multiple anatomic areas.[32]
- For larger lesions, interventional radiology may be helpful in embolizing feeding vessels. This will decrease or limit the amount of open exposure necessary in the first stage.
- In this approach, the extremity is not exsanguinated completely to facilitate identification of the vessels.
- Several key principles must be adhered to when dealing with malformations of the upper extremity: (1) rigorous hemostasis with tourniquet control, (2) staged dissection within well-defined anatomic areas, (3) careful identification and preservation of all anatomic structures, (4) complete removal of well-localized lesions, and (5) delay of next stage until after return of function and softening of scar tissue.[32]
- When excising these lesions, all feeding and draining vessels must be ligated proximal and distal to the tumor. It is possible that ligation of these vessels may induce distal ischemia. The authors' preference is to temporarily occlude feeding and draining vessels with vascular clamps and assess distal perfusion. If distal ischemia is observed, the surgeon should be prepared to bypass the anatomic defect with autogenous vein grafts. Alternatively, the vessels in question may be selectively preserved, with the understanding that multiple staged procedures may be necessary and reexpansion of the tumor may occur.
- If the tumor is adherent to the skin, that portion of tissue is excised as well and the area is covered with grafts or flaps.[24]

Amputation

- Amputation is the treatment choice for highly aggressive malignancies such as hemangiosarcoma, lymphangiosarcoma, aggressive hemangioendothelioma, and massive arteriovenous malformations that have created a nonfunctional extremity.
- This should be performed with a proximal tourniquet for operative hemostasis.
- If the lesion is too proximal for a tourniquet, an internal vascular balloon can be used to occlude the feeding vessel or vessels.
- Guillotine amputation is an option if infection is present; otherwise, closure should be performed at the time of amputation.
- The most common error we have seen after amputation of a digit or hand is failure to obtain adequate, tension-free soft tissue coverage.
- Wide local excision may be considered for less aggressive hemangioendothelioma, hemangiopericytomas, malformations, and hemangiomas that have not involuted.

TECHNIQUES

Transungual Excision

- Transungual excision is an approach to subungual lesions, such as glomus tumors.
- Make small radial and ulnar corner incisions over the nail fold (**TECH FIG 1A,B**).
- Half the nail is then elevated and folded over, allowing for visualization of the nail matrix (**TECH FIG 1C**).
  - The nail can be completely removed with a Freer elevator if necessary for access to the tumor (**TECH FIG 1D**).
- Make a longitudinal incision with a no. 15 blade into the nail matrix, directly over the tumor, and excise the lesion circumferentially down to the phalanx (**TECH FIG 1E,F**).
- Curette the bone before the nail bed is closed with 6-0 plain gut.
- Replace the nail into the eponychial fold as a dressing for the nail bed and suture the corner incision closed (**TECH FIG 1G**).[21,29]

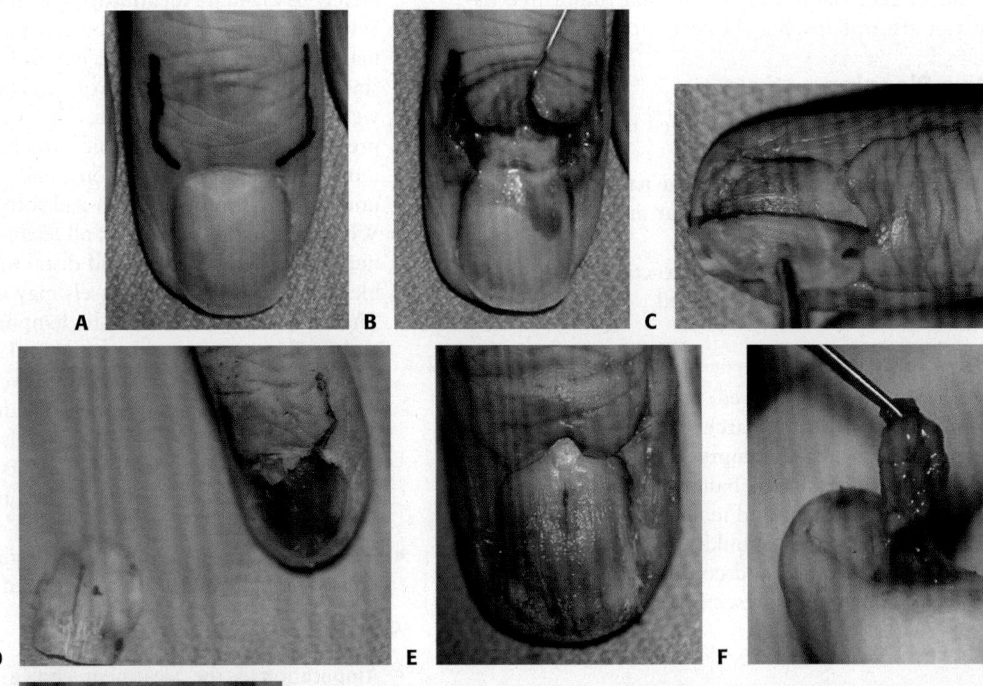

TECH FIG 1 • A. Radial and/or ulnar incisions of the nail fold are drawn. If the lesion is proximal in the nail bed, one or both of these incisions may be necessary to access the lesion. **B.** The incisions are at oblique angles to the nail fold to avoid contracture of the area. **C,D.** The nail plate is elevated off the nail bed with a Freer elevator. Half the nail is elevated primarily (**C**), but the entire nail may be removed to allow for access to the lesion (**D**). Incision(s) are then extended, if necessary, to allow for visualization. **E,F.** A longitudinal incision is made in the nail bed to allow for removal of the lesion. The bone is curetted to remove any tumor, and the nail bed is then closed with 6-0 or 7-0 plain gut. **G.** The nail plate is then replaced as the dressing and the incision(s) are closed with 5-0 or 6-0 nylon or chromic.

Lateral Incision

- This is an alternative to the transungual excision and allows exposure of the dorsal distal phalanx without violating the nail matrix. Because the view of the tumor is narrower, we do not recommend this approach.[21]
- If this approach is to be used, then a longitudinal midaxial incision slightly dorsal to the neurovascular bundle is used (**TECH FIG 2A**).
  - The incision is placed on the radial or ulnar surface of the digit, based on the location of the lesion.
- Sharp dissection is carried out to the distal phalanx without manipulating the surrounding soft tissue.
- A small, sharp elevator is used to create a subperiosteal dorsal flap (**TECH FIG 2B**).
- A small curette or elevator is used to excise the lesion.
- The flap is replaced, and the incision is closed with interrupted or running nylon suture.[29,34]

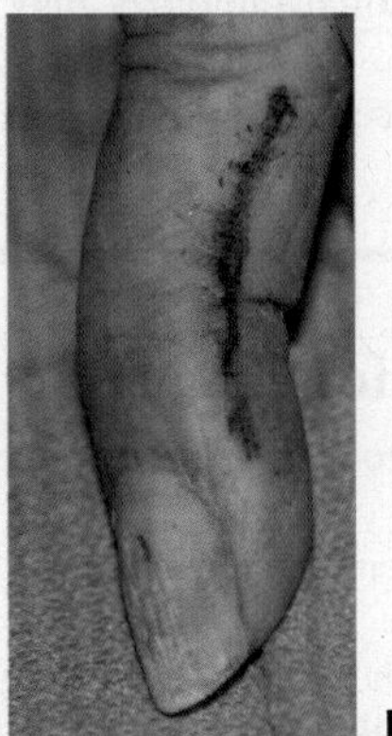

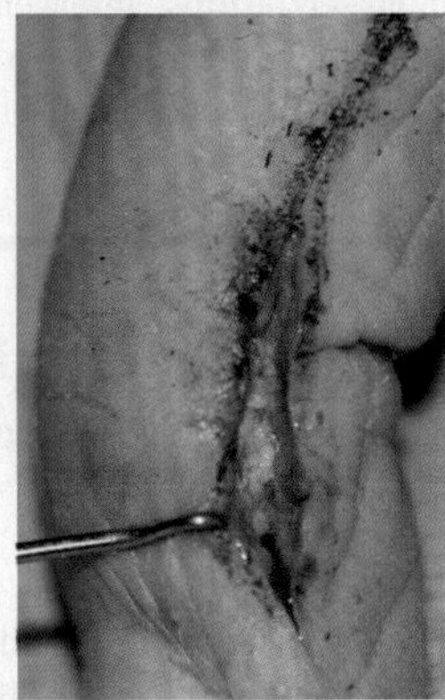

TECH FIG 2 • A. A midlateral incision is drawn just dorsal to the midaxial line. The incision is carried sharply down to the bone, keeping the neurovascular bundle volar to the incision and dissection. **B.** A Freer elevator is then used to create a subperiosteal flap to allow removal of the lesion.[2,4–8,10–12,14–16,20–26,29–36]

Epiphysiodesis

- Epiphysiodesis, destroying the growth plate by scraping or drilling, may help to diminish hypertrophy in patients whose digits have reached adult size.
- Make a midaxial incision sharply, with dissection continued to the bone.
  - Retract the neurovascular bundle volarly to avoid injury (**TECH FIG 3A**).
- The dorsal branches may be transected if it is necessary to gain access to the dorsal aspect of the phalanx.
- Use a burr to destroy the growth plate of the phalanx (**TECH FIG 3B**).
- Close the incision with 5-0 or 6-0 nylon.

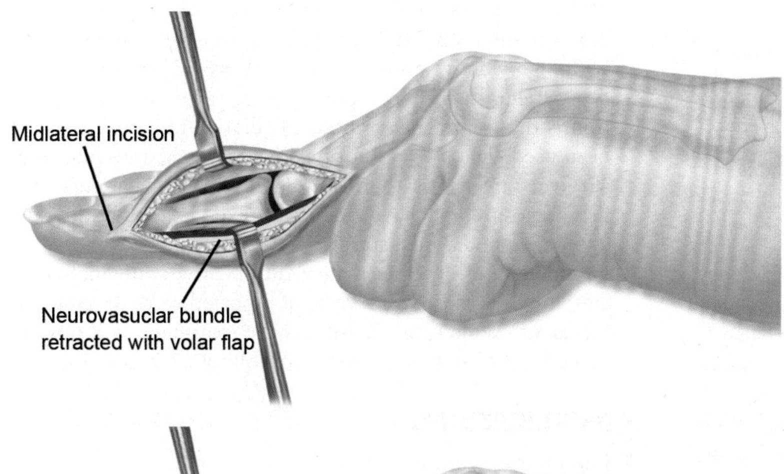

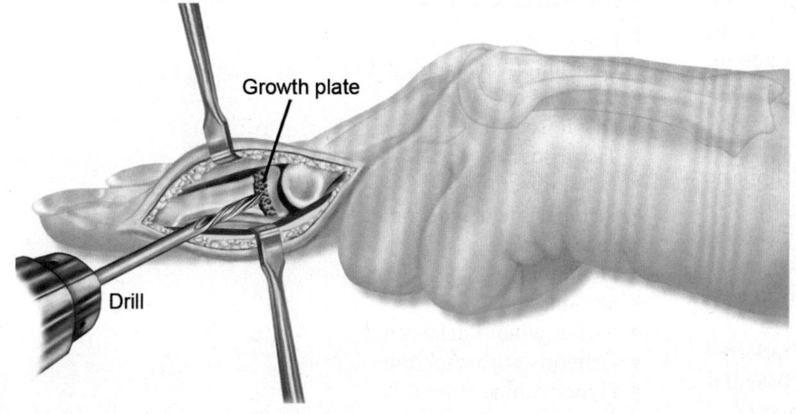

TECH FIG 3 • **A.** A midlateral incision is made sharply and dissection continues to the level of the bone. The neurovascular bundle is retracted with the volar flap to ensure that it is not injured during dissection. The dorsal branches may be ligated or left intact, if it does not interfere with the exposure of the phalanx. **B.** A drill is used to annihilate the growth plate of the phalanx to halt its growth. The incision is then closed with 5-0 or 6-0 nylon.

PEARLS AND PITFALLS

Have a tourniquet on the extremity before the incision for arteriovenous malformations.	■ Avoid overly aggressive resection of lesions.
Make the family aware of the guarded prognosis for complete removal of arteriovenous malformations and possibility of overgrowth or recurrence of the lesions.	■ Exsanguination of an arteriovenous malformation may lead to incomplete excision.
Insist on multiple high-quality imaging studies to evaluate the lesions.	■ For small lesions, imaging may not fully show the lesion.
Check patient for associated syndromic abnormalities.	

POSTOPERATIVE CARE

- After excision of the lesion, most patients will require a conforming dressing and will be able to return to their normal activity within 1 to 6 weeks, depending on the size and location of the lesion.
  - Patients with partial resection of arteriovenous malformations may need to continue wearing compressive garments postoperatively when the dressings are removed.
- If a skin graft or flaps is required, dressings and splints should be left in place to keep the patient from shearing the graft or pulling at the flap until the incisions are healed.
  - Graft bolsters or splints should be left in place for about 4 to 7 days to allow the graft to adhere.
- For patients who require amputations, prosthetics may be helpful, depending on the patient and level of amputation. These are more readily available for patients who have below- or above-elbow amputations, although patients who have forequarter amputations may also be candidates for specialized prosthetics.

OUTCOMES

- The prognosis of hemangiomas is not affected by race, gender, tumor site, size, or presence at birth.[16]
- Attempts to excise arteriovenous malformations may lead to serious complications.
  - Complications are seen in about 22% of slow-flow lesions and 28% of fast-flow lesions. Wound dehiscence, seromas, and hematomas are noted early on. Partial skin loss and incision site infection are seen in the late postoperative period.
  - In fast-flow malformations, episodic bleeding and wound breakdown are more common.[23]
  - After resection of venous malformations and lymphatic malformations, persistent edema and swelling are frequent. Patients with type C arteriovenous malformations (see section on Vascular Malformations) more consistently require multiple operative procedures due to complications.
  - Disseminated intravascular coagulation has been reported in venous and arteriovenous malformations, and coagulation studies should be obtained before any intervention.
  - In the study by Mendel and Louis,[22] 13 of 17 lesions persisted after excision through extension or recurrence. Ten of these lesions were diffuse. Thus, two-fifths of lesions that are thought to be localized are diffuse and will require more than one procedure for complete excision.
  - In view of the high recurrence rate after excision, excision should be considered in selected situations. Partial resection might be chosen to provide relief of symptoms but as a balance between aggressive resection and preservation of function.[22]
- Patients who had wide local excision of venous malformations were found to have a 2% recurrence rate.[20]
  - It is generally accepted that primary tumor excision is the treatment of choice in all adults with venous malformations and children who have been observed for 1 year without regression of the lesion.
- Glomus tumors recur in 15% to 24% of patients, with an average time before recurrence of 2.9 years.
  - Late presentation of recurrence is thought to be due to a new tumor near the site of excision. Patients who had incomplete excisions had recurrence of the tumor within weeks of surgery.
  - In patients who had transungual excisions, nail deformities were noted in 26% of patients.
- The prognosis of hemangioendothelioma depends on the grade of the tumor. Patients with low-grade lesions have a good long-term survival rate, and those with aggressive tumors may not survive longer than 2 years.
- Kaposi sarcoma in elderly non-HIV patients may be cured with wide local excision; however, the accepted treatment for these patients is chemoradiation and alpha-interferon therapy. The 5-year survival rate of these patients is only 19%. In patients with HIV/AIDS, the mortality rate of Kaposi sarcoma was 80% at 2 years, but this has improved with highly active antiretroviral therapy (HAART).[24]
- For patients with hemangiosarcoma, early radical amputation is the treatment of choice. Palliative radiation has also been used. The average survival is 2.5 years, and the 5-year survival rate is less than 20%. One-third of patients with hemangiosarcoma have hemorrhage or coagulopathy, and 45% have nodal metastases.[24]
- Glomangiosarcomas are believed to be low-grade malignancies; however, more than 25% of reported cases develop metastases.[16] Wide local excision is the treatment of choice for these lesions, and close long-term follow-up is necessary.

COMPLICATIONS

- High-output cardiac failure
- Consumptive coagulopathy
- Bacterial endocarditis
- Distal ischemia
- Tissue loss
- Local infection
- Compartment syndrome
- Arterial steal
- Hematoma
- Seroma
- Partial wound dehiscence
- Cellulitis at the operative site
- Hypertrophic scarring
- Joint contracture
- Neuromas
- Reflex sympathetic dystrophy
- Pain
- Extremity gangrene
- Vesicle formation
- Recurrence

REFERENCES

1. Allen EV. Thromboangiitis obliterans (methods of diagnosis of chronic occlusive arterial lesions distal to the wrist with illustrative cases). Am J Med Sci 1929;178:237–244.
2. Al-Qattan MM, Al-Namla A, Al-Thunayan A, et al. Magnetic resonance imaging in the diagnosis of glomus tumours of the hand. J Hand Surg Br 2005;30(5):535–540.
3. Belov S. Anatomopathological classification of congenital vascular defects. Semin Vasc Surg 1993;6(4):219–224.
4. Boyd JB, Mulliken JB, Kaban LB, et al. Skeletal changes associated with vascular malformations. Plast Reconstr Surg 1984;74(6):789–797.
5. Burrows PE, Mulliken JB, Fellows KE, et al. Childhood hemangiomas and vascular malformations: angiographic differentiation. AJR Am J Roentgenol 1983;141(3):483–488.

6. Coleman SS, Anson BJ. Arterial patterns in the hand based upon a study of 650 specimens. Surg Gynecol Obstet 1961;113:409–424.
7. DiFazio F, Mogan J. Intravenous pyogenic granuloma of the hand. J Hand Surg Am 1989;14(2 pt 1):310–312.
8. Disa JJ, Chung KC, Gellad FE, et al. Efficacy of magnetic resonance angiography in the evaluation of vascular malformations of the hand. Plast Reconstr Surg 1997;99(1):136–144; discussion 145–147.
9. Enjolras O, Mulliken JB. The current management of vascular birthmarks. Pediatr Dermatol 1993;10(4):311–313.
10. Frappaz D, Rigal D, Valla JS, et al. Multiple vascular thromboses in severe acute autoimmune hemolytic anemia with Mycoplasma pneumoniae serology treated by plasma exchange and immunosuppressive agents [in French]. Pediatrie 1983;38(6):411–419.
11. Giele H. Hildreth's test is a reliable clinical sign for the diagnosis of glomus tumours. J Hand Surg Br 2002;27(2):157–158.
12. Griffin JM, Vasconez LO, Schatten WE. Congenital arteriovenous malformations of the upper extremity. Plast Reconstr Surg 1978;62(1):49–58.
13. Hall GW. Kasabach-Merritt syndrome: pathogenesis and management. Br J Haematol 2001;112(4):851–862.
14. Hassanein AH, Mulliken JB, Fishman SJ, et al. Evaluation of terminology for vascular anomalies in current literature. Plast Reconstr Surg 2011;127(1):347–351.
15. Hauswald KR, Kasdan ML, Weiss DL. Vascular leiomyoma of the hand. Case report. Plast Reconstr Surg 1975;55(1):89–91.
16. Khoury T, Balos L, McGrath B, et al. Malignant glomus tumor: a case report and review of literature, focusing on its clinicopathologic features and immunohistochemical profile. Am J Dermatopathol 2005;27(5):428–431.
17. Léauté-Labrèze C, Dumas de la Roque E, Hubiche T, et al. Propranolol for severe hemangiomas of infancy. N Engl J Med 2008;358(24):2649–2651.
18. Legiehn GM, Heran MK. Classification, diagnosis, and interventional radiologic management of vascular malformations. Orthop Clin North Am 2006;37(3):435–474, vii–viii.
19. Mac-Moune Lai F, To KF, Choi PC, et al. Kaposiform hemangioendothelioma: five patients with cutaneous lesion and long follow-up. Mod Pathol 2001;14(11):1087–1092.
20. McClinton MA. Tumors and aneurysms of the upper extremity. Hand Clin 1993;9(1):151–169.
21. McDermott EM, Weiss AP. Glomus tumors. J Hand Surg Am 2006;31(8):1397–1400.
22. Mendel T, Louis DS. Major vascular malformations of the upper extremity: long-term observation. J Hand Surg Am 1997;22(2):302–306.
23. Palmieri TJ. Subcutaneous hemangiomas of the hand. J Hand Surg Am 1983;8(2):201–204.
24. Palmieri TJ. Vascular tumors of the hand and forearm. Hand Clin 1987;3(2):225–240.
25. Park JH, Oh SH, Yang MH, et al. Glomangiosarcoma of the hand: a case report and review of the literature. J Dermatol 2003;30(11):827–833.
26. Pérez de la Fuente T, Vega C, Gutierrez Palacios A, et al. Glomangiosarcoma of the hypothenar eminence: a case report. Chir Main 2005;24(3–4):199–202.
27. Richter GT, Friedman AB. Hemangiomas and vascular malformations: current theory and management. Int J Pediatr 2012;2012:645678.
28. Sun BG, Yun-tao W, Jia-zhen L. Glomus tumours of the hand and foot. Int Orthop 1996;20(6):339–341.
29. Takata H, Ikuta Y, Ishida O, et al. Treatment of subungual glomus tumour. Hand Surg 2001;6(1):25–27.
30. Trop I, Dubois J, Guibaud L, et al. Soft-tissue venous malformations in pediatric and young adult patients: diagnosis with Doppler US. Radiology 1999;212(3):841–845.
31. Upton J, Coombs C. Vascular tumors in children. Hand Clin 1995;11(2):307–337.
32. Upton J, Coombs CJ, Mulliken JB, et al. Vascular malformations of the upper limb: a review of 270 patients. J Hand Surg Am 1999;24(5):1019–1035.
33. Upton J, Sampson C, Havlik R, et al. Acquired arteriovenous fistulas in children. J Hand Surg Am 1994;19(4):656–658.
34. Vasisht B, Watson HK, Joseph E, et al. Digital glomus tumors: a 29-year experience with a lateral subperiosteal approach. Plast Reconstr Surg 2004;114(6):1486–1489.
35. Vathana P. Primary hemangiopericytoma of bone in the hand: a case report. J Hand Surg Am 1984;9(5):761–764.
36. Walsh JJ IV, Eady JL. Vascular tumors. Hand Clin 2004;20(3):261–268, v–vi.
37. Willard KJ, Cappel MA, Kozin SH, et al. Congenital and infantile skin lesions affecting the hand and upper extremity, part 1: vascular neoplasms and malformations. J Hand Surg Am 2013;38(11):2271–2283.

144

CHAPTER

Squamous Cell Carcinoma and Melanoma of the Hand

Patrick Cole, Yoav Kaufman, and Jason Petrungaro

DEFINITION

- Squamous cell carcinoma (SCC) and melanoma are malignant transformations of normal epidermal cells in either cutaneous or noncutaneous regions of the body.
- Both SCC and melanoma demonstrate the ability to extend locally, involve regional lymph node basins, and metastasize to distant sites. SCC is also prone to locally extending along nerves sheaths.
- Early diagnosis, accurate histopathologic evaluation, detailed staging, appropriate surgical, and medical management as well as appropriate follow-up are critical to the management of SCC and melanoma of the hand.

ANATOMY

- Intact skin is composed of epidermis and dermis. These act as physiologic barriers to infection and malignant spread. SCC and melanoma develop from different epidermal layers.
  - SCCs develop from epidermal keratinocytes.
  - Melanomas derive from dendritic (neural crest) cells within the epidermis. Melanomas are typically pigmented; however, amelanotic melanomas (nonpigmented melanoma) represent 5% of all melanomas.

PATHOGENESIS

- The typical SCC lesion is a firm, scaly papule or nodule containing a central ulcer surrounded by an indurated raised border (**FIG 1**).
- Risk factors include the following:
  - Repetitive damage from sun, heat, and wind
  - Severe burns and chronic ulcers
  - Advanced age
- Immune compromise (organ transplantation and AIDS)
- Major risks for melanoma include the following:
  - Personal or family history of melanoma
  - Propensity for sunburn with excessive sun exposure
  - Immune compromise
  - Previous skin cancers
  - Exposure to coal tar, radiation, or radium

NATURAL HISTORY

- SCC is the second most common type, behind basal cell carcinoma (BCC).
- The American Cancer Society estimates more than 1 million new diagnoses of cutaneous BCC and SCC are made annually. However, BCC and SCC account for less than 0.1% of patient deaths caused by all cancers.
- The American Cancer Society anticipates approximately 60,000 new melanoma cases each year, with an estimated 8110 deaths.
- The probability of developing melanoma from birth to death is 2.04 (1 in 49) in males and 1.38 (1 in 73) in females.
- Nail matrix SCC or melanoma account for less than 1% of their respective cutaneous malignancies. The histologic features of the epidermis and dermis, including physiologic barriers, are absent in the nail complex. In the nail complex, the matrix is adherent to the underlying phalanx.

PATIENT HISTORY AND PHYSICAL FINDINGS

- Patients typically present for evaluation after noting the recent appearance of, or changes to, an existing lesion.
- Change in size, shape, coloration, the presence of satellite lesions, or ulceration of a lesion should prompt a thorough evaluation and possible biopsy with histopathologic analysis (**FIG 2**).
- Melanoma and SCC can metastasize. Regional lymph node beds (axillary) should be routinely examined in all suspected cases of upper extremity skin cancer.
- The presence of a Hutchinson sign (extension of brown-black pigment from the nail bed, matrix, or nail plate onto the adjacent cuticle and proximal or lateral nail folds) is consistent with a subungual melanoma (**FIG 3**). Subungual melanoma should also be suspected when the nail bed contains a new or enlarging pigmented streak wider than 3 mm (**FIG 4**).

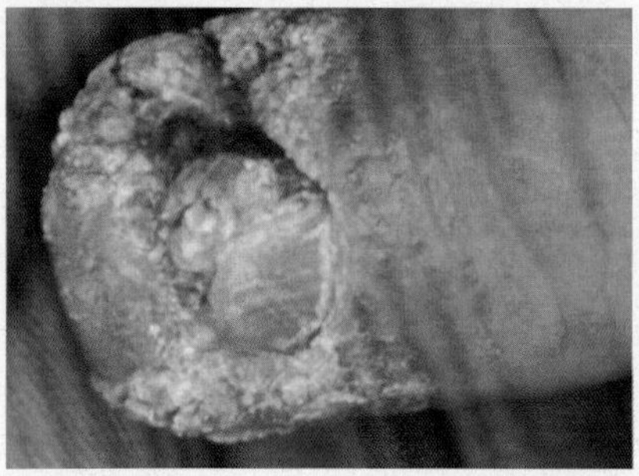

FIG 1 • The typical SCC lesion is a firm, scaly papule or nodule containing a central ulcer surrounded by an indurated raised border.

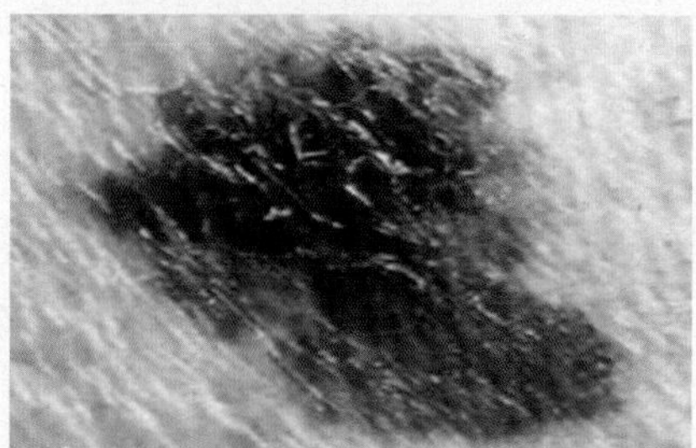

FIG 2 • Change in size, shape, border irregularity, coloration, the presence of satellite lesions, or ulceration should prompt a thorough evaluation and biopsy.

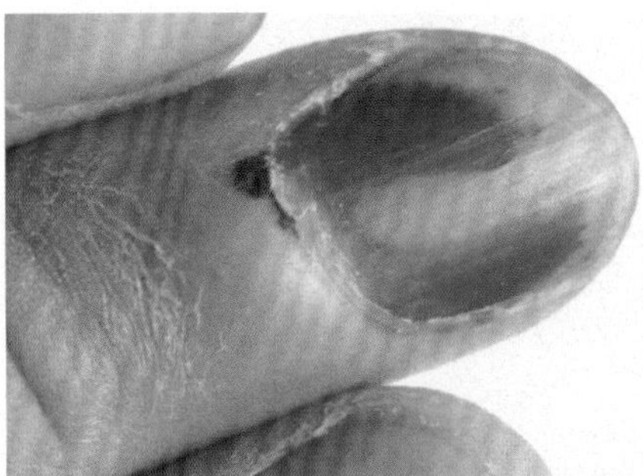

FIG 3 • A Hutchinson sign, extension of brown-black pigment from the nail bed, matrix, and nail plate onto the adjacent cuticle and proximal or lateral nail folds, is consistent with a subungual melanoma.

- Although there have been reports of amelanotic melanoma of the nail bed, the actual incidence is unknown.

IMAGING AND OTHER DIAGNOSTIC STUDIES

- Radiographic evaluation of the hand with plain view x-rays are helpful and may reveal bone involvement (**FIG 5**).
- For both SCC and melanoma, a chest radiograph, complete blood count, and liver panel may be obtained. If these labs reveal abnormality, prompt evaluation by an internist or oncologist is appropriate.
- More detailed imaging studies (computed tomography [CT], magnetic resonance imaging [MRI], and positron emission tomography [PET]) may be performed to evaluate specific organ systems (central nervous system, pulmonary, gastrointestinal, and others) if indicated.
- The diagnosis of skin cancer requires adequate histopathologic evaluation with a full-thickness (surface to full depth) specimen.
  - Suspicious pigmented lesions must never be shaved, cauterized, or vaporized for fear of losing the opportunity to accurately identify the lesion depth.
- SCC is *graded* 1 to 4 based on the proportion of differentiating cells present and the frequency of atypical tumor cells.
- Melanoma subtypes include the following:
  - Superficial spreading: most common, 70%
  - Nodular: 15% to 30%, more aggressive
  - Lentigo maligna: most common subtype among Asians and African Americans
  - Acral lentiginous (palmar–plantar and subungual)
  - Miscellaneous unusual types are as follows:
    - Mucosal lentiginous (oral and genital)

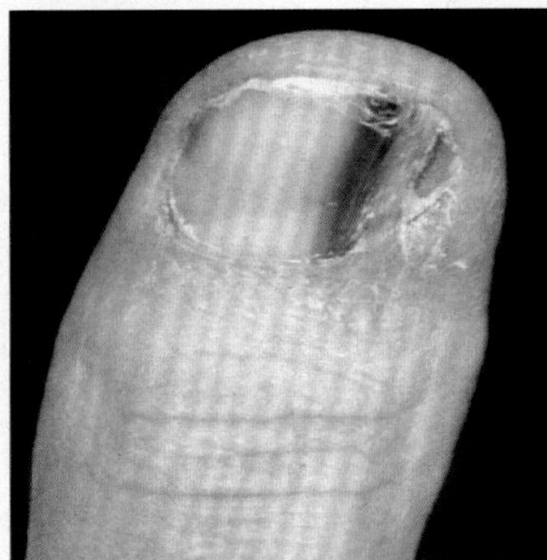

FIG 4 • Subungual melanoma should also be suspected when the nail bed contains a new or enlarging pigmented streak wider than 3 mm.

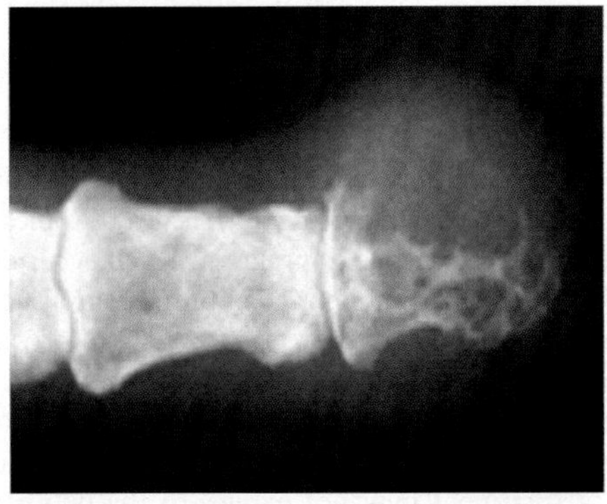

FIG 5 • Radiographic evaluation of the hand with plain view x-rays are helpful and may reveal bone involvement.

    - Desmoplastic
    - Verrucous
- Malignant melanoma staging is determined by histopathologic evaluation of the vertical thickness of the lesion in millimeters (Breslow classification) or the anatomic level of local invasion (Clark classification).
- Along with the presence of ulceration, Breslow thickness more accurately predicts melanoma behavior in lesions thicker than 1.5 mm. Estimates of prognosis should be modified by sex and anatomic site in coordination with clinical and histologic evaluation.
- The Clark classification ranges from level I (in situ lesions involving only the epidermis) to level V (invasion through the reticular dermis into the subcutaneous tissue).
  - Micrometastases are diagnosed by elective sentinel lymphadenectomy.
  - Macrometastases are defined as clinically detectable lymph node metastases confirmed by therapeutic lymphadenectomy or when any lymph node metastasis exhibits gross extracapsular extension.
- Clinical staging includes microstaging of the primary melanoma and clinical or radiologic evaluation of potential metastases. With the exception of clinical stage 0 or stage IA patients (who have a low risk of lymphatic involvement and do not require pathologic evaluation of the lymph nodes), pathologic staging includes microstaging of the primary melanoma and pathologic information about the regional lymph nodes after sentinel node biopsy and, if indicated, complete lymphadenectomy.

DIFFERENTIAL DIAGNOSIS OF SQUAMOUS CELL CARCINOMA AND MELANOMA

- Seborrheic keratosis
- Pigmented actinic keratosis
- Hemangioma
- Dermatofibroma
- Blue nevus
- Basal cell carcinoma
- Cutaneous T-cell lymphomas (eg, mycosis fungoides)
- Kaposi sarcoma
- Extramammary Paget disease
- Apocrine carcinoma of the skin
- Metastatic malignancies from various primary sites
- The differential diagnosis of subungual lesions includes chronic paronychia and onychomycosis, subungual hematoma, pyogenic granuloma, and glomus tumor.

NONOPERATIVE MANAGEMENT

Squamous Cell Carcinoma

- Topical fluorouracil (5-FU) may be helpful in the management of selected preinvasive, in situ SCC (Bowen disease).
- The deepest lesion extent may not be reached by topical 5-FU. In these instances, recurrence or progression can occur despite the belief that adequate treatment has been accomplished. Therefore, close follow-up with thorough evaluation is required.
- Electrodesiccation and curettage and cryosurgery may be useful for small (<2 cm), well-defined in situ tumors in patients with medical conditions limiting excisional surgery.
- Depth of treatment may not extend to the depth of tumor and therefore may be inadequate.
- Cryosurgery and electrodessication and curettage should not be used for SCC with suspected extension through the dermis.
- Carbon dioxide (CO_2) laser treatment may be useful in a subset of medically compromised patients with small SCC in situ.
- Because the CO_2 laser coagulates, this technique is also valuable for patients with a bleeding diathesis.
- Radiation therapy is a logical treatment option and is particularly useful when treating poor operative candidates, locally challenging lesions, or tumors extending over large areas.
- Radiation therapy can also be used for recurrent lesions after a primary surgical removal.
- Radiation therapy is contraindicated for use in patients with prior radiation to the affected site, xeroderma pigmentosum, epidermodysplasia verruciformis, or basal cell nevus syndrome.

SURGICAL MANAGEMENT

- The fundamental oncologic principle of tumor clearance first, *then* reconstruction must be followed without compromise. As always, tumor clearance must be prioritized over any eventual coverage/reconstruction.
- Wide local excision +/− lymph node sampling is recommended for melanomas.
- Melanoma in situ requires a 5 mm negative margin. Melanomas of less than 1 mm thickness require a 1 cm clear margin. Melanomas of 1 to 4 mm in thickness require a 2 cm clear margin. Finally, melanomas of greater than 4 mm thickness require a 3 cm clear margin.
- Clinical appearance of lymph node involvement or evidence of lymphatic bed extension as shown by sentinel lymph node biopsy should prompt lymphadenectomy.

Cutaneous Squamous Cell Carcinoma

- The two primary methods of SCC treatment are surgical excision with frozen or permanent histopathologic sections and Mohs micrographic surgery (**FIG 6**).
- When surgically excising SCC of the hand, the surgeon should maintain at least a 3 mm margin of disease-free tissue.
- Mohs resection of hand SCC results in the highest cure rate (98%) with maximal preservation of normal tissue.

Nail Matrix Squamous Cell Carcinoma

- For SCC of the nail matrix *without* bone involvement, tumor resection with 3 mm clear margins and tumor-free deep margins containing subcutaneous fat is appropriate. Mohs resection has also proven useful (**FIG 7**).

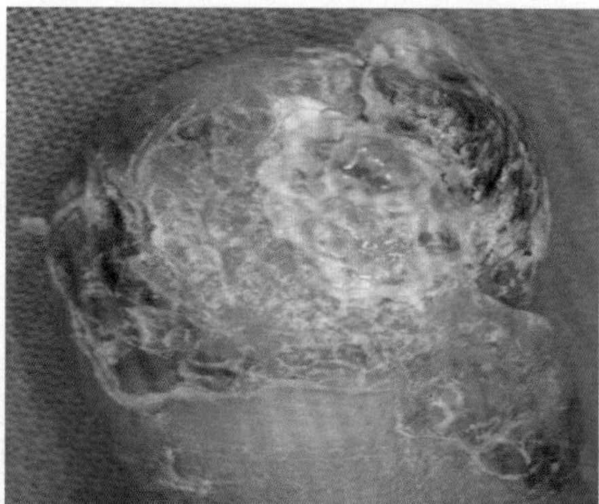

FIG 6 • Excision of digital SCC may be accomplished with either excisional biopsy or Mohs micrographic surgery.

- For SCC of the nail matrix *involving bone*, the appropriate technique is amputation at the distal joint.

Melanoma

- Malignant melanoma can spontaneously regress, but the incidence of spontaneous, complete regressions is less than 1%.
- Without nail matrix involvement, invasion of osseous cortices or perineural invasion, wide local excision should be directed by Breslow depth.
- Melanoma of the hand with less than 1.5 mm thickness has a low incidence of nodal metastases and is treated effectively with wide local excision of the primary tumor with a 1- to 2-cm margins.
- Thicker melanomas are associated with more than 50% rate of regional or systemic spread. In the absence of metastatic disease, these individuals should undergo local excision with a 2-cm margins and sentinel lymph node biopsy followed by lymphadenectomy if the sentinel node is positive (**FIG 8A,B**).
- Melanomas of the nail complex are especially concerning due to the absence of the usual skin barrier as well as proximity of the underlying phalanx and tendons. Due to these circumstances, Breslow depth and Clark levels are irrelevant.
- Total digital (ray) amputation of the fingers results in significant functional deficits without significant survival benefit.
- The respective digit is amputated at the joint level proximal to the lesion. In the case of nail matrix melanomas, amputation of the digit just proximal to the distal interphalangeal joint (DIPJ) is appropriate.

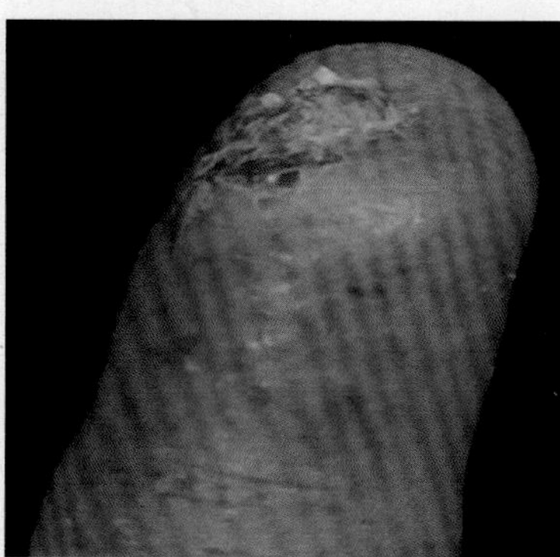

FIG 7 • For SCC of the nail matrix *without* bone involvement, tumor resection with 3-mm clear margins and tumor-free deep margins containing subcutaneous fat is appropriate.

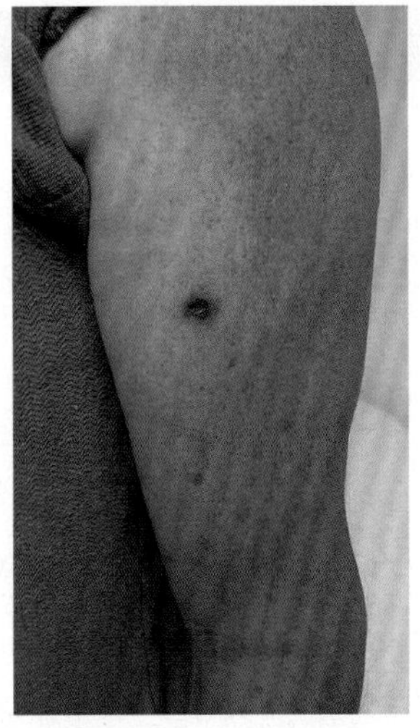

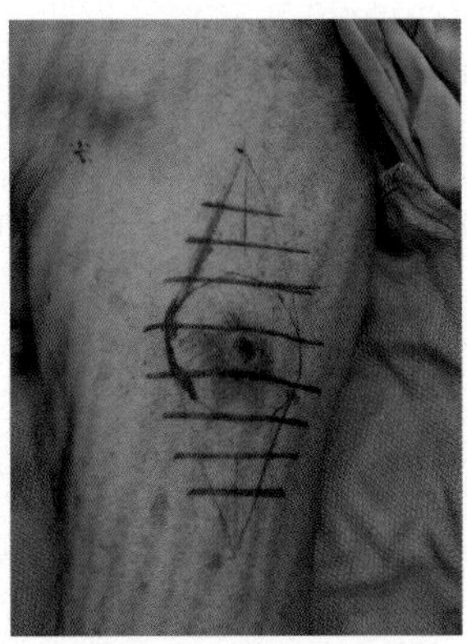

FIG 8 • **A.** Invasive melanoma treated initially with cutaneous laser ablation. **B.** Intraoperative invasive melanoma lesion with margins marked out and after injection of isosulfan blue. Note visible adenopathy in anterior superior axilla.

- For more proximal digital melanoma with bone involvement or perineural invasion, either complete digital (ray) amputation is indicated.
- Specific recommendations are individualized for each patient. Other significant factors, such as the primary tumor anatomic location, specific tumor features, healing ability, and medical risk factors, must be considered. The surgical goal is to minimize local and regional recurrence and metastasis while maintaining acceptable risks to minimize morbidity and mortality.

Coverage and Reconstruction

- After wide local excision, most wounds can be closed primarily without tension using minimal perimeter undermining and closure.
- If an extended time period is required to establish final histopathology, local wound care using clean dressings or negative pressure wound system can temporarily be used.
- Coverage options include allowing secondary closure, primary closure, skin graft, local flap, regional flap, and free flap coverage. Use of alloplasts, such as Integra, may also be helpful.
- Exposed vessels, nerves, tendons, and bone should prompt flap coverage or use of alloplast materials.
- Skin grafting can be either split or full thickness depending on the wound bed vascularity, anatomic area, and aesthetics. Typically, split-thickness skin grafts are useful on the dorsal surface of the hand. Full-thickness skin grafts are helpful on the volar surface.
- Digital V-Y flaps, cross-finger flaps, hypothenar flaps, flag flaps, dorsal metacarpal artery flaps, and radial forearm flaps are common flap options as well.

Preoperative Planning

- To direct management of local tumor, regional lymph nodes, and metastatic disease, the patient must be staged. The histopathology of the primary tumor is determined by an accurate histopathologic diagnosis.
- Mohs micrographic surgery requires the assistance of a trained surgeon or physician, such as a dermatologist.
- Before resection, plans must be made for coverage.

Positioning

- Positioning should allow access to the primary tumor and the regional lymph node basin if necessary.
- A sterile tourniquet is used. When access to the axillary lymph nodes is required, the tourniquet is removed.

Approach

- For wide local excision, the primary lesion is marked and the indicated margin is measured around the lesion using calipers and/or a ruler.
- Wide local excision includes the intact tumor or biopsy site en bloc with a defined perimeter of normal skin and underlying subcutaneous tissue. The underlying muscular fascia is not included.
- For primary closure, an ellipse is marked out incorporating the required margins for wide local excision.
- The excised length-to-lesion diameter is at least 3:1.
- For amputation, the appropriate joint level is marked, along with planned fish-mouth dorsal and volar flaps.
- For selective lymph node sampling, a grid is marked over the axillary area. The point of highest radioactivity is marked on the grid.

Mohs Micrographic Surgery

- Mohs micrographic surgery is performed by a Mohs-trained surgeon (often a dermatologist) who both excises the lesion as well as performs immediate histopathologic staining and analysis.
- Excise a thin layer of tissue with 2- to 3-mm margins.
- Map the tissue with color-coded three-dimensional orientation.
- Both the deep and peripheral margins are examined in one horizontal plane by frozen section analysis with theoretically 100% margin control.
- With immediate performance of histologic interpretation, the precise anatomic location of any residual tumor is identified and re-excised until tumor-free three-dimensional margins are obtained.
- Multiple excisions with immediate staining and evaluation may be performed multiple times in order to obtain clear tissue margins.

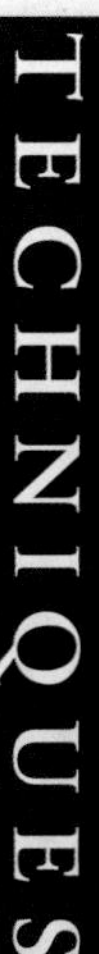

PEARLS AND PITFALLS

Chronic or nonhealing skin or matrix lesion	■ Send tissue biopsy for histopathologic evaluation and culture (bacterial, fungal, and tuberculosis).
Patient referred for treatment with histopathologic report	■ Obtain and review original histopathologic slides before treatment.
Nonpigmented chronic or nonhealing skin or matrix lesion	■ Remember amelanotic melanoma. Send tissue biopsy for histopathologic evaluation and culture (bacterial, fungal, and tuberculosis).

POSTOPERATIVE CARE

- Initial postoperative care focuses on pain control and surgical site wound care.
- Occupational therapy is by protocol, depending primarily on the coverage performed.
- Patients must be monitored.
- Both SCC and melanoma have metastatic potential. Patients should be reexamined every 3 months for the first several years, then every 6 months for 3 years, and then yearly indefinitely. Evaluation should focus on the potential for local recurrence, lymph node involvement, metastasis, and the appearance of additional skin cancers.
- For melanoma, the follow-up schedule for patients who have surgically resected disease is based on the primary lesion's thickness and nodal involvement. Patients with thin primary melanoma and negative nodes are followed with clinical examination every 6 months for the first 2 to 3 years, then yearly for 2 to 3 years. Patients with intermediate or thick melanomas and negative regional nodes are followed every 3 to 6 months for the first 2 to 3 years and every 6 to 12 months for the next 2 to 3 years. Patients with resected regional disease require follow-up every 3 to 4 months for the first 2 years, then every 6 months up to year 5, and yearly beyond that.
- All patients diagnosed with SCC or melanoma should maintain routine lifelong dermatologic screening. Patients with prior SCC or melanoma remain at higher than average risk for a second skin cancer.

OUTCOMES

- SCC is the second most common type of skin malignancy behind BCC. Although the BCC and SCC are the most common of all malignancies, they account for less than 0.1% of cancer deaths.
- The overall cure rate for SCC is directly related to the stage of the disease and the type of treatment used.
- Melanoma 5-year survival rates are related to stage and range from 18% for stage IV to 99% for stage IA.

COMPLICATIONS

- The most common complications of sentinel lymph node biopsy are hematoma and seroma. The rate of lymphedema after sentinel lymph node biopsy is 0.7% to 1.7%, compared with 4.6% (axillary) and 31.5% (inguinal) with complete lymphadenectomy.
- Positive margins on final pathology for SCC or melanoma must be addressed by reexcision.

SUGGESTED READINGS

1. Abide JM, Nahai F, Bennett RG. The meaning of surgical margins. Plast Reconstr Surg 1984;73:492–497.
2. Balch CM, Urist MM, Karakousis CP, et al. Efficacy of 2-cm surgical margins for intermediate-thickness melanomas (1 to 4 mm): results of a multi-institutional randomized surgical trial. Ann Surg 1993;218:262–269.
3. Cottel WI. Perineural invasion by squamous-cell carcinoma. J Dermatol Surg Oncol 1982;8:589–600.
4. Essner R, Conforti A, Kelley MC, et al. Efficacy of lymphatic mapping, sentinel lymphadenectomy, and selective complete lymph node dissection as a therapeutic procedure for early-stage melanoma. Ann Surg Oncol 1999;6:442–449.
5. Gershenwald JE, Thompson W, Mansfield PF, et al. Multi-institutional melanoma lymphatic mapping experience: the prognostic value of sentinel lymph node status in 612 stage I or II melanoma patients. J Clin Oncol 1999;17:976–983.
6. Hochwald SN, Coit DG. Role of elective lymph node dissection in melanoma. Semin Surg Oncol 1998;14:276–282.
7. Lee ML, Tomsu K, Von Eschen KB. Duration of survival for disseminated malignant melanoma: results of a meta-analysis. Melanoma Res 2000;10:81–92.
8. Leo F, Cagini L, Rocmans P, et al. Lung metastases from melanoma: when is surgical treatment warranted? Br J Cancer 2000;83:569–572.
9. Morton DL, Cochran AJ, Thompson JF, et al. Sentinel node biopsy for early-stage melanoma: accuracy and morbidity in MSLT-I, an international multicenter trial. Ann Surg 2005;242:302–313.
10. Mraz-Gernhard S, Sagebiel RW, Kashani-Sabet M, et al. Prediction of sentinel lymph node micrometastasis by histological features in primary cutaneous malignant melanoma. Arch Dermatol 1998;134:983–987.
11. Ollila DW, Hsueh EC, Stern SL, et al. Metastasectomy for recurrent stage IV melanoma. J Surg Oncol 1999;71:209–213.
12. Preston DS, Stern RS. Nonmelanoma cancers of the skin. N Engl J Med 1992;327:1649–1662.
13. Thomas JM, Newton-Bishop J, A'Hern R, et al. Excision margins in high-risk malignant melanoma. N Engl J Med 2004;350:757–766.
14. Thomas RM, Amonette RA. Mohs micrographic surgery. Am Fam Physician 1988;37:135–142.
15. Veronesi U, Cascinelli N. Narrow excision (1-cm margin): a safe procedure for thin cutaneous melanoma. Arch Surg 1991;126:438–441.
16. Veronesi U, Cascinelli N, Adamus J, et al. Thin stage I primary cutaneous malignant melanoma: comparison of excision with margins of 1 or 3 cm. N Engl J Med 1988;318:1159–1162.
17. Wagner JD, Gordon MS, Chuang TY, et al. Current therapy of cutaneous melanoma. Plast Reconstr Surg 2000;105:1774–1801.

Open and Arthroscopic Excision of Ganglion Cysts and Related Tumors

145 CHAPTER

Mitchell E. Nahra and John S. Bucchieri

DEFINITION

Ganglion Cysts

- Ganglion cysts, although not true cysts, are the most common tumors of the hand and wrist.
- These fluid-filled cysts are a frequent cause of hand and wrist pain.
- Ganglion cysts typically arise from either a joint or tendon sheath.
- Most ganglion cysts occur in the wrist. Dorsal wrist ganglion cysts account for 60% to 70% of all ganglion cysts, with volar wrist ganglion cysts accounting for about 18% to 20%.[1]
- Ganglion cysts may also arise from a tendon sheath (volar retinacular cyst) or occur in association with arthritis (degenerative mucous cyst).

Giant Cell Tumors

- Giant cell tumors of the tendon sheath—also referred to as *localized nodular synovitis*,[11] *fibrous xanthoma*, and *pigmented villonodular synovitis*—are benign, slow-growing soft tissue tumors.
- After ganglion cyst cysts, these lesions are the second most common tumor in the hand.[6]

Epidermal Inclusion Cysts

- Epidermal inclusion cysts are benign, slow-growing soft tissue tumors.
- They are the third most common type of hand tumor.

ANATOMY

Ganglion Cysts

- Ganglion cysts typically consist of a cyst sac that communicates through a stalk to an underlying joint or tendon sheath (**FIG 1**).
- The cyst sac may have a single cavity or be multilobulated.
- Although not a true cyst, lacking an epithelial lining, ganglion cysts are typically filled with a clear, viscous, jelly-like mucinous fluid made up of glucosamine, albumin, globulin, and a high concentration of hyaluronic acid.[17]

Giant Cell Tumors

- The tumor is usually a multilobular, well-circumscribed mass, ranging in size from 0.5 to 7 cm.[6]
- The color ranges from yellow to deep brown depending on the amount of hemosiderin, histiocytes, and collagen present in the lesion.
- These lesions have a thin pseudocapsule. Aggressive lesions may invade adjacent soft tissue, tendon, and capsular structures and can envelop neurovascular bundles. A large study showed joint involvement in one-fifth of all cases.[7] Long-standing lesions may erode into cortical bone but will not involve cartilage or the medullary canal of bone. Satellite lesions may occur.
- Histologically, giant cell tumors contain collagen-producing polyhedral-shaped histiocytes, scattered multinucleated giant cells, and hemosiderin deposits.[6]

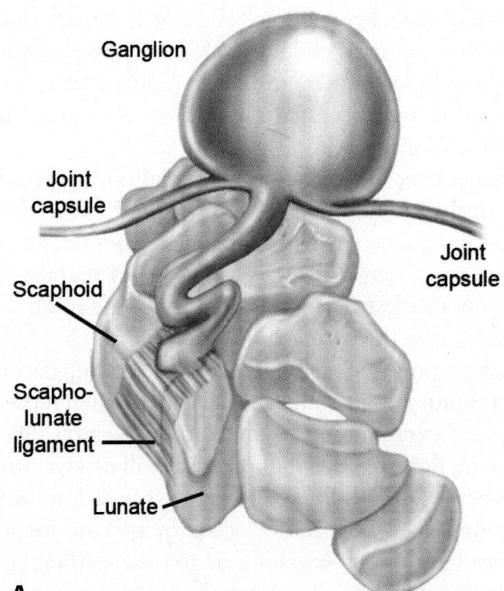

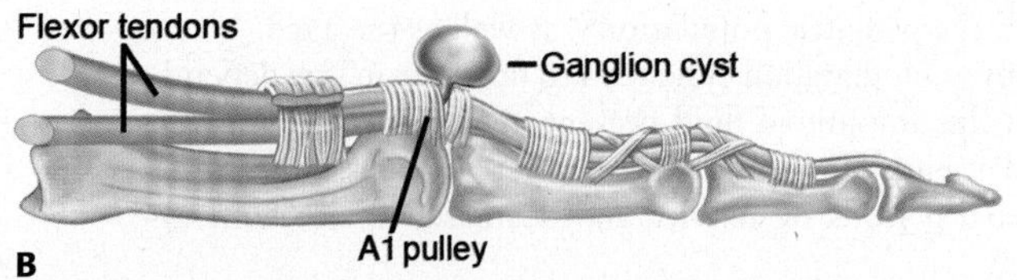

FIG 1 • **A.** Ganglion cyst arising from dorsal scapholunate joint. **B.** Ganglion cyst arising from flexor sheath.

Epidermal Inclusion Cysts

- Epidermal inclusion cysts are well-circumscribed, firm, and slightly mobile lesions.
- They are often superficial and adherent to overlying skin.
- They may be flesh-colored, yellow, or white.
- They contain a thick, white, keratinous material.
- Cysts in the fingertip may erode into the distal phalanx, causing a lytic lesion.
- Histologically, they are cysts filled with keratin and lined with epithelial cells.

PATHOGENESIS

Ganglion Cysts

- The true causes of ganglion cysts remain unclear, although multiple theories have been proposed.
- Some early investigators theorized that ganglion cysts occurred as the result of synovial herniation and others felt that ganglion cysts resulted from mucoid degeneration.
- A more recent theory proposes that ganglion cysts arise from stress at the synovial capsular interface. This stress, such as stretching of the capsular and ligamentous structures, stimulates the production of mucin from modified synovial, mesenchymal, and fibroblast cells, all of which have been shown to produce hyaluronic acid. The mucin then dissects through the capsular and ligamentous tissues, forming the main cyst. The fluid may enter the cyst from the capsular ligamentous interface via a one-way valve type of mechanism and then decrease as the water component is resorbed, accounting for the often-fluctuating cyst size.[1]

Giant Cell Tumors

- The cause of giant cell tumors is not known. There is a strong association of giant cell tumors with rheumatoid arthritis. There are no clinical studies associating these tumors with trauma.[6]
- Although these tumors are histologically similar to the pigmented villonodular synovitis seen in large joints in the lower extremity, they are thought to be clinically distinct lesions.

Epidermal Inclusion Cysts

- Epidermal inclusion cysts occur as a result of trauma when epithelial cells are introduced into the underlying subcutaneous tissues or bone. These cells slowly grow to produce a cyst lined with epithelial cells and filled with keratin.

NATURAL HISTORY

Ganglion Cysts

- Ganglion cysts typically arise spontaneously and are most common in the second through the fourth decade but may arise in the pediatric population[19] as well as the aged.
- Once present, ganglion cysts tend to fluctuate in size depending on the amount of fluid present in the cyst at any given time. Patients often note that the cyst becomes larger after increased periods of activity and decreases in size with inactivity.
- Ganglion cysts tend to be self-limiting and do not typically continue to expand in size.
- If left untreated, ganglion cysts can persist for years. They may resolve or rupture spontaneously. One cannot predict how long that they will persist or if and when they will resolve.
- Resolution is far more common in the pediatric population.

Giant Cell Tumors

- The lesion begins as a single nodule, becoming multinodular as it enlarges.
- Malignant transformation of giant cell tumor of the tendon sheath in the hand has not been reported.[6]

Epidermal Inclusion Cysts

- These lesions occur months to years after a traumatic event. They grow slowly to produce a painless mass, most commonly seen in the fingertip.
- Malignant transformation of these lesions in the hand has not been reported.[12]

PATIENT HISTORY AND PHYSICAL FINDINGS

Ganglion Cysts

- Patients often present with an asymptomatic mass that has been present for weeks to years.
- A history of trauma is often absent.
- Pain if present is often described as a dull ache. Nocturnal pain is uncommon and pain is more common with active hand use.
- Paresthesias are rare but can occur if the ganglion cyst compresses any local nerves.
- Patients often report that the mass tends to fluctuate in size, a characteristic typical of ganglion cysts and not typical of other types of soft tissue tumors.
- Patients with wrist ganglion cysts—particularly dorsal wrist cysts—will often complain of weakness of grip.
- Patients with dorsal wrist ganglion cysts most commonly note a mass over the dorsum of the wrist, typically over the dorsal scapholunate region. In contrast, patients with volar wrist ganglion cysts typically note a mass over the volar aspect of the wrist in the interval between the flexor carpi radialis (FCR) and first extensor compartment tendons.
- Volar retinacular cysts or ganglion cysts of tendon sheath usually present as a mass in the palm in the region of the first and second annular pulleys. The cyst is typically fluctuant but may feel like a firm nodule. The cyst is usually slightly mobile but does not often glide with flexor tendon movement.
  - These types of cysts are often painless at rest but become painful when patients perform activities that involve forceful grip.
- Degenerative mucous cysts are ganglion cysts that arise from the distal interphalangeal joint, usually in association with underlying osteoarthritis.[4] Patients often note a painless soft tissue mass that arises from the dorsal surface of the joint, radially or ulnarly (less commonly in the midline), often extending into the eponychial fold region.
  - Commonly, the cyst will thin the overlying dermis, resulting in rupture of the skin, and the patient often reports drainage.
- Physical examination begins with inspection (**FIG 2**).
  - Being fluid-filled, ganglion cysts will often transilluminate, whereas other more solid soft tissue lesions will not.
  - Ganglion cysts usually occur in specific locations in the hand and wrist. Swelling or masses in these locations are diagnostic clues that a ganglion cyst may be present.

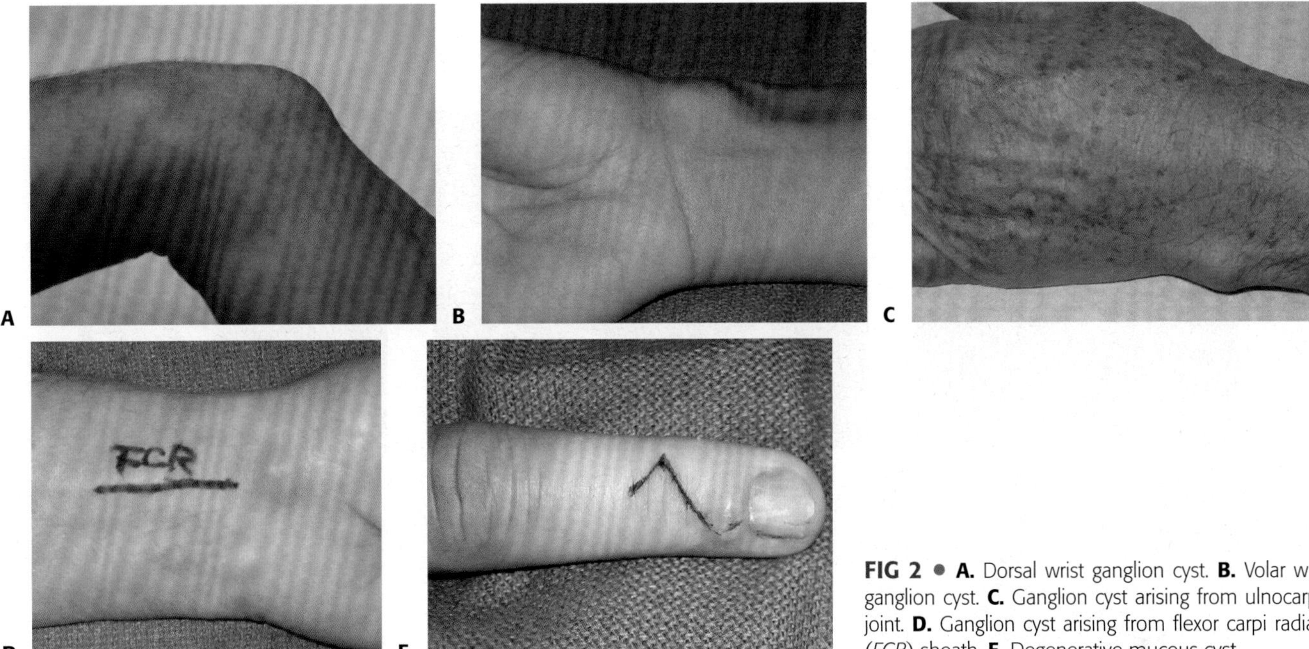

FIG 2 • **A.** Dorsal wrist ganglion cyst. **B.** Volar wrist ganglion cyst. **C.** Ganglion cyst arising from ulnocarpal joint. **D.** Ganglion cyst arising from flexor carpi radialis (*FCR*) sheath. **E.** Degenerative mucous cyst.

- The examiner should palpate the mass for fluctuance and mobility and assess tenderness.
  - Ganglion cysts are generally fluctuant and slightly mobile. When they become more distended with fluid, they may feel more firm and less fluctuant. Firm, less mobile masses suggest the possibility of other soft tissue lesions.
  - Ganglion cysts of tendon sheath do not usually glide with tendon motion, but less common ganglion cysts, such as those that arise in the fourth extensor compartment, are often adherent and do glide with tendon motion.
- The examiner should assess joint mobility through the range of motion. With the exception of dorsal wrist ganglion cysts, which may cause some loss of wrist dorsiflexion secondary to impingement, loss of joint range of motion suggests the possibility of an underlying joint abnormality.

Giant Cell Tumors

- Giant cell tumors are most common in the fourth to sixth decade, with a slight predominance in women.
- Patients typically present with a slow-growing, multilobulated, firm, painless mass present for several months to years.
- Lesions usually occur in the radial three digits of the hand on the volar surface. Dorsal involvement, particularly around the distal interphalangeal joint, is not uncommon.[7]
- These lesions are typically firmer than ganglion cysts and do not transilluminate.
- Large lesions may limit range of motion or result in neuropathic symptoms as a result of compression of digital nerves.
- Direct palpation typically reveals a firm, multinodular, nontender lesion.
- Loss of range of motion may occur when large lesions occur near the interphalangeal joints.
- Patients may have sensory deficits secondary to digital nerve compression. These can be revealed by testing two-point discrimination.

Epidermal Inclusion Cysts

- Epidermal inclusion cysts are more common in men than in women and occur in the third to fourth decade.[2]
- Patients commonly present with a painless, slow-growing mass after a laceration, puncture wound, or traumatic amputation of the finger.[2]
- These lesions should be suspected in laborers who have a painless mass in the palm.[12]
- Erythematous and painful lesions have been reported. One study reported two cases mimicking a collar-button abscess resulting from rupture of the cyst in the palmar soft tissues.[20]
- These lesions are typically firmer than ganglion cysts and do not transilluminate.
- Direct palpation will reveal a lesion that is firm, nontender, superficial, and mobile.
- Loss of range of motion may occur when large lesions occur near the interphalangeal joints.
- Two-point discrimination testing may reveal sensory deficits secondary to digital nerve compression.

IMAGING AND OTHER DIAGNOSTIC STUDIES

Ganglion Cysts

- Radiographs are obtained if there is clinical suspicion of an underlying bony abnormality noted on physical examination, such as joint crepitation, swelling, carpal instability, or a history of trauma.
  - Radiographs are also useful in identifying an intraosseous ganglion cyst in patients with wrist pain of uncertain cause (**FIG 3A**).
  - Radiographs are also often obtained in patients with a degenerative mucous cyst of the digit because the cysts typically arise as the result of degenerative arthritis of the distal interphalangeal joint.
- If the clinical findings suggest the possibility of an occult ganglion cyst, or if there is suspicion that the patient may

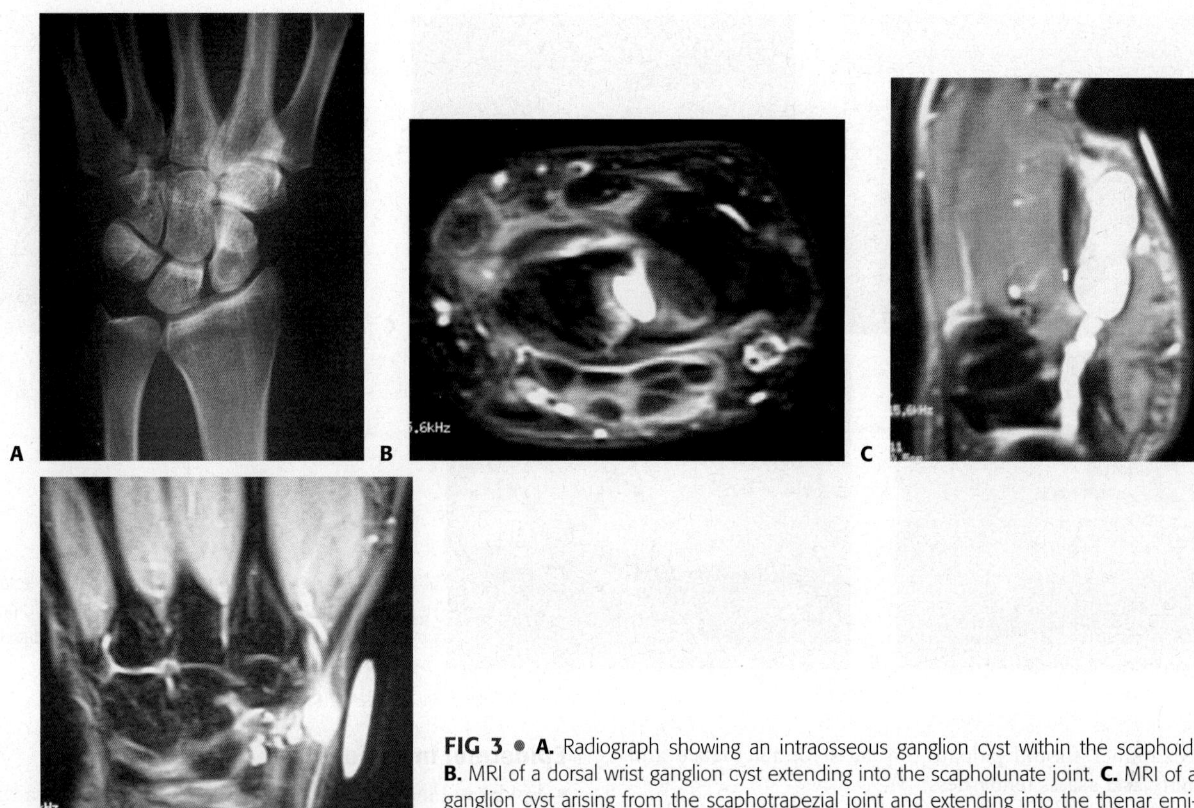

FIG 3 • **A.** Radiograph showing an intraosseous ganglion cyst within the scaphoid. **B.** MRI of a dorsal wrist ganglion cyst extending into the scapholunate joint. **C.** MRI of a ganglion cyst arising from the scaphotrapezial joint and extending into the thenar eminence. **D.** MRI of a ganglion cyst in the snuffbox but arising from the dorsal scapholunate ligament.

have a symptomatic intraosseous ganglion cyst, magnetic resonance imaging (MRI) can be a useful tool to confirm the diagnosis (**FIG 3B**).
  - MRI can also be used to better localize the site of origin as part of preoperative planning in ganglion cysts that occur in atypical locations (**FIG 3C,D**).
- Ultrasound can also be used to diagnose ganglion cysts, but this test is examiner dependent and less sensitive and specific than MRI.
- Computed tomography (CT) scans are generally obtained only for preoperative planning to better localize and evaluate the bony architecture of intraosseous ganglion cysts.

Giant Cell Tumors

- Plain radiographs show a soft tissue mass. Juxtacortical lesions may show bony erosion.
- MRI demonstrates a benign-appearing encapsulated mass, with decreased signal on T1- and T2-weighted images.

Epidermal Inclusion Cysts

- Plain radiographs show a soft tissue mass.
- A lytic lesion may be seen in the distal phalanx if it erodes into bone.

DIFFERENTIAL DIAGNOSIS

Ganglion Cysts

- Epidermoid inclusion cyst
- Giant cell tumor of tendon sheath
- Lipoma
- Synovial cyst

Giant Cell Tumors

- Fibroma of the tendon sheath, synovial chondromatosis, synovial hemangioma, tophaceous gout, foreign body granuloma, periosteal chondroma

Epidermal Inclusion Cysts

- Tophaceous gout, foreign body granuloma, giant cell tumor, ganglion cyst, sebaceous cyst
- Bony destruction may mimic a malignant or infectious process.[11] Some patients with these lesions have been treated with primary amputation before pathologic diagnosis.[6]

NONOPERATIVE MANAGEMENT

- Of the three tumors discussed in this chapter, only ganglion cysts can be managed without surgery.
- Ganglion cysts are benign cysts that may resolve spontaneously. Treatment often depends on the level of a patient's symptoms. Many patients seek medical care because they are concerned about the presence of a soft tissue mass and possibility of malignancy.[21] Once a diagnosis of a ganglion cyst is made, with proper counseling as to the nature of these lesions, many patients will be satisfied with a course of observation.
- In patients who are symptomatic, typical nonoperative treatments include rest and immobilization, oral analgesics such as nonsteroidal anti-inflammatories and acetaminophen, and aspiration of the cyst with or without injection.[3,13,14,21]

- In wrist ganglion cysts, the results of aspiration have variable cure rates in the literature, ranging from 15% to 89%.[12] Various agents have been injected into the ganglion cyst after aspiration, including hyaluronidase and methylprednisolone.[15]
  - On average, injection does not seem to increase the cure rate after aspiration, and we now typically perform aspiration alone. We generally inform patients that aspiration has about a 50% cure rate. The use of sclerosing agents is frowned on because these agents may cause articular damage.[10]
- Traditional methods of traumatic rupture of the cyst from a direct blow with an object such as a large book (hence the term *Bible cyst*) are mostly of historical significance.
- Ganglion cysts of tendon sheath (volar retinacular cysts) when symptomatic often respond to aspiration and injection and rarely require surgery when not associated with stenosing tenosynovitis. When they occur in association with stenosing tenosynovitis (trigger finger, de Quervain tendinitis), they often resolve with successful treatment of the underlying tendinitis.
  - We typically do not aspirate ganglion cysts of tendon sheath but have had great success by injecting these cysts with local anesthetic and a small amount of corticosteroid (1.5 to 2 mL of 1% lidocaine and 10 mg of Depo-Medrol). The cyst is entered with a 25-gauge needle and then distended to the point of rupture. The remaining fluid in the syringe is then injected into the tendon sheath. If necessary, gentle digital massage can be used to rupture the cyst after injection if the cyst fails to rupture with distention.

SURGICAL MANAGEMENT

Indications

Ganglion Cysts

- Surgery is generally indicated in patients who have symptoms and who either have failed nonoperative treatment or choose to proceed directly with surgery.
- In patients who have been diagnosed with a symptomatic wrist ganglion cyst, we generally describe the nature of the condition and outline the available forms of treatment, allowing the patient to decide which treatment is best for him or her. Some patients will choose observation, others will elect to undergo an aspiration, and some will chose to proceed directly with surgical excision.
- In the case of symptomatic ganglion cysts of tendon sheath, most of these will resolve with a corticosteroid injection and surgery is reserved for cysts that continue to recur.
- Degenerative mucous cysts that are draining or have a history of draining should be treated operatively because these cysts are at risk for infection that may extend into the distal interphalangeal joint and result in septic arthritis. If not draining, these cysts can be treated nonoperatively or surgically, depending on the patient's symptoms and choice of treatment.
- Intraosseous ganglion cysts that are symptomatic or have resulted in pathologic fracture or may exhibit an impending pathologic fracture are often treated operatively.

Giant Cell Tumors

- Indications for surgery include appearance, neuropathic symptoms, or loss of function.
- Careful, meticulous marginal excision of the lesion is the treatment of choice.
- Care must be taken to protect the neurovascular structures.
- Satellite lesions must be identified and carefully removed to minimize the chance of recurrence.

Epidermal Inclusion Cysts

- Indications for surgery include appearance, diagnosis, pain, and loss of function.
- Marginal excision of the lesion is the treatment of choice.

Preoperative Planning

Ganglion Cysts

- When removing ganglion cysts arising in atypical locations, MRI studies can help to identify the cyst origin and plan appropriate surgical exposure.
- MRI and CT scans, along with plain radiographs, are valuable to determine the ideal exposure and for treating intraosseous ganglion cysts with curettage and bone grafting.
- Plain radiographs are reviewed before excising degenerative mucous cysts to determine the extent of underlying osteophytes that may need to be addressed.

Giant Cell Tumors

- Although the diagnosis of giant cell tumor is primarily made based on history and clinical examination, radiographic studies should be reviewed to rule out other conditions.
- The patient should be advised that even with careful surgical techniques, the recurrence rate can be as high as 5% to 50%. Risk factors for local recurrence include proximity to the distal interphalangeal joint, degenerative joint disease, and bony erosion.[16]
- Temporary digital nerve neurapraxias may also occur after extrication of these tumors during surgery.

Epidermal Inclusion Cysts

- Although the diagnosis of epidermal inclusion cyst is primarily made based on history and clinical examination, radiographic studies should be reviewed to rule out other conditions.
- If a lytic lesion is present in the distal phalanx, a biopsy should be considered before surgical removal.
- The recurrence rate after marginal excision is low.

Positioning

- Patients undergoing hand or wrist surgery are positioned supine on the operating table with the operative extremity resting on a hand table. This position allows for circumferential access to the hand and wrist.
- The procedure is performed under regional anesthesia with a tourniquet applied to the upper arm or under a digital block with a tourniquet applied to the digit.
- For arthroscopic procedures, a traction tower or longitudinal finger trap traction is used (**FIG 4**).

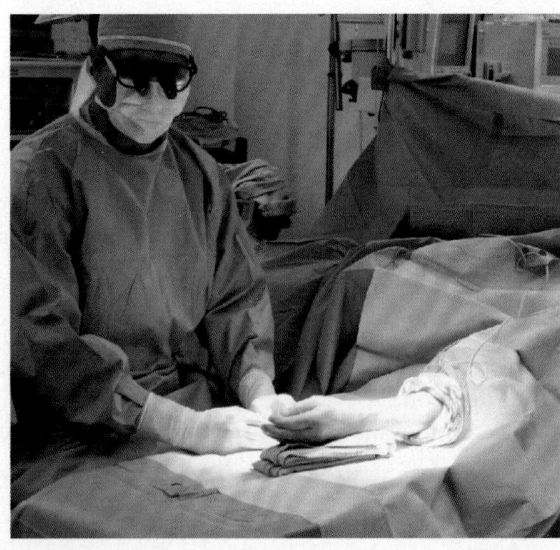

FIG 4 • The patient is positioned supine with an arm board attached to the operating table and the upper extremity is prepared and draped in a standard manner. The surgeon is generally seated in the axilla with full access to the hand and wrist.

Approach

Ganglion Cysts

- Standard approaches to the hand and wrist are used, depending on the location of the cyst.
- It is important to have a good understanding of the anatomy and the most likely origin of the cyst to best plan the incision and dissection to avoid injury to important neurovascular structures.
- When treating ganglion cysts in atypical locations, preoperative studies can aid in determining the best surgical approach because the origin of the cyst can be remote from the cyst (see **FIG 3D**).
- Volar giant cell tumors and epidermal inclusion cysts are approached through Brunner zigzag incisions (**FIG 5A**).
- Dorsal giant cell tumors require dorsal midline or curvilinear incisions, whereas dorsal epidermal inclusion cysts can be approached through small longitudinal incisions directly over the lesion (**FIG 5B**).
- Incisions should be designed for a possible extensile exposure, which may be necessary for complete excision of the lesion.

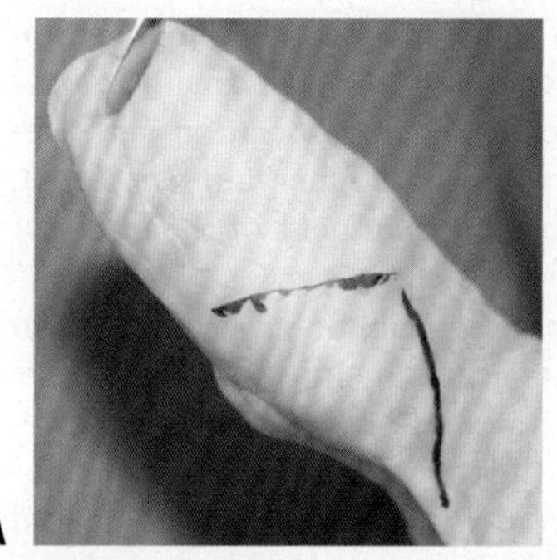

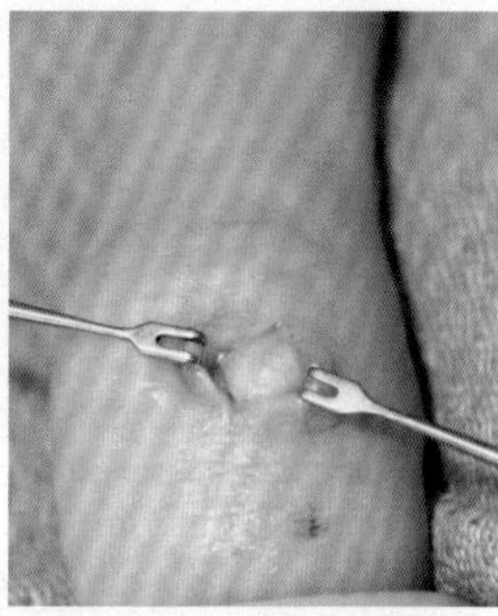

FIG 5 • **A.** A Brunner incision is made for a volar multilobular mass. **B.** A dorsal epidermal inclusion cyst is approached through a small longitudinal incision directly over the lesion.

TECHNIQUES

Open Excision of a Dorsal Wrist Ganglion Cyst

- The location of the cyst is typically dorsal to the scapholunate interosseous ligament. The incision needs to provide access to this ligament. The scapholunate ligament is found just distal to the tubercle of Lister in the third and fourth extensor compartment interval (**TECH FIG 1A**).
- We generally perform a transverse skin incision centered over the scapholunate ligament region and cyst. This incision heals with the best appearance (**TECH FIG 1B**).

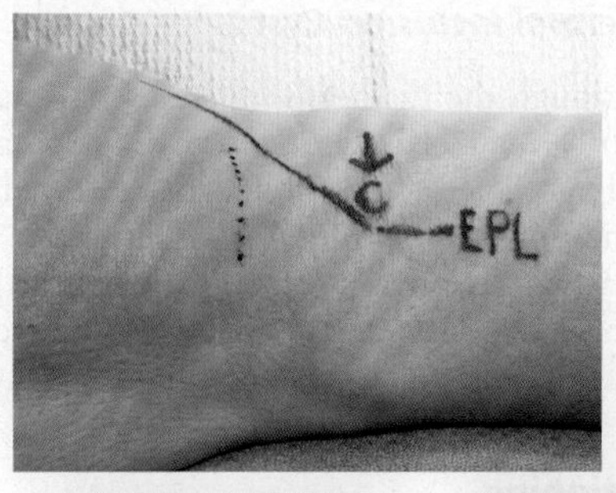

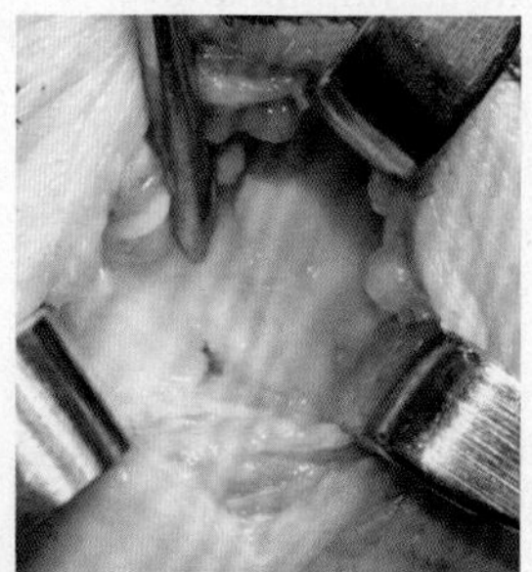

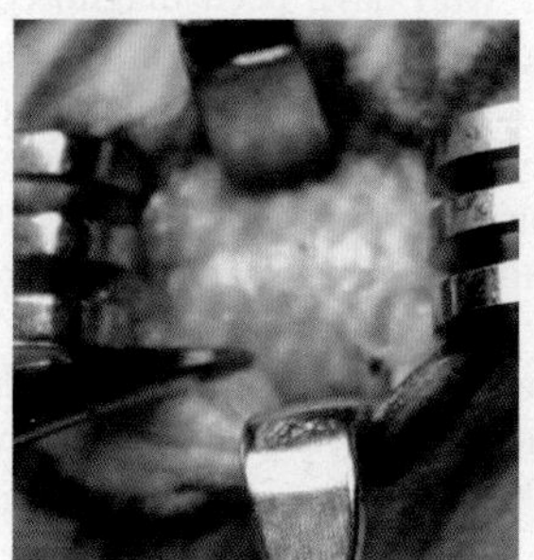

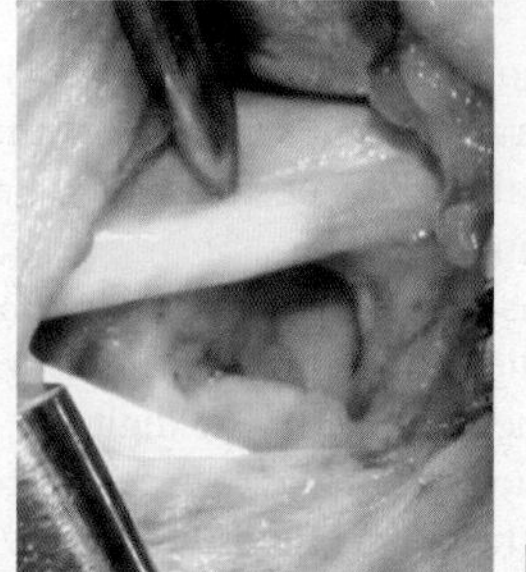

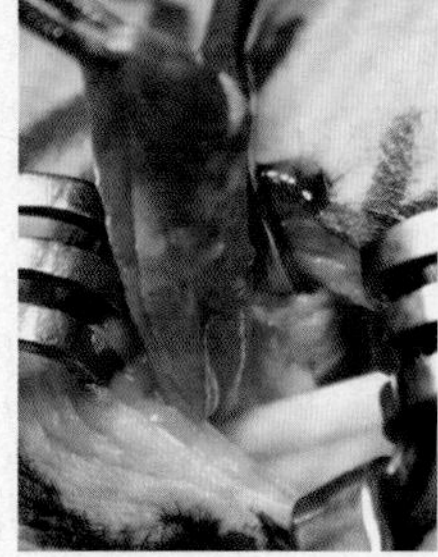

TECH FIG 1 • **A.** The dorsal scapholunate ligament is found just distal to the tubercle of Lister. *EPL*, extensor pollicis longus. **B.** Dorsal ganglion cysts typically arise from the dorsal scapholunate ligament. **C.** The extensor retinaculum is incised transversely. **D.** The extensor tendons are retracted, allowing visualization of the cyst. **E.** Cyst stalk arising from the dorsal scapholunate ligament. *(continued)*

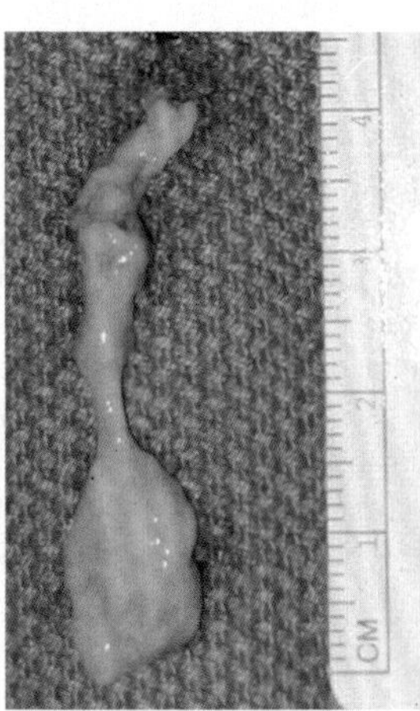
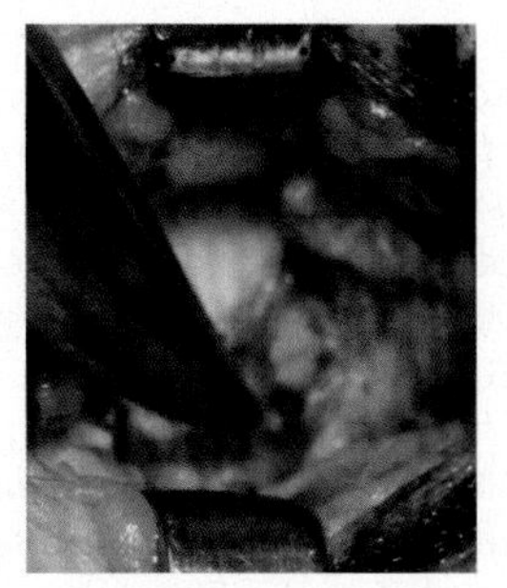
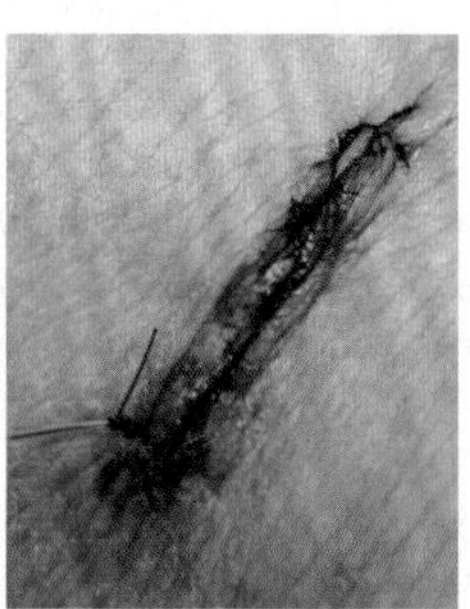

TECH FIG 1 • *(continued)* **F.** Excised cyst and stalk. **G.** The area of origin of the cyst is cauterized, taking care to preserve the ligament and interosseous membrane. **H.** Closure with running subcuticular suture.

- Dissect the subcutaneous tissues with blunt dissection, taking care to protect and preserve any branches of the dorsal radial and ulnar sensory nerves. Loupe magnification is often helpful.
- The extensor retinaculum is generally not well developed at this level and is incised transversely as the cyst is dissected from the surrounding soft tissues (**TECH FIG 1C**).
- The cyst is identified typically in the interval between the third and fourth extensor compartments. Retract the second and third extensor compartment tendons radially and the fourth extensor compartment tendons ulnarly (**TECH FIG 1D**).
- The dorsal wrist capsule is also incised transversely as the cyst is traced to a stalk, which usually arises from the dorsal aspect of the scapholunate interosseous membrane, just proximal to the dorsal scapholunate ligament (**TECH FIG 1E**).
- Excise the cyst at the base of the stalk and send it for pathologic examination (**TECH FIG 1F**).
- Although excision of a small window of tissue at the site of cyst origin has been previously recommended, we have concern that overzealous excision may lead to injury to the scapholunate ligamentous complex. We recommend the use of a bipolar cautery to precisely cauterize the site of origin (**TECH FIG 1G**).
- After excision of the cyst, inspect the joint for any abnormalities.
- Allow the capsular tissues and tendons to return to their anatomic position. Avoid capsular closure, as this may lead to joint stiffness.
- Skin closure is usually accomplished with a running subcuticular nonabsorbable monofilament suture (**TECH FIG 1H**).
- We prefer to dress the wound with an antibiotic ointment and petroleum gauze, and a bulky hand dressing is applied with a plaster palmar splint maintaining the wrist in a neutral position.
  - The dressing is removed along with the sutures at about 1 week postoperatively and Steri-Strips are applied to the wound.

Open Excision of a Volar Wrist Ganglion Cyst

- Volar wrist ganglion cysts most often arise from the volar radiocarpal ligaments. They may also arise from the scaphotrapezial joint[8] or at times from the FCR sheath. The cysts are typically located in the interval between the FCR sheath and first extensor compartment tendons, just proximal to the wrist flexion crease.
- Under tourniquet control, we prefer to use a zigzag type of incision that begins at the wrist flexion crease and extends proximally over the cyst in the FCR and first extensor compartment interval. This incision provides access in both the longitudinal and transverse planes. A longitudinal incision may heal with scar contracture, whereas a transverse incision may not provide adequate exposure in the longitudinal plane (**TECH FIG 2A**).

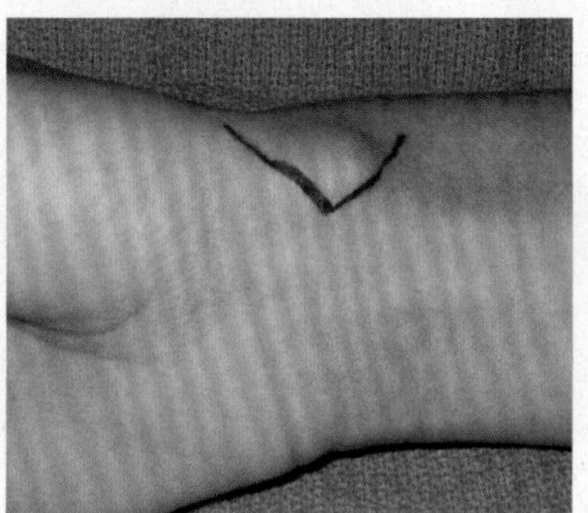
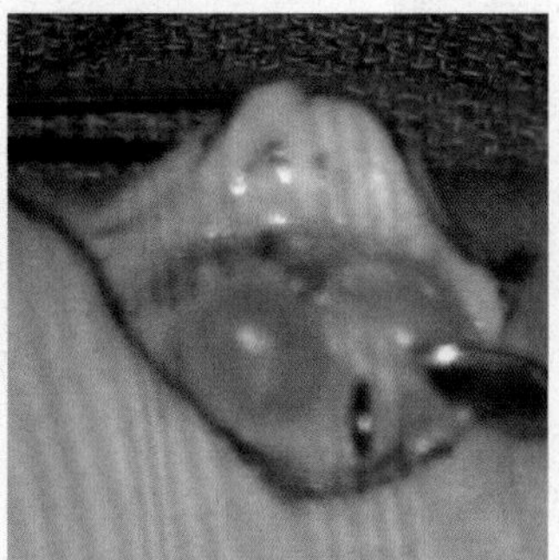
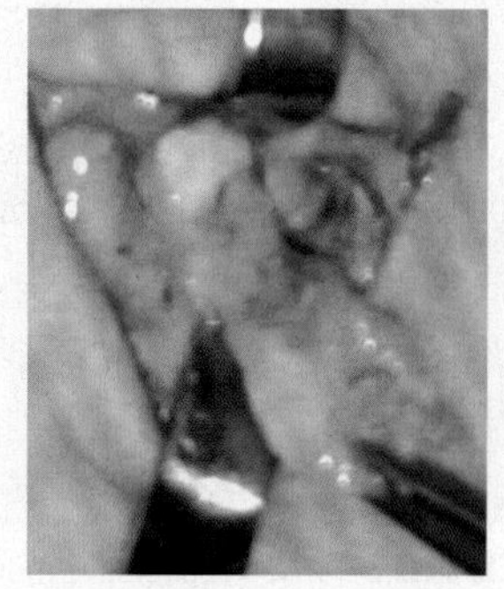

TECH FIG 2 • **A.** A Brunner type of incision allows for more exposure and avoids contracture associated with straight longitudinal incisions in this location. **B.** A volar cyst adherent to the radial artery and venae comitantes. **C.** A volar wrist ganglion stalk arising from the volar radiocarpal ligaments.

- Under loupe magnification, the subcutaneous tissues are carefully dissected and branches of the lateral antebrachial cutaneous nerve and dorsal radial sensory nerve are carefully protected. If dissection ulnar to the FCR tendon is required, the palmar cutaneous branch of the median nerve must also be identified and protected.
- Ganglion cysts in this location are commonly adherent to the radial artery and its venae comitantes (**TECH FIG 2B**). Take care to avoid injury to the artery. If the cyst cannot be freely dissected from the artery, a small cuff of cyst wall can be left adherent to the artery without a significant increase in recurrence.[9]
- The cyst is traced to a stalk that most often arises from the volar radiocarpal ligaments (**TECH FIG 2C**). The cyst is excised at the base of the stalk. We routinely send the cyst for pathologic evaluation.
- As with dorsal ganglion cysts, we cauterize the site of origin of the cyst with a bipolar electrocautery.
- After excision of the cyst, the tourniquet is deflated to ensure that the radial artery is uninjured. Satisfactory hemostasis is achieved.
- We generally close the wound with a running subcuticular suture, removed about 7 to 10 days after surgery.
- We prefer to dress the wound with antibiotic ointment and petroleum gauze, and a bulky hand dressing is applied with a plaster palmar splint, maintaining the wrist in a neutral position.
  - The dressing is removed along with the sutures at about 1 week postoperatively and Steri-Strips are applied to the wound.

Open Curettage and Bone Grafting of an Intraosseous Ganglion Cyst

- The patient is positioned supine on the operating table with the operative hand resting on a hand table.
- Symptomatic intraosseous ganglion cysts most often involve the carpal bones. Surgical incisions are planned according to the preoperative studies (MRI and CT scans) to identify the best location for creating a cortical window and avoiding injury to cartilaginous surfaces.
- Under tourniquet control, make an appropriate incision and carry dissection to the level of the wrist capsule. Loupe magnification is often helpful during the dissection. Enter the wrist capsule, preserving important capsular ligaments.
- The bony cortex is generally weakened in the area of the cyst and access is easily accomplished with a handheld curette. If the cortex is not weak, a small cortical window can be created using 0.045-inch Kirschner wires to create small drill holes to create a cortical window.
- Curette the cyst cavity along with any mucinous material. Remove the cyst membrane.
- Pack the cyst cavity with bone graft or a bone graft substitute.
- Wound closure is accomplished in the usual manner.
- We usually immobilize the patient in a plaster splint for 1 week and then a cast for 3 to 5 weeks, depending on the cyst size and bone integrity.
- Obtain postoperative radiographs to monitor and ensure incorporation of the bone graft.

Excision of a Degenerative Mucous Cyst

- Mucous cysts can be excised under local digital block anesthesia.
- The hand is prepared in the standard fashion.
- A finger tourniquet is applied to the involved digit.
- We usually use a Brunner type of incision or a simple transverse incision incorporating the cyst and allowing access to the origin of the cyst, which arises from the distal interphalangeal joint capsule between the terminal extensor tendon and collateral ligament (**TECH FIG 3A**).
- During the dissection, take care to avoid injury to the germinal matrix of the nail bed (**TECH FIG 3B**).
- Excise the cyst at the base of its stalk along with a portion of the joint capsule (**TECH FIG 3C**).

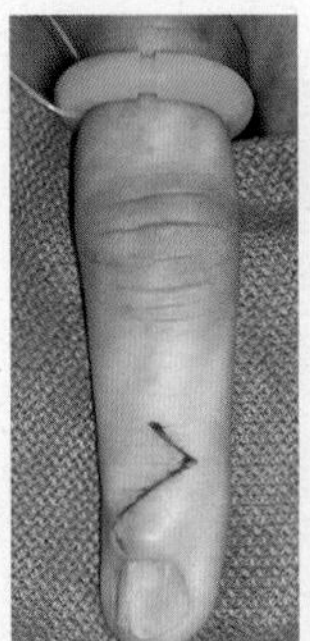
A
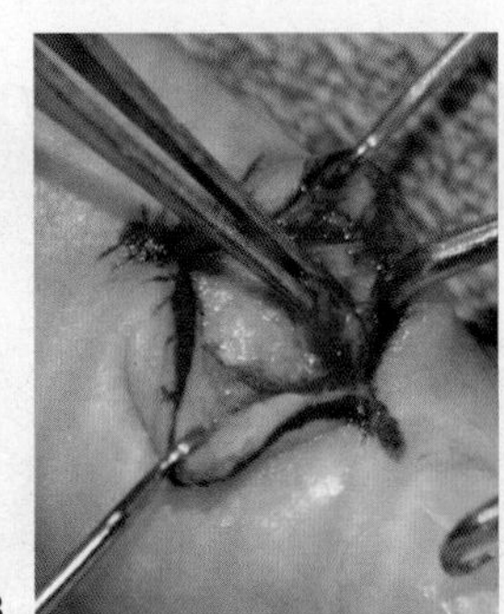
B
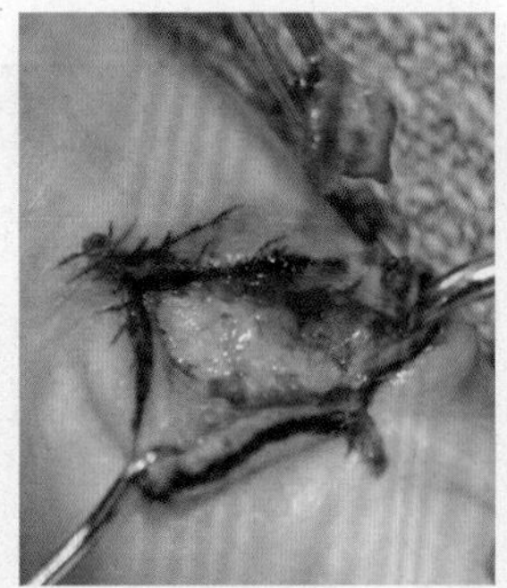
C
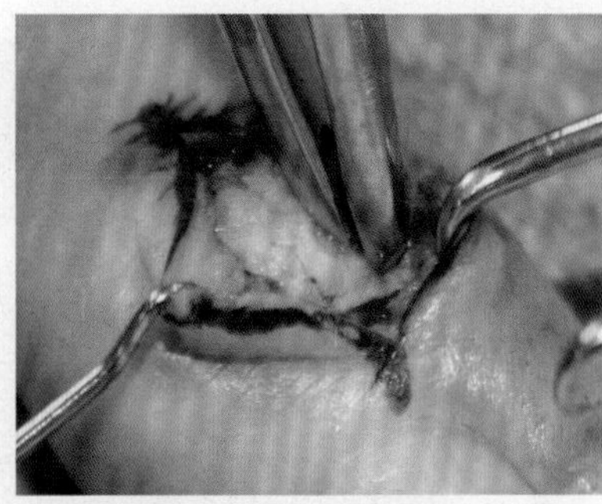
D

TECH FIG 3 • **A.** Degenerative mucous cyst in the eponychial region resulting in nail plate deformity. **B.** Aggressive dissection is avoided distally to protect the nail germinal matrix. The cyst is traced proximally to its origin at the distal interphalangeal joint. **C.** The cyst is excised along with a portion of the joint capsule at its point of origin between the central tendon and collateral ligament. **D.** A rongeur is used to débride underlying osteophytes.

- Excising underlying osteophytes and hypertrophic synovial tissue is the key to preventing recurrence of the cyst (**TECH FIG 3D**).
- The wound is irrigated, the tourniquet is removed, and hemostasis is achieved with bipolar cautery.
- Wound closure is accomplished with nonabsorbable monofilament sutures.
- The wound is dressed with antibiotic ointment, petroleum gauze, gauze fluff, and tube gauze dressing.
- The patient is instructed to remove the dressing in 3 to 5 days, and then cleanse the wound daily with antibacterial soap and water.
- Sutures are removed at 7 to 10 days.

Excision of a Ganglion Cyst of Tendon Sheath (Volar Retinacular Cyst)

- The patient is supine on the operating table with the involved upper extremity resting on a hand table.
- Anesthesia is usually accomplished with local anesthetic.
- Under tourniquet control (well tolerated by most awake patients for the 10 to 15 minutes required), a skin incision is made over the suspected ganglion cyst.
- Loupe magnification aids in limiting the size of the incision and identifying important anatomic structures. Retract the soft tissues and the digital neurovascular bundles.
- The ganglion cyst is commonly identified arising from the first or second annular pulley region.
- Dissect the ganglion cyst from the surrounding soft tissues and excise it at its base. We usually cauterize the site of origin with the bipolar cautery, which lowers the chance of a recurrence.
- The tourniquet is released, hemostasis is achieved, and wound closure is performed.
- A light hand dressing is applied for 7 to 10 days.

Arthroscopic Excision of a Dorsal Wrist Ganglion Cyst

- The patient is positioned supine on the operating room table with the operative upper extremity positioned in an arthroscopic traction tower (**TECH FIG 4**).
- Identify the standard wrist arthroscopic and anatomic landmarks.
- The 3-4, 4-5, 6R, and 6U portals are typically used.
- Under tourniquet control, insert a 2.7-mm small joint arthroscope into the 3-4 or 4-5 portal sites to inspect the joint and identify the ganglion stalk. The stalk in the typical dorsal wrist ganglion cysts is found arising from the dorsal distal margin of the scapholunate intraosseous membrane just proximal to the dorsal scapholunate intraosseous ligament. The stalk is not always identifiable or visualized.[17]
- Introduce a 2.9-mm resector shaver into the joint and excise the stalk (when visible) along with a 1-cm portion of dorsal wrist capsule and ganglion cyst.
- Use extreme caution when resecting the ganglion stalk and capsule to avoid injury to the scapholunate ligament and intraosseous membrane as well as the overlying extensor carpi radialis brevis and extensor digitorum communis tendons.
- Midcarpal arthroscopy is performed if indicated, but routine inspection is not necessary when treating a dorsal wrist ganglion cyst.
- The portal sites are typically closed with a removable monofilament suture.
- A light hand dressing is applied with a plaster palmar splint, which is left in place for about 5 to 7 days.

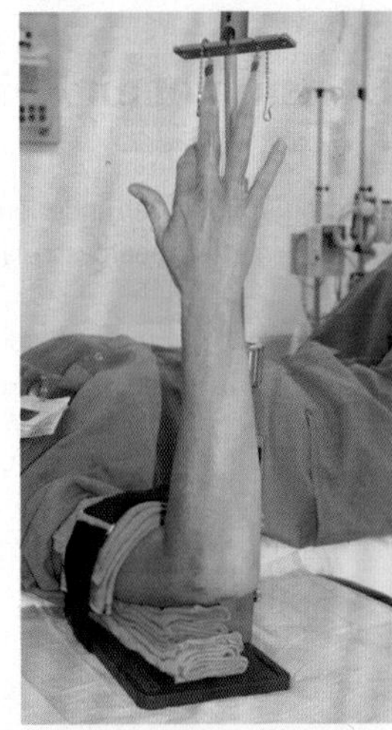

TECH FIG 4 • Standard arthroscopic setup using a traction tower. The traction tower, which can be sterilized, is typically positioned in this manner on a hand table after standard preparation and draping.

Excision of a Giant Cell Tumor of the Tendon Sheath

- The standard treatment is complete surgical removal.
- Careful surgical dissection is performed under loupe magnification (**TECH FIG 5A**).
- After initial exposure, isolate the neurovascular bundle proximal and distal to the lesion (**TECH FIG 5B**).
- Once the pseudocapsule is identified, it can be bluntly dissected or teased away from underlying structures with a Freer elevator, with care taken not to seed the surrounding tissues.[6] Alternatively, a small portion of the tendon sheath may be

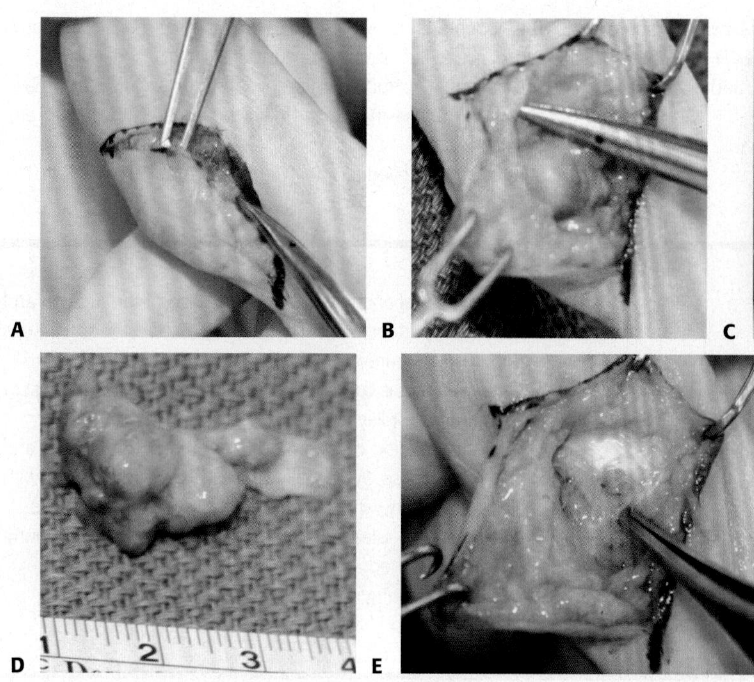

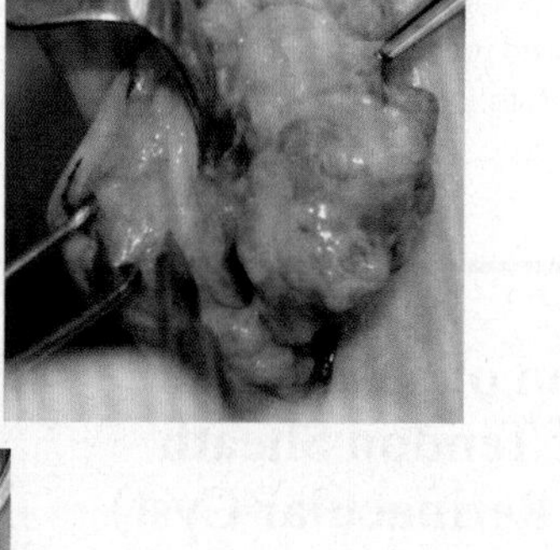

TECH FIG 5 • **A.** Careful surgical dissection of the subcutaneous tissues through a Brunner incision. **B.** The digital nerve is identified distal to the lesion and protected throughout the procedure. **C.** The tumor should be carefully removed from surrounding soft tissues. **D.** Excision demonstrates a firm, multinodular lesion. **E.** Any satellite lesions should be carefully identified and removed.

excised with the tumor origin and the area cauterized with bipolar electrocautery[12] (**TECH FIG 5C,D**).

- Carefully examine the local tissues for satellite lesions, which may be only a few millimeters in size. These lesions need to be completely excised (**TECH FIG 5E**).
- If the extensor tendon is involved, surgical excision of a portion of the tendon may be required. In rare cases, tendon reconstruction may be necessary. Lesions eroding into bone may require local curettage.
- If the tumor appears to arise from an underlying joint, it is important to perform a capsulotomy to inspect the joint and débride any pigmented tissue.[11]
- Arthrodesis of the distal interphalangeal joint may be necessary to completely excise some lesions.

Marginal Excision of an Epidermal Inclusion Cyst

- Careful surgical dissection is undertaken under loupe magnification.
- After initial exposure, isolate the neurovascular bundles in the area of the lesion.
- Once the capsule is identified, it can be sharply dissected from overlying skin and bluntly dissected from deeper soft tissues (**TECH FIG 6**).
- Take care to remove the entire capsule.
- Lesions eroding into bone may require local curettage and bone graft.
- In rare cases with advanced bony destruction, amputation is an alternative.

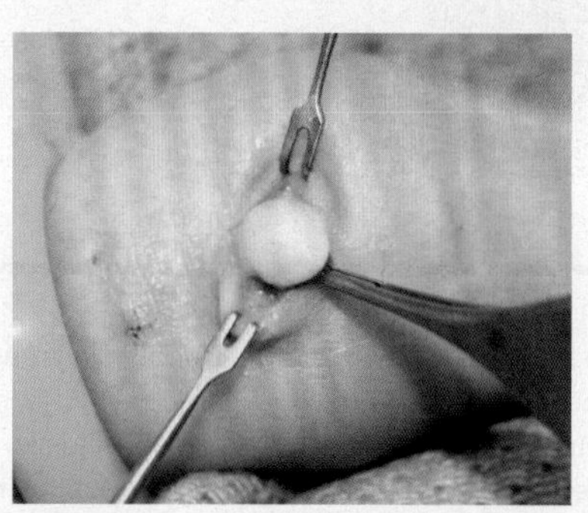

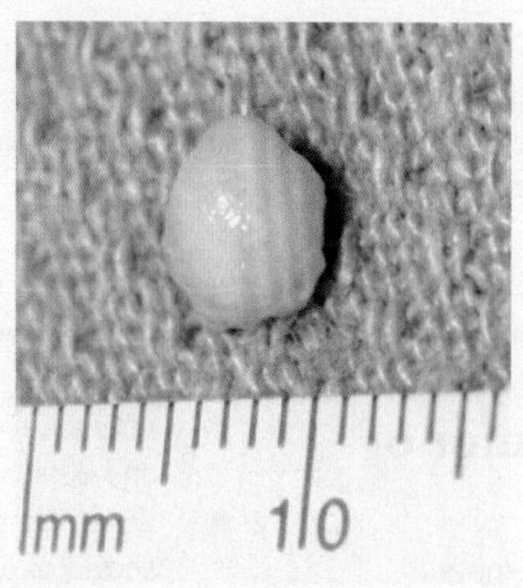

TECH FIG 6 • **A.** Through a small longitudinal incision directly over the lesion, the cyst is bluntly excised from surrounding soft tissues. **B.** Excision of the lesion demonstrates a firm, white, encapsulated mass.

PEARLS AND PITFALLS

Dorsal ganglion cysts	■ The scapholunate ligament is just distal to the tubercle of Lister. Dorsal ganglion cysts almost always arise from the distal margin of the dorsal scapholunate intraosseous membrane, just proximal to the dorsal scapholunate ligament. ■ Excise the cyst at the base of the stalk, which is the site of origin. ■ Cauterize the site of origin with a bipolar cautery to decrease the chances of recurrence. ■ Take care to avoid injury to the dorsal scapholunate ligament. ■ If the ganglion cyst recedes in size before surgery, dissect to identify the scapholunate ligament, which will often reveal the cyst.
Volar wrist ganglion cysts	■ Always identify both superficial and deep branches of the radial artery when excising these cysts. These vessels are often adherent to the artery. ■ Take care to avoid injury to branches of the lateral antebrachial cutaneous and dorsal radial sensory nerves when exposing the cysts.
Degenerative mucous cysts	■ Perform a small capsulectomy at the site of cyst origin and débride underlying osteophytes and hypertrophic synovium to prevent recurrence. ■ Take care to avoid injury to the extensor origin and germinal matrix of the nail bed. ■ Even when the cyst thins the overlying dermis, preserve the skin for closure. Rarely, skin grafts are required. A portion of the cyst wall attached to the skin can be left behind as long as the cyst origin is excised and osteophytes are débrided.
Giant cell tumors	■ The patient should be advised of the high recurrence rate after excision. ■ Neurovascular structures should be carefully isolated. ■ Satellite lesions should be completely excised. ■ An arthrotomy should be performed for suspected joint involvement.
Epidermal inclusion cysts	■ Biopsy should be considered for cases where a lytic bony lesion is present to rule out neoplasm or infection. ■ Neurovascular structures should be carefully protected. ■ Bony lesions may require curettage and bone graft.

POSTOPERATIVE CARE

Ganglion Cysts of the Wrist

- The splint and sutures are removed about 1 week postoperatively and Steri-Strips applied to the wound.
- Range-of-motion exercises and light use of the hand are initiated at 1 week, with gradual advancement of activities as tolerated.
- Scar massage is encouraged at 2 weeks.

Ganglion Cyst of Tendon Sheath and Degenerative Mucous Cyst

- Patients are instructed to remove their postoperative dressing 4 to 5 days after surgery. We prefer to have the patients clean their wound at least twice daily with antibacterial soap and water. The wound is redressed with light gauze or an adhesive bandage.
- Sutures are generally removed at 1 week and Steri-Strips applied to the wound.
- Range-of-motion exercises and light use of the hand are initiated, with gradual advancement of activities as tolerated.
- Scar massage is encouraged at 2 weeks.

Intraosseous Ganglion Cysts

- Postoperative dressing and sutures are removed at 1 week and Steri-Strips applied to the wound.
- We generally apply a short-arm cast for 3 to 5 weeks. The cast is removed and range-of-motion exercises and light hand use are initiated.
- Incorporation of the bone graft is monitored with use of serial radiographs. If the intraosseous ganglion cyst has weakened the bone, a protective splint may be used once the cast is removed until incorporation of the bone graft.

Giant Cell Tumors and Epidermal Inclusion Cysts

- Patients should be instructed about the high rate of recurrence of giant cell tumors.
- Range-of-motion exercises and antiedema techniques should be started immediately after surgery.
- Sutures can be removed at 8 to 10 days.

OUTCOMES

Ganglion Cysts

- Symptomatic relief is often accomplished after excision of most ganglion cysts.
- Recurrence rates after ganglion cyst surgery have been reported to range from 4% to 40%.[18] With adherence to the preceding principles, however, the recurrence rate in our experience is less than 5%.
- Complications of ganglion cyst removal are infrequent.
- The recurrence rate of giant cell tumors has varied from 5% to 50%. The high rate of recurrence is due to incomplete excision or satellite lesions.[6]
- Recurrence rates are even higher after excision of a recurrent tumor.[16]
- In contrast, the recurrence rate after epidermal inclusion cyst excision, even with bony involvement, is low.

COMPLICATIONS

- Wound complications (eg, painful or unsightly scar), infection, digital neurapraxia, or recurrence can occur.
- Ganglion cyst excision can result in a neurovascular injury. This complication is rare with adherence to good surgical technique and a good understanding of the local anatomy. Volar wrist ganglion cysts are adherent to the radial artery and can be difficult to dissect free from the artery. If necessary, a cuff of the cyst is left attached to the artery. If injury to the artery does occur, a repair should be performed.
- Stiffness is a complication of ganglion cyst excision. Avoiding direct capsular closure reduces the risk of this complication.
- Complications associated with degenerative mucous cysts include extensor lag, joint stiffness, infection, nail plate deformity, and distal interphalangeal joint deformity.[5]

REFERENCES

1. Angelides AC. Ganglions of the hand and wrist. In: Green DP, Hotchkiss RN, Pederson WC, eds. Operative Hand Surgery, vol 2, ed 4. New York: Churchill Livingstone, 1999:2171–2183.
2. Athanasian EA. Bone and soft tissue tumors. In: Green DP, Hotchkiss RN, Pederson WC, et al, eds. Operative Hand Surgery, vol 2, ed 5. New York: Churchill Livingstone, 2005:2211–2264.
3. Burge P. Aspiration of ganglia. J Hand Surg Br 1993;18(3):409–410.
4. Dodge LD, Brown RL, Niebauer JJ, et al. The treatment of mucous cysts: long-term follow-up in sixty-two cases. J Hand Surg Am 1984;9(6):901–904.
5. Fritz GR, Stern PJ, Dickey M. Complications following mucous cyst excision. J Hand Surg Br 1997;22(2):222–225.
6. Glowacki KA. Giant cell tumors of the tendon sheath. J Am Soc Surg Hand 2003;3:100–107.
7. Glowacki KA, Weiss AP. Giant cell tumor of the tendon sheath. Hand Clin 1995;11(2):245–253.
8. Greendyke SD, Wilson M, Shepler TR. Anterior wrist ganglia from the scaphotrapezial joint. J Hand Surg Am 1992;17(3):487–490.
9. Lister GD, Smith RR. Protection of the radial artery in the resection of adherent ganglions of the wrist. Plast Reconstr Surg 1978;61:127–129.
10. Mackie IG, Howard CB, Wilkins P. The dangers of sclerotherapy in the treatment of ganglia. J Hand Surg Br 1984;9(2):181–184.
11. Moore JR, Weiland AJ, Curtis RM. Localized nodular tenosynovitis: experience with 115 cases. J Hand Surg Am 1982;9(3):412–417.
12. Nahra ME, Bucchieri JS. Ganglion cysts and other tumor related conditions of the hand and wrist. Hand Clin 2004;20:249–260.
13. Nield DV, Evans DM. Aspiration of ganglia. J Hand Surg Br 1986;11(2):264.
14. Oni JA. Treatment of ganglia by aspiration alone. J Hand Surg Br 1992;17(6):660.
15. Paul AS, Sochart DH. Improving the results of ganglion aspiration by the use of hyaluronidase. J Hand Surg Br 1997;22(2):219–221.
16. Reilly KE, Stern PJ, Dale A. Recurrent giant cell tumors of the tendon sheath. J Hand Surg Am 1999;24(6):1298–1302.
17. Rizzo M, Berger RA, Steinman SP, et al. Arthroscopic resection in the management of dorsal wrist ganglions: results with a minimum 2-year follow-up period. J Hand Surg Am 2004;29(1):59–62.
18. Thornburg LE. Ganglions of the hand and wrist. J Am Acad Orthop Surg 1999;7:231–238.
19. Wang AA, Hutchinson DT. Longitudinal observation of pediatric hand and wrist ganglia. J Hand Surg Am 2001;26(4):599–602.
20. Ward WA, Labosky DA. Ruptured epidermal inclusion cyst in the palm presenting as a collar-button abscess. J Hand Surg Am 1985;10(6 pt 1):899–901.
21. Zubowicz VN, Ishii CH. Management of ganglion cysts of the hand by simple aspiration. J Hand Surg Am 1987;12(4):618–620.

SUGGESTED READINGS

Soren A. Pathogenesis and treatment of ganglion. Clin Orthop Relat Res 1996;48:173–179.

Westbrook AP, Stephen AB, Oni J, et al. Ganglia: the patient's perception. J Hand Surg Br 2000;25(6):566–567.

Surgical Treatment of Nerve Tumors in the Distal Upper Extremity

146

CHAPTER

Christopher L. Forthman, Susanne Roberts, and Philip E. Blazar

DEFINITION

- Nerve tumors make up less than 5% of tumors about the hand and wrist.[13]
- Most nerve tumors are benign and grow without causing neural dysfunction. As a result, the neural origin of a mass is often not anticipated and unexpected loss of function may occur after surgery.
- The key is to prepare for excision of any mass by discussing the possibility of a nerve tumor with the patient, by recognizing patients and masses with a high likelihood of a nerve tumor, and by being familiar with surgical techniques that allow preservation or, if necessary, reconstruction of the affected nerve.

ANATOMY

- Peripheral nerves consist of axons surrounded by a nerve sheath (**FIG 1**).
- The epineurium is a thin outer layer of connective tissue containing blood vessels that supply the nerve.
- Perineural cells form a strong cellular layer, the perineurium, surrounding each fascicle (bundle) of axons.
- An endoneurial layer of protective Schwann cells surrounds each individual axon.

PATHOGENESIS

- Tumors of the peripheral nerve arise from and resemble components of the nerve sheath.
- Most nerve tumors arise from the Schwann cell and are informally called *schwannomas* (or neurilemomas). Schwannomas surround the nerve.[11]

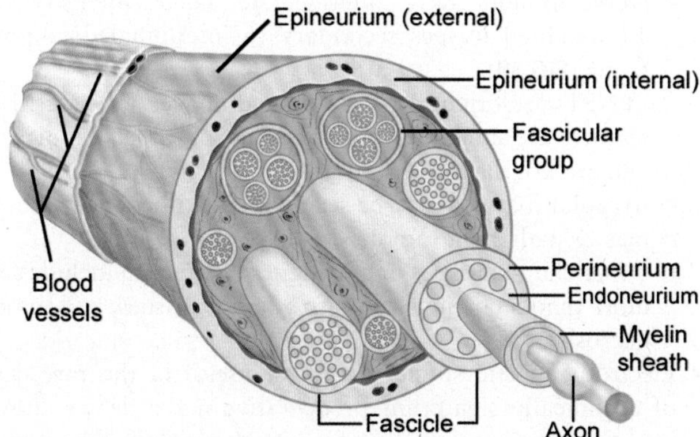

FIG 1 • Peripheral nerve anatomy. Individual axons travel together within a well-organized nerve sheath. The cells of the nerve sheath (not the axons) form the nerve tumor.

- Neurofibromas also arise from nonmyelinating Schwann cells but are found within the substance of the nerve and cannot be enucleated from the fascicles.[11]
- Other benign peripheral nerve sheath tumors (BPNSTs) include the granular cell tumor, neurothekeoma, nerve sheath myxoma, and perineurioma. Electron microscopy and immunohistochemistry may be necessary to determine the type of tumor and cell of origin in some cases.[3]
- Malignant peripheral nerve sheath tumors (MPNSTs) arise de novo or from malignant change within a BPNST, usually a neurofibroma.
  - About half of MPNSTs occur in patients with neurofibromatosis (NF) type I (von Recklinghausen disease).
  - The incidence of a MPNST in patients with NF type I is 2%[8] (compared to 0.001% in general population[4]), although the lifetime risk rises to 13%.[2]

NATURAL HISTORY

- Upper extremity BPNSTs are usually solitary and occur most in middle-aged adults.[5,7]
  - Pediatric nerve tumors are uncommon.[1]
- BPNSTs are typically painless and slow-growing, with malignant degeneration being exceedingly rare. Most tumors are relatively small (<2.5 cm), although they may cause nerve dysfunction due to focal impingement on the adjacent axons.
- Patients with NF type I often have multiple schwannomas, neurofibromas, or both of major upper extremity nerves. Thick tortuous "plexiform" neurofibromas are common in NF type I and have a high risk of progression to malignancy.

PATIENT HISTORY AND PHYSICAL FINDINGS

- The history should include the duration, growth characteristics, and local effects of the mass. Mild discomfort is common with nerve tumors, but pain is more consistent with MPNST than BPNST. Paresthesias are the exception rather than the rule. Hence, the possibility of a nerve tumor must often be entertained for the sake of completeness alone. Similarly, physical examination may suggest but cannot definitively diagnose a nerve tumor.
- A complete examination of a distal upper extremity soft tissue mass should evaluate other nonneural possibilities within the differential diagnosis.
  - Ganglia: arise from joint and tendon sheaths in characteristic locations. The mass will typically transilluminate and the diagnosis can be confirmed by aspiration of highly viscous mucinoid material. Ganglia may mimic nerve tumors by causing compression of an adjacent nerve (eg, a ganglion in the canal of Guyon may cause ulnar neuropathy) (**FIG 2**).

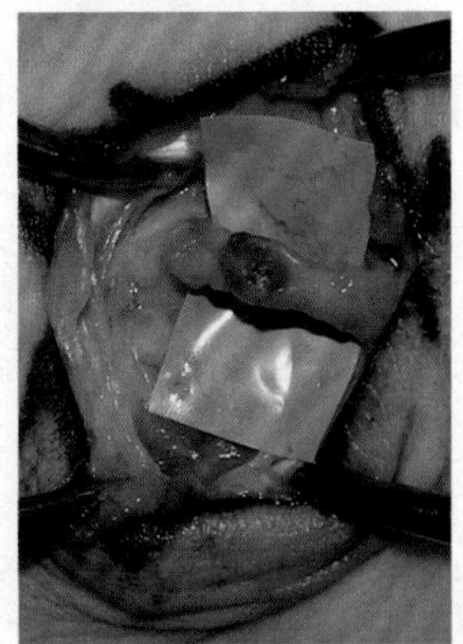
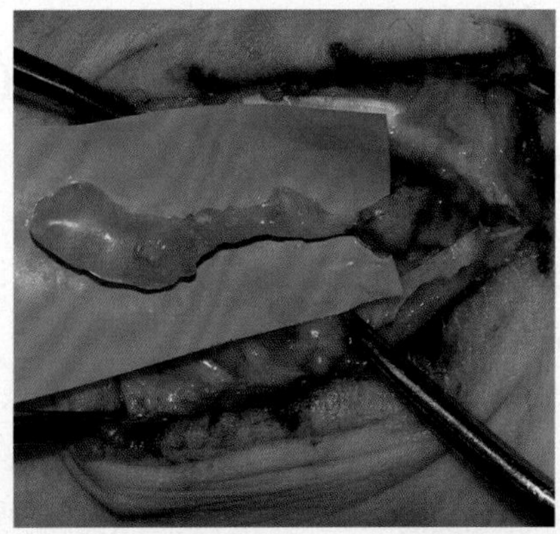
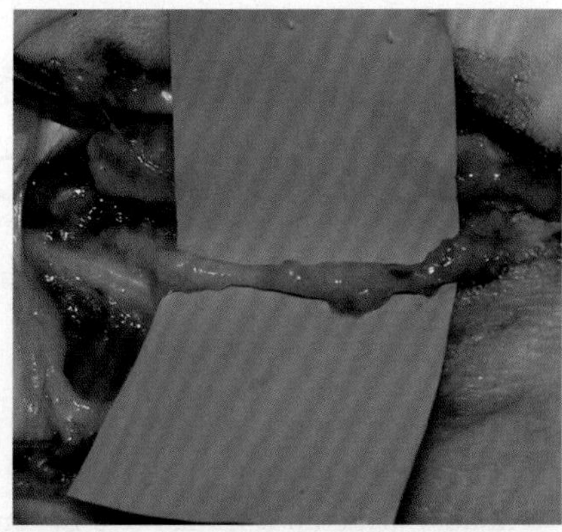

FIG 2 • **A.** Hypesthesia of the thenar eminence caused by an apparent tumor of the palmar cutaneous branch (PCB) of the median nerve. **B.** Careful dissection reveals a ganglion arising from the radioscaphoid articulation. **C.** The PCB is freed from the compressive mass.

- Giant cell tumors (GCTs) of the tendon sheath: reactive lesions of synovium that occur about the palm and fingers in similar locations to nerve tumors. GCTs are often palpably nodular compared to the smooth margins of a nerve tumor.
- Lipomas: These fatty tumors are usually more superficial and mobile than a nerve tumor. Rarely, lipomas grow in the carpal canal, causing median neuropathy.
- Epidermal inclusion cysts: should be suspected when examination reveals evidence of prior penetrating trauma. Unlike neuromas, these cysts do not cause nerve symptoms and a Tinel sign is not present.
- Nodular fasciitis: a firm, reactive soft tissue proliferation that may grow rapidly on the volar surface of the forearm or hand. The location may suggest a nerve tumor and the aggressive spread mimics sarcoma. Although most nerve tumors are mobile in the transverse plane, palpation of nodular fasciitis reveals dense adhesions to the adjacent subcutaneous tissue.

- Patients with NF type I may have multiple nerve tumors, along with features such as café-au-lait spots, freckling in the axilla or groin, optic pathway tumors, iris hamartomas, and bone dysplasias. In patients with NF type 1, rapid growth of a neurofibroma, severe pain, and a new neurologic deficit often herald malignant degeneration.
- Examination techniques include the following:
  - Palpation: The examiner moves the mass transversely and longitudinally. Nerve tumors may be translated transversely but are tethered in the longitudinal plane.
  - Sensory testing using Semmes-Weinstein monofilament. Early nerve compression increases threshold, whereas innervation density (two-point) remains normal. In a busy clinical practice, light moving touch may be as reliable (Stauch).[12]
  - The examiner assesses visible atrophy and weakness in motor units innervated by the affected nerve. Manual strength testing is usually normal.
  - Direct pressure is applied over the nerve just proximal to the mass. Nerves under compression by a mass are sometimes sensitive to touch and may produce paresthesias when manipulated.
  - The nerve is percussed immediately adjacent to the mass. A positive result is paresthesias in the cutaneous distribution of the nerve. The Tinel sign is positive only when an injured nerve is attempting to regenerate. Most nerve tumors do not have a positive Tinel sign.

IMAGING AND OTHER DIAGNOSTIC STUDIES

- Plain radiographs should be obtained to look for intralesional calcification or invasion of adjacent bony architecture.
  - Intralesional calcification is rarely seen in BPNST and should alert the surgeon to the more likely possibility of a lipoma, hemangioma, GCT of tendon sheath, synovial chondromatosis, calcific tendonitis, myositis ossificans, or synovial sarcoma.
  - A malignant nerve tumor may invade nearby osseous structures.
- Ultrasound is another good screening modality that can provide information about cystic or solid character, size, and an associated traceable nerve. Ultrasound cannot readily distinguish schwannomas, neurofibromas, and MPNST.
- A magnetic resonance imaging (MRI) is the gold standard imaging modality and is useful for evaluating tumor characteristics, delineating the surrounding anatomy, and planning a surgical approach.
  - Localization of the tumor to the vicinity of a large nerve trunk suggests a peripheral nerve tumor (**FIG 3A**).
  - MRI may also occasionally demonstrate subtle muscle atrophy of the distally innervated musculature. Tumor margins are smooth and there is mild intralesional inhomogeneity.
  - Nerve tumors have intermediate signal intensity on T1-weighted images secondary to intermingled adipose tissue (**FIG 3B**).
  - BPNSTs are bright on T2-weighted images.[14] These MRI features are similar to those of other soft tissue neoplasms and are not diagnostic.[9]
  - Irregular margins may be seen with plexiform neurofibromas or malignant tumors.
  - Other characteristics of a malignant neoplasm include size more than 5 cm, invasion into adjacent tissues, and tumor necrosis.
- Electrodiagnostic studies are most useful in the rare case of a clinically significant preoperative nerve deficit. Slowing of the nerve conduction velocity at the site of the tumor manifests as increases in the distal motor and sensory latencies, whereas electromyography will detect subtle muscle denervation.

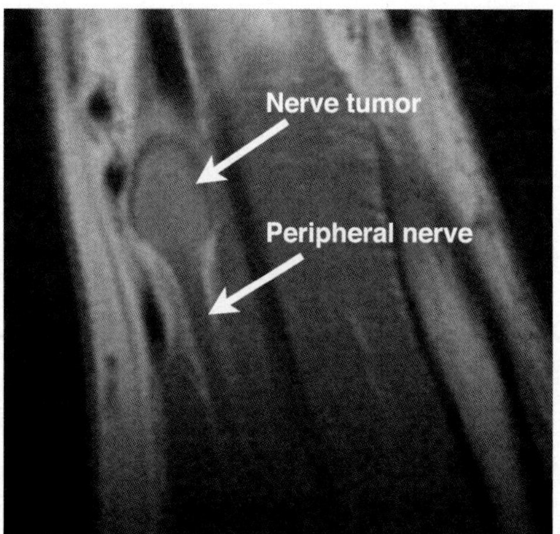

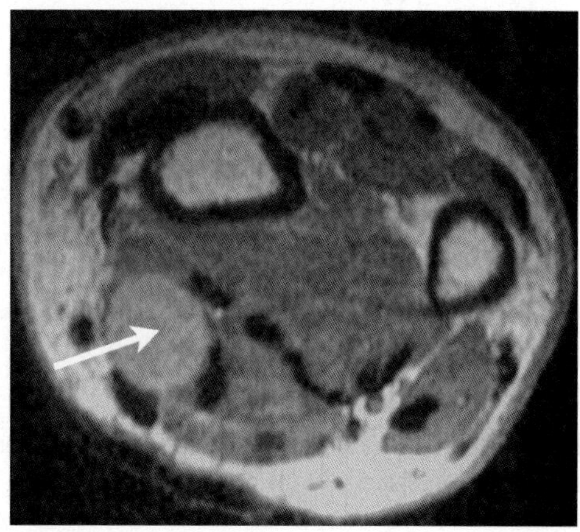

FIG 3 ● **A.** Cross-sectional imaging of a BPNST reveals the mass to be contiguous with normal axons proximally. **B.** MRI of a benign nerve sheath tumor (*arrow*) often demonstrates a high fat content, seen best on T1-weighted images.

DIFFERENTIAL DIAGNOSIS

- Neuroma
- Lipofibromatous hamartoma (fibrofatty infiltration)
- Nerve sheath ganglion
- Intraneural tumors of nonneural origin
  - Intraneural lipoma
  - Intraneural hemangioma

NONOPERATIVE MANAGEMENT

- In the absence of rapid growth, pain, or nerve dysfunction, it is reasonable to observe a distal upper extremity mass. An MRI may be obtained to identify features consistent with a BPNST and to exclude signs of malignancy (see earlier).
- Patients with NF type I often have multiple neurofibromas, including dermal and plexiform types.
  - Dermal neurofibromas grow through the dermis and subcutaneous tissue to form plaque-like swellings. Although sometimes unsightly, these tumors are routinely observed, as the surgical defects are no more cosmetically pleasing.
  - Plexiform neurofibromas are visible as nodular masses lying longitudinally along the course of peripheral nerves. These tumors must be carefully followed as progression to a MPNST (neurofibrosarcoma) is common.
  - Pain is the most predictive symptom of malignant change. If there is no concern for malignancy, surgical excision is generally avoided, as it frequently results in nerve deficits postoperatively.
- Children and young adults may develop masses of fibrofatty tissue infiltrating major nerves and their branches, particularly the median nerve.
  - These lipofibromatous hamartomas cause slow progressive nodular swelling and, at times, distal soft tissue overgrowth (macrodactyly).
  - When asymptomatic, nonoperative management may be preferred, particularly if MRI shows pathognomonic features of this lesion.[15]
  - Carpal tunnel symptoms may be treated with limited surgery, including an open carpal tunnel release and a definitive biopsy of a small cutaneous branch of the nerve.

SURGICAL MANAGEMENT

- An isolated distal upper extremity mass is treated surgically for definitive diagnosis, to control symptoms, or to exclude malignancy.

Preoperative Planning

- MRI is reviewed to confirm characteristics of a BPNST and to plan a surgical approach.
- Nerve reconstruction options are discussed with the patient.
- We consider synthetic absorbable nerve conduits for defects of up to 2 cm, particularly in the palm.
  - We avoid conduits when there is any concern of extrusion (eg, about joints in the digits) or in superficial sites where foreign body reaction may be confused with a tumor recurrence.
  - The medial antebrachial cutaneous nerve (MABC) is a suitable graft for the common and proper digital nerves.
  - A sural nerve cable graft may be necessary for major peripheral nerve defects.
- If significant nerve dysfunction is present before surgery (or is expected afterward), consideration should be given to performing concomitant tendon transfers, particularly in adults.

Positioning

- The patient is positioned supine with the affected extremity placed on a hand table. A brachial tourniquet is applied proximally, allowing access to the medial elbow for MABC nerve harvest if necessary.
- If sural nerve harvest is considered a possibility, we place a proximal thigh tourniquet and prepare and drape the contralateral lower extremity so that a second team may operate unencumbered.

Approach

- The surgical approach varies with tumor location.
  - A midlateral approach to digital nerve lesions allows excellent visualization of the tumor, protection of the adjacent digital artery, and good soft tissue coverage of the adjacent flexor tendon sheath.

- Lesions in the palm are approached with a Brunner zigzag type of skin incision, which provides excellent visualization and minimizes restrictive postoperative longitudinal scar formation.
- An open carpal tunnel approach is included for tumors close to the median nerve to decrease nerve compression from postoperative edema.
- Any suspected malignancy is managed according to the principles described in the oncology section of this text: A biopsy incision must allow optimal definitive resection options later. For example, a biopsy of a possible neurofibrosarcoma of the radial sensory nerve should be made through the mobile wad compartment as opposed to the more familiar Henry approach to this region.

Enucleation

- Most isolated BPNSTs are schwannomas and arise eccentrically from the nerve sheath (**TECH FIG 1A**). The tumor is encapsulated and can be safely enucleated without removing nerve fascicles.
- The nerve is exposed and fascicles are seen to drape over the mass, sometimes with a pedicled or multilobulated appearance. Inspect the nerve circumferentially for the window of splayed fascicles that affords the best resection plane (**TECH FIG 1B**).
- Incise the nerve sheath longitudinally, preserving the vessels running in the epineurium. Expand the window by carefully peeling away the fascicles and, ultimately, delivering the tumor out of the nerve (**TECH FIG 1C**).
- The resected specimen contains no nerve fascicles (**TECH FIG 1D**).

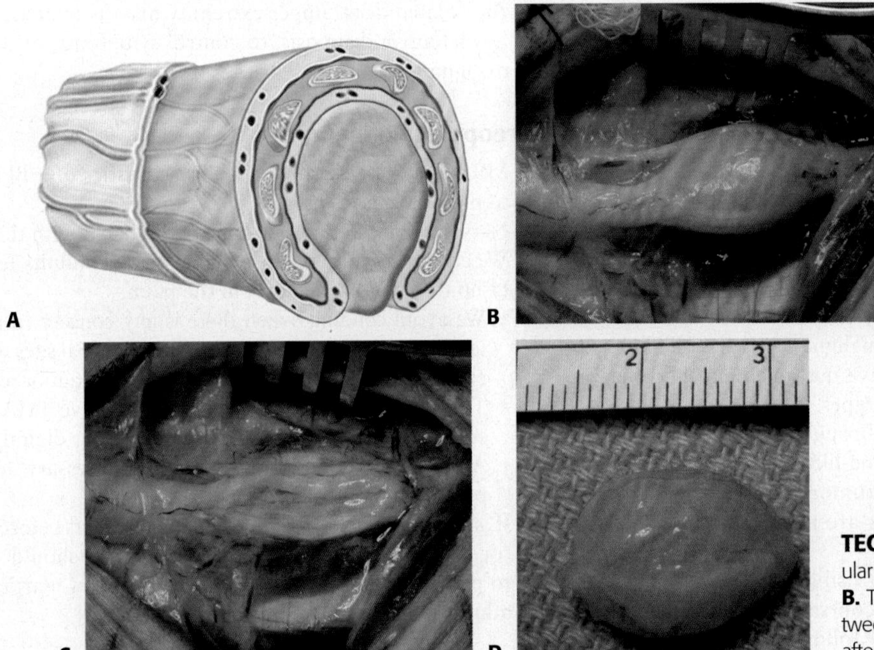

TECH FIG 1 • **A.** Nerve fascicles and fascicular groups are displaced by a schwannoma. **B.** The tumor may be "shelled out" from between the splayed fascicles. **C.** Intact fascicles after tumor resection. **D.** Specimen.

Nerve Repairs, Grafts, and Conduits

- Surgical exploration of a nerve tumor may reveal a centrally placed expansile lesion with characteristic incorporation of nerve fascicles within the mass—the neurofibroma (**TECH FIG 2A**). Although poorly encapsulated within the nerve, these tumors are typically free of adhesions to the adjacent soft tissues. Complete excision may require resection of the involved section of the nerve.
- The neurofibroma is exposed similar to the schwannoma. In this case, fusiform expansion of the posterior interosseous nerve is identified. Fascicles are seen entering the lesion at its proximal and distal extent, confirming the diagnosis of a neurofibroma (**TECH FIG 2B**).
- A microscope may allow identification of a prominent fascicular group that can be microdissected from the adjacent normal fascicles. If no prominent fascicular group or groups can be identified, then tumor resection will require nerve transection through normal fascicles at each end of the mass.
  - Direct reapproximation of the nerve ends is optimal but should be done only with minimal joint flexion and tension. Direct repairs done with significant joint flexion or high tension have poor results.

- The MABC is harvested if an autologous nerve graft is required (**TECH FIG 2C**). The nerve exits the brachial fascia adjacent to the basilic vein at the junction of the middle and distal third of the forearm.
  - The length of the nerve may be harvested for a nerve cable graft if a major peripheral nerve has been sacrificed.
- The small anterior branch of the MABC may be harvested an inch anterior and distal to the medial epicondyle. The anterior branch is generally a good size match for a digital nerve, as seen in this case of a nerve tumor with iatrogenic soft tissue loss (**TECH FIG 2D**).
  - Alternatively, a nerve tube may be used to bridge an intercalary nerve defect (**TECH FIG 2E**).
- A digital neurofibroma can be resected and the defect bridged with a nerve tube (**TECH FIG 2F**). Studies suggest that nerve conduits are best suited for defects of 2 cm or less.

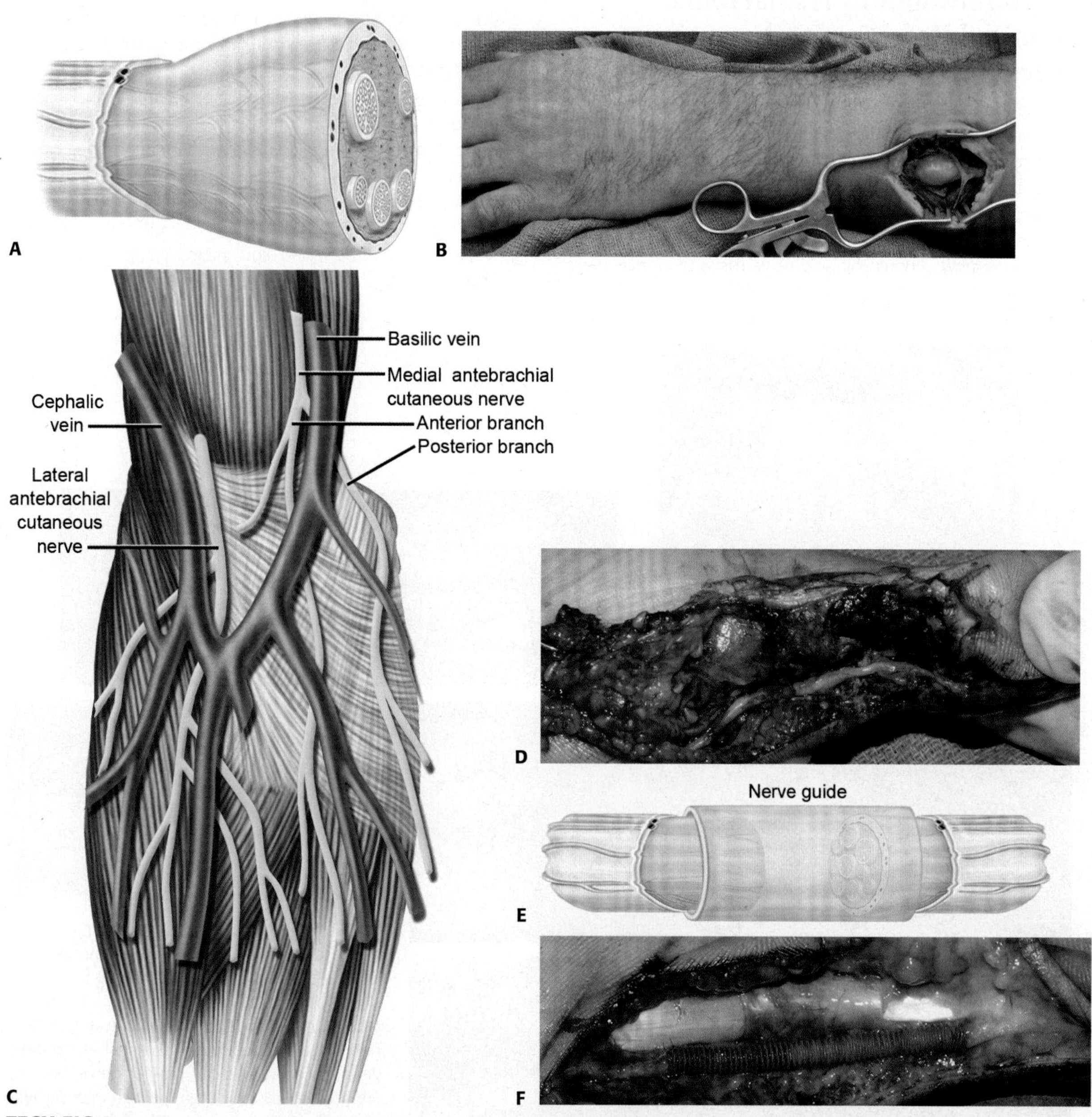

TECH FIG 2 • **A.** Fascicles are intertwined with tumor cells in a neurofibroma; tumor resection often requires excising a segment of nerve. **B.** A neurofibroma of the posterior interosseous nerve (PIN). This tumor was inseparable from normal nerve fascicles and excision resulted in permanent loss of finger extension. **C.** Branches of the MABC run with the basilic vein. The anterior branch is a good match for a digital nerve and can be harvested near the elbow. **D.** The ulnar digital nerve of the thumb has been grafted with the MABC in this patient, with prior nerve tumor resection and iatrogenic soft tissue loss. **E.** Nerve conduits provide an environment for nerve regeneration and have been shown to be as good as or better than nerve grafts in many situations. **F.** A digital neurofibroma was resected and a nerve conduit placed to bridge the intercalary defect. The soft tissues were slow to heal due to motion about the conduit at the metacarpophalangeal joint. Newer, less rigid collagen nerve guides may be better suited for use around the finger joints; however, human trials are lacking.

Microdissection

- Digital nerve schwannomas may sometimes require microdissection to preserve axons.
- The nerve is isolated under loupe magnification.
- The operating microscope facilitates identification of normal nerve fibers proximally. These axon bundles are traced distally and carefully dissected free of the mass.
- Occasionally, microdissection will allow the surgeon to identify and preserve normal fascicles from a neurofibroma of a large peripheral nerve.[13]

Lipofibromatous Hamartoma: Limited Resection and Sural Nerve Grafting

- A lipofibromatous hamartoma of the median nerve is most apparent about the proximal and distal extent of the transverse carpal ligament (**TECH FIG 3A**). The contained space of the carpal canal limits outward expansion of the hamartoma, causing compression of nerve fascicles. Open carpal tunnel release may improve pain and nerve dysfunction. However, a mass that continues to grow, causing pain and nerve dysfunction, may need to be resected. Nerve grafts should be considered, especially in young patients.[6] Management in adults is controversial.
- Sagittal plane MRI images will show the extent of the lesion (**TECH FIG 3B**).
- Surgical exposure begins with an open carpal tunnel release to identify the transition zone between normal and abnormal nerve. The incision is carried distally in a Brunner zigzag type of fashion to find the end of the lesion (**TECH FIG 3C**).
- The hamartoma is excised en bloc at healthy-appearing fascicular margins (**TECH FIG 3D**).
- A sural nerve is harvested and interposed as a cable graft (**TECH FIG 3E**).

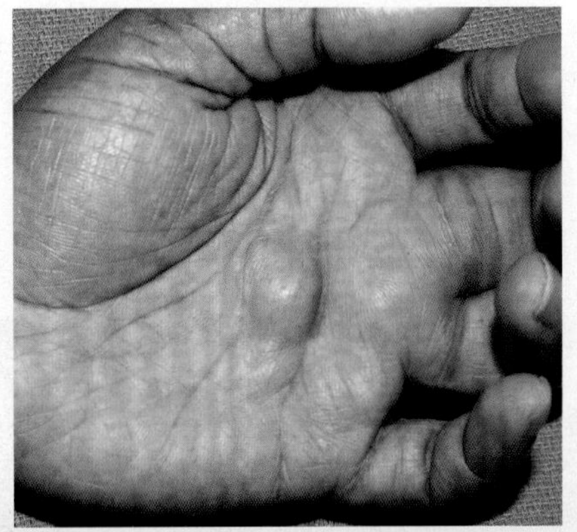
A

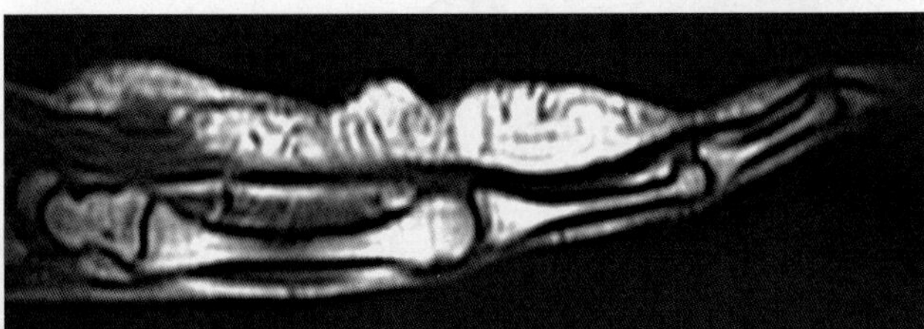
B

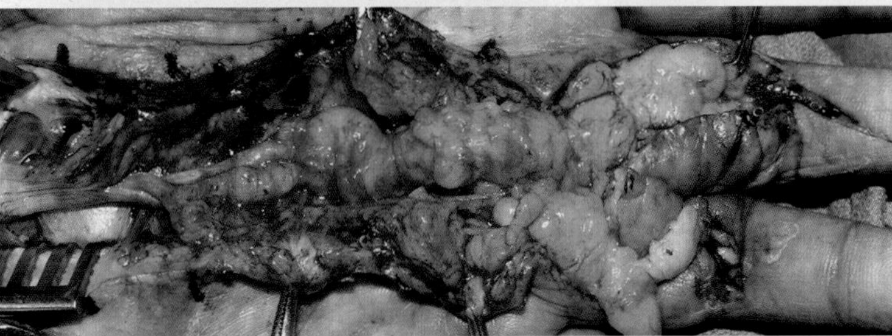
C

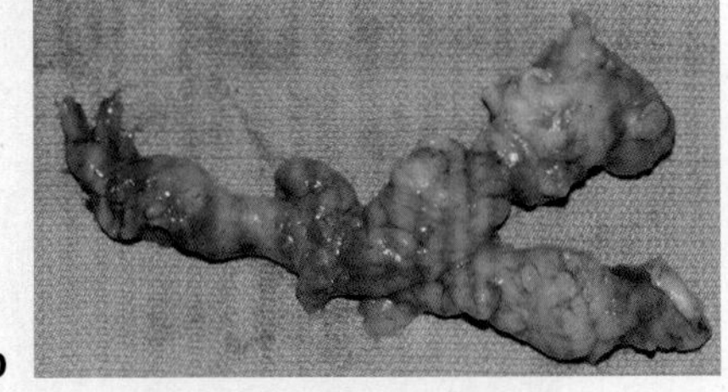
D

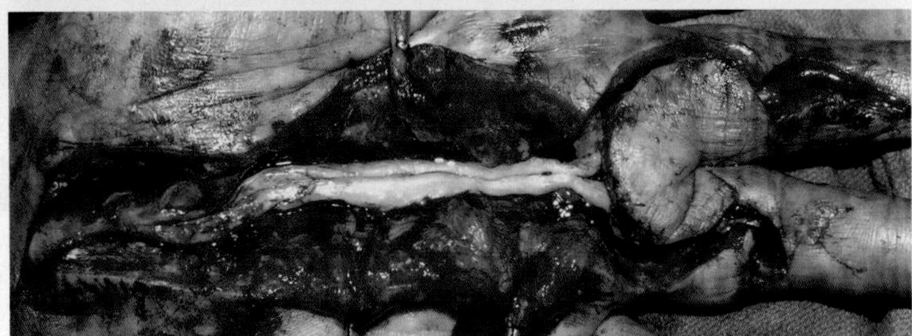
E

TECH FIG 3 • **A.** Painful expanding soft tissue mass along the common digital nerve to the third web space. The middle and ring fingers had slowly lost sensibility on the affected sides. **B.** MRI shows that the mass originates from the median nerve and extends to the proximal interphalangeal joint. Low-intensity normal nerve fascicles are seen coursing through the high-intensity fatty mass. **C.** At surgery, normal fascicles cannot be distinguished from the fibrofatty proliferation. **D.** Specimen. **E.** Sural nerve graft to the middle and ring finger proper digital nerves.

PEARLS AND PITFALLS

Diagnosis	■ A nerve tumor must be part of the differential diagnosis for any distal upper extremity mass. ■ Anticipation allows for appropriate preoperative planning and discussions with the patient.
Nonsurgical management	■ Watch for signs of malignancy, including increasing nerve dysfunction, rapid growth, and pain. ■ Plexiform neurofibromas seen in patients with NF type 1 have a high risk for malignant change.
Surgical approach	■ Masses should be resected through an extensile approach; avoid transverse incisions. ■ Tumors that are invasive into the adjacent tissue are likely malignant. An incisional biopsy should be performed and the wound closed.
Tumor resection	■ Loupe magnification and microinstruments facilitate enucleation of a tumor (schwannoma). ■ A microscope should be available should microdissection or nerve resection and reconstruction become necessary (neurofibroma).

POSTOPERATIVE CARE

- At a minimum, short arcs of joint motion are initiated early to discourage adhesion formation between the cutaneous scar and the underlying nerve.
- If necessary, the end range of motion may be avoided for up to 1 month to protect nerve repairs or reconstructions.
- When axons have been injured, a hand therapist may assist with desensitization or sensory reeducation.
- A Tinel sign may be followed for reinnervation along the course of the affected nerve.
- Late changes in nerve function or swelling suggest the possibility of recurrence.

OUTCOMES

- Transient paresthesias, numbness, or weakness are common after enucleation of a schwannoma (75%); however, long-term nerve function is generally the same as or improved compared to the preoperative state with a recovery rate of 95%.[10] Tumor recurrence is rare.
- Permanent neurologic deficits follow en bloc resection of a neurofibroma, thus limiting the surgical indications for this procedure. Microdissection preserves nerve function[13] but likely has an increased risk of recurrence.
- Resection of a lipofibromatous hamartoma of the median nerve (including partial excision or interfascicular dissection) often results in permanent nerve deficits. There is limited long-term follow-up for nerve grafting of these lesions.

COMPLICATIONS

- Loss of nerve function after tumor resection. Although this is more common in excision of neurofibromas, it is possible in enucleation of schwannomas (18%). The risk of major neurologic deficit or severe neuropathic pain and the fact that these complications may warrant reexploration with or without grafting should be discussed with the patient.[10]
- Loss of motion due to prolonged immobilization
- Neuroma formation at a nerve donor site (eg, MABC neuroma)
- Wound breakdown over a nerve conduit, especially in the digits

REFERENCES

1. Colon F, Upton J. Pediatric hand tumors. A review of 349 cases. Hand Clin 1995;11:223–243.
2. Evans DG, Baser ME, McGaughran J, et al. Malignant peripheral nerve sheath tumours in neurofibromatosis 1. J Med Genet 2002;39:311–314.
3. Forthman CL, Blazar PE. Nerve tumors of the hand and upper extremity. Hand Clin 2004;20:233–242.
4. Hajdu SI. Peripheral nerve sheath tumors. Histogenesis, classification, and prognosis. Cancer 1993;72:3549–3552.
5. Holdsworth BJ. Nerve tumours in the upper limb. A clinical review. J Hand Surg Br 1985;10(2):236–238.
6. Houpt P, Storm van Leeuwen JB, van den Bergen HA. Intraneural lipofibroma of the median nerve. J Hand Surg Am 1989;14(4):706–709.
7. Kehoe NJ, Reid RP, Semple JC. Solitary benign peripheral-nerve tumours. Review of 32 years' experience. J Bone Joint Surg Br 1995;77(3):497–500.
8. King AA, Debaun MR, Riccardi VM, et al. Malignant peripheral nerve sheath tumors in neurofibromatosis 1. Am J Med Genet 2000;93:388–392.
9. Kransdorf MJ, Jelinek JS, Moser RP Jr. Imaging of soft tissue tumors. Radiol Clin North Am 1993;31:359–372.
10. Park MJ, Seo KN, Kang HJ. Neurological deficit after surgical enucleation of schwannomas of the upper limb. J Bone Joint Surg Br 2009;91(11):1482–1486.
11. Rinaldi E. Neurilemomas and neurofibromas of the upper limb. J Hand Surg Am 1983;8(5 pt 1):590–593.
12. Strauch B, Lang A, Ferder M, et al. The ten test. Plast Reconstr Surg 1997;99:1074–1078.
13. Strickland JW, Steichen JB. Nerve tumors of the hand and forearm. J Hand Surg Am 1977;2(4):285–291.
14. Stull MA, Moser RP Jr, Kransdorf MJ, et al. Magnetic resonance appearance of peripheral nerve sheath tumors. Skeletal Radiol 1991;20:9–14.
15. Toms AP, Anastakis D, Bleakney RR, et al. Lipofibromatous hamartoma of the upper extremity: a review of the radiologic findings for 15 patients. AJR Am J Roentgenol 2006;186:805–811.

Treatment of Enchondroma, Bone Cyst, and Giant Cell Tumor of the Distal Upper Extremity

Edward A. Athanasian

DEFINITION

- Enchondromas are benign cartilaginous neoplasms that are commonly seen in the medullary cavity of phalanges and metacarpals and less commonly in the radius and ulna. Enchondroma is the most common neoplasm of bone arising in the hand.
- Unicameral bone cysts are benign endothelial-lined fluid-filled cavities arising in metaphyseal bone; they are occasionally seen in the distal radius and rarely seen in the hand.
- Giant cell tumor of bone is an uncommon neoplasm of bone, which is locally aggressive and can metastasize. Although its histology suggests a benign process, is behaves as a low-grade malignancy.

ANATOMY

- Enchondroma most commonly arises in the proximal phalanx or metacarpal when seen in the hand (**FIG 1A**). It can be seen in metaphyseal and epiphyseal regions and is typically confined to the bone. The enchondroma may distend the bone and pathologic fracture may be seen.
- Unicameral bone cysts are rarely seen in the hand. When presenting in the radius, they are often metaphyseal and may be in continuity with the distal radial physis (**FIG 1B**). Unicameral bone cysts are typically confined to bone and pathologic fracture may be seen.
- Giant cell tumor of bone most commonly arises in the epiphyseal region except in the skeletally immature patient, in whom it may arise in the metaphysis. The distal radius is the third most frequent location for these tumors (**FIG 1C**), after the distal femur and the proximal tibia. Hand lesions account for 2% of giant cell tumors of bone.

PATHOGENESIS

- The pathogenesis of enchondroma, unicameral bone cyst, and giant cell tumor of bone is uncertain. Enchondroma and unicameral bone cysts may be associated with bone development and growth.
- Enchondroma, unicameral bone cyst, and giant cell tumor of bone can weaken the bone and predispose the patient to pathologic fracture.

NATURAL HISTORY

- Enchondromas are most commonly identified incidentally during unrelated evaluation. They also can present after pathologic fracture. On occasion, a patient may complain of painful swelling in the bone.
  - Enchondromas found incidentally and not causing considerable mechanical weakness may be observed if typical radiographic findings are seen.
  - Enchondromas causing substantial fracture risk and those presenting after pathologic fracture can be treated surgically with a low risk of recurrence.[7]
  - Enchondromas can extremely rarely transform to chondrosarcomas.
- Unicameral bone cysts are most commonly seen during adolescence or childhood. They are most commonly identified after pathologic fracture. Proximal humerus lesions may be seen.
  - Unicameral bone cysts with a low risk of fracture may be observed with activity modification.
  - Unicameral bone cysts causing substantial weakness and fracture risk may be treated with surgery or injection.
  - Suspected unicameral bone cysts in the bones of the hand are sufficiently rare that strong consideration should be given to biopsy when this lesion is suspected.

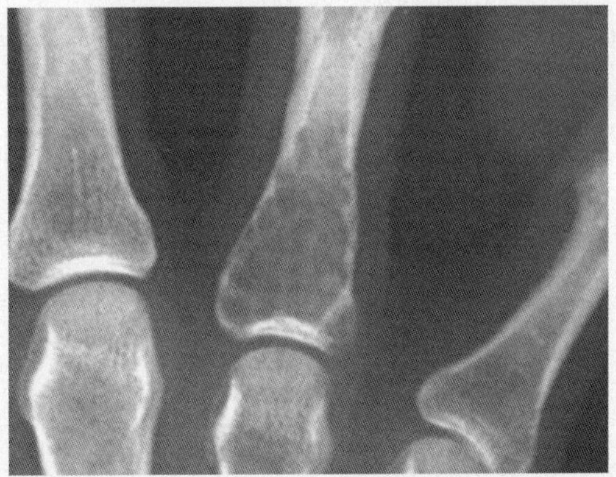
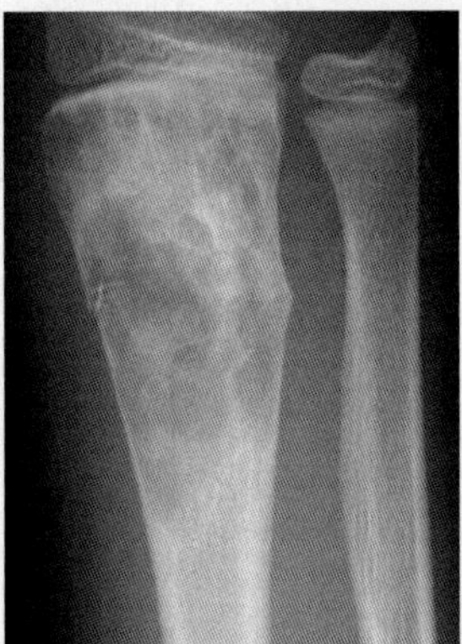
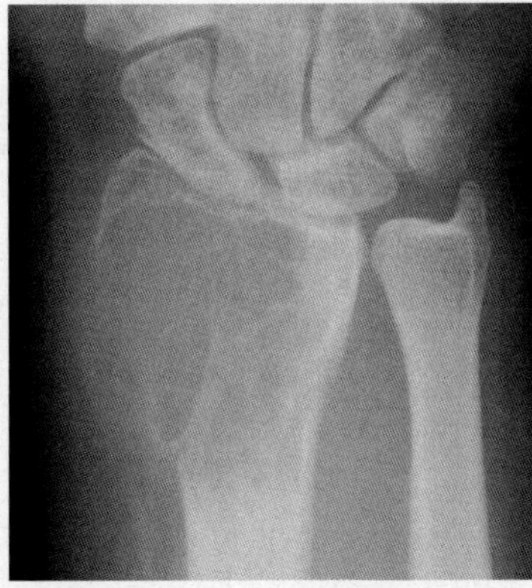

FIG 1 • **A.** Enchondroma of the proximal phalanx. **B.** Unicameral bone cyst of the distal radius. **C.** Giant cell tumor of the distal radius.

- Giant cell tumor of bone is locally aggressive. Patients may present with pain and swelling or after pathologic fracture.
  - Giant cell tumor of bone metastasizes 2% to 10% of the time, with metastasis more frequently seen with distal radius and hand lesions.[1,2,4–6] Metastasis most frequently occurs concurrent with or after a local recurrence.
  - Patients with giant cell tumor of bone require systemic staging, treatment, and long-term surveillance, as recurrence may be seen late.

PATIENT HISTORY AND PHYSICAL FINDINGS

- Enchondroma is most often an incidental finding and is asymptomatic. Pain and deformity can be seen after pathologic fracture. On occasion, there will be bone distention and tenderness with palpation.
- Unicameral bone cysts are most commonly seen after pathologic fracture. On occasion, there will be swelling and tenderness.
- Giant cell tumor of bone may cause swelling, pain, tenderness, and a sense of weakness. Loss of range of motion is common, as these lesions are typically periarticular. Pathologic fracture may be seen.

IMAGING AND OTHER DIAGNOSTIC STUDIES

- Plain radiographs are indispensable in the initial evaluation of primary bone tumors (**FIG 2A**).
- Magnetic resonance imaging (MRI) is useful when an aggressive lesion or soft tissue extension is suspected. MRI may allow better identification of the local extent of disease and may assist in operative planning (**FIG 2B**).
  - Campanacci et al's[3] grading system or Kang et al's[4] modification may be used:
    - Grade 1 lesions are confined to the intramedullary cavity without distention or distortion of the cortex.
    - Grade 2 lesions distend the cortex but do not extend into the surrounding soft tissues.
    - Grade 3 lesions destroy the cortex and extend into the surrounding soft tissues.
- Total body bone scan and lung computed tomography (CT) scan are required for staging patients with giant cell tumor of bone.
- Incision or needle biopsy may be required when radiographs and MRI are not diagnostic.

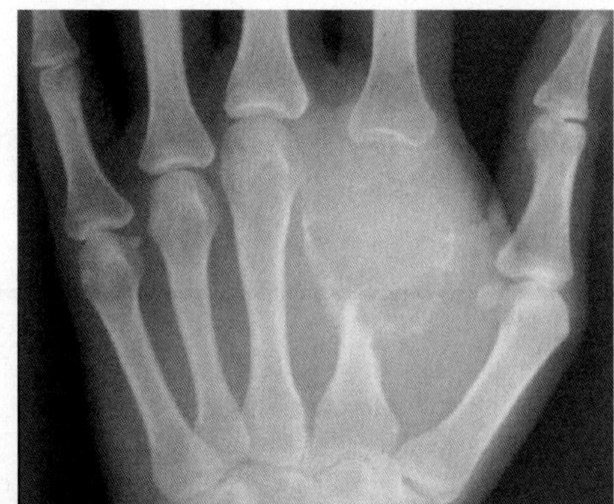

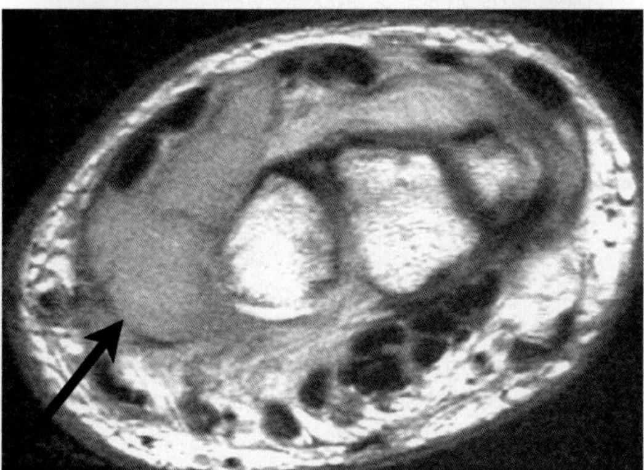

FIG 2 • A. Radiograph showing giant cell tumor of the metacarpal. **B.** MRI axial image of grade 3 giant cell tumor of the distal radius (*arrow*).

DIFFERENTIAL DIAGNOSIS

- Enchondroma
- Chondromyxoid fibroma
- Chondrosarcoma
- Unicameral bone cyst
- Infection
- Aneurysmal bone cyst
- Giant cell tumor of bone
- Primary malignant bone neoplasms
- Acrometastasis

NONOPERATIVE MANAGEMENT

- Enchondromas and unicameral bone cysts may be observed provided radiographic assessment is diagnostic or the differential diagnoses are limited to benign, nonaggressive lesions with an indolent natural history. The assessment of risk of pathologic fracture is paramount. Lesions with a substantial risk of pathologic fracture in the context of the patient's activity level are best treated operatively.
- The rare risk of malignant degeneration of enchondromas should be considered and discussed with the patient.
- Suspected giant cell tumor of bone requires biopsy. Rarely, these can be treated with radiation alone; however, this approach is the exception and should not be considered first-line treatment. Radiation is associated with a risk of subsequent true malignant degeneration to a highly malignant giant cell tumor of bone.

SURGICAL MANAGEMENT

- All suspected giant cell tumors of bone and those enchondromas and unicameral bone cysts with a high risk of fracture are best treated surgically.

Preoperative Planning

- The radiographic extent of disease must be assessed.
- The approach will vary depending on the anatomic location.
- Bone graft source (autologous or allograft) must be considered.
- Precautions to prevent donor site cross-contamination must be considered and reviewed with the operating room team.
- The surgeon must determine the anticipated need for frozen section and discuss this with the pathologist and review radiographs before any anticipated frozen section.
- The surgeon must secure and confirm the availability of any necessary grafting materials, instruments, implants, or adjuvants (ie, liquid nitrogen).

- The surgeon must confirm the availability of intraoperative imaging. Radiographs will give better resolution than fluoroscopy.

Positioning

- Surgery is typically done in the supine position with the arm extended on a radiolucent arm board.
- Proximal humerus lesions may be approached in a modified beach-chair position.

Approach

- Phalanx lesions may be approached from the dorsal or lateral approach.
- Metacarpal lesions are best approached dorsally in most instances.
- Carpal lesions are usually best approached dorsally.
- Distal radius lesions may be approached at the tubercle of Lister or at the interval between the radial border of the pronator quadratus and the first dorsal compartment, proximal to the radial styloid.
- Ulnar lesions are usually best approached dorsally or ulnarly.
- Proximal humerus lesions are best approached just lateral to the deltopectoral interval.
- Biopsy must always take into consideration the potential for malignancy. It must be done in a way that does not compromise the potential need for a subsequent limb-sparing procedure.

TECHNIQUES

Curettage and Excision of Proximal Phalangeal Enchondroma

- The midaxial approach from the ulnar side is preferred whenever possible (**TECH FIG 1A**).
- After making the incision under tourniquet control, identify the lateral band and retract it dorsally.
- Reflect the periosteum and create a bone window using curettes, rongeur, or drill (**TECH FIG 1B**).
- Curette the lesion in its entirety. The use of flexible fiberoptic lights may improve visualization.
- Pack the cavity with preferred bone grafting material.
- Obtain plain radiographs in the operating room to confirm complete excision and appropriate grafting.

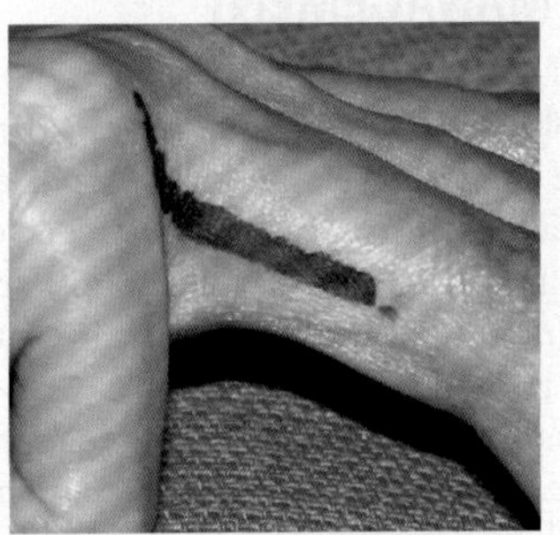
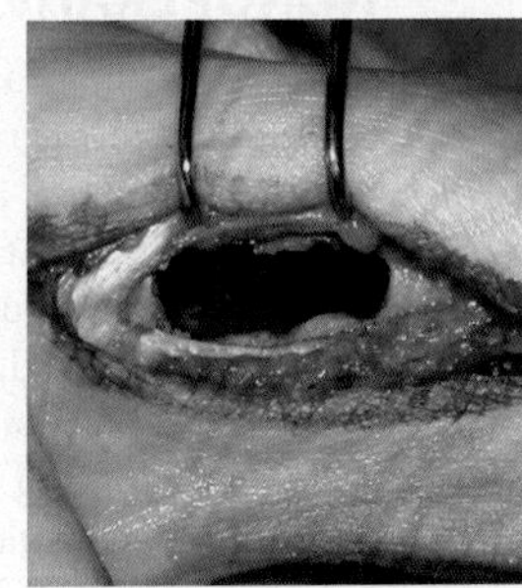

TECH FIG 1 • **A.** Midaxial approach to proximal phalanx enchondroma. **B.** The lateral band is retracted and a bone window is created before curettage.

Curettage and Excision of Metacarpal Enchondroma

- Metacarpal lesions are approached dorsally through longitudinal incisions.
- Reflect the periosteum and create a bone window using curettes, rongeur, or drill.
- Curette the lesion in its entirety. Ensure adequate visualization through a longitudinal bone trough.
- Pack the cavity with preferred bone grafting material.
- Obtain plain radiographs in the operating room to confirm complete excision and appropriate grafting.

Curettage, Cryosurgery, and Cementation of Distal Radius Giant Cell Tumor of Bone

- Preoperative preparation includes confirming the availability of liquid nitrogen, proper storage containers, cryosurgery instruments, and trained operative staff.
- Grades 1, 2, or 3 lesions with a single plane of palmar perforation can be approached from a palmar radial incision between the first dorsal compartment and the radial artery (**TECH FIG 2A,B**).
  - A branch of the superficial radial nerve may be encountered and should be retracted and protected. The radial 50% of the pronator quadratus is exposed.

- When palmar soft tissue perforation is present, it will commonly be contained by the pronator quadratus. The pronator overlying the region of perforation should be excised en bloc with the bone window, effectively converting a grade 3 lesion to a grade 2 lesion with a palmar bone window.
- Wide exteriorization of the lesion with a window roughly two-thirds the maximum dimension of the lesion is needed to ensure adequate visualization.
- Thoroughly curette the lesion. Fiberoptic lighting may assist in viewing the extent of radial styloid involvement.
- Burr the endosteal surface if it is sufficiently thick. Irrigate and dry the cavity.
- The argon beam coagulator may be used to achieve hemostasis in the cavity and may have a beneficial effect as an adjuvant causing surface necrosis.
- Perform cryosurgery using three separate freeze–thaw cycles with either the direct pour technique or the spray gun (**TECH FIG 2C**).
- Fill the cavity with polymethylmethacrylate bone cement. Reinforcing Rush pins (Rush Pin, Meridian, MS) may be used (**TECH FIG 2D**).
- Apply a bulky compressive bandage and volar splint.

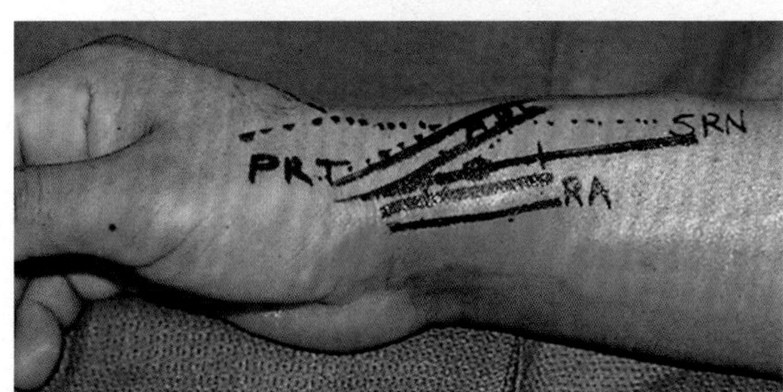

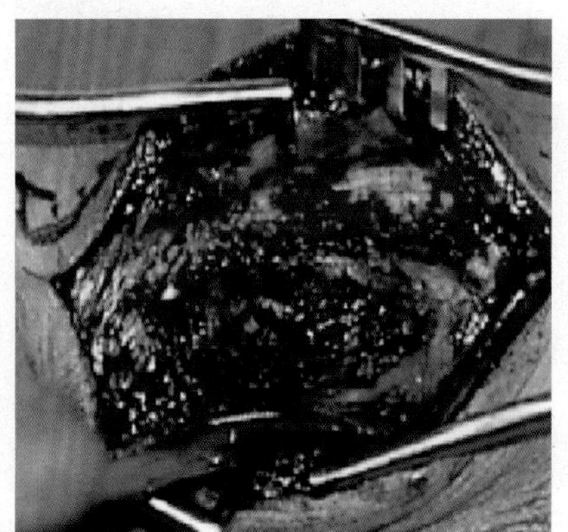

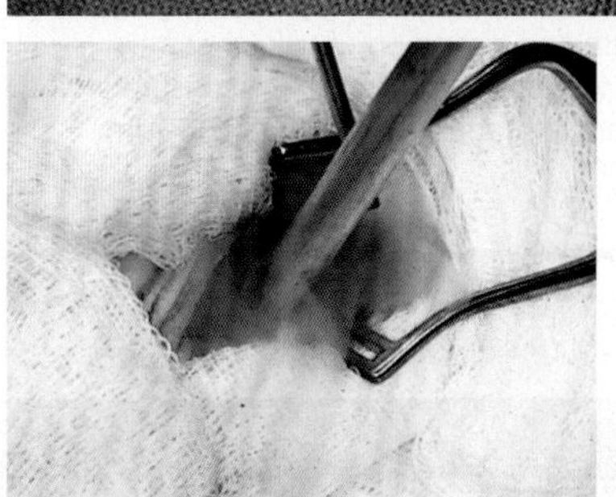

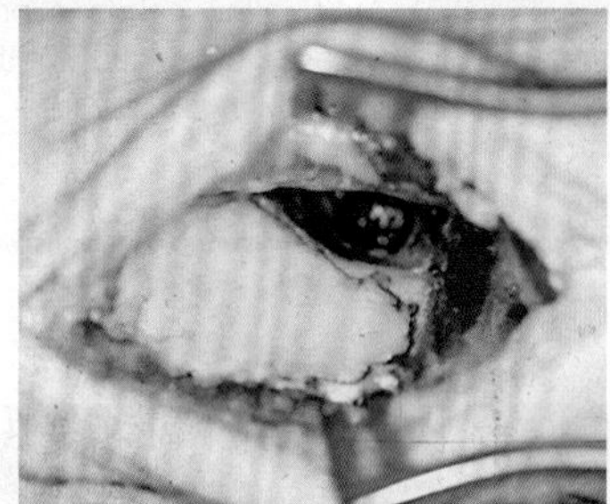

TECH FIG 2 • **A.** The right radius is approached from the palmar radial aspect between the first dorsal compartment and the radial artery. *SRN*, superficial radial nerve; *RA*, radial artery. **B.** The radial border of the pronator quadratus is exposed to gain access to the lesion for creation of the bone window. **C.** Cryosurgery is performed after wide retraction and soft tissue protection. **D.** The defect is filled with bone cement.

Wide En Bloc Extra-articular Distal Radius Resection

- Wide extra-articular excision of the distal radius may be indicated for grade 3 giant cell tumors with extensive cortical destruction, recurrent lesions, and those with pathologic fracture into the radiocarpal articulation.
- A dorsal approach maximizes exposure and facilitates subsequent intercalary arthrodesis.
- Finger extensors are released from the retinaculum, whereas wrist extensors and often thumb extensors or abductors may need to be sacrificed.
- Cut the radius proximal to the tumor. Cut the ulna proximal to the distal radioulnar joint, away from the ulnar extent of the lesion (**TECH FIG 3A**).
- "Evert" the radius and ulna into the wound while the interosseous membrane is transected (**TECH FIG 3B**). Dissect the flexor pollicis longus and the radial artery away from the tumor-bearing segment.
- Mobilize the flexor tendons, median nerve, and ulnar nerve away from the tumor-bearing segment.
- The midcarpal articulation can be disarticulated initially from a dorsal approach and then circumferentially to complete the resection (**TECH FIG 3C**).
- Alternatively, the midcarpal articulation can be excised en bloc with the tumor-bearing segment by cutting with an oscillating saw from dorsal to palmar through the distal aspect of the distal carpal row bones.
- Reconstruction is readily accomplished by means of a vascularized or nonvascularized fibula graft (**TECH FIG 3D**).
- Spanning rigid internal fixation with a 3.5-mm dynamic compression plate lowers the risk of nonunion.

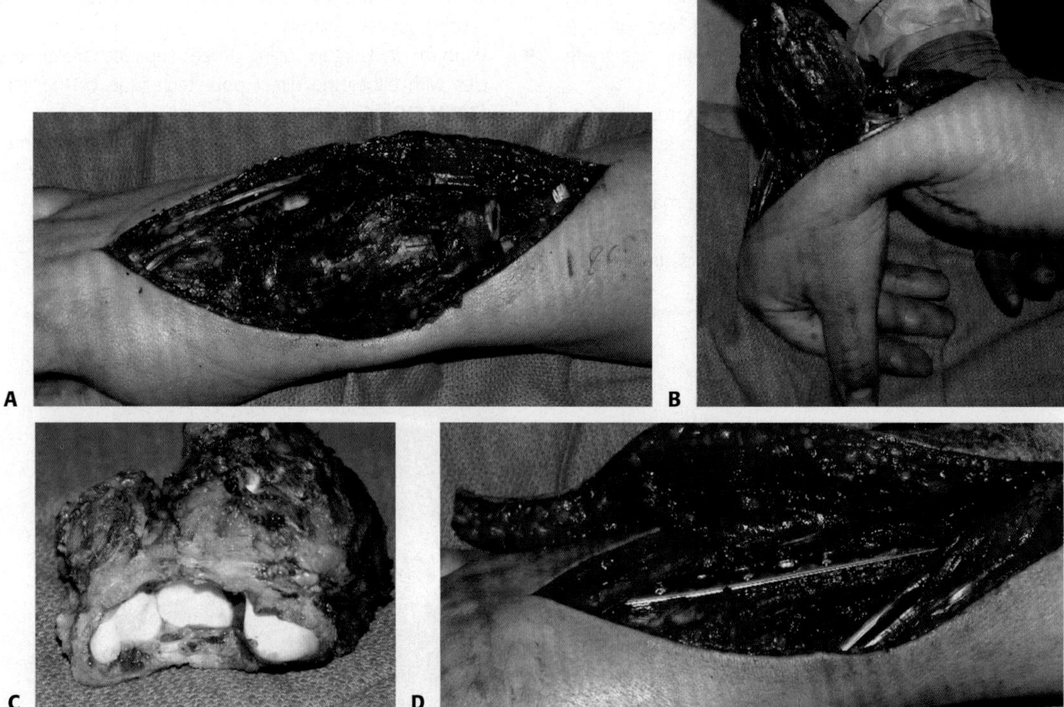

TECH FIG 3 • **A.** Dorsal exposure of the distal radius and ulna with transection of the radius and ulna proximally. **B.** The radius and ulna are everted into the dorsal wound to allow palmar exposure and dissection of palmar soft tissues. **C.** The resection specimen, demonstrating the midcarpal articulation of the proximal carpal row. **D.** Reconstruction is by means of an osteoseptocutaneous vascularized fibula graft for intercalary arthrodesis. A spanning 3.5-mm compression plate is used for fixation.

PEARLS AND PITFALLS

"Exteriorization"	▪ Make the bone window to the lesion two-thirds the greatest dimension of the lesion to allow adequate visualization of the cavity.
Pathology consultation	▪ Consult the pathologist in advance. Frozen section analysis of cartilaginous lesions is notoriously difficult.
Approach	▪ A lateral approach to phalanx lesions provides more rapid return to normal motion and a better appearance. A volar radial approach for distal radius grade 1 and 2 giant cell tumors of bone allows excellent visualization and limits local contamination risk. ▪ The dorsal approach for large grade 3 giant cell tumor distal radius lesions is best when wide excision and reconstruction or arthrodesis is anticipated.
Monitoring	▪ Surveillance monitoring is mandatory, particularly for giant cell tumor of bone, which can recur late and metastasize.

POSTOPERATIVE CARE

- Phalanx or metacarpal enchondroma
  - Bulky protective dressings are applied and range of motion is initiated at the first dressing change, usually 8 to 10 days postoperatively.
  - Protective splinting is continued for 6 weeks after surgery. High-risk activities are restricted for 12 to 16 weeks.
  - Periodic surveillance continues for 3 to 5 years.
- Curettage, cryosurgery, and cementation of distal radius giant cell tumor of bone
  - Dressings are changed 10 days postoperatively. Sutures are removed and the patient is fitted with a removable splint.
  - Active range-of-motion exercises are initiated. Active-assisted and passive range-of-motion exercises are added at week 6.

- Activities are gradually increased, with high-risk activities being restricted for up to 2 years due to cryonecrosis of bone caused by cryosurgery.
- Wide en bloc extra-articular distal radius resection
  - Patients are dressed in a bulky compressive dressing, most commonly with a volar splint.
  - Elevation is encouraged for the first 48 hours, and digit range of motion is encouraged.
  - Formal supervised therapy is initiated at the first dressing change, typically 8 to 10 days after surgery.
    - At that time, bandages are removed and sutures can be removed.
- Most commonly, active and active-assisted range-of-motion exercises are initiated. When not exercising, patients are asked to use a protective splint for an additional month. Activities are progressively increased as soft tissue and bone healing allows.
- Range-of-motion exercises are initiated no later than 10 days after surgery.
- Protective splinting continues a total of 6 weeks minimum after intralesional procedures and until bone healing is confirmed after arthrodesis.
- Sporting activities are typically restricted for 12 to 18 weeks. High-risk activities are avoided for longer periods.
- Surveillance for local recurrence should continue for 5 years for benign lesions and 10 years for giant cell tumor of bone.

OUTCOMES

- Local recurrence
  - The local recurrence rate after curettage and bone grafting of enchondromas is about 5%. When recurrence is seen, the question of malignant transformation should be considered.[7]
  - The local recurrence rate after curettage and bone grafting of giant cell tumor of bone in the distal radius is about 50% and adjuvants such as liquid nitrogen can lower this to about 20%. Intralesional treatment (curettage) is best reserved for lesions without soft tissue extension or extension limited to a single plane of palmar perforation bound by pronator quadratus (grade 1 and 2 lesions).[4–6]
  - Wide excision of distal radius lesions is associated with local recurrence rates of less than 10%; however, reconstruction in the form of articular allograft or intercalary arthrodesis results in inferior function, motion, and strength and higher levels of pain.[4–6,9]
  - The local recurrence rate after curettage and bone grafting of giant cell tumor of bones of the hand is about 80%. Isolated curettage without the use of adjuvants cannot be advocated in this setting. There are several successful examples of curettage, cryosurgery, and cementation of giant cell tumor of the small bones of the hand. This type of procedure is best done at a tumor referral center.[1,2]
  - Wide excision or amputation has been advocated for giant cell tumor of bone when it arises in the phalanges or metacarpals. Local recurrence may still be seen, but the rate is probably less than 10%.[1,2]
  - The local recurrence rate after curettage of enchondromas arising in the hand is about 5%.[7]
  - The local recurrence rate after wide excision or amputation for giant cell tumor of the bones of the hand is less than 10%.
  - The local recurrence rate after curettage, cryosurgery, and cementation of distal radius giant cell tumor of bone is about 20% to 25% and correlates with soft tissue extension.[4,6]
  - The local recurrence rate after wide excision of distal radius giant cell tumor of bone is likely less than 10%.[8]
- Metastasis
  - Benign giant cell tumor of bone metastasizes in 2% to 8% in general case series.[1,2,5]
- Motion and strength
  - Range of digit motion is typically excellent after curettage for enchondroma.
  - Range of motion of the wrist may be slightly diminished after curettage of enchondromas in the distal radius.
  - Grip strength is reduced to 60% of normal after wide excision of the distal radius for giant cell tumor with intercalary segmental arthrodesis. Forearm rotation is typically preserved.

COMPLICATIONS

- Infection, hematoma, nerve injury, intraoperative fracture, postoperative fracture, nonunion, limited range of motion, and tendon gliding problems may be seen after treatment of enchondroma or giant cell tumor of bone when arising in the upper extremity.
- Delayed complications include extensor tendon rupture due to prominent residual ulna, nonunion, and fracture after hardware removal.

REFERENCES

1. Athanasian EA, Wold LE, Amadio PC. Giant cell tumors of the bones of the hand. J Hand Surg Am 1997;22(1):91–98.
2. Averill RA, Smith RJ, Campbell CJ. Giant-cell tumors of the bones of the hand. J Hand Surg Am 1980;5(1):39–50.
3. Campanacci M, Laus M, Boriani S. Resection of the distal end of the radius. Ital J Orthop Traumatol 1979;5:145–152.
4. Kang L, Manoso MW, Boland PJ, et al. Features of grade 3 giant cell tumors of the distal radius associated with successful intralesional treatment. J Hand Surg Am 2010;35(11):1850–1857.
5. O'Donnell RJ, Springfield DS, Motwani HK, et al. Recurrence of giant-cell tumors of the long bones after curettage and packing with cement. J Bone Joint Surg Am 1994;76(12):1827–1833.
6. Sheth DS, Healey JH, Sobel M, et al. Giant cell tumor of the distal radius. J Hand Surg Am 1995;20(3):432–440.
7. Takigawa K. Chondroma of the bones of the hand. A review of 110 cases. J Bone Joint Surg Am 1971;53(8):1591–1600.
8. Vander Griend RA, Funderburk CH. The treatment of giant-cell tumors of the distal part of the radius. J Bone Joint Surg Am 1993;75(6):899–908.
9. Weiland AJ, Kleinert HE, Kutz JE, et al. Free vascularized bone grafts in surgery of the upper extremity. J Hand Surg Am 1979;4(2):129–144.

Above-Elbow and Below-Elbow Amputations

148 CHAPTER

Jacob Bickels, Yair Gortzak, Yehuda Kollender, and Martin M. Malawer

BACKGROUND

- Tumors of the upper extremity may cause extensive soft tissue and bone destruction and extend into the main neurovascular bundle. In those extreme situations, limb sparing may not be feasible, and amputation is required to achieve wide margins of resection and local tumor control.
- Above-elbow amputations may be required for advanced soft tissue and bone sarcomas of the forearm and around the elbow (**FIG 1A**); below-elbow amputations are performed for such tumors of the forearm and the hand (**FIG 1B**).
- Above- and below-elbow amputations are rarely done because the upper arm, elbow, and forearms are rare location for musculoskeletal tumors and because tumors at that site are noticed in relatively early stages and in most cases are resectable. Furthermore, administration of preoperative chemotherapy and availability of isolated limb perfusion have allowed to control the majority of patients that present with a large tumor.
- Nonetheless, above- and below-elbow amputations retain a definitive role in the management of soft tissue and bone tumors of the upper extremity.

ANATOMIC CONSIDERATIONS

- Above-elbow amputations can be metaphyseal (high), diaphyseal, or supracondylar (see **FIG 1A**).
- High above-elbow amputations are those proximal to the deltoid tuberosity. Patients who undergo amputation proximal to the insertions of the deltoid and pectoralis major muscles have far greater difficulties adjusting to their prosthesis than do those who have undergone a more distal amputation.
- Below-elbow amputations should preserve the maximal length of both radius and ulna. Although tumors of the hand are treated by a standard below-elbow amputation, performed through the distal third of the forearm, tumors of the distal forearm require a higher amputation and warrant special consideration. A minimum of 2.5 to 3 cm of bony stump, measured from the radial tuberosity, is required to preserve function. Additional length in a very short stump can be obtained by releasing the biceps tendon; adequate flexion of the stump will be provided by the brachialis muscle.

INDICATIONS

- Extensive soft tissue and bone tumor extension with no option for reconstruction and reasonable function following resection (**FIGS 2** to **4**)
- Local recurrence was once considered a primary indication for amputation. The mere presence of a recurrent sarcoma is no longer an immediate indication for an amputation.

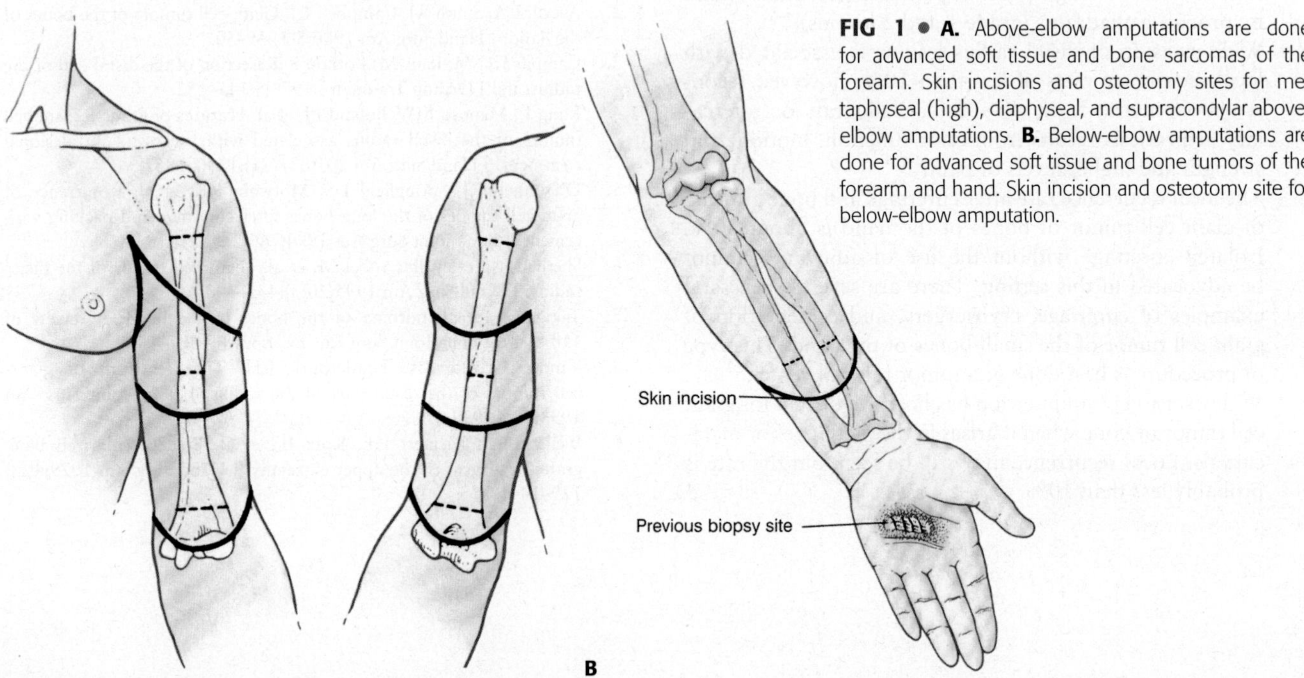

FIG 1 • **A.** Above-elbow amputations are done for advanced soft tissue and bone sarcomas of the forearm. Skin incisions and osteotomy sites for metaphyseal (high), diaphyseal, and supracondylar above-elbow amputations. **B.** Below-elbow amputations are done for advanced soft tissue and bone tumors of the forearm and hand. Skin incision and osteotomy site for below-elbow amputation.

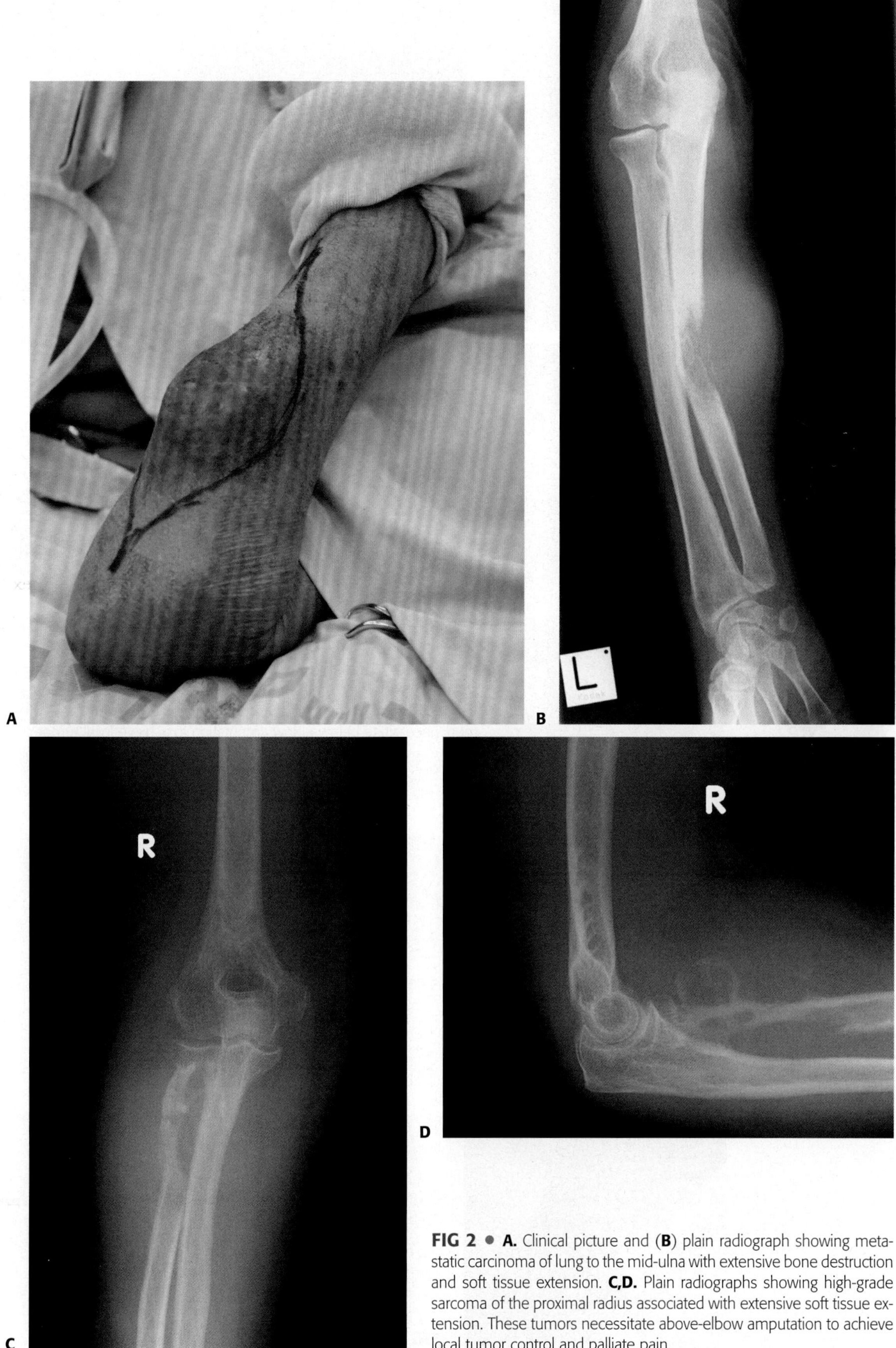

FIG 2 • **A.** Clinical picture and (**B**) plain radiograph showing metastatic carcinoma of lung to the mid-ulna with extensive bone destruction and soft tissue extension. **C,D.** Plain radiographs showing high-grade sarcoma of the proximal radius associated with extensive soft tissue extension. These tumors necessitate above-elbow amputation to achieve local tumor control and palliate pain.

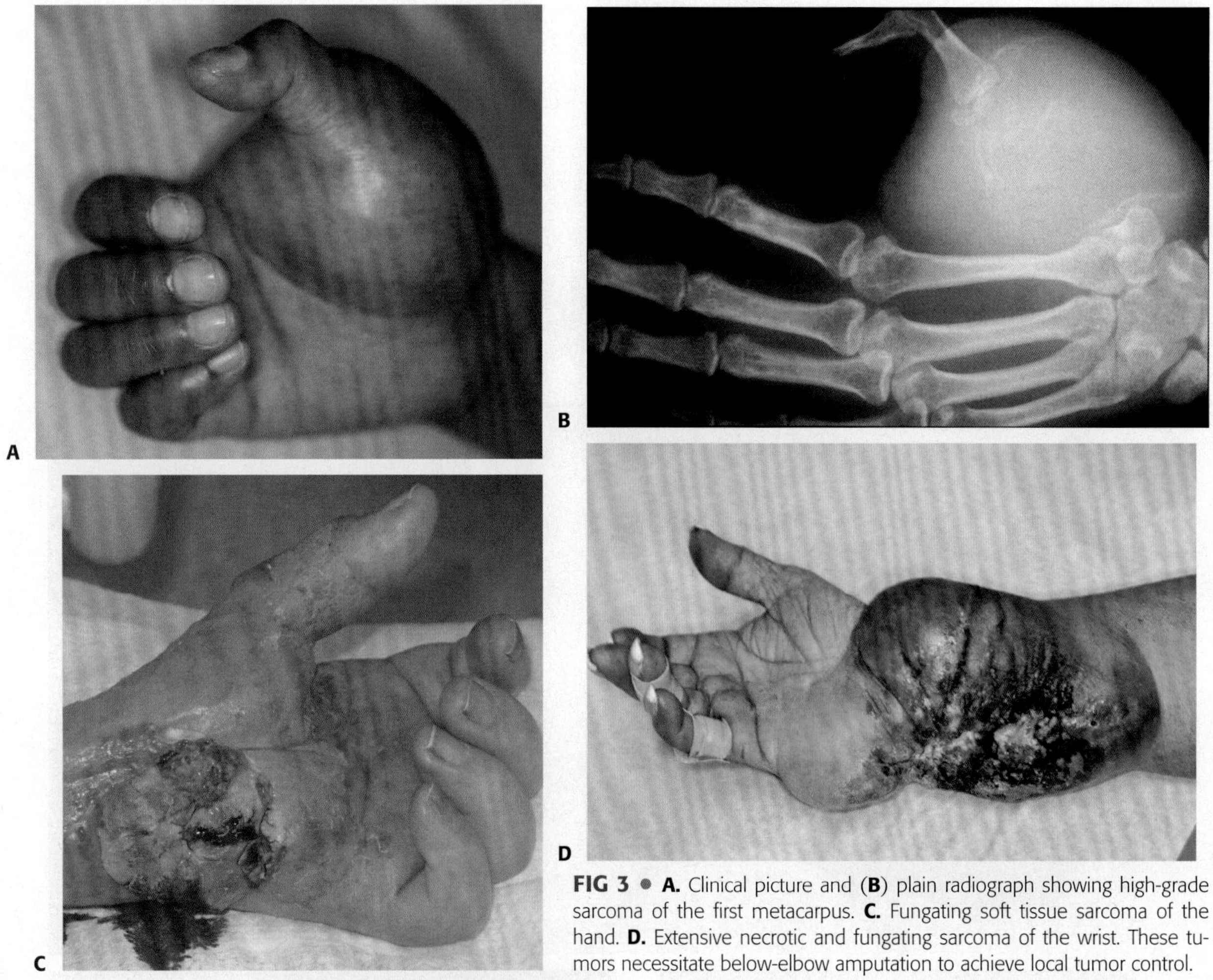

FIG 3 • **A.** Clinical picture and (**B**) plain radiograph showing high-grade sarcoma of the first metacarpus. **C.** Fungating soft tissue sarcoma of the hand. **D.** Extensive necrotic and fungating sarcoma of the wrist. These tumors necessitate below-elbow amputation to achieve local tumor control.

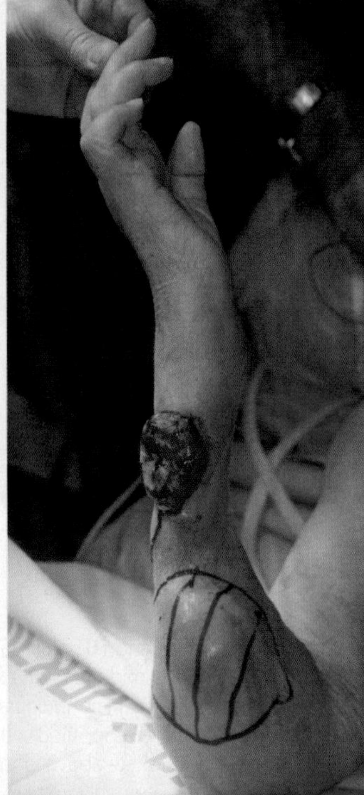

FIG 4 • Extensive squamous cell carcinomatosis of the forearm. Above-elbow amputation was done.

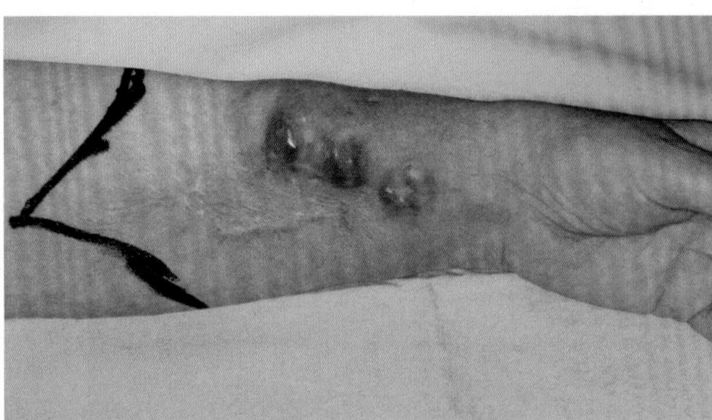

FIG 5 • Recurrent high-grade sarcoma of the distal forearm. The recurrent disease is diffused and wide resection would result in loss of neurovascular structures and all flexor tendons and would end with an extensive soft tissue defect in a previously irradiated surgical field. Below-elbow amputation was, therefore, done (planned incision is outlined).

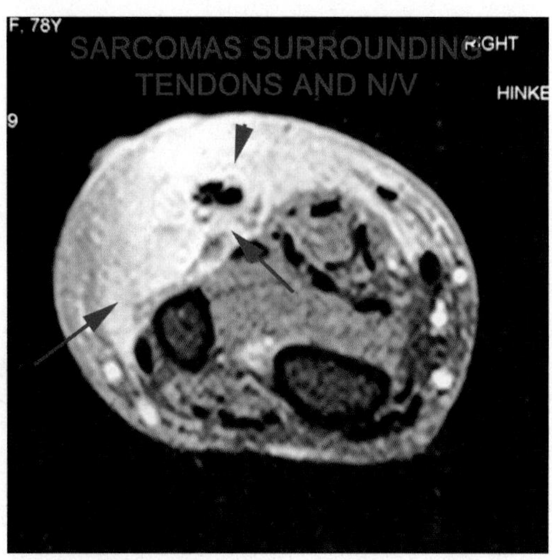

FIG 6 • MRI demonstrating tendon and neurovascular involvement, a true indication for amputation.

The capability to resect the recurrent tumor without compromising the function of the extremity is the determining factor on which the decision to amputate is based (**FIG 5**).

- Major vascular involvement. The neurovascular bundle within the arm is tightly integrated in a closed anatomic space. The cephalic vein usually provides sufficient collateral flow if the brachial or the axillary vein has to be sacrificed. However, although occasionally the tumor mass can be delicately dissected off the brachial artery, in most cases of vascular involvement, the brachial artery is extensively encased and amputation is inevitable (**FIG 6**). The compact nature of the vascular supply to the wrist makes involvement of the radial and ulnar arteries likely when a large tumor invades the volar aspect of the distal forearm. In this instance, the incidence of morbidity and failure associated with resection and reconstruction using a vascular graft of one of these vessels is prohibitively high.
- Major nerve involvement. In general, one nerve around the arm can be sacrificed and a two-nerve deficit is tolerated. Sacrifice of the three major nerves leaves the patient with a functionless extremity that is better off amputated. Nerve grafting for replacement of a section of the median, radial, or ulnar nerves is still not associated with satisfactory function.

IMAGING AND OTHER STAGING STUDIES

- Patients requiring above- or below-elbow amputations for a soft tissue or primary bone sarcoma must undergo complete staging in order to allow the surgeon to determine the level of amputation and extent of soft tissue resection.
  - Complete staging allows determination of full tumor extent and, as a result, the site for skin incision, shape of the flaps, and site of osteotomy.
- The combined use of plain radiography, computerized tomography (CT), and magnetic resonance imaging (MRI) is necessary to determine the proximal extent of the intraosseous and soft tissue components of the tumor. In general, the more proximal of the two levels of involvement (ie, bone or soft tissue) determines the level of amputation.

SURGICAL MANAGEMENT

Positioning

- The patient is supine with the ipsilateral shoulder slightly elevated.

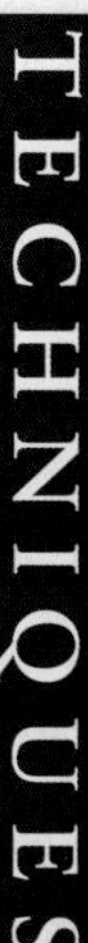

Amputations at the Elbow

- Standard anterior/posterior "fish-mouth" flaps are used. However, medial–lateral flaps may occasionally be needed because of local tumor anatomy. Because of the excellent blood supply to the upper extremity, wound healing is rarely a problem, regardless of flap configuration. The skin and superficial fascia are divided perpendicular to the skin surface (**TECH FIG 1**).
- Large blood vessels are ligated in continuity and then suture ligated. The nerves are handled delicately. They are pulled approximately 2 cm from their muscular bed, doubly ligated with nonabsorbable monofilament suture, and cut with a knife.
- Muscles are transected according to the flap design and the humerus or the radius and ulna are cut at the appropriate location, as determined by the preoperative imaging studies (**TECH FIG 2**). The radius and ulna are transected at equal lengths.
- For optimal function and mobility of the stump, it is important that muscle groups will be positioned tightly and securely over the cut ends of the bones (**TECH FIG 3**).
- Myodesis is reinforced by Dacron tapes passed through drill holes made in the cut end of the bone.
- Superficial fascia and skin are closed over closed suction drains (**TECH FIG 4**).

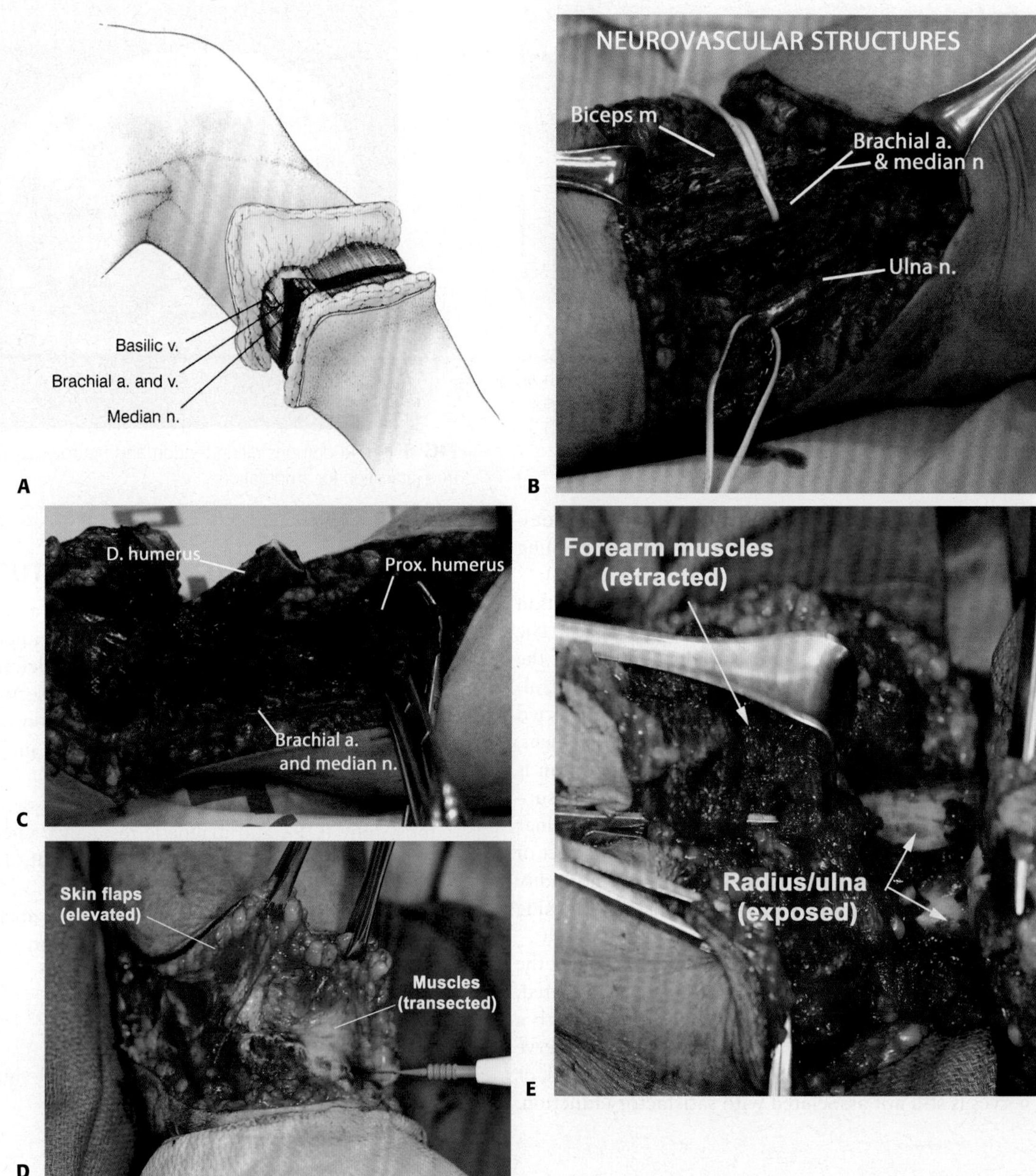

TECH FIG 1 • **A.** Anterior/posterior fish-mouth flaps are used. **B.** The skin and superficial fascia are divided perpendicular to the skin surface. **C–E.** Intraoperative photographs representing the flap development and exposure of the soft tissues and neurovasculature prior to osteotomy.

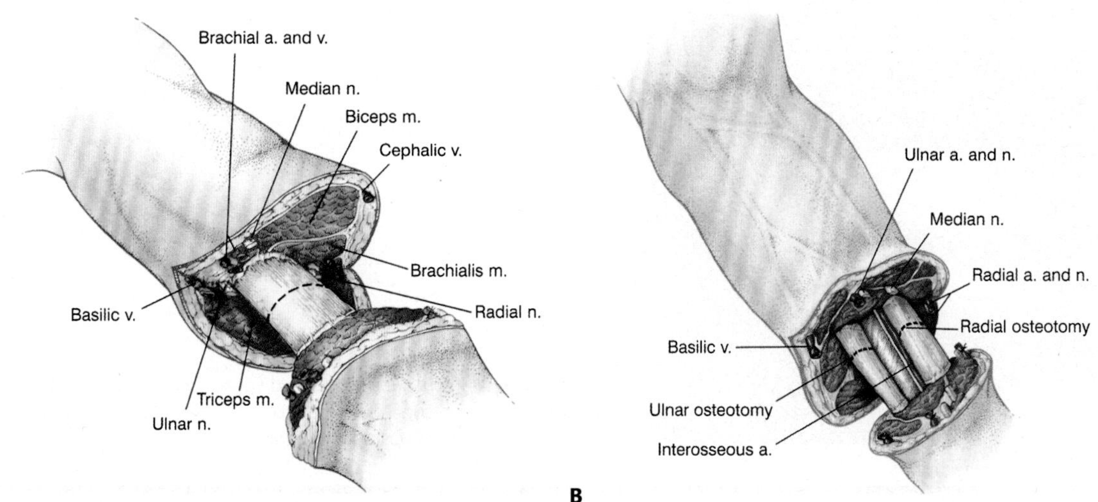

TECH FIG 2 • Osteotomies are performed at the appropriate location, as determined by the preoperative imaging studies: (**A**) above-elbow amputation and (**B**) below-elbow amputation. For above-elbow amputation, the osteotomy is done at the distal third of the humerus; for below-elbow amputation, the radius and ulna are transected at equal lengths at the appropriate level.

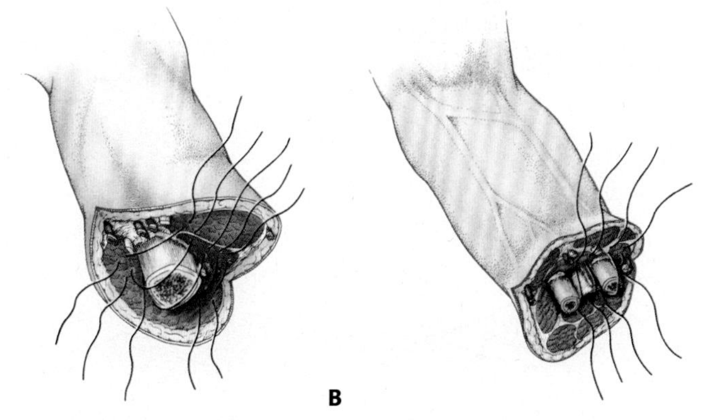

TECH FIG 3 • Muscle groups are positioned tightly and securely over the transected bone ends: (**A**) above-elbow amputation and (**B**) below-elbow amputation.

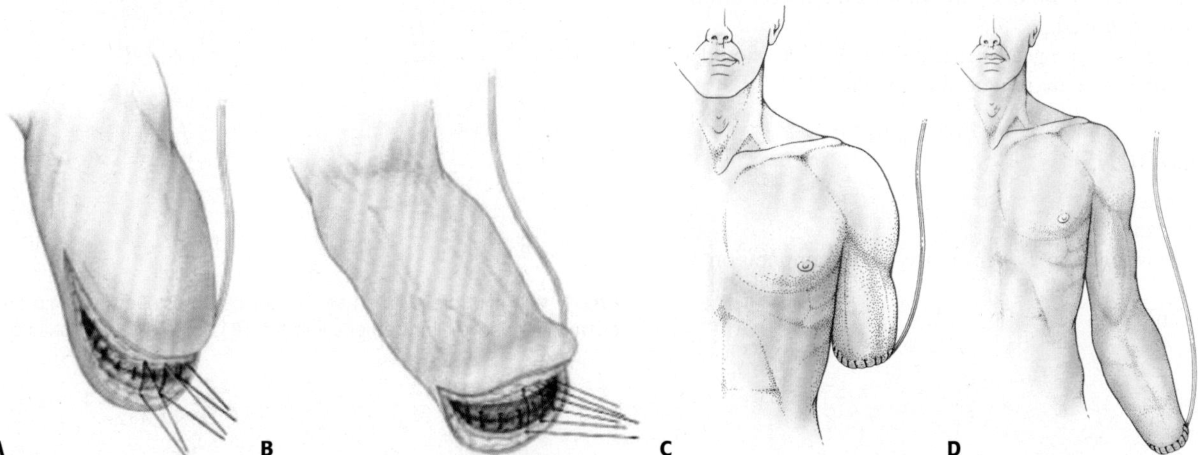

TECH FIG 4 • Superficial fascia and skin are closed over closed suction drains: (**A**) above-elbow amputation and (**B**) below-elbow amputation. Final closure for above-elbow amputation (**C**) and below-elbow amputation (**D**) with closed suction drains. *(continued)*

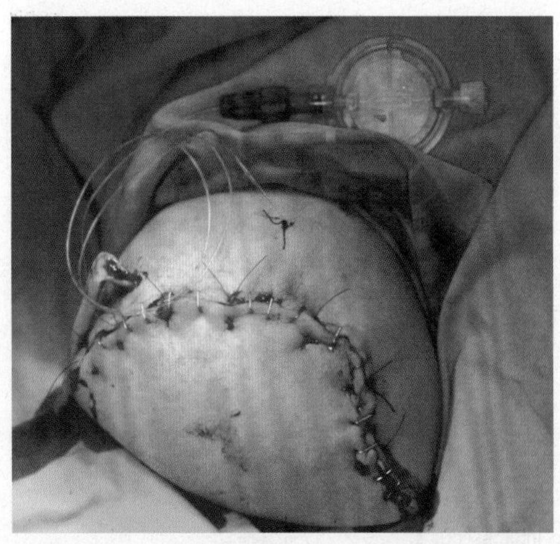

TECH FIG 4 • *(continued)* **E.** Closed surgical wound over an epineural catheter which provides continuous flow of local analgesics was installed into the nerve sheath to control postoperative pain.

PEARLS AND PITFALLS

Radiology	■ Detailed preoperative imaging for evaluation of tumor extent
Operative procedure	■ Functional and tight myodesis over the cut ends of the bones
Postoperative care and rehabilitation	■ Rigid dressing and early range-of-motion exercises

POSTOPERATIVE CARE

- A rigid dressing is applied immediately postoperatively to decrease pain and edema and facilitate maturation of the stump (**FIG 7**). Care must be taken to adequately protect the skin that directly overlies the bone.
- Stump edema is rarely a significant problem in the upper extremity, and prosthesis training should begin as soon as possible after surgery.
- Continuous suction is required for 3 to 5 days, and perioperative intravenous antibiotics are continued until the drainage tubes are removed.
- Active and passive ranges of motion around the shoulder and elbow (if exists) are practiced as tolerated.

COMPLICATIONS

- Wound dehiscence
- Deep infection
- Loss of elbow motion (when above-elbow amputation is done)
- Phantom limb pain

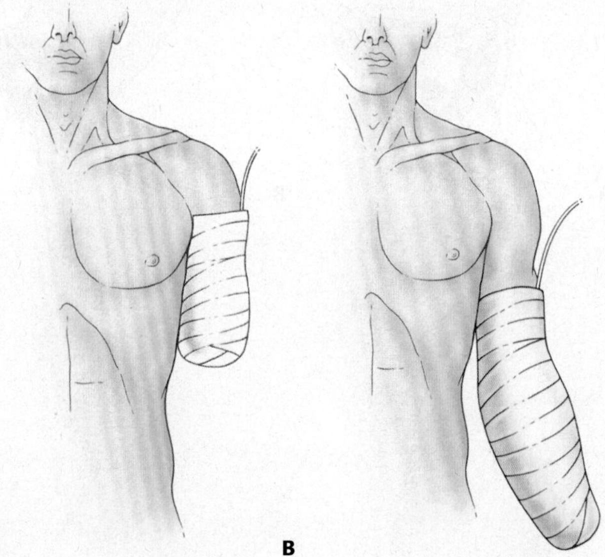

FIG 7 • A rigid dressing is used to decrease postoperative pain and edema: (**A**) above-elbow amputation and (**B**) below-elbow amputation.

Congenital Forearm, Wrist, and Hand Disorders

Forearm Osteotomy for Multiple Hereditary Exostoses

149 CHAPTER

Carley Vuillermin, Carla Baldrighi, and Scott N. Oishi

DEFINITION

- Multiple hereditary exostoses (MHE), first described by Boyer[3] in 1814, is a familial disorder with an autosomal dominant mode of inheritance exhibiting very high penetrance and variable expressivity.[12]
- Also known as *multiple osteochondromatosis*, *multiple osteochondromata*, *multiple cartilage exostoses*, *diaphyseal aclasis*, or *metaphyseal aclasis*[5,23]

ANATOMY

- Knowledge of the normal anatomy and biomechanics of the forearm in the immature individual is instrumental in understanding the pathogenesis of the deformity and ultimately in planning appropriate treatment.
- During forearm pronation–supination, the relationship between the radius and ulna changes. This rotational movement requires near-anatomic alignment of both as well as integrity of the proximal and distal radioulnar joints and the interosseous membrane. Minimal axial or rotational bone deformity, asymmetric bone shortening, or ligament instability can hinder this function.
- The ulna acts like a swivel hinge around which the radius rotates. The axis of forearm rotation is oblique.

PATHOGENESIS

- The most common genetic mutations are in the *EXT-1* and *EXT-2* genes.[6]
- Approximately 10% of individuals with manifestations of multiple exostoses have no family history of MHE.[22]
- The prevalence of MHE in the general population is estimated to be at least one in 50,000, with a median age of first diagnosis of 2 to 3 years of age (exostoses rarely develop before age 2 years).[22] An average of five or six exostoses, involving both upper and lower extremities, is found at the time of the first consultation.[9]
  - The presence of exostoses is almost always evident by the age of 12 years.
- Osteochondromas develop at numerous sites in the immature skeleton, they may affect any bone except the skull. They most commonly affect the ends of long bones and flat bones including the scapula and pelvis.
- Osteochondromas consist of a base or stalk covered by a cartilaginous cap. They arise from the peripheral aspect of the growth plate of bones that undergo endochondral ossification.[14]
  - They are the product of abnormal proliferation of chondroblasts and subsequent defective remodeling of the metaphysis. This leads to the two main characteristics of this condition: skeletal metaphyseal exostoses and retardation of longitudinal bone growth.
  - They migrate away from the physis with longitudinal growth.[14]
- In MHE, the exostoses vary greatly in number, location, size, and configuration. They tend to have a more irregular and bizarre shape than solitary osteochondromas.
  - Should always be continuous with the medullary cavity of the bone from which they arise
  - Once skeletal maturity is reached, the lesions will become quiescent.[22] Lesions that enlarge after skeletal maturity should be investigated to exclude malignant change.

NATURAL HISTORY

- Deformity of the forearm is seen in 30% to 60% of the individuals with MHE.[22] The forearm deformities can be progressive and result in a variable amount of weakness, pain,[4] functional limitation, and aesthetic deformity.
  - The deformities are almost always accompanied by discrepancy in length between the two bones. Asynchronous longitudinal growth between paired bones leads to a greater risk of anatomic distortion. Most of the longitudinal growth of the ulna occurs at the distal physis,[15] which is also the more commonly affected physis (30% to 85% of the cases).[22,23]
  - The affected ulna typically remains relatively shortened and curved, and this often leads to significant bowing of the radius. When the ulna is shorter, the ulnar-sided soft tissue acts as a tether, causing bowing of the radius. In addition, the local presence of the exostosis itself causes radial bowing by disturbing hemiepiphyseal growth.[15]
- A serious risk associated with MHE is the potential for malignant transformation of an exostosis into chondrosarcoma. This can occur at any age, but it is exceedingly rare during childhood.[22]
- Patients affected by MHE have a normal life expectancy unless malignant degeneration and metastasis develop.[9] The risk of malignant degeneration in adults with MHE has been reported to range from 0.57% to 5%.[12,22,31]
- MHE can have a serious influence on the quality of life of affected individuals, affecting sporting participation, occupation, and daily activities.[8]

HISTORY AND PHYSICAL FINDINGS

- The diagnosis is rarely difficult as 90% of affected individuals have a positive family history, and therefore initial history taking should focus on the symptoms and functional impairment that exist.

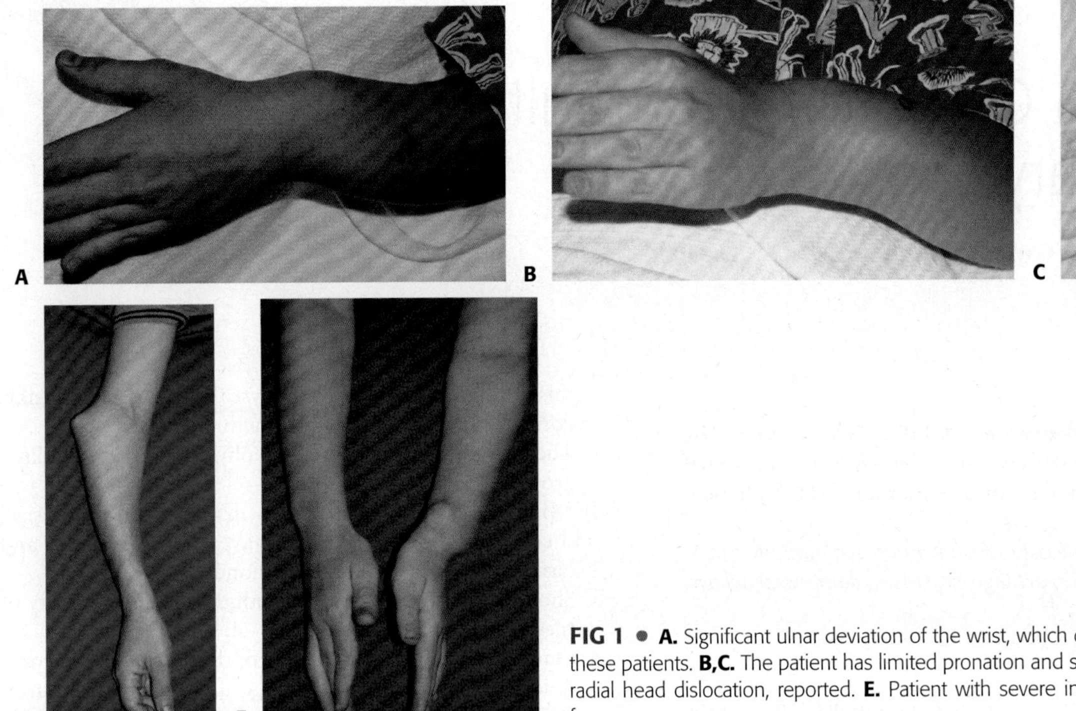

FIG 1 ● **A.** Significant ulnar deviation of the wrist, which can also be present in these patients. **B,C.** The patient has limited pronation and supination. **D.** Obvious radial head dislocation, reported. **E.** Patient with severe involvement of the left forearm.

- Physical examination of the upper extremity should assess for location of disease burden and common associated findings.
  - It is a common finding that the deformity is quite asymmetric. One forearm may be heavily affected, whereas the other relatively spared.
- Shortening of the forearm, specifically relative shortening of the ulna, increased radial bow and possible radial head dislocation.
- A mild flexion deformity of the elbow is often present.
- At the wrist level, an increased ulnar tilt of the radial epiphysis, ulnar deviation of the hand, and progressive ulnar translocation of the carpus are often present. These deformities can lead to a loss of radial deviation of the hand and loss of pronation–supination of the forearm (**FIG 1**).
- The loss of forearm pronation–supination may develop early and become progressively more severe as the child ages.[26] Pronation–supination may be limited due to altered mechanical alignment, osteochondroma blocking motion, or radial head dislocation. The greater the number of osteochondromas and shorter the ulna, the greater the loss of motion.[10,32]
- Radial head dislocation is reported to occur in 22% of the affected forearms.[23] It may present as pain, a mass on the lateral side of the elbow, altered carrying angle, decreased elbow range of motion or decreased pronation–supination, or catching.
- It is possible to have neurologic impingement from either direct compression by an osteochondroma or through deformity including radial head dislocation.

IMAGING AND OTHER DIAGNOSTIC STUDIES

- Plain radiographic evaluation is usually sufficient to confirm the diagnosis and to determine the number, location, and morphology of the exostoses (**FIG 2**).
- Like solitary osteochondromas, the exostoses may be described as sessile or pedunculated; they nearly always point away from the physis, however in the hand they may not. In MHE, the lesions tend to be larger and have a more bizarre shape (see **FIG 2**).
- At least two full views of the forearm (true anteroposterior and lateral containing both the elbow and the wrist) are necessary to properly assess the ulnar variance, the radial articular angle (RAA), the carpal slip, and the relative radial bow. These radiographic measurements are useful in the surgical planning phase (**FIG 3**).[2]

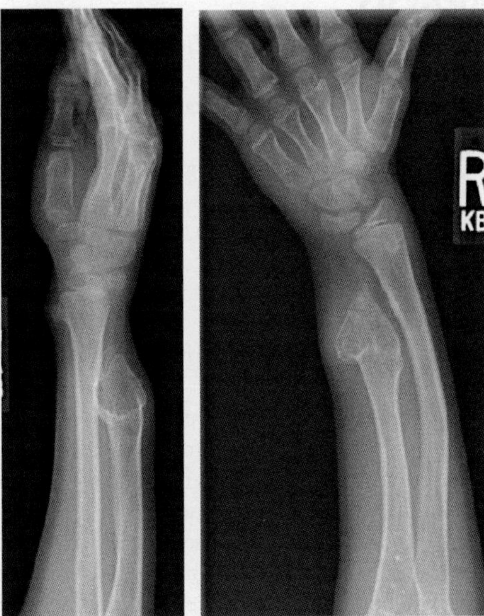

FIG 2 ● Radiographs showing large osteochondroma of distal ulna affecting the epiphysis and causing significant tethering of the radius. Characteristically, the distal ulna is narrow with a pointed end.

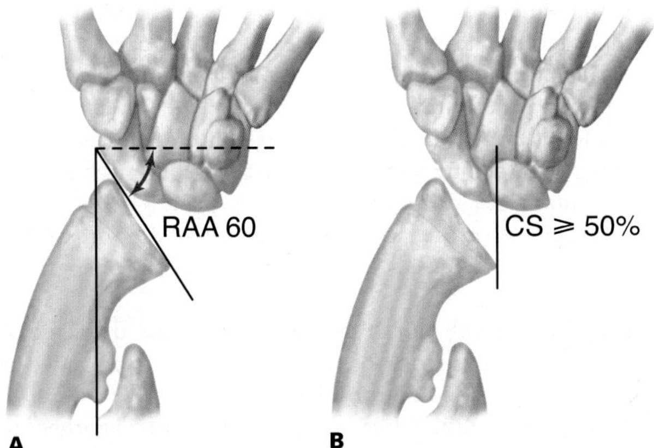

FIG 3 • The RAA and carpal slip (*CS*). **A.** The RAA is defined as the angle between a line running along the articular surface of the radius and another line that is perpendicular to a line joining the center of the radial head to the radial border of the distal radial epiphysis (the radial styloid in skeletally mature individuals). The normal range of the angle is 15 to 30 degrees. **B.** CS is measured by determining the percentage of the lunate that is in contact with the radius. First, a line is drawn from the center of the olecranon through the ulnar border of the radial epiphysis (the radial articular surface in skeletally mature individuals).[1] This line normally bisects the lunate. An abnormal CS is defined as being present when ulnar displacement of the lunate exceeds 50%. (Adapted from Akita S, Mursae T, Yonenobu K, et al. Long-term results of surgery for forearm deformities in patients with multiple cartilaginous exostoses. J Bone Joint Surg Am 2007;89:1993–1999.)

- Alterations of the radial head on radiographs must always be assessed. They range from flattening to subluxation and complete radial head dislocation.
- Masada et al[15] morphologically classified the involvement of the forearm in MHE into three types (**FIG 4**). This classification is also used for treatment planning.
- Computed tomography (CT), magnetic resonance imaging (MRI), and magnetic resonance angiography are performed at times for specific and symptomatic lesions. These can be especially helpful to detail the anatomic position relative to soft tissue structures or when malignant transformation is suspected.[27]
  - In older children and teenagers, irregular areas of calcification of the cartilaginous cap may be present. Extensive calcification with changes in the shape, thickness of the cartilaginous cap, or a lesion enlarging more rapidly than the growth of the child should raise suspicion of possible chondrosarcoma transformation.

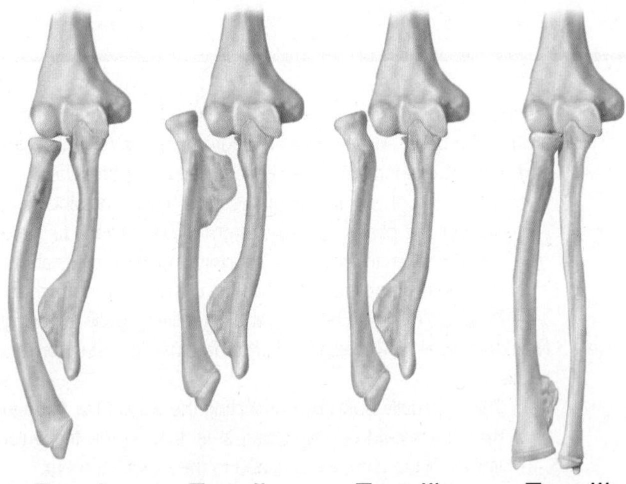

FIG 4 • Masada classification of the involvement of the forearm in MHE. (Adapted from Masada K, Tsuyuguchi Y, Kawai H, et al. Operations for forearm deformity caused by multiple osteochondromas. J Bone Joint Surg Br 1989;71:24–29.)

DIFFERENTIAL DIAGNOSIS

- Langer-Giedion syndrome
- Madelung deformity
- Chondrosarcoma

NONOPERATIVE MANAGEMENT

- Patients with MHE can often be managed successfully using a conservative approach.
  - Exostoses alone can often be surprisingly well tolerated and result in minimal loss of function.[26] It has been reported that forearm function in untreated adults with MHE is subjectively greater than the one objectively measured.[17]
  - The conspicuous number of lesions and the fact that they are mostly asymptomatic warrant a cautious surgical approach.
  - A dislocated radial head that is not symptomatic should be left alone.
    - Attempts at relocating a dislocated radial head have been unsuccessful.[2,19]

SURGICAL MANAGEMENT

- Surgical treatment of forearm deformities in MHE remains controversial. A number of operative techniques have been proposed.[5,10,15,20,24]
- The main surgical indications are to
  - Improve forearm function (pronation–supination)[2]
  - Relieve pain from external trauma or irritation of the surrounding soft tissue[4]
  - Improve appearance[10]
  - Exclude malignancy when there is a rapid increase in size of a lesion[18]
- When evaluating the surgical indications in an individual patient, it is important to distinguish between the functional deficit and the cosmetic appearance.
  - The postoperative appearance of the forearm has been shown to be unrelated to the functional outcome.[17]
- Despite many maintaining good function even without treatment,[2,17] a percentage of patients find the appearance of the shortening, angulation, and deformities unacceptable.[17] If surgery is being undertaken for aesthetic rather than functional purposes, the hopes, concerns, and expectations of patient and parents must be thoroughly discussed and accurately outlined.
  - A mass or deformation may be removed; however, a scar shall be added.
  - Restoration of range of motion and improvement of radiographic parameters are unpredictable but may occur.[2,11]
- Some[5,15,18] advocate an aggressive approach based on the rationale that forearm deformities may lead to functional impairment especially if radial head dislocation occurs.[2,26]

Surgical treatment employed includes excision of the exostoses and ulnar lengthening and associated radial osteotomy when indicated.

- Radiographic indications cited include relative ulnar shortening (with or without bowing) of more than 1.5 cm, RAA of greater than 30 degrees, carpal slip of more than 60%, and bowing of the radius or the ulna (or both).[5]
- Predication of radial head dislocation has remained one of the most difficult aspects of MHE forearm care.
  - The most common association with radial head dislocation is isolated distal ulnar osteochondromas.[7]
- However, our approach reflects that the presence of forearm deformities alone is relatively unrelated to functional impairment,[2,17,26] and therefore we do not recommend surgical correction of the deformities only to prevent a possible, but not predictable, future functional impairment.

- Symptomatic dislocation of the radial head is an indication for surgical intervention when it interferes with joint motion or causes significant pain.

Procedures

- Exostosis excision alone is indicated when a lesion becomes symptomatic or when it directly causes limitation of forearm pronation–supination.
  - This procedure alone does not necessarily correct the forearm deformity.
  - Excision of a distal ulnar osteochondroma may lead to remodeling of the radius.[11]
- Ulnar tether release is indicated when there is significant wrist deformity present secondary to ulnar shortening.
  - When the distal epiphyseal plate of the ulna has lost its growth potential and resultant significant radial bowing exists, extensive ulnar tether release is our preferred technique to improve wrist position and potentially decrease the risk of radial head subluxation/dislocation. Lengthening may temporarily level the joint; however, the physis will not provide growth and recurrent deformity is common.
  - May be combined with osteochondroma excision or radial osteotomy
  - If the patient has significant growth potential remaining, ulnar tether release alone can lead to radial correction.
- Ulnar lengthening with or without radial osteotomy remains a common procedure.
  - Acute[10,30] and gradual[1,13,16,20,28] lengthenings have been used.
  - Ulnar lengthening levels the joint and relieves tension on the ulnar-sided soft tissues.
  - Anatomic structure, alignment, and potential for remodeling of the DRUJ needs to be considered prior to lengthening the ulna.
  - Lengthening will not restore growth to the distal ulna, the remaining growth potential and possible recurrence of deformity needs to be considered.
  - There are incumbent risks associated with lengthening procedures. The risks and benefits must be considered. The time to union or consolidation of bone regenerate is commonly 2 to 3 months.
- Radial osteotomy is performed in the skeletally mature or nearly skeletally mature patient.
  - Significant remodeling of the radius is unlikely in the older patient.
  - Radial osteotomy acutely corrects the radial deformity.
  - Combination with osteochondroma excision and ulnar-sided procedures is common.
  - Consider staging procedures if the level of surgery is similar on the radius and ulna to minimize the risk of synostosis or loss of correction.
- Distal radial hemiepiphysiodesis with stapling has been used in the past.[15,25] It has not gained widespread use.
- Treatment for symptomatic radial head dislocation is usually limited to salvage procedures.
  - Surgical excision may be performed once the patient is skeletally mature. Excision before this time may lead to instability, growth disturbance, and possible worsening of the wrist or elbow deformity.
- Formation of a single-bone forearm has been successfully used in the skeletally immature and skeletally mature patient.[19,21,29]
- In rare instances, exostosis excision with osteotomy or ulnar lengthening may be effective in relocating the radial head.[16]

TECHNIQUES

Exostosis Excision and Ulnar Tethering Release

- The location of the incision in the distal forearm varies depending on where the osteochondroma is located. Planning of this is important, as the ability to access the distal ulna is imperative whether the osteochondroma is located on the distal ulna or radius.
  - If the patient has ulnar involvement only, the incision can be placed on the subcutaneous border of the ulna between the flexor carpi ulnaris and the extensor carpi ulnaris (ECU). Care must be taken to identify and preserve the dorsal branch of the ulnar nerve.
  - If the patient has osteochondroma of both the radius and ulna, the incision has to be modified to allow exposure of both bones as well as the distal ulna.
- A tourniquet of appropriate size is used.
- Once the initial incision is made, the soft tissues are cleared from around the base, and the osteochondroma is carefully exposed and excised, ensuring that the cartilage cap is not breeched.
  - If near the physis, resection should proceed from the base nearest the physis and away from it (**TECH FIG 1**). Care must be taken to preserve satisfactory bony cortex for stability.
  - Bone wax is applied to the base of the resected osteochondroma to minimize bleeding and potential for bone regrowth.
- Next, the distal ulna is exposed and the ulnar tethering force is released.
  - This is usually done by transecting the distal ulna through the ulna styloid or epiphyseal area, leaving the triangular fibrocartilage complex attached to the distal fragment.
  - The ECU subsheath needs to be released for a maximal correction.
  - A radiocarpal wire can be used to maintain radiocarpal alignment in addition to a long-arm cast in the early postoperative period.

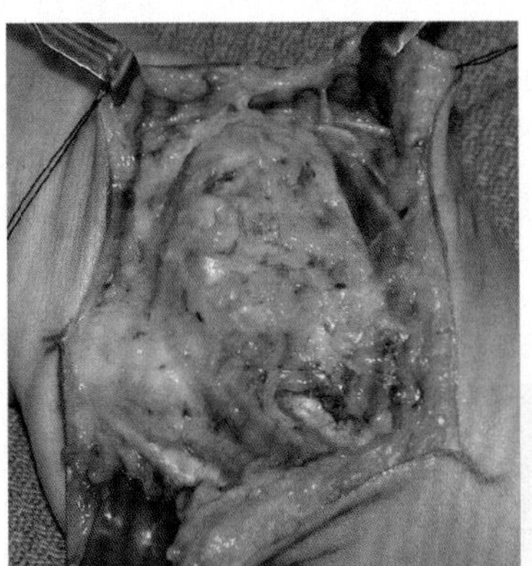
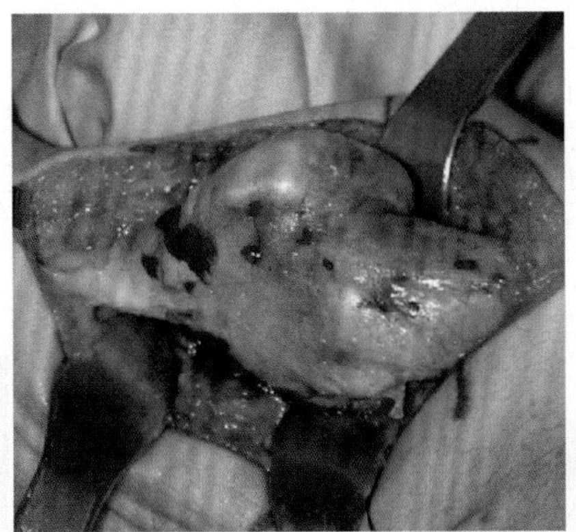
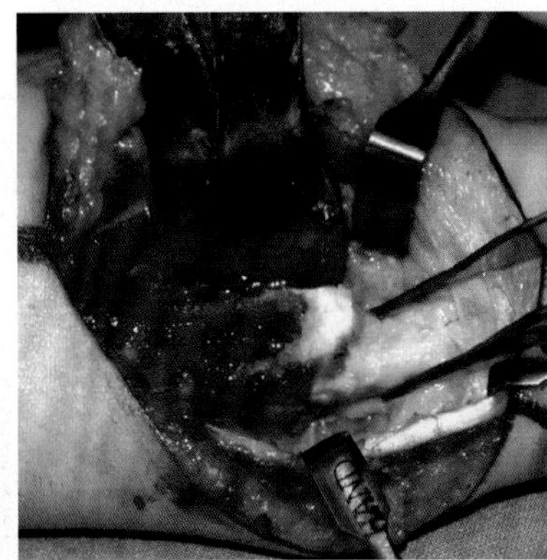

TECH FIG 1 • A. Exposure of large osteochondroma of the distal ulna. **B.** Dissection and exposure of the osteochondroma. Significant tethering is present distally. **C.** After excision of osteochondroma and release of ulnar tethering.

Distal Radial Osteotomy

- Radial osteotomy can be performed if the forearm bowing and deformity is severe, especially close to skeletal maturity (**TECH FIG 2A**).
- Preoperative radiographs are used for osteotomy planning. The site and magnitude of correction are determined, aiming for normalization of the RAA.
- A volar flexor carpi radialis (FCR) bed approach is made (unless another appropriate approach has been used for osteochondroma excision).
- Pronator quadratus is reflected, leaving a small cuff of tissue along the radial border for later repair.
- A closing wedge osteotomy is normally selected. A closing wedge osteotomy reduces radial height; however, this is not problematic when ulnar shortening has occurred.
  - A dome osteotomy is selected when there is no significant ulnar shortening.
  - Wire fixation is usually adequate for the osteotomy (either two stout K-wires or multiple smaller caliber wires).
    - Wires may be preplaced in the radial styloid before completion and displacement of the osteotomy. They are inserted percutaneously into the radial styloid.
  - Once the osteotomy is displaced, the wires are driven across until they obtain bicortical fixation.
- Adequacy of correction and final alignment is checked using fluoroscopy (**TECH FIG 2B,C**).
- Pronator quadratus is repaired using interrupted absorbable sutures.

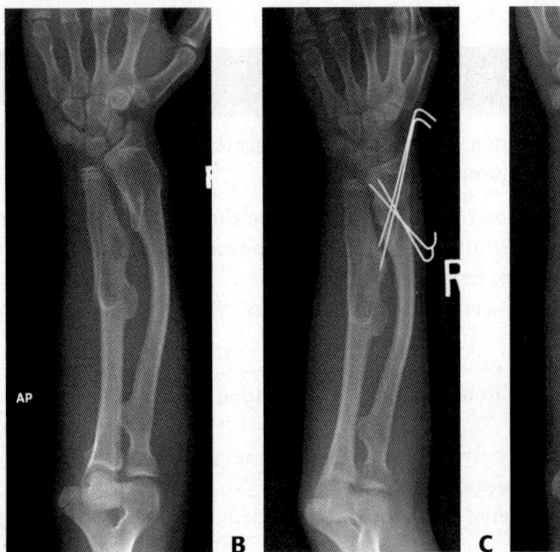

TECH FIG 2 • A. Prior to distal radial dome osteotomy. **B.** Early postoperative radiograph. **C.** Postoperative outcome at skeletal maturity.

Radial Head Excision

- An incision is made over the prominent radial head with the forearm in pronation to protect the posterior interosseous nerve.
- Dissection is then carried down in the interval between the anconeus muscle and ECU.
- The radial head is then exposed and excised (**TECH FIG 3**).
- Layered closure is then performed and the extremity is immobilized for 2 weeks, followed by institution of range-of-motion exercises.

A
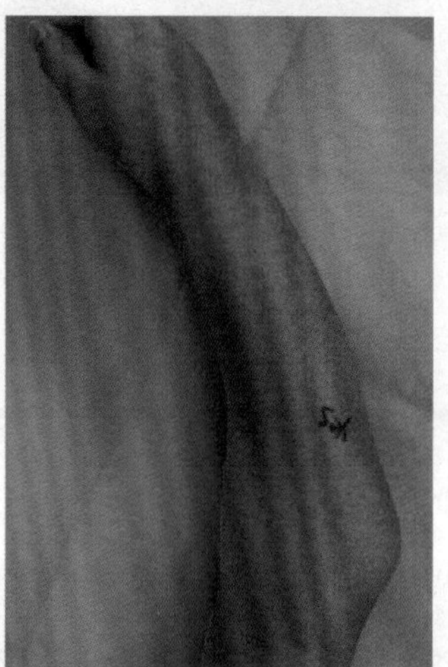
B
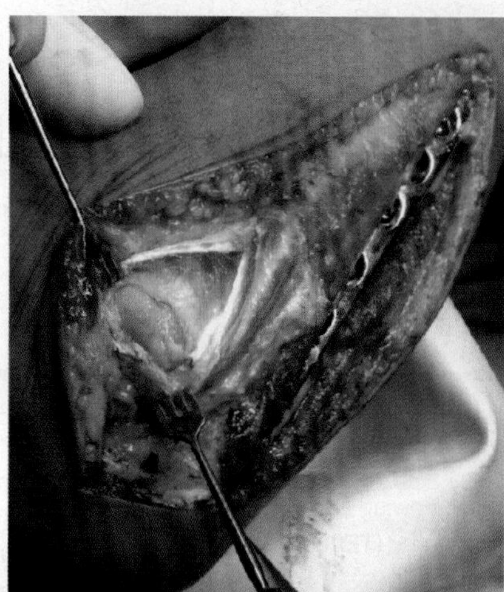
C
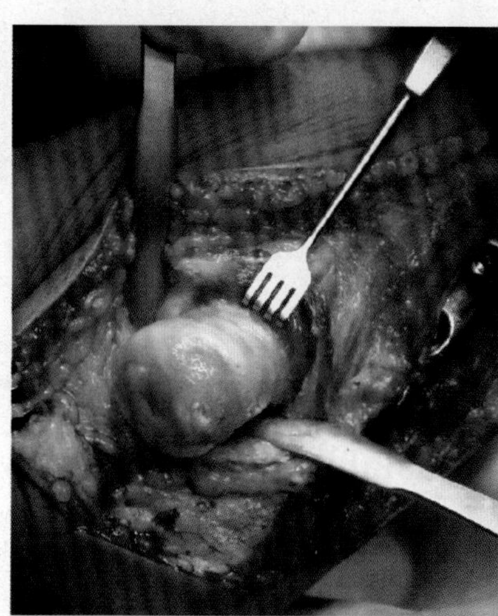
D
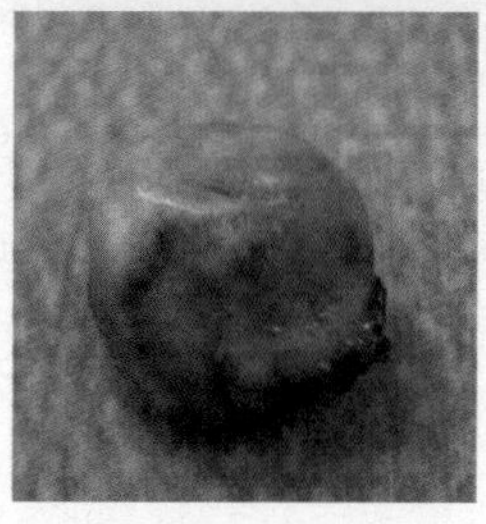

TECH FIG 3 • A. Patient with painful radial head dislocation. **B.** Exposure of the radial head. Forearm is in a pronated position to protect the posterior interosseous nerve. **C.** Radial head exposed before excision. **D.** Excised radial head. Significant degenerative changes are present.

PEARLS AND PITFALLS

Surgical approach	■ Be aware of the risk of creating a synostosis. Use separate approaches or staged procedures if both sides of the distal radius and ulna require surgical treatment.
Excision of osteochondromas	■ When resecting pedunculated osteochondromas, ensure that the axilla is clear of soft tissue—this is particularly so in the proximal radius as the radial nerve may become entrapped. Cutaneous nerves are also commonly draped over the surface of symptomatic lesions around the wrist. ■ Be aware of the physis when resecting osteochondromas. Minimize any additional trauma.
Ulnar tether release	■ Ensure that the ECU subsheath is completely released for maximal correction.
Radial osteotomy	■ Preplaced K-wires need to be almost parallel to the radial cortex to be correctly aligned once the osteotomy is displaced. ■ If using a dome osteotomy for correction of increased radial inclination, orient the concavity of the dome toward the joint to avoid excess translation. ■ Have a low threshold for a limited fasciotomy if a forearm osteotomy has been performed.
Radial head excision	■ Distorted anatomy means the radial/posterior interosseous nerve may be in a location that you do not expect it to be. ■ Avoid posterior dissection and further disruption of the lateral ulnar collateral ligament (LUCL). Repair the soft tissue envelope to minimize secondary instability.

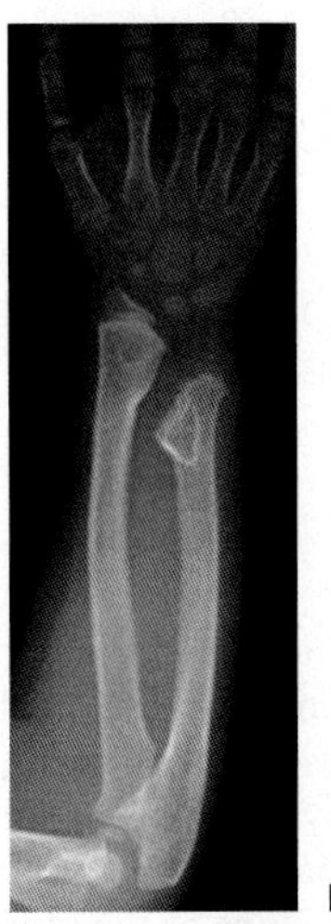
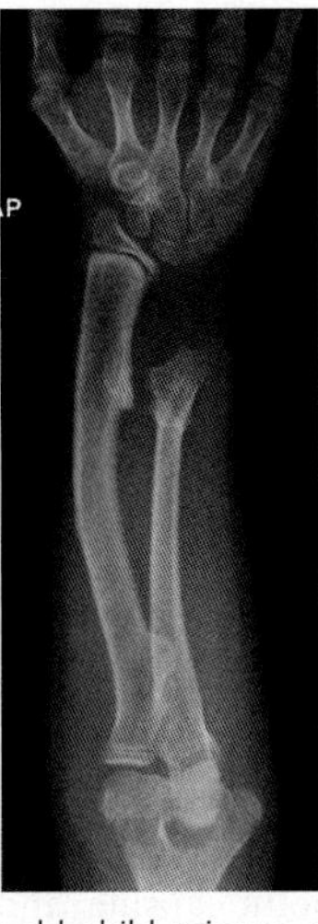

FIG 5 • **A.** Radiograph of a 5-year-old child prior to ulnar tether release with increased radial slope and severely affected distal ulnar physis. **B.** Seven years after ulnar tether release.

POSTOPERATIVE CARE

- Exercises to maintain the range of motion of the fingers are encouraged immediately after surgery regardless of the technique used.
- In cases of ulnar tethering release, casting is performed for 4 weeks, followed by range-of-motion exercises and splinting.
- If an osteotomy was performed, casting is continued until radiographic evidence of healing is seen.

OUTCOMES

- Many MHE patients do not need surgery. In patients who require surgery, ulnar tether release, with or without exostoses excision, with or without radial osteotomy, provides reliable results with the few complications (**FIG 5**). In selected patients, this can greatly improve function in addition to the improved cosmesis of the extremity.
- Ulnar lengthening is reserved for select patients.
- For symptomatic radial head dislocations, radial head excision usually leads to a consistent, reproducible result; however, formation of single-bone forearm can certainly be beneficial, especially in the skeletally immature patient.

REFERENCES

1. Abe M, Shirai H, Okamoto M, et al. Lengthening of the forearm by callus distraction. J Hand Surg Br 1996;21:151–163.
2. Akita S, Murase T, Yonenobu K, et al. Long-term results of surgery for forearm deformities in patients with multiple cartilaginous exostoses. J Bone Joint Surg Am 2007;89:1993–1999.
3. Boyer A. Traite des Maladies Chirurgicales et des Operations qui Leur Conviennent. Paris: Chez l'Auteur, 1814.
4. Darilek S, Wicklund C, Novy D, et al. Hereditary multiple exostoses and pain. J Pediatr Orthop 2005;25:369–376.
5. Fogel GR, McElfresh EC, Peterson HA, et al. Management of deformities of the forearm in multiple hereditary osteochondromas. J Bone Joint Surg Am 1984;66:670–680.
6. Francannet C, Cohen-Tanugi A, LeMerrer M, et al. Genotype–phenotype correlation in hereditary multiple exostoses. J Med Genet 2001;38:430–434.
7. Gottschalk HP, Kanauchi Y, Bednar MS, et al. Effect of osteochondroma location on forearm deformity in patients with multiple hereditary osteochondromatosis. J Hand Surg Am 2012;37:2286–2293.
8. Goud AL, de Lange J, Scholtes VA, et al. Pain, physical and social functioning, and quality of life in individuals with multiple hereditary exostoses in The Netherlands: a national cohort study. J Bone Joint Surg 2012;94:1013–1020.
9. Herring JA. Tachdjian's Pediatric Orthopaedics. ed 4. Philadelphia: WB Saunders, 2007.
10. Ip D, Li YH, Chow W, et al. Reconstruction of the forearm deformities in multiple cartilaginous exostoses. J Pediatr Orthop B 2003;12:17–21.
11. Ishikawa J, Kato H, Fujioka F, et al. Tumor location affects the results of simple excision for multiple osteochondromas in the forearm. J Bone Joint Surg Am 2007;89:1238–1247.
12. Legeai-Mallet L, Munnich A, Maroteaux P, et al. Incomplete penetrance and expressivity skewing in hereditary multiple exostoses. Clin Genet 1997;52:12–16.
13. Mader K, Gausepohl T, Pennig D. Shortening and deformity of radius and ulna in children: correction of axis and length by callus distraction. J Pediatr Orthop B 2003;12:183–191.
14. Mansoor A, Beals RK. Multiple exostosis: a short study of abnormalities near the growth plate. J Pediatr Orthop B 2007;16:363–365.
15. Masada K, Tsuyuguchi Y, Kawai H, et al. Operations for forearm deformity caused by multiple osteochondromas. J Bone Joint Surg Br 1989;71:24–29.
16. Matsubara H, Tsuchiya H, Sakurakichi K, et al. Correction and lengthening for deformities of the forearm in multiple cartilaginous exostoses. J Orthop Sci 2006;11:459–466.
17. Noonan KJ, Levenda A, Snead J, et al. Evaluation of the forearm in untreated adult subjects with multiple hereditary osteochondromatosis. J Bone Joint Surg Am 2002;84:397–403.
18. Peterson HA. Deformities and problems of the forearm in children with multiple hereditary osteochondromata. J Pediatr Orthop 1994;14:92–100.
19. Peterson HA. The ulnius: a one-bone forearm in children. J Pediatr Orthop B 2008;17:95–101.
20. Pritchett JW. Lengthening the ulna in patients with hereditary multiple exostoses. J Bone Joint Surg Br 1986;68:561–565.
21. Rodgers WB, Hall JE. One-bone forearm as a salvage procedure for recalcitrant forearm deformity in hereditary multiple exostoses. J Pediatr Orthop 1993;13:587–591.
22. Schmale GA, Conrad EU III, Raskind WH. The natural history of hereditary multiple exostoses. J Bone Joint Surg Am 1994;76:986–992.
23. Shapiro F, Simon G, Glimcher MJ. Hereditary multiple exostoses. Anthropometric, roentgenographic, and clinical aspect. J Bone Joint Surg Am 1979;61:815–824.
24. Shin EK, Jones NF, Lawrence JF. Treatment of multiple hereditary osteochondromas of the forearm in children: a study of surgical procedures. J Bone Joint Surg Br 2006;88:255–260.
25. Siffert RS, Levy RN. Correction of the wrist deformity in diaphyseal aclasis by stapling. Report of a case. J Bone Joint Surg Am 1965;47:1378–1380.
26. Stanton RP, Hansen MO. Function of the upper extremities in hereditary multiple exostoses. J Bone Joint Surg Am 1996;78:568–573.
27. Vanhoenacker FM, Van Hul W, Wuyts W, et al. Hereditary multiple exostoses: from genetics to clinical syndrome and complications. Eur J Radiol 2001;40:208–217.
28. Vogt B, Tretow HL, Daniilidis K, et al. Reconstruction of forearm deformity by distraction osteogenesis in children with relative shortening of the ulna due to multiple cartilaginous exostosis. J Pediatr Orthop 2011;31:393–401.
29. Waters PM. Forearm rebalancing in osteochondromatosis by radioulnar fusion. Tech Hand Up Extrem Surg 2007;11:236–240.
30. Waters PM, Van Heest AE, Emans J. Acute forearm lengthenings. J Pediatr Orthop 1997;17:444–449.
31. Watts AC, Ballantyne JA, Fraser M, et al. The association between the ulnar length and the forearm movement in patients with multiple osteochondromas. J Hand Surg Am 2007;32(5):667–673.
32. Wicklund CL, Pauli RM, Johnston D, et al. Natural history study of hereditary multiple exostoses. Am J Med Genet 1995;55:43–46.

Radial Dysplasia Reconstruction

Carley Vuillermin, Marybeth Ezaki, and Scott N. Oishi

DEFINITION

- Radial dysplasia represents a spectrum of longitudinal deficiency in radial growth.
- This deficiency can be mild or severe based on the deficiency in the radius.

ANATOMY

- The anatomic relations of the radial aspect of the wrist are altered due to the variable absence of the radius.
  - The higher the degree of radial dysplasia, the more divergent from normal anatomic relationships the findings will be. This is critically important when undertaking surgical intervention.
  - A consistent but highly abnormal brachiocarpalis muscle has been described in thrombocytopenia–absent radius (TAR) syndrome.[14] This muscle spans from just distal to the deltoid insertion directly into the radial side of the carpus and inserts as a broad aponeurotic fan into the carpus, joint capsule, and tendons of the radial wrist.
- Many patients have associated thumb hypoplasia.[10]
- Bayne and Klug[2] have provided a classification based on radiographic findings (Table 1).
  - Several authors have proposed alterations to this classification in order to better describe the spectrum of presentation. James et al[12] added N and 0 categories. N represents patients with a normal radius and carpus but hypoplastic thumb and 0 for patients with carpal abnormalities and

Table 1 Bayne and Klug Classification of Radial Dysplasia

Type	Radiograph	Description
I	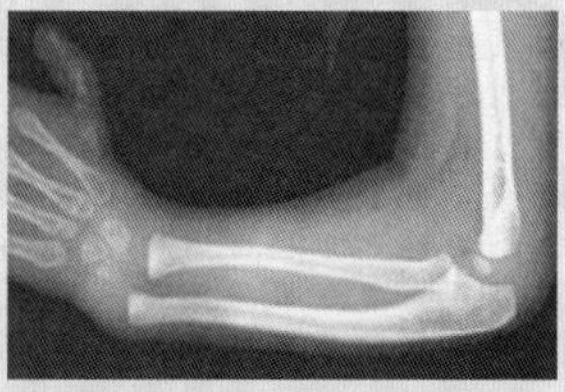	Short distal radius; distal epiphysis present, delayed; mild radial deviation
II	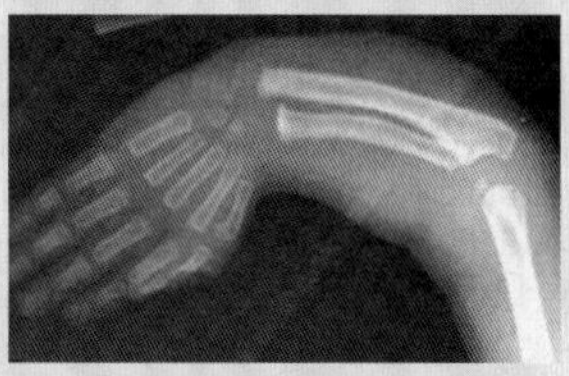	Defective growth proximal–distal epiphyses; radius in miniature
III	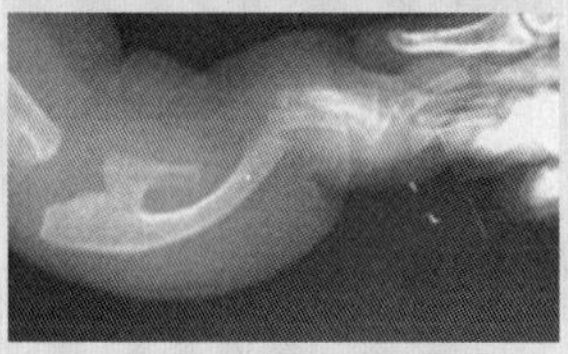	Partial absence of radius; wrist unsupported
IV	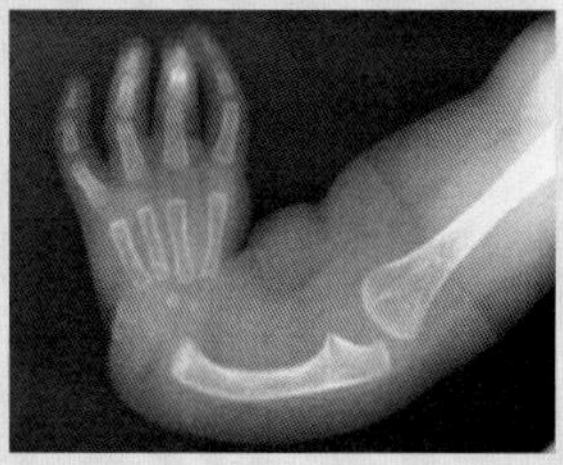	Total absence of radius

Adapted from Bayne CG, Klug MS. Long-term review of the surgical treatment of radial deficiencies. J Hand Surg Am 1987;12(2):169–179.

normal radial length. Goldfarb et al[9] proposed a type V for more proximal deficiencies.

PATHOGENESIS

- Radial dysplasia develops during the period of embryogenesis. During this period, other organ systems are developing and may also be affected, as discussed later in this chapter.

NATURAL HISTORY

- The natural history of patients with radial dysplasia clearly depends on the type of dysplasia present and the associated conditions.
  - Patients with isolated type I or II radial dysplasia usually do not require surgical intervention to address the wrist and radial deformity.
  - Patients with more severe dysplasia can frequently benefit from surgical intervention.
- Many times radial dysplasia is part of a syndrome, and the associated sequelae clearly affect these patients more than the underlying radial dysplasia. The most common associations are with Holt-Oram syndrome, TAR syndrome, Fanconi anemia, and VACTERL (vertebral anomalies, anal atresia, cardiovascular anomalies, tracheoesophageal fistula, esophageal atresia, renal or radial anomalies, limb anomalies).[10,11]
- An association with several craniofacial syndromes has been well documented.[8]
- No matter what procedure is used for treating the radial dysplasia, the patients all have a high incidence of recurrent deformity as they get older.[2,4,17]

PATIENT HISTORY AND PHYSICAL FINDINGS

- The most significant finding is radial deviation at the wrist (**FIG 1**).
- If the patient is older, the affected forearm will also be short.
- Assessment of adjacent joints is essential. Frequently, there will be associated thumb hypoplasia or absence, and in more severe cases (especially Holt-Oram syndrome), the other digits may be stiff. Elbow range of motion is important and the ability to bring the hand to the mouth once the wrist is in a corrected position should be assessed. Radioulnar synostosis is also sometimes present especially in children with Holt-Oram syndrome.
- Because of its frequent association with systemic conditions, all patients require careful examination of their spine and cardiac, renal, and hematologic systems.

IMAGING AND OTHER DIAGNOSTIC STUDIES

- Radiographs should be taken of both forearms to assess stage of radial dysplasia (see Table 1).
- In addition, all patients warrant a workup for syndromes and associated conditions, such as Holt-Oram syndrome, Fanconi anemia, TAR syndrome, and VACTERL.
  - This may require echocardiogram, renal ultrasound, hematologic studies (complete blood count [CBC] and chromosomal fragility studies), and spinal evaluation.
  - Each treating physician should consider these associations and not assume they have already been worked up, especially if surgical care of the limb is contemplated.

NONOPERATIVE MANAGEMENT

- All patients warrant stretching and splinting before consideration of any surgical intervention.
  - The splints should be large enough to be effective and also to minimize any choking hazard.

SURGICAL MANAGEMENT

- Patients with type I or II radial dysplasia usually do not require surgical intervention.
- Surgical treatment has generally ranged from soft tissue rebalancing alone to full centralization of the wrist with or without external fixation.
  - Before any procedure is contemplated, the surgeon must remember that the patient must maintain the ability to get his or her fingers to the mouth with the wrist in the surgically altered position.
  - Very severe radial dysplasia associated with poor elbow function or poor fingers is a contraindication to surgical intervention. The patient may rely on the radial deviation to reach their mouth or use radial wrist pinch for function.
- Many different surgical procedures have been described (**FIG 2**).
  - Soft tissue procedures have traditionally been combined with skeletal rearrangement. Local rotational flaps allow for redistribution of tissue from the ulnar side of the wrist. Evans et al[7] first described the bilobed flap in 1995.

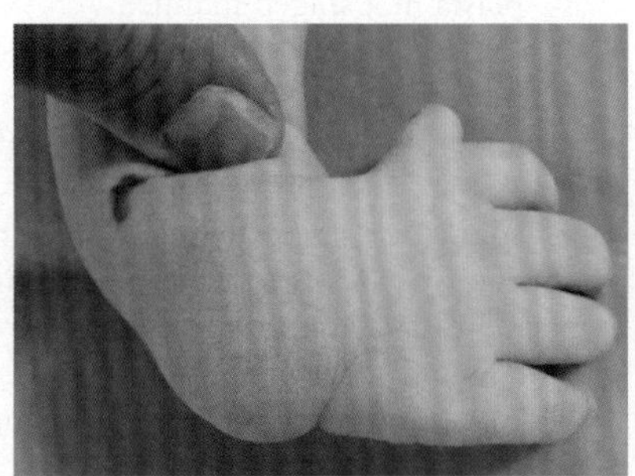
A

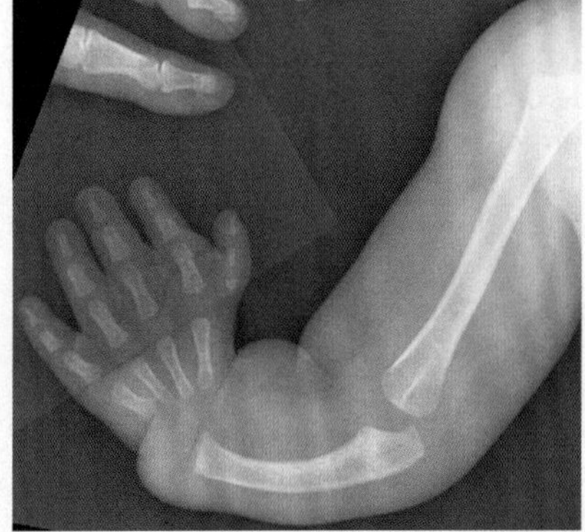
B

FIG 1 • **A.** Preoperative photo showing radial deviation of the wrist. **B.** Anteroposterior (AP) radiograph of the same child demonstrating type IV radial deficiency.

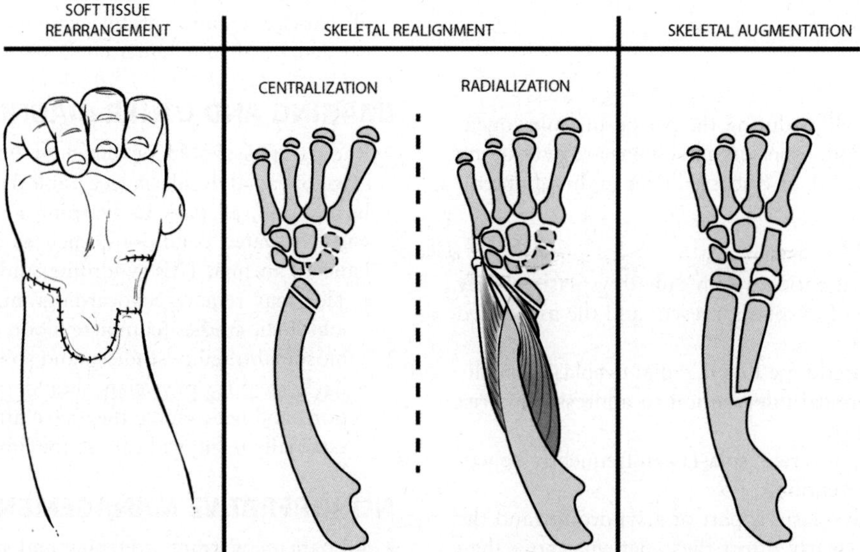

FIG 2 • Surgical options for correction of radial dysplasia.

Manske and others[13] previously described simple excision of the ulnar redundancy without the addition of tissue to the radial side.

- Centralization has been the most common procedure and was first described by Sayre in 1893.[15] These procedures bring the carpus in line with the distal ulna and many create a notch to stabilize the carpus in a mortise and tenon fashion. Buck-Gramcko[3] described radialization, where the carpus is brought across to the ulnar side of the ulna and the extensor carpi radialis (ECR) and flexor carpi radialis (FCR) muscle are transposed. This was proposed to improve balance and limit the recurrence seen after centralization.
  - Ulnar growth disturbance has been found to be increased in patients who have undergone centralization procedures.[16]
- Nonvascularized bone transfer has been tried with or without epiphyseal transfer[1,18] and largely abandoned due to a lack of ongoing growth leading to recurrent deformity.
- Vascularized bone transfer can be used in selective cases to provide stabilization of the radial side of the wrist.[19] A vascularized second toe metatarsophalangeal (MTP) joint as described by De Jong et al[5] and Vilkki[20] or proximal fibular transfer, provide structural support to the deficient radial side of the wrist and allow for continued growth with the growth of the child. These potentially limit recurrence while maintaining wrist motion.
- The long-term problem for any surgical procedure is the recurrence rate.
- Interventions should aim to minimize risk of further growth abnormality and preserve motion. Total range of motion of the fingers and wrist are more important to activity and participation than the angulation at the wrist.[6] Preservation of range of motion should be the goal of any selected surgical procedure.
- We have had experience with various procedures for the treatment of radial dysplasia, including centralization, free toe MTP transfer for stabilization of the radial wrist, and soft tissue release alone. We no longer use formal centralization procedures, as we have found the recurrence rate to be similar to our soft tissue release procedure. In addition, this procedure jeopardizes the ulnar epiphysis, which can lead to an extraordinarily short forearm. Also, loss of mobility results when a centralization procedure is successful.
  - For our patients, soft tissue release with a bilobed flap reconstruction has provided the most reliable, effective results. This maintains motion, improves position, and minimizes injury to the distal ulnar physis. This does not preclude vascularized free joint transfer or other procedures at a subsequent juncture.

Preoperative Planning

- Timing of surgery. Younger patients have the most to gain from soft tissue release with bilobed flap. Our preference is to perform this procedure between 12 months and 2 years of age; however, older patients will also benefit.
  - May be combined with other indicated surgical procedures, including flexor digitorum superficialis (FDS) opponensplasty
  - We prefer to perform pollicization or thumb reconstructive procedures for associated types IIIB to V thumb hypoplasia in a staged manner.
  - Others have combined centralization procedures with bilobed flaps.
- Radiographs are performed to confirm clinical findings (see **FIG 1B**).
- Clearance of associated comorbidities—appropriate consultation or investigation in particular to exclude cardiac and hematologic abnormalities that may influence safety of anesthesia and surgical complications.
- Before surgery, the patient must have undergone adequate soft tissue stretching.
  - In the first few months, this is accomplished by splinting. In severe cases, serial casting may be necessary.

- After about 6 months of age, active stretching is started by the parents with use of nighttime splinting.
- External fixator–assisted soft tissue distraction is reserved for the most severe cases and, in our experience, is uncommonly indicated prior to a bilobed flap; it may be beneficial in older children.

Positioning

- The patient is placed in the standard supine position, and a general anesthetic is used in all cases.
- We do not use a standard tourniquet, as we have found this to be inadequate in young children. Instead, we use the elastic Esmarch bandage as a tourniquet on the upper arm.

Approach

- The bilobed flap design must be drawn appropriately to take advantage of the redundant tissue on the ulnar side of the wrist.
- A dorsal or volar surgical approach and flap design may be used, our experience with the volar approach is that it allows more direct access and release of the tight structures on the volar radial aspect of the wrist and places the scars in an aesthetically less prominent position without compromising the surgical outcome.

Volar Bilobed Flap

- After induction of general anesthesia, the upper extremity is prepared and draped to allow access to the entire arm.
- The volar bilobed flap is then carefully designed using a marking pen (**TECH FIG 1**).
  - Key points in marking out the flap:
    - Point for insetting of the flap on the radial side of the wrist is at the maximal concavity of the deformity. This is the point of maximal tension when the wrist is ulnarly deviated.
    - Mark the first lobe of the flap on the volar surface of the wrist with the apex proximal (starting at the inset point). The base of the flap is perpendicular to the long axis of the forearm.
    - The second lobe of the flap is identical in geometry to the first however perpendicular to it on the ulnar side of the wrist. This flap uses the redundant ulnar skin.
    - Finally, the inset incision on the radial side of the wrist is marked to correspond to the height of the lobes.
  - The Esmarch bandage is used to exsanguinate the limb; it is then wrapped three times around the upper arm for use as a tourniquet.

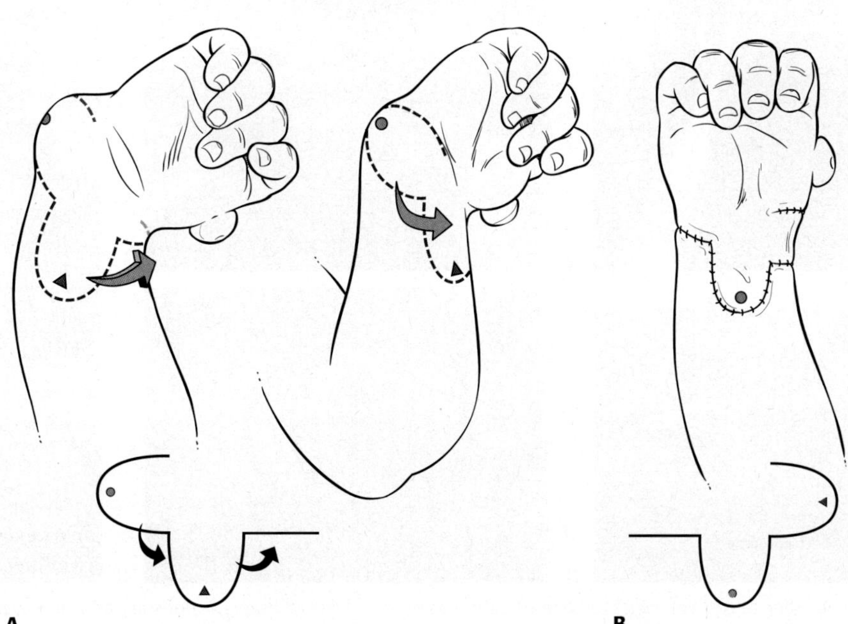

TECH FIG 1 • **A.** Flap design. **B.** Flap rotation and final positioning. *(continued)*

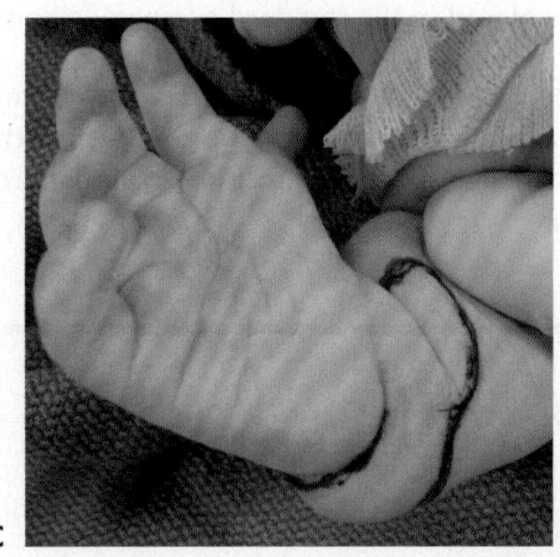

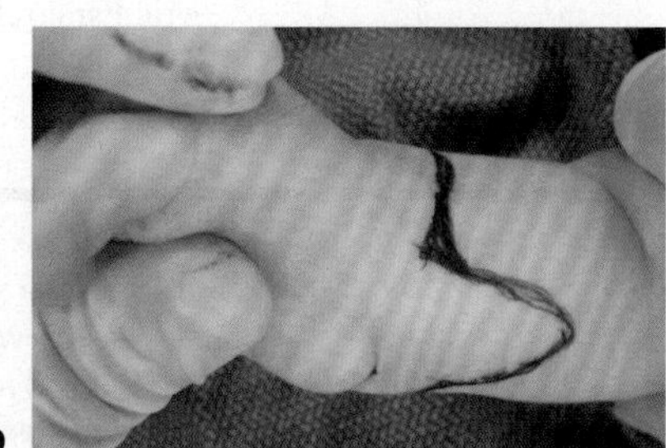

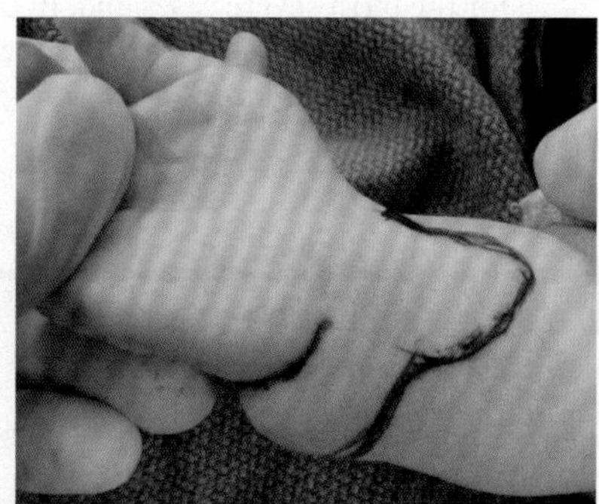

TECH FIG 1 • *(continued)* **C–E.** Markings for bilobed flap.

Release of the Radial Deviation of the Wrist

- After careful incision and elevation of full-thickness skin flaps, the finger and flexor tendons, as well as the median and superficial radial nerves, are carefully identified and preserved. A vascular loop may be used for protection (**TECH FIG 2A**).
- All other tissues in the radial wrist are released including fascial bands and tendons with pure radial deviation wrist moments.
  - Rebalancing of radial wrist flexors to an ulnar insertion or extensor may be performed.
  - Care must be taken not to dissect excessively near the ulnar epiphysis to prevent injury to the vascular supply to this area.
- After release is accomplished, the wrist is placed in a neutral position and pinned with a 0.062-inch Kirschner wire.
  - The Kirschner wire is temporary and is put across the joint from either direction (ie, there is no specific location for the exit or entrance site). Our preferred trajectory is one which avoids crossing the ulnar physis.
- The flaps are then rotated and sutured in place (**TECH FIG 2B–E**).
- The tourniquet is removed to ensure perfusion to the fingers, and a long-arm cast is placed.

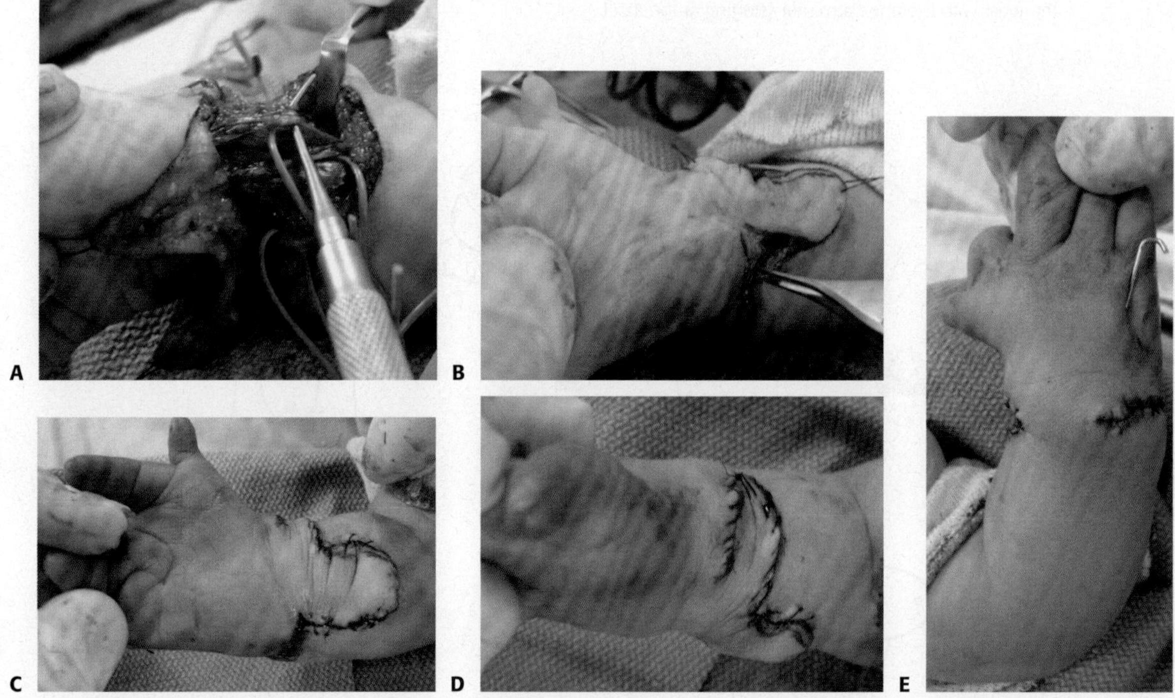

TECH FIG 2 • **A.** After release of radial tethering tissue, protection of finger flexors, extensors, and neurovascular structures. **B.** Rotation of flaps. **C,D.** Skin is sutured. **E.** Dorsal view with protective pin.

PEARLS AND PITFALLS

Adequate preoperative stretching of soft tissues	■ If not adequate, this may lead to a suboptimal result.
Identification of median nerves and tendons, as these structures tend to be in very aberrant locations	■ There is the potential for injury to nerve or tendon during soft tissue release if this is not done.
Careful dissection around the distal ulna	■ If too aggressive, it can lead to injury to the epiphyseal region, leading to growth problems in the ulna.
Pinning of ulnocarpal joint after release	■ Failure to do this can lead to partial flap loss because of motion at the joint.

POSTOPERATIVE CARE

- The long-arm cast is left on for 3 to 4 weeks.
- At that point, the pin is removed and the patient is changed to a removable splint.

OUTCOMES

- The bilobed flap procedure is an effective procedure for treating radial dysplasia (**FIG 3**).
- Deformity tends to recur, although the incidence of this appears to be similar to that for other procedures used to treat radial dysplasia.

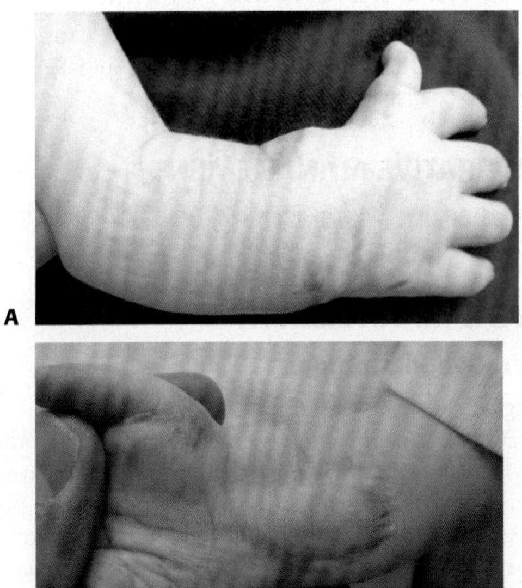

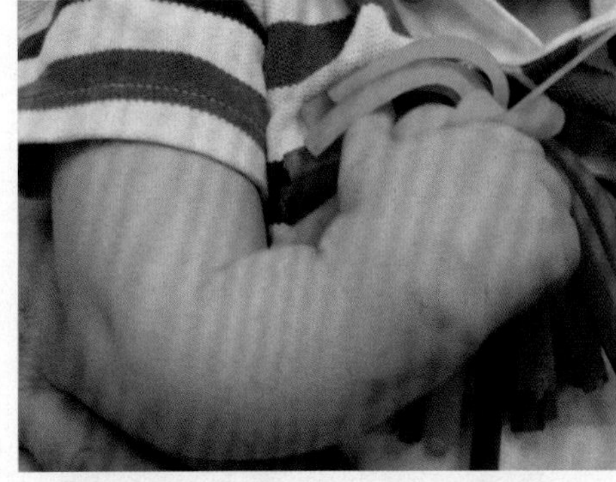

FIG 3 • Postoperative results. **A.** Early healing and resting wrist position. **B.** Volar bilobed flap, post staged pollicization procedure. **C.** Functional positioning post pollicization.

COMPLICATIONS

- Few complications are associated with this procedure.
- Partial flap loss can occur, but the risk seems to be minimized by appropriate flap design, transfixion with a Kirschner wire, and immobilization after the procedure.

REFERENCES

1. Albee FH. Formation of radius congenitally absent: condition seven years after implantation of bone graft. Ann Surg 1928;87(1):105–110.
2. Bayne LG, Klug MS. Long-term review of the surgical treatment of radial deficiency. J Hand Surg Am 1987;12(2):169–179.
3. Buck-Gramcko D. Radialization as a new treatment for radial club hand. J Hand Surg Am 1985;10(6 pt 2):964–968.
4. Damore E, Kozin SH, Thoder JJ, et al. The recurrence of deformity after surgical centralization for radial clubhand. J Hand Surg Am 2000;25(4):745–751.
5. De Jong JP, Moran SL, Vilkki SK. Changing paradigms in the treatment of radial club hand: microvascular joint transfer for correction of radial deviation and preservation of long-term growth. Clin Orthop Surg 2012;4(1):36–44.
6. Ekblom AG, Dahlin LB, Rosberg HE, et al. Hand function in children with radial longitudinal deficiency. BMC Musculoskelet Disord 2013;14:116.
7. Evans DM, Gateley DR, Lewis JS. The use of a bilobed flap in the correction of radial club hand. J Hand Surg Br 1995;20(3):333–337.
8. Goldberg MJ, Bartoshesky LE. Congenital hand anomaly: etiology and associated malformations. Hand Clin 1985;1(3):405–415.
9. Goldfarb CA, Manske PR, Busa R, et al. Upper-extremity phocomelia reexamined: a longitudinal dysplasia. J Bone Joint Surg Am 2005;87(12):2639–2648.
10. Goldfarb CA, Wall L, Manske PR. Radial longitudinal deficiency: the incidence of associated medical and musculoskeletal conditions. J Hand Surg Am 2006;31(7):1176–1182.
11. James MA, Green HD, McCarroll HR, et al. The association of radial deficiency with thumb hypoplasia. J Bone Joint Surg Am 2004;86-A(10):2196–2205.
12. James MA, McCarroll HR Jr, Manske PR. The spectrum of radial longitudinal deficiency: a modified classification. J Hand Surg Am 1999;24(6):1145–1155.
13. Manske PR, McCarroll HR Jr, Swanson K. Centralization of the radial club hand: an ulnar surgical approach. J Hand Surg Am 1981;6(5):423–433.
14. Oishi SN, Carter P, Bidwell T, et al. Thrombocytopenia absent radius syndrome: presence of brachiocarpalis muscle and its importance. J Hand Surg Am 2009;34(9):1696–1699.
15. Sayre RH. A contribution to the study of club-hand. Trans Am Orthop Assn 1893;6:208–216.
16. Sestero AM, Van Heest A, Agel J. Ulnar growth patterns in radial longitudinal deficiency. J Hand Surg Am 2006;31(6):960–967.
17. Shariatzadeh H, Jafari D, Taheri H, et al. Recurrence rate after radial club hand surgery in long term follow up. J Res Med Sci 2009;14(3):179–186.
18. Starr DE. Congenital absence of the radius: a method of surgical correction. J Bone Joint Surg Am 1945;27(4):572–577.
19. Vilkki SK. Distraction and microvascular epiphysis transfer for radial club hand. J Hand Surg Br 1998;23(4):445–452.
20. Vilkki SK. Vascularized metatarsophalangeal joint transfer for radial hypoplasia. Semin Plast Surg 2008;22(3):195–212.

CHAPTER

Preaxial and Postaxial Polydactyly

Robert Carrigan

DEFINITION

- Polydactyly refers to having greater than the normal number of digits.
- Preaxial polydactyly is duplication or splitting of the thumb.
- Central polydactyly is duplication of the central digits (index, middle, and ring).
- Postaxial polydactyly is duplication of the small finger.

ANATOMY

- In cases of digit duplication, one may observe duplication in some or all of the elements of the finger (bone, nail, joints, and tendon). The duplicate finger may be well formed and near normal in appearance or underdeveloped and rudimentary in appearance.
- Wassel published a classification of thumb duplication based on the work of Adrian Flatt, MD (Table 1).
- Postaxial polydactyly classification
  - Type A: well-formed duplicate small finger with bone or tendon attachments (**FIG 1**)
  - Type B: small pediculated nubbin

PATHOGENESIS

- Duplication of the digits occurs early in embryogenesis.
- Patterning of the limb is demonstrated in three axis: proximodistal axis (modulated by the apical ectodermal ridge [AER]), anteroposterior axis (modulated by the zone of polarizing activity [ZPA]), and the dorsoventral axis regulated by the Engrailed 1 protein (EN1).
- Abnormal or ectopic presence of sonic hedgehog protein is implicated in preaxial polydactyly.
- Familial cases of postaxial polydactyly demonstrate a defect in the *GLI3* gene.

Table 1 Wassel Classification of Thumb Duplication

Type	Description
I	Bifid distal phalanx
II	Duplicate distal phalanx
III	Bifid proximal phalanx
IV	Duplicate proximal phalanx
V	Bifid metacarpal
VI	Duplicate metacarpal
VII	Triphalangeal thumb

From Wassel HD. The results of surgery for polydactyly of the thumb. Clin Orthop Relat Res 1969;64:175–193.

PATIENT HISTORY AND PHYSICAL FINDINGS

- The diagnosis of polydactyly is straightforward, clinical examination and radiographs are sufficient to make the diagnosis.

IMAGING AND OTHER DIAGNOSTIC STUDIES

- Standard radiographs (three views—anteroposterior, lateral, and oblique) of the hand and affected digit are sufficient to determine the area of involvement (**FIG 2**).
- Advanced imaging such as magnetic resonance imaging (MRI) and computed tomography (CT) is rarely needed.

DIFFERENTIAL DIAGNOSIS

- Associated syndromes should be screened for, including trisomy 21 and Rubinstein-Taybi, Apert, and Russell-Silver syndrome.

NONOPERATIVE MANAGEMENT

- Observation may be considered for duplicated digits that do not impair function of the hand.

SURGICAL MANAGEMENT

Preoperative Planning

- Timing of surgery is variable.
- Type B postaxial polydactyly may be removed in the office under local anesthesia, when the child is just a few weeks old.
- Preaxial polydactyly reconstruction and type A postaxial reconstructions are elective procedures and are generally performed after 1 year of age and before the start of school.

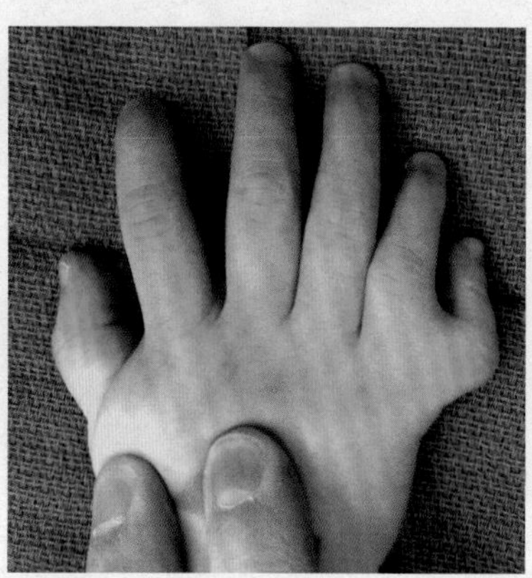

FIG 1 • Type A postaxial polydactyly.

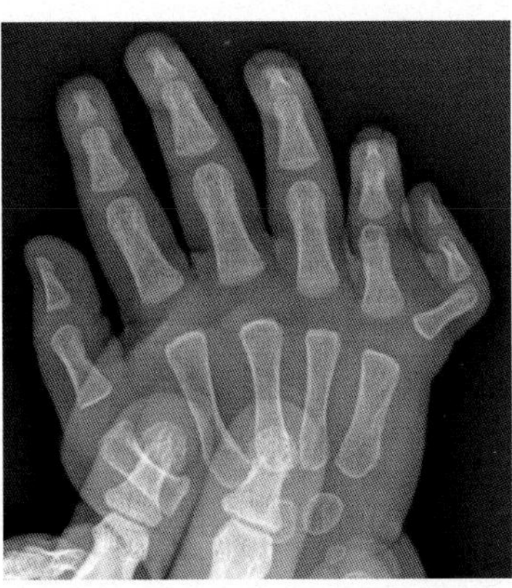

FIG 2 • Preoperative radiograph of the patient in **FIG 1** with type A postaxial polydactyly, depicting the bifacet metacarpal head.

Positioning

- The patient is positioned supine on the table and the body is pulled over to the affected side.
- The arm is placed on a radiolucent hand table and an arm tourniquet is applied.

Approach

- Deletion and reconstruction of a polydactyly is not simply an amputation. The surgeon should be aware of protecting and preserving vital structures such as the collateral ligaments and tendon insertions for reattachment to the preserved digit.
- Several approaches may be considered for the management of pre- and postaxial polydactyly.
- Skin incisions must take in to consideration preservation of nail folds where appropriate.

TECHNIQUES

Type A Postaxial Polydactyly

- A racquet-type incision is made around the digit to be deleted. Skin flaps are developed.
- The adductor digiti minimi (ADQ) is identified and detached from its insertion and tagged.
- The ulnar collateral ligament (UCL) from the metacarpophalangeal joint (MCP) is released from the proximal phalanx with a large sleeve of periosteum and tagged.
- The digital nerves and vessels are identified and ligated.
- The duplicated digit is removed (**TECH FIG 1**).
- The ADQ and UCL are reinserted with 4-0 nonabsorbable suture (Ethibond).
- Skin is closed with absorbable suture (5-0 fast absorbing chromic gut).
- The hand is dressed and casted with the fingertips exposed for 2 weeks.

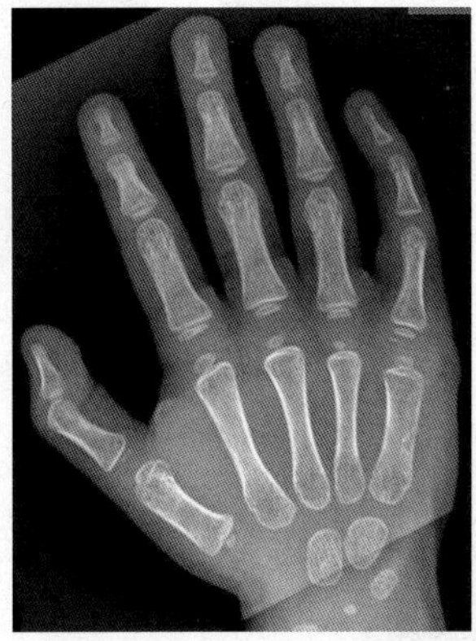

TECH FIG 1 • Postoperative radiograph of the patient in **FIGS 1** and **2** demonstrating well-aligned MCP joint.

Type B Postaxial Polydactyly

- These rudimentary supernumerary digits can be addressed by simple ligature or excision.
- Ligature of the rudimentary digit can be accomplished via a surgical tie such as 2-0 silk or hemaclip.
  - Application of the ligature should be tight enough to occlude the digital artery. A loose ligature will simple occlude the venous outflow and cause congestion, which can be painful for the child and prolong the time for the digit to become ischemic and fall off. A ligature placed too distal on the pedicle stalk will leave a stump and often a painful neuroma.
- Surgical excision can be performed in the office under local anesthetic.
- The child is placed in a papoose. A digital block is performed and the hand is prepped.
- The base of the supernumerary is pinched between the surgeon's index finger and thumb, and the stalk is cut with a pair of iris scissors. The vessel is identified and cauterized.
- The base is then sutured with interrupted locking absorbable 5-0 fast absorbing gut suture.
- Soft compressive dressings are applied with the tips available for the parents to observe.
- Dressings are removed in 3 days and bathing can be initiated after that.
- No follow-up is usually necessary.

Wassel I or II Preaxial Polydactyly

- Reconstruction of the duplicated thumb involving the distal phalanx may be accomplished in one of two ways.

Bilhaut-Cloquet Procedure

- The Bilhaut-Cloquet procedure has been historically advocated for treatment of Wassel I or II thumb duplication.
- This involves a central wedge resection and reapproximation of the radial and ulnar structures (**TECH FIGS 2** and **3**).
- This procedure has fallen out of favor due to residual nail irregularities.

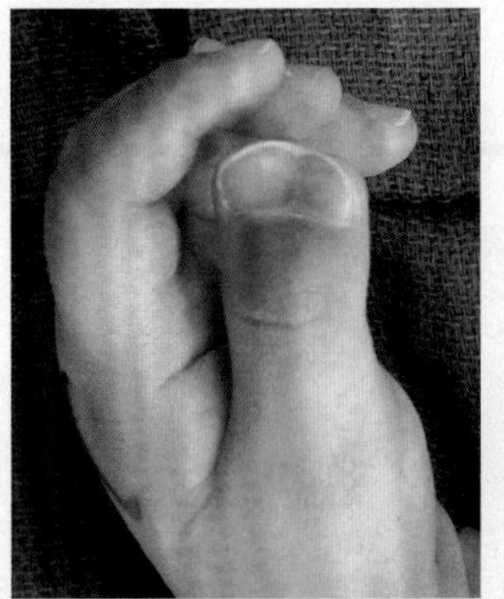

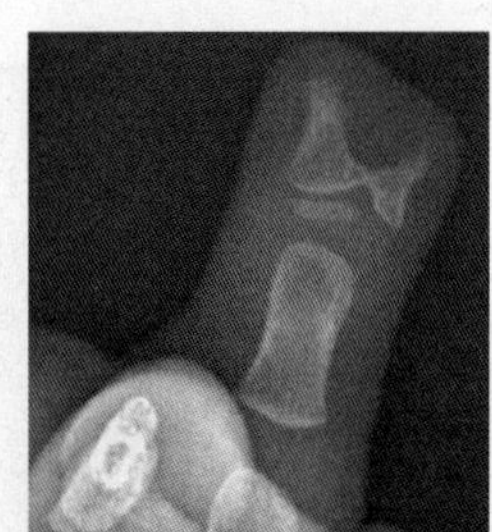

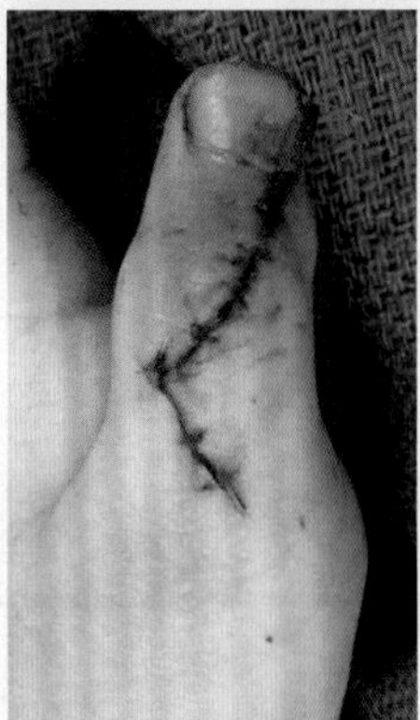

TECH FIG 2 • **A.** Clinical photograph demonstrating conjoined nails in a Wassel I thumb. **B.** Preoperative radiograph. **C.** Postoperative photograph demonstrates normal IP alignment and nail fold following resection of small duplicated thumb.

Removal of Duplicate Thumb

- Duplication of the thumb is rarely symmetric. One of the two duplicated thumb parts is usually larger. Deletion of the smaller thumb part is favorable.
- Racquet-shaped incisions are made about the thumb to excise the desired duplication. Careful attention is made to preserve the appropriate nail elements.
- Skin flaps are developed and the extensor tendons and flexor tendons are identified. Tendon insertions to the intended deleted digit are transected and tagged for reinsertion.
- The collateral ligament to the interphalangeal (IP) joint is elevated with a sleeve of periosteum.
- The duplicated digit is excised; if the head of the proximal phalanx has two facets, a chondroplasty (reshaping of the head) with a no. 15 blade may be necessary.
- The collateral ligament is reinserted and the joint is tested for stability.
- The flexor and extensor tendons are rebalanced.
- Skin is closed with 5-0 fast absorbing gut suture.
- Sterile dressings and a long-arm thumb spica cast are applied.
- Follow-up in 2 weeks for cast removal.

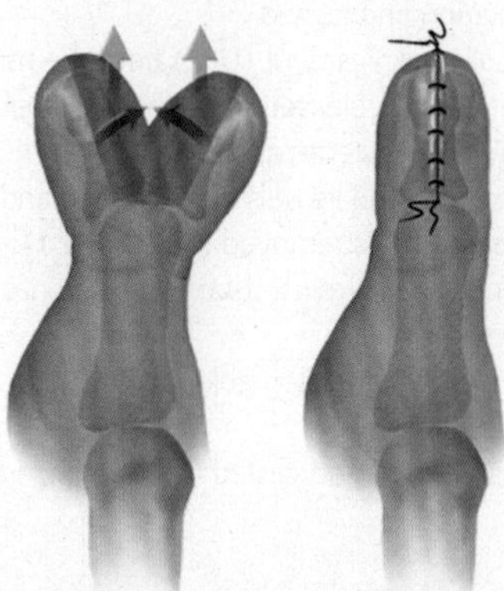

TECH FIG 3 • Diagram depicting the Bilhaut-Cloquet procedure. (From Waters PM, Bae DS. Preaxial polydactyly. In: Pediatric Hand and Upper Limb Surgery: A Practical Guide. Philadelphia: Lippincott Williams & Wilkins, 2012:32–42.)

Wassel Type III or IV Preaxial Polydactyly

- Duplication of the thumb is rarely symmetric. One of the two duplicated thumb parts is usually larger. Deletion of the smaller thumb part is favorable (**TECH FIG 4**).
- In most cases, the radial digit is the smaller of the two, and deletion is favored as it preserves the native UCL, which is important for pinch (**TECH FIG 5A,B**).
- Racquet-shaped incisions are made about the thumb to excise the desired duplication.
- Skin flaps are developed and the extensor tendons and flexor tendons are identified.
- Tendon insertions to the intended deleted digit are transected and tagged for reinsertion.

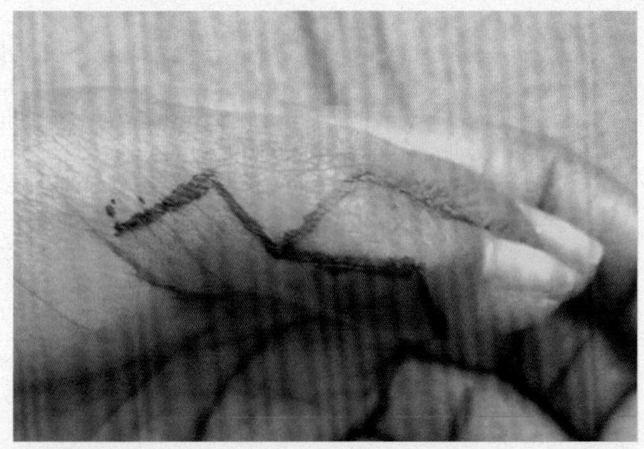

TECH FIG 4 • Skin incisions for resection of Wassel III duplicate.

- The intrinsic musculature is elevated from its insertion and tagged.
- The collateral ligament to the MCP joint is elevated with a sleeve of periosteum.
- The duplicated digit is excised; if the head of metacarpal has two facets, a chondroplasty (reshaping of the head) with a no.15 blade may be necessary.
- If angulation of the thumb is present at the MCP joint, a closed wedge osteotomy of the metacarpal neck may be necessary to align the thumb. This can be accomplished with a small rongeur, removing bone on the radial side of the metacarpal, leaving the ulnar cortex intact, and closing the osteotomy and securing with wire.
- The collateral ligament is reinserted, and the joint is tested for stability.
- The intrinsic musculature is reinserted (**TECH FIG 5C**).
- The flexor and extensor tendons are rebalanced.
- Skin is closed with 5-0 fast absorbing gut suture (**TECH FIG 5D**).
- Sterile dressings and a long-arm thumb spica cast are applied.

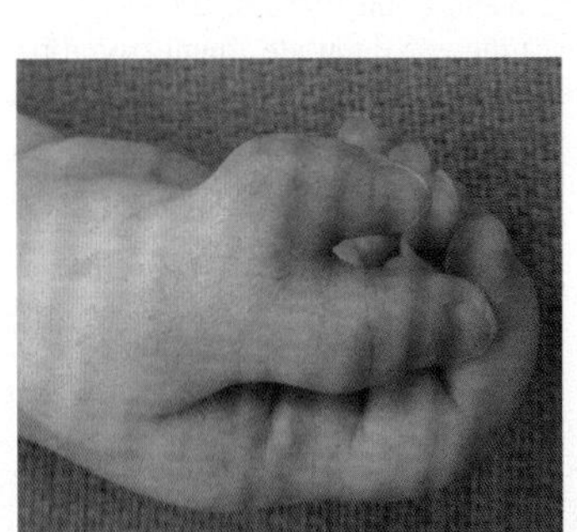
A

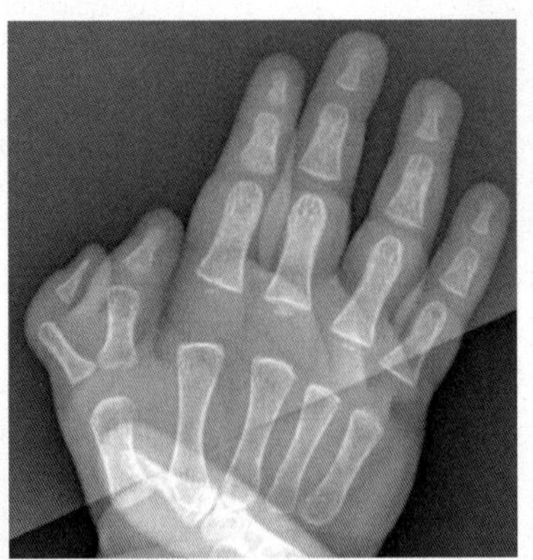
B

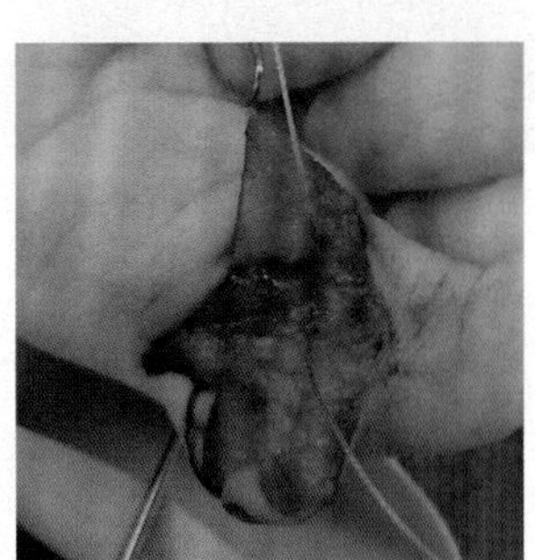
C

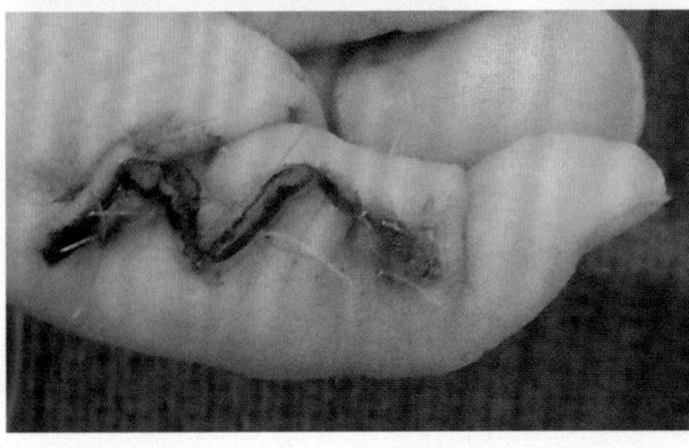
D

TECH FIG 5 • **A,B.** Preoperative photograph and radiography, respectively, of Wassel IV duplicate thumb. **C.** Intraoperative photograph depicting reinsertion of intrinsic musculature following deletion of radial duplicate thumb. **D.** Postoperative skin closure following deletion of radial duplicate thumb.

PEARLS AND PITFALLS

Persistent joint angulation	■ Failure to recognize deforming factors, such as misaligned tendons and residual bony deformity
Persistent joint instability	■ Collateral ligaments must be properly reinserted.
Painful neuromas (see FIG 3)	■ Digital nerves must be identified and cut short to retract away from the skin surface.

POSTOPERATIVE CARE

- The first postoperative visit is 2 weeks from surgery, 4 weeks if an osteotomy is performed.
- The cast is removed and digit is inspected.
- Radiographs are obtained to evaluate healing in the case of and osteotomy.
- Pins are pulled where appropriate.
- The family is instructed about wound care and scar massage.
- Occupational therapy is not instituted unless there is concern for persistent joint stiffness.

OUTCOMES

- Outcomes from polydactyly reconstruction correction are generally good with most patients reporting good function and aesthetics.

COMPLICATIONS

- Irregularities with the nail fold and residual IP joint angulation are common following thumb reconstruction.
- Neuroma sometimes occurs after suture ligation of postaxial polydactyly (**FIG 3**).

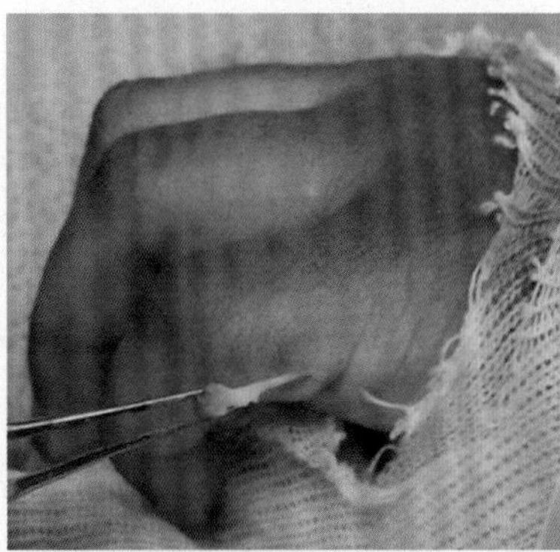

FIG 3 ● Painful neuroma following suture ligation of postaxial polydactyly.

- Failure to reinsert collateral ligaments or intrinsic musculature may lead to joint incompetence or weakness, respectively.

SUGGESTED READINGS

1. Al-Qattan MM, Kozin SH. Update on embryology of the upper limb. J Hand Surg Am 2013;38:1835–1844.
2. Dobyns JH, Lipscomb PR, Cooney WP. Management of thumb duplication. Clin Orthop Relat Res 1985:(195):26–44.
3. Ezaki M. Radial polydactyly. Hand Clin 1990;6:577–588.
4. Ganley TJ, Lubahn JD. Radial polydactyly: an outcome study. Ann Plast Surg 1995;35:86–89.
5. Goldfarb CA, Patterson JM, Maender A, et al. Thumb size and appearance following reconstruction of radial polydactyly. J Hand Surg Am 2008;33:1348–1353.
6. Manske PR. Treatment of duplicated thumb using a ligamentous/periosteal flap. J Hand Surg Am 1989;14:728–733.
7. Mih AD. Complications of duplicate thumb reconstruction. Hand Clin 1998;14:143–149.

152

CHAPTER

Correction of Thumb-in-Palm Deformity in Cerebral Palsy

Thanapong Waitayawinyu, Carley Vuillermin, and Scott N. Oishi

DEFINITION

- The thumb-in-palm deformity is a fixed adduction–flexion posture in the affected hand of the patient with spastic cerebral palsy. This influences both hand function and hygiene.

ANATOMY

- Imbalance of the spastic thumb flexor–adductor and the paretic thumb extensor results in thumb-in-palm deformity (**FIG 1A**).
- The adductor pollicis (AP) is the most commonly involved muscle; the abductor pollicis brevis (APB) is usually not involved.[17]
- The spastic AP, the first dorsal interosseous muscle, or both adduct the thumb and index metacarpals and cause first web space contracture.
- If the flexor pollicis brevis (FPB) is spastic, the thumb metacarpophalangeal (MCP) joint will develop a flexion deformity.
- Involvement of both the AP and FPB results in a thumb flexion and adduction posture with the thumb lying across the palm.
- Involvement of the flexor pollicis longus (FPL) results in added thumb interphalangeal (IP) joint flexion (**FIG 1B**).
- Weak thumb extensor and abductor pollicis longus (APL) may also contribute to the deformity.
- Active function of the extensor pollicis longus (EPL) and extensor pollicis brevis (EPB) may result in hyperextension of the thumb MCP joint.

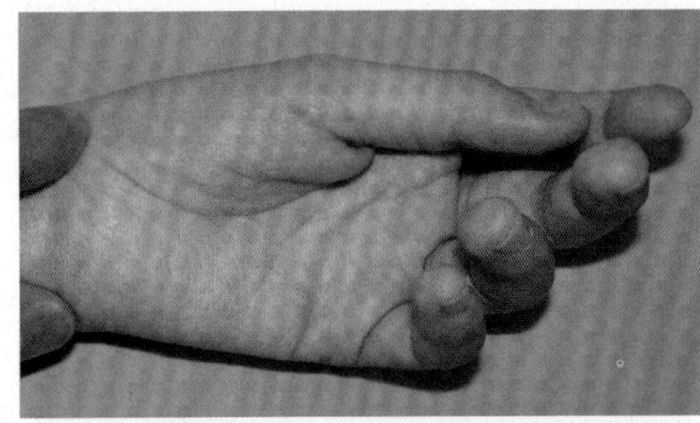

A

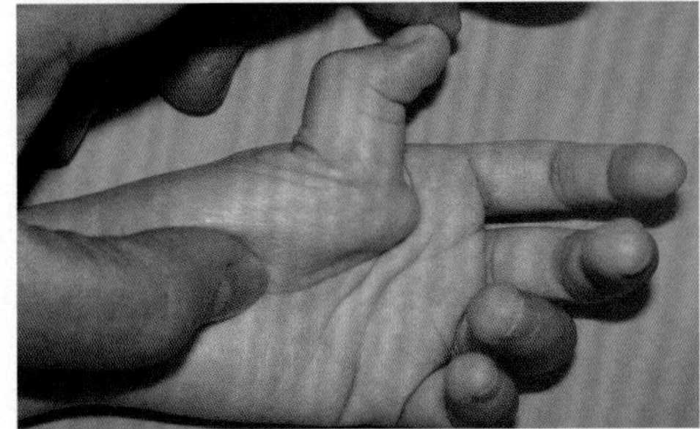

B

FIG 1 • Thumb-in-palm deformity (**A**) demonstrating MCP laxity and hyperextension (**B**).

PATHOGENESIS

- Cerebral palsy is permanent disorder of the development of movement and posture, causing activity limitation, attributed to a nonprogressive neurologic disturbance that occurred in the developing fetal or infant brain. The disorders of cerebral palsy are often accompanied by disturbances of sensation, perception, and cognition.[11]
- The musculoskeletal findings develop secondarily. Spasticity initially results in shortening of the myotendinous unit and ultimately secondary contractures.
  - Paresis of muscles may contribute to greater deformity when spastic muscles are unopposed. The ultimate deformity depends on the overall imbalance.

NATURAL HISTORY

- A supple thumb-in-palm posture is a normal finding in infants during the first year. Persistence of a tightly closed thumb in palm longer than 1 year is abnormal and should be evaluated.[3]
- The deformity is usually correctable at first and then progresses to a fixed deformity as myostatic contracture develops.
- A progressive and variable-size discrepancy of the involved limb may develop, resulting in a smaller thumb.[1]
- The lack of thumb extension and abduction can impair hand grip, function, appearance, and hygiene.

PATIENT HISTORY AND PHYSICAL FINDINGS

- A complete history and physical examination of a child with cerebral palsy should be done carefully and thoroughly.
- Input from other professionals such as neurologists and occupational therapists is often helpful.
- Associated deformities of the spastic upper extremity such as finger and wrist flexion, forearm pronation, elbow flexion, and shoulder adduction and internal rotation should also be evaluated. Surgical treatment of thumb-in-palm deformity may be only one part of surgical care of the involved extremity.
- Thumb muscle involvement, motion, and stability should be evaluated in the physical examination before organizing the treatment plan.
  - Individual muscle involvement is detected by observing thumb position and palpating spastic or contracted muscles (Table 1). As spasticity is rate-dependent tone, slow gradual stretch should be able to overcome this force, unlike a contracture which is a fixed shortening of a muscle tendon unit or joint.
  - Motion and stability are assessed by passive and active range of thumb abduction–adduction, flexion–extension, and palmar abduction and opposition.

Table 1 Grading of Thumb-in-Palm Deformity

Degree of Deformity	Illustration	Classification: House (1981)	Classification: Tonkin (2001)	Description
Simple deformity		Type I		Spastic or contracted AP, first dorsal interosseous muscle, or both
Intrinsic deformity		Type II	Type 1	Spastic or contracted AP, first dorsal interosseous, or both Spastic or contracted FPB
		Type III		Spastic or contracted AP, first dorsal interosseous, or both Compensatory action of EPL and EPB to the unstable MCP joint Absence of spastic FPL
Extrinsic deformity			Type 2	Spastic or contracted FPL Paretic EPL
Most severe: combined intrinsic and extrinsic deformity		Type IV	Type 3	Spastic or contracted AP, first dorsal interosseous, or both Spastic or contracted FPB and FPL

AP, adductor pollicis longus; FPB, flexor pollicis brevis; EPL, extensor pollicis longus; EPB, extensor pollicis brevis; MCL, metacarpophalangeal; FPL, flexor pollicis longus.

- The pattern of voluntary grasp and release of large objects and manipulation of small objects should be determined by observing the child during functional activities.
- Sensory deficits impair function. Assessment of sensation should include stereognosis.
- Repeated observation or videotaping of the child during various activities can also be useful for accurate evaluation. This can be particularly valuable in detecting dystonia.
- Lower extremity function and need for intervention should be considered and coordinated appropriately.

IMAGING AND OTHER DIAGNOSTIC STUDIES

- Electrophysiologic testing and selective nerve blocks may help in localizing involved muscles and identifying muscles available for tendon transfers.
- Select nerve blocks may help differentiate between spastic, spared, and fibrotic muscles.
- Dynamic electromyography (EMG) with motion analysis may offer important information for planning tendon transfer surgery.[5]
- Radiographs may reveal thumb joint instability or growth disturbance.

DIFFERENTIAL DIAGNOSIS

- Clasped thumb
- Distal arthrogryposis
- Apparent absence of thumb extensor (faux extensor agenesis)

MANAGEMENT

- The goals of treatment need to be clearly defined.
- No peripheral intervention will overcome the fundamental central nervous system etiology.

- For many patients, the goal will be to improve thumb position for function; however, there is a subset of highly involved patients for whom improved hygiene alone may the goal.

NONOPERATIVE MANAGEMENT

- Use of tone-reducing medication such as botulinum toxin to the AP can soften the deformities and improve joint range of motion for nonoperative management.[4]
- In mild, nonrigid deformity, nonoperative treatment with orthoses may help in maintaining thumb abduction and improve hand function,[13] but too-rigid splinting may result in limited thumb motion.

SURGICAL MANAGEMENT

- The principles of surgery for thumb-in-palm deformity are the following[2]:
  - Release of spastic muscles or contractures
  - Augmentation of paretic muscles
  - Stabilization of unstable thumb joints
- Release of contracture with or without augmentation of weak muscles aims to rebalance the thumb muscles, depending on the pattern of motor dysfunction of the thumb and the patient's degree of voluntary control.
- Release of spastic muscle or myostatic contractures can be performed by intrinsic muscle release of the AP, FPB, APB, and first dorsal interosseous.
  - Extrinsic muscle release of the FPL may be considered if it is affected.
  - Secondary skin and fascial contracture of the first web space need to be addressed by four-flap or double-opposing Z-plasty.
- Augmentation of paretic thumb abduction and extension can be accomplished by a combination of tenodesis and tendon rerouting or transfers and depends on the specific deficit, the muscles available, and the extent of voluntary control of selected muscles.
- Thumb MCP joint arthrodesis or sesamoid capsulodesis should be considered for stabilizing the thumb MCP joints when the joint remains unstable.[2]
  - These joint stabilization procedures can also enhance tendon transfer procedures for extension–abduction.
- Thumb MCP joint arthrodesis is considered when tendon transfer fails to correct the deformities or when sesamoid capsulodesis cannot control the hyperextension of the MCP joint.[1]
- Thumb carpometacarpal (CMC) joint stabilization is indicated when metacarpal adduction cannot be controlled. CMC fusion, which preserves scaphotrapezial motion, is preferable to the rigid intermetacarpal fusion.[2]
- Thumb IP joint fusion is usually not necessary, but this procedure may be indicated when the IP joint flexion contracture is severe or in the rare event of an FPL rupture after lengthening.[2]
- Neurectomy may be an adjunct procedure for a clenched fist deformity in a hand with no active movement and difficulty with passive hand function including hygiene[9]; however, its role is limited.
- Table 2 lists surgical options for treating thumb-in-palm deformity.[14]

Table 2 Surgical Options for Correcting Thumb-in-Palm Deformity

Releases
Adductor release in palm
Adductor tenotomy
First dorsal interosseous release
FPB release
FPL slide
First web skin and fascia release
Augmentation of APL, EPL, EPB using
Brachioradialis
FDS
PL
EPL to EPB
FCR or FCU
ECRL
APL tenodesis
Through radius to brachioradialis, ECRL, FCR through first dorsal compartment
Joint stabilization
CMC joint fusion
MCP joint sesamoid capsulodesis
MCP joint fusion
IP joint fusion

FPB, flexor pollicis brevis; FPL, flexor pollicis longus; APL, adductor pollicis longus; EPL, extensor pollicis longus; EPB, extensor pollicis brevis, FDS, flexor digitorum superficialis; PL, pollicis longus; FCR, flexor carpi radialis; FCU, flexor carpi ulnaris; ECRL, extensor carpi radialis longus; CMC, carpometacarpal; MCP, metacarpophalangeal; IP, interphalangeal. (Adapted from Tonkin MA. Thumb deformity in the spastic hand: classification and surgical techniques. Tech Hand Up Extrem Surg 2003;7:18–25.)

Preoperative Planning

- Comprehensive evaluation is necessary with a multispecialty approach.
- Surgery should be done when the central nervous system has matured and the child is old enough to cooperate with postoperative therapy—usually at least 5 to 6 years old.[6]
- Associated abnormalities (eg, seizures, mental status problems) should be assessed and the management optimized before surgery is contemplated.
- Patient understanding and emotional readiness as well as family and social support should be addressed before surgery.
- Physical examination under anesthesia is crucial. This can differentiate spastic from myostatic conditions and can accurately evaluate the stability of thumb joints.

Positioning

- The patient is placed in the supine position, and surgery is performed under general anesthesia and tourniquet control.

Approach

- Surgical approaches for thumb-in-palm deformity depend on the objectives.
- Release of static or long-standing intrinsic contracture is usually performed through a curved incision located over the line of the thenar crease to release the origin of the AP with or without the origin of the FPB.[8]
- Release of a simple intrinsic contracture may be performed through the first web space approach to release the AP and the first dorsal interosseous muscle, combined with four-flap

or double-opposing Z-plasty to release the secondary web space contracture.[2]

- A surgical approach by a small incision over the volar aspect of the distal forearm is used for extrinsic release of the FPL tendon, if necessary.
- A dorsal approach to the thumb and a dorsoradial approach over the wrist is used for augmentation of thumb extensors, with a volar-radial approach being used for augmentation of the thumb abductor.

Release of Contractures

Release of Static Intrinsic Contracture

- A curved skin incision is performed next to the line of the thenar crease, extending distally from the carpal tunnel area (**TECH FIG 1A**).
- The superficial palmar arch and median nerve, including its motor branch to the thenar muscle, distal to the transverse carpal ligament are identified and protected. Careful dissection must be performed because occasionally, the motor branch comes through the transverse carpal ligament instead of being distal to this structure (**TECH FIG 1B**).
- The flexor digitorum sublimis and profundi are identified and retracted ulnarly with the neurovascular bundle.
- The transverse head of AP is identified and divided from its origin on the third metacarpal (**TECH FIG 1C,D**).
- The motor branch of the ulnar nerve and the deep palmar arch are identified and protected.
- Release of the oblique head of the AP from its origin at the bases of the second and third metacarpal, capitate, and trapezoid is performed.
- The FPB origin at the transverse carpal ligament and trapezium may also be released if this muscle limits abduction and extension of the thumb ray.
- The first dorsal interosseous may be released at the distal portion of the muscle from the ulnar aspect of the first metacarpal if needed to obtain adequate passive abduction and extension of the thumb.

Release of Simple Intrinsic Contracture

- A four-flap Z-plasty over the contracted first web space is designed (**TECH FIG 2A,B**).
- After the skin incision, the dorsal fascia is incised while protecting the neurovascular bundles.
- The first dorsal interosseous is released at its origin from the thumb metacarpal.
- The AP is lengthened by release in an oblique cut at its intramuscular tendon; the surgeon should aim to preserve some adductor function (**TECH FIG 2C**).
- Four skin flaps are rearranged to increase the first web space (**TECH FIG 2D**).

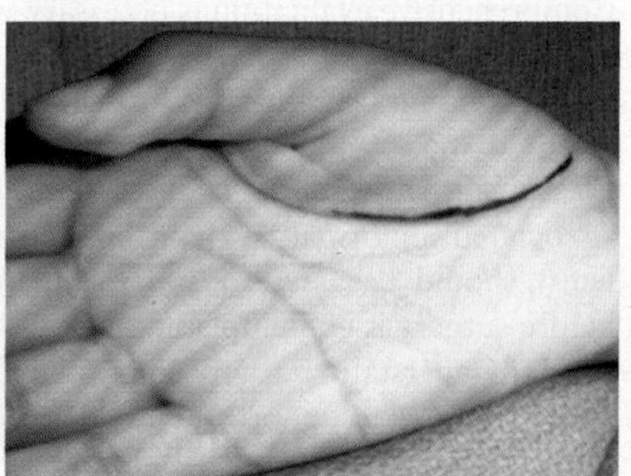

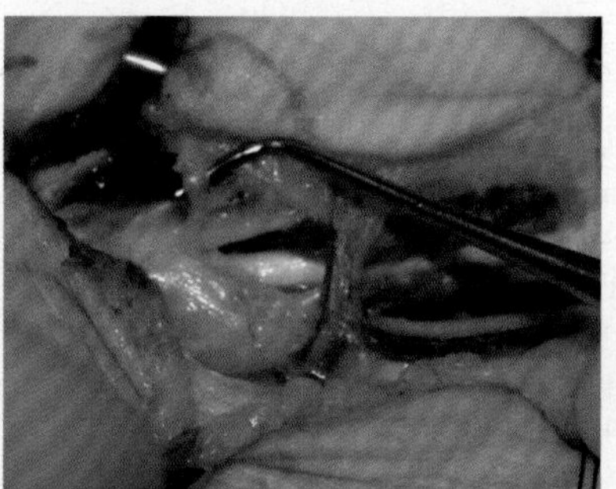

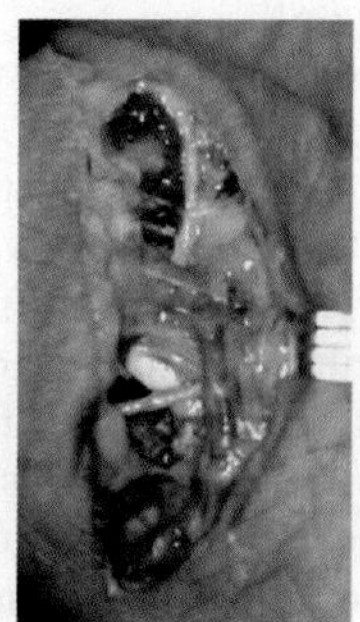

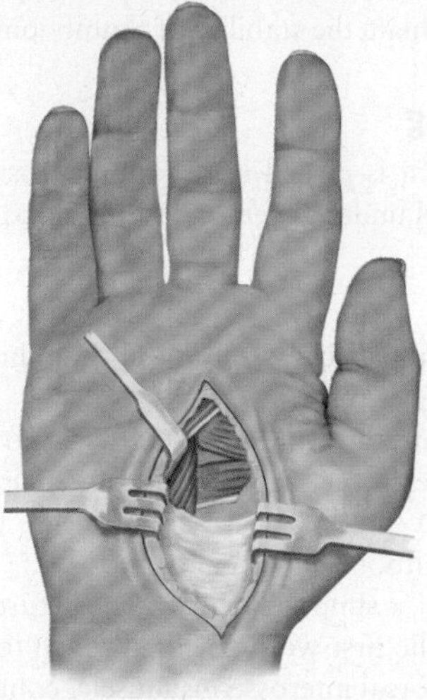

TECH FIG 1 • Intrinsic release. **A.** A curved incision is made over the thenar crease. **B.** Thenar release showing motor branch. **C,D.** Thumb intrinsics are released.

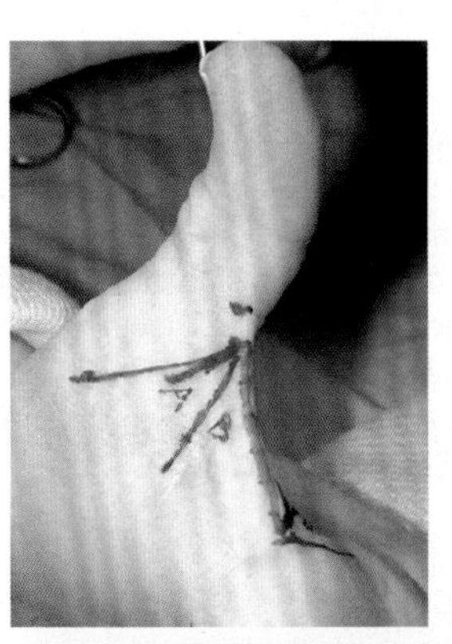
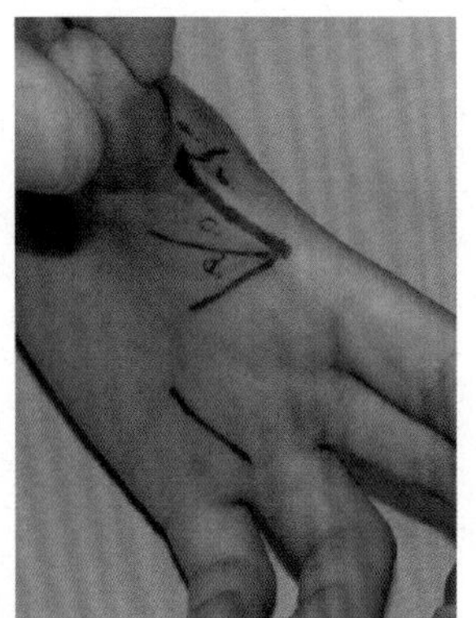
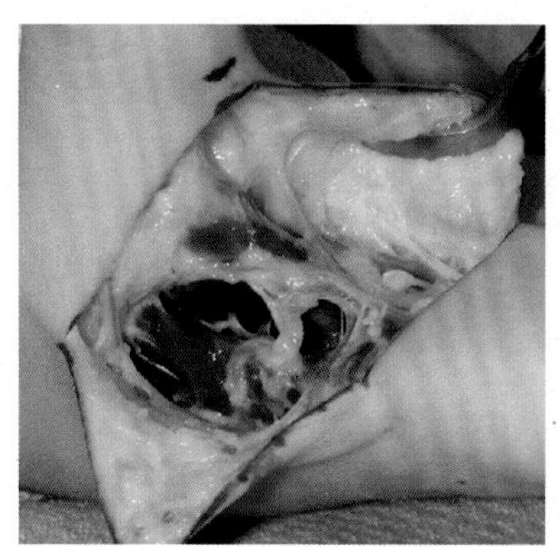
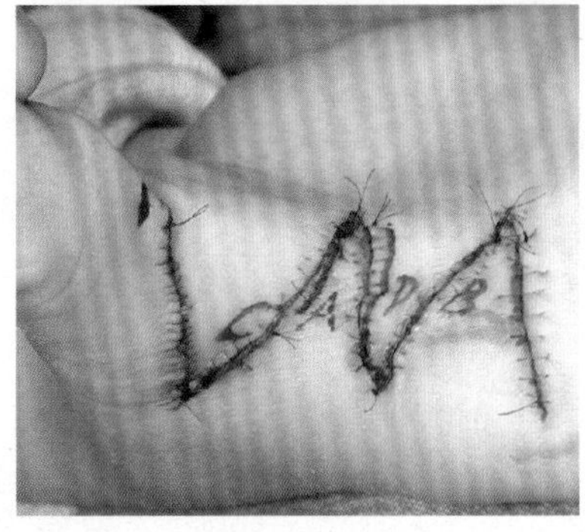

TECH FIG 2 • Four-flap Z-plasty over first web space. **A,B.** Skin markings. **C.** Elevation of flaps and adductor exposure. **D.** After rotation of skin flaps.

Release of Extrinsic Contracture

- A small longitudinal incision over the distal-volar aspect of the forearm is performed.
- The FPL tendon is exposed and incised over the musculotendinous portion.
- The thumb IP joint is hyperextended until 1 cm of distal sliding of the FPL tendon is identified.
- The FPL may be lengthened by Z-lengthening of the FPL tendon, with 0.5 mm of lengthening for each degree of correction.[1]

Augmentation of Weak Muscles

Abductor Pollicis Longus Augmentation

- Two small transverse incisions over the volar wrist crease and the first extensor compartment are made, aiming to expose the palmaris longus (PL) or flexor carpi radialis (FCR) and APL, respectively.
- The superficial branch of the radial nerve is identified and protected.
- The first extensor compartment is then opened, and the APL is identified. Each slip of the APL tendon should be pulled into tension to show the best slip for CMC joint abduction.
- At the volar incision, the palmar branch of the median nerve is identified and protected. The PL tendon is then divided.
- The selected APL tendon slip is translocated volarly until acceptable thumb metacarpal abduction is achieved.
- The PL tendon is passed through a subcutaneous tunnel to the volar-radial incision.
- End-to-side tendon weave of the PL to the translocated APL is then performed under sufficient tension to obtain appropriate thumb abduction (**TECH FIG 3A**).
- Alternatively, the APL tendon may be cut and the distal segment rerouted volarly and woven with end-to-end PL or end-to-side FCR. The proximal segment of the APL may be used to augment thumb MCP joint extension by end-to-side anastomosis with the EPB (**TECH FIG 3B**).

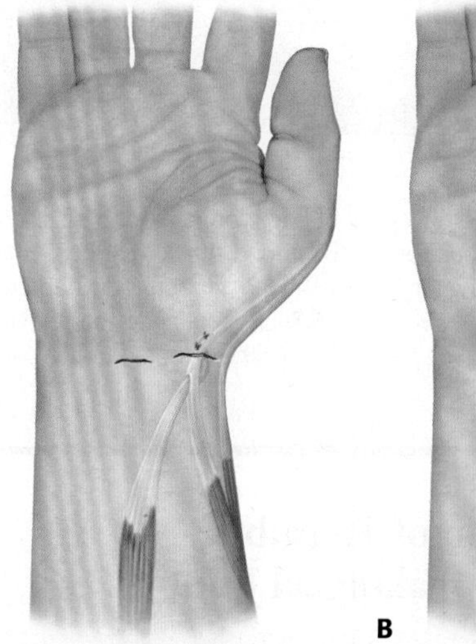
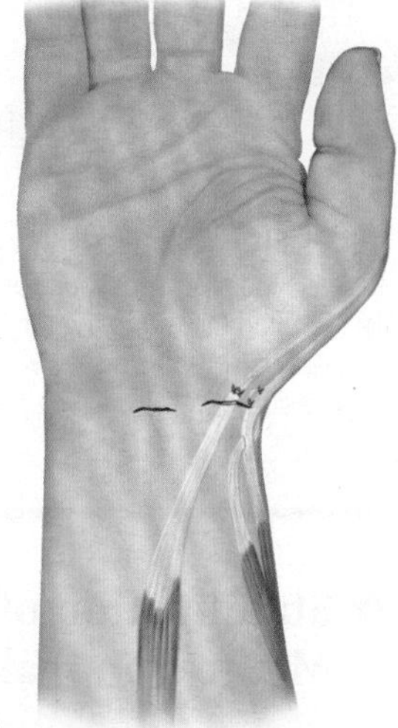

TECH FIG 3 • **A.** Transfer of PL to translocated APL by end-to-side anastomosis. **B.** APL augmentation by rerouting of the distal segment and anastomosis with end-to-end pollicis longus or end-to-side FCR. Thumb MCP joint extension is augmented by anastomosis of the proximal segment of APL with end-to-side EPB.

Extensor Pollicis Longus Rerouting

- A dorsal skin incision over the thumb MCP and IP joint and another small longitudinal incision just ulnar to the Lister tubercle are used for this procedure.[7]
- The EPL tendon is identified and divided 10 mm distal to the MCP joint. The tendon is then retracted out to the second incision (**TECH FIG 4A**).
- The EPL tendon is rerouted to the radial aspect of the Lister tubercle and passed subcutaneously around the APL and EPB tendon (**TECH FIG 4B**).
- The tendon is then passed through the MCP joint capsule (**TECH FIG 4C**).
- The thumb is set in appropriate abduction and IP extension. The rerouted EPL is sutured back to the extensor mechanism 10 mm distal to the defect.
- The rerouted EPL may be reinforced by the transfer of the PL, FCR, or brachioradialis.
- The EPL may be divided proximal to the Lister tubercle, leaving the tendon attached to its insertion. Rerouting is then performed from distal to proximal (**TECH FIG 4D**).[10]
- The EPL may be rerouted to the new pulley created from the extensor retinaculum (**TECH FIG 4E,F**).[1]

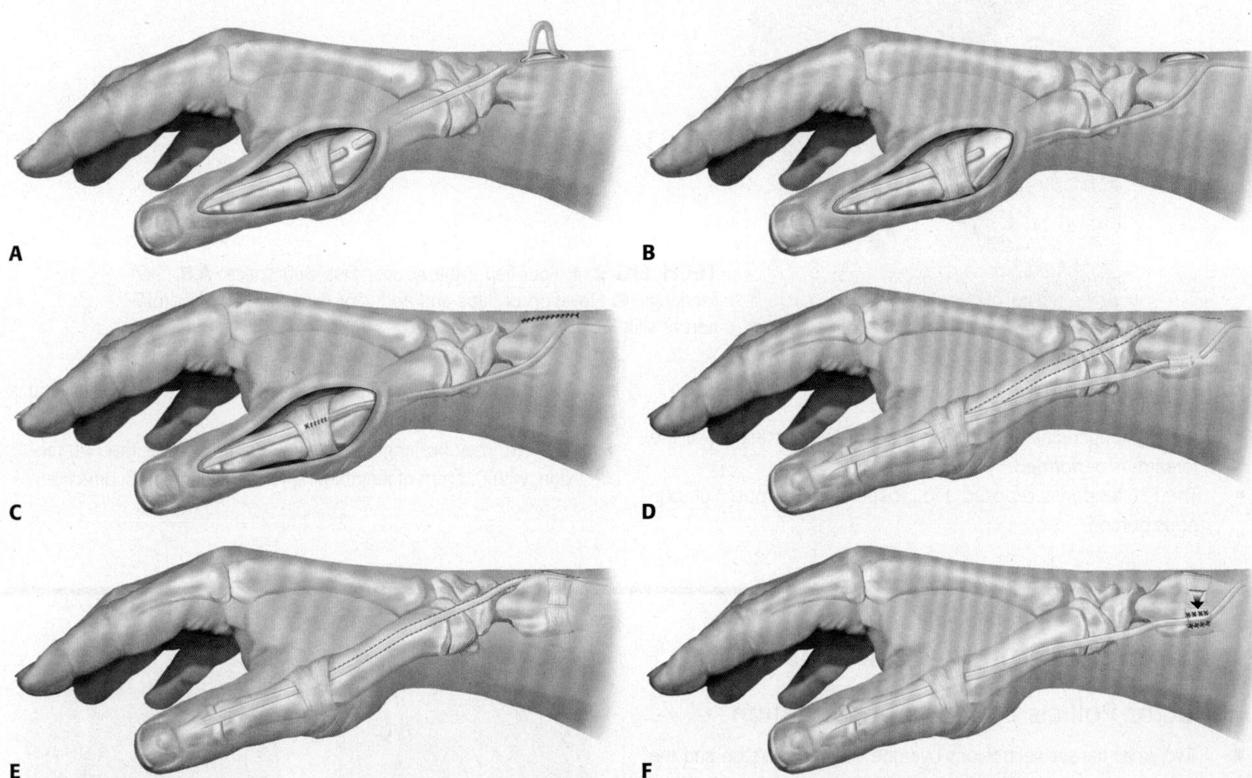

TECH FIG 4 • EPL rerouting. **A.** EPL tendon is divided distally and mobilized. **B.** The tendon is rerouted to the radial aspect of the Lister tubercle and passed subcutaneously around the APL and EPB tendon. **C.** The rerouted EPL is sutured back to the extensor mechanism. **D.** Modified EPL rerouting technique. The EPL tendon is divided proximal to the Lister tubercle, rerouted to the first extensor compartment, and sutured back to the proximal stump. **E,F.** EPL routing to the retinaculum. **E.** The EPL tendon is released from the third extensor compartment and rerouted radially. **F.** The new pulley for the rerouted EPL is created from the extensor retinaculum.

■ Stabilization of Thumb Metacarpophalangeal Joint

Thumb Metacarpophalangeal Joint Arthrodesis

- A dorsoulnar incision is made over the thumb MCP joint.
- The extensor mechanism is split longitudinally, and the ulnar collateral ligament is then detached from the metacarpal head to expose the joint (**TECH FIG 5A**).
- The articular cartilage of the metacarpal head is removed with a scalpel, and the proximal phalanx epiphysis is shaved until the secondary center of ossification is exposed (**TECH FIG 5B**). This allows fusion of the epiphyses and preserves the physis.
- The joint is set in 10 degrees of flexion, 10 degrees of abduction, and slight pronation,[12] and a small (1 mm in diameter), smooth Kirschner wire is passed through the joint centrally to minimize epiphyseal damage (**TECH FIG 5C**).

Sesamoid Capsulodesis

- A curved dorsoradial incision is made over the thumb MCP joint.[15]
- The accessory collateral ligament is divided at its insertion into the volar plate.

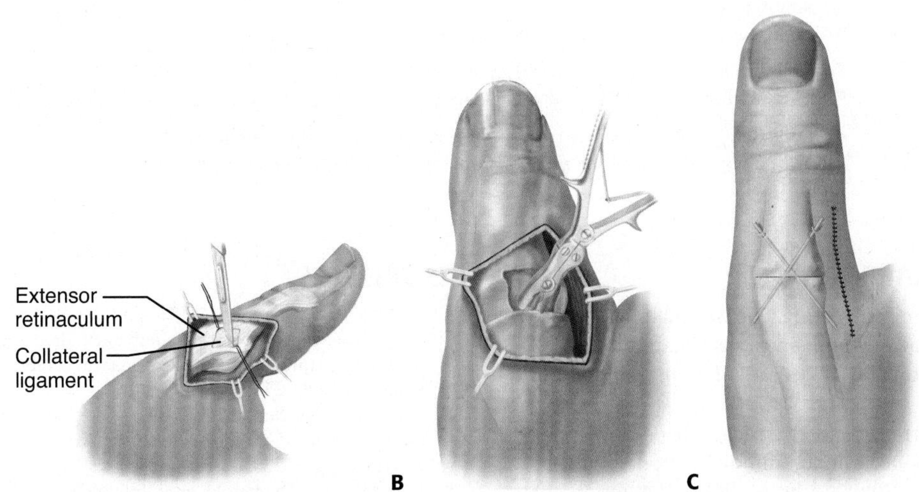

TECH FIG 5 • Thumb MCP arthrodesis. **A.** After the extensor mechanism over the MCP joint is split longitudinally, the ulnar collateral ligament is detached from the metacarpal head. **B.** The articular cartilage of the metacarpal head is removed. The epiphyseal plate of the proximal phalanx is preserved. **C.** After the joint is set, smooth Kirschner wires are used to maintain the joint position.

- The volar plate is then mobilized to expose the radial sesamoid.
- The articular cartilage of the sesamoid is denuded. A cortical defect is created at the head–neck junction of the metacarpal.
- The suture is passed through the sesamoid–volar plate and metacarpal defect with straight needles by using a Kirschner wire driver (**TECH FIG 6A**).
- The MCP joint is set to 30 degrees of flexion. The intraosseous suture is then tied over the dorsal surface of the metacarpal under the extensor tendons to secure the sesamoid to the metacarpal neck.
- A Kirschner wire is passed through the joint to maintain the joint position for 6 weeks (**TECH FIG 6B**).

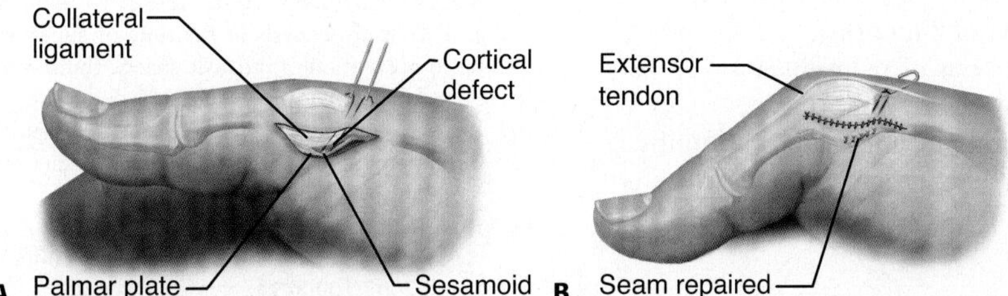

TECH FIG 6 • Sesamoid capsulodesis. The volar plate is mobilized to expose the radial sesamoid. The articular cartilage of the sesamoid is denuded corresponding with the cortical defect created at the head–neck junction of the metacarpal. **A.** The suture is passed through the sesamoid–volar plate and metacarpal defect. **B.** The intraosseous suture is tied over the dorsal surface of the metacarpal under the extensor tendons. A Kirschner wire is used to maintain the joint position.

PEARLS AND PITFALLS

General approach	■ A comprehensive history and physical examination, including appropriate investigations with other professionals, should be done for accurate diagnosis and treatment planning.
Patient selection	■ Voluntary control of the selected muscle, which indicates the potential active use of the hand postoperatively, is important for selection of surgical candidates.
Procedure selection	■ The procedures must be individualized because of variation in deformities in each patient.

Release of spastic muscle and contractures	■ Selective release of the deforming forces is performed in sequential order to obtain adequate, functional thumb positions. ■ Adjacent neurovascular structures must be protected with care.
Augmentation of paretic muscles	■ The muscle selected for transfer depends on the availability and the extent of voluntary control. ■ The stability of the MCP joint is evaluated before performing any augmentation procedures across it.
Joint stabilization	■ Joint stabilization is the key to success of rebalancing the thumb-deforming forces. ■ The epiphyseal plate of the proximal phalanx must be preserved with care.

POSTOPERATIVE CARE

- Postoperative care for contracture releases includes immobilization in a short-arm thumb spica cast maintaining full thumb radial abduction and 20 degrees of palmar abduction for 4 weeks.
- Removable splinting is then continued for another 4 to 6 weeks.
- If tendon transfer has been done, immobilization should be extended to 6 weeks, followed by additional splinting for 6 weeks. Dynamic splinting may be considered.
- Immobilization of the MCP arthrodesis with a thumb spica cast should be continued until radiographic healing is detected.

OUTCOMES

- The functional outcome of thumb-in-palm deformity should be assessed before and after surgery by the physician, therapist, parent, and patient.
- House et al[2] demonstrated improved functional grade in all 56 patients postoperatively. Half of patients improved three or more grades.
- Tonkin et al[16] found good results in 32 patients after surgical correction of thumb-in-palm deformity. The average follow-up was 32 months (range, 10 to 88 months).
  - The thumb was maintained out of palm in 29 of 32 patients (30 of 33 thumbs).
  - Patients could perform lateral pinch in 26 of 33 thumbs.
  - Many patients improved function, but no patient improved from dependent to independent functioning.

COMPLICATIONS

- Inadequate release of contracted or fibrotic muscle may result in insufficient release of the thumb out of the palm.
- Adhesions along the transferred tendon may cause loss of excursion postoperatively.
- Improper techniques such as overlengthening and an incorrect vector of transfer may result in limited active abduction and extension of the thumb.
- Untreated or inadequate treatment of an unstable MCP joint may result in failed tendon transfer.
- Avoiding neurovascular injury is crucial. Care should be taken to properly identify and protect neurovascular bundles throughout surgery.
- An improper rehabilitation program and social support may result in failed treatment.

REFERENCES

1. Goldner JL, Koman LA, Gelberman R, et al. Arthrodesis of the metacarpophalangeal joint of the thumb in children and adults. Adjunctive treatment of thumb-in-palm deformity in cerebral palsy. Clin Orthop Relat Res 1990;(253):75–89.
2. House JH, Gwathmey FW, Fidler MO. A dynamic approach to the thumb-in-palm deformity in cerebral palsy. J Bone Joint Surg Am 1981;63(2):216–225.
3. Jaffe M, Tal Y, Dabbah H, et al. Infants with a thumb-in-fist posture. Pediatrics 2000;105(3):E41.
4. Koman LA, Mooney JF III, Smith B, et al. Management of cerebral palsy with botulinum A toxin: preliminary investigation. J Pediatr Orthop 1993;13:489–495.
5. Kozin SH, Keenan MA. Using dynamic electromyography to guide surgical treatment of the spastic upper extremity in the brain-injured patient. Clin Orthop Relat Res 1993;(288):109–117.
6. Lawson RD, Tonkin MA. Surgical management of the thumb in cerebral palsy. Hand Clin 2003;19:667–677.
7. Manske PR. Redirection of extensor pollicis longus in the treatment of spastic thumb-in-palm deformity. J Hand Surg Am 1985;10(4):553–560.
8. Matev IB. Surgical treatment of flexion–adduction contracture of the thumb in cerebral palsy. Acta Orthop Scand 1970;41:439–445.
9. Pappas N, Baldwin K, Keenan MA. Efficacy of median nerve recurrent branch neurectomy as an adjunct to ulnar motor nerve neurectomy and wrist arthrodesis at the time of superficialis to profundus transfer in prevention of intrinsic spastic thumb-in-palm deformity. J Hand Surg Am 2010;35(8):1310–1316.
10. Rayan GM, Saccone PG. Treatment of spastic thumb-in-palm deformity: a modified extensor pollicis longus tendon rerouting. J Hand Surg Am 1996;21(5):834–839.
11. Rosenbaum P, Paneth N, Leviton A, et al. A report: the definition and classification of cerebral palsy April 2006. Dev Med Child Neurol Suppl 2007;109:8–14.
12. Swanson AB. Surgery of the hand in cerebral palsy. In: Flynn JE, ed. Hand Surgery. Baltimore: Williams & Wilkins, 1982:476–488.
13. Ten Berge SR, Boonstra AM, Dijkstra PU, et al. A systematic evaluation of the effect of thumb opponens splints on hand function in children with unilateral spastic cerebral palsy. Clin Rehabil 2012;26(4):362–371.
14. Tonkin MA. Thumb deformity in the spastic hand: classification and surgical techniques. Tech Hand Up Extrem Surg 2003;7:18–25.
15. Tonkin MA, Beard AJ, Kemp SJ, et al. Sesamoid arthrodesis for hyperextension of the thumb metacarpophalangeal joint. J Hand Surg Am 1995;20(2):334–338.
16. Tonkin MA, Hatrick NC, Eckersley JR, et al. Surgery for cerebral palsy part 3: classification and operative procedures for thumb deformity. J Hand Surg Br 2001;26(5):465–470.
17. Zancolli EA, Zancolli E Jr. Surgical rehabilitation of the spastic upper limb in cerebral palsy. In: Lamb DW, ed. The Paralyzed Hand. Edinburgh: Churchill Livingstone, 1987:153–168.

Release of Simple Syndactyly

Donald S. Bae

DEFINITION

- *Syndactyly* refers to the failure of separation between adjacent digits, resulting in "webbed" fingers.
- Congenital syndactyly is classified according to the extent of digital involvement and the character of the conjoined tissue.
  - *Complete syndactyly* extends to the digital tips (**FIG 1A**), whereas *incomplete syndactyly* ends proximal to the fingertips (**FIG 1B**).
  - *Simple syndactyly* refers to digits connected only by skin and soft tissue. *Complex syndactyly* denotes bony fusions between adjacent phalanges.
  - *Complicated syndactyly* refers to the interposition of accessory phalanges or abnormal bones between digits.

ANATOMY

- Understanding of normal digital web space anatomy guides surgical reconstructive efforts.
- Typically, the index–long and ring–small finger commissures are U-shaped, whereas the long–ring web is V-shaped.
- The nonglabrous skin of the normal web space is sloped about 45 degrees from proximal–dorsal to distal–volar, extending to roughly the midpoint of the proximal phalanx.
- The natatory ligaments (or superficial transverse metacarpal ligament) help form the web contour and join adjacent lateral digital sheets.
- Normally, each digit is vascularized in part via a radial and an ulnar digital artery, which arise from the bifurcation of the common digital arteries.
- In simple syndactyly, adjacent digits are joined by varying amounts of skin and soft tissue.
  - The nail plates may or may not be fused.
  - The joints, ligaments, and tendons of the affected digits usually are normal.
- It is of critical surgical importance that the bifurcation of the digital arteries and nerves may be abnormally distal in cases of syndactyly.

PATHOGENESIS

- Syndactyly represents a failure of differentiation and is so classified by the embryologic classification of congenital anomalies adopted by the International Federation for Societies for Surgery of the Hand.
- Embryologically, the digits arise from condensations of mesoderm within the rudimentary hand paddle of the developing upper limb.
- During the fifth and sixth weeks of gestation, interdigital clefts form through the process of apoptosis, or programmed cell death, beginning at the digital tips and proceeding in a distal to proximal direction.
- The apical ectodermal ridge regulates this embryologic process, in conjunction with fibroblast growth factors, bone morphogenetic proteins, transforming growth factors, homeobox gene products, and the sonic hedgehog protein.
- Interruption of this precise and highly regulated process results in syndactyly.

NATURAL HISTORY

- There is no potential for spontaneous resolution.
- Given the importance of independent digit function in today's world, surgical release is recommended for simple complete syndactyly, with few exceptions.
- When digits of differing lengths are joined, the syndactyly may lead to deformity and growth disturbance, with the longer digit typically developing a flexion contracture and angular deviation toward the shorter digit.
- Simple complete syndactyly of the long–ring interspace may be well tolerated and may not significantly compromise growth or function in young patients.
- Simple incomplete syndactylies may be aesthetically subtle and cause little functional compromise. In these situations, observation may be considered.

A 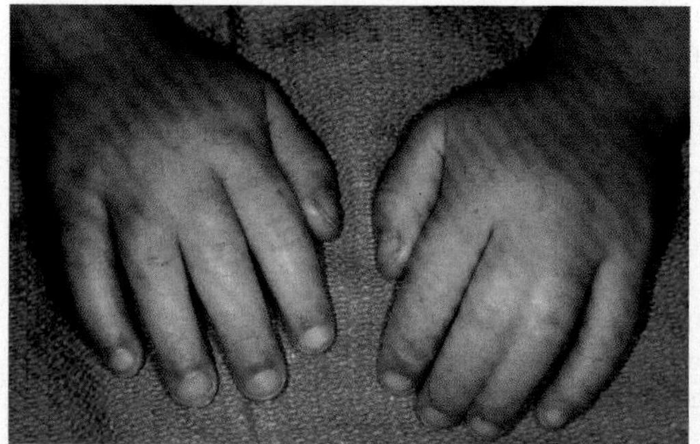

B 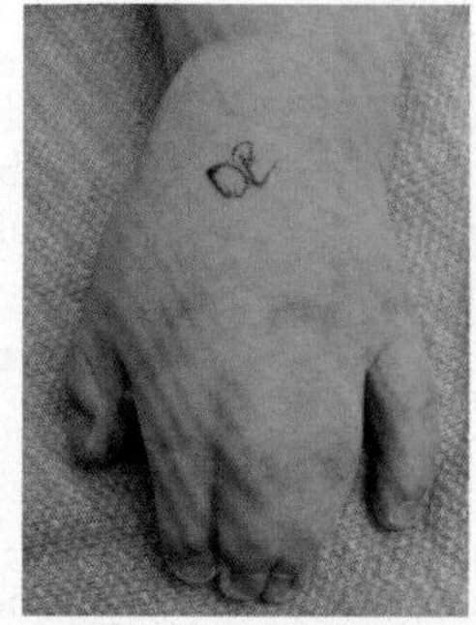

FIG 1 • **A.** Simple incomplete syndactylies of the bilateral third web spaces, with the left hand more severely affected. **B.** Simple complete syndactyly of the second and third web spaces is seen in another patient. Observe the conjoined fingernail (synonychia) between the long and ring fingers. (Copyright © 2006 Children's Orthopaedic Surgery Foundation.)

PATIENT HISTORY AND PHYSICAL FINDINGS

- The diagnosis of syndactyly usually is not subtle, and the extent of digital involvement typically is readily apparent.
- Syndactyly is the most common congenital hand anomaly, with an estimated incidence of 1 in 2000 to 2500 live births.
  - The true incidence of syndactyly is unknown, in part because of the difficulty distinguishing mild simple syndactylies from normal web spaces.
- The third web space is most commonly affected (50%), followed by the fourth (30%), second (15%), and first (5%) web spaces.
- Males tend to be more commonly affected than females and whites more than blacks or Asians.
- Inheritance is thought to be autosomal dominant with incomplete penetrance and variable expression.
- The absence of differential motion of the affected digits suggests a complex or complicated syndactyly.
- Because the joints and tendons usually are normal, patients typically have flexion and extension creases over the interphalangeal joints and active digital motion.
- Syndactyly may exist in isolation or may be seen in the context of associated clinical syndromes, including Poland syndrome, Apert syndrome, and constriction band syndrome. For this reason, careful evaluation of the entire upper extremity, contralateral upper limb, chest, and feet is advised.

IMAGING AND OTHER DIAGNOSTIC STUDIES

- Plain radiographs of the affected digits or hand are routinely obtained to accurately classify the syndactyly and assess for bony fusions or interposed or accessory bones (**FIG 2**).
- Magnetic resonance imaging (MRI), angiography, or other diagnostic studies are not typically obtained because they do not assist surgical decision making or operative treatment.

NONOPERATIVE MANAGEMENT

- Nonoperative management may be considered for mild, simple incomplete syndactyly.
- Nonoperative treatment also may be favored in cases of complicated syndactyly with the so-called "superdigit" or in cases of complex polysyndactyly because of the difficulty in achieving reproducible functional improvement with surgical release.

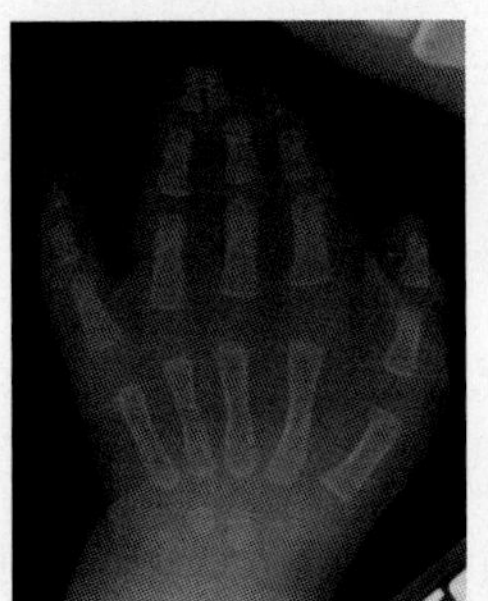

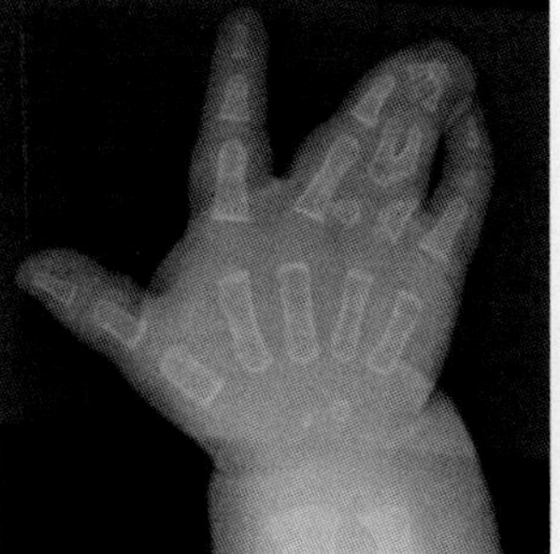

FIG 2 • **A.** Anteroposterior (AP) radiograph of the patient depicted in **FIG 1B**. Note the simple complete syndactyly between the index and long fingers and a complex complete syndactyly between the long and ring fingers. **B.** AP radiograph depicting a complicated polysyndactyly in another patient.

- However, given the importance of independent digital motion—particularly in the current keyboard-driven digital age—nonoperative treatment of simple complete syndactyly is not recommended.

SURGICAL MANAGEMENT

- General surgical principles include the following:
  - Digits of differing lengths should be released early to prevent deformity and growth disturbance of the affected digits.
  - Digits should be operated upon on only one side at the same time to avoid vascular embarrassment.
  - Local skin flaps should be used to recreate the commissure to avoid scar contracture and "web creep."
  - Zigzag lateral flaps should be created to avoid longitudinal scar contracture.
  - Judicious defatting of the skin flaps should be performed to facilitate skin closure, reduce tension across the flaps, and improve the aesthetics of the reconstructed fingers.
  - Full-thickness skin grafts typically are used to cover "bare areas" after syndactyly release. (In cases of simple complete syndactyly, the combined circumference of the separated digits is 22% greater than the original circumference of the syndactylized digits.)[7,8]

Preoperative Planning

- The timing of surgery must be considered in preoperative planning.
- There is great variability in recommendations of when releases should be performed.
  - Flatt[8] wrote, "I believe one should ask not how soon the operation can be done but rather how late the functional demands of the hand will allow postponement of surgery."
  - In general, releases are performed between 6 and 24 months of age.
- As mentioned, digits of differing lengths (eg, thumb–index syndactyly) should be released earlier to avoid secondary deformity.
- There is some evidence that releases performed after 18 months have better long-term outcomes with lower incidence of web creep.[9,10]

Positioning

- The patient is positioned supine with the affected limb supported on a hand table.
- Placement of a sterile or nonsterile tourniquet must be sufficiently proximal to allow access to the antecubital fossa, if full-thickness skin graft is to be taken from that site.
- If the skin graft is to be harvested from the inguinal region, the ipsilateral groin is prepared and draped to allow for easy access.
- Before draping, a surgical pen may be used to mark the inguinal skin fold when the hip is flexed; graft harvest along this axis will allow for a more aesthetic skin closure.
- Care should be taken to harvest the skin graft lateral to the femoral artery to avoid transfer of hair-bearing skin.

Approach

- The principles of separation for simple complete syndactyly are well accepted; however, there is tremendous variation in the surgical incisions and skin flap designs used for these operations.

- All use local tissue to reconstruct the interdigital commissure, and all employ interdigitating zigzag lateral flaps. Dorsal skin flaps are preferred for commissure reconstruction because of their pliability and ability to recreate the normal dorsal–proximal to volar–distal slope of the web.
- When dorsal skin is used to create the commissure, the length of the dorsal flap should approximate two-thirds of the length of the proximal phalanx to create an appropriate slope to the web. The proximal extent of the volar incision will become the new palmodigital crease (**FIG 3A**).
- Furthermore, flaps are designed to interdigitate during closure; to achieve this, palmar triangular flaps are based at the level corresponding to the apex of the dorsal flaps. These flaps usually are fashioned to traverse between the midlines of the syndactylized digits.
- **FIG 3B** shows examples of skin incisions for simple complete syndactyly releases.[17]

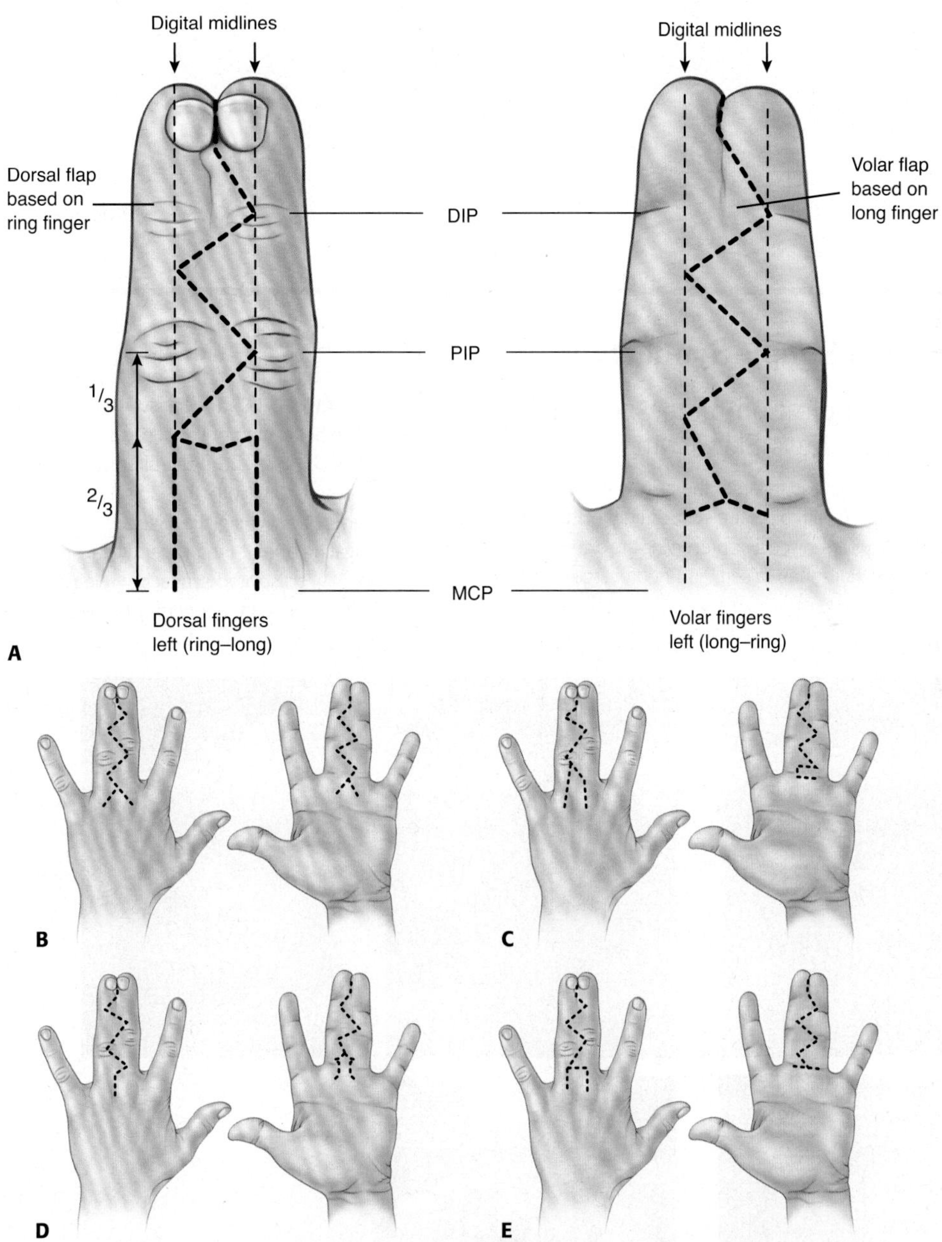

FIG 3 • **A.** Skin incision design. The dorsal skin flap measures approximately two-thirds the length of the proximal phalanx, and the zigzag incisions are fashioned between the midlines of the syndactylized digits. **B–I.** Skin incisions used for release of simple complete syndactyly. (**B:** Cronin, 1943; **C:** Flatt, 1962; **D:** Blauth, 1970; **E:** Hentz, 1977; **F:** Upton, 1984; **G:** Gilbert, 1986; **H:** Wood, 1998; **I:** James, 2005.) *(continued)*

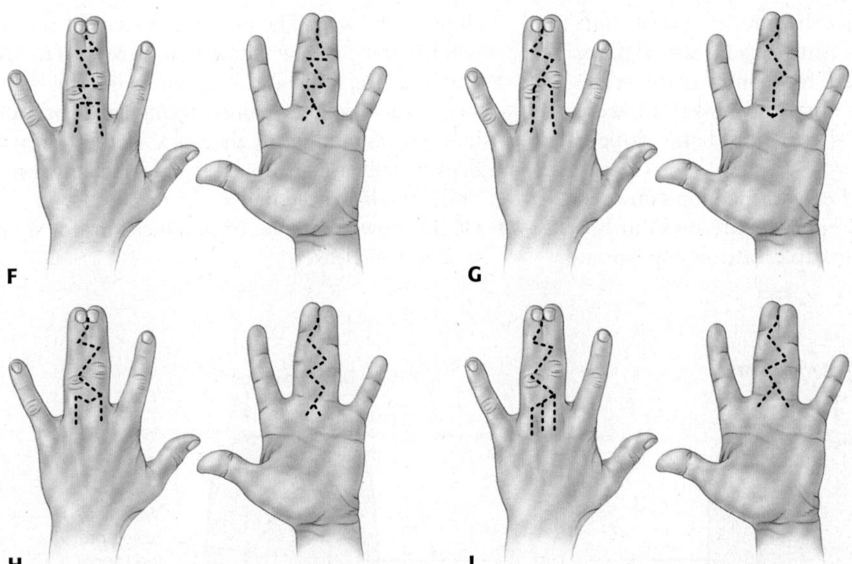

FIG 3 • (continued)

Release of Simple Syndactyly

Release of Simple Complete Syndactyly Using Full-Thickness Skin Graft

- After the tourniquet is inflated, the skin is incised, and hemostasis is achieved with bipolar electrocautery (**TECH FIG 1A,B**).
- Dorsal skin flaps are raised first, preserving the extensor paratenon.
- Volar skin flaps are then raised, and neurovascular bundles are identified.
- Digits are carefully separated distal to proximal, releasing the interdigital fascia that often connects the syndactylized digits (**TECH FIG 1C**). The transverse metacarpal ligament is not divided.
- The bifurcation of the common digital artery and nerve is identified; if there is a distal bifurcation precluding restoration of the commissure with the dorsal skin flap, consideration may be given to splitting the fascicles of the common digital nerve or ligating one of the proper digital arteries.
  - For isolated syndactyly release, the smaller caliber or nondominant artery may be taken.

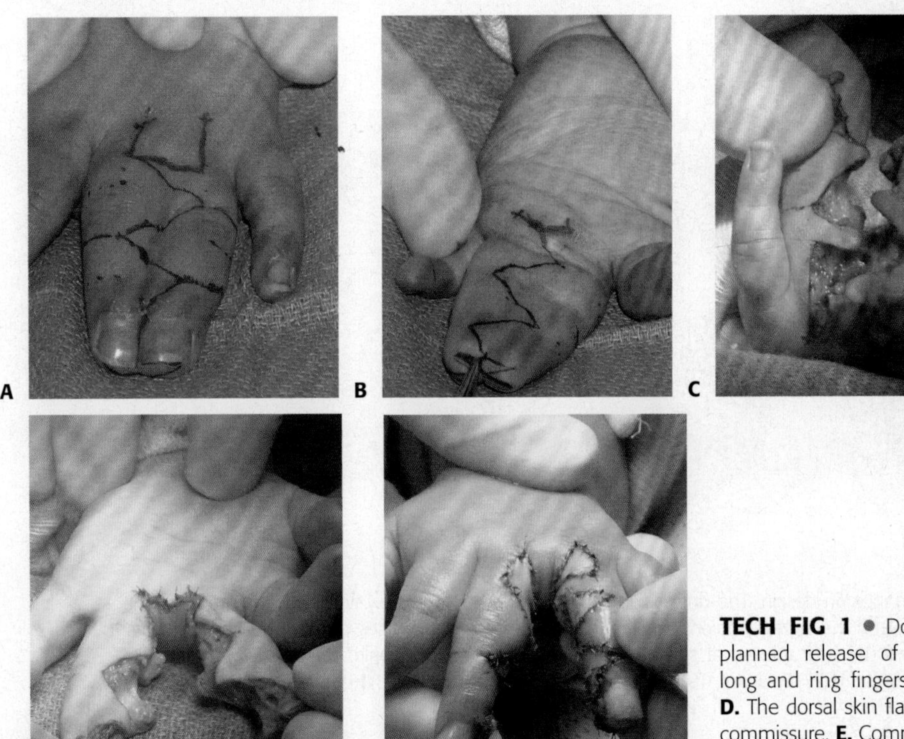

TECH FIG 1 • Dorsal (**A**) and volar (**B**) incisions for planned release of simple complete syndactyly of the long and ring fingers. **C.** The digits have been separated. **D.** The dorsal skin flap is sewn in to recreate the interdigital commissure. **E.** Completion of the release with full-thickness skin grafting. (Copyright 2006 Children's Orthopaedic Surgery Foundation.)

- If a syndactyly release is planned on the other side of one of the digits, its proper digital artery should be preserved.
- Skin flaps are then defatted and allowed to interdigitate.
- The dorsal skin flap is then advanced to the palmodigital crease and secured with multiple interrupted 5-0 absorbable sutures (eg, chromic or polyglactin; **TECH FIG 1D**).
- Interdigitated skin flaps are similarly reapproximated with multiple interrupted 5-0 absorbable suture.
- Skin defects are identified and covered with full-thickness skin graft, which may be harvested from the hypothenar eminence, antecubital fossa, or inguinal region (**TECH FIG 1E**).
- The tourniquet is deflated, and vascularity of the digits and flaps is confirmed.
- A nonadherent gauze bolstered with moist cotton is then placed into the newly formed web space, applying gentle compression to the skin graft sites.
  - Care should be taken to place the dressing deep within the commissure to avoid resyndactylization during the healing process.
- An above-elbow cast is then applied with the elbow in 90 degrees of flexion, with liberal use of casting material to protect the surgical dressing.

Reconstruction of the Paronychium

- In cases of simple complete syndactyly, the nail plates of the involved digits are conjoined, a phenomenon known as *synonychia.*
- Although division of the midportion of the nail plate is easily performed, care must be made to reconstitute the nail folds.
  - Ideally, this is performed using local tissue from the digital pulp.[2]
  - Laterally based flaps are incorporated into the skin incisions, raised from the shared hyponychium at the digital tips (**TECH FIG 2**).
  - The length of the flaps should equal the length of the nail plate.
  - Once these flaps are raised and the digits separated, the flaps are easily rotated and reapproximated adjacent to the new nail plates, recreating a paronychial fold.
  - Alternative solutions, including the use of skin graft, thenar or hypothenar flaps, or free composite toe grafts, are more involved and may provide less pleasing aesthetic results.

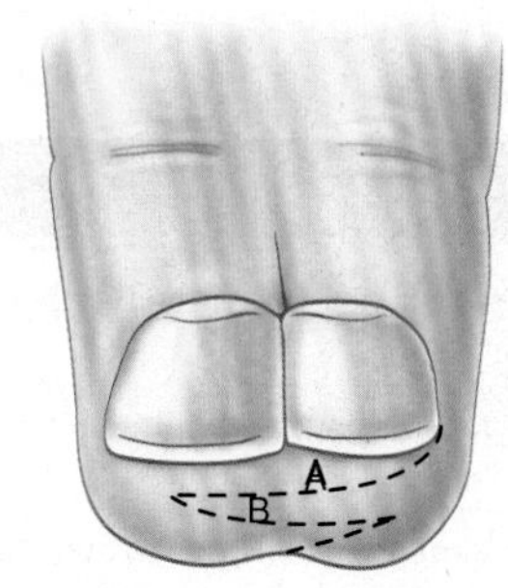

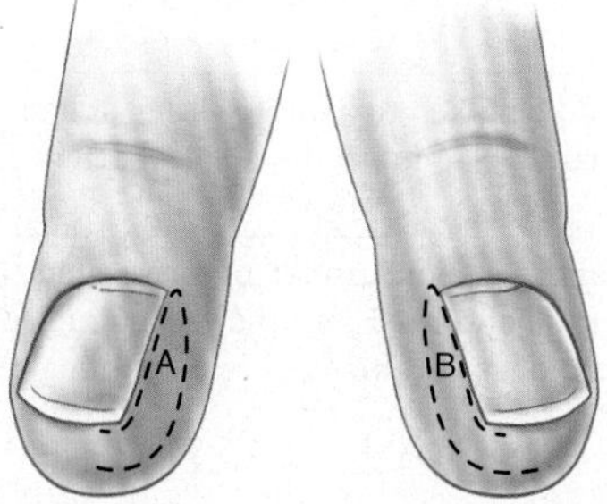

TECH FIG 2 • Schematic diagram depicting the incisions used to release a synoncychia, using local tissue to reconstitute the nail folds.

Technique of "Graftless" Syndactyly Release

- Simple complete syndactyly releases may also be performed without the need for full-thickness skin grafting.[1,5,11,12]
- In general, principles of syndactyly release mentioned earlier apply.
- In graftless techniques, however, dorsal skin is raised from the dorsum of the hand and advanced to recreate the interdigital commissure. The resulting defect is closed primarily in the fashion of a V-Y advancement flap (**TECH FIG 3**).
- Because proximal skin is used to recreate the web, more tissue is available to allow for primary closure of the digits following judicious defatting of the flaps, obviating the need for skin grafting.
- The use of preoperative tissue expansion to avoid the need for skin grafting for syndactyly release has been proposed. Results have been unpredictable at best, however, and this approach currently is not widely accepted.

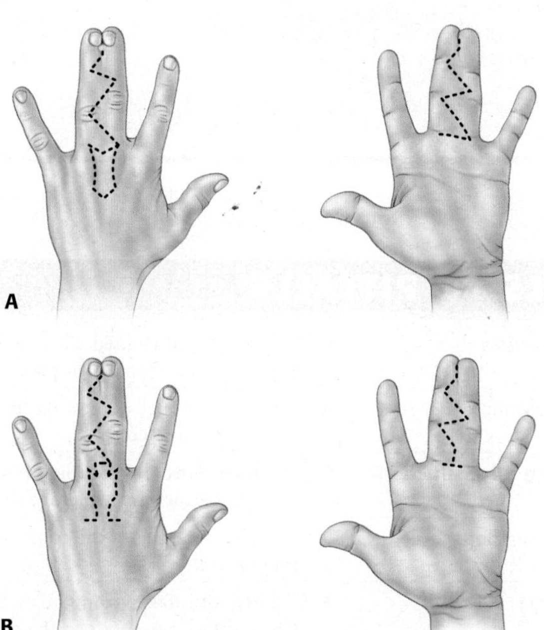

TECH FIG 3 • **A,B.** Schematic diagram depicting incisions used to perform graftless syndactyly releases. (**A:** From Sherif MM. V-Y dorsal metacarpal flap: a new technique for the correction of syndactyly without skin graft. Plast Reconstr Surg 1998;101:1861–1866; **B:** From Niranjan NS, DeCarpentier J. A new technique for the division of syndactyly. Eur J Plast Surg 1990;13:101–104; Ekerot L. Syndactyly correction without skin-grafting. J Hand Surg Br 1996;21:330–337.)

Local Skin Flaps for Simple Incomplete Syndactyly

- In cases of simple incomplete syndactyly in which the web does not extend beyond the level of the proximal interphalangeal joint (ie, the length of the syndactyly does not exceed the desired depth of the reconstructed interdigital commissure), release may be performed using local skin flaps without the need for full-thickness skin grafting.
- Multiple flap designs have been proposed, and, in general, all are variations of double opposing Z-plasties[13,15] (**TECH FIG 4**).
- In these situations, brief postoperative cast immobilization is recommended until skin flaps have healed.

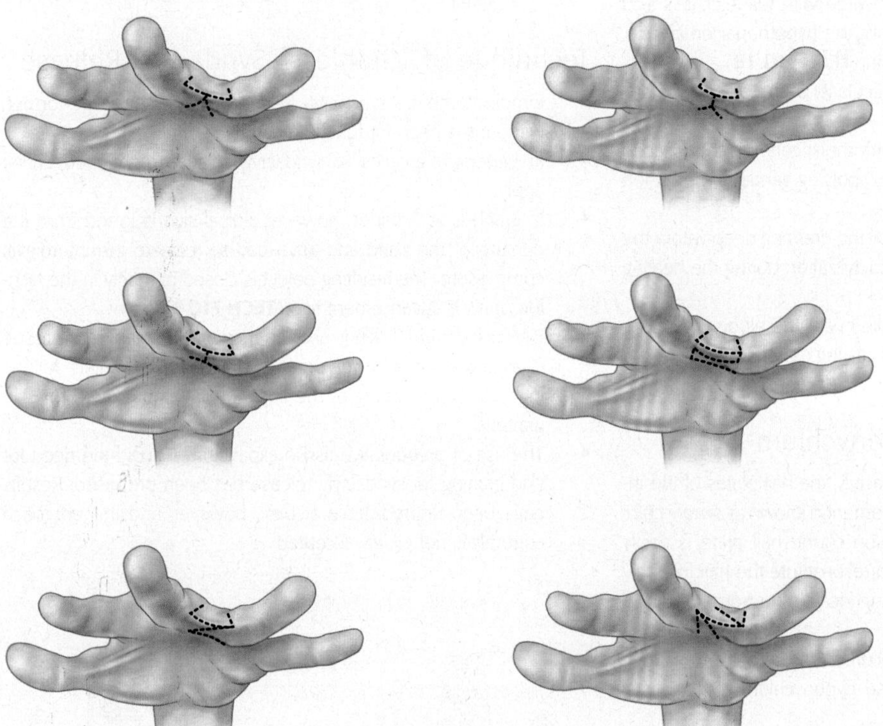

TECH FIG 4 • Schematic diagram depicting incisions used to perform release of simple incomplete syndactyly.

PEARLS AND PITFALLS

Patient selection	■ Caution should be used when considering release of the superdigit or polysyndactyly because functional results are mixed and postoperative deformity may ensue.
Surgical approach	■ The proximal edge of the volar incision may be placed proximal to the palmodigital crease to account for possible late web creep.
Commissure reconstruction	■ Zigzag closure of the interdigital commissure is preferred over transverse incisions to avoid scar contracture and subsequent narrowing of the web space.
Interdigitating flaps	■ Judicious defatting of the triangular flaps will allow for tension-free closure and reduce the area of skin graft needed.
Graft harvest	■ If skin graft is taken from the inguinal region, care should be taken to avoid transfer of hair-bearing skin. This is difficult to assess in the young child; however, harvest lateral to the femoral artery can serve as a helpful guide.
Postoperative care	■ The importance of the postoperative dressing and immobilization cannot be overstated. Nonadherent gauze with appropriate bolsters placed over the skin grafts and deep into the reconstructed commissure will optimize skin graft "take" and lessen the risk of resyndactylization during the healing period.

POSTOPERATIVE CARE

- Cast immobilization usually is discontinued after 2 to 4 weeks.
- The wound is kept dry until the scabs desiccate and fall off.
- Silicone gel sheets, elastomer, or scar molds may be used to minimize hypertrophic scar formation.
- Formal occupational therapy for motion and strengthening is not typically required because most children will use their hands quite readily with activities of daily living.

OUTCOMES

- Very little has been published regarding long-term outcomes following surgical release of syndactyly.
- Furthermore, interpretation of the available literature is difficult given the diversity of clinical presentations, surgical techniques, and methods of evaluation.
- In general, syndactyly release can be expected to provide excellent independent digital function with acceptable aesthetic results when performed according to the principles outlined in this chapter.
- Colville[3] reported the results of 57 simple syndactyly releases performed over a 10-year period with minimum 2-year follow-up.
  - Two patients required reoperation for early graft failure, and three others demonstrated slight angular deformity due to scar contracture, but they did not require additional surgery.
- D'Arcangelo et al[4] published their results of 122 releases in 50 patients with minimum 8 years of follow-up.
  - Satisfactory functional and aesthetic results were seen in most patients, but eight patients demonstrated web creep and three patients developed scar contractures.
- DeSmet et al[6] reported their results of 50 syndactyly releases in 24 patients.
  - A normal or near-normal web was seen in 74% of cases, and cosmesis was deemed satisfactory in 64%.
- In their review of 218 releases performed in 100 patients, Percival and Sykes[14] noted that 42 patients required secondary surgery for web creep (22%) and contracture (26%).
- Toledo and Ger[16] published their results of 176 releases performed in 61 patients with average 14-year follow-up.
  - Secondary procedures were performed in 30% of patients with simple syndactylies.
  - The need for secondary surgery was associated with operations performed before the age of 18 months, the use of split-thickness skin grafts, and the presence of complex or complicated syndactyly.

COMPLICATIONS

- With adherence to the principles presented in this chapter and meticulous surgical technique, the risk of complications may be minimized; however, up to one-third of patients may require secondary procedures following simple complete syndactyly release.
- Digital necrosis is the most serious potential complication of syndactyly release. Careful identification and preservation of the digital arteries—in addition to avoidance of surgical release of both the radial and ulnar sides of a single digit at the same time—is critical to avoid vascular embarrassment and digital loss.
- Skin graft failure may result from hematoma formation beneath the graft or shear stresses imposed on the graft during the healing process.
  - This risk may be greater in younger patients, in whom appropriate graft tensioning is more difficult and in whom postoperative immobilization is a greater challenge.
  - If allowed to heal by secondary intention, subsequent hypertrophic scar formation may lead to suboptimal aesthetic and functional results.
- Skin flap failure due to devascularization is less common but also may lead to scarring and secondary contracture.
  - Triangular skin flaps should be designed with tip angles greater than 45 degrees to prevent tip necrosis.
  - Careful defatting of the flaps and primary closure without excess tension, in addition to assessment of flap viability after tourniquet release, will further aid in preventing skin flap complications.
- Contractures and angular deformity of the released digits may occur owing to linear scars on the radial or ulnar aspects of the fingers.
  - Use of zigzag incisions and interdigitating flap designs will minimize this risk.
- Nail plate deformity is common after simple complete syndactyly release in the presence of a synonychia.
  - Although techniques of nail fold reconstruction using distal pulp tissue will optimize aesthetic results, patients and families should be counseled in advance regarding this common occurrence.
- Web creep refers to the distal migration of the reconstructed interdigital commissure with continued growth and is a common occurrence following syndactyly release, with a variously reported incidence of between 7% and 60% of cases.
  - Some evidence suggests that the risk of web creep may be diminished if release is performed after 18 months of age.
  - Other factors that may contribute to web creep include inappropriate flap design for commissure reconstruction, the use of split-thickness rather than full-thickness skin grafts, skin graft loss, and creation of a transverse linear scar in the reconstituted web space.
  - In cases of clinically significant web creep, secondary releases may be required.

REFERENCES

1. Aydin A, Ozden BC. Dorsal metacarpal island flap in syndactyly treatment. Ann Plast Surg 2004;52:43–48.
2. Buck-Gramcko D. Congenital malformations: syndactyly and related deformities. In: Nigst H, Buck-Gramcko D, Millesi H, et al, eds. Hand Surgery. New York: Thieme Medical Publishers, 1988:12.
3. Colville J. Syndactyly correction. Br J Plast Surg 1989;42:12–16.
4. D'Arcangelo M, Gilbert A, Pirrello R. Correction of syndactyly using a dorsal omega flap and two lateral and volar flaps. A long-term review. J Hand Surg Br 1996;21:320–324.
5. D'Arcangelo M, Maffulli N. Tissue expanders in syndactyly: a brief review. Acta Chir Plast 1996;38:11–13.
6. DeSmet L, Van Ransbeeck H, Deneef G. Syndactyly release: results of the Flatt technique. Acta Orthop Belg 1998;64:301–305.
7. Eaton CJ, Lister GD. Syndactyly. Hand Clin 1990;6:555–575.
8. Flatt AE. The Care of Congenital Ha nd Anomalies, ed 2. St Louis: Quality Medical Publishing, 1994:228–275.
9. Keret D, Ger E. Evaluation of a uniform operative technique to treat syndactyly. J Hand Surg Am 1987;12:727–729.

10. Kettelkamp DB, Flatt AE. An evaluation of syndactylia repair. Surg Gynecol Obstet 1961;113:471–478.
11. Niranjan NS, Azad SM, Fleming AN, et al. Long-term results of primary syndactyly correction by the trilobed flap technique. Br J Plast Surg 2005;58:14–21.
12. Niranjan NS, DeCarpentier J. A new technique for the division of syndactyly. Eur J Plast Surg 1990;13:101–104.
13. Ostrowski DM, Feagin CA, Gould JS. A three-flap web-plasty for release of short congenital syndactyly and dorsal adduction contracture. J Hand Surg Am 1991;16:634–641.
14. Percival NJ, Sykes PJ. Syndactyly: a review of the factors which influence surgical treatment. J Hand Surg Br 1989;14:196–200.
15. Shaw DT, Li CS, Richey DG, et al. Interdigital butterfly flap in the hand (the double-opposing Z-plasty). J Bone Joint Surg Am 1973;55(8):1677–1679.
16. Toledo LC, Ger E. Evaluation of the operative treatment of syndactyly. J Hand Surg Am 1979;4(6):556–564.
17. Upton J. Congenital anomalies of the hand and forearm. In: McCarthy JG, May JW, Littler JW, eds. Plastic Surgery. Philadelphia: WB Saunders, 1990:5279–5309.

Amniotic Band Syndrome

Joshua M. Abzug and Scott H. Kozin

154

CHAPTER

DEFINITION

- Amniotic band syndrome is a nonhereditary congenital difference. The entire fetal limb or a portion of it becomes entangled in amniotic membrane leading to partial or complete circumferential constriction, deformity, or amputation of the entire part.
- Multiple other terms are used to describe the condition including constriction band syndrome, Streeter dysplasia, and amniotic disruption sequence among others (Table 1).
- Bands affecting the upper extremities vary from mild with only appearance being an issue to severe with substantial deformity and functional limitations (**FIG 1**). The worst-case scenario is complete deletion or amputation of a part. Each case is different and requires individualized treatment.

ANATOMY

- The bands may affect the soft tissue and involve partial or complete circumferential constriction of part or all of the following structures: skin, subcutaneous tissue, tendons/muscles, nerves, and bone.
- The bands may entangle any part of the upper or lower extremity. Proximal constricture can lead to loss of the entire arm or leg. Distal involvement is more common and presentation varies with degrees of constriction.
- The presence of a cleft proximal to acrosyndactyly (connection of the digit tips) is diagnostic of amniotic band syndrome as this represents normal apoptosis leading to development of the web and subsequent syndactylization due to scarring from the bands (**FIG 2**).

PATHOGENESIS

- Numerous theories exist regarding the underlying cause of amniotic band syndrome. The most common theory is that amniotic disruption causes release of bands (free-floating strands of membrane) that encircle the affected part, causing circumferential constrictions that strangle the affected limb or digit.[5] Rupture also leads to oligohydramnios with resultant external compression on the developing limb.
- Protruding fetal structures are more likely to be involved due to entrapment by the bands.
  - Most common location is digits (56%), followed by hand/wrist (24%), then foot/ankle (10%).[3]
  - Most commonly affected digits are the central digits due to their increased length—long finger (28%), ring finger (27%), and index finger (23%).

Table 1 Terms Used to Describe Amniotic Band Syndrome

Constriction band syndrome
Streeter dysplasia
Amniotic disruption sequence
Constriction ring syndrome
Limb-body wall malformation complex
Annular band syndrome
Amniotic deformity, adhesions, and mutations complex
Simonart band
Early amnion rupture sequence
Intrauterine or fetal amputation

NATURAL HISTORY

- Amniotic band syndrome is nonprogressive.
- Recognition of the limb difference occurs either in utero via ultrasonography or is readily apparent at birth.
- Ultrasound will show a progressive enlargement of the digit distal to the band (Francisco).
- Peripheral nerve palsy, distal anesthesia, vascular insufficiency, venous congestion, or lymphedema may occur due to the presence of a band affecting the neurovascular structures.[8,10]

PATIENT HISTORY AND PHYSICAL FINDINGS

- Examination of the child at birth will demonstrate the location and extent of the band(s).
- Digital constriction will dictate the clinical scenario.
  - Mild to moderate damage initiates an embryonic repair process and yields variable amounts of circumferential stricture with or without resultant distal lymphedema.
  - Inflammatory response may cause adjacent digits to merge distal to the rudimentary web.

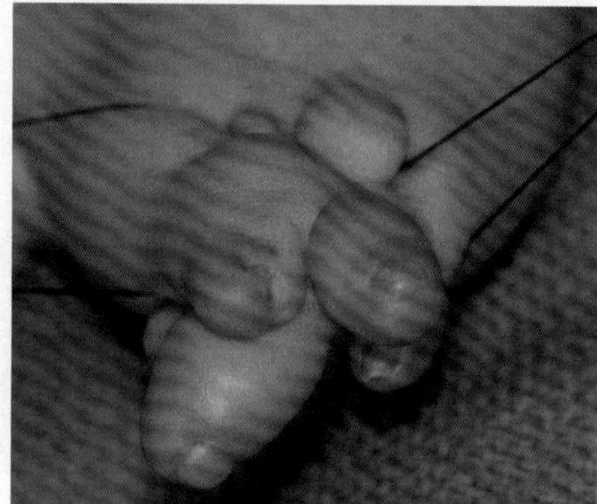

FIG 1 • Photograph of a severe case of amniotic band syndrome that caused substantial deformity and functional limitations. (Courtesy of Shriners Hospital for Children, Philadelphia, PA.)

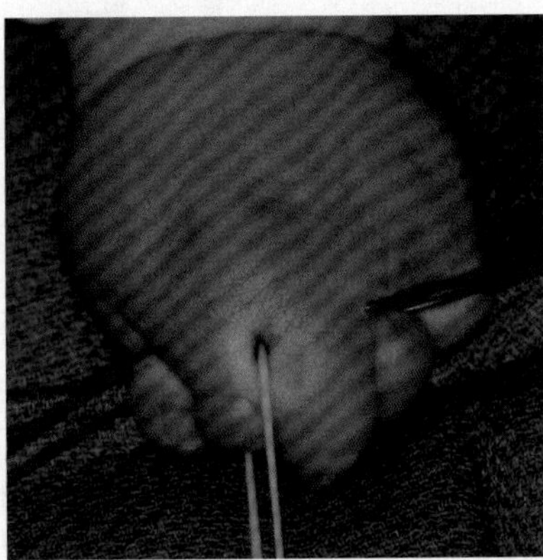

FIG 2 • Dorsal view of brachysyndactyly that occurred due to amniotic band syndrome. The presence of the clefts proximally, that vessel loops are traversing is diagnostic of amniotic band syndrome. (Courtesy of Shriners Hospital for Children, Philadelphia, PA.)

  - A large fusion mass may occur, making it difficult to decipher precise orientation of the digits.
- Severe constrictions may result in digit(s)/limb(s) amputation.
- Ulceration at the base of a ring or with firm skin protuberances on the dorsum of the finger may occur.[2]

IMAGING AND OTHER DIAGNOSTIC STUDIES

- No imaging is required to manage simple bands or bands that are proximal.
- Plain radiographs are sufficient to evaluate digits when there are multiple digits fused.
  - Typically, only a posteroanterior (PA) view is needed (**FIG 3**).

DIFFERENTIAL DIAGNOSIS

- Brachysyndactyly
- Transverse deficiency
- Apert syndrome
- Vasculocutaneous catastrophe of the newborn (also known as *neonatal gangrene, neonatal Volkmann contracture*)

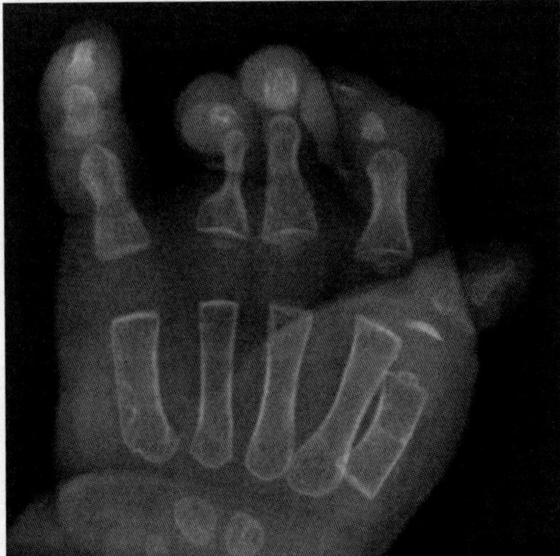

FIG 3 • PA radiograph of a hand with multiple syndactylized digits due to amniotic band syndrome. Note the compression of the proximal phalanx of the ring and long fingers due to the band. (Courtesy of Shriners Hospital for Children, Philadelphia, PA.)

NONOPERATIVE MANAGEMENT

- Observation is the nonoperative management of amniotic band syndrome.
- As with all congenital differences, priority should be given to function over appearance. In other words, function trumps form. Therefore, it may be better in certain circumstances to leave digits syndactylized if they function better together than apart.

SURGICAL MANAGEMENT

- Surgical management is the most common management for amniotic band syndrome to maximize function and appearance. Once again, form trumps function in operative planning, and amputation of one or more digits may be the best course of action (**FIG 4**).
- Strategies are to prioritize the thumb, thumb–index web space, and digits with adequate separation, motion, and length.
  - Bands in sequence are released in stages beginning with release of the most distal band.[3,11]
- Release of bands requires complete excision of the invaginating band and subcutaneous tissue.
  - The void is covered with a Z-plasty, using the surrounding tissue.[11]
  - Traditional treatment is release of one-half of a circumferential band at a time; however, complete circumferential excision can be safely performed if the surgeon is confident that the artery and vein are preserved.[7,11,12]
- Timing is dictated by the depth of the band.
  - Mild to moderate bands and digital masses from amputations can be treated electively. However, bands causing tethering of adjacent digits should be released early following the principles of traditional syndactyly release (**FIG 5**).
  - A deep band jeopardizing limb viability requires immediate release if the limb is salvageable.
  - In utero release has been successfully performed, but there are noteworthy risks including the risk of spontaneous abortion.[9]

Preoperative Planning

- Discussion with the family regarding the possibility of staged reconstruction and the need for skin grafting must occur.
  - In digits syndactylized, separate only one side of a digit at a time.

Positioning

- Supine positioning on a standard operating room table.
  - A hand table can be used for older/larger children.
- A tourniquet is applied to the upper arm.

Approach

- No standard approach is used, as the bands are circumferential and excision requires a circumferential incision.
  - Knowledge of the anatomy of the area is essential to avoid damaging neurovascular structures that may be tethered.
- Release of syndactylized digits uses a similar technique to traditional syndactyly release by typically using zigzag-type flaps as well as flaps to recreate the commissure.
- Synonychia release requires re-creation of paronychial folds with flaps such as Buck-Gramcko flaps.

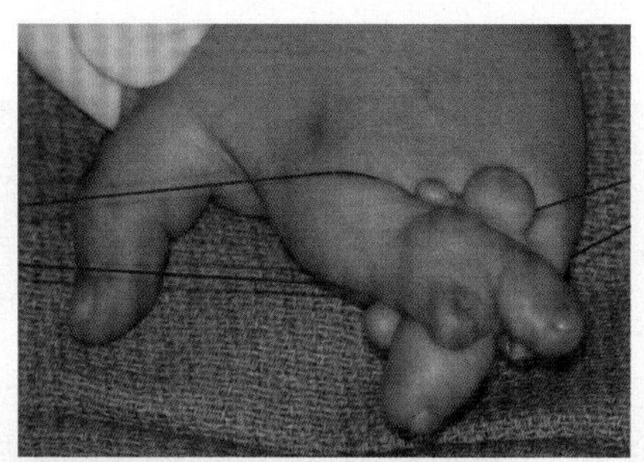
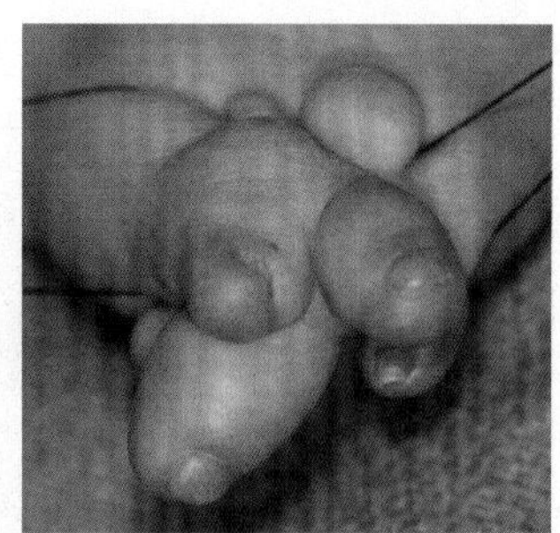
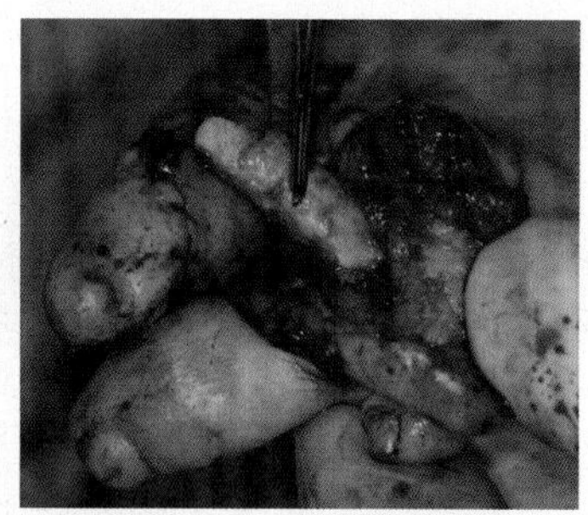
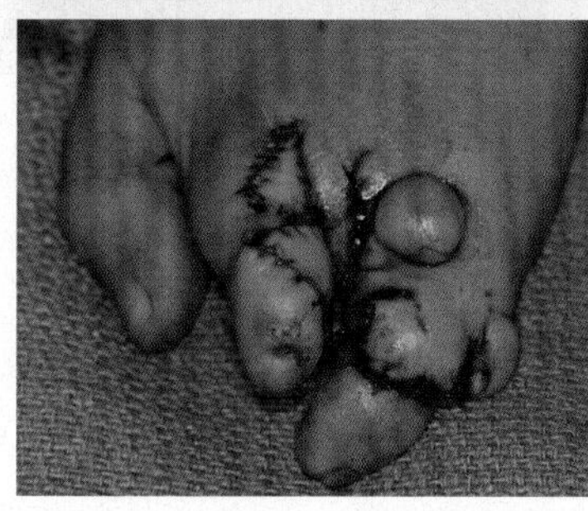

FIG 4 • Three-year-old boy with complex banding of his left hand requiring long-finger amputation and commissure reconstruction. **A.** Preoperative dorsal view. **B.** Close-up of digital conglomeration. **C.** Amputation of long finger. **D.** Commissure reconstruction with flap and adjacent skin graft. (Courtesy of Shriners Hospital for Children, Philadelphia, PA.)

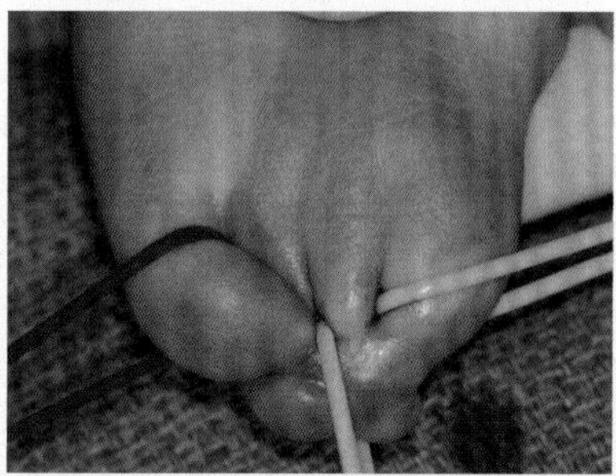
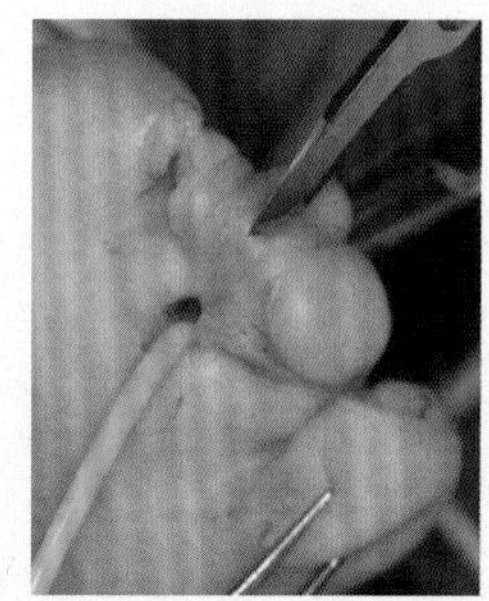
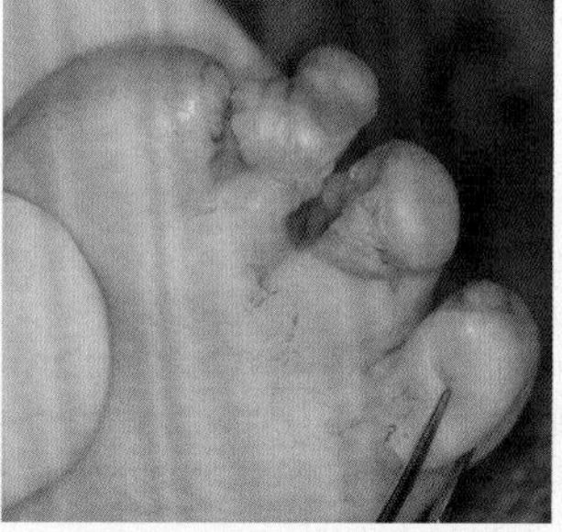

FIG 5 • Three month-old boy with bands of his left hand requiring early release to prevent tethering. **A.** Preoperative dorsal view. **B.** Separation of connected fingertips with scalpel blade. **C.** Fingers liberated to allow unimpeded growth. (Courtesy of Shriners Hospital for Children, Philadelphia, PA.)

TECHNIQUES

Simple Constriction Ring Release

- Make a circumferential incision to excise band (**TECH FIG 1A,B**), including skin and subcutaneous adipose tissue.
  - Can mark sidewalls of band with marking pen and then bring proximal and distal skin edges together such that they touch. The painted area is the appropriate amount to excise.[11]
  - Failure to excise the entirety of a band, including the abnormal subcutaneous tissue, may result in scar contracture and "recurrence."
- Mobilize surrounding skin and subcutaneous adipose tissue (**TECH FIG 1C**).
  - Preserve deep subcutaneous veins and neurovascular bundles to prevent postoperative venous congestion.
- Reapproximate adipose tissue over muscle/fascia.
- Perform Z-plasty closure of band (**TECH FIG 1D**).

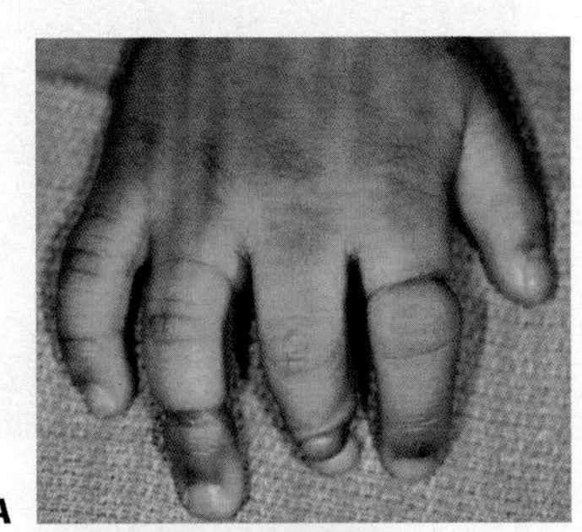

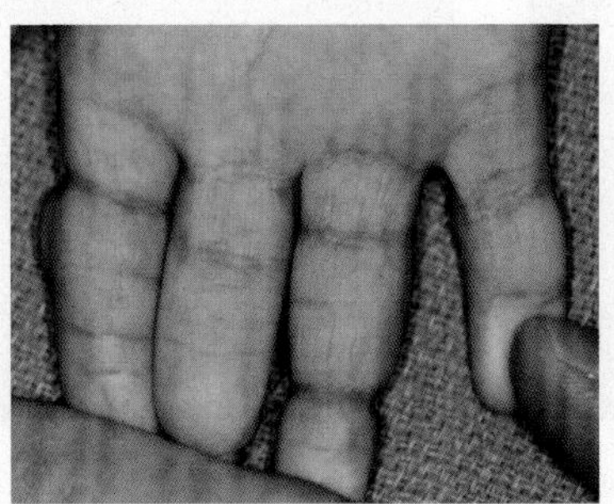

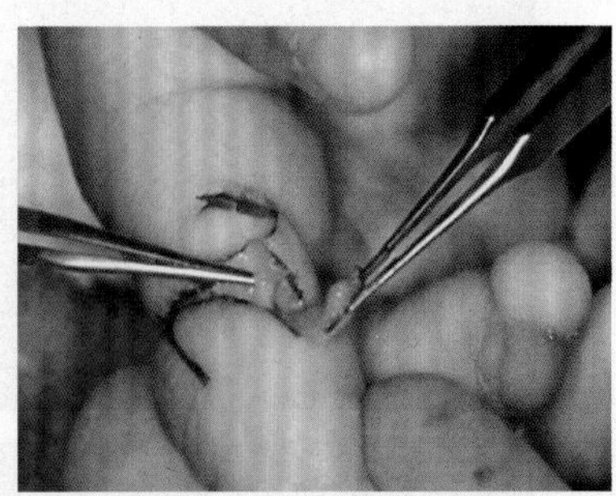

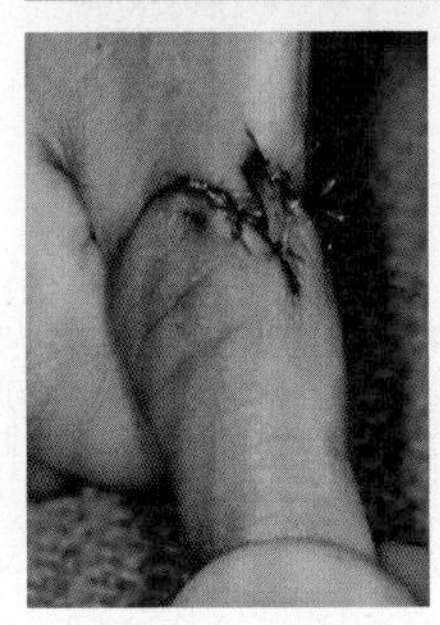

TECH FIG 1 • Simple constriction rings present on multiple digits. **A.** Dorsal view. **B.** Palmar view. **C.** Elevation of skin flaps following excision of a band. Note the full-thickness nature of the flap by the presence of adipose tissue. **D.** Closure of the Z-plasty. (Courtesy of Shriners Hospital for Children, Philadelphia, PA.)

Acrosyndactyly Release

- Draw flap designs.
  - Create new broad commissure using dorsal skin that ends approximately two-thirds of the way up the proximal phalanx from the metacarpophalangeal joint to the proximal interphalangeal joint (**TECH FIG 2A**).
  - Zigzag incisions to minimize the amount of necessary skin graft. The points of the zigzag should be opposite the base from the other side.
  - On the volar side, fashion a pattern such as a three-sided box to have a place for the commissure flap to set into (**TECH FIG 2B**).
  - In cases with a connected common nail, Buck-Gramcko flaps are needed to generate paronychial folds.
- Exsanguinate limb loosely and inflate tourniquet.
- Begin with dorsal skin incision to elevate commissure flap.
  - Start thin (full-thickness dermis) distally and progress to thick (full thickness including subcutaneous fat).

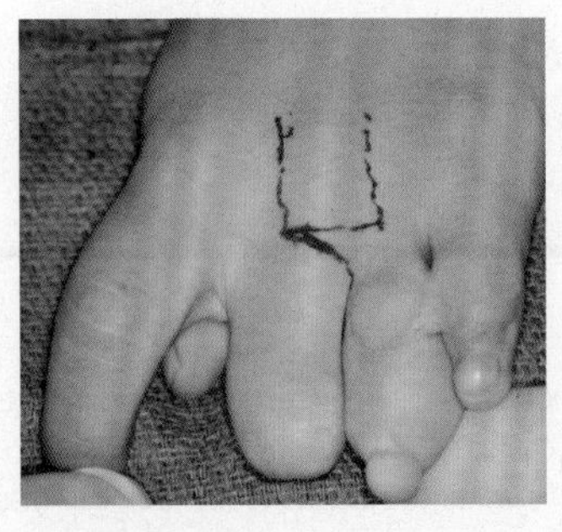

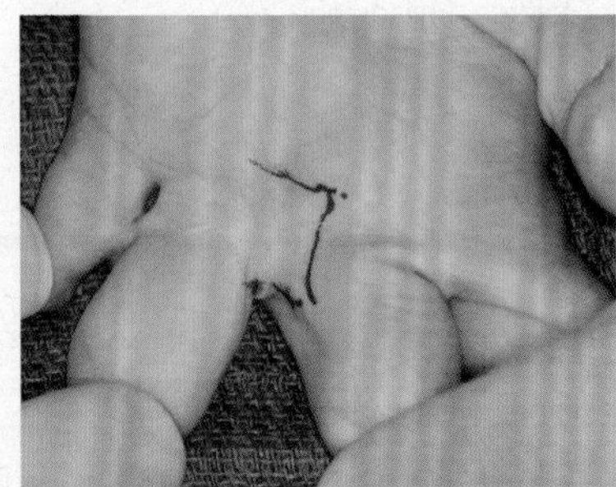

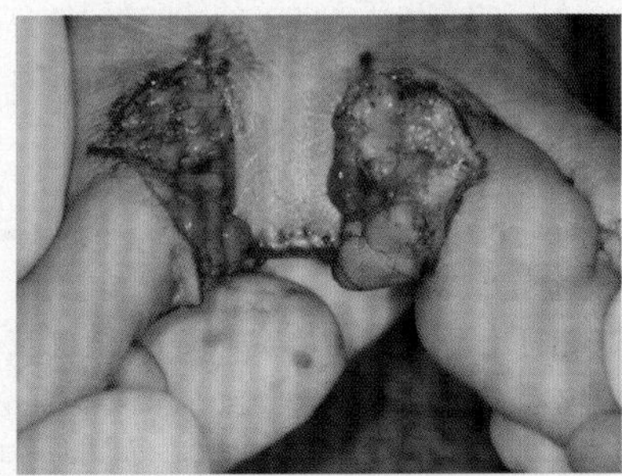

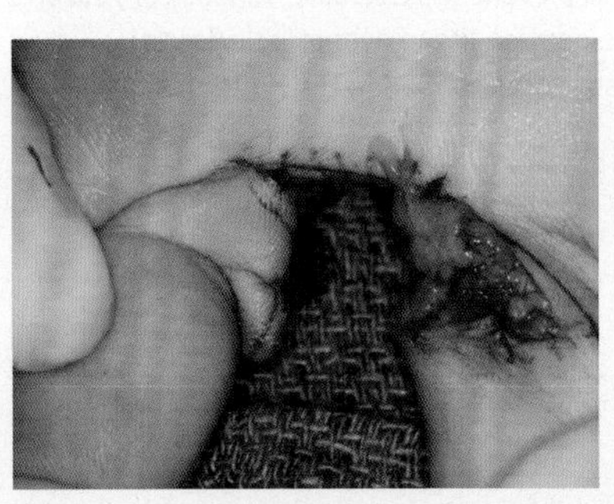

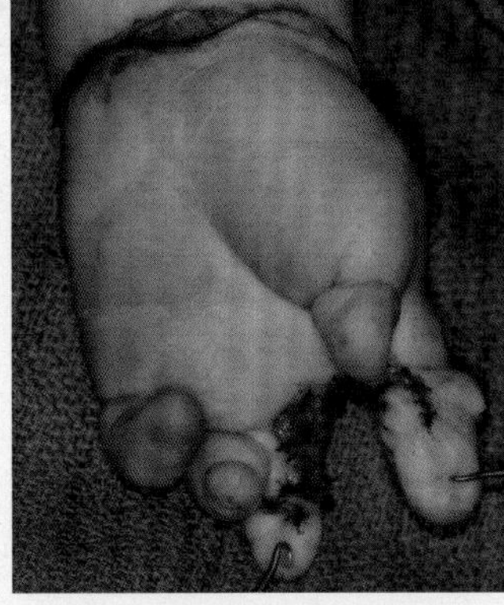

TECH FIG 2 • **A.** Flap design of digital commissure using dorsal skin. **B.** Flap design on volar side to receive commissure. Note the ability of the three-sided box to wrap onto the ring finger. **C,D.** Dorsal and palmar views, respectively, of insertion of the commissure flap. **E.** Use of wrist flexion crease to obtain skin graft. Note the closure obtained which will leave a scar that is difficult to visualize. (Courtesy of Shriners Hospital for Children, Philadelphia, PA.)

- Incise dorsal zigzag template in a full-thickness skin manner.
  - Minimize fat present on this skin.
- Following raising of the flaps, spread transversally to separate digits.
- From dorsal side, identify neurovascular bundles.
- Raise volar flaps with minimal fat.
  - Ensure the Buck-Gramcko flaps are not damaged as you dissect distally.
- Raise Buck-Gramcko flaps.
- Separate bone/synonychia with knife as needed.
- Begin closing flaps by first insetting commissure flap (**TECH FIG 2C,D**).
  - Use 5-0 plain gut to close flaps.
- Obtain full-thickness skin graft to close remaining areas.
  - Make ellipse centered on wrist flexion crease.
  - Incise skin only and raise flap.
  - Can defat as you dissect with knife parallel to skin
  - Close donor site with subcutaneous and subcuticular closure (**TECH FIG 2E**).
- Deflate tourniquet and ensure brisk capillary refill is present.
  - Remove a few sutures if capillary refill is sluggish.
- Apply bulky dressing to prevent shear followed by a cast application.
- **TECH FIG 3** shows a complete acrosyndactyly release.

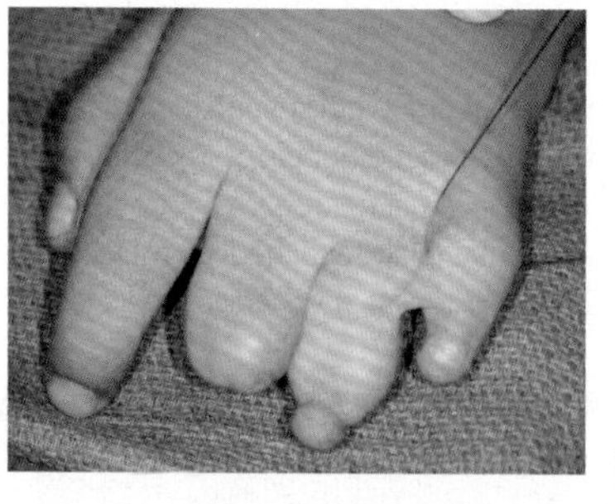
A

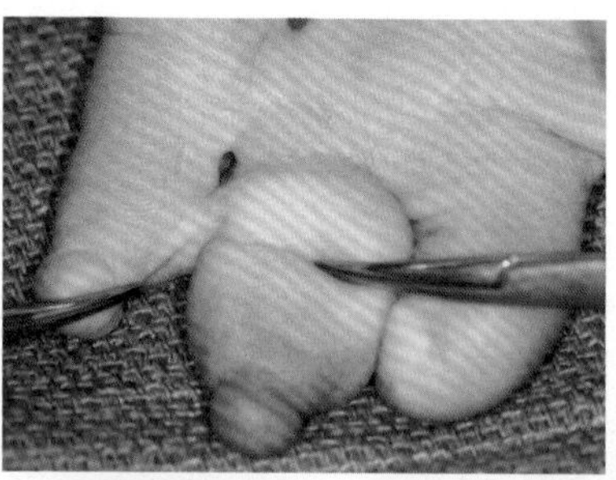
B

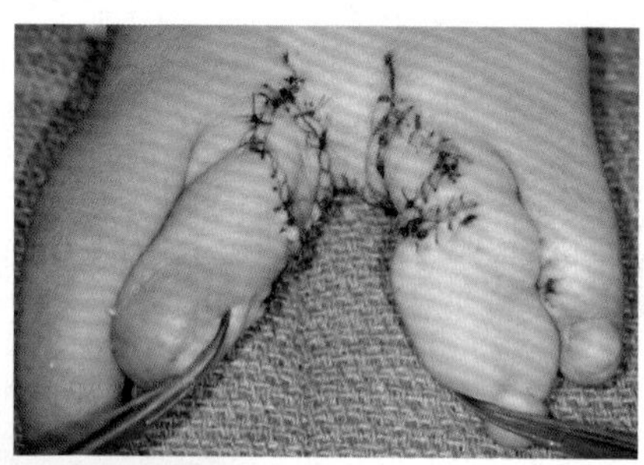
C

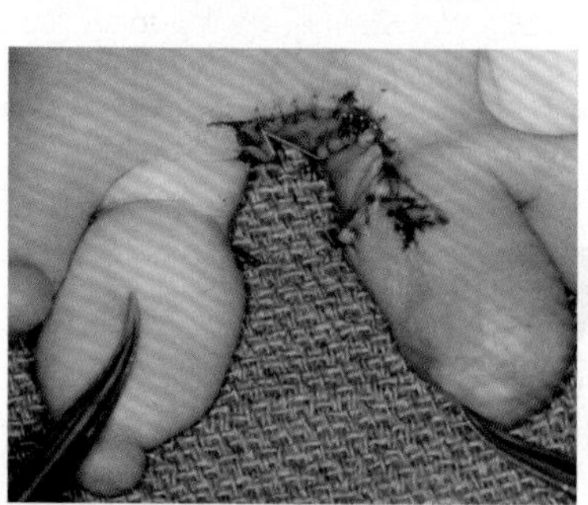
D

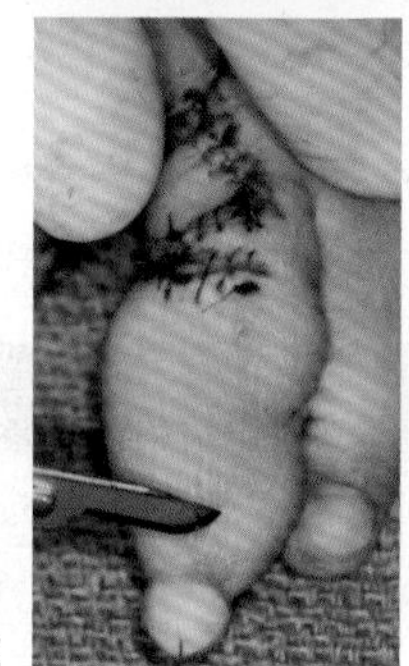
E

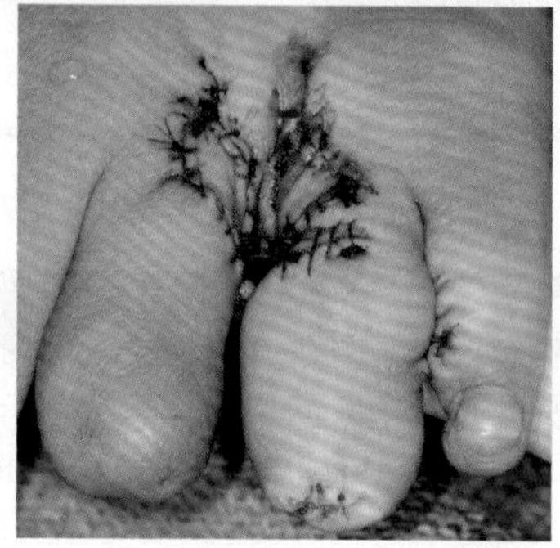
F

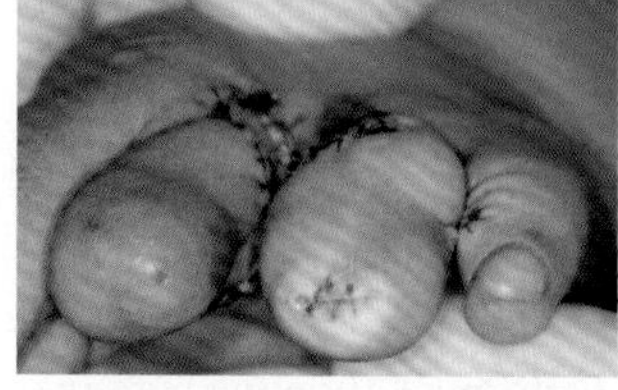
G

TECH FIG 3 • A 5-year-old boy with amniotic band syndrome affecting his left hand. **A.** Dorsal view. **B.** Palmar view. **C.** Dorsal view following syndactyly release and skin grafting. **D.** Palmar view following syndactyly release and skin grafting. **E.** Presence of nonfunctional portion of distal ring finger. **F.** Excision of distal ring finger tip to improve appearance. **G.** Distal view following excision of tip of ring finger. (Courtesy of Shriners Hospital for Children, Philadelphia, PA.)

Nonvascularized Toe Phalangeal Transfer

- Exsanguinate limb and inflate tourniquet.
- Dorsal zigzag incision on affected digit down to level of extensor mechanism
- Incise extensor mechanism longitudinally.
- Perform gentle longitudinal spreading to create a soft tissue pocket to accept toe.
- Attention now turned to foot where the proximal phalanx of second toe is now exposed through a chevron/longitudinal incision (**TECH FIG 4A**).
  - Proximal phalanx of third and fourth toes can be used if needed.
- Toe extensor mechanism is split longitudinally.
- Collateral ligaments released from distal extent of toe.
- Extraperiosteal dissection performed from distal to proximal.

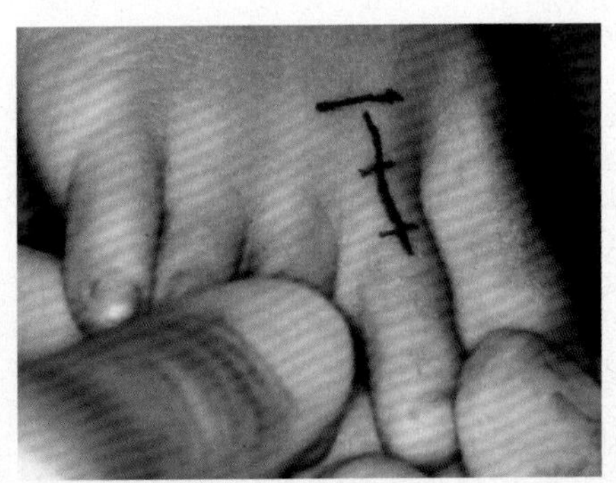
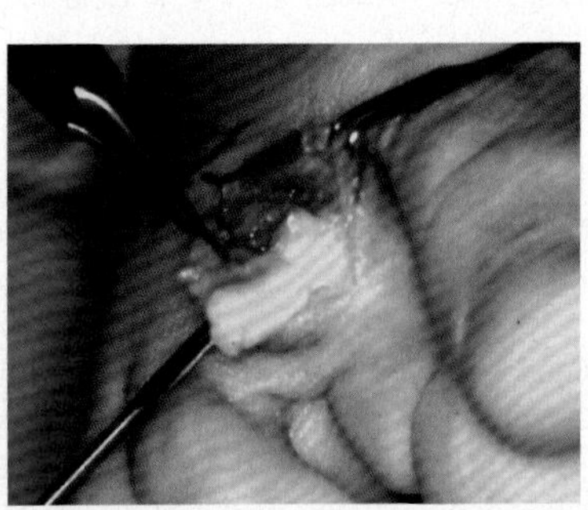
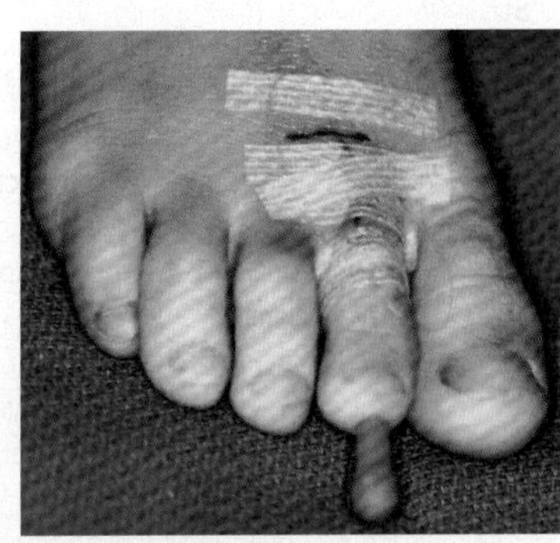

TECH FIG 4 • **A.** Incision used to obtain proximal phalanx of second toe for nonvascularized toe transfer. **B.** Extraperiosteal excision of proximal phalanx. **C.** Appearance of second toe following excision of proximal phalanx and placement of a smooth wire. (Courtesy of Shriners Hospital for Children, Philadelphia, PA.)

- Plantar plate and then pulleys are released.
  - Be careful to protect and preserve the toe flexor tendons and neurovascular bundles.
- Toe phalanx now released while preserving the proximal collateral ligaments and plantar plate which are used for attachment to the metacarpal (**TECH FIG 4B**).
- Toe extensor tendon sewn to flexor tendon to close the defect and preserve length and alignment.[1]
- Smooth pin placed in a longitudinal direction across excised toe phalanx (**TECH FIG 4C**).
- Toe phalanx placed in finger soft tissue pocket and pin advanced antegrade out the tip of the soft tissue nubbin.
- Pin driven retrograde into metacarpal head.
- Collateral ligaments and plantar plate attached to metacarpophalangeal joint capsule and extensor mechanism attached to toe phalanx.
- Skin closed with simple interrupted sutures.
- Long-arm mitten cast applied over a bulky dressing.

PEARLS AND PITFALLS

Timing	▪ If connected digits are unequal in length, early tip separation is warranted to prevent a tether and restricted growth.
Skin graft	▪ Use of the volar wrist flexion crease skin allows for a hidden scar and avoids the potential for hair growth seen when using groin skin.
Flap design	▪ If possible, wrap the three-sided box from the volar flap onto the ring finger to permit ring wear that does not overlie a potentially painful scar (see **TECH FIGS 2B** and **3C,D**).
Postoperative care	▪ Use whirlpool to remove postoperative dressings at 2 weeks.

POSTOPERATIVE CARE

- Children are typically admitted for 24 hours for pain control and observation including regular neurovascular checks to ensure digit viability.
- Elevate limb for 48 hours to aid with venous return.
- Remove cast and dressings at 2 to 3 weeks postoperatively for band excisions or syndactyly releases.
- Remove cast and pins at 4 to 6 weeks for nonvascularized toe transfers.

OUTCOMES

- Successful release of bands is the anticipated outcome following excision and Z-plasties. Specific results of band excision and syndactyly release are directly related to the extent of the constricture. Published results are limited.
- Nonvascularized toe transfers performed at young ages (before 12 to 18 months) yield good results exhibiting open physes that permits longitudinal and appositional growth.[1,5]
- Vascularized toe to hand transfers have been performed for amniotic band syndrome and can achieve 95% or greater success rates of viability in experienced hands.[4,6]
- However, this is a technically challenging procedure that requires substantial experience.

COMPLICATIONS

- Flap/graft necrosis
- Hematoma formation
- Venous congestion
- Infection
- Web creep

- Circulatory compromise
- Stiffness
- Ugly/painful scar formation

REFERENCES

1. Buck-Gramcko D. The role of nonvascularized toe phalanx transplantation. Hand Clin 1990;6:643–659.
2. Emmett AJ. The ring constriction syndrome. Handchir Mikrochir Plast Chir 1992;24:3–15.
3. Flatt AE. Constriction ring syndrome. In: The Care of Congenital Hand Anomalies. St. Louis: CV Mosby, 1977:214.
4. Foucher G, Medina J, Navarro R, et al. Toe transfer in congenital hand malformations. J Reconstr Microsurg 2001;17:1–7.
5. Goldberg NH, Watson HK. Composite toe (phalanx and epiphysis) transfers in the reconstruction of the aphalangic hand. J Hand Surg Am 1982;7:454–459.
6. Jones NF, Hansen SL, Bates SJ. Toe-to-hand transfers for congenital anomalies of the hand. Hand Clin 2007;23:129–136.
7. Miura T. Congenital constriction band syndrome. J Hand Surg Am 1984;9A(1):82–88.
8. Moran SL, Jensen M, Bravo C. Amniotic band syndrome of the upper extremity: diagnosis and management. J Am Acad Orthop Surg 2007;15:397–407.
9. Soldado F, Aguirre M, Peiró JL, et al. Fetoscopic release of extremity amniotic bands with risk of amputation. J Pediatr Orthop 2009;29:290–293.
10. Uchida Y, Sugioka Y. Peripheral nerve palsy associated with congenital constriction band syndrome. J Hand Surg Br 1991;16:109–112.
11. Upton J, Tan C. Correction of constriction rings. J Hand Surg 1991;(1695):947–953.
12. Wiedrich TA. Congenital constriction band syndrome. Hand Clin 1998;14:29–38.

155

CHAPTER

Clinodactyly

Robert Carrigan

DEFINITION

- *Clinodactyly* refers to an abnormal about of radioulnar angulation of a digit (>15 degrees).
- The small finger is most commonly observed.
- This condition is often bilateral.

ANATOMY

- The finger consists of three phalanges (proximal, middle, and distal).
- The normal phalangeal physis is located at the proximal portion of each phalanx.

PATHOGENESIS

- The angulation is result of abnormal development of one of the phalanges (most often the middle phalanx [p2]).
- Abnormal development of the phalanx may be due to an irregular physis (longitudinal bracket epiphysis). This may also be referred to as a *delta phalanx*.
- The tethering effect of the bracket epiphysis on the radial side of the finger causes abnormal growth of the phalanx resulting in a triangular or trapezoidal shape.
- Extra bones may be encountered.

NATURAL HISTORY

- The natural history of clinodactyly is variable and poorly documented, owing to the great number of cases that are asymptomatic and do not require treatment.
- Angulation may be stable or rapidly progressive at times of growth, depending on the extent of the involvement of the physis and/or presence of extra phalanges.

PATIENT HISTORY AND PHYSICAL EXAM FINDINGS

- Clinodactyly may be present at birth or develop during a period of growth (**FIG 1**).
- Clinodactyly is often bilateral in the small finger.
- Clinodactyly is an autosomal dominant condition with variable penetration.
- Involvement of the thumb is rare and is associated with varying syndromes.

IMAGING AND OTHER DIAGNOSTIC STUDIES

- Standard radiographs (three views: anteroposterior[AP], lateral [LAT], and oblique [OBL]) of the hand and affected digit are sufficient to determine the area of involvement.
- Contralateral images are useful for comparison.
- Advanced imaging such as computed tomography (CT) is rarely needed. Magnetic resonance imaging (MRI) may be useful to delineate the shape of a bracket diaphysis.

DIFFERENTIAL DIAGNOSIS

- The diagnosis of clinodactyly is straightforward; clinical examination and radiographs are sufficient to make the diagnosis.
- Associated syndrome should be screened for, these include Down, Rubinstein-Taybi, Apert, and Russell-Silver.

NONOPERATIVE MANAGEMENT

- Observation may be considered for angulated digits that do not impair function. Splinting is not effective.
- Most cases can be treated nonoperatively; surgery should be considered for significant angular deformity that compromises hand function.

SURGICAL MANAGEMENT

Preoperative Planning

- Timing of surgery is variable, depending on the degree of angulation and how much growth potential remains.
- Small amounts of angulation with little remaining growth potential may be addressed when the child is older.
- Larger amounts of angulation or children with the potential for worsening angulation may consider earlier intervention.

Positioning

- The patient is positioned supine on the operating room table and the body is pulled over to the affected side.

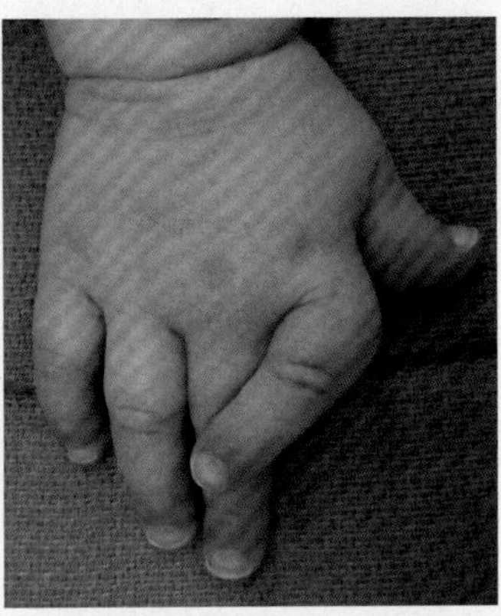

FIG 1 • Clinodactyly of the index finger from osteochondroma in a child with multiple hereditary exostosis.

- The arm is placed on a radiolucent hand table and an arm tourniquet is applied.
- Prepping and draping are performed in the standard fashion.

Approach

- Several approaches may be considered for clinodactyly correction, but the principles remain consistent regardless of surgical approach.
- Skin incisions must address the excess skin on the convex side of the angulation and the lack of skin on the concave side.
- Extensile incisions are preferred.
- Bony correction of the angulation can be accomplished via osteotomy, physiolysis of the bracket diaphysis, excision of extra phalanx, or a combination of all three.

TECHNIQUES

Physiolysis

- This technique is favored for the younger child with significant growth potential.
- Skin incisions are made over the radial aspect of the digit.
- Flaps are developed and the flexor and extensor tendons are identified and protected.
- Fluoroscopy is used to identify the physis.
- The physis is incised with a no. 15 blade transversely and the central portion of the physis is removed with a small curette. Local fat may be placed in the void but may not be necessary.
- The skin is closed and a cast is applied.

Phalanx Excision

- Elliptical skin incisions along the convex side of the angulation are favored. These incisions allow for excision of redundant skin, aiding the cosmetic appearance on completion of the case (**TECH FIG 1**).
- The extensor tendons are protected and the extra phalanx is identified.
- The phalanx is excised and the collateral ligaments are preserved.
- The joint is inspected and reduced.
- The collateral ligaments are tightened with interrupted suture and the joint is pinned with a single K-wire along the long axis of the joint.
- Skin is closed with absorbable suture and a cast is applied.

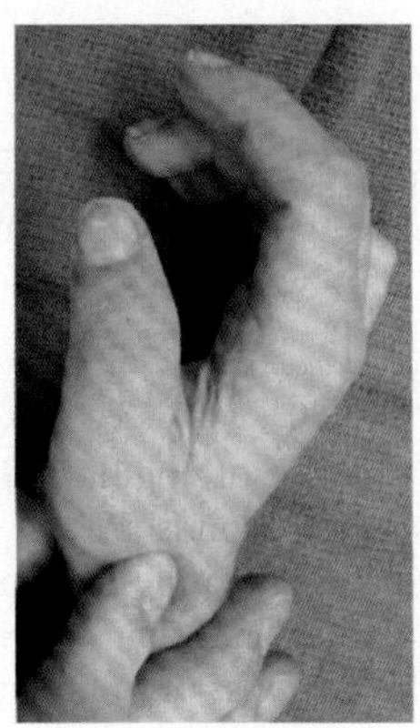

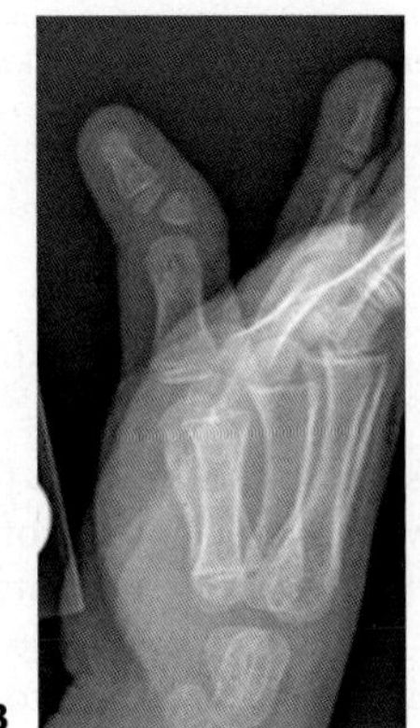

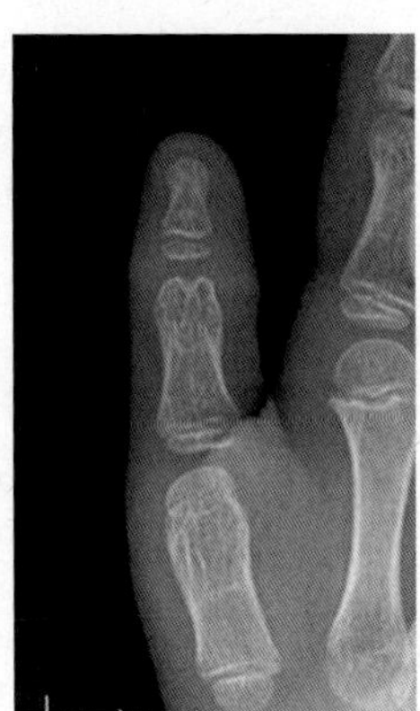

TECH FIG 1 • Clinodactyly of the thumb. **A.** Clinical photograph. **B.** Radiograph demonstrating triangular phalanx. **C.** Postoperative photograph after excision of triangular phalanx and pinning.

Osteotomy

- Closing wedge, opening wedge, or reverse wedge osteotomy can be strongly considered for large amounts of angulation in patients who are close to or skeletally mature (**TECH FIG 2**).
- Incisions are made along the convex side (ulnar side of the finger) for closing wedge osteotomies and along the concave side (radial side of the finger) for opening wedge ostetomies.
- Skin flaps are developed.
- The digital neurovascular bundles are protected as well as the extensor tendons.
- The periosteum is elevated off the phalanx and the osteotomy is templated.
- The closing wedge osteotomy can be performed with either thin narrow rongeur or oscillating saw.
    - A rongeur is favorable in smaller children where the bone is small.
    - Using this method, the far cortex is left in place and the finger is bent back to a neutral alignment using the far cortex as hinge.
    - The osteotomy is stabilized with one or two K-wires.

- The opening wedge osteotomy is performed in a similar fashion as the closing wedge, only the incision is made on the radial border of the digit; no wedge of bone is removed.
  - A single osteotomy is made in the radial aspect of the phalanx, leaving the ulnar cortex intact.
  - The osteotomy is opened and stabilized with one or two K-wires.
  - Bone graft is often not necessary in young children.
- The reverse wedge is useful when large amounts of angulation correction are necessary. This technique allows for correction of angulation with preservation of length.
  - This osteotomy is performed with an oscillating saw.
  - A wedge of bone is taken from the near side and flipped and inserted in the far side.
  - The osteotomy is stabilized with one or two K-wires.

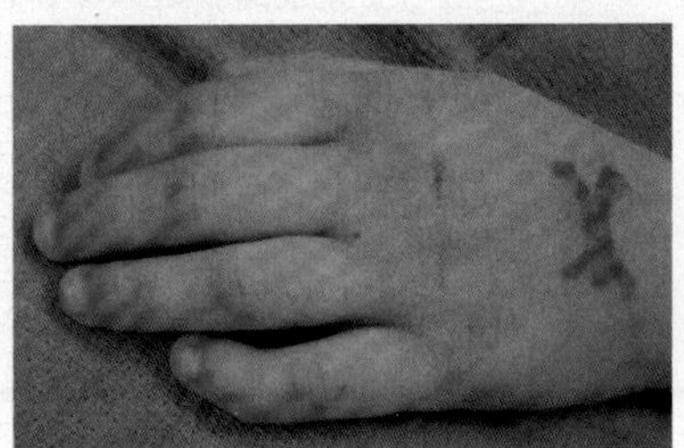
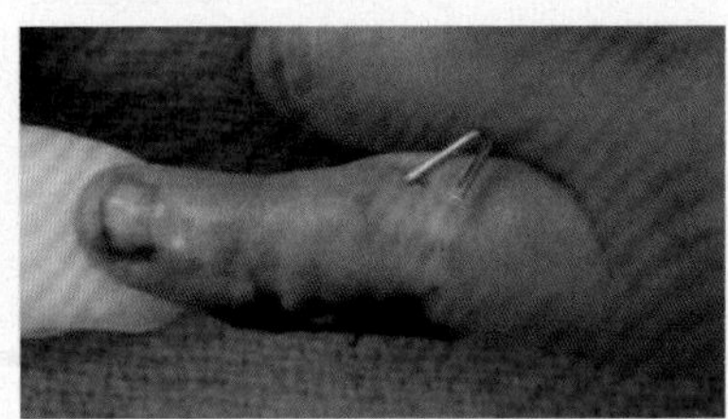
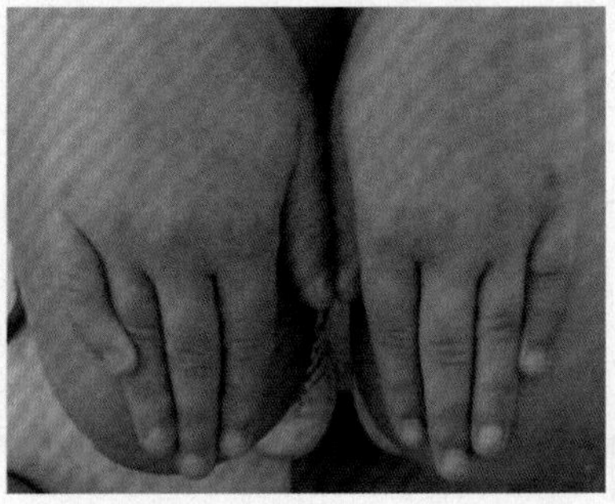

TECH FIG 2 • Small finger clinodactyly. **A.** Preoperative clinical photograph. **B.** Intraoperative photograph after osteotomy and pinning. **C.** Postoperative photograph demonstrating surgical correction of the left and no correction on the right.

PEARLS AND PITFALLS

Undercorrection or overcorrection of angular deformity	■ Precise surgical planning with good radiographs and measured correction
Redundant skin causing uneven appearance of finger after phalanx excision	■ Elliptical skin incisions can reduce redundant skin on the convex side when excising a phalanx.
Lack of motion after angular correction	■ Excessive periosteal stripping leading to tendon adhesions. Limit soft tissue dissection.

POSTOPERATIVE CARE

- Occupational therapy is started after the first postoperative visit. The parents are instructed to wash and clean the hand. A progressive active and passive range of motion program is initiated.
- In cases where an osteotomy is performed, the patient is placed in a cast until the osteotomy has healed (typically 4 weeks). At this time, the pins are removed and occupational therapy is initiated.
- Patients are followed until full range of motion has been achieved, typically 6 to 8 weeks.

OUTCOMES

- Outcomes from clinodactyly correction are generally good.
- Patient satisfaction is correlated to the degree of preoperative angulation and degree of correction.

COMPLICATIONS

- Residual angulation may persist, usually due to initial undercorrection or continued abnormal growth. This usually is not an issue especially when the amount of angulation is mild and when the magnitude of the correction is great.
- Digital stiffness may be encountered. Tendon adhesions and scar tissue are usually the cause. Occupational therapy and parental education are helpful to address a loss of full digital motion.

SUGGESTED READINGS

1. Ali M, Jackson T, Rayan GM. Closing wedge osteotomy of abnormal middle phalanx for clinodactyly. J Hand Surg Am 2009;34:914–918.
2. Al-Qattan MM. Congenital sporadic clinodactyly of the index finger. Ann Plast Surg 2007;59:682–687.
3. Bednar MS, Bindra RR, Light TR. Epiphyseal bar resection and fat interposition for clinodactyly. J Hand Surg Am 2010;35:834–837.
4. Strauss NL, Goldfarb CA. Surgical correction of clinodactyly: two straightforward techniques. Tech Hand Up Extrem Surg 2010;14:54–57.
5. Ty JM, James MA. Failure of differentiation: part II (arthrogryposis, camptodactyly, clinodactyly, Madelung deformity, trigger finger, and trigger thumb). Hand Clin 2009;25:195–213.

Exam Table for Hand, Wrist, and Elbow Surgery

Examination	Technique	Illustration	Grading & Significance
Hand and Wrist			
Abductor pollicis brevis muscle test	Abduction of thumb against resistance with palpation of thenar muscle	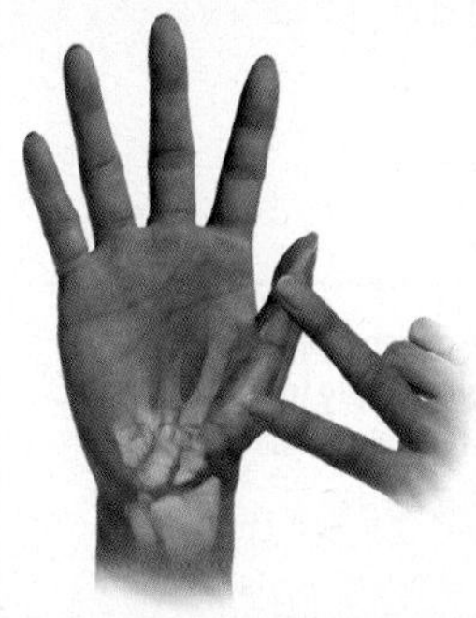	MRC grading. If weak, the surgeon should consider a median nerve lesion.
Advancing Tinel sign	Percussion along course of a nerve in a distal to proximal direction	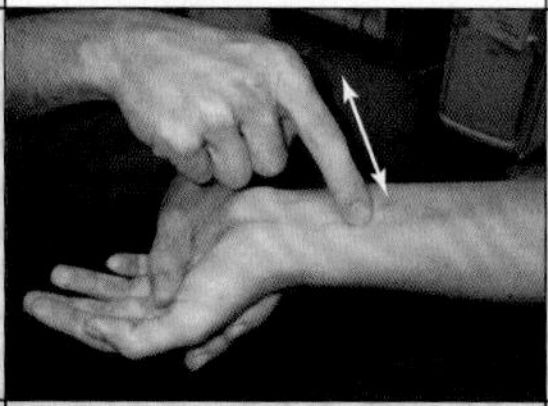	During percussion, the patient notes a tingling sensation in the sensory distribution of the nerve. Detects regenerating (unmyelinated) axons. Serial progression of a Tinel sign distally is useful to monitor axon progression after nerve repair or injury.
Allen test	The patient is asked to actively open and close the hand to create blanching in the palm. With the hand tightly closed, the examiner occludes the radial and ulnar arteries. The examiner releases one artery and watches for reperfusion and then repeats, releasing the other artery.	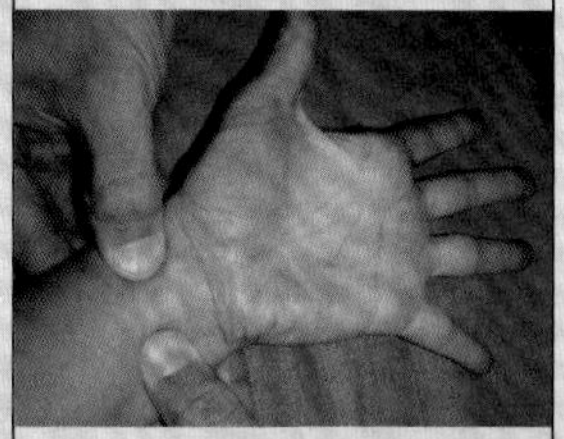	Reperfusion should occur within a few seconds. If it does not, then that artery does not provide good flow to the hand. If, for example, the radial artery is dominant (ie, the ulnar artery does not reperfuse the hand), then injury to this vessel during the procedure could lead to ischemia of the hand.
Anatomic snuffbox palpation	The examiner palpates the anatomic snuffbox between the first and third extensor compartment tendons while moving the wrist from radial to ulnar deviation.	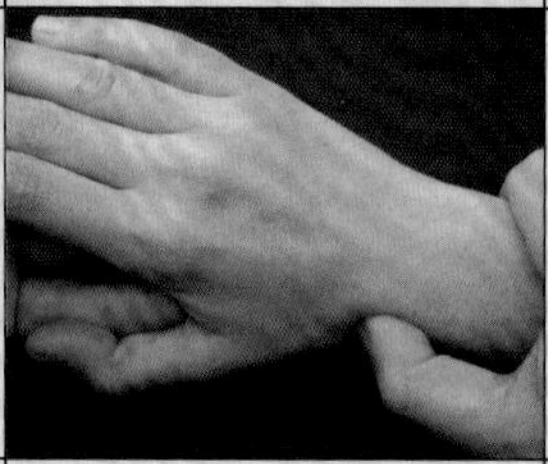	Pain at the articular–nonarticular junction of the scaphoid may be the result of periscaphoid synovitis, scaphoid instability, radial styloid arthrosis, or scaphoid fracture or nonunion.
Boyes oblique retinacular ligament tightness test	The examiner passively extends the proximal interphalangeal (PIP) joint and evaluates distal interphalangeal (DIP) motion. Tightness of the oblique retinacular ligaments of Landsmeer is evaluated by assessing the relative degree of resistance to active and passive DIP joint flexion with the PIP joint held in maximum extension by the examiner.	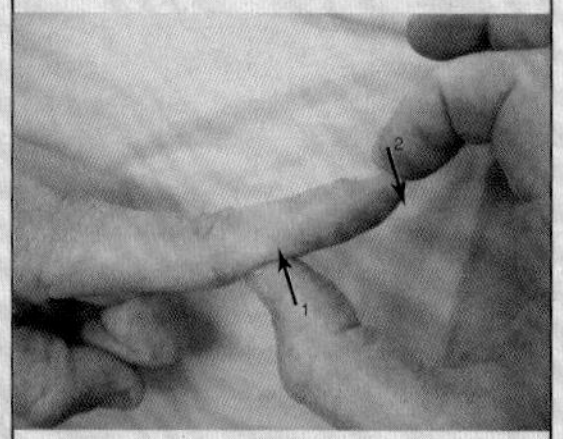	In a positive test, passive extension of the PIP joint will result in extension of the DIP joint. Increased resistance to active and passive DIP joint flexion with the PIP joint held in extension signifies relative tightness of the oblique retinacular ligaments (ORLs) of Landsmeer, signifying a potential subacute or chronic central slip injury. Continued shortening of the ORLs will result in a boutonnière deformity.

(continued)

Examination	Technique	Illustration	Grading & Significance
Bunnell intrinsic tightness test	While holding the metacarpophalangeal (MCP) joint in extension, the examiner assesses the degree of resistance to passive PIP joint flexion. The test is repeated with the MCP joint held in flexion.	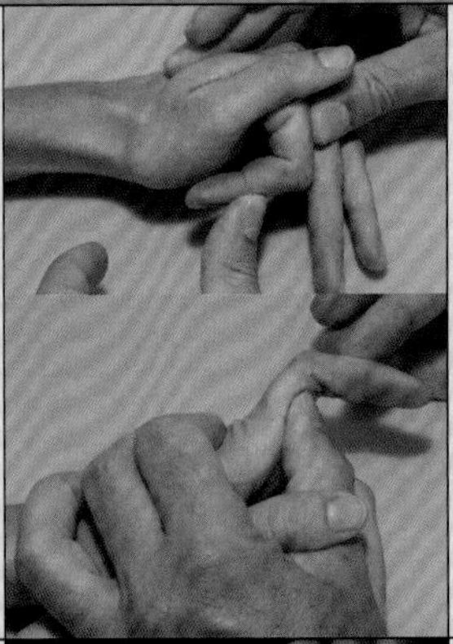	Intrinsic tightness results in limited passive flexion of the PIP joint when the MCP joint is held extended. Extrinsic tightness results in limited PIP joint passive flexion when the MCP joint is held flexed.
Carpal supination reduction test	The examiner applies dorsally directed pressure to the volar aspect of the supinated ulnar carpus.	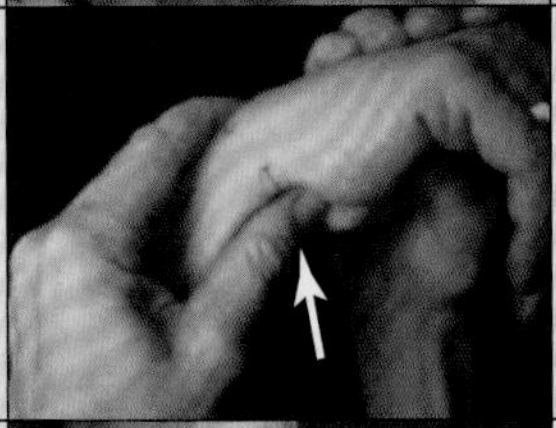	The ulnar carpus will be supinated and the distal ulna prominent, signifying an ulnar extrinsic ligament injury. Reduction is noted visually after application of the force.
Carpal tunnel compression test	The examiner applies direct compression to the median nerve at the level of the carpal tunnel for 60 seconds or until symptomatic.	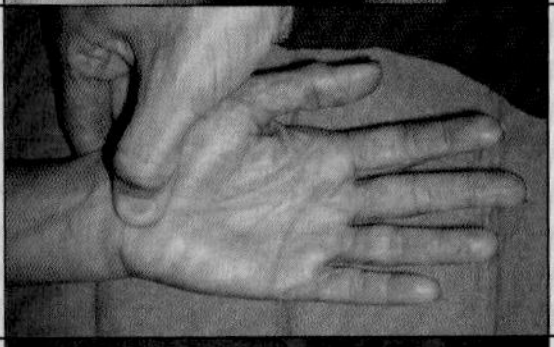	Reproduction of symptoms in the median nerve distribution is consistent with carpal tunnel syndrome.
Carpometacarpal (CMC) distraction test	The examiner distracts the thumb and palpates the CMC joint.	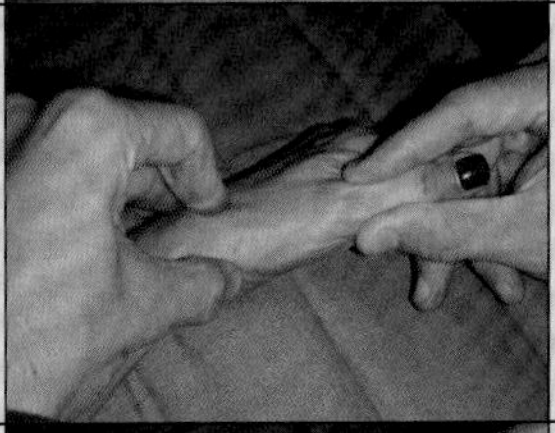	Reproduction of pain confirms the CMC joint as a site of disease or inflammation.
CMC grind test	The examiner axially compresses the thumb and applies flexion, extension, circumduction, and rotation.	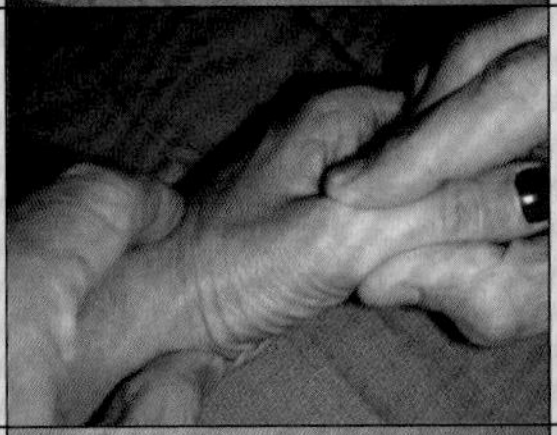	Usually crepitus is appreciated starting with stage II disease, but it is more predictable in stage III or IV disease. A positive test is suggestive of degenerative thumb CMC joint disease.
Cross-finger test	The patient is asked to cross the long and index fingers.	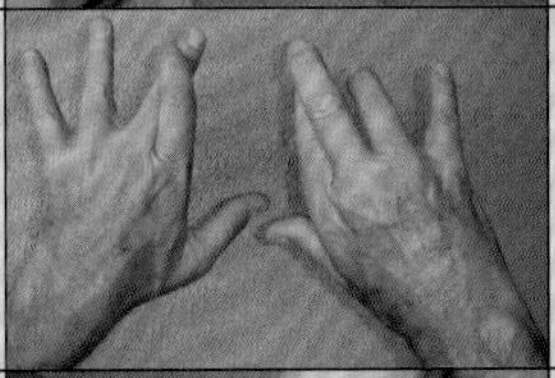	The test is positive if the patient cannot cross the fingers. This test demonstrates weakness of dorsal and palmar interossei.
Cubital tunnel Tinel sign	The ulnar nerve is percussed around the elbow.	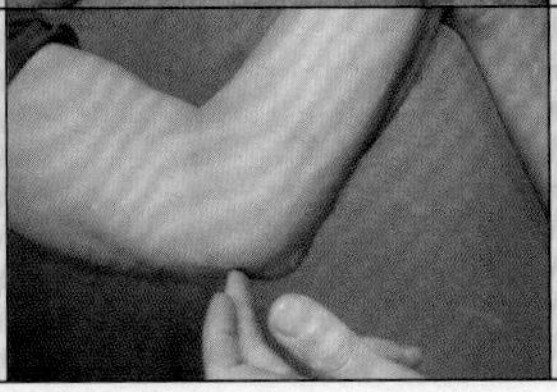	A positive test results in radiating paresthesias into the ulnar nerve distribution of the hand. This test may not be specific for ulnar nerve pathology.

Examination	Technique	Illustration	Grading & Significance
Distal radioulnar joint (DRUJ) compression test	The examiner compresses the ulnar head against the sigmoid notch while holding the patient's mid-forearm and passively rotating.		Positive or negative. A positive test is exacerbation of pain, which suggests arthritis or instability; dorsal or palmar subluxation may be noted.
DRUJ press test	With both wrists pronated, the patient rises from a chair using the affected hand and wrist or pushes downward on a tabletop.		Increased depression of the ulnar head on the affected side results in a "dimple sign" indicating instability. Pain without increased ulnar head depression may indicate a triangular fibrocartilage complex tear.
DRUJ stability test	With the elbow flexed 90 degrees, the examiner grasps the radius over its distal third with one hand and holds the ulna head between the index finger and thumb with the other hand. The examiner displaces the ulna volarly and dorsally in neutral rotation, full supination, and full pronation. The sides are compared.		Substantially less stability than is noted on the opposite side or pain at extremes of rotation may correlate with symptomatic DRUJ instability related to triangular fibrocartilage complex or ligamentous instability. Palpable crepitus at the DRUJ may be indicative of DRUJ arthrosis. Instability Grading Scale: 0: normal; about 1 cm of motion in neutral, no motion at extremes of rotation I: $<$0.5 cm of motion at extremes. Firm endpoint. II: $>$0.5 cm of motion at extremes with soft endpoint but no dislocation III: reduced joint before stress with dislocation of the DRUJ at extremes IV: dislocated joint. "Mushy" feeling with stressing joint.
Extensor carpi ulnaris (ECU) subluxation test	The patient is asked to ulnarly deviate the wrist while actively pronating and supinating. The examiner palpates the ECU tendon at and just proximal to the ulnar groove with the patient's wrist in supination, mild flexion, and ulnar deviation. The sides are compared.		Passively subluxatable versus actively subluxatable. Click versus no click. Pain with subluxation versus no significant pain with subluxation. If the tendon dislocates with passive supination, palmar flexion, and ulnar deviation the ECU is grossly unstable. If the addition of ECU contraction is required for frank dislocation, some inherent stability remains. Pain with subluxation is a critical finding when contemplating surgical treatment.

(continued)

Examination	Technique	Illustration	Grading & Significance
Elbow flexion test	The elbow is fully flexed with the forearm supinated for 60 seconds or until symptoms develop.	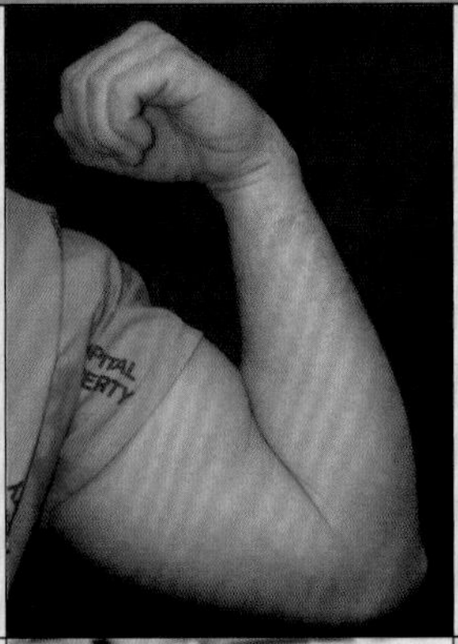	The test is positive for cubital tunnel syndrome if the patient's symptoms are reproduced in the ulnar nerve distribution while holding this position.
Elsen test	The patient's injured PIP joint is flexed 90 degrees over the edge of a table. The patient is asked to actively extend the PIP joint against resistance. The examiner palpates for active middle phalanx extension and simultaneous extension rigidity of the DIP joint.	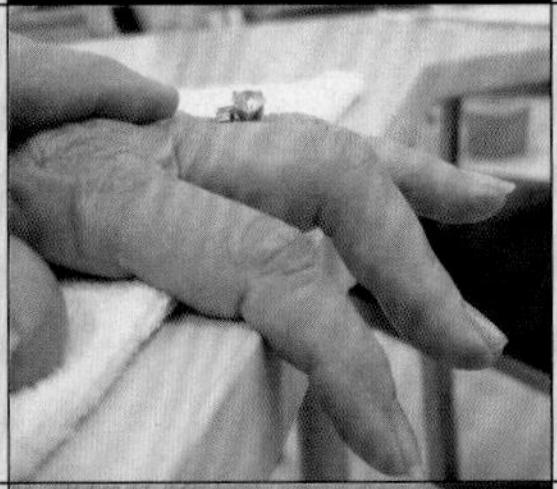	A positive test is consistent with a complete central slip disruption at any time frame. No extension force is felt associated with the middle phalanx but DIP joint rigidity is readily perceived secondary to the effects of the lateral bands. This test will not necessarily detect a partial central slip injury.
Extensor apparatus examination	The examiner observes and palpates the extensor tendon and sagittal bands at MCP and PIP.	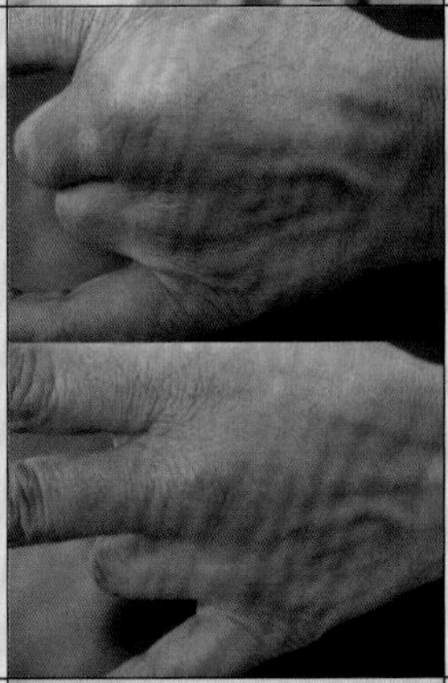	The examiner should look for: 1. Tenderness adjacent to MCP 2. Tendon subluxation at MCP 3. Swan-neck deformity Rules out extensor mechanism abnormalities, which may cause overlapping signs or symptoms.
Flexor digitorum profundus (FDP) examination	The patient is asked to flex the DIP with the PIP joint blocked in extension.	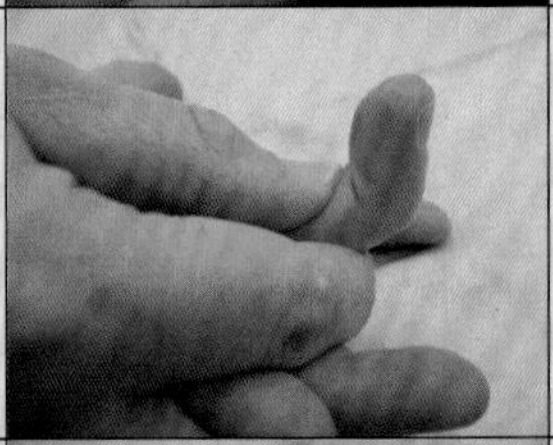	FDP function present or absent. Loss of active DIP flexion suggests disruption or loss of FDP function.
Flexor digitorum superficialis (FDS) examination	The patient is asked to flex the finger with the adjacent digits held in extension.	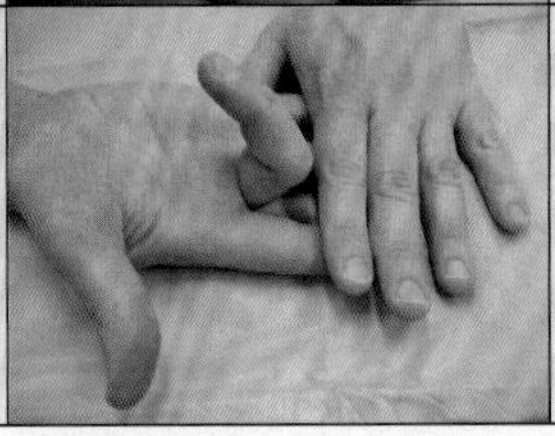	FDS function present or absent. Loss of active PIP flexion suggests disruption or loss of FDS function.

Examination	Technique	Illustration	Grading & Significance
Finger cascade	The examiner observes the position of the fingers with the patient at rest.		Loss of the normal cascade suggests disruption or loss of function of the flexor tendons.
Finkelstein maneuver	With palpation along the first dorsal compartment, the thumb is flexed and the wrist is ulnarly deviated.		Pain indicates DeQuervain tenosynovitis.
Flexor tendon contracture	The wrist and metacarpophalangeal joints are extended, and the examiner assesses extension of the interphalangeal joints.		With flexor tendon contracture there will be limited extension of the interphalangeal joints.
Foveal sign	The examiner palpates the ulnocarpal joint in the interval between the ulnar styloid and the flexor carpi ulnaris tendon.		Pain is indicative of triangular fibrocartilage complex pathology.
Froment sign	The patient is asked to pinch a piece of paper between the index and thumb. Then the examiner attempts to pull the paper out. Both hands are tested simultaneously.		Positive if paper is held only by flexing the thumb interphalangeal joint. This results from recruitment of the flexor pollicis longus and paralysis of the adductor pollicis, usually from an ulnar nerve disorder.

(continued)

Examination	Technique	Illustration	Grading & Significance
Grip strength	The Jamar Dynometer can be used to objectively measure grip strength. The patient's elbow is placed in 90 degrees of flexion and the forearm and wrist in neutral. The recorded value is the average of three maximal attempts with the dynamamometer set on the third station.		Findings are compared to the contralateral side. Decreased strength in association with physical findings can be indicative of wrist pathology. The presence of pain in the central aspect of the wrist with attempted grip has been associated with scapholunate ligament disruption. Mean grip strength for males is 103 to 104 for the dominant extremity and 92 to 99 for the non-dominant extremity. Mean grip strength for females is 62 to 63 for the dominant extremity and 53 to 55 for the non-dominant extremity.
Lichtman Midcarpal Shift Test	With the hand pronated and the forearm stabilized, the examiner positions the wrist in 15 degrees ulnar deviation. The examiner grabs the patient's hand and exerts palmar pressure on the distal capitate. The examiner axially loads and ulnarly deviates the wrist. The procedure is repeated for radial deviation.		No characteristic clunk to severe clunk with pain. Midcarpal instability.
Love pin test	The head of a pin or paperclip is gently pressed against the tender area to localize the pain.		Locates a glomus tumor. In subungual tumors, the pin is placed on the nail plate at various locations to find the tumor.
Lunotriquetral (LT) compression test	Compression is applied in the ulnar snuffbox to give a radially directed force across the LT joint.		Pain with this maneuver may indicate pathology at the LT or triquetral hamate joints.
Lumbrical muscle contracture	An intrinsic tightness test is performed with the fingers radially or ulnarly deviated. Alternatively, the test can be performed with the DIP joint flexed as well as the PIP joint.		With lumbrical contracture, there is less passive flexion of the PIP joint with the finger deviated or with the DIP joint flexed in comparison to intrinsic testing. If present, this suggests lumbrical muscle contracture as part of the pathology.

Examination	Technique	Illustration	Grading & Significance
LT ballottement (Reagan) test	The examiner secures the lunate between the thumb and index finger of one hand and the pisotriquetral unit with the other hand. Anterior and posterior stress is applied across the LT joint.		The test is positive if increased anteroposterior laxity and pain are present. Pain and instability are indicative of LT ligament tear or arthrosis.
LT shear (Kleinman) test	The forearm is placed in neutral rotation and the elbow on the examination table. The examiner's contralateral thumb is placed over the dorsum of the lunate. With the lunate supported, the examiner's ipsilateral thumb loads the pisotriquetral joint from the palmar aspect, creating a shear force at the LT joint.		Positive with pain, crepitance, and abnormal mobility of the LT joint
LT Shuck test	The examiner stabilizes the pisotriquetral joint while passively ulnarly and radially deviating the wrist. Findings are compared with the contralateral wrist.		In a positive test the patient experiences a painful click as the lunate and triquetrum slide abnormally. It signifies a LT ligament injury.
Metacarpophalangeal (MCP) and proximal interphalangeal (PIP) joint instability testing	The individual MCP or PIP joints are tested by the examiner grasping the patient's finger and then applying a valgus and then a varus stress with the joint extended and flexed. The resultant motion is compared to the contralateral side. Differences in laxity indicate ligamentous instability.		Grade 1: No difference in joint line opening compared to the contralateral joint Grade 2: Notable opening of the joint line compared to the contralateral joint, but a solid "endpoint" is reached Grade 3: Complete opening of the radial or lateral joint line with valgus or varus stress. No endpoint can be discerned. Attempts at hyperextension of the digit at the PIP of the MCP joints can identify volar plate instability and the propensity of the digit to subluxate or dislocate.
Mill test	With the elbow flexed, the forearm slightly pronated, and the wrist slightly extended, the patient actively supinates against resistance.		Pain either at the epicondyle or radiating distally along the extensor carpi radialis brevis represents a positive test. Increasing strain in an inflamed or degenerative tendon causes pain.
Palpation of LT interval	The LT joint is deeply palpated dorsally and slightly distal to the site of the 4–5 arthroscopy portal.		Point tenderness indicates LT interosseous ligament injury or triangular fibrocartilage complex pathology.

(continued)

Examination	Technique	Illustration	Grading & Significance
Palpation of scapholunate (SL) interval	The SL joint is deeply palpated dorsally and 1.5 cm distal to the tubercle of Lister (slightly distal to the 3–4 arthroscopy portal). Alternatively, the examiner palpates the third metacarpal, moving proximally until a depression is felt. Just proximal to this cavity is the SL joint, which is palpable between the second and fourth dorsal extensor compartments.	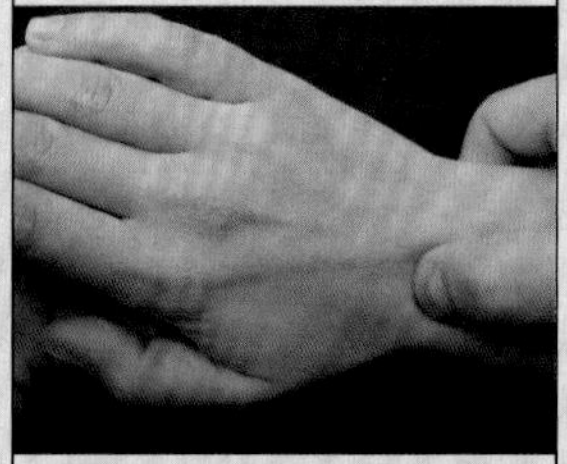	Point tenderness may indicate SL interosseous ligament injury, scaphoid injury, ganglion cyst, or Kienbock disease.
Phalen test	The patient's wrist is placed in maximum flexion and the elbow in extension for 60 seconds or until symptomatic.	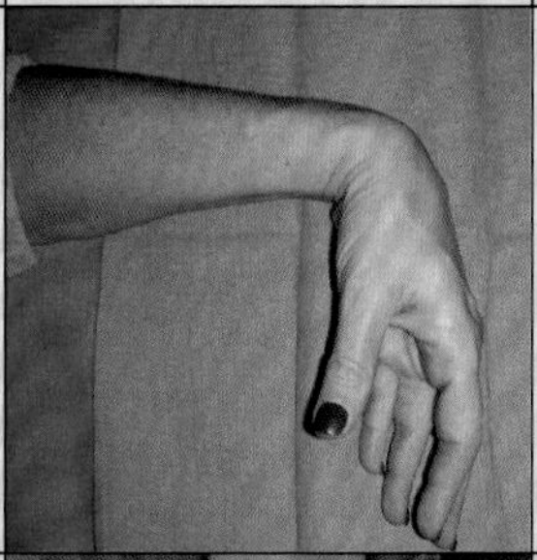	Reproduction of symptoms in the median nerve distribution indicates carpal tunnel syndrome.
Piano key sign	The radius is stabilized with one hand. The ulna is passively translated dorsally and volarly with the opposite hand. This test is performed in pronation, neutral, and supination, and findings are compared to the opposite side.	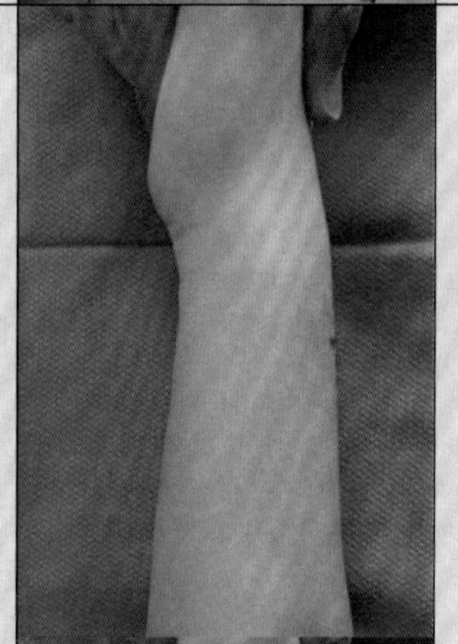 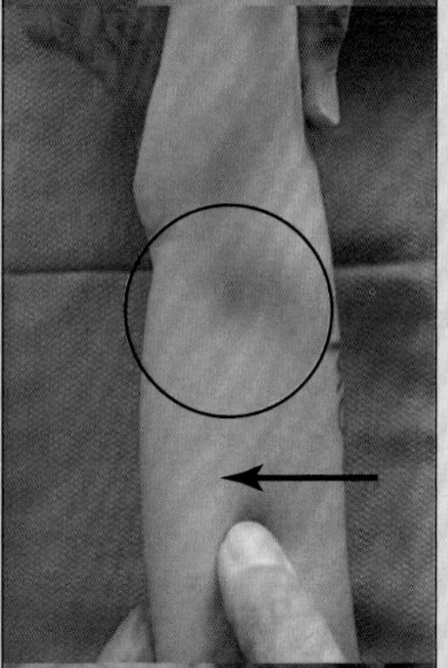 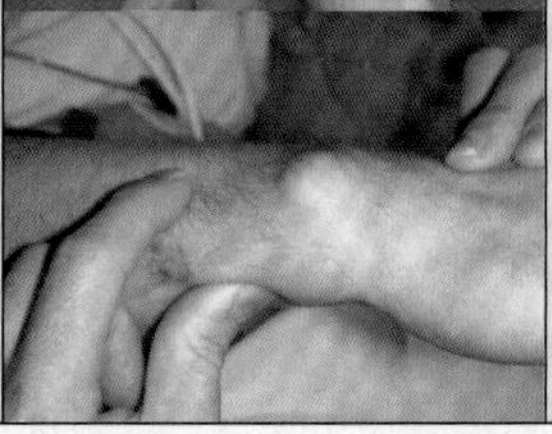	A positive result is characterized by painful laxity in the affected wrist compared with the contralateral wrist, suggesting DRUJ synovitis related to instability. "Winging" is associated with loss of structural support at the DRUJ and may indicate a complete peripheral tear of the triangular fibrocartilage complex. Depression and rebounding of the ulnar head is a positive finding.

Examination	Technique	Illustration	Grading & Significance
Pisotriquetral shear test	The examiner's thumb is placed over the pisiform and a circular grinding motion and dorsally directed pressure are applied.	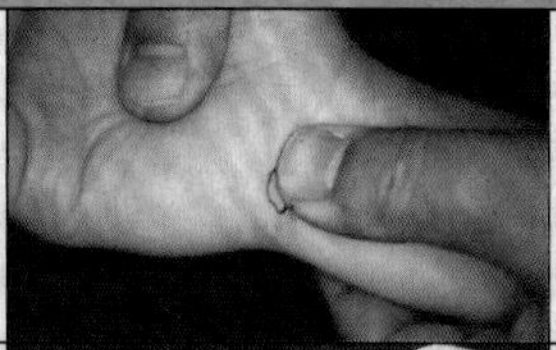	Crepitus and pain over pisotriquetral joint. Pisotriquetral arthritis.
Scaphoid ballottement test	The scaphoid is grasped with one hand and the lunate with the other. The scaphoid is then balloted anteroposteriorly. Anteroposterior translation is compared to the contralateral side.	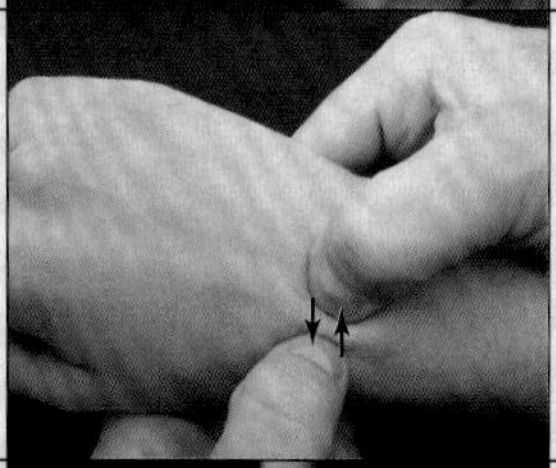	Pain and increased anteroposterior laxity are highly suggestive of SL instability.
Scaphoid shift test (Watson)	Dorsally directed pressure is exerted on the patient's volar scaphoid tuberosity (distal pole) by the examiner's ipsilateral thumb while the wrist is passively moved from ulnar to radial deviation by the examiner's contralateral hand. The distal pole of the scaphoid is stabilized with the wrist in ulnar deviation, and then the examiner passively radially deviates the wrist. Next the pressure on the distal pole is removed and the examiner feels for relocation of the scaphoid into the scaphoid facet of the distal radius. Findings are compared with the contralateral wrist.	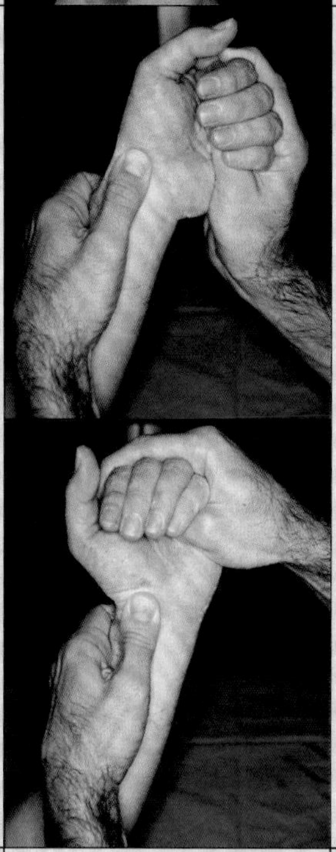	The scaphoid normally flexes as the wrist goes from ulnar to radial deviation. The examiner's thumb prevents scaphoid flexion and in scapholunate dissociation, the proximal scaphoid pole subluxates dorsally out of the scaphoid fossa, causing pain. When the thumb is released from the distal pole of the scaphoid, there may be a palpable or audible clunk, signifying spontaneous reduction of the scaphoid back into the scaphoid fossa. This clunk may be present in 11% of asymptomatic wrists. It is the presence of pain along with the clunk that is diagnostic for scapholunate ligament disruption. If only pain is present and no clunk is felt, a sprain or a partial tear of the scapholunate ligament is likely. This test is not terribly specific and may be positive in patients with hyperlaxity, synovitis, occult ganglia, and radioscaphoid impingement or arthritis
Supination test (Ouellette)	With the forearm mildly pronated, the examiner uses their contralateral hand to stabilize the distal ulna and their ipsilateral hand to secure the pisotriquetral unit and with that hand exert a supination force on the ulnar carpus along with compression across the ulnocarpal joint. The examiner listens for clicks and clunks.	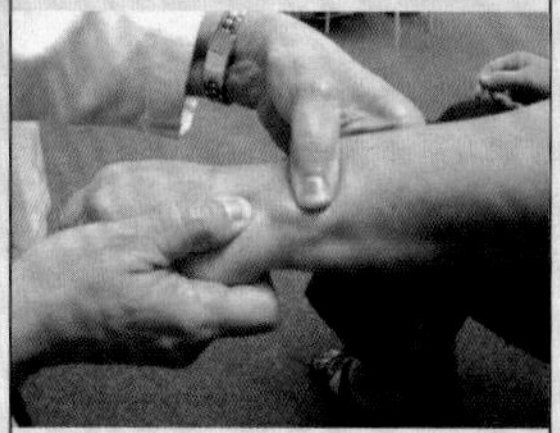	Pain, instability and the presence of clicks or clunks are compared to the contralateral wrist. Graded from stable to unstable. The examiner should note the presence of clicks and clunks in both wrists. Abnormal supination of carpus in relation to the forearm.
Thompson test	With the elbow extended, the wrist in slight extension, and the digits in a fist, the patient extends the wrist against the examiner.	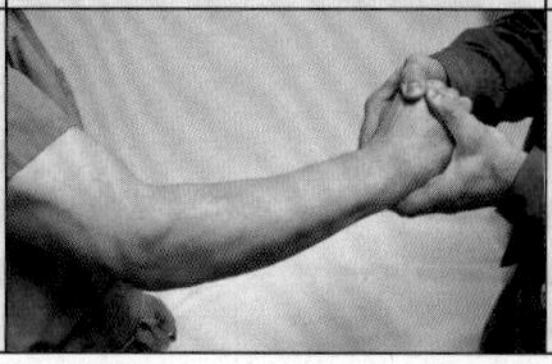	Pain either at the lateral epicondyle or radiating distally along the extensor carpi radialis brevis is indicative of inflamed or degenerative tendon.

(continued)

Examination	Technique	Illustration	Grading & Significance
Thumb MCP joint collateral ligament stability test	The metacarpal is stabilized between the examiner's thumb and index finger of one hand and the proximal phalanx is stabilized between the examiner's thumb and index finger of the other hand. Radially or ulnarly directed forces are applied with the joint flexed 30 to 35 degrees and with the joint extended. Findings are compared with the uninjured thumb. Use of a digital block is sometimes helpful to obtain an accurate assessment.	*	Grade 0: No significant instability Grade 1, Mild: <25 degrees of opening Grade 2, Moderate: <30 degrees of difference versus the contralateral thumb Grade 3, Severe: Gross instability, without a solid endpoint in both flexion and extension. Consistent with a complete disruption of the proper and accessory collateral ligaments. Severe collateral ligament injury is uncommon in conjunction with volar plate instability but must be recognized and treated where indicated.
Trigger digit evaluation	A digit is placed along the volar aspect of the thumb or finger, proximal to the MP joint, and the patient is asked to flex and extend the digit.		Reproduction of pain, triggering, or locking of the thumb indicates trigger thumb as a cause.
Ulnocarpal (triangular fibrocartilage complex) compression test	The examiner ulnarly deviates, pronates, and axially loads the wrist. Passive pronation and supination may be added.		A click or snap reproducing pain and symptoms is a positive test and consistent with triangular fibrocartilage complex, LT, and midcarpal pathology. This maneuver will also be painful if ulna impaction syndrome is present.
Volar plate stability	The metacarpal is stabilized between the examiner's thumb and index finger of one hand and the proximal phalanx is stabilized between the examiner's thumb and index finger of other hand. Hyperextension force is applied.		0 = No hyperextension; 1 = Mild, definite endpoint; 2 = moderate, soft endpoint; 3 = severe, gross instability. Volar instability must be recognized and treated appropriately to maximize outcomes.
Wartenberg sign	The patient is asked to extend the fingers.		The sign is considered positive if the small finger assumes an abducted posture with finger extension. This sign is the result of palmar interossei weakness resulting in unopposed ulnar pull of the extensor digiti quinti.

Examination	Technique	Illustration	Grading & Significance
Elbow			
Range of motion (ROM), elbow	Active and passive ROM (flexion–extension of the elbow, rotation of the forearm) is compared to the uninjured side. Palpable and auditory crepitus should be noted.		Normal values: 0 to 145 degrees of flexion–extension, 85 degrees of supination, and 80 degrees of pronation. The examiner should check for perching on the lateral view. Locking of the elbow could represent loose bodies. Stiffness may indicate intrinsic capsular contracture.
Effusion	The examiner palpates the anconeus triangle (radial head [RH], lateral epicondyle [L], and olecranon tip [O]) and lateral gutter, noting prominence of lateral epicondyle, gutter effusion, or subcutaneous atrophy from prior corticosteroid injections.	RH L O	It is difficult to estimate the amount of fluid, but the presence of an effusion should be noted and may represent hemarthrosis due to intra-articular fracture, radiocapitellar wear, or ligamentous disruption. In acute injuries an effusion should be present; in more chronic situations it may be absent.
Capitellum tenderness	Examiner's thumb pushes against the posterior capitellum while taking the elbow through a range of motion of flexion to extension.	Capitellum Radial head	Most clinicians just grade this as none, mild, moderate, or significant pain. Tenderness may be present with osteochondritis dissecans.

(continued)

Examination	Technique	Illustration	Grading & Significance
Active radiocapitellar compression test	Forearm pronation and supination with the elbow in full extension is performed.	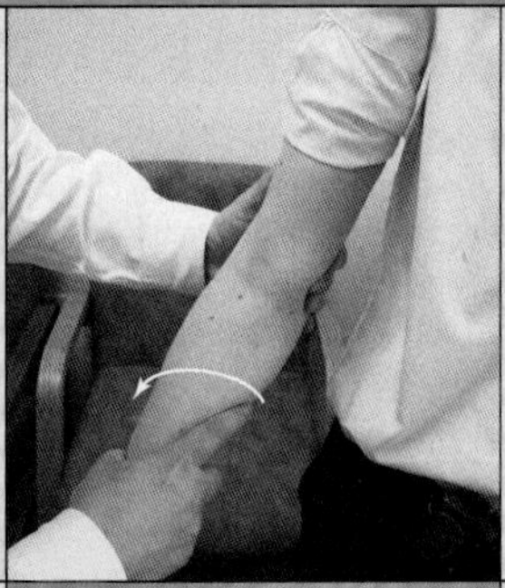	Most clinicians just grade this as none, mild, moderate, or significant pain. This test loads the radiocapitellar joint in pronation. Pain on pronation that is reduced in supination may be present in osteochondritis dissecans.
Supine lateral pivot-shift test	Patient is supine, with arm extended overhead and supinated. The examiner stabilizes the humerus with one hand and applies a valgus force with the other as the elbow is taken from extension to flexion.	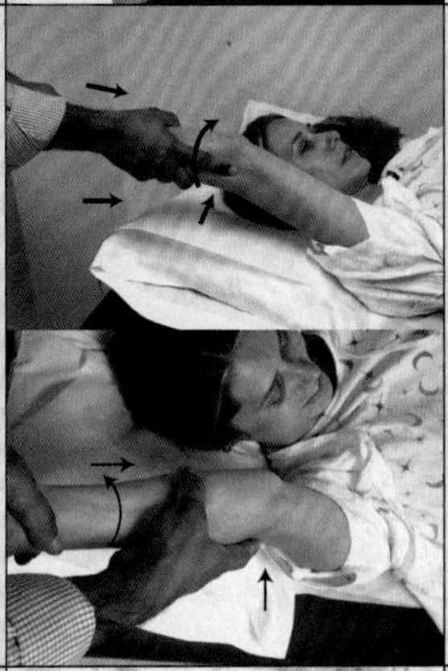	When the elbow is slightly flexed the radial head can be palpated to subluxate or frankly dislocate; as the elbow flexes past 40 degrees, it will relocate, often with a palpable clunk. This test is difficult to perform on an awake patient; often apprehension will be felt and the patient will not allow the test to continue. Examination under anesthesia may be required.
Prone pivot-shift test	Placing the patient prone with the arm hanging over the table stabilizes the humerus and leaves one of the examiner's hands free to palpate the radial head.	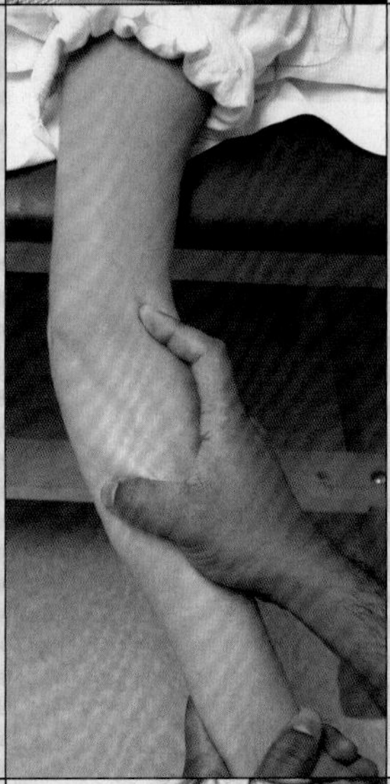	A positive test reveals radial head or ulnohumeral subluxation. Same as pivotshift test.
Elbow drawer test	With the patient in prone position, the humerus is stabilized with one arm while a distraction force is placed on the forearm to sublux the ulnohumeral joint.	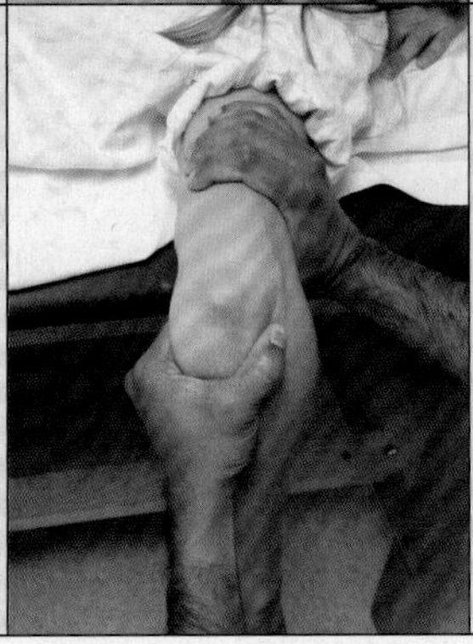	A positive test reveals ulnohumeral subluxation.

Examination	Technique	Illustration	Grading & Significance
Push-off test	From a seated position the patient attempts to push off from the armrests. Pain or apprehension is suggestive of lateral ligamentous insufficiency.	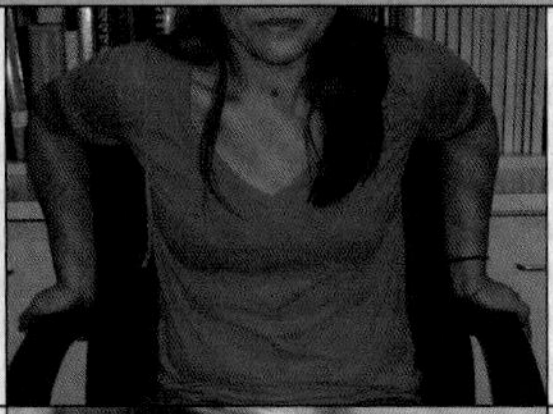	A positive test will reproduce the patient's symptoms of apprehension during supination and not pronation. Inability to complete the push-up is a positive test. A positive test indicates a posterolateral rotatory insufficiency.
Table-top relocation test	The symptomatic hand/arm is placed on the lateral edge of a table. The patient is asked to perform push-up with the elbow pointing laterally. The maneuver is repeated with the examiner's thumb stabilizing the radial head during press-up. The maneuver is once again repeated without the examiner's thumb in place.	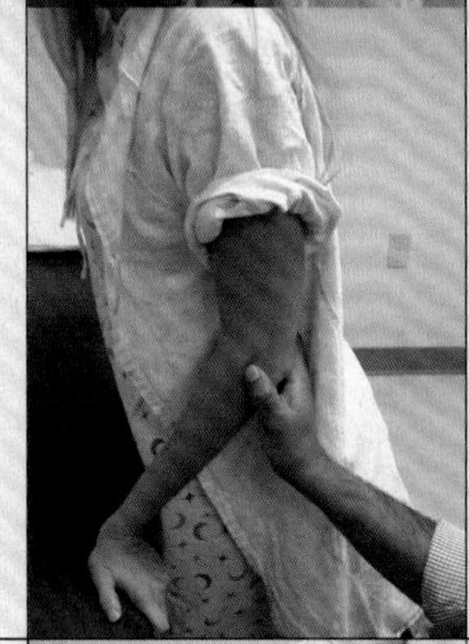 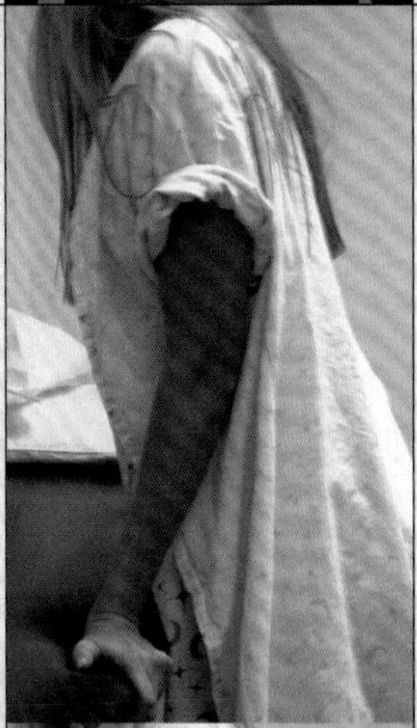	A positive test elicits pain or apprehension as the elbow reaches 40 degrees.
Varus stress test	Stabilize the humerus and stress the elbow in supination and slight flexion.	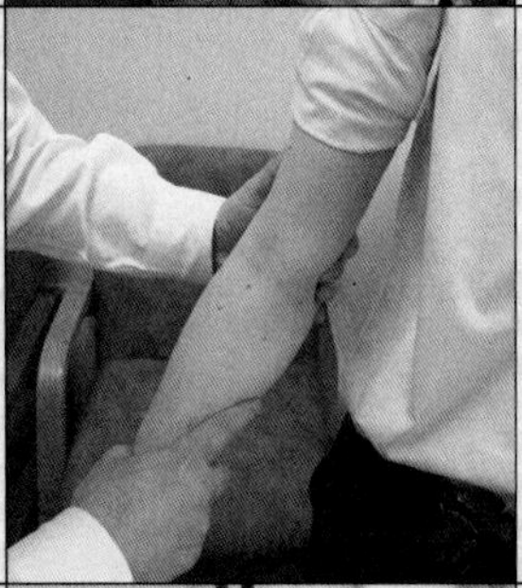	A positive test indicates injury to the anterior band of the medial collateral ligament.
Valgus stress test	The examiner stabilizes the humerus and stresses the lateral ulnar collateral ligament in slight flexion.	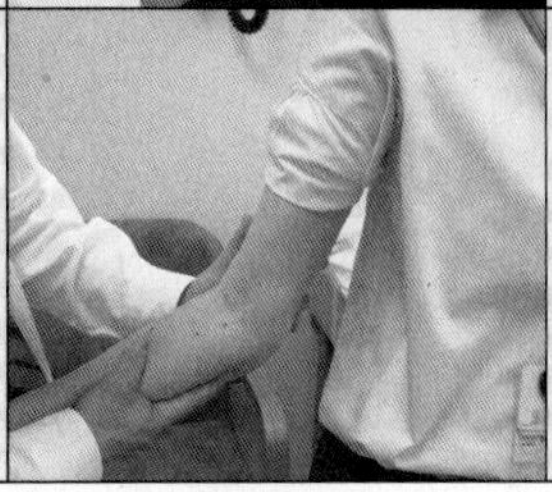	A positive test indicates injury to the lateral ulnar collateral ligament.

(continued)

Examination	Technique	Illustration	Grading & Significance
Medial collateral ligament shear test	Patient places the contralateral arm under the injured elbow and grasps the thumb of the symptomatic extremity. With the elbow maximally flexed the patient applies a valgus load to the elbow as he or she brings it out into extension.	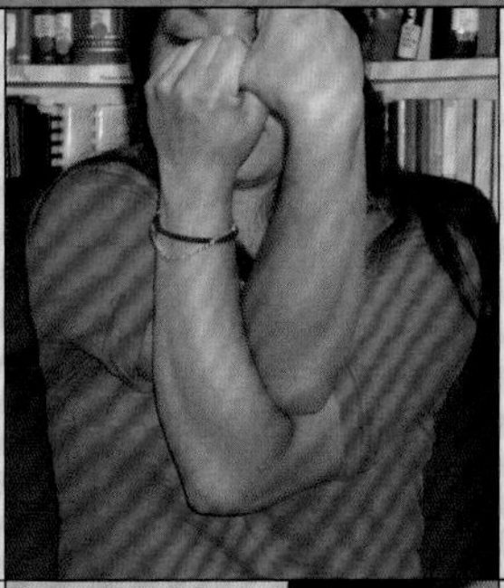	A positive test will localize pain to the medial elbow, suggesting an incompetent ulnar collateral ligament.
Milking maneuver	With forearm fully supinated, elbow is placed in greater than 90 degrees of flexion. The examiner pulls on the patient's thumb.	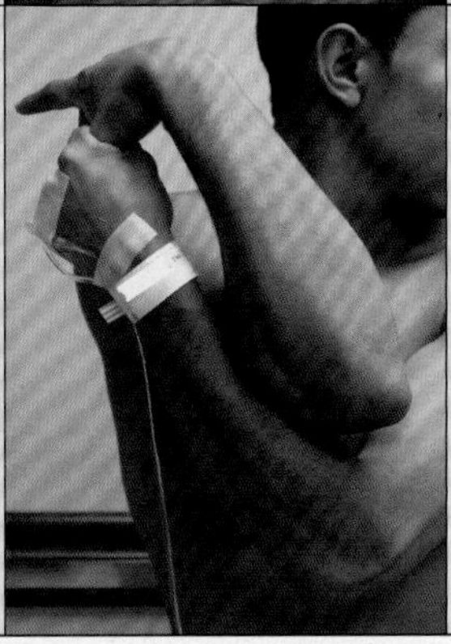	Maneuver eliciting pain, apprehension, or instability is indicative of ulnar collateral ligament (UCL) insufficiency. Posterior bundle of anterior band of UCL.

Index

Page numbers followed by *f* and *t* indicate figures and tables, respectively.

G

M

T

U